D0578248

HEARD DISEASE

A Textbook of Cardiovascular Medicine

5TH EDITION

HEART DISEASE

A Textbook of Cardiovascular Medicine

VOLUME 2

Edited by

EUGENE BRAUNWALD A.B., M.D., M.A. (hon.), M.D. (hon.), Sc.D. (hon.), F.R.C.P.

Vice President for Academic Programs, Partners HealthCare System; Distinguished Hersey Professor of Medicine, Faculty Dean for Academic Programs at Brigham and Women's Hospital and Massachusetts General Hospital, Harvard Medical School, Boston, Massachusetts

W.B. SAUNDERS COMPANY
A Division of Harcourt Brace & Company
PHILADELPHIA / LONDON / TORONTO / MONTREAL / SYDNEY / TOKYO

W.B. SAUNDERS COMPANY
A Division of Harcourt Brace & Company

The Curtis Center
Independence Square West
Philadelphia, Pennsylvania 19106

Library of Congress Cataloging-in-Publication Data

Heart disease: a textbook of cardiovascular medicine /
[edited by] Eugene Braunwald.—5th ed.

p. cm.

Includes bibliographical references and index.

ISBN 0–7216–5666–8 (single v.).—ISBN 0–7216–5663–3 (set).
ISBN 0–7216–5664–1 (v. 1).—ISBN 0–7216–5665–X (v. 2)

1. Heart—Diseases. 2. Cardiovascular system—Diseases.
I. Braunwald, Eugene
[DNLM: 1. Heart Diseases. WG 200 H4364 1997]

RC681.H362 1997 616.1′2—dc20

DNLM/DLC 95-24767

HEART DISEASE: A Textbook of
Cardiovascular Medicine, Fifth Edition

ISBN 0–7216–5666–8 (single vol.)
ISBN 0–7216–5663–3 (2-vol. set)
ISBN 0–7216–5664–1 (vol. 1)
ISBN 0–7216–5665–X (vol. 2)

Printed in the United States of America

Last digit is the print number: 9 8 7 6 5 4 3 2 1

CONTENTS 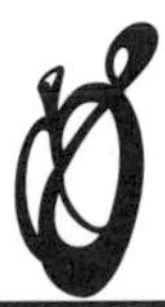

PART I EXAMINATION OF THE PATIENT

CHAPTER 1 THE HISTORY 1
EUGENE BRAUNWALD

CHAPTER 2 PHYSICAL EXAMINATION OF THE HEART AND CIRCULATION 15
JOSEPH K. PERLOFF and EUGENE BRAUNWALD

CHAPTER 3 ECHOCARDIOGRAPHY 53
HARVEY FEIGENBAUM

CHAPTER 4 ELECTROCARDIOGRAPHY 108
CHARLES FISCH

CHAPTER 5 EXERCISE STRESS TESTING........ 153
BERNARD R. CHAITMAN

CHAPTER 6 CARDIAC CATHETERIZATION........ 177
CHARLES J. DAVIDSON, ROBERT F. FISHMAN, and ROBERT O. BONOW

CHAPTER 7 RADIOLOGY OF THE HEART........ 204
ROBERT M. STEINER and DAVID C. LEVIN

CHAPTER 8 CORONARY ARTERIOGRAPHY........ 240
JOHN A. BITTL and DAVID C. LEVIN

CHAPTER 9 NUCLEAR CARDIOLOGY........ 273
FRANS J. TH. WACKERS, ROBERT SOUFER, and BARRY L. ZARET

CHAPTER 10 NEWER CARDIAC IMAGING TECHNIQUES: MAGNETIC RESONANCE IMAGING AND COMPUTED TOMOGRAPHY........ 317
CHARLES B. HIGGINS

CHAPTER 11 RELATIVE MERITS OF IMAGING TECHNIQUES 349
DAVID J. SKORTON, BRUCE H. BRUNDAGE, HEINRICH R. SCHELBERT, and GERALD L. WOLF

PART II NORMAL AND ABNORMAL CIRCULATORY FUNCTION

CHAPTER 12 MECHANISMS OF CARDIAC CONTRACTION AND RELAXATION 360
LIONEL H. OPIE

CHAPTER 13 PATHOPHYSIOLOGY OF HEART FAILURE 394
WILSON S. COLUCCI and EUGENE BRAUNWALD

CHAPTER 14 ASSESSMENT OF CARDIAC FUNCTION 421
WILLIAM C. LITTLE and EUGENE BRAUNWALD

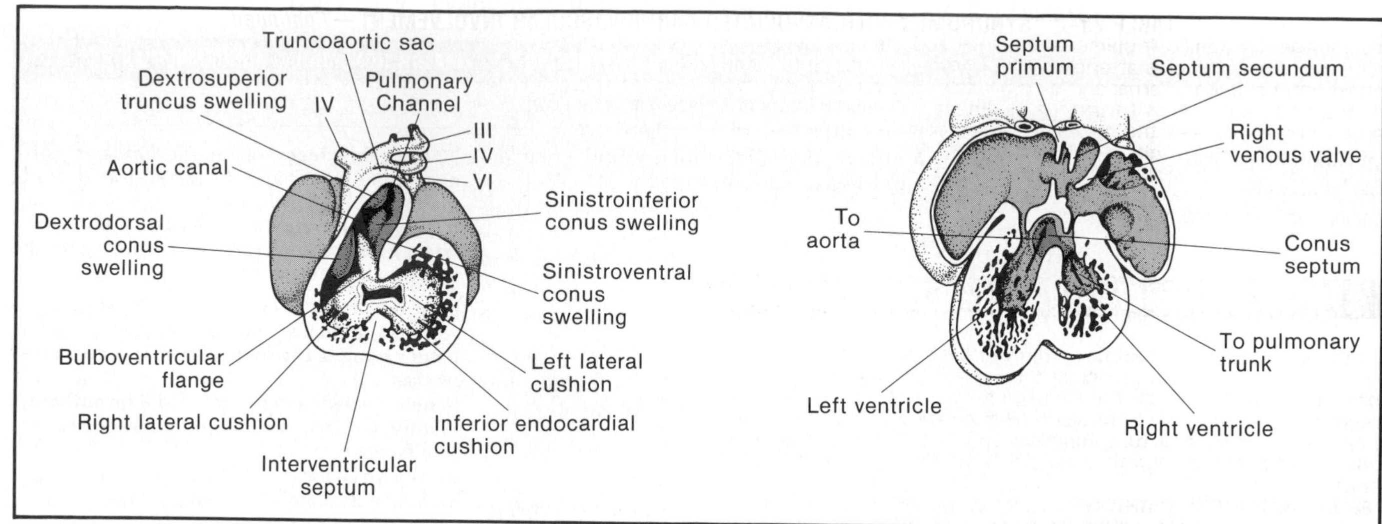

FIGURE 29–2. Frontal section through the heart of a 9-mm embryo (left panel) and 15-mm embryo (right panel). At 9 mm, development is noted of the cushions in the atrioventricular canal, and the truncus and conus swellings are visible. At 15 mm, the conus septum is completed; note the septation in the atrial region. (From Clark, E. B., and Van Mierop, L. H. S.: Development of the cardiovascular system. *In* Moss' Heart Disease in Infants, Children, and Adolescents. Baltimore, © Williams and Wilkins, 1989.)

THE LUNGS. These structures arise from the primitive foregut and are drained early in embryogenesis by channels from the splanchnic plexus to the cardinal and umbilicovitelline veins. An outpouching from the posterior left atrium forms the common pulmonary vein, which communicates with the splanchnic plexus, establishing pulmonary venous drainage to the left atrium. The umbilicovitelline and anterior cardinal vein communications atrophy as the common pulmonary vein is incorporated into the left atrium. Anomalous pulmonary venous connections (see p. 946) to the umbilicovitelline (portal) venous system or to the cardinal system (superior vena cava) result from failure of the common pulmonary vein to develop or establish communications to the splanchnic plexus. Cor triatriatum (see p. 923) results from a narrowing of the common pulmonary vein–left atrial junction.

THE GREAT ARTERIES. The truncus arteriosus is connected to the dorsal aorta in the embryo by six pairs of aortic arches. Partition of the truncus arteriosus into two great arteries is a result of the fusion of tissue arising from the back wall of the vessel and the truncus septum. Rotation of the truncus coils the aorticopulmonary septum and creates the normal spiral relation between aorta and pulmonary artery. Semilunar valves and their related sinuses are created by absorption and hollowing out of tissue at the distal side of the truncus ridges. Aorticopulmonary septal defect (see p. 906) and persistent truncus arteriosus (see p. 907) represent varying degrees of partitioning failure.

Although the six aortic arches appear sequentially, portions of the arch system and dorsal aorta disappear at different times during embryogenesis (Fig. 29–3). The first, second, and fifth sets of paired

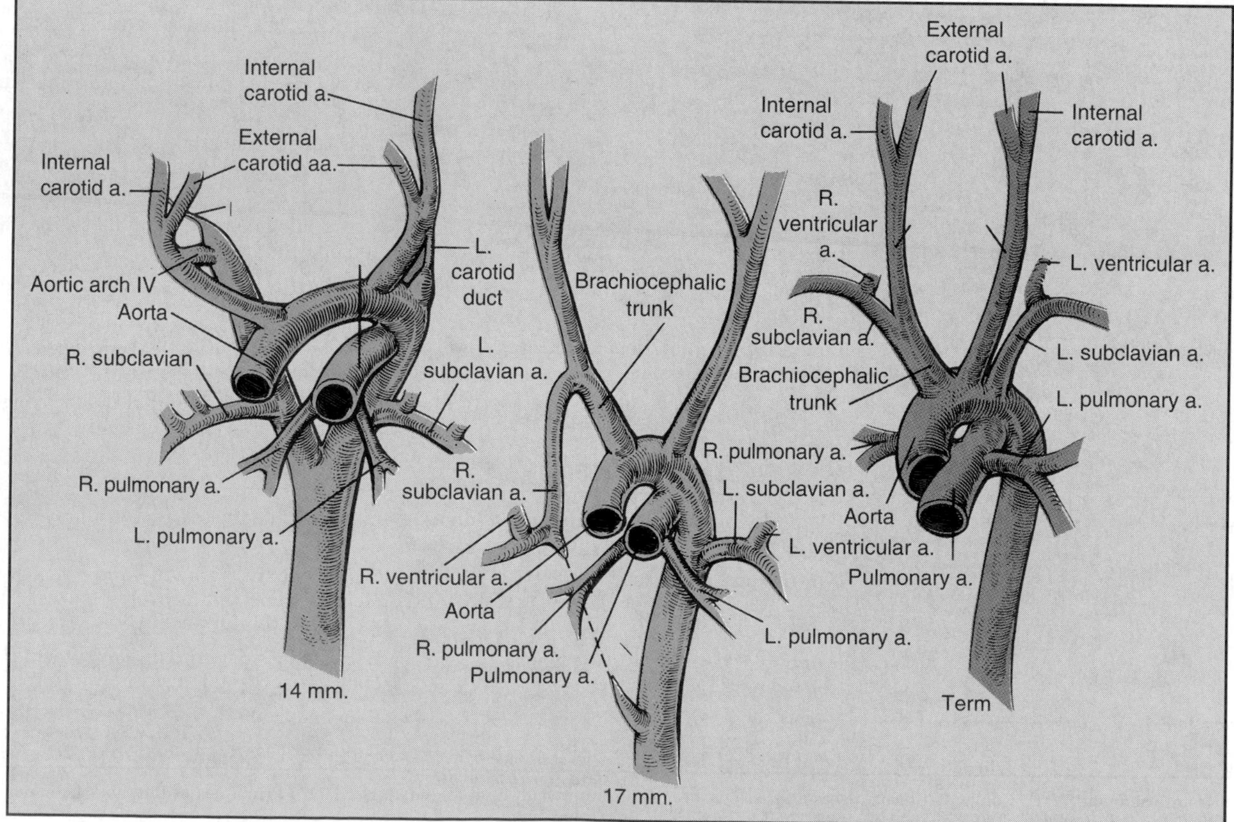

FIGURE 29–3. Transformation of the aortic arches and dorsal aortae into the definitive vascular pattern is a process of fusion and segmental resorption of the paired first to sixth branchial arches with the paired dorsal aortae. (From Castaneda, A., et al.: Cardiac Surgery of the Neonate and Infant. Philadelphia, W.B. Saunders Company, 1994, p. 398.)

arches regress completely. The proximal portions of the sixth arches become the right and left pulmonary arteries and the distal left sixth arch becomes the ductus arteriosus. The third aortic arch forms the connection between internal and external carotid arteries, while the left fourth arch becomes the arterial segment between left carotid and subclavian arteries; the proximal portion of the right subclavian artery forms from the right fourth arch. An abnormality in regression of the arch system in a number of sites can produce a wide variety of arch anomalies, whereas a failure of regression usually results in a double aortic arch malformation.

FETAL AND TRANSITIONAL CIRCULATIONS

Although the illness created by the presence of a cardiac malformation is almost always recognized only after an affected baby is born, important effects on the circulation have existed from early in pregnancy until the time of delivery. Thus knowledge of the changes in cardiocirculatory structure, function, and metabolism that accompany development is central to a systematic comprehension of congenital heart disease.

FETAL CIRCULATORY PATHWAYS. Dynamic alterations occur in the circulation during the transition from fetal to neonatal life when the lungs take over the function of gas exchange from the placenta. The single fetal circulation consists of parallel pulmonary and systemic pathways (Fig. 29–4) in contrast to the two-circuit system in the newborn and adult, in whom the pulmonary vasculature exists in series with the systemic circulation. Prenatal survival is not endangered by major cardiac anomalies as long as one side of the heart can drive blood from the great veins to the aorta; in the fetus, blood can bypass the nonfunctioning lungs both proximal and distal to the heart.

Oxygenated blood returns from the placenta through the umbilical vein and enters the portal venous system. A variable amount of this stream bypasses the hepatic microcirculation and enters the inferior vena cava by way of the ductus venosus. Inferior vena caval blood is composed to flow from the ductus venosus, hepatic vein, and lower

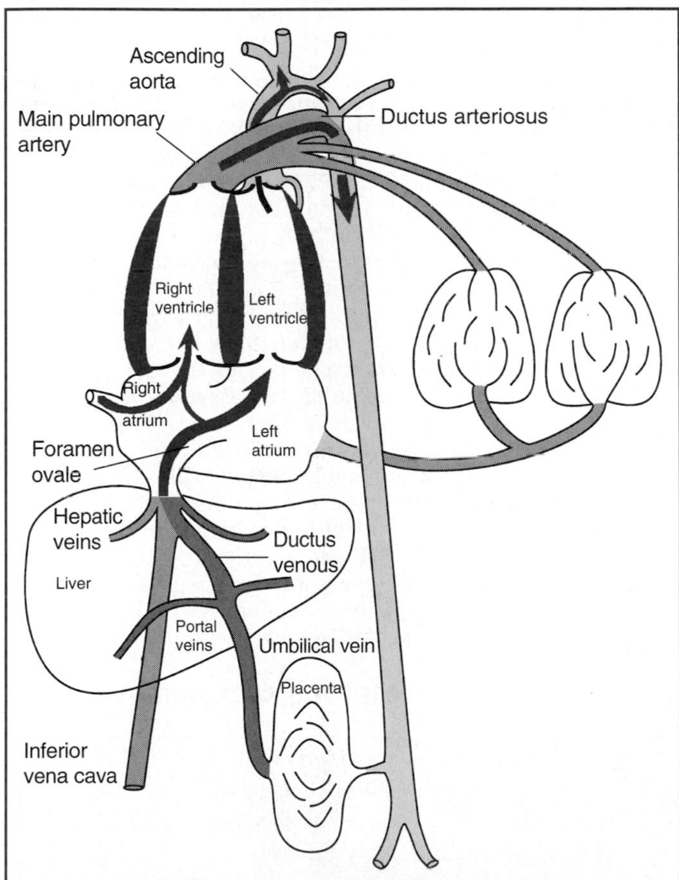

FIGURE 29–4. The fetal circulation with arrows indicating the directions of flow. A fraction of umbilical venous blood enters the ductus venosus and bypasses the liver. This relatively low-oxygenated blood flows across the foramen ovale to the left heart, preferentially perfusing the coronary arteries, head, and upper trunk. The output of the right ventricle flows preferentially across the ductus arteriosus and circulates to the placenta as well as to the abdominal viscera and lower trunk. (Courtesy of David Teitel, M.D.)

body venous drainage, which is summarily deflected to a significant extent across the foramen ovale into the left atrium. Almost all superior vena caval blood passes directly through the tricuspid valve entering the right ventricle. Most of the blood that reaches the right ventricle bypasses the high-resistance, unexpanded lungs and passes through the ductus arteriosus into the descending aorta. The right ventricle contributes about 55 per cent and the left 45 per cent to the total fetal cardiac output. The major portion of blood ejected from the left ventricle supplies the brain and upper body, with lesser flow to the coronary arteries; the balance passes across the aortic isthmus to the descending aorta, where it joins with the large stream from the ductus arteriosus before flowing to the lower body and placenta.

FETAL PULMONARY CIRCULATION. In fetal life, pulmonary arteries and arterioles are surrounded by a fluid medium, have relatively thick walls and small lumina, and resemble comparable arteries in the systemic circulation. The low pulmonary blood flow in the fetus (7 to 10 per cent of the total cardiac output) is the result of high pulmonary vascular resistance. Fetal pulmonary vessels are highly reactive to changes in oxygen tension or in the pH of blood perfusing them as well as to a number of other physiological and pharmacological influences.

EFFECTS OF CARDIAC MALFORMATIONS ON THE FETUS. Although fetal somatic growth may be unimpaired, the hemodynamic effects in utero of many cardiac malformations may alter the development and structure of the fetal heart and circulation.[21] Thus, total anomalous pulmonary venous connection in utero may result in underdevelopment of the left atrium and left ventricle (see p. 944), and premature closure of the foramen ovale may result in hypoplasia of the left ventricle. Moreover, postnatally, the caliber of the aortic isthmus may be reduced (see p. 913) in the presence of lesions in utero that create left ventricular hypertrophy and impede filling because of reduced compliance of that chamber. It may also be reduced in the presence of a lesion that interferes with left ventricular filling directly (e.g., mitral stenosis) or indirectly by diverting a proportion of left ventricular output away from the ascending aorta while increasing right ventricular output and ductus arteriosus flow (e.g., atrioventricular septal defect with left ventricular–right atrial shunt or aortic or subaortic stenosis with ventricular septal defect). Similarly, obstruction in utero to right ventricular outflow is associated with an increase in proximal aortic flow and diameter and almost never with aortic coarctation (see p. 965). In these and other examples it is important to recognize that malformations compatible with fetal survival may nonetheless result in abnormal development of the circulation in utero and also affect circulatory adjustments after birth.

FUNCTION OF THE FETAL HEART. Compared with the adult heart, the fetal and newborn heart is unique with respect to its ultrastructural appearance,[22] its mechanical and biochemical properties,[23–27] and its autonomic innervation.[24,27] During late fetal and early neonatal development there is maturation of the excitation-contraction coupling process[25,26,30,31] and the biochemical composition of the heart's energy-utilizing myofibrillar proteins and of adenosine triphosphate and creatine phosphate energy-producing proteins.[27] Moreover, fetal and neonatal myocardial cells are small in diameter and reduced in density, so that the young heart contains relatively more noncontractile mass (primarily mitochondria, nuclei, and surface membranes) than later in postnatal life. As a result, force generation and the extent and velocity of shortening are decreased, and stiffness and water content of ventricular myocardium are increased in the fetal and early newborn periods.

The diminished function of the young heart is reflected in its limited ability to increase cardiac output in the presence of either a volume load or a lesion that increases resistance to emptying.[32] Although functional integrity exists of efferent and afferent cardiac autonomic pathways early in life, fetal and newborn myocardium lacks the complete development of sympathetic but not cholinergic innervation. Thus, adaptation to cardiocirculatory stress in fetal or early newborn life may be less effective than in adulthood.

CHANGES AT BIRTH. The fundamental change that normally occurs at birth is a division of the single parallel fetal circulation into separate, independent circulations. Inflation of the lungs at the first inspiration produces a marked reduction in pulmonary vascular resistance owing partly to the sudden suspension in air of fetal pulmonary vessels previously supported by fluid media. The reduced extravascular pressure assists new vessels to open and already patent vessels to enlarge. The rapid decrease in pulmonary vascular resistance is related more importantly to vasodilatation owing to the increase in oxygen tension to which pulmonary vessels are exposed rather than to physical expansion of alveoli with gas. Great interest exists currently in defining the role of nitric oxide in the mediation of changes in pulmonary vascular tone in these events.[22,33] Pulmonary arterial pressure falls, and pulmonary blood flow increases greatly. Systemic vascular resistance rises when clamping of the umbilical cord removes the low-resistance placental circulation. Increased pulmonary blood flow increases the return of blood to the left atrium and raises left atrial pressure, which in turn closes the foramen ovale.

The shift in oxygen dependence from the placenta to the lungs produces a sudden increase in arterial blood oxygen tension, which, in concert with alterations in the local prostaglandin milieu, initiates constriction of the ductus arteriosus.[35] Pulmonary pressure falls further as the ductus constricts. In healthy mature infants the ductus arteriosus is profoundly constricted at 10 to 15 hours and is closed functionally by 72 hours, with total anatomical closure following within a few weeks by a process of thrombosis, intimal proliferation, and fibrosis. A high incidence exists in preterm infants of persistent patency of the ductus arteriosus because of an immaturity of those mechanisms responsible for constriction (see p. 905). In surviving preterm infants the ductus arteriosus spontaneously closes within 4 to 12 months of birth.

The ductus venosus, ductus arteriosus, and foramen ovale remain potential channels for blood flow after birth. Thus persistent patency of the ductus venosus may mask the most marked signs of pulmonary venous obstruction in infants with total anomalous pulmonary venous connection below the diaphragm (see p. 944). Similarly, lesions producing right or left atrial volume or pressure overload may stretch the foramen ovale and render incompetent the flap valve mechanism for its closure. Anomalies that depend on patency of the ductus arteriosus for preserving pulmonary or systemic blood flow remain latent until the ductus arteriosus constricts. A common example is the rapid intensification of cyanosis observed in the infant with tetralogy of Fallot when the magnitude of pulmonary hypoperfusion is unmasked by spontaneous closure of the ductus arteriosus. Moreover, there is increasing evidence that ductal constriction is a key factor in the postnatal development of coarctation of the aorta (see p. 965). Lastly, it should be recognized that because the ductus arteriosus is potentially patent after birth and the pulmonary resistance vessels are hyperreactive, hypoxic pulmonary vasoconstriction of diverse causes may result in a right-to-left shunt through the ductus.

PATHOLOGICAL CONSEQUENCES OF CONGENITAL CARDIAC LESIONS

CONGESTIVE HEART FAILURE

Although the basic mechanisms of cardiac failure, as outlined in Chapter 13, are similar for all ages, the pediatric cardiologist should clearly recognize that the common causes, time of onset, and often the approach to treatment vary with age.[36–38] The development of fetal echocardiography has allowed the diagnosis of intrauterine cardiac failure.[39–41] The cardinal findings of fetal heart failure are scalp edema, ascites, pericardial effusion, and decreased fetal movements. Although abnormalities in several organ systems may result in nonimmunological fetal hydrops, cardiac causes include a host of structural, functional, rhythm, and metabolic disturbances of the heart. Infants under 1 year of age with cardiac malformations account for 80 to 90 per cent of pediatric patients who develop congestive failure. Moreover, cardiac decompensation in the infant is a medical emergency necessitating immediate treatment if the patient is to be saved.

CAUSES OF HEART FAILURE. In the preterm infant, especially under 1500 gm birthweight, persistent patency of the ductus arteriosus is the most common cause of cardiac decompensation, and other forms of structural heart disease are rare.[42] In the full-term newborn the earliest important causes of heart failure are the hypoplastic left heart and coarctation of the aorta syndromes, sustained tachyarrythmia, cerebral or hepatic arteriovenous fistula, and myocarditis. Among the lesions commonly producing heart failure beyond age 1 to 2 weeks, when diminished pulmonary vascular resistance allows substantial left-to-right shunting, are ventricular septal and atrioventricular septal defects, transposition of the great arteries, truncus arteriosus, and total anomalous pulmonary venous connection, often with pulmonary venous obstruction. Although heart failure usually is the result of a structural defect or of myocardial disease, it should be recognized that the newborn myocardium may be severely depressed by such abnormalities as hypoxemia and acidemia, anemia, septicemia, marked hypoglycemia, hypocalcemia, and polycythemia. In the older child, heart failure often is due to acquired disease (Chap. 31) or is a complication of open-heart surgical procedures. In the acquired category are rheumatic and endomyocardial diseases, infective endocarditis, hematological and nutritional disorders, and severe cardiac arrhythmias.

CLINICAL MANIFESTATIONS IN THE INFANT. The clinical expression of cardiac decompensation in the infant consists of distinctive signs of pulmonary and systemic venous congestion and altered cardiocirculatory performance that resemble, but often are not identical to, those of the older child or adult (Table 29–3).[36,43] These reflect the interplay between the hemodynamic burden and adaptive responses. Common symptoms and signs are feeding difficulties and failure to gain weight and grow, tachypnea, tachycardia, pulmonary rales and rhonchi, liver enlargement, and cardiomegaly. Less frequent manifestations include peripheral edema, ascites, pulsus alternans, gallop rhythm, and inappropriate sweating. Pleural and pericardial effusions are exceedingly rare. The distinction between left and right heart failure is less obvious in the infant than in the older child or adult because most lesions that create a left ventricular pressure or volume overload also result in left-to-right shunting of blood through the foramen ovale and/or patent ductus arteriosus as well as pulmonary hypertension owing to elevated pulmonary venous pressures. Conversely, augmented filling or elevated pressure of the right ventricle in the infant reduces left ventricular compliance disproportionately when compared with the older child or adult and gives rise to signs of both systemic and pulmonary venous congestion.[37]

Fatigue and dyspnea on exertion express themselves as a feeding problem in the infant. Characteristically, the respiratory rate in heart failure is rapid (50 to 100 breaths/min). In the presence of left ventricular failure, interstitial pulmonary edema reduces pulmonary compliance and results in tachypnea and retractions. Excessive pulmonary blood flow by way of significant left-to-right shunts may further decrease lung compliance. Moreover, upper airway obstruction may be produced by selective enlargement of cardiovascular structures. In patients with large left-to-right shunts and left atrial and main pulmonary artery enlargement, the left main stem bronchus may be compressed, resulting in emphysematous expansion of the left upper or lower lobe or left lower lobe collapse.[44] Respiratory distress with grunting, flaring of the alae nasi, and intercostal retractions is observed when failure is severe and especially when pulmonary infection precipitates cardiac decompensation, which often is the case. Under these circumstances pulmonary rales may be due to the infection or failure, or both. A resting heart rate with little variability is also characteristic of heart failure. Hepatomegaly is regularly seen in infants in failure, although liver tenderness is uncommon. Cardiomegaly may be assessed roentgenographically, but it

TABLE 29–3 FEATURES OF HEART FAILURE IN INFANTS

Poor feeding and failure to thrive
Respiratory distress—mainly tachypnea
Rapid heart rate (160 to 180 beats/min)
Pulmonary rales or wheezing
Cardiomegaly and pulmonary edema on radiogram
Hepatomegaly (peripheral edema unusual)
Gallop sounds
Color—ashen pale or faintly cyanotic
Excessive perspiration
Diminished urine output

must be recognized that in the normal newborn infant, the cardiac diameter may be as much as 60 per cent of the thoracic diameter, and the large thymus gland in infants occasionally interferes with evaluation of heart size. Two-dimensional and Doppler echocardiography provide a good estimate of cardiac performance and chamber dimensions, and values may be compared with data derived from normal infants.[45–49]

Cardiac decompensation may progress with extreme rapidity in the first hours and days of life, producing a clinical picture of advanced cardiogenic shock and a profoundly obtunded infant. The presence of marked hepatomegaly and gross cardiomegaly usually allows distinction from noncardiac causes of diminished systemic perfusion.

The management of the infant with congenital heart disease and heart failure is described on p. 889.

CYANOSIS

Cyanosis is produced by reduced hemoglobin in cutaneous vessels in excess of approximately 3 gm/dl (see p. 891). Peripheral cyanosis usually reflects an abnormally great extraction of oxygen from normally saturated arterial blood, commonly the result of peripheral cutaneous vasoconstriction. Central cyanosis is a result of arterial blood oxygen unsaturation, most often in patients with congenital heart disease caused by shunting of systemic venous blood into the arterial circuit. Infants especially (as compared with adults) may appear cyanotic when in heart failure because of both peripheral and central factors[50]; the latter may include severe impairment of pulmonary function that commonly exists with alveolar hypoventilation, ventilation-perfusion inequality, or impaired oxygen diffusion.

In patients with central cyanosis owing to arterial oxygen unsaturation, the degree of cutaneous discoloration depends on the absolute amount of reduced hemoglobin, the magnitude of the right-to-left shunt relative to systemic flow, and the oxyhemoglobin saturation of venous blood. The last of these depends in turn on the tissue extraction of oxygen. Commonly, cyanosis appears or intensifies with physical activity or exercise as the saturation of systemic venous blood declines concurrent with an increase in right-to-left shunting across a defect as peripheral vascular resistance decreases. Oxygen transfer to the tissues is affected by shifts in the oxygen hemoglobin dissociation relation, which may be altered by blood pH and levels of red blood cell 2,3-diphosphoglycerate concentration.

The clinical approach to the infant with cyanosis is discussed on pp. 890 to 894.

CLUBBING AND POLYCYTHEMIA/ERYTHROCYTOSIS. Prominent accompaniments of arterial hypoxemia are polycythemia and clubbing of the digits. The latter is associated with an increased number of capillaries with increased blood flow through extensive arteriovenous aneurysms and an increase of connective tissue in the terminal phalanges of the fingers and toes. Polycythemia is a physiological response to chronic hypoxemia that stimulates erythrocytosis. The extremely high hematocrits observed in patients with arterial oxygen unsaturation cause a progressive increase in blood viscosity. Because the relationship is nonlinear between hematocrit and blood viscosity, relatively small increases beyond packed blood cell volumes of 60 per cent result in large increases in viscosity. Also, the apparent viscosity of blood increases in the microcirculation where lower shear rates exist, an increasingly important factor as the hematocrit exceeds 70 per cent.

Both the hematocrit and the circulating whole blood volume are increased in polycythemia accompanying cyanotic congenital heart disease; the hypervolemia is the result of an increase in red cell volume. The augmented red blood cell volume provoked by hypoxemia provides an increased oxygen-carrying capacity and enhanced oxygen supply to the tissues. The compensatory polycythemia often is of such severity that it becomes a liability and produces such adverse physiological effects as hyperviscosity, cellular aggregation, and thrombotic lesions in diverse organs and a hemorrhagic diathesis.[51] In this regard, oral steroid contraceptives are contraindicated in the adolescent cyanotic female because of the enhanced risk of cerebral thrombosis.

Management. Red cell volume reduction and replacement with plasma or albumin (erythrophoresis) lower blood viscosity and increase systemic blood flow and systemic oxygen transport, and thus may be helpful in the management of patients with severe hypoxic polycythemia (hematocrit $\geq$ 65 per cent). A final hematocrit of 55 to 63 per cent should be achieved; the higher level is necessary in patients with low initial oxygen saturation to avoid a severe reduction in arterial oxygen content. Acute phlebotomy without fluid replacement is contraindicated.

CEREBRAL AND PULMONARY COMPLICATIONS. Cerebrovascular accidents and brain abscesses occur particularly in cyanotic patients with substantial arterial desaturation.[52,53] *Cerebral thrombosis* is most common under age 2 years in severely cyanotic children, even in the presence of relatively low hematocrits, and occurs especially in a clinical setting in which oxygen requirements are raised by fever or, if blood viscosity is increased, dehydration.

Brain Abscess. This is an important complication of cyanotic heart disease.[53] Such abscesses are rare under 18 months of age and commonly are of insidious onset marked by headache, low-grade fever, vomiting, and a change in personality. Seizures or paralysis less frequently herald the onset of a brain abscess. Abscess must be suspected in any cyanotic child with focal neurological signs. Morbidity and mortality are related inversely to oxygen saturation levels. Brain abscess is thought to occur in about 2 per cent of the population with cyanotic congenital heart disease; a mortality rate of 30 to 40 per cent often is related to delay in diagnosis and treatment.

Paradoxical Embolus. This is a rare complication of cyanotic heart disease, usually observed only at necropsy.[54] Emboli arising in systemic veins may pass directly to the systemic circulation, because right-to-left intracardiac shunts allow venous blood to bypass the normal filtering action of the lungs.

Retinopathy. Dilated tortuous vessels progressing to papilledema, and retinal edema occasionally are observed in cyanotic patients, and appear to be related to decreased arterial oxygen saturation and/or to erythrocytosis but not to hypercapnia.

Hemoptysis. This is an uncommon but major complication in cyanotic patients with congenital heart disease, and occurs most often in the presence of pulmonary vascular obstructive disease or in patients with an extensive bronchial collateral circulation or pulmonary venous congestion.[55] Massive hemoptysis almost always represents rupture of a dilated bronchial artery.

SQUATTING. After exertion, patients with cyanotic heart disease, especially tetralogy of Fallot, typical assume a squatting posture to obtain relief from breathlessness.[56] Squatting appears to improve arterial oxygen saturation by increasing systemic vascular resistance, thereby diminishing the right-to-left shunt, and also by the pooling of markedly desaturated blood in the lower extremities. In addition, systemic venous return, and therefore pulmonary blood flow, may increase.

HYPOXIC SPELLS. Hypercyanotic or hypoxemic spells commonly complicate the clinical course in younger children with certain types of cyanotic heart disease, especially tetralogy of Fallot (see p. 929).[56] The spells are characterized by anxiety, hyperpnea, and a sudden marked increase in cyanosis; they are the result of an abrupt reduction in pulmonary blood flow. Unless terminated, the hypercyanotic episodes may lead to convulsions and may even be fatal. The sudden reduction in pulmonary blood flow may be precipitated by fluctuations in arterial pCO_2 and pH, a sudden fall in systemic or increase in pulmonary vascular resistance, or an acute increase in the severity of right ventricular outflow tract obstruction either by augmented contraction of the hypertrophied muscle in the right ventricular outflow tract or by a decrease in right ventricular cavity volume owing to tachycardia.

Treatment. This consists of oxygen administration, placing the child in the knee-chest position, and administration of morphine sulfate. Additional medications that may prove of value include the intravenous administration of sodium bicarbonate to correct the accompanying acidemia, alpha-adrenoceptor stimulants such as phenylephrine hydrochloride (Neo-Synephrine) or methoxamine to raise peripheral resistance and diminish right-to-left shunting, and beta-adrenoceptor blocking agents, which reduce cardiac sympathetic tone and depress cardiac contractility directly and increase ventricular volume by reducing heart rate.

ACID-BASE IMBALANCE

Disturbances in blood gas and acid-base equilibrium are noted particularly in infants with either congestive heart failure or cyanosis.[57] Large-volume left-to-right shunts, especially with pulmonary edema, may be associated with moderate respiratory acidemia and a lowering of arterial oxygen tensions, reflecting an increase in the alveolar-arterial oxygen tension gradient and ventilation-perfusion imbalance. Interference with carbon dioxide transport implies moderate to severe failure in these infants. Lesions associated with a reduced systemic cardiac output, such as severe coarctation of the aorta or critical aortic stenosis in infancy, often present as cardiac failure complicated by a severe metabolic acidemia and relatively high values of arterial oxygen tension. The latter finding, even in the presence of right-to-left shunting across a patent ductus arteriosus, is a result of diminished systemic perfusion and an elevated pulmonary-systemic blood flow ratio.

Respiratory acidemia and depressed levels of oxygen tension are observed in infants with obstruction to pulmonary venous return and right-to-left atrial shunting. Many infants with severe hypoxemia caused by lesions such as transposition of the great arteries or pulmonic atresia show metabolic acidemia and marked reductions in carbon dioxide tension secondary to hyperventilation, resulting from hypoxic stimulation of peripheral chemoreceptors.

IMPAIRED GROWTH

Impaired growth and physical development and delayed onset of adolescence are common features of many cyanotic and, to a lesser extent, acyanotic forms of congenital heart disease.[58–60] Mental development seldom is affected. The severity of growth disturbance depends on the anatomical lesion and its functional effect. Most children with mild defects grow normally. Weight gain is commonly slower than linear growth in acyanotic patients with large left-to-right shunts, whereas in cyanotic congenital heart disease, height and weight usually parallel each other. Boys appear to be more retarded in growth than girls, especially in the second decade. Skeletal maturity (i.e., bone age) is delayed in cyanotic children in relation to the severity of hypoxemia.

In some children, prenatal factors such as intrauterine infection and chromosomal or other hereditary and nonhereditary syndromes are responsible for growth retardation. In other patients, extracardiac malformations may contribute to poor weight gain and linear growth. Additional explanations for the mechanisms of growth interference have implicated malnutrition as a result of anorexia and inadequate nutrient and caloric intake, hypermetabolic state, acidemia and cation imbalance, tissue hypoxemia, diminished peripheral blood flow, chronic cardiac decompensation, malabsorption or protein loss, recurrent respiratory infections, and endocrine or genetic factors. In some instances, the underdevelopment is influenced little by operative correction of the underlying cardiac anomaly.

Among factors that may be responsible for persistent growth retardation postoperatively are age at operation, hemodynamically significant residual lesions, and sequelae or complications of operation. As a general rule, it is unwise preoperatively to guarantee to the parents of a child with heart disease that surgery will result in accelerated growth and development.

PULMONARY HYPERTENSION

(See also Chap. 25)

Pulmonary hypertension is a common accompaniment of many congenital cardiac lesions, and the status of the pulmonary vascular bed often is the principal determinant of the clinical manifestations, the course, and whether surgical treatment is feasible.[61] Increases in pulmonary arterial pressure result from elevations of pulmonary blood flow and/or resistance, the latter sometimes caused by an increase in vascular tone, but usually the result of underdevelopment and/or obstructive, obliterative structural changes within the pulmonary vascular bed.[62–64]

Pulmonary vascular resistance normally falls rapidly immediately after birth, owing to onset of ventilation and subsequent release of hypoxic pulmonary vasoconstriction. Subsequently the medial smooth muscle of pulmonary arterial resistance vessels thins gradually.[65] This latter process often is delayed by several months in infants with large aorticopulmonary or ventricular communications, at which time levels of pulmonary vascular resistance are still somewhat elevated. In patients with high pulmonary arterial pressure from birth, failure of normal growth of the pulmonary circulation may occur, and anatomical changes in the pulmonary vessels in the form of proliferation of intimal cells and intimal and medial thickening often progress, so that in the older child or adult vascular resistance ultimately may become fixed by obliterative changes in the pulmonary vascular bed. The causes of pulmonary vascular obstructive disease remain unknown, although increased pulmonary arterial blood pressure, elevated pulmonary venous pressure, polycythemia, systemic hypoxia, acidemia, and the nature of the bronchial circulation have all been implicated. Quite likely, injury to pulmonary vascular endothelial cells initiates a cascade of events that involve the release or activation of factors that alter the extracellular matrix, induce hypertrophy, cause proliferation of vascular smooth muscle cells, and promote connective tissue protein synthesis. Taken together these may permanently alter vessel structure and function.[66,67]

There are many patients with pulmonary vascular obstruction whose cardiac anomaly places them at particular risk quite early in life, precluding survival to adulthood. Patients at particularly high risk for the development of significant pulmonary vascular obstruction are those with certain forms of cyanotic congenital heart disease, such as complete transposition of the great arteries with or without ventricular septal defect or patent ductus arteriosus, single ventricle without pulmonary stenosis, double-outlet right ventricle, and truncus arteriosus. Other conditions in which pulmonary vascular obstruction appears to progress rapidly include large ventricular septal defect, as well as the less common conditions of unilateral pulmonary artery absence, congenital left-to-right shunts in an environment of high altitude or in association with the Down syndrome of trisomy 21, and complete atrioventricular canal defects, even those unassociated with a chromosomal anomaly.

MECHANISMS OF DEVELOPMENT. Intimal damage appears to be related to shear stresses because endothelial cell damage occurs at high-flow shear rates. A reduction in pulmonary arteriolar lumen size due to either thickened medial muscle or vasoconstriction increases the velocity of flow. Shear stress also increases as blood viscosity rises; therefore, infants with hypoxemia and high hematocrits as well as increased pulmonary blood flow are at increased risk of developing pulmonary vascular disease. In patients with left-to-right shunts, pulmonary arterial hypertension, if not present in infancy or childhood, may never occur or may not develop until the third or fourth decade or later. Once developed, intimal proliferative changes with hyalinization and fibrosis are not reversible by repair of the underlying cardiac defect. In severe pulmonary vascular obstructive disease, arteriovenous malformations may develop and predispose to massive hemoptysis.

Most vexing is the variability among patients with the same or similar cardiac lesions in both the time of appearance and rate of progression of their pulmonary vascular obstructive process. Although genetic influences may be operative (an example is the apparent acceleration of pulmonary vascular disease in patients with congenital heart disease and trisomy 21), evidence is now accumulating for important prenatal and postnatal modifiers of the pulmonary vascular bed that appear, at least in part, to be lesion-dependent. Thus a quantitative variability exists in the pulmonary vascular bed related to the *number*, not just the size and wall structure, of arterial vessels within the pulmonary circulation.[68,69]

Modeling of the blood vessels occurs proximal to and within terminal bronchioles (preacinar and intraacinar vessels, respectively) continuously from before birth. The intraacinar vessels, in particular, increase in size and number from late fetal life throughout childhood with minimal muscularization of their walls. The ensuing increase in the cross-sectional area of the pulmonary arterial circulation allows the cardiac output to rise substantially without an increase in pulmonary arterial pressure. If, however, the presence of a cardiac lesion interferes with the normal growth and multiplication of these most peripheral arteries, the resulting elevation of pulmonary vascular resistance may first be related to failure of the intraacinar pulmonary circulation to develop fully, and then secondarily to the morphological changes of obliterative vascular disease—medial thickening, intimal proliferation, hyalinization and fibrosis, angiomatoid and plexiform lesions, and ultimately, arterial necrosis.[64,70]

In essence, the morphometric framework adds an important dimension, that of growth and development of the pulmonary circulation, to the traditional view of pulmonary vascular obstructive disease occurring primarily as a result of anatomical changes in the individual pulmonary arterioles. Research attention currently focuses on the cellular and molecular biology of the vessel wall and abnormalities in endothelial cell–smooth muscle interactions in pulmonary hypertension.[62,66,67,69,70]

ASSESSMENT OF THE PATIENT WITH PULMONARY HYPERTENSION. It is important to understand the difficulties that exist with standard methods of assessing the severity of pulmonary vascular obstructive disease. Clinical and electrocardiographic observations do not distinguish between reversible and irreversible elevations in pulmonary vascular resistance. Echocardiography and Doppler interrogation of the heart may enable one to diagnose the presence of pulmonary hypertension but do not provide an accurate estimate of pressure or a reliable calculation of pulmonary vascular resistance.[71] Thus, hemodynamic measurements at cardiac catheterization are the mainstay in assessing the pulmonary vascular bed, especially its reactivity. The premium on accuracy is high because the presence, degree, and reactivity of pulmonary vascular obstruction determine the feasibility and long-term outcome of operation. Surgery must not be offered to patients with severe, fixed pulmonary vascular obstruction, even when the cardiac defect is anatomically correctable. Such patients either do not survive operation or, if they do, are not benefited and more often than not are harmed.

The aims of hemodynamic study are to quantify and compare the pulmonary and systemic flows and resistances and to determine the reactivity of the pulmonary vascular bed in patients with pulmonary hypertension. Because resistance to pulmonary blood flow cannot be measured directly, it is calculated from the ratio of pressure gradient to flow across the pulmonary bed according to Poiseuille's equation, which refers to steady flow of a newtonian fluid through straight, rigid tubes. There are potential errors in applying the equation and errors inherent in the methods of measurement. Furthermore, it is not possible in every patient to catheterize the pulmonary artery; when this is the case pulmonary venous wedge pressures may be used, but they are not always reliable indicators of pulmonary artery pressure, and the moment of hemodynamic evaluation may not be representative of potentially variable states of the pulmonary circulation. Nonetheless, a practical index of pulmonary vascular resistance can be established from measurements of pulmonary and systemic arterial pressures and calculated flows. One can then determine whether administration of drugs or oxygen or nitric oxide reduces the pulmonary vascular resistance, implying that the resistance is not fixed and therefore may decrease or at least not progress after successful operation.[72] A reduction in calculated pulmonary vascular resistance in response to oxygen or nitric oxide inhalation or pharmacological invention does not exclude coexisting anatomical pulmonary vascular disease but does imply a component of potentially reversible vasoconstriction contributing to the high resistance.

Other Diagnostic Methods. Because of the aforementioned shortcomings, additional methods have been developed to study the morphology of the small pulmonary arteries in patients with pulmonary hypertension. An example is the use of high-resolution magnification for *pulmonary wedge angiography* to determine the presence and extent of obstructive pulmonary vascular changes.[73] Pulmonary wedge angiograms, assessed quantitatively, appear to correlate well with both hemodynamic findings and histological observations of the structural state of the pulmonary vascular bed. Of additional interest is the current practical application of morphometric structural analyses that attempt to identify for operation patients whose postoperative pulmonary hemodynamics might be expected to improve, if not normalize.[74] Thus, *lung biopsy* at surgery has been proposed in patients with equivocal hemodynamic data to aid in determining whether to proceed with operation in reasonable anticipation of postoperative regression of elevated pulmonary vascular resistance.

THE MORPHOMETRIC APPROACH. Decisions on optimal timing of operations often are difficult because of the varying rates of development of pulmonary vascular disease in different patients with the same anomaly and because the evaluation of pulmonary vascular resistance and reactivity in the catheterization laboratory is a less than perfect science. Preoperative lung biopsy using the Heath-Edwards criteria has enjoyed little popularity, especially because sampling errors may result from the scatter of different grades of lesion in different parts of the lung. Accordingly, it is attractive to seek an alternative method that would obviate these problems. In this regard, application of a morphometric approach holds promise because the described changes in pulmonary vessel morphological characteristics are more uniformly distributed throughout the lung and, importantly, lend themselves to quantification.

Three abnormalities have been identified as anatomical markers of elevated pulmonary vascular resistance: (1) an excessive and premature extension of vascular smooth muscle into intraacinar pulmonary arteries, (2) failure of preacinar arterial wall thickness to regress normally, and (3) failure of pulmonary arteries to grow and proliferate normally during postnatal development. Frozen-section lung biopsy provides a firmer basis for judgment of whether reparative or palliative operation should proceed. The technique has proved useful in patients with univentricular hearts or tricuspid atresia in determining the feasibility of a Fontan procedure (see p. 933) and in patients with lesions known to exhibit early and rapidly progressive pulmonary vascular disease, such as complete transposition of the great arteries, complete atrioventricular canal defect, and nonrestrictive ventricular septal defect.[75]

CLINICAL MANIFESTATIONS OF PULMONARY HYPERTENSION. When this condition is associated with a large left-to-right shunt, the clinical manifestations reflect the specific malformation responsible. When pulmonary vascular resistance is elevated and a significant right-to-left shunt exists, the patient is cyanotic, and polycythemia and clubbing are noted. A dominant *a* wave in the jugular venous pulse may be seen, reflecting vigorous right atrial contraction caused by diminished compliance of the right ventricle. In some instances there are large systolic *c-v* waves, which suggest tricuspid regurgitation. A prominent right ventricular parasternal lift and palpable systolic expansion of the pulmonary artery are present. A soft pulmonary systolic ejection murmur preceded by an ejection sound and followed by a markedly accentuated pulmonic component of the second heart sound often is audible on auscultation; an early diastolic decrescendo blowing murmur of pulmonary regurgitation may be heard. If right ventricular failure and dilatation supervene, the systolic murmur of tricuspid regurgitation may be audible at the lower left sternal border. Right ventricular enlargement may be evident on the chest roentgenogram and electrocardiogram. The former examination also reveals a conspicuously enlarged pulmonary artery, prominent hilar pulmonary vascular markings, and attenuated peripheral vessels. The presence of pulmonary hypertension is suggested by analysis of Doppler waveforms of right and left ventricular ejection.[76,77] The site of the underlying defect may be localized by means of two-dimensional and Doppler echocardiography and/or cardiac catheterization and angiocardiography. Pressures in the right side of the heart are essentially identical to systemic pressures in cyanotic patients if the shunt is at the ventricular or aorticopulmonary levels, but they usually are lower than systemic pressures in patients with an intraatrial shunt. No specific treatment has proved beneficial for obstructive pulmonary vascular disease.

This fact underscores the importance of efforts to define the optimal age at operation to provide the highest probability of postoperative normalization of the pulmonary vascular bed. It is important to emphasize that almost all congenital cardiovascular defects are amenable to surgical repair in infancy, and it is likely that the surgical art will progress to the point that virtually all patients with lesions associated with pulmonary hypertension will be operated on within the first 3 to 18 months of life. When this goal is reached without increased operative mortality, the incidence of postoperative pulmonary vascular obstruction may well achieve the status of a bygone concern.

OTHER CONSEQUENCES OF CONGENITAL HEART DISEASE

INFECTIVE ENDOCARDITIS (see also Chap. 33). Infective endocarditis is uncommon under age 2 years and thereafter most often affects children with tetralogy of Fallot (especially after systemic-pulmonary anastomosis), ventricular septal defect, aortic stenosis, and patent ductus arteriosus. Postsurgical patients with prosthetic heterograft or homograft valves or conduits are at particular risk. Infants and children with normal cardiac anatomy are at increased risk now that the use of central venous catheters is routine, and drug addiction in adolescents is an emerging risk factor.[78,79]

A causative organism can be isolated in about 90 per cent of children, usually either alpha-streptococci (usually *Streptococcus viridans*) or *Staphylococcus aureus*, although uncommon organisms may also be identified.[78,80,81] Fungal endocarditis is quite rare in the pediatric age group. Mortality appears to be highest when coagulase-positive *Staphylococcus* is the offending organism and when the endocarditis involves the left, rather than the right, side of the heart. Most recent data suggest 75 to 80 per cent overall survival.[80] Factors predisposing to endocarditis may be identified in about one-third of cases. These include cardiovascular surgery with infection during the perioperative period, respiratory tract infections, and ear, nose, throat, and dental procedures. Less often, contamination during a surgical procedure or cardiac catheterization or an infection involving the skin, genitourinary tract, or other organ system has been the cause.

Although routine antimicrobial prophylaxis is recommended for all children with congenital heart disease and for the majority of patients after operative repair of the lesion,[82] it should be recognized that many different microbes are responsible for the disease and that an effective preventive approach ultimately may center on active immunization rather than antibiotics. Antibiotic prophylaxis currently is recommended for all dental procedures known to induce gingival or mucosal bleeding, including cleaning, oral trauma, and other procedures such as tonsillectomy, gastrointestinal surgery, genitourinary surgery, and incision and drainage of infected tissue (Table 29–4). The risk of endocarditis is undoubtedly related both to the magnitude of bacteremia and to the type of underlying heart disease. Because infection on a prosthetic heart valve or conduit may be devastating, combinations of antibiotics given parenterally are advisable in these patients.

CHEST PAIN (see also pages 3 and 1291). *Angina pectoris* is an uncommon symptom of cardiac disease in infants and children, occurring in association with anomalous pulmonary origin of a coronary artery or, occasionally, in association with severe aortic stenosis, pulmonic stenosis, or pulmonary hypertension owing to pulmonary vascular obstruction. Cardiac pain in the infant with anomalous coronary artery (see p. 909) usually takes the form of irritability and crying during feeding or straining at bowel movement. In children with severe or right ventricular outflow tract obstruction, chest pain commonly follows effort and is identical to angina observed in adults. Cardiac pain associated with *pulmonary vascular obstruction* may be anginal in nature but often is evanescent and pleuritic in type. Atypical forms of chest pain associated with the syndrome of *mitral valve prolapse* are much less usual in children than in adults. A sensation of chest discomfort or cardiac awareness frequently is interpreted as pain by the parents of children with cardiac arrhythmias. Careful questioning serves to identify palpitations rather than pain as the symptom and often elicits an additional history of anxiety, pallor, and sweating. Pain caused by *pericarditis* is commonly of acute onset and associated with fever, and can be identified by specific physical, roentgenographic, and echocardiographic findings.

Most commonly, chest pain in children is *musculoskeletal* in origin and may be reproduced on upper-extremity movement or by palpation; chest wall pain often is the result of *costochondritis*.[83] Finally, children, like adults, may suffer chest pain of nonspecific form owing to *anxiety*, with or without hyperventilation; a history often is elicited of a family member or friend who had recently died from or suffered myocardial infarction.

SYNCOPE (see also Chap. 28). Syncope is an unusual feature of heart disease in children; its presence suggests specific diagnoses, the most common being an arrhythmia. The symptom is observed in patients with long QT syndrome and in children with complete atrioventricular block that is less often of congenital origin than a sequela of cardiac operation. Syncope caused by abrupt episodes of either bradycardia or tachcyardia occurs in association with the sick sinus syndrome. The latter is most commonly produced in children after surgical procedures that involve the region of the sinoatrial node, e.g., atrial septal defect closure or Mustard's venous switch procedure for transposition of the great arteries (see p. 835). Syncope is an occasional but ominous symptom if associated with severe aortic stenosis, pulmonary vascular obstruction, or a left atrial myxoma that transiently occludes left ventricular inflow.[84]

In children with an anatomically normal heart, transient episodes of vasovagally mediated hypotension and bradycardia (neurocardiogenic syncope) may be diagnosed by autonomic function testing and head-upright tilt table testing (see p. 584). The latter is especially helpful in assessing the adequacy of prophylactic therapy, usually by volume expansion (e.g., salt and fludrocortisone), or by beta-adrenergic blockade or alpha-adrenergic agonist or serotonin reuptake inhibitor therapy.[85–87]

SUDDEN DEATH (see also Chap. 24). The sudden infant death syndrome is not likely due to a cardiac cause but rather to pulmonary and/or central nervous system causes. In contrast to adults, children seldom die suddenly and unexpectedly from cardiovascular disease. Arrhythmias, hypoxemia, and coronary insufficiency secondary to left ventricular outflow tract obstruction are the most frequent causes of death.[88–91] Sudden death most often is reported in patients with postoperative heart disease or dilated cardiomyopathy. It is also observed in patients with aortic stenosis or hypertrophic obstructive cardiomyopathy, primary pulmonary hypertension, the Eisenmenger syndrome of pulmonary vascular obstruction, myocarditis, congenital complete heart block, primary endocardial fibroelastosis, anomalies of the coronary arteries, and cyanotic congenital heart disease with pulmonic stenosis or atresia. A relation exists between strenuous exercise and sudden death in patients with aortic stenosis or obstructive cardiomyopathy, thus providing justification for restricting patients with these lesions from gymnastic activities and strenuous competitive sports.

TABLE 29–4 PROPHYLACTIC ANTIBIOTICS FOR PROTECTION FROM BACTERIAL ENDOCARDITIS

I. STANDARD PROPHYLACTIC REGIMEN FOR DENTAL/ORAL/UPPER RESPIRATORY TRACT PROCEDURES

Amoxicillin 3.0 gm orally 1 hour before procedure, then 1.5 gm 6 hours after initial dose.

For amoxicillin/penicillin-allergic individuals:

Erythromycin ethylsuccinate 800 mg or erythromycin stearate 1 gm orally 2 hours before a procedure, then one-half the dose 6 hours after the initial administration.

-OR-

Clindamycin 300 mg 1 hour before a procedure, and 150 mg 6 hours after initial dose.

II. ALTERNATIVE PROPHYLACTIC REGIMENS FOR DENTAL/ORAL/UPPER RESPIRATORY TRACT PROCEDURES

For patients unable to take oral medications:

Ampicillin 2.0 gm IV (or IM) 30 minutes before procedure, then 1.0 gm ampicillin IV (or IM) or 1.5 gm amoxicillin orally 6 hours after initial dose.

For ampicillin/amoxicillin/penicillin-allergic patients unable to take oral medications:

Clindamycin 300 mg IV 1 hour before a procedure and 150 mg IV (or orally) 6 hours after initial dose.

Optional regimen for individuals considered to be at very high risk who are not candidates for the standard regimen:

Ampicillin 2.0 gm IV (or IM) plus gentamicin 1.5 mg/kg IV (or IM) (not to exceed 80 mg) one-half hour before procedure, followed by 1.5 gm oral amoxicillin 6 hours after the initial dose. Alternatively, the parenteral regimen may be repeated 8 hours after the initial dose.

Optional regimen for amoxicillin/ampicillin/penicillin-allergic patients:

Vancomycin 1.0 gm IV administered over 1 hour, starting 1 hour before the procedure. No repeat dose is necessary.

III. REGIMENS FOR GENITOURINARY/GASTROINTESTINAL PROCEDURES

Standard regimen:

Ampicillin 2.0 gm IV (or IM) plus gentamicin 1.5 mg/kg IV (or IM) (not to exceed 80 mg) one-half hour before procedure, followed by 1.5 gm oral amoxicillin 6 hours after the initial dose. Alternatively, the parenteral regimen may be repeated once 8 hours after the initial dose.

For amoxicillin/ampicillin/penicillin-allergic patients:

Vancomycin 1.0 gm IV administered over 1 hour plus gentamicin 1.5 mg/kg IV (or IM) (not to exceed 80 mg) 1 hour before the procedure. May be repeated once 8 hours after initial dose.

Alternative oral regimen in low-risk patients:

Amoxicillin 3.0 gm orally 1 hour before the procedure, then 1.5 gm 6 hours after the initial dose.

Note: Initial pediatric dosages are listed below. Follow-up doses should be one-half the initial dose. Total pediatric dose should not exceed total adult dose.

Amoxicillin:	50 mg/kg
Ampicillin:	50 mg/kg
Clindamycin:	10 mg/kg
Gentamicin:	2.0 mg/kg
Vancomycin:	20 mg/kg
Erythromycin ethylsuccinate or stearate:	20 mg/kg

Adapted from Dajani, A. S., et al.: Prevention of bacterial endocarditis. Recommendations by the American Heart Association. JAMA *264*:2919, 1990.

THE HIGH-RISK INFANT WITH CONGENITAL HEART DISEASE

Without prompt recognition, accurate diagnosis, and treatment, about one-third of all infants born with congenital heart disease die in the first months of life. Heart failure and cyanosis are the two cardinal signs in the high-risk infant with heart disease, and this section provides an approach for the management of each.

HEART FAILURE

The causes and clinical manifestations of heart failure in the infant with congenital heart disease are discussed on p. 884. Care of the infant with heart failure must include careful consideration of the underlying structural or functional disturbance. The general aims of treatment are to achieve an increase in cardiac performance, augment peripheral perfusion, and decrease pulmonary and systemic venous congestion.[36,37] It must be emphasized, however, that under many conditions medical management cannot control the effects of the abnormal loads imposed by a host of congenital cardiac lesions. Under these circumstances cardiac diagnosis and interventional catheter or operative intervention may be urgently required.[28,68] Thus initial therapy is aimed at stabilizing the infant's condition for diagnostic ultrasonography or hemodynamic or angiocardiographic study as soon as possible. In almost all situations the decision to intervene surgically or to continue medical management requires a definitive anatomical diagnosis.

RESERVE MECHANISMS IN THE NEONATAL HEART

Pediatricians in particular should be aware of the important concept of cardiac reserve because it is in this regard that important differences exist between the young heart (of the preterm or newborn infant) and the fully developed heart of the older child, adolescent, and adult (Fig. 29–5).

Clinicians have long recognized the unique fragility and lability of the neonatal circulation in response to disease states and various physiological stimuli. Moreover, it often is apparent that newborns may exhibit suboptimal therapeutic responses to drugs such as digitalis, which directly stimulate cardiac contractility. The age dependency of these observations have their basis in the reduced ability of the hearts of premature and full-term newborns, when compared with the hearts and circulation of older children or adults, to call on a functional reserve capacity to adapt to stress.[36,92,93]

Studies from the author's and other laboratories have shown that structural, functional, biochemical, and pharmacological properties of the young heart differ considerably from those of its older counterpart.[22–32] The young heart contains fewer myofilaments to generate force with and to shorten during contraction. In addition, the chamber stiffness of the young heart's ventricles is greater than that seen later in life.

PRELOAD RESERVE. Any increase in ventricular filling or volume in the small, young heart results in a disproportionately greater rise in ventricular wall tension or stress. Similarly, it takes a smaller increase in ventricular filling to reach the limits of assistance given to cardiac pump and muscle function by stretching the myofilaments; that is, *preload or diastolic reserve is limited.*

The young heart generates relatively less force; it cannot generate the same ventricular systolic pressure or wall tensions, or obtain the same stroke volume augmentation from any initial stretch, as can the older heart. With these facts in mind, it must be remembered that the oxygen consumption of the normal newborn is considerably higher than later in life; accordingly, the newborn at rest has a much higher cardiac output/m^2 than the child or adult. Thus, even in the absence of stress, the young heart must function near peak performance just to satisfy the normal demands of the peripheral tissues. Because newborn cardiac performance at rest is so close to its ceiling, or limits of function, little *systolic reserve* is available to adapt to an acute or chronic stress such as pressure or volume load from an obstructive lesion or left-to-right circulatory shunt, respectively, or asphyxia.

HEART RATE RESERVE. This consists of the ability of the heart to change its rate of pumping to raise the level of cardiac output. In this regard the newborn also is limited because in this age group the intrinsic heart rate normally is quite high. In addition, heart failure per se raises the frequency of contraction even further, primarily as a result of high circulating levels of catecholamines. In this sense, the newborn's heart rate also is closer than the child's or adult's to its ceiling, or upper limits of effectiveness. Furthermore, increases in heart rate occur largely at the expense of diastolic filling time. Thus, at very rapid heart rates, there is a disproportionately diminished diastolic time and therefore diminished time for perfusion of the myocardium by its own coronary arterial system. In addition, rapid heart rates result in elevated myocardial energy expenditure and increased myocardial demand for oxygen. The sum of these considerations indicates that newborn *heart rate reserve* is reduced.

TREATMENT (see also Chap. 17). Table 29–5 lists supportive and pharmacological measures in the treatment of the newborn with heart failure. The supportive measures are designed to increase tissue oxygen supply, decrease tissue oxygen consumption, and correct metabolic abnormalities. Digitalis glycosides and certain diuretic agents provide the most important elements of medical therapy, but it is important to recognize that the dosage regimen of drugs administered to young patients must be adjusted to take into account the age and size of the patient and the maturity-dependent pharmacological properties of cardioactive drugs.[92,94] Because this is especially true in early in-

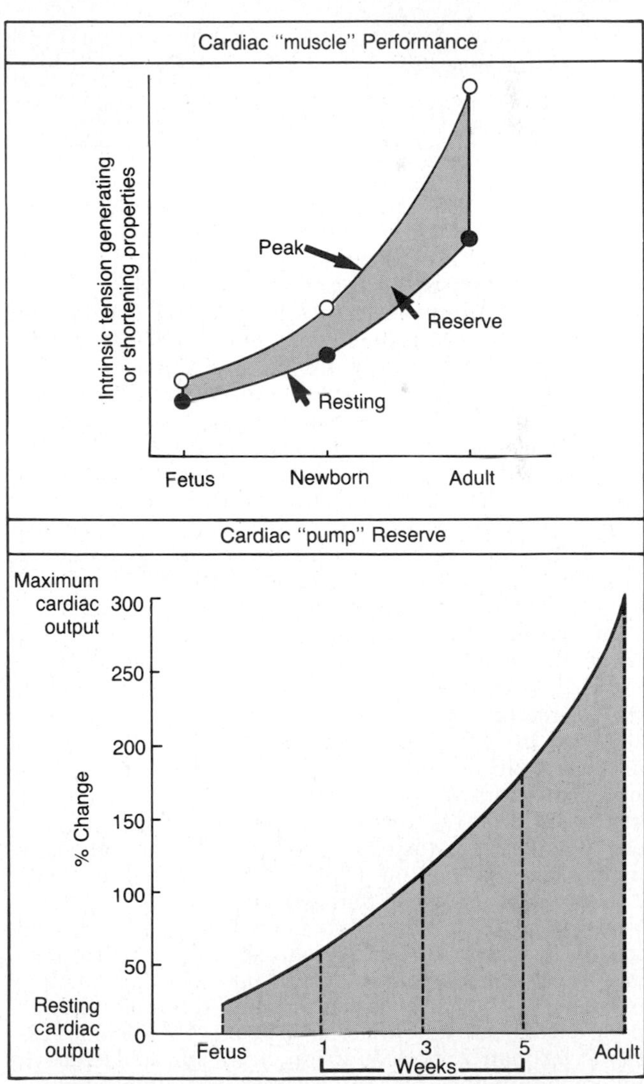

FIGURE 29–5. Schema of reduced cardiac reserve in fetal and newborn hearts compared with the adult's. In the newborn infant, resting cardiac muscle performance *(top panel)* is close to the peak of ventricular function because of limitations in diastolic, systolic, and heart rate reserve. Similarly, pump reserve *(bottom panel)* early in life is limited by these factors, as well as by a much higher resting cardiac output relative to body weight, compared with the adult.

TABLE 29–5 TREATMENT OF CONGESTIVE HEART FAILURE

I. GENERAL INTERVENTIONS
- Rest (occasional sedation)
- Semi-Fowler position
- Temperature and humidity control
- Oxygen
- Decrease sodium load
- Avoid aspiration
- Treat infection, if present

II. SPECIFIC INTERVENTIONS
- Preload manipulation
  - Move ventricular function curve up by volume infusion to increase venous return
  - Move ventricular function curve down with diuretics, venodilators
- Afterload reduction
  - Facilitate ventricular emptying by reducing wall tension
  - Reduce blood viscosity
  - Drugs, arteriolar dilators, mechanical counterpulsation
- Inotropic stimulation
  - Improve physical and metabolic milieu: pH, PaO_2, glucose, calcium, hemoglobin
  - Inotropic drugs: digitalis, catecholamines, dobutamine, dopamine
- Heart rate
  - Control rhythm disturbances with pacing, drugs
- Other
  - Mechanical ventilation
  - Prostaglandin manipulation
  - Peritoneal dialysis

III. INTERVENTIONAL CATHETER-DIRECTED THERAPY or SURGERY (may include transplantation)

fancy, Table 29–6 provides the dosages of digoxin and diuretics commonly used for infants.

Digitalis and Diuretics. Digoxin is the glycoside used exclusively to treat pediatric patients in most cardiac centers because it is readily absorbed, available in convenient dosage form, and excreted rapidly from the body. Premature infants are more sensitive to digitalis than are full-term newborns, who, in turn, are more sensitive than older infants. Infants absorb and excrete digoxin as well as adults do, and their relative distribution of the glycoside to different body tissues is also similar. The prevailing dose schedules for digoxin produce higher serum concentrations in infants than would be considered optimal for adults.[95] The basis for the higher digitalis requirement in infancy is unclear, although it may relate to an age-dependent alteration in the sensitivity of the myocardium per se to the glycosides. In this regard, infants tolerate higher serum digoxin concentrations than adults without developing signs of toxicity. In the adult, the usual therapeutic concentrations of digoxin are less than 2 ng/ml blood, and toxicity commonly occurs above that level. In contrast, in infants, therapeutic levels of digoxin range from 1 to 5 ng/ml (mean = 3.5), while toxicity is associated with concentrations in excess of 3 ng/ml. Older children have therapeutic and toxic levels similar to those of adults.

A restricted fluid intake (65 ml/kg/day) and a low-sodium diet (1 to 2 mEq/kg/day) should accompany diuretic therapy in the most seriously ill infants with heart failure. Furosemide is the agent of choice when the rapid elimination of excess salt and water is needed. Hydrochlorothiazide, occasionally in conjunction with spironolactone or triamterene to reduce potassium loss and sodium retention, is convenient for long-term therapy.

Other Pharmacological Approaches. These may prove to be of significant benefit in selected instances in which digitalis and diuretics are relatively ineffective. In situations in which cardiac decompensation is not the result of an obstructive lesion, catecholamines may be used temporarily to alleviate cardiac failure while the patient is awaiting more definitive operative treatment (Table 29–7).[92] In infants with the coarctation of the aorta syndrome, in whom ductal constriction unmasks the aortic branch point producing aortic narrowing (see p. 911), or with aortic arch interruption, heart failure may be reversed dramatically by the intravenous infusion of prostaglandin E_1 (0.03–0.1 mg/kg/min), which results in dilatation of the ductus arteriosus and relief of the obstruction.[96,97] Conversely, in preterm infants in whom patent ductus arteriosus is responsible for profound cardiopulmonary deterioration, constriction of the ductus arteriosus may be accomplished by inhibition of prostaglandin synthesis with the nonsteroidal anti-inflammatory agent indomethacin (0.2 mg/kg IV).[98,99]

Vasodilator therapy also is used in infants or children with heart disease in whom preload or afterload alterations may be expected to improve cardiac performance (Table 29–8).[36,37,92,100] Moreover, treatment of severe cardiac failure often requires combining inotropic and afterload-reducing agents (see p. 495). Combinations of dopamine, dobutamine, and nitroprusside have been used extensively and effectively in the pediatric population, primarily in the setting of low cardiac output after open-heart surgery.[92] Use of oral afterload-reducing agents, e.g., hydralazine or captopril, in association with digoxin is worthwhile in the long-term therapy of outpatients with congestive cardiomyopathy and/or significant mitral or aortic regurgitation.

Rapid developments in molecular biology have begun to revolutionize our understanding of cardiovascular regulation, both before and after birth and at all ages. As knowledge is gained about the mechanisms responsible for the variability of gene expression in the heart, it is apparent that the future holds the opportunity for clinicians to modify gene expression in ways that will importantly enhance the heart's ability to respond to both the heart failure state

TABLE 29–6 DIURETIC AND DIGITALIS DOSAGES FOR INFANTS

PREPARATION	DOSAGE AND ROUTE OF ADMINISTRATION	
Furosemide	IV, 1 mg/kg/dose; oral, 2 to 6 mg/kg/day	
Ethacrynic acid	IV, 1 mg/kg/dose; oral, 2 to 3 mg/kg/day	
Hydrochlorothiazide	Oral, 2 to 5 mg/kg/day	
Spironolactone	Oral, 1 to 3 mg/kg/day	
Triamterene	Oral, 2 to 4 mg/kg/day	
Digoxin		
Elixir	0.05 mg/ml	
Parenteral	0.10 mg/ml	
	DOSE AND ROUTE*	
AGE AND WEIGHT	Acute Digitalization	Maintenance
Prematures <1.5 kg	10–20 μg/kg IV TDD: ½, ¼, ¼ of dose q 8h	4 μg/kg/day IV (may increase to 4 μg/kg q 12h at age 1 month)
1.5–2.5 kg	Same as above	4 μg/kg q 12h IV
Full-term newborns	30 μg/kg IV, TDD	4–5 μg/kg q 12h IV
Infants (1–12 months)	35 μg/kg IV, TDD	5–10 μg/kg q 12h IV
>12 months	40 μg/kg IV, TDD (maximum 1.0 mg)	5–10 μg/kg q 12h IV
Older children (over 20 kg)	1.0–2.0 mg IV, TDD over 48 hours	0.125–0.250 mg IV q day

* po = Oral dose approximately 20 per cent greater than IV dose except in "older children." In older children, IV = oral dose.
TDD = Total digitalizing dose.

TABLE 29–7 DOSAGE REGIMENS: INOTROPIC AGENTS

DRUG	DOSE	COMMENTS
Epinephrine (Adrenalin)	0.05–1.0 μg/kg/min IV	May cause hypertension and cardiac arrhythmias; inactivated in alkaline solution
Isoproterenol (Isuprel)	0.05–0.5 μg/kg/min IV	May decrease coronary blood flow; results in peripheral and pulmonary vasodilation
Norepinephrine (Levophed)	0.05–0.5 μg/kg/min IV	Causes significant vasoconstriction
Dobutamine (Dobutrex)	2–10 μg/kg/min IV (Max 40 μg/kg/min)	No direct effect on renal perfusion, little or no peripheral vasodilatation or tachycardia
Dopamine (Intropin)	2–20 μg/kg/min IV (Max 50 μg/kg/min) 2–5 μg/kg/min 5–8 μg/kg/min >8 μg/kg/min >10 μg/kg/min 15–20 μg/kg/min	Significant renal vasodilatation Inotropic ± heart rate acceleration Significant heart rate acceleration ± Vasoconstriction Significant vasoconstriction
	(Above dose/effect relations speculative in neonates)	
Amrinone	Dose schedule not established for infants and children Adults: 40 μg/kg/min IV for 1 hr, then 6–10 μg/kg/min; 50–450 mg/day po divided TID	May cause thrombocytopenia, hepatic and GI disturbance, fever, and arrhythmias

From Friedman, W. F., and George, B. L.: New concepts and drugs in the treatment of congestive heart failure. Pediatr. Clin. North Am. *31*:1197, 1984.

and those diseases that are responsible for the abnormalities leading to cardiac disease.[101,102]

CYANOSIS

Cyanosis in the infant (see p. 885) often presents as a diagnostic emergency, necessitating prompt detection of the underlying cause. The schema in Figure 29–6 outlines a general approach to diagnosis. The cardiologist must distinguish between three types of cyanosis—peripheral, differential, and central—while recognizing that cyanosis may accompany diseases of the central nervous, hematological, respiratory, and cardiac systems.

PERIPHERAL CYANOSIS. Peripheral cyanosis (normal arterial oxygen saturation and widened arteriovenous oxygen differences) usually indicates stasis of blood flow in the periphery. The level of reduced hemoglobin in the capillaries of the skin usually exceeds 3 gm/100 dl. The most prominent causes of peripheral cyanosis in the newborn are autonomically controlled alterations in the cutaneous distribution of capillary blood flow (acrocyanosis) and septicemia associated with evidence of a low cardiac output, i.e., hypotension, weak pulse, and cold extremities. In many instances, peripheral cyanosis is clearly the result of a cold environment or high hemoglobin content. When cyanosis is caused by the former, vasodilatation produced by immersing the extremity in warm water for several minutes reverses the cyanosis.

CENTRAL CYANOSIS. Oxygen unsaturation in central cyanosis may result from inadequately oxygenated pulmonary venous blood, in which case inhalation of 100 per cent oxygen may diminish or clear the discoloration (see below). Conversely, in instances in which cyanosis is due to an intracardiac or extracardiac right-to-left shunt, pulmonary venous blood is fully saturated, and inhalation of 100 per cent oxygen usually does not improve the infant's color. It is necessary to qualify the latter statement because oxygen may act directly in infants with elevated pulmonary vascular resistance to dilate the pulmonary blood vessels and thus reduce the magnitude of the venoarterial shunt. Central cyanosis also may be due to the replacement of normal by abnormal hemoglobin, as in methemoglobinemia.

Several factors influence the oxygen saturation produced at any given arterial pO_2. These include temperature, pH, ratio of fetal to adult hemoglobin, and erythrocyte concentration of 2,3-diphosphoglycerate. For example, fetal hemoglobin has a higher affinity for oxygen than does adult hemoglobin and therefore would be more highly saturated at any given pO_2. Thus, determination of the systemic arterial oxygen tension may provide a more accurate picture of the underlying pathophysiology than simply measuring the oxygen saturation.[50,103]

DIFFERENTIAL CYANOSIS. Differential cyanosis virtually always indicates the presence of congenital heart disease, often with patency of the ductus arteriosus and coarctation of the aorta as components of the abnormal anatomical complex. If the upper part of the body is pink and the lower part of the body blue, coarctation of the aorta or interruption of the aortic arch is probable, with oxygenated blood supplying the upper body and desaturated blood supplying the lower body by way of right-to-left flow through the ductus arteriosus. The latter also occurs in patients with patent ductus arteriosus and markedly elevated pulmonary vascular resistance. A patient with transposition of the great arteries and coarctation of the aorta with retrograde flow through a patent ductus arteriosus demonstrates the reverse situation, i.e., the lower part of the body is pink and the upper part blue. Simultaneous determinations of oxygen saturation in the temporal or right brachial artery and the femoral artery are helpful in confirming the presence of differential cyanosis.

TABLE 29–8 DOSAGE REGIMENS: VASODILATORS IN INFANTS AND CHILDREN

DRUG	DOSE AND ROUTE OF ADMINISTRATION	COMMENTS
Nitroglycerin	0.5–20 μg/kg/min IV (Max 60 μg/kg/min IV)	Dosage schedule for IV and other routes of administration not well established for children
Hydralazine (Apresoline)	0.5 mg/kg/day po q 6–8h (Max 200 mg/day or 7 mg/kg/day) 1.5 μg/kg/min IV or 0.1–0.5 mg/kg/dose IV q 6h (Max 2 mg/kg q 6h)	May cause tachycardia, GI symptoms, neutropenia, lupus-like syndrome
Captopril (Capoten)	0.1–0.4 mg/kg/dose po given q 6–24h as needed	May cause neutropenia/proteinuria
Nitroprusside (Nipride)	0.5–8 μg/kg/min IV	May result in thiocyanate or cyanide toxicity if used in high doses or for prolonged periods of time; light-sensitive
Prazosin (Minipress)	1st dose: 5 μg/kg/po (Max 25 μg/kg/dose q 6h)	Initial dose used to elevate hypotensive effects; orthostatic hypotension, attenuation of hemodynamic effects may occur.

From Friedman, W. F., and George, B. L.: New concepts and drugs in the treatment of congestive heart failure. Pediatr. Clin. North Am. *31*:1197, 1984.

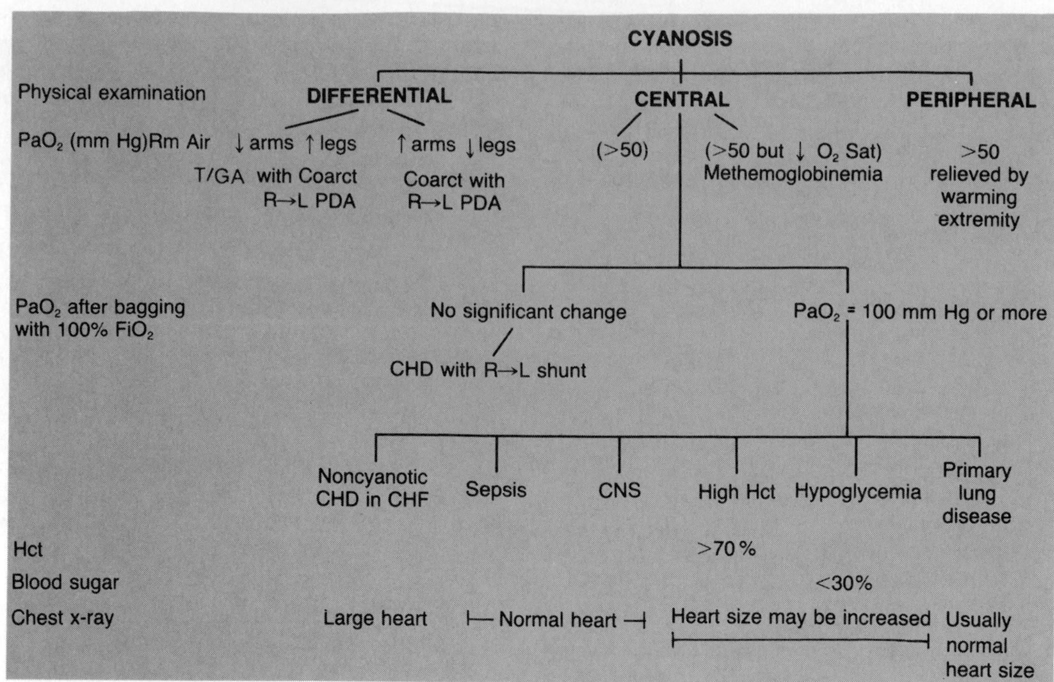

FIGURE 29–6. Flow chart for the evaluation of cyanotic infants. Tests to be done are listed at the left. The response to each of these tests leads along the line to the proper diagnostic category. CHD = congenital heart disease, CHF = congestive heart failure, CNS = central nervous system, Hct = hematocrit, PDA = patent ductus arteriosus, T/GA = transposition of great arteries. (From Kirkpatrick, S. E., et al.: Differential diagnosis of congenital heart disease in the newborn—University of California, San Diego, School of Medicine, and University Hospital, San Diego [Specialty Conference]. West. J. Med. *128*:127, 1978.)

Differentiating Between Pulmonary and Cardiac Causes of Cyanosis

The distinction between respiratory signs and symptoms arising from cyanotic cardiac disease and those associated with a primary pulmonary disorder is an important challenge to the cardiologist.[43] Upper airway obstruction precipitates cyanosis by producing alveolar hypoventilation owing to reduced pulmonary ventilation. Mechanical obstruction may occur from the nares to the carina, and the important diagnostic possibilities among congenital abnormalities are choanal atresia, vascular ring, laryngeal web, and tracheomalacia. Acquired causes include vocal cord paresis, obstetrical injury to the cricothyroid cartilage, and foreign body. Structural abnormalities in the lungs resulting from intrapulmonary disease are more frequently a basis for cyanosis among newborns than is upper airway obstruction. Hyaline membrane disease, atelectasis, or pneumonitis causing inflammation, collapse, and fluid accumulation in the alveoli results in reduction of the oxygenation of blood reaching the systemic circulation.

Successfully distinguishing between these various causes of cyanosis depends on interpretation of the respiratory pattern, the cardiac physical examination, evaluation of arterial blood gases (Table 29–9), and interpretation of the electrocardiogram, chest x-ray, and echocardiogram.

RESPIRATORY PATTERNS. The key to differential diagnosis at the bedside commonly is the proper evaluation of the pattern of respiration. Term infants normally exhibit a progressive reduction in respiratory rate during the first day of life from 60 to 70 per minute to 35 to 55 per minute. Moreover, mild intercostal retractions and minimal expiratory grunting disappear within several hours of birth. An increased depth of respiration in the presence of cyanosis, but without other signs of respiratory distress, often is associated with congenital cardiac disease in which inadequate pulmonary blood flow is the most important functional component.

Apnea. The most important variations from normal respiratory patterns are apnea and bradypnea, and tachypnea. Intermittent apneic episodes are common in premature infants with central nervous system immaturity or disease. In addition, higher centers may be depressed as a result of severe hypoxemia, acidemia, or the administration of pharmacological agents to mother or baby. The association of apneic episodes, lethargy, hypotonicity, and a reduction of spontaneous movement most often points to intracranial disease as an underlying cause.

Tachypnea. Diverse conditions result in tachypnea in the newborn period. Tachypnea in the presence of intrinsic pulmonary disease with upper or lower airway obstruction usually is accompanied by flaring of the alae nasi, chest-

TABLE 29–9 ARTERIAL BLOOD GAS PATTERNS IN VARIOUS DISORDERS CAUSING CYANOSIS IN INFANTS

PATTERN	pH	pO_2	pCO_2	RESPONSE TO O_2	VENOUS pH	SUGGESTED CONDITION
1	↓	↓↓	↑	↑↑	↓	Hyaline membrane or other pulmonary parenchymal disease
2	↓	↓	↑↑↑	↑	↓	Hypoventilation
3	–	↓	–	↑	–	Venous admixture
4	↓	↓↓	–	–	↓	Decreased or ineffective pulmonary blood flow
5	↓↓↓	↓	–↑	–↑	↓↓↓↓	Systemic hypoperfusion

– = no effect. For description of patterns, see p. 893.

wall retractions, and grunting. In contrast, tachypnea associated with intense cyanosis in the absence of obvious respiratory distress suggests the presence of cyanotic congenital heart disease. In general, highest respiratory rates (80 to 110/min) are seen in association with primary lung, and not heart, disease. Initial chest radiography frequently is diagnostic, especially if the problem is aspiration, mucous plug, adenomatoid malformation, lobar emphysema, diaphragmatic hernia, pneumothorax, lung agenesis, pulmonary hemorrhage, or an abnormal thoracic cage configuration. Choanal atresia may be excluded by passing a feeding tube through the nares, and the more common types of esophageal atresia and tracheoesophageal fistula may be excluded by passing the tube farther into the stomach.

CARDIAC EXAMINATION. Specific findings on cardiovascular examination may direct attention to a cardiac cause for cyanosis. Peripheral perfusion is poor in the presence of severe primary myocardial disease or the hypoplastic left heart syndrome. In contrast, peripheral pulses are bounding and the dorsalis pedis and palmar pulses are easily palpable in infants with patent ductus arteriosus, truncus arteriosus, or aorticopulmonary window. A marked discrepancy between upper- and lower-extremity blood pressures helps to identify the infant with coarctation of the aorta. Inspection and palpation of the precordium allow an overall estimate of cardiac activity. A thrill in the suprasternal notch and/or over the precordium occasionally may be felt in the infant with patent ductus arteriosus, critical aortic stenosis, or coarctation of the aorta. Characterization of the second heart sound may be of help because it often is single in infants with a hypoplastic left heart complex, pulmonary atresia with or without an intact ventricular septum, or truncus arteriosus. Wide splitting of the second heart sound may occur in infants with total anomalous pulmonary venous return. Ejection sounds often are detectable in infants with persistent truncus arteriosus and occasionally with critical aortic or pulmonic stenosis. The presence of a third heart sound is normal, but a gallop rhythm may provide a clue to myocardial failure. Wide splitting of the first and second heart sounds may produce the characteristically rhythmic auscultatory cadence of Ebstein's anomaly of the tricuspid valve (see p. 934). The presence of a cardiac murmur may point clearly to underlying cardiac disease, but the absence of a murmur does not exclude the presence of a cardiac malformation. Moreover, cardiac murmurs of specific anomalies often are atypical in the newborn period. However, certain cardiac murmurs such as the decrescendo holosystolic murmur of tricuspid regurgitation in Ebstein's anomaly or the transient tricuspid regurgitation of infancy may point clearly to an accurate diagnosis. Auscultation of the head and abdomen may detect the murmur of an arteriovenous malformation at those sites in infants who present with findings of severe heart failure.

BLOOD GAS AND pH PATTERNS. Arterial blood gas analysis may be a reliable method of evaluating cyanosis, suggesting the type of altered physiology, and assessing responses to therapeutic maneuvers.[57] Specimens for blood gas analysis should be obtained in room air and in 100 per cent oxygen. Stick capillary samples from the patient's warmed heel may be used, although determinations obtained by arterial puncture are preferable for evaluation of oxygenation because they are less susceptible to alterations in regional blood flow in the critically ill infant. Sampling of right radial or temporal arterial blood is preferable because these sites are proximal to flow through a ductus arteriosus and do not reflect right-to-left ductal shunting, as would a sample from the descending aorta obtained by means of an umbilical artery catheter. A trial of continuous positive airway pressure may improve oxygenation in infants with either hyaline membrane disease or pulmonary edema.

Arterial blood gas patterns in various pathophysiological conditions are listed in Table 29–9. Pattern 1 typically is observed in infants with ventilation-perfusion abnormalities resulting from primary respiratory disease, often associated with elevated pulmonary vascular resistance and venoarterial shunting across a patent foramen ovale or patent ductus arteriosus. Pulmonary hypoventilation with CO_2 retention produces pattern 2. In the presence of a lesion causing obligatory venous admixture, such as total anomalous pulmonary venous connection (pattern 3), the response to oxygen may reflect an increase in pulmonary venous return secondary to a fall in pulmonary vascular resistance. Pattern 4 typically is seen in infants with a cardiac malformation that results in reduced pulmonary blood flow. Oxygen administration in these infants does not alter the arterial pO_2. The alterations of pattern 5 are observed when systemic hypoperfusion is the principal hemodynamic problem. In these babies the arteriovenous oxygen difference is high, and the acidemia may be progressive and unrelenting.

ELECTROCARDIOGRAM (see also Chap. 4). This is less helpful in suggesting a diagnosis of heart disease in the premature and newborn infant than in the older child. Right ventricular hypertrophy is a normal finding in the neonate, and the range of normal voltages is wide. However, specific observations may offer major clues to the presence of a cardiovascular anomaly. A counterclockwise, superiorly oriented frontal QRS loop with absent or reduced right ventricular forces suggests the diagnosis of tricuspid atresia (see p. 932). In contrast, when the QRS axis is normal but left ventricular forces predominate, the diagnosis of pulmonic atresia must be considered (see p. 926). The counterclockwise, superior QRS orientation also is observed in infants with an endocardiac cushion defect (see p. 898) and in some with double-outlet right ventricle (see p. 941); right ventricular forces in these babies are increased.

The initial septal vector should be assessed from the electrocardiogram. Often Q waves are not clearly seen in the lateral precordial leads in the first 72 hours of life. A leftward, posteriorly directed septal vector giving rise to Q waves in the right precordial leads is abnormal and suggests the presence of marked right ventricular hypertrophy, single ventricle (see p. 947), or inversion of the ventricles. T-wave alterations may be seen in a normal neonatal electrocardiogram and may be of no particular consequence. However, by 72 hours of age the T waves should be inverted in V_3 and V_1 and upright in the lateral precordium; persistently upright T waves in the right precordial leads are a sign of right ventricular hypertrophy. Depressed or flattened T waves in the lateral precordium may suggest subendocardial ischemia and a left heart outflow tract obstructive lesion, electrolyte disturbance, acidosis, or hypoxemia. An electrocardiographic pattern of myocardial infarction suggests a diagnosis of anomalous pulmonary origin of the coronary artery (see p. 909). Finally, rhythm disturbances such as complete heart block or supraventricular tachycardia can be detected readily by electrocardiography.

RADIOGRAPHIC EXAMINATION (see also Chap. 7). Chest radiography often is useful in differentiating between respiratory and cardiac causes of cyanosis in the newborn period. Determination of a normal cardiac and abdominal situs aids in ruling out several kinds of complex cyanotic cardiac malformations associated with asplenia or polysplenia with abdominal heterotaxy and dextrocardia (see p. 966). The distinct appearance of pulmonary parenchymal disease, such as the classic reticulogranular pattern of hyaline membrane disease, may allow a specific radiological diagnosis. In those premature infants with a large ductus arteriosus the radiographic appearance often evolves from the typical findings of hyaline membrane disease to increased pulmonary vascular markings and finally to perihilar and generalized pulmonary edema.

Most important, the pediatric cardiologist depends heavily on the evaluation of pulmonary vascular markings to categorize congenital cardiac malformations in the newborn infant according to function. In the presence of cyanosis, diminished pulmonary vascular markings call attention to the group of anomalies that includes tetralogy of Fallot, pulmonic stenosis with intact ventricular septum, pulmonic atresia, tricuspid atresia, and Ebstein's malformation of the tricuspid valve. Reduced pulmonary blood flow is responsible for the systemic arterial desaturation in these babies. Increased pulmonary vascular markings in the cyanotic infant are associated with lesions in which an obligatory admixture of systemic venous and pulmonary venous blood occurs. The more common anomalies in this category include transposition of the great arteries, hypoplastic left heart syndrome, truncus arteriosus, and total anomalous pulmonary venous drainage.

As mentioned earlier, overall heart size in the normal newborn infant is greater than in the older child, and cardiothoracic ratios up to 0.60 are within normal limits. The thymus shadow occasionally obscures the cardiac silhouette and prohibits accurate estimation of heart size. An enlarged heart on x-ray examination suggests a cardiac disorder. However, in the presence of severe respiratory difficulties with an increase in carbon dioxide tension and a decrease in both pH and arterial oxygen tension, cardiomegaly may be only moderate. A right aortic arch suggests the presence of either tetralogy of Fallot or persistent truncus arteriosus. An ovoid heart with a narrow base associated with increased pulmonary vascular marking is typical of transposition of the great arteries. A boot-shaped heart with concavity of the pulmonary outflow tract suggests tetralogy of Fallot, pulmonic atresia, or tricuspid atresia.

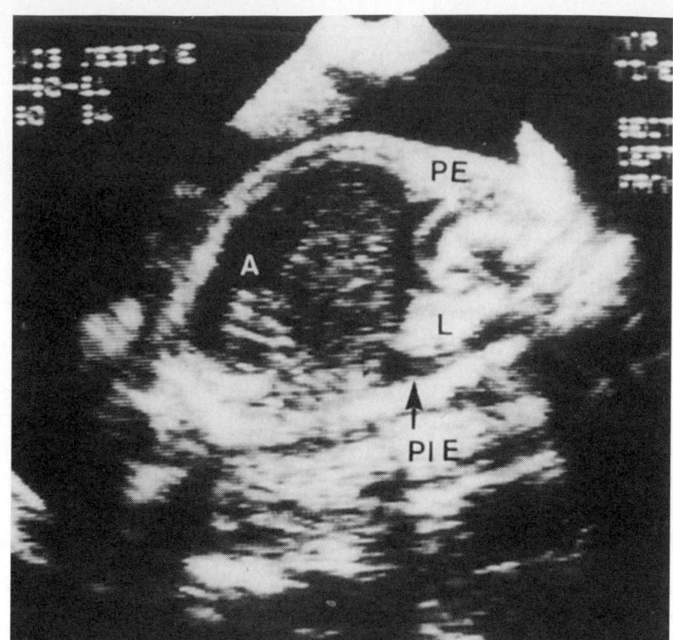

FIGURE 29–7. Abdominal ultrasound examination of a 28-week fetus with nonimmunological hydrops fetalis. A = ascites, PE = pericardial effusion, L = lung, PIE = pleural effusion. The fetal heart is to the right and inferior of the arrow showing the pericardial effusion.

LABORATORY STUDIES IN CONGENITAL HEART DISEASE

FETAL ECHOCARDIOGRAPHY (see also p. 54). Ultrasound technology now allows examination of human fetal cardiac development and function in utero.[39–41,104–106] Diagnostic-quality images of the fetal heart in utero can be obtained as early as 16 weeks of gestation. Cardiac structures are imaged primarily by cross-sectional echocardiography and augmented by a combination of range-gated pulse Doppler ultrasonography and M-mode echocardiography. The analysis of the structure and function of the fetal heart during the second and third trimesters of pregnancy has allowed cardiologists to counsel prospective parents, and in a number of instances to formulate management plans for pregnancy, delivery, and the immediate postnatal period. Using fetal echocardiography, major forms of congenital heart disease have been diagnosed in utero, and cardiac rhythm abnormalities have been detected, permitting direct efforts at transplacental therapy. In particular, it has been established that a high incidence exists of cardiac pathology in the presence of nonimmune fetal hydrops. It appears clear that hydrops fetalis often represents end-stage fetal cardiac decompensation (Fig. 29–7). Atrioventricular valve insufficiency often causes fetal right ventricular volume overload and systemic venous hypertension leading to hydrops fetalis.

Pulsed Doppler ultrasound examination of the fetus importantly supplements the echocardiographic findings in identifying the responsible defects, such as Ebstein's malformation of the tricuspid valve, atrial isomerism with atrioventricular septal defects, and the absent pulmonary valve and hypoplastic left heart syndromes.

Fetal cardiac ultrasonography is of special importance in analyzing disturbances of fetal cardiac rhythm, which usually are first suspected on the basis of auscultatory findings. Transabdominal electrocardiography cannot identify atrial depolarization and is of limited value in the analysis of cardiac arrhythmias in utero. However, M-mode recordings of cardiac motion versus time allow conclusions regarding electrical events in the fetal heart, as they are reflected by the mechanical responses that are recorded echocardiographically. Supraventricular tachyarrhythmias are a common cause of nonimmune fetal hydrops (Fig. 29–8). Detection is of practical use in the management of these patients because the arrhythmia is treatable with use of various antiarrhythmic drugs, such as digoxin, procainamide, propranolol, and flecainide, administered to the mother and reaching the fetus transplacentally or, rarely, under sonographic guidance, by means of injection of drugs, such as amiodarone, into the umbilical vein.[107]

ECHOCARDIOGRAPHY IN THE NEONATE. Echocardiography is of immense value in differentiating between heart dis-

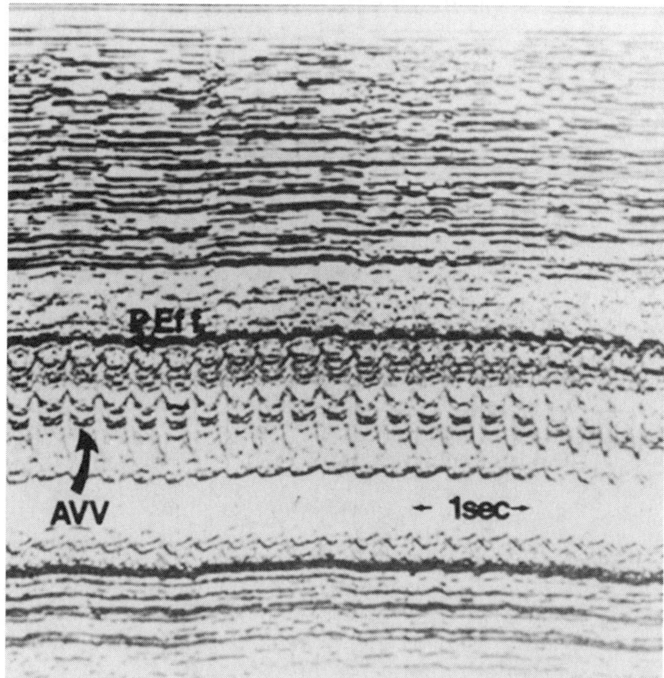

FIGURE 29–8. M-mode echocardiogram at 35 weeks' gestation, showing fetal supraventricular tachycardia and pericardial effusion (PEff). The tracing, taken at the midventricular level, allows the heart rate to be calculated from atrioventricular valve (AVV) motion (250 beats/min). (Courtesy of Charles Kleinman, M.D.)

ease and lung disease in the newborn.[108] Echocardiographic diagnoses that often can be made with certainty include hypoplastic left heart syndrome, aortic valve stenosis, membranous and fibromuscular subvalvular aortic stenosis, aortic coarctation, hypertrophic cardiomyopathy, cor triatriatum, atrial septal defect, tricuspid atresia, Ebstein's anomaly of the tricuspid valve, valvular pulmonic stenosis, atrioventricular septal defect, single ventricle, double-outlet right ventricle, transposition of the great arteries, and patent ductus arteriosus. The echocardiogram provides suggestive and often conclusive evidence for tetralogy of Fallot, truncus arteriosus, total anomalous pulmonary venous connection, and pulmonary atresia with an intact ventricular septum.

Doppler ultrasonography (see p. 56) supplements the two-dimensional echocardiographic examination by its ability to quantify valve gradients, cardiac output, blood flow patterns in the cardiac chambers and great arteries, and often shunt size.[108–111] For example, the pulmonary-systemic blood flow ratio can be calculated by multiplying the square of the ratio of the great vessel diameters by the ratio of the peak systolic flow velocities, the pulmonary variable being the numerator in each ratio.[109] The coupling of Doppler ultrasonographic techniques with the two-dimensional echocardiogram, and the representation in color of abnormalities in flow, volume, and direction (see p. 63), greatly improve diagnostic accuracy.

CARDIAC CATHETERIZATION (see also Chap. 6). If certain cardiac anomalies are identified by noninvasive studies or if a clear-cut differentiation cannot be made between cardiac and pulmonary disease, heart catheterization and angiocardiography may be necessary to define the underlying state precisely. However, fewer cardiac catheterizations have been performed in infants and children of all ages since the beginning of aggressive pursuit of preoperative diagnoses by noninvasive imaging modalities, particularly two-dimensional Doppler flow echocardiography.[111,112] Hemodynamic study of the newborn infant carries a small but distinct risk.[113] As a general rule, cardiac catheterization is not performed unless the information sought is central to the management of the infant. Most infants with serious heart disease require therapeutic intervention, and thus catheterization should be performed only when surgical support is readily available. Cardiac catheterization usually is indicated in most newborns who experience congestive heart failure in the first days after birth if the cause is an anatomical abnormality rather than an arrhythmia or a metabolic disturbance. Preferably, medical measures will have been instituted to stabilize the clinical state before a hemodynamic study is performed.

It is generally agreed that some newborns with cyanotic congenital heart disease require prompt cardiac catheterization because of the considerable risk of rapid deterioration.[21] Under these circumstances hemodynamic and angiographic study may not only provide the anatomical diagnosis required before emergency operation but also allow the opportunity for therapeutic maneuvers such as balloon atrial septostomy to facilitate intercirculatory mixing in patients with complete transposition of the great arteries or to augment interatrial shunting in patients with a restrictive patent foramen ovale and either tricuspid, pulmonic, or mitral atresia, or total anomalous pulmonary venous connection. The selective infusion of low doses of prostaglandin E_1 (0.05–0.1 μg/kg/min) intravenously has been used before and at cardiac catheterization for the emergency palliation of ductus-dependent cardiac lesions such as pulmonary atresia, aortic coarctation, and interruption of the aortic arch.[96] Because a patent ductus arteriosus maintains pulmonary and systemic blood flow, respectively, in these infants, dilatation of the ductus with vasodilatory prostaglandins may retard their clinical deterioration. Thus, prostaglandin E_1 infusion has been shown to be an effective short-term measure to correct hypoxemia and acidemia and to improve the preoperative and intraoperative status of infants who require surgical relief of the congenital cardiac lesion that is causing pulmonary or systemic hypoperfusion.

Therapeutic Catheterization (see also Chap. 39). Balloon atrial septostomy was the first catheter intervention that proved useful to treat congenital heart disease, and it remains the standard initial palliation in infants with complete transposition of the great arteries unless the arterial switch operation is performed imminently.[114] Many additional transcatheter techniques are now used successfully to treat congenital heart disease. These include knife blade atrial septostomy, umbrella or coil closure of patent ductus arteriosus, umbrella closure of atrial septal defect,[112,115] balloon-expandable intravascular stents for peripheral pulmonary artery and selected postoperative stenoses, and balloon and coil embolization of large systemic pulmonary artery collateral vessels and arteriovenous fistulas. Other procedures that have expanded the role of the cardiac catheter from a diagnostic tool to a therapeutic instrument include transvenous or transarterial pacemaker insertion and retrieval of foreign bodies from the cardiovascular system. Transluminal balloon angioplasty currently is used principally in pediatrics for dilation of pulmonic and aortic valve stenosis, native and recoarctation of the aorta, and peripheral pulmonary artery stenosis. Unresolved questions continue to exist about transluminal angioplasty in native neonatal coarctation and congenital subaortic and mitral stenosis. Lastly, electrode catheter radiofrequency ablative techniques for the treatment of tachycardias are now performed routinely in centers with pediatric electrophysiology programs.[116,117]

Electrophysiological Studies (see also Chap. 21). The cardiac catheterization laboratory also is being used with increasing frequency to define the anatomical and physiological diagnoses of arrhythmias, thus facilitating an accurate prognosis and providing a rational basis for pharmacological, catheter ablative, or surgical treatment.[118–121] The invasive electrophysiological approach provides unique information that cannot be obtained noninvasively. These include determination of conduction times of individual components of the conducting system and measurement of refractory periods for structures such as the atrioventricular node, His bundle, and bundle branches. In addition, one can determine the origin or anatomical circuit, sustaining mechanisms, and possible perturbations that terminate the arrhythmia. This last maneuver is particularly important because it may enable the planning of effective drug treatment. It also may determine the advisability of catheter ablation, pacemaker control, or surgical treatment of the rhythm disturbance.

SPECIFIC CARDIAC DEFECTS

Many classifications of congenital cardiovascular lesions have been proposed on the basis of hemodynamic, anatomical, and radiographic factors. Although there is overlapping between groups, the following arrangement of cardiac anomalies is used in this chapter: (1) communications between the systemic and pulmonary circulations without cyanosis (left-to-right shunts), (2) obstructing valvular and vascular lesions with or without associated right-to-left shunt, (3) abnormalities in the origins of the great arteries and veins (the transposition complexes), (4) malpositions of the heart and cardiac apex, and (5) miscellaneous anomalies.

Atrial Septal Defect

(See also p. 1660)

MORPHOLOGY. Atrial septal defect is one of the most commonly recognized congenital cardiac anomalies in adults but is very rarely diagnosed and even less commonly results in disability in infants.[122] The anatomical sites of interatrial defects are shown in Figure 29–9. Defects of the sinus venosus type are high in the atrial septum near the entry of the superior vena cava and may be created by a deficiency in the wall that normally separates the pulmonary veins from the right lung and the superior vena cava and right atrium, thereby also resulting in partial anomalous pulmonary venous drainage.[99,123] Most often the atrial septal defect involves the fossa ovalis, is midseptal in location, and is of the ostium secundum type. This type of defect is a true deficiency of the atrial septum and should not be confused with a patent foramen ovale. Embryologically the left side of the atrial septum is derived from the septum primum, which possesses an opening—the interatrial ostium secundum (Fig. 29–1). The ostium secundum lies forward and superior to the position of the foramen ovale. The latter is formed by the septum secundum and occupies the right side of the atrial septum. Tissue of the septum primum lying to the left of the foramen ovale serves as a flap valve that usually becomes fused postnatally with the side of the foramen ovale, yielding an anatomically closed or sealed foramen. "Probe patency," or an incomplete seal of the foramen ovale, occurs in about 25 per cent of adults. A widely patent foramen ovale may be considered an acquired form of atrial septal defect that occurs especially when a disproportion exists between the size of the foramen ovale and the effective length of its valve. Enlargement of the foramen ovale per se is commonly associated with obstructive lesions on the right side of the heart, whereas a short valve relative to the size of the foramen often is seen in large-volume left-to-right shunts in which left atrial dilatation is prominent.

Ostium primum atrial septal anomalies are a form of atrioventricular septal defect and are dealt with in the next section. Lutembacher's syndrome is a designation applied to the rare combination of atrial septal defect and mitral stenosis, which is almost invariably the result of acquired rheumatic valvulitis.[124] Ten to 20 per cent of patients with ostium secundum atrial septal defect also have prolapse of the mitral valve as an associated anomaly.[125]

HEMODYNAMICS. The magnitude of the left-to-right shunt through an atrial septal defect depends on the size of the defect and the relative compliance of the ventricles, and the relative resistance in both the pulmonary and the systemic circulation.[126] In patients with a small atrial septal defect or patent foramen ovale, the left atrial pressure may exceed the right by several millimeters of mercury, whereas the mean pressures in both atria are nearly identical when the defect is large. Left-to-right shunting occurs predominantly in late ventricular systole and early diastole with some augmentation during atrial contraction. The shunt results in diastolic overloading of the right ventricle and increased pulmonary blood flow. During the first few days and weeks of life, pulmonary resistance falls and systemic resistance rises, facilitating right ventricular emptying and impeding left ventricular emptying; the left-to-right shunt rises. Early in infancy left-to-right flow through even a large interatrial communication commonly is limited by both the reduced chamber compliance of the thick neonatal right ventricle and the elevated pulmonary and reduced systemic vascular resistance of the neonate. The pulmonary vascular resistance commonly is normal or low in the older infant or child with atrial septal defect, and the volume load usually is well tolerated, even though pulmonary blood flow may be two to five times greater than systemic. A transient and small right-to-left shunt occurring with the onset of left ventricular contraction and especially during respiratory periods of decreasing intrathoracic pressure is common in patients with ostium secundum defect, even in the absence of pulmonary hypertension.

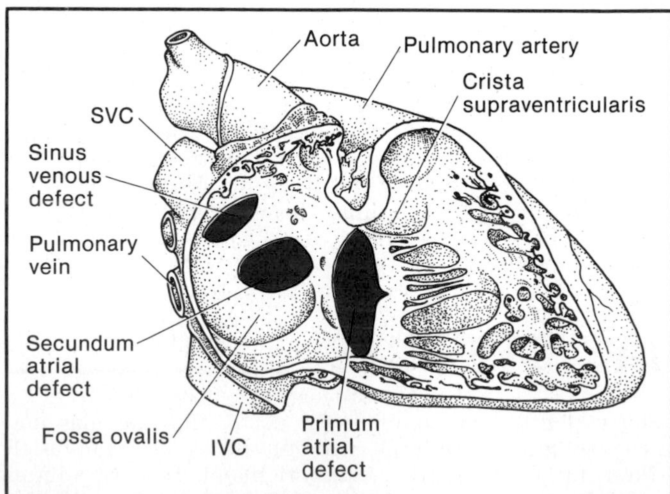

FIGURE 29–9 Composite locations of atrial defects. SVC = superior vena cava, IVC = inferior vena cava.

CLINICAL FINDINGS. Patients with atrial septal defect usually are asymptomatic early in life, although occasional reports exist of congestive heart failure and recurrent pneumonia in infancy.[122] Children with atrial septal defect may experience easy fatigability and exertional dyspnea. They tend to be somewhat underdeveloped physically and prone to respiratory infection. Atrial arrhythmias, pulmonary arterial hypertension, development of pulmonary vascular obstruction, and heart failure are exceedingly uncommon in the pediatric age range, in contrast to their common appearance in adults with atrial septal defect. In the former group, diagnosis often is entertained after detection of a heart murmur on routine physical examination prompts a more extensive cardiac evaluation.

Physical Examination. Common findings include a prominent right ventricular cardiac impulse and palpable pulmonary artery pulsation. The first heart sound is normal or split, with accentuation of the tricuspid valve closure sound. Increased flow across the pulmonic valve is responsible for a midsystolic pulmonary ejection murmur. After the normal postnatal drop in pulmonary vascular resistance, the second heart sound is split widely and is relatively fixed in relation to respiration in patients with normal pulmonary pressures and low pulmonary vascular impedance because of a delay in pulmonic valve closure. With pulmonary hypertension the splitting interval is a function of the electromechanical intervals of each ventricle; wide splitting occurs with shortening of the left and/or lengthening of the right ventricular electromechanical interval.[127] If the shunt is large, increased blood flow across the tricuspid valve is responsible for a mid-diastolic rumbling murmur at the lower left sternal border. In patients with associated prolapse of the mitral valve, an apical holosystolic or late systolic murmur radiating to the axilla often is heard, but a midsystolic click may be difficult to discern. Moreover, left ventricular precordial overactivity usually is absent because mitral regurgitation is mild in most patients.

In the teenage patient, the physical findings may be altered when an increase in pulmonary vascular resistance results in diminution of the left-to-right shunt. Both the pulmonary and the tricuspid murmurs decrease in intensity, whereas the pulmonic component of the second heart sound becomes accentuated and the two components of the second heart sound may fuse; a diastolic murmur of pulmonic incompetence appears. Cyanosis and clubbing accompany development of a right-to-left shunt.

Electrocardiogam. In patients with an ostium secundum defect, the electrocardiogram usually shows right-axis deviation, right ventricular hypertrophy, and rSR'or rsR' pattern in the right precordial leads with a normal QRS duration (Fig. 29–10). It is not clear whether the delay in right ventricular activation is a manifestation of right ventricular volume overload or a true conduction delay in the right bundle branch and peripheral Purkinje system.[128] Left-axis deviation of the P wave in the frontal plane (manifested by a negative P wave in lead III) suggests the presence of a sinus venosus rather than an ostium secundum type of atrial septal defect. Left-axis deviation and superior orientation and counterclockwise rotation of the QRS loop in the frontal plane suggests the presence of either an ostium primum defect or a secundum atrial septal defect in association with mitral valve prolapse. Prolongation of the P-R interval may be seen with all types of atrial septal defects; the prolonged internodal conduction time may be related to both the increased size of the atrium and the increased distance for internodal conduction produced by the defect itself.[128]

Chest Roentgenogram (Figs. 7–43, p. 232). This usually reveals enlargement of the right atrium and ventricle, dilatation of the pulmonary artery and its branches, and increased pulmonary vascular markings. Dilatation of the proximal portion of the superior vena cava occasionally is noted in patients with a sinus venosus defect. Left atrial dilatation is extremely rare but may be observed when significant mitral regurgitation exists.

Echocardiographic Features. These include pulmonary arterial and right ventricular dilatation and anterior systolic (paradoxical) or "flat" interventricular septal motion if significant right ventricular volume overload is present.[108] The defect may be visualized directly by two-dimensional echo imaging, particularly from a subcostal view of the interatrial septum[46] (Fig. 29–11; also see Fig. 3–77, p. 82). Transesophageal color-coded Doppler echocardiography provides excellent visualization of defects of the atrial septum.[129,130] Associated mitral valve prolapse also may be identified by echocardiographic examination (Figs. 3–51, p. 73 and 3–52, p. 74). Findings on ultrafast computed tomographic scanning are discussed on page 342.

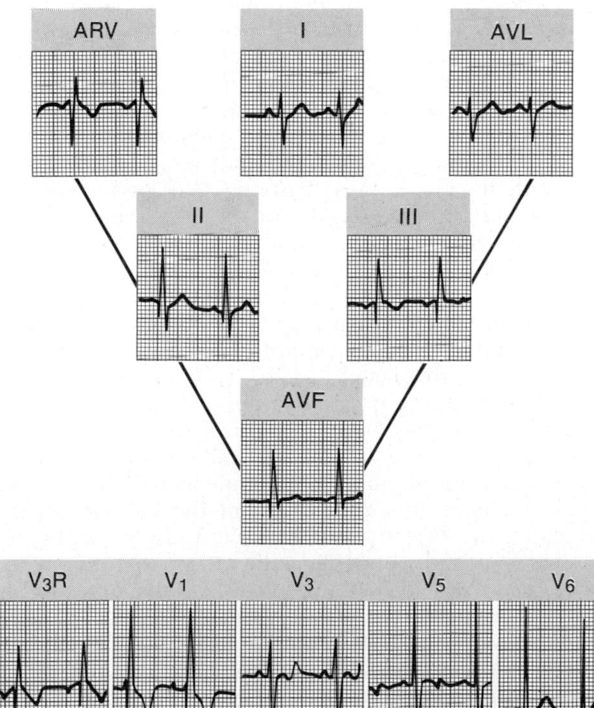

FIGURE 29–10. Typical electrocardiographic tracing in secundum atrial septal defect showing right axis deviation, rSR' in the right pericordial leads, and right ventricular hypertrophy. (Courtesy of Delores A. Danilowicz, M.D.)

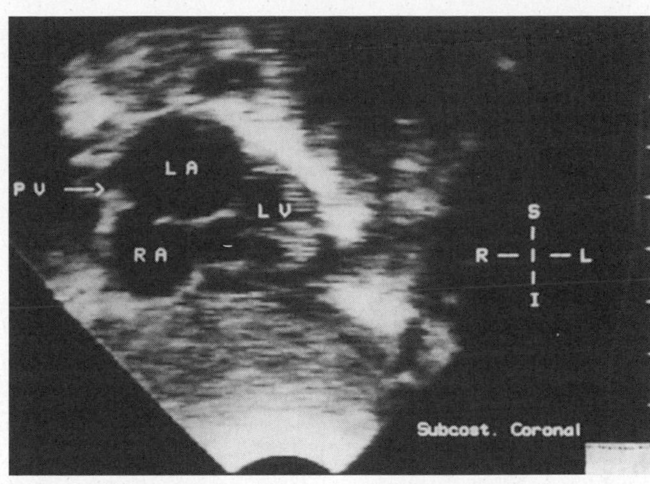

FIGURE 29–11. Subcostal coronal view showing a secundum atrial septal defect between the left atrium (LA) and the right atrium (RA). The right upper pulmonary vein (PV) is seen entering the left atrium. This view is posterior to the major portion of the ventricles; the left ventricle (LV) is seen, but only a small portion of the right ventricle (unlabeled) is apparent. I = inferior, L = left, R = right, S = superior. (Courtesy of Norman Silverman, M.D.)

Two-dimensional echocardiography, supplemented by conventional or color-coded Doppler flow and/or contrast echocardiography, has supplanted cardiac catheterization as the confirmatory test for atrial septal defect.[131,132] Cardiac catheterization is then used if inconsistencies exist in the clinical data or if significant pulmonary hypertension is suspected.

Cardiac Catheterization. Diagnosis may be readily confirmed by passage of the catheter across the atrial defect. The site at which the catheter crosses, if high in the cardiac silhouette, may suggest a sinus venosus defect; if midseptal, a patent foramen ovale or ostium secundum defect; or, if low, a primum defect.[133] Serial determinations of the oxygen saturation or indicator dilution curve techniques may be used to estimate the magnitude of the shunt. In the absence of pulmonary hypertension, pressures on the right side of the heart often are normal, despite a large shunt. When a high oxygen saturation is found in the superior vena cava or when the catheter enters pulmonary veins directly from the right atrium, a sinus venosus defect is likely, and indicator dilution curves and selective angiography aid in identifying the number and location of the anomalous veins. *Partial anomalous pulmonary venous connection,* although usually associated with sinus venosus defect, may accompany secundum defects. Selective left ventricular angiography identifies prolapse of the mitral valve and allows assessment of the magnitude of mitral regurgitation that may be present in such patients.

MANAGEMENT. In contrast to adults, children with sinus venosus or secundum types of atrial septal defect seldom require treatment for heart failure or antiarrhythmic medications for atrial fibrillation or supraventricular tachycardia. Respiratory tract infections should be treated promptly. Although the risk of infective endocarditis is low, antibiotics should be administered prophylactically before dental procedures.

Operative Repair. This should be advised for all patients with uncomplicated atrial septal defects in whom there is evidence of significant left-to-right shunting, i.e., with pulmonary-systemic flow ratios exceeding about 1.5:1.0. Ideally, this should be carried out in those 2 to 4

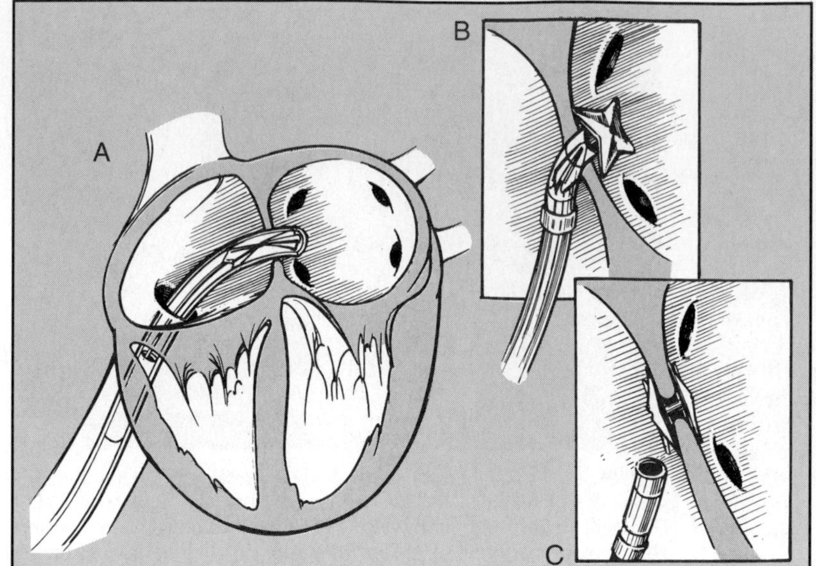

FIGURE 29–12. Clam-shell umbrella occlusion of an ostium secundum atrial septal defect. A long sheath is positioned in the left atrium (*A*). *B*, The distal umbrella arms are opened in the left atrium and the umbrella and sheath are pulled back together to the atrial septum. *C*, The proximal set of arms is then delivered on the right atrial side of the atrial septum. The correct position of the device is confirmed by fluoroscopy, angiography, and echocardiography before it is released. (From Castaneda, A., et al.: Cardiac Surgery of the Neonate and Infant. Philadelphia, W.B. Saunders Company, 1994, p. 136.)

years of age. Rarely, an atrial septal aneurysm is seen in association with a secundum-type atrial septal defect.[134] Such patients may experience spontaneous closure and may be followed more conservatively until an older age before advising operation. The defect is closed by suture or with a patch of prosthetic material with the patient on cardiopulmonary bypass. Earlier surgical repair is definitive treatment for the small number of infants and young children with significant symptoms or congestive failure. The surgical mortality rate is less than 1 per cent, and results usually are excellent. Although the mitral valve may be examined directly at operation, it seldom is necessary in childhood to attempt plication or replacement of a ballooning or prolapsing mitral valve.

Operation should *not* be carried out in patients with small defects and trivial left-to-right shunts (pulmonary-systemic flow ratio $\leq 1.5:1.0$) or in those with severe pulmonary vascular disease (pulmonary-systemic resistance ratio $\geq 0.7:1.0$) without a significant left-to-right shunt.[135] Still investigational is the use of transcatheter closure by way of a clam-shell-configuration double umbrella or a buttoned device using fluoroscopic or transesophageal echocardiographic imaging guidance[114,136–138a] (Fig. 29–12). Limitations include difficulties in centering the device, the need to use a large sheath delivery system, the need to have more than a 4-mm separation between the edges of the defect and other important cardiac structures, and the inability to close defects whose stretched diameter exceeds 22 mm.[114,136–138a]

Subtle evidence of left ventricular dysfunction may be observed preoperatively at cardiac catheterization in children with isolated large atrial septal defects but without overt left or right ventricular failure.[139] Thus decreased left ventricular stroke volume and cardiac output have been observed in children with both low and normal left ventricular end-diastolic volumes. In routine catheterization studies carried out on patients whose atrial septal defects were closed during preadolescence or later, a residual reduced cardiac output response to intense upright exercise in the absence of residual shunts, arrhythmias, or pulmonary arterial hypertension has been observed.[140] Normal myocardial function is preserved in patients in whom the defects were closed in early childhood.[141]

Electrophysiological Abnormalities. Intracardiac electrophysiological studies reveal a high incidence of intrinsic dysfunction of the sinoatrial and atrioventricular nodes, which persists after surgical repair. These intrinsic nodal abnormalities are more common in sinus venosus than in ostium secundum defects[142,143] but occur in both varieties. There also is evidence that the type of venous cannulation at the time of operative repair may contribute to the incidence and severity of arrhythmias observed at long-term follow-up.[144]

Atrioventricular (AV) Septal Defect

AV septal defects account for 4 to 5 per cent of congenital heart defects and comprise a range of malformations characterized by varying degrees of incomplete development of the inferior portion of the atrial septum, the inflow portion of the ventricular septum, and the AV valves (Fig. 29–1). These anomalies also have been called endocardial cushion defects and AV canal defects. The basic defect is a deficiency of the AV septum which separates the left ventricular inlet from the right atrium; it causes anomalies that range in severity from a small ostium primum atrial defect to a complete AV septal malformation that also involves defects in the interventricular septum and the mitral and tricuspid valves. The latter often are abnormal to varying degrees, with five or six leaflets present of variable size, and variability also in the completeness of their commissures. Often AV septal defects are encountered in association with other congenital abnormalities, such as asplenia or polysplenia syndromes, trisomy 21 (Down syndrome), and Ellis–van Creveld syndrome of ectodermal dysplasia and polydactyly.

OSTIUM PRIMUM DEFECT (PARTIAL AV CANAL). Ostium primum atrial septal defects lie immediately adjacent to the AV valves, either of which may be deformed and incompetent. Most often only the anterior or septal leaflet of the mitral valve is displaced, and it commonly is cleft; the tricuspid valve usually is not involved. A cleft often is considered to be present in the mitral valve, although it is likely that the valve is in fact a trileaflet structure, with the cleft representing an abnormal commissure. The interatrial defect often is large, and the size of the left-to-right interatrial shunt in these patients is controlled by the same factors that exist in patients with ostium secundum atrial septal defect. Moreover, the clinical features are quite similar and principally consist of right ventricular precordial hyperactivity, a wide and persistently split second heart sound, a right ventricular outflow tract systolic ejection murmur, and a mid-diastolic tricuspid flow rumble. The murmurs of AV valve regurgitation may be audible if either valve is significantly abnormal; however, serious AV valve regurgitation usually is absent. In the occasional patient, mitral regurgitation is substantial and creates prominent signs of left ventricular overload.

Chest roentgenography usually reveals right atrial and ventricular cardiomegaly, prominence of the right ventricular outflow tract, and increased pulmonary vascular markings. The *electrocardiogram* is characteristic, and shows a right ventricular conduction defect accompanied by left anterior division block, left-axis deviation, and superior orientation and counterclockwise rotation of the QRS loop in the frontal plane (Fig. 4–21, p. 123).[145] Hemodynamic factors do not appear to be important in producing the characteristic electrocardiogram. Rather, the superior QRS vector in patients with a shortened H-V interval appears to be related to early activation of the posterobasal left ventricular wall; in other patients with a normal conduction time between the bundle of His and the ventricles, the counterclockwise superior inscription of the frontal plane vector appears to be related to late activation of the anterolateral left ventricular wall.[146] A prolonged P-R interval is observed in many patients with an ostium primum atrial septal defect; prolonged internodal conduction may be related to displacement of the AV node in a posteroinferior direction in some patients or to the enlarged right atrium, or both.[147]

Echocardiography. Two-dimensional echocardiography is considered the standard for the diagnosis of all forms of AV septal defect (Fig. 3–77, p. 82). Important features include enlargement of both the right ventricle and the pulmonary artery, systolic anterior ventricular septal motion, prolonged mitral-septal apposition in diastole, and various abnormalities in mitral valve motion.[148,149] The defect is easily visualized from the precordial apical and subxiphoid positions, with the latter views best demonstrating the relation between the atrial defect, AV valves, and the interventricular septum (Figs. 29–13 and 3–81, p. 83, color plate No. 4). Interatrial septal tissue is absent in the region of the crest of the interventricular septum; the trileaflet configuration of the mitral valve also may be identified. The subxiphoid long-axis view of the left ventricular outflow tract exhibits the "gooseneck" deformity in a manner similar to that with a right anterior oblique left ventricular angiogram. Echocardiography is particularly useful for detecting and characterizing double-orifice mitral valve, an association in about 3 per cent of patients with ostium primum atrial defect. It also allows detection of single left ventricular papillary muscle, hypoplasia of the left ventricle, and coarctation of the aorta, seen especially in symptomatic infants with an ostium primum atrial defect but without trisomy 21.[150] The *angiographic features* resemble those in the complete form of AV septal defect and are discussed below.

COMPLETE AV SEPTAL DEFECT

Morphology. The complete form of the AV septal defect includes, in addition to the ostium primum atrial septal defect, a ventricular septal defect in the posterior basal inlet portion of the ventricular septum and a common AV orifice. The common AV valve usually has six leaflets: left superior and inferior, left and right lateral, and right superior and inferior. The left and right superior leaflets together often are referred to as the "anterior" bridging leaflet. No attachment exists between the left superior and inferior leaflets and the right superior and inferior leaflets. The left superior leaflet may cross the crest of the ventricular septum to reside partially on the right ventricular side. A classification of complete AV canal defect into types A, B, and C reflects the variability and the degree of anterior leaflet bridging of the ventricular septum (Fig. 29–14). Thus in type A the anterior leaflet is almost entirely committed to the left ventricle and is attached by chordae tendineae to the crest of the ventricular septum. In type C there is marked rightward displacement of the anterior bridging leaflet, which floats freely over the crest of the ventricular septum and is not attached to it by chordae tendineae. In type B chordal attachments extend medially to an anomalous papillary muscle adjacent to the septum in the right ventricle.

A high incidence (about 35 per cent) of additional cardiovascular lesions exists in patients with common AV canal. Principal among those associated with type C are tetralogy of Fallot, double-outlet right ventricle, transposition of the great arteries, and asplenia and polysplenia syndromes. Moreover, the type A complete AV septal anomaly commonly is seen in patients with Down syndrome.

The designation *unbalanced atrioventricular canal* is applied to the condition in which one ventricle is hypoplastic and the other receives most of the common AV valve. Subaortic obstruction may be due to abnormal features of the left side of the common AV valve or to hypoplasia of the left ventricle. The left-sided (mitral) component may also be the site of a potential form of double orifice mitral stenosis postoperatively.

Diagnosis. Patients with common AV septal defects present clinically under age 1 year with a history of frequent respiratory infections and poor weight gain. Heart failure in infancy is extremely common. The *physical findings* are similar to those observed in patients with ostium primum atrial septal defect but may include as well the holosystolic, lower left sternal border murmur of an interventricular communication and/or the decrescendo, holosystolic apical murmur of mitral regurgitation. The *electro-*

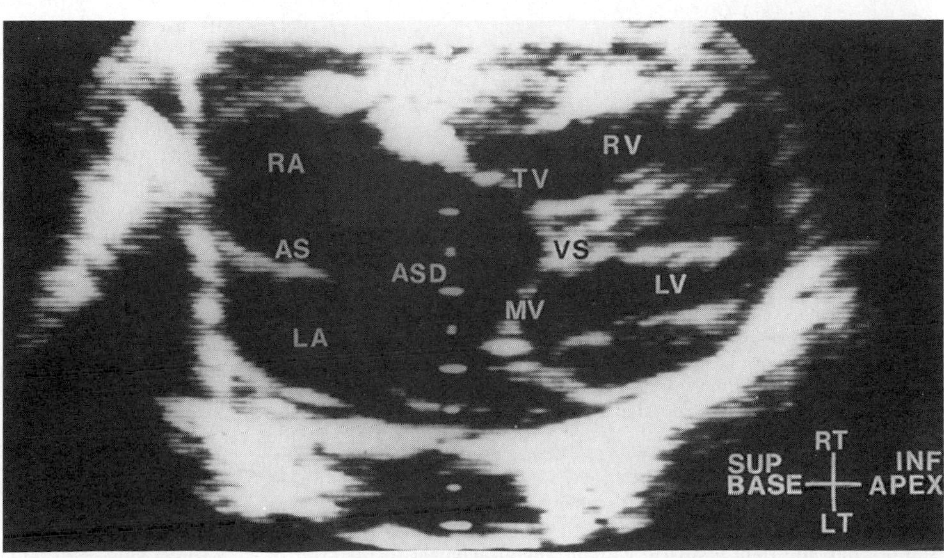

FIGURE 29–13. Subcostal four-chamber view showing an ostium primum atrial septal defect (ASD). There is echo dropout in the inferior portion of the atrial septum (AS). RA = right atrium, LA = left atrium, TV = tricuspid valve, MV = mitral valve, VS = ventricular septum, RV = right ventricle, LV = left ventricle. (Courtesy of Thomas DiSessa, M.D.)

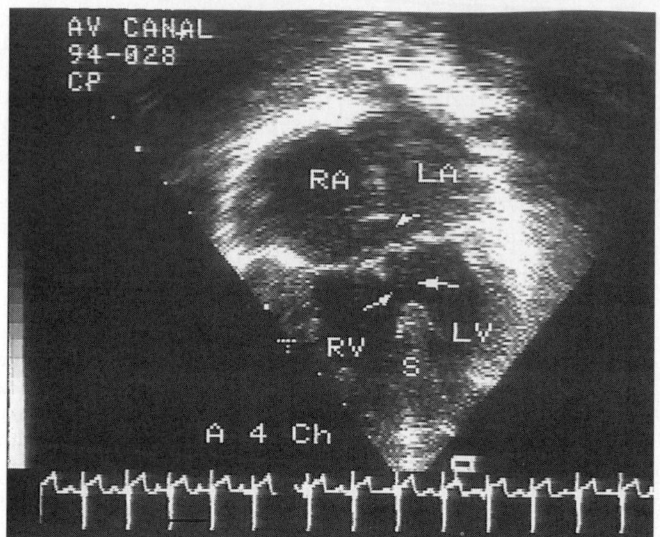

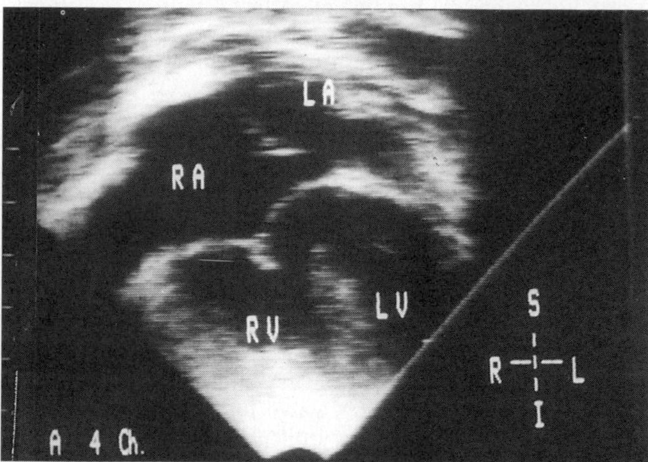

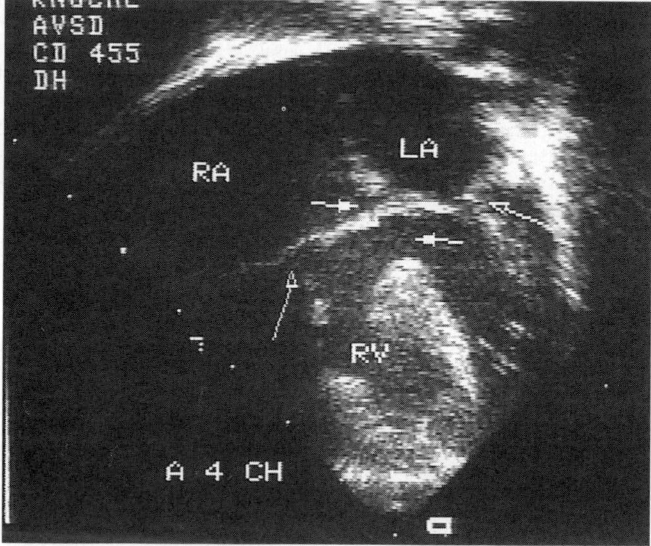

FIGURE 29–14. Composite of atrioventricular septal defects in apical four chamber views. *Top,* Atrioventricular septal defect of Rastelli type A variety. The arrows indicate the positions of the interatrial and interventricular communications. A common atrioventricular valve leaflet can be seen to straddle the defects, and the arrows in the ventricle identify the position of the chordae tendineae attached to the crest of the septum from the anterior superior bridging leaflet. *Middle,* Atrioventricular septal defect, Rastelli type B, in which the anterior superior bridging leaflet is not attached to the crest of the septum, but rather attaches to a papillary muscle within the right ventricle. *Bottom,* Rastelli type C, the so-called free-floating anterior superior bridging leaflet, indicated by the arrows. The leaflet arises from a papillary muscle within the left ventricle and straddles the septum into the right ventricle without any attachment to the crest of the ventricular septum and attaches to the anterior papillary muscle lying within the right ventricle. Orientation: S = superior, I = inferior, R = right, L = left. LA = left atrium, LV = left ventricle, RA = right atrium, RV = right ventricle, S = ventricular septum. (Courtesy of Norman Silverman, M.D.)

cardiographic features of complete AV canal defects resemble those in the partial ostium primum variety of AV septal anomalies (Fig. 29–11). *Radiographically,* the usual findings are generalized cardiomegaly and engorged pulmonary vessels.

Two-dimensional echocardiography is diagnostic (Figs. 29–14 and 3–79, p. 83).[148,149] Apical and subcostal views are used to determine the size of the septal defects, the commitment of valve tissue and chordal attachments to the ventricles, ventricular size, the magnitude of AV valve insufficiency, and the anatomy of the left ventricular outflow tract. The subcostal oblique coronal view is often best to evaluate the commitment of AV valve tissue to each ventricle. Patterns of shunting and the number and magnitude of regurgitant jets are best evaluated by using pulsed, continuous-wave, and color flow Doppler imaging. On *hemodynamic study,* patients with persistent common AV canal invariably have elevated pulmonary arterial pressures; beyond age 2 years a significant number of these patients have progressively severe pulmonary vascular obstructive disease.

Diagnosis also is reliably established by selective left ventricular *angiocardiography* using rapid injection of relatively large quantities of contrast material.[151] The findings include an absence of the AV septum and a deficiency of the inlet portion of the ventricular septum, with elongation of the left ventricular outflow tract in relation to the inflow tract. The aortic valve is elevated and displaced anteriorly relative to the AV valves, changing the relation between the anterior components of the left AV valve and the aorta, which produces a pathognomonic "gooseneck" deformity seen angiographically in diastole.

Management. In patients with complete AV canal, cardiac decompensation should be controlled initially. Even if there is an adequate response to medical therapy early in life, operation should be considered before age 6 months because infants with a complete form of the AV septal defect are at high risk of obstructive pulmonary vascular disease. The level of major shunting should be determined by echocardiographic–Doppler data, or less often during initial hemodynamic and angiographic study because if it is mainly at the ventricular level, pulmonary artery banding occasionally may be advised for intractable heart failure and failure to thrive. Often, however, there is a significant left ventricular–right atrial shunt either directly or indirectly by way of mitral regurgitation and left-to-right interatrial shunting, which will be unaffected by pulmonary artery banding and requires complete surgical correction.

SURGICAL REPAIR. In most centers primary repair in patients who have intractable heart failure, growth failure, or severe pulmonary hypertension is the preferred approach at any age.[152] Mild to moderate regurgitation often persists after surgical repair, particularly if significant AV valve incompetence existed preoperatively.[153] Rarely, if left AV leaflet tissue is remarkably deficient or deformed, mitral valve replacement may be required. Recent advances in the surgical approach to complex forms of AV septal defects have greatly improved the outlook for patients born with this malformation.[154,155] These include better reconstruction of the mitral valve (Fig. 29–15) and a more precise preoperative detection of such anatomical features as additional muscular ventricular septal defects, malalignment of the complete AV septum, and left ventricular hypoplasia. Operative improvement is primarily related to a clearer understanding of the anatomy of this complex lesion and to the ability to reconstruct the left AV valve, often by splitting of

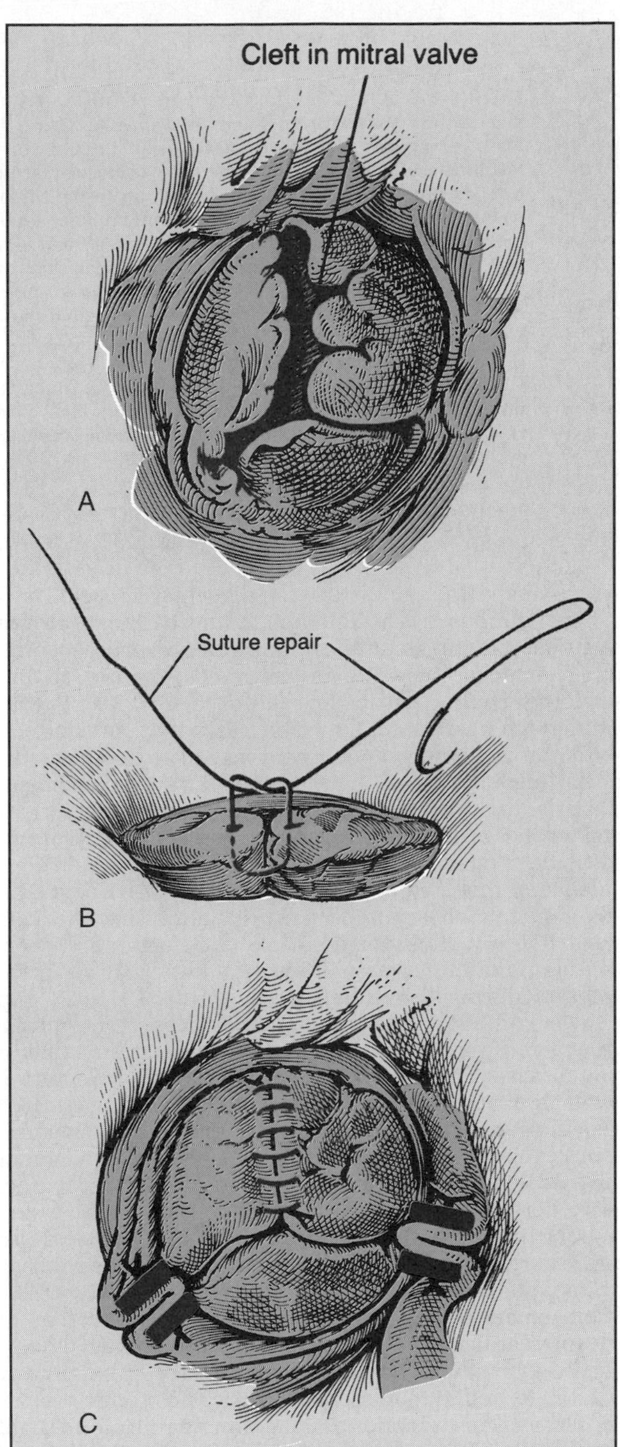

FIGURE 29–15. A suture technique is illustrated for repair of a cleft mitral valve *(A)*. Absolute alignment of the cleft in all its dimensions is of critical importance with placement of the sutures where the edges naturally coapt *(B)*. *C*, The cleft repair is accompanied by annuloplasty. (From Castaneda, A., et al.: Cardiac Surgery of the Neonate and Infant. Philadelphia, W.B. Saunders Company, 1994, p. 174.)

papillary muscles and shortening of cordae tendineae, with or without annuloplasty. Many surgeons prefer to close the septal defects with a single patch rather than separating ventricular and atrial patches. Suture placement is avoided in the region of the AV node and the bundle of His.

Ventricular Septal Defect

(See also p. 967)

MORPHOLOGY. Among the most prevalent of cardiac malformations, defects of the ventricular septum occur commonly, both as isolated anomalies and in combination with other anomalies. The ventricular septum is made up of four compartments: the membranous septum, the inlet septum, the trabecular septum, and the outlet, or infundibular, septum. Defects result from a deficiency of growth or a failure of alignment or fusion of component parts. Defects most commonly are classified as occurring in or adjacent to one or more of the septal components (Fig. 29–16).[156–159]

The most common defects occur in the region of the membranous septum, and are referred to as *paramembranous* or *perimembranous defects* because they are larger than the membranous septum itself and are associated with a muscular defect at a portion of their perimeter. They also are known as infracristal, subaortic, or conoventricular defects. These perimembranous defects also can be defined by their adjacent areas as inlet, trabecular, or outlet. A second type of defect is one with an entirely muscular rim. Such muscular defects also can be defined as inlet, trabecular, central, apical, marginal or "Swiss cheese," or outlet and vary greatly in size, shape, and number. A third type of defect occurs when the outlet septum is deficient and commonly is referred to as supracristal, subpulmonary, outlet, infundibular, or conoseptal. Because the aortic and pulmonary valves are in fibrous continuity, this type of defect also may be referred to as doubly committed subarterial. A septal deficiency of the site of the atrioventricular septum characterizes defects called atrioventricular septal, atrioventricular canal, or inlet septal defects.

The other feature of any defect may be a malalignment of the septal components. Either the inlet or the outlet septum can be malaligned. Malalignment of the inlet septum produces either mitral or tricuspid valve override and/or straddle. Malalignment of the outlet septum can be to the right or the left of the trabecular septum; when to the left of the trabecular septum, the ventricular septal defect is characteristic of tetralogy of Fallot, double-outlet ventricle, truncus arteriosus, and, in some cases, transposition of the great arteries.

ECHOCARDIOGRAPHY. Two-dimensional and Doppler echocardiography identify the type of defect in the ventricular septum.[160–163] Perimembranous ventricular septal defects are identified by septal dropout in the area behind the septal leaflet of the tricuspid valve and below the right border of the aortic annulus. The subaortic or anterior malalignment type of ventricular septal defect appears just below the posterior semilunar valve cusps, entirely superior to the tricuspid valve. The subpulmonary ventricular septal defect appears as echo dropout within the outflow septum, which extends to the pulmonary annulus. One or two of the aortic cusps may be visualized protruding through the defect into the right ventricular outflow tract. The inlet atrioventricular septal–type of ventricular septal defect extends from the fibrous annulus of the tricuspid valve into the muscular septum and often is entirely beneath the septal tricuspid leaflet. Muscular defects may appear anywhere throughout the ventricular septum and may be either large and single or small and multiple. Anatomical localization of all ventricular septal defects is facilitated by coupling two-dimensional ultrasound images (Fig. 3–75, p. 82) with a Doppler system and also by superimposing a color-coded direction and velocity of blood flow on the real-time images.[163–167]

Pulmonary and systemic blood flow can be calculated from arterial velocity profiles and cross-sectional areas of the great vessels. The calculation of pulmonary/systemic flow ratios is reasonably accurate. The detection of jets within the right ventricle allows determination of right ventricular pressure by subtracting the product using the Bernoulli equation, which gives the pressure difference, from the systemic systolic blood pressure. Continuous-wave Doppler has been helpful in determining the right ventricular pressure from tricuspid insufficiency which is found fairly often with ventricular septal defects. Many other techniques of Doppler measurement have been used with

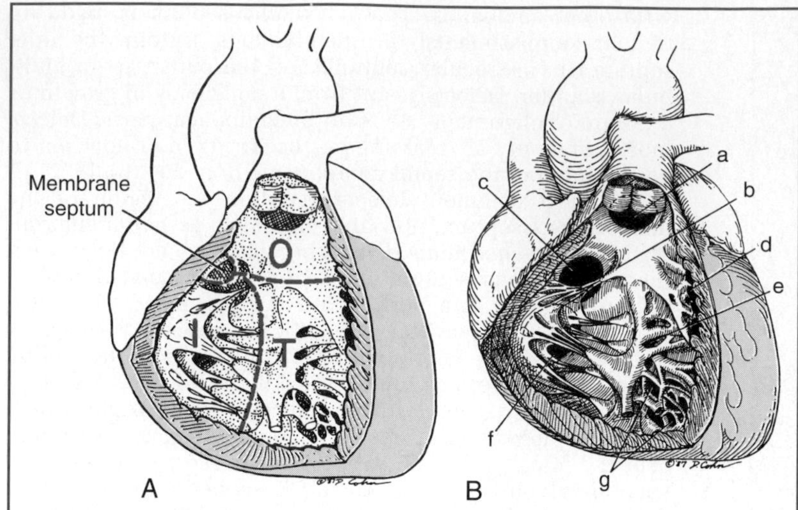

FIGURE 29-16. *A,* The four components of the ventricular septum viewed from the right ventricular side. I = inlet component extends from tricuspid annulus to attachments of the tricuspid valve, T = trabecular septum extends from inlet out to the apex and up to the smooth-walled outlet, O = outlet septum or infundibular septum extends up to the pulmonary valve and membranous septum. *B,* The anatomical position of ventricular septal defects. a = outlet defect, b = papillary muscle of the conus, c = perimembranous defect, d = marginal muscular defects, e = central muscular defects, f = inlet defect, g = apical muscular defects. (From Graham, T. P., Jr., and Gutgesell, H. P.: Ventricular septal defects. *In* Emmanouilides, G. C., Allen, H. D., et al. (eds.): Moss and Adams' Heart Disease in Infants, Children and Adolescents. 5th ed. Baltimore, © Williams and Wilkins, 1994, p. 724.)

varying success in efforts to accurately determine pulmonary arterial pressure.

PATHOPHYSIOLOGY. The functional disturbance caused by a ventricular septal defect depends primarily on its size and the status of the pulmonary vascular bed rather than on the location of the defect. A small ventricular septal defect with high resistance to flow permits only a small left-to-right shunt. A large interventricular communication allows a large left-to-right shunt only if there is no pulmonic stenosis or high pulmonary vascular resistance because these factors also determine shunt flow. Resistance to left ventricular emptying also affects shunt flow because it is an important factor in determining left ventricular pressure. Large defects allow both ventricles to function hemodynamically as a single pumping chamber with two outlets, equalizing the pressure in the systemic and pulmonary circulations. In such patients the magnitude of the left-to-right shunt varies inversely with pulmonary vascular resistance.

A wide spectrum exists in the natural history of ventricular septal defects, ranging from spontaneous closure to congestive cardiac failure and death in early infancy. Within this spectrum are possible development of pulmonary vascular obstruction, right ventricular outflow tract obstruction, aortic regurgitation, and infective endocarditis.[167-176]

INFANTS. It is unusual for a ventricular septal defect to cause difficulties in the immediate postnatal period, although congestive heart failure during the first 6 months of life is a frequent occurrence. Early diagnosis is helpful to ensure more careful observation of the affected infant.[172] The examining physician usually suspects the diagnosis because of a harsh systolic murmur at the lower left sternal border. The electrocardiogram and chest roentgenogram are within normal limits in the immediate neonatal period because appreciable left-to-right shunting occurs only after the pulmonary vascular resistance decreases as the pulmonary vessels lose their fetal characteristics. It is desirable to follow these infants closely.

A ventricular septal defect that either decreases in size or closes completely during the first year of life presents no problems to the practicing physician. Spontaneous closure occurs by age 3 years in about 45 per cent of patients born with ventricular septal defect; occasional patients, however, do not experience spontaneous closure until age 8 to 10 years or even later.[170] Closure is more common in patients born with a small ventricular septal defect; nonetheless, about 7 per cent of infants with a large defect and congestive heart failure early in life also may experience spontaneous closure. Partial rather than complete closure is common in patients with both large and small ventricular septal defects. Anatomically, reduction of the ventricular septal defect often is based on adherence of the tricuspid valve to the defect, hypertrophy of septal muscle, or ingrowth of fibrous tissue. Rarely, closure of the ventricular septal defect is the result of prolapse of an aortic cusp[173] or infective endocarditis.[176] Some defects close when an aneurysm forms in the ventricular septum.[171] On auscultation a click may be heard in early systole as the aneurysm tenses toward the right; the septal aneurysm may be detected by echocardiography as an anterior systolic bulge in the right ventricular outflow tract. A persistent minute ventricular septal defect is not life-threatening unless infective endocarditis develops. With proper precautions (see p. 974), the incidence of this complication is less than 1 per cent.

If a moderate or large defect maintains its size after birth, the net left-to-right shunt increases during the first month of life as pulmonary vascular resistance falls. *Physical examination* during this time usually reveals a thrill along the lower left sternal border, and the holosystolic murmur of flow across the interventricular defect is accompanied by a low-pitched diastolic rumble at the apex, reflecting increased flow across the mitral valve. *Chest roentgenograms* reveal increased pulmonary vascular markings; evidence of left or biventricular hypertrophy may be observed on the electrocardiogram. Infants with a large left-to-right shunt tend to do poorly, with recurrent upper and lower respiratory tract infections, failure to gain weight, and congestive heart failure. Congestive heart failure may be severe and intractable despite intensive medical management.

Management. This author currently recommends primary intracardiac repair of the ventricular septal defect at any age rather than surgical banding of the pulmonary artery[177,178] to reduce pulmonary blood flow and alleviate heart failure. An exception is made for the rare infant with multiple ventricular septal defects and a sievelike septum, who is at higher risk for complications following operative repair. Operation usually is deferred, along with debanding of the pulmonary artery, until the child reaches 3 to 5 years. Primary closure of the ventricular septal defect, preferably through the right atrium, may be performed in infancy using cardiopulmonary bypass, profound hypothermia and cardiocirculatory arrest, or a combination of the two techniques. Mortality approaches zero in major centers if the defect is isolated and uncomplicated but approaches 10 per cent if multiple anomalies are present.[179]

Fortunately, medical treatment often is successful in controlling congestive heart failure. Nevertheless, these infants should be referred for cardiac catheterization to evaluate pulmonary vascular resistance and to detect associated defects that may require operation, such as patent ductus arteriosus and coarctation of the aorta.

CHILDREN. Beyond the first year of life a variable clinical picture emerges in children with ventricular septal defect.[170-172,176] If a small defect is present, the child usually is asymptomatic, the electrocardiogram usually is normal, and the chest roentgenogram shows normal or only a mild increase in pulmonary vascular markings. Effort intolerance and fatigue are associated with moderate left-to-right shunts. These children exhibit cardiomegaly with a forceful left ventricular impulse and a prominent systolic thrill along the lower left sternal border. The second heart sound normally is split, with moderate accentuation of the pulmonic component; a third heart sound and rumbling diastolic murmur that reflects increased flow across the mitral valve are audible at the cardiac apex. The characteristic murmur resulting from flow across the defect is harsh and holosystolic, is best heard along the third and fourth interspaces to the left of the sternum, and is widely transmitted over the precordium. A basal midsystolic ejection murmur due to increased flow across the pulmonic valve also may be heard. The electrocardiogram reveals left or combined ventricular hypertrophy, and the chest roentgenogram and CT scan (Fig. 7–43, p. 232) show cardiomegaly, left atrial enlargement, and vascular engorgement.

PULMONARY HYPERTENSION. It is of utmost importance to identify patients who may develop irreversible pulmonary vascular obstructive disease (the Eisenmenger reaction).[180–182] Retrospective analyses of children who develop this complication indicate that infants with systemic or near systemic pressures in the pulmonary artery at the time of initial hemodynamic study are most at risk. If early primary closure is not recommended, recatheterization before age 18 months and a second determination of pulmonary vascular resistance should be performed in these patients to decide whether surgical intervention is obligatory to prevent development of fixed obliterative changes in the pulmonary vessels.

Mechanisms. It is likely that multiple factors are involved in the development of pulmonary vascular disease (Chap. 25, p. 781).[61–69] The anatomically large ventricular septal defect allows some or all of the systemic pressure to be transmitted to the pulmonary arteries, thereby retarding regression of their muscular media. Medial hypertrophy in the first months of life is responsible for higher pulmonary vascular resistance than would be anticipated for the amount of pulmonary blood flow. The shearing forces created by the high velocity of flow through narrowed pulmonary arterioles cause endothelial damage that is progressive.

Although an elevation in left atrial pressure may contribute to the rise in pulmonary vascular resistance, it is not an essential factor because pulmonary venous pressures can be low in patients who later develop pulmonary vascular disease. Nonetheless, pulmonary venous hypertension also may contribute to pulmonary arterial vasoconstriction and thus to increased shear forces. In this same regard, pulmonary vasoconstriction enhancing the risk of pulmonary vascular obstruction also may be caused by hypoxia due to either high altitude or lung disease. At high altitudes, large ventricular septal defects have higher pulmonary vascular resistances and smaller shunts than at low altitudes.

Clinical Features. If a child who previously had a loud murmur and thrill associated with poor growth suddenly has a growth spurt, fewer respiratory infections, and a diminution of the intensity of the cardiac murmur and disappearance of the thrill, he or she may be developing severe obliterative changes in the pulmonary vascular bed. An increase in intensity of the pulmonic component of the second heart sound, a reduction in heart size on the chest roentgenogram, and more pronounced right ventricular hypertrophy on the electrocardiogram also are noted. These changes occur because the increased pulmonary vascular resistance causes a decrease in the left-to-right shunt. If these changes are suspected, cardiac catheterization should be repeated; if they are confirmed, prompt surgical repair is indicated before an inoperable predominant right-to-left shunt ensues. If operation is performed under age 2 years, pulmonary vascular resistance may be expected to fall to normal levels.[182]

In older patients the degree to which pulmonary vascular resistance is elevated before operation is a critical factor determining prognosis. If the pulmonary vascular resistance is one-third or less of the systemic value, progressive pulmonary vascular disease after operation is unusual. However, if a moderate-to-severe increase in pulmonary vascular resistance exists preoperatively, either no change or progression of pulmonary vascular disease is common postoperatively. Moreover, the presence of increased pulmonary vascular resistance results in a higher immediate postoperative mortality rate for surgical closure of ventricular septal defect. These observations make it clear that a large ventricular septal defect should be approached surgically very early in life when pulmonary vascular disease is still reversible or has not yet developed (Fig. 29–17).

RIGHT VENTRICULAR OUTFLOW TRACT OBSTRUCTION. With time, the clinical picture changes in 5 to 10 per cent of patients with ventricular septal defect and a moderate to large left-to-right shunt early in life. It begins to resemble more closely the tetralogy of Fallot (see p. 929); i.e., subvalvular right ventricular outflow tract obstruction develops owing to progressive hypertrophy of the crista supraventricularis. Depending on the severity of the latter process, it ultimately may result in reduced blood flow and a right-to-left shunt across the ventricular septal defect. As right ventricular outflow tract obstruction develops, the holosystolic murmur is replaced by the crescendo-decrescendo ejection systolic murmur of pulmonic stenosis, and the pulmonary closure sound becomes softer. Right ventricular hypertrophy is evident on the electrocardiogram, and the chest roentgenogram shows a reduction in pulmonary vascular markings and a smaller heart size with a right ventricular configuration. Infundibular hypertrophy may progress quite rapidly within the first year of life, but the typical evolution to a clinical picture of cyanotic tetralogy of Fallot often takes 1 to 4 years. In those infants who develop right ventricular outflow obstruction the incidence of spontaneous closure or reduction in size of a ventricular septal defect is low.

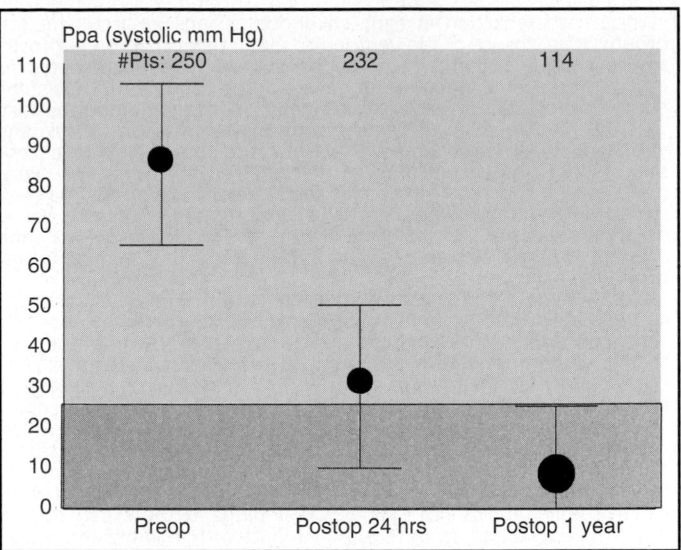

FIGURE 29–17. Early and late postoperative changes of pulmonary artery pressure after closure of ventricular septal defects in infants. (From Castaneda, A., et al.: Cardiac Surgery of the Neonate and Infant. Philadelphia, W.B. Saunders Company, 1994, p. 200.)

VENTRICULAR SEPTAL DEFECT WITH AORTIC REGURGITATION. This well-described complication of ventricular septal defect occurs in about 5 per cent of patients.[183,184] It usually is noted after age 5 years when a physician detects the early diastolic blowing murmur and wide pulse pressure of aortic regurgitation while following a patient with a ventricular septal defect. The diagnosis is readily confirmed by Doppler echocardiography. In such patients aortic regurgitation may become the predominant hemodynamic abnormality. It is of interest that ventricular septal defect with aortic regurgitation is rare in Europe and the United States, with an incidence of about 4 per cent of all cases of isolated ventricular septal defect, whereas in Japan the incidence is substantially higher (about 10 per cent). In the Japanese, in particular, aortic regurgitation is the result of herniation of an aortic leaflet (usually the right coronary) through a subpulmonic supracristal ventricular septal defect. In these patients, closure of the ventricular septal defect may be all that is required to relieve aortic regurgitation. In many patients, however, especially in the Western world, the ventricular septal defect is below the infundibular septum (crista supraventricularis). Although aortic leaflet herniation, especially of the right or noncoronary cusp, may occur in some of these patients, quite often aortic regurgitation results from a primary abnormality of the valve, usually one defective commissure. In the latter situation, plication of the elongated leaflet may lessen, but not abolish, the aortic regurgitation; in some patients prosthetic aortic valve replacement may be necessary to provide hemodynamic relief.

In most patients with ventricular septal defect and aortic regurgitation, the ventricular septal defect is small to moderate in size, and mild right ventricular outflow tract obstruction exists. The latter is caused by either subpulmonic infundibular stenosis or projection of the herniated aortic cusp into the right ventricular outflow tract. The distinction between types of ventricular septal defect with aortic regurgitation usually can be made by two-dimensional and Doppler echocardiography and by selective left ventricular angiocardiography to define the site of the interventricular communication in combination with retrograde aortography to assess the anatomy and competence of the aortic valve.[184,185]

Management. Treatment of the patient with ventricular septal defect and aortic regurgitation is controversial. In patients with a large, hemodynamically significant left-to-right shunt, repair of the ventricular septal defect is indicated, but aortic regurgitation is repaired only if at least moderate aortic regurgitation exists. If a supracristal ventricular septal defect without aortic regurgitation is identified at cardiac catheterization in early childhood, a sensible argument for prophylactic closure of the ventricular septal defect can be put forth to prevent the potential complication of aortic valve incompetence. In the presence of moderate or severe aortic regurgitation, valvuloplasty is preferred to valve replacement, in recognition of the fact that the severity of aortic regurgitation may increase in subsequent years and that reoperation with valve replacement may be necessary.[186] Operation should probably be deferred in asymptomatic patients with a subcristal ventricular septal defect and an insignificant left-to-right shunt in whom aortic regurgitation is not severe. If the defect is supracristal in the same clinical setting, its closure may not alleviate the mild degree of aortic incompetence but may retard its progression.

OTHER FORMS OF VENTRICULAR DEFECT. Unusual forms of ventricular septal defect include multiple muscular defects and left ventricular–right atrial communications. Defects in the muscular ventricular septum frequently are multiple small fenestrations that produce a large net left-to-right shunt.[168,187] Their recognition is a necessary preliminary to successful operation because incomplete repair may result in postoperative cardiac failure and death. A shunt from the left ventricle to right atrium may occur with a ventricular septal defect in the most superior portion of the ventricular septum because the tricuspid valve is lower than the mitral valve. The clinical, electrocardiographic, and radiological findings in these patients do not differ appreciably from those in patients with a simple ventricular septal defect, although right atrial enlargement may provide a clue to correct diagnosis of left ventricular–right atrial communication.[188]

The pathophysiology of a single or common ventricle (p. 947) may resemble that of a large ventricular septal defect, although these defects are dissimilar embryologically. The single chamber frequently is the morphological left ventricle; malposition of the great arteries is quite common. There may be no detectable cyanosis if selective streaming and increased pulmonary blood flow rather than complete mixing occurs. Pulmonary hypertension invariably is present unless pulmonic stenosis exists. It is imperative to differentiate a single ventricle from a large ventricular septal defect by echocardiography[162] and angiography[151] because the operative approaches to the former malformation require the atriopulmonary Fontan connection.

MANAGEMENT OF VENTRICULAR SEPTAL DEFECT. It is rarely necessary to restrict the activities of a child with an isolated ventricular septal defect. Infective bacterial endocarditis is always a threat, and antibiotic prophylaxis for dental procedures and minor surgery is indicated (Table 29–4).[189] Respiratory infections require prompt evaluation and treatment. These children should be seen at least once or twice yearly to detect changes in the clinical picture that suggest the development of pulmonary vascular obliterative changes.

Surgical Treatment. When clinical findings suggest a moderate shunt but no pulmonary hypertension, elective hemodynamic evaluation should be advised between ages 3 and 6 years. Of prime importance in the hemodynamic evaluation is a determination of pressure and blood flow in the pulmonary artery.[190] Surgical treatment is not recommended for children who have normal pulmonary arterial pressures with small shunts (pulmonary-systemic flow ratios of less than 1.5 to 2.0:1).[191] In such patients the remaining risk of infective endocarditis does not exceed the risk of operation. Moreover, although the inherent risk of operation is small, the possibility of postoperative heart block, infection, or other complications of operation and cardiopulmonary bypass dictates a conservative approach when the cardiac defect may be well tolerated for life.

In some centers, the use of intraoperative transesophageal echocardiography has provided an accurate assessment of patch integrity and the presence of additional muscular defects after termination of cardiopulmonary bypass.[192,193]

With larger shunts, elective operation may be advised before the child enters school, thus minimizing any subsequent distinction of these patients from their normal classmates. A total assessment of the psychosocial dynamics of the family and child is helpful in determining the proper age for elective operation in each patient.

Under investigation is transcatheter closure by umbrella or clamshell occluder devices (see p. 898) inserted by crossing the ventricular defect by way of the left ventricle to guide a venous catheter through a long sheath, and, ultimately, placing the device across the ventricular septum from the right ventricular side.[194]

Complete heart block is the most significant surgically induced conduction system abnormality, occurring immediately after surgery in fewer than 1 per cent of patients. Late-onset complete heart block occasionally is a problem, especially in the 10 to 25 per cent of patients whose postoperative electrocardiographic findings show complete right bundle branch block with left anterior hemiblock.[195] When the latter electrocardiographic pattern is observed in patients with transient complete heart block in the early postoperative period, electrophysiological studies should be conducted at postoperative cardiac catheterization. Patients presenting postoperatively with right bundle block and left anterior hemiblock appear to fall into two populations, defined by either peripheral damage to the conduction system or damage to the bundle of His or its proximal branches.[195] The former has not been associated with transient postoperative complete heart block, and these patients usually have a benign course. Trifascicular damage may be demonstrated in the latter population by a prolonged H-V interval, which implies a higher risk of complete heart block later in life. Although the prophylactic use of permanent pacemakers in asymptomatic patients with evidence of trifascicular damage is not currently recommended, this group certainly requires careful follow-up and continued study.

Treadmill exercise studies in patients who preoperatively had normal or only moderately elevated pulmonary vascular resistance and essentially normal postoperative cardiac catheterization data may uncover late abnormalities in circulatory function.[196,197] Despite normal cardiac output at rest, an impaired cardiac output response to exercise is noted in some. Moreover, despite a normal pulmonary arterial pressure at rest, markedly abnormal increases in pulmonary arterial pressure may be noted during exercise. These findings may be related to abnormal left ventricular function after closure of the ventricular septal defect and/or to persistent pathological changes in the pulmonary arterioles or to abnormal pulmonary vascular reactivity.[198] A direct relation exists between age at operation and the magnitude of the pulmonary arterial pressure response to intense exercise, suggesting that early operation may prevent permanent impairment of the functional capacity of the myocardium and pulmonary vascular bed.

Occasionally a child may come to medical attention who has already developed pulmonary vascular obstruction and a net right-to-left shunt across the ventricular septal defect. Symptoms may consist of exertional dyspnea, chest pain, syncope, and hemoptysis; the right-to-left shunt leads to cyanosis, clubbing, and polycythemia. There currently is little to offer this group of patients other than continuing support to the patient and family.

Patent Ductus Arteriosus

(See also p. 966)

The ductus arteriosus normally exists in the fetus as a widely patent vessel connecting the pulmonary trunk and the descending aorta just distal to the left subclavian artery (Fig. 29–4). In the fetus most of the output of the right ventricle bypasses the unexpanded lungs by way of the ductus arteriosus and enters the descending aorta, where it travels to the placenta, the fetal organ of oxygenation.

It was earlier assumed that during fetal life the ductus arteriosus was a passively open channel that constricted postnatally by means of undefined molecular mechanisms in response to the abrupt rise in arterial pO_2 accompanying the first breath of life.[199] Even in utero the lumen of the ductus arteriosus may be influenced by vasoactive substances, particularly prostaglandins.[98,99,200–202] Thus inhibition of prostaglandin synthesis causes profound constriction of the ductus arteriosus in the mammalian fetus that may be reversed by administration of vasodilatory E-type prostaglandins. Initial contraction and functional closure of the ductus arteriosus shortly after birth is related both to the sudden increase in the partial pressure of oxygen that accompanies ventilation and to changes in the synthesis and metabolism of vasoactive eicosanoids. Intimal proliferation and fibrosis proceed more gradually, so that anatomical closure may take as long as several weeks for completion.[203]

The ductus arteriosus is a unique structure after birth because its patency may, on the one hand, result in cardiac decompensation but may, on the other hand, provide the only life-sustaining conduit to preserve systemic or pulmonary arterial blood flow in the presence of certain cardiac malformations.[96] Appreciable left-to-right shunting across the patent ductus arteriosus frequently complicates the clinical course of infants born prematurely.[204] The ductal shunt has been implicated specifically in the deterioration of pulmonary function in infants with the respiratory distress syndrome in whom severe congestive heart failure often is unresponsive to digitalis and diuretics.[99]

A distinction should be made between patency of the ductus arteriosus in the *preterm* infant, who lacks the normal mechanisms for postnatal ductal closure because of immaturity, and the full-term newborn, in whom patency of the ductus is a true congenital malformation, probably related to a primary anatomical defect of the elastic tissue within the wall of the ductus.[203] In the former circumstance, delayed spontaneous closure of the ductus may be anticipated if the infant does not succumb to the cardiopulmonary difficulties caused by the ductus itself or to some lethal complication of prematurity, such as hyaline membrane disease, intraventricular hemorrhage, or necrotizing enterocolitis. In a similar manner, some full-term newborns have persistent patency of the ductus arteriosus for weeks or months because their relative hypoxemia contributes to vasodilatation of the channel. In the latter category are infants born at high altitude; those born with congenital malformations causing hypoxemia, such as pulmonary atresia with or without ventricular septal defect; or malformations in which ductal flow supplies the systemic circulation, such as hypoplastic left heart syndrome, interruption of the aortic arch, or some examples of coarctation of the aorta syndrome.

In the clinical settings in which the ductus preserves pulmonary blood flow, the essentially inevitable spontaneous closure of the vessel is associated with profound clinical deterioration. The latter may be reversed medically within the first 4 to 5 days of life by infusion of prostaglandin E_1 intravenously. By dilating the constricted ductus arteriosus, a temporary increase occurs in arterial blood oxygen tension and oxygen saturation and correction of acidemia.[96] These infants can then undergo operative repair or a palliative systemic-pulmonary anastomosis, under more optimal circumstances. Pharmacological dilation of the ductus arteriosus also is effective in the preoperative restoration of systemic blood flow and the alleviation of heart failure, especially in infants with aortic coarctation or hypoplastic left heart syndrome, and in infants with complete transposition of the great arteries in whom intercirculatory mixing is augmented.[96]

PREMATURE INFANTS. In most, if not all, preterm infants under 1500 gm birthweight, persistence of a patent ductus arteriosus is prolonged, and in about one-third of these infants a large aortico-pulmonary shunt is responsible for significant cardiopulmonary deterioration.[204–206] Radiographic, echocardiographic, and Doppler ultrasound signs of significant left-to-right shunting usually precede the appearance of physical findings suggesting ductal patency.[42,203,207,208] A significant increase in the cardiothoracic ratio is seen on sequential roentgenograms as well as increased pulmonary arterial markings progressing to perihilar and generalized pulmonary edema. Serial echocardiographic evaluations that demonstrate increases in left ventricular end-diastolic and left atrial dimensions, especially when correlated with the aforementioned radiographic signs, are highly suggestive of a large shunt.[207] Two-dimensional and Doppler echocardiography directly visualize and define the flow characteristics of the ductus arteriosus with great accuracy (Fig. 3–82, p. 84).[42,208,209]

Clinical Findings. These include bounding peripheral pulses, an infraclavicular and interscapular systolic murmur (occasionally a continuous murmur), precordial hyperactivity, hepatomegaly, and either multiple episodes of apnea and bradycardia or respiratory dependency. Cardiac catheterization carries a high risk in the preterm infant and seldom is indicated unless the diagnosis is obscure.

Treatment. Management of the preterm infant with a patent ductus arteriosus varies with the magnitude of shunting and the severity of hyaline membrane disease because the ductus may contribute importantly to mortality in the respiratory distress syndrome. Intervention in an asymptomatic infant with a small left-to-right shunt is unnecessary because the patent ductus arteriosus almost invariably undergoes spontaneous closure and does not require late surgical ligation and division. Those infants who demonstrate unmistakable signs of a significant ductal left-to-right shunt during the course of the respiratory distress syndrome often are unresponsive to medical measures to control congestive heart failure and require closure of the patent ductus arteriosus to survive. These infants are best managed within the first 2 to 7 days of life by pharmacological inhibition of prostaglandin synthesis with indomethacin to constrict and close the ductus[204,210–214]; surgical ligation is required in the estimated 10 per cent of infants who are unresponsive to indomethacin.[210,215] Early intervention is advised to reduce the likelihood of necrotizing enterocolitis and of bronchopulmonary dysplasia related to prolonged respirator and oxygen dependency.[214] Less often, indications for pharmacological or surgical closure of the ductus consist of life-threatening episodes of apnea and bradycardia or a prolonged failure to gain weight and grow.

FULL-TERM INFANTS AND CHILDREN. In full-term newborns and older infants and children, patency of the ductus arteriosus occurs particularly in females and in the offspring of pregnancies complicated by first-trimester rubella. Although most frequent in isolated form, the anomaly may coexist with other malformations, particularly coarctation of the aorta, ventricular septal defect, pulmonic stenosis, and aortic stenosis. Flow across the ductus is determined by the pressure relation between the aorta and the pulmonary artery and by the cross-sectional area and length of the ductus itself.[216] Pulmonary pressures most commonly are normal, and a persistent gradient and shunt from aorta to pulmonary artery exist throughout the cardiac cycle.

Physical examination reveals a characteristic thrill and a continuous "machinery" murmur with a late systolic accentuation at the upper left sternal border. The left atrium and left ventricle enlarge to accommodate the increased pulmonary venous return, and flow murmurs across the mitral and aortic valves may be detected. With significant left-to-right shunting, the runoff of blood through the ductus causes a widened systemic pulse pressure and bounding peripheral pulses. The hemodynamic abnormality is reflected in the electrocardiogram by left ventricular and occasionally left atrial hypertrophy, and in the chest roentgenogram by left atrial and ventricular enlargement, prominent ascending aorta and pulmonary artery, and pulmonary vascular engorgement (Fig. 7–43, p. 232 and Fig. 30–6, p. 967).

The clinical diagnosis may be difficult when the findings do not conform to the classic presentation.[217] As mentioned above, disappearance of the diastolic component of the murmur is common in premature infants because higher pulmonary arterial diastolic pressures exist at that age. In older patients both heart failure and pulmonary hypertension are associated with a reduction in the pressure gradient across the ductus arteriosus and result in atypical systolic murmurs. When severe pulmonary vascular obstructive disease results in reversal of flow through the ductus and preferential shunting of unoxygenated blood to

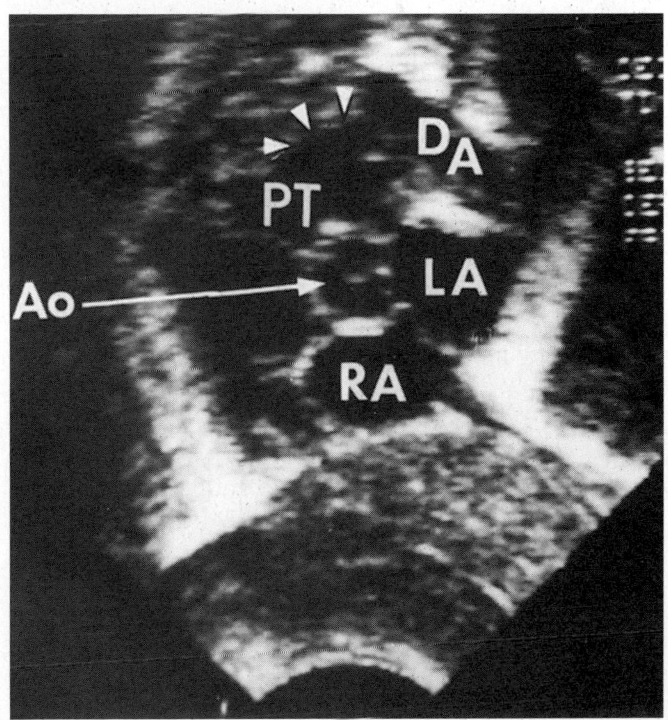

FIGURE 29–18. Parasternal short-axis view of a patent ductus arteriosus (arrowheads) in an infant. The pulmonic valve is the linear echo just beneath the pulmonary trunk (PT). AO = aortic valve, DA = descending aorta, RA = right atrium, LA = left atrium. (From Perloff, J.: The Clinical Recognition of Congenital Heart Disease. 3rd ed. Philadelphia, W.B. Saunders Company, 1986.)

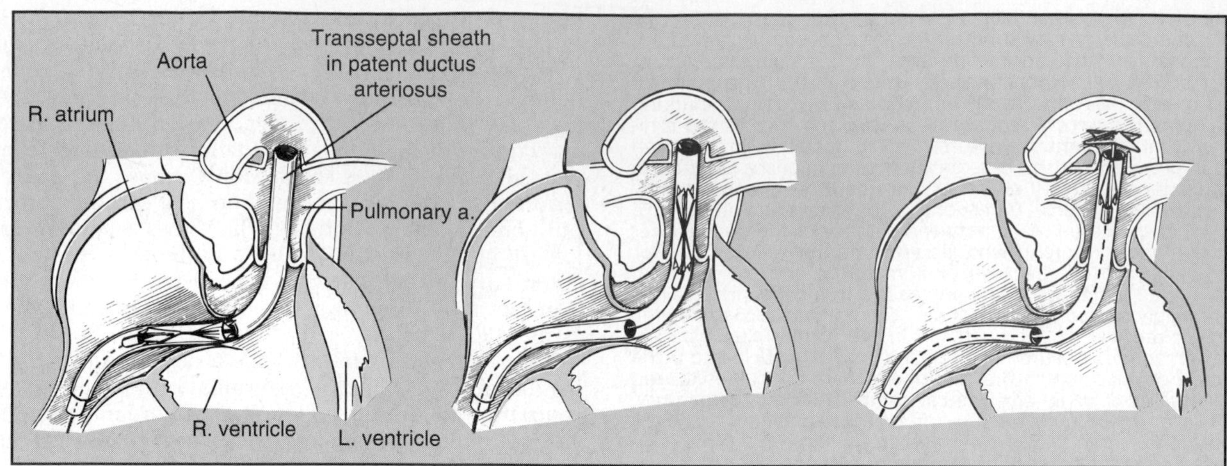

FIGURE 29–19. Transcatheter closure of a patent ductus arteriosus is illustrated using the Rashkind double-umbrella technique. The catheter approaches the ductus via a long sheath advanced from the femoral vein. The right panel shows expansion of the distal umbrella. (From Castaneda, A., et al.: Cardiac Surgery of the Neonate and Infant. Philadelphia, W.B. Saunders Company, 1994, p. 136.)

the descending aorta, the toes, rather than the fingers, may show cyanosis and clubbing.

The full-term infant with patent ductus arteriosus may survive for a number of years, although occasionally a large defect results in heart failure and pulmonary edema early in life. The leading causes of death in older children are infective endocarditis and heart failure. Beyond the third decade severe pulmonary vascular obstruction has been known to cause aneurysmal dilatation, calcification, and rupture of the ductus.[217]

The patent ductus usually can be directly visualized by two-dimensional echocardiography (Fig. 29–18); range-gated pulse Doppler echocardiography shows the characteristic flow abnormalities across the ductus, as well as a continuous flow disturbance in the pulmonary artery. Cardiac catheterization may be indicated when additional lesions or pulmonary vascular obstruction is suspected.

Management. In the absence of severe pulmonary vascular disease with predominant right-to-left shunting, the anatomical presence of a patent ductus usually is considered sufficient indication for operation. Ligation or division of the ductus carries a low risk, whether performed electively in the asymptomatic child or at any age if symptoms are present. The operative risk is reduced if heart failure can be compensated by medical measures before surgery. Operation should be deferred for several months in patients treated successfully for infective endarteritis because the ductus may remain somewhat edematous and friable. Rarely, when the infection does not subside with intensive antibiotic treatment, surgical ligation may be necessary to eradicate the infection.

Although still investigational, substantial experience exists with transcatheter closure of the patent ductus using a variety of approaches, including coils, buttons, plugs, and umbrellas, with each occluder device introduced through a relatively large-diameter sheath from the femoral vein (Fig. 29–19).[218–224a] The approach is especially feasible in patients who weigh more than 10 kg, and with neither a long tubular ductus nor a ductus with a long, narrow aortic end. In experienced hands, initial occlusion is successful in 85 to 90 per cent of patients; reocclusion adds 5 to 7 per cent to the overall success rate. Potential complications in 5 to 10 per cent of patients include embolization of the device, endocarditis, and hemolysis.[114,224] Ductal closure by thoracoscopy will undoubtedly undergo future evaluation.

Aorticopulmonary Septal Defect

Aorticopulmonary window or fenestration, partial truncus arteriosus, and aortic septal defect are other designations applied to this relatively uncommon anomaly. Septation of the aortopulmonary trunk occurs by fusion of the conotruncal ridges (Fig. 29–2). The right and left sixth aortic arches, destined to become the pulmonary arteries, join the pulmonary artery to complete great artery development (Fig. 29–5). Congenital defects between the ascending aorta and the pulmonary artery result from faulty development of this area during embryonic life. The typical aortopulmonary septal defect results because of incomplete fusion of the distal aortopulmonary septum.[225] Malalignment of the conotruncal ridges results in unequal partitioning of the aortopulmonary trunk, which may result in partial or complete fusion of the right pulmonary artery to the aorta.

The usual defect consists of a communication between the aorta and pulmonary artery just above the semilunar valves. Persistent patency of the ductus arteriosus is an associated lesion in 10 to 15 per cent of cases. Less common accompanying cardiovascular lesions include ventricular septal defect, aortic origin of the right pulmonary artery, aortic arch interruption, coarctation of the aorta, and right aortic arch. Aorticopulmonary septal defects usually are large and are accompanied by severe pulmonary arterial hypertension and early-onset pulmonary vascular obstruction.

PHYSICAL EXAMINATION. The pulses typically are bounding, like those of a large patent ductus arteriosus. The murmur, however, seldom is continuous, and a basal systolic murmur is most common. Cardiomegaly is present, and pulmonary hypertension is reflected in a loud and palpable sound of pulmonary valve closure. Aorticopulmonary septal defect should be suspected whenever a large shunt into the pulmonary artery is demonstrated at catheterization. Diagnosis of the anomaly and its distinction from patent ductus and persistent truncus arteriosus usually can be done by two-dimensional echocardiography, but definitive identification of the aortopulmonary window and associated malformations requires hemodynamic study and selective angiocardiography with the injection of contrast mate-

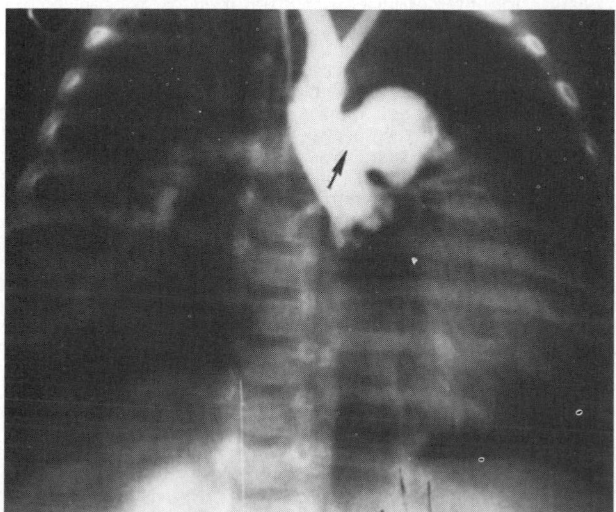

FIGURE 29–20. Aortic root injection of contrast material in the frontal view produces simultaneous opacification of aorta and pulmonary artery through a large aorticopulmonary septal defect (arrow). (Courtesy of Robert White, M.D.)

rial into the left ventricle and/or the root of the aorta (Fig. 29–20). Although some patients may survive to adulthood with uncorrected aorticopulmonary septal defect, most die early in life unless surgical treatment is undertaken. Operative correction is indicated in all symptomatic infants when the diagnosis is made. Elective repair is advised at 3 to 6 months. Profound hypothermic total circulatory arrest or total cardiopulmonary bypass is required, and the defect is closed by way of a transaortic approach, usually with a prosthetic or xenograft pericardial patch.[226,227]

Persistent Truncus Arteriosus

MORPHOLOGY. Persistent truncus arteriosus is a rare but serious anomaly in which a single vessel forms the outlet of both ventricles and gives rise to the systemic, pulmonary, and coronary arteries.[228] The defect results from failure of septation of the embryonic truncus by the infundibular truncal ridges (Fig. 29–4). It is always accompanied by a ventricular septal defect, frequently with a right-sided aortic arch. The ventricular septal defect is due to the absence or underdevelopment of the distal portion of the pulmonary infundibulum. The truncal valve usually is tricuspid but is quadricuspid in about one-third of patients and rarely can be bicuspid. Truncal valve regurgitation and truncal valve stenosis are each seen in 10 to 15 per cent of patients. There may be a single coronary artery, displacement of the coronary ostia (usually the left ostium posteriorly), or a single posterior descending coronary artery arising from the right coronary or, less often, from the left circumflex artery, especially in patients with a single coronary artery.[229,230]

Truncus malformations may be classified either anatomically according to the mode of origin of pulmonary vessels from the common trunk or from a functional point of view, based on the magnitude of blood flow to the lungs.[231] In the common type (type I) of truncus arteriosus malformation a partially separate pulmonary trunk of variable length exists because of the presence of an incompletely formed aorticopulmonary septum. The pulmonary trunk usually is very short and gives rise to left and right pulmonary arteries. When the aorticopulmonary septum is absent, there is no discrete main pulmonary artery component, and both pulmonary artery branches arise directly from the truncus.

In type II, each pulmonary artery arises separately but close to the other from the posterior aspect of the truncus (Fig. 29–21). In type III, each pulmonary artery arises from the lateral aspect of the truncus. Less commonly, one pulmonary artery branch may be absent, with collateral arteries supplying the lung that does not receive a pulmonary artery branch from the truncus. Truncus arteriosus malformation should not be confused with "pseudotruncus arteriosus," which is the severe form of tetralogy of Fallot with pulmonary atresia in which the single aorta arises from the heart accompanied by a remnant of atretic pulmonary artery.

HEMODYNAMICS. Pulmonary blood flow is governed by the size of the pulmonary arteries and the pulmonary vascular resistance. In infancy, pulmonary blood flow is usually excessive because pulmonary vascular resistance is not greatly increased. Thus, despite an obligatory admixture of systemic and pulmonary venous blood in the common trunk, only minimal cyanosis is present. Rarely, pulmonary blood flow is restricted by hypoplastic or stenotic pulmonary arteries arising from the truncus. Pulmonary vascular obstruction usually does not restrict pulmonary blood flow before 1 year of age.[232]

CLINICAL FEATURES. The infant with truncus arteriosus usually presents with mild cyanosis coexisting with the cardiac findings of a large left-to-right shunt. Symptoms of heart failure and poor physical development usually appear in the first weeks or months of life. The most frequent physical findings include cardiomegaly, a systolic ejection sound accompanied by a thrill, a loud single second heart sound, a harsh systolic murmur, and a low-pitched mid-diastolic rumbling murmur and bounding pulses. Truncus arteriosus often is a measure of the *DiGeorge syndrome* (Table 29–2); thus facial dysmorphism, a high incidence of extracardiac malformations (particularly of the limbs, kidneys, and intestines), atrophy or absence of the thymus gland, T-lymphocyte deficiency, and predilection to infection also may be features of the clinical presentation.[233] Recent evidence suggests that embryonic abnormalities in the cardiac neural crest play a major role in the creation of the cardiovascular malformation as well as the other components of the syndrome.[234]

Truncal valve incompetence is suggested by the presence of a diastolic decrescendo murmur at the base of the heart.[235] The physical findings are quite different if pulmonary blood flow is restricted by either high pulmonary vascular resistance or pulmonary arterial stenosis: Cyanosis is prominent, congestive failure is rare, and only a short systolic ejection may be audible occasionally accompanied by continuous murmurs posteriorly of bronchial collateral flow.

ECG AND RADIOGRAPHY. Left ventricular hypertrophy alone or in combination with right ventricular hypertrophy is present electrocardiographically when a prominent left-to-right shunt exists; right ventricular hypertrophy is observed in patients with restricted pulmonary blood flow. The radiographic findings depend on the hemodynamic circumstances. Gross cardiomegaly with left or combined ventricular enlargement, left atrial enlargement, and a small or absent main pulmonary artery segment with pulmonary vascular engorgement are the usual radiographic features. A right aortic arch is common (25 to 30 per cent of patients). When pulmonary blood flow is reduced, both heart size and pulmonary vascular markings are less prominent.

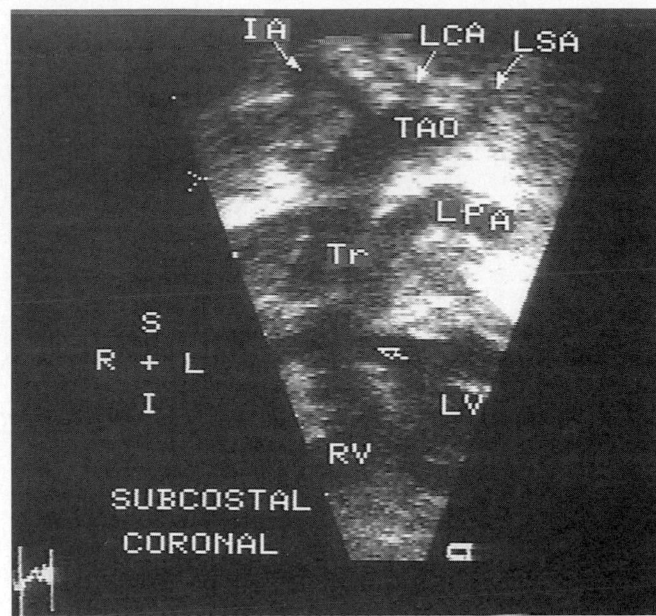

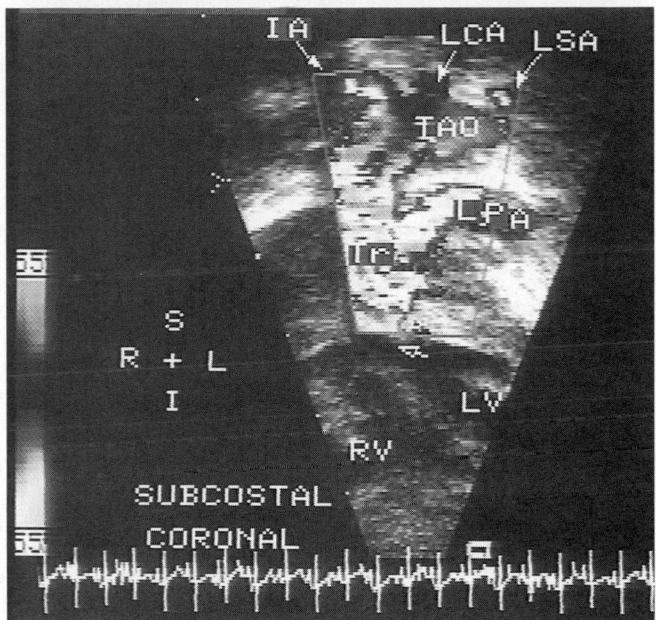

FIGURE 29–21. *Top,* Subcostal coronal view of truncus arteriosus (Tr). The truncal valve lies above the ventricular septal defect (open arrow), which appears above the left ventricle (LV) and right ventricle (RV). The truncus arteriosus (Tr) is seen dividing into the transverse aortic arch (TAO), which gives rise to the vessels supplying the head and neck: the innominate artery (IA), the left carotid artery (LCA), and the left subclavian artery (LSA). *Bottom,* Doppler color flow image showing the superimposition of color flow into the truncus arteriosus, left pulmonary artery, transverse aorta, and branches to the head and neck. Orientation: S = superior, I = inferior, R = right, L = left. (Courtesy of Norman Silverman, M.D.)

The *echocardiographic* features of truncus arteriosus (Fig. 29–21) include the detection of a large truncal root overriding the ventricular septum, truncal valve abnormalities, an increase in the right ventricular dimension, and mitral valve–truncal root continuity. Differentiation be-

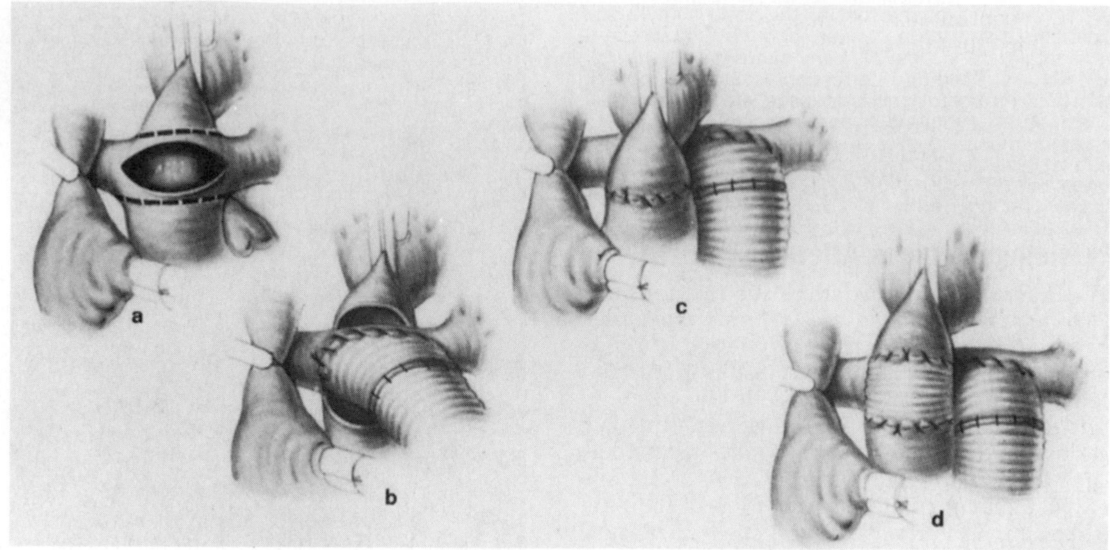

FIGURE 29–22. Operative correction of truncus arteriosus, type III. The pulmonary arteries arise separately from the truncus. An anterior incision is made and a segment of aorta containing the orifices of both pulmonary arteries is excised from the truncus (a). The cuff of tissue containing the two pulmonary arteries is anastomosed to an extracardiac valved conduit (b). Aortic continuity is restored by direct suture (c) or by interposing a preclotted graft (d). The diagram does not show closure of the ventricular septal defect. (From Stark, J., and DeLaval, M.: Surgery for Congenital Heart Defects. New York, Grune and Stratton, 1983, p. 420.)

tween truncus arteriosus and tetralogy of Fallot by ultrasonography may be difficult unless either the separate origin of the pulmonary arteries or a single trunk from the ascending portion of a single arterial root can be identified. The origin of the pulmonary arteries is detected best from high short-axis views, scanning superiorly from the semilunar valve. Diagnosis should be suspected at cardiac catheterization if the catheter fails to enter the central pulmonary arteries from the right ventricle. Selective angiocardiography and retrograde aortography are necessary to establish a precise diagnosis and to reveal the common trunk arising from the heart and the origin of the pulmonary arteries from the truncus.[236]

The early fatal course as well as early development of pulmonary vascular obstructive disease in patients surviving infancy is responsible for the poor prognosis associated with truncus arteriosus. In infants and young children with large left-to-right shunts, surgical banding of one or both pulmonary arteries to reduce pulmonary flow has been used with little success. Corrective operation is indicated before age 3 months to avoid the development of severe pulmonary vascular obstructive disease.[237]

SURGICAL TREATMENT. Operation consists of closure of the ventricular septal defect, leaving the aorta arising from the left ventricle; the pulmonary arteries are excised from their truncus origin and a valve-containing prosthetic conduit or aortic homograft valve conduit is used to establish continuity between the right ventricle and the pulmonary arteries (Fig. 29–22). Important risk factors for perioperative death are severe truncal valve regurgitation, interrupted aortic arch, coronary artery anomalies, and age at operation greater than 100 days.[238] Patients with only one pulmonary artery are especially prone to early development of severe pulmonary vascular disease but otherwise are not at increased risk from surgery.

With truncus arteriosus defects, the possible inequalities of pressure and flow between the two pulmonary arteries often make precise calculation of pulmonary resistance difficult. Corrective operation may be performed in patients with at least one adequate pulmonary artery having low distal pressure or arteriolar resistance. Conversely, significant systemic arterial desaturation in a patient with two pulmonary arteries and with neither pulmonary artery stenosis nor a previous pulmonary artery band signifies that high pulmonary vascular resistance exists and that the condition is probably inoperable. It is not yet clear how often and at what age the conduit between the right ventricle and pulmonary artery must be replaced with a larger prosthesis because of either growth of the patient, in whom a small conduit causes eventual obstruction, heterograft valve degeneration, or obstruction created by neointimal proliferation within a prosthetic conduit.[239] When operation is carried out within a conduit in the first year of life, conduit replacement often is required within 3 to 5 years.

Coronary Arteriovenous Fistula

Coronary arteriovenous fistula (see also p. 967) is an unusual anomaly that consists of a communication between one of the coronary arteries and a cardiac chamber or vein. The right coronary artery, or its branches, is the site of the fistula in about 55 per cent of cases; the left coronary artery is involved in about 35 per cent, and both coronary arteries in 5 per cent. Connections between the coronary system and a cardiac chamber appear to represent persistence of embryonic intertrabecular spaces and sinusoids. Most of these fistulas drain into the right ventricle, right atrium, or coronary sinus; fistulous communication to the pulmonary artery, left atrium, or left ventricle is much less frequent. Most often the shunt through the fistula is of small magnitude, and myocardial blood flow is not compromised.[240] Rarely, spontaneous closure may occur. Potential complications include pulmonary hypertension and congestive heart failure if a large left-to-right shunt exists, bacterial endocarditis, rupture or thrombosis of the fistula or an associated arterial aneurysm, and myocardial ischemia distal to the fistula due to decreased coronary blood flow.

Most pediatric patients are asymptomatic and are referred because of a cardiac murmur that is loud, superficial, and continuous at the lower or midsternal border. The site of maximal intensity of the murmur is related to the site of drainage and usually is different from the second left intercostal space—the classic site of the continuous murmur of persistent ductus arteriosus—except when the fistula drains into the pulmonary artery or right ventricle. In the latter situation the murmur is louder in diastole than in systole because of compression of the fistula by contracting myocardium. The electrocardiogram and chest roentgenogram quite often are normal and seldom show selective chamber enlargement or myocardial ischemia. Significantly enlarged coronary arteries may be detected by two-dimensional echocardiography, and the actual diagnosis of an arteriovenous fistula occasionally can be made by combining two-dimensional echocardiography and Doppler techniques to detect the entrance site of the shunt, which is characterized by a continuous turbulent systolic and diastolic flow pattern (Fig. 30–8, p. 968).[241,242]

Standard retrograde thoracic aortography, balloon occlusion angiography of the aortic root with a 45-degree caudal tilt of the frontal camera ("laid back" aortogram),[243] or coronary arteriography can be used reliably to identify the size and anatomical features of the fistulous tract, which can be closed by transcatheter coil embolization or suture obliteration in most cases.[243,244] In the presence of a large left-to-right shunt and symptoms of heart failure, the decision to operate is clearly justified. Most often the fistula is closed in asymptomatic patients to prevent future symptoms or complications, such as infective endocarditis. The prognosis after successful closure of a coronary artery–cardiac chamber fistula is excellent.

Anomalous Pulmonary Origin of the Coronary Artery

This rare malformation occurs in about 0.4 per cent of patients with congenital cardiac anomalies. In almost all patients the left coronary artery originates from the posterior sinus of the pulmonary artery.[246]

Unusual cases have been reported in which the right coronary artery, or the entire coronary artery system, originates from the main pulmonary trunk. Embryologically the distal coronary artery system is formed by 9 weeks from solid angioblastic buds that extend throughout the epicardium to form the major coronary artery branches. Proximally the coronary network forms a ring around the truncus arteriosus, joining with coronary buds from the primitive aortic sinuses as the truncus partitions to form the great arteries. The varieties of anomalous pulmonary origin of the coronary artery are the result of displacement in this proximal process.

PATHOPHYSIOLOGY. During fetal life pulmonary artery pressure is slightly greater than aortic pressure, and perfusion of the left coronary artery is antegrade (Fig. 29–23*A*). After birth, when pulmonary artery pressure falls below aortic pressure, perfusion of the left coronary artery from the pulmonary artery ceases, and the direction of flow in the anomalous vessel reverses. Blood flows from the aorta to the right coronary artery, then through collateral channels to the left coronary artery, and finally to the pulmonary artery (Fig. 29–23*B*). In effect, the left coronary artery behaves as a fistulous communication between the aorta and pulmonary artery.[245] If adequate collateral channels exist or develop between the two coronary artery circulations, total myocardial perfusion through the right coronary artery increases (Fig. 29–23*C*). In 10 to 15 per cent of patients myocardial ischemia never develops because extensive intercoronary collaterals allow survival to adolescence or adulthood.[245] In fact, if collateral blood flow is considerable, the patient may develop the clinical manifestations of a large arteriovenous shunt and a continuous or diastolic murmur.

By far the most common clinical presentation is that of the infant who suffers a myocardial infarction and develops congestive heart failure.[247–249] The infant syndrome usually becomes manifested at age 2 to 4 months with angina-like symptoms that may be misinterpreted as colic. Feeding and defecation often are accompanied by dyspnea, irritability and crying, pallor, diaphoresis, and occasional loss of consciousness. Older children or adults usually present with a continuous murmur or with mitral regurgitation resulting from dysfunction of ischemic or infarcted papillary muscles. In some instances the coronary anomaly is unsuspected until a previously well adolescent or adult experiences angina, heart failure, or sudden death.

DIAGNOSIS. The diagnosis of anomalous origin of the coronary artery is supported by the electrocardiographic demonstration of deep Q waves in association with ST-segment alterations and T-wave inversions in leads I, aV_L, V_5, and V_6 (Fig. 29–24). These findings greatly assist the distinction of this anomaly from myocarditis and dilated cardiomyopathy.[250] Chest roentgenograms show moderate to severe enlargement of the left atrium and ventricle. Echocardiography with Doppler color-flow mapping is replacing cardiac catheterization as the standard method of diagnosis. The color flow mapping demonstrates retrograde flow in the left coronary system and an abnormal flow jet from the left coronary artery into the pulmonary trunk. Moreover, detection of antegrade flow in the left coronary system helps to exclude the diagnosis.[251] The origin of the anomalous left coronary artery occasionally may be visualized echocardiographically from long- or short-axis views of the pulmonary artery.[252] Absence of the left coronary artery from its usual origin in the left sinus of Valsalva does not distinguish this lesion from single coronary artery. Color-flow Doppler examination may also reveal associated mitral regurgitation. Ischemia or infarction is suggested by the echocardiographic findings of segmental wall motion abnormalities, particularly involving the anterolateral free wall of the left ventricle. Stress thallium scintigraphy shows a characteristic defect of the anterolateral wall of the left ventricle. Positron emission tomography reveals both

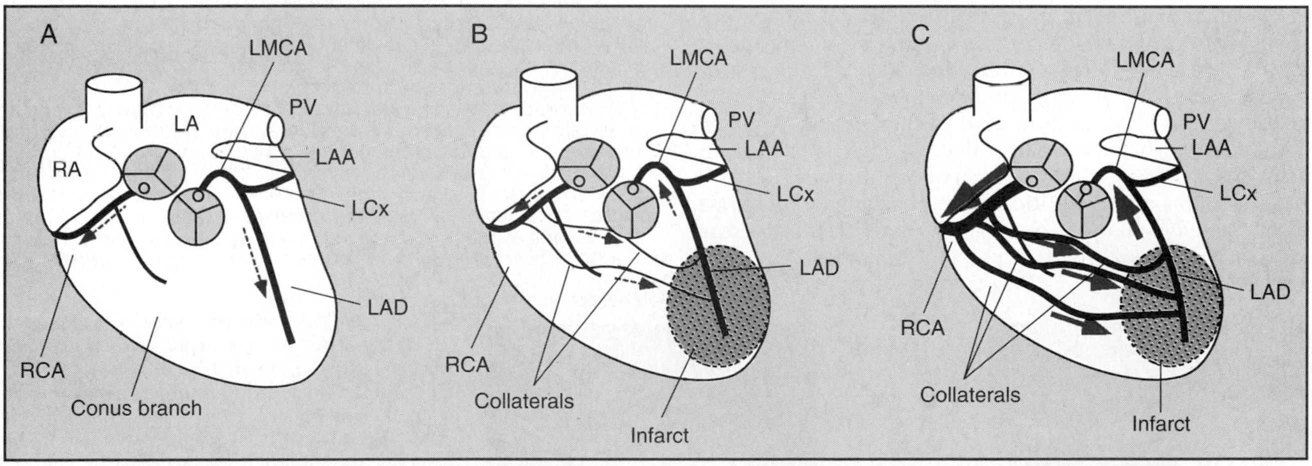

FIGURE 29–23. Anomalous origin of left main coronary artery from pulmonary artery. *A,* In fetus, both right and left coronary arteries receive forward flow from their respective great arteries. *B,* Early after birth, before collaterals are well developed, there may be an anterolateral infarct and slight retrograde flow from the left coronary artery to the pulmonary artery. *C,* After collaterals have enlarged, there is high flow in the enlarged right coronary artery and the collaterals and significant retrograde flow into the pulmonary artery. Dotted arrows indicate direction and approximate magnitude of flow in the right and left coronary arteries and the collaterals between them. SVC = superior vena cava, PV = pulmonary vein, LA = left atrium, LAA = left atrial appendage, RA = right atrium, LMCA = left main coronary artery, LCx = left circumflex coronary artery, LAD = left anterior descending coronary artery, RCA = right coronary artery, RVI = right ventricular infundibulum (outflow tract). (From Hoffman, J. I. E.: *In* Moss and Adams' Heart Disease in Infants, Children, and Adolescents. 5th ed. Baltimore, © Williams and Wilkins, 1994, p. 776.)

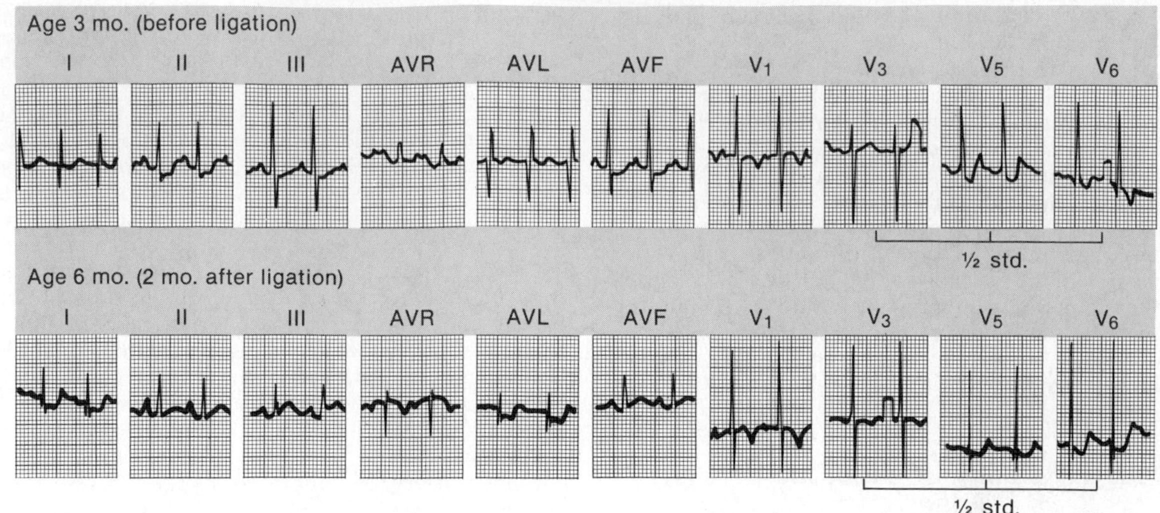

FIGURE 29–24. **Typical electrocardiogram of an infant with anomalous left coronary artery before *(above)* and after *(below)* ligation of the anomalous left coronary artery. Note the abnormal Q waves in I, AV_L, and V_6. (Courtesy of Delores A. Danilowicz, M.D.)**

the perfusion defect and its metabolic consequences (Fig. 29–25).

Aortography or coronary angiography demonstrates the retrograde drainage of the coronary vessel into the pulmonary artery. It should be recognized that ventricular arrhythmias may complicate the course of hemodynamic study. The magnitude of shunting into the pulmonary artery may be determined by oximetry, indicator dilution curves, or angiography.

MANAGEMENT. *Medical treatment* is indicated in infants with myocardial infarction for congestive heart failure, arrhythmias, and cardiogenic shock. In patients with a small left-to-right shunt or no shunt at all, the prognosis is exceedingly poor with conservative management, justifying an attempt to reestablish a two–coronary artery system. The *operations* that have been used include reimplanting the left coronary artery into the aortic root, surgically creating an aortopulmonary window and a tunnel to convey blood from the window across the back of the pulmonary trunk to the origin of the anomalous left coronary artery, with reconstruction of the anterior wall of the pulmonary trunk, and anastomosis of the left coronary artery with the subclavian artery or with the aorta by means of a graft.[253–255] If clinical deterioration occurs in infants in whom a sizable left-to-right shunt into the pulmonary artery exists, simple ligation of the left coronary artery at its origin prevents retrograde flow and allows perfusion of the left ventricle with blood supplied through anastomoses with the right coronary artery. If medical management stabilizes the infant with significant intercoronary collaterals, operation may be postponed to allow the patient to grow, because increased size of the vessels enhances the likelihood of successful reimplantation or coronary arterial bypass surgery. The outcome of surgery and ultimate prognosis are significantly influenced by the degree of myocardial damage suffered preoperatively.[256] Uncommonly, it is necessary to consider aneurysmectomy or mitral valve replacement.

Aortic Sinus Aneurysm and Fistula

Congenital aneurysm of an aortic sinus of Valsalva (see also p. 967), particularly the right coronary sinus, is an uncommon anomaly that occurs three times more often in males than in females. The malformation consists of a separation, or lack of fusion, between the media of the aorta and the annulus fibrosis of the aortic valve.[257] The receiving chamber of the aorticocardiac fistula usually is the right ventricle, but occasionally, when the noncoronary cusp is involved, the fistula drains into the right atrium.

Five to 15 per cent of aneurysms originate in the posterior or noncoronary sinus; seldom is the left aortic sinus involved. Associated anomalies are common and include bicuspid aortic valve, ventricular septal defect, and coartation of the aorta.

The deficiency in the aortic media appears to be congenital. Reports in infants are exceedingly rare[258] and are infrequent in children, because progressive aneurysmal dilatation of the weakened area develops but may not be recognized until the third or fourth decade of life, when rupture into a cardiac chamber occurs.

The *unruptured aneurysm* usually does not produce a hemodynamic abnormality, although pressure on the intracardiac conduction system by an unruptured aneurysm may be a rare cause of complete atrioventricular block; rarely, myocardial ischemia may be caused by coronary arterial compression. Rupture is often of abrupt onset, causes chest pain, and creates continuous arteriovenous shunting and volume loading of both right and left heart chambers, which results in heart failure. An additional complication is infective endo-

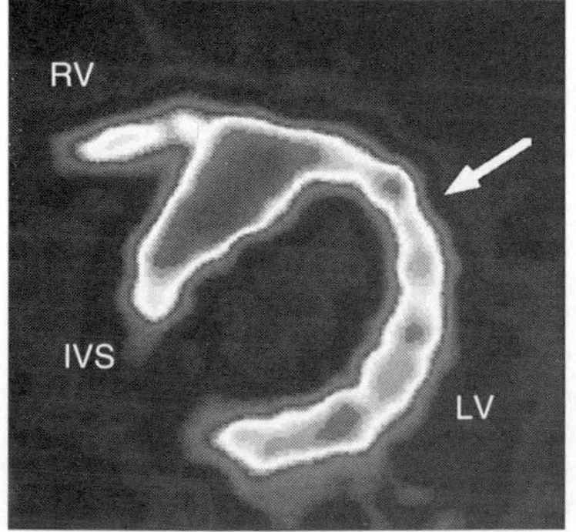

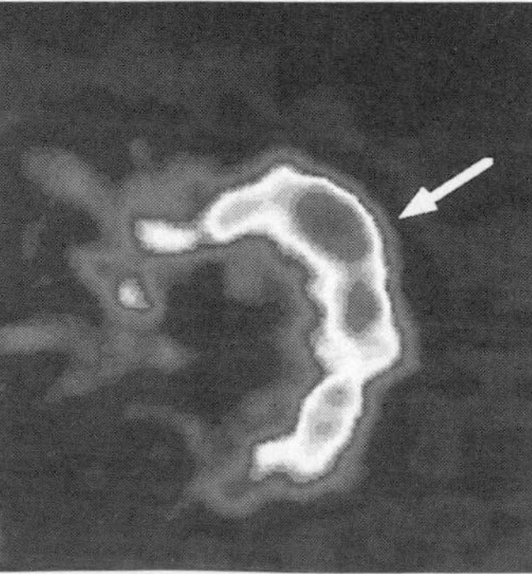

FIGURE 29–25. **Positron emission tomography (PET) transaxial images depict myocardial perfusion and glucose metabolism in a 7-month-old infant with anomalous origin of left coronary artery from the pulmonary artery. The ammonia (NH_3) scan demonstrates hypoperfusion *(left panel),* whereas the fluorodeoxyglucose scan shows increased glucose metabolism *(right panel)* in the anterior lateral left ventricular wall (arrows) in the region perfused by left coronary artery (LCA). Under fasting conditions, normal myocardium has minimal glucose (FDG) uptake, whereas, in this figure, hypoperfused myocardium preferentially metabolizes glucose. The "mismatch" pattern in this figure indicates ischemic but viable myocardium. This patient underwent reimplantation of the LCA with subsequent complete recovery of cardiac function and normalization of PET perfusion and metabolism. RV = right ventricle, LV = left ventricle, IVS = interventricular septum, A = anterior, L = lateral, P = posterior, R = right.**

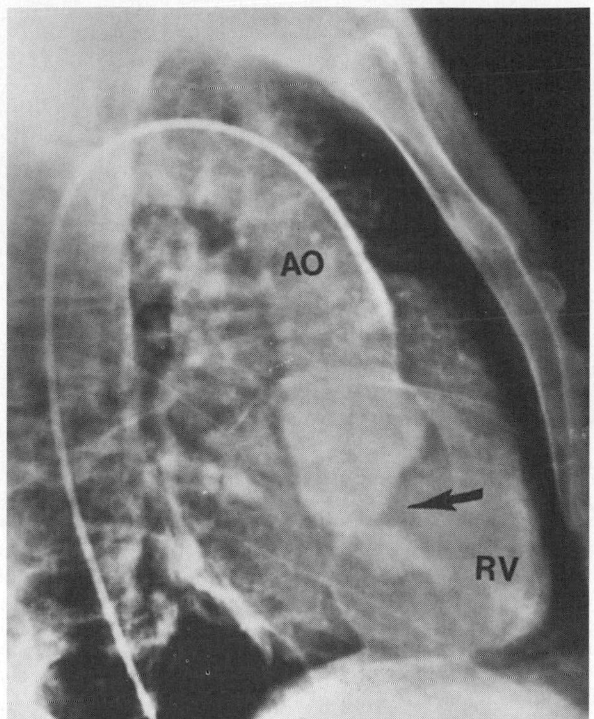

FIGURE 29–26. A retrograde aortogram shows the fistulous connection between the noncoronary sinus of Valsalva and the right ventricle (RV) (arrow). AO = aorta. (Courtesy of Robert White, M.D.)

carditis, which may originate either on the edges of the aneurysm or on those areas in the right side of the heart that are traumatized by the jet-like stream of blood flowing through the fistula.

DIAGNOSIS. The presence of this anomaly should be suspected in a patient with a history of chest pain of recent onset, symptoms of diminished cardiac reserve, bounding pulses, and a loud superficial continuous murmur accentuated in diastole when the fistula opens into the right ventricle, as well as a thrill along the right or left lower parasternal border. The *physical findings* may be difficult to distinguish from those produced by a coronary arteriovenous fistula. *Electrocardiography* shows biventricular hypertrophy, and chest roentgenography demonstrates generalized cardiomegaly. Two-dimensional and pulsed Doppler *echocardiographic* studies may detect the walls of the aneurysm and disturbed flow within the aneurysm or at the site of perforation, respectively.[259] *Transesophageal echocardiography* may provide more precise information than the transthoracic approach. *Cardiac catheterization* reveals a left-to-right shunt at the ventricular or, less commonly, the atrial level; the diagnosis may be established definitively by retrograde thoracic aortography (Fig. 29–26).

MANAGEMENT. Preoperative medical management consists of measures to relieve cardiac failure and to treat coexistent arrhythmias or endocarditis, if present. At operation the aneurysm is closed and amputated, and the aortic wall is reunited with the heart, either by direct suture or with a prosthesis.[260] Every effort should be made to preserve the aortic valve in children because patch closure of the defect combined with prosthetic valve replacement greatly enhances the risk of operation in small patients.

VALVULAR AND VASCULAR LESIONS WITH OR WITHOUT RIGHT-TO-LEFT SHUNT

Aortic Arch Obstruction

The conventional anatomical and clinical divisions into preductal and postductal coarctation or infantile and adult types, respectively, are misleading because the anatomical localization is inaccurate and the age-dependency of the clinical presentation does not hold true (i.e., the adult type often is seen in the first weeks of life). A spectrum of anatomical lesions exists, causing obstruction of the aortic arch or proximal portion of the descending aorta. These range from a localized coarctation or constriction of the lumen, most commonly located just distal to the origin of the left subclavian artery and closely related to the attachment of the ductus arteriosus with the aorta, to diffuse narrowing or interruption of a portion of the aortic arch. In this chapter, aortic arch obstruction is divided into three types: (1) localized juxtaductal coarctation, (2) hypoplasia of the aortic isthmus, and (3) aortic arch interruption. *Pseudocoarctation* is used synonymously with "kinking" or "buckling" of the aorta, which is a subclinical form of localized juxtaductal coarctation of the aorta.[261]

Localized Juxtaductal Coarctation

(See also p. 965)

MORPHOLOGY. This lesion consists of a localized shelf-like thickening and infolding of the media of the posterolateral aortic wall opposite the ductus arteriosus; the wall of the aorta into which the ductus or ligamentum arteriosum inserts is not involved.[262] Juxtaductal coarctation occurs two to five times more commonly in males than in females, and there is a high degree of association with gonadal dysgenesis (Turner syndrome) and bicuspid aortic valve. Other common associated anomalies include ventricular septal defect and mitral stenosis or regurgitation. The most important extracardiac anomaly is aneurysm of the circle of Willis.

PATHOGENESIS. Juxtaductal coarctation is probably related to an abnormality in the pattern of ductus arteriosus blood flow in utero, which, in turn, may be the result of associated intracardiac anomalies.[262,263] Thus, in fetal life, blood flow through the aortic isthmus constitutes only 12 to 17 per cent of the total cardiac output, while blood flow through the ductus arteriosus exceeds that across the aortic valve. The dorsal aortic wall directly opposite the ductus arteriosus resembles morphologically the apex of a normal branch point of the aorta if ductal flow pathways in utero diverge, with some flow directed cephalad into the aortic isthmus and the remainder proceeding into the descending aorta. The aortic branch point is identical histologically to the posterior shelf of juxtaductal aortic coarctation. A divergence of ductal flow is fostered by the presence of lesions in the fetus that create an imbalance between left and right ventricular outputs, with right-sided flow predominating (e.g., bicuspid aortic valve, mitral valve anomaly). In the absence of an anomaly fostering augmented ductal flow, a branch point may be created by an alteration in the angle at which the ductus arteriosus meets the aorta, pointing the ductal stream directly against the posterior aortic wall rather than obliquely down into the descending aorta. Cardiac anomalies that cause augmented ascending aortic blood flow (e.g., pulmonic atresia or stenosis, tetralogy of Fallot) prevent development of a branch point and indeed are almost never seen in association with juxtaductal coarctation of the aorta.

During fetal life the posterior aortic shelf is not obstructive because blood may pass readily from the ascending aorta to the descending aorta by traversing the anterior aortic segment and the aortic end of the ductus arteriosus. Postnatally, however, when the ductus undergoes obliteration at its aortic end, the shelf-like projection of the posterior aortic wall unmasks the obstruction to aortic flow (Fig. 29–27). After pharmacological interventions that dilate the ductus arteriosus (prostaglandin E_1 infusion) the pressure difference may be obliterated across the site of coarctation because the fetal flow pattern is reestablished.[96,264]

The pathogenesis of juxtaductal coarctation already described explains the prevalence of associated intracardiac anomalies that foster reduced ascending aortic flow and augmented ductus arteriosus flow in utero, and the absence of associated intracardiac anomalies in which the converse flow conditions exist in utero. The dependence of aortic obstruction on constriction of the ductus arteriosus postnatally explains the variable onset after birth of the clinical manifestations of coarctation, as well as the dramatic alleviation of the obstruction produced pharmacologically by dilatation of the ductus arteriosus.

CLINICAL FINDINGS. The manifestations of juxtaductal coarctation of the aorta depend on the prominence of the posterolateral aortic shelf, which determines the intensity of obstruction and on the rapidity with which obstruction develops.

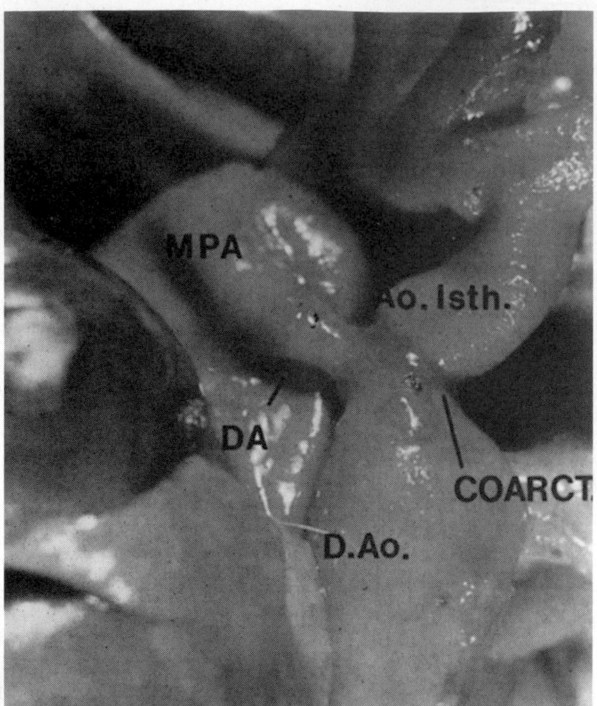

FIGURE 29–27. Juxtaductal coarctation (COARCT) unmasked by constriction of the ductus arteriosus (DA). MPA = main pulmonary artery, D.Ao. = descending aorta, Ao.Isth. = aortic isthmus. (Courtesy of Norman Talner, M.D.)

NEONATES AND INFANTS. Rapid, severe obstruction in infancy is a prominent cause of left ventricular failure and systemic hypoperfusion. Substantial left-to-right shunting across a patent foramen ovale and pulmonary venous hypertension secondary to heart failure cause pulmonary arterial hypertension. Because little or no aortic obstruction existed during fetal life, the collateral circulation in the newborn period is often poorly developed. Characteristically in these infants, peripheral pulses are weak throughout the body until left ventricular function is improved with medical management; a significant pressure difference then develops between the arms and the legs, allowing detection of a pulse discrepancy. Cardiac murmurs are nonspecific in infancy and commonly are derived from associated lesions.

The *electrocardiogram* shows the right-axis deviation and right ventricular hypertrophy; the *chest radiograph* shows generalized cardiomegaly and pulmonary arterial and venous engorgement. Two-dimensional and Doppler echocardiography provide an accurate noninvasive assessment of the anatomy and physiology in most patients. Hemodynamic study also allows delineation of the site and extent of aortic obstruction and the detection of associated cardiac malformations. Most infants with early-onset severe heart failure respond poorly to medical management, and balloon angioplasty, surgical excision of the coartation, or a subclavian flap angioplasty often is required.

Aortic obstruction may develop slowly in infants in whom the posterolateral aortic shelf is not prominent at birth and in whom ductus arteriosus constriction is gradual. In these babies compensatory myocardial hypertrophy and an extensive collateral circulation have time to develop. If the obstruction does not intensify and cardiac failure does not occur by age 6 or 9 months, circulatory compensation is likely until adult life.

CHILDREN. Most children with isolated juxtaductal coarctation are asymptomatic. Complaints of headache, cold extremities, and claudication with exercise may be noted, although attention usually is directed to the cardiovascular system by detection of a heart murmur of upper-extremity hypertension on routine physical examination. Mechanical factors rather than those of renal origin play the primary role in the production of hypertension. Absent, markedly diminished, or delayed pulsations in the femoral arteries and a low or unobtainable arterial pressure in the lower extremities with hypertension in the arms are the basic clues to the diagnosis. A midsystolic murmur over the anterior chest, back, and spinous processes is most frequent, becoming continuous if the lumen is sufficiently narrowed to result in a high-velocity jet across the lesion

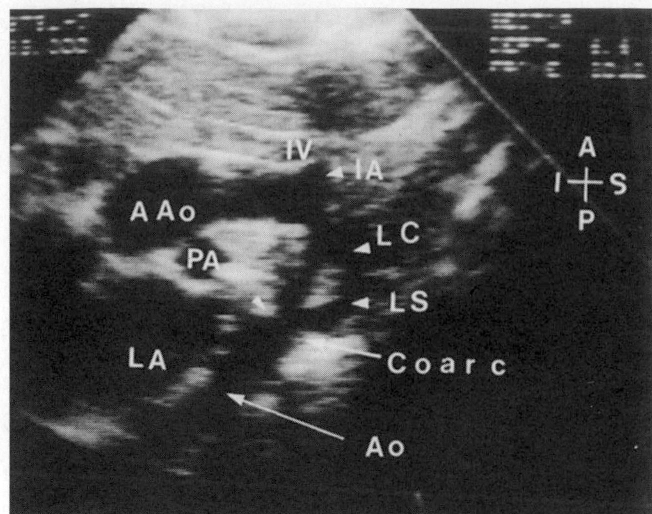

FIGURE 29–28. Aortic coarctation (Coarc) is visualized from the suprasternal notch. The aorta (Ao) can be traced from the ascending aorta (AAo). The aortic arch is somewhat narrowed, and the relationship of the left subclavian artery (LS) to the coarctation is identified clearly. LA = left atrium, PA = pulmonary artery, IA = innominate artery, LC = left carotid artery. (Courtesy of Norman Silverman, M.D.)

throughout the cardiac cycle. Additional systolic and continuous murmurs over the lateral thoracic wall may reflect increased flow through dilated and tortuous collateral vessels.

Electrocardiography reveals left ventricular hypertrophy of varying degrees, depending on the height of arterial pressure above the obstruction and the patient's age. Combined with right ventricular hypertrophy, this usually implies a complicated lesion. *Chest roentgenograms* (Fig. 7–42, p. 232) may show a dilated left subclavian artery high on the left mediastinal border and a dilated ascending aorta. Indentation of the aorta at the site of coarctation and prestenotic and poststenotic dilatation (the "3" sign) along the left premediastinal shadow is almost pathognomonic. Poststenotic dilation also may be detected by indentation of the barium-filled esophagus. Notching of the ribs, an important radiographic sign, is due to erosion by dilated collateral vessels, increases with age, and usually becomes apparent between the 4th and 12th years of life. The aortic coarctation may be visualized directly by two-dimensional

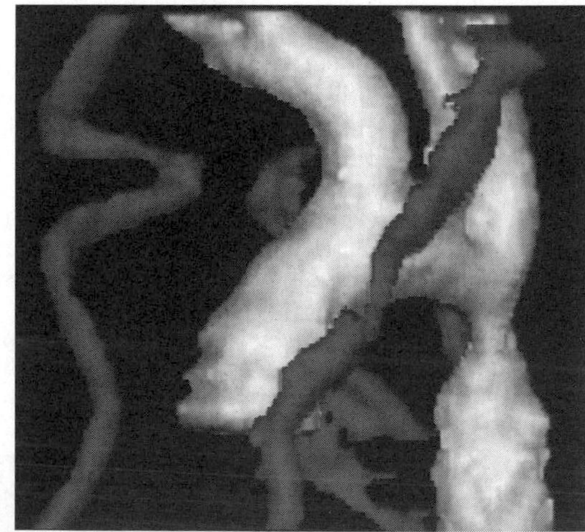

FIGURE 29–29. Three-dimensional computer reconstruction of magnetic resonance images in a child with discrete coarctation and numerous large collateral vessels, displayed in a lateral projection. Dilated brachiocephalic and internal mammary arteries are evident. (Courtesy of W. James Parks, M.D., The Children's Heart Center, Emory University, Atlanta, Georgia.)

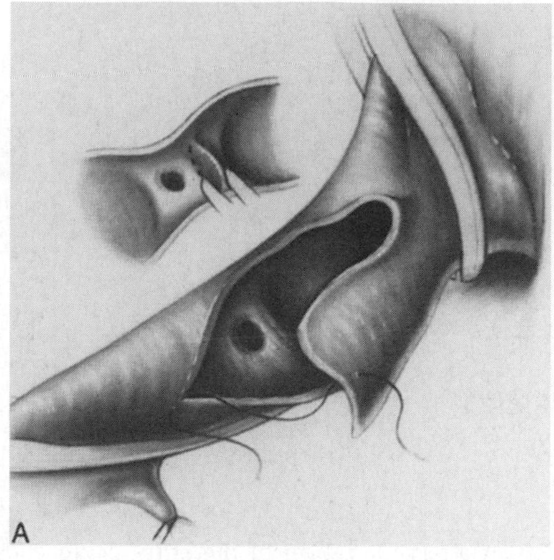

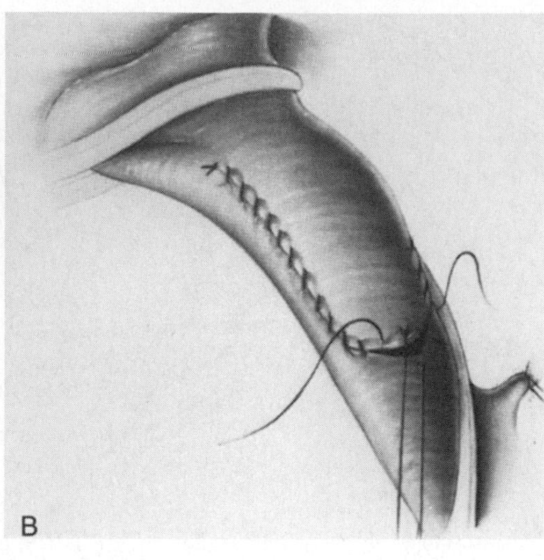

FIGURE 29–30. Subclavian flap aortoplasty repair of aortic coarctation. *A,* The left subclavian artery has been ligated and divided; the aorta is incised from below the coarctation ridge of tissue, which is carefully excised. *B,* The distal end of the subclavian artery forms a flap, which is sutured to the aortotomy. (From Stark, J., and DeLaval, M.: Surgery for Congenital Heart Defects. New York, Grune and Stratton, 1983, p. 216.)

echocardiography from high parasternal or suprasternal notch views with short focused transducers and from the subxiphoid window with extended focal range transducers (Fig. 29–28). Doppler examination reveals a flow disturbance and high-velocity jet at the site of obstruction and provides a reasonable estimate of the transcoarctation pressure gradient.[265,266] Computed tomography,[267] magnetic resonance imaging[268] (Fig. 29–29 and Fig. 10–22, p. 328), or cardiac catheterization and aortography also accurately localizes the site of obstruction, determines the length of coarctation, and, particularly, identifies associated malformations. Preoperative catheterization is avoided for selected patients with typical clinical and two-dimensional and Doppler echocardiographic findings.[269] Intravascular ultrasonography provides interesting morphological images suitable especially for comparison to postoperative status.[270,271]

MANAGEMENT. Controversy exists concerning the role of balloon angioplasty (see p. 1366) in the treatment of native coarctation, especially in neonates.[271–274] There is concern about residual pressure gradients, aneurysm formation, aortic dissection and rupture, and femoral arterial complications, especially late after angioplasty. It is clear that angioplasty can effectively reduce obstruction in many patients, albeit with an unpredictable late outcome.

Subclavian flap aortoplasty (Fig. 29–30), particularly in neonates and infants, or surgical resection and end-to-end anastomosis of uncomplicated juxtaductal coarctation of the aorta can be accomplished with excellent results in most patients[275,276]; some surgeons prefer an on-lay patch across the site of obstruction. In children who are asymptomatic it is preferable to delay surgery until age 4 to 6 years, at which time coarctation seldom recurs.[277] Paradoxical hypertension of short duration often is noted in the immediate postoperative period, a phenomenon much less common after balloon angioplasty.[278] A resetting of carotid baroreceptors and increased catecholamine secretion appears to be responsible for the initial phase of postoperative systemic hypertension with a later, second phase of prolonged elevation of systolic and particularly diastolic blood pressure related to activation of the renin-angiotensin system.[279] A necrotizing panarteritis of the small vessels of the gastrointestinal tract of uncertain cause occasionally complicates the course of recovery.

A 5 to 10 per cent risk of recurrent narrowing exists after repair of coarctation in infancy. Such narrowing is best detected by magnetic resonance imaging or Doppler ultrasonography.[280] This problem is treated most effectively by transcutaneous balloon angioplasty,[281,281a] which may be expected to markedly reduce, but not abolish entirely, the pressure differences across the site of recoarctation.

In those patients who survive the first 2 years of life, complications of juxtaductal coarctation are uncommon before the second or third decade. The chief hazards to patients with coarctation result from severe hypertension and include the development of cerebral aneurysms and hemorrhage, hypertensive encephalopathy, rupture of the aorta, left ventricular failure, and infective endocarditis. Systemic hypertension in the absence of residual coarctation has been observed in resting or exercise-stressed patients postoperatively and appears to be related to the duration of preoperative hypertension.[282–284] Lifelong observation is desirable because of the late onset of hypertension in some postoperative patients.[285–288]

Hypoplasia of the Aortic Arch

MORPHOLOGY. The aortic isthmus, the portion of the aorta between the left subclavian artery and the ductus arteriosus, normally is narrowed in the fetus and newborn. The lumen of the aortic isthmus is about two-thirds that of the ascending and descending portions of the aorta until age 6 to 9 months, when the physiological narrowing disappears.[289] Pathological tubular hypoplasia of the aortic arch usually is noted in the aortic isthmus and often is referred to as preductal or infantile coarctation of the aorta.[290] Associated major cardiac malformations occur in virtually all such infants and include large ventricular septal defect, atrioventricular septal defect, transposition of the great arteries, the Taussig-Bing type of anomaly, and double-outlet right ventricle. The ventricular septal defect most often is subpulmonary, lying within the substance of the infundibular septum. Thus, muscle persists between the aortic and pulmonary valve leaflets, which, when displaced leftward, produces subaortic stenosis. Persistent patency of the ductus arteriosus commonly coexists, and right-to-left flow across the ductus arteriosus usually provides filling of the descending aorta. The adequacy of blood flow to the lower body depends on the degree of aortic hypoplasia, the caliber of the ductus arteriosus, and the relationship between pulmonary and systemic vascular resistance. Substantial right-to-left shunting through a wide-open ductus arteriosus minimizes the arterial blood pressure difference between the upper and lower body.

CLINICAL FINDINGS. Differential cyanosis of the toes and feet with normal color of the fingers and hands may be difficult to discern because intracardiac left-to-right shunting and pulmonary edema attenuate the differences in oxygen saturation in the ascending and descending aorta. Clinical deterioration is associated with ductal constriction or a fall in pulmonary vascular resistance. Moreover, the clinical presentation often is dictated by the hemodynamic effects of complex associated intracardiac malformations. Infants most often present with findings of a large left-to-right intracardiac shunt, pulmonary hypertension, and marked cardiac decompensation. Although tubular hypoplasia is detectable by two-dimensional echocardiography, cardiac catheterization may be required to evaluate the full extent of intracardiac and extracardiac lesions.[291] Surgical repair of aortic arch hypoplasia usually must be accompanied by operative palliation or correction of associated intracardiac lesions. An extended end-to-end anastomosis (Fig. 29-31), classic or reversed subclavian flap angioplasty, patch aortography, and bypass grafting are among the operative approaches to correct long segment narrowing.[292–294] Recoarctation is common and often necessitates transcatheter balloon aortoplasty and/or a second operation later in life to relieve anastomotic stenosis.

AORTIC ARCH INTERRUPTION

Aortic arch interruption is a rare and usually lethal anomaly; unless treated surgically almost all infants die within the first

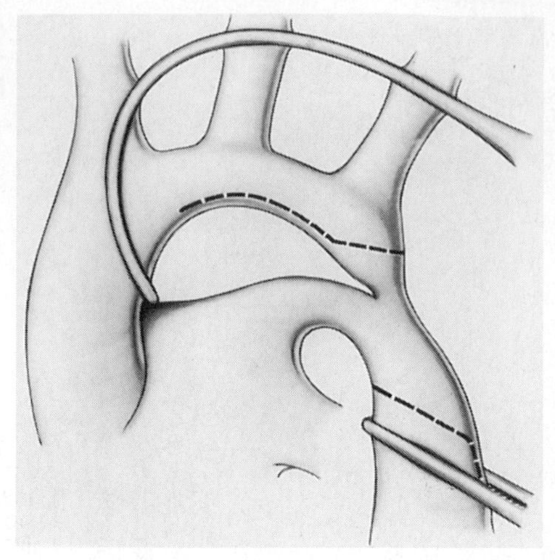

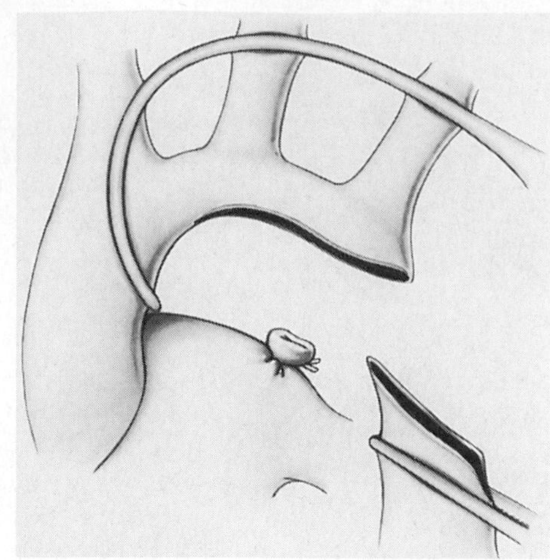

FIGURE 29–31. An extended repair of aortic coarctation is employed in the presence of a hypoplastic aortic arch. The dashed lines in the left panel delineate resection sites of the coarcted segment. In the right panel, the ductus arteriosus has been ligated and the incisions are extended to the undersurface of the aortic arch and onto the distal aorta. When the suture line is completed, the reconstruction of the arch is generally excellent. (From Stark, J., and DeLaval, M.: Surgery for Congenital Heart Defects. 2nd ed. Philadelphia, W.B. Saunders Company, 1994, p. 292.)

month of life.[295] Interruptions distal to the left subclavian artery (Type A) occur with almost equal frequency to interruptions distal to the left common carotid artery (Type B); interruptions distal to the innominate artery (Type C) are extremely uncommon. The right subclavian artery often is of variable origin, frequently arising from the descending aortic segment distal to the interruption. The clinical presentation resembles that seen in tubular hypoplasia or severe juxtaductal coarctation of the aorta with a patent ductus arteriosus.

Virtually all patients have associated intracardiac anomalies. A patent ductus arteriosus almost always connects the main pulmonary artery with the descending aorta. With rare exceptions, patients with interrupted aortic arch have either a ventricular septal defect (80 to 90 per cent of cases) or an aorticopulmonary window (10 to 20 per cent). Because the ductus arteriosus provides lower-body blood flow, its spontaneous constriction results in profound clinical deterioration. The latter may be temporarily ameliorated by prostaglandin E_1 infusion.[96,264] The ventricular septal defect most often is subpulmonary, lying within the substance of the infundibular septum. Thus, muscle persists between the aortic and pulmonary valve leaflets, which, when displaced leftward, produces subaortic stenosis. Other complex intracardiac malformations, such as transposition of the great arteries, aortopulmonary window, and truncus arteriosus, are common.[296]

CLINICAL FEATURES. An association is frequent with DiGeorge syndrome, a constellation of cardiac, parathyroid, thymic, and facial anomalies attributed to disruption of the interaction of premigratory neural crest cells with endodermal pharyngeal pouch cells. In this syndrome thymic hypoplasia or aplasia is accompanied by immunological and hypocalcemia problems.[297,298] The major clinical problem is severe congestive heart failure as a consequence of volume overload of the left ventricle resulting from an associated intracardiac left-to-right shunt and of pressure overload imposed by systemic hypertension.

Management. The perioperative clinical condition of most patients can be improved by intensive medical management with mechanical ventilation, inotropic support, and prostaglandin infusion. Various forms of palliative operative techniques have fair to poor results. There has been increasing success with complete primary repair in infancy as the procedure of choice.[299–301] In some circumstances, a two-stage approach with initial arch repair and pulmonary artery banding is followed by later repair of the intracardiac lesion. Recurrent narrowing at the aortic suture line can be treated by balloon angioplasty or reoperation.

Congenital Valvular Aortic Stenosis

(See also p. 1035)

MORPHOLOGY. Congenital valvular aortic stenosis is a relatively common anomaly, estimated to occur in 3 to 6 per cent of patients with congenital cardiovascular defects. However, it must be appreciated that the true incidence of the malformation is probably grossly underestimated because the congenital bicuspid aortic valve may be undetected in early life and becomes stenotic and of clinical significance only in adult life, at a time when it may be indistinguishable from the acquired forms of aortic stenosis (Fig. 30–1, p. 964). Congenital valvular aortic stenosis occurs much more frequently in males than in females, with the gender ratio approximating 4:1. Associated cardiovascular anomalies have been noted in as many as 20 per cent of patients.[302] Patent ductus arteriosus and coarctation of the aorta occur most frequently with valvular aortic stenosis; all three of these lesions may coexist.

The basic malformation consists of thickening of valve tissue with varying degrees of commissural fusion. The valve most commonly is bicuspid with a single fused commissure and an eccentrically place orifice. Sometimes a third commissure, incomplete or rudimentary, is apparent. Less commonly, the valve has three fused cusps with a stenotic central orifice. In some patients the stenotic aortic valve is unicuspid and dome-shaped with no or one lateral attachment to the aorta at the level of the orifice. In infants and young children with severe aortic stenosis the aortic valve ring may be relatively underdeveloped. This lesion forms a continuum with the hypoplastic left heart syndrome and the aortic atresia and hypoplasia complexes. Secondary calcification of the valve is extremely rare in childhood, but the dynamics of blood flow associated with the congenitally deformed aortic valve ultimately lead to thickening of the cusps and calcification in adult life. When the obstruction is hemodynamically significant, concentric hypertrophy of the left ventricular wall and dilatation of the ascending aorta occur.

HEMODYNAMICS (see also Figs. 6–12, p. 194, and 32–27, p. 1036). The hemodynamic abnormalities produced by obstruction to left ventricular outflow are discussed on p. 1036. A peak systolic gradient exceeding 75 mm Hg in association with a normal cardiac output or an effective aortic orifice less than 0.5 cm^2/m^2 body surface area is considered to reflect critical or severe obstruction to left ventricular outflow.[302,303] The normal outflow orifice approximates 2.0 cm^2/m^2 body surface area; areas of 0.5 to 0.8 cm^2/m^2 signify moderate obstruction; when the area is larger than 0.8 cm^2/m^2, the obstruction is considered to be mild.

The resting cardiac output and stroke volume usually are within normal limits. During exercise, most children with critical stenosis show an elevation of the cardiac output and an associated elevation in the transvalvular pressure gradient.[304,305] When left ventricular failure occurs, the cardiac output decreases, and the left atrial, left ventricular end-diastolic, and pulmonary vascular pressures increase.

Studies of left ventricular performance in children with aortic stenosis often indicate that supernormal pump function exists, as indicated by increases in ejection fraction and circumferential fiber shortening.[306] Despite high left ventricular systolic pressures, left ventricular wall stress appears to be lower than normal throughout systole, presumably because increases in wall thickness provide overcompensation for the pressure overload. Undoubtedly, a spectrum exists, from well-compensated patients at one end, who have supernormal pump function and normal contractile function, to patients with heart failure at the opposite end, who have both impaired pump function and a reduced contractile state.

Whereas pressure overload hypertrophy may preserve systolic function, it may also result in abnormal left ventricular early diastolic filling.[307,308] Thus, clinical studies seeking to analyze the determinants of left ventricular filling by a separate assessment of dynamic (elastic recoil, ventricular relaxation rate, and atrial driving pressure) and static (chamber stiffness and left ventricular hypertrophy) determinants suggest that diastolic function most importantly varies according to the severity of left ventricular hypertrophy and systolic function. Studies in children suggest that hypertrophy is a more important factor than excessive wall stress and depressed ejection performance in accounting for abnormal diastolic filling.

The blood supply to the myocardium may be significantly compromised in infants and children with aortic stenosis, despite normal patency of the coronary arteries.[309] Coronary blood flow and arterial oxygen content are critical determinants of oxygen supply to the myocardium. Because intramyocardial compressive forces are greatest in the subendocardium, blood flow to that region of the left ventricle is entirely diastolic in the presence of elevated left ventricular systolic pressure. In patients with left ventricular outflow tract obstruction, coronary vasodilatation may give an inadequate response to an increase in the demands of the myocardium for oxygen at rest or with exercise. When subendocardial vessels are maximally dilated, the coronary artery driving pressure and the duration of diastole determine the magnitude of subendocardial flow. When the duration of systolic ejection lengthens across the stenotic orifice, diastole is shortened, especially at high heart rates. Moreover, a reduction occurs in coronary driving pressure if left ventricular end-diastolic pressure is high or if aortic diastolic pressure is low, e.g., with aortic regurgitation or heart failure. In patients with severe aortic stenosis the redistribution of flow away from the subendocardium and the ischemia that results in that portion of ventricular muscle may be estimated by relating the diastolic pressure–time index (DPTI) (i.e., the area between the aortic and left ventricular pressures in diastole) to the systolic pressure–time index (SPTI) (a measure of myocardial oxygen demands). Inadequate subendocardial oxygen delivery has been shown to exist when the ratio [DPTI × arterial oxygen content/SPTI] falls below 10.[309]

NEONATES AND INFANTS. Reports exist of cardiac dysfunction and even nonimmunological fetal hydrops fetalis in association with severe aortic stenosis.[310] The hydrops may be the result of in utero left ventricular myocardial infarction or profound left ventricular systolic and diastolic dysfunction. Balloon dilation using coronary balloon catheters has been attempted via transabdominal echo guided needle puncture of the fetal left ventricle. This approach is not established and it remains conjectural whether it will become a management option.[311]

Fortunately, isolated aortic valvular stenosis seldom causes symptoms in infancy.[312–314] This lesion, however, occasionally may be responsible for profound and intractable heart failure. Despite normal coronary arterial anatomy, infarction of left ventricular papillary muscles may occur, resulting in an acquired form of mitral valvular regurgitation that intensifies the heart failure state. In addition, endocardial fibroelastosis may result from limited subendocardial oxygen delivery, and myocardial degeneration may be significant.[314] The symptomatic infant with isolated valvular aortic stenosis is irritable, pale, and hypotensive and presents with tachycardia, cardiomegaly, and pulmonary congestion manifested by dyspnea, tachypnea, subcostal retractions, and diffuse rales. Cyanosis may be observed secondary to pulmonary venous desaturation. The systolic murmur in infants often is atypical; it is best heard at the apex or along the lower left sternal border and may be confused with that caused by a ventricular septal defect. In infants with heart failure the murmur occasionally may be absent or extremely soft, becoming louder when myocardial contractility is improved with digitalis and other medical measures. The response to medical management of the infant with heart failure is frequently poor.

The *electrocardiographic findings* may not be characteristic; left ventricular hypertrophy and/or strain as well as right atrial enlargement and right ventricular hypertrophy may be detected shortly after birth.[312] The latter signs of right heart involvement result from both pulmonary hypertension secondary to elevated left ventricular diastolic and left atrial pressures and from volume loading of the right ventricle caused by left-to-right shunting across the foramen ovale. Survival past the early neonatal period does not preclude subsequent difficulties, and clinical deterioration may recur with the onset of physiological anemia.

MANAGEMENT. Congenital aortic stenosis must be considered a medical emergency in the seriously ill newborn, and echocardiography, and sometimes cardiac catheterization and angiocardiography, may be indicated in the first 24 hours of life. Two-dimensional echocardiographic studies show a severe immobility of the aortic valve, with little or no systolic opening, poststenotic dilation of the aorta, left ventricular hypertrophy, right ventricular enlargement, and a severely disturbed Doppler-determined pattern of ascending aortic flow velocity. The echo-Doppler examination must also identify associated intracardiac and extracardiac anomalies, one of the most important of which is severe aortic arch obstruction.

In many centers, expeditious balloon aortic valvuloplasty follows the echo-Doppler examination in infants who are unstable and markedly symptomatic.[315–316b] A number of approaches have been reported for performing this procedure, including the use of a carotid artery cutdown, which thus far does not appear to result in any abnormalities of the carotid pulse or any neurological sequelae.[317] A transumbilical technique of balloon valvuloplasty can be performed quickly, safely, and effectively with preservation of the femoral artery.[314] Because of a high risk of iliofemoral artery complications in infants with the transfemoral route to valvuloplasty, when this route is employed it is advisable to use double-balloon techniques to allow insertion of small valvuloplasty catheters. The complications of balloon valvuloplasty are related to the small size and young age of the patient. Accordingly, if arterial access is a problem, and in infants less than 1 month of age, surgical valvotomy remains a satisfactory option. Open repair under direct vision is the preferred type of operation.

Hemodynamic findings in neonates and infants frequently include left-to-right shunting at the atrial level, an elevated left atrial and left ventricular end-diastolic pressure, and a small pressure drop across the aortic valve as a result of markedly reduced cardiac output. Right-to-left shunting across a patent ductus arteriosus is encountered occasionally. The lesion may be distinguished from the hypoplastic left heart syndrome echocardiographically and angiographically by the presence of normal or enlarged left ventricular cavity and normal or dilated ascending aorta. Establishment of the diagnosis and prompt catheter valvuloplasty or surgical valvotomy are justified because prolonged periods of stabilization are uncommon with medical therapy. Poor myocardial performance resulting from endocardial fibroelastosis, subendocardial ischemia, reduced left ventricular compliance, and inadequate relief of obstruction with or without aortic insufficiency are some of the factors accounting for high mortality and morbidity following catheter-directed treatment or operation.

At the extreme end of the spectrum of critical valvar aortic stenosis in the newborn are patients with multiple small left-sided structures in whom the adverse effects of small inflow, outflow, and/or cavity size of the left ventricle appear to be cumulative.[318–320] It is in this group that traditional treatment by aortic valvuloplasty or valvotomy, which is a two-sided ventricle repair, may be less effective than a multistaged Norwood approach.[321] The latter consists of an initial single-ventricle repair in which the main pulmonary artery is anastomosed to the aorta with creation of a systemic-to-pulmonary arterial shunt, followed later by a Fontan-type operation that creates an atriopulmonary connection, with or without a prior superior cava–pulmonary connection. The single-ventricle repair results in the functional sacrifice of the left ventricle and the right ventricle supporting the systemic circulation without a pulmonary ventricle.

CHILDREN. Congenital aortic stenosis may be responsible for severe obstruction to left ventricular outflow in the absence of clinical symptoms of diminished cardiac reserve that are so frequent in other forms of congenital heart disease.[322] Most children with congenital aortic stenosis grow and develop normally and are asymptomatic. Attention usually is called to these children when a murmur is detected on routine examination. When symptoms occur, those noted most commonly are fatigability, exertional dyspnea, angina pectoris, and syncope. Less often described are abdominal pain, profuse sweating, and epistaxis. The symptomatic child usually has critical stenosis. There is a distinct threat of sudden death in patients with severe obstruction[303] (p. 885). Although the precise cause is poorly understood, ventricular arrhythmias, perhaps initiated by acute myocardial ischemia, are probably the most common inciting event. It has been speculated that an abrupt rise in intracavity left ventricular systolic pressure elicits a reflex hypotensive syncope that promotes acute ischemia and ventricular fibrillation.[323] Bacterial endocarditis occurs in about 4 per cent of patients with congenital valvular aortic stenosis.[324]

DIAGNOSIS. Physical Findings. When the magnitude of obstruction is significant, a left ventricular lift usually is palpable, and a precordial systolic thrill often is palpated over the base of the heart with transmission to the jugular notch and along the carotid arteries; presystolic expansion often is palpable. The obstruction usually is mild if neither a left ventricular lift nor a thrill is present.

Opening of the aortic valve produces a systolic aortic ejection sound that typically is present at the cardiac apex when the valve is mobile, particularly in patients with mild to moderate stenosis. A delay in closure of the stenotic aortic valve leads to a single or a closely split second heart sound, and paradoxical splitting may be present. A fourth heart sound normally is associated with severe obstruction. A loud, harsh, rhomboid-shaped systolic murmur starts after completion of left ventricular isometric contraction and is best heard at the base of the heart. The murmur, like the thrill, radiates to the suprasternal notch and carotid vessel as well as to the apex. An early diastolic blowing murmur of aortic regurgitation is present in some patients, but unless the valve leaflets have been eroded by bacterial endocarditis, the regurgitation usually is not hemodynamically significant; uncommonly, in patients with a congenitally bicuspid valve, aortic regurgitation may be severe and may predominate.

Electrocardiography. There is a tendency for electrocardiographic signs of left ventricular hypertrophy to vary with the severity of obstruction, although a normal or near-normal electrocardiogram does not exclude severe aortic stenosis, and excessive left ventricular voltages may be observed in children with mild obstruction.[322] The lack of a good correlation between the ECG and the transvalvular pressure gradient emphasizes the potential hazard of relying on the ECG in patient management. The most reliable index of the severity of obstruction is the presence of a left ventricular "strain pattern," consisting of left ventricular hypertrophy combined with ST-segment depressions and T-wave inversion in the left precordial leads (Fig. 29–32).

Roentgenography. Overall heart size is normal or the degree of enlargement is slight in most children with congenital valvular aortic stenosis. Concentric left ventricular hypertrophy accompanies moderate or severe obstruction and is manifested by rounding of the cardiac apex in the frontal projection and posterior displacement in the lateral view.

Echocardiography. Two-dimensional and Doppler echocardiography are the current methods of choice for defining the anatomy and the hemodynamic severity of valvular aortic stenosis.[325–328] Real-time cross-sectional echocardiography reveals impaired mobility of cusp tissue, an alteration in the phasic movement of the aortic valve with reduced lateral and increased superior excursions of valve echoes, and an increase in the internal aortic root dimension beyond the level of the valve annulus.[302] Imaging of the valve must be performed many times in order to display the valve through the long axis of the left ventricular outflow tract and then through a plane parallel to the valve annulus. The long-axis view of the left ventricular outflow tract allows evaluation of the valve mobility and cusp separation; it is the best view for demonstrating doming of the aortic valve. The parasternal short-axis view bisects the face of the valve, demonstrating the anatomy of the commissures (Fig. 29–33).

The echocardiogram also reveals associated left ventricular hypertrophy and the presence of endocardial fibroelastosis (seen as bright endocardial echoes). Further, the measurement of mitral valve diameter, left ventricular end-diastolic dimension, and left ventricular cross-sectional area serve to distinguish those infants with critical aortic stenosis from those with a hypoplastic left ventricle.[326] Among these calculations suggesting the latter are an end-

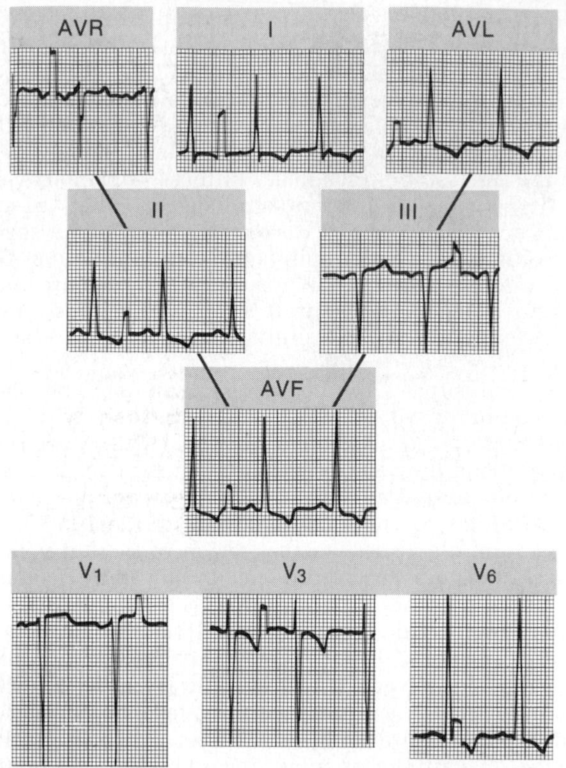

FIGURE 29–32. Electrocardiogram in congenital aortic stenosis. This tracing shows left ventricular hypertrophy and the typical left ventricular "strain" pattern (V_6, *arrow*). (Courtesy of Delores A. Danilowicz, M.D.)

diastolic volume less than 20 ml/m^2, an inflow dimension of 25 mm, a narrow ventricular aortic junction less than 5 mm, or a small mitral orifice less than 9 mm. Pulse-Doppler echocardiography allows inspection of the pattern of flow velocity within the circulation.[325,327] This technique detects the altered and disturbed turbulence of flow in patients with aortic stenosis. A highly accurate noninvasive approach to quantifying the severity of obstruction combines continuous-wave Doppler flow analysis with the cross-sectional echocardiographic determination of the area of the orifice.[329] A simplified Bernoulli equation uses the measurement of the maximum velocity of the aortic jet and time-averaged pressure drop obtained from planimetry of the maximal velocity spectral reading. A simpler estimate of the transvalvular gradient (in mm Hg) may be calculated as four times the square of the peak Doppler velocity (m/sec).

The Doppler method records a peak instantaneous pressure difference, which may differ importantly from the gradient recorded by a cardiac catheter, which is a peak-to-peak pressure difference.[330] Doppler mean gradient is more accurate than the instantaneous gradient when compared with the pressures found at cardiac catheterization. Management decisions often depend on the estimation of the severity of obstruction, and all pressure gradient estimations depend on flow velocity across the valve, which may be confounded by low cardiac output or concomitant valvar regurgitation. Thus, an important argument can be made that the determination of the stenotic valve systolic area is often more important than calculation of a systolic gradient.[327–329]

The most widely accepted technique for correcting the gradient for flow is to use the continuity equation, which measures the flow velocity ratio across the aortic valve and, therefore, corrects for high and low flow rates. The continuity equation presumes that for flow in a series, the product of mean velocity and cross-sectional area is constant at all points in the flow circuit. In patients with aortic stenosis, the area of the left ventricular outflow tract is deter-

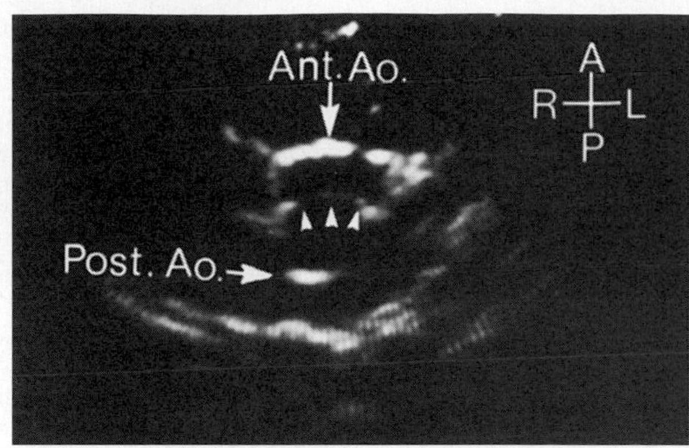

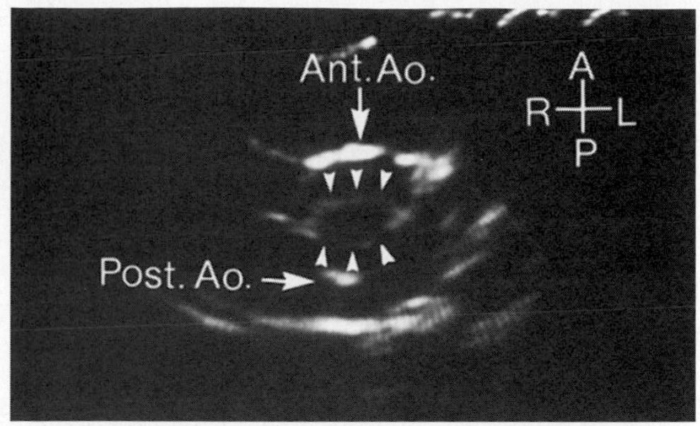

FIGURE 29–33. **Short-axis view at the base of the heart of a bicuspid aortic valve. In the left panel the valve is imaged as a single diastolic echo (arrows) in the aortic root. In systole *(right panel)*, the valve opens (arrows) with a typical fish-mouth appearance. Ant.Ao. = anterior aorta, Post.Ao. = posterior aorta. (From DiSessa, T. G., and Friedman, W. F.: Cardiovascular Clinics. Fowler, N. [ed.], Philadelphia, F. A. Davis Co., 1983.)**

mined by two-dimensional echocardiography, the flow velocity of the outflow tract by pulse-Doppler, and the flow velocity immediately above the valve by continuous wave Doppler, all of which, taken together, allow the determination of the valve area by the continuity equation: Aortic valve area (area) LVOT × (V)LVOT/(V)AV (obtained by converting the diameter to area and assuming that it is circular); (V)LVOT = peak outflow tract velocity, and (V)AV = peak velocity across the aortic valve.

Transesophageal two-dimensional echocardiographic determination of aortic valve area has been applied in adults with aortic stenosis.[331,332] The approach offers considerably better resolution of cardiac anatomy than does conventional transthoracic two-dimensional echocardiography and may also prove to be more accurate in estimating pressure gradients and aortic valve areas. The approach has not yet been reported in children in sufficient detail to make specific recommendations.

Diagnostic Cardiac Catheterization. Cardiac catheterization is now rarely used to establish the site and severity of obstruction to left ventricular outflow because the malformation is readily diagnosed and the evaluation of the intensity of stenosis is accurate by echo-Doppler examination.[333] Instead, catheterization is undertaken when therapeutic interventional transcatheter balloon aortic valvuloplasty is indicated.

During the catheterization procedure, cardiac output is measured by the indicator-dilution, thermodilution, or Fick technique. Retrograde left heart catheterization allows withdrawal pressure recordings across the site of stenosis, and left ventricular angiocardiography can be carried out, permitting an evaluation of the size of the left ventricular cavity, the thickness of the wall, the competency of the mitral valve, the patency of the coronary arteries, and the diameter of the aortic root and ascending aorta. If aortic insufficiency is thought to be present, cineaortography is performed with injection of contrast material into the aortic root. The severity of aortic insufficiency can be assessed qualitatively by cineaortography and quantitatively by ventriculography with calculation of regurgitant volume by subtraction of net forward flow (calculated by the Fick method) from angiographically determined total forward flow.[336] The typical angiocardiographic features of valvar stenosis are thickening of the aortic cusps, poststenotic dilation of the ascending aorta, and, occasionally, a jet of contrast material entering the ascending aorta through a central or eccentric narrowed valve orifice (Fig. 29–34). The leaflets of the bicuspid valve are domed in systole, and

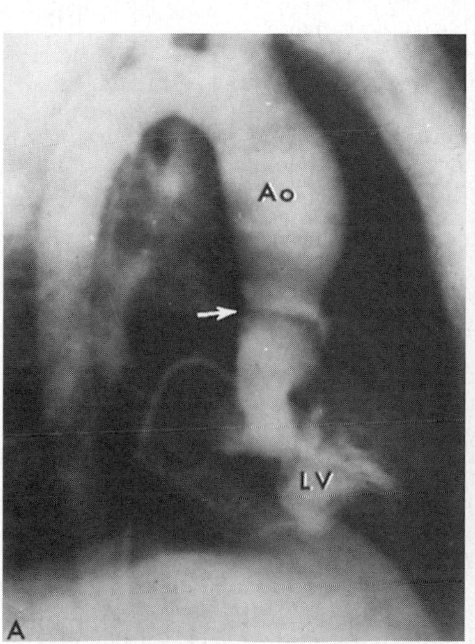

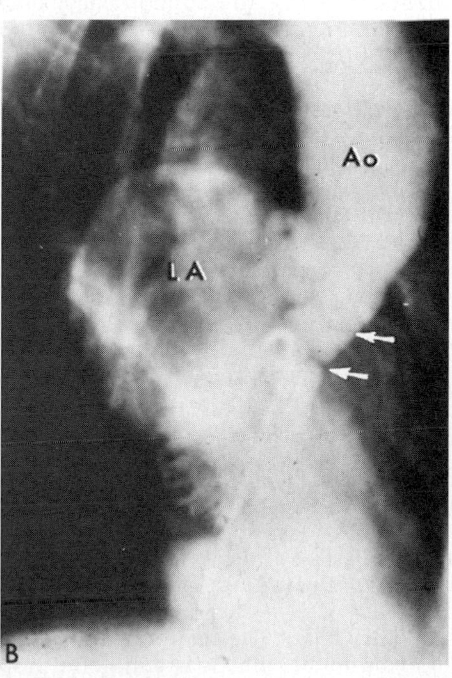

FIGURE 29–34. ***A,*** **Left ventricular angiocardiogram obtained by the transseptal method in a patient with congenital valvular aortic stenosis. Ao = poststenotic dilatation of the aorta; LV = left ventricle. Arrow denotes the thickened valve cusp.** ***B,*** **Selective angiocardiogram in a patient with discrete subvalvular stenosis (bottom arrow). Associated mitral regurgitation is evident from the reflux of contrast into an enlarged left atrium (LA). The aortic valve (top arrow) is normal, and the right coronary artery is visualized. (From Friedman, W. F., Kirkpatrick, S. E.: Congenital aortic stenosis.** ***In*** **Moss, A. J., Adams, F. H., and Emmanouilides, G. C. [eds.]: Heart Disease in Infants, Children and Adolescents. 2nd ed. Baltimore, © Williams and Wilkins, 1977.)**

a central jet corresponds to the orifice of the stenotic valve. In contrast, the stenotic orifice of the unicommissural valve can be visualized by the systolic jet in contact with the posterior wall of the aorta, with leaflet tissue and valve motion seen only anteriorly.[302]

Balloon Valvuloplasty. Balloon dilatation may be indicated in any child with a clinical diagnosis of aortic stenosis in whom the clinical examination, roentgenogram, resting or exercise ECG, or Doppler echocardiogram suggests the possibility of severe obstruction.[334,335] Even in the absence of such findings, balloon valvuloplasty may be performed if symptoms that might be related to AS exist, such as dizziness, fainting, or angina.

This author prefers to catheterize the left side of the heart via a retrograde approach by femoral percutaneous puncture. The goals of the study are to analyze the severity of obstruction and assess the function of the left ventricle. In most centers, balloon valvuloplasty is recommended if the severity of the AS would otherwise require surgical treatment, that is, a peak systolic pressure gradient exceeding 70 mm Hg measured in the basal state or a calculated effective orifice less than 0.5 cm^2/m^2 of body surface area. In the presence of symptoms or left ventricular strain pattern on the ECG or an abnormal exercise ECG, there is less rigid regard to the hemodynamic assessment of the severity of stenosis. Further, some centers go forward with balloon valvuloplasty with peak systolic gradients greater than or equal to 50 mm Hg. There is general agreement that there be no significant aortic regurgitation (less than grade 2 of 4) and that other associated cardiac anomalies be absent, except aortic coarctation.

Balloon dilatation of the aortic valve began in the mid-1980s; truly long-term follow-up studies are not yet available. Early studies and the experience of the author suggest that the diameter of the balloon should not exceed that of the aortic valve ring. Most centers prefer a balloon with a diameter 80 to 100 per cent that of, or at least 1 mm smaller than, the aortic annulus. The expected hemodynamic result is a reduction in the catheterization-measured peak-to-peak ejection gradient of about 60 to 70 per cent. The appearance of aortic regurgitation or its progression is the major complication of valvuloplasty, although the aortic regurgitation is mild in the great majority of patients.[316b,334] Significant aortic regurgitation appears to accompany the development of aortic valve prolapse, which is likely due to tearing of the valve cusp or its raphe or partial detachment of the valve from the valve ring, all of which undermine the support mechanism of the valve.[335] In those patients whose balloon valvuloplasty has resulted in very significant aortic regurgitation, valve surgery may be required to either replace the valve or repair a tear in the valve. Other complications from balloon aortic valvuloplasty include bleeding, arrhythmias, cerebral vascular accidents, iliofemoral arterial complications, injury to the mitral valve, and, rarely beyond infancy, death.[334]

Natural History. Congenital aortic stenosis frequently is a progressive disorder, even early in life, in a significant fraction of patients presenting initially with mild obstruction.[337–340] Thus, clinical deterioration may be anticipated because of an intensification in the severity of stenosis rather than the development of significant aortic regurgitation. Progression of obstruction usually is the result of the increase in cardiac output that occurs concurrent with increased body growth. Less often, a decrease in the area of the orifice is an added factor in the intensification of obstruction. The onset of symptoms or changes in the phonocardiogram or graphic pulse tracings, chest roentgenograms, electrocardiograms, or vectorcardiograms cannot be depended on to indicate progressive obstruction in the individual patient; Doppler echocardiography is most reliable.

MANAGEMENT. The malformed aortic valve is a potential site of bacterial infection; antibiotic prophylaxis is recommended for all patients, regardless of the severity of obstruction. Strict avoidance of strenuous physical activity is advised if severe aortic stenosis is present. Participation in competitive sports also should probably be restricted in patients with milder degrees of obstruction. Digitalis should be administered to patients who have symptoms of diminished cardiac reserve and also should be considered in patients with left ventricular hypertrophy, even if they are not in heart failure.

Surgery. Percutaneous balloon aortic valvuloplasty is a useful palliation to delay open valvulotomy or valve replacement. For those patients in whom balloon valvuloplasty is unsuccessful, operation is carried out under direct vision after institution of cardiopulmonary bypass, and the fused commissures are opened. When this is done precisely and judiciously, the commissural incision enlarges the valve orifice and does not result in significant aortic insufficiency.[341] When operation is performed in childhood, a mortality rate of less than 2 per cent can be expected.[341,342] Among the factors influencing the indications, techniques, and results of operation are the patient's age, the nature of the valvar deformity, and the experience of the surgical team.

Long-term follow-up studies indicate that aortic valvotomy is a safe and effective means of palliative treatment with excellent relief of symptoms.[341–343] Occasionally, aortic insufficiency may be progressive and require valve replacement. Moreover, following commissurotomy, the valve leaflets remain somewhat deformed; and it is likely that further degenerative changes, including calcification, will lead to significant stenosis in later years.[302] Thus, prosthetic valve replacement is required in approximately 35 per cent of patients within 15 to 20 years of the original operation.[342,343] Because the valve is not rendered normal, antibiotic prophylaxis is indicated in the postoperative patient, even if the systolic pressure gradient has been abolished.[342] For those patients eventually requiring aortic valve replacement, the surgical options include replacement with a prosthetic aortic valve, an aortic homograft, or a pulmonary autograft in the aortic position.[344–347a] Evidence is beginning to accumulate that the pulmonary autograft may ultimately be preferable to the aortic homograft for aortic reconstruction. Neither homografts nor autografts require anticoagulation. There is a finite incidence of valve degeneration of approximately 2 per cent per patient per year with the former, whereas primary tissue failure has not been observed among pulmonary autografts.

Discrete Subaortic Stenosis

This malformation accounts for 8 to 10 per cent of all cases of congenital aortic stenosis and occurs twice as frequently in males as in females. The lesion consists of a membranous diaphragm or fibrous ring encircling the left ventricular outflow tract or a long fibromuscular narrowing just beneath the base of the aortic valve. Subaortic stenosis is rarely diagnosed in infancy, when it is usually the result of a malalignment ventricular septal defect with deviation posteriorly of the outlet septum into the left ventricular outflow tract, often associated with coarctation of the aorta or interruption of the aortic arch.

Distinction of subvalvular from valvular aortic stenosis is extremely difficult by means of clinical findings alone.[302] Rarely, a systolic ejection sound is heard, and the diastolic murmur of aortic regurgitation is more common than it is in valvular aortic stenosis. Dilatation of the ascending aorta is common, but valvular calcification is not observed.

Echocardiography is useful in the differentiation between valvular and subvalvular stenosis (Figs. 3–71, p. 80, and 3–72, p. 81).[348,349] The criterion for diagnosis of the latter is the demonstration of a localized subvalvar discrete ridge or long segment narrowing in the left ventricular outflow tract. Further, because of the possibility of recurrence of subvalvular aortic stenosis, careful postoperative follow-up echocardiography is required. Two-dimensional echocardiographic studies from the apical two-chamber and left parasternal and subxiphoid long-axis views demonstrate persistent, prominent echoes in the subaortic left ventricle in both systole and diastole (Fig. 29–35). Doppler sampling proximal to the aortic valve shows increased flow velocity.[348] Most important, echocardiography also can identify hypertrophic subaortic stenosis when it coexists with fixed subaortic stenosis and can differentiate between the two forms of obstruction.

Definitive distinction between valvular and subvalvular obstruction is also provided by transesophageal Doppler echocardiography[350] and by recording pressure tracings as a catheter is withdrawn across the outflow tract and valve, or by localizing the site of obstruction with selective left ventricular angiocardiography (Fig. 29–34).

Mild degrees of aortic valvular regurgitation commonly are observed in patients with discrete subaortic stenosis and appear to be caused by thickening of the valve and impaired mobility of the cusps secondary to the trauma created by the high-velocity jet passing through the subaortic diaphragm. Further deformation of these abnormal valve cusps by the vegetations of bacterial endocarditis often results in severe aortic regurgitation.

MANAGEMENT. Because of the likelihood of both progressive obstruction and aortic regurgitation, the presence of even mild or moderate subaortic stenosis warrants consideration of elective operation.[351,352] Reports exist of transluminal balloon dilation for discrete subaortic stenosis. This palliative approach may be an acceptable alternative in selected patients,[353] but the relief of obstruction is not likely to be as complete or as long as in those patients undergoing surgical resection. It is clear that further study is required to delineate which forms of subaortic stenosis are most favorable for balloon dilation in comparing the long-term results of this approach with those of surgical treatment.

The risks of operation in patients with discrete subaortic stenosis and valvular aortic stenosis are essentially the same. The surgical treatment of discrete subaortic stenosis has evolved from simply excising the membrane or fibrous ridge to adding a generous ventricular myotomy and myectomy to the membranectomy.[354] Operation may be expected to improve the hemodynamic state substantially; it frequently is totally curative.[361]

Recent evidence indicates that muscle resection combined with membrane excision lowers the risk of reoperation for recurrent subaortic stenosis.[355] A tendency appears to exist for discrete membranous subaortic stenosis to recur after operation, although this author and others consider these recurrences to be often related, at least in part, to incomplete removal of the lesion at initial operation. Intraoperative echocardiography has been used as an adjunct to operation to enable immediate assessment of the adequacy of relieving obstruction.[356] Studies have suggested that abnormal flow patterns may predispose to pathological proliferation of subvalvar aortic tissue, which reinforces the requirement that careful echocardiographic and surgical exploration of the outflow tract, even well below the subvalvar stenosis, be undertaken to detect and resect structures that cause turbulence.[357]

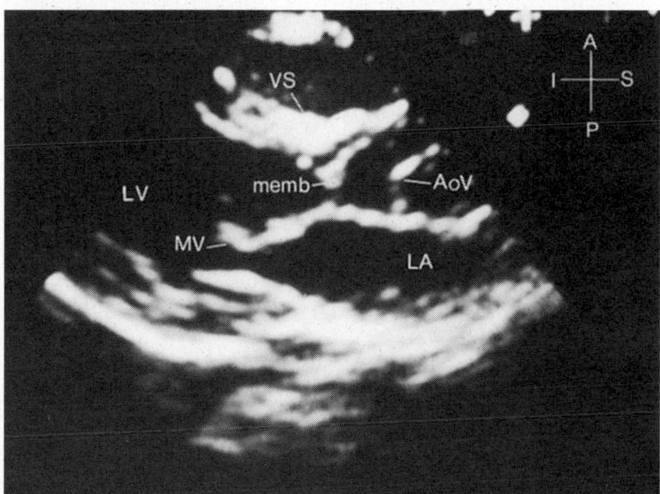

FIGURE 29–35. Long-axis view of discrete membranous subaortic stenosis. A discrete membrane (memb) is imaged in the left ventricular (LV) outflow tract beneath and parallel to the aortic valve (AoV), extending from the ventricular septum (VS) to the anterior leaflet of the mitral valve (MV). LA = left atrium.

UNCOMMON FORMS OF SUBAORTIC STENOSIS

Combined Valvular and Subvalvular Stenosis

In some patients, valvular and subvalvular aortic stenosis coexist with hypoplasia of the aortic valve ring and thickened valve leaflets, producing a tunnel-like narrowing of the left ventricular outflow tract. Additional findings often include a small ascending aorta. The subvalvular fibrous process usually extends onto the aortic valve cusps and almost always makes contact with the ventricular aspect of the anterior mitral leaflet at its base. The presence of "tunnel stenosis" may be suspected echocardiographically or angiographically from the appearance of the outflow tract and the aortic root. Operative treatment often is complicated by the need for an aortoventriculoplasty, consisting of prosthetic or homograft replacement of the aortic valve as well as enlarging the aortic annulus, proximal aorta, and left ventricular outlet tract (the Konno-Rastan operation). The *modified* Konno-Rastan operation preserves the native aortic valve if the annulus is normal or near normal. Alternatively, a conal enlargement technique may be used.[358–360]

Various anatomical lesions other than a discrete membrane or ridge may produce subaortic stenosis.[362–364] Among these are abnormal adherence of the anterior leaflet of the mitral valve to the left septal surface, and the presence in the left ventricular outflow tract of accessory endocardial cushion tissue. In some patients with atrioventricular canal, the part of the ventricular septum that contributes to the wall of the left ventricular outflow tract is deficient, and the ventricular aspect of the anterior leaflet of the common atrioventricular valve is adherent to the posterior edge of the deficient septum, resulting in a narrow left ventricular outflow tract. Malalignment of the conoventricular septum, resulting in an inferior ventricular septal defect, produces a leftward superior deviation and insertion of the conal septum, obstructing left ventricular outflow.[364] In patients with a single ventricle and an outflow chamber, the bulboventricular foramen serves as a potential site of aortic outflow obstruction. Additionally, rarer causes of subaortic stenosis include redundant dysplastic left atrioventricular valve tissue in patients with congenitally corrected transposition of the great arteries and anomalous muscle bundles of the left ventricular outflow tract.

MUSCULAR SUBAORTIC STENOSIS. A muscular type of subaortic stenosis may result from a convergence of all the mitral chordae into one or two fused papillary muscles; a "parachute" deformity of the mitral valve is produced that often is seen in association with supravalvular stenosis of the left atrium and coarctation of the aorta. In some of these patients, discrete membranous subvalvular aortic obstruction also has been noted.

In patients with ventricular septal defect, muscular subaortic stenosis has been shown to develop after surgical banding of the pulmonary artery, possibly as a result of hypertrophy of the conal septum or crista supraventricularis encroaching on the left ventricular outflow tract above the septal defect.

Subaortic muscular hypertrophy secondary to diffuse involvement of the myocardium by glycogen storage disease (Pompe's disease) is an extremely rare cause of obstruction to left ventricular outflow. A positive family history, symptoms of muscle weakness, heart failure in infancy, and the characteristic electrocardiographic findings of a short PR interval, high-voltage QRS and T waves, and left ventricular hypertrophy warrant skeletal muscle biopsy or fibroblast culture, permitting an antemortem diagnosis.

The last, relatively uncommon form of subaortic stenosis to be mentioned occurs infrequently in patients with congenitally corrected transposition of the great arteries in whom an anomalous muscle bundle in the subaortic area of the arterial ventricle obstructs outflow.

Supravalvular Aortic Stenosis

Supravalvular aortic stenosis is a congenital narrowing of the ascending aorta that may be localized or diffuse, originating at the superior margin of the sinuses of Valsalva just above the levels of the coronary arteries.

The clinical picture of supravalvular obstruction usually differs in major respects from that observed in the other forms of aortic stenosis. Chief among these differences is the association of supravalvular aortic stenosis with idiopathic infantile hypercalcemia, a disease that occurs in the first years of life and may be related to deranged vitamin D metabolism.[365–368]

It is helpful to classify patients according to their clinical presentation into nonfamilial, sporadic cases with normal facies and intelligence; autosomal dominant familial cases with normal facies and intelligence; and the Williams syndrome with abnormal facial appearance and mental retardation (Fig. 29–36). In contrast to the other forms of aortic stenosis, there appears to be no gender predilection in any of these three categories.

WILLIAMS SYNDROME. The designations supravalvular aortic stenosis syndrome or Williams syndrome or Williams-Beuren syndrome[369,370] have been applied to the distinctive picture produced by coexistence of the cardiac and multiple-system disorder. Beyond infancy in these patients, a challenge with vitamin D or calcium loading tests unmask abnormalities in the regulation of circulating 25-hydroxyvitamin D.[371,372] Unanimity of opinion does not exist of the exact relation between Williams syndrome and calcium metabolism. Some have suggested that the abnormalities of calcium metabolism might be explained by a defect in synthesis or release of calcitonin, whereas others have concluded recently that calcitonin deficiency is not present in patients with Williams syndrome.[373]

Infants with Williams syndrome often exhibit feeding difficulties, failure to thrive, and gastrointestinal problems in the form of vomiting, constipation, and colic. The entire spectrum of clinical manifestations includes auditory hyperacusis, inguinal hernia, a hoarse voice, and a typical personality that is outgoing and engaging. Other manifestations of this syndrome include mental retardation, "elfin facies" (Fig. 29–33), narrowing of peripheral systemic and pulmonary arteries, strabismus, and abnormalities of dental development consisting of microdontia, enamel hypoplasia, and malocclusion.

Many medical conditions can complicate the course of Williams syndrome,[372] including systemic hypertension, gastrointestinal problems, and urinary tract abnormalities. Particularly in the older child or adult, progressive joint limitation and hypertonia may become a problem. Adult patients are usually handicapped by their developmental disabilities.

Hypervitaminosis D in the pregnant rabbit has resulted in craniofacial and dental abnormalities and malformations resembling supravalvular aortic stenosis in the offspring.[365–367] Skin fibroblast cultures from patients with Williams syndrome show enhanced metachromasia upon addition of vitamin D and calcium.[371] In humans, chromosome studies have revealed normal karyotypes, with the exception of one patient who demonstrated a 46/47 mosaic pattern with an extra chromosome resembling the 19 to 20 group.

Until recently, Williams syndrome was considered to be nonfamilial. Interestingly, three families have been identified in which parent-to-child transmission of Williams syndrome has occurred. These are not families with autosomal dominant supravalvular aortic stenosis whose members are normal in appearance and intelligence. All of these families show a parent and child to be affected with Williams syndrome, including one instance of male-to-male transmission. This supports autosomal dominant inheritance as the likely pattern, with most cases of Williams syndrome probably occurring as the result of a new mutation.

FAMILIAL AUTOSOMAL DOMINANT PRESENTATION. Most commonly, supravalvular aortic stenosis is a feature of the distinctive Williams syndrome described above.[374] However, the aortic anomaly and peripheral pulmonary arterial stenosis are also seen in familial and sporadic forms *unassociated* with the other features of the syndrome.[375] Thus, affected patients have normal intelligence and are normal in facial appearance. Genetic studies suggest that when the anomaly is familial, it is transmitted as autosomal dominant with variable expression. Some family members may have peripheral pulmonary stenosis either as an isolated lesion or in combination with the supravalvular aortic anomaly.

Recently, linkage analyses in two unrelated families with autosomal dominant supravalvular aortic stenosis were performed. Linkage was identified between the supravalvular aortic stenosis phenotype and polymorphic markers on the long arm of chromosome 7.[376] These findings indicate that a gene for supravalvular aortic stenosis may be located in the same chromosomal subunit as elastin. Further, a family has been identified with autosomal dominant supravalvular aortic stenosis in which a balanced translocation was identified, which disrupts the elastin gene and cosegregates with the disease in this family, supporting the hypothesis that mutations in the elastin gene may cause supravalvular aortic stenosis.[377] Hemizygosity at the elastin locus is likely responsible for the vascular pathology in Williams syndrome, although it is unlikely that elastin deletions account for all features of the syndrome. Because the deletions responsible for Williams syndrome extend well beyond the elastin locus, it is probable that the syndrome is a contiguous gene disorder.[377a]

MORPHOLOGY. Three anatomical types of supravalvular aortic stenosis are recognized, although some patients may have findings of more than one type. Most common is the hourglass type, in which marked thickening and disorganization of the aortic media produce a constricting annular ridge at the superior margin of the sinuses of Valsalva. The membranous type is the result of fibrous or fibromuscular semicircular diaphragm with a small central opening stretched across the lumen of the aorta. Uniform hypoplasia of the ascending aorta characterizes the hypoplastic type.[378]

Because the coronary arteries arise proximal to the site of outflow obstruction in supravalvular aortic stenosis, they are subjected to the elevated pressure that exists within the left ventricle. These vessels often are dilated and tortuous, and premature coronary arteriosclerosis has been observed. Moreover, if the free edges of some or all of the aortic cusps adhere to the site of supravalvular stenosis, coronary artery inflow may be reduced. The formation of thoracic aortic aneurysms has been described in several patients.

CLINICAL FEATURES. Patients with Williams syndrome are mentally retarded and resemble one another in their facial features. The typical appearance is similar to that of the elfin facies observed in the severe form of idiopathic infantile hypercalcemia and is characterized by a high prominent forehead, stellate or lacy iris patterns, epicanthal folds, underdeveloped bridge of the nose and mandible, overhanging upper lip, strabismus, and anomalies of dentition (Fig. 29–36). Recognition of this distinctive appearance, even in infancy, should alert the physician to the

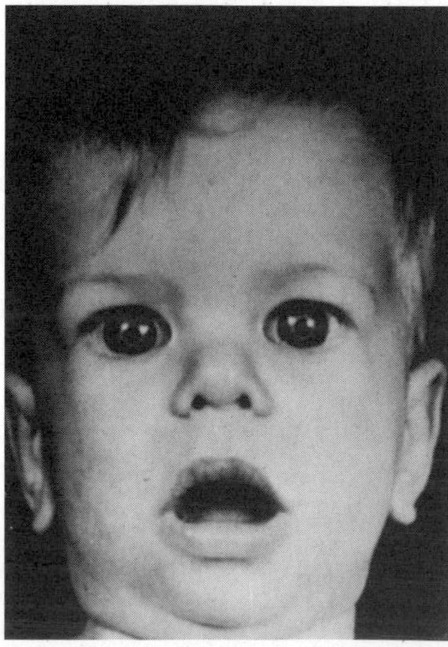
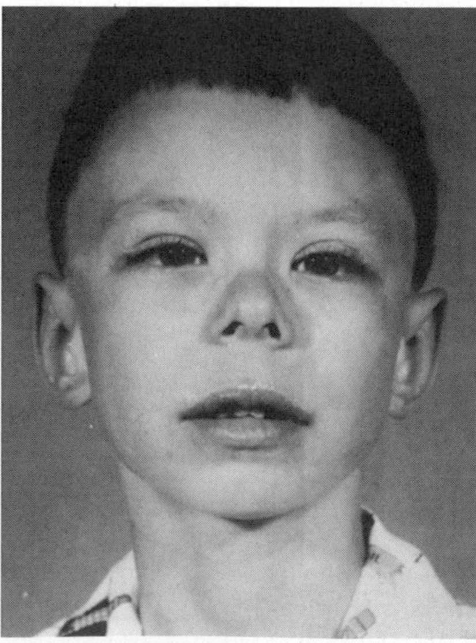
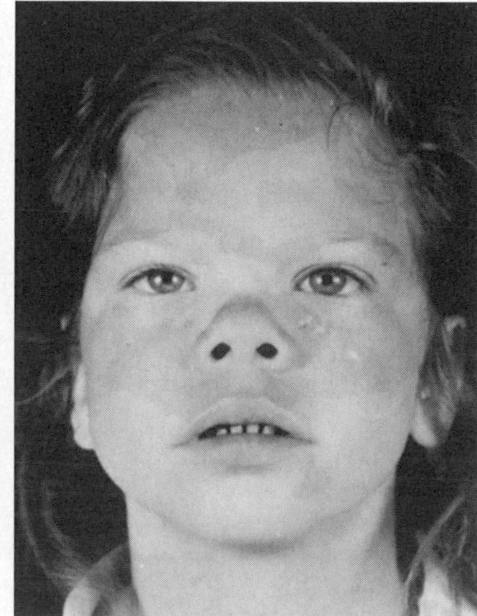

FIGURE 29–36. Typical elfin facies in three patients with supravalvular aortic stenosis. (Friedman, W. F., Kirkpatrick, S. E.: Congenital aortic stenosis. *In* Moss, A. J., Adams, F. H., and Emmanouilides, G. C. [eds.]: Heart Disease in Infants, Children and Adolescents. 2nd ed. Baltimore, © Williams and Wilkins, 1977.)

possibility of underlying multisystem disease. In addition, a positive family history in a patient with a normal appearance and clinical signs suggesting left ventricular outflow obstruction should lead to the suspicion of either supravalvular aortic stenosis or hypertrophic obstructive cardiomyopathy.[291]

Patients with supravalvular aortic obstruction appear to be subject to the same risks of unexpected sudden death [in some of whom myocardial infarction has been found at autopsy[379]] and endocarditis as those with valvular aortic stenosis. Studies of the natural history of the principal vascular lesions in these patients[380,381]—supravalvular aortic stenosis and peripheral pulmonary artery stenosis—indicate that the aortic lesion is usually progressive, with an increase in the intensity of obstruction related often to poor growth of the ascending aorta. In contrast, the patients with pulmonary branch stenosis, whether or not associated with the aortic lesion, tend to show no change or a reduction in right ventricular pressure with time.

With few exceptions, the major *physical findings* resemble those observed in patients with valvular aortic stenosis. Among these exceptions are accentuation of aortic valve closure due to elevated pressure in the aorta proximal to the stenosis, an infrequent systolic ejection sound, and the especially prominent transmission of a thrill and murmur into the jugular notch and along the carotid vessels. Uncommonly, there is an early diastolic, decrescendo, blowing murmur of aortic regurgitation caused by the fusion of one or more cusps to the area of stenosis. The narrowing of the peripheral pulmonary arteries that often coexists in these patients frequently produces a late systolic or continuous murmur that may help to distinguish this anomaly from valvular aortic stenosis. This differentiation is reinforced by the frequent finding of a significant disparity between the arterial pressures in the upper extremities in supravalvular aortic stenosis; the systolic pressure in the right arm tends to be the higher of the two and occasionally exceeds that in the femoral arteries. The disparity in pulses may relate to the tendency of a jet stream to adhere to a vessel wall (Coanda effect) and selective streaming of blood into the innominate artery.[382,383]

Electrocardiography usually reveals left ventricular hypertrophy when obstruction is severe. Biventricular, or even right ventricular, hypertrophy may be found if significant narrowing of peripheral pulmonary arteries coexists. Radiographically, in contrast to valvular and discrete subvalvular aortic stenosis, poststenotic dilation of the ascending aorta seldom is seen. The sinuses of Valsalva usually are dilated, and the ascending aorta and aortic arch are of normal size or appear small.

Echocardiography is the most valuable technique for localizing the site of obstruction to the supravalvular area (Fig. 29–37). Most often the sinuses of Valsalva are dilated and the ascending aorta and arch are of normal size or appear small. A useful ratio can be constructed of the measurements of the aortic annulus and the sinotubular junction, in which the latter is always less than the former in patients with supravalvular stenosis, a finding not present in normals.[384] Recently, intraluminal ultrasound imaging has been used to visualize the vascular pathology in Williams syndrome.[385] Doppler examination and retrograde aortic catheterization can determine the degree of hemodynamic abnormality.[386]

Because of the nature of the anatomical defect, this author does not think that transcatheter balloon angioplasty will be an effective treatment option. For several reasons, depending primarily on the anatomical variant of the lesion, supravalvular aortic stenosis may be less amenable to operative treatment than either valvular or discrete subvalvular stenosis. The lumen of the aorta at the supravalvular level may be widened by the insertion of an oval- or diamond-shaped fabric prosthesis in those patients with a normal or near normal ascending aorta.[387] However, if the

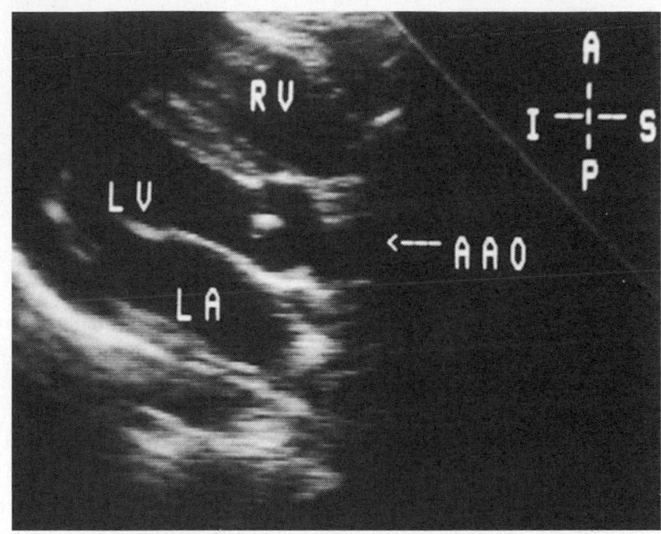

FIGURE 29–37. Supravalvar aortic stenosis is seen in a parasternal long-axis view. The constriction is distal to the sinuses of Valsalva in the ascending aorta (AAO). RV = right ventricle, LV = left ventricle, LA = left atrium. (Courtesy of Norman Silverman, M.D.)

aorta is markedly hypoplastic, this operation merely displaces the pressure gradient distally without abolishing the obstruction. Under these circumstances, repair may require replacement or widening of the entire hypoplastic aorta with an appropriate prosthesis.[387]

Hypoplastic Left Heart Syndrome

This designation is used to describe a group of closely related cardiac anomalies characterized by underdevelopment of the left cardiac chambers, atresia or stenosis of the aortic and/or the mitral orifices, and hypoplasia of the aorta.[388] These anomalies are an especially common cause of heart failure in the first week of life. The left atrium and ventricle often exhibit *endocardial fibroelastosis.* Pulmonary venous blood traverses a patent foramen ovale, and a dilated and hypertrophied right ventricle acts as the systemic, as well as pulmonary, ventricle; the systemic circulation receives blood by way of a patent ductus arteriosus (Fig. 29–38).

The diagnosis should be considered in infants, particularly males, with the sudden onset of heart failure, systemic hypoperfusion, and nonspecific murmur. *Electrocardiography* frequently reveals right axis deviation, right atrial and ventricular enlargement, and ST and T-wave abnormalities in the left precordial leads. Chest roentgenography may show only slight enlargement shortly after birth, but with clinical deterioration there are marked cardiomegaly and increased pulmonary venous and arterial vascular markings. The *echocardiographic* findings usually are diagnostic (Fig. 29–39), and include a diminutive aortic root and left ventricular cavity and absence or poor visualization of aortic and mitral valve echoes, which, when seen, are of diminished amplitude and mobility.[389] *Retrograde aortography* shows hypoplasia of the ascending aorta.

MANAGEMENT. Medical therapy directed at cardiac decompensation, hypoxemia, and metabolic acidemia seldom prolongs survival beyond the first days of life. Constriction of the patent ductus arteriosus and limited flow through a restrictive patent foramen ovale are the principal factors responsible for early death. Prostaglandin E_1 infusion is effective in maintaining ductal patency.

SURGICAL TREATMENT. Some centers are attempting staged surgical management in an effort to provide long-term palliation.[388,390–392] The first stage, often referred to as the *Norwood procedure*, consists of creating an unobstructed communication between the right ventricle and aorta, and enlargement of the ascending aorta. The right ventricular–aortic connection has been accomplished with homograft or prosthetic conduits from the right ventricle or pulmonary trunk to

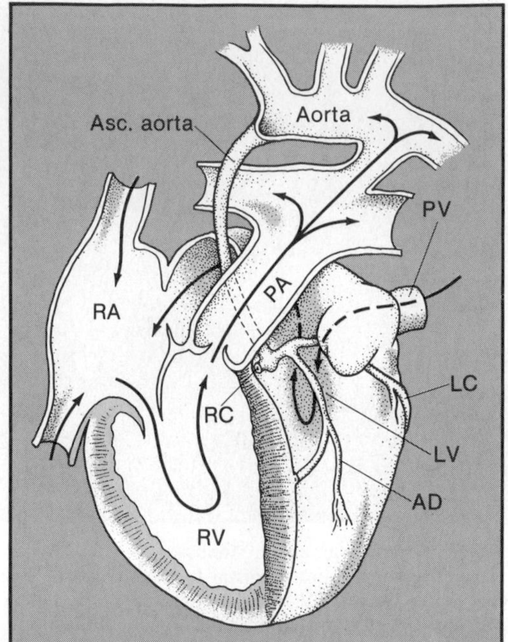

FIGURE 29–38. Hypoplastic left heart with aortic hypoplasia, aortic valve atresia, and a hypoplastic mitral valve and left ventricle. RA = right atrium, RV = right ventricle, RC = right coronary artery, PA = pulmonary artery, PV = pulmonary vein, LC = left coronary artery, LV = left ventricle, AD = anterior descending coronary artery. (From Neufeld, H. N., et al.: Diagnosis of aortic atresia by retrograde aortography. Circulation *25*:278, 1962. Copyright American Heart Association.)

the descending aorta, or by direct connection between the proximal pulmonary trunk and ascending aorta, which also enlarges the ascending aorta. Pulmonary blood flow and pressure are controlled by a tubed interposition systemic-pulmonary shunt to the distal pulmonary artery. The patent ductus arteriosus is ligated. A large interatrial communication also must be assured in stage 1 to allow free access of pulmonary venous blood to the tricuspid valve.

In stage 2 an interatrial baffle is created to provide continuity between left atrium and tricuspid valve; the pulmonary arterial circulation is provided by direct anastomosis of the right atrium to the pulmonary arteries (the Fontan connection).[393] Many surgeons prefer to perform a modified superior vena cava–pulmonary artery shunt (bidirectional Glenn operation) as an intermediate step before the Fontan procedure. In some centers, the preferred operation is cardiac transplantation.[394,395,395a] Stenting of the ductus arteriosus may be used as an ambulatory bridge to transplantation.[396]

Congenital Aortic Regurgitation

Congenital aortic valve regurgitation is a rare isolated congenital cardiac lesion.[397,398] Aortic regurgitation most often occurs in association with congenital valvular aortic stenosis in which the valve commissures are fused, inhibiting cusp mobility; subvalvular aortic stenosis in which the aortic ring is dilated and the valve cusps are deformed; coarctation of the aorta when the aortic ring is dilated and the aortic valve is bicuspid; ventricular septal defect (see p. 901); and endocardial fibroelastosis. Aortic valve regurgitation also may accompany aortic sinus aneurysm or be secondary to dilatation of the ascending aorta in patients with Marfan syndrome, Turner syndrome, cystic medial necrosis, or osteogenesis imperfecta, in which the aortic lesions are manifestations of the underlying connective tissue disorder.

Severe aortic regurgitation also may occur through channels other than the aortic valve.[399,400] Thus aortico–left ventricular tunnel is a rare anomaly that must be distinguished from congenital aortic valve regurgitation, because the approach to management of the former usually does not include consideration for prosthetic valve replacement. The aortico–left ventricular tunnel is an abnormal channel beginning in the ascending aorta above the right coronary orifice and ending in the left ventricle below the right aortic cusp. The channel usually passes behind the right ventricular infundibulum and through the ventricular septum.

Echocardiography, Doppler studies, and aortography combine to establish a precise diagnosis. Exercise testing[401] and magnetic resonance velocity mapping[402] are useful to assess the severity of the lesion. In infants and children with congenital aortic regurgitation the severity of regurgitation increases with time, and valve replacement, rather than plication, is almost always necessary to correct the lesion. Operation should be deferred until symptoms, signs, and noninvasive assessment dictate its necessity. Conversely, closure of an aortic–left ventricular communication is advisable before progressive dilation of the aortic annulus creates secondary changes in the aortic valve itself which may necessitate aortic valve replacement.

Pulmonary Vein Atresia and Stenosis

Pulmonary vein atresia is a rare anomaly in which the pulmonary veins do not connect with the heart or with a major systemic vein.[403] The lesion is incompatible with life, but infants may survive for days, probably because communications exist between the pulmonary veins and the bronchial or esophageal veins that allow limited egress for pulmonary venous blood. Pulmonary vein stenosis may occur as a focal stenosis at the atrial junction or generalized hypoplasia of one

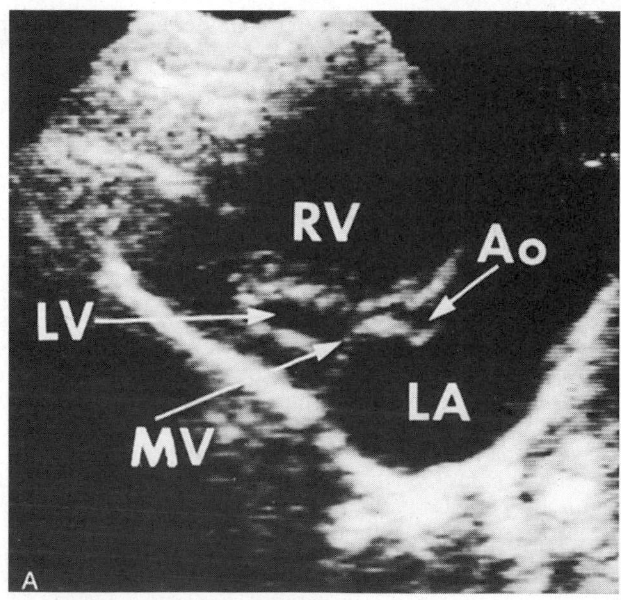

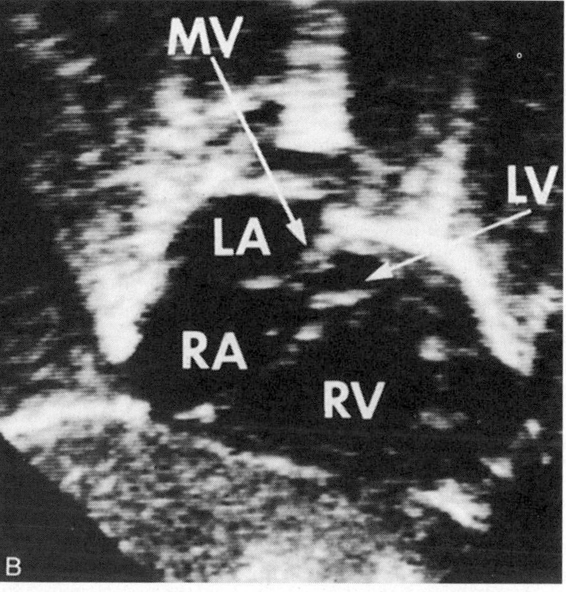

FIGURE 29–39. ***A,*** **Hypoplastic left heart in a parasternal long-axis view in a newborn with aortic atresia, intact ventricular septum, and patent but hypoplastic mitral valve (MV). The left ventricular (LV) cavity is diminutive and the ascending aorta (Ao) is hypoplastic. Right ventricular (RV) dilation is noted.** ***B,*** **In the subcostal four-chamber view dilatation of the right atrium (RA) and right ventricle (RV) is noted. The endocardial echoes are very bright owing to fibroelastosis. (From Perloff, J.: The Clinical Recognition of Congenital Heart Disease. 3rd ed. Philadelphia, W.B. Saunders Company, 1986.)**

or more pulmonary veins. There is an extremely high incidence of associated cardiac malformations, including atrial septal defect, tetralogy of Fallot, tricuspid and mitral atresia, and endocardial cushion defect. The severe pulmonary vein obstruction imposed by pulmonary vein abnormalities causes severe cyanosis, congestive cardiac failure, and early death. Focal stenosis of one or more pulmonary veins at the atrial junction, recognized by two-dimensional echocardiography or angiography, may be relieved surgically.[404] Results of transcutaneous balloon angioplasty have been disappointing.

Cor Triatriatum

In this malformation failure of resorption of the common pulmonary vein results in a left atrium divided by an abnormal fibromuscular diaphragm into a posterosuperior chamber receiving the pulmonary veins and an anteroinferior chamber giving rise to the left atrial appendage and leading to the mitral orifice.[405] The communication between the divided atrial chambers may be large, small, or absent, depending on the size of the opening in the subdividing diaphragm, which determines the degree of obstruction to pulmonary venous return. Elevations of both pulmonary venous pressure and pulmonary vascular resistance result in severe pulmonary artery hypertension.

The diagnosis is established by two-dimensional or transesophageal echocardiography; cardiac catheterization and angiography are necessary only if major associated cardiac anomalies are suspected.[406–406b] The obstructive membrane is visualized in the parasternal long- and short-axis and four-chamber (Fig. 29–40) views and can be distinguished from a supravalvular mitral ring[406a] by its position superior to the left atrial appendage, which forms part of the distal chamber. Also present are diastolic fluttering of the mitral leaflets and high-velocity flow detected by Doppler examination in the distal atrial chamber and at the mitral orifice.

The diagnosis should be suspected at cardiac catheterization if the pulmonary arterial wedge pressure is higher than a simultaneous left atrial pressure. The diagnosis also may be established by visualizing the obstructing lesion angiographically. Although rare, it is important to recognize the malformation because it may be easily correctable at operation.[407]

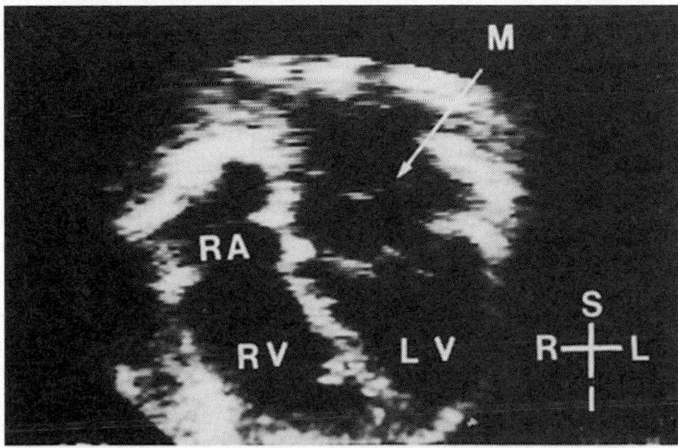

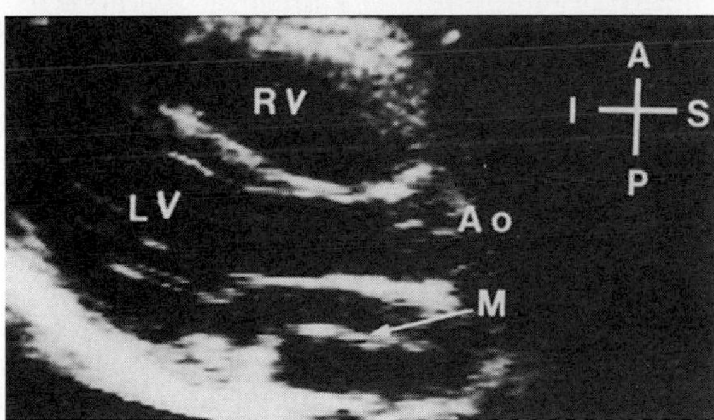

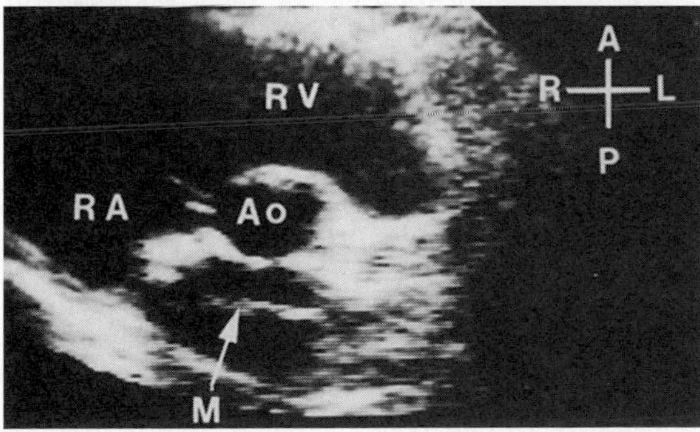

FIGURE 29–40. Echocardiograms demonstrating the membrane (M) of cor triatriatum. The apical four-chamber view *(top panel)* shows the membrane lying within the left atrial chamber. The atrial appendage is distal to the membrane and the pulmonary veins drain into the proximal portion. The parasternal long-axis view *(center panel)* shows the membrane posterior to the aortic root (AO) and mitral valve, dividing the left atrium into two chambers. In the parasternal short-axis view *(bottom panel),* the membrane is within the left atrium close to the posterior aortic root. RA = right atrium, RV = right ventricle, LV = left ventricle. (Courtesy of Norman Silverman, M.D.)

Congenital Mitral Stenosis

Anatomical types of mitral stenosis include the parachute deformity of the valve, in which shortened chordae tendineae converge and insert into a single large papillary muscle; thickened leaflets with shortening and fusion of the chordae tendineae; an anomalous arcade of obstructing papillary muscles; accessory mitral valve tissue; and a supravalvular circumferential ridge of connective tissue arising at the base of the atrial aspect of the mitral leaflets.[408,409] Associated cardiac defects are common, including endocardial fibroelastosis, coarctation of the aorta, patent ductus arteriosus, and left ventricular outflow tract obstruction. Two-dimensional echocardiography, combined with Doppler studies, often provides a complete analysis of the anatomy and function of congenital left ventricular inflow lesions.[410,411] The clinical and hemodynamic consequences of isolated congenital mitral stenosis are similar to those of acquired mitral obstruction with modifications imposed by coexisting anomalies.

The prognosis is poor; symptoms attributable to pulmonary vein obstruction begin usually in infancy and the majority of patients expire before age 1 year unless catheter balloon dilation or operation is successful.[411–412a] Conduit bypass of the mitral valve and prosthetic valve replacement are required if a reparative operation is not possible.[413,414] The use of a porcine bioprosthesis is contraindicated because of its rapid degeneration in the infant or young child.

Congenital Mitral Regurgitation

The syndrome of *mitral valve prolapse* is discussed on p. 1029. This condition usually is quite benign in children. However, occasional difficulties exist with infective endocarditis, arrhythmias, atypical chest pain, and sudden death.[415] *Isolated congenital mitral regurgitation* of hemodynamic significance is an unusual lesion in infants and children.

MORPHOLOGY. Congenital malformations of the mitral valve producing insufficiency most often are encountered in association with endocardial cushion defect, congenitally corrected transposition of the great arteries, endocardial fibroelastosis, anomalous pulmonary origin of the coronary artery, congenital subaortic stenosis, hypertrophic obstructive cardiomyopathy, and coarctation of the aorta. Mitral valve dysfunction also commonly is seen in various metabolic disorders (e.g., the mucopolysaccharidoses), primary and secondary cardiomyopathies, connective tissue disease (e.g., rheumatoid arthritis, Marfan syndrome, Ehlers-Danlos syndrome, pseudoxanthoma elasticum), and rheumatic and nonrheumatic inflammatory diseases of the myocardium.[416]

The various anatomical lesions that result in isolated congenital mitral regurgitation include prolapse of one or both mitral leaflets, cleft or perforated mitral leaflet, inadequate leaflet tissue, double orifice of the mitral valve, anomalous insertion of chordae tendineae (anomalous mitral arcade), redundant leaflet tissue, displacement inferiorly of the ring of the inferior leaflet into the left ventricle, and abnormal length of the chordae tendineae.[416]

CLINICAL FINDINGS. The clinical, echocardiographic, and hemodynamic findings in patients with isolated congenital mitral incompetence resemble those observed in acquired mitral regurgitation.[417] Mitral annuloplasty (which is preferred) and prosthetic valve replacement are procedures reserved for infants and children who are at least moderately symptomatic despite comprehensive medical management, often with repeated episodes of pulmonary infection, or cardiac failure with anorexia and retarded growth and development.[416] Operative condidates are shown by echocardiographic, Doppler, hemodynamic, and angiographic studies to have pulmonary hypertension, a regurgitant fraction in excess of 50 per cent, and a marked increase in left ventricular end-diastolic volume.[418]

Pulmonary Arteriovenous Fistula

Abnormal development of the pulmonary arteries and veins in a common vascular complex is responsible for this rare congenital anomaly (see also p. 967). A variable number of pulmonary arteries communicate directly with branches of the pulmonary veins; in some cases the fistula receives systemic arterial branches.[419] Most patients have an associated Weber-Osler-Rendu syndrome; additional associated problems include bronchiectasis and other malformations of the bronchial tree, and absence of the right lower lobe. Venoarterial shunting depends on the extent of the fistulous communications and may result in cyanosis and secondary polycythemia. Paradoxical emboli and brain abscess may cause major neurological deficits.

Patients with hereditary hemorrhagic telangiectasis often are anemic owing to repeated blood loss and may have less obvious cyanosis. Systolic and continuous murmurs are audible over areas of the fistula. Rounded opacities of variable size in one or both lungs on chest roentgenogram may suggest the presence of the lesion. Pulmonary angiography reveals the site and extent of the abnormal communication (Fig. 30–8, p. 968). Unless the lesions are widespread throughout both lungs, surgical treatment aimed at removing the lesions with preservation of healthy lung tissue commonly is indicated to avoid the complications of massive hemorrhage, bacterial endocarditis, and rupture of arteriovenous aneurysms.

Transcatheter balloon or plug or coil occlusion embolotherapy may prove to be the therapeutic procedure of choice.[420,421]

Peripheral Pulmonary Artery Stenosis

Stenosis of the pulmonary artery may occur as single or multiple lesions located anywhere from the main pulmonary trunk to the smaller peripheral arterial branches.[422] Associated defects are observed in most patients and include pulmonic valvular stenosis, ventricular septal defect, tetralogy of Fallot, and supravalvular aortic stenosis.

ETIOLOGY. The most important cause of significant pulmonary artery stenoses producing symptoms in the newborn is intrauterine rubella infection.[423] Diagnosis is facilitated in these infants by finding elevations of the IgM fraction and rubella antibody titer. Other cardiovascular malformations commonly seen in association with congenital rubella include patent ductus arteriosus, pulmonic valve stenosis, and atrial septal defect. Generalized systemic arterial stenotic lesions also may be a feature of the rubella embryopathy, often involving large and medium-sized vessels such as the aorta and coronary, cerebral, mesenteric, and renal arteries. Cardiovascular lesions are but one manifestation of intrauterine rubella infection because cataracts, microphthalmia, deafness, thrombocytopenia, hepatitis, and blood dyscrasias also are common. Thus, the clinical picture in infants with rubella syndrome depends on the severity of the cardiovascular lesions and the associated abnormalities of other organs and systems. Peripheral pulmonary stenosis also often is associated with supravalvular aortic stenosis in patients with the familial form of the latter anomaly or in patients with the Williams syndrome (see also p. 920).

MORPHOLOGY. Obstruction within the pulmonary arterial tree may be classified into four types: (1) stenosis of the main pulmonary trunk or the main left or right branch; (2) narrowing at the bifurcation of the pulmonary artery, extending into both right and left branches; (3) multiple sites of peripheral branch stenosis; and (4) a combination of main and peripheral stenosis. Pulmonary artery obstruction may be produced by localized narrowing, diffuse constrictions, or, rarely, a membrane or diaphragm. Poststenotic dilatation is usual when the stenosis is localized but may be absent or minimal with elongated constriction. It should be recognized that a physiological branch pulmonary artery stenosis often is present in the normal newborn in whom both right and left main pulmonary arteries are small and arise almost perpendicular from a large main pulmonary artery.[424] The branch vessels increase in size with growth and become less angulated in their take-off from the main pulmonary artery.

CLINICAL FINDINGS. The degree of obstruction is the principal determinant of clinical severity; the type of obstruction determines the feasibility of direct surgical relief. The clinical features vary; most infants and children are asymptomatic.[425] An ejection systolic murmur at the upper left sternal border that is well transmitted to the axillae and back is most common. The presence of an ejection sound suggests that pulmonic valve stenosis coexists. The pulmonic component of the second heart sound may be slightly accentuated, but occasionally is extremely loud if multiple peripheral stenoses exist. A continuous murmur is audible, especially in patients with main or branch stenosis, and particularly if an associated cardiovascular anomaly produces increased pulmonary blood flow. Electrocardiography shows right ventricular hypertrophy when obstruction is severe; left-axis deviation with counterclockwise orientation of the frontal QRS vector is common in the rubella syndrome and when the lesion coexists with supravalvular aortic stenosis. Mild or moderate stenosis usually produces a normal chest roentgenogram; detectable differences in vascularity between regions of the lungs or dilated pulmonary artery segments are uncommon. When obstruction is bilateral and severe, right atrial and ventricular enlargement may be observed.

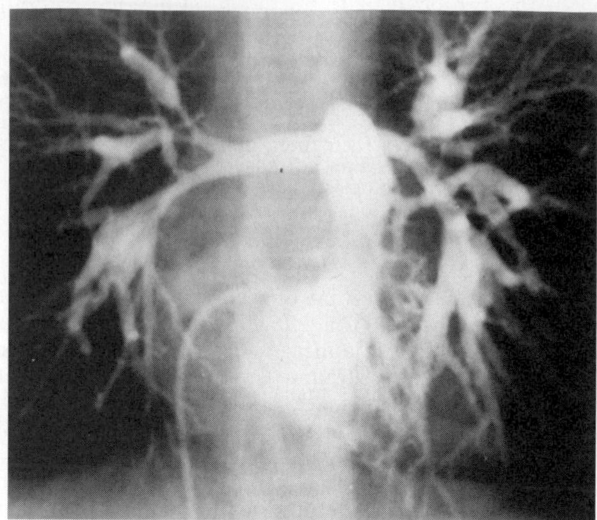

FIGURE 29–41. Right ventricular angiocardiogram showing multiple sites of peripheral pulmonic stenosis and poststenotic dilatation of the peripheral pulmonic arteries.

Diagnosis. This is confirmed by observing pressure gradients within the pulmonary arterial system at cardiac catheterization; digital subtraction and/or selective pulmonary angiography defines the exact location, extent, and distribution of the lesion (Fig. 29–41). Mild to moderate unilateral or bilateral stenosis does not require surgical relief; numerous stenotic areas are not amenable to correction, even with intraoperative balloon angioplasty. Well-localized obstruction of severe degree in the main pulmonary artery or its major branches may be alleviated by percutaneous transcatheter balloon angioplasty (see p. 1313),[426] often accompanied by endovascular stent implantation,[427] or with a patch graft or bypassed with a tubular conduit. The natural history of peripheral pulmonary stenosis is not clear. Obstruction may increase by discrepant growth between a stenotic area and normal portions of the pulmonary artery tree, or as a result of an increase in cardiac output, especially during adolescence. Rarely, hypertrophy of right ventricular infundibular muscle is progressive and results in hypercyanotic spells.

Pulmonic Stenosis with Intact Ventricular Septum

Valvular pulmonic stenosis, resulting from fusion of the valve cusps during mid to late intrauterine development, is the most common form of isolated right ventricular obstruction and occurs in about 7 per cent of patients with congenital heart disease. Hypertrophy of the septal and parietal bands narrowing the right ventricular infundibulum often accompanies the pulmonic valve lesion, especially if it is severe. Fused cusps of varying thickness and rigidity form a fibrous dome in the severest forms. Pulmonic valve dysplasia, especially common in patients with Noonan syndrome (see p. 1663), produces obstruction in the absence of adherent leaflets because leaflets are thickened, rigid, and myxomatous and are limited in their lateral movement because of the presence of tissue pads within the pulmonic valve sinuses.[428]

NEONATES AND INFANTS. The clinical presentation and course of circulation in the newborn with pulmonic stenosis depends on the severity of obstruction and the degree of development of the right ventricle and its outflow tract, the tricuspid valve, and the pulmonary arterial tree. The greater the degree of pulmonic valve stenosis, the more closely the manifestations resemble those observed with pulmonary atresia and intact ventricular septum (see p. 922). Severe pulmonic stenosis is characterized by cyanosis caused by right-to-left shunting through the foramen ovale, cardiomegaly, and diminished pulmonary blood flow in the absence of persistent patency of the ductus arteriosus. Hypoxemia and metabolic acidemia, rather than right ventricular failure, are the main clinical disturbances in the symptomatic neonate and can be alleviated temporarily by infusion of prostaglandin E_1 to dilate the ductus arteriosus and increase pulmonary blood flow. Distinction of these babies from those with tetralogy of Fallot or tricuspid or pulmonary atresia usually is possible because infants with tetralogy usually do not have roentgenographic evidence of cardiomegaly; infants with tricuspid and pulmonary atresia show a preponderance of left ventricular forces by electrocardiography in contrast to the right ventricular hypertrophy usually observed with critical pulmonic stenosis in the absence of right ventricular hypoplasia.

Combined two-dimensional echocardiographic and continuous-wave Doppler examination (Fig. 3–68, p. 79) characterizes the anatomical valve abnormality and its severity, and has essentially eliminated the requirement for cardiac catheterization and angiographic studies to establish a precise diagnosis (Fig. 29–42).[429,430]

Balloon Valvuloplasty. Balloon dilatation of the pulmonary valve (see p. 968) is the therapeutic procedure of choice,[430a,430b] but a pulmonary valvotomy and systemic-to-pulmonary arterial shunt may be necessary in infants with underdevelopment of the right ventricular cavity.[431] In this group, recent success has been achieved by modification of balloon valvuloplasty with predilation initially using a coronary dilatation catheter to facilitate introduction of a definitive balloon catheter.[432] Transcatheter balloon valvuloplasty may be expected to reduce, but not abolish, the pressure difference in neonates with mobile doming valves. This approach is of lesser efficacy in those patients with dysplastic valves, and is contraindicated if valve dysplasia is associated with annular hypoplasia.[433,434]

CHILDREN. The clinical profile of patients with valvular pulmonic stenosis beyond infancy usually is distinctive.[435] The severity of obstruction is the most important determinant of the clinical course. In the presence of a normal cardiac output a peak systolic transvalvular pressure gradient between 50 and 80 mm Hg or a peak systolic right ventricular pressure between 75 and 100 mm Hg is considered to be indicative of moderate stenosis; levels below and above that range are classified as mild and severe, respectively. Most patients with mild pulmonic stenosis are asymptomatic, and the condition is discovered during routine examination. In patients with more significant obstruction the severity of stenosis may increase with time. Progression may be relative and reflect disproportional physical growth of the patient, infundibular narrowing due to progressive hypertrophy of the right ventricular outflow tract, or fibrosis of the valve cusps. Symptoms, when present, vary from mild exertional dyspnea and mild cyanosis to signs and symptoms of heart failure, depending on the degree of obstruction and the level of myocardial compensation. Exertional fatigue, syncope, and chest pain are related to an inability to augment pulmonary blood flow during exercise in some patients with moderate or severe obstruction.

Physical Examination. The severity of obstruction often is suggested by the physical findings. Right ventricular hypertrophy reduces compliance of that chamber, and a forceful right atrial contraction is necessary to augment right ventricular filling. Prominent *a* waves in the jugular venous pulse, a fourth heart sound, and, occasionally, presystolic pulsations of the liver reflect a vigorous atrial contraction and suggest the presence of severe stenosis. Cardiomegaly and a right ventricular parasternal lift accompany moderate or severe obstruction. A systolic thrill is palpable along the upper left sternal border in all but the mildest forms of stenosis. The first heart sound is normal and is followed by a systolic ejection sound at the upper left sternal edge produced by sudden opening of the stenotic valve; an ejection sound is not heard in patients with pulmonic valve dysplasia. The ejection sound typically is louder during expiration; when it is inaudible or occurs less than 0.08 second from the onset of the Q wave on electrocardiogram, severe obstruction is suggested. Right ventricular ejection is prolonged in patients with moderate or severe stenosis, and the sound of pulmonic valve closure is delayed and soft. The characteristic feature of valvular pulmonic stenosis on auscultation is a harsh, diamond-shaped systolic ejection murmur heard best at the upper left sternal border. The systolic murmur becomes louder and its crescendo occurs later in systole, obscuring the aortic component of the second sound with more severe degrees of valvular obstruction because these patients have a greater prolongation of right ventricular systole. The holosystolic decrescendo murmur of tricuspid regurgitation may accompany severe pulmonic stenosis, especially in the presence of congestive heart failure. Cyanosis, reflecting venoarterial shunting through a patent foramen ovale, is absent with mild stenosis and infrequent with moderate obstruction. Cyanosis may not be apparent in patients with severe obstruction if the atrial septum is intact.

Electrocardiography (Fig. 30–9, p. 969). This technique may be helpful in assessing the degree of obstruction to right ventricular output.[436] In mild cases the electrocardiogram often is normal, whereas moderate and severe steno-

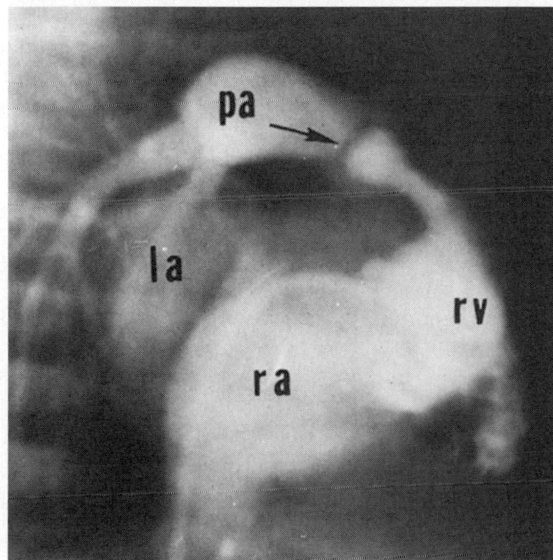

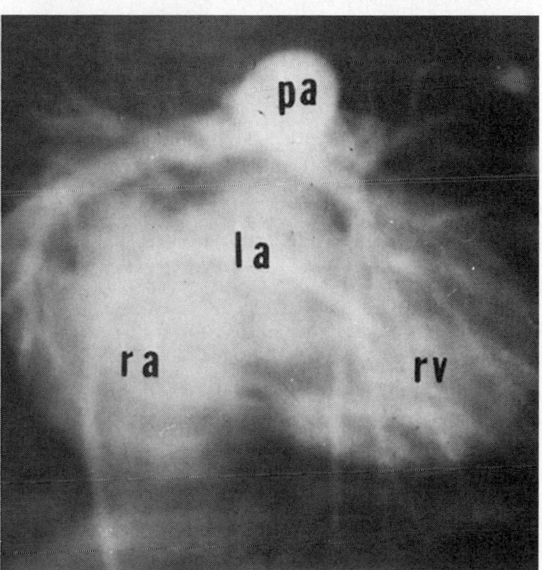

FIGURE 29–42. Right ventriculogram in an infant with critical pulmonic stenosis shows the thickened, nonmobile pulmonic valve (arrow) in the lateral projection *(left)*. Both the lateral and frontal *(right)* projections show regurgitation of contrast material across the tricuspid valve into the right atrium (ra), with subsequent shunting across the foramen ovale to the left atrium (la). rv = right ventricle; pa = pulmonary artery. (Courtesy of Norman Talner, M.D.)

ses are associated with right axis deviation and right ventricular hypertrophy. In the latter patients between ages 2 and 20 years, an estimate of right ventricular pressure can be made by multiplying the height of the R wave in lead V_{4R} or V_1 by 5.[436] A tall QR wave in the right precordial leads with T-wave inversion and ST-segment suppression (right ventricular "strain") reflects severe stenosis. When an rSR′ pattern is observed in lead V_1 (20 per cent of patients) lower right ventricular pressures are found than in patients with a pure R wave of equal amplitude. High-amplitude P waves in leads II and V_1 indicating right atrial enlargement are associated with severe stenosis.

Chest Roentgenography. In patients with mild or moderate pulmonic stenosis chest roentgenography often shows a heart of normal size and normal pulmonary vascularity (Fig. 7–20, p. 218). Poststenotic dilatation of the main and left pulmonary arteries often is evident. Right atrial and right ventricular enlargement are observed in patients with severe obstruction and resultant right ventricular failure. The pulmonary vascularity may be reduced in patients with severe stenosis, right ventricular failure, and/or a venoarterial shunt at the atrial level (see p. 983).

Echocardiography. Reliable localization of the site of obstruction and assessment of its severity are obtained by combined continuous-wave or pulsed Doppler and two-dimensional echocardiography[429–431,437] (Figs. 3–68, p. 79, 30–4, p. 965, and Fig. 29–43). The latter usually shows quite prominent pulmonary valve echoes with restricted systolic motion as well as poststenotic dilation of the main pulmonary artery and its branches. In contrast to these findings in classical valvular pulmonic stenosis, patients with a dysplastic valve show thickened and immobile leaflets with hypoplasia of the pulmonary valve annulus and absent poststenotic dilatation of the pulmonary artery. Parasternal and subcostal views are required to detect most accurately maximal pulmonary artery blood flow velocity, which is converted to a pressure difference across the valve utilizing a modified Bernoulli equation (pressure difference [mm Hg] = 4 × the squared peak Doppler velocity [m/s]). A semiquantitative estimation of pulmonary and tricuspid regurgitation can be obtained. The peak systolic velocity of the tricuspid regurgitant jet provides a reliable indirect measurement of the severity of obstruction because the reverse gradient between the right ventricle and right atrium allows derivation of the ventricular peak systolic pressure. The constant value of 14 is used for right atrial pressure in the calculation.

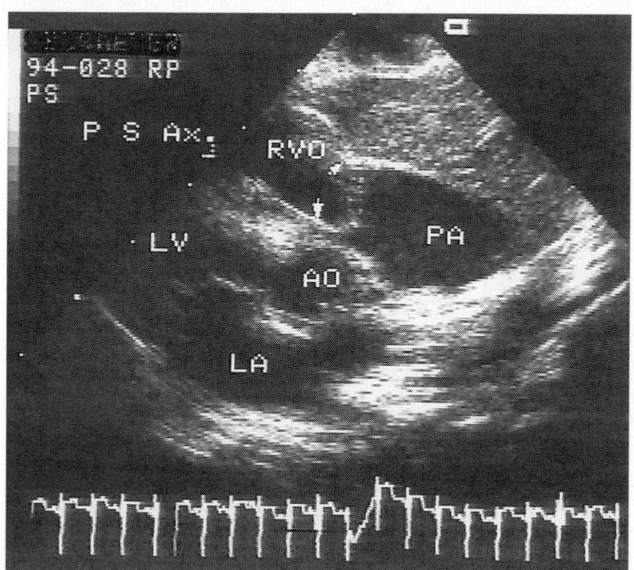

FIGURE 29–43. Severe valvular pulmonic stenosis seen from a parasternal short-axis view. The thickened pulmonary valve can be seen lying between the right ventricular outflow tract (RVO) and a dilated pulmonary artery (PA). The arrows are at the annulus of the pulmonary valve; the thickened, domed valve can be identified clearly. LV = left ventricle, AO = aorta, LA = left atrium. (Courtesy of Norman Silverman, M.D.)

Cardiac Catheterization and Angiocardiography. These techniques are now used only rarely to establish or exclude other diagnostic possibilities. The usual indication for cardiac catheterization is to provide definitive therapy for the lesion. Cardiac catheterization, however, may also localize the site of obstruction, evaluate its severity, and document the coexistence of additional cardiac malformations. The resting cardiac output usually is normal, even in cases of severe stenosis, and most children show the ability to increase cardiac output with exercise.[438] Right ventricular dysfunction occurs especially when venoarterial shunting is significant and produces systemic arterial desaturation. In patients with critical stenosis, care must be taken during hemodynamic study that the cardiac catheter does not dangerously occlude the stenotic valve opening. The angiographic appearance of a typical valvular pulmonic stenosis differs from that of a dysplastic valve. The former is thickened and domes during systole, returning to normal configuration in diastole. Poststenotic dilatation of the main pulmonary trunk and sometimes of the left pulmonary artery is usual. The leaflets of the dysplastic valve are not fused anatomically but are thickened and immobile, creating little change in the angiographic picture during the cardiac cycle. Moreover, a small annulus and narrow sinuses of Valsalva are common accompaniments of valve dysplasia. With either type of valve, systolic narrowing of the right ventricular infundibulum usually is associated with moderate or severe obstruction.

Natural History. Mild and moderate pulmonic valve stenoses have a generally favorable course; uncommonly, progression occurs in the severity of obstruction.[439,440] Serial hemodynamic studies reveal unchanged pressure gradients over 4- to 8-year intervals in three-fourths of patients. Equal percentages of the remainder have an increase or a decrease in the severity of obstruction; significant increases in the pressure gradient occur especially in children with a gradient in excess of 50 mm Hg at initial examination.[435]

Management. Percutaneous transluminal balloon valvuloplasty (see p. 1313) is the initial procedure of choice in patients with typical pulmonary valve stenosis and moderate to severe degrees of obstruction (Fig. 29–44).[114,434] This approach provides palliative improvement with the great likelihood that the improvement is permanent. In these same patients *surgical relief* also can be accomplished at extremely low risk.[441] The valve is approached through an incision in the pulmonary arterial trunk, and resection of infundibular muscle, if necessary, may be accomplished through the pulmonic valve. Reoperation or subsequent balloon valvuloplasty is seldom required. In patients with a dysplastic valve, in whom transcatheter valvuloplasty is ineffective, the thickened valve tissue is removed and a patch often is required to widen the annulus and proximal main pulmonary artery. In children with mild pulmonic valve stenosis, prophylaxis against infective endocarditis is recommended; these patients need not restrict their physical activities.

Pulmonic Atresia with Intact Ventricular Septum

MORPHOLOGY. This anomaly is an uncommon and highly lethal cause of cyanosis in the neonatal period that may respond well to aggressive medical and surgical treatment.[442–444] In almost all infants the pulmonic valve is atretic; in the majority both the valve ring and the main pulmonary artery are hypoplastic. The right ventricular infundibulum occasionally may be atretic or extremely narrowed. A spectrum exists in right ventricular cavity size and configuration, from a diminutive right ventricular chamber, often with tricuspid stenosis, to a large right ventricle, frequently with tricuspid regurgitation (Fig. 29–45). In most infants the right ventricle is hypoplastic, and

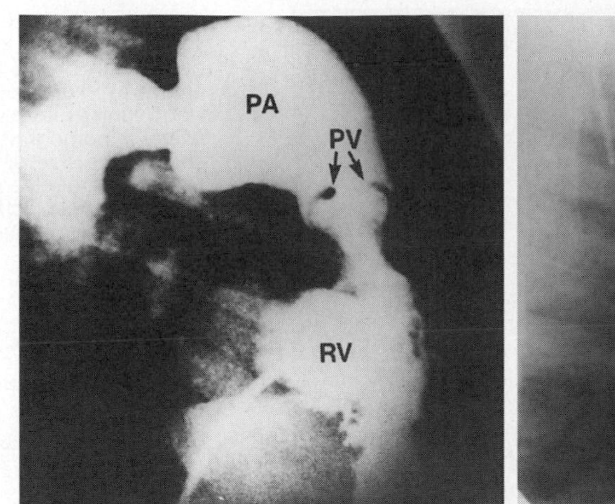

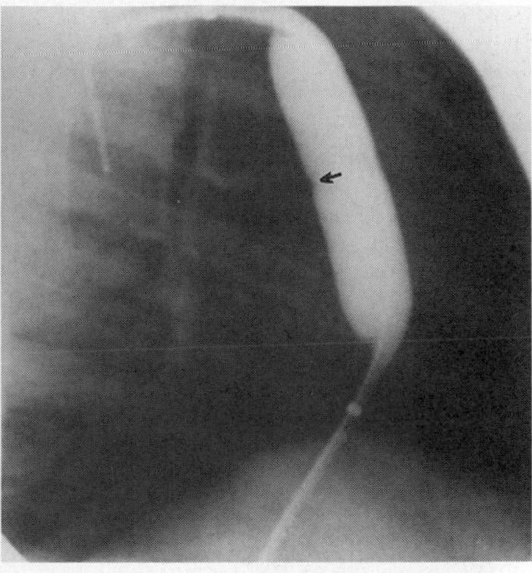

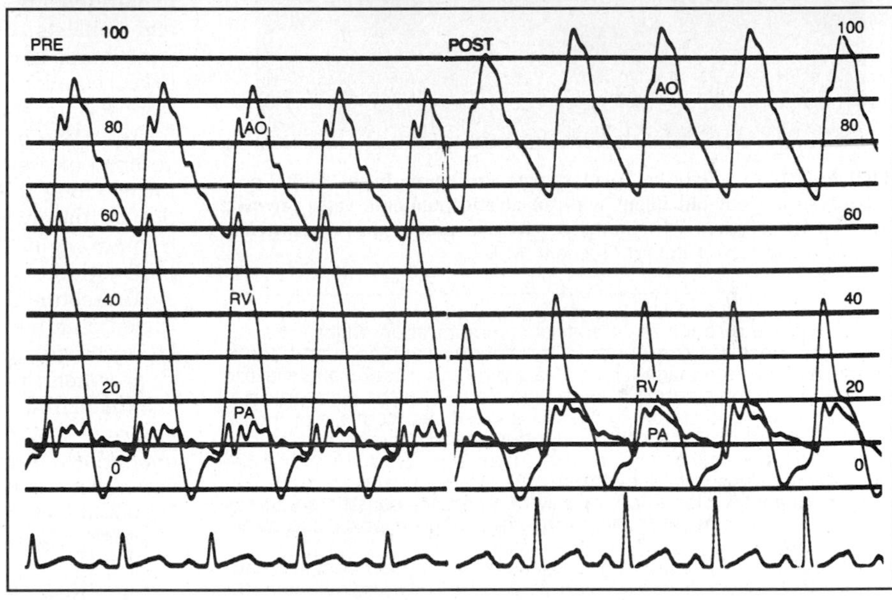

FIGURE 29–44. Right ventriculogram (RV) in the lateral projection *(top left)* from a patient with valvular pulmonic stenosis. The pulmonary valve (PV) is thickened and domes in systole. There is poststenotic dilatation of the pulmonary artery (PA). At the top right, successful balloon valvuloplasty shows almost complete disappearance of the stenotic waist (arrow). The bottom panel shows the pre *(left)* and post *(right)* valvuloplasty hemodynamics, showing a reduction from moderately severe to mild pulmonic stenosis. Ao = aorta. (Courtesy of Dr. Thomas G. DiSessa.)

sinusoidal communications exist in half the patients between the right ventricular cavity and the coronary circulation.[444,445]

The intramyocardial sinusoids may end blindly or communicate with coronary arteries. Further, these communications may be multiple and feed both the left and right coronary systems, or they may be fed via a single, dilated vessel. The proximal coronary arteries in some patients may be atrophic, proximal to a communication between the sinusoids and the distal coronary artery, particularly in hearts with severe hypoplasia of the right ventricle. In these circumstances, the distal coronary vessels are supplied by communications with the right ventricle, and the coronary circulation is, therefore, right ventricle–dependent. In this group, decompression of the right ventricle by a surgical procedure would be associated with a high risk of myocardial ischemia and death.[448]

Because the pulmonic valve is imperforate and completely obstructed, systemic venous blood returning to the heart bypasses the

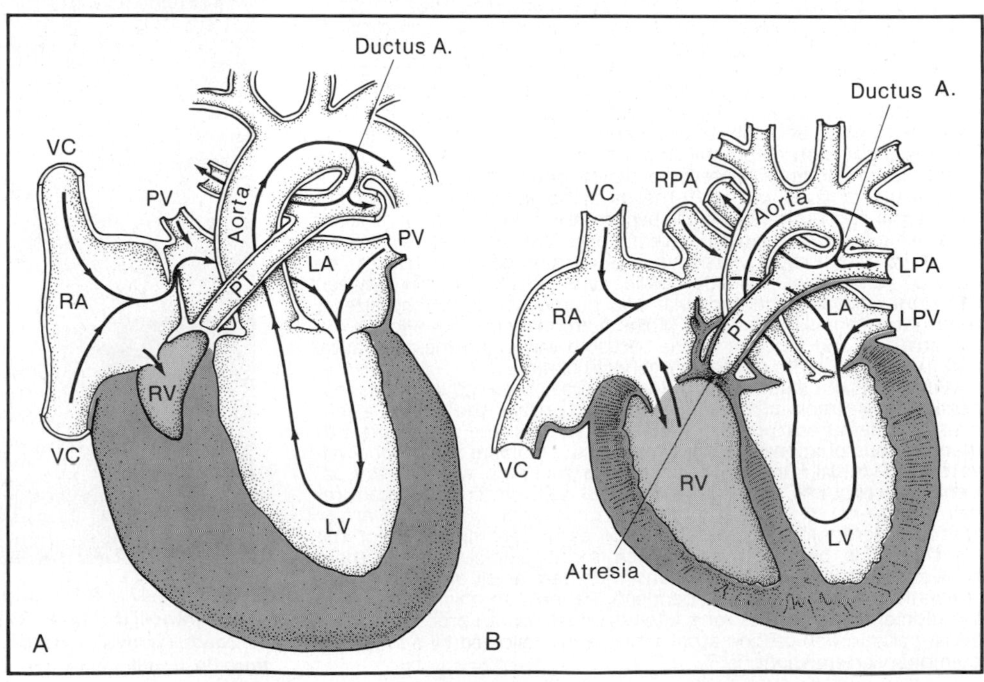

FIGURE 29–45. Pulmonic atresia with intact ventricular septum. With a competent tricuspid valve the right ventricular chamber is diminutive (*A*); Significant tricuspid regurgitation is associated with a normal or large right ventricular cavity (*B*). VC = vena cava, RA = right atrium, RV = right ventricle, PT = pulmonary trunk, PV = pulmonary vein, LA = left atrium, LV = left ventricle, Ductus A. = ductus arteriosus, LPA = left pulmonary artery, RPA = right pulmonary artery, LPV = left pulmonary vein. (From Edwards J. E.: Congenital malformations of the heart and great vessels. *In* Gould, S. E. [ed.]: Pathology of the Heart. 2nd ed. Springfield, Ill., Charles C Thomas, 1960.)

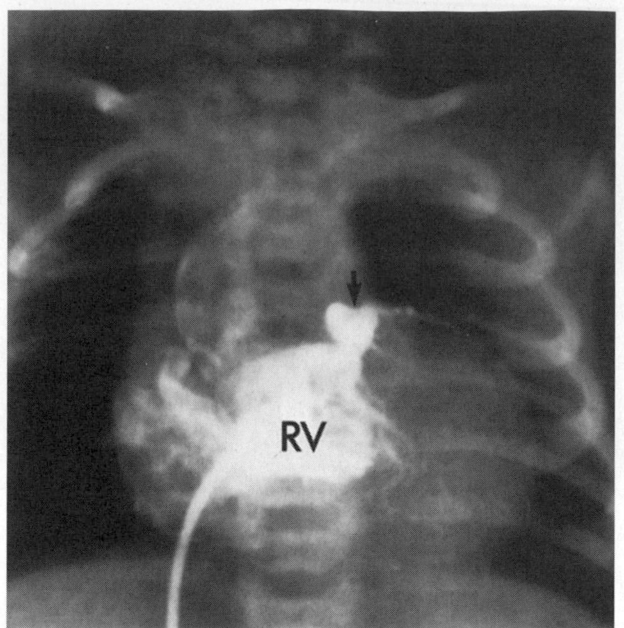

FIGURE 29–46. Right ventricular angiocardiogram in the frontal projection in a 1-day-old infant with an atretic pulmonic valve (arrow). The cavity of the right ventricle (RV) is small and eccentrically shaped. (Courtesy of Robert Freedom, M.D.)

right ventricle through an interatrial communication. Right ventricular output does not contribute to the effective cardiac output and is proportional to the magnitude of tricuspid regurgitation and the size and extent of the sinusoidal communications with the coronary arterial tree. The blood supply to the lungs is derived from the bronchial circulation and from flow through a persistently patent ductus arteriosus. The size and patency of the ductus arteriosus are critical determinants in postnatal survival; ductus closure results in death. Reduced pulmonary blood flow by way of a partially constricted ductus arteriosus results in profound hypoxemia, tissue hypoxia, and metabolic acidemia.

DIAGNOSIS. The diagnosis is suggested by roentgenographic findings of pulmonary hypoperfusion and the electrocardiographic observation of a normal QRS axis, absent or diminished right ventricular forces, and/or dominant left ventricular forces. In the minority of infants with marked tricuspid regurgitation, the right ventricle and right atrium are massively enlarged. The echocardiogram in the usual infant shows a small right ventricular cavity and diminutive or absent pulmonic valve echoes.[446,447] Doppler examination shows continuous retrograde flow to the pulmonary artery and/or its branches through a patent ductus arteriosus, which usually is narrow and tortuous. Only if tricuspid valve echoes are imaged by ultrasound examination can tricuspid atresia be distinguished from pulmonic atresia.

Although the diagnosis of this entity can be made by echocardiography, angiocardiography is required to assess treatment options because key determinants are the identification and nature of ventriculocoronary connections, which are not well characterized by echocardiography. Cardiac catheterization usually is performed on an emergency basis. Because survival depends on patency of the ductus arteriosus, infusion of prostaglandin E_1 (0.05 – 0.1 μg/kg/min) intravenously may dramatically reverse clinical deterioration and improve arterial blood gases and pH.[96] The usual hemodynamic findings are right atrial and right ventricular hypertension, with right ventricular pressure often greater than systemic pressure, and a massive right-to-left interatrial shunt. Selective angiocardiography establishes the diagnosis and allows evaluation of the degree of separation between the right ventricular infundibular and pulmonary trunk, the size of the right ventricular cavity and of the pulmonary arteries (Fig. 29–46), the anatomy and function of the tricuspid valve, and the anatomical and functional details of the coronary circulation.

MANAGEMENT. Initial stabilization is usually required in infants, necessitating infusion of prostaglandin E_1 to dilate the ductus arteriosus and measures to correct metabolic acidosis. The rare infant with membranous pulmonary atresia may be a candidate for balloon valvotomy.[447a] Initial surgical considerations focus on whether the patient is a candidate for a biventricular or univentricular (Fontan) repair (Fig. 29–46).[448–456] The angiographic delineation of coronary artery anatomy determines the feasibility of early decompression of the right ventricle, because this approach is contraindicated when there are ventriculocoronary connections with part or all of the coronary circulation right ventricle-dependent. Patients in this latter group are ultimately candidates for a lateral tunnel Fontan procedure, after initial palliation by balloon atrial septostomy followed by a systemic-pulmonary artery shunt.[457,458]

At the other end of the spectrum, babies with only mild hypoplasia of the right ventricle and tricuspid valve are candidates for a transventricular closed pulmonary valvotomy, followed later by balloon angioplasty or repeat surgical valvotomy. In infants with moderate right ventricular hypoplasia, a biventricular repair is preferred, often using a homograft valve in the outflow tract. In this group, the smaller the size of the right ventricle and tricuspid valve, the more likely a partial biventricular repair will be necessary, relieving the outflow tract obstruction with insertion of a valve, coupled with a bidirectional cavopulmonary (Glenn) shunt to ensure obligatory pulmonary blood flow.

Intraventricular Right Ventricular Obstruction

Infundibular pulmonic stenosis with an intact ventricular septum and the presence of anomalous muscle bundles are the two principal causes of intraventricular right ventricular obstruction (Fig. 29–47).[459]

SUBPULMONIC INFUNDIBULAR STENOSIS. This anomaly usually occurs at the proximal portion of the infundibulum and consists of a fibrous band at the junction of the right ventricular cavity and outflow tract. The clinical manifestations, course, and prognosis of patients with infundibular stenosis are similar to those of patients with valvular stenosis, although the former diagnosis is suggested by the absence of a systolic ejection sound and a systolic murmur lower along the left sternal border. Doppler echocardiography, withdrawal pressure tracings, and selective right ventricular angiocardiography permit localization of the site of obstruction and assessment of its extent and severity. Surgical treatment consists of resection of the fibrotic narrowed area and hypertrophied muscle. Occasionally it may be necessary to widen the outflow tract with a pericardial or prosthetic patch.

ANOMALOUS MUSCLE BUNDLES. A two-chambered right ventricle is formed by right ventricular obstruction due to anomalous muscle bundles; most of the patients have an associated malalignment or perimembranous ventricular septal defect, and about 5 per cent have subaortic stenosis.[459,460] Aberrant hypertrophied muscle bands traverse the

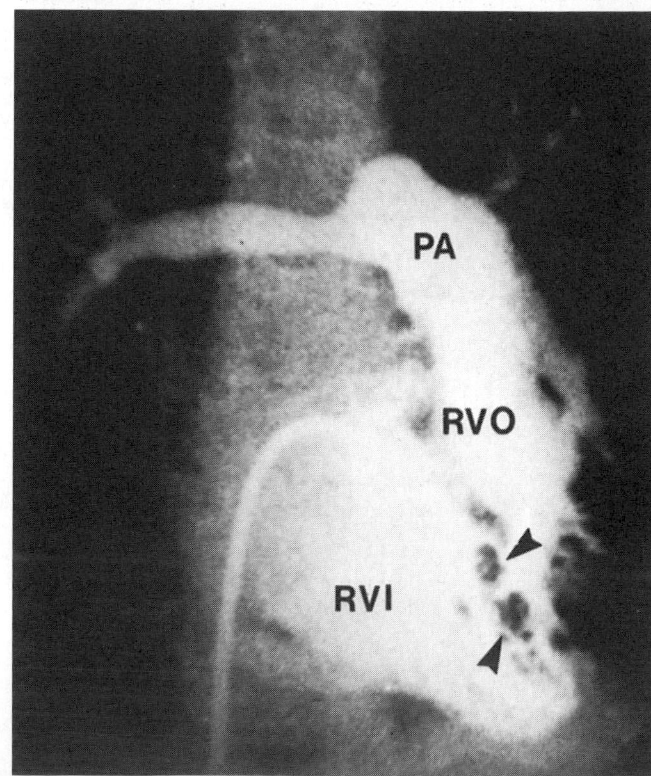

FIGURE 29–47. Intraventricular right ventricular obstruction. The right ventricular inflow (RVI) and outflow (RVO) tracts are separated by bands (arrows), creating intraventricular right ventricular obstruction. PA = pulmonary artery.

right ventricular cavity, extending from its anterior wall to the crista supraventricularis and/or the portion of the adjacent interventricular septum. The anomalous pyramid-shaped muscle mass obstructs blood flow through the body of the right ventricle and produces a proximal high-pressure inflow chamber and a distal low-pressure chamber. Thus this type of obstruction is distinguishable from that in tetralogy of Fallot, in which hypertrophied infundibular muscle protrudes into but does not cross the cavity of the right ventricle.

The clinical, electrocardiographic, and chest roentgenographic findings resemble those observed in pulmonic valvular or subvalvular infundibular obstruction, although the systolic thrill and murmur may be displaced lower along the left sternal border. Progressive obstruction occurs in some patients. The diagnosis may be established by two-dimensional echocardiography.[460] Selective right ventricular angiocardiography provides the most accurate diagnosis and reveals a filling defect in the midportion of the right ventricle which often does not change significantly with systole and diastole.

Management. The treatment for anomalous muscle bundles consists of surgical removal.[461] In the absence of preoperative recognition of the anomaly, the surgeon should be alerted to the correct diagnosis by the presence of a dimple during contraction on the ordinarily smooth anterior surface of the right ventricle and/or the inability to view the tricuspid valve through a longitudinal ventriculotomy because of the presence of the abnormal muscle mass.

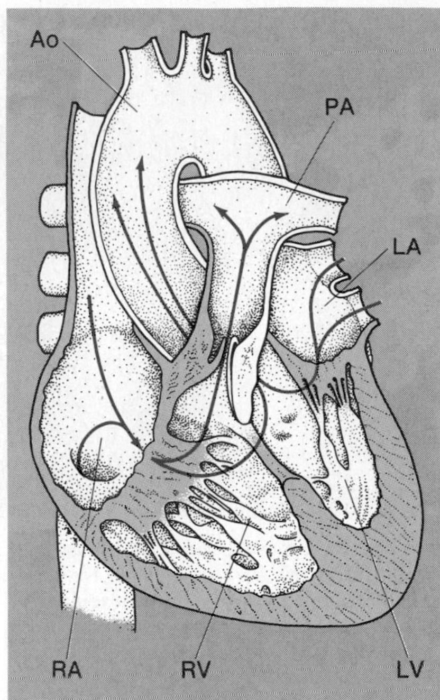

FIGURE 29–48. Tetralogy of Fallot with infundibular and valvular pulmonic stenosis. The arrows indicate direction of blood flow. A substantial right-to-left shunt exists across the ventricular septal defect. RA = right atrium, LA = left atrium, RV = right ventricle, LV = left ventricle, Ao = aorta, PA = pulmonary artery.

Tetralogy of Fallot

DEFINITION. The overall incidence of this anomaly approaches 10 per cent of all forms of congenital heart disease, and it is the most common cardiac malformation responsible for cyanosis after 1 year of age.[462] The four components of this malformation are (1) ventricular septal defect, (2) obstruction to right ventricular outflow, (3) overriding of the aorta, and (4) right ventricular hypertrophy. The basic anomaly is the result of an anterior deviation of the septal insertion of the infundibular ventricular septum from its usual location in the normal heart between the limbs of the trabecular septum. The interventricular malalignment defect usually is large, approximating the aortic orifice in size, and is located high in the septum just below the right cusp of the aortic valve, separated from the pulmonic valve by the crista supraventricularis. The aortic root may be displaced anteriorly and straddle or override the septal defect, but, as in the normal heart, it lies to the right of the origin of the pulmonary artery. In most cases no dextroposition of the aorta exists; overriding of the aorta is a phenomenon secondary to the subaortic location of the ventricular septal defect.

HEMODYNAMICS. The degree of obstruction to pulmonary blood flow is the principal determinant of the clinical presentation. The site of obstruction is variable[463–465]; infundibular stenosis is the only major obstruction in about 50 per cent of patients and coexists with valvular obstruction in another 20 to 25 per cent (Fig. 29–48). Supravalvular and peripheral pulmonary arterial narrowing may be observed, and unilateral absence of a pulmonary artery (usually the left) is found in a small number of patients. Circulation to the abnormal lung is accomplished by bronchial and other collateral arteries.[465–467] Atresia of the pulmonic valve, infundibulum, or main pulmonary artery occasionally is referred to as "pseudotruncus arteriosus." True truncus arteriosus with absent pulmonary arteries (Type 4) differs from Fallot's tetralogy, in which pulmonary artery branches are present but are fed by a patent ductus arteriosus and/or bronchial arteries (see Fig. 29–51).[462] A right-sided aortic knob, aortic arch, and descending aorta occur in about 25 per cent of patients with tetralogy of Fallot. The coronary arteries may have surgically important variations[468]: the anterior descending artery may originate from the right coronary artery; a single right coronary artery may give off a left branch that courses anterior to the pulmonary trunk; a single left coronary artery may give off a right branch that crosses the infundibulum of the right ventricle. Enlargement of the infundibulum branch of the right coronary artery often presents a problem with respect to a right ventriculotomy.

Associated cardiac anomalies exist in about 40 per cent of patients. Major associated cardiac anomalies include patent ductus arteriosus, multiple (usually muscular) ventricular septal defects, and complete atrioventricular septal defects. Localized single or multiple peripheral pulmonary arterial stenotic lesions are common; rarely, the right or left pulmonary artery may arise anomalously from the ascending aorta. Infrequently, aortic valve regurgitation results from aortic cusp prolapse. Associated extracardiac anomalies are present in 20 to 30 per cent of patients.

The relation between the resistance of blood flow from the ventricles into the aorta and into the pulmonary vessels plays a major role in determining the hemodynamic and clinical picture.[469] Thus, the severity of obstruction to right ventricular outflow is of fundamental significance. When right ventricular outflow tract obstruction is severe, the pulmonary blood flow is markedly reduced, and a large volume of unsaturated systemic venous blood is shunted from right to left across the ventricular septal defect. Severe cyanosis and polycythemia occur, and symptoms and sequelae of systemic hypoxemia are prominent. At the opposite end of the spectrum, the term "acyanotic" or "pink" tetralogy of Fallot often is used to describe an interventricular communication and a milder degree of obstruction to right ventricular outflow with little or no venoarterial shunting. In many infants and children the obstruction to right ventricular outflow is mild but progressive, so that early in life pulmonary exceeds systemic blood flow, and the symptoms resemble those produced by a simple ventricular septal defect.

CLINICAL MANIFESTATIONS. Few children with tetralogy of Fallot remain asymptomatic or acyanotic. Most are cyanotic from birth or develop cyanosis before age 1 year. In general, the earlier the onset of systemic hypoxemia, the

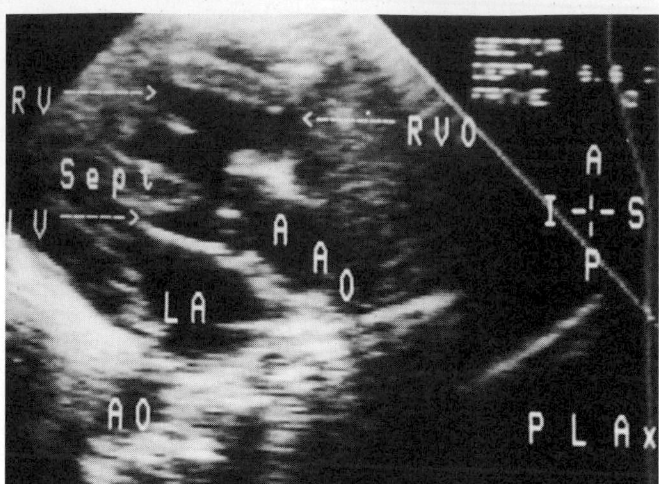

FIGURE 29–49. Tetralogy of Fallot in a parasternal long-axis (PLAx) view, which demonstrates the aorta overriding the ventricular septum (Sept). RV = right ventricle, RVO = right ventricular outflow tract, LV = left ventricle, LA = left atrium, AO = ascending aorta. (Courtesy of Norman Silverman, M.D.)

more likely the possibility that severe pulmonary outflow tract stenosis or atresia exists. Dyspnea with exertion, clubbing, and polycythemia is common. When resting after exertion, children with tetralogy characteristically assume a squatting posture (see p. 885). The latter may be obvious even in infancy; many cyanotic infants prefer to lie in a knee-chest position. Spells of intense cyanosis related to a sudden increase in venoarterial shunting and a reduction in pulmonary blood flow most often have their onset between 2 and 9 months of age and constitute an important threat to survival.[470–472] The attacks are not restricted to patients with severe cyanosis; they are most common in the morning after awakening and are characterized by hyperpnea and increasing cyanosis that progresses to limpness and syncope and occasionally terminates in convulsions, a cerebrovascular accident, and death.

Physical Examination. This reveals variable degrees of underdevelopment and cyanosis. Clubbing of the terminal digits may be prominent after the first year of life. The heart is not hyperactive or enlarged; a right ventricular impulse and systolic thrill often are palpable along the left sternal border. An early systolic ejection sound that is aortic in origin may be heard at the lower left sternal border and apex; the second heart sound is single, the pulmonic component rarely being audible. A systolic ejection murmur is produced by flow across the narrowed right ventricular infundibulum or pulmonic valve. The intensity and duration of the murmur vary inversely with the severity of obstruction—the opposite of the relation that exists in patients with pulmonic stenosis and an intact ventricular septum. Polycythemia, decreased systemic vascular resistance, and increased obstruction to right ventricular outflow may all be responsible for a decrease in intensity of the murmur; with extreme outflow tract stenosis or pulmonic atresia and during an attack of paroxysmal hypoxemia, there may be no or only a very short, faint murmur. A continuous murmur faintly audible over the anterior or posterior chest reflects flow through enlarged bronchial collateral vessels. A loud continuous murmur of flow through a patent ductus arteriosus occasionally may be heard at the upper left sternal border.

LABORATORY EXAMINATIONS. The *electrocardiogram* ordinarily shows right ventricular and, less frequently, right atrial hypertrophy. In a patient with acyanotic tetralogy, combined ventricular hypertrophy may be noted initially, progressing to right ventricular hypertrophy as cyanosis develops. *Roentgenographic* examination characteristically reveals a normal-sized, boot-shaped heart (coeur en sabot) with prominence of the right ventricle and a concavity in the region of the underdeveloped right ventricular outflow tract and main pulmonary artery. The pulmonary vascular markings typically are diminished, and the aortic arch and knob may be on the right side; the ascending aorta usually is large. A uniform, diffuse, fine reticular pattern of vascular markings is noted in the presence of prominent collateral vessels.

Echocardiography. Findings include aortic enlargement, aortic–septal discontinuity, and aortic overriding of the ventricular septum.[473] Two-dimensional echocardiography (Fig. 3–84, p. 84) shows the right ventricular outflow tract to be narrowed and in a more horizontal orientation than normal. The main pulmonary artery and its branches are mildly to severely hypoplastic. The usual ventricular septal malalignment defect lies superior to the tricuspid valve and immediately below the aortic valve cusps. These findings are best displayed in views of the long axis of the right ventricular outflow tract, which are the subxiphoid short axis and the high transverse parasternal echo windows. Echo views that show the anteroposterior coordinates best indicate the overriding of the aorta; these are the parasternal long-axis, apical two-chamber, and subxiphoid views (Fig. 29–49). The echocardiographic examination also reveals the origin of the main pulmonary artery from the right ventricle, and continuity of the main pulmonary artery with its right and left branches, and is accurate for diagnosing coronary abnormalities, although the latter are identified best by angiography.[467,471] The demonstration of mitral–semilunar valve continuity helps to distinguish tetralogy from double-outlet right ventricle with pulmonic stenosis, in which discontinuity of the mitral valve echo and the aortic cusp echo is a critical feature.

Cardiac Catheterization and Angiocardiography (Fig. 29–50). Despite the accuracy of noninvasive approaches, many centers still consider invasive study necessary to

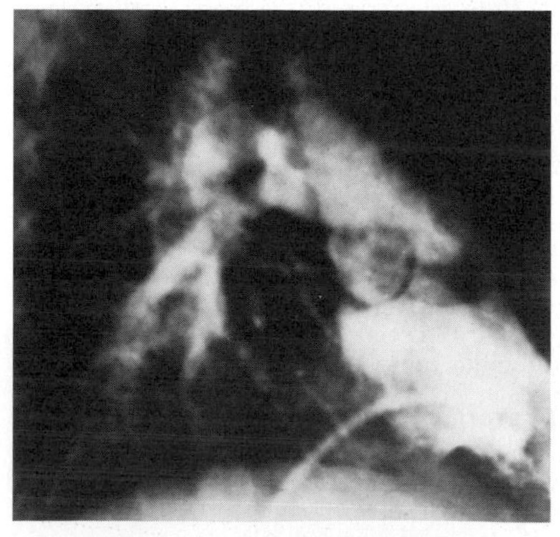

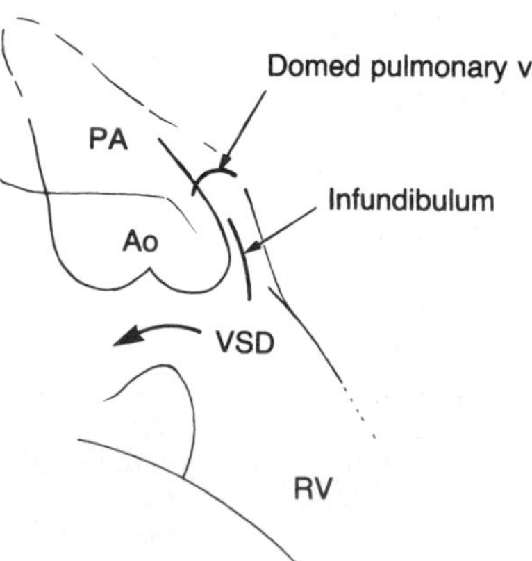

FIGURE 29–50. Lateral view of a right ventriculogram in a child with tetralogy of Fallot showing simultaneous opacification of the pulmonary artery (PA) and aorta (Ao). PV = pulmonic valve, VSD = ventricular septal defect, RV = right ventricle.

confirm the diagnosis; assess the magnitude of right-to-left shunting; provide details of additional muscular ventricular septal defects, if present; evaluate the architecture of the right ventricular outflow tract, pulmonic valve, and annulus and the morphology and caliber of the main branches of the pulmonary arteries; and analyze the anatomy of the coronary arteries. *Axial cineangiography,* utilizing the sitting-up projection, greatly facilitates evaluation of the pulmonary outflow tract and arteries.[151] The preoperative assessment of tetralogy with pulmonic atresia must include delineation of the arterial supply to both lungs by selective catheterization and visualization of bronchial collateral arteries with late serial filming; pulmonary arteries may be opacified only after the bronchial collateral arteries have cleared of contrast material (Fig. 29–51).[463] A patient with pulmonic atresia should not be ruled out as a candidate for surgical correction unless an inadequate pulmonary arterial supply to the lungs is clearly demonstrated.[466] Rarely, injection of contrast through a catheter in the pulmonary venous capillary wedge position is required to assess the possibility that anatomical pulmonary arteries are present. Computer-assisted axial tomography may visualize central pulmonary arteries when conventional angiography cannot.

MANAGEMENT. Among the factors that may complicate the management of patients with tetralogy are iron deficiency anemia, infective endocarditis, paradoxical embolism, polycythemia, coagulation disorders, and cerebral infarction or abscess. Paroxysmal hypercyanotic spells may respond quickly to oxygen, placing the child in the knee-chest position, and morphine. If the spell persists, metabolic acidosis will develop from prolonged anaerobic metabolism, and infusion of sodium bicarbonate may be necessary to interrupt the attack. Vasopressors, beta-adrenoceptor receptor blockade, or general anesthesia occasionally may be necessary.[472]

Total Surgical Correction. This operation is advisable ultimately for almost all patients with tetralogy of Fallot.[474–479] Early definitive repair, even in infancy, currently is advocated in most centers that are experienced in intracardiac surgery in infants. Successful early correction appears to prevent the consequences of progressive infundibular obstruction and acquired pulmonic atresia, delayed growth and development, and complications secondary to hypoxemia and polycythemia with bleeding tendencies. The anatomy of the right ventricular outflow tract and the size of the pulmonary arteries, rather than the age or size of the infant or child, are the most important determinants in assessing candidacy for primary repair; a transannular patch may be used in infants with severe outflow narrowing.[479] Marked hypoplasia of the pulmonary arteries is a relative contraindication for early corrective operation.

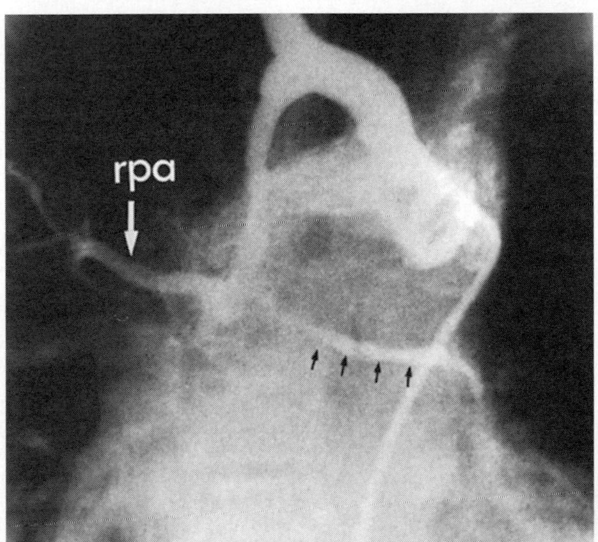

FIGURE 29–51. Selective systemic collateral bronchial arteriogram demonstrates "gull-wing" configuration of the hypoplastic right pulmonary artery (rpa) and left pulmonary artery (arrows) in a patient with tetralogy of Fallot and pulmonic atresia. (Courtesy of Robert Freedom, M.D.)

Palliative Surgery. When marked hypoplasia of the pulmonary arteries exists, a palliative operation designed to increased pulmonary blood flow is recommended and usually consists in the smallest infants of a systemic-pulmonary arterial anastomosis.[480] A transventricular infundibulectomy or valvulotomy is an alternative palliative procedure that may be considered. Balloon dilatation of the pulmonary valve may afford palliation in selected infants.[481,481a] Total correction can then be carried out at a lower risk later in childhood. The palliative procedures relieve hypoxemia caused by diminished pulmonary blood flow and reduce the stimulus to polycythemia. Because pulmonary venous return is augmented, the left atrium and ventricle are stimulated to enlarge their capacity in anticipation of total correction. In the most severe forms of tetralogy of Fallot with pulmonic atresia, the goals of operation include establishment of nonstenotic continuity between the right ventricle and pulmonary arteries, closure of the intracardiac shunt, and interruption of surgically created shunts or major collateral arteries to the lungs. When atresia is confined to the infundibulum or pulmonic valve, repair may be accomplished by infundibular resection and reconstruction of the outflow tract with a pericardial patch. If a long segment of pulmonary arterial atresia exists, a valve-containing conduit is inserted from the right ventricle to the distal pulmonary artery.[482] The presence of a single pulmonary artery in the hilus of either lung is a prerequisite for repair of pulmonic atresia. Prior unifocalization to incorporate multiple systemic to pulmonary artery collaterals into a neo–pulmonary artery may be required in selected patients. A conduit also may be necessary in less severe forms of right ventricular outflow tract obstruction when an anomalous coronary artery crosses the right ventricular outflow tract.

Postoperative Complications. A variety of complications are common in the postoperative period after palliative or corrective operation. Mild-to-moderate left ventricular decompensation may be secondary to the sudden increase in pulmonary venous return; varying degrees of pulmonic valvular regurgitation increase right ventricular cavity size further.[483] Patients with progressive pulmonary insufficiency and severe right ventricular dilatation are candidates for prosthetic pulmonary valve insertion.[484,485]

Bleeding problems frequently are seen, especially in older polycythemic patients. Complete right bundle branch block or the pattern of left anterior hemiblock often is seen, but disabling dysrhythmias are infrequent.[486] Restricted pulmonary arterial flow is the greatest cause for early and late mortality and poor late results.[462] After convalescence from intracardiac repair, symptoms of hypoxemia and severe exercise intolerance are relieved even in the presence of some residual right ventricular outflow tract obstruction, pulmonic valve incompetence, and/or cardiomegaly.[479,487] However, cardiovascular performance at rest or during exercise may remain below normal,[488,489] and major complications, such as trifascicular block, complete heart block, ventricular arrhythmias, and sudden death, may rarely occur many years after surgical treatment.

Late ventricular arrhythmias are rare in patients with successful early correction of the malformation unless complex or multiple operations were performed. Because widespread use of ambulatory electrocardiographic monitoring has resulted in greater detection of ventricular arrhythmias, usually isolated ventricular extrasystoles or nonsustained tachycardia, some have suggested that the asymptomatic patients in this category should have pharmacological suppression of their arrhythmias. Most recent studies, how-

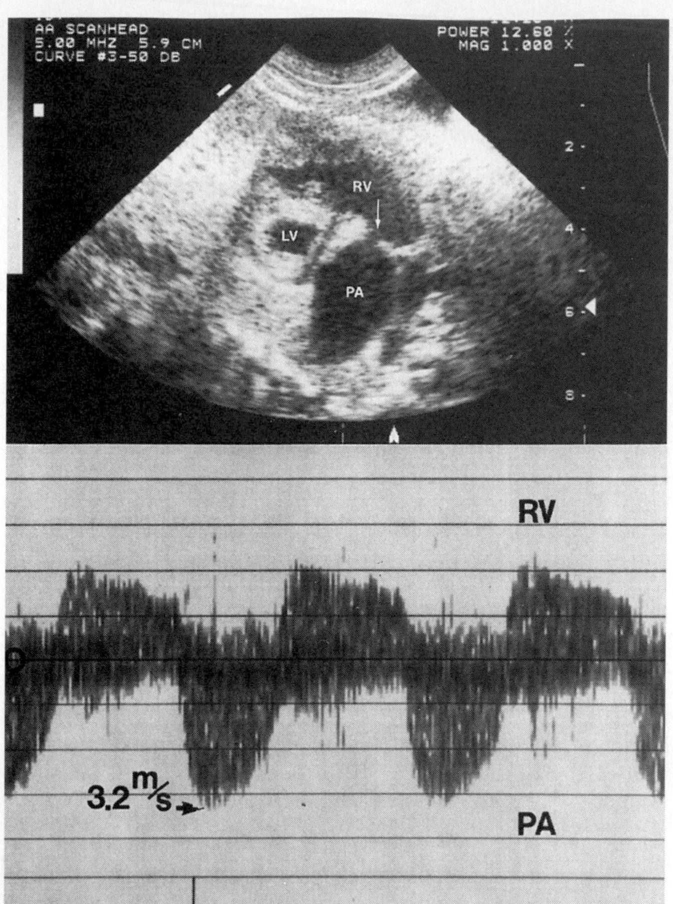

FIGURE 29–52. Two-dimensional *(top panel)* and Doppler *(lower panel)* echocardiogram of a 30-week gestation fetus with tetralogy of Fallot and absent pulmonary valve. The pulmonary artery (PA) is aneurysmally dilated and the right ventricle (RV) is also dilated. The arrow points to the stenotic pulmonary valve annulus. Pulmonary valve leaflets are not detectable. The Doppler study at the level of the pulmonary valve annulus demonstrates to-and-fro flow with increased forward velocity in systole. LV = left ventricle. (Courtesy of James C. Huhta, M.D.)

ever, do not support the use of potentially dangerous long-term antiarrhythmic treatment for asymptomatic postoperative patients.[490–494a]

Congenital Absence of the Pulmonic Valve

PATHOLOGY AND PATHOGENESIS. In the majority of cases of this rare malformation the lesion is associated with a ventricular septal defect, a narrowed obstructive annulus of the pulmonic valve, and marked aneurysmal dilatation of the pulmonary arteries. The combination of anomalies often is referred to as tetralogy of Fallot with absent pulmonic valve. The obstructing lesion principally consists of underdeveloped, primitive valve tissue within a hypoplastic annulus; infundibular obstruction and the ventricular septal defect do not differ from classic tetralogy of Fallot. Recent reports indicate that deletion within chromosome 22 is common in patients with this anomaly.[494b]

The massively dilated pulmonary arteries often are the major determinant of the clinical course because they frequently result in upper airway obstruction and severe respiratory distress in infancy.[495] Smaller intrapulmonary bronchi may also be compressed by abnormally branching distal pulmonary arteries, and in some cases a reduction exists in the number of bronchial generations or alveolar multiplications.[496,497] Poststenotic pulmonary artery aneurysms develop in utero, and their size and location appear to be related to the magnitude of pulmonic regurgitation in fetal life, the orientation of the right ventricular infundibulum to the right or left, and the size of the ductus arteriosus.[498]

CLINICAL AND LABORATORY FINDINGS. The *clinical* features often are distinctive, with an early onset of severe respiratory distress caused by tracheobronchial compression accompanied by a systolic ejection and a widely transmitted low-pitched, decrescendo diastolic murmur at the upper left sternal border. In the absence of pulmonary complications cyanosis is commonly mild. *Roentgenographically* the heart is moderately enlarged; hyperinflated lung fields are observed with large hilar densities representing the aneurysmally dilated pulmonary arteries. The *echocardiographic* features are similar to those seen in classic tetralogy of Fallot, in addition to massive dilatation of the main pulmonary artery and branch pulmonary arteries. Remnants of pulmonary cusps may be visible. Right ventricular dilatation is produced by significant pulmonary regurgitation; the latter is identified by retrograde diastolic flow in the pulmonary arteries and right ventricle at Doppler examination. These findings may be detected before birth (Fig. 29–52). Definitive diagnosis is established by cardiac catheterization and selective angiocardiography.

NATURAL HISTORY AND MANAGEMENT. Prognosis is related to the intensity of upper airway obstruction; pulmonary complications are the usual cause of death in infancy. If survival beyond infancy is accomplished, the respiratory symptoms usually diminish, probably because of maturational changes in the structure of the tracheobronchial tree. The surgical approach in infancy often is unsatisfactory; a variety of procedures have been attempted, ranging from aneurysmorrhaphy to pulmonary artery suspension to transection and reanastomosis of pulmonary artery segments to homograft insertion.[499,500] Also suggested are ligation of the main pulmonary artery and creation of a systemic-pulmonary shunt, and primary repair of the ventricular septal defect with pulmonary arterial plication. In older patients the stenotic annulus may be widened with a patch and the ventricular septal defect closed. It seldom is necessary to replace the pulmonic valve.

Tricuspid Atresia

MORPHOLOGY. This anomaly is characterized by absence of the tricuspid orifice, an interatrial communication, hypoplasia of the right ventricle, and the presence of a communication between the systemic and pulmonary circulations, usually a ventricular septal defect.[501] Thus there is a univentricular atrioventricular connection, consisting of a left-sided mitral valve between the morphological left

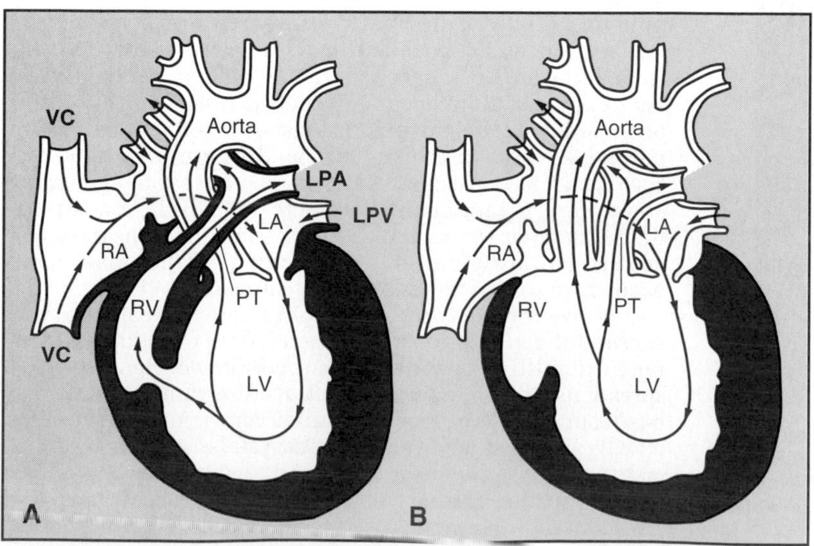

FIGURE 29–53. *A,* Tricuspid atresia with normally related great arteries, a small ventricular septal defect, diminutive right ventricular chamber, and narrowed outflow tract. *B,* An example of tricuspid atresia and complete transposition of the great arteries in which the left ventricular chamber is essentially a common ventricle, with the aorta arising from an infundibular component (RV) of the common ventricle. VC = vena cava, RA = right atrium, LA = left atrium, RV = right ventricle, LV = left ventricle, LPV = left pulmonary vein, LPA = left pulmonary artery. (Modified from Edwards, J. E., and Burchell, H. B.: Congenital tricuspid atresia: Classification. Med. Clin. North Am. *33*:1177, 1949.)

atrium and left ventricle. Unequal division of the atrioventricular canal by fusion of the right-sided endocardial cushions has been proposed as the embryological fault. Patients may be subdivided into those with normally related great arteries (70 to 80 per cent of cases) and those with D-transposition of the great arteries; further classification depends on the presence of pulmonic stenosis or atresia and the absence or size of the ventricular septal defect (Fig. 29–53). Additional cardiovascular malformations often are present, especially in patients with D-transposition of the great arteries, and include persistent left superior vena cava, patent ductus arteriosus, coarctation of the aorta, and juxtaposition of the atrial appendages.

PATHOPHYSIOLOGY. The association with other cardiac malformations determines whether or not pulmonary blood flow is decreased, normal, or increased and therefore the degree of systemic hypoxemia.[502] The clinical picture usually is dominated by symptoms resulting from greatly diminished pulmonary blood flow with severe cyanosis. Cyanosis results from an obligatory admixture of systemic and pulmonary venous blood in the left atrium, and its intensity primarily depends on the magnitude of pulmonary blood flow. Heart failure, rather than cyanosis, is the predominant problem in infants with torrential pulmonary blood flow, which results when D-transposition of the great arteries, a ventricular septal defect, and an unobstructed pulmonary outflow tract coexist. If these patients survive infancy, they are candidates for pulmonary vascular obstructive disease; a favorable response to pulmonary arterial banding is common early in life.

CLINICAL FEATURES. The diagnosis is easily established in the vast majority of infants with tricuspid atresia and pulmonary hypoperfusion. The *electrocardiographic* findings of left-axis deviation, right atrial enlargement, and left ventricular hypertrophy in a cyanotic infant strongly suggest tricuspid atresia.[502] *Echocardiography* reveals a small or absent right ventricle, large left ventricle, and absent tricuspid valve echoes (Figs. 29–54 and 3–19, p. 60); further, it may demonstrate the relation of the great arteries unless pulmonic atresia is present. Color flow and pulsed Doppler echocardiography reveals the abnormal flow patterns; apical and subxiphoid cross-sectional views best reveal the atretic tricuspid orifice. *Roentgenographically,* there are diminished pulmonary vascular markings and a concavity in the region of the cardiac silhouette usually occupied by the main pulmonary artery. The right atrial shadow may be prominent unless left-sided juxtaposition of the atrial appendages exists, which produces a straight and flattened right heart border.

CARDIAC CATHETERIZATION AND ANGIOGRAPHY. The right ventricle cannot be entered directly from the right atrium. When the great arteries are related normally, pulmonary blood flow is found to be derived from shunting through a ventricular septal defect or by way of a patent ductus arteriosus; the latter and the bronchial collaterals are the source of pulmonary flow if the ventricular septum is intact. In complete transposition the pulmonary artery fills directly from the left ventricle and the aorta indirectly through a ventricular septal defect and the hypoplastic right ventricle. Because complete admixture exists in the left atrium of pulmonary and systemic venous return, the degree of systemic arterial hypoxemia depends on the pulmonary-systemic flow ratio. Right atrial angiography does not opacify the right ventricle unless by way of a ventricular septal defect. Selective left ventricular *angiography* permits identification of the hypoplastic right ventricle, the size and location of the ventricular septal defect, the type of pulmonary obstruction, the relation between the great arteries, and the size of the distal pulmonary arterial tree.

MANAGEMENT. *Balloon atrial septostomy* in those infants with a restrictive interatrial communication and palliative operations designed to increase pulmonary blood flow (systemic arterial—or venous—pulmonary artery anastomosis)

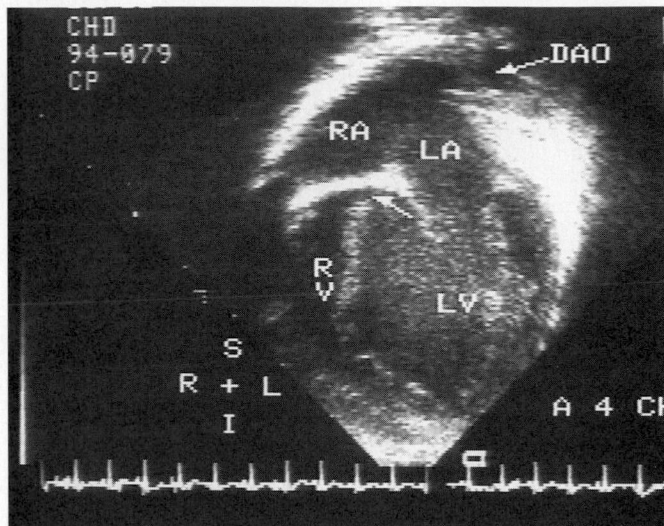

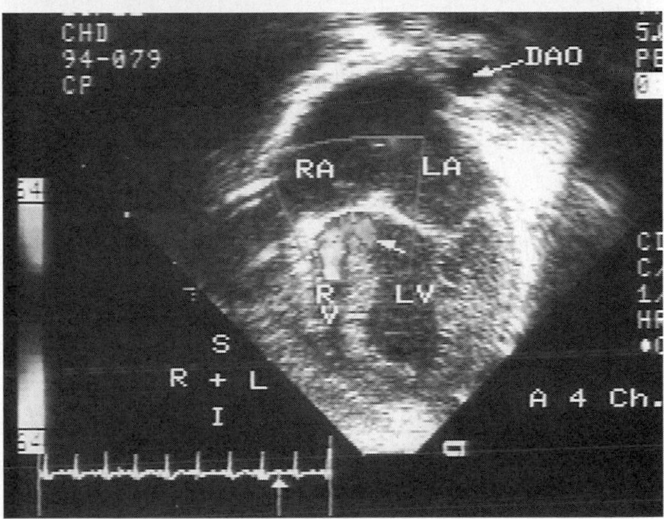

FIGURE 29–54. Apical four-chamber views of a patient with tricuspid atresia. In these views the right atrium (RA) and left atrium (LA) can be seen above, and the small right ventricle (RV) and large left ventricle (LV) can be seen below. *Top,* Diastole with the mitral valve in the open position. Note the intense tissue echoes from the right atrioventricular groove between the right atrium (RA) and right ventricle (RV), indicating the absence of the tricuspid valve. The descending aorta (DAO) can be identified posterior to the left atrium (LA). *Bottom,* Doppler color flow map of the same patient taken toward end-systole, showing the passage of blood across the ventricular septal defect (arrow). Orientation: S = superior, I = inferior, R = right, L = left. (Courtesy of Norman Silverman, M.D.)

are capable of producing clinical improvement of significant duration in patients with diminished blood flow.[502]

Functional correction of the anomaly has been accomplished in children beyond age 12 months by an intraatrial cavopulmonary baffle (lateral tunnel Fontan) (Fig. 29–55) or connection of the left pulmonary artery to the superior vena cava and inferior vena cava to the right pulmonary artery.[502a] An adjustable snare around the atrial septal defect or a fenestrated cavocaval baffle with later transcatheter closure appears to prevent acute increases in systemic venous pressure, improve cardiac output, and enhance surgical survival.[503–504a] In patients with tricuspid atresia and complete transposition of the great arteries, subaortic obstruction can be anticipated when the ventricular septal defect becomes restrictive, also referred to as an obstructive bulboventricular foramen. In most patients, the subaortic tissue must be resected, or preferably, a main pulmonary artery to ascending aorta anastomosis (Damus-Stansel-Kaye procedure) is performed at the time of the Fontan operation.[505] Candidates for these corrective procedures must

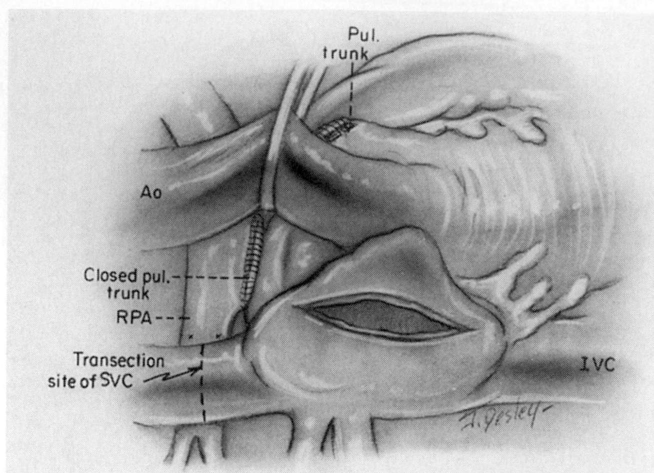

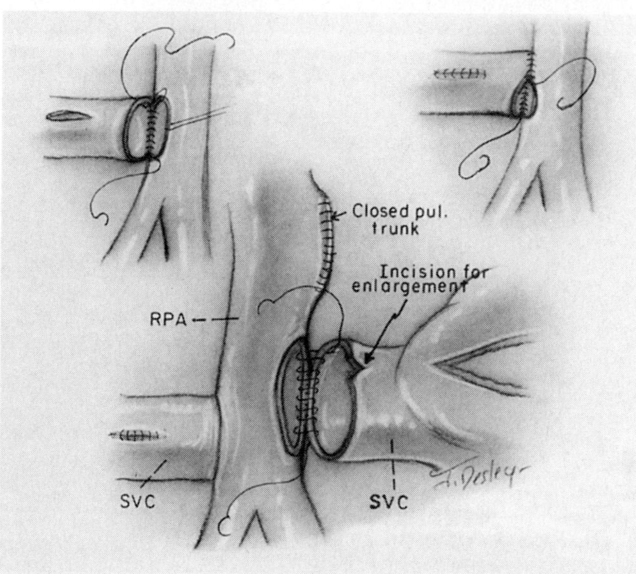

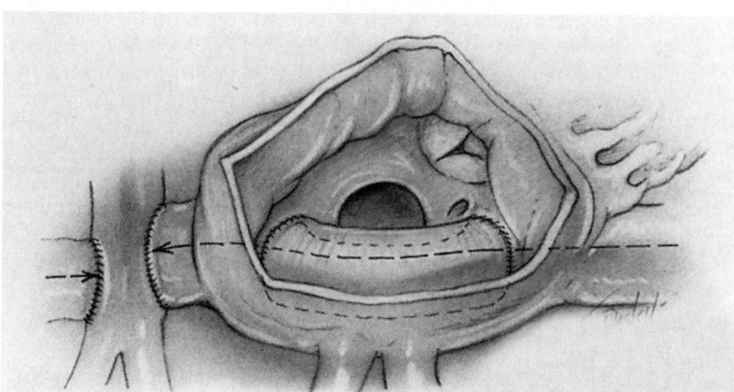

FIGURE 29–55. The Fontan operation by total cavopulmonary connection. *Top,* The pulmonary trunk has been divided close to the pulmonary valve and both ends closed. The right atrium is opened and a pump sump sucker is placed across the foramen ovale and into the left atrium (not shown). Marking stitches are placed at the proposed site of transection of the superior vena cava and at the proposed sites of the two longitudinal incisions on the superior and inferior aspects of the right pulmonary artery. *Middle,* The anastomosis made between the distal end of the divided superior vena cava and the incision in the superior aspect of the right pulmonary artery. The cardiac end of the superior vena cava is rarely enlarged; anastomosis is made to an incision in the inferior aspect of the right pulmonary artery. *Bottom,* A tunnel is created from a cylinder of either Dacron, Gore-Tex, or pericardium connecting the inferior vena cava to the atrial orifice of the superior vena cava. The right pulmonary veins drain behind the tunnel. (From Kirklin, J. W., and Barratt-Boyes, B. G.: Cardiac Surgery. 2nd ed. New York, Churchill Livingstone, 1993, p. 1068.)

have normal pulmonary vascular resistance and a mean pulmonary artery pressure less than 20 mm Hg, pulmonary arteries of adequate size, and good left ventricular function.[506–508] The postoperative period usually is characterized transiently by a superior vena cava syndrome with right heart failure, edema, ascites, and hepatomegaly. Long-term results have been good.[509–511a] Late atrial arrhythmias may be a consequence of adverse preoperative hemodynamic function.[512]

Ebstein's Anomaly of the Tricuspid Valve

(See also p. 966)

This malformation is characterized by a downward displacement of the tricuspid valve into the right ventricle due to anomalous attachment of the tricuspid leaflets (Fig. 29–56).[513] Case-control studies suggest that maternal exposure in the first trimester to lithium carbonate, used in the management of manic-depressive psychosis, is associated with a greatly increased risk of this anomaly in exposed offspring.[514] Tricuspid valve tissue is dysplastic, and a variable portion of the septal and inferior cusps adhere to the right ventricular wall some distance away from the atrioventricular junction. Because of the abnormally situated tricuspid orifice, a portion of the right ventricle lies between the atrioventricular ring and the origin of the valve, which is continuous with the right atrial chamber. This proximal segment is "atrialized," and a distal, functionally small ventricular chamber exists. The degree of impairment of right ventricular function depends primarily on the extent to which the right ventricular inflow portion is atrialized and on the magnitude of tricuspid valve regurgitation.

CLINICAL MANIFESTATIONS. These are variable because the spectrum of pathology varies widely and because of the presence of associated malformations.[515,516] If the tricuspid valve is deformed severely, neonatal heart failure or even

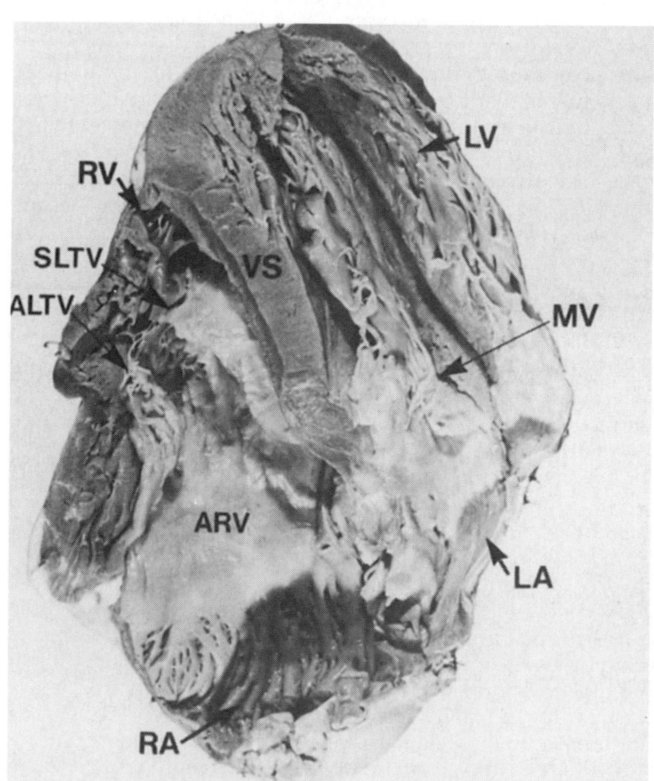

FIGURE 29–56. Anatomical specimen of Ebstein's anomaly of the tricuspid valve, cut in the same place as an apical four-chamber echocardiographic view (Fig. 29–57). The septal and anterior leaflets of the tricuspid valve (SLTV, ALTV) are displaced into the right ventricle (RV), producing a large atrialized right ventricle (ARV). VS = ventricular septum, RA = right atrium, LA = left atrium, MV = mitral valve, LV = left ventricle. (Courtesy of Thomas DiSessa, M.D.)

fetal hydrops and intrauterine death may occur.[517] At the other end of the spectrum, patients with a mildly deformed tricuspid valve may remain symptom free well into adulthood. The severity of symptoms also depends upon the presence or absence of associated malformations. An interatrial communication consisting of a patent foramen ovale or an ostium secundum atrial septal defect is present in more than half the cases. The most common important associated defect is pulmonic stenosis or atresia. Other coexistent anomalies may include an ostium primum type of atrial septal defect and ventricular septal defect alone or in combination with other lesions. The Ebstein's lesion commonly is observed in association with congenitally corrected transposition of the great arteries, in which the tricuspid valve is in the left atrioventricular orifice (see p. 940). The usual manifestations in infancy are cyanosis, a cardiac murmur, and severe congestive heart failure. The magnitude of tricuspid regurgitation in the neonate is enhanced because the pulmonary vascular resistance is normally high early in life.[518] In this regard, newborn infants with Ebstein's anomaly and massive tricuspid regurgitation must be distinguished by two-dimensional and Doppler echocardiography from those with organic pulmonary atresia and the presence of elevated perinatal pulmonary vascular resistance.[519]

The tricuspid regurgitation in infants with Ebstein's anomaly may lessen substantially, and cyanosis may disappear early in life as pulmonary vascular resistance falls, only to occur at a later age when right ventricular dysfunction and/or paroxysmal arrhythmias develop. In some infants with Ebstein's malformation, cyanosis is suddenly intensified as the degree of pulmonary hypoperfusion is unmasked by spontaneous closure of a patent ductus arteriosus.

Beyond infancy the onset of symptoms is insidious; the most common complaints are exertional dyspnea, fatigue, and cyanosis. About 25 per cent of patients suffer episodes of paroxysmal atrial tachycardia. A prominent systolic pulsation of the liver and a large *v* wave in the jugular venous pulse accompany the systolic thrill and murmur of tricuspid regurgitation. Wide splitting of the first and second heart sounds and prominent third and fourth heart sounds may produce a characteristically rhythmic auscultatory cadence with a triple, quadruple, and quintuple combination of sounds.

LABORATORY FINDINGS. The electrocardiographic abnormalities commonly fall into two categories—those with a right bundle branch block pattern and those with a Wolff-Parkinson-White syndrome (Fig. 4–28, p. 126). The pattern in the latter is always Type B, resembling left bundle branch block with predominant S waves in the right pericardial leads. The presence of a preexcitation (Fig. 30–7, p. 968) pattern increases the risk of supraventricular paroxysmal tachycardia.[520] The electrocardiogram most often shows giant P waves, a prolonged P-R interval, and prolonged terminal QRS depolarization, producing variable degrees of right bundle branch block. These distinctive findings help to distinguish Ebstein's anomaly from other forms of right ventricular dysplasia whose presenting problem often is an arrhythmia. *Roentgenographic* studies (Fig. 7–46, p. 234) usually demonstrate an enlarged right atrium, a small right ventricle, and a pulmonary artery with reduced pulsations; the pulmonary vascularity may be reduced if a large right-to-left shunt is present.

Echocardiographic Findings. The principal echocardiographic findings observed in patients with this anomaly, as well as in those with other forms of right ventricular volume overload, are an increase in right ventricular dimension, paradoxical ventricular septal motion, an increase in tricuspid valve excursion, and an abnormal closing velocity of the tricuspid valve. More specific findings for Ebstein's anomaly include a delay in tricuspid valve closure relative to mitral closure and a decrease in the E-F slope of the tricuspid valve, an abnormal anterior position of the tricuspid valve during diastole, and the detection of tricuspid valve echoes with more lateral placement of the transducer than usual.[521] Two-dimensional echocardiographic techniques are superior for observation of the inferior and leftward displacement of the tricuspid valve and simultaneously demonstrate the abnormal positional relation between the tricuspid and mitral valves (Figs. 29–57 and 3–69, p. 80). Moreover, the boundaries of the atrialized right ventricle may be defined.

Specific diagnosis requires identification, usually from an apical four-chamber view, of displacement of the septal tricuspid leaflet.[522]

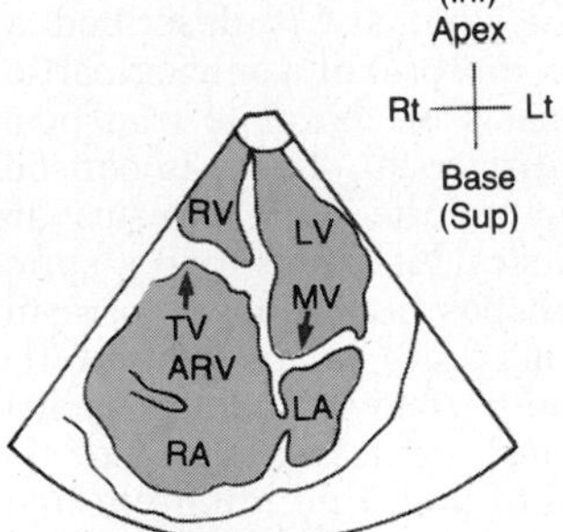

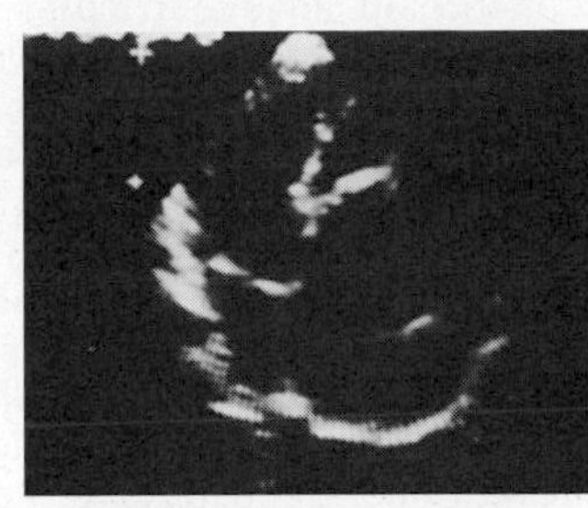

FIGURE 29–57. Apical four-chamber view of Ebstein's anomaly, corresponding to the anatomical specimen in Figure 29–56. RA = right atrium, LA = left atrium, MV = mitral valve, LV = left ventricle, TV = tricuspid valve, ARV = atrialized right ventricle, RV = right ventricle. (Courtesy of Thomas DiSessa, M.D.)

Tricuspid regurgitation, if present, is detected by Doppler examination.

Invasive Study. These are rarely necessary. When *cardiac catheterization* is performed, the intracavitary electrocardiogram recorded just proximal to the tricuspid valve shows a right ventricular type of complex, while the pressure recorded is that of the right atrium. A right-to-left atrial shunt normally is present. The hemodynamic findings depend on the degree of tricuspid regurgitation. The cardiac muscle is unusually irritable, and a high incidence of significant arrhythmias during catheterization has been noted. Selective right ventricular *angiocardiography* shows the position of the displaced tricuspid valve, the size of the right ventricle, and the configuration of the outflow portion of the right ventricle.

MANAGEMENT. Ebstein's anomaly may be compatible with a relatively long and active life, with most patients surviving into the the third decade.[515,523,524] In symptomatic infants with severe cardiomegaly, the initial surgical approach is similar to that in patients with tricuspid atresia, creating a systemic pulmonary shunt, and at a later age the Fontan approach. Consideration may be given in some of these patients to the creation of a bidirectional Glenn shunt from the superior vena cava to the pulmonary arteries, to divert systemic venous return from the right atrium and to increase pulmonary blood flow. In older patients, significant benefit has resulted from reconstruction of the tricuspid valve, closure of the atrial septal defect, plication of the free wall of the right ventricle, posterior tricuspid annuloplasty, and a reduction in right atrial size.[515] Because late results of this latter approach are encouraging, we now recommend operation for all symptomatic patients and even asymptomatic patients if their heart size is increasing significantly. In patients with a preexcitation syndrome (see p. 673) that is producing life-threatening rhythm disturbances, the accessory conduction pathways are either catheter ablated or surgically divided.

TRANSPOSITION COMPLEXES

The term *transposition* identifies a group of malformations that have in common an abnormal relation between the cardiac chambers and great arteries. In this chapter the term is used to include both anomalous insertion of the pulmonary veins and cardiac malpositions.

Complete Transposition of the Great Arteries

MORPHOLOGY. This is a common and potentially lethal form of heart disease in newborns and infants.[525] The malformation consists of the origin of the aorta arising from the morphological right ventricle and that of the pulmonary artery from the morphological left ventricle. With rare exceptions there is no fibrous continuity between the aortic and mitral valves. The origin of the aorta usually is to the right and anterior to, but may be lateral to, the main pulmonary artery. Thus, dextro- or D-transposition is a term often used interchangeably with complete transposition. In other classifications the anomaly is described as concordant atrioventricular and discordant ventriculoarterial connections. The embryogenesis of complete transposition of the great arteries is controversial. There is consensus that the ventricular origins of the great arteries are reversed after development of a straight rather than a spiral infundibulotruncal septum. Transposition appears to result from a transfer of the pulmonary artery, instead of the aorta, from the heart tube's outlet zone to the left ventricle.[526] The latter may result from maldevelopment of the infundibulum, or a combination of both infundibulum maldevelopment and truncal malseptation; the former results if the subpulmonary, rather than the subaortic, infundibulum is absorbed.

The anatomical arrangement results in two separate and parallel circulations. Some communication between the two circulations must exist after birth to sustain life; otherwise, unoxygenated systemic venous blood is directed inappropriately to the systemic circulation and oxygenated pulmonary venous blood is directed to the pulmonary circulation. Almost all patients have an interatrial communication (Fig. 29–58). Two-thirds have a patent ductus arteriosus, and about one-third have an associated ventricular septal defect. Complete transposition occurs more frequently in the offspring of diabetic mothers and more often in males than in females. Without treatment, about 30 per cent of these infants die within the first week of life, 50 per cent within the first month, 70 per cent within 6 months, and 90 per cent within the first year.[525] Those who live beyond infancy have, as a general rule, either an isolated large atrial septal defect or a single ventricle, or ventricular septal defect and pulmonic stenosis. Current aggressive medical and surgical approaches to this group of patients have transformed the prognosis for an infant with this malformation from hopeless to very good.

HEMODYNAMICS. The *clinical course* is determined by the degree of tissue hypoxia, the ability of each ventricle to sustain an increased workload in the presence of reduced coronary arterial oxygenation, the nature of the associated cardiovascular anomalies, and the anatomical and functional status of the pulmonary vascular bed.[525] A bidirectional shunt is always present because continuous unidirectional shunting would result in a progressive depletion of the circulating volume in either the pulmonary or the systemic vascular bed.

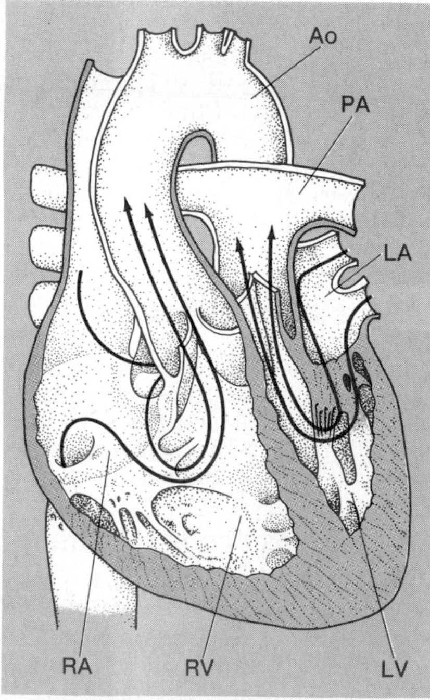

FIGURE 29–58. Complete transposition of the great arteries. Intercirculatory mixing occurs only at the atrial level. RA = right atrium, LA = left atrium, RV = right ventricle, LV = left ventricle, Ao = aorta, PA = pulmonary artery.

A major determinant of the systemic arterial oxygen saturation is the amount of blood exchanged between the two circulations by intercirculatory shunts. The net volume of blood passing left to right from the pulmonary to the systemic circulation represents the anatomical left-to-right shunt and is in fact the effective systemic blood flow (i.e., the amount of oxygenated pulmonary venous return reaching the systemic capillary bed). Conversely, the volume of blood passing right to left from the systemic to the pulmonary circulation constitutes the anatomical right-to-left shunt and is in fact the effective pulmonary blood flow (i.e., the net volume of unsaturated systemic venous return perfusing the pulmonary capillary bed).

The net volume exchange between the two circulations per unit time is equal. The magnitude of the intercirculatory mixing volume is modified by the number of intercirculatory communications that exist, the presence of associated obstructive intracardiac and extracardiac anomalies, the extent of the bronchopulmonary circulation, and the relation between pulmonary and systemic vascular resistance. For example, in the newborn with an intact ventricular septum and a constricted or closed patent ductus arteriosus, inadequate mixing through a small patent foramen ovale often is the cause of severe hypoxemia. If a large interatrial communication or a ventricular septal defect exists, systemic arterial oxygen saturation is influenced more importantly by the pulmonary–systemic blood flow relation than by the adequacy of mixing; augmented pulmonary blood flow produces a higher systemic arterial saturation if the left ventricle can sustain a high-output state without the intervention of congestive heart failure and pulmonary edema. The systemic arterial oxygen saturation is quite low, despite adequate intercirculatory mixing sites, if pulmonary blood flow is reduced by left ventricular outflow tract obstruction or increased pulmonary vascular resistance.

Pulmonary Vascular Changes. Infants with complete transposition of the great arteries are particularly susceptible to the early development of *pulmonary vascular obstructive disease*.[63,527] Moderately severe morphological alterations develop in the pulmonary vascular bed by the age of 6 to 12 months in many infants and by 2 years in almost all patients with an associated large ventricular septal defect or large patent ductus arteriosus in the absence of obstruction to left ventricular outflow. Advanced pulmonary vascular disease also is seen within this same time frame in 15 to 30 per cent of patients without a patent ductus arteriosus and with an intact ventricular septum. Systemic arterial hypoxemia, increased pulmonary blood flow, and pulmonary hypertension contribute to the development of pulmonary vascular obstruction in these patients as they do in other forms of congenital heart disease. Among the additional factors implicated in the accelerated and more widespread pulmonary vascular obstruction found in patients with complete transposition is the presence of extensive bronchopulmonary anastomotic channels, which enter the pulmonary vascular bed proximal to the pulmonary capillary bed; thus, oxygen tension is reduced at the precapillary level, causing pulmonary vasoconstriction.[528]

Beyond the early neonatal period many patients have an abnormal distribution pattern of pulmonary blood flow, with preferential flow to the right lung.[529] The asymmetrical distribution of pulmonary blood flow in these individuals results from an abnormal rightward inclination of the main pulmonary artery in the transposition malformation that favors flow from the main to the right pulmonary artery. Persistently increased pulmonary blood flow to the right lung would be expected to contribute to pulmonary vascular obstructive changes within the lung; in the left pulmonary vascular bed, thrombotic changes may occur because of the combination of reduced flow and polycythemia. Finally, it should be recognized that a prenatal alteration in pulmonary vascular smooth muscle may exist because blood perfusing the fetal lungs in complete transposition of great arteries has a higher than normal pO_2 and may serve to dilate pulmonary vessels in utero. Postnatally such vessels may have an enhanced capacity to constrict in response to vasoactive stimuli and suffer anatomical, obliterative changes.

CLINICAL FINDINGS. Average birthweight and size of infants born with complete transposition of the great arteries are greater than normal. The usual clinical manifestations are dyspnea and cyanosis from birth, progessive hypoxemia, and congestive heart failure. Early in postnatal life the clinical manifestations and course are influenced principally by the magnitude of intercirculatory mixing. The most severe cyanosis and hypoxemia are observed in infants with only a small patent foramen ovale or ductus arteriosus and an intact ventricular septum in whom mixing is inadequate, or in those infants with relatively reduced pulmonary blood flow because of left ventricular outflow tract obstruction.[530] With a large persistent patent ductus arteriosus or a large ventricular septal defect, cyanosis may be minimal and heart failure is the usual dominant problem after the first few weeks of life.[525] It should be recognized that a patent ductus arteriosus is present in about half of newborn infants with transposition, although it closes functionally and anatomically soon after birth in almost all cases. If the ductus arteriosus remains open, better mixing of the venous and arterial circulations usually is at the expense of pulmonary artery hypertension.[531]

Cardiac murmurs are of little diagnostic significance and are absent or insignificant in about 30 to 50 per cent of infants with complete transposition of the great arteries and an intact ventricular septum. In infants with a large persistent patent ductus arteriosus, fewer than half exhibit physical signs typical of ductus arteriosus, such as continuous murmur, bounding pulses, or a prominent mid-diastolic rumble. Moreover, *differential cyanosis* caused by reversed pulmonary-to-systemic shunting across the ductus arteriosus is difficult to detect because of generalized arterial desaturation. In those infants with a large ventricular septal defect, a pansystolic murmur usually emerges within the first 7 to 10 days of life. In newborns with transposition and severe pulmonic stenosis or atresia, the clinical findings are similar to those in the infant with tetralogy of Fallot.

ELECTROCARDIOGRAPHY AND ROENTGENOGRAPHY. The most usual *electrocardiographic findings* include right-axis deviation, right atrial enlargement, and right ventricular hypertrophy, reflecting that the right ventricle is the systemic pumping chamber. Combined ventricular hypertrophy may be present in those patients with a large ventricular septal defect and elevated pulmonary blood flow. Isolated left ventricular hypertrophy is encountered rarely in patients with a ventricular septal defect and a hypoplastic right ventricle, in many of whom the tricuspid valve is displaced abnormally and straddles a ventricular septal defect. In the first days of life the chest radiogram may appear normal, particularly in infants with an intact ventricular septum. Thereafter, roentgenographic findings often are highly suggestive of the diagnosis,[532] and consist of (1) progressive cardiac enlargement in early infancy; (2) a characteristic oval or egg-shaped cardiac configuration in the anteroposterior view, and a narrow vascular pedicle created by superimposition of the aortic and pulmonary artery segments; and (3) increased pulmonary vascular markings (Fig. 29–59). A right aortic arch is seen in about 4 per cent of infants with an intact ventricular septum and 11 per cent of infants with a ventricular septal defect.

CT scanning (see p. 342) and MR imaging (Fig. 10–20, p. 327) are also capable of establishing the diagnosis.

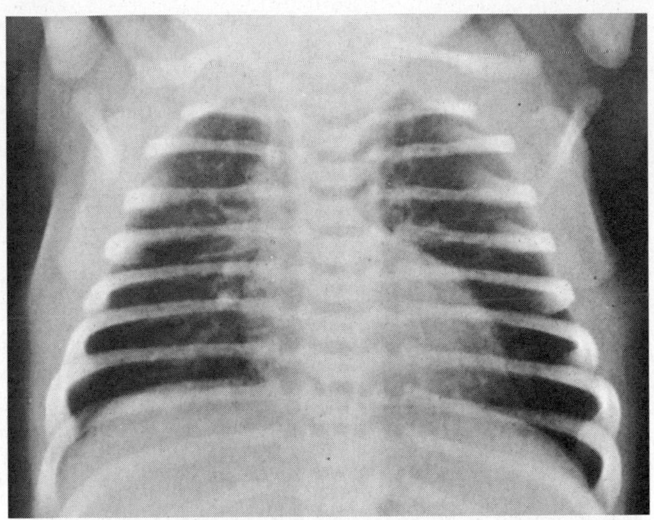

FIGURE 29–59. Chest roentgenogram in a 4-day-old infant with complete transposition of the great arteries showing an oval-shaped heart with a narrow base and increased pulmonary vascular markings.

ECHOCARDIOGRAPHY. Two-dimensional echocardiography is the procedure of choice in the diagnosis of complete transposition of the great arteries and the detection of significant associated cardiac anomalies[533–535] (Figs. 29–60 and 29–61). In sagittal cross sections the aorta is observed to ascend retrosternally, in contrast to the normal posterior sweep of the pulmonary artery. With transverse short-axis cross-sectional imaging, the diagnosis is confirmed by demonstrating that the anterior great artery (the aorta) is to the right of the posterior great artery (pulmonary) or that the two arteries are visualized side by side (Fig. 29–60). Moreover, from subcostal views (Fig. 29–61) the course of the two great arteries may be traced to delineate their ventricle of origin, demonstrating that the anterior rightward vessel (aorta) originates from the right ventricle and the posterior leftward vessel (pulmonary artery) originates from the left ventricle (Fig. 29–61). Echocardiography also may assist in identifying associated defects. Ventricular septal defects may be localized to the membranous, atrioventricular, and trabecular muscular septa, and malalignment types of ventricular septal defects may be identified if the infundibular septum is shifted either anteriorly or posteriorly.[536] A subaortic obstruction may be created by anterior shifting of the infundibular septum, whereas a posterior shift may narrow the subpulmonary area. The nature of left ventricular outflow tract obstruction may be further identified as a fixed obstruction caused by a fibromuscular ridge or as a dynamic obstruction caused by deviation of the interventricular septum toward the left ventricular cavity and the apposition between a thickened interventricular septum and systolic anterior motion of the mitral valve.

Ultrasound imaging may also be used to guide catheter placement and manipulation during balloon atrial septostomy and to assess the anatomical adequacy of the septostomy.

CARDIAC CATHETERIZATION AND ANGIOCARDIOGRAPHY. The major abnormal hemodynamic findings include right ventricular pressure at systemic levels and either a high or low left ventricular pressure, depending on pulmonary blood flow, pulmonary vascular resistance, and the presence or absence of left ventricular outflow tract obstructive lesions. Oxygen saturation in the aorta is lower than that in the pulmonary artery. Application of the Fick principle to the calculation of pulmonary and systemic blood flow rates in these patients is an important source of error. Assumed values of oxygen consumption are unreliable in the severely hypoxemic infant. Moreover, because systemic and

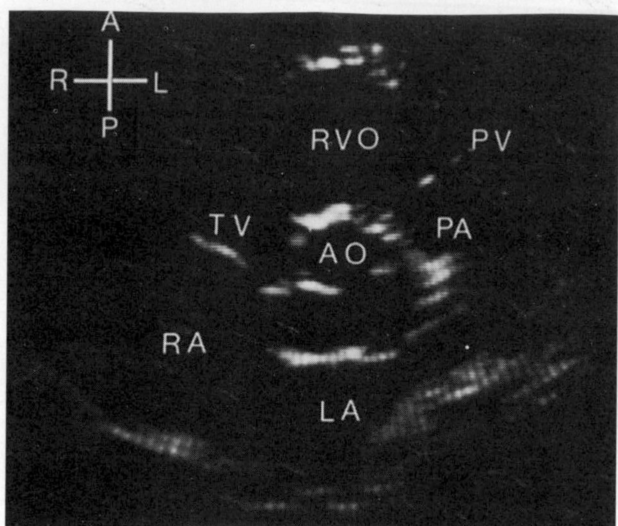

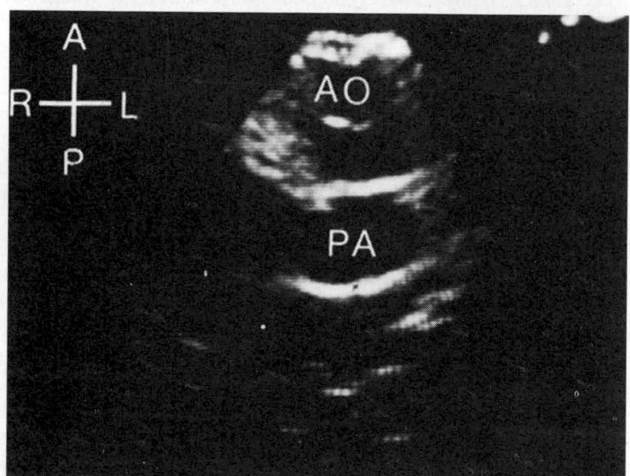

FIGURE 29–60. *Top,* A two-dimensional echocardiographic short-axis scan demonstrates normal great artery relations. The right ventricular outflow tract (RVO) wraps around the aorta (AO) in a clockwise manner. The pulmonic valve (PV) is to the left of the aortic valve. *Bottom,* Short-axis scan shows the abnormal great artery relations in an infant with transposition of the great arteries. The aorta (AO) is directly anterior and slightly to the right of the pulmonary artery (PA). The clockwise partial encirclement of the aorta by the right ventricular outflow tract is no longer observed. A = anterior, L = left, P = posterior, R = right, LA = left atrium, RA = right atrium, TV = tricuspid valve.

particularly pulmonary arteriovenous oxygen differences may be quite reduced, small errors in oxygen saturation values result in large errors in flow calculations. Furthermore, because bronchial collaterals enter the pulmonary circuit at the precapillary level, a true mixed pulmonary artery saturation cannot be sampled; pulmonary blood flow is therefore overestimated when one uses a sample from the central pulmonary artery, and pulmonary vascular resistance values often are underestimated.

Infants with simple, complete transposition of the great arteries who present in the first few weeks of life to a center prepared to correct the anomaly by the arterial switch operation (see below) often are taken to the operating room shortly after two-dimensional echocardiography and Doppler examination are performed.[535] In these cases, transcatheter balloon atrial septostomy is not performed unless a delay is expected in taking the patient to the operating room. In essentially all other patients, cardiac catheterization and balloon septostomy are components of the initial approach to the patient.

The diagnostic portion of the cardiac catheterization allows confirmation of the anatomical derangement of the great arteries and establishes the presence of associated lesions; in the newborn, unless prompt arterial switch repair is planned, it should always be accompanied by a palliative balloon atrial septostomy, which serves to enlarge the interatrial communication and improve oxygenation. In the older neonate, usually beyond age 3 weeks, thickening of the atrial septum may preclude satisfactory balloon septostomy. In those instances, transcatheter blade septostomy is the preferred approach to palliation. Two-dimensional echocardiography, with or without fluoroscopy, may be used as the imaging mode for both balloon and blade creation of an atrial septal defect.[536] Subcostal four-chamber and sagittal views image cardiac anatomy and catheter position during the procedure, substantially reducing radiation dosage.[537]

Both the diagnostic and the palliative procedures can be performed by percutaneous entry into the femoral vein, umbilical vein catheterization, or direct cutdown into the femoral or saphenous vein. The catheter passes easily across the foramen ovale into the left atrium and left ventricle and may be manipulated into the pulmonary artery by means of a flow-directed balloon-guided catheter or by manipulation of a standard catheter bent in the form of a J loop within the left ventricle, with the tip pointed posteriorly to the pulmonary artery. When a large ventricular septal defect is present, the catheter often can be manipulated directly across it from the right ventricle into the pulmonary artery.[538]

Selective Ventricular Angiography. This is diagnostic and demonstrates that the anteriorly placed aorta arises from the right ventricle and that the posteriorly placed pulmonary artery in continuity with the mitral valve arises from the left ventricle. The status of the ductus arteriosus and the site and size of a ventricular septal defect can be well visualized by angiography. Interventricular defects posterior and inferior to the crista supraventricularis occur in about half of these patients; less often the defects are anterior and superior to the crista supraventricularis or are of the atrioventricular septal type.[539] A variety of lesions may be identified as the cause of left ventricular outflow tract obstruction, including ventricular septal hypertrophy with systolic anterior movement of the mitral valve, discrete or tunnel fibromuscular subpulmonic stenosis, valvular and supravalvular stenosis, and, rarely, an aneurysm of the membranous ventricular septum or redundant tricuspid valve tissue protruding through a ventricular septal defect.

Both angiographic and echocardiographic imaging may be required to detect the coronary arterial patterns that are seen in patients with complete transposition of the great arteries.[540–542a] In the majority, the left coronary artery originates in the left sinus and the right coronary artery originates in the posterior sinus, with a single ostium above both the left and the posterior sinus. In almost 20 per cent of patients the left circumflex artery arises as a branch of the right coronary artery; a single coronary artery is present in about 6 per cent; in 3 to 4 per cent of patients either the right coronary and anterior descending arteries originate in the left sinus, with the left circumflex originating in the posterior sinus, or two ostia are present above one sinus, one giving rise to the right and the other to the left coronary artery. To avoid the danger of excision during transfer of the coronary arteries as part of the arterial switch corrective operation, the intramural course of the left coronary artery or the left anterior descending coronary artery should be identified, a finding in up to 5 per cent of patients. An intramural course should be assumed when the vessel has an aberrant origin from the right sinus or when it is in intimate relationship with the commissure between the right and left sinuses and courses between the great arteries.[542]

MANAGEMENT. Medical treatment often is of limited help but should be vigorous because both functional and anatomical corrections of the malformation achieve good results. Conservative measures include the use of oxygen,

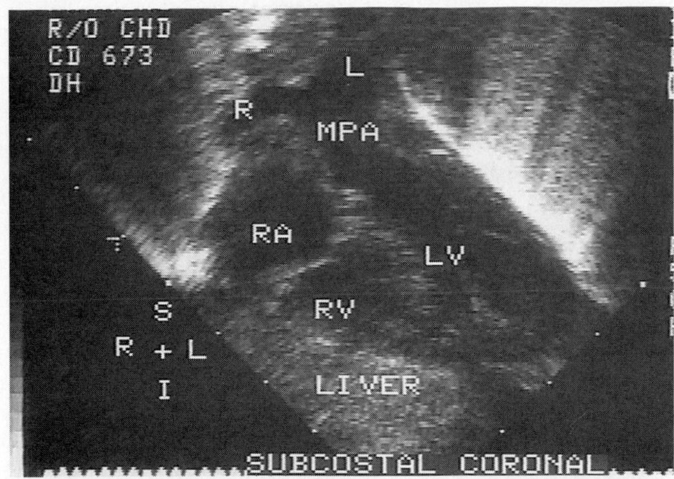

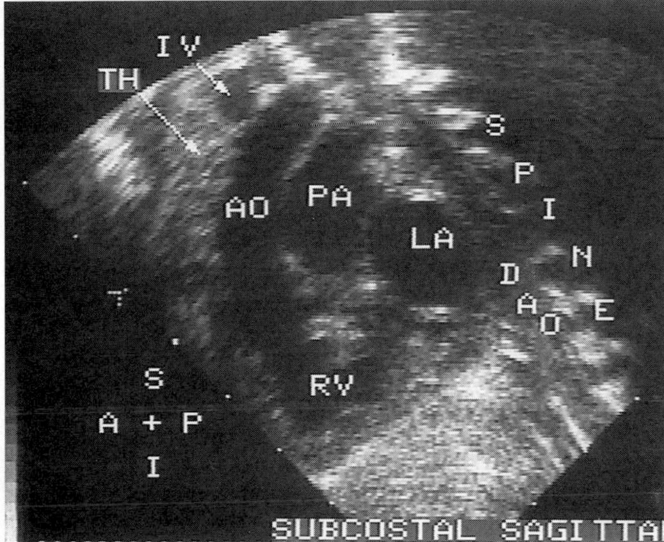

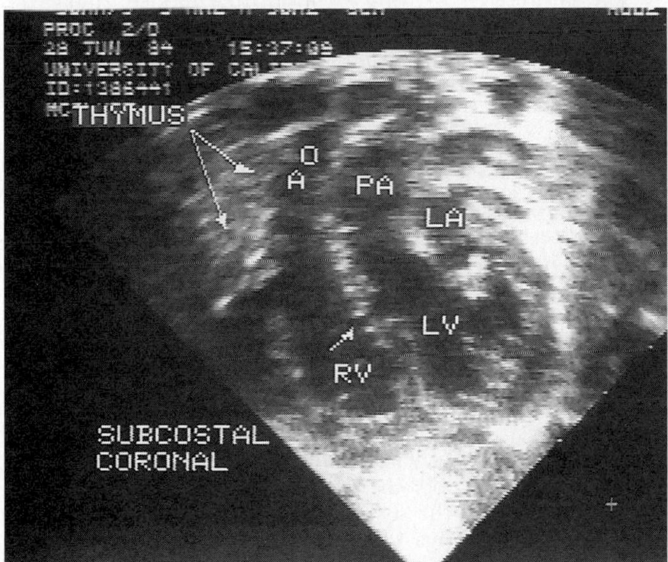

FIGURE 29–61. Composite subcostal views of transposition of the great arteries. *Top,* Subcostal coronal view showing the main pulmonary artery (MPA) arising directly from the left ventricle (LV) and dividing into the right (R) and left (L) pulmonary arteries. The right atrium (RA) and right ventricle (RV) lie adjacent in this view to the liver. *Middle,* The scan plane has been rotated 90 degrees clockwise (note the change in spatial orientation and the position of the spine). The thymus (TH) is seen anteriorly, and the innominate vein (IV) lies anterior to the aortic arch. The right ventricle (RV) lies anteriorly above the diaphragm and behind the thymus and gives rise to the aorta (AO), its arch, and the descending aorta (DAO). The main pulmonary artery (PA) lies in the crux of the aortic arch. *Bottom,* An intermediate subcostal view, lying oblique in a plane between the top two panels. The entire ventriculoarterial connection is imaged in this plane, showing the right ventricle connecting to the aortic arch, a small ventricular septal defect (VSD) indicated by the small arrow, and the pulmonary artery (PA) arising from the left ventricle (LV). The left atrium (LA) can be seen below the pulmonary artery. (Courtesy of Norman Silverman, M.D.)

digitalis, diuretics, iron (if an associated iron-deficiency anemia is present), and intravenous sodium bicarbonate for severe hypoxemic metabolic acidosis. Dilatation of the ductus arteriosus by prostaglandin E_1 in the early neonatal period both augments pulmonary blood flow and enhances intercirculatory mixing.

Atrial Septostomy. The creation or enlargement of an interatrial communication is the simplest procedure for providing increased intracardiac mixing of systemic and pulmonary venous blood; preferably this is achieved by rupturing the valve of the foramen ovale by balloon catheter during transseptal catheterization of the left side of the heart (Rashkind's procedure), or by blade septostomy. Surgical atrial septectomy seldom is required. The balloon should be inflated to a diameter of about 15 mm before pullback to the right atrium. Salutary results consist of a fall in left atrial pressure, equalization of mean left and right atrial pressures, and an increase in the systemic arterial oxygen saturation. When the foramen ovale is stretched by the balloon without accomplishing rupture of the septum primum valve of the fossa ovalis, the improvement in oxygenation is short-lived. Infusion or reinfusion intravenously of prostaglandin E_1 (0.05 to 0.1 mg/kg/min) has been shown to improve systemic oxygenation temporarily in the latter situation, by dilating the ductus arteriosus and thereby facilitating intercirculatory mixing.[96] Although balloon atrial septostomy usually is successful in stabilizing the infant's condition and allowing survival in the neonatal period, the initial rise in systemic arterial oxyen saturation to 65 to 75 per cent often is not sustained beyond 6 to 9 months of age.

SURGICAL TREATMENT

The development of *corrective operations* for infants born with transposition of the great arteries has greatly improved prognosis.[543,544]

ATRIAL (VENOUS) SWITCH OPERATION. This correction, by the *Mustard* technique, is accomplished by excision of the interatrial septum and creation of a new interatrial septum with a pericardial baffle diverting the systemic venous return into the left ventricle through the mitral valve and thence to the left ventricle and pulmonary artery, while the pulmonary venous blood is diverted through the tricuspid valve and right ventricle to the aorta.[545,545a] The *Senning* procedure is based on a similar principle and consists of diversion of left pulmonary venous blood by a coronary sinus flap and rerouting of caval flow by the use of an atrial wall flap.[546]

After physiological correction by atrial switch, postoperative complications are observed that are directly related to the intraatrial repair (shunts across the intraatrial patch and obstruction to either systemic or pulmonary venous return or both).[547–550] There is a high incidence of early and late postoperative dysrhythmias that are more likely to have their basis in injury to the sinoatrial node and/or its arterial supply than in disruption of internodal tracts or damage to the atrioventricular node.[551] Tricuspid regurgitation is a less common complication of operation and may be related in some patients to a preexisting abnormality of the tricuspid valve, whereas in most it is related to right ventricular dysfunction. Although the assessment of right ventricular contractility is difficult, the right ventricular pump function appears to be impaired before Mustard operation and does not return to normal after successful surgery.[552–554] It seems likely that the right ventricle can perform as a systemic pumping chamber for the duration of a normal life span.

ARTERIAL SWITCH OPERATION. A one-stage anatomical correction is now the approach of choice in major centers that care for infants with congenital heart disease.[555–557] In this operation both coronary arteries are transposed to the posterior artery; the aorta and pulmonary arteries are transsected, contraposed, and anastomosed (Jatene operation) (Fig. 29–62). The arterial switch anatomical correction may be complicated by coronary ostial stenosis, acquired supravalvular aortic and/or pulmonary stenosis, and pulmonic and/or aortic incompetence. The major advantages of the arterial switch procedure,

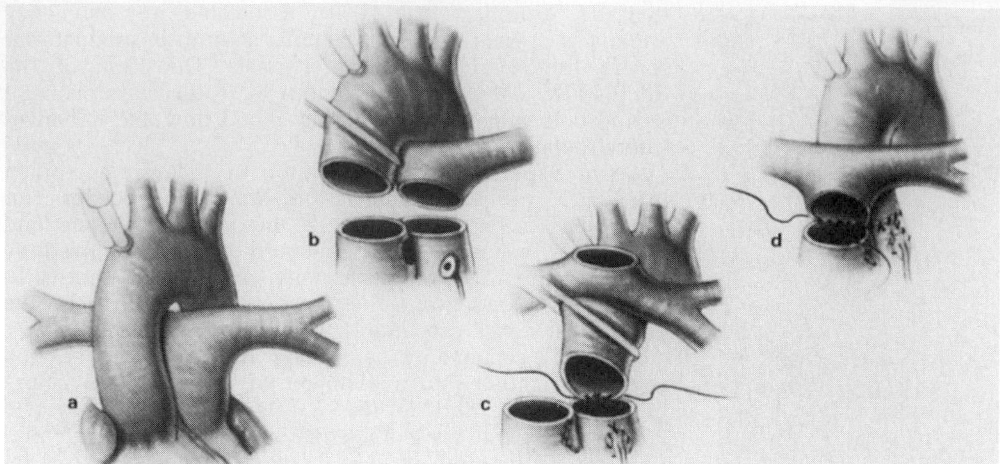

FIGURE 29–62. Complete transposition of the great arteries, corrected by a modified arterial switch operation. The aorta and pulmonary artery are transected and the orifices of the coronary arteries are excised with a rim of adjacent aortic wall (b). The aorta is brought under the bifurcation of the pulmonary artery, and the proximal pulmonary artery and the aorta are anastomosed without necessitating graft interposition. The coronary arteries are transferred to the pulmonary artery (c). The mobilized pulmonary artery is directly anastomosed to the proximal aortic stump (d). (From Stark, J., and DeLaval, M.: Surgery for Congenital Heart Defects. New York, Grune and Stratton, 1983, p. 379.)

when compared with the atrial switch procedure, are the restoration of the left ventricle as the systemic pump and the potential for long-term maintenance of sinus rhythm.[558–561]

Within the first month of life the arterial switch operation may be performed as a single-stage repair. In such patients, the origin and branching patterns of the coronary arteries are defined reliably preoperatively by two-dimensional echocardiography.[525] In older infants it appears necessary to prepare the left ventricle to withstand the systemic pressure that is produced after switching the great arteries because, if the ventricular septum is intact, left ventricular pressure and left ventricular wall thickness diminish normally in relation to the postnatal reduction in pulmonary artery pressure. In these infants a two-stage approach is used, the first of which consists of banding the pulmonary artery; the arterial switch is performed soon thereafter, in some centers as early as 1 to 2 weeks later.[562,563]

In the unusual infant with an intact ventricular septum and a significant patent ductus arteriosus, an early neonatal arterial switch corrective operation with closure of the ductus is indicated. The optimal management of patients with a large ventricular septal defect is a one-stage intraarterial switch anatomical correction as early in life as possible.

In some patients after early arterial repair of transposition of the great arteries, abnormally enlarged bronchial arteries are identified at postoperative catheterization and they explain continuous murmurs or persistent cardiomegaly. When these vessels are large enough to produce a volume load to the systemic ventricle, catheter-directed coil embolization is indicated.[564] Follow-up studies after the arterial switch operation have demonstrated good left ventricular function and normal exercise capacity. Potential sequelae of the operation include supravalvular pulmonary stenosis, which may be treated either by reoperation or balloon angioplasty, supravalvular aortic stenosis, and neo–aortic regurgitation, usually mild.[565,566] Long-term patency and growth of the coronary arteries appear satisfactory.[557–570] Infants with transposition of the great arteries plus a ventricular septal defect and left ventricular outflow tract obstruction may require a systemic–pulmonary artery anastomosis when a pronounced diminution in pulmonary blood flow exists. A later corrective procedure for these patients bypasses the left ventricular outflow obstruction and uses an intracardiac ventricular baffle connecting the left ventricle to the aorta and an extracardiac prosthetic conduit between the right ventricle and the distal end of a divided pulmonary artery (Rastelli procedure).[571] An alternative approach (the Lecompte procedure) couples an intraventricular tunnel and the arterial switch operation, avoiding the use of an extracardiac conduit.[572]

In patients with significant pulmonary vascular obstructive disease the risk associated with definitive repair (anatomical correction or intraatrial baffle and closure of the ventricular septal defect) is great. In this group of patients a "palliative" Mustard or Senning procedure leaving the ventricular septal defect open often provides good, short-term, symptomatic improvement by increasing arterial oxygen tension and reducing the stimulus to progressive polycythemia.[573]

Congenitally Corrected Transposition of the Great Arteries

This term is applied to two distinctly different anomalies: anatomically corrected transposition or malposition of the great arteries and physiologically corrected levo- or L-transposition of the great arteries.

MORPHOLOGY. Anatomically corrected malposition of the great arteries is a rare form of congenital heart disease in which the great arteries are abnormally related to each other and to the ventricles but arise, nonetheless, above the anatomically correct ventricles.[574,575] Because of this, the term *malposition,* rather than *transposition,* is preferable. The anomaly results from either leftward looping of the ventricular segment of the embryonic heart tube in the situs solitus heart, or rightward looping in the situs inversus heart. In this unusual malformation the aorta is anterior and to the left (levo- or L-malposition) and the pulmonary artery is posteromedial and to the right, presumably because of a subaortic conus which causes mitral-aortic discontinuity.

When no other defect exists, the circulation proceeds normally. When an associated lesion prompts echocardiographic examination, the diagnosis is indicated by the finding of atrioventricular concordance in association with wide mitral-aortic discontinuity with an anteriorly placed aorta. At cardiac catheterization, the diagnosis of the abnormal relation between the great arteries may be made by biplane angiocardiography. Anomalies commonly associated with anatomically corrected malposition of the great arteries include ventricular septal defect, left juxtaposition of the atrial appendages, tricuspid atresia or stenosis, and valvular and subvalvular pulmonic stenosis.

DEFINITION. Invariably, the term *congenitally corrected transposition* is applied to the heart in which a functional correction of the circulation exists by virtue of the relation between the ventricles and great arteries.[576,577] Corrected or L-transposition occurs when the primitive cardiac tube loops to the left, instead of to the right, during embryogenesis. The anatomical right ventricle comes to lie on the left and receives oxygenated blood from the left atrium; this blood is ejected into an anteriorly placed, left-sided aorta. The anatomical left ventricle lies to the right and connects the right atrium to a posteriorly placed pulmonary artery. Thus, there are both ventriculoarterial and atrioventricular discordant connections, with ventricular inversion. This arrangement of the great arteries and ventricles (in contrast to the uncorrected, complete, or D-transposition) permits functional correction, so that systemic venous blood passes into the pulmonary trunk while arterialized pulmonary venous blood flows into the aorta. In the heart with congenitally corrected transposition, the venae cavae and coronary sinus drain into a right atrium that is normal in position and structure.

PHYSIOLOGY. Venous blood flows from the right atrium, designated as the "venous atrium," across an atrioventricular valve that has the structure of a normal mitral valve and into the right-sided "venous ventricle." The venous ventricle, however, has the morphological characteristics of a normal left ventricle; i.e., its interior lining is trabeculated, it has no crista supraventricularis, and the atrioventricular valve is in continuity with the posteriorly placed semilunar valve. It ejects blood into the pulmonary trunk, which arises posterior to the ascending aorta. Oxygenated blood returns from the lungs to the left atrium, which is normal in position and structure; from there it flows into the left-sided "arterial ventricle" across an atrioventricular valve that has the structure of a normal tricuspid valve. The interior lining of the arterial ventricle has the morphological characteristics of a normal right ventricle (i.e., it has coarse trabeculations and a crista supraventricularis), and the tricuspid atrioventricular valve is not in continuity with the anteriorly placed semilunar valve. The arterial ventricle ejects blood into the aorta, which arises anterior to the pulmonary trunk. In addition to inversion of the cardiac ventricles, there is inversion of the conduction system and coronary arteries. Commonly associated anatomical lesions include atrial and ventricular septal defects, often accompanied by valvular or subvalvular pulmonary stenosis; single ventricle with an outlet chamber with or without pulmonic stenosis; left atrioventricular valve regurgitation, usually because of an Ebstein's malformation of the left-sided tricuspid valve; and abnormalities of visceral and atrial situs.[578]

CLINICAL MANIFESTATIONS. The clinical presentation, course, and prognosis of patients with congenital functionally corrected transposition vary, depending on the nature and severity of the complicating intracardiac anomalies.[579,579a] Patients in whom corrected transposition exists as an isolated anomaly present no functional alterations and have no symptoms. Asymptomatic children with an increase in the size of the systemic ventricle, due to significant left-to-right shunting or tricuspid regurgitation, usually develop symptoms of systemic ventricular dysfunction by the third or fourth decade.[580]

The *physical findings* in congenitally corrected transposition are those of the associated lesions with two exceptions: (1) a single accentuated second heart sound usually is present in the second left intercostal space, representing closure of the aortic valve lying lateral and anterior to the pulmonic valve; and (2) there is a high incidence of cardiac dysrhythmias.

LABORATORY EXAMINATION. Because of the inversion of the heart's conduction system, the *electrocardiogram* may provide important clues in the diagnosis. An abnormal direction of initial (septal) depolarization from right to left causes leftward, anterior, and superior orientation of the initial QRS forces and reversal of the precordial Q-wave pattern (Q waves are present in the right precordial leads and absent in the left). In addition to inversion of the conduction system, the His bundle is elongated because of the greater distance between the atrioventricular node and the base of the ventricular septum.[581] The His bundle is located beneath the pulmonic valve in the position of mitral pulmonary continuity; thus, it is subject to significant excursions during mitral valve closure. This arrangement may be a causal factor in the arrhythmias and atrioventricular conduction disturbances commonly observed in these patients. First-degree atrioventricular (AV) block occurs in about 50 per cent, and complete AV block occurs in 10 to 15 per cent of patients. Other degrees of AV dissociation may be observed as well as paroxysmal supraventricular tachycardia and ventricular extrasystoles. In some patients, Kent bundle connections provide the anatomical substrate for preexcitation.[582]

Roentgenographic examination characteristically reveals absence of the normal pulmonary artery segment and a smooth convexity of the left supracardiac border produced by the displaced ascending aorta (Fig. 7–45, p. 233). The latter may be visualized by radionuclide scintillation scans of the central circulation. The main pulmonary trunk is medially displaced and absent from the cardiac silhouette; the right pulmonary hilus often is prominent and elevated compared with the left, producing a right-sided "waterfall" appearance.

Two-dimensional echocardiography seeks to identify the morphology of each ventricle by defining the characteristics of the inflow and outflow tracts and papillary and trabecular muscle morphology, ventricular shape, and great artery position.[583] By tracing the great arteries back to their ventricles of origin in subxiphoid and parasternal short-axis planes, one would find that the anterior leftward great artery (the aorta) arises from the left-sided ventricle and is not in continuity with the left-sided atrioventricular valve. The great arteries exit the heart in parallel fashion; the position, origin, and branching pattern of the great arteries are observed in subxiphoid and suprasternal views, while the anteroposterior and right-left positions of the great arteries can be seen from the parasternal short-axis view. Because the ventricular septum lies in the anteroposterior plane parallel to the echo beam, it may not be visualized from a left parasternal view. In apical-basal or subxiphoid, four-chamber echocardiographic views, the right and left ventricular morphology and the inverted position of the atrioventricular valves may be ascertained correctly. The latter views also demonstrate the level of attachment of the atrioventricular valves and allow detection of inferior displacement of the left-sided tricuspid valve when Ebstein's anomaly coexists.

At *cardiac catheterization* the diagnosis should be suspected when the venous catheter enters a posterior and midline main pulmonary trunk. Retrograde arterial catheter passage establishes the typical position of the ascending aorta at the upper left cardiac border. Hemodynamic abnormalities depend on the lesions associated with corrected transposition. Selective *angiocardiography* allows visualization of the transposed great arteries and morphological differentiation of the two ventricles (Fig. 29–63). The ventricles usually lie side by side, with the ventricular septum oriented in an anteroposterior direction. Selective aortography demonstrates the inverted coronary arterial pattern that is invariably present in corrected transposition. The competence of the left atrioventricular valve may be determined by injection of contrast material into the arterial ventricle.[584] When a left-sided Ebstein's malformation exists, the leaflets are displaced distal to the true valve annulus. The level of the annulus may be determined by visualization of the circumflex branch of the left coronary artery, which courses posteriorly in the AV groove.

Specific problems have attended operative repair of the lesions associated with congenitally corrected transposition, owing primarily to the course of the atrioventricular conduction system and the coronary arterial pattern.[585–587] Intraoperative electrophysiological mapping of the course of the conduction system has been proposed to reduce, but not abolish, the risk of surgically induced heart block. The AV bundle is located anteriorly and in relation to the anterolateral quadrant of the pulmonary outflow tract. Thus, when a ventricular septal defect is present, the bundle usually is related to the anterior and superior margins of the defect and lies beneath the pulmonic valve. In corrected transposition, the coronary arteries have a course appropriate to their ventricles; i.e., the anterior descending and circumflex arteries supply the morphological left ventricle, and the right coronary artery supplies the morphological right ventricle. However, because the great arteries are transposed, the noncoronary sinus is the anterior sinus of the aortic valve.

The inversion of the coronary arterial system occasionally may limit and preclude an incision into the venous ventricle, thereby interfering with exposure of intracardiac defects in the usual manner. The disadvantage in approaching intracardiac anomalies using an incision in the morphological right ventricle is that this is the systemic ventricle. When significant pulmonary stenosis exists within a ventricular septal defect, a valved extracardiac conduit often is a required part of the surgical repair. Surgical risks are especially high in patients in whom significant regurgitation exists from the arterial ventricle to the arterial atrium. In these patients, annuloplasty, or more usually valve replacement, is required. In all operative approaches, if complete heart block has been present intermittently or permanently preoperatively or intraoperatively, permanent epicardial atrial and ventricular pacemaker leads are implanted.

Double-Outlet Right Ventricle

MORPHOLOGY. Other designations applied to this lesion include origin of both great arteries from the right ventricle, partial transposition, complete transposition of the aorta and levo-position of the pulmonary artery, complete dextroposition of the aorta, and the Taussig-Bing complex. This is an extremely heterogeneous category of malformations in which an abnormal relation exists between the aorta and the pulmonary trunk, which arise wholly or in large part from the right ventricle.[588]

DEFINITIONS. A uniform definition or classification of double-outlet right ventricle does not exist. To some, double-outlet right ventricle means origin of one great artery and at least 50 per cent of the other over the right ventricle; others require the presence of bilateral conus muscle between both great arteries and the atrioventricular annulus. One or both great arteries may arise from an infundibular chamber; there may be considerable variability in the amount of subarterial conus muscle. Thus, the semilunar valves may lie side by side, or with the pulmonary valve more anterior and superior, or with a more anterior and superior aortic valve. Commonly, neither semilunar valve is in fibrous continuity with either atrioventricular valve, and usually a ventricular septal defect is present and represents the

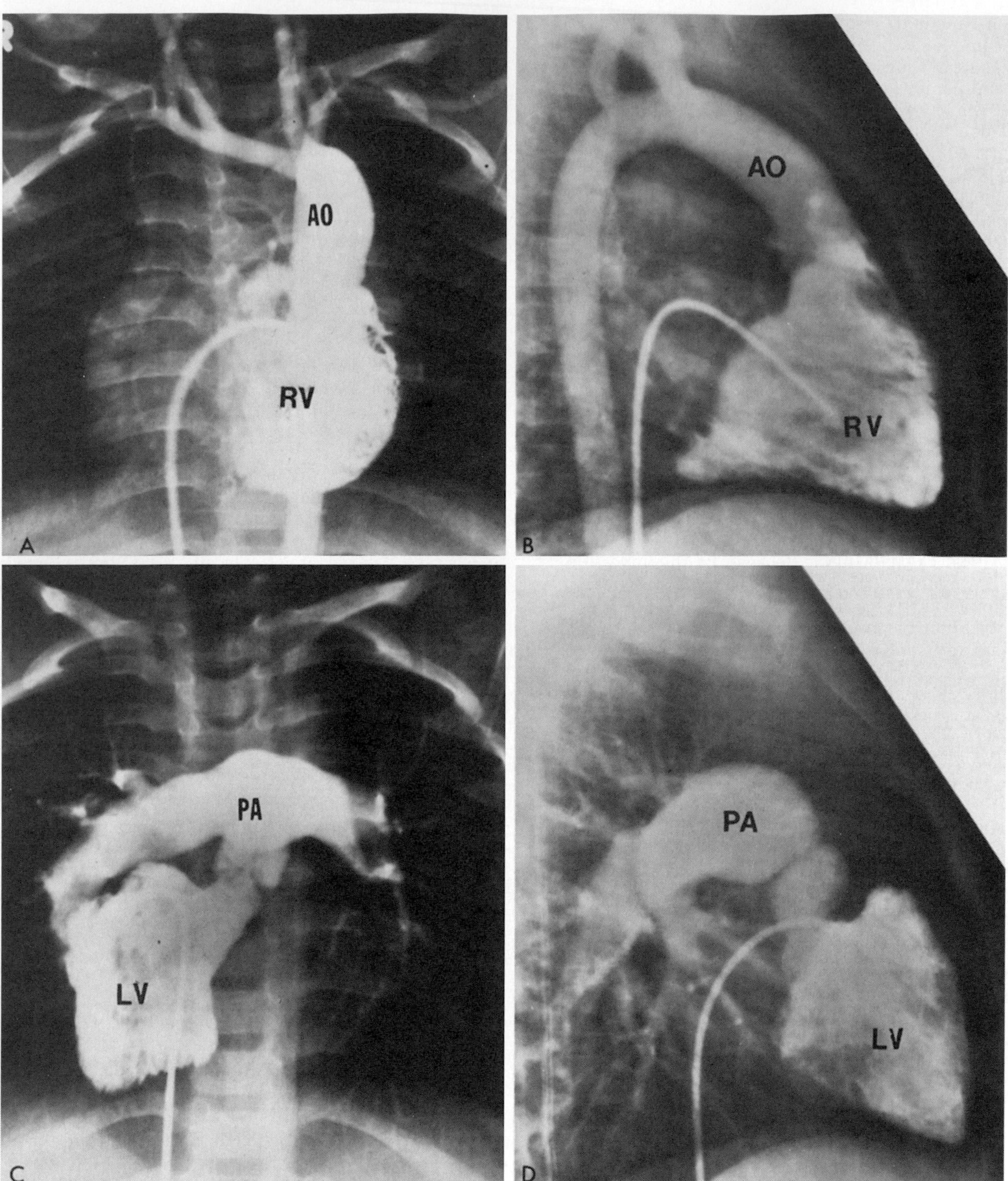

FIGURE 29–63. Congenitally corrected (levo-)transposition of the great arteries in a 4-year-old boy. *A*, Anteroposterior ventriculogram in left-sided ventricle with mesocardia. The morphological right ventricle (RV) is left-sided, indicating an L-ventricular loop (inverted ventricles in *situs solitus*). The aorta (AO) originates above the morphological right ventricle and is thus transposed and in classic levo-transposition. *B*, Lateral ventriculogram in left-sided ventricle (same frame as *A*). The aorta originates anteriorly above the morphological right ventricle (RV). *C*, Anteroposterior ventriculogram in right-sided morphological left ventricle (LV). The transposed pulmonary artery (PA) arises from this ventricle, and the ventricular septum appears intact. Pulmonic valve thickening is also evident. The aorta (*A*) is to the left of the pulmonary artery. Note that the ventricular septum in the L-ventricular loop is visualized best in the anteroposterior views. *D*, Lateral ventriculogram in right-sided ventricle (same frame as *C*). The pulmonary artery is posterior to the aorta, and supravalvular pulmonic narrowing is seen. (Reproduced with permission from Freedom, R. M., et al.: The differential diagnosis of levo-transposed or malposed aorta. An angiocardiographic study. Circulation *50*:1040, 1974. Copyright 1974 the American Heart Association.)

only outlet from the left ventricle. The ventricular septal defect is of the malalignment type because the infundibular septum is positioned abnormally.

When the amount of conus muscle beneath the two great arteries varies, the ventricular septal defect commonly is positioned beneath the more posterior semilunar valve, which in fact usually overrides the interventricular septum through this ventricular septal defect. The amount of conus muscle underneath the valve determines the position of the semilunar root in relation to the ventricles below. Thus double-outlet right ventricle resides within the spectrum of conotruncal abnormalities ranging from tetralogy of Fallot to transposition of the great arteries. The ventricular septal defect occasion-

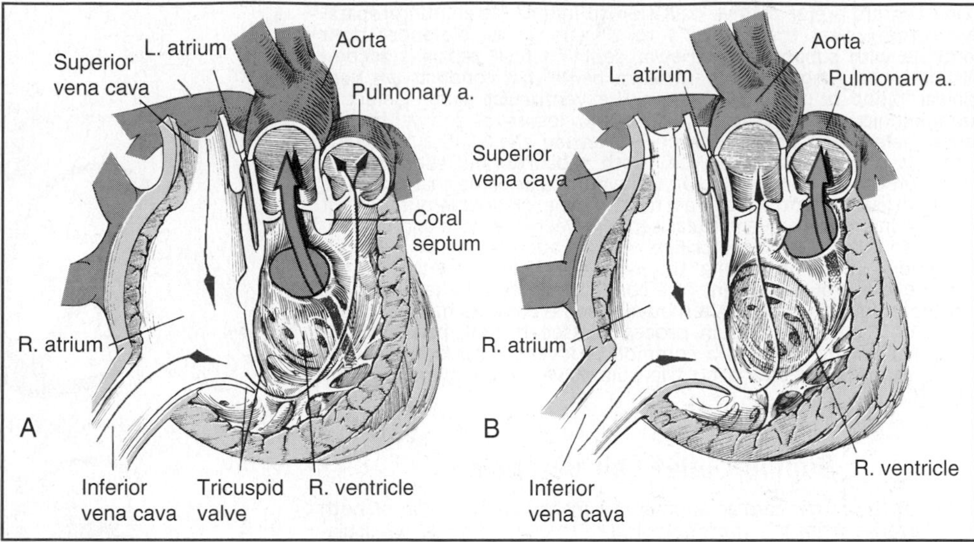

FIGURE 29–64. Double-outlet right ventricle (RV) with side-by-side relation of great arteries is illustrated in both panels. A subaortic ventricular septal defect (VSD) below the crista supraventricularis *(left)* favors delivery of left ventricular blood to the aorta *(A)*. Subpulmonary location of the VSD above the crista *(right)* favors streaming to the pulmonary trunk *(B)*. (From Castaneda, A., et al.: Cardiac Surgery of the Neonate and Infant. Philadelphia, W.B. Saunders Company, 1994, p. 446.)

ally extends beneath both great arteries and is referred to as doubly committed. In some instances, the ventricular septal defect is remote to both great arteries, or is considered uncommitted, in which case the defect often lies in the inlet or muscular portion of the interventricular septum.

ASSOCIATED LESIONS. More than half of patients with double-outlet right ventricle have associated anomalies of the right atrioventricular valves.[588] Mitral atresia associated with a hypoplastic left ventricle is common; less often observed are tricuspid stenosis, Ebstein's anomaly of the tricuspid valve, complete atrioventricular septal defect, and overriding or straddling of either atrioventricular valve. Aortic coarctation may be associated with double-outlet right ventricle, particularly when the subaortic area is narrowed by malalignment of the infundibular septum. Double-outlet right ventricle also may be a component of the multiple cardiovascular anomalies of the splenic dysgenesis or heterotaxy syndromes. An increased incidence of the anomaly occurs in infants with the trisomy 18 syndrome.

The pathological features in most patients include side-by-side pulmonic and aortic valves and discontinuity between the mitral and aortic valves. The latter exists because muscular infundibulum is usual beneath both semilunar valves. The ventricular septal defect may be remote from or closely related to one or both semilunar valves (Fig. 29–64).[588] When the interventricular defect is subpulmonic, with or without a straddling pulmonary trunk, the complex is designated "Taussig-Bing." In most patients the interventricular septal defect is below the crista supraventricularis and is subaortic in location. Least often the defect either is remote from both semilunar valves ("uncommitted") or underlies both ("doubly committed").

CLINICAL MANIFESTATIONS. The clinical and physiological picture is determined by the size and location of the ventricular septal defect and the presence or absence of pulmonic stenosis. In the Taussig-Bing form of double-outlet right ventricle, the malformation resembles physiologically and clinically complete transposition with ventricular septal defect and pulmonary hypertension. When the ventricular septal defect is subaortic, the stream of blood from the left ventricle is directed preferentially to the aorta. Thus, there may be little or no detectable cyanosis, and these patients usually clinically resemble those with an isolated, large ventricular septal defect and pulmonary hypertension.

The most important determinant of the natural history in both these types of double-outlet right ventricle is the progression of pulmonary vascular obstruction. In contrast, when there is pulmonary outflow tract obstruction, which often is severe and found commonly in these patients in whom the ventricular septal defect is subaortic, clinical findings are similar to those of cyanotic tetralogy of Fallot. In some patients, especially without pulmonic stenosis, the electrocardiogram shows a superiorly oriented counterclockwise frontal plane QRS loop in addition to right ventricular hypertrophy.[589] The pattern appears to result from relative hypoplasia of the anterosuperior left bundle and preferential activation of the posteroinferior left ventricular wall. The presence of the latter electrocardiographic pattern in patients with double-outlet right ventricle should raise the possibility of a coexistent atrioventricular septal defect or abnormality of the mitral valve.

DIAGNOSIS. Two-dimensional *echocardiography* may reliably distinguish double-outlet right ventricle from other lesions causing cyanosis, such as tetralogy of Fallot and transposition of the great arteries.[590] The three key imaging features are origin of both great arteries from the anterior right ventricle, mitral-semilunar valve discontinuity, and absence of left ventricular outflow other than the ventricular septal defect. The relative anteroposterior positions of the great arteries can be determined from the parasternal short-axis view. The parasternal long-axis view shows the position of the more posterior semilunar root relative to the interventricular septum and anterior mitral leaflet and is the best view for demonstrating the presence of subarterial conus muscle. Subxiphoid views best demonstrate the position of both great arteries over the ventricles. Each great artery is displayed on long- and short-axis subxiphoid sweeps.

In reporting echocardiographic results, it is imperative to state each component's anatomical feature, i.e., the position of both great arteries, the presence and amount of infundibulum under each semilunar valve, the anatomy of both subpulmonary and subaortic outflow tracts, the position and size of the associated ventricular septal defect, and the presence of all other associated lesions, particularly atrioventricular valve anomalies and coarctation of the aorta.

In each of the different types of double-outlet right ventricle, precise delineation of the malformation also depends on careful angiocardiographic analysis. The diagnosis can be established with confidence when the angiographic findings include simultaneous opacification of both great vessels from the right ventricle, aortic and pulmonic valves at the same transverse level, and separation of the aortic valve from the aortic leaflet of the mitral valve by the crista supraventricularis (Fig. 29–65).[591] The position of the ventricular septal defect and the relation between the great arteries must be defined to plan surgical procedures appropriately.

Experience is growing with the application of transesophageal echocardiography in analyzing the complex anatomical and spatial relationships encountered in double-outlet right ventricle, requiring a biplane or multiplane format for adequate assessment.

SURGICAL TREATMENT. The goals of operative treatment are to establish left ventricle-to-aorta continuity, create adequate right ventricle–to-pulmonary continuity and repair associated lesions.[592] Because of the complexity of intracardiac repair of these anomalies,

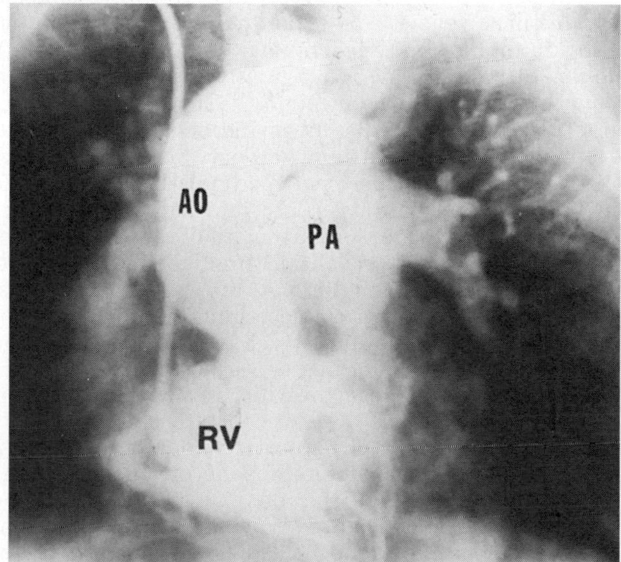

FIGURE 29–65. Simultaneous opacification of both great arteries from a right ventricular injection of contrast material in a patient with double-outlet right ventricle (RV). The aortic and pulmonic valves are at the same transverse level. AO = aorta, PA = pulmonary artery. (Courtesy of Robert White, M.D.)

many centers prefer to give palliation to infants, attempting reparative surgery after the age of 1 to 2 years. In double-outlet right ventricle with subaortic ventricular septal defect, repair is accomplished by creating an intraventricular baffle that conducts left ventricular blood to the aorta. When the ventricular septal defect is subpulmonic, repair is accomplished by closure of the ventricular septal defect and arterial switch.[592,593] When the ventricular septal defect is doubly committed, i.e., both subaortic and subpulmonic, operation consists of creating an intraventricular baffle that conducts left ventricular blood to the aorta. The type of double-outlet right ventricle in which the ventricular septal defect is remote and uncommitted to either semilunar orifice may be approached by a venous switch operation, permitting the right ventricle to eject into the aorta, followed by placement of a conduit between the left ventricle and the pulmonary trunk. Alternatively, some patients may be candidates for a modified Fontan procedure (see p. 933), particularly if additional findings include a common atrioventricular orifice, hypoplastic ventricles, a straddling tricuspid valve, or a straddling mitral valve.[594]

Double-Outlet Left Ventricle

One of the rarest cardiac anomalies consists of the origin of both great arteries from the morphological left ventricle. Conal musculature or an infundibulum usually is absent or deficient beneath the orifices of both semilunar valves.[595] A broad spectrum of associated malformations exists. A ventricular septal defect and valvular or subvalvular pulmonic stenosis have been present in most patients. Supportive diagnostic information is provided by magnetic resonance imaging.[596] Echocardiographic[597] and angiocardiographic assessment of the spatial relations of the origins of the great arteries is essential to an accurate diagnosis and to evaluating the possibility of operative repair. In most patients, the latter consists of closure of the ventricular septal defect and placement of a right ventricle–pulmonary artery conduit.

Total Anomalous Pulmonary Venous Connection

This anomaly has been estimated to account for 1 to 3 per cent of all cases of congenital heart disease and 2 per cent of deaths therefrom in the first year of life.[403,598] The anomaly is the result of persistence during embryogenesis of communications between the pulmonary portion of the foregut plexus and the cardinal or umbilicovitelline system of veins, resulting in the connection of all the pulmonary veins either to the right atrium directly or to the systemic veins and their tributaries. Because all venous blood returns to the right atrium, an interatrial communication is an integral part of this malformation. Additional major cardiac malformations occur in about 30 per cent of patients.[598] Among these are common atrium, single ventricle, truncus arteriosus, and anomalies of the systemic veins. Extracardiac malformations, particularly of the alimentary, endocrine, and genitourinary systems, are present in 25 to 30 per cent of cases.

MORPHOLOGY. The anatomical varieties of total anomalous pulmonary venous connection may be subdivided, depending on the level of the abnormal drainage (Fig. 29–66). Table 29–10 provides average figures of the distribution of the sites of anomalous connection.[403] The anomalous connection usually is supradiaphragmatic and to the left brachiocephalic vein, right atrium, coronary sinus, or superior vena cava. In about 13 per cent, particularly in males, the distal site of connection is below the diaphragm. In this situation a common trunk originates from the confluence of pulmonary veins and descends in front of the esophagus, penetrating the diaphragm through the esophageal hiatus. The anomalous trunk then connects into the portal vein or one of its tributaries, the ductus venosus, or, rarely, to one of the hepatic veins. In rare cases various combinations of anomalous connection occur in which drainage is to multiple levels.

HEMODYNAMICS. The physiological consequences and, accordingly, the clinical picture depend on the size of the interatrial communication and on the magnitude of the pulmonary vascular resistance. When the interatrial communication is small, systemic blood flow is markedly limited.[599] Right atrial and systemic venous pressures are elevated, and hepatic enlargement and peripheral edema are present. The size of the interatrial communication also is an important determinant in the development in utero and postnatally of the left atrium and left ventricle. Left atrial

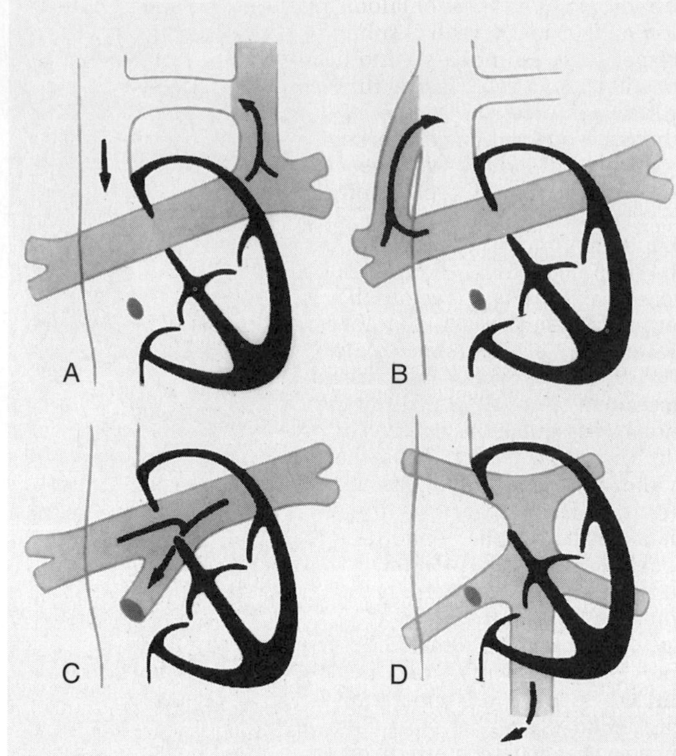

FIGURE 29–66. Anatomical types of total anomalous pulmonary venous return. Supracardiac, in which the pulmonary veins drain either via the vertical vein to the anomalous vein *(A)* or directly to the superior vena cava with the orifice close to the orifice of the azygos vein *(B)*. *C* shows drainage directly into the right atrium or into the coronary sinus. *D* shows infracardiac drainage via a vertical vein into the portal vein or the inferior vena cava. (From Stark, J., and DeLeval, M.: Surgery for Congenital Heart Defects. 2nd ed. Philadelphia, W.B. Saunders Company, 1994, p. 330.)

cavity size usually is somewhat reduced, whereas left ventricular volumes may be reduced or normal. The magnitude of pulmonary blood flow and therefore the ratio of oxygenated to unoxygenated blood that returns to the right atrium are a function of pulmonary vascular resistance. The arterial oxygen saturation, which ranges from markedly reduced to normal values, is inversely related to the pulmonary vascular resistance. In this regard, in most patients the principal determinant of pulmonary pressures and resistance is related less to augmented pulmonary blood flow and pulmonary arteriolar vascular obstruction than to the presence and intensity of pulmonary venous obstruction.[600–602]

Obstruction to pulmonary venous return and pulmonary venous hypertension are invariably present in patients with

TABLE 29–10 SITE OF CONNECTION IN TOTAL ANOMALOUS PULMONARY VENOUS CONNECTION

Site	%
1. Connection to right atrium	15%
2. Connection to common cardinal system	
a. (Right) superior vena cava	11%
b. Azygos vein	1%
3. Connection to left common cardinal system	
a. Left innominate vein	36%
b. Coronary sinus	16%
4. Connection to umbilicovitelline system	
a. Portal vein	6%
b. Ductus venosus	4%
c. Inferior vena cava	2%
d. Hepatic vein	1%
5. Multiple sites	7%
6. Unknown	1%

infradiaphragmatic anomalous pulmonary venous connection and in many with a subdiaphragmatic pathway. In the former type, pulmonary venous obstruction results from the length and narrowness of the common pulmonary venous trunk, compression at the esophageal hiatus of the diaphragm, constriction at the subdiaphragmatic site of insertion, or pulmonary venous return that must pass first through the portal-hepatic circulation before returning to the right atrium. When venous obstruction occurs in supradiaphragmatic types of drainage, constriction may exist at the entrance site of the anomalous veins into the systemic venous circulation, and/or the anomalous venous channel may be kinked or situated abnormally and compressed between the left pulmonary artery and left bronchus.[602,603] The presence of a small, restrictive patent foramen ovale occasionally results in pulmonary venous obstruction. Pulmonary vascular obstructive disease is rare during infancy, although exceptions have been reported.[604] In patients without pulmonary venous obstruction the risk of developing the Eisenmenger reaction is comparable to that in patients with an atrial septal defect.

CLINICAL MANIFESTATIONS. The majority of patients with total anomalous pulmonary venous connection have symptoms during the first year of life, and 80 per cent die before age 1 year if left untreated.[598] The few who remain asymptomatic have a relatively good prognosis; once the condition is detected, operation may be elected later in childhood. Symptomatic infants with total anomalous pulmonary venous connection present with signs of heart failure and/or cyanosis. Infants with pulmonary venous obstruction present with the early onset of severe dyspnea, pulmonary edema, cyanosis, and right heart failure. Cardiac murmurs often are not prominent. In the unobstructed forms of total anomalous pulmonary venous connection the characteristic physical findings include right ventricular precordial overactivity and minimal cyanosis unless congestive heart failure intervenes. Multiple heart sounds often are audible, consisting of a first heart sound followed by an ejection sound; a fixed, widely split second heart sound with an accentuated pulmonic component; and a third and often a fourth heart sound. A soft systolic ejection murmur is usual along the left sternal border, and a mid-diastolic murmur of flow across the tricuspid valve commonly is audible at the lower left sternal border.

LABORATORY FINDINGS. The *electrocardiogram* shows right-axis deviation and right atrial and right ventricular hypertrophy. *Roentgenograms* of the chest reveal increased pulmonary blood flow; the right atrium and ventricle are dilated and hypertrophied, and the pulmonary artery segment is enlarged (Fig. 29–67). In addition, the specific site of anomalous connection may cause a characteristic appearance of the cardiac silhouette. Thus, in patients with total anomalous pulmonary venous connection to the left brachiocephalic vein, the superior vena cava on the right, left brachiocephalic vein superiorly, and vertical vein on the left produce a cardiac shadow that resembles a snowman or figure of eight. The upper right cardiac border may be prominent when the anomalous connection is to the right superior vena cava.

Echocardiography demonstrates marked enlargement of the right ventricle and a small left atrium.[605] The objective of ultrasound imaging in these patients is to confirm the clinical diagnosis and to locate the site of connection of the common pulmonary vein. Doppler studies are required to assess the presence of obstruction within individual pulmonary veins and along the vertical vein. An echo-free space representing the common pulmonary venous chamber occasionally may be seen to lie behind the left atrium on ultrasound examination. Diagnostic echocardiographic findings include an absence of pulmonary vein connections and a small left atrium in the presence of right to left bulging of the septum primum at the foramen ovale. Positive diagnosis is made by identifying pulmonary venous connection to the systemic veins, coronary sinus, or right atrium, rather than to the left atrium. All four pulmonary veins and their connections must be identified to diagnose mixed types accurately.[605] There is no standard echocardiographic method for tracing pulmonary venous pathways because of their diverse anatomical positions.

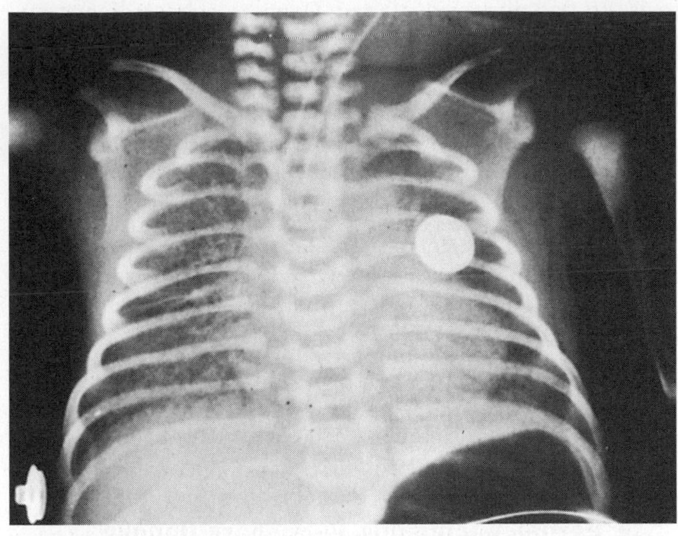

FIGURE 29–67. Chest roentgenogram in an infant with total anomalous pulmonary venous connection below the diaphragm shows normal overall heart size but diffuse pattern of pulmonary venous hypertension in both lung fields.

Infradiaphragmatic total anomalous pulmonary venous connection usually connects to the portal venous system but can connect to the hepatic veins. Doppler is utilized to distinguish between the abdominal vessels. Thus, the flow pattern in the inferior vena cava is phasic, nearly continuous, and toward the heart, in contrast to flow in the descending aorta, which has a laminar profile in systole in a direction away from the heart. Flow in the common pulmonary vein resembles that of the inferior vena cava except that its direction is away from the heart. Although not often employed, especially in infants, magnetic resonance imaging may also delineate the site of connections of the various types of total anomalous pulmonary venous return.

At *cardiac catheterization* those patients found to have systemic arterial saturations below 70 per cent and with pulmonary artery pressure at or above systemic levels are likely to have pulmonary venous obstruction. Variations in oxygen saturation in the systemic venous circulation may be helpful. In the subdiaphragmatic type, a step-up may not be apparent in inferior vena caval oxygen saturations obtained by way of femoral vein cannulation because of the contribution of highly oxygenated renal venous blood to the caval stream. In contrast, sampling of the hepatic or portal vein by way of a catheter inserted through the umbilical vein yields diagnostically higher oxygen saturations, indicating anomalous return to those vessels. If the cardiac catheter can be manipulated directly into the anomalous trunk through its site of connection, selective injection of contrast material into the common channel provides anatomical definition of the pulmonary venous tree. If the pulmonary veins cannot be entered directly, selective right and left main pulmonary artery injection of contrast material often is more helpful than is injection into a main pulmonary artery because many infants have a persistent patent ductus arteriosus through which the contrast agent flows right to left. Moreover, the drainage from both lungs must be outlined clearly to exclude a mixed type of anomalous venous drainage. Pulmonary venous obstruction may be detected by noting a pressure difference between the pulmonary artery wedge pressure and the right atrium.

MANAGEMENT. Corrective surgery for the sick infant should be performed as soon as possible, usually on the basis of two-dimensional and Doppler echocardiography, avoiding the additional stress of invasive diagnostic study. Before age 1 month, survival greater than 75 per cent is anticipated. Infants with the worst prognosis are those in whom individual pulmonary vein sizes are smallest, measurements that can be made preoperatively by echocardiogram.[606] Unless pulmonary vascular disease is present, results of operation for total anomalous pulmonary venous connection in patients beyond infancy are generally good.[607] The procedure consists of creating an anastomosis between the common pulmonary venous channel and left atrium and closing the atrial defect and the anomalous venous pathway. Improved results of operation in infancy require that postoperative pulmonary venous hypertension be averted by construction of a generally large anastomosis with or without enlargement of the left atrium. Normal hemodynamics and cardiac function have been demonstrated after surgical correction.

Partial Anomalous Pulmonary Venous Connection

In this condition one or more of the pulmonary veins, but not all, are connected to the right atrium or to one or more of its venous tributaries (see p. 944). An atrial septal defect, particularly one of the sinus venosus type, commonly accompanies this anomaly; the usual connection involves the veins of the right upper and middle lobes and the superior vena cava.[598] Exclusive of atrial septal defects, major additional cardiac malformations occur in about 20 per cent of patients; these include ventricular septal defect, tetralogy of Fallot, and a variety of complex anomalies.

In the absence of associated anomalies the physiological disturbance is determined by the number of anomalous veins and their site of connection, the presence and size of an atrial septal defect, and the state of the pulmonary vascular bed.[608] In the usual patient with isolated partial pulmonary venous connection the hemodynamic state and physical findings are similar to those in atrial septal defect. Rarely, venous drainage of the right lung is into the inferior vena cava. This condition often is associated with hypoplasia of the right lung, dextroposition of the heart, pulmonary parenchymal abnormalities, and anomalous system supply to the lower lobe of the right lung from the abdominal aorta or its main branches. This complex has been designated the "scimitar syndrome" because of the characteristic roentgenographic finding of a crescent-like shadow in the right lower lung field that is produced by the anomalous venous channel.[609,610]

At *cardiac catheterization,* partial anomalous pulmonary venous connection to the coronary sinus, azygos vein, or superior vena cava may be identified by careful and frequent oximetry sampling. Oximetry is of limited value when the anomalous connection is to the inferior vena cava because of both reduced flow through the right lung and the contribution to the vena caval stream of highly oxgenated blood from the renal veins. Selective angiography is most helpful in cases in which the anomalous veins connect far away from the right atrium. Surgical repair offers definitive therapy at low risk if pulmonary vascular obliterative disease has not yet developed.

Malpositions of the Heart and Cardiac Apex

Positional anomalies of the heart are conditions in which the cardiac apex is located in the right side of the chest (dextrocardia) or is centrally located (mesocardia) or in which there is a normal location of the heart in the left side of the chest but abnormal position of the viscera (isolated levocardia). Such hearts commonly are abnormal with respect to chamber localization and great artery attachments; associated complex intracardiac and extracardiac lesions are common.

Problems of terminology abound in the literature describing these complex cardiac anomalies, although sensible and uniform systems of classification are available.[611, 612]

ANATOMICAL FEATURES. Defining the cardiac anatomy in instances of cardiac malposition requires a description of three cardiac segments—the visceroatrial situs, the ventricular loop, and the conotruncus (the atria, ventricles, and great arteries, respectively). In addition to defining positional interrelation, the description of the malposed heart also must include the connections of the ventricles to the atria and great arteries as well as chamber identification, both morphologically and functionally.

DIAGNOSIS. To accomplish accurate diagnosis may require a synthesis of findings from noninvasive tests such as two-dimensional echocardiography, computed tomography, and magnetic resonance imaging, as well as hemodynamic and cineangiographic findings obtained at cardiac catheterization. Expert echocardiographers analyze, separately and independent of adjacent segments, each cardiac segment (atria, atrioventricular canal, ventricles, infundibulum, and great arteries) in terms of both situs and alignments.[613–616]

In general, the determination of the body situs indicates the position of the atria. The visceral situs usually can be determined by the location of the stomach bubble and liver on a routine roentgenogram and of the inferior vena cava by means of echocardiography or the position of a cardiac catheter, or by means of a computed axial tomogram or venous or radioisotope angiocardiogram. Atrial anatomy is best investigated noninvasively by using subxiphoid long- and short-axis and apical four-chamber echocardiographic views. Venous contrast injections may be useful to define systemic venous connections.

Situs solitus is the normal arrangement of viscera and atria, with the right atrium right-sided and the left atrium left-sided. Situs solitus is further characterized by a trilobed right lung and eparterial bronchus (i.e., the right upper lobe bronchus passes above the right pulmonary artery), a bilobed left lung and hyparterial bronchus (i.e., the left bronchus passes below the left pulmonary artery), the major lobe of the liver on the right, a left-sided stomach and spleen, and right-sided venae cavae. *Situs inversus* is a mirror image of normal. *Situs ambiguus* or visceral heterotaxy refers to an anatomically uncertain or indeterminate body configuration. The latter often is seen in association with congenital asplenia, which resembles bilateral right-sidedness, and congenital polysplenia, which resembles bilateral left-sidedness.[617–620]

ASPLENIA. Cardiac anomalies associated commonly with asplenia include anomalous systemic venous connection, atrial septal or complete endocardial cushion defect, common ventricle, transposition of the great arteries, severe pulmonic stenosis or atresia, and anomalous pulmonary venous connection. Polysplenia commonly is associated with absence of the hepatic portion of the inferior vena cava with azygos continuation, bilateral superior venae cavae, anomalous pulmonary venous connection, and atrial septal defect (either ostium secundum or endocardial cushion). Pulmonic stenosis and double-outlet right ventricle are each observed in about 25 per cent of cases. It is important to recognize these complex syndromes to distinguish them from forms of cyanotic heart disease that may be more amenable to corrective surgical therapy. In many of these patients, improvement results from palliation by modifications of the Fontan procedure, despite anomalies of systemic and pulmonary venous return in association with single ventricle anatomy.[621,622] Diagnosis is suggested by a symmetrical liver shadow roentgenographically and, in asplenia, by the presence of Howell-Jolly and Heinz bodies in red blood cells demonstrated on blood smear, and it is confirmed by a negative or abnormal radioactive spleen scan.

Once the type of visceral situs is defined, it is necessary to describe the bulboventricular loop. The primitive cardiac tune normally bends to the right (D-loop), which brings the anatomical right ventricle to the right of the anatomical left ventricle. An L-loop brings the morphological right ventricle left-sided relative to the morphological left ventricle. The L-loop is normal in the presence of situs inversus, but in situs solitus it is synonymous with inverted ventricles.

VENTRICULAR MORPHOLOGY. The number, morphology, and size of the ventricles can be ascertained by using a variety of echocardiographic views. The morphological features of each ventricle also can be identified angiographically. The anatomical right ventricle is equipped with a tricuspid valve, is highly trabeculated, and contains the septal band of the single papillary muscle; its infundibulum lies anterior to and superiorly beyond the outlet of the left ventricle. The anatomical right ventricle usually connects with whichever of the two great arteries is the more anterior. The anatomical left ventricle is smooth-walled and contains an outlet that lies posterior to the right ventricular infundibulum; its entrance is guarded by a bicuspid mitral valve, the anterior leaflet of which is normally in continuity with elements of the semilunar valve at its outlet.

GREAT ARTERIES. The great arteries are described in terms of their positional interrelations and their ventricular connections. Each outflow tract and semilunar valve should be examined in both long- and short-axis echocardiographic views.[613,615] The ventriculoarterial alignments may be determined by direct visualization from the subxiphoid window. The relation between the great arteries can best be demonstrated noninvasively using parasternal short-axis echocardiographic views, which display the semilunar roots. The aortic arch and brachiocephalic arteries are seen well using suprasternal notch views. The pulmonary artery is seen from high parasternal or suprasternal notch short-axis sections. The ventricular attachments may be normal or may form the anomalies of double-outlet right or left ventricle or transposition. The arterial interrelations are described as D (dextro), in which the ascending aorta sweeps toward the right and lies to the right of the main pulmonary artery; L (levo), in which the ascending aorta sweeps toward the left and lies to the left of the main pulmonary artery; or A (antero), which is the rare situation in which the aorta lies directly in front of the pulmonary artery. The D, L, and A descriptions of the aorticopulmonary artery interrelations should not be confused with the D- or L-loop designation of the ventricular interrelations.[612]

Using segmental sets composed of descriptive units of visceroatrial situs/ventricular loop/great artery relations greatly simplifies expression of the type of cardiac anatomy present in cardiac malposition. For example, the normal heart in a patient with situs inversus and dextrocardia is referred to as inversus/L loop/L normal; complete transposition of the great arteries in a patient with situs inversus is referred to as inversus/L loop/L transposition; functionally corrected transposition in a patient with situs solitus is referred to as solitus/L loop/L transposition; dextrocardia and functionally corrected transposition is designated solitus/D loop/D transposition with dextrocardia.

After the cardiac chambers are diagnosed functionally (arterial and venous), the positional and morphological relations are understood, and the presence of associated anomalies is established, the principles of medical and surgical treatment apply to these cardiac malpositions as they do to normally located hearts.

OTHER CONDITIONS

Congenital Pericardial Defects

Isolated pericardial defects (see p. 1522) are rare. They most commonly occur in males and usually are left-sided, although they may be right-sided, diaphragmatic, or total.[623] The anomaly is produced by deficient formation of the pleuropericardial membrane, or, if diaphragmatic, defective formations of the septum transversum. Associated congenital anomalies of the heart and lungs occur in about 30 per cent of cases. Most patients with the isolated defect are asymptomatic. Nonspecific anterior chest pain may be the result of torsion of the great arteries due to absence of the stabilizing forces of the left pericardium.

With complete absence of the left pericardium a conspicuous apical impulse may be noted shifted leftward to the anterior or midaxillary line. Electrocardiographic changes may be related to levo-position of the heart; a leftward displacement of the QRS transition in the precordial leads and vertical or right-axis deviation are usual. The diagnosis may be suggested by chest roentgenograms.[624] With complete left pericardial absence, the heart is levo-posed, and the aortic knob, pulmonary artery, and ventricles form three prominent left heart border convexities.

A partial left pericardial defect may be suspected on the basis of varying degrees of prominence of the pulmonary artery and/or the left atrial appendage. Echocardiographic findings often mimic those observed in patients with right ventricular volume overload (enlarged right ventricle and abnormal ventricular septal motion), probably owing to the altered cardiac position and motion with the thorax.[625] Other echocardiographic clues include lateral extension of the left atrial appendage as it herniates through the pericardial defect; this is best seen in short-axis views. The anomaly can be definitively diagnosed by computed tomography or magnetic resonance imaging. Cardiac catheterization is of little diagnostic value.

Complete absence of the left pericardium requires no treatment. However, partial defects may impose serious risks, including herniation and strangulation of the ventricles or left atrial appendage with left-sided defects, or the possibility of a superior vena cava obstructive syndrome with right-sided defects.[626] In the diaphragmatic type, cardiac compression by abdominal contents requires surgical repair.[627] Partial left or right defects may be closed with a patch of mediastinal pleura.

Single Atrium

Single or common atrium is a rare, isolated defect. The anomaly consists of an absent atrial septum, usually with a cleft in the anteromedial leaflet of the mitral valve and, occasionally, with a cleft tricuspid valve as well. The lesion may be seen as one component of the Ellis–van Creveld syndrome (Table 29–2) or of the complex cardiac anomalies seen in patients with asplenia or polysplenia.

Single atrium may be suspected clinically by the presence of cardiac murmurs of an atrial septal defect and mitral regurgitation associated with mild cyanosis, roentgenographic evidence of cardiac enlargement and increased pulmonary blood flow, and electrocardiographic features of atrioventricular septal defect. An absence of echoes from any part of the atrial septum is the essential feature of two-dimensional echocardiographic examination, which also may show a cleft anterior mitral leaflet, increased right ventricular end-diastolic dimension, paradoxical ventricular septal motion, and dilated, pulsatile pulmonary trunk. Angiographically, the absence of the atrial septum produces a large, globe-shaped single atrial structure. Selective left ventricular angiocardiography shows the characteristic gooseneck appearance seen in the various forms of atrioventricular septal defect. In the absence of pulmonary vascular obstructive disease surgical correction is indicated by means of a prosthetic patch.

Single Ventricle (Univentricular Atrioventricular Connection)

Hearts with univentricular atrioventricular connection constitute a family of complex lesions in which both atrioventricular valves, or a common atrioventricular valve, open into a single ventricular chamber.[628] Terminology is varied, and the anomaly often is referred to as single or common ventricle, which is imprecise but useful shorthand for the entity. The definition excludes examples of tricuspid or mitral atresia. Single ventricle is almost always accompanied by abnormal great artery positional relations; the incidence of L-malposition of the great arteries is about equal to that of D-malposition. Associated anomalies are common, and include, in particular, pulmonic valvular or subvalvular stenosis, subaortic stenosis, total or partial anomalous pulmonary venous connection, and coarctation of the aorta.

MORPHOLOGY. In about 80 per cent of patients the single ventricle morphologically resembles a left ventricular chamber that is separated from an infundibular outlet chamber by a bulboventricular septum.[629] The opening is variously called the bulboventricular foramen and ventricular septal defect. The infundibular chamber is considered to represent developmentally the outflow tract of the right ventricle. When the great arteries are malposed the infundibulum lying anterior at the basal position of the single ventricle communicates with the aorta and may be in one of two positions: noninverted (D-malposition), when it is situated at the right basal aspect of the heart, or inverted (L-malposition), when it is located at the left base of the heart. In the unusual situation in which the great arteries are normally related, the infundibulum communicates with the pulmonary trunk.[629] *Double-inlet left ventricle* is a term used synonymously to describe the most frequently encountered single ventricular chamber that has the anatomical characteristics of the left ventricle. Less commonly the single ventricular chamber resembles a right ventricle (double-inlet right ventricle) or contains features suggestive of both ventricles or neither one; the latter two situations occasionally have been designated common ventricle and single ventricle of the primitive type, respectively.

CLINICAL FINDINGS. Depending on the associated anomalies, the clinical presentation of single ventricle mimics other conditions in which cyanosis and decreased or increased pulmonary blood flow coexist, e.g., tetralogy of Fallot or tricuspid atresia in the former instance or complete transposition of the great arteries and double-outlet right ventricle in the latter. The *electrocardiogram* in double-inlet left ventricle without inversion of the infundibulum (D-malposition) usually shows features of left ventricular hypertrophy. With infundibular inversion (L-malposition) the electrical forces are directed anteriorly and rightward, as they are in ventricular inversion without associated defects. In patients with the more primitive types of common or single ventricle there is a repetitious rS pattern in all the precordial electrocardiographic leads. *Chest roentgenographic* findings resemble those observed in patients with complete (dextro-) transposition of the great arteries or functionally corrected (levo-) transposition of the great arteries without features distinctive for single ventricle.

ECHOCARDIOGRAPHY. Two-dimensional and Doppler echocardiography are extremely important to demonstrate ventricular anatomy and to recognize associated intra- and extracardiac anomalies (Fig. 29–68). A segmental approach should be employed for accurate and complete echocardiographic evaluation. Thus, precise details are required of the basic anatomy of atrial and visceral situs, location of the cardiac apex, the extracardiac course of the great arteries, and systemic and pulmonary venous connections.

In those patients in whom two separate atrioventricular valves communicate with the single ventricular chamber, *echocardiography* (Fig. 3–85, p. 85) suggests the correct diagnosis when echoes are visualized from the two valves without an intervening interventricu-

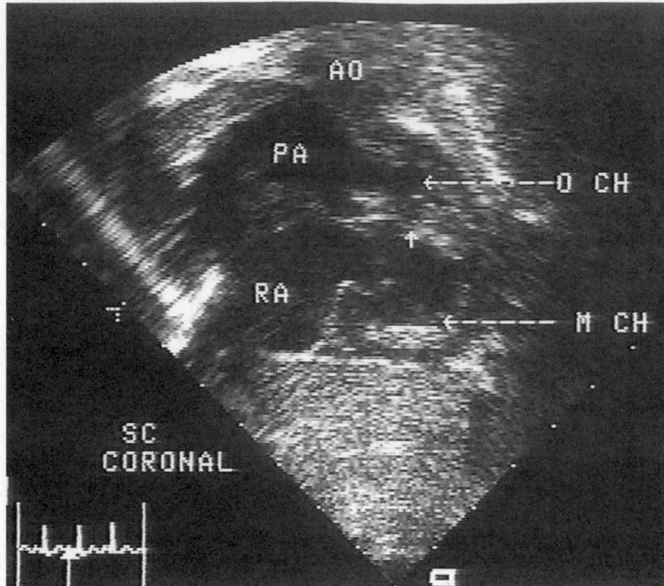

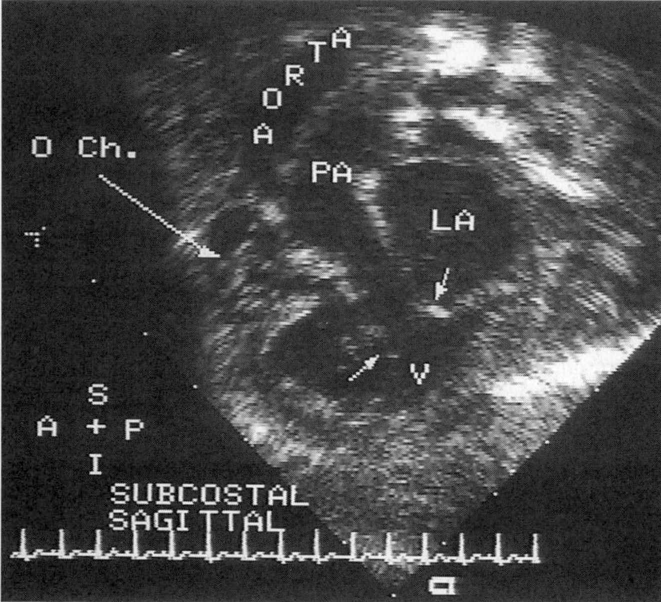

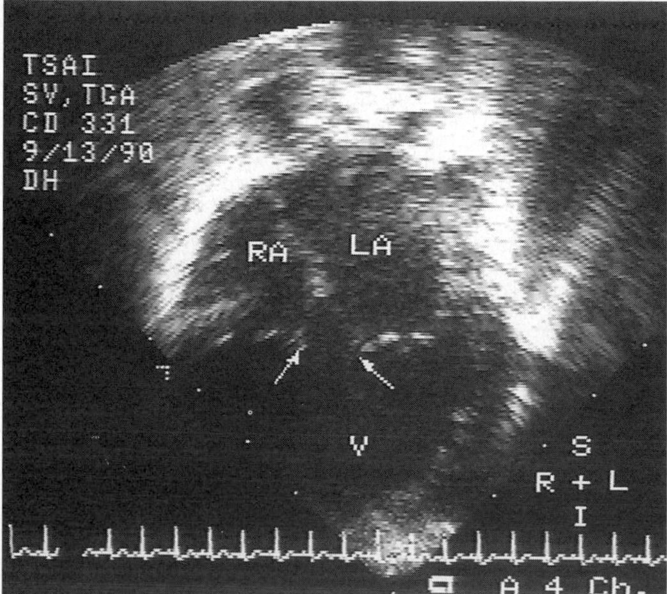

FIGURE 29–68. Echo images of a double-inlet left ventricle type of univentricular heart. *Top,* Subcostal coronal view shows the right atrium (RA) giving rise to a tricuspid valve guarding entry into a main chamber (M CH) of left ventricular morphology from which the pulmonary artery (PA) arises. The arrow indicates the small ventricular septal defect (bulboventricular foramen) entering into an outflow chamber (O CH) which gives rise to the aorta (AO). *Middle,* Orthogonal subcostal sagittal equivalent to the top frame. The left atrium (LA) is seen above the main chamber of left ventricular morphology (V). The arrows indicate the origin of the left and right atrioventricular valves within the same ventricular chamber. The pulmonary artery (PA) arises from the main chamber and the long narrow bulboventricular foramen is shown to enter the outlet chamber (O CH) with its connection to the aorta. *Bottom,* Apical four-chamber view shows the right atrium (RA) and the left atrium (LA) with their corresponding valves (arrows) entering into the common large ventricle (V). (Courtesy of Norman Silverman, M.D.)

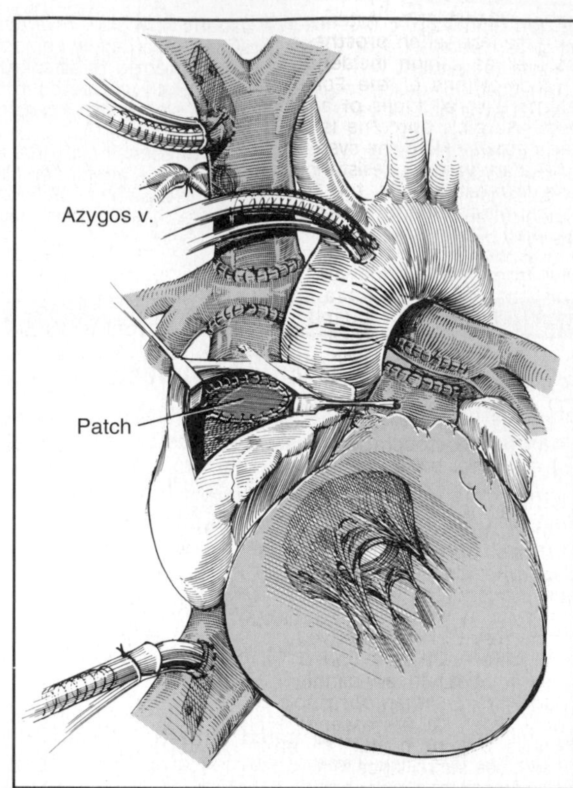

FIGURE 29–69. A bidirectional cavopulmonary artery shunt with patch occlusion of the superior vena cava right atrial junction (hemi-Fontan procedure) using direct cannulation of the superior and inferior venae cavae and a single arterial cannula. The main pulmonary artery is shown divided and oversewn, but in some cases it may be allowed to remain patent. Connections are made between both ends of the divided superior vena cava and the pulmonary artery. A subsequent Fontan operation involves only removal of the patch at the junction of the superior vena cava and the right atrium and placement of the intraatrial baffle to divert the inferior vena caval blood up to the superior vena cava orifice. (From Castaneda, A., et al.: Cardiac Surgery of the Neonate and Infant. Philadelphia, W.B. Saunders Company, 1994, p. 263.)

lar septum.[630,631] In the absence of ventricular septal echoes when the two valves are not visualized simultaneously, they may be identified separately with a careful long-axis sweep of the ventricle. It is possible to detect the presence of a small outflow chamber anterior to the atrioventricular valves by using subcostal or parasternal short-axis views, and a plane orthogonal to the long-axis plane (Fig. 29–64).

The single ventricle with a single atrioventricular valve is suspected when the excursion of echoes from the single valve located posteriorly in the ventricular chamber is of large amplitude. Enhanced assessment of the atrioventricular valve in patients with single ventricle is provided by Doppler echocardiography.[632] Magnetic resonance imaging provides valuable complementary information to echocardiographic study.[630,631] Selective ventriculography is necessary to delineate with certainty the anatomical type of single ventricle and to diagnose the associated great artery interrelations and the presence or absence of additional lesions.[633]

SURGICAL TREATMENT. Attempts to partition the single ventricle with a Dacron or Teflon prosthetic patch have met with limited success as well as a high incidence of postoperative complete heart block. Modifications of the Fontan approach are generally applied to patients with all types of anatomical and functional single ventricle.[634–636] Surgical outcome is related to the creation of an unobstructed pathway from the systemic veins to the pulmonary arteries, low pulmonary vascular resistance, and a compliant, well-functioning ventricle. In most centers, the Fontan procedure is divided into two stages, an initial superior vena cava–pulmonary artery anastomosis (bidirectional Glenn shunt or hemi-Fontan procedure; Fig. 29–69, p. 948), followed later by completion of the Fontan procedure directing flow from the inferior vena cava to the amalgamation of the superior vena cava and the branch pulmonary arteries. At first-stage operation, prior systemic–pulmonary shunts are eliminated and any areas of distortion or narrowing of the pulmonary arteries are repaired, particularly if a prior pulmonary artery banding was performed to limit pulmonary blood flow.

At the author's center, the complete Fontan procedure is accompanied by placement of a snare around the atrial septal defect to control its size postoperatively, whereas in other centers, fenestrations in the atrial baffle may be used. These procedures appear to reduce significantly postoperative morbidity from pericardial effusions and significantly improve survival. Results of early bidirectional cavopulmonary shunting in young infants are encouraging. The objective of this approach early in life is to yield a more suitable Fontan candidate while reducing ventricular volume overload and repeated palliative procedures. Subaortic stenosis, a common occurrence in patients with univentricular heart and malposed great arteries, occurs as a result of a restrictive bulboventricular foramen (ventricular septal defect) or as a consequence of ventricular hypertrophy from a previous pulmonary banding operation.

The *Damus-Kaye-Stansel operation*, consisting of anastomosis of the pulmonary artery to the ascending aorta, is a generally successful approach to this problem.[637–641] After operation, all patients need continued close surveillance.[642–646] Complications include thromboembolic phenomena and atrial arrhythmias. Survivors generally lead active lives with exercise levels less than normal, but relevant to ordinary daily life.

VASCULAR RINGS

MORPHOLOGY. The normal development of the aortic arch system is described on page 882 (Fig. 29–3). The term *vascular ring* is used for those aortic arch or pulmonary artery malformations that exhibit an abnormal relation with the esophagus and trachea, causing compression, dysphagia, and/or respiratory symptoms.[647] The most common and serious vascular ring is produced by a double aortic arch in which both the right and left fourth embryonic aortic arches persist. In the most common type of double aortic arch there is a left ligamentum arteriosum or ductus arteriosus, and both arches are patent, the right being larger than the left. A right aortic arch with a left ductus or ligamentum arteriosum connecting the left pulmonary artery and the upper part of the descending aorta, and with an anomalous right subclavian artery arising from the left descending aorta, are additional important vascular ring arrangements.[648] The latter anomaly frequently exists in cases of tetralogy of Fallot and otherwise uncomplicated coarctation of the aorta. An unusual cause of tracheal compression is the "vascular sling" created by an anomalous left pulmonary artery that arises from a rightward, elongated pulmonary trunk and courses between the trachea and esophagus before it branches normally within the left lung.[649] This arrangement commonly is associated with other cardiac and extracardiac anomalies.

CLINICAL FINDINGS. The symptoms produced by vascular rings depend on the tightness of anatomical constriction of the trachea and esophagus and consist principally of respiratory difficulties, cyanosis (associated especially with feeding), stridor, and dysphagia. The electrocardiogram is normal unless associated cardiovascular anomalies are present. The barium esophagogram is a useful screening procedure. Prominent posterior indentation of the esophagus is observed in the common vascular ring arrangements, although the pulmonary artery "vascular sling" produces an anterior indentation. Unusual and rare aortic arch anomalies may create rings that impinge on the trachea but do not compress the esophagus and are detected not by this simple radiographic procedure but rather by bronchoscopy. Selective contrast angiography delineates the anatomy of the aorta and its branches or the course of the main pulmonary arteries. Computed axial tomography and magnetic resonance imaging offer excellent imaging alternatives.[650,651]

MANAGEMENT. The severity of symptoms and the anatomy of the malformation are the most important factors in determining treatment. Patients, particularly infants, with respiratory obstruction require prompt surgical intervention. Operative repair of the double aortic arch requires division of the minor arch (usually the left).[652] A reported 20 to 30 per cent operative mortality is related, in part, to problems in postoperative respiratory care, especially when there is coexistent residual anatomical tracheal narrowing. Patients with a right aortic arch and a left ductus or ligamentum arteriosum require division of the ductus or ligamentum and/or ligation and division of the left subclavian artery, which is the posterior component of the ring. Operation seldom is indicated for patients with an aberrant right subclavian artery derived from a left aortic arch and left descending aorta. In patients with a pulmonary artery vascular sling, operation consists of detachment of the left pulmonary artery at its origin and anastomosis to the main pulmonary artery directly or by way of a conduit of its proximal end brought anterior to the trachea.[652] Some patients with persistent respiratory symptoms require postoperative evaluation of residual anatomical obstruction, tests of pulmonary function, and bronchodilator therapy.[653]

CONGENITAL ARRHYTHMIAS

This classification refers to arrhythmias that are present in infancy, whose causes, when known, relate to a structural malformation or defect of the conduction system or to an acquired prenatal condition such as myocarditis, hypoxia acidosis, or transplacental passage of a drug or substance from mother to fetus. In these latter examples, the substrate for the postnatal expression of the rhythm disturbance existed before birth and the arrhythmia is therefore designated "congenital." Complete heart block and supraventricular and ventricular tachycardias are the most common important congenital arrhythmias.[654] The electrophysiological and electrocardiographic features of these arrhythmias are discussed elsewhere in the text (Chaps. 22 and 23).

Congenital Complete Heart Block

(See also p. 966)

The atrioventricular node and the His bundle originate during fetal development as separate structures and later join together. Anatomical studies have shown the basic lesion in congenital complete heart block to consist of discontinuity between the atrial musculature and the AV node or the His bundle, if the AV node is absent. The anatomical interruption occasionally may be situated between the AV node and the main His bundle, or within the bundle itself.[655] No cause is known for the vast majority of cases of congenital heart block in infants, who usually have otherwise anatomically normal hearts. However, fetal myocarditis, idiopathic hemorrhage and necrosis involving conduction tissue, and degeneration and fibrosis related in some instances to the transplacental passage of anti-Ro/ss-A antibody and other immune complexes from mothers with systemic lupus erythematosus are all entities capable of causing congenital heart block.[656,657] Less often, congenital heart block may be associated with various forms of congenital heart disease, the most common malformation being congenitally corrected transposition of the great arteries.[655a]

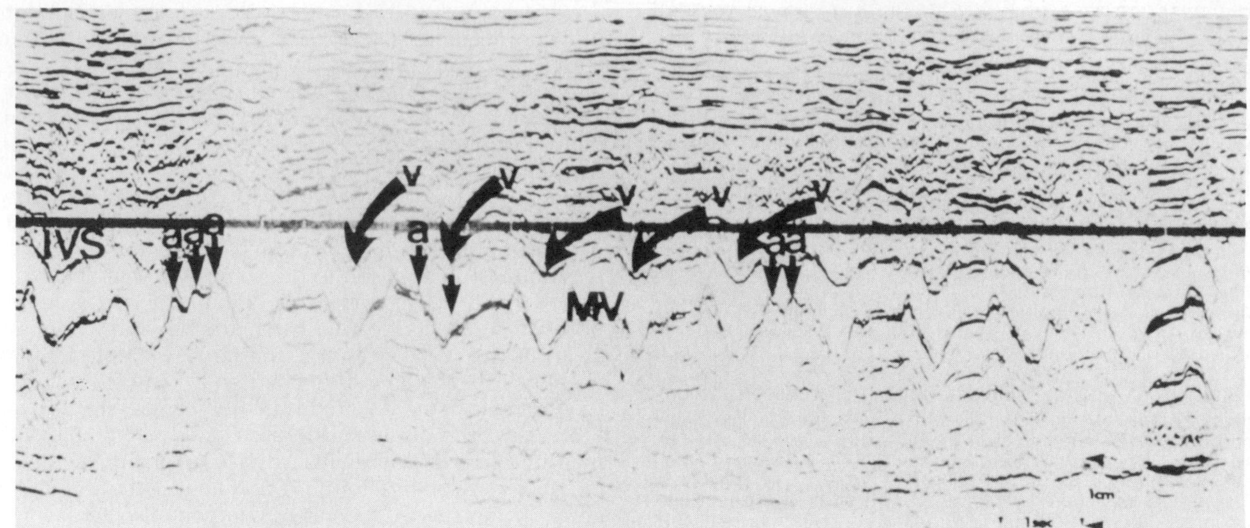

FIGURE 29–70. Fetal M-mode echocardiogram of complete heart block at 28 weeks' gestation. A slow ventricular rate of 45 to 50 beats/min is seen by the undulations (v, *curved arrows*) of the interventricular septum (IVS). Atrial contractions (a, *straight vertical arrows*) cause regular undulations of the mitral valve (MV) at a rate of 120 to 130 beats/min. The atrial activity has no fixed relationship to the idioventricular rhythm. (Courtesy of Charles Kleinman, M.D.)

Detection of consistent fetal bradycardia (heart rate 40 to 80 beats/min) by auscultation, fetal echocardiography (Fig. 29–70), or electronic monitoring allows anticipation of the correct diagnosis. The newborn, especially with a ventricular rate less than 50 beats/min and atrial rate in excess of 150 beats/min, is at highest risk; the presence of an associated cardiovascular anomaly greatly lessens the chances of survival. Treatment is not required for the asymptomatic infant. Digitalization is recommended for the baby in congestive heart failure, irrespective of complete heart block. Isoproterenol and other sympathomimetic drugs and atropine do not have permanent or beneficial effect. Congestive heart failure and Stokes-Adams attacks require pacemaker treatment at any age. This requires transvenous or transatrial placement of endocardial leads in the older child or permanent epicardial pacemaker insertion in infants and small children. A variety of problems may be anticipated after pacemaker implantation related to growth of the patient, which stresses the electrical lead system; the fragility of the lead system in a physically active young patient; and the limited life span of the pulse generator. Patients with congenital complete heart block who survive infancy usually remain asymptomatic until late in childhood or adolescence.[662]

Supraventricular Tachycardia

Paroxysmal tachycardia of supraventricular origin may have its origin in utero or in the immediate postnatal period. The most frequent arrhythmias producing symptoms are paroxysmal atrial tachycardia with or without ventricular preexcitation, atrial flutter, and junctional tachycardia. The arrhythmia may cause intrauterine cardiac failure; its detection and persistence prenatally should prompt consideration of administration of digitalis, or if that fails, of propranolol, quinidine, flecainide, or amiodarone to the mother if amniocentesis indicates surfactant deficiency and fetal lung immaturity because early delivery is not indicated if the baby will have hyaline membrane disease. Experience is limited with antiarrhythmic drugs, delivered by umbilical venous infusion.[107] Cesarean delivery or induced labor may be indicated if the fetus is close to term. No cause is recognized for the disorder in the majority of infants. The transplacental passage of long-acting thyroid-stimulators (LATS) and immune gamma 2 globulin from hyperthyroid mothers, hypoglycemia, and Ebstein's anomaly of the tricuspid valve occasionally are causative.[665] Wolff-Parkinson-White syndrome (see p. 667) is present in 10 to 50 per cent of infants with supraventricular tachycardia.[666] Symptoms produced by the tachyarrhythmia after birth are subtle and often go undetected until signs of heart failure have been present for 24 to 36 hours. Conversion to normal sinus rhythm usually is accomplished by administration of digitalis or adenosine, direct-current cardioversion, transesophageal atrial pacing, or a diving reflex elicited by covering the face with an ice-cold wet washcloth for 4 to 5 seconds.[667] Conversion should be followed by digitalization on a prophylactic basis. Common practice consists of digitalis treatment for 9 to 12 recurrence-free months followed by its abrupt cessation. Recurrence of tachycardia, particularly in those infants with ventricular preexcitation, is not uncommon; maintenance of normal rhythm may require the administration, alone or in combination, of digitalis, phenytoin sodium, flecainide, and propranolol.[667] The rate of recurrence falls substantially between ages 2 and 10 years, with a slight rise during adolescence. In general, the prognosis is excellent.[668]

ELECTROPHYSIOLOGICAL STUDIES. Beyond infancy, patients whose condition is refractory to medical treatment are candidates for electrophysiological catheter evaluation, which facilitates differentiation of a causative ectopic anatomical focus within the atria from accessory conduction pathways.[654,669] Endocardial mapping is performed to specifically localize the site of earliest activation in the atrium, or to identify multiple foci of ectopic impulses. Electrophysiological studies should include measurement of resting intervals and sinus and atrioventricular node function, including recovery times, effective refractory period, and Wenckebach conduction. Premature atrial stimulation may be used to interrupt tachycardia. Premature ventricular stimulation is used to measure retrograde conduction and localize the site of earliest atrial activation, and to assess the effective refractory period of the accessory pathway. Coronary sinus and right atrial catheters provide localization of the site of earliest atrial activation during tachycardia, and allow measurement of the antegrade effective refractory period of the accessory pathway.

If the tachyarrhythmia is refractory to pharmacological therapy, it may be treated definitively by radiofrequency catheter ablation of accessory pathways (see p. 621). This procedure has become the primary treatment modality for most symptomatic rhythm disturbances in children.[670–674]

Among the advantages of this approach is that successful ablation represents a cure; the heart is left structurally normal, and the cause of the arrhythmia is eliminated. Further, the need for antiarrhythmic agents with the concomitant risk of side effects or proarrhythmia is eliminated. This author has used transesophageal biplanar cross-sectional imaging during ablation procedures to precisely localize the ablation catheter tip and its stability.

ATRIAL FLUTTER. Uncommonly, atrial flutter is the cause of supraventricular tachycardia,[675–677] especially in the setting of newborn infants with hydrops fetalis, whose intrauterine tachyarrhythmia is an alternation between supraventricular tachycardia with Wolff-Parkinson-White syndrome and atrial flutter. Another common clinical setting for atrial flutter is in the infant under age 6 months with an otherwise normal heart, who shows frequent premature atrial contractions. In infants, classic flutter waves may not be present on a surface electrocardiogram or rhythm strip; detection may require recordings of transesophageal atrial electrograms. Acute treatment with electrical conversion or transesophageal overdrive pacing effectively terminates the rhythm disturbance.[677,678] If synchronized direct-current electrocardioversion is used, standby pacing should be available; if overdrive pacing is used, the same pacing catheter can be used to pace the heart in the event of asystole. Uncommonly, chronic drug treatment with digitalis, digitalis plus quinidine, or amiodarone may be required.

Junctional automatic tachycardia is characterized by a narrow QRS complex and AV dissociation, with the ventricular rate faster than the normal atrial rate. Ventricular dysfunction and congestive heart failure occur early, and the rhythm disturbance usually is not convertible to sinus rhythm by any medical treatment. When the latter fails and because sudden death is a risk, pacemaker implantation is recommended with subsequent catheter ablation.

VENTRICULAR TACHYCARDIA. Ventricular tachycardia is defined as three or more consecutive premature ventricular contractions. The definition, however, fails to identify a high-risk group. Infants or children who meet this criterion but seldom require treatment and seem to be at little risk have no symptoms and no evidence of anatomical heart disease. Potentially serious ventricular tachycardia in the newborn is associated with Q-T prolongation, mitral valve prolapse, and Marfan syndrome. In these settings the tachycardia is potentially life-threatening and always merits treatment.[654]

The genes have been mapped for the long Q-T syndrome (see p. 685). The two most effective treatments are beta blockade and high thoracic left sympathectomy, which reduce the incidence of syncope and sudden death without affecting the Q-T interval.

The treatment of ventricular tachycardia (see p. 619) consists of intravenous administration of lidocaine, followed by direct-current electrical cardioversion. In the absence of Q-T prolongation but in the presence of mitral prolapse or other cardiac abnormalities, chronic treatment should be undertaken of multiform premature ventricular contractions, couplets, or ventricular tachycardia. In infants and children unresponsive to conventional or investigational antiarrhythmic drugs, consideration should be given to pacemaker implantation, cardiac sympathetic denervation, and perhaps implantation of a defibrillator.[680]

REFERENCES

1. Hoffman, J. I. E.: Congenital heart disease. Ped. Clin. North Am. *37*:45, 1990.
2. Roberts, W. C.: Anatomically isolated aortic valvular disease: The case against its being of rheumatic etiology. Am. J. Cardiol. *49*:151, 1970.
3. Warth, D. C., King, M. E., Cohen, J. M., et al.: Prevalence of mitral valve prolapse in normal children. J. Am. Coll. Cardiol. *5*:1173, 1985.
4. Fontana, R. S., and Edwards, J. E.: Congenital Cardiac Disease: A Review of 357 Cases Studied Pathologically. Philadelphia, W.B. Saunders Company, 1962.
5. Bankl, H.: Congenital Malformations of the Heart and Great Vessels: Synopsis of Pathology, Embryology and Natural History. Baltimore-Munich, Urban and Schwarzenberg, 1977.
5a. Gerlis, L. M.: Covert congenital cardiovascular malformations discovered in an autopsy series of nearly 5000 cases. Cardiovasc. Pathol. *5*:11, 1996.
6. Samanek, M.: Boy:girl ratio in children born with different forms of cardiac malformation: A population-based study. Pediatr. Cardiol. *15*:53, 1994.
7. Greenwood, R. D.: Cardiovascular malformations associated with extracardiac anomalies and malformation syndromes. Clin. Pediatr. *23*:145, 1984.
8. Ferencz, C., and Villasenor, A. C.: Epidemiology of cardiovascular malformations: The state of the art. Cardiol. Young. *1*:264, 1991.
9. de la Cruz, M. V., Munoz-Castellanos, L., and Nadal-Ginard, S.: Extrinsic factors in the genesis of congenital heart disease. Br. Heart J. *33*:203, 1971.
10. Ruttenberg, H. D.: Concerning the etiology of congenital cardiac disease. Am. Heart J. *84*:437, 1972.
11. Ouelette, E. M., Rossett, H. L., Rossman, M. P., and Wiener, L.: Adverse effects on offspring of maternal alcohol abuse during pregnancy. N. Engl. J. Med. *297*:528, 1977.
12. Stevens, C. A., Carey, J. C., and Shigeoka, A. O.: DiGeorge anomaly and velocardiofacial syndrome. Pediatrics *85*:526, 1990.
13. Dietz, H. C., and Pyeritz, R. E.: Molecular genetic approaches to the study of human cardiovascular disease. Annu. Rev. Physiol. *56*:763, 1994.
14. Noonan, J.: Twins, conjoined twins, and cardiac defects. Am. J. Dis. Child. *132*:17, 1978.
15. Burn, J.: Consequences of chromosome 22q11.2 deletions. Circulation *90*:II–ID, 1994.
16. Corone, P., Bonaiti, C., Feingold, J., et al.: Familial congenital heart disease: How are the various types related? Am. J. Cardiol. *51*:942, 1983.
17. Whittemore, R., Wells, J. A., and Castellsague, X.: A second-generation study of 427 probands with congenital heart defects and their 837 children. J. Am. Coll. Cardiol. *23*:1459, 1994.
18. Anderson, R. H., and Ashley, G. T.: Anatomic development of the cardiovascular system. *In* Davies, J., and Dobbing, J. (eds.): Scientific Foundations of Paediatrics. London, Heinemann, 1974, p. 165.
19. Langman, J., and van Mierop, L. H. S.: Development of the cardiovascular system. *In* Moss, A. J., and Adams, F. H. (eds.): Heart Disease in Infants, Children, and Adolescents. Baltimore, Williams and Wilkins, 1968, p. 3.
20. Los, J. A.: Embryology. *In* Watson, H. (ed.): Pediatric Cardiology. London, Lloyd Luke Ltd., 1968, p. 1.
21. Rudolph, A. M.: Congenital Diseases of the Heart. Chicago Year Book Medical Publishers, 1974.
22. Sheldon, C. A., Friedman, W. F., and Sybers, H. D.: Scanning electron microscopy of fetal and neonatal lamb cardiac cells. J. Mol. Cell. Cardiol. *8*:853, 1976.
23. McPherson, R. A., Kramer, M. F., Covell, J. W., and Friedman, W. F.: A comparison of the active stiffness of fetal and adult cardiac muscle. Pediatr. Res. *10*:660, 1976.
24. Friedman, W. F.: The intrinsic physiologic properties of the developing heart. Prog. Cardiovasc. Dis. *15*:87, 1972.
25. Huynh, T. V., Wetzel, G. T., Friedman, W. F., and Klitzner, T. S.: Developmental changes in membrane Ca^{2+} and K^+ currents in fatal, neonatal, and adult heart cells. Circ. Res. *70*:508, 1992.
26. Chen, F., Wetzel, G. T., Friedman, W. F., and Klitzner, T. S.: ATP sensitive potassium channels in isolated neonatal and adult rabbit ventricular myocytes. Pediatr. Res. *32*:230, 1992.
27. Ingwall, J. S., Kramer, M. F., Woodman, D., and Friedman, W. F.: Maturation of energy metabolism in the lamb: Changes in myosin ATPase and creatine kinase activities. Pediatr. Res. *15*:1128, 1981.
28. Friedman, W. F.: Physiological properties of the developing heart. Paediatric Cardiology. Vol. 6. New York, Churchill Livingstone, 1987, p. 3.
29. Geis, W. P., Tatooles, C. J., Priola, D. V., and Friedman, W. F.: Factors influencing neurohumoral control of the heart and newborn. Am. J. Physiol. *228*:1685, 1975.
30. Klitzner, T. S., and Friedman, W. F.: Excitation contraction coupling in developing mammalian myocardium. Pediatr. Res. *23*:428, 1988.
31. Klitzner, T. S., and Friedman, W. F.: A diminished role for the sarcoplasmic reticulum in newborn myocardial contraction. Pediatr. Res. *26*:98, 1989.
32. Romero, T. E., and Friedman, W. F.: Limited left ventricular response to volume overload in the neonatal period. Pediatr. Res. *13*:910, 1979.
33. Finer, N. N., Etches, P. C., Kamstra, B., et al.: Inhaled nitric oxide in infants referred for extracorporeal membrane oxygenation: Dose response. J. Pediatr. *124*:302, 1994.
34. Geggel, R. L.: Inhalational nitric oxide: A selective pulmonary vasodilator for treatment of persistent pulmonary hypertension of the newborn. J. Pediatr. *123*:76, 1993.
35. Friedman, W. F., Printz, M. P., Kirkpatrick, S. E., and Hoskins, E. J.: The vasoactivity of the fetal lamb ductus arteriosus studied in utero. Pediatr. Res. *17*:331, 1983.

PATHOLOGICAL CONSEQUENCES

36. Friedman, W. F., and George, B. L.: Medical progress—Treatment of congestive heart failure by altering loading conditions of the heart. J. Pediatr. *106*:697, 1985.
37. Friedman, W. F., and George, B. L.: Treatment of cardiac failure in infants. Compr. Ther. *12*:8, 1986.
38. Artman, M., Parrish, M. D., and Graham, T. P., Jr.: Congestive heart failure in childhood and adolescence: Recognition and management. Am. Heart J. *105*:471, 1983.
39. Schmidt, K. G., Araujo, L., and Silverman, N. H.: Evaluation of structural and functional abnormalities of the fetal heart by echocardiography. Am. J. Cardiol. Imag. *2*:57, 1988.
40. Wyllie, J., Wren, C., and Stewart, H.: Screening for fetal cardiac malformations. Br. Heart J. *71*:20, 1994.
41. Meijboom, E. J., Van Engelen, A. D., Van de Beek, E. W., et al.: Fetal arrhythmias. Curr. Opin. Cardiol. *9*:97, 1994.
42. Milne, M. J., Sung, R. Y. T., Fok, T. F., and Crozier, I. G.: Doppler echocardiographic assessment of shunting via the ductus arteriosus in newborn infants. Am. J. Cardiol. *64*:102, 1989.
43. Sahn, D. J., and Friedman, W. F.: Difficulties in distinguishing cardiac from pulmonary disease in the neonate. Pediatr. Clin. North Am. *20*:293, 1973.
44. Stanger, P., Lucas, R. V., Jr., and Edwards, J. E.: Anatomic factors causing respiratory distress in acyanotic congenital cardiac disease: Special reference to bronchial obstruction. Pediatrics *43*:760, 1969.

45. DiSessa, T. G., and Friedman, W. F.: Echocardiographic evaluation of cardiac performance. Cardiol. Clin. *1*:487, 1983.
46. DiSessa, T. G., and Friedman, W. F.: Echocardiographic evaluation of cardiac performance. *In* Friedman, W. F., and Higgins, C. B. (eds.): Pediatric Cardiac Imaging. Philadelphia, W. B. Saunders Company, 1984, p. 219.
47. Mercier, J. C., DiSessa, T. G., Jarmakani, J., and Friedman, W. F.: Two dimensional echocardiographic assessment of left ventricular volumes and ejection fraction. Circulation *65*:962, 1982.
48. Huwez, F. U., Houston, A. B., Watson, J., et al.: Age and body surface area related normal upper and lower limits of M mode echocardiographic measurements and left ventricular volume and mass from infancy to early adulthood. Br. Heart J. *72*:276, 1994.
49. Wessel, A., Schüller, W. C., Yelbuz, T. M., and Bürsch, J. H.: Effect of increased wall thickness on indices of left ventricular pump function in children. Br. Heart J. *72*:182, 1994.
50. Teitel, D., and Rudolph, A. M.: Perinatal oxygen delivery and cardiac function. Adv. Pediatr. *32*:321, 1985.
51. Rosenthal, A., Nathan, D. G., Marty, A. T., et al.: Acute hemodynamic effects of red cell volume reduction, polycythemia of cyanotic congenital heart disease. Circulation *42*:297, 1970.
52. Voigt, G. C., and Wright, J. R.: Cyanotic congenital heart disease and sudden death. Am. Heart J. *87*:773, 1974.
53. Fischbein, C. A., Rosenthal, A., Fischer, E. G., et al.: Risk factors for brain abscess in patients with congenital heart disease. Am. J. Cardiol. *34*:97, 1974.
54. Corrin, C.: Paradoxical embolism. Br. Heart J. *26*:549, 1964.
55. Haroutunian, L. M., and Neill, C. A.: Pulmonary complications of congenital heart disease: Hemoptysis. Am. Heart J. *84*:540, 1972.
56. Guntheroth, W. G., Morgan, B. C., and Mullens, G. L.: Physiologic studies of paroxysmal hyperpnea in cyanotic congenital heart disease. Circulation *31*:70, 1965.
57. Talmer, N. S.: Congestive heart failure in the infant. Pediatr. Clin. North Am. *18*:1011, 1971.
58. Rosenthal, A., and Castaneda, A. R.: Growth and development after cardiovascular surgery in infants and children. *In* Rosenthal, A., Sonnenblick, E. H., and Lesch, M. (eds.): Postoperative Congestive Heart Disease. New York, Grune and Stratton, 1975, p. 110.
59. Gingell, R. I., and Hornung, M. G.: Growth problems associated with congenital heart disease in infancy. *In* Lebenthal, E. (ed.): Textbook of Gastroenterology and Nutrition in Infancy. New York, Raven Press, 1989, p. 639.
60. Salzer, H. R., Haschke, F., Wimmer, M., et al.: Growth and nutritional intake of infants with congenital heart disease. Pediatr. Cardiol. *10*:17, 1989.
61. Friedman, W. F., Heiferman, M. F., and Perloff, J. K.: Late postoperative pulmonary vascular disease—Clinical concerns. *In* Engle, M. A., and Perloff, J. K. (eds.): Congenital Heart Disease After Surgery. New York, York Medical Publishers, 1983, p. 151.
62. Rabinovitch, M.: Structure and function of the pulmonary vascular bed: An update. Cardiol. Clin. *7*:227, 1989.
63. Rabinovitch, M., Keane, J. F., and Norwood, W. I.: Vascular structure and lung biopsy tissue correlated with pulmonary hemodynamic findings after repair of congenital heart defects. Circulation *69*:655, 1984.
64. Heath, D., and Edwards, J. E.: The pathology of hypertensive pulmonary vascular disease. Circulation *18*:533, 1958.
65. Levin, D. L., Rudolph, A. M., Heymann, M. A., and Phibbs, R. H.: Morphological development of the pulmonary vascular bed in the fetal lamb. Circulation *53*:144, 1976.
66. Burchenal, J. E. B., and Loscalzo, J.: Endothelial dysfunction and pulmonary hypertension. Primary Cardiol. *20*:28, 1994.
67. Celermajer, D. S., Dollery, C., Burch, M., and Deanfield, J. E.: Role of endothelium in the maintenance of low pulmonary vascular tone in normal children. Circulation *89*:2041, 1994.
68. Rabinovitch, M., and Reid, L. M.: Quantitative structural analysis of the pulmonary vascular bed in congenital heart defects. *In* Engle, M. A. (ed.): Pediatric Cardiovascular Disease. Philadelphia, F. A. Davis, 1981, p. 149.
69. Friedman, W. F.: Proceedings of the National Heart, Lung and Blood Institute Pediatric Cardiology Workshop: Pulmonary Hypertension. Pediatr. Res. *20*:8, 1986.
70. Aiello, V. D., Higuchi, M., Lopes, E. A., et al.: An immunohistochemical study of arterial lesions due to pulmonary hypertension in patients with congenital heart defects. Cardiol Young *4*:37, 1994.
71. Hopkins, W., and Waggoner, A. D.: Right and left ventricular area and function determined by two-dimensional echocardiography in adults with the Eisenmenger syndrome from a variety of congenital anomalies. Am. J. Cardiol. *72*:90, 1993.
72. Roberts, J. D., Lang, P., Bigatello, L. M., et al.: Inhaled nitric oxide in congenital heart disease. Circulation *87*:447, 1992.
73. Rabinovitch, M., Keane, J. F., Fellows, K. E., et al.: Quantitative analysis of the pulmonary wedge angiogram in congenital heart defects. Circulation *63*:152, 1981.
74. Rabinovitch, M., Castaneda, A. R., and Reid, L.: Lung biopsy with frozen section as a diagnostic aid in patients with congenital heart defects. Am. J. Cardiol. *47*:77, 1981.
75. Rabinovitch, M.: Pathophysiology of pulmonary hypertension. *In* Emmanouilides, G. C., et al. (eds.): Moss and Adams' Heart Disease in Infants, Children, and Adolescents. 5th ed. Baltimore, Williams and Wilkins, 1994, p. 1659.
76. Zeller, S. T., and Gutgesell, H. P.: Noninvasive estimation of pulmonary artery pressure. J. Pediatr. *114*:735, 1989.
77. Morera, J., Hoadley, S. D., Roland, J. M., et al.: Estimation of the ratio of pulmonary to systemic pressures by pulsewave Doppler echocardiography for assessment of pulmonary artery pressures. Am. J. Cardiol. *63*:862, 1989.
78. Awadallah, S. M., Kavey, R. E., Byrum, C. J., et al.: The changing pattern of infective endocarditis in childhood. Am. J. Cardiol. *68*:90, 1991.
79. Saiman, L., Prince, A., and Gersony, W. M.: Pediatric infective endocarditis in the modern era. J. Pediatr. *122*:847, 1993.
80. Van Hare, G. F., Ben-Shachar, G., Liebman, J., et al.: Infective endocarditis in infants and children during the past 10 years: A decade of change. Am. Heart J. *107*:1235, 1984.
81. Dajani, A. S.: Prevention of bacterial endocarditis. Pediatr. Infect. Dis. *4*:349, 1985.
82. Dajani, A. S., Bisno, A. L., Chung, K. J., et al.: Prevention of bacterial endocarditis: Recommendations by the American Heart Association. JAMA *264*:2919, 1990.
83. Selbst, S. M., Ruddy, R. M., Clark, B. J., et al.: Pediatric chest pain: A prospective study. Pediatrics *82*:319, 1988.
84. Graham, T. P., Gessner, I. H., Friedman, W. F., et al.: Recommendations for use of laboratory studies for pediatric patients with suspected or proven heart disease: A statement of the Committee on Congenital Cardiac Defects of the Council on Cardiovascular Disease in the Young of the AHA. Circulation *74*:443a, 1986.
85. Strieper, M. J., and Campbell, R. M.: Efficacy of alpha-adrenergic agonist therapy for prevention of pediatric neurocardiogenic syncope. J. Am. Coll. Cardiol. *22*:594, 1993.
86. Grubb, B. P., Samoil, D., Kosinski, D., et al.: Use of sertraline hydrochloride in the treatment of refractory neurocardiogenic syncope in children and adolescents. J. Am. Coll. Cardiol. *24*:490, 1994.
87. Perry, J., and Garson, A.: The child with recurrent syncope: Autonomic function testing and beta-adrenergic hypersensitivity. J. Am. Coll. Cardiol. *17*:1168, 1991.
88. Driscoll, D. J., and Edwards, W. D.: Sudden unexpected death in children and adolescents. J. Am. Coll. Cardiol. *5*:118B, 1985.
89. Denfield, S. W., and Garson, A., Jr.: Sudden death in children and young adults. Ped. Clin. North Am. *37*:215, 1990.
90. Klitzner, T. S.: Sudden cardiac death in children. Circulation *82*:629, 1990.
91. Gillette, P. C., and Garson, A.: Sudden cardiac death in the pediatric population. Circulation *85*:I, 1992.

APPROACH TO THE HIGH-RISK INFANT

92. Friedman, W. F., and George, B. L.: New concepts and drugs in the treatment of congestive heart failure. Pediatr. Clin. North Am. *31*:1197, 1984.
93. Anderson, P. A. W.: Maturation in cardiac contractility. Cardiol. Clin. *7*:209, 1989.
94. Talner, N. S., and Lister, G.: Perioperative care of the infant with congenital heart disease. Cardiol. Clin. *7*:419, 1989.
95. Park, M. K.: Use of digoxin in infants and children, with specific emphasis on dosage. J. Pediatr. *108*:871, 1986.
96. Freed, M. D., Hegmann, M. A., Lewis, A. B., et al.: Prostaglandin E_1 in infants with ductus arteriosus dependent congenital heart disease. Circulation *64*:899, 1981.
97. Lewis, A. B., Freed, M. D., Hegmann, M. A., et al.: Side effects of therapy with prostaglandin E_1 in infants with critical congenital heart disease. Circulation *64*:893, 1981.
98. Friedman, W. F., Kurlinski, J., Jacob, J., et al.: Inhibition of prostaglandin and prostacyclin synthesis in clinical management of PDA. Semin. Perinatol. *4*:125, 1980.
99. Friedman, W. F.: Patent ductus arteriosus in respiratory distress syndrome. Pediatr. Cardiol. *4*(Suppl. 2):3, 1983.
100. Montigny, M., Davignon, A., Fouron, J. C., et al.: Captopril in infants for congestive heart failure secondary to a large ventricular to right shunt. Am. J. Cardiol. *63*:631, 1989.
101. Schwartz, K., Chassagne, C., and Boheler, K. R.: The molecular biology of heart failure. J. Am. Coll. Cardiol. *22*:30A, 1993.
102. Carter, L. F., and Rubin, S. A.: The molecular and cellular biology of heart failure. Curr. Opin. Cardiol. *8*:361, 1993.
103. Snyder, J. V.: Assessment of systemic oxygen transport. *In* Snyder, J. V. (ed.): Oxygen Transport in the Clinically Ill. Chicago, Year Book Medical Publishing Co., 1987, p. 179.
104. Kleinman, C. S., and Donnerstein, R. L.: Ultrasonic assessment of cardiac function in the intact human fetus. J. Am. Coll. Cardiol. *5*:84S, 1985.
105. Silverman, N. H., Kleinman, C. S., Rudolph, A. M., et al.: Fetal atrioventricular valve insufficiency associated with nonimmune hydrops: A two-dimensional echocardiographic and pulsed Doppler ultrasound study. Circulation *72*:825, 1985.
106. Reed, K. L., Appelton, C. P., Anderson, C. F., et al.: Doppler studies of venacaval flows in human fetuses. Circulation *81*:498, 1990.
107. Gembruch, U., Manz, M., Bald, R., et al.: Repeated intravascular treatment with amiodarone in a fetus with refractory supraventricular tachycardia and hydrops fetalis. Am. Heart J. *118*:1335, 1989.
108. Silverman, N. H., and Schmidt, K. G.: The current role of Doppler echocardiography in the diagnosis of heart disease in children. Cardiol. Clin. *7*:265, 1989.
109. Cloez, J. L., Schmidt, K. G., Birk, E., and Silverman, N. H.: Determina-

tion of pulmonary systemic blood flow ratio in children by simplified Doppler echocardiographic method. J. Am. Coll. Cardiol. *11*:825, 1988.
110. Sahn, D. J.: Applications of color flow mapping in pediatric cardiology. Cardiol. Clin. *7*:255, 1989.
111. Krabill, K. A., Ring, W. S., Foker, J. E., et al.: Echocardiographic versus cardiac catheterization diagnosis of infants with congenital heart disease requiring cardiac surgery. Am. J. Cardiol. *60*:351, 1987.
112. Beekman, R. P., Filippini, L. H. P. M., and Meijboom, E. J.: Evolving usage of pediatric cardiac catheterization. Curr. Opin. Cardiol. *9*:721, 1994.
113. Stanger, P., Heymann, M. A., Tarnoff, H., et al.: Complications of cardiac catheterization of neonates, infants and children. Circulation *50*:595, 1974.
114. Allen, H. D., Driscoll, D. J., Fricker, F. J., et al.: Guidelines for pediatric therapeutic cardiac catheterization. Circulation *84*:2248, 1991.
115. Tynan, M., and Qureshi, S.: Interventional catheterization in congenital heart disease. Curr. Opin. Cardiol. *8*:114, 1993.
116. Hebe, J., Schluter, M., and Kuck, K. H.: Catheter ablation in children with supraventricular tachycardia mediated by accessory pathways—use of radiofrequency current as a first line of therapy. Cardiol. Young *4*:28, 1994.
117. Kugler, J. D., Danford, D. A., and Deal, B. J.: Radiofrequency catheter ablation for tachyarrhythmias in children and adolescents. N. Engl. J. Med. *330*:1481, 1994.
118. Zipes, D. P., Akthar, M., Denes, P., et al.: Guidelines for clinical intracardiac electrophysiologic studies: A report of the American College of Cardiology/AHA Task Force on assessment of diagnostic and therapeutic cardiovascular procedures. J. Am. Coll. Cardiol. *14*:1827, 1989.
119. Klitzner, T. S., Wetzel, G. T., Saxon, L. A., and Stevenson, W. G.: Radiofrequency ablation: A new era in the management of pediatric arrhythmias. Am. J. Dis. Child. *147*:769, 1993.
120. Van Hare, G. F., Lesh, M. D., and Stanger, P.: Radiofrequency catheter ablation of supraventricular arrhythmias in patients with congenital heart disease: Results and technical considerations. J. Am. Coll. Cardiol. *22*:883, 1993.
121. Dhala, A., Bremner, S., Deshpande, S., et al.: Efficacy and safety of atrioventricular nodal modification for atrioventricular nodal reentrant tachycardia in the pediatric population. Am. Heart J. *128*:903, 1994.

SPECIFIC CARDIAC DEFECTS

122. Hunt, C. E., and Lucas, R. V., Jr.: Symptomatic atrial septal defect in infancy. Circulation *42*:1042, 1973.
123. Van Praagh, S., Carrera, M. E., Sanders, S. P., et al.: Sinus venosus defects: Unroofing of the right pulmonary veins—anatomic and echocardiographic findings and surgical treatment. Am. Heart J. *128*:365, 1994.
124. Bashi, V. V., Ravikumar, E., Jairaj, P. S., et al.: Coexistent mitral valve disease with left-to-right shunt at the atrial level: Clinical profile, hemodynamics, and surgical considerations in 67 consecutive patients. Am. Heart J. *114*:1406, 1987.
125. Leachman, R. D., Cokkinos, D. V., and Cooley, D. A.: Association of ostium secundum atrial septal defects with mitral valve prolapse. Am. J. Cardiol. *38*:167, 1976.
126. Levin, A. R., Spach, M. S., Boineau, J. P., et al.: Atrial pressure flow dynamics and atrial septal defects (secundum type). Circulation *37*:476, 1968.
127. O'Toole, J. D., Reddy, I., Curtiss., E. I., and Shaver, J. A.: The mechanism of splitting the second heart sound in atrial septal defect. Circulation *41*:1047, 1977.
128. Clark, E. B., and Kugler, J. D.: Preoperative secundum atrial septal defect with coexisting sinus node and atrioventricular node dysfunction. Circulation *65*:976, 1982.
129. Konstantinides, S., Kasper, W., Geibel, A., et al.: Detection of left-to-right shunt in atrial septal defect by negative contrast echocardiography: A comparison of transthoracic and transesophageal approach. Am. Heart J. *126*:909, 1993.
130. Ishii, M., Kato, H., Inoue, O., et al.: Biplane transesophageal echo-Doppler studies of atrial septal defects: Quantitative evaluation and monitoring for transcatheter closure. Am. Heart J. *125*:1363, 1993.
131. Shub, C., Tajik., A. J., Seward, J. B., et al.: Surgical repair of uncomplicated atrial septal defect without "routine" preoperative cardiac catheterization. J. Am. Coll. Cardiol. *6*:49, 1985.
132. Freed, M. D., Nadas, A. S., Norwood, W. I., and Castaneda, A. R.: Is routine preoperative cardiac catheterization necessary before repair of secundum and sinus venosus atrial septal defects? J. Am. Coll. Cardiol. *4*:333, 1984.
133. Taketa, R. M., Sahn, D. J., Simon, A. L., et al.: Catheter positions in congenital cardiac malformations. Circulation *51*:749, 1975.
134. Brand, A., Keren, A., Branski, D., et al.: Natural course of atrial septal aneurysm in children and the potential for spontaneous closure of associated septal defect. Am. J. Cardiol. *64*:996, 1989.
135. Steele, P. M., Fuster, V., Cohen, M., et al.: Isolated atrial septal defect with pulmonary vascular obstructive disease—long term follow up and prediction of outcome after surgical correction. Circulation *76*:1037, 1987.
136. Lloyd, T. R., Rao, P. S., Beekman, R. H., et al.: Atrial septal defect occlusion with the buttoned device (a multi-institutional U.S. trial). Am. J. Cardiol. *73*:286, 1994.
137. Hausdorf, G., Schneider, M., Franzbach, B., et al.: Transcatheter closure of secundum atrial septal defects with the atrial septal defect occlusion system (ASDOS): Initial experience in children. Heart *75*:83, 1996.
138. Reddy, S. C. B., Rao, P. S., Ewenko, J., et al.: Echocardiographic predictors of success of catheter closure of atrial septal defect with the buttoned device. Am. Heart J. *129*:76, 1995.
138a. Auslender, M., Beekman, R. H., and Lloyd, T. R.: Transcatheter closure of atrial septal defects. J. Interven. Cardiol. *8*:533, 1995.
139. Levin, A. R., Liebson, P. R., Ehlers, K. H., and Daimant, B.: Assessment of left ventricular function in atrial septal defect. Pediatr. Res. *9*:894, 1975.
140. Epstein, S. E., Beiser, G. D., Goldstein, R. E., et al.: Hemodynamic abnormalities in response to mild and intense upright exercise following operative correction of an atrial septal defect or tetralogy of Fallot. Circulation *42*:1065, 1973.
141. Murphy, J. G., Gersh, B. J., McGoon, M. D., et al.: Long term outcome after surgical repair of isolated atrial septal defect. N. Engl. J. Med. *323*:1645, 1990.
142. Karpawich, P. P., Antillon, J. R., Cappola, P. R., and Agarwal, K. C.: Pre- and postoperative electrophysiologic assessment of children with secundum atrial septal defect. Am. J. Cardiol. *55*:519, 1985.
143. Bink-Boelkens, M. T. E., Bergstra, A., and Landsman, M. L. J.: Functional abnormalities of the conduction system in children with an atrial septal defect. Int. J. Cardiol. *20*:263, 1988.
144. Bink-Boelkens, M. T. E., Meuzelaar, K. J., and Eygelaar, A.: Arrhythmias after repair of secundum atrial septal defect: The influence of surgical modification. Am. Heart J. *115*:629, 1988.
145. Borkon, A. M., Pieroni, D. R., Varghese, P. J., et al.: The superior QRS axis in ostium primum ASD. Am. Heart J. *92*:15, 1975.
146. Jacobsen, J. R., Gillette, P. C., Corbett, B. N., et al.: Intracardiac electrography in endocardial cushion defects. Circulation *54*:599, 1976.
147. Waldo, A. L., Kaiser, G. A., Bowman, F. O., Jr., and Malm, J. R.: Etiology of prolongation of the PR interval in patients with an endocardial cushion defect. Circulation *43*:19, 1973.
148. Zellers, T. M., Zehr, R., Weinstein, E., et al.: Two-dimensional and Doppler echocardiography alone can adequately define preoperative anatomy and hemodynamic status before repair of complete atrioventricular septal defect in infants <1 year old. J. Am. Coll. Cardiol. *24*:1565, 1994.
149. Minich, L. A., Snider, A. R., Bove, E. L., et al.: Echocardiographic evaluation of atrioventricular orifice anatomy in children with atrioventricular septal defect. J. Am. Coll. Cardiol. *19*:149, 1992.
150. DeBia, S. E. L., DiCommo, V., Ballerini, L., et al.: Prevalence of left-sided obstructive lesions in patients with atrial ventricular canal without Down's syndrome. J. Thorac. Cardiovasc. Surg. *91*:467, 1986.
151. Elliott, L. P., Bargeron, L. M., Jr., and Green, C. E.: Angled angiography: General approach and findings. *In* Friedman, W. F., and Higgins, C. B. (eds.): Pediatric Cardiac Imaging. Philadelphia, W. B. Saunders Company, 1984, p. 1.
152. Merrill, W. H., Hammon, J. W., Jr., and Bender, H. W., Jr.: Technique of repair of atrioventricular septal defect with a common atrioventricular orifice. Cardiol. Young *1*:379, 1991.
153. Kadoba, K., and Jonas, R. A.: Replacement of the left atrioventricular valve after repair of atrioventricular septal defect. Cardiol. Young *1*:383, 1991.
154. DeLeon, S. Y., Ilbawi, M. N., Wilson, W. R., et al.: Surgical options in subaortic stenosis associated with endocardial cushion defects. Ann. Thorac. Surg. *52*:1076, 1991.
155. Gatzoulis, M. A., Yacoub, M., and Shinebourne, E. A.: Complete atrioventricular septal defect with tetralogy of Fallot: Diagnosis and management. Br. Heart J. *71*:579, 1994.
156. Soto, B., Ceballos, R., and Kirklin, J. W.: Ventricular septal defects: A surgical viewpoint. J. Am. Coll. Cardiol. *14*:1291, 1989.
157. Van Praagh, R., Geva, T., and Kreutzer, J.: Ventricular septal defects: How shall we describe, name and classify them? J. Am. Coll. Cardiol. *14*:1298, 1989.
158. Hagler, D. J., Edwards, W. D., Seward, J. B., and Tajik, A. J.: Standardized nomenclature of the ventricular septum and ventricular septal defects, with applications for two-dimensional echocardiography. Mayo Clin. Proc. *60*:741, 1985.
159. Baker, E. J., Leung, M. P., Anderson, R. H., et al.: The cross-sectional anatomy of ventricular septal defects: A reappraisal. Br. Heart J. *69*:339, 1988.
160. Helmcke, F., Souza, A., Nanda, N. C., et al.: Two-dimensional and color Doppler assessment of ventricular septal defect of congenital origin. Am. J. Cardiol. *63*:1112, 1989.
161. Sharif, D. S., Huhta, J. C., Marantz, P., et al.: Two-dimensional echocardiographic determination of ventricular septal defect size: Correlation of autopsy. Am. Heart J. *117*:1333, 1989.
162. Ortiz, E., Robinson, P. J., Deanfield, J. E., et al.: Localisation of ventricular septal defects by simultaneous display of superimposed colour Doppler and cross sectional echocardiographic images. Br. Heart J. *54*:53, 1985.
163. Pieroni, D. R., Nishimura, R. A., Bierman, F. Z., et al.: Second natural history study of congenital heart defects: Ventricular septal defect: Echocardiography. Circulation *87*:I, 1993.
164. Murphy, D. J., Ludomirsky, A., and Huhta, J. C.: Continuous-wave Doppler in children with ventricular septal defect: Noninvasive estimation of interventricular pressure gradient. Am. J. Cardiol. *57*:428, 1986.
165. Kurokawa, S., Takahashi, M., Katoh, Y., et al.: Noninvasive evaluation of the ratio of pulmonary to systemic flow in ventricular septal defect

by means of Doppler two-dimensional echocardiography. Am. Heart J. *116:*1033, 1988.
166. Williams, R. G.: Doppler color-flow mapping and prediction of ventricular defect outcome. J. Am. Coll. Cardiol. *13:*1119, 1989.
167. Hornberger, L. K., Sahn, D. J., Krabill, K. A., et al.: Elucidation of the natural history of ventricular septal defects by serial Doppler color-flow mapping studies. J. Am. Coll. Cardiol. *13:*1111, 1989.
168. Friedman, W. F., Mehrizi, A., and Pusch, A. L.: Multiple muscular ventricular septal defects. Circulation *32:*35, 1964.
169. Dickinson, D. F., Arnold, R., and Wilkinson, J. L.: Ventricular septal defects in children born in Liverpool: Evaluation of natural course and surgical implications in an unselected population. Br. Heart J. *46:*47, 1981.
170. Weidman, W. H., Blount, S. G., Jr., DuShane, J. W., et al.: Clinical course in ventricular septal defect: Natural history study. Circulation *56*(Suppl.):I, 1977.
171. Ramaciotti, C., Keren, A., and Silverman, N. H.: Importance of (perimembranous) ventricular septal aneurysm in the natural history of isolated perimembranous ventricular septal defect. Am. J. Cardiol. *57:*268, 1986.
172. Friedman, W. F., and Pitlick, P. T.: Ventricular septal defect in infancy —University of California, San Diego (Specialty Conference). West. J. Med. *120:*295, 1974.
173. Moe, D. J., and Guntheroth, W. G.: Spontaneous closure of uncomplicated ventricular septal defect. Am. J. Cardiol. *60:*674, 1987.
174. Neutze, J. M., Ishikawa, T., Clarkson, P. M., et al.: Assessment and follow up of patients with ventricular septal defect and elevated pulmonary vascular resistance. Am. J. Cardiol. *63:*327, 1989.
175. Van Den Heuvel, F., Timmers, T., and Hess, J.: Morphological, haemodynamic, and clinical variables as predictors for management of isolated ventricular septal defect. Br. Heart J. *73:*49, 1995.
176. Kidd, L., Driscoll, D. J., Gersony, W. M., et al.: Second natural history study of congenital heart defects: Results of treatment of patients with ventricular septal defects. Circulation *87:*I, 1993.
177. Yeager, S. B., Freed, M. D., Keane, J. F., et al.: Primary surgical closure of ventricular septal defect in the first year of life: Results in 128 infants. J. Am. Coll. Cardiol. *3:*1269, 1984.
178. Kirkllin, J. W., and Barrett-Boyes, B. J. (eds.): Cardiac Surgery. 2nd ed. New York, Churchill Livingstone, 1993, p. 798.
179. McDaniel, N., Gutgesell, H. P., Nolan, S. P., and Kron, I. L.: Repair of large muscular ventricular septal defects in infants employing left ventriculotomy. Ann. Thorac. Surg. *47:*593, 1989.
180. Gheen, K. M., and Reeves, J. T.: Effects of size of ventricular septal defect and age on pulmonary hemodynamics at sea level. Am. J. Cardiol. *75:*66, 1995.
181. Hislop, A., Haworth, S. G., Shinebourne, E. A., and Reid, L.: Quantitative structural analysis of pulmonary vessels in isolated ventricular septal defect in infancy. Br. Heart J. *37:*1014, 1975.
182. DuShane, J. W., and Kirklin, J. W.: Late results of the repair of ventricular septal defect on pulmonary vascular disease. *In* Kirklin, J. W. (ed.): Advances in Cardiovascular Surgery. New York, Grune and Stratton, 1973, p. 9.
183. Rhodes, L. A., Keane, J. F., Keane, J. P., et al.: Long-term follow up (up to 43 years) of ventricular septal defect with audible aortic regurgitation. Am. J. Cardiol. *66:*340, 1990.
184. Schmidt, K. G., Cassidy, S. C., Silverman, N. H., and Stanger, P.: Doubly committed subarterial ventricular septal defects: Echocardiographic features and surgical implications. J. Am. Coll. Cardiol. *12:*1538, 1988.
185. Wang, J. K., Lue, H. C., Wu, M. H., et al.: Assessment of ventricular septal defect with aortic valvar prolapse by means of echocardiography and angiography. Cardiol. Young *4:*44, 1994.
186. Bonhoeffer, P., Fabbrocini, M., Lecompte, Y., et al.: Infundibular septal defect with severe aortic regurgitation: A new surgical approach. Ann. Thorac. Surg. *53:*851, 1992.
187. Ramaciotti, C., Vetter, J. M., Bornemeier, R. A., and Chin, A. J.: Prevalence, relation to spontaneous closure, and association of muscular ventricular septal defects with other cardiac defects. Am. J. Cardiol. *75:*61, 1995.
188. Leung, M. P., Mok, C. K., Lo, R. N. S., and Lau, K. C.: An echocardiographic study of perimembranous ventricular septal defect with left ventricular to right atrial shunting. Br. Heart J. *55:*45, 1986.
189. Gersony, W. M., and Hayes, C. J.: Bacterial endocarditis in patients with pulmonary stenosis, aortic stenosis, or ventricular septal defect: Natural history study. Circulation *56*(Suppl.):I, 1977.
190. deLeval, M.: Ventricular septal defects. *In* Stark, J., and deLeval, M. (eds.): Surgery for Congenital Heart Defects. New York, Grune and Stratton, Inc., 1983, p. 271.
191. Waldman, J. D.: Why not close a small ventricular septal defect? Ann. Thorac. Surg. *56:*1011, 1993.
192. Van Der Velde, M. E., Sanders, S. P., Keane, J. F., et al.: Transesophageal echocardiographic guidance of transcatheter ventricular septal defect closure. J. Am. Coll. Cardiol. *23:*1660, 1994.
193. Tee, S. D. C., Shiota, T., Weintraub, R., et al.: Evaluation of ventricular septal defect by transesophageal echocardiography: Intraoperative assessment. Am. Heart J. *127:*585, 1994.
194. Rigby, M., and Redington, A. N.: Primary transcatheter umbrella closure of perimembranous ventricular septal defect. Br. Heart J. *72:*368, 1994.
195. Okarama, E. O., Guller, B., Molony, J. D., and Weidman, W. H.: Etiology of right bundle-branch block pattern after surgical closure of ventricular-septal defects. Am. Heart J. *90:*14, 1975.
196. Otterstad, J. E., Simonsen, S., and Erikssen, J.: Hemodynamic findings at rest and during mild supine exercise in adults with isolated uncomplicated ventricular septal defects. Circulation *71:*650, 1985.
197. Maron, B. J., Redwood, D. R., Hirschfield, J. W., Jr., et al.: Postoperative assessment of patients with ventricular septal defect and pulmonary hypertension: Response to intense upright exercise. Circulation *48:*864, 1973.
198. Graham, T. P., Jr., Atwood, G. F., Boucek, R. J., Jr., et al.: Right ventricular volume characteristics in ventricular septal defect. Circulation *54:*800, 1976.
199. Heymann, M. A., and Rudolph, A. M.: Control of the ductus arteriosus. Physiol. Rev. *55:*62, 1975.
200. Friedman, W. F., Printz, M. P., Kirkpatrick, S. E., and Hoskins, E. J.: The vasoactivity of the fetal lamb ductus arteriosus studied in utero. Pediatr. Res. *17:*331, 1983.
201. Skidgel, R. A., Friedman, W. F., and Printz, M. P.: Prostaglandin biosynthetic activities of the fetal lamb ductus arteriosus, other blood vessels and fetal lung. Pediatr. Res. *18:*12, 1984.
202. Printz, M. P., Skidgel, R. A., and Friedman, W. F.: Studies of pulmonary prostaglandin biosynthetic and catabolic enzymes as factors in ductus arteriosus patency and closure: Evidence for a shift in products with gestational age. Pediatr. Res. *18:*19, 1984.
203. Gittenberger-DeGroot, A. C.: Persistent ductus arteriosus: Most probably a primary congenital malformation. Br. Heart J. *39:*610, 1977.
204. Friedman, W. F., Hirschklau, M. J., Printz, M. P., et al.: Pharmacologic closure of patient ductus arteriosus in the premature infant. N. Engl. J. Med. *295:*526, 1976.
205. Douidar, S. M., Richardson, J., and Snodgrass, W. R.: Use of indomethacin in ductus closure: An update evaluation. Dev. Pharmacol. Ther. *11:*196, 1988.
206. Shimada, S., Kasai, T., Konishi, M., et al.: Effects of patent ductus arteriosus on left ventricular output and organ blood flows in preterm infants with respiratory distress syndrome treated with surfactant. J. Pediatr. *125:*270, 1994.
207. Sahn, D. J., Vaucher, Y., Williams, D. E., et al.: Echocardiographic detection of large left to right shunts and cardiomyopathies in infants and children. Am. J. Cardiol. *38:*73, 1976.
208. Liao, P. K., Su, W. J., and Hung, J. S.: Doppler echocardiographic flow characteristics of isolated patent ductus arteriosus: Better delineation by Doppler color-flow mapping. J. Am. Coll. Cardiol. *12:*1285, 1988.
209. Hiraishi, S., Horiguchi, Y., Misawa, H., et al.: Noninvasive Doppler echocardiographic evaluation of shunt flow dynamics of the ductus arteriosus. Circulation *75:*1146, 1987.
210. Yeh, T. F., Achanti, B., Patel, H., and Pildes, R. S.: Indomethacin therapy in premature infants with patent ductus arteriosus—determination of therapeutic plasma levels. Dev. Pharmacol. Ther. *12:*169, 1989.
211. Jacob, J., Gluck, L., DiSessa., T. G., et al.: The contribution of PDA in the neonate with severe RDS. J. Pediatr. *96:*79, 1980.
212. Merritt, T. A., Harris, J. P., and Roghmann, K.: Early closure of the patent ductus arteriosus in very low birth weight infants: A controlled trial. J. Pediatr. *99:*281, 1981.
213. Gersony, W. M., Peckham, G. J., Ellison, R. C., et al.: Effects of indomethacin in premature infants with patent ductus arteriosus: Results of a national collaborative study. J. Pediatr. *102:*895, 1983.
214. Cassady, G., Crouse, D. T., Kirklin, J. W., et al.: A randomized control trial of very early prophylactic ligation of the ductus arteriosus in babies who weighed 1000 g or less at birth. N. Engl. J. Med. *320:*1511, 1989.
215. Wagner, H. R., Ellison, R. C., Zierler, S., et al.: Surgical closure of patent ductus arteriosus in 268 preterm infants. J. Thorac. Cardiovasc. Surg. *87:*870, 1984.
216. Jarmakini, M. M., Graham, T. P., Jr., Canent, R. V., Jr., et al.: Effect of site of shunt on left heart volume characteristics in children with ventricular septal defect and patent ductus arteriosus. Circulation *40:*411, 1969.
217. Bessenger, F. B., Jr., Blieden, L. C., and Edwards, J. E.: Hypertensive pulmonary vascular disease associated with patent ductus arteriosus. Circulation *52:*157, 1975.
218. Moore, J. W., George, L., Kirkpatrick, S. E., et al.: Percutaneous closure of the small patent ductus arteriosus using occluding spring coils. J. Am. Coll. Cardiol. *23:*759, 1994.
219. Magee, A. G., Stumper, O., Burns, J. E., et al.: Medium-term follow up of residual shunting and potential complications after transcatheter occlusion of the ductus arteriosus. Br. Heart J. *71:*63, 1994.
220. Verin, V. E., Saveliev, S. V., Kolody, S. M., et al.: Results of transcatheter closure of the patent ductus arteriosus with the Botallooccluder. J. Am. Coll. Cardiol. *22:*1509, 1993.
221. Schräder, R., Kneissl, G. D., Sievert, H., et al.: Nonoperative closure of the patent ductus arteriosus: The Frankfurt experience. J. Interven. Cardiol. *5:*89, 1992.
222. Galal, O., de Moor, M., Al-Fadley, F., and Hijazi, Z. M.: Transcatheter closure of the patent ductus arteriosus: Comparison between the Rashkind occluder device and the anterograde Gianturco coils technique. Am. Heart J. *131:*368, 1996.
223. Gray, D. T., Fyler, D. C., Walker, A. M., et al.: Clinical outcomes and costs of transcatheter as compared with surgical closure of patent ductus arteriosus. N. Engl. J. Med. *329:*1517, 1993.
224. Gray, D. T., Walker, A. M., Fyler, D. C., et al.: Examination of the early "learning curve" for transcatheter closure of patent ductus arteriosus using the Rashkind occluder. Circulation *90:*36, 1994.

224a. Moore, J. W., and Cambier, P. A.: Transcatheter occlusion of patent ductus arteriosus. J. Interven. Cardiol. *8*:517, 1995.
225. Kutsche, L. M., and Van Mierop, L. H. S.: Anatomy and pathogenesis of aorticopulmonary septal defect. Am. J. Cardiol. *59*:443, 1987.
226. Matsuki, O., Yagihara, T., Yamamoto, F., et al.: New surgical technique for total-defect aortopulmonary window. Ann. Thorac. Surg. *54*:991, 1992.
227. Prasad, T. R., Valiathan, M. S., Chyamakrishnan, K. G., et al.: Surgical management of aortopulmonary septal defect. Ann. Thorac. Surg. *47*:877, 1989.
228. Crupi, G., Macartney, F. J., and Anderson, R. H.: Persistent truncus arteriosus: A study of 66 autopsy cases with special reference to definition and morphogenesis. Am. J. Cardiol. *40*:569, 1977.
229. Shrivastava, F., and Edwards, J. E.: Coronary arterial origin and persistent truncus arteriosus. Circulation *55*:551, 1977.
230. Suzuki, A., Ho, S. Y., Anderson, R. H., and Deanfield, J. E.: Coronary arterial and sinusal anatomy in hearts with a common arterial trunk. Ann. Thorac. Surg. *48*:792, 1989.
231. Calder, L., Van Praagh, R., Sears, W. P., et al.: Truncus arteriosus communis. Am. Heart J. *92*:23, 1976.
232. Juaneda, E., and Haworth, S. G.: Pulmonary vascular disease in children with truncus arteriosus. Am. J. Cardiol. *54*:1314, 1984.
233. Radford, D. J., Perkins, L., Lachman, R., and Thong, Y. H.: Spectrum of DiGeorge syndrome in patients with truncus arteriosus: Expanded DiGeorge syndrome. Pediatr. Cardiol. *9*:95, 1988.
234. Kirby, M. L., and Waldo, K. L.: Role of neural crest in congenital heart disease. Circulation *82*:332, 1990.
235. Gelband, H., Van Meter, S., and Gersony, W. M.: Truncal valve abnormalities in infants with persistent truncus arteriosus. Circulation *45*:397, 1972.
236. Yoshizato, T., and Julsrud, P. R.: Truncus arteriosus revisited: An angiographic demonstration. Pediatr. Cardiol. *11*:36, 1990.
237. Bove, E. L., Beekman, R. H., Snider, A. R., et al.: Repair of truncus arteriosus in the neonate and young infant. Ann. Thorac. Surg. *47*:499, 1989.
238. Hanley, F. L., Heinemann, M. K., Jonas, R. A., et al.: Repair of truncus arteriosus in the neonate. J. Thorac. Cardiovasc. Surg. *105*:1047, 1993.
239. Heinemann, M. K., Hanley, F. L., Fenton, K. N., et al.: Fate of small homograft conduits after early repair of truncus arteriosus. Ann. Thorac. Surg. *55*:1409, 1993.
240. Davis, J. T., Allen, H. D., Wheler, J. J., et al.: Coronary artery fistula in the pediatric age group: A 19-year institutional experience. Ann. Thorac. Surg. *58*:760, 1994.
241. Yoshikawa, J., Katao, H., Yanagihara, K., et al.: Noninvasive visualization of the dilated main coronary arteries in coronary artery fistulas by cross-sectional echocardiography. Circulation *65*:600, 1993.
242. Miyatake, K., Okamoto, M., Kinoshita, N., et al.: Doppler echocardiographic features of coronary arteriovenous fistula: Complementary roles of cross sectional echocardiography and the Doppler technique. Br. Heart J. *51*:508, 1984.
243. Hofbeck, M., Wild, F., and Singer, H.: Improved visualisation of a coronary artery fist by the "laid-back" aortogram. Br. Heart J. *70*:272, 1993.
244. Perry, S. B., Rome, J., Keane, J. F., et al.: Transcatheter closure of coronary artery fistulas. J. Am. Coll. Cardiol. *20*:205, 1992.
245. Ruttenhouse, E. A., Doty, D. B., and Ehrenhaft, J. L.: Congenital coronary artery-cardiac chamber fistula: Review of operative management. Ann. Thorac. Surg. *20*:468, 1975.
246. Angelini, P.: Normal and anomalous coronary arteries: Definitions and classification. Am. Heart J. *117*:418, 1989.
247. Celermajer, D. S., Sholler, G. F., Howman-Giles, R., and Celermajer, J. M.: Myocardial infarction in childhood: Clinical analysis of 17 cases and medium term follow up of survivors. Br. Heart J. *65*:332, 1991.
248. Hurwitz, R. A., Caldwell, R. L., Girod, D. A., et al.: Clinical and hemodynamic course of infants and children with anomalous left coronary artery. Am. Heart J. *118*:1176, 1989.
249. Menahem, S., and Venables, A. W.: Anomalous left coronary artery from the pulmonary artery: A 15-year sample. Br. Heart J. *58*:378, 1987.
250. Johnsrude, C. L., Perry, J. C., Cecchin, F., et al.: Differentiating anomalous left main coronary artery originating from the pulmonary artery in infants from myocarditis and dilated cardiomyopathy by electrocardiogram. Am. J. Cardiol. *75*:71, 1995.
251. Karr, S. S., Parness, I. A., Spevak, P. J., et al.: Diagnosis of anomalous left coronary artery by Doppler color flow mapping: Distinction from other causes of dilated cardiomyopathy. J. Am. Coll. Cardiol. *19*:1271, 1992.
252. Schmidt, K. G., Cooper, M. J., Silverman, N. H., and Stanger, P.: Pulmonary artery origin of the left coronary artery: Diagnosis by two-dimensional echocardiography, pulsed Doppler ultrasound and color-flow mapping. J. Am. Coll. Cardiol. *11*:396, 1988.
253. Vouhe, P. R., Tamisier, D., Sidi, D., et al.: Anomalous left coronary artery from the pulmonary artery: Results of isolated aortic reimplantation. Ann. Thorac. Surg. *54*:621, 1992.
254. Fernandes, E. D., Kadivar, H., Hallman, G. L., et al.: Congenital malformations of the coronary arteries: The Texas Heart Institute experience. Ann. Thorac. Surg. *54*:732, 1992.
255. Francois, K., Provenier, F., Jordaens, L., and Van Nooten, G. J.: Anomalous origin of the left coronary artery from the pulmonary artery. Ann. Thorac. Surg. *56*:1168, 1993.
256. Dua, R., Smith, J. A., Wilkinson, J. L., et al.: Long-term follow-up after two coronary repair of anomalous left coronary artery from the pulmonary artery. J. Cardiovasc. Surg. *8*:384, 1993.
257. Boutefeu, J. M., Morat, P. R., Hahn, C., and Hauf, E.: Aneurysms of the sinus of Valsalva: Report of seven cases in review of the literature. Am. J. Med. *65*:18, 1978.
258. Perry, L. W., Martin, G. R., Galioto, F. M., Midgley, F. M.: Rupture of congenital sinus of valsalva aneurysm in a newborn. Am. J. Cardiol. *68*:1255, 1991.
259. Holdright, D. R., Brecker, S., and Sheppard, M.: Ruptured aneurysm of the aortic sinus of Valsalva—difficulties in establishing the diagnosis. Cardiol. Young *5*:75, 1995.
260. Barragry, T. P., Ring, W. S., Moller, J. H., and Lillehei, C. W.: 15 to 30 year follow up of patients undergoing repair of ruptured congenital aneurysms of the sinus of Valsalva. Ann. Thorac. Surg. *46*:515, 1988.
261. Smyth, P. T., and Edwards, J. E.: Pseudocoarctation, kinking or buckling of the aorta. Circulation *46*:1027, 1972.
262. Hutchins, G. M.: Coarctation of the aorta explained as a branch point of the ductus arteriosus. Am. J. Pathol. *63*:203, 1971.
263. Talner, N. S., and Berman, M. A.: Postnatal development of obstruction in coarctation of the aorta: Role of the ductus arteriosus. Pediatrics *56*:562, 1975.
264. Heymann, M. A., Berman, W., Jr., Rudolph, A. M., and Whitman, V.: Dilatation of the ductus arteriosus by prostaglandin E_1 in aortic arch abnormalities. Circulation *59*:169, 1979.
265. Van Son, J. A. M., Skotnicki, S. H., Van Asten, W. N., et al.: Quantitative assessment of coarctation in infancy by Doppler spectral analysis. Am. J. Cardiol. *63*:1282, 1989.
266. Rao, P. S., and Carey, P.: Doppler ultrasound in the prediction of pressure gradients across aortic coarctation. Am. Heart J. *118*:299, 1989.
267. Godwin, C. D., Herfkens, R. L., Brundage, D. H., and Lipton, N. J.: Evaluation of coarctation of the aorta by computed tomography. J. Comput. Assist. Tomogr. *5*:153, 1981.
268. Mohiaddin, R. H., Kilner, P. J., Rees, S., et al.: Magnetic resonance volume flow and jet velocity mapping in aortic coarctation. J. Am. Coll. Cardiol. *22*:1515, 1993.
269. George, B., DiSessa, T. G., Williams, R. G., et al.: Coarctation repair without cardiac catheterization in infants. Am. Heart J. *114*:1421, 1987.
270. DeGroff, C. G., Rice, M. J., Reller, M. D., et al.: Intravascular ultrasound can assist angiographic assessment of coarctation of the aorta. Am. Heart J. *128*:836, 1994.
271. Rao, P. S., Galal, O., Smith, P. A., and Wilson, A. D.: Five- to nine-year follow-up results of balloon angioplasty of native aortic coarctation in infants and children. J. Am. Coll. Cardiol. *27*:462, 1996.
271a. Ino, T., Nishimoto, K., Akimoto, K., et al.: Prospective study on a new therapeutic strategy for infants and children with aortic coarctation. Cardiol. Young *5*:36, 1995.
271b. Fletcher, S., Nihill, M. R., Grifka, R. G., et al.: Balloon angioplasty of native coarctation of the aorta: Midterm follow-up and prognostic factors. J. Am. Coll. Cardiol. *25*:730, 1995.
271c. Mendelsohn, A. M.: Balloon angioplasty for native coarctation of the aorta. J. Interven. Cardiol. *8*:487, 1995.
272. Johnson, M. C., Canter, C. E., Strauss, A. W., et al.: Repair of coarctation of the aorta in infancy: Comparison of surgical and balloon angioplasty. Am. Heart J. *125*:464, 1993.
273. Rao, P. S., Chopra, P. S., Koscik, R., et al.: Surgical versus balloon therapy for aortic coarctation in infants ≤3 months old. J. Am. Coll. Cardiol. *23*:1479, 1994.
274. Shaddy, R. E., Boucek, M. M., Sturtevant, J. E., et al.: Comparison of angioplasty and surgery for unoperated coarctation of the aorta. Circulation *87*:793, 1993.
275. Merrill, W. H., Hoff, S. J., Stewart, J. R., et al.: Operative risk factors and durability of repair of coarctation of the aorta in the neonate. Ann. Thorac. Surg. *58*:399, 1994.
276. Kopf, G. S., Hellenbrand, W., Kleinman, C., et al.: Repair of aortic coarctation in the first three months of life: Immediate and long-term results. Ann. Thorac. Surg. *41*:425, 1986.
277. Beekman, R. H., Rocchini, A. P., Behrendt, D. M., and Rosenthal, A.: Reoperation for coarctation of the aorta. Am. J. Cardiol. *48*:1108, 1981.
278. Choy, M., Rocchini, A. P., Beekman, R. H., et al.: Paradoxical hypertension after repair of coarctation of the aorta in children: Balloon angioplasty versus surgical repair. Circulation *75*:1186, 1987.
279. Gidding, S. S., Rocchini, A. P., Beekman, R., et al.: Therapeutic effect of propranolol on paradoxical hypertension after repair of coarctation of the aorta. N. Engl. J. Med. *312*:1224, 1985.
280. Mühler, E. G., Neuerburg, J. M., Rüben, A., et al.: Evaluation of aortic coarctation after surgical repair: Role of magnetic resonance imaging and Doppler ultrasound. Br. Heart J. *70*:285, 1993.
281. Fawzy, M. E., Dunn, B., Galal, O., et al.: Balloon coarctation angioplasty in adolescents and adults: Early and intermediate results. Am. Heart J. *124*:167, 1992.
281a. Hijazi, A. M., Geggel, R. L.: Balloon angioplasty for postoperative recurrent coarctation of the aorta. J. Interven. Cardiol. *8*:509, 1995.
282. Kimball, T. R., Reynolds, J. M., Mays, W. A., et al.: Persistent hyperdynamic cardiovascular state at rest and during exercise in children after successful repair of coarctation of the aorta. J. Am. Coll. Cardiol. *24*:194, 1994.
283. Balderston, S. M., Daberkow, E., Clarke, D. R., et al.: Maximal voluntary exercise variables in children with postoperative coarctation of the aorta. J. Am. Coll. Cardiol. *19*:154, 1992.
284. Murphy, A. M., Blades, M., Daniels, S., and James, F. W.: Blood pres-

sure in cardiac output during exercise: A longitudinal study of children undergoing repair of coarctation. Am. Heart J. *117*:1327, 1989.
285. Krogmann, O. N., Rammos, S., Jakob, M., et al.: Left ventricular diastolic dysfunction late after coarctation repair in childhood: Influence of left ventricular hypertrophy. J. Am. Coll. Cardiol. *21*:1454, 1993.
286. Johnson, M. C., Gutierrez, F. R., Sekarski, D. R., et al.: Comparison of ventricular mass and function in early versus late repair of coarctation of the aorta. Am. J. Cardiol. *73*:698, 1994.
287. Mathew, P., Moodie, D., Blechman, G., et al.: Long-term follow-up of aortic coarctation in infants, children and adults. Cardiol. Young *3*:20, 1993.
288. Gardiner, H. M., Celermajer, D. S., Sorensen, K. E., et al.: Arterial reactivity is significantly impaired in normotensive young adults after successful repair of aortic coarctation in childhood. Circulation *89*:1745, 1994.
289. Van Woezik, E. V. M., Kline, H. W., and Krediet, P.: Normal internal calibers of ostia, great arteries and aortic isthmus in children. Br. Heart J. *39*:860, 1977.
290. Bharati, S., and Lev, M.: The surgical anatomy of the heart in tubular hypoplasia of the transverse aorta (preductal coarctation). J. Thorac. Cardiovasc. Surg. *91*:79, 1986.
291. Graham, T. P., Jr., Atwood, G. F., Boerth, R. C., et al.: Right and left heart size and function in infants with symptomatic coarctation. Circulation *56*:641, 1977.
292. Zannini, L., Gargiulo, G., Albanese, S. B., et al.: Aortic coarctation with hypoplastic arch in neonates: A spectrum of anatomic lesions requiring different surgical options. Ann. Thorac. Surg. *56*:288, 1993.
293. Hoff, S. J., Stewart, J. R., and Bender, H. W., Jr.: Aortic obstructions in infants and children: Surgery for complex aortic coarctation. Prog. Pediatr. Cardiol. *3*:62, 1994.
294. Ino, T., Nishimoto, K., Akimoto, K., et al.: Prospective study on a new therapeutic strategy for infants and children with aortic coarctation. Cardiol. Young *5*:36, 1995.
295. Johns, J. A., and Graham, T. P., Jr.: Aortic obstructions in infants and children: Pathophysiology and clinical presentation of interrupted aortic arch. Prog. Pediatr. Cardiol. *3*:87, 1994.
296. Dekker, A. O., Gittenberger-DeGroot, A. C., and Roozendaal, H.: The ductus arteriosus and associated cardiac anomalies in interruption of the aortic arch. Pediatr. Cardiol. *2*:185, 1982.
297. Stevens, C. A., Carey, J. C., and Shigeoka, A. O.: DiGeorge anomaly and velocardiofacial syndrome. Pediatrics *85*:526, 1990.
298. Buck, S. H., Graham, T. P., Jr., and Lawton, A. R.: DiGeorge syndrome: Implications for aortic arch obstruction. Prog. Pediatr. Cardiol. *3*:94, 1994.
299. Hoff, S. J., Merrill, W. H., and Bender, H. W., Jr.: Aortic obstructions in infants and children: Surgery for interrupted aortic arch. Prog. Pediatr. Cardiol. *3*:100, 1994.
300. Matsuki, O., Yagihara, T., Yamamoto, F., et al.: One-stage repair for intracardiac malformations associated with interrupted aortic arch or aortic coarctation in the first year of life. Cardiol. Young *5*:15, 1995.
301. Foker, J. E.: Surgical repair of aortic arch interruption. Ann. Thorac. Surg. *53*:369, 1992.
302. Friedman, W. F.: Congenital aortic stenosis. *In* Emmanoulides, G., et al. (eds.): Moss and Adams' Heart Disease in Infants, Children, and Adolescents. 5th ed. Baltimore, Williams and Wilkins, 1994, p. 1087.
303. Friedman, W. F., and Pappelbaum, S. J.: Indications for hemodynamic evaluation and surgery in congenital aortic stenosis. Pediatr. Clin. North Am. *18*:1207, 1971.
304. Kveselis, D. A., Rocchini, A. P., Rosenthal, A., et al.: Hemodynamic determinants of exercise-induced ST-segment depression in children with valvar aortic stenosis. Am. J. Cardiol. *55*:1133, 1985.
305. Driscoll, D. J., Wolfe, R. R., Gersony, W. M., et al.: Cardiorespiratory responses to exercise of patients with aortic stenosis, pulmonary stenosis, and ventricular septal defect. Circulation *87*(Suppl. I):I, 1993.
306. Graham, T. P., Louis, B. J., Jarmakani, J. M., et al.: Left heart volume and mass quantification in children with left ventricular pressure overload. Circulation *41*:203, 1970.
307. Fifer, M. A., Borow, K. M., Colan, S. D., et al.: Early diastolic left ventricular function in children and adults with aortic stenosis. J. Am. Coll. Cardiol. *5*:1147, 1985.
308. Villari, B., Hess, O. M., Kaufmann, P., et al.: Effect of aortic valve stenosis (pressure overload) and regurgitation (volume overload) on left ventricular systolic and diastolic function. Am. J. Cardiol. *69*:927, 1992.
309. Lewis, A. L., Heymann, M. A., Stanger, P., et al.: Evaluation of subendocardial ischemia in valvar aortic stenosis in children. Circulation *49*:978, 1974.
310. Strasburger, J. F., Kugler, J. D., Cheatham, J. P., and McManus, B. M.: Nonimmunologic hydrops fetalis associated with congenital aortic valvular stenosis. Am. Heart J. *108*:1380, 1984.
311. Maxwell, D., Allan, L., and Tynan, M. J.: Balloon dilation of the aortic valve in the fetus: A report of two cases. Br. Heart J. *55*:53, 1991.
312. Lakier, J. B., Lewis, A. B., Heymann, M. A., et al.: Isolated aortic stenosis of the neonate: Natural history and hemodynamic considerations. Circulation *50*:801, 1974.
313. Karl, T. R., Sano, S., Brawn, W. J., and Mee, R. B. B.: Critical aortic stenosis in the first month of life: Surgical results in 26 infants. Ann. Thorac. Surg. *50*:105, 1990.
314. Broderick, T. W., Higgins, C. B., and Friedman, W. F.: Critical aortic stenosis in neonates. Radiology *129*:393, 1978.
315. Donti, A., Bonvicini, M., Gargiulo, G., et al.: Criteria for selection of balloon valvoplasty for treatment of aortic stenosis in neonates. Cardiol. Young *5*:31, 1995.
316. Beekman, R. H., Rocchini, A. P., and Andes, A.: Balloon valvuloplasty for critical aortic stenosis in the newborn: Influence of new catheter technology. J. Am. Coll. Cardiol. *17*:1172, 1991.
316a. Donti, A., Bonvicini, M., Gargiulo, G., et al.: Criteria for selection of balloon valvuloplasty for treatment of aortic stenosis in neonates. Cardiol. Young *5*:31, 1995.
316b. Sandhu, S. K., Silka, M. J., and Reller, M. D.: Balloon aortic valvuloplasty for aortic stenosis in neonates, children, and young adults. J. Interven. Cardiol. *8*:477, 1995.
317. Fischer, D. R., Ettedgui, J. A., Park, S. C., et al.: Carotid artery approach for balloon dilation of aortic valve stenosis in the neonate: A preliminary report. J. Am. Coll. Cardiol. *14*:1633, 1990.
318. Rhodes, L. A., Colan, S. D., Perry, S. B., et al.: Predictors of survival in neonates with critical aortic stenosis. Circulation *84*:2325, 1991.
319. Leung, M. P., McKay, R., Smith, A., et al.: Critical aortic stenosis in early infancy. J. Thorac. Cardiovasc. Surg. *101*:526, 1991.
320. Vogel, M., Sebening, F., Sauer, U., and Buhlmeyer, K.: Left ventricular function and myocardial mass after aortic valvotomy in infancy. Pediatr. Cardiol. *13*:5, 1992.
321. Rychik, K., Murdison, K. A., Chin, A. J., and Norwood, W. I.: Surgical management of severe aortic outflow obstruction in lesions other than the hypoplastic left heart syndrome: Use of the pulmonary artery to aorta anastomosis. J. Am. Coll. Cardiol. *18*:809, 1991.
322. Braunwald, E., Goldblatt, A., Aygen, M. M., et al.: Congenital aortic stenosis. I. Clinical and hemodynamic findings in 100 patients. Circulation *27*:426, 1963.
323. Johnson, A. M.: Aortic stenosis, sudden death, and the left ventricular baroreceptors. Br. Heart J. *33*:1, 1971.
324. Gersony, W. M., Hayes, C. J., Driscoll, D. J., et al.: Bacterial endocarditis in patients with aortic stenosis, pulmonary stenosis, or ventricular septal defect. Circulation *87*(Suppl. I):I, 1993.
325. Bengur, A. R., Snider, A. R., Serwer, G. A., et al.: Usefulness of the Doppler mean gradient in evaluation of children with aortic valve stenosis in comparison to gradient at catheterization. Am. J. Cardiol. *64*:756, 1989.
326. Parsons, N. K., Moreau, G. A., Graham, T. P., Jr., et al.: Echocardiographic estimation of critical left ventricular size in infants with isolated aortic valve stenosis. J. Am. Coll. Cardiol. *18*:1049, 1991.
327. Bengur, A. R., Snider, A. R., Meliones, J. M., and Vermilion, R. P.: Doppler evaluation of aortic valve area in children with aortic stenosis. J. Am. Coll. Cardiol. *18*:1499, 1991.
328. Nishimura, R. A., Pieroni, D. R., Bierman, F. Z., et al.: Second natural history study of congenital heart defects: Aortic stenosis: Echocardiography. Circulation *87*:I, 1993.
329. Gutgesell, H. P., and French, M.: Echocardiographic determination of aortic and pulmonary valve areas in subjects with normal hearts. Am. J. Cardiol. *68*:773, 1991.
330. Beekman, R. H., Rocchini, A. P., Gillon, J. H., et al.: Hemodynamic determinants of the peak systolic left ventricular–aortic pressure gradient in children with valvar aortic stenosis. Am. J. Cardiol. *69*:813, 1992.
331. Stoddard, M. F., Arce, J., and Liddell, N. E.: Kupersmith two-dimensional transesophageal echocardiographic determination of aortic valve area in adults with aortic stenosis. Am. Heart J. *122*:1415, 1991.
332. Tribouilloy, C., Shen, W. F., Pelrier, M., et al.: Quantitation of aortic valve area in aortic stenosis with multiplane transesophageal echocardiography: Comparison with monoplane transesophageal approach. Am. Heart J. *128*:526, 1994.
333. Shah, P. M., and Graham, B. M.: Management of aortic stenosis: Is cardiac catheterization necessary? Am. J. Cardiol. *67*:1031, 1991.
334. McCrindle, B. W., for the Valvuloplasty and Angioplasty of Congenital Anomalies (VACA) Registry Investigators: Independent predictors of immediate results of percutaneous balloon aortic valvotomy in childhood. Am. J. Cardiol. *77*:286, 1996.
335. Witsenburg, M., Cromme-Dijkhuis, A., Frohn-Mulder, I. M. E., and Hess, J.: Short and midterm results of balloon valvuloplasty for valvular aortic stenosis in children. Am. J. Cardiol. *69*:945, 1992.
336. Kennedy, J. W., Twiss, R. D., Blackmon, J. R., et al.: Quantitative angiography. III. Relationships of left ventricular pressure, volume and mass in aortic valve disease. Circulation *38*:838, 1968.
337. El-Said, G., Gallioto, F. J., Mullens, C. E., and McNamara, D. G.: Natural hemodynamic history of congenital aortic stenosis in childhood. Am. J. Cardiol. *30*:6, 1972.
338. Hurwitz, R. A.: Aortic valve stenosis in childhood: Clinical and hemodynamic history. J. Pediatr. *82*:228, 1973.
339. Friedman, W. F., Modlinger, J., and Morgan, J.: Serial hemodynamic observations in asymptomatic children with valvar aortic stenosis. Circulation *43*:91, 1971.
340. Cohen, L. S., Friedman, W. F., and Braunwald, E.: Natural history of mild congenital aortic stenosis elucidated by serial hemodynamic studies. Am. J. Cardiol. *30*:1, 1972.
341. DeBoer, B. A., Robbins, R. C., Maron, B. J., et al.: Late results of aortic valvotomy for congenital valvular aortic stenosis. Ann. Thorac. Surg. *50*:69, 1990.
342. Keane, J. F., Driscoll, D. J., Gersony, W. M., et al.: Second natural history study of congenital heart defects. Circulation *87*(Suppl. I):I, 1993.
343. Kitchiner, D., Sreeram, N., Malaiya, N., et al.: Long-term follow-up of treated clinical aortic stenosis. Cardiol. Young *5*:9, 1995.
344. Gerosa, G., McKay, R., Davies, J., and Ross, O. N.: Comparison of the

aortic homograft and the pulmonary autograft for aortic valve or root replacement in children. J. Thorac. Cardiovasc. Surg. *102*:51, 1991.
345. Gerosa, G., McKay, R., and Ross, D. N.: Replacement of the aortic valve or root with a pulmonary autograft in children. Ann. Thorac. Surg. *51*:424, 1991.
346. Ross, D. B., Trusler, G. A., Coles, J. G., et al.: Small aortic root in childhood: Surgical options. Ann. Thorac. Surg. *58*:1617, 1994.
347. Elkins, R. C., Knott-Craig, C. J., Ward, K. E., et al.: Pulmonary autograft in children: Realized growth potential. Ann. Thorac. Surg. *57*:1387, 1994.
347a. Westaby, S.: Pulmonary autograft replacement of the aortic valve. Br. Heart J. *74*:1, 1995.
348. Kinney, E. L., Machado, H., Cortada, X., and Galbut, D. L.: Diagnosis of discrete subaortic stenosis by pulsed and continuous wave echocardiography. Am. Heart J. *110*:1069, 1985.
349. Frommelt, M. A., Snider, A. R., Bove, E. L., and Lupinetti, F. M.: Echocardiographic assessment of subvalvular aortic stenosis before and after operation. J. Am. Coll. Cardiol. *19*:1018, 1992.
350. Mugge, A., Daniel, W. G., Wolpers, H. G., et al.: Improved visualization of discrete subvalvular aortic stenosis by transesophageal color-coded Doppler echocardiography. Am. Heart J. *117*:474, 1989.
351. Choi, J. Y., and Sullivan, I. D.: Fixed subaortic stenosis: Anatomical spectrum and nature of progression. Br. Heart J. *65*:280, 1991.
352. DeVries, A. G., Hess, J., Witsenburg, M., et al.: Management of fixed subaortic stenosis: A retrospective study of 57 cases. J. Am. Coll. Cardiol. *19*:1013, 1992.
353. Ritter, S. B.: Discrete subaortic stenosis and balloon dilation: The four questions revisited. J. Am. Coll. Cardiol. *18*:1316, 1991.
354. Drinkwater, D. C., and Laks, H.: Surgery for subvalvular aortic stenosis. Prog. Pediatr. Cardiol. *3*:189, 1994.
355. Lupinetti, F. M., Pridjian, A. K., Callow, L. B., et al.: Optimum treatment of discrete subaortic stenosis. Ann. Thorac. Surg. *54*:467, 1992.
356. Sreeram, N., Sutherland, G. R., Bogers, A. J. J. C., et al.: Subaortic obstruction: Intraoperative echocardiography as an adjunct to operation. Ann. Thorac. Surg. *50*:579, 1990.
357. Gewillig., M., Daenen, W., Dumoulin, M., and Van Der Hauwaert, L.: Rheologic genesis of discrete subvalvular aortic stenosis: A Doppler echocardiographic study. J. Am. Coll. Cardiol. *19*:818, 1992.
358. Frommelt, P. C., Lupinetti, F. M., and Bove, E. L.: Aortoventriculoplasty in infants and children. Circulation *86*:II, 1992.
359. DeLeon, S. Y., Iobawi, M. N., Robertson, D. A., et al.: Conal enlargement for diffuse subaortic stenosis. J. Thorac. Cardiovasc. Surg. *102*:814, 1991.
360. Van Son, J. A. M., Schaff, H. V., Danielson, G. K., et al.: Surgical treatment of discrete and tunnel subaortic stenosis. Circulation *88*:159, 1993.
361. Coleman, D. M., Smallhorn, J. F., McCrindle, B. W., et al.: Postoperative follow-up of fibromuscular subaortic stenosis. J. Am. Coll. Cardiol. *24*:1558, 1994.
362. Waldman, J. D., Schneeweiss, A., Edwards, W. D., et al.: The obstructive subaortic conus. Circulation *70*:339, 1984.
363. Ow, E. P., DeLeon, S. Y., Freeman, J. E., et al.: Recognition and management of accessory mitral tissue causing severe subaortic stenosis. Ann. Thorac. Surg. *57*:952, 1994.
364. Reeder, G. S., Danielson, G. K., Seward, J. B., et al.: Fixed subaortic stenosis in atrioventricular canal defect: A Doppler echocardiographic study. J. Am. Coll. Cardiol. *20*:386, 1992.
365. Friedman, W. G., and Roberts, W. C.: Vitamin D and the subvalvular aortic stenosis syndrome: The transplacental effects of vitamin D on the aorta of the rabbit. Circulation *34*:77, 1966.
366. Friedman, W. F.: Vitamin D embryopathy. Adv. Teratol. *3*:85, 1968.
367. Friedman, W. F., and Mills, L. F.: The relationship between vitamin D and the craniofacial and dental anomalies of the supraventricular aortic stenosis syndrome. Pediatrics *43*:12, 1969.
368. Garcia, R. C., Friedman, W. F., Kaback, M. M., and Rowe, R. D.: Idiopathic hypercalcemia and supravalvular aortic stenosis: Documentation of a new syndrome. N. Engl. J. Med. *271*:117, 1964.
369. Williams, J. C. P., Barrett-Boyes, B. G., and Low, J. B.: Supravalvular aortic stenosis. Circulation *24*:1311, 1961.
370. Zalzstein, E., Moes, C. A. F., Musewe, N. N., and Freedom, R. M.: Spectrum of cardiovascular anomalies in Williams-Beuren syndrome. Pediatr. Cardiol. *12*:219, 1991.
371. Becroft, D. M., and Chamber, D.: Supravalvular aortic stenosis—infantile hypercalcemia syndrome: In vitro hypersensitivity to vitamin D and calcium. J. Med. Genet. *13*:223, 1976.
372. Taylor, A. B., Stern, P. H., and Bell, N. H.: Abnormal regulation of circulating 25-hydroxy vitamin D in the Williams syndrome. N. Engl. J. Med. *306*:972, 1982.
373. Kruse, K., Pankau, R., Gosch, A., and Wohlfahrt, K.: Calcium metabolism in Williams-Beuren syndrome. J. Pediat. *121*:902, 1992.
374. Morris, C. A., Demsey, S. A., Leonard, C. O., et al.: Natural history of Williams syndrome: Physical characteristics. J. Pediatr. *113*:318, 1988.
375. Kahler, R. L., Braunwald, E., Plauth, W. H., Jr., and Morrow, A. G.: Familial congenital heart disease. Am. J. Med. *40*:384, 1966.
376. Ewart, A. K., Morris, C. A., Ensing, G. J., et al.: A human vascular disorder, supravalvular aortic stenosis, maps to chromosome 7. Proc. Natl. Acad. Sci. *90*:3226, 1993.
377. Curran, M., Atkinson, D. L., Ewart, A. K., et al.: The elastin gene is disrupted by a translocation associated with supravalvular aortic stenosis. Cell *73*:159, 1993.
377a. Keating, M. T.: Genetic approaches to cardiovascular disease, supravalvular aortic stenosis, Williams syndrome, and long-QT syndrome. Circulation *92*:142, 1995.
378. Zalzstein, E., Moes, C. A. F., Musewe, N. N., and Freedom, R. M.: Spectrum of cardiovascular anomalies in Williams-Beuren syndrome. Pediatr. Cardiol. *12*:219, 1991.
379. Conway, E. E., Noonan, J., Marion, R. W., and Steeg, C. N.: Myocardial infarction leading to sudden death in the Williams syndrome: Report of three cases. J. Pediatr. *117*:593, 1990.
380. Ino, T., Nishimoto, K., Iwahara, M., et al.: Progressive vascular lesions in Williams-Beuren syndrome. Pediatr. Cardiol. *9*:55, 1988.
381. Wren, C., Oslizlok, P., and Bull, C.: Natural history of supravalvular aortic stenosis and pulmonary artery stenosis. J. Am. Coll. Cardiol. *15*:1625, 1990.
382. French, J. W., and Guntheroth, W. G.: An explanation of asymmetric upper extremity blood pressure in supravalvular aortic stenosis: The Coanda effect. Circulation *42*:31, 1970.
383. Goldstein, R. E., and Epstein, S. E.: Mechanism of elevated innominate artery pressures in supravalvular aortic stenosis. Circulation *42*:23, 1970.
384. Masura, J., Bzduch, J., Lolan, M., et al.: Diagnosis of supravalvular aortic stenosis by means of two-dimensional echocardiography (in Slovak). Bratisl. Lek. Listy. *90*:895, 1989.
385. Rein, A. J. J. T., Preminger, T. J., Perry, S. B., et al.: Generalized arteriopathy in Williams syndrome: An intravascular ultrasound study. J. Am. Coll. Cardiol. *21*:1727, 1993.
386. Brand, A., Keren, A., Reifen, R. M., et al.: Echocardiographic and Doppler findings in the Williams syndrome. Am. J. Cardiol. *63*:633, 1989.
387. Permut, L. C., and Laks, H.: Surgery for valvar and supravalvar aortic stenosis. Prog. Pediatr. Cardiol. *3*:177, 1994.
388. Sade, R. M., Crawford, F. A., Jr., and Fyfe, D. A.: Symposium on hypoplastic left heart syndrome. J. Thorac. Cardiovasc. Surg. *91*:937,1986.
389. Bash, S. E., Huhta, J. C., Vick, G. W., III, et al.: Hypoplastic left heart syndrome: Is echocardiography accurate enough to guide surgical palliation? J. Am. Coll. Cardiol. *7*:610, 1986.
390. Rossi, A. F., Sommer, R. J., Lotvin, A., et al.: Usefulness of intermittent monitoring of mixed venous oxygen saturation after stage I palliation for hypoplastic left heart syndrome. Am. J. Cardiol. *73*:1118, 1994.
391. Norwood, W. I., Jacobs, M. L., and Murphy, J. D.: Fontan procedure for hypoplastic left heart syndrome. Ann. Thorac. Surg. *54*:1025, 1992.
392. Guntheroth, W. G.: Fontan procedure for hypoplastic left heart syndrome. Circulation *86*:1662, 1992.
393. Rossi, A. F., Sommer, R. J., Steinberg, L. G., et al.: Effect of older age on outcome for stage one palliation of hypoplastic left heart syndrome. Am. J. Cardiol. *77*:319, 1996.
394. Bailey, L. L., and Gundry, S. R.: Hypoplastic left heart syndrome. Pediatr. Clin. North Am. *37*:137, 1990.
395. Canter, C. E., Moorhead, S., Huddleston, C. B., and Spray, T. L.: Restrictive atrial septal communication as a determinant of outcome of cardiac transplantation for hypoplastic left heart syndrome. Circulation *88*:456, 1993.
395a. Gutgesell, H. P., and Massaro, T. A.: Management of hypoplastic left heart syndrome in a consortium of university hospitals. Am. J. Cardiol. *76*:809, 1995.
396. Slack, M. C., Kirby, W. C., Towbin, J. A., et al.: Stenting of the ductus arteriosus in the hypoplastic left heart syndrome as an ambulatory bridge to cardiac transplantation. Am. J. Cardiol. *74*:636, 1994.
397. Frahm, C. J., Braunwald, E., and Morrow, A. G.: Congenital aortic regurgitation. Am. J. Med. *31*:63, 1961.
398. Donofrio, M. T., Engle, M. A., O'Loughlin, J. E., et al.: Congenital aortic regurgitation: Natural history and management. J. Am. Coll. Cardiol. *20*:336, 1992.
399. Tuna, I. C., and Edwards, J. E.: Aortico-left ventricular tunnel and aortic insufficiency. Ann. Thorac. Surg. *45*:5, 1988.
400. Hovaguimian, H., Cobanoglu, A., and Starr, A.: Aortico-left ventricular tunnel: A clinical review and new surgical classification. Ann. Thorac. Surg. *45*:106, 1988.
401. Goforth, D., James, F. W., Kaplan, S., and Donner, R.: Maximal exercise in children with aortic regurgitation: An adjunct to noninvasive assessment of disease severity. Am. Heart J. *108*:1306, 1984.
402. Sondergaard, L., Lindvig, K., Hildebrandt, P., et al.: Quantification of aortic regurgitation by magnetic resonance velocity mapping. Am. Heart J. *125*:1081, 1993.
403. Lucas, R. V., Jr.: Anomalous venous connection, pulmonary and systemic. *In* Adams, F. H., and Emmanouilides, G. C. (eds.): Moss' Heart Disease in Infants, Children and Adolescents. 4th ed. Baltimore, Williams and Wilkins, 1989, p. 580.
404. Pacifico, A. D., Mandke, N. V., McGrath, L. B., et al.: Repair of congenital pulmonary venous thrombosis with living autologous atrial tissue. J. Thorac. Cardiovasc. Surg. *89*:604, 1985.
405. Marin-Garcia, J., Tandon, R., Lucas, R. V., Jr., and Edwards, J. E.: Cor triatriatum: Study of 20 cases. Am. J. Cardiol. *35*:59, 1975.
406. Burton, D. A., Chin, A., Weinberg, P. M., and Pigott, J. D.: Identification of cor triatriatum dexter by two-dimensional echocardiography. Am. J. Cardiol. *59*:409, 1987.
406a. Tulloh, R. M. R., Bull, C., Elliott, M. J., and Sullivan, I. D.: Supravalvar mitral stenosis: Risk factors for recurrence or death after resection. Br. Heart J. *73*:164, 1995.
406b. Shuler, C. O., Fyfe, D. A., Sade, R., and Crawford, F. A.: Transesophageal echocardiographic evaluation of cor triatriatum in children. Am. Heart J. *129*:507, 1995.

407. Oglietti, J., Cooley, D. A., Izquierdo, J. P., et al.: Cor triatriatum: Operative results in 25 patients. Ann. Thorac. Surg. *35*:415, 1983.
408. Ruckman, R. N., and Van Praagh, R.: Anatomic types of congenital mitral stenosis: Report of 49 autopsy cases with consideration of diagnosis and surgical implications. Am. J. Cardiol. *42*:592, 1978.
409. Parr, G. V. S., Fripp, R. A., Whitman, V., et al.: Anomalous mitral arcade: Echocardiographic and angiographic reception. Pediatr. Cardiol. *4*:163, 1983.
410. Ortiz, E., and Somerville, J.: Assessment by cross-sectional echocardiography of surgical mitral valve disease in children and adolescents. Br. Heart J. *56*:267, 1986.
411. Moore, P., Adatia, I., Spevak, P. J., et al.: Severe congenital mitral stenosis in infants. Circulation *89*:2099, 1994.
412. Fawzy, M. E., Mimish, L., Awad, M., et al.: Mitral balloon valvotomy in children with Inoue balloon technique: Immediate and intermediate-term result. Am. Heart J. *127*:1559, 1994.
412a. Tulloh, R. M. R., Bull, C., Elliott, M. J., and Sullivan, I. D.: Supravalvular mitral stenosis: Risk factors for recurrence or death after resection. Br. Heart J. *73*:164, 1995.
413. Mazzera, E., Corno, A., Di Donato, R., et al.: Surgical bypass of the systemic atrioventricular valve in children by means of a valve conduit. J. Thorac. Cardiovasc. Surg. *96*:321, 1988.
414. Zweng, T. N., Bluett, M. K., Mosca, R., et al.: Mitral valve replacement in the first 5 years of life. Ann. Thorac. Surg. *47*:720, 1989.
415. Perloff, J. K.: Evolving concepts of mitral valve prolapse. N. Engl. J. Med. *307*:369, 1982.
416. Carpentier, A.: Congenital malformations of the mitral valve. *In* Stark, J., and deLeval, M. (eds.): Surgery for Congenital Heart Defects. New York, Grune and Stratton, 1983, p. 467.
417. Wu, Y. T., Chang, A. C., and Chin, A. J.: Semiquantitative assessment of mitral regurgitation by Doppler color flow imaging in patients aged <20 years. Am. J. Cardiol. *71*:727, 1993.
418. Lamberti, J. J., Gensen, T. S., Grehl, T. M., et al.: Late reoperation for systemic atrioventricular valve regurgitation after repair of congenital heart defects. Ann. Thorac. Surg. *47*:517, 1989.
419. Gonzalez, V. R., Pieper, W. M., and Kap-herr, S. H.: Pulmonary arteriovenous fistula in childhood. Z. Kinderchir. *40*:101, 1985.
420. Grady, R. M., Sharkey, A. M., and Bridges, N. D.: Transcatheter coil embolisation of a pulmonary arteriovenous malformation in a neonate. Br. Heart J. *71*:370, 1994.
421. Puskas, J. D., Allen, M. S., Moncure, A. C., et al.: Pulmonary arteriovenous malformations: Therapeutic options. Ann. Thorac. Surg. *56*:253, 1993.
422. D'Cruz, I. A., Agustssou, M. M., Bicoff, J. P., et al.: Stenotic lesions of the pulmonary arteries: Clinical hemodynamic findings in 84 cases. Am. J. Cardiol. *13*:441, 1964.
423. Venables, A. W.: The syndrome of pulmonary stenosis complicating maternal rubella. Br. Heart J. *27*:49, 1965.
424. Friedman, D. M., Fernandes, J., Rutkowski, M., and Danilowicz, D.: Doppler evaluation of physiologic peripheral pulmonic stenosis in newborns. Cardiol. Young *2*:179, 1992.
425. Eldredge, W. J., Tingelstad, J. B., Robertson, L. W., et al.: Observations on the natural history of pulmonary artery coarctation. Circulation *45*:404, 1972.
426. Kan, J. S., Marvin, W. J., Jr., Bass, J. L., et al.: Balloon angioplasty-branch pulmonary artery stenosis: Results from the valvuloplasty and angioplasty of congenital anomalies registry. Am. J. Cardiol. *65*:798, 1990.
427. O'Laughlin, M. P., Slack, M. C., Grifka, R. G.: Implantation and intermediate-term follow-up of stents in congenital heart disease. Circulation *88*:605, 1993.
428. Burch, M., Sharland, M., Shinebourne, E., et al.: Cardiologic abnormalities in Noonan syndrome: Phenotypic diagnosis and echocardiographic assessment of 118 patients. J. Am. Coll. Cardiol. *22*:1189, 1993.
429. Aldousany, A. W., DiSessa, T. G., Dubois, R., et al.: Doppler estimation of pressure gradient in pulmonary stenosis: Maximal instantaneous vs peak-to-peak, vs mean catheter gradient. Pediatr. Cardiol. *10*:145, 1989.
430. Frantz, E. G., and Silverman, N. H.: Doppler ultrasound evaluation of valvular pulmonary stenosis from multiple transducer positions in children requiring pulmonary valvuloplasty. Am. J. Cardiol. *61*:844, 1988.
430a. Fedderly, R. T., and Beekman, R. H.: Balloon valvuloplasty for pulmonary valve stenosis. J. Interven. Cardiol. *8*:451, 1995.
430b. Tabatabaei, H., Boutin, C., Nykanen, D. G., et al.: Morphologic and hemodynamic consequences after percutaneous balloon valvotomy for neonatal pulmonary stenosis: Medium-term follow-up. J. Am. Coll. Cardiol. *27*:473, 1996.
431. Srinivasan, V., Konyer, A., Broda, J. J., and Subramanian, S.: Critical pulmonary stenosis in infants less than three months of age: A reappraisal of closed transventricular pulmonary valvotomy. Ann. Thorac. Surg. *34*:46, 1982.
432. Burzynski, J. B., Kveselis, D. A., Byrum, C. J., et al.: Modified technique for balloon valvuloplasty of critical pulmonary stenosis in the newborn. J. Am. Coll. Cardiol. *22*:1944, 1993.
433. Radtke, W., and Lock, J.: Balloon dilation. Pediatr. Clin. North Am. *37*:193, 1990.
434. Fedderly, R. T., Lloyd, T. R., Mendelsohn, A. M., et al.: Determinants of successful balloon valvotomy in infants with critical pulmonary stenosis or membranous pulmonary atresia with intact ventricular septum. J. Am. Coll. Cardiol. *25*:460, 1995.
435. Lange, P. E., Onnasch, G. W., and Heintzen, P. H.: Valvular pulmonary stenosis: Natural history and right ventricular function in infants and children. Eur. Heart J. *6*:706, 1985.
436. Mahra-Pour, M., Whitney, A., Liebman, J., et al.: Quantification of the Frank and MacFee-Parungao orthogonal electrocardiogram in valvular pulmonic stenosis: Correlation with hemodynamic measurements. J. Electrocardiol. *12*:69, 1979.
437. Nishimura, R. A., Pieroni, D. R., Bierman, F. Z., et al.: Second natural history of congenital heart defects: Pulmonary stenosis: Echocardiography. Circulation *87*:I, 1993.
438. Krabill, K. A., Wang, Y., Einzig, S., and Moller, J. H.: Rest and exercise hemodynamics in pulmonary stenosis: Comparison of children and adults. Am. J. Cardiol. *56*:360, 1985.
439. Danilowicz, D., Hoffman, J. I. E., and Rudolph, A. M.: Serial studies of pulmonary stenosis in infancy and childhood. Br. Heart J. *37*:808, 1975.
440. Wennevold, A., and Jacobsen, J. R.: Natural history of valvular pulmonary stenosis in children below the age of two years: Long-term follow-up with serial heart catheterizations. Eur. J. Cardiol. *8*:371, 1978.
441. Hayes, C. J., Gersony, W. M., Driscoll, D. J., et al.: Second natural history study of congenital heart defects: Results of treatment of patients with pulmonary valvar stenosis. Circulation *87*:I, 1993.
442. Laks, H., and Billingsley, A. M.: Advances in the treatment of pulmonary atresia with intact ventricular septum: Palliative and definitive repair. Cardiol Clin. *7*:387, 1989.
443. Coles, J. G., Freedman, R. M., Lightfoot, N. E., et al.: Long-term results in neonates with pulmonary atresia and intact ventricular septum. Ann. Thorac. Surg. *47*:213, 1989.
444. Vosa, C., Arciprete, P., Caianiello, G., and Palma, G.: Pulmonary atresia with intact ventricular septum: Is it possible to improve survival? Cardiol. Young *2*:391, 1992.
445. Daliento, L., Scognamiglio, R., Thiene, G., et al.: Morphologic and functional analysis of myocardial status in pulmonary atresia with intact ventricular septum—an angiographic, histologic and morphometric study. Cardiol. Young *2*:361, 1992.
446. Hanseus, K., Bjorkhem, G., Lundstrom, N. R., and Laurin, S.: Cross-sectional echocardiographic measurements of right ventricular size and growth in patients with pulmonary atresia and intact ventricular septum. Pediatr. Cardiol. *12*:135, 1991.
447. Leung, M. P., Mok, C. K., and Hui, P. W.: Echocardiographic assessment of neonates with pulmonary atresia and intact ventricular septum. J. Am. Coll. Cardiol. *12*:719, 1988.
447a. Fedderly, R. T., Lloyd, T. R., Mendelsohn, A. M., et al.: Determinants of successful balloon valvulotomy in infants with critical pulmonary stenosis or membranous pulmonary atresia with intact ventricular septum. J. Am. Coll. Cardiol. *25*:460, 1995.
448. Freedom, R. M., Wilson, G., Trusler, G., et al.: Pulmonary atresia and intact ventricular septum: A review of the anatomy, myocardium and factors influencing right ventricular growth and guidelines for surgical intervention. Scand. J. Thorac. Cardiovasc. Surg. *17*:1, 1983.
449. Leung, M. P., Mok, C. K., Lee, J., et al.: Management evolution of pulmonary atresia and intact ventricular septum. Am. J. Cardiol. *71*:1331, 1993.
450. Giglia, T. M., Jenkins, K. J., Matitiau, A., et al.: Influence of right heart size on outcome in pulmonary atresia with intact ventricular septum. Circulation *88*:22, 1993.
451. Laks, H., Pearl, J. M., Drinkwater, D. C., et al.: Partial biventricular repair of pulmonary atresia with intact ventricular septum: Use of an adjustable atrial septal defect. Circulation *86*:II, 1992.
452. Hanley, F. L., Sade, R. M., Blackstone, E. H., et al.: Outcomes in neonatal pulmonary atresia with intact ventricular septum: A multi-institutional study. J. Thorac. Cardiovasc. Surg. *105*:406, 1993.
453. Pawade, A., Capuani, A., Penny, D. J., et al.: Pulmonary atresia with intact ventricular septum: Surgical management based on right ventricular infundibulum. J. Cardiovasc. Surg. *8*:371, 1993.
454. Steinberger, J., Berry, J. M., Bass, J. L., et al.: Results of a right ventricular outflow patch for pulmonary atresia with intact ventricular septum. Circulation *86*:II, 1992.
455. Gentles, T. L., Colan, S. D., Giglia, T. M., et al.: Right ventricular decompression and left ventricular function in pulmonary atresia with intact ventricular septum. Circulation *88*:II, 1993.
456. Schmidt, K. G., Cloe, J-L., and Silverman, N. H.: Changes of right ventricular size and function after valvotomy for pulmonary atresia or critical pulmonary stenosis and intact ventricular septum. J. Am. Coll. Cardiol. *19*:1032, 1992.
457. Latson, L. A.: Nonsurgical treatment of a neonate with pulmonary atresia and intact ventricular septum by transcatheter puncture and balloon dilation of the atretic valve. Am. J. Cardiol. *68*:277, 1991.
458. Leung, M. P., Lo, R. N. S., Cheung, H., et al.: Balloon valvuloplasty after pulmonary valvotomy for babies with pulmonary atresia and intact ventricular septum. Ann. Thorac. Surg. *53*:864, 1992.
459. Danilowicz, D., and Ishmael, R.: Anomalous right ventricular muscle bundle: Clinical pitfalls and extracardiac anomalies. Clin. Cardiol. *4*:146, 1981.
460. Wong, P. C., Sanders, S. P., Jonas, R. A., et al.: Pulmonary valve–moderator band distance and association with development of double-chambered right ventricle. Am. J. Cardiol. *68*:1681, 1991.
461. Ford, D. K., Bollaboy, C. A., Derkac, W. M., et al.: Transatrial repair of double-chambered right ventricle. Ann. Thorac. Surg. *46*:412, 1988.
462. Pinsky, W. W., and Arciniegas, E.: Tetralogy of Fallot. Pediatr. Clin. North Am. *37*:179, 1990.

463. Soto, B., and McConnell, M. E.: Tetralogy of Fallot: Angiographic and pathological correlation. Semin. Thorac. Cardiovasc. Surg. *2*:12, 1990.
464. Rabinovitch, M.: Pathology and anatomy of pulmonary atresia and ventricular septal defect. Prog. Pediatr. Cardiol. *1*:9, 1992.
465. Castaneda, A. R., Mayer, J. E., Jr., and Lock, J. E.: Tetralogy of Fallot pulmonary atresia and diminutive pulmonary arteries. Prog. Pediatr. Cardiol. *1*:50, 1992.
466. Barbero-Marcial, M., and Jatene, A. D.: Surgical management of the anomalies of the pulmonary arteries in the tetralogy of Fallot with pulmonary atresia. Semin. Thorac. Cardiovasc. Surg. *2*:93, 1990.
467. Hiraishi, S., Misawa, H., Hirota, H., et al.: Noninvasive quantitative evaluation of the morphology of the major pulmonary artery branches in cyanotic congenital heart disease. Angiocardiographic and echocardiographic correlative study. Circulation *89*:1306, 1994.
468. Carvalho, J. S., Silva, C. M. C., Rigby, M. L., et al.: Angiographic diagnosis of anomalous coronary artery in tetralogy of Fallot. Br. Heart J. *70*:75, 1993.
469. Feldt, R. H., Liao, P., and Puga, F. J.: Clinical profile and natural history of pulmonary atresia and ventricular septal defect. Prog. Pediatr. Cardiol. *1*:18, 1992.
470. Santoro, G., Marino, B., Di Carlo, D., et al.: Echocardiographically guided repair of tetralogy of Fallot. Am. J. Cardiol. *73*:808, 1994.
471. Morgan, B. C., Guntheroth, W. G., Blume, R. S., and Fyler, D. C.: A clinical profile of paroxysmal hyperpnea in cyanotic congenital heart disease. Circulation *31*:66, 1965.
472. Shaddy, R. E., Viney, J., Judd, V. E., and McGough, E. C.: Continuous intravenous phenylephrine infusion for treatment of hypoxemic spells in tetralogy of Fallot. J. Pediatr. *114*:468, 1989.
473. McConnell, M. E.: Echocardiography in classical tetralogy of Fallot. Semin. Thorac. Cardiovasc. Surg. *2*:2, 1990.
474. Castaneda, A. R.: Classical repair of tetralogy of Fallot: Timing, technique, and results. Semin. Thorac. Cardiovasc. Surg. *2*:70, 1990.
475. Pacifico, A. D., Kirklin, J. K., Colvin, E. V., et al.: Transatrial-transpulmonary repair of tetralogy of Fallot. Semin. Thorac. Cardiovasc. Surg. *2*:76, 1990.
476. Puga, F. J.: Surgical treatment of pulmonary atresia and ventricular septal defect. Prog. Pediatr. Cardiol. *1*:37, 1992.
477. Groh, M. A., Meliones, J. N., Bove, E., et al.: Repair of tetralogy of Fallot in infancy: Effect of pulmonary artery size on outcome. Circulation *84*(Suppl. III):206, 1991.
478. Permut, L. C., Laks, H., Haas, G. S., et al.: Surgical management of pulmonary atresia and ventricular septal defect with major systemic-pulmonary collaterals. J. Am. Coll. Cardiol. *15*:79A, 1990.
479. Kirklin, J. W., Blackstone, E. H., Jonas, R. A., et al.: Morphologic and surgical determinants of outcome events after repair of tetralogy of Fallot and pulmonary stenosis. J. Thorac. Cardiovasc. Surg. *103*:706, 1992.
480. Rosankranz, E. R.: Modified Blalock-Taussig shunts in the treatment of tetralogy of Fallot. Semin. Thorac. Cardiovasc. Surg. *2*:27, 1990.
481. Sreeram, N., Saleem, M., Jackson, M., et al.: Results of balloon pulmonary valvuloplasty as a palliative procedure in tetralogy of Fallot. J. Am. Coll. Cardiol. *18*:59, 1991.
481a. Sluysmans, T., Neven, B., Rubay, J., et al.: Early balloon dilatation of the pulmonary valve in infants with tetralogy of Fallot. Circulation *91*:1506, 1995.
482. Chan, K. C., Fyfe, D. A., McKay, C. A., et al.: Right ventricular outflow reconstruction with cryopreserved homografts in pediatric patients: Intermediate-term follow-up with serial echocardiographic assessment. J. Am. Coll. Cardiol. *24*:483, 1994.
483. Naito, Y., Fujita, T., Yagihara, T., et al.: Usefulness of left ventricular volume in assessing tetralogy of Fallot for total correction. Am. J. Cardiol. *56*:356, 1985.
484. Rebergen, S. A., Chin, J. G. J., Ottenkamp, J., et al.: Pulmonary regurgitation in the late postoperative follow-up of tetralogy of Fallot: Volumetric quantitation by nuclear magnetic resonance velocity mapping. Circulation *88*:2257, 1993.
485. Warner, K. G, Anderson, J. E., Fulton, D. R., et al.: Restoration of the pulmonary valve reduces right ventricular volume overload after previous repair of tetralogy of Fallot. Circulation *88*:189, 1993.
486. Garson, A., Jr., Randall, D. C., Gillette, P. C., et al.: Prevention of sudden death after repair of tetralogy of Fallot: Treatment of ventricular arrhythmias. J. Am. Coll. Cardiol. *6*:221, 1985.
487. Oku, H., Shirotani, H., Sunakawa, A., and Yokoyama, T.: Postoperative long-term results in total correction of tetralogy of Fallot: Hemodynamics and cardiac function. Ann. Thorac. Surg. *41*:413, 1986.
488. Rosenthal, A., Behrendt, D., Sloan, H., et al.: Long-term prognosis (15 to 26 years) after repair of tetralogy of Fallot: I. Survival and symptomatic status. Ann. Thorac. Surg. *38*:151, 1984.
489. Sandor, G. G. S., Patterson, M. W. H., Tipple, M., et al.: Left ventricular systolic and diastolic function after total correction of tetralogy of Fallot. Am. J. Cardiol. *60*:1148, 1987.
490. Cullen, S., Celermajer, D. S., Franklin, R. C. G., et al.: Prognostic significance of ventricular arrhythmia after repair of tetralogy of Fallot: A 12-year prospective study. J. Am. Coll. Cardiol. *23*:1151, 1994.
491. Joffe, H., Georgakopoulos, D., Celermajer, D. S., et al.: Late ventricular arrhythmia is rare after early repair of tetralogy of Fallot. J. Am. Coll. Cardiol. *23*:1146, 1994.
492. Ross, B. A.: From the bedside to the basic science laboratory: Arrhythmias in Fallot's tetralogy. J. Am. Coll. Cardiol. *21*:1738, 1993.
493. Vaksmann, G., Kohen, M. E., Lacroix, D., et al.: Influence of clinical and hemodynamic characteristics on signal-averaged electrocardiogram in postoperative tetralogy of Fallot. Am. J. Cardiol. *71*:317, 1993.
494. Misaki, T., Tsubota, M., Watanabe, G., et al.: Surgical treatment of ventricular tachycardia after surgical repair of tetralogy of Fallot: Relation between intraoperative mapping and histological findings. Circulation *90*:264, 1994.
494a. Bricker, J. T.: Sudden death and tetralogy of Fallot. Risks, markers, and causes. Circulation *92*:162, 1995.
494b. Johnson, M. C., Strauss, A. W., Dowton, S. B., et al.: Deletion within chromosome 22 is common in patients with absent pulmonary valve syndrome. Am. J. Cardiol. *76*:66, 1995.
495. Fouron, J. C.: Tetralogy of Fallot with absent pulmonary valve: Clarification of a complex malformation and of its therapeutic challenge. Circulation *82*:1531, 1990.
496. Rabinovich, M., Grady, S., David, J., et al.: Compression of intrapulmonary bronchi by abnormally branching pulmonary valves. Am. J. Cardiol. *50*:804, 1982.
497. Milanesi, O., Talenti, E., Pallegrino, P. A., and Thiene, G.: Abnormal pulmonary artery branching in tetralogy of Fallot with absent pulmonary valve. Int. J. Cardiol. *6*:375, 1984.
498. Fischer, D. R., Neches, W. H., Beerman, L. B., et al.: Tetralogy of Fallot with absent pulmonic valve: Analysis of 17 patients. Am. J. Cardiol. *53*:1433, 1984.
499. Dunnigan, A., Oldham, H. N., and Benson, D. W.: Absent pulmonary valve syndrome in infancy: Surgery reconsidered. Am. J. Cardiol. *48*:117, 1981.
500. Kron, I. L., Johnson, A. M., Carpenter, M. A., et al.: Treatment of absent pulmonary valve syndrome with homograft. Ann. Thorac. Surg. *46*:579, 1988.
501. Rigby, M. L., Carvalho, J. S., Anderson, R. H., and Redington, A.: The investigation and diagnosis of tricuspid atresia. Int. J. Cardiol. *27*:1, 1990.
502. Sade, R. M., and Fyfe, D. A.: Tricuspid atresia: Current concepts in diagnosis and treatment. Pediatr. Clin. North Am. *7*:151, 1990.
502a. Laks, H., Ardehali, A., Grant, P. W., et al.: Modification of the Fontan procedure. Superior vena cava to left pulmonary artery connection and inferior vena cava to right pulmonary artery connection with adjustable atrial septal defect. Circulation *91*:2943, 1995.
503. Pearl, J. M., Laks, H., Drinkwater, D. C., et al.: Modified Fontan procedure in patients less than 4 years of age. Circulation *86*:II, 1992.
504. Bridges, N. D., Mayer, J. E., Lock, J. E., et al.: Effect of baffle fenestration on outcome of the modified Fontan operation. Circulation *86*:1762, 1992.
504a. Kuhn, M. A., Jarmakani, J. M., Laks, H., et al.: Effect of late postoperative atrial septal defect closure on hemodynamic function in patients with a lateral tunnel Fontan procedure. J. Am. Coll. Cardiol. *26*:259, 1995.
505. Carter, T., Mainwaring, R. D., and Lamberti, J. J.: Damus-Kaye-Stansel procedure: Midterm follow-up and technical considerations. Ann. Thorac. Surg. *58*:1603, 1994.
506. Gross, G. J., Jonas, R. A., Castaneda, A. R., et al.: Maturational and hemodynamic factors predictive of increased cyanosis after bidirectional cavopulmonary anastomosis. Am. J. Cardiol. *74*:705, 1994.
507. Senzaki, H., Isoda, T., Ishizawa, A., and Hishi, T.: Reconsideration of criteria for the Fontan operation: Influence of pulmonary artery size on postoperative hemodynamics of the Fontan operation. Circulation *89*:1196, 1994.
508. Sandor, G. G. S., Patterson, M. W. H., and LeBlanc, J. G.: Systolic and diastolic function in tricuspid valve atresia before the Fontan operation. Am. J. Cardiol. *73*:292, 1994.
509. Frommelt, P. C., Snider, R., Meliones, J. N., and Vermilion, R. P.: Doppler assessment of pulmonary artery flow patterns and ventricular function after the Fontan operation. Am. J. Cardiol. *68*:1211, 1991.
510. Mair, D. D., Puga, F. J., and Danielson, G. K.: Late functional status of survivors of the Fontan procedure performed during the 1970s. Circulation *86*:II, 1992.
511. Driscoll, D. J., Offord, K. P., Feldt, R. H., et al.: Five- to fifteen-year follow-up after Fontan operation. Circulation *85*:469, 1992.
511a. Rosenthal, M., Bush, A., Deanfield, J., et al.: Comparison of cardiopulmonary adaptation during exercise in children after the atriopulmonary and total cavopulmonary connection Fontan procedures. Circulation *91*:372, 1995.
512. Gewillig, M., Wyse, R. K., de Leval, M. R., and Deanfield, J. E.: Early and late arrhythmias after the Fontan operation: Predisposing factors and clinical consequences. Br. Heart J. *67*:72, 1992.
513. Gussenhoven, E. J., Stewart, P. A., Becker, A. E., et al.: "Offsetting" of the septal tricuspid leaflet in normal hearts and in hearts with Ebstein's anomaly. Am. J. Cardiol. *53*:172, 1984.
514. Zalzstein, E., Koran, G., Einarson, T., and Freedom, R. M.: A case control study on the association between first trimester exposure to lithium and Ebstein's anomaly. Am. J. Cardiol. *65*:817, 1990.
515. Mair, D. D.: Ebstein's anomaly: Natural history and management. J. Am. Coll. Cardiol. *19*:1047, 1992.
516. Celermajer, D. S., Bull, C., Till, J. A., et al.: Ebstein's anomaly: Presentation and outcome from fetus to adult. J. Am. Coll. Cardiol. *23*:170, 1994.
517. Oberhoffer, R., Cook, A. C., Lang, D., et al.: Correlation between echocardiographic and morphological investigations of lesions of the tricuspid valve diagnosed during fetal life. Br. Heart J. *68*:580, 1992.
518. Boucek, R. J., Jr., Graham, T. P., Jr., Morgan J. P., et al.: Spontaneous

resolution of massive congenital tricuspid insufficiency. Circulation *54:*795, 1976.
519. Freedom, R. M., Culham, J. A. G., Olley, P. M., et al.: The differentiation of functional from organic pulmonary atresia: The role of aortography. Am. J. Cardiol. *41:*914, 1978.
520. Kastor, J. A., Goldreier, B. N., Josephson, M. E., et al.: Electrophysiologic characteristics of Ebstein's anomaly of the tricuspid valve. Circulation *52:*987, 1975.
521. Gussenhoven, W. J., Spitaels, S. E. C., Bom, N., and Becker, A. E.: Echocardiographic criteria for Ebstein's anomaly of tricuspid valve. Br. Heart J. *43:*31, 1980.
522. Hirschklau, M. J., Sahn, D. J., Hagan, A. D., et al.: Cross-sectional echocardiographic features of Ebstein's anomaly of the tricuspid valve. Am. J. Cardiol. *40:*400, 1977.
523. Hong, Y. M., and Moller, J. H.: Ebstein's anomaly: A long-term study of survival. Am. Heart J. *125:*1419, 1993.
524. Hurwitz, R. A.: Left ventricular function in infants and children with symptomatic Ebstein's anomaly. Am. J. Cardiol. *73:*716, 1994.
525. Paul, N. H., and Wernodsky, G.: Transposition of the great arteries. *In* Emmanoulides, G. C., Allen, H. D., et al. (eds.): Moss and Adams' Heart Disease in Infants, Children and Adolescents. 5th ed. Baltimore, Williams and Wilkins, 1994, p. 1154.
526. Anderson, R. H., Henry, G. W., and Becker, A. E.: Morphologic aspects of complete transposition. Cardiol. Young *1:*41, 1991.
527. Lakier, J. B., Stanger, P., Heymann, M. A., et al.: Early onset of pulmonary vascular obstruction in patients with aortopulmonary transposition and intact ventricular septum. Circulation *51:*875, 1975.
528. Aziz, K. U., Paul, M. H., and Rowe, R. D.: Bronchopulmonary circulation in D-transposition of the great arteries: Possible role and genesis of accelerated pulmonary vascular disease. Am. J. Cardiol. *39:*432, 1977.
529. Muster, A. J., Paul, M. H., Van Grondell, E. A., and Conway, J. J.: Asymmetric distribution of the pulmonary blood flow between the right and left lungs in D-transposition of the great arteries. Am. J. Cardiol. *38:*352, 1976
530. Chiu, I., Anderson, R. H., Macartney, F. J., et al.: Morphologic features of an intact ventricular septum susceptible to subpulmonary obstruction in complete transposition. Am. J. Cardiol. *53:*1633, 1984.
531. Waldman, J. D., Paul, M. H., Newfeld, E. A., et al.: Transposition of the great arteries with intact ventricular septum and patent ductus arteriosus. Am. J. Cardiol. *39:*232, 1977.
532. Tonkin, I. L., Kelley, M. J., Bream, P. R., and Elliott, L. P.: The frontal chest film as a method of suspecting transposition complexes. Circulation *53:*1016, 1976.
533. Deal, B. J., Chin, A. J., Sanders, S. P., et al.: Subxiphoid two-dimensional echocardiographic identification of tricuspid valve abnormalities in transposition of the great arteries with ventricular septal defect. Am. J. Cardiol. *55:*1146, 1985.
534. Chin, A. J., Yeager, S. B., Sanders, S. P., et al.: Accuracy of prospective two-dimensional echocardiographic evaluation of left ventricular outflow tract in complete transposition of the great arteries. Am. J. Cardiol. *55:*759, 1985.
535. Rigby, M. L., and Chan, K-Y.: The diagnostic evaluation of patients with complete transposition. Cardiol. Young *1:*26, 1991.
536. Pasquini, L., Sanders, S. P., Parness, I. A., et al.: Conal anatomy in 119 patients with D-loop transposition of the great arteries and ventricular septal defect: An echocardiographic and pathologic study. J. Am. Coll. Cardiol. *21:*1712, 1993.
537. DiSessa, T. G., Childs, W., Ti, C. C., and Friedman, W. F.: Systolic anterior motion of the mitral valve in a one day old infant with transposition of the great vessels. J. Clin. Ultrasound *6:*186, 1978.
538. Lin, A. E., DiSessa, T. G., Williams, R. G., et al.: Balloon and blade atrial septostomy facilitated by two-dimensional echocardiography. Am. J. Cardiol. *57:*273, 1986.
539. Moene, R. J., Oppenheimer-Dekker, A., Wenink, A. C. G., et al.: Morphology of ventricular septal defect in complete transposition of the great arteries. Am. J. Cardiol. *55:*1566, 1985.
540. Amato, J. J., Zelen, J., and Bushong, J.: Coronary arterial patterns in complete transposition—classification in relation to the arterial switch procedure. Cardiol. Young *4:*329, 1994.
541. Sim, E. K. W., van Son, J. A. M., Edwards, W. D., et al.: Coronary artery anatomy in complete transposition of the great arteries. Ann. Thorac. Surg. *57:*890, 1994.
542. Pasquini, L., Parness, I. A., Colan, S. D., et al.: Diagnosis of intramural coronary artery in transposition of the great arteries using two-dimensional echocardiography. Circulation *88:*1136, 1993.
542a. Chiu, I. S., Chu, S. H., Wang, J. K., et al.: Evolution of coronary artery pattern according to short-axis aortopulmonary rotation: A new categorization for complete transposition of the great arteries. J. Am. Coll. Cardiol. *26:*250, 1995.
543. Kirklin, J. W., Colvin, E. V., McConnell, M. E., and Bargeron, L. M.: Complete transposition of the great arteries: Treatment in the current era. Pediatr. Clin. North Am. *37:*171, 1990.
544. Kirklin, J. W.: The surgical repair for complete transposition. Cardiol. Young *1:*13, 1991.
545. Oelert, H.: Modification of the Mustard operation for surgical treatment of complete transposition by creating a confluence of the caval veins. Cardiol. Young *1:*71, 1991.
545a. Sagin-Saylam, G., and Somerville, J.: Palliative Mustard operation for transposition of the great arteries: Late results after 15–20 years. Heart *75:*72, 1996.
546. Merrill, W. H., Stewart, J. R., Hammon, J. W., Jr., et al: The Senning operation for complete transposition: Mid-term physiologic, electrophysiologic, and functional results. Cardiol. Young *1:*80, 1991.
547. Wong, K. Y., Venables, A. W., Kelly, M. J., and Kalff, V.: Longitudinal study of ventricular function after the Mustard operation for transposition of the great arteries: A long-term follow up. Br. Heart J. *60:*316, 1988.
548. Dihmis, W. C., Hutter, J. A., Joffe, H. S., et al.: Medium-term clinical results after the Senning procedure with haemodynamic and angiographic evaluation of the venous pathways. Br. Heart J. *69:*436, 1993.
549. Hochreiter, C., Snyder, M. S., Borer, J. S., et al.: Right and left ventricular performance 10 years after Mustard repair of transposition of the great arteries. Am. J. Cardiol. *74:*478, 1994.
550. Reybrouck, T., Gewillig, M., Dumoulin, M., et al.: Cardiorespiratory exercise performance after Senning operation for transposition of the great arteries. Br. Heart J. *70:*175, 1993.
551. Deanfield, J. E., Cullen, S., and Gewillig, M.: Arrhythmias after surgery for complete transposition: Do they matter? Cardiol. Young *1:*91, 1991.
552. Hurwitz, R. A., Caldwell, R. L., Girod, D. A., and Brown, J.: Right ventricular systolic function in adolescents and young adults after Mustard operation for transposition of the great arteries. Am. J. Cardiol. *77:*294, 1996.
553. Ensing, G. J., Heise, C. T., and Driscoll, D. J.: Cardiovascular response to exercise after the Mustard operation for simple and complex transposition of great arteries. Am. J. Cardiol. *62:*617, 1988.
554. Turina, M. I., Siebenmann, R., Von Segesser, L., et al.: Late functional deterioration after atrial correction for transposition of the great arteries. Circulation *80*(Suppl. I):162, 1989.
555. Gutgesell, H. P., Massaro, T. A., and Kron, I. L.: The arterial switch operation for transposition of the great arteries in a consortium of university hospitals. Am. J. Cardiol. *74:*959, 1994.
556. Castaneda, A. R., Mayer, J. E., Jonas, R. A., et al.: Transposition of the great arteries: The arterial switch operation. Cardiol. Clin. *7:*369, 1989.
557. Planche, C., Serraf, A., Lacour-Gayet, F., et al.: Anatomic correction of complete transposition with ventricular septal defect in neonates: Experience with 42 consecutive cases. Cardiol. Young *1:*101, 1991.
558. Colan, S. D., Trowitz, S. C. H. E., Wernvosky, G., et al.: Myocardial performance after arterial switch operation for transposition of the great arteries with intact ventricular septum. Circulation *78:*132, 1988.
559. Gleason, M. M., Chin, A., Andrews, B. A., et al.: Two-dimensional and Doppler echocardiographic assessment of neonatal arterial repair for transposition of the great arteries. J. Am. Coll. Cardiol. *13:*1320, 1989.
560. Martin, M. M., Snider, R., Bove, E. L., et al.: Two-dimensional and Doppler echocardiographic evaluation after arterial switch repair in infancy for complete transposition of the great arteries. Am. J. Cardiol. *63:*332, 1989.
561. Villafane, J., White, S., Elbl, F., et al.: An electrocardiographic midterm follow up study after anatomic repair of transposition of the great arteries. Am. J. Cardiol. *66:*350, 1990.
562. Boutin, C., Wernovsky, G., Sanders, S. P., et al.: Rapid two-stage arterial switch operation: Evaluation of left ventricular systolic mechanics late after an acute pressure overload stimulus in infancy. Circulation *90:*1294, 1994.
563. Boutin, C., Jonas, R. A., Sanders, S. P., et al.: Rapid two-stage arterial switch operation: Acquisition of left ventricular mass after pulmonary artery banding in infants with transposition of the great arteries. Circulation *90:*1304, 1994.
564. Wernovsky, G., Bridges, N. D., and Mandell, V. S.: Enlarged bronchial arteries after early repair of transposition of the great arteries. J. Am. Coll. Cardiol. *21:*465, 1993.
565. Nakanishi, T., Matsumoto, Y., Seguchi, M., et al.: Balloon angioplasty for postoperative pulmonary artery stenosis in transposition of the great arteries. J. Am. Coll. Cardiol. *22:*859, 1993.
566. Martin, R. P., Ettedgui, J. A., Qureshi, S. A., et al.: A quantitative evaluation of aortic regurgitation after anatomic correction of transposition of the great arteries. J. Am. Coll. Cardiol. *12:*1281, 1988.
566a. Redington, A. N.: Functional assessment of the heart after corrective surgery for complete transposition. Cardiol. Young *1:*84, 1991.
567. Hourihan, M., Colan, S. D., Wernovsky, G., et al.: Growth of the aortic anastomosis, annulus, and root after the arterial switch procedure performed in infancy. Circulation *88:*615, 1993.
568. Weindling, S. N., Wernovsky, G., Colan, S. D., et al.: Myocardial perfusion, function and exercise tolerance after the arterial switch operation. J. Am. Coll. Cardiol. *23:*424, 1994.
569. Lupinetti, F. M., Bove, E. L., Minich, L. L., et al.: Intermediate-term survival and functional results after arterial repair for transposition of the great arteries. J. Thorac. Cardiovasc. Surg. *103:*421, 1992.
570. Elkins, R. C., Knott-Craig, C. J., Ahn, J. H., et al.: Ventricular function after the arterial switch operation for transposition of the great arteries. Ann. Thorac. Surg. *57:*826, 1994.
571. Corno, A., George, B., Pearl, J., and Laks, H.: Surgical options for complex transposition of the great arteries. J. Am. Coll. Cardiol *14:*742, 1989.
572. Lecompte, Y., Neveux, J. Y., Leca, F., et al.: Reconstruction of the pulmonary outflow tract without prosthetic conduit. J. Thorac. Cardiovasc. Surg. *87:*727, 1982.
573. Corno, A. F., Parisi, F., Marino, B., et al.: Palliative Mustard operation: An expanded horizon. Eur. J. Cardiothorac. Surg. *1:*144, 1987.
574. Colli, A. M., De Leval, M., and Somerville, J.: Anatomically corrected malposition of the great arteries. Am. J. Cardiol. *55:*1367, 1985.
575. Kirklin, J. W., Pacifico, A. D., Bargeron, L. M., Jr., and Soto, B.: Cardiac

repair and anatomically corrected malposition of the great arteries. Circulation *48*:153, 1973.
576. Berry, W. B., Roberts, W. C., Morrow, A. G., and Braunwald, E.: Corrected transposition of the aorta and pulmonary trunk: Clinical, hemodynamic, and pathologic findings. Am. J. Med. *36*:35, 1964.
577. Freedberg, D. Z., and Nadas, A. S.: Clinical profile of patients with congenital corrected transposition of the great arteries. N. Engl. J. Med. *282*:1053, 1970.
578. Bjarke, B. B., and Kidd, B. S. L.: Congenitally corrected transposition of the great arteries: A clinical study of 101 cases. Acta Paediatr. Scand. *65*:153, 1976.
579. Lundstrom, U., Bull, C., Wyse, R. K. H., et al.: The natural and "unnatural" history of congenitally corrected transposition. Am. J. Cardiol. *65*:1222, 1990.
579a. Presbitero, P., Somerville, J., Rabajoli, F., et al.: Corrected transposition of the great arteries without associated defects in adult patients: Clinical profile and follow up. Br. Heart J. *74*:57, 1995.
580. Dimas, A. P., Moodie, D. S., Strba, R., and Gill, C. C.: Long-term function of the morphologic right ventricle in adult patients with corrected transposition of the great arteries. Am. Heart J. *118*:526, 1989.
581. Waldo, A. L., Pacifico, A. D., Bargeron, L. M., Jr., et al.: Electrophysiological delineation of specialized AV conduction system in patients with corrected transposition of the great vessels and ventricular septal defect. Circulation *52*:435, 1975.
582. Bharati, B., Rosen, K., Steinfield, L., et al.: The anatomic substrate for pre-excitation in corrected transposition. Circulation *62*:831, 1980.
583. Meissner, M. D., Panidis, I. P., Eshaghpour, E., et al.: Corrected transposition of the great arteries: Evaluation by two-dimensional and Doppler echocardiography. Am. Heart J. *111*:599, 1986.
584. Freedom, R. M., Harrington, D. P., and White, R. I., Jr.: The differential diagnosis of levotransposed or malposed aorta: An angiocardiographic study. Circulation *50*:1040, 1974.
585. Russo, P., Danielson, G. K., and Driscoll, D. J.: Transaortic closure of ventricular septal defect in patients with corrected transposition with pulmonary stenosis or atresia. Circulation *76*(Suppl. III):88, 1987.
586. McGrath, L. B., Kirklin, J. W., Blackstone, E. H., et al.: Death and other events after cardiac repair in discordant atrioventricular connection. J. Thorac. Cardiovasc. Surg. *90*:711, 1985.
587. Yoshimura, N., Yamaguchi, M., Oshima, Y., et al.: Systemic atrioventricular valve replacement in an infant with corrected transposition of the great arteries. Ann. Thorac. Surg. *54*:573, 1992.
588. Hagler, D. J.: Double-outlet right ventricle. *In* Emmanoulides, G. C., Allen, H. D., et al. (eds.): Moss and Adams' Heart Disease in Infants, Children and Adolescents. 5th ed. Baltimore, Williams and Wilkins, 1994, p. 1246.
589. Goitein, K. J., Neches, W. H., Park, S. C., et al.: Electrocardiogram in double chamber right ventricle. Am. J. Cardiol. *45*:604, 1980.
590. Roberson, D. A., and Silverman, N. H.: Malaligned outlet septum with subpulmonary ventricular septal defect and abnormal ventriculoarterial connection: A morphologic spectrum defined echocardiographically. J. Am. Coll. Cardiol. *16*:459, 1990.
591. Sridaromont, S., Ritter, D. G., Feldt, R. H., et al.: Double outlet right ventricle: Anatomic and angiocardiographic correlations. Mayo Clin. Proc. *53*:555, 1978.
592. Kirklin, J. W., Pacifico, A. D., Blackstone, E. H., et al.: Current risks and protocols for operations for double-outlet right ventricle. J. Thorac. Cardiovasc. Surg. *92*:913, 1986.
593. Russo, P., Danielson, G. K., Puga, F. J., et al.: Modified Fontan procedure for biventricular hearts with complex forms of double-outlet right ventricle. Circulation *78*(Suppl. III):20, 1988.
594. Day, R., Laks, H., Milgalter, E., et al.: Partial biventricular repair for double-outlet right ventricle with left ventricular hypoplasia. Ann. Thorac. Surg. *49*:1003, 1990.
595. Van Praagh, R., Weinberg, P. M., and Srebro, J. P.: Double-outlet left ventricle. *In* Emmanouilides, G. C., et al. (eds.): Moss and Adams' Heart Disease in Infants, Children, and Adolescents. 4th ed. Baltimore, Williams and Wilkins, 1989, p. 461.
596. Rebergen, S. A., Guit, G. L., and de Roos, A.: Double outlet left ventricle: Diagnosis with magnetic resonance imaging. Br. Heart J. *66*:381, 1991.
597. Marino, B., and Bevilacqua, M.: Double-outlet left ventricle: Two-dimensional echocardiographic diagnosis. Am. Heart J. *123*:1075, 1992.
598. Krabill, K. A., and Lucas, R. V., Jr.: Abnormal pulmonary venous connections. *In* Emmanouilides, G. C., Allen, H. D., et al. (eds.): Moss and Adams' Heart Disease in Infants, Children, and Adolescents. 5th ed. Baltimore, Williams and Wilkins, 1994, p. 838.
599. Ward, K. E., Mullins, C. E., Huhta, J. C., et al.: Restrictive interatrial communication in total anomalous pulmonary venous connection. Am. J. Cardiol. *57*:1131, 1986.
600. Lucas, R. V., Jr., Lock, J. E., Tandon, R., and Edwards, J. E.: Gross and histologic anatomy of total anomalous pulmonary venous connections. Am. J. Cardiol. *62*:292, 1988.
601. Lincoln, C. R., Rigby, M. L., Marcanti, C., et al.: Surgical risk factors in total anomalous pulmonary venous connection. Am. J. Cardiol. *61*:608, 1988.
602. Wang, J. K., Lue, H. C., Wu, M. H., et al.: Obstructed total anomalous pulmonary venous connection. Pediatr. Cardiol. *14*:28, 1993.
603. Elliott, L. P., and Edwards, J. E.: The problem of pulmonary venous obstruction in total anomalous pulmonary venous connection to the left innominate vein. Circulation *25*:913, 1962.
604. Newfeld, E. A., Wilson, A., Paul, M. H., and Reisch, J. S.: Pulmonary vascular disease in total anomalous pulmonary venous drainage. Circulation *61*:103, 1980.
605. Chin, A. J., Sanders, S. P., Sherman, F., et al.: Accuracy of subcostal two-dimensional echocardiography in prospective diagnosis of total anomalous pulmonary venous connection. Am. Heart J. *113*:1153, 1987.
606. Jenkins, K. J., Sanders, S. P., Orav, E. J., et al.: Individual pulmonary vein size and survival in infants with totally anomalous pulmonary venous connection. J. Am. Coll. Cardiol. *22*:201, 1993.
607. Lamb, R. K., Qureshi, S. A., Wilkinson, J. L., et al.: Total anomalous pulmonary venous drainage: 17-year surgical experience. J. Thorac. Cardiovasc. Surg. *96*:368, 1988.
608. Van Meter, C., Jr., LeBlanc, J. G., Culpepper, W. S., III, and Ochsner, J. L.: Partial anomalous pulmonary venous return. Circulation *82*(Suppl. IV):195, 1990.
609. Gao, Y. A., Burrows, P. E., Benson, L. N., et al.: Scimitar syndrome in infancy. J. Am. Coll. Cardiol. *22*:873, 1993.
610. Dupuis, C., Charaf, L. A. C., Breviere, G. M., and Abou, P.: "Infantile" form of the scimitar syndrome with pulmonary hypertension. Am. J. Cardiol. *71*:1326, 1993.
611. Stanger, P., Rudolph, A. M., and Edwards, J. E.: Cardiac malpositions: An overview based on a study of 65 necropsy specimens. Circulation *56*:159, 1977.
612. Van Praagh, R.: Diagnosis of complex congenital heart disease: Morphologic-anatomic method and terminology. Cardiovasc. Intervent. Radiol. *7*:115, 1984.
613. Silverman, N. H.: An ultrasonic approach to the diagnosis of cardiac situs, connections, and malposition. *In* Friedman, W. F., and Higgins, C. B. (eds.): Pediatric Cardiac Imaging. Philadelphia, W. B. Saunders Company, 1984, p. 188.
614. Geva, T., Vick, W., Wendt, R., and Rokey, R.: Role of spin echo and cine magnetic resonance imaging in presurgical planning of heterotaxy syndrome: Comparison with echocardiography and catheterization. Circulation *90*:348, 1994.
615. Geva, T., Sanders, S. P., Ayres, N. A., et al.: Two-dimensional echocardiographic anatomy of atrioventricular alignment discordance with situs concordance. Am. Heart J. *125*:459, 1993.
616. Wang, J. K., Li, Y. W., Chiu, I. S., et al.: Usefulness of magnetic resonance imaging in the assessment of venoatrial connections, atrial morphology, bronchial situs, and other anomalies in right isomerism. Am. J. Cardiol. *74*:701, 1994.
617. Anderson, C., Devine, W. A., Anderson, R. H., et al.: Abnormalities of the spleen in relation to congenital malformations of the heart: Survey of necropsy findings in children. Br. Heart J. *63*:122, 1990.
618. Peoples, W. M., Moller, J. H., and Edwards, J. E.: Polysplenia: A review of 146 cases. Pediatr. Cardiol. *4*:129, 1983.
619. Phoon, C. K., and Neill, C. A.: Asplenia syndrome—risk factors for early unfavorable outcome. Am. J. Cardiol. *73*:1235, 1994.
620. Phoon, C. K., and Neill, C. A.: Asplenia syndrome: Insight into embryology through an analysis of cardiac and extracardiac anomalies. Am. J. Cardiol. *73*:581, 1994.
621. Culbertson, C. B., George, B. L., Day, R. W., et al.: Factors influencing survival of patients with heterotaxy syndrome undergoing the Fontan procedure. J. Am. Coll. Cardiol. *20*:678, 1992.
622. Oku, H., Iemura, J., Kitayama, H., et al.: Bivalvation with bridging for common atrioventricular valve regurgitation in right isomerism. Ann. Thorac. Surg. *57*:1324, 1994.
623. Gehlman, H. R., and Van Ingen, G. J.: Symptomatic congenital complete absence of the left pericardium: Case report and review of the literature. Eur. Heart J. *10*:670, 1989.
624. Pernot, C., Hoeffel, J. C., and Henry, M.: Radiologic patterns of congenital malformation of the pericardium. Radiol. Clin. (Basel) *44*:505, 1975.
625. Rowland, T. W., Twible, E. A., Norwood, W. I., Jr., and Keane, J. F.: Partial absence of the left pericardium: Diagnosis by two-dimensional echocardiography. Am. J. Dis. Child. *136*:628, 1982.
626. Jones, J. W., and McManus, B. M.: Fatal cardiac strangulation by congenital partial pericardial defect. Am. Heart J. *107*:183, 1984.
627. Rowland, T. W., Twible, E. A., Norwood, W. J., Jr., and Keane, J. F.: Partial absence of the left pericardium. Am. J. Dis. Child. *136*:628, 1982.
628. Anderson, R. H., Macartney, F. J., Tynan, M., et al.: Univentricular atrioventricular connection: The single ventricle trap unsprung. Pediatr. Cardiol. *4*:273, 1983.
629. Thies, W. R., Soto, B., Diethelm, E., et al.: Angiographic anatomy of hearts with one ventricular chamber: The true single ventricle. Am. J. Cardiol. *55*:1363, 1985.
630. Change, A. C., Hanley, F. L., Wernovsky, G., et al.: Early bidirectional cavopulmonary shunt in young infants. Circulation *88*:149, 1993.
631. Calderon-Colmenero, J., Ramirez, S., Rijlaarsdam, M., et al.: Use of bidirectional cavopulmonary shunt in patients under one year of age. Cardiol. Young *5*:28, 1995.
632. Moak, J. P., and Gersony, W. M.: Progressive atrioventricular valvular regurgitation in single ventricle. Am. J. Cardiol. *59*:656, 1987.
633. Mair, D. D., Hagler, D. J., Julsrud, P. R., et al.: Early and late results of the modified Fontan procedure for double-inlet left ventricle: The Mayo Clinic experience. J. Am. Coll. Cardiol. *18*:1727, 1991.
634. DiSessa, T. G., Isabel-Jones, J. G., Heins, H., et al.: Two dimensional echocardiographic features of the univentricular heart. Cardiovasc. Ultrason. *3*:89, 1984.
635. Jacobs, M. I., and Norwood, W. I.: Fontan operation: Influence of modifications on morbidity and mortality. Ann. Thorac. Surg. *58*:945, 1994.
636. Bevilacqua, M., Sanders, S. P., and van Praagh, S.: Double-inlet single

left ventricle: Echocardiographic anatomy with emphasis on the morphology of the atrioventricular valves and ventricular septal defect. J. Am. Coll. Cardiol. *18*:559, 1991.
637. Fogel, M. A., Weinberg, P. M., Fellows, K. E., and Hoffman, E. A.: Magnetic resonance imaging of constant total heart volume and center of mass in patients with functional single ventricle before and after staged Fontan procedure. Am. J. Cardiol. *72*:1435, 1993.
638. Matitiau, A., Geva, T., Colan, S. D., et al.: Bulboventricular foramen size in infants with double-inlet left ventricle or tricuspid atresia with transposed great arteries: Influence on initial palliative operation and rate of growth. J. Am. Coll. Cardiol. *19*:142, 1992.
639. Huggon, I. C., Baker, E. J., Maisey, M. N., et al.: Magnetic resonance imaging of hearts with atrioventricular valve atresia or double inlet ventricle. Br. Heart J. *68*:313, 1992.
640. Mayer, J. E.: Surgical aortico-pulmonary anastomosis for a complex aortic obstruction with single ventricle. Prog. Pediatr. Cardiol. *3*:106, 1994.
641. Lui, R. C., Williams, W. G., Trusler, G. A., et al.: Experience with the Damus-Kaye-Stansel procedure for children with Taussig-Bing hearts or univentricular hearts with subaortic stenosis. Circulation *88*:170, 1993.
642. Gewillig, M., Wyse, R. K., De Leval, M. R., et al.: Early and late arrhythmias after the Fontan operation: Predisposing factors and clinical consequences. Br. Heart J. *67*:72, 1992.
643. Parikh, S. R., Hurwitz, R. A., Caldwell, R. L., and Girod, D. A.: Ventricular function in the single ventricle before and after Fontan surgery. Am. J. Cardiol. *67*:1390, 1991.
644. Kurer, C. C., Tanner, C. S., and Vetter, V. L.: Electrophysiologic findings after Fontan repair of functional single ventricle. J. Am. Coll. Cardiol. *17*:174, 1991.
645. Sluysmans, T., Sanders, S. P., van der Velde, M., et al.: Natural history and patterns of recovery of contractile function in single left ventricle after Fontan operation. Circulation *86*:1753, 1992.
646. Rosenthal, M., Bush, A., Deanfield, J., and Redington, A.: Comparison of cardiopulmonary adaptation during exercise in children after the atriopulmonary and total cavopulmonary connection Fontan procedures. Circulation *91*:372, 1995.
647. Stevenson, O., Soderlund, S., Thoren, C., and Wallgren, G.: Arterial anomalies causing compression of the trachea and/or the esophagus. Acta Paediatr. Scand. *60*:81, 1971.
648. Park, C. D., Waldhausen, J. A., Friedman, S., et al.: Tracheal compression by the great arteries in the mediastinum: Report of 39 cases. Arch. Surg. *103*:626, 1971.
649. Ashwinikumar, P., de Leval, M. R., Elliott, M. J., et al.: Pulmonary artery sling. Ann. Thorac. Surg. *54*:967, 1992.
650. Baron, R. L., Gutierrez, F. R., and McKnight, R. C.: Computed tomographic evaluation of the great arteries and aortic arch malformations. *In* Friedman, W. F., and Higgins, C. B. (eds.): Pediatric Cardiac Imaging. Philadelphia, W. B. Saunders Company, 1983, p. 135.
651. Azarow, K. S., Pearl, R. H., Hoffman, M. A., et al.: Vascular ring: Does magnetic resonance imaging replace angiography? Ann. Thorac. Surg. *53*:882, 1992.
652. deLeval, M.: Vascular rings. *In* Stark, J., and deLeval, M. (eds.): Surgery for Congenital Heart Defects. New York, Grune and Stratton, 1983, p. 227.
653. Anand, R., Dooley, K. J., Williams, W. H., et al.: Follow-up of surgical correction of vascular anomalies causing tracheobronchial compression. Pediatr. Cardiol. *15*:58, 1994.
654. Perry, J. C., and Garson, A., Jr.: Diagnosis and treatment of arrhythmias. Adv. Pediatr. *36*:177, 1989.
655. Anderson, R. H., Wenick, A. C. G., Losekoot, T. G., and Becker, A. E.: Congenitally complete heart block. Circulation *56*:90, 1977.
655a. Michaelsson, M.: Congenital complete atrioventricular block. Progr. Pediatr. Cardiol. *4*:1, 1995.
656. Derksen, R. H., and Meilof, J. F.: Anti-Ro/SS-A and anti-La/SS-B autoantibody levels in relation to systemic lupus erythematosus disease activity and congenital heart block. Arthritis Rheum. *35*:953, 1992.
657. Horsfall, A. C., and Rose, L. M.: Cross-reactive maternal autoantibodies and congenital heart block. J. Autoimmun. *5*:479, 1992.
658. Ross, B. A.: Congenital complete atrioventricular block. Pediatr. Clin. North Am. *37*:69, 1990.
659. Kugler, J. D., and Danford, D. A.: Pacemakers in children: An update. Am. Heart J. *117*:665, 1989.
660. Hoyer, M. H., Beerman, L. B., Ettedgui, J. A., et al.: Transatrial lead placement for endocardial pacing in children. Ann. Thorac. Surg. *58*:97, 1994.
661. Dreifus, L. S., Fisch, C., Griffin, J. C., et al.: Guidelines for implantation of cardiac pacemakers and antiarrhythmia devices: A report of the American College of Cardiology/American Heart Association Task Force on assessment of diagnostic and therapeutic cardiovascular procedures (Committee on Pacemaker Implantation). J. Am. Coll. Cardiol. *18*:1, 1991.
662. Michaelsson, M., and Engle, M. A.: Congenital complete heart block: An international study of the natural history. Cardiovasc. Clin. *4*:85, 1982.
663. Ko, J. K., Deal, B. J., Strasburger, J. F., et al.: Supraventricular tachycardia mechanisms and their age distribution in pediatric patients. Am. J. Cardiol. *69*:1028, 1992.
664. Kleinman, C. S., Donnerstein, R. L., DeVore, G. R., et al.: Fetal echocardiography for evaluation of in utero congestive heart failure. N. Engl. J. Med. *306*:568, 1982.
665. Radford, D. J., Izukawa, T., and Rowe, R. D.: Congenital paroxysmal atrial tachycardia. Arch. Dis. Child. *51*:613, 1976.
666. Deal, B. J., Keane, J. F., Gillette, P. C., and Gardon, A., Jr.: Wolff-Parkinson-White syndrome and supraventricular tachycardia during infancy: Management and follow-up. J. Am. Coll. Cardiol. *5*:130, 1985.
667. Klitzner, T. S., and Friedman, W. F.: Cardiac arrhythmias: The role of pharmacologic intervention. Cardiol. Clin. *7*:299, 1989.
668. Benson, D. W., Jr., Dunnigan, A., and Benditt, D. G.: Follow-up evaluation of infant paroxysmal atrial tachycardia: Transesophageal study. Circulation *75*:542, 1987.
669. Zipes, D. P., et al.: Guidelines for clinical intracardiac electrophysiologic studies: A report of the American College of Cardiology/American Heart Association Task Force on Assessment of Diagnostic and Therapeutic Cardiovascular Procedures. J. Am. Coll. Cardiol. *14*:1827, 1989.
670. Klitzner, T. S., Wetzel, G. T., Saxon, L. A., et al.: Radiofrequency ablation: A new era in the treatment of pediatric arrhythmias. Am. J. Dis. Child. *147*:769, 1993.
671. Lai, W. W., Al-Khatib, Y., Klitzner, T. S., et al.: Biplanar transesophageal echocardiographic direction of radiofrequency catheter ablation in children and adolescents with the Wolff-Parkinson-White syndrome. Am. J. Cardiol. *71*:872, 1993.
672. Dhala, A., Bremner, S., Deshpande, S., et al.: Efficacy and safety of atrioventricular nodal modification for atrioventricular nodal reentrant tachycardia in the pediatric population. Am. Heart J. *128*:903, 1994.
673. Hebe, J., Schlüter, M., and Kuck, K. H.: Catheter ablation in children with supraventricular tachycardia mediated by accessory pathways—use of radiofrequency current as a first line of therapy. Cardiol. Young *4*:28, 1994.
674. Kugler, J. D., Danford, D. A., Deal, B. J., et al.: Radiofrequency catheter ablation for tachyarrhythmias in children and adolescents. N. Engl. J. Med. *330*:1481, 1994.
675. Garson, A., Jr., Bink-Boelkens, M., Hesslein, P. S., et al.: Atrial flutter in the young: A collaborative study of 380 cases. J. Am. Coll. Cardiol. *6*:871, 1985.
676. Mendelsohn, A., Dick, M., and Serwer, G. A.: Natural history of isolated atrial flutter in infancy. J. Pediatr. *119*:386, 1991.
677. Dunnigan, A., Benson, W., Jr., and Benditt, D. G.: Atrial flutter in infancy: Diagnosis, clinical features and treatment. Pediatrics *75*:725, 1985.
678. Dick, M., Scott, W. A., Serwer, G. S., et al.: Acute termination of supraventricular tachyarrhythmias in children by transesophageal atrial pacing. Am. J. Cardiol. *61*:925, 1988.
679. Jiang, C., Atkinson, D., Towbin, J. A., et al.: Two long QT syndrome loci map to chromosomes 3 and 7 with evidence for further heterogeneity. Nature Genetics *8*:141, 1994.
680. Garson, A., Jr., Dick, M., II, Fournier, A., et al.: The long QT syndrome in children: An international study of 287 patients. Circulation *87*:1866, 1993.

Chapter 30
Congenital Heart Disease in Adults

JOSEPH K. PERLOFF

SURVIVAL PATTERNS 964
Unoperated Patients 964
Common Defects in Which Unoperated Adult Survival is Expected 964
Uncommon Defects in Which Unoperated Adult Survival is Expected 966
Common Defects in Which Unoperated Adult Survival is Exceptional 967
Late Survival After Cardiac Surgery or Interventional Catheterization 968
MEDICAL MANAGEMENT OF ADULT CONGENITAL HEART DISEASE 971
Cyanotic 971
Infective Endocarditis 974
Pregnancy and Congenital Heart Disease: Mother and Fetus 975
Medical Management of the Pregnant Woman with Congenital Heart Disease 976
Medical Management of the Fetus 977
Exercise Before and After Surgery or Interventional Catheterization 978
Surgical Considerations 980
Cardiac Catheterization as a Therapeutic Intervention 980
Noncardiac Surgery in Adults with Congenital Heart Disease 981
Postoperative Residua and Sequelae 982
REFERENCES 984

Advances in diagnostic techniques and in the surgical and medical management of infants and children with congenital malformations of the heart and circulation have had a major impact upon longevity.[1–3] The number of older patients with congenital heart disease is steadily increasing, and the trend promises to continue. Congenital heart disease in adults has emerged as a special area of cardiovascular interest[4] that includes patients who have never undergone cardiac surgery, those who have undergone cardiac surgery and require no further operation, those who have had palliation with or without anticipation of reparative surgery, and those whose condition is inoperable apart from organ transplantation. This chapter begins with a brief historical perspective and then focuses upon the multidisciplinary facilities for comprehensive care, survival patterns (without operation and postoperative), medical considerations, surgical considerations, and postoperative residua and sequelae.[2]

HISTORICAL PERSPECTIVES

Congenital heart disease is, by definition, present at birth (*con,* together; *genitus,* born), but survival patterns vary widely.[2,5] In 1888, Etienne-Louis Arthur Fallot wrote, "We have seen from our observations that cyanosis, especially in the adult, is the result of a small number of cardiac malformations well determined."[6] Fallot referred to the tetralogy that still bears his name as one of the most familiar eponyms in cardiovascular medicine.

In the first half of the twentieth century, the untiring work of Maude Abbott culminated in her remarkable *Atlas of Congenital Heart Disease,* which was based upon 1000 pathology specimens personally studied.[7] The atlas was not only a landmark in the classification of congenital malformations of the heart but also provided invaluable information on survival patterns before the advent of cardiac surgery. The seminal contributions of Gross, Blalock, and Crafoord appreciably modified those survival patterns, and the sense of despair that had surrounded congenital cardiac anomalies—those "hopeless futilities"—began to dissipate.

In 1939, Robert Gross, a pediatric surgeon in Boston, ligated a patent ductus arteriosus in a 7½-year-old girl.[8] A few years later, Helen Brooke Taussig, a pediatric cardiologist in Baltimore, conceived the idea of "creating" a patent ductus in cyanotic children suffering from deficient pulmonary blood flow, and in 1945, Alfred Blalock, a vascular surgeon at Johns Hopkins Hospital, implemented Taussig's idea by suturing the end of a subclavian artery to the side of a pulmonary artery in a patient with Fallot's tetralogy, thus establishing the Blalock-Taussig anastomosis.[9] Before this operation, ". . . a blue baby with a malformed heart was considered beyond the reach of surgical aid." In the early 1940's, Clarence Crafoord, at the Karolinska Institute in Sweden, while operating on patients with patent ductus arteriosus, "began to wonder whether it might not also be possible to treat coarctation of the aortic isthmus by surgical means."[10] The introduction of cardiac catheterization after World War II, a technique for which Andre F. Cournand and Dickenson W. Richards in the United States and Werner Forssman in Germany received the Nobel Prize in 1956, was a major step forward both diagnostically and in the study of circulatory physiology.[2] The development of extracorporeal circulation in the early to mid-1950's was destined to make virtually all congenital malformations of the heart accessible to the skills of cardiac surgeons. The stage was set for "accurate visualization of structures within the heart for a period sufficient to permit precise corrective measures."[11]

The culmination of these historical landmarks was one of the most successful diagnostic and therapeutic achievements that medicine has witnessed. Formidable technical resources became accessible, permitting remarkably accurate anatomical and physiological diagnoses and astonishing feats of reparative surgery. Survival patterns were affected, often profoundly. Congenital heart disease should therefore be considered not only in terms of age of onset but also in terms of the age range that survival now permits—an uninterrupted continuum from fetal life to senescence.[2,4] Although long-term management remains concerned with unoperated patients, medical management increasingly focuses on the growing numbers of postoperative patients who need surveillance. The quality of care provided by pediatric cardiologists from birth to maturity must be matched with care of equal quality for adults.

Unoperated adults experience improved longevity because of refinements in the management of arrhythmias and conduction disturbances, ventricular failure, pulmonary vascular disease, hematological disorders, renal function, urate metabolism, infective endocarditis, pregnancy, and noncardiac surgery. The management of patients *after* cardiac surgery or interventional catheterization requires knowledge of the intrinsic congenital cardiac or vascular malformation, the nature and effects of the therapeutic intervention, and the presence, type, and extent of postinterventional residua and sequelae. The ideal of cure in the literal sense is rarely achieved, however, so that a broad range of residua and sequelae are left behind and require prolonged, if not indefinite, medical attention that is essential if the concerns inherent in this new and increasing patient population are to be addressed properly.[2,4]

MULTIDISCIPLINARY CARE OF ADULTS WITH CONGENITAL HEART DISEASE

In the United States and abroad, increasing numbers of specialized facilities are emerging for the care of adults with congenital heart disease.[2,4] Relevant to these facilities are staffing, diagnostic laboratories, criteria for patient entry, referral patterns, outpatient and inpatient management, multidisciplinary consultants, and educational, training, and research commitments.[2]

Patients are best managed, at least for the foreseeable future, by collaboration between medical and pediatric cardiologists and cardiac surgeons with the assistance of cardiovascular nurse specialists or physician assistants. Cardiac surgeons who have the knowledge and skills needed to deal with congenital heart disease can, as a rule, adapt those skills to coexisting acquired cardiac diseases and obviate the need for two cardiac surgeons to perform one operation. An adult congenital heart disease facility should be a collaborative effort, especially in the setting of a university hospital in which intellectual interchange, teaching, and research are as paramount as optimal patient care. Cardiologists with special expertise in this area are now recognized as part of the profile of cardiovascular specialists.[12]

Consultative needs should be anticipated rather than solicited as ad hoc opinions. Noncardiac consultants are best incorporated into the adult congenital heart disease facility and include electrophysiologists, hematologists, nephrologists, rheumatologists, transplant cardiologists, pulmonologists, high-risk pregnancy obstetricians, gynecologists, psychiatrists, cardiac anesthesiologists, cardiac pathologists, and social service personnel for insurance and vocational counseling.

Criteria for patient entry into the specialized facilities are based on age and psychological and physical maturity. Adolescents are neither children nor adults, and adolescent medicine, at least at present, is best dealt with by the more knowledgeable pediatricians or by medical cardiologists with pediatric experience. In some centers, adolescent patients remain the province of pediatric cardiologists, whereas in others, adolescents are included within the adult congenital heart disease facility, provided that facility has a pediatric cardiologist on its staff.[4]

Tertiary centers for congenital heart disease in adults do not compete with practicing physicians or community hospitals but instead offer services that are difficult if not impossible to duplicate. Broadly speaking, the base of the referral pyramid is the primary care physician in the community (general pediatrician, general physician). The next level (stratum) is the cardiologist in the community (pediatric, medical) who provides both consultative and primary care. Tertiary care depends upon regional specialized facilities that have experience even with rare and complex malformations.

There is a mounting consensus that adults with congenital heart disease are best managed in an adult setting, both outpatient and inpatient. Pediatric cardiology clinics tend to reinforce a sense of dependency that patients must overcome if they are to function as mature adults. Inpatient policy depends in part on whether medicine and pediatrics share the same hospital. When that is the case, adults with congenital heart disease are admitted to adult inpatient facilities under the care of the cardiologist with inpatient privileges. Hospitalized adults are an important part of the educational experience of house staff and fellows. Admissions are for cardiac or noncardiac surgery, for labor and delivery, for cardiac intensive care (generally arrhythmias), for heart failure, or for coexisting general medical disorders.

Noninvasive, exercise, catheterization, angiographic, and magnetic resonance imaging (MRI) laboratories must provide the same high quality of care for adults with congenital heart disease as that provided by pediatric laboratories for infants and children. Quality cannot be compromised for expediency.

Medical records serve multiple purposes. The goal should be a quality standard appropriate for the use of records for research purposes. Reports to referring physicians should be both practical and educational. It is useful to have a dual record system, with one set for hospital files and a second for the congenital heart disease facility. When patients move to another area, copies of their records should be carried for delivery to their new cardiologist. Patients have proved to be responsible emissaries.

The educational and training commitments of an adult congenital heart disease facility extend to community physicians, house staff, fellows, medical students, visiting physicians, nurses (especially nurse specialists), and the patients themselves. Tertiary care centers should assume responsibility for informing community physicians that adults with congenital heart disease require special expertise seldom available in local hospitals. That level of awareness is important in channeling patients to tertiary facilities.

Adult congenital heart disease centers, especially in university hospitals, should be committed to research prompted by a desire to address unresolved questions posed by this patient population. A rich harvest is in store if advantage is taken of collaboration with colleagues in other disciplines. A research base must be provided for fellows with career interests in adult congenital heart disease.

SURVIVAL PATTERNS

Unoperated Patients

The term *natural history* is a misnomer, because mortality and morbidity for patients who have not undergone cardiac surgery have been materially influenced by advances in *medical* management. Accordingly, "natural history" should be replaced by "unoperated survival."

Unoperated patients include those with malformations that do not require surgery, malformations that are amenable to operation in adulthood, and malformations that are inoperable except for heart, lung, or heart-lung transplantation. Management of unoperated adults must take into account not only the congenital disorder per se but also the medical disorders that are inherent components of certain types of congenital heart disease, as well as acquired disorders of the heart and circulation that coexist with and modify the physiological expressions of the congenital malformation. This section deals chiefly with common or uncommon defects in which unoperated adult survival is expected and with certain defects that are common and therefore familiar but for which adult survival is exceptional.

Common Defects in Which Unoperated Adult Survival is Expected

BICUSPID AORTIC VALVE (see also p. 914, and Fig. 3–67, p. 79, and Fig. 29–33, p. 917). This malformation is the most

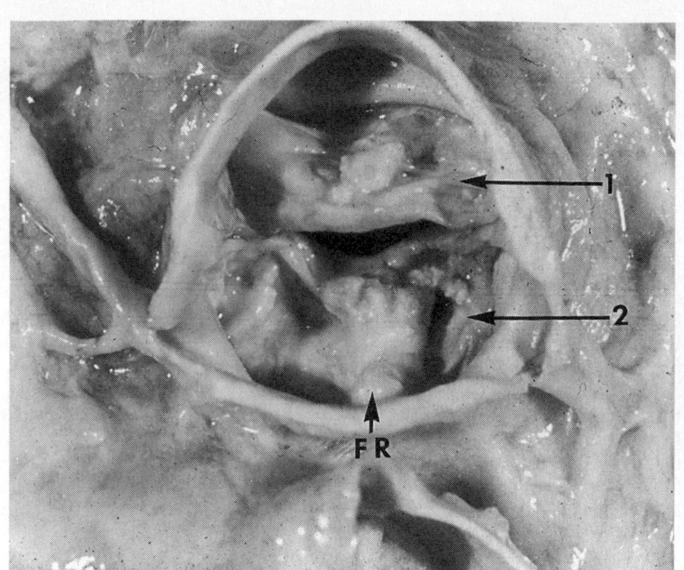

FIGURE 30–1. Necropsy specimen from an adult with bicuspid aortic stenosis. The first arrow points to one calcified leaflet, the second arrow points to a second calcified leaflet, and the vertical arrow points to calcium in the false raphe (FR). (Courtesy of Dr. William C. Roberts.

frequent congenital anomaly to which that structure is subject and is one of the most common gross morphological congenital anomalies of the heart or great arteries.[13] Bicuspid aortic valves that are functionally normal at birth can remain so throughout a normal life span. Progressive stenosis results from fibrocalcific thickening, a substrate that accounts for about one-half of surgical cases of isolated calcific aortic valve stenosis in adults (Fig. 30–1).[14] Conversely, a functionally normal bicuspid aortic valve may develop progressive incompetence and is an important cause of anatomically isolated aortic regurgitation in adults.[5] A bicuspid aortic valve may be modified, sometimes suddenly and appreciably, by infective endocarditis, to which the malformation is highly susceptible.[15] An inherent relationship exists between a congenital bicuspid aortic valve and an abnormality of the aortic root that takes the form of cystic medial necrosis related to the bicuspid

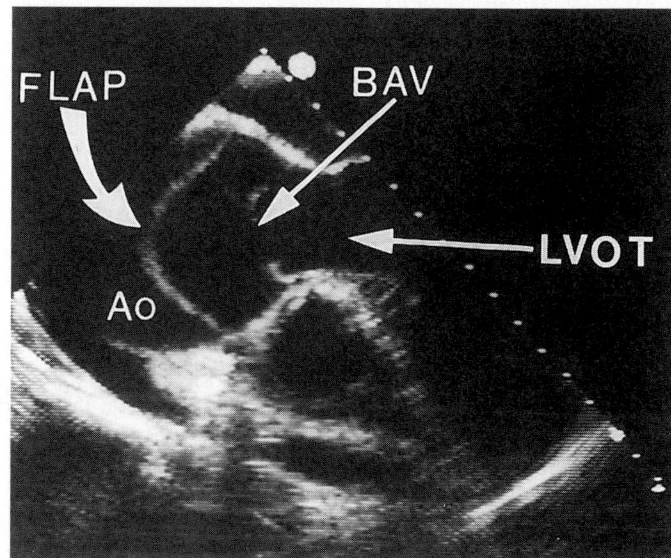

FIGURE 30–2. Transesophageal echocardiogram from a 37-year-old man with a bicuspid aortic valve, aortic regurgitation, and a dissecting aneurysm of the ascending aorta. The flap of the aortic dissection (FLAP) moved freely within the dilated aortic root (Ao). The dissection began just distal to the bicuspid aortic valve (BAV). LVOT = left ventricular outflow tract.

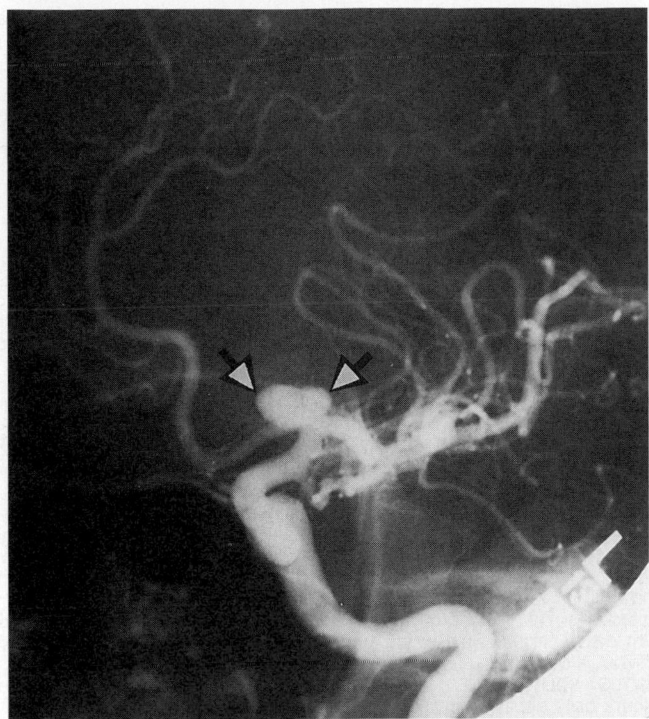

FIGURE 30–3. Congenital berry aneurysm of the circle of Willis in a 28-year-old woman with Fallot's tetralogy and pulmonary atresia. This type of congenital cerebral aneurysm is usually found in conjunction with coarctation of the aorta.

valve, whether functionally normal, stenotic, or incompetent.[5,16,16a] This aortic root disease can express itself in older adults as an aneurysm with aortic regurgitation or can announce itself dramatically in younger adults as aortic dissection (Fig. 30–2).

COARCTATION OF THE AORTA (see also p. 911). This malformation is likely to produce significant symptoms either in early infancy or after age 20 to 30 years.[5,17] The majority of patients who survive early life live to reach adulthood, but sporadic examples of exceptional longevity should not obscure the inherent risks that shorten life span.[5] Half of unoperated patients die by age 30, and more than three-quarters by age 50.[17] The oldest recorded survivor was a 92-year-old man reported by Reynaud in 1828.[18]

Survival and morbidity in adults with aortic coarctation are influenced by coexisting congenital and acquired cardiac and vascular diseases. The most common associated congenital malformation is the bicuspid aortic valve[5] (see above). Infective endocarditis is more likely to involve the bicuspid aortic valve than the site of coarctation.[5] A less common but potentially lethal coexisting malformation is a congenital aneurysm of the circle of Willis (Fig. 30–3), which typically becomes manifested by sudden rupture.[19] Dissection or rupture of the aorta itself is a dramatic complication with peak incidence in the third and fourth decades.[5] The proximal ascending aorta is the most common site, a susceptibility influenced in part by a coexisting bicuspid aortic valve or by XO Turner's syndrome.[5] The second site of rupture or dissection is in the postcoarctation aorta, which, like the aortic root, histologically resembles cystic medial necrosis.[20] Left ventricular failure in unoperated patients with coarctation of the aorta occurs either before the first year of life or after age 40 but seldom in between.[5] Systemic hypertension predisposes to premature coronary artery disease.[21]

PULMONARY VALVE STENOSIS (see also p. 968, and Fig. 29–42, p. 925). Represented by a pliant conical or dome-shaped valve with a narrow outlet at its apex, this malformation typically occurs as an isolated anomaly and is the most common variety of congenital obstruction to right ventricular outflow.[5] Survival into adolescence and adulthood is the rule, except for pinpoint pulmonary stenosis in neonates. Longevity depends chiefly on three variables: (1) the initial severity of obstruction, (2) whether a given degree of obstruction remains constant or progresses, and (3) the functional adequacy of the pressure-overloaded right ventricle.[22–24] The orifice size of isolated pulmonary valve stenosis usually increases appropriately with body growth. However, the development of secondary hypertrophic subpulmonary stenosis (Fig. 30–4) or fibrocalcific thickening in older patients may augment the degree of obstruction. Although subjective complaints become more prevalent as years go by, equivalent degrees of stenosis may limit one patient in childhood yet leave another relatively unencumbered as an adult.[5] Right ventricular failure is the most common cause of death. Infective endocarditis is a risk, except perhaps in mild pulmonary valve stenosis.

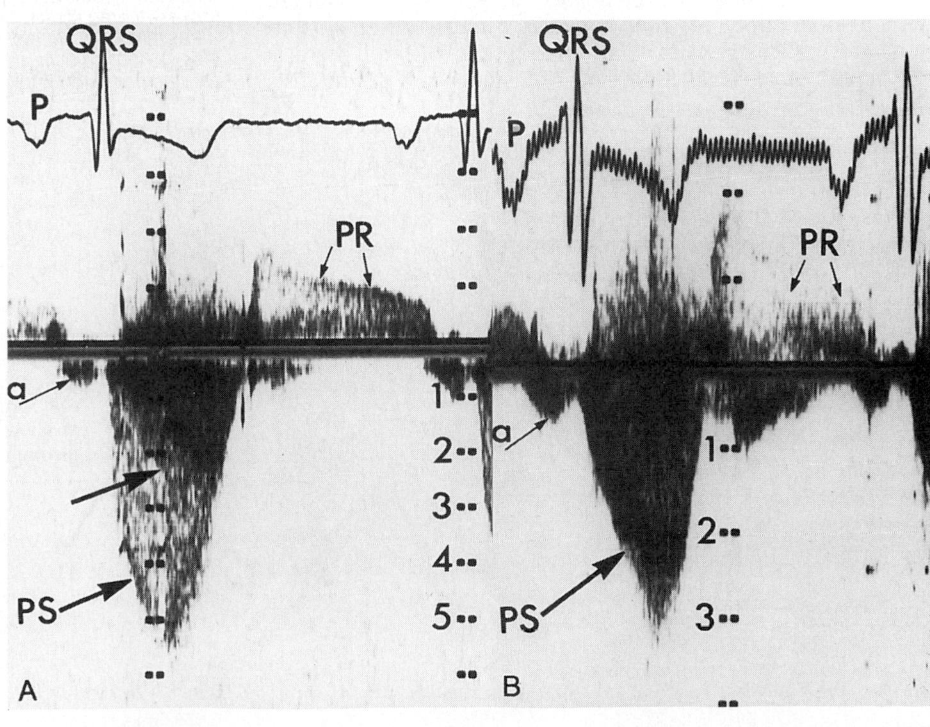

FIGURE 30–4. *A,* Continuous-wave Doppler across the right ventricular outflow tract of a 33-year-old man with severe pulmonary valve stenosis (PS) and secondary hypertrophic subpulmonary stenosis. The peak instantaneous gradient across the valve was 120 mm Hg. Within the major symmetrical flow disturbance envelope, there is an asymmetrical, lower-velocity pattern (unmarked arrow) caused by the hypertrophic subpulmonary stenosis. a = presystolic flow in response to an increased force of right atrial contractions; PR = pulmonary regurgitation. *B,* After balloon dilatation, the gradient at valve level was virtually abolished, leaving only the subpulmonary (PS) gradient, which subsequently resolved.

OSTIUM SECUNDUM ATRIAL SEPTAL DEFECT (see also p. 896 and Figs. 3–80, p. 83, and 29–11, p. 897). This anomaly is among the most common congenital cardiac malformations in unoperated adults and is by far the most common shunt lesion.[25–27] Although life expectancy is not normal, survival into adulthood is the rule.[5] Ostium secundum atrial septal defects are sporadically found in patients beyond age 70 years and occasionally in patients in their 80's or 90's.[26–28] One of the author's patients died at age 87 (Fig. 30–5), and another lived relatively comfortably until 3 months before his 95th birthday.[29]

Almost all patients who survive beyond the sixth decade are symptomatic. Death may be unrelated to the malformation, but when a relationship exists, cardiac failure is the most common cause of death. Older patients deteriorate chiefly on three counts[5]: (1) A decrease in left ventricular distensibility (acquired coronary artery disease, systemic hypertension) augments the left-to-right shunt; (2) atrial tachyarrhythmias, especially fibrillation, less commonly flutter or atrial tachycardia, increase in frequency after the fourth decade and serve to precipitate right ventricular failure; (3) the majority of symptomatic adults beyond age 40 have mild to moderate pulmonary hypertension despite the presence of a persistent, large left-to-right shunt, so the aging right ventricle is doubly beset by both pressure and volume overload.

The incidence, extent, and degree of associated mitral valve disease increase with age and the disease is characterized morphologically by thick, fibrotic leaflets and short, fibrotic chordae tendineae.[30,31] These mitral valve abnormalities have been attributed to abnormal cusp movement (trauma) caused by the effects of left ventricular cavity deformity (abnormal position and motion of the ventricular septum in response to volume overload of the right ventricle).[32,33] The abnormalities are believed to be the basis for the mitral regurgitation that tends to develop with age in about 15 per cent of patients.[29–31]

PATENT DUCTUS ARTERIOSUS (see also p. 971 and Fig. 29–19, p. 906). A large ductus is a relatively common cause of congestive heart failure in term infants, but after the first year of life, most patients with patent ductus arteriosus are asymptomatic.[34] In the second decade, the risk of infective endarteritis exceeds the risk of heart failure.[34] Beginning with the third decade (occasionally earlier), more patients with significant left-to-right shunts develop heart failure,[35] whereas those with small shunts remain asymptomatic. One of the author's patients was an 84-year-old woman with a moderately restrictive patent ductus, atrial fibrillation, and congestive heart failure (Fig. 30–6), and there is one report of survival to age 90.[36] A significant cumulative risk of infective endarteritis exists, especially if the ductus is restrictive. Patients with nonrestrictive patent ductus arteriosus seldom reach adulthood unless a rise in pulmonary vascular resistance relieves the left ventricle of excessive volume overload.[37] Survival to adulthood is then the rule, with differential cyanosis a distinctive feature of the reversed shunt.[5]

Uncommon Defects in Which Unoperated Adult Survival is Expected

SITUS INVERSUS WITH DEXTROCARDIA (see also p. 946). This cardiac malposition usually occurs with an otherwise structurally and functionally normal heart.[5] Symptoms related to *acquired* cardiac or noncardiac disease may lead to the discovery of the hitherto unsuspected malposition. If angina pectoris or myocardial infarction occurs with complete situs inversus, the pain is located in the *right* anterior chest with radiation to the right shoulder and right arm.[38] The pain of appendicitis is referred to the *left* lower quadrant, and the pain of biliary colic presents in the *left* upper quadrant, owing to the mirror image positions of abdominal viscera. The cardiac malposition is occasionally associated with sinusitis and bronchiectasis—Kartagener's triad.[5] Symptoms of bronchiectasis usually develop in early adulthood and may prompt investigations that lead to the discovery of the malposition. Situs inversus is common in men with infertility secondary to sperm immotility,[39] an observation that led to identification of a generalized disorder of ciliary motility in Kartagener's triad.[40] When situs inversus with dextrocardia coexists with congenital malformations of the heart, survival is determined by the associated anomalies.[5]

SITUS SOLITUS WITH DEXTROCARDIA. This cardiac malposition occurs only occasionally with a structurally normal heart, which permits adult survival but delays clinical recognition.[5] A routine chest radiograph may provide the first evidence of the malposition. Coexisting congenital cardiac anomalies, which are usually present, determine survival.

CONGENITAL COMPLETE HEART BLOCK (see also pp. 691 and 904). Adult survival is the rule, although the ultimate fate of large numbers of older patients with congenital complete heart block dampens optimism, and mortality even in infancy and childhood is not negligible.[41–43] A substantial majority of young patients are asymptomatic, but mild, serious, or even fatal sequelae sometimes occur.[5] Key determinants of clinical stability in uncomplicated congenital complete heart block are the ventricular rate, the hemodynamic adjustments at rest and with exercise, and the presence of intrinsically normal myocardium.[5]

CONGENITALLY CORRECTED TRANSPOSITION OF THE GREAT ARTERIES (see also p. 940 and Fig 29–62, p. 940). When this malformation is isolated (uncomplicated), survival is good but not normal because of the vulnerability of a morphological right ventricle in the systemic location.[44–47] A major variable that decreases long-term survival is the presence and degree of incompetence of the inverted left atrioventricular valve (Ebstein-like anomaly) that may be mistaken for acquired mitral regurgitation.[5] Survival into the sixth or seventh decade is uncommon, but not unknown, with an occasional patient reaching the eighth decade.[48] Complete atrioventricular block accrues at a rate of about 2 per cent per year and may become manifested with a Stokes-Adams attack or sudden death.[49]

EBSTEIN'S ANOMALY OF THE TRICUSPID VALVE (see also p. 969 and Figs. 29–56, p. 934, and 29–57, p. 935). Longevity ranges from intrauterine or neonatal death to asymptomatic survival into late

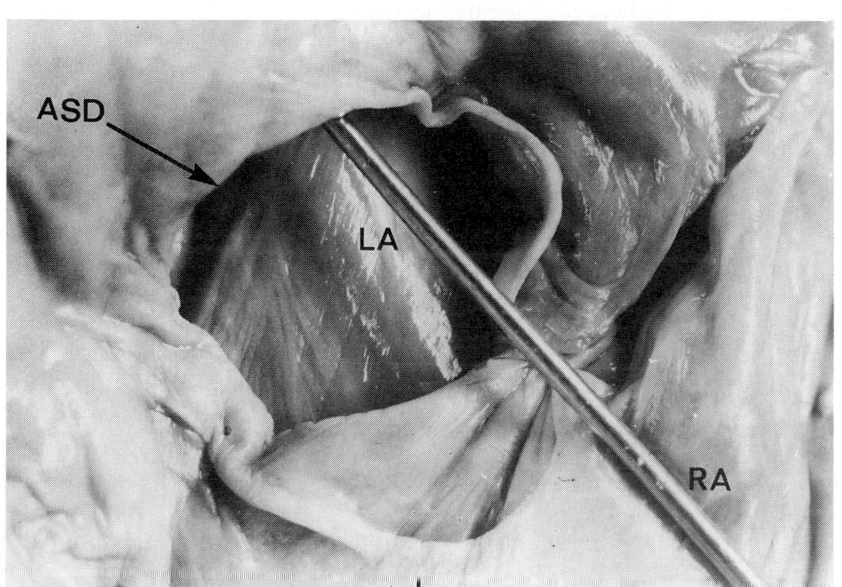

FIGURE 30–5. Necropsy specimen from an 87-year-old woman with a nonrestrictive ostium secundum atrial septal defect (ASD). The left atrium (LA) is seen through the defect. RA = right atrium.

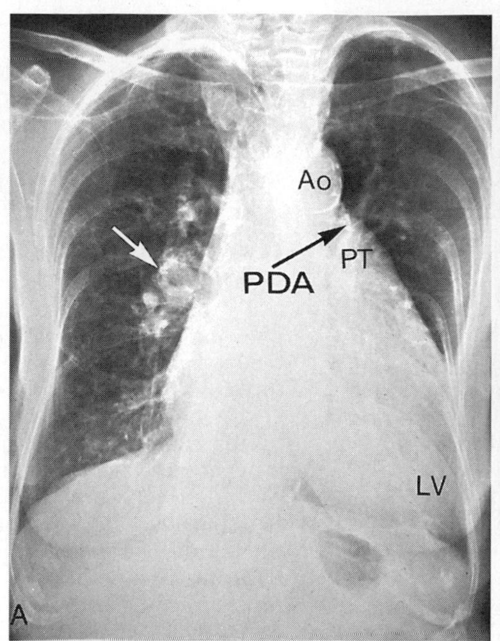

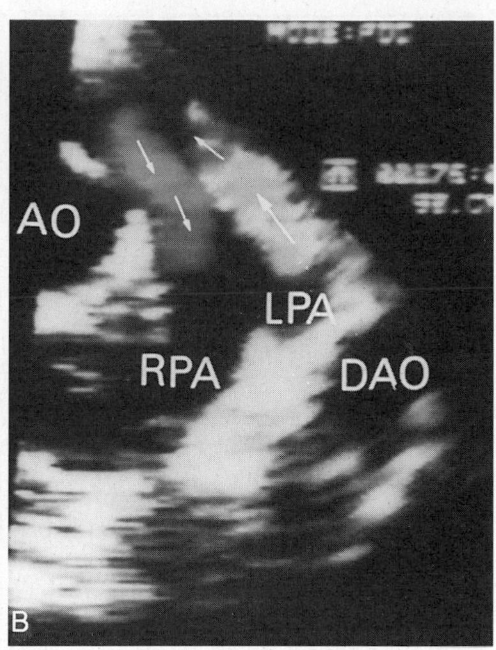

FIGURE 30–6. *A,* Radiograph from an 84-year-old woman with a moderately restrictive calcified patent ductus arteriosus (PDA). The pulmonary trunk (PT) and its right branch (unmarked white arrow) are dilated. Pulmonary arterial pressure was 90/40 mm Hg. The enlarged left ventricle (LV) occupies the apex. The aortic knuckle (Ao) is calcified. *B,* Black and white print of a color flow image (parasternal short axis). Arrows trace the direction of ductal flow, moving first down the left lateral wall of the pulmonary trunk, then up the opposite wall. LPA = left pulmonary artery; RPA = right pulmonary artery; DAo = descending aorta.

adulthood.[50–52] The majority of patients fall between these extremes. Factors chiefly limiting survival in adults are functional class, marked increase in cardiac size, cyanosis, and recurrent paroxysmal rapid heart action, especially when accompanied by accelerated conduction through accessory pathways (Fig. 30–7).[53,54] Left ventricular function is an additional matter of concern.[55,56] Syncope heightens suspicion of accelerated bypass conduction (rapid atrial fibrillation or one-to-one atrial flutter). The rapid ventricular response has been responsible for sudden death. For patients who survive the first year of life, there is a cumulative mortality of approximately 12 per cent, which is distributed about evenly throughout childhood and adolescence.[53,54] Nevertheless, there are accounts of patients with Ebstein's anomaly who have survived into their eighth decade.[57,58] The oldest patient recorded with the anomaly lived to age 85 and had no cardiac symptoms until age 79.[59]

CONGENITAL PULMONARY VALVE REGURGITATION (see also p. 1059). Because the degree of regurgitation is seldom more than moderate, and because the right ventricle readily adapts to low pressure volume overload, most patients tolerate this anomaly into adulthood, through middle age, and occasionally into their sixth, seventh, or even eighth decade.[60–62] However, right heart failure may occur in older adults after decades of stability, because acquired cardiopulmonary disorders serve to increase the amount of regurgitation across the congenitally incompetent pulmonary valve.[5]

LUTEMBACHER'S SYNDROME. The disorder consists of a congenital atrial septal defect upon which *acquired* mitral stenosis is imposed.[5] Mitral stenosis augments the left-to-right interatrial shunt, while the atrial septal defect decompresses the left atrium and reduces the mean left atrial pressure and the gradient across the stenotic mitral valve. Lutembacher's patient was a 61-year-old woman who had seven pregnancies,[63] and Firkett's patient was a 74-year-old woman who had 11 pregnancies.[64] The oldest recorded patient was an 81-year-old woman who experienced no cardiac symptoms until her 75th year.[65] These favorable reports should not obscure the fact that survival in patients with ostium secundum atrial septal defects is unfavorably influenced by mitral stenosis that augments the left-to-right shunt and predisposes to atrial fibrillation and right ventricular failure.[5]

SINUS OF VALSALVA ANEURYSM (see also p. 910). The malformation begins as a blind pouch or diverticulum that takes origin from a localized site in one aortic sinus.[66] A substantial majority of ruptures occur before age 30 (rarely in infancy or early childhood), generally in men, at an average age of 34 years with a range of 11 to 67 years.[66,67] The physiological consequences and clinical course depend upon the rapidity with which the rupture develops, the amount of blood flowing through the abnormal communication, and the chamber (site) that receives the shunt.[68] Complete heart block is an occasional cause of syncope or sudden death when a ruptured or unruptured aneurysm penetrates the base of the ventricular septum.[69] Small perforations may come to light because of an asymptomatic continuous murmur, because of a right ventricular outflow tract systolic murmur (subpulmonary obstruction by the aneurysm), or because of aortic regurgitation.[5] Small chronic perforations are susceptible to infective endocarditis. About 20 per cent of congenital sinus of Valsalva aneurysms are unperforated and are discovered at necropsy, cardiac surgery, or operation for ventricular septal defect, which sometimes coexists with an aortic sinus aneurysm.[68] In one of our patients, an 85-year-old man, an unsuspected unperforated aortic sinus aneurysm was diagnosed by echocardiography.

CORONARY ARTERIAL FISTULAS. These anomalies represent one of the most common major congenital malformations of the coronary circulation that permit adult survival.[70] Both coronary arteries arise from the aorta at their normal sites, but a fistulous branch of one or more arteries communicates directly with a cardiac chamber or with the pulmonary trunk, coronary sinus, vena cava, or a pulmonary vein. Clinically occult coronary arterial fistulas, generally to the pulmonary artery, have been found in a small but consistent percentage of adults undergoing diagnostic coronary angiography for other reasons.[71] Survival into adulthood is the rule, although life span is not normal.[70] Longevity depends upon the amount of blood traversing the communication, the chamber or vessel into which the fistula drains, and the presence and degree of myocardial ischemia that might result when the fistula causes a coronary steal.[72] Occasional survivals have been recorded in the seventh and eighth decades, with one report of a patient living to age 84.[73] Death, when it comes, may be due to noncardiac causes or to acquired coronary artery disease.

CONGENITAL PULMONARY ARTERIOVENOUS FISTULA. These fistulas can be solitary or multiple, unilateral or bilateral, or minute and diffuse throughout both lungs, and are usually associated with hereditary hemorrhagic telangiectasia (Rendu-Osler-Weber syndrome).[74] A substantial majority go unrecognized until adulthood.[5] Dyspnea and fatigue are often related to anemia caused by bleeding telangiectases rather than to the pulmonary arteriovenous fistulas per se. Two of the author's patients without telangiectasia were siblings aged 71 and 73 years (Fig. 30–8).[75]

Common Defects in Which Unoperated Adult Survival is Exceptional

VENTRICULAR SEPTAL DEFECT (see also p. 901, Fig. 29–16, p. 902). These defects are among the most common congenital cardiac malformations at birth but are seldom found in adulthood.[76,77] Adult survivors comprise two widely disparate groups[78–80]: (1) those with defects that have either closed spontaneously or decreased to a small or moderately restrictive size, and (2) those with nonrestrictive defects with elevated pulmonary vascular resistance that relieves the left ventricle of volume overload while imposing no additional afterload upon the systemic right ventricle (Eisenmenger's complex).

The chief reason for adult survival in patients with ventricular septal defects is spontaneous closure.[81] Paul Wood asked, "Where's the maladie de Roger? Assuming it does not provide immortality, it must either close spontaneously in middle life or have long since run its mortal course."[82] Early spontaneous closure by formation of septal aneurysm leaves the patient with a functionally normal heart that still harbors a morphological abnormality.[83] The occasional adult survivor with persistent patency of a small perimembranous ventricular septal defect confronts a cumulative risk of infective endocarditis.[84]

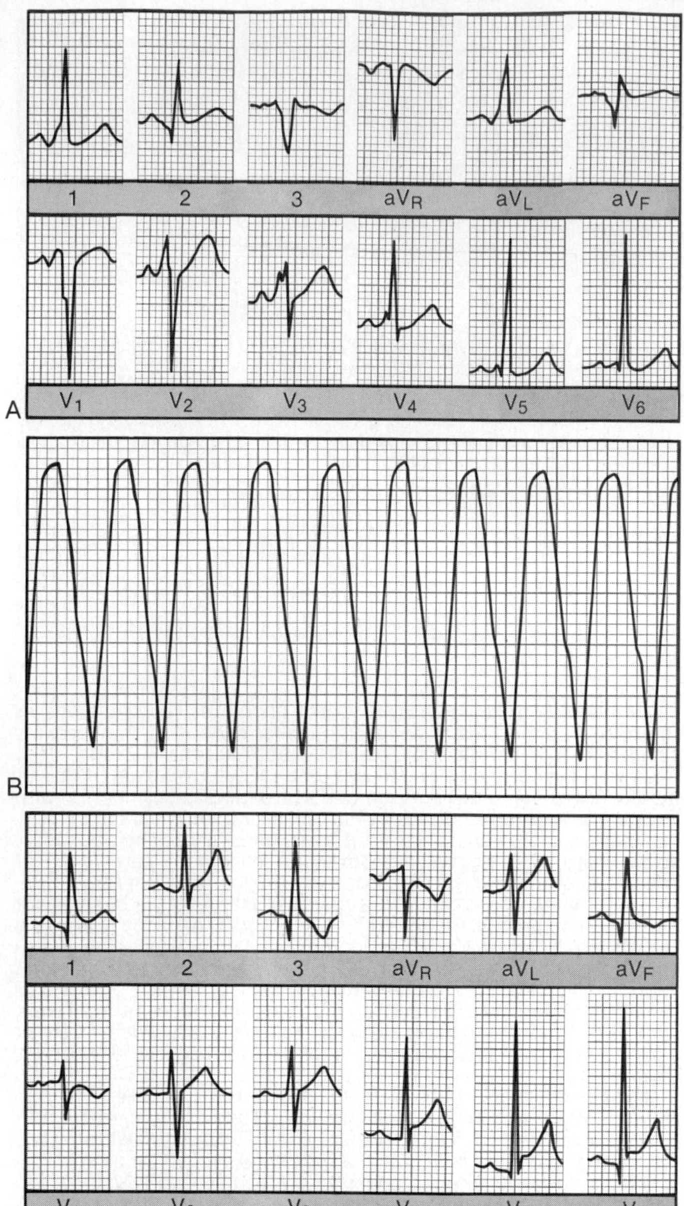

FIGURE 30–7. *A,* Twelve-lead electrocardiogram from a patient with Ebstein's anomaly of the tricuspid valve. There are typical fusion beats due to a right atrioventricular bypass tract. The delta wave is directed to the left, superior and posterior. *B,* Lead V_1 showing antegrade wide QRS tachycardia via the right bypass tract. *C,* Twelve-lead electrocardiogram after tricuspid valve reconstruction with interruption of the bypass tract by surgical dissociation between right atrium and right ventricle. The delta wave is absent.

It is the rule rather than the exception for patients with Eisenmenger's complex to reach adulthood. The author's oldest patient died from noncardiac causes at age 69 years.

FALLOT'S TETRALOGY (see also p. 929). Arthur Fallot recognized that ". . . cyanosis, especially in the adult, is the result of a small number of cardiac malformations. . . . One of these cardiac malformations is much more frequent than others . . ."[6] namely, the tetralogy to which he referred. Fallot's tetralogy represents the largest proportion of adults with cyanotic congenital heart disease, but only 6 per cent of unoperated patients are alive at age 30 and 3 per cent at age 40.[85,86] There are individual reports of survival into the seventh decade.[85] Fallot's tetralogy with pulmonary atresia and adequate but not excessive aortic-to-pulmonary collateral circulation occasionally permits survival not only to adolescence but to adulthood.[87] One of the author's patients lived to age 55, despite acquired calcific aortic stenosis.

Systemic hypertension is a special problem in adult survivors, because the increase in afterload is imposed on both the left and right ventricles (biventricular aorta).[5] The rise in right ventricular systolic pressure may augment pulmonary blood flow and reduce cyanosis but at the price of right ventricular (or biventricular) failure. Infective endocarditis on an incompetent biventricular aortic valve may incur catastrophic acute severe aortic regurgitation into both right and left ventricles.

Late Survival After Cardiac Surgery or Interventional Catheterization

An understanding of long-term outcomes requires knowledge of the preoperative or preinterventional congenital malformation, the nature and effects of the therapeutic intervention, and the subsequent residua and sequelae.[2] Success is measured not only by the length of survival but also by the quality of life and the need for reoperation. Surgical refinements affect long-term outcome, often significantly. Techniques have evolved and will continue to do so. Patients who underwent cardiac surgery decades ago benefited from the anatomical repairs but often suffered from deleterious effects of inadequate intraoperative myocardial protection.[2] Prosthetic materials—valves, patches, conduits—that were previously state of the art have been superseded by many generations of improved devices and materials.

Congenitally Malformed Cardiac Valves

ISOLATED PULMONARY VALVE STENOSIS (see also pp. 965 and 924). Balloon dilatation has largely replaced surgery for typical isolated congenital pulmonary valve stenosis, provided that the stenotic valve is thin, pliant, and mobile (Fig. 30–9).[88,89] Secondary hypertrophic subpulmonary stenosis tends to regress after successful dilatation of the stenotic valve (Fig. 30-4). Long-term results of balloon valvuloplasty have thus far been as good as those of surgical valvotomy.[87] If pulmonary stenosis is relieved during childhood, long-term survival patterns are similar to those in age- and sex-matched controls.[87] Exemplary results are qualified by age at intervention and by the severity of the stenosis before relief. The more severe and protracted the obstruction, the less optimal the long-term outcome, including late death from right ventricular failure. These con-

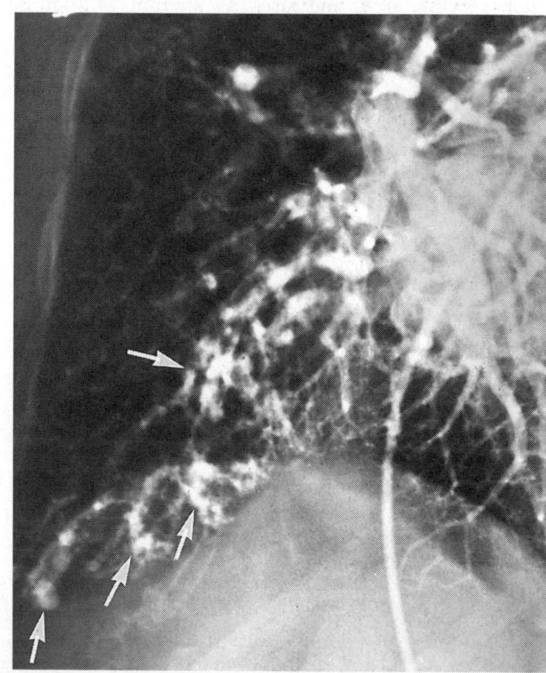

FIGURE 30–8. Selective right pulmonary arteriogram from a 71-year-old man with congenital bilateral pulmonary arteriovenous fistulas (arrows). His 73-year-old sister was similarly afflicted. Neither had telangiectasia.

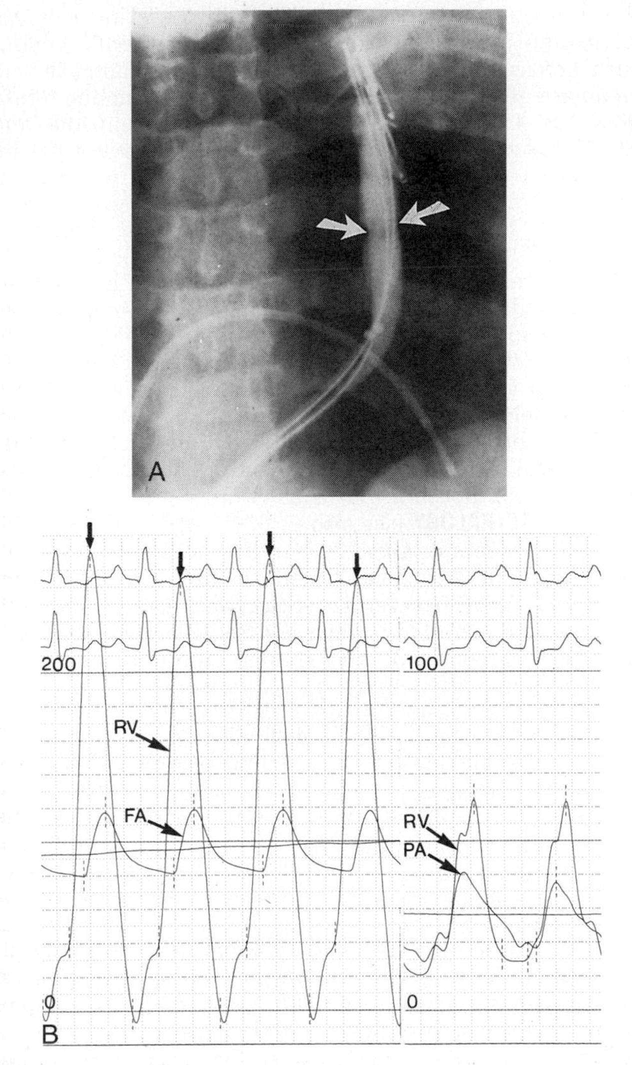

FIGURE 30–9. *A*, Single balloon across a severely stenotic mobile pulmonary valve of an 18-year-old pregnant woman near term. *B*, Pressure pulses before *(left)* and after *(right)* balloon dilatation. The right ventricular (RV) pressure fell from 280 to 60 mm Hg. The right ventricular to pulmonary arterial gradient fell to 40 mm Hg. Right ventricular pulsus alternans was present before dilatation, indicating depressed right ventricular systolic function. Three days after balloon dilatation, the patient went into spontaneous uncomplicated labor. FA = femoral arteries; PA = pulmonary artery.

clusions support the practice of relieving hemodynamically significant pulmonary valve stenosis during childhood but underscore the desirability of surveillance through adolescence and adulthood. With few exceptions, postinterventional or postoperative pulmonary regurgitation is no more than mild to moderate. Residual dilatation of the pulmonary trunk is of no clinical significance even when marked. Susceptibility to infective endocarditis is believed to be low if not absent if the postinterventional gradient is small and if pulmonary regurgitation is absent or mild.

CONGENITAL AORTIC VALVE STENOSIS (see also pp. 964 and 914). Balloon dilatation in young patients with congenital bicuspid aortic stenosis is feasible provided the valve is thin and mobile, with no calcific deposits (Fig. 30–10*A*). The best that can be achieved, however, is separation of the fused commissures that results in a functionally normal bicuspid aortic valve (Fig. 30–10*B*) with an outlook analogous to that of surgical reconstruction.[90,91] The repaired valve has at least the same tendency as an unoperated, functionally normal bicuspid aortic valve to develop regurgitation or to thicken, calcify, and become stenotic with the passage of time (Fig. 30–1). The risk of infective endocarditis is not affected by either balloon dilatation or surgical reconstruction. The enhanced ejection performance of the left ventricle in young patients with congenital aortic stenosis[92] tends to be maintained after relief of the obstruction, provided relief is achieved before contractility begins to decline.[92,93] If the aortic valve is replaced, the fate of the prosthesis and the need for anticoagulants are important determinants of late postoperative outcome. The inherent risk of aortic root dissection (Fig. 30–2) persists after either balloon dilatation, direct reconstruction, or aortic valve replacement.

A functionally normal bicuspid aortic valve may develop gradually progressive *aortic regurgitation* that requires surgical relief using a prosthetic valve. Prime objectives of valve replacement are removal of left ventricular volume overload and preservation or restoration of satisfactory left ventricular systolic function. Even if these objectives are achieved, a minority of patients die late after operation, not because of heart failure but because of what is presumed to be a disturbance in ventricular rhythm (sudden death). Infective endocarditis can convert a bicuspid aortic valve that is functionally normal into the catastrophic hemodynamic fault of acute severe aortic regurgitation that, with few exceptions, requires emergency valve replacement.[15]

EBSTEIN'S ANOMALY (see also pp. 934 and 966). This malformation is the most common cause of surgically important congenital tricuspid regurgitation.[94] The timing and success of operation in large part depend on whether or not the malformed valve can be reconstructed rather than replaced. Transesophageal echocardiography provides a se-

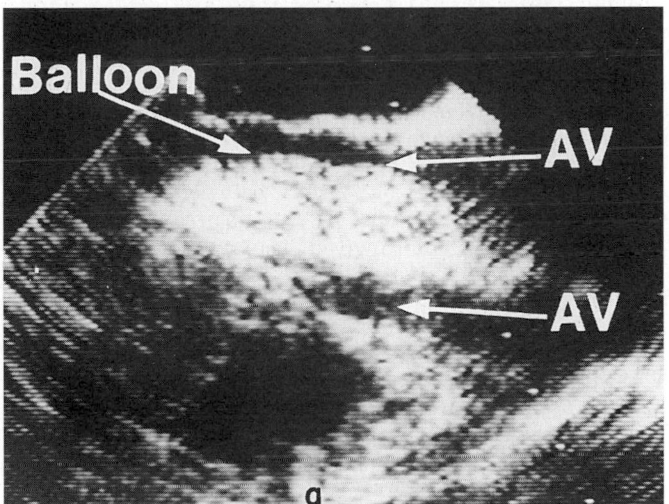

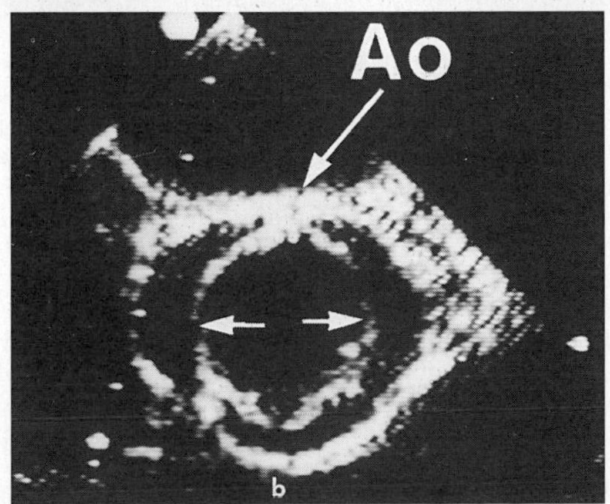

FIGURE 30–10. *A*, Balloon dilatation of bicuspid aortic stenosis using transesophageal echocardiographic monitoring in a 32-year-old man. The inflated balloon is across the stenotic bicuspid aortic valve (AV). *B*, A short-axis image after balloon dilatation showing a mobile functionally normal bicuspid aortic valve (Ao) with no commissural fusion. There was mild residual aortic regurgitation.

cure basis for judging whether a large mobile anterior tricuspid leaflet can be used to create a competent unicuspid valve. Successful operation relieves right ventricular volume overload, improves right ventricular function, removes the risk of paradoxical emboli through an interatrial communication, and interrupts right atrioventricular bypass tracts, eliminating the hazard of rapid ventricular response to atrial flutter or fibrillation (Fig. 30–7). Supraventricular arrhythmias may recur postoperatively, but if the accessory pathways have been divided, the ventricular response is not accelerated, and the arrhythmias are more likely to respond to pharmacological management. Tissue valves are used for tricuspid replacement because mechanical prostheses function poorly in the tricuspid location in addition to posing the risk of pulmonary embolization even with anticoagulation.

ISOLATED INCOMPETENCE OF THE LEFT-SIDED ATRIOVENTRICULAR VALVE IN CONGENITALLY CORRECTED TRANSPOSITION OF THE GREAT ARTERIES. The Ebstein-like anomaly that causes incompetence of the tricuspid valve in the systemic (inverted) position is analogous to, but not identical to, Ebstein's anomaly as just described.[5] The anterior leaflet is smaller in size than in right-sided Ebstein's anomaly and is usually malformed. Accordingly, when surgical relief of regurgitation is indicated, the left-sided tricuspid valve almost always requires replacement. Long-term outcome is then determined by the duration of preoperative regurgitation, the functional adequacy (or inadequacy) of a morphological right ventricle in the systemic location, and an accrued incidence of high-degree atrioventricular heart block.

ATRIAL SEPTAL DEFECT (OSTIUM SECUNDUM) (see also pp. 896 and 966). Children, adolescents, and young adults with this malformation usually have few or no symptoms.[5] An assessment of asymptomatic or minimally symptomatic patients with ostium secundum or sinus venosus atrial septal defects who were over 25 at the time of presentation disclosed no difference in survival or symptoms and no difference in the incidence of new arrhythmias, stroke, embolic phenomena, or cardiac failure between medically and surgically managed patients after a mean follow-up of 25 years.[95] The study confirmed that progressive pulmonary vascular disease does not develop in this patient population, so its anticipation is not a rationale for operation.[95,96] Long-term observations after closure of atrial septal defects found that actuarial 27-year rates of survival in patients 12 to 24 years of age at operation were the same as for normal patients; operation at 25 to 41 years of age was followed by long-term survival that was good but not normal, whereas closure after age 41 years was associated with a significant increase in late mortality and in the frequency of late cardiac failure, stroke, and atrial fibrillation.[97] The age beyond which surgery should not be offered has been questioned.[95,98] However, in patients older than age 40 years, a recent multivariate analysis of 84 postoperative patients with atrial septal defects was compared with results in 95 patients who had been treated medically; there was a significant reduction in overall mortality and considerable improvement in long-term functional status of the surgically treated patients.[99] Long-term functional improvement was sustained in 69 per cent of patients who had suffered from severe heart failure before surgery.[99] In contrast to the clear benefit of surgery with respect to long-term survival and symptomatic improvement, repair later in life did not significantly reduce the prevalence of atrial fibrillation or flutter or morbidity associated with thromboembolic complications.[99]

COMPLETE TRANSPOSITION OF THE GREAT ARTERIES (see also p. 935). A relatively large number of patients with this malformation have reached adulthood because of a Rashkind balloon atrial septostomy as neonates followed by intraatrial redirection of venous return (Mustard or Senning atrial switch operations).[2] Twenty-year survival after atrial switch has been reported at 80 to 90 per cent, but major late postoperative sequelae are the rule.[100,101] Intraatrial repair involves excision of the atrial septum and insertion of a pericardial or Dacron baffle that directs systemic venous return across the mitral valve into the left ventricle and pulmonary artery and that directs pulmonary venous return across the tricuspid valve into the right ventricle and aorta.[102] Electrophysiological sequelae of this extensive reconstruction are damage to the sinus node, atrial arrhythmias (atrial fibrillation or flutter), and damage to the atrioventricular node (Fig. 30–11).[103,104] During long-term follow-up, 2 to 8 per cent of patients die suddenly due to bradyarrhythmias, atrial tachyarrhythmias, or high-degree atrioventricular block. A second major postoperative concern is the long-term performance of a morphological right ventricle in the systemic location.[105,106] Progressive systolic dysfunction is not uncommon, and there is a relatively high incidence of coexisting left ventricular dysfunction.[106,107] Aortic regurgitation, still another late postoperative concern, exerts a negative impact on already depressed function of the morphological right ventricle.

FALLOT'S TETRALOGY (see also p. 929). Assessment of the postoperative course must take into account the morphological variations of the basic malformation, previous shunt procedures, age at intracardiac repair, and the presence and degree of postoperative residua and sequelae.[108,110] Patients who had undergone palliative shunts, followed by intracardiac repair in early childhood, experienced 87 per cent survival 10 to 20 years after operation.[109] All but a minority were free from significant cardiac or vascular symptoms and were leading normal lives. Some patients who reach adulthood after successful shunt operations in infancy or early childhood maintain improvement for decades and ultimately benefit from intracardiac repair as adults. The outlook for patients who had a Waterston or Potts shunt before intracardiac repair is more guarded, because these shunts lend themselves to the risk of excessive pulmonary blood flow, pulmonary vascular disease, or kinking of a pulmonary artery.[109] A technically good intracardiac repair in infancy substantially improves cumulative survival, reduces incidence of complications, and improves quality of life.[109,110] Older age at the time of intraventricular repair was a powerful predictor of poor late survival.[109,111,112]

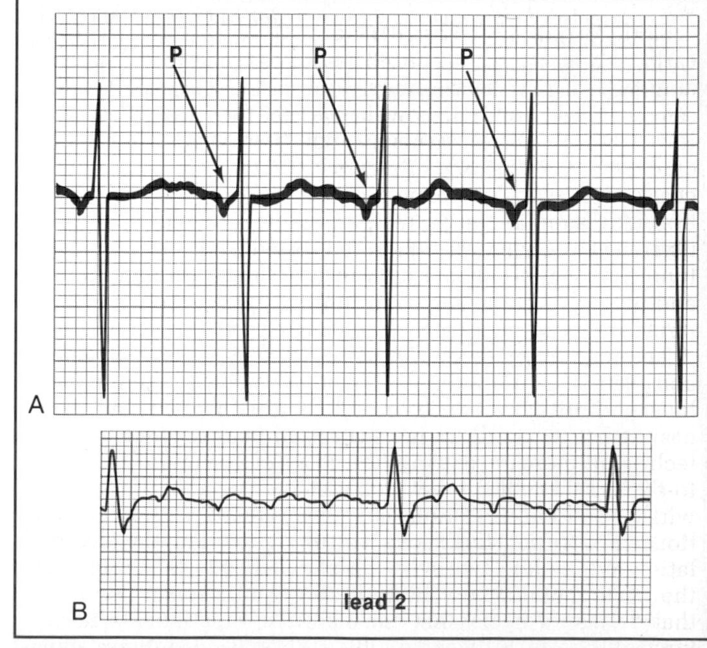

FIGURE 30–11. *A,* Junctional ectopic rhythm early after a Mustard repair for complete transposition of the great arteries. *B,* Late-onset atrial flutter with a slow ventricular response (impaired atrioventricular conduction) in a 25-year-old man who had a Mustard repair in infancy. The patient developed sinus node dysfunction in addition to atrial tachyarrhythmias.

The effectiveness of surgery must take into account not only survival but symptomatic status, postoperative residua and sequelae, and the need for reoperation.[113] Late postoperative sudden death has been a legitimate concern. Ventricular electrical instability, rather than high-degree heart block, is now considered the major risk factor.[108,109,109a] Ventricular ectopic rhythms correlate with older age at intracardiac repair, with postoperative right ventricular pressure or volume overload, and with depressed right ventricular function.[108,109] Postoperative *left* ventricular dysfunction is related to age at the time of intracardiac repair and to previous shunt procedures. A decrease in *left* ventricular volume and ejection fraction is a feature of severe cyanotic Fallot's tetralogy because of reduced pulmonary arterial blood flow (underloading).[114] A shunt operation increases left ventricular volume, sometimes excessively, setting the stage for late postoperative electrical instability. If primary intracardiac repair is undertaken after 2 years of age, left heart volumes approach normal, but left ventricular function may remain subnormal.[114,115]

The emphasis on disturbances in ventricular rhythm after intracardiac repair of Fallot's tetralogy should not obscure the importance of disturbances in atrial rhythm.[116] Atrial fibrillation, atrial flutter, and supraventricular tachycardia were important determinants of morbidity in approximately one-third of patients. Attention was also called to the incidence of sinus node dysfunction, with pacemakers needed twice as often for sinus bradycardia as for atrioventricular block.[116]

PATENT DUCTUS ARTERIOSUS (see also p. 905). Division of an isolated restrictive patent ductus arteriosus in childhood represents one of the few literal cures of congenital malformations of the heart and circulation. Transcatheter ductal occlusion must compete with this record, which is ideal except for the thoracotomy.[117] The risk of infective endocarditis is eliminated. When a ductus is moderately restrictive or nonrestrictive, division in early childhood usually results in regression of left atrial and left ventricular enlargement and normalization of pulmonary arterial and right ventricular systolic pressures. Adult survival of patients with a nonrestrictive patent ductus depends on a rise in pulmonary vascular resistance that relieves the left ventricle of volume overload but incurs inoperability when the shunt is reversed.

COARCTATION OF THE AORTA (see also p. 911). Repair in early childhood results in 89 per cent survival at 15 years and 83 per cent at 25 years.[118] Postoperative residua and sequelae are common, however, and require long-term follow-up.[119,120] Three principal postoperative concerns include residual systolic hypertension despite absence of a coarctation gradient, bicuspid aortic valve, and recoarctation. A major risk factor for persistent postoperative hypertension is older age at repair: i.e., the duration of preoperative hypertension that results in baroreceptor abnormalities and compliance changes in the walls of the major arteries.[121,122]

The fate of a coexisting functionally normal bicuspid aortic valve is the same as that of an isolated congenitally bicuspid aortic valve as described earlier. Recurrence of coarctation after reparative surgery is related chiefly to the technique used for the initial repair.[123] Resection with end-to-end anastomosis, when technically feasible, is associated with the lowest incidence of recoarctation. Balloon dilatation has been a step forward in the management of recoarctation, but *not* of the native obstruction.[124] The histology of the aorta immediately distal to the coarctation resembles that of the Marfan syndrome. Balloon dilatation further injures this inherently vulnerable segment.[20] Conversely, resection with end-to-end anastomosis removes the vulnerable segment, an advantage to women during subsequent pregnancy. Premature coronary artery atherosclerosis, myocardial infarction, and congestive heart failure were causes of death in 12 per cent of patients 11 to 25 years after coarctectomy.[119] Early successful repair promises to minimize these late complications. Congenital aneurysms of the circle of Willis (Fig. 30–3) are uncommon but well-established coexisting malformations in patients with coarctation of the aorta and set the stage for catastrophic cerebral hemorrhage. Rupture of an aneurysm has been reported in normotensive patients long after successful coarctation repair.[125] Abnormalities of the mitral apparatus occur in 26 to 58 per cent of patients with coarctation and vary from clinically occult and functionally benign to overt stenosis or incompetence of the mitral orifice.[126]

CONGENITAL SINUS OF VALSALVA ANEURYSMS (see also p. 910). An acute large rupture announces itself dramatically, whereas as a small perforation that develops gradually or an unruptured aneurysm may go unnoticed, at least initially.[5] In any event, surgical mortality is low, and late results of repair are excellent, especially when aortic valve regurgitation is absent.

THE FONTAN PROCEDURE (see Figs. 29–55, p. 934, and 29–69, p. 948). In 1971, Fontan and Baudet reported a new operation for tricuspid atresia (caval-to-pulmonary artery anastomosis)[127] that bears the first author's name as an eponym. The Fontan operation has emerged as a landmark in the surgical treatment of congenital heart disease.[128] Complete bypass of the right ventricle was a logical extension of its predecessor, the partial right heart bypass procedure introduced by Glenn.[129] The original Glenn shunt consisted of an anastomosis of the superior vena cava to the right pulmonary artery that was divided from the pulmonary trunk.[129] Acquired right lower-lobe pulmonary arteriovenous fistulas were late postoperative complications.[130] The procedure has now been modified as the "bidirectional Glenn shunt," represented by anastomosis of the superior vena cava to an undivided right pulmonary artery.[130] The bidirectional Glenn shunt is used as palliation in patients for whom a Fontan operation is not considered feasible or as the first stage in anticipation of total caval-to-pulmonary arterial connection, which is the most recent modification of the Fontan repair.[130–132,132a] Among 352 patients who had a Fontan operation prior to 1995, the 10-year survival was 60 per cent.[132] Survival was adversely affected by depressed ventricular function, increased pulmonary arterial pressure, and atrioventricular valve dysfunction.[132] Meticulous selection of patients increases late survival and reduces morbidity. As experience has accumulated, operative risk has declined, survival has improved, morbidity has decreased, and the quality of life has improved, sometimes appreciably.[132–134]

The Fontan operation for patients 18 years or older has also been successful, occasionally achieving remarkable degrees of rehabilitation.[133] There are, however, a number of caveats. Because of the importance of ventricular function, postoperative afterload reduction using angiotensin-converting enzyme inhibitors is common practice, and the importance of maintaining sinus rhythm has been emphasized.[133,134] Atrial arrhythmias, especially atrial flutter or fibrillation, adversely affect ventricular function and may precipitate congestive heart failure. Thrombotic and thromboembolic events are additional concerns and do not appear to be related to ventricular function or disturbances in atrial rhythm.[132] Thrombi have been identified in the superior vena cava, inferior vena cava, lateral tunnel, right atrium, and the ventricular chamber, setting the stage for pulmonary and systemic emboli. Anticoagulation is an important consideration.

MEDICAL MANAGEMENT OF ADULT CONGENITAL HEART DISEASE

Cyanotic

Cyanotic congenital heart disease can be viewed as a multisystem, systemic disorder that affects red blood cells and hemostasis, the kidneys, urate metabolism, the digits and long bones, bilirubin kinetics, respiration and ventilation, the coronary and systemic vascular beds, and the central nervous system.[135]

REGULATION OF RED CELL MASS

Erythrocytosis is a physiologically appropriate response to a decrease in tissue oxygenation (arterial hypoxemia) that stimulates elaboration of erythropoietin from specialized sensor cells in the kidney, resulting in an increase in the number of circulating red blood cells and in an expanded blood volume.[136,137] The increase in erythrocyte mass offsets the deficit in tissue oxygenation. When erythrocytosis is sufficient to raise the tissue oxygen concentration above the threshold for release of erythropoietin by the renal oxygen sensors, a new equilibrium is established at a higher hematocrit level.[138] Should tissue oxygen concentration fail to reach that threshold, or should the renal oxygen sensors fail to respond appropriately, a stable equilibrium at a higher hematocrit level is not achieved.[138] Erythropoietin secretion and red blood cell mass continue to rise (negative feedback inhibition does not seem to occur) despite potentially harmful effects that accompany a further increase in hematocrit level.[138]

The adaptive increase in red blood cell mass of cyanotic congenital heart disease is fundamentally different from polycythemia rubra vera (primary polycythemia), which is an idiopathic clonal disorder of the bone marrow characterized by autonomous overproduction of red blood cells, thrombocytosis, leukocytosis, an increase in leukocyte alkaline phosphatase, and basophilia (see Chap. 57). To make that distinction clear, the increase in red blood cell mass prompted by the hypoxemia of cyanotic congenital heart disease is properly called "erythrocytosis" rather than "polycythemia."[135]

The erythrocytosis of cyanotic congenital heart disease falls into two categories: compensated and decompensated, defined in terms of erythrocyte indices and hyperviscosity symptoms.[138,139] *Compensated* erythrocytosis refers to patients who establish equilibrium hematocrit levels in iron-replete states and who have absent, mild, or moderate hyperviscosity symptoms, even at high hematocrit levels, even in excess of 70 per cent. *Decompensated* erythrocytosis refers to patients who fail to establish equilibrium conditions, who manifest unstable, rising hematocrit levels that are uncontrolled by negative feedback inhibition and who experience marked-to-severe hyperviscosity symptoms. Hematocrit levels should be determined by automated techniques, because microhematocrit centrifugation results in plasma trapping and falsely elevated levels.[135]

IRON AND IRON DEFICIENCY. The role of iron and the effects of iron deficiency are important clinical aspects of the erythrocytosis of cyanotic congenital heart disease. Iron is an integral part of myoglobin and of certain mitochondrial enzymes and plays a pivotal role in oxidative metabolism. Iron deficiency decreases work capacity in both experimental animals and in human subjects.[140,141] The consequences of iron deficiency are related not only to anemia per se but also to a decrease in the activity or concentration of iron-containing enzymes in muscle mitochondria and to impaired red cell deformability.[135,140] During iron repletion, muscle oxidases approach control values, reflecting a shift to greater dependence upon oxidative metabolism. An important effect of iron deficiency is on red blood cell shape.[140]

Whole-blood viscosity is a function of hematocrit level and of a number of other variables including deformability of erythrocytes, aggregation and dispersion of cellular elements, flow velocity (shear rate), temperature, vessel bore, endothelial integrity, and plasma viscosity. The normal biconcave disc-shaped erythrocyte is a flexible membrane partially filled with a viscous, noncompressible hemoglobin solution that allows deformation into an infinite variety of shapes with little or no change in cell volume or surface area. Conversely, iron-deficient red blood cells are relatively rigid microspherocytes that resist deformation in the microcirculation, thus increasing whole-blood viscosity. Accordingly, for an equivalent red blood cell mass, whole-blood viscosity is higher in an iron-deficient state.[140]

PHLEBOTOMIES. Adults with cyanotic congenital heart disease and erythrocytosis are frequently phlebotomized and occasionally anticoagulated. The rationale for phlebotomy assumes an inherent increase in the risk of cerebral arterial thrombotic stroke, a risk that has not withstood scrutiny in a study of 112 adults with cyanotic congenital heart disease observed for a total of 748 patient years.[142]

In cyanotic adults, cerebrovascular accidents are often associated with excessive, injudicious phlebotomies or with the use of antiplatelet agents (aspirin) or anticoagulants that reinforce intrinsic hemostatic defects and risk intracranial bleeding.[134,142] As the risk of stroke due to cerebral arterial thrombosis has not materialized, because the circulatory effects of phlebotomy are transient and because the result of phlebotomy-induced iron deficiency is an increase in whole-blood viscosity, phlebotomy is not recommended on the basis of hematocrit level per se.[134,142] For patients with *compensated* erythrocytosis, phlebotomy is not advised, even when the hematocrit level exceeds 70 per cent, as long as symptoms attributed to hyperviscosity are absent, mild, or moderate. Hyperviscosity symptoms at hematocrit levels less than 65 per cent are almost always due to iron deficiency. Phlebotomy further depletes iron stores and aggravates rather than alleviates the symptoms that respond instead to iron repletion. Iron therapy must be monitored closely, because hematocrit levels tend to rise rapidly.[134]

The firmest indication for phlebotomy is marked-to-severe symptomatic hyperviscosity in patients with hematocrit levels exceeding 65 per cent, provided that dehydration is not the cause. The objective of phlebotomy is temporary alleviation of intrusive hyperviscosity symptoms while minimizing the degree of phlebotomy-induced iron deficiency. A comparatively simple and safe outpatient method of phlebotomy for adults involves removal of 500 ml of blood over 30 to 45 minutes followed by quantitative replacement of the volume with isotonic saline. Saline is as efficacious as albumin for volume replacement, but if saline is clinically undesirable, isovolumetric repletion can be achieved with dextran 40 (5 per cent dextrose in water), which is salt free.

HEMOSTASIS. Bleeding tendencies tend to be mild to moderate in cyanotic adults, and are principally mucocutaneous.[143] However, epistaxis and hemoptysis vary from occasional and mild to copious and recurrent. In addition, serious and sometimes fatal bleeding can occur with accidental trauma or with surgical procedures. A decrease or absence of high molecular weight forms of the von Willebrand factor in plasma has recently been established and correlated with cyanosis, pulmonary vascular disease, and turbulent blood flow.[143] The von Willebrand abnormality in congenital heart disease is believed to be acquired, and the types and prevalence of bleeding are similar to the patterns in other forms of acquired von Willebrand disease.[143] Platelet counts are generally in the low range of normal in cyanotic adults but occasionally are moderately to markedly reduced.[134]

The hemostatic defect(s), especially in cyanotic patients, tend to be reinforced by an increase in tissue vascularity.[143] Aspirin, oral anticoagulants, and nonsteroidal antiinflammatory agents increase these intrinsic bleeding tendencies. Bronchoscopy should not be used to investigate hemoptysis, because the procedure is accompanied by risks while providing no additional basis for therapeutic judgment.

Hematocrit levels above 65 per cent incur an increased likelihood of perioperative hemorrhage. Preoperative phlebotomy designed to reduce the hematocrit level to just below 65 per cent serves to improve hemostasis and decrease the perioperative risk.[134] Phlebotomized units should be stored for potential postoperative autologous transfusion.

Another therapeutic issue in cyanotic adults is the use of nasal oxygen. From both the hematological and respiratory points of view, there is little evidence that oxygen is beneficial,[144] and the drying effect on nasal mucous membranes increases the risk of epistaxis.

RENAL INVOLVEMENT. Involvement of the kidneys in cyanotic congenital heart disease has been known for over four decades, but the pathogenesis of the lesion has only recently been clarified.[145] Renal histopathology resides chiefly in the glomerulus.[146] The abnormality takes the form of a vascular response including dilatation of hilar arterioles, dilatation and engorgement of capillaries and enlargement of the glomerular tuft, and also a nonvascular response characterized by an increase in mesangial matrix and cellularity, and an increase in endothelial cell proliferation.[145] The *vascular* response has been ascribed to release of L-arginine–derived nitric oxide that acts as an autocrine hormone, modulating the increased glomerular vascular resistance incurred by erythrocytosis.[145] The *nonvascular* response has been assigned to local release of platelet-derived growth factor from the cytoplasm of circulating systemic venous megakaryocytes that are delivered into the systemic arterial circulation through the right-to-left shunt.[145]

URATE METABOLISM. Hyperuricemia and proteinuria are common features of cyanotic congenital heart disease.[147] The mechanism of proteinuria is unclear, but a relationship appears to exist between proteinuria and hyperviscosity.[147] High plasma uric acid levels are secondary to inappropriately low renal fractional uric acid excretion rather than to urate overproduction.[147] Hyperuricemia therefore serves as a marker of abnormal intrarenal hemodynamics but appears to exert little or no deleterious effect on renal function and is not routinely treated.[134] Acute gouty arthritis is relatively uncommon, despite elevated uric acid levels, an observation similar to that in other forms of secondary hyperuricemia.[147,148]

Intravenous colchicine, the preferred treatment for acute gouty arthritis in cyanotic adults, is followed by a rapid clinical response and minimizes the undesirable dehydrating gastrointestinal side effects of oral colchicine. Prophylaxis after resolution of acute gouty arthritis is best achieved with low-dose oral colchicine (0.6 mg once or twice daily), a dose schedule that prevents recurrences in 75 to 90 per cent of patients and is usually tolerated without gastrointestinal side effects. Recurrent gouty arthritis is treated with allopurinol, probenicid, sulfinpyrazone, or combined therapy.

CLUBBING OF THE DIGITS AND HYPERTROPHIC OSTEOARTHROPATHY (Fig. 2–4, p. 17). These abnormalities are also believed to be responses to local release of platelet-derived growth factor from the cytoplasm of megakaryotyes that are shunted from right to left and that impact in the capillary beds of the fingers, toes, and periosteum.[149] Clubbing is asymptomatic, but hypertrophic osteoarthropathy not uncommonly causes arthralgias over long bones. If therapy is indicated, salsalate is sometimes helpful. The drug is a nonacetylated analog of aspirin but does not interfere with normal platelet function.

GALLSTONES. Cyanotic adults with erythrocytosis are at risk for cholelithiasis caused by calcium bilirubinate gallstones[134] (Fig. 30–12*A*). An expanded red blood cell mass provides the substrate for an in-

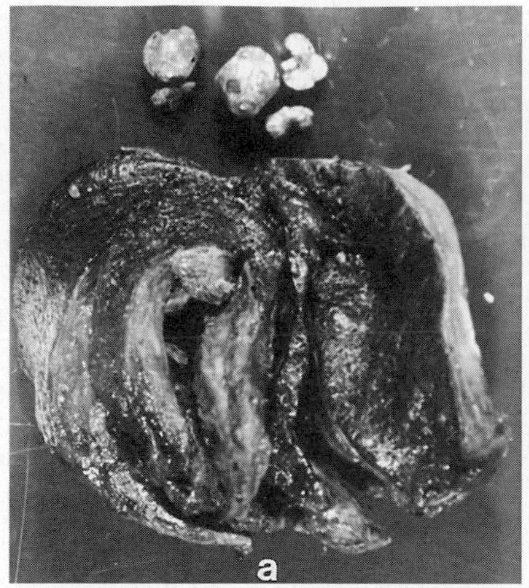

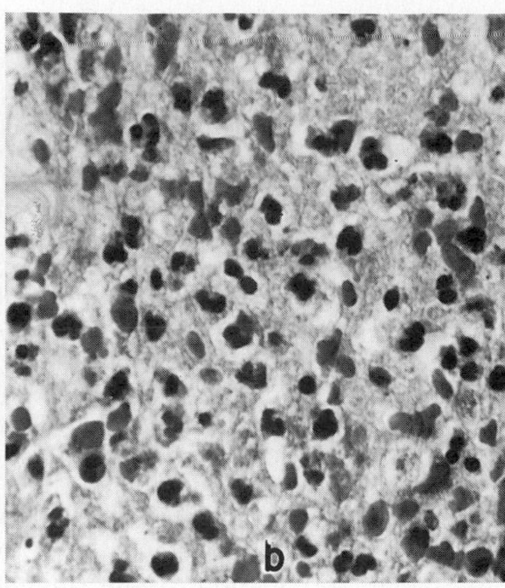

FIGURE 30–12. *A,* Thick-walled gallbladder with calcium bilirubinate gallstones shown above the specimen which was removed from a 47-year-old cyanotic man with Eisenmenger's complex and acute cholecystitis. *B,* Microscopic section of the gallbladder showing acute inflammatory cells.

crease in unconjugated bilirubin, which is believed to cause pigment stones because the compound is largely insoluble in water. Biliary colic may become clinically overt years after surgical relief of the cyanosis. An additional hazard of acute cholecystitis is infective endocarditis caused by bacteremia associated with septic inflammation of the gallbladder (Fig. 30–12*B*).

OXYGEN UPTAKE AND CONTROL OF VENTILATION. Diversion of venous blood into the systemic arterial circulation is a basic pathological fault in cyanotic congenital heart disease. Exercise serves to increase significantly the degree of venoarterial shunting and materially influences the dynamics of oxygen uptake ($\dot{V}O_2$) and ventilation.[150,151] Patients with cyanotic congenital heart disease experience markedly abnormal responses in achieving a steady state for $\dot{V}O_2$ after the onset of dynamic (isotonic) exercise. The prolonged onset and recovery of $\dot{V}O_2$ kinetics result in large O_2 deficits and hypoxemia, even with low levels of isotonic exercise; this suggests that patients with significant right-to-left shunts rely to an unusual degree on anaerobic metabolism. Unlike in the prolonged $\dot{V}O_2$ kinetics, cyanotic patients exhibit large increases in ventilation in phase I of exercise, and, in contrast to normal subjects, ventilation increases much more rapidly than $\dot{V}O_2$ in phase II (Fig. 30–13).[150,151] Ventilatory stimuli that are augmented by exercise in patients with right-to-left shunts include hypoxemia, metabolic acidosis, and shunting of CO_2 into the systemic arterial circulation. Because these patients have a

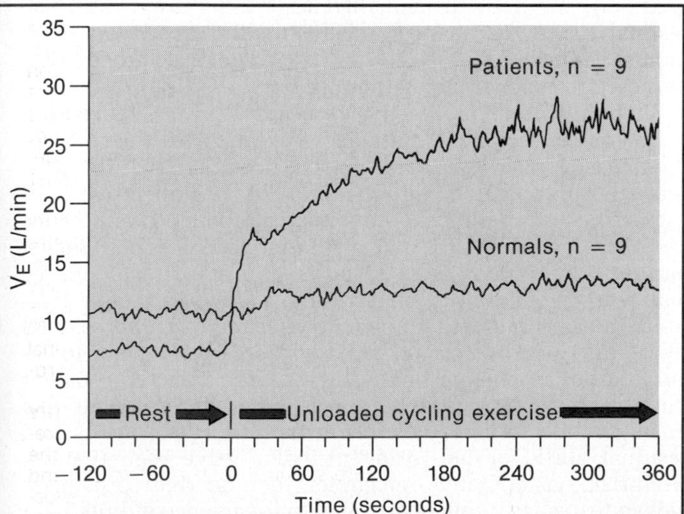

FIGURE 30–13. The increase in ventilation in response to unloaded cycle ergometric exercise in nine adults with right-to-left shunts and in nine normal subjects. The patients had higher minute ventilation both at rest and in response to exercise. (From Sietsema, K. E., et al.: Control of ventilation during exercise in patients with central venous to systemic arterial shunts. J. Appl. Physiol. *64*:234, 1988.)

substantially greater increase in ventilation during isotonic exercise than do normal subjects, "dyspnea" may be a prominent subjective complaint.[134] The New York Heart Association functional class is inappropriate because "dyspnea" is, in fact, hyperventilation unrelated to heart failure. The functional classification shown in Table 30–1 is recommended for patients with congenital heart disease.

THE CORONARY VASCULAR BED. It has long been known that the extramural coronary arteries in older patients with cyanotic congenital heart disease tend to become enlarged and tortuous, sometimes dramatically so.[152] The reason may lie in the dilating effects of nitric oxide and perhaps of prostaglandins that are elaborated by endothelium in response to the viscosity-induced increase in shear stress.[143] Of potentially greater functional importance is the effect of cyanotic congenital heart disease on myocardial perfusion. Recent studies using positron emission tomography (PET) disclosed that myocardial perfusion at rest is normal, but perfusion reserve is reduced after pharmacological stress, implying a perfusion deficit during physical exercise.[153]

DISORDERS OF THE CENTRAL NERVOUS SYSTEM. Prominent among these in adults with congenital heart disease are brain abscess, cerebral emboli, subclavian steal, syncope, intracerebral and subarachnoid hemorrhage, and seizures.[154]

The pathogenesis of a brain abscess is not always clear. Right-to-left shunts in patients with cyanotic congenital heart disease bypass the pulmonary filter, permitting bacteria to enter the systemic and therefore cerebral circulations. However, a focal zone of cerebral vulnerability appears to be necessary for formation of abscess.[154] Brain abscess should be suspected when adults with cyanosis experience headache, focal neurological signs, seizures, and fever. The diagnosis of a recent brain abscess can be established by computed tomography (CT), which identifies the lesion and the distinctive ring enhancement. Seizures may accompany the fresh abscess and may persist or recur years later because of focal brain injury at the site of the healed abscess.

Paradoxical Emboli. Cerebral emboli (see p. 885) can be bland or infected. Relatively unique to congenital heart

TABLE 30–1 CONGENITAL HEART DISEASE FUNCTIONAL CLASSIFICATION (PRESENCE AND DEGREE OF SYMPTOMS)

Class 1	Asymptomatic at all levels of activity
Class 2	Symptoms are present but do not curtail average everyday activity
Class 3	Symptoms significantly curtail most but not all average everyday activity
Class 4	Symptoms significantly curtail virtually all average everyday activity and may be present at rest

disease—usually, but not necessarily, cyanotic—are paradoxical emboli.[154] In cyanotic patients, paradoxical emboli originate in lower-extremity or pelvic veins and reach the brain by peripheral venous blood that has direct access to the systemic arterial circulation due to the right-to-left shunt. Anticoagulants may reduce the risk of paradoxical embolization, but reinforce the intrinsic hemostatic defects in cyanotic patients and increase the risk of cerebral hemorrhage.

A potential source of paradoxical embolization in hospitalized cyanotic patients is an intravenous line inserted for infusions or drugs.[155] Particles or air accidentally introduced into peripheral veins may be delivered into the systemic circulation through the right-to-left shunt.

Paradoxical emboli in acyanotic patients occur when an interatrial communication—ostium secundum atrial septal defect or patent foramen ovale—permits inferior caval blood to stream across the atrial septum into the left atrium and systemic circulation. Recent interest has focused upon young adults with stroke ascribed to paradoxical emboli through a patent foramen ovale,[156] a pathway analogous to that of an ostium secundum atrial septal defect. Platelet/fibrin particles that circulate in the systemic nervous bed are removed by the efficient lytic system in the lungs. Isometric exercise, the Valsalva maneuver, or vigorous coughing may provoke transient venoarterial mixing that delivers clusters of these particles through a patent foramen ovale into the systemic circulation and into a cerebrovascular bed that lacks a lytic system. The Valsalva maneuver is used diagnostically to initiate a transient right-to-left shunt through a foramen ovale during contrast echocardiography or transcranial contrast ultrasound.[156]

An atrial septal aneurysm may be the source of fibrin/platelet thrombi and embolic strokes, generally manifested by transient ischemic attacks in acyanotic patients.[157] The aneurysm can be suspected in a transthoracic echocardiogram but is best established by transesophageal echocardiography (see Fig. 3–16, p. 59).

Cerebral Hemorrhage. This complication tends to occur in adults with congenital heart disease under a limited number of circumstances. One cause is the injudicious use of anticoagulants or antiplatelet agents in cyanotic patients. An uncommon but potentially catastrophic cause of a hemorrhagic cerebrovascular accident is rupture of a congenital aneurysm of the circle of Willis, especially but not exclusively in patients with coarctation of the aorta (Fig. 30–3).

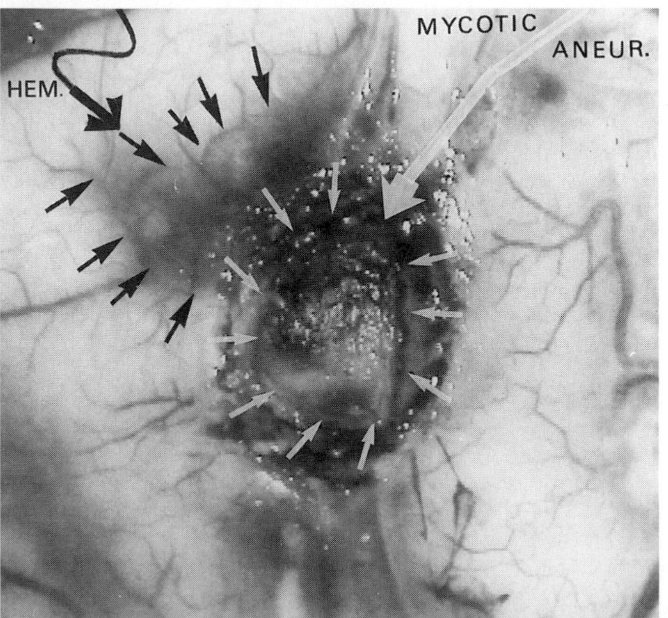

FIGURE 30–14. Mycotic aneurysm photographed at craniotomy in a 27-year-old man with *Streptococcus viridans* infective endocarditis, status postintracardiac repair of congenitally corrected transposition of the great arteries, ventricular septal defect, and pulmonary stenosis. Hemorrhage (HEM) adjacent to the aneurysm indicated impending rupture had surgery not intervened.

Mycotic aneurysms (better termed *septic aneurysms*) (Fig. 30–14) result from inflammatory weakening of the wall of a cerebral artery caused by septic microemboli to vasa vasora or by impaction of an infected embolus in the lumen of the artery.[154] Cerebral mycotic aneurysms may enlarge and rupture despite antibiotic eradication of the offending organism. Headaches or seizures announce an enlarging or perforating aneurysm, which can be diagnosed by CT scan and cerebral angiography. Aneurysms approaching 1 cm in diameter are treated by surgical excision to prevent catastrophic rupture.

Other Neurological Complications. The subclavian steal is an occasional neurological complication of a Blalock-Taussig anastomosis.[158] The classic shunt operation may create an anatomical and physiological substrate analogous to that of an atherosclerotic subclavian steal. Symptoms of the steal may appear decades after the shunt is established, depending on the development of cervical and intrathoracic collaterals. The steal is not necessarily corrected by intracardiac repair, even though the anastomosis is ligated. Congenital subclavian steal is rare.

In patients with congenital aortic stenosis, cerebral symptoms may consist of mere giddiness, faintness, or lightheadedness with effort. Conversely, syncopal episodes are sometimes recurrent and potentially dangerous.

Infective Endocarditis: Risks and Prophylaxis

(See also Chap. 33)

The clinical and bacteriological profiles of infective endocarditis changed significantly after the advent of cardiac surgery and prosthetic devices. Certain operations (division of a patent ductus arteriosus) eliminate the risk, whereas other operations (shunts, prosthetic valves or conduits) materially increase the risk.[2] However, certain general principles still prevail: namely, that the two major predisposing factors that increase the risk of infective endocarditis are a susceptible cardiac or vascular substrate and the presence of bacteremia. Susceptible lesions are those associated with high-velocity turbulent flow, jet impact, and focal increases in the rate of shear. An exception is the peculiar lack of susceptibility associated with the high-velocity diastolic flow accompanying pulmonary hypertensive pulmonary regurgitation. Portals of entry include the oral cavity, the genitourinary tract in men, the upper and lower gastrointestinal tracts, the airways and respiratory tract, and treatments such as obstetrical and gynecological procedures, and certain types of noncardiac surgery.

Susceptibility to infective endocarditis in congenital heart disease has been classified according to low-risk unoperated anomalies, low- or no-risk postoperative, intermediate-risk unoperated, intermediate-risk postoperative, and high-risk postoperative.[2] Low-risk unoperated anomalies are represented by ostium secundum atrial septal defect and mild pulmonary valve stenosis. A no-risk postoperative lesion is typified by a patent ductus arteriosus after ligation. Intermediate-risk unoperated lesions are represented by a functionally normal bicuspid aortic valve, aortic regurgitation, restrictive ventricular septal defect, or patent ductus arteriosus, especially restrictive. Intermediate-risk postoperative lesions include bicuspid aortic stenosis and residual aortic or left atrioventricular valve regurgitation. High-risk postoperative substrates include rigid prosthetic valves (especially left-sided), external-valved conduits, and aortopulmonary shunts.

Prophylaxis for infective endocarditis consists of both nonchemotherapeutic and chemotherapeutic (antimicrobial) measures. Nonchemotherapeutic prophylaxis involves day-to-day oral hygiene, skin care, nail care, and female contraception. The spongy, fragile gums of patients with cyanotic congenital heart disease are of special concern. A soft-bristled toothbrush should be used. Dental appointments for prophylaxis should be at least twice yearly. Meticulous skin care is important, especially in adolescents and young adults with acne that may be distributed beyond the face. Biting or picking of fingernails risks injury to contiguous skin and predisposes to paronychial infection with staphylococci. Intrauterine devices are best avoided because of the risk of bacteremia.

Pregnancy and Congenital Heart Disease: The Mother and the Fetus

(See also pp. 1846–1848)

Central to this topic is the intricate interplay between maternal circulatory and respiratory physiology and maternal congenital heart disease and the effects of this interplay upon the fetus. The fetus is exposed to risks that threaten its intrauterine viability and to risks that subsequently express themselves as developmental defects or transmitted congenital malformations of the heart or circulation.[159]

An important aspect of congenital heart disease and pregnancy is contraception.[159] Barrier methods include the condom (male) and the diaphragm with spermicide for the female. Tubal ligation can be accomplished safely, even in relatively high-risk women. The levonorgestrel implant (controlled release of progestin) is a safe and efficacious contraceptive for cyanotic women with pulmonary vascular disease. Retention of fluid is modest and does not preclude use of the implant for patients with controlled heart failure. Progestin injections are not recommended for patients with heart failure because of the associated retention of fluid. Low estrin is the lowest estrogen-containing oral contraceptive, and is considered safe and nonthrombogenic with a low rate of failure if no dose is missed. Use of the intrauterine device within a monogamous relationship probably does not increase the risk of infection or of infective endocarditis, but endometrial irritation may induce excessive bleeding, especially in patients with cyanotic congenital heart disease and hemostatic defect(s).

THE UNOPERATED PATIENT

There are a number of common congenital malformations that are found in unoperated adult women (Table 30–2).

OSTIUM SECUNDUM ATRIAL SEPTAL DEFECT. This malformation is of special relevance because the history without operation spans the reproductive years and because the majority of affected patients are female.[5] Young women with uncomplicated ostium secundum atrial septal defects generally tolerate pregnancy with no ill effects. An important risk, however, is a paradoxical embolus that originates in pelvic and leg veins and is carried by inferior vena caval blood across the atrial septal defect into the systemic circulation.[160] Accordingly, meticulous leg care and early ambulation after delivery are mandatory. Acute blood loss poses a potential risk because hemorrhage provokes a rise in systemic vascular resistance and a fall in systemic venous return, augmenting the left-to-right shunt, sometimes appreciably.[159]

PATENT DUCTUS ARTERIOSUS. This anomaly predominates in women but is of limited practical importance as a complication of pregnancy, because the clinical diagnosis is simple, and division of the ductus in childhood is curative. A small or moderate-sized patent ductus with normal pulmonary arterial pressure poses no risk apart from susceptibility to infective endocarditis during delivery. In the presence of a moderately restrictive patent ductus (Fig. 30–15), the gestational fall in systemic vascular resistance serves to decrease

TABLE 30–2 COMMON MALFORMATIONS WITH EXPECTED ADULT SURVIVAL (ORDER OF FEMALE PREVALENCE)

Acyanotic
Atrial septal defect (secundum)
Patent ductus arteriosus
Pulmonary valve stenosis
Coarctation of the aorta
Aortic valve disease
Cyanotic
Fallot's tetralogy

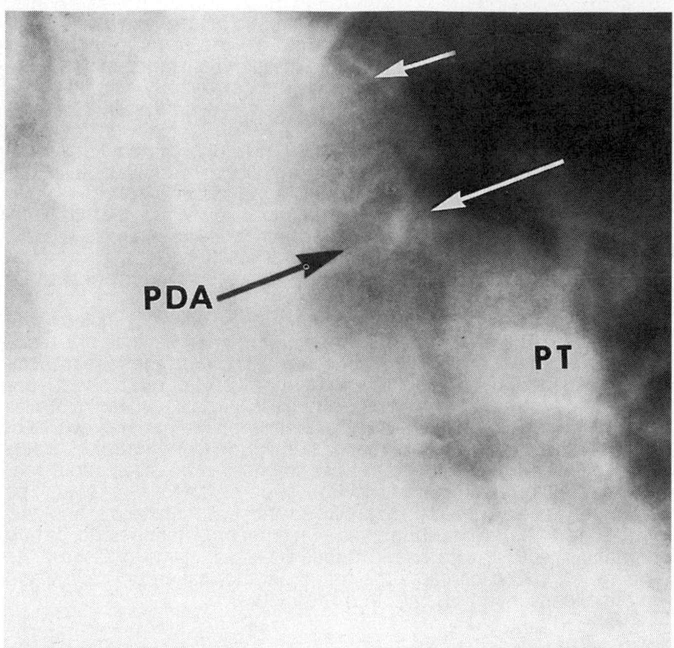

FIGURE 30–15. Chest radiograph (closeup) from a 57-year-old woman with a calcified patent ductus arteriosus (PDA, dark arrow) that was moderately restrictive. She had 20 pregnancies with 12 live births. The pulmonary trunk (PT) is dilated. The aorta also contains calcium (top white arrow).

ductal flow, but if the shunt is large, that benefit is unlikely to compensate for the hemodynamic burden of pregnancy. At highest risk is the patient with a nonrestrictive patent ductus, pulmonary vascular disease, and reversed shunt.[159] The gestational decline in systemic vascular resistance augments the right-to-left shunt through the ductus, further lowering uterine arterial oxygen saturation, which poses potential harm to the fetus.

ISOLATED PULMONARY VALVE STENOSIS. Fifty per cent of patients with this malformation are women and adult survival is the rule, even in the presence of significant obstruction to right ventricular outflow.[5] Severe pulmonary stenosis is occasionally tolerated despite gestational volume overload imposed upon an already pressure-loaded right ventricle. Infective endocarditis prophylaxis is advisable during delivery, although the probability of infection in patients with mild obstruction to right ventricular outflow is believed to be negligible.

COARCTATION OF THE AORTA. The malformation occurs chiefly in men but is dealt with here because maternal morbidity—cardiovascular complications without death—is relatively high.[159,161] The hypertension of coarctation is accompanied by a comparatively low incidence of toxemia compared to other forms of systemic hypertension.[5] Connective tissue changes in the walls of systemic arteries during normal pregnancy[162] increase the risk of aortic rupture or dissection, especially in the vulnerable postcoarctation segment and in the aortic root,[20] and increase the risk of cerebral hemorrhage from rupture of an aneurysm of the circle of Willis (Fig 30–3). Left ventricular failure is exceptional, despite augmented volume imposed upon the pressure-loaded left ventricle. Susceptibility to infective endocarditis is determined chiefly by coexistence of a bicuspid aortic valve.

BICUSPID AORTIC STENOSIS. Because of the low incidence of this malformation among women, bicuspid aortic stenosis is only an occasional complication of pregnancy. The increased cardiac output tends to be tolerated in women with mild-to-moderate bicuspid aortic stenosis, but severe obstruction encroaches on limited circulatory reserve. Dyspnea, angina pectoris, or cerebral symptoms that precede conception or appear early in gestation are matters of grave concern.

BICUSPID AORTIC REGURGITATION. Moderate-to-severe chronic bicuspid aortic regurgitation is generally well tolerated during pregnancy, provided that the adaptive response of the left ventricle preserves normal function. The gestational fall in systemic vascular resistance, together with a more rapid heart rate (shorter diastole), results in a decrease in regurgitant flow.[159] The risk of infective endocarditis is high; therefore, antibiotic prophylaxis is obligatory during labor and delivery.

FALLOT'S TETRALOGY. About half of patients with this anomaly are women, and Fallot's tetralogy is the most common cyanotic malformation that might permit unoperated survival into reproductive age. A gestational fall in systemic vascular resistance and augmented venous return to an obstructed right ventricle result in an increase in the right-to-left shunt and a fall in systemic arterial oxygen saturation, changes that are especially harmful to the fetus. During labor and delivery, a sudden fall in systemic vascular resistance may precipitate intense cyanosis, syncope, and death. Conversely, bearing down during labor may abruptly and dangerously reduce systemic arterial blood flow.

CONGENITAL COMPLETE HEART BLOCK. This uncommon congenital conduction defect permits survival into childbearing age, and about one-half of the patients are female.[5] Asymptomatic young women usually experience an uneventful pregnancy, provided that the QRS duration is not prolonged and the rate response to exercise is satisfactory.[159,163,164] Stokes-Adams attacks occasionally occur during gestation, and the heart and circulation may not respond appropriately to the volatile demands of labor and delivery.

EBSTEIN'S ANOMALY OF THE TRICUSPID VALVE. About half of the patients with this malformation are women, and the majority reach adulthood.[5] The functionally inadequate right ventricle, already volume-overloaded by tricuspid regurgitation, copes poorly with the gestational increase in cardiac output.[165] Atrial tachyarrhythmias occur in approximately one-third of nonpregnant patients with Ebstein's anomaly and are potential hazards during pregnancy.[166] Wolff-Parkinson-White bypass tracts set the stage for excessively rapid ventricular rates in response to atrial fibrillation or flutter (Fig. 30–7). The consequences can be catastrophic. Cyanosis in Ebstein's anomaly (right-to-left interatrial shunt) may first become manifested during pregnancy because of a rise in right ventricular filling pressure. The right-to-left shunt increases the risk of paradoxical embolization, and the hypoxemia increases the risk to the fetus.

THE POSTOPERATIVE PATIENT

There is a consensus that successful surgery before gestation can be pivotal in reducing maternal risks of congenital heart disease. Surgery should therefore be anticipatory. The objectives of reparative surgery are to increase the safety and success of pregnancy, to preserve the health of the mother, and to reduce the risk to the fetus. Closure of an *ostium secundum atrial septal defect* in children or young adults permits pregnancy without maternal risk. The complication of paradoxical embolization from the inferior vena cava is eliminated. However, an increase in incidence of atrial tachyarrhythmias should be considered when the defect is closed after young adulthood.

Division of a small nonpulmonary hypertensive *patent ductus* early in life is curative. Division of a nonrestrictive or moderately restrictive ductus is sometimes followed by incomplete resolution of elevated pulmonary vascular resistance or by less than adequate functional recovery of the volume-overloaded left ventricle, important residua that might confront the pregnant woman. In any event, division of a patent ductus eliminates the risk of infective endocarditis.

Successful response of congenital *pulmonary valve stenosis* to balloon dilatation or to direct repair permits the pregnant woman to anticipate a normal pregnancy except for a low, if not altogether absent, risk of infective endocarditis. Mild-to-moderate low-pressure postinterventional pulmonary regurgitation is not a concern, with few exceptions. Balloon dilatation has proven efficacious during pregnancy (Fig. 30–9).

After repair of *coarctation of the aorta,* the risk of pregnancy depends on relief of the isthmic obstruction (and reduction of systemic blood pressure), the surgical technique, and whether or not a bicuspid aortic valve coexists. To what extent correction of coarctation reduces the hazard of gestational rupture of an aneurysm of the circle of Willis is open to question. The histology of the aorta immediately distal to the coarctation resembles that of cystic medionecrosis, and balloon dilatation injures this already vulnerable aortic segment.[20] Relief of the isthmic obstruction by partial resection and roofing with a graft leaves the vulnerable postcoarctation aortic segment largely in place. The procedure of choice in women is resection that includes the segment of aorta distal to the coarctation, with end-to-end anastomosis. Should a bicuspid aortic valve coexist, two additional postoperative concerns persist: susceptibility to infective endocarditis and the risk inherent in the histological abnormalities of the aortic root.

Surgical relief or balloon dilatation of congenital bicuspid *aortic stenosis* (Fig. 30–10) significantly lowers the risk of pregnancy (see earlier), but not the risk of infective endocarditis. In the presence of hemodynamically significant bicuspid aortic regurgitation, it is usually better to advise pregnancy before aortic valve replacement, provided that left ventricular function is normal or nearly normal. If a stenotic or incompetent aortic valve requires replacement in a woman of childbearing age, a tissue valve has the advantage of good hemodynamics without the need for anticoagulants (but with the caveats commented upon later).

Pregnancy after repair of *Fallot's tetralogy* is accompanied by a gratifyingly small risk, especially when outflow obstruction is relieved without inducing significant low-pressure pulmonary regurgitation. Elimination of cyanosis increases the probability of successful conception,[167] improves the stability of pregnancy, and results in normal fetal growth and development. Postoperative electrophysiological sequelae cannot be ignored but are comparatively infrequent when successful repair is accomplished at a young age (see p. 982).

Closure of a nonrestrictive or moderately restrictive perimembranous *ventricular septal defect* in infancy or early childhood serves to preclude the development of pulmonary vascular disease and to relieve the left ventricle of volume overload. Pregnancy can be anticipated with optimism. Postoperative electrophysiological sequelae are exceptional.

A pacemaker is occasionally required in young women with *congenital complete heart block,* but with relative confidence that pregnancy can then safely proceed if ventricular function is normal, which is usually the case. Although a dual-chamber pacemaker is preferable, a fixed-rate system provides satisfactory physiological support.

Surgical repair of *Ebstein's anomaly of the tricuspid valve* ideally takes the form of reconstruction using the large mobile anterior tricuspid leaflet to create a competent unicuspid atrioventricular valve. Active or potential bypass tracts are eliminated by surgical dissociation of right atrium from right ventricle (Fig. 30–7). The maternal risk of pregnancy, including susceptibility to infective endocarditis, is reduced but not eliminated.

Pregnancy after repair of certain forms of *complex cyanotic congenital heart disease* is now a practical objective. However, menstrual patterns of women who were cyanotic before operation differ significantly from normal women, implying abnormalities of gynecological endocrinology that may influence fertility.[167] After a *Fontan procedure,* a twofold increment in cardiac index can usually be achieved in response to isotonic exercise.[168] The corollary is that women who have undergone successful Fontan repairs and have good if not normal ventricular function confront the physiological burden of pregnancy with circulations that potentially possess adequate hemodynamic reserve. However, other variables may influence outcome.[133]

Medical Management of the Pregnant Woman with Congenital Heart Disease

PRENATAL CARE. A major objective of medical management is to minimize the factors that encroach upon the limited circulatory reserve of pregnant women with heart disease. Cardiac reserve is encroached upon by the hemodynamic burden of pregnancy and by the heart disease itself. Anxiety is a special concern in the primigravida as she anticipates her first gestational experience. The expectant mother should be prepared for what awaits her during pregnancy, labor, delivery, and puerperium in order to decrease if not eliminate fear of the unknown. Diuretics can be used judiciously for the edema of cardiac failure but should not be used for the edema of normal pregnancy.[159] The pregnant woman with heart disease should limit herself to moderate isotonic exercise. Heat and humidity add to the hemodynamic burden; a dry cool atmosphere is therapeutic. The physiological anemia of pregnancy must be distinguished from pathological anemia, and the latter assiduously addressed. Meticulous leg care reduces the gestational tendency for lower-extremity venous stasis and the attendant risk of thromboembolism. Passive standing should be avoided, the supine position minimized (compression of the inferior vena cava by the enlarged uterus), and the pregnant woman should minimize or avoid sitting with knees flexed and legs dependent. As term approaches, an important element in reducing anxiety is assurance that the pain of labor and delivery will be minimized.

The efficacy of oxygen administration during gestation in cyanotic women is open to question, with little or no convincing evidence of benefit to the mother. There is less-than-convincing evidence that oxygen administration exerts a favorable effect on growth retardation of the fetus in cyanotic women.

Maternal mortality in pregnant women with heart disease has been coupled with functional class. Symptoms associated with congenital heart disease, especially cyanotic, have prompted the use of the functional classification shown in Table 30–1. In addition to and apart from symptoms and functional limitations, certain congenital cardiac malformations impose such a formidable threat to maternal survival that pregnancy is proscribed or should be interrupted. Of the two major maternal cardiac risks—pulmonary vascular disease and pulmonary edema—the former is more relevant to congenital heart disease. Primary pulmonary hypertension epitomizes this risk (see Chap.

25), but pulmonary vascular disease in any context is a major hazard, limiting if not precluding rapid adaptive responses to the circulatory changes of pregnancy and to the volatile changes during labor, delivery, and the puerperium.

LABOR AND DELIVERY. In women with functionally mild unoperated lesions and in patients after successful cardiac surgery, management of labor and delivery is the same as for normal pregnant women. The need for infective endocarditis prophylaxis during routine delivery in pregnant cardiac patients has been questioned because of the low incidence of bacteremia that accompanies a normal uncomplicated vaginal delivery.[169] It should not be assumed, however, that a given delivery will be uncomplicated. An episiotomy and vacuum extraction are, strictly speaking, not "normal." Accordingly, pregnant women with cardiac lesions susceptible to infective endocarditis should receive appropriate antibiotic prophylaxis from the onset of labor through the third or fourth postpartal day.[170]

For pregnant women with functionally important congenital cardiac disease—unoperated or operated—the management of labor, delivery, and the puerperium is crucial if risk is to be minimized. The first necessity is to underscore the beneficial effects of induced vaginal delivery. Cesarean section should be reserved for cephalopelvic disproportion, for breech presentation, or for preterm labor in a woman receiving coumadin anticoagulation. Cesarean section results in about twice the blood loss as vaginal delivery, in addition to the risks of wound and uterine infection, thrombophlebitis (delayed ambulation), and potential postoperative complications.

Amniocentesis around the 37th week determines whether or not fetal lung maturity has been achieved and whether induced delivery can safely proceed. The pregnant woman is then admitted for induction, with delivery planned as far as possible during the working day so that a high-risk obstetrician, neonatologist, and cardiologist can more readily be available. On admission, prostaglandin vaginal gel is applied to soften and dilate the cervix.[159] *Laminaria*, derived from the stems of a special seaweed, can be used for the same purpose because of its hydrophilic properties. Oxytocin may be required for augmentation of uterine contractions that are usually initiated by absorbed prostaglandin. The sequence of cervical softening and dilatation precedes the onset of uterine contractions, as in normal spontaneous vaginal delivery.

After contractions are under way, artificial rupture of the membranes is performed. The woman should labor in a lateral decubitus position in order to attenuate the hemodynamic fluctuations provoked by major uterine contractions in the supine position. Meperidine is used selectively for relief of pain and apprehension. The anesthetic of choice is a lumbar epidural preparation, such as fentanyl, that exquisitely controls pain without reducing the strength of uterine contractions, which are monitored together with fetal rate (Fig. 30–9*A*). The fetus is allowed to pass through the pelvis in response to the force of uterine contractions unsupplemented by straining in order to avoid the undesirable circulatory effects of the Valsalva maneuver. Delivery is assisted by vacuum extraction and low forceps.

Systemic arterial pressure should be monitored during labor, because lumbar epidural anesthetics may cause hypotension. In patients with Fallot's tetralogy or Eisenmenger's complex, a sudden fall in systemic vascular resistance poses a special threat. Use of a flotation catheter for hemodynamic monitoring is an individual cardiological decision, rather than routine policy. In Eisenmenger's complex, for example, the risks of a flotation catheter far outweigh the benefits.[171] Oxygen is often intuitively administered during labor, especially in cyanotic women, although without proven efficacy.

After expulsion of the placenta, bleeding is reduced by uterine massage. If intravenous oxytocin is used, the drug should be administered slowly because of its potential hypotensive effect. In the postpartum period, meticulous leg care, use of elastic support stockings, and early ambulation are important preventive measures that reduce the risk of thromboembolism.

BREAST FEEDING. This practice may encroach upon cardiac reserve and increase the risk of mastitis and bacteremia. Nursing should therefore be advised with caution in patients with congenital cardiac disease, and its duration should be minimized. Engorgement of the breasts and suppression of lactation are managed with binding, cold packs, and analgesics rather than with bromocriptine, which can cause hypotension.

Medical Management of the Fetus

Maternal congenital heart disease exposes the fetus to risks that threaten its intrauterine viability and to risks of potential congenital and developmental malformations.[172] Intrauterine viability is influenced by the functional class of the mother (with the qualifications noted above), by maternal cyanosis, and by oral anticoagulants. Maternal cyanosis threatens the growth, development, and viability of the fetus and materially increases fetal wastage, dysmaturity, and prematurity. The risk to the fetus of oral anticoagulants has not been satisfactorily resolved, so the need for anticoagulation should be minimized (see p. 1066). Valve reconstruction is recommended in women of childbearing age. A bioprosthetic valve obviates the need for anticoagulants but subjects the patient to subsequent reoperation. In addition, there is concern that pregnancy itself might accelerate degeneration of a bioprosthetic valve because of the inherent gestational changes in connective tissue. Aspirin is not a viable alternative to anticoagulants because of its potential for closing the fetal ductus and because of low efficacy.

There is no consensus on how best to administer anticoagulants. It is currently believed that the risk of fetal wastage from heparin is not of the same order as from coumadin,[173] previous reports notwithstanding. Whichever regimen of heparin and/or coumadin is chosen, the patient and her partner should be so advised before conception. There is a mounting consensus that warfarin should be replaced with heparin before conception in order to avoid the teratogenic risk of coumadin in early gestation.

The change from coumadin to heparin is best accomplished in the hospital. A nurse specialist instructs the patient and her partner on the technique of subcutaneous administration of heparin using a short 25-gauge needle and an abdominal site for injection at right angles to the elevated skin surface. The needle should be withdrawn slowly, and the site should not be massaged.

Heparin can either be continued throughout gestation (provided that the anticoagulant response is carefully monitored) or replaced with warfarin in the second trimester, returning to heparin in the 36th week. Because of harmful effects that coumadin might exert on the fetal central nervous system—which continues to develop throughout gestation—it has been argued that heparin is the preferred drug because it does not cross the placental barrier and is therefore not teratogenic either during initial organogenesis or during subsequent maturation of the higher centers of the brain. That is, the risk of coumadin lies not only in warfarin embryopathy but potentially in the effect of the oral anticoagulant on central nervous system development.[174] In light of concern that the risk of embryopathy varies directly with blood level, warfarin dosage should be monitored using the International Normalized Ratio (INR) in order to achieve a therapeutic range at the lowest possible dose.[175]

Preterm labor in a pregnant woman taking warfarin threatens the fetus with fatal hemorrhage because fetal anticoagulation cannot be promptly reversed. Emergency cesarean section is required if the fetus is to be saved. Maternal administration of vitamin K and infusion of fresh frozen plasma do not reverse fetal anticoagulation quickly enough to obviate fatal hemorrhage, but fresh frozen plasma should be administered to the newborn. There are, however, four concerns regarding the administration of heparin throughout pregnancy[173]: (1) greater difficulty in achieving a stable therapeutic response; (2) the inconvenience of parenteral administration, an inconvenience that the woman may not be prepared to sustain; (3) the risk of heparin-induced thrombocytopenia; and (4) the risk of bone demineralization.

Extracorporeal circulation is associated with a high incidence of fetal wastage, but cardiac surgery is rarely employed during gestation, especially in the pregnant woman with congenital heart disease. Should cardiac surgery be necessary, it is best to await the 25th to 26th week of gestation.

In addition to threats to its intrauterine viability, the fetus is exposed to risks that take the form of genetic parental transmission, teratogenic effects of certain cardiac drugs, and the harmful effects of certain environmental toxins. A substantial majority of congenital heart diseases cannot be attributed to either a syndrome or a single-gene defect that exhibits mendelian inheritance.[172] A number of studies have concluded that the risk of recurrence of congenital cardiac defects in offspring is greater if the mother rather than the father is the affected parent.[172] A hypothesis that might account for this pattern is cytoplasmic or maternal inheritance based on the observation that mitochondrial DNA is inherited only from the mother.[172] A second hypothesis, "parental imprinting" or "genomic imprinting," refers to gene expression that varies according to its maternal or paternal origin.[176] The imprinting factor is believed to be DNA methylation.

Exercise Before and After Surgery or Interventional Catheterization

Certain types of congenital disorders of the heart or circulation expose patients to the risk of complications or sudden death during strenuous exercise or competitive sports.[177] Consideration must be given to (1) the type, intensity, and duration of exercise; (2) the risk of body collision inherent in a given type of athletic activity; (3) the training program (conditioning) required for a given sport; (4) the emotional stress that the participant experiences in anticipation of or during a particular sport event; (5) the risk of injury to either the participant or spectators if the athletic activity induces loss of consciousness; and (6) the sometimes arbitrary distinction between competitive and recreational athletics.[178]

Two general types of exercise are recognized: isotonic (dynamic) and isometric (static).[2] *Isotonic exercise* is associated with changes in muscle length and with rhythmic muscular contractions that develop comparatively little force. A steady state can be achieved. *Isometric exercise* results in sudden development of a comparatively large force with little or no change in muscle length; a steady state cannot be achieved, even temporarily. There is usually a continuum between the two types, with most physical activity incorporating isotonic and isometric components. The risk incurred by conditioning (training) may equal or exceed the risk of the competitive event itself. The heightened emotional response of an athlete before or during a sporting event may trigger a disturbance in cardiac rhythm and a loss of consciousness, putting the athlete, as well as bystanders, at risk of injury. Central to the following discussion are the type and severity of a given congenital malformation, whether or not the patient had undergone cardiac surgery, and, if so, the type and success of the operation.

CONGENITAL HEART BLOCK. Patients with congenital complete heart block occasionally perform optimally,[5] but prolonged, high-intensity isotonic exercise is ill advised, and strenuous isometric exercise is unwise, even if tolerated. If a pacemaker is required, patients are allowed isotonic or isometric exercise within the limits of sensible moderation and according to the type of pacemaker used. Contact sports risk damage to the pacemaker.

ABERRANT CORONARY ARTERY BETWEEN THE AORTA AND RIGHT VENTRICULAR OUTFLOW TRACT (see Fig. 8–28, p. 262). This uncommon anomaly can cause angina pectoris, myocardial infarction, and sudden death.[179] The risk is greatest, especially in men, when the *left* coronary artery arises from the right aortic sinus and passes between the aorta and right ventricular outflow tract (Fig. 30–16). Sudden death typically accompanies or immediately follows relatively strenuous physical effort. Expansion of the aortic root and pulmonary trunk during exercise is believed to increase preexisting acute angulation of the proximal course of the aberrant coronary artery and to reduce its lumen, especially if the lumen is slit-like.[180,181] If the coronary anomaly is identified and surgically corrected, subsequent athletic activity is not restricted, provided that flow is unobstructed and myocardial ischemia is absent.

COARCTATION OF THE AORTA. In this condition the proximal aorta is less distensible than is the postcoarctation aorta, accounting, in part, for the disproportionate rise in systolic blood pressure in the proximal compartment.[5] The excessive rise in systolic blood pressure during isotonic exercise represents an exaggeration of the disproportionate systolic hypertension in the resting state. A disproportionate exercise-induced postoperative rise in systolic pressure

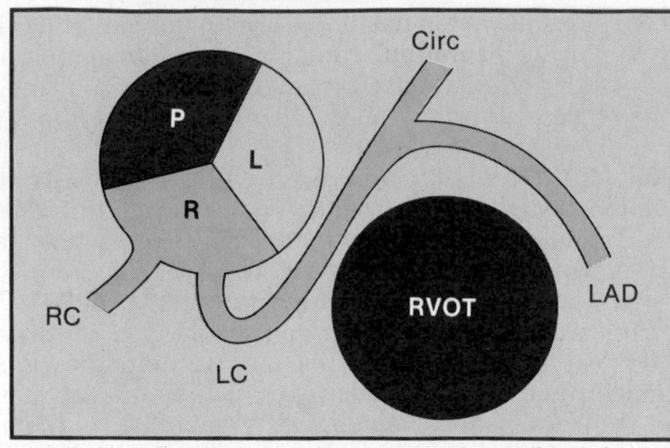

FIGURE 30–16. Illustration of the left coronary artery (LC) arising from a right aortic sinus (R) and coursing between the aorta and the right ventricular outflow tract (RVOT). P = posterior aortic sinus; L = left aortic sinus; RC = right coronary artery; Circ = circumflex coronary artery; and LAD = left anterior descending artery.

is in large part related to age at the time of repair and the adequacy of repair.

CONGENITAL AORTIC STENOSIS. Unoperated patients with *mild* congenital aortic valve stenosis (resting gradient 20 mm Hg or less) are not restricted, provided that the electrocardiogram (ECG) is normal, the response to exercise stress testing is normal, left ventricular function is normal or supernormal, and no significant disturbances in rhythm are recorded during 24-hour ambulatory electrocardiography. Patients with *moderate* congenital aortic stenosis (resting gradients higher than 20 but less than 50 mm Hg), especially those at the upper range, should confine athletics to low-intensity isotonic exercise. Isometric exercise, by increasing aortic root systolic pressure, reduces the gradient, but increases an already elevated left ventricular afterload. Peak systolic gradients in excess of 50 mm Hg warn against high-intensity isotonic or isometric exercise or competitive sports.

The potential risk of sudden death is a legitimate concern when advising exercise limitations in patients with aortic stenosis. Syncope that precedes sudden death is believed to be initiated by left ventricular baroreceptors activated by an exercise-induced increase in left ventricular pressure or stretch, which causes vasodilatation in skeletal muscle followed by systemic hypotension.[182] Malignant ventricular arrhythmias seldom *initiate* syncope but are thought to be the chief cause of death *after* a faint. Syncope-induced hypotension is more likely to provoke disturbances in ventricular rhythm in adults with coexisting coronary artery disease than in younger patients with normal coronary arteries and no myocardial ischemia.

After valvotomy or valvuloplasty for congenital aortic stenosis, recommendations based on the above criteria do not necessarily apply, because risk is not determined by the gradient, even when it is relatively small. Athletic activity should be limited to low or moderate intensity when left ventricular internal dimensions at end diastole are increased, when aortic regurgitation is more than mild, when the scalar ECG shows residual abnormalities of repolarization at rest or with exercise, or when important disturbances in ventricular rhythm are present at rest, with exercise, or on 24-hour ambulatory ECG. These recommendations are appropriate even if left ventricular systolic function is within normal range.

PULMONARY STENOSIS. Patients with mild pulmonary valve stenosis (peak systolic gradient <25 mm Hg) are allowed unrestricted athletic activity. When obstruction is moderate (gradient between 25 and 50 mm Hg), high-intensity competitive sports are unwise even if tolerated, because right ventricular systolic pressure can rise appreciably. When the resting peak systolic gradient exceeds 50 mm Hg—especially if there is impaired right ventricular function—isotonic exercise should be limited to mild intensity and short duration. After successful balloon dilatation or valvotomy, patients generally need few restrictions, and, as a rule, may safely participate in high-intensity competitive athletics, provided that right ventricular size, wall thickness, and function are normal. If postinterventional obstruction to right ventricular outflow is moderate or greater, athletic activity should be limited to noncompetitive low-to-moderate–intensity exercise, especially if right ventricular internal dimensions are increased and systolic function is less than normal.

ATRIAL SEPTAL DEFECT. The majority of young adults with uncomplicated ostium secundum atrial septal defect are asymptomatic and often have relatively normal tolerance to exercise. High-intensity competitive sports may be tolerated but are probably unwise. When surgery abolishes the shunt in childhood or young adulthood, long-term outlook is excellent, and athletic activity is unrestricted, provided that pulmonary vascular resistance is normal, sinus node function and atrioventricular conduction are normal, and the right atrial and right ventricular volumes are normal or nearly so.

VENTRICULAR SEPTAL DEFECT. A restrictive ventricular septal defect with a functionally normal heart imposes no exercise limitations. Although patients can safely participate in competitive sports without restriction, adults in this category are uncommon. An important variation on the theme is the adult who had a moderately restrictive perimembranous ventricular septal defect that decreased in size or closed spontaneously in infancy. There is consensus that such patients are physiologically normal and should be permitted unrestricted physical activity. However, two-dimensional echocardiography with Doppler interrogation and color flow imaging should be performed to determine whether the defect closed by formation of a "septal aneurysm."[5] Although there is no evidence that strenuous athletic exercise, especially isotonic, risks rupturing a septal aneurysm, it is prudent to be aware of the morphological substrate.

After surgical closure of a moderate-to-large ventricular septal defect, recommendations regarding physical activity and competitive sports depend on the postoperative pulmonary arterial pressure; the absence of significant disturbances in ventricular rhythm during maximal exercise stress testing and during 24-hour ambulatory electrocardiography; and two-dimensional echocardiographic evidence of an intact ventricular septum together with normalization of left ventricular and left atrial size and left ventricular function. It is also desirable that the 12-lead scalar ECG exhibit little or no evidence of left ventricular volume overload or right ventricular pressure overload. If these criteria are met, patients are permitted unrestricted exercise. Persistent postoperative elevation of pulmonary arterial pressure, especially if accompanied by exercise-induced right ventricular ectopic rhythms, requires limitation to isotonic physical activity of low intensity and short duration.

PATENT DUCTUS ARTERIOSUS. A small patent ductus arteriosus is of little or no physiological significance, and there are no postoperative limitations after division of an isolated restrictive patent ductus. Recommendations after division of a moderately restrictive or nonrestrictive patent ductus with large left-to-right shunt and variable elevations of pulmonary arterial pressure depend upon the guidelines just set forth for postoperative moderately restrictive to nonrestrictive ventricular septal defect.

Pulmonary vascular disease in these cyanotic patients is a contraindication to strenuous exercise. In patients with suprasystemic pulmonary vascular resistance and right-to-left shunts, even low levels of isotonic exercise tend to be accompanied by decrements in systemic arterial oxygen content and the development of tissue lactic acidosis. The exercise-induced increase in right-to-left shunt poses a special problem regarding the elimination of metabolically produced carbon dioxide, resulting in high ventilatory requirements, subjective dyspnea (Fig. 30–13), and occasionally, respiratory acidosis.[150,151] In nonrestrictive patent ductus arteriosus with suprasystemic pulmonary vascular resistance and reversed shunt, exercise may cause leg fatigue but comparatively little dyspnea, because the ventilatory stimuli of hypoxemia, hypercapnia, and acidemia circumvent the respiratory center. (Venous blood is delivered to the lower body but not to the vital centers of the head and neck.[5])

FALLOT'S TETRALOGY. In patients with this anomaly isotonic exercise provokes a fall in systemic vascular resistance and an augmentation of venous return to a right ventricle with fixed obstruction to outflow, so the right-to-left shunt increases. The subjective sensation of breathlessness is caused chiefly by the response of the respiratory center to the sudden change and blood gas composition and pH as just described. The relief of effort-induced dyspnea by squatting (see p. 885), a time-honored hallmark of Fallot's tetralogy in children, is seldom seen in adults.[5] Squatting exerts its salutary effect by countering the exercise-induced fall in systemic vascular resistance and by decreasing the amount of low oxygen content inferior vena caval blood that is received by the right ventricle and shunted into the aorta during exercise. High-intensity *isometric* exercise in Fallot's tetralogy abruptly reduces flow from the right ventricle into the aorta in the face of fixed obstruction to right ventricular outflow, so systemic flow suddenly falls, risking syncope and occasionally sudden death. All but low-intensity isometric exercise is proscribed.

After repair of Fallot's tetralogy, recommendations regarding physical activity and participation in athletics depend upon patient age at operation and the presence and degree of postoperative residua and sequelae.[183] After repair of Fallot's tetralogy, patients should undergo two-dimensional echocardiography with Doppler interrogation and color flow imaging, exercise stress testing, and 24-hour ambulatory electrocardiography. If obstruction to right ventricular outflow is mild or absent, if the shunt is absent or trivial, if low-pressure pulmonary regurgitation is no more than mild to moderate, if there are no significant disturbances in ventricular rhythm, and if right ventricular size and function are normal or nearly so, limitations are not imposed upon athletic activity, either isotonic or isometric.[183] Of particular concern are residual right ventricular outflow gradients that increase significantly during exercise and are accompanied by right ventricular ectopic rhythms believed to originate at the site of the ventriculotomy scar. Postoperative bifascicular block (Fig. 30–17) is uncommon with current surgical techniques. Bifascicular block without the aforementioned residua or sequelae does not in itself preclude unrestricted physical activity, provided that the 24-hour ambulatory ECG records no additional evidence of impaired atrioventricular conduction.

COMPLETE TRANSPOSITION OF THE GREAT ARTERIES. Data regarding this anomaly are derived chiefly from patients who have undergone atrial switch operations in early life. With few exceptions, important postoperative residua and sequelae require that isotonic physical activity be restricted to mild or moderate intensity and limited duration. Recommendations regarding athletic activity after the *arterial* switch operation cannot currently be made. However, there is an air of cautious optimism that uncomplicated arterial switch repairs may circumvent the electrophysiological sequelae so common after atrial switch operations (Fig. 30–11), while allowing the morphological left ventricle to serve as the systemic pump.

The *Fontan operation* permits study of the human circulation in which total right atrial or total caval flow is channeled directly into the pulmonary artery or into a small right ventricle that serves only as a conduit. Exercise per-

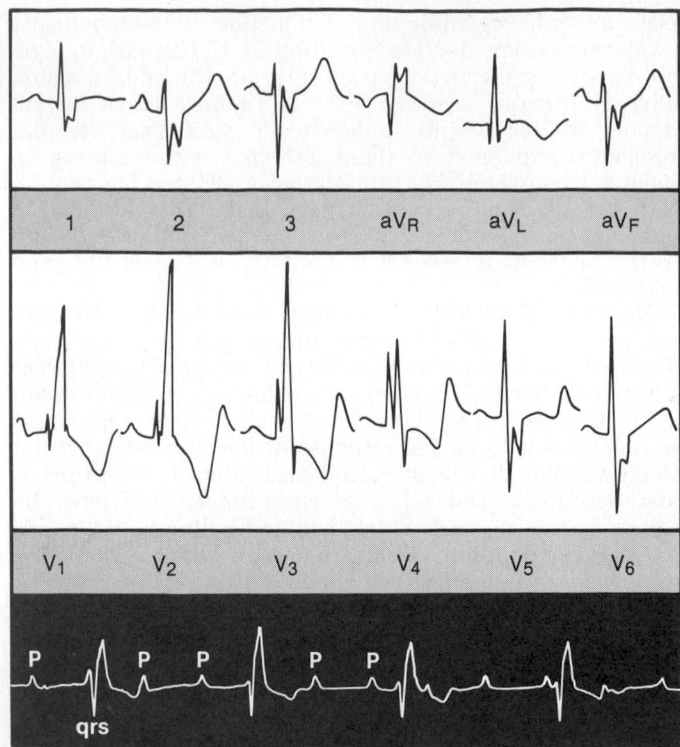

FIGURE 30–17. **Twelve-lead electrocardiogram *(top and center panels)* and single-channel electrocardiogram from a patient with Fallot's tetralogy after intracardiac repair. Bifascicular block (right bundle branch block with left anterior fascicular block) *(top)* progressed to complete atrioventricular block *(bottom).***

formance improves but remains subnormal and the cardiac index increases, but seldom more than twofold.[132a,168,184] Patients with optimal repairs are permitted moderate-intensity isotonic exercise if the following criteria are met: (1) a satisfactory working capacity as judged by exercise stress testing, (2) stable sinus rhythm with no significant disturbances in atrial or ventricular rhythm in response to exercise or on 24-hour ambulatory electrocardiography, (3) normal ventricular function as determined by two-dimensional echocardiography or radionuclide imaging, and (4) normal systemic arterial oxygen saturation.

Employability and Psychosocial Considerations

EMPLOYABILITY. Opportunities for employment of adults with congenital heart defects are influenced by the type of cardiac lesion, cardiac surgery, job discrimination, and educational level.[185] Legislation has been enacted to protect the rights of patients and to provide assistance in seeking employment. Overprotective attitudes of parents and teachers combined with absence of self-discipline may seriously reduce competitive spirit and curtail educational achievement. Job discrimination is one of the most important factors affecting employment opportunities for patients with congenital heart disease. The smaller the company, the greater the reluctance to hire an employee with a thoracotomy scar or with preexisting cardiac disease.

In selected occupations (bus drivers and airline pilots, for example), the safety of others is in the hands of a single individual. To make sensible recommendations regarding fitness for these occupations, the patient's risk of incapacity or sudden death must be defined. The National Rehabilitation Act of 1973 and the Vocational Rehabilitation Act of 1920 offer a wide range of services that are significantly underutilized, especially by cardiac patients.

PSYCHOSOCIAL CONSIDERATIONS. Special if not unique psychological problems confront patients who have experienced dramatic and sometimes traumatic diagnostic and therapeutic interventions during key developmental phases of their lives.[186] The trend toward early diagnosis and reparative surgery in congenital heart disease has made it difficult to generalize from results of studies done 10 to 20 years ago. Despite methodological difficulties and a number of constraints, a reasonable understanding has been achieved by critical assessment of available data combined with clinical experience.

Most patients with congenital heart disease function within normal psychological range, although low self-esteem, insecurity, and feeling of vulnerability are matters of concern.[186] Parental knowledge, understanding, and attitude significantly affect psychosocial adjustments. Difficulty in accepting illness may be manifested by denial and by potentially self-destructive behavior, especially in adolescents. Adults with congenital heart disease face problems in the workplace, in dating, in marriage, and in parenthood. Cyanosis impairs intellectual function, although the degree of impairment is generally mild and often overestimated by IQ tests that depend upon gross motor function at a young age. Early surgery in cyanotic patients appears to improve intellectual and psychological development.[187] Circulatory arrest with deep hypothermia may have subtle adverse effects upon intellectual function, especially if the circulatory arrest and hypothermia are prolonged.[188]

Surgical Considerations

Operation or reoperation for adults with congenital heart disease involves special surgical considerations peculiar to an older patient population.[2] When preoperative phlebotomy is required to improve hemostasis in cyanotic patients, the blood should be stored for potential autologous transfusion. Reoperation after palliative procedures involves revision of Blalock-Taussig shunts, Glenn shunts, Potts or Waterston shunts, and pulmonary arterial bands. Important considerations at reoperation after reparative surgery are reconstruction of cardiac valves and replacement of conduits or prosthetic valves. Operative planning requires knowledge of the basic congenital malformation, of the initial surgical procedure, and of postoperative residua, sequelae, and complications. Perhaps the most important variable that precludes reparative or palliative surgery or reoperation is pulmonary vascular disease. Depressed ventricular function, which is the second major impediment to operability or reoperability, is a consequence of volume or pressure overload, myocardial ischemia, and inherent ventricular morphology.

Certain important principles apply intraoperatively, including myocardial protection, cardioplegia, and hypothermia. Intraoperative salvage of red blood cells and platelet-rich plasma before cardiopulmonary bypass has diminished the need for nonautologous blood and blood products. Minimizing the need for donor blood and blood products is more important at reoperation because of the greater risk of bleeding. The sternotomy incision at reoperation is a technical problem, posing a significant risk when an enlarged right ventricle is apposed to the sternum and when right ventricular outflow conduits adhere. The risk can be reduced materially if reoperation is anticipated at the time of initial repair with placement of an anterior patch of synthetic pericardium.

There are three categories of prostheses: patches, valves, and conduits. The devices and materials selected must achieve an immediately successful technical result, while taking into account the long-term postoperative effects on morbidity and mortality. The choice of materials is based on the patient's age and size, the nature of the congenital malformation, the type of repair, whether or not subsequent repairs are anticipated, the availability of various synthetic and biological materials and devices, complications of long-term anticoagulation, and the risk of infection.

Cardiac Catheterization as a Therapeutic Intervention

(See also Chap. 39)

Therapeutic cardiac catheterization, like cardiac surgery, has three principal objectives: (1) preservation or improvement of cardiac function, (2) an increase in longevity, and (3) maintenance or improvement of the quality of life. When the catheterization technique achieves these ends, surgical morbidity and mortality are circumvented. *Corrective* or *reparative* interventional catheterization procedures currently apply to pulmonary valve stenosis (Fig. 30–9), recoarctation of the aorta, patent ductus arteriosus, and selected patients with atrial septal defect. *Palliative* interventions can be either in lieu of surgery or as adjuncts to surgery. Procedures performed in lieu of surgery apply to lesions such as aortic valve stenosis (Fig. 30–10), postoperative systemic or pulmonary venous obstruction, native coarctation of the aorta, obstructed bioprosthetic valves, and pulmonary arteriovenous fistulas (Fig. 30–8). Palliative procedures that are adjuncts to surgery deal with systemic-to-pulmonary arterial collaterals, systemic-to-pulmonary arterial surgical shunts, pulmonary or systemic venous obstruction, certain intraatrial communications, and selected patients with pulmonary artery stenosis.

Noncardiac Surgery in Adults with Congenital Heart Disease

(See also Chap. 54)

When adults with congenital heart disease require noncardiac surgery, perioperative risks can be reduced, often appreciably, if problems inherent in that patient population are anticipated.[2,155] The following discussion includes patients with cyanotic or acyanotic congenital heart disease who have *not* undergone cardiac surgery, and patients who have undergone reparative cardiac surgery.

SITUS INVERSUS WITH DEXTROCARDIA (see p. 946). This cardiac malposition may go unrecognized until an illness that requires noncardiac surgery brings the adult to medical attention.[5] Accompanying symptoms are likely to be misconstrued and diagnostic conclusions incorrect unless the mirror-image visceral positions are known. In acute appendicitis, the abdominal pain is in the *left* lower quadrant, whereas biliary colic is in the *left* upper quadrant. The risk of noncardiac surgery is the same in the presence of situs inversus as in patients with normal situs, provided no congenital malformations coexist in the mirror-image heart.

CONGENITAL COMPLETE HEART BLOCK (see p. 949). This conduction defect requires electrocardiographic monitoring during and immediately after noncardiac surgery. Intraoperative vagotonic stimuli during ophthalmic or gastrointestinal surgery should be minimized and treated with intravenous atropine expectantly or if there is a sudden decrease in heart rate.[155] If the preoperative scalar ECG shows wide QRS complexes and a relatively slow ventricular rate, especially if there is a history of syncope or near syncope, a temporary right ventricular pacemaker should be inserted.

BICUSPID AORTIC VALVE (see p. 914). If the valve is functionally normal, or nearly normal, noncardiac surgery incurs nothing more than the risk of infective endocarditis. When emergency noncardiac surgery is required in an adult with severe calcific bicuspid aortic stenosis and marginal left ventricular function, hemodynamic monitoring with a flotation catheter should be used. If surgery is elective, consideration should be given to preemptive aortic valve replacement. Balloon valvuloplasty is problematic, even more so if stenosis is due to calcification of a congenitally *bicuspid* aortic valve rather than to calcification of a *trileaflet* aortic valve. Coronary angiography may shed light on whether or not angina pectoris is caused by coexisting coronary artery disease or by augmented oxygen demands of the afterloaded left ventricle. The margin of safety during noncardiac surgery is sometimes improved by preoperative coronary angioplasty. Intraoperative monitoring of systemic blood pressure is important because a sudden fall in systemic vascular resistance may not be associated with an adequate increase in stroke volume, owing to fixed obstruction to left ventricular outflow. An attempt to correct hypotension with rapid infusion of intravenous fluids may cause pulmonary edema.[155] Pharmacological support of systemic resistance is safer than an intravenous infusion and just as efficacious.

Patients with hemodynamically significant *bicuspid aortic regurgitation* confront noncardiac surgery with risks determined by left ventricular function and susceptibility to infective endocarditis. If ventricular function is normal, the risk of noncardiac surgery is small. Moderate intraoperative anesthetic hypotension is not a hazard, serving instead to decrease regurgitant flow and reduce the volume overload of the left ventricle. If left ventricular function is depressed, elective noncardiac surgery raises the question of preemptive replacement of the aortic valve. A tissue valve is preferred to avoid anticoagulants if subsequent noncardiac surgery is anticipated. Emergency noncardiac operation in the presence of depressed left ventricular function calls for hemodynamic monitoring and reduction of postoperative pharmacological afterload.

EBSTEIN'S ANOMALY OF THE TRICUSPID VALVE (see p. 934). Patients with the acyanotic form of the anomaly confront noncardiac surgery with four risks: (1) the functionally inadequate right ventricle, (2) atrial tachyarrhythmias with or without accessory pathways, (3) paradoxical embolism through an intraatrial communication, and (4) infective endocarditis on the malformed tricuspid valve. Right ventricular failure is less a perioperative risk than sudden atrial flutter or fibrillation, especially with rapid antegrade conduction through bypass tracts. Patients with histories of rapid heart action or fusion beats (type B Wolff-Parkinson-White) on scalar ECG require electrocardiographic monitoring. Postoperative thrombophlebitis and the attendant risk of paradoxical embolization are reduced by the use of support hose and early ambulation.

OSTIUM SECUNDUM ATRIAL SEPTAL DEFECT (see p. 896). Young adults with uncomplicated defects experience comparatively little risk during noncardiac surgery, with two exceptions. In response to hemorrhage, systemic resistance rises and venous return diminishes, a combination that augments the left-to-right interatrial shunt, sometimes considerably. An additional concern is the risk of paradoxical emboli from leg veins because thrombi carried by the inferior vena cava tend to stream across the atrial septal defect into the systemic circulation. Meticulous leg care and early ambulation minimize venous stasis.

CYANOTIC CONGENITAL HEART DISEASE. Cyanotic adults have an increased incidence of acute cholecystitis caused by *calcium bilirubinate gallstones* (Fig. 30–12). Perioperative improvement in *hemostasis* in cyanotic patients can be addressed if surgery is elective, with guidelines set forth earlier. Inhalation of oxygen may raise arterial oxygen saturation even in the presence of a right-to-left shunt, but there is little evidence that its routine perioperative use is beneficial. *Intravenous lines, infusions,* and *drugs* must be managed with special care in cyanotic patients. Introduction of air or particles into peripheral veins risks delivery into the systemic circulation because of the right-to-left shunt. Use of an air/particle filter obviates the risk.

Older patients with *Fallot's tetralogy* may come to noncardiac surgery without intracardiac repair or with only a shunt inserted in infancy or childhood. Meticulous perioperative monitoring of oxygen saturation (pulse oximeter) and blood pressure is important, because a sudden fall in systemic resistance may precipitate intense cyanosis and occasionally death, or a sudden rise in systemic resistance may abruptly and dangerously depress systemic blood flow.[155] The risk of postoperative postural hypotension is mentioned below. Susceptibility to infective endocarditis requires prophylaxis.

Cyanotic patients with *elevated pulmonary vascular resistance* face noncardiac surgery with risks inherent in the cyanosis itself in addition to the formidable risks of pulmonary vascular disease. Fixed pulmonary resistance precludes rapid adaptive responses to labile intraoperative or postoperative hemodynamic changes. In Eisenmenger's complex or physiologically analogous lesions, a sudden fall or a sudden rise in systemic vascular resistance precipitates responses similar to those already described in Fallot's tetralogy. Every effort should be made to minimize the postural hypotension that tends to occur during early convalescence in patients having general anesthesia.[155] Because the attendant drop in systemic vascular resistance suddenly augments the right-to-left shunt, convalescent cyanotic patients with pulmonary vascular disease should change positions slowly until the risk of postoperative postural hypotension has abated.

Noncardiac Surgery in Adults with Repaired Congenital Heart Disease

Adults who have undergone reparative surgery for congenital heart disease comprise an increasing percentage of patients who require subsequent noncardiac operations. If cardiac surgery is curative (division of a small patent ductus arteriosus), there is no added risk of a noncardiac surgical procedure. Early correction of simple pulmonary valve stenosis is also close to a cure. Subsequent noncardiac surgery imposes little or no risk, including, in all probability, susceptibility to infective endocarditis. Closure of an ostium secundum atrial septal defect in childhood is close to a cure.

Valvular residua and *sequelae* after cardiac surgery or therapeutic catheterization are relevant in the medical management of patients who undergo noncardiac surgery in adulthood.[189] Successful repair of coarctation of the aorta may leave behind a functionally normal bicuspid aortic valve that is susceptible to infective endocarditis. After complete relief of congenital pulmonary valve stenosis by direct repair or balloon dilatation, the risk of infective endocarditis is low if not absent, but the functional adequacy of the right ventricle is an important perioperative variable. In Fallot's tetralogy, reconstruction of the right ventricular outflow tract may largely or entirely abolish the gradient. If the function of the right ventricle is satisfactory, and if postoperative pulmonary regurgitation is no more than moderate, the risk of noncardiac surgery is small. Infective endocarditis prophylaxis is advisable even though susceptibility is relatively low.

After surgical repair of *Ebstein's anomaly of the tricuspid valve* (tricuspid reconstruction and division of bypass tracts), atrial arrhythmias remain a concern during noncardiac surgery, but without fear of accelerated conduction (Fig. 30–7). Closure of the intraatrial communication eliminates cyanosis, so the hematological derangements are no longer issues, and the potential for paradoxical embolization is eliminated. The postoperative right ventricle is not functionally normal, but the hemodynamic risk during subsequent noncardiac surgery is small. If residual tricuspid regurgitation is more than mild, prophylaxis for infective endocarditis is advisable.

PROSTHETIC MECHANICAL VALVES. These devices (see p. 1066) complicate the management of noncardiac surgery. The immediate issue is anticoagulation in addition to and apart from the risk of infective endocarditis. If noncardiac surgery is elective, and if the prosthesis carries a high thromboembolic risk (mitral location with atrial fibrillation), warfarin should be replaced with an in-hospital continuous infusion of heparin that is discontinued 4 to 6 hours before the elective surgery, restarted within 48 hours after surgery, and then replaced by warfarin. For a lower-risk prosthetic valve in the aortic location, it is relatively safe to discontinue warfarin 2 to 3 days before noncardiac surgery and resume the drug 2 to 3 days after surgery.

Emergency noncardiac surgery in an anticoagulated patient with a mechanical prosthesis is managed differently. Prompt restitution of hemostasis requires infusion of fresh frozen plasma. Cessation of warfarin and administration of vitamin K do not achieve immediate reversal of the anticoagulant effects, which persist for 24 hours or more. If vitamin K is used, the preoperative response to readministration of warfarin is blunted.

ELECTROPHYSIOLOGICAL SEQUELAE. Electrophysiological sequelae after reparative surgery are important concerns during management of subsequent noncardiac surgery. The most diverse and complex sequelae are incurred by intraatrial repairs (Mustard or Senning operations) for complete transposition of the great arteries, and require monitoring during noncardiac surgery. Intraventricular surgery may result in electrophysiological sequelae that are potentially important. Awareness of the presence or potential presence of these sequelae decreases perioperative risk.

After repair of coarctation of the aorta, *systemic hypertension* may persist or recur even if the obstruction has been completely relieved, but the incidence is declining owing to the success of early operation. Nevertheless, pharmacological control of perioperative hypertension is sometimes necessary during noncardiac surgery. The greater the duration of systemic hypertension before repair, the greater the likelihood of premature coronary artery disease—a point to be considered in subsequent perioperative management.

VENTRICULAR FUNCTION. The adequacy of ventricular function (left, right, or single ventricle) is a major determinant of risk during noncardiac surgery in adults. Excessive intravenous fluids should be avoided, and hemodynamic monitoring used when the morphological substrate permits insertion of a flotation catheter.[155]

Medical management during noncardiac surgery must also take into account acquired diseases of the heart and circulation, especially coronary artery disease and systemic hypertension, as well as noncardiac acquired medical disorders such as renal, respiratory, gastrointestinal, or endocrinological.

Postoperative Residua and Sequelae

Residua are defined as cardiac, vascular, or noncardiovascular disorders that are unavoidably left behind at the time of reparative heart surgery[189] (Table 30-3). With few exceptions, residua do not result from surgery having fallen short of its goal, at least in a technical sense.[190] By contrast, *sequelae* are defined as alterations or disorders that are intentionally incurred—occasionally or invariably—at the time of reparative surgery and are looked upon as necessary and acceptable consequences of surgery[189] (Table 30–4). *Complications* are unintentional aftermaths of reparative surgery that range in degree from inconsequential to fatal. Complications and sequelae imperceptibly merge. Surgery is *curative* if there are no cardiac or vascular residua, sequelae, or complications after surgery. "Curative" means that normal cardiovascular structure and function are achieved and maintained, life expectancy is normal, and further medical or surgical treatment for the congenital heart disease is unnecessary. This ideal seldom is realized, and even curative cardiac surgery does not preclude noncardiac residua.[189]

Residua

ELECTROPHYSIOLOGICAL RESIDUA. With some exceptions, these residua are inherent components of certain congenital cardiac malformations.[189] The abnormalities are often evident in standard preoperative 12-lead ECG's, and persist—sometimes harmlessly, sometimes not so harmlessly—after reparative surgery. Electrophysiological residua include (1) axis deviation, especially left; (2) conduction defects, especially atrioventricular; (3) disorders of impulse formation, especially of the sinus node; and (4) arrhythmias, especially atrial.

RESIDUAL ABNORMALITIES OF CARDIAC VALVES. These residua fall into three general categories: (1) congenitally malformed cardiac valves that are functionally normal and

TABLE 30–3 RESIDUA AFTER REPARATIVE SURGERY FOR CONGENITAL HEART DISEASE

1. Electrophysiological
2. Valvular
3. Ventricular
   a. Chamber morphology
   b. Chamber mass
   c. Chamber function
   d. Myocardial connective tissue
4. Vascular
   a. Anatomical (morphological) vascular anomalies or defects
   b. Elevated resistance and/or pressure: systemic, pulmonary
5. Noncardiovascular
   a. Developmental abnormalities
   b. Somatic defects
   c. Medical disorders

TABLE 30–4 SEQUELAE OF REPARATIVE SURGERY FOR CONGENITAL HEART DISEASE

A. Electrophysiological
  1. Atriotomy
    a. Intraatrial repair
    b. Intraventricular repair
  2. Ventriculotomy
    a. Incision site
    b. Intracardiac repair
B. Native valves
  1. Left ventricular or right ventricular *outflow* repair
  2. Left ventricular or right ventricular *inflow* repair
C. Prosthetic materials
  1. Patches
  2. Valves
  3. Conduits
D. Myocardial and endocardial sequelae

do not require attention during reparative surgery; (2) intrinsically normal cardiac valves that are rendered incompetent because of the physiological stress imposed by the congenital malformation that prompted surgical repair; and (3) residually incompetent or stenotic congenitally malformed cardiac valves that do not lend themselves to complete repair. Aortic valve abnormalities that represent unimportant residua include functionally normal bicuspid aortic valve with coarctation of the aorta and mild aortic regurgitation that may accompany Fallot's tetralogy. Residual congenital mitral valve abnormalities that are functionally unimportant include the "cleft" but competent anterior mitral leaflet of an atrioventricular septal defect and the reduction in interpapillary muscle distance associated with coarctation of the aorta. Postoperative residual incompetence of an intrinsically normal pulmonary or tricuspid valve is usually the result of pulmonary hypertension or obstruction to right ventricular outflow.

RESIDUAL VENTRICULAR ABNORMALITIES. Certain ventricular abnormalities are obligatory and permanent after reparative surgery, such as the morphology of a chamber, or may change with the passage of time, such as alterations in chamber mass and function. In patients undergoing either an atrial switch operation for complete transposition of the great arteries, or operation for congenitally corrected transposition of the great arteries, a postoperative residuum of fundamental importance is the presence of a morphological right ventricle in the systemic location. A pivotal question is whether that right ventricle, perfused by a right coronary artery, can, in the long term, perform as a systemic chamber as well as a morphological left ventricle perfused by a left coronary artery.

The development of increased ventricular mass and its regression after reparative surgery are important properties of ventricular myocardium.[190–192] An increase in ventricular mass in excess of the normal process of growth is determined by the nature of the inciting stimulus (hemodynamic or hypoxic), the duration and type of the hemodynamic stimulus (pressure or volume overload), myocardial age (maturity) at the time the stimulus is imposed, and the cell type that is involved.[191–193] The response of a given cell type to a hemodynamic or hypoxic stimulus depends chiefly upon myocyte maturity. If overload or hypoxia is imposed on the immature heart, the cellular response is characterized by replication (hyperplasia) of myocytes and fibroblasts.[194] If the stimulus continues beyond immaturity, myocytes respond by hypertrophy (enlargement) and fibroblasts by hyperplasia (replication).[192] An unresolved concern is the cellular basis for the regression in mass after surgical relief from ventricular overload or hypoxia (Fig. 30–18). The fate of myocytes that replicate in excess of their genetically regulated numbers has not been established.[195] A postoperative reduction in ventricular mass in the setting of hyperplasia implies, at least in part, that the numerically excessive myocytes become smaller in size, not fewer in number. If this contention is valid, its long-term functional significance is unknown. The response of connective tissue cell hyperplasia to operative removal of the overload or hypoxic stimulus is also unknown, although there is evidence that connective tissue cells do not regress as readily as myocytes.[196]

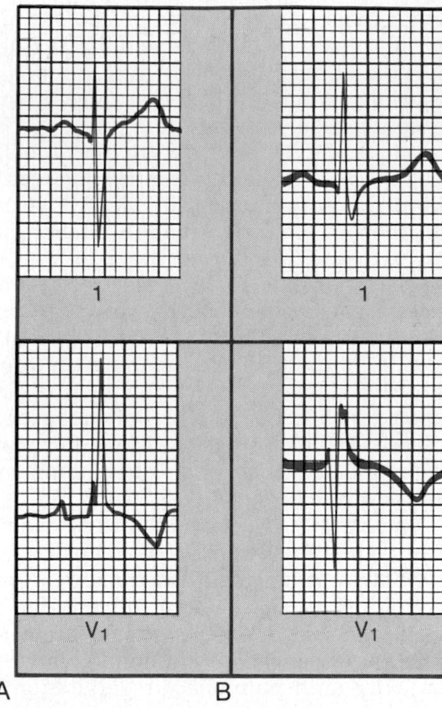

FIGURE 30–18. *A,* Leads 1 and V_1 from a 2-year-old boy with severe pulmonary valve stenosis. *B,* Leads 1 and V_1, 7 years after surgical pulmonary valvotomy. Right axis deviation has resolved and the rR′ in lead V_1 has been replaced with an rSr′. These are electrocardiographic features of regression of right ventricular hypertrophy.

VASCULAR RESIDUA. Vascular residua consist of anatomical anomalies or defects or elevated resistance and/or pressure in the systemic or pulmonary circulation. Examples include the relationship between aortic root disease and bicuspid aortic valve and rupture of an aneurysm of the circle of Willis associated with coarctation of the aorta.

Congenital anomalies of the coronary arteries coexist with a number of congenital malformations of the heart.[5] Examples include Fallot's tetralogy and the residual coronary artery disease (intimal proliferation, medial thickening, premature atherosclerosis) initiated by the hypertension of coarctation of the aorta. The preoperative status of the pulmonary vascular bed, especially the resistance vessels, is a major determinant of the presence and degree of residual postoperative pulmonary vascular disease. Refinements and improved safety that currently permit surgical repairs within the first 6 to 12 months of life make it likely that postoperative pulmonary vascular disease will become less and less a postoperative residuum.

NONCARDIOVASCULAR RESIDUA. These can be important long-term concerns after reparative surgery.[189] Developmental abnormalities such as the mental retardation of Down syndrome or the physical abnormalities of Turner's or the Ellis-van Creveld syndrome are examples. Residual somatic defects include dysmorphism and limb abnormalities. Psychosocial disorders may exist as important postoperative residua, and a healed brain abscess can serve as a focus of a seizure disorder. Cataracts and deafness persist as residua after division of the patent ductus in children with the rubella syndrome.

Sequelae

Sequelae relate to electrophysiological disturbances, native cardiac valves, prosthetic materials, myocardium, and endocardium (Table 30–4). *Electrophysiological sequelae* after intraatrial repair are represented by disturbances in rhythm and conduction, sinoatrial dysfunction, junctional rhythm, atrial fibrillation, atrial flutter, and impaired atrioventricular conduction varying from prolongation of the P-R interval to complete atrioventricular block. Electrophysiological sequelae after intraventricular repair through a right atrial incision result from injury to internodal pathways and to the proximal right bundle branch alone or in combination with the left anterior fascicle.[197] A right ventriculotomy is responsible for two electrophysiological sequelae: an alteration in the sequence of ventricular activation and electrical instability of the incised right ventricle. The surface ECG is useful in determining the proximal origin of abnormal right ventricular activation when right bundle branch block coexists with left anterior fascicular block.[197] Bifascicular block sets the stage for postoperative complete heart block, which is an uncommon but hazardous electrophysiological sequel (Fig. 30–17).

Sequelae involving native cardiac valves occur after left ventricular or right ventricular *outflow* repairs, or left ventricular or right ventricular *inflow* repairs. Postoperative aortic regurgitation as a sequel of surgery for congenital bicuspid aortic stenosis is an example. Surgical repair or balloon dilatation of congenital pulmonary valve stenosis is often followed by mild pulmonary regurgitation, a physiologically minor and therefore acceptable sequel. Repair of complex obstruction to right ventricular outflow, as in Fallot's tetralogy, usually induces pulmonary regurgitation, the importance of which depends on the degree of regurgitant flow and the functional state of the right ventricle.

Sequelae associated with left ventricular *inflow* repairs accompany operations for congenital mitral regurgitation or congenital obstruction to left ventricular inflow. Assuming complete relief of the mitral regurgitation associated with an atrioventricular septal defect, morphological abnormalities intrinsic to the congenitally malformed valve leave the left ventricular inflow guarded by an abnormal mitral apparatus. Reconstruction of the tricuspid valve in Ebstein's anomaly is somewhat analogous. Repair is necessarily followed by sequelae intrinsic to the basic tricuspid valve malformation, even if competence is established.

PROSTHETIC MATERIALS. Insertion of these materials represents a special category of sequelae after reparative surgery for congenital heart disease. Certain materials are exceptions, such as an endogenous pericardial patch for closure of an ostium secundum atrial septal defect or a synthetic patch that is entirely covered by a neointimal layer. Valve replacement results in sequelae that vary in significance according to the physical and hemodynamic characteristics of the prosthetic device (bioprosthetic or rigid), the site of insertion, and patient age at the time of operation. Reoperation is required when an infant or child outgrows the original valve prosthesis. Bioprosthetic valves degenerate at rates determined chiefly by patient age at the time of insertion, and by the tissue characteristics of the device (endogenous or exogenous materials, homografts or xenografts). Susceptibility to infective endocarditis varies from negligible with aortic homografts to high with mechanical prostheses. The incidence of thromboembolic complications is low with an aortic homograft and high with a rigid mitral prosthesis. Anticoagulants reduce but do not eliminate thromboembolic complications and carry the inherent risk of anticoagulant-induced bleeding and the risk of teratogenicity during pregnancy.

Conduits can be nonvalved (usually synthetic) or valved (bioprosthetic or mechanical) and pose the risks of degeneration, thrombogenicity, anticoagulation, and infective endocarditis. In addition, conduits—especially valved—are subject to pseudointimal proliferation (peel).[2] Conduit obstruction can therefore result from both nongrowth of the device and pseudointimal proliferation.

MYOCARDIAL SEQUELAE. Morphological or mechanical sequelae at the site of the ventriculotomy or atriotomy are usually negligible unless there is formation of an aneurysm, which is more properly considered a complication. Electrophysiological sequelae were discussed earlier. Certain *endocardial sequelae* after intraventricular repair have been called "surgical fibroelastosis."[198,199] The cause and functional significance of these endocardial lesions, which are not necessarily confined to the chamber in which the intracardiac repair was done, have not been established.

REFERENCES

1. Perloff, J. K.: Pediatric congenital cardiac becomes a postoperative adult. The changing population of congenital heart disease. Circulation *47*:606, 1973.
2. Perloff, J. K., and Child, J. S.: Congenital Heart Disease in Adults. Philadelphia, W. B. Saunders Company, 1991.
3. Perloff, J. K.: Congenital heart disease in adults: A new cardiovascular subspecialty. Circulation *84*:1881, 1991.
4. Perloff, J. K. (Chairman): 22nd Bethesda Conference: Congenital heart disease after childhood: An expanding patient population. J. Am. Coll. Cardiol. *18*:311, 1991.
5. Perloff, J. K.: The Clinical Recognition of Congenital Heart Disease. 4th ed. Philadelphia, W. B. Saunders Company, 1994.
6. Fallot, A.: Contribution a l'anatomie pathologique de la maladie bleue (cyanose cardiaque). Marseillеméd. *25*:418, 1888.
7. Abbott, M. E.: Atlas of Congenital Heart Disease. New York, The American Heart Association, 1936.
8. Gross, R. E., and Hubbard, J. P.: Surgical ligation of a patent ductus arteriosus: report of first successful case. JAMA *112*:729, 1939.
9. Blalock, A., and Taussig, H. B.: Surgical treatment of malformations of the heart in which there is pulmonary stenosis or pulmonary atresia. JAMA *128*:189, 1945.
10. Crafoord, C., and Nylin, G.: Congenital coarctation of the aorta and its surgical treatment. J. Thorac. Surg. *14*:347, 1945.
11. Kirklin, J. W., DuShane, J. W., Patrick, R. T., et al.: Intracardiac surgery with the aid of a mechanical pump-oxygenator system (Gibbon type): Report of eight cases. Proc. Staff Meet. Mayo Clin. *30*:201, 1955.
12. Ritchie, J. L., Cheitlin, M. D., Hlatky, M. A., et al.: Task Force 5: Profile of the cardiovascular specialist: Trends in needs and supply and implications for the future. J. Am. Coll. Cardiol. *24*:313, 1994.
13. Roberts, W. C.: The congenitally bicuspid aortic valve: a study of 85 autopsy cases. Am. J. Cardiol. *26*:72, 1970.

SURVIVAL PATTERNS

14. Subramanian, R., Olson, L. J., and Edwards, W. D.: Surgical pathology of pure aortic stenosis: A study of 374 cases. Mayo Clin. Proc. *59*:683, 1984.
15. Morganroth, J., Perloff, J. K., Zeldes, S. M., and Dunkman, W. B.: Acute severe aortic regurgitation. Ann. Intern. Med. *87*:223, 1977.
16. Larson, E. W., and Edwards, W. D.: Risk factors for aortic dissection: A necropsy study of 161 cases. Am. J. Cardiol. *53*:849, 1984.
16a. Hahn, R. T., Roman, M. J., Maftader, A. H., and Devereux, R. B.: Association of aortic dilatation with regurgitant, stenotic and functionally normal bicuspid aortic values. J. Am. Coll. Cardiol. *19*:283, 1992.
17. Campbell, M.: Natural history of coarctation of the aorta. Br. Heart J. *32*:633, 1970.
18. Jarcho, S.: Coarctation of the aorta (Reynaud, 1828). Am. J. Cardiol. *9*:591, 1962.
19. Hodes, H. L., Steinfeld, L., and Blumenthal, S.: Congenital cerebral aneurysms and coarctation of the aorta. Arch. Pediatr. *76*:28, 1959.
20. Isner, J. M., Donaldson, R. F., Fulton, D., et al.: Cystic medial necrosis in coarctation of the aorta. Circulation *75*:689, 1987.
21. Vladover, Z., and Neufeld, H. N.: Coronary arteries in coarctation of the aorta. Circulation *37*:449, 1968.
22. Campbell, M.: The natural history of congenital pulmonic stenosis. Br. Heart J. *31*:394, 1969.
23. Nugent, E. W., Freedom, R. M., Nora, J. J., et al.: Clinical course in pulmonary stenosis. Circulation *56*(Suppl. 1):38, 1977.
24. Moller, J. H., and Adams, P. Jr.: Natural history of pulmonary valvular stenosis: Serial cardiac catheterization in 21 children. Am. J. Cardiol. *16*:654, 1965.
25. Campbell, M.: Natural history of atrial septal defect. Br. Heart J. *32*:820, 1970.
26. Craig, R. J., and Selzer, A.: Natural history and prognosis of atrial septal defect. Circulation *37*:805, 1968.
27. Markman, P. G., Horvitt, E. G., and Wade, E. G.: Atrial septal defect in the middle-aged and elderly. Q. J. Med. *34*:409, 1965.
28. Colmers, R. E.: Atrial septal defects in elderly patients: Report of three patients aged 68, 72, and 78. Am. J. Cardiol. *1*:768, 1958.
29. Perloff, J. K.: Ostium secundum atrial septal defect—survival for 87 and 94 years. Am. J. Cardiol. *53*:388, 1984.
30. Nagata, S., Yasuharu, N., Sakakibara, H., et al: Mitral valve lesion associated with secundum atrial septal defect. Br. Heart J. *49*:51, 1983.
31. Boucher, C. A., Liberthson, R. R., and Buckley, M. J.: Secundum atrial

septal defect and significant mitral regurgitation: Incidence, management and morphologic basis. Chest *75*:697, 1979.
32. Popio, K. A., Gorlin, R., Teichholz, L., et al.: Abnormalities of left ventricular function and geometry in adults with an atrial septal defect. Am. J. Cardiol. *36*:302, 1975.
33. Wanderman, K. L., Ovsyheer, I., and Gueron, M.: Left ventricular performance in patients with atrial septal defect: Evaluation with noninvasive methods. Am. J. Cardiol. *41*:487, 1978.
34. Campbell, M.: Natural history of persistent ductus arteriosus. Br. Heart J. *30*:4, 1968.
35. Marquis, R. M., Miller, H. C., McCormack, R. J. M., et al: Persistence of ductus arteriosus with left to right shunt in the older patient. Br. Heart J. *48*:469, 1982.
36. White, P. D., Maxurkie, S. J., and Boschetti, A. E.: Patency of the ductus arteriosus at 90. N. Engl. J. Med. *280*:146, 1969.
37. Wood, P.: The Eisenmenger syndrome or pulmonary hypertension with reversed central shunt. Br. Med. J. *2*:701 and 755, 1958.
38. Hynes, K. M., Gau, G. T., Titus, J. L.: Coronary heart disease in situs inversus totalis. Am. J. Cardiol. *31*:666, 1973.
39. Afzlius, B. A.: Genetical and ultrastructural aspects of the immobile cilia syndrome. Am. J. Human Genet. *33*:852, 1981.
40. Davey, R. D., Nadol, J. B., Holmes, L. B., et al.: Kartagener's syndrome: A blinded, controlled study of cilia ultrastructure. Arch. Otolaryngol. Head Neck Surg. *112*:646, 1986.
41. McHenry, M. M.: Factors influencing longevity in adults with congenital complete heart block. Am. J. Cardiol. *29*:416, 1972.
42. Reybrouck, T., Vanden Eynde, B. B., Dumoulin, M., and Van der Hauwaert, L. G.: Cardiorespiratory response to exercise in congenital complete atrioventricular block. Am. J. Cardiol. *64*:896, 1989.
43. Dewey, R. C., Capeless, M. A., and Levy, A. M.: Use of ambulatory electrocardiographic monitoring to identify high-risk patients with congenital complete heart block. N. Engl. J. Med. *316*:835, 1987.
44. Bjarke, B. B., and Kidd, B. S. L.: Congenitally corrected transposition of the great arteries: a clinical study of 101 cases. Acta Paediatr. Scand. *65*:153, 1976.
45. Cumming, G. R.: Congenital corrected transposition of the great vessels without associated intracardiac anomalies. Am. J. Cardiol. *10*:605, 1962.
46. Nagle, J. P., Cheitlin, M. D., and McCarty, R. J.: Corrected transposition of the great vessels without associated anomalies. Chest *60*:363, 1971.
47. Schiebler, G. L., Edwards, J. E., Burchell, H. B., et al.: Congenital corrected transposition of the great vessels. Pediatrics *27*:851, 1961.
48. Lieberson, A. D., Schumacker, R., and Childress, D.: Corrected transposition of the great vessels in a 73-year-old man. Circulation *39*:96, 1969.
49. Huhta, J. C., Danielson, G. K., Ritter, D. G., and Ilstrup, D. M.: Survival in atrioventricular discordance. Pediatr. Cardiol. *6*:57, 1985.
50. Anderson, K. R., Zuberbuhler, J. R., Anderson, R. H., et al.: Morphologic spectrum of Ebstein's anomaly of the heart. Mayo Clin. Proc. *54*:174, 1979.
51. Watson, H.: Natural history of Ebstein's anomaly of tricuspid valve in childhood and adolescence: An international cooperative study of 505 cases. Br. Heart J. *36*:417, 1974.
52. Radford, D. J., Graff, R. F., and Neilson, G. H.: Diagnosis and natural history of Ebstein's anomaly. Br. Heart J. *54*:517, 1985.
53. Giuliani, E. R., Fuster, V., Brandenburg, R. O., and Mair, D. D.: Ebstein's anomaly: the clinical features and natural history of Ebstein's anomaly of the tricuspid valve. Mayo Clin. Proc. *54*:163, 1979.
54. Leung, M. P., Baker, E. J., Anderson, R. H., and Zuberbuhler, J. R.: Cineangiographic spectrum of Ebstein's malformations: Its relevance to clinical presentation and outcome. J. Am. Coll. Cardiol. *11*:154, 1988.
55. Benson, L. N., Child, J. S., Schwaiger, M., Perloff, J. K., et al.: Left ventricular geometry and function in adults with Ebstein's anomaly of the tricuspid valve. Circulation *75*:353, 1987.
56. Saxena, A., Fona, L. V., Tristam, M., et al.: Left ventricular function in patients >20 years of age with Ebstein's anomaly of the tricuspid valve. Am. J. Cardiol. *67*:217, 1991.
57. Makous, N., and Vander Veer, J. B.: Ebstein's anomaly and life expectancy: Report of a survival to over seventy-nine. Am. J. Cardiol. *18*:100, 1966.
58. Adams, J. C. L., and Hudson, R.: Case of Ebstein's anomaly surviving to age 79. Br. Heart J. *18*:129, 1956.
59. Seward, J. B., Tajik, A. J., Feist, D. J., and Smith, H. C.: Ebstein's anomaly in an 85 year old man. Mayo Clin. Proc. *54*:193, 1979.
60. Collins, N. P., Braunwald, E., and Morrow, A. G.: Isolated congenital pulmonary valvular regurgitation. Am. J. Med. *28*:159, 1960.
61. Cortes, F. M., and Jacoby, W. J.: Isolated congenital pulmonary valvular insufficiency. Am. J. Cardiol. *10*:287, 1962.
62. Pouget, J. M., Kelly, C. E., and Pilz, C. G.: Congenital absence of the pulmonic valve: Report of a case in a 73 year old man. Am. J. Cardiol. *19*:732, 1967.
63. Lutembacher, R.: De la stenose mitrale avec communication interauriculaire. Arch. Mal. Coeur *9*:237, 1916.
64. Firkett, C. H.: Examen anatomique d'un cas de pesistence du trou ovale de botal, avec lesions valvulaires considerables du coueur gauche, chez une femme de 74 ans. Ann. Soc. Med. Chir. Liege *19*:188, 1880.
65. Rosenthal, L.: Atrial septal defect with mitral stenosis (Lutembacher's syndrome) in a woman of 81. Br. Med. J. *2*:1351, 1956.
66. Botefeu, J. M., Moret, P. R., Hahn, C., and Hauf, E.: Aneurysms of the sinus of Valsalva: Report of seven cases and review of the literature. Am. J. Med. *65*:18, 1983.
67. Mayer, E. D., Ruffman, K., Saggau, W., et al.: Ruptured aneurysms of the sinus of Valsalva. Ann. Thorac. Surg. *42*:81, 1986.
68. Sakakibara, S., and Konno, S.: Congenital aneurysm of the sinus of Valsalva: A clinical study. Am. Heart J. *63*:708, 1962.
69. Onat, A., Ersanli, O., Kanuni, A., and Aykan, T. B.: Congenital aortic sinus aneurysms with particular reference to dissection of the interventricular septum. Am. Heart J. *72*:158, 1966.
70. Liberthson, R. R., Sagar, K., Berkoben, J. P., et al.: Congenital coronary arteriovenous fistula: Report of 13 patients, review of the literature and delineation of management. Circulation *59*:849, 1979.
71. Gillebert, C., Van Hoof, R., Van de Werf, F, et al.: Coronary artery fistulas in an adult population. Eur. Heart J. *7*:437, 1986.
72. Cheng, T. O.: Left coronary artery-to-left ventricular fistula: Demonstration of coronary steal phenomenon. Am. Heart J. *104*:870, 1982.
73. Paul, O., Sweet, R. H., and White, P. D.: Coronary arteriovenous fistula case report. Am. Heart J. *37*:441, 1949.
74. Dines, D. E., Seward, J. B., and Bernatz, P. E.: Pulmonary arteriovenous fistula. Mayo Clin. Proc. *58*:176, 1983.
75. Wong, L. B., and Perloff, J. K.: Familial occurrence of congenital pulmonary arteriovenous fistulae in octogenarian siblings. Am. J. Cardiol. *62*:1149, 1988.
76. Corone, P., Doyon, F., Gaudeau, S., et al.: Natural history of ventricular septal defect: A study involving 790 cases. Circulation *55*:908, 1977.
77. Campbell, M.: Natural history of ventricular septal defect. Br. Heart J. *33*:246, 1971.
78. Weidman, W. H., DuShane, J. W., and Ellison, R. C.: Clinical course in adults with ventricular septal defect. Circulation *56*(Suppl. I):78, 1977.
79. Ellis, J. H. IV, Moodie, D. S., Sterba, R., and Gill, C. C.: Ventricular septal defect in the adult: Natural and unnatural history. Am. Heart J. *114*:115, 1987.
80. Otterstad, J. E., Nitter-Hauge, S., and Myhre, E.: Isolated ventricular septal defect in adults: Clinical and haemodynamic findings. Br. Heart J. *50*:343, 1983.
81. Moe, D. G., and Guntheroth, W. G.: Spontaneous closure of uncomplicated ventricular septal defect. Am. J. Cardiol. *60*:674, 1987.
82. Wood, P.: Foreword. Bedford, E. D., and Caird, F. L.: Valvular Diseases of the Heart in Old Age. Boston, Little, Brown, and Co., 1960.
83. Ramaciotti, C., Keren, A., and Silverman, N. H.: Importance of (perimembranous) ventricular septal aneurysm in the natural history of isolated perimembranous ventricular septal defect. Am. J. Cardiol. *57*:268, 1986.
84. Shah, P., Singh, W. S. A., Rose, V., and Keith, J. D.: Incidence of bacterial endocarditis in ventricular septal defects. Circulation *34*:127, 1966.
85. Abraham, K. A., Cherian, G., Rao, V. D., et al.: Tetralogy of Fallot in adults: A report on 147 patients. Am. J. Med. *66*:811, 1979.
86. Bertranou, E. G., Blackstone, E. H., Hazelrig, J. B., et al.: Life expectancy without surgery in tetralogy of Fallot. Am. J. Cardiol. *42*:458, 1978.
87. Marelli, A. J., Perloff, J. K., Child, J. S., and Laks, H.: Pulmonary atresia with ventricular septal defect in adults. Circulation *89*:243, 1994.
88. Stanger, P., Cassidy, S. C., Girod, D. A., et al.: Balloon pulmonary angioplasty: Results of the Valvuloplasty and Angioplasty of Congenital Anomalies Registry. Am. J. Cardiol. *65*:775, 1990.
89. Nishimura, R. A., Holmes, D. R., and Reeder, G. S.: Percutaneous balloon valvuloplasty. Mayo Clin. Proc. *65*:198, 1990.
90. Sandor, G. G. S., Olley, P. M., Trusler, G. A., et al.: Long-term follow-up of patients after valvotomy for congenital valvular aortic stenosis in children. J. Thorac. Cardiovasc. Surg. *80*:171, 1980.
91. Hsieh, K., Keane, J. F., Nadas, A. S., et al.: Long-term follow-up of valvulotomy before 1968 for congenital aortic stenosis. Am. J. Cardiol. *58*:338, 1986.
92. Donner, R. M., Carabello, B. A., Black, I., and Spann, J. F.: Left ventricular wall stress in compensated aortic stenosis in children. Am. J. Cardiol. *51*:946, 1983.
93. Assey, M. E., Wisenbaugh, T., Spann, J. F., et al.: Unexpected persistence into adulthood of low wall stress in patients with congenital aortic stenosis: Is there a fundamental difference in the hypertrophic response to a pressure overload present from birth? Circulation *75*:973, 1987.
94. Danielson, G. K., and Fuster, V.: Surgical repair of Ebstein's anomaly. Ann. Surg. *196*:499, 1982.
95. Shah, D., Azhar, M., Oakley, C. M., et al.: Natural history of secundum atrial septal defect in adults after medical or surgical treatment: A historical prospective study. Br. Heart J. *71*:224, 1994.
96. Steele, P. M., Fuster, V., Cohen, M., et al.: Isolated atrial septal defect with pulmonary vascular obstructive disease: Long-term follow-up and prediction of outcome after surgical correction. Circulation *76*:1037, 1987.
97. Murphy, J. G., Gersh, B. J., McGoon, D. C., et al.: Long-term outcome after surgical repair of isolated atrial septal defect. N. Engl. J. Med *323*:1645, 1990.
98. Ward, C.: Secundum atrial septal defect: Routine surgical treatment is not of proven benefit. Br. Heart J. *71*:219, 1994.
99. Konstantinides, S., Gerbel, A., Olschewski, M., et al.: Clinical course of atrial septal defect in patients older than 40 years: Benefits of surgical repair compared with medical treatment. N. Engl. J. Med. *333*:469, 1995.
100. Williams, W. G., Trusler, G. A., Kirklin, J. W., et al.: Early and late

results of a protocol for simple transposition leading to an atrial switch (Mustard) repair. J. Thorac. Cardiovasc. Surg. *45*:717, 1988.

101. Turina, M., Siebenmann, R., Nussbaumer, P., and Senning, A.: Long-term outlook after atrial correction of transposition of the great arteries. J. Thorac. Cardiovasc. Surg. *95*:828, 1988.
102. Mustard, W. T.: Successful two-stage correction of transposition of the great vessels. Surgery *55*:469, 1964.
103. Gillette, P. C., Kugler, J. D., Garson, A., et al.: Mechanism of the cardiac arrhythmias after the Mustard operation for transposition of the great arteries. Am. J. Cardiol. *45*:1225, 1980.
104. Vetter, V. L., Tanner, C. S., Horowitz, L. N.: Inducible atrial flutter after the Mustard repair of complete transposition of the great arteries. Am. J. Cardiol. *61*:428, 1988.
105. Musewe, N. N., Reisman, J., Benson, L. N., et al.: Cardiopulmonary adaptation at rest and during exercise 10 years after Mustard atrial repair for transposition of the great arteries. Circulation *77*:1055, 1988.
106. Parrish, M. D., Graham, T. P., Bender, H. W., et al.: Radionuclide angiographic evaluation of right and left ventricular function during exercise after repair of transposition of the great arteries. Circulation *67*:178, 1983.
107. Ramsay, J. M., Venables, A. W., Kelly, M. J., and Kalff, V.: Right and left ventricular function at rest and with exercise after the Mustard operation for transposition of the great arteries. Br. Heart J. *51*:364, 1984.
108. Waien, S. A., Liu, P. P., Ross, B. L., et al.: Serial follow-up of adults with repaired tetralogy of Fallot. JAMA *20*:295, 1992.
109. Murphy, J. G., Gersh, B. J., Mair, D. D., et al.: Long-term outcome in patients undergoing surgical repair of tetralogy of Fallot. N. Engl. J. Med. *329*:593, 1993.
109a. Gatzoulis, M. A., Till, J. A., Somerville, J., and Redington, A. N.: Mechanoelectrical interaction in tetralogy of Fallot. Circulation *92*:231, 1995.
110. Walsh, E. P., Rockenmacher, S., Keane, J. F., et al.: Late results in patients with tetralogy of Fallot repaired during infancy. Circulation *77*:1062, 1988.
111. Hu, D. C. K., Seward, J. B., Puga, F. J., et al: Total correction of tetralogy of Fallot at age 40 years or older: Long-term follow-up. J. Am. Coll. Cardiol. *5*:40, 1985.
112. Hughes, C. F., Lim, Y. C., Cartmill, T. B., et al.: Total intracardiac repair for tetralogy of Fallot in adults. Ann. Thorac. Surg. *43*:634, 1987.
113. Zhao, H., Miller, D. C., Reitz, B. A., and Shumway, N. E.: Surgical repair of tetralogy of Fallot: Long-term follow-up with particular emphasis on late death and reoperation. J. Thorac. Cardiovasc. Surg. *89*:204, 1985.
114. Jarmakani, J. M., Graham, T. P., and Canent, R. V.: Left heart function in children with tetralogy of Fallot before and after palliative or corrective surgery. Circulation *46*:478, 1972.
115. Borow, K. M., Green, L. H., Castenada, A. R., and Keane, J. F.: Left ventricular function after repair of tetralogy of Fallot and its relationship to age of surgery. Circulation *61*:1150, 1980.
116. Roos-Hesselink, J., Perlroth, M. G., McGhie, J., and Spitaels, S.: Atrial arrhythmias in adults after repair of tetralogy of Fallot: Correlations with clinical, exercise and echocardiographic findings. Circulation *91*:2214, 1995.
117. Fisher, R. G., Moodie, D. S., Sterba, R., and Gill, C. G.: Patent ductus arteriosus in adults—long-term follow-up: Nonsurgical versus surgical treatment. J. Am. Coll. Cardiol. *8*:280, 1986.
118. Kirklin, J. W., and Barratt-Boyes, B. G.: Cardiac Surgery. New York, John Wiley and Sons, 1986, p. 1059.
119. Koller, M., Rothlin, M., and Senning, A.: Coarctation of the aorta: Review of 362 operated patients. Long-term follow-up and assessment of prognostic variables. Eur. Heart J. *8*:670, 1987.
120. Presbitero, P., Demarie, D., Villani, M., et al.: Long-term results (15 to 30 years) of surgical repair of aortic coarctation. Br. Heart J. *57*:462, 1987.
121. Daniels, S. R., James, F. W., Loggie, J. M. H., and Kaplan, S.: Correlates of resting and maximal exercise systolic blood pressure after repair of coarctation of the aorta: a multivariate analysis. Am. Heart J. *113*:349, 1987.
122. Clarkson, P. M., Nicholson, M. R., Barratt-Boyes, B. G., et al.: Results after repair of coarctation of the aorta beyond infancy: A 10 to 28 year follow-up with particular reference to late systemic hypertension. Am. J. Cardiol. *51*:1481, 1983.
123. Hesslein, P. S., McNamara, D. G., Morriss, M. J. H., et al.: Comparison of resection versus patch aortoplasty for repair of coarctation in infants and children. Circulation *64*:164, 1981.
124. Hellenbrand, W., Allen, H., Golinko, R., et al.: Balloon angioplasty for aortic recoarctation: Results of the valvuloplasty and angioplasty of congenital anomalies Registry. Am. J. Cardiol. *65*:793, 1990.
125. Liberthson, R. L., Pennington, D. G., Jacobs, M. L., and Daggett, W. M.: Coarctation of the aorta: Review of 234 patients and clarification of management problems. Am. J. Cardiol. *43*:835, 1979.
126. Celano, V., Pieroni, D. R., Morera, J. A., et al.: Two-dimensional echocardiographic examination of mitral valve abnormalities associated with coarctation of the aorta. Circulation *69*:924, 1984.
127. Fontan, F., and Baudet, E.: Surgical repair of tricuspid atresia. Thorax *26*:240, 1971.
128. Cowgill, L. D.: The Fontan procedure: A historical review. Ann. Thorac. Surg. *51*:1026, 1991.
129. Glenn, W. W. L.: Circulatory bypass of the right side of the heart. IV Shunt between superior vena cava and distal right pulmonary artery: Report of clinical application. N. Engl. J. Med. *259*:117, 1958.
130. Kopf, G. S., Laks, H., Stansel, H. C., et al.: Thirty-year follow-up of superior vena cava-pulmonary artery (Glenn) shunts. J. Thorac. Cardiovasc. Surg. *100*:662, 1990.
131. de Leval, M. R., Kilner, P., Gewillig, M., and Bull, C.: Total cavopulmonary connection: A logical alternative to atriopulmonary connection for complex Fontan operations. Experimental studies and early clinical experience. J. Thorac. Cardiovasc. Surg. *96*:682, 1988.
132. Stein, D. G., Laks, H., Drinkwater, D. C., et al.: Results of total cavopulmonary connection in the treatment of patients with a functional single ventricle. J. Thorac. Cardiovasc. Surg. *102*:280, 1991.
132a. Rosenthal, M., Bush, A., Deanfield, J., and Redington, A.: Comparison of cardiopulmonary adaptation during exercise in children after the atriopulmonary and total cavopulmonary connection Fontan procedures. Circulation *91*:372, 1995.
133. Driscoll, D. J., Offord, K. P., Feldt, R. H., et al.: Five-to-fifteen follow-up after Fontan operation. Circulation *85*:469, 1992.
134. Humes, R. A., Mair, D. D., Porter, C. J., et al.: Results of the modified Fontan operation in adults. Am. J. Cardiol. *61*:602, 1988.

MEDICAL MANAGEMENT OF ADULT CONGENITAL HEART DISEASE

135. Perloff, J. K.: Systemic complications of cyanosis in adults with congenital heart disease. Cardiol. Clin. *11*:689, 1993.
136. Berman, W., Jr., Wood, S. C., Yabek, S. M., et al.: Systemic oxygen transport in patients with congenital heart disease. Circulation *75*:360, 1987.
137. Tyndall, M. R., Teitel, D. F., Lutin, W. A., et al.: Serum erythropoietin levels in patients with congenital heart disease. J. Pediatr. *110*:538, 1987.
138. Rosove, M. H., Perloff, J. K., Hocking, W. G., et al.: Chronic hypoxaemia and decompensated erythrocytosis in cyanotic congenital heart disease. Lancet *2*:313, 1986.
139. Perloff, J. K., Rosove, M. H., Child, J. S., and Wright, G. B.: Adults with cyanotic congenital heart disease: Hematologic management. Ann. Intern. Med. *109*:406, 1988.
140. Linderkamp, O., Klose, H. J., Betke, K., et al.: Increased blood viscosity in patients with cyanotic congenital heart disease and iron deficiency. J. Pediatr. *95*:567, 1979.
141. Giddings, S. S., and Stockman, J. A.: Effect of iron deficiency on tissue oxygen delivery in cyanotic congenital heart disease. Am. J. Cardiol. *61*:605, 1988.
142. Perloff, J. K., Marelli, A. J., and Miner, P. D.: Risk of stroke in adults with cyanotic congenital heart disease. Circulation *87*:1954, 1993.
143. Territo, M. C., Perloff, J. K., Rosove, M. H., and Moake, J.: von Willebrand factor abnormalities in adults with congenital heart disease: A hematologic/pathophysiologic correlative study. *(In preparation.)*
144. Bowyer, J. J., Busst, C. M., Denison, D. M., and Shinebourne, E. A.: Effect of long-term oxygen treatment at home in children with pulmonary vascular disease. Br. Heart J. *55*:385, 1986.
145. Perloff, J. K., Latta, H., and Barsotti, P.: Pathogenesis of the abnormal glomerulus in cyanotic congenital heart disease *(in preparation).*
146. Spear, G. S.: The glomerular lesion of cyanotic congenital heart disease. Bull. Johns Hopkins Hosp. *140*:185, 1977.
147. Ross, E. A., Perloff, J. K., Danovitch, G. M., et al.: Renal function and urate metabolism in late survivors with cyanotic congenital heart disease. Circulation *73*:396, 1986.
148. German, D. C., and Holmes, E. W.: Hyperuricemia and gout. Med. Clin. North Am. *70*:419, 1986.
149. Martinez-Lavin, M.: Cardiogenic hypertrophic osteoarthropathy. Clin. Exp. Rheum. *10*:19, 1992.
150. Sietsema, K. E., Cooper, D. M., Perloff, J. K., et al.: Dynamics of oxygen uptake during exercise in adults with cyanotic congenital heart disease. Circulation *73*:1137, 1986.
151. Sietsema, K. E., Cooper, D. M., Perloff, J. K., et al.: Control of ventilation during exercise in patients with central venous-to-systemic arterial shunts. J. Appl. Physiol. *64*:234, 1988.
152. Perloff, J. K., Urschell, C. W., Roberts, W. C., and Caulfield, W. H.: Aneurysmal dilatation of the coronary arteries in cyanotic congenital heart disease. Am. J. Med. *45*:802, 1968.
153. Czernin, J., Brunken, R. C., Perloff, J. K., et al.: Myocardial perfusion and perfusion reserve in adults with cyanotic congenital heart disease. *(In preparation.)*
154. Perloff, J. K., and Marelli, A. J.: Neurological and psychosocial disorders in adults with congenital heart disease. Heart Dis. Stroke *1*:218, 1992.
155. Baum, V. C., and Perloff, J. K.: Anesthetic implications of adults with congenital heart disease. Anesth. Analg. *76*:1342, 1993.
156. Karnik, R., Stollberger, C., Valentin, A., et al.: Detection of patent foramen ovale by transcranial contrast Doppler ultrasound. Am. J. Cardiol. *69*:560, 1992.
157. Pearson, A. C., Nagelhout, D., Castello, R., et al.: Atrial septal aneurysm and stoke: A transesophageal echocardiographic study. JAMA *18*:1223, 1991.
158. Kurlan, R., Krall, R. L., and Deweese, J. A.: Vertebrobasilar ischemia after total repair of tetralogy of Fallot: Significance of subclavian steal created by Blalock-Taussig anastomosis. Stroke *15*:359, 1984.

159. Perloff, J. K.: Congenital heart disease and pregnancy. Clin. Cardiol. *17*:579, 1994.
160. Loscalzo, J.: Paradoxical embolization: Clinical presentation, diagnostic strategies, and therapeutic options. Am. Heart J. *112*:141, 1986.
161. Pitkin, R. M., Perloff, J. K., Koos, B. J., and Beall, M. H.: Pregnancy and congenital heart disease. Ann. Intern. Med. *112*:445, 1990.
162. Manalo-Estrella, P., and Barker, A. E.: Histopathologic findings in human aortic media associated with pregnancy. Arch. Pathol. *83*:336, 1967.
163. Esscher, E. B.: Congenital complete heart block in adolescence and adult life: A follow-up study. Eur. Heart J. *2*:281, 1981.
164. Esscher, E. B.: Congenital complete heart block (Review). Acta Paediatr. Scand. *70*:131, 1981.
165. Waickman, L. A., Skorton, D. J., Varner, M. W., et al.: Ebstein's anomaly and pregnancy. Am. J. Cardiol. *53*:357, 1984.
166. Saxon, L. A., and Perloff, J. K.: Arrhythmias and conduction disturbances associated with pregnancy. *In* Podrid, P. J. and Kowey, P. R. (eds.): Cardiac Arrhythmia. Baltimore, Williams and Wilkins, 1995, p. 1161.
167. Canobbio, M. M., Rapkin, A. J., Perloff, J. K., et al.: Menstrual patterns in women with congenital heart disease. Pediatr. Cardiol. *16*:12, 1995.
168. Barber, G., DiSessa, T., Child, J. S., et al.: Hemodynamic responses to isolated increments in heart rate by atrial pacing after a Fontan procedure. Am. Heart J. *115*:837, 1988.
169. Baker, T. H., Machikawa, J. H., Stapleton, J. J.: Asymptomatic peripheral bacteremia. Am. J. Obstet. Gynecol. *94*:903, 1966.
170. Child, J. S., and Perloff, J. K.: Infective endocarditis: Risks and prophylaxis. *In* Perloff, J. K., and Child, J. S. (eds.): Congenital Heart Disease in Adults. Philadelphia, W. B. Saunders Company, 1991.
171. Devitt, J. H., Noble, W. H., and Byrick, R. J.: A Swan-Ganz catheter-related complication in a patient with Eisenmenger's syndrome. Anesthesiology *57*:335, 1982.
172. Clarke, C. F., Beall, M. H., Perloff, J. K.: Genetics, epidemiology, counseling, and prevention. *In* Perloff, J. K., and Child, J. S. (eds.): Congenital Heart Disease in Adults. Philadelphia, W. B. Saunders Company, 1991.
173. Ginsberg, J. S., Kowalchuk, G., Hirsh, J., et al.: Heparin therapy during pregnancy: Risks to mothers and fetus. Arch. Intern. Med. *149*:2233, 1989.
174. Zakzouk, M. S.: The congenital warfarin syndrome. J. Laryngol. Otol. *100*:215, 1986.
175. Hirsh, J., and Fuster, V.: AHA medical/scientific statement. Guide to anticoagulant therapy part 2: Oral anticoagulants. Circulation *89*:1469, 1994.
176. Barlow, D. P.: Methylation and imprinting: From host defense to gene regulation? Science *260*:309, 1993.
177. Maron, B. J., Epstein, S. E., and Mitchell, J. H.: Sixteenth Bethesda Conference: Cardiovascular abnormalities in the athlete: Recommendations regarding eligibility for competition. J. Am. Coll. Cardiol. *6*:1189, 1985.
178. Mitchell, J. H., Blomqvist, G., Haskell, W. L., et al.: Classification of sports. Am. J. Coll. Cardiol. *6*:1189, 1985.
179. Barth, C. W., and Roberts, W. C.: Left main coronary artery originating from the right sinus of Valsalva and coursing between the aorta and pulmonary trunk. J. Am. Coll. Cardiol. *7*:366, 1986.
180. Cheitlin, M. D., De Castro, C. M., and McAllister, H. A.: Sudden death as a complication of anomalous left coronary origin from the anterior sinus of Valsalva: A not so minor congenital anomaly. Circulation *50*:780, 1974.
181. Maron, B. J., Roberts, W. C., McAllister, H. A., et al.: Sudden death in young athletes. Circulation *62*:218, 1980.
182. Mark, A. L., Abboud, F. M., Schmidt, P. G., and Heistad, D. D.: Reflex vascular responses to left ventricular outflow obstruction and activation of ventricular baroreceptors in dogs. J. Clin. Invest. *52*:1147, 1982.
183. Garson, A., Gillette, P. C., Gutgesell, H. P., and McNamara, D. G.: Stress-induced ventricular arrhythmias after repair of tetralogy of Fallot. Am. J. Cardiol. *46*:1006, 1980.
184. Driscoll, D. J., Danielson, O. K., Puga, F. J., et al.: Exercise tolerance and cardiorespiratory response to exercise after the Fontan operation for tricuspid atresia or functional single ventricle. J. Am. Coll. Cardiol. *7*:1087, 1986.
185. Manning, J. A.: Insurability and employability of young cardiac patients. *In* Engle, M. A. (ed.): Pediatric Cardiovascular Disease. Philadelphia, F. A. Davis Co., 1981.
186. Sillanpaa, M.: Social adjustment and functioning of chronically ill and impaired children and adolescents. Acta. Paediatr. Scand. *340*[Suppl]:1, 1987.
187. Baer, P. E., Freedman, D. A., and Garson, A.: Long-term psychological follow-up of patients after corrective surgery for tetralogy of Fallot. J. Am. Acad. Child Psychiatry *5*:622, 1984.
188. Dickinson, D. F., and Sambrooks, J. E.: Intellectual performance in children after circulatory arrest with profound hypothermia in infancy. Arch. Dis. Child. *54*:1, 1979.
189. Perloff, J. K.: Residua and sequelae. *In* Perloff, J. K., and Child, J. S. (eds.): Congenital Heart Disease in Adults. Philadelphia, W. B. Saunders Company, 1991, p. 251.
190. Stark, J.: Do we really correct congenital heart defects? J. Thorac. Cardiovasc. Surg. *97*:1, 1989.
191. Grossman, W.: Cardiac hypertrophy: useful adaptation or pathologic process? Am. J. Med. *69*:576, 1980.
192. Zak, R., Kizu, A., and Bugaisay, L.: Cardiac hypertrophy: its characteristics as a growth process. Am. J. Cardiol. *44*:941, 1979.
193. Anversa, P., Ricci, R., and Olivetti, G.: Quantitative structural analysis of the myocardium during physiologic growth and induced cardiac hypertrophy: A review. J. Am. Coll. Cardiol. *7*:1140, 1986.
194. Ghani, Q. P., and Hollenberg, M.: Poly-adenosine biphosphate ribose metabolism and regulation of myocardial cell growth by oxygen. Biochem. J. *170*:378, 1978.
195. Hathaway, D. R., and March, K. L.: Molecular cardiology: New avenues for the diagnosis and treatment of cardiovascular disease. J. Am. Coll. Cardiol. *13*:265, 1989.
196. Cutilleta, A. F., Bowell, R. T., Rudnik, M., et al.: Regression of myocardial hypertrophy: I. Experimental model, changes in heart weight, nucleic acids and collagen. J. Molec. Cell. Cardiol. *7*:67, 1975.
197. Horowitz, L. N., Alexander, J. A., and Edmunds, L. H.: Postoperative right bundle branch block: Identification of three levels of block. Circulation *62*:319, 1980.
198. Bharati, S., and Lev, M.: Sequelae of atriotomy on the endocardium, conduction system and coronary arteries. *In* Engle, M. A. and Perloff, J. K. (eds.): Congenital Heart Disease after Surgery. New York, Yorke Medical Books, 1983.
199. Miller, A. J., Pick, R., and Katz, L. N.: Ventricular endomyocardial change after impairment of cardiac lymph flow in dogs. Br. Heart J. *25*:182, 1963.

Chapter 31
Acquired Heart Disease in Infancy and Childhood

WILLIAM F. FRIEDMAN

NONRHEUMATIC INFLAMMATORY DISEASE .988
Infective Myocarditis 988
Infective Pericarditis 990
Postpericardiotomy Syndrome 990

PRIMARY CARDIOMYOPATHIES 990
Idiopathic Dilated Cardiomyopathy 990
Endocardial Fibroelastosis 991

SECONDARY CARDIOMYOPATHIES 992
Cardiomyopathy in Infants of Diabetic Mothers..........................992
Glycogen Storage Disease 992
Neonatal Thyrotoxicosis 993
Infantile Beriberi 993
Protein-Calorie Malnutrition 994
Tropical Endomyocardial Fibrosis 994
Kawasaki Disease (Mucocutaneous Lymph Node Syndrome)....................994
Anthracycline Toxicity 997

SYSTEMIC HYPERTENSION 997

HYPERLIPIDEMIAS 1003

REFERENCES 1004

Because many of the topics discussed in this chapter are given more substantial coverage elsewhere in this text, the emphasis herein is placed on features of acquired heart disease that are relatively unique to or common in infancy and childhood, although the disease processes per se may not recognize age-related boundaries. Acute rheumatic fever and rheumatic heart disease are discussed in Chapter 55. The hyperlipidemias are discussed in Chapter 35.

NONRHEUMATIC INFLAMMATORY DISEASE

Infective Myocarditis

(See also Chapter 41)

Infectious processes that cause inflammatory disease of the heart may occur at any age, including fetal life. Causative agents include viruses, ricketsiae, bacteria, spirochetes, fungi, protozoa, and helminths. As a general rule, few of the generalized illnesses caused by these agents feature significant involvement of the heart. Myocardial involvement may be demonstrated histologically, but in most cases little or no expression of cardiac inflammation is detected clinically. Important exceptions are infections caused by certain viruses, diphtheria, and trypanosomes; these are discussed individually below.

VIRAL MYOCARDITIS. Coxsackie B and rubella viruses are the most common causative agents in infective myocarditis of the newborn. The rubella embryopathy and its associated cardiovascular malformations are discussed on page 878. Active *rubella myocarditis* occurs in utero, and may cause varying degrees of myocardial damage.[1] Invariably, however, other cardiovascular manifestations of the rubella syndrome dominate the clinical picture.

Coxsackie B typically causes outbreaks of epidemic myocarditis but may occur in the isolated infant in the newborn nursery, commonly with a fatal outcome.[2] The illness is of sudden onset and is characterized by fever, tachycardia, signs of systemic hypoperfusion, cyanosis, and, occasionally, cardiac failure. In some infants signs and symptoms of encephalomyelitis and hepatitis predominate. The diagnosis is suggested by electrocardiographic findings of atrial and/or ventricular arrhythmias, generalized ST-segment and T-wave changes, and low-voltage QRS complexes, accompanied by the appearance of marked generalized cardiomegaly and pulmonary vascular congestion on the chest roentgenogram. Echocardiography reveals dilatation of both ventricles and depressed indices of cardiac performance. Echocardiography is especially helpful in excluding congenital cardiac structural anomalies. The diagnosis is strongly suggested or confirmed when the virus can be isolated from pericardial fluid, pharyngeal secretions, or feces and when elevations occur in type-specific–neutralizing, hemagglutination-inhibiting, or complement-fixing antibody.[3] The immune system plays a role in the pathogenesis of myocarditis, and pathogenic autoantibodies to cardiac sarcolemma and myofibrils (known antigens in various anti-inflammatory heart diseases) have been identified.[4] These antibodies are up-regulated by viral stimulation, fix complement, and exert cytolytic and cytotoxic effects in vitro. Digitalis, diuretics, and general supportive measures are of limited benefit. Although increased sensitivity to the toxic effects of the glycosides is common, digitalis should be administered cautiously and continued until heart size is normal because cardiac failure may recur when the drug is discontinued.

Numerous viral agents have been identified as a cause of myocarditis in childhood beyond infancy.[5–7] The most common are Coxsackie A and B, influenza, adenovirus, and ECHO virus. Moreover, myocarditis, usually of mild degree, may be associated with the common viral infectious diseases of childhood, including mumps, measles, infectious mononucleosis, varicella, and variola. Although the diagnosis usually is one of exclusion, it may be suggested by the presence of sustained tachycardia out of proportion to fever, cardiomegaly without significant murmurs, poor-quality heart sounds, a gallop rhythm, an unexplained arrhythmia, and the electrocardiographic findings already mentioned.

Radionuclide gallium-67 scanning of the heart, showing a dense gallium uptake, provides suggestive evidence of active myocarditis.[8] Technetium-labeled leukocyte scanning may also prove useful in evaluation.[9] Magnetic resonance imaging holds promise for the noninvasive diagnosis of acute myocarditis, showing consistently greater than normal myocardial/skeletal muscle signal intensity ratios.[10] Although endomyocardial biopsy is a reasonably safe procedure in infants, children, and adolescents, a poor correlation exists between clinical and endomyocardial biopsy diagnoses of acute myocarditis in these age groups.[11–14] However, the recent development of in situ hybridization and polymerase chain reaction gene amplification technology may provide direct evidence by detecting enterovirus genome in the myocardium, greatly facilitating etiological diagnosis.[14a] Important differential diagnostic possibilities include endocardial fibroelastosis, glycogen storage disease with cardiac involvement, anomalous pulmonary origin of a coronary artery, critical aortic stenosis in infancy, and coarctation of the aorta or hypoplastic left heart syndromes.

The vast majority of these children recover from the acute episode of myocarditis with few or no sequelae. The results of treating patients with antiviral therapy or with immunosuppressants and antiinflammatory drugs have been inconclusive or disappointing.[13,15,16] Evidence that viral persistence in the myocardium may signify a poor prognosis raises the hope that antiviral therapy may prove beneficial in the future.[17] In some centers, high-dose intravenous gamma-globulin is administered to all children with presumed acute myocarditis. Results suggest that this approach results in better survival and improved recovery of left ventricular function.[18] Some patients may retain a permanent conduction defect or mild cardiac enlargement as a result of the acute illness. Moreover, a child may progress from the acute episode to a chronic dilated cardiomyopathy, characterized by signs of left ventricular dysfunction and mitral valve insufficiency. Unfortunately there are no predictive criteria to identify the latter situation.[19] Cardiac transplantation has been successful in some of these children with cardiomyopathy and a chronic, relentless, and refractory course of heart failure. However, cardiac transplantation in children, especially in infants or very young children, is complicated by growth suppression related to the required corticosteroid doses, and the complexity and severity of the immunosuppression in these infection-prone age groups.

DIPHTHERITIC CARDIOMYOPATHY

Diphtheria usually occurs in unimmunized children, especially in the western United States. Cardiac involvement is the result of the bacterial endotoxin rather than cardiac invasion by the bacillus.[20] Cardiac dysfunction appears to be related to abnormal fat metabolism because diphtheria toxin causes marked depletion of myocardial carnitine, a cofactor required for the beta-oxidation of fats.[21] Thus, what was formerly designated a form of myocarditis is now considered an acute metabolic cardiomyopathy. The pathology includes extensive intracellular fat vacuolization and glycogen depletion. Plasma carnitine deficiences have also been found in children with other forms of dilated cardiomyopathy.[22]

Cardiac involvement occurs in about 10 per cent of affected patients and is the most common cause of death from this disease. Heart disease is most reliably indicated by electrocardiographic changes, which range from ST-segment and T-wave changes to arrhythmias and conduction disturbances, including complete heart block.[23] Occasionally, the electrocardiographic pattern of myocardial infarction may emerge. The electrocardiogram is a fair indicator of the extent of myocardial involvement and of prognosis. The latter usually is favorable if only ST-segment and T-wave changes are observed in the absence of conduction system disturbances. Right or left bundle branch block and complete atrioventricular block are associated with mortality rates of 50 to 80 per cent. The electrocardiographic findings may be accompanied by evidence of myocardial dysfunction and ventricular chamber dilatation on cardiac ultrasound.

MANAGEMENT. Treatment of diphtheritic cardiomyopathy usually is unsatisfactory. All patients should receive diphtheria anti-toxin and intravenous penicillin after appropriate skin testing. Corticosteroid therapy is of no value. Digitalis should be administered cautiously because it may increase atrioventricular block. Diuretics and antiarrhythmic medications usually are indicated; transvenous pacemaker therapy is instituted for complete AV block.[23a] Parenteral administration of carnitine (100 mg/kg/day) has been found to partially reverse diphtheritic cardiac dysfunction and reduce the risk of cardiac death.[24] This observation requires confirmation. If the child recovers from the acute episode of diphtheritic cardiomyopathy, the prognosis is quite good.

MYOCARDITIS CAUSED BY TRYPANOSOMAL INFECTION

Chagas' disease (p. 1442) is a chronic parasitosis caused by *Trypanosoma cruzi*, transmitted to humans by the bite of insects in the reduviid family. In the United States the disease is seen mostly in the southern states; endemic infection occurs in Latin America. Its most important clinical manifestation is a late-developing, chronic myocarditis and, much less frequently, an early acute myocarditis that is fatal in up to 10 per cent of cases.[25] In approximately 30 per cent of patients who survive the acute stage, cardiomyopathy may occur after an interval of 10 to 30 years.

DIAGNOSIS. The cardiac findings are often accompanied by digestive and autonomic disorders. It has been suggested that parasitic neuroaminodase may alter cell membrane gangliosides in target tissues.[26]

Diagnosis of the acute illness is supported by findings of edema and adenitis in the region of the insect bite, associated with low-grade intermittent fever, sweating, muscle pain, and, at times, diarrhea and vomiting; weeks or months later cardiomegaly, gallop rhythm, and conduction disturbances may be noted. Xenodiagnosis (examination of the excreta of laboratory-bred insects fed on the patient) or complement-fixation tests provide confirmation. Newer approaches are promising to improve direct detection of parasites by polymerase chain reaction amplification techniques.[27–29]

Endomyocardial biopsy reveals mitochondrial, nuclear, and cell membrane abnormalities early in the myocardial degenerative process. Late stages are characterized by severe myofibrillar lysis and variable amounts of fibrous tissue and cellular infiltrates.[30]

There is no satisfactory treatment.[30a] Administrtion of mixed gangliosides intramuscularly may be beneficial in reducing arrhythmias.[31] Treatment of ventricular tachycardia with drugs guided by electrophysiological study may improve survival in chronic chagasic patients with this complication.[32] Prophylaxis consists of control of the carrier of the parasites, reduviid bugs, by benzene hexachloride. Nitrofuran compounds, nifurtimox and benznidazole, appear effective in the acute stage of infection but not during the intracellular parasitic infection period.[33] Recently, binary and tertiary combinations of sterol biosynthesis inhibitors (ketoconazole, terbinafine, mevanolin) have shown strong antiproliferative, synergistic action in vitro on *T. cruzi* and in a murine model,[34,35] suggesting that this novel approach may achieve clinical significance.

Trypanosoma rhodesiense, which causes African sleeping sickness, may also produce myocardial hemorrhage, interstitial edema, mononuclear infiltration, and myocardial degeneration.[36] Cardiac involvement is usually relatively mild, and the clinical picture is dominated by evidence of encephalitis.

MYOCARDITIS CAUSED BY HUMAN IMMUNODEFICIENCY VIRUS (see also p. 1438). In infants and children, the cardiac complications of the acquired immunodeficiency syndrome (AIDS) range from incidental microscopic inflammatory findings at necropsy to clinically significant, extensive, and chronic cardiac dysfunction.[37–39] In most children infected with the human immunodeficiency virus (HIV), the virus appears to have been transmitted from mother to child; other routes of transmission include contaminated blood products. Older children or adolescents also can be infected by routes more commonly associated with adults, such as sharing needles used for the injection of drugs, and sexual activity.

Cardiovascular abnormalities have been observed in as many as 65 per cent of infants or children with AIDS, whether induced by opportunistic infection or by the HIV infection itself.[40] As the prevalence of AIDS escalates, it is predictable that the cardiac involvement in infants and children with this disease will become better defined. Ventricular dysfunction, pericardial effusion, dilated cardiomyopathy, and rhythm disturbances (including high-grade atrial and ventricular ectopy and sudden death) provide evidence that HIV infection may have multiple direct or indirect effects on the heart. The latter may be due to infection with a variety of opportunistic organisms as well as to toxins, drugs, and autoimmunity.[40a] Other possible contributors to the cardiomyopathy include the myocardial depressant action of overwhelming noncardiac infection, the hypoxic and ischemic influence of severe lung disease, renal failure, autonomic dysfunction, chronic anemia, malnutrition, elevated endogenous catecholamines, vasoactive substances related to stress, and therapeutic interventions, including the use of steroids. Serial noninvasive assessment of this patient population, particularly by echocardiography, will, it is hoped, enable early or even anticipatory medical therapy, improving the cardiovascular status of children with HIV infection.

MYOCARDITIS IN LYME DISEASE (see also p. 1440). Transmitted to humans via the saliva of the deer tick *Ixodes dammini*, Lyme disease is caused by the spirochete, *Borrelia burgdorferi*. The disease is endemic in the northeastern United States, Wisconsin, and Minnesota and is associated with carditis in approximately 10 per cent of cases. Lyme disease occurs usually in stages, manifested initially by a characteristic skin lesion (erythema chronicum migrans) and flulike symptoms. If left untreated, it may progress to neurological, arthritic, and cardiac manifestations. Attempts to culture the organism are usually unsuccessful; an enzyme-linked immunosorbent assay is commonly employed to detect antibody to *B. burgdorferi*.[41] Cardiac involvement is usually a late manifestation expressed as various degrees of atrioventricular block, myopericarditis, and myocardial dysfunction. Nuclear isotope testing showing increased gallium-67 uptake, or by means of indium-111 antimyosin antibody scintigraphy, supports but is not specific for cardiac involvement. Early antibiotic treatment with penicillin, amoxicillin, doxycline, or ceftriaxone may prevent Lyme carditis.[42] Despite scattered reports of possible benefit from corticosteroids or salicylates, their therapeutic role has not been established. In children with high degrees of atrioventricular block, a finding that usually resolves with treatment, temporary transvenous pacing may be necessary.

Infective Pericarditis

(See also p. 1505)

Numerous infectious agents may be responsible for infective pericarditis. Viral and tuberculous inflammatory pericardial diseases are discussed in detail in Chapter 43. Of special concern in infancy and childhood is disease caused by pyogenic bacteria.[43,44] Purulent pericarditis occurs most often in the first two decades of life and is especially common in children under 6 years of age. Acute bacterial pericarditis usually is fatal if misdiagnosed or incorrectly treated. The most common pathogens are *Staphylococcus aureus, Streptococcus pneumoniae, Haemophilus influenzae*, and *Neisseria meningitides*. Unusual organisms that cause purulent pericarditis include *Escherichia coli, Pseudomonas, Salmonella, Klebsiella*, Proteus, and *Bacteroides. H. influenzae*, in particular, affects infants and young children, usually in association either with upper respiratory tract infection and croup, with lower respiratory tract pneumonia, bronchitis, or, occasionally, with meningitis.

Presenting clinical signs and symptoms vary, depending on the age of the patient, the responsible organism, and the site(s) of associated infection. The latter two require identification if therapy is to be effective. Fever, tachycardia, dyspnea, and chest pain are invariably present. Pericardial exudate resulting from the acute suppurative process commonly produces signs of life-threatening cardiac tamponade. Physical findings suggestive of purulent pericarditis include neck vein distention and hepatomegaly, pulsus paradoxus, and/or systemic hypotension with a narrow pulse pressure, muffled and distant heart sounds, marked cardiomegaly, and a point of maximal cardiac impulse well within the area of percussed dullness. Although the presence of a pericardial friction rub clearly points to pericardial involvement, this sign occurs infrequently.

An enlarged, globular cardiac configuration on chest radiography, electrocardiographic findings of diminished QRS amplitude, and abnormalities of the ST segment (usually elevated) and T waves (often inverted) usually focus attention on the pericardium. Echocardiographic evaluation (see p. 93) is reliable for establishing the diagnosis of significant pericardial effusion and for directing and guiding pericardiocentesis.[45] Culture and examination of pericardial fluid obtained by pericardiocentesis are essential for diagnosis and treatment.[46] Unless effective surgical drainage is combined with antibiotic treatment, the mortality rate is high. Operation should consist of creation of a subxiphoid pericardial window with placement of a drainage tube, or anterior pericardiectomy with tube drainage.[47] Early aggressive diagnosis and treatment reduce the risk of death substantially (10 to 20 per cent).[46] Pericardial constriction is uncommon, but all patients should be followed carefully for this complication.[48]

Postpericardiotomy Syndrome

(See also p. 1520)

In the first year after cardiac operation in which the pericardium is opened, and seldom in the second or third postoperative year, a febrile illness may occur, consisting of a pericardial and pleural inflammatory reaction with effusion and often with pulmonary parenchymal involvement. The illness occurs in 25 to 30 per cent of children undergoing pericardiotomy and usually is self-limiting; infants undergoing open-heart surgery are seldom affected. It is characterized by fever; chest, neck, or shoulder pain that becomes worse with inspiration; anorexia; and laboratory findings of leukocytosis and an elevated erythrocyte sedimentation rate.[49] Recurrences are uncommon and usually mild. Physical, electrocardiographic, and roentgenographic signs of pericardial involvement vary with the magnitude of the effusion. Echocardiographic detection of the effusion is common between 4 and 10 days postoperatively.[50] Cardiac tamponade, although not usual, occurs with sufficient frequency to warrant careful observation of the patient.

Viral infection and an autoimmune reaction have been implicated in the pathogenesis. Serum antibodies and a rise in titer frequently are found in reaction to adenovirus, Coxsackievirus, and cytomegalovirus. Elevations in levels of heart-reactive antibody are common.

An association recently has been shown between antinuclear antibodies, which are immunoglobulins directed toward antigenic nuclear material, and postpericardiotomy syndrome.[51]

The syndrome must be distinguished from infective endocarditis and the postperfusion syndrome of atypical lymphocytosis and hepatosplenomegaly, which occurs about 3 to 6 weeks after extracorporeal circulation and is caused by cytomegalovirus infection.[52]

.Treatment of the postpericardiotomy syndrome depends on the degree of patient discomfort and the magnitude of pericardial and/ or pleural effusion. In some patients signs of cardiac tamponade require pericardiocentesis. Bed rest and salicylates or indomethacin lessen patient discomfort and diminish the production of pleural or pericardial fluid. Corticosteroids are employed by some in all cases; most consider them indicated for severe illness because steroids promptly relieve fever and symptoms.[53] Antibiotics are not useful in the treatment. Prolonged therapy is seldom necessary because of the self-limited nature of this postoperative complication. Late or recurrent tamponade, although rare, may require reinstitution of treatment.[54]

PRIMARY CARDIOMYOPATHIES

(See also Chap. 41)

The important *nonobstructive* cardiomyopathies, of special concern in infants and children, are idiopathic dilated (congestive) cardiomyopathy and the familial forms of endocardial fibroelastosis,[55,56] which afflict many of the patients also designated as having *dilated cardiomyopathy*.[57–61] By definition these diagnostic terms exclude patients whose myocardial dysfunction is caused by active infection, a congenital cardiac anomaly, or increased preload or afterload. Dilated (congestive) cardiomyopathy often is a disease of infants, with most cases becoming manifested before the age of 1 year, with a history of respiratory or diarrheal illness preceding the onset of cardiac symptoms. Severely ill patients may have endocardial fibroelastosis, although the latter can be confirmed definitely only after myocardial biopsy or autopsy.[62] Beyond age 2 years, dilated cardiomyopathy, like the condition in adults, is characterized by an unobstructed, dilated, and poorly contracting left ventricle.[63] For this group of children, debate exists as to whether endocardial fibroelastosis should be categorized as a separate entity under dilated or congestive cardiomyopathy, and whether it is an end stage of dilated cardiomyopathy of *any* cause.

Idiopathic Dilated Cardiomyopathy in Childhood

Approximately 90 per cent of all children presenting with dilated cardiomyopathy have no clearly identifiable cause, although it has long been speculated that a viral disease is a pivotal factor in the pathogenesis of the entity.[64–67] The application of molecular biology to clinical diagnosis, particularly techniques for gene amplification, have strengthened this hypothesis. Viral cytotoxicity, immunological responses, viral RNA persistence, and spasm of the coronary microvasculature have all been implicated in the development of the cardiomyopathy.

Dilated cardiomyopathy is characterized by a large dilated heart with poor biventricular systolic function. Signs and symptoms of congestive heart failure prevail. Symptoms consisting most often of fatigue and breathlessness are usually rapidly progressive. Examination reveals tachycardia, cardiomegaly, gallop rhythm, and hepatosplenomegaly. Cardiac murmurs are present in about half of patients, most of whom have the characteristic apical systolic murmur of mitral regurgitation.[68]

Chest roentgenography reveals marked generalized cardiomegaly with normal or congested pulmonary vascular markings. Most children have abnormal electrocardiograms showing hypertrophy, conduction disturbance, or ST-segment and T-wave abnormalities. Approximately 20 per cent of patients have arrhythmias, most of which are ventricular in origin. Two-dimensional echocardiography is virtually diagnostic of cardiomyopathy (Fig. 31–1). Dilated cardiac chambers are observed with generalized poor ventricular function. Mitral valve closure may be delayed, and aortic valve closure may occur earlier than normal. Valve regurgitation is detected readily by Doppler echocardiography. Calculations of left ventricular shortening fraction are helpful in both initial diagnosis and following the course of the disease, although measures of shortening fraction, left ven-

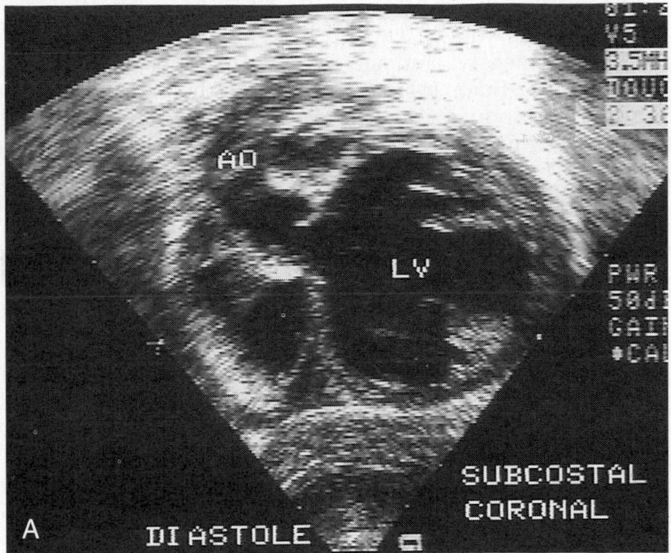

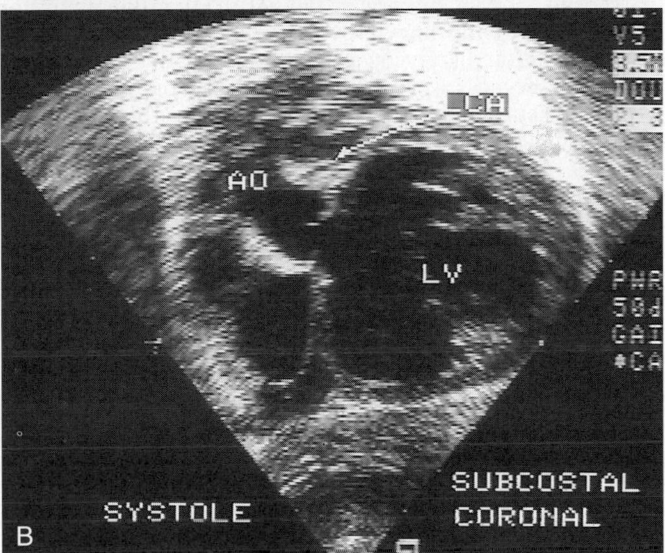

FIGURE 31–1. **Subcostal coronal echocardiographic views at end-diastole *(top)* and end-systole *(bottom)* from a 4-year-old with idiopathic dilated cardiomyopathy, demonstrating minimal contraction of the left ventricle (LV). Identification at end-systole of the left coronary artery (LCA) from the aortic root (AO) indicates this is not an example of anomalous pulmonary origin of the left coronary artery. (Courtesy of Norman H. Silverman, M.D.)**

tricular diastolic diameter, and wall mass have not been predictive of ultimate clinical outcome.[69–72,72a–c]

DIAGNOSIS. The diagnosis of dilated cardiomyopathy is generally one of exclusion. Differential diagnosis includes anomalous pulmonary origin of the left coronary artery, myocarditis, hypertrophic obstructive cardiomyopathy, anomalies that cause left ventricular outflow tract obstruction, and glycogen storage disease of the heart. The first four of these entities differ appreciably from dilated cardiomyopathy in their electrocardiographic or echocardiographic features; the skeletal muscle biopsy in glycogen storage disease is diagnostic.

Hemodynamic studies reveal evidence of left ventricular dysfunction. This includes elevations in left ventricular end-diastolic and left atrial pressures, moderate pulmonary hypertension, widened arteriovenous oxygen differences, and reduced left ventricular stroke volume and cardiac output. Angiography usually demonstrates a markedly dilated left ventricle, a reduced ejection fraction, and varying degrees of mitral regurgitation.

MANAGEMENT. This is directed at alleviating the signs and symptoms of congestive heart failure and includes the use of diuretics, inotropic support, afterload reduction, and antiarrhythmic therapy when indicated.[73–76] Heart transplantation is an acceptable therapy for end-stage cardiomyopathy.[77,78] The overall 2-year survival for children between the ages of 1 and 18 years exceeds 72 per cent. Identifying the child who is most gravely ill is the biggest problem in determining the timing of transplantation. The overall mortality of dilated cardiomyopathy approaches 35 per cent, the vast majority of fatal cases occurring during the first episode of cardiac failure.

Endocardial Fibroelastosis (EFE)

Various designations have been applied to this condition, including endocardial sclerosis, fetal endocarditis, fetal endomyocardial fibrosis, and elastic tissue hyperplasia.[58] In recent years familial cases have been encountered more commonly than has the isolated form. The data provided by family studies fit neither an autosomal recessive nor a multifactorial mode of inheritance. Although the reasons are obscure, a marked reduction has been observed in the past decade of isolated, nonfamilial EFE. No definite cause for this condition has been established, although a host of theories have been proposed; inadequate subendocardial blood flow and/or prenatal or postnatal inflammation or infection currently are considered the most likely pathogenetic pathways.[62,79]

A distinction has been made between primary EFE, in which there is no cardiac malformation, and EFE secondary to congenital malformations of the heart.[55] In the *secondary* variety, focal areas of opaque fibroelastotic thickening of the mural endocardium or cardiac valves are observed in association with cardiac malformations. Underlying cardiovascular anomalies are almost always obstructive lesions, particularly of the left side of the heart, and these create cardiac hypertrophy and an imbalance in the myocardial oxygen supply-demand relation. Thus, secondary EFE quite commonly occurs in aortic stenosis, coarctation of the aorta, and hypoplastic left heart syndrome.

The *primary* form of EFE invariably involves the left ventricle and mitral and aortic valves without significant associated cardiac defects. Although the use of the term "primary" implies that this form of EFE is a specific disease entity, most would agree that it is the end result of many different diseases.[62] Further, as already discussed, clear separation may not exist clinically between primary EFE and dilated cardiomyopathy. Primary EFE commonly produces a marked dilatation of the left ventricle; rarely, a "contracted" type of primary EFE is observed, in which the left ventricle is relatively hypoplastic or normal in size. In the latter situation the right and left atria and the right ventricle are markedly enlarged and hypertrophied, with minimal or no endocardial sclerosis. In the common, dilated type of primary EFE, microthrombi may be found adherent to the endocardium. The diffuse endocardial hyperplasia may be several millimeters thick (Fig. 31–2). The aortic and mitral valve leaflets are thickened and distorted; mitral regurgitation is especially common. The papillary muscles and chordae tendineae are involved in the fibroelastic process and are shortened and distorted.

Primary EFE is a disease of infancy; symptoms usually develop between 2 and 12 months of age, although rarely they may be present shortly after birth. Clinical features reflect left ventricular dysfunction and congestive heart failure.[80]

Echocardiographic features include an increase in left atrial and left ventricular dimensions, reduced left ventricular septal and posterior wall motion, reduced ejection fraction, and abnormal mitral valve motion. Dense echoes along the endocardium of the left ventricle are a diagnostic clue. *Endomyocardial biopsy* shows a diagnostic invasion of the endocardium and subendocardium by fibroelastic tissue.[11,14,81] The *contracted form* of primary EFE produces a clinical picture of left-sided obstructive disease, particu-

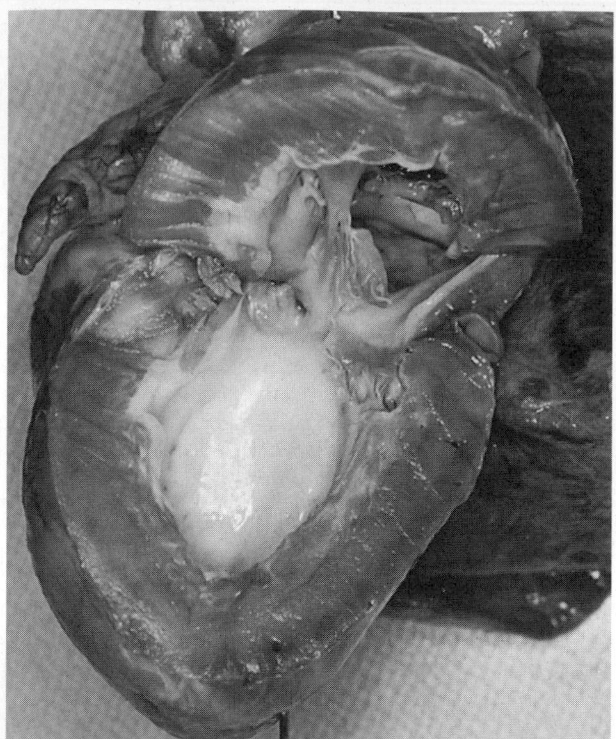

FIGURE 31–2. Diffuse left ventricular endocardial fibroelastosis. There is myocardial hypertrophy and obliteration of the papillary muscles as well as encroachment of the sclerotic subendocardial process onto the base of the aortic cusps. (From Tingelstaad, J. B., et al.: The electrocardiogram in the contracted type of primary endocardial fibroelastosis. Am. J. Cardiol. *27*:304, 1971.)

larly if the mitral valve is small. Left atrial pressure is elevated, with pulmonary artery pressures at or near systemic arterial levels.

The optimal management of patients with primary EFE consists of early and prolonged treatment with digitalis. Glycoside therapy should be continued for many years after the disappearance of symptoms, because cessation of the drug may result in acute cardiac failure, even when the heart size has returned to normal. The results of pericardial poudrage and mitral valve replacement in seriously afflicted infants have been disappointing. Cardiac transplantation may be recommended for those patients with end-stage disease.

SECONDARY CARDIOMYOPATHIES

The designation "secondary" cardiomyopathy refers to intrinsic myocardial disease that is secondary to or associated with systemic disease or diseases of other organs or in other systems. Myocardial disease coexisting with collagen vascular disorders (Chap. 56), neuromuscular disorders (Chap. 60), neoplasms (Chap. 57), acute glomerulonephritis (Chap. 62), and thalassemia and sickle cell disease (Chap. 57) are discussed elsewhere in this text. An abbreviated list of secondary cardiomyopathies in children is provided in Table 31–1. Of special interest to those caring for infants and children are the conditions seen in infants of diabetic mothers, and associated with glycogen storage disease, neonatal thyrotoxicosis, infantile beriberi, protein-calorie malnutrition, tropical endomyocardial fibrosis, anthracycline toxicity, and the mucocutaneous lymph node syndrome. Attention is directed to each of these latter disorders.

Cardiomyopathy in Infants of Diabetic Mothers

Infants born of gestational or established diabetic mothers are exposed to chronic hyperinsulinism in utero and to reactive hypoglycemia after birth. They are large for gestational age, often weighing more than 4 kg at birth, have organomegaly, and are subject to hypocalcemia and polycythemia. Such infants occasionally display two basic forms of cardiomyopathy, both of which usually are transient.[82–85] Evidence exists that suboptimal metabolic control of maternal diabetes during pregnancy increases the incidence of these abnormalities.[85] In some of these infants, hypertrophy and hyperplasia of myocardial cells constitute a diffuse process, producing reversible signs and symptoms that resemble those of congestive cardiomyopathy. In other infants, the clinical findings are indistinguishable from those of hypertrophic obstructive cardiomyopathy.[86] The natural history in this latter group has been one of gradual spontaneous regression within 1 to 12 months of obstructive murmurs, cardiomegaly, and electrocardiographic and echocardiographic abnormalities typical of hypertrophic obstructive cardiomyopathy.

Glycogen Storage Disease

Glycogen storage disease is the result of a deficiency of one or more of the enzymes involved in the biosynthesis and degradation of glycogen. Cardiomyopathy is rare but may be observed in types III, IV, and VI of this disease, each representing an enzymatic defect on the glycolytic pathway.[87] The heart is importantly involved in type II (Pompe's disease), which results from a deficiency of alpha-1,4-glucosidase (acid maltase), a lysosomal enzyme that hydrolyzes glycogen into glucose.[88] This disease is a hereditary error of metabolism transmitted through a single recessive gene. Generalized glycogenesis takes place, occurring especially in the heart, the skeletal muscles, and the liver. The glycogen within cardiac muscle cells is biochemically normal but is present in excessive amounts, both within lysosomes and free in the cytoplasm. As a result, the heart enlarges, often to a marked degree, and congestive heart failure supervenes. Glycogen deposition within the myocardium usually is uniform, although occasionally the

TABLE 31–1 COMMON SECONDARY CARDIOMYOPATHIES IN CHILDREN

Inflammatory
Postinfectious (viral, bacterial, fungal, protozoal, rickettsial, spirochetal)
Hypersensitivity
Giant cell
Neuromuscular
Muscular dystrophy
Myotonic dystrophy
Toxic
Alcohol
Anthracyclines (doxorubicin)
Lead
Cyclophosphamide
Vincristine
Infiltrative/fibrotic
Glycogen storage
Mucopolysaccharidoses
Hemochromatosis
Endomyocardial fibrosis
Metabolic
Infants of diabetic mothers
Carnitine deficiency
Nutritional deficiency (thiamine, kwashiorkor, selenium)
Thyroid disease
Catecholamine cardiomyopathy
Ischemic/anemic
Kawasaki disease
Familial hypercholesterolemia
Congenital coronary artery malformation
Sickle cell anemia

interventricular septum is especially involved, producing subpulmonic obstruction or a constellation of features indistinguishable from hypertrophic obstructive cardiomyopathy. Selective angiography has revealed a distinctive trabeculation of the left ventricle in some infants.[89]

Clinical signs of type II glycogen storage disease usually become prominent in the early neonatal period.[90,91] Characteristic symptoms include failure to thrive, progressive hypotonia, lethargy, and a weak cry. Prominent early features include nonspecific cardiac murmurs, cardiomegaly, signs of congestive heart failure, macroglossia, poor skeletal muscle tone, and weakness. The electrocardiogram shows extremely tall, broad QRS complexes with a short P-R interval (commonly less than 0.09 sec) (Fig. 31–3).

The short P-R interval may be the result of facilitated atrioventricular conduction owing to myocardial glycogen deposition. Less often, deep Q waves are observed over the mid or left precordium as are T-wave inversion and ST-segment elevation. Chest roentgenograms show an enlarged globular heart associated with pulmonary vascular congestion (Fig. 31–4). In rare patients with cardiac glycogenosis the cardiac murmur suggests left ventricular outflow tract obstruction and/or mitral regurgitation; the echocardiographic, hemodynamic, and angiographic features in this subgroup are indistinguishable from those in infants with hypertrophic obstructive cardiomyopathy. Diagnosis is confirmed by demonstrating the enzymatic deficiency in lymphocytes, skeletal muscle, or liver. Skeletal muscle biopsy reveals histological and histochemical evidence of glycogen deposition.

Cardiac glycogenosis may be confused with other entities that cause cardiac failure in the early months of life, including idiopathic dilated cardiomyopathy and endocardial fibroelastosis, anomalous pulmonary origin of the left coronary artery, fixed and dynamic forms of left ventricular outflow tract obstruction, coarctation of the aorta, and myocarditis. The short P-R interval and the skeletal muscle hypotonia in glycogen storage disease help to distinguish this disorder from dilated cardiomyopathy and *endocardial fibroelastosis*. Infants with an anomalous pulmonary origin of the *left coronary artery* usually have a distinctive electrocardiographic pattern of anterolateral myocardial infarction. In infants with *coarctation of the aorta* the pulse and blood pressure discrepancies between the upper and lower extremities point to the proper diagnosis (see p. 965). *Myocarditis* usually is of abrupt onset in a previously healthy child and is not associated with marked hypotonia; the generally low-voltage electrocardiogram does not show the short P-R interval. The skeletal muscle hypotonia and the macroglossia in infants with glycogen storage disease occasionally raise the possibilities of amyotonia congenita and cretinism or mongolism, respectively.

Cardiac glycogenosis leads to progressive impairment of myocardial function; Pompe's disease is uniformly fatal, usually within the first year of life. Death quite often is the result of either cardiac failure or complications of respiratory management such as pneumonia or aspiration.

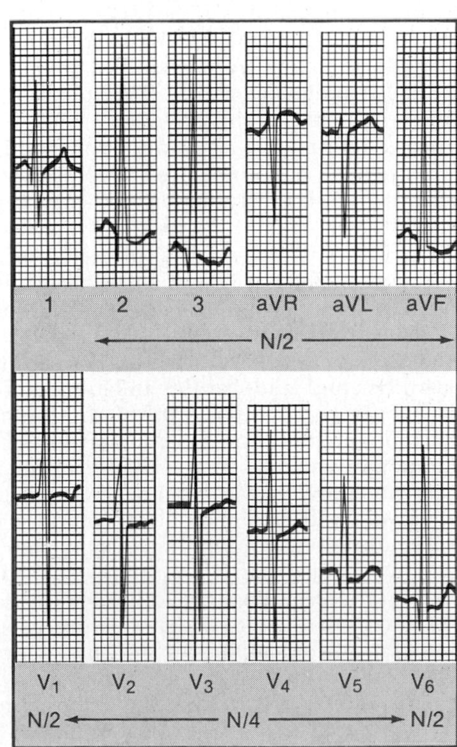

FIGURE 31–3. Electrocardiogram of an infant with glycogen storage disease showing a short PR interval and left ventricular hypertrophy.

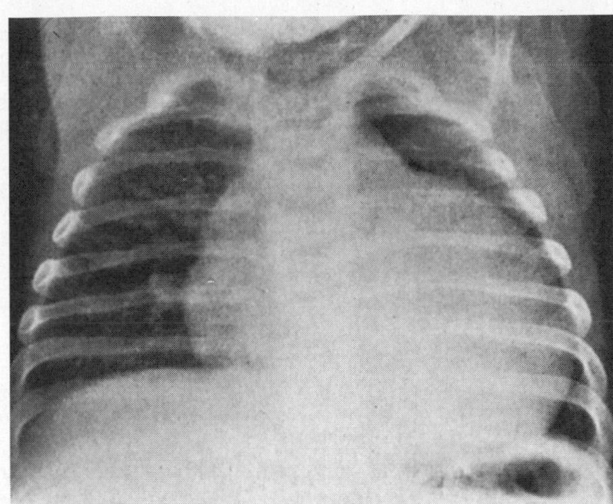

FIGURE 31–4. Chest roentgenogram of an infant with glycogen storage disease showing massive cardiomegaly and pulmonary edema. (From Taussig, H.: Congenital Malformations of the Heart. Vol. 2. 2nd ed. Boston, Commonwealth Fund, Harvard University, 1960, p. 901.)

Neonatal Thyrotoxicosis

Thyroid-stimulating immunoglobulin traverses the placental barrier and stimulates the fetal thyroid gland when maternal hyperthyroidism exists. Many infants are born prematurely or are small for gestational age. Jitteriness and irritability are noted early. Thyroid hormone has both direct and indirect effects on the heart and circulation.[92] Cardiac findings include tachycardia, bounding pulses, systolic hypertension, and a precordial systolic murmur. Congestive heart failure frequently is present, and the presenting finding occasionally is an episode of paroxysmal atrial tachycardia. A neonatal goiter may be observed, especially if the mother received iodine therapy during pregnancy.

Diagnosis should be anticipated whenever a history of hyperthyroidism exists in the mother. Neonatal thyrotoxicosis occurs in the offspring of about 1 to 2 per cent of these women. A maternal level of thyroid-stimulating immunoglobulin should be obtained before delivery in anticipation of the problem arising in the newborn infant because high levels often are observed in both mother and offspring. The serum levels of thyroxine are increased in the newborn.

The infant who has heart failure may be treated with digitalis and propylthiouracil or carbimazole. The latter two drugs are not completely effective for many weeks; a beta blocker usually is helpful in addition to these agents. Supportive measures such as sedation and minimal stimulation may be helpful. Exchange transfusion or corticosteroid treatment is of no proven benefit.

Infants usually improve between the second and third month of life, although lack of attention to the problem or inadequate therapy may result in a fatal outcome.

Infantile Beriberi

(See also p. 461)

Thiamine (vitamin B_1) deficiency mainly occurs in regions of Southeast Asia, India, Brazil, and Africa, in which the dietary staple is polished rice or cassava. Thiamine functions as a coenzyme in decarboxylation of alpha-keto acids and in the utilization of pentose in the hexose monophosphate shunt. A reduction in myocardial energy production causes symptoms in the infant, usually between 1 and 4 months of age, who is breast fed by a thiamine-deficient mother.[93] Rarely, improper and ill-advised parental feeding practices lead to the vitamin deficiency.[93a] Such infants usually are edematous, irritable, pale, and anorectic. Hoarseness or aphonia is common, owing to involvement of the recurrent laryngeal nerve; blepharoptosis occurs in one-third of infants. Typically, cardiac involvement manifests as dilation of the right ventricle and prominent signs of systemic venous congestion. Electrocardiographic findings are nonspecific, and radiological findings principally consist of right ventricular dilatation. Infantile beriberi may be rapidly fatal but responds quickly and well to administration of thiamine (25 to 50 mg intravenously initially, with reduction of the dose to 10 mg/day for several days, and then orally for several weeks). Dramatic amelioration occurs within a few days of the cardiac findings. Cure is complete with no known sequelae.

Protein-Calorie Malnutrition

(See also p. 1907)

This is a major public health problem in underdeveloped areas of the tropics.[94] In infants inadequate diet results in a state of emaciation termed "marasmus"; "kwashiorkor" is a designation applied to this syndrome in children beyond 1 year of age. The disease results from a deficiency of protein relative to calories, although the latter and other essential nutrients often are lacking as well. General muscle wasting, loss of subcutaneous fat, and atrophy of most organs, including the heart, are typical in marasmic infants. In both marasmus and kwashiorkor, thinning and atrophy of cardiac muscle fibers and interstitial edema or vacuolization of the myocardial fibers are noted.[95] As the condition progresses, listlessness becomes prominent. Cardiovascular collapse is easily precipitated in these infants by the stress of infection.

In both infancy and childhood the principal physical findings reflect systemic hypoperfusion and principally consist of hypothermia, hypotension, tachycardia, and low-amplitude peripheral arterial pulsations. Peripheral usually nonpitting edema is prominent, as are wasting of the skeletal musculature, exfoliative dermatitis, and gray or red discoloration of the hair. Changes seen on electrocardiogram and on radiographic examination are nonspecific.

Treatment should be directed at correction of fluid and electrolyte imbalance, eradication of infection, and management of such associated problems as anemia and parasitic infestation. Care is required in the correction of dehydration or severe anemia because volume overload of the heart is easily produced. Supplements of potassium and magnesium often are required, and because of deficiencies in these elements, digitalis should probably be avoided or used with extreme caution. If the infant or child survives the initial phase, a well-balanced diet effects an impressive recovery over several months' duration.

Tropical Endomyocardial Fibrosis

(See also p. 1431)

Endomyocardial fibrosis (endomyocardial disease) is a rare, acquired, progressive disease, usually involving children and young adults from Africa, Southeast Asia, and South America. This cardiomyopathy of unknown cause is characterized by focal endocardial fibrosis of one or, rarely, both ventricles.[96] Controversy exists as to whether or not endomyocardial fibrosis, which is not associated with eosinophilia, and Löffler's endocarditis with eosinophilia (Chap. 41) are the same disorder described from temperate climates.[97] Endocardial fibrosis is located almost exclusively in the inflow tracts of the ventricles and commonly involves one or the other atrioventricular valve. Partial obliteration of either cardiac chamber results in reduced ventricular compliance with impairment of filling. The fibrotic process often involves the chordae tendineae, resulting in mitral and/or tricuspid regurgitation. Plaques of heaped-up fibrous tissue without elastic fibers are especially common within the left ventricle. Endomyocardial fibrosis involving the right ventricle may have to be differentiated from Ebstein's anomaly of the tricuspid valve (see p. 934), and endomyocardial fibrosis involving the left ventricle may have to be differentiated from rheumatic mitral regurgitation.

When left ventricular disease predominates, the clinical findings often resemble those of mitral stenosis or regurgitation. When endocardial involvement of the right ventricle is more severe than that of the left ventricle, the patient usually presents with findings of markedly elevated systemic venous pressure and tricuspid regurgitation.

Treatment is supportive. Survival usually depends on the extent of endocardial and valvular involvement and is better when right ventricular disease predominates.[98] Mean survival after the onset of symptoms is about 24 months. Specific treatment does not exist, and corticosteroid therapy has not proved efficacious. Surgical excision (decortication) of affected tissue with prosthetic valve replacement has been associated with clinical improvement.[99] However, children most severely affected by this disease commonly reside in regions of the tropics and subtropics where cardiac surgery is not readily available.

Kawasaki Disease (Mucocutaneous Lymph Node Syndrome)

Kawasaki disease was first described in Japan in 1967. It is a generalized vasculitis of unknown etiology and a leading cause of acquired heart disease in the United States. Eighty per cent of cases occur in children less than 5 years of age, and most are under 2. Fewer than 2 per cent of patients have recurrences.

The syndrome presents with fever and ocular and oral manifestations followed in 5 days by a rash and indurative edema of the hands and feet, with palmar and plantar erythema. Finally, after about 2 weeks, cutaneous desquamation occurs. Diagnostic criteria include (1) a fever lasting for 5 or more days that is unresponsive to antibiotics; (2) bilateral congestion of the ocular conjunctiva; (3) peripheral limb changes that include an indurative peripheral edema and erythema of the palms and feet, followed later in the course of the illness by a membranous desquamation of the fingertips; (4) changes in the lips and mouth, including dry, erythematous, and fissured lips, injected oropharyngeal mucosa, and a strawberry tongue; (5) a polymorphous exanthema of the trunk without crusts or vesicles; and (6) cervical lymphadenopathy. Diagnosis is accepted when the first criterion and at least four of the remainder are present.[100]

In addition to the mucous membrane and cutaneous effects, multiple organ system involvement has been noted. Noncardiovascular complications of the illness include arthritis, cerebrospinal fluid pleocytosis, pulmonary infiltrates, hepatic dysfunction, and hydrops of the gallbladder. The illness often is accompanied by diarrhea, vomiting and abdominal pain, leukocytosis with a predominance of neutrophils, thrombocytosis, sterile pyuria and proteinuria, elevated liver transaminases, an elevation in the erythrocyte sedimentation rate, $alpha_1$-antitrypsin and serum immunoglobulin E, and a positive C-reactive protein.[100]

An extensive search for the cause of Kawasaki disease has been unproductive. The epidemiology and clinical presentation are highly suggestive of an infectious agent; person-to-person transmission is highly unlikely. Multiple immunoregulatory abnormalities have been suggested to be involved in the pathogenesis of the illness, with speculation that they result from profound superantigenic stimulation from microbial toxins. Abnormalities include marked polyclonal B-cell expansion; T-cell, monocyte, and macrophage activation; increased interleukins-1, -2, -6, and -8, tumor necrosis factor-alpha, and antibodies against endothelial cell antigens; and increased expression of heat shock protein.[101,102] Recent studies do not support a retroviral etiology.[103]

NATURAL HISTORY. On the basis of pathological data, progression of the disease may be divided into four stages.[104] In stage I, lasting for 1 to 9 days, acute perivasculitis of the small arteries is evident and involves the vasa vasorum of the major coronary arteries. Pericarditis, interstitial myocarditis, and endocardial inflammation also are seen; these changes chiefly consist of neutrophilic, eosinophilic, and lymphocytic infiltrations. In stage II, of 12 to 25 days' duration, panvasculitis involves the major coronary arteries. It affects the intima, media, and adventitia and results in aneurysm and thrombus formation. In stage III, of 28 to 31 days' duration, granulating thrombi and marked intimal thickening cause partial or total occlusion of the major coronary arteries. Stage IV follows and may be of many years' duration, during which healing occurs, consisting of scarring, calcification, and recanalization of occluded arteries.

The syndrome has an associated acute mortality of less than 1 per cent, secondary to complications from coronary artery involvement, myocarditis, or pericarditis, with a majority of deaths occurring in the third or fourth week of

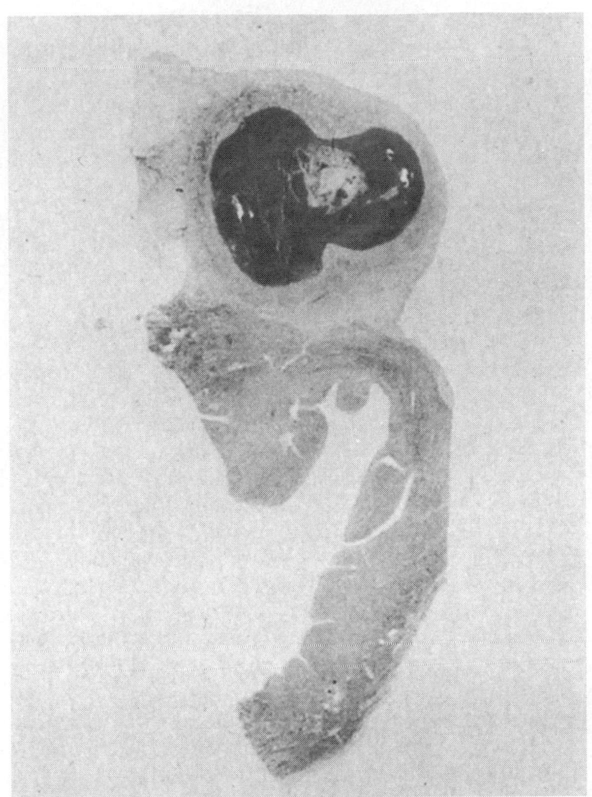

FIGURE 31–5. Low-power photomicrograph of a coronary artery aneurysm with recent occlusive thrombosis in a patient with mucocutaneous lymph node syndrome. (From Landing, B. H., and Larson, E. J.: Are infantile periarteritis nodosa with coronary artery involvement and fatal mucocutaneous lymph node syndrome the same? Comparison of 20 patients from North America with patients from Hawaii and Japan. Pediatrics *59*:651, 1977. Copyright American Academy of Pediatrics, 1977.)

illness.[105] Other children may die later in life as a result of myocardial infarction.[106,107] Autopsy examination has almost uniformly demonstrated coronary arterial aneurysms, with occlusion caused by thromboendarteritis (Fig. 31–5). The clinical and laboratory features are shown in Table 31–2 and the spectrum of cardiovascular involvement is outlined in Table 31–3. The factors associated with increased risk of developing coronary aneurysms include male gender, age less than 1 year, signs of pancarditis including arrhythmias, prolonged period of inflammation including fever lasting for more than 10 days, and recurrence of fever after an afebrile period of at least 24 hours.

The disease often has been misdiagnosed in the United States as scarlet fever, drug reaction, measles or other febrile viral exanthems, Stevens-Johnson syndrome, Rocky Mountain spotted fever, staphylococcal scalded skin syndrome, leptospirosis, or mercury poisoning.[100]

CARDIAC MANIFESTATIONS. Infants and children with this syndrome should be closely watched for signs of cardiac involvement. A significant number of patients show evidence of myocarditis or pericarditis, or both, in the early phases of the disease.[104] Pericardial effusion is detected by echocardiography in approximately 30 per cent of patients. It rarely progresses to tamponade and usually resolves without specific therapy. Electrocardiographic evidence of myocarditis with low voltage and nonspecific ST-T wave changes is seen in 45 per cent of patients, echocardiographic evidence of poor left ventricular function in 25 per cent, cardiomegaly on chest radiographs in 25 per cent, and a gallop rhythm in 12 per cent. Coronary arterial abnormalities develop in approximately 20 per cent of untreated patients and are the most common case of both short- and long-term morbidity and mortality.[107a] In these children aneurysms of the coronary arteries with narrowing, tortuosity, and obstruction are detected by two-dimensional echocardiography, aortography, and coronary angiography (Fig. 31–6).[107–112] The appearance more than 6 weeks after the onset of illness is uncommon.

Echocardiography is the primary tool for evaluation and follow-up of coronary abnormalities (Fig. 31–7). Detailed examination displays the left main, anterior descending, and left circumflex coronary arteries as well as the proximal, middle, and distal segments of the right and posterior coronary arteries. These vessels are seen in multiple planes using a combination of view windows. A conclusion that the coronary arteries are normal should not be reached until all major vessel segments have been visualized and determined to be normal.[107a] Intravascular imaging may

TABLE 31–2 CLINICAL AND LABORATORY FEATURES OF KAWASAKI DISEASE

Diagnostic criteria (principal clinical findings*)
Fever of at least 5 days' duration†
Presence of four of the following principal features:
Changes in extremities
Polymorphous exanthem
Bilateral conjunctival injection
Changes in the lips and oral cavity
Cervical lymphadenopathy
Exclusion of other diseases with similar findings
Other clinical and laboratory findings
Cardiac findings
Pancarditis, in early stages of disease
Coronary artery abnormalities, usually beyond 10 days of onset of illness
Noncardiac findings
Musculoskeletal system
Arthritis, arthralgia
Gastrointestinal tract
Diarrhea, vomiting, abdominal pain
Hepatic dysfunction
Hydrops of the gallbladder
Central nervous system
Extreme irritability
Aseptic meningitis
Respiratory tract
Post-respiratory illness
Otitis media
Pulmonary infiltrates
Other findings
Erythema and induration at Bacille Calmette-Guérin (BCG) inoculation site
Auditory abnormalities
Testicular swelling
Peripheral gangrene
Aneurysms of medium-sized noncoronary arteries
Laboratory findings
Neutrophilia with immature forms
Elevated erythrocyte sedimentation rate
Positive C-reactive protein
Elevated serum alpha$_1$-antitrypsin
Anemia
Hypoalbuminemia
Elevated serum immunoglobulin E
Thrombocytosis
Proteinuria
Sterile pyuria
Elevated serum transaminases

* Patients with fever and fewer than four principal clinical features can be diagnosed as having Kawasaki disease when coronary artery disease is detected by two-dimensional echocardiography or coronary angiography.

† Many experts believe that, in the presence of classic features, the diagnosis of Kawasaki disease can be made by experienced practitioners before the fifth day of fever.

From Dajani, A. S., Taubert, K. A., Gerber, M. A., et al.: Diagnosis and therapy of Kawasaki disease in children. Circulation *87*:1776–1780, 1993. Copyright 1993 American Heart Association.

TABLE 31–3 SPECTRUM OF CARDIOCIRCULATORY FINDINGS IN KAWASAKI DISEASE

CARDITIS (myocarditis, pericarditis)
- Congestive heart failure
- Arrhythmias

CORONARY ANGIITIS
- Thromboendarteritis—aneurysms
  - Regression
  - Thrombosis—recanalization
  - Obstruction—stenosis
  - Collaterals
  - Rupture
- Myocardial ischemia or infarction
  - Ventricular aneurysm
  - Papillary muscle dysfunction—mitral regurgitation

ARTERIAL INVOLVEMENT
- Pulmonary/renal angiitis—pulmonary/renal hypertension
- Arteritis, aneurysms: Femoral, iliac, brachial, cerebral, hepatic, etc.

allow more detailed visualization of coronary wall morphology and the healing process, as well as the analysis of coronary artery distensibility.[113]

About half of the children with coronary aneurysms diagnosed shortly after the acute phase of the disease subsides have normal-appearing vessels by angiography 1 or 2 years later.[114–116] Patients with giant aneurysms (internal diameter ≥8 mm) have the worst prognosis and greatest chance of developing coronary thrombosis, stenosis, or myocardial infarction. In those patients with residual cardiac abnormalities after recovery from the acute illness phase, a variety of findings have been described. These include impairment of left ventricular function secondary to the coronary arterial involvement, papillary muscle dysfunction with mitral regurgitation,[117] impaired left ventricular function,[118] and abnormalities of the distensibility of the coronary arteries (even after aneurysms have disappeared and no morphological abnormalities are recognized by coronary arteriography).[119]

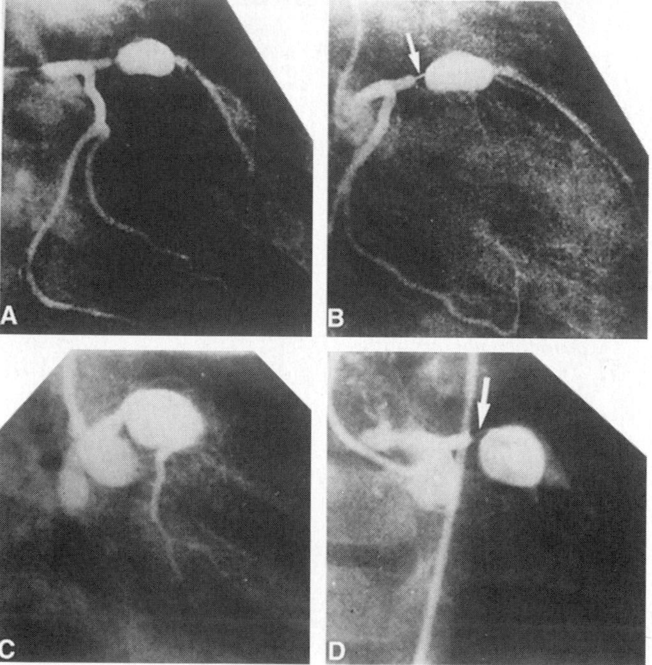

FIGURE 31–6. *A,* Left selective coronary angiogram at 30 degrees right anterior oblique projection, showing localized stenosis of about 75 per cent. *B,* Selective coronary angiogram, inclining to 60 degrees right anterior oblique, shows a 99 per cent stenosis (white arrow). *C,* Left selective coronary angiogram failed to demonstrate a localized stenosis because the catheter tip had been pushed into the aneurysm. *D,* In this selective coronary angiogram, the catheter tip at the ostium shows a localized 99 per cent stenosis at the inlet of the aneurysm *(arrow).* (From Tsubata, S., Suzuki, A., Ono, Y. et al.: Coronary arterial lesions due to Kawasaki disease: Selective coronary angiography in five cases with difficult-to-detect localized stenosis. Pediatr. Cardiol. *14:*169, 1993.)

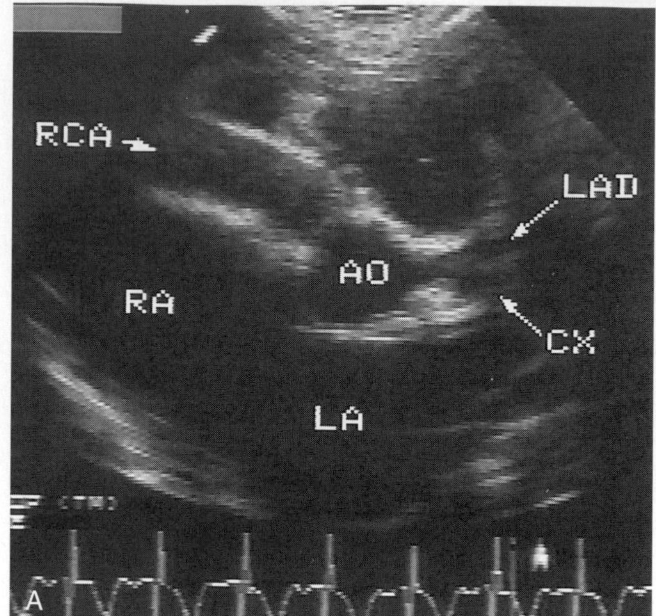

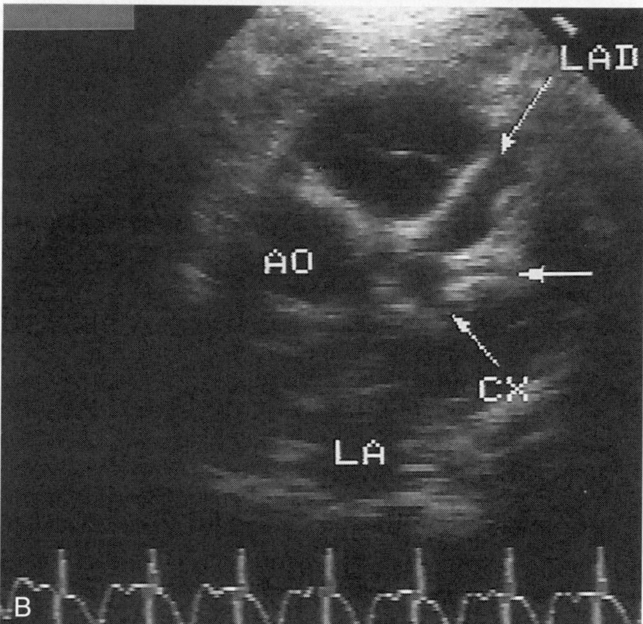

FIGURE 31–7. Parasternal short-axis echocardiographic views of the coronary arteries in a 2-year-old boy with Kawasaki disease. *A,* At the level of the aortic root (AO), a giant fusiform coronary aneurysm of the right coronary artery (RCA) and enlargement of the left anterior descending (LAD) and circumflex (Cx) coronary arteries. *B,* A close-up view of the left coronary artery system demonstrating a fusiform aneurysm of the left anterior descending coronary artery (LAD) and a proximal aneurysm of the circumflex coronary artery (Cx). The arrow between the LAD and Cx indicates a prominent obtuse marginal branch. RA = right atrium, LA = left atrium. (Courtesy of Norman H. Silverman, M.D.)

MANAGEMENT. Initial therapy during the acute stage for Kawasaki disease is directed at reducing inflammation, especially in the coronary arterial tree and myocardium. Later, treatment is directed toward preventing coronary thrombosis by inhibiting platelet aggregation. Specific treatment awaits discovery of the etiological agent.[100]

Current therapy is outlined in Table 31–4. It appears that corticosteroid therapy is detrimental during the acute ill-

TABLE 31–4 TREATMENT FOR ACUTE STAGE OF KAWASAKI DISEASE

Intravenous gamma-globulin (IVGG)
2 gm/kg as single infusion over 12 hours
PLUS
Aspirin
80–100 mg/kg/day orally in four equally divided doses until patient is afebrile
THEN
3–5 mg/kg orally once daily up to 6–8 weeks*

* Discontinue 6–8 weeks after onset of illness if no coronary artery abnormalities are present by echocardiography. Continue indefinitely if there are coronary artery abnormalities.

ness. Many children with Kawasaki disease fail to achieve therapeutic serum concentrations of salicylate despite high oral dosage because of impaired gastrointestinal absorption.[120,121] Therefore, monitoring of serum salicylate levels is advisable.

All children diagnosed with Kawasaki disease within 10 days of onset of fever should receive intravenous gamma-globulin and high-dose aspirin as early as possible.[100] Trials comparing single with multiple dose gamma-globulin schedules favor the former.[122,123] Intravenous gamma-globulin reduces the likelihood of development of giant coronary artery aneurysms and appears to have a direct beneficial effect on abnormalities in cardiac function associated with the acute phase of Kawasaki disease. Intravenous gamma-globulin should also be considered for patients in whom a diagnosis of Kawasaki disease is made after day 10 of the illness if they have signs of ongoing inflammation or evolving coronary artery disease. Also, some patients already have coronary arterial abnormalities within 10 days of onset of fever. These patients should receive aspirin and intravenous gamma-globulin. It should be recognized that the mechanism of action of intravenous gamma-globulin in Kawasaki disease is unknown. Although the costs of intravenous gamma-globulin are high, studies have shown that lower rates of coronary artery involvement result in lower overall medical costs.[124]

In some patients with acute coronary thrombosis, especially those with giant coronary aneurysms, intracoronary thrombolytic therapy may prevent total occlusion of the artery.[125] The prognosis of children with vascular involvement should be guarded[125a]; some are candidates for percutaneous transluminal coronary angioplasty, bypass grafting, and cardiac transplantation.[126–128] The patency rate of saphenous vein grafts is generally unsatisfactory; bypasses using the internal mammary artery and gastroepiploic artery grafts appear to offer better long-term patency and growth in caliber than saphenous vein grafts.[129]

The approach to follow-up of patients with coronary involvement employs the judicious use of exercise testing,[129a] echocardiography, and radionuclide and angiographic studies to detect and evaluate occlusive lesions.

Anthracycline Toxicity

(See also p. 1800)

Anthracycline drugs such as doxorubicin and daunorubicin and the newer derivatives, used as cancer chemotherapeutic agents, cause a dose-related cardiomyopathy.[130,131] The risk of cardiac involvement increases significantly with doses in excess of 400 mg/m². The onset of cardiac symptoms often is delayed, occurring 2 to 3 months after the anthracycline dose. Cardiac dysfunction usually presents first as unexplained tachycardia, progressing to dyspnea, congestive heart failure, hepatomegaly, and, often, death. The cardiomyopathy most often is reversible only in its early stages.[132] Later, it usually is poorly responsive to digitalis, diuretics, and afterload-reducing agents. Quite often patients are in remission from their neoplasm when the drug's cardiotoxicity proves lethal. Sequential monitoring of cardiac function of patients undergoing chemotherapy allows identification of subclinical cardiotoxicity.[131] Guidelines have been formulated for cardiac monitoring for both modifying therapy and long-term assessment (Fig. 31–8).[131] Long-term follow-up has disclosed elevated levels of left ventricular wall stress and impairment of diastolic function in children without overt cardiomyopathy. Further, there are occasional reports of late-onset heart failure in previously asymptomatic children many years after their cancer chemotherapy.

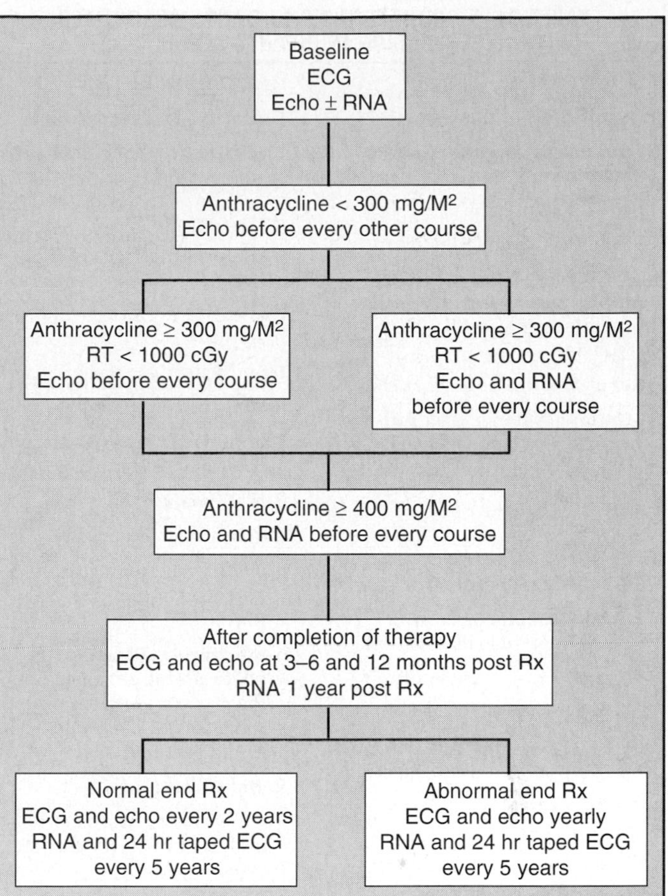

FIGURE 31–8. The monitoring of patients receiving anthracycline. ECG = electrocardiogram; Echo = echocardiogram; RNA = radionuclide angiocardiogram; RT = radiation therapy; Rx = therapy. (From Steinherz, L. J., Graham, T., Hurwitz, R., et al.: Guidelines for cardiac monitoring of children during and after anthracycline therapy: Report of the Cardiology Committee of the Children's Cancer Study Group. Pediatrics *89*:942–949, 1992. Copyright American Academy of Pediatrics, 1992.)

SYSTEMIC HYPERTENSION

(See also p. 822)

Unfortunately, many physicians consider hypertension a disease of adults and not children. Thus, all too frequently, blood pressure is not recorded during the pediatric physical examination. It should be emphasized that elevations in systemic blood pressure may occur in as many as 2 per cent of children, and it has been well documented that undetected or untreated hypertension may lead to unfortunate consequences.[133] Three points in particular require recognition[134]:

1. Causes of hypertension in infants and children differ markedly from those in adults. Most children have secondary rather than essential forms of hypertension (Table 31–5); therefore, it is important to search for a remedial cause.
2. Offspring of hypertensive parents are known to have an increased susceptibility to blood pressure elevation.
3. Children with elevated blood pressure require the same surveillance and treatment as adults.

Accurate blood pressure measurements require cuffs of different sizes because of the variation in arm size from infancy through adolescence. To measure blood pressure

TABLE 31–5 CONDITIONS AND DRUGS ASSOCIATED WITH HYPERTENSION IN INFANTS AND CHILDREN

CONGENITAL
- Coarctation of the aorta
- Gonadal dysgenesis (Turner syndrome)
- Rubella syndrome
- Pseudoxanthoma elasticum (Ehlers-Danlos syndrome)
- Ask-Upmark syndrome (segmental renal artery dysplasia)
- Renal arterial abnormalities
- Multiple systemic and pulmonary artery stenoses
- Solitary renal cyst
- Hydronephrosis

GENETIC
- Diabetes mellitus
- Neurofibromatosis (von Recklinghausen's disease)
- Adrenogenital syndrome
- Pheochromocytoma
- Polycystic kidney disease (infantile and adult forms)
- Familial nephritis (Alport syndrome)
- Little syndrome
- Fabry's disease (angiokeratoma corporis diffusum)
- Familial dysautonomia (Riley-Day syndrome)
- Essential hypertension
- Tuberous sclerosis with angiolipomas
- Primary hyperparathyroidism
- Porphyria

PHARMACOLOGICAL
- Sympathomimetics: ephedrine, epinephrine, isoproterenol
- Adrenal steroids
- Heavy metals: mercury, lead
- Licorice

ACQUIRED, RENAL
- Unilateral hydronephrosis
- Unilateral pyelonephritis
- Renal trauma
- Renal tumors
- Unilateral multicystic kidney
- Unilateral ureteral occlusion
- Renal artery stenosis
- Renal arteritis
- Fibromuscular dysplasia of the renal artery
- Renal fistula
- Renal artery aneurysm
- Chronic pyelonephritis superimposed on abnormal kidneys
- Nephritis: shunt nephritis, acute poststreptococcal disease, anaphylactoid purpura, disseminated lupus erythematosus
- Renal tuberculosis
- Renal cortical necrosis: hemolytic uremic syndrome; sepsis
- Renal vein thrombosis
- Radiation nephritis
- Postrenal transplantation

ACQUIRED, OTHER THAN RENAL
- Hyperthyroidism
- Retrosternal goiter
- Guillain-Barré syndrome or poliomyelitis
- Cerebral edema
- Stevens-Johnson syndrome
- Neuroblastoma
- Hypercalcemia or hypernatremia
- Adrenal adenoma or hyperplasia: primary aldosteronism or Cushing's syndrome
- Hyperuricemic nephropathy
- Burns

Modified from Lieberman, E.: Diagnostic evaluation of hypertensive children. Pediatr. Ann. *6*:390, 1977.

correctly, width of the inner rubber cuff bladder should be 40 per cent of the circumference of the upper arm or thigh while leaving the antecubital or popliteal fossa free. A cuff that is too small is likely to produce spuriously high readings. In infants under age 2 years the flush technique may be used, although a Doppler instrument is preferred.[135] Because disappearance of the Korotkoff sound may cause underestimation of the diastolic pressure, both muffling (the fourth phase of the Korotkoff sound) and disappearance (fifth phase) should be recorded. The fourth phase is the more accurate measure of diastolic pressure in most prepubertal children; beyond adolescence the fifth phase sound more closely reflects diastolic pressure.[136]

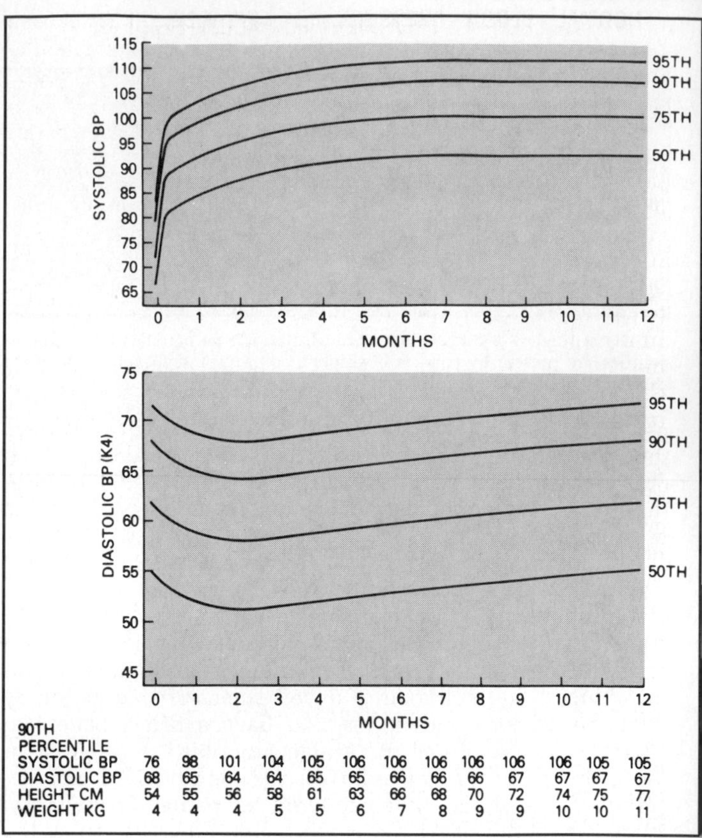

90TH PERCENTILE	0	1	2	3	4	5	6	7	8	9	10	11	12
SYSTOLIC BP	76	98	101	104	105	106	106	106	106	106	106	105	105
DIASTOLIC BP	68	65	64	64	65	65	66	66	66	67	67	67	67
HEIGHT CM	54	55	56	58	61	63	66	68	70	72	74	75	77
WEIGHT KG	4	4	4	5	5	6	7	8	9	9	10	10	11

FIGURE 31–9. Age-specific percentiles of blood pressure measurements in girls—birth to 12 months of age. Korotkoff phase IV used for diastolic blood pressure. (From Horan, M. J., et al.: Report of the second task force on blood pressure control in children—1987. Pediatrics *79*:1, 1987. Copyright American Academy of Pediatrics, 1987.)

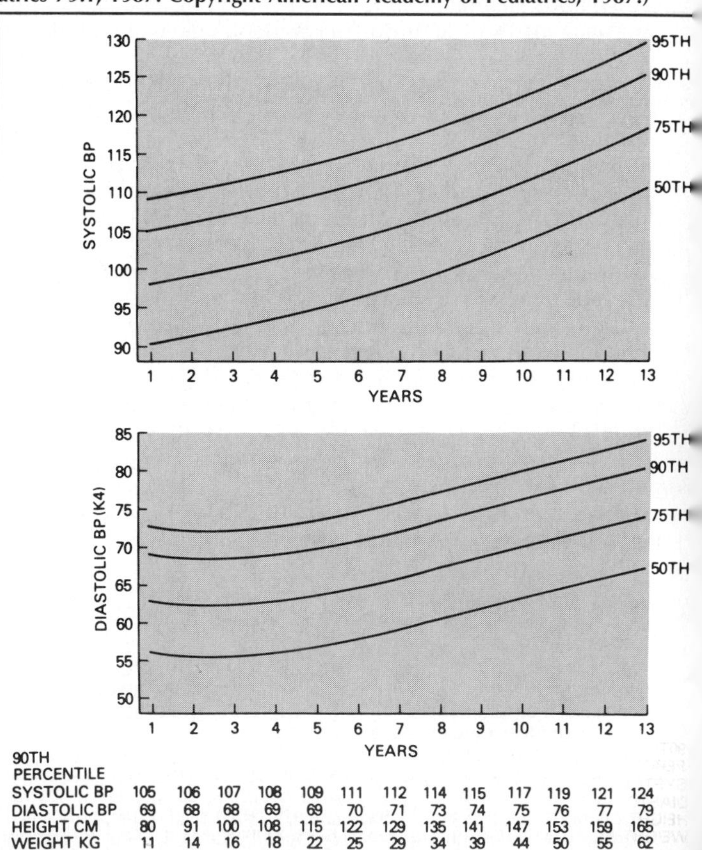

90TH PERCENTILE	1	2	3	4	5	6	7	8	9	10	11	12	13
SYSTOLIC BP	105	106	107	108	109	111	112	114	115	117	119	121	124
DIASTOLIC BP	69	68	68	69	69	70	71	73	74	75	76	77	79
HEIGHT CM	80	91	100	108	115	122	129	135	141	147	153	159	165
WEIGHT KG	11	14	16	18	22	25	29	34	39	44	50	55	62

FIGURE 31–10. Age-specific percentiles of blood pressure measurements in boys—1 to 13 years of age. Korotkoff phase IV used for diastolic blood pressure. (From Horan, M. J., et al.: Report of the second task force on blood pressure control in children—1987. Pediatrics *79*:1, 1987. Copyright American Academy of Pediatrics, 1987.)

NORMAL BLOOD PRESSURE IN CHILDREN. The normal ranges of blood pressure relative to age are shown in Figures 31–9 through 31–13 and serve as a guide in judging unsafe levels. Because considerable variation exists in most children's pressures, it should be recognized that a single blood pressure recording at or higher than the 90th percentile at a single point in time may not be an abnormal finding. In an apparently healthy child measurements should be repeated serially; further investigation is warranted if the blood pressure persists at or above the 90th percentile.[137,138] In contrast, definite or severe hypertension (i.e., pressures repeatedly well beyond the broad limits of normal) requires prompt investigation and treatment.[139,140] Particularly urgent attention must be paid to those children whose systolic and diastolic pressures are remarkably high (i.e., equal to or greater than 180 and 110 mm Hg, respectively). Other findings identifying the patient at acute risk include localized neurological signs and/or generalized seizures; blurred vision or such eye ground changes as retinal hemorrhage, exudate, papilledema, or retinal arterial constriction; renal or abdominal pain; evidence of left ventricular hypertrophy or cardiac decompensation; renal dysfunction; palpation of an abdominal mass or enlargement of the kidneys; or auscultation of an abdominal bruit.

ASSESSMENT. Evaluation of the asymptomatic child or adolescent with a blood pressure level above the 90th percentile on three or more occasions includes a careful history focusing on conditions or drugs known to be associated with or to predispose to high blood pressure. These include oral contraceptives (see p. 823), use of glucocorticoids, renal disease, and symptoms that suggest aldosteronism (see p. 827) (i.e., spells, weakness, polyuria, muscle cramps) or pheochromocytoma (see p. 1897) (i.e., excessive sweating, palpitations). The family history should be re-

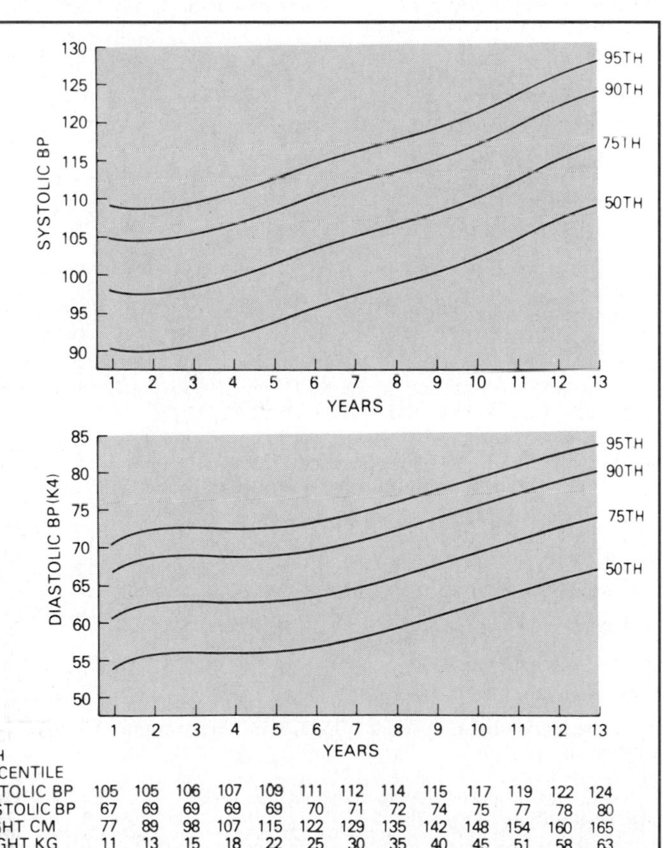

90TH PERCENTILE	1	2	3	4	5	6	7	8	9	10	11	12	13
SYSTOLIC BP	105	105	106	107	109	111	112	114	115	117	119	122	124
DIASTOLIC BP	67	69	69	69	69	70	71	72	74	75	77	78	80
HEIGHT CM	77	89	98	107	115	122	129	135	142	148	154	160	165
WEIGHT KG	11	13	15	18	22	25	30	35	40	45	51	58	63

FIGURE 31–11. Age-specific percentiles of blood pressure measurements in girls—1 to 13 years of age. Korotkoff phase IV used for diastolic blood pressure. (From Horan, M. J., et al.: Report of the second task force on blood pressure control in children—1987. Pediatrics *79*:1, 1987. Copyright American Academy of Pediatrics, 1987.)

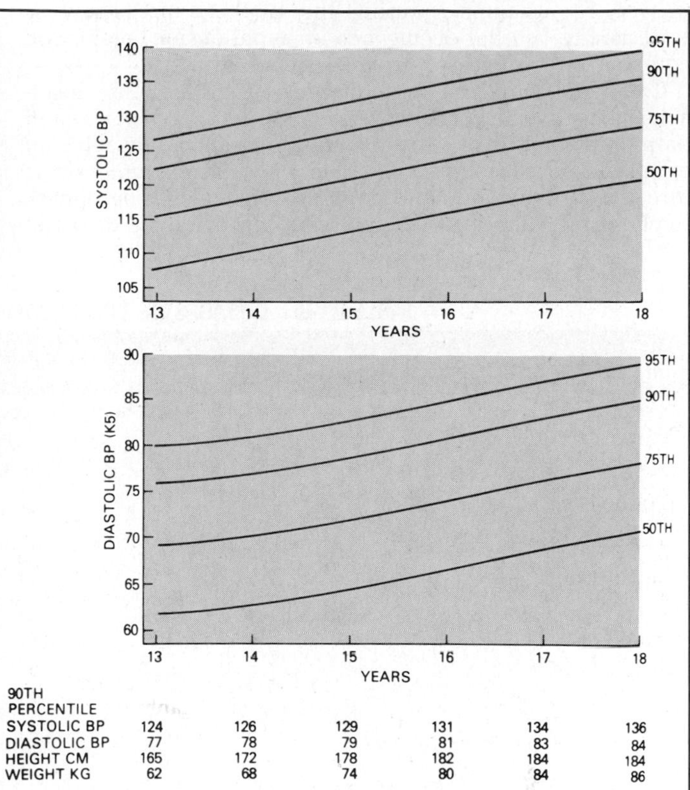

90TH PERCENTILE	13	14	15	16	17	18
SYSTOLIC BP	124	126	129	131	134	136
DIASTOLIC BP	77	78	79	81	83	84
HEIGHT CM	165	172	178	182	184	184
WEIGHT KG	62	68	74	80	84	86

FIGURE 31–12. Age-specific percentiles of blood pressure measurements in boys—13 to 18 years of age. Korotkoff phase V used for diastolic blood pressure. (From Horan, M. J., et al.: Report of the second task force on blood pressure control in children—1987. Pediatrics *79*:1, 1987. Copyright American Academy of Pediatrics, 1987.)

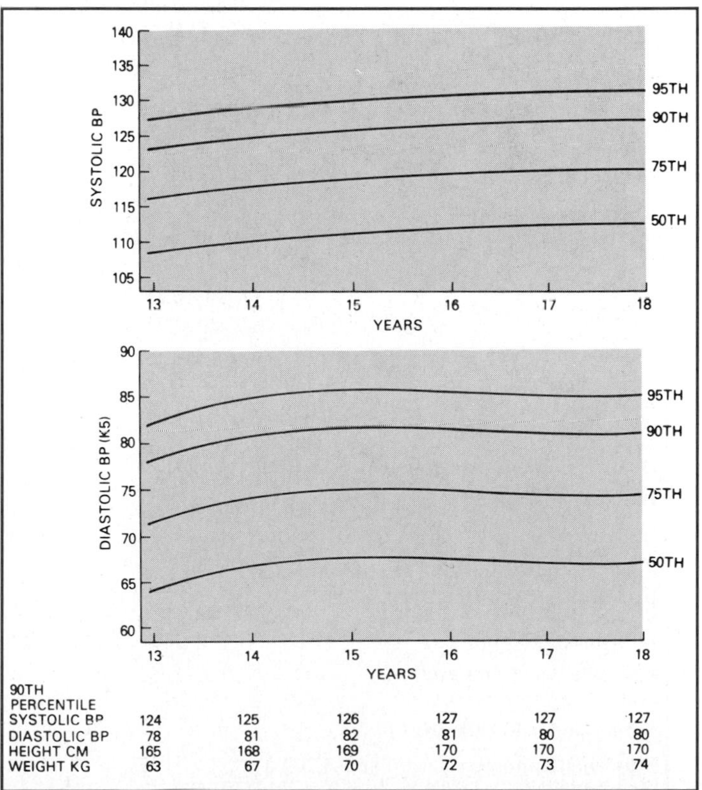

90TH PERCENTILE	13	14	15	16	17	18
SYSTOLIC BP	124	125	126	127	127	127
DIASTOLIC BP	78	81	82	81	80	80
HEIGHT CM	165	168	169	170	170	170
WEIGHT KG	63	67	70	72	73	74

FIGURE 31–13. Age-specific percentiles of blood pressure measurements in girls—13 to 18 years of age. Korotkoff phase V used for diastolic blood pressure. (From Horan, M. J., et al.: Report of the second task force on blood pressure control in children—1987. Pediatrics *79*:1, 1987. Copyright American Academy of Pediatrics, 1987.)

viewed for eclampsia during the mother's pregnancy as well as any familial occurrence of hypertension, premature coronary artery disease, stroke, or renal failure.

Common *symptoms* in hypertensive children are headache, nausea and vomiting, loss of appetite, epistaxis, and palpitation. A dietary history should be obtained with an emphasis on sodium intake. The *physical examination* is directed at detecting conditions associated with secondary hypertension (Table 31–5) and finding evidence of target organ damage on funduscopic and cardiac examination. Typically, the physical findings in hypertensive disorders in children reflect the underlying cause of the elevated pressure; distinctive physical findings accompany many of the conditions listed in Table 31–5 (see also Chap. 26).

LABORATORY STUDIES. These are aimed primarily at identifying secondary causes of hypertension.[139] The minimal laboratory tests required are a urinalysis, complete blood count, serum electrolytes, blood urea nitrogen, serum

TABLE 31–6 DOSAGES OF DRUGS COMMONLY USED IN PEDIATRIC CARDIOLOGY

DRUG	ROUTE OF ADMINISTRATION	DOSAGE
Acetaminophen (Tylenol)	PO or PR	<1 year 60 mg (q4h); 1 to 3 years 120 mg (q4h); >3 years 120 to 240 mg (q4h)
Acetylsalicylic acid (aspirin)	PO or PR	30 to 100 mg/kg/day (q4h)
ϵ-Aminocaproic acid (Amicar)	IV	Total 100 mg/kg/dose (q6h)
Aminophylline	PO, PR, or IV	12 mg/kg/day (q6h)
Amiodarone	PO	10 mg/kg/day for 10 to 14 days, then 5 mg/kg/day for 1 to 2 mo, then 2.5 mg/kg/day
Ammonium chloride	PO	75 mg/kg/day (q6h)
Atropine	IV, SC, or PO	0.01 to 0.03 mg/kg (q4–6h)
Bicarbonate sodium	IV	1 to 2 mEq/kg/5 min
Bishydroxycoumarin (Dicumarol)	PO	Loading dose: 50 to 100 mg Maintenance: 10 to 50 mg/day (regulate according to prothrombin times)
Bretylium	IV	5 mg/kg/dose over 10 minutes, then 50 to 100 μg/kg/min
Calcium chloride	IV	1 to 4 ml of 10% solution; for cardiac arrest, 10 mg/kg/dose
Calcium gluconate	IV PO	2 to 6 ml of 10% solution; for cardiac arrest, 10 mg/kg/dose 500 mg/kg/day (q6h)
Captopril	PO	0.1 to 0.4 mg/kg/day (infants) 0.5 to 1.0 mg/kg/day (q8h) (children)
Chlorothiazide (Diuril)	PO	20 to 40 mg/kg/day (q12h)
Chlorthalidone	PO	1 to 2 mg/kg/day (q12h)
Cholestyramine (Questran)	PO	250 to 1500 mg/kg/day (q6–12h)
Clonidine (Catapres)	PO	0.002 to 0.008 mg/kg/day in divided doses
Codeine	PO	0.5 to 1.5 mg/kg/dose (q3h)
Dexamethasone (Decadron)	IV	0.2 to 0.5 mg/kg/dose (q6h) for cerebral edema
Diazoxide	IV	1 to 3 mg/kg/dose over 30 sec (q2–6h) (careful of severe hypotension)
Digitalis (Digoxin)		Loading dose: Premature infants 0.01–0.02 mg/kg IV or IM Term infants Parenteral: Up to 4 wk: 0.03 mg/kg; 4 wk to 12 mo: 0.035 mg/kg; over 12 mo: 0.040 mg/kg; beyond 2 yr: 0.03 mg/kg Oral: Approximately 20% greater than IV dose Maintenance: ⅓ to ¼ of loading dose, given in two divided doses/24 hr
Digoxin immune Fab fragments (Ovine)	IV	0.6 mg digoxin bound by 40 mg Fab fragments
Dobutamine	IV	2 to 15 μg/kg/min
Dopamine	IV	1 gm in 250 ml D_5W; 2 to 20 μg/kg/min
Edrophonium chloride (Tensilon)	IV	0.05 to 0.2 mg/kg/dose
Enalapril maleate (Vasotec)	PO	0.1 to 0.4 mg/kg/day
Ephedrine sulfate	IM or PO	0.8 to 1.6 mg/kg/day (q6h)
Epinephrine (Adrenalin)	IV	For cardiac arrest: single dose: 0.1 to 1.0 ml of 1:1000; 0.1 to 1.0 μg/min infusion
Ethacrynic acid (Edecrin)	IV	1.0 mg/kg/day
Ethylenediaminetetraacetic acid (EDTA) disodium salt	IV	20 mg/ml: 10 to 50 mg/kg (q12h)
Flecainide acetate (Tambocor)	PO	3 to 6 mg/kg/day (q8h)
Furosemide (Lasix)	IV or IM PO	1 to 2 mg/kg/dose 1 to 4 mg/kg/day
Glucagon	IV	0.05 to 0.10 mg/kg/hr

DRUG	ROUTE OF ADMINISTRATION	DOSAGE
Glucose 50%	IV	1 mg/kg/dose
Glucose 50% + Insulin	IV	1 gm glucose/kg (50% solution) with insulin, 1 unit/3 gm glucose
Heparin	IV	100 units/kg (q4h)
Hydralazine hydrochloride (Apresoline)	IV PO	0.8 to 3.0 mg/kg/day (q4–6h) 0.75 to 7.5 mg/kg/day (q6–8h)
Hydrochlorothiazide	PO	1 to 3 mg/kg/day (q12h)
Hydrocortisone sodium succinate (Solu-Cortef)	IV	For shock: 50 to 75 mg/kg (q6h)
Indomethacin	IV	0.1 to 0.25 mg/kg/dose (premature, for ductal closure)
Innovar (fentanyl citrate & droperidol)	IV	0.01 to 0.02 ml/kg
Isoproterenol hydrochloride (Isuprel hydrochloride)	IV	0.05 to 0.25 μg/kg/min
Lidocaine (Xylocaine hydrochloride)	IV	Single dose: 1 mg/kg; 10 to 50 μg/kg/min infusion
Magnesium sulfate, 3%	IV	For neonatal seizure: single dose: 2 to 6 ml
Mannitol	IV	For cerebral edema: 1 to 2 gm/kg Repeated doses: 250 mg/kg (q4h) For hemoglobinuria: single dose: 0.5 gm/kg; 5% solution infusion if necessary
Meperidine hydrochloride (Demerol)	IM or IV	1 mg/kg/dose (q3h)
Metaraminol (Aramine metaraminol bitartrate)	IV	Single dose: 0.1 mg/kg or 50 mg/500 ml; titrate to effect infusion
Methyldopa (Aldomet)	PO or IV	10 to 40 mg/kg/day (q6–8h)
Methylprednisolone (Solu-Medrol)	IV	For shock: 30 mg/kg/dose; for cerebral edema: 4 to 5 mg/kg/dose
Mexiletine	PO	4 to 20 mg/kg/day (q8h)
Minoxidil	PO	0.05 to 2.0 mg/kg/day
Morphine sulfate	SC	0.1 to 0.2 mg/kg/dose (q3h)
Naloxone hydrochloride (Narcan)	IM or IV	0.01 to 0.1 mg/kg/dose
Nifedipine (Procardia)	PO	0.25 to 0.5 mg/kg/dose (hypertension) 0.6 to 0.9 mg/kg/day (q6–8h) (hypertrophic cardiomyopathy)
Nitroglycerine	IV	1 to 3 μg/kg/min
Nitroprusside, sodium	IV	0.5 to 0.8 μg/kg/min initial rate; titrate to effect
Norepinephrine (Levophed bitartrate)	IV	0.1 to 1.0 μg/kg/min
Pentobarbital (Nembutal)	PO or IM	2 to 3 mg/kg/dose
Phenobarbital	PO or IM	3 to 5 mg/kg/day (q8h)
Phenoxybenzamine	IV	0.5 to 1.0 mg/kg
Phentolamine	IV	0.05 to 0.10 mg/kg
Phenylephrine (Neo-Synephrine hydrochloride)	IV	10 mg/100 ml D_5W; 0.1 to 0.5 μg/kg/min, titrate to effect
Phenytoin (Dilantin)	PO or IV	For seizures: 5 to 10 mg/kg/day (q8h); for arrhythmias: 1 to 5 mg/kg/5 min, not to exceed 15 mg/kg
Potassium chloride	PO IV	1 to 4 mEq/kg/day 0.5 mEq/kg/hr not to exceed 2 mEq/kg, as 40 to 80 mEq/liter solution
Potassium gluconate (Kaon) and potassium triplex	PO	1 to 2 mEq/kg/day
Prazosin HCl (Minipress)	PO	25 to 150 μg/kg/day (q6h)
Procainamide hydrochloride (Pronestyl)	PO IM IV	15 to 50 mg/kg/day (q4–6h), not to exceed 4 g/day 20 to 30 mg/kg (q6h) 2 to 6 mg/kg/dose over 5 min, maintenance 20 to 80 μg/kg/min
Promethazine	PO	0.5 to 2 mg/kg/day (q6–8h)

Table continues on following page

DRUG	ROUTE OF ADMINISTRATION	DOSAGE
Propranolol hydrochloride (Inderal)	PO IV IM	1.0 to 6.0 mg/kg/day (divided q6h) 0.01 to 0.15 mg/kg (q6–8h) 0.5 to 1.0 mg/kg (q4–6h)
Prostaglandin E_1	IV	0.1 μg/kg/min, reduce to 0.01 μg/kg/min to maintain effect
Protamine sulfate	IV	1 mg for every 100 units of heparin
Quinidine gluconate	IV	2 to 10 mg/kg/dose (q3–6h), not recommended
Quinidine sulfate	PO	15 to 60 mg/kg/dose (q6h)
Sodium polystyrene sulfonate (Kayexalate)	PO, PR	1 gm/kg mixed with sorbitol
Spironolactone (Aldactone)	PO	1 to 3 mg/kg/day (q6–12h)
Succinylcholine chloride (Anectine chloride)	IV	1 to 2 mg/kg dose
Tolazoline (Priscoline)	IV	1 mg/kg/dose, then 1 to 3 mg/kg/hr
Triamterene (Dyrenium)	PO	2–4 mg/kg/day
Trimethaphan camsylate (Arfonad)	IV	50 mg in 100 ml D_5W, titrate to effect
Tris buffer (THAM) (Tromethamine)	IV	(0.3M) weight (kg) × base deficit = dose in ml
Tubocurarine chloride (curare)	IM or IV	Initial dose: 0.3 to 0.5 mg/kg; subsequent dose: 0.1 mg/kg
Verapamil (Isopten)	IV	0.1 to 0.2 mg/kg/dose over 2 min
Vitamin K (AquaMEPHYTON)	IM or IV	Single dose (neonate): 1 mg
Warfarin sodium crystalline (Coumadin)	PO or IM	Initial dose: 0.5 mg/kg Maintenance: 1 to 5 mg/day (regulate according to prothrombin times)

creatinine, uric acid, echocardiogram, electrocardiogram, and chest roentgenogram. Because the most common cause of secondary hypertension in children is renal disease, evaluation often proceeds to include plasma renin activity with 24-hour urinary sodium excretion[141] or plasma renin in response to captopril (see p. 827), rapid-sequence intravenous pyelogram, ultrasonography of the kidneys, and isotopic or angiographic analysis of the kidneys and/or their blood supply. Fortunately, most identifiable causes of correctable hypertension in children and adolescents are associated with clinical findings that direct attention to a particular organ system (renal, endocrine, central nervous, and cardiovascular). Less often, hypertension may result from tumors (ganglioneuroma, pheochromocytoma, Wilms', and neuroblastoma) or collagen vascular disease. Laboratory studies should be as specific as possible to avoid an unselected analysis of every organ system theoretically associated with hypertension. In general, the younger the child and the higher the blood pressure elevation, the more vigorous should be the laboratory evaluation. It should be recognized that although essential hypertension often is a diagnosis by exclusion in prepubertal children, it is a viable diagnosis, particularly in adolescents.[137,142,143] In the author's opinion the need for extensive laboratory investigations has been overemphasized in children or adolescents with mild sustained elevations in blood pressure.

MANAGEMENT. Asymptomatic children and adolescents with borderline or only mildly elevated blood pressure (<5 to 10 mm Hg beyond the 90th percentile values for age) may not require antihypertensive pharmacological agents but should receive counseling regarding weight control, salt abuse, and avoidance of agents with pressor effects (e.g., caffeine, some bronchoconstrictors, nicotine). These patients should be encouraged to be physically active, especially in exercises improving cardiovascular fitness. Isometric or static exercise such as wrestling and weight lifting should be avoided, especially in children with evidence of left ventricular hypertrophy. If the latter exists or if these conservative measures do not result in normalization of blood pressure, treatment with antihypertensive drugs is indicated.

Drug therapy (Table 31–6) is aimed at prescribing the least complex regimen with the fewest side effects (see also Chap. 27). Pharmacological management is usually undertaken if diastolic blood pressure is greater than 85 mm Hg in children less than age 12 years, and greater than 90 mm Hg in children older than 12 years. If left ventricular hypertrophy is evident by echocardiogram, drug treatment is advisable at lower diastolic pressures. An oral thiazide diuretic usually is the initial drug of choice and may be combined with a potassium-sparing drug or with a dietary regimen that provides adequate potassium. If blood pressure control is not achieved, an angiotensin-converting en-

TABLE 31–7 FASTING LIPID AND LIPOPROTEIN LEVELS (mg/dl) IN CHILDREN BY AGE

	MALES			FEMALES		
	5%	50%	95%	5%	50%	95%
Cholesterol						
0–4 yr	114	155	203	112	156	200
5–9 yr	121	160	203	126	164	205
10–14 yr	119	158	202	124	160	201
15–19 yr	113	150	197	120	158	203
Triglycerides						
0–4 yr	29	56	98	34	64	112
5–9 yr	30	56	101	32	60	105
10–14 yr	32	66	125	37	75	131
15–19 yr	37	78	148	39	75	132
HDL Cholesterol						
5–9 yr	38	56	74	36	53	73
10–14 yr	37	55	74	37	52	70
15–19 yr	30	46	63	35	52	74
LDL Cholesterol						
5–9 yr	63	93	129	68	100	140
10–14 yr	64	100	140	68	97	132
15–19 yr	62	94	130	59	96	137

Data from Lipid Research Clinics: Population Studies Data Book. Dept. of Health and Human Services (NIH) 80-1527, Vol. I: The Prevalence Study.

zyme inhibitor may be added to the regimen. Occasionally it is necessary to use a beta-adrenergic blocking agent such as atenolol, a calcium channel blocker such as nifedipine, or a central sympathetic inhibitor such as clonidine.

Acute, life-threatening episodes of hypertension occur rarely and in a variety of clinical situations.[144] Encephalopathy is the most severe complication of an acute hypertensive crisis; its presence demands immediate lowering of the systemic arterial blood pressure. Diazoxide is the agent of choice as a first drug for the patient with encephalopathy. If diazoxide is ineffective, catecholamine-producing tumors must be suspected and consideration given to using alpha-adrenergic blocking agents such as phentolamine or phenoxybenzamine. Sodium nitroprusside usually is considered the agent to be administered when all others have failed. If a cause for sustained hypertension has been detected, medical and/or surgical treatment should be directed at the underlying disease process.

HYPERLIPIDEMIAS

(See also Chap. 35)

The importance of prevention of arteriosclerosis in childhood is widely accepted.[145,146] Hyperlipidemic children are at high risk of becoming hyperlipidemic adults and are therefore at greater risk of future atherosclerotic disease.[147,148] Although opinions vary about the feasibility of maintaining low serum lipid levels in normal children by dietary modification, there is consensus that children whose serum cholesterol or triglyceride levels are beyond the 95th percentile for their age and gender should be treated. Guidelines for abnormal levels in the first two decades of life are provided in Table 31–7.

Controversy exists concerning the value of selective versus universal cholesterol and lipid screening strategies for children.[147–151] The National Cholesterol Education Pro-

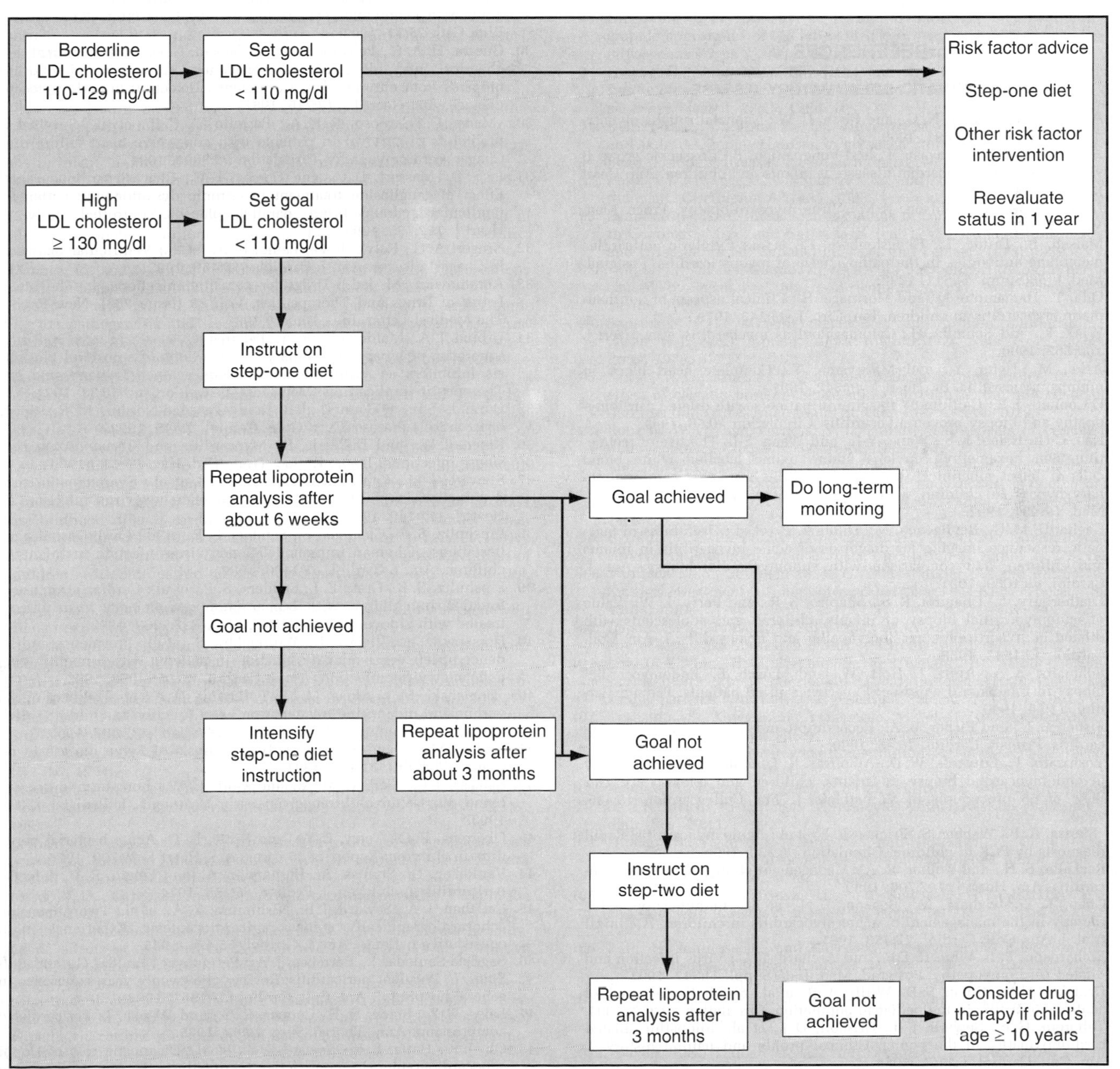

FIGURE 31–14. The National Cholesterol Education Program recommendation for dietary treatment of hypercholesterolemia in children. LDL = low density lipoprotein. (From The Report of the Expert Panel on Blood Cholesterol Levels in Children and Adolescents. Pediatrics *89*:525–584, 1992. Copyright American Academy of Pediatrics, 1992.)

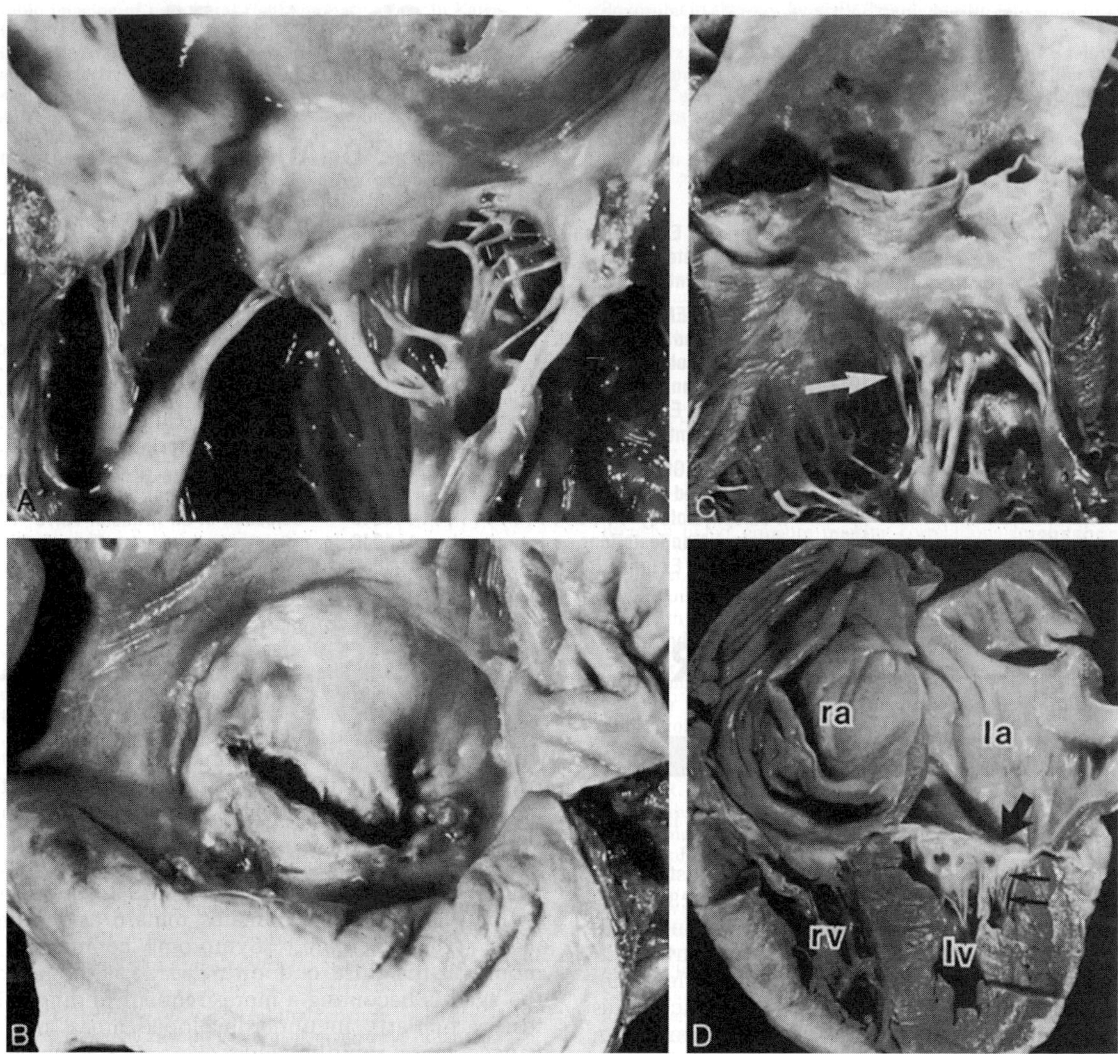

FIGURE 32–1. Rheumatic mitral stenosis. *A*, Moderate valvular changes including diffuse leaflet fibrosis, commissural fusion, and chordal thickening and fusion. In another case, atrial view *(B)* and subvalvular and aortic aspects *(C)* show prominent subvalvular involvement; severe subvalvular distortion is evident (arrow). *D*, Severe rheumatic mitral stenosis with specimen shown in apical four-chamber echocardiographic view, demonstrating small left ventricle (lv) and enlarged left atrium (la), right ventricle (rv), and right atrium (ra). Note the calcified stenotic valve (arrow) and prominent subvalvular changes (double arrows). (*A* and *D* from Schoen, F. J., and St. John Sutton, M.: Contemporary issues in the pathology of valvular heart disease. Hum. Pathol. *18:*568, 1987.)

increase the rate of blood flow across the mitral orifice and result in further elevation of the left atrial pressure.[14,15]

In order to assess the severity of obstruction of the mitral valve (and, for that matter, of any valve), it is essential to measure both the transvalvular pressure gradient and the flow rate.[15a] The latter depends not only on cardiac output but on heart rate as well. An increase in heart rate shortens diastole proportionately more than systole and diminishes the time available for flow across the mitral valve. Therefore, at any given level of cardiac output, tachycardia augments the transmitral valvular pressure gradient and elevates left atrial pressures further.[16] This explains the sudden occurrence of dyspnea and pulmonary edema in previously asymptomatic patients with MS who develop atrial fibrillation with a rapid ventricular rate[17]; it also accounts for the equally rapid improvement in these patients when the ventricular rate is slowed by means of cardiac glycosides and/or beta-adrenoceptor blocking agents, even when the cardiac output per minute remains constant. Hydraulic considerations dictate that at any given orifice size the transvalvular gradient is a function of the square of the transvalvular flow rate (see p. 194).[18] Thus, a doubling of flow rate will quadruple the pressure gradient, so that a stress such as exercise in patients with moderate or severe MS will cause marked elevation of left atrial pressure.[18a] Pregnancy, hypervolemia, and hyperthyroidism all increase mitral valve flow and thereby the transvalvular pressure gradient. Although the Gorlin formula has been the benchmark for evaluating stenotic valvular orifices since 1951[18] (see p. 194), there is increasing evidence that valvular orifices are not rigid and that, in fact, as transvalvular flow increases, the orifice becomes distended. Accordingly, it has been proposed that stenosis be expressed as valvular resistance, the quotient of the mean transvalvular pressure gradient and the mean transvalvular flow.[19]

Atrial contraction augments the presystolic transmitral valvular gradient by approximately 30 per cent in patients with MS. Withdrawal of atrial transport when atrial fibrillation develops decreases cardiac output by about 20 per cent. The more rapid ventricular rate that occurs in atrial fibrillation until it is pharmacologically controlled raises the transvalvular pressure gradient. Thus, hemodynamic considerations indicate the desirability of maintaining sinus rhythm in patients with MS.

Intracardiac and Intravascular Pressures

Left ventricular diastolic pressure is normal in patients with pure MS; coexisting MR, aortic valve lesions, systemic hypertension, ischemic heart disease, and cardiomyopathy may all be responsible for elevations of left ventricular diastolic pressure. In approximately 85 per cent of patients

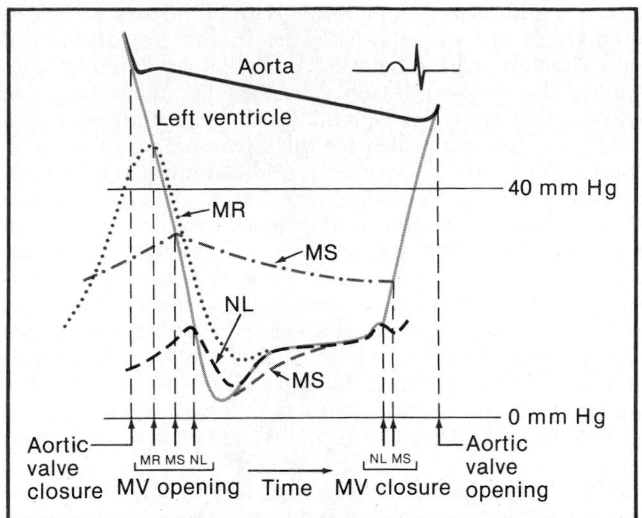

FIGURE 32–2. Schematic relationship of left ventricular (———), aortic (▬▬▬), and pulmonary atrial wedge (PAW) pressures. Note that the higher the left atrial *v* wave, the earlier the pressure crossover, and the earlier the mitral valve (MV) opening. The higher left atrial end-diastolic pressure with severe mitral stenosis (MS) also results in later closure of the mitral valve. PAW pressures in severe mitral regurgitation (MR) (· · · · ·), mitral stenosis (— · — · — ·), and normal (— — — —). The LV diastolic pressure in mitral stenosis (▪ ▪ ▪ ▪ ▪ ▪) rises slowly, denoting the absence of a rapid filling wave. (From Braunwald, E., and Turi, Z. G.: Pathophysiology of mitral valve disease. *In* Wells, F. C., and Schapiro, L. M. [eds.]: Mitral Valve Disease. London, Butterworths, 1996.)

with pure MS, the end-diastolic volume is within the normal range, whereas it is reduced in the remainder.[20] In approximately one-fourth of patients with pure MS the ejection fraction and other ejection indices of systolic performance (see p. 425) are below normal, most likely resulting from chronic reduction in preload and elevated afterload, the latter related to a chronically depressed cardiac output.[21] Regional hypokinesis is common,[22] perhaps caused by extension of the scarring process from the mitral valve into the adjacent posterior basal myocardium or by associated ischemic heart disease. Leftward displacement of the interventricular septum secondary to more rapid early filling of the right ventricle may be responsible for a reduction of left ventricular distensibility.[23] The left ventricular mass is normal or slightly reduced.[20] It has long been postulated that persistent myocardial dysfunction, perhaps caused by smoldering rheumatic myocarditis, may be responsible for the poor results following surgical treatment of some patients with pure MS.[24] The bulk of available evidence suggests that myocardial *contractility* is normal or slightly impaired in the majority of patients.[25] Associated ischemic heart disease may be responsible for myocardial dysfunction.[26] Most patients with MS show a normal elevation of ejection fraction and reduction of end-systolic volume during exercise.[27]

In MS and sinus rhythm, the *left atrial pressure pulse* generally exhibits a prominent atrial contraction (*a*) wave (Fig. 6–13, p. 194) and a gradual pressure decline after mitral valve opening (*y* descent); the mean left atrial pressure is elevated. In patients with mild to moderate MS without elevation of pulmonary vascular resistance, pulmonary arterial pressure may be normal or only slightly elevated at rest and may rise only during exercise. However, in patients with severe MS and/or those in whom the pulmonary vascular resistance is significantly increased, pulmonary arterial pressure is elevated when the patient is at rest, and in rare cases of extreme elevation of the pulmonary vascular resistance it may exceed the systemic arterial pressure. Further elevations of left atrial and pulmonary vascular pressures occur during exercise or tachycardia or both. With moderate elevation of pulmonary artery pressure (systolic pressure 30 to 60 mm Hg), right ventricular performance is usually maintained.[28] However, an elevation of pulmonary arterial systolic pressure exceeding 60 mm Hg represents a serious impedance to emptying of the right ventricle and may cause right ventricular failure with elevations of the right ventricular end-diastolic and right atrial pressures. During exercise, patients with MS and pulmonary hypertension commonly fail to exhibit normal elevation of right ventricular ejection fraction.[24]

The *clinical and hemodynamic features* of MS of any given severity are dictated largely by the levels of cardiac output and pulmonary vascular resistance. The response to a given degree of mitral obstruction may be characterized at one end of the hemodynamic spectrum by a normal cardiac output and a high left atrioventricular pressure gradient or, at the opposite end of the spectrum, by a markedly reduced cardiac output and low transvalvular pressure gradient. Thus, in some patients with moderately severe stenosis (mitral valve area = 1.0 to 1.5 cm^2) cardiac output at rest may be normal and it rises normally during exertion as well. In these patients, marked elevation of left atrial and pulmonary capillary pressures and the high transvalvular pressure gradient together lead to severe pulmonary congestion during exertion. In contrast, in the majority of patients with severe MS, cardiac output rises subnormally during exertion, thus reducing the pulmonary venous pressure and the severity of symptoms of pulmonary congestion more than would be the case if the output rose normally. In patients with severe stenosis (mitral valve area < 1.0 cm^2), particularly when pulmonary vascular resistance is elevated, cardiac output is usually depressed at rest and may fail to rise at all during exertion. These patients frequently have prominent symptoms secondary to a low cardiac output, e.g., severe weakness and fatigue.

Pulmonary hypertension in patients with MS results from (1) passive backward transmission of the elevated left atrial pressure; (2) pulmonary arteriolar constriction, which presumably is triggered by left atrial and pulmonary venous hypertension (reactive pulmonary hypertension)[29]; and (3) organic obliterative changes in the pulmonary vascular bed, which may be considered to be a complication of longstanding and severe MS[30] (Chap. 25). In time, severe pulmonary hypertension results in right-sided failure, with dilatation of the right ventricle and its annulus, and secondary tricuspid and sometimes pulmonic regurgitation. It has been suggested that these changes in the pulmonary vascular bed may also exert a protective effect; the elevated precapillary resistance makes the development of symptoms of pulmonary congestion less likely by tending to prevent blood from surging into the pulmonary capillary bed and damming up behind the stenotic mitral valve, although this protection occurs at the expense of a reduced cardiac output. In patients with severe MS, pulmonary vein–bronchial vein shunts occur.[31] Patients with severe MS manifest a marked reduction in lung compliance, an increase in the work of breathing, and a redistribution of pulmonary blood flow from the bases to the apices.

The combination of mitral valve disease and atrial inflammation secondary to rheumatic carditis causes (1) left atrial dilatation, (2) fibrosis of the atrial wall, and (3) disorganization of the atrial muscle bundles. The third condition leads to disparate conduction velocities and inhomogeneous refractory periods. Premature atrial activation, due either to an automatic focus or to reentry, may stimulate the left atrium during the vulnerable period and may thus precipitate atrial fibrillation. Often this is episodic at first, but then it becomes more persistent. Atrial fibrillation per se causes diffuse atrophy of atrial muscle, further atrial enlargement,[32] and further inhomogeneity of refractoriness and conduction; these changes, in turn, lead to irreversible atrial fibrillation.

CLINICAL MANIFESTATIONS

History

The principal symptom of MS is dyspnea, largely the result of reduced compliance of the lungs. Cough and wheezing may be accompanying symptoms. Vital capacity is reduced, presumably owing to the presence of engorged pulmonary vessels and interstitial edema. Patients with critical obstruction to left atrial emptying and dyspnea with ordinary activity (functional Class III) generally have orthopnea and are at risk of experiencing attacks of frank pulmonary edema. The latter may be precipitated by effort, emotional stress, respiratory infection, fever, sexual intercourse, pregnancy, atrial fibrillation with a rapid ventricular rate or other tachyarrhythmia, or, indeed, by any condition that increases blood flow across the stenotic mitral valve, either by increasing total cardiac output or by reducing the time available for this flow of blood to occur. In patients with a markedly elevated pulmonary vascular resistance, right ventricular function is often impaired.[32a]

HEMOPTYSIS. Wood has differentiated between several kinds of *hemoptysis* complicating MS.[14]

1. Sudden hemorrhage (sometimes called pulmonary apoplexy), while often profuse, is only rarely life-threatening.[33] It results from the rupture of thin-walled, dilated bronchial veins,[31,34] usually as a consequence of a sudden rise in left atrial pressure. With persistence of pulmonary venous hypertension, the walls of these veins thicken appreciably, and this form of hemoptysis tends to disappear.
2. Blood-stained sputum associated with attacks of paroxysmal nocturnal dyspnea.
3. Pink, frothy sputum characteristic of acute pulmonary edema with rupture of alveolar capillaries.
4. Pulmonary infarction, a late complication of MS associated with heart failure.
5. Blood-stained sputum complicating chronic bronchitis; the edematous bronchial mucosa in patients with chronic MS increases the likelihood of chronic bronchitis, a common complication of MS, particularly in Great Britain.

CHEST PAIN. A small fraction, perhaps 15 per cent, of patients with MS experience chest discomfort that is indistinguishable from angina pectoris.[14,15] This symptom may be caused by right ventricular hypertension or by coincidental coronary atherosclerosis,[26] or it may be secondary to coronary obstruction caused by coronary embolization.[35] In many such patients, however, a satisfactory explanation cannot be uncovered even after complete hemodynamic and angiographic studies.

THROMBOEMBOLISM. Prior to the advent of surgical treatment, this serious complication of MS developed in at least 20 per cent of patients at some time during the course of their disease, and as many as 10 to 15 per cent of this group died as a consequence.[36] Before the era of anticoagulant therapy and surgical treatment, approximately one-fourth of all fatalities in patients with mitral valve disease were secondary to embolism. The tendency for embolization correlates inversely with cardiac output and directly with the patient's age and the size of the left atrial appendage; 80 per cent of patients with MS in whom systemic emboli develop are in atrial fibrillation. When embolization occurs in patients in sinus rhythm, the possibility of transient atrial fibrillation and underlying infective endocarditis should be considered. There is no simple correlation between the incidence of embolism on one hand and the size of the mitral orifice on the other. Indeed, embolism may be the first symptom of MS and may occur in patients with mild MS even before the development of dyspnea. Patients older than 35 with atrial fibrillation, especially with a low cardiac output and dilation of the left atrial appendage, are at the highest risk for emboli and therefore should receive prophylactic anticoagulant treatment.

Because thrombi are found in the left atrium at operation in only a minority of patients with a history of recent embolism, it is likely that only fresh clots are discharged. Approximately half of all clinically apparent emboli are found in the cerebral vessels. Coronary embolism may lead to myocardial infarction, angina pectoris, or both, and renal emboli may be responsible for the development of systemic hypertension. Emboli are recurrent and multiple in approximately 25 per cent of patients subject to this complication. Rarely, massive thrombosis develops in the left atrium, resulting in a pedunculated ball-valve thrombus, which may suddenly aggravate obstruction to left atrial outflow when a specific body position is assumed, or it may cause sudden death.[5,37] Similar consequences occur in patients with free-floating thrombi in the left atrium. These two conditions are usually characterized by variability in the physical findings, often on a positional basis; they are very hazardous and require surgical treatment, often on an emergent basis.

INFECTIVE ENDOCARDITIS (see also Chap. 33). This complication tends to occur *less frequently* on rigid, thickened, calcified valves and is therefore more common in patients with mild than with severe MS.

OTHER SYMPTOMS. Compression of the left recurrent laryngeal nerve by a greatly dilated left atrium, enlarged tracheobronchial lymph nodes, and dilated pulmonary artery may cause hoarseness (Ortner's syndrome).[38] A history of repeated hemoptysis is common in patients with pulmonary hemosiderosis, and longstanding elevation of pulmonary venous pressure is present in patients with pulmonary ossification. Systemic venous hypertension, hepatomegaly, edema, ascites, and hydrothorax are all signs of severe MS with elevated pulmonary vascular resistance and right heart failure.

Physical Examination[39,40]

Patients with severe MS, a low cardiac output, and systemic vasoconstriction may exhibit the so-called mitral facies, characterized by pinkish-purple patches on the cheeks.[14] The *arterial pulse* is usually normal, but in patients in whom the stroke volume is reduced, it may be small in volume. The *jugular venous pulse* usually exhibits a prominent *a* wave in patients with sinus rhythm (Fig. 2–6*A*, p. 19) and elevated pulmonary vascular resistance. In atrial fibrillation, the *x* descent of the jugular pulse disappears, and there is only one crest, a prominent *v* or *c-v* wave, per cardiac cycle. *Palpation* of the cardiac apex usually reveals an inconspicuous left ventricle; the presence of either a palpable presystolic expansion wave or an early diastolic rapid filling wave speaks strongly against significant MS. A readily palpable, tapping first heart sound (S_1) suggests that the anterior mitral valve leaflet is pliable. When the patient is in the left lateral recumbent position, the low-pitched diastolic rumbling murmur of MS may be palpable as a thrill at the apex. Often a right ventricular lift is felt in the left parasternal region in patients with pulmonary hypertension. A markedly enlarged right ventricle may displace the left ventricle posteriorly and produce a prominent apex beat that can be confused with a left ventricular lift. A loud pulmonic closure sound (P_2) may be palpable in the second left intercostal space in patients with MS and pulmonary hypertension.

AUSCULTATION. The auscultatory (and phonocardiographic) features of MS (some of which are illustrated in Fig. 2–38, p. 42) include an accentuated S_1 with prolongation of the Q-S_1 interval, correlating with the level of the left atrial pressure. Accentuation of S_1 occurs when the mitral valve leaflets are flexible.[41] It is caused, in part, by the rapidity with which left ventricular pressure rises at the time of mitral valve closure as well as by the wide closing excursion of the valve leaflets.[42] Marked calcification or thickening of the mitral valve leaflets or both reduce the amplitude of S_1, probably because of diminished motion of the leaflets. As pulmonary artery pressure rises, P_2 at first becomes accentuated and widely transmitted and can often be readily heard and recorded at both the mitral and the aortic areas. With further elevation of pulmonary artery pressure, splitting of S_2 narrows because of reduced compliance of the pulmonary vascular bed, which shortens the "hangout interval." Finally, S_2 becomes single and accentuated. Other signs of pulmonary hypertension include a nonvalvular pulmonic ejection sound that diminishes during inspiration, owing to dilation of the pulmonary artery; the systolic murmur of tricuspid regurgitation; a Graham Steell murmur of pulmonic regurgitation; and an S_4 originating from the right ventricle.[43] An S_3 originating from the left ventricle is absent, unless significant mitral or aortic regurgitation coexists.

The *opening snap* (OS) of the mitral valve appears to be due to a sudden tensing of the valve leaflets after the valve cusps have completed their opening excursion. OS occurs when the movement of the mitral dome into the left ventricle suddenly stops.[42] It is most readily audible at the apex and with the diaphragm of the stethoscope and can usually be differentiated from P_2 because the OS occurs later, unless right bundle branch block is present. The mitral valve cannot be totally rigid if it produces an OS, which is usually accompanied by an accentuated S_1. The OS and the delayed S_1 are "reciprocal sounds," both caused by abrupt termination of movement of the fused mitral complex.[42] Calcification confined to the tip of the mitral valve leaflets does not preclude an OS, although calcification of the body and tip does. In patients with combined MS and regurgitation, the OS may be followed by an S_3. The mitral OS follows A_2 by 0.04 to 0.12 sec; this interval varies inversely with left atrial pressure.[41] Although a short A_2-OS interval is a reliable indicator of severe MS, the converse is not necessarily the case. (Q-S_1)–(A_2-OS) correlates better with the height of the left atrial pressure than does either term alone.

The diastolic murmur of MS is a low-pitched, rumbling murmur, best heard at the apex and with the bell of the stethoscope (Fig. 2–38, p. 42). When this murmur is soft, it is limited to the apex, but when louder, it may radiate to the axilla or the lower left sternal area. Although the intensity of the diastolic murmur is not closely related to the severity of stenosis, the *duration* of the murmur is a guide to the severity of mitral narrowing. The murmur persists for as long as the left atrioventricular pressure gradient exceeds approximately 3 mm Hg. The murmur usually commences immediately after the mitral OS. In mild MS, the early diastolic murmur is brief but it resumes in presystole. In severe stenosis, the murmur is holodiastolic, with presystolic accentuation in patients with sinus rhythm.

Although a *presystolic murmur* is usually present in patients with sinus rhythm in whom transvalvular blood flow is accelerated by atrial contraction, a presystolic murmur may also occur in patients with atrial fibrillation, in whom it results from the increased velocity of blood flow across a mitral valve orifice that begins to narrow after the onset of left ventricular contraction. Because in patients with atrial fibrillation, this murmur results from motion of the mitral valve leaflets, a flexible mitral valve is required for its generation.

The *diastolic rumbling murmur* of MS may be masked by the presence of obesity, pulmonary emphysema, and a low cardiac output with a low flow rate across the mitral valve. This murmur may be sharply localized and thus missed unless palpation is used to detect the apex of the left ventricle and to pinpoint the area at which auscultation should be carried out. In so-called "silent" MS, there is usually marked right ventricular enlargement, so that the right ventricle occupies the cardiac apex, the left ventricle is rotated posteriorly, and cardiac output is reduced, so that the murmur either is not audible at all or can be heard only in the mid- or posterior axillary line. Auscultation of the murmur is facilitated by placing the patient in the left lateral position and auscultating during expiration after a few sit-ups, walking up a flight of stairs, or other maneuvers described later.

Dynamic Auscultation. The diastolic murmur and OS of MS are often reduced during inspiration and augmented during expiration[39,40]—the opposite of what occurs when these findings are secondary to tricuspid stenosis (see p. 1054). During inspiration the A_2-OS interval widens, and three sequential sounds (A_2, P_2, and OS) are frequently audible. Sudden standing and the resultant reduction of venous return lower left atrial pressure and widen the A_2-OS interval; this maneuver is useful in distinguishing an A_2-OS combination from a split S_2, which narrows on standing. In contrast, A_2-OS is significantly narrowed during exercise as left atrial pressure rises. The diastolic rumbling murmur of MS is reduced during the strain of a Valsalva maneuver and in any condition in which transmitral valve flow rate declines. Amyl nitrite, coughing, isometric or isotonic exercise, and sudden squatting are all useful in accentuating a faint or equivocal murmur of MS. Progressive narrowing of A_2-OS on serial examinations suggests an increase in the severity of stenosis, whereas widening of A_2-OS after mitral commissurotomy indicates that the severity of stenosis has been reduced significantly.

DIFFERENTIAL DIAGNOSIS. A number of conditions other than MS may exhibit auscultatory findings that can be confused with MS. In addition to the findings listed in the table, the *Carey-Coombs murmur* of acute rheumatic fever is a sign of active mitral valvulitis and can be confused with the murmur of MS. The Carey-Coombs murmur is a soft, early diastolic murmur, usually varies from day to day, and is higher pitched than the diastolic rumbling murmur of established MS. In pure, severe MR—indeed, in any condition in which there is increased flow across a nonstenotic mitral valve—there may also be a short diastolic murmur following an S_3. *Left atrial myxoma* may produce auscultatory findings similar to those in rheumatic valvular MS (see p. 1466). A high-frequency early systolic murmur is audible along the lower left sternal border in one-third of patients with MS.[42] This should be distinguished from the apical (often holosystolic or late systolic) murmur of MR. In addition, a *pansystolic murmur of tricuspid regurgitation* and an S_3 originating from the right ventricle may be audible in the fourth intercostal space in the left parasternal region in patients with severe mitral stenosis. These signs, secondary to pulmonary hypertension, may be confused with the findings of MR. However, the inspiratory augmentation of the murmur and of the S_3 and the prominent *v* wave in the jugular venous pulse aid in establishing that the murmur originates from the tricuspid valve. A decrescendo diastolic murmur along the left sternal border in patients with MS and pulmonary hypertension is usually due to aortic regurgitation but occasionally represents a Graham Steell murmur of pulmonary regurgitation[43] (see p. 41); the latter, when present, characteristically increases during inspiration.

LABORATORY EXAMINATION

ELECTROCARDIOGRAPHY. The ECG and vectorcardiogram are relatively insensitive techniques for the detection of mild MS, but they do show characteristic changes in moderate or severe obstruction.[44,45] Left atrial enlargement (P-wave duration in lead II > 0.12 sec, terminal negative P force in lead $V_1 > 0.003$ mV/sec, P-wave axis between $+45$ and -30 degrees) is a principal electrocardiographic feature of MS and is found in 90 per cent of patients with significant MS and sinus rhythm.[46] The ECG signs of left atrial enlargement correlate more closely with left atrial volume than with left atrial pressure and often regress following successful valvulotomy.[14] When atrial fibrillation is present, the fibrillatory waves are usually coarse, i.e., greater than 0.1 mV in amplitude in V_1, also suggesting the presence of atrial enlargement.[47] Atrial fibrillation usually develops in the presence of preexistent ECG evidence of left atrial enlargement and is related to the size and the extent of fibrosis of the left atrial myocardium, the duration of atriomegaly, and the age of the patient.[48]

Whether or not there is ECG evidence of right ventricular hypertrophy depends largely on the height of right ventricular systolic pressure; an incomplete right bundle branch block pattern with an rSr pattern in V_1 is not usual. It is infrequent in patients with right ventricular systolic pressures less than 70 mm Hg.[46] Approximately half of all patients with right ventricular systolic pressures between 70 and 100 mm Hg manifest the electrocardiographic criteria for right ventricular hypertrophy, including both a mean QRS axis greater than 80 degrees in the frontal plane and an R:S ratio greater than 1.0 in V_1.[49] In other patients with this degree of pulmonary hypertension there is no frank evidence of right ventricular hypertrophy, but the R:S ratio fails to increase from right to midprecordial leads. When right ventricular systolic pressures exceed 100 mm Hg, electrocardiographic evidence of right ventricular hypertrophy is found quite consistently.

The *QRS axis in the frontal plane* often correlates with the severity of valve obstruction and with the level of pulmonary vascular resistance in pure MS; thus, a mean frontal axis between 0 and +60 degrees suggests that the mitral valve area exceeds 1.3 cm², whereas an axis greater than 60 degrees suggests that the valve area is less than 1.3 cm². In patients in whom pulmonary vascular resistance is greater than 650 dynes · sec · cm^{-5}, the mean axis usually exceeds +110 degrees. In patients whose pulmonary artery systolic pressures approach systemic levels, the mean axis averages +150 degrees.[50]

VECTORCARDIOGRAPHY. The characteristic *vectorcardiographic finding* in MS is right ventricular hypertrophy Type C characterized by counterclockwise rotation in the horizontal plane and a terminal deflection directed to the right, posteriorly, and superiorly.[46,50,51]

RADIOLOGICAL FINDINGS (see also Figs. 7–8*B*, p. 209; 7–16, p. 215 and 7–35, p. 226). Although in patients with hemodynamically significant MS the cardiac silhouette may be normal in the frontal projection, with the exception of an enlarged atrial appendage, left atrial enlargement is almost invariably evident on the lateral and left anterior oblique views. The size of the left atrium does *not* correlate with the severity of obstruction. Extreme left atrial enlargement rarely occurs in pure MS; when it is present, MR is usually severe. Enlargement of the pulmonary artery, right ventricle, and right atrium (as well as the left atrium) is commonly seen in severe MS (Fig. 7–35, p. 226). Occasionally, calcification of the mitral valve is evident on the chest roentgenogram (Fig. 7–29, p. 222), but, more commonly, fluoroscopy is required to detect valvular calcification.

Radiological changes in the lung fields (Fig. 7–35, p. 226) are useful in estimating the height of pulmonary venous pressure and thereby the severity of MS. Interstitial edema, an indication of severe obstruction, is manifested as Kerley B lines (dense, short, horizontal lines most commonly seen in the costophrenic angles).[52] This finding is present in 30 per cent of patients with resting pulmonary artery wedge pressures below 20 mm Hg and in 70 per cent of patients with pressures exceeding 20 mm Hg. Severe, longstanding mitral obstruction often results in Kerley A lines (straight, dense lines up to 4 cm in length running toward the hilum) as well as the findings of pulmonary hemosiderosis (Fig. 7–35, p. 226) and rarely of parenchymal ossification. Pulmonary edema is rarely evident.

ANGIOGRAPHY. Angiograms exposed in the right and left anterior oblique projections afford the best views of the mitral valve. Although ideally contrast medium should be injected into the left atrium, it is often possible to achieve good visualization of the left side of the heart by injecting a large volume into the main pulmonary artery. Such angiograms provide an assessment of left atrial size, may demonstrate thickening and reduced motion of the valve leaflets, and may outline large intraluminal thrombi.[53] Left cine ventriculography is useful in the assessment of mitral valve motion. Although this technique allows visualization of only the ventricular aspect of the leaflet in patients with pure MS, it makes possible simultaneous assessment of left ventricular contractile function and of the subvalvular mitral apparatus. Angiography in the evaluation of patients with MS or suspected MS has been largely superseded by echocardiography.

ECHOCARDIOGRAPHY (see also p. 71). MS can ordinarily be readily diagnosed by M-mode echocardiography (Fig. 3–45, p. 71), but this technique does not allow a precise determination of its severity. Echocardiograms of a thickened, calcified stenotic rheumatic valve demonstrate increased acoustic impedence and fusion of the mitral valve leaflets and poor leaflet separation in diastole.[54] The leaflets fail to close normally in mid-diastole and may not reopen widely during atrial contraction. Normally, the posterior leaflet of the mitral valve moves posteriorly during early diastole, but in more than 90 per cent of patients with MS, both leaflets move anteriorly at this time. The left atrium is usually enlarged, and in isolated MS the left ventricular cavity is normal or reduced in size. Two-dimensional echocardiography may be helpful in the preoperative recognition of left atrial thrombus and in assessing mitral valve calcification and left ventricular contractility.

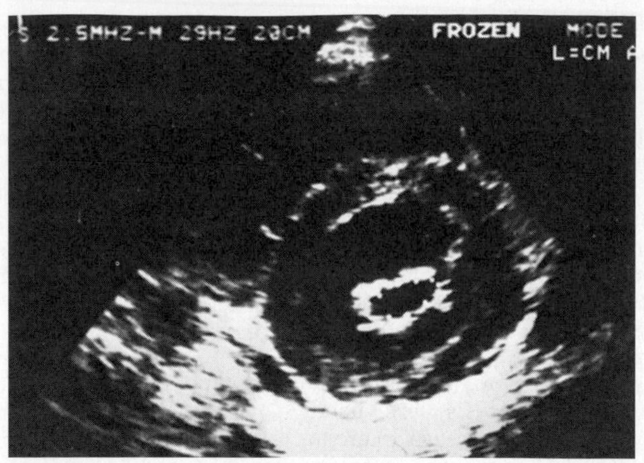

FIGURE 32–3. Two-dimensional parasternal short-axis view of the mitral valve orifice during diastole, demonstrating the echocardiographic method of mitral valve area calculation. The innermost border of the mitral orifice was planimetered with the use of a light-pen system to obtain the area (in cm²). (Reproduced with permission from Smith, M. D., et al.: Comparative accuracy of two-dimensional echocardiography and Doppler pressure half-time methods in assessing severity of mitral stenosis in patients with and without prior commissurotomy. Circulation *73*:100, 1986. Copyright 1986 American Heart Association.)

Two-dimensional echocardiography (Fig. 32–3 and Fig. 3–46, p. 72) is more accurate than M-mode echocardiography in determining mitral orifice size.[55] It reveals restricted motion and doming of the valve leaflets. With progressive thickening and fibrosis of the leaflets, the orifice becomes fixed and can then often be imaged directly and measured. This technique also provides information on the pliability and extent of calcification of the valve, thickening of the subvalvular apparatus, and fusion and retraction of the chordae as well as calcification of the mitral annulus. The echocardiogram is helpful in determining whether the patient with MS is a suitable candidate for balloon mitral valvuloplasty (see p. 1385).

Doppler echocardiography is the most accurate noninvasive technique available for quantifying the severity of MS[55,56] (Fig. 3–47, p. 72). This technique is also useful for estimating pulmonary arterial pressure. Doppler color flow imaging can be used to enhance the accuracy of the Doppler data by guiding the position of the beam[56] and to determine whether mitral regurgitation and other valvular abnormalities coexist. Transesophageal two-dimensional echocardiography provides superior images of the mitral valve and may show thrombus in the left atrium. Pedunculated and free-floating thrombi are also usually readily detected by this technique.

A detailed echocardiographic examination including two-dimensional echocardiography, a Doppler study, and Doppler color flow imaging in a patient with MS can frequently provide sufficient information to allow development of a therapeutic plan without the need for cardiac catheterization. Of course, it provides no information on the state of the coronary arteries. If surgery is planned, it is important to ascertain whether or not bypass grafting is indicated in patients at risk of having coexisting coronary artery disease.

MANAGEMENT

Medical Treatment

Patients with rheumatic heart disease should receive penicillin prophylaxis for beta-hemolytic streptococcal infections and prophylaxis for infective endocarditis (see p.

1098). Anemia and infections should be treated promptly and aggressively in patients with valvular heart disease. Adolescents and young adults with serious valvular heart disease should be advised to avoid entering occupations requiring strenuous exertion.

In symptomatic patients with mitral valve disease, considerable improvement occurs with oral diuretics and the restriction of sodium intake. Digitalis glycosides do not alter the hemodynamics and usually do not benefit patients with MS and sinus rhythm[54,57] but are of great value in slowing the ventricular rate in patients with atrial fibrillation and in the treatment of right-sided heart failure. Measures designed to reduce pulmonary venous pressure, including sedation, assumption of the upright posture, and aggressive diuresis, are used to treat hemoptysis. Beta blockers may increase exercise capacity by reducing heart rate in patients with sinus rhythm[58] but especially in patients with atrial fibrillation.

In patients with rheumatic heart disease and heart failure, anticoagulant therapy is helpful in preventing venous thrombosis and pulmonary embolism in those who have experienced one or more previous embolic episodes, in those who are at high risk of embolization, i.e., with atrial fibrillation, and in those with mechanical prosthetic heart valves. However, no firm evidence exists that anticoagulant therapy reduces the incidence of pulmonary or systemic embolism in patients in sinus rhythm in whom such episodes have not previously occurred.

TREATMENT OF ARRHYTHMIAS. Frequent premature atrial contractions often presage atrial fibrillation, and the administration of antiarrhythmic drugs, as outlined on page 593, may be effective in preventing this complication. However, once atrial fibrillation has developed, these agents may be ineffective in restoring sinus rhythm or even in maintaining sinus rhythm following electrical cardioversion, because of the pathological changes that occur in the atrium secondary to the arrhythmia itself. After electrical cardioversion, sinus rhythm can often be maintained with antiarrhythmic drugs in young patients with mild MS without marked left atrial enlargement who have been in atrial fibrillation less than 6 months and who are maintained by adequate doses of quinidine. If elective cardioversion (pharmacological or electrical) is to be attempted in the patient with MS and atrial fibrillation, a preparatory 3-week course of anticoagulation should be given to minimize the risk of systemic embolism when sinus rhythm resumes (see Ch. 46). Immediate treatment of atrial fibrillation should be directed toward reducing the ventricular rate by means of digitalis and, if possible, toward reestablishing sinus rhythm by a combination of pharmacological treatment and cardioversion. Paroxysmal atrial fibrillation and repeated conversions, spontaneous or induced, carry the risk of embolization. In patients who cannot be converted or maintained in sinus rhythm, the ventricular rate at rest should be maintained at approximately 60 to 65 beats/min with digitalis. If this is not possible, small doses of a beta blocker, such as atenolol (25 mg daily), may be added. Multiple repeat cardioversions are *not* indicated if the patient has not sustained sinus rhythm while on adequate doses of quinidine. Patients with chronic atrial fibrillation who undergo open mitral repair or valve replacement may undergo the Cox maze procedure (atrial compartment operation). More than 80 per cent of such patients can be maintained in sinus rhythm postoperatively[59] and regain normal atrial function.[60,61]

Natural History

The development of effective surgical treatment has obscured our understanding of the natural history of MS (Fig. 32–4) and, for that matter, of all valvular lesions.[53] Although few meaningful data are available, it appears that in temperate zones such as the United States and Europe, after an attack of rheumatic fever there is an asymptomatic period of approximately 15 to 20 years before symptoms set in. It then takes approximately 3 years for most patients to progress from mild disability (i.e., early Class II) to severe disability (i.e., Class III or IV). The progression is much more rapid in patients in tropical and subtropical areas,[62] in Polynesians, as well as in Alaskan Eskimos. Economic as well as genetic conditions may play a role. In India, critical MS may be present in children as young as 6 to 12 years.

In the *presurgical era,* Olesen found 62 per cent 5-year and 38 per cent 10-year survival rates among patients in New York Heart Association functional Class III but only 15 per cent 5-year survival rate in patients in Class IV.[63] Among asymptomatic patients (Class I) with MS treated medically, 40 per cent had a worsened course or had died within 10 years. Among mildly symptomatic patients (Class II), the comparable number was 80 per cent.[64] In medically treated patients with MS or with combined MS and MR, Munoz et al. found a 45 per cent 5-year survival rate.[65] In a comparable group of patients subjected to mitral commissurotomy, the 5-year survival rate was substantially better. In an unselected mix of patients with MS of varying severity, 80 per cent were alive after 5 years and 60 per cent after 10 years of medical treatment.[66]

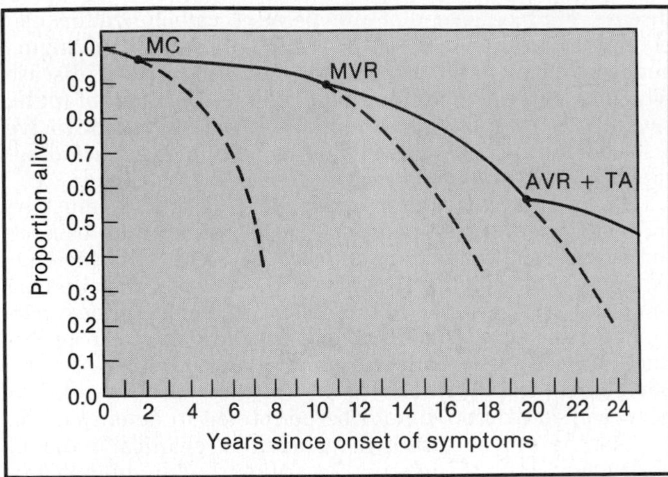

FIGURE 32–4. Schematic representation of the subsequent life history after the initial development of symptoms in a large group of patients with mitral stenosis. The colored solid circles and colored lines indicate a surgical procedure. The dashed lines represent estimated survival of patients not receiving the surgical procedure. MC = mitral commissurotomy, MVR = mitral valve replacement, TA = tricuspid annuloplasty, AVR = aortic valve replacement. (From Kirklin, J. W., and Barratt-Boyes, B. G. [eds.]: Cardiac Surgery. New York, John Wiley and Sons, 1986, p. 328.)

Surgical Treatment

INDICATIONS FOR OPERATION. Patients with MS who are asymptomatic or minimally symptomatic frequently remain so for years. However, once moderate symptoms (Class II) develop, if the stenosis is not relieved mechanically, the disease may progress relatively rapidly, as already discussed. Operation (or balloon valvuloplasty) should therefore be carried out in symptomatic patients with moderate to severe MS (i.e., a mitral valve orifice size less than approximately 1.0 cm^2/m^2 body surface area [BSA]—less than 1.5 to 1.7 cm^2 in normal-sized adults).

There has been considerable debate concerning the need for routine cardiac catheterization in determining whether operation is indicated.[67–69] A careful clinical evaluation and noninvasive assessment, particularly using two-dimensional and Doppler echocardiography, can provide sufficient information to permit an informed decision in the majority of patients. However, the consequences of valvular surgery, particularly valve replacement, are so profound that I recommend preoperative catheterization and angiography in the following groups of patients with MS: (1) patients with heart murmurs and other findings suggesting the presence of valve lesions in addition to MS, (2) patients with associated chronic obstructive pulmonary disease in which it is important to determine the contribution of MS to the symptoms, (3) patients in whom left atrial myxoma should be excluded, and (4) patients who have angina or angina-like chest pain or who have risk factors for coronary artery disease in whom associated coronary artery disease must be excluded. Critical narrowing of one or more coronary vessels occurs in approximately one-fourth of all adults with severe MS. It is more common in men over 45 years who have angina and risk factors for coronary artery disease.[26,70] I believe that preoperative catheterization can be omitted in the young (<40 years) patient without angina and significant risk factors for coronary artery disease who has typical symptoms and classic findings of pure, severe MS on physical examination and by noninvasive tests, including two-dimensional and Doppler echocardiography.

Care of mildly symptomatic patients (Class II) must be individualized. It is necessary to consider and balance three important factors: (1) the size of the mitral orifice, (2) the degree to which the patient's life style is impaired by the mitral obstruction, (3) the history of complications, particularly systemic embolism, and (4) the risk of the procedure (operation or balloon valvuloplasty). If there are no obvious contraindications to one of these procedures, left heart catheterization should be performed to determine the size of the valve orifice. In general, mechanical relief of obstruction can be deferred in patients with mild symptoms and mild stenosis (i.e., mitral valve orifice size > approximately 1.0 cm^2/m^2 BSA), whereas it should be recommended for those with mild symptoms and more severe stenosis (i.e., mitral valve orifice size < approximately 1.0 cm^2/m^2 BSA). However, this plan is subject to qualification. For instance, mechanical relief of obstruction might well be deferred in a retired, sedentary septuagenarian with a mitral valve orifice of 0.8 cm^2/m^2 BSA. On the other hand, a 30-year-old laborer whose family's economic well-being depends on his continued physical exertion might be an excellent candidate for mechanical relief of obstruction, although his mitral valve orifice size is 1.2 cm^2/m^2 BSA.

Because of the high rate of recurrence, mechanical relief of obstruction is also indicated in patients with MS in whom systemic embolism has previously occurred, even if they are otherwise asymptomatic and even though there is no definitive evidence that the incidence of recurrent emboli will be significantly reduced. Anticoagulants should be administered up to the time of operation. Although the risk of operation is higher in patients with advanced disease characterized by severe pulmonary hypertension and right-sided heart failure, surviving patients nearly always show striking clinical and hemodynamic improvement, with a marked reduction in pulmonary vascular pressures. In the pregnant patient with MS, operative treatment should be carried out only if serious pulmonary congestion occurs despite intensive medical treatment including bed rest (p. 1849).

There is no evidence that surgical treatment improves the prognosis of patients with no or only slight functional impairment. Therefore, valvotomy is not indicated in patients who are entirely asymptomatic, except in unusual circumstances. For example, some years ago I saw a 33-year-old woman with MS who had had hemoptysis and pulmonary edema during the second trimester of a pregnancy 2 years previously. She then became asymptomatic but wished to have another child. Hemodynamic study showed a pulmonary wedge pressure of 17 mm Hg and a mitral orifice area of 1.7 cm^2/m^2 BSA. Prophylactic mitral valvotomy was undertaken in this patient because it was virtually certain that another pregnancy would have resulted in serious heart failure. At present I would recommend balloon mitral valvuloplasty for such a patient (see p. 1016).

SURGICAL TECHNIQUES. Three basically different operative approaches are available for the treatment of rheumatic MS: (1) closed mitral valvotomy[71,72]; (2) open valvotomy, i.e., valvotomy carried out under direct vision with the aid of cardiopulmonary bypass; and (3) mitral valve replacement.[73] *Closed mitral valvotomy,* performed with the aid of a transventricular dilator,[72] is an effective operation, provided that MR, atrial thrombosis, or valvular calcification is not serious and that chordal fusion and shortening are not severe. Echocardiographic examination is an important prerequisite. Unfortunately, few patients satisfy all these criteria, and they are difficult to identify preoperatively. In one large series,[72] hospital mortality was 1.5 per cent, and 0.3 per cent of patients developed severe MR. Marked symptomatic improvement occurred in 86 per cent of survivors. Actuarial survival rate was 89.5 per cent after 18 years. Closed valvotomy for restenosis was carried out with a 6.7 per cent mortality. Long-term follow-up has shown that the results are best if the operation is carried out before chronic atrial fibrillation and/or heart failure has occurred.[71] If possible, closed mitral valvotomy should be carried out with "pump standby"; if the surgeon is unable to achieve a satisfactory result, the patient can be placed on cardiopulmonary bypass, and the valvotomy carried out under direct vision or the valve replaced. Closed mitral valvotomy is rarely used in the United States today, having been replaced by balloon valvuloplasty, which is of similar effectiveness in patients who are candidates for closed mitral valvotomy (see p. 1016). Closed mitral valvotomy is more popular in developing nations, where the expense of open-heart surgery is a more important factor and where patients with mitral valve disease are younger. In any event, echocardiography is useful in selecting suitable candidates for closed mitral valvotomy by identifying patients without valvular calcification or dense fibrosis.

Most surgeons in North America and Western Europe now prefer to carry out *direct-vision* or *open valvotomy.*[73–75] Cardiopulmonary bypass is established, and in order to obtain a dry, quiet heart, body temperature is usually lowered, the heart is arrested, and the aorta is occluded intermittently. Thrombi are removed from the left atrium and its appendage, and the latter is often amputated in order to remove a potential source of postoperative emboli. The commissures are incised, and when necessary, fused chordae are separated, the underlying papillary muscle is split, and the valve leaflets are debrided of calcium; mild or even moderate mitral regurgitation may be corrected. Left atrial and ventricular pressures are measured after bypass has been discontinued to confirm that the valvotomy has in fact been effective. In patients with atrial fibrillation, conversion to sinus rhythm is carried out at the completion of the operation. In a series of open mitral valve reconstructive procedures for MS at Brigham and Women's Hospital, the actuarial probability of survival at 10 years was 95 per cent. The annual reoperation rate was 1.7 per cent.[76] A survival rate of 75 per cent over 20 years after surgical repair of MS has been reported.[7]

The mortality rate after mitral valvotomy, whether open or closed, ranges from 1 to 3 per cent, depending on the condition of the patient and the skill and experience of the surgical team.[74–76] Five-year survival rates are 90 to 96 per cent and event-free survival rates 72 to 94 per cent.[77–79] In general, open valvotomy provides better hemodynamic relief of mitral valve obstruction than does the closed procedure,[75,80,81] and the risk of dislodging thrombi from the atrium or calcium from the mitral valve is also less.[76] Left atrial size, the need for mitral or tricuspid annuloplasty, and the presence of left atrial thrombus are all "risk factors" for a less than optimal outcome.[81] However, it must be recognized that mitral valvotomy, whether open or closed, and valvuloplasty are *palliative* rather than curative procedures, and even when successful they merely "turn the clock back." (The generally more effective open valvulotomy turns the clock farther back than does the closed valvulotomy or balloon mitral valvuloplasty.) Thus, valvulotomy does not result in a normal mitral valve but, at best, results in one resembling the valve as it existed perhaps a decade earlier. Because the valve is not normal postoperatively, turbulent flow usually persists in the paravalvular region, and the resultant trauma may well play a role in restenosis. These changes are analogous to the gradual development of obstruction in a congenitally bicuspid aortic valve (see p. 964) and are not usually the result of recurrent rheumatic fever. When commissurotomy is attempted and the results are inadequate—most commonly due to severe distortion and calcification of the valve and subvalvular apparatus with the accompanying regurgitation that cannot be corrected—mitral valve replacement is carried out (see p. 1027).[82]

Although a contemporary control series of medically and surgically treated patients is not available (nor is it likely ever to be), appropriate surgical treatment appears to prolong survival substantially in patients with MS (Fig. 32–4).

Mitral Restenosis

This condition can be diagnosed with certainty only on the basis of three satisfactory hemodynamic or echocardiographic investigations: a preintervention study, a second study following a successful intervention in which an increase in the size of the valvular orifice has been demonstrated, and a third when a reduction in size relative to the earlier postintervention study is noted. On clinical grounds alone, i.e., based on the reappearance of symptoms, the incidence of "restenosis" has been estimated to range widely, from 2 to 60 per cent[83]; approximately 10 per cent of patients who have undergone mitral valvotomy require reoperation within 5 years, but that fraction increases to 60 per cent by 10 years.[84] The recurrence of symptoms is *not necessarily* due to restenosis. Recurrent symptoms may be due to one of four other conditions: (1) an inadequate first operation with residual stenosis; (2) the presence or development of MR, either at operation or as a consequence of infective endocarditis; (3) the progression of aortic valve disease; and (4) the development of symptoms due to an unrelated illness, such as ischemic heart disease or chronic obstructive lung disease. In a study in which the size of the mitral valve orifice was estimated using two-dimensional echocardiography in 18 patients who had undergone successful surgical valvotomy, no change in the mitral valve area occurred over a 10- to 14-year period in 13 patients, whereas in 5 (28 per cent) true restenosis developed.[84] The rate of restenosis is approximately 10 per cent within 6 years.[85]

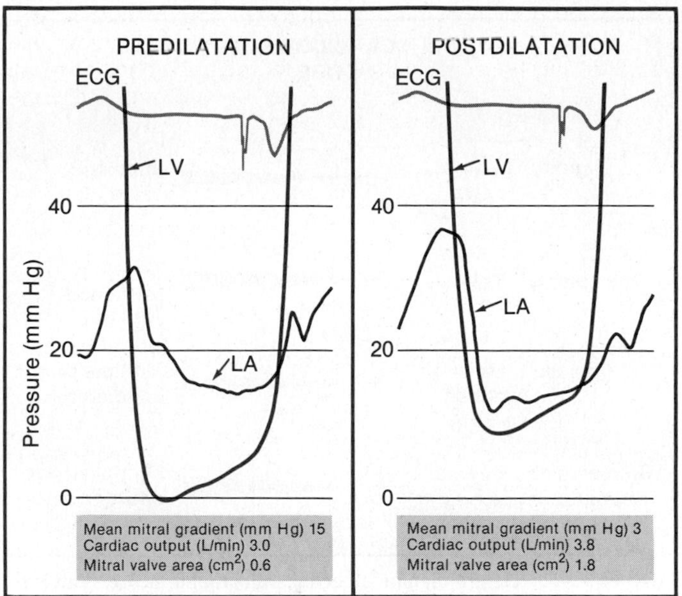

FIGURE 32–6. Simultaneous left atrial (LA) and left ventricular (LV) pressure before and after balloon valvuloplasty of the mitral valve in a patient with severe mitral stenosis. (Courtesy of Raymond G. McKay, M.D.)

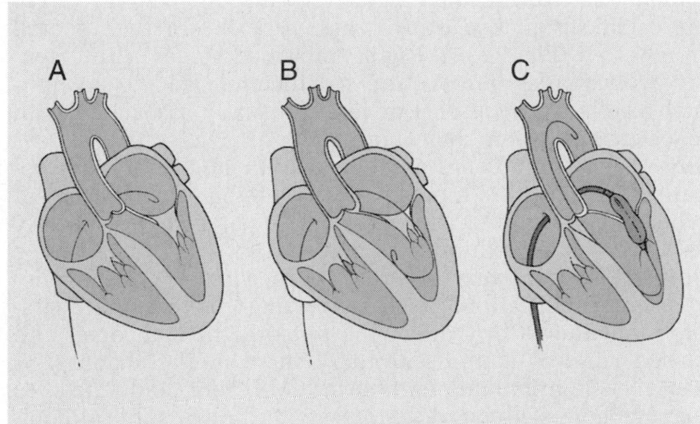

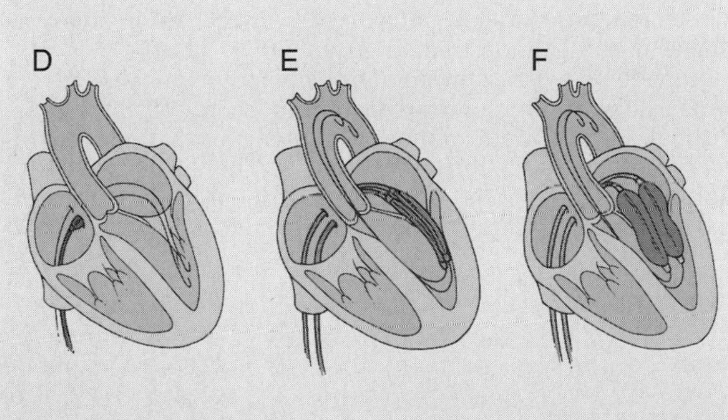

FIGURE 32–5. Technique of double-balloon mitral valvuloplasty. *A,* The position of the guidewire in the left atrium after left atrial puncture using the Brockenbrough needle. *B,* The position of the guidewire as it is advanced into the left ventricle across the stenotic mitral valve. *C,* Partial inflation of a single-balloon catheter across the stenotic mitral valve when a single-balloon valvuloplasty is to be performed. Notice that the guidewire may be advanced into the aorta in an antegrade fashion to provide greater stabilization. *D,* Dilatation of the atrial septum using an Olbert catheter in anticipation of performing a two-balloon mitral valvuloplasty. *E,* The two valvuloplasty catheters across the stenotic mitral valve. *F,* The appearance of the two simultaneously inflated balloons as the two-balloon valvuloplasty is being performed. (From Srebro, J. P., and Ports, T. A.: Catheter balloon valvuloplasty. *In* Chatterjee, K., et al. [eds.]: Cardiology: An Illustrated Text. Philadelphia, J.B. Lippincott, 1991, p. 9.54.)

Thus, in properly selected patients, mitral valvotomy results in a significant increase in the size of the mitral orifice and, at a low risk, favorably alters the clinical course of an otherwise progressive disease. Pulmonary artery pressure falls promptly and decisively when mitral obstruction is effectively relieved.[86,87] Some patients maintain clinical improvement for many (10 to 15) years of follow-up. When a second operation is required because of symptomatic deterioration, the valve is usually calcified and more seriously deformed than at the time of the first operation, and adequate reconstruction is not always possible. Accordingly, mitral valve replacement is often necessary at that time.

Also, in patients with combined MS and MR, and in those with extensive calcification involving the commissures of the valve, mitral replacement rather than valvotomy is often required. The operative mortality following mitral valve replacement ranges from 3 to 8 per cent in most hospitals. As described below (see p. 1027), the long-term fate of the prosthetic valves is not yet clear; also, the hazards of lifelong anticoagulant treatment in patients with mechanical prostheses cannot be neglected. Therefore, in patients in whom preoperative evaluation suggests that valve replacement may be required, the threshold for operation should be higher than in patients believed to require commissurotomy alone.

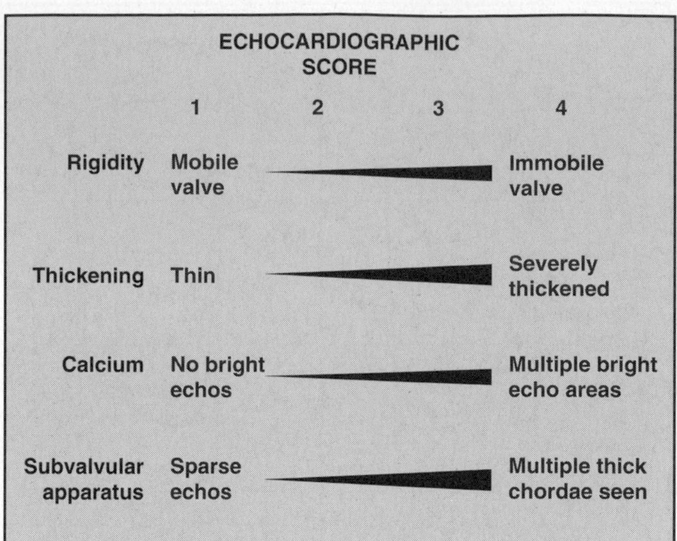

FIGURE 32–7. Determination of echocardiographic score. Valve rigidity, thickening, calcification, and the amount of subvalvular disease are graded 1 to 4 depending on severity of abnormality. The sum of the four factors equals the echo score. (From Block, P. C.: Mitral balloon valvotomy: Why, when and how? Cardiol. Rev. *2*:19, 1994.)

Balloon Mitral Valvuloplasty

(See also Chap. 39)

This procedure represents an alternative to surgical treatment of MS. The technique consists of advancing a small balloon flotation catheter across the interatrial septum (after transseptal puncture), enlarging the opening and advancing one large (23 to 25 mm) or two smaller (12 to 18 mm) balloons across the mitral orifice, and inflating them within the orifice[54,77,88–90a] (Fig. 32–5 and Fig. 39–14, p. 1385). Commissural separation and fracture of nodular calcium appear to be the mechanisms responsible for improvement in valvular function. In several series the hemodynamic results have been quite favorable (Fig. 32–6), with reduction of the transmitral pressure gradient from an average of approximately 18 to 6 mm Hg, a small (average 20 per cent) increase in cardiac output, and, on the average, a doubling of the calculated mitral valve area from 1.0 to 2.0 cm^2. The reported mortality averages 0.5 per cent. Complications include cerebral embolic events (despite absence of detectable thrombus on two-dimensional echocardiography) and cardiac perforation, each in approximately 1 per cent, and the development of mitral regurgitation severe enough to require operation in another 2 per cent (approximately 15 per cent develop lesser, but still undesirable, degrees of regurgitation). Results are especially impressive in younger patients without valvular thickening or calcification. Improvement in exercise tolerance has paralleled the favorable hemodynamic changes.

Approximately 10 per cent of patients are left with a small residual atrial septal defect, but this closes or decreases in size in the majority. Rarely, the defect is large enough to cause right heart failure.[91] Elevated pulmonary vascular resistance declines rapidly (but usually not completely) following mitral balloon valvuloplasty,[92] and pulmonary function improves as well. In follow-up studies over 3 years, hemodynamic benefit has been maintained in the majority of patients, and they have not required surgical treatment, i.e., with commissurotomy or mitral valve replacement. Approximately 10 per cent have developed restenosis.

The combination of significant symptoms and documented MS generally serves as an indication for balloon valvulotomy. The skill and experience of the operator (interventional cardiologist) must be considered. Detailed two-dimensional and Doppler echocardiographic studies are indicated before a decision is made. Left atrial thrombus must be excluded by echocardiography.

An echocardiographic scoring system developed by Wilkins et al.[93] has been found to be particularly valuable in patient selection. Leaflet rigidity, leaflet thickening, valvular calcification, and subvalvular disease are each scored from 0 to 4 (Fig. 32–7). Rigid, thickened valves with extensive subvalvular fibrosis and calcification lead to suboptimal results. A score of 8 or less is usually associated with an excellent immediate and long-term result, whereas scores exceeding 8 are associated with less impressive results (Fig. 32–8). Fluoroscopically visible calcium is another important predictor of outcome; patients with heavily calcified valves exhibit less increase in valve area and a poorer long-term survival than those with no or lesser degrees of calcification.[94,94a] The findings on echocardiography and fluoroscopy affect the outcome of both open and closed surgical commissurotomy in a similar manner. A trial in which patients with severe MS were randomized to percutaneous balloon valvuloplasty and open surgical commissurotomy resulted in similar clinical results from the two techniques. Indeed, after 3 years, mitral valve area was greater in the balloon-treated group[95] (Fig. 32–9).

In patients with symptomatic, hemodynamically severe stenosis, with an echocardiographic score of 8 or less, without left atrial thrombus, percutaneous balloon angioplasty is the procedure of choice.[89] The lower cost and morbidity are obvious advantages. The procedure is optimal for treating young patients with noncalcific MS in de-

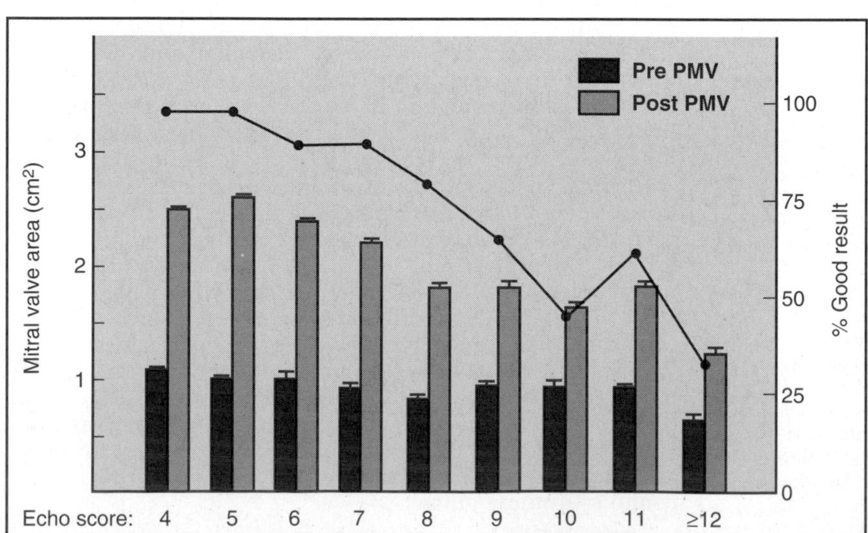

FIGURE 32–8. Relationship between echocardiographic score (X axis), the increase in mitral valve area produced by percutaneous mitral valvotomy (left Y axis), and the per cent of patients having a good result (mitral valve area > 1.5 cm^2) (right Y axis). (From Block, P. C., and Palacios, I. F.: Aortic and mitral balloon valvuloplasty: The United States experience. *In* Topol, E. J. [ed.]: Textbook of Interventional Cardiology. Philadelphia, W.B. Saunders Company, 1990, p. 831.)

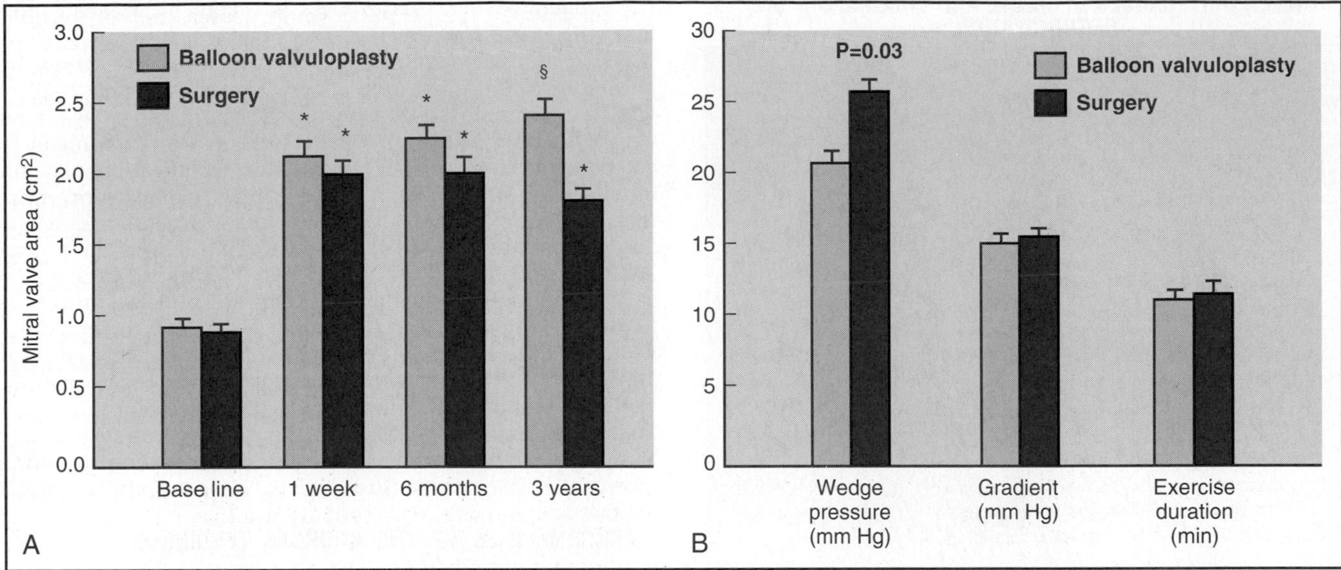

FIGURE 32–9. *A,* Hemodynamic variables at baseline and 1 week, 6 months, and 3 years after balloon mitral valvuloplasty or open surgical commissurotomy. The asterisk indicates $P < 0.001$ for the comparison with the baseline value. The section mark (§) indicates $P < 0.001$ for the comparison with the surgery group. The bars indicate the standard errors. *B,* Pulmonary artery wedge pressure and mitral valve gradient during exercise and duration of exercise at the 3-year follow-up examination. The bars indicate the standard errors. (From Reyes, V. P., Raju, B. S., Wynne, J., et al.: Percutaneous balloon valvuloplasty compared with open surgical commissurotomy for mitral stenosis. N. Engl. J. Med. *331:*961, 1994. Copyright Massachusetts Medical Society.)

veloping nations with limited facilities for open heart surgery.[90] It may also be used in patients with less favorable valves who are unsuitable for surgery because of high risk.[96,96a] These include very elderly patients and patients with associated severe ischemic heart disease, as well as patients in whom MS is complicated by pulmonary, renal, or neoplastic disease, women of childbearing age in whom valve replacement is undesirable, and pregnant women with MS.[97] Balloon angioplasty can also be the initial procedure in patients with symptomatic, severe MS and unfavorable valves (echocardiographic score >8 and/or dense calcification on fluoroscopic examination)[94,98] without any of these characteristics but with the appreciation that the failure rate is considerable and that the patient may require follow-up surgical treatment, ordinarily mitral valve replacement.

MITRAL REGURGITATION

ETIOLOGY AND PATHOLOGY

The mitral valve apparatus involves the mitral leaflets per se, the chordae tendineae, the papillary muscles, and the mitral annulus. Abnormalities of any of these structures may cause mitral regurgitation (MR)[98a] (Table 32–1). The mitral valve prolapse syndrome, an important cause of MR, is discussed in a separate section (see p. 1029).

ABNORMALITIES OF VALVE LEAFLETS. MR due to predominant involvement of the valve leaflets occurs most commonly in chronic rheumatic heart disease and is more frequent in men than in women. It is a consequence of shortening, rigidity, deformity, and retraction of one or both cusps of the mitral valve, associated with shortening and fusion of the chordae tendineae and papillary muscles.[99,99a] Infective endocarditis can cause MR by perforating valve leaflets; vegetations can prevent leaflet coaptation, and valvular retraction during the healing phase of endocarditis can cause MR. Destruction of the mitral valve leaflets can also occur in penetrating and nonpenetrating trauma (see p. 1541). When severe MR accompanies acute rheumatic fever in children or in adolescents in developing countries, regurgitation is usually secondary to a combination of prolapse of the anterior leaflet, elongation of the chordae, and dilatation of the annulus.[100] Left ventricular submitral aneurysm has been reported as a cause of MR in sub-Saharan Africa. It appears to be caused by a congenital defect in the posterior portion of the annulus. Diagnosis by transesophageal echocardiography[101] and surgical repair have been reported.

ABNORMALITIES OF THE MITRAL ANNULUS. Dilatation. In a normal adult the mitral annulus measures approximately 10 cm in circumference; it is soft and flexible, and during systole contraction of the surrounding left ventricular muscle causes the annulus to constrict. This constriction contributes importantly to valve closure. MR secondary to dilatation of the mitral annulus can occur in any form of heart disease characterized by severe dilatation of the left ventricle,[102] especially dilated ischemic cardiomyopathy.[103] It is often difficult to differentiate this secondary from the primary form of MR, but it is notable that primary valvular regurgitation is often more severe than is regurgitation secondary to annular dilatation.

Calcification. Idiopathic (degenerative) calcification of the mitral annulus is one of the most common cardiac abnormalities found at autopsy; in most hearts it is of little functional consequence. However, when it is severe it may be an important cause of MR,[103a] and in contrast to MR secondary to rheumatic fever, this cause is more common in women than in men. The development of degenerative calcification of the mitral annulus is accelerated by systemic hypertension, aortic stenosis, and diabetes, as well as by an intrinsic defect in the fibrous skeleton of the heart, such as occurs in the Marfan and Hurler syndromes. In these two conditions, the mitral annulus is not only calcified but is also dilated, further contributing to MR. The incidence of mitral annular calcification is also increased in patients with chronic renal failure with secondary hyperparathyroidism.[104] The annulus may also become thick, rigid, and calcified secondary to rheumatic

TABLE 32–1 CAUSES OF ACUTE AND CHRONIC MITRAL REGURGITATION

ACUTE

Mitral Annulus Disorders
- Infective endocarditis (abscess formation)
- Trauma (valvular heart surgery)
- Paravalvular leak due to suture interruption (surgical technical problems or infective endocarditis)

Mitral Leaflet Disorders
- Infective endocarditis (perforation or interfering with valve closure by vegetation)
- Trauma (tear during percutaneous mitral balloon valvotomy or penetrating chest injury)
- Tumors (atrial myxoma)
- Myxomatous degeneration
- Systemic lupus erythematosus (Libman-Sacks lesion)

Rupture of Chordae Tendineae
- Idiopathic, e.g., spontaneous
- Myxomatous degeneration (mitral valve prolapse, Marfan syndrome, Ehlers-Danlos syndrome)
- Infective endocarditis
- Acute rheumatic fever
- Trauma (percutaneous balloon valvotomy, blunt chest trauma)

Papillary Muscle Disorders
- Coronary artery disease (causing dysfunction and rarely rupture)
- Acute global left ventricular dysfunction
- Infiltrative diseases (amyloidosis, sarcoidosis)
- Trauma

Primary Mitral Valve Prosthetic Disorders
- Porcine cusp perforation (endocarditis)
- Porcine cusp degeneration
- Mechanical failure (strut fracture)
- Immobilized disc or ball of the mechanical prosthesis

CHRONIC

Inflammatory
- Rheumatic heart disease
- Systemic lupus erythematosus
- Scleroderma

Degenerative
- Myxomatous degeneration of mitral valve leaflets (Barlow's click-murmur syndrome, prolapsing leaflet, mitral valve prolapse)
- Marfan syndrome
- Ehlers-Danlos syndrome
- Pseudoxanthoma elasticum
- Calcification of mitral valve annulus

Infective
- Infective endocarditis affecting normal, abnormal, or prosthetic mitral valves

Structural
- Ruptured chordae tendineae (spontaneous or secondary to myocardial infarction, trauma, mitral valve prolapse, endocarditis)
- Rupture or dysfunction of papillary muscle (ischemia or myocardial infarction)
- Dilatation of mitral valve annulus and left ventricular cavity (congestive cardiomyopathies, aneurysmal dilatation of the left ventricle)
- Hypertrophic cardiomyopathy
- Paravalvular prosthetic leak

Congenital
- Mitral valve clefts or fenestrations
- Parachute mitral valve abnormality in association with:
  - Endocardial cushion defects
  - Endocardial fibroelastosis
  - Transposition of the great arteries
  - Anomalous origin of the left coronary artery

Data from Jutzy, K. R., and Al-Zaibag, M.: Acute mitral and aortic valve regurgitation. *In* Al-Zaibag, M., and Duran, C. M. G. (eds.): Valvular Heart Disease. New York, Marcel Dekker, 1994, pp. 345–382 (top portion) and Haffajee, C. I.: Chronic mitral regurgitation. *In* Dalen, J. E., and Alpert, J. S. (eds.): Valvular Heart Disease. 2nd ed. Boston, Little, Brown and Co., 1987, p. 112 (lower portion).

involvement; when this process is severe, it also can interfere with valve closure.

When annular calcification is severe, a rigid, curved bar or ring of calcium encircles the mitral orifice (Fig. 7–28, p. 222), and calcific spurs may project into the adjacent left ventricular myocardium.[105] The bulk of the calcium is located in the subvalvular region. The calcification may immobilize the basal portion of the mitral leaflets, preventing their normal excursion in diastole and coaptation in systole and aggravating the MR that results from loss of the normal sphincteric action of the mitral ring.[106] Rarely, when severe calcification encroaches on or protrudes into the mitral orifice, obstruction to left ventricular filling may occur. Calcification of the aortic valve cusps is an associated finding in approximately 50 per cent of patients with severe annular calcification, but this rarely causes aortic stenosis. In patients with severe calcification the conduction system may be invaded by calcium, leading to atrioventricular and/or intraventricular conduction defects.[105] Occasionally, calcific deposits extend into the coronary arteries.

ABNORMALITIES OF THE CHORDAE TENDINEAE. These are important causes of MR. The chordae may be congenitally abnormal; rupture may be spontaneous ("primary")[106] or may occur as a consequence of infective endocarditis, trauma, rheumatic fever, or rarely, osteogenesis imperfecta.[107,108] Lengthening and rupture of chordae tendineae are cardinal features of the mitral valve prolapse syndrome (see p. 1029). In most cases no cause for chordal rupture is apparent, other than increased mechanical strain. Chordae to the posterior leaflet rupture more frequently than those to the anterior leaflet. Patients with idiopathic rupture of mitral chordae tendineae frequently exhibit pathological fibrosis of the papillary muscles. It is possible that the dysfunction of the papillary muscles may have caused stretching and ultimately rupture of the chordae. Chordal rupture may also result from acute left ventricular dilatation, regardless of etiology. Depending on the number of chordae involved in rupture and rate at which rupture occurs, the resultant MR may be mild, moderate, or severe and acute, subacute, or chronic, respectively.

INVOLVEMENT OF THE PAPILLARY MUSCLES. Diseases of the left ventricular papillary muscles frequently cause MR.[109] Because these muscles are perfused by the terminal portion of the coronary vascular bed, they are particularly vulnerable to ischemia, and any disturbance in coronary perfusion may result in papillary muscle dysfunction (Fig. 32–10). When ischemia is transient, it results in temporary papillary muscle dysfunction and may cause transient episodes of MR sometimes associated with attacks of angina pectoris. When ischemia of papillary muscles is severe and prolonged, it causes papillary muscle dysfunction and scarring and chronic MR. The posterior papillary muscle, which is supplied by the posterior descending branch of the right coronary artery, becomes ischemic and infarcted more frequently than does the anterolateral papillary muscle, which is supplied by diagonal branches of the left anterior descending coronary artery and often by marginal branches from the left circumflex artery as well. Ischemia of the papillary muscle is caused most commonly by coronary artery disease, but it may also occur in severe anemia, shock, coronary arteritis of any etiology, and anomalous left coronary artery. MR occurs frequently in patients with healed myocardial infarcts, and is caused by dyskinesis of the left ventricular myocardium at the base of a papillary muscle.[110]

Left ventricular dilatation of any cause, including ischemia, can alter the spatial relationships between the papillary muscles and the chordae tendineae and thereby result in MR.[111] Although *necrosis of a papillary muscle* is a frequent complication of myocardial infarction,[112] frank rupture is far less common; the latter is usually fatal because of the extremely severe MR that it produces. However, rupture of one or two of the apical heads of a

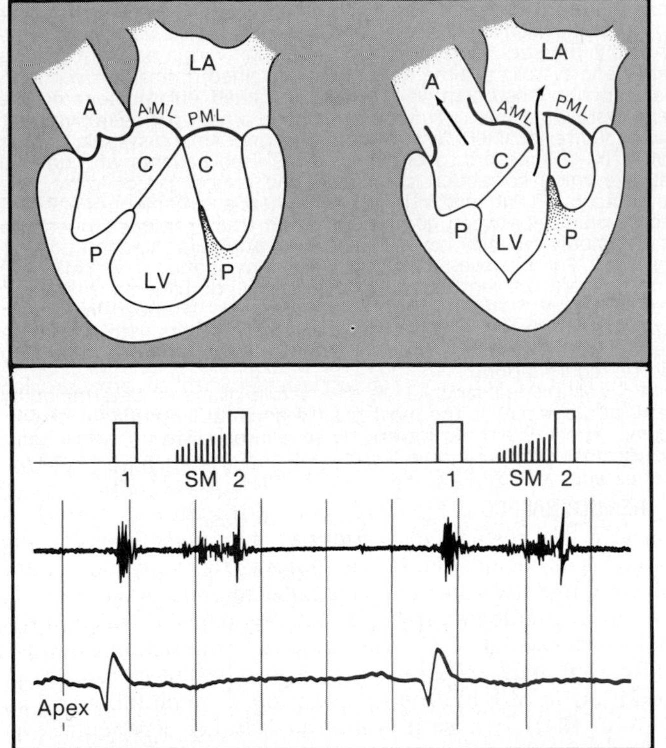

FIGURE 32–10. *Top,* Mitral regurgitation due to papillary muscle dysfunction. At the onset of systole (left), the anterior and posterior mitral valve leaflets (AML and PML) approximate. Later in systole (right), the anterior papillary muscle (P, nonhatched) contracts while the posterior papillary muscle (P, hatched) fails to contract because of ischemia or infarction. Part of the posterior leaflet is allowed to prolapse into the left atrium (LA) during systole, producing regurgitation. This process may involve either papillary muscle. C = chordae tendineae, LV = left ventricle, A = aorta. *Bottom,* Late systolic murmur (SM) that developed in a patient following an inferior myocardial infarction and is probably due to weakening of the posterior papillary muscle with prolapse of the mitral leaflet into the atrium during late systole. (From Ravin, A., et al.: Auscultation of the Heart. 3rd ed. Chicago, Year Book Medical Publishers, 1977, p. 99. Copyright © 1977 by Year Book Medical Publishers, Inc., Chicago.)

muscle, which results in a lesser degree of MR, makes survival possible, usually with surgical therapy (see p. 1243).

Some degree of MR is found in approximately 30 per cent of patients with coronary artery disease who are being considered for coronary bypass surgery,[110] and in them it is secondary to ischemic damage of the papillary muscles, dilatation of the mitral valve ring, or both. In most of these patients MR is mild, but in the small percentage in whom MR is severe (3 per cent in one large series of patients with coronary artery disease proved by coronary arteriography), it is associated with a poor prognosis.[113] The incidence and severity of regurgitation vary inversely with the left ventricular ejection fraction and directly with the left ventricular end-diastolic pressure.

A variety of other disorders of papillary muscles may also be responsible for the development of mitral regurgitation (Table 32–1). These include congenital malposition, absence of one papillary muscle, resulting in the so-called parachute mitral valve syndrome, and involvement or infiltration of papillary muscles by a variety of processes, including abscesses, granulomas, neoplasms, amyloidosis, and sarcoidosis.

Other causes of MR, discussed in greater detail elsewhere, include obstructive cardiomyopathy (see p. 1404), mitral valve prolapse (see p. 1029), the hypereosinophilic syndrome,[114] endomyocardial fibrosis,[115] trauma affecting the leaflets[116] and/or papillary muscles[117] (see p. 1541), Kawasaki disease[118] (see p. 994), left atrial myxoma, a variety of congenital anomalies including cleft anterior leaflet,[119] and ostium secundum atrial septal defect.[120]

PATHOPHYSIOLOGY

Because the regurgitant mitral orifice is functionally in parallel with the aortic valve, the impedance to ventricular emptying is reduced in MR. Consequently, MR enhances left ventricular emptying. Almost half of the regurgitant volume is ejected into the left atrium before the aortic valve opens.[121] The volume of MR depends on the impedance to left ventricular emptying and is increased by hypertension and aortic stenosis and reduced in shock.

The volume of mitral regurgitation flow depends on a combination of the instantaneous size of the regurgitant orifice and the (reverse) pressure gradient between the left ventricle and left atrium[18a,122–124]; both of these factors—orifice size and pressure gradient—are labile. Left ventricular systolic pressure and therefore the left ventricular–left atrial gradient depends on systemic vascular resistance[122] and in patients in whom the mitral annulus is normally flexible, the cross-sectional area of the mitral annulus may be altered by many interventions. Thus, increases of both preload and afterload and depressions of contractility increase left ventricular size and enlarge the mitral annulus and thereby the regurgitant orifice.[124] When ventricular size is reduced by treatment with positive inotropic agents, diuretics, and particularly vasodilators, the volume of regurgitant flow declines, as reflected in the height of the *v* wave in the left atrial pressure pulse and in the intensity and duration of the systolic murmur. Conversely, left ventricular dilatation may increase MR.

In canine experiments in which the acute effects of equally severe MR and aortic regurgitation (AR) on the left ventricle were compared, left ventricular end-diastolic pressure, volume, and radius rose with both lesions, but far *less* so with MR.[125] Peak left ventricular wall tension rose markedly when AR was induced but either did not change greatly or actually declined with MR. According to Laplace's law, myocardial wall tension is related to the product of intraventricular pressure and ventricular radius. Because *acute* MR reduces both late systolic ventricular pressure and radius, left ventricular wall tension declines markedly (and proportionately to a greater extent than left ventricular pressure), permitting a reciprocal increase in both the extent and velocity of myocardial fiber shortening. Thus, the reduced left ventricular afterload allows a greater proportion of the contractile energy of the myocardium to be expended in shortening than in tension development and explains how the left ventricle can adapt to the load imposed by MR. The ratio of wall thickness (h) to ventricular radius (r) is lower and the fractional shortening of myocardium greater in patients with MR than AR.[126,127]

The left ventricle initially compensates for the development of acute MR in part by emptying more completely and in part by increasing preload, i.e., by use of the Frank-Starling principle. As regurgitation, particularly severe regurgitation, becomes chronic, the left ventricular end-diastolic volume increases. By the Laplace principle, this increases wall tension to normal or supranormal levels.[128] The resultant increase in left ventricular volume and mitral annular diameter may create a vicious circle in which "MR begets more MR." [129]

For many years it was thought that when heart failure occurred in patients with severe rheumatic MR and acute rheumatic fever, it was caused, at least in part, by the accompanying rheumatic myocarditis. However, the normalization of hemodynamics following valve replacement in such patients makes this unlikely and instead suggests that the heart failure is secondary to the valvular lesion itself.[130]

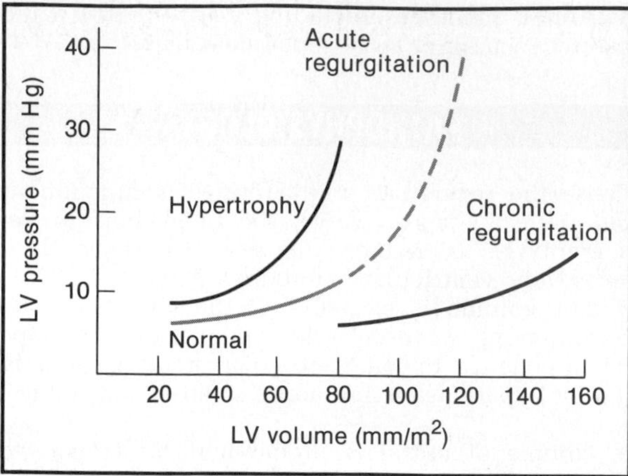

FIGURE 32–11. Diagrammatic representation of the changes in the diastolic pressure-volume relationship that occur in valve disease. Hypertrophy without significant ventricular dilatation (e.g., in aortic stenosis) produces a somewhat steeper curve than normal. Acute regurgitation produces a sudden volume load on the ventricle without time for other changes to occur and the ventricle operates at the upper (steep) end of the normal curve (broken line). Chronic aortic and mitral regurgitation with volume overload produces a flattened curve so that large volumes are accommodated without the large rise in end-diastolic pressure which occurs in acute regurgitation. (From Hall, R. J., and Julian, D. G.: Diseases of the Cardiac Valves. New York, Churchill Livingstone, 1989, p. 291.)

A large volume of MR induced experimentally produces only slightly increased myocardial oxygen consumption,[131] because myocardial fiber shortening, which is elevated in MR, is not one of the principal determinants of myocardial oxygen consumption.[132] One of these, mean left ventricular wall tension, may actually be reduced in MR whereas the other two, contractility and heart rate, may be little affected. These experimental observations correlate with the low incidence of clinical manifestations of myocardial ischemia in patients with severe MR compared with that occurring in aortic stenosis or aortic regurgitation, conditions in which myocardial oxygen demands are augmented.

In patients with chronic MR, both left ventricular end-diastolic volume and mass are increased; i.e., typical volume overload (eccentric) hypertrophy develops. The degree of hypertrophy is usually appropriate to the left ventricular dilatation, so that the ratio of left ventricular mass to end-diastolic volume is normal (Fig. 13–10, p. 401). A shift to the right occurs in the left ventricular diastolic pressure-volume curve with chronic MR (Fig. 32–11).[133]

ASSESSMENT OF MYOCARDIAL CONTRACTILITY IN MITRAL REGURGITATION

(See also p. 430)

Because the ejection phase indices of myocardial contractility are inversely correlated with afterload, patients with early MR (with reduced left ventricular afterload) often exhibit elevations in ejection phase indices of myocardial contractility, such as ejection fraction (EF), fractional fiber shortening (FS), and velocity of circumferential fiber shortening (VCF).[134] However, by the time patients become seriously symptomatic, EF, FS, and mean VCF have usually declined to *normal* levels or below. As MR persists, the reduction in afterload, which increases myocardial shortening and the above-mentioned ejection phase indices, is opposed by the impairment of myocardial function characteristic of severe chronic diastolic overload. However, even in patients with overt heart failure secondary to MR, the EF and FS may be only slightly reduced.[183,184,188] Therefore, *normal* values for the ejection phase indices of myocardial performance in patients with acute MR may actually reflect impaired myocardial function,[135,136] whereas moderately reduced values (e.g., an ejection fraction of 40 to 50 per cent) generally signify severe, often irreversible, impairment of contractility. An ejection fraction under 40 per cent in patients with severe MR usually represents advanced myocardial dysfunction; such patients are high operative risks and may not experience marked improvement following mitral valve replacement (see p. 1026). Indeed, long-term survival following replacement or repair of regurgitant mitral valves is reduced if the ejection fraction declines below 60 per cent.[136]

END-SYSTOLIC VOLUME. Preoperative myocardial contractility is an important determinant of the risk of operative death and of cardiac failure in the perioperative period and of the level of left ventricular function postoperatively. Therefore, it is not surprising that the end-systolic pressure (or stress/dimension) relation has emerged as a useful index for evaluating left ventricular function in patients with valvular regurgitation.[137] Indeed, the simple measurement of end-systolic volume has been found to be more useful as a predictor of outcome than the ejection fraction, end-diastolic volume, or end-diastolic pressure.[138] Patients with severe MR with a normal preoperative end-systolic volume (<40 ml/m²) retained normal left ventricular function postoperatively, whereas marked enlargement of the end-systolic volume (>80 ml/m²) signified a high perioperative mortality and residual left ventricular dysfunction. An end-systolic volume of 55 ml/m² appears to discriminate between patients who do well after surgical correction and those who are at risk of irreversible dysfunction.[139] Patients with MR and modest enlargement of end-systolic volume (between 40 and 80 ml/m²) usually tolerate operation satisfactorily but may have reduced left ventricular function postoperatively. For any level of end-systolic volume, patients with MR have more severe left ventricular dysfunction than do patients with aortic regurgitation.[140] This finding reflects the lower afterload in MR and correlates with the clinical observation that patients with MR have a less favorable response to surgical intervention than do those with aortic regurgitation.[138]

A closely related variable, the end-systolic diameter, determined by echocardiography, is the most reliable noninvasive predictor of outcome (survival without severe heart failure) following mitral valve replacement. The outcome is excellent until the end-systolic diameter exceeds approximately 45 mm or 26 ml/m² (Fig. 32–12).[141]

HEMODYNAMICS. Effective (forward) *cardiac output* is usually depressed in seriously symptomatic patients, whereas *total* left ventricular output (the sum of forward and regurgitant flow, which can be measured by radionuclide ventriculography)[142] is usually elevated until quite late in the patient's course. The atrial contraction (*a*) wave in the left atrial pressure pulse is usually not as prominent in MR as in MS, but the *v* wave is often much taller[123] (Fig. 6–5, p. 184), because it is inscribed during ventricular systole, when the left atrium is being filled with blood from the pulmonary veins as well as from the left ventricle (Fig. 32–13). Occasionally, backward transmission of the tall *v* wave into the pulmonary arterial bed may result in an early diastolic "pulmonary arterial *v* wave."[143] In patients with pure MR, the *y* descent is particularly rapid as the distended left atrium empties rapidly during early systole. However, in patients with combined MS and MR, the *y* descent is gradual. Although a left atrioventricular pressure gradient persisting throughout diastole signifies the

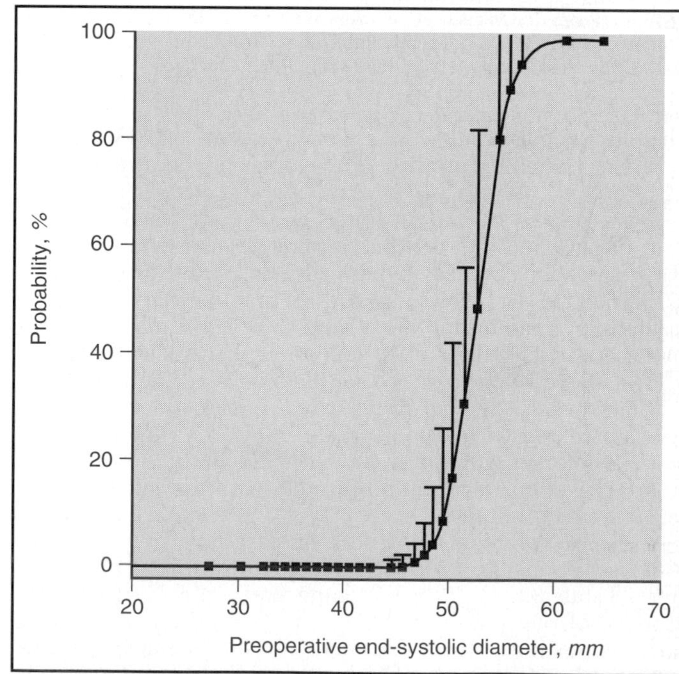

FIGURE 32–12. The probability of postoperative death or persistence of severe heart failure in patients with mitral regurgitation plotted against preoperative echocardiographic end-systolic diameter. As end-systolic diameter exceeded 45 mm, the incidence of a poor postoperative outcome increased abruptly. (Reproduced with permission from Wisenbaugh, T., et al.: Prediction of outcome after valve replacement for rheumatic mitral regurgitation in the era of chordal preservation. Circulation *89*:191, 1994. Copyright 1994 American Heart Association.)

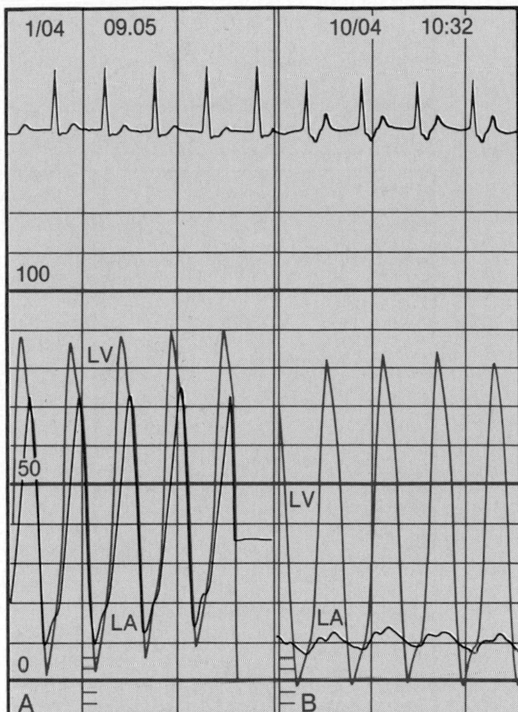

FIGURE 32–13. Intraoperative simultaneous left ventricular (LV) and left atrial (LA) pressures (mm Hg) before (*A*) and after (*B*) mitral valvuloplasty for correction of severe acute mitral regurgitation. Note the height of the *v* wave in the preoperative tracing. (From Barlow, J. B.: Perspectives on the Mitral Valve. Philadelphia, F. A. Davis Co., 1987, p. 257.)

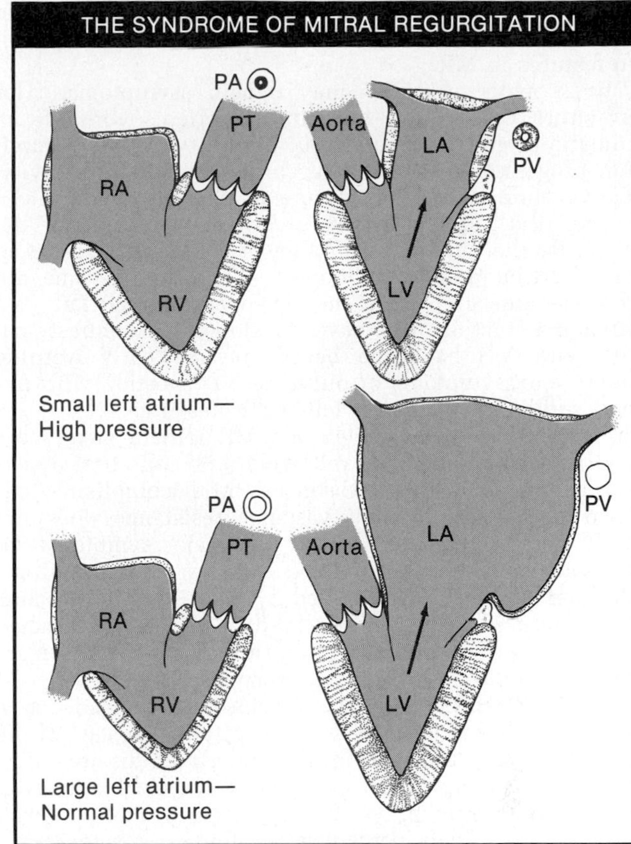

FIGURE 32–14. Diagram depicting the two extremes of the spectrum in pure mitral regurgitation. When severe mitral regurgitation appears suddenly in individuals with previously normal or near-normal hearts *(top)*, the left atrium (LA) is relatively small and the high pressure within it is reflected back into the pulmonary vessels and right ventricle (RV). The anatomical indicator of this latter physiological event is severe hypertrophy of the left atrial and right ventricular walls and marked intimal proliferation and medial hypertrophy of the pulmonary arteries (PA), arterioles, and veins (PV). At the other extreme with severe chronic mitral regurgitation *(bottom)*, the left atrial cavity is of giant size and its wall is thin. It is thus able to "absorb" the left ventricular (LV) pressure without reflecting it back into the pulmonary vessels or right ventricle. As a consequence, pulmonary vessels remain normal, and the right ventricular wall does not thicken. PT = pulmonary trunk; RA = right atrium. (From Roberts, W. C., et al.: Nonrheumatic valvular cardiac disease. A clinicopathologic survey of 27 different conditions causing valvular dysfunction. *In* Likoff, W. [ed.]: Cardiovascular Clinics. Vol. 5, No. 2, Valvular Heart Disease. Philadelphia, F. A. Davis Co., 1973, p. 403.)

presence of significant associated MS, a brief early diastolic gradient may occur in patients with isolated, severe regurgitation as a result of the torrential flow of blood across a normal-sized mitral orifice[143a] (Fig. 32–2).

LEFT ATRIAL COMPLIANCE

The compliance of the left atrium (and pulmonary venous bed) is an important determinant of the hemodynamic[144,145] and clinical picture in MR. Three major subgroups of patients with severe MR based on left atrial compliance have been identified[125,146,147] (Fig. 32–14) and are characterized as follows:

NORMAL OR REDUCED COMPLIANCE. There is little enlargement of the left atrium but marked elevation of the mean left atrial pressure, particularly of the *v* wave,[148,149] and pulmonary congestion is a prominent symptom. In most cases, severe MR has developed suddenly, as occurs with rupture of chordae tendineae, infarction of one of the heads of a papillary muscle, or perforation of a mitral leaflet as a consequence of trauma or endocarditis. Initially in acute MR the left atrium operates on the steep portion of its pressure-volume curve. Sinus rhythm is usually present; with the passage of weeks or a few months the left atrial wall frequently exhibits striking hypertrophy, is capable of contracting vigorously, and facilitates left ventricular filling.[144] The thicker atrium is less compliant than normal, increasing further the height of the *v* wave. Thickening of the walls of the pulmonary veins and proliferative changes in the pulmonary arteries as well as marked elevation of pulmonary vascular resistance usually develop over the course of 6 to 12 months.

MARKEDLY INCREASED COMPLIANCE. At the opposite end of the spectrum from patients in the first group are those with severe, longstanding MR with massive enlargement of the left atrium and normal or only slightly elevated left atrial pressure.[147] The atrial wall contains only a small remnant of muscle surrounded by a great deal of fibrous tissue. Longstanding MR in these patients has altered the physical properties of the left atrial wall and thereby displaced the atrial pressure-volume curve, allowing a normal or almost normal pressure to exist in a greatly enlarged left atrium. (This shift in the left atrial pressure-volume curve with persistent MR has been documented in animal experiments.[144]) Pulmonary artery pressure and pulmonary vascular resistance are normal or only slightly elevated at rest. Atrial fibrillation and a low cardiac output are almost invariably present.[147]

MODERATELY INCREASED COMPLIANCE. This, the most common subgroup, consists of patients between the ends of the spectrum represented by groups 1 and 2; these patients have severe chronic MR and exhibit variable degrees of enlargement of the left atrium, associated with significant elevation of the left atrial pressure.

CLINICAL MANIFESTATIONS

History

The nature and severity of the symptoms of patients with chronic MR are functions of its severity, rate of progression, the level of pulmonary artery pressure, and the presence of associated valvular, myocardial, or coronary artery disease. Because symptoms usually do not develop in patients with chronic MR until the left ventricle fails, the time interval between the initial attack of rheumatic fever (when one has occurred) and the development of symptoms tends to be longer in MR than in MS and often exceeds two decades. The course in patients with chronic MR tends to be less dramatic and is punctuated with fewer acute complications than in patients with MS. Acute pulmonary edema occurs less frequently in chronic MR than in MS, presumably because sudden surges in left atrial pressure are less common.[15] Similarly, although hemoptysis and systemic embolization do occur in MR, they are less common than in MS. The development of atrial fibrillation affects the course adversely but perhaps not as dramatically as it does in MS. On the other hand, chronic weakness and fatigue secondary to a low cardiac output are more prominent features in MR.

Patients with mild MR may remain asymptomatic for their entire lives.[41] The majority of patients with MR of rheumatic origin have only mild disability, unless regurgitation progresses as a result of chronic rheumatic activity, infective endocarditis, or rupture of chordae tendineae.[147] However, the indolent course of MR may, in fact, be deceptive. By the time that symptoms secondary to a reduced cardiac output and/or pulmonary congestion become apparent, serious and sometimes even irreversible left ventricular dysfunction may have developed. In contrast, patients with MS have the benefit of an "early warning system," i.e., symptoms of pulmonary congestion with frequent, sudden elevations of left atrial pressure.

In patients with severe chronic MR with a greatly enlarged left atrium and with relatively mild left atrial hypertension (group 2 with increased left atrial compliance, described above), pulmonary vascular resistance does not usually rise appreciably. Instead, the major symptoms, fatigue and exhaustion, are related to a low cardiac output. Right heart failure, characterized by congestive hepatomegaly, edema, and ascites, is observed in patients with acute MR and elevated pulmonary vascular resistance. Angina pectoris is rare unless coronary artery disease coexists.

NATURAL HISTORY. This is variable and depends on a combination of the volume of regurgitation, the state of the myocardium, and the cause of the underlying disorder. The condition in asymptomatic patients with mild MR usually remains stable for many years[150]; severe regurgitation develops in only a small percentage of these, in some cases because of intervening infective endocarditis or rupture of chordae tendineae or both. Regurgitation tends to progress more rapidly in patients with connective tissue diseases, such as Marfan syndrome, than in those with chronic MR on a rheumatic basis. Isolated severe MR secondary to acute rheumatic fever occurs frequently in adolescents in developing nations. The course is often rapidly progressive. Because the natural history of severe MR has been altered greatly by surgical intervention, it is difficult now to predict the course of patients on medical therapy alone. However, in an unselected group of patients with MR who were treated medically before surgical treatment of severe MR became commonplace, approximately 80 per cent survived 5 years after the diagnosis and almost 60 per cent survived 10 years.[66] Patients with combined MS and MR had a poorer prognosis, with only 67 per cent surviving 5 years and 30 per cent surviving 10 years after diagnosis. Munoz et al., in studying a group of patients with greater disability, found that medically treated patients with severe MR had a 5-year survival rate of only 45 per cent.[65] Among medically treated patients with MR, the arteriovenous oxygen difference and ventricular end-diastolic volume were significant (inverse) predictors of survival.[148]

Physical Examination

Palpation of the arterial pulse is helpful in differentiating aortic stenosis from MR; both may produce a prominent systolic murmur at the base of the heart.[32a] The carotid arterial upstroke is sharp in severe MR[151] and delayed in aortic stenosis; the volume of the pulse may be normal or reduced in the presence of heart failure.

The cardiac impulse, like the arterial peel, is brisk and hyperdynamic, and it is displaced to the left[15] (Table 2–1, p. 24 and Fig. 32–15), and a prominent left ventricular filling wave is frequently palpable in early diastole. Systolic expansion of the enlarged left atrium may result in a late systolic thrust in the parasternal region, which may be confused with right ventricular enlargement.[152]

AUSCULTATION. With severe, chronic MR due to defective valve cusps, S_1, produced by valve closure, is usually

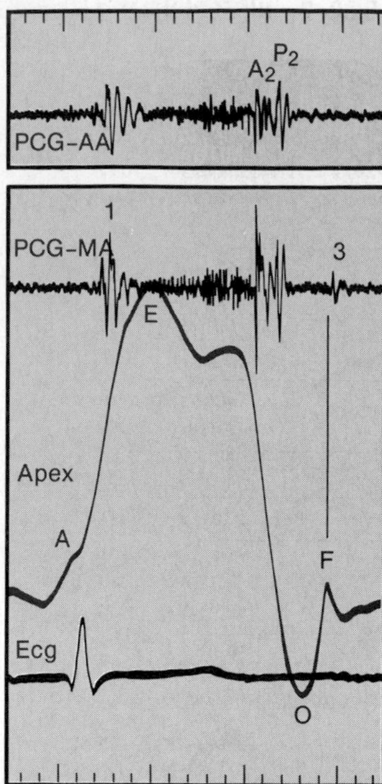

FIGURE 32–15. Hyperdynamic apexcardiogram in mitral regurgitation. The configuration of the tracing in systole is qualitatively similar to a normal curve, although the amplitude was clearly exaggerated by palpation. The rapid filling wave (F) is higher than normal and terminates in a sharp point coincident with its audible counterpart, the third heart sound (3). (From Craige, E., and Smith, D.: Heart sounds. *In* Braunwald, E. [ed.]: Heart Disease: A Textbook of Cardiovascular Medicine. 3rd ed, Philadelphia, W. B. Saunders Company, 1988, p. 58.)

diminished.[153,154] Wide splitting of S_2 is common and results from the shortening of left ventricular ejection and an earlier A_2 as a consequence of reduced resistance to left ventricular outflow. In the presence of MR with severe pulmonary hypertension, P_2 is louder than A_2. The abnormal increase in the flow rate across the mitral orifice during the rapid filling phase is usually associated with an S_3 (Fig. 32–15), the auscultatory counterpart of a palpable rapid filling wave. A left ventricular S_3, i.e., one that is not augmented by inspiration, excludes predominant MS (unless aortic regurgitation, ischemic heart disease, or another cause of an S_3 is present).

The *systolic murmur* is the most prominent physical finding in MR; it must be differentiated from the systolic murmur heard in aortic stenosis, tricuspid regurgitation, ventricular septal defect, and sometimes MS (Table 32–2). In most cases of severe MR the systolic murmur commences immediately after the soft S_1 and continues beyond and may obscure A_2 because of the persistence of the pressure difference between the left ventricle and left atrium (Figs. 2–31, p. 38, and 2–32, p. 39). The holosystolic murmur of chronic MR is usually constant in intensity, blowing, high-pitched, and loudest at the apex with radiation to the axilla and left infrascapular area; however, radiation toward the sternum or the aortic area may occur with abnormalities of the posterior leaflet. The murmur shows little change even in the presence of large beat-to-beat variations of left ventricular stroke volume, as occur in atrial fibrillation, in contrast to most midsystolic (ejection) murmurs, such as in aortic stenosis, which vary greatly in intensity with stroke volume and therefore with the duration of diastole.[155] There is little correlation between the intensity of the systolic murmur and the severity of MR. Indeed, in patients with severe MR due to left ventricular dilatation, acute myocardial infarction, or paraprosthetic valvular regurgitation, or in those who have marked emphysema, obesity,

TABLE 32–2 DIFFERENTIAL DIAGNOSIS OF MITRAL REGURGITATION, VENTRICULAR SEPTAL DEFECT, TRICUSPID REGURGITATION, AND AORTIC STENOSIS

PHYSICAL, ROENTGENOGRAPHIC, OR ELECTROCARDIOGRAPHIC FEATURE	MITRAL REGURGITATION	VENTRICULAR SEPTAL DEFECT	TRICUSPID REGURGITATION	AORTIC STENOSIS
Systolic murmur	Harsh and pansystolic	Harsh and pansystolic	Pansystolic	Ejection, crescendo-decrescendo
Primary location of murmur	Apex	Left sternal border	Left sternal border	Base of heart; occasionally apical
Radiation of murmur	Axilla; occasionally base and neck	Left precordium	Little	Carotids
Thrill	Occasionally present at apex	Usually present at left sternal border	Rare	Occasionally present at base
Murmur with inspiration	No change	No change	Increases	No change
Valsalva maneuver	May increase	Increases or no change	No change	Decreases
Venous pressure	Often normal	Slightly elevated with prominent A and V waves	Elevated, with very prominent V waves	Usually normal
Pulsatile liver	No	No	Yes	No
Pulmonary component of S_2	Normal; occasionally increased	Normal or loud; usually delayed	Usually increased	Normal
Apical impulse	Hyperkinetic; occasional heaving	Hyperkinetic	Weak or normal	Forceful and sustained
ECG	Left ventricular hypertrophy; left atrial hypertrophy	Biventricular hypertrophy (Katz-Wachtel phenomenon)	Right ventricular hypertrophy, occasional right atrial hypertrophy	Left ventricular hypertrophy with associated ST-T changes
Chest roentgenogram	Moderately enlarged heart, marked left atrial enlargement	Enlarged left and right ventricle	Enlarged right ventricle	Often normal heart size or left ventricular hypertrophy

From Haffajee, C. I.: Chronic mitral regurgitation. *In* Dalen, J. E., and Alpert, J. S. (eds.): Valvular Heart Disease. 2nd ed. Boston, Little, Brown and Company, 1987, p. 141.

chest deformity, or a prosthetic heart valve, the systolic murmur may be barely audible or even absent, a condition referred to as "silent MR."[156]

Pansystolic and late systolic murmurs (and pansystolic murmurs with late systolic accentuation) are characteristic of MR. When the murmur is confined to late systole, the regurgitation is usually mild and may be secondary to prolapse of the mitral valve or papillary muscle dysfunction. These causes of MR are frequently associated with a normal S_1 because initial closure of the mitral valve cusps may be unimpaired. The murmur of papillary muscle dysfunction is particularly variable; it may become accentuated or holosystolic during acute myocardial ischemia and often disappears when ischemia is relieved. The response of a mid- to late-systolic murmur to a number of maneuvers, as described on page 1032, helps to establish the diagnosis of prolapse of the mitral valve.

Dynamic Auscultation (Table 2–4, p. 46; Fig. 2–40, p. 42). The holosystolic murmur of rheumatic MR varies little during respiration. However, sudden standing and amyl nitrite inhalation usually diminish the murmur (Table 32–3), whereas squatting and methoxamine or phenylephrine augment it. The murmur is reduced during the strain of the Valsalva maneuver and shows a left-sided response, i.e., a transient overshoot, six to eight beats following release. The murmur of MR is usually intensified by isometric exercise, differentiating it from the systolic murmurs of valvular aortic stenosis and hypertrophic obstructive cardiomyopathy, both of which are reduced by this intervention. The murmur due to left ventricular dilatation *decreases* in intensity and duration with effective therapy with cardiac glycosides, diuretics, rest, and particularly vasodilators.

Differential Diagnosis. The holosystolic murmur of MR resembles that produced by a ventricular septal defect.

TABLE 32–3 EFFECT OF VARIOUS INTERVENTIONS ON SYSTOLIC MURMURS

INTERVENTION	HYPERTROPHIC OBSTRUCTIVE CARDIOMYOPATHY	AORTIC STENOSIS	MITRAL REGURGITATION	MITRAL PROLAPSE
Valsalva	↑	↓	↓	↑ or ↓
Standing	↑	↑ or unchanged	↓	↑
Handgrip or squatting	↓	↓ or unchanged	↑	↓
Supine position with legs elevated	↓	↑ or unchanged	Unchanged	↓
Exercise	↑	↑ or unchanged	↓	↑
Amyl nitrite	↑↑	↑	↓	↑
Isoproterenol	↑↑	↑	↓	↑

↑↑ = Markedly increased.

Modified from Paraskos, J. A.: Combined valvular disease. *In* Dalen, J. E., and Alpert, J. S. (eds.): Valvular Heart Disease. 2nd ed. Boston, Little, Brown and Company, 1987, p. 365.

However, the latter is usually loudest at the sternal border rather than the apex and is usually accompanied by a parasternal, rather than an apical, thrill. The murmur of MR may also be confused with that of tricuspid regurgitation, which is usually heard best along the left sternal border, is augmented during inspiration, and is accompanied by a prominent *v* wave and *y* descent in the jugular venous pulse.

When the chordae tendineae to the posterior leaflet of the mitral valve rupture, the regurgitant jet is often directed anteriorly, so that it impinges on the atrial septum adjacent to the aortic root and causes a systolic murmur most prominent at the base of the heart, which can be confused with that of aortic stenosis. The acoustic energy derived from the mitral regurgitant jet may be transmitted to the aorta by the impact of the jet on the portion of the left atrial wall adjacent to the aortic root.[157] On the other hand, when the chordae to the anterior leaflet rupture, the jet is usually directed to the posterior wall of the left atrium, and the murmur may be transmitted to the spine or even to the top of the head.[158]

Patients with rheumatic disease of the mitral valve exhibit a spectrum of abnormalities, ranging from pure MS to pure MR. The presence of an S_3, a rapid left ventricular filling wave and left ventricular impulse on palpation, and a soft S_1 all favor predominant MR. In contrast, an accentuated S_1, a prominent OS with a short A_2-OS interval, and a soft, short systolic murmur all point to predominant MS. Elucidation of the predominant valvular lesion may be complicated by the presence of a holosystolic murmur of tricuspid regurgitation in patients with pure MS and pulmonary hypertension; this murmur, as has already been noted, may sometimes be heard at the apex when the right ventricle is greatly enlarged and may therefore be mistaken for the murmur of MR. Many patients with severe tricuspid regurgitation have a low cardiac output and an inaudible or barely audible diastolic murmur of MS, further complicating the clinical diagnosis. An S_3 originating from the right ventricle in patients with MS and pulmonary hypertension may falsely suggest the presence of MR. On the other hand, systolic expansion of the left atrium, as occurs in severe MR, often produces a late systolic parasternal expansion that may be confused with right ventricular hypertrophy and falsely attributed to mitral stenosis.

LABORATORY EXAMINATION

ELECTROCARDIOGRAPHY. The principal *electrocardiographic* findings in patients with MR are left atrial enlargement and atrial fibrillation.[46,153,159] Electrocardiographic evidence of left ventricular enlargement occurs in about one-third of patients with severe MR. Approximately 15 per cent can exhibit electrocardiographic evidence of right ventricular hypertrophy, a change that reflects the presence of pulmonary hypertension of sufficient severity to counterbalance even the hypertrophied left ventricle of MR.

RADIOLOGICAL FINDINGS (Figs. 7–37, p. 227, and 7–38, p. 228). Cardiomegaly with left ventricular and particularly with left atrial enlargement is a common finding in patients with chronic severe MR.[160] However, there is little correlation between left atrial size and pressure. Changes in the lung fields are less prominent in MR than in MS, but interstitial edema with Kerley B lines is frequently seen with acute regurgitation or with progressive left ventricular failure.

In patients with combined MS and MR, overall cardiac enlargement and particularly left atrial dilatation are prominent findings. However, it is often difficult to determine which lesion is predominant from the plain chest roentgenogram because it may be difficult to distinguish between right and left ventricular enlargement. Predominant MS is suggested by relatively mild cardiomegaly, principally straightening of the left cardiac border with significant changes in the lung fields, whereas predominant MR is more likely when the heart is greatly enlarged and the changes in the lungs are relatively inconspicuous. When the left atrium is aneurysmally dilated, chronic MR is almost always the dominant lesion. Calcification of the mitral valve occurs in patients with stenosis, regurgitation, or mixed lesions.

Calcification of the mitral annulus, an important cause of MR in the elderly, is most prominent in the posterior third of the cardiac silhouette and is best visualized on films exposed in the lateral or right anterior oblique projection, in which it appears as a dense, coarse, C-shaped opacity (Fig. 7–28, p. 222).

LEFT VENTRICULAR ANGIOCARDIOGRAPHY. The diagnosis of MR can be established definitively by means of left ventricular angiocardiography.[161] The prompt appearance of contrast material in the left atrium following its injection into the left ventricle indicates the presence of MR (Fig. 32–16). The injection should be rapid enough to permit left ventricular opacification but slow enough to avoid the development of premature ventricular contractions, which can induce spurious regurgitation.

The regurgitant volume can be determined from the difference between the total left ventricular stroke volume, estimated angiocardiographically, and the simultaneous measurement of the effective forward stroke by Fick's method (see p. 192). The results of such studies suggest that in patients with severe regurgitation, the regurgitant volume may approach and in rare instances may even exceed the effective forward stroke volume.

Qualitative but clinically useful estimates of the severity of MR may be made by cineangiographic observation of the degree of opacification of the left atrium and pulmonary veins following the injection of contrast material into the left ventricle. MR secondary to rheumatic heart disease is characterized angiographically by a central regurgitant jet and by thickened leaflets that exhibit reduced motion, whereas in regurgitation due to other causes, particularly dilatation or calcification of the mitral annulus or ruptured chordae and papillary muscles, the systolic jet may be eccentric, and the valves consist of thin filaments that display excessive motion. The cause of the regurgitation, e.g., prolapse of the mitral valve, and a flail leaflet are often distinguishable angiographically.

MAGNETIC RESONANCE IMAGING. This technique, described on p. 319, is effective in measuring regurgitant flow and is the most accurate noninvasive technique that can provide these measurements[162,162a] (Fig. 10–28, p. 333).

ECHOCARDIOGRAPHY (see also p. 72). Two-dimensional transthoracic echocardiography is more useful in evaluating left ventricular function and in determining the etiology of MR than in estimating the severity of MR. Severe MR results in enlargement of the left atrium and left ventricle, with increased systolic motion of both of these chambers. The underlying cause of the regurgitation—e.g., rupture of chordae tendineae, mitral valve prolapse (Figs. 3–51, p. 73 and

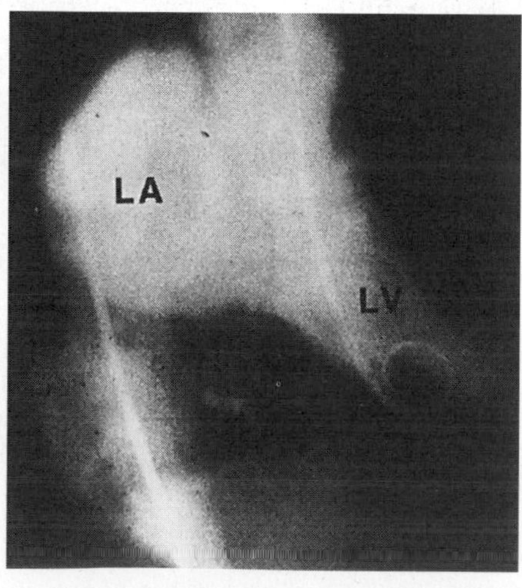

FIGURE 32–16. Diastolic *(left)* and systolic *(right)* frames of a left ventricular cineangiogram from a patient with severe mitral regurgitation. Dense opacification of the left atrium was seen in the first systolic frame. Left ventricular contraction is excellent. (From Hall, R. J., and Julian, D. G.: Diseases of the Cardiac Valves. New York, Churchill Livingstone, 1989, p. 66.)

3–52, p. 74), a flail leaflet[163] (Fig. 3–53, p. 74), and vegetation (Fig. 33–4, p. 1084)—can often be determined on the transthoracic echocardiogram, which may also show calcification of the mitral annulus as a band of dense echoes between the mitral apparatus and the posterior wall of the heart.[164] This technique is also useful for estimating the hemodynamic consequences of MR; with left ventricular dysfunction, end-diastolic and end-systolic volumes are increased. Doppler assessment of mitral regurgitant flow is provided by the difference between transmitral and transaortic flow.[165]

Doppler echocardiography in MR reveals a high-velocity jet in the left atrium during systole. The severity of the regurgitation is a function of the distance from the valve that the jet can be detected (Fig. 3–11, p. 57) and the size of the left atrium. Both color flow Doppler (Fig. 3–49, p. 73 color plate No. 2, and Fig. 3–50, p. 73, color plate No. 2) and pulsed techniques have been found to correlate well with angiographic methods in estimating the severity of MR. Other methods of assessing the severity of MR include measurement of the absolute mitral jet (>8 cm^2 specifies severe MR). However, color flow jet areas are influenced importantly by the cause of the regurgitation and jet eccentricity, limiting the accuracy of this approach.[166] However, the width of the proximal jet appears to correlate with established measures of MR.[167]

Transesophageal echocardiography is superior to transthoracic echocardiography in assessing the detailed anatomy of the regurgitant mitral valve, and therefore it is useful in the preoperative determination of whether valve replacement is necessary or repair is feasible.[168,169] Also, color flow mapping obtained by the transesophageal technique correlates better with angiographic grading of MR than does the transthoracic technique.[169a]

RADIONUCLIDE ANGIOGRAPHY. Gated pool imaging or first-pass angiography may reveal an increased end-diastolic volume; the regurgitant fraction can be estimated from the ratio of left ventricular to right ventricular stroke volume[142]; in patients with MR and impaired left ventricular function, ejection fraction fails to rise normally during exercise. Radionuclide angiograms are useful for interval follow-up of patients. Progressive increases in ventricular end-diastolic or end-systolic volume often suggest that surgical treatment is necessary (discussed later).

Acute Mitral Regurgitation

The causes of acute MR are shown in Table 32–1 *(bottom).* They are diverse and represent acute manifestations of disease processes that may, under other circumstances, cause chronic MR. Especially important causes of acute MR are infective endocarditis with disruption of valve leaflets or rupture of chordae tendineae, ischemic dysfunction or rupture of a papillary muscle, and malfunction of a prosthetic valve.

One major hemodynamic difference between acute and chronic MR derives from the differences in the compliance of the left atrium, as discussed on page 1020 and as illustrated in Figure 32–14. As shown in Table 32–4 *(top),* acute severe MR causes a marked reduction of forward stroke volume, a slight reduction of end-systolic volume, and an increase in end-diastolic volume. The differences in the clinical features between acute and chronic MR are summarized in Table 32–4 *(bottom).* Patients who develop acute MR usually have a normal-sized left atrium (group 1 with normal or reduced left atrial compliance, p. 1021). The left atrial pressure rises abruptly, possibly leading to pulmonary edema, marked elevation of pulmonary vascular resistance, and right-sided heart failure. Because the *v* wave is markedly elevated in acute MR, the pressure gradient between the left ventricle and atrium declines at the end of systole (Fig. 32–13), and the murmur may not be holosystolic but decrescendo, ending well before A_2. It is usually lower-pitched and softer than the murmur of chronic MR. A left-sided S_4 is common.[148] Pulmonary hypertension, common in acute MR, may increase the intensity of P_2 and the murmurs of pulmonary and tricuspid regurgitation, and a right-sided S_4 may also develop. Rarely in patients with severe acute MR, a *v* wave (late systolic pressure rise) in the pulmonary artery pressure pulse may cause premature

TABLE 32–4 DIFFERENTIAL DIAGNOSIS OF ACUTE VERSUS CHRONIC SEVERE MITRAL REGURGITATION

FINDING	CHRONIC SEVERE	ACUTE SEVERE
Clinical		
Onset	Chronic and gradual dyspnea	Acute
Appearance	Normal/mildly dyspneic	Severely ill
Blood pressure	Variable	Variable
Tachycardia	Variable/not striking	Almost always
Apical impulse	Displaced and forcible (large heart)	Not displaced
Apical systolic thrill	Common	No
S_1	Normal or soft	Usually normal or mildly increased
S_2	Wide splitting	Usually normal
S_3	Common	Common
S_4	Rare	Common
Apical mitral murmur	Harsh parasystolic	Soft or absent early systolic and decrescendo
X-radiation of murmur	Axilla	Axilla, spine, or base
Basal ejection systolic murmur	No	With posterior leaflet chordal rupture (not aortic in origin)
Apical rumbling diastolic murmur	Infrequent	Common and short
ECG/LVH	Almost always	No
Chest X-ray	Severe cardiomegaly	No cardiomegaly
Lung fields	Pulmonary venous congestion	Pulmonary edema
Echocardiography		
LV size	Dilated	Normal
LV function	Variable	Hyperactive
LA size	Dilated	Normal
Look for clues of underlying etiology		
Myocardial infarction	History, ECG, and echo	
Endocarditis	Peripheral signs, echo (vegetation)	
Leaking mitral prosthesis	Transesophageal echo and fluoroscopy (clots, vegetation)	

From Jutzy, K. R., and Al-Zaibag, M.: Acute mitral and aortic valve regurgitation. *In* Al-Zaibag, M., and Duran, C. M. G. (eds.): Valvular Heart Disease. New York, Marcel Dekker, 1994, pp. 345–382.

closure of the pulmonary valve, early P_2, and paradoxical splitting of S_2.[153] Acute MR, even if severe, often does not increase overall cardiac size of the chest roentgenogram and may produce only mild left atrial enlargement despite marked elevation of left atrial pressure. With acute MR, there may be little increase in the internal diameter of either of these chambers of the echocardiogram, but increased systolic motion of the ventricle is prominent.

Acute vs. Chronic Mitral Regurgitation

Both the clinical features and hemodynamic findings differ between acute and chronic MR. These differences are summarized in Table 32–4.

MANAGEMENT

Medical Treatment

This includes all the measures used in the treatment of heart failure, as outlined in Chapter 17. Afterload reduction is of particular benefit in the management of MR—both the acute and the chronic forms.[170,171] By reducing the impedance to ejection into the aorta, the volume of blood regurgitating into the left atrium is reduced. In addition, decreasing left ventricular volume reduces the diameter of the mitral annulus and thereby the regurgitant orifice.[170] Mean left atrial pressure and, in particular, the elevated *v* wave decline. Thus, in the management of MR, vasodilator therapy is actually directed at relieving the physiological abnormality rather than simply dealing with its consequences. Afterload reduction with intravenous nitroprusside may be lifesaving in acute MR due to rupture of the head of a papillary muscle occurring in the course of an acute myocardial infarction. It may permit stabilization of the patient's condition and thereby allow coronary arteriography and operation to be carried out with the patient in optimal condition. When surgical treatment is contraindicated, chronic afterload reduction with an angiotensin inhibitor[171] or oral hydralazine may improve the clinical state for months or even years in patients with severe, chronic MR. Digitalis glycosides play a more important role in the management of MR than of MS. Like diuretics, they are indicated in patients with severe MR and clinical evidence of heart failure. Cardiac glycosides are particularly helpful in patients with established atrial fibrillation. These patients should also receive anticoagulants.

Appropriate prophylaxis to prevent infective endocarditis (see p. 1097) is indicated in MR as in all valvular lesions. In patients with functional disability despite optimal medical management and/or in patients with only mild symptoms but progressively deteriorating left ventricular function on noninvasive examination, surgical treatment should be considered. Two-dimensional or transesophageal echocardiography with Doppler echocardiography and color flow Doppler imaging provide detailed assessment of mitral valve structure and function. However, left-sided cardiac catheterization, selective left ventricular angiocardiography, and coronary arteriography are indicated when surgery is considered. The objectives of these studies are to (1) confirm the presence of MR and estimate its severity; (2) aid in the identification of patients with primary myocardial disease and functional MR secondary to ventricular dilatation who are not likely to benefit from operation and in whom the operative risk is relatively high; (3) detect and assess the severity of any associated valve lesions; and (4) determine the presence and assess the extent of coronary artery disease. Because of the additional risks when surgical treatment is carried out in patients with severe left ventricular dysfunction, these left heart studies and consideration of surgical treatment should be carried out before the patient has developed severe heart failure.

Surgical Treatment

When operative treatment is under consideration, the chronic and often slowly but relentlessly progressive nature of MR must be weighed against the immediate risks and long-term uncertainties attendant upon surgery (Fig. 32–17). Surgical mortality depends on the patient's clinical and hemodynamic state (particularly the function of the left ventricle), on the presence of comorbid conditions such as renal, hepatic, or pulmonary disease, and on the skill and experience of the surgical team. The decision to replace (Fig. 32–18) or reconstruct (Figs. 32–19 and 32–20) the valve is of critical importance because replacement carries with it the risk of thromboembolism and anticoagulation in the case of mechanical prostheses and of valve deterioration in the case of bioprostheses (see p. 1061). Surgical mortality does not depend significantly on *which* of the currently used tissue or mechanical valve prostheses is used (see p. 1028).

The reconstructive procedure consists of annuloplasty, often with the use of a rigid (Carpentier) or a flexible prosthetic (Duran) ring (Fig. 32–19), or reconstruction of the valve[172–177] (Fig. 32–20). Prolapsed valves causing severe MR are usually treated with resection of the prolapsing

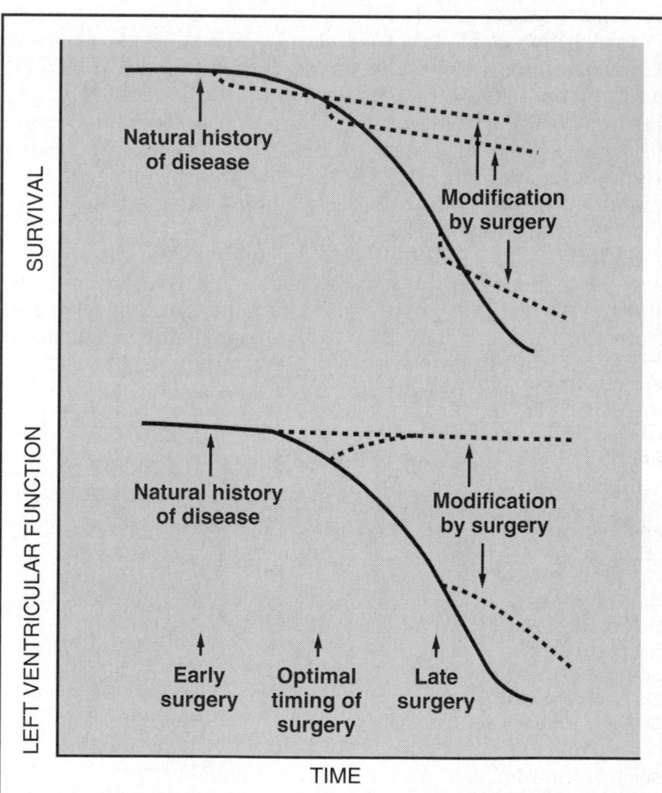

FIGURE 32–17. Schematic representation of the concept of optimal timing of valve replacement surgery. Early surgery yields low operative mortality and preservation of ventricular function. However, because of a finite postoperative risk of prosthesis-associated complications (the major determinant of the slope of the postoperative survival curve in either early or optimally timed surgery), postoperative risk exceeds that of pure medical treatment at this early phase of the disease. In contrast, if surgery is done too late, operative mortality is increased and ventricular function may progressively deteriorate after surgery. Thus, following late surgery, postoperative survival is primarily determined by both prosthesis-associated complications and congestive heart failure. Optimal timing of surgery balances the risks of maintained medical management with the new risks associated with postoperative complications. With optimally timed surgical intervention, operative mortality is relatively low, ventricular function is almost completely preserved, and postoperative risk is determined, as in early surgery, predominantly in the risk of prosthesis-associated complications. (From Schoen, F. J., and St. John Sutton, M.: Contemporary issues in the pathology of valvular disease. Hum. Pathol. *18*:568, 1987.)

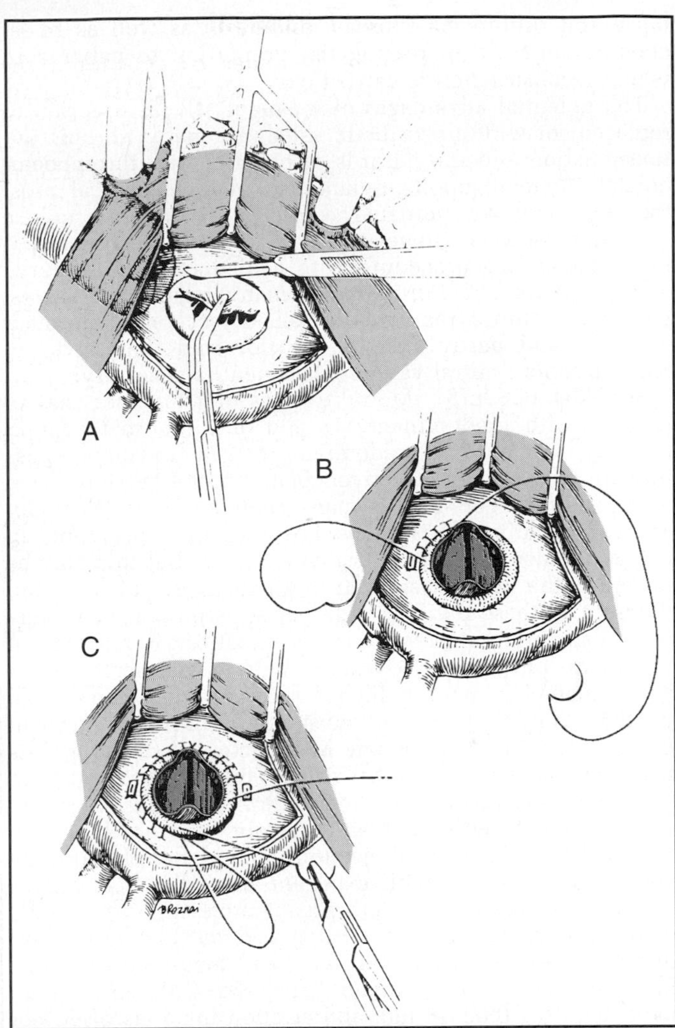

FIGURE 32–18. Continuous technique for mitral valve replacement. *A,* The excision of the valve is facilitated by applying traction to the anterior leaflet. A knife incision in the midportion of the leaflet allows precise initiation of the excision, which is usually completed by scissors. Position of the aorta, circumflex coronary artery, and conduction system should always be kept in mind. *B,* A 0-polypropylene double-armed pledgetted mattress suture is started in the anterolateral commissure. The valve without the holder is lowered in place at this point. *C,* The second 0-polypropylene pledgetted mattress suture is started at the posteromedial commissure. The two suture lines meet at one-half the distance in the anterior and posterior leaflet. The sutures are tied behind the pillar guard of the SJM prosthesis. (From Albertucci, M., and Karp, R. B.: Prosthetic valve replacement. *In* Al-Zaibag, M., and Duran, C. M. G. [eds.]: Valvular Heart Disease. New York, Marcel Dekker, 1994, pp. 601–634.)

segment and plication of the annulus (see p. 1029). Replacement,[178] reimplantation, elongation or shortening of chordae tendineae, splitting of the papillary muscle, and repair of the subvalvular apparatus have been successful in selected patients with pure or predominant MR.[173] Reconstruction of the mitral valve is often successful in patients with noncalcific MR who have pliable valves and a dilated mitral annulus and whose MR is secondary to ruptured chordae to the posterior leaflet or perforation of a mitral leaflet due to infective endocarditis but who do *not* have severe subvalvular chordal thickening and major loss of leaflet substance.[179] The results of these reconstructive operations have, in general, been more favorable in children and adolescents with pliable valves and in patients with MR secondary to mitral valve prolapse, annular dilatation, papillary muscle secondary to ischemia, dysfunction or rupture, or chordal rupture than they have been in older patients with the rigid, calcified, deformed valves of rheumatic heart disease. Many of the latter require mitral valve replacement, which is also usually the procedure of choice in patients with badly scarred mitral valves who have previously undergone mitral commissurotomy. Young patients in developing countries with severe rheumatic MR in the absence of active carditis may undergo successful repair.[172]

Ischemic MR following acute myocardial infarction may be managed by reattaching the papillary muscle to adjacent myocardium[175] or by valve replacement. Ischemic MR secondary to severe annular dilatation may be treated with direct or ring annuloplasty. Episodic MR due to transient ischemia is often eliminated by coronary revascularization, whereas severe chronic MR secondary to fibrotic infarcted papillary muscle usually requires valve replacement.

Although mitral valve replacement[179a]—with mechanical or bioprostheses—has been used successfully in the treatment of MR for three and a half decades, there has been some dissatisfaction with the results of this operation. First, left ventricular function often deteriorates following this procedure, contributing to early and late mortality and late disability. The increase in afterload consequent to abolition of the low impedance leak was first believed to be responsible, but now it is clear that the loss of annular-chordal-papillary muscle continuity interferes with left ventricular function in patients who have undergone mitral valve replacement. This does not occur after mitral valve reconstruction.[178] Indeed, animal experiments have shown convincingly that the normal function of the mitral valve apparatus "primes" the left ventricle for normal contraction and that this is prevented when operation causes discontinuity of this apparatus. There is evidence, both from animal experiments[181] and patients,[182–185] that preservation of the papillary muscle and its chordal attachments to the mitral annulus is beneficial for postoperative left ventricular function, even when the mitral valve is replaced.

A second disadvantage of prosthetic mitral valve replacement results from the prosthesis itself: thromboembolism or hemorrhage in the case of mechanical prostheses, late mechanical dysfunction of bioprostheses, and the hazard of infective endocarditis with all prostheses. For these reasons, increasing efforts are being made to reconstruct the mitral valve whenever possible, especially in patients with pure and predominant regurgitation. Indeed, these procedures, widely employed in Europe since the early 1960's, are now frequently used by U.S. surgeons as well. In many centers in the United States, approximately half of all patients requiring operation for pure or predominant MR re

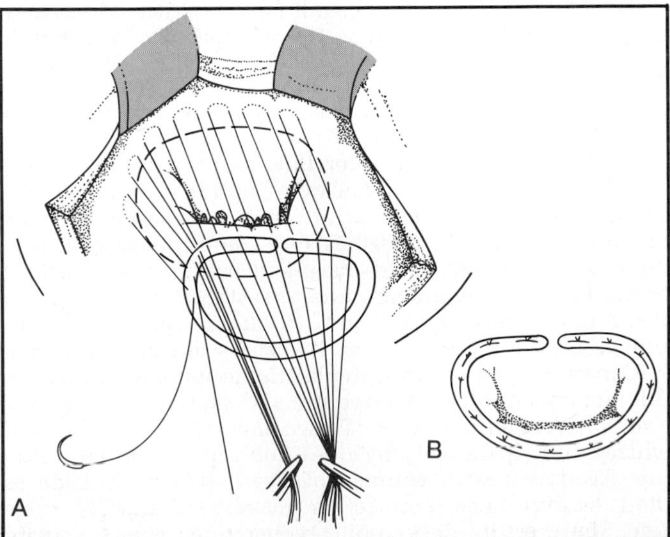

FIGURE 32–19. Illustration of insertion of annuloplasty ring. (Reproduced with permission from Galloway, A. C., Colvin, S. B., Baumann, F. G., et al.: Current concepts of mitral valve reconstruction for mitral insufficiency. Circulation *78:*1087, 1988. Copyright 1989 American Heart Association.)

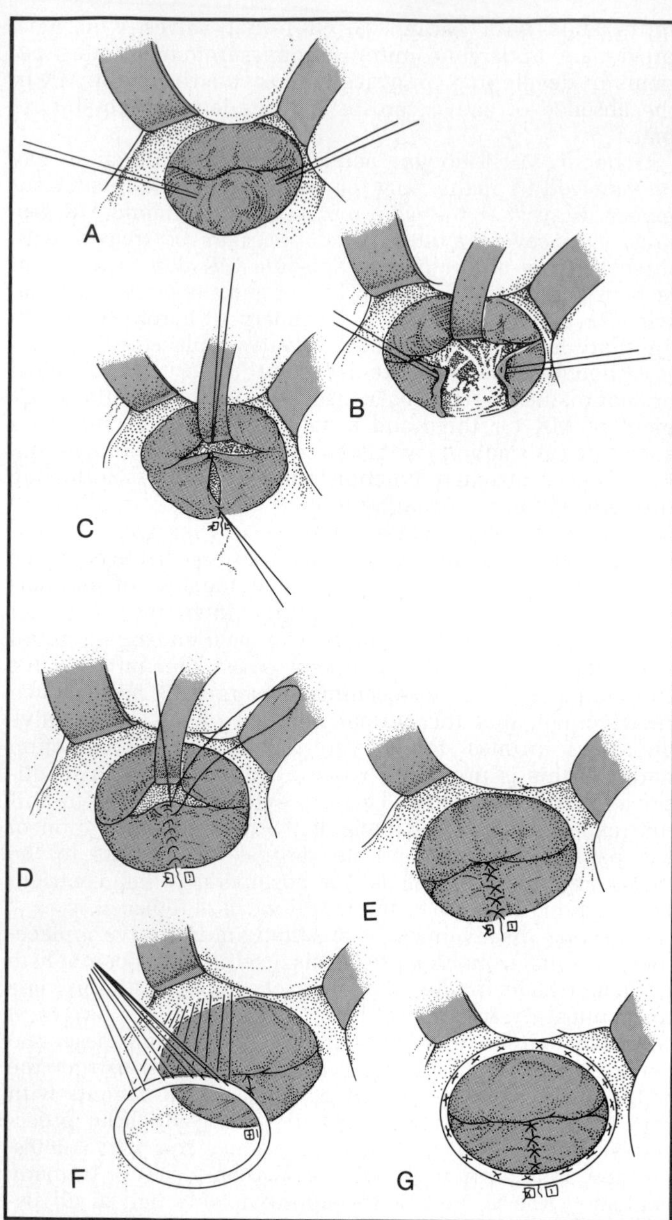

FIGURE 32–20. Valve repair techniques for quadrilateral resection of posterior leaflet of mitral valve. (From Cohn, L. H., DiSesa, V. J., Couper, G. S., et al.: Mitral valve repair for myxomatous degeneration and prolapse of the mitral valve. J. Thorac. Cardiovasc. Surg. *98*:987, 1989.)

ceive reconstructive procedures and the other half valve replacement.

Intraoperative Doppler color flow mapping is extremely useful in assessing the adequacy of mitral valve repair. In the minority of patients with persistent severe MR in whom the results are unsatisfactory, the problem can usually be corrected before the chest is closed.[178] Left ventricular outflow tract obstruction due to systolic anterior motion of the mitral valve occurs in 5 to 10 per cent of patients following mitral valve repair. Its causes are not clear, but they may include excess valvular tissue with severe leaflet redundancy and/or an interventricular septum bulging into a small left ventricle.[176–186] This complication may be recognized intraoperatively by transesophageal echocardiography. Treatment with volume loading and beta-blockade is often helpful. The obstruction usually disappears with time, but if it does not, reoperation and re-repair or replacement may be necessary.

Progressive reduction in the prevalence of rheumatic heart disease—in which damaged valves often are not suitable for reconstructive surgery—with a simultaneous rise in degenerative causes of MR (including mitral valve prolapse and rupture of chordae tendineae) as well as in ischemic causes is increasing the proportion of patients in whom reconstruction is carried out.

The potential advantages of repair of MR (as opposed to replacement with a prosthetic valve) are many; chronic anticoagulation and the hazards of bleeding and thromboembolism attendant upon implantation of a mechanical prosthesis are largely eliminated, as are the risks of late failure of a bioprosthesis. However, mitral repair is technically a more demanding procedure with a distinct learning curve for the surgeon.[187] Furthermore, many regurgitant valves, particularly those that are thickened, severely deformed, calcified, and partly stenotic, do not lend themselves to reconstruction: mitral valve replacement is necessary.

SURGICAL RESULTS. Mortality rates of 1 to 4 per cent in patients with predominant MS and of 2 to 7 per cent in patients with pure or predominant MR in functional Class II or III, who undergo elective isolated mitral valve replacement, are now common in many centers.[131,141,174,188,189] Operative mortality tends to be lower (1 to 4 per cent) in patients undergoing reconstructive surgery, but this may be related to the younger age and lower incidence of comorbid illnesses in these patients. Age per se is no barrier to successful surgery; mitral valve replacement can be carried out in patients older than 75 years if their general health status is adequate but with a higher risk than in younger patients.[183] Surgical treatment substantially improves survival in patients with symptomatic MR. Factors such as age less than 60 years, a preoperative New York Heart Association functional Class of II, a cardiac index exceeding 2.0 liters/min/m^2, a left ventricular end-diastolic pressure less than 12 mm Hg, and a normal ejection fraction and end-systolic volume all correlate with excellent immediate as well as long-term survival rates. Both preoperative and end-systolic diameter (Fig. 32–12) and ejection fraction (Fig. 32–21) are important predictors of short-term and long-term outcome. Excellent survival is observed in patients with end-systolic diameters less than 45 mm and ejection fractions of 60 per cent or more. Intermediate outcomes are seen in patients with diameters between 45 and 52 mm and ejection fractions between 50 and 60 per cent, with poor outcomes beyond these limits. In some series, only age and preoperative ejection fraction predicted long-term survival following mitral valve replacement.[190]

In a large proportion of survivors of operation, the clinical state and quality of life improve following valve replacement or repair. Severe pulmonary hypertension is re-

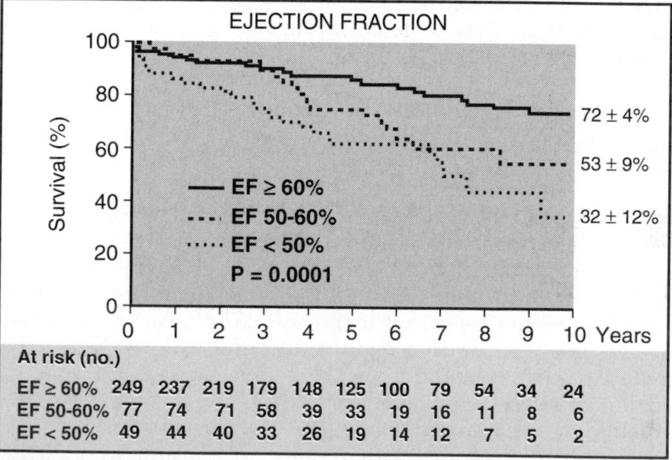

FIGURE 32–21. Graph of the late survival of operative survivors of surgical correction of MR according to preoperative echocardiographic ejection fraction (EF). Number at risk for each interval is indicated at bottom. (Reproduced with permission from Enriquez-Sarano, M., et al.: Echocardiographic prediction of survival after surgical correction of organic mitral regurgitation. Circulation *90*:833, 1994. Copyright 1994 American Heart Association.)

lieved almost uniformly,[53] and left ventricular end-diastolic volume and mass are reduced. Depressed contractile function due to mitral regurgitation improves, especially after mitral valve reconstruction (or mitral valve repair if the chordae attachment to the annulus remains intact). However, patients with MR with marked left ventricular dysfunction preoperatively sometimes remain symptomatic with a depressed ejection fraction[192] after a technically satisfactory operation. Indeed, progressive left ventricular dysfunction and death from heart failure may occur. Long-term survival in patients with predominant MR who undergo mitral valve replacement may be poorer than in those with pure stenosis or mixed stenotic and regurgitant lesions, presumably because left ventricular dysfunction may be quite advanced and largely irreversible by the time patients with pure regurgitation become seriously symptomatic.[191,192] However, even though it is clearly desirable to operate on patients with MR before they develop marked left ventricular dysfunction, and despite the limitations of the results of surgical treatment in these patients, operation is still indicated in the majority of these patients because conservative therapy has little to offer.

The cause of MR also plays an important role in the outcome following surgical treatment. In patients in whom mitral dysfunction is secondary to ischemic heart disease, the 5-year survival rate is about 40 per cent, whereas in rheumatic mitral regurgitation it is much better, approximately 75 per cent. Occlusive coronary artery disease coexisting with, but not the primary cause of, mitral dysfunction requires simultaneous coronary artery bypass grafting and mitral valve replacement or repair. This is associated with decreased perioperative and long-term postoperative survival. Some improvement from mitral valve reconstruction or replacement can be expected even in patients with MR secondary to ischemic heart disease who are medically unresponsive and in congestive heart failure, as long as the cardiac index and ejection fraction exceed 1.8 liters/min/m^2 and 40 per cent, respectively. When left ventricular dysfunction is more severe, however, the risk of perioperative death becomes prohibitive.[195]

Surgical Treatment of Acute Mitral Regurgitation. Emergency surgical treatment of acute left ventricular failure caused by acute MR due to myocardial infarction and rupture of the head of a papillary muscle, by trauma to the mitral valve, or by endocarditis is associated with higher mortality rate than is the elective surgical treatment of chronic MR. However, unless such patients with acute, severe MR and heart failure are treated aggressively, a fatal outcome is almost certain. If the condition of patients with MR secondary to acute infarction can be stabilized by medical treatment, it is preferable to defer operation until 4 to 6 weeks after infarction. Vasodilator treatment may be useful during this period. However, medical management should not be prolonged if multisystem (renal or pulmonary or both) failure occurs. Surgical mortality is also higher in patients with refractory heart failure (functional Class IV), in those in whom a previously implanted prosthetic valve must be replaced because of thromboembolism or valve dysfunction, and in those with active infective endocarditis (of a natural or prosthetic valve). Despite the higher surgical risks, the efficacy of early operation has been established in patients with infective endocarditis complicated by medically uncontrollable congestive heart failure, recurrent emboli, or both (see p. 1096). Because fungal endocarditis responds poorly to medical management, it is now the practice to recommend valve replacement in these cases *before* the onset of heart failure or embolization.

INDICATIONS FOR OPERATION. In view of the reductions in operative mortality, and the improvements both in mitral reconstructive procedures and in artificial valves, as well as the poor long-term results in many patients whose MR is corrected after a long history of heart failure, a more aggressive stance concerning the desirability of operation is in order. Only a few years ago, I, along with many cardiologists, recommended operation for patients with chronic severe MR only if they were in functional Class III or IV, i.e., with symptoms at rest or on ordinary activity despite medical treatment. However, it is now my policy to recommend operation also for patients with severe MR who are in Class II, i.e., who become distinctly symptomatic only on heavy exertion, and if end-systolic volume and diameter are elevated (>50 ml/m^2 BSA and >45 mm, respectively).

The asymptomatic patient with severe MR presents a particularly challenging problem.[139,196,196a] Careful history and performance of an exercise test often reveal that these patients are not, in fact, truly asymptomatic, and if they are symptomatic they should be considered for operation, as indicated as above. However, patients with severe MR who are asymptomatic and perform well on an exercise test and have normal ventricular function (ejection fraction >70 per cent, end-systolic diameter <40 mm, end-systolic volume <40 ml/m^2) are followed by echocardiography every 6 to 12 months. Operation should be considered even in asymptomatic patients if they are under age 70, if they are likely to be candidates for mitral valve repair, and if ventricular function as reflected in end-systolic volume and/or diameter shows *progressive* deterioration. If valve replacement is likely to be necessary, a somewhat higher threshold for clinical and hemodynamic impairment is employed than if valvular reconstruction is contemplated. Because of the higher operative mortality, older patients (>75 years) should, in general, be operated on only for symptoms.

MITRAL VALVE PROLAPSE

ETIOLOGY AND PATHOLOGY

(Fig. 32–22)

DEFINITION. The mitral valve prolapse (MVP) syndrome has been given many names, including the systolic click-murmur syndrome, Barlow syndrome, billowing mitral cusp syndrome, myxomatous mitral valve, floppy valve syndrome, and redundant cusp syndrome.[197–202,202a] It is a common but variable clinical syndrome that results from diverse pathogenic mechanisms of one or more portions of the mitral valve apparatus, the valve leaflets, chordae tendineae, papillary muscle, and valve annulus. The MVP syndrome has become recognized as one of the most prevalent cardiac valvular abnormalities, affecting as much as 3 to 5 per cent of the population.[203,204] It is twice as frequent in females as in males. In 1963 Barlow et al. demonstrated that midsystolic clicks and late systolic murmurs, the auscultatory hallmarks of this syndrome, are frequently associated with prolapse of the mitral valve, often associated with regurgitation.[205]

Normally, the mitral valve billows slightly into the left atrium, and an exaggeration should be termed "billowing mitral valve." A "floppy valve" is regarded as an extreme form of billowing. MVP occurs when the leaflet edges of the valve do not coapt, causing MR. With chordal rupture, the prolapsed mitral valve is "flail." Obviously, these conditions blend into one another, and it is often difficult to distinguish them.

Perloff et al. have proposed specific clinical criteria for the diagnosis of MVP.[199] They have divided the findings into three groups (Table 32–5): (1) major criteria, the pres-

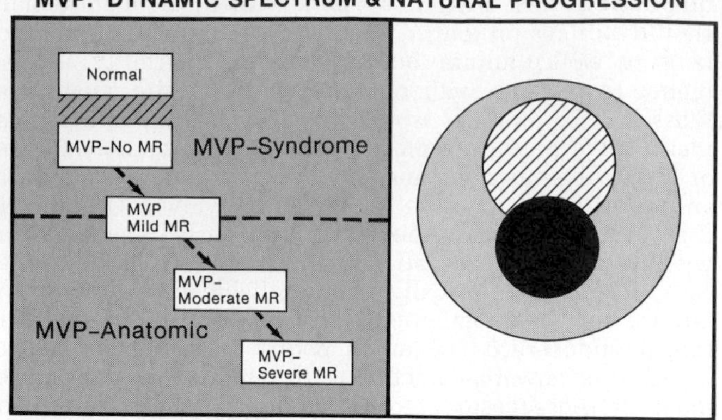

FIGURE 32–22. *Left panel,* The dynamic spectrum, time in years, and the progression of mitral valve prolapse (MVP) are shown. A subtle gradation (cross-hatched area) exists between the normal mitral valve and valves that produce mild MVP without mitral regurgitation (no MR). Progression from the level MVP–no MR to another level may or may not occur. Most of the MVP syndrome cases occupy the area above the dotted line, while progressive mitral valve dysfunction cases occupy the area below the dotted line. *Right panel,* The large circle represents the total number of patients with MVP. Patients with MVP may be symptomatic or asymptomatic. Symptoms may be directly related to mitral valve dysfunction (black circle), or to autonomic dysfunction (cross-hatched circle). Certain patients with symptoms directly related to mitral valve dysfunction may present with and continue to have symptoms secondary to autonomic dysfunction. (From Boudoulas, H., and Wooley, C. F.: Mitral Valve Prolapse and the Mitral Valve Prolapse Syndrome. Mount Kisco, NY, Futura Publishing Co., Inc., 1988.)

ence of one or more of which establishes the diagnosis of MVP; (2) minor criteria, which cannot be discounted and which raise the suspicion of MVP but which by themselves are not sufficient to establish the diagnosis; and (3) nonspecific findings which, although often present in patients with MVP, are quite nonspecific. Although they may alert the clinician, they do not aid in establishing the diagnosis. When rigorous two-dimensional echocardiography criteria (extension of leaflet tissue located cephalad to the plane of the mitral annulus) were employed, only 2 of 100 healthy young women displayed MVP.[200] In addition, Marks et al. have emphasized the importance of systolic displacement of one or both mitral leaflets into the left atrium in the *parasternal view* in the diagnosis of MVP. Such an approach avoids overdiagnosis, which may occur with posterior bowing of the mitral valve on the M-mode echocardiogram and even in the four-chamber view on two-dimensional echocardiography.

ETIOLOGY. Most frequently MVP occurs as a primary condition unassociated with other disease.[197,206] However, it has been reported to be associated with many conditions.[206–216] It is not clear how many of these are chance associations. MVP occurs quite commonly in heritable disorders of connective tissue that increase the size of the mitral leaflets and apparatus, including the Marfan syndrome (see p. 1669). Ehlers-Danlos syndrome[217,218] (see p. 1672), osteogenesis imperfecta, pseudoxanthoma elasticum,[219] and periarteritis nodosa, as well as with myotonic dystrophy,[210] von Willebrand's disease,[209] hyperthyroidism,[208] and congenital malformations such as Ebstein's anomaly of the tricuspid valve, atrial septal defect of the ostium secundum variety,[218] and the Holt-Oram syndrome (see p. 1661).[212] There appears to be a high incidence of MVP in patients with asthenic habitus[220] and a variety of congenital thoracic deformities, including a straight back, a pectus excavatum, and a shallow chest.[212,214] In these cases the association may be with a left ventricle that is small in relation to the mitral valve apparatus.

PATHOLOGY (Fig. 32–23). There is myxomatous proliferation of the mitral valve, in which the spongiosa component of the valve, i.e., the middle layer of the leaflet composed of loose, myxomatous material, is unusually prominent[221] and the quantity of acid mucopolysaccharide is increased secondary to a fundamental abnormality of collagen metabolism.[222,223] The concordance between inadequate production of type III collagen and echocardiographic findings of MVP in patients with type IV Ehlers-Danlos syndrome suggests that this abnormality of collagen is responsible for this subgroup.[222] Although the majority of patients with MVP exhibit myxomatous degeneration of the valve, postinflammatory changes also may be responsible for prolapse.[224]

Electron microscopy has shown haphazard arrangement, disruption, and fragmentation of collagen fibrils (Fig. 32–24). In mild cases, the valvular myxoid stroma is enlarged on histological examination but the leaflets are grossly normal. However, with increasing quantities of myxoid stroma, the leaflets become grossly abnormal and redundant and prolapse. Regions of endothelial disruption, possible sites of endocarditis or thrombus formation, are common.[225] The

TABLE 32–5 DIAGNOSTIC CRITERIA AND NONSPECIFIC FINDINGS IN MITRAL VALVE PROLAPSE

MAJOR CRITERIA

Auscultation
- Mid- to late systolic clicks and late systolic murmur or "whoop" alone or in combination at the cardiac apex

Two-dimensional echocardiogram
- Marked superior systolic displacement of mitral leaflets with coaptation point at or superior to annular plane
- Mild to moderate superior systolic displacement of mitral leaflets with:
  - Chordal rupture
  - Doppler mitral regurgitation
  - Annular dilatation

Echocardiogram plus auscultation
- Mild to moderate superior systolic displacement of mitral leaflets with:
  - Prominent mid- to late systolic clicks at the cardiac apex
  - Apical late systolic or holosystolic murmur in the young
  - Late systolic "whoop"

MINOR CRITERIA

Auscultation
- Loud first heart sound with an apical holosystolic murmur

Two-dimensional echocardiogram
- Isolated mild to moderate superior systolic displacement of the posterior mitral leaflet
- Moderate superior systolic displacement of both mitral leaflets

Echocardiogram plus history of:
- Mild to moderate superior systolic displacement of mitral leaflets with:
  - Focal neurologic attacks or amaurosis fugax in the young
  - First-degree relatives with major criteria

NONSPECIFIC FINDINGS

Symptoms
- "Atypical" chest pain, dyspnea, fatigue, lassitude, giddiness, dizziness, syncope
- Psychological disturbances

Physical appearance
- Thoracic bony abnormalities
- Hypomastia

Electrocardiogram
- T-wave inversions in inferior limb leads or lateral precordial leads
- Premature ventricular beats at rest, during exercise, or on ambulatory ECG
- Supraventricular tachycardia

X-ray
- Scoliosis, pectus excavatum or carinatum, or loss of thoracic kyphosis

Two-dimensional echocardiogram
- Mild superior systolic displacement of anterior or anterior and posterior mitral leaflets

From Perloff, J. K., Child, J. S., and Edwards, J. E.: New guidelines for the clinical diagnosis of mitral valve prolapse. Am. J. Cardiol. *57*:1124, 1986.

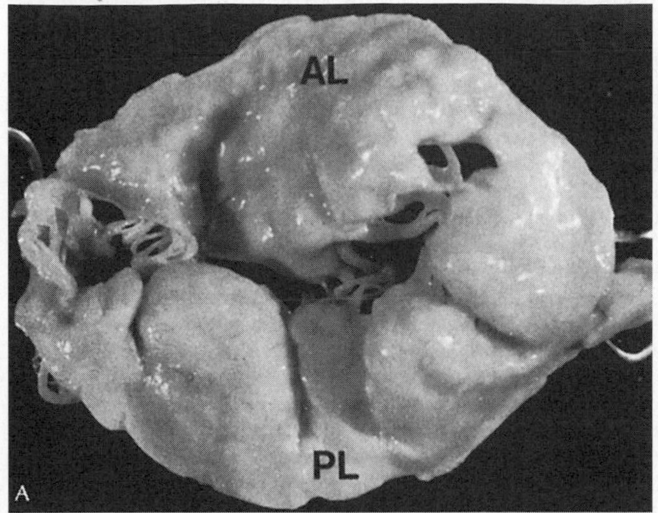

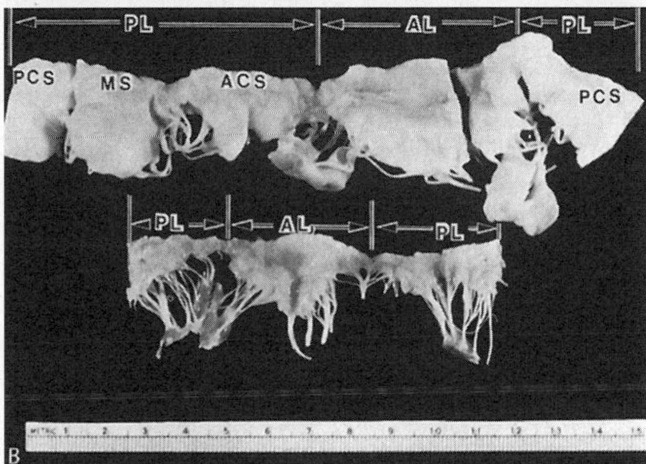

FIGURE 32–23. *A,* Myxomatous mitral valve, atrial view, from a patient with severe mitral regurgitation. The surface area of the valve is increased, with increased folding of the valve surface. The widths of the anterior leaflet (AL) and the posterior leaflet (PL) are almost equal. Individual scallops of the posterior leaflet are enlarged and redundant. *B,* Comparison of an excised myxomatous mitral valve from a patient with severe mitral regurgitation (top) with a normal mitral valve from a patient who died of noncardiac causes (bottom), showing the increased surface area of both anterior leaflets (AL) and posterior leaflets (PL) of the myxomatous valve with enlarged and redundant posterior leaflet scallops, enlarged mitral annulus, and elongated chordae tendineae. PCS = posteromedial commissural scallops; MS = middle scallop; ACS = anterolateral commissural scallop. (From Boudoulas, H., and Wooley, C. F.: Mitral valve prolapse and the mitral valve prolapse syndrome. *In* Yu, P., and Goodwin, J. [eds.]: Progress in Cardiology. Philadelphia, Lea and Febiger, 1986.)

severity of MR depends on the extent of the prolapse. The cusps of the mitral valve, the chordae tendineae, and the annulus may all be affected by myxomatous proliferation. Degeneration of collagen within the central core of the chordae tendineae is primarily responsible for chordal rupture, which occurs commonly in this syndrome and may intensify the severity of MR, although increased chordal tension resulting from the enlarged area of the valve cusps may play a contributory role.[226] Myxomatous changes in the annulus may result in annular dilatation and calcification—contributing to the severity of MR.

Myxomatous proliferation, although most commonly affecting the mitral valve, is not limited to this valve but has been described in the tricuspid,[215] aortic, and pulmonic valves, particularly in patients with Marfan syndrome, and may lead to regurgitation of these valves. The MVP syndrome appears to exhibit a strong hereditary component[197,221] and in some cases is transmitted as an autosomal dominant trait, with varying penetrance. Genetic segregation analyses of familial MVP have shown *no* linkage to fibrillar collagen genes.[227]

The MVP syndrome can coexist with rheumatic MS, and it may develop following mitral commissurotomy for this lesion. In hypertrophic obstructive cardiomyopathy, prolapse of the posterior leaflet of the mitral valve may accompany the usual anterior displacement of the anterior mitral valve leaflet.

Ischemic heart disease and MVP are both common disorders and coexist not infrequently; MVP may also occur secondary to papillary muscle dysfunction. In some patients, MVP has been documented to develop for the first time *following* myocardial infarction.[228] MVP may cause myocardial ischemia by increasing tension on the base of the involved muscle. During systole the tips of the papillary muscles move basally instead of apically. It has also been proposed that coronary artery spasm occurs as a reflex

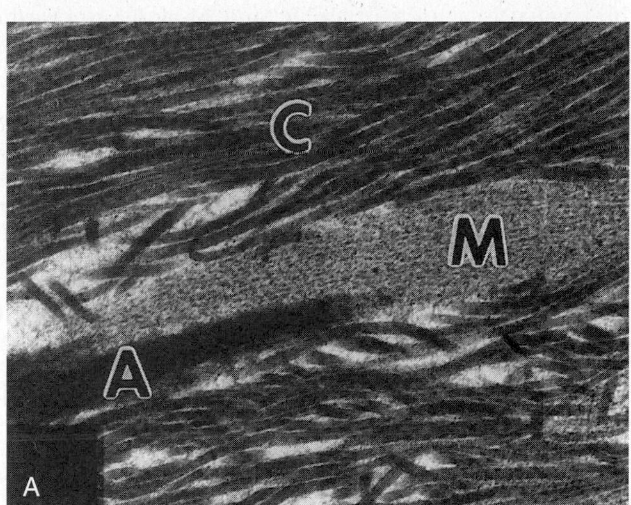

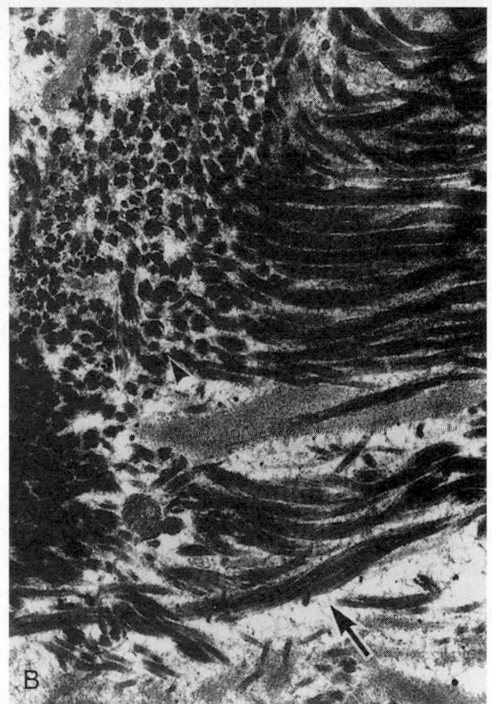

FIGURE 32–24. Electron micrographs of mitral valve. *A,* Normal valve: Elastic fiber is composed of amorphous component (A), associated with microfibrils (M) oriented in parallel. Collagen fibrils (C) are compactly arranged (Kajikawa stain; original magnification ×22,000). *B,* Prolapsed mitral valve. Collagen fibrils show spiraling appearance in longitudinal section (arrow) and flower-like appearance (arrowhead) in transverse section (Kajikawa stain; original magnification ×27,000). (From Tamura, K., Fukuda, Y., Ishizaki, M., et al.: Abnormalities in elastic fibers and other connective-tissue components of floppy mitral valve. Am. Heart J. *129:*1149, 1995.)

response to prolapse of the posterior mitral leaflet and that the resultant ischemia may be responsible for angina or angina-like pain, myocardial infarction, arrhythmias, and sudden death in this syndrome.

CLINICAL MANIFESTATIONS

The clinical presentations of the MVP syndrome are diverse.[197,229] The condition has been observed in patients of all ages and in both sexes. It is a common syndrome; indeed, prolapse of the mitral valve has been reported to occur in 6 per cent of healthy young women surveyed by echocardiography.[230] One series of 100 presumably healthy young women revealed that 17 had a midsystolic click or late systolic murmur or both and that 10 of these 17 had evidence of prolapse of the mitral valve on echocardiography.[231] However, as already noted, because billowing of the mitral valve is a normal variant and M-mode echocardiographic findings may be nonspecific, more rigorous criteria for diagnosis based on two-dimensional echocardiography will indicate a much lower prevalence.[199] Indeed, MVP is now the most common cause of isolated MR requiring surgical treatment.[202] Echocardiographic evidence of MVP has been found in more than 90 per cent of patients with Marfan syndrome[232] and in many of their first-degree relatives.

History

A large majority of patients with MVP are asymptomatic[233,234] (Fig. 32–22). In many cases, otherwise asymptomatic patients with MVP suffer from undue anxiety, perhaps precipitated by their having been informed of the presence of heart disease. Boudoulas et al. have called attention to an "MVP syndrome" with a characteristic systolic nonejection click and a variety of nonspecific symptoms, such as fatigability, palpitations, postural orthostasis, and neuropsychiatric symptoms, as well as symptoms of autonomic dysfunction.[234] How, and indeed whether, these symptoms relate to the presence of MVP is not clear. However, it has been suggested that many of the symptoms are related to dysfunction of the autonomic nervous system, which occurs frequently in the MVP syndrome.[235]

Patients may complain of syncope, presyncope, palpitations, chest discomfort, and, when MR is severe, symptoms of diminished cardiac reserve. Chest discomfort may be typical of angina but most often it is atypical in that it is prolonged, not clearly related to exertion, and punctuated by brief attacks or severe stabbing pain at the apex. The discomfort may be secondary to abnormal tension on papillary muscles.

Physical Examination

The body weight is often low. The blood pressure is usually normal or low; orthostatic hypotension may be present. As already mentioned, patients with MVP have a higher than expected prevalence of "straight back syndrome," scoliosis, and pectus excavatum.[195] MR ranges from nonexistent to severe and in the latter case palpation of the precordium and of the carotid pulses is characteristic (see p. 18).

The auscultatory findings are best elicited with the diaphragm of the stethoscope. The patient should be examined in the supine, left decubitus, and sitting positions. The physical findings unique to the MVP syndrome are detected by auscultation and can be corroborated by phonocardiography.[196] The most important is a systolic click at least 0.14 sec after S_1 (Fig. 2–34, p. 39). This can be differentiated from a systolic ejection click because it occurs distinctly after the beginning of the upstroke of the carotid pulse. Occasionally, multiple mid- and late-systolic clicks are audible most readily along the lower left sternal border and are believed to be produced by sudden tensing of the elongated chordae tendineae and of the prolapsing leaflets. The click is often, although not invariably, followed by a mid- to late-crescendo systolic murmur that continues to A_2. This murmur is similar to that produced by papillary muscle dysfunction (Fig. 32–10, p. 1019), which is readily understandable because both result from mid- to late-systolic MR. In general, the duration of the murmur is a function of the severity of the MR, and when the murmur is confined to the latter portion of systole, MR usually is not severe. However, as MR becomes more severe, the murmur commences earlier and becomes holosystolic.

It is important to emphasize the variability of the physical findings in the MVP syndrome. Some patients exhibit both a midsystolic click and a mid- to late-systolic murmur; others present with one or the other of these two findings; still others have only a click on one occasion and only a murmur on another, both on a third examination, and no abnormality at all on a fourth. MVP may also cause an early diastolic sound or murmur, best heard at the apex or left sternal border 70 to 110 msec following A_2, at a time when the prolapsed posterior leaflet descends into the left ventricle. Conditions other than MVP cause midsystolic clicks; these include tricuspid valve clicks, atrial septal aneurysms,[236] and extracardiac causes.

DYNAMIC AUSCULTATION. The auscultatory and phonocardiographic findings are exquisitely sensitive to physiological and pharmacological interventions, and recognition of the changes induced by these interventions is of great value in the diagnosis of the MVP syndrome (Fig. 2–21, p. 31, and Fig. 2–29, p. 37; Table 32–3).[196] The mitral valve begins to prolapse when the reduction of left ventricular volume during systole reaches a critical point at which the valve leaflets no longer coapt; at that instant, the click occurs and the murmur commences. Any maneuver that decreases left ventricular volume, such as a reduction of impedance to left ventricular outflow, a reduction in venous return, or an augmentation of contractility, results in an earlier occurrence of prolapse during systole. As a consequence, the click and onset of the murmur move closer to S_1. When prolapse is severe or left ventricular size is markedly reduced or both, prolapse may begin with the onset of systole, and as a consequence, the click may not be audible and the murmur may be holosystolic. On the other hand, when left ventricular volume is augmented by an increase in venous return, a reduction of myocardial contractility, bradycardia, or an increase in the impedance to left ventricular emptying, both the click and the onset of the murmur will be delayed. Indeed, if the left ventricle becomes extremely large, prolapse may not occur at all, and the abnormal auscultatory features may disappear entirely.

During the straining phase of the Valsalva maneuver, upon sudden standing, and early during the inhalation of amyl nitrite, cardiac size decreases, and both the click and the onset of the murmur occur earlier in systole. In contrast, a sudden change from the standing to the supine position, leg-raising, squatting, maximal isometric exercise, and, to a lesser extent, expiration will delay the click and the onset of the murmur (Fig. 2–21, p. 31). During the overshoot phase of the Valsalva maneuver (i.e., six to eight cycles following release) and with prolongation of the R-R interval, either following a premature contraction or in atrial fibrillation, the click and onset of the murmur are usually delayed, and the intensity of the murmur is reduced. Maneuvers that elevate arterial pressure, such as isometric exercise, increase the intensity of the click and murmur.

In general, when the onset of the murmur is delayed, both its duration and intensity are diminished, reflecting a reduction in the severity of MR. With some maneuvers, however, there is a discrepancy between changes in the intensity and duration of the murmur. Following amyl nitrite inhalation, for example, the reduced left ventricular size results in an earlier click and longer murmur, but the lower left ventricular systolic pressure diminishes the severity of regurgitation and the intensity of the murmur. Conversely, phenylephrine and methoxamine delay the click and the onset of the murmur, but the larger volume of regurgitation consequent to the elevated left ventricular systolic pressure increases regurgitation and the intensity of the murmur.

There may be confusion between the systolic murmurs of hypertrophic cardiomyopathy (HCM) and of MVP, particularly because midsystolic clicks and a late systolic murmur have been reported in HCM and because the murmur may increase in intensity and duration with standing and decrease with squatting in both conditions (see p. 1420). However, the response to several interventions may be helpful in differentiating these two conditions. During the strain of the Valsalva maneuver, the murmur of HCM increases in intensity in contrast to that of MVP, which becomes longer but usually not louder. The murmur of HCM becomes louder after amyl nitrite inhalation, whereas that of MVP does not. Following a premature beat, the murmur of HCM increases in intensity and duration, whereas that due to MVP usually remains unchanged or decreases.

LABORATORY EXAMINATION

Electrocardiography

The electrocardiogram is usually normal in asymptomatic patients with typical auscultatory and echocardiographic findings. In a minority of asymptomatic patients and in many symptomatic patients, the electrocardiogram shows inverted or biphasic T waves and nonspecific ST-segment changes in leads II, III, and aV_f and occasionally in the anterolateral leads as well.[196] The ST- and T-wave changes may become exaggerated during amyl nitrite inhalation and exercise. These electrocardiographic findings may be related to ischemia of the papillary muscles or of the left ventricle at their bases, resulting from increased tension on these structures produced by the prolapsing valve acting on the chordae. Alternatively, it is possible that the electrocardiographic abnormality reflects an underlying cardiomyopathy.

ARRHYTHMIAS. A spectrum of arrhythmias, including atrial and ventricular premature contractions and supraventricular and ventricular tachyarrhythmias[236–239] as well as bradyarrhythmias due to sinus node dysfunction or varying degrees of atrioventricular block,[239] have been observed. The mechanism of the arrhythmias is not clear. Diastolic depolarization of muscle fibers in the anterior mitral leaflet in response to stretch has been demonstrated experimentally, and the abnormal stretch of the prolapsed leaflet may be of pathogenetic significance. Wit et al. have shown that mitral valve leaflets contain atrium-like muscle fibers in continuity with left atrial myocardium. It is possible that mechanical stimulation of these fibers generates slow-response action potentials and sustained rhythmic action that penetrates the cardiac chambers.[240] Although most of these arrhythmias are of little clinical importance, recurrent ventricular tachycardia, refractory to the usual agents, and even ventricular fibrillation have been reported. These serious ventricular arrhythmias are significantly more frequent in patients with ST-segment and T-wave abnormalities on the resting electrocardiogram.

Paroxysmal supraventricular tachycardia is the most common sustained tachyarrhythmia in patients with MVP and may be related to what may be an increased incidence of left atrioventricular bypass tracts in this condition.[237] In the general population only 20 per cent of patients with paroxysmal supraventricular tachycardia have such bypass tracts, whereas the incidence in patients with MVP is three times as great. Conversely, there is evidence that the incidence of MVP among patients with the Wolff-Parkinson-White syndrome is increased.[241] Patients with MVP who develop paroxysmal supraventricular tachycardia should be subjected to electrophysiological investigation. The outcome of such studies may be important, because digitalis or propranolol, which may be useful in reentry tachycardias, may be hazardous in the presence of antegrade conduction over an atrioventricular bypass tract. There is also an increased association between MVP and prolongation of the Q-T interval, and this association may play a role in the genesis of ventricular arrhythmias.[237] Patients with MVP have an increased incidence of abnormal late potentials on signal-averaged electrocardiograms, as well as reduced heart rate variability[239]; the latter is a predictor of early mortality or of future need for valve surgery.

MVP AND SUDDEN DEATH. The relation between the MVP syndrome and sudden death is not clear.[238] However, the best evidence suggests that MVP increases the risk of sudden death slightly,[197] especially in patients with severe MR[240] or severe valvular deformity.[241] The immediate cause of the sudden, unexpected death is probably ventricular fibrillation,[242] although complete heart block with prolonged asystole has also been reported in this syndrome.[237]

Kligfield et al. have identified the following as potential risks for sudden death in MVP: the presence of significant MR, complex ventricular arrhythmias, prolongation of Q-T interval, and a history of syncope and palpitations.[237]

Echocardiography

(See also p. 73)

Echocardiography plays a key role in the diagnosis of MVP and has been most useful in the delineation of this syndrome (Figs. 3–51, p. 73, and 3–52, p. 74). The most common electrocardiographic finding on M-mode echocardiography is abrupt posterior movement of the posterior leaflet or of both mitral leaflets in mid-systole with the leaflet interface greater than 2 mm posterior to the C-D line; this movement occurs simultaneously with the systolic click; a second finding is pansystolic posterior prolapse of one or both leaflets, giving rise to a U- or hammock-shaped configuration 3 mm or more posterior to the C-D segment. This is the opposite of what is seen in hypertrophic obstructive cardiomyopathy, in which the anterior leaflet of the mitral valve moves toward the ventricular septum in midsystole.

The two-dimensional echocardiogram shows one or both mitral valve leaflets billowing into the left atrium during systole (Fig. 32–25).[243,244] It is also helpful in the identification of patients at significant risk of developing severe MR or infective endocarditis; the leaflets are distinctly thickened or redundant[245] and the mitral annular diameter is abnormally increased in these patients.[243,246] Doppler echocardiography frequently reveals mild MR that is not always associated with an audible murmur. Color flow Doppler is useful in identifying the location and severity of the regurgitant jets. MR is moderate or severe in 10 per cent of patients, most commonly in men over the age of 50.[246,247] Transesophageal echocardiography provides additional details regarding the mitral valve apparatus and may demonstrate rupture of chordae tendineae.

The variability in physical findings in this syndrome, already commented upon, extends to the echocardiogram.[248] Thus, some patients have a systolic click with or without a murmur and show no evidence of MVP on the echocardiogram. Conversely, the echocardiographic findings of MVP may be observed in patients without the click or murmur. Others have both the typical echocardiographic and auscultatory features. The echocardiographic findings of MVP have been reported to occur in a large number of first-degree relatives of patients with established MVP.[249]

Two-dimensional echocardiography has also revealed prolapse of the tricuspid and aortic valves in approximately one-fifth of patients with MVP.[249,250] Conversely, however, prolapse of the tricuspid and aortic valves occurs *uncommonly* in patients without prolapse of the mitral valve.[250]

Stress Scintigraphy

The differential diagnosis between two common conditions—MVP associated with atypical chest pain and electrocardiographic abnormalities, and primary coronary artery disease associated with MVP—may be aided by exercise electrocardiography, but myocardial perfusion scintigraphy using thallium-201 or sestamibi during exercise pharmacological stress (see p. 290) is more specific. When findings are normal, i.e., when there is no evidence of stress-induced regional myocardial ischemia, the diagnosis of MVP unrelated to ischemic heart disease is favored.[251] Ejection fraction at rest determined by radionuclide angiography is usually normal in patients having MVP without associated MR.

Angiography

The configuration of the left ventriculogram during systole is helpful in the diagnosis of MVP. The right anterior oblique projection is most useful for defining the posterior leaflet of the mitral valve and

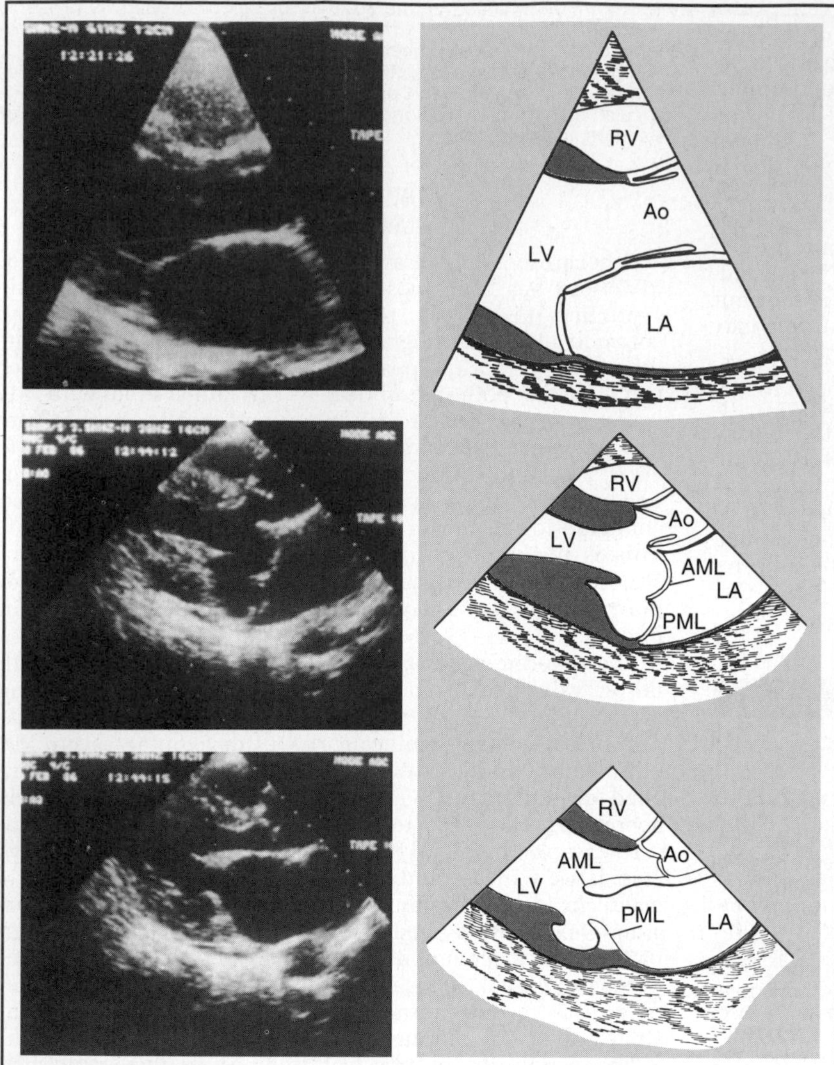

FIGURE 32–25. *Top,* Parasternal long-axis view of normal mitral valve leaflets during systole. RV = right ventricle, LV = left ventricle, Ao = aorta, and LA = left atrium. *Center,* Classic mitral valve prolapse. The parasternal long-axis view shows the mitral leaflets prolapsing into the left atrium during systole. Note the relation of the mitral leaflets to the mitral annulus. RV denotes right ventricle; LV = left ventricle, Ao = aorta, LA = left atrium, AML = anterior mitral leaflet, and PML = posterior mitral leaflet. *Bottom,* Classic mitral valve prolapse with leaflet thickening. The parasternal long-axis view of the same mitral valve as in center figure is shown during diastole. This view was used to measure the thickness of the leaflets. RV denotes right ventricle, LV = left ventricle, Ao = aorta, AML = anterior mitral leaflet, PML = posterior mitral leaflet, and LA = left atrium. (Reprinted by permission from Marks, A. R., Choong, C. Y., Sanfilippo, A. J., et al.: Identification of high-risk and low-risk subgroups of patients with mitral valve prolapse. N. Engl. J. Med. *320:*1031, 1989. Copyright 1989 Massachusetts Medical Society.)

the left anterior oblique projection for studying the anterior leaflet. The most helpful sign is extension of the mitral leaflet tissue inferiorly and posteriorly to the point of attachment of the mitral leaflets to the mitral annulus.[252] Angiography may also reveal scalloped edges of the leaflets, reflecting redundancy of tissue.

Other abnormalities noted on angiography of some patients with MVP include dilatation, decreased systolic contraction, and calcification of the mitral annulus and poor contraction of the basal portion of the left ventricle.[253] There may be an indentation at the base of the posteromedial papillary muscle associated with prolapse of the posterior leaflet and resulting from abnormal traction on this muscle. With involvement of both papillary muscles, there may be an indentation of the anterior as well as the inferior wall of the left ventricle, giving the cardiac silhouette an hourglass appearance. These left ventricular contraction abnormalities are secondary to redundancy of the mitral valve leaflets and transmission of the abnormal tension on these leaflets to the papillary muscles and underlying left ventricle.

NATURAL HISTORY

The outlook for MVP in children is excellent, a large majority remaining asymptomatic for many years without any change in clinical or laboratory manifestations.[197,233,254]

Progressive MR is the most frequent serious complication,[233,255,256] occurring in about 15 per cent of patients over a 10- to 15-year period; the incidence of this complication is significantly greater in patients with both murmurs and clicks than in those with an isolated click. In many patients, rupture of chordae tendineae is responsible for the intensification of the MR.[252] Severe MR occurs more frequently in men older than 50 years with MVP.[256] Patients with the MVP syndrome are also at risk of developing infective endocarditis,[257,258] although the incidence appears to be extremely low in patients with a midsystolic click only; the incidence rises in patients with a systolic murmur.[258] It is higher in men than in women and in those more than 50 years of age. Endocarditis often aggravates the severity of MR and therefore the need for surgical treatment. Zuppiroli et al. followed 316 patients with MVP for an average of more than 8 years; 70 per cent were women and 29 per cent had familial MVP. Serious complications (cardiac death, need for cardiac surgery, acute infective endocarditis, or cerebral embolic events) occurred at a rate of 1 per 100 patient years.[233]

Acute hemiplegia, transient ischemic attacks, cerebellar infarcts, amaurosis fugax, and retinal arteriolar occlusions all appear to occur more frequently in patients with the MVP syndrome, suggesting that cerebral emboli are unusually common in this condition.[259,260] These neurological complications are often associated with shortened platelet survival. Loss of endothelial continuity and tearing of the endocardium overlying the myxomatous valve may initiate platelet aggregation and the formation of mural platelet-fibrin complexes.[259] The paroxysmal arrhythmias that occur in the MVP syndrome may contribute to the likelihood of embolization. Indeed, it is possible that cerebral embolization secondary to MVP may be a significant cause for unexplained strokes and other cerebral and retinal complications in young people without cerebrovascular disease. Similarly, myocardial infarction in patients with MVP and normal coronary arteries may be secondary to embolization.[261]

TABLE 32–6 MATCHING RISK AND MANAGEMENT IN PATIENTS WITH MITRAL VALVE PROLAPSE

RISK LEVEL	PATIENTS	MANAGEMENT
Lowest	Subjects without mitral regurgitant murmurs or regurgitation revealed by Doppler echocardiography, especially women younger than age 45	Reassurance; peridental antibiotics not clearly necessary and if used should not include medication with risk of allergic reactions; reevaluation and echocardiography at moderate intervals (5 years)
Moderate	Subjects with intermittent or persistent mitral murmurs and mild regurgitation revealed by Doppler echocardiography	Antibiotic prophylaxis with erythromycin or amoxicillin; treatment of even mild established hypertension; reevaluation and echocardiography more frequently (2 to 3 years)
High	Subjects with moderate or severe mitral regurgitation	Antibiotic prophylaxis with amoxicillin (unless allergic); optimization of afterload (arterial pressure); reevaluation with Doppler echocardiography and other tests if needed annually; consider valve repair or replacement for exertional dyspnea or decline of left ventricular function into low-normal range

From Devereux, R. B.: Recent developments in the diagnosis and management of mitral valve prolapse. Curr. Opin. Cardiol. *10*:107, 1995. Modified from Devereux, R. B., and Kligfield, P.: Mitral valve prolapse. *In* Rakel, R.: Current Therapy. Philadelphia, W. B. Saunders Company, 1992, p. 237, 241.

MANAGEMENT

(Table 32–6)

Asymptomatic patients (or those whose principal complaint is anxiety) with no arrhythmias evident on a routine extended electrocardiographic tracing and on prolonged auscultation, with normal ST segments and without evidence of MR, have an excellent prognosis. They should be reassured about the favorable prognosis but should have follow-up examinations every 3 to 5 years. This should include a two-dimensional echocardiogram and a Doppler study. Patients with a long systolic murmur may show progression of MR and should be examined more frequently, at intervals of approximately 12 months. Mitral valve surgery, most commonly mitral valve repair,[202] should be carried out for patients with MVP and severe MR (see p. 1026). *Endocarditis prophylaxis* is advisable in patients with a typical systolic murmur and characteristic echocardiographic features of MVP and some evidence of MR. Prophylaxis does not appear to be necessary in patients, particularly women, with a midsystolic click without a systolic murmur.[257] Some, however, recommend prophylaxis when such patients are subjected to instrumentation of the upper respiratory or genitourinary tract (see p. 1097).

Patients with a history of palpitations, lightheadedness, dizziness, or syncope or those who have ventricular arrhythmias or Q-T prolongation on a routine electrocardiogram should undergo ambulatory (24-hour) electrocardiographic monitoring or exercise electrocardiography or both to detect arrhythmias. Because of the risk—albeit low—of sudden death,[237,238] electrophysiological studies should be carried out to characterize arrhythmias in symptomatic patients. Beta-adrenoceptor blockers are useful in the treatment of palpitations secondary to frequent ventricular premature contractions and for self-terminating episodes of supraventricular tachycardias. These drugs may also be useful in the treatment of chest discomfort, both in patients with associated coronary artery disease and in those with normal coronary vessels in whom the symptoms may be due to regional ischemia secondary to MVP. Radiofrequency ablation of atrioventricular bypass tracts is useful for frequent or prolonged episodes of supraventricular tachycardia.

In patients with MVP who have had any of the aforementioned cerebral events and in whom no other cause is apparent, anticoagulant therapy and/or aspirin should be given.

Patients with MVP and symptoms of left ventricular failure attributable to MR should be treated as are other patients with severe MR (see p. 1026), and those with severe regurgitation who are not responsive to medical management may require mitral valve surgery. Reconstructive surgery without valve replacement is often possible (Fig. 32–20).[202] Approximately half of all mitral valve reconstructions for MR are now carried out in patients with MVP. Among 252 such patients operated upon at the Brigham and Women's Hospital, resection of the most deformed leaflet segment and insertion of an annuloplasty ring to reduce the dilated annulus was the most commonly employed procedure. Rupture of the chords to the anterior leaflet could sometimes be treated by chordal transfer from the posterior leaflet. In other cases, shortening of the chordae and/or papillary muscle was necessary. The operative mortality was 2 per cent; structural valve degeneration occurred in 15 per cent at 5 years.

Coronary arteriography should be performed in patients with angina on effort and/or ischemic electrocardiographic changes or abnormalities on a thallium perfusion scan during exercise, and treatment should take into account both the responsiveness of symptoms to medical management and the coronary anatomy.

Although this discussion has focused attention on complications of the MVP syndrome, it should not be forgotten that, on the whole, this is a benign condition and that the *vast majority* of patients with this syndrome remain asymptomatic for their entire lives and require, at most, observation every few years and reassurance.[262]

AORTIC STENOSIS

ETIOLOGY AND PATHOLOGY

Obstruction to left ventricular outflow is localized most commonly at the aortic valve and is discussed in this section. However, obstruction may also occur above the valve (supravalvular stenosis [see p. 919]) or below the valve (discrete subvalvular aortic stenosis [see p. 918]) or may be caused by hypertrophic obstructive cardiomyopathy (see p. 1414). Valvular aortic stenosis (AS) *without accompanying mitral valve disease* is more common in men and very rarely occurs on a rheumatic basis but instead is usually either congenital or degenerative in origin[263–264a] (Figs. 32–26 and 32–27).

CONGENITAL AORTIC STENOSIS (see also pp. 914 and 969). Congenital malformations of the aortic valve may be

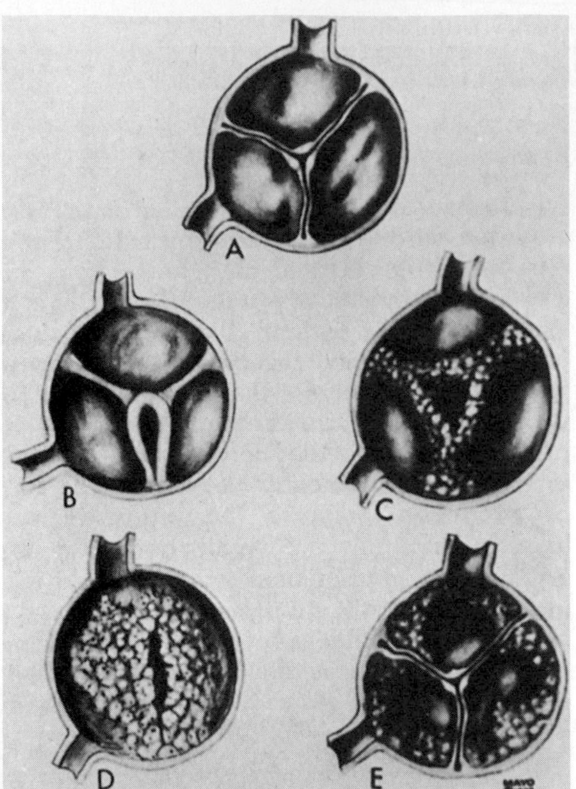

FIGURE 32–26. Types of aortic valve stenosis. *A*, Normal aortic valve. *B*, Congenital aortic stenosis. *C*, Rheumatic aortic stenosis. *D*, Calcific aortic stenosis. *E*, Calcific senile aortic stenosis. (From Brandenburg, R. O., et al.: Valvular heart disease—When should the patient be referred? Pract. Cardiol. *5*:50, 1979.)

unicuspid, bicuspid, or tricuspid, or there may be a dome-shaped diaphragm. *Unicuspid valves* produce severe obstruction in infancy and are the most frequent malformations found in fatal valvular aortic stenosis in children under the age of 1 year. Congenitally *bicuspid valves* may be stenotic with commissural fusion at birth, but more commonly they are not responsible for serious narrowing of the aortic orifice during childhood; their abnormal architecture induces turbulent flow, which traumatizes the leaflets and ultimately leads to fibrosis, increased rigidity, and calcification of the leaflets and narrowing of the aortic orifice[265,266] (Fig. 32–28). Infective endocarditis may develop on a congenitally bicuspid valve, which then becomes regurgitant. Rarely, a congenitally bicuspid valve is purely regurgitant in the absence of antecedent infection. It should be emphasized that in a majority of cases, a bicuspid valve is not stenotic at birth and the changes causing stenosis resemble those occurring in senile, degenerative calcific stenosis of a tricuspid aortic valve except that in the congenitally bicuspid valve these changes occur several decades earlier.

A third form of a congenitally malformed valve is *tricuspid*, with the cusps of unequal size and some commissural fusion. Although many of these valves retain normal function throughout life, it has been postulated that the turbulent flow produced by the mild congenital architectural abnormality may lead to fibrosis and ultimately to calcification and stenosis. Tricuspid stenotic aortic valves in adults may be congenital, rheumatic, or degenerative in origin.

ACQUIRED AORTIC STENOSIS. Rheumatic AS results from adhesions and fusions of the commissures and cusps and vascularization of the leaflets of the valve ring, leading to retraction and stiffening of the free borders of the cusps, with calcific nodules present on both surfaces and an orifice that is reduced to a small round or triangular opening. As a consequence, the rheumatic valve is often regurgitant as well as stenotic.[263] The heart frequently exhibits other stigmata of rheumatic heart disease, especially mitral valve involvement. Rheumatic AS appears to be decreasing in frequency in industrialized nations with the decline in rheumatic fever.

In degenerative (senile) calcific AS, the cusps are immobilized by a deposit of calcium along their flexion lines at their bases. This most common cause of AS in adults (which is now the most frequent in patients with AS requiring aortic valve replacement)[267] appears to result from years of normal mechanical stress on the valve. Although degenerative calcification may extend in the direction of the cusps, no commissural fusion is present. Degenerative "wear and tear" appears to be the most likely cause of this form of AS, which is commonly accompanied by calcifications of the mitral annulus and coronary arteries but rarely by aortic regurgitation. Both diabetes mellitus and hypercholesterolemia are risk factors for the development of this lesion.[268] The stenosis is produced by the calcific deposits that prevent the cusps from opening normally during systole (Fig. 32–28).

In atherosclerotic aortic valvular stenosis, severe atherosclerosis involves the aorta and other major arteries; this form of AS occurs most frequently in patients with severe hypercholesterolemia and is observed in children with homozygous type II hyperlipoproteinemia, an extremely rare condition (see Ch. 35). Calcific aortic stenosis is observed in Paget's disease of bone[269] as well as in end-stage renal disease.[270] *Rheumatoid involvement* of the valve is a rare cause of AS and results in nodular thickening of the valve leaflets and involvement of the proximal part of the aorta (see p. 1776). *Ochronosis* is another rare cause of aortic stenosis.[271]

Roberts studied hearts with AS obtained at autopsy from patients between 15 and 65 years of age and found that almost 40 per cent were tricuspid. Because thickening of the mitral valve and a history of acute rheumatic fever were present in half of these cases, it is likely that the AS was rheumatic in etiology; in the remainder it was either congenital or degenerative in origin. In 90 per cent of hearts of patients with AS who were older than 65 years and who were examined at autopsy, the valves were tricuspid, with nodular calcific deposits on the aortic aspects of the cusps, but without commissural fusion,[264] indicative of degenerative disease.

Hemodynamically significant AS leads to severe concentric left ventricular hypertrophy,[272] with heart weights as great as 1000 gm. The interventricular septum often bulges into and encroaches on the right ventricular cavity. When

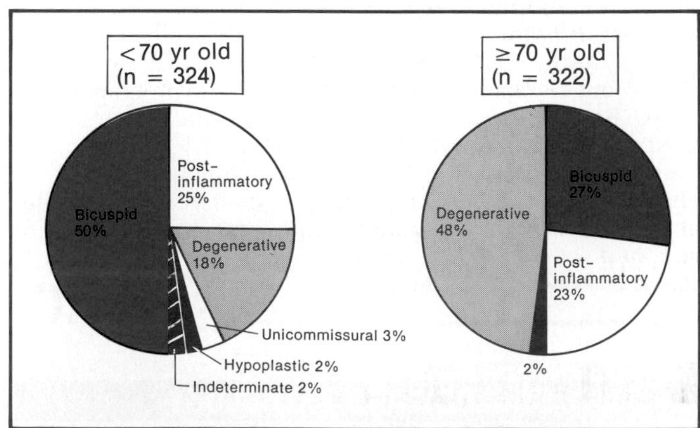

FIGURE 32–27. Causes of aortic stenosis, shown for two age groups. Among patients younger than 70 years *(left)*, calcification of congenitally bicuspid valves accounted for half of the surgical cases. In contrast, in those 70 years of age or older *(right)*, degenerative calcification accounted for almost half of the cases. (From Passik, C. S., et al.: Temporal changes in the causes of aortic stenosis: A surgical pathologic study of 646 cases. Mayo Clin. Proc. *62*:119, 1987.)

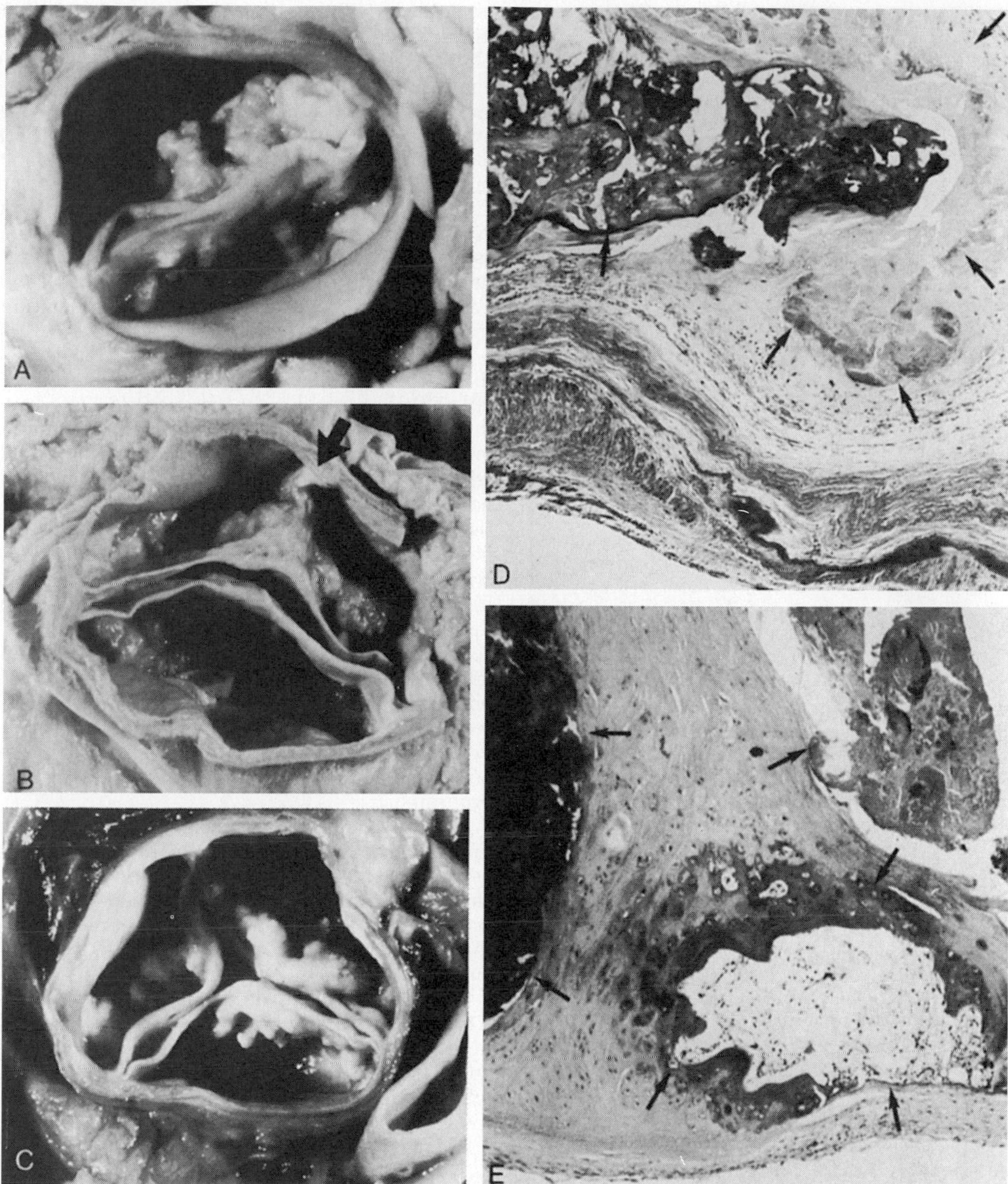

FIGURE 32–28. Calcific aortic stenosis. *A*, Congenitally bicuspid aortic valve, characterized by two equal cusps with basal mineralization. *B*, Congenitally bicuspid aortic valve having two unequal cusps, the larger with a central raphe (arrow). *C*, Otherwise anatomically normal tricuspid aortic valve in an elderly patient, characterized by isolated cusps with calcification localized to basilar aspect; cuspal free edges are not involved. *D* and *E*, Photomicrographs of calcific deposits in calcific aortic stenosis; deposits are rimmed by arrows (hematoxylin and eosin, ×15). *D*, Deposits with underlying cusp largely intact; transmural calcific deposits are shown in *E* (*A* and *C* from Schoen, F. J., and St. John Sutton, M.: Contemporary issues in the pathology of valvular heart disease. Hum. Pathol. *18*:568, 1987.)

left ventricular failure supervenes, the left ventricle dilates,[272] the left atrium enlarges, and changes secondary to backward failure occur in the pulmonary vascular bed, right side of the heart, and systemic venous bed.

PATHOPHYSIOLOGY

(Fig. 32–29)

The left ventricle responds to *sudden* severe obstruction to outflow by dilatation and reduction of stroke volume.[273] However, in adults with AS, the obstruction usually develops and increases gradually over a prolonged period. In infants and children with congenital AS, the valve orifice shows little change as the child grows, thereby intensifying the relative obstruction quite gradually. Left ventricular function can be well maintained in experimentally produced, chronic, gradually developing subcoronary AS.[274] Left ventricular output is maintained by the presence of left ventricular hypertrophy, which may sustain a large pressure gradient across the aortic valve for many years without a reduction in cardiac output, left ventricular dilatation, or the development of symptoms. A peak systolic pressure gradient exceeding 50 mm Hg in the presence of a normal cardiac output or an effective aortic orifice less than about 0.8 cm^2 in an average-sized adult, i.e., 0.5 cm^2/m^2 of body surface area (less than approximately one-fourth of the normal orifice), is generally considered to represent critical obstruction to left ventricular outflow.[275]

As contraction of the left ventricle becomes progressively more isometric, the left ventricular pressure pulse exhibits

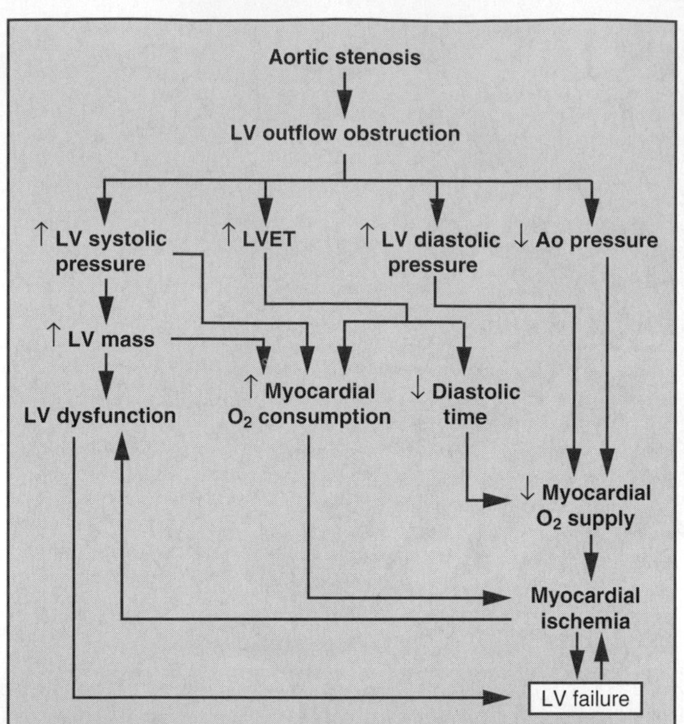

FIGURE 32–29. Pathophysiology of aortic stenosis. Left ventricular (LV) outflow obstruction results in an increased LV systolic pressure, increased left ventricular ejection time (LVET), increased left ventricular diastolic pressure, and decreased aortic (Ao) pressure. Increased LV systolic pressure with LV volume overload increases LV mass, which may lead to LV dysfunction and failure. Increased LV systolic pressure, LV mass, and LVET increase myocardial oxygen (O_2) consumption. Increased LVET results in a decrease of diastolic time (myocardial perfusion time). Increased LV diastolic pressure and decreased Ao diastolic pressure decrease coronary perfusion pressure. Decreased diastolic time and coronary perfusion pressure decrease myocardial O_2 supply. Increased myocardial O_2 consumption and decreased myocardial O_2 supply produce myocardial ischemia, which further deteriorates LV function (↑ = increased, ↓ = decreased). (From Boudoulas, H., and Gravanis, M. B.: Valvular heart disease. *In* Gravanis, M. B.: Cardiovascular Disorders: Pathogenesis and Pathophysiology. St. Louis, C. V. Mosby, 1993, p. 64.)

a rounded, rather than flattened, summit. The elevated left ventricular end-diastolic pressure, which is characteristic of severe AS, does not necessarily signify the presence of left ventricular dilatation or failure but often reflects diminished compliance of the hypertrophied left ventricular wall; usually it results from a combination of both processes.[276,277]

In patients with severe AS, large *a* waves usually appear in the left atrial pressure pulse because of the combination of enhanced contraction of a hypertrophied left atrium and diminished left ventricular compliance. Atrial contraction plays a particularly important role in filling of the left ventricle in AS. It raises left ventricular end-diastolic pressure without producing a concomitant elevation of mean left atrial pressure.[278] This "booster pump" function of the left atrium prevents the pulmonary venous and capillary pressures from rising to levels that would produce pulmonary congestion, while at the same time maintaining left ventricular end-diastolic pressure at the elevated level necessary for effective left ventricular contraction. Loss of appropriately timed, vigorous atrial contraction, as occurs in atrial fibrillation or atrioventricular dissociation, may result in rapid clinical deterioration in patients with severe AS.

Although the *cardiac output* at rest is within normal limits in the majority of patients with severe AS,[275] it often fails to rise normally during exertion. Late in the course of the disease the cardiac output, stroke volume, and therefore the left ventricular–aortic pressure gradient all decline, whereas the mean left atrial, pulmonary capillary, pulmonary arterial, right ventricular systolic and diastolic, and right atrial pressures rise, often sequentially.[275a] AS intensifies the severity of any existing mitral regurgitation by increasing the pressure gradient responsible for driving blood from the left ventricle to the left atrium. In addition, the dilatation of the left ventricle, which occurs late in the course of aortic valve disease, may produce mitral regurgitation, superimposing the hemodynamic changes associated with this lesion on those produced by AS. Also, as a consequence of pulmonary hypertension or bulging of the hypertrophied septum into the right ventricular cavity or both, the *a* wave in the right atrial pressure pulse becomes prominent.

Left ventricular end-diastolic volume usually remains normal until quite late in the course of the disease, but left ventricular mass increases in response to the chronic pressure overload, resulting in an increase in the mass/volume ratio. However, the increase in mass may not be as great as that seen with aortic regurgitation (AR) or combined AS and AR.

Gender differences in the response of the left ventricle to AS have been reported.[279–280a] Women more frequently exhibit normal or even supernormal ventricular performance and smaller, thicker-walled concentrically hypertrophied left ventricles whereas men more frequently have eccentric hypertrophy and ventricular dilatation (Fig. 32–30).

MYOCARDIAL FUNCTION IN AORTIC STENOSIS

In experimental animals, when the aorta is suddenly constricted, left ventricular pressure rises, and there is a large increase in wall stress, whereas both extent and velocity of shortening decline. As pointed out in Chapter 13, the development of ventricular hypertrophy is one of the principal mechanisms by which the heart adapts

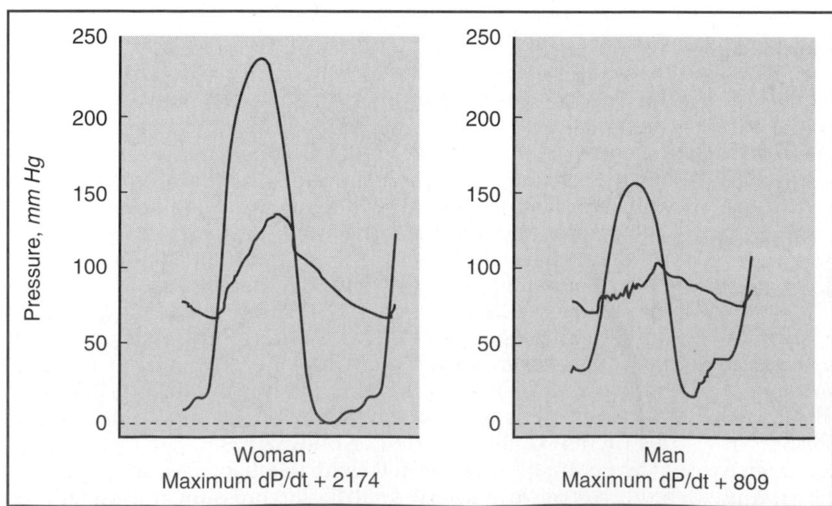

FIGURE 32–30. The difference in pressure-generating capabilities of the left ventricle in an 83-year-old woman and a 60-year-old man with a similar degree of aortic stenosis is shown. dP/dt—rate of pressure increase. (Reproduced with permission from Carroll, J. D., Carroll, E. P., Felman, T., et al.: Sex-associated differences in left ventricular function in aortic stenosis of the elderly. Circulation *86:*1099, 1992. Copyright 1992 American Heart Association.)

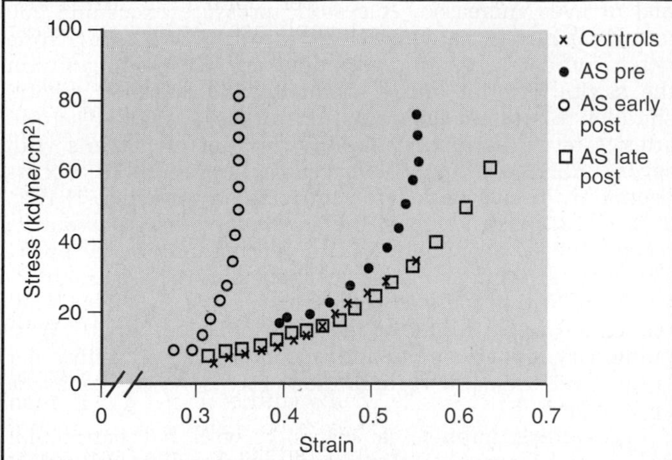

FIGURE 32–31. **Representative plot of the diastolic stress-strain relation in a control subject and a patient with severe aortic stenosis (AS) before surgery (pre) as well as early and late after valve replacement (post). Early after surgery (early post), the curve is shifted to the left compared with the preoperative evaluation, and the constant of myocardial stiffness is increased. Late after valve replacement (late post) the curve is shifted to the right, and the constant of myocardial stiffness is normalized. (Reproduced with permission from Villari, B., et al.: Normalization of diastolic dysfunction in aortic stenosis late after valve replacement. Circulation *91*:2353, 1995. Copyright 1995 American Heart Association.)**

to such an increased hemodynamic burden.[281] The increased systolic wall stress induced by AS apparently leads to parallel replication of sarcomeres and concentric hypertrophy (Fig. 13–10, p. 401), and the increase in left ventricular wall thickness is often sufficient to counterbalance the increased pressure so that peak systolic wall tension returns to normal or remains so if the obstruction develops slowly.[281–284] An inverse correlation between wall stress and ejection fraction exists in patients with AS.[284] This suggests that the depressed ejection fraction and velocity of fiber shortening that occur in *some* patients are a consequence of inadequate wall thickening,[285] resulting in "afterload mismatch."[286] Patients having AS with compensated pressure overload as well as some patients with depressed left ventricular ejection fraction and overt congestive failure may have normal values of intraventricular stress ($d\sigma/dt$)[287] and pressure (dP/dt) development, indicative of normal contractility.[279,280] In others, the lower ejection fraction is secondary to a depression of contractility; in the latter, surgical treatment is less effective.[288] Thus, both increased afterload and altered contractility are operative in depressing left ventricular performance.[279,280]

In order to evaluate myocardial function in patients with AS, the ejection phase indices, such as ejection fraction and myocardial fiber shortening, should be related to the existing wall tension. Wall thickness is a critical determinant of ventricular performance in patients with AS; inadequate hypertrophy, an intrinsic depression of myocardial contractility, or a combination of these two defects may lead to a depression of ventricular performance.[289] Impaired systolic function also occurs in prolonged, severe AS with massive hypertrophy (LV mass > 300 g/m²). It is associated with degenerative changes in the ultrastructure, including disruption of sarcomeres and increased interstitial fibrosis.

DIASTOLIC PROPERTIES (see p. 402). Although ventricular hypertrophy is a key adaptive mechanism to the pressure load imposed by AS, it has an adverse pathophysiological consequence; i.e., it increases diastolic stiffness (Figs. 32–11, and 32–31). As a result, greater intracavitary pressure is required for ventricular filling.[276,277,289a] Some patients with AS manifest an increase in stiffness of the left ventricle (chamber stiffness) due simply to an increase in muscle mass but with no alteration in the diastolic properties of each unit of myocardium (muscle stiffness); others exhibit increases in both chamber and muscle stiffness, which contribute to the elevation of ventricular diastolic filling pressure at any level of ventricular diastolic volume.[290,291] The diastolic dysfunction may be responsible for flash pulmonary edema in AS. Chamber stiffness may revert toward normal as hypertrophy regresses following relief of AS,[276,277] and at least in some patients muscle stiffness may also revert to normal. Whether this occurs in all patients is not clear. It is expected that this regression of stiffness would not occur in patients with extensive myocardial fibrosis. Indeed, in some patients stiffness increases postoperatively as ventricular hypertrophy regresses, while interstitial fibrosis remains unchanged.[292] The rate of ventricular thinning in diastole is slowed in AS.

STRUCTURE. A variety of changes in the myocardial ultrastructure have been documented in patients with severe AS. These include unusually large nuclei, loss of myofibrils, accumulation of mitochondria, large cytoplasmic areas devoid of contractile material, and proliferation of fibroblasts and collagen fibers in the interstitial space.[293] The depression of cardiac function that occurs late in the course of the disease may well be related to these morphological alterations. In adults with AS, both myocardial cellular hypertrophy and relative and absolute increases in connective tissue occur.[294] An inverse correlation between left ventricular ejection fraction and myocardial fiber diameter has been reported.[294]

ISCHEMIA. In AS, coronary blood flow at rest is elevated in absolute terms but is normal when corrected for myocardial mass.[295] There may be inadequate myocardial oxygenation in severe AS, even in the absence of coronary artery disease. The hypertrophied left ventricular muscle mass, the increased systolic pressure, and the prolongation of ejection all elevate myocardial oxygen consumption,[296] and the abnormally heightened pressure compressing the coronary arteries exceeds the coronary perfusion pressure, thereby interfering with coronary blood flow,[297,298] thus leading to a potential imbalance between myocardial oxygen supply and demand. Myocardial perfusion is also impaired by the relative decrease in myocardial capillary density and by the elevation of left ventricular end-diastolic pressure, which lowers the aortic–left ventricular pressure gradient in diastole, i.e., the coronary perfusion pressure gradient. The subendocardium in severe AS in particular is susceptible to ischemia, and this underperfusion may be responsible for the development of subendocardial ischemia.[297] Marcus et al. have demonstrated a reduction in the velocity of coronary blood flow during reactive hyperemia at the time of operation in patients with severe AS,[299] and this may correlate with the angina commonly observed in these patients. Metabolic evidence of myocardial ischemia, i.e., lactate production, can be demonstrated when myocardial oxygen needs are stimulated by exercise or isoproterenol in patients with AS, in both the presence and the absence of coronary arterial narrowing.

CLINICAL MANIFESTATIONS

History

In the natural history of adults with AS, a long latent period exists during which there is gradually increasing obstruction and an increase in the pressure load on the myocardium while the patient remains asymptomatic.[300] The cardinal manifestations of AS, which commence most commonly in the sixth decade of life, are angina pectoris, syncope, and heart failure.[301] In patients in whom the obstruction remains unrelieved, once these symptoms become manifested, the prognosis is poor; survival curves show that the interval from the onset of symptoms to the time of death is approximately 2 years in patients with heart failure, 3 years in those with syncope, and 5 years in those with angina.[302,303] *Angina* occurs in approximately two-thirds of patients with critical AS (about half of whom have associated significant coronary artery obstruction)[304] and usually resembles that observed in patients with coronary artery disease, in that it is commonly precipitated by exertion and relieved by rest. In patients without coronary artery disease it results from the combination of increased oxygen needs by the hypertrophied myocardium and reduction of oxygen delivery secondary to the excessive compression of coronary vessels[295,299] (see Ischemia, above). In patients with coronary artery disease, angina is caused by a combination of the epicardial coronary obstruction and the above-described oxygen imbalance characteristic of AS. Rarely, angina results from calcium emboli to the coronary vascular bed.[306]

Syncope is most commonly due to the reduced cerebral perfusion that occurs during exertion when arterial pressure declines consequent to systemic vasodilatation in the presence of a fixed cardiac output. Syncope has also been attributed to malfunction of the baroreceptor mechanism[266,308] and to vasodepressor response to a greatly elevated left ventricular systolic pressure during exercise.[309] Premonitory symptoms are common. Exertional hypotension may also be manifested as "graying out" spells or dizziness on effort. Syncope at rest may be due to transient ventricular fibrillation,[307] from which the patient recovers spontaneously; from transient atrial fibrillation with loss of the atrial contribution to left ventricular filling causing a precipitous decline in cardiac output; or transient atrioventricular block due to extension of the calcification of the valve into the conduction system. Exertional dyspnea with orthopnea, paroxysmal nocturnal dyspnea, and pulmonary edema reflect varying degrees of pulmonary venous hypertension. These are relatively late symptoms in AS, and their presence for more than 5 years should suggest the possibility of associated mitral valvular disease.

Gastrointestinal bleeding, idiopathic or due to angiodysplasia (most commonly of the right colon) or other vascular malformations, occurs more often in patients with calcific AS than in persons without this condition; it may cease after aortic valve replacement.[310] Infective endocarditis is a greater risk in younger patients with milder valvular deformity than in older patients with rocklike calcific aortic deformities. Cerebral emboli resulting in stroke or transient ischemic attacks may result from microthrombi on thickened bicuspid valves.[311] Calcific AS may cause embolization of calcium to a variety of organs, including the heart, kidney, and brain. Abrupt loss of vision has been reported when calcific emboli occluded the central retinal artery.[312]

Because cardiac output is usually well maintained for many years in patients with severe AS, marked fatigability, debilitation, peripheral cyanosis, and other manifestations of a low cardiac output are usually not prominent until quite late in the natural history of the disease. Atrial fibrillation, pulmonary hypertension, and systemic venous hypertension in patients with isolated AS are often preterminal findings. Although AS may be responsible for sudden death (see p. 749), this usually occurs in patients who had previously been symptomatic.

Physical Examination

The arterial pulse characteristically rises slowly and is small and sustained (pulsus parvus et tardus) (Fig. 2–8*B*, p. 21).[313,314] In the advanced stage, systolic and pulse pressures are both reduced. However, in patients with mild AS with associated AR and in older patients with an inelastic arterial bed, both systolic and pulse pressures may be normal or even increased. A systolic pressure exceeding 200 mm Hg is rare in patients with critical AS.[313] The anacrotic notch and coarse systolic vibrations are felt most readily in the carotid arterial pulse, producing the so-called carotid shudder. Simultaneous palpation of the apex and carotid arteries reveals a distinct lag in the latter in patients with severe AS.[315] Although left ventricular alternans occurs commonly in AS with left ventricular dysfunction[316] (Fig. 2–9, p. 23), obstruction of the aortic valve may prevent its recognition by examination of the peripheral arterial pulse. The jugular venous pulse usually shows prominent *a* waves, reflecting reduced right ventricular compliance consequent to hypertrophy of the ventricular septum.[317] With pulmonary hypertension and secondary right ventricular failure and tricuspid regurgitation, *v* or *c-v* waves may be prominent.

The cardiac impulse is sustained with left ventricular failure; it becomes displaced inferiorly and laterally (Fig. 2–11*C*). Presystolic distention of the left ventricle, i.e., a prominent precordial *a* wave, is often both visible and palpable. A hyperdynamic left ventricle suggests concomitant aortic and/or mitral regurgitation. A systolic thrill is usually best appreciated when the patient leans forward in full expiration. It is palpated most readily in the second left intercostal space on either side of the sternum or in the suprasternal notch and is frequently transmitted along the carotid arteries.

Rarely, right ventricular failure with systemic venous congestion, hepatomegaly, and edema precedes left ventricular failure. Probably this is caused by the so-called Bernheim effect, which results from the hypertrophied ventricular septum's bulging into and encroaching on the right ventricular cavity and leads to impairment of right ventricular filling. In such cases, the jugular venous pressure is elevated and the *a* wave is prominent.

AUSCULTATION (Tables 32–2 and 32–7). S_1 is normal or soft and S_4 is prominent, presumably because atrial contraction is vigorous and the mitral valve is partially closed during presystole.[318] S_2 may be single because calcification and immobility of the aortic valve make A_2 inaudible, be-

TABLE 32–7 DIFFERENTIAL DIAGNOSIS OF AORTIC STENOSIS: PHYSICAL FINDINGS

TYPE OF STENOSIS	MAXIMUM MURMUR AND THRILL	AORTIC EJECTION SOUND	AORTIC COMPONENT OF SECOND SOUND	REGURGITANT DIASTOLIC MURMUR	ARTERIAL PULSE
Acquired nonrheumatic or rheumatic	Second right sternal border to neck; may be at apex in the aged	Uncommon	Decreased or absent	Common	Delayed upstroke; anacrotic notch; ± small amplitude
Hypertrophic subaortic	Fourth left sternal border to apex (± regurgitant systolic murmur at apex)	Rare	Normal or decreased	Very rare	Brisk upstroke, sometimes bisferiens
Congenital valvular	Second right sternal border to neck (along left sternal border in some infants)	Very common in children, disappearing with decrease in valve mobility with age	Normal or increased in childhood; decreased with decrease in valve mobility with age	Uncommon in child; not uncommon in adult	Delayed upstroke; anacrotic notch; ± small amplitude
Congenital subvalvular	Discrete: like valvular; tunnel: left sternal border	Rare	Not helpful (normal, increased, decreased or absent)	Almost all	
Congenital supravalvular	First right sternal border to neck and sometimes to medial aspect of right arm; occasionally greater in neck than in chest	Rare	Normal or decreased	Uncommon	Rapid upstroke in right carotid, delayed in left carotid; right arm pulse pressure greater than left

From Levinson, G. E.: Aortic stenosis. *In* Dalen, J. E., and Alpert, J. S. (eds.): Valvular Heart Disease. 2nd ed. Boston, Little, Brown and Company, 1987, p. 202.

cause P_2 is buried in the prolonged aortic ejection murmur, or because prolongation of left ventricular systole makes A_2 coincide with P_2. Paradoxical splitting of S_2, which suggests associated left ventricular dysfunction, may also occur. With left ventricular failure and secondary pulmonary hypertension, P_2 may become accentuated. When the valve is rigid, A_2 may be inaudible, but when the valve is flexible, A_2 may be snapping and accentuated.

An aortic ejection sound (see p. 30) occurs simultaneously with the halting upward movement of the aortic valve (Fig. 2–17, p. 30). It is dependent on mobility of the valve cusps and disappears when they become severely calcified. Thus, it is common in children with congenital AS but is rare in elderly adults with acquired calcific AS and rigid valves. This sound occurs approximately 0.06 sec after the onset of S_1 and has a frequency similar to that of S_1. The ejection sound is heard most readily with the diaphragm of the stethoscope along the left sternal border, although it is often well transmitted to the apex, where it may be confused with S_1 (and the S_1 may be mistaken for an S_4). In contrast to a pulmonic ejection sound, aortic ejection sounds usually do not vary with respiration.

The *systolic murmur* of AS is usually late-peaking and heard best at the base of the heart but is often well transmitted along the carotid vessels and to the apex (Fig. 2–27, p. 36). Cessation of the murmur before A_2 is usually helpful in differentiating it from a pansystolic mitral murmur, but it may be falsely considered to be a pansystolic murmur because it may end with S_2, which represents pulmonic valve closure while A_2 is soft or even inaudible. In patients with calcified aortic valves, the murmur is harsh and rasping at the base, but high-frequency components selectively radiate to the apex (the so-called Gallavardin phenomenon [Fig. 2–28, p. 37]), where it may actually be more prominent and where it may be mistaken for the murmur of MR. Frequently, there is a "quiet area" between the base and apex where the murmur is diminished in intensity, supporting the erroneous impression that the apical and basal murmurs have different origins. In general, the more severe the stenosis, the longer the duration of the murmur[319] and the more likely that it peaks in mid-systole.[320]

In patients with degenerative AS, there may be heavy valvular calcification, but obstruction may not be severe because the commissural fusion characteristic of congenital and rheumatic AS is absent. The nonfused calcified cusps vibrate freely, resulting in a softer, more musical murmur, more prominent at the apex than the murmur of congenital or rheumatic AS.[319] High-pitched decrescendo diastolic murmurs secondary to AR are common in many patients with dominant AS.

In hypertrophic cardiomyopathy (HCM), the murmur is delayed in onset and may continue up to A_2 (see p. 1418); the carotid artery characteristically rises sharply and is bisferious. Palpation of the carotid pulse is also extremely helpful in differentiating between valvular AS on the one hand and HCM and MR on the other, because the arterial pulse generally rises slowly in AS but sharply in the other two conditions. However, confusion can arise in young patients with congenital AS, in whom sudden upward displacement ("doming") of the pliant aortic leaflet or leaflets with ventricular systole may result in a brisk initial upstroke in the carotid pulse, coincident with the systolic ejection click.

When the left ventricle fails and the cardiac output falls in AS, the murmur becomes softer or disappears altogether. The slow rise is more difficult to recognize. Stated simply, the clinical picture changes to that of severe left ventricular failure with a low cardiac output. Thus, occult AS may be a cause of intractable heart failure, and critical AS should be ruled out by echocardiography in patients with severe heart failure of unknown cause because operative treatment may be life-saving and may result in substantial clinical improvement.[321]

Dynamic Auscultation (Table 32–3). The murmur of valvular AS is augmented by the inhalation of amyl nitrite and by squatting, which increase stroke volume. It is reduced in intensity during the Valsalva strain (which increases the murmur of HCM), with vasopressors, moderate isometric exercise, or standing, all of which reduce transvalvular flow.[322] The intensity of the systolic murmur varies from beat to beat when the duration of diastolic filling varies, as in atrial fibrillation or following a premature contraction. This characteristic is helpful in differentiating AS from MR, in which the murmur is usually unaffected.

LABORATORY EXAMINATION

ELECTROCARDIOGRAPHY

The principal electrocardiographic change is left ventricular hypertrophy, which is found in approximately 85 per cent of patients with severe AS. The absence of left ventricular hypertrophy does not exclude the presence of critical AS, and the correlation between the absolute voltages in precordial leads and the severity of obstruction, which is quite good in children with congenital AS, is not as good in adults. However, a good correlation has been reported between the sum of the QRS amplitudes in 12 leads and the height of the left ventricular systolic pressure.[323] T-wave inversion and ST-segment depression in leads with upright QRS complexes are common. ST-segment depressions greater than 0.2 mV in patients with AS (left ventricular "strain") suggest that severe ventricular hypertrophy is present. The progressive development of ST-segment and T-wave abnormalities suggests that hypertrophy has progressed. Occasionally, a "pseudoinfarction" pattern is present, characterized by a loss of *r* waves in the right precordial leads. There is evidence of left atrial enlargement in more than 80 per cent of patients with severe isolated AS[324]; the principal manifestation is prominent late negativity of the P wave in V_1 rather than an increased duration in lead II, suggesting hypertrophy rather than dilatation. Atrial fibrillation is an uncommon and late sign of pure AS, and its presence in a patient who does not appear to have end-stage aortic disease should suggest the coexistence of mitral valvular disease.

The extension of calcific infiltrates from the aortic valve into the conduction system may cause various forms and degrees of atrioventricular and intraventricular block in 5 per cent of patients with calcific AS.[325] Conduction defects are more common in patients who have associated mitral annular calcium.[325] Almost 10 per cent of all instances of left anterior hemiblock are secondary to aortic valvular disease.

Ambulatory electrocardiography frequently shows complex ventricular arrhythmias,[326] particularly in patients with myocardial dysfunction.

RADIOLOGICAL FINDINGS

Routine radiological examination may be entirely normal despite the presence of critical AS. The heart is usually of normal size or slightly enlarged, with a rounding of the left ventricular border and apex (Fig. 7–10*A*, p. 210), unless regurgitation or left ventricular failure is present and causes substantial cardiomegaly. Poststenotic dilatation of the ascending aorta is a common finding. Calcification of the aortic valve is found in almost all adults with hemodynamically significant AS;[327] it is more readily detected on fluoroscopy (or echocardiography) rather than on the roentgenogram. The *absence* of calcium in the region of the aortic valve on careful fluoroscopic examination in a patient older than 35 essentially rules out severe valvular AS. The converse is not true, however, and in patients over the age of 65 with degenerative AS, severe calcification of the valve may occur with only mild obstruction. The left atrium may be slightly enlarged, and there may be radiological signs of pulmonary venous hypertension. However, when left atrial enlargement is marked, particularly if the atrial appendage is prominent, the presence of associated mitral valvular disease should be suspected.

ANGIOGRAPHY. Angiographic studies of the aortic valve are best performed by injecting contrast medium into the left ventricle and filming in the 30-degree right anterior oblique and 60-degree left anterior oblique projections. These examinations often make it possible to ascertain the number of cusps of the stenotic valve and to demonstrate doming of a thickened valve and a systolic jet. There is some hazard associated with the rapid injection of a large volume of contrast material into a high-pressure left ventricle, and this is ordinarily not indicated in patients with AS, critical obstruction, and/or left ventricular failure.

ECHOCARDIOGRAPHY (see also p. 74). The normal range of opening of the aortic valve is 1.6 to 2.6 cm, and the normal aortic valve leaflets are barely visible in systole on the M-mode echogram. Two-dimensional transthoracic echocardiography may be helpful in the detection of valvular calcification, in outlining the valve leaflets, and sometimes in determining the severity of the stenosis, by imaging the orifice. The orifice may be more clearly defined by transesophageal echocardiography, which offers a precise short-axis view of the aortic valve[328] (Fig. 3–54, p. 74). Multiplanar transesophageal echocardiography is particularly useful.[329] Two-dimensional transthoracic echocardiography is invaluable in detecting associated mitral valve disease and in assessing left ventricular performance, dilatation, and hypertrophy. Doppler echocardiography allows calculation of the left ventricular-aortic pressure gradient[330,331] (Figs. 3–42, p. 70, and 3–55, p. 75) using a modified Bernoulli equation (Fig. 3–4, p. 69). The gradients noninvasively determined by this method correlate well with those determined by left heart catheterization.[332,333] Color flow Doppler imaging is helpful in the detection and determination of the severity of any accompanying aortic regurgitation.

NATURAL HISTORY

In contrast to MS, which leads to symptoms almost immediately after its development, patients with severe AS may be asymptomatic for many years despite the presence of severe obstruction.[300,305,334] The systolic pressure gradient can exceed 150 mm Hg, and the peak left ventricular systolic pressure can reach approximately 300 mm Hg with relatively little increase in overall heart size on radiographic examination and with normal left ventricular end-diastolic and end-systolic volumes.

Patients with severe chronic AS tend to be free of cardiovascular symptoms until relatively late in the course of the disease. In Rapaport's series, 40 per cent of patients treated medically survived for 5 years and 20 per cent for 10 years after diagnosis.[66] In another series of patients with hemodynamically significant valvular AS treated medically, the 5-year survival rate was 64 per cent. However, once patients with AS become symptomatic with angina or syncope, the average survival is 2 to 3 years, whereas with congestive heart failure it is 1.5 years[302,303] (Fig. 32–32). In an analysis of elderly patients with severe AS and symptoms of heart failure who declined surgery, 50 per cent had died by 18 months of follow-up; the ejection fraction correlated inversely with survival.[335]

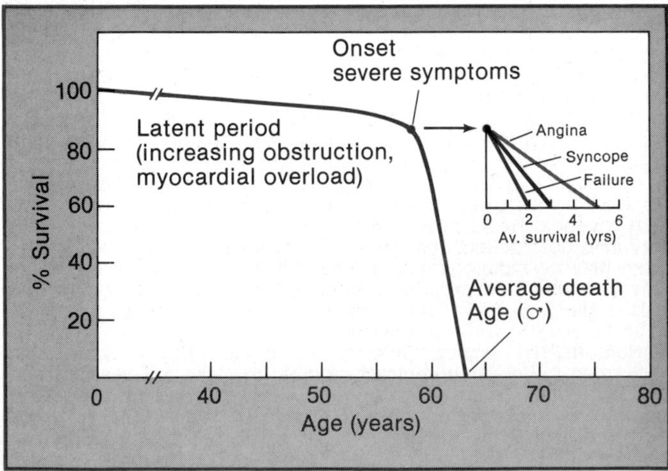

FIGURE 32–32. Natural history of aortic stenosis without operative treatment. (Reproduced with permission from Ross, J., Jr., and Braunwald, E.: Aortic stenosis. Circulation *38*[Suppl. V]:61, 1968. Copyright 1968 American Heart Association.)

Asymptomatic patients have an excellent prognosis.[336,337] Sudden death, like syncope, in patients with severe AS may be due to cerebral hypoperfusion followed by arrhythmia. Although severe AS is a potentially lethal disease, death, even when sudden, usually occurs in *symptomatic* patients. A number of authors have followed asymptomatic patients with critical AS,[338] and sudden death is extremely rare. Of 229 asymptomatic patients with critical aortic stenosis, only 5 (2 per cent) died suddenly (certainly not higher than the mortality from operation).[339]

MANAGEMENT

Medical Treatment

Patients with known severe AS who are asymptomatic should be advised to report promptly the development of any symptoms possibly related to AS. Patients with critical obstruction should be cautioned to avoid vigorous athletic and physical activity. However, such restrictions do not apply to patients with mild obstruction. The necessity for endocarditis prophylaxis should be explained (see p. 1097). Because of the gradual increase in the severity of obstruction, noninvasive assessment of the severity of obstruction by Doppler echocardiography should be carried out at intervals. In patients with mild obstruction, this measurement should be repeated every 2 years. Doppler-derived gradients have been shown to increase by 4 to 8 mm Hg per year.[339–341] The rate of increase is greater in patients with coexisting coronary artery disease and lower in patients with rheumatic AS. In asymptomatic patients with severe obstruction, repeat echocardiography should be carried out every 6 to 12 months, with particular attention to possible changes in left ventricular function.

Digitalis glycosides are indicated if there is an increase in ventricular volume or reduced ejection fraction. Although diuretics are beneficial when there is abnormal accumulation of fluid, they must be used with caution, because hypovolemia may reduce the elevated left ventricular end-diastolic pressure, lower cardiac output, and produce orthostatic hypotension. Beta-adrenoceptor blockers can depress myocardial function and induce left ventricular failure and should be used only with great caution, if at all, in patients with AS.

Atrial flutter or fibrillation occurs in fewer than 10 per cent of patients with severe AS, perhaps because of the late occurrence of left atrial enlargement in this condition. When such an arrhythmia is observed in a patient with AS, the possibility of associated mitral valve disease should be considered. In light of the adverse hemodynamic effects of the loss of atrial booster pump function with atrial fibrillation in patients with AS,[278] an effort should be made to prevent the development of this arrhythmia by prophylaxis with an antiarrhythmic agent when premature atrial contractions are frequent. When atrial fibrillation does occur, the rapid ventricular rate may cause angina or electrocardiographic evidence of myocardial ischemia or both; the loss of the atrial contribution to ventricular filling and a sudden fall in cardiac output may cause serious hypotension. Therefore, this arrhythmia should be treated promptly (see p. 654), and a search for previously unrecognized mitral valve disease should be undertaken. If symptoms develop, adults considered to have severe AS should undergo left heart catheterization. In men over 35 years and women over 45 years, coronary arteriography is indicated. The purpose of catheterization is to confirm the site and document the severity of the obstruction, to determine the state of left ventricular function, and to ascertain the presence or absence of associated valvular disease and coronary artery disease.

Surgical Treatment

INDICATIONS FOR OPERATION. The most critical decision in the management of patients with AS—indeed, of all patients with valvular heart disease—concerns the advisability and timing of surgical treatment.[300,342] The indications for surgery as well as the techniques and results of operation depend on the patient's age and the nature of the valvular deformity. In children and adolescents with noncalcific congenital AS, who most commonly have bicuspid aortic valves, simple commissural incision under direct vision usually leads to substantial hemodynamic improvement at low risk, i.e., a mortality rate of less than 1 per cent (see p. 915).[343] Therefore, this procedure (or aortic balloon valvuloplasty) is indicated not only in symptomatic patients but also in asymptomatic children and adolescents with critical aortic stenosis, i.e., a calculated effective orifice less than 0.8 cm^2 or 0.5 cm^2/m^2 BSA. Despite the salutary hemodynamic results following this procedure, the valve is not rendered entirely normal anatomically, and the turbulent blood flow through it may lead to further deformation, calcification, the development of regurgitation, and restenosis after 10 to 20 years, probably requiring reoperation and valve replacement later.

In most adults with calcific AS, satisfactory valvular function cannot be restored, even by careful sculpturing procedures carried out under direct vision, and valve replacement is the surgical treatment of choice.[344] Ultrasonic decalcification and other repairs may be effective immediately in a fraction of patients, but restenosis is a serious problem.[345] The aortic valve should, in general, be replaced (Fig. 32–33) in patients who have hemodynamic evidence of severe obstruction (aortic valve orifice <0.8 cm^2 or <0.5 cm^2/m^2 BSA) and symptoms believed to result from AS. (Prosthetic valves are discussed on pp. 1061 to 1066). Surgical treatment should also be carried out in asymptomatic patients with progressive left ventricular dysfunction and/or significant ventricular ectopic activity at rest or an abnormal hemodynamic response (inadequate elevation of systolic arterial pressure) to exercise.[338] Although a prospective randomized controlled study has not been done, the long-term mortality in asymptomatic patients with critical AS and left ventricular dysfunction undergoing operation appears to be lower than that in medically treated patients without operation.[346] As artificial valves and surgical skills continue to improve, it is likely that patients with severe AS will become candidates for operation at progressively earlier stages in the natural history of their disease. At the present time, however, I do not recommend prophylactic replacement of a critically narrow calcific aortic valve in *asymptomatic* adults unless they exhibit progressive left ventricular dysfunction.

RESULTS. Successful replacement of the aortic valve results in substantial clinical and hemodynamic improvement in patients with AS, AR, or combined lesions.[347] In patients without frank left ventricular failure, the operative risk ranges from 2 to 8 per cent in most centers, and in patients under the age of 70 years it has been reported to be as low as 1 per cent.[280] Risk factors for higher mortality include high New York Heart Association (NYHA) class, impairment of left ventricular function, age, and the presence of associated AR.[343] The 5-year actuarial survival rate of hospital survivors is approximately 85 per cent. Risk factors for late death include higher preoperative NYHA class, advanced age, concomitant untreated coronary artery disease, preoperative impaired left ventricular function, preoperative ventricular arrhythmias, and associated significant AR. Symptoms secondary to elevations of left atrial pressure and myocardial ischemia are relieved in almost every patient. Hemodynamic results are equally impressive; elevated end-diastolic and end-systolic volumes show significant reduction. Impaired ventricular performance returns to normal more frequently in patients with AS than in those with aortic or mitral regurgitation. Diastolic function is normalized (Fig. 32–31).[276,277]

However, the finding that the strongest predictor of postoperative left ventricular dysfunction is preoperative dysfunction[346,348] suggests that patients should, if possible, be operated on before left ventricular function becomes seriously impaired. The increased left ventricular mass is reduced toward (but not to) normal within 18 months after aortic valve replacement in patients with AS.[349] When restudied 5 years postoperatively, left ventricular mass had returned to normal.[350] Myocyte hypertrophy regresses before fibrous tissue is resorbed.

When operation is carried out in patients with frank left

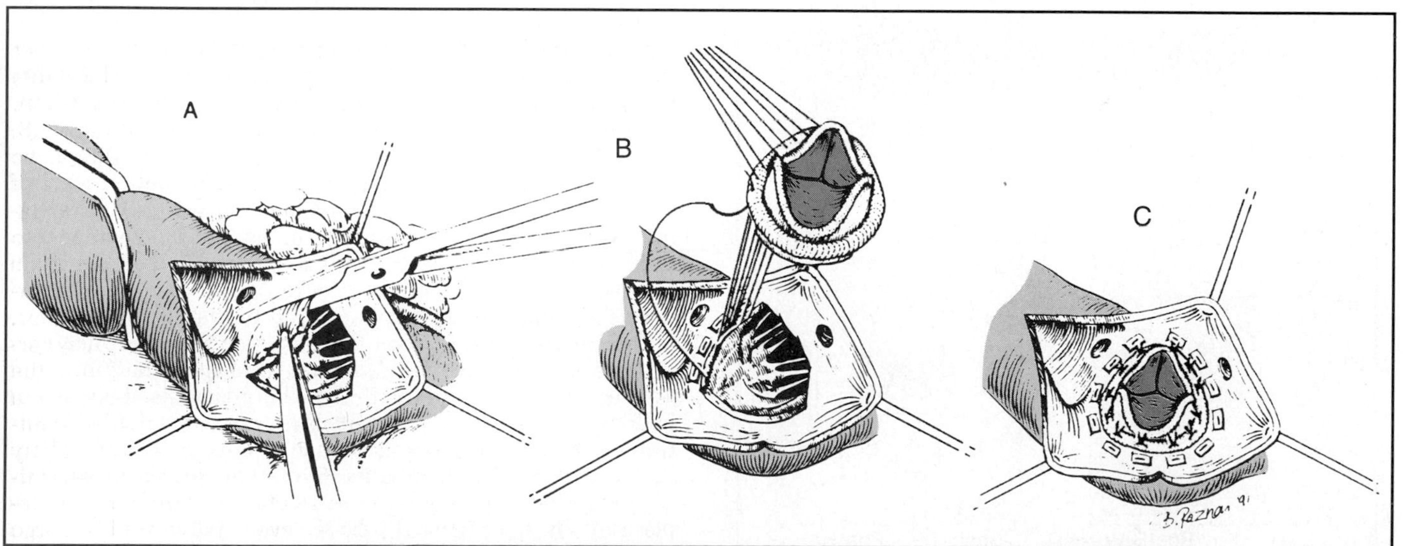

FIGURE 32–33. Interrupted suture technique for aortic valve replacement. *A,* The aortic valve is excised, leaving 1 or 2 mm of annular tissue as a sewing cuff. *B,* Pledgetted Tyeron mattress sutures (2-0) are placed with the pledget on the aortic side. Sutures are placed in the aortic ring and passed directly onto the prosthetic valve sewing ring held at a distance. *C,* After all sutures are placed, the valve is lowered in place and the sutures tied. The valve is then inspected for proper function and fit. (From Albertucci, M., and Karp, R. B.: Prosthetic valve replacement. *In* Al-Zaibag, M., and Duran, C. M. G. [eds.]: Valvular Heart Disease. New York, Marcel Dekker, 1994, pp. 601–634.)

ventricular failure or a depressed ejection fraction, the operative risk is higher, and the mortality ranges from 10 to 25 per cent, depending on the skill of the surgical team and the severity of depression of left ventricular function. A depressed relation between ejection fraction and wall stress is a poor prognostic index, as is a depressed level of dP/dt max at any given left ventricular end-diastolic pressure.[351] Obviously, it is desirable to perform surgery before the development of heart failure, but emergency operation is sometimes lifesaving even in the most desperate situations. In view of the extremely poor prognosis of such patients when they are treated medically, there is usually little choice but to advise immediate mechanical relief of obstruction, i.e., balloon angioplasty (see later discussion) or emergency surgery.[352] Many symptomatic patients with calcific AS are elderly, in whom particular attention must be directed to the adequacy of hepatic, renal, and pulmonary functions. However, the results of aortic valve replacement are satisfactory in patients older than 70[353] or even 80.[354] Age per se, while adding to the risk, should not be considered a contraindication to operation.

In patients with AS and obstructive coronary artery disease (a relatively common combination), aortic valve replacement and myocardial revascularization should be performed together.[354] Although the risk of aortic valve surgery is increased by the association of coronary artery disease, the operative mortality in patients undergoing the combined procedure is not necessarily higher than that of isolated aortic valve replacement in this group.[343] Indeed, the surgical risk rises if severe coronary artery disease is left untreated. The ability to avoid serious myocardial ischemia in the perioperative period is a major factor that has served to reduce operative mortality. After the patient has been placed on cardiopulmonary bypass, the heart is protected by means of hypothermic cardiac arrest alone or combined with cardioplegia. The calcified valve must be removed with great care to avoid embolization of calcified fragments into the systemic circulation.

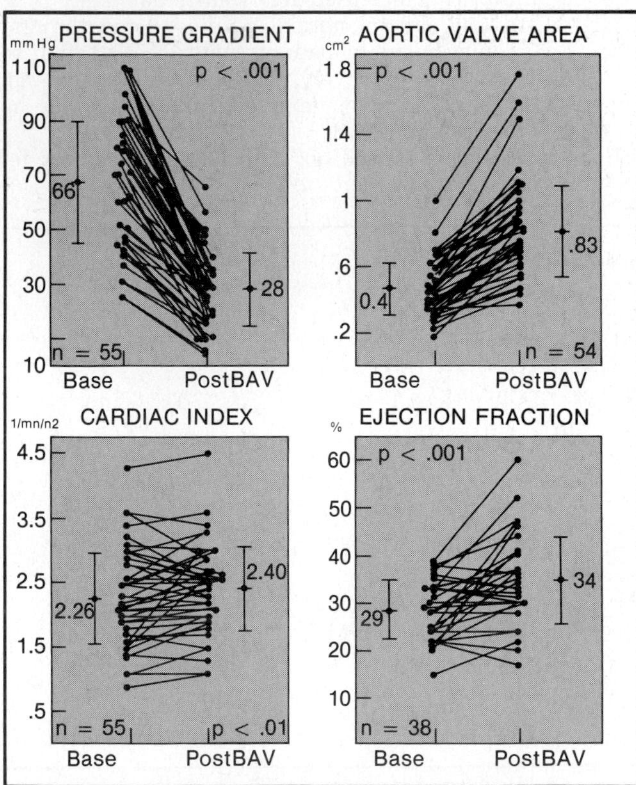

FIGURE 32–34. Plots of changes in pressure gradient, valve area, cardiac index, and ejection fraction at baseline (Base) after balloon aortic valvuloplasty (BAV). (Reproduced with permission from Berland, J., et al.: Percutaneous balloon valvuloplasty in patients with severe aortic stenosis and low ejection fraction. Circulation *79*:1189, 1989. Copyright 1989 American Heart Association.)

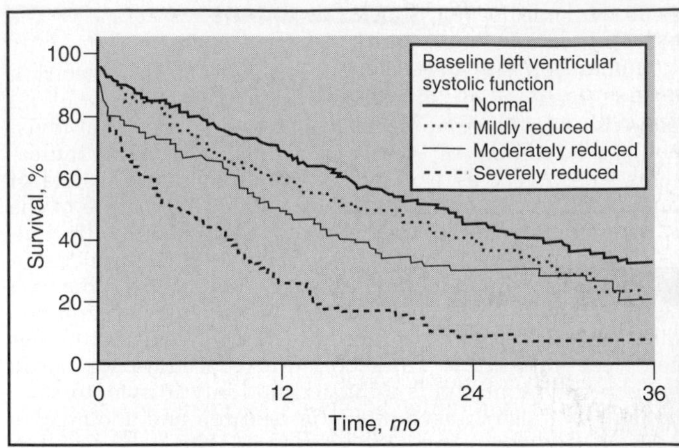

FIGURE 32–35. Kaplan-Meier survival curves following balloon aortic valvuloplasty for aortic stenosis, grouped according to left ventricular function. (Reproduced with permission from Otto, C. M., Mickel, M. C., Kennedy, J. W., et al.: Three-year outcome after balloon aortic valvuloplasty: Insights into prognosis of valvular aortic stenosis. Circulation *89*:642, 1994. Copyright 1994 American Heart Association.)

Balloon Aortic Valvuloplasty

(See also Chap. 39)

This technique represents an increasingly attractive alternative to aortic valvotomy in children, adolescents, and young adults with congenital noncalcific AS (see p. 1385), but its value is limited in adults with calcific AS. A series of balloon dilatation catheters are advanced along a guidewire positioned at the left ventricular apex. In balloon dilatation of calcified stenotic aortic valves carried out on postmortem specimens and in the operating room, fracture of calcified nodules and/or separation of fused commissures were found to be responsible for the relief of obstruction[355]; stretching of the aortic valve ring is probably also involved.[356] There is considerable variation in patient response. However, balloon aortic valvuloplasty results initially in relief of obstruction in most patients[357–359] (Fig. 32–34). In a report of a multicenter registry involving 674 elderly (average age = 78 years) seriously ill patients treated at 24 centers, the procedural mortality was 3 per cent and the 30-day mortality 14 per cent. One-year mortality was 45 per cent. Valve area initially increased from 0.50 to 0.80 cm², and the mean gradient declined from approximately 55 to 29 mm Hg. Better survival was seen in patients with higher preoperative pressure gradients, in those with better preserved left ventricular systolic function (Fig. 32–35), and in women.[360] Left ventricular ejection fraction tends to rise in patients with depressed left ventricular function. In addition to the procedural mortality, another 6 per cent develop serious complications such as myocardial perforation, myocardial infarction, and severe aortic regurgitation.[362–364] The major disadvantage of balloon valvuloplasty in adults with critical, calcified AS is restenosis due to scarring, which occurs in about half of the patients within 6 months. Symptoms lessen in severity in the majority of patients but recur in approximately 30 per cent by 6 months. In most series, patients have been elderly, have had heart failure, and have been considered poor operative risks.

Although the overall intermediate-term (6 to 12 months) results of balloon aortic valvuloplasty have been disappointing, largely because of restenosis, the procedure does have a role in the management of severe calcific AS in patients who are not surgical candidates. This includes patients with cardiogenic shock due to critical AS,[365] patients with critical AS who require an urgent noncardiac operation, as a "bridge" to aortic valve replacement in patients with severe heart failure who are at extremely high operative risk, in pregnant women with critical AS,[366] and in patients with critical AS who refuse surgical treatment. However, in the adult with calcified AS, balloon aortic valvuloplasty is *not* a substitute for surgery (as balloon mitral valvuloplasty may be in the case of MS [see p. 1013]).

AORTIC REGURGITATION

ETIOLOGY AND PATHOLOGY

Aortic regurgitation (AR) may be caused by primary disease of either the aortic valve leaflets or the wall of the aortic root or both (Fig. 32–36).[367] Among patients with *pure* AR coming to valve replacement, the percentage with aortic root disease has been increasing steadily during the past few decades and now accounts for more than one-half of the patients.[263]

Valvular Disease

Rheumatic fever is a common cause of primary disease of the valve leading to regurgitation.[368,368a] The cusps become infiltrated with fibrous tissues and retract, a process that prevents cusp apposition during diastole and usually leads to regurgitation into the left ventricle through a defect in the center of the valve.[8] The associated fusion of the commissures may also restrict the opening of the valve, resulting in combined AS and AR; some associated mitral valve

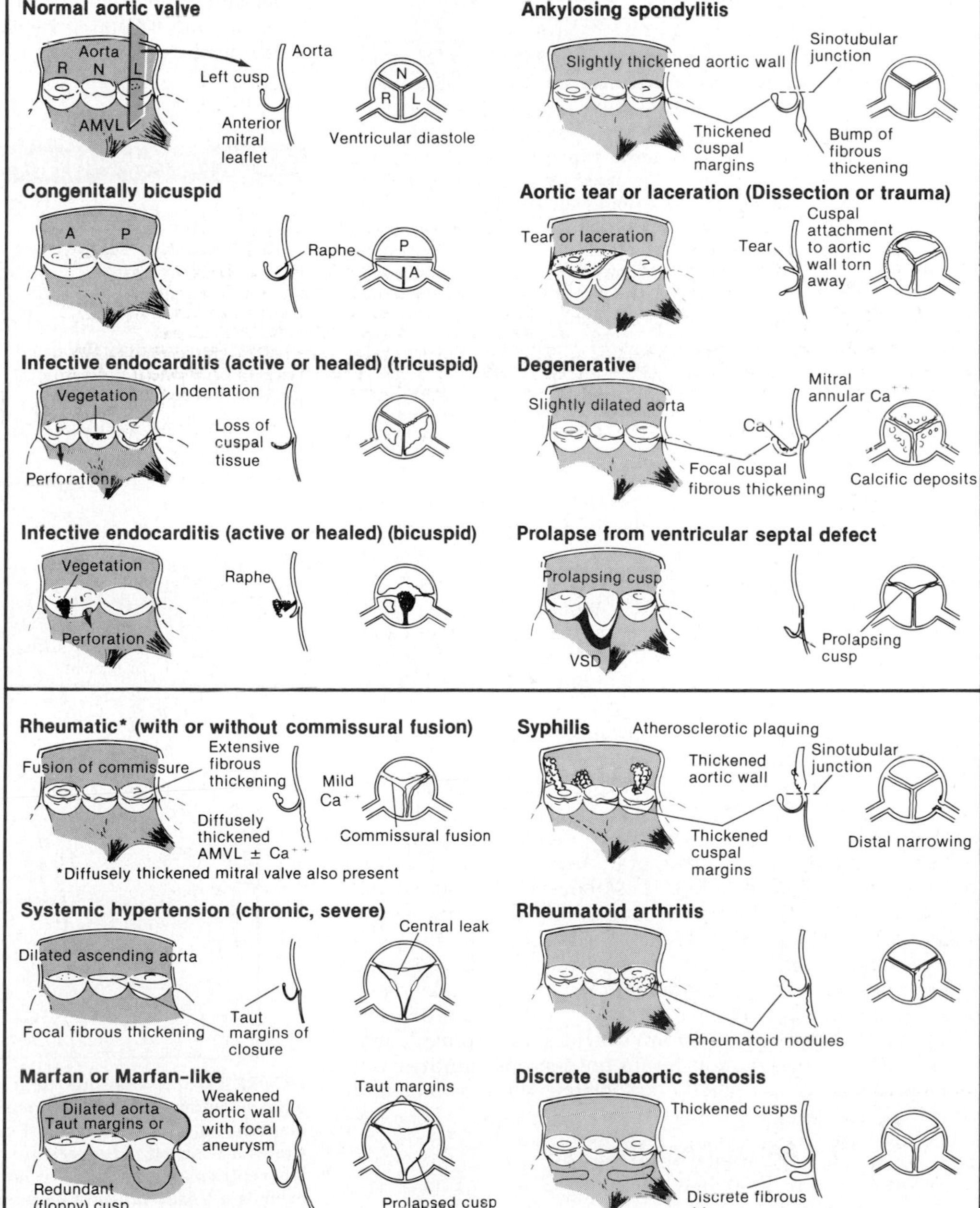

FIGURE 32–36. Diagram of various causes of pure aortic regurgitation. (From Waller, B. F.: Rheumatic and nonrheumatic conditions producing valvular heart disease. *In* Frankl, W. S., and Brest, A. N. [eds.]: Cardiovascular Clinics. Valvular Heart Disease: Comprehensive Evaluation and Management. Philadelphia, F. A. Davis Co., 1986, pp. 30–31.)

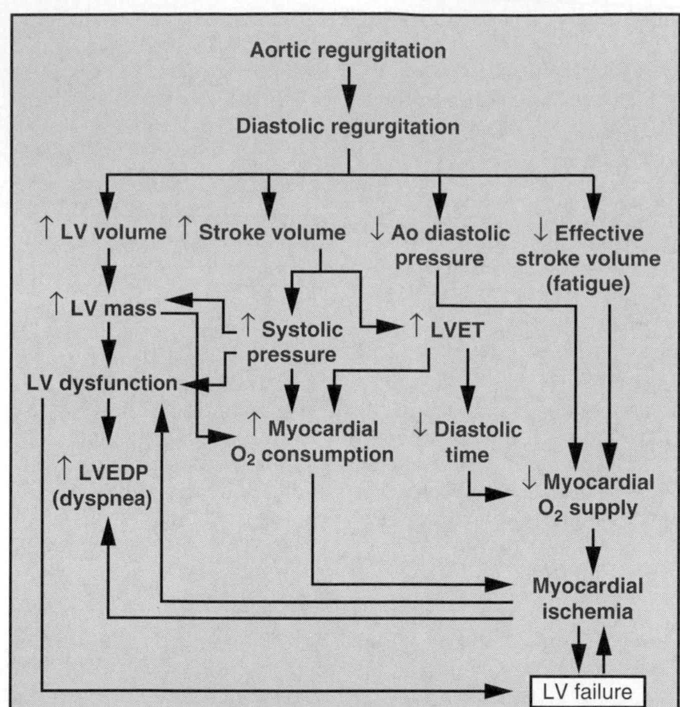

FIGURE 32–37. Pathophysiology of aortic regurgitation. Aortic regurgitation results in an increased left ventricular (LV) volume, increased stroke volume, increased aortic (Ao) systolic pressure, and decreased effective stroke volume. Increased LV volume results in an increased LV mass, which may lead to LV dysfunction and failure. Increased LV stroke volume increases systolic pressure and prolongation of left ventricular ejection time (LVET). Increased LV systolic pressure results in a decrease in diastolic time. Decreased diastolic time (myocardial perfusion time), diastolic aortic pressure, and effective stroke volume reduce myocardial O_2 supply. Increased myocardial O_2 consumption and decreased myocardial O_2 supply produce myocardial ischemia, which further deteriorates LV function (↑ = increased, ↓ = decreased). (From Boudoulas, H., and Gravanis, M. B.: Valvular heart disease. *In* Gravanis, M. B.: Cardiovascular Disorders: Pathogenesis and Pathophysiology. St. Louis, C. V. Mosby, 1993, p. 64.)

involvement is common. Other primary valvular causes of AR include *infective endocarditis* (Chap. 33), in which the infection may destroy or cause perforation of a leaflet, or the vegetations may interfere with proper coaptation of the cusps. *Trauma* (Fig. 44–9, p. 1542) resulting in a tear of the ascending aorta and loss of commissural support can cause prolapse of an aortic cusp. Although the most common complication of a congenitally *bicuspid valve* in adult life is stenosis, incomplete closure and/or prolapse of a bicuspid valve may cause isolated regurgitation or a combination of stenosis and regurgitation.[368–370] AR may develop in patients with large ventricular septal defects. Progressive regurgitation may also occur in patients with myxomatous proliferation of the aortic valve.[371] An increasingly common cause of valvular AR is structural deterioration of a bioprosthetic valve (see p. 1063). Less common causes of AR include a variety of forms of congenital AR: rupture of a congenitally fenestrated valve,[372] particularly in the presence of hypertension[373]; AR in association with systemic lupus erythematosus[374]; rheumatoid arthritis[375]; ankylosing spondylitis[376]; Jaccoud's arthropathy[377]; Takayasu's disease; Whipple's disease[378]; and Crohn's disease.[379] Isolated congenital AR is an uncommon lesion on necropsy studies, but when present, it is usually associated with a bicuspid valve.[380]

Aortic Root Disease

(See also Chap. 45)

A variety of diseases produce AR by causing marked dilatation of the ascending aorta (Fig. 32–36). AR secondary to root disease is now more common than primary valve disease in patients undergoing aortic root replacement.[263] These conditions include age-related (degenerative) aortic dilatation, cystic medial necrosis of the aorta (either isolated or associated with classic Marfan syndrome), aortic dissection, osteogenesis imperfecta, syphilitic aortitis, ankylosing spondylitis, Behçet's syndrome, psoriatic arthritis, arthritis associated with ulcerative colitis, relapsing polychondritis, Reiter's syndrome, giant cell arteritis, and systemic hypertension.[373,381–385]

When the aortic annulus becomes greatly dilated, the aortic leaflets separate, and AR may ensue. Dissection of the diseased aortic wall may occur and may aggravate the AR. Dilatation of the aortic root may also have secondary effects on the aortic valve, because it results in tension and bowing of the individual cusps, which may thicken, retract, and become too short to close the aortic orifice. This leads to intensification of the AR, which increases left ventricular stroke volume, further dilating the ascending aorta and thus leading to a vicious circle in which, just as is the case for MR, "regurgitation begets regurgitation."

AR, regardless of its cause, produces dilatation and hypertrophy of the left ventricle, dilatation of the mitral valve ring, and sometimes hypertrophy and dilatation of the left atrium. Endocardial pockets frequently develop in the left ventricular cavity at sites of impact of the regurgitant jet.

PATHOPHYSIOLOGY

(Fig. 32–37)

In contrast to MR, in which a fraction of the left ventricular stroke volume is ejected into the low-pressure left atrium, in AR the entire left ventricular stroke volume is ejected into a high-pressure chamber, i.e., the aorta (although the low aortic diastolic pressure does facilitate ventricular emptying during early systole). Whereas in MR the reduction of wall tension (i.e., reduced afterload) allows more complete systolic emptying, in AR the increase in left ventricular end-diastolic volume (i.e., increased preload) provides major hemodynamic compensation.[386,387]

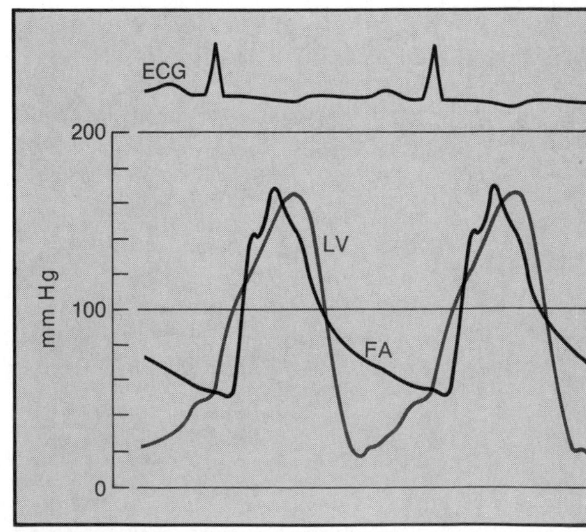

FIGURE 32–38. Pressure curves obtained from a 63-year-old man with symptoms of left ventricular failure and a loud decrescendo diastolic murmur. The femoral arterial (FA) pressure tracing demonstrates a widened pulse pressure of 115 mm Hg and equalization with left ventricular (LV) pressure late in diastole. The LV pressure curve exhibits a steady pressure increase throughout diastole, culminating in a markedly elevated end-diastolic pressure of 45 mm Hg. These findings are indicative of severe aortic regurgitation.

Severe AR may occur with a normal effective forward stroke volume and a normal ejection fraction (total [forward plus regurgitant] stroke volume/end-diastolic volume), together with an elevated left ventricular end-diastolic volume, pressure, and stress[388] (Figs. 32–38 and 32–39). In accord with Laplace's law (which indicates that wall tension is related to the product of intraventricular pressure and radius divided by wall thickness), left ventricular dilatation also increases the left ventricular systolic tension required to develop any level of systolic pressure. The increased end-diastolic wall stress leads to volume overload (eccentric) hypertrophy, with replication of sarcomeres largely in series, elongation of fibers, and sufficient wall thickening so that the ratio of ventricular wall thickness to cavity radius remains normal to maintain or return end-diastolic wall stress to normal levels.[389] This contrasts with the events in AS, in which there is pressure overload (concentric) hypertrophy with replication of sarcomeres largely in parallel and an increased ratio of wall thickness to radius. In AR, left ventricular mass is usually greatly elevated, often to levels even higher than in isolated AS[272] and sometimes exceeding 1000 gm.

Patients with severe chronic AR have the largest end-diastolic volumes of those with any form of heart disease (resulting in so-called *cor bovinum*). However, end-diastolic pressure is not uniformly elevated (i.e., left ventricular compliance often becomes increased [Fig. 32–11]).[392]

In the more severe cases of AR, the regurgitant flow may exceed 20 liters/min, so that the total left ventricular output at rest approaches 25 liters/min, a level that can be achieved acutely only by a trained endurance runner during maximal exercise. Thus, the adaptive response to gradually increasing, chronic AR permits the ventricle to function as an effective high-compliance pump, handling large end-diastolic and stroke volumes, often with little increase in filling pressure (Fig. 32–11). During exercise, peripheral vascular resistance declines, and with an increase in heart rate, diastole shortens and the regurgitation per beat decreases,[390,391] facilitating an increment in effective forward cardiac output without substantial increases in end-diastolic volume and pressure. The ejection fraction (total stroke volume/end-diastolic volume) and related ejection phase indices (see p. 425) are often within normal limits, both at rest and during exercise, even though myocardial function, as reflected in the slope of the end-systolic pressure-volume relation, is depressed. Thus, the latter appears to be a more sensitive index of contractility than the former (see p. 430).

LEFT VENTRICULAR FUNCTION. As left ventricular function deteriorates, the left ventricle dilates (Fig. 32–39*D*). Ventricular end-diastolic volume increases without further elevation of the aortic regurgitant volume; the ratio of left ventricular end-diastolic thickness to radius declines,[392] systolic wall tension rises, reducing ejection fraction, forward stroke volume, and ventricular emptying, while end-systolic volume rises. As the left ventricle decompensates, interstitial fibrosis increases and compliance may decline and left ventricular end-diastolic pressure rises. In advanced stages there may be considerable elevation of the left atrial, pulmonary artery wedge, pulmonary arterial, right ventricular, and right atrial pressures and lowering of the effective cardiac output, first during exercise[391] and then even at rest. There is failure of the normal decline in end-systolic volume or rise in ejection fraction during exercise.[393] Symptoms of heart failure, particularly those secondary to pulmonary congestion, develop.

As is the case in MR (see p. 1017), the end-systolic volume provides a useful overall index of myocardial function in patients with AR and

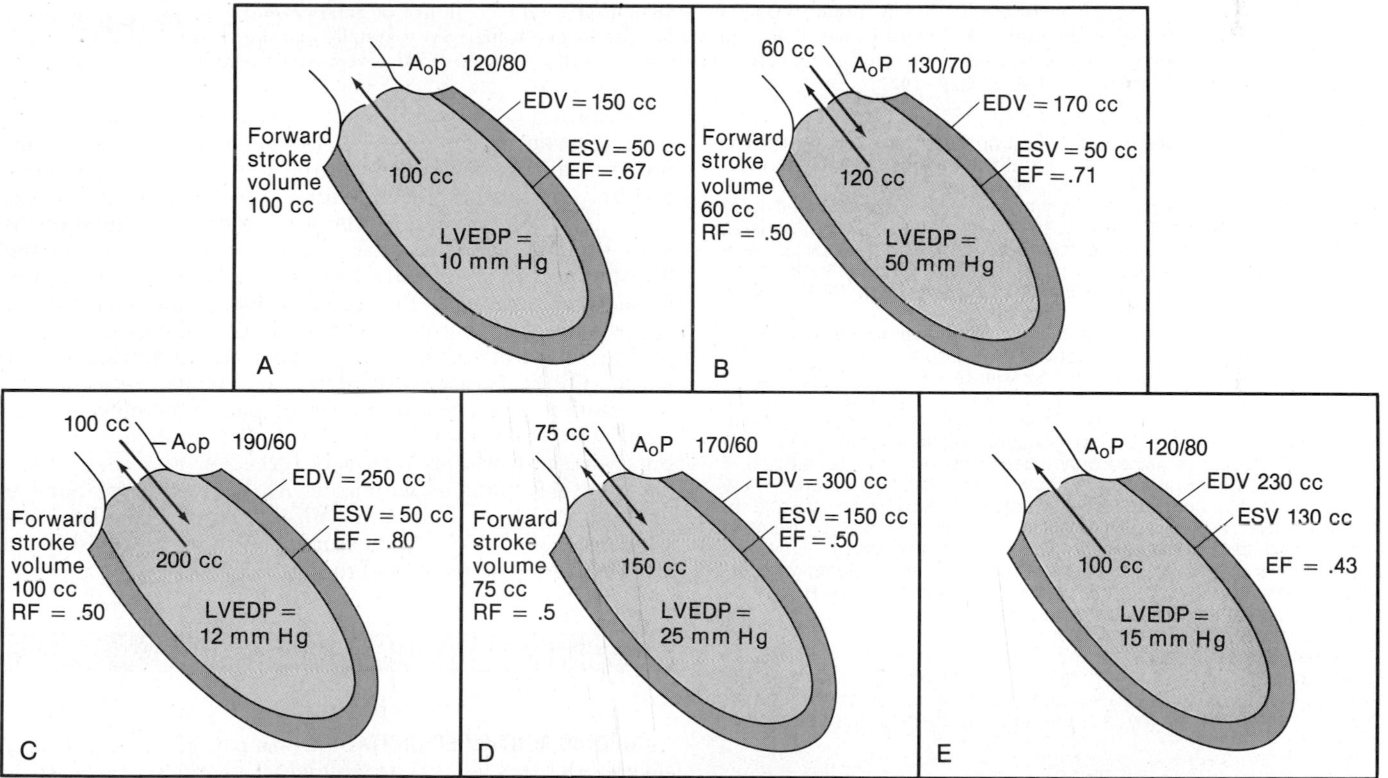

FIGURE 32–39. Hemodynamics of aortic regurgitation. *A,* Normal conditions. *B,* The hemodynamic changes that occur in severe acute aortic regurgitation. Although total stroke volume is increased, forward stroke volume is reduced. Left ventricular end-diastolic pressure rises dramatically. *C,* Hemodynamic changes occurring in chronic compensated aortic regurgitation are shown. Eccentric hypertrophy produces increased end-diastolic volume, which permits an increase in total as well as forward stroke volume. The volume overload is accommodated and left ventricular filling pressure is normalized. Ventricular emptying and end-systolic volume remain normal. *D,* In chronic decompensated aortic regurgitation, impaired left ventricular emptying produces an increase in end-systolic volume and a fall in ejection fraction, total stroke volume, and forward stroke volume. There is further cardiac dilatation and reelevation of left ventricular filling pressure. *E,* Immediately following valve replacement, preload estimated by end-diastolic volume decreases, as does filling pressure. End-systolic volume also is decreased but to a lesser extent. The result is an initial fall in ejection fraction. Despite these changes, elimination of regurgitation leads to an increase in forward stroke volume. AoP = aortic pressure; EDV = end-diastolic volume; ESV = end-systolic volume; EF = ejection fraction; LVEDP = left ventricular end-diastolic pressure; RF = regurgitant fraction. (From Carabello, B. A.: Aortic regurgitation: Hemodynamic determinants of prognosis. *In* Cohn, L. H., and DiSesa, V. J. [eds.]: Aortic Regurgitation: Medical and Surgical Management. New York, Marcel Dekker, Inc., 1986.)

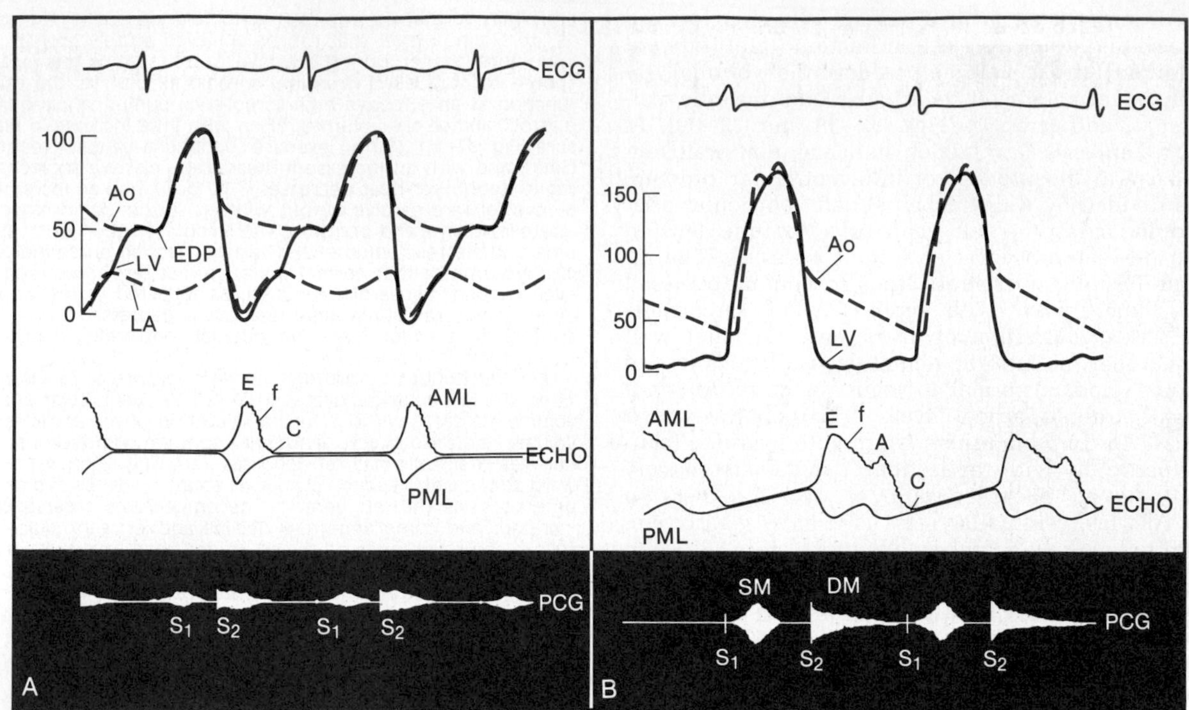

FIGURE 32–40. Schematic representations contrasting the hemodynamic, echocardiographic (ECHO), and phonocardiographic (PCG) manifestations of acute severe *(A)* and chronic severe *(B)* aortic regurgitation. Ao = aorta; LV = left ventricle; LA = left atrium; EDP = end-diastolic pressure; f = flutter of anterior mitral valve leaflet; AML = anterior mitral valve leaflet; PML = posterior mitral valve leaflet; SM = systolic murmur; DM = diastolic murmur; C = closure point of mitral valve. (From Morganroth, J., et al.: Acute severe aortic regurgitation. Ann. Intern. Med. *87*:225, 1977.)

correlates with operative mortality and postoperative left ventricular dysfunction.[138] Both the immediate and the long-term results are excellent in patients with normal left ventricular end-systolic volumes (<40 ml/m^2), poor in patients in whom the index is elevated (>80 ml/m^2), and variable in patients with intermediate values. In general, however, for any given preoperative level of impairment of left ventricular function, the outlook for left ventricular function in the postoperative period is somewhat better in patients with AR than with MR.

When *acute* AR is induced experimentally, preload, wall tension, and myocardial oxygen consumption all rise substantially,[131] secondary to an increase in wall tension. In patients with chronic, severe AR, total myocardial oxygen requirements are also augmented by the increase in left ventricular mass. Because the major portion of coronary blood flow occurs during diastole, when arterial pressure is lower than normal in AR, coronary perfusion pressure is reduced.[393] Studies in experimental AR have shown a reduction in coronary flow reserve with a change in forward coronary flow from diastole to systole.[394] The result—a combination of increased oxygen demand and reduced supply—sets the stage for the development of myocardial ischemia, especially during exercise.[395] Indeed, patients with severe AR exhibit a reduction of coronary reserve,[396] which may be responsible for myocardial ischemia, which in turn may play a role in the deterioration of left ventricular function.

The heightened activity of the adrenergic nervous system as a compensatory mechanism in patients with chronic AR is reflected in an abnormal increase in plasma catecholamine concentration during exercise, accompanied by a reduction in cardiac norepinephrine stores.[397]

Acute Aortic Regurgitation

In contrast to the pathophysiological events in chronic AR described above, in which the left ventricle has had the opportunity to adapt to the increased load, in acute AR (caused most commonly by infective endocarditis, aortic dissection, or trauma) the regurgitant volume fills a ventricle of normal size that cannot accommodate the combined large regurgitant volume and inflow from the left atrium.[398] Because the ability of total stroke volume to rise acutely is limited, forward stroke volume declines. The sudden increase in left ventricular filling causes the left ventricular diastolic pressure to rise rapidly to high levels, as the ventricle operates on a steep portion of its pressure-volume curve (Fig. 32–11).[386]

As left ventricular pressure rises rapidly above left atrial pressure during early diastole, the mitral valve closes prematurely in diastole (Fig. 32–40).[399] Preclosure of the mitral valve is accompanied by diastolic mitral regurgitation.[400] This protects the pulmonary venous bed from backward transmission of the greatly elevated end-diastolic pressure. Premature closure of the mitral valve, together with the tachycardia that shortens diastole, reduces the time interval during which the mitral valve is open. Left ventricular and aortic systolic pressures exhibit little change. Because aortic diastolic pressure cannot decline below the elevated left ventricular end-diastolic pressure, the systemic arterial pulse pressure widens relatively little. For a similar severe degree of AR, patients with acute AR have a lower effective forward stroke volume and pulse pressure, smaller end-diastolic and end-systolic volumes, and a more rapid heart rate than the patient with chronic AR.[409]

CLINICAL MANIFESTATIONS

History

CHRONIC AORTIC REGURGITATION. In patients with chronic, severe AR, the left ventricle gradually undergoes enlargement while the patient remains asymptomatic or almost so.[367] Symptoms of reduced cardiac reserve or myocardial ischemia develop, most often in the fourth or fifth decade and usually only *after* considerable cardiomegaly and myocardial dysfunction have occurred. Exertional dyspnea, orthopnea, and paroxysmal nocturnal dyspnea are the principal complaints. Syncope is rare, and although angina pectoris is less frequent than it is in patients with AS, nocturnal angina, often accompanied by diaphoresis that occurs when the heart rate slows and arterial diastolic pressure falls to extremely low levels, may be troublesome. These episodes are occasionally accompanied by abdominal discomfort, presumably caused by splanchnic ischemia. Patients with severe AR often complain of an uncomfortable awareness of the heartbeat, especially on lying down,

TABLE 32–8 DIFFERENTIAL DIAGNOSIS OF ACUTE VERSUS CHRONIC SEVERE AORTIC REGURGITATION

	CHRONIC SEVERE	ACUTE SEVERE
Clinical		
Onset	Chronic and gradual dyspnea	Acute
Appearance	Normal/mildly dyspneic	Severely ill
Blood pressure	Wide pulse pressure (very low diastolic and high systolic BP)	Not striking, normal, or even low
Tachycardia	Variable/not striking	Always
Peripheral arterial signs	Obvious	No
Apical impulse	Displaced and forcible (very large heart)	No
Basal diastolic thrill	Rare	More common (perforation)
Basal systolic thrill	Common	No
S_1	Usually normal	Soft
S_2	Usually normal (soft calcific valve)	Soft
S_3	Common with LV failure	Common
Basal ejection systolic murmur	Common and harsh	Common and soft
Basal early diastolic murmur	Long, blowing, and decresendo	Short, soft, or loud and musical with perforation
Apical rumbling diastolic murmur	Common	Common but with no presystolic accentuation
ECG/LVH	Almost always	No
Chest X-ray		
Cardiomegaly	Severe	No
Lung fields	Usually normal	Pulmonary edema
Echocardiograph		
LV size	Severely dilated	Normal
LV function (EF)	Variable	Hyperactive
Premature closure of mitral valve	No	Common
Diastolic mitral regurgitation	No	Common
Late mitral valve opening	No	Common
Look for clues of underlying etiology		
Marfan's syndrome		
Aortic dissection		
Prosthetic aortic valve dysfunction		
Infective endocarditis		

From Jutzy, K. R., and Al-Zaibag, M.: Acute mitral and aortic valve regurgitation. *In* Al-Zaibag, M., and Duran, C. M. G. (eds.): Valvular Heart Disease. New York, Marcel Dekker, 1994, pp. 345–382.

and disagreeable thoracic pain due to pounding of the heart against the chest wall. Tachycardia, occurring with emotional stress or exertion, may produce palpitations and head pounding; premature ventricular contractions are particularly distressing because of the great heave of the volume-loaded left ventricle during the postpremature beat. These complaints may be present for many years before symptoms of overt left ventricular dysfunction develop.

ACUTE AORTIC REGURGITATION. In light of the limited ability of the left ventricle to tolerate severe, acute AR, patients with this valvular lesion often develop sudden clinical manifestations of cardiovascular collapse, with weakness, severe dyspnea, and hypotension secondary to the reduced stroke volume and elevated left atrial pressure, as discussed above (Table 32–8).

Physical Examination

In patients with chronic, severe AR, the head frequently bobs with each heartbeat *(de Musset's sign)*,[401] and the pulses are of the water-hammer or collapsing type with abrupt distention and quick collapse (*Corrigan's pulse*, p. 22). The arterial pulse is often prominent in the carotid arteries and can be best appreciated by palpation of the radial artery with the patient's arm elevated. A *bisferious pulse* may be present (Fig. 2–8*C*, p. 21) and is more readily recognized in the brachial and femoral than in the carotid arteries. A variety of auscultatory findings provide confirmation of a wide pulse pressure. *Traube's sign* (also known as "pistol shot sounds"[402]) refers to booming systolic and diastolic sounds heard over the femoral artery, *Müller's sign* consists of systolic pulsations of the uvula, and *Duroziez's sign* consists of a systolic murmur heard over the femoral artery when it is compressed proximally and a diastolic murmur when it is compressed distally. Capillary pulsations, i.e., *Quincke's sign*, can be detected by pressing a glass slide on the patient's lip or by transmitting a light through the patient's fingertips.

Systolic arterial pressure is elevated, and diastolic pressure is abnormally low. *Hill's sign* refers to popliteal cuff systolic pressure exceeding brachial cuff pressure by more than 60 mm Hg. Korotkoff sounds often persist to zero even though intraarterial pressure rarely falls below 30 mm Hg. The point of change in Korotkoff sounds, i.e., the muffling of these sounds in phase IV, correlates with the diastolic pressure. As heart failure develops, peripheral vasoconstriction may occur and arterial diastolic pressure may rise. This finding should not be interpreted as the presence of mild AR.

The apical impulse is diffuse and hyperdynamic and is displaced laterally and inferiorly; there may be systolic retraction over the parasternal region. A rapid ventricular filling wave is often palpable at the apex, as is a *systolic* thrill at the base of the heart or suprasternal notch and over the carotid arteries, resulting from the augmented stroke volume. In many patients, a carotid shudder is palpable or may be recorded.[403]

AUSCULTATION. In *chronic,* severe AR, there may be prolongation of the P-R interval, causing a soft S_1. A_2 is soft or absent, and P_2 may be obscured by the early diastolic murmur.[404] Thus, S_2 may be absent or single or exhibit narrow or paradoxical splitting. A systolic ejection sound, presumably related to abrupt distention of the aorta by the augmented stroke volume, is frequently audible. An S_3 gallop correlates with an increased left ventricular end-systolic volume and its development has been suggested as a sign of impaired left ventricular function, useful in identifying patients with severe regurgitation for surgical treatment.[405]

The aortic regurgitant murmur is one of high frequency that begins immediately after A_2 (Figs. 2–37, p. 41 and 2–41, p. 42). It may be distinguished from the murmur of pulmonic regurgitation (see p. 1059) by its earlier onset, i.e., immediately after A_2 rather than after P_2, and usually by the presence of a widened pulse pressure. The murmur is heard best with the diaphragm of the stethoscope while the patient is sitting up and leaning forward, with the breath held in deep expiration. In severe AR, the murmur reaches an early peak and then has a dominant decrescendo pattern throughout diastole.

The severity of the regurgitation correlates better with the *duration* than with the *intensity* of the murmur. In mild AR, the murmur may be limited to early diastole and is typically high-pitched and blowing; in severe regurgitation, the murmur is holodiastolic and may have a rough quality. When the murmur is musical ("cooing dove" murmur), it usually signifies eversion or perforation of an aortic cusp. In severe AR and left ventricular decompensation, equilibration of aortic and left ventricular pressures in late diastole (Fig. 32–38) abolishes this component of the regurgitant murmur. When regurgitation is due to primary valvular disease, the diastolic murmur is best heard along the left sternal border in the third and fourth intercostal spaces. However, when it is due mainly to dilatation of the ascending aorta,[406] the murmur is often more readily audible along the right sternal border.

A mid- and late-diastolic apical rumble, the *Austin Flint murmur,* is common in severe AR and may occur in the presence of a normal mitral valve (Fig. 2–41, p. 42). This murmur appears to be created by rapid antegrade flow across a mitral orifice that is narrowed by the rapidly rising left ventricular diastolic pressure caused by severe aortic reflux.[407] The Austin Flint murmur may be difficult to differentiate from that due to MS, but the presence of an opening snap and a loud S_1 in MS and the absence of these findings in AR are helpful clues. As the left ventricular end-diastolic pressure rises, the Austin Flint murmur commences and terminates earlier, and in acute AR with premature diastolic closure of the mitral valve, the presystolic portion of the Austin Flint murmur is eliminated. A short, midsystolic murmur, grades 1 to 4/6, related to the increased ejection rate and stroke volume, may be audible at the base of the heart and transmitted to the carotid vessels. It may be higher pitched and less rasping than the murmur of aortic stenosis but is often accompanied by a systolic thrill.

Dynamic Auscultation. The diastolic murmur of AR may be accentuated when the patient sits up and leans forward or by interventions that raise the arterial pressure, such as infusion of a vasopressor drug, squatting, or isometric exercise. The intensity of the murmur is reduced by interventions that lower the systolic pressure, such as amyl nitrite inhalation and the strain of the Valsalva maneuver.[408] The Austin Flint murmur, like that of AR, is augmented by isometric exercise and vasopressors and is reduced by amyl nitrite inhalation (Fig. 2–41, p. 42).[408]

ACUTE AORTIC REGURGITATION. When acute AR is severe, these patients appear gravely ill, with tachycardia, severe peripheral vasoconstriction and cyanosis, and sometimes pulmonary congestion and edema.[398,409,410] The peripheral signs of AR are often not impressive and certainly not as dramatic as in patients with chronic AR.[399] Duroziez's murmur, pistol shot sounds over the peripheral arteries (Traube's sign), and bisferious pulses are usually *absent* in acute AR. The normal or only slightly widened pulse pressure may lead to serious underestimation of the severity of the valvular lesion. The left ventricular impulse is normal or nearly so, and the rocking motion of the chest characteristic of chronic AR is not apparent. S_1 may be soft or absent because of premature closure of the mitral valve.[411] Instead, the sound of mitral valve closure is occasionally audible. However, closure of the mitral valve may be incomplete, and diastolic mitral regurgitation may occur.[412] Evidence of pulmonary hypertension, with an accentuated P_2 and an S_3 and S_4, is frequently present. The early diastolic murmur of acute AR is lower pitched and shorter than that of chronic AR, because as left ventricular diastolic pressure rises, the pressure gradient between the aorta and the left ventricle is rapidly reduced. The Austin Flint murmur, if present, is brief and ceases when left ventricular pressure exceeds left atrial pressure in diastole.

LABORATORY EXAMINATION

ELECTROCARDIOGRAM. *Chronic* AR results in left axis deviation and a pattern of left ventricular diastolic volume overload, characterized by an increase in initial forces (prominent Q waves in leads I, aV_1, and V_3 to V_6) and a relatively small *r* wave in V_1 (Fig. 32–41). With the passage of time, these initial forces diminish, but the total QRS amplitude increases. The T waves may be tall and upright in left precordial leads early in the course, but more commonly they are inverted, with ST-segment depressions.[413] Left intraventricular conduction defects occur late in the course and are usually associated with left ventricular dysfunction. The electrocardiogram is not an accurate predictor of the severity of AR or cardiac weight.[414] When AR is caused by an inflammatory process, P-R prolongation may be present.[414]

In *acute* AR, the electrocardiogram may or may not show left ventricular hypertrophy, despite the presence of left ventricular failure, depending upon the severity and duration of the regurgitation. However, nonspecific ST-segment and T-wave changes are common.

RADIOLOGICAL FINDINGS (see also p. 225). Cardiac size is a function of the duration and severity of regurgitation and the state of left ventricular function. In acute AR, there may be little cardiac enlargement, but marked enlargement is a common finding in chronic AR. Typically, the left ventricle enlarges in an inferior and leftward direction, causing a significant increase in the long axis (Fig. 7–34, p. 226) but sometimes little or no increase in the transverse diameter of the heart. Calcification of the aortic valve is uncommon in patients with pure AR but is often present in patients with combined AS and AR. As in the case with AS, the presence of distinct left atrial enlargement in the absence of heart failure should suggest the possibility of associated mitral valve disease. Dilatation of the ascending aorta is usually more marked than in AS and may involve the entire aortic arch, including the aortic knob. Severe, aneurysmal dilatation of the aorta should suggest that aortic root disease (e.g., Marfan syndrome, cystic medionecrosis, or annuloaortic ectasia) is responsible for the AR. Linear calcifications in the wall of the ascending aorta are seen in syphilitic aortitis but are nonspecific and are observed in degenerative disease as well.

For angiographic assessment of AR, contrast material should be injected rapidly (i.e., 25 to 35 ml/sec) into the aortic root, and filming should be carried out in the right and left anterior oblique projections. Opacification may be improved by filming during a Valsalva maneuver. In acute AR, there is only a slight increase in ventricular end-diastolic volume, but with the passage of time both the end-diastolic volume and the thickness of the ventricular wall increase, usually in parallel.

ECHOCARDIOGRAPHY (Figs. 3–57 to 3–59, p. 76). Echocardiography is helpful in identifying the cause of AR. It may show thickening of the valve cusps, prolapse of the valve, a flail leaflet, vegetations, or dilatation of the aortic root.[415] Although transthoracic imaging is usually satisfactory, transesophageal echocardiography often provides more detail. Two-dimensional studies are useful for the measurement of left ventricular end-diastolic and end-systolic dimensions and volumes, shortening fractions, and ejection fractions. These measurements, when made serially, are of great value in selecting the optimal time for surgical intervention (see p. 1052).

In acute AR (Table 32–8; Fig. 3–59, p. 76), the echocardiogram reveals a reduction in amplitude of the opening

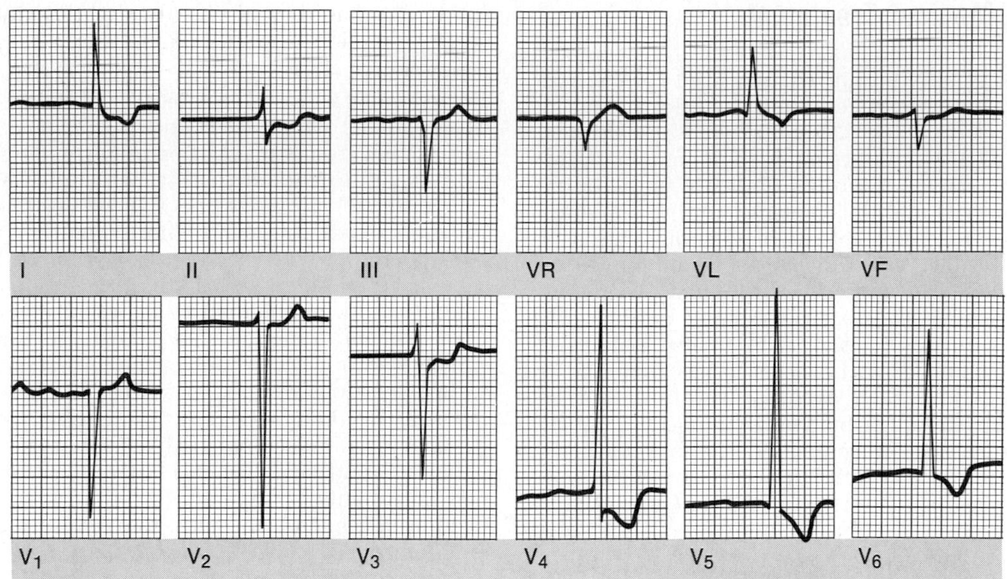

FIGURE 32–41. Atrial fibrillation and left ventricular hypertrophy. The most prominent features are the gross increase in precordial voltage (RV5 + SV2 = 70 mm) and the marked anterolateral ST/T wave changes (leads I, aVL, and V4-6). The patient had aortic regurgitation and normal coronary arteries and was not taking digitalis. (Normal standardization, i.e., 1 mV = 10 mm.) (From Hall, R. J., and Julian, D. G.: Diseases of the Cardiac Valves. New York, Churchill Livingstone, 1989, p. 39.)

movement of the mitral valve, premature closure and delayed opening of the mitral valve,[416] and, on the M-mode study, a reduction in the E-F slope, indicating that the left ventricle is operating on the steep portion of its pressure-volume curve. Left ventricular end-diastolic dimensions are not markedly increased, and fractional shortening is normal. This contrasts with the findings in chronic AR, in which end-diastolic dimensions and wall motion are increased. Occasionally, with equilibration of aortic and left ventricular pressures in diastole, premature opening of the aortic valve may be detected.[417]

High-frequency diastolic fluttering of the anterior leaflet of the mitral valve during diastole is an important echocardiographic finding in both acute and chronic AR; however, it does not occur when the mitral valve is rigid. This sign, which, unlike the Austin Flint rumble, occurs even in mild AR, results from the movement imparted to the anterior leaflet of the mitral valve by the jet of blood regurgitating from the aorta.

Doppler echocardiography and color flow Doppler imaging are the most sensitive and accurate noninvasive techniques in the detection of AR.[418,418a] They readily detect mild degrees of AR that may be inaudible by auscultation. In addition, by measuring the rate of decrease in velocity of the regurgitant jet in the left ventricle (see p. 332), they allow estimation of the severity. The aortic regurgitant orifice can be estimated, as can aortic regurgitant flow, from the difference between flow through the aortic and either the pulmonic or mitral valve orifice determined by continuous Doppler echocardiography.[419]

RADIONUCLIDE IMAGING. Radionuclide angiography, by allowing determination of the regurgitant fraction and of the left ventricular/right ventricular stroke volume ratio, provides an accurate noninvasive assessment of the severity of AR.[420] This technique is nonspecific because the ratio is increased by associated MR and reduced by tricuspid or pulmonary regurgitation. However, in the absence of these complicating lesions, a left ventricular/right ventricular stroke volume ratio of 2.0 or more denotes severe AR. Radionuclide angiography is of value in the assessment of left ventricular function in patients with AR.[393] Serial measurements are useful in the early detection of deterioration of left ventricular function.

NUCLEAR MAGNETIC RESONANCE IMAGING (Figs. 10–26 and 10–27, p. 332). This technique provides accurate measurements of regurgitant volumes, ventricular end-systolic and diastolic volumes, and the regurgitant orifice.[421] Although expensive, NMR imaging appears to be the most accurate noninvasive technique for assessing the patient with AR.[162,305]

MANAGEMENT

ACUTE AORTIC REGURGITATION. Since early demise due to left ventricular failure is frequent in patients with *severe acute* AR despite intensive medical management, prompt surgical intervention is indicated. Even a normal ventricle cannot sustain the burden of acute severe volume overload; therefore, the risk of *acute* AR is much greater than that of chronic AR.[398,409,410] While the patient is being prepared for surgery, intravenous treatment with a positive inotropic agent (dopamine or dobutamine) and/or vasodilator (nitroprusside) may be necessary. The agent and dosage should be selected on the basis of arterial pressure (Chap. 17). In hemodynamically stable patients with acute AR secondary to active infective endocarditis, operation may be deferred to allow 5 to 7 days of intensive antibiotic therapy.[410] However, aortic valve replacement should be undertaken at the earliest sign of hemodynamic instability, or if echocardiographic evidence of diastolic closure of the mitral valve develops.[422]

NATURAL HISTORY OF CHRONIC AORTIC REGURGITATION. Management must take into account the natural history of the lesion.[423] Moderately severe or even severe chronic AR may be associated with a generally favorable prognosis for many years. Approximately 75 per cent of patients survive for 5 years and 50 per cent for 10 years after diagnosis.[66] However, as is the case for AS, once the patient becomes symptomatic, the condition often deteriorates rapidly, and sudden death may occur, usually in previously symptomatic patients. Without surgical treatment, death usually occurs within 4 years after the development of angina and within 2 years after the onset of heart failure. Even during the asymptomatic period gradual deterioration of left ventricular function may occur; it is important, therefore, to intervene surgically before these changes have become irreversible.[423a]

Medical Treatment

Patients with mild or moderate AR who are asymptomatic with normal or only minimally increased cardiac size require no therapy but should be followed clinically and by echocardiography every 12 or 24 months if their clinical condition and echocardiogram remain stable, and with antibiotic prophylaxis for endocarditis. Patients with limitations of cardiac reserve and/or left ventricular dysfunction secondary to AR should not engage in vigorous sports or heavy exertion.[4] Cardiac glycosides may be employed in patients with severe AR and left ventricular dilatation, even in the absence of symptoms. Systemic arterial diastolic hypertension, if present, should be treated because it increases the regurgitant flow; however, drugs that impair left ventricular function, such as propranolol, should be avoided. Atrial fibrillation and bradyarrhythmias are poorly tolerated and should be prevented if possible. Because these and other cardiac arrhythmias and infections are poorly tolerated in patients with severe AR, such complications must be treated promptly and vigorously. Even though nitroglycerin and other nitrates are not as helpful in relieving anginal pain in patients with AR as they are in patients with coronary artery disease or AS, they are worth a trial. Although patients with left ventricular failure secondary to AR require surgical treatment, they respond, at least temporarily, to treatment with digitalis glycosides, salt restriction, and diuretics. The response to vasodilator therapy is often impressive. Hemodynamic studies have shown beneficial effects of intravenous hydralazine,[424] sublingual nifedipine,[425] and oral prazosin.[426] This form of therapy may be particularly helpful in stabilizing patients with acute lesions or those with decompensated chronic AR who are awaiting operation. However, because of the high incidence of side effects of hydralazine, attention has focused on nifedipine.[427] In a comparison of digoxin with nifedipine in asymptomatic patients with severe AR, the latter delayed the need for operation (the development of symptoms or of left ventricular dysfunction).[428]

Asymptomatic patients with severe chronic AR and normal left ventricular function should be examined at intervals of approximately 6 months. In addition to clinical examination, serial echocardiographic assessments of left ventricular size and ejection fraction should be made.

Surgical Treatment

INDICATIONS FOR OPERATION. Operative correction is usually deferred in patients with severe chronic AR who are asymptomatic, have good exercise tolerance, and have normal left ventricular function. Similarly, there is a consensus that in the absence of contraindications surgical treatment is advisable in patients with severe AR who are symptomatic as a result of this lesion and who have impaired left ventricular function. Between these two ends of the clinical-hemodynamic spectrum are many patients in whom it may be quite difficult to balance the immediate risks of operation and, in cases when it is required, the continuing risks of an implanted prosthetic valve on the one hand, against the hazards of allowing a severe volume overload to damage the left ventricle on the other.[429–432]

Postoperative left ventricular function is usually excellent in patients who have normal systolic function preoperatively.[433] However, changes in left ventricular function can develop in some patients with AR so that, even after successful correction of AR, they may have persistent cardiomegaly and depressed left ventricular function.[434,435] In such patients, symptoms of impaired left ventricular function present preoperatively may persist and occasionally even get worse despite successful valve replacement. Therefore, it is highly desirable to operate on patients *before* irreversible left ventricular changes have occurred. Patients whose ventricular function does not return to normal after aortic valve replacement often exhibit histological changes in the left ventricle, including massive fiber hypertrophy and increased interstitial fibrous tissue. However, even patients with irreversible left ventricular dysfunction may benefit from surgical treatment, whereas medical treatment has little to offer them.

In order to minimize the risk of postoperative left ventricular dysfunction, every effort should be made to operate on patients *before* serious left ventricular dysfunction occurs. Serial echocardiograms or radionuclide ventriculograms should be obtained to detect changes in left ventricular size and function. These examinations can provide valuable information concerning progressive deterioration in left ventricular function at rest. Both techniques allow repeated evaluation of ejection fraction and end-systolic volume (or dimensions) both at rest and during exercise. Impaired ventricular function at *rest* is the basis for selection of patients for operation; failure of a normal ejection fraction to respond normally to *exercise* portends impaired function at rest.

Because AR has complex effects on both preload and afterload, the selection of appropriate indices of ventricular contractility is a challenge.[436] Simple left ventricular end-diastolic volume and the ejection phase indices such as ejection fraction and ventricular fraction shortening are too strongly influenced by loading to be accurate indicators of ventricular contractility but may be useful empirical predictors of postoperative function.[348] On the other hand, preoperative left ventricular end-systolic volume and dimensions are largely preload dependent and are good predictors of postoperative left ventricular function.[437] The relationship between end-systolic wall stress and ejection fraction or per cent[438] fractional shortening may be even more useful. However, in the absence of such measurements, *serial* changes in ventricular end-diastolic and end-systolic volumes or dimensions can be employed to detect *relative* deterioration of ventricular function.

Patients with *severely* impaired left ventricular systolic function preoperatively are at high risk of developing irreversible left ventricular dysfunction and, indeed, of dying of congestive heart failure postoperatively. Other patients with impaired left ventricular function preoperatively, improve postoperatively—both symptomatically and insofar as left ventricular function is concerned. Bonow et al. have reported that, after valve replacement, survival was excellent in patients with normal resting ejection fractions preoperatively. However, patients with subnormal ejection fractions and only a relatively brief (<1 year) duration of left ventricular dysfunction also did well postoperatively and maintained their preoperative levels of exercise tolerance. Asymptomatic patients with severe AR but normal left ventricular function have an excellent prognosis and do not warrant operation.[429] Less than 4 per cent per year require operation because of the development of symptoms of left ventricular dysfunction. On the other hand, patients with prolonged left ventricular dysfunction exhibited poor postoperative survival.[430] The end-systolic dimension determined by two-dimensional echocardiography is valuable in predicting outcome in asymptomatic patients. Patients with severe AR and an end-systolic diameter less than 40 mm almost invariably remain stable without cardiac failure or death, whereas those with an end-systolic diameter greater than 55 mm (Fig. 32–42), an end-systolic volume greater than 55 ml/m^2, an end-diastolic volume greater than 200 ml/m^2, or an ejection fraction less than 50 per cent have an increased risk of death secondary to left ventricular dysfunction.

Thus, the decision to recommend surgical treatment in some patients with severe AR remains difficult. Operation should be deferred in asymptomatic patients with normal and stable left ventricular function and should be recom-

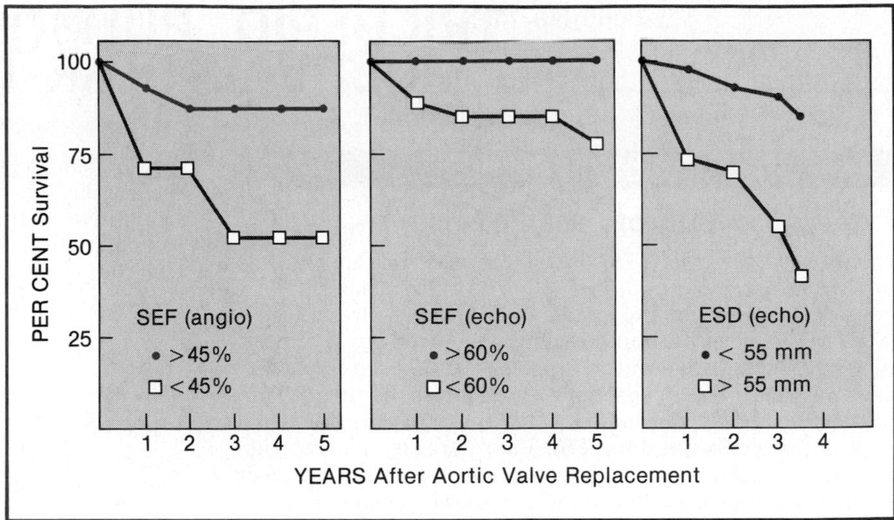

FIGURE 32–42. Relation of preoperative ventricular function to postoperative survival. Data of Greves et al. *(left)* and those of Bonow et al. *(right)* show remarkable agreement: Both groups incorporated limits clearly in abnormal range. Cunha et al. *(center)* selected a limit that was well within normal range. These and other published data indicate that preoperative ventricular function is an important determinant of postoperative survival. SEF = systolic ejection fraction; ESD = echocardiographically measured dimension at end-systole; angio = angiography; echo = echocardiography. (From Errichetti, A., et al.: Is valve replacement indicated in asymptomatic patients with aortic stenosis or aortic regurgitation? *In* Cheitlin, M. [ed.]: Dilemmas in Clinical Cardiology. Philadelphia, F. A. Davis Co., 1990, p. 204.)

mended in symptomatic patients regardless of the status of their left ventricular function. Asymptomatic patients with impaired left ventricular function must be treated individually, taking into account associated medical conditions and coronary artery disease that may add to the surgical risk, as well as the experience and results of the surgical team. A decision should be based not on a single abnormal measurement of impaired left ventricular function but rather on several observations of depressed performance and impaired exercise tolerance, carried out at intervals of 3 to 6 months. If abnormalities are progressive or consistent—i.e., if the left ventricular ejection fraction declines to 50 per cent, the left ventricular end-systolic diameter exceeds 45 to 50 mm, or the left ventricular end-systolic volume exceeds 55 ml/m^2—operation should be carried out. If evidence of left ventricular dysfunction is borderline or is not consistent, continued close follow-up is indicated. The threshold for surgery may be lower when the surgeon believes that valve replacement will not be necessary (see below), but this prediction may be difficult.

OPERATIVE PROCEDURES. Because an increasing proportion of patients with severe, isolated AR coming to surgery now have primary aortic root rather than primary valve disease, an increasing proportion can be treated surgically by correcting the dilated aortic root.[439] One of two annuloplasty procedures may be employed—an encircling suture of the aorta or subcommissural annuloplasty. Aneurysmal dilatation of the ascending aorta requires excision, replacement with a graft, and reimplantation of the coronary arteries.[440] In patients with AR secondary to prolapse of an aortic leaflet, aortic cusp resuspension or cusp resection may be employed.[441,442] When AR is caused by leaflet perforation resulting from healed infective endocarditis, a pericardial patch can be used for repair.[443]

A large majority of patients with severe AR due to primary valve disease and almost all patients with combined AS and AR and calcific disease require placement with a prosthetic valve (see p. 1061). Because the aortic annulus in patients with severe AR is usually not as narrow as it is in patients with AS, a larger artificial valve can be inserted, and mild postoperative obstruction to left ventricular outflow is less of a problem than it is in some patients with AS. Occasionally, when a leaflet has been torn from its attachments to the aortic annulus by trauma, surgical replacement without repair may be possible.

In general, the results of aortic valve replacement in patients with AR are similar to those in patients with AS, with a large percentage of patients exhibiting striking improvement in symptoms. Reductions in heart size and in left ventricular diastolic volume and mass occur in the majority of patients.[344,439] However, as already indicated, the extent of improvement in left ventricular function may not be as salutary in patients with AR as it is in patients with AS, perhaps because the ventricular dysfunction is more advanced and less reversible in patients with volume overload by the time they become symptomatic and are referred for surgical treatment[440] than it is in patients with pressure overload. As is the case of AS, the operative risk of aortic valve replacement in patients with AR depends on the general condition of the patient, the state of left ventricular function, and the skill and experience of the surgical team; the mortality rate ranges from 3 to 8 per cent in most medical centers. A late mortality of approximately 5 to 10 per cent per year is observed in survivors in whom cardiac enlargement was marked and prolonged left ventricular dysfunction was present preoperatively (Fig. 32–42). Follow-up studies have shown both early rapid and then slower long-term reductions of ventricular mass, ejection fraction, myocyte hypertrophy, and ventricular fibrous content.[294,350] By extending the indications for operation to symptomatic patients with normal left ventricular function as well as to asymptomatic patients with early left ventricular dysfunction, both early and late results are improving. It is likely that with the continued improvement of surgical techniques and results, it will become possible to extend the recommendation for operative treatment to asymptomatic patients with severe regurgitation and normal cardiac function. However, given the risks of operation and the long-term complications of artificial valves, I believe that the time for such a policy has not yet arrived.

TRICUSPID, PULMONIC, AND MULTIVALVULAR DISEASE

TRICUSPID STENOSIS

Etiology and Pathology

Tricuspid stenosis (TS) is almost always rheumatic in origin.[8] Other causes of obstruction to right atrial emptying are unusual and include congenital tricuspid atresia (see p. 932), right atrial tumors (which may produce a clinical picture suggesting rapidly progressive TS [see p. 1066]), and the carcinoid syndrome (which more frequently produces tricuspid regurgitation [TR] [see p. 1056] but which may occasionally produce TS). Rarely, obstruction to right ventricular inflow can be due to endomyocardial fibrosis, tricuspid valve vegetations, and extracardiac tumors.

The majority of cases of rheumatic tricuspid valve disease present with tricuspid regurgitation or a combination of stenosis and regurgitation. Rheumatic TS is uncommon and *almost* never occurs as an isolated lesion but generally accompanies mitral valve disease[442–444]; in many patients with TS, the aortic valve is also involved, i.e., trivalvular stenosis is present. TS is found at autopsy in about 15 per cent of patients with rheumatic heart disease but is of clinical significance in only about 5 per cent.[445]

Organic tricuspid valve disease is more common in India than in North America or Western Europe; it has been reported to occur in the hearts of more than one-third of patients with rheumatic heart disease studied at autopsy on the subcontinent.[446] The anatomical changes of rheumatic TS resemble those of MS, with fusion and shortening of the chordae tendineae and fusion of the leaflets at their edges producing a diaphragm with a fixed central aperture. However, valvular calcification is rare. As is the case with MS, TS is more common in women and, in the United States, TS is seen most commonly in persons between the ages of 20 and 60. Again, as in mitral valve disease, stenosis, regurgitation, or some combination of the two may exist.

The right atrium is often greatly dilated, and its walls are thickened. There may be evidence of severe passive congestion, with enlargement of the liver and spleen.

Pathophysiology

A diastolic pressure gradient between the right atrium and ventricle—the hemodynamic expression of TS—is augmented when the transvalvular blood flow increases during exercise or inspiration and is reduced when flow declines during expiration. A relatively modest diastolic pressure gradient, i.e., a mean gradient exceeding only 5 mm Hg, is usually sufficient to elevate mean right atrial pressure to levels that result in systemic venous congestion and, unless sodium intake has been restricted or diuretics have been given, is associated with jugular venous distention, ascites, and edema.

In patients with sinus rhythm, the right atrial *a* wave may be extremely tall (Fig. 32–43) and may even approach the level of the right ventricular systolic pressure. Resting cardiac output is usually markedly reduced and fails to rise during exercise, accounting for the normal or only slightly elevated left atrial, pulmonary arterial, and right ventricular systolic pressures, despite the presence of accompanying mitral valve disease.

A *mean* diastolic pressure gradient across the tricuspid valve as low as 2 mm Hg is sufficient to establish the diagnosis of TS. However, exercise, deep inspiration, and the rapid infusion of fluid or the administration of atropine may enhance greatly a borderline gradient in the presence of TS; expiration reduces or abolishes the gradient. Therefore, whenever this diagnosis is suspected, right atrial and ventricular pressures should be recorded simultaneously, using two catheters or a single catheter with a double lumen, with one lumen opening on either side of the tricuspid valve. The effects of respiration on any pressure difference should be examined.

Clinical Manifestations

(Table 32–9)

HISTORY. The low cardiac output characteristic of TS causes fatigue, and patients often complain of discomfort due to hepatomegaly, swelling of the abdomen, and anasarca.[447] The severity of these symptoms, which are secondary to an elevated systemic venous pressure, is out of proportion to the degree of dyspnea.[446] Some patients complain of a fluttering discomfort in the neck, caused by giant *a* waves in the jugular venous pulse. Despite the coexistance of MS, the symptoms characteristic of this valve lesion, i.e., hemoptysis, paroxysmal nocturnal dyspnea, and acute pulmonary edema, are usually absent in the presence of severe TS because the TS prevents surges of blood into the pulmonary circulation behind the stenotic mitral valve. Indeed, the *absence* of the symptoms of pulmonary congestion in a patient with obvious MS should suggest the possibility of TS.

PHYSICAL EXAMINATION. Because of the high frequency with which MS occurs in patients with TS and the similarity in the physical findings between the two valvular lesions, the diagnosis of TS is commonly missed. The physical findings are mistakenly attributed to MS, which is, of course, more common and may be more obvious. Therefore, a high index of suspicion is required to detect the tricuspid valve lesion. In the presence of sinus rhythm (which is surprisingly common in patients with TS), the *a* wave in the jugular venous pulse is tall, sharp, and flicking and on first impression may be confused with an arterial pulsation; a presystolic hepatic pulsation is often palpable. The *y* descent is slow and barely appreciable, indicating

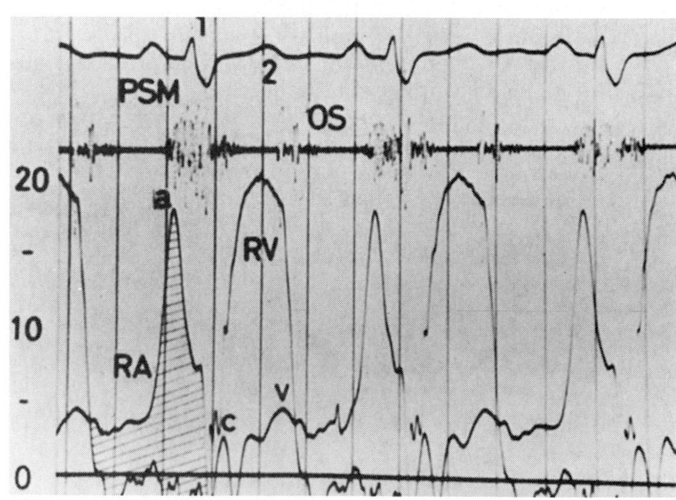

FIGURE 32–43. Phonocardiogram and right heart pressures in a patient with tricuspid stenosis. The giant right atrial *a* wave (a) nearly equals right ventricular (RV) systolic pressure and produces a large diastolic gradient (shaded area). A presystolic murmur (PSM), loud first heart sound (1), and early diastolic opening snap (OS) simulate the findings in mitral stenosis. (Time lines = 0.2 sec.) (From Criley, J. M., et al.: Departures from the expected auscultatory events in mitral stenosis. *In* Likoff, W. [ed.]: Valvular Heart Disease. Philadelphia, F. A. Davis Co., 1973, p. 214.)

TABLE 32–9 CLINICAL AND LABORATORY FEATURES OF RHEUMATIC TRICUSPID STENOSIS

HISTORY
Long history
Progressive fatigue, edema, anorexia
Minimal orthopnea, paroxysmal nocturnal dyspnea
Rheumatic fever in two-thirds of patients
Female preponderance
Orthopnea and paroxysmal nocturnal dyspnea are unusual
Pulmonary edema and hemoptysis are rare
PHYSICAL FINDINGS
Signs of multivalvular involvement
Wasting
Peripheral cyanosis
Neck vein distention, with prominent *v* waves
Right ventricular lift
Associated murmurs of mitral and aortic valve disease
Holosystolic murmur maximal at left lower sternal border, accentuating with inspiration
Hepatic pulsation
Ascites, peripheral edema
LABORATORY FINDINGS
Normal sinus rhythm is frequently present with large *a* waves in the neck veins
Absent right ventricular lift
Auscultation reveals a diastolic rumble at lower left sternal edge, increasing in intensity with inspiration
Electrocardiogram shows tall right atrial P waves and no right ventricular hypertrophy
Roentgenogram shows a dilated right atrium without an enlarged pulmonary artery segment

Modified from Ockene, I. S.: Tricuspid valve disease. *In* Dalen, J. E., and Alpert, J. S. (eds.): Valvular Heart Disease. 2nd ed. Boston, Little, Brown and Company, 1987, pp. 356, 390.

the absence of normal rapid early right ventricular filling. The lung fields are clear, and despite engorgement of the neck veins and the presence of ascites and anasarca, the patient may be comfortable while lying flat. A parasternal (right ventricular) lift is inconspicuous, and pulmonic valve closure is *not* palpable, but occasionally the pulsations of a greatly enlarged right atrium may be felt to the right of the sternum. Thus, the diagnosis of TS may be suspected from inspection and palpation from the combination of a prominent *a* wave in the jugular venous pulse in a patient with MS without evidence of pulmonary hypertension or right ventricular enlargement. This suspicion is strengthened when a diastolic thrill is felt at the lower left sternal edge, particularly if it appears or becomes more prominent during inspiration.[15]

The auscultatory findings of the accompanying MS are usually prominent and often overshadow the more subtle signs of TS. A tricuspid valvular opening snap (OS) may be audible but is often difficult to distinguish from a mitral OS. However, the tricuspid OS usually follows the mitral OS, and is localized to the lower left sternal border, whereas the mitral OS is usually most prominent at the apex and radiates more widely. The diastolic murmur of TS (Fig. 32–43) is commonly heard best along the lower left parasternal border in the fourth intercostal space and is usually softer, higher pitched, and shorter in duration than the murmur of MS. The presystolic component has a scratchy quality, commences earlier (0.06 sec after the P wave in TS compared with 0.12 in MS), and has a crescendo-decrescendo configuration, diminishing before S_1.[444] The diastolic murmur and OS of TS are both augmented by maneuvers that increase transtricuspid valve flow, including inspiration (Fig. 2–44, p. 44), the Mueller maneuver, assumption of the right lateral decubitus position, leg-raising, inhalation of amyl nitrite, squatting, and isotonic exercise. They are reduced during expiration or the strain of the Valsalva maneuver and return to control levels immediately (i.e., within two to three beats) after Valsalva release.

Laboratory Examination

ELECTROCARDIOGRAM. In a patient with valvular heart disease in the absence of atrial fibrillation, TS is suggested by the presence of ECG evidence of right atrial enlargement disproportionate to the degree of right ventricular hypertrophy. The P-wave amplitude in leads II and V exceeds 0.25 mV (see p. 115), and there may be depression of the P-R segment resulting from increased magnitude of the atrial T wave. Because most patients with TS have mitral valve disease, the ECG signs of biatrial enlargement (see p. 116) with abnormally tall, broad P waves in leads II, III, and aV_f and prominent positive and negative deflections in V_f are commonly found. Right atrial dilatation may rotate the ventricular septum and affect QRS morphology in a manner so that the large volume of the right atrium between the exploring electrode and the ventricles reduces the amplitude of the QRS complex in lead V_1 (which often has a Q wave), whereas the QRS complex is much taller in V_2.

RADIOLOGICAL FINDINGS. The key radiological findings in TS are marked cardiomegaly, with conspicuous enlargement of the right atrium (i.e., prominence of the right heart border), which extends into a dilated superior vena cava and azygos vein, but without dilatation of the pulmonary artery. The vascular changes in the lungs characteristic of mitral valve disease may be masked, with little or no interstitial edema or vascular redistribution, but left atrial enlargement may be present.

Angiography carried out following injection of contrast material into the right atrium and filming in the 30-degree right anterior oblique projection is useful for evaluating the appearance of the tricuspid valve. Thickening and decreased mobility of the leaflets, a jet through the constricted orifice, and thickening of the right atrial wall are characteristic findings.

ECHOCARDIOGRAM (see also p. 76). Although the motion of the normal tricuspid valve is similar to that of the normal mitral valve, it is more difficult to image. Not surprisingly, the changes in the echocardiogram of the tricuspid valve in TS resemble those observed in the mitral valve in MS (see p. 1012). Two-dimensional echocardiography characteristically shows diastolic doming of the leaflets, especially the anterior tricuspid valve leaflet, thickening and restriction of motion of the other leaflets, reduced separation of the tips of the leaflets,[448,449] and a reduction in diameter of the tricuspid orifice (Fig. 32–44). Transesophageal echocardiography allows added delineation of the details of valve structure.[450] Doppler echocardiography shows a prolonged slope of antegrade flow and compares well with cardiac catheterization in the quantification of TS and in the assessment of associated tricuspid regurgitation.[451]

Management

Although the fundamental approach to the management of severe TS is surgical treatment, intensive sodium restriction and diuretic therapy may diminish the symptoms secondary to the accumulation of excess salt and water. A prolonged preparatory period of diuresis may diminish hepatic congestion and thereby improve hepatic function sufficiently to diminish the risks of subsequent operation.

Most patients with TS have coexisting valvular disease that requires surgery. In patients with combined TS and MS, the former alone must not be corrected surgically because pulmonary congestion or edema may ensue.[452] Surgical treatment of TS should be carried out in patients with TS in whom the mean diastolic pressure gradients exceed 5 mm Hg and the tricuspid orifice is less than approximately 2.0 cm² at the time of mitral valve repair or replacement. The final decision concerning surgical treatment is often made at the operating table.[453] Because TS is almost always accompanied by some TR, simple finger fracture commissurotomy may not result in significant hemodynamic improvement but may merely substitute severe regurgitation for stenosis. However, open valvulotomy in which the stenotic tricuspid valve is converted into a functionally bicuspid one may result in substantial improvement. The commissures between the anterior and septal leaflets and between the posterior and septal leaflets are opened; it is not advisable to open the commissure between the anterior and posterior leaflets for fear of producing severe regurgitation. If open commissurotomy does not restore reasonable

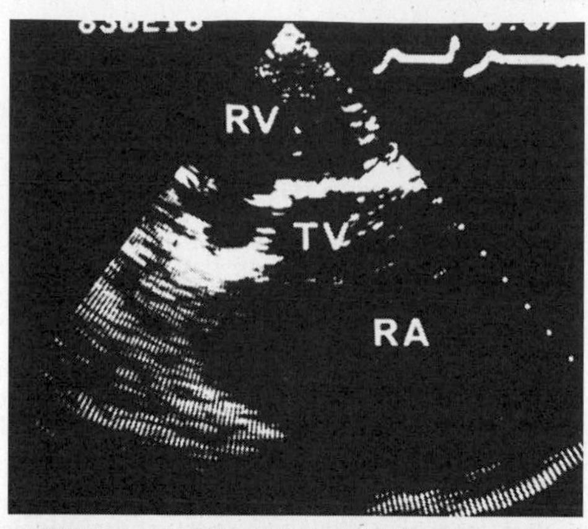

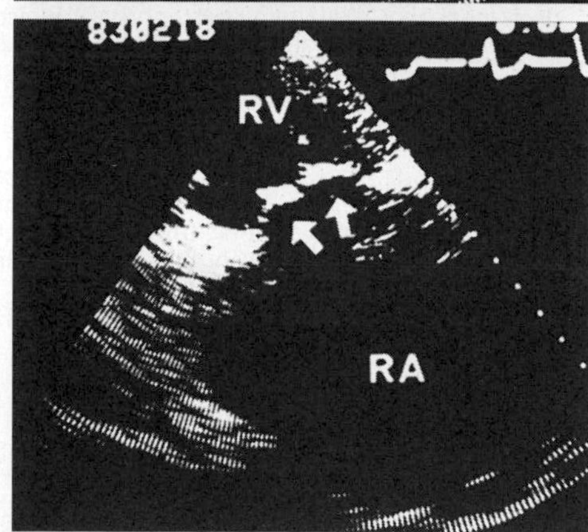

FIGURE 32–44. Two-dimensional echocardiograms in the long-axis view in a patient with tricuspid stenosis. ***Top,*** **Systolic frame.** ***Bottom,*** **Diastolic frame that shows doming of both leaflets of the tricuspid valve (TV) (arrows). RA = right atrium; RV = right ventricle. (From Shimada, R., et al.: Diagnosis of tricuspid stenosis by M-mode and two-dimensional echocardiography. Am. J. Cardiol.** ***53:*****164, 1984.)**

normal valve function, the tricuspid valve may have to be replaced.[454] A porcine bioprosthesis (see p. 1066) is preferred to a mechanical prosthesis in the tricuspid position because of the high risk of thrombosis of the latter[455] and the long-term durability of bioprostheses in the tricuspid position.[456–460] The feasibility of tricuspid balloon valvuloplasty has been demonstrated,[461] but it is not clear how this procedure will be used most effectively.

TRICUSPID REGURGITATION

Etiology and Pathology

(Table 32–10)

The most common cause of tricuspid regurgitation (TR) is not intrinsic involvement of the valve itself but *dilatation of the right ventricle* and of the tricuspid annulus, which may be complications of right ventricular failure of any cause and which cause secondary, functional TR. This is observed in patients with right ventricular hypertension secondary to any form of cardiac and pulmonary vascular disease, most commonly mitral valve disease,[454,461–464] right ventricular infarction[465] (see p. 1192), congenital heart disease (e.g., pulmonic stenosis and pulmonary hypertension secondary to Eisenmenger's syndrome), primary pulmonary hypertension, and rarely cor pulmonale. Severe TR has been reported to be the presenting manifestation in thyrotoxicosis.[466] In infants, TR may complicate right ventricular failure secondary to neonatal pulmonary diseases and pulmonary hypertension with persistence of the fetal pulmonary circulation.[467] In all of these cases, TR reflects the presence of, and in turn aggravates, severe right ventricular failure. Functional regurgitation may diminish or disappear as the right ventricle decreases in size with the treatment of heart failure. TR can also occur as a consequence of dilatation of the annulus in Marfan syndrome, in which it is not associated with right ventricular dilatation secondary to pulmonary hypertension.

TABLE 32–10 CAUSES AND MECHANISMS OF PURE TRICUSPID REGURGITATION

CAUSES

Anatomically ABNORMAL valve
- Rheumatic
- Nonrheumatic
  - Infective endocarditis
  - Ebstein's anomaly
  - Floppy (prolapse)
  - Congenital (non-Ebstein's)
  - Carcinoid
  - Papillary muscle dysfunction
  - Trauma
  - Connective tissue disorders (Marfan)
  - Rheumatoid arthritis
  - Radiation injury

Anatomically NORMAL valve (functional)
- Elevated right ventricular systolic pressure (dilated annulus)

MECHANISMS

Condition	Leaflet Area	Annular Circumference	Leaflet Insertion
Floppy	↑	↑	Normal
Ebstein's anomaly	↑	↑	Abnormal
Pulmonary/right ventricular systolic hypertension	Normal	↑	Normal
Papillary muscle dysfunction	Normal	Normal	Normal
Carcinoid	↓/Normal	Normal	Normal
Rheumatic	↓/Normal	Normal	Normal
Infective endocarditis	↓/Normal	Normal	Normal

Modified from Waller, B. F.: Rheumatic and nonrheumatic conditions producing valvular heart disease. *In* Frankl, W. S., and Brest, A. N. (eds.): Cardiovascular Clinics. Valvular Heart Disease: Comprehensive Evaluation and Management. Philadelphia, F. A. Davis Co., 1989, pp. 35, 95.

A variety of disease processes can affect the tricuspid valve apparatus *directly* and lead to regurgitation. Thus, organic TR may occur on a congenital basis, as part of *Ebstein's anomaly* (see p. 934), in atrioventricular canal, and when the tricuspid valve is involved in the formation of an aneurysm of the ventricular septum,[468] or it may occur as an isolated congenital lesion.[469] Rheumatic fever may involve the tricuspid valve directly,[460] and when it does so, it usually causes scarring of the valve leaflets and/or chordae, leading to limited leaflet mobility, pure TR, and/or a combination of TR and TS.

TR or the combination of TR and TS is an important feature of the *carcinoid syndrome* (Fig. 32–45), which leads to focal or diffuse deposits of fibrous tissue on the endocardium of the valvular cusps and cardiac chambers and on the intima of the great veins and coronary sinus.[470,471] The white, fibrous carcinoid plaques are most extensive on the right side of the heart, where they are usually deposited on the ventricular surfaces of the tricuspid valve and cause the cusps to adhere to the underlying right ventricular wall, thereby producing TR.

TR may result from prolapse of the tricuspid valve caused by myxomatous changes in the valve and chordae tendineae; this condition usually, but not always, accompanies prolapse of the mitral valve.[472,473] Prolapse of the tricuspid valve occurs in about one-third of all patients with mitral valve prolapse.[446] Tricuspid valve prolapse may also be associated with atrial septal defect. Other causes of TR include penetrating and nonpenetrating trauma,[474] dilated

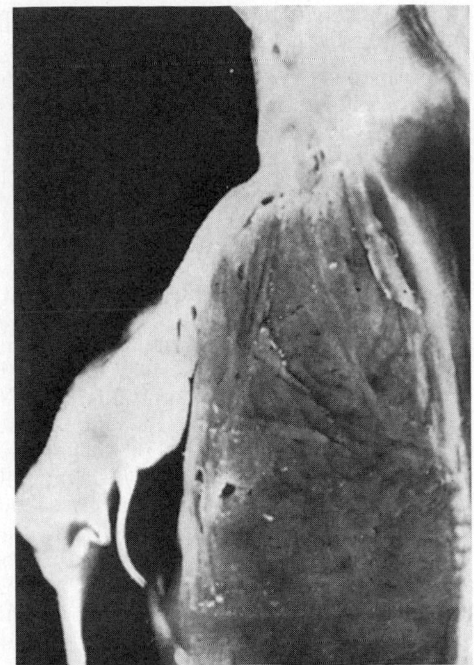

FIGURE 32–45. Septal tricuspid leaflet thickened by carcinoid plaques and fused to underlying ventricular septum. (From Callahan, J. A., et al.: Echocardiographic features of carcinoid heart disease. Am. J. Cardiol. *50*:766, 1982.)

cardiomyopathy,[475] infective endocarditis,[476] particularly staphylococcal endocarditis in narcotics addicts (see p. 1078), and surgical excision of the tricuspid valve that has been necessary in patients with infective endocarditis unresponsive to medical management.[477] Less common causes of TR include cardiac tumors, particularly right atrial myxoma; endomyocardial fibrosis; methysergide-induced valvular disease[478]; and systemic lupus erythematosus involving the tricuspid valve.[479]

Clinical Manifestations

HISTORY. In the absence of pulmonary hypertension, TR is generally well tolerated. However, when pulmonary hypertension and TR coexist, cardiac output declines, and the manifestations of right-sided heart failure become intensified.[480] Thus, the symptoms of TR result from a reduced cardiac output and from ascites, painful congestive hepatomegaly, and massive edema. Occasionally, patients complain of throbbing pulsations in the neck due to jugular venous distention, which intensify on effort,[15] and systolic pulsations of the eyeballs are sometimes noted.[481] In the many patients with TR who have mitral valve disease, the symptoms of the latter usually predominate. Symptoms of pulmonary congestion may abate as TR develops, but they are replaced by weakness, fatigue, and other manifestations of a depressed cardiac output.

PHYSICAL EXAMINATION (Fig. 2–7, p. 21). Evidence of weight loss and cachexia, cyanosis, and jaundice is often present on inspection. Atrial fibrillation is common. There is jugular venous distention,[482] the normal *x* and *x'* descents disappear, and a prominent systolic *("s")* wave, i.e., a *c-v* wave, is apparent. The descent of this wave, the *y* descent, is sharp and becomes the most prominent feature of the venous pulse (unless there is a coexisting TS, in which case it is slowed). The *s* waves and *y* descents become more prominent during inspiration.[483] A venous systolic thrill and murmur in the neck may be present in severe TR.[484] The right ventricular impulse is hyperdynamic and thrusting in quality. Rarely, a right atrial systolic impulse may be observed or palpated along the right lower sternal edge.[15] In patients with combined mitral valve disease and TR, a relatively quiet zone may be present between the apex and the left sternal edge. Systolic pulsations of an enlarged tender liver are commonly present initially, but in chronic TR with congestive cirrhosis, the liver may be firm and nontender. Ascites and edema are frequent.

Auscultation (Table 32–2). This usually reveals an S_3 originating from the right ventricle, i.e., one accentuated by inspiration; when TR is associated with pulmonary hypertension, P_2 is accentuated as well. When TR occurs in the presence of pulmonary hypertension, the murmur is usually high-pitched, pansystolic, and loudest in the fourth intercostal space in the parasternal region but occasionally in the subxiphoid area. When TR is mild, the murmur may be short. When TR occurs in the absence of pulmonary hypertension, as for example in infective endocarditis or following trauma, the murmur is usually of low intensity and limited to the first half of systole. When the right ventricle is greatly dilated and occupies the anterior surface of the heart, the murmur may be the most prominent at the apex and difficult to distinguish from that produced by MR.

The response of the murmur to respiration and other maneuvers is of considerable aid in establishing the diagnosis of tricuspid regurgitation (Table 2–4, p. 46). It is usually augmented during inspiration (Carvallo's sign, p. 38). However, when the failing ventricle can no longer increase its stroke volume, the inspiratory augmentation may be elicited by standing and thereby reducing venous return. The murmur also increases during inspiration, the Mueller maneuver (forced inspiration against a closed glottis), exercise, leg-raising, hepatic compression, and amyl nitrite inhalation as well as after a prolonged diastole. It demonstrates an immediate overshoot after release of the Valsalva strain but is reduced in intensity and duration in the standing position and during the strain of the Valsalva maneuver. Rarely, TR is silent except for the selective appearance of a soft systolic murmur during inspiration.[485] Increased atrioventricular flow may cause a short early diastolic flow rumble in the left parasternal region following S_3. Tricuspid valve prolapse, like MVP, causes nonejection systolic clicks and late systolic murmurs. These findings are more prominent at the lower left sternal border. With inspiration the clicks occur later and the murmurs intensify and become shorter in duration.

Laboratory Examination

ELECTROCARDIOGRAM. This is usually nonspecific and characteristic of the lesion causing TR. Incomplete right bundle branch block, Q waves in lead V_1, and atrial fibrillation are commonly found.

RADIOLOGICAL FINDINGS. In patients with functional TR, marked cardiomegaly secondary to the condition responsible for the dilatation of the right ventricle is usually evident. The right atrium is prominent.[483] Evidence of elevated right atrial pressure may include distention of the azygos vein and the presence of pleural effusion. Ascites with upward displacement of the diaphragm may be present. Rarely, with prolonged elevation of right ventricular pressure, the tricuspid ring may calcify. The findings of pulmonary arterial and venous hypertension are common. Systolic pulsations of the right atrium may be present on fluoroscopy.

ECHOCARDIOGRAM (see also p. 76). The goal of echocardiography is to detect TR, estimate its severity, and assess pulmonary artery pressure and right ventricular function. In patients with TR secondary to dilation of the tricuspid annulus, usually associated with right ventricular systolic hypertension, the right atrium, right ventricle, and tricuspid annulus are all usually greatly dilated on echocardiography.[486,487] There is evidence of right ventricular diastolic overload with paradoxical motion of the ventricular septum similar to that observed in atrial septal defect. Exaggerated motion and delayed closure of the tricuspid valve are evident in patients with Ebstein's anomaly. In patients with TR secondary to right ventricular dilatation and pulmonary hypertension, the pulmonic valve echogram shows a diminished or absent *a* deflection. *Prolapse of the tricuspid valve* due to myxomatous degeneration may be evident on M-mode and two-dimensional echocardiography[472,473] (Fig. 3–60, p. 77). Simultaneous echocardiographic studies of the tricuspid valve and phonocardiography may reveal a nonejection systolic click originating from the right side of the heart that occurs at the onset of prolapse. Echocardiographic indications of tricuspid valve abnormalities, especially TR by Doppler examination, can be detected in the majority of patients with carcinoid heart disease.[470]

Contrast Echocardiography. This involves rapid ejection of saline or indocyanine green dye into an antecubital vein made while a two-dimensional echocardiogram is being recorded (see p. 58). It is both sensitive and specific for TR.[488] The injection produces microcavities that are readily visible on echocardiography and normally travel as a bolus through the circulation. In TR, these microcavities can be seen to travel back and forth across the tricuspid orifice and to pass into the inferior vena cava and hepatic veins during systole. TR secondary to carcinoid heart disease shows thickened, retracted valve leaflets, fixed in a semiopen position throughout the cardiac cycle,[489] whereas that due to endocarditis may reveal vegetations on the valve, or a flail valve. Transesophageal echocardiography enhances detection of TR.

Pulsed Doppler Echocardiography. This reveals systolic flow from right ventricle to right atrium and is an exquisitely sensitive technique for detecting TR.[490] Reverse flow can also be recorded in the inferior vena cava[491] and hepatic veins.[492] The peak velocity of TR flow is useful in the noninvasive estimation of right ventricular (and pulmonary artery) systolic pressure. Color Doppler imaging is an extremely accurate, sensitive, and specific method for assessing TR[493] and is helpful in selecting patients for surgical treatment and in assessing postoperative results.

HEMODYNAMIC AND ANGIOGRAPHIC FINDINGS. The right atrial and right ventricular end-diastolic pressures are characteristically elevated in TR, whether the condition is due to organic disease of the tricuspid valve or is secondary to right ventricular systolic overload (e.g., pulmonary hypertension and pulmonic stenosis). The right atrial pressure tracing reveals absence of the *x* descent and a prominent *v* or *c-v* wave ("ventricularization" of the atrial pressure). Therefore, as the severity of TR increases, the contour of the right atrial pressure pulse increasingly resembles that of the right ventricular pressure pulse (Fig. 32–46). A rise or no change in right atrial pressure on deep inspiration, rather than the usual fall, is characteristic.[483,494] Pulmonary artery (or right ventricular) systolic pressure may be helpful in determining whether the TR is primary (i.e., due to disease of the valve or its supporting structures) or functional (i.e., secondary to right ventricular dilatation). A pulmonary artery or right ventricular systolic pressure less than 40 mm Hg favors a primary etiology, whereas a pressure greater than 60 mm Hg suggests that TR is secondary.

Diagnosis and quantitative assessment of TR can be aided in many instances by right ventriculography, but the fact that the catheter must be positioned across the tricuspid valve cannot exclude the possibility of a false-positive diagnosis of TR. Modifications of previous angiographic techniques have been introduced in which a special, preformed catheter is positioned in the right ventricle, and angiography is carried out at low injection rates[495] or a special balloon catheter is employed to minimize the induction of extrasystoles, which can also cause spurious regurgitation.[496]

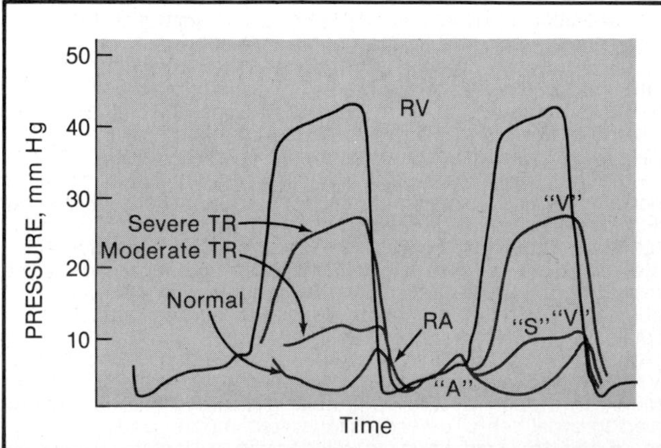

FIGURE 32–46. Appearance of right atrial (RA) pressure contour in patients with severe tricuspid regurgitation (TR), moderate TR, and no TR (normal). Note the regurgitant systolic ("S") wave that blends with the normal filling ("V") wave in severe TR. The resultant RA pressure waveform resembles a right ventricular (RV) pressure recording. (From Grossman, W. [ed.]: Cardiac Catheterization and Angiography. 3rd ed. Philadelphia, Lea and Febiger, 1986, p. 378.)

Management

TR in the absence of pulmonary hypertension usually does not require surgical treatment. Indeed, both patients and experimental animals with normal pulmonary artery pressure may tolerate total excision of the tricuspid valve, as long as right ventricular systolic pressure is normal for a period of time.[496] Dilatation of the right side of the heart usually occurs months or years after tricuspid valvectomy (usually carried out for acute infective endocarditis), and annuloplasty with insertion of a prosthetic valve can then be carried out after adequate sterilization of the valve ring. *Surgical treatment* of acquired regurgitation secondary to annular dilatation was greatly improved when Carpentier introduced the concept of suturing the annulus to a right prosthetic ring of appropriate dimensions.[497,498] Annuloplasty without insertion of a prosthetic ring (so-called DeVega annuloplasty) has also been found to be effective in patients with annular dilatation. This technique is now widely employed.[453,480,499–501]

At the time of mitral valve surgery in patients with TR secondary to pulmonary hypertension, the severity of the regurgitation should be assessed by palpation of the valve and a determination made whether the TR is functional (secondary) or organic (primary). Patients with mild TR usually do not require surgical treatment[501]; pulmonary vascular pressures decline following successful mitral valve surgery, and the mild TR tends to disappear. Excellent results have been reported in patients with moderate TR with the use of suture annuloplasty of the posterior (unsupported) portion of the annulus.[453,502] Patients with severe TR and primary (organic) rheumatic valve disease with commissural fusion require commissurotomy and ring annuloplasty.[499,503] However, management of severe functional TR is more controversial. Although it is not clear whether severe TR should be treated by annuloplasty or valve replacement, most surgeons prefer the former approach and utilize a rigid (Carpentier) ring.[501] If it does not provide a good functional result at the operating table, as assessed by transesophageal echocardiography, they resort to valve replacement.

Organic disease of the tricuspid valve responsible for TR, as in Ebstein's anomaly[504] or carcinoid heart disease,[457] when severe enough to require surgery, usually requires valve replacement. The risk of thrombosis of mechanical prostheses is greater in the tricuspid than in the mitral or aortic positions, presumably because pressure and flow rates are lower in the right side of the heart. For this reason, the artificial valve of choice for the tricuspid position in adults at present is a large porcine heterograft.[458,459] Anticoagulants are not required, and a durability of more than 10 years has been established.

In treating the difficult problem of tricuspid endocarditis in heroin addicts, it has been noted that total excision of the tricuspid valve *without immediate replacement* can be tolerated by these patients, who usually do not have associated pulmonary hypertension. When antibiotic therapy is unsuccessful, valvular replacement frequently results in reinfection or continued infection. Therefore, diseased valvular tissue should be excised to eradicate the endocarditis, and antibiotic treatment can then be continued. Initially, most patients tolerate loss of the tricuspid valve without great difficulty, although a reduction in left ventricular ejection fraction may occur.[505] Later, right ventricular dysfunction usually occurs. Therefore, a bioprosthetic valve may be inserted 6 to 9 months after valve excision and control of the infection.

PULMONIC VALVE DISEASE

Etiology and Pathology

PULMONIC STENOSIS (PS). The *congenital* form is the most common cause of pulmonic stenosis.[506] Its manifestations in children are discussed on page 924 and in adults on page 965. *Rheumatic* inflammation of the pulmonic valve is very uncommon, is usually associated with involvement of other valves, and rarely leads to serious deformity. However, a high incidence of significant pulmonic valve involvement secondary to rheumatic fever has been reported in Mexico City, perhaps related to the pulmonary hypertension that occurs at high altitudes and the resultant greater stress on the pulmonic valve.[507] *Carcinoid* plaques, similar to those involving the tricuspid valve, are often present in the outflow tract of the right ventricle in patients with malignant carcinoid and result in constriction of the pulmonic valve ring, retraction and fusion of the valve cusps, and either PS or the combination of PS and pulmonic regurgitation (PR) (Fig. 32–47).[508,509] Obstruction in the region of the pulmonic valve may be extrinsic to the valve apparatus and may be produced by cardiac tumors or aneurysm of the sinus Valsalva.[510]

PULMONIC REGURGITATION (PR). By far the most common cause of PR is dilatation of the valve ring secondary to pulmonary hypertension (of any etiology) or to dilatation of the pulmonary artery, either idiopathic[511,512] or consequent to a connective tissue disorder such as Marfan syndrome. The second most common cause of PR is infective endocarditis.[508,513] Less frequently, it is iatrogenic and is induced at the time of surgical treatment of congenital PS or tetralogy of Fallot. PR may also result from a variety of lesions directly affecting the pulmonic valve. These include congenital malformations, such as absent, malformed, fenestrated, or supernumerary leaflets. These anomalies may occur as isolated lesions[514] but more often are associated with other congenital anomalies, particularly tetralogy of Fallot, ventricular septal defect, and pulmonic valvular stenosis. Less common causes include trauma, carcinoid syndrome,[500] rheumatic involvement,[515] injury produced by a pulmonary artery flow-directed catheter,[516] syphilis,[517] and chest trauma.[518]

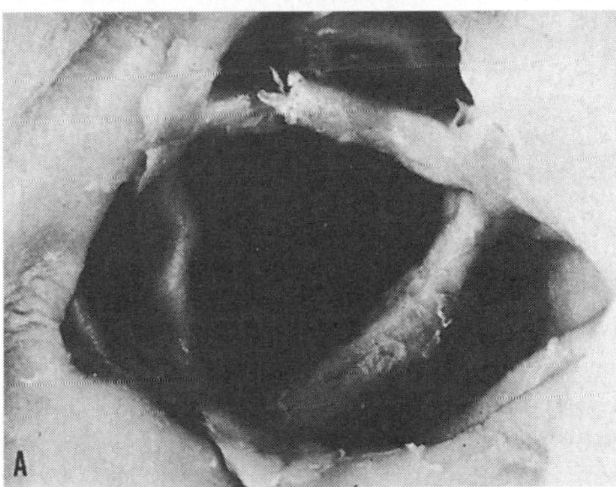

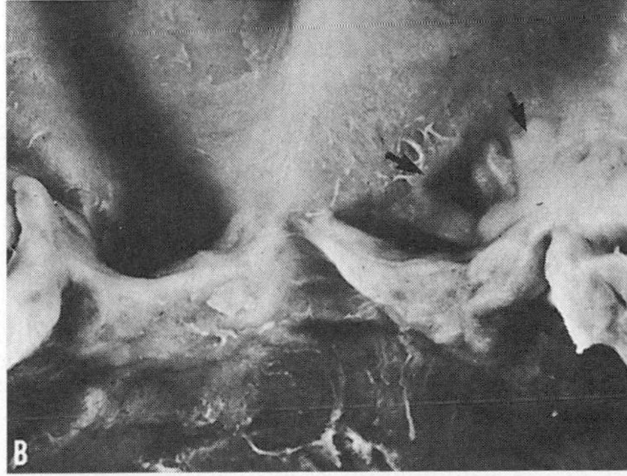

FIGURE 32–47. Carcinoid heart disease; pulmonary valve viewed from above *(A)* and opened *(B)*. The thickened and retracted cusps result in valvular incompetence. The constricted annulus results in valvular stenosis. Carcinoid plaques (arrows) extend onto the pulmonary trunk. (From Callahan, J. A., et al.: Echocardiographic features of carcinoid heart disease. Am. J. Cardiol. *50:*767, 1982.)

Clinical Manifestations

Like TR, isolated PR causes right ventricular volume overload and may be tolerated for many years without difficulty unless it complicates or is complicated by pulmonary hypertension, in which case it is usually accompanied by and aggravates right ventricular failure. Patients with PR caused by infective endocarditis who develop septic pulmonary emboli and pulmonary hypertension often exhibit severe right ventricular failure.[518] In most patients the clinical manifestations of the primary disease are severe and usually overshadow the PR, which often results only in incidental auscultatory findings. *Physical examination* reveals a hyperdynamic right ventricle, producing palpable systolic pulsations in the left parasternal area and an enlarged pulmonary artery that often results in palpable systolic pulsations in the second left intercostal space; sometimes systolic and diastolic thrills are felt in the same area. A tap reflecting pulmonic valve closure is usually easily palpable in the second intercostal space in patients with pulmonary hypertension and secondary PR.

AUSCULTATION. In patients with congenital absence of the pulmonic valve, P_2 is not audible, but this sound is accentuated in patients with PR secondary to pulmonary hypertension, particularly when the dilated pulmonary artery is near the chest wall. There may be wide splitting of S_2 due to prolongation of right ventricular ejection accompanying the augmented right ventricular stroke volume.[515] A nonvalvular systolic ejection click due to the sudden expansion of the pulmonary artery by the augmented right ventricular stroke volume frequently initiates a midsystolic ejection murmur, most prominent in the second left intercostal space. An S_3 and S_4 originating from the right ventricle are often audible, most readily in the fourth intercostal space at the left parasternal area, and are augmented by inspiration.

In the absence of pulmonary hypertension, the diastolic murmur of PR is low-pitched and is usually heard best at the third and fourth left intercostal spaces adjacent to the sternum (Fig. 2–42, p. 43). The murmur commences when pressures in the pulmonary artery and right ventricle diverge, approximately 0.04 sec after P_2. It is diamond-shaped in configuration and brief, reaching a peak intensity when the gradient between these pressures is maximal and ending with equilibration of the pressures.[517] The murmur becomes louder during inspiration and following inhalation of amyl nitrite.

Graham Steell Murmur. When pulmonary artery systolic pressure exceeds approximately 60 mm Hg, dilatation of the pulmonic annulus results in a regurgitant jet of high velocity that is responsible for the so-called Graham Steell murmur of PR. (Doppler ultrasound reveals pulmonary regurgitation at much lower pulmonary arterial pressures.)[518] The Graham Steell murmur is a high-pitched, blowing decrescendo murmur beginning immediately after P_2 and is most prominent in the left parasternal region in the second to fourth intercostal spaces. Thus, although it resembles the murmur of AR, it is usually accompanied by the findings of severe pulmonary hypertension, i.e., an accentuated P_2 or fused S_2, an ejection sound, and a systolic murmur of tricuspid regurgitation, and not by a widened arterial pulse pressure. Sometimes a low-frequency presystolic murmur is present, i.e., a right-sided Austin Flint murmur originating from the mitral valve.[519]

The Graham Steell murmur of PR secondary to pulmonary hypertension usually increases in intensity with inspiration, exhibits little change after amyl nitrite inhalation or vasopressors, is diminished during the Valsalva strain, and returns to baseline intensity almost immediately after release of the Valsalva strain. This murmur resembles and may be confused with the diastolic blowing murmur of AR. However, indicator dilution studies[520] and aortography have established that a diastolic blowing murmur along the left sternal border in patients with rheumatic heart disease and pulmonary hypertension—even in the absence of peripheral signs of AR—is usually due to AR and not PR.

Laboratory Examination

ELECTROCARDIOGRAM. In the absence of pulmonary hypertension, PR often results in an ECG that reflects right ventricular diastolic overload, i.e., an rSr′ (or rsR′) configuration in the right precordial leads. PR secondary to pulmonary hypertension is usually associated with ECG evidence of right ventricular hypertrophy.

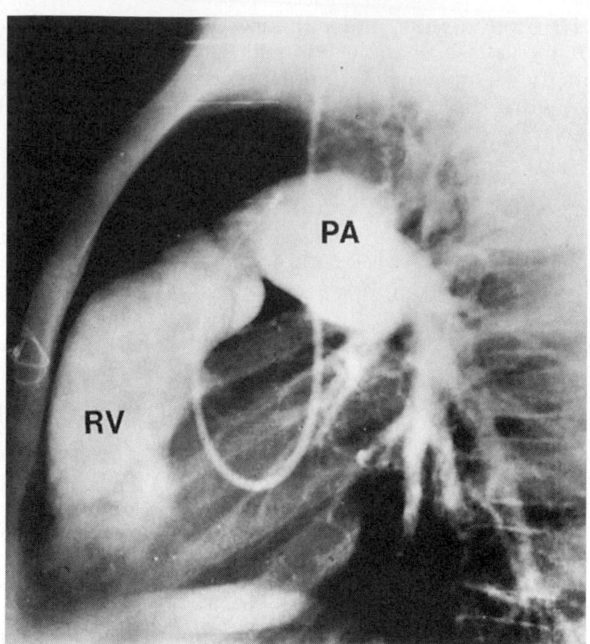

FIGURE 32–48. Pulmonic valvular regurgitation. Contrast medium has been injected into the main pulmonary artery (PA) and regurgitates back into an enlarged right ventricle (RV). (Reproduced with permission from Carlsson, E., et al.: The radiological diagnosis of cardiac valvular insufficiency. Circulation *55*:921, 1977. Copyright 1977 American Heart Association.)

RADIOLOGICAL FINDINGS. Both the pulmonary artery and the right ventricle are usually enlarged, but these signs are nonspecific. Fluoroscopy may demonstrate pronounced pulsation of the main pulmonary artery. PR can be diagnosed by observing opacification of the right ventricle following injection of contrast material into the main pulmonary artery (Fig. 32–48). The diagnosis is supported by noting superimposition of the pulmonary artery and right ventricular pressure curves during mid and late diastole. Indicator dilution techniques with injections into the pulmonary artery and sampling from the right ventricle,[521] as well as intracardiac phonocardiography, can also be helpful in establishing the diagnosis in mild cases.

ECHOCARDIOGRAM. This shows right ventricular dilatation and, in patients with pulmonary hypertension, right ventricular hypertrophy as well. Abnormal motion of the septum characteristic of volume overload of the right ventricle in diastole and/or septal flutter[522] may be evident. The motion of the pulmonic valve may point to the cause of the pulmonic regurgitation.[523] Absence of *a* waves and systolic notching of the posterior leaflet suggest pulmonary hypertension; large *a* waves indicate pulmonic stenosis. PR can be detected by contrast echocardiography. The pulsed Doppler technique is extremely accurate in detecting PR. Abnormal Doppler signals in the right ventricular outflow tract whose velocity is sustained throughout diastole are generally observed in patients in whom dilatation of the valve ring (functional regurgitation) secondary to pulmonary hypertension is the cause. When the velocity falls during diastole, the pulmonary artery pressure is usually normal, and the regurgitation is caused by an abnormality of the valve itself.[523]

MANAGEMENT. PR per se is seldom severe enough to require specific treatment. Cardiac glycosides are useful in the management of right ventricular dilatation or failure. Treatment of the primary condition, such as infective endocarditis, or the lesion responsible for the pulmonary hypertension, such as surgical treatment of mitral valvular disease, often ameliorates the PR. Surgical treatment of *primary* PR directed specifically at the pulmonic valve is required only occasionally because of intractable right heart failure, and under such circumstances valve replacement may be carried out,[524] preferably with a porcine bioprosthesis.

MULTIVALVULAR DISEASE

Multivalvular involvement is caused most frequently by rheumatic fever, and a variety of clinical and hemodynamic syndromes can be produced by different combinations of valvular abnormalities. The Marfan syndrome and other connective tissue disorders may cause prolapse and dilatation of more than one valve annulus, causing multivalvular regurgitation. Degenerative calcification of the aortic valve may be associated with degenerative mitral annular calcification and cause AS and MR. Different pathological conditions may affect each valve, such as infective endocarditis on the aortic valve and ischemic mitral regurgitation. Development of PR and TR secondary to dilatation of the pulmonic valve ring and tricuspid annulus, respectively, as a consequence of pulmonary hypertension secondary to disease involving the mitral or aortic valve or both, has already been discussed (see p. 1056), as has the combination of *organic* rheumatic tricuspid and mitral valvular disease (see p. 1011). In patients with multivalvular disease, the clinical manifestations depend on the relative severities of each the lesions. When the valvular abnormalities are of approximately equal severity, as a general rule, clinical manifestations produced by the more proximal (upstream) of two valvular lesions, i.e., the mitral valve in patients with combined mitral and aortic valvular disease and the tricuspid valve in patients with combined tricuspid and mitral valvular disease, are more prominent than those produced by the distal lesion. Thus, the proximal lesion masks the distal lesion.

It is important to recognize multivalvular involvement preoperatively because failure to correct all significant valvular disease at the time of operation increases mortality considerably. In patients with multivalvular disease, the relative severity of each lesion may be difficult to estimate by clinical examination and noninvasive techniques, because one lesion may mask the manifestations of the other. For this reason, patients suspected of multivalvular involvement and in whom surgical treatment is under consideration should undergo (in addition to careful clinical examination and noninvasive workup, with emphasis on two-dimensional and Doppler echocardiography), right- and left-sided cardiac catheterization and angiography. If there is any question concerning the presence of significant AS in patients undergoing an operation on the mitral valve, the aortic valve should be inspected because overlooking this condition can lead to a high perioperative mortality. Similarly, it is useful to palpate the tricuspid valve at the time of operation on the mitral valve.

MITRAL STENOSIS AND AORTIC REGURGITATION

Approximately two-thirds of patients with severe MS have an early blowing diastolic murmur along the left sternal border with a normal pulse pressure; in 90 per cent of these the murmur is due to mild or moderate AR and is usually of little clinical importance. However, approximately 10 per cent of patients with MS have severe rheumatic AR,[525] which can usually be recognized by the peripheral signs of a widened pulse pressure, left ventricular dilatation and increased wall motion on echocardiography, and signs of left ventricular enlargement on radiological and electrocardiographic examinations.

In keeping with the general observation that a proximal lesion may mask a distal lesion, significant AR may be missed in patients with severe MS. The widened pulse pressure, in particular, may be absent. On the other hand, on clinical examination of patients with obvious AR, MS may be missed or, conversely, may be falsely diagnosed. An accentuated S_1 and an opening snap in a patient with AR should suggest the possibility of mitral valve disease. On the other hand, an Austin Flint murmur is often inappropriately considered to be the diastolic rumbling murmur of MS. These two murmurs may be distinguished at the bedside by means of amyl nitrite inhalation, which diminishes the Austin Flint murmur (Fig. 2–41, p. 42) but augments the murmur of MS; isometric handgrip and squatting augment both the diastolic murmur of AR and the Austin Flint murmur. Echocardiography, particularly pulsed Doppler echocardiography, is of decisive value in the detection of both lesions.

MITRAL STENOSIS AND AORTIC STENOSIS

The left ventricles of patients with these two lesions are usually small, stiff, and hypertrophied. When severe MS and AS coexist, the former masks many of the manifestations of the latter.[526] The cardiac output tends to be reduced further than in patients with isolated AS, and the atrial booster pump mechanism, so important in filling the ventricle in AS (see p. 1035), has little impact when MS is present. The reduction in cardiac output lowers both the transaortic valvular pressure gradient and the left ventricular systolic pressure, diminishes the incidence of angina, and retards the development of aortic valvular calcification and left ventricular hypertrophy.[527] On the other hand, clinical manifestations associated with MS, such as pulmonary congestion and hemoptysis, atrial fibrillation, and systemic embolization, occur more frequently than in patients with isolated AS.

On *physical examination,* presystolic distention of the left ventricle and an S_4, common in pure AS, are usually not present. The midsystolic murmur characteristic of AS may be reduced in intensity and duration because of stroke volume reduced by the MS. The *electrocardiogram* may fail to demonstrate left ventricular hypertrophy, but left atrial enlargement is common in patients in sinus rhythm. The *chest roentgenogram* is usually typical of MS except that calcium may be present in the region of the aortic valve. The two-dimensional and Doppler *echocardiograms* are of the greatest value because stenosis of both valves may be evident. However, the low cardiac output characteristic of the combination of lesions may reduce the transvalvular gradients estimated by Doppler echocardiography. The indirect *carotid pulse* tracing reveals a delayed upstroke.

It is vital to recognize the presence of hemodynamically significant aortic valvular disease (stenosis and/or regurgitation) preoperatively in patients who are to undergo surgical correction of MS because isolated mitral valvulotomy may be hazardous in such patients; this operation can impose a sudden hemodynamic load on the left ventricle that was previously protected by the MS and may lead to acute pulmonary edema.

AORTIC STENOSIS AND MITRAL REGURGITATION

The combination of severe AS and MR is a hazardous one, but fortunately it is relatively uncommon. Obstruction to left ventricular outflow augments the volume of MR flow,[122] whereas the presence of MR diminishes the ventricular preload necessary for maintenance of the left ventricular stroke volume in AS. The result is a reduced forward cardiac output and marked left atrial and pulmonary venous hypertension. The physical findings may be confusing because the delayed arterial pulse of AS may be counteracted by the sharp upstroke of MR, and it may be difficult to recognize two distinct systolic murmurs. Amyl nitrite tends to increase the intensity of the murmur of AS and to reduce that of MR. On echocardiography and roentgenography the left atrium and ventricle are usually larger than in isolated AS. Usually both valves must be treated surgically in patients with severe AS and MR.

AORTIC REGURGITATION AND MITRAL REGURGITATION

This relatively frequent combination of lesions[528] may be caused by rheumatic heart disease or by prolapse of both the aortic and mitral valves due to myxomatous degeneration,[529] or dilatation of both annuli in connective tissue disorders. The left ventricle is usually greatly dilated. The clinical features of AR usually predominate, and it sometimes is difficult to determine whether the MR is due to organic involvement of this valve or dilatation of the mitral valve ring secondary to left ventricular enlargement. When both valvular leaks are severe, this combination of lesions is poorly tolerated. The normal mitral valve ordinarily serves as a "backup" to the aortic valve, and premature (diastolic) closure of the mitral valve limits the volume of reflux that occurs in patients with acute AR.[386] With combined regurgitant lesions, regardless of the cause of the mitral lesion, blood may reflux from the aorta through both chambers of the left side of the heart into the pulmonary veins. Physical and laboratory examination will usually show evidence of both lesions. Both lesions are frequently associated with an S_3 and a brisk arterial pulse. The relative severity of each lesion can be assessed best by contrast angiography.

When MR occurs in patients with AR secondary to left ventricular dilatation, it often regresses following aortic valve replacement. If severe, it may be corrected by annuloplasty at the time of aortic valve replacement. An intrinsically normal mitral valve that is regurgitant due to a dilated annulus should not be replaced.

SURGICAL TREATMENT OF MULTIVALVULAR DISEASE

Combined aortic and mitral valve replacement is usually associated with a higher risk and poorer survival than is replacement of either of the two valves alone.[452] The operative risk of double-valve replacement is about 50 per cent higher than it is for single-valve replacement and, like the latter, has been slowly but steadily declining[530] and now ranges from 5 to 10 per cent. Kirklin reported a 5-year survival rate of 63 per cent after double-valve replacement compared with 80 per cent for single-valve replacement.[452] The long-term survival depends strongly on the preoperative functional status.[531] Patients operated on for the combination of AR and MR fare worse than patients receiving double-valve replacement for any of the other combinations, presumably because both of these valvular abnormalities may produce irreversible left ventricular damage. Mitral repair in combination with aortic valve replacement is preferable to double-valve replacement. Risk factors reducing long-term survival include advanced age, higher New York Heart Association class, greater left ventricular enlargement, and accompanying ischemic heart disease requiring coronary bypass surgery.[452]

Given the higher risks, a higher threshold is required for multivalve versus single-valve surgery. Thus, patients are generally not advised to undergo multivalve surgery until they reach late Class II or Class III (NY Heart Association). Despite detailed noninvasive and invasive workup, the decision to treat more than one valve is often made by palpation or direct inspection at the operating table.

THREE-VALVE DISEASE. Hemodynamically significant disease involving the mitral, aortic, and tricuspid valves is uncommon. Patients with trivalvular disease may present in advanced heart failure with marked cardiomegaly, and surgical correction of all three valvular lesions is imperative. However, triple-valve replacement is a long and complex operation. Early in the experience with this procedure, the mortality rate was 20 per cent in patients in functional Class III and 40 per cent in Class IV. More recently, it has declined to 5 per cent.[531,532] In some patients with trivalvular disease, it is possible to replace the mitral and aortic valves and carry out a tricuspid valvuloplasty.

Patients who survive three-valve surgery usually show substantial clinical improvement in the early postoperative period,[533,534] and postoperative catheterization studies show marked reductions in pulmonary arterial and capillary pressures. However, some patients succumb to arrhythmias[534] or congestive heart failure in the late postoperative period despite three normally functioning prostheses. The cause of cardiac failure in this situation is not known, but it may be related to intraoperative myocardial ischemia, microemboli from the multipole prosthesis, or continued subclinical episodes of rheumatic myocarditis.

When multiple prosthetic valves must be inserted, it is logical to select either two bioprostheses or mechanical prostheses for the left side of the heart. If the patient is to be exposed to the hazards of anticoagulants for one mechanical prosthesis, it seems unreasonable to add the potential risks of early failure of a bioprosthesis. However, if two mechanical prostheses on the left side of the heart are selected, the use of a bioprosthesis in the tricuspid position is suggested.[531]

PROSTHETIC CARDIAC VALVES

The first successful replacements of cardiac valves in the human were accomplished by Nina Braunwald,[535] Harken et al.,[536] and Starr[537] in 1960. Two major groups of artificial (prosthetic) valves are currently available in models designed for both the atrioventricular (mitral and tricuspid) and the aortic positions: mechanical prostheses and bioprostheses (tissue valves).[537a]

MECHANICAL PROSTHESES

Mechanical prosthetic valves are classified into two major groups: caged-ball and tilting-disc valves. The *Starr Edwards* caged-ball valve, the oldest prosthetic valve in continuous use (Figs. 32–49 and 32–50), has the longest record of predictable performance of any artificial valve.[538,539] The poppet is made of silicone rubber, the cage of stellite alloy, and the sewing ring of Teflon/polypropylene cloth. A disadvantage is its bulky cage design; it is not suitable in patients with a small left ventricular cavity or a small aortic annulus or in a valve–aortic arch composite graft. In a small number of patients it induces hemolysis, which may be greatly exaggerated and become of clinical importance if a perivalvular leak develops. In small sizes, this valve may cause mild obstruction, and the incidence of thromboembolism is slightly higher than with the tilting-disc valve.[540]

Several types of tilting-disc valves are widely employed; these are less bulky and have a lower profile than the caged-ball valve. The *St. Jude* valve (Fig. 32–49*D*), currently the most widely used prosthesis on a worldwide basis, is coated with pyrolytic carbon and has two semicircular discs that pivot between open and closed positions without the need for supporting struts (Fig. 32–50). It possesses favorable flow characteristics and causes a lower transvalvular gradient at any outer diameter and cardiac output than the caged-ball or tilting valves.[541,542] The St. Jude valve appears to have particularly favorable hemodynamic characteristics in the smaller sizes; therefore, it is especially useful in children. Thrombogenicity in the mitral position *may* be less than for other prosthetic valves. However, as with other mechanical prostheses, permanent anticoagulation is needed—antiplatelet agents alone are not sufficient.[541] A variation of the St. Jude valve, the *Carbomedics* prosthesis (Fig. 32–49*E*), is also a bileaflet valve composed of pyrolytic carbon with a titanium housing that can be rotated so as to avoid interference with disc excursion by subvalvular tissue.

The *Omniscience* valve (Fig. 32–49*B*), the successor to the *Lillehei-Kaster* pivoting-disc valve, consists of a titanium valve housing with a polyester knit sewing ring in which a pyrolytic disc is suspended. In the open position, the disc swings to an angle of 80 degrees, providing a large central flow orifice.[543,544] A closely related valve is the

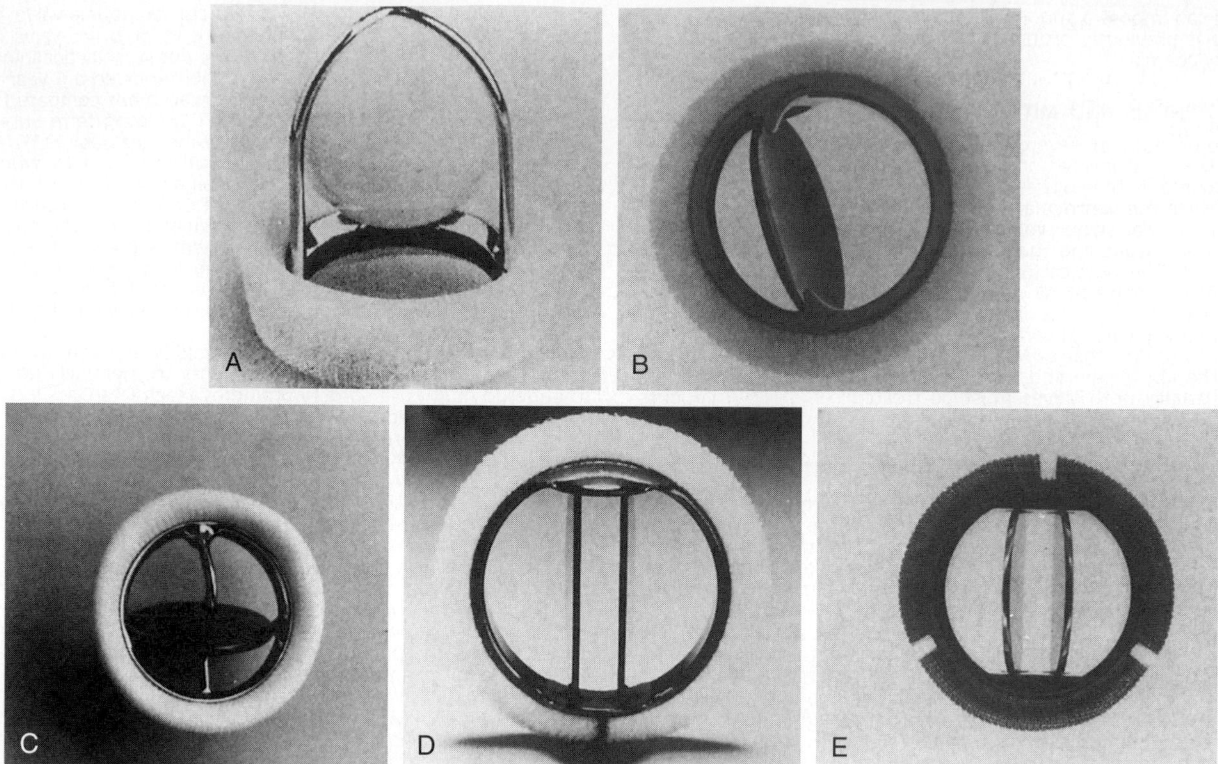

FIGURE 32–49. *A,* The Starr-Edwards ball and cage valve. *B,* The Omniscience valve. *C,* The Medtronic-Hall valve. *D,* The St. Jude valve. *E,* The Carbomedics bileaflet valve. (From Cohn, L. H.: Aortic valve prostheses. Cardiol. Rev. *2*:219, 1995.)

Medtronic-Hall valve (Fig. 32–49*C*), which has a Teflon sewing ring and titanium housing, and its thin, carbon-coated pivoting disc has a central perforation that allows improved hemodynamics. Thrombogenicity appears to be quite low—less than one episode per 100 patient-years in the mitral position[545]—and mechanical performance is excellent over the long term.

DURABILITY AND THROMBOGENICITY. Mechanical prosthetic valves all have an excellent record of durability—up to 35 years in the case of the Starr-Edwards valve. In the mitral position, perivalvular regurgitation appears to occur more frequently with mechanical than with tissue valves.[546] However, patients with any mechanical prosthesis—regardless of design or site of placement—require long-term anticoagulation because of the hazard of thromboembolism, which is greatest in the first postoperative year. Without anticoagulation, the incidence of thromboembolism is three- to sixfold higher than with proper doses. Very rarely, thrombosis of the mechanical valve occurs. This may be a fatal event, but when nonfatal it interferes with prosthetic valve function and may sometimes be managed by thrombolytic therapy (see p. 1596).

Anticoagulation in patients with prosthetic valves is discussed on p. 1066. Sodium warfarin should begin about 2 days after operation, and the INR should be in the range of 2.5 to 3.5.[547] This relatively conservative approach reduces the risk of anticoagulant hemorrhage yet does not appear to be associated with a greater frequency of thromboembolism than an INR of 3.0 to 4.0, which was used in the past. Antiplatelet agents without anticoagulants do not provide adequate protection. However, the addition of 100 mg aspirin daily with coumadin may reduce the risk of embolism.[548]

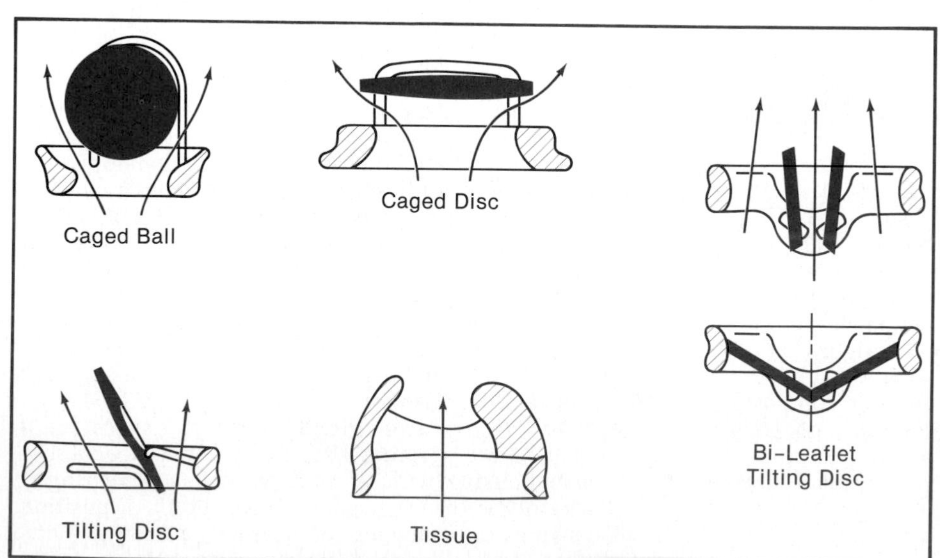

FIGURE 32–50. Designs and flow patterns of major categories of prosthetic heart valves: caged-ball, caged-disc, tilting-disc, bileaflet tilting-disc, and bioprosthetic (tissue) valves. Whereas flow in mechanical valves must course along both sides of the occluder, bioprostheses have a central flow pattern. (Reproduced by permission from Schoen, F. J., et al.: Bioengineering aspects of heart valve replacement. Ann. Biomed. Eng. *10*:97, 1982. Copyright 1983, Pergamon Press Limited, 1983; and from Schoen, F. J.: Pathology of cardiac valve replacement. *In* Morse, D., Steiner, R. M., and Fernandez, J. [eds.]: Guide to Prosthetic Cardiac Valves. New York, Springer-Verlag, 1985, p. 209. Copyright 1985 Springer-Verlag, Inc.)

It must be recognized that (1) the administration of warfarin carries its own mortality and morbidity, estimated at 0.2 and 2.2 per 100 patient-years, respectively; and (2) despite treatment with anticoagulants, the incidence of thromboembolic complications with the best mechanical prosthesis is still about 0.2 (fatal) and 1 to 2 (nonfatal) per 100 patient-years for aortic valves and 2 to 3 for mitral valves.[549] Valve thrombosis, a particularly hazardous complication, occurs at an incidence of about 0.1 per cent per year in the aortic and 0.35 per cent per year in the mitral position. Thrombosis of mechanical prostheses in the tricuspid position is quite high, and for this reason bioprostheses are preferred at this site. The incidence of embolization in patients who have experienced repeated emboli from a prosthetic valve despite anticoagulants may be reduced by replacement with a tissue valve.

Mechanical prostheses regularly cause mild hemolysis,[550] but this is not severe enough to be of clinical importance unless the patient develops periprosthetic regurgitation.

TISSUE VALVES

Tissue valves (bioprostheses) have been developed largely to overcome the risk of thromboembolism that is inherent in all mechanical prosthetic valves and the attendant hazards and inconvenience of permanent anticoagulant therapy. The first of these to be widely used were chemically sterilized aortic homografts obtained from cadavers. However, these exhibited a high incidence of breakdown within 3 years, and antibiotic-treated cryopreserved frozen-irradiated homografts were then developed. These are more durable[551–554] but, although they have many desirable properties, their use has been restricted by the problems inherent in their procurement (see below).

PORCINE HETEROGRAFTS. Porcine aortic heterografts were developed for both the mitral and the aortic positions and have been used clinically since 1965. Three porcine heterografts are widely used today.[544,551–554] (1) The *Hancock* valve (Fig. 32–51*A*) is fixed and preserved in glutaraldehyde and is mounted on a Dacron cloth–covered flexible polypropylene strut. In the smaller aortic models, the right coronary cusp is replaced by a posterior cusp from another valve to reduce obstruction resulting from the septal shelf of the valve. (2) The *Carpentier-Edwards* valve[551] (Fig. 32–51*B*) is pressure-fixed and then preserved in glutaraldehyde and is mounted on a Teflon-covered Eljiloy strut in a manner as to minimize the septal shelf. (3) The *Intact* valve is also glutaraldehyde-treated but at a fixation pressure of zero and with toluidine in an attempt to inhibit calcium deposition.

The hemodynamic profiles of the porcine heterografts are similar to those of comparably sized low-profile mechanical prostheses.[555,556] In contrast to the latter, however, the valve orifice is blood flow–dependent, with greater orifice size as transvalvular flow increases. The Hancock valve has been reported to have slightly better hemodynamics than the Carpentier-Edwards valve.[557]

During the first 3 postoperative months, while the sewing ring becomes endothelialized, the thromboembolic rate is high enough that anticoagulation is extremely desirable.

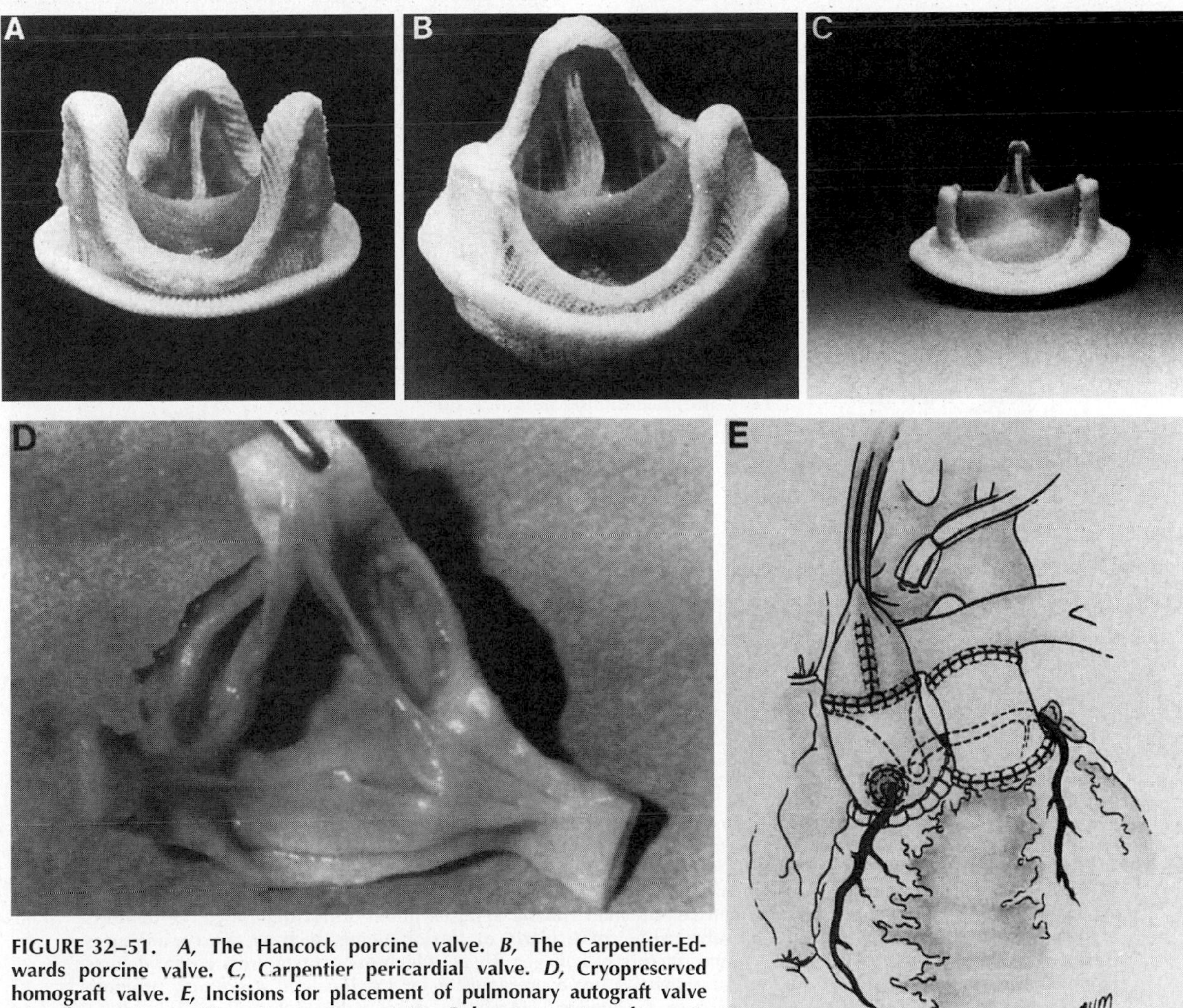

FIGURE 32–51. *A,* The Hancock porcine valve. *B,* The Carpentier-Edwards porcine valve. *C,* Carpentier pericardial valve. *D,* Cryopreserved homograft valve. *E,* Incisions for placement of pulmonary autograft valve into the aortic position. (From Oury, J. H.: Pulmonary autograft—past, present and future. J. Heart Valve Dis. *2:*366, 1993.)

Thereafter, anticoagulants are not required for porcine valves in the aortic position, and the thromboembolic rate is approximately 1 to 2 episodes per 100 patient-years without these drugs.[558] When these valves have been placed in mitral position in patients who are in sinus rhythm, without heart failure, without thrombus in the left atrium or the left atrial appendage, and without a history of embolism preoperatively, anticoagulants are not needed (after the first 3 postoperative months), and the thromboembolic rate is also approximately 1 to 2 per 100 patient-years. This rate is comparable to that observed in patients with the St. Jude or other mechanical valves receiving anticoagulants and therefore subject to the risks of hemorrhage. It is unlikely that any replacement of the mitral valve can be associated with a thromboembolic rate much below 0.5 per 100 patient-years because some of the emboli in patients with longstanding mitral disease are derived from the left atrium rather than from the valve itself.[556] In patients undergoing mitral valve replacement who have experienced a previous embolus, in whom thrombus is found in the left atrium at operation, or who remain in atrial fibrillation postoperatively (approximately one-third of all patients receiving mitral valve replacements), the hazard of thromboembolism persists. Indeed, in patients with atrial fibrillation the incidence of postoperative emboli following implantation of a porcine bioprosthesis into the mitral position is three times as high as in patients in sinus rhythm. Therefore, anticoagulants are indicated in those patients with these three risk factors. The need for anticoagulants negates the principal advantage of the tissue valves.

The major problem with porcine bioprostheses is their limited durability (Fig. 32–52). Cuspal tears, degeneration, fibrin deposition, disruption of the fibrocollagenous structure, perforation, fibrosis, and calcification sufficiently severe to require reoperation begin to appear in some patients in the fourth or fifth postoperative year, and by 10 years the rate of primary tissue failure averages 30 per cent. It then accelerates, and by 15 years the actuarial freedom from bioprosthetic primary tissue failure has ranged from 30 to 60 per cent in several series.[552] Structural valve deterioration is more frequent in patients with bioprostheses in the mitral than in the aortic position, presumably because of the higher closing pressure. It is likely that with the passage of time even more of these valves will fail, and essentially all valves implanted into patients aged less than 60 years may have to be replaced.[559] Fortunately, however, these valves usually do not fail suddenly (as is often the case for structural failure or thrombosis of mechanical prostheses). Rereplacement of a bioprosthetic valve should be carried out when significant and/or progressive deterioration is evident before it becomes an emergency, and the second operation, when carried out on an elective basis, may be associated with a surgical mortality in the range of 10 to 15 per cent. Color Doppler echocardiography with two-dimensional imaging is extremely helpful in the early detection of bioprosthetic malfunction.[555] Transesophageal echocardiography is more sensitive than transthoracic imaging in detecting bioprosthetic valve deterioration. Even patients without new murmurs or other physical findings of valve dysfunction should have routine echocardiographic studies to look for early bioprosthetic valve dysfunction every year for 5 years after valve replacement and every 6 months beginning 8 years after surgery.

The time after implantation at which tissue valves fail varies inversely with age: It is prohibitively rapid in children and adults under 35 to 40 years of age. Therefore, bioprostheses are not advisable in these patient groups. On the other hand, degeneration is extremely rare when these valves are implanted into patients older than 70 years.[558] Bioprostheses also have extremely limited desirability in patients with chronic renal failure and hypercalcemia related to secondary hyperparathyroidism.

Prosthetic valve endocarditis, discussed on pp. 1079 to 1080, is a serious, often grave illness.

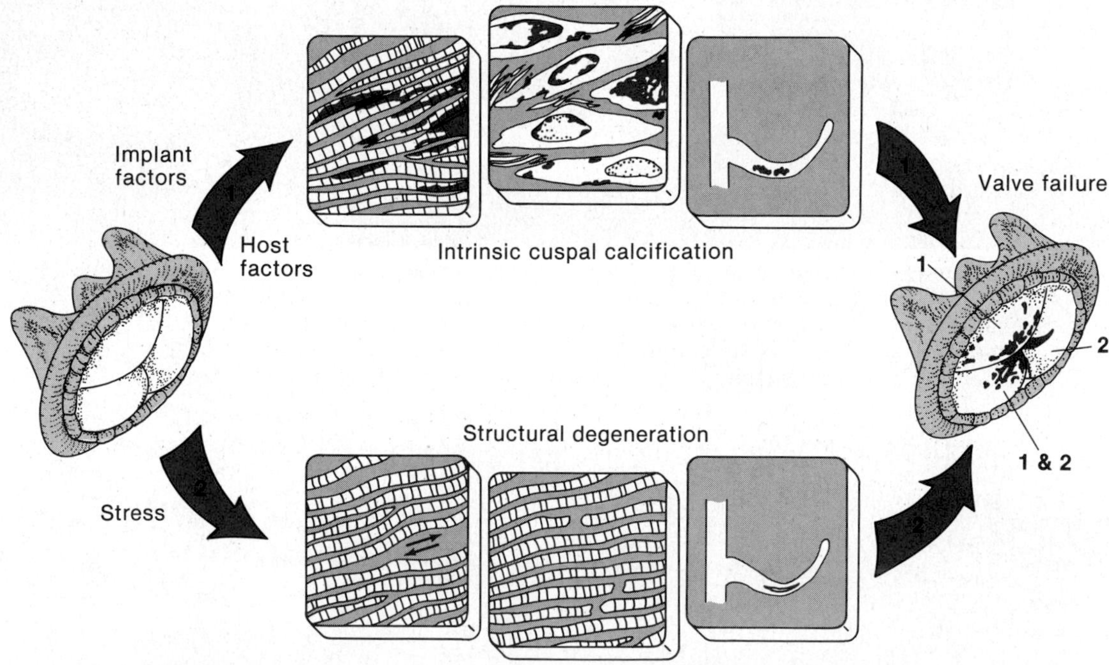

FIGURE 32–52. Unified model for bioprosthetic heart valve failure relating isolated tissue processes of mineralization and collagen degeneration to gross clinical failures. Such failures have calcification with cuspal stiffening (1), cuspal defects without calcific deposits (2), or cuspal tears associated with mineralization (1 and 2). These processes may occur independently or they may be synergistic. Specifically, implant and host factors interact to induce the collagen-oriented and cell-oriented calcific deposits noted ultrastructurally. The deposits predominate in the central portions of valve cusps, particularly at flexion points such as the commissures (Pathway 1). Stress causes shear between and fracture of collagen fibers, which may create gross cuspal defects (Pathway 2). Although dynamic mechanical activity is not a prerequisite for calcification, stress may promote (i.e., accelerate) this process through unknown mechanisms. (Amended from Schoen, F. I., and Levy, R. J.: Bioprosthetic heart valve failure: Pathology and pathogenesis. Cardiol. Clin. 2:717, 1984.)

HOMOGRAFT (ALLOGRAFT) AORTIC VALVES. These are harvested from cadavers, often along with kidneys, and are now usually preserved at −196°C (Fig. 32–51*D*). They are inserted directly—usually in the aortic position—without being placed into a prosthetic stent. Their hemodynamics are superior to those of stented porcine valves. Like porcine xenografts, their thrombogenicity is low, but they appear to be subject to a similar rate of structural deterioration.[552] Homograft aortic valves are indicated in the presence of native or prosthetic valve endocarditis, but they are difficult to use when the aortic root and ascending aorta are greatly enlarged. Availability is often limited.[560,561]

PULMONARY AUTOGRAFTS. The patient's own pulmonary valve and adjacent main pulmonary artery are removed and used to replace the diseased aortic valve and often the neighboring aorta with reimplantation of the coronary arteries into the graft[562–564] (Fig. 32–51*E*). A human pulmonary or aortic homograft is then inserted into the pulmonary position. The autograft is nonthrombogenic and there is evidence in children and adolescents that it grows along with the patient; the risk of endocarditis is very low, anticoagulants are not required, and perhaps most important the long-term durability appears to be excellent.[565–567] While the pulmonary autograft is the replacement valve of choice in children, adolescents, and younger adults who have a long (>20 year) life expectancy, its use has been limited because the operation is technically much more complex than a simple aortic valve replacement. It should be carried out only by experienced surgeons.

HEMODYNAMICS OF VALVE REPLACEMENTS

The most commonly used prosthetic valves, mechanical prostheses and stented porcine xenografts, have an effective in vitro orifice size that is *smaller* than the normal valve at the same site.[568] (Unstented, i.e., free, homografts and pulmonary autografts have this problem.) After implantation, tissue ingrowth and endothelialization reduce the size of the in vivo effective orifice further. Therefore, the valves currently available must be considered to be mildly stenotic. However, postoperative hemodynamic measurements of the rigid prostheses show reasonably good function, with effective mitral valve orifice areas averaging 1.7 to 2.0 cm^2 and mitral valve gradients of 4 to 8 mm Hg at rest. The cloth-covered Starr-Edwards valve appears to be intrinsically slightly more stenotic than the Medtronic-Hall or Omniscience tilting-disc valves. The bileaflet St. Jude and Carbomedics valves, in turn, may be slightly superior to the latter. In hemodynamic studies, the porcine mitral valves behave in a manner similar to that of a mechanical prosthetic valve of the same diameter. Serious hemodynamic obstruction of an artificial valve (most commonly Starr-Edwards) in the mitral position is quite uncommon, unless the valve is placed into a small left ventricular cavity or into an unusually small mitral annulus or unless the prosthesis chosen is inappropriate in size.

The problem of intrinsic stenosis may be more serious in patients who undergo aortic valve replacements for AS. The annulus into which the prosthesis is inserted in these patients is usually smaller than it is in patients with AR, and the surgeon may be forced to select an artificial valve of relatively small size. As a consequence, aortic valve replacement may not abolish obstruction in AS but may merely convert severe obstruction to a mild or moderate type. When the smaller models of the porcine xenograft or mechanical prosthesis are placed into the aortic position, effective orifice areas of about 1.1 to 1.3 cm^2 are common. In such patients, peak transvalvular gradients as high as 40 mm Hg during exercise have been recorded. It is possible that the poor late results observed in a minority of patients undergoing replacement of stenotic aortic valves may be the delayed effects of moderate stenosis of the prosthesis. In patients with AS who do not exhibit clinical improvement postoperatively, it is important to evaluate the function of both the prosthetic valve and the left ventricle. Rarely, reoperation to correct a malfunctioning prosthesis may be necessary.

SELECTION OF AN ARTIFICIAL VALVE

Most comparisons of mechanical and bioprostheses indicate similar overall results in terms of early and late mortality, prosthetic valve endocarditis and other complications, and the need for reoperation, at least for the first 5 years postoperatively. As indicated, there appear to be no significant differences insofar as hemodynamics are concerned, except that in patients with an unusually small left ventricular cavity or mitral or aortic annulus, the low-profile (tilting-disc) St. Jude or Carbomedics prosthesis or a tissue valve may perform better than other valves.[568,569] Patients with small aortic annuli may be better candidates for unstented homografts, heterografts, or pulmonary autografts.

The major task in selection of an artifical valve is to weigh the advantage of durability and the disadvantages of the risk of thromboembolism and of anticoagulant treatment inherent in mechanical prostheses on the one hand with the advantage of low thrombogenicity and the serious disadvantage of abbreviated durability of the bioprostheses on the other. Hammermeister et al.[570] has compared the outcome in 575 men who were randomized to replacement of the mitral or aortic valve with a mechanical versus a bioprosthetic valve. There was no difference in survival or in the probability of developing a valve-related complica-

TABLE 32–11 PROBABILITY OF DEATH DUE TO ANY CAUSE, ANY VALVE-RELATED COMPLICATION, AND INDIVIDUAL VALVE-RELATED COMPLICATIONS 11 YEARS AFTER RANDOMIZATION, ACCORDING TO TYPE AND LOCATION OF REPLACEMENT VALVE

	AORTIC VALVE		MITRAL VALVE	
EVENT	Mechanical Prosthesis (N = 198)	Bioprosthesis (N = 196)	Mechanical Prosthesis (N = 88)	Bioprosthesis (N = 93)
Death from any cause	0.53	0.59	0.64	0.67
Any valve-related complication	0.62	0.64	0.71	0.79
Systemic embolism	0.16	0.15	0.18	0.15
Bleeding	0.43	0.24*	0.41	0.28†
Endocarditis	0.07	0.08	0.11	0.17
Valve thrombosis	0.02	0.01	0.01	0.01
Perivalvular regurgitation	0.04	0.02	0.17	0.09†
Reoperation	0.07	0.16	0.21	0.47
Structural valve failure	0.00	0.15*	0.00	0.36*

P values are for the difference in the probability of event-free survival between patients with a mechanical prosthesis and those with a bioprosthesis at each site: $*P < 0.001$; $†P < 0.05$.

From Hammermeister, K. E., Sethi, G. K., Henderson, W. G., et al.: A comparison of outcomes in men 11 years after heart-valve replacement with a mechanical valve or bioprosthesis. N. Engl. J. Med. *328*:1289, 1993.

tion, including endocarditis, valve thrombosis, and systemic embolism. The rate of structurally-related valve failure requiring reoperation (which is associated with about twice the mortality of the initial procedure) was much higher in patients receiving tissue as opposed to mechanical valves. On the other hand, as anticipated, anticoagulant-related bleeding was higher in patients receiving mechanical valves. The latter also had a higher incidence of perivalvular regurgitation in the mitral position (Table 32–11). In the Edinburgh randomized trial, which also compared a mechanical with a porcine xenograft valve,[571] actuarial survival tended to be better and the freedom from all valve-related adverse events was significantly better with mechanical valves. Therefore, mechanical prostheses, usually of the bileaflet variety, are the valves of choice in the majority of patients. However, the following groups of patients should receive bioprostheses: (1) patients with coexisting disease who are prone to hemorrhage, such as those with bleeding disorders, intestinal polyposis, and angiodysplasia; (2) patients who are noncompliant with permanent anticoagulant treatment, who are unwilling to take anticoagulants on a regular basis, or who live in developing nations and cannot be monitored; (3) patients over the age of 65 to 70 years, in whom bioprosthetic valves deteriorate very slowly, who are unlikely to outlive their bioprostheses and who by reason of their age may also be at greater risk of hemorrhage while taking anticoagulants; (4) patients with a small aortic annulus in whom an unstented (free) autograft may provide superior hemodynamics; and (5) younger (<40 years) patients, especially women wishing to bear children, who require aortic valve replacement and in whom a pulmonary autograft may be preferable. However, the technical difficulties associated with the latter procedure must be taken into account.

Special Situations

PREGNANCY (see also p. 1856). Women with artificial valves can tolerate the hemodynamic burden of pregnancy well, but the hypercoagulable state of pregnancy increases the risk of thromboembolism in such patients with mechanical prostheses. Anticoagulation must not be interrupted, although an increased risk of fatal fetal hemorrhage is seen in those in whom it is continued. There is also a risk of fetal malformation caused by the probable teratogenic effect of warfarin. Although these problems represent arguments for the use of tissue valves in all women of childbearing age,[570,571] their limited durability in young adults makes their use unacceptable. Therefore, unless a pulmonary autograft can be employed (for patients who require aortic valve replacement), every effort should be made to defer valve replacement until after childbirth. In pregnant women with critical mitral or aortic stenosis, balloon valvuloplasty should be considered, and, if at all possible, mitral valve repair should be undertaken for patients with MR. Women of childbearing potential with a mechanical prosthesis should be counseled against pregnancy. When a woman in whom a mechanical prosthetic valve is already in place becomes pregnant, the risk to the fetus if the mother receives oral anticoagulants appears to be lower than the risk to the mother if anticoagulants are discontinued. Therefore, coumarin derivatives should be continued and the INR maintained between 2 and 3 until 2 weeks before expected delivery, when the patient should be switched to intravenous heparin.[570–572] Heparin should be discontinued at the onset of labor but may be restarted, along with coumarin, several hours after delivery.

NONCARDIAC SURGERY. When this is required in patients with prosthetic valves who are receiving anticoagulants, the risk is minimal when the drug regimen is stopped 1 to 3 days preoperatively and for a similar period postoperatively. It may be desirable, however, to protect the patient with low molecular weight dextran during the perioperative period.

PATIENTS DESTINED TO RECEIVE ANTICOAGULANTS. Patients with earlier implantation of a mechanical prosthesis, chronic atrial fibrillation in the presence of an enlarged left atrium, a history of thromboembolism, or a thrombus in the left atrium at operation (and who therefore are destined to receive anticoagulants) should receive a mechanical prosthesis because the potential advantage of a tissue valve is negated.

CHILDREN AND PATIENTS RECEIVING CHRONIC HEMODIALYSIS. The high incidence of bioprosthetic valve failure in children and adolescents[573,574] and in patients on chronic hemodialysis virtually prohibits their use in these groups. In young adults between the ages of 25 and 35, the failure of bioprosthetic valves is somewhat higher than it is in older adults; this serves as a relative, but not an absolute, contraindication to their use in this age group.

In children, a mechanical prosthesis (generally the St. Jude valve) with its favorable hemodynamics is preferred despite the disadvantages inherent in anticoagulants in this age group.[575] Similarly, mechanical prostheses should be used in patients with chronic renal failure and/or hypercalcemia. Alternatively, if an experienced surgical team is available and the patient requires an aortic valve replacement, a pulmonary autograft may be employed.

TRICUSPID POSITION. The risk of thrombosis for all valves is highest in the tricuspid position because of the lower pressures and velocity of blood flow; this complication appears to be highest for tilting-disc valves, intermediate for caged-ball valves, and lowest for the bioprostheses, which are the valves of choice as tricuspid replacements. In the tricuspid position bioprostheses exhibit a much slower rate of mechanical deterioration than in the mitral or aortic position.

Detection of Prosthetic Valve Dysfunction

Artificial valves have distinctive auscultatory and phonocardiographic characteristics.[576] Transthoracic and transesophageal echocardiography, phonocardiography, and cineradiography are extremely useful in the identification of artificial valve dysfunction.[577,578] Two-dimensional and Doppler echocardiography are particularly useful in the follow-up of patients who demonstrate clinical deterioration in the postoperative period following porcine heterograft implantation. These techniques may prove capable of distinguishing between failure of a bioprosthesis (abnormal valve motion) and left ventricular dysfunction.

REFERENCES

MITRAL STENOSIS

1. Olson, L. J., Subramanian, R., and Ackermann, D. M.: Surgical pathology of the mitral valve: A study of 712 cases spanning 21 years. Mayo Clin. Proc. *62*:22, 1987.
2. Bortolotti, U., Valente, M., Agozzino, L., et al.: Rheumatoid mitral stenosis requiring valve replacement. Am. Heart J. *107*:1049, 1984.
3. Ladefoged, C., and Rohr, N.: Amyloid deposits in aortic and mitral valves. Virchows Arch. (A) *404*:301, 1984.
4. Misch, K. A.: Development of heart valve lesions during methylsergide therapy. Br. Med. J. *2*:365, 1974.
5. Wrisley, D., Giambartolomei, A., Lee, I., and Brownlee, W.: Left atrial ball thrombus: Review of clinical and echocardiographic manifestations with suggestions for management. Am. Heart. J. *121*:1784, 1991.
6. Kumar, A., Sinha, M., and Sinha, D. N. P.: Chronic rheumatic heart diseases in Ranchi. Angiology *33*:141, 1982.
7. Delahaye, F., Delahaye, J., Ecochard, R., et al.: Influence of associated valvular lesions on long-term prognosis of mitral stenosis: A 20-year follow-up of 202 patients. Eur. Heart J. *12*(Suppl B):77, 1991.
8. Schoen, F. J., and St. John Sutton, M.: Contemporary pathologic considerations in valvular disease. *In* Virmani, R., Atkinson, J. B., and Feuoglio, J. J. (eds.): Cardiovascular Pathology. Philadelphia, W. B. Saunders Co., 1991, p. 334.
9. Wells, F. C., and Shapiro, L. M. (eds.): Mitral Valve Disease. 2nd ed. London, Butterworths, 1996, 204 pp.
10. Bowe, J. C., Bland, F., Sprague, H. B., and White, P. D.: Course of mitral stenosis without surgery: 10 and 20 year perspectives. Ann. Intern. Med. *52*:741, 1960.

11. Bell, M. H., and Mintz, G. S.: Mitral valve disease in the elderly. *In* Frankl, W. S., and Brest, A. N. (eds.): Cardiovascular Clinics. Valvular Heart Disease: Comprehensive Evaluation and Management. Philadelphia, F. A. Davis, 1986, pp. 313–324.
12. Chopra, P., Tandon, H. D., Raizada, V., et al.: Comparative studies in mitral valves in rheumatic heart disease. Arch. Intern. Med. *143*:661, 1983.
12a. Kawanishi, D. T., and Rahimtoola, S. H.: Mitral stenosis. *In* Rahimtoola, S. H. (ed.): Valvular Heart Disease and Endocarditis. Atlas of Heart Diseases. Vol. 11. St. Louis, Mosby, 1996.
13. Dalen, J. E., and Alpert, J. S. (eds.): Valvular Heart Disease. 2nd ed. Boston, Little, Brown and Co., 1987, 600 pp.
14. Wood, P.: An appreciation of mitral stenosis. Br. Med. J. *1*:1051, and 1113, 1954.
15. Reichek, N., Shelburne, J. D., and Perloff, J. R.: Clinical aspects of rheumatic valvular disease. Prog. Cardiovasc. Dis. *15*:491, 1973.
15a. Grossman, W.: Profiles in valvular heart disease. *In* Baim, D. S., and Grossman, W. (eds.): Cardiac Catheterization, Angiography and Interventions. 5th ed. Baltimore, Williams and Wilkins, 1996, pp. 735–756.
16. Leavitt, J. L., Coats, M. H., and Falk, R. H.: Effects of exercise on transmitral gradient and pulmonary artery pressure in patients with mitral stenosis or a prosthetic mitral valve: A Doppler echocardiographic study. J. Am. Coll. Cardiol. *17*:1520, 1991.
17. Selzer, A.: Effects of atrial fibrillation upon the circulation in patients with mitral stenosis. Am. Heart J. *59*:518, 1960.
18. Gorlin, R., and Gorlin, S. G.: Hydraulic formula for calculation of the area of stenotic mitral valve, other cardiac valves and central circulatory shunts. Am. Heart J. *41*:1, 1951.
18a. Braunwald, E., and Turi, Z. G.: Pathophysiology of mitral valve disease. *In* Wells, F. C., and Shapiro, L. M. (eds.): Mitral Valve Disease. 2nd ed. London, Butterworths, 1996, pp. 28–36.
19. Ford, L. E., Feldman, T., and Carroll, J. D.: Valve resistance. Circulation *89*:893, 1994.
20. Kennedy, J. W.: The use of quantitative angiocardiography in mitral valve disease. *In* Duran, C., Angell, W. W., Johnson, A. D., and Oury, J. H. (eds.): Recent Progress in Mitral Valve Disease. London, Butterworths, 1984, pp. 149–159.
21. Gash, A. K., Carabello, B. A., Cepin, D., and Spann, J. F.: Left ventricular ejection performance and systolic muscle function in patients with mitral stenosis. Circulation *67*:148, 1983.
22. Colle, J. P., Rahal, S., Ohayon, J., et al.: Global left ventricular function and regional wall motion in pure mitral stenosis. Clin. Cardiol. *7*:573, 1984.
23. Gaasch, W. H., and Folland, E. D.: Left ventricular function in rheumatic mitral stenosis. Eur. Heart J. *12*(Suppl. B):66, 1991.
24. Harvey, R. M., Ferrer, M. I., Samet, P., et al.: Mechanical and myocardial factors in rheumatic heart disease in mitral stenosis. Circulation *11*:531, 1955.
25. Mohan, J. C., Khalilullah, M., and Arora, R.: Left ventricular intrinsic contractility in pure rheumatic mitral stenosis. Am. J. Cardiol. *64*:240, 1989.
26. Reis, R. N., and Roberts, W. C.: Amounts of coronary arterial narrowing by atherosclerotic plaques in clinically isolated mitral valve stenosis: Analysis of 76 necropsy patients older than 30 years. Am. J. Cardiol. *57*:1117, 1986.
27. Johnston, D. L., and Kotsuk, W. J.: Left and right ventricular function during symptom-limited exercise in patients with isolated mitral stenosis. Chest *89*:186, 1986.
28. Wroblewski, E., Spann, J. F., and Bove, A. A.: Right ventricular performance in mitral stenosis. Am. J. Cardiol. *47*:51, 1981.
29. Halperin, J. L., Brooks, K. M., Rothlauf, E. B., et al.: Effect of nitroglycerin on the pulmonary venous gradient in patients after mitral valve replacement. J. Am. Coll. Cardiol. *5*:34, 1985.
30. Haworth, S. G., Hall, S. M., and Patel, M.: Peripheral pulmonary vascular and airway abnormalities in adolescents with rheumatic mitral stenosis. Int. J. Cardiol. *18*:405, 1988.
31. Babic, U. U., Popovic, Z., Grujicic, S., et al.: Systemic and pulmonary flow in mitral stenosis: Evidence for a bronchial vein shunt. Cardiology *78*:311, 1991.
32. Keren, G., Etzion, T., Sherez, J., et al.: Atrial fibrillation and atrial enlargement in patients with mitral stenosis. Am. Heart J. *114*:1146, 1987.
32a. Leatham, A.: Assessment of mitral valve function: clinical presentation, assessment and prognosis. *In* Wells, F. C., and Shapiro, L. M. (eds.): Mitral Valve Disease. 2nd ed. London, Butterworths, 1996, pp. 37–46.
33. Scarlat, A., Bodner, G., and Liron, M.: Massive haemoptysis as the presenting symptom in mitral stenosis. Thorax *41*:413, 1986.
34. Ohmichi, M., Tagaki, S., Nomura, N., et al.: Endobronchial changes in chronic pulmonary venous hypertension. Chest *94*:1127, 1988.
35. Baxter, R. H., Reid, J. M., McGuiness, J. B., and Stevenson, J. G.: Relation of angina to coronary artery disease in mitral and aortic valve disease. Br. Heart J. *40*:918, 1978.
36. Nielson, G. H., Galea, E. G., and Houssack, K. F.: Thromboembolic complications of mitral valve disease. Aust. N. Z. J. Med. *8*:372, 1978.
37. Lie, J. T., and Entmann, M. L.: "Hole-in-one" sudden death: Mitral stenosis and left atrial thrombus. Am. Heart J. *91*:798, 1976.
38. Sharma, N. G. K., Kapoor, C. P., Mahambre, L., and Borkar, M. P.: Ortner's syndrome. J. Indian Med. Assoc. *60*:427, 1973.
39. Horwitz, L. D., and Groves, B. M. (eds.): Signs and Symptoms in Cardiology. Philadelphia, J.B. Lippincott, 1985, 506 pp.
40. Abrams, J.: Mitral stenosis. *In* Essentials of Cardiac Physical Diagnosis. Philadelphia, Lea and Febiger, 1987, pp. 275–306.
41. Longhini, C., Baracca, E., Aggio, S., et al.: The first heart sound in mitral stenosis. Acta Cardiol. (Brux.) *46*:73, 1991.
42. Barrington, W. W., Boudoulas, J., Bashore, T., et al.: Mitral stenosis: Mitral dome excursion and M_1 and the mitral opening snap—the concept of reciprocal heart sounds. Am. Heart J. *115*:1280, 1988.
43. Perloff, J. K.: Auscultatory and phonocardiographic manifestations of pulmonary hypertension. Prog. Cardiovasc. Dis. *9*:303, 1967.
44. Saunders, J. L., Calatayud, J. B., Schultz, K. J., et al.: Evaluation of ECG criteria for P-wave abnormalities. Am. Heart J. *74*:757, 1967.
45. Walston, A., Harley, A., and Pipberger, H. V.: Computer analysis of the orthogonal electrocardiogram and vectorcardiogram in mitral stenosis. Circulation *50*:472, 1974.
46. Cooksey, J. D., Dunn, M., and Massie, E.: Clinical Vectorcardiography and Electrocardiography. 2nd ed. Chicago, Year Book Medical Publishers, 1977, p. 272.
47. Mounsey, P.: The atrial electrocardiogram as a guide to prognosis after mitral valvulotomy. Br. Heart J. *21*:617, 1961.
48. Probst, P., Goldschlager, N., and Selzer, A.: Left atrial size and atrial fibrillation in mitral stenosis: Factors influencing their relationship. Circulation *48*:1281, 1973.
49. Cueto, J., Toshima, J., Armyo, G., et al.: Vectorcardiographic studies in acquired valvular disease with reference to the diagnosis of right ventricular hypertrophy. Circulation *33*:588, 1967.
50. Taymor, R. C., Hoffman, I., and Henry, E.: The Frank vectorcardiogram in mitral stenosis. Circulation *30*:865, 1964.
51. Donoso, E., Jick, S., Braunwald, E., et al.: The spatial vectorcardiogram in mitral valve disease. Am. Heart J. *53*:760, 1957.
52. Melhem, R. E., Dunbar, J. D., and Booth, R. W.: "B" lines of Kerley and left atrial size in mitral valve disease: Their correlation with mean atrial pressure as measured by left atrial puncture. Radiology *76*:65, 1961.
53. Parker, B. M., Friedenberg, M. J., Templeton, A. W., and Burford, T. H.: Preoperative angiocardiographic diagnosis of left atrial thrombi in mitral stenosis. N. Engl. J. Med. *273*:136, 1965.
54. Rahimtoola, S. H.: Perspective on valvular heart disease: An update. J. Am. Coll. Cardiol. *14*:1, 1989.
55. Shapiro, L. M.: Echocardiography of the mitral valve. *In* Wells, F. C., and Shapiro, L. M. (eds.): Mitral Valve Disease. 2nd ed. London, Butterworths, 1996, pp. 47–50.
56. Shandheria, B. K., Tajik, A. J., Reeder, G. S., et al.: Doppler color flow imaging: A new technique for visualization and characterization of the blood flow jet in mitral stenosis. Mayo Clin. Proc. *61*:623, 1986.
57. Beiser, G. D., Epstein, S. E., Braunwald, E., et al.: Studies on digitalis. XVIII. Effects of ouabain on the hemodynamic response to exercise in patients with mitral stenosis in normal sinus rhythm. N. Engl. J. Med. *278*:131, 1968.
58. Klein, H. O., Sareli, P., Schamroth, C. L., et al.: Effects of atenolol on exercise capacity in patients with mitral stenosis with sinus rhythm. Am. J. Cardiol. *56*:598, 1985.
59. Kosakai, Y., Kawaguchi, A. T., Isobe, F., et al.: Cox maze procedure for chronic atrial fibrillation associated with mitral valve disease. J. Thorac. Cardiovasc. Surg. *108*:1049, 1994.
60. Shyu, K. G., Cheng, J. J., Chen, J. J., et al.: Recovery of atrial function after atrial compartment operation for chronic atrial fibrillation in mitral valve disease. J. Am. Coll. Cardiol. *24*:392, 1994.
61. Chua, Y. L., Schaff, H. V., Orszulak, T. A., and Morris, J. J.: Outcome of mitral valve repair in patients with preoperative atrial fibrillation: Should the maze procedure be combined with mitral valvuloplasty? J. Thorac. Cardiovasc. Surg. *107*:408, 1994.
62. Joswig, B. C., Glover, M. U., Handler, J. B., et al.: Contrasting progression of mitral stenosis in the Malayans versus American-born Caucasians. Am. Heart J. *104*:1400, 1982.
63. Olesen, K. H.: The natural history of 271 patients with mitral stenosis under medical treatment. Br. Heart J. *24*:349, 1962.
64. Rowe, J. C., Bland, E. F., Sprague, H. B., and White, P. D.: The course of mitral stenosis without surgery: Ten- and twenty-year perspectives. Ann. Intern. Med. *52*:741, 1960.
65. Munoz, S., Gallardo, J., Diaz-Gorrin, J. R., and Medina, O.: Influence of surgery on the natural history of rheumatic mitral and aortic valve disease. Am. J. Cardiol. *35*:234, 1975.
66. Rapaport, E.: Natural history of aortic and mitral valve disease. Am. J. Cardiol. *35*:221, 1975.
67. Sutton, M. J. St. J., Oldershaw, P., Sacchetti, R., et al.: Valve replacement without preoperative cardiac catheterization. N. Engl. J. Med. *305*:1233, 1981.
68. Slater, J., Gindea, A. J., Freedberg, R. S., et al.: Comparison of cardiac catheterization and Doppler echocardiography in the decision to operate in aortic and mitral valve disease. J. Am. Coll. Cardiol. *17*:1026, 1991.
69. O'Rourke, R. A.: Preoperative cardiac catheterization. Its need in most patients with valvular heart disease. JAMA *248*:745, 1982.
70. Ramsdale, D. R., Faragher, E. B., Bennett, D. H., et al.: Preoperative prediction of significant coronary artery disease in patients with valvular heart disease. Br. Med. J. *284*:223, 1982.
71. Gautam, P. C., Coulshed, N., Epstein, E. J., et al.: Preoperative clinical predictors of long-term survival in mitral stenosis: Analysis of 200 cases followed for up to 27 years after closed mitral valvotomy. Thorax *41*:401, 1986.

72. English, T.: Closed mitral valvotomy. *In* Wells, F. C., and Shapiro, L. M. (eds.): Mitral Valve Disease. 2nd ed. London, Butterworths, 1996, pp. 107–113.
73. de Vivie, E. R., and Hellberg, K.: Closed transventricular mitral commissurotomy. *In* Ionescu, M. I., and Cohn, L. H. (eds.): Mitral Valve Disease: Diagnosis and Treatment. London, Butterworths, 1985, pp. 139–152.
74. Duran, C.: Mitral reconstruction in predominant mitral stenosis. *In* Duran, C., Angell, W. W., Johnson, A. D., and Oury, J. H. (eds.): Recent Progress in Mitral Valve Disease. London, Butterworths, 1984, pp. 255–264.
75. Farhat, M. B., Boussadia, H., Gandjbakhch, I., et al.: Closed versus open mitral commissurotomy in pure noncalcific mitral stenosis: Hemodynamic studies before and after operation. J. Thorac. Cardiovasc. Surg. *99*:639, 1990.
76. Cohn, L. H., Allred, E. N., Cohn, L. A., et al.: Long-term results of open mitral valve reconstruction for mitral stenosis. Am. J. Cardiol. *55*:731, 1985.
77. John, S., Bashi, V. V., Jairaj, P. S., et al.: Closed mitral valvotomy: Early results and long-term follow-up of 3724 consecutive patients. Circulation *68*:891, 1983.
78. Cohen, D. J., Kuntz, R. E., Gordon, S. P. F., et al.: Predictors of long-term outcome after percutaneous balloon mitral valvuloplasty. N. Engl. J. Med. *327*:1329, 1992.
79. Hickey, M. S., Blackstone, E. H., Kirklin, J. W., and Dean, L. S.: Outcome probabilities and life history after surgical mitral commissurotomy: Implications for balloon commissurotomy. J. Am. Coll. Cardiol. *17*:29, 1991.
80. Eguaras, M. G., Luque, I., Montero, A., et al.: Conservative operation for mitral stenosis: Independent determinants of late results. J. Thorac. Cardiovasc. Surg. *95*:1031, 1988.
81. Gross, R. J., Cunningham, J. N., Jr., Snively, S. L., et al.: Long-term results of open radical mitral commissurotomy: Ten year follow-up study of 202 patients. Am. J. Cardiol. *47*:821, 1981.
82. Kirklin, J. W., and Barrat-Boyes, B. G.: Mitral commissurotomy. *In* Cardiac Surgery. 2nd ed. New York, Churchill-Livingstone, 1993, p. 444.
83. Aora, R., Khalilullah, M., Gupta, M. P., and Padmavati, S.: Mitral restenosis. Incidence and epidemiology. Indian Heart J. *30*:265, 1978.
84. Heger, J. J., Wann, L. S., Weyman, A. E., et al.: Long-term changes in mitral valve area after successful mitral commissurotomy. Circulation *59*:443, 1979.
85. Higgs, L. M., Glancy, D. L., O'Brien, K. P., et al.: Mitral restenosis: An uncommon cause of recurrent symptoms following mitral commissurotomy. Am. J. Cardiol. *26*:34, 1970.
86. Braunwald, E., Braunwald, N. S., Ross, J., Jr., and Morrow, A. G.: Effects of mitral valve replacement on the pulmonary vascular dynamics of patients with pulmonary hypertension. N. Engl. J. Med. *273*:509, 1965.
87. Foltz, B. D., Hessel, E. A., and Ivey, T. D.: The early course of pulmonary artery hypertension in patients undergoing mitral valve replacement with cardioplegic arrest. J. Thorac. Cardiovasc. Surg. *88*:238, 1984.
88. Shapiro, L. M.: Balloon dilatation of the stenotic mitral valve. *In* Wells, F. C., and Shapiro, L. M. (eds.): Mitral Valve Disease. 2nd ed. London, Butterworths, 1996, pp. 181–186.
89. Palacios, I. F., Tuzeu, M. E., Weyman, A. E., et al.: Clinical follow-up of patients undergoing percutaneous mitral balloon valvotomy. Circulation *91*:671, 1995.
90. Chen, C-R., and Cheng, T. O.: Percutaneous balloon mitral valvuloplasty by the Inoue technique: A multicenter study of 4832 patients in China. Am. Heart J. *129*:1197, 1995.
90a. Berman, A. D., McKay, R. G., and Grossman, W.: Balloon valvuloplasty. *In* Baim, D. S., and Grossman, W. (eds.): Cardiac Catheterization, Angiography and Intervention. 2nd ed. Baltimore, Williams and Wilkins, 1996, pp. 659–688.
91. L'Epine, Y., Drobinski, G., Sotirov, Y., et al.: Right heart failure due to an inter-atrial shunt after percutaneous mitral balloon dilatation. Eur. Heart J. *10*:285, 1989.
92. Fawzy, M. E., Mimish, L., Sivanandam, V., et al.: Immediate and long-term effect of mitral balloon valvotomy on severe pulmonary hypertension in patients with mitral stenosis. Am. Heart J. *131*:89, 1996.
93. Wilkins, G. T., Weyman, A. E., Abascal, V. M., et al.: Percutaneous mitral valvotomy: An analysis of echocardiographic variables related to outcome and the mechanism of dilatation. Br. Heart. J. *60*:299, 1988.
94. Tuzcu, E. M., Block, P. C., Griffin, B., et al.: Percutaneous mitral balloon valvotomy in patients with calcific mitral stenosis: Immediate and long-term outcome. J. Am. Coll. Cardiol. *23*:1604, 1994.
95. Reyes, V. P., Raju, B. S., Wynne, J., et al.: Percutaneous balloon valvuloplasty compared with open surgical commissurotomy for mitral stenosis. N. Engl. J. Med. *331*:961, 1994.
96. Post, J. R., Feldman, T., Isner, J., and Herrmann, H. C.: Inoue balloon mitral valvotomy in patients with severe valvular and subvalvular deformity. J. Am. Coll. Cardiol. *25*:1129, 1995.
96a. Trevino, A. J., Ibarra, M., Garcia, A., et al.: Immediate and long-term results of balloon mitral commissurotomy for rheumatic mitral stenosis: Comparison between Inoue and double-balloon techniques. Am. Heart J. *131*:530, 1996.
97. Iung, B., Cormier, B., Elias, J., et al.: Usefulness of percutaneous balloon commissurotomy for mitral stenosis during pregnancy. Am. J. Cardiol. *73*:398, 1994.
98. Zhang, H. P., Allen, J. W., Lau, F. Y. K., and Ruiz, C. E.: Immediate and late outcome of percutaneous balloon mitral valvotomy in patients with significantly calcified valves. Am. Heart J. *129*:501, 1995.
98a. Carabello, B.: Mitral regurgitation. *In* Rahimtoola, S. H. (ed.): Valvular Heart Disease and Endocarditis. Atlas of Heart Diseases. Vol. 11. St. Louis, Mosby, 1996.

MITRAL REGURGITATION

99. Davies, M. J.: Aetiology and pathology of the diseased mitral valve. *In* Ionescu, M. I., and Cohn, L. H. (eds.): Mitral Valve Disease: Diagnosis and Treatment. London, Butterworths, 1985, pp. 27–42.
99a. Anderson, R. H., and Wilcox, B. R.: The anatomy of the mitral valve. *In* Wells, F. C., and Shapiro, L. M. (eds.): Mitral Valve Disease. 2nd ed. London, Butterworths, 1996, pp. 4–13.
100. Marcus, R. H., Sareli, P., Pocock, W. A., and Barlow, J. B.: The spectrum of severe rheumatic mitral valve disease in a developing country: Correlations among clinical presentation, surgical pathologic findings, and hemodynamic sequelae. Ann. Intern. Med. *120*:177, 1994.
101. Essop, M. R., Skoularigis, J., and Sareli, P.: Transesophageal echocardiography in congenital submitral aneurysm. Am. J. Cardiol. *71*:481, 1993.
102. Boltwood, C. M., Tei, C., Wong, M., and Shah, P. M.: Quantitative echocardiography of the mitral complex in dilated cardiomyopathy: The mechanism of functional mitral regurgitation. Circulation *68*:498, 1983.
103. Keren, G., Sonnenblick, E. H., and LeJemtel, T. H.: Mitral annulus motion: Relation to pulmonary venous and transmitral flows in normal subjects and in patients with dilated cardiomyopathy. Circulation *78*:621, 1988.
103a. Mann, J. M., and Davies, M. J.: The pathology of the mitral valve. *In* Wells, F. C., and Shapiro, L. M. (eds.): Mitral Valve Disease. 2nd ed. London, Butterworths, 1996, pp. 16–27.
104. Nestico, P. F., DePace, N. L., Kotler, M. N., et al.: Calcium phosphorus metabolism in dialysis patients with and without mitral anular calcium. Analysis of 30 patients. Am. J. Cardiol. *51*:497, 1983.
105. Mellino, M., Salcedo, E. E., Lever, H. M., et al.: Echographic-quantified severity of mitral annulus calcification: Prognostic correlation to related hemodynamic, valvular, rhythm, and conduction abnormalities. Am. Heart J. *103*:222, 1982.
106. Scott-Jupp, W., Barnett, N. L., Gallagher, P. J., et al.: Ultrastructural changes in spontaneous rupture of mitral chordae tendineae. J. Pathol. *133*:185, 1981.
107. Oliveira, D. B. G., Dawkins, K. D., Kay, P. H., and Paneth, M.: Chordal rupture I: Aetiology and natural history. Br. Heart J. *50*:312, 1983.
108. Hickey, A. J., Wilcken, D. E. L., Wright, J. S. and Warren, B. A.: Primary (spontaneous) chordal rupture: Relation to myxomatous valve disease and mitral valve prolapse. J. Am. Coll. Cardiol. *5*:1341, 1985.
109. Godley, R. W., Wann, L. S., Rogers, E. W., et al.: Incomplete mitral leaflet closure in patients with papillary muscle dysfunction. Circulation *63*:565, 1981.
110. Izumi, S., Miyatake, K., Beppu, S., et al.: Mechanism of mitral regurgitation in patients with myocardial infarction: A study using real-time two-dimensional Doppler flow imaging and echocardiography. Circulation *76*:777, 1987.
111. Ballester, M., Jajoo, J., Rees, S., et al.: The mechanism of mitral regurgitation in dilated left ventricle. Clin. Cardiol. *6*:333, 1983.
112. Tcheng, J. E., Jackman, J. D., Nelson, C. L., et al.: Outcome of patients sustaining acute ischemic mitral regurgitation during myocardial infarction. Ann. Intern. Med. *117*:18, 1992.
113. Hickey, M. St. J., Smith, L. R., Muhlbaier, L. H., et al.: Current prognosis of ischemic mitral regurgitation: Implications for future management. Circulation *78*(Suppl. I):I51, 1988.
114. Gottdiener, J. S., Maron, B. J., Schooley, R. T., et al.: Two-dimensional echocardiographic assessment of the idiopathic hypereosinophilic syndrome. Anatomic basis of mitral regurgitation and peripheral embolization. Circulation *67*:572, 1983.
115. Metras, D., Ouezzin-Coulibaly, A., Ouattara, K., et al.: Endomyocardial fibrosis masquerading as rheumatic mitral incompetence. A report of six surgical cases. J. Thorac. Cardiovasc. Surg. *86*:753, 1983.
116. Mazzucco, A., Rizzoli, G., Faggian, G., et al.: Acute mitral regurgitation after blunt chest trauma. Arch. Intern. Med. *143*:2326, 1983.
117. Jolly, D. T.: Traumatic rupture of a papillary muscle of the mitral valve due to blunt thoracic trauma. Can. Fam. Phys. *29*:1960, 1983.
118. Gidding, S. S., Shulman, S. T., Ibawi, M., et al.: Mucocutaneous lymph node syndrome (Kawasaki disease): Delayed aortic and mitral insufficiency secondary to active valvulitis. J. Am. Coll. Cardiol. *7*:894, 1986.
119. DiSegni, E., and Edwards, J. E.: Cleft anterior leaflet of the mitral valve with intact septa. A study of 20 cases. Am. J. Cardiol. *51*:919, 1983.
120. Nagata, S., Nimura, Y., Sakakibara, H., et al.: Mitral valve lesion associated with secundum atrial septal defect. Analysis of real-time two-dimensional echocardiography. Br. Heart J. *49*:151, 1983.
121. Eckberg, D. L., Gault, J. H., Bouchard, R. L., et al.: Mechanics of left ventricular contraction in chronic severe mitral regurgitation. Circulation *47*:1252, 1973.
122. Braunwald, E., Welch, G. H., Jr., and Sarnoff, S. J.: Hemodynamic effects of quantitatively varied experimental mitral regurgitation. Circ. Res. *5*:539, 1957.
123. Braunwald, E., and Turi, Z. G.: Pathophysiology of mitral valve disease. *In* Ionescu, M. I., and Cohn, L. H. (eds.): Mitral Valve Disease: Diagnosis and Treatment. London, Butterworths, 1985, pp. 3–10.

124. Yellin, E. L., Yoran, C., Frater, R. W. M., and Sonnenblick, E. H.: Dynamics of acute experimental mitral regurgitation. *In* Ionescu, M. I., and Cohn, L. H. (eds.): Mitral Valve Disease: Diagnosis and Treatment. London, Butterworths, 1985, pp. 11–26.
125. Braunwald, E.: Mitral regurgitation: Physiological, clinical and surgical considerations. N. Engl. J. Med. *281*:425, 1969.
126. Corin, W. J., Monrad, E. S., Murakami, T., et al.: The relationship of afterload to ejection performance in chronic mitral regurgitation. Circulation *76*:59, 1987.
127. Nwasokwa, O., Camesas, A., Weg, I., and Bodenheimer, M. M.: Differences in left ventricular adaptation to chronic mitral and aortic regurgitation. Chest *95*:106, 1989.
128. Knotos, G. J., Jr., Schaff, H. V., Gersh, B. J., and Bove, A. A.: Left ventricular function in subacute and chronic mitral regurgitation: Effect on function early postoperatively. J. Thorac. Cardiovasc. Surg. *98*:163, 1989.
129. Keren, G., Katz, S., Strom, J., et al.: Dynamic mitral regurgitation: An important determinant of the hemodynamic response to load alterations and inotropic therapy in severe heart failure. Circulation *80*:306, 1989.
130. Essop, M. R., Wisenbaugh, T., and Sareli, P.: Evidence against a myocardial factor as the cause of left ventricular dilation in active rheumatic carditis. J. Am. Coll. Cardiol. *22*:826, 1993.
131. Urschel, C. W., Covell, J. W., Graham, T. P., et al.: Effects of acute valvular regurgitation on the oxygen consumption of the canine heart. Circ. Res. *23*:33, 1968.
132. Braunwald, E.: Control of myocardial oxygen consumption: Physiologic and clinical considerations. Am. J. Cardiol. *27*:416, 1971.
133. Corin, W. J., Murakami, T., Monrad, E. S., et al.: Left ventricular passive diastolic properties in chronic mitral regurgitation. Circulation *83*:797, 1991.
134. Ross, J., Jr.: Left ventricular function and the timing of surgical treatment in valvular heart disease. Ann. Intern. Med. *94*:498, 1981.
135. Mirsky, I., Corin, W. J., Murakami, T., et al.: Correction for preload in assessment of myocardial contractility in aortic and mitral valve disease: Application of the concept of systolic myocardial stiffness. Circulation *78*:68, 1988.
136. Enriquez-Sarano, M., Tajik, A. K., Schaff, H. V., et al.: Echocardiographic prediction of survival after surgical correction of organic mitral regurgitation. Circulation *90*:830, 1994.
137. Ramanthan, K. B., Knowles, J., Connor, M. J., et al.: Natural history of chronic mitral insufficiency: Relation of peak systolic pressure/end-systolic volume ratio to morbidity and mortality. J. Am. Coll. Cardiol. *3*:1412, 1984.
138. Borow, K., Green, L. H., Mann, T., et al.: End-systolic volume as a predictor of postoperative left ventricular performance in volume overload from valvular regurgitation. Am. J. Med. *68*:655, 1980.
139. Mudge, G. H.: Asymptomatic mitral regurgitation. J. Cardiovasc. Surg. *9*(Suppl.):248, 1994.
140. Wisenbaugh, T., Spann, J. F., and Carabello, B. A.: Differences in myocardial performance and load between patients with similar amounts of chronic aortic versus chronic mitral regurgitation. J. Am. Coll. Cardiol. *3*:913, 1984.
141. Wisenbaugh, T., Skudicky, D., and Sareli, P.: Prediction of outcome after valve replacement for rheumatic mitral regurgitation in the era of chordal preservation. Circulation *89*:191, 1994.
142. Boucher, C. A., Bingham, J. B., Osbakken, M. D., et al.: Early changes in left ventricular size and function after correction of left ventricular volume overload. Am. J. Cardiol. *47*:991, 1981.
143. Grose, R., Strain, J., and Cohen, M. V.: Pulmonary arterial V waves in mitral regurgitation. Clinical and experimental observations. Circulation *69*:214, 1984.
143a. Schofield, P. M.: Invasive investigation of the mitral valve. *In* Wells, F. C., and Shapiro, L. M. (eds.): Mitral Valve Disease. 2nd ed. London, Butterworths, 1996, pp. 84–91.
144. Kihara, Y., Sasayama, S., Miyazaki, S., et al.: Role of the left atrium in adaptation of the heart to chronic mitral regurgitation in conscious dogs. Circ. Res. *62*:543, 1988.
145. Pape, L. A., Price, J. M., Alpert, J. S., et al.: Relation of left atrial size to pulmonary capillary wedge pressure in severe mitral regurgitation. Cardiology *78*:297, 1991.
146. Braunwald, E., and Awe, W. C.: The syndrome of severe mitral regurgitation with normal left atrial pressure. Circulation *27*:29, 1963.
147. Roberts, W. C., Braunwald, E., and Morrow, A. G.: Acute severe mitral regurgitation secondary to ruptured chordae tendineae. Clinical, hemodynamic and pathologic considerations. Circulation *33*:58, 1966.
148. Cohen, L. S., Mason, D. T., and Braunwald, E.: Significance of an atrial gallop sound in mitral regurgitation: A clue to the diagnosis of ruptured chordae tendineae. Circulation *35*:112, 1966.
149. Rippe, J. M., and Howe, J. P., III: Acute mitral regurgitation. *In* Dalen, J. E., and Alpert, J. S. (eds.): Valvular Heart Disease. 2nd ed. Boston, Little, Brown and Co., 1987, pp. 151–176.
150. Rosen, S. F., Borer, J. S., Hochreiter, C., et al.: Natural history of the asymptomatic patient with severe mitral regurgitation secondary to mitral valve prolapse and normal right and left ventricular performance. Am. J. Cardiol. *74*:374, 1994.
151. Elkins, R. C., Morrow, A. G., Vasko, J. S., and Braunwald, E.: The effects of mitral regurgitation on the pattern of instantaneous aortic blood flow. Clinical and experimental observations. Circulation *36*:45, 1967.
152. Basta, L. L., Wolfson, P., Eckberg, D. L., and Abboud, F. M.: The value of left parasternal impulse recordings in the assessment of mitral regurgitation. Circulation *48*:1055, 1973.
153. Barlow, J. B.: Mitral regurgitation. *In* Perspectives on the Mitral Valve. Philadelphia, F. A. Davis Co., 1987, pp. 113–131.
154. Haffajee, C. I.: Chronic mitral regurgitation. *In* Dalen, J. E., and Alpert, J. S. (eds.): Valvular Heart Disease. 2nd ed. Boston, Little, Brown and Co., 1987, pp. 111–150.
155. Karliner, J. S., O'Rourke, R. A., Kearney, D. J., and Shabetai, R.: Haemodynamic explanation of why the murmur of mitral regurgitation is independent of cycle length. Br. Heart J. *35*:397, 1973.
156. Schreiber, T. L., Fisher, J., Mangla, A., and Miller, D.: Severe "silent" mitral regurgitation: A potentially reversible cause of refractory heart failure. Chest *96*:242, 1989.
157. Antman, E. M., Angoff, G. H., and Sloss, J. J.: Demonstration of the mechanism by which mitral regurgitation mimics aortic stenosis. Am. J. Cardiol. *42*:1044, 1978.
158. Merendino, K. A., and Hessel, E. A.: The murmur on top of the head in acquired mitral insufficiency. JAMA. *199*:392, 1967.
159. Morris, J. J., Estes, E. H., Whalen, R. E., et al.: P wave analysis in valvular heart disease. Circulation *29*:242, 1964.
160. Priest, E. A., Finlayson, J. K., and Short, D. S.: The x-ray manifestations in the heart and lungs of mitral regurgitation. Prog. Cardiovasc. Dis. *5*:219, 1962.
161. Wexler, L., Silverman, J. F., DeBusk, R. F., and Harrison, D. C.: Angiographic features of rheumatic and nonrheumatic mitral regurgitation. Circulation *44*:1080, 1971.
162. Globits, S., and Higgins, C. B.: Assessment of valvular heart disease by magnetic resonance imaging. Am. Heart J. *129*:369, 1995.
162a. Manzara, C. C., Pennell, D. J., and Underwood, S. R.: Assessment of the mitral valve by magnetic resonance imaging. *In* Wells, F. C., and Shapiro, L. M. (eds.): Mitral Valve Disease. 2nd ed. London, Butterworths, 1996, pp. 71–83.
163. Himelman, R. B., Kusumoto, F., Oken, K., et al.: The flail mitral valve: Echocardiographic findings by precordial and transesophageal imaging and Doppler color flow mapping. J. Am. Coll. Cardiol. *17*:272, 1991.
164. Nair, C. K., Aronow, W. S., Sketch, M. H., et al.: Clinical and echocardiographic characteristics of patients with mitral annular calcification. Am. J. Cardiol. *51*:992, 1983.
165. Jenni, R., Ritter, M., Eberli, F., et al.: Quantification of mitral regurgitation with amplitude-weighted mean velocity from continuous wave Doppler spectra. Circulation *79*:1294, 1989.
166. Krivovkapich, J.: Echocardiography in valvular heart disease. Curr. Opin. Cardiol. *9*:158, 1994.
167. Mele, D., Vandervoort, P., Palacios, I., et al.: Proximal jet size by Doppler color flow mapping predicts severity of mitral regurgitation. Circulation *91*:746, 1995.
168. Shyu, K., Lei, M., Hwang, J., et al.: Morphologic characterization and quantitative assessment of mitral regurgitation with ruptured chordae tendineae by transesophageal echocardiography. Am. J. Cardiol. *70*:1152, 1992.
169. Smith, M. D., Cassidy, J. M., Gurley, J. C., et al.: Echo Doppler evaluation of patients with acute mitral regurgitation: Superiority of transesophageal echocardiography with color flow imaging. Am. Heart. J. *129*:967, 1995.
169a. Bach, D.-S., Deeb, G. M., and Bolling, S. F.: Accuracy of intraoperative transesophageal echocardiography for estimating the severity of functional mitral regurgitation. Am. J. Cardiol. **76**:508, 1995.
170. Yoran, C., Yellin, E. L., Becker, R. M., et al.: Mechanism of reduction of mitral regurgitation with vasodilator therapy. Am. J. Cardiol. *43*:773, 1979.
171. Shimoyama, H., Sabbah, H. N., Roman, H., et al.: Effects of long-term therapy with enalapril on severity of functional mitral regurgitation in dogs with moderate heart failure. J. Am. Coll. Cardiol. *25*:768, 1995.
172. Skoularigis, J., Sinovich, V., Joubert, G., and Sareli, P.: Evaluation of the long-term results of mitral valve repair in 254 young patients with rheumatic mitral regurgitation. Circulation *90*:II–167, 1994
173. Wells, F. C.: Conservation and surgical repair of the mitral valve. *In* Wells, F. C., and Shapiro, L. M. (eds.): Mitral Valve Disease. 2nd ed. London, Butterworths, 1996, pp. 114–134.
174. Straub, U., Feindt, P., Huwer, H., et al.: Mitral valve replacement with preservation of the subvalvular structures where possible: An echocardiographic and clinical comparison with cases where preservation was not possible. Thorac. Cardiovasc. Surg. *42*:2, 1994.
175. David, T. E.: Techniques and results of mitral valve repair for ischemic mitral regurgitation. J. Cardiovasc. Surg. *9*:274, 1994.
176. Odell, J. A., and Orszulak, T. A.: Surgical repair and reconstruction of valvular lesions. Curr. Opin. Cardiol. *10*:135, 1995.
177. Oury, J. H., Cleveland, J. C., Duran, C. G., and Angell, W. W.: Ischemic mitral valve disease: Classification and systemic approach to management. J. Cardiovasc. Surg. *9*(Suppl.):262, 1994.
178. Frater, R. W. M., Vetter, O., Zussa, C., and Dahm, M: Chordal replacement in mitral valve repair. Circulation *82*(Suppl. IV):125, 1990.
179. Craver, J. M., Cohen, C., and Weintraub, W. S.: Case-matched comparison of mitral valve replacement and repair. Ann. Thorac. Surg. *49*:964, 1990.
179a. Colon, R., and Frazier, O. H.: Mitral valve replacement techniques. *In* Wells, F. C., and Shapiro, L. M. (eds.): Mitral Valve Disease. 2nd ed. London, Butterworths, 1996, pp. 135–147.
180. Rozich, J. D., Carabello, B. A., and Usher, B. W.: Mitral valve replacement with and without chordal preservation in patients with chronic mitral regurgitation. Circulation *86*:1718, 1992.

181. Nakano, K., Swindler, M. M., Spinale, F. B., et al.: Depressed contractile function due to canine mitral regurgitation improves after correction of the volume overload. J. Clin. Invest. *87*:2077, 1991.
182. Duran, C. M., Gometza, B., and Saad, E.: Valve repair in rheumatic mitral disease: An unsolved problem. J. Cardiovasc. Surg. *9*(Suppl.): 282, 1994.
183. Enriquez-Sarano, M., Schaff, H. V., Orszulak, T. A., et al.: Valve repair improves the outcome of surgery for mitral regurgitation. Circulation *91*:1022, 1995.
184. Corin, W. J., Sutsch, G., Murakami, T., et al.: Left ventricular function in chronic mitral regurgitation. Preoperative and postoperative comparison. J. Am. Coll. Cardiol. *25*:113, 1995.
185. Stewart, W. J., Currie, P. J., Salcedo, E. E., et al.: Intraoperative Doppler color flow mapping for decision-making in valve repair for mitral regurgitation. Circulation *81*:556, 1990.
186. Lee, K. S., Stewart, W. J., Lever, H. M., et al.: Mechanism of outflow tract obstruction causing failed mitral valve repair: Anterior displacement of leaflet coaptation. Circulation *88*:24, 1993.
187. Rankin, J. S., Feneley, M. P., Hickey, M. St. J., et al.: A clinical comparison of mitral valve repair versus valve replacement in ischemic mitral regurgitation. J. Thorac. Cardiovasc. Surg. *95*:165, 1988.
188. Wisenbaugh, T., Skucicky, D., and Sarelli, P.: Prediction of outcome after valve replacement for rheumatic mitral regurgitation in the era of chordal preservation. Circulation *89*:191, 1994.
189. Lee, S. J. K., and Bay, K. S.: Mortality risk factors associated with mitral valve replacement: A survival analysis of 10 year follow-up data. Can. J. Cardiol. *7*:11, 1991.
190. Phillips, H. R., Levine, F. H., Carter, J. E., et al.: Mitral valve replacement for isolated mitral regurgitation: Analysis of clinical course and late postoperative left ventricular ejection fraction. Am. J. Cardiol. *48*:647, 1981.
191. Peterson, K. L.: The timing of surgical intervention in chronic mitral regurgitation. Cathet. Cardiovasc. Diagn. *9*:433, 1983.
192. Huikuri, H.: Effect of mitral valve replacement on left ventricular function in mitral regurgitation. Br. Heart J. *49*:328, 1983.
193. Oury, J. H., Cleveland, J. C., Duran, C. G., and Angell, W. W.: Ischemic mitral valve disease: Classification and systemic approach to management. J. Cardiovasc. Surg. *9*(Suppl.):262, 1994.
194. Akins, C. W., Hilgenberg, A. D., Buckley, M. J., et al.: Mitral valve reconstruction versus replacement for degenerative ischemic mitral regurgitation. Ann. Thorac. Surg. *58*:668, 1994.
195. Connolly, M. W., Gelbfish, J. S., Jacobowitz, I. J., et al.: Surgical results for mitral regurgitation from coronary artery disease. J. Thorac. Cardiovasc. Surg. *91*:379, 1986.
196. Gaasch, W. H., and Aurigemma, G. P.: Is corrective surgery ever indicated in the asymptomatic patient with mitral regurgitation? Cardiol. Rev. *2*:138, 1994.
196a. Treasure, T.: Timing of surgery in chronic mitral regurgitation. *In* Wells, F. C., and Shapiro, L. M. (eds.): Mitral Valve Disease. 2nd ed. London, Butterworths, 1996, pp. 187–196.

THE MITRAL VALVE PROLAPSE SYNDROME

197. Devereux, R. B.: Recent developments in the diagnosis and management of mitral valve prolapse. Curr. Opin. Cardiol. *10*:107, 1995.
198. Pocock, W. A.: Mitral leaflet billowing and prolapse. *In* Barlow, J. B. (ed.): Perspectives on the Mitral Valve. Philadelphia, F. A. Davis Co., 1987, pp. 45–112.
199. Perloff, J. K., Child, J. S., and Edwards, J. E.: New guidelines for the clinical diagnosis of mitral valve prolapse. Am. J. Cardiol. *57*:1124, 1986.
200. Wann, L. S., Grove, J. R., Hess, T. R., et al.: Prevalence of mitral prolapse by two-dimensional echocardiography in healthy young women. Br. Heart J. *49*:334, 1983.
201. Fontana, M. E., Sparks, E. A., Boudoulas, H., and Wooley, C. F.: Mitral valve prolapse and the mitral valve prolapse syndrome. Curr. Probl. Cardiol. *16*:311, 1991.
202. Cohn, L. H., Couper, G. S., Aranki, S. F., et al.: Long-term results of mitral valve reconstruction for the regurgitating myxomatous mitral valve. J. Thorac. Cardiovasc. Surg. *107*:143, 1994.
202a. Prabhu, S., and O'Rourke, R. A.: Mitral valve prolapse. *In* Rahimtoola, S. H. (ed.): Valvular Heart Disease and Endocarditis. Atlas of Heart Diseases. Vol. 11. St. Louis, Mosby, 1996.
203. Devereux, R. B., Hawkins, I., Kramer-Fox, R., et al.: Complications of mitral valve prolapse: Disproportionate occurrence in men and older patients. Am. J. Med. *81*:751, 1986.
204. Levy, D., and Savage, D. D.: Prevalence and clinical features of mitral valve prolapse. Am. Heart J. *113*:1281, 1987.
205. Barlow, J. B., Pocock, W. A., Marchand, P., and Denny, M.: The significance of the late systolic murmurs. Am. Heart J. *66*:443, 1963.
206. Devereux, R. B., Kramer-Fox, R., and Kligfield, P.: Mitral valve prolapse: Etiology, clinical manifestations and management. Ann. Intern. Med. *111*:305, 1989.
207. Goldhaber, S. Z., Brown, W. D., and St. John Sutton, M. G.: High frequency of mitral valve prolapse and aortic regurgitation among asymptomatic adults with Down's syndrome. J. A. M. A. *258*:1793, 1987.
208. Noah, M. S., Sulimani, R. A., Famuyiwa, F. O., et al.: Prolapse of the mitral valve in hyperthyroid patients in Saudi Arabia. Int. J. Cardiol. *19*:217, 1988.
209. [illegible], P., Margulis, T., Grenadier, E., et al.: Von Willebrand factor and mitral valve prolapse. Thromb. Haemost. *60*:230, 1988.
210. Streib, E. W., Meyers, D. G., and Sun, S. F.: Mitral valve prolapse in myotonic dystrophy. Muscle Nerve *8*:650, 1985.
211. Johnson, G. L., Humphries, L. L., Shirley, P. B., et al.: Mitral valve prolapse in patients with anorexia nervosa and bulimia. Arch. Intern. Med. *146*:1525, 1986.
212. Waite, P., and McCallum, C. A.: Mitral valve prolapse in craniofacial skeletal deformities. Oral Surg. Oral Med. Oral Pathol. *61*:15, 1986.
213. Comens, S. M., Alpert, M. A., Sharp, G. C., et al.: Frequency of mitral valve prolapse in systemic lupus erythematosus, progressive systemic sclerosis and mixed connective tissue disease. Am. J. Cardiol. *63*:59, 1989.
214. Chan, F. L., Chen, W. W., Wong, P. H. C., and Chow, J. S. F.: Skeletal abnormalities in mitral valve prolapse. Clin. Radiol. *34*:207, 1983.
215. Zuppiroli, A., Roman, M. J., O'Gardy, M., and Devereux, R. B.: Lack of association between mitral valve prolapse and history of rheumatic fever. Am Heart J. *131*:525, 1996.
216. Lu-Li, S., Guang-Gen, C., and Ru-Lian, L.: Valve prolapse in Behçet's disease. Br. Heart J. *54*:100, 1985.
217. Levine, R. A., Handschumacher, M. D., Sanfilippo, A. J., et al.: Three-dimensional echocardiographic reconstruction of the mitral valve, with implications for the diagnosis of mitral valve prolapse. Circulation *80*:589, 1989.
218. Cabeen, W. R., Jr., Reza, M. J., Kovick, R. B., and Stern, M. S.: Mitral valve prolapse and conduction defects in Ehlers-Danlos syndrome. Arch. Intern. Med. *137*:1227, 1977.
219. Lebwohl, M. G., Distefano, D., Prioleau, P. G., et al.: Pseudoxanthoma elasticum and mitral valve prolapse. N. Engl. J. Med. *307*:228, 1982.
220. Zema, M. J., Chiaramida, S., DeFilipp, G. J., et al.: Somatotype and idiopathic mitral valve prolapse. Cathet. Cardiovasc. Diagn. *8*:105, 1982.
221. Malcolm, A. D.: Mitral valve prolapse associated with other disorders. Causal coincidence, common link, or fundamental genetic disturbance? Br. Heart J. *53*:353, 1985.
222. Jaffe, A. S., Geltman, E. M., Rodey, G. E., and Uitto, J.: Mitral valve prolapse: A consistent manifestation of Type IV Ehlers-Danlos syndrome. The pathogenetic role of the abnormal production of Type III collagen. Circulation *64*:121, 1981.
223. King, B. D., Clark, M. A., Baba, N., et al.: "Myxomatous" mitral valves: Collagen dissolution as the primary defect. Circulation *66*:288, 1982.
224. Tomaru, T., Uchida, Y., Mohri, N., et al.: Postinflammatory mitral and aortic valve prolapse: A clinical and pathological study. Circulation *76*:68, 1987.
225. Stein, P. D., Wang, C.-H., Riddle, J. M., et al.: Scanning electron microscopy of operatively excised severely regurgitant floppy mitral valves. Am. J. Cardiol. *64*:392, 1989.
226. Baker, P. B., Bansal, G., Boudoulas, H., et al.: Floppy mitral valve chordae tendineae: Histopathologic alterations. Hum. Pathol. *19*:507, 1988.
227. Wordsworth, P., Ogilvie, D., Akhras, F., et al.: Genetic segregation analysis of familial mitral valve prolapse shows no linkage to fibrillar collagen genes. Br. Heart J. *61*:300, 1989.
228. Sanfilippo, A. J., Harrigan, P., Popovic, A. D., et al.: Papillary muscle traction in mitral valve prolapse: Quantitation by two-dimensional echocardiography. J. Am. Coll. Cardiol. *19*:564, 1992.
229. Devereux, R. B., Kramer-Fox, R., and Kligfield, P.: Mitral valve prolapse: Causes, clinical manifestations, and management. Arch. Intern. Med. *111*:305, 1989.
230. Procacci, P. M., Savran, S. V., Schreiter, S. L., and Bryson, A. L.: Prevalence of clinical mitral valve prolapse in 1,169 young women. N. Engl. J. Med. *294*:1086, 1976.
231. Markiewicz, W., Stoner, J., London, E., et al.: Mitral valve prolapse in one hundred presumably healthy young females. Circulation *53*:464, 1976.
232. Pan, C. W., Chen, C. C., Wang, S. P., et al.: Echocardiographic study of cardiac abnormalities in families of patients with Marfan's syndrome. J. Am. Coll. Cardiol. *6*:1016, 1985.
233. Zuppiroli, A., Rinaldi, M., Kramer-Fox, R., et al.: Natural history of mitral valve prolapse. Am. J. Cardiol. *75*:1028, 1995.
234. Boudoulas, H., Kolibash, A. J., Jr., Baker, P., et al.: Mitral valve prolapse and the mitral valve prolapse syndrome: A diagnostic classification and pathogenesis of symptoms. Am. Heart J. *118*:796, 1989.
235. Davies, A. O., Mares, A., Pool, J. L., and Taylor, A. A.: Mitral valve prolapse with symptoms of beta-adrenergic hypersensitivity. $Beta_2$-adrenergic receptor supercoupling with desensitization on isoproterenol exposure. Am. J. Med. *82*:193, 1987.
236. Alexander, M. D., Bloom, K. R., Hart, P., et al.: Atrial septal aneurysm: A cause of midsystolic click. Report of a case and review of the literature. Circulation *63*:1186, 1981.
237. Kligfield, P., and Devereux, R. B.: Arrhythmia in mitral valve prolapse. *In* Podrid, P. R., and Kowey, P. R. (eds.): Cardiac Arrhythmia: Mechanisms, Diagnosis and Management. Baltimore, Williams and Wilkins Co., 1995, p. 1253.
238. Kligfield, P., Hochreiter, C., Niles, N., et al.: Relation of sudden death in pure mitral regurgitation with and without mitral valve prolapse, to repetitive ventricular arrhythmias and right and left ventricular ejection fraction. Am. J. Cardiol. *60*:397, 1987.
239. Stein, K. M., Borer, J. S., Hochreiter, C., et al.: Prognostic value and physiological correlates of heart rate variability in chronic severe mitral regurgitation. Circulation *88*:127, 1993.
240. Wit, A. L., Fenoglio, J. J., Hordof, A. J., and Reemtsma, K.: Ultrastructure and transmembrane potentials of cardiac muscle in the human anterior mitral valve leaflet. Circulation *59*:1283, 1979.

241. Gallagher, J. J., Gilbert, M., and Svenson, R. H.: Wolff-Parkinson-White syndrome. The problem, evaluation and surgical correction. Circulation *57*:767, 1975.
242. Pocock, W. A., Bosman, C. K., Chesler, E., et al.: Sudden death in primary mitral valve prolapse. Am. Heart J. *107*:378, 1984.
243. Levine, R. A., Stathogiannis, E., Newell, J. B., et al.: Reconsideration of echocardiographic standards for mitral valve prolapse: Lack of association between leaflet displacement isolated to the apical four chamber view and independent echocardiographic evidence of abnormality. J. Am. Coll. Cardiol. *11*:1010, 1988.
244. Alpert, M. A., Carney, R. J., Flaker, G. C., et al.: Sensitivity and specificity of two-dimensional echocardiographic signs of mitral valve prolapse. Am. J. Cardiol. *54*:792, 1984.
245. Marks, A. R., Choong, C. Y., Sanfilippo, A. J., et al.: Identification of high-risk and low-risk subgroups of patients with mitral valve prolapse. N. Engl. J. Med. *320*:1031, 1989.
246. Panidis, I. P., McAllister, M., Ross, J., and Mintz, G. S.: Prevalence and severity of mitral regurgitation in the mitral valve prolapse syndrome: A Doppler echocardiographic study of 80 patients. J. Am. Coll. Cardiol. *7*:975, 1986.
247. Weissman, N. J., Pini, R., Roman, M. J., et al.: In vivo mitral valve morphology and function in mitral valve prolapse. Am. J. Cardiol. *73*:1080, 1994.
248. Arvan, S., and Tunick, S.: Relationship between auscultatory events and structural abnormalities in mitral valve prolapse: A two-dimensional echocardiographic evaluation. Am. Heart J. *108*:1298, 1984.
249. Sahn, D. J., Wood, J., Allen, H. D., et al.: Echocardiographic spectrum of mitral valve motion in children with and without mitral valve prolapse: The nature of false-positive diagnosis. Am. J. Cardiol. *39*:422, 1977.
250. Rodger, J. C., and Morley, P.: Abnormal aortic valve echoes in mitral prolapse. Echocardiographic features of floppy aortic valve. Br. Heart J. *47*:337, 1982.
251. Klein, G. J., Kostuk, W. J., Boughner, D. R., and Chamberlain, M. J.: Stress myocardial imaging in mitral leaflet prolapse syndrome. Am. J. Cardiol. *42*:746, 1978.
252. Cohen, M. V., Shah, P. K., and Spindola-Franco, H.: Angiographic-echocardiographic correlation of mitral valve prolapse. Am. Heart J. *97*:43, 1979.
253. Cipriano, P. R., Kline, S. A., and Baltaxe, H. A.: An angiographic assessment of left ventricular-function in isolated mitral valvular prolapse. Invest. Radiol. *15*:293, 1980.
254. Mills, P., Rose, J., Hollingsworth, J., et al.: Long-term prognosis of mitral valve prolapse. N. Engl. J Med *297*:13, 1977.
255. Olson, L. J., Subramanian, R., Ackermann, D. M., et al.: Surgical pathology of the mitral valve: A study of 712 cases spanning 21 years. Mayo Clin. Proc. *62*:22, 1987.
256. Wilcken, D. E., and Hickey, A. J.: Lifetime risk for patients with mitral prolapse of developing severe valve regurgitation requiring surgery. Circulation *78*:10, 1988.
256a. Fakuda, N., Oki, T., Iuchi, A., et al.: Predisposing factors for severe mitral regurgitation in idiopathic mitral valve prolapse. Am. J. Cardiol. *76*:503, 1995.
257. Hickey, A. J., MacMahon, S. W., and Wilcken, D. E. L.: Mitral valve prolapse and bacterial endocarditis: When is antibiotic prophylaxis necessary? Am. Heart J. *109*:431, 1985.
258. Danchin, N., Briancon, S., Mathieu, P., et al.: Mitral valve prolapse as a risk factor for infective endocarditis. Lancet *1*:743, 1989.
259. Schnee, M. A., and Bucal, A. A.: Fatal embolism in mitral valve prolapse. Chest *83*:285, 1983.
260. Barletta, G. A., Gagliardi, R., Benvenuti, L., and Fantini, F.: Cerebral ischemic attacks as a complication of aortic and mitral valve prolapse. Stroke *16*:219, 1985.
261. Makino, H., and Al-Sadir, J.: Myocardial infarction in patients with mitral valve prolapse and normal coronary arteries. J. Am. Coll. Cardiol. *1*:661, 1983.

AORTIC STENOSIS

262. Levinson, G. E.: Aortic stenosis. *In* Dalen, J. E., and Alpert, J. S. (eds.): Valvular Heart Disease. 2nd ed. Boston, Little, Brown and Co., 1987, pp. 197–282.
263. Dare, A. J., Veinot, J. P., Edwards, W. D., et al.: New observations on the etiology of aortic valve disease. Hum. Pathol. *24*:1330, 1993.
264. Roberts, W. C.: Valvular, subvalvular and supravalvular aortic stenosis. Morphologic features. Cardiovasc. Clin. *5*:97, 1973.
264a. Rahimtoola, S. H.: Aortic stenosis. *In* Rahimtoola, S. H. (ed.): Valvular Heart Disease and Endocarditis. Atlas of Heart Diseases. Vol. 11. St. Louis, Mosby, 1996.
265. Braunwald, E., Goldblatt, A., Aygen, M. M., et al.: Congenital aortic stenosis: Clinical and hemodynamic findings in 100 patients. Circulation *27*:426, 1963.
266. Selzer, A.: Changing aspects of the natural history of valvular aortic stenosis. N. Engl. J. Med. *317*:91, 1987.
267. Passik, C. S., Ackermann, D. M., Pluth, J. R., and Edwards, W. D.: Temporal changes in the causes of aortic stenosis: A surgical pathologic study of 646 cases. Mayo Clin. Proc. *62*:119, 1987.
268. Deutscher, S., Rockette, H. E., and Krishnaswami, V.: Diabetes and hypercholesterolemia among patients with calcific aortic stenosis. J. Chron. Dis. *37*:407, 1984.
269. Strickberger, S. A., Schulman, S. P., and Hutchings, G. M.: Association of Paget's disease of bone with calcific aortic valve disease. Am. J. Med. *82*:953, 1987.
270. Maher, E. R., Young, G., Smyth-Walsh, B., et al.: Aortic and mitral valve calcification in patients with end stage renal diseases. Lancet *1*:875, 1987.
271. Dereymacker, L., Van Parijs, G., Bayart, M., et al.: Ochronosis and alkaptonuria: Report of a new case with calcified aortic valve stenosis. Acta Cardiol. *45*:98, 1990.
272. Kennedy, J. W., Twiss, R. D., and Blackmon, J. R.: Quantitative angiography. III. Relationships of left ventricular pressure volume and mass in aortic valve disease. Circulation *38*:838, 1968.
273. Carabello, B. A.: Aortic stenosis. Cardiol. Rev. *1*:59, 1993.
274. Carabello, B. A., Mee, R., Collins, J. J., Jr., et al.: Contractile function in chronic gradually developing subcoronary aortic stenosis. Am. J. Physiol. *240*:H80, 1981.
275. Grossman, W.: Profiles in valvular heart disease. *In* Grossman, W., and Baim, D. (eds.): Cardiac Catheterization and Angiography. 4th ed. Philadelphia, Lea and Febiger, 1991.
275a. Laskey, W. K., Kussmaul, W. G., and Noordergraaf, A.: Valvular and systemic arterial hemodynamics in aortic valve stenosis. Circulation *9*:1473, 1995.
276. Hess, O. L., Villari, B., and Krayenbuehl, H.: Diastolic dysfunction in aortic stenosis. Circulation *87*(Suppl. 5):IV-73, 1993.
277. Villari, B., Vassalli, G., Monrad, E. S., et al.: Normalization of diastolic dysfunction in aortic stenosis late after valve replacement. Circulation *91*:2353, 1995.
278. Braunwald, E., and Frahm, C. J.: Studies on Starling's law of the heart. IV. Observations on the hemodynamic functions of the left atrium in man. Circulation *24*:633, 1961.
279. Carroll, J. D., Carroll, E. P., Feldman, T., et al.: Sex-associated differences in left ventricular function in aortic stenosis of the elderly. Circulation *86*:1099, 1992.
280. Morris, J. J., Schaff, H. V., Mullany, C. J., et al.: Gender differences in left ventricular functional response to aortic valve replacement. Circulation *90*:II-183, 1994.
280a. Legget, M. E., Kuusisto, J., Healy, N. L., et al.: Gender differences in left ventricular function at rest and with exercise in asymptomatic aortic stenosis. Am. Heart J. *131*:94, 1996.
281. Donner, R., Carabello, B. A., Black, I., and Spann, J. F.: Left ventricular wall stress in compensated aortic stenosis in children. Am. J. Cardiol. *51*:946, 1983.
282. Spann, J. F., Bove, A. A., Natarajan, G., and Kreulens, T.: Ventricular performance, pump function, and compensatory mechanisms in patients with aortic stenosis. Circulation *62*:576, 1980.
283. Brouwer, C. B., Verwers, F. A., Alpert, J. S., and Goldberg, R. J.: Isolated aortic stenosis: Analysis of clinical and hemodynamic subsets. J. Appl. Cardiol. *4*:565, 1989.
284. Krayenbuehl, H. P., Hess, O. M., Ritter, M., et al.: Left ventricular systolic function in aortic stenosis. Eur. Heart J. *9*(Suppl. E):19, 1988.
285. Gunther, S., and Grossman, W.: Determinants of ventricular function in pressure overload hypertrophy in man. Circulation *59*:679, 1979.
286. Ross, J., Jr.: Afterload mismatch and preload reserve: A conceptual framework for the analysis of ventricular function. Prog. Cardiovasc. Dis. *18*:255, 1976.
287. Fifer, M. A., Gunther, S., Grossman, W., et al.: Myocardial contractile function in aortic stenosis as determined from the rate of stress development during isovolumic systole. Am. J. Cardiol. *44*:1318, 1979.
288. Carabello, B. A., Green, L. H., Grossman, W., et al.: Hemodynamic determinants of prognosis of aortic valve replacement in critical aortic stenosis and advanced congestive heart failure. Circulation *62*:42, 1980.
289. Huber, D., Grimm, J., Koch, R., and Krayenbuehl, H. P.: Determinants of ejection performance in aortic stenosis. Circulation *64*:126, 1981.
289a. Movsowitz, C., Kussmaul, W. G., and Laskey, W. K.: Left ventricular diastolic response to exercise in valvular aortic stenosis. Am. J. Cardiol. *77*:275, 1996.
290. Dineen, E., and Brent, B. N.: Aortic valve stenosis: Comparison of patients to those without chronic congestive heart failure. Am. J. Cardiol. *57*:419, 1986.
291. Fifer, M. A., Borow, K. M., Colan, S. D., and Lorell, B. H.: Early diastolic left ventricular function in children and adults with aortic stenosis. J. Am. Coll. Cardiol. *5*:1147, 1985.
292. Hess, O. M., Ritter, M., Schneider, J., et al.: Diastolic stiffness and myocardial structure in aortic valve disease before and after replacement. Circulation *69*:855, 1984.
293. Schwarz, F., Flameng, W., Schaper, J., et al.: Myocardial structure and function in patients with aortic valve disease and their relation to postoperative results. Am. J. Cardiol. *41*:661, 1978.
294. Krayenbuehl, H. P., Hess, O. M., Monrad, E. S., et al.: Left ventricular myocardial structure in aortic valve disease before, intermediate, and later after aortic valve replacement. Circulation *79*:744, 1989.
295. Bertrand, M. E., LaBlanche, J. M., Tilmant, P. Y., et al.: Coronary sinus blood flow at rest and during isometric exercise in patients with aortic valve disease. Mechanism of angina pectoris in presence of normal coronary arteries. Am. J. Cardiol. *47*:199, 1981.
296. Smucker, M. L., Tedesco, C. L., and Manning, S. B.: Demonstration of an imbalance between coronary perfusion and excessive load as a mechanism of ischemia during stress in patients with aortic stenosis. Circulation *78*:573, 1988.
297. Vinten-Johansen, J., and Weiss, H. R.: Oxygen consumption in subepicardial and subendocardial regions of the canine left ventricle—The

effect of experimental acute valvular aortic stenosis. Circ. Res. *46*:139, 1980.
298. Matsuo, S., Tsuruta, M., Hayano, M., et al.: Phasic coronary artery flow velocity determined by Doppler flowmeter catheter in aortic stenosis and aortic regurgitation. Am. J. Cardiol. *62*:917, 1988.
299. Marcus, M. L., Dot, D. B., Hiratzka, L. F., et al.: Decreased coronary reserve. A mechanism for angina pectoris in patients with aortic stenosis and normal coronary arteries. N. Engl. J. Med. *307*:1362, 1982.
300. Oakley, C. M.: Management of valvular stenosis. Curr. Opin. Cardiol. *10*:117, 1995.
301. Kennedy, K. D., Nishimura, R. A., Holmes, D. R., et al.: Natural history of moderate aortic stenosis. J. Am. Coll. Cardiol. *17*:313, 1991.
302. Ross, J., Jr., and Braunwald, E.: The influence of corrective operations on the natural history of aortic stenosis. Circulation *37*(Suppl. V):61, 1968.
303. Frank, S., Johnson, A., and Ross, J., Jr.: Natural history of valvular aortic stenosis. Br. Heart J. *35*:41, 1973.
304. Hakki, A.-H., Kimbiris, D., Iskandrian, A. S., et al.: Angina pectoris and coronary artery disease in patients with severe aortic valvular disease. Am. Heart. J. *100*:441, 1980.
305. Baxley, W. A.: Aortic valve disease. Curr. Opin. Cardiol. *9*:152, 1994.
306. Holley, K. E., Bahn, R. C., McGoon, D. C., and Mankin, H. T.: Spontaneous calcific embolization associated with calcific aortic stenosis. Circulation *27*:197, 1963.
307. Grech, E. D., and Ramsdale, D. R.: Exertional syncope in aortic stenosis: Evidence to support inappropriate left ventricular baroreceptor response. Am. Heart J. *121*:603, 1991.
308. Carabello, B. A.: Aortic stenosis. Cardiol. Rev. *1*:59, 1993.
309. Schwartz, L. S., Goldfischer, J., Sprague, G. J., and Schwartz, S. P.: Syncope and sudden death in aortic stenosis. Am. J. Cardiol. *23*:647, 1969.
310. Love, J. W.: The syndrome of calcific aortic stenosis and gastrointestinal bleeding: Resolution following aortic valve replacement. J. Thorac. Cardiovasc. Surg. *83*:779, 1982.
311. Pleet, A. B., Massey, E. W., and Vengrow, M. E.: TIA, stroke, and the bicuspid aortic valve. Neurology *31*:1540, 1981.
312. Brockmeier, L. B., Adolph, R. J., Gustin, B. W., et al.: Calcium emboli to the retinal artery in calcific aortic stenosis. Am. Heart J. *101*:32, 1981.
313. Wood, P.: Aortic stenosis. Am. J. Cardiol. *1*:553, 1958.
314. Aortic stenosis. *In* Fowler, N. O.: Diagnosis of Heart Disease. New York, Springer-Verlag, 1991, p. 134–145.
315. Abrams, J.: Aortic stenosis. *In* Essentials of Cardiac Physical Diagnosis. Philadelphia, Lea and Febiger, 1987, pp. 205–224.
316. Cooper, T., Braunwald, E., and Morrow, A. G.: Pulsus alternans in aortic stenosis: Hemodynamic observations in 50 patients studied by left heart catheterization. Circulation *18*:64, 1958.
317. Perloff, J. K.: Clinical recognition of aortic stenosis. The physical signs and differential diagnosis of the various forms of obstruction to left ventricular outflow. Prog. Cardiovasc. Dis. *10*:323, 1968.
318. Goldblatt, A., Aygen, M. M., and Braunwald, E.: Hemodynamic-phonocardiographic correlations of the fourth heart sound in aortic stenosis. Circulation *26*:92, 1962.
319. Morton, B. C.: Natural history and management of chronic aortic valve disease. Can. Med. Assoc. J. *126*:477, 1982.
320. Forssell, G., Jonasson, R., and Orinius, E.: Identifying severe aortic valvular stenosis by bedside examination. Acta Med. Scand. *218*:397, 1985.
321. Dymond, D. S., Wolf, F. G., and Schmidt, D. H.: Severe left ventricular dysfunction in critical aortic stenosis—reversal following aortic valve replacement. Postgrad. Med. J. *59*:781, 1983.
322. Delman, A. J., and Stein, E.: Valvular aortic stenosis. *In* Dynamic Cardiac Auscultation and Phonocardiography. Philadelphia, W. B. Saunders Co., 1979, p. 795.
323. Siegel, R. J., and Roberts, W. C.: Electrocardiographic observations in severe aortic valve stenosis: Correlative necropsy study of clinical, hemodynamic, and ECG variables demonstrating relation of 12-lead QRS amplitude to peak systolic transaortic pressure gradient. Am. Heart J. *103*:210, 1982.
324. Gooch, A. S., Calatayud, J. B., Rogers, P. A., and Garman, P. A.: Analysis of the P wave in severe aortic stenosis. Dis. Chest *49*:459, 1966.
325. Nair, C. K., Aronow, W. S., Stokke, K., et al.: Cardiac conduction defects in patients older than 60 years with aortic stenosis and without mitral annular calcium. Am. J. Cardiol. *53*:169, 1984.
326. Klein, R. C.: Ventricular arrhythmias in aortic valve disease: Analysis of 102 patients. Am. J. Cardiol. *53*:1079, 1984.
327. Szamosi, A., and Wassberg, B.: Radiologic detection of aortic stenosis. Acta Radiol. Diagn. *24*:201, 1983.
328. Hoffmann, R., Flachskampf, F. A., and Hanrath, P.: Aortic stenosis using multiplane transesophageal echocardiography. J. Am. Coll. Cardiol. *22*:529, 1993.
329. Tribouilloy, C., Shen, W. F., Peltier, M., et al.: Quantitation of aortic valve area in aortic stenosis with multiplane transesophageal echocardiography: Comparison with monoplane transesophageal approach. Am. Heart J. *128*:526, 1994.
330. Galan, A., Zoghbi, W. A., and Quiñones, M. A.: Determination of severity of valvular aortic stenosis by Doppler echocardiography and relation of findings to clinical outcome and agreement with hemodynamic measurements determined at cardiac catheterization. Am. J. Cardiol. *67*:1007, 1991.
331. Currie, P. J., Hagler, D. J., Seward, J. B., et al.: Instantaneous pressure gradient: A simultaneous Doppler and dual catheter correlative study. J. Am. Coll. Cardiol. *7*:800, 1986.
332. Agatston, A. S., Chengot, M., Rao, A., et al.: Doppler diagnosis of valvular aortic stenosis in patients over 60 years of age. Am. J. Cardiol. *56*:106, 1985.
333. Yeager, M., Yock, P. G., and Popp, R. L.: Comparison of Doppler-derived pressure gradient to that determined at cardiac catheterization in adults with aortic valve stenosis: Implications for management. Am. J. Cardiol. *57*:644, 1986.
334. Stone, P. H.: Management of the patient with asymptomatic aortic stenosis. J. Cardiovasc. Surg. *9*(Suppl.):139, 1994.
335. Aronow, W. S., Ahn, C., Kronson, I., and Nanna, M.: Prognosis of congestive heart failure in patients aged ≥62 years with unoperated severe valvular aortic stenosis. Am. J. Cardiol. *72*:846, 1993.
336. Cheitlin, M. D.: Should an asymptomatic patient with hemodynamically severe aortic stenosis ever have aortic valve surgery? Cardiol. Rev. *1*:344, 1993.
337. Braunwald, E.: On the natural history of severe aortic stenosis (editorial). J. Am. Coll. Cardiol. *15*:1018, 1990.
338. Pellikka, P. A., Nishimura, R. A., Bailey, K. R., and Tajik, A. J.: The natural history of adults with asymptomatic hemodynamically significant aortic stenosis. J. Am. Coll. Cardiol. *15*:1012, 1990.
339. Davies, S. W., Gershlick, A. H., and Balcon, R.: The progression of valvular aortic stenosis: A long-term retrospective study. Eur. Heart J. *12*:10, 1991.
340. Peter, M., Hoffman, A., Parker, C., et al.: Progression of aortic stenosis: Role of age and concomitant coronary artery disease. Chest *103*:1715, 1993.
341. Brener, S. J., Duffy, C. I., Thomas, J. U. D., and Stewart, W. J.: Progression of aortic stenosis in 394 patients: Relation to changes in myocardial and mitral valve dysfunction. J. Am. Coll. Cardiol. *25*:305, 1995.
342. Usher, B. W.: Valve surgery: Indications and long-term results. Curr. Opin. Cardiol. *6*:219, 1991.
343. Kirklin, J. W., and Barratt-Boyes, B. G.: Congenital aortic stenosis. *In* Cardiac Surgery. 2nd ed. New York, Churchill-Livingstone, 1993, pp. 1195–1238.
344. Kirklin, J. W., and Barratt-Boyes, B. G.: Aortic valve disease. *In* Cardiac Surgery. 2nd ed. New York, Churchill-Livingstone, 1993, pp. 491–571.
345. McBride, L. R., Naunheim, K. S., Fiore, A. C., et al.: Aortic valve decalcification. J. Thorac. Cardiovasc. Surg. *100*:36, 1990.
346. Lund, O.: Preoperative risk evaluation and stratification of long-term survival after valve replacement for aortic stenosis. Circulation *82*:124, 1990.
347. Monrad, E. S., Hess, O. M., Murakami, T., et al.: Abnormal exercise hemodynamics in patients with normal systolic function late after aortic valve replacement. Circulation *77*:613, 1988.
348. Hwang, M. H., Hammermeister, K. E., Oprian, C., et al.: Preoperative identification of patients likely to have left ventricular dysfunction after aortic valve replacement. Participants in the Veterans Administration Cooperative Study on Valvular Heart Disease. Circulation *80*(Suppl. I):165, 1989.
349. Kennedy, J. W., Doces, J., and Stewart, D. K.: Left ventricular function before and following aortic valve replacement. Circulation *56*:944, 1977.
350. Monrad, E. S., Hess, O. M., Murakami, T., et al.: Time course of regression of left ventricular hypertrophy after aortic valve replacement. Circulation *77*:1345, 1988.
351. Mirsky, I., Henschke, C., Hess, O. M., and Krayenbuehl, H. P.: Prediction of postoperative performance in aortic valve disease. Am. J. Cardiol. *48*:295, 1981.
352. Smith, N., McAnulty, J. H., and Rahimtoola, S. H.: Severe aortic stenosis with impaired left ventricular function and clinical heart failure: Results of valve replacement. Circulation *58*:255, 1978.
353. Culliford, A. T., Galloway, A. C., Colvin, S. B., et al.: Aortic valve replacement for aortic stenosis in persons aged 80 years and over. Am. J. Cardiol. *67*:1256, 1991.
354. Iung, B., Drissi, M. F., Michel, P-L., et al.: Prognosis of valve replacement for aortic stenosis with or without coexisting coronary heart disease: A comparative study. J. Heart Valve Dis. *2*:430, 1993.
355. Safian, R. D., Mandell, V. S., Thurer, R. E., et al.: Postmortem and intraoperative balloon valvuloplasty of calcific aortic stenosis in elderly patients: Mechanisms of successful dilation. J. Am. Coll. Cardiol. *9*:655, 1987.
356. Beatt, K. J.: Balloon dilatation of the aortic valve in adults: A physician's view. Br. Heart J. *63*:207, 1990.
357. Nishimura, R. A., Holmes, D. R., Jr., Michela, M. A., et al.: Follow-up of patients with low output, low gradient hemodynamics after percutaneous balloon aortic valvuloplasty: The Mansfield Scientific Aortic Valvuloplasty Registry. J. Am. Coll. Cardiol. *17*:828, 1991.
358. Otto, C. M., Mickel, M. C., Kennedy, J. W., et al.: Three-year outcome after balloon aortic valvuloplasty: Insights into prognosis of valvular aortic stenosis. Circulation *89*:642, 1994.
359. Elliott, J. M., and Tuzcu, E. M.: Recent developments in balloon valvuloplasty techniques. Curr. Opin. Cardiol. *10*:128, 1995.
360. Otto, C. M., Mickel, M. C., Kennedy, J. W., et al.: Three-year outcome after balloon aortic valvuloplasty: Insights into prognosis of valvular aortic stenosis. Circulation *89*:642, 1994.
361. Lieberman, E. B., Wilson, J. S., Harrison, J. K., et al.: Aortic valve replacement in adults after balloon aortic valvuloplasty. Circulation *90*:II-205, 1994.
362. Berland, J., Cribier, A., Savin, T., et al.: Percutaneous balloon valvulo-

plasty in patients with severe aortic stenosis and low ejection fraction. Circulation *79:*1189, 1989.
363. Isner, J. A., and the Mansfield Scientific Aortic Valvuloplasty Registry Investigators: Acute catastrophic complications of balloon aortic valvuloplasty. J. Am. Coll. Cardiol. *17:*1436, 1991.
364. Holmes, D. R., Jr., Nishimura, R. A., and Reeder, G. S.: In-hospital mortality after balloon aortic valvuloplasty: Frequency and associated factors. J. Am. Coll. Cardiol. *17:*189, 1991.
365. Moreno, P. R., Jang, I.-K., Newell, J. B., et al.: The role of percutaneous aortic balloon valvuloplasty in patients with cardiogenic shock and critical aortic stenosis. J. Am. Coll. Cardiol *23:*1071, 1994.
366. Angel, J. L., Chapman, C., and Knuppel, R. A.: Percutaneous balloon aortic valvuloplasty in pregnancy. Obstet. Gynecol. *72:*438, 1988.

AORTIC REGURGITATION

367. Alpert, J. S.: Chronic aortic regurgitation. *In* Dalen, J. E., and Alpert, J. S. (eds.): Valvular Heart Disease. 2nd ed. Boston, Little, Brown and Co., 1987, pp. 283–318.
368. Stewart, W. J., King, M. E., Gillam, L. D., et al.: Prevalence of aortic valve prolapse with bicuspid aortic valve and its relation to aortic regurgitation: A cross-sectional echocardiographic study. Am. J. Cardiol. *54:*1277, 1984.
368a. Rahimtoola, S. H.: Aortic regurgitation. *In* Rahimtoola, S. H. (ed.): Valvular Heart Disease and Endocarditis. Atlas of Heart Diseases. Vol. 11. St. Louis, Mosby, 1996.
369. Frahm, C. J., Braunwald, E., and Morrow, A. G.: Congenital aortic regurgitation. Clinical and hemodynamic findings in four patients. Am. J. Med. *31:*63, 1961.
370. Roberts, W. C., Morrow, A. G., McIntosh, C. L., et al.: Congenitally bicuspid aortic valve causing severe, pure aortic regurgitation without superimposed infective endocarditis. Am. J. Cardiol. *47:*206, 1981.
371. Tonnemacher, D., Reid, C., Kawanishi, D., et al.: Frequency of myxomatous degeneration of the aortic valve as a cause of isolated aortic regurgitation severe enough to warrant aortic valve replacement. Am. J. Cardiol. *60:*1194, 1987.
372. Morain, S. V., Casanegra, P., Maturana, G., and Dubernet, J.: Spontaneous rupture of a fenestrated aortic valve. Surgical treatment. J. Thorac. Cardiovasc. Surg. *73:*716, 1977.
373. Waller, B. F., Kishel, J. C., and Roberts, W. C.: Severe aortic regurgitation from systemic hypertension. Chest *82:*365, 1982.
374. Chartash, E. K., Lans, D. M., Paget, S. A., et al.: Aortic insufficiency and mitral regurgitation in patients with severe systemic lupus erythematosus and the antiphospholipid syndrome. Am. J. Med. *86:*407, 1989.
375. Kramer, P. H., Imboden, J. B., Jr., Waldman, F. M., et al.: Severe aortic insufficiency in juvenile chronic arthritis. Am. J. Med. *74:*1088, 1983.
376. Demoulin, J. C., Lespagnard, J., Bertholet, M., and Soumagne, D.: Acute fulminant aortic regurgitation in ankylosing spondylitis. Am. Heart J. *105:*859, 1983.
377. Tahakur, R., Gupta, L. C., Misra, M., et al.: Jaccoud's arthropathy—diagnostic and therapeutic implications. Postgrad. Med. J. *64:*809, 1988.
378. Bostwick, D. G., Bensch, K. G., Burke, J. S., et al.: Whipple's disease presenting as aortic insufficiency. N. Engl. J. Med. *305:*995, 1981.
379. Burdick, S., Tresch, D. D., and Komokowski, R. A.: Cardiac valvular dysfunction associated with Crohn's disease in the absence of ankylosing spondylitis. Am. Heart J. *118:*174, 1989.
380. Darvill, F. R., Jr.: Aortic insufficiency of unusual etiology. J.A.M.A. *184:*753, 1963.
381. Emanuel, R., Ng, R. A. L., Marcomichelakis, J., et al.: Formes frustes of Marfan's syndrome presenting with severe aortic regurgitation. Clinicogenetic study of 18 families. Br. Heart J. *39:*190, 1977.
382. Reid, G. D., Patterson, M. W. H., Patterson, A. C., and Cooperberg, P. L.: Aortic insufficiency in association with juvenile ankylosing spondylitis. J. Pediatr. *95:*78, 1979.
383. Paulus, H. E., Pearson, C. M., and Pitts, W., Jr.: Aortic insufficiency in five patients with Reiter's syndrome: A detailed clinical and pathologic study. Am. J. Med. *53:*404, 1972.
384. Heppner, R. L., Babitt, H. I., Blanchine, J. W., and Warbasse, J. R.: Aortic regurgitation and aneurysm of sinus of Valsalva associated with osteogenesis imperfecta. Am. J. Cardiol. *31:*654, 1973.
385. Esdah, J., Hawkins, D., Gold, P., et al.: Vascular involvement in relapsing polychondritis. Can. Med. Assoc. J. *116:*1019, 1977.
386. Welch, G. H., Jr., Braunwald, E., and Sarnoff, S. J.: Hemodynamic effects of quantitatively varied experimental aortic regurgitation. Circ. Res. *5:*546, 1957.
387. Iskandrian, A. S., Hakki, A-H., Manno, B., et al.: Left ventricular function in chronic aortic regurgitation. J. Am. Coll. Cardiol. *1:*1374, 1983.
388. Borow, K. M., and Marcus, R. H.: Aortic regurgitation: The need for an integrated physiologic approach. J. Am. Coll. Cardiol. *17:*898, 1991.
389. Grossman, W., Jones, D., and McLaurin, L. P.: Wall stress and patterns of hypertrophy in the human left ventricle. J. Clin. Invest. *56:*56, 1975.
390. Kawanishi, D. T., McKay, C. R., Chandraratna, A. N., et al.: Cardiovascular response to dynamic exercise in patients with chronic symptomatic mild-to-moderate and severe aortic regurgitation. Circulation *73:*62, 1986.
391. Massie, B. M., Kramer, B. L., Loge, D., et al.: Ejection fraction response to supine exercise in asymptomatic aortic regurgitation: Relation to simultaneous hemodynamic measurements. J. Am. Coll. Cardiol. *5:*847, 1985.
392. Scognamiglio, R., Roelandt, J., Fasoli, G., et al.: Relation between myocardial contractility, hypertrophy and pump performance in patients with chronic aortic regurgitation: An echocardiographic study. Int. J. Cardiol. *6:*473, 1984.
393. Dehmer, G. J., Firth, E. G., Hillis, L. D., et al.: Alterations in left ventricular volumes and ejection fraction at rest and during exercise in patients with aortic regurgitation. Am. J. Cardiol. *48:*17, 1981.
394. Ardehall, A., Segal, J., and Cheitlin, M. D.: Coronary blood flow reserve in acute aortic regurgitation. J. Am. Coll. Cardiol. *25:*1387, 1995.
395. Uhl, G. S., Boucher, C. A., Oliveros, R. A., and Murgo, J. P.: Exercise-induced myocardial oxygen supply-demand imbalance in asymptomatic or mildly symptomatic aortic regurgitation. Chest *80:*686, 1981.
396. Nitenberg, A., Foult, J-M., Antony, I., et al.: Coronary flow and resistance reserve in patients with chronic aortic regurgitation, angina pectoris, and normal coronary arteries. J. Am. Coll. Cardiol. *11:*478, 1988.
397. Maurer, W., Ablasser, A., Tschada, R., et al.: Myocardial catecholamine metabolism in patients with chronic aortic regurgitation. Circulation *66*(Suppl. I):139, 1982.
398. Benotti, J. R.: Acute aortic insufficiency. *In* Dalen, J. E., and Alpert, J. S. (eds.): Valvular Heart Disease. 2nd ed. Boston, Little, Brown and Co., 1987, pp. 319–352.
399. Downes, T. R., Nomeir, A-M., Hackshaw, B. T., et al.: Diastolic mitral regurgitation in acute but not chronic aortic regurgitation: Implications regarding the mechanism of mitral closure. Am. Heart J.*117:*1106, 1989.
400. Eusebio, J., Louie, E. K., Edwards, D. C., et al.: Alterations in transmitral flow dynamics in patients with early mitral valve closure and aortic regurgitation. Am. Heart J. *128:*941, 1994.
401. Sapira, J. D.: Quincke, DeMusset, Duroziez and Hill: Some aortic regurgitations. South. Med. J. *74:*459, 1981.
402. Boudoulas, H., Triposkiadis, F., Dervenagas, J., et al.: Mechanisms of pistol shot sounds in aortic regurgitation. Acta Cardiol. *46:*139, 1991.
403. Alpert, J. S., Veiweg, W. V. R., and Hagan, A. D.: Incidence and morphology of carotid shudders in aortic valve disease. Am. Heart J. *92:*435, 1976.
404. Aortic insufficiency. *In* Fowler, N. O.: Diagnosis of Heart Disease. New York, Springer-Verlag, 1991, pp. 123–133.
405. Abdulla, A. M., Frank, M. J., Erdin, R. A., Jr., and Canedo, M. I.: Clinical significance and hemodynamic correlates of the third heart sound gallop in aortic regurgitation. A guide to optimal timing of cardiac catheterization. Circulation *64:*464, 1981.
406. Harvey, W., Corrado, M. A., and Perloff, J. K.: "Right-sided" murmurs of aortic insufficiency. Am. J. Med. Sci. [illegible]
407. Fortuin, N. J., and Craige, E.: On the mechanism of the Austin Flint murmur. Circulation *45:*558, 1972.
408. Delman, A. J., and Stein, E.: Aortic regurgitation. *In* Dynamic Cardiac Auscultation and Phonocardiography. Philadelphia, W. B. Saunders Co., 1979, pp. 811–824.
409. Perloff, J. K.: Acute severe aortic regurgitation: Recognition and management. J. Cardiovasc. Med. *8:*209, 1983.
410. Benotti, J. R., and Dalen, J. E.: Aortic valvular regurgitation: Natural history and medical treatment. *In* Cohn, L. H., and DiSesa, V. J. (eds.): Aortic Regurgitation: Medical and Surgical Management. New York, Marcel Dekker, 1986, pp. 1–54.
411. Spring, D. A., Folts, J. D., Young, W. P., and Rowe, G. G.: Premature closure of the mitral and tricuspid valves. Circulation *45:*663, 1972.
412. Wong, M.: Diastolic mitral regurgitation. Hemodynamic and angiographic correlation. Br. Heart J. *31:*468, 1969.
413. Estes, E. H.: Left ventricular hypertrophy in acquired heart disease: A comparison of the vectorcardiogram in aortic stenosis and aortic insufficiency. *In* Hoffman, I. (ed.): Vectorcardiography. Amsterdam, North Holland Publishing Co., 1976.
414. Roberts, W. C., and Day, P. J.: Electrocardiographic observations in clinically isolated, pure, and chronic, severe aortic regurgitation: Analysis of 30 necropsy patients aged 19 to 65 years. Am. J. Cardiol. *55:*431, 1985.
415. DePace, N. L., Nestico, P. F., Kotler, M. N., et al.: Comparison of echocardiography and angiography in determining the cause of severe aortic regurgitation. Br. Heart J. *51:*36, 1984.
416. Meyer, T., Sareli, P., Pocock, W. A., et al.: Echocardiographic and hemodynamic correlates of diastolic closure of mitral valve and diastolic opening of aortic valve in severe regurgitation. Am. J. Cardiol. *59:*1144, 1987.
417. Weaver, W. F., Wilson, C. S., Rourke, T., and Caudill, C. C.: Mid-diastolic aortic valve opening in severe acute aortic regurgitation. Circulation *55:*112, 1977.
418. Dolan, M. S., Castello, R., St. Vrain, J. A., et al.: Quantitation of aortic regurgitation by Doppler echocardiography: A practical approach. Am. Heart J. *129:*1014, 1995.
418a. Shiota, T., Jones, M., Yamada, I., et al.: Effective regurgitant orifice area by the color Doppler flow convergence method for evaluating the severity of chronic aortic regurgitation: An animal study. Circulation *93:*594, 1996.
419. Masuyama, T., Kodama, K., Kitabatake, A., et al.: Noninvasive evaluation of aortic regurgitation by continuous-wave Doppler echocardiography. Circulation *73:*460, 1986.
420. Manyari, D. E., Nolewajka, A. J., and Kostuk, W. J.: Quantitative assessment of aortic valvular insufficiency by radionuclide angiography. Chest *81:*170, 1982.
421. Reimold, S. C., Maier, S. E., Fleischmann, K. E., et al.: Dynamic nature of the aortic regurgitant orifice area during diastole in patients with chronic aortic regurgitation. Circulation *89:*2085, 1994.

422. Sareli, P., Klein, H. O., Schamroth, C. L., et al.: Contribution of echocardiography and immediate surgery to the management of severe aortic regurgitation from active infective endocarditis. Am. J. Cardiol. *57*:413, 1986.
423. Goldschlager, N., Pfeifer, J., Cohn, K., et al.: The natural history of aortic regurgitation. A clinical and hemodynamic study. Am. J. Med. *54*:577, 1973.
423a. Klodas, E., Enriquez-Sarano, M., Tajik, A. J., et al.: Aortic regurgitation complicated by extreme left ventricular dilatation: Long-term outcome after surgical correction. J. Am. Coll. Cardiol. *27*:670, 1996.
424. Elkayam, U., McKay, C. R., Weber, L., et al.: Favorable effects of hydralazine on the hemodynamic response to isometric exercise in chronic severe aortic regurgitation. Am. J. Cardiol. *54*:1603, 1984.
425. Fioretti, P., Benussi, B., Scardi, S., et al.: Afterload reduction with nifedipine in aortic insufficiency. Am. J. Cardiol. *49*:1728, 1982.
426. Jebavy, P., Koudelkova, E., and Henzlova, M.: Unloading effects of prazosin in patients with chronic aortic regurgitation. Am. Heart J. *105*:567, 1983.
427. Rothlisberger, C., Sareli, P., and Wisenbaugh, T.: Comparison of single-dose nifedipine and captopril for chronic severe aortic regurgitation. Am. J. Cardiol. *71*:799, 1993.
428. Scognamiglio, R., Rahimtoola, S. H., Fasoli, G., et al.: Nifedipine in asymptomatic patients with severe aortic regurgitation and normal left ventricular function. N. Engl. J. Med. *331*:689, 1994.
429. Bonow, R. O.: Asymptomatic aortic regurgitation: Indications for operation. J. Cardiovasc. Surg. *9*(Suppl):170, 1994.
430. Bonow, R. O., Lakatos, E., Maron, B. J., and Epstein S. E.: Serial long-term assessment of the natural history of asymptomatic patients with chronic aortic regurgitation and normal left ventricular systolic function. Circulation *84*:1625, 1991.
431. Hancock, E. W.: When is the best time to operate for aortic regurgitation? Cardiol. Rev. *1*:301, 1993.
432. Nishimura, R., McGoon, M. D., Schaff, H. V., and Giuliani, E. R.: Chronic aortic regurgitation: Indications for operation—1988. Mayo Clin. Proc. *63*:270, 1988.
433. Bonow, R. O., Rosing, D. R., Kent, K. M., and Epstein, S. E.: Timing of operation for chronic aortic regurgitation. Am. J. Cardiol. *50*:325, 1982.
434. Taniguchi, K., Nakano, S., Matsuda, H., et al.: Depressed myocardial contractility and normal ejection performance after aortic valve replacement in patients with aortic regurgitation. J. Thorac. Cardiovasc. Surg. *98*:258, 1989.
435. Borow, K. M.: Surgical outcome in chronic aortic regurgitation: A physiologic framework for assessing preoperative predictors. J. Am. Coll. Cardiol. *10*:1165, 1987.
436. Bonow, R. O., Dodd, J. T., Maron, B. J., et al.: Long-term serial changes in left ventricular function and reversal of ventricular dilatation after valve replacement for chronic aortic regurgitation. Circulation *78*:1108, 1988.
437. Carabello, B. A., Usher, B. W., Hedrik, G. H., et al.: Predictors of outcome for aortic valve replacement in patients with aortic regurgitation and left ventricular dysfunction: A change in the measuring stick. J. Am. Coll. Cardiol. *10*:991, 1987.
438. Wisenbaugh, T., Booth, D., DeMaria, A., et al.: Relationship of contractile state to ejection performance in patients with chronic aortic valve disease. Circulation *73*:47, 1986.
439. Odell, J. A., and Orszulak, T. A.: Surgical repair and reconstruction of valvular lesions. Curr. Opin. Cardiol. *10*:135, 1995.
440. David, T. E.: Aortic valve repair in patients with Marfan syndrome and ascending aorta aneurysms due to degenerative disease. J. Cardiovasc. Surg. *9*(Suppl.):182, 1994.
441. Cosgrove, M., Rosenkranz, E. R., Hendren, W. G., et al.: Valvuloplasty for aortic insufficiency. J. Thorac. Cardiovasc. Surg. *102*:571, 1991.
442. Duran, C. M.: Present status of reconstructive surgery for aortic valve disease. J. Cardiovasc. Surg. *8*:443, 1993.
443. Duran, C. M. G.: Conservative valve surgery. *In* Al-Zaibag, M., and Duran, C. M. G. (eds.): Valvular Heart Disease. New York, Marcel Dekker, 1994, p. 569.

TRICUSPID, PULMONIC, AND MULTIVALVULAR DISEASE

444. Wooley, C. F., Fontana, M. E., Kilman, J. W., and Ryan, J. M.: Tricuspid stenosis: Atrial systolic murmur, tricuspid opening snap and right atrial pressure pulse. Am. J. Med. *78*:375, 1985.
445. Kitchin, A., and Turner, R.: Diagnosis and treatment of tricuspid stenosis. Br. Heart J. *26*:354, 1964.
446. Ewy, G. A.: Tricuspid valve disease. *In* Chatterjee, K., Cheitlin, M. D., Karliner, J., et al. (eds.): Cardiology: An Illustrated Text Reference, Vol. 2. Philadelphia, J. B. Lippincott, 1991, p. 991.
447. Tricuspid valve disease. *In* Fowler, N. O.: Diagnosis of Heart Disease. New York, Springer-Verlag, 1991, pp. 181–186.
448. Pillai, M. G., Sharma, S., Munsi, S. C., et al.: Value of echocardiography in detecting rheumatic tricuspid stenosis. J. Cardiovasc. Ultrasonogr. *4*:185, 1985.
449. Ribeiro, P. A., Al-Zaibag, M., and Sawyer, W.: A prospective study comparing the haemodynamic with the cross-sectional echocardiographic diagnosis of rheumatic tricuspid stenosis. Eur. Heart J. *10*:120, 1989.
450. Lundin, L., Landelius, J., Adren, B., and Oberg, K.: Transesophageal echocardiography improves the diagnostic value of cardiac ultrasound in patients with carcinoid heart disease. Br. Heart J. *64*:190, 1990.
451. Fawzy, M. E., Mercer, E. N., Dunn, B., et al.: Doppler echocardiography in the evaluation of tricuspid stenosis. Eur. Heart J. *10*:985, 1989.
452. Kirklin, J. W., and Barratt-Boyes, B. G.: Combined aortic and mitral valve disease with or without tricuspid valve disease. *In* Cardiac Surgery. 2nd ed. New York, Churchill-Livingstone, 1993, pp. 573–588.
453. Kirklin, J. W., and Barratt-Boyes, B. G.: Tricuspid valve disease. *In* Cardiac Surgery. 2nd ed. New York, Churchill-Livingstone, 1993, pp. 589–608.
454. Throburn, C. W., Morgan, J. J., Shanahan, M. X., and Chang, V. P.: Long-term results of tricuspid valve replacement and the problem of prosthetic valve thrombosis. Am. J. Cardiol. *51*:1128, 1983.
455. Boskovic, D., Elezovic, I., Boskovic, D., et al.: Late thrombosis of the Björk-Shiley tilting disc valve in the tricuspid position. J. Thorac. Cardiovasc. Surg. *91*:1, 1986.
456. Treasure, T.: Which prosthetic valve should we choose? Curr. Opin. Cardiol. *10*:144, 1995.
457. Robiolio, P. A., Rigolin, V. H., Harrison, J. K., et al.: Predictors of outcome of tricuspid valve replacement in carcinoid heart disease. Am. J. Cardiol. *75*:485, 1995.
458. Jegaden, O. L., Perinetti, M., Barthelet, M., et al.: Long-term results of porcine bioprostheses in the tricuspid position. Cardiothorac. Surg. *6*:256, 1992.
459. McGrath, L. B., Chen, C., Bailey, B. M., et al.: Early and late phase events following bioprosthetic tricuspid valve replacement. J. Cardiovasc. Surg. *7*:245, 1992.
460. Guerra, F., Bortolotti, U., Thiene, G., et al.: Long-term performance of the Hancock porcine bioprosthesis in the tricuspid position. A review of 45 patients with 14-year follow-up. J. Thorac. Cardiovasc. Surg. *99*:838, 1990.
461. Goldenberg, I. F., Pedersen, W., Olson, J., et al.: Percutaneous double balloon valvuloplasty for severe tricuspid stenosis. Am. Heart J. *118*:417, 1989.
462. Shafie, M. Z., Hayat, N., and Majid, O. A.: Fate of tricuspid regurgitation after closed valvotomy for mitral stenosis. Chest *88*:870, 1985.
463. Cohen, S. R., Sell, J. E., McIntosh, C. L., and Clark, R. E.: Tricuspid regurgitation in patients with acquired, chronic, pure mitral regurgitation. 1. Prevalence, diagnosis, and comparison of preoperative clinical and hemodynamic features in patients with and without tricuspid regurgitation. J. Thorac. Cardiovasc. Surg. *94*:481, 1987.
464. Morrison, D. A., Ovitt, T., and Hammermeister, K. E.: Functional tricuspid regurgitation and right ventricular dysfunction in pulmonary hypertension. Am. J. Cardiol. *62*:108, 1988.
465. Vatterott, P. J., Nishimura, R. A., Gersh, B. J., and Smith, H. C.: Severe isolated tricuspid insufficiency in coronary artery disease. Int. J. Cardiol. *14*:295, 1987.
466. Dougherty, M. J., and Craige, E.: Apathetic hyperthyroidism presenting as tricuspid regurgitation. Chest *63*:767, 1973.
467. Scheck-Krejca, H., Zulstra, F., Roelandt, J., and Vletter-McGhie, J.: Diagnosis of tricuspid regurgitation: Comparison of jugular venous and liver pulse tracings with combined two-dimensional and Doppler echocardiography. Eur. Heart J. *7*:973, 1986.
468. Esaghpour, E., Kawai, N., and Linhart, J. W.: Tricuspid insufficiency associated with aneurysm of the ventricular septum. Pediatrics *61*:586, 1978.
469. Sakai, K., Inoue, Y., and Osawa, M.: Congenital isolated tricuspid regurgitation in an adult. Am. Heart J. *110*:680, 1985.
470. Ohri, S. K., Schofield, J. B., Hodgson, H., et al.: Carcinoid heart disease: Early failure of an allograft valve replacement. Ann. Thorac. Surg. *58*:1161, 1994.
471. Lundin, L., Norheim, I., Landelius, J., et al.: Carcinoid heart disease: Relationship of circulating vasoactive substances to ultrasound-detectable cardiac abnormalities. Circulation *77*:264, 1988.
472. Jackson, D., Gibbs, H. R., and Zee-Cheng, C. S.: Isolated tricuspid valve prolapse diagnosed by echocardiography. Am. J. Med. *80*:281, 1986.
473. Schlamowitz, R. A., Gross, S., Keating, E., et al.: Tricuspid valve prolapse: A common occurrence in the click-murmur syndrome. J. Clin. Ultrasound *10*:435, 1982.
474. Gayet, C., Pierre, B., Delahaye, J-P., et al.: Traumatic tricuspid insufficiency: An underdiagnosed disease. Chest *92*:429, 1987.
475. Dickerman, S. A., and Rubler, S.: Mitral and tricuspid valve regurgitation in dilated cardiomyopathy. Am. J. Cardiol. *63*:629, 1989.
476. Ginzton, L. E., Siegel, R. J., and Criley, J. M.: Natural history of tricuspid valve endocarditis: A two-dimensional echocardiographic study. Am. J. Cardiol. *49*:1853, 1982.
477. Arbulu, A., and Asfaw, I.: Tricuspid valvulectomy without prosthetic replacement. Ten years of clinical experience. J. Thorac. Cardiovasc. Surg. *82*:684, 1981.
478. Mason, J. W., Billingham, M. E., and Friedman, J. P.: Methysergide induced heart disease: A case of multivalvular and myocardial fibrosis. Circulation *56*:889, 1977.
479. Laufer, J., Frand, M., and Milo, S.: Valve replacement for severe tricuspid regurgitation caused by Libman-Sacks endocarditis. Br. Heart J. *48*:294, 1982.
480. Pellegrini, A., Columbo, T., Donatelli, E., et al.: Evaluation and treatment of secondary tricuspid insufficiency. Eur. J. Cardiothorac. Surg. *6*:288, 1992.
481. Allen, S. J., and Naylor, D.: Pulsation of the eyeballs in tricuspid regurgitation. Can. Med. Assoc. J. *133*:119, 1985.
482. Abrams, J.: Tricuspid regurgitation. *In* Essentials of Cardiac Physical Diagnosis. Philadelphia, Lea and Febiger, 1987, pp. 375–400.

483. Cha, S. D., and Gooch, A. S.: Diagnosis of tricuspid regurgitation: Current status. Arch. Intern. Med. *143*:1763, 1983.
484. Amidi, M., Irwin, J. M., Salerni, R., et al.: Venous systolic thrill and murmur in the neck: A consequence of severe tricuspid insufficiency. J. Am. Coll. Cardiol. *7*:942, 1986.
485. Maisel, A. S., Atwood, J. E., and Goldberger, A. L.: Hepatojugular reflux: Useful in the bedside diagnosis of tricuspid regurgitation. Ann. Intern. Med. *101*:781, 1984.
486. Come, P. C., and Riley, M. F.: Tricuspid annular dilatation and failure of tricuspid leaflet coaptation in patients with tricuspid regurgitation. Am. J. Cardiol. *55*:599, 1985.
487. Popp, R. L.: When is tricuspid regurgitation important? Cardiol. Rev. *2*:183, 1994.
488. Meltzer, R. S., van Hoogenhuyze, D., Serruys, P. W., et al.: Diagnosis of tricuspid regurgitation by contrast echocardiography. Circulation *63*:1093, 1981.
489. Forman, M. B., Byrd, B. F., Oates, J. A., and Robertson, R. M.: Two-dimensional echocardiography in the diagnosis of carcinoid heart disease. Am. Heart J. *107*:492, 1984.
490. Curtius, J. M., Thyssen, M., Breuer, H. W. M., and Loogen, F.: Doppler versus contrast echocardiography for diagnosis of tricuspid regurgitation. Am. J. Cardiol. *56*:333, 1985.
491. Diebold, B., Touati, R., Blanchard, D., et al.: Quantitative assessment of tricuspid regurgitation using pulsed Doppler echocardiography. Br. Heart J. *50*:443, 1983.
492. Pennestri, F., Loperfido, F., Salvatori, M. F., et al.: Assessment of tricuspid regurgitation by pulsed Doppler ultrasonography of the hepatic veins. Am. J. Cardiol. *54*:363, 1984.
493. Suzuki, Y., Kambara, H., Kadota, K., et al.: Detection and evaluation of tricuspid regurgitation using a real-time, two-dimensional, color-coded, Doppler flow imaging system: Comparison with contrast two-dimensional echocardiography and right ventriculography. Am. J. Cardiol. *57*:811, 1986.
494. Lingameni, R., Cha, S. D., Maranhao, V., et al.: Tricuspid regurgitation: Clinical and angiographic assessment. Cathet. Cardiovasc. Diagn. *5*:7, 1979.
495. Cheitlin, M., and MacGregor, J. S.: Acquired tricuspid and pulmonary valve disease. *In* Rahimtoola, S. H. (ed.): Valvular Heart Disease and Endocarditis. Atlas of Heart Diseases. Vol. 11. St. Louis, Mosby, 1996.
496. Ubago, J. L., Figueroa, A., Colman, T., et al.: Right ventriculography as a valid method for the diagnosis of tricuspid insufficiency. Cathet. Cardiovasc. Diagn. *7*:433, 1981.
497. Carpentier, A., Deloche, A., and Dauptain, J.: A new reconstructive operation for correction of mitral and tricuspid insufficiency. J. Thorac. Cardiovasc. Surg. *61*:1, 1971.
498. Lambertz, H., Minale, C., Flachskampf, F. A., et al.: Long-term follow-up after Carpentier tricuspid valvuloplasty. Am. Heart J. *117*:615, 1989.
499. Duran, C. M., Kumar, N., Prabhakar, G., et al.: Vanishing De Vega annuloplasty for functional tricuspid regurgitation. J. Thorac. Cardiovasc. Surg. *106*:609, 1993.
500. Prabhakar, G., Kumar, N., Gometza, B., et al.: Surgery for organic rheumatic disease of the tricuspid valve. J. Heart Valve Dis. *2*:561, 1993.
501. Cohn, L. H.: Tricuspid regurgitation secondary to mitral valve disease: When and how to repair. J. Cardiovasc. Surg. *9*(Suppl.):237, 1994.
502. Chidambaram, M., Abdulali, S. A., Baliga, B. G., and Ionescu, M. I.: Long-term results of DeVega tricuspid annuloplasty. Ann. Thorac. Surg. *43*:185, 1987.
503. Duran, C. M.: Tricuspid valve surgery revisited. J. Cardiovasc. Surg. *9*(Suppl.):242, 1994.
504. Silver, M. A., Cohen, S. R., McIntosh, C. L., et al.: Late (5 to 132 months) clinical and hemodynamic results after either tricuspid valve replacement or annuloplasty for Ebstein's anomaly of the tricuspid valve. Am. J. Cardiol. *54*:627, 1984.
505. Lin, S. S., Reynerstonm, S. I., Louie, E. K., and Levitsky, S.: Right ventricular volume overload results in depression of left ventricular ejection fraction. Circulation *90*:II-209, 1994.
506. Kirshenbaum, H. D.: Pulmonary valve disease. *In* Dalen, J. E., and Alpert, J. S. (eds.): Valvular Heart Disease. 2nd ed. Boston, Little, Brown and Co., 1987, pp. 403–438.
507. Vela, J. E., Conteras, R., and Sosa, F. R.: Rheumatic pulmonary valve disease. Am. J. Cardiol. *23*:12, 1969.
508. Altrichter, P. M., Olson, L. J., Edwards, W. D., et al.: Surgical pathology of the pulmonary valve: A study of 116 cases spanning 15 years. Mayo Clin. Proc. *64*:1352, 1989.
509. Ohri, S. K., Schofield, J. B., Hodgson, H., et al.: Carcinoid heart disease: Early failure of an allograft valve replacement. Ann. Thorac. Surg. *58*:1161, 1994.
510. Seymour, J., Emanuel, R., and Patterson, N.: Acquired pulmonary stenosis. Br. Heart J. *30*:776, 1968.
511. Brayshaw, J. R., and Perloff, J. K.: Congenital pulmonary insufficiency complicating idiopathic dilatation of the pulmonary artery. Am. J. Cardiol. *10*:282, 1962.
512. Runco, V., and Levin, H. S.: The spectrum of pulmonic regurgitation. *In* Physiologic Principles of Heart Sounds and Murmurs. American Heart Association Monograph No. 46, 1975, p. 175.
513. Cassling, R. S., Rogler, W. C., and McManus, B. M.: Isolated pulmonic valve infective endocarditis: A diagnostically elusive entity. Am. Heart J. *109*:558, 1985.
514. Collins, N. P., Braunwald, E., and Morrow, A. G.: Isolated congenital pulmonic valvular regurgitation. Am. J. Med. *28*:159, 1960.
515. Jacoby, W. J., Tucker, D. H., and Sumner, R. G.: The second heart sound in congenital pulmonary valvular insufficiency. Am. Heart J. *69*:603, 1965.
516. O'Toole, J. D., Wurtzbacher, J. J., Wearner, N. E., and Jain, A. C.: Pulmonary valve injury and insufficiency during pulmonary-artery catheterization. N. Engl. J. Med. *301*:1167, 1979.
517. Bousvaros, G. A., and Deuchar, D. C.: The murmur of pulmonary regurgitation which is not associated with pulmonary hypertension. Lancet *2*:962, 1961.
518. DePace, N. L., Nestico, P. F., Iskandrian, A. S., and Morganroth, J.: Acute severe pulmonic valve regurgitation: Pathophysiology, diagnosis and treatment. Am. Heart J. *108*:567, 1984.
519. Green, E. W., Agruss, N. S., and Adolph, R. J.: Right-sided Austin Flint murmur. Documentation by intracardiac phonocardiography, echocardiography and postmortem findings. Am. J. Cardiol. *32*:370, 1973.
520. Braunwald, E., and Morrow, A. G.: A method for detection and estimation of aortic regurgitant flow in man. Circulation *17*:505, 1958.
521. Collins, N. P., Braunwald, E., and Morrow, A. G.: Detection of pulmonic and tricuspid valvular regurgitation by means of indicator solutions. Circulation *20*:561, 1959.
522. Van Meurs-Van Woezik, H., McGhie, J., and Roelandt, J.: Septal flutter in pulmonary insufficiency. J. Cardiovasc. Ultrasonogr. *3*:159, 1984.
523. Miyatake, K., Okamoto, M., Kinoshita, N., et al.: Pulmonary regurgitation studied with the ultrasonic pulsed Doppler technique. Circulation *65*:969, 1982.
524. Emery, R. W., Landes, R. G., Moller, J. H., and Nicoloff, D. M.: Pulmonary valve replacement with a porcine aortic heterograft. Ann. Thorac. Surg. *27*:148, 1979.
525. Segal, J., Harvey, W. P., and Hufnagel, C. A.: Clinical study of one hundred cases of severe aortic insufficiency. Am. J. Med. *21*:200, 1956.
526. Zitnik, R. S.: The masking of aortic stenosis by mitral stenosis. Am. Heart J. *69*:22, 1965.
527. Schattenberg, T. T., Titus, J. L., and Parkin, T. W.: Clinical findings in acquired aortic valve stenosis. Effect of disease of other valves. Am. Heart J. *73*:322, 1967.
528. Melvin, D. B., Tecklenberg, P. L., Hollingsworth, J. F., et al.: Computer-based analysis of preoperative and postoperative prognostic factors in 100 patients with combined aortic and mitral valve replacement. Circulation *48*(Suppl. III):58, 1973.
529. Rippe, J. M.: Multiple floppy valves. An echocardiographic syndrome. Am. J. Med. *66*:817, 1979.
530. Nitter-Hauge, S., and Horstkotte, D.: Management of multivalvular heart disease. Eur. Heart J. *8*:643, 1987.
531. Coll-Mazzei, J. V., Jegaden, O., Janody, P., et al.: Results of triple valve replacement: Perioperative mortality and long-term results. J. Cardiovasc. Surg. *28*:369, 1987.
532. Michel, P. L., Houdart, E., Ghanem, G., et al.: Combined aortic mitral and tricuspid surgery: Results in 78 patients. Eur. Heart J. *8*:457, 1987.
533. MacManus, Q., Grunkemeier, G., and Starr, A.: Late results of triple valve replacement: A 14-year review. Ann. Thorac. Surg. *25*:402, 1978.
534. Vatterott, P. J., Gersh, B. J., Fuster, V., et al.: Long-term followup (2–20 years) of patients with triple valve replacement. J. Am. Coll. Cardiol. *1*(Abs.):586, 1983.

PROSTHETIC CARDIAC VALVES

535. Braunwald, N. S., Cooper, T. S., and Morrow, A. G.: Complete replacement of the mitral valve. J. Thorac. Cardiovasc. Surg. *40*:1, 1960.
536. Harken, D. E., Soroff, M. S., and Taylor, M. C.: Partial and complete prostheses in aortic insufficiency. J. Thorac. Cardiovasc. Surg. *40*:744, 1960.
537. Starr, A., and Edwards, M. L.: Mitral replacement: Clinical experience with a ball-valve prosthesis. Ann. Surg. *154*:726, 1961.
537a. Grunkemeier, G. L., Starr, A., and Rahimtoola, S. H.: Performance of prosthetic heart valves. *In* Rahimtoola, S. H. (ed.): Valvular Heart Disease and Endocarditis. Atlas of Heart Diseases. Vol. 11. St. Louis, Mosby, 1996.
538. Grunkemeier, G. L., and Starr, A.: Twenty-five year experience with Starr-Edwards heart valves: Follow-up methods and results. Can. J. Cardiol. *4*:381, 1988.
539. Pilegaard, H. K., Lund, O., Nielsen, T. T., et al.: Twenty-two-year experience with aortic valve replacement: Starr-Edwards ball valves versus disc valves. Texas Heart Inst. J. *18*:24, 1991.
540. Cohn, L. H.: Aortic valve prosthesis. Cardiol. Rev. *2*:219, 1994.
541. Nair, C., Mohiuddin, S. M., Hilleman, D. E., et al.: Ten-year results with the St. Jude medical prosthesis. Am. J. Cardiol. *65*:217, 1990.
542. Burckhardt, D., Streibel, D., Vogt, S., et al.: Heart valve replacement with St. Jude medical valve prosthesis: Long-term experience in 743 patients in Switzerland. Circulation *78*(Suppl. I):I18, 1988.
543. Stewart, S., Cianciotta, D., Hicks, G. L., and DeWeese, J. A.: The Lillehei-Kaster aortic valve prosthesis. J. Thorac. Cardiovasc. Surg. *95*:1023, 1988.
544. Starek, P. J. K., Beaudet, R. L., and Hall, K.-V.: The Medtronic-Hall valve: Development and clinical experience. *In* Crawford, F. A. (ed.): Cardiac Surgery: Current Heart Valve Prostheses. Vol. 1. Philadelphia, Hanley and Belfus, 1987, pp. 223–236.
545. Beaudet, R. L., Nakhle, G., Beaulieu, C. R., et al.: Medtronic-Hall prosthesis: Valve related deaths and complications. Can. J. Cardiol. *4*:376, 1988.
546. Hammermeister, K. E., Sethi, G. K., Henderson, W. G., et al.: A compar-

ison of outcomes in men 11 years after heart-valve replacement with a mechanical valve or bioprosthesis. N. Engl. J. Med. *328*:1289, 1993.

547. Horstkotte, D., Schulte, H., Bircks, W., et al.: Lower intensity anticoagulation therapy results in lower complication rates with the St. Jude medical prosthesis. J. Thorac. Cardiovasc. Surg. *107*:1136, 1994.
548. Turpie, A. G., Gent, M., Laupacis, A., et al.: A comparison of aspirin with placebo in patients treated with warfarin after heart-valve replacement. N. Engl. J. Med. *329*:524, 1993.
549. Turina, J., Hess, O. M., Turina, M., and Krayenbuehl, H. P.: Cardiac bioprosthesis in the 1990s. Circulation *88*:775, 1993.
550. Skoularigis, J., Essop, M. R., Skucicky, D., et al.: Frequency and severity of intravascular hemolysis after left-sided cardiac valve replacement with Medtronic-Hall, St. Jude Medical Protheses and influence of prosthetic type, position, size and number. Am. J. Cardiol. *71*:587, 1993.
551. Glower, D. D., White, W. D., Hatton, A. C., et al.: Determinants of reoperation after 960 valve replacements with Carpentier-Edwards prostheses. J. Thorac. Cardiovasc. Surg. *107*:381, 1994.
552. Grunkemeier, G. L., and Bodnar, E.: Comparison of structural valve failure among different "models" of homograft valves. J. Heart Valve Dis. *3*:556, 1994.
553. Barratt-Boyes, B. G., and Christie, G. W.: What is the best bioprosthetic operation for the small aortic root? Allograft, autograft, porcine, pericardial? Stented or unstented? J. Cardiovasc. Surg. *9*(Suppl.):158, 1994.
554. Bloomfield, P., Wheatley, D. J., Prescott, R. J., and Miller, H. C.: Twelve-year comparison of a Björk-Shiley mechanical heart valve with porcine bioprostheses. N. Engl. J. Med. *324*:573, 1991.
555. Khuri, S. F., Folland, E. D., Sethi, G. K., et al.: Six month postoperative hemodynamics of the Hancock heterograft and the Björk-Shiley prosthesis: Results of a Veteran's Administration cooperative prospective randomized trial. J. Am. Coll. Cardiol. *12*:8, 1988.
556. Janusz, M. T., Jamieson, W. R. E., Burr, L. H., et al.: Thromboembolism risks and role of anticoagulants in patients in chronic atrial fibrillation following mitral valve replacement with porcine bioprostheses. J. Am. Coll. Cardiol. *1*:587, 1983.
557. Khan, S. S., Mitchell, R. S., Derby, G. C., et al.: Differences in Hancock and Carpentier-Edwards porcine xenograft aortic valve hemodynamics: Effect of valve size. Circulation *82*(Suppl. IV):117, 1990.
558. Cohn, L. H., Collins, J. J., DiSesa, V. J., et al.: Fifteen-year experience with 1678 Hancock porcine bioprosthetic heart valve replacements. Ann. Surg. *210*:435, 1989.
559. Jamieson, W. R. E., Tyers, G. F. O., Janusz, M. T., et al.: Age as a determinant for selection of porcine bioprostheses for cardiac valve replacement: Experience with Carpentier-Edwards standard bioprosthesis. Can. J. Cardiol. *7*:181, 1991.
560. Kirklin, J. K., Smith, D., and Novick, W.: Long-term function of cryopreserved aortic homografts: A ten year study. J. Thorac. Cardiovasc. Surg. *106*:154, 1993.
561. Doty, D. B., Michielon, G., Wang, N-D., et al.: Replacement of the aortic valve with cryopreserved aortic allograft. Ann. Thorac. Surg. *56*:228, 1993.
562. Treasure, T.: The pulmonary autograft as aortic valve replacement. Lancet *343*:1308, 1994.
563. Kouchoukos, N. T., Davila-Roman, V. G., Spray, T. L., et al.: Replacement of the aortic root with a pulmonary autograft in children and young adults with aortic-valve disease. N. Engl. J. Med. *330*:1, 1994.
564. Elkins, R. C.: Pulmonary autograft—The optimal substitute for the aortic valve? N. Engl. J. Med. *330*:59, 1994.
565. Ross, D., Jackson, M., and Davies, J.: The pulmonary autograft: A permanent aortic valve. Eur. J. Cardiothorac. Surg. *6*:113, 1992.
566. Oury, J. H., Angell, W. W., Eddy, A. C., and Cleveland, J. C.: Pulmonary autograft—Past, present, and future. J. Heart Valve Dis. *2*:365, 1993.
567. Doty, D. B.: Replacement of the aortic valve with cryopreserved aortic allograft: The procedures of choice for young patients. J. Cardiac Surg. *9*(Suppl.):192, 1994.
568. Bloomfield, P., Wheatley, D. J., Prescott, R. J., and Miller, H. C.: Twelve-year comparison of a Björk-Shiley mechanical heart valve with porcine bioprostheses. N. Engl. J. Med. *324*:573, 1991.
569. Nashof, S. A. M., Sethia, B., Turner, M. A., et al.: Björk-Shiley and Carpentier-Edwards valves: A comparative analysis. J. Thorac. Cardiovasc. Surg. *93*:394, 1987.
570. Hammond, G. I., Geha, A. S., Klopf, G. S., and Hashim, S. W.: Biological versus mechanical valves: Analysis of 1116 valves inserted in 1012 adult patients with a 4818 patient-year and a 5327 valve-year followup. J. Thorac. Cardiovasc. Surg. *93*:182, 1987.
571. Sareli, P., England, M. J., Berk, M. R., et al.: Maternal and fetal sequelae of anticoagulation during pregnancy in patients with mechanical heart valve prostheses. Am. J. Cardiol. *63*:1462, 1989.
572. Iturbe-Alessio, I., Fonesca, M. D. C., Mutchinik, O., et al.: Risks of anticoagulant therapy in pregnant women with artificial heart valves. N. Engl. J. Med. *315*:1390, 1986.
573. John, S.: Valve replacement in the young patients with rheumatic heart disease: Review of a twenty year experience. J. Thorac. Cardiovasc. Surg. *99*:631, 1990.
574. Selwyn, L., Rao, S., Mardin, M. K., et al.: Prosthetic valves in children and adolescents. Am. Heart J. *121*:557, 1991.
575. Gardner, T. J.: Anticoagulants for children requiring heart valve replacement. *In* Dunn, J. M. (ed.): Cardiac Valve Disease in Children. New York, Elsevier, 1988, p. 359.
576. Smith, N. D., Raizada, V., and Abrams, J.: Auscultation of the normally functioning prosthetic valve. Ann. Intern. Med. *95*:594, 1981.
577. Klein, H. O., Schamroth, C. L., Marcus, B. D., et al.: Echo-phonocardiographic assessment of the Medtronic-Hall mitral valve prosthesis: Observations on normal and abnormal function. J. Cardiovasc. Ultrasonogr. *5*:115, 1986.
578. Alam, M., Serwin, J. B., Rosman, H. S., et al.: Transesophageal echocardiographic features of normal and dysfunctioning bioprosthetic valves. Am. Heart J. *121*:1149, 1991.

Chapter 33
Infective Endocarditis

ADOLF W. KARCHMER

DEFINITION 1077
CLINICAL CLASSIFICATION 1078
Etiological Microorganisms 1080
PATHOGENESIS 1082
PATHOPHYSIOLOGY 1083
CLINICAL FEATURES 1084
DIAGNOSIS 1086
Laboratory Tests 1087
Echocardiography 1088
TREATMENT 1089
Antimicrobial Therapy for Specific Organisms 1089
Surgical Treatment of Intracardiac Complications 1094
Treatment of Extracardiac Complications . . 1095
Response to Therapy and Outcome 1096
PREVENTION 1097
REFERENCES 1099

DEFINITION

Infective endocarditis (IE) is the condition in which there is microbial infection of the endothelial surface of the heart. The characteristic lesion, the vegetation, is a variably sized amorphous mass of platelets and fibrin in which abundant microorganisms and scant inflammatory cells are enmeshed. Heart valves are most commonly involved; however, infection may occur at the site of a septal defect or on chordae tendineae or mural endocardium. Infection of arteriovenous shunts, arterioarterial shunts (patent ductus arteriosus), or coarctation of the aorta, although actually an endarteritis, is clinically and pathologically similar to IE. Many diverse species of bacteria, fungi, mycobacteria, rickettsiae, chlamydiae, and mycoplasma cause IE; nevertheless, streptococci, staphylococci, enterococci, and fastidious gram-negative coccobacilli that reside in the oral cavity and upper respiratory tract cause the majority of cases of IE.

IE has traditionally been classified as *acute* or *subacute*. Originally, these terms were applied to untreated patients and denoted a disease resulting in marked systemic toxicity and death in days to less than 6 weeks or an indolent, less toxic illness resulting in death in 6 weeks to 6 months or more, respectively. Today acute IE presents with marked toxicity and progresses over days to several weeks to valvular destruction and metastatic infection. In contrast, subacute IE evolves over weeks to months with only modest toxicity and rarely causes metastatic infection. Acute IE is caused typically, although not exclusively, by *Staphylococcus aureus,* whereas the subacute syndrome is more likely caused by viridans streptococci, enterococci, coagulase-negative staphylococci, or gram-negative coccobacilli. Classifications that indicate not only the temporal-toxicity aspects but also the etiology, the anatomical site of infection, and the relevant pathogenetic risk factors, if any, are preferred because they imply therapeutic and prognostic considerations.

EPIDEMIOLOGY

The incidence of IE is remarkably similar in developed countries. From 1950 through 1987, in Olmstead County, Minnesota, the incidence of IE remained relatively constant; it was 4.2 per 100,000 patient-years from 1970 to 1987.[1,2] During the 1980's, the yearly incidence of IE per 100,000 population was 2.0 in the United Kingdom and Wales, 1.9 in the Netherlands, and 1.7 in Louisiana.[3–5] Endocarditis occurred more frequently in men; gender derived ratios range from 1.6 to 2.5.[1,2,4] The age-specific incidence of endocarditis increased progressively after 30 years of age and exceeded 15 to 30 cases per 100,000 person-years in the sixth through eighth decades of life.[1,2,4] From 55 to 75 per cent of patients with native valve endocarditis (NVE) have predisposing conditions: rheumatic heart disease, congenital heart disease, mitral valve prolapse, degenerative heart disease, asymmetrical septal hypertrophy, or intravenous drug abuse.[2,6–8] From 7 to 25 per cent of cases involve prosthetic valves.[2,4,5,7,8] Predisposing conditions cannot be identified in 25 to 45 per cent of patients. The nature of predisposing conditions and, in part, the microbiology of IE correlate with the age of patients (Table 33–1).

CHANGE IN PATIENTS WITH IE. Infective endocarditis is an evolving disease. Changes in some aspects appear incontestable in spite of the hazard of referral bias in available data. As a consequence of changes in the population at risk for IE, the median age of patients has gradually increased from 30 to 40 years of age in the preantibiotic and early antibiotic eras to 47 to 64 years in recent decades.[1,4,7–10] Rheumatic fever with subsequent rheumatic heart disease in children and young adults has been markedly reduced in developed countries. Patients with congenital and acquired valvular disease, who are vulnerable to IE, enjoy greater longevity. Additionally, during their later years many of these patients require valve replacement, which places them at greater risk for endocarditis. The increasing life span of the general population results in the emergence of degenerative heart disease as a major substrate for IE. Finally, nosocomial endocarditis presents with increased frequency among the elderly, who experience high rates of hospitalization for underlying illnesses.[9,11,12] In recent years, only the increasing role of intravenous drug abuse as predisposition for IE favors the occurrence of infection in younger patients.[10]

Changes have also occurred in the relative frequency of conditions that predispose to IE; the redistribution of predisposing conditions impacts on the age distribution of IE. Intravenous drug abuse, prosthetic heart valves, and nosocomial bacteremia have altered the epidemiological picture of IE over the past three decades. During this period mitral valve prolapse with a murmur of mitral regurgitation has been recognized as an important predisposition for endocarditis.[6,13–16]

CHANGES IN THE MICROBIOLOGY OF IE. The microbiology of IE is affected by the alterations in predisposing conditions and the age of patients with IE. Coagulase-negative staphylococci, previously a minor cause of NVE, are an important cause of prosthetic valve endocarditis (PVE) and nosocomial IE.[16–18] *S. aureus* is the predominant cause of IE among intravenous drug abusers, particularly of infection involving the tricuspid valve. In addition, *Pseudomonas aeruginosa,* other gram-negative bacilli, and *Candida* species, unusual causes of NVE in

TABLE 33–1 PREDISPOSING CONDITIONS AND MICROBIOLOGY OF NATIVE VALVE ENDOCARDITIS

	CHILDREN (%)		ADULTS (%)	
	Neonates	2 mo–15 yr	15–60 yr	> 60 yr
PREDISPOSING CONDITIONS				
RHD		2–10	25–30	8
CHD	28	75–90*	10–20	2
MVP		5–15	10–30	10
DHD			Rare	30
Parenteral drug abuse			15–35	10
Other			10–15	10
None	72†	2–5	25–45	25–40
MICROBIOLOGY				
Streptococci	15–20	40–50	45–65	30–45
Enterococci		4	5–8	15
S. aureus	40–50	25	30–40	25–30
Coagulase-negative staphylococci	10	5	3–5	5–8
GNB	10	5	4–8	5
Fungi	10	1	1	Rare
Polymicrobial	4		1	Rare
Other			1	2
Culture negative	4	0–15	3–10	5

RHD = Rheumatic heart disease; CHD = congenital heart disease; MVP = mitral valve prolapse; DHD = degenerative heart disease; GNB = gram-negative bacteria, frequently *Haemophilus* species, *Actinobacillus actinomycetemcomitans, Cardiobacterium hominis.*

* 50% of cases follow surgery and may involve implanted devices and foreign material.

† Often tricuspid valve IE.

other settings, are important causes of IE in drug abusers.[19] IE caused by enterococci, which are associated with genitourinary tract manipulations, and by *Streptococcus bovis,* which is associated with gastrointestinal malignancy and colonic polyps, occurs more frequently in the elderly, the population likely to experience these precipitating conditions.[1,3,9]

CLINICAL CLASSIFICATION

Cases of IE occurring in defined populations or settings often share clinical features and microbiology. Accordingly, it is useful to classify IE in terms of the population involved or a predisposing condition.

CHILDREN. The incidence of IE among hospitalized children ranges from 1 in 4500 to 1 in 1280.[20] In the Netherlands, IE was noted in 1.7 and 1.2 per 100,000 male and female children less than 10 years old, respectively.[4] Recently, IE has been noted in neonates with increasing frequency. Among neonates, IE typically involves the tricuspid valve of structurally normal hearts and is associated with very high mortality rates. It is likely that many of these episodes arise as a consequence of infected intravenous and right-heart catheters as well as cardiac surgery.[20–22]

The vast majority of children with IE occurring after the neonatal period have identifiable structural cardiac abnormalities (Table 33–1). In recent series, rheumatic heart disease was an infrequent predisposition for IE (≤4 per cent).[22–24] Congenital heart abnormalities, particularly those involving the aortic valve; ventricular septal defects; tetralogy of Fallot; and other complex structural anomalies associated with cyanosis are found in 75 to 90 per cent of cases. Of children with IE on congenital defects, 50 per cent develop infection after cardiac surgery; in these children, infection frequently involves prosthetic valves, valved conduits, or synthetic patches.[22–24] Secundum atrial septal defects are not associated with an increased risk for IE.[25] Since 1990 mitral valve prolapse has been recognized as a predisposition for IE in children; it, generally in association with a regurgitant murmur, was the predisposing cardiac abnormality in 15 per cent and 5 per cent of cases in two series.[23,24]

Endocarditis among neonates is caused primarily by *S. aureus,* coagulase-negative staphylococci, and group B streptococci.[20,21] Occasionally, infection is caused by gram-negative bacilli and *Candida* species.[20,22] Among older children, streptococci, the predominant cause, account for at least 40 per cent of cases, and *S. aureus* occurring as a nosocomial or community-acquired acute infection is the second most common cause of IE.[20,22–24] *Streptococcus pneumoniae,* a common cause of bacteremia in children, is nevertheless an uncommon cause of IE. Like *S. aureus, S. pneumoniae* may involve normal or abnormal valves, present as acute fulminant IE, cause rapid valve destruction and heart failure, and often result in death.[20] Although *Haemophilus influenzae* type B is also a frequent cause of bacteremia and meningitis in young children, it rarely causes IE.[20]

The clinical features and echocardiographic findings of IE in children are similar to those noted among adults with NVE or PVE, respectively.[20,23] In contrast, IE among neonates is more cryptic; the clinical picture is dominated by bacteremia, and classic signs of IE are rare.[20]

ADULTS. Some of the common features and evolving aspects of IE occurring in adults have been noted in considering the epidemiology of IE. Mitral valve prolapse has emerged as a predominant predisposing structural cardiac abnormality and accounts for 7 to 30 per cent of NVE in adults which is not related to drug abuse or nosocomial infection.[2,4,6–8,13] The frequency of mitral prolapse in IE is not a direct reflection of risk, however, because as many as 2 to 4 per cent of healthy persons have mitral valve prolapse, and rates increase to 20 per cent among young women.[26,27]

In case-control studies, the relative risk of endocarditis among patients with mitral valve prolapse ranges from 3.5 to 8.2.[13–17] This increased risk of endocarditis is almost entirely confined to patients with both prolapse and a mitral regurgitation murmur. Risk is also increased among men and patients over age 45.[14,16] Valve redundancy and thickened leaflets (>5 mm) by echocardiography also identify a population at increased risk for IE.[19,28] Among patients with mitral valve prolapse and a systolic murmur, the incidence of IE is 52 per 100,000 person-years, compared with a rate of 4.6 per 100,000 person-years among those with prolapse and no murmur or among the general population.[16] Among 110 episodes of IE involving prolapsing mitral valves, infection was caused by streptococci in 53 per cent, *S. aureus* in 10 per cent, coagulase-negative staphylococci in 9 per cent, enterococci in 9 per cent, and *Haemophilus* species in 6 per cent.[29] The mortality rate was 14 per cent, similar to rates noted in NVE in general.[29]

Rheumatic heart disease was the predisposing cardiac lesion for IE in 20 to 25 per cent of cases in the 1970's and 1980's.[25] In reports from community hospitals in the United States in the 1980's, rheumatic heart disease predisposed to IE in only 7 and 10 per cent of cases.[7,8] In patients with rheumatic heart disease, endocarditis occurs most frequently on the mitral valve, a site at which women are more commonly infected. The aortic valve is the next most common site for IE; infection in this setting occurs more commonly in men.

Congenital heart disease is the substrate for IE in 10 to 20 per cent of younger adults and 8 per cent of older adults. Among adults, the common predisposing lesions are patent ductus arteriosus, ventricular septal defects, and bicuspid aortic valves, the latter seen particularly among older men (>60 years).

In settings where NVE among adults is not skewed dramatically by infection occurring among intravenous drug abusers and nosocomial disease, the microbiology is notably similar to that shown in Table 33–1.[2–4,30] *Coxiella burnetii,* an uncommon cause of IE in the United States, caused 3 per cent of all cases in the United Kingdom from 1976 to 1985 and is a prominent cause of IE in France.[3,31]

INTRAVENOUS DRUG ABUSERS. The risk for IE among intravenous drug abusers, 2 to 5 per cent per patient-year, is estimated to be severalfold greater than that of patients with rheumatic heart disease or prosthetic valves.[32] In one study IE was diagnosed in 74 (6.4 per cent) of 1150 intravenous drug abusers who were hospitalized during 12 months.[33] The ratio of men to women with IE in this study was 5.4:1, similar to that seen in other reports, and the average age of IE patients was 32.5 years. Intravenous cocaine use has been associated with an increased risk for endocarditis, and the intravenous use of pentazocine mixed with tripelennamine was associated with IE caused by *Pseudomonas aeruginosa* sero group 011 in both Detroit and Chicago.[34–36]

Endocarditis occurring in intravenous drug abusers has a unique propensity to infect right heart valves.[32,33] On postmortem examination of 80 addicts with active or healed IE involving 103 valves, evidence of infection was seen on the tricuspid valve in 44 per cent, the mitral valve in 43 per cent, the aortic valve in 40 per cent, and the pulmonic valve in 3 per cent.[37] Because mortality rates are higher in patients with left-sided versus right-sided IE, this distribution is undoubtedly skewed. In clinical series the typical distribution of valve involvement is tricuspid in 78 per cent, mitral in 24 per cent, and aortic in 8 per cent (8 patients had infection of multiple sites).[33] In intravenous drug abusers the valves were normal prior to infection in 75 to 93 per cent of patients.[32,33,37] The remaining patients have preexisting aortic or mitral valve abnormalities, resulting primarily from rheumatic heart disease, congenital heart disease, or prior episodes of IE. Intravenous drug abuse is a risk factor for recurrent NVE.[38]

The microbiology of IE occurring in intravenous drug abusers is unique in several respects (Table 33–2). In contrast to NVE among adults in general, *S. aureus* causes more than 50 per cent of these infections overall and more than 70 per cent of those involving the tricuspid valve. The well-established predilection for *S. aureus* to infect normal as well as abnormal left heart valves is seen in addicts. Although the phenomenon of *S. aureus* infection of normal tricuspid valves is not unique to addicts, the high frequency is characteristic.[32,39] Streptococcal and enterococcal infection of previously abnormal mitral or aortic valves in

TABLE 33–2 MICROBIOLOGY OF ENDOCARDITIS ASSOCIATED WITH INTRAVENOUS DRUG ABUSE

ORGANISM	PER CENT* Right-sided (N = 346)	Left-sided (N = 204)	All Cases (N = 550)
Staphylococcus aureus	77	23	57
Streptococci	5	15	9
Enterococci	2	24	10
Gram-negative bacilli†	5	12	7
Fungi (predominantly *Candida* species)	0	12	5
Polymicrobial	6	7	6
Culture-negative	3	3	3
Miscellaneous	2	3	3

Data from references 32, 33, and 219.
* 10 cases with right- and left-sided IE are each counted twice.
† *P. aeruginosa, S. marcescens,* and Enterobacteriaceae.

addicts is comparable to that noted generally in NVE. In contrast, infection of right and left heart valves by *P. aeruginosa* and other gram-negative bacilli and left heart valves by fungi occurs with increased frequency among drug abusers. In addition, unusual organisms, some of which are likely related to injection of contaminated materials, cause endocarditis in these patients, e.g., *Corynebacterium* species, *Lactobacillus, Bacillus cereus,* and non-pathogenic *Neisseria* species. Polymicrobial endocarditis occurs with increased frequency in intravenous drug abusers. Among 85 cases of polymicrobial IE reported during the 1980's, intravenous drug abuse was a risk factor in 72 per cent.[40]

The clinical manifestations of IE in intravenous drug abusers depend on the valve(s) involved and, to a lesser degree, upon the infecting organism. Tricuspid valve endocarditis, particularly when caused by *S. aureus,* presents with pleuritic chest pain, shortness of breath, cough, and hemoptysis. In 75 per cent of patients, chest roentgenograms contain abnormalities due to septic pulmonary emboli. Murmurs of tricuspid regurgitation are noted in less than half of these patients. Infection of the aortic or mitral valve in addicts clinically resembles IE seen in other patients. That caused by *S. aureus* generally presents as acute endocarditis with marked systemic toxicity. Symptoms and signs of left heart failure, neurologic injury, systemic emboli, metastatic infections, and the classic peripheral stigmata of IE are strongly associated with left-sided endocarditis.[32]

Thirty-four human immunodeficiency virus (HIV)–infected and 12 HIV seronegative intravenous drug abusers were studied with 40 and 14 episodes of IE, respectively. Endocarditis in the two groups was similar in clinical presentation, microbiology, complications, and overall survival. Among HIV-infected patients, death attributed to IE was more frequent in CDC group IV patients (40 per cent) than in the non–group IV patients (10 per cent).[41]

PROSTHETIC VALVE ENDOCARDITIS (PVE). Epidemiologic studies suggest that PVE comprises 10 to 20 per cent of all cases of IE in developed countries.[2,4] In four studies with careful follow-up of valve recipients, the cumulative incidence of PVE estimated actuarially was 1.4 to 3.1 per cent at 12 months, 4.1 to 5.4 per cent at 4 years, and 3.2 to 5.7 per cent at 5 years.[42–45] The risk of PVE over time, however, is not uniform. The risk is greatest during the initial 6 months after valve surgery (particularly during the initial 5 to 6 weeks) and thereafter declines to a lower but persistent risk (0.2 to 0.35 per cent per year).[42–46]

PVE has been called "early" when symptoms begin within 60 days of valve surgery and "late" with onset thereafter. These terms were established to distinguish early PVE that arose as a complication of valve surgery from late infection that was more likely community acquired. In fact, many cases with onset between 60 days and 1 year after surgery are likely to be nosocomial and in spite of their delayed presentation derive from events during the surgical admission.[47] Studies to identify risk factors for PVE have not resulted in a coherent picture. Data suggest that during the initial months after valve implantation mechanical prostheses are at greater risk of infection than bioprosthetic valves but that after 12 months the risk for infection of bioprostheses exceeds that of mechanical valves.[43–46] Patients with antecedent native valve endocarditis, particularly if active, are at increased risk for PVE.[43,44,46]

Microbiology of PVE. The microbiology of PVE is relatively predictable and reflects in part the presumed nosocomial or community acquisition of infection (Table 33–3). Coagulase-negative staphylococci, which when speciated are primarily *Staphylococcus epidermidis,* are the predominant causes of PVE diagnosed within 60 days after surgery. *S. aureus,* gram-negative bacilli, diphtheroids, and fungi (particularly *Candida* species) are also common causes of PVE during this period. Occasional cases of nosocomial PVE caused by *Legionella* species, atypical mycobacteria, mycoplasma, and fungi other than *Candida* have been reported. The spectrum and frequency of microorganisms causing PVE that occurs between 2 and 12 months after cardiac surgery and within the initial 60 postoperative days are similar. More than 80 per cent of the coagulase-negative staphylococci from either of these time periods are resistant to methicillin and all other beta-lactam antibiotics. In contrast, 30 per cent or fewer of the coagulase-negative staphylococci causing PVE with onset more than 1 year after valve surgery are methicillin-resistant.[45,48] PVE with onset 1 year or more postoperatively presumably results from transient bacteremia arising from dental, gastrointestinal, and genitourinary manipulations, breaks in the skin barrier, and intercurrent infections.[46,47] Consequently, the microbiology of these cases resembles that seen in community-acquired NVE in non-addicts: streptococci, *S. aureus,* enterococci, and fastidious gram-negative coccobacilli (*Haemophilus* species, *Actinobacillus actinomycetemcomitans, Cardiobacterium hominis, Eikenella,* and *Kingella*—the so-called HACEK group). Coagulase-negative staphylococci cause 15 per cent of these cases of PVE.

Pathology of PVE. The intracardiac pathology of PVE differs notably from the largely leaflet-confined pathology of NVE. Infection on mechanical prostheses commonly extends beyond the valve ring into the annulus and periannular tissue as well as the mitral-aortic intravalvular fibrosa, resulting in ring abscesses, septal abscesses, fistulous tracts, and dehiscence of the prosthesis with hemodynami-

TABLE 33–3 MICROBIOLOGY OF PROSTHETIC VALVE ENDOCARDITIS, 1975–1989

ORGANISM	TIME OF ONSET AFTER CARDIAC SURGERY (%) < 2 Months (N = 73)	2–12 Months (N = 38)	> 12 Months (N = 94)
Coagulase-negative staphylococci	38	50	15
Staphylococcus aureus	14	11	13
Gram-negative bacilli	11	5	1
Streptococci	0	3	33
Enterococci	7	5	11
Diphtheroids	12	3	2
Fastidious gram-negative coccobacilli	0	3	12
Fungi	10	5	3
Miscellaneous	4	5	1
Culture-negative	4	11	10

Data from references 47 and 257–260.

cally significant paravalvular regurgitation (Fig. 33–1). In autopsy experience with 74 patients, which is clearly biased toward the most severe pathology, annular invasion was noted in 85 per cent, myocardial abscess in 32 per cent, and valve obstruction by vegetation overgrowth, a phenomenon of PVE at the mitral site, in 19 per cent.[47] Erosion through the aortic annulus to cause pericarditis occurred in 5 per cent.[47] In clinical series encompassing 85 patients, the rate of annulus invasion was 42 per cent, myocardial abscess 14 per cent, valve obstruction 4 per cent, and pericarditis 2 per cent.[47] The intracardiac pathology of bioprosthetic valve IE is more heterogeneous and includes invasive disease, comparable to that noted when PVE involves mechanical valves, as well as leaflet destruction (Figs. 33–1 and 33–2). Among 85 patients with bioprosthetic PVE, 29 (59 per cent) of 49 with infection within a year after surgery had invasive disease, in contrast to only 9 (25 per cent) of 36 patients with infection occurring more than 1 year postoperatively. Infection confined to the leaflets was proven in another 9 (25 per cent) with late onset and was assumed in the majority of the remaining 18 patients who survived without surgical intervention.[47] In a study of PVE involving either mechanical or bioprosthetic valves, aortic site and clinical onset within a year of valve surgery were significantly correlated with an increased risk for invasive infection.[49] Other studies have noted increased invasive disease with PVE at the aortic versus the mitral site.[50,51]

The clinical features of PVE resemble those found in non-drug abuse–associated NVE. Signs and symptoms in patients developing PVE within 60 days of cardiac surgery may be obscured by surgery or other postoperative complications. Peripheral signs of endocarditis (5 to 14 per cent) and central nervous system emboli (10 per cent) occur less frequently in these patients than in those with PVE occurring later after surgery. Among patients with later onset PVE, congestive heart failure occurs in 40 per cent, cerebrovascular complications in 26 to 28 per cent, and peripheral signs in 15 to 28 per cent.[47,52,53]

NOSOCOMIAL ENDOCARDITIS. Hospital-acquired endocarditis unrelated to concurrent cardiac surgery comprises 5 to 29 per cent of all cases of IE in various series.[7,8,11,12,54] Nosocomial IE has involved abnormal native cardiac valves, normal valves including the tricuspid, and prosthetic valves and occurs with similar frequency among patients with NVE and PVE (unrelated to valve surgery).[4,7,11] Infected intravascular devices and catheters give rise to 45 to 65 per cent of the bacteremia that results in nosocomial IE.[11,12,54] Other sources of bacteremia include genitourinary and gastrointestinal tract instrumentation or surgery. In 141 bone marrow transplant recipients, prolonged placement (mean 98 days) of central venous catheters extending into or near the right atrium was associated with eight episodes of endocarditis, of which seven were right-sided.[55] In an autopsy study of 55 patients who had been managed using flow-directed pulmonary artery catheters, four were found to have right-sided endocarditis.[56]

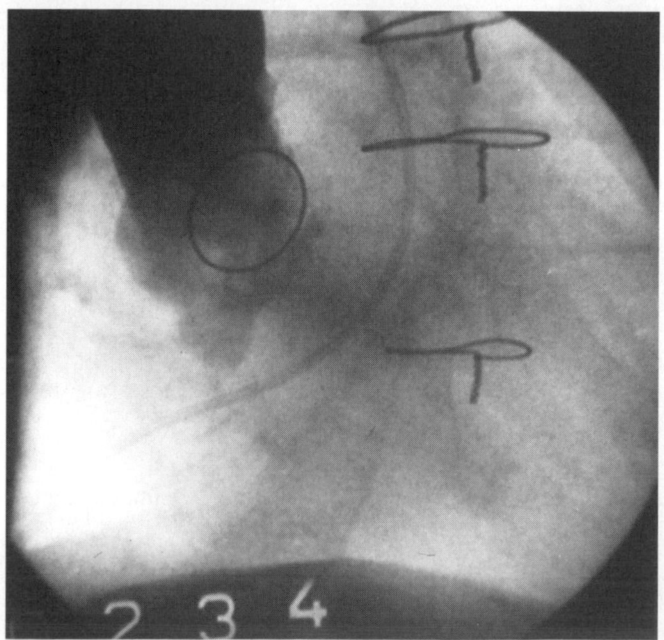

FIGURE 33–1. *S. epidermidis* infection of a bioprosthetic aortic valve 3 months after surgery. Contrast material injected supravalvularly fills a paravalvular abscess and regurgitates into the left ventricle.

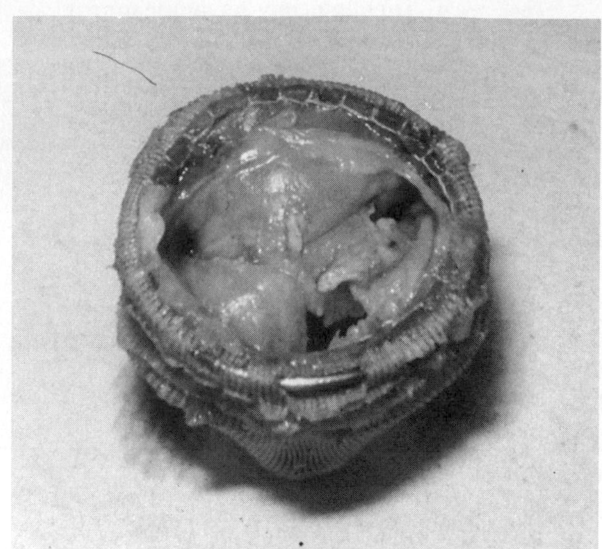

FIGURE 33–2. A bioprosthetic valve removed from the aortic position 18 months after insertion because of enterococcal PVE causing severe leaflet destruction and aortic regurgitation.

Microbiology of Nosocomial IE. Gram-positive cocci are the predominant cause of nosocomial IE. Among 45 episodes from two series, *S. aureus* caused 44 per cent, coagulase-negative staphylococci 22 per cent, enterococci 18 per cent, streptococci and *Candida* species and gram-negative bacilli each 4 per cent. One patient (2 per cent) had negative cultures.[11,12] The frequency of endocarditis or other deep-seated *S. aureus* infections after catheter-related bacteremia ranges from 3 to 8 per cent; nevertheless, catheter-associated *S. aureus* bacteremia occurs with sufficient frequency to be the predominant predisposition for nosocomial IE.[11,12,57–60] IE complicates 0.85 to 3.1 per cent of nosocomial enterococcal bacteremia; although the risk of nosocomial enterococcal IE is increased in patients with abnormal valves, it remains small, relative to that for nosocomial *S. aureus* bacteremia.[11,12,61,62] Among 115 patients with prosthetic valves and a nosocomial bacteremia that was not the index test for PVE, 18 patients (15.6 per cent) subsequently developed PVE that was the apparent consequence of the bacteremia. *S. aureus* and *S. epidermidis* were that most common organisms in these cases of PVE, although gram-negative bacilli and fungi also caused episodes of PVE.[63] Bacteremia persisting for days prior to treatment or for 72 hours or more after removal of an infected catheter and initiation of treatment, especially in patients with abnormal heart valves or prosthetic valves, suggests the diagnosis of IE.[12,54,60]

The onset of nosocomial IE is usually acute and although a changing murmur may be heard, other classical signs of endocarditis are infrequent.[11,64] Mortality rates among these patients, many of whom are elderly and have serious underlying diseases, are high (40 to 56 per cent).[11,12,54]

Etiological Microorganisms

VIRIDANS STREPTOCOCCI. These streptococci, which cause 30 to 65 per cent of NVE unrelated to drug abuse, are normal inhabitants of the oropharynx, characteristically produce alpha-hemolysis when grown on sheep blood agar, and are usually nontypable using the Lancefield system. The viridans streptococci are not a species but rather a group of organisms composed of multiple species, many of which have recently undergone taxonomic redefinition. Using the previous classification, the species causing streptococcal NVE were distributed as follows: *Streptococcus mitior* (31 per cent of cases), *Streptococcus sanguis* (24 per cent), *Streptococcus bovis* (27 per cent), *Streptococcus mutans* (7 per cent), *Streptococcus milleri* (4 per cent), *Streptococcus faecalis* (now *Enterococcus faecalis*) (7 per cent), and *Streptococcus salivarius* and other species (2 per cent).[62] Another study, adjusted for the new taxonomy, has reported a similar distribution of streptococci causing IE.[65] Nutritionally variant streptococci, strains that require media supplemented with either pyridoxal hydrochloride or L-cysteine for growth and are now speciated as *Streptococcus adjacens* or *Streptococcus defectivus,* cause 5 per cent of streptococcal NVE.[62,66]

The viridans streptococci, other than the nutritionally variant organisms, are in general highly susceptible to penicillin (minimum inhibitory concentration [MIC] $\leq$ 0.1 μg/ml for 83 per cent) and are killed in an enhanced manner (synergistically) by penicillin plus gentamicin.[62,66,67] *S. adjacens* and *S. defectivus* appear more resistant to penicillin (MIC > 0.12 μg/ml in more than 30 per cent of strains).[66] Although penicillin-aminoglycoside synergy was not demonstrated in vitro with *S. adjacens* and *S. defectivus*, in therapy of experimental endocarditis caused by these organisms, penicillin-aminoglycoside combinations were more effective than penicillin alone; also, therapy with vancomycin alone was comparable to that with the penicillin-aminoglycoside combination.[66]

***STREPTOCOCCUS BOVIS* AND OTHER STREPTOCOCCI.** *S. bovis,* part of the gastrointestinal tract normal flora, causes 27 per cent of the episodes of streptococcal NVE.[62] Although superficially resembling the enterococci, this species can be easily distinguished by its biochemical characteristics. The distinction is important because *S. bovis* is highly penicillin susceptible, in contrast to the relative penicillin resistance of enterococci. *S. bovis* NVE is frequently associated with coexistent colonic polyps or malignancy.[9,10,68]

Group A streptococci, which can infect normal valves, cause rare episodes of endocarditis. Among intravenous drug abusers, group A streptococci have caused tricuspid valve IE similar to that noted with *S. aureus.*[69] Group B organisms, *Streptococcus agalactiae,* are part of the normal flora of the mouth, genital tract, and gastrointestinal tract. Group B streptococci infect normal and abnormal valves and cause a very morbid NVE syndrome with a high incidence of systemic emboli.[70,71] The organisms' failure to produce fibrinolysin may result in large vegetations and a high rate of systemic emboli. Endocarditis caused by this organism may be associated with villous adenomas and colonic neoplasms.[72] Group G streptococci also produce a destructive, highly morbid left-sided NVE.[73] The *Streptococcus milleri* group, now divided into three species—*Streptococcus intermedius, Streptococcus constellatus,* and *Streptococcus anginosus*—are highly pyogenic organisms, some of which type as Lancefield group F.[74] These penicillin-susceptible organisms, which cause destructive infections similar to those caused by *S. aureus,* have accounted for 2 to 5 per cent of streptococcal NVE cases.[62,65]

STREPTOCOCCUS PNEUMONIAE. Although pneumococcal bacteremia occurs frequently, *S. pneumoniae* accounts for only 1 to 3 per cent of NVE cases. When causing IE, *S. pneumoniae* frequently involves a previously normal aortic valve and progresses rapidly with valve destruction, myocardial abscess formation, and acute congestive heart failure. Mortality rates range from 30 to 50 per cent.[75–77] Alcoholism is a risk factor for pneumococcal IE, and concurrent pneumonia or meningitis is common.[75,77] Although pneumococci causing endocarditis have been highly susceptible to penicillin, strains that are relatively penicillin-resistant (MIC $\geq$ 0.1 μg/ml to $\leq$ 1.0 μg/ml) and highly penicillin-resistant (MIC > 1.0 μg/ml) are increasingly common causes of pneumococcal infection, particularly in children.[78] Many of the highly resistant strains are also resistant to erythromycin, trimethoprim-sulfamethoxazole, and cephalosporins, including ceftriaxone. These strains remain susceptible to vancomycin. In the future these penicillin-resistant strains are likely to cause sporadic cases of IE.[79]

ENTEROCOCCI. These organisms, once considered Lancefield group D streptococci, have recently been accorded their own genus, *Enterococcus.* Although there are at present 12 species of enterococci, *Enterococcus faecalis* and *Enterococcus faecium* cause 85 per cent and 10 per cent of cases of enterococcal IE, respectively. Enterococci are part of the normal gastrointestinal flora and cause genitourinary tract infection. Enterococci account for 5 to 15 per cent of cases of NVE and a similar percentage of PVE cases (Tables 33–2 and 33–3).[47,80] Occasional cases occur in young women as a consequence of genitourinary tract manipulation or infection. The majority of cases occur, however, in older, predominantly male, patients and have the urinary tract as a likely portal of entry.[81] Enterococci infect either normal or previously abnormal valves and present as either acute or subacute IE.[80]

Enterococci are overtly resistant to cephalosporins, semisynthetic penicillinase-resistant penicillins (oxacillin and nafcillin), and therapeutic concentrations of aminoglycosides. Most enterococci are inhibited by modest concentrations of the cell wall–active antibiotics—penicillin, ampicillin, vancomycin, and teicoplanin (not licensed in the United States). Bactericidal anti-enterococcal activity can be achieved by combining an inhibitory cell wall–active agent and an appropriate aminoglycoside. This bactericidal activity, called synergy, is essential for optimal treatment of enterococcal IE.[80] Strains of enterococci that are highly resistant to penicillin and ampicillin, resistant to vancomycin, and highly resistant to all aminoglycosides have been identified as causes of nosocomial infections.[80,82] Although these resistant strains have caused only sporadic cases of IE, their wide distribution and frequency as nosocomial pathogens have increased the complexity of treating enterococcal IE (see Antimicrobial Therapy).[80–83]

STAPHYLOCOCCI. The coagulase-positive staphylococci are a single species, *S. aureus.* Of the 13 species of coagulase-negative staphylococci that colonize humans, one, *S. epidermidis,* has emerged as an important pathogen in the setting of implanted devices and hospitalized patients. *S. aureus* and *S. epidermidis* have surface receptors that bind to host proteins, including fibronectin and fibrinogen. These proteins, in turn, may be present at sites of endocardial injury and coat implanted foreign devices. Although the pathogenesis is undoubtedly far more complex, these receptors, by binding to host proteins, may facilitate the adherence of staphylococci to sites where they proliferate to generate endocarditis.[84,85] Coagulase-negative staphylococci are coated with a slime or glycocalyx layer that favors their survival on foreign devices. Embedded in this material, large populations of coagulase-negative staphylococci accumulate on the surface of foreign devices; these organisms in turn have altered phenotypes, including increased resistance to the bactericidal effects of many antibiotics.[86,87] A capsular polysaccharide/adhesin of *S. epidermidis* has increased the organism's resistance to eradication by host granulocytes and thus may allow an initial small inoculum to proliferate and ultimately cause IE.[88,89]

Antibiotic Resistance. In excess of 90 per cent of *S. aureus,* whether acquired in the hospital or community, produce beta-lactamase and thus are resistant to penicillin, ampicillin, and the ureidopenicillins. These organisms are, however, susceptible to the penicillinase-resistant beta-lactam antibiotics (oxacillin, nafcillin, cefazolin, and other first-generation cephalosporins). Resistance of *S. aureus* to methicillin and other beta-lactam antibiotics is based upon production of an altered penicillin-binding protein (called 2a or 2′) with decreased affinity for beta-lactam antibiotics. Methicillin-resistant strains are increasingly prevalent in nosocomial settings and among selected, nonhospitalized populations (intravenous drug abusers, nursing home residents); methicillin-resistant strains must be considered when selecting initial empirical therapy for IE in patients from these groups.[33,90] Coagulase-negative staphylococci frequently produce beta-lactamase; furthermore, strains causing community-acquired infections are frequently methicillin-susceptible, while those causing nosocomial infections, including IE, are commonly methicillin-resistant.[48,91] Coagulase-negative staphylococci may not always phenotypically express methicillin resistance (a property called heteroresistance). Consequently, special testing may be required to detect this resistance.[48,90,91] Resistance to aminoglycosides and to fluoroquinolones is increasingly common among staphylococci, particularly those that are methicillin-resistant.[90,91] Most staphylococci are susceptible to rifampin; however, resistant strains are rapidly selected when rifampin is used alone to treat staphylococcal infections.[48,90] Staphylococci, including most strains that are resistant to methicillin, remain susceptible to vancomycin and teicoplanin.[48,90]

Clinical Features. *S. aureus* is a major cause of IE in all population groups (Tables 33–1 to 33–3). *S. aureus* IE is characterized by a highly toxic febrile illness, frequent focal metastatic infection, and a 30 to 50 per cent rate of central nervous system complications.[90] A cerebrospinal fluid polymorphonuclear pleocytosis, with or without *S. aureus* cultured from the cerebrospinal fluid, is common.[90] Heart murmurs are heard in 30 to 45 per cent of patients on initial evaluation and are ultimately heard in 75 to 85 per cent as a consequence of intracardiac damage. The mortality rate in nonaddicts with left-sided *S. aureus* endocarditis is 34 per cent overall and increases in those over 50 years of age, in those with significant underlying diseases, and when IE is complicated by a major neurologic event, valve dysfunction, or congestive heart failure.[90] Among addicts left-sided *S. aureus* IE resembles that seen in nonaddicts. In contrast, in patients with IE limited to the tricuspid valve, complications are rare, and mortality rates are only 2 to 4 per cent.[90,92] Occasionally tricuspid staphylococcal IE results in overwhelming septic pulmonary emboli, pyopneumothorax, and severe respiratory insufficiency.

Coagulase-Negative Staphylococci. These are a major cause of PVE, particularly during the initial year after valve surgery, an important cause of nosocomial IE, and the cause of 3 to 8 per cent of NVE, usually in the setting of prior valve abnormalities (Tables 33–1 and 33–3).[90,91] The vast majority of coagulase-negative staphylococci causing PVE, when speciated, are *S. epidermidis.*[48,90] In contrast, when infection involves native valves, only 50 per cent of isolates are *S. epidermidis.*[90,91] *Staphylococcus lugdunensis,* a coagulase-negative species, has caused highly destructive, often fatal NVE and PVE.[93,94] *S. lugdunensis* IE is usually community-acquired and the organism is often susceptible to many antistaphylococcal antibiotics, including penicillin.[94] Coagulase-negative staphylococcal NVE is generally subacute, and occasional patients have minimal or no fever throughout their illness. Nevertheless, destruction of intracardiac structures, metastatic infection including vertebral osteomyelitis, and central nervous system complications occur frequently in NVE caused by species other than *S. lugdunensis.*[90,91]

GRAM-NEGATIVE BACTERIA. Organisms of the so-called HACEK group, which are part of the upper respiratory tract and oropharyngeal flora, infect abnormal cardiac valves, causing subacute NVE, and cause PVE that occurs a year or more after valve surgery.[95–97] In NVE, the HACEK organisms have been associated with large vegetations and a high incidence of systemic emboli.[97] These organisms are fastidious and slow growing; when they are suspected, blood cultures should be incubated for 3 weeks. *Haemophilus* species, primarily *H. aphrophilus* followed by *H. parainfluenzae* and *H. influenzae,* account for 0.5 to 1.0 per cent of all IE. Among the other organisms in this group, *A. actinomycetemcomitans* and *C. hominis* are the next most common causes of IE, followed by *E. corrodens,* which is microaerophilic, and *Kingella* species. The HACEK group have been susceptible to penicillin, ampicillin, aminoglycosides, quinolones, and third-generation cephalosporins. Some recent isolates have produced a beta-lactamase; thus, penicillin and ampicillin must be used with caution when treating HACEK endocarditis.[29,95]

P. aeruginosa is the gram-negative bacillus that most commonly causes endocarditis. The proclivity of *P. aeruginosa*, as opposed to Enterobacteriaceae, to cause IE correlates with its resistance to the bactericidal activity of human sera and its adherence to cardiac valves and platelet-fibrin thrombi. Pseudomonal IE involves normal and abnormal valves on both sides of the heart and often causes valve destruction and heart failure (Fig. 33–3).[35,36,97]

The Enterobacteriaceae, in spite of causing frequent episodes of bacteremia, are implicated in only sporadic cases of IE. *Escherichia coli, Klebsiella-Enterobacter* species, and *Salmonella* species have infected normal as well as abnormal valves. *Salmonella* species also infect mural endocardial thrombi and atherosclerotic arterial aneurysms. Gram-negative bacillus IE is noted with increased frequency among intravenous drug abusers and during the initial year after prosthetic valve placement.[32,47] *Serratia marcescens* has caused regional epidemics of IE among addicts.[32,97]

Neisseria gonorrhoeae, a common cause of IE during the preantibiotic era, rarely causes endocarditis today.[98,99] Gonococci, similar to pneumococci, infect the aortic valve of young patients, resulting in valve destruction, abscess formation, and a probable need for valve replacement.[99] Penicillinase production and intrinsic resistance to penicillin are common among gonococci; however, all strains remain susceptible to ceftriaxone. Nonpathogenic *Neisseria* cause sporadic cases of IE.[99] *Brucella*, small aerobic slow-growing coccobacillary organisms, cause subacute IE in patients with valvular abnormalities, particularly among men exposed to infected foods and animals.[99,100] High antibody titers against *Brucella* can suggest the diagnosis when cultures are negative.

OTHER ORGANISMS. *Corynebacterium* species and other coryneform bacteria, often called diphtheroids, are commensals on the skin and mucous membranes. Prolonged incubation of blood cultures is often required to isolate these slow-growing, fastidious organisms from patients with IE. Although often contaminants in blood cultures, diphtheroids in multiple blood cultures cannot be ignored. They are an important cause of PVE occurring during the initial year after valve surgery and a surprisingly common cause of endocarditis involving abnormal valves.[47,101] Diphtheroids are often killed by the synergistic interaction of penicillin and an effective aminoglycoside as well as by vancomycin.[102] *Listeria monocytogenes*, a small gram-positive rod, causes occasional cases of IE involving abnormal left heart valves and prosthetic devices.[103] *Bartonella* species, formerly called *Rochalimaea*, can be isolated from patients with IE by prolonged incubation of blood cultures (2 weeks) followed by blind subculturing to fresh chocolate agar or sheep blood agar, which is in turn incubated for 2 to 3 weeks in 5 to 8 per cent CO_2.[104,105] *Bartonella quintana, Bartonella elizabethae*, and *Bartonella henselae* have caused subacute endocarditis with valvular damage. In the absence of special efforts in culturing, these cases would have been "culture negative."[104,105] Although *B. quintana* causes trench fever vectored by the body louse and cat-scratch disease, the role of ectoparasites and cats in the epidemiology of *Bartonella* endocarditis is not known.

The rickettsia *Coxiella burnetii*, a weakly gram-negative obligate intracellular organism, infects humans after inhalation of desiccated materials from infected animals or contact with infected parturient animals. At variable intervals after acute infection by *C. burnetii* (Q fever), persons with abnormal mitral or aortic valves who have not been able to eradicate the organism develop subacute IE with typical manifestations and often with valve dysfunction causing heart failure.[31,106] The diagnosis is typically based on high antibody titers to phase I and II *C. burnetii* antigens. However, the organism can be grown from blood (buffy coat) or valve tissue on human embryonic lung fibroblast cell culture and can be demonstrated in excised cardiac valves by immunohistological staining.[31,106] *Chlamydia psittaci*, the agent of psittacosis, has caused occasional episodes of subacute IE and has resulted in hemodynamically significant valve damage. There may be concurrent pneumonia, and a history of contact with birds is often noted. The diagnosis can be suspected when routine blood cultures are negative and there is a strong serologic response. The organism can be cultured on cell monolayers from blood, the respiratory tract, or valve; it also can be demonstrated immunohistologically in excised valve tissue.[107] The many other organisms that have caused IE are beyond the scope of this chapter; some have been discussed in recent reviews.[99,108]

FUNGI. *Candida albicans*, non-albicans *Candida* species, *Torulopsis glabrata*, and *Aspergillus* species are the most common of the many fungal organisms identified as causing IE. Fungal endocarditis arises in specific settings. Valve replacement cardiac surgery and intravenous drug abuse are major predispositions. The most frequent fungi causing PVE are *C. albicans, Aspergillus* species, and non-albicans *Candida* species, while addict-associated fungal IE is most commonly caused by non-*albicans Candida* species, particularly *C. parapsilosis*.[109,110] Fungal IE resulting from prolonged intravenous antimicrobial therapy and parenteral alimentation is caused predominantly by *C. albicans* and *T. glabrata*. Patients who are severely immunodepressed occasionally experience IE caused by *Candida* species, *Aspergillus* species, or opportunistic mycelia fungi. Blood cultures frequently are positive when *Candida* species or *T. glabrata* cause IE but rarely yield organisms when IE is caused by mycelial organisms. Bulky vegetations, which embolize frequently, are common in fungal IE. Removal and careful microbiological evaluation of an embolic vegetation may provide an etiological diagnosis in fungal IE.[109,110]

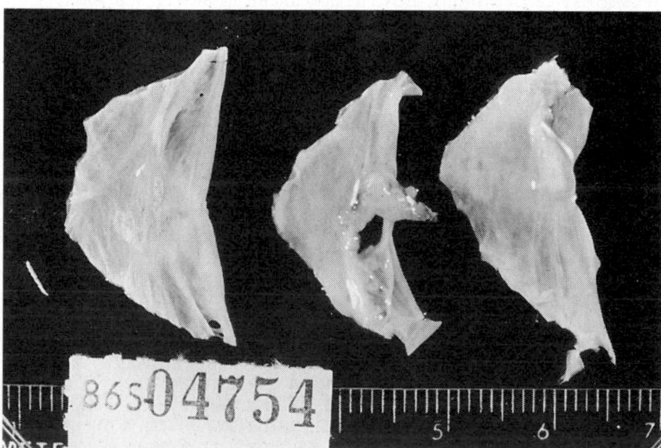

FIGURE 33–3. Aortic valve with multiple vegetations and valve destruction caused by *P. aeruginosa*. Surgery was required because of uncontrolled infection and congestive heart failure.

PATHOGENESIS

The interactions between the human host and selected microorganisms that culminate in IE involve the vascular endothelium, hemostatic mechanisms, the host immune system, gross anatomic abnormalities in the heart, surface properties of microorganisms, and peripheral events that initiate bacteremia. Each component of these interactions is in itself complex, influenced by many factors and not fully elucidated. The rarity of endocarditis and endarteritis in the face of frequent transient asymptomatic and symptomatic bacteremia indicates that the intact endothelium is resistant to infection. The normal cardiac valve endothelium in rabbits is resistant to colonization by bacteria even with injection of 10^9 to 10^{10} organisms. If the endothelium on the valve surface is damaged, hemostasis is stimulated, leading to deposition of platelets and fibrin.[111] This resulting platelet-fibrin complex is more receptive to colonization by bacteria than is the intact endothelium.[112,113] It is hypothesized that platelet-fibrin deposition occurs spontaneously in persons vulnerable to endocarditis and that these deposits, called nonbacterial thrombotic endocarditis (NBTE), are the sites at which microorganisms adhere to initiate IE. Bacteremia allows organisms access to the NBTE. The relative uniformity of organisms causing IE, as contrasted with the variety of organisms causing overt and asymptomatic bacteremia, and the infectiousness of specific organisms in animal models of endocarditis, indicates that certain microorganisms are advantaged in their ability to colonize and infect NBTE. The events after colonization that lead to IE entail survival and multiplication of microorganisms and accrual of vegetation and are complex interactions as well. (Space limitations require that this summary of pathogenesis be abbreviated and incompletely referenced. For detailed reviews see references 114 to 119.)

DEVELOPMENT OF NONBACTERIAL THROMBOTIC ENDOCARDITIS. Two major mechanisms appear pivotal in the formation of NBTE: endothelial injury and a hypercoagulable state. NBTE has been found in 1.3 per cent of patients at autopsy and, while present at all ages, is more common with increasing age.[120] These lesions have also been noted frequently in patients with malignancy, disseminated intravascular coagulation, uremia, burns, systemic lupus erythematosus, valvular heart disease, and intracardiac catheters.[114,116,120] The platelet-thrombin deposits are found at the valve closure-contact line on the atrial surfaces of the mitral and tricuspid valves and the ventricular surfaces of the aortic and pulmonic valves. The sites of these NBTE correspond closely with the location of infected vegetations in patients with IE.[120]

Three hemodynamic circumstances may injure the endothelium, initiating NBTE: (1) a high-velocity jet impacting endothelium; (2) flow from a high- to a low-pressure chamber; (3) flow across a narrow orifice at high velocity. Rodbard demonstrated that flow through a narrowed orifice, as a consequence of the Venturi effect, deposited bacteria maximally at the low-pressure sink immediately beyond an orifice or at the site where a jet stream impacts a surface. These are the same sites where NBTE forms as a result of hemodynamic circumstances. The superimposition of NBTE formation and preferential deposition of bacteria help explain the distribution of infected vegetations when IE complicates cardiac valvular abnormalities, septal defects, arteriovenous fistulas, coartation of the aorta, and a patent ductus arteriosus.[119,121,122] Additionally, the attenuation of these circumstances when intracardiac defects are associated with low flow and reduced turbulence (secundum atrial septal defect, atrial fibrillation, congestive heart failure) correlates with the observed reduction in frequency of IE in the respective circumstance.[119,121,122]

CONVERSION OF NBTE TO IE. The initiating event that ultimately converts NBTE to IE is the entry of microorganisms into the circulation as a consequence of localized infection or trauma to a body surface. The frequency and magnitude of bacteremia associated with daily activities and health care procedures appear related to specific mucosal surfaces and skin, the density of colonizing bacteria, the disease state of the surface, and the extent of the local trauma. Bacteremia rates are highest for events that traumatize the oral mucosa, particularly the gingiva, and progressively decrease with procedures involving the genitourinary tract and the gastrointestinal tract.[123,124] A diseased mucosal surface, particularly one that is infected, is associated with an increased risk of bacteremia. Thus, oral irrigation devices, prostate surgery, and urinary tract manipulation are associated with higher rates of bacteremia when there is severe gingivitis and poor dentition or infected urine, respectively, than when these states are absent.[123] In studies of rats with periodontitis and after teeth were extracted, the likelihood of endocarditis was not related to the magnitude of bacteremia by a specific organism; instead, the occurrence of endocarditis correlated with the capacity of bacterial organisms to adhere in vitro to platelet-fibrin aggregates.[125] The relationship between the magnitude of bacteremia with infection or after a procedure and the risk of endocarditis in humans is not known.

Although IE develops when circulating microorganisms are deposited at a site of NBTE, the coincidence of bacteremia and NBTE does not uniformly result in IE. To cause IE the organism must be able to persist and propagate on the endothelium. This requires resistance to host defenses. The impact of serum bactericidal activity is illustrated by the reduced frequency of IE caused by aerobic gram-negative bacilli. Only strains resistant to the complement-mediated bactericidal activity of serum, e.g., selected *E. coli, P. aeruginosa,* and *S. marcescens,* cause IE with significant frequency or are virulent in the rabbit model of endocarditis.[114,116] The precise role of granulocytes in eradicating early colonizing organisms is not clear. Platelet-released microbicidal material has been shown to eliminate recently adherent, susceptible viridans streptococci from valves in experimental endocarditis.[126]

The adherence of microorganisms to the NBTE is a pivotal early event in the development of IE. Those organisms that most frequently cause endocarditis adhere more vigorously in vitro to cardiac valves than do organisms that rarely cause IE. Multiple mechanisms promote this adherence, including the surface carbohydrates of bacteria.[116] Bacteremic streptococci that produce extracellular dextran cause endocarditis more frequently than do strains that do not produce dextran. Dextran on the surface of streptococci can be shown to mediate adherence to platelet fibrin lattices and injured valves. Dextran production, however, is not universal among the major microbial causes of IE; thus, other mechanisms of adherence are likely. Fibronectin has been identified as an important factor in this process.[84] Fibronectin has been identified in lesions on heart valves and is produced by endothelial cells, platelets, and fibroblasts in response to vascular injury; a soluble form binds to exposed subendothelial collagen. Receptors for fibronectin are present on the surface of *S. aureus,* viridans streptococci, group A, C, and G streptococci, enterococci, *S. pneumoniae,* and *C. albicans.* Fibronectin has multiple binding domains and thus can bind simultaneously to fibrin, collagen, cells, and microorganisms and serve to facilitate adherence of bacteria to the valve at the site of injury or NBTE. Soluble fibronectin may coat circulating bacteria and subsequently bind to injured endothelium, or uncoated bacteria may adhere specifically to fibronectin bound to platelets, fibroblasts, and collagen at the endothelial surface. The glycocalyx or slime on the surface of *S. epidermidis* has been considered an adhesin in the pathogenesis of PVE. Other studies, however, have questioned the adhesin function, and recent observations suggest that the polysaccharide material may render organisms more virulent by virtue of enhancing their ability to avoid eradication by host defenses.[85,88,89]

The mechanism whereby virulent organisms colonize and infect intact valvular endothelium is less clearly understood. Endothelial cells in monolayers in vitro can phagocytize *S. aureus* and *Candida.* Multiplication of the organism intracellularly results in cell death, which in turn disrupts the endothelial surface and initiates formation of platelet-fibrin deposits.[127,128] Alternatively, fibronectin may facilitate the adherence of *S. aureus* to intact endothelium.[84]

After adherence to the NBTE or endothelium (in the case of virulent organisms), persistence and multiplication result in a complex dynamic process during which the infected vegetation increases in size by platelet-fibrin aggregation, microorganisms are shed into the blood, and vegetation fragments embolize. Staphylococci and streptococci promote platelet aggregation and growth of the vegetation. Surface antigens that promote platelet adhesion (Class I antigen) and aggregation (Class II antigen that functionally mimics a platelet interactive domain of collagen) are expressed by *S. aureus.* Strains of *S. sanguis* with the aggregation antigen cause more severe endocarditis in the rabbit model than do antigen-negative strains.[129] Fibrin deposition is enhanced by tissue factor (a tissue thromboplastin that binds to Factor VII) elaborated by endothelial cells, fibroblasts, or monocytes interacting with bacteria.[130,131] The vegetation has been considered a sheltered site wherein bacteria were protected from polymorphonuclear leukocytes. Recent studies indicate that platelet-fibrin deposits may do more than shield microorganisms from host defenses. Platelets elaborate a potent platelet microbicidal protein that kills some strains of streptococci and *S. aureus* and thus kills organisms in vegetations.[126,132,133]

PATHOPHYSIOLOGY

Aside from the constitutional symptoms of infection, which are likely mediated by cytokines, the clinical manifestations of IE result from (1) the local destructive effects of intracardiac infection; (2) the embolization of bland or septic fragments of vegetations to distant sites, resulting in infarction or infection; (3) the hematogenous seeding of remote sites during continuous bacteremia; and (4) an antibody response to the infecting organism with subsequent tissue injury due to deposition of preformed immune complexes or antibody-complement interaction with antigens deposited in tissues.

The intracardiac consequences of IE range from trivial, characterized by an infected vegetation with no attendant tissue damage, to catastrophic, when infection is locally destructive or extends beyond the valve leaflet. Distortion or perforation of valve leaflets, rupture of chordae tendineae, and perforations or fistulas between major vessels and cardiac chambers or between chambers themselves as a consequence of burrowing infection may result in congestive heart failure that is progressive (Figs. 33–3 and 33–4).[134–136] Infection, particularly that involving the aortic valve or prosthetic valves, may extend into paravalvular tissue and result in abscesses and persistent fever due to antibiotic unresponsive infection, disruption of the conduction system with electrocardiographic conduction abnor-

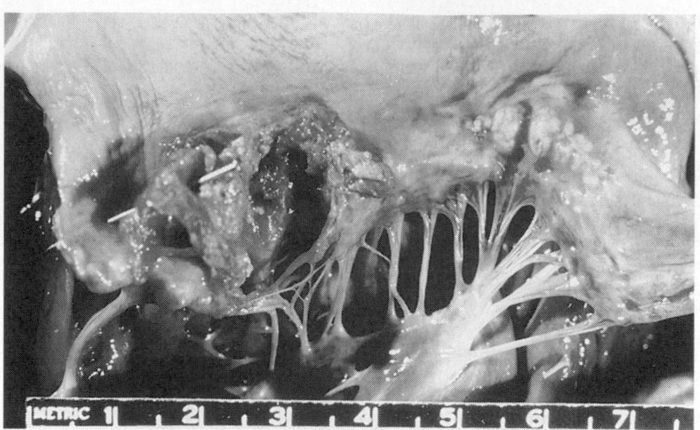

FIGURE 33–4. A large vegetation deforming and perforating the mitral valve. The nail probes an abscess that burrowed into the mitral valve annulus.

malities and clinically relevant arrhythmias, or purulent pericarditis.[30,137,138] Large vegetations, particularly at the mitral valve, can result in functional valvular stenosis and hemodynamic deterioration.[47,139] In general, intracardiac complications involving the aortic valve evolve more rapidly than those associated with the mitral valve; nevertheless, the progression is highly variable and unpredictable in individual patients.

Embolization of fragments from vegetations is clinically evident in 11 to 43 per cent of patients.[119,122,140,141] However, pathologic evidence of emboli at autopsy is found more frequently (45 to 65 per cent). Emboli from left-sided IE produce symptoms by infection or infarction at the site of lodgment, depending upon whether the vegetative material contains viable virulent organisms or is bland (sterile or contains avirulent organisms). Although not demonstrated in all studies, pooled data suggest that larger vegetations (>10 mm) are associated with a higher frequency of emboli, as are hypermobile vegetations.[142–144] Pulmonary emboli, which are often septic, occur in 75 per cent of intravenous drug abusers with tricuspid valve IE.[32]

The persistent bacteremia of IE, with or without septic emboli, may result in metastatic infection. In general, these infections originate before initiation of antimicrobial therapy; however, clinical manifestation may be delayed. These infections may present as local signs and symptoms or as persistent fever during therapy.[137,145] IE caused by virulent organisms, particularly *S. aureus,* is complicated more frequently by metastatic infection than is that due to avirulent bacteria, e.g., viridans streptococci. Virtually any organ or tissue may be hematogenously infected, including the spleen, kidney, brain, meninges, pericardium, bone (especially the vertebrae), synovium, and even vitreous humor. Metastatic abscesses are often small and miliary. Metastatic infection assumes particular importance when the required therapy is more than the antibiotics indicated for IE or when these infections constitute a focus that engenders relapse.[145]

The humoral and cell-mediated arms of the immune system are stimulated in patients with IE. Antibodies to the infecting organism in the three major classes—IgM, IgG, and IgA—with functional capacity including opsonization, agglutination, and complement fixation have been noted. Additionally, hypergammaglobulinemia and cryoglobulins have been noted. Cellular responses are suggested by activated circulating macrophages and splenomegaly.

Circulating immune complexes in high titer have been detected in most patients with bacteremic IE and PVE. The frequency and titer of the circulating immune complexes are highest in IE of long duration, in the presence of extravalvular manifestation, and in right-sided IE.[146] Although circulating immune complex titers fall with effective antibiotic therapy and rise or reappear with failure of therapy, the finding of a fall in titers not widely used to monitor therapy. Immune complexes are clinically relevant when, with complement, they deposit subepithelially along the glomerular basement membrane to cause diffuse or focal glomerulonephritis.[122,147] Histological examination of affected glomeruli stained with fluorescent-labeled antibody to human globulin reveals a "lumpy-bumpy" pattern. The immunoglobulin eluted from the glomerular lesions reacts with bacterial antigens.[148] Rheumatological manifestations of IE and some peripheral manifestations of IE, such as Osler's nodes, have been attributed to local deposition of immune complexes.[122] Osler's nodes, however, have also been associated with septic embolization in *S. aureus* IE.

Rheumatoid factor (an IgM antibody directed against IgG) is present in half of the patients with IE of greater than 6 weeks' duration.[122,149] The titer of rheumatoid factor decreases slowly with effective antimicrobial therapy. Rheumatoid factor does not appear to play a role in the immune complex glomerulonephritis of IE.

CLINICAL FEATURES

The interval between the presumed initiating bacteremia and the onset of symptoms of IE is short. It is estimated that more than 80 per cent of patients with NVE develop symptoms within 2 weeks.[150] Interestingly, in some patients with intraoperative or perioperative infection of prosthetic valves, the incubation period may be prolonged (2 to 5 or more months).[47]

Fever is the most common symptom and sign in patients with IE (Table 33–4). In patients with subacute IE, fevers are low grade, rarely exceeding 39.4°C, remittent, and usually not associated with rigors. Fever may be absent or minimal in the elderly or in those with congestive heart failure, severe debility, or chronic renal failure and occasionally in patients with NVE caused by coagulase-negative staphylococci.[9,91]

Heart murmurs are noted in 80 to 85 per cent of patients with NVE and are emblematic of the lesion predisposing to IE. Murmurs are commonly not audible in patients with tricuspid valve IE. Similarly, in acute NVE due to *S. aureus,* murmurs are heard in only 30 to 45 per cent of patients on initial evaluation but are ultimately noted in 75 to 85 per cent. The new or changing murmurs (alterations

TABLE 33–4 CLINICAL FEATURES OF INFECTIVE ENDOCARDITIS

SYMPTOMS	PER CENT	SIGNS	PER CENT
Fever	80–85	Fever	80–90
Chills	42–75	Murmur	80–85
Sweats	25	Changing/new murmur	10–40
Anorexia	25–55	Neurological abnormalities†	30–40
Weight loss	25–35	Embolic event	20–40
Malaise	25–40	Splenomegaly	15–50
Dyspnea	20–40	Clubbing	10–20
Cough	25	Peripheral manifestation	
Stroke	13–20	Osler's nodes	7–10
Headache	15–40	Splinter hemorrhage	5–15
Nausea/vomiting	15–20	Petechiae	10–40
Myalgia/arthralgia	15–30	Janeway lesion	6–10
Chest pain*	8–35	Retinal lesion/Roth spot	4–10
Abdominal pain	5–15		
Back pain	7–10		
Confusion	10–20		

* More common in intravenous drug abusers.
† Central nervous system.

unrelated to heart rate or cardiac output) are relatively infrequent in subacute NVE and are more prevalent in acute IE and PVE.[47,151] They are frequently important harbingers of congestive heart failure.

Enlargement of the spleen is noted less commonly in recent reports than previously; in recent series splenomegaly has been noted in 15 to 50 per cent of patients and is more common in subacute IE of long duration.

Although 50 per cent of patients with IE were reported to have one or more of the classic peripheral manifestations of this illness, these findings are encountered less frequently today and are absent in IE restricted to the tricuspid valve.[1,7,9,32] *Petechiae* (Fig. 33–5), the most common of these manifestations, are found on the palpebral conjunctiva, the buccal and palatal mucosa, and the extremities. They are not specific for endocarditis even on the conjunctiva. *Splinter or subungual hemorrhages* (Fig. 33–6) are dark red, linear, or occasionally flame-shaped streaks in the nail bed of the fingers or toes. Distal lesions are likely due to trauma, whereas the more proximal ones are more likely related to IE. *Osler's nodes* are small, tender subcutaneous nodules that develop in the pulp of the digits or occasionally more proximally in the fingers and persist for hours to several days. These are not pathognomonic for this diagnosis. Osler's nodes have been described in patients with systemic lupus erythematosus, marantic endocarditis, and disseminated gonococcal disease and distal to infected arterial catheters.[151] Janeway lesions are small erythematous or hemorrhagic macular nontender lesions on the palms and soles and are the consequence of septic embolic events. Roth spots (Fig. 33–7), oval retinal hemorrhages with pale centers, are infrequent findings in patients with IE. They have been noted in patients with collagen vascular disease and hematologic disorders, including severe anemia.

Musculoskeletal symptoms, unrelated to focal infection, are relatively common in patients with IE.[152] These include arthralgias and myalgias, occasional true arthritis with nondiagnostic but inflammatory synovial fluid findings, and prominent back pain without evidence of vertebral body, disc space, or sacroiliac joint infection.[151,152] In patients with arthritis or back pain, focal infection must be excluded because additional therapy may be required.

Systemic emboli are among the most common clinical sequelae of IE, occurring in up to 40 per cent of patients, and are frequent subclinical events found only at autopsy.[119,122,140,141] Emboli often antedate diagnosis. Although embolic events may occur during or after antimicrobial therapy, the incidence decreases promptly during the administration of effective antibiotic therapy.[153,154] Embolic splenic infarction may cause left upper quadrant abdominal pain, left shoulder pain, and a small left pleural effusion and must be distinguished from the less common splenic abscess (see Treatment of Extracardiac Complications). Renal emboli may occur asymptomatically or with flank pain and may cause gross or microscopic hematuria but rarely result in clinically significant renal dysfunction. Embolic stroke syndromes, predominantly involving the middle cerebral artery territory, occur in 15 to 20 per cent of patients with NVE and PVE.[47,155–158] IE caused by *S. aureus* is associated with an increased risk of embolic complications.[153,158] Coronary artery emboli are common findings at autopsy but rarely result in transmural infarction. Emboli to the extremities may produce pain and overt ischemia, and those to mesenteric arteries may cause abdominal pain, ileus, and guaiac-positive stools. Embolic occlusion of a central retinal artery, which occurs in less than 3 per cent of IE cases, presents as sudden monocular blindness.[140,157]

Neurological symptoms and signs occur in 30 to 40 per cent of patients with IE, are more frequent when IE is

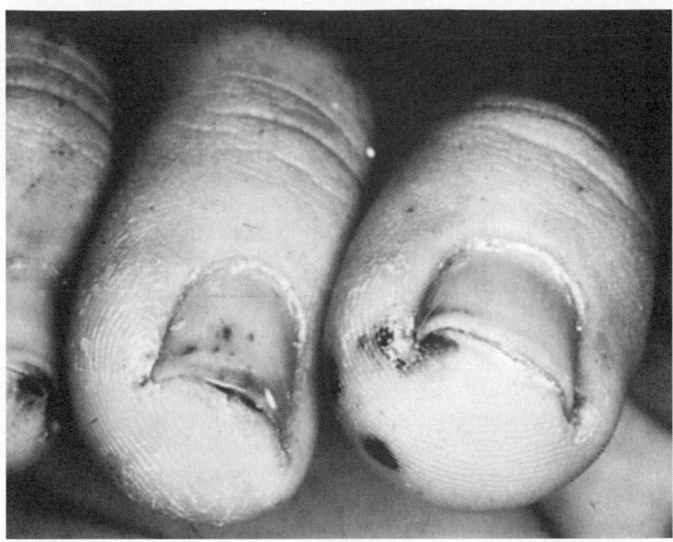

FIGURE 33–6. Subungual hemorrhages (splinter hemorrhages) and digital petechiae in a patient with IE. (From Korzeniowski, O. M., and Kaye, D.: Infective endocarditis. *In* Braunwald, E. (ed.): Heart Disease. 4th ed. Philadelphia, W. B. Saunders Company, 1992.)

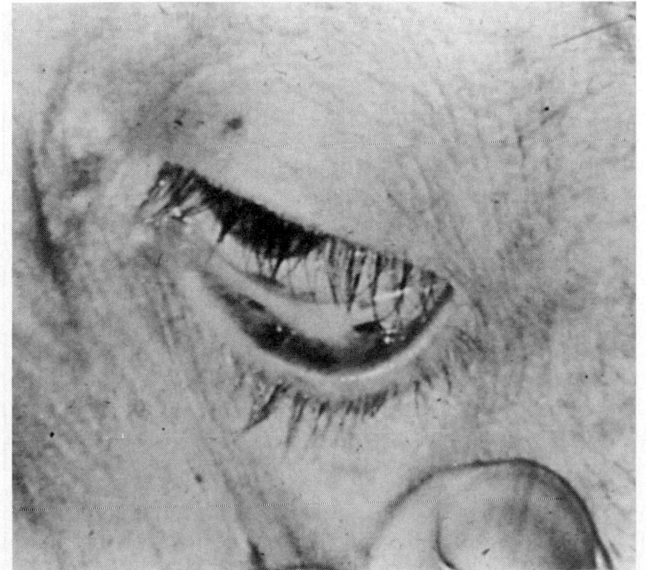

FIGURE 33–5. Conjunctival petechiae in a patient with IE. (From Kaye, D.: Infective Endocarditis. Baltimore, University Park Press, 1976.)

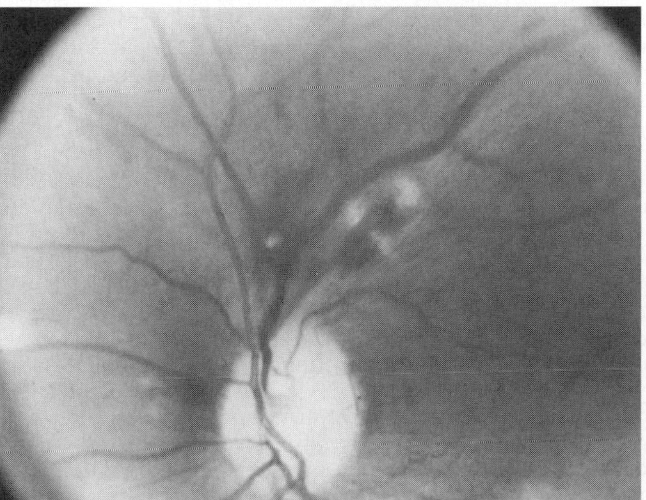

FIGURE 33–7. Roth spot (retinal hemorrhage with a clear center) in a patient with IE. (From Korzeniowski, O. M., and Kaye, D.: Infective endocarditis. *In* Braunwald, E. (ed.): Heart Disease. 4th ed. Philadelphia, W. B. Saunders Company, 1992.)

caused by *S. aureus,* and are associated with increased mortality rates.[140,151,155,157,158] Neurological manifestations, such as a stroke, intracerebral hemorrhage, or subarachnoid hemorrhage occurring at presentation, may be so dramatic that the diagnosis of IE is obscured. Embolic stroke is the most common and clinically important of the neurological manifestations. Intracranial hemorrhage occurs in 5 per cent of patients with IE. Bleeding results from rupture of a mycotic aneurysm, rupture of an artery due to septic arteritis at the site of embolic occlusion, or hemorrhage into an infarct.[159,160] Mycotic aneurysms, with or without rupture, occur in 2 to 10 per cent of patients with IE; approximately half of these involve intracranial arteries. Cerebritis with microabscesses complicates IE caused by invasive pathogens such as *S. aureus,* but large brain abscesses are rare.[155,158] Purulent meningitis complicates some episodes of IE caused by *S. aureus* or *S. pneumoniae,* but more typically the cerebrospinal fluid has an aseptic profile. Other neurological manifestations include severe headache (a potential clue to a mycotic aneurysm), seizure, and encephalopathy.

Congestive heart failure (CHF) complicating IE is primarily the result of valve destruction or distortion or rupture of chordae tendineae. Occasionally intracardiac fistulas, myocarditis, or coronary artery embolization may contribute to the genesis of CHF, as obviously can underlying cardiac disease. In the absence of surgery to correct valvular dysfunction, CHF, particularly that due to aortic insufficiency, was associated with very high mortality rates.[135,161] With appropriately-timed surgery, this increased mortality can be largely avoided.[135,140,161]

Renal insufficiency as a result of immune complex–mediated glomerulonephritis occurs in less than 15 per cent of patients with IE. Azotemia as a result of this process may develop or progress during initial therapy; it usually improves with continued administration of effective antibiotic therapy.[151] Focal glomerulonephritis and renal infarcts cause hematuria but rarely result in azotemia. Renal dysfunction in patients with IE is most commonly a manifestation of impaired hemodynamics or toxicities associated with antimicrobial therapy (interstitial nephritis or aminoglycoside-induced injury).

DIAGNOSIS

The symptoms and signs of endocarditis are often constitutional and, when localized, often result from a complication of IE rather than reflect the intracardiac infection itself (Table 33–4). Consequently, if physicians are to avoid overlooking the diagnosis of IE, a high index of suspicion must be maintained. The diagnosis must be investigated when patients with fever present with one or more of the cardinal elements of IE: a predisposing cardiac lesion or behavior pattern, bacteremia, embolic phenomenon, and evidence of an active endocardial process.

IE must be considered in a patient with significant valvular heart disease and a persistent unexplained fever, in the intravenous drug abuser with fever especially if there is cough and pleuritic chest pain, or in the young patient with an unexpected stroke or subarachnoid hemorrhage. The development of a new regurgitant murmur, which is indicative of an active endocardial process, must raise the possibility of IE. Because patients with prosthetic heart valves are always at risk for PVE, the presence of fever or new prosthesis dysfunction at any time warrants considering this diagnosis. In patients at risk for endocarditis, concurrent illnesses or iatrogenic events may create clusters of symptoms and signs that superficially mimic IE and require careful consideration to arrive at a correct diagnosis. For example, in an elderly patient with a murmur, low-grade fever, weight loss, myalgias and arthralgias, anemia, and elevated erythrocyte sedimentation rate, it may be difficult to distinguish IE from polymyalgia rheumatica. Even when the illness seems typical of endocarditis, the definitive diagnosis requires positive blood cultures or positive cultures (or histology) from the vegetation or embolus. There are many culture-negative mimics of IE: atrial myxoma, acute rheumatic fever, systemic lupus erythematosus or other collagen-vascular disease, marantic endocarditis, the antiphospholipid syndrome, carcinoid syndrome, renal cell carcinoma with increased cardiac output, and thrombotic thrombocytopenic purpura.

BACTEREMIA. Positive blood cultures may stimulate consideration of IE as a possible diagnosis. Sustained low-level (<100 organisms/ml) bacteremia is typical of IE. In evaluating positive blood cultures, sustained bacteremia (persisting over more than 1 hour) should be distinguished from transient bacteremia. When multiple blood cultures obtained over 24 hours or more are positive, the diagnosis of IE must be considered. The identity of the organism is also helpful in determining the intensity with which the diagnosis is entertained. Organisms can be divided into those that commonly cause IE, those that rarely cause IE, and the intermediate-behaving organisms, e.g., *S. aureus,* which, when in the blood, may or may not indicate IE. Lastly, the presence or absence of alternative sources for the bacteremia aids in the assessment of bacteremia. These considerations are embodied in the diagnostic criteria for IE (see Table 33–5).[162]

Among patients with *S. aureus* bacteremia, the risk of IE has been greatest in those with community-acquired infection, those who lack a peripheral site of infection, those who are intravenous drug abusers, those who have evidence of valvular disease, and those who are diabetic with chronic cutaneous infections. Screening of patients with community-acquired *S. aureus* bacteremia using transthoracic echocardiography demonstrated 20 per cent of the patients to have either occult IE or valve lesions predisposing to IE.[163,164] In contrast, among patients with catheter-associated nosocomial *S. aureus* bacteremia, the frequency of IE is 3 to 8 per cent.[57–60] Screening the latter group of patients with transthoracic echocardiography is not cost effective. Screening with transthoracic echocardiography is recommended for patients with *S. aureus* bacteremia acquired in a community setting or in a nosocomial setting, when patients have known underlying valvular heart disease, have a new significant heart murmur, or have persistent fever or bacteremia for 3 days or more after removal of the presumed primary focus of infection (intravascular catheter or drainage of an abscess) and initiation of therapy.[60,163,164]

When used judiciously over the entire evaluation sequence, i.e., not limited to initial findings, recently published criteria provide a sensitive and specific approach to the diagnosis of IE (Table 33–5).[162,165,166] Erroneous rejection of the diagnosis of endocarditis is unlikely. When using these diagnostic criteria to guide therapy, patients who are categorized with possible endocarditis should be treated as if they have IE. To use bacteremia due to coagulase-negative staphylococci or diphtheroids (organisms that may cause IE but more often contaminate blood cultures) to support the diagnosis of endocarditis, blood cultures must be persistently positive or the organisms recovered in multiple sporadically positive cultures must be proved to represent a single clone.[93,162]

Inclusion of echocardiographic evidence of endocardial infection in these criteria recognizes the high sensitivity of two-dimensional echocardiography with color Doppler, especially if the transesophageal approach is used, and the relative infrequency of false-positive studies when experienced operators use specific definitions for vegetations.[167–170] Although the sensitivity of transesophageal echocardiography to detect vegetations in patients with suspected infective endocarditis is 82 to 94 per cent (or higher if a follow-up study is performed), a negative study does not exclude the diagnosis or the need for therapy if

TABLE 33–5 DIAGNOSIS OF INFECTIVE ENDOCARDITIS

DEFINITIVE INFECTIVE ENDOCARDITIS
Pathological criteria
Microorganisms: demonstrated by culture or histology in a vegetation, *or* in a vegetation that has embolized, *or* in an intracardiac abscess, *or*
Pathological lesions: vegetation or intracardiac abscess present, confirmed by histology showing active endocarditis
Clinical criteria, using specific definitions listed below
Two major criteria, *or*
One major and three minor criteria, *or*
Five minor criteria

POSSIBLE INFECTIVE ENDOCARDITIS
Findings consistent with infective endocarditis that fall short of definite endocarditis but are not rejected

REJECTED
Firm alternative diagnosis for manifestations of endocarditis, *or*
Sustained resolution of manifestations of endocarditis, with antibiotic therapy for 4 days or less, *or*
No pathological evidence of infective endocarditis at surgery or autopsy, after antibiotic therapy for 4 days or less

CRITERIA FOR DIAGNOSIS OF INFECTIVE ENDOCARDITIS

MAJOR CRITERIA
Positive blood culture
Typical microorganism for infective endocarditis from two separate blood cultures
Viridans streptococci, *Streptococcus bovis,* HACEK group, *or*
Community-acquired *Staphylococcus aureus* or enterococci, in the absence of a primary focus, *or*
Persistently positive blood culture, defined as recovery of a microorganism consistent with infective endocarditis from:
Blood cultures drawn more than 12 hours apart, *or*
All of three or a majority of four or more separate blood cultures, with first and last drawn at least 1 hour apart
Evidence of endocardial involvement
Positive echocardiogram
Oscillating intracardiac mass, on valve or supporting structures, *or* in the path of regurgitant jets, *or* on implanted material, in the absence of an alternative anatomical explanation, *or*
Abscess, *or*
New partial dehiscence of prosthetic valve, *or*
New valvular regurgitation (increase or change in preexisting murmur not sufficient)

MINOR CRITERIA
Predisposition: predisposing heart condition *or* intravenous drug use
Fever ≥ 38.0°C (100.4°F)
Vascular phenomena: major arterial emboli, septic pulmonary infarcts, mycotic aneurysm, intracranial hemorrhage, conjunctival hemorrhages, Janeway lesions
Immunological phenomena: glomerulonephritis, Osler's nodes, Roth spots, rheumatoid factor
Microbiological evidence: positive blood culture but not meeting major criterion as noted previously* *or* serologic evidence of active infection with organism consistent with infective endocarditis
Echocardiogram: consistent with infective endocarditis but not meeting major criterion

* Excluding single positive cultures for coagulase-negative staphylococci and organisms that do not cause endocarditis.

Adapted from Durack, D. T., Lukes, A. S., and Bright, D. K.: New criteria for diagnosis of infective endocarditis: Utilization of specific echocardiographic findings. Am. J. Med. *96*:200, 1994.

the clinical suspicion is high.[169,170] In this population the false-negative rate for detection of vegetations on a single transesophageal echocardiogram ranges from 6 to 18 per cent; with repeat examinations, the likelihood of false-negative transesophageal studies is 4 to 13 per cent. Thus, these studies help to exclude the diagnosis when the clinical suspicion is low.[169,170] These guidelines are vulnerable to misidentifying as culture-negative infective endocarditis the entity of NBTE that complicates marasmus, cryptic collagen-vascular disease, or the antiphospholipid antibody syndrome.

A microbial cause for infective endocarditis is established by recovering the infecting agent from the blood or from surgically removed endocardial vegetations or embolic material. Bacteremia in patients with endocarditis is continuous; hence, there is no advantage to obtaining blood cultures in relationship to fever. Furthermore, blood obtained from arterial and venous sources are culture positive at similar rates. In patients who have not received prior antibiotics and who will ultimately have blood culture–positive IE, it is likely that 95 to 100 per cent of all cultures obtained will be positive. In a study of 206 patients with IE who had not received prior antibiotics, among those with streptococcal IE, the first culture was positive in 96 per cent of patients and one of the first two cultures was positive in 98 per cent. Among patients with nonstreptococcal IE, the first culture was positive in 86 per cent of patients and the first or second culture was positive in all cases.[171] Prior antibiotic therapy is a major cause of blood culture–negative IE, particularly when the causative microorganism is highly antibiotic susceptible. In a recent study of 620 cases of IE, 88 (14 per cent) were culture-negative. In 31 (35 per cent) of the 88 culture-negative cases, the failure to isolate the causative agent from blood was attributed to prior antimicrobial therapy.[172] After subtherapeutic antibiotic exposure the time required for reversion to positive cultures is directly related to the duration of antimicrobial therapy and the susceptibility of the causative agent; days to a week or more may be required.

OBTAINING BLOOD CULTURES. Three separate sets of blood cultures, each from a separate venipuncture, obtained over 24 hours, are recommended to evaluate patients with suspected endocarditis.[173] Each set should include two flasks, one containing an aerobic medium and the other containing thioglycollate broth (anaerobic medium) into which at least 10 ml of blood should be placed. The laboratory should be advised that endocarditis is a possible diagnosis and which, if any, unusual bacteria are suspected (*Legionella* species, *Bartonella* species, HACEK organisms). If alerted, the laboratory can both hold the culture for a prolonged period and use special isolation techniques. If a clinically stable patient has received an antimicrobial agent during the past several weeks, it is prudent to delay therapy so that repeat cultures can be obtained on successive days. If fungal endocarditis is suspected, blood cultures should be obtained using the lysis-centrifugation method. The laboratory should be asked to save the organism causing endocarditis until successful therapy has been completed. Occasionally, serologic tests are used to make the presumptive etiological diagnosis of endocarditis caused by *Brucella* species, *Legionella* species, *Bartonella* species, *Coxiella burnetii,* or *Chlamydia* species. By special techniques these agents can be identified in or recovered from blood or vegetations.[31,104–107]

Laboratory Tests

Blood cultures are the crucial laboratory tests used in the diagnosis of IE (see Diagnosis). Other tests are inevitably obtained and merit mention.[174] Hematological parameters are commonly abnormal. Anemia, with normochromic normocytic red cell indices, a low serum iron, and low serum iron-binding capacity, is seen in 70 to 90 per cent of patients. Anemia worsens with increased duration of illness and thus in acute IE may be absent. In subacute IE the white blood cell count is usually normal; in contrast, a leukocytosis with increased segmented granulocytes is common in acute IE. Thrombocytopenia occurs only rarely.

The *erythrocyte sedimentation rate* (ESR) is elevated (average approximately 55 mm/hr) in almost all patients with IE; the exceptions are those with congestive heart failure, renal failure, or disseminated intravascular coagulation. Although a nonspecific test, the absence of an increased ESR, other than in selected circumstances, argues against the diagnosis of IE. Other tests often indicate immune stimulation or inflammation (see Pathophysiology): circulating immune complexes, rheumatoid factor, quantitative immune globulin determinations, cryoglobulins, and C-reactive protein. Although the results of these tests parallel disease activity, the tests are costly and not efficient ways to diagnose IE or monitor response to therapy. Very high serum concentrations of circulating immune complexes can help to distinguish transient bacteremia from endocarditis.[175] This test might, therefore, be useful when the results of blood cultures and echocardiography have not differentiated transient bacteremia from IE. Measurement of circulating immune complexes and complement may be useful in evaluating azotemia. Azotemia due to diffuse immune complex glomerulonephritis is associated with increased circulating immune complexes and hypocomplementemia.[146,147,174]

The *urine analysis* is often abnormal, even when renal function remains normal. Proteinuria and microscopic hematuria are noted in 50 per cent of patients. The urinalysis plays a standard role in the evaluation of azotemia.

Serological tests are used to evaluate blood culture–negative IE (see Diagnosis). Tests to detect antibodies to ribitol teichoic acids from staphylococci were developed in an attempt to distinguish uncomplicated *S. aureus* bacteremia from that associated with IE or other deep-seated infection. In clinical applications these tests have not been sufficiently specific or predictive.[164]

Echocardiography

(See also pp. 77 to 78)

Evaluation of patients with clinically suspected IE by this technique frequently allows the morphologic confirmation of infection and increasingly aids in decisions regarding management.[142,144,167–170] Echocardiography is not a useful screening test for the diagnosis of IE in unselected patients with positive blood cultures or in patients with fevers of unknown origin.[168,176] Nevertheless, echocardiographic evaluation should be performed in all patients with clinically suspected IE, including those with negative blood cultures. Although many patients with NVE involving the aortic or mitral valve can be imaged adequately by transthoracic echocardiography (TTE), transesophageal echocardiography (TEE) using biplane technology with incorporated color flow and continuous as well as pulsed Doppler is the state of the art.[168,177] TEE allows visualization of smaller vegetations and provides improved resolution compared with TTE. Not only is TEE the preferred approach in patients with clinically suspected IE in whom TTE is suboptimal, it is also the procedure of choice for imaging the pulmonic valve, patients with PVE (especially at the mitral site), and patients with signs of persistent or invasive infection in spite of adequate antimicrobial therapy.[167,168,177–179]

The sensitivity of echocardiographic detection of vegetations depends upon the technique and portal for the examination; M-mode is less sensitive than two-dimensional echocardiography and TTE is less sensitive than TEE. In two large studies of patients with proven IE examined by both approaches, the sensitivity of TEE was 100 and 90 per cent and that of TTE was 63 and 58 per cent, respectively.[142,180] In the setting of clinically suspected IE, the sensitivity of TEE ranges from 82 to 94 per cent (see Diagnosis).[169,170] In patients with PVE, TTE is limited by the shadowing effect of mitral valve prostheses. In two studies of PVE involving mechanical and bioprosthetic devices, the sensitivity of TEE to detect vegetations was 82 and 96 per cent, while that of TTE was 36 and 16 per cent.[178,181]

In spite of the sensitivity of TEE in detecting vegetations in patients with proven IE, echocardiography does not provide a specific diagnosis. Vegetations and valve dysfunction may be demonstrated, but determination of causality requires clinical or direct anatomical and microbiological confirmation. Infectious vegetations cannot be distinguished from marantic lesions on native valves, nor can vegetations be distinguished from thrombus or pannus on prostheses. Furthermore, it is usually not possible to distinguish active from healed vegetations in NVE.[168,182,183] Thickened valves, ruptured chordae or valves, valve calcification, and nodules may be mistaken for vegetations, indicating the specificity limitations of echocardiography.[142,168]

The natural history of vegetations during therapy is variable. On repeat echocardiogram 3 weeks to 3 months after initiation of ultimately effective antimicrobial therapy, 29 per cent of 41 initial vegetations were no longer detectable. Of the 29 vegetations that remained detectable, 58 per cent were unchanged, 24 per cent were smaller, and 17 per cent were larger. Mobility and extent (valves involved) of vegetations were unchanged in 86 and 65 per cent, respectively. The evolution of these vegetations was unrelated to the duration of therapy or initial vegetation size, nor did it predict late complications of IE.[183] In another study among patients, not all of whom were responding to therapy, persistence or increase in vegetation size during therapy was associated with an increased rate of complications.[184] Accordingly, changes in vegetations must be interpreted in a clinical context and do not in themselves reflect the efficacy of therapy. Vegetations persisting after effective therapy must not be misinterpreted as recurrence of IE unless there is supportive clinical and microbiological evidence.

Valve dysfunction due to tissue disruption or large obstructing vegetations can be visualized and quantitated by echocardiogram with Doppler.[143,168] Some degree of regurgitation by Doppler is almost universal early in the course of NVE and PVE and does not necessarily predict subsequent hemodynamic deterioration.[142,168,185,186] Extension of infection beyond the valve leaflet into surrounding tissue is an ominous step in the progression of IE. It can result in abscesses in various areas of the annulus or adjacent structures, mycotic aneurysms of the sinus of Valsalva or mitral valve, intracardiac fistulas, and purulent pericarditis. Using the knowledge of the anatomical relationships between the valve cusps and adjacent structures, the echocardiographer can define these perivalvular extensions of infection.[134,143] Myocardial abscesses are more readily detected by TEE than TTE in patients with NVE or PVE.[167,178] The sensitivity and specificity for abscess detection were 28 per cent and 98 per cent for TTE, compared with 87 per cent and 95 per cent for TEE.[167] Other studies have reported similar findings, especially in recognizing subaortic invasive disease.[187]

The stratification of patients into groups that are at high and low risk for congestive heart failure, systemic embolization, need for surgical intervention, and death based upon the presence or absence of vegetations remains controversial.[143,168] The heterogeneous nature of the patients examined, the technologies used, and the lack of correlation with other features of IE, as well as the increasing ability to visualize vegetations in most patients with IE using TEE, undermines this debate. Although not demonstrated in all individual studies, pooled data from two-dimensional echocardiographic studies suggest that patients with larger vegetations (>10 mm in diameter) are at increased risk for embolic complications (20 per cent versus 40 per cent).[143,168,186] This increased risk appears to be particularly associated with large vegetations involving the mitral valve and with the mobility of vegetations.[142,144,168] The correlation of aortic or mitral valve vegetation size, extent, mobility, and site with congestive heart failure, need for surgical intervention, and mortality (other than that associated with embolic events) has not been fully established.[142,144,168,186,188]

Among patients with right-sided IE, the visualization of vegetations by TTE has been correlated with prolonged fever during therapy and increased right ventricular end-diastolic dimensions. These findings were not related to vegetation size, nor did the presence of vegetations or their size predict the failure of medical therapy and a need for surgical intervention.[92]

MAGNETIC RESONANCE IMAGING. This technique has identified paravalvular extension of infection, aortic root aneurysms, and fistulas; however, its utility relative to echocardiography has not been established.[134,189]

SCINTIGRAPHY. Efforts to identify vegetations and intracardiac abscess in patients with IE and animal models have utilized scintigraphy with gallium-67 citrate, indium-111–labeled granulocytes, and indium-111–labeled platelets. These efforts have not been sufficiently sensitive nor anatomically localizing to be useful clinically.[134,190]

TREATMENT

Two major objectives must be addressed to effectively treat IE. The infecting microorganism must be eradicated. Failure to accomplish this results in relapse of infection. Also, the invasive, destructive intracardiac and focal extracardiac complications of infection must be addressed if morbidity and mortality are to be minimized. The second objective often exceeds the capacity of effective antimicrobial therapy and requires cardiac or other surgical intervention.

The principles that guide current treatment of endocarditis derive from observations made in vitro, in animal models of endocarditis, and in clinical studies. Bacteria in vegetations are able to multiply to population densities approaching 10^9 to 10^{10} organisms per gram of tissue.[116] Under the conditions in the vegetation, bacteria become metabolically dormant and less vulnerable to the killing action of antimicrobial agents, particularly the penicillins, cephalosporins, and vancomycin, which are the cornerstones of antibiotic therapy for IE. These observations, supplemented by clinical experience, suggest that optimal therapy should use bactericidal antibiotics or antibiotic combinations rather than bacteriostatic agents. Additionally, antibiotics reach the central areas of avascular vegetations by passive diffusion. To reach effective antibiotic concentrations in vegetations, high serum concentrations must be achieved, and even then penetration by some agents is limited.[191] Parenteral antimicrobial therapy is used whenever feasible in order to achieve suitable serum antibiotic concentrations and to avoid the potentially erratic absorption of orally administered therapy. Treatment is continued for prolonged periods to ensure the eradication of dormant microorganisms.

In selecting antimicrobial therapy for patients with IE, the ability of potential agents to kill the causative organism as well as the minimum inhibitory concentration (MIC) and minimum bactericidal concentration (MBC) of these antibiotics for the organism must be considered. The MIC is the lowest concentration that inhibits growth and the MBC is the lowest concentration that decreases a standard inoculum of organisms 99.9 per cent during 24 hours. For the vast majority of streptococci and staphylococci, the MIC and MBC of penicillins, cephalosporins, or vancomycin are the same or differ by only a factor of two to four. Occasionally, organisms are encountered for which the MBC for these antibiotics is 10-fold or greater than the MIC. This phenomenon has been termed tolerance.[108] Most of the tolerant strains are simply killed more slowly than nontolerant strains, and with prolonged incubation (48 hours) their MICs and MBCs are similar. Enterococci exhibit what superficially appears to be tolerance when tested against penicillins and vancomycin; however, these organisms are, in fact, not killed by these agents but are merely inhibited, even after longer incubation times. Enterococci can be killed by the combined activity of selected penicillins or vancomycin and an aminoglycoside. This enhanced antibiotic activity of the combination against enterococci, if of sufficient magnitude, is called synergy or a synergistic bactericidal effect.[80,108] A similar effect can be seen with these combinations against streptococci and staphylococci; this effect overcomes tolerance.[67,108]

A synergistic bactericidal effect is required for the optimal therapy of enterococcal endocarditis and has been employed to achieve more effective therapy or effective short-course therapy of IE caused by other organisms. The finding of tolerance in streptococci or staphylococci causing endocarditis has not been correlated with decreased cure rates or delayed responses to treatment with penicillins, cephalosporins, or vancomycin. Accordingly, the presence of tolerance in streptococci or staphylococci has not required combination therapy and, in fact, regimens are designed using the MICs of these organisms.[83]

The regimens recommended for the treatment of IE caused by specific organisms are designed to provide high concentrations of antibiotics (relative to the MIC of the target organism) in serum as well as concentrations deep in vegetations that exceed the organism's MIC throughout most, if not all, of the interval between doses. Although antibiotic concentrations in vegetations of patients with IE have been measured infrequently, the success of the recommended regimens suggests that this goal has been achieved. Accordingly, for optimal therapy, it is important that the recommended regimens be followed carefully.

Antimicrobial Therapy for Specific Organisms

The antimicrobial therapy for endocarditis should not only eradicate the causative agent but should do so while causing little or no toxicity. Therapy for a given patient requires modification to accommodate end-organ dysfunction, existing allergies, and other anticipated toxicities. With the exception of staphylococcal endocarditis, the antimicrobial regimens recommended for the treatment of patients with NVE and PVE are similar, although more prolonged treatment is often advised for patients with PVE.[47,83]

PENICILLIN-SUSCEPTIBLE VIRIDANS STREPTOCOCCI OR *STREPTOCOCCUS BOVIS*. Four regimens provide highly effective, comparable therapy for patients with endocarditis caused by penicillin-susceptible streptococci and *S. bovis* (Table 33–6).[83] The 4-week regimens yield bacteriologic cure rates of 98 per cent among patients who complete therapy. Treatment with the synergistic combination of penicillin plus gentamicin for 2 weeks is as effective in selected cases as treatment with the 4-week regimens. The combination regimen is recommended for patients with uncomplicated native valve endocarditis who are not at increased risk for aminoglycoside toxicity. Patients with endocarditis caused by nutritionally variant streptococci, endocarditis involving a prosthetic valve, or endocarditis complicated by a mycotic aneurysm, myocardial abscess, perivalvular infection, or an extracardiac focus of infection should not be treated with this short-course regimen. From 2 to 8 per cent of viridans streptococci and *S. bovis* causing endocarditis are highly resistant to streptomycin (MIC $> 2000\ \mu g/ml$) and are not killed synergistically by penicillin plus streptomycin. These highly streptomycin-resistant strains are, however, killed synergistically by penicillin plus gentamicin.[67] Consequently, unless a causative streptococcus can be evaluated to exclude high-level resistance to streptomycin, gentamicin is recommended for use in the short-course combination regimen.[192] The nutritionally variant streptococci, *S. adjacens* and *S. defectivus,* are generally more resistant to penicillin than are other viridans streptococci.[62,66] Patients with endocarditis caused by these streptococci are treated with regimens recommended for enterococcal endocarditis (Table 33–8); however, outcome remains unsatisfactory.[193]

TABLE 33–6 TREATMENT FOR NATIVE VALVE ENDOCARDITIS DUE TO PENICILLIN-SUSCEPTIBLE VIRIDANS STREPTOCOCCI AND *STREPTOCOCCUS BOVIS* (MINIMUM INHIBITORY CONCENTRATION ≤0.1 μg/ml)*

ANTIBIOTIC	DOSAGE AND ROUTE†	DURATION (WEEKS)
Aqueous penicillin G	12–18 million U/24 hours IV either continuously or every 4 hours in six equally divided doses	4
Ceftriaxone	2 gm once daily IV or IM	4
Aqueous penicillin G *plus*	12–18 million U/24 hours IV either continuously or every 4 hours in six equally divided doses	2
Gentamicin	1 mg/kg IM or IV every 8 hours	2
Vancomycin	30 mg/kg per 24 hours IV in two equally divided doses, not to exceed 2 gm/24 hours unless serum levels are monitored	4

* For nutritionally variant streptococci (*Streptococcus adjacens, Streptococcus defectivus*), see Table 33–8.

† Dosages given are for patients with normal renal function. Vancomycin and gentamicin doses must be reduced for treatment of patients with renal dysfunction. Vancomycin and gentamicin doses are calculated using ideal body weight (men = 50 kg + 2.3 kg per inch over 5 feet; women = 45.5 kg + 2.3 kg per inch over 5 feet).

Modified from Wilson, W. R., Karchmer, A. W., Dajani, A. S., et al.: Antibiotic treatment of adults with infective endocarditis due to streptococci, enterococci, staphylococci, and HACEK microorganisms. JAMA *274*:1706, 1995. Copyright 1995 American Medical Association.

For the treatment of streptococcal endocarditis in patients with a history of immediate allergic reactions (urticarial or anaphylactic reactions) to a penicillin or cephalosporin antibiotic, vancomycin is recommended (Table 33–6). Patients with other forms of penicillin allergy (delayed maculopapular skin rash) may be treated cautiously with the ceftriaxone regimen (Table 33–6) or with cefazolin, 2 gm IV every 8 hours for 4 weeks.

For patients with PVE caused by penicillin-susceptible streptococci, treatment with 6 weeks of penicillin is recommended, with gentamicin given during the initial 2 weeks.[47]

RELATIVELY PENICILLIN-RESISTANT STREPTOCOCCI. Approximately 15 per cent of streptococci that cause endocarditis are relatively resistant to penicillin (MIC > 0.1 μg/ml).[62] Four weeks of high-dose parenteral penicillin plus an aminoglycoside (primarily gentamicin for the reasons noted previously) during the initial 2 weeks is recommended for treatment of patients with endocarditis caused by streptococci with MICs for penicillin between 0.2 and 0.5 μg/ml (Table 33–7). Patients who cannot tolerate penicillin because of immediate hypersensitivity reactions can be treated with vancomycin alone (Table 33–7). For those with nonimmediate penicillin hypersensitivity, effective treatment can be accomplished with either vancomycin alone or by adding gentamicin to the initial 2 weeks of the ceftriaxone regimen (Table 33–6). Patients with endocarditis caused by streptococci that are highly resistant to penicillin (MIC > 0.5 μg/ml) should be treated with one of the regimens recommended for enterococcal endocarditis (Table 33–8).

TABLE 33–7 TREATMENT FOR NATIVE VALVE ENDOCARDITIS DUE TO STRAINS OF VIRIDANS STREPTOCOCCI AND *STREPTOCOCCUS BOVIS* RELATIVELY RESISTANT TO PENICILLIN G (MINIMUM INHIBITORY CONCENTRATION > 0.1 μg/ml AND < 0.5 μg/ml)

ANTIBIOTIC	DOSAGE AND ROUTE*	DURATION (WEEKS)
Aqueous penicillin G *plus*	18 million U/24 h IV either continuously or every 4 hours in 6 equally divided doses	4
Gentamicin	1 mg/kg IM or IV every 8 hours	2
Vancomycin	30 mg/kg per 24 hours IV in 2 equally divided doses, not to exceed 2 gm/24 hours unless serum levels are monitored	4

* Dosages are for patients with normal renal function; see Table 33–6 footnote.

Modified from Wilson, W. R., Karchmer, A. W., Dajani, A. S., et al.: Antibiotic treatment of adults with infective endocarditis due to streptococci, enterococci, staphylococci, and HACEK microorganisms. JAMA *274*:1706, 1995. Copyright 1995 American Medical Association.

***STREPTOCOCCUS PYOGENES, STREPTOCOCCUS PNEUMONIAE,* AND GROUP B, C, AND G STREPTOCOCCI.** Endocarditis caused by these streptococci has been either refractory to antibiotic therapy or associated with extensive valvular damage. Penicillin G in a dose of 3 million units intravenously every 4 hours for 4 weeks is recommended for the treatment of group A streptococcal and pneumococcal endocarditis. Pneumococci that are relatively resistant (MIC > 0.1 μg/ml to 1.0 μg/ml) and highly resistant (MIC > 1.0 μg/ml) to penicillin are widely distributed and likely to cause sporadic cases of endocarditis.[79] Although serum concentrations of penicillin G or ceftriaxone, using doses recommended for treatment of endocarditis, markedly exceed the MICs of these penicillin-resistant pneumococci, the efficacy of treatment with these antibiotics is not established. Treatment with vancomycin may be preferable. IE caused by group G, C, or B streptococci is more difficult to treat than that caused by penicillin-susceptible viridans streptococci. Consequently, the addition of gentamicin to the first 2 weeks of a 4-week regimen using high doses of penicillin is often advocated (Table 33–7).

ENTEROCOCCI. Optimal therapy for enterococcal endocarditis requires the synergistic bactericidal interaction of an antimicrobial targeted against the bacterial cell wall (penicillin, ampicillin, or vancomycin) and an aminoglycoside that is able to exert a lethal effect (primarily streptomycin or gentamicin). High-level resistance, defined as the inability of high concentrations of streptomycin (2000 μg/ml) or gentamicin (500 to 2000 μg/ml) to inhibit the growth of an enterococcus, is predictive of the agent's inability to exert this lethal effect and participate in the bactericidal synergistic interaction in vitro and in vivo.[80,82]

The standard regimens recommended for the treatment of enterococcal endocarditis (Table 33–8) are designed to achieve bactericidal synergy. Synergistic combination therapy has resulted in cure rates of approximately 85 per cent, compared with 40 per cent with single-agent, nonbactericidal treatment.[80,81] Some authorities prefer gentamicin doses of 1.5 mg/kg every 8 hours; however, because this dose may be associated with an increased frequency of nephrotoxicity, others advocate doses of 1 mg/kg every 8 hours. Peak serum gentamicin concentrations of approximately 5 μg/ml and 3.5 μg/ml are sought with these doses, respectively. In the absence of high-level resistance to streptomycin in a causative strain, streptomycin 9.5 mg/kg IM or IV, every 12 hours, to achieve a peak serum concentration of approximately 20 μg/ml, can be substituted for gentamicin in the standard regimens. For patients allergic to penicillin, the vancomycin-aminoglycoside regimen (Table 33–8) is recommended; alternatively, patients can be desensitized to penicillin. Desensitization may be desirable when pre-existing renal dysfunction favors avoiding the potentially more nephrotoxic vancomycin-aminoglycoside combination. Cephalosporins are not effective in the treatment of enterococcal endocarditis. Therapy is administered for 4 to 6 weeks, with the longer course used to treat patients with IE that was symptomatic for more than 3 months, with complicated disease, and when there is enterococcal PVE. During treatment, careful clinical follow-up of patients and aminoglycoside levels is required to prevent nephrotoxicity and ototoxicity.

Previously, 40 per cent of enterococci demonstrated high-level resistance to streptomycin, and none was highly resistant to gentamicin. Furthermore, penicillin, ampicillin, and vancomycin inhibited all

TABLE 33–8 STANDARD THERAPY FOR ENDOCARDITIS DUE TO ENTEROCOCCI*

ANTIBIOTIC	DOSAGE AND ROUTE†	DURATION (WEEKS)
Aqueous penicillin G	18–30 million U/24 hours IV given continuously or every 4 hours in six equally divided doses	4–6
plus Gentamicin	1 mg/kg IM or IV every 8 hours	4–6
Ampicillin	12 gm/24 hours IV given continuously or every 4 hours in six equally divided doses	4–6
plus Gentamicin	1 mg/kg IM or IV every 8 hours	4–6
Vancomycin‡	30 mg/kg per 24 hours IV in two equally divided doses not to exceed 2 gm/24 hours unless serum levels are monitored	4–6
plus Gentamicin	1 mg/kg IM or IV every 8 hours	4–6

* All enterococci causing endocarditis must be tested for antimicrobial susceptibility in order to select optimal therapy. These regimens are for treatment of endocarditis caused by enterococci that are susceptible to vancomycin or ampicillin and not highly resistant to gentamicin. These may also be used for treatment of endocarditis caused by penicillin-resistant (MIC > 0.5) viridans streptococci and nutritionally variant streptococci (*S. defectivus, S. adjacens*), or enterococcal PVE.

† Dosages are for patients with normal renal function. See Table 33–6, footnote.

‡ Cephalosporins are not alternatives to penicillin/ampicillin in penicillin-allergic patients.

Modified from Wilson, W. R., Karchmer, A. W., Dajani, A. S., et al.: Antibiotic treatment of adults with infective endocarditis due to streptococci, enterococci, staphylococci, and HACEK microorganisms. JAMA *274*:1706, 1995. Copyright 1995 American Medical Association.

enterococci at concentrations achieved in the serum with standard intravenous doses. Accordingly, one of the standard regimens could be selected for treatment with confidence that bactericidal synergy would be achieved. Antimicrobial resistance among enterococci is now complex and cannot be predicted without in vitro testing. High-level resistance to gentamicin has been noted in 10 to 25 per cent of *E. faecalis* and 45 to 50 per cent of *E. faecium*, and resistance to penicillin, ampicillin, and vancomycin has become commonplace, especially in *E. faecium*. Resistance to these antibiotics is most commonly seen among enterococci isolated from hospitalized or previously hospitalized persons.[194]

Nevertheless, all enterococci causing endocarditis must be evaluated carefully in order to select effective therapy (Table 33–9). The strain causing endocarditis must be tested for high-level resistance to both streptomycin and gentamicin, as well as to determine its susceptibility to penicillin, ampicillin, and vancomycin. If the strain is either resistant to achievable serum concentrations of the cell wall–active agent or highly resistant to the aminoglycosides, synergy and optimal therapy cannot be obtained with a standard regimen that includes the inactive antimicrobial. Furthermore, high-level resistance to gentamicin predicts resistance to all other aminoglycosides except streptomycin. These susceptibility data allow the selection of a bactericidal synergistic regimen, if one is possible, or alternative treatment (Table 33–9).[82]

STAPHYLOCOCCI. More than 90 per cent of coagulase-positive and coagulase-negative staphylococci are penicillin resistant. Methicillin resistance is common among coagulase-negative staphylococci and is a less frequent but important characteristic among *S. aureus*. Methicillin-resistant strains are resistant to all beta-lactam antibiotics but remain susceptible to vancomycin. Although staphylococci are killed by cell wall–active antibiotics, the bactericidal effects of these agents can be enhanced by aminoglycosides. Combinations of semisynthetic penicillinase-resistant penicillins or vancomycin with rifampin do not result in predictable bactericidal synergism; nevertheless, rifampin has unique activity against staphylococcal infections that involve foreign material.[195,196] Staphylococcal infections involving prosthetic heart valves are treated differently from native valve endocarditis caused by the same species (Table 33–10).[47,83,91]

STAPHYLOCOCCAL NATIVE VALVE ENDOCARDITIS. The semisynthetic penicillinase-resistant penicillins are the cornerstones of the treatment of endocarditis caused by methicillin-susceptible staphylococci. When patients have a penicillin allergy that does not induce urticaria or anaphylaxis, a first-generation cephalosporin can be used. The synergistic interaction of beta-lactam antibiotics with an aminoglycoside has not increased the cure rates for staphylococcal endocarditis; however, treatment with these combinations has modestly accelerated the eradication of staphylococci in vegetations and from the blood. To achieve this potential benefit, gentamicin may be added to beta-lactam antibiotic therapy for *S. aureus* during the initial 3 to 5 days of treatment.[83] More prolonged administration of gentamicin has been associated with nephrotoxicity and should be avoided. The role for combination therapy is less well defined in NVE caused by coagulase-negative staphylococci; pooled data suggest improved cure rates with combination therapy.[91] Methicillin-susceptible *S. aureus* endocarditis in intravenous drug addicts that is apparently uncomplicated and limited to the right heart valves has been effectively treated with 2 weeks of semisynthetic penicillinase-resistant penicillin (but not vancomycin) plus an aminoglycoside (doses as noted in Table 33–10).[197,198] However, a significant proportion of patients with right-sided *S. aureus* endocarditis remain febrile and toxic after completing 2 weeks of combination therapy.[92] Hence, clinical judgment must be exercised when this abbreviated regimen is used. Therapy should be extended in those patients who remain febrile after 1 week of treatment or who develop signs suggesting left-sided infection. Endocarditis caused by methicillin-resistant staphylococci requires treatment with vancomycin (Table 33–10). Trimethoprim-sulfamethoxazole treatment of right-sided endocarditis caused by *S. aureus* susceptible to this antimicrobial has been only moderately successful.[199] Truly suitable alternatives to vancomycin are not available. Teicoplanin, a glycopeptide antibiotic similar to vancomycin but not available

TABLE 33–9 STRATEGY FOR SELECTING THERAPY FOR ENTEROCOCCAL ENDOCARDITIS CAUSED BY STRAINS RESISTANT TO COMPONENTS OF THE STANDARD REGIMEN

I. Ideal therapy includes a cell wall–active agent plus an effective aminoglycoside to achieve bactericidal synergy
II. Cell wall–active antimicrobial
   A. Determine MIC for ampicillin and vancomycin; test for beta-lactamase production (nitrocefin test)
   B. If ampicillin and vancomycin susceptible, use ampicillin
   C. If ampicillin resistant (MIC ≥ 16 μg/ml), use vancomycin
   D. If beta-lactamase produced, use vancomycin or consider ampicillin-sulbactam
   E. If ampicillin-resistant and vancomycin-resistant (MIC ≥ 16 μg/ml), consider teicoplanin*
   F. If ampicillin-resistant and highly resistant to vancomycin and teicoplanin (MIC ≥ 256 μg/ml), see alternatives in IV.
III. Aminoglycoside to be used with cell wall–active antimicrobial
   A. If no high-level resistance to streptomycin (MIC < 2000 μg/ml) or gentamicin (MIC < 500–2000 μg/ml), use gentamicin or streptomycin
   B. If high-level resistance to gentamicin (MIC > 500–2000 μg/ml), test streptomycin. If no high-level resistance to streptomycin, use streptomycin
   C. If high-level resistance to gentamicin and streptomycin, omit aminoglycoside therapy; use prolonged therapy with cell wall–active antimicrobial (8 to 12 weeks)
IV. Alternative regimens and approaches
   A. Consider ampicillin, vancomycin (or teicoplanin), and gentamicin (or streptomycin based on absence of high-level resistance)
   B. Treatment with fluoroquinolones, rifampin, or trimethoprim-sulfamethoxazole is of questionable efficacy
   C. Consider suppressive therapy with chloramphenicol or tetracycline and surgical intervention
   D. Consider quinupristin/dalfopristin* therapy for IE due to susceptible *E. faecium*
   E. Single drug therapy (III, C) and surgical intervention

* Not approved by the Food and Drug Administration for use in the United States; may be available through compassionate-use protocol.

TABLE 33–10 TREATMENT FOR STAPHYLOCOCCAL ENDOCARDITIS IN THE ABSENCE OF PROSTHETIC MATERIAL

ANTIBIOTIC	DOSAGE AND ROUTE*	DURATION (WEEKS)
METHICILLIN-SUSCEPTIBLE STAPHYLOCOCCI†		
Nafcillin or oxacillin	2 gm IV every 4 hours	4–6
With optional addition of gentamicin	1 mg/kg IM or IV every 8 hours	3–5 days
Cefazolin (or other first-generation cephalosporins in equivalent dosages)‡	2 gm IV every 8 hours	4–6
With optional addition of gentamicin	1 mg/kg IM or IV every 8 hours	3–5 days
Vancomycin‡	30 mg/kg per 24 hours IV in two equally divided doses, not to exceed 2 gm/24 hours unless serum levels are monitored	4–6
METHICILLIN-RESISTANT STAPHYLOCOCCI		
Vancomycin	30 mg/kg per 24 hours IV in two equally divided doses, not to exceed 2 gm/24 hours unless serum levels are monitored	4–6

* Dosages are for patients with normal renal function. See Table 33–6, footnote.

† For treatment of endocarditis due to penicillin-susceptible staphylococci (minimum inhibitory concentration ≤ 0.1 μg/ml), aqueous penicillin G (18 to 24 million U/24 hours) can be used for 4 to 6 weeks instead of nafcillin or oxacillin.

‡ Cefazolin, other first-generation cephalosporins, or vancomycin may be used in selected penicillin-allergic patients.

Modified from Wilson, W. R., Karchmer, A. W., Dajani, A. S., et al.: Antibiotic treatment of adults with infective endocarditis due to streptococci, enterococci, staphylococci, and HACEK microorganisms. JAMA *274*:1706, 1995. Copyright 1995 American Medical Association.

in the United States, has been considered a possible alternative; however, some strains of *S. aureus* have become resistant to teicoplanin.[200] If the methicillin-resistant strain is susceptible to gentamicin, the aminoglycoside can be used in combination with vancomycin to enhance activity against these organisms. However, the frequency of renal toxicity may also be increased by this combination. The addition of rifampin to vancomycin for treatment of methicillin-resistant *S. aureus* endocarditis has not been beneficial.[201] Right-sided endocarditis caused by methicillin-resistant *S. aureus* is not treated with a 2-week regimen.

STAPHYLOCOCCAL PROSTHETIC VALVE ENDOCARDITIS. Evidence from in vitro studies, experimental animal models of infection, and clinical studies suggests that staphylococcal infections involving foreign bodies, such as prosthetic heart valves, should be treated with two or three antibiotics in combination. Rifampin provides unique antistaphylococcal activity when infection involves foreign bodies.[195,196] However, rifampin-resistant staphylococci emerge rapidly when rifampin is used alone or in combination with vancomycin to treat staphylococcal PVE.[47] Consequently, staphylococcal prosthetic valve endocarditis is treated with two antimicrobials plus rifampin.[47] This author prefers to delay rifampin therapy briefly until treatment with two effective antistaphylococcal agents is in place.

For PVE caused by methicillin-resistant staphylococci, treatment is initiated with vancomycin plus gentamicin, with rifampin added if the organism is susceptible to gentamicin. If the organism is resistant to gentamicin, an alternative aminoglycoside to which the organism is susceptible should be sought. Alternatively, for treatment of PVE caused by an organism resistant to all aminoglycosides, a quinolone to which it is susceptible may be used in lieu of an aminoglycoside.[47] For treatment of PVE caused by methicillin-susceptible staphylococci, a semisynthetic penicillinase-resistant penicillin should be substituted for vancomycin in the combination regimen (Table 33–11).

Patients with a nonimmediate penicillin allergy can be treated with a first-generation cephalosporin in lieu of the semisynthetic penicillin. PVE caused by coagulase-negative staphylococci that occurs within the initial year after valve placement is often complicated by perivalvular extension of infection, and valve replacement surgery is often required to eradicate infection and maintain suitable valve function.[47] Patients with *S. aureus* PVE have frequent intracardiac complications and exceptionally high mortality rates; they should be considered for early surgical intervention if antimicrobial therapy response is not prompt.[47,202]

***HAEMOPHILUS PARAINFLUENZAE, HAEMOPHILUS APHROPHILUS, ACTINOBACILLUS ACTINOMYCETEMCOMITANS, CARDIOBACTERIUM HOMINIS, EIKENELLA CORRODENS,* AND *KINGELLA KINGII* (HACEK ORGANISMS).** Endocarditis caused by the HACEK group has in the past been treated with ampicillin administered alone or in combination with gentamicin. Occasional HACEK organisms that are ampicillin-resistant by virtue of beta-lactamase production have been isolated. Given the marked susceptibility of both beta-lactamase–producing and non-beta-lactamase–producing HACEK strains to third-generation cephalosporins, ceftriaxone or a comparable third-generation cephalosporin is recommended for treatment of NVE or PVE caused by these organisms (Table 33–12).[83] For endocarditis caused by strains that do not produce beta-lactamase, ampicillin combined with gentamicin can be used in lieu of ceftriaxone (Table 33–12).

OTHER PATHOGENS. The antimicrobial therapy for patients with IE caused by unusual organisms is based upon very limited clinical experience and data from animal models and in vitro studies. Therapeutic regimens for most of these infections are beyond the scope of this chapter; in fact, physicians are urged to review the published experience with a specific causative agent as well as to seek assistance from experienced infectious disease consultants when treating these patients. Among the more common of the unusual agents causing endocarditis are *P. aeruginosa*, *Candida* species, and *Corynebacterium* species. The preferred treatment for patients with endocarditis caused by *P. aeruginosa* is an antipseudomonal penicillin (ticarcillin or piperacillin) plus high doses of tobramycin (8 mg/kg/day

TABLE 33–11 TREATMENT OF STAPHYLOCOCCAL ENDOCARDITIS IN THE PRESENCE OF A PROSTHETIC VALVE OR OTHER PROSTHETIC MATERIAL

ANTIBIOTIC	DOSAGE AND ROUTE*	DURATION (WEEKS)
REGIMEN FOR METHICILLIN-RESISTANT STAPHYLOCOCCI		
Vancomycin	30 mg/kg per 24 hours IV in two equally divided doses, not to exceed 2 gm/24 hours unless serum levels are monitored	≥6
plus Rifampin *and*	300 mg p.o. every 8 hours	≥6
Gentamicin†	1.0 mg/kg IM or IV every 8 hours	2
REGIMEN FOR METHICILLIN-SUSCEPTIBLE STAPHYLOCOCCI		
Nafcillin or Oxacillin *plus*	2 gm IV every 4 hours	≥6
Rifampin *and*	300 mg p.o. every 8 hours	≥6
Gentamicin†	1.0 mg/kg IM or IV every 8 hours	2

* Dosages are for patients with normal renal function. See Table 33–6, footnote.

† Use during initial 2 weeks of treatment. If strain is gentamicin-resistant, see text for alternatives.

Modified from Wilson, W. R., Karchmer, A. W., Dajani, A. S., et al.: Antibiotic treatment of adults with infective endocarditis due to streptococci, enterococci, staphylococci, and HACEK microorganisms. JAMA *274*:1706, 1995. Copyright 1995 American Medical Association.

TABLE 33–12 TREATMENT FOR ENDOCARDITIS DUE TO HACEK MICROORGANISMS*

ANTIBIOTIC	DOSAGE AND ROUTE†	DURATION (WEEKS)
Ceftriaxone‡	2 gm once daily IV or IM	4
Ampicillin	12 gm/24 hours IV given continuously or every 4 hours in six equally divided doses	4
plus		
Gentamicin	1 mg/kg IM or IV every 8 hours	4

* HACEK microorganisms are ***Haemophilus parainfluenzae, Haemophilus aphrophilus, Actinobacillus actinomycetemcomitans, Cardiobacterium hominis, Eikenella corrodens,*** and ***Kingella kingii.***

† Dosages are for those with normal renal function. (Table 33–6, footnote.)

‡ Cefotaxime or ceftizoxime in comparable doses may be substituted for ceftriaxone.

Modified from Wilson, W. R., Karchmer, A. W., Dajani, A. S., et al.: Antibiotic treatment of adults with infective endocarditis due to streptococci, enterococci, staphylococci, and HACEK microorganisms. JAMA *274*:1706, 1995. Copyright 1995 American Medical Association.

IM or IV in divided doses every 8 hours to achieve peak serum concentrations of 15 μg/ml).[203] Endocarditis caused by *P. aeruginosa* is often both destructive and poorly responsive to antibiotic therapy (Fig. 33–2). As a result, many patients with *P. aeruginosa* endocarditis require cardiac surgery.

Amphotericin at full doses is recommended for treatment of *Candida* endocarditis. Several patients with *Candida* endocarditis are reported to have been cured by prolonged treatment with fluconazole.[204] Nevertheless, surgical intervention shortly after beginning amphotericin treatment remains the standard treatment for *Candida* endocarditis.

The antimicrobial susceptibility of corynebacteria causing endocarditis must be carefully evaluated. Many remain susceptible to penicillin, vancomycin, and aminoglycosides. Strains susceptible to aminoglycosides are killed synergistically by penicillin in combination with the aminoglycoside.[102] *Corynebacterium jeikeium,* while often resistant to penicillin and aminoglycosides, is killed by vancomycin.[102] NVE or PVE caused by *Corynebacterium* species can be treated with the combination of penicillin plus an aminoglycoside or vancomycin, contingent upon the susceptibilities of the causative strain.[101,102,205]

The Enterobacteriaceae (*E. coli* and *Klebsiella, Enterobacter, Serratia,* and *Proteus* species) are highly susceptible to third-generation cephalosporins, imipenem, and aztreonam. One of these antimicrobial agents in high doses is combined with an aminoglycoside to treat IE caused by an Enterobacteriaceae.

The optimal treatment of IE caused by *Coxiella burnetii* has not been established. Prolonged therapy (3 years) using doxycycline (100 mg twice daily) or another tetracycline is used but is not curative.[31,206] Adding a quinolone to doxycycline therapy is advocated.[206] Surgery is important in effective treatment.

CULTURE-NEGATIVE ENDOCARDITIS. Special studies to diagnose IE caused by fastidious bacteria and other organisms must be performed (see Diagnosis). Thereafter, unless clinical or epidemiologic clues suggest an etiologic diagnosis, the recommended treatment for culture-negative NVE is ampicillin plus gentamicin (see standard regimen for enterococcal endocarditis, Table 33–8); for patients with culture-negative PVE, vancomycin is added to this regimen.[47,207] Mortality rates are lower for patients with culture-negative endocarditis who received antibiotics prior to obtaining blood cultures and those who become afebrile during the initial week of antimicrobial treatment.[172,207] Surgical intervention should be considered for those who do not fully respond to empirical antimicrobial therapy. If surgical intervention is undertaken, a detailed microbiological and pathological examination of excised material must be performed in order to establish an etiologic diagnosis.

TIMING THE INITIATION OF ANTIMICROBIAL THERAPY. Current cost-containment pressures frequently result in initiation of antimicrobial therapy for suspected endocarditis immediately after blood cultures have been obtained. This practice is appropriate in the management of patients with acute IE in whom infection is highly destructive and rapidly progressive and of patients presenting with hemodynamic decompensation requiring urgent or emergent surgical intervention. Immediate therapy may have a favorable impact on outcome in these patients. In contrast, precipitous initiation of therapy in hemodynamically stable patients with suspected subacute endocarditis does not prevent early complications and may, by compromising subsequent blood cultures, obscure the etiological diagnosis of endocarditis. In these latter patients, it is prudent to briefly delay antibiotic therapy pending the results of the initial blood cultures. If these cultures are not positive promptly, this delay provides an important opportunity to obtain additional blood cultures without the confounding effect of empirical treatment. This opportunity is particularly important when patients have received antibiotics recently.

MONITORING THERAPY FOR ENDOCARDITIS. Patients must be monitored carefully during therapy and for several months thereafter to detect complications of endocarditis or therapy. Failure of antimicrobial therapy, myocardial or metastatic abscess, emboli, hypersensitivity to antimicrobial agents, and other complications of therapy (catheter-related infection, thrombophlebitis) or intercurrent illness may be manifested by persistent or recurrent fever. Clinical events may indicate a need for potentially life-saving revision of antimicrobial therapy or adjunctive surgical therapy.

The serum bactericidal titer (SBT), the highest dilution of the patient's serum during therapy that in vitro kills 99.9 per cent of a standard inoculum of the patient's infecting organism, has been used to assess the adequacy of antimicrobial therapy. The use of this test has, however, become controversial. The SBT has correlated poorly with outcome of therapy. These poor correlations can be attributed to performance of the test in a nonstandardized manner and the marked impact of complications on outcome. Several studies suggested, however, that peak and trough titers of at least 1:64 or 1:32 and 1:32, respectively, obtained with a standardized SBT method correlate with bacteriological cure.[208,209] When using regimens considered optimal on the basis of clinical experience, monitoring therapy with this test is not recommended.[83] The SBT may be useful when treating patients with endocarditis caused by organisms for which optimal therapy is not established or when using unconventional antimicrobial regimens.

The serum concentration of vancomycin or aminoglycosides should be measured periodically. This allows dose adjustment to ensure optimal therapy and avoid adverse events. Additionally, renal function should be monitored in patients receiving these two antimicrobials, and the complete blood count should be checked at least weekly in patients receiving high-dose beta-lactam antibiotics or vancomycin.

Repeat blood cultures should be obtained during the initial days of therapy or if fever persists to determine if the bacteremia has been controlled. It is common practice to confirm the eradication of infection by obtaining several blood cultures 2 to 8 weeks after completion of therapy. However, in patients with recrudescent fever after treatment, prompt cultures are essential to assess possible relapse of endocarditis.

OUTPATIENT ANTIMICROBIAL THERAPY. Technical advances allowing the safe administration of complex antimicrobial regimens, combined with well-developed home care systems that provide supplies and monitor outpatient treatment, make it feasible to treat patients with endocarditis on an outpatient basis. Doing so can reduce the cost of therapy significantly. However, only those patients who have responded to initial therapy and are free of fever, who are not experiencing threatening complications, who will be compliant with therapy, and who have a home situation that is physically suitable should be considered for outpatient treatment. Furthermore, patients being treated at home must be apprised of the potential complications of endocarditis, instructed to seek advice promptly when encountering unexpected or untoward clinical events, and have assiduous clinical and laboratory monitoring. Lastly, outpatient therapy must not result in compromises of antimicrobial therapy leading to suboptimal treatment.

Surgical Treatment of Intracardiac Complications

Cardiac surgical intervention plays an increasingly important role in the treatment of patients with intracardiac complications of endocarditis. Retrospective data suggest that mortality is unacceptably high when patients with these complications are treated with antibiotics alone, whereas mortality is reduced when treatment combines antibiotics and surgical intervention.[64,135,161,210–213] Accordingly, these complications have become indications for cardiac surgery (Table 33–13).

VALVULAR DYSFUNCTION. Medical therapy of patients with NVE that is complicated by moderate to severe (New York Heart Association Class III and IV) congestive heart failure due to new or worsening valvular dysfunction results in mortality rates of 50 to 90 per cent. Survival rates for a similar group of patients treated with antibiotics and cardiac surgery are 60 to 80 per cent.[64,135,210–213] Although survival rates among surgically treated patients with PVE complicated by valvular dysfunction and congestive heart failure are 45 to 64 per cent, few PVE patients with these complications are alive at 6 months when treated with antibiotics alone.[47] Worsening aortic valve incompetence is associated with more severe and more rapidly progressive congestive heart failure than is mitral valve incompetence. Hence, patients with aortic valve endocarditis not only account for the majority of surgically treated patients but also require surgery on a more urgent basis when heart failure supervenes. Severe mitral valve insufficiency, nevertheless, results in inexorable heart failure and ultimately requires surgical intervention. Doppler echocardiography and color flow mapping indicating significant valvular regurgitation during the initial week of endocarditis treatment does not reliably predict those patients who will require valve replacement during active endocarditis. Alternatively, despite the absence of significant valvular regurgitation on early echocardiography, marked congestive heart failure may still develop. Decisions regarding surgical intervention should not be made solely on the basis of echocardiographic findings but rather by integrating clinical data during careful serial monitoring.[185] On occasion, very large vegetations on the mitral valve, particularly a mitral valve prosthesis, result in significant obstruction and require surgery.[47]

UNSTABLE PROSTHESES. Dehiscence of an infected prosthetic valve is a manifestation of perivalvular infection and often results in hemodynamically significant valvular dysfunction. Surgical intervention is recommended for PVE patients with these complications.[47,210] The risk of invasive infection is increased among patients with onset of PVE within the year after valve implantation and those with infection of an aortic valve prosthesis.[49] Endocarditis in these patients is often caused by invasive antimicrobial-resistant organisms; consequently, the benefit of combined medical-surgical therapy is enhanced further. Patients who appear clinically stable but who have overtly unstable and hypermobile prostheses, a finding indicative of dehiscence in excess of 40 per cent of the circumference, are likely to experience progressive valve instability and warrant surgical treatment. Occasional patients with PVE caused by noninvasive, highly antibiotic-susceptible organisms, e.g., streptococci, despite a favorable clinical course during antibiotic therapy, late in treatment experience minor valve dehiscence without prosthesis instability or hemodynamic deterioration. Surgical treatment of these patients can be deferred unless clear indications arise.

TABLE 33–13 CARDIAC SURGERY IN PATIENTS WITH INFECTIVE ENDOCARDITIS

ABSOLUTE INDICATIONS
Moderate to severe congestive heart failure due to valve dysfunction
Unstable prosthesis
Uncontrolled infection: Persistent bacteremia, ineffective antimicrobial therapy, fungal endocarditis
Relapse after optimal therapy (prosthetic valves)
RELATIVE INDICATIONS
Perivalvular extension of infection
Staphylococcus aureus endocarditis (aortic, mitral, prosthetic valve)
Relapse after optimal antimicrobial therapy (native valves)
Culture-negative endocarditis with persistent unexplained fever (≥ 10 days)
Large (> 10 mm) vegetations

UNCONTROLLED INFECTION. Surgical intervention has improved the outcome of several forms of endocarditis when maximal antibiotic therapy fails to eradicate infection and, in some instances, even to suppress bacteremia. Amphotericin B is inadequate therapy for fungal endocarditis, including that caused by *Candida* species, and surgical intervention is recommended shortly after initiation of full doses of antifungal therapy. Endocarditis caused by some gram-negative bacilli, e.g., *P. aeruginosa, Achromobacter xylosoxidans,* may not be eradicated by maximum tolerable antibiotic therapy and may require surgical excision of the infected tissue to achieve cure. Similarly, standard therapy of endocarditis caused by *Brucella* species includes surgery because medical therapy is rarely successful.[100] Surgical intervention is recommended when patients with enterococcal endocarditis caused by a strain resistant to synergistic bactericidal therapy (see Antimicrobial Therapy for Specific Organisms—Enterococci) do not respond to initial therapy or relapse. Perivalvular invasive infection is in some instances a form of ineradicable infection. Relapse of PVE after optimal antimicrobial therapy reflects invasive disease. Patients with relapse of PVE are treated surgically.[47,49] In contrast, patients with NVE who relapse, unless it is associated with a highly resistant microorganism or demonstrable perivalvular infection, often are treated again with an intensified, prolonged course of antimicrobial therapy.[47,49,214]

PERIVALVULAR INVASIVE INFECTION. NVE at the aortic site and PVE are most commonly associated with perivalvular invasion with abscess or intracardiac fistula formation.[30,47,49,134,188] Invasive infection occurs in 10 to 14 per cent of patients with NVE and 45 to 60 per cent of those with PVE.[30,47,188] Persistent, otherwise unexplained fever in spite of appropriate antimicrobial therapy or pericarditis in patients with aortic valve endocarditis suggests infection extending beyond the valve leaflet.[137,167,215] New-onset and persistent electrocardiographic conduction abnormalities, although not a sensitive indicator of perivalvular infection (28 per cent), are relatively specific (85 to 90 per cent).[30,134] TEE is superior to TTE for detecting invasive infection in patients with NVE and PVE.[167] Doppler and color flow Doppler or contrast two-dimensional echocardiography optimally define fistulas.[134] Patients with IE in whom an abscess is suspected but not detected by TEE should undergo MRI, including MR angiography.[134] Cardiac catheterization may add little to these imaging studies and is not recommended unless coronary angiography is needed for patients undergoing valve surgery but also suspected of having significant coronary artery disease.[64,134]

In patients with endocarditis complicated by perivalvular extension of infection, cardiac surgery should be considered to debride invasive infection, ablate abscesses, and reconstruct anatomical damage. In patients with invasive disease that significantly disrupts cardiac structures, is associated with congestive heart failure, results in instability of a prosthetic valve, or renders infection uncontrolled (persistent fever), surgery is warranted. However, it is likely that increasingly sensitive imaging techniques will elucidate invasive infections that do not require immediate surgery. Patients with perivalvular infection detected by MRI have been effectively treated with antibiotics alone.[134] Also, conservative medical management has been effective for selected patients with perivalvular infection detected by TEE.[216]

LEFT-SIDED *S. AUREUS* ENDOCARDITIS. Because this infection is difficult to control, highly destructive, and associated with high mortality, some authors have suggested that these patients should be considered for surgical treatment when the response to antimicrobial therapy is not prompt and complete.[212,217,218] *S. aureus* PVE is associated with mortality rates exceeding 80 per cent and thus is an even stronger indication for surgical treatment.[47,202] In contrast, intravenous drug abusers with *S. aureus* endocarditis limited to the tricuspid or pulmonary valves often experience prolonged fever during antimicrobial therapy; nevertheless, the vast majority of these patients respond to antimicrobial therapy and do not require surgery.[92,219]

UNRESPONSIVE CULTURE-NEGATIVE ENDOCARDITIS. Patients with culture-negative endocarditis who experience unexplained persistent fever during empirical antimicrobial therapy, particularly those with PVE, should be considered for surgical intervention. Persistent fever in these patients represents either unrecognized perivalvular infection or ineffective antimicrobial therapy.

LARGE VEGETATIONS (>10 MM) AND THE PREVENTION OF SYSTEMIC EMBOLI. A meta-analysis suggested that the risk of systemic embolization was increased in patients with vegetations greater than 10 mm versus those with smaller or no detectable vegetations, 33 per cent versus 19 per cent.[143] The association of larger mitral valve vegetations (>10 mm) with systemic emboli was confirmed when sizing used transesophageal imaging; however, vegetation size was not related to development of congestive heart failure or increased mortality.[142] Although a relationship may exist between vegetation characteristics—including size, mobility, and extent (number of leaflets involved)—and complications, the implications for surgical intervention are not clear. Yet to be performed are multivariate analyses examining the relationship between outcome or the need for surgical intervention and variables including not only vegetation characteristics but also valve dysfunction, perivalvular invasion by infection, organism, and infection site. Nevertheless, some authors have concluded that vegetation characteristics alone might warrant surgery.[64,142] This recommendation can be questioned, even if it is focused on prevention of emboli as the complications that correlate best with vegetation size.

The rate of systemic or cerebral emboli in patients with NVE and PVE decreases during the course of effective antibiotic therapy.[153,154,156,157,220] Additionally, it is not clear that surgical intervention reduces the frequency of systemic emboli.[135,210] Finally, the morbidity and mortality of cerebral and coronary emboli are rarely compared to the immediate and long-term risks of valve replacement surgery. The latter include perioperative mortality, recrudescent endocarditis on the prosthesis, thromboembolic complications, early and late valve dysfunction requiring repeat valve replacement, the hazards of warfarin anticoagulation (including its contraindication during pregnancy), and the risk and morbidity of late-onset PVE.[210] In the author's opinion, vegetation size alone is rarely an indication for surgery. The clinical findings and echocardiographic evidence for other intracardiac complications must be weighed against the immediate and remote hazards of cardiac surgery when recommending therapy.[143,186] Thus, the risk for systemic embolization as related to vegetation size is only one of many factors to be considered when planning treatment. Prior systemic embolization should be considered in a manner analogous to vegetation size and not as an independent indication for surgical intervention.[153,154,156,157,220]

TECHNIQUES FOR REPAIR OF INTRACARDIAC DEFECTS. New surgical techniques to address severe tissue destruction in NVE and PVE have been developed. Although these are beyond the scope of this discussion, examples include valve composite graft replacement of the aortic root, use of sewing skirts attached to the prostheses, and homograft replacement of the aortic valve and root with coronary artery reimplantation.[221–225] Furthermore, repair of the mitral valve in patients with acute or healed endocarditis avoids insertion of prosthetic materials and the associated hazards.[226,227] Although tricuspid valvulectomy without valve replacement has been advocated for treatment of uncontrolled tricuspid valve infection in intravenous drug abusers at high risk of recidivism and recurrent endocarditis,[228] the likelihood of refractory right-heart failure with time after valvulectomy makes tricuspid valve repair preferable.[64] Cardiac transplantation has been used to salvage an occasional patient with refractory endocarditis.[229]

TIMING OF SURGICAL INTERVENTION. When endocarditis is complicated by valvular regurgitation and significant impairment of cardiac function, surgical intervention before the development of severe intractable hemodynamic dysfunction is recommended, regardless of the duration of antimicrobial therapy.[210,211,230] Postoperative mortality correlates with the severity of preoperative hemodynamic dysfunction; consequently, this approach is justified. In patients with valvular dysfunction in whom infection is controlled and cardiac function is compensated, surgery may be delayed until antimicrobial therapy has been completed. However, if infection is not controlled, surgery should be performed promptly. Similarly, if a patient who requires valve replacement in the near future has a large vegetation, indicating a high risk for systemic embolization, early cardiac surgery is appropriate.

In order to avoid intracranial hemorrhagic complications in patients who have sustained recent neurological injury, the timing of surgical intervention may require modification. Where cardiac function permits, surgery should be delayed for patients who have had prior embolic infarcts until at least 4 and ideally 10 postinfarction days have elapsed[158,231–234] and for those who have sustained an intracranial hemorrhagic event until at least 21 days have elapsed.[232,234] It is prudent to evaluate the cerebral vasculature in patients who have sustained an embolic infarct or who have persistent headaches prior to cardiac surgery. If a mycotic aneurysm is found, the timing of cardiac surgery should be reconsidered and prostheses that require postoperative anticoagulant therapy should be avoided.

DURATION OF ANTIMICROBIAL THERAPY AFTER SURGICAL INTERVENTION. Inflammatory changes and bacteria are commonly seen in culture-negative vegetations removed from patients who have received most or all of the standard antibiotic therapy recommended for endocarditis caused by the specific microorganism.[235] This does not indicate that antimicrobial therapy has failed nor a need for a full course of antibiotic therapy postoperatively. The duration of antimicrobial therapy after surgery depends upon the length of preoperative therapy, antibiotic susceptibility of the causative organism, the presence of paravalvular invasive infection, and the culture status of the vegetation. In general, for endocarditis caused by relatively antibiotic-resistant organisms with negative cultures of operative specimens, preoperative plus postoperative therapy should at least equal a full course of recommended therapy; for those patients with positive intraoperative cultures, a full course of therapy should be given postoperatively. Patients with PVE should be treated conservatively and receive a full course of antimicrobial therapy postoperatively when organisms are seen in resected material.[47]

Treatment of Extracardiac Complications

SPLENIC ABSCESS. Three to 5 per cent of patients with IE develop a splenic abscess; these abscesses most commonly occur in patients with IE caused by *S. aureus*, streptococci, and gram-negative bacilli.[140,145] Although splenic defects can be identified by ultrasonography and CT, these tests usually cannot discriminate between abscess and infarct. Progressive enlargement of the lesion during antimicrobial therapy suggests that it is an abscess; this can be confirmed by percutaneous needle aspiration. Successful therapy of splenic abscesses generally requires drainage, which can often be accomplished by percutaneous placement of a catheter.[145] In patients with endocarditis complicated by multiple splenic abscesses or in whom percutaneous drainage is unsuccessful, splenectomy is required.[145] Splenic abscesses should be effectively treated prior to valve replacement surgery in order to avoid recrudescent infection and seeding of the valve prosthesis.

MYCOTIC ANEURYSMS AND SEPTIC ARTERITIS. From 2 to 10 per cent of patients with endocarditis have mycotic aneurysms; in 1 to 5 per cent the aneurysms involve cerebral vessels.[157,158] Cerebral mycotic aneurysms occur at the branch points in cerebral vessels, are generally located distally over the cerebral cortex, and are found most commonly in branches of the middle cerebral artery. The aneurysms arise either from occlusion of vessels by septic emboli with secondary arteritis and vessel wall destruction or from bacteremic seeding of the vessel wall through the vasa vasorum. *S. aureus* is commonly implicated in the former and viridans streptococci in the latter.[159,160] Although many patients with mycotic aneurysms or septic arteritis present with devastating intracranial hemorrhage, focal deficits from embolic events and persistent focal headache may be premonitory symptoms. Cerebral angiography is required to evaluate patients with subarachnoid hemorrhage and has been recommended for patients experiencing premonitory symptoms or for those with neurologic symptoms in whom anticoagulant therapy is planned.[157,158] Mycotic aneurysms may resolve during antimicrobial therapy[157]; however, where anatomically feasible, aneurysms that have ruptured should be repaired surgically. Aneurysms that have not leaked should be followed angiographically during antimicrobial therapy. Surgery should be considered for a single lesion that enlarges during or following antimicrobial therapy. Anticoagulant therapy should be avoided in patients with a persisting mycotic aneurysm. Although persistent stable aneurysms may rupture after completion of standard antimicrobial therapy, there is no accurate estimation of risk for late rupture, and recommendations for surgical intervention are arbitrary. Nevertheless, prevaling opinion favors, whenever possible without serious neurological injury, the resection of single aneurysms that persist after therapy.[236] The potential existence of occult aneurysms in patients without neurological symptoms or those who have had a negative angiographic evaluation is not considered a contraindication to anticoagulant therapy after completion of antimicrobial therapy.[157]

Extracranial mycotic aneurysms should be followed during antibiotic therapy of IE in a manner analogous to that outlined for cerebral aneurysms. Those that leak, are expanding during therapy, or persist after therapy should be repaired. Particular attention should be given to aneurysms that involve intraabdominal arteries, rupture of which could result in life-threatening hemorrhage.

ANTICOAGULANT THERAPY. Patients with PVE involving devices that would usually warrant maintenance anticoagulation are continued on anticoagulant therapy.[47] Prothrombin times should be maintained at 1.5 times the control (INR = 3.0). Anticoagulation is not initiated as prophylaxis against thromboembolism in patients with PVE involving devices that do not usually require this therapy. Among patients with NVE there is no evidence that anticoagulant therapy prevents embolization, and in some instances it may contribute to intracranial hemorrhage, particularly in the presence of a recent cerebral infarct or a mycotic aneurysm.[157–159] Anticoagulant therapy in patients with NVE is limited to those patients for whom there is a clear indication for this therapy and for whom there is not a known increased risk for intracranial hemorrhage. If central nervous system complications occur in patients with IE who are receiving anticoagulant therapy, anticoagulation should be reversed immediately.[47]

Response to Therapy and Outcome

Temperature returns to normal in most patients with IE, including those with PVE, within a week after initiation of effective antimicrobial therapy.[47,137,237] Almost 75 per cent of patients are afebrile at the end of 1 week of therapy, and 90 per cent have defervesced by the end of the second week of treatment.[215,237] Prolonged fever during therapy is associated with IE due to *S. aureus, P. aeruginosa,* and culture-negative IE as well as IE characterized by microvascular phenomena and major embolic complications.[137,215,237] Persistence or recurrence of fever more than 7 to 10 days after initiation of antibiotic therapy identified patients with increased mortality rates and with complications of infection or therapy.[47,137,215,237] Those patients with prolonged or recurrent fever should be evaluated for intracardiac complications, focal extracardiac septic complications, intercurrent nosocomial infections, recurrent pulmonary emboli (patients with right-sided IE), drug-associated fever, additional underlying illnesses, and, if appropriate, in-hospital substance abuse.

Blood cultures should be repeated in search of persistent bacteremia or the presence of additional pathogens, e.g., previously unrecognized polymicrobial IE. The antimicrobial susceptibility of the causative organism should be re-evaluated, as should the adequacy of antibiotic therapy. Drug reactions have accounted for fever in 17 to 19 per cent of these patients.[137,215] Drug fever attributed to the antimicrobial therapy itself may warrant revision of treatment if a suitable alternative is available. In the absence of effective alternative therapy, treatment can be continued with an antibiotic that is causing fever but is not causing significant end-organ toxicity. In 33 to 45 per cent of patients, persistent fever was associated with significant intracardiac complications, many of which required surgical intervention.[137,215]

Many clinical and laboratory features of IE are slow to resolve in spite of effective antimicrobial therapy. Peripheral manifestations of endocarditis and systemic emboli occur during the early weeks of treatment, although with decreasing frequency. Splenomegaly is slow to resolve, and murmurs may change throughout treatment. Normalization of the sedimentation rate and other inflammatory parameters, as well as correction of the anemia, may not occur until after therapy has been completed.

Mortality rates for large series of NVE treated between 1975 and 1990 range from 16 to 27 per cent.[4,7,8,30,238] Death due to IE has been associated with increased age (>65 to 70 years old), underlying diseases, infection involving the aortic valve, development of congestive heart failure, and central nervous system complications.[1,4,8,30] The treatment of heart failure due to valve dysfunction by early surgical intervention has decreased the mortality associated with congestive heart failure; but subsequently, neurological events and septic complications, e.g., uncontrolled infection and myocardial abscess, have accounted for a larger proportion of deaths and have been associated with high mortality rates.[140]

Mortality rates among patients with IE caused by viridans streptococci and *S. bovis* have ranged from 4 to 9 per cent.[1,4,7] Higher mortality rates are reported with left-sided NVE caused by other organisms: enterococci, 15 to 20 per cent[4,7,81]; *S. aureus,* 25 to 47 per cent[1,4,7,90]; nonviridans streptococci (groups B, C, and G), 50 per cent[239]; *C. burnetti,* 37 per cent[31]; *P. aeruginosa,* Enterobacteriaceae, and fungi, greater than 50 per cent.[35,97,109]

In a retrospective study of NVE patients with either Class III or IV heart failure (New York Heart Association), persistent hypotension, uncontrolled infection for over 21 days, aortic root abscess, or pericarditis, mortality rates for those treated with antibiotics plus surgery and those treated with antibiotics alone were 9 and 51 per cent, respectively.[135] Mortality rates among patients with NVE, particularly involving the aortic valve, who were treated surgically, have ranged from 5 to 26 per cent, with rates toward the high end of this range reported more frequently.[218,230,240–242] Severity of heart failure, abscess, *S. aureus* infection, and decreased renal function (possibly related to heart failure) have been associated with increased postoperative mortality.[218,242]

Outcome for patients with PVE, as contrasted with NVE, has been less desirable. Prior to 1980, mortality rates among patients with onset less than 60 days after surgery and later-onset PVE averaged 70 and 45 per cent, respectively.[47] With the recognition that PVE was frequently complicated by invasive infection and that patients would benefit from surgical intervention, mortality rates have decreased.[47,49] Long-term survival was adversely affected by the presence of moderate or severe heart failure at discharge.[49] Survival rates after aggressive surgery for PVE ranged from 75 to 80 per cent and were not related to time of onset after cardiac surgery.[49,243]

Among patients with NVE (nonaddicts) discharged after medical or medical-surgical therapy, long-term survival was

88 per cent at 5 years and 81 per cent at 10 years.[238] Among patients treated surgically for NVE, survival at 5 years ranged from 70 to 80 per cent.[64,240,241,243] Among patients with PVE treated surgically, survival rates at 4 to 6 years range from 50 to 80 per cent.[64,69,75,225]

RELAPSE AND RECURRENCE. Relapse of IE usually occurs within 2 months of discontinuing antibiotic treatment. Of patients with NVE caused by penicillin-susceptible viridans streptococci who receive a recommended course of therapy, less than 2 per cent relapse. From 8 to 20 per cent of patients with enterococcal IE relapse after standard therapy.[81,214] Patients with IE caused by *S. aureus,* Enterobacteriaceae, or fungi are more likely to experience overt failure of therapy rather than relapse; nevertheless, 4 per cent of patients with *S. aureus* IE relapse.[214] Relapse of fungal endocarditis at long intervals after treatment has been reported. At least 10 per cent of patients with PVE relapse.[49]

Among nonaddicts with an initial episode of NVE or PVE, 4.5 to 7 per cent experience one or more additional episodes.[49,214,238] Among these patients, recurrent IE shares the clinical, microbiological, and response to therapy noted in primary episodes of IE. Intravenous drug abuse is now the most common predisposition for recurrent IE (43 per cent of patients). This population is at increased risk for recurrence within the year after the initial episode.[38]

PREVENTION

A rationale for prophylaxis for endocarditis can be derived by considering the pathogenesis, epidemiology, and microbiology of the illness. This rationale, even in the absence of supporting clinical trials, has generated recommendations for prophylaxis against endocarditis that are routinely applied in developed countries.[244–246] During bacteremia provoked by daily activities, infections, or health care procedures, bacteria adhere to and colonize the platelet fibrin aggregates, NBTE, that have formed on the valve endothelium as a consequence of preexisting congenital or acquired cardiac disease. If the adherence and the subsequent multiplication of bacteria in the vegetation exceed the capacity of host defenses for bacterial eradication, IE results. Although many bacteria enter the bloodstream, those uniquely suited to adhere to NBTE cause the majority of cases of endocarditis. These organisms and the cardiac abnormalities resulting in vulnerable NBTE are evident from reported cases of IE. Events that predispose to bacteremia by organisms causing endocarditis have been identified.[123] By identifying the patients at risk, the causative bacteria and their respective antimicrobial susceptibility, and the events that induce bacteremia, strategies for prevention of some episodes of IE have been formulated. For practical consideration, these strategies have been focused on procedures inducing bacteremia by organisms frequently implicated as causes of IE.

Viridans streptococci, the most common cause of NVE and late-onset PVE, are the predominant aerobic flora of the oral cavity and the most frequent blood isolates after dental extractions and other procedures involving the oral cavity and upper respiratory tract.[123,247] Although gram-negative enteric bacilli are the organisms most commonly recovered from the blood after procedures involving the genitourinary tract, these organisms rarely cause IE.[123] In contrast, procedures involving the genitourinary and gastrointestinal tracts commonly precede the development of enterococcal endocarditis.[81,244] The prophylaxis for endocarditis used in conjunction with procedures involving these mucosal surfaces is targeted against the bacteremic isolates that are common causes of endocarditis. When incision and drainage of skin or soft tissue infections are undertaken, prophylaxis is focused on *S. aureus.* In identifying procedures for which IE prophylaxis is recommended, clinical evidence that a procedure is associated with IE is also considered.

Procedures for which IE prophylaxis is recommended or not recommended have been identified by the American Heart Association and others (Table 33–14).[124,244,245] Although prophylaxis is advised for all patients at risk who undergo dental procedures that cause gingival bleeding, extractions are the most strongly associated with subsequent IE.[150,248] Prophylaxis is recommended when patients at high or intermediate risk for endocarditis (Table 33–15) undergo esophageal dilatation, sclerotherapy for esophageal varices, and retrograde cholangiography when the bile ducts are obstructed. Because endocarditis has been reported only rarely in association with other gastrointestinal endoscopic procedures with or without biopsy, prophylaxis is not routinely recommended in this situation. However, some physicians may elect to give prophylaxis to high-risk patients who undergo these or other low-risk procedures.[244,245] Prophylaxis is not recommended with routine cardiac catheterization or TEE.[124,244,249]

The relative risk associated with specific cardiac lesions is reflected in the increased frequency of the lesion among

TABLE 33–14 PROCEDURES FOR WHICH PROPHYLAXIS AGAINST ENDOCARDITIS IS CONSIDERED

PROPHYLAXIS RECOMMENDED	PROPHYLAXIS NOT RECOMMENDED
Dental procedures known to induce gingival or mucosal bleeding, including professional cleaning and scaling	Dental procedures not likely to cause bleeding, such as adjustment of orthodontic appliances and simple fillings above the gum line
Tonsillectomy or adenoidectomy	Intraoral injection or local anesthetic
Surgery involving gastrointestinal or upper respiratory mucosa	Shedding of primary teeth
Bronchoscopy with rigid bronchoscope	Tympanostomy tube insertion
Sclerotherapy for esophageal varices	Endotracheal tube insertion
Esophageal dilation	Bronchoscopy with flexible bronchoscope, with or without biopsy†
Gallbladder surgery	Cardiac catheterization
Cytoscopy, urethral dilation	Gastrointestinal endoscopy, with or without biopsy†
Uretheral catheterization if urinary infection is present	Cesarean section
Urinary tract surgery, including prostate surgery	In the absence of infection: Urethral catheterization, dilatation and curettage, uncomplicated vaginal delivery, therapeutic abortion, insertion or removal of intrauterine device, sterilization procedures, laparoscopy†
Incision and drainage of infected tissue*	
Vaginal hysterectomy	
Vaginal delivery complicated by infection	

* Antibiotic prophylaxis should be directed against the most likely endocarditis-associated pathogen(s), often staphylococci.
† In patients at highest risk physicians may elect to use prophylaxis for these procedures.
Adapted from Dajani, A. S., Bisno, A. L., Chung, K. S, et al.: Prevention of bacterial endocarditis: Recommendations of the American Heart Association. JAMA *264*:2919, 1990.

TABLE 33–15 RELATIVE RISK OF INFECTIVE ENDOCARDITIS ASSOCIATED WITH PREEXISTING CARDIAC DISORDERS

RELATIVELY HIGH RISK	INTERMEDIATE RISK	VERY LOW OR NEGLIGIBLE RISK*
Prosthetic heart valves†	Mitral valve prolapse with regurgitation (murmur)	Mitral valve prolapse without regurgitation (murmur)
Previous infective endocarditis†	Pure mitral stenosis	Trivial valvular regurgitation on echocardiography without structural abnormality
Cyanotic congenital heart disease†	Tricuspid valve disease	Isolated atrial septal defect (secundum)
Patent ductus arteriosus	Pulmonary stenosis	Arteriosclerotic plaques
Aortic regurgitation	Asymmetrical septal hypertrophy	Coronary artery disease
Aortic stenosis	Bicuspid aortic valve or calcific aortic sclerosis with minimal hemodynamic abnormality	Cardiac pacemaker, implanted defibrillators
Mitral regurgitation	Degenerative valvular disease in elderly patients	Surgically repaired intracardiac lesions, with minimal or no hemodynamic abnormality, more than 6 months after operation
Mitral stenosis and regurgitation	Surgically repaired intracardiac lesions with minimal or no hemodynamic abnormality, less than 6 months after operation	Prior coronary bypass graft surgery
Ventricular septal defect		Prior Kawasaki disease or rheumatic fever without valvular dysfunction
Coarctation of the aorta		
Surgically repaired intracardiac lesion with residual hemodynamic abnormality		
Surgically constructed systemic-pulmonary shunts†		

* Prophylaxis against endocarditis not recommended.
† Lesions considered at highest risk for endocarditis.
Adapted from Durack, D. T.: Prevention of infective endocarditis. N. Engl. J. Med. *332*:38, 1995; and Dajani, A. S., Bisno, A. L., Chung, K. J., et al.: Prevention of bacterial endocarditis: Recommendations of the American Heart Association. JAMA *264*:2919, 1990. Copyright 1990 American Medical Association.

patients with endocarditis compared with the general population. Accordingly, lesions have been assigned to high, intermediate, low, and negligible risk categories (Table 33–15).[25,124,250,251] The American Heart Association and the Expert Group of the International Society for Chemotherapy have identified patients with prosthetic valves, uncorrected cyanotic congenital heart disease, prior infective endocarditis, and surgically constructed systemic-pulmonary shunts or conduits as being at the highest risk for IE.[244,245] Currently, rheumatic heart disease is a less common predisposition for IE in most of the developed countries; however, the attack rate of IE among persons with rheumatic valvular disease approaches that seen with prosthetic valves and suggests that these lesions entail a high risk also.[251]

The risk of IE for patients with mitral valve prolapse and the resulting role of prophylaxis among these patients have been controversial. Mitral valve prolapse has been identified frequently among patients with IE. However, the risk of endocarditis among patients with mitral valve prolapse and a murmur of mitral regurgitation is still relatively low. It is 5- to 10-fold higher than that noted in the general population but 100-fold less than that among patients with rheumatic valvular heart disease.[251] As a result, mitral valve prolapse with a murmur of mitral regurgitation defines a patient with an intermediate risk for IE and one for whom prophylaxis against endocarditis is recommended when undergoing an endocarditis-prone procedure (Table 33–14). In the absence of a mitral regurgitation murmur, prophylaxis is not recommended.[244,245]

GENERAL METHODS. The incidence of IE can be significantly reduced by total surgical correction of some congenital lesions that otherwise predispose patients to IE, e.g., patent ductus arteriosus, atrial septal defect, ventricular septal defect, pulmonary stenosis, and tetralogy of Fallot.[250] Patients with persisting congenital lesions and those with acquired valvular heart disease who remain at risk for IE should be instructed regarding their risk for endocarditis and the potential benefits of antibiotic prophylaxis. Although the recommendations for chemoprophylaxis are

TABLE 33–16 REGIMENS FOR PROPHYLAXIS AGAINST ENDOCARDITIS FOR USE WITH DENTAL, ORAL, AND UPPER RESPIRATORY TRACT PROCEDURES

SETTING	REGIMEN*
Standard regimen†	Amoxicillin, 3.0 gm orally 1 hour before procedure; then 1.5 gm 6 hours after initial dose
Regimen for amoxicillin/penicillin–allergic patients	Erythromycin ethylsuccinate, 800 mg, or erythromycin stearate, 1.0 gm, orally 2 hours before procedure; then half the dose 6 hours after initial dose *OR* Clindamycin, 300 mg orally 1 hour before procedure and 150 mg 6 hours after initial dose
Regimen for patients unable to take oral medications	Ampicillin, 2.0 gm IM or IV 30 minutes before procedure; then either ampicillin, 1.0 g IM or IV, or amoxicillin, 1.5 gm orally, 6 hours after initial dose
Regimens for ampicillin/amoxicillin/penicillin–allergic patients unable to take oral medications	Clindamycin, 300 mg IV 30 minutes before procedure then 150 mg 6 hours after initial dose
Regimen for patients considered at highest risk and not candidates for standard regimen	Use standard regimen for genitourinary and gastrointestinal procedures
Regimen for ampicillin/amoxicillin/penicillin–allergic patients considered at highest risk	Use regimen for allergic patients undergoing genitourinary and gastrointestinal procedures

* Dosages for adults. Initial pediatric dosages are as follows: Ampicillin or amoxicillin, 50 mg/kg; clindamycin, 10 mg/kg; erythromycin ethylsuccinate or erythromycin stearate, 20 mg/kg; gentamicin, 2.0 mg/kg; and vancomycin, 20 mg/kg. Follow-up doses should be one-half the initial dose. **Total pediatric dose should not exceed total adult dose.**
† Generally recommended for patients at highest risk, including those with prosthetic heart valves; physician may elect more vigorous regimens.
Adapted from Dajani, A. S., Bisno, A. L., Chung, K. J., et al.: Prevention of bacterial endocarditis: Recommendations of the American Heart Association. JAMA *264*:2919, 1990. Copyright 1990 American Medical Association.

TABLE 33–17 PROPHYLAXIS AGAINST ENDOCARDITIS: REGIMENS FOR USE WITH GENITOURINARY/GASTROINTESTINAL PROCEDURES

SETTING	REGIMEN*
Standard regimen†	Ampicillin, 2.0 gm IV plus gentamicin, 1.5 mg/kg (not to exceed 80 mg) IV or IM 30 minutes before procedure; followed by amoxicillin, 1.5 gm orally 6 hours after initial dose Alternatively, the parenteral regimen may be repeated once 8 hours after initial dose
Regimen for ampicillin/amoxicillin/ penicillin–allergic patients†	Vancomycin, 1.0 gm IV infused over 1 hour plus gentamicin, 1.5 mg/kg (not to exceed 80 mg) IV or IM, 1 hour before procedure May be repeated once 8 hours after initial dose
Alternative regimen for low-risk patient/ low-risk procedure	Amoxicillin, 3.0 gm orally 1 hour before procedure; then 1.5 gm 6 hours after initial dose

* Dosages for adults. Repeat doses of vancomycin or gentamicin require adjustment for renal dysfunction. Initial pediatric dosages, see Table 33–16, footnote.

† Regimens identical to those of Expert Group of the International Society for Chemotherapy, reference 245.

Adapted from Dajani, A. S., Bisno, A. L., Chung, K. J., et al.: Prevention of bacterial endocarditis: Recommendations of the American Heart Association. JAMA *264*:2919, 1990. Copyright 1990 American Medical Association.

often known to patients at risk, dentists, and physicians, compliance with these guidelines is poor.[18,248,252] Patients should be given written documentation of their predisposing cardiac lesion and the recommended prophylaxis.

Maintenance of good oral hygiene may be a more important preventive than procedure-focused chemoprophylaxis. Good oral hygiene decreases the frequency of bacteremias that accompany daily activities (chewing, tooth brushing), events that may entail more risks than the occasional defined endocarditis-prone procedure.[248,252] Oral hygiene should be addressed before prosthetic valves are placed electively.

Among patients at risk for IE, some activities or procedures likely to induce bacteremia should be avoided. Oral irrigating devices, which may produce bacteremia even in patients with normal gingiva, are not recommended. Similarly, the use of central intravascular catheters and urinary catheters should be minimized. Infections associated with bacteremia must be treated promptly and if possible eradicated before the involved tissues are incised or manipulated.[244,245]

CHEMOPROPHYLAXIS. The widely promulgated recommendations of antimicrobial prophylaxis for endocarditis are based upon circumstantial evidence supplemented by studies of prophylaxis using animal models.

Initial experiments in animal models demonstrated that bactericidal antibiotics could prevent endocarditis even in the face of a nonphysiological large inoculum of bacteria and with a foreign body at the target site. Recent studies, however, suggest that prophylactic antibiotics prevent endocarditis by inhibiting growth of the bacteria adherent to NBTE sufficiently to allow their subsequent complete elimination by host defenses.[124,125] With more numerous bacteria adherent to the valve, a longer period of antibiotic inhibitory activity is required to prevent endocarditis.[125] Although experimental studies that mimic single-dose amoxicillin prophylaxis in humans suggest adequate margins of efficacy, the more sustained inhibitory effect achieved through a postprocedure dose of antibiotics is likely to provide an even higher degree of efficacy.[125,253]

Clinical studies supporting the efficacy of antibiotic prophylaxis for endocarditis are limited. The frequency of viridans streptococcal bacteremia immediately after dental extractions is not reduced by prophylactic antibiotics.[247] This, however, is not inconsistent with effective prophylaxis as demonstrated in animal models.[125] A retrospective study of patients with prosthetic valves who underwent dental and surgical procedures suggested that antibiotic prophylaxis prevented PVE.[254] A small case-control study with several major design limitations suggested a 91 per cent protective effect for prophylaxis.[255] However, a second case-control study suggested only a 49 per cent protective effect for antibiotic prophylaxis.[256] Additionally, failures of antibiotic prophylaxis unrelated to resistant bacteria have been noted.[124]

Risk-benefit and cost-benefit analyses have raised significant questions regarding antibiotic prophylaxis for patients with mitral valve prolapse. The conclusions of these studies depend highly upon initial assumptions. Nevertheless, it is clear that unless both the cost and risks of prophylaxis are very low, the cost per case of IE prevented is high and mortality or morbidity may not be reduced. From a population perspective, prophylaxis in low- to intermediate-risk settings may not be cost- or risk-beneficial, and prophylaxis might be reserved for patients with high-risk cardiac lesions who are undergoing high-risk procedures.[124]

Even if antibiotic prophylaxis is effective as well as safe and inexpensive, only a small percentage of the cases are preventable. For example, only 55 to 75 per cent of patients with NVE have preexisting endocarditis-prone valvular disease, and many are not aware of the lesion before the onset of NVE.[2,6–8,124,248] Additionally, among patients with IE, only a small fraction (5 per cent) had both a known valve lesion and a procedure within 30 days of onset of IE that would have warranted prophylaxis.[248] Nevertheless, the morbidity and mortality associated with IE justify the use of the recommended prophylaxis regimens (Tables 33–16 and 33–17) in patients with high- and intermediate-risk cardiac lesions (Table 33–15) who are to undergo bacteremia-inducing procedures (Table 33–14). Penicillin-resistant flora may emerge among patients who are receiving continuous penicillin for prevention of rheumatic fever. Consequently, a non–penicillin prophylaxis regimen is preferred for these patients. Similarly, when serial dental procedures are anticipated, resistance may emerge to a repetitively used antibiotic. Varying the regimens used or extending the intervals between dental procedures may reduce the emergence of resistant oral flora. Prophylactic antibiotics should be administered as recommended. Initiation of prophylaxis several days before a procedure encourages the emergence of antibiotic-resistant organisms at the mucosal site.

REFERENCES

EPIDEMIOLOGY

1. Steckelberg, J. M., Melton, L. J., III, Ilstrup, D. M., et al.: Influence of referral bias on the apparent clinical spectrum of infective endocarditis. Am. J. Med. *88*:582, 1990.
2. Griffin, M. R., Wilson, W. R., Edwards, W. D., et al.: Infective endocarditis: Olmstead County, Minnesota, 1950 through 1981. JAMA *254*:1199, 1985.
3. Young, S. E. J.: Aetiology and epidemiology of infective endocarditis in England and Wales. J. Antimicrob. Chemother. *20*(Suppl. A):7, 1987.
4. van der Meer, J. T. M., Thompson, J., Valkenburg, H. A., and Michel, M. F.: Epidemiology of bacterial endocarditis in the Netherlands. I. Patient Characteristics. Arch. Intern. Med. *152*:1863, 1992.
5. King, J. W., Nguyen, V. Q., and Conrad, S. A.: Results of a prospective statewide reporting system for infective endocarditis. Am. J. Med. Sci. *295*:517, 1988.

6. McKinsey, D. S., Ratts, T. E., and Bisno, A. L.: Underlying cardiac lesions in adults with infective endocarditis: The changing spectrum. Am. J. Med. *82*:681, 1987.
7. Watanakunakorn, C., and Burkert, T.: Infective endocarditis at a large community teaching hospital, 1980–1990: A review of 210 episodes. Medicine *72*:90, 1993.
8. Kazanjian, P.: Infective endocarditis: Review of 60 cases treated in community hospitals. Infect. Dis. Clin. Pract. *2*:41, 1993.
9. Terpenning, M. S., Buggy, B. P., and Kauffman, C. A.: Infective endocarditis: Clinical features in young and elderly patients. Am. J. Med. *83*:626, 1987.
10. Kaye, D.: Changing pattern of infective endocarditis. Am. J. Med. *78*(Suppl. 6B):157, 1985.
11. Terpenning, M. S., Buggy, B. P., and Kauffman, C. A.: Hospital-acquired infective endocarditis. Arch. Intern. Med. *148*:1601, 1988.
12. Fernandez-Guerrero, M. L., Verdejo, C., Azofra, J., and de Gorgolas, M.: Hospital-acquired infectious endocarditis not associated with cardiac surgery: An emerging problem. Clin. Infect. Dis. *20*:16, 1995.
13. Clemens, J. D., Horwitz, R. I., Jaffe, C. C., et al.: A controlled evaluation of the risk of bacterial endocarditis in persons with mitral-valve prolapse. N. Engl. J. Med. *307*:776, 1982.
14. Hickey, A. J., MacMahon, S. W., and Wilcken, D. E. L.: Mitral valve prolapse and bacterial endocarditis: When is antibiotic prophylaxis necessary? Am. Heart J. *109*:431, 1985.
15. McMahon, S. W., Hickey, A. J., Wilcken, D. E. L., et al.: Risk of infective endocarditis in mitral valve prolapse with and without precordial systolic murmurs. Am. J. Cardiol. *58*:105, 1986.
16. MacMahon, S. W., Roberts, J. K., Kramer-Fox, R., et al.: Mitral valve prolapse and infective endocarditis. Am. Heart J. *113*:1291, 1987.
17. Danchin, N., Briancon, S., Mathieu, P., et al.: Mitral valve prolapse as a risk factor for infective endocarditis. Lancet *1*:743, 1989.
18. van der Meer, J. T. M., van Wijk, W., Thompson, J., et al.: Awareness of need and actual use of prophylaxis: Lack of patient compliance in the prevention of bacterial endocarditis. J. Antimicrob. Chemother. *29*:187, 1992.
19. Nishimara, R. A., McGoon, M. D., Shub, C., et al.: Echocardiographically documented mitral-valve prolapse: Long-term follow-up of 237 patients. N. Engl. J. Med. *313*:1305, 1985.

CLINICAL CLASSIFICATION

20. Stull, T. L., and LiPuma, J. J.: Endocarditis in children. *In* Kaye, D. (ed.): Infective Endocarditis. 2nd ed. New York, Raven Press, 1992, p. 313.
21. Millard, D. D., and Shulman, S. T.: The changing spectrum of neonatal endocarditis. Clin. Perinatol. *15*:587, 1988.
22. Baltimore, R. S.: Infective endocarditis in children. Pediatr. Infect. Dis. J. *11*:907, 1992.
23. Awadallah, S. M., Kavey, R. E. W., Byrum, C. J., et al.: The changing pattern of infective endocarditis in childhood. Am. J. Cardiol. *68*:90, 1991.
24. Normand, J., Bozio, A., Etienne, J., et al.: Changing patterns and prognosis of infective endocarditis in childhood. Eur. Heart J. *16*(Suppl. B):28, 1995.
25. Michel, P. L., and Acar, J.: Native cardiac disease predisposing to infective endocarditis. Eur. Heart J. *16*(Suppl. B):2, 1995.
26. Lavie, C. J., Khandheria, B. K., Seward, J. B., et al.: Factors associated with the recommendation for endocarditis prophylaxis in mitral valve prolapse. JAMA *262*:3308, 1989.
27. Savage, D. D., Garrison, R. J., Devereux, R. B., et al.: Mitral valve prolapse in the general population. I. Epidemiologic features: The Framingham study. Am. Heart J. *106*:571, 1983.
28. Marks, A. R., Choong, C. Y., Sanfilippo, A. J., et al.: Identification of high-risk and low-risk subgroups of patients with mitral-valve prolapse. N. Engl. J. Med. *320*:1031, 1989.
29. Baddour, L. M., and Bisno, A. L.: Infective endocarditis complicating mitral valve prolapse: Epidemiologic, clinical, and microbiologic aspects. Rev. Infect. Dis. *8*:117, 1986.
30. DiNubile, M. J., Calderwood, S. B., Steinhaus, D. M., and Karchmer, A. W.: Cardiac conduction abnormalities complicating native valve active infective endocarditis. Am. J. Cardiol. *58*:1213, 1986.
31. Stein, A., and Raoult, D.: Q fever endocarditis. Eur. Heart J. *16*(Suppl. B):19, 1995.
32. Sande, M. A., Lee, B. L., Mills, J., et al.: Endocarditis in intravenous drug users. *In* Kaye, D. (ed.): Infective Endocarditis. 2nd ed. New York, Raven Press, 1992, p. 345.
33. Levine, D. P., Crane, L. R., and Zervos, M. J.: Bacteremia in narcotic addicts at the Detroit Medical Center. II. Infectious endocarditis: A prospective comparative study. Rev. Infect. Dis. *8*:374, 1986.
34. Chambers, H. F., Morris, D. L., Tauber, M. G., and Modin, G.: Cocaine use and the risk for endocarditis in intravenous drug users. Ann. Intern. Med. *106*:833, 1987.
35. Komshain, S. V., Tablan, O. C., Palutke, W., and Reyes, M. P.: Characteristics of left-sided endocarditis due to *Pseudomonas aeruginosa* in the Detroit Medical Center. Rev. Infect. Dis. *12*:693, 1990.
36. Levin, M. H., Weinstein, R. A., Nathan, C., et al.: Association of infection caused by *Pseudomonas aeruginosa* serotype 011 with intravenous abuse of pentazocine mixed with tripelennamine. J. Clin. Microbiol. *20*:758, 1984.
37. Dressler, F. A., and Roberts, W. C.: Infective endocarditis in opiate addicts: Analysis of 80 cases studied at necropsy. Am. J. Cardiol. *63*:1240, 1989.
38. Baddour, L. M.: Twelve-year review of recurrent native-valve infective endocarditis: A disease of the modern antibiotic era. Rev. Infect. Dis. *10*:1163, 1988.
39. Clifford, C. P., Eykyn, S. J., and Oakley, C. M.: Staphylococcal tricuspid valve endocarditis in patients with structurally normal hearts and no evidence of narcotic abuse. Q. J. Med. *87*:755, 1994.
40. Baddour, L. M.: Polymicrobial infective endocarditis in the 1980's. Rev. Infect. Dis. *13*:963, 1991.
41. Nahass, R. G., Weinstein, M. P., Bartels, J., and Gocke, D. J.: Infective endocarditis in intravenous drug users: A comparison of human immunodeficiency virus type 1–negative and –positive patients. J. Infect. Dis. *162*:967, 1990.
42. Rutledge, R., Kim, J., and Applebaum, R. E.: Actuarial analysis of the risk of prosthetic valve endocarditis in 1,598 patients with mechanical and bioprosthetic valves. Arch. Surg. *120*:469, 1985.
43. Ivert, T. S. A., Dismukes, W. E., Cobbs, C. G., et al.: Prosthetic valve endocarditis. Circulation *69*:223, 1984.
44. Arvay, A., and Lengyel, M.: Incidence and risk factors of prosthetic valve endocarditis. Eur. J. Cardiothorac. Surg. *2*:340, 1988.
45. Calderwood, S. B., Swinski, L. A., Waternaux, C. M., et al.: Risk factors for the development of prosthetic valve endocarditis. Circulation *72*:31, 1985.
46. Horskotte, D., Piper, C., Niehues, R., et al.: Late prosthetic valve endocarditis. Eur. Heart J. *16*(Suppl. B):39, 1995.
47. Karchmer, A. W., and Gibbons, G. W.: Infections of prosthetic heart valves and vascular grafts. *In* Bisno, A. L., and Waldvogel, F. A. (eds): Infections Associated with Indwelling Devices. 2nd ed. Washington, D.C., American Society for Microbiology, 1994, p. 213.
48. Karchmer, A. W., Archer, G. L., and Dismukes, W. E.: *Staphylococcus epidermidis* causing prosthetic valve endocarditis: Microbiologic and clinical observations as guides to therapy. Ann. Intern. Med. *98*:447, 1983.
49. Calderwood, S. B., Swinski, L. A., Karchmer, A. W., et al.: Prosthetic valve endocarditis: Analysis of factors affecting outcome of therapy. J. Thorac. Cardiovasc. Surg. *92*:776, 1986.
50. Ismail, M. B., Hannachi, N., Abid, F., et al.: Prosthetic valve endocarditis: A survey. Br. Heart J. *58*:72, 1987.
51. Kuyvenhoven, J. P., van Rijk-Zwickker, G. L., Hermans, J., et al.: Prosthetic valve endocarditis: Analysis of risk factors for mortality. Eur. J. Cardiothorac. Surg. *8*:420, 1994.
52. Chastre, J., and Trouillet, J. L.: Early infective endocarditis on prosthetic valves. Eur. Heart J. *16*(Suppl. B):32, 1995.
53. Douglas, J. L., and Cobbs, C. G.: Prosthetic valve endocarditis. *In* Kaye, D. (ed.): Infective Endocarditis. 2nd ed. New York, Raven Press, 1992, p. 375.
54. Sobel, J. D.: Nosocomial infective endocarditis. *In* Kaye, D. (ed.): Infective Endocarditis. 2nd ed. New York, Raven Press, 1992, p. 361.
55. Martino, P., Micozzi, A., Venditti, M., et al.: Catheter-related right-sided endocarditis in bone marrow transplant recipients. Rev. Infect. Dis. *12*:250, 1990.
56. Rowley, K. M., Clubb, K. S., Smith, G. J. W., and Cabin, M. S.: Right-sided infective endocarditis as a consequence of flow-directed pulmonary artery catheterization: A clinicopathological study of 55 autopsies. N. Engl. J. Med. *311*:1152, 1984.
57. Jernigan, J. A., and Farr, B. M.: Short-course therapy of catheter-related *Staphylococcus aureus* bacteremia: A meta-analysis. Ann. Intern. Med. *119*:304, 1993.
58. Ehni, W. F., and Reller, L. B.: Short-course therapy for catheter-associated *Staphylococcus aureus* bacteremia. Arch. Intern. Med. *149*:533, 1989.
59. Mylotte, J. M., McDermott, C., and Spooner, J. A.: Prospective study of 114 consecutive episodes of *Staphylococcus aureus* bacteremia. Rev. Infect. Dis. *9*:891, 1987.
60. Raad, I. I., and Sabbagh, M. F.: Optimal duration of therapy for catheter-related *Staphylococcus aureus* bacteremia: A study of 55 cases and review. Clin. Infect. Dis. *14*:75, 1992.
61. Maki, D. G., and Agger, W. A.: Enterococcal bacteremia: Clinical features, the risk of endocarditis, and management. Medicine *67*:248, 1988.
62. Roberts, R. B., Krieger, A. G., Schiller, N. L., and Gross, K. C.: Viridans streptococcal endocarditis: The role of various species, including pyridoxal-dependent streptococci. Rev. Infect. Dis. *1*:955, 1979.
63. Fang, G., Keys, T. F., Gentry, L. O., et al.: Prosthetic valve endocarditis resulting from nosocomial bacteremia: A prospective, multicenter study. Ann. Intern. Med. *119*:560, 1993.
64. Larbalestier, R. I., Kinchla, N. M., Aranki, S. F., et al.: Acute bacterial endocarditis: Optimizing surgical results. Circulation *86*(Suppl. II):II68, 1992.

Etiologic Microorganisms

65. Douglas, C. W. I., Heath, J., Hampton, K. K., and Preston, F. E.: Identity of viridans streptococci isolated from cases of infective endocarditis. J. Med. Microbiol. *39*:179, 1993.
66. Bouvet, A.: Human endocarditis due to nutritionally variant streptococci: *Streptococcus adjacens* and *Streptococcus defectivus*. Eur. Heart J. *16*(Suppl. B):24, 1995.
67. Enzler, M. J., Rouse, M. S., Henry, N. K., et al.: In vitro and in vivo

studies of streptomycin-resistant, penicillin-susceptible streptococci from patients with infective endocarditis. J. Infect. Dis. *155*:954, 1987.
68. Ruoff, K. L., Miller, S. I., Garner, C. V., et al.: Bacteremia with *Streptococcus bovis* and *Streptococcus salivarius:* Clinical correlates of more accurate identification of isolates. J. Clin. Microbiol. *27*:305, 1989.
69. Burkert, T., and Watanakunakorn, C.: Group A streptococcus endocarditis: Report of five cases and review of the literature. J. Infect. *23*:307, 1991.
70. Gallagher, P. G., and Watanakunakorn, C.: Group B streptococcal endocarditis: Report of seven cases and review of the literature, 1962–1985. Rev. Infect. Dis. *8*:175, 1986.
71. Scully, B. E., Spriggs, D., and Neu, H. C.: *Streptococcus agalactiae* (group B) endocarditis—A description of twelve cases and review of the literature. Infection *15*:169, 1987.
72. Wiseman, A., Rene, P., and Crelinsten, G. L.: *Streptococcus agalactiae* endocarditis: An association with villous adenomas of the large intestine. Ann. Intern. Med. *103*:893, 1985.
73. Venezio, F. R., Gullberg, R. M., Westenfelder, G. O., et al.: Group G streptococcal endocarditis and bacteremia. Am. J. Med. *81*:29, 1986.
74. Shlaes, D. M., Lerner, P. I., Wolinsky, E., and Gopalakrishna, K. V.: Infections due to Lancefield group F and related streptococci *(S. milleri, S. anginosus).* Medicine *60*:197, 1981.
75. Ugolini, V., Pacifico, A., Smitherman, T. C., and Mackowiak, P. A.: Pneumococcal endocarditis update: Analysis of 10 cases diagnosed between 1974 and 1984. Am. Heart J. *112*:813, 1986.
76. Powderly, W. G., Stanley, S. L., Jr., and Medoff, G.: Pneumococcal endocarditis: Report of a series and review of the literature. Rev. Infect. Dis. *8*:786, 1986.
77. Finley, J. C., Davidson, M., Parkinson, A. J., and Sullivan, R. W.: Pneumococcal endocarditis in Alaska natives: A population-based experience, 1978 through 1990. Arch. Intern. Med. *152*:1641, 1992.
78. Friedland, I. R., and McCracken, G. H., Jr.: Management of Infections caused by antibiotic-resistant *Streptococcus pneumoniae.* N. Engl. J. Med. *331*:377, 1994.
79. Okumura, A., Ito, K., Kondo, M., et al.: Infective endocarditis caused by highly penicillin-resistant *Streptococcus pneumoniae:* Successful treatment with cefuzonam, ampicillin and imipenem. Pediatr. Infect. Dis. J. *14*:327, 1995.
80. Eliopoulos, G. M.: Enterococcal endocarditis. *In* Kaye, D. (ed.): Infective Endocarditis. 2nd ed. New York, Raven Press, 1992, p. 209.
81. Rice, L. B., Calderwood, S. B., Eliopoulos, G. M., et al.: Enterococcal endocarditis: A comparison of prosthetic and native valve disease. Rev. Infect. Dis. *13*:1, 1991.
82. Eliopoulos, G. M.: Aminoglycoside resistant enterococcal endocarditis. Infect. Dis. Clin. North Am. *7*:117, 1993.
83. Wilson, W. R., Karchmer, A. W., Dajani, A. S., et al.: Antibiotic treatment of adults with infective endocarditis due to streptococci, enterococci, staphylococci, and HACEK microorganisms. JAMA *274*:1706, 1995.
84. Hamill, R. J.: Role of fibronectin in infective endocarditis. Rev. Infect. Dis. *9*(Suppl. 4):S360, 1987.
85. Vaudaux, P. E., Lew, D. P., and Waldvogel, F. A.: Host factors predisposing to and influencing therapy of foreign body infections. *In* Bisno, A. L., and Waldvogel, F. A. (eds.): Infections Associated with Indwelling Medical Devices. 2nd ed. Washington, D.C., American Society for Microbiology, 1994, p. 1.
86. Chuard, C., Vaudaux, P., Waldvogel, F. A., and Lew, D. P.: Susceptibility of *Staphylococcus aureus* growing on fibronectin-coated surfaces to bactericidal antibiotics. Antimicrob. Agents Chemother. *37*:625, 1993.
87. Anwar, H., Strap, J. L., and Costerton, J. W.: Establishment of aging biofilms: Possible mechanism of bacterial resistance to antimicrobial therapy. Antimicrob. Agents Chemother. *36*:1347, 1992.
88. Takeda, S., Pier, G. B., Kojima, Y., et al.: Protection against endocarditis due to *Staphylococcus epidermidis* by immunization with capsular polysaccharide/adhesin. Circulation *84*:2539, 1991.
89. Shiro, H., Muller, E., Gutierrez, N., et al.: Transposition mutants of *Staphylococcus epidermidis* deficient in elaboration of capsular polysaccharide/adhesin and slime are avirulent in a rabbit model of endocarditis. J. Infect. Dis. *169*:1042, 1994.
90. Karchmer, A. W.: Staphylococcal endocarditis. *In* Kaye, D. (eds.): Infective Endocarditis. 2nd ed. New York, Raven Press, 1992, p. 225.
91. Whitener, C., Caputo, G. M., Weitekamp, M. R., and Karchmer, A. W. Endocarditis due to coagulase-negative staphylococci: Microbiologic, epidemiologic, and clinical considerations. Infect. Dis. Clin. North Am. *7*:81, 1993.
92. Bayer, A. S., Blomquist, I. K., Bello, E., et al.: Tricuspid valve endocarditis due to *Staphylococcus aureus:* Correlation of two-dimensional echocardiography with clinical outcome. Chest *93*:247, 1988.
93. Breen, J. D., and Karchmer, A. W.: Usefulness of pulsed-field gel electrophoresis in confirming endocarditis due to *Staphylococcus lugdunensis.* Clin. Infect. Dis. *19*:985, 1994.
94. Vandenesch, F., Etienne, J., Reverdy, M. E., and Eykyn, S. J.: Endocarditis due to *Staphylococcus lugdunensis:* Report of 11 cases and review. Clin. Infect. Dis. *17*:871, 1993.
95. Grace, C. J., Levitz, R. E., Katz-Pollak, H., and Brettman, L. R.: *Actinobacillus actinomycetemcomitans* prosthetic valve endocarditis. Rev. Infect. Dis. *10*:922, 1988.
96. Meyer, D. J., and Gerding, D. N.: Favorable prognosis of patients with prosthetic valve endocarditis caused by gram-negative bacilli of the HACEK group. Am. J. Med. *85*:104, 1988.
97. Hessen, M. T., and Abrutyn, E.: Gram-negative bacterial endocarditis. *In* Kaye, D. (ed.): Infective Endocarditis. 2nd ed. New York, Raven Press, 1992, p. 251.
98. Jackman, J. D., Jr., and Glamann, D. B.: Southwestern Internal Medicine Conference: Gonococcal endocarditis: Twenty-five year experience. Am. J. Med. Sci. *301*:221, 1991.
99. Siller, K. A., and Johnson, W. D., Jr.: Unusual bacterial causes of endocarditis. *In* Kaye, D. (ed.): Infective Endocarditis. 2nd ed. New York, Raven Press, 1992, p. 265.
100. Jacobs, F., Abramowicz, D., Vereerstraeten, P., et al.: Brucella endocarditis: The role of combined medical and surgical treatment. Rev. Infect. Dis. *12*:740, 1990.
101. Petit, A. I. C., Bok, J. W., Thompson, J., et al.: Native-valve endocarditis due to CDC coryneform group ANF-3: Report of a case and review of corynebacterial endocarditis. Clin. Infect. Dis. *19*:897, 1994.
102. Murray, B. E., Karchmer, A. W., and Moellering, R. C., Jr.: Diphtheroid prosthetic valve endocarditis: A study of clinical features and infecting organisms. Am. J. Med. *69*:838, 1980.
103. Lamothe, M., Simmons, B., Gelfand, M., and Schoettle, P.: *Listeria monocytogenes* causing endovascular infection. South. Med. J. *85*:193, 1992.
104. Drancourt, M., Mainardi, J. L., Brouqui, P., et al.: *Bartonella (Rochalimaea) quintana* endocarditis in three homeless men. N. Engl. J. Med. *332*:419, 1995.
105. Spach, D. H., Kanter, A. S., Daniels, N. A., et al.: *Bartonella (Rochalimaea)* species as a cause of apparent "culture-negative" endocarditis. Clin. Infect. Dis. *20*:1044, 1995.
106. Brouqui, P., Dumler, J. S., and Raoult, D.: Immunohistologic demonstration of *Coxiella burnetii* in the valves of patients with Q fever endocarditis. Am. J. Med. *97*:451, 1994.
107. Shapiro, D. S., Kenney, S. C., Johnson, M., et al.: Brief report: *Chlamydia psittaci* endocarditis diagnosed by blood culture. N. Engl. J. Med. *326*:1192, 1992.
108. Scheld, W. M., and Sande, M. A.: Endocarditis and intravascular infections. *In* Mandell, G. L., Bennett, J. E., and Dolin, R. (eds.): Mandel, Douglas and Bennett's Principles and Practice of Infectious Diseases. 4th ed. New York, Churchill Livingstone, 1995, p. 740.
109. Rubinstein, E., and Lang, R.: Fungal endocarditis. Eur. Heart J. *16*(Suppl. B):84, 1995.
110. Moyer, D. V., and Edwards, J. E., Jr.: Fungal endocarditis. *In* Kaye, D. (ed.): Infective Endocarditis. 2nd ed. New York, Raven Press, 1992, p. 299.

PATHOGENESIS

111. Richardson, M., Kinlough-Rathbone, R. L., and Groves, H. M.: Ultrastructural changes in re-endothelialized and non-endothelialized rabbit aorta neo-intima following reinjury with a balloon catheter. Br. J. Exp. Pathol. *65*:597, 1984.
112. Ferguson, D. J. P., McColm, A. A., and Savage, T. J.: A morphologic study of experimental rabbit staphylococcal endocarditis and aortitis. I. Formation and effect of infected and uninfected vegetations on the aorta. Br. J. Exp. Pathol. *67*:667, 1986.
113. Ferguson, D. J. P., McColm, A. A., and Savage, T. J.: A morphologic study of experimental rabbit staphylococcal endocarditis and aortitis. II. Interrelationship of bacteria, vegetation and cardiovasculature in established infections. Br. J. Exp. Pathol. *67*:679, 1986.
114. Livornese, L. L., Jr., and Korzeniowski, O. M.: Pathogenesis of infective endocarditis. *In* Kaye, D. (ed.): Infective Endocarditis. 2nd ed. New York, Raven Press, 1992, p. 19.
115. Baddour, L. M., Christensen, G. D., Lowrance, J. H., and Simpson, W. A.: Pathogenesis of experimental endocarditis. Rev. Infect. Dis. *11*:452, 1989.
116. Scheld, W. M.: Pathogenesis and pathophysiology of infective endocarditis. *In* Sande, M. A., Kaye, D., and Root, R. K. (eds.): Endocarditis. New York, Churchill Livingstone, 1984, p. 1.
117. Freedman, L. R.: The pathogenesis of infective endocarditis. J. Antimicrob. Chemother. *20*(Suppl. A):1, 1987.
118. Freedman, L. R.: Infective Endocarditis and Other Intravascular Infections. New York, Plenum Medical Book Company, 1982, p. 5.
119. Weinstein, L., and Schlesinger, J. J.: Pathoanatomic, pathophysiologic and clinical correlations in endocarditis (first of two parts). N. Engl. J. Med. *291*:832, 1974.
120. Lopez, J. A., Ross, R. S., Fishbein, M. C., and Siegel, R. J.: Nonbacterial thrombotic endocarditis: A review. Am. Heart J. *113*:773, 1987.
121. Rodbard, S.: Blood velocity and endocarditis. Circulation *27*:18, 1963.
122. Weinstein, L., and Schlesinger, J. J.: Pathoanatomic, pathophysiologic and clinical correlations in endocarditis (second of two parts). N. Engl. J. Med. *291*:1122, 1974.
123. Everett, E. D., and Hirschmann, J. V.: Transient bacteremia and endocarditis prophylaxis: A review. Medicine *56*:61, 1977.
124. Durack, D. T.: Prevention of infective endocarditis. N. Engl. J. Med. *332*:38, 1995.
125. Blatter, M., and Francioli, P.: Endocarditis prophylaxis: From experimental models to human recommendation. Eur. Heart J. *16*(Suppl. B):107, 1995.
126. Dankert, J., van der Werff, J., Zaat, S. A. J., et al.: Involvement of bactericidal factors from thrombin-stimulated platelets in clearance of adherent viridans streptococci in experimental infective endocarditis. Infect. Immun. *63*:663, 1995.

127. Hamill, R. J., Vann, J. M., and Proctor, R. A.: Phagocytosis of *Staphylococcus aureus* by cultured bovine aortic endothelial cells: Model for postadherence events in endovascular infections. Infect. Immun. *54*:833, 1986.
128. Rotrosen, D., Edwards, J. E., Jr., Gibson, T. R., et al.: Adherence of *Candida* to cultured vascular endothelial cells: Mechanisms of attachment and endothelial cell penetration. J. Infect. Dis. *152*:1264, 1985.
129. Herzberg, M. C., MacFarlane, G. D., Gong, K., et al.: The platelet interactivity phenotype of *Streptococcus sanguis* influences the course of experimental endocarditis. Infect. Immun. *60*:4809, 1992.
130. Drake, T. A., Rodgers, G. M., and Sande, M. A.: Tissue factor is a major stimulus for vegetation formation in enterococcal endocarditis in rabbits. J. Clin. Invest. *73*:1750, 1984.
131. Bancsi, M. J. L. M. F., Thompson, J., and Bertina, R. M.: Stimulation and monocyte tissue factor expression in an in vitro model of bacterial endocarditis. Infect. Immun. *62*:5669, 1994.
132. Sullam, P. M., Frank, U., Yeaman, M. R., et al.: Effect of thrombocytopenia on the early course of streptococcal endocarditis. J. Infect. Dis. *168*:910, 1993.
133. Yeaman, M. R., Puentes, S. M., Norman, D. C., and Bayer, A. S.: Partial characterization and staphylocidal activity of thrombin-induced platelet microbicidal protein. Infect. Immun. *60*:1202, 1992.

PATHOPHYSIOLOGY

134. Carpenter, J. L.: Perivalvular extension of infection in patients with infective endocarditis. Rev. Infect. Dis. *13*:127, 1991.
135. Croft, C. H., Woodward, W., Elliott, A., et al.: Analysis of surgical versus medical therapy in active complicated native valve infective endocarditis. Am. J. Cardiol. *51*:1650, 1983.
136. Watanabe, G., Haverich, A., Speier, R., et al.: Surgical treatment of active infective endocarditis with paravalvular involvement. J. Thorac. Cardiovasc. Surg. *107*:171, 1994.
137. Blumberg, E. A., Robbins, N., Adimora, A., and Lowy, F. D.: Persistent fever in association with infective endocarditis. Clin. Infect. Dis. *15*:983, 1992.
138. Arnett, E. N., and Roberts, W. C.: Valve ring abscess in active infective endocarditis: Frequency, location, and clues to clinical diagnosis from the study of 95 necropsy patients. Circulation *54*:140, 1976.
139. Douglas, J. L., and Dismukes, W. E.: Surgical therapy of infective endocarditis on natural valves. *In* Kaye, D. (ed.): Infective Endocarditis. 2nd ed. New York, Raven Press, 1992, p. 397.
140. Mansur, A. J., Grinberg, M., Lemos da Luz, P., and Bellotti, G.: The complications of infective endocarditis: A reappraisal in the 1980's. Arch. Intern. Med. *152*:2428, 1992.
141. Steckelberg, J. M., Murphy, J. G., and Wilson, W. R.: Management of complications of infective endocarditis. *In* Kaye, D. (ed.): Infective Endocarditis. 2nd ed. New York, Raven Press, 1992, p. 435.
142. Mugge, A., Daniel, W. C., Frank, G., and Lichtlen, P. R.: Echocardiography in infective endocarditis: Reassessment of prognostic implications of vegetation size determined by the transthoracic and transesophageal approach. J. Am. Coll. Cardiol. *14*:631, 1989.
143. Aragam, J. R., and Weyman, A. E.: Echocardiographic findings in infective endocarditis. *In* Weyman, A. E. (ed.): Principles and Practice of Echocardiography. 2nd ed. Philadelphia, Lea & Febiger, 1994, p. 1178.
144. Sanfilippo, A. J., Picard, M. H., Newell, J. B., et al.: Echocardiographic assessment of patients with infectious endocarditis: Prediction of risk for complications. J. Am. Coll. Cardiol. *18*:1191, 1991.
145. Allan, J. D., Jr.: Splenic abscess: Pathophysiology, diagnosis and management. *In* Remington, J. S., and Swartz, M. N. (eds.): Current Clinical Topics in Infectious Diseases. Boston, Blackwell Scientific Publications, 1994, p. 23.
146. Bayer, A. S., Theofilopoulos, A. N., Eisenberg, R., et al.: Circulating immune complexes in infective endocarditis. N. Engl. J. Med. *295*:1500, 1976.
147. Gutman, R. A., Striker, G. E., Gilliland, B. C., and Cutler, R. E.: The immune complex glomerulonephritis of bacterial endocarditis. Medicine *51*:1, 1972.
148. Levy, R. L., and Hong, R.: The immune nature of subacute bacterial endocarditis (SBE) nephritis. Am. J. Med. *54*:645, 1973.
149. Williams, R. C., Jr., and Kunkel, H. G.: Rheumatoid factor, complement, and conglutinin aberrations in patients with subacute bacterial endocarditis. J. Clin. Invest. *41*:666, 1962.

CLINICAL FEATURES

150. Starkebaum, M., Durack, D., and Beeson, P.: The "incubation period" of subacute bacterial endocarditis. Yale J. Biol. Med. *50*:49, 1977.
151. Bush, L. M., and Johnson, C. C.: Clinical syndrome and diagnosis. *In* Kaye, D. (ed.): Infective Endocarditis. 2nd ed. New York, Raven Press, 1992, p. 99.
152. Churchill, M. A., Jr., Geraci, J. E., and Hunder, G. G.: Musculoskeletal manifestations of bacterial endocarditis. Ann. Intern. Med. *87*:754, 1977.
153. Steckelberg, J. M., Murphy, J. G., Ballard, D., et al.: Emboli in infective endocarditis: The prognostic value of echocardiography. Ann. Intern. Med. *114*:635, 1991.
154. Paschalis, C., Pugsley, W., John, R., and Harrison, M. J. G.: Rate of cerebral embolic events in relation to antibiotic and anticoagulant therapy in patients with bacterial endocarditis. Eur. Neurol. *30*:87, 1990.
155. Pruitt, A. A., Rubin, R. H., Karchmer, A. W., and Duncan, G. W.: Neurologic complications of bacterial endocarditis. Medicine *57*:329, 1978.
156. Hart, R. G., Foster, J. W., Luther, M. F., and Kanter, M. C.: Stroke in infective endocarditis. Stroke *21*:695, 1990.
157. Salgado, A. V., Furlan, A. J., Keys, T. F., et al.: Neurologic complications of endocarditis: A 12-year experience. Neurology *39*:173, 1989.
158. Kanter, M. C., and Hart, R. G.: Neurologic complications of infective endocarditis. Neurology *41*:1015, 1991.
159. Hart, R. G., Kagan-Hallet, K., and Joerns, S. E.: Mechanisms of intracranial hemorrhage in infective endocarditis. Stroke *18*:1048, 1987.
160. Masuda, J., Yutani, C., Waki, R., et al.: Histopathological analysis of the mechanisms of intracranial hemorrhage complicating infective endocarditis. Stroke *23*:843, 1992.
161. Griffin, F. M., Jones, G., and Cobbs, C. G.: Aortic insufficiency in bacterial endocarditis. Ann. Intern. Med. *76*:23, 1972.

DIAGNOSIS

162. Durack, D. T., Lukes, A. S., and Bright, D. K.: New criteria for diagnosis of infective endocarditis: Utilization of specific echocardiographic findings. Am. J. Med. *96*:200, 1994.
163. Mortara, L. A., and Bayer, A. S.: *Staphylococcus aureus* bacteremia and endocarditis: New diagnostic and therapeutic concepts. Infect. Dis. Clin. North Am. *7*:53, 1993.
164. Bayer, A. S., Lam, K., Ginzton, L., et al.: *Staphylococcus aureus* bacteremia: Clinical, serologic, and echocardiographic findings in patients with and without endocarditis. Arch. Intern. Med. *147*:457, 1987.
165. Bayer, A. S., Ward, J. I., Ginzton, L. E., and Shapiro, S. M.: Evaluation of new clinical criteria for the diagnosis of infective endocarditis. Am. J. Med. *96*:211, 1994.
166. von Reyn, C. F., and Arbeit, R. D.: Case definitions for infective endocarditis. Am. J. Med. *96*:220, 1994.
167. Daniel, W. G., Mugge, A., Martin, R. P., et al.: Improvement in the diagnosis of abscesses associated with endocarditis by transesophageal echocardiography. N. Engl. J. Med. *324*:795, 1991.
168. Mugge, A.: Echocardiographic detection of cardiac valve vegetations and prognostic implications. Infect. Dis. Clin. North Am. *7*:877, 1993.
169. Shively, B. K., Gurule, F. T., Roldan, C. A., et al.: Diagnostic value of transesophageal compared with transthoracic echocardiography in infective endocarditis. J. Am. Coll. Cardiol. *18*:391, 1991.
170. Sochowski, R. A., and Chan, K. L.: Implication of negative results on a monoplane transesophageal echocardiographic study in patients with suspected infective endocarditis. J. Am. Coll. Cardiol. *21*:216, 1993.
171. Werner, A. S., Cobbs, C. G., Kaye, D., and Hook, E. W.: Studies on the bacteremia of bacterial endocarditis. JAMA *202*:127, 1967.
172. Hoen, B., Selton-Suty, C., Lacassin, F., et al.: Infective endocarditis in patients with negative blood cultures: Analysis of 88 cases from a one-year nationwide survey in France. Clin. Infect. Dis. *20*:501, 1995.
173. Washington, J. A.: The microbiologic diagnosis of infective endocarditis. J. Antimicrob. Chemother. *20*(Suppl. A):29, 1987.
174. Kaye, K. M., and Kaye, D.: Laboratory findings including blood cultures. *In* Kaye, D. (ed.): Infective Endocarditis. 2nd ed. New York, Raven Press, 1992, p. 117.
175. Kauffmann, R. H., Thompson, J., Valentijn, R. M., et al.: The clinical implications and the pathogenic significance of circulating immune complexes in infective endocarditis. Am. J. Med. *71*:17, 1981.
176. Stratton, J. R., Werner, J. A., Pearlman, A. S., et al.: Bacteremia and the heart: Serial echocardiographic findings in 80 patients with documented or suspected bacteremia. Am. J. Med. *73*:851, 1982.
177. Daniel, W. G., and Mugge, A.: Transesophageal echocardiography. N. Engl. J. Med. *332*:1268, 1995.
178. Vered, Z., Mossinson, D., Peleg, E., et al.: Echocardiographic assessment of prosthetic valve endocarditis. Eur. Heart J. *16*(Suppl. B):63, 1995.
179. Pedersen, W. R., Walker, M., Olson, J. D., et al.: Value of transesophageal echocardiography as an adjunct to transthoracic echocardiography in evaluation of native and prosthetic valve endocarditis. Chest *100*:351, 1991.
180. Lindner, J. R., Case, R. A., Dent, J. M., et al.: Diagnostic value of echocardiography in suspected endocarditis: An evaluation based on the pretest probability of disease. Circulation *93*:730, 1996.
181. Daniel, W. G., Mugge, A., Grote, J., et al.: Comparison of transthoracic and transesophageal echocardiography for detection of abnormalities of prosthetic and bioprosthetic valves in the mitral and aortic positions. Am. J. Cardiol. *71*:210, 1993.
182. Tak, T., Rahimtoola, S. H., and Kamar, A.: Value of digital image processing of two dimensional echocardiograms in differentiating active from chronic vegetations of infective endocarditis. Circulation *78*:116, 1988.
183. Vuille, C., Nidorf, M., Weyman, A. E., and Picard, M. H.: Natural history of vegetations during successful medical treatment of endocarditis. Am. Heart J. *128*:1200, 1994.
184. Rohmann, S., Erbel, R., and Darius, H.: Prediction of rapid versus prolonged healing of infective endocarditis in monitoring vegetation size. J. Am. Soc. Echocardiogr. *4*:465, 1991.
185. Karalis, D. G., Blumberg, E. A., Vilaro, J. F., et al.: Prognostic significance of valvular regurgitation in patients with infective endocarditis. Am. J. Med. *90*:193, 1991.
186. Jaffe, W. M., Morgan, D. E., Pearlman, A. S., and Otto, C. M.: Infective endocarditis, 1983–1988: Echocardiographic findings and factors in-

fluencing morbidity and mortality. J. Am. Coll. Cardiol. *15*:1227, 1990.
187. Karalis, D. G., Bansal, R. C., Hauck, A. J., et al.: Transesophageal echocardiographic recognition of subaortic complications in aortic valve endocarditis: Clinical and surgical implications. Circulation *86*:353, 1992.
188. Omari, B., Shapiro, S., Ginzton, L., et al.: Predictive risk factors for periannular extension of native valve endocarditis: Clinical and echocardiographic analyses. Chest *96*:1273, 1989.
189. Akins, E. W., Slone, R. M., Wiechmann, B. N., et al.: Perivalvular pseudoaneurysm complicating bacterial endocarditis: MR detection in five cases. Am. J. Roentgenol. *156*:1155, 1991.
190. Sokil, A. B.: Cardiac imaging in infective endocarditis. *In* Kaye, D. (ed.): Infective Endocarditis. 2nd ed. New York, Raven Press, 1992, p. 125.

TREATMENT

191. Cremieux, A. C., Maziere, B., Vallois, J. M., et al.: Evaluation of antibiotic diffusion into cardiac vegetations by quantitative autoradiography. J. Infect. Dis. *159*:938, 1989.

Antimicrobial Therapy

192. Roberts, S. A., Lang, S. D. R., and Ellis-Pegler, R. B.: Short-course treatment of penicillin-susceptible viridans streptococcal infective endocarditis with penicillin and gentamicin. Infect. Dis. Clin. Pract. *2*:191, 1993.
193. Stein, D. S., and Nelson, K. E.: Endocarditis due to nutritionally deficient streptococci: Therapeutic dilemma. Rev. Infect. Dis. *9*:908, 1987.
194. Coque, T. M., Arduino, R. C., and Murray, B. E.: High-level resistance to aminoglycosides: Comparison of community and nosocomial fecal isolates of enterococci. Clin. Infect. Dis. *20*:1048, 1995.
195. Chuard, C., Herrmann, M., Vaudaux, P., et al.: Successful therapy of experimental chronic foreign-body infection due to methicillin-resistant *Staphylococcus aureus* by antimicrobial combinations. Antimicrob. Agents Chemother. *35*:2611, 1991.
196. Drancourt, M., Stein, A., Argenson, J. N., et al.: Oral rifampin plus ofloxacin for treatment of *Staphylococcus*-infected orthopedic implants. Antimicrob. Agents Chemother. *37*:1214, 1993.
197. Chambers, H. F., Miller, T., and Newman, M. D.: Right-sided *Staphylococcus aureus* endocarditis in intravenous drug abusers: Two-week combination therapy. Ann. Intern. Med. *109*:619, 1988.
198. Torres-Tortosa, M., de Cueto, M., Vergara, A., et al.: Prospective evaluation of a two-week course of intravenous antibiotics in intravenous drug addicts with infective endocarditis. Eur. J. Clin. Microbiol. Infect. Dis. *13*:559, 1994.
199. Markowitz, N., Quinn, E. L., and Saravolatz, L. D.: Trimethoprim-sulfamethoxazole compared with vancomycin for the treatment of *Staphylococcus aureus* infection. Ann. Intern. Med. *117*:390, 1992.
200. Mainardi, J. L., Shlaes, D. M., Goering, R. V., et al.: Decreased teicoplanin susceptibility of methicillin-resistant strains of *Staphylococcus aureus*. J. Infect. Dis. *171*:1646, 1995.
201. Levine, D. P., Fromm, B. S., and Reddy, B. R.: Slow response to vancomycin or vancomycin plus rifampin in methicillin-resistant *Staphylococcus aureus* endocarditis. Ann. Intern. Med. *115*:674, 1991.
202. Sett, S. S., Hudon, M. P. J., Jamieson, W. R. E., and Chow, A. W.: Prosthetic valve endocarditis: Experience with porcine bioprostheses. J. Thorac. Cardiovasc. Surg. *105*:428, 1993.
203. Reyes, M. P., and Lerner, A. M.: Current problems in the treatment of infective endocarditis due to *Pseudomonas aeruginosa*. Rev. Infect. Dis. *5*:314, 1983.
204. Venditti, M., DeBernardis, F., Micozzi, A., et al.: Fluconazole treatment of catheter-related right-sided endocarditis caused by *Candida albicans* and associated endophthalmitis and folliculitis. Clin. Infect. Dis. *14*:422, 1992.
205. Morris, A., and Guild, I.: Endocarditis due to *Corynebacterium pseudodiphtheriticum:* Five case reports, review, and antibiotic susceptibility of nine strains. Rev. Infect. Dis. *13*:887, 1991.
206. Levy, P. Y., Drancourt, M., Etienne, J., et al.: Comparison of different antibiotic regimens for therapy of 32 cases of Q fever endocarditis. Antimicrob. Agents Chemother. *35*:533, 1991.
207. Tunkel, A. R., and Kaye, D.: Endocarditis with negative blood cultures. N. Engl. J. Med. *326*:1215, 1992.
208. Stratton, C. W.: The role of the microbiology laboratory in the treatment of infective endocarditis. J. Antimicrob. Chemother. *20*(Suppl. A):41, 1987.
209. Weinstein, M. P., Stratton, C. W., Ackley, A., et al.: Multicenter collaborative evaluation of a standardized serum bactericidal test as a prognostic indicator in infective endocarditis. Am. J. Med. *78*:262, 1985.

Surgical Treatment of Intracardiac Complications

210. Alsip, S. G., Blackstone, E. H., Kirklin, J. W., and Cobbs, C. G.: Indications for cardiac surgery in patients with active infective endocarditis. Am. J. Med. *78*(Suppl. 6B):138, 1985.
211. DiNubile, M. J.: Surgery in active endocarditis. Ann. Intern. Med. *96*:650, 1982.
212. Mullany, C. J., McIsaacs, A. I., Rowe, M. H., and Hale, G. S.: The surgical treatment of infective endocarditis. World J. Surg. *13*:132, 1989.
213. Al Jubair, K., Al Fagih, M., Ashmeg, A., et al.: Cardiac operations during active endocarditis. J. Thorac. Cardiovasc. Surg. *104*:487, 1992.
214. Santoro, J., and Ingerman, M.: Response to therapy: Relapses and reinfections. *In* Kaye, D. (ed.): Infective Endocarditis. 2nd ed. New York, Raven Press, 1992, p. 423.
215. Douglas, A., Moore-Gillon, J., and Eykyn, S.: Fever during treatment of infective endocarditis. Lancet *1*:1341, 1986.
216. Chan, K. L., and Sochowski, R. A.: Conservative medical treatment can be appropriate in the management of perivalvular abscess: Diagnosis and follow-up by transesophageal echocardiography. J. Am. Coll. Cardiol. *50*(Abs.):322A, 1994.
217. Richardson, J. V., Karp, R. B., Kirklin, J. W., and Dismukes, W. E.: Treatment of infective endocarditis: A 10-year comparative analysis. Circulation *58*:589, 1978.
218. D'Agostino, R. S., Miller, C., Stinson, E. B., et al.: Valve replacement in patients with native valve endocarditis: What really determines operative outcome? Ann. Thorac. Surg. *40*:429, 1985.
219. Hecht, S. R., and Berger, M.: Right-sided endocarditis in intravenous drug users: Prognostic features in 102 episodes. Ann. Intern. Med. *117*:560, 1992.
220. Davenport, J., and Hart, R. G.: Prosthetic valve endocarditis 1976–1987: Antibiotics, anticoagulation, and stroke. Stroke *21*:993, 1990.
221. Ergin, M. A., Raissi, S., Follis, F., et al.: Annular destruction in acute bacterial endocarditis: Surgical techniques to meet the challenge. J. Thorac. Cardiovasc. Surg. *97*:755, 1989.
222. Miller, D. C.: Predictors of outcome in patients with prosthetic valve endocarditis (PVE) and potential advantages of homograft aortic root replacement for prosthetic ascending aortic valve-graft infections. J. Cardiac Surg. *5*:53, 1990.
223. Ross, D.: Allograft root replacement for prosthetic endocarditis. J. Cardiac Surg. *5*:68, 1990.
224. McGiffin, D. C., Galbraith, A. J., McLachian, G. J., et al.: Aortic valve infection: Risk factors for death and recurrent endocarditis after aortic valve replacement. J. Thorac. Cardiovasc. Surg. *104*:511, 1992.
225. Jault, F., Gandjbakheh, I., Chastre, J. C., et al.: Prosthetic valve endocarditis with ring abscesses: Surgical management and long-term results. J. Thorac. Cardiovasc. Surg. *105*:1106, 1993.
226. Dreyfus, C., Serraf, A., Jebara, V. A., et al.: Valve repair in acute endocarditis. Ann. Thorac. Surg. *49*:706, 1990.
227. Hendren, W. G., Morris, A. S., Rosenkranz, E. R., et al.: Mitral valve repair for bacterial endocarditis. J. Thorac. Cardiovasc. Surg. *103*:124, 1992.
228. Arbulu, A., Holmes, R. J., and Asfaw, I.: Tricuspid valvulectomy without replacement: Twenty years' experience. J. Thorac. Cardiovasc. Surg. *102*:917, 1991.
229. DiSesa, V. J., Sloss, L. J., and Cohn, L. H.: Heart transplantation for intractable prosthetic valve endocarditis. J. Heart Transplant. *9*:142, 1990.
230. Middlemost, S., Wisenbaugh, T., Meyerowitz, C., et al.: A case for early surgery in native left-sided endocarditis complicated by heart failure: Results in 203 patients. J. Am. Coll. Cardiol. *18*:663, 1991.
231. Maruyama, M., Kuriyama, Y., Sawada, T., et al.: Brain damage after open heart surgery in patients with acute cardioembolic stroke. Stroke *20*:1305, 1989.
232. Ting, W., Silverman, N., and Levitsky, S.: Valve replacement in patients with endocarditis and cerebral septic emboli. Ann. Thorac. Surg. *51*:18, 1991.
233. Zisbrod, Z., Rose, D. M., Jacobowitz, I. J., et al.: Results of open heart surgery in patients with recent cardiogenic embolic stroke and central nervous system dysfunction. Circulation *76*(Suppl. V):V109, 1987.
234. Matsushita, K., Kuriyama, Y., Sawada, T., et al.: Hemorrhagic and ischemic cerebrovascular complications of active infective endocarditis of native valve. Eur. Neurol. *33*:267, 1993.
235. Morris, A., Strickett, A., and MacCulloch, D.: Gram stain culture and histology results of heart valves removed during active bacterial endocarditis (Abs. 1174). Programs of the 31st Interscience Conference on Antimicrobial Agents and Chemotherapy, 1991.
236. Ojemann, R. G.: Surgical management of bacterial intracranial aneurysms. *In* Schmidek, H. H., and Sweet, W. H. (eds.): Operative Neurosurgical Techniques. 2nd ed. Orlando, Grune and Stratton, 1988, p. 997.

RESPONSE TO THERAPY AND OUTCOME

237. Lederman, M. M., Sprague, L., Wallis, R. S., and Ellner, J. J.: Duration of fever during treatment of infective endocarditis. Medicine *71*:52, 1992.
238. Tornos, M. P., Permanyer-Miralda, G., Olona, M., et al.: Long-term complications of native valve infective endocarditis in non-addicts: A 15-year follow-up study. Ann. Intern. Med. *117*:567, 1992.
239. Roberts, R. B.: Streptococcal endocarditis: The viridans and beta hemolytic streptococci. *In* Kaye, D. (ed.): Infective Endocarditis. 2nd ed. New York, Raven Press, 1992, p. 191.
240. Acar, J., Michel, P. L., Varenne, O., et al.: Surgical treatment of infective endocarditis. Eur. Heart J. *16*(Suppl. B):94, 1995.
241. Amrani, M., Schoevaerdts, J. C., Eucher, P., et al.: Extension of native aortic valve endocarditis: Surgical considerations. Eur. Heart J. *16*(Suppl. B):103, 1995.
242. Mullany, C. J., Chua, Y. L., Schaff, H. V., et al.: Early and late survival after surgical treatment of culture-positive active endocarditis. Mayo Clin. Proc. *70*:517, 1995.
243. Lytle, B. W.: Surgical treatment of prosthetic valve endocarditis. Semin. Thorac. Cardiovasc. Surg. *7*:13, 1995.

244. Dajani, A. S., Bisno, A. L., Chung, K. J., et al.: Prevention of bacterial endocarditis: Recommendations by the American Heart Association. J.A.M.A. *264*:2919, 1990.
245. Leport, C., Horstkotte, D., Burckhardt, D., and Group of Experts of the International Society for Chemotherapy: Antibiotic prophylaxis for infective endocarditis from an international group of experts towards a European consensus. Eur. Heart J. *16*(Suppl. B):126, 1995.
246. Hay, D. R., Chambers, S. T., Ellis-Pegler, R. B., et al.: Prevention of infective endocarditis associated with dental treatment and other medical interventions. N. Z. Med. J. *105*:192, 1992.
247. Hall, G., Hedstrom, S. A., Heimdahl, A., and Nord, C. E.: Prophylactic administration of penicillins for endocarditis does not reduce the incidence of postextraction bacteremia. Clin. Infect. Dis. *17*:188, 1993.
248. van der Meer, J. T. M., Thompson, J., Valkenburg, H. A., and Michel, M. F.: Epidemiology of bacterial endocarditis in the Netherlands. II. Antecedent procedures and use of prophylaxis. Arch. Intern. Med. *152*:1869, 1992.
249. Melendez, L. J., Chan, K. L., Cheung, P. K., et al.: Incidence of bacteremia in transesophageal echocardiography: A prospective study of 140 consecutive patients. J. Am. Coll. Cardiol. *18*:1650, 1991.
250. DeGevigney, G., Pop, C., and Delahaye, J. P.: The risk of infective endocarditis after cardiac surgical and interventional procedures. Eur. Heart J. *16*(Suppl. B):7, 1995.
251. Steckelberg, J. M., and Wilson, W. R.: Risk factors for infective endocarditis. Infect. Dis. Clin. North Am. *7*:9, 1993.
252. Wahl, M. J.: Myths of dental-induced endocarditis. Arch. Intern. Med. *154*:137, 1994.
253. Fluckiger, U., Moreillon, P., Blaser, J., et al.: Simulation of amoxicillin pharmacokinetics in humans for the prevention of streptococcal endocarditis in rats. Antimicrob. Agents Chemother. *38*:2846, 1994.
254. Horstkotte, D., Friedrichs, W., Pippert, H., et al.: Nutzen der endokarditisprophylaxe bei patienten mit prothetischen herzklappen. Kardiologie *75*:8, 1986.
255. Imperiale, T. F., and Horwitz, R. I.: Does prophylaxis prevent postdental infective endocarditis? A controlled evaluation of protective efficacy. Am. J. Med. *88*:131, 1990.
256. van der Meer, J. T., van Wuk, W., Thompson, J., et al.: Efficacy of antibiotic prophylaxis for prevention of native-valve endocarditis. Lancet *339*:135, 1992.
257. Tornos, P., Sanz, E., Permanyer-Miralda, G., et al.: Late prosthetic valve endocarditis: Immediate and long-term prognosis. Chest *101*:37, 1992.
258. Grover, F. L., Cohen, D. J., Oprian, C., et al.: Determinants of the occurrence of and survival from prosthetic valve endocarditis. J. Thorac. Cardiovasc. Surg. *108*:207, 1994.
259. Keys, T. F.: Early-onset prosthetic valve endocarditis. Cleve. Clin. J. Med. *60*:455, 1993.
260. Chen, S. C., Sorrell, T. C., Dwyer, D. E., et al.: Endocarditis associated with prosthetic cardiac valves. Med. J. Aust. *152*:458, 1990.

Chapter 34
The Pathogenesis of Atherosclerosis

RUSSELL ROSS

RISK FACTORS .1105
THE NORMAL ARTERY 1105
The Intima 1105
The Media 1106
The Adventitia 1106
CELLS OF THE ARTERY AND FROM THE BLOOD POTENTIALLY INVOLVED IN ATHEROGENESIS 1106
Endothelium 1106
Smooth Muscle 1108
Macrophages .1110
Platelets 1110
T-Lymphocytes 1111
THE LESIONS OF ATHEROSCLEROSIS 1111
The Fatty Streak (Lesion Types I to III) .1112
Diffuse Intimal Thickening (Lesion Type IV) 1113
The Fibrous Plaque (Lesion Types V and VI) 1113
HYPOTHESES OF ATHEROGENESIS 1114
The Response-to-Injury Hypothesis 1114
LIPIDS, LIPOPROTEINS, AND MODIFIED LDL IN ATHEROSCLEROSIS 1116
GROWTH FACTORS AND CYTOKINES 1116
CELLULAR EVENTS THAT OCCUR DURING ATHEROGENESIS 1117
REGRESSION OF ATHEROSCLEROSIS 1121
THROMBOSIS .1121
IMAGING ATHEROSCLEROSIS. 1122
CONCLUSIONS. 1122
REFERENCES .1122

Atherosclerosis, the principal cause of death in Western civilization,[1] is a progressive disease process that generally begins in childhood and has clinical manifestations in middle to late adulthood. Two decades ago, atherosclerosis was considered to be a degenerative process because of the accumulation of lipid and necrotic debris in the advanced lesions. We now recognize that it is a multifactorial process which, if it leads to clinical sequelae, requires extensive accumulation of smooth muscle cells within the intima of the affected artery. The form and content of the advanced lesions of atherosclerosis demonstrate the results of three fundamental biological processes. These are: (1) accumulation of intimal smooth muscle cells, together with variable numbers of accumulated macrophages and T-lymphocytes; (2) formation by the proliferated smooth muscle cells of large amounts of connective tissue matrix, including collagen, elastic fibers, and proteoglycans; and (3) accumulation of lipid, principally in the form of cholesteryl esters and free cholesterol within the cells as well as in the surrounding connective tissues.[2–5,5a] Despite the fact that the term "atherosclerosis" is derived from the Greek "athero" (gruel or porridge) and "sclerosis" (hardening), it is important to note that there may be great variability in the relative amounts of tissue formed by each of these processes in the lesions. Consequently, many lesions of atherosclerosis are dense and fibrous, whereas others may contain large amounts of lipid and necrotic debris, with most demonstrating combinations and variations of each of these characteristics. The distribution of lipid and connective tissue in these lesions determines whether they are stable or are at risk of rupture, thrombosis, and clinical sequelae.

RISK FACTORS

(See also Chap. 35)

The development of the concept of "risk factors" and their relationships to the incidence of coronary artery disease evolved from prospective epidemiological studies in the United States and Europe.[6–9] These studies demonstrated a consistent association among characteristics observed at one point in time in apparently healthy individuals with the subsequent incidence of coronary artery disease in those individuals. These associations include an increase in the concentration of plasma cholesterol, the incidence of cigarette smoking, hypertension, clinical diabetes, obesity, age, or male gender, and the occurrence of coronary artery disease.[10–12] As a result of these associations, each characteristic has been termed a risk factor for coronary artery disease, and this terminology has been generally accepted and has become part of the scientific literature associated with this problem.

It is important to remember, however, that the presence of a risk factor does not necessarily imply a direct causal relationship. In most instances, a risk factor is the trait that predicts the risk of development of clinically significant disease within a population. In some cases, it may be involved in the causation of the disease; however, to achieve the latter requires a proven epidemiological association that is statistically valid. The risk factor concept has been extremely useful because it permits one to assess the importance not only of the aforementioned risk factors but also of genetic traits in given individuals, such as a family history of premature coronary artery disease. Using such information, it has become possible to determine whether modification of a given risk factor will result in modification of the risk of a particular disease.

Thus, a risk factor may be defined broadly as "any habit or trait that can be used to predict an individual's probability of developing that disease."[9] A risk factor so defined may be a causative agent but is not necessarily one. A more limited and specific definition is that a risk factor is a causative agent or condition that can be used to predict an individual's probability of developing disease. Used in this fashion, there are at least three independent predictors of risk for individuals within a population of the incidence of atherosclerosis: plasma cholesterol concentration,[13–15] cigarette smoking,[16,17] and elevated blood pressure.[17–19]

THE NORMAL ARTERY

The normal artery (Fig. 34–1) consists of an intima lined by endothelium on the inner (luminal) aspect of the vessel and bounded by the internal elastic lamina on its outer aspect. The media is bounded by the internal elastic lamina and, in well-developed muscular and elastic arteries, by an external elastic lamina. The adventitia is bounded by the external elastic lamina and the exterior of the vessel itself.

The Intima

At birth, the intima consists of a relatively thin layer of connective tissue which contains occasional solitary smooth muscle cells. Most of the connective tissue at birth consists of basement membrane. With increasing age, the amount of connective tissue increases, principally as a result of thickening of the basement membrane and formation of collagen fibrils and new elastic fibers. With increasing age, there appears to be a concentric increase in the numbers of intimal smooth muscle cells.

The intima is the site at which the lesions of atherosclerosis form. The lesions of atherosclerosis appear to be able to form in two ways in different individuals. In those who develop clinical sequelae, the lesions form by a generally asymmetrical thickening of the intima which continually encroaches upon the lumen, resulting in a decrease in the flow of blood. The second form of intimal thickening is one in which the increase in the intima may be associated with

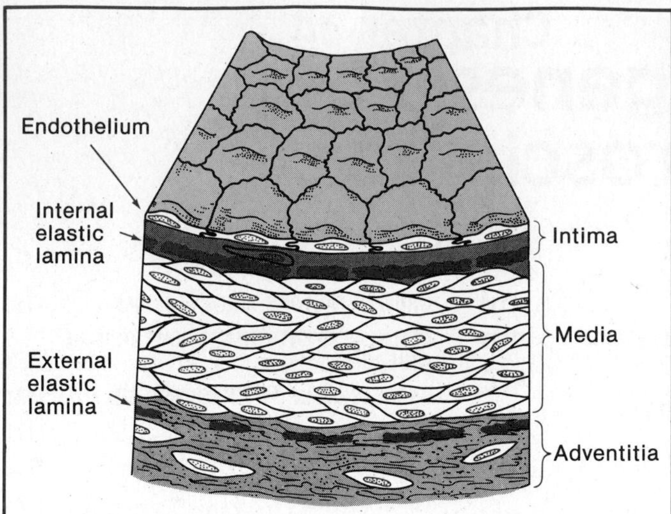

FIGURE 34–1. Structure of a normal muscular artery. (Reprinted by permission from Ross, R., and Glomset, J.: The pathogenesis of atherosclerosis. N. Engl. J. Med. *295*:369, 1976. Copyright Massachusetts Medical Society.)

continued dilation of the artery so that the actual lumen changes little, if at all, in diameter. In the latter case, although lesions of atherosclerosis may form, they are generally more symmetrical and concentric; few if any clinical sequelae appear to result.

The Media

The media is the muscular wall of the artery, bounded by the internal and external elastic laminae (Fig. 34–1). These laminae consist of fenestrated sheets of elastic fibers with numerous openings large enough to permit both substances and cells to pass in either direction. The media of muscular arteries consists of spiraling layers of smooth muscle cells attached to one another, each cell surrounded by a discontinuous basement membrane and by interspersed collagen fibrils and proteoglycan. Elastic arteries contain multiple lamellae of smooth muscle cells, each equivalent to a single media in a small muscular artery, or arteriole. Each lamella is bounded by an elastic lamina on its inner and outer aspects. The number of lamellar units present in elastic arteries has been shown to be highly predictable in relation to the size of the animal and to other factors, such as the anatomical position of the artery. Twenty-nine lamellar units have been suggested to represent the thickest amount of artery wall capable of transporting oxygenated metabolites from the lumen of the aorta to the outermost lamella. When more than 29 lamellar units are present, vasa vasorum that are derived from the adventitia appear to be necessary. These can provide nutrients to the remaining outer lamellar units.[20,21]

The Adventitia

The adventitia consists of a dense collagenous structure containing numerous bundles of collagen fibrils, elastic fibers, and many fibroblasts, together with some smooth muscle cells (Fig. 34–1). It is a highly vascular tissue and contains many nerve fibers as well. As indicated earlier, the adventitia provides the outermost portion of the media of large elastic arteries with much of their nutrition via vasa vasorum, as well as with lymphatic channels and innervation. Wolinsky and Glagov[21] have observed that the abdominal aorta in humans lacks vasa vasorum in its outermost aspects and have suggested that this may be one of the reasons the abdominal aorta is particularly vulnerable to atherogenesis. Barger et al. have observed an increase in adventitial microvessels opposite fibrous plaques in the intima of the coronary artery.[22,23] Using postmortem cinematography and silicon polymers injected into the lumen of the coronary artery, they noted not only an increase in adventitial vessels but in microvessels within the plaque itself. These may play an important role in hemorrhage and thrombosis should the plaques become unstable (see below).

CELLS OF THE ARTERY AND FROM THE BLOOD POTENTIALLY INVOLVED IN ATHEROGENESIS

Endothelium

The endothelial cells probably represent the largest and most extensive tissue in the body because they line the entire vascular tree. In the arterial system, the endothelial cells form a continuous, smooth, uninterrupted surface and represent the principal barrier between the elements of the blood and the artery wall (Fig. 34–2). In adulthood, the turnover of endothelial cells in those arteries that have been studied is relatively low; however, Schwartz and Benditt[24,25] have observed that there are "hot spots" where turnover of endothelium is high in the aorta, even in adults. These hot spots do not appear to be necessarily located at particular anatomical sites. The endothelium forms a highly selective permeability barrier,[26–30] is usually thought to be a nonthrombogenic surface,[31] is a highly active metabolic tissue,[32] and is capable of forming several

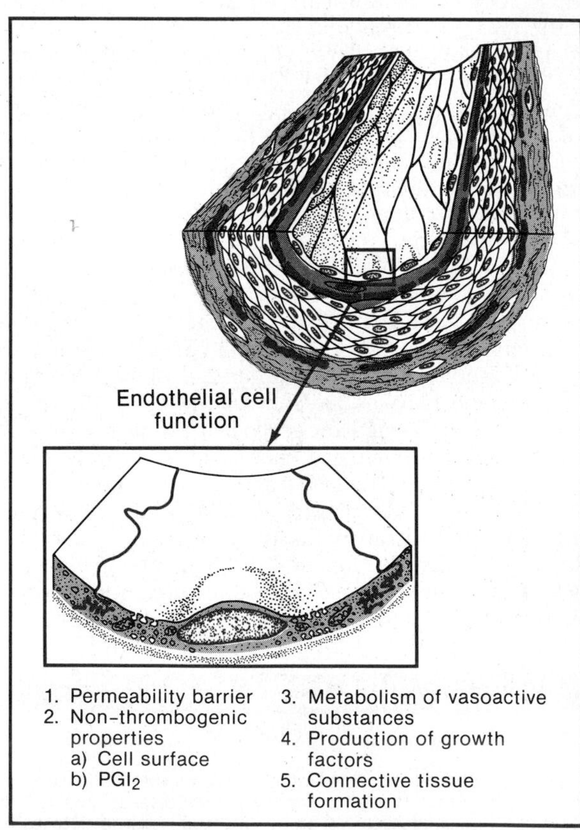

FIGURE 34–2. The endothelial barrier present in the normal artery wall. In the higher magnification inset, the borders between the endothelial cells are irregular, allowing the cells to interdigitate. Vesicles and infoldings at either cell surface permit the cells to transport materials from the lumen of the artery to the tissue by pinocytosis. Transport also occurs below the cell junctions, demonstrated by vesicles that fuse in these regions. In the artery, the cell rests on a connective tissue matrix that consists of a basement membrane intermixed with collagen fibrils. (Reprinted by permission from Ross, R., and Glomset, J.: The pathogenesis of atherosclerosis. N. Engl. J. Med. *295*:371, 1976. Copyright Massachusetts Medical Society.)

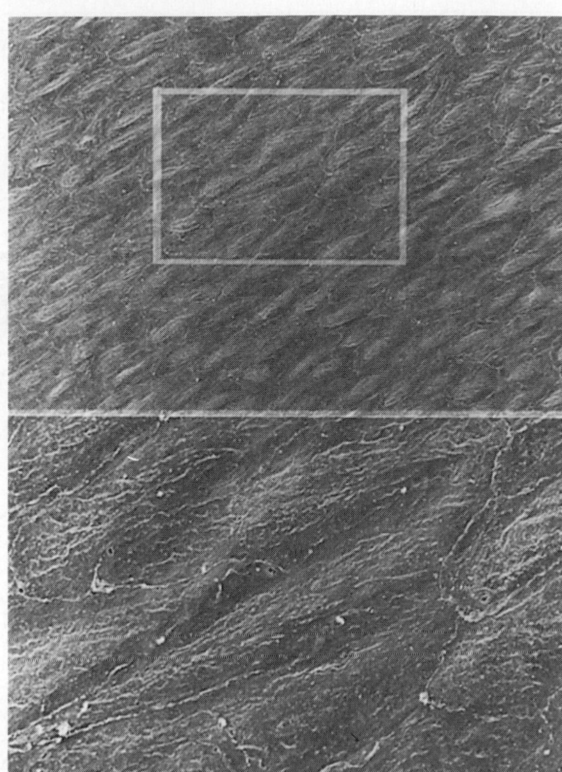

FIGURE 34–3. Scanning electron micrographs of the thoracic aorta endothelium from normal monkey *(Macaca nemestrina)*. ×540. At somewhat higher magnification, the overlapping folds of the endothelial cells can be clearly visualized. The elongated and elliptical appearance of the endothelium can also be seen. The long axes of the cells appear to be diagonal and are oriented in the main direction of the flow of blood in the artery. ×2100. (Reproduced with permission from Ross, R.: Atherosclerosis: A problem of the biology of arterial wall cells and their interactions with blood components. Arteriosclerosis *1*:297, 1981. Copyright 1981 American Heart Association.)

vasoactive substances[31,33,34,36] and connective tissue macromolecules.[35] Endothelial cells examined in culture also have procoagulant properties[37]; however, it is probable that these procoagulant properties are manifested at times of "injury" to the endothelium and are probably not present in situ in the normal artery.

Although the endothelial cells, as seen *en face* by light and scanning electron microscopy (Fig. 34–3) and in cross section by light and transmission electron microscopy (Fig. 34–4), appear to be highly similar morphologically in different parts of the arterial tree, there may be functional differences in these lining cells in different anatomical sites. For example, capillary endothelial cells contain receptors on their surfaces for a potent growth-regulatory peptide, platelet-derived growth factor (PDGF), whereas these receptors are absent on arterial endothelium.[38] Other differences are likely to be found, not only between capillary and arterial endothelium, but among endothelial cells in different parts of the arterial tree itself. With these differences, one might anticipate that there might be differences in the way in which endothelial cells respond to injury after exposure to various injurious agents in different parts of the arterial tree. Endothelial cells are normally attached to each other by tight junctions and by gap junctions. They transport substances in both directions via the process of endocytosis, sometimes called *transcytosis*. Transendothelial channels have been observed in capillary endothelium; however, it is not clear whether they play a role in macromolecular transport in arterial tissue. It has also been suggested that the junctions between endothelial cells may serve as potential sites of increased endothelial transport, particularly when the endothelium has been injured.

Endothelial cells rest on a basement membrane that consists of a particular form of collagen (type IV collagen) intermixed with particular types of proteoglycan molecules. The endothelial cells are undoubtedly responsible for the synthesis of these connective tissue molecules.[35] The base-

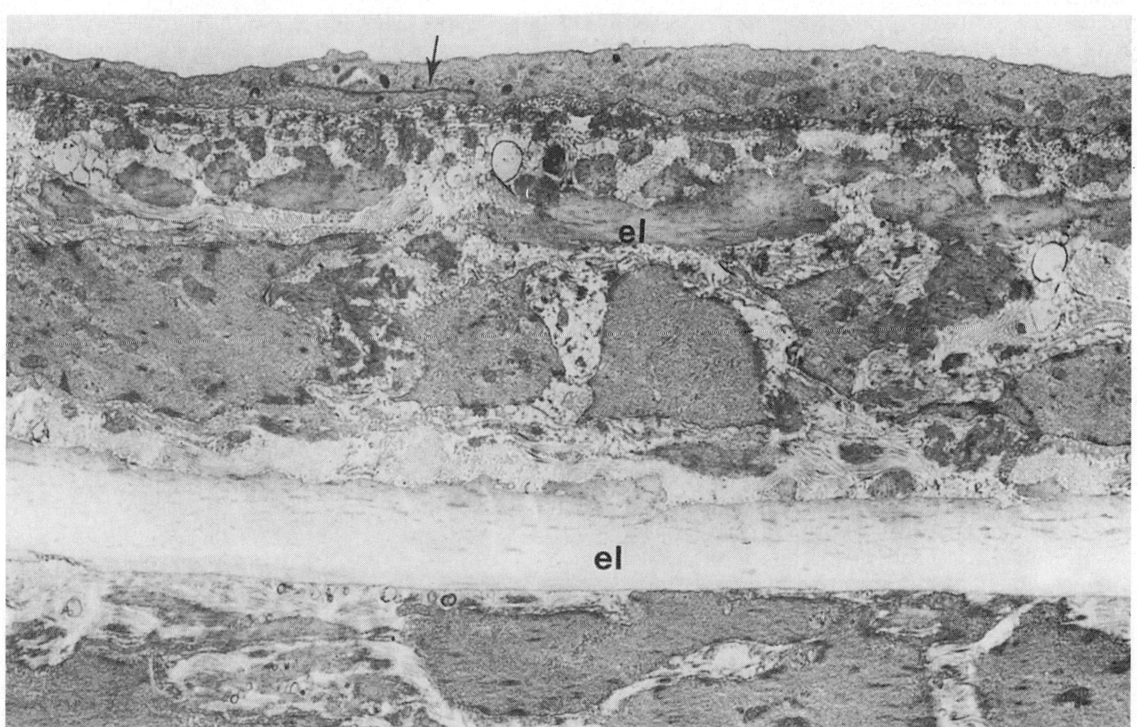

FIGURE 34–4. Transmission electron micrograph of a developing monkey aorta. Two endothelial cells can be seen at the lumen with a junction between them (arrow). Beneath the endothelial cells are newly forming elastic fibers (el) that are separated from the endothelium by basement membrane and collagen fibrils. Beneath the newly forming elastic fibers is a layer of smooth muscle cells separated from another layer by a well-formed elastica (el). No nuclei are apparent in the endothelial cells in this particular thin section.

ment membrane probably also serves as a crude form of filter.

Endothelial cells have receptors for many different molecules on their surface, including receptors for low-density lipoprotein (LDL),[39] for growth factors, and probably for a number of pharmacological agents. A special capacity of endothelium that may be particularly important in atherogenesis is its ability to modify lipoproteins. LDLs appear to be "modified" by a process of low-level oxidation when they are bound to LDL receptors, internalized, and transported through the endothelium. Such modified LDLs can bind to a specific type of receptor, termed a scavenger receptor, on the surface of macrophages, where they are ingested and contribute to the formation of foam cells. This activity is probably important in atherogenesis (see below). The endothelium normally provides a nonthrombogenic surface because of its capacity to form prostaglandin derivatives, particularly prostacyclin (PGI_2) (Chap. 59), a potent vasodilator that is an effective inhibitor of platelet aggregation,[31,34] and because of its surface coat of heparan sulfate. Endothelial cells also make the most potent vasodilator thus far discovered, endothelial-derived relaxing factor (EDRF), a thiolated form of nitric oxide (Chap. 36). EDRF formation by endothelium may be critical in maintaining a balance between vasoconstriction and vasodilation in the process of arterial homeostasis.[33,36] Endothelial cells can also secrete agents that are effective in lysing fibrin clots, including plasminogen, as well as procoagulant materials such as von Willebrand factor.[37] They also secrete a number of vasoactive agents, such as endothelin,[40] angiotensin-converting enzyme, and platelet-derived growth factor, which may be important in vasoconstriction.

A particular characteristic of the endothelium that may be of great importance is the fact that endothelial cells grow in an obligate monolayer. Such growth is representative of cells that line most body surfaces, including epithelial surfaces, and is characterized by the fact that the endothelial cells cannot crawl over one another at sites of injury to facilitate repair of a surface that has been deendothelialized. In other words, only the cells at the margin of an injury can participate in the regenerative response. Thus if a particular anatomical site is repeatedly injured over a prolonged period, and if the endothelial cells that regenerate lose their replication capacity, cells distal to the site, capable of replicating, may not be able to participate simply because they cannot reach the site to do so.

Arterial endothelial cells are capable of synthesizing and secreting several mitogens, one of which is a form of PDGF.[41–43] PDGF is a growth factor for mesenchymally derived, connective tissue–forming cells such as fibroblasts and smooth muscle, but not for arterial endothelial cells. The capacity of endothelium, when it has been appropriately "activated," to form such growth factors may be important in atherogenesis. This is discussed further in the section concerning the response-to-injury hypothesis of atherosclerosis (see p. 1114) (Fig. 34–5).

Thus, the endothelium forms an obligate monolayer that lines the entire arterial tree, is metabolically active, produces vasoactive substances, has a nonthrombogenic surface, and can form procoagulant materials.[44,45] It also serves as the permeability barrier that controls the passage of molecules into the artery. It can oxidize LDL and form nitric oxide (NO), the principal means by which vasodilation is maintained.[46] All of these activities demonstrate the dynamic nature of the endothelial lining and how potentially important this cell layer is in the maintenance of arterial homeostasis. If the endothelium forms oxLDL, the endothelium itself as well as the underlying cells in the artery wall may be injured. OxLDL may play an important initiating role in inducing increased adherence and migration of monocytes and T-lymphocytes from the lumen into the artery wall. OxLDL can induce the formation of at least two adhesive molecules on the surface of the endothelium, vascular cell adhesion molecule-1 (VCAM-1) and intercellular adhesion molecule-1 (ICAM-1). These two molecules can participate in the increased adhesion of monocytes and T cells to the endothelium through receptor-ligand–type interactions with appropriate molecules on the surface of the leukocytes. The roles of these molecules are discussed below.

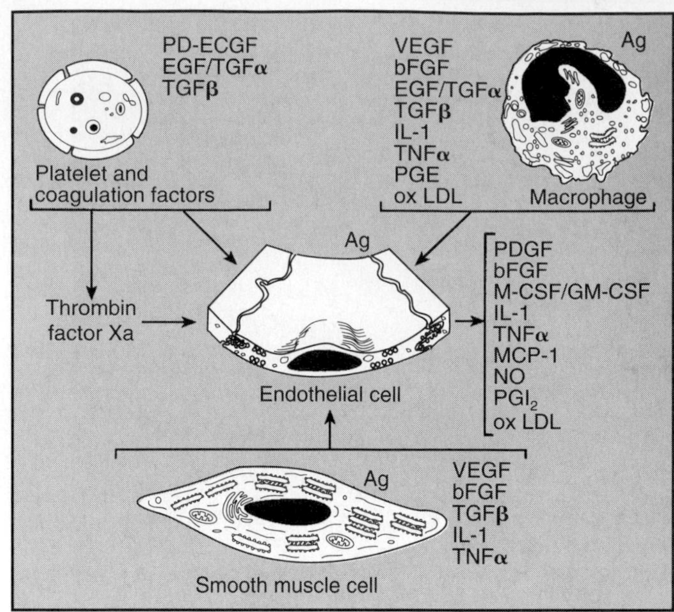

FIGURE 34–5. The endothelial cells normally present a barrier to the artery wall, have nonthrombogenic properties, and are capable of metabolizing numerous vasoactive substances, such as prostacyclin (PGI_2) and nitric oxide (NO). They are capable of producing growth factors and forming connective tissue matrix. The endothelial cells can also interact with platelets, monocytes, T-lymphocytes, and smooth muscle cells. The principal products of platelets, macrophages, and smooth muscle cells that may affect the endothelium are shown in this figure. Endothelial mitogens that can be produced by macrophages include vascular endothelial growth factor (VEGF), fibroblast growth factor (FGF), and transforming growth factor α (TGFα). Transforming growth factor β (TGFβ), as well as interleukin-1 (IL-1) and tumor necrosis factor α (TNFα), is capable of inhibiting endothelial proliferation and can also induce secondary gene expression of other growth-regulatory molecules by the endothelium. TGFβ is a potent inducer of connective tissue matrix synthesis.

Oxidized LDL (oxLDL), produced by endothelium, macrophages, or smooth muscle cells, can profoundly injure neighboring endothelial and smooth muscle cells. Platelets can provide a host of vasoactive substances, coagulation factors, and mitogens. Thrombin and Factor Xa from plasma may also stimulate the endothelium to a procoagulant state. Endothelial cells can also synthesize a number of growth-regulatory molecules, as noted to the right of the endothelial cell, that can induce proliferation of neighboring cells and their formation of connective tissue. Such cellular interactions are discussed in this chapter. Because oxLDL may be a principal cause of atherogenesis, it is important to note that the endothelial cells represent the first potential site of oxidation of LDL as it is transported into the artery wall. (From Ross, R.: The pathogenesis of atherosclerosis: A perspective for the 1990s. Nature *362*:801, 1993. Copyright 1993 Macmillan Magazines Limited.)

Smooth Muscle

The cell that proliferates in the arterial intima to form the intermediate and advanced lesions of atherosclerosis, the smooth muscle cell, is originally derived from the media.[46a] In his early work, Wissler[47] described this cell as a "multifunctional medial mesenchymal cell." It is now widely accepted that accumulation of smooth muscle cells in the intima represents the sine qua non of the lesions of advanced atherosclerosis (Fig. 34–6).

Twenty-five years ago, the only functional capacity attributed to the smooth muscle cell was its ability to con-

PLATE 9

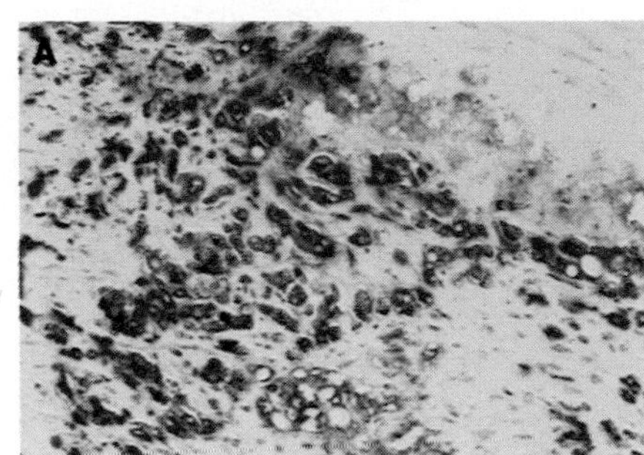

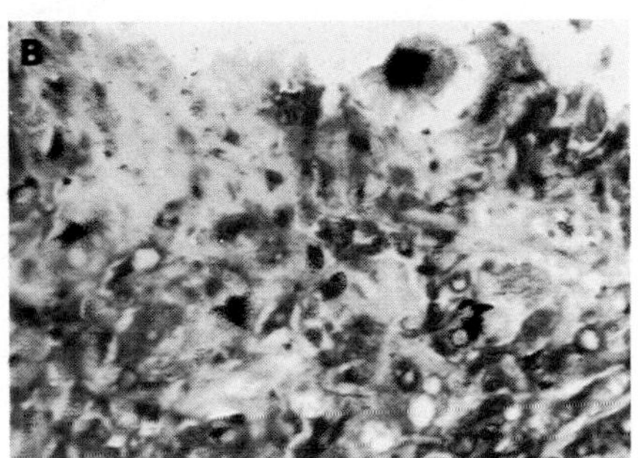

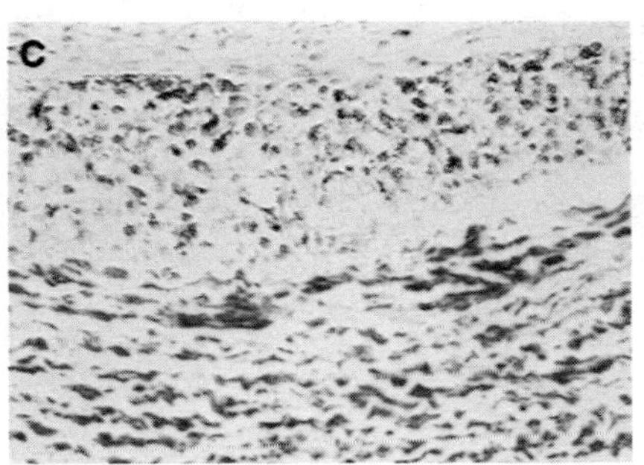

FIGURE 34–13. Double-immunostained preparations demonstrating the distribution of PDGF-B chain in methacarn-fixed, deparaffinized sections of advanced lesions of atherosclerosis from a high-level hypercholesterolemic nonhuman primate fed a hypercholesterolemic diet for 1 year. The sections were stained with a monoclonal antibody specific for PDGF-B-chain protein, and with cell-type-specific monoclonal antibodies for macrophages *(A, B)* or smooth muscle *(C)*, with IGSS and avidin-biotin immunoalkaline-phosphatase procedures. *A,* PDGF-B chain (black, granular reaction product) is localized to HAM56-positive macrophages (red reaction product). *B,* Positive cells at higher magnification. *C,* PDGF-B chain (black, granular reaction product) and HHF35–positive smooth muscle cells (red reaction product) are identified in nonoverlapping cell populations. All sections were counterstained with methyl green. *A* and *C* original magnifications, ×250; *B* original magnification, ×400. (From Ross, R., et al.: Localization of PDGF-B protein in macrophages in all phases of atherogenesis. Science *248:*1009, 1990. © Copyright 1990 by the American Association for the Advancement of Science.)

tract. In 1971, it became possible to maintain and propagate pure populations of smooth muscle cells in culture and to demonstrate that this cell, like the fibroblast, is one of the principal connective tissue–forming cells in the body.[48] It is capable of synthesizing and secreting several forms of collagen, both elastic fiber proteins and several different types of proteoglycans.[49] The principal role of the smooth muscle cell in the fully formed adult artery is presumably to maintain the tone of the arterial wall by its capacity to maintain the slow contractions peculiar to smooth muscle. The smooth muscle cell responds to numerous vasoactive agents, such as epinephrine and angiotensin, which induce contraction and vasoconstriction, and prostacyclin and NO, which can induce relaxation and vasodilation. Smooth muscle cells, like fibroblasts, contain specific high-affinity receptors for a number of ligands. These ligands include LDL[50] (see p. 1134) (which is the principal cholesterol-carrying plasma lipoprotein that participates in regulation of cholesterol metabolism), insulin (which is involved in glucose metabolism), and growth stimulators such as PDGF[51] and growth inhibitors such as transforming growth factor beta (TGF β) (which help to regulate cell multiplication). Arterial smooth muscle cells of the newborn rat, in contrast to adult rat smooth muscle, have been shown to be capable of synthesizing and secreting PDGF.[52] These observations suggest possible roles for smooth muscle in growth and development and possibly in atherosclerosis as well (to be discussed below).

Smooth muscle cells appear to be capable of presenting two different phenotypes in culture.[53,54] The first of these, the *contractile phenotype,* is generally thought to be associated with cell contractility because the cells contain extensive myofibrils throughout their cytoplasm consisting of actin and myosin filaments. These contractile filaments bind to one another and to the subplasmalemmal surface of the cell by dense bodies. Such cells do *not* appear to be capable of responding to mitogens such as PDGF. When a smooth muscle cell becomes appropriately stimulated, it loses its contractile phenotype and changes to a cell that has decreased content of myofilaments and that contains an extensively developed rough endoplasmic reticulum and Golgi complex. Such a cell has been described as being in a *synthetic phenotype.* Smooth muscle cells in the synthetic phenotype appear to be involved in the formation of numerous secretory proteins, including connective tissue matrix macromolecules.

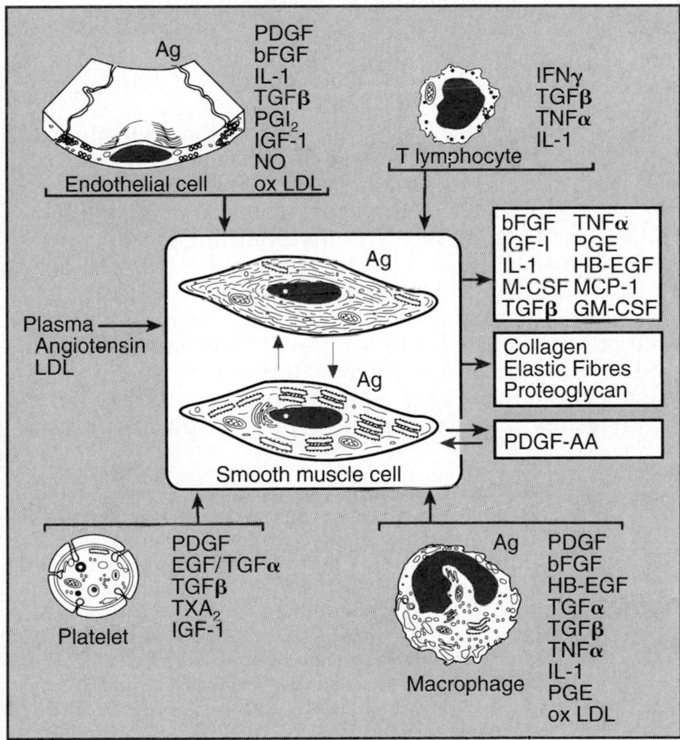

FIGURE 34–6. In the synthetic phenotype it is presumed that smooth muscle cells can form connective tissue molecules, as well as growth factors such as PDGF-AA and can stimulate themselves, as well as their neighbors. In their interactions with the overlying endothelium and neighboring T-lymphocytes, platelets, and macrophages, smooth muscle cells can respond to the different cytokines, growth-regulatory molecules, and vasodilator and vasoconstrictor substances that can be generated from these cells, as well as substances from the plasma, such as angiotensin. Thus, the genes that are expressed in the different phenotypic states by the smooth muscle (listed to the right), as well as those expressed by the neighboring cells (listed next to each cell) in the artery wall that result from these cellular interactions, determine whether a lesion progresses or regresses. (From Ross, R.: The pathogenesis of atherosclerosis: A perspective for the 1990s. Nature *362*:801, 1993. Copyright 1993 Macmillan Magazines Limited.)

Smooth muscle cells rich in contractile elements can respond to agents that can induce vasoconstriction, such as endothelin (ET), catecholamines, or angiotensin II (AII). Agents that can induce vasodilation such as prostaglandin E, prostacyclin (PGI_2), neuropeptides, leukotrienes, or NO, can also have profound effects upon these cells. When the cells are rich in rough endoplasmic reticulum and Golgi complex (synthetic state), they can express genes for a number of the growth-regulatory molecules and cytokines (noted in Fig. 34–6). If smooth muscle cells are sufficiently injured, they can release growth factors such as FGF. In so doing they could stimulate neighboring smooth muscle or adjacent endothelium. The smooth muscle cell is the principal contributor to the reparative, fibroproliferative process in the development of the lesions of atherosclerosis.

It has been suggested that the phenotypic differentiation of the smooth muscle cell may be important in terms of its capacity to respond to mitogens such as PDGF and thus to form the proliferative lesions of atherosclerosis. Smooth muscle cells in the contractile phenotype have been described as nonresponsive to mitogens, whereas those in the synthetic phenotype have been described as responsive.[53,54] For the lesions of atherosclerosis to form, the smooth muscle cells must, in most cases, migrate from the media into the intima, where they can respond mitogenically. Consequently, control of the phenotypic state of smooth muscle cells could be important in understanding and preventing atherogenesis (Fig. 34–6).

Smooth muscle cells are derived locally from individual organ parenchyma during embryogenesis in contrast with the endothelium, which appears to be derived from the embryonic vasculature that invades the organ.[55] As a consequence, smooth muscle cells in different arteries may respond differently to agonists presented to them, which may explain in part why different arterial beds respond differently to local stimuli associated with the process of atherogenesis.[56]

One characteristic feature of the smooth muscle cells found in the lesions of atherosclerosis is the accumulation of lipid that results in formation of vacuolated cells, or foam cells.

Although smooth muscle cells were originally conceived of as only the receiver of signals such as those derived from mitogens, it has now been demonstrated not only that they can respond to mitogens such as PDGF but that they can synthesize and secrete substances such as PDGF and other growth-regulatory molecules so that they may stimulate themselves and their neighbors. Thus, smooth muscle cells may respond in autocrine fashion to molecules they themselves form. For example, it is well known that a marked intimal smooth muscle proliferative lesion can be induced by passing an intraarterial balloon embolectomy catheter through an artery. The pressure exerted by the balloon is sufficient to strip off the lining endothelium, expand the artery, and damage many of the smooth muscle cells in the wall of the artery. The exposed subendothelial connective tissue attracts platelets to adhere and degranulate, and many of the injured subendothelial smooth muscle cells undergo a change and migrate from the media into the intima, where they proliferate and form a myointimal hyperplastic fibrotic lesion. If the smooth muscle cells are cultured from such a lesion and are compared with those cultured from a contralateral uninjured artery, the cells from the proliferative lesion secrete a form of PDGF (see section on Growth Factors) and thus may participate in further enlargement of the lesion by autocrine stimulation. Similarly, when smooth muscle cells derived from lesions of atherosclerosis are grown in culture, they secrete PDGF into the culture medium. Interestingly, data suggest that smooth muscle cells derived from human occlusive fibrous plaques of the superficial femoral arteries have a limited capacity to divide in culture. When placed in culture, these cells respond less well to mitogens and act like senescent cells that have already undergone numerous cell doublings.[57] Although the cells may secrete mitogens in culture, it remains to be determined whether they are capable of secreting mitogens and responding to them in vivo.

Some data relevant to these observations have come from studies in nonhuman primates where Northern blots of advanced lesions of atherosclerosis, using cDNA probes for different growth-regulatory peptides, have demonstrated increased messenger RNA for PDGF-B chain, and for both receptors of PDGF. Recent studies (see below), however, show that the principal source of the PDGF-B chain in these lesions is the macrophage. The smooth muscle cells appear to be the principal recipient of the growth regulatory peptides. Thus the regulation of smooth muscle cells via cellular interaction in the lesions of atherosclerosis needs to be further explored.

Macrophages

Macrophages in all tissues, whether they are resident macrophages or cells that have entered the tissue during an inflammatory response, are derived at some point in their life span from circulating monocytes.[58] When the monocyte enters a tissue, it appears to take on characteristics peculiar to the host tissue. In most inflammatory sites, the macrophage acts as a scavenger cell to remove foreign substances by phagocytosis and intracellular hydrolysis and as a second line of defense after the neutrophil against microbial organisms.[59] As a scavenger cell, the macrophage attempts to remove injurious materials such as oxLDL via scavenger receptors[60] and can oxidize LDL by such means as lipoxygenase enzymes (e.g., 15-lipoxygenase).[61] OxLDL can be taken up by the same macrophages or by neighboring macrophages. The importance of oxLDL in atherogenesis was first established in studies of the antioxidant drug probucol in hypercholesterolemic rabbits (discussed in greater detail below; see Lipids, Lipoproteins, and Modified LDL in Atherosclerosis). It has been recognized that not only do smooth muscle cells replicate in lesions of atherosclerosis, but macrophages may do so as well. Macrophage replication may represent as great, if not greater, source than smooth muscle cells in cell accumulation within the lesions. Thus, factors associated with their turnover, their replication, and programmed cell death (apoptosis) are all-important in determining whether macrophages accumulate in lesions (discussed in greater detail below; see The Response-to-Injury Hypothesis).

Macrophages are capable of secreting a large number of biologically important substances, including chemotactic agents such as leukotriene B4[62] and interleukin 1,[63] and oxygen metabolites such as superoxide anion,[64] which can be toxic to other cells. Macrophages have recently been shown to be capable of synthesizing and secreting at least six different growth factors.[65] These include (1) PDGF,[66] a growth factor for mesenchymal cells such as smooth muscle and fibroblasts; (2) interleukin 1, a cytokine that induces PDGF gene expression in fibroblasts[63,67]; (3) fibroblast growth factor (FGF),[68] a mitogen for endothelial cells and thus a potentially important angiogenic agent; (4) epidermal growth factor (EGF) and EGF-like molecules (e.g., transforming growth factor alpha [TGF α]), both of which bind to the same receptor and are capable of stimulating the growth of epithelial cells; (5) TGF β, a substance that participates in a synergistic way with some of the aforementioned growth factors in aiding the proliferation of many cells in different tissues and in many instances in inhibiting cell growth; and (6) M-CSF, a growth factor for monocyte macrophages[69] (Fig. 34–7).

As a result of its scavenging capacity and its ability to form and secrete growth factors, the macrophage is probably the key cell responsible for the promotion of connective tissue proliferation so commonly associated with chronic inflammatory responses. Macrophages, like smooth muscle, are a major source of foam cells in the lesions of atherosclerosis. In fact, they are the principal cells in the fatty streak, the initial lesion of atherosclerosis. They accumulate large amounts of lipid in the form of droplets that contain large amounts of cholesteryl ester. The role of the macrophage in atherogenesis is discussed below.

Platelets

(See also Chap. 58)

Although they may be uninvolved in the generation of many lesions, platelets are clearly implicated in the genesis of some of the lesions of atherosclerosis. (This is discussed in greater detail below.) However, platelets are also important because they are regularly involved in one of the principal sequelae of atherosclerosis, thrombosis. It is usually a mural or occlusive thrombus or both that lead to infarction.

Platelets are amazing cells in that, although they are capable of little to no protein synthesis, they contain, sequestered in their granules, numerous prepacked extraordinarily potent molecules[70,71] (Fig. 34–8). Among these are a number of factors that participate in the coagulation cascade

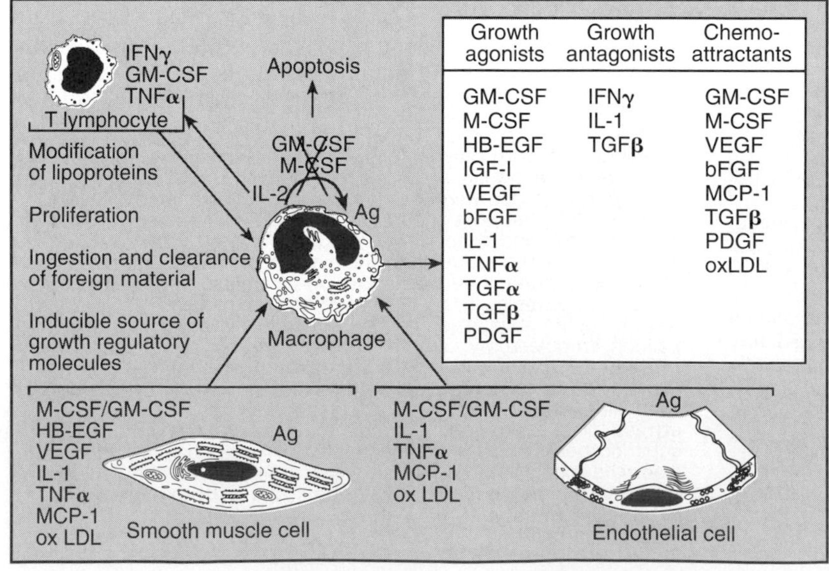

FIGURE 34–7. The reverse arrows between the T-lymphocyte and macrophage suggest that some form of immune response may occur during atherogenesis. Interactions between T cells and macrophages can result in proliferation of each of these cell types through IL-2 and CSFs, respectively. All of the cells with which the macrophage can interact, namely, the T-lymphocyte, smooth muscle, and endothelium, can present CSF to the macrophages to maintain cell viability and prevent apoptosis and cell death, and participate in further macrophage activation and replication. In addition, smooth muscle and endothelium can present antigens (Ag) at their surfaces and secrete chemoattractants for macrophages, including MCP-1 and oxLDL, as well as factors that can alter macrophage metabolism such as IL-1 or TNFα.

When macrophages are activated, they can produce an extraordinary number of biologically relevant molecules, some of which are listed in the box in relation to their capacity to induce or inhibit replication of endothelium, smooth muscle, or macrophages themselves, as well as their capacity to make chemoattractants for each of these cell types. (From Ross, R.: The pathogenesis of atherosclerosis: A perspective for the 1990s. Nature *362*:801, 1993. Copyright 1993 Macmillan Magazines Limited.)

and, in addition, at least four extremely potent growth factors or mitogens. These are the same growth factors that can be formed by the activated macrophage, namely, PDGF,[72] FGF, EGF[73] or TGF α, and TGF β.[74] It appears that each of these growth factors is present in a class of granules, the alpha granules, which were originally thought to represent a single class on the basis of cell fractionation studies. They may, however, represent several different granules that are similar in morphological and flotation characteristics. Thus, when they are separated by cell fractionation and density gradient centrifugation, they appear to sequester into a single population.

When the platelet is exposed to substrates that induce platelet adherence, aggregation, and degranulation, each of these growth factors is potentially released and thus is capable of eliciting a proliferative response by essentially all of the resident cells in a particular tissue. In other words, platelets contain growth factors potentially stimulatory for each of the cell types present in any tissue in which platelet aggregation and release may occur. Thus, at sites of injury in which collagen exposure, thrombin and fibrin formation, or adenosine diphosphate release occur, platelet aggregation and thrombosis can occur, leading to release of the numerous vasoactive, stimulatory, and proliferative agents carried by the platelets. Each of these agents may play an important role in stimulating an early vasoconstrictive and proliferative response.[75] This early reparative response to injury may be important in the initiation of the lesions of atherosclerosis as well.

Numerous factors may increase platelet activation in vitro, which could have profound effects on lesion formation or progression. High levels of circulating catecholamines, such as norepinephrine, may be associated with increased platelet activity and ability to aggregate.[76] Furthermore, chronic emotional stress, a history of cigarette smoking, or a strong family history of increased ability for platelets to aggregate have been shown to activate platelets in patients with coronary artery disease and thus decrease platelet survival.[77,78]

A lipid particle, lipoprotein (a) (Lp[a]), may also play an important role in atherogenesis and its progression. Lp(a) (see Chap. 35) consists of an LDL particle with a protein highly homologous to plasminogen covalently bound to the LDL moiety. It has been suggested that high levels of Lp(a) interfere with plasminogen by competing for plasminogen, and thus create a hyperthrombotic state. Potentially thrombogenic or high levels of Lp(a) have not yet been documented as a cause of an increase in the incidence of myocardial infarction. Nevertheless, children with high Lp(a) levels retrospectively show an increased incidence of myocardial infarction at a young age.[79–81] Thus, platelets may play an important role in atherogenesis but a potentially critical role in the progression of lesions and in the clinical sequelae of advanced lesions that may be susceptible to rupture and thrombosis (see below).

T-Lymphocytes

T-lymphocytes, both CD-8+ and CD-4+, have been observed in all phases of atherogenesis in humans and in nonhuman primates.[82–85] Their involvement in the lesions of atherosclerosis supports the notion that these lesions may develop, at least in part, as a result of an immune or possibly autoimmune response. Experimentally induced autoimmunity has been shown to induce rampant proliferative lesions of atherosclerosis in rabbits.[86] In humans, rejected cardiac transplants characteristically have extensive occlusive lesions of atherosclerosis in the coronary arteries. However, in contrast to the lesions observed in common atherosclerosis, the majority of which are eccentric lesions, those observed in the rejected hearts are concentric in appearance. The nature of the antigen(s) that may play a role in common atherosclerosis is unknown. However, interac-

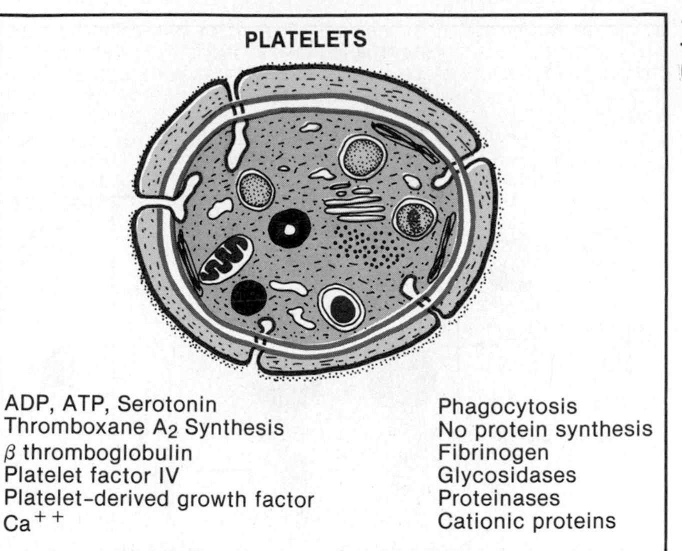

FIGURE 34–8. A platelet demonstrating its principal constituents which are listed beneath the figure. (Reproduced with permission from Ross, R.: Atherosclerosis: A problem of the biology of arterial wall cells and their interactions with blood components. Arteriosclerosis *1*:301, 1981. Copyright 1981 American Heart Association.)

tions between T-lymphocytes and activated macrophages, both of which are prominent in the lesions, suggest that antigen presentation and the release of cytokines and growth factors between the activated macrophages and T cells may be important in this process.[87,88]

Libby and Hansson demonstrated that oxLDL may serve as one of the potential major antigens that stimulate macrophage–T-cell interactions. Many T cells and lesions are shown to be activated based upon their expression of the histocompatibility antigen HLA-DR. Nevertheless, clonal expansion of these lymphocytes does not appear to take place.[89] If oxLDL proves to be the antigen principally responsible for T-cell activation, this would provide a new approach to therapy and to the immune response in the process of atherogenesis.

THE LESIONS OF ATHEROSCLEROSIS

Although atherosclerosis has been known for centuries, its clinical effects are manifested principally in medium-sized muscular arteries, including the coronary, carotid, basilar, and vertebral arteries, as well as several arteries affecting the lower extremities, particularly the iliac and superficial femoral arteries. Larger arteries, such as the aorta and the iliac arteries, can also be involved, and the principal clinical sequelae in these large arteries is usually aneurysmal dilatation and its related effects.[90]

The earliest lesions of atherosclerosis can be found in young children and infants in the form of a lesion called the *fatty streak,* whereas the advanced lesion, the fibrous plaque, generally appears during early adulthood and progresses with age.[91–96] Until recently, most tissues that had been prepared for examination were derived from autopsy specimens and were sufficiently poorly preserved so that when the cells became laden with lipid and appeared as foam cells, it was virtually impossible to determine the origin of the cell. Advances in tissue fixation and embedding have permitted new modes of preservation. Furthermore, monoclonal antibodies have been developed that are specific for smooth muscle cells, for macrophages, and for lymphocytes. With the use of these antibodies and with improved preservation techniques, it has been possible to identify specifically the origin of the cells in the different lesions of atherosclerosis.

Studies of advanced complicated lesions of atherosclero-

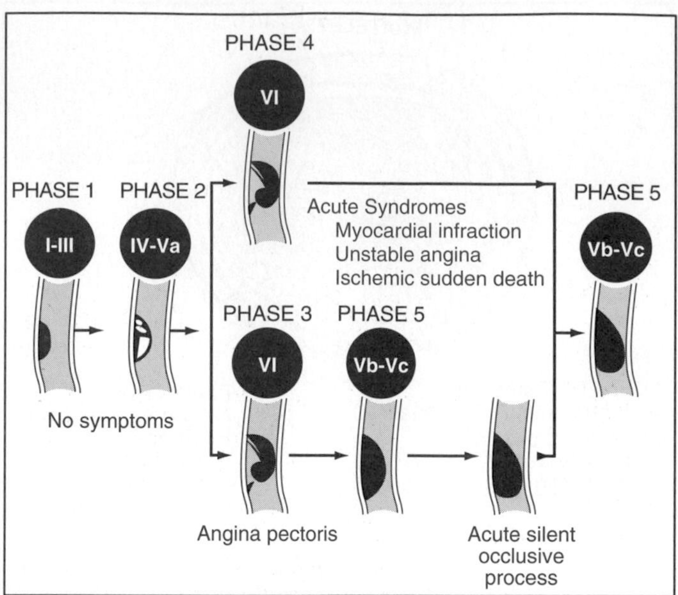

FIGURE 34–9. This figure shows the stages (phases) and lesion morphology of the progression of coronary atherosclerosis according to gross pathological and clinical findings. (Reproduced with permission from Fuster V.: Lewis A. Conner Memorial Lecture. Mechanisms leading to myocardial infarction: Insights from studies of vascular biology. Circulation *90*:2126, 1994. Copyright 1994 American Heart Association.)

sis have recently been aided by the use of the atherectomy catheter. Examination of atherectomy specimens has demonstrated virtually all of the cellular and structural features of atherosclerosis described in experimental animals and autopsy specimens. The use of freshly derived tissues and cells has demonstrated the nature and diversity of the connective tissue matrix and provided new data concerning proteoglycan constituents. Studies in progress use antibodies to PCNA, a nuclear marker of cells in cell cycle traverse, to determine cell replication in human lesions, which can be compared with lesions obtained from experimental studies.

A redefinition of lesion staging and phases of lesion progression has been completed by a committee of the American Heart Association. Fatty streaks have been included in Phase 1 lesions, which include types I to III (Fig. 34–9). The different types of fatty streaks (I and II) are based on the relative numbers of smooth muscle cells and macrophages and the amount of lipid contained within the lesions.[94] Lesions that progress to phase 2, which includes types IV and Va, can evolve into more stenotic, fibrotic lesions. Fibrotic lesions include types Vb and Vc, either of which can thrombose and lead to acute clinical sequelae. Type IV lesions can also rapidly progress to type VI, a complicated lesion, which can disrupt, thrombose, and lead to myocardial infarction or ischemic sudden death. Phase 3 lesions can also progress through phase 4 to phase 5 silently and gradually while developing collateral circulation (Fig. 34–9). This approach to categorizing lesions relates their progression with the clinical sequelae that may result.[95]

The Fatty Streak

(Lesion Types I to III)

Fatty streaks were observed by Stary[96] in his studies of a series of children and young adults. He demonstrated that by the age of 10 years, the fatty streaks consisted principally of lipid-laden macrophages, together with varying (but usually small) numbers of lipid-filled smooth muscle cells that accumulated beneath them as the lesions increased in size. Grossly, the fatty streak appears as an area of yellow discoloration due to the large amount of lipid deposited in the foam cells. The bulk of this lipid is in the form of cholesterol and cholesteryl ester, which probably enters the fatty streak by transport of lipoproteins from the plasma via the endothelial cells, after which it is taken up by macrophages and smooth muscle cells. The plasma lipids present in the intima are ingested by macrophages and are hydrolyzed and reesterified once they have been taken up by these cells.

Stary also studied fatty streaks in the coronary arteries of a series of children and young adults and observed that they were localized at anatomical sites that were the same as the sites in other older individuals that were occupied by advanced fibromuscular lesions or fibrous plaques. His data and that of others suggested that over a time, fatty

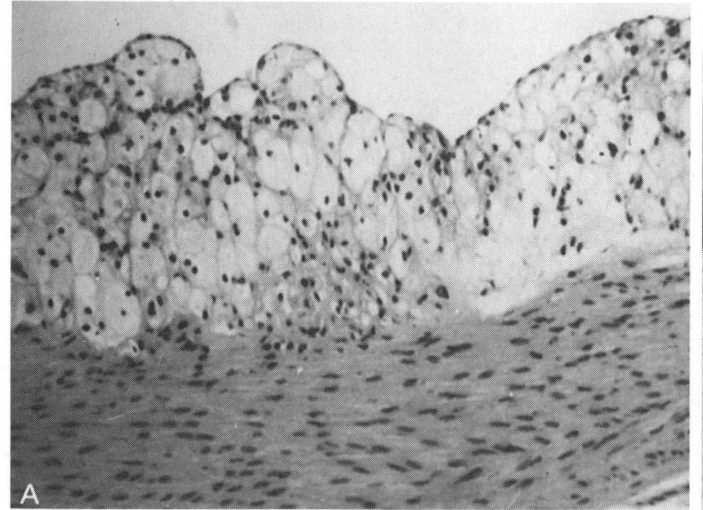

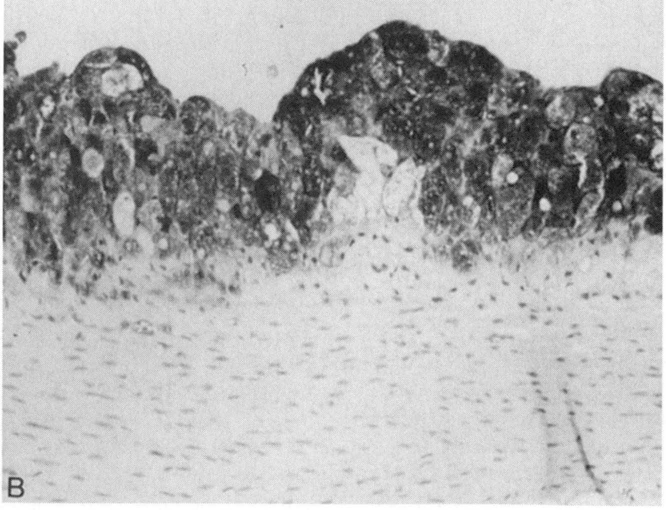

FIGURE 34–10. Light micrographs demonstrating portions of a fatty streak obtained from an aorta of a hypercholesterolemic monkey. This particular fatty streak contains several layers of macrophages. *A* is a routinely fixed and embedded paraffin section that has been stained with hematoxylin and eosin. The macrophage-rich areas are seen as clear because they are lipid-containing and the lipid has been extracted during the process of dehydration and embedding. *B* demonstrates an adjacent section that has been stained with immunoperoxidase coupled to an antibody specific for a cytoplasmic antigen present within the macrophage. The macrophages stain densely black in this micrograph, demonstrating that the large majority of the lipid-rich cells in the fatty streak are macrophages. Such antibodies make it possible to recognize cell type, even after the cells have become distorted by inclusions.

streaks at particular sites are converted by a series of changes into the more advanced fibroproliferative lesions of atherosclerosis, whereas fatty streaks at other anatomical sites either remain the same or regress and disappear. McGill[97] has gone on to review data to demonstrate that with time, fatty streaks occupy increasing surface areas of the coronary arteries and that these sites also precede the formation of advanced lesions. Thus, although it is difficult to derive firm conclusions from these types of data, such observations suggest that the fatty streak in many instances, if not the large majority, is the precursor lesion that becomes converted into the advanced occlusive form of atherosclerosis.

Once foam cells have formed in fatty streaks and in advanced lesions, it may become extremely difficult to define the cell of origin. The cells become filled with lipid droplets that appear as empty vacuoles in paraffin-embedded tissues which are often surrounded by a very thin rim of cytoplasm (Fig. 34–10). Electron microscopic examination may permit identification of some of these cells; however, large numbers remain difficult if not impossible to identify using standard techniques of tissue staining.

Several monoclonal antibodies have been developed, at least two of which appear to be specific for cell type. Tsudaka et al.[98] have developed monoclonal antibodies against smooth muscle–alpha actin and against a cytoplasmic antigen present in macrophages. Fortunately, these antigens resist some modes of fixation and embedding in paraffin. With these monoclonal antibodies, it has been possible to positively identify macrophages, T-lymphocytes, and smooth muscle cells in lesions of atherosclerosis. Thus it can be said definitively that the fatty streak consists principally of lipid-laden macrophages and T-lymphocytes, together with small and variable numbers of smooth muscle cells (Fig. 34–10).

Diffuse Intimal Thickening

(Lesion Type IV)

One form of lesion, described as a diffuse intimal thickening, consists of increased numbers of intimal smooth muscle cells surrounded by variable amounts of connective tissue. It is not entirely clear whether these sites of thickened intima represent developmental thickenings or whether such multilayered cushions of intimal smooth muscle cells are sites that formed because of increased stress on the artery wall but do not progress to advanced lesions of atherosclerosis. This is a somewhat poorly understood and controversial subject. These lesions may also have diffusely extracellular lipid intermixed with smooth muscle, macrophages, T cells, and connective tissue.

The Fibrous Plaque

(Lesion Types V and VI)

The advanced lesion of atherosclerosis is generally called a fibrous plaque. When the fibrous plaque becomes involved with thrombosis, hemorrhage, and/or calcification, it is often called a *complicated lesion.*

Fibrous plaques are grossly white in appearance and are usually elevated. In many cases they protrude into the lumen of the artery and, if sufficiently large, compromise the flow of blood. These lesions consist of large numbers of intimal smooth muscle cells, together with numerous macrophages and T-lymphocytes. When the macrophages and smooth muscle contain lipid, the lipid is primarily in the form of cholesterol and cholesteryl ester. The proliferated smooth muscle cells are surrounded by collagen and elastic fibers, by large amounts of proteoglycan, and, in individuals who are hypercholesterolemic, by varying amounts of lipid deposited in the cells and in the connective tissue. Fibrous plaques characteristically are covered by a fibrous cap.

In a study of a large series of male patients who had advanced occlusive lesions of the superficial femoral artery, we observed that the fibrous cap of each lesion consisted largely of a particular form of smooth muscle cell that is thin and pancake shaped and is surrounded by numerous lamellae of basement membrane, proteoglycan, and large numbers of collagen fibrils. The connective tissue in the fibrous cap is exceedingly dense. Beneath the fibrous cap lies a mixture of smooth muscle cells, macrophages, and numerous lymphocytes, principally CD-8+ and some CD-4+ T cells. Using the monoclonal antibodies already described, as well as antibodies to lymphocytes, it has been possible to identify definitively each of these cell types in the advanced lesions of atherosclerosis. In this highly cellular portion of the fibrous plaque, there are also large amounts of connective tissue. Beneath the cell-rich region, a zone of necrotic tissue and debris may contain cholesterol crystals and regions of calcification as well as numerous enlarged foam cells (Fig. 34–11).

Some plaques are densely fibrous and contain relatively little lipid, whereas others are rich in lipid deposits. Such differences can be found in different arteries within a given individual but are often associated with different risk factors. For example, it is common that the fibrous plaques observed in the superficial femoral arteries of those who are heavy cigarette smokers are extremely fibrous and contain relatively little lipid. On the other hand, individuals who are hypercholesterolemic and have advanced lesions in the coronary arteries often have large amounts of lipid within the lesions.[57]

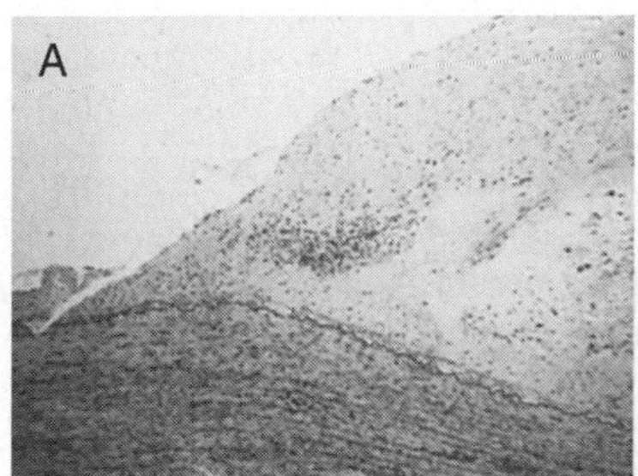

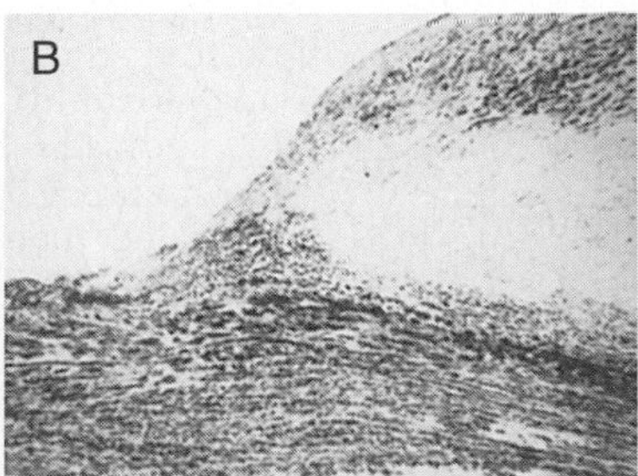

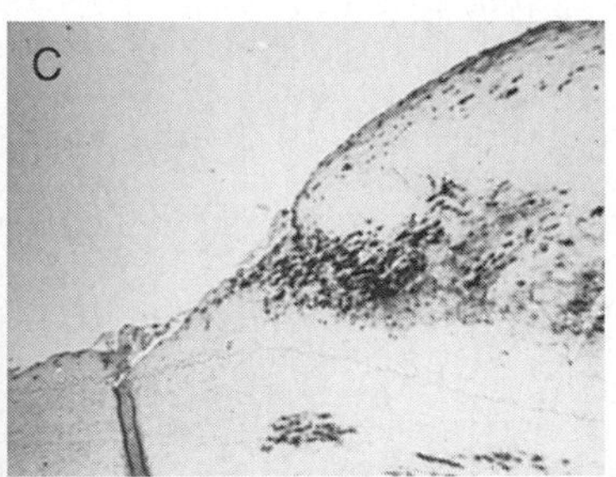

FIGURE 34–11. Three light micrographs demonstrating adjacent sections of a human fibrous plaque from a carotid endarterectomy specimen. *A* was stained with hematoxylin (H) and eosin (E). In the elevated portion of the lesion, the area adjacent to the lumen consists of a fibrous cap of parallel layers of smooth muscle cells covering a mixture of cells. With H & E it is impossible to determine cell type. *B* is an adjacent section that has been stained using immunoperoxidase coupled to an anti–smooth muscle actin antibody. The smooth muscle cells in the fibrous cap, in the media underlying the lesion, and in patches and individual cells located throughout the lesion are stained black. *C* is an adjacent section stained with immunoperoxidase coupled to an anti-macrophage antibody. Individual macrophages can be seen dispersed among the smooth muscle cells in the fibrous cap but are found principally in the area deep to the fibrous cap between the fibrous cap and the media, where most of the lipid-containing cells in this particular lesion can be found.

There appears to be a general pattern in the distribution of advanced lesions of atherosclerosis in humans. Generally, the abdominal aorta is more extensively involved than the thoracic aorta.[20] Lesions in the aorta are usually most prominent near the ostia of major branches that leave the aorta. Some arteries such as the renal arteries appear to be spared from atherosclerosis, except at their ostia.[99] The coronary arteries generally demonstrate the most intense involvement, with lesions of atherosclerosis located within the first 6 cm of the artery.[100] In hypertensive patients, lesions of the carotid, cerebral, and basilar arteries are more common. It has been suggested that the severity of lesion formation in a given artery may be related in part to the particular nature of the characteristics of the blood flow in the artery, and that rheological forces play a major role in determining the localization, extent, and severity of lesions in susceptible individuals.[101,102]

The principal clinical results of advanced lesions of atherosclerosis are derived either from the fact that they partially or totally occlude the lumen of the affected artery or because cracks and fissures develop in the lesions, leading to thrombosis and embolism or to aneurysmal dilatation (which usually occurs in large arteries such as the aorta). Many advanced lesions appear to be quite unstable, subject to rupture and thrombosis, and represent the principal cause of myocardial infarction and sudden ischemic death (discussed in detail below; see Thrombosis).

HYPOTHESES OF ATHEROGENESIS

Current theories of the pathogenesis of the lesions of atherosclerosis relate back to early proposals made by Virchow,[103] von Rokitansky,[104] and Duguid.[105] Virchow believed that a form of low-grade injury to the artery wall resulted in a type of inflammatory insudation, which in turn caused increased passage and accumulation of plasma constituents in the intima of the artery.[103] Rokitansky's belief, subsequently elaborated upon by Duguid, was that an encrustation of small mural thrombi existed at sites of arterial injury, that these thrombi went on to organize by the growth of smooth muscle cells into them, and that they would become incorporated into the lesions and thus serve as sites where the lesions would progress.[104,105]

In 1973, these two notions about atherogenesis were combined with new knowledge of the cellular and molecular biology of the artery wall in a hypothesis termed the *response-to-injury hypothesis of atherosclerosis*.[2] This hypothesis has been modified as new data have come forth. It now takes into account many aspects of the behavior of arterial and blood cells described above, as well as the numerous risk factors that have been associated with atherogenesis, including hyperlipidemia, hormone dysfunction, altered rheological forces as may occur in hypertension, and alteration of the endothelial barrier by factors associated with cigarette smoking, diabetes, and so on.[3,4,28,29,106]

A second hypothesis that was also formulated in 1973, the *monoclonal hypothesis*, suggests that the lesions of atherosclerosis may represent some form of neoplasia.[107] For further discussion of this hypothesis, the reader is referred to the review in reference number 3.

The Response-to-Injury Hypothesis

The response-to-injury hypothesis of atherosclerosis states that some form of "injury" may occur to the lining endothelial cells at particular anatomical sites in the artery wall. Injury to the endothelium is a key event in this hypothesis, and defining and understanding the subtleties of the nature of the various possible forms of injury are paramount in both testing the hypothesis and developing means of prevention and intervention. Sources of injury could include not only modified forms of lipoproteins but also viruses, such as herpesvirus,[108] and possibly other organisms, such as chlamydia, which have been observed in lesions.[109] However, the presence of organisms does not establish a causal relation. Thus, their role in the etiology and pathogenesis of the lesions remains to be determined.

Endothelial injury may be manifested as a number of forms of endothelial dysfunction.[108a] For example, interference with the permeability barrier role of the endothelium, alterations in the nonthrombogenic properties of the endothelial surface, promotion of the procoagulant properties of the endothelium, or increased release of vasoconstrictor or vasodilator molecules would all represent forms of dysfunction and injury that could result in some of the changes to be discussed below. Furthermore, maintenance of the continuity of the endothelial surface and maintenance of the normal low rates of turnover of the endothelial cells at most sites in the arterial tree are important in maintaining homeostasis. When turnover of the endothelium increases, it is possible that such turnover may be related to a series of changes in the endothelium, including the synthesis and secretion of vasoactive substances, of lipolytic enzymes, and of growth factors by the endothelial cells. Thus, endothelial injury could potentially lead to a host of changes in the functional activities of the lining endothelial cells, which could then lead to a critical sequence of cellular interactions, culminating in formation of lesions of atherosclerosis (Fig. 34–12).

In the case of chronic hyperlipidemia, the response-to-injury hypothesis proposes that an increase in plasma lipoproteins, principally oxidized LDL's and cholesterol, would result in toxic injury to the endothelium. It would also change the surface characteristics of both the endothelial cells and the circulating leukocytes, particularly circulating monocytes and possibly platelets as well. Hypercholesterolemia also somehow leads to increased adhesion of monocytes to endothelium at sites throughout the arterial tree.[110–113] When these monocytes adhere, they probe and are chemotactically attracted to migrate between endothelial cells and localize subendothelially, where they can become active as scavenger cells and are converted to macrophages. When they become macrophages, these cells take up lipid, principally modified, or oxidized LDL via receptors called scavenger receptors.[114–117] The lipid may enter the subendothelium in large quantities in the hypercholesterolemic state, resulting in the formation of foam cells and in the development of fatty streaks. The oxidized LDL may be toxic to the endothelium and to other cells in the microenvironment. The accumulation of macrophages in the intimal space would then establish conditions that could lead to further alterations in the endothelium.

Macrophages are well known to be capable of synthesizing and secreting numerous injurious agents that normally could play a role in killing ingested microorganisms or in nullifying toxic substances.[59] In this instance, the macrophages could potentially secrete oxidative metabolites such as oxidized LDL and superoxide anion, which could further injure the overlying endothelial cells. It has been demonstrated that lipid-laden macrophages are capable of oxidizing LDL and of forming peroxide and superoxide anion in vitro,[64] suggesting that this may occur in vivo as well.

An additional and potentially important reaction of the macrophage is related to its capacity to form growth regulatory molecules. Activated macrophages can, as already noted, synthesize and secrete at least four potent growth factors: PDGF, FGF, an EGF-like factor, and TGF β. PDGF is a potent mitogen for smooth muscle cells, as is FGF under some circumstances. The combination of these growth factors, together with TGF β, has been shown in vivo to be extremely potent in stimulating the migration and proliferation of fibroblasts and potentially of smooth muscle cells, and in stimulating formation of new connective tissue by these cells.[118]

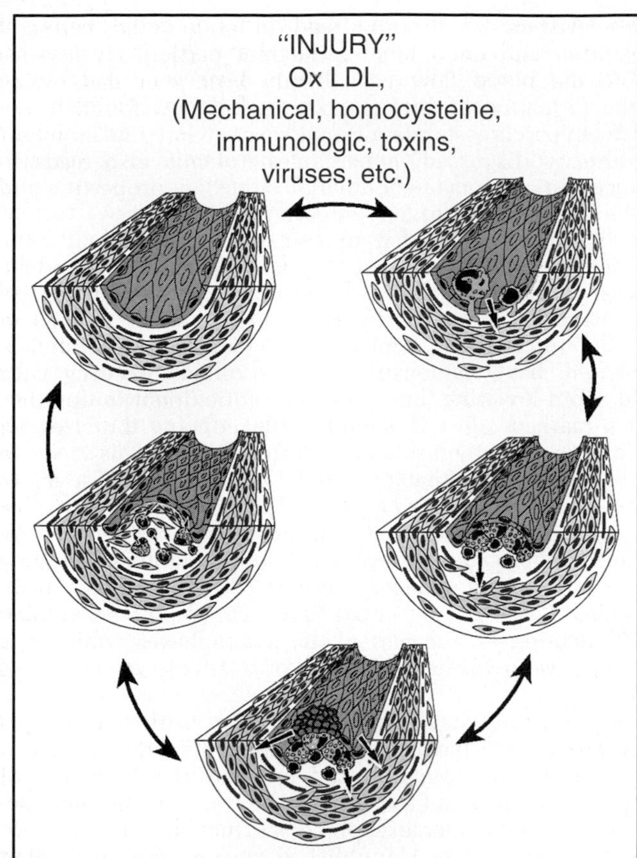

FIGURE 34–12. The response-to-injury hypothesis of atherosclerosis. Several different sources of injury to the endothelium can lead to endothelial cell dysfunction. One of the parameters associated with endothelial cell dysfunction that results from exposure to agents, such as oxLDL, is increased adherence of monocytes/macrophages and T-lymphocytes. These cells then migrate between the endothelium and localize subendothelially. The macrophages become large foam cells due to lipid accumulation and, with the T cells and smooth muscle, form a fatty streak. The fatty streak can then progress to an intermediate, fibrofatty lesion and ultimately to a fibrous plaque.

As the lesions accumulate increasing numbers of cells and the macrophages scavenge the lipid, some of the lipid-laden macrophages may emigrate back into the bloodstream by pushing apart the endothelial cells. Upon doing so, those at sites such as branches and bifurcations where blood flow is irregular with eddy currents and back currents may become thrombogenic sites that lead to formation of platelet mural thrombi. Such thrombi can release many potent growth-regulatory molecules from the platelets that can join with those released by the activated macrophages and possibly by lesion smooth muscle cells into the artery wall. Platelet thrombi can also form at sites where endothelial dysjunction may have occurred. Ultimately, the formation and release of numerous growth-regulatory molecules and cytokines from a network established between cells in the lesion, consisting of activated macrophages, smooth muscle, T cells, and endothelium, lead to progression of the lesions of atherosclerosis to a fibrous plaque or advanced, complicated lesion.

Each of the stages of lesion formation is potentially reversible. Thus, lesion regression can occur if the injurious agents are removed, or when protective factors intervene to reverse the inflammatory and fibroproliferative processes. (From Ross, R.: The pathogenesis of atherosclerosis: A perspective for the 1990s. Nature *362*:801, 1993. Copyright 1993 Macmillan Magazines Limited.)

TGF β is not only a potent stimulator of connective tissue synthesis but is also the most potent inhibitor of smooth muscle proliferation thus far discovered.[119] It is ubiquitous in the sense that most cells have the capacity to form it, and rich sources of this molecule are the platelet and the activated macrophage. Much of the TGF β that is secreted by these cells is in a latent form that requires decreased pH or proteolytic cleavage for activity. Nevertheless, the balance between inhibitors such as TGF β and stimulators of smooth muscle proliferation such as PDGF is probably critical in determining whether a net proliferative response of smooth muscle cells will occur, resulting in the formation of an atherosclerotic lesion. Thus, if the macrophage-derived foam cells are appropriately activated in the subendothelial space, they could potentially be involved in the secretion of growth factors that could chemotactically attract smooth muscle cells to migrate from the media into the intima, to proliferate within the intima, and to set up a series of conditions that could lead to the formation of an intimal, fibromuscular, proliferative lesion.

It has been demonstrated that PDGF-B-chain–containing protein is present in approximately 20 percent of the macrophages in both human and nonhuman atherosclerotic lesions in all phases of development. PDGF is present in the non–foam-cell macrophages that are distributed throughout the lesion, as well as in macrophages present among the smooth muscle cells in the fibrous cap portion of the fibrous plaque[120] (Fig. 34–13). The presence of PDGF-B protein in the macrophages in these lesions provides the first convincing basis for assigning the macrophage a key role in the induction and maintenance of the smooth muscle proliferative response during atherogenesis because PDGF-BB is one of the most potent growth factors, capable of stimulating smooth muscle migration, chemotaxis, and proliferation. Thus macrophage-derived PDGF-BB (Fig. 34–7) could be involved not only in the appearance of smooth muscle cells that migrate into macrophage-rich fatty streaks, but in the progression of these fatty streaks to intermediate or fibro-fatty lesions, which may ultimately become advanced occlusive lesions, or fibrous plaques. If the cycle of "endothelial injury" and macrophage accumulation and stimulation is repeated, at least two cells capable of releasing growth factors into the intima—the activated endothelial cell and the activated macrophage—may continue to contribute to progression of the lesions.

The response-to-injury hypothesis also provides an opportunity for the interaction of a third cell, the platelet. The hypothesis suggests that if the flow properties of the blood at particular anatomical sites are such that these properties participate in the endothelial injury, endothelial cell–cell attachment may be affected and cell disjunction may occur, leading to retraction of endothelial cells and exposure of the underlying foam cells or connective tissue or both. In either case, this would permit opportunities for platelets to interact, adhere, aggregate, and form mural thrombi.[121–125] Should this occur, the platelet could provide a third potent source of growth factors, including the same four factors that can be released by the activated macrophage. Thus, there are numerous opportunities for mitogens to be deposited in the artery wall, which, under proper circumstances, could play critical roles in the genesis of proliferative smooth muscle lesions of atherosclerosis (Fig. 34–13).

It is important to point out that injury to the endothelium need not result in denudation of the endothelial cells. Endothelial injury may simply be manifested by relatively rapid replacement of individual endothelial cells that are lost and is principally reflected in endothelial dysfunction such as alterations in endothelial permeability, increased adhesion of leukocytes to the endothelium, and release of vasoactive substances and growth factors.

Finally, it has been shown that human arterial smooth muscle cells removed from lesions of atherosclerosis have the capacity to express one of the PDGF genes and secrete a form of PDGF when they are grown in cell culture.[126] If this were to occur in vivo, then as the smooth muscle cells

FIGURE 34–13. See color plate 9.

proliferate in developing lesions, they could participate in inducing further progression of the lesions by release of PDGF. Thus a vicious circle might be established that would have to be stopped if one hoped to stop lesion progression and induce lesion regression.

LIPIDS, LIPOPROTEINS, AND MODIFIED LDL IN ATHEROSCLEROSIS

Because hypercholesterolemia is the major risk factor associated with the increased incidence of atherosclerosis in the United States and Western Europe, it is important to understand the role that lipids play in this process. Although many lesions of atherosclerosis are fibrous and contain relatively little lipid, the effects of lipid on endothelium, monocytes, and smooth muscle and the accumulation of lipid in the lesions of hypercholesterolemic individuals are critical components of the process of atherogenesis. Consequently, it is important to understand specifically how elevated levels of cholesterol-bearing lipoproteins are related to the process of atherogenesis. These subjects are discussed in detail on pp. 1127 to 1143.

The Lipid Research Clinic Trials have provided data suggesting that it would be beneficial to lower plasma LDL levels.[14,15] Those studies showed that the decrease in plasma cholesterol can be correlated with a reduction in the incidence of myocardial infarction and presumably atherosclerosis. The genetic basis for the increase in plasma LDL is not known for most individuals in the population who are hypercholesterolemic, although some may be heterozygous for the familial hypercholesterolemia (FH) trait. Nevertheless, our understanding of the LDL receptor control of HMG CoA reductase, and thus cholesterol synthesis, has been critical in permitting us to understand how cholesterol metabolism is regulated. As important as these studies are, however, they do not provide data that permit us to understand how the lesions of atherosclerosis form. In other words, although the LDL receptor pathway provides an understanding of the control of cholesterol metabolism, it yields no information concerning the basis of the cellular changes and interactions that occur when elevated plasma cholesterol leads to atherosclerosis.

To answer this question, it has been necessary to devise experiments using appropriate animal models and appropriate cell culture systems. These tests provide opportunities to determine how smooth muscle cells proliferate and under what circumstances, what cellular interactions occur during the pathogenesis of this disease process, and what factors are elaborated by the cells that control not only smooth muscle multiplication but also connective tissue formation and lipid accumulation.

The response-to-injury hypothesis of atherosclerosis already discussed can be taken one step further in terms of asking how chronic hypercholesterolemia may "injure" endothelium. Jackson and Gotto[127] have suggested that one form of endothelial injury which may occur upon exposure to chronically elevated levels of LDL may result from the effects of an increase in the number of cholesterol molecules in the plasma membranes of cells, including the endothelial cells. When the cholesterol/phospholipid ratio of endothelial plasma membranes is elevated, this could theoretically lead to an increase in the viscosity of the membranes. Changes such as these would decrease the malleability of the endothelial cell surface and, should this occur, could have critical effects at particular anatomical sites such as branches of bifurcations in the arterial tree, where the endothelial cells are exposed to changes in the flow of blood. Such rheological changes could cause an otherwise normally malleable endothelial surface, if it becomes more viscous and thus more rigid, to be incapable of dealing with the stresses caused by these changes in the flow characteristics. This could lead to endothelial cell–cell separation and endothelial retraction, particularly at sites where the blood flow has already been modified owing to the formation of fatty streaks, as has been found to occur in hypercholesterolemic monkeys, swine, and humans. As already discussed, hypercholesterolemia also leads to changes in monocyte-endothelial adhesion properties and to the development of fatty streaks themselves.

It is also possible that hypercholesterolemia may alter the endothelial cells so that they are stimulated to produce increased amounts of growth factor. Recent studies with the Watanabe heritable hyperlipemic (WHHL) rabbit, an animal model of homozygous familial hypercholesterolemia, have demonstrated that probucol, a drug with mild lipid-lowering but powerful antioxidant properties, had a marked effect in significantly reducing the size and incidence of atherosclerotic lesions.[128,129] This led to studies suggesting that oxidized LDL might play a major role as an injurious agent responsible for many of the early events associated with atherogenesis, particularly because macrophages have scavenger receptors that can bind and permit phagocytosis of these oxidized lipid particles. The ingestion of oxidized LDL could lead to foam cell formation on the part of the macrophages, which can also engage in further oxidation of available molecules of LDL.

Recent studies in nonhuman primates with the antioxidant probucol[130] have further demonstrated that probucol decreases lesion formation and prevents the formation of fatty streaks. This antioxidant appears to have an early effect on the inflammatory processes that are required for lesion development. Unpublished data also suggest that there is a decreased turnover of both macrophages and smooth muscle cells in the lesions of the probucol-treated animals. Clinical trials are under way to determine the effectiveness of antioxidant therapy using oral antioxidants, including vitamins C, E, and beta-carotene. Results of these studies should provide further insight into the role of oxidation and other modifications of LDL, such as glycation, in the process of atherogenesis. Oxidized LDL is injurious to both endothelium and smooth muscle in vitro and has been found in both human and experimental lesions of atherosclerosis.[131] Thus the presence of this modified lipoprotein in the lesions suggests that it is the principal culprit in atherogenesis in hypercholesterolemic individuals and that interference with its formation could be an important step in lesion prevention.

GROWTH FACTORS AND CYTOKINES

As discussed earlier, growth factors and cytokines can be elaborated by all four cells potentially involved in the lesions of atherosclerosis: endothelium, monocyte/macrophages, platelets, and smooth muscle (Figs. 34–5 to 34–7). Although the first three of these cells can produce more than one growth factor, PDGF could play a critical role in the genesis of atherosclerosis because of its chemotactic and mitogenic effects on smooth muscle cells.

PDGF is a two-chain molecule of approximately 30,000 molecular weight that is highly cationic and highly disulfide bonded. It is an extraordinarily potent mitogen that binds with very high affinity to responsive cells[132] and is chemotactic for the same cells for which it is mitogenic.[133,134] When it binds to its high-affinity cell-surface receptor, it induces a series of biological events, some of which are probably related to induction of DNA synthesis and cell division. These cellular responses include phosphorylation of the PDGF receptor through the activation of a tyrosine kinase on the receptor, and the activation of C-kinase in the subplasmalemmal cytoplasm resulting from phospholipase activation at the cell surface. C-kinase activation could ultimately lead to calcium transfer from intracellular compartments, which in itself may possibly be important in induction of the mitogenic signal.[65]

PDGF also induces increased binding of LDL to cells by increasing the numbers of LDL receptors,[50,135] increased cholesterol synthesis, increased endocytosis, increased flux of ions into the cell, reorganization of actin cables within the cells, and change in cell shape. It also has recently been found to be a potent vasoactive agent, even more potent than angiotensin II.[65] Thus, if PDGF is released from platelets when they adhere to the artery wall at sites of injury, from activated macrophages where it is now known to present in these cells[120] after they enter the artery wall (particularly during fatty streak formation), from activated endothelial cells if they are appropriately stimulated, and perhaps in some special instances from appropriately activated smooth muscle cells, then such responses would enhance lesion formation.

PDGF has an extremely short half-life when it is injected into the circulation.[136] This short half-life suggests that PDGF that is not bound locally to tissue would be cleared rapidly and thus would be unavailable at sites distant from its release. Furthermore, PDGF binds to a number of proteins in the plasma, including alpha$_2$-macroglobulin. These binding proteins could serve to increase further the capacity of PDGF to act as a tissue mitogen at local sites where PDGF has been released and is bound to the tissue.[137]

There is a striking homology between the amino acid sequence of purified PDGF and that of a transforming protein derived from an oncogene of the simian sarcoma virus. This homology suggests that PDGF may be important in proliferation of cells transformed by the simian sarcoma virus.[138,139] Furthermore, numerous lines of transformed cells secrete a form of PDGF and have downregulated receptors for PDGF, suggesting that a form of PDGF may play a role in the proliferation of cells that are neoplastically transformed in other ways.[140] Both chains of PDGF and their receptors have been cloned. cDNA probes are available for each chain of PDGF and for both receptors. Investigations of these receptors have demonstrated a high degree of specificity of binding of the three different isomeric forms of PDGF (PDGF-AA, PDGF-AB, PDGF-BB) for the three different forms of the receptor (PDGF receptor $\alpha\alpha$, $\alpha\beta$, $\beta\beta$). For example, the A chain of PDGF can bind only to the alpha-receptor subunit; thus PDGF-AA can bind only to PDGF receptor $\alpha\alpha$. In contrast, PDGF-BB can bind to any one of the three forms of the PDGF receptor.[141] It therefore becomes important to understand the relative numbers of receptors on the different smooth muscle cells in different regions of the artery wall if one is to determine how effective the specific form of PDGF will be on these cells in a given site in the arterial tree. Our increased understanding of these degrees of specificity and responsivity will increase opportunities to make effective agents that can either induce smooth muscle proliferation or, potentially, prevent such a proliferative response.

CELLULAR EVENTS THAT OCCUR DURING ATHEROGENESIS

Several animals form lesions of atherosclerosis similar to humans when they develop hypercholesterolemia from eating a fatty diet. This has made it possible to study the effects of hypercholesterolemia in terms of understanding the cellular interactions which occur that lead to the lesions of atherosclerosis. Such studies have been performed by Faggiotto et al.[142,143] and by Masuda and Ross[144,145] on nonhuman primates, by Gerrity[146–148] and his colleagues on swine, and by Rosenfeld et al.[149] on fat-fed rabbits and the WHHL rabbit. The latter studies have provided highly detailed observations concerning the sequence of cellular events that occur in endogenous hypercholesterolemia (the WHHL rabbit, a model of familial homozygous hypercholesterolemia) as compared with those that take place during diet-induced hypercholesterolemia.

Recently, genetically modified mice, in particular, the homozygous apoprotein E- (ApoE-) deficient transgenic mouse, have provided small murine models of atherosclerosis. The ApoE-deficient mouse, for example, develops lesions at anatomical sites similar to those found in humans. A sequence of cellular interactions and events similar to that in nonhuman primates and humans has been observed.[150,151] This model and other genetically modified mice provide opportunities to study which appropriate genetic combinations can be made by adding or removing specific molecules to determine their roles in the process of atherogenesis. An important new frontier of research has been opened in this area.

EARLY CHANGES. The data of Faggiotto et al.,[142,143] Masuda and Ross,[144,145] and Nakashima et al.[150] show that the first and most striking event occurs after 7 to 14 days of diet-induced hypercholesterolemia. This consists of the attachment of large numbers of leukocytes, principally monocytes, to the surface of the arterial endothelium (Fig. 34–14). The monocytes attach to the endothelial cells in clus-

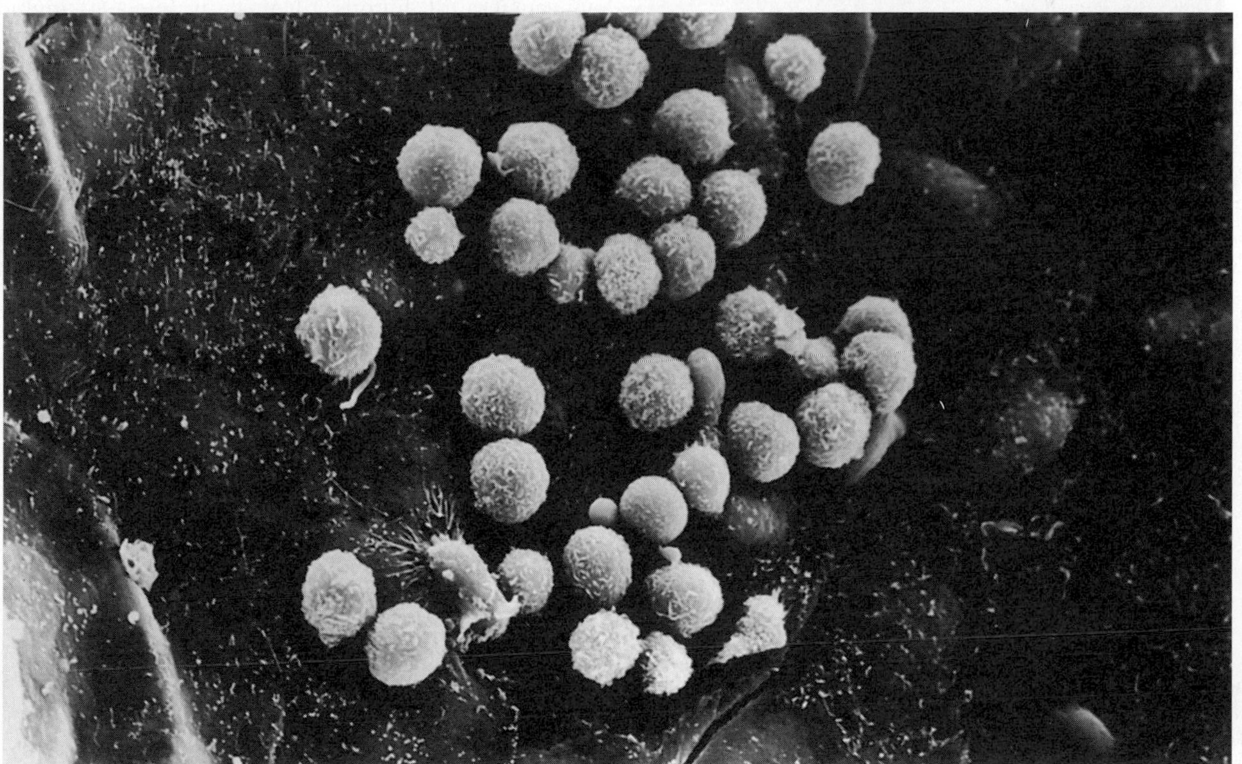

FIGURE 34–14. Electron micrograph demonstrating leukocytes adherent to the endothelium of the aorta of a hypercholesterolemic monkey after 14 days of an atherogenic diet. Adherent leukocytes (mostly monocytes) were found scattered in patches such as these randomly distributed at all levels of the aortic tree. Some of the cells appear spread on the surface, whereas others are rounded.

ters that appear to be located at branches and bifurcations throughout the arterial tree in all large and medium-sized arteries. The attached monocytes then migrate over the surface of the endothelium, where they probe, find a junction between the endothelial cells, and use this junctional site to slip between the cells and localize in the subendothelial space (Fig. 34–15). This process, as viewed in cell culture, appears to occur very rapidly and presumably does so in vivo as well. After finding their way into the subendothelial intimal space, the monocytes become converted into macrophages, so that within less than 1 month large numbers of foam cells, or lipid-filled macrophages, are found beneath an intact endothelium. These cells continue to enlarge as they fill with lipid. Such accumulations of foam cells represent the establishment of the first and ubiquitous lesion of atherosclerosis, the fatty streak (Fig. 34–16).

The fatty streaks continue to expand in hypercholesterolemic animals by continuing the process of monocyte adherence, subendothelial migration and localization, and lipid accumulation. As the fatty streaks expand, the surface of the artery becomes highly irregular and convoluted (Fig. 34–17). With increasing time, small numbers of smooth muscle cells begin to appear beneath the accumulated macrophages within the intima and also begin to accumulate deposits of lipid and take on the appearance of foam cells. As discussed earlier, monoclonal antibodies specific for

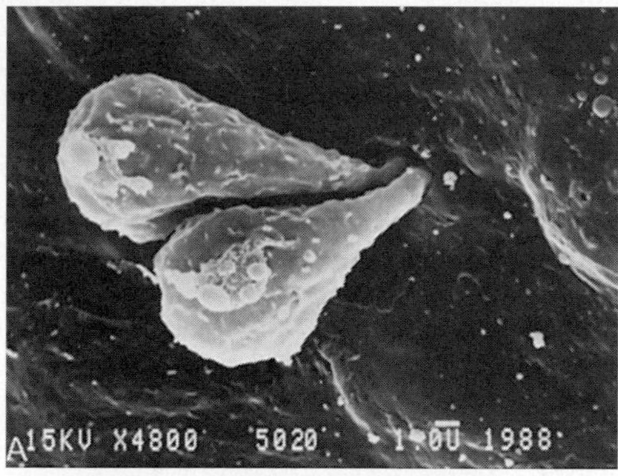

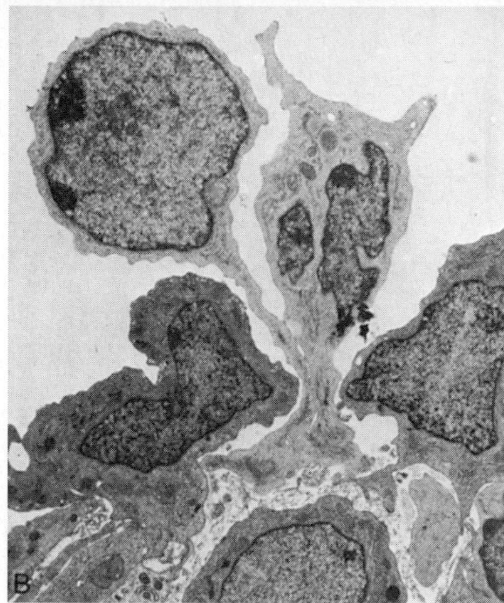

FIGURE 34–15. Scanning and transmission electron micrographs demonstrating leukocytes entering into the artery wall between endothelial junctions after 6 months and 1 year, respectively, of an atherogenic diet in nonhuman primates. *A*, Thoracic aorta, 6 months. ×4000. *B*, Thoracic aorta, 1 year. ×4700. (Reproduced with permission from Masuda, J., and Ross, R.: Atherogenesis during low level hypercholesterolemia in the nonhuman primate: I. Fatty streak formation. Arteriosclerosis *10*:164, 1990. Copyright 1990 American Heart Association.)

smooth muscle and macrophages have made it possible to show that both types of cell become foam cells as the lesions expand. The cholesterol levels in the plasma of the fat-fed animals ranged between 500 and 1000 mg/dl, which are not dissimilar from the levels of plasma cholesterol found in humans with FH disease.

LATER CHANGES. After approximately 5 to 6 months at the very high cholesterol and LDL levels and after 1 year at levels closer to those observed in humans, a second series of changes occurred in the monkeys, initially at branches and bifurcations in the iliac arteries and subsequently at higher regions in the arterial tree. The changes that were found at branches and bifurcations suggest that they may be associated with the flow characteristics at these particular sites in the vessel. They consist of retraction of the endothelial cells covering some of the fatty streaks caused by endothelial cell-cell detachment. Endothelial retraction exposes the numerous lipid-filled macrophages to the circulation (Fig. 34–18) and permits them to remove the lipid they have ingested from the lesion by taking it with them into the circulation to the spleen and to lymph nodes. In this fashion, the macrophages play a role in the lesions of atherosclerosis similar to their role at sites of injury, where they are the principal scavenger cells. Thus, in a very real sense, the progressing lesions of atherosclerosis represent a special kind of inflammatory response in which macrophages (and perhaps T-lymphocytes) attempt initially to protect the tissues. With the continuing insult (hypercholesterolemia, diabetes, and so on), the response becomes excessive, and the resultant fibroproliferative events themselves become the disease process.

When the macrophages become exposed to the circulation they can serve as sites for platelet adherence and for microthrombi to form, demonstrating that the macrophages may represent a potent site for platelet interactions (Fig. 34–19). In these cases in which platelet interactions such as those just described occurred, similar anatomical sites were observed 1 to 2 months later to be occupied by space-filling lesions of advanced atherosclerosis, or fibrous plaques. These fibrous plaques had all of the characteristic appearances of fibrous plaques in humans, including a dense fibrous cap that overlay areas of extensive proliferation of smooth muscle cells intermixed with lipid-filled macrophages, beneath which were found areas of cell debris, lipid accumulation, and sometimes calcification (Fig. 34–20). The same changes occurred at the iliac bifurcation after approximately 7 months, in the abdominal aorta after 9 months, in the thoracic aorta by 11 months, and in the coronary arteries after 12 to 13 months. By analyzing the distribution of these changes and correlating this distribution with the levels of cholesterol in the animals with time, Faggiotto et al.[142,143] and Masuda and Ross[144,145] were able to demonstrate a correlation among three factors: the level of plasma cholesterol, the duration of the maintenance of this increased level of cholesterol, and the changes that occur at particular anatomical sites with time.

Another important observation was that many advanced lesions of atherosclerosis also occurred at sites where fatty streaks were present but where there was no clear evidence of endothelial cell–cell separation and exposure of the subendothelium.[143] Thus, one has to conclude that proliferative lesions of atherosclerosis can occur at sites where the endothelium remains intact over preexisting lesions such as fatty streaks. This can undoubtedly be explained by the fact that both activated macrophages and endothelium can serve as sources of growth factors so that platelet interactions are not required for smooth muscle proliferation to occur.

This leads to the need to determine what constitutes endothelial injury. It also suggests that nondenuding forms of injury or endothelial dysfunction are more important than the denuding forms described above. Reidy and

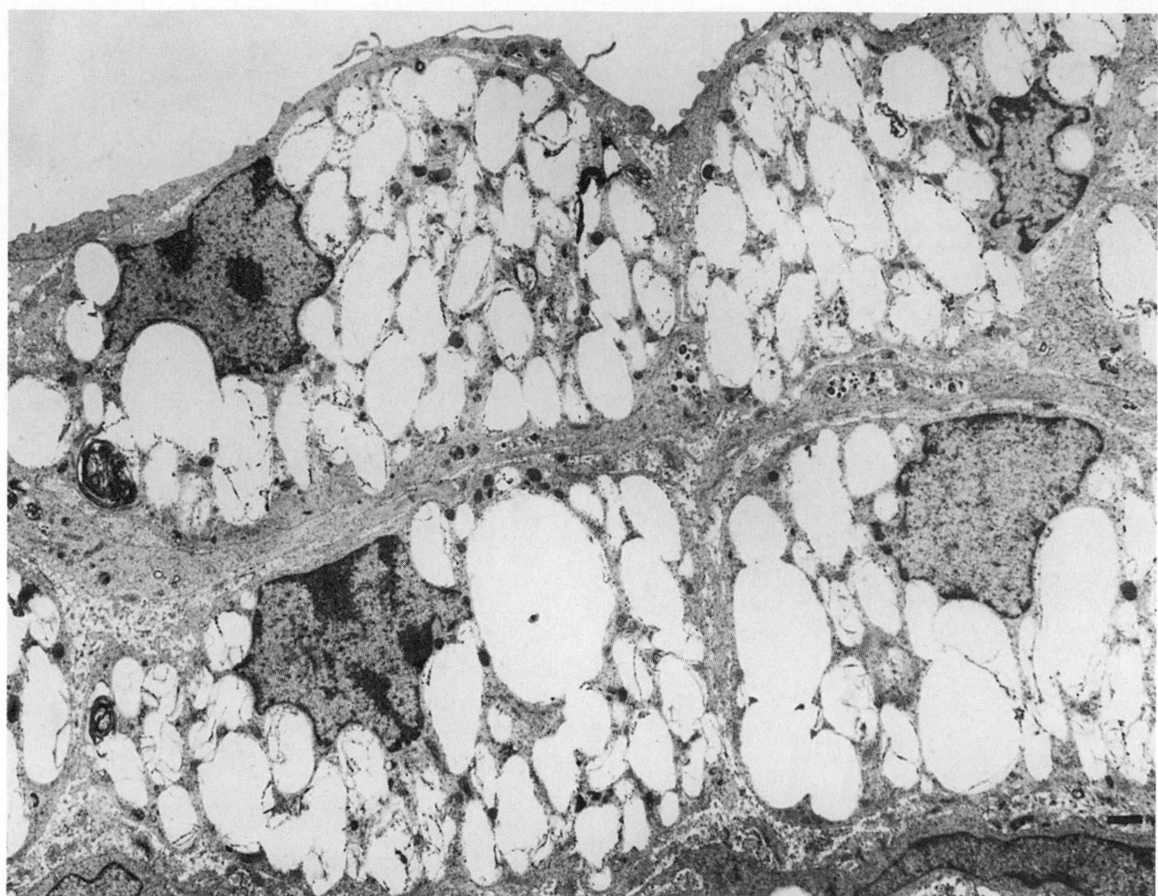

FIGURE 34–16. Transmission electron micrograph showing a fatty streak containing two layers of subendothelial foam cells after 2 months of hypercholesterolemia in a fat-fed nonhuman primate. The large lipid-filled macrophages are distributed focally in multilayers. The cells are four- to six-fold larger than lipid-laden macrophages observed in control animals. There is a small amount of intercellular matrix and some lipid debris. The macrophages maintain a close relationship to the intact endothelium. The endothelium is markedly stretched so that the endothelial cells have become very thin. (Reproduced with permission from Faggiotto, A., Ross, R., and Harker, L.: Studies of hypercholesterolemia in the nonhuman primate: I. Changes that lead to fatty streak formation. Arteriosclerosis *4*:332, 1984. Copyright 1984 American Heart Association.)

Schwartz[152,153] have indicated that one of the most common results of endothelial injury may be detachment of individual endothelial cells, which are rapidly replaced by neighboring cells so that endothelial continuity is maintained. Several markers have been developed that can be used to

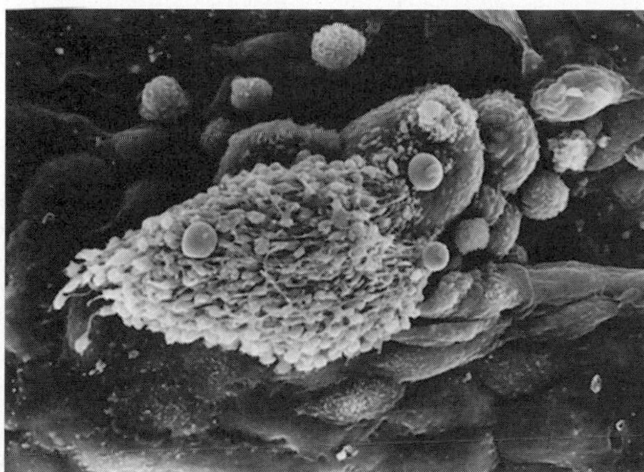

FIGURE 34–17. Scanning electron micrograph providing a surface view of a fatty streak from a fat-fed monkey after 2 months of hypercholesterolemia. The surface of the fatty streak has become highly irregular and has a striking nodular pattern with deep crevices between the nodules. Such a pattern forms by continuing adherence of monocytes to the endothelial cells that probe and migrate subendothelially between cells to continually expand the fatty streak.

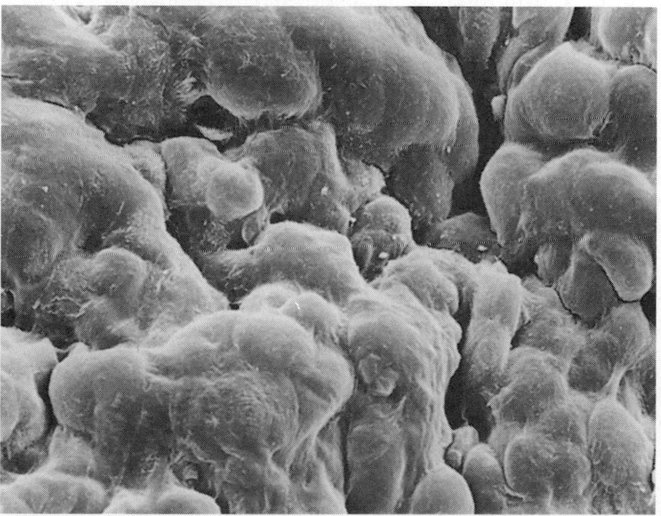

FIGURE 34–18. A scanning electron micrograph of the thoracic aorta of a nonhuman primate, showing the irregular surface of a fatty streak after 2 years of an atherogenic diet. Platelet microthrombi adherent to exposed macrophages are visible at a site of endothelial retraction. Many adherent leukocytes are also seen on the intact endothelial cells. ×720. (Reproduced with permission from Masuda, J., and Ross, R.: Atherogenesis during low level hypercholesterolemia in the nonhuman primate: II. Fatty streak conversion to fibrous plaque. Arteriosclerosis *10*:178, 1990. Copyright 1990 American Heart Association.)

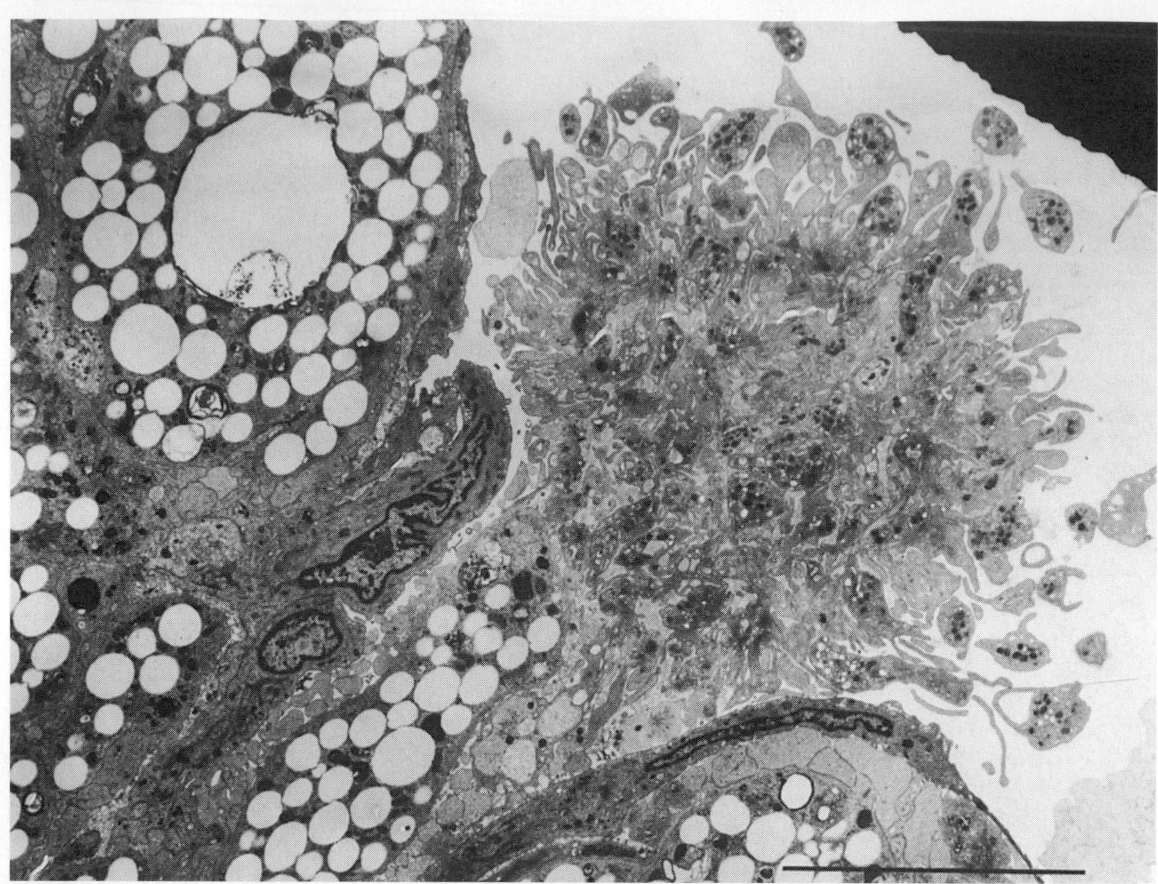

FIGURE 34–19. Transmission electron micrograph of platelets adherent to an exposed macrophage from a fatty streak in a fat-fed monkey that had been hypercholesterolemic for 6 months. The platelets in this thrombus are generally adherent to exposed foam cells and penetrate into the depth of a crevice in the fatty streak. Many of the platelets have undergone degranulation and have released their contents. Bar = 10 μ. (Reproduced with permission from Faggiotto, A., and Ross, R.: Studies of hypercholesterolemia in the nonhuman primate: II. Fatty streak conversion to fibrous plaque. Arteriosclerosis *4*:349, 1984. Copyright 1984 American Heart Association.)

identify sites of endothelial injury. Hansson et al.[154] demonstrated that injured endothelial cells take up IgG whereas normal endothelium does not, and that such IgG uptake can be correlated with increased replication of the endothelium. Furthermore, Reidy and Schwartz[155] showed that a linear correlation exists between the extent of endothelial injury (the number of denuded cells) and the localization of indium-111–labeled platelets at these sites. Platelets would adhere because injured endothelium appears to have lost its nonthrombogenic properties.

Thus, there may be several different forms of endothelial injury and more subtle techniques may be necessary to uncover them. This raises the interesting question, as suggested earlier, whether one subtle form of endothelial injury may be the stimulation of these cells to synthesize and secrete growth factors, including PDGF, that could then

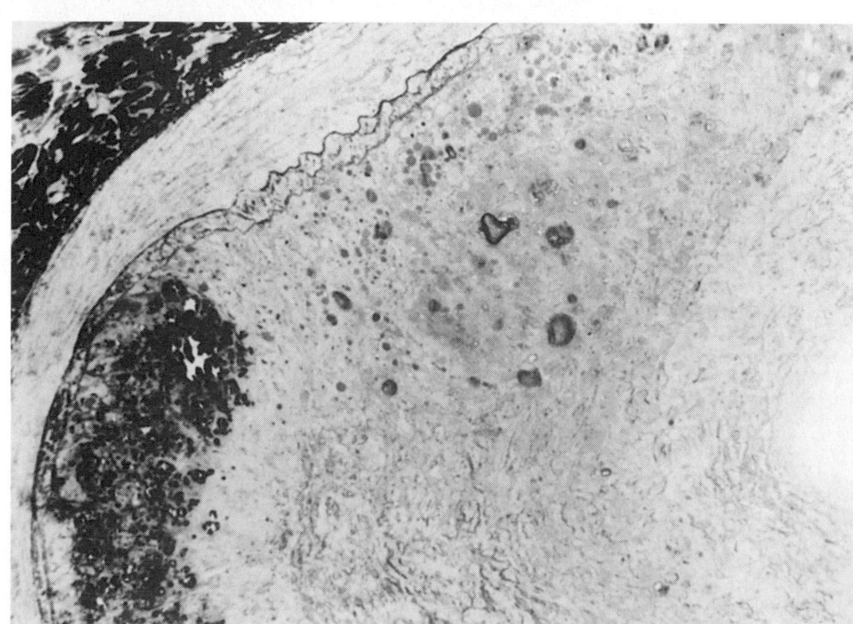

FIGURE 34–20. Light micrograph demonstrating an advanced fibrous plaque that formed in the internal iliac artery of a monkey that was hypercholesterolemic for 7 months. The lesion has occluded approximately 70 per cent of the arterial lumen and consists of numerous layers of smooth muscle cells surrounded by fibrous connective tissue. An area of lipid and necrotic tissue occupies the left side and upper portion of this lesion. (Reproduced with permission from Faggiotto, A., and Ross, R.: Studies of hypercholesterolemia in the nonhuman primate: II. Fatty streak conversion to fibrous plaque. Arteriosclerosis *4*:345, 1984. Copyright 1984 American Heart Association.)

play a critical role in the genesis of the events previously described. If this were the case, then endothelial disjunction, retraction, and subendothelial exposure are clearly not necessary for lesions of atherosclerosis to develop because both activated endothelium and macrophages could be sufficient in themselves to provide a mitogenic stimulus for smooth muscle cells to form lesions of atherosclerosis.

REGRESSION OF ATHEROSCLEROSIS

ANIMAL STUDIES. A number of studies have demonstrated that lesions of experimentally induced atherosclerosis can in fact regress. When hypercholesterolemic swine and nonhuman primates that have developed severe lesions are fed a normocholesterolemic diet, these lesions can regress. Fatty streaks formed in the monkeys receiving the high-fat, high-cholesterol diet of Faggiotto et al.[142] were found to regress completely within 1 month after the animals resumed a normal diet. Most of the studies of regression of the advanced lesions of atherosclerosis have been performed in nonhuman primates, principally in different strains of macaques and in squirrel monkeys. The studies were performed by providing the monkeys with atherogenic diets that took them through stages of fatty streak development and on to fibrous plaque formation. When cholesterol was removed from the diet and plasma cholesterol concentrations returned to normal, Faggiotto et al.[142] observed that reasonably rapid regression of fatty streaks occurred. Of greater potential interest, significant reduction in the size of the smooth muscle proliferative lesions has been observed by several different investigators. Some of the earliest studies were performed by Armstrong et al.,[156] who demonstrated that coronary atherosclerosis could regress. These studies were subsequently confirmed by Wissler and Vesselinovitch.[157] Perhaps the largest number of studies have been performed by Clarkson and his colleagues.[158] They demonstrated the clear therapeutic benefit of lowering plasma cholesterol concentrations after having induced fibrous plaques in animals on hypercholesterolemic regimens for periods of 12 months and longer. Regression occurred principally in lesions in the abdominal aorta and in the coronary arteries, in contrast to those that formed at the carotid bifurcation, which appeared, on some occasions, to develop lesions relatively independently of plasma lipid concentrations. When regression occurs and plasma cholesterol levels return to baseline, the lesions of atherosclerosis become smaller, contain less lipid, and demonstrate marked decreases in their content of cholesterol and cholesteryl esters. Remodeling of connective tissue proteins also appears to take place, as shown by decreases in both collagen and elastic fiber proteins in these lesions. Thus it seems that, over a sufficiently long period, advanced lesions can in some cases also regress.

By decreasing lipid deposition or enhancing removal of lipids from the artery wall, for example, by reducing fat intake or increasing plasma HDL levels, it has been possible to show that lesion regression can be induced.[159] Similarly, as described above, antioxidants can induce lesion regression in the WHHL rabbit.[128,129]

HUMAN STUDIES. It has been demonstrated that advanced, semiocclusive lesions of human coronary atherosclerosis also can regress. In a quantitative image analysis study of coronary angiograms from a series of patients being aggressively treated with lipid-lowering regimens of either niacin and colestipol or lovastatin and colestipol, Brown and colleagues[160] have demonstrated statistically significant regression in association with decreases in plasma cholesterol and LDL. This provides clear evidence that the lesions of atherosclerosis are able to regress at apparently all stages of lesion development.

Various approaches have been used in clinical trials to induce lesion regression in humans. These trials have included lipid-lowering agents, including HMG–CoA reductase inhibitors, cholestyramine, colestipol/niacin therapy, as well as dietary and lifestyle changes, and even surgical approaches.[163–171] All of these trials have demonstrated decrease in incidence of acute cardiac events and, in some cases, extensive reduction with detectable, but minimal, lesion regression as determined angiographically. These approaches may increase the stability of advanced lesions of atherosclerosis without necessarily reducing their size as imaged angiographically. Because angiograms do not provide information on actual lesion size but only on lumen dimensions, it is not entirely clear what changes may have occurred in the lesions. Nevertheless, several trials have demonstrated substantial reduction in angina by reducing lipid levels.

A number of investigators have probed the capability of fish oils, which contain large amounts of omega-3 fatty acids, to decrease plasma cholesterol levels and potentially to induce lesion regression when added to the diet of hypercholesterolemic individuals.[172] Not only do these diets lead to decrease in plasma cholesterol levels, they also change the balance of prostaglandins that are formed by the cells. It is well known that platelets have the capacity to use arachidonic acid to form the prostaglandin derivative thromboxane A_2, a proaggregating factor for platelets. On the other hand, endothelial cells and smooth muscle use the same fatty acid to form, via cyclo-oxygenase, the prostaglandin metabolite prostacyclin (PGI_2), an extraordinarily potent antiaggregant and vasodilator. When the omega-3 fatty acids are fed to animals (and if they are particularly rich in eicosapentaenoic acid), they shift the balance because thromboxane A_3 derived from this fatty acid is inactive as a platelet aggregant, whereas PGI_3 is as active as PGI_2, thus favoring antiaggregant, vasodilator effects over effects that might lead to platelet aggregation and thrombosis.

Unstable Lesions and Sudden Death. The work of Davies and Thomas and Falk has provided evidence that many cases of sudden death result from lesion fissures or ruptures, which can induce hemorrhage or thrombosis and stenosis of the lumen.[161,162] Such lesions, discussed above, represent a new classification of lesions, which at present are extremely difficult to diagnose. Fibrous plaques susceptible to rupture are unstable in part due to the relative thinness of their fibrous cap, which may be partially explained by decreased formation of connective tissue by the smooth muscle cells of the lesion or by increased degradation of the matrix in the cap due to collections of macrophages often located at the shoulders of advanced lesions, which can provide connective tissue hydrolytic enzymes. If matrix removal exceeds that of deposition, then the fibrous cap that overlies the lipid-rich necrotic core of the fibrous plaque can become unstable. Stress increases on the fibrous cap of lesions located at branches and bifurcations where changes in blood flow may lead to induction of plaque rupture, hemorrhage, thrombosis, and either myocardial infarction or sudden death.

THROMBOSIS

(See also Chap. 58)

As described at the beginning of this chapter, thrombosis was originally considered to be an important component in the initiation and progression of the lesions of atherosclerosis. It now appears that thrombosis may play several roles. One prominent and potentially important clinical role is that of thrombi which become incorporated into existing advanced lesions of atherosclerosis, rapidly resulting in lumen narrowing and increase in lesion dimensions. Perhaps one of the most persistent and common complications of atherosclerosis is the formation of cracks and fissures in the advanced lesions of atherosclerosis that can act as sites for platelet attachment and formation of mural and potentially occlusive thrombi, which could lead to unstable angina or myocardial infarction.

As discussed earlier, there is good evidence in nonhuman primates and in rabbits that mural thrombi can contribute to the initiation and development of lesions of atherosclerosis.[121–125] This has also been demonstrated in humans at the perianastomotic site of coronary bypass surgery, where new lesions of atherosclerosis form in approximately 30 per cent of all bypass grafts.[173] In monkeys or rabbits receiving a hyperlipemic diet, intraarterial balloon catheter deendothelialization can lead to intimal smooth muscle proliferative lesions that appear very much like those found in hypercholesterolemic patients.

Thrombi have been observed in the coronary arteries of the vast majority of individuals who die of transmural myocardial infarction. However, thrombi are much less common in individuals who die of subendothelial infarction. Thrombosis is even less common in individuals who die of sudden cardiac death, although both thrombosis and embolism are well recognized as complications of cerebrovascular disease as well as peripheral vascular disease.

The role of the endothelium in the process of thrombosis is not entirely clear because, as discussed earlier, endothelial cells have both nonthrombogenic and procoagulant activities. Endothelial cells produce von Willebrand factor as well as plasminogen activator and prostacyclin. The development of agents that can alter thromboxane formation and thus prevent platelet interaction, or alter prostacyclin formation and thus promote platelet interactions, should make it possible to obtain a clearer idea of the role of these agents compared with others that can be produced by the endothelial cells in the process of thrombosis in general.

IMAGING ATHEROSCLEROSIS

Detection of occlusive lesions of atherosclerosis has until the present time required invasive methodology such as angiography and intravascular ultrasonography. For some peripheral arteries, it has been possible to use Doppler ultrasound techniques. However, the only current method that provides any information on the artery wall, the area occupied by the lesion, is intravascular ultrasonography (Fig. 3–95, p. 89), which is invasive and requires catheterization, possibly inducing some injury to the artery itself. Recently, Skinner et al. have taken advantage of magnetic resonance imaging (MRI) to visualize occlusive and aneurysmal lesions of atherosclerosis in rabbits[174] and more recently in nonhuman primates (unpublished observations).

With MRI not only is it possible to visualize the lumen using a procedure called "time of flight," but it also provides images similar to those seen on angiograms. This method also provides information on artery walls once they are thicker than 0.4 mm (the resolution of MRI), so that it is possible to see the lesion and fine structure of advanced lesions of atherosclerosis, such as a fibrous plaque containing a fibrous cap, necrotic core, and even fissuring. This method even allows serial imaging of experimental animals and, if used in patients, lesion progression and regression.

At present MRI can be used for peripheral arteries such as the iliac and superficial femoral arteries and for the abdominal aorta or the carotid artery. Because of motion due to breathing or heartbeat, it is not possible to use this method to visualize the thoracic aorta or the coronary arteries. However, new developments may make it feasible in the near future. Thus, on the immediate horizon is the advent of methodology to permit visualization of stenotic lesions that can be followed during therapy. Potentially dangerous lesions, which may have thin fibrous caps and may be subject to fissure, can be seen using this method, which could then permit intervention at a time prior to the disastrous consequences that can occur from rupture or fissuring of lesions.

CONCLUSIONS

Knowledge in the field of atherosclerosis has exploded and is changing rapidly. The opportunity to use the tools of cell and molecular biology, as well as new noninvasive methods for examining individuals at the clinical level, has broadened our understanding of the roles of the cells in atherogenesis. Cell and molecular biology has rapidly increased our understanding of the principal cells involved in atherosclerosis: endothelium, smooth muscle, platelets, and monocytes/macrophages and T-lymphocytes. How the risk factors that are commonly associated with an increased incidence of atherosclerosis are related to these cellular interactions is beginning to be understood, particularly in relation to hypercholesterolemia. Unfortunately, there are no good animal models that permit us to study the questions related to cigarette smoking, hypertension, diabetes, or some of the other risk factors that are epidemiologically associated with atherosclerosis. Without these, it is difficult to know the nature of the cellular interactions that occur during the genesis of the disease process as it is associated with each of these important risk factors.

Perhaps the most critical aspect of this problem is the need to understand the basis of the genetic susceptibility of individuals to these risk factors and thus to circumstances that can lead to these increased cellular interactions. Once the genetic loci for the various apoproteins are identified, and once it is possible to demonstrate altered genetic loci for these and other factors important in atherogenesis in individuals who are at increased risk for heart attack and/or stroke, it should be possible to begin to probe this question using these new tools.

Acknowledgments

This work was supported in part by US Public Health Service Grant HL-18645 and NIH grant RR-00166 to the Northwest Regional Primate Center. The author is particularly indebted to Elaine Raines, Agostino Faggiotto, Junichi Masuda, Michael Rosenfeld, Toyohiro Tsukada, Masakiyo Sasahara, Shogo Katsuda, Allen Gown, Daniel Bowen-Pope, Michael Skinner, and Yutaka Nakashima, with whom work reported from the author's laboratory was performed.

REFERENCES

RISK FACTORS

1. WHO-MONICA Project: Myocardial infarction and coronary deaths in the World Health Organization Monica Project: Registration procedures, event rates, and case-fatality rates in 38 populations from 21 countries in four continents. Circulation *90*:583, 1994.
2. Ross, R., and Glomset, J. A.: Atherosclerosis and the arterial smooth muscle cell. Science *180*:1332, 1973.
3. Ross, R., and Glomset, J. A.: The pathogenesis of atherosclerosis. N. Engl. J. Med. *295*:369, 420, 1976.
4. Ross, R., and Harker, L.: Hyperlipidemia and atherosclerosis. Science *193*:1094, 1976.
5. Fuster, V., Badimon, L., Badimon, J. J., and Chesebro, J. H.: The pathogenesis of coronary artery disease and the acute coronary syndromes. N. Engl. J. Med. *326*:242, 1992.

5a. Ross, R., and Fuster, V.: The pathogenesis of atherosclerosis. *In* Fuster, V., Ross, R., and Topol, E. J. (eds.): Atherosclerosis and Coronary Artery Disease. Philadelphia, Lippincott–Raven, 1996, pp. 441–462.

6. Dawber, T. R., Moore, F. E., and Mann, G. V.: Measuring the risk of coronary heart disease in adult population groups: II. Coronary heart disease in the Framingham study. Am. J. Public Health *47*:4, 1957.
7. American Heart Association: Heart and stroke facts. Dallas, American Heart Association National Center, 1992.
8. Cooper, E. S.: Prevention: The key to progress. Circulation *24*:629, 1993.
9. Report of the Working Group on Arteriosclerosis of the National Heart, Lung, and Blood Institute: DHEW Publication No. (NIH) 82–2035, Vol. 2. Washington, DC, US Government Printing Office, 1981.

10. Report of the Inter-Society Commission for Heart Disease Resources: Primary prevention of the atherosclerotic disease. Circulation *42*:55, 1970.
11. Stamler, J., Berkson, D. M., and Lindberg, H. A.: Risk factors: Their role in the etiology and pathogenesis of the atherosclerotic diseases. *In* Wissler, R. W., Geer, J. C., and Kaufman, N. (eds.): The Pathogenesis of Atherosclerosis. Baltimore, Williams and Wilkins Co., 1972, p. 41.
12. Kuller, L. H.: Epidemiology of cardiovascular disease: Current perspectives. Am. J. Epidemiol. *104*:425, 1976.
13. Inkeles, S., and Eisenberg, D.: Hyperlipidemia and coronary atherosclerosis: A review. Medicine *70*:110, 1981.
14. Lipid Research Clinics Program: The Lipid Research Clinics Coronary Primary Prevention Trial Results: I. Reduction in incidence of coronary heart disease. JAMA *251*:351, 1984.
15. Lipid Research Clinics Program: The Lipid Research Clinics Coronary Primary Prevention Trial Results: II. The relationship of reduction in incidence of coronary heart disease to cholesterol lowering. JAMA *251*:365, 1984.
16. Smoking and Health, Ch. 3: Criteria for Judgment. DHEW Publication No. (NIH) 1103, Washington, DC, U.S. Government Printing Office, 1964.
17. The Pooling Project Research Group: Relationship of blood pressure, serum cholesterol, smoking habit, relative weight, and ECG abnormalities to incidence of major coronary events: Final report of the pooling project. J. Chronic Dis. *31*:201, 1978.
18. Oberman, A., Harlan, W. R., Smith, M., and Graybiel, A.: The cardiovascular risk associated with different levels and types of elevated blood pressure. Minn. Med. *52*:1283, 1969.

THE NORMAL ARTERY

19. 1988 Joint National Committee: The 1988 report of the Joint National Committee on detection, evaluation and treatment of high blood pressure. Arch. Intern. Med. *148*:1023, 1988.
20. Glagov, S.: Hemodynamic risk factors: Mechanical stress, mural architecture, medial nutrition and the vulnerability of arteries to atherosclerosis. *In* Wissler, R. W., and Geer, J. C., (eds.): The Pathogenesis of Atherosclerosis. Baltimore, Williams and Wilkins, 1972, p. 164.
21. Wolinsky, H., and Glagov, S.: Comparison of abdominal and thoracic aortic medial structure in mammals: Deviation of man from the usual pattern. Circ. Res. *25*:677, 1969.
22. Barger, A. C., Beeuwkes, R., Lainey, L. L., and Silverman, K. J.: Hypothesis: Vasa vasorum and neovascularization of human coronary arteries. N. Engl. J. Med. *310*:175, 1984.
23. Barger, A. C., and Beeuwkes, R., III: Rupture of coronary vasa vasorum as a trigger of acute myocardial infarction. Am. J. Cardiol. *66*:41G, 1990.

CELLS OF THE ARTERY AND FROM THE BLOOD POTENTIALLY INVOLVED IN ATHEROGENESIS

24. Schwartz, S. M., and Benditt, E. P.: Clustering of replicating cells in aortic endothelium. Proc. Natl. Acad. Sci. U.S.A. *73*:651, 1976.
25. Schwartz, S. M., and Benditt, E. P.: Aortic endothelial cell replication. Effects of age and hypertension in the rat. Circ. Res. *41*:248, 1977.
26. Simionescu, N., Simionescu, M., and Palade, G. E.: Permeability of muscle capillaries to small heme-peptides: Evidence for the existence of patent transendothelial channels. J. Cell. Biol. *64*:586, 1975.
27. Gimbrone, M. A., Jr.: Culture of vascular endothelium. Prog. Hemost. Thromb. *3*:1, 1976.
28. Ross, R.: The pathogenesis of atherosclerosis—an update. N. Engl. J. Med. *314*:488, 1986.
29. Ross, R.: The pathogenesis of atherosclerosis: A perspective for the 1990s. Nature *362*:801, 1993.
30. Renkin, E. M.: Multiple pathways of capillary permeability. Circ. Res. *41*:735, 1977.
31. Moncada, S., Herman, A. G., Higgs, E. A., and Vane, J. R.: Differential formation of prostacyclin (PGX or PGI_2) by layers of the arterial wall: An explanation for the antithrombotic properties of vascular endothelium. Thromb. Res. *11*:323, 1977.
32. Fielding, C. J.: Metabolism of cholesterol-rich chylomicrons: Mechanism of binding and uptake of cholesteryl esters by the vascular bed of the perfused rat heart. J. Clin. Invest. *62*:141, 1978.
33. Furchgott, R. F.: Role of endothelium in responses of vascular smooth muscle. Circ. Res. *53*:557, 1983.
34. Gimbrone, M. A., Jr., and Alexander, R. W.: Angiotensin II stimulation of prostaglandin production in cultured human vascular endothelium. Science *189*:219, 1975.
35. Jaffe, E. A., Minick, C. R., Adelman, B., et al.: Synthesis of basement membrane by cultured human endothelial cells. J. Exp. Med. *144*:209, 1976.
36. Lüscher, T. F.: Imbalance of endothelium-derived relaxing and contracting factors: A new concept in hypertension? Am. J. Hypertens. *3*:317, 1990.
37. Jaffe, E. A., Hoyer, L. W., and Nachman, R. L.: Synthesis of antihemophilic factor antigen by cultured human endothelial cells. J. Clin. Invest. *52*:2757, 1973.
38. Rubin, K., Tingström, A., Hansson, G. K., et al.: Induction of B-type receptors for platelet-derived growth factor in vascular inflammation: Possible implications for development of vascular proliferative lesions. Lancet *1*:1353, 1988.
39. Steinberg, D.: Lipoproteins and atherosclerosis: A look back and a look ahead. Arteriosclerosis *3*:283, 1983.
40. Yanagisawa, M., Kurihara, H., Kimura, S., et al.: A novel potent vasoconstrictor peptide produced by vascular endothelial cells. Nature *332*:411, 1988.
41. Gajdusek, D. M., DiCorleto, P. E., Ross, R., and Schwartz, S. M.: An endothelial cell–derived growth factor. J. Cell Biol. *85*:467, 1980.
42. DiCorleto, P. E., Gajdusek, C. M., Schwartz, S. M., and Ross, R.: Biochemical properties of the endothelium-derived growth factor: Comparison to other growth factors. J. Cell Physiol. *114*:339, 1983.
43. DiCorleto, P. E., and Bowen-Pope, D. F.: Cultured endothelial cells produce a platelet-derived growth factor–like protein. Proc. Natl. Acad. Sci. U.S.A. *80*:1919, 1983.
44. Loskutoff, D. J., and Curriden, S. A.: The fibrinolytic system of the vessel wall and its role in the control of thrombosis. Ann. N. Y. Acad. Sci. *598*:238, 1990.
45. Sawdey, M. S., and Loskutoff, D. J.: Regulation of murine type 1 plasminogen activator inhibitor gene expression in vivo tissue specificity and induction by lipopolysaccharide tumor necrosis factor-alpha and transforming growth factor-beta. J. Clin. Invest. *88*:1346, 1991.
46. Moncada, S., and Higgs, E. A.: Nitric oxide from L-arginine: A bioregulatory system. Amsterdam, Excerpta Medica, 1990.
46a. Owens, G. K.: Role of alterations in the differentiated state of smooth muscle cell in atherogenesis. *In* Fuster, V., Ross, R., and Topol, E. J. (eds.): Atherosclerosis and Coronary Artery Disease. Philadelphia, Lippincott–Raven, 1996, pp. 401–420.
47. Wissler, R. W.: The arterial medial cell, smooth muscle, or multifunctional mesenchyme? J. Atheroscler. Res. *8*:201, 1968.
48. Ross, R.: The smooth muscle cells. II. Growth of smooth muscle in culture and formation of elastic fibers. J. Cell Biol. *50*:172, 1971.
49. Burke, J. M., and Ross, R.: Synthesis of connective tissue macromolecules by smooth muscle. Int. Rev. Connect. Tissue Res. *8*:119, 1979.
50. Chait, A., Ross, R., Albers, J. J., and Bierman, E. L.: Platelet-derived growth factor stimulates activity of low density lipoprotein receptors. Proc. Natl. Acad. Sci. U.S.A. *77*:4084, 1980.
51. Bowen-Pope, D. F., Seifert, R. A., and Ross, R.: The platelet-derived growth factor receptor. *In* Boynton, A. L., and Leffert, H. L. (eds.): Control of Animal Cell Proliferation: Recent Advances, Vol. 1. New York, Academic Press, 1985, p. 281.
52. Seifert, R. A., Schwartz, S. M., and Bowen-Pope, D. F.: Developmentally regulated production of platelet-derived growth factor–like molecules. Nature *311*:669, 1984.
53. Chamley-Campbell, J., Campbell, G., and Ross, R.: Phenotype-dependent response of cultured aortic smooth muscle to serum mitogens. J. Cell Biol. *89*:379, 1981.
54. Thyberg, J., Palmberg, L., Nilsson, J., et al.: Phenotype modulation in primary cultures of arterial smooth muscle cells: On the role of platelet-derived growth factor. Differentiation *25*:156, 1983.
55. Schwartz, S. M., Heimark, R. L., and Majesky, M. W.: Developmental mechanisms underlying pathology of arteries. Physiol. Rev. *70*:1177, 1990.
56. Hultgardh-Nilsson, A., Krondahl, U., Querol-Ferrer, V., and Ringertz, N. R.: Differences in growth factor response in smooth muscle cells isolated from adult and neonatal rat arteries. Differentiation *47*:99, 1991.
57. Ross, R., Wight, T. N., Strandness, E., and Thiele, B.: Human atherosclerosis. I. Cell constitution and characteristics of advanced lesions of the superficial femoral artery. Am. J. Pathol. *114*:79, 1984.
58. Van Furth, R.: Current view on the mononuclear phagocyte system. Immunobiology *161*:178, 1982.
59. Nathan, C. F., Murray, H. W., and Cohn, Z. A.: Current concepts: The macrophage as an effector cell. N. Engl. J. Med. *303*:622, 1980.
60. Goldstein, J. L., Ho, Y. K., Basu, S. K., and Brown, M. S.: Binding site of macrophages that mediates uptake and degradation of acetylated low density lipoprotein, producing massive cholesterol deposition. Proc. Natl. Acad. Sci. U.S.A. *76*:333, 1979.
61. Rosenfeld, M. E., Khoo, J. C., Miller, E., et al.: Macrophage-derived foam cells freshly isolated from rabbit atherosclerotic lesions degrade modified lipoproteins, promote oxidation of low-density lipoproteins, and contain oxidation-specific lipid-protein adducts. J. Clin. Invest. *87*:90, 1990.
62. Martin, T. R., Altman, L. C., Albert, R. K., and Henderson, W. R.: Leukotriene B4 production by human alveolar macrophage: A potential mechanism for amplifying inflammation in the lung. Am. Rev. Respir. Dis. *129*:106, 1984.
63. Bevilacqua, M. P., Pober, J. S., Cotran, R. S., and Gimbrone, M. A., Jr.: Interleukin 1 (IL 1) acts upon vascular endothelium to stimulate procoagulant activity and leukocyte adhesion. J. Cell. Biochem. *9A*(Suppl. A):148, 1985.
64. Cathcart, M. K., Morel, D. W., and Chisolm, G. M.: Monocytes and neutrophils oxidize low-density lipoprotein making it cytotoxic. J. Leukoc. Biol. *38*:341, 1985.
65. Ross, R., Raines, E. W., and Bowen-Pope, D. F.: The biology of platelet-derived growth factor. Cell *46*:155, 1986.
66. Shimokado, K., Raines, E. W., Madtes, D. K., et al.: A significant part of macrophage-derived growth factor consists of at least two forms of PDGF. Cell *43*:277, 1985.
67. Raines, E. W., Dower, S. K., and Ross, R.: Il-1 mitogenic activity for fibroblasts and smooth muscle cells is due to PDGF-AA. Science *243*:393, 1989.
68. Baird, A., Mormede, P., and Bohlen, P.: Immunoreactive fibroblast-

growth factor in cells of peritoneal exudate suggests its identity with macrophage-derived growth factor. Biochem. Biophys. Res. Commun. *126*:358, 1985.

69. Ralph, P.: Colony stimulating factors. *In* Zembala, M., and Asherson, G. (eds.): Human Monocytes. New York, Academic Press, 1989, p. 228.
70. Holmsen, H., and Weiss, H. J.: Secretable storage pools in platelets. Annu. Rev. Med. *30*:119, 1979.
71. Pepper, D. S.: Macromolecules released from platelet storage organelles. Thromb. Haemost. *42*:1667, 1980.
72. Ross, R., Glomset, J., Kariya, B., and Harker, L.: A platelet-dependent serum factor that stimulates the proliferation of arterial smooth muscle cells in vitro. Proc. Natl. Acad. Sci. U.S.A. *71*:1207, 1974.
73. Oka, Y., and Orth, D. N.: Human plasma epidermal growth factor/beta-urogastrone is associated with blood platelets. J. Clin. Invest. *72*:249, 1983.
74. Assoian, R. K., Komoriya, A., Meyers, C. A., et al.: Transforming growth factor-β in human platelets: Identification of a major storage site, purification, and characterization. J. Biol. Chem. *258*:7155, 1983.
75. Baumgartner, H. R.: Platelet interaction with vascular structures. Thromb. Diath. Haemorrh. *51* (Suppl.):161, 1972.
76. Larsson, P. T., Wallen, N. H., and Hjemdahl, P.: Norepinephrine-induced human platelet activation in vivo is only partly counteracted by aspirin. Circulation *89*:1951, 1994.
77. Grignani, G., Soffiantino, F., Zucchella, M., et al.: Platelet activation by emotional stress in patients with coronary artery disease. Circulation *83* (Suppl. II):II128, 1991.
78. Fuster, V., Chesebro, J. H., Frye, R. L., and Elveback, L. R.: Platelet survival and the development of coronary artery disease in the young adult: Effects of cigarette smoking, strong family history, and medical therapy. Circulation *63*:546, 1981.
79. Ridker, P. M., Hennekens, C. H., and Stampfer, J. J.: A prospective study of lipoprotein(s) and the risk of myocardial infarction. JAMA *270*:2195, 1993.
80. Kostner, G. M., Czinner, A., Pfeiffer, K. H., and Bihari-Varga, M.: Lipoprotein(a) concentrations as indicators for atherosclerosis. Arch. Dis. Child. *66*:1054, 1991.
81. Bogalusa Heart Study: Racial (black/white) differences in serum lipoprotein(a) distribution and its relation to parental myocardial infarction in children: Bogalusa Heart Study. Circulation *84*:160, 1991.
82. Jonasson, L., Holm, J., Skalli, O., et al.: Regional accumulations of T cells, macrophages, and smooth muscle cells in the human atherosclerotic plaque. Arteriosclerosis *6*:131–138, 1986.
83. Gown, A. M., Tsukada, T., and Ross, R.: Human atherosclerosis. II. Immunocytochemical analysis of the cellular composition of human atherosclerotic lesions. Am. J. Pathol. *125*:191–207, 1986.
84. Munro, J. M., van der Walt, J. D., Munro, C. S., et al.: An immunohistochemical analysis of human aortic fatty streaks. Hum. Pathol. *18*:375, 1987.
85. Emeson, E. E., and Robertson, A. L., Jr.: T lymphocytes in aortic and coronary intimas: Their potential role in atherogenesis. Am. J. Pathol. *130*:369, 1988.
86. Minick, C. R., and Murphy, G. E.: Experimental induction of atheroarteriosclerosis by the synergy of allergic injury to arteries and lipid-rich diet. II. Effect of repeated injections of horse serum in rabbits fed a lipid-rich, cholesterol-poor diet. Am. J. Pathol. *73*:265, 1973.
87. Hansson, G. K., Holm, J., and Jonasson, L.: Detection of activated T lymphocytes in the human atherosclerotic plaque. Am. J. Pathol. *135*:169, 1989.
88. Hansson, G. K., Jonasson, L., Holm, J., and Clasesson-Welsh, L.: MHC antigen expression in the atherosclerotic plaque: Smooth muscle cells express HLA-DR, HLA-DQ, and the invariant gamma chain. Clin. Exp. Immunol. *64*:261, 1986.
89. Libby, P., and Hansson, G. K.: Involvement of the immune system in human atherogenesis: Current knowledge and unanswered questions. Lab. Invest. *64*:5, 1991.

THE LESIONS OF ATHEROSCLEROSIS

90. McGill, H. C., Jr. (ed.): The Geographic Pathology of Atherosclerosis. Baltimore, Williams and Wilkins Co., 1968.
91. Geer, J. C., McGill, H. C., Jr., and Strong, J. P.: The fine structure of human atherosclerotic lesions. Am. J. Pathol. *38*:263, 1961.
92. Geer, J. C.: Fine structure of human aortic intimal thickening and fatty streaks. Lab. Invest. *14*:1764, 1965.
93. Ghidoni, J. J., and O'Neal, R. M.: Recent advances in molecular pathology: A review: Ultrastructure of human atheroma. Exp. Mol. Pathol. *7*:378, 1967.
94. Stary, H. C., Chandler, A. B., Glagov, S., et al.: A definition of initial, fatty streak and intermediate lesions of atherosclerosis: A report from the Committee on Vascular Lesions of the Council on Arteriosclerosis, American Heart Association. Circulation *89*:2462, 1994.
95. A report from the Committee on Vascular Lesions of the Council on Arteriosclerosis, American Heart Association: Definitions of advanced types of atherosclerotic lesions and a historical classification of atherosclerosis. Circulation *15*:1512, 1995.
96. Stary, H. C.: Evolution of atherosclerotic plaques in the coronary arteries of young adults. Arteriosclerosis *3*:471a, 1983.
97. McGill, H. C., Jr.: Persistent problems in the pathogenesis of atherosclerosis. Arteriosclerosis *4*:443, 1984.
98. Tsudaka, T., Rosenfeld, M., Ross, R., and Gown, A. M.: Immunocytochemical analysis of cellular components in atherosclerotic lesions: Use of monoclonal antibodies with the Watanabe and fat-fed rabbit. Arteriosclerosis *6*:601, 1986.
99. Glagov, S., and Ozoa, A.: Significance of the relatively low incidence of atherosclerosis in the pulmonary, renal and mesenteric arteries. Ann. N. Y. Acad. Sci. *149*:940, 1968.
100. Strong, J. P., Eggen, D. A., and Oalmann, M. C.: The natural history, geographic pathology, and epidemiology of atherosclerosis. *In* Wissler, R. W., and Geer, J. C. (eds.): The Pathogenesis of Atherosclerosis. Baltimore, Williams and Wilkins Co., 1972, p. 20.
101. Glagov, S., Rowley, D. A., Cramer, D. B., and Page, R. G.: Heart rate during 24 hours of usual activity in 100 normal men. J. Appl. Physiol. *29*:799, 1970.
102. Wissler, R. W., and Vesselinovitch, D.: Atherosclerosis—relationship to coronary blood flow. Am. J. Cardiol. *52*:2A, 1983.

HYPOTHESES OF ATHEROGENESIS

103. Virchow, R.: Phlogose und thrombose in gefassystem. *In* Virchow, R. (ed.): Gesammelte Abhandlungen zur Wissenschaftlichen Medicin. Berlin, Meidinger Sohn and Co., 1856, p. 458.
104. von Rokitansky, C.: A Manual of Pathological Anatomy, translated by Day, G. E. Vol. 4. London, The Sydenham Society, 1852.
105. Duguid, J. B.: Thrombosis as a factor in the pathogenesis of coronary atherosclerosis. J. Pathol. Bacteriol. *58*:207, 1946.
106. Ross, R.: Atherosclerosis—a problem of the biology of arterial wall cells and their interaction with blood components. Arteriosclerosis *1*:293, 1981.
107. Benditt, E. P., and Benditt, J. M.: Evidence for a monoclonal origin of human atherosclerotic plaques. Proc. Natl. Acad. Sci. U.S.A. *70*:1753, 1973.
108. Hajjar, D. P., Fabricant, C. G., Minick, C. R., and Fabricant, J.: Virus-induced atherosclerosis: Herpes virus infection alters arterial cholesterol metabolism and accumulation. Am. J. Pathol. *122*:62, 1986.
108a. Glasser, S. P., Selwyn, A. F., and Ganz, P.: Atherosclerosis: Risk factors and the vascular endothelium. Am. Heart J. *131*:379, 1996.
109. Kuo, C. C., Gown, A. M., Benditt, E. P., and Grayston, J. T.: Detection of *Chlamydia pneumoniae* in aortic lesions of atherosclerosis by immunocytochemical stain. Arterioscler. Thromb. *13*:1501, 1993.
110. Leary, T.: The genesis of atherosclerosis. Arch. Pathol. *32*:507, 1941.
111. Springer, T. A.: Adhesion receptors of the immune system. Nature *346*:425, 1990.
112. Cybulsky, M. I., and Gimbrone, M. A., Jr.: Endothelial expression of a mononuclear leukocyte adhesion molecule during atherogenesis. Science *251*:788, 1991.
113. Navab, M., Hama, S. Y., Nguyen, T. B., and Fogelman, A. M.: Monocyte adhesion and transmigration in atherosclerosis. Cor. Art. Dis. *5*:198, 1994.
114. Parthasarathy, S., Quinn, M. T., Schwenke, D. C., et al.: Oxidative modification of beta-very low density lipoprotein: Potential role in monocyte recruitment and foam cell formation. Arteriosclerosis *9*:398, 1989.
115. Goldstein, J. L., Ho, Y. K., Basu, S. K., and Brown, M. S.: Binding site of macrophages that mediates uptake and degradation of acetylated low density lipoprotein, producing massive cholesterol deposition. Proc. Natl. Acad. Sci. U.S.A. *76*:333, 1979.
116. Steinberg, D.: Antioxidants and atherosclerosis: A current perspective. Circulation *86*:1420, 1991.
117. Kodama, T., Freeman, M., Rohrer, L., et al.: Type I macrophage scavenger receptor contains α-helical and collagen-like coiled coils. Nature *343*:531, 1990.
118. Assoian, R. K., Grotendorst, G. R., Miller, D. M., and Sporn, M. B.: Cellular transformation by coordinated action of three peptide growth factors from human platelets. Nature *309*:804, 1984.
119. Sporn, M. B., Roberts, A. B., Wakefield, L. M., and de Crombrugghe, B.: Some recent advances in the chemistry and biology of transforming growth factor-beta. J. Cell. Biol. *105*:1039, 1987.
120. Ross, R., Masuda, J., Raines, E. W., et al.: Localization of PDGF-B protein in macrophages in all phases of atherogenesis. Science *248*:1009, 1990.
121. Stemerman, M. B., and Ross, R.: Experimental arteriosclerosis. I. Fibrous plaque formation in primates, an electron microscope study. J. Exp. Med. *136*:769, 1972.
122. Shepard, B. L., and French, J. E.: Platelet adhesion in the rabbit abdominal aorta following the removal of the endothelium: A scanning and transmission electron microscopical study. Proc. R. Soc. Lond. (Biol.) *176*:427, 1971.
123. More, S.: Thromboatherosclerosis in normolipemic rabbits: A result of continued endothelial damage. Lab. Invest. *29*:478, 1973.
124. Friedman, R. J., Moore, S., and Singal, D. P.: Repeated endothelial injury and induction of atherosclerosis in normolipemic rabbits by human serum. Lab. Invest. *32*:404, 1975.
125. Harker, L. A., Ross, R., Slichter, S. J., and Scott, C. R.: Homocystine-induced arteriosclerosis: The role of endothelial cell injury and platelet response in its genesis. J. Clin. Invest. *58*:731, 1976.
126. Libby, P., Warner, S. J. C., Salomon, R. N., and Birinyi, L. K.: Production of platelet-derived growth factor–like mitogen by smooth-muscle cells from human atheroma. N. Engl. J. Med. *318*:1493, 1988.

LIPIDS AND LIPOPROTEINS AND MODIFIED LDL IN ATHEROSCLEROSIS

127. Jackson, R. L., and Gotto, A. M., Jr.: Hypothesis concerning membrane structure, cholesterol, and atherosclerosis. *In* Paoletti, R., and Gotto,

A. M., Jr. (eds.): Atherosclerosis Reviews. Vol. 1. New York, Raven Press, 1976, p. 1.
128. Carew, T. E., Schwenke, D. C., and Steinberg, D.: Antiatherogenic effect of probucol unrelated to its hypocholesterolemic effect: Evidence that antioxidants in vivo can selectively inhibit low density lipoprotein degradation in macrophage-rich fatty streaks and slow the progression of atherosclerosis in the Watanabe heritable hyperlipidemic (WHHL) rabbit. Proc. Natl. Acad. Sci. U.S.A. *84*:7725, 1987.
129. Kita, T., Nagano, Y., Yokode, M., et al.: Probucol prevents the progression of atherosclerosis in Watanabe heritable hyperlipidemic rabbit, an animal model for familial hypercholesterolemia. Proc. Natl. Acad. Sci. U.S.A. *84*:5928, 1987.
130. Sasahara, M., Raines, E. W., Chait, A., et al.: Inhibition of hypercholesterolemia-induced atherosclerosis in the nonhuman primate by probucol. I. Is the extent of atherosclerosis related to resistance of LDL to oxidation? J. Clin. Invest. *94*:155, 1994.
131. Boyd, H. C., Gown, A. M., Wolfbauer, G., and Chait, A.: Direct evidence for a protein recognized by a monoclonal antibody against oxidatively modified LDL in atherosclerotic lesions from a Watanabe heritable hyperlipidemic rabbit. Am. J. Pathol. *135*:815, 1989.

GROWTH FACTORS AND CYTOKINES

132. Bowen-Pope, D. F., and Ross, R.: Platelet-derived growth factor. II. Specific binding to cultured cells. J. Biol. Chem. *257*:5161, 1982.
133. Grotendorst, G., Seppa, H. E. J., Kleinman, H. K., and Martin, G.: Attachment of smooth muscle cells to collagen and their migration toward platelet-derived growth factor. Proc. Natl. Acad. Sci. U.S.A. *78*:3669, 1981.
134. Grotendorst, G. R., Chang, T., Seppa, H. E. J., et al.: Platelet-derived growth factor is a chemoattractant for vascular smooth muscle cells. J. Cell. Physiol. *113*:261, 1982.
135. Witte, L. D., and Cornicelli, J. A.: Platelet-derived growth factor stimulates low density lipoprotein receptor activity in cultured human fibroblasts. Proc. Natl. Acad. Sci. U.S.A. *77*:5962, 1986.
136. Bowen-Pope, D. F., Malpass, T. W., Foster, D. M., and Ross, R.: Platelet-derived growth factor in vivo: Levels, activity, and rate of clearance. Blood *64*:458, 1984.
137. Raines, E. W., Bowen-Pope, D. F., and Ross, R.: Plasma binding proteins for platelet-derived growth factor that inhibit its binding to cell-surface receptors. Proc. Natl. Acad. Sci. U.S.A. *81*:3424, 1984.
138. Doolittle, R. F., Hunkapiller, M. W., Hood, L. E., et al.: Simian sarcoma virus onc gene, v-sis, is derived from the gene (or genes) encoding a platelet-derived growth factor. Science *221*:275, 1983.
139. Waterfield, M. D., Scrace, G. T., Whittle, N., et al.: Platelet-derived growth factor is structurally related to the putative transforming protein $p28^{sis}$ of simian sarcoma virus. Nature *304*:35, 1983.
140. Bowen-Pope, D. F., Vogel, A., and Ross, R.: Production of platelet-derived growth factor–like molecules and reduced expression of platelet-derived growth factor receptors accompany transformation by a wide spectrum of agents. Proc. Natl. Acad. Sci. U.S.A. *81*:2396, 1984.
141. Seifert, R. A., Hart, C. E., Phillips, P. E., et al.: Two different subunits associate to create isoform-specific platelet-derived growth factor receptors. J. Biol. Chem. *264*:8771, 1989.

CELLULAR EVENTS THAT OCCUR DURING ATHEROGENESIS

142. Faggiotto, A., Ross, R., and Harker, L.: Studies of hypercholesterolemia in the nonhuman primate. I. Changes that lead to fatty streak formation. Arteriosclerosis *4*:323, 1984.
143. Faggiotto, A., and Ross, R.: Studies of hypercholesterolemia in the nonhuman primate. II. Fatty streak conversion to fibrous plaque. Arteriosclerosis *4*:341, 1984.
144. Masuda, J., and Ross, R.: Atherogenesis during low-level hypercholesterolemia in the nonhuman primate. I. Fatty streak formation. Arteriosclerosis *10*:164, 1990.
145. Masuda, J., and Ross, R.: Atherogenesis during low-level hypercholesterolemia in the nonhuman primate. II. Fatty streak conversion to fibrous plaque. Arteriosclerosis *10*:178, 1990.
146. Gerrity, R. G., Naito, H. K., Richardson, M., and Schwartz, C. J.: Dietary induced atherogenesis in swine: Morphology of the intima in prelesion stages. Am. J. Pathol. *95*:775, 1979.
147. Gerrity, R. G.: The role of the monocyte in atherogenesis. I. Transition of blood-borne monocytes into foam cells in fatty lesions. Am. J. Pathol. *103*:181, 1981.
148. Gerrity, R. G., Goss, J. A., and Soby, L.: Control of monocyte recruitment by chemotactic factor(s) in lesion-prone areas of swine aorta. Arteriosclerosis *5*:55, 1985.
149. Rosenfeld, M. E., Tsukada, T., Chait, A., et al.: Fatty streak expansion and maturation in Watanabe heritable hyperlipemic and comparably hypercholesterolemic fat-fed rabbits. Arteriosclerosis *7*:24, 1987.
150. Nakashima, Y., Plump, A. S., Raines, E. W., et al.: ApoE-deficient mice develop lesions of all phases of atherosclerosis throughout the arterial tree. Arterioscler. Thromb. *14*:133, 1994.
151. Reddick, R. L., Zhang, S. H., and Maeda, N.: Atherosclerosis in mice lacking apo E: Evaluation of lesional development and progression. Arterioscler. Thromb. *14*:141, 1994.
152. Reidy, M. A., and Schwartz, S. M.: Endothelial regeneration. III. Time course of intimal changes after small defined injury to rat aortic endothelium. Lab. Invest. *44*:301, 1981.
153. Reidy, M. A., and Schwartz, S. M.: Endothelial regeneration. IV. Endotoxin: A nondenuding injury to aortic endothelium. Lab. Invest. *48*:25, 1983.
154. Hansson, G. K., Bondjers, G., Bylock, A., and Hjalmarsson, L.: Ultrastructural studies on nonatherosclerotic rabbits. Exp. Mol. Pathol. *33*:301, 1980.
155. Reidy, M. A., and Schwartz, S. M.: Recent advances in molecular pathology: Arterial endothelium—assessment of in vivo injury. Exp. Mol. Pathol. *41*:419, 1984.

REGRESSION OF ATHEROSCLEROSIS

156. Armstrong, M. L., Warner, E. D., and Conner, W. E.: Regression of coronary atheromatosis in rhesus monkeys. Circ. Res. *27*:59, 1970.
157. Wissler, R. W., and Vesselinovitch, D.: Studies of regression of advanced atherosclerosis in experimental animals and man. Ann. N. Y. Acad. Sci. *275*:363, 1976.
158. Clarkson, T. B., Bond, M. G., Bullock, B. C., et al.: A study of atherosclerosis regression in *Macaca mulatta*. V. Changes in abdominal aorta and carotid and coronary arteries from animals with atherosclerosis induced for 38 months and then regressed for 24 or 48 months at plasma cholesterol concentrations of 300 or 200 mg/dl. Exp. Mol. Pathol. *41*:96, 1984.
159. Badimon, J. J., Badimon, L., and Fuster, V.: Regression of atherosclerotic lesions by high density lipoprotein plasma fraction in the cholesterol-fed rabbit. J. Clin. Invest. *85*:1234, 1990.
160. Brown, B. G., Albers, J. J., Fisher, L. D., et al.: Treatment study: A randomized trial demonstrating coronary disease regression and clinical benefit from lipid altering therapy among men with high apolipoprotein B. N. Engl. J. Med. *323*:1289, 1990.
161. Davies, M. J., and Thomas, A. C.: Plaque fissuring: The cause of acute myocardial infarction, sudden ischemic death and crescendo angina. Br. Heart J. *53*:363, 1985.
162. Falk, E.: Unstable angina with fatal outcome: Dynamic coronary thrombosis leading to infarction and/or sudden death: Autopsy evidence of recurrent mural thrombosis with peripheral embolization culminating in total vascular occlusion. Circulation *71*:699, 1985.
163. Blankenhorn, D. H., and Hodis, H. N.: Arterial imaging and atherosclerosis reversal. Arterioscler. Thromb. *14*:177, 1994.
164. Brown, B. G., Zhao, X.-Q., Sacco, D. E., and Albers, J. J.: Lipid lowering and plaque regression: New insights into prevention of plaque disruption and clinical events in coronary disease. Circulation *87*:1781, 1993.
165. Brensike, J. F., Levy, R. I., Kelsey, S. F., et al.: Effects of therapy with cholestyramine on progression of coronary arteriosclerosis: Results of the NHLBI Type II Coronary Intervention Study. Circulation *69*:313, 1984.
166. Blankenhorn, D. H., Selzer, R. H., Mack, W. J., et al.: Evaluation of colestipol/niacin therapy with computer-derived coronary end point measures: A comparison of different measures of treatment effect. Circulation *86*:1701, 1992.
167. Ornish, D., Brown, S. E., Scherwitz, L. W., et al.: Can lifestyle changes reverse coronary heart disease? The lifestyle heart trial. Lancet *336*:129, 1990.
168. Buchwald, H., Matts, J. P., Fitch, L. L., et al., for the Program on the Surgical Control of the Hyperlipidemias (POSCH) Group: Changes in sequential coronary arteriograms and subsequent coronary events. JAMA *268*:1429, 1992.
169. Kane, J. P., Malloy, M. J., Ports, T. A., et al.: Regression of coronary atherosclerosis during treatment of familial hypercholesterolemia with combined drug regimens. JAMA *264*:3007, 1990.
170. Watts, G. F., Lewis, B., Brunt, J. N., et al.: Effects on coronary artery disease of lipid-lowering diet, or diet plus cholestyramine, in the St. Thomas' Atherosclerosis Regression Study (STARS). Lancet *339*:563, 1992.
171. Haskell, W. L., Alderman, E. L., Fair, J. M., et al.: Effects of intensive multiple risk factor reduction on coronary atherosclerosis and clinical cardiac events in men and women with coronary artery disease: The Stanford Coronary Risk Intervention Project (SCRIP). Circulation *89*:975, 1994.
172. Cannon, P. J.: Eicosanoids and the blood vessel wall. Circulation *70*:523, 1984.

THROMBOSIS

173. Chesebro, J. H., Clements, I. P., Fuster, V., et al.: A platelet-inhibitor–drug trial in coronary-artery bypass operations: Benefit of perioperative dipyridamole and aspirin therapy on early postoperative vein-graft patency. N. Engl. J. Med. *307*:73, 1982.
174. Skinner, M. P., Yuan, C., Mitsumori, L., et al.: Serial magnetic resonance imaging of experimental atherosclerosis detects lesion fine structure, progression, and complications in vivo. Nature Med. *1*:69, 1995.

Chapter 35
Dyslipidemia and Other Risk Factors for Coronary Artery Disease

JOHN A. FARMER, ANTONIO M. GOTTO, Jr.

DECLINING MORTALITY AND THE RISK FACTOR CONCEPT 1126
DYSLIPIDEMIA 1126
Hypercholesterolemia 1127
Low High-Density Lipoprotein Cholesterol .1143
Hypertriglyceridemia 1144
Elevated Lipoprotein(a) 1146
TOBACCO USE 1147
HYPERTENSION 1148
DIABETES MELLITUS 1150
PHYSICAL INACTIVITY 1151
OBESITY 1152
NONMODIFIABLE RISK FACTORS 1152
Family History 1152
Age 1152
Gender 1153
OTHER RISK FACTORS 1153
REFERENCES 1155

DECLINING MORTALITY AND THE RISK FACTOR CONCEPT

Coronary artery disease (CAD) is the single most important disease entity in the United States and many other industrialized nations in terms of both mortality and morbidity. In the United States, CAD accounts for fully one-half of the nearly 1 million deaths each year from cardiovascular disease and is the leading cause of death in both genders.[1] Each year, about 1.5 million Americans suffer acute myocardial infarction, and almost all myocardial infarctions are due to atherosclerosis of the coronary arteries. Among the two-thirds who survive the myocardial infarction, about two-thirds do not make a full recovery; in 19 per cent of Americans aged 15 years or older who are categorized as disabled, the disability is from CAD or other cardiovascular disease.[1] CAD often strikes at the height of working careers. About 45 per cent of myocardial infarctions occur in people under age 65, and about 37 per cent of American males and 29 per cent of American females who die of CAD are younger than 55.[1] The economic burden of CAD to the nation is also enormous: An estimated $50 billion to $100 billion per year in medical interventions and lost wages.[2,3]

Nevertheless, an encouraging downward trend in CAD death rates in the United States began in the early 1960's and has continued. The CAD mortality rate fell 54 per cent between 1963 and 1990, accounting for 49 per cent of the decline in the total mortality rate.[4] In 1950, the annual age-adjusted death rate from myocardial infarction was 226.4 per 100,000; in 1991, it was 108.0.[1] The period of 1982 to 1992 alone saw a 31 per cent decline in myocardial infarction death rate.[1] These decreases have coincided with national risk reduction efforts—beginning in the 1960's, 1970's, and 1980's, respectively—against the major CAD risk factors of smoking, hypertension, and hypercholesterolemia, as well as with the improvement of therapies for myocardial infarction. The percentage of Americans who smoke has declined 37 per cent since 1965,[1] although there may now be a leveling off and even an increase in some groups, notably young women. The annual death rate from hypertension was 56.0 per 100,000 in 1950, compared with 6.5 in 1991.[1] Between 1960 and 1991, the average plasma cholesterol level decreased from 220 mg/dl to 205 mg/dl in Americans aged 20 to 74 years.[4] Nevertheless, these risk factors remain common: estimates are that 28 per cent of American men and 22 per cent of American women smoke,[5] 25 and 23 per cent have hypertension,[6] and 32 and 27 per cent have hypercholesterolemia[7] that requires dietary therapy by current National Cholesterol Education Program (NCEP) clinical guidelines.[2,3]

Risk factor reduction is the primary clinical approach to preventing CAD morbidity and mortality. Epidemiological studies have clearly demonstrated that risk factors such as dyslipidemia, hypertension, and the use of tobacco products act in a synergistic manner.[8] The concept of risk factor identification and modification is based on the premise that exposure to certain host and environmental factors increases the statistical risk for developing a disease and that alteration of these conditions decreases the risk. However, a given factor may not stand in a cause-and-effect relation to the disease but may be simply a nonspecific marker of the disease process. Criteria for determining whether an observed statistical association reflects causality include strength of the association, expressed by the relative risk of individuals exposed to a certain factor compared with individuals not exposed; whether the association represents a dose–response relation, so that relative risk is progressively increased at increasing levels of exposure to the factor; precedence of exposure to clinical onset of disease; consistency of results in different populations; independence of the association when controlling for other known risk factors; predictivity of disease incidence in different populations; and biological plausibility.[9]

Major CAD risk factors established by these criteria are dyslipidemia, hypertension, tobacco use, and diabetes mellitus. Other CAD risk factors include physical inactivity, obesity, family history of CAD, age, gender, hemostatic factors, homocysteinemia, alcohol consumption, and psychological factors. The identification of risk factors provides a means for decreasing CAD risk, through the reduction of modifiable risk factors, and for informing treatment decisions, through more accurate determination of overall risk status.

DYSLIPIDEMIA

Lipids are transported through the plasma compartment in lipoproteins, complex water-soluble molecules consisting of a core of cholesteryl ester and triglyceride covered by a surface monolayer of phospholipids, free cholesterol, and apolipoproteins. The major plasma lipoproteins—chylomicrons, very-low-density lipoprotein (VLDL), intermediate-density lipoprotein (IDL), low-density lipoprotein (LDL), and high-density lipoprotein (HDL)—are distinguished by lipid content, density on ultracentrifugation, size, mobility on electrophoresis, and the proteins on their

TABLE 35–1 CLASSIFICATION AND PROPERTIES OF PLASMA LIPOPROTEINS

LIPOPROTEIN CLASS	MAJOR LIPIDS	APOLIPOPROTEINS	DENSITY (g/ml)	DIAMETER (Å)	ELECTROPHORETIC MOBILITY
Chylomicrons	Dietary triglyceride, cholesteryl ester	A-I, A-II, A-IV, B-48, C-I, C-II, C-III, E	<0.95	800–5000	Origin
Chylomicron remnants	Dietary cholesteryl ester	B-48, E	<1.006	>300	Origin
VLDL	Endogenous triglyceride	B-100, C-I, C-II, C-III, E	<1.006	300–800	Pre-beta
IDL	Cholesteryl ester, triglyceride	B-100, E	1.006–1.019	250–350	Broad-beta
LDL	Cholesteryl ester	B-100	1.019–1.063	180–280	Beta
HDL_2	Cholesteryl ester	A-I, A-II, C-I, C-II, C-III, E	1.063–1.125	90–120	Alpha
HDL_3	Cholesteryl ester	A-I, A-II, C-I, C-II, C-III, E	1.125–1.210	50–90	Alpha

Abbreviations: HDL = high-density lipoprotein; IDL = intermediate-density lipoprotein; LDL = low-density lipoprotein; VLDL = very-low-density lipoprotein.

surfaces (Table 35–1). The lipoproteins vary in their contribution to atherosclerotic risk: The triglyceride-rich lipoproteins—chylomicrons and VLDL—are not thought to be atherogenic, but the remnants of their lipolysis—chylomicron remnants and IDL, respectively—are believed to be atherogenic. The atherogenicity of LDL—the metabolic end product of VLDL—and lipoprotein(a) [Lp(a)] has been established, as has the cardioprotective effect of HDL (see below).

In dyslipidemia, circulating levels of lipid or lipoprotein fractions are abnormal because of genetic and/or environmental conditions that alter the production, catabolism, or clearance of plasma lipoproteins from the circulation. Dyslipidemias may be classified according to which lipoprotein levels are abnormal, as in the Fredrickson classification system (Table 35–2). The Fredrickson classification system is not diagnostic and does not consider HDL or Lp(a).

Hypercholesterolemia

The dyslipidemia most clearly associated with increased risk for CAD is hypercholesterolemia, particularly elevated plasma levels of cholesterol carried in LDL. LDL contains approximately 70 per cent of cholesterol in the blood and is the primary target of intervention in the guidelines of the second Adult Treatment Panel of the NCEP.[2,3]

The association between elevated blood cholesterol and CAD has been established in observational and interventional epidemiological studies, examples of which are presented here. These data support the lipid hypothesis: CAD risk is increased at increasing plasma cholesterol levels and can be decreased by decreasing plasma cholesterol.

Observational Studies

A continuous and graded positive relation was demonstrated between total cholesterol level and CAD mortality in the more than 350,000 men screened for the Multiple Risk Factor Intervention Trial (MRFIT).[10] The relation between total cholesterol level and coronary disease is not limited by nationality or ethnicity, as demonstrated in the Seven Countries Study, which determined that in areas such as Japan and countries surrounding the Mediterranean Sea, where the dietary intake of saturated fat is low and average plasma cholesterol level is relatively low, the mortality rate for CAD is also low, compared with countries such as Finland and the United States, where both the average plasma cholesterol level and the coronary mortality rate are higher.[11] Similarly, in the Ni-Hon-San Study, men of Japanese descent living in the United States consumed a diet higher in fat and cholesterol than Japanese men living in Japan[12] and had higher total cholesterol levels[13] and a higher age-adjusted incidence of myocardial infarction and CAD death.[14]

Interventional Studies in Primary Prevention

Although observational data lend credence to the lipid hypothesis, they do not demonstrate the effect of cholesterol lowering on coronary morbidity and mortality. Consequently, randomized, controlled clinical trials have employed a variety of interventions to determine the efficacy of cholesterol lowering in preventing CAD events in individuals free of known CAD, or primary prevention, and in preventing subsequent CAD events in subjects with known CAD, or secondary prevention.

Cholesterol-lowering interventions used to prevent CAD in subjects without known CAD have included pharmacological monotherapy and life style modification. Clinical events such as myocardial infarction and CAD death are typical endpoints in these studies.

LIPID RESEARCH CLINICS CORONARY PRIMARY PREVENTION TRIAL. The Lipid Research Clinics Coronary Primary Prevention Trial (LRC-CPPT) randomized 3806 hypercholesterolemic men (total cholesterol ≥265 mg/dl, LDL cholesterol ≥190 mg/dl, triglyceride ≤300 mg/dl), aged 35 to 59 years, to receive either the bile-acid sequestrant cholestyramine at a prescribed dosage of 24 gm/day or a placebo.[15] All subjects were to follow a moderate cholesterol-lowering diet (cholesterol 400 mg/day, polyunsaturated fat: saturated fat ratio 0.8). The study design predicted a 28 per cent decrease in total cholesterol in cholestyramine subjects ad-

TABLE 35–2 FREDRICKSON CLASSIFICATION OF THE HYPERLIPIDEMIAS*

PHENOTYPE	LIPOPROTEIN(S) ELEVATED	PLASMA CHOLESTEROL LEVEL	PLASMA TRIGLYCERIDE LEVEL	ATHEROGENICITY	RELATIVE FREQUENCY†
I	Chylomicrons	Normal to ↑	↑↑↑↑	None seen	<1%
IIa	LDL	↑↑	Normal	+++	10%
IIb	LDL and VLDL	↑↑	↑↑	+++	40%
III	IDL	↑↑	↑↑↑	+++	<1%
IV	VLDL	Normal to ↑	↑↑	+	45%
V	VLDL and chylomicrons	↑ to ↑↑	↑↑↑↑	+	5%

* The Fredrickson classification does not consider levels of high-density lipoprotein (HDL) cholesterol. It is not an etiological classification and does not differentiate primary and secondary hyperlipidemias.

† Approximate percentages of US patients with hyperlipidemia.

Abbreviations: IDL = intermediate-density lipoprotein; LDL = low-density lipoprotein; VLDL = very-low-density lipoprotein.

(From International Lipid Information Bureau: The ILIB Lipid Handbook for Clinical Practice: Blood Lipids and Coronary Heart Disease. Houston, International Lipid Information Bureau, 1995.)

hering to the prescribed dosage, but adherence was lower than expected because of gastrointestinal side effects and poor palatability of the drug. The actual cholestyramine dosage averaged 14 gm/day. The average time on trial was 7.4 years.

In the placebo group, diet alone decreased total cholesterol 5 per cent. Total cholesterol decreased 13 per cent from baseline in the group treated with diet and cholestyramine, and LDL cholesterol decreased 8 per cent and 20 per cent in the respective groups. In the cholestyramine group, the primary endpoint of nonfatal myocardial infarction and CAD death was significantly reduced 19 per cent. Development of new-onset angina pectoris was significantly reduced 20 per cent in the cholestyramine group, and incidence of new positive exercise stress test results was significantly reduced 25 per cent. Incidence of coronary bypass surgery was reduced 21 per cent, which was not statistically significant. CAD mortality was reduced 24 per cent, but total mortality was reduced only 7 per cent because of an increase in noncardiovascular deaths, particularly accidental and violent deaths; neither of these reductions in mortality was significant.

In the cholestyramine group, 32 per cent of subjects achieved a reduction in LDL cholesterol that was greater than 25 per cent. In this subgroup, the incidence of nonfatal myocardial infarction and CAD death was reduced 64 per cent.[16]

The LRC-CPPT provided the first major clinical substantiation of the lipid hypothesis. Its results were the first to give rise to the rule of thumb that a 1 per cent decrease in total cholesterol reduces the incidence of CAD events 2 to 3 per cent.

WORLD HEALTH ORGANIZATION COOPERATIVE TRIAL. The World Health Organization (WHO) Cooperative Trial randomized more than 10,000 men, aged 30 to 59 years, with total cholesterol level in the upper tertile of those screened for the trial, in which they received either the fibric-acid derivative clofibrate, 1600 mg/day, or a placebo.[17] Mean duration of treatment was 5.3 years. Results were not initially analyzed on an intent-to-treat basis, and data on subjects who dropped out of the trial because of morbid events, including nonfatal myocardial infarction, were not included in the original analysis.

In the group receiving clofibrate, total cholesterol decreased 9 per cent from baseline, and CAD incidence was significantly reduced 20 per cent. However, total mortality was increased in this group, largely due to an increase in noncardiovascular deaths. An analysis conducted almost 8 years after the trial ended indicated that the excess in mortality with clofibrate decreased from 47 per cent during the trial to 11 per cent during the entire 13 years of follow-up and was no longer statistically significant.[18]

HELSINKI HEART STUDY. The Helsinki Heart Study randomized 4081 men, aged 40 to 55 years, with non-HDL cholesterol greater than 200 mg/dl to receive the fibric-acid derivative gemfibrozil, 1200 mg/day, or placebo for 5 years.[19] Included in the trial were hypertriglyceridemic as well as hypercholesterolemic subjects. All subjects also received dietary counseling.

Compared with the placebo group, the gemfibrozil group had a 10 per cent decrease in total cholesterol, an 11 per cent decrease in LDL cholesterol, an 11 per cent increase in HDL cholesterol, and a 35 per cent decrease in triglyceride. The primary endpoint, incidence of cardiac events, defined as fatal and nonfatal myocardial infarction and cardiac death, was significantly reduced 34 per cent in the gemfibrozil group. CAD mortality was 26 per cent lower in the gemfibrozil group, but total mortality was slightly higher because of an increase in noncardiovascular deaths, particularly deaths due to accidents, violence, or intracranial hemorrhage; none of these differences was statistically significant.[20]

OSLO STUDY DIET AND ANTISMOKING TRIAL. The Oslo Study Diet and Antismoking Trial randomized 1232 men, aged 40 to 49 years, with total cholesterol of 290 to 380 mg/dl, systolic blood pressure below 150 mm Hg, and a coronary risk score, based on cholesterol, smoking, and blood pressure, in the highest quartile of the distribution.[21] Subjects in the intervention group were given dietary and antismoking advice. Approximately 80 per cent of each group were smokers.

During the 5-year trial, total cholesterol in the intervention group decreased approximately 13 per cent compared with the control group, and triglyceride decreased 20 per cent. Although the quantity of cigarettes smoked decreased 45 per cent more in the intervention group than in the control group, only 25 per cent of smokers in the intervention group stopped smoking, compared with 17 per cent of smokers in the control group. Incidence of fatal and nonfatal myocardial infarction and sudden coronary death was significantly reduced 47 per cent in the intervention group. The difference in CAD incidence between treatment groups was thought to be largely due to the reduction in total cholesterol, and 25 per cent was attributed to reduced cigarette consumption. Coronary mortality was reduced 55 per cent and total mortality was reduced 33 per cent in the intervention group, but these differences were not statistically significant.

At 102-month follow-up, 3 years after the trial was completed, the reduction in total cholesterol achieved by the intervention group during the trial was maintained.[22] Total cholesterol in the control group was reduced but remained higher than in the intervention group. Cigarette consumption in the intervention group was higher than at the end of the trial, although not as high as baseline; cigarette consumption in the control group remained about the same as at the end of the trial and only slightly higher than in the intervention group. Although the differences in risk factors between treatment groups were less than during the trial, between-group differences in incidence of fatal and nonfatal myocardial infarction and sudden coronary death remained the same as during the trial. Sudden death, coronary death, and total coronary events occurred significantly less frequently in the intervention group. Total mortality was reduced 40 per cent in the intervention group, which was a marginally significant difference.

WEST OF SCOTLAND CORONARY PREVENTION STUDY. The benefit of lipid-lowering with a 3-hydroxy-3-methylglutaryl coenzyme A (HMG-CoA) reductase inhibitor was extended to primary prevention in the West of Scotland Coronary Prevention Study (WOSCOPS), which randomized 6595 men, aged 45 to 64 years, with no history of myocardial infarction to receive pravastatin, 40 mg/day, or placebo.[22a] Eligible subjects had an LDL cholesterol level of at least 155 mg/dl on two assessments despite dietary therapy, at least 174 mg/dl on at least one assessment, and no more than 232 mg/dl on one assessment. Individuals with stable angina were not excluded if they had not been hospitalized within the previous year. The primary endpoint was either definite nonfatal myocardial infarction or CAD death as a first event. Mean follow-up was 4.9 years.

Lipid changes by intent-to-treat analysis are not available, but in subjects who actually received pravastatin, total plasma cholesterol was decreased 20 per cent, LDL cholesterol was decreased 26 per cent, triglyceride was decreased 12 per cent, and HDL cholesterol was increased 5 per cent.

For the primary endpoint, the relative risk in the group randomized to pravastatin was reduced 31 per cent compared with the group randomized to placebo, which was a significant difference. Noncardiovascular mortality was not significantly different between treatment groups. The group randomized to pravastatin had a 22 per cent reduction in death resulting from any cause compared with the group randomized to placebo, but this difference was of borderline statistical significance ($P = .051$).

TABLE 35–3 MAJOR ANGIOGRAPHICALLY MONITORED LIPID-LOWERING TRIALS IN PATIENTS WITH CORONARY ATHEROSCLEROSIS: LIPID AND ANGIOGRAPHIC RESULTS

TRIAL*	SUBJECTS†	TRIAL PERIOD (YR)	INTERVENTION‡	PER CENT LIPID RESPONSE (RX/CONTROL) TC	LDL-C	ASSESSMENT§	PER CENT PATIENTS WITH CORONARY LESION Progression (Rx/Control)	Regression (Rx/Control)	EVENTS (RX/CONTROL)‖
NHLBI	143 M + F	5	Ch	−17/−1	−26/−5	P	32/49	7/7	8/12
CLAS I	188 M	2	C + N	−26/−4	−43/−5	P	39/61	16/4	25/25
CLAS II	103 M	4	C + N	−25/−6	−40/−6	P	48/85	18/6	15/14
FATS	120 M	2.5	C + N	−23/−3	−32/−7	Q	25/46	39/11	2/10
			C + L	−34/−3	−46/−7	Q	21/46	32/11	3/10
UCSF-SCOR	72 M + F	2	C/N/L¶	−31/−9	−39/−12	Q	20/41	32/13	0/1
STARS	90 M	3	Ch	−25/−2	−36/−3	Q	12/46	33/4	1/10
			Diet alone	−14/−2	−16/−3	Q	15/46	38/4	3/10
POSCH	838 M + F	5**	PIB	−28/−5	−42/−7	P	37/65	13/5	
		10**		−22/−4	−39/−6	P	55/85	6/4	82/125
LHT	48 M + F	1	Life style	−24/−5	−37/−6	Q	18/53	82/42	Not available
MARS	270 M + F	2	L	−32/−2	−45/−3	Q	29/41	23/12	22/31
						P	47/65	23/11	
CCAIT	331 M + F	2	L	−21/−1	−29/−2	Q	33/50	10/7	15/20
REGRESS	885 M	2	P	−20/+2	−29/+2	Q	45/55	17/9	59/93
MAAS	381 M + F	4	S	−22/+3	−31/+7	Q	41/54	33/20	53/74

TC = total cholesterol; LDL-C = low-density lipoprotein cholesterol.

* NHLBI: National Heart, Lung, and Blood Institute Type II Coronary Intervention Study[30]; CLAS I: Cholesterol Lowering Atherosclerosis Study I[33]; CLAS II[35]; FATS: Familial Atherosclerosis Treatment Study[36]; UCSF SCOR: University of California, San Francisco, Arteriosclerosis Specialized Center of Research Intervention Trial[37]; STARS: St. Thomas' Atherosclerosis Regression Study[38]; POSCH: Program on the Surgical Control of the Hyperlipidemias[39]; LHT: Lifestyle Heart Trial[41]; MARS: Monitored Atherosclerosis Regression Study[42]; CCAIT: Canadian Coronary Atherosclerosis Intervention Trial[44]; REGRESS: Regression Growth Evaluation Statin Study[46]; MAAS: Multicentre Anti-Atheroma Study.[47]

† M = male; F = female.

‡ All interventions included diet. C = colestipol; Ch = cholestyramine; L = lovastatin; N = nicotinic acid; P = pravastatin; PIB = partial ileal bypass; S = simvastatin.

§ P = panel assessment of lesion change (viewer estimation); Q = assessment by quantitative coronary angiography.

‖ Events variably defined among trials; generally, coronary death, myocardial infarction, unstable ischemia requiring revascularization.

¶ Various binary and ternary drug combinations.

** Follow-up rather than trial period (intervention was surgery).

Adapted from Jones, P. H., and Gotto, A. M., Jr.: Prevention of coronary heart disease in 1994: Evidence for intervention. Heart Dis. Stroke *3*:290, 1994.

Interventional Studies in Secondary Prevention

Individuals with existing CAD or other clinical atherosclerotic disease are at the highest short-term risk for a CAD event. However, aggressive intervention has been shown to reduce that risk. Secondary-prevention trials using dietary, pharmacological, and/or surgical interventions have demonstrated a decrease in the progression of atherosclerotic lesions (Table 35–3) and a reduction in CAD morbidity and mortality with lipid-regulating therapy.[23] Recently published data also establish the beneficial effect of aggressive intervention on total mortality.

Early studies with angiographic endpoints were hampered by the limitation of visual interpretation as the only available means of assessing progression, regression, or stabilization of atherosclerotic lesions. The anatomical changes induced by therapeutic interventions are often quite modest and may be better assessed by computer-based quantitative techniques, which are more reproducible than visual assessment because they are not subject to the large interobserver and intraobserver variability that may occur in visual interpretation.[24] Quantitative coronary angiography can be used to evaluate a variety of parameters, including cross-sectional area and minimum lumen diameter. However, these measurements may not accurately reflect the clinical significance or overall severity of disease.[25] B-mode ultrasonography has been used in the carotid arteries to measure intima–media thickness, which has been suggested as a more accurate measurement of early atherosclerosis.[26] Positron emission tomography is now being used not only to quantify anatomic changes but also to determine the functional impact of these lesions on coronary flow reserve and myocardial viability.[27]

CORONARY DRUG PROJECT. The Coronary Drug Project tested the effects of pharmacological monotherapy with various agents in men, aged 30 to 64 years, with previous myocardial infarction.[28] Although 8341 men were randomized for the 5-year trial, three treatment arms were discontinued because of adverse effects. Conjugated estrogens, 5 mg/day, produced excess incidence of nonfatal myocardial infarction and insufficient efficacy; dextrothyroxine, 6 mg/day, produced excess mortality; and conjugated estrogens, 2.5 mg/day, produced excess incidence of thromboembolism, excess cancer mortality, and a small increase in total mortality.

Clofibrate, 1800 mg/day, was prescribed in 1103 subjects. In this treatment arm, total cholesterol decreased 6 per cent, and total triglyceride decreased 22 per cent. Combined incidence of CAD death and nonfatal myocardial infarction was reduced 9 per cent, but the difference was not statistically significant. Clofibrate treatment did not affect total mortality.

Nicotinic acid, 3 gm/day, was prescribed in 1119 subjects. In this treatment group, total cholesterol decreased 10 per cent, and total triglyceride decreased 26 per cent. During the trial period, there was a statistically significant 27 per cent decrease in incidence of nonfatal myocardial infarction compared with the placebo group but no difference in total mortality or CAD death. However, 15-year follow-up demonstrated an 11 per cent reduction in total mortality that was highly statistically significant and provided evidence that short-term reduction of coronary events translates into long-term mortality benefits.[29]

NATIONAL HEART, LUNG, AND BLOOD INSTITUTE TYPE II CORONARY INTERVENTION STUDY. The National Heart, Lung, and Blood Institute (NHLBI) Type II Coronary Intervention Study was the first major randomized trial to examine the effect of cholesterol lowering on angiographic parameters. This trial randomized 143 men and women, aged 21 to 55 years, to receive cholestyramine at a prescribed dosage of 24 gm/day or placebo for 5 years.[30] Entry criteria included angiographic evidence of CAD and an LDL cholesterol level above the 90th percentile for the general population despite dietary therapy (polyunsaturated fat : saturated fat ratio 2 : 1, cholesterol < 300 mg/day).[31] All subjects were to continue on the diet.

Total cholesterol decreased 17 per cent from baseline in

the cholestyramine group, and LDL cholesterol decreased 26 per cent, compared with respective decreases of 1 and 5 per cent in the placebo group. In the respective groups, HDL cholesterol increased 8 and 2 per cent, and triglyceride increased 28 and 26 per cent.

Angiograms taken at baseline and at 5-year follow-up were assessed visually to determine the primary endpoint of change in severity of CAD. Regression without progression was seen in approximately 7 per cent of both treatment groups. Progression without regression was seen in 32 per cent of subjects in the cholestyramine group and 49 per cent of subjects in the placebo group, which was a statistically significant difference. The benefit of cholestyramine treatment was most dramatic in lesions causing 50 per cent or greater stenosis at baseline: Progression in these lesions was seen in 12 per cent of subjects in the cholestyramine group compared with 33 per cent in the placebo group, which was a significant difference. The cholestyramine group had a 40 per cent reduced risk for progression, death, or nonfatal myocardial infarction, but this difference was not statistically significant.

Changes in HDL cholesterol: total cholesterol ratio and HDL cholesterol: LDL cholesterol ratio were the best predictors of angiographic change.[32] A significant inverse relation was found between lesion progression at 5 years and a combined increase in HDL cholesterol and decrease in LDL cholesterol.

CHOLESTEROL LOWERING ATHEROSCLEROSIS STUDY. The Cholesterol Lowering Atherosclerosis Study (CLAS) evaluated the effects of intensive combination-drug therapy on atherosclerosis in native coronary vessels and saphenous vein bypass grafts in a two-phase study. CLAS I randomized 188 nonsmoking men, aged 40 to 59 years, with previous coronary bypass surgery, progressive atherosclerosis, and total cholesterol of 185 to 350 mg/dl to receive either the bile-acid sequestrant colestipol, 30 gm/day, and nicotinic acid, 3 to 12 gm/day, or placebo for 2 years.[33] Both treatment groups were to follow a cholesterol-lowering diet, but that of the group randomized to combination-drug therapy was somewhat more restrictive (total fat 22 per cent, polyunsaturated fat 10 per cent, and saturated fat 4 per cent of total calories; cholesterol <125 mg/day) than that of the placebo group (total fat 26 per cent, polyunsaturated fat 10 per cent, and saturated fat 5 per cent of total calories; cholesterol <250 mg/day). All subjects received both study drugs for a 6-week pretrial period to ensure adequate compliance and a response of at least a 15 per cent decrease in total cholesterol.

In the group receiving combination-drug therapy, total cholesterol decreased 27 per cent, LDL cholesterol decreased 43 per cent, triglyceride decreased 22 per cent, and HDL cholesterol increased 37 per cent. The placebo group had decreases of 4 per cent, 5 per cent, and 5 per cent, and an increase of 2 per cent in the respective lipid levels.

A coronary global change score determined by visual assessment of angiograms obtained at baseline and 2-year follow-up was the primary endpoint. By this determination, progression was demonstrated in 39 per cent of subjects in the drug-treated group and 60 per cent of subjects in the placebo group. Regression was demonstrated in 16 per cent and 4 per cent of the respective groups, which was a statistically significant difference. Both native coronary arteries and saphenous vein bypass grafts showed improvement. Mean global change score in the drug-treated group was 0.3, compared with 0.8 in the placebo group, which represented a significant reduction in progression with combination-drug therapy. In each quartile of increased fat and polyunsaturated fat consumption, risk for new lesions was significantly increased.[34] Cardiovascular events occurred at similar rates in both treatment groups.

In CLAS II, 103 men completed an additional 2 years of treatment.[35] Lipid changes were maintained in the drug-treated group, and at 4-year follow-up, nonprogression or regression was seen in significantly more subjects in the drug-treated group. Coronary global change score indicated progression in 48 per cent of subjects in the drug-treated group and 85 per cent of subjects in the placebo group. Regression was demonstrated in 18 per cent and 6 per cent of the respective groups, which was a significant difference.

FAMILIAL ATHEROSCLEROSIS TREATMENT STUDY. In the Familial Atherosclerosis Treatment Study (FATS), combination-drug therapy with the HMG-CoA reductase inhibitor lovastatin, 40 to 80 mg/day, and colestipol, 30 gm/day, or with nicotinic acid, 4 to 6 gm/day, and colestipol, 30 gm/day, was compared with placebo in 120 men, aged 62 years or less, with elevated plasma apolipoprotein (apo) B (>125 mg/dl), family history of CAD, and at least one coronary lesion causing 50 per cent or greater stenosis or three coronary lesions causing 30 per cent or greater stenosis.[36] All subjects received dietary therapy. Subjects randomized to placebo who had LDL cholesterol above the 90th percentile for age (43 per cent of the placebo group) also received colestipol, 30 gm/day. Average time on trial was 2.5 years.

Total cholesterol decreased 34 per cent in the group receiving lovastatin plus colestipol, 23 per cent in the group receiving nicotinic acid plus colestipol, and 3 per cent in the group receiving conventional therapy. In the respective groups, LDL cholesterol decreased 46, 32, and 7 per cent; HDL cholesterol increased 15, 43, and 5 per cent; and triglyceride decreased 9 and 30 per cent and increased 15 per cent. The large increase in HDL cholesterol reflects the use of nicotinic acid.

The primary endpoint, mean change in per cent stenosis of the worst lesion in each of nine proximal segments as assessed by quantitative coronary angiography, decreased 0.7 percentage point in the group receiving lovastatin plus colestipol and 0.9 percentage point in the group receiving nicotinic acid plus colestipol, indicative of lesion regression, and increased 2.1 percentage points in the group receiving conventional therapy, indicative of progression (Fig. 35–1). The change in the conventional-therapy group was significantly different from the changes in the combination-drug groups.

In the group receiving lovastatin plus colestipol, progression as the only angiographic change was seen in 21 per cent of subjects, and regression only was seen in 32 per cent of subjects. In the group receiving nicotinic acid plus colestipol, progression only was seen in 25 per cent of subjects, and regression only was seen in 39 per cent of subjects. In the group receiving conventional therapy, progression only was seen in 46 per cent of subjects, and regression only was seen in 11 per cent of subjects.

Cardiovascular events were defined as death, myocardial infarction, and need for peripheral or coronary bypass or angioplasty. These occurred in three subjects in the group receiving lovastatin plus colestipol, two subjects in the group receiving nicotinic acid plus colestipol, and ten subjects in the group receiving conventional therapy. Relative risk for a cardiovascular event was significantly greater in the conventional-therapy group than in the combination-drug groups.

UNIVERSITY OF CALIFORNIA, SAN FRANCISCO, ARTERIOSCLEROSIS SPECIALIZED CENTER OF RESEARCH INTERVENTION TRIAL. In the University of California, San Francisco, Arteriosclerosis Specialized Center of Research (UCSF-SCOR) Intervention Trial, 72 men and women aged 19 to 72 years with heterozygous familial hypercholesterolemia (FH) (described below) were randomized to receive combination-drug therapy consisting of colestipol, 15 to 30 gm/day; nicotinic acid, up to 7.5 gm/day; and lovastatin, 40 to 60 mg/day in various binary and ternary combinations or placebo.[37] During the 26-month trial, when the LRC-CPPT results were reported, UCSF-SCOR subjects randomized to placebo were given the option of receiving colestipol

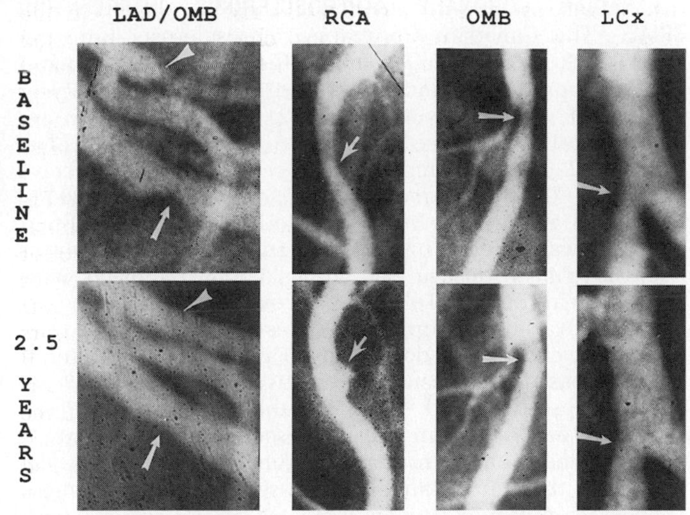

FIGURE 35–1. Regression of coronary atherosclerotic lesions with lipid-regulating therapy: The Familial Atherosclerosis Treatment Study. LAD = left anterior descending artery; LCx = left circumflex artery; OMB = obtuse marginal branch; RCA = right coronary artery. Angiograms taken at baseline and after 2.5 years of treatment reflected improvement with aggressive lipid-regulating therapy. From left to right, stenosis decreased from 100 per cent to 28 per cent in the LAD and from 39 per cent to 18 per cent in the OMB, from 48 per cent to 30 per cent in the RCA, from 69 per cent to 37 per cent in the OMB, and from 44 per cent to 30 per cent in the LCx. (From Brown, G., Albers, J. J., Fisher, L. D., et al.: Regression of coronary artery disease as a result of intensive lipid-lowering therapy in men with high levels of apolipoprotein B. N. Engl. J. Med. *323:*1289, 1990. Copyright Massachusetts Medical Society.)

15 gm/day; 44 per cent of UCSF-SCOR subjects in the placebo group took colestipol.

In the combination-drug group, total cholesterol decreased 31 percent, LDL cholesterol decreased 39 per cent, HDL cholesterol increased 25 per cent, and triglyceride decreased 21 per cent. Respective changes in the placebo group were decreases of 9 and 12 per cent and increases of 1 and 4 per cent.

The primary endpoint was mean within-patient change in per cent area stenosis as assessed by quantitative coronary angiography. This endpoint decreased 1.53 percentage points in the combination-drug group, indicative of lesion regression, and increased 0.80 percentage point in the placebo group, indicative of progression. The difference between groups was statistically significant. In subgroup analysis of women, the primary endpoint remained significantly different between treatment groups; the difference was not statistically significant in subgroup analysis of men.

In the combination-drug group, progression was reported in 20 per cent of subjects, and regression was reported in 32.5 per cent of subjects. In the placebo group, progression was reported in 41 per cent of subjects, and regression was reported in 12.5 per cent of subjects. Although the trend was toward more regression and less progression with combination-drug therapy, the difference was not significant.

ST THOMAS' ATHEROSCLEROSIS REGRESSION STUDY. The St Thomas' Atherosclerosis Regression Study (STARS) randomized 90 men with CAD, aged less than 66 years and with total cholesterol greater than 230 mg/dl, to receive a lipid-lowering diet plus cholestyramine, the same diet alone, or usual care.[38] The diet restricted total fat to 27 per cent and saturated fat to 8 to 10 per cent of total calories and increased omega-6 and omega-3 polyunsaturated fatty acids to 8 per cent of total calories; cholesterol was limited to 100 mg per 1000 kcal, and soluble fiber was increased to the equivalent of 3.6 gm polygalacturonate per 1000 kcal. Angiograms obtained at baseline and after an average of 39 months on trial were assessed quantitatively to determine the primary endpoint of change in the mean absolute width of coronary artery segments.

In the diet-plus-cholestyramine group, total cholesterol decreased 25 per cent, and LDL cholesterol decreased 36 per cent. Respective decreases in the diet-only group were 14 and 16 per cent, and respective decreases in the usual-care group were 2 and 3 per cent.

The primary endpoint was significantly improved in the active-treatment groups compared with the usual-care group. The mean absolute width of coronary artery segments increased 0.103 mm in the diet-plus-cholestyramine group and 0.003 mm in the diet-only group, indicative of lesion regression, but decreased 0.201 mm in the usual-care group, indicative of progression.

Significant improvement in clinical events was also demonstrated in the active-treatment groups. Cardiovascular events, defined as CAD death, myocardial infarction, coronary surgery, angioplasty, or stroke, were reported in one subject in the diet-plus-cholestyramine group, three subjects in the diet-only group, and ten subjects in the usual-care group.

PROGRAM ON THE SURGICAL CONTROL OF THE HYPERLIPIDEMIAS. The Program on the Surgical Control of the Hyperlipidemias (POSCH) randomized 838 men and women, aged 30 to 64 years, with one prior MI and hypercholesterolemia to receive partial ileal bypass surgery or usual care.[39] All subjects received dietary instruction (total fat <25 per cent of calories; saturated, monounsaturated, and polyunsaturated fat each one-third of fat calories; cholesterol <250 mg/day). Entry criteria included total cholesterol of at least 220 mg/dl or LDL cholesterol of at least 140 mg/dl after 6 weeks on diet. The primary endpoint was death of any cause. Angiograms were obtained at baseline and at 3-, 5-, and 7- or 10-year follow-up.

Compared with the control group, the surgery group had a 23 per cent decrease in total cholesterol, a 38 per cent decrease in LDL cholesterol, a 4 per cent increase in HDL cholesterol, and a 20 per cent increase in triglyceride at 5-year follow-up. Lesion progression as determined by a global change score was significantly reduced in the surgery group at each follow-up: 28 per cent compared with 41 per cent in the control group at 3 years, 37 per cent compared with 65 per cent of the control group at 5 years, 48 per cent compared with 77 per cent in the control group at 7 years, and 55 per cent compared with 85 per cent in the control group at 10 years. During the 10 years of the trial, total mortality was reduced 22 per cent and CAD mortality was reduced 28 per cent in the surgery group, but neither of these differences was significant. However, risk for CAD death or nonfatal myocardial infarction was significantly reduced 35 per cent in the surgery group. Changes between angiograms taken at baseline and at 3-year follow-up were significantly associated with total mortality and CAD mortality during the course of the study.[40]

POSCH demonstrated the effects of lipid lowering by a method that ensured compliance. Since the initiation of that trial, however, the availability of pharmacological agents with increased potency has reduced the need for such radical intervention.

LIFE STYLE HEART TRIAL. The Life style Heart Trial randomized 48 men and women aged 35 to 75 years and with angiographically documented CAD to a comprehensive life style-modification program, which included a low-fat vegetarian diet (as prescribed, total fat 10 per cent of calories, polyunsaturated fat:saturated fat ratio >1, protein 15 to 20 per cent of calories, carbohydrate 70 to 75 per cent of calories and predominantly complex carbohydrates, cholesterol ≤ 5 mg/day), smoking cessation, stress management training, and moderate physical exercise, or to usual care.[41] Angiograms made at baseline and at 1-year follow-up were evaluated quantitatively.

In the life style-modification group, total cholesterol decreased 24 per cent and LDL cholesterol decreased 37 per cent. Respective decreases in the usual-care group were 5 and 6 per cent. The average per cent diameter stenosis in all detectable lesions decreased from 40 to 38 per cent in the life style-modification group and increased from 43 to 46 per cent in the usual-care group, which was a significant difference. In addition to the anatomical improvement, the life style-modification group had a significant 91 per cent decrease in frequency of angina, a nonsignificant 42 per cent decrease in duration of angina, and a significant 28 per cent reduction in severity of angina; respective increases in the control group were 165, 95, and 39 per cent. Although life style modifications of this magnitude require considerable dedication, this small trial demonstrated that substantial clinical benefit can be achieved by aggressive nonpharmacological intervention in highly motivated individuals.

MONITORED ATHEROSCLEROSIS REGRESSION STUDY. Monotherapy with an HMG-CoA reductase inhibitor has been evaluated in a number of angiographically monitored studies. The Monitored Atherosclerosis Regression Study (MARS) randomized 270 men and women, aged 37 to 67 years, to receive maximum-dosage lovastatin (80 mg/day) or placebo for 2 years.[42] Subjects were selected on the basis of angiographic evidence of CAD rather than dyslipidemia; total cholesterol could range from 190 to 295 mg/dl. All subjects were to follow a low-fat, low-cholesterol diet (total fat ≤27 per cent, saturated fat ≤7 per cent, monounsaturated fat ≤10 per cent, and polyunsaturated fat ≤10 per cent of total calories; cholesterol ≤250 mg/day).

Lovastatin therapy decreased total cholesterol 32 per cent, LDL cholesterol 45 per cent, and triglyceride 22 per cent and increased HDL cholesterol 8.5 per cent, compared with decreases of 2 and 3 per cent and increases of 3.5 and 2 per cent in the respective lipid levels in the placebo group.

Quantitative assessment of angiograms obtained at baseline and at 2-year follow-up did not demonstrate a significant improvement with lovastatin therapy in the primary endpoint of mean per-patient change in per cent diameter stenosis. Both groups showed lesion progression: Mean per cent diameter stenosis increased 1.6 per cent in the lovastatin group and 2.2 per cent in the placebo group. By this assessment, 29 per cent of lovastatin subjects and 41 per cent of placebo subjects demonstrated progression, and 23 and 12 per cent of the respective groups demonstrated regression; both of these differences were statistically significant. In lesions causing 50 per cent or greater stenosis at baseline, the lovastatin group showed a 4.1 per cent decrease in per cent diameter stenosis compared with a 0.9 per cent increase in the placebo group, which was a significant improvement. In the lovastatin group, the predominant predictor of progression in mild and moderate lesions was apo C-III, whereas the predominant predictor of progression in severe lesions was the LDL cholesterol:HDL cholesterol ratio; the predominant predictor of progression in both lesion categories in the placebo group was the total cholesterol:HDL cholesterol ratio.[43]

However, by a visually assessed global change score, there was significantly less progression in the lovastatin group, which had an average global change score of 0.41, than in the placebo group, which had an average score of 0.88. By this assessment, 47 per cent of lovastatin subjects and 65 per cent of placebo subjects demonstrated progression, and 23 per cent of lovastatin subjects and 11 per cent of placebo subjects demonstrated regression; both of these differences were statistically significant.

Between-group comparison of clinical coronary events—myocardial infarction, percutaneous transluminal coronary angioplasty, coronary artery bypass surgery, coronary death, and hospitalization for unstable angina—showed a slight reduction in events in the lovastatin group, which had 22 events compared with 31 in the placebo group, but this difference was not statistically significant.

CANADIAN CORONARY ATHEROSCLEROSIS INTERVENTION TRIAL. The Canadian Coronary Atherosclerosis Intervention Trial (CCAIT) also evaluated the benefit of lovastatin monotherapy in secondary prevention.[44] In this 2-year study, 331 men and women aged 21 to 70 years with angiographically demonstrated diffuse CAD and total cholesterol of 220 to 300 mg/dl were randomized to receive lovastatin dosed to reduce LDL cholesterol to 90 to 130 mg/dl or placebo. Initial lovastatin dosage was 20 mg/day and was titrated up to a maximum of 80 mg/day as necessary; mean dosage was 36 mg/day. All subjects were instructed in the Step I diet (see below).

In the lovastatin group, total cholesterol decreased 21 per cent, LDL cholesterol decreased 29 per cent, HDL cholesterol increased 7 per cent, and triglyceride decreased 8 per cent. Respective lipid levels in the placebo group decreased 1 and 2 per cent and increased 3 and 4 per cent.

The primary endpoint was a coronary change score defined as the quantitatively assessed mean per-patient change in minimum lumen diameter for all lesions measured. Although this assessment demonstrated lesion progression in both groups, the lovastatin group had significantly less progression than the placebo group: Mean lumen diameter decreased 0.05 mm and 0.09 mm in the respective groups. Progression as the only angiographic change was reported in 33 per cent of subjects in the lovastatin group and 50 per cent of subjects in the placebo group, which was a significant improvement. New lesion formation was significantly decreased in the lovastatin group, in which new lesions were seen in 16 per cent of subjects, compared with 32 per cent of subjects in the placebo group. Regression as the only angiographic change was not significantly different between treatment groups, occurring in 10 per cent of subjects in the lovastatin group and 7 per cent of subjects in the placebo group.

Fewer clinical coronary events, defined as cardiac death, myocardial infarction, and unstable angina, were reported in the lovastatin group, in which 14 subjects had 15 events, compared with the placebo group, in which 18 subjects had 20 events, but the difference was not statistically significant.

PRAVASTATIN LIMITATION OF ATHEROSCLEROSIS IN THE CORONARY ARTERIES. The Pravastatin Limitation of Atherosclerosis in the Coronary Arteries (PLAC I) study assessed the effect of pharmacological monotherapy with the HMG-CoA reductase inhibitor pravastatin on angiographic and clinical endpoints in 408 men and women with angiographic evidence of CAD (≥50 per cent stenosis in one or more coronary arteries) and LDL cholesterol of 130 to 190 mg/dl.[45] Subjects were randomized to receive pravastatin, 40 mg/day, or placebo for 3 years.

In the pravastatin group, the primary endpoint—mean change in diameter of 10 predetermined coronary artery segments as assessed by quantitative coronary angiography—decreased 0.02 mm/year, which was not significantly different from the 0.04 mm/year decrease in the placebo group. Pravastatin decreased total cholesterol 19 per cent, triglyceride 8 per cent, and LDL cholesterol 28 per cent and increased HDL cholesterol 7 per cent. Clinical cardiovascular events—fatal and nonfatal myocardial infarction, other cardiac death, stroke, bypass surgery, and coronary angioplasty—were significantly reduced in the pravastatin group.

REGRESSION GROWTH EVALUATION STATIN STUDY. In the Regression Growth Evaluation Statin Study (REGRESS), 885 men aged less than 70 years with total cholesterol between 155 mg/dl and 310 mg/dl and at least one coronary lesion causing at least 50 per cent stenosis in a major coronary artery were randomized to receive pravastatin, 40 mg/day, or placebo.[46] All subjects were to follow a diet that derived 10 to 15 per cent of total calories from protein, 30 to 35 per cent from lipid, and 50 to 55 per cent from carbohydrate. In subjects whose total cholesterol level was greater than

310 mg/dl on repeated assessments, cholestyramine was administered in addition to the study drug. Quantitative coronary angiography was performed at baseline and after 2 years of treatment.

In the pravastatin group, total cholesterol decreased 20 per cent, LDL cholesterol decreased 29 per cent, HDL cholesterol increased 10 per cent, and triglyceride decreased 7 per cent. All lipid values increased slightly in the placebo group.

Primary angiographic endpoints were the per-patient change in average mean segment diameter and the per-patient change in average minimum obstruction diameter. Both groups showed progression by both of these determinations. However, the pravastatin group showed significantly less decrease in the mean segment diameter (0.06 mm) than the placebo group (0.10 mm) and significantly less decrease in the minimum obstruction diameter (0.03 mm) than the placebo group (0.06 mm).

In the pravastatin group, 59 clinical events (fatal or nonfatal myocardial infarction, CAD death, unscheduled percutaneous transluminal coronary angioplasty or coronary artery bypass grafting, stroke or transient ischemic attack, and death of any other cause) were reported, compared with 93 in the placebo group.

MULTICENTRE ANTI-ATHEROMA STUDY. The effect of HMG-CoA reductase inhibitor monotherapy with simvastatin on known coronary atherosclerotic lesions was evaluated in the Multicentre Anti-Atheroma Study (MAAS).[47] In this study, 381 men and women, aged 30 to 67 years, were randomized to receive simvastatin, 20 mg/day, or placebo for 4 years. Entry criteria included angiographic evidence of atherosclerosis in at least two coronary artery segments, total cholesterol of 210 to 310 mg/dl, and triglyceride less than 350 mg/dl. Dietary instruction according to the usual practice of each center was given to all subjects.

Compared with placebo, simvastatin decreased total cholesterol 23 per cent, LDL cholesterol 31 per cent, and triglyceride 18 per cent and increased HDL cholesterol 9 per cent.

Angiograms obtained at baseline and at 2- and 4-year follow-up were assessed quantitatively. Change in diffuse coronary atherosclerosis was determined by the per-patient average of mean lumen diameter of all coronary artery segments, and change in focal coronary atherosclerosis was determined by the per-patient average of minimum lumen diameter of all segments that were atheromatous at baseline and/or follow-up. In both treatment groups, progression was seen in both measures of atherosclerotic disease, although there was significantly less progression by both determinations with simvastatin therapy. In the simvastatin group, mean lumen diameter decreased 0.02 mm and minimum lumen diameter decreased 0.04 mm; respective decreases in the placebo group were 0.08 mm and 0.13 mm. Progression as the only angiographic change was seen in 23 per cent of subjects in the simvastatin group and 32 per cent of subjects in the placebo group. Regression as the only angiographic change was seen in 19 per cent and 12 per cent of the respective groups.

Clinical event rates were similar between treatment groups. Myocardial infarction was reported in 11 subjects randomized to simvastatin and 7 subjects randomized to placebo. Cardiac death was reported in 4 subjects in each group.

SCANDINAVIAN SIMVASTATIN SURVIVAL STUDY. The Scandinavian Simvastatin Survival Study (4S) provided strong evidence that intensive lipid lowering improves survival in patients with coronary disease. This multicenter trial randomized 4444 men and women, aged 35 to 60 years, with a history of angina pectoris or myocardial infarction to receive placebo or simvastatin dosed to reduce total cholesterol to 115 to 200 mg/dl.[48] Other entry criteria were total cholesterol of 210 to 310 mg/dl and triglyceride of 220 mg/dl or less after dietary instruction. Simvastatin dosage was increased from the initial 20 mg/day to 40 mg/day in 37 per cent of simvastatin subjects and decreased to 10 mg/day in 2 subjects. Median time on trial was 5.4 years. Analysis was intent to treat.

Simvastatin therapy decreased total cholesterol 25 per cent, LDL cholesterol 35 per cent, and triglyceride 10 per cent and increased HDL cholesterol 8 per cent. In the placebo group, respective lipid levels increased 1 per cent, 1 per cent, 7 per cent, and 1 per cent. Total mortality, the primary endpoint, was significantly decreased 30 per cent in the simvastatin group. Coronary mortality decreased 42 per cent, and there was no increase in noncardiovascular deaths, including deaths caused by violence or cancer, in the simvastatin group. Incidence of major coronary events, defined as coronary death, nonfatal myocardial infarction, and resuscitated cardiac arrest, was significantly decreased 34 per cent in the simvastatin group. Risk for major coronary events was similarly reduced in each quartile of baseline total cholesterol, LDL cholesterol, and HDL cholesterol distribution.[49]

Predetermined subgroup analyses compared clinical event rates by age and gender. In subjects aged 60 years or older, total mortality and incidence of major coronary events were significantly reduced with simvastatin treatment, although these reductions were less than in the overall study population. In women, total mortality was similar between treatment groups, but the incidence of major coronary events was significantly decreased 35 per cent in the simvastatin group.

Low Cholesterol and Mortality

Some epidemiological studies have found an increase in mortality at the lowest cholesterol levels,[50] and, as noted above, some early interventional trials of lipid lowering showed no improvement in total mortality, despite a reduction in coronary mortality, because of an increase in noncardiac mortality. These results have raised questions about a potential adverse effect of cholesterol lowering and about the causality of increased death rates at the lowest cholesterol levels reported in some studies.[51] The major controversy is whether the association between low cholesterol and increased mortality is causal or is attributable to confounding factors not adequately evaluated in epidemiological studies.[52]

The definition of low cholesterol has not been established, but many experts consider total cholesterol less than 160 mg/dl to be low. However, populations that consume low-fat, low-cholesterol diets have average total cholesterol levels in this general range. For example, in Shanghai, the mean total cholesterol level is 162 mg/dl, but no increase in cancer mortality or other causes of death has been demonstrated.[53]

In addition to diet, a variety of genetic and environmental conditions can decrease total cholesterol.[54] Genetic diseases characterized by low cholesterol include abetalipoproteinemia,[55] an autosomal recessive disorder characterized by a marked decrease or absence of apo B–containing lipoproteins and total cholesterol of 20 to 45 mg/dl, and hypobetalipoproteinemia,[56] an autosomal dominant disorder that in its homozygous form resembles abetalipoproteinemia and in its heterozygous form is characterized by total cholesterol of 90 to 140 mg/dl and LDL cholesterol of 30 to 50 mg/dl. Abnormalities associated with these conditions include peripheral neuropathies and fat malabsorption. However, patients with these disorders do not appear to have increased rates of death of malignancy or a shortened life span, despite lifelong exposure to cholesterol levels far below those obtained in clinical trials. Nongenetic factors associated with decreased plasma cholesterol include chronic disease states such as chronic obstructive pulmonary disease, bronchogenic carcinoma, and alcoholic cirrhosis. Preclinical malignancies may be the cause rather than the result of hypocholesterolemia.[57]

The Honolulu Heart Program demonstrated a definite U-shaped association between quintile of cholesterol and total mortality rate.[58] Subjects in quintile 3 (total cholesterol 210 to 239 mg/dl) had the lowest age-adjusted mortality rate (66.4 per 1000), subjects in quintiles 2 (total cholesterol 180 to 209 mg/dl) and 4 (total cholesterol 240 to 269 mg/dl) had slightly increased total mortality (69.5 per 1000 and 67.5 per 1000, respectively), and subjects in the lowest quintile (total cholesterol <180 mg/dl) and the highest quintile (total cholesterol 270 mg/dl or greater) had increased total mortality (97.3 per 1000 and 100.9 per 1000, respectively). However, in a reassessment of the Honolulu Heart Program data, excess mortality at low cholesterol levels was limited to subjects with confounding health problems, such as heavy alcohol consumption, heavy smoking, gastrectomy, cirrhosis, colectomy, or intestinal disease.[59] In additional analysis of traumatic deaths and suicides during 23 years of follow-up in the Honolulu Heart Program, total cholesterol at any level was found to be directly related to risk for suicide, and multivariate analysis did not find a relation between total cholesterol level and risk for traumatic death.[60]

Similarly, in the Whitehall Study, age-adjusted total mortality rate was slightly higher in the lowest quintile of total cholesterol (<129 mg/dl) than in the second-lowest quintile (129 to 174 mg/dl)—13.78 compared with 13.29 per 1000 person-years—but this difference was not statistically significant.[61] CAD mortality increased with each quintile of total cholesterol. The increase in noncardiovascular mortality was largely accounted for by confounding factors such as recent unexplained weight loss, respiratory symptoms, body mass index, marital status, and employment grade.

In a 30-year follow-up of subjects in the Framingham Heart Study who were without cancer or cardiovascular disease at initial assessment, total cholesterol level was directly related to total mortality and cardiovascular mortality in both men and women aged less than 50 years.[62] No association was found between cholesterol level and total mortality in subjects aged 50 years or older, presumably because of confounding by diseases that decrease cholesterol level.

When the increases in accidental and violent deaths reported in the LRC-CPPT and the Helsinki Heart Study were reanalyzed for potential confounding factors, it was noted that the two victims of homicide were both innocent victims and not offenders, and one had not been taking the study drug for more than 1 year.[63] The eight suicides include five subjects who had withdrawn from the trials and had not been taking the study drug for months or years. Of the ten accidental deaths, two were in subjects who had withdrawn from the study, three were in subjects with high blood alcohol concentrations at autopsy, and three were in subjects with a history of psychiatric disorders. Additionally, in both the LRC-CPPT and the Helsinki Heart Study, cholesterol lowering did not decrease cholesterol levels to what would be considered low.

Low cholesterol has been hypothesized to increase violent behavior because of a decrease in serotonin receptor activity in the brain.[64] However, lowering plasma cholesterol may not alter cholesterol level within the central nervous system, because essentially all the cholesterol in the central nervous system is produced locally, and the exchangeable pool of cholesterol is much lower in the central nervous system than in other organs.[65]

In 4S, cholesterol lowering decreased both coronary mortality and total mortality, demonstrating that noncoronary death rates did not offset improvement in cardiovascular mortality. Specifically, there was no increase in deaths due to violence or cancer.

In a prospectively planned pooled analysis of PLAC I, REGRESS, and two other regression studies using pravastatin 40 mg/day monotherapy for 2 or 3 years, combined incidence of nonfatal or fatal myocardial infarction was significantly reduced 62 per cent; this benefit was demonstrated in men and women and in patients older and younger than 65 years.[66] In this analysis, total mortality was decreased 46 per cent with pravastatin, but this difference was not significant.

Low-Density Lipoprotein Metabolism

LDL is the major carrier of cholesterol to the periphery and supplies the cholesterol essential for the integrity of nerve tissue, steroid synthesis, and cell membranes. Apo B-100 on the surface of LDL allows recognition, binding, and removal of the lipoprotein by the B/E (LDL) receptor, which removes approximately 75 per cent of LDL particles from the circulation and is downregulated as intracellular cholesterol increases. Scavenger receptors on macrophages and non–receptor-mediated pathways account for the clearance of the remaining LDL particles.

SMALL, DENSE LOW-DENSITY LIPOPROTEIN. In addition to LDL cholesterol level, LDL composition influences CAD risk. Triglyceride may be transferred from chylomicrons and VLDL to LDL, through the action of cholesteryl ester transfer protein (CETP), and subsequently hydrolyzed by hepatic lipase to produce LDL particles that are smaller and denser than normal. Large, buoyant LDL particles predominate in LDL subclass pattern A, and small, dense LDL particles predominate in LDL subclass pattern B.[67] LDL subclass pattern B is associated with a threefold-increased risk for myocardial infarction,[68] and LDL particles in individuals with angiographic evidence of CAD have been reported to be smaller and denser than LDL in individuals without angiographic evidence of CAD.[69] Although LDL subclass pattern B has been reported in approximately 37 per cent of males and 25 per cent of females, it is present in only 17 per cent of males aged 6 to 19 years and only 13 per cent of premenopausal females.[70] Genetic influences appear to account for 33 per cent to 50 per cent of the variation in LDL subclass,[71] indicating substantial environmental and thus potentially modifiable factors. Small, dense LDL frequently occurs in conjunction with elevated triglyceride level, low HDL cholesterol level, truncal obesity, and hypertension. Individuals with LDL subclass pattern B have been found to be more insulin resistant than individuals with LDL subclass pattern A,[72] suggesting that complex metabolic factors may also affect LDL subclass.

LDL subclass pattern can be altered to a potentially less atherogenic pattern. Pharmacological therapy, for example, with gemfibrozil[73] or bezafibrate,[74] has been shown to shift LDL particles toward a larger, more buoyant species.

The mechanism by which small, dense LDL confers increased atherosclerotic risk has not been totally determined and may be a combination of mechanisms. Compared with large, buoyant LDL, small, dense LDL has a lower sialic acid content, which may increase the binding capacity of LDL for proteoglycans localized to the arterial wall.[75] Hemostatic variables may be shifted to a more atherogenic pattern in the presence of small, dense LDL. A dose-dependent increase in thromboxane synthesis has been reported with increasing density of LDL particles.[76] Small, dense LDL appears to be more susceptible to in vitro oxidation than large, buoyant LDL.[77]

OXIDIZED LOW-DENSITY LIPOPROTEIN. LDL may be oxidized as a result of exposure to endothelial cells, smooth muscle cells, or macrophages.[78,78a] Oxidized LDL attracts circulating monocytes, which then adhere to the arterial wall, and precipitates their activation as macrophages, which are then prevented from leaving the arterial wall[79] (see Chap. 34). Scavenger receptors on macrophages recognize and bind oxidized LDL and, unlike the B/E receptor, are not downregulated as intracellular cholesterol accumulates. As uptake continues, the macrophages can become lipid-laden foam cells, the components of the fatty streak, which is the precursor atherosclerotic lesion.

Diagnosis and Treatment of Dyslipidemia

In the NCEP adult guidelines, the determination of lipid levels and estimation of the need for and intensity of lipid-regulating treatment are influenced by the individual's overall risk for CAD. Because, as noted above, individuals with existing CAD or other atherosclerotic disease, such as peripheral arterial disease or symptomatic carotid artery disease, are at the highest short-term risk for a CAD event, the initial risk stratification of the NCEP adult guidelines is according to the presence or absence of atherosclerotic disease. But it should be borne in mind that the distinction between primary and secondary prevention is at times semantic because many high-risk asymptomatic individuals have significant atherosclerosis.

Separate recommendations have been issued by the Expert Panel on Blood Cholesterol Levels in Children and Adolescents of the NCEP.[80] These guidelines, developed for individuals aged 2 to 19 years, recommend screening for dyslipidemia in children and adolescents who are from families with premature cardiovascular disease or dyslipidemia. LDL cholesterol of 170 mg/dl or greater should be treated by dietary therapy. If, after 6 months to 1 year of dietary therapy, LDL cholesterol remains 190 mg/dl or greater, or 160 mg/dl or greater in the presence of either a positive family history of cardiovascular disease before age 55 or two other risk factors that have not been successfully controlled, drug therapy should be considered in patients aged at least 10 years. Bile-acid sequestrant therapy is appropriate in this age group.

DETECTION OF DYSLIPIDEMIA. The NCEP adult guidelines recommend that all individuals aged 20 years or older without CAD or other atherosclerotic disease have their total cholesterol and, if accuracy can be assured, HDL cholesterol levels measured at least once every 5 years. These measurements can be obtained from nonfasting samples. At the discretion of the physician, a full fasting lipoprotein analysis may be performed instead. Lipoprotein analysis is the initial assessment in individuals with CAD or other atherosclerotic disease.

Primary Prevention. In individuals without atherosclerotic disease, estimation of risk status at a given cholesterol level is guided by the number of other risk factors present, although clinical judgment is required to evaluate the severity of each risk factor and the overall risk status of the individual. The following additional risk factors (besides LDL cholesterol elevation) are included in the NCEP's algorithm:

Positive risk factors
- Age (45 years or older in men; 55 years or older, or premature menopause without estrogen-replacement therapy, in women)
- Family history of premature CAD (myocardial infarction or sudden death before the age of 55 in father or other male first-degree relative, or before the age of 65 in mother or other female first-degree relative)
- Current cigarette smoking
  Hypertension (≥140/90 mm Hg, or on antihypertensive medication)
- Low HDL cholesterol (<35 mg/dl)
- Diabetes mellitus

Negative risk factor (subtract 1 of the additional risk factors if present)
- High HDL cholesterol (≥60 mg/dl)

Obesity is not included in the algorithm because it is usually found in conjunction with hypertension, hyperlipidemia, low HDL cholesterol, and diabetes mellitus, which are listed; nevertheless, it should be a target for intervention, as should physical inactivity. A concerted effort should be made to reduce all modifiable risk factors.

In primary prevention, total cholesterol less than 200 mg/dl is considered desirable, 200 to 239 mg/dl is considered borderline high, and 240 mg/dl or greater is considered high (Fig. 35–2). At a total cholesterol level of 240 mg/dl, CAD risk is approximately twice that at a total cholesterol level of 200 mg/dl. However, because the relation between cholesterol level and CAD risk is continuous and graded, this categorization of cholesterol provides not absolute cutpoints but a guide for risk assessment.

In individuals without CAD whose total cholesterol is desirable and HDL cholesterol is 35 mg/dl or greater, no lipid-regulating intervention is required. These individuals should receive instruction in following dietary recommendations for the general population (Step I Diet) and in risk factor reduction. Retesting should be performed in 5 years. Individuals without CAD whose total cholesterol is borderline high and HDL cholesterol is 35 mg/dl or greater in the presence of fewer than two other risk factors should receive similar instruction and should be reevaluated in 1 to 2 years, at which time dietary instruction should be reinforced.

Individuals with low HDL cholesterol, borderline-high total cholesterol in the presence of two or more other risk factors, or high total cholesterol require full fasting lipoprotein analysis to help determine CAD risk. The analysis is performed on a sample obtained after a 12-hour fast to allow clearance of chylomicrons. Total cholesterol, HDL cholesterol, and total triglyceride levels are measured, and LDL cholesterol is calculated by the Friedewald formula:

$$\text{LDL cholesterol (mg/dl)} = \text{Total cholesterol} - \text{HDL cholesterol} - (\text{triglyceride}/5)$$

The formula is not accurate if triglyceride is greater than 400 mg/dl or if the patient has type III hyperlipidemia or is homozygous for apo E_2; in these instances, LDL cholesterol needs to be determined by ultracentrifugation at a specialized laboratory.

The NCEP adult guidelines classify LDL cholesterol less than 130 mg/dl as desirable, 130 to 159 mg/dl as borderline high, and 160 mg/dl or greater as high in primary prevention (Fig. 35–3). Patients whose LDL cholesterol is desirable should receive instruction in dietary recommendations for the general population and in risk factor reduction. Low HDL cholesterol and hypertriglyceridemia require treatment as described below.

Patients who have borderline-high LDL cholesterol and fewer than two other risk factors should receive instruction in dietary modification and recommended physical activity. Retesting by lipoprotein analysis should be performed in 1 year. In patients who have borderline-high LDL cholesterol and two or more other risk factors, and in patients who have high LDL cholesterol, lipoprotein analysis should be repeated within 1 to 8 weeks. If the LDL cholesterol values vary by more than 30 mg/dl, the analysis should be repeated a third time. Treatment decisions should be based on the average of two, or, if necessary, three, LDL cholesterol values. Confirmation of borderline-high or high LDL cholesterol indicates the need for clinical evaluation and lipid-regulating intervention.

Secondary Prevention. Full fasting lipoprotein analysis should be performed at least once every year in individuals with CAD. Because LDL cholesterol may be decreased in patients recovering from an acute coronary event, analyses performed during the weeks immediately following the event may not accurately reflect the baseline LDL cholesterol level. However, elevated LDL cholesterol during this period suggests an even greater elevation upon recovery.

In patients with CAD, an LDL cholesterol level of 100 mg/dl or less is considered optimal (Fig. 35–4). Patients who have optimal LDL cholesterol should be given individualized instruction in dietary recommendations (Step II Diet) and physical activity. Retesting by lipoprotein analysis should be repeated annually. Low HDL cholesterol and hypertriglyceridemia require treatment as described below. Patients who have LDL cholesterol higher than opti-

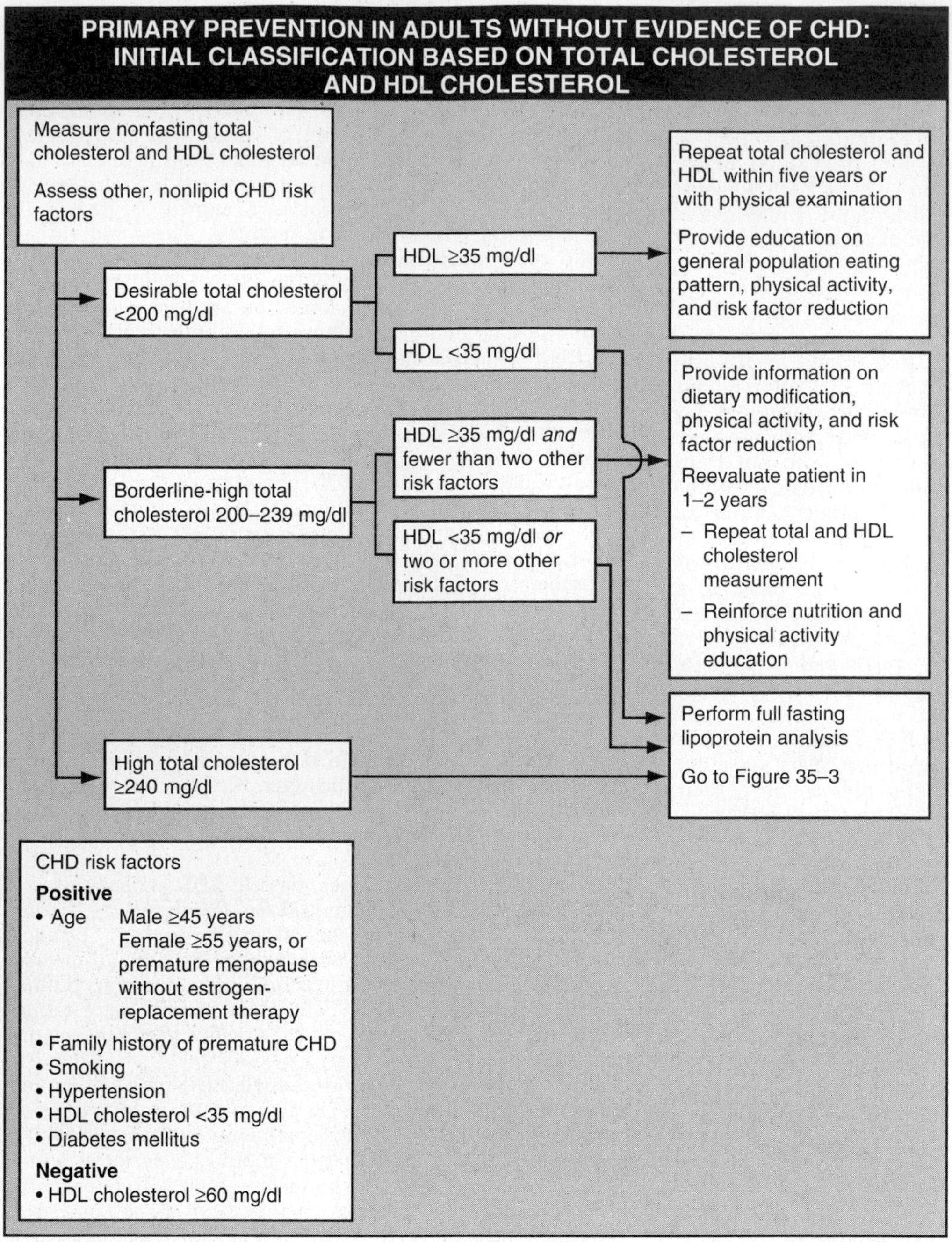

PRIMARY PREVENTION IN ADULTS WITHOUT EVIDENCE OF CHD: INITIAL CLASSIFICATION BASED ON TOTAL CHOLESTEROL AND HDL CHOLESTEROL

Measure nonfasting total cholesterol and HDL cholesterol

Assess other, nonlipid CHD risk factors

Desirable total cholesterol <200 mg/dl

HDL ≥35 mg/dl → Repeat total cholesterol and HDL within five years or with physical examination. Provide education on general population eating pattern, physical activity, and risk factor reduction

HDL <35 mg/dl → Perform full fasting lipoprotein analysis. Go to Figure 35–3

Borderline-high total cholesterol 200–239 mg/dl

HDL ≥35 mg/dl *and* fewer than two other risk factors → Provide information on dietary modification, physical activity, and risk factor reduction. Reevaluate patient in 1–2 years
- Repeat total and HDL cholesterol measurement
- Reinforce nutrition and physical activity education

HDL <35 mg/dl *or* two or more other risk factors → Perform full fasting lipoprotein analysis. Go to Figure 35–3

High total cholesterol ≥240 mg/dl → Perform full fasting lipoprotein analysis. Go to Figure 35–3

CHD risk factors

Positive
- Age Male ≥45 years
  Female ≥55 years, or premature menopause without estrogen-replacement therapy
- Family history of premature CHD
- Smoking
- Hypertension
- HDL cholesterol <35 mg/dl
- Diabetes mellitus

Negative
- HDL cholesterol ≥60 mg/dl

FIGURE 35–2. Primary prevention classification by total cholesterol. In patients without coronary artery disease or other atherosclerotic disease, initial assessment for dyslipidemia is by total cholesterol and high-density lipoprotein cholesterol levels (minimum approach). The physician may choose the full fasting lipoprotein analysis as the first assessment. (From National Cholesterol Education Program.[2,3])

mal, as confirmed by multiple assessments as detailed above, should receive clinical evaluation and lipid-lowering intervention.

CLINICAL EVALUATION. The clinical evaluation estimates overall risk for CAD and attempts to determine whether the dyslipidemia is caused by a genetic disorder or is secondary to diet, to another condition such as diabetes mellitus, hypothyroidism, nephrotic syndrome, or obstructive liver disease, or to the use of drugs such as progestins, anabolic steroids, corticosteroids, beta blockers, or diuretics.

Essential components of the evaluation are personal and family history, physical examination, and basic laboratory tests. The physical examination should include careful assessment for manifestations of dyslipidemia, such as corneal arcus, xanthelasmas or xanthomas, and hepatosplenomegaly, and for manifestations of atherosclerosis, such as decreased peripheral pulses and vascular bruits. The clinical evaluation further refines estimation of the patient's CAD risk and provides additional targets for intervention through the identification of other risk factors. If genetic dyslipidemia is suspected, family members should be assessed. If dyslipidemia does not respond to treatment of underlying conditions or removal or reduction of drugs that can cause dyslipidemia, it should be treated as a primary dyslipidemia.

Dietary Therapy

In the NCEP guidelines, the primary therapy for dyslipidemia is dietary. Reduction of saturated fat and cholesterol consumption is part of a triad of life style modifications that should also include weight loss if necessary and increased physical activity as appropriate. Dietary therapy judiciously employed is a risk-free intervention whose efficacy has been demonstrated in clinical trials.[81] The synergistic effects of dietary modification, regular exercise, and weight control are beneficial in reducing CAD risk by improving not only the lipid profile but also blood pressure and glucose tolerance.

In primary prevention in patients with fewer than two other risk factors, dietary therapy should be initiated if LDL cholesterol is 160 mg/dl or greater (Table 35–4). The goal of treatment in these patients is LDL cholesterol less than 160 mg/dl. In primary prevention in patients with two or more other risk factors, dietary therapy should be initiated

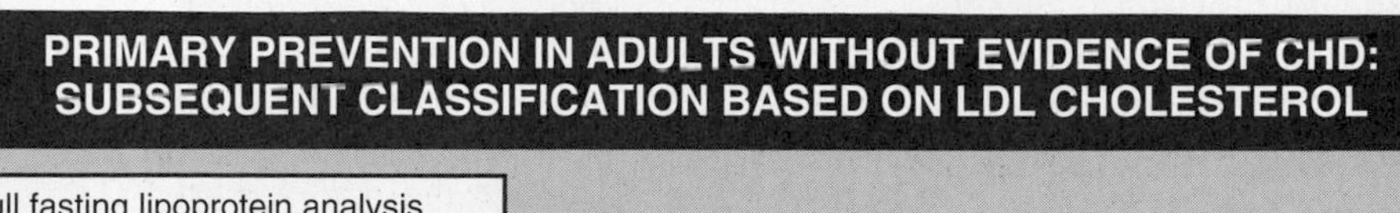

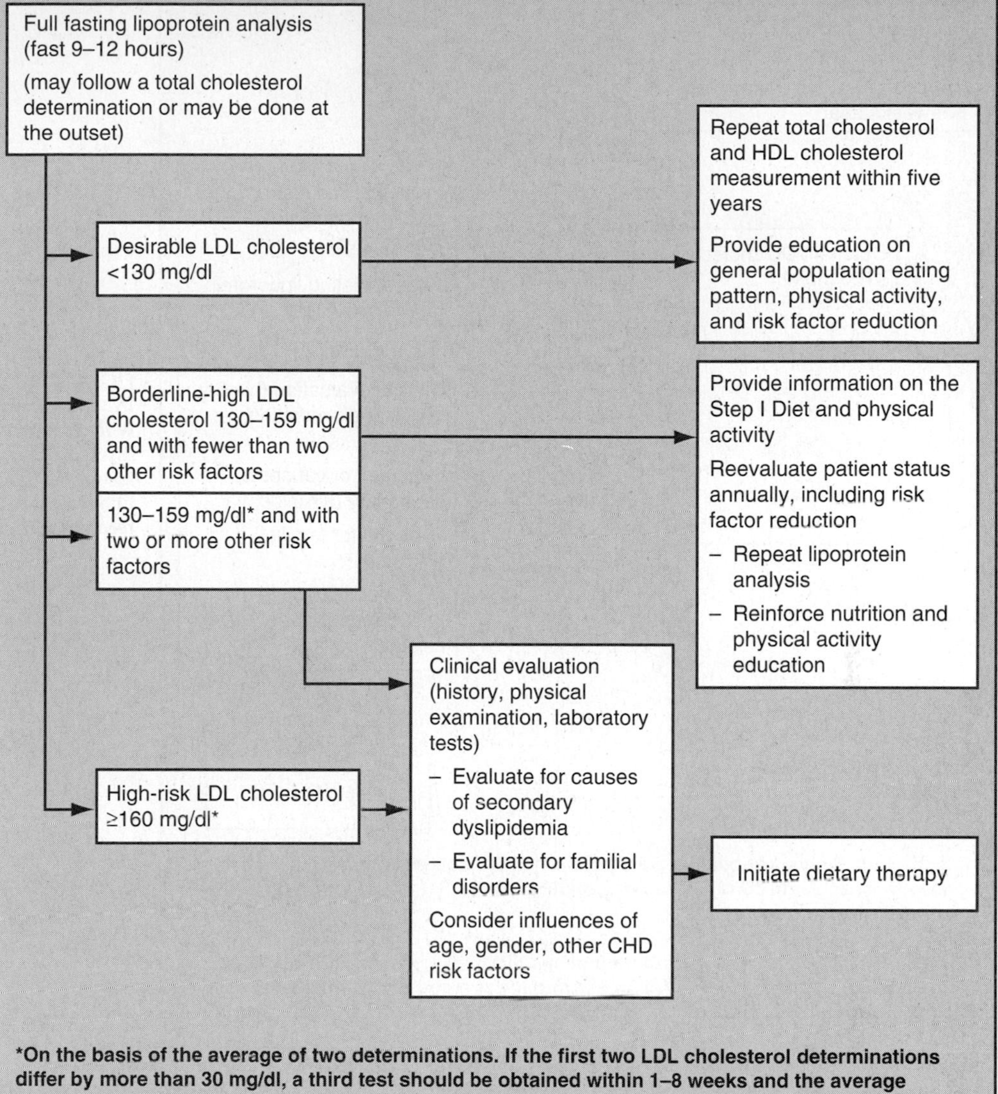

FIGURE 35–3. Primary prevention classification by low-density lipoprotein cholesterol. In patients without coronary artery disease or other atherosclerotic disease who have low high-density lipoprotein cholesterol, borderline-high total cholesterol in the presence of two or more other risk factors, or high total cholesterol, full fasting lipoprotein analysis is required to determine low-density lipoprotein cholesterol level. (From National Cholesterol Education Program.[2,3])

if LDL cholesterol is 130 mg/dl or greater. The goal of treatment in these patients is LDL cholesterol less than 130 mg/dl. The lower initiation level and goal reflect the additive impact of multiple risk factors on coronary disease, which justifies a more aggressive approach. In secondary prevention, dietary therapy should be initiated if LDL cholesterol is greater than 100 mg/dl. The goal of treatment in these patients is LDL cholesterol of 100 mg/dl or less.

TABLE 35–4 DIETARY THERAPY TREATMENT LEVELS IN ADULTS

RISK	LDL CHOLESTEROL LEVEL (mg/dl) Initiation Level	Goal
Without CHD, fewer than two other risk factors	≥160	<160
Without CHD, two or more other risk factors	≥130	<130
With CHD or other atherosclerotic disease	>100	≤100

CHD = coronary heart disease; LDL = low-density lipoprotein.

From National Cholesterol Education Program: Second report of the Expert Panel on Detection, Evaluation, and Treatment of High Blood Cholesterol in Adults (Adult Treatment Panel II). Circulation *89*:1329, 1994 Copyright American Heart Association.

STEP I DIET. In primary prevention in patients following a typical Western diet, the initial diet is the Step I Diet (Table 35–5), which is recommended for the general population aged at least 2 years. The Step I Diet derives no more than 30 per cent of total calories from fat, 8 to 10 per cent of total calories from saturated fat, no more than 10 per cent of total calories from polyunsaturated fat, and no more than 15 per cent of total calories from monounsaturated fat.[81a] Cholesterol is limited to less than 300 mg/day, and total calories should be sufficient to achieve and maintain desirable weight.

STEP II DIET. In patients whose LDL cholesterol remains elevated despite adherence to the Step I Diet for 3 months, the Step II Diet should be instituted. The Step II Diet reduces saturated fat to less than 7 per cent of total calories and reduces cholesterol to less than 200 mg/day. In patients with CAD and in patients following the Step I Diet at the time of assessment, the Step II Diet is the initial therapy.

In patients previously consuming a typical Western diet, institution of the Step I Diet generally decreases total cholesterol 5 to 7 per cent, and institution of the Step II

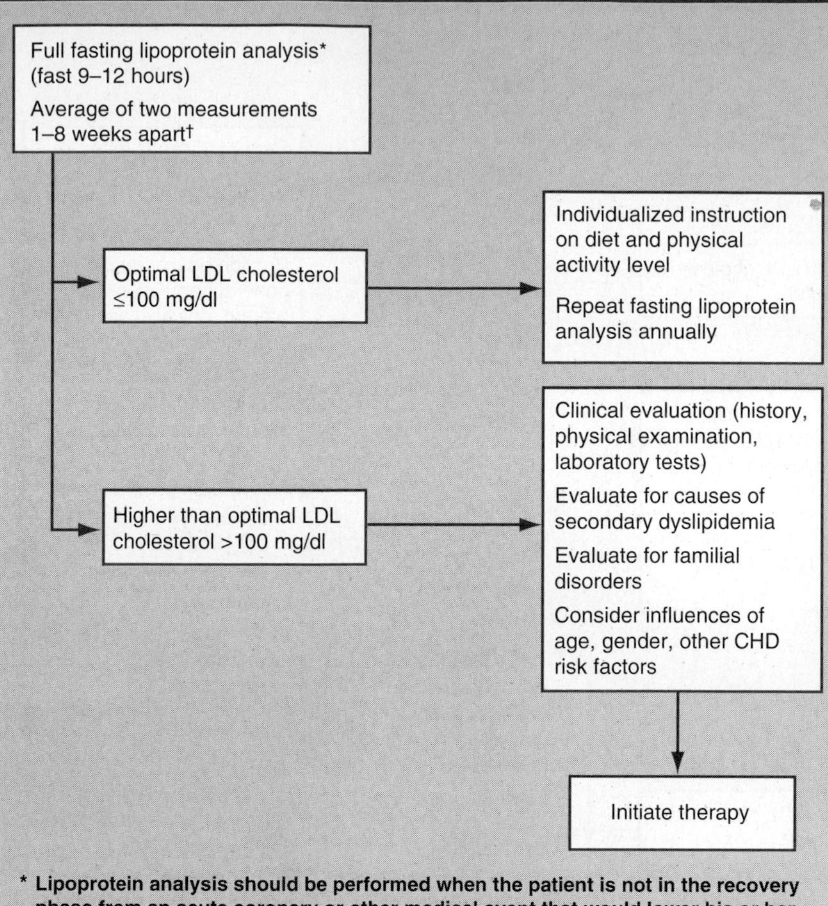

FIGURE 35–4. Secondary prevention classification by low-density lipoprotein cholesterol. In patients with coronary artery disease or other atherosclerotic disease, initial assessment for dyslipidemia is by full fasting lipoprotein analysis to determine low-density lipoprotein cholesterol level. (From National Cholesterol Education Program.[2,3])

Diet decreases total cholesterol an additional 5 to 13 per cent.[82]

MONITORING DIETARY THERAPY. Total cholesterol may be used to monitor response to diet. In patients prescribed the Step I Diet, initial monitoring should occur 4 to 6 weeks and 3 months after the institution of therapy. Initial monitoring in patients prescribed the Step II Diet should occur 3 to 4 weeks and 3 months after the institution of therapy. Adherence to both diets should be assessed at 3 months. Some patients may require a longer trial before response to diet can be ascertained. More frequent follow-up may increase adherence. In most cases, an adequate trial of diet requires a minimum of 6 months' adherence. After LDL cholesterol goals have been achieved, long-term monitoring can be performed at 6-month intervals, providing an opportunity for continual reinforcement of dietary counseling.

Instituting and maintaining appropriate dietary therapy is a complex and frequently time-consuming process. Consultation with a dietitian provides an efficient means of assessing the patient's dietary habits. In addition, involvement of a dietitian is helpful in promoting adherence and ensuring adequate nutrition, particularly in patients prescribed the Step II Diet. A concerted effort should be made to maximize the effectiveness of dietary therapy, and the importance of this treatment should be stressed by the physician.

TABLE 35–5 DIETARY THERAPY OF HIGH BLOOD CHOLESTEROL

NUTRIENT	STEP I DIET*	STEP II DIET
Total fat	≤30% of total calories†	
Saturated fat	8–10% of total calories	<7% of total calories
Polyunsaturated fat	≤10% of total calories†	
Monounsaturated fat	≤15% of total calories†	
Carbohydrates	≥55% of total calories†	
Protein	~15% of total calories†	
Cholesterol	<300 mg/d	<200 mg/d
Total calories	Sufficient to achieve and maintain desirable weight	

* Recommended eating pattern for all healthy Americans aged 2 years or older.

† for both Step I and Step II Diet.

From National Cholesterol Education Program: Second report of the Expert Panel on Detection, Evaluation, and Treatment of High Blood Cholesterol in Adults (Adult Treatment Panel II). Circulation *89*:1329, 1994. Copyright American Heart Association.

Drug Therapy

If, after an adequate trial of maximal dietary therapy, LDL cholesterol level remains above the initiation level for drug therapy (Table 35–6), pharmacological treatment of dyslipidemia should be considered in addition to dietary therapy (Table 35–7). Although an adequate trial of diet usually requires 6 months, a shorter time may be warranted in patients with CAD and in patients with severely ele-

TABLE 35–6 DRUG THERAPY TREATMENT LEVELS IN ADULTS

RISK	LDL CHOLESTEROL LEVEL (mg/dl)	
	Consideration Level	Goal
Without CHD, fewer than two other risk factors	≥190*	<160
Without CHD, two or more other risk factors	≥160	<130
With CHD or other atherosclerotic disease	≥130†	≤100

CHD = coronary heart disease; LDL = low-density lipoprotein.

* In younger patients (men aged <35 years and premenopausal women) with LDL cholesterol 190–220 mg/dl, drug therapy may be delayed if other risk is absent.

† In patients with CHD and LDL cholesterol 100–130 mg/dl, the physician should exercise clinical judgment in deciding whether to initiate drug therapy.

From National Cholesterol Education Program: Second report of the Expert Panel on Detection, Evaluation, and Treatment of High Blood Cholesterol in Adults (Adult Treatment Panel II). Circulation *89*:1329, 1994.

vated cholesterol levels that would not be expected to be corrected by diet alone. The decision to initiate drug therapy requires careful weighing of the expected benefits and costs of potentially lifelong therapy, including possible adverse effects. Once drug therapy has been initiated, discontinuation quickly returns LDL cholesterol to pretreatment levels.

In primary prevention, drug therapy should be considered in patients with fewer than two other risk factors whose LDL cholesterol remains 190 mg/dl or greater on maximal dietary therapy. The goal of treatment in these patients is to reduce LDL cholesterol to less than 160 mg/dl. Because younger patients are at lower risk for CAD events, the NCEP guidelines recommend that drug therapy be delayed in men aged less than 35 years and in premenopausal women unless LDL cholesterol is 220 mg/dl or greater or unless additional risk is present. Clinical judgment is required to assess the patient's overall risk.

In patients without CAD who have two or more other risk factors, drug therapy should be considered if LDL cholesterol remains 160 mg/dl or greater on maximal dietary therapy. In these patients, the goal of treatment is to reduce LDL cholesterol to less than 130 mg/dl.

In secondary prevention, the high rate of recurrence of acute ischemic events warrants more intensive therapy. Drug therapy should be considered if maximal dietary therapy does not lower LDL cholesterol to 130 mg/dl or less. However, clinical judgment should be used in deciding whether drug therapy is needed in patients whose LDL cholesterol is 100 to 129 mg/dl. Clinical judgment is also required to recognize patients in whom lipid-regulating pharmacological therapy is not appropriate, such as patients with a very advanced age, poor cardiac prognosis, or severe concomitant medical conditions. In general, even high-risk patients with limited life expectancy would not be expected to receive sufficient benefit from lipid-regulating drug therapy to justify its initiation.

Response to drug therapy should be monitored 6 to 8 weeks after initiation or, if nicotinic acid is used, 4 to 6 weeks after dosage stabilization; response should be reevaluated 6 weeks later. A minimum of two fasting lipoprotein analyses should be used to determine response, and adherence should be ascertained before adjusting dosage or considering another agent.

If 3 months' adherence to pharmacological monotherapy does not reduce LDL cholesterol to target levels, combination-drug therapy may be considered (Table 35–7). Although the addition of a second agent may increase the potential for side effects and drug interactions, combination therapy often decreases side effects and costs and increases adherence, because a lower dosage of each agent is required. In secondary prevention, clinical judgment is required to determine whether to add a second agent if LDL cholesterol is 100 to 129 mg/dl with pharmacological monotherapy.

Available lipid-regulating agents are bile-acid sequestrants, nicotinic acid, HMG-CoA reductase inhibitors, fibric-acid derivatives, and probucol (Table 35–8).[83a] In some postmenopausal women, estrogen-replacement therapy may provide an alternative to drug therapy.

BILE-ACID SEQUESTRANTS. The bile-acid sequestrants are quaternary ammonium salts, usually dispensed as a powdered preparation that requires mixing with liquids or foods prior to administration. However, a caplet and confectionery bar have been developed to increase ease of administration and palatability. The bile-acid sequestrants have a long history of clinical use, and their mechanisms of action, side effects, and clinical efficacy are well established. The use of bile-acid sequestrant monotherapy has declined in recent years because of the advent of more palatable and more potent drugs.

The mechanisms of action of the two available agents, cholestyramine and colestipol, are similar. These agents interrupt the enterohepatic circulation of bile acids by acting as polycationic exchange resins that bind the bile acids in the intestinal lumen and increase fecal loss.[83] Normally, approximately 97 per cent of the endogenously produced bile acids are reabsorbed and recycled in the enterohepatic circulation, and only 3 per cent are excreted. The increased excretion of bile acids with bile-acid sequestrant therapy causes an increase in the activity of 7-alpha-hydroxylase, the rate-limiting enzyme of bile acid synthesis, thereby increasing the conversion of cholesterol into bile acids. The resulting decrease in intrahepatic cholesterol causes increased activity of the B/E receptor and therefore the enhanced removal of apo B– and apo E–containing lipoproteins from the circulation. However, HMG-CoA reductase activity is also increased in response to the decrease in intrahepatic cholesterol, so that plasma cholesterol returns toward pretreatment levels.[84]

TABLE 35–7 DRUG SELECTION IN ADULTS: NATIONAL CHOLESTEROL EDUCATION PROGRAM RECOMMENDATIONS

HYPERLIPIDEMIA	SINGLE DRUG	COMBINATION DRUG
Elevated LDL cholesterol and triglyceride <200 mg/dl	Bile-acid sequestrant	Bile-acid sequestrant + HMG-CoA reductase inhibitor
	HMG-CoA reductase inhibitor	Bile-acid sequestrant + nicotinic acid
	Nicotinic acid	HMG-CoA reductase inhibitor + nicotinic acid*
Elevated LDL cholesterol and triglyceride 200–400 mg/dl	Nicotinic acid	Nicotinic acid + HMG-CoA reductase inhibitor*
	HMG-CoA reductase inhibitor	HMG-CoA reductase inhibitor + gemfibrozil†
	Gemfibrozil	Nicotinic acid + bile-acid sequestrant
		Nicotinic acid + gemfibrozil

HMG-CoA = 3-hydroxy-3-methylglutaryl coenzyme A; LDL = low-density lipoprotein.

* Possible increased risk for myopathy or liver dysfunction.

† Increased risk for myopathy; must be used with caution.

From National Cholesterol Education Program: Second report of the Expert Panel on Detection, Evaluation, and Treatment of High Blood Cholesterol in Adults (Adult Treatment Panel II). Circulation *89*:1329, 1994.

TABLE 35–8 LIPID-LOWERING AGENTS: MECHANISMS, LIPID EFFECTS, AND SIDE EFFECTS

DRUG CLASS AND AGENTS	MECHANISM OF ACTION AND LIPID EFFECTS	SELECTED BIOCHEMICAL SIDE EFFECTS	SELECTED SYSTEMIC SIDE EFFECTS
Bile-acid sequestrants (resins) Cholestyramine (4–24 gm/day) Colestipol (5–30 gm/day)	Increase excretion of bile acids in the stool; increase LDL-receptor activity. Effectively decrease LDL cholesterol; HDL cholesterol increases slightly; may increase triglyceride	Binding and decreased absorption of certain other drugs; may prevent absorption of fat-soluble vitamins	No systemic toxicity; upper and lower gastrointestinal complaints common, such as constipation, bloating
Nicotinic acid (niacin) (1.5–6 gm/day)	Decreases plasma levels of free fatty acids; decreases hepatic VLDL synthesis; possibly inhibits cholesterol synthesis. Effectively decreases both LDL cholesterol and triglyceride; effectively increases HDL cholesterol	Altered liver function tests, increased uric acid, increased glucose intolerance	Cutaneous flushing, pruritus, gastrointestinal upset; side effects tend to limit compliance
HMG-CoA reductase inhibitors (statins) Fluvastatin (20–40 mg/day) Lovastatin (10–80 mg/day) Pravastatin (10–40 mg/day) Simvastatin (5–40 mg/day)	Inhibit HMG-CoA reductase, the rate-limiting step in cholesterol biosynthesis; increase LDL-receptor activity. Effectively decrease LDL cholesterol; moderate effect in decreasing triglyceride and in increasing HDL cholesterol	Elevated transaminase levels can occur (minor and usually transient); increased creatine kinase (uncommon)	Mild gastrointestinal symptoms; myositis syndrome (rare)
Fibric-acid derivatives (fibrates) Gemfibrozil (1.2 gm/day) Clofibrate (2 gm/day)	Decrease hepatic VLDL synthesis; increase lipoprotein lipase activity. Decrease triglyceride effectively; increase HDL cholesterol effectively; effect on LDL cholesterol variable, but may increase, especially in hypertriglyceridemia	Transient transaminase increases not infrequent; can potentiate effects of oral anticoagulants	Increased incidence of cholelithiasis; diarrhea, nausea, skin rash, myositis (rare)
Probucol (1 gm/day)	Enhances scavenger pathway removal of LDL. Slightly to moderately decreases LDL cholesterol; usually no effect on triglyceride; substantially decreases HDL cholesterol	Prolongation of QT interval and serious ventricular arrhythmias have occurred but are rare	Side effects usually infrequent and of short duration; chiefly, diarrhea, nausea, flatulence

HDL = high-density lipoprotein; HMG-CoA = 3-hydroxy-3-methylglutaryl coenzyme A; LDL = low-density lipoprotein; VLDL = very-low-density lipoprotein.

From Jones P. H., and Gotto, A. M., Jr.: Hyperlipidemia. *In* Hurst, J. W. (ed.): Medicine for the Practicing Physician, 4th ed. Norwalk, CT, Appleton & Lange 1996.

Cholestyramine dosed at 4 to 16 gm/day, up to a maximum of 24 gm/day, or colestipol dosed at 5 to 20 gm/day, up to a maximum of 30 gm/day, decreases LDL cholesterol 15 to 30 per cent on average. HDL cholesterol may increase 3 to 5 per cent, although it has not been determined if bile-acid sequestrants alter HDL synthesis or catabolic rates. Plasma triglyceride is not usually affected but may increase; this increase is more common in patients who are hypertriglyceridemic before therapy.

The major side effects of cholestyramine and colestipol are gastrointestinal disorders such as constipation, reflux esophagitis, and nausea. Because these drugs are not absorbed into the circulation, systemic side effects are uncommon. The same nonspecific binding by which the bile-acid sequestrants bind bile acids may cause decreased absorption of other drugs, including warfarin,[85] digitalis preparations,[86] thiazide diuretics,[87] and beta blockers.[88]

NICOTINIC ACID. Nicotinic acid is a B vitamin that was discovered to have lipid-regulating effects at high doses. Although nicotinic acid is a coenzyme in intermediary carbohydrate metabolism, this role is not related to its lipid-regulating action.

The mechanisms of action of nicotinic acid are complex and result in favorable changes in all lipoprotein fractions except chylomicrons. The primary action is a decrease in the hepatic synthesis and release of VLDL, thus also decreasing the circulating levels of IDL and LDL because of decreased production of precursor particles.[89] In addition, nicotinic acid causes a decrease in the release of free fatty acids from adipocytes, thereby decreasing hepatic production of triglyceride by decreasing the availability of the substrates for triglyceride synthesis. However, the long-term impact of this peripheral effect on the lipid profile has been questioned.[90]

Crystalline nicotinic acid dosed at 1.5 to 6 gm/day decreases LDL cholesterol 10 to 25 per cent. Triglyceride decreases 20 to 50 per cent, and HDL cholesterol increases 15 to 35 per cent. The increase in HDL cholesterol is caused by decreased catabolism of HDL and apo A-I.[91] Nicotinic acid has been shown to decrease Lp(a) levels,[92] which are not usually affected by lipid-regulating drugs. Nicotinic acid is also available in sustained-release preparations, which are administered at lower doses, but increased side effects and safety concerns have limited their use (see below).

Side effects of nicotinic acid include mild clinical irritations and potentially life-threatening complications. The rapid absorption of crystalline nicotinic acid from the gastrointestinal tract after oral administration may account for the agent's vasodilatory effects. Flushing is seen in virtually all patients and is secondary to the release of prostaglandin by the endothelium. Preadministration of prostaglandin inhibitors, such as aspirin, may decrease flushing. Hepatic toxicity, perhaps due to the high first-pass extraction of nicotinic acid by the liver, ranges from mild elevations of transaminase levels to fulminant hepatic failure,[93] although the latter is reported more often with sustained-release preparations.[94] Mild elevations of liver enzymes may be seen in as many as 5 per cent of patients receiving nicotinic acid[90] and are not in and of themselves indications for discontinuation of this drug. However, close clinical monitoring is warranted; an increase in liver enzymes to three times normal or greater requires discontinuation of nicotinic acid. On the other hand, a sudden decline in liver enzyme levels may indicate significant clinical deterioration and decreased synthetic ability and constitutes a medical emergency. Other gastrointestinal side effects include activation of peptic ulcer disease.[95] Nicotinic acid has also been reported to worsen glucose tolerance, precipitate gout, and cause ophthalmological complications that include worsening of glaucoma and cystic maculopathy secondary to increased fluid retention within the retina. Myositis is rare with nicotinic acid monotherapy[96] but may be somewhat more common when nicotinic acid is combined with an HMG-CoA reductase inhibitor.[97]

HMG-COA REDUCTASE INHIBITORS. The HMG-CoA reductase inhibitors represent a major therapeutic advance in lipid-regulating pharmacological therapy because of their increased efficacy, tolerability, and ease of administration. Fluvastatin, lovastatin, pravastatin, and simvastatin are the currently available agents.

Despite structural differences, the HMG-CoA reductase inhibitors appear to share a common mechanism of action, the partial inhibition of HMG-CoA reductase, the rate-limiting enzyme in cholesterol biosynthesis. The resultant reduction in intracellular cholesterol in the liver stimulates the upregulation of the B/E receptor and increases clearance of lipoproteins containing apo B or apo E from the plasma compartment. Although the predominant effect is to decrease circulating LDL cholesterol, VLDL and IDL particles are also removed. Inhibition of the synthesis of apo B–containing lipoproteins has also been postulated as a potential mechanism for these agents,[98] but this hypothesis remains controversial. Potential beneficial nonlipid effects include a reduction in plasminogen activator inhibitor 1 (PAI-1) in patients with hypercholesterolemia, reported with lovastatin[99] and pravastatin,[100] which provides a hemostatic mechanism for clinical improvement with HMG-CoA reductase inhibitor therapy.

Fluvastatin dosed at 20 to 40 mg/day, lovastatin dosed at 10 to 80 mg/day, pravastatin dosed at 10 to 40 mg/day, or simvastatin dosed at 5 to 40 mg/day may be expected to decrease LDL cholesterol 20 to 40 per cent. The dose–response effect of the HMG-CoA reductase inhibitors is log-linear: At higher doses, the cholesterol-lowering effect increases in smaller increments. HDL cholesterol increases 5 to 15 per cent, although the precise mechanism has not been elucidated, and triglyceride decreases 10 to 20 per cent, presumably because of increased clearance of VLDL by the B/E receptor.[101] Lp(a) level does not appear to be affected by HMG-CoA reductase inhibitor therapy.[102]

Because of their high patient acceptance rate and lipid-regulating efficacy, the HMG-CoA reductase inhibitors are frequently used as first-line pharmacological monotherapy. In addition, recently published clinical trial data have demonstrated improvements in clinical and anatomical endpoints. However, these agents are too new to have accumulated the long-term safety and efficacy data recorded for agents such as the bile-acid sequestrants; consequently, the NCEP does not recommend HMG-CoA reductase inhibitors as first-line drug therapy in primary prevention in young adults unless the underlying dyslipidemia is severe.

The side effects of the HMG-CoA reductase inhibitors are minimal. The major clinical problems that have been reported are hepatotoxicity and myopathy. Serum liver enzyme levels were greater than three times the upper limit of normal in less than 2 per cent of subjects who received maximum-dosage lovastatin in the 1-year Expanded Clinical Evaluation of Lovastatin (EXCEL) study, and at the usual dosage, the incidence was less than 1 per cent.[103] Most cases of transaminase elevation appear to occur within the first 3 months of therapy. Rhabdomyolysis has been documented in approximately 0.1 per cent of subjects receiving lovastatin monotherapy[104] and appears to occur at about the same frequency for all the HMG-CoA reductase inhibitors. However, the exact incidence of myopathy, as defined by creatine kinase elevation, that is attributable to HMG-CoA reductase inhibitor use is difficult to establish: In subjects who continued in the EXCEL study a second year, creatine kinase elevations above the upper limit of normal were reported in 50 to 67 per cent of the groups receiving various dosages of lovastatin and 54 per cent of the placebo group.[105] Risk for myopathy may be increased when an HMG-CoA reductase inhibitor is combined with a fibric-acid derivative,[106] nicotinic acid,[107] cyclosporine,[108] or erythromycin.[109] Despite initial concern based on inhibitors of enzymes of cholesterol synthesis other than HMG-CoA, no evidence of increased lens opacity has been reported with the use of HMG-CoA reductase inhibitors.[110] Although it has been postulated that the lipophilic agents, lovastatin and simvastatin, may have a greater potential for sleep disturbances than the hydrophilic fluvastatin and pravastatin, because the former cross the blood–brain barrier, the incidence of sleep disturbances is uncommon with either lipophilic or hydrophilic agents.[111]

FIBRIC-ACID DERIVATIVES. The fibric-acid derivatives have been used clinically in a variety of lipoprotein disorders, and their efficacy and safety have been demonstrated. Clofibrate, which is little used, and gemfibrozil are currently available in the United States, and bezafibrate, ciprofibrate, and fenofibrate are available in other countries. Fenofibrate has been approved in the United States but is not yet available.

The mechanism of action of the fibric-acid derivatives is complex and has not been completely elucidated. The major effect is a decrease in VLDL secondary to increased lipoprotein lipase activity; lipoprotein lipase hydrolyzes triglyceride from VLDL to form IDL, which is either removed by the B/E receptor through apo E–mediated recognition and binding or further hydrolyzed by hepatic lipase to form LDL. The fibrates may also exert a peripheral effect by decreasing plasma levels of free fatty acids.[112]

Gemfibrozil dosed at 1200 mg/day or clofibrate dosed at 2000 mg/day decreases triglyceride 20 to 50 per cent and increases HDL cholesterol 10 to 15 per cent. LDL cholesterol is typically decreased 10 to 15 per cent but may increase in patients with hypertriglyceridemia, perhaps because of the inability of the B/E receptor to remove the increased number of LDL particles that result from enhanced VLDL catabolism. A decrease in Lp(a) has been reported with bezafibrate administration.[113]

In addition to their effects on lipoprotein levels, fibric-acid derivatives may alter the composition of lipoproteins. As noted above, gemfibrozil and bezafibrate have been shown to decrease the concentration of small, dense LDL. The fibrates may thus protect against coronary atherosclerosis not only by reducing LDL cholesterol level but also by shifting LDL particles to a less atherogenic phenotype.

Additionally, the fibric-acid derivatives provide nonlipid benefits, such as improvements in coagulation and fibrinolysis. A reduction in platelet aggregability and reactivity in response to epinephrine has been documented with gemfibrozil.[114] Gemfibrozil has also been shown to decrease the activity of PAI-1, thereby potentially improving fibrinolytic efficacy.[115] Bezafibrate has been reported to decrease circulating levels of fibrinogen[116]; fibrinogen has been directly associated with CAD risk in epidemiological studies (see below).

The side effects of the fibric-acid derivatives are generally mild and are encountered in approximately 5 to 10 per cent of patients treated with these agents. The majority of complaints are of nonspecific gastrointestinal symptoms such as nausea, flatulence, bloating, and dyspepsia. Increased lithogenicity of bile has been reported with clofibrate therapy[28] but has not been clearly demonstrated with the other fibrates. Fibrate monotherapy rarely results in muscle toxicity,[117] although mild elevations of creatine kinase may occasionally occur. However, the risk for myopathy is increased when a fibrate is used in combination with an HMG-CoA reductase inhibitor, as described above. Although recent studies have demonstrated that this combination may be used without severe muscle toxicity,[118] great caution is required, and careful patient education and surveillance are prerequisites.

PROBUCOL. Probucol is a complex agent that cannot be readily classified with the other lipid-regulating drugs in terms of structure or mechanism of action. It is a bisphenol derivative that is similar in structure to butylated hydroxytoluene, a compound with powerful antioxidant activity that has also been demonstrated to decrease the early microcirculatory changes induced by hypercholesterolemia in rabbits.[119]

The mechanism of action by which probucol lowers lipid levels has not been completely elucidated. Probucol does not appear to decrease the production of lipoproteins nor does it alter plasma clearance through the B/E receptor pathway. In the Watanabe heritable hyperlipidemic rabbit, which serves as an animal model for FH because it lacks functioning B/E receptors, the decreased rate of progression of atherosclerotic lesions with probucol administration appears to be predominantly attributable to the inhibitory effect of probucol on LDL oxidation.[120] In patients with FH, regression of tendinous xanthomas has been reported with probucol use.[121]

Probucol dosed at 1 gm/day decreases LDL cholesterol 5 to 15 per cent and decreases HDL cholesterol 20 to 30 per cent. Triglyceride is usually not affected. The effect on HDL cholesterol appears to be greater in patients with higher pretreatment levels of HDL cholesterol[122] and is of concern because of the inverse relation between HDL cholesterol level and CAD incidence established in epidemiological studies (see below). The composition of HDL particles is also altered by probucol therapy: The triglyceride content of HDL is increased, and the concentration of cholesteryl ester in HDL is decreased, apparently owing to increased CETP activity.[123] The clinical impact of the probucol-induced reduction in HDL cholesterol is controversial, but evidence suggests that probucol administration may enhance reverse cholesterol transport secondary to increased CETP activity and increased hepatic uptake of HDL.[124]

The side effects of probucol appear to be minimal. Probucol is highly lipophilic, so its absorption is enhanced after a fatty meal; therefore, administration should be separated from meals to prevent drug toxicity. Mild gastrointestinal symptoms are occasionally reported. The main clinical concern with probucol use is the possible potentiation of rhythm disorders associated with prolongation of repolarization. In experimental animals, increased incidence of sudden cardiac death with probucol administration was thought to be caused by induced ventricular arrhythmias.[125] Although no clear correlation between probucol use and sudden cardiac death has been established in humans, the Q-T interval should be monitored, especially in patients with baseline prolongation or receiving concomitant sotalol, quinidine, procainamide, tricyclic antidepressants, phenothiazines, or other agents known to increase the Q-T interval.

ESTROGEN. Women lose their relative protection against coronary atherosclerosis at menopause, when decreased estrogen production causes a gradual rise in LDL cholesterol levels. In a study in 542 healthy women, postmenopausal women had 14 per cent higher total cholesterol, 12 per cent higher triglyceride, and 27 per cent higher LDL cholesterol; HDL cholesterol was 7 per cent lower.[126] These potentially atherogenic alterations in the lipid profile have prompted an increased interest in estrogen-replacement therapy in postmenopausal women.

Estrogen-replacement therapy has been shown to decrease CAD morbidity and CAD mortality in observational epidemiological studies.[127] In a meta-analysis of case–control, cross-sectional, and prospective studies, the relative risk for CAD in postmenopausal subjects taking estrogen was 0.56 compared with postmenopausal subjects not taking estrogen.[128]

The precise mechanisms by which estrogen decreases CAD risk are not known. Increased HDL cholesterol and decreased LDL cholesterol have been demonstrated,[129] and other possible benefits include improved coronary tone and altered platelet aggregation. A decreased accumulation of LDL in the arterial wall has been reported in animal studies.[130] Circulating Lp(a) may also be decreased.[131]

Conjugated estrogen dosed at 0.625 mg/day or micronized estradiol dosed at 2 mg/day, administered orally, decreases LDL cholesterol 15 per cent and increases HDL cholesterol up to 15 per cent. Plasma triglyceride may increase, particularly if it is elevated before initiation of therapy. Transcutaneous or percutaneous administration of estrogen generally appears to have less effect on lipid levels than oral administration. Estrogen does not have a U.S. Food and Drug Administration indication for lipid regulation or CAD risk reduction.

Unopposed estrogen use increases risk for endometrial cancer and possibly increases risk for breast cancer. However, coadministration with progesterone moderates the risk for endometrial cancer without nullifying the lipid-regulating benefits of estrogen.[132]

Primary Dyslipidemias Characterized by Hypercholesterolemia

Fredrickson phenotypes in which hypercholesterolemia is the major dyslipidemia are types IIa and IIb. In type IIa, hypercholesterolemia is the only dyslipidemia, and in type IIb, triglyceride is also elevated. Both of these phenotypes are associated with increased risk for atherosclerotic disease. Among causes of secondary type II hyperlipidemia, which should be ruled out before a primary cause is considered, are diet, myxedema, obstructive liver disease, and nephrosis.

FAMILIAL HYPERCHOLESTEROLEMIA. The most clearly delineated familial disorder presenting as a type IIa and rarely as a type IIb phenotype is FH, an autosomal dominant disorder caused by a defect in the gene for the B/E receptor that results in decreased production or function of B/E receptors.[133,133a] Heterozygous FH occurs in approximately 1 in 500 individuals in the United States but has a higher frequency in Lebanon and in the Afrikaner population in South Africa, where the gene frequency is thought to be 1 per cent. Affected individuals have approximately half the number of functioning B/E receptors, and total cholesterol, which is elevated at birth, may reach 350 to 500 mg/dl. Symptomatic CAD typically develops by age 50 in men and age 60 in women. Clinical features include tendon xanthomas and corneal arcus. Heterozygous FH may be difficult to diagnose[134]; familial combined hyperlipidemia (FCH) and familial defective apo B-100 (see below) should be considered in the differential diagnosis. Treatment consists of dietary and drug therapy; combination-drug therapy is usually required.

Homozygous FH occurs in approximately 1 in 1 million individuals in the United States. Affected individuals have virtually no competent B/E receptors, and total cholesterol, which is elevated at birth, reaches 700 to 1200 mg/dl. Symptomatic CAD typically develops before age 20; premature atherosclerosis is the rule, and myocardial infarctions have been reported before the age of 2 years. Clinical features include cutaneous xanthomas, tendinous xanthomas, corneal arcus, and severe, diffuse atherosclerosis. The presence of xanthomas, which frequently occur in the buttocks, tongue, eyelid, and buccal mucosa, strongly suggests a diagnosis of FH, although tendinous xanthomas are not specific to FH but are also seen in other rare diseases such as cerebrotendinous xanthomatosis and sitosterolemia. Similarly, corneal arcus is a nonspecific finding for the diagnosis of FH; the presence of corneal arcus in a white patient aged less than 35 years suggests the presence of an underlying metabolic defect, but this sign loses its specificity in older patients and in black patients.

Low-Density Lipoprotein Apheresis. Because FH is usually resistant to dietary and pharmacological therapy, special techniques may be required to reduce circulating LDL cholesterol. LDL apheresis removes apo B–containing lipoproteins from blood by extracorporeal binding to dextran sulfate–cellulose columns, heparin precipitation, or immunoabsorption. In the LDL-Apheresis Regression Study, conducted in 37 subjects (7 patients with homozygous FH, 25 patients with heterozygous FH, and 5 hypercholesterolemic patients not diagnosed with FH), LDL cholesterol was reduced 78 per cent immediately after apheresis, and, after 1 year of apheresis treatments, regression was reported in 38 per cent of subjects.[135] The reduction in LDL cholesterol is only temporary, so the procedure must be repeated at 2- to 4-week intervals. In the Familial Hypercholesterolaemia Regression Study, 39 men and women with heterozygous FH were followed up by quantitative coronary angiography after a mean of 2.1 years of receiving either LDL apheresis every 2 weeks and simvastatin 40 mg/day or colestipol 20 gm/day and simvastatin 40 mg/day.[136] Entry criteria included total cholesterol of 310 mg/dl or greater plus either tendon xanthomas in the subject or a first-degree relative or total cholesterol of at least 310 mg/dl or myocardial infarction before age 60 in a first-degree relative or before age 50 in a second-degree relative, at least two abnormal coronary segments on angiographic assessment, and age of 20 to 64 years. Despite greater lowering of LDL cholesterol with apheresis plus simvastatin (53 per cent compared with 44 per cent with colestipol plus simvastatin), the primary angiographic endpoint of mean change in per cent diameter stenosis of the worst lesion in diseased segments was not significantly different between treatment groups, and the other primary endpoint—the number of patients demonstrating progression, regression, and no change or a mixed response—was also similar between groups. LDL apheresis is expensive and currently available only in selected centers.

Liver Transplantation. This procedure has been performed in patients with homozygous FH. In a 6-year-old patient, transplantation of a liver and heart from a normal donor decreased plasma LDL cholesterol 81 per cent and increased the fractional catabolic rate of radiolabeled LDL 2.5 times.[137]

Gene Therapy. This technique has recently been employed to introduce functioning B/E receptors in a patient with homozygous FH.[138] The ex vivo technique used requires partial hepatectomy, and the isolated hepatocytes are infected with retroviruses that express the normal B/E receptor. After the treated hepatocytes were infused into the patient, LDL cholesterol decreased 17 per cent. However, liver resection may cause a decrease in circulating LDL, because of decreased secretion of VLDL, and it has been suggested that gene therapy experiments demonstrate that LDL reductions are the result of increased B/E receptor activity, which should then be demonstrated to result from the exogenous gene.[139]

POLYGENIC HYPERCHOLESTEROLEMIA. The most common genetic cause of type IIa hyperlipidemia is polygenic hypercholesterolemia.[140] Although the prevalence of this disorder is unknown, it is thought to be between 1 in 20 and 1 in 100 in the United States. Total cholesterol level is usually less than in heterozygous FH, and xanthomas are absent. Severe cases may require treatment similar to that of heterozygous FH but may not require combination-drug therapy.

FAMILIAL COMBINED HYPERLIPIDEMIA. FCH[141] may present as type IIa, type IIb, or type IV hyperlipidemia. In type II presentations, total cholesterol is usually 250 to 350 mg/dl. In type IIb and type IV presentations, triglyceride elevations are typically mild to moderate but may be severe. Presentation may vary within a family and within an individual. The disorder is relatively common in the United States, occurring in approximately 1 in 100 individuals. It is not known whether transmission is monogenic or polygenic; inheritance is autosomal dominant. The underlying mechanism is thought to be overproduction of apo B-100. Clinically, this disease may be distinguished from FH by a lack of tendinous xanthomas. Expression may or may not occur before adulthood. Premature coronary atherosclerosis is associated with FCH, and early recognition and treatment are required. The primary treatment is dietary; if diet proves inadequate, drug therapy should be added as appropriate for the dyslipidemia.

FAMILIAL DEFECTIVE APOLIPOPROTEIN B-100. Familial defective apo B-100 is an autosomal dominant disorder caused by a mutation in the gene for apo B-100 that results in apo B-100 with an abnormal structure and decreased binding by the B/E receptor.[142] Prevalence varies but is approximately 1 in 700 in whites. Cholesterol levels are similar to those in heterozygous FH but may be more moderate. In general, familial defective apo B-100 may be distinguished from heterozygous FH by the lack of tendinous xanthomas and by less severe hypercholesterolemia, but accurate diagnosis may require molecular analysis. Treatment is as for heterozygous FH and should begin with dietary therapy, to which may be added an HMG-CoA reductase inhibitor or a bile-acid sequestrant. Nicotinic acid is also useful in treating familial defective apo B-100.[143]

Low High-Density Lipoprotein Cholesterol

An inverse association has been established between HDL cholesterol level and CAD incidence in numerous epidemiological studies. For example, in the Framingham Heart Study, men and women with HDL cholesterol of 35 mg/dl or less had an eightfold increase in CAD incidence compared with men and women with HDL cholesterol of 65 mg/dl or greater.[144] Each 1 mg/dl increase in HDL cholesterol is estimated to decrease CAD risk 2 per cent in men and 3 per cent in women.[145]

Primary hypoalphalipoproteinemia may occur in up to 5 per cent of the general population. HDL cholesterol levels may also be lowered by cigarette smoking, the use of drugs such as anabolic steroids or beta blockers, and a diet very high in polyunsaturated fat.

High-Density Lipoprotein Metabolism

HDL is believed to be secreted by the liver and intestine as a discoidal precursor particle of phospholipid, cholesterol, and apolipoproteins. Through the activity of lecithin:cholesterol acyltransferase (LCAT), a core of cholesteryl ester is generated from the phospholipid and cholesterol, and the disk is transformed into mature, spherical HDL_3. HDL_3 acquires additional phospholipid and cholesterol from cell membranes and from the excess surface components of hydrolyzed triglyceride-rich lipoproteins. Through continued LCAT activity, HDL_3 is converted to HDL_2, which is larger and more cholesterol rich than HDL_3. Women have significantly higher plasma levels of HDL_2 than men[146]; increased levels of these larger, less dense particles may be partially responsible for the relative cardioprotection seen in premenopausal women.

The mechanism by which HDL confers decreased risk for CAD is complex and poorly understood. One proposed mechanism is as the possible vehicle of reverse cholesterol transport, the posited process by which cholesterol is returned from peripheral cells to the liver for excretion into the bile acid pool or for reconstitution into cell membranes or VLDL. Although the process by which cholesterol leaves the peripheral cell and is scavenged by HDL has not been clarified, a number of potential mechanisms have been proposed, including cholesterol efflux.[147]

Through the action of CETP, triglyceride from the triglyceride-rich lipoproteins is exchanged for cholesteryl ester in HDL. The transferred triglyceride then becomes a substrate for hepatic lipase, and the transferred cholesteryl ester continues with the triglyceride-rich lipoproteins in their respective lipolytic cascades and is removed with chylomicron remnants, IDL, and LDL. Because of the metabolic interrelation between HDL and the triglyceride-rich lipoproteins, high HDL cholesterol level may reflect rapid clearance of these triglyceride-rich particles, thereby decreasing the exposure of the vessel wall to potentially atherogenic remnant particles.[148] HDL levels would then serve as a marker of the efficiency of this metabolic process, rather than conferring direct protection against CAD.

Other potential mechanisms by which HDL may confer cardioprotection include enhancement of endothelial repair[149] and prostacyclin stabilization.[150] HDL has also demonstrated dose-dependent protection against peroxidation of LDL.[151]

Diagnosis and Treatment of Low High-Density Lipoprotein Cholesterol

As stated above, HDL cholesterol less than 35 mg/dl is considered low in the NCEP guidelines. The primary therapy for low HDL cholesterol is life style modification, emphasizing diet, regular exercise, smoking cessation, and weight reduction as appropriate. Intense efforts should also be made to control blood pressure and diabetes mellitus. If feasible, drugs that lower HDL cholesterol should be discontinued.

None of the available lipid-regulating agents acts exclusively to increase HDL cholesterol, and the NCEP does not recommend introducing a drug solely for this purpose in primary prevention in patients who are otherwise at low risk for CAD. However, if drug therapy is indicated to lower LDL cholesterol, a secondary goal of increasing HDL cholesterol should guide in selection of the agent. Lipid-regulating agents that are particularly effective in increasing HDL cholesterol are the fibric-acid derivatives, which have a greater effect in patients who also have increased plasma triglyceride, and nicotinic acid. In general, the same treatment plan should be used in secondary prevention, although the NCEP does recommend the consideration of nicotinic acid to increase HDL cholesterol even in patients whose LDL cholesterol is below the initiation level for drug therapy.

Primary Dyslipidemias Characterized by Low High-Density Lipoprotein Cholesterol

TANGIER DISEASE. Tangier disease, which was initially thought to be a lipid storage disorder, is a rare autosomal recessive disorder marked by low levels of both HDL cholesterol and apo A-I.[152] Cholesteryl ester is deposited in the tissues of the reticuloendothelial system, causing orange tonsils that in combination with low total cholesterol are diagnostic of this disease. Other symptoms include splenomegaly, peripheral neuropathy, and ocular abnormalities. Atherosclerotic risk does not appear to be increased.[153] This disorder results from markedly increased catabolism of HDL, apo A-I, and apo A-II[154] instead of from decreased synthesis.

LECITHIN:CHOLESTEROL ACYLTRANSFERASE DEFICIENCY. In familial LCAT deficiency disorder, LCAT activity is absent, resulting in increased plasma levels of cholesterol and lecithin and decreased plasma levels of cholesteryl ester and lysolecithin.[155] Composition, structure, and concentration of all lipoprotein fractions are altered.[156] HDL may remain as discoidal precursor particles or small, spherical particles. Clinical features include corneal opacities, anemia, renal failure, and proteinuria. Despite decreased HDL cholesterol, CAD risk is not usually increased, but atherosclerosis and tendon and planar xanthomas may result from hyperlipidemia and hypertension secondary to renal failure.

FISH-EYE DISEASE. Fish-eye disease resembles LCAT deficiency, but only LCAT activity toward HDL is decreased.[157] HDL particles are similar to those in LCAT deficiency, and triglyceride may be elevated. Corneal opacities are characteristic of this disease, and corneal transplantation is required in older patients. Atherosclerotic risk does not appear to be increased.

APO A-I$_{Milano}$. Individuals who have the apo A-I$_{Milano}$ mutation have low HDL cholesterol and hypertriglyceridemia. In a comparison of 29 affected individuals with age- and gender-matched controls, HDL cholesterol was decreased 67 per cent and triglyceride was increased 75 per cent.[158] Apo A-I$_{Milano}$ results from a mutation in the gene for apo A-I that has been shown to increase plasma clearance of apo A-I: Apo A-I$_{Milano}$ was catabolized more rapidly than normal apo A-I in normal subjects, and both apo A-I$_{Milano}$ and normal apo A-I were catabolized more rapidly in subjects with apo A-I$_{Milano}$ than in normal subjects.[159] Apo A-I$_{Milano}$ may also be more easily dissociated from HDL, thus potentially increasing the role of free apo A-I in cholesterol efflux. Despite low HDL cholesterol levels in these patients, CAD risk does not appear to be increased.[160]

APO A-I/APO C-III DEFICIENCY. A genetic disorder in which low HDL cholesterol is associated with increased atherosclerotic risk was reported in two sisters aged 29 and 31 years, who had HDL cholesterol levels of 4 mg/dl and 7 mg/dl and severe coronary atherosclerosis.[161] Apo A-I was not detectable on electrophoresis, and only traces were detectable on radioimmunoassay. Apo C-III was not detectable. The half-life of infused HDL was about half that in normal individuals. First-degree relatives also had low HDL cholesterol and low apo A-I. The underlying genetic abnormality is an inversion of the DNA i.e., DNA that contains parts of the genes for apo A-I and apo C-III.[162]

HIGH-DENSITY LIPOPROTEIN DEFICIENCY WITH XANTHOMAS. HDL deficiency with xanthomas has been described in a Turkish kindred with repetitive consanguinity.[163] The proband had HDL cholesterol of only 2 mg/dl and no apo A-I. Apo A-II level was approximately 15 per cent of normal, but apo A-IV and apo C-III levels were normal. Apo B and LDL cholesterol levels were increased, VLDL and IDL were decreased, and triglyceride level was normal. The underlying genetic defect, which has an autosomal dominant transmission, is a mutation in the apo A-I gene.

Hypertriglyceridemia

Although the relation between plasma triglyceride and CAD is not as well established as the relation between plasma cholesterol and CAD, epidemiological evidence suggests that triglyceride plays an important role in determining CAD risk. In prospective studies, univariate analyses have established a direct association between triglyceride level and CAD incidence, but the association often weakens in multivariate analyses and may disappear in analyses controlling for HDL cholesterol.[164]

In part, the weakening of association may be due to the metabolic interrelation between the triglyceride-rich lipoproteins and HDL. Variability of triglyceride measurements both within an individual and between individuals may also account for the uncertain relation between triglyceride and CAD.[165] Subjects may be misclassified in epidemiological and clinical trials, and controlling for more accurately measured lipids such as HDL cholesterol may cause the association of triglyceride and CAD to disappear.[166]

Triglyceride concentration is ordinarily determined from a fasting sample, but postprandial lipemia may also contribute to CAD risk. Recent studies have correlated the magnitude of elevation of remnants of triglyceride-rich lipoproteins with CAD, although fasting triglyceride level may be normal.[167] In one study, postprandial triglyceride level but not fasting triglyceride level was shown to be an independent predictor of CAD even in multivariate analysis controlling for HDL cholesterol.[168] These studies suggest that the inability to clear these lipid-rich and potentially cytotoxic remnant particles may play a role in atherogenesis. Gemfibrozil and lovastatin have been shown to decrease postprandial triglyceride levels.[169]

Epidemiological Evidence

A meta-analysis of 16 population-based, prospective studies, 12 that together enrolled 33,214 men and 4 that together enrolled 5836 women, with follow-up ranging from 3 to 14.5 years, triglyceride was established as a CAD risk factor even after adjusting for HDL cholesterol.[170] Although controlling for HDL cholesterol weakened the relation between triglyceride and CAD risk, the relation remained significant.

PROSPECTIVE CARDIOVASCULAR MÜNSTER STUDY. Among 4576 men in the observational Prospective Cardiovascular Münster (PROCAM) study, 39 per cent of subjects with myocardial infarction or CAD death, compared with 21 per cent of surviving subjects without myocardial infarction or stroke, had a triglyceride level of at least 200 mg/dl.[171] Triglyceride level was significantly related to CAD events in univariate analysis, but the association disappeared in multivariate analysis controlling for total cholesterol or HDL cholesterol. However, the combination of triglyceride level of at least 200 mg/dl and LDL cholesterol:HDL cholesterol ratio of at least 5 identified the subgroup at highest risk for a CAD event. Almost 25 per cent of CAD events occurred in this subgroup, which accounted for less than 4 per cent of subjects in this analysis.

CHOLESTEROL LOWERING ATHEROSCLEROSIS STUDY. Multivariate analysis of 2-year CLAS data (see p. 1130) found that the primary predictor of atherosclerotic lesion progression in subjects in the drug-treated group was the apo C-III content of HDL, and the primary predictor of atherosclerotic progression in subjects in the placebo group was non-HDL cholesterol.[172] In univariate analysis, apo C-III, which is thought to inhibit lipoprotein lipase activity, was a significant predictor of progression in both treatment groups. These findings indicate the importance of triglyceride-rich lipoprotein metabolism in atherosclerosis. Sequestration of apo C-III within HDL would presumably leave apo C-II unopposed, thereby increasing the catabolism of triglyceride-rich particles and decreasing the exposure of the vascular endothelium to their potentially atherogenic remnants.

HELSINKI HEART STUDY. Subsequent analysis of the Helsinki Heart Study (see p. 1128) determined that the relative risk for cardiac events was 3.8 in the subgroup with triglyceride higher than 200 mg/dl and LDL cholesterol:HDL cholesterol ratio greater than 5 compared with the subgroup with triglyceride of 200 mg/dl or less and LDL cholesterol:HDL cholesterol ratio of 5 or less.[173] In this high-risk subgroup, which accounted for approximately 10 per cent of study subjects, risk for cardiac events was reduced 71 per cent with gemfibrozil treatment.

Triglyceride-Rich Lipoprotein Metabolism

Chylomicrons are the largest lipoprotein particles and are produced in the endoplasmic reticulum of the gastrointestinal tract after a fatty meal. Apo B-48, which is produced by the insertion of a stop codon in the gene for apo B-100, is unique to chylomicrons and their metabolic remnants. VLDL particles are produced by the liver and contain apo B-100, which is characteristic of all particles in the endogenous lipolytic cascade. Chylomicrons and VLDL also contain C apolipoproteins, which modulate the metabolism of the triglyceride-rich lipoproteins, and apo E, which enables the metabolized remnant particle to be removed from the circulation.

As triglyceride from chylomicrons and VLDL is hydrolyzed through the action of lipoprotein lipase, which is activated by apo C-II on the lipoprotein surface, the surface components made redundant by the shrinking lipoprotein core are transferred to HDL. The C apolipoproteins transferred to HDL are subsequently transferred to newly secreted VLDL.

Unlike their precursor particles, chylomicron remnants and IDL are believed to increase CAD risk. Cholesterol from chylomicron remnants suppresses B/E receptor activity, thereby decreasing the removal of LDL from the circulation, and IDL was found to be predictive of atherosclerotic lesion progression in both the NHLBI Type II Coronary Intervention Study[174] and the nicardipine study of the Montreal Heart Institute.[175]

Hypertriglyceridemia

DETECTION. In the NCEP guidelines, triglyceride less than 200 mg/dl is normal, 200 to 400 mg/dl is borderline high, 400 to 1000 mg/dl is high, and greater than 1000 mg/dl is very high. As in hypercholesterolemia, treatment is influenced by the degree of CAD risk. Particularly in patients with CAD, FCH, diabetes, or a family history of premature CAD, elevated triglyceride should be reduced to decrease CAD risk. Causes of secondary hypertriglyceridemia include diabetes mellitus, obesity, hypothyroidism, dysglobulinemia, and use of beta blockers, diuretics, and estrogen. Underlying conditions should be treated and, as possible, offending drugs discontinued or decreased. High and very high triglyceride levels are usually caused by a combination of primary and secondary factors.

TREATMENT. The primary treatment for hypertriglyceridemia is life style modification, which should include weight control, a diet low in saturated fat and cholesterol, regular exercise, smoking cessation, and, in some patients, alcohol restriction. Frequent concomitants of elevated triglyceride are obesity, physical inactivity, and glucose intolerance.

The NCEP guidelines recommend the consideration of drug therapy in patients with borderline-high triglyceride in conjunction with CAD, family history of premature CAD, high total cholesterol combined with low HDL cholesterol, or a genetic hypertriglyceridemia known to increase CAD risk, such as dysbetalipoproteinemia (see below) or FCH. The agent should decrease LDL cholesterol, increase HDL cholesterol, and decrease VLDL and remnant particles. Suggested agents are nicotinic acid and fibric-acid derivatives.

High triglyceride may require drug therapy, especially in patients with a history of acute pancreatitis, to prevent an increase in triglyceride to a level that can cause pancreatitis. Treatment is as for borderline hypertriglyceridemia, but emphasis should be placed on controlling secondary causes, the most common of which is obesity.

Patients with very high triglyceride are at increased risk for pancreatitis and so require vigorous immediate intervention. Drugs that increase triglyceride should be discontinued, diabetes mellitus should be controlled, alcohol intake should be restricted, and dietary fat should be limited to 10 to 20 per cent of total calories. If triglyceride remains above 1000 mg/dl despite these measures, drug therapy should be initiated. Suggested agents are fibric-acid derivatives and, in patients who do not have diabetes mellitus, nicotinic acid. Triglyceride levels seldom return to normal in these patients; a reasonable treatment goal is triglyceride less than 500 mg/dl. There is no drug treatment for chylomicronemia (see below).

Fish Oil. In addition to the lipid-regulating drugs described above that affect triglyceride as well as cholesterol, omega-3 polyunsaturated fatty acids—predominantly eicosapentaenoic acid and docosahexaenoic acid—exert a triglyceride-lowering effect. In observational epidemiological studies, a diet rich in these compounds has been associated with decreased prevalence of atherosclerosis in populations such as Greenland Eskimos,[176] and in MRFIT, CAD mortality was found to be inversely related to the consumption of omega-3 polyunsaturated fatty acids.[177] However, the effect of long-term exposure to high doses of these compounds is not known, and the administration of fish oil supplements is not recommended by the NCEP.

Although the precise mechanism by which these compounds confer cardioprotection is not clear, high consumption of omega-3 fatty acids has been demonstrated to decrease the production of VLDL.[178] Fish oil also increases the proportion of HDL_2 to HDL_3,[179] thereby increasing the amount of cholesterol carried in HDL. Nonlipid benefits include a dose–response hypotensive effect, strongest in subjects with hypertension, hypercholesterolemia, or CAD, that was reported in a meta-analysis of placebo-controlled trials.[180] Prolonged bleeding has been reported with increased fish oil intake, but the alteration in hemostatic parameters may be less than previously suggested.[181] In some studies, fish oil supplementation has been shown to reduce restenosis after coronary angioplasty.[182]

Primary Dyslipidemias Characterized by Hypertriglyceridemia

FAMILIAL CHYLOMICRONEMIA. Familial chylomicronemia[183] is a rare disorder characterized by an elevation of circulating chylomicrons that persists in fasting plasma (Fredrickson phenotype I). The presence of chylomicrons is indicated by a creamy supernatant on plasma refrigerated for 12 hours. Blood cholesterol is normal to slightly elevated, and blood triglyceride is greatly increased. However, atherosclerotic risk does not appear to be increased.

Familial chylomicronemia results from decreased activity of lipoprotein lipase caused by genetic deficiency of lipoprotein lipase or of its activator apo C-II[184] or by the presence of an inhibitor to lipoprotein lipase.[185] Diagnosis is by determination of postheparin lipoprotein lipase activity. In patients with homozygous lipoprotein lipase deficiency or homozygous apo C-II deficiency, plasma triglyceride may exceed 1000 mg/dl. Inheritance of lipoprotein lipase and apo C-II deficiencies is autosomal recessive; the former genetic defect is more common than the latter.

Chylomicronemia usually causes diffuse abdominal pain and pancreatitis. Diagnosis is typically in childhood. Dermatological abnormalities include eruptive xanthomas that may be diffused over the entire body. These yellow, papular lesions consist of triglyceride-laden macrophages and may be controlled by lowering triglyceride levels. Lipemia retinalis may occur with more severe hypertriglyceridemia and is detected on funduscopic examination of the retina by diffuse pink discoloration caused by the dispersion of light by chylomicrons. Visual acuity is not affected, and there are no long-term ophthalmological sequelae.

The primary treatment for chylomicronemia is dietary and should include restriction of dietary fat to less than 10 per cent of total calories. Dietary fat should be in the form of short- and medium-chain triglycerides, which are absorbed directly into the portal vein instead of being formed into chylomicrons in the gastrointestinal tract. Agents that increase triglyceride production, such as estrogen and alcohol, should be avoided. Drug therapy is usually not effective in patients with this dyslipidemia.

DYSBETALIPOPROTEINEMIA (TYPE III HYPERLIPIDEMIA). Dysbetalipoproteinemia, or type III hyperlipidemia, is characterized by an elevation in IDL particles. Both cholesterol and triglyceride levels are elevated, and atherosclerotic risk is increased. Inheritance is most commonly autosomal recessive. This disorder, which occurs in approximately 1 in 5000 individuals in the United States, is most often found in individuals homozygous for apo E_2 but usually requires other metabolic or environmental factors for full clinical expression. Because the B/E receptor and possibly the putative chylomicron remnant receptor have decreased affinity for apo E_2, chylomicron and VLDL remnants accumulate instead of being cleared from the circulation by apo E–mediated removal. These remnant particles, which are known as beta-VLDL because they have beta electrophoretic mobility instead of the pre-beta mobility characteristic of normal VLDL, are enriched in cholesteryl ester.[186] Beta-VLDL particles can be taken up by macrophages, and because this uptake is not downregulated as intracellular cholesterol accumulates, the macrophages can become lipid-laden foam cells.[187]

Total cholesterol is typically 300 to 600 mg/dl, and total triglyceride is typically 400 to 800 mg/dl but may be much higher. Clinical signs of dysbetalipoproteinemia may include palmar xanthomas and tuberoeruptive xanthomas. Definitive diagnosis is by identification of apo E isoform, which requires special laboratory analysis. However, a VLDL cholesterol: plasma triglyceride ratio of 0.3 or greater supports the diagnosis of dysbetalipoproteinemia.[188] This disorder is not usually expressed in childhood and may be exacerbated by obesity, diabetes mellitus, hypothyroidism, myxedema, and excessive alcohol consumption.

Dysbetalipoproteinemia is extremely sensitive to dietary therapy, and reduction in saturated fat intake combined with weight reduction as necessary frequently corrects the dyslipidemia. If drug therapy is required, recommended agents are fibric-acid derivatives, HMG-CoA reductase inhibitors, and in patients who do not have diabetes or a prediabetic condition, nicotinic acid.

FAMILIAL ENDOGENOUS HYPERTRIGLYCERIDEMIA. Familial endogenous hypertriglyceridemia characterized by elevated VLDL (Fredrickson phenotype IV) occurs in approximately 1 in 300 individuals in the United States. In the type IV phenotype, blood triglyceride level is typically 200 to 500 mg/dl, and HDL cholesterol is usually decreased. Premature CAD is a feature in some kindreds but not in others. Treatment is as for hypertriglyceridemia, outlined above.

Rarely, this disease presents as type V hyperlipidemia, which may be recognized by a creamy supernatant of chylomicrons overlying a turbid layer of VLDL-rich fasting plasma. In this presentation, plasma triglyceride is typically greater than 1000 mg/dl, HDL cholesterol is usually decreased, and total cholesterol is normal to elevated. Atherosclerotic risk is increased. Triglyceride-lowering treatment, as outlined above, frequently alters the phenotype to type IV or IIb.

FAMILIAL COMBINED HYPERLIPIDEMIA. As noted above, FCH may present as type IV hyperlipidemia. Treatment should then be directed at triglyceride reduction.

Elevated Lipoprotein(a)

Lp(a) level has been shown in a number of clinical studies, primarily retrospective, to be an independent risk factor for CAD.[189] Structurally, Lp(a) is identical to LDL with the addition of a single apo(a) molecule attached by a disulfide bond to the apo B-100. The distribution of Lp(a) concentration is bell shaped in blacks but skewed in whites, who typically have levels below 20 mg/dl. A level above 30 mg/dl is generally considered elevated.

The primary determinant of Lp(a) level has been shown to be genetic. In one study in white families, more than 90 per cent of the variation in Lp(a) level was attributable to variation in the gene for apo(a).[190] Less than 10 per cent of the inherited variation in Lp(a) level may be attributable to variations in genes at other loci, such as the B/E receptor gene. Lp(a) concentration was reported to be three times higher in patients with heterozygous FH than in controls.[191] About 4 per cent of the variation in Lp(a) level may be attributable to variation in the gene for apo E: Compared with individuals with the gene for apo E_3, Lp(a) concentration was 25 per cent lower in individuals with the gene for apo E_2 and 25 per cent higher in individuals with the gene for apo E_4.[192]

The mechanism by which Lp(a) may increase risk for

CAD is complex. Lp(a) may interfere with the generation of plasmin because of structural similarity between apo(a) and plasminogen.[193] Lp(a) has been demonstrated to be deposited in the arterial wall, particularly in areas with atherosclerotic plaque, and apo(a) has been found co-localized with fibrinogen in the arterial wall.[194] Lp(a) that has been modified by malondialdehyde was reported to be removed by scavenger receptors on macrophages at a rate 20 times higher than that of native Lp(a).[195] Lp(a) appears to be more susceptible to oxidative modification than LDL[196] and thus may be preferentially taken up by scavenger receptors.

Treatment of elevated Lp(a) is problematic. Most lipid-regulating agents do not seem to lower Lp(a), except, as noted above, nicotinic acid, bezafibrate, and estrogen. Neomycin[197] and stanozolol[198] have also been reported to decrease Lp(a). Although lowering Lp(a) level is theoretically attractive, the clinical impact has not been determined. Because Lp(a) measurement is not a widely available laboratory determination and the clinical significance of alterations in Lp(a) level is not known, the NCEP does not recommend the routine measurement of this lipoprotein at this time.

TOBACCO USE

The use of tobacco products continues to be a major public health hazard in the United States[199,199a] and is one of the primary modifiable risk factors for CAD. In the United States, 46 million adults, or 25 per cent of the population aged 18 years or older, smoke.[5] Cigarette smoking is the leading preventable cause of premature death in the United States, and it is estimated that in 1990, approximately 417,000 Americans died of smoking-related causes.[1] Tobacco use is the largest single cause of premature death in the developed world among individuals aged 35 to 69 years, estimated to account for approximately 30 per cent of all deaths in this age group in the 1990s.[200] Cardiovascular diseases linked with tobacco use include CAD and cerebrovascular disease. Smoking multiplies the effect of other coronary risk factors and is estimated to be the cause of approximately 20 per cent of all deaths of cardiovascular disease in the United States in 1990.[201]

Epidemiological Evidence

In the Framingham Heart Study, cardiovascular mortality increased 18 per cent in men and 31 per cent in women for each 10 cigarettes smoked per day.[202] In addition, the use of tobacco products in individuals with other cardiac risk factors was found to have a synergistic effect on CAD morbidity and mortality: Smoking was found to increase the risk for CAD, stroke, heart failure, and peripheral vascular disease at every level of blood pressure (Table 35–9). Smoking cessation in hypertensive patients who smoke 1 pack per day was estimated to reduce cardiovascular risk by 35 to 40 per cent.

Low-tar cigarettes and smokeless tobacco are *not* effective substitutes for discontinuing the use of tobacco products, despite claims to the contrary. In a multicenter case–control study, the relative risks for myocardial infarction in patients who smoked cigarettes with tar yield less than 10 mg, 10 to 15 mg, 15 to 20 mg, and greater than 20 mg were 3.8, 4.3, 3.2, and 3.7, respectively, compared with nonsmokers.[203] Compared with patients who smoked cigarettes with tar yield in the lowest category, the relative risks for myocardial infarction in patients who smoked cigarettes with tar yield in the subsequent categories were 1.2, 0.8, and 1.0. Smokeless tobacco is also associated with an increased risk for cardiovascular disease. In a 12-year observational epidemiological study conducted in 135,036 men, the age-adjusted relative risk for death of cardiovascular disease was 1.4 in users of smokeless tobacco, 1.8 in smokers of less than 15 cigarettes per day, and 1.9 in smokers of 15 or more cigarettes per day, compared with subjects who did not use any tobacco products.[204]

Passive exposure to smoke in individuals who have never smoked may also increase risk for CAD. In an analysis of nine epidemiological studies, the relative risk for heart disease death among individuals who had never smoked was as much as 3.0 in subjects who lived with current or former smokers compared with those who lived with nonsmokers.[205] In this analysis, among men who had never smoked, subjects who lived with a current or former smoker were estimated to have a 9.6 per cent chance of dying of ischemic heart disease by the age of 74, compared with a 7.4 per cent chance in subjects who lived with a nonsmoker; the respective risks in women were estimated to be 6.1 per cent and 4.9 per cent.

Mechanisms of Increased Risk

The use of tobacco products decreases HDL cholesterol. In an observational epidemiological study, HDL cholesterol was 12 per cent lower in male smokers and 7 per cent lower in female smokers than in nonsmokers.[206] Tobacco smoke may adversely affect HDL metabolism and structure by modifying the activity of LCAT. In an in vitro study, LCAT activity in human plasma exposed to the gas phase of cigarette smoke for only 15 minutes was reduced 7 per cent, and at 6 hours of exposure, LCAT activity was only 22 per cent of that in plasma exposed to filtered air.[207] Additionally, plasma exposure to cigarette smoke resulted in cross-linking between apo A-I and apo A-II, which may alter the function of HDL. Because of the cardioprotective

TABLE 35–9 RISK FOR CARDIOVASCULAR DISEASE BY SYSTOLIC BLOOD PRESSURE AND SMOKING STATUS: FRAMINGHAM 26-YEAR FOLLOW-UP OF MEN AGED 50 YEARS*

	8-YEAR RATES PER 1000 SUBJECTS							
	Any Cardiovascular Disease		Intermittent Claudication		Myocardial Infarction		Stroke	
SBP	*Nonsmokers*	*Smokers*	*Nonsmokers*	*Smokers*	*Nonsmokers*	*Smokers*	*Nonsmokers*	*Smokers*
105	37	64	3	10	17	26	7	11
120	47	81	4	12	21	32	8	13
135	60	102	5	15	26	39	9	15
150	76	128	6	19	31	47	11	18
165	96	160	7	23	39	58	13	21
180	121	198	9	29	47	70	15	25
195	151	242	11	36	58	86	18	29

Abbreviation: SBP = systolic blood pressure.
* Cholesterol 185 mg/dl; no glucose intolerance; no left ventricular hypertrophy.
From Kannel, W. B., and Higgins, M.: Smoking and hypertension as predictors of cardiovascular risk in population studies. J. Hypertens. Suppl. 8:S3, 1990.

effect of HDL, these alterations may provide a mechanism by which cigarette smoke increases risk for CAD.

Smoking may also have a detrimental effect on coronary flow. In a case–control study, smoking significantly increased the risk for vasospasm; the adjusted odds ratio for smoking as a risk factor for vasospasm was 2.41.[208] In addition, smoking adversely affects endothelial function,[209] fibrinogen level,[210] and platelet aggregation.[211]

Risk Factor Reduction

A computer model designed to measure the effect of risk factor modification on life expectancy in Americans who became 35 years old in 1990 predicted that the population-wide increase in life expectancy that would be gained with smoking cessation was 0.8 year in men and 0.7 year in women.[212] By comparison, reduction of cholesterol to 200 mg/dl, blood pressure control, and achievement of ideal body weight was predicted to increase life expectancy 0.7 year, 1.1 years, and 0.6 year, respectively, in men and 0.8 year, 0.4 year, and 0.4 year, respectively, in women. However, in individuals with a given risk factor, the effects of risk factor reduction are more impressive. Smoking cessation in smokers was estimated to increase life expectancy 2.3 years in men and 2.8 years in women. The elimination of CAD mortality in this age group was estimated to increase the average life expectancy 3.1 years in men and 3.3 years in women.

Smoking cessation improves other cardiovascular risk factors as well. In a recent study, LDL cholesterol decreased 5.6 per cent and HDL cholesterol increased 3.4 per cent in subjects who stopped smoking and stopped chewing nicotinic gum for at least 12 weeks.[213] Smoking cessation decreased platelet volume and increased the platelet cyclic adenosine monophosphate response to stimulation of adenylate cyclase by prostaglandin E_1. Elevation of platelet cyclic adenosine monophosphate levels has been associated with platelet reactivity, implying that the antiaggregating effect of vasoprotective prostaglandins may be increased after smoking cessation. Amounts of epinephrine and norepinephrine excreted in urine were decreased by smoking cessation, which may reflect improvement in vascular reactivity. Smoking cessation did not affect systolic blood pressure, but diastolic blood pressure was significantly increased.

Although smoking cessation has been reported to increase blood pressure in some studies, in the 3470 subjects in the interventional group in MRFIT who reported smoking at the initial screening and also attended the 72-month follow-up visit, the significantly increased incidence of hypertension, which occurred in 35 per cent of subjects who stopped smoking compared with 27 per cent of subjects who did not stop smoking, was found to be at least partially attributable to increased weight gain after smoking cessation.[214] At 72-month follow-up, weight gain of 2.7 kg (6 lb) occurred in 47 per cent of subjects who quit smoking, compared with 25 per cent of subjects who did not stop smoking. Stepped-care antihypertensive therapy was similarly effective in lowering diastolic blood pressure in hypertensive subjects who did or did not stop smoking.

Smoking cessation produces clinical benefits in a short period of time. In a population-based case–control study in which 1282 cases were compared with 2068 controls, the risk for myocardial infarction or coronary death in current smokers was 2.7 in men and 4.7 in women compared with the respective risks in nonsmokers.[215] After smoking cessation, the risk for CAD quickly declined and at approximately 3 years after smoking cessation became similar to that of subjects who had never smoked.

Smoking cessation, which is cost-free and has minimal adverse effects, should be encouraged in all patients. Approximately 70 per cent of current smokers report a desire to stop smoking completely.[5] However, data from the 1991 National Health Interview Survey of the Centers for Disease Control indicate that only slightly more than half of the smokers who had at least one outpatient visit with a physician or other health-care professional during a 1-year period were advised to quit.[216] It has been estimated that each year an additional 1 million individuals could be helped to stop smoking if all primary-care providers gave brief counseling to their smoking patients.[217] Brief counseling should include determining whether the patient smokes, advising any patient who smokes to quit, assisting the patient in quitting, for example, by setting a quit date and providing self-help material, and scheduling follow-up visits to reinforce adherence.[218]

HYPERTENSION

(See also Chaps. 25 and 26)

In the United States and other Western countries, the prevalence of hypertension is high and increases with age. The third and most recent National Health and Nutrition Examination Survey (NHANES III), conducted between 1988 and 1991, documented an overall prevalence of hypertension in adult Americans of 24 per cent, representing more than 43 million individuals[6] and ranging from 4 per cent of Americans aged 18 to 29 years to 65 per cent of Americans aged more than 80 years.[219]

Epidemiological Evidence

Numerous observational epidemiological studies in geographically and ethnically diverse populations have established a direct relation between blood pressure elevation and incidence of CAD and stroke. In a meta-analysis of nine prospective studies that together included almost 420,000 individuals without prior myocardial infarction or stroke who were followed up for an average of 10 years, baseline blood pressure level correlated with subsequent incidence rates of CAD death and nonfatal myocardial infarction.[220] The relative risk for CAD events in subjects in the highest quintile of diastolic blood pressure (mean, 105 mm Hg) was approximately 5 to 6 times that in subjects in the lowest quintile (mean, 76 mm Hg). Each 7.5 mm Hg difference in diastolic blood pressure was associated with an estimated 29 per cent difference in CAD risk. No threshold level of blood pressure was identified below which the association with CAD events changed.

In a meta-analysis of 14 randomized trials of hypotensive drug therapy, together enrolling almost 37,000 subjects, blood pressure was 6 mm Hg lower in treated subjects than in control subjects, and CAD event rate was 14 per cent lower,[221] which was a smaller improvement in CAD events than would have been expected on the basis of observational data. However, some of the hypotensive agents used in these interventional trials may adversely affect the lipid profile and may offset, at least partially, the reduction in risk obtained by lowering blood pressure. Thiazide diuretics and beta blockers without intrinsic sympathomimetic activity increase plasma triglyceride levels and may produce other metabolic adverse effects.[222]

Some studies have found a J-shaped relation between blood pressure and CAD events. In one study, in which this effect was limited to patients with evidence of CAD, the lowest incidence of fatal myocardial infarction was in patients whose diastolic blood pressure was 85 to 90 mm Hg; risk for fatal myocardial infarction was increased in patients whose blood pressure was either lower or higher than this range.[223] The precise clinical role of the J-shaped curve remains controversial but may be related to overzealous reduction of blood pressure in subjects with ostial coronary lesions, severe diastolic abnormalities that cause subendocardial ischemia, or potential adverse metabolic effects of hypotensive agents. In addition, left ventricular dysfunction may affect blood pressure and increase risk for coronary events immediately after a myocardial infarction.

TABLE 35–10 EFFECTS OF ANTIHYPERTENSIVE DRUGS ON OTHER CORONARY ARTERY DISEASE RISK FACTORS

RISK FACTORS	DIURETICS	INDAPAMIDE	BETA-BLOCKERS WITHOUT ISA	BETA-BLOCKERS WITH ISA	LABETALOL	GUANETHIDINE GUANADREL	CENTRAL ALPHA-AGONISTS	METHYLDOPA	DIRECT VASODILATORS	ALPHA-BLOCKERS	ACE INHIBITORS	CALCIUM BLOCKERS	RESERPINE
Hypertension	Reduced	Reduced	Reduced	Decreased	Decreased	Decreased	Decreased	Decreased	Decreased	Decreased	Decreased	Decreased	Decreased
Dyslipidemia	Increased	Neutral	Increased	No change	No change	No change	Decreased	Increased	No change	Decreased	No change	Decreased	Increased
Glucose intolerance	Increased	Neutral Increased	Increased	Increased	Increased	No change	No change No change	No change No change	No change No change	Decreased Decreased	Decreased Decreased	No change No change	No change Unknown
Insulin resistance	Increased	No change	Increased	Increased	Unknown	Unknown						Decreased	
LVH	No change Increased	Reduced	No change	Increased	Decreased	Decreased	Decreased No change	Decreased No change	Increased No change	Decreased No change	Decreased No change	Decreased No change	Decreased Decreased
Exercise	No change Decreased	No change	Decreased	Decreased	No change Decreased	Decreased	No change	No change	No change	No change	Increased	No change	No change
Potassium	Decreased	Decreased	No change Increased	No change	No change	No change	No change	No change	No change	No change	No change Increased	No change	No change
Magnesium	Decreased	Decreased	No change	No change	No change	No change	No change	No change	No change	No change	Decreased	No change	No change
Uric acid	Increased	Increased	Increased	Increased	Increased	No change	Decreased	Decreased				Decreased	
Blood viscosity	Increased	No change	No change	No change	No change	No change	No change	No change	Decreased	Decreased	No change	Unknown	Unknown
Blood velocity	No change Increased	No change	Decreased	No change	No change	No change	Decreased	Increased	Increased	Decreased	Decreased	Decreased	Decreased
Catecholamines	Increased	Decreased	Increased	Increased	No change	Decreased	Decreased	Decreased	Increased	No change	Decreased	Decreased	Decreased
Angiotensin II	Increased	No change Decreased	Decreased	No change	Decreased	Increased				Decreased			
Arrhythmia potential	Increased	No change	Decreased	No change Increased	No change	Increased	Decreased	Decreased	Increased	No change Decreased	Decreased	Decreased	Decreased
Fibrinogen	Increased	No change	Unknown	Unknown	Unknown	Unknown	Decreased	Decreased	Increased	No change	Decreased	Decreased	Increased
Platelet function	Increased	Decreased	No change Decreased	Unknown	Unknown	Unknown	Unknown Decreased	Unknown No change	Unknown Unknown	Unknown Unknown	Unknown Decreased	Unknown Decreased	Unknown Unknown
Thrombogenic potential	Increased	Decreased	Unknown	Unknown	Unknown	Unknown	Unknown	Unknown	Unknown	Unknown	Unknown	Decreased	Unknown
Antiatherogenic	No	Neutral	Yes (animal studies)	Unknown	Unknown	Yes	Unknown	Unknown	Unknown	Unknown	Decreased (animals)	Decreased (animals, humans)	Yes (animals)
CHD relative risk ratio Unfavorable/total	16/18	3–4/18	6/18	7/18	3/18	3/18	0/18	2/18	5/18	0/18	0/18	0/18	3/18

From Houston, M. C.: The management of hypertension and associated risk factors for the prevention of long-term cardiac complications. J. Cardiovasc. Pharmacol. *21*(Suppl. 2):S2, 1993.

Large-scale prospective interventional trials are under way to clarify this issue.[224]

Risk Factor Reduction

Elevated blood pressure frequently coexists with other risk factors.[225] The insulin-resistance syndrome (or metabolic syndrome X) described by Reaven[226] is characterized by resistance to insulin-mediated glucose intake, glucose intolerance, hyperinsulinemia, hypertension, increased triglyceride and decreased HDL cholesterol levels, and possibly microvascular angina, hyperuricemia, and increased PAI-1 level.[227] In addition, truncal obesity and coagulation abnormalities often coexist with hypertension. Evaluation of other risk factors that occur with hypertension is of special clinical importance because controlling blood pressure with certain antihypertensive medications may adversely affect other risk factors (Table 35–10).

DIABETES MELLITUS

(See also Chap. 61)

Almost 14 million individuals in the United States are estimated to have diabetes mellitus, although more than half have not been diagnosed.[228] Approximately 700,000 have insulin-dependent diabetes mellitus (IDDM), which occurs more often in whites and tends to cluster in families. More than 95 per cent of Americans with diabetes have non–insulin-dependent diabetes mellitus (NIDDM), which typically develops after age 30 but often is not recognized until serious complications occur. Risk for NIDDM increases with age, and among Americans aged 65 to 74 years, 17 per cent of whites, 25 per cent of blacks, and 33 per cent of Hispanics have NIDDM.[229]

Epidemiological Evidence

CAD is a major complication of both IDDM and NIDDM. In 14-year follow-up of the Rancho Bernardo Study, in which 334 men and women with NIDDM were compared with 2137 men and women without diabetes, the relative risk for CAD death was 1.9 in diabetic men and 3.3 in diabetic women compared with nondiabetic men and women after adjustment for other CAD risk factors.[230] CAD, cerebrovascular disease, or peripheral vascular disease is the cause of death in 75 to 80 per cent of adults with diabetes.[231] Atherosclerosis occurs earlier and more often in diabetic patients, and women with diabetes do not share the relative gender-mediated premenopausal protection against CAD of women without diabetes.

The relation between diabetes and cardiovascular disease is not uniform in all populations. In the WHO Multinational Study of Vascular Disease in Diabetics, the incidence of death in diabetic patients that was attributable to circulatory disease ranged from 32 per cent in men and 0 per cent in women in Tokyo to 67 per cent in men and 47 per cent in women in London.[232]

Mechanisms of Increased Risk

Diabetes frequently exists in the presence of other, often modifiable CAD risk factors. Hypertension and obesity are common in patients with diabetes, and the typical dyslipidemia in diabetes is increased plasma triglyceride and decreased HDL cholesterol, often in conjunction with small, dense LDL particles. Postprandial lipemia may also contribute to atherosclerotic risk in patients with diabetes. In a study in patients with NIDDM, VLDL level was increased but chylomicron level was similar compared with corresponding levels in subjects with normal glucose tolerance.[233] In the same study, significant correlations were found between postprandial insulin response and triglyceride response and between postprandial triglyceride response and fasting HDL cholesterol level. However, even taken together, these other risk factors do not explain all of the increased risk associated with diabetes.[234]

Resistance to the action of circulating insulin may play a role in the dyslipidemia of diabetes.[235] Insulin normally suppresses plasma concentration of free fatty acids, and in insulin-resistance syndromes, the decreased suppression results in an increase in circulating levels of free fatty acids, which in turn stimulates triglyceride synthesis. Although elevated plasma triglyceride frequently occurs in conjunction with decreased HDL cholesterol, in part because of the metabolic interrelation of the triglyceride-rich lipoproteins and HDL, increased urinary loss of HDL has been demonstrated in patients with IDDM and albuminuria.[236]

In diabetic patients, lipoproteins may be altered by glycation, which affects their recognition and binding by receptors.[237] Glycation of LDL causes its accumulation in the circulation and may increase cholesteryl ester accumulation in macrophages.[238] Glycation of HDL may also promote cholesteryl ester accumulation in the arterial wall.[239] In addition to glycation, oxidation of LDL may be increased in diabetic individuals,[240] although extensive studies have not been performed.

The role of Lp(a) in diabetes is controversial and appears to be related at least in part to the type of diabetes. In a recent analysis of available data, patients with NIDDM generally did not have elevated Lp(a), nor was Lp(a) level a function of metabolic control; however, patients with IDDM tended to have increased Lp(a), especially patients with microalbuminuria or poor glycemic control.[241]

Atherosclerosis in diabetics is often complicated by a procoagulant state caused by increased platelet aggregability[242] and increased PAI-1.[243] Insulin may contribute to atherogenesis by promoting smooth muscle cell proliferation and cholesteryl ester accumulation in the arterial wall.[244]

Risk Factor Reduction

The relation between glycemic control and prevention of diabetic complications remains controversial. Epidemiological studies have estimated that approximately 25 per cent of patients with diabetes do not develop complications regardless of the degree of glycemic control; however, clinical trials have demonstrated decreased retinopathy and microalbuminuria with improved glycemic control, and blood lipoprotein levels show significant improvement when blood glucose is controlled near normal levels.[245] In addition, glycosylated hemoglobin, used as a marker of poor glycemic control, has been significantly correlated with death from diabetes and death from ischemic heart disease.[246]

The Diabetes Control and Complications Trial (DCCT) addressed the role of tight glycemic control in preventing complications of diabetes by analyzing 1441 patients with IDDM, aged 13 to 39 years, who were randomized to receive intensive insulin therapy or conventional treatment.[247] The intensive therapy consisted of administration of insulin by an external insulin pump three or more times daily as indicated by frequent blood glucose monitoring; conventional therapy consisted of one to two daily injections of insulin. After a mean of 6.5 years, intensive therapy significantly reduced risk for retinopathy, microalbuminuria, and clinical neuropathy. LDL cholesterol was lowered 34 per cent, and the combined occurrence of all major cardiovascular and peripheral vascular events was reduced 41 per cent, but this reduction in macrovascular events was not significant. However, the young cohort was not expected to produce enough macrovascular events to allow distinction of the treatment groups. The major adverse event was a significant threefold increase in incidence of severe hypoglycemia. Additional studies are needed to determine whether intensive glycemic control decreases risk for macrovascular complications without an offsetting increase in risk for hypoglycemia.

In risk factor reduction in patients with diabetes, great care must be taken not to exacerbate one condition while treating another. For example, as noted above, antihypertensive agents may adversely affect glucose tolerance, lipid levels, or both.[248,249] Thiazide diuretics have been implicated in worsening glucose control and in provoking dyslipidemia, and noncardioselective beta blockers that inhibit the adrenergic-mediated activation of lipoprotein lipase have been shown to worsen both glucose tolerance and triglyceride metabolism and, thus, should be used with caution in patients with brittle diabetes.

In treating dyslipidemia in patients with diabetes, the report of the American Diabetes Association (ADA) Consensus Development Conference on the Detection and Management of Lipid Disorders in Diabetes emphasizes the benefits of ideal body weight, appropriate diet, and a moderate exercise program.[231] Physical exercise may also decrease the risk for atherosclerotic disease in patients with diabetes by decreasing hyperinsulinemia, improving insulin resistance, and/or preventing increased intraabdominal adiposity.[250] If hygienic methods do not control the lipid abnormality, pharmacological therapy may be indicated. Many authorities, including the ADA consensus panel, recommend more stringent intervention levels and therapeutic goals in the diabetic patient. The ADA consensus panel recommends screening for dyslipidemia annually in all patients with diabetes by full fasting lipoprotein analysis and initiating treatment if LDL cholesterol is elevated (130 mg/dl or greater without evidence of macrovascular disease, greater than 100 mg/dl with evidence of macrovascular disease), if triglyceride is elevated (200 mg/dl or greater without macrovascular disease, greater than 150 mg/dl with macrovascular disease), or if HDL cholesterol is low (35 mg/dl or less).

PHYSICAL INACTIVITY

Almost 60 per cent of U.S. adults reported little or no leisure-time physical activity in the 1991 Behavioral Risk Factor Surveillance System of the Centers for Disease Control.[251] In this survey, prevalence of sedentary life style was similar in men and women and lower in whites (57 per cent) than in other races (64 per cent). Physical inactivity was directly related to age, ranging from 55 per cent in subjects aged 18 to 34 years to 62 per cent in subjects aged 55 years or older, and inversely related to income and education.

Epidemiological Evidence

Regular physical activity has been shown to reduce risk for CAD events in a number of observational epidemiological studies.[252] A meta-analysis of studies that compared CAD incidence in occupations with different activity levels determined that the relative risk for CAD death was 1.9 in sedentary occupations compared with active occupations.[253] In 10-year follow-up of MRFIT subjects, subjects in both treatment groups who engaged in moderate physical activity had a 27 per cent lower CAD mortality rate than less active subjects.[254]

Because of the methodological problems encountered in quantitating exercise and because of the potential for unreliability in self-reported estimates of physical activity, the level of physical fitness may provide a more accurate predictor of CAD risk. In the Lipid Research Clinics Mortality Follow-up Study, heart rate at stage 2 of a treadmill exercise test was used to determine physical fitness in 3106 healthy men and 649 men with symptoms suggestive of cardiovascular disease or taking antihypertensive medication.[255] Stage 2 heart rate ranged from 112 beats/min in subjects in the fittest quartile to 156 beats/min in subjects in the least fit quartile. Compared with the fittest quartile, cardiovascular disease mortality was 8.5 times higher and CAD mortality was 6.5 times higher in the least fit quartile.

In a study in 1960 healthy men, physical fitness, measured as total work on a bicycle ergometer, and other coronary risk factors were assessed at baseline, and subjects were followed up for 16 years.[256] After adjustment for other cardiovascular risk factors, a graded, independent, inverse correlation was seen between physical fitness and cardiovascular mortality. Compared with subjects in the least fit quartile, relative risk for cardiovascular death in subjects in the fittest quartile was 0.41; relative risk in the second fittest quartile was 0.45, and relative risk in the third fittest quartile was 0.59. Compared with subjects in the least fit quartile, subjects in the fittest quartile had a 0.54 adjusted relative risk for death of any cause, but the relative risk for death of any cause was similar in the three fittest quartiles.

In addition to measurements of physical activity, maximum oxygen uptake during a monitored exercise test may be used as a marker for cardiorespiratory fitness. In 5-year follow-up of 1453 men, aged 42 to 60 years, with no history of cardiovascular disease, age-adjusted relative risk for myocardial infarction in subjects in the highest tertile of physical activity was 0.31 compared with subjects in the lowest tertile.[257] Similarly, the relative risk for myocardial infarction in subjects in the highest tertile of maximal oxygen uptake was 0.26 compared with subjects in the lowest tertile of maximal oxygen uptake, after adjustment for age, weight, height, and other variables. After controlling for 17 confounding variables, the relative risks for myocardial infarction in subjects in the highest tertile of physical activity and subjects in the highest tertile of maximal oxygen uptake were 0.34 and 0.35 compared with subjects in the lowest tertiles, which were statistically significant differences.

Risk Factor Reduction

The mechanisms by which increased exercise decreases risk for CAD events may include improvements in HDL cholesterol level,[258] insulin resistance,[259] body weight,[260] and blood pressure.[261] Exercise also increases maximal cardiac output and the amount of oxygen extracted from blood.[262] In addition to these direct benefits, exercise has been shown to increase the lipid-regulating effects of dietary therapy in moderately overweight, sedentary subjects.[263]

The optimal intensity and duration of exercise to produce cardiovascular benefit have not been firmly established and appear to relate to baseline activity level (Fig. 35–5). In 8-year follow-up of more than 10,000 Harvard University alumni, the self-reported initiation of moderately vigorous sports activity, defined as activity requiring 4.5 or more metabolic equivalents, was associated with a significant 41 per cent reduction in CAD mortality and a significant 23 per cent reduction in all-cause mortality.[264] Subjects who increased physical activity to 2000 kcal per week had a 17 per cent reduction in CAD mortality, but this reduction was not statistically significant.

Cardioprotective benefits may be obtained from a regular program of 30 minutes of moderate aerobic physical activity three times a week. Some experts recommend 30 minutes or more of moderately intensive physical activity daily for all adults.[265] Prudent exercise programs are cost-effective and have a low risk for adverse events in either primary or secondary prevention.[266] Exercise should be individualized to accommodate the patient's level of physical fitness, cardiac status, and preferred activities. In secondary prevention, a limited treadmill exercise test is required at discharge after an acute coronary event to determine prognostic stratification; a symptom-limited treadmill exercise test should be performed 6 weeks later to determine exercise recommendations.

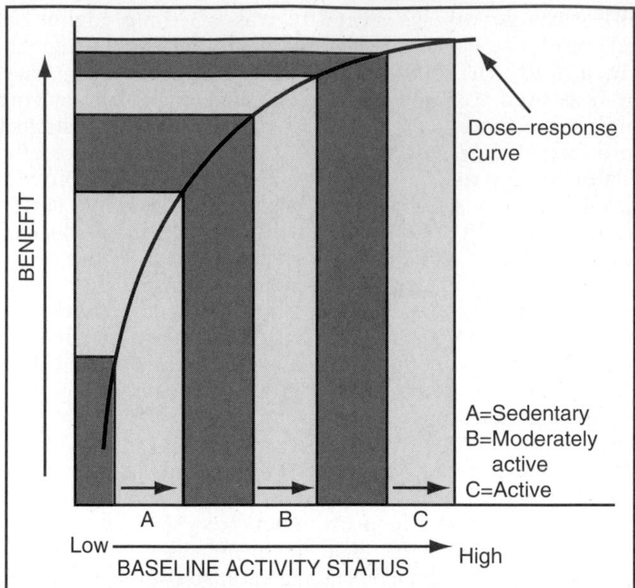

FIGURE 35–5. Dose–response relation between baseline physical activity and health benefit. The intensity and duration of physical activity required to produce a health benefit are related to the level of physical activity at baseline. In sedentary patients, even a modest increase in physical activity is beneficial. (From Pate, R. R., Pratt, M., Blair, S. N., et al.: Physical activity and public health: A recommendation from the Centers for Disease Control and Prevention and the American College of Sports Medicine. JAMA *273*: 402–407, 1995. Copyright 1995 American Medical Association.)

OBESITY

In the third and most recent National Health and Nutrition Examination Survey (NHANES III), approximately 58 million U.S. adults—one-third of Americans aged 20 years or older—were estimated to be overweight, defined as a body mass index (weight in kg/height in m^2) of 27.8 or greater in men and 27.3 or greater in women.[267] This increase in prevalence of 8 per cent since NHANES II was completed in 1988 reflects increases in all age groups and both genders. Prevalence ranges from a low of 31.2 per cent in black men to a high of 48.6 per cent in black women. The largest increase in prevalence occurred in white men and women, in whom prevalence of overweight increased 8 to 9 per cent.

The health risks of obesity not only increase with its severity but also may be affected by the distribution of body fat.[268] Visceral obesity, characterized by excessive adipose fat in the abdomen, appears to impart greater risk for CAD.[269] Recommended waist:hip ratios are less than 0.9 in men and less than 0.8 in middle-aged and elderly women.[270]

Epidemiological Evidence

In the Framingham Heart Study, obesity was found to be an independent risk factor for cardiovascular disease in both men and women. Among subjects aged less than 50 years, incidence of cardiovascular disease was two times higher in men and almost 2.5 times higher in women in the most obese tertile compared with the leanest tertile.[271]

Even individuals with a high-normal body mass index appear to be at increased risk for CAD. In a prospective cohort study conducted in 115,818 middle-aged women, the relative risk for a nonfatal myocardial infarction or fatal CAD was 1.46 in subjects with a body mass index of 23.0 to 24.9 and 2.06 in subjects with a body mass index of 25.0 to 28.9, compared with subjects with a body mass index less than 21.0, which were statistically significant increases.[272] Relative risk in subjects with a body mass index of 21 to 22.9 was 1.19, which was not significant, and relative risk in subjects with a body mass index of 29 or more, which would be considered obese by the definition used in NHANES, was 3.56.

Risk Factor Reduction

Obesity frequently accompanies other cardiovascular risk factors such as hypercholesterolemia,[273] low HDL cholesterol,[274] hypertension,[275] and diabetes mellitus.[276] To improve lipid levels, blood pressure, and glucose tolerance, a concerted effort should be made to obtain ideal body weight by a combination of exercise and dietary interventions.

NONMODIFIABLE RISK FACTORS

Although risk factors such as a positive family history of CAD, age, and gender cannot be modified, their identification can help refine assessment of the patient's CAD risk profile.

Family History

Coronary atherosclerosis tends to aggregate in families. In studies that controlled for other risk factors, a family history of CAD has been shown to be a strong independent risk factor for CAD. For example, a study in relatives of 223 patients with angiographically demonstrated CAD and 57 control subjects found that, after stratification by age, gender, blood pressure, total cholesterol, smoking, diabetes, and left ventricular hypertrophy, relatives of patients had a significantly greater risk for CAD than relatives of controls, as reflected in odds ratios of 2.0 to 3.9 for various CAD endpoints.[277] In a 2-year study in 45,317 men, aged 40 to 75 years, without known CAD at baseline, relative risk for myocardial infarction was 2.2 in subjects whose parent had a myocardial infarction before the age of 70, compared with subjects without a family history of premature myocardial infarction.[278] In addition, risk for myocardial infarction was inversely related to the age at which myocardial infarction occurred in the parent.

Although symptomatic CAD typically does not occur until middle age, family history of CAD may influence atherosclerotic risk beginning in infancy. In an autopsy study of 136 infants aged less than 1 year, mean luminal narrowing in the left coronary artery was 1.4 times greater in infants with a family history of CAD than in infants with no family history of CAD, which was a statistically significant difference; there was no statistically significant difference in narrowing in the right coronary artery between groups.[279]

The increased CAD risk associated with a positive family history may be mediated by genetic effects on other risk factors such as obesity, hypertension, dyslipidemia, and diabetes.[280] Assessment of family history of these other risk factors may provide additional information about an individual's CAD risk and inform treatment decisions.

Age

Approximately four-fifths of fatal myocardial infarctions are in patients aged 65 years and older.[1] Because of the increased short-term risk for a CAD event in middle-aged and elderly patients, reduction of modifiable risk factors in this population is more likely to decrease CAD events in a shorter period of time than in younger patients with otherwise similar risk factors. For example, excess CAD mortality attributable to hypercholesterolemia increased more than five times with age in the observational Kaiser Permanente Coronary Heart Disease in the Elderly Study, conducted in 2746 men without CAD, aged 60 to 79 years.[281] Similarly, major cardiovascular events were reduced 32 per cent with antihypertensive drug therapy in men and women, aged 60 years or older, in the Systolic Hypertension in the Elderly Program (SHEP).[282]

Although older patients should not be excluded from aggressive risk factor reduction simply on the basis of age, overall health status and concomitant illnesses should be assessed in making treatment decisions. If pharmacological intervention is indicated, consideration must be given to the increased susceptibility to adverse drug effects in older patients. The patient's life expectancy should also guide treatment because risk factor reduction may not produce clinical benefit until after a few years of treatment. For example, in clinical trials, lipid-regulating therapy usually requires approximately 2 years before clinical benefit is demonstrated.

Gender

In the Framingham Heart Study, 26-year follow-up of men and women aged 35 to 84 years indicated that CAD morbidity was twice as high in men as in women, and 60 per cent of coronary events occurred in men.[283] The onset of symptomatic CAD is typically about 10 years earlier in men, but CAD incidence in women increases rapidly at menopause. Women have the same modifiable risk factors as men,[284] although diabetes appears to confer greater risk in women than in men,[285] as may low HDL cholesterol and elevated plasma triglyceride.[286]

OTHER RISK FACTORS

Hemostatic Factors

Thrombogenic factors have been demonstrated to predict CAD events. Although levels of coagulation factors, PAI-1, and fibrinolytic activity are not routinely measured to determine risk, their predictive power has been the subject of increasing research.

FIBRINOGEN. Fibrinogen levels vary among populations. Among blacks and whites in the United States, age-adjusted fibrinogen levels are 23 to 40 mg/dl higher in men and 25 to 67 mg/dl higher in women than in their counterparts in Japan, suggesting that low cholesterol levels in Japan may not fully explain the lower prevalence of CAD.[287]

Although elevated plasma fibrinogen occurs in conjunction with other CAD risk factors, such as age, cigarette smoking, hypertension, and obesity, fibrinogen has been demonstrated to be an independent CAD risk factor.[288] In 6-year follow-up of 2116 men in the PROCAM study, mean plasma fibrinogen level was significantly higher in men who had coronary events (2.88 gm/liter) than in men who did not have events (2.63 gm/liter), and the incidence of coronary events was 2.4 times higher in subjects in the highest tertile of plasma fibrinogen distribution (>2.77 gm/liter) than in subjects in the lowest tertile (<2.36 gm/liter).[289] In combined analysis of the Caerphilly and Speedwell prospective studies, which together evaluated almost 5000 men, age-adjusted relative risk for ischemic heart disease events was 4.1 for men in the highest quintile of fibrinogen distribution compared with men in the lowest quintile.[290]

COAGULATION FACTOR VII. Coagulation factor VII has been shown to increase CAD risk in a number of epidemiological studies.[291] factor VII levels are higher in individuals with a high intake of dietary fat,[292] and a direct association has been established between factor VII and total cholesterol level.[293] Elevated factor VII activity may increase thrombin production,[294] further leading to a hypercoagulant state.

FIBRINOLYTIC ACTIVITY. Decreased fibrinolytic activity has been reported in patients with coronary atherosclerosis. In the Northwick Park Heart Study, a difference of 1 standard deviation in fibrinolytic activity was significantly associated with a difference of 40 per cent in risk for ischemic heart disease events in men aged 40 to 54 years at entry into the study (mean follow-up, 16 years).[295] The association persisted after adjustment for plasma fibrinogen level, which was also directly associated with ischemic heart disease events. These results suggest that the decreased ability to lyse a clot and clear fibrin debris may play a role in atherosclerosis.

PLASMINOGEN ACTIVATOR INHIBITOR 1. Decreased fibrinolytic activity may result from elevated levels of PAI-1. In many case–control and cross-sectional studies, plasma PAI-1 has been reported to be increased in patients with CAD.[296] For example, in a study of men and women who had a myocardial infarction before age 45, PAI-1 level was higher than in healthy subjects.[297] This study also found PAI-1 level to be directly related to triglyceride level. In a study of almost 1500 men and women with angina pectoris, PAI-1 was found to be directly related to insulin level, confirming the role of PAI-1 in the insulin-resistance syndrome.[298] Increased PAI-1 has also been shown to be a risk factor for reinfarction in a prospective study of men whose first myocardial infarction occurred before age 45.[299] In addition to systemic increases in PAI-1, atherosclerotic lesions have been found to contain higher levels of PAI-1 than the normal arterial wall.[300]

Homocysteine

Plasma homocysteine is elevated in patients with homozygous homocystinuria, a rare autosomal recessive disorder, but levels are also increased in patients with CAD who do not have homocystinuria.[301,301a] Homocysteinemia has been established as an independent risk factor for coronary vascular disease, cerebrovascular disease, and peripheral vascular disease.[302]

In a study conducted in 482 hyperlipidemic men and women, 72 per cent of subjects with elevated serum homocysteine, defined as 16.2 nmol/ml or greater, had atherosclerotic vascular disease, compared with 44 per cent of those with normal serum homocysteine, which was a significant difference.[303] Compared with subjects in the lowest quintile of serum homocysteine (<6.9 nmol/ml), relative risk for atherosclerotic events was 2.8 in subjects in the highest quintile of serum homocysteine (≥11.4 nmol/ml).

In 271 men in the Physicians' Health Study who had a myocardial infarction during the 5-year study, plasma homocysteine level was significantly higher (mean, 11.1 nmol/ml) than in controls matched for age and smoking habits (mean, 10.5 nmol/ml).[304] Compared with subjects with plasma homocysteine no higher than the 90th percentile, relative risk for subjects with plasma homocysteine above the 95th percentile was 3.4 after adjustment for other cardiovascular risk factors.

Although the precise mechanism by which elevated plasma homocysteine increases risk for CAD has not been determined, possibilities include endothelial damage and altered anticoagulant activity.[305] Deficiency of vitamins B_6 and B_{12} and folic acid can cause elevated plasma homocysteine, and supplementation with these vitamins can decrease plasma homocysteine.

Alcohol

The role of alcohol in CAD risk is complicated by difficulties in obtaining accurate data on individual alcohol consumption. In a number of studies, moderate alcohol intake has been associated with decreased coronary risk,[306] and this protective effect may be mediated by an increase in HDL cholesterol.[307] In an analysis of subjects in the Honolulu Heart Program, approximately 50 per cent of the cardioprotection demonstrated with moderate alcohol consumption was attributable to increased HDL cholesterol, and 18 per cent was attributable to decreased LDL cholesterol, although the latter was offset by an increase in CAD risk of 17 per cent caused by increased systolic blood pressure.[308]

The mechanism responsible for the remaining cardioprotection is not known but may relate to decreased thrombogenicity. Alcohol may inhibit thrombosis[309] and may increase plasma levels of fibrinogen and decrease fibrinolytic activity.[310] Alcohol has been shown to increase tissue-type plasminogen activator (t-PA) secretion by endothelial cells.[311] In 631 men in the Physicians' Health Study, a direct relation was established between alcohol consumption and plasma level of t-PA antigen.[312] In subjects who drank alcohol daily, weekly, monthly, rarely, and never, mean t-PA antigen levels were 10.9, 9.7, 9.1, and 8.1 ng/ml, respectively. The relation persisted after controlling for other cardiovascular risk factors, including HDL cholesterol, supporting the hypothesis that alteration in fibrinolytic activity may contribute to alcohol-mediated protection against CAD.

In France, CAD incidence is relatively low despite mean plasma HDL cholesterol levels similar to those in other countries and fairly high intake of saturated fat. Suggested explanations for this so-called French paradox include alcohol-induced inhibition of platelet aggregation[313] and antioxidant effects of red wine.[314]

Type A Personality and Stress

The role of personality type[315] and emotional stress[316] in risk stratification for CAD remains controversial. Type A personalities are highly competitive, ambitious, and in constant struggle with their environment, whereas type B personalities are passive and less disturbed by environmental stress. Type A personality was reported to be an independent risk factor for CAD in 8.5-year follow-up of 3154 men, aged 39 to 59 years and without CAD at baseline, in the Western Collaborative Group Study: Type A subjects were twice as likely to have angina or myocardial infarction as type B subjects.[317] However, in 20 years of follow-up in 1289 men and women in the Framingham Heart Study, there was a significant twofold excess in risk for angina pectoris in both men and women with type A behavior but no association between personality type and risk for either myocardial infarction or fatal coronary events.[318] Similarly, in MRFIT subjects, type A behavior was not significantly associated with risk for first major coronary events, defined as coronary death and nonfatal myocardial infarction.[319] One possible explanation for the variable association between type A behavior and CAD risk is the use of different methods to determine behavior type.[320]

The mechanism by which personality types may predispose to increased coronary risk is not known but may include increased cardiovascular reactivity,[321] which may lead to increased endothelial injury and platelet aggregation, and increased sympathetic nervous system activity,[322] which increases blood pressure and heart rate.

Studies have been conducted to determine whether anger affects CAD risk. Findings indicate that the expression of anger may increase risk, because of increased cardiovascular reactivity, but that neither the experience nor the repression of anger has such an effect.[323] In a study in 12 patients undergoing cardiac catheterization for symptomatic myocardial ischemia, recalling a recent anger-provoking event significantly increased vasoconstriction, measured as decreases in mean and minimal diameters, in narrowed arteries but not in nonnarrowed arteries.[324]

Low Circulating Levels of Antioxidants

Blood concentrations of antioxidants may affect the susceptibility of LDL and Lp(a) to oxidation. Because lipoprotein oxidation is thought to be prerequisite to the recognition of these particles by the scavenger receptor on macrophages, decreased levels of substances that protect against oxidation may increase atherosclerotic risk.

Observational epidemiological studies have demonstrated an inverse relation between vitamin E intake and CAD events.[325] In the Health Professionals Follow-up Study, in which 39,910 American male health professionals aged 40 to 75 years were followed up for 4 years, risk for a CAD event (fatal coronary disease, nonfatal myocardial infarction, coronary artery bypass grafting, percutaneous transluminal coronary angioplasty) in subjects in the highest quintile of vitamin E intake (median, 419.0 IU/day) was significantly reduced 41 per cent, after adjustment for age, compared with subjects in the lowest quintile of vitamin E intake (median, 6.4 IU/day).[326] Similarly, in the Nurses' Health Study, in which 87,247 American female registered nurses aged 34 to 59 years were evaluated for 8 years, risk for major coronary disease (nonfatal myocardial infarction or CAD death) in subjects in the highest quintile of vitamin E intake (median, 208.0 IU/day) was significantly reduced 41 per cent, after adjustment for age, compared with subjects in the lowest quintile of vitamin E intake (median, 2.8 IU/day).[327] In both of these studies, vitamin E supplementation and not dietary sources alone appeared necessary to reduce risk for CAD events.

Additional observational data have come from information collected in interventional studies. During 13 years of follow-up of 1883 men in the placebo group of the LRC-CPPT, risk for a CAD event (nonfatal myocardial infarction or CAD death) in subjects in the highest quartile of serum carotenoid concentration (>3.16 μmol/L) was significantly reduced 36 per cent compared with subjects in the lowest quartile of serum carotenoid concentration (<2.33 μmol/L).[328] Among 156 CLAS subjects with 2-year angiograms evaluable by quantitative coronary angiography, evenly divided between drug and placebo groups, per cent stenosis in all coronary artery lesions decreased 0.8 percentage point, indicative of regression, in subjects with supplementary vitamin E intake of 100 IU/day or more, whereas per cent stenosis increased 2.0 percentage points, indicative of progression, in subjects with supplementary vitamin E intake less than 100 IU/day; this difference was statistically significant.[329] Lesion progression was not affected by supplementary intake of vitamin C or by dietary intake of vitamin E or vitamin C. In a case–control study of 270 subjects in the Helsinki Heart Study, the level of antibodies to oxidized LDL was significantly associated with an increased risk for a clinical event, defined as cardiac death or nonfatal myocardial infarction.[330] Compared with subjects in the lowest tertile of antibody level, subjects in the highest tertile had a 2.5-fold increased risk for a cardiac event after adjustment for age, smoking status, blood pressure, and HDL cholesterol level.

Few interventional data on the effect of antioxidants on CAD risk are available. In the Alpha-Tocopherol, Beta Carotene Cancer Prevention Study, 29,133 Finnish male smokers aged 50 to 69 years were randomized to receive alpha-tocopherol, 50 mg/day; beta-carotene, 20 mg/day; the combination; or placebo and followed up for a median of 6 years.[331] Although the study was designed to evaluate incidence of lung cancer, cardiovascular events were also recorded. Lung cancer incidence was reduced 2 per cent in subjects who received alpha-tocopherol, which was not a significant reduction, but was significantly increased 18 per cent in subjects who received beta-carotene. In subjects who received alpha-tocopherol, CAD mortality rate was 71.0 per 10,000 person-years, compared with 75.0 per 10,000 person-years in subjects who did not receive alpha-tocopherol, but total mortality increased 2 per cent, which was not a significant increase. In subjects who received beta-carotene, CAD mortality rate was 77.1 per 10,000 person-years, compared with 68.9 per 10,000 person-years in subjects who did not receive beta-carotene, and total mortality was significantly increased 8 per cent. These results, which appear to be in conflict with observational findings, may reflect the low dosages of the agents administered as well as the deleterious effects of tobacco use in the study population.

The NCEP does not recommend the use of antioxidant vitamin supplements to reduce CAD risk because of insufficient data supporting their cardiovascular benefits.[3] In addition, the effects of long-term use of antioxidants in large doses are not known.[332] Studies in progress, notably the Physicians' Health Study and the Women's Health Initiative, should help clarify this issue.

REFERENCES

DECLINING MORTALITY AND THE RISK FACTOR CONCEPT

1. American Heart Association: Heart and Stroke Facts: 1995 Statistical Supplement. Dallas, American Heart Association, 1994.
2. Expert Panel on Detection, Evaluation, and Treatment of High Blood Cholesterol in Adults: Summary of the second report of the National Cholesterol Education Program (NCEP) Expert Panel on Detection, Evaluation, and Treatment of High Blood Cholesterol in Adults (Adult Treatment Panel II). J. A. M. A. *269:*3015, 1993.
3. National Cholesterol Education Program: Second report of the Expert Panel on Detection, Evaluation, and Treatment of High Blood Cholesterol in Adults (Adult Treatment Panel II). Circulation *89:*1329, 1994.
4. Johnson, C. L., Rifkind, B. M., Sempos, C. T., et al.: Declining serum total cholesterol levels among US adults: The National Health and Nutrition Examination Surveys. J. A. M. A. *269:*3002, 1993.
5. Cigarette smoking among adults—United States, 1993. M. M. W. R. *43:*925, 1994.
6. Burt, V. L., Whelton, P., Roccella, E. J., et al.: Prevalence of hypertension in the US adult population: Results from the third National Health and Nutrition Examination Survey, 1988–1991. Hypertension *25:*305, 1995.
7. Sempos, C. T., Cleeman, J. I., Carroll, M. D., et al.: Prevalence of high blood cholesterol among US adults: An update based on guidelines from the second report of the National Cholesterol Education Program Adult Treatment Panel. J. A. M. A. *269:*3009, 1993.
8. Anderson, K. M., Wilson, P. W. F., Odell, P. M., and Kannel, W. B.: An updated coronary risk profile: A statement for health professionals. Circulation *83:*356, 1991.
9. Stamler, J.: Epidemiology, established major risk factors, and the primary prevention of coronary heart disease. *In* Chatterjee, K., Cheitlin, M. P., Karlines, J., et al. (eds.): Cardiology: An Illustrated Text/Reference. Vol. 2, p. 1. Philadelphia, J. B. Lippincott, 1991.

DYSLIPIDEMIA

10. Stamler, J., Wentworth, D., and Neaton, J. D., for the MRFIT Research Group: Is relationship between serum cholesterol and risk of premature death from coronary heart disease continuous and graded? Findings in 356 222 primary screenees of the Multiple Risk Factor Intervention Trial (MRFIT). J. A. M. A. *256:*2823, 1986.
11. Keys, A. (ed.): Coronary Heart Disease in Seven Countries. American Heart Association Monograph 29. Circulation *41*(Suppl. 1):1, 1970.
12. Kagan A., Harris, B. R., Winkelstein, W., Jr., et al.: Epidemiologic studies of coronary heart disease and stroke in Japanese men living in Japan, Hawaii and California: Demographic, physical, dietary and biochemical characteristics. J. Chronic Dis. *27:*345, 1974.
13. Marmot, M. G., Syme, S. L., Kagan, A., et al.: Epidemiologic studies of coronary heart disease and stroke in Japanese men living in Japan, Hawaii and California: Prevalence of coronary and hypertensive heart disease and associated risk factors. Am. J. Epidemiol. *102:*514, 1975.
14. Robertson, T. L., Kato, H., Rhoads, G. G., et al.: Epidemiologic studies of coronary heart disease and stroke in Japanese men living in Japan, Hawaii and California: Incidence of myocardial infarction and death from coronary heart disease. Am. J. Cardiol. *39:*239, 1977.
15. Lipid Research Clinics Program: The Lipid Research Clinics Coronary Primary Prevention Trial results. I. Reduction in incidence of coronary heart disease. J. A. M. A. *251:*351, 1984.
16. Lipid Research Clinics Program: The Lipid Research Clinics Coronary Primary Prevention Trial results. II. The relationship of reduction in incidence of coronary heart disease to cholesterol lowering. J. A. M. A. *251:*365, 1984.
17. Committee of Principal Investigators: A co-operative trial in the primary prevention of ischaemic heart disease using clofibrate. Br. Heart J. *40:*1069, 1978.
18. Committee of Principal Investigators: WHO cooperative trial on primary prevention of ischaemic heart disease with clofibrate to lower serum cholesterol: Final mortality follow-up. Lancet *2:*600, 1984.
19. Huttunen, J. K., Manninen, V., Mänttäri, M., et al.: The Helsinki Heart Study: Central findings and clinical implications. Ann. Med. *23:*155, 1991.
20. Frick, M. H., Elo, O., Haapa, K., et al.: Helsinki Heart Study: Primary-prevention trial with gemfibrozil in middle-aged men with dyslipidemia: Safety of treatment, changes in risk factors, and incidence of coronary heart disease. N. Engl. J. Med. *317:*1237, 1987.
21. Hjermann, I., Velve Byre, K., Holme, I., and Leren, P.: Effect of diet and smoking intervention on the incidence of coronary heart disease: Report from the Oslo Study Group of a randomised trial in healthy men. Lancet *2:*1303, 1981.
22. Hjermann, I., Holme, I., and Leren, P.: Oslo Study Diet and Antismoking Trial: Results after 102 months. Am. J. Med. *80*(Suppl. 2A):7, 1986.

22a. Shepherd, J., Cobbe, S. M., Ford, I., et al., for the West of Scotland Coronary Prevention Study Group: Prevention of coronary heart disease with provastatin in men with hypercholesterolemia. N. Engl. J. Med. *333:*1301, 1995.

23. Brown, B. G., Zhao, X. -Q., Sacco, D. E., and Albers, J. J.: Lipid lowering and plaque regression: New insights into prevention of plaque disruption and clinical events in coronary disease. Circulation *87:*1781, 1993.
24. Brown, B. G., Bolson, E. L., and Dodge, H. T.: Arteriographic assessment of coronary atherosclerosis: Review of current methods, their limitations, and clinical applications. Arteriosclerosis *2:*2, 1982.
25. de Feyter, P. J., Serruys, P. W., Davies, M. J., et al.: Quantitative coronary angiography to measure progression and regression of coronary atherosclerosis: Value, limitations, and implications for clinical trials. Circulation *84:*412, 1991.
26. Blankenhorn, D. H., and Hodis, H. N.: Arterial imaging and atherosclerosis reversal. Arterioscler. Thromb. *14:*177, 1994.
27. Gould, K. L.: Reversal of coronary atherosclerosis: Clinical promise as the basis for noninvasive management of coronary artery disease. Circulation *90:*1558, 1994.
28. Coronary Drug Project Research Group: Clofibrate and niacin in coronary heart disease. J. A. M. A. *231:*360, 1975.
29. Canner, P. L., Berge, K. G., Wenger, N. K., et al., for the Coronary Drug Project Research Group: Fifteen year mortality in Coronary Drug Project patients: Long-term benefit with niacin. J. Am. Coll. Cardiol. *8:*1245, 1986.
30. Brensike, J. F., Levy, R. I., Kelsey, S. F., et al.: Effects of therapy with cholestyramine on progression of coronary arteriosclerosis: Results of the NHLBI Type II Coronary Intervention Study. Circulation *69:*313, 1984.
31. Brensike, J. F., Kelsey, S. F., Passamani, E. R., et al.: National Heart, Lung, and Blood Institute Type II Coronary Intervention Study: Design, methods, and baseline characteristics. Controlled Clin. Trials *3:*91, 1982.
32. Levy, R. I., Brensike, J. F., Epstein, S. E., et al.: The influence of changes in lipid values induced by cholestyramine and diet on progression of coronary artery disease: Results of the NHLBI Type II Coronary Intervention Study. Circulation *69:*325, 1984.
33. Blankenhorn, D. H., Nessim, S. A., Johnson, R. L., et al.: Beneficial effects of combined colestipol-niacin therapy on coronary atherosclerosis and coronary venous bypass grafts. J. A. M. A. *257:*3233, 1987.
34. Blankenhorn, D. H., Johnson, R. L., Mack, W. J., et al.: The influence of diet on the appearance of new lesions in human coronary arteries. J. A. M. A. *263:*1646, 1990.
35. Cashin-Hemphill, L., Mack, W. J., Pogoda, J. M., et al.: Beneficial effects of colestipol-niacin on coronary atherosclerosis: A 4-year follow-up. J. A. M. A. *264:*3013, 1990.
36. Brown, G., Albers, J. J., Fisher, L. D., et al.: Regression of coronary artery disease as a result of intensive lipid-lowering therapy in men with high levels of apolipoprotein B. N. Engl. J. Med. *323:*1289, 1990.
37. Kane, J. P., Malloy, M. J., Ports, T. A., et al.: Regression of coronary atherosclerosis during treatment of familial hypercholesterolemia with combined drug regimens. J. A. M. A. *264:*3007, 1990.
38. Watts, G. F., Lewis, B., Brunt, J. N. H., et al.: Effects on coronary artery disease of lipid-lowering diet, or diet plus cholestyramine, in the St Thomas' Atherosclerosis Regression Study (STARS). Lancet *339:*563, 1992.
39. Buchwald, H., Varco, R. L., Matts, J. P., et al.: Effect of partial ileal bypass surgery on mortality and morbidity from coronary heart disease in patients with hypercholesterolemia: Report of the Program on the Surgical Control of the Hyperlipidemias (POSCH). N. Engl. J. Med. *323:*946, 1990.
40. Buchwald, H., Matts, J. P., Fitch, L. L., et al., for the Program on the Surgical Control of the Hyperlipidemias (POSCH) Group: Changes in sequential coronary arteriograms and subsequent coronary events. J. A. M. A. *268:*1429, 1992.
41. Ornish, D., Brown, S. E., Scherwitz, L. W., et al.: Can lifestyle changes reverse coronary heart disease? The Lifestyle Heart Trial. Lancet *336:*129, 1990.
42. Blankenhorn, D. H., Azen, S. P., Kramsch, D. M., et al.: Coronary angiographic changes with lovastatin therapy: The Monitored Atherosclerosis Regression Study (MARS). Ann. Intern. Med. *119:*969, 1993.
43. Hodis, H. N., Mack, W. J., Azen, S. P., et al.: Triglyceride- and cholesterol-rich lipoproteins have a differential effect on mild/moderate and severe lesion progression as assessed by quantitative coronary angiography in a controlled trial of lovastatin. Circulation *90:*42, 1994.
44. Waters, D., Higginson, L., Gladstone, P., et al.: Effects of monotherapy with an HMG-CoA reductase inhibitor on the progression of coronary atherosclerosis as assessed by serial quantitative arteriography: The Canadian Coronary Atherosclerosis Intervention Trial. Circulation *89:*959, 1994.
45. Pitt, B., Mancini, G. B. J., Ellis, S. G., et al., for the PLAC I Investigators: Pravastatin Limitation of Atherosclerosis in the Coronary Arteries

(PLAC I): Reduction in atherosclerosis progression and clinical events. J. Am. Coll. Cardiol. *26*:1133, 1995.

46. Jukema, J. W., Bruschke, A. V. G., van Boven, A. J., et al., on behalf of the REGRESS Study Group: Effects of lipid lowering by pravastatin on progression and regression of coronary artery disease in symptomatic men with normal to moderately elevated serum cholesterol levels: The Regression Growth Evaluation Statin Study (REGRESS). Circulation *91*:2528, 1995.
47. MAAS Investigators: Effect of simvastatin on coronary atheroma: The Multicentre Anti-Atheroma Study (MAAS). Lancet *344*:633, 1994.
48. Scandinavian Simvastatin Survival Study Group: Randomised trial of cholesterol lowering in 4444 patients with coronary heart disease: The Scandinavian Simvastatin Survival Study (4S). Lancet *344*:1383, 1994.
49. Scandinavian Simvastatin Survival Study Group: Baseline serum cholesterol and treatment effect in the Scandinavian Simvastatin Survival Study (4S). Lancet *345*:1274, 1995.
50. Neaton, J. D., Blackburn, H., Jacobs, D., et al.: Serum cholesterol level and mortality findings for men screened in the Multiple Risk Factor Intervention Trial. Arch. Intern. Med. *152*:1490, 1992.
51. Lewis, B., Paoletti, R., Tikkanen, M. J. (eds.): Low Blood Cholesterol: Health Implications: Proceedings of a workshop held in Milan, July 1993, under the auspices of the International Task Force for the Prevention of Coronary Heart Disease, International Society and Federation of Cardiology, Giovanni Lorenzini Foundation. London, Current Medical Literature Ltd., 1993.
52. Rossouw, J. E., and Gotto, A. M., Jr.: Does low cholesterol cause death? (editorial) Cardiovasc. Drugs Ther. *7*:789, 1993.
53. Chen, Z., Peto, R., Collins, R., et al.: Serum cholesterol concentration and coronary heart disease in population with low cholesterol concentrations. B. M. J. *303*:276, 1991.
54. Ettinger, W. H., Jr., and Harris, T.: Causes of hypocholesterolemia. Coron. Artery Dis. *4*:854, 1993.
55. Kane, J. P., and Havel, R. J.: Disorders of the biogenesis and secretion of lipoproteins containing the B apolipoproteins. *In* Scriver, C. R., Beaudet, A. L., Sly, W. S., and Valle, D. (eds.): The Metabolic and Molecular Bases of Inherited Disease, 7th ed. New York, McGraw-Hill, 1995, p. 1853.
56. Linton, M. F., Farese, R. V., and Young, S. G.: Familial hypobetalipoproteinemia. J. Lipid Res. *34*:521, 1993.
57. Rose, G., and Shipley, M.: Plasma lipids and mortality: A source of error. Lancet *1*:523, 1980.
58. Kagan, A., McGee, D. L., Yano, K., et al.: Serum cholesterol and mortality in a Japanese-American population: The Honolulu Heart Program. Am. J. Epidemiol. *114*:11, 1981.
59. Iribarren, C., Dwyer, J. H., Burchfiel, C. M., and Reed, S. M.: Can the U-shaped relation between mortality and serum cholesterol be explained by confounding? (abstract) Circulation *87*:684, 1993.
60. Iribarren, C., Reed, D. M., Wergowske, G., et al.: Serum cholesterol level and mortality due to suicide and trauma in the Honolulu Heart Program. Arch. Intern. Med. *155*:695, 1995.
61. Davey Smith, G., Shipley, M. J., Marmot, M. G., and Rose, G.: Plasma cholesterol concentration and mortality: The Whitehall Study. J. A. M. A. *267*:70, 1992.
62. Anderson, K. M., Castelli, W. P., and Levy, D.: Cholesterol and mortality: 30 years of follow-up from the Framingham Study. J. A. M. A. *257*:2176, 1987.
63. Wysowski, D. K., and Gross, T. P.: Deaths due to accidents and violence in two recent trials of cholesterol-lowering drugs. Arch. Intern. Med. *150*:2169, 1990.
64. Engelberg, H.: Low serum cholesterol and suicide. Lancet *339*:727, 1992.
65. Hawton, K., Cowen, P., Owens, D., et al.: Low serum cholesterol and suicide. Br. J. Psychiatry *162*:818, 1993.
66. Byington, R. P., Jukema, J. W., Salonen, J. T., et al.: Reduction in cardiovascular events during pravastatin therapy: Pooled analysis of clinical events of the pravastatin atherosclerosis intervention program. Circulation *92*:2419, 1995.
67. Krauss, R. M.: The tangled web of coronary risk factors. Am. J. Med. *90*(Suppl. 2A):2A–36S, 1991.
68. Austin, M. A., Breslow, J. L., Hennekens, C. H., et al.: Low-density lipoprotein subclass patterns and risk of myocardial infarction. J. A. M. A. *260*:1917, 1988.
69. Coresh, J., Kwiterovich, P. O., Jr., Smith, H. H., and Bachorik, P. S.: Association of plasma triglyceride concentration and LDL particle diameter, density, and chemical composition with premature coronary artery disease in men and women. J. Lipid Res. *34*:1687, 1993.
70. Austin, M. A., King, M-C., Vranizan, K. M., et al.: Inheritance of low-density lipoprotein subclass patterns: Results of complex segregation analysis. Am. J. Hum. Genet. *43*:838, 1988.
71. Austin, M. A.: Genetic epidemiology of low-density lipoprotein subclass phenotypes. Ann. Med. *24*:477, 1992.
72. Reaven, G. M., Chen, Y-D. I., Jeppesen, J., et al.: Insulin resistance and hyperinsulinemia in individuals with small, dense low density lipoprotein particles. J. Clin. Invest. *92*:141, 1993.
73. Tilly-Kiesi, M., and Tikkanen, M. J.: Low density lipoprotein density and composition in hypercholesterolaemic men treated with HMG CoA reductase inhibitors and gemfibrozil. J. Intern. Med. *229*:427, 1991.
74. Eisenberg, S., Gavish, D., Oschry, Y., et al.: Abnormalities in very low, low, and high density lipoproteins in hypertriglyceridemia: Reversal toward normal with bezafibrate treatment. J. Clin. Invest. *74*:470, 1984.
75. La Belle, M., and Krauss, R. M.: Differences in carbohydrate content of low density lipoproteins associated with low density lipoprotein subclass patterns. J. Lipid Res. *31*:1577, 1990.
76. Weisser, B., Locher, R., de Graaf, J., et al.: Low density lipoprotein subfractions increase thromboxane formation in endothelial cells. Biochem. Biophys. Res. Commun. *192*:1245, 1993.
77. Dejager, S., Bruckert, E., and Chapman, M. J.: Dense low density lipoprotein subspecies with diminished oxidative resistance predominate in combined hyperlipidemia. J. Lipid Res. *349*:295, 1993.
78. Steinberg, D., and Witztum, J. L.: Lipoproteins and atherogenesis: Current concepts. J. A. M. A. *264*:3047, 1990.
78a. Thorne, S. A., Abbot, S. E., Winyard, P. G., et al.: Extent of oxidative modification of low density lipoprotein determines the degree of cytotoxicity to human coronary artery cells. Heart *75*:11, 1996.
79. Schwartz, C. J., Valente, A. J., and Sprague, E. A.: A modern view of atherogenesis. Am. J. Cardiol. *71*:9B, 1993.
80. National Cholesterol Education Program: Report of the Expert Panel on Blood Cholesterol Levels in Children and Adolescents. Pediatrics *39*(3 pt 2):525, 1992.
81. Denke, M. A.: Cholesterol-lowering diets: A review of the evidence. Arch. Intern. Med. *155*:17, 1995.
81a. Grundy, S. M.: Lipids, nutrition, and coronary heart disease. *In* Fuster, V., Ross, R., and Topol, E. J. (eds.): Atherosclerosis and Coronary Artery Disease. Philadelphia, Lippincott-Raven, 1996, pp. 45–68.
82. Kris-Etherton, P. M., Krummel, D., Russell, M. E., et al.: The effect of diet on plasma lipids, lipoproteins, and coronary heart disease. J. Am. Diet. Assoc. *88*:1373, 1988.
83. Moore, R. B., Crane, C. A., and Frantz, I. D., Jr.: Effect of cholestyramine on the fecal excretion of intravenously administered cholesterol-4-^{14}C and its degradation products in a hypercholesterolemic patient. J. Clin. Invest. *47*:1664, 1968.
83a. Witztum, J. L.: Drugs used in the treatment of hyperlipoproteinemias. *In* Hardman, J. G., et al. (eds.): Goodman & Gilman's The pharmacological basis of therapeutics, 9th ed. New York, McGraw-Hill, 1996, pp. 875–898.
84. Grundy, S. M., Ahrens, E. H., Jr., and Salen, G.: Interruption of the enterohepatic circulation of bile acids in man: Comparative effects of cholestyramine and ileal exclusion on cholesterol metabolism. J. Lab. Clin. Med. *78*:94, 1971.
85. Gallo, D. G., Bailey, K. R., and Sheffner, A. L.: The interaction between cholestyramine and drugs. Proc. Soc. Exp. Biol. Med. *120*:60, 1965.
86. Bazzano, G., and Bazzano, G. S.: Digitalis intoxication: Treatment with a new steroid-binding resin. J. A. M. A. *220*:828, 1972.
87. Hunninghake, D. B., King, S., and LaCroix, K.: The effect of cholestyramine and colestipol on the absorption of hydrochlorothiazide. Int. J. Clin. Pharmacol. Ther. Toxicol. *20*:151, 1982.
88. Hibbard, D. M., Peters, J. R., and Hunninghake, D. B.: Effects of cholestyramine and colestipol on the plasma concentrations of propranolol. Br. J. Clin. Pharmacol. *18*:337, 1984.
89. Grundy, S. M., Mok, H. Y. I., Zech, L., and Berman, M.: Influence of nicotinic acid on metabolism of cholesterol and triglycerides in man. J. Lipid Res. *22*:24, 1981.
90. Brown, W. V., Howard, W. J., and Field, L.: Nicotinic acid and its derivatives. *In* Rifkind, B. M. (ed.): Drug Treatment of Hyperlipidemia. New York, Marcel Dekker, 1991, p. 189.
91. Shepherd, J., Packard, C. J., Patsch, J. R., et al.: Effects of nicotinic acid therapy on plasma high density lipoprotein subfraction distribution and composition and on apolipoprotein A metabolism. J. Clin. Invest. *63*:858, 1979.
92. Carlson, L. A., Hamsten, A., and Asplund, A.: Pronounced lowering of serum levels of lipoprotein Lp(a) in hyperlipidaemic subjects treated with nicotinic acid. J. Intern. Med. *226*:271, 1989.
93. Mullin, G. E., Greenson, J. K., and Mitchell, M. C.: Fulminant hepatic failure after ingestion of sustained-release nicotinic acid. Ann. Intern. Med. *111*:253, 1989.
94. Rader, J. I., Calvert, R. J., and Hathcock, J. N.: Hepatic toxicity of unmodified and time-release preparations of niacin. Am. J. Med. *92*:77, 1992.
95. Charman, R. C., Matthews, L. B., and Braeuler, C.: Nicotinic acid in the treatment of hypercholesterolemia: A long term study. Angiology *23*:29, 1972.
96. Litin, S. C., and Anderson, C. F.: Nicotinic acid–associated myopathy: A report of three cases. Am. J. Med. *86*:481, 1989.
97. Reaven, P., and Witztum, J. L.: Lovastatin, nicotinic acid, and rhabdomyolysis (letter). Ann. Intern. Med. *109*:597, 1988.
98. Arad, Y., Ramakrishnan, R., and Ginsberg, H. N.: Lovastatin therapy reduces low density lipoprotein apoB levels in subjects with combined hyperlipidemia by reducing the production of apoB-containing lipoproteins: Implications for the pathophysiology of apoB production. J. Lipid Res. *31*:567, 1990.
99. Isaacsohn, J. L., Setaro, J. F., Nicholas, C., et al.: Effects of lovastatin therapy on plasminogen activator inhibitor-1 antigen levels. Am. J. Cardiol. *74*:735, 1994.
100. Wada, H., Mori, Y., Kaneko, T., et al.: Elevated plasma levels of vascular endothelial cell markers in patients with hypercholesterolemia. Am. J. Hematol. *44*:112, 1993.
101. Gianturco, S. H., Bradley, W. A., Nozaki, S., et al.: Effects of lovastatin on the levels, structure, and atherogenicity of VLDL in patients with moderate hypertriglyceridemia. Arterioscler. Thromb. *13*:472, 1993.
102. Kostner, G. M., Gavish, D., Leopold, B., et al.: HMG CoA reductase inhibitors lower LDL cholesterol without reducing Lp(a) levels. Circulation *80*:1313, 1989.

103. Bradford, R. H., Shear, C. L., Chremos, A. N., et al.: Expanded Clinical Evaluation of Lovastatin (EXCEL) Study results. I. Efficacy in modifying plasma lipoproteins and adverse event profile in 8245 patients with moderate hypercholesterolemia. Arch. Intern. Med. *151*:43, 1991.
104. Tobert, J. A., Shear, C. L., Chremos, A. N., and Mantell, G. E.: Clinical experience with lovastatin. Am. J. Cardiol. *65*:23F, 1990.
105. Bradford, R. H., Shear, C. L., Chremos, A. N., et al.: Expanded Clinical Evaluation of Lovastatin (EXCEL) Study results: Two-year efficacy and safety follow-up. Am. J. Cardiol. *74*:667, 1994.
106. Pierce, L. R., Wysowski, D. K., and Gross, T. P.: Myopathy and rhabdomyolysis associated with lovastatin-gemfibrozil combination therapy. J. A. M. A. *264*:71, 1990.
107. Tobert, J. A.: Efficacy and long-term adverse effect pattern of lovastatin. Am. J. Cardiol. *62*:28J, 1988.
108. Corpier, C. L., Jones, P. H., Suki, W. N., et al.: Rhabdomyolysis and renal injury with lovastatin use: Report of two cases in cardiac transplant recipients. J. A. M. A. *260*:239, 1988.
109. Spach, D. H., Bauwens, J. E., Clark, C. D., and Burke, W. G.: Rhabdomyolysis associated with lovastatin and erythromycin use. West. J. Med. *154*:213, 1991.
110. Laties, A. M., Shear, C. L., Lippa, E. A., et al.: Expanded Clinical Evaluation of Lovastatin (EXCEL) Study results. II. Assessment of the human lens after 48 weeks of treatment with lovastatin. Am. J. Cardiol. *67*:447, 1991.
111. Illingworth, D. R., and Tobert, J. A.: A review of clinical trials comparing HMG-CoA reductase inhibitors. Clin. Ther. *16*:366, 1994.
112. Levy, R. I., Morganroth, J., and Rifkind, B. M.: Treatment of hyperlipidemia. N. Engl. J. Med. *290*:1295, 1976.
113. Bimmermann, A., Boerschmann, C., Schwartzkopff, W., et al.: Effective therapeutic measures for reducing lipoprotein (a) in patients with dyslipidemia: Lipoprotein (a) reduction with sustained-release bezafibrate. Current Therapeutic Research: Clinical and Experimental *49*:635, 1991.
114. Todd, P. A., and Ward, A.: Gemfibrozil: A review of its pharmacodynamic and pharmacokinetic properties, and therapeutic use in dyslipidaemia. Drugs *36*:314, 1988.
115. Andersen, P., Smith, P., Seljeflot, I., et al.: Effects of gemfibrozil on lipids and haemostasis after myocardial infarction. Thromb. Haemost. *63*:174, 1990.
116. Bo, M., Bonino, F., Neirotti, M., et al.: Hemorrheologic and coagulative pattern in hypercholesterolemic subjects treated with lipid-lowering drugs. Angiology *42*:106, 1991.
117. Langer, T., and Levy, R. I.: Acute muscular syndrome associated with administration of clofibrate. N. Engl. J. Med. *279*:856, 1968.
118. Wiklund, O., Angelin, B., Bergman, M., et al.: Pravastatin and gemfibrozil alone and in combination for the treatment of hypercholesterolemia. Am. J. Med. *94*:13, 1993.
119. Xiu, R. J., Freyschuss, A., Ying, X., et al.: The antioxidant butylated hydroxytoluene prevents early cholesterol-induced microcirculatory changes in rabbits. J. Clin. Invest. *93*:2732, 1994.
120. Carew, T. E., Schwenke, D. C., and Steinberg, D.: Antiatherogenic effect of probucol unrelated to its hypocholesterolemic effect: Evidence that antioxidants *in vivo* can selectively inhibit low density lipoprotein degradation in macrophage-rich fatty streaks and slow the progression of atherosclerosis in the Watanabe heritable hyperlipidemic rabbit. Proc. Natl. Acad. Sci. U. S. A. *84*:7725, 1987.
121. Yamamoto, A., Matsuzawa, Y., Yokoyama, S., et al.: Effects of probucol on xanthomata regression in familial hypercholesterolemia. Am. J. Cardiol. *57*:29H, 1986.
122. Mellies, M. J., Gartside, P. S., Glatfelder, L., et al.: Effects of probucol on plasma cholesterol, high and low density lipoprotein cholesterol, and apolipoproteins A1 and A2 in adults with primary familial hypercholesterolemia. Metabolism *29*:956, 1980.
123. Franceschini, G., Sirtori, M., Vaccarino, V., et al.: Mechanisms of HDL reduction after probucol: Changes in HDL subfractions and increased reverse cholesteryl ester transfer. Arteriosclerosis *9*:462, 1989.
124. McPherson, R., and Marcel, Y.: Role of cholesteryl ester transfer protein in reverse cholesterol transport. Clin. Cardiol. *14*:131, 1991.
125. Buckley, M. M-T., Goa, K. L., Price, A. H., and Brogden, R. N.: Probucol: A reappraisal of its pharmacological properties and therapeutic use in hypercholesterolaemia. Drugs *37*:761, 1989.
126. Stevenson, J. C., Crook, D., and Gosland, I. F.: Influence of age and menopause on serum lipids and lipoproteins in healthy women. Atherosclerosis *98*:83, 1993.
127. Stampfer, M. J., Colditz, G. A., Willett, W. C., et al.: Postmenopausal estrogen therapy and cardiovascular disease: Ten-year follow-up from the Nurses' Health Study. N. Engl. J. Med. *325*:756, 1991.
128. Stampfer, M. J., and Colditz, G. A.: Estrogen replacement therapy and coronary heart disease: A quantitative assessment of the epidemiologic evidence. Prev. Med. *20*:47, 1991.
129. Granfone, A., Campos, H., McNamara, J. R., et al.: Effects of estrogen replacement on plasma lipoproteins and apolipoproteins in postmenopausal, dyslipidemic women. Metabolism *41*:1193, 1992.
130. Wagner, J. D., St. Clair, R. W., Schwenke, D. C., et al.: Regional differences in arterial low density lipoprotein metabolism in surgically postmenopausal cynomolgus monkeys: Effects of estrogen and progesterone replacement therapy. Arterioscler. Thromb. *12*:717, 1992.
131. Gotto, A. M., Jr.: Postmenopausal hormone-replacement therapy, plasma lipoprotein[a], and risk for coronary heart disease (editorial). J. Lab. Clin. Med. *123*:800, 1994.
132. Writing Group for the PEPI Trial: Effects of estrogen or estrogen/progestin regimens on heart disease risk factors in postmenopausal women: The Postmenopausal Estrogen/Progestin Interventions (PEPI) trial. JAMA *273*:199, 1995.
133. Goldstein, J. L., Hobbs, H. H., and Brown, M. S.: Familial hypercholesterolemia. *In* Scriver, C. R., Beaudet, A. L., Sly, W. S., and Valle, D. (eds.): The Metabolic and Molecular Bases of Inherited Disease, 7th ed. New York, McGraw-Hill, 1995, p. 1981.
133a. Brewer, H. B. Jr., Santamarina-Fojo, S., and Hoeg, J. M.: Genetic dyslipoproteinemias. *In* Fuster, V., Ross, R., and Topol, E. J. (eds.): Atherosclerosis and Coronary Artery Disease. Philadelphia, Lippincott-Raven, 1996, pp. 69–88.
134. Bild, D. E., Williams, R. R., Brewer, H. B., et al.: Identification and management of heterozygous familial hypercholesterolemia: Summary and recommendations from an NHLBI workshop. Am. J. Cardiol. *72*:1D, 1993.
135. Tatami, R., Inoue, N., Itoh, H., et al., for the LARS Investigators: Regression of coronary atherosclerosis by combined LDL-apheresis and lipid-lowering drug therapy in patients with familial hypercholesterolemia: A multicenter study. Atherosclerosis *95*:1, 1992.
136. Thompson, G. R., Maher, V. M. G., Matthews, S., et al.: Familial Hypercholesterolaemia Regression Study: A randomised trial of low-density-lipoprotein apheresis. Lancet *345*:811, 1995.
137. Bilheimer, D. W., Goldstein, J. L., Grundy, S. M., et al.: Liver transplantation to provide low-density-lipoprotein receptors and lower plasma cholesterol in a child with homozygous familial hypercholesterolemia. N. Engl. J. Med. *311*:1658, 1984.
138. Grossman, M., Raper, S. E., Kozarsky, K., et al.: Successful *ex vivo* gene therapy directed to liver in a patient with familial hypercholesterolaemia. Nat. Genet. *6*:335, 1994.
139. Brown, M. S., Goldstein, J. L., Havel, R. J., and Steinberg, D.: Gene therapy for cholesterol (letter). Nat. Genet. *7*:349, 1994.
140. Grundy, S. M.: Multifactorial etiology of hypercholesterolemia: Implications for prevention of coronary heart disease. Arterioscler. Thromb. *11*:1619, 1991.
141. Kwiterovich, P. O., Jr.: Genetics and molecular biology of familial combined hyperlipidemia. Curr. Opin. Lipidol. *4*:133, 1993.
142. Myant, N. B.: Familial defective apolipoprotein B-100: A review, including some comparisons with familial hypercholesterolaemia. Atherosclerosis *104*:1, 1993.
143. Schmidt, E. B., Illingworth, D. R., Bacon, S., et al.: Hypolipidemic effects of nicotinic acid in patients with familial defective apolipoprotein B-100. Metabolism *42*:137, 1993.
144. Gordon, T., Castelli, W. P., Hjortland, M. C., et al.: High density lipoprotein as a protective factor against coronary heart disease: The Framingham Study. Am. J. Med. *62*:707, 1977.
145. Gordon, D. J., Probstfield, J. L., Garrison, R. J., et al.: High-density lipoprotein cholesterol and cardiovascular disease: Four prospective American studies. Circulation *79*:8, 1989.
146. James, R. W., and Pometta, D.: Immunofractionation of high density lipoprotein subclasses 2 and 3: Similarities and differences of fractions isolated from male and female populations. Atherosclerosis *83*:35, 1990.
147. Eisenberg, S.: High density lipoprotein metabolism. J. Lipid Res. *25*:1017, 1984.
148. Patsch, J. R.: Triglyceride-rich lipoproteins and atherosclerosis. Atherosclerosis *110*:S23, 1994.
149. Kuhn, F. E., Mohler, E. R., Satler, L. F., et al.: Effects of high-density lipoprotein on acetylcholine-induced coronary vasoreactivity. Am. J. Cardiol. *68*:1425, 1991.
150. Aoyama, T., Yui, Y., Morishita, H., and Kawai, C.: Prostacyclin stabilization by high density lipoprotein is decreased in acute myocardial infarction and unstable angina pectoris. Circulation *81*:1784, 1990.
151. Mackness, M. I., Abbott, C., Arrol, S., and Durrington, P. N.: The role of high-density lipoprotein and lipid-soluble antioxidant vitamins in inhibiting low-density lipoprotein oxidation. Biochem. J. *294*:829, 1993.
152. Assmann, G., von Eckardstein, A., and Brewer, H. B., Jr.: Familial high density lipoprotein deficiency: Tangier disease. *In* Scriver, C. R., Beaudet, A. L., Sly, W. S., and Valle, D. (eds.): The Metabolic and Molecular Bases of Inherited Disease, 7th ed. New York, McGraw-Hill, 1995, p. 2053.
153. Schaefer, E. J., Zech, L. A., Schwartz, D. E., and Brewer, H. B., Jr.: Coronary heart disease prevalence and other clinical features in familial high-density lipoprotein deficiency (Tangier disease). Ann. Intern. Med. *93*:261, 1980.
154. Schaefer, E. J., Blum, C. B., Levy, R. I., et al.: Metabolism of high density lipoprotein apoproteins in Tangier disease. N. Engl. J. Med. *299*:905, 1978.
155. Glomset, J. A., and Norum, K. R.: The metabolic role of lecithin:cholesterol acyltransferase: Perspectives from pathology. Adv. Lipid Res. *11*:1, 1973.
156. Glomset, J. A., Assmann, G., Gjone, E., and Norum, K. R.: Lecithin: cholesterol acyltransferase deficiency and fish eye disease. *In* Scriver, C. R., Beaudet, A. L., Sly, W. S., and Valle, D. (eds.): The Metabolic and Molecular Bases of Inherited Disease, 7th ed. New York, McGraw-Hill, 1995, p. 1933.
157. Carlson, L. A., and Holmquist, L.: Paradoxical esterification of plasma cholesterol in fish eye disease. Acta Med. Scand. *217*:491, 1985.
158. Breslow, J. L.: Familial disorders of high density lipoprotein metabolism. *In* Scriver, C. R., Beaudet, A. L., Sly, W. S., and Valle, D. (eds.): The Metabolic and Molecular Bases of Inherited Disease, 7th ed. New York, McGraw-Hill, 1995, p. 2031.
159. Roma, P., Gregg, R. E., Meng, M. S., et al.: In vivo metabolism of a

mutant form of apolipoprotein A-I, apo A-I_{Milano}, associated with familial hypoalphalipoproteinemia. J. Clin. Invest. *91*:1445, 1993.
160. Franceschini, G., Sirtori, C. R., Capurso, A., et al.: A-I_{Milano} apoprotein: Decreased high density lipoprotein cholesterol levels with significant lipoprotein modifications and without clinical atherosclerosis in an Italian family. J. Clin. Invest. *66*:892, 1980.
161. Norum, R. A., Lakier, J. B., Goldstein, S., et al.: Familial deficiency of apolipoproteins A-I and C-III and precocious coronary-artery disease. N. Engl. J. Med. *306*:1513, 1982.
162. Karathanasis, S. K., Ferris, E., and Haddad, I. A.: DNA inversion within the apolipoproteins AI/CIII/AIV-encoding gene cluster of certain patients with premature atherosclerosis. Proc. Natl. Acad. Sci. U. S. A. *84*:7198, 1987.
163. Lackner, K. J., Dieplinger, H., Nowicka, G., and Schmitz, G.: High density lipoprotein deficiency with xanthomas: A defect in reverse cholesterol transport caused by a point mutation in the apolipoprotein A-I gene. J. Clin. Invest. *92*:2262, 1993.
164. Austin, M. A.: Plasma triglyceride and coronary heart disease. Arterioscler. Thromb. *11*:2, 1991.
165. Austin, M. A.: Plasma triglyceride as a risk factor for coronary heart disease: The epidemiologic evidence and beyond. Am. J. Epidemiol. *129*:249, 1989.
166. Criqui, M. H., Heiss, G., Cohn, R., et al.: Plasma triglyceride level and mortality from coronary heart disease. N. Engl. J. Med. *328*:1220, 1993.
167. Groot, P. H. E., van Stiphout, W. A. H. J., Krauss, X. H., et al.: Postprandial lipoprotein metabolism in normolipemic men with and without coronary artery disease. Arterioscler. Thromb. *11*:653, 1991.
168. Patsch, J. R., Miesenböck, G., Hopferwieser, T., et al.: Relation of triglyceride metabolism and coronary artery disease: Studies in the postprandial state. Arterioscler. Thromb. *12*:1336, 1992.
169. Simo, I. E., Yakichuk, J. A., and Ooi, T. C.: Effect of gemfibrozil and lovastatin on postprandial lipoprotein clearance in the hypoalphalipoproteinemia and hypertriglyceridemia syndrome. Atherosclerosis *100*:55, 1993.
170. Hokanson, J. E., and Austin, M. A.: Triglyceride is a risk factor for coronary disease in men and women: A meta-analysis of population-based prospective studies. Circulation *88*(Abs.):I-510, 1993.
171. Assmann, G., and Schulte, H.: Role of triglycerides in coronary artery disease: Lessons from the Prospective Cardiovascular Münster study. Am. J. Cardiol. *70*:10H, 1992.
172. Blankenhorn, D. H., Alaupovic, P., Wickham, E., et al.: Prediction of angiographic change in native human coronary arteries and aortocoronary bypass grafts: Lipid and nonlipid factors. Circulation *81*:470, 1990.
173. Manninen, V., Tenkanen, L., Koskinen, P., et al.: Joint effects of serum triglyceride and LDL cholesterol and HDL cholesterol concentrations on coronary heart disease risk in the Helsinki Heart Study: Implications for treatment. Circulation *85*:37, 1992.
174. Krauss, R. M., Lindgren, F. T., Williams, P. T., et al.: Intermediate-density lipoproteins and progression of coronary artery disease in hypercholesterolaemic men. Lancet *2*:62, 1987.
175. Phillips, N. R., Waters, D., and Havel, R. J.: Plasma lipoproteins and progression of coronary artery disease evaluated by angiography and clinical events. Circulation *88*:2762, 1993.
176. Bang, H. O., and Dyerberg, J.: Plasma lipids and lipoproteins in Greenlandic west coast Eskimos. Acta Med. Scand. *192*:85, 1972.
177. Dolecek, T. A.: Epidemiological evidence of relationships between dietary polyunsaturated fatty acids and mortality in the Multiple Risk Factor Intervention Trial. Proc. Soc. Exp. Biol. Med. *200*:177, 1992.
178. Nestel, P. J., Connor, W. E., Reardon, M. F., et al.: Suppression by diets rich in fish oil of very low density lipoprotein production in man. J. Clin. Invest. *74*:82, 1984.
179. Abbey, M., Clifton, P., Kestin, M., et al.: Effect of fish oil on lipoproteins, lecithin:cholesterol acyltransferase, and lipid transfer protein activity in humans. Arteriosclerosis *10*:85, 1990.
180. Morris, M. C., Sacks, F., and Rosner, B.: Does fish oil lower blood pressure? A meta-analysis of controlled trials. Circulation *88*:523, 1993.
181. Braden, G. A., Knapp, H. R., and FitzGerald, G. A.: Suppression of eicosanoid biosynthesis during coronary angioplasty by fish oil and aspirin. Circulation *84*:679, 1991.
182. Bairati, I., Roy, L., and Meyer, F.: Double-blind, randomized, controlled trial of fish oil supplements in prevention of recurrence of stenosis after coronary angioplasty. Circulation *85*:950, 1992.
183. Chait, A., and Brunyell, J. D.: Chylomicronemia syndrome. Adv. Intern. Med. *37*:249, 1991.
184. Santamarina-Fojo, S., and Brewer, H. B., Jr.: The familial hyperchylomicronemia syndrome: New insights into underlying genetic defects. JAMA *265*:904, 1991.
185. Brunzell, J. D., Miller, N. E., Alaupovic, P., et al.: Familial chylomicronemia due to a circulating inhibitor of lipoprotein lipase activity. J. Lipid Res. *24*:12, 1983.
186. Kane, J. P., Chen, G. C., Hamilton, R. L., et al.: Remnants of lipoproteins of intestinal and hepatic origin in familial dysbetalipoproteinemia. Arteriosclerosis *3*:47, 1983.
187. Mahley, R. W., Innerarity, T. L., Weisgraber, K. H., and Rall, S. C., Jr.: Genetic defects in lipoprotein metabolism: Elevation of atherogenic lipoproteins caused by impaired catabolism. JAMA *265*:78, 1991.
188. Mahley, R. W., and Rall, S. C., Jr.: Type III hyperlipoproteinemia (dysbetalipoproteinemia): The role of apolipoprotein E in normal and abnormal lipoprotein metabolism. *In* Scriver, C. R., Beaudet, A. L., Sly, W. S., and Valle, D. (eds.): The Metabolic and Molecular Bases of Inherited Disease, 7th ed. New York, McGraw-Hill, 1995, p. 1953.
189. Loscalzo, J.: Lipoprotein(a): A unique risk factor for atherothrombotic disease. Arteriosclerosis *10*:672, 1990.
190. Boerwinkle, E., Leffert, C. C., Lin, J., et al.: Apolipoprotein(a) accounts for greater than 90% of the variation in plasma lipoprotein(a) concentrations. J. Clin. Invest. *90*:52, 1992.
191. Utermann, G., Hoppichler, F., Dieplinger, H., et al.: Defects in the low density lipoprotein receptor gene affect lipoprotein(a) levels: Multiplicative interaction of two gene loci associated with premature atherosclerosis. Proc. Natl. Acad. Sci. U. S. A. *86*:4171, 1989.
192. De Knijff, P., Kaptein, A., Boomsma, D., et al.: Apolipoprotein E polymorphism affects plasma levels of lipoprotein(a). Atherosclerosis *90*:169, 1991.
193. Loscalzo, J., Weinfeld, M., Fless, G. M., and Scanu, A. M.: Lipoprotein(a), fibrin binding, and plasminogen activation. Arteriosclerosis *10*:240, 1990.
194. Beisiegel, U., Niendorf, A., Wolf, K., et al.: Lipoprotein(a) in the arterial wall. Eur. Heart J. *11*(Suppl. E):174, 1990.
195. Haberland, M. E., Fless, G. M., Scanu, A. M., and Fogelman, A. M.: Malondialdehyde modification of lipoprotein(a) produces avid uptake by human monocyte–macrophages. J. Biol. Chem. *267*:4143, 1992.
196. Naruszewicz, M., Selinger, E., and Davignon, J.: Oxidative modification of lipoprotein(a) and the effect of β-carotene. Metabolism *41*:1215, 1992.
197. Gurakar, A., Hoeg, J. M., Kostner, G., et al.: Levels of lipoprotein Lp(a) decline with neomycin and niacin treatment. Atherosclerosis *57*:293, 1985.
198. Albers, J. J., Taggart, H. M., Appelbaum-Bowden, D., et al.: Reduction of LCAT, apo D, and the Lp(a) lipoprotein with the anabolic steroid stanozolol. Biochim. Biophys. Acta *795*:293, 1984.

TOBACCO USE

199. Bartecchi, C. E., MacKenzie, T. D., and Schrier, R. W.: The human costs of tobacco use (first of two parts). N. Engl. J. Med. *330*:907, 1994.
199a. Stafford, R. S., and Becker, C. G.: Cigarette smoking and atherosclerosis. *In* Fuster, V., Ross, R., and Topol, E. J. (eds.): Atherosclerosis and Coronary Artery Disease. Philadelphia, Lippincott-Raven, 1996, pp. 303–326.
200. Peto, R., Lopez, A. D., Boreham, J., et al.: Mortality from tobacco in developed countries: Indirect estimation from national vital statistics. Lancet *339*:1268, 1992.
201. Smoking-Related Deaths and Financial Costs: Estimates for 1990, rev. ed. Washington, D.C., Office of Technology Assessment, 1993.
202. Kannel, W. B., and Higgins, M.: Smoking and hypertension as predictors of cardiovascular risk in population studies. J. Hypertens. Suppl. *8*:S3, 1990.
203. Negri, E., Franzosi, M. G., La Vecchia, C., et al.: Tar yield of cigarettes and risk of acute myocardial infarction. B. M. J. *306*:1567, 1993.
204. Bolinder, G., Alfredsson, L., Englund, A., and de Faire, U.: Smokeless tobacco use and increased cardiovascular mortality among Swedish construction workers. Am. J. Public Health *84*:399, 1994.
205. Steenland, K.: Passive smoking and the risk of heart disease. JAMA *267*:94, 1992.
206. Sigurdsson, G., Jr., Gudnason, V., Sigurdsson, G., and Humphries, S. E.: Interaction between a polymorphism of the apo A-I promoter region and smoking determines plasma levels of HDL and apo A-I. Arterioscler. Thromb. *12*:1017, 1992.
207. McCall, M. R., van den Berg, J. J., Kuypers, F. A., et al.: Modification of LCAT activity and HDL structure: New links between cigarette smoke and coronary heart disease risk. Arterioscler. Thromb. *14*:248, 1994.
208. Sugiishi, M., and Takatsu, F.: Cigarette smoking is a major risk factor for coronary spasm. Circulation *87*:76, 1993.
209. Pittilo, R. M., Mackie, I. J., Rowles, P. M., et al.: Effects of cigarette smoking on the ultrastructure of rat thoracic aorta and its ability to produce prostacyclin. Thromb. Haemost. *48*:173, 1982.
210. Ogston, D., Bennett, N. B., and Ogston, C. M.: The influence of cigarette smoking on the plasma fibrinogen concentration. Atherosclerosis *11*:349, 1970.
211. FitzGerald, G. A., Oates, J. A., and Nowak, J.: Cigarette smoking and hemostatic function. Am. Heart J. *115*:267, 1988.
212. Tsevat, J., Weinstein, M. C., Williams, L. W., et al.: Expected gains in life expectancy from various coronary heart disease risk factor modifications. Circulation *83*:1194, 1991.
213. Terres, W., Becker, P., and Rosenberg, A.: Changes in cardiovascular risk profile during the cessation of smoking. Am. J. Med. *97*:242, 1994.
214. Gerace, T. A., Hollis, J., Ockene, J. K., and Svendsen, K.: Smoking cessation and change in diastolic blood pressure, body weight, and plasma lipids: MRFIT Research Group. Prev. Med. *20*:602, 1991.
215. Dobson, A. J., Alexander, H. M., Heller, R. F., and Lloyd, D. M.: How soon after quitting smoking does risk of heart attack decline? J. Clin. Epidemiol. *44*:1247, 1991.
216. Physician and other health-care professional counseling of smokers to quit—United States, 1991. M. M. W. R. *42*:854, 1993.
217. Public Health Service: Healthy People 2000: National health promotion and disease prevention objectives—full report, with commentary. [DHHS publication no. (PHS)91-50212.] Washington, D.C., U.S. Department of Health and Human Services, Public Health Service, 1991.
218. Glynn, T. J., and Manley, M. W.: How to Help Your Patients Stop Smoking: A National Cancer Institute manual for physicians. [DHHS

publication no. (PHS)92-3064.] Bethesda, Md., U.S. Department of Health and Human Services, Public Health Service, National Institutes of Health, National Cancer Institute, 1992.

HYPERTENSION

219. National High Blood Pressure Education Program Working Group: Report on primary prevention of hypertension. Arch. Intern. Med. *153*:186, 1993.
220. MacMahon, S., Peto, R., Cutler, J., et al.: Blood pressure, stroke, and coronary heart disease. Part 1. Prolonged differences in blood pressure: Prospective observational studies corrected for the regression dilution bias. Lancet *335*:765, 1990.
221. Collins, R., Peto, R., MacMahon, S., et al.: Blood pressure, stroke, and coronary heart disease. Part 2. Short-term reductions in blood pressure: Overview of randomised drug trials in their epidemiological context. Lancet *335*:827, 1990.
222. Black, H. R.: Metabolic considerations in the choice of therapy for the patient with hypertension. Am. Heart J. *121*:707, 1991.
223. Samuelsson, O. G., Wilhelmsen, L. W., Pennert, K. M., et al.: The J-shaped relationship between coronary heart disease and achieved blood pressure level in treated hypertension: Further analyses of 12 years of follow-up of treated hypertensives in the Primary Prevention Trial in Gothenburg, Sweden. J. Hypertens. *8*:547, 1990.
224. Hansson, L., and Zanchetti, A.: The Hypertension Optimal Treatment (HOT) Study—patient characteristics: Randomization, risk profiles, and early blood pressure results. Blood Press. *3*:322, 1994.
225. Houston, M. C.: The management of hypertension and associated risk factors for the prevention of long-term cardiac complications. J. Cardiovasc. Pharmacol. *21*(Suppl. 2):S2, 1993.
226. Reaven, G. M.: Role of insulin resistance in human disease (syndrome X): An expanded definition. Annu. Rev. Med. *44*:121, 1993.
227. DeFronzo, R. A., and Ferrannini, E.: Insulin resistance: A multifaceted syndrome responsible for NIDDM, obesity, hypertension, dyslipidemia, and atherosclerotic cardiovascular disease. Diabetes Care *14*:173, 1991.

DIABETES MELLITUS

228. American Diabetes Association: Diabetes Facts: The Dangerous Toll of Diabetes. Alexandria, Va., American Diabetes Association, 1994.
229. American Diabetes Association: Diabetes Facts: Profile of the Diagnosed. Alexandria, Va., American Diabetes Association, 1993.
230. Barrett-Connor, E. L., Cohn, B. A., Wingard, D. L., and Edelstein, S. L.: Why is diabetes mellitus a stronger risk factor for fatal ischemic heart disease in women than in men? The Rancho Bernardo Study. JAMA *265*:627, 1991.
231. American Diabetes Association: Detection and management of lipid disorders in diabetes. Diabetes Care *16*(Suppl. 2):106, 1993.
232. Head, J., and Fuller, J. H.: International variations in mortality among diabetic patients: The WHO Multinational Study of Vascular Disease in Diabetics. Diabetologia *33*:477, 1990.
233. Chen, Y. D., Swami, S., Skowronski, R., et al.: Differences in postprandial lipemia between patients with normal glucose tolerance and non-insulin-dependent diabetes mellitus. J. Clin. Endocrinol. Metab. *76*:172, 1993.
234. Pyörälä, K., Laakso, M., and Uusitupa, M.: Diabetes and atherosclerosis: An epidemiologic view. Diabetes Metab. Rev. *3*:463, 1987.
235. Reaven, G. M., and Chen, Y-D. I.: Role of insulin in regulation of lipoprotein metabolism in diabetes. Diabetes Metab. Rev. *4*:639, 1988.
236. Haaber, A. B., Deckert, M., Stender, S., and Jensen, T.: Increased urinary loss of high density lipoproteins in albuminuric insulin-dependent diabetic patients. Scand. J. Clin. Lab. Invest. *53*:191, 1993.
237. Witztum, J. L., Mahoney, E. M., Branks, M. J., et al.: Nonenzymatic glycosylation of low-density lipoprotein alters its biologic activity. Diabetes *31*:283, 1982.
238. Lopes-Virella, M. F., Klein, R. L., Lyons, T. J., et al.: Glycosylation of low-density lipoprotein enhances cholesteryl ester synthesis in human monocyte-derived macrophages. Diabetes *37*:550, 1988.
239. Duell, P. B., Oram, J. F., and Bierman, E. L.: Nonenzymatic glycosylation of HDL and impaired HDL-receptor–mediated cholesterol efflux. Diabetes *40*:377, 1991.
240. Morel, D. W., and Chisolm, G. M.: Antioxidant treatment of diabetic rats inhibits lipoprotein oxidation and cytotoxicity. J. Lipid Res. *30*:1827, 1989.
241. Haffner, S. M.: Lipoprotein(a) and diabetes: An update. Diabetes Care *16*:835, 1993.
242. Colwell, J. A., Winocour, P. D., Lopes-Virella, M., and Halushka, P. V.: New concepts about the pathogenesis of atherosclerosis in diabetes mellitus. Am. J. Med. *75*:67, 1983.
243. Juhan-Vague, I., Roul, C., Alessi, M., et al.: Increased plasminogen activator inhibitor activity in non insulin dependent diabetic patients: Relationship with plasma insulin. Thromb. Haemost. *61*:370, 1989.
244. Bierman, E. L.: Atherogenesis in diabetes. Arterioscler. Thromb. *12*:647, 1992.
245. Strowig, S., and Raskin, P.: Glycemic control and diabetic complications. Diabetes Care *15*:1126, 1992.
246. Moss, S. E., Klein, R., Klein, B. E., and Meuer, S. M.: The association of glycemia and cause-specific mortality in a diabetic population. Arch. Intern. Med. *154*:2473, 1994.
247. Diabetes Control and Complications Trial Research Group: The effect of intensive treatment of diabetes on the development and progression of long-term complications in insulin-dependent diabetes mellitus. N. Engl. J. Med. *329*:977, 1993.
248. Pandit, M. K., Burke, J., Gustafson, A. B., et al.: Drug-induced disorders of glucose tolerance. Ann. Intern. Med. *118*:529, 1993.
249. Lardinois, C. K., and Neuman, S. L.: The effects of antihypertensive agents on serum lipids and lipoproteins. Arch. Intern. Med. *148*:1280, 1988.
250. Ruderman, N. B., and Schneider, S. H.: Diabetes, exercise and atherosclerosis. Diabetes Care *15*:1787, 1992.

PHYSICAL INACTIVITY

251. Prevalence of sedentary lifestyle—Behavioral Risk Factor Surveillance System, United States, 1991. M. M. W. R. *42*:576, 1993.
252. Powell, K. E., Thompson, P. D., Caspersen, C. J., et al.: Physical activity and the incidence of coronary heart disease. Annu. Rev. Public Health *8*:253, 1987.
253. Berlin, J. A., and Colditz, G. A.: A meta-analysis of physical activity in the prevention of coronary heart disease. Am. J. Epidemiol. *132*:612, 1990.
254. Leon, A. S., Connett, J., for the MRFIT Research Group: Physical activity and 10.5 year mortality in the Multiple Risk Factor Intervention Trial (MRFIT). Int. J. Epidemiol. *20*:690, 1991.
255. Ekelund, L-G., Haskell, W. L., Johnson, J. L., et al.: Physical fitness as a predictor of cardiovascular mortality in asymptomatic North American men: The Lipid Research Clinics Mortality Follow-up Study. N. Engl. J. Med. *319*:1379, 1988.
256. Sandvik, L., Erikssen, J., Thaulow, E., et al.: Physical fitness as a predictor of mortality among healthy, middle-aged Norwegian men. N. Engl. J. Med. *328*:533, 1993.
257. Lakka, T. A., Venalainen, J. M., Rauramaa, R., et al.: Relation of leisure-time physical activity and cardiorespiratory fitness to the risk of acute myocardial infarction. N. Engl. J. Med. *330*:1549, 1994.
258. Blair, S. N., Cooper, K. H., Gibbons, L. W., et al.: Changes in coronary heart disease risk factors associated with increased treadmill time in 753 men. Am. J. Epidemiol. *118*:352, 1983.
259. Helmrich, S. P., Ragland, D. R., Leung, R. W., and Paffenbarger, R. S., Jr.: Physical activity and reduced occurrence of non-insulin-dependent diabetes mellitus. N. Engl. J. Med. *325*:147, 1991.
260. Desprès, J-P., Pouliot, M-C., Moorjani, S., et al.: Loss of abdominal fat and metabolic response to exercise training in obese women. Am. J. Physiol. *261*:E159, 1991.
261. Arroll, B., and Beaglehole, R.: Does physical activity lower blood pressure: A critical review of the clinical trials. J. Clin. Epidemiol. *45*:439, 1992.
262. Fletcher, G. F., Blair, S. N., Blumenthal, J., et al.: Statement on exercise: Benefits and recommendations for physical activity programs for all Americans: A statement for health professionals by the Committee on Exercise and Cardiac Rehabilitation of the Council on Clinical Cardiology, American Heart Association. Circulation *86*:340, 1992.
263. Wood, P. D., Stefanick, M. L., Williams, P. T., and Haskell, W. L.: The effects on plasma lipoproteins of a prudent weight-reducing diet, with or without exercise, in overweight men and women. N. Engl. J. Med. *325*:461, 1991.
264. Paffenbarger, R. S., Jr., Hyde, R. T., Wing, A. L., et al.: The association of changes in physical-activity level and other lifestyle characteristics with mortality among men. N. Engl. J. Med. *328*:538, 1993.
265. Pate, R. R., Pratt, M., Blair, S. N., et al.: Physical activity and public health: A recommendation from the Centers for Disease Control and Prevention and the American College of Sports Medicine. J. A. M. A. *273*:402, 1995.
266. Levine, G. N., and Balady, G. J.: The benefits and risks of exercise training: The exercise prescription. Adv. Intern. Med. *38*:57, 1993.

OBESITY

267. Kuczmarski, R. J., Flegal, K. M., Campbell, S. M., and Johnson, C. L.: Increasing prevalence of overweight among US adults: The National Health and Nutrition Examination Surveys, 1960 to 1991. J. A. M. A. *272*:205, 1994.
268. Bjorntorp, P.: Obesity and adipose tissue distribution as risk factors for the development of disease—a review. Infusiontherapie *17*:24, 1990.
269. Larsson, B., Bengtsson, C., Bjorntorp, P., et al.: Is abdominal body fat distribution a major explanation for the sex difference in the incidence of myocardial infarction? The study of men born in 1913 and the study of women. Am. J. Epidemiol. *135*:266, 1992.
270. Freedman, D. S., Jacobsen, S. J., Barboriak, J. J., et al.: Body fat distribution and male/female differences in lipids and lipoproteins. Circulation *81*:1498, 1990.
271. Hubert, H. B., Feinleib, M., McNamara, P. M., and Castelli, W. P.: Obesity as an independent risk factor for cardiovascular disease: A 26-year follow-up of participants in the Framingham Heart Study. Circulation *67*:968, 1983.
272. Willett, W. C., Manson, J. A. E., Stampfer, M. J., et al.: Weight, weight change, and coronary heart disease in women: Risk within the 'normal' weight range. J. A. M. A. *273*:461, 1995.
273. Denke, M. A., Sempos, C. T., and Grundy, S. M.: Excess body weight: An underrecognized contributor to high blood cholesterol levels in white American men. Arch. Intern. Med. *153*:1093, 1993.
274. Garrison, R. J., Wilson, P. W., Castelli, W. P., et al.: Obesity and lipoprotein cholesterol in the Framingham Offspring Study. Metabolism *29*:1053, 1980.

275. Berchtold, P., Jorgens, V., Finke, C., and Berger, M.: Epidemiology of obesity and hypertension. Int. J. Obes. *5*(Suppl. 1):1, 1981.
276. Hartz, A. J., Rupley, D. C., Kalkhoff, R. D., and Rimm, A. A.: Relationship of obesity to diabetes: Influence of obesity level and body fat distribution. Prev. Med. *12*:351, 1983.

NONMODIFIABLE RISK FACTORS

277. Shea, S., Ottman, R., Gabrieli, C., et al.: Family history as an independent risk factor for coronary artery disease. J. Am. Coll. Cardiol. *4*:793, 1984.
278. Colditz, G. A., Rimm, E. B., Giovannucci, E., et al.: A prospective study of parental history of myocardial infarction and coronary artery disease in men. Am. J. Cardiol. *67*:933, 1991.
279. Kaprio, J., Norio, R., Pesonen, E., and Sarna, S.: Intimal thickening of the coronary arteries in infants in relation to family history of coronary artery disease. Circulation *87*:1960, 1993.
280. Slyper, A., and Schectman, G.: Coronary artery disease risk factors from a genetic and developmental perspective. Arch. Intern. Med. *154*:633, 1994.
281. Rubin, S. M., Sidney, S., Black, D. M., et al.: High blood cholesterol in elderly men and the excess risk for coronary heart disease. Ann. Intern. Med. *113*:916, 1990.
282. SHEP Cooperative Research Group: Prevention of stroke by antihypertensive drug treatment in older persons with isolated systolic hypertension: Final results of the Systolic Hypertension in the Elderly Program (SHEP). J. A. M. A. *265*:3255, 1991.
283. Lerner, D. J., and Kannel, W. B.: Patterns of coronary heart disease morbidity and mortality in the sexes: A 26-year follow-up of the Framingham population. Am. Heart J. *111*:383, 1986.
284. Brezinka, V., and Padmos, I.: Coronary heart disease risk factors in women. Eur. Heart J. *15*:1571, 1994.
285. Kannel, W. B., and McGee, D. L.: Diabetes and glucose tolerance as risk factors for cardiovascular disease: The Framingham Study. Diabetes Care *2*:120, 1979.
286. Castelli, W. P.: Epidemiology of triglycerides: A view from Framingham. Am. J. Cardiol. *70*:3H, 1992.

OTHER RISK FACTORS

287. Iso, H., Folsom, A. R., Sato, S., et al.: Plasma fibrinogen and its correlates in Japanese and US population samples. Arterioscler. Thromb. *13*:783, 1993.
288. Ernst, E.: Plasma fibrinogen—an independent cardiovascular risk factor. J. Intern. Med. *227*:365, 1990.
289. Heinrich, J., Balleisen, L., Schulte, H., et al.: Fibrinogen and factor VII in the prediction of coronary risk: Results from the PROCAM study in healthy men. Arterioscler. Thromb. *14*:54, 1994.
290. Yarnell, J. W. G., Baker, I. A., Sweetnam, P. M., et al.: Fibrinogen, viscosity, and white blood cell count are major risk factors for ischemic heart disease: The Caerphilly and Speedwell collaborative heart disease studies. Circulation *83*:836, 1991.
291. Miller, G. J.: Hemostasis and cardiovascular risk: The British and European experience. Arch. Pathol. Lab. Med. *116*:1318, 1992.
292. Miller, G. J.: Environmental influences on hemostasis and thrombosis: Diet and smoking. Ann. Epidemiol. *2*:387, 1992.
293. Kelleher, C. C.: Plasma fibrinogen and factor VII as risk factors for cardiovascular disease. Eur. J. Epidemiol. *8*(Suppl. 1):79, 1992.
294. Meade, T. W.: Hypercoagulability and ischaemic heart disease. Blood Rev. *1*:2, 1987.
295. Meade, T. W., Ruddock, V., Stirling, Y., et al.: Fibrinolytic activity, clotting factors, and long-term incidence of ischaemic heart disease in the Northwick Park Heart Study. Lancet *342*:1076, 1993.
296. Juhan-Vague, I., and Alessi, M. C.: Plasminogen activator inhibitor 1 and atherothrombosis. Thromb. Haemost. *70*:138, 1993.
297. Hamsten, A., Wiman, B., de Faire, U., and Blomback, M.: Increased plasma levels of a rapid inhibitor of tissue plasminogen activator in young survivors of myocardial infarction. N. Engl. J. Med. *313*:1557, 1985.
298. Juhan-Vague, I., Thompson, S. G., Jespersen, J., on behalf of the ECAT Angina Pectoris Study Group: Involvement of the hemostatic system in the insulin resistance syndrome: A study of 1500 patients with angina pectoris. Arterioscler. Thromb. *13*:1865, 1993.
299. Hamsten, A., de Faire, U., Walldius, G., et al.: Plasminogen activator inhibitor in plasma: Risk factor for recurrent myocardial infarction. Lancet *2*:3, 1987.
300. Schneiderman, J., Sawdey, M. S., Keeton, M. R., et al.: Increased type 1 plasminogen activator inhibitor gene expression in atherosclerotic human arteries. Proc. Natl. Acad. Sci. U. S. A. *89*:6998, 1992.
301. Robinson, K., Mayer, E., and Jacobsen, D. W.: Homocysteine and coronary artery disease. Cleve. Clin. J. Med. *61*:438, 1994.
301a. Mayer, E. L., Jacobsen, D. W., and Robinson, K.: Homocysteine and coronary atherosclerosis. J. Am. Coll. Cardiol. *27*:517, 1996.
302. Clarke, R., Daly, L., Robinson, K., et al.: Hyperhomocysteinemia: An independent risk factor for vascular disease. N. Engl. J. Med. *324*:1149, 1991.
303. Glueck, C. J., Shaw, P., Lang, J. E., et al.: Evidence that homocysteine is an independent risk factor for atherosclerosis in hyperlipidemic patients. Am. J. Cardiol. *75*:132, 1995.
304. Stampfer, M. J., Malinow, M. R., Willett, W. C., et al.: A prospective study of plasma homocyst(e)ine and risk of myocardial infarction in US physicians. J. A. M. A. *268*:877, 1992.
305. Rodgers, G. M., and Conn, M. T.: Homocysteine, an atherogenic stimulus, reduces protein C activation by arterial and venous endothelial cells. Blood *75*:895, 1990.
306. Pohorecky, L. A.: Interaction of alcohol and stress at the cardiovascular level. Alcohol *7*:537, 1990.
307. Gaziano, J. M., Buring, J. E., Breslow, J. L., et al.: Moderate alcohol intake, increased levels of high-density lipoprotein and its subfractions, and decreased risk of myocardial infarction. N. Engl. J. Med. *329*:1829, 1993.
308. Langer, R. D., Criqui, M. H., and Reed, D. M.: Lipoproteins and blood pressure as biological pathways for effect of moderate alcohol consumption on coronary heart disease. Circulation *85*:910, 1992.
309. Criqui, M. H., Cowan, L. D., Heiss, G., et al.: Frequency and clustering of non-lipid coronary risk factors in dyslipoproteinemia. Circulation *73*:I-40, 1986.
310. Meade, T. W., Vickers, M. V., Thompson, S. G., et al.: Epidemiological characteristics of platelet aggregability. B. M. J. *290*:428, 1985.
311. Laug, W. E.: Ethyl alcohol enhances plasminogen activator secretion by endothelial cells. J. A. M. A. *250*:772, 1983.
312. Ridker, P. M., Vaughan, D. E., Stampfer, M. J., et al.: Association of moderate alcohol consumption and plasma concentration of endogenous tissue-type plasminogen activator. J. A. M. A. *272*:929, 1994.
313. Renaud, S., and de Lorgeril, M.: Wine, alcohol, platelets, and the French paradox for coronary heart disease. Lancet *339*:1523, 1992.
314. Frankel, E. N., Kanner, J., German, J. B., et al.: Inhibition of oxidation of human low-density lipoprotein by phenolic substances in red wine. Lancet *341*:454, 1993.
315. Lachar, B. L.: Coronary-prone behavior: Type A behavior revisited. Tex. Heart Inst. J. *20*:143, 1993.
316. Littman, A. B.: Review of psychosomatic aspects of cardiovascular disease. Psychother. Psychosom. *60*:148, 1993.
317. Rosenman, R. H., Brand, R. J., Jenkins, C. D., et al.: Coronary heart disease in the Western Collaborative Group Study: Final follow-up experience of 8½ years. J. A. M. A. *233*:872, 1975.
318. Eaker, E. D., Abbott, R. D., and Kannel, W. B.: Frequency of uncomplicated angina pectoris in type A compared with type B persons (the Framingham Study). Am. J. Cardiol. *63*:1042, 1989.
319. Shekelle, R. B., Hulley, S. B., Neaton, J. D., et al.: The MRFIT Behavior Pattern Study. II. Type A behavior and incidence of coronary heart disease. Am. J. Epidemiol. *122*:559, 1985.
320. Matthews, K. A., and Haynes, S. G.: Type A behavior pattern and coronary disease risk: Update and critical evaluation. Am. J. Epidemiol. *123*:923, 1986.
321. O'Rourke, D. F., Houston, B. K., Harris, J. K., and Snyder, C. R.: The type A behavior pattern: Summary, conclusions, and implications. *In* Houston, B. K., and Snyder, C. R. (eds.): Type A Behavior Pattern. Research, Theory, and Intervention. New York, John Wiley and Sons, 1988, p. 312.
322. Williams, R. B., Jr.: Biological mechanisms mediating the relationship between behavior and coronary heart disease. *In* Siegman, A. W., and Dembroski, T. M. (eds.): In Search of Coronary-Prone Behavior. Beyond Type A. Hillsdale, N. J., Lawrence Erlbaum Associates, 1989, p. 195.
323. Siegman, A. W.: Cardiovascular consequences of expressing, experiencing, and repressing anger. J. Behav. Med. *16*:539, 1993.
324. Boltwood, M. D., Taylor, C. B., Burke, M. B., et al.: Anger report predicts coronary artery vasomotor response to mental stress in atherosclerotic segments. Am. J. Cardiol. *72*:1361, 1993.
325. Hoffman, R. M., and Garewal, H. S.: Antioxidants and the prevention of coronary heart disease. Arch. Intern. Med. *155*:241, 1995.
326. Rimm, E. B., Stampfer, M. J., Ascherio, A., et al.: Vitamin E consumption and the risk of coronary heart disease in men. N. Engl. J. Med. *328*:1450, 1993.
327. Stampfer, M. J., Hennekens, C. H., Manson, J. E., et al.: Vitamin E consumption and the risk of coronary disease in women. N. Engl. J. Med. *328*:1444, 1993.
328. Morris, D. L., Kritchevsky, S. B., and Davis, C. E.: Serum carotenoids and coronary heart disease: The Lipid Research Clinics Coronary Primary Prevention Trial and Follow-up Study. J. A. M. A. *272*:1439, 1994.
329. Hodis, H. N., Mack, W. J., LaBree, L., et al.: Serial coronary angiographic evidence that antioxidant vitamin intake reduces progression of coronary artery atherosclerosis. J. A. M. A. *273*:1849, 1995.
330. Puurunen, M., Mänttäri, M., Manninen, V., et al.: Antibody against oxidized low-density lipoprotein predicting myocardial infarction. Arch. Intern. Med. *154*:2605, 1994.
331. Alpha-Tocopherol, Beta Carotene Cancer Prevention Study Group: The effect of vitamin E and beta carotene on the incidence of lung cancer and other cancers in male smokers. N. Engl. J. Med. *330*:1029, 1994.
332. Steinberg, D.: Antioxidant vitamins and coronary heart disease (editorial). N. Engl. J. Med. *328*:1487, 1993.

Chapter 36
Coronary Blood Flow and Myocardial Ischemia

Peter Ganz, Eugene Braunwald

HYPOXIA AND ISCHEMIA 1161
DETERMINANTS OF MYOCARDIAL OXYGEN CONSUMPTION 1161
REGULATION OF CORONARY BLOOD FLOW 1163
Metabolic Regulation 1163
Endothelial Control of Coronary Vascular Tone 1164
Autoregulation of Coronary Blood Flow . . . 1168
Extravascular Compressive Forces 1169
Transmural Distribution of Myocardial Blood Flow 1169
Neural and Neurotransmitter Control 1170
Effects of Coronary Stenoses 1171
Coronary Collateral Circulation 1174
CONSEQUENCES OF MYOCARDIAL ISCHEMIA 1176
Myocardial Stunning and Hibernation 1176
Hemodynamic Consequences of Ischemia 1176
The "Wavefront" of Ischemic Necrosis . . . 1177
Effects of Ischemia on Myocardial Metabolism 1178
Reperfusion Injury 1179
REFERENCES 1179

HYPOXIA AND ISCHEMIA

Definitions

Hypoxia is the condition in which oxygen supply is reduced despite adequate perfusion; *anoxia* is the absence of oxygen supply despite adequate perfusion. These conditions should be distinguished from *ischemia,* in which oxygen deprivation is accompanied by inadequate removal of metabolites consequent to reduced perfusion. Although clinical manifestations of coronary insufficiency generally reflect the effects of ischemia, under selected experimental and clinical conditions, deprivation of oxygen can be separated from reduced washout of metabolites.[1] For example, cyanotic congenital heart disease, cor pulmonale, severe anemia, asphyxiation, and carbon monoxide poisoning are characterized by anoxia without ischemia because washout of metabolites is not hindered.

During ischemia an imbalance occurs between myocardial oxygen supply and demand (Fig. 36–1). Ischemia may be manifest as anginal discomfort, deviation of the ST segment on the electrocardiogram, reduced uptake of thallium-201 in myocardial perfusion images, or regional or global impairment of ventricular function. In the presence of coronary obstruction, an increase of myocardial oxygen requirements by exercise, tachycardia, or emotion leads to a transitory imbalance. This condition is frequently termed "demand ischemia" and is responsible for most episodes of chronic stable angina. In other situations the imbalance is caused by a reduction of oxygen supply secondary to increased coronary vascular tone or by platelet aggregates or thrombi; this condition, termed "supply ischemia," is responsible for myocardial infarction and most episodes of unstable angina. In many circumstances, ischemia results from both an increase in oxygen demand and a reduction in supply.

In this chapter we consider first the determinants of myocardial oxygen consumption, then the control of coronary blood flow, and finally, the hemodynamic and biochemical consequences of ischemia.

DETERMINANTS OF MYOCARDIAL OXYGEN CONSUMPTION

The heart is an aerobic organ; that is, it relies almost exclusively on the oxidation of substrates for the generation of energy, and it can develop only a small oxygen debt. Therefore, in a steady state, determination of the rate of myocardial oxygen consumption (MVO_2) provides an accurate measure of its total metabolism.[2] It has been known for many years that the total metabolism of the arrested, quiescent heart is only a small fraction of that of the working organ. The MVO_2 of the beating canine heart ranges from 8 to 15 ml/min/100 gm, whereas the MVO_2 of the noncontracting heart is approximately 1.5 ml/min/100 gm. The latter is required for those physiological processes not directly associated with contraction. Increases in the frequency of depolarization of the noncontracting heart are accompanied by only small increases of MVO_2[2-4] (Tables 36–1 and 36–2).

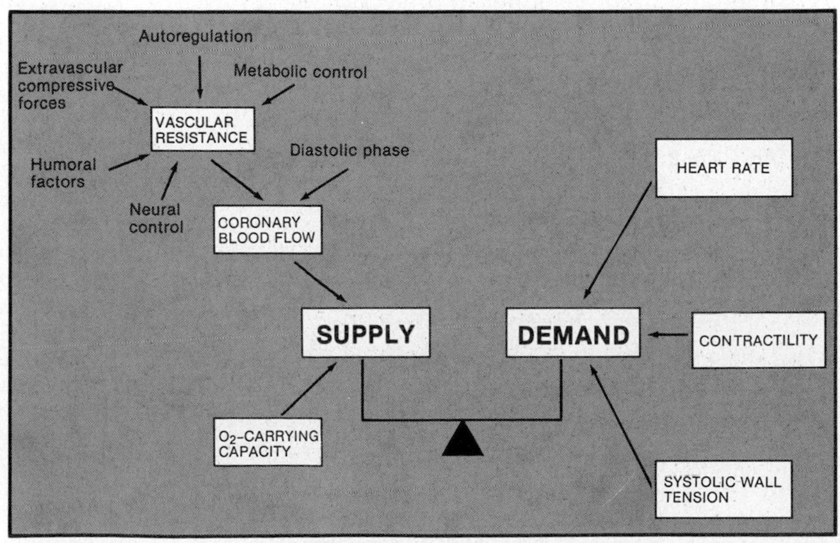

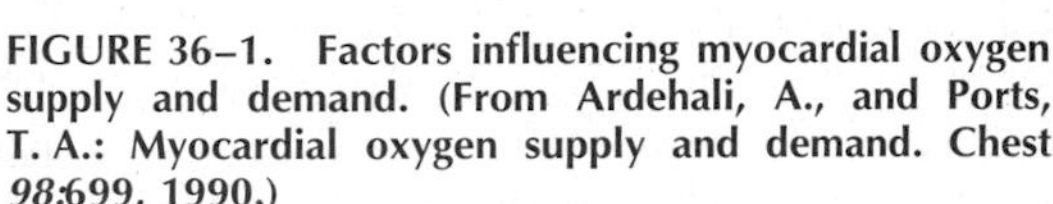
FIGURE 36–1. Factors influencing myocardial oxygen supply and demand. (From Ardehali, A., and Ports, T. A.: Myocardial oxygen supply and demand. Chest *98*:699, 1990.)

TABLE 36–1 MYOCARDIAL O_2 CONSUMPTION COMPONENTS

TOTAL: 6–8 cc/min/100 gm			
DISTRIBUTION			
Basal	20%	Volume work	15%
Electrical	1%	Pressure work	64%
EFFECTS ON MVO_2 of 50% INCREASES IN			
Wall stress	25%	Heart rate	50%
Contractility	45%	Volume work	4%
Pressure work	50%		

The table demonstrates the dominant contribution to MVO_2 made by pressure work and prominent effects of increasing pressure work and heart rate on MVO_2.

From Gould, K. L.: Coronary Artery Stenosis, New York, Elsevier, 1991, p. 8.

MYOCARDIAL TENSION. As early as 1915 Evans and Matsuoka concluded from studies of the Starling heart-lung preparation that "there is a relation between the tension set up on contraction and the metabolism of the contractile tissue."[5] In a systematic investigation of the relative effects of ventricular pressure, stroke volume, and heart rate on MVO_2, it was found that ventricular pressure development is a key determinant of MVO_2. These investigations suggested that MVO_2 per beat correlates well with the area under the left ventricular pressure curve, termed the "tension-time index." Subsequently, it was emphasized that the myocardial wall tension time integral is a more definitive determinant of MVO_2 than is the developed pressure.[6,7] Later studies demonstrated that frequency of contraction is an important determinant as well. An augmentation of heart rate elevates the MVO_2 by increasing the frequency of tension development per unit of time, as well as by increasing contractility.[6,8]

Rooke and Feigl have provided evidence that MVO_2 is influenced by stroke volume—that is, myocardial shortening—although less so than by tension development.[9] They have also provided an experimental basis for the use of the systolic pressure-rate product (plus an estimate of the oxygen requirements of the noncontracting heart) as a clinically useful index of MVO_2. Reexamination of the determinants of MVO_2 has emphasized that they correlate closely with the left ventricular systolic pressure volume area,[10,11] which consists of the sum of the area within the systolic pressure-volume loop (see Fig. 14-14, p. 431), that is, the external mechanical work and the end-systolic elastic potential energy in the ventricular wall, the area enclosed by the systolic pressure-volume trajectory and the E_{max} line (Fig. 36–2).[10a,11]

MYOCARDIAL CONTRACTILITY. In addition to the systolic pressure-volume area and heart rate, myocardial contractility is the third major determinant of MVO_2. The net effect of positive inotropic stimuli (such as Ca^{++} and catecholamines) on MVO_2 is the end result of their influence on two of its major determinants that change in opposite directions in the intact heart.[2] These are wall tension, which declines as a consequence of reduction in heart size, and myocardial contractility, which, by definition, is augmented by inotropic stimuli. In the failing, dilated ventricle, the increased contractility reduces the left ventricular end-diastolic pressure and volume. On the basis of the Laplace relation, the reduction in ventricular volume leads to a reduction in myocardial tension, which reduces MVO_2. However, the decrease in MVO_2 that might be expected to result from falling ventricular wall tension is opposed by the increase in contractility, which tends to augment MVO_2. Thus, the change in MVO_2 consequent to an inotropic stimulus depends on the extent to which intramyocardial tension is reduced in relation to the extent to which contractility is augmented. In the absence of heart failure, drugs that stimulate myocardial contractility elevate MVO_2 because heart size and therefore wall tension are not reduced substantially and do not offset the effect on metabolism of the simulation of contractility.

TABLE 36–2 DETERMINANTS OF MYOCARDIAL OXYGEN CONSUMPTION

1. Tension development
2. Contractile state
3. Heart rate
4. Shortening against a load (Fenn effect)
5. Maintenance of cell viability in basal state
6. Depolarization
7. Activation
8. Maintenance of active state
9. Direct metabolic effect of catecholamines
10. Fatty acid uptake

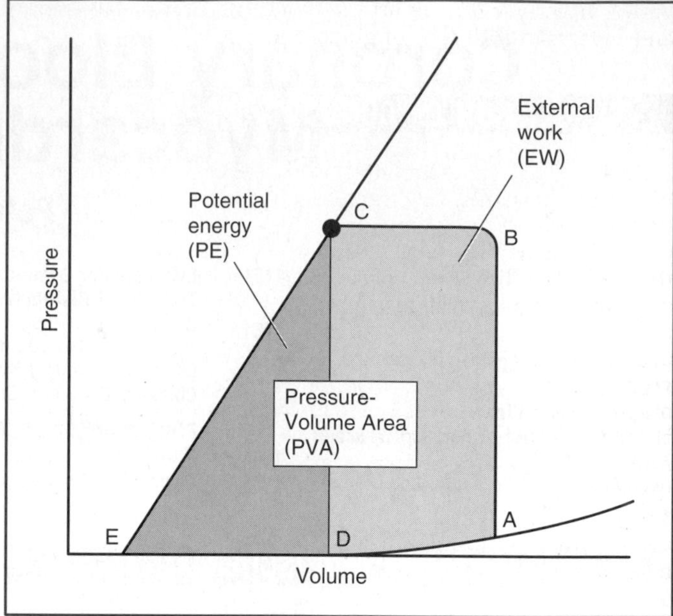

FIGURE 36–2. Myocardial oxygen consumption correlates with the left ventricular pressure–volume area (PVA). PVA is the area in the P-V diagram that is circumscribed by the end-systolic P-V line (E-C), the end-diastolic P-V relation curve (D-A), and the systolic segment of P-V trajectory (E-A-B-C-E). PVA consists of the external work (EW) performed during systole and the end-systolic elastic potential energy (PE) stored in the ventricular wall at end-systole. EW is the area within the P-V loop trajectory (A-B-C-D-A), and PE is the area between end-systolic P-V line and end-diastolic P-V relation curve to the left of EW (E-C-D-E). (Reproduced with permission from Kameyama, T., et al.: Energy conversion efficiency in human left ventricle. Circulation *85:*988, 1992. Copyright American Heart Association.)

It has been suggested by Suga that almost the entire increase in MVO_2 produced by the administration of positive inotropic agents such as Ca^{++} and epinephrine results from the energy costs of enhanced excitation-contraction coupling.[10] Specifically, the increased energy costs result from the greater and more rapid Ca^{++} uptake by the sarcoplasmic reticulum as well as from the increased contractile activity, rather than from a direct stimulating effect of positive inotropic agents on basal myocardial metabolism. In experiments in which the relative effects of changes in tension development and in myocardial contractility on MVO_2 were assessed in the same heart, the quantitative effects of MVO_2 of changes in contractility and tension development were found to be both substantial and of the same order of magnitude.[12]

MVO_2 is also influenced by the substrate utilized. Specifically, it correlates directly with the fraction of energy derived from the metabolism of fatty acids, which in turn varies directly with the arterial concentration of fatty acids and inversely with that of glucose and insulin.[13]

REGULATION OF CORONARY BLOOD FLOW

During diastole, when the aortic valve is closed, aortic diastolic pressure is transmitted without impediment through the dilated sinuses of Valsalva to the coronary ostia. The aortic arch and sinuses then act as a miniature reservoir, facilitating maintenance of relatively uniform coronary inflow through diastole. The major coronary arteries and their principal branches course across the epicardial surface of the heart. They serve as conductance vessels and normally offer little resistance to coronary blood flow. The epicardial conductance vessels can constrict in response to alpha-adrenergic stimuli and dilate to nitroglycerin.[14] These vessels give rise to smaller penetrating vessels approximately at right angles (see Fig. 36–13, p. 1169). A large pressure drop occurs in these intramural vessels and in the coronary arterioles—hence their designation as "resistance vessels." The dense network of about 4000 capillaries per square millimeter is not uniformly patent because precapillary sphincters appear to serve a regulatory function[15] in accordance with the flow needs of the myocardium. This capillary density is reduced in the presence of ventricular hypertrophy.

As in any vascular bed, blood flow in the coronary bed depends on the driving pressure and the resistance offered by this bed. Coronary vascular resistance, in turn, is regulated by several control mechanisms that will be reviewed: myocardial metabolism (metabolic control), endothelial (and other humoral) control, autoregulation, myogenic control, extravascular compressive forces, and neural control. These individual control mechanisms may be impaired in a variety of conditions and contribute to the development of myocardial ischemia.

Metabolic Regulation

RELATIONSHIP BETWEEN CORONARY BLOOD FLOW AND MYOCARDIAL OXYGEN CONSUMPTION. Coronary blood flow is closely coupled to MVO_2 in normal hearts.[8,16] This linkage is necessary because the myocardium depends almost completely on aerobic metabolism. The oxygen content of coronary venous blood is low, permitting little additional oxygen extraction (baseline coronary venous oxygen saturation is 25 to 30 per cent), and oxygen stores in the heart are sparse.

Changes in myocardial oxygen balance lead to alterations in coronary vascular resistance with great rapidity, generally in less than 1 second. For example, occlusion of a coronary artery for less than 1 second produces an increase in coronary blood flow above baseline immediately following release of the occlusion.[17–19] This response is called coronary reactive hyperemia. In the dog, peak flow response follows coronary occlusion of 15 to 20 seconds.[20] The mechanisms that link metabolic activity and coronary vascular resistance have been extensively investigated. Investigations have focused on adenosine, other nucleotides, nitric oxide, prostaglandins, CO_2, and H^+ as the most likely potential mediators.

ADENOSINE. Degradation of adenine nucleotides under conditions in which ATP utilization exceeds the capacity of myocardial cells to resynthesize high-energy phosphate compounds (a process dependent on oxidative phosphorylation in mitochondria) results in the production of adenosine monophosphate (AMP). The enzyme 5′-nucleotidase is responsible for the formation of adenosine from AMP.[21] Accordingly, adenosine and its metabolites, inosine and hypoxanthine, appear in interstitial fluid and in the coronary sinus venous effluent. Adenosine is a powerful vasodilator that is considered to be an important, perhaps the critical, mediator linking metabolically induced vasodilation to diminished coronary perfusion[22] (Fig. 36–3). Its production increases at times of an imbalance in the supply-to-demand ratio for oxygen,[23] and the rise in the interstitial concentration of adenosine parallels the increase in coronary blood flow.[24]

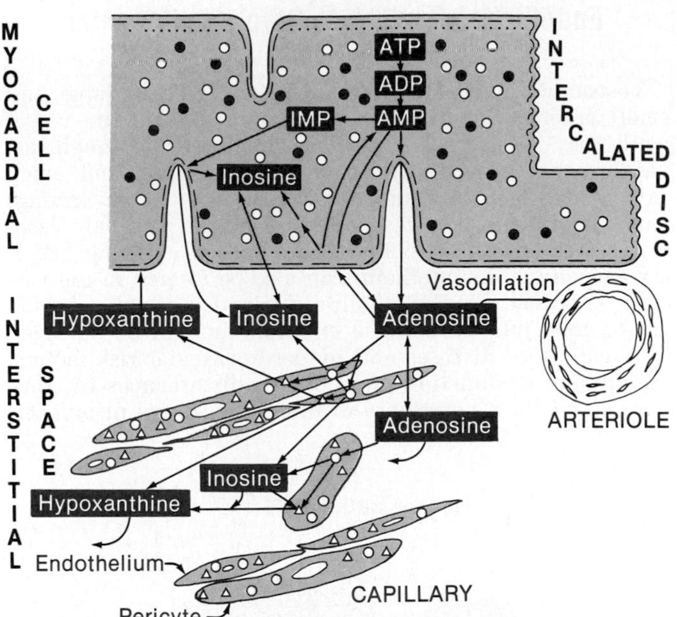

FIGURE 36–3. Schematic drawing depicting a myocardial interstitial space, an arteriole, and a capillary with the localization of enzymes involved in the formation and fate of adenosine. Adenosine formed by 5′-nucleotidase from AMP (which in turn arises from ATP) can enter the interstitial space. There it can induce arteriolar dilation and reenter the myocardial cell, where it is either phosphorylated to AMP by adenosine kinase or deaminated to inosine by adenosine deaminase, or it can enter the capillaries and leave the tissue. A large fraction of adenosine that crosses the capillary wall is deaminated to inosine, which in turn is split to hypoxanthine and ribose-1-PO_4 by nucleoside phosphorylase located in the endothelial cells, pericytes, and erythrocytes. Most of the adenosine is taken up by the myocardial cells, and that escaping into the circulation is largely in the form of inosine and hypoxanthine. Since adenylic acid deaminase (which deaminates AMP to IMP) is in low concentration in heart muscle, the major degradative pathway from AMP is via dephosphorylation to adenosine. ○, Adenosine deaminase; ●, adenylic acid deaminase; △, nucleoside phosphorylase; (---), 5′-nucleotidase; (···), adenosine kinase. (From Berne, R. M., and Rubio, R.: Coronary circulation. *In* Berne, R. M., Sperelakis, N., and Geiger, S. R. [eds.]: Handbook of Physiology, Section 2. The Cardiovascular System. Bethesda, Md., American Physiological Society, 1979, p. 924.)

Many investigators believe that adenosine fulfills most of the criteria for the metabolic regulation of blood flow.[22] Thus, it has been demonstrated that adenosine plays a significant role in the regulation of coronary blood flow during reactive hyperemia, hypoxia, inotropic stimulation with isoproterenol, dobutamine, and mental stress.[25–29] On the other hand, it has been reported that adenosine plays no significant role in the coronary vasodilation associated with inotropic stimulation with norepinephrine or the metabolic stress induced by rapid atrial pacing.[30,31] Thus, despite its acknowledged importance, adenosine is almost certainly not the *only* vasoactive factor involved in the metabolic regulation of coronary blood flow. Others include nitric oxide (see below) and prostanoids.

It is likely that vasoactive factors act in concert to regulate coronary flow in response to metabolic needs. Thus the reactive hyperemia following 10 to 20 seconds of occlusion can be reduced by approximately 30 per cent each by inhibitors of adenosine and nitric oxide. Simultaneous administration of these inhibitors attenuates reactive hyperemia by nearly 60 per cent.[32]

Endothelial Control of Coronary Vascular Tone

Vasoactive agents that influence the tone of large and small coronary vessels can arise from outside the vessel wall; they can circulate in the blood (e.g., epinephrine, vasopressin) or be derived from circulating elements such as platelets (e.g., serotonin, ADP) or from nerve endings (e.g., norepinephrine, vasoactive intestinal peptide). Vasoactive factors such as endothelium-derived relaxing factor, prostacyclin, and endothelin can also be formed in the vascular endothelium. Endothelium-derived vasoactive factors are of great interest because endothelium can be damaged by a variety of diseases and by cardiovascular risk factors. Endothelial dysfunction may lead to disturbances in coronary blood flow, contribute to the pathogenesis of myocardial ischemia, and is a central feature in the evolution of atherosclerosis, thrombosis, inflammation, and atherogenesis[32a] (Fig. 36–4).

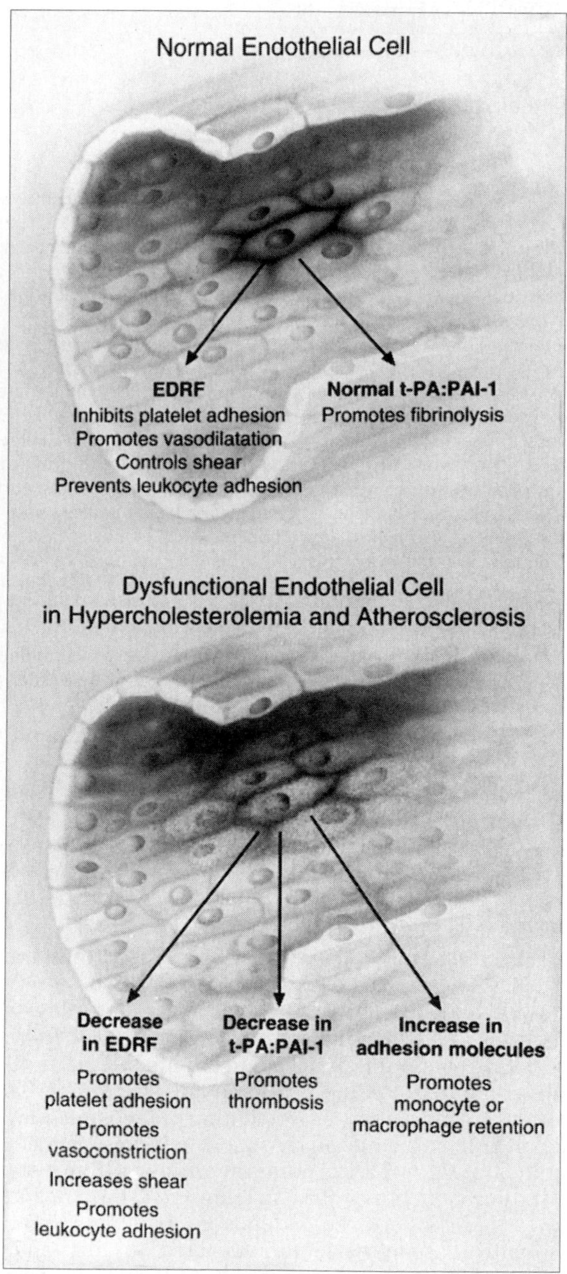

FIGURE 36–4. Normal and dysfunctional endothelial cells, with some of the functions adversely influenced by hypercholesterolemia and atherosclerosis that may contribute to acute coronary syndromes. The abbreviation t-PA : PAI-1 denotes the ratio of tissue plasminogen activator to plasminogen-activator inhibitor type 1. EDRF = endothelial derived relaxing factor. (From Levine, G. N., Keaney, J. F., and Vita, J. A.: Cholesterol reduction in cardiovascular disease. N. Engl. J. Med. *332*:312, 1995. Copyright Massachusetts Medical Society.)

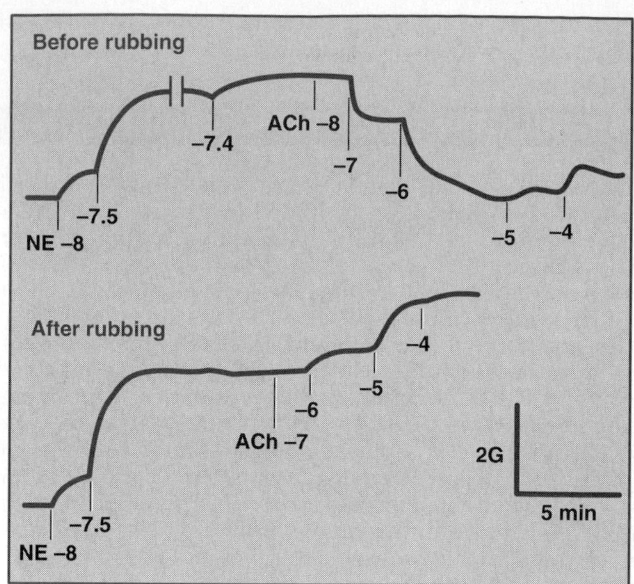

FIGURE 36–5. Relaxation by acetylcholine (ACh) of rings of rabbit thoracic aorta precontracted by norepinephrine (NE). Aortic rings were exposed to increasing concentrations of ACh with endothelium either intact or removed by rubbing with a wooden applicator stick. This representative tracing shows loss of relaxation in response to ACh with removal of endothelium and appearance of mild constriction. (Reproduced with permission from Furchgott, R. F.: Role of endothelium in responses of vascular smooth muscle. Circ. Res. *53*:557, 1983. Copyright American Heart Association.)

ENDOTHELIUM-DERIVED RELAXING FACTOR. The endothelium synthesizes several powerful vasodilators, including endothelium-derived relaxing factor (EDRF),[33] prostacyclin,[34] and endothelium-derived hyperpolarizing factor.[35] The discovery of these substances has changed the view that the vascular endothelium is simply an inert nonthrombogenic barrier separating the blood from the vascular smooth muscle.

The discovery of EDRF by Furchgott and Zawadzki[33] resulted from the observation that intact endothelium is a prerequisite for acetylcholine-induced vasodilation. In the presence of endothelium, acetylcholine produces dose-dependent vasodilation. When the endothelium is removed, only constriction is induced by acetylcholine (Fig. 36–5). It became apparent that acetylcholine has two distinct and opposite actions on blood vessels: a direct vasoconstrictor action and an indirect vasodilator action that is mediated by endothelium. In any blood vessel, the net response is related to the sum of these two actions. In most normal arteries, endothelium-dependent vasodilation predominates over direct vasoconstriction.

EDRF has been identified to be the nitric oxide (NO) radical[36,37] or a sulfhydryl complex containing it.[38] Nitric oxide is synthesized from the amino acid L-arginine[39] by the actions of the enzyme nitric oxide synthase.[40] Aside from acetylcholine, the release of nitric oxide is stimulated by aggregating platelets (serotonin, ADP), thrombin, the products of mast cells (histamine), and increased shear stress resulting from an increase in blood flow; the latter is responsible for so-called flow-mediated vasodilation[41] (Fig. 36–6). Vasoconstrictors such as alpha-adrenergic agonists may also stimulate the release of EDRF.[42] Although their net effect on the blood vessel may be vasoconstriction, the presence of an endothelium-dependent vasodilating influence attenuates this action. Only a few vasodilators can act independently of the endothelium and directly on vascular smooth muscle. These include the nitrovasodilators (e.g., nitroglycerin, nitroprusside), prostacyclin, and adenosine.

FIGURE 36–6. Endothelium-derived vasoactive substances. The endothelium is a source of relaxing (see bottom right) and contracting (see bottom left) factors. ACE = angiotensin converting enzyme; Ach = acetylcholine; ADP = adenosine diphosphate; BK = bradykinin; cAMP/cGMP = cyclic adenosine/guanosine monophosphate; ECE = endothelin converting enzymes; EDHF = endothelium-derived hyperpolarizing factor; ET-1 = endothelin-1; 5HT = 5-hydroxytryptamine (serotonin); L-arg = L-arginine; NO = nitric oxide; PGH_2 = prostaglandin H_2; PGI_2 = prostacyclin; $TGF\beta_1$ = transforming growth factor β_1; Thr = thrombin; TXA_2 = thromboxane A_2; Circles represent receptors (AT = angiotensinergic; B = bradykinergic; M = muscarinic; P = purinergic; T = thrombin receptor). (From Lüscher, T. F., and Noll, G.: The endothelium in coronary vascular control. *In* Braunwald, E. (ed.): Heart Disease—Update 3. Philadelphia, W.B. Saunders Company, 1995, p. 2.)

ENDOTHELIUM-DEPENDENT VASODILATION IN EPICARDIAL ARTERIES. The importance of endothelium-dependent vasodilation to vascular control has been established in many species and most vascular beds tested.[43–45] Intracoronary administration of acetylcholine, an endothelium-dependent agonist, has been shown to dilate normal coronary arteries in humans[46] (Fig. 36–7). Compelling evidence indicates that this is mediated by nitric oxide; inhibitors of nitric oxide such as N^G-monomethyl-L-arginine, hemoglobin and methylene blue abolish vasodilation and may even convert the vasodilator response to acetylcholine to vasoconstriction.[47,47a] Other substances that have been shown to dilate healthy human coronary arteries and increase blood flow by acting on the endothelium to release EDRF include serotonin, histamine, and substance P.[48–51]

One of the functions of the normal endothelium is to synthesize and release EDRF. It has been suggested that the tendency to vasoconstriction that characterizes atherosclerosis may be related to vasodilator dysfunction of the endothelium, resulting in the unopposed stimulation of vascular smooth muscle. Augmented vasoconstrictor responses resulting from an impairment of endothelium-dependent relaxation have been demonstrated in experimental models of atherosclerosis in several species.[52,53] Responses to endothelium-dependent stimuli that dilate healthy human coronary arteries have been found to be markedly impaired in patients with both early and advanced atherosclerosis. Acetylcholine constricts atherosclerotic coronary arteries,[46,54,55] presumably reflecting the loss of EDRF and acetylcholine's unopposed direct constrictor effects on vascular smooth muscle (Fig. 36–7). Although the role of acetylcholine in the physiological regulation of vascular tone has not been established, abnormal vasomotor responses to acetylcholine have served as convenient functional markers of endothelial dysfunction in atherosclerosis. This demonstration of endothelial vasodilator dysfunction has been confirmed using other stimuli that release EDRF, including serotonin,[48,56] ADP, and increased coronary blood flow (flow-mediated dilation).[50,57] For example, whereas serotonin, which is released by aggregating platelets, dilates normal human coronary arteries, it constricts atherosclerotic arteries.[48]

ENDOTHELIUM-DEPENDENT VASODILATION IN CORONARY RESISTANCE VESSELS. Endothelium-dependent vasodilation operates not only in large (conductance) arteries, but it is also an important mechanism that controls resistance in small vessels.[58–62] Studies in the human forearm have suggested that *continuous* basal release of nitric oxide is an important determinant of resting vascular resistance.[60] When a specific inhibitor of nitric oxide synthesis was infused into the forearm, resting flow was reduced by half.

Atherosclerosis and hypercholesterolemia markedly im-

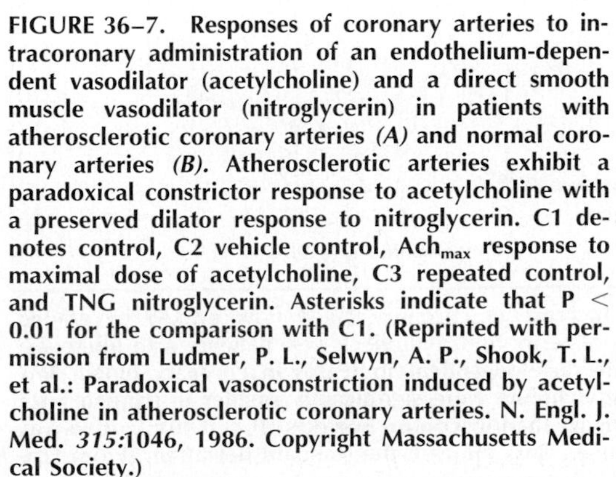

FIGURE 36–7. Responses of coronary arteries to intracoronary administration of an endothelium-dependent vasodilator (acetylcholine) and a direct smooth muscle vasodilator (nitroglycerin) in patients with atherosclerotic coronary arteries *(A)* and normal coronary arteries *(B)*. Atherosclerotic arteries exhibit a paradoxical constrictor response to acetylcholine with a preserved dilator response to nitroglycerin. C1 denotes control, C2 vehicle control, Ach_{max} response to maximal dose of acetylcholine, C3 repeated control, and TNG nitroglycerin. Asterisks indicate that $P < 0.01$ for the comparison with C1. (Reprinted with permission from Ludmer, P. L., Selwyn, A. P., Shook, T. L., et al.: Paradoxical vasoconstriction induced by acetylcholine in atherosclerotic coronary arteries. N. Engl. J. Med. *315*:1046, 1986. Copyright Massachusetts Medical Society.)

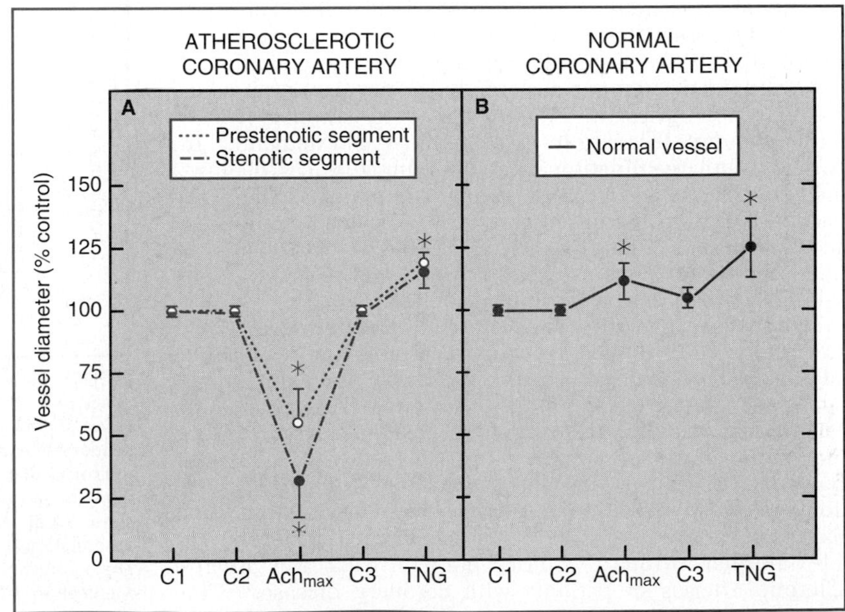

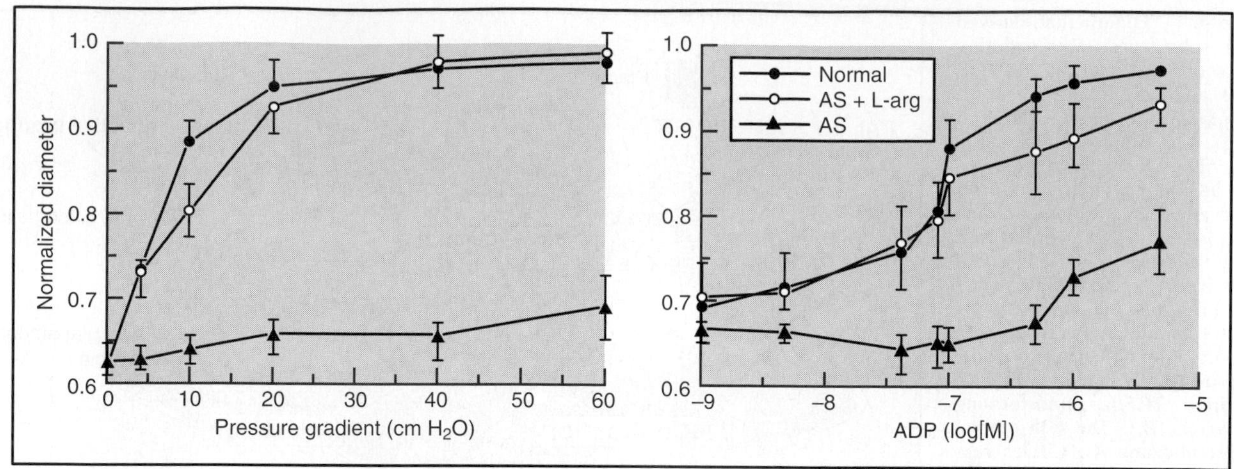

FIGURE 36–8. The effects of atherosclerosis on flow-dependent and pharmacological vasodilatation (adenosine diphosphate, ADP) in coronary arterioles. Pressure gradient (left) is proportional to blood flow. In vessels from normal control animals, both flow and ADP produced vasodilatation, whereas in atherosclerotic animals, this response was absent. Administration of L-arginine restored the responses in the atherosclerotic animals. (Reproduced with permission from Jones, C. J. H., Kuo, L., Davis, M. J., and Chilian, W. M.: Regulation of coronary blood flow: Coordination of heterogeneous control mechanisms in vascular microdomains. Cardiovasc. Res. *29*:585, 1995. Adapted from Kuo, L., et al.: Pathophysiological consequences of atherosclerosis extend into the coronary microcirculation. Restoration of endothelium-dependent responses by L-arginine. Circ. Res. *70*:465, 1992. Copyright American Heart Association.)

pair the responses of resistance vessels to endothelium-dependent vasodilators[61,63,64] (Fig. 36–8). The close correlation between the extent of endothelial dysfunction in resistance vessels and the failure of coronary blood flow to respond appropriately to metabolic stimuli suggests that endothelial dysfunction in resistance vessels may be an important factor in preventing coronary blood flow from rising appropriately during times of increased metabolic stress.[64a] An inappropriate increase in the tone of resistance vessels in the presence of an increase in metabolic demand may represent one of the mechanisms by which disturbances in endothelial function can lead to the development of myocardial ischemia in atherosclerosis.

ENDOTHELIAL DYSFUNCTION AND MYOCARDIAL ISCHEMIA. Several studies have demonstrated that reduced endothelium-dependent relaxation may play a role in the pathogenesis of myocardial ischemia in patients with stable angina. In such patients, mental stress caused dilation of the arteries with normal endothelium (evidenced by a normal response to acetylcholine) but constriction of vessels with evidence of endothelial dysfunction.[65] A similar pattern of dilation of normal coronary arteries and paradoxical constriction of atherosclerotic coronary arteries with dysfunctional endothelium has been observed with exercise,[66] the cold pressor test,[55] and an increase in heart rate.[67] These stimuli are normally accompanied by activation of the sympathetic nervous system, by an increase in circulating catecholamines, and by increases in coronary blood flow secondary to a rise in myocardial oxygen demand.[68] In patients with dysfunctional endothelium, the loss of flow-mediated[50,55,57] and catecholamine-stimulated EDRF release[69,70] allows the constrictor effects of catecholamines to act unopposed. Thus, the loss of EDRF may contribute to impaired dilator responses of epicardial and resistance vessel and thereby to myocardial ischemia.[68,71]

Plaque fissuring with superimposed platelet aggregation and occlusive thrombus formation is a hallmark of unstable angina,[72,72a] but coronary constriction also plays an important pathogenetic role in this condition[71,73] (see p. 1333). Endothelial vasodilator dysfunction has been implicated in the pathogenesis of coronary constriction, which is triggered by thrombosis and the products of platelet aggregation. As already mentioned, intracoronary administration of serotonin, a product released by aggregating platelets, dilates normal coronary arteries but constricts the atherosclerotic arteries of patients with coronary disease.[48] The clinical significance of these findings is supported by the observations that patients with unstable coronary syndromes and complex plaques demonstrate augmented release of serotonin into the coronary circulation[74] and that aspirin is an effective agent in the treatment of this condition.

Patients with a recent history of myocardial infarction show evidence of endothelial vasodilator dysfunction in the infarct-related artery which is more pronounced than in patients with stable stenoses of similar severity. Available evidence suggests that endothelium damaged by the atherosclerotic process and by plaque fissuring contributes to coronary constriction in response to a variety of substances that would normally elicit vasodilation.

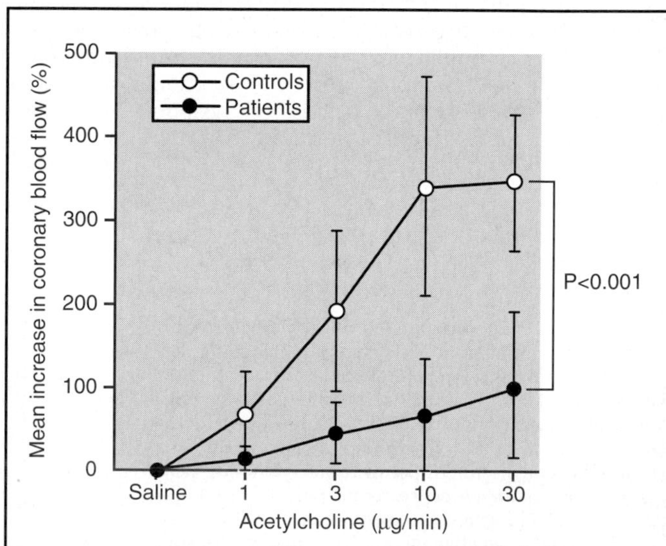

FIGURE 36–9. Increase in coronary blood flow evoked by graded doses of acetylcholine in control subjects and patients with microvascular angina. The dose-dependent increases in coronary blood flow produced by acetylcholine were significantly smaller in patients with microvascular angina than in control subjects ($P < 0.001$ by two-way analysis of variance). Bars indicate the standard deviation. (From Egashira, K., et al.: Evidence of impaired endothelium-dependent coronary vasodilatation in patients with angina pectoris and normal coronary angiograms. N. Engl. J. Med. *328*:1659, 1993. Copyright Massachusetts Medical Society.)

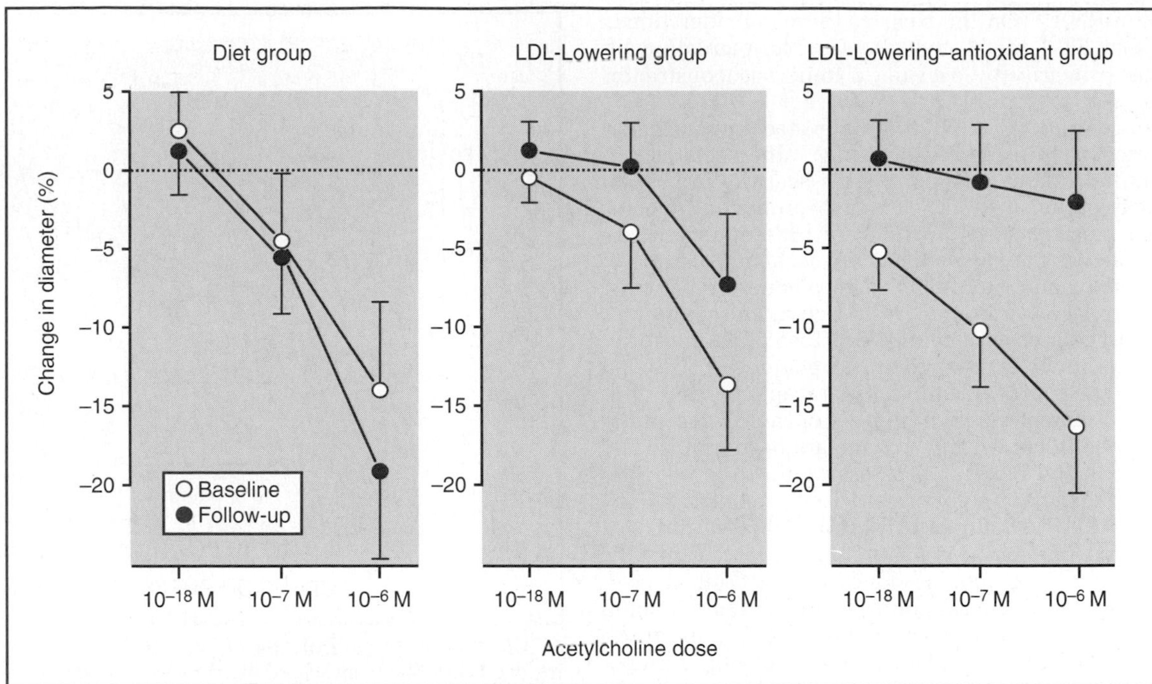

FIGURE 36–10. Mean (± SE) change in coronary artery diameter in response to serial infusions of acetylcholine at baseline and after 1 year of therapy in the three study groups. The improvement in the response from baseline to follow-up in the LDL-lowering–antioxidant group was significantly greater than that in the diet group ($P > 0.05$). Negative numbers indicate vasoconstriction. (From Anderson, T. J., et al.: The effect of cholesterol-lowering and antioxidant therapy on endothelium-dependent coronary vasomotion. N. Engl. J. Med. *332*:488, 1995. Copyright Massachusetts Medical Society.)

Endothelial dysfunction may involve the coronary resistance vessels in the *absence* of obstructive epicardial artery disease.[67,75] Impaired endothelium-dependent dilation of coronary resistance vessels has been demonstrated in patients with syndrome X, that is, anginal discomfort, evidence of myocardial ischemia on exercise testing, and angiographically normal coronary arteries (see p. 1343)[77–79] (Fig. 36–9). Impairment of endothelium-dependent vasodilation has also been observed in patients with coronary risk factors but without angiographic evidence of coronary artery disease. Lipid abnormalities, smoking, hypertension, and advanced age all may be associated with endothelial dysfunction.[68,80–81a]

Management. The use of cholesterol-lowering agents (lovastatin, pravastatin, or cholestyramine) for a period of 6 to 12 months has been associated with significantly improved responses to the endothelium-dependent vasodilator acetylcholine in both the epicardial arteries and resistance arterioles.[82–84a] The addition of the antioxidant probucol to lovastatin may yield an added benefit[82] (Figs. 36–10 and 36–11). These studies suggest that disturbances in vascular regulation associated with atherosclerosis may be reversible if coronary risk factors are aggressively treated.

ENDOTHELIUM-DERIVED CONSTRICTING FACTORS. The endothelium not only mediates vasodilation but is a source of vasoconstrictor factors as well (Fig. 36–6). The best characterized of these are the endothelins (see p. 415). Endothelin-1 (ET-1) is a 21-amino-acid peptide that has potent vasoconstrictor activity.[85] Two other forms of endothelin have been discovered (ET-2 and ET-3), but endothelium produces only ET-1.[86] Synthesis of ET-1 is complex, with a large precursor molecule, preproendothelin, which is first processed to "big endothelin" and finally converted by the action of endothelin-converting enzyme to the fully active ET-1.

Unlike nitric oxide, which is released rapidly in response to vasodilator stimuli and then inactivated in a few seconds, ET-1 has actions that last minutes to hours.[85] In addition, agents that stimulate ET-1, such as thrombin, angiotensin II, epinephrine, or vasopressin do so by *de novo*

Initial Study

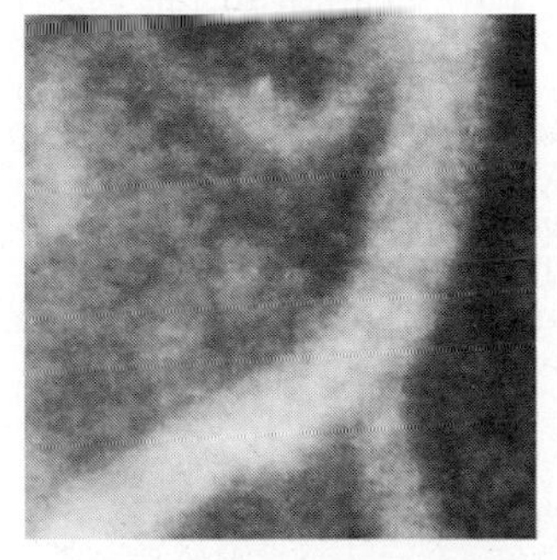
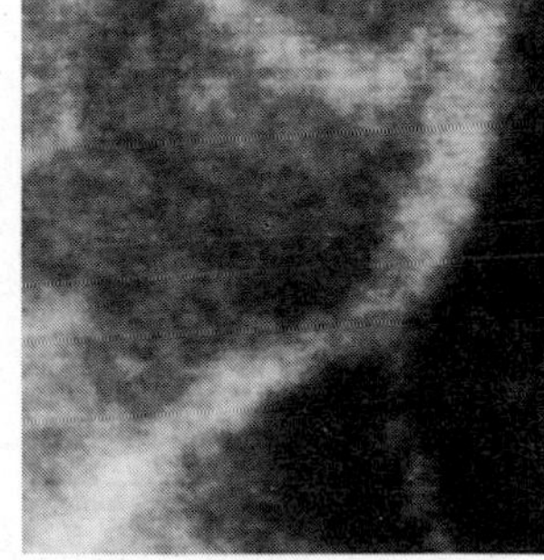

Follow-up Study

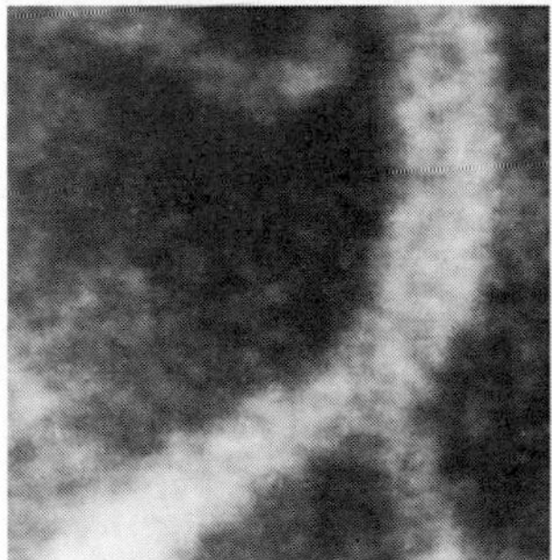
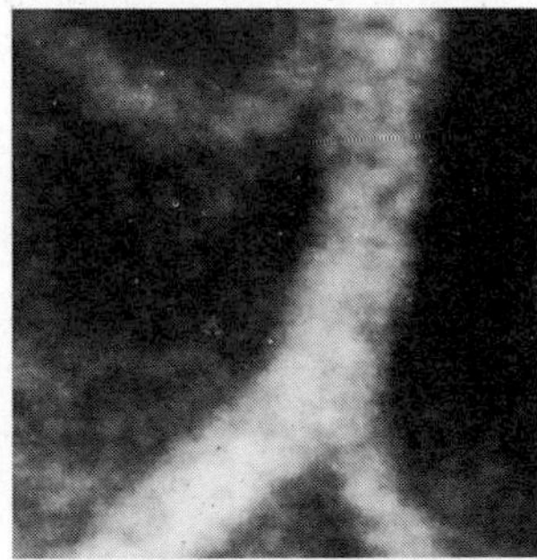

Control — Peak Acetylcholine

FIGURE 36–11. Segment of the circumflex coronary artery at the initial and follow-up (5.5 months) studies in a patient with coronary atherosclerosis assigned to lovastatin. Both left panels demonstrate baseline (control) arteriograms; both right panels demonstrate post-acetylcholine arteriograms. Substantial vasoconstriction occurs in response to the peak infusion of acetylcholine in the initial study, with marked improvement (a mild vasodilator response) in the follow-up study. (From Treasure, C. B., et al.: Beneficial effects of cholesterol-lowering therapy on the coronary endothelium in patients with coronary artery disease. N. Engl. J. Med. *332*:481, 1995. Copyright Massachusetts Medical Society.)

synthesis of m-RNA.[87] On the basis of these considerations, it is likely that ET-1 might contribute to the regulation of vascular tone primarily by exerting a tonic vasoconstrictor influence.

Plasma concentrations of ET-1 are elevated in a number of cardiovascular disorders, including atherosclerosis,[88] acute myocardial infarction,[89] congestive heart failure[90] (see p. 415), and hypertension.[91] ET-1 is also produced by activated human macrophages,[92] which are present in atherosclerotic lesions of patients with acute ischemic coronary syndromes and plaque rupture.[93,94] The plaques of patients with acute coronary syndromes (rest angina, crescendo angina, and post-infarction angina) expressed significantly greater ET-1 immunoreactivity than did plaques of patients with stable angina.[76] Two endothelin receptors, ET_A and ET_B, have been characterized. Inhibitors of the ET receptors or of the endothelin-converting enzyme are becoming available[95] and should be helpful in assessing the role of ET-1 in diseases associated with abnormal vascular constrictions.

CLINICAL IMPLICATIONS OF ENDOTHELIAL DYSFUNCTION. It is now clear that the coronary anatomy as revealed by coronary angiography is a poor predictor of the clinical presentation and of the long-term course of individual patients with myocardial ischemia.[68] Many patients with only moderate stenoses but unstable plaques may develop serious complications, including unstable angina, myocardial infarction, or sudden death, whereas others with severe stenoses may have a stable pattern of symptoms.

Reductions of myocardial blood flow may be triggered by coronary vasoconstriction, by platelet aggregation and thrombosis, or by a combination of these factors. Normally functioning endothelium is important not only in the regulation of vascular tone but also in providing a nonthrombogenic surface and in preventing inflammation in the vessel wall that might lead to fissuring of a plaque. It is likely that endothelial dysfunction is a common link responsible for vasoconstrictor, inflammatory, and thrombotic manifestations of atherosclerosis. Reversal of endothelial dysfunction, as may be accomplished with the aggressive treatment of hypercholesterolemia (Fig. 36–10 and 36–11) may address the abnormal biology of atherosclerosis by improving coronary perfusion as well as other clinical sequelae of atherosclerosis.[96]

Autoregulation of Coronary Blood Flow

When sudden alterations in perfusion pressure are imposed in many arterial beds (including the coronary), the resulting abrupt changes in blood flow are only transitory, with flow returning promptly to the previous steady state level[97] (Fig. 36–12). This ability to maintain myocardial perfusion at constant levels in the face of changing driving pressure is termed *autoregulation.* Demonstration of autoregulation in the coronary bed is difficult in intact animals because modification of coronary perfusion pressure also changes myocardial oxygen demand and the extrinsic compression of the coronary vessels. However, under controlled experimental conditions in which perfusion pressure is altered but ventricular pressure, cardiac contractility, and heart rate—the principal determinants of myocardial oxygen demand—are maintained constant, autoregulation is clearly evident. Thus, in normal dogs, autoregulation is maintained at pressures as low as 60 mm Hg and as high as 130 mm Hg.[98] That is to say, when mean aortic pressure is within this range, coronary perfusion is relatively constant. When aortic pressure falls below 60 mm Hg, coronary blood flow declines. When aortic pressure exceeds 130 mm Hg, coronary flow rises sharply.

Although autoregulation cannot be studied in detail in humans, it does appear to play an important role in patients with coronary artery disease. Most patients with demand-induced angina have severe stenoses in epicardial

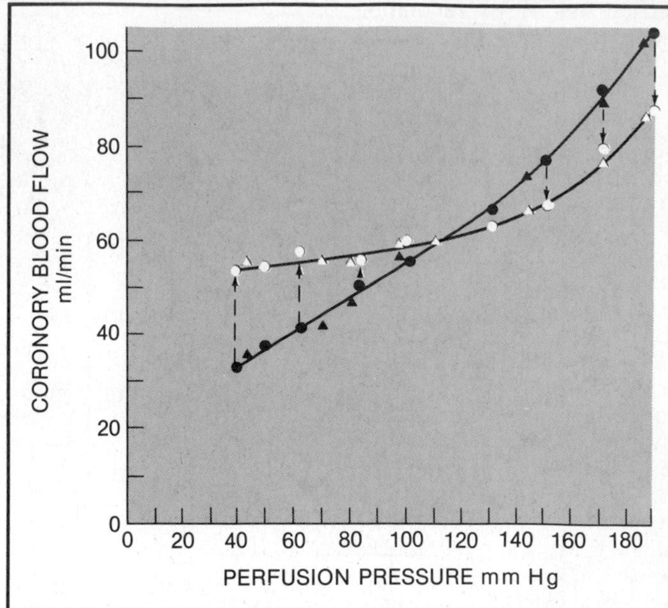

FIGURE 36–12. Autoregulation of coronary blood flow in the beating dog heart. The point where the curves cross represents the control steady-state pressure and flow. A sudden, sustained charge in perfusion pressure caused an abrupt change in flow represented by the filled symbols and black line (transient flow). The open symbols and red line represents the steady-state flows obtained at each perfusion pressure. The points represented by triangles were obtained after blockade of cardiac prostaglandin synthesis with indomethacin. (Reproduced by permission from Rubio, K., and Berne, K. M.: Regulation of coronary blood flow. Prog. Cardiovasc. Dis. *18:*105, 1975.)

coronary arteries but no evidence of a resting perfusion deficit or myocardial ischemia. Reductions in perfusion pressure distal to stenoses are compensated for by autoregulatory dilation of the resistance vessels. However, in the presence of a critical stenosis, the ability of autoregulation to compensate for the effect of a proximal epicardial obstruction may be compromised by a reduction of aortic pressure. The latter can lower distal perfusion pressure below the critical levels at which autoregulation is no longer effective, thereby lowering myocardial perfusion, intensifying myocardial ischemia, and increasing left ventricular filling pressure, which decreases the perfusion pressure gradient further. These events may cause a vicious circle, especially in patients with extensive coronary artery disease. Insertion of an intraaortic balloon pump in this setting raises diastolic perfusion pressure and restores distal coronary pressure so that autoregulation is reestablished and myocardial ischemia is lessened.

Chronic hypertension and left ventricular hypertrophy narrow the range of autoregulation, especially in the subendocardium, in which autoregulation is ordinarily more limited than in the subepicardium.[99] This amplifies the detrimental effects of coronary stenoses on myocardial perfusion and in patients with severe hypertrophy may lead to subendocardial ischemia even in the absence of coronary stenosis.

Conditions that alter the function of vascular smooth muscle in coronary arteries can also attenuate autoregulation. Dilators of resistance vessels such as adenosine and dipyridamole reduce perfusion pressure distal to a stenosis by increasing subepicardial flow, abolish subendocardial autoregulation,[100,101] and reduce subendocardial perfusion, a phenomenon termed "transmural coronary steal." In the presence of coronary occlusion, perfusion of the ischemic myocardium is markedly pressure-dependent because coronary collaterals do not exhibit autoregulation.[102] This explains why patients with extensive collateral-dependent segments of myocardium tolerate hypotension poorly.

Mechanisms of Autoregulation

NITRIC OXIDE. Evidence strongly suggests a role for EDRF in coronary autoregulation. Inhibition of nitric oxide in conscious dogs raises the lower autoregulatory threshold by about 15 mm Hg.[103] Autoregulation is also impaired in guinea pig hearts when production of nitric oxide is inhibited but not with inhibition of the cyclooxygenase pathway.[104] These observations suggest that the endothelium modulates coronary autoregulation through the production of nitric oxide but not of prostanoids. The involvement of nitric oxide may be related to the ability of the endothelium to sense changes in perfusion pressure through specific pressure-sensitive channels.[105]

MYOGENIC CONTROL. Arteriolar smooth muscle reacts to increased intraluminal pressure by contracting.[106] The consequent augmentation of resistance tends to return blood flow toward normal despite the higher perfusion pressure. This regulatory mechanism, referred to as *myogenic control*,[106,107] is an important mechanism of autoregulation. Myogenic contraction can be demonstrated in organ chamber experiments; a stretch on a vascular ring or an increase in intravascular pressure in isolated perfused microvessels is followed by active contraction.[20]

Myogenic mechanisms are particularly prominent in arterioles smaller than 100 microns and less important in larger arterioles, in which other autoregulatory mechanisms play a greater role.[108] They are also more important in subepicardial than subendocardial arterioles.

Extravascular Compressive Forces

SYSTOLIC COMPRESSIVE FORCES. Because systolic ventricular wall tension compresses intramyocardial vessels, most of the coronary blood flow to the left ventricle occurs during diastole. Thus, the contracting heart obstructs its own blood supply. At peak systole, there is even backflow in the coronary arteries, particularly in the intramural and small epicardial vessels.[109] The extravascular systolic compressive force has two components. The first is left ventricular systolic intracavitary pressure, which is transmitted fully to the subendocardium but falls off to almost zero at the epicardial surface. The second, and perhaps even more important, is the vascular narrowing caused by compression and bending of small arterioles coursing through the ventricular wall as the heart contracts.[20,110]

The important resistance to coronary blood flow caused by left ventricular systolic compression can be demonstrated experimentally in a beating heart perfused at constant pressure in which transient asystole is induced by vagal stimulation. At that point, coronary blood flow suddenly increases by approximately 50 per cent because of the relief of the compressive effect.[111]

The "throttling" effect of systole on myocardial perfusion is particularly important when systolic intraventricular pressure is elevated to levels exceeding coronary perfusion pressure, as occurs with obstruction to left ventricular outflow by valvular or subvalvular aortic stenosis[111a] or with severe aortic regurgitation.[112] Because an increase in heart rate augments the total duration of systolic time per minute during which coronary vascular compression occurs, while augmenting myocardial oxygen demand, tachycardia may cause myocardial ischemia. The importance of extravascular compressive forces in limiting coronary blood flow is magnified when coronary vascular tone is diminished,[113] as may occur during the administration of arteriolar vasodilators or during metabolic vasodilation associated with physical activity.

Because compressive forces exerted by the right ventricle are ordinarily far smaller than those of the left ventricle, ventricular perfusion is reduced but not interrupted during systole. However, when right ventricular pressure is elevated, the phasic blood flow pattern of the arteries perfusing the right ventricle resembles those of the left ventricle.[20]

DIASTOLIC COMPRESSIVE FORCES. The coronary perfusion or effective driving pressure has been assumed to be the pressure gradient between the coronary arteries and the pressure in either the right atrium or the left ventricle in diastole, because coronary flow drains primarily into these two chambers during this phase of the cardiac cycle. When coronary perfusion pressure is lowered, diastolic blood flow ceases when coronary driving pressure reaches approximately 50 mm Hg, the so-called pressure at zero flow (P_{zf}).[114,115] This pressure is determined largely by diastolic compressive forces.

Transmural Distribution of Myocardial Blood Flow

Extravascular compressive forces are greater in subendocardial than in subepicardial zones (Fig. 36–13). Subendocardial arterioles may be particularly susceptible to compression as they arborize from long, transmural vessels.[116] Therefore, *systolic* flow is more reduced in the subendocardium than the subepicardium. Nevertheless, in conscious dogs under resting physiological conditions, the ratio of endocardial to epicardial flow averaged throughout the cardiac cycle is approximately 1.25:1 as a consequence of preferential dilatation of the subendocardial vessels, causing a large increase in diastolic flow in the subendocardium.[117] The greater subendocardial blood flow appears to be secondary to the higher wall stress (and therefore oxygen consumption per unit weight), which is normally about 20 per cent greater than that of subepicardial muscle.[118]

SUBENDOCARDIAL ISCHEMIA. The subendocardium is more vulnerable to ischemic damage than the midmyocardium or subepicardium.[119] Epicardial coronary stenoses are associated with reductions in the subendocardial to subepicardial flow ratio.[120,122] When coronary arteries are constricted sufficiently to reduce total coronary flow to approximately 40 per cent of control, endocardial to epicardial flow ratio falls from 1.16 at baseline to 0.37.[121] This pattern of redistribution of flow away from the endocardium is further exaggerated during exercise and during pacing-induced tachycardia (Fig. 36–14).[120,122] Potent arteriolar vasodilators,

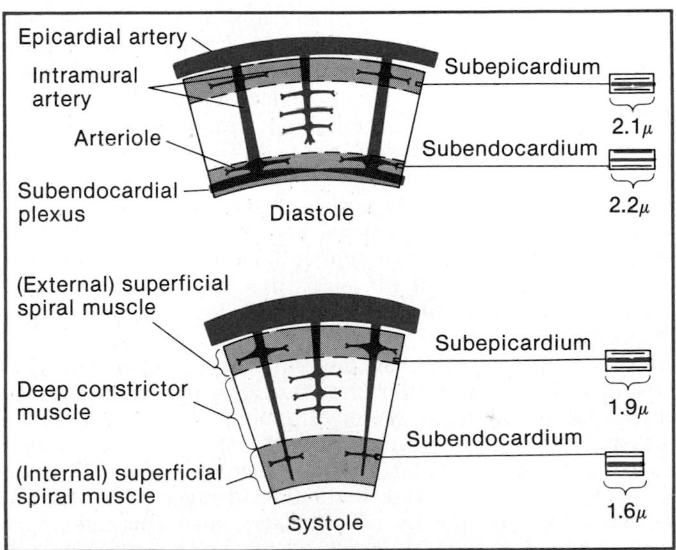

FIGURE 36–13. Cross-section of the left ventricular wall in diastole and systole. Factors involved in the susceptibility of the subendocardium to the development of ischemia include the greater dependence of this region on diastolic perfusion and the greater degree of shortening, and therefore of energy expenditure, of this region during systole. (From Bell, J. R., and Fox, A. C.: Pathogenesis of subendocardial ischemia. Am. J. Med. Sci. *268*:2, 1974.)

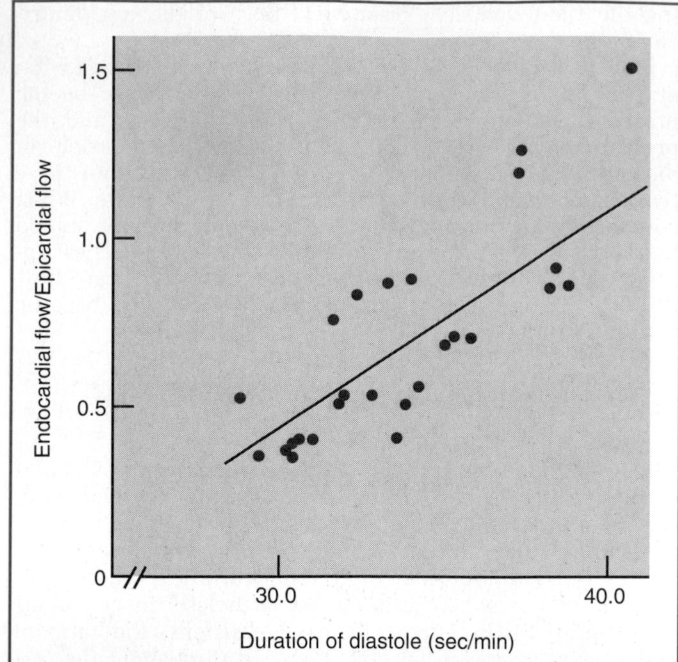

FIGURE 36–14. Relationship between subendocardial : subepicardial flow ratios and the duration of diastole during ventricular pacing at 100, 150, 200, and 250 beats per minute in seven dogs with maximal coronary vasodilation produced by intravenous infusion of adenosine, 4 μg/kg of body weight per minute. As heart rate is increased (shorter diastole), endocardial : epicardial flow falls. (Reproduced with permission from Bache, R. J., and Cobb, F. R.: Effect of maximal coronary vasodilation on transmural myocardial perfusion during tachycardia in the awake dog. Circ. Res. *41*:648, 1977. Copyright American Heart Association.)

such as adenosine, especially in the presence of an epicardial stenosis, can similarly affect transmural myocardial perfusion, causing an "intramural steal."[123,124] Severe pressure-induced left ventricular hypertrophy,[125] as well as heart failure with elevated left ventricular end-diastolic pressure, may also reduce the endocardial : epicardial flow ratio[126,127] (Fig. 36–15). When the markedly elevated left ventricular end-diastolic pressure in heart failure is corrected, subendocardial coronary flow reserve is restored and the endocardial : epicardial ratio is normalized.[127] Thus, impairment of endocardial perfusion in heart failure may be a direct consequence of the elevated left ventricular diastolic pressure and the diastolic compressive forces exerted on subendocardial perfusion (see p. 404).

A low subendocardial : subepicardial flow ratio can be increased by elevation of aortic pressure, which increases perfusion of the subendocardial region whose arterioles are maximally dilated and in which flow is pressure dependent. Overperfusion of the epicardial region is prevented by autoregulatory arteriolar constriction. Alpha-adrenergic arteriolar constrictors[128] or inhibitors of adenosine-induced arteriolar dilation such as theophylline[129] cause constriction of subepicardial arterioles, resulting in a reduction of epicardial blood flow, thereby reducing the transstenotic pressure gradient and increasing pressure distal to the stenosis. This rise in distal pressure augments blood flow to the subendocardial region. Reduction of myocardial oxygen demand, for example by beta-blockers, also decreases epicardial blood flow and increases perfusion pressure and thereby flow to ischemic subendocardial region.[130,131]

Neural and Neurotransmitter Control

The coronary arteries are richly innervated by adrenergic and parasympathetic nerves,[14] and their activation can exert important influences on coronary vasomotor tone. Both $alpha_1$ and $alpha_2$ adrenoceptors are present in coronary arteries,[132] and when activated by neuronally released or circulating norepinephrine both cause vasoconstriction,[133–135] which appears to be mediated by an increased concentration of calcium in coronary vascular smooth muscle.[134–136] When inotropic and chronotropic effects of norepinephrine are blocked[137] and the production of metabolic vasodilator stimuli inhibited, stimulation of sympathetic cardiac nerves causes coronary vasoconstriction. The activation of $alpha_1$ receptors induced by the infusion of methoxamine reduces the diameter of coronary arteries, despite increasing intraluminal pressure.[138] Activation of the carotid chemoreceptor reflex causes marked coronary constriction, which can be blocked by surgical denervation or by the alpha blocker phentolamine.[138] On the other hand, $beta_2$ adrenoceptors in the large and small coronary arteries mediate vasodilation.[139] Beta blockade induces coronary constriction, but this effect appears not to be a direct action on the coronary arteries. Instead, it results from blockade of beta-adrenoceptor mediated increase in myocardial oxygen demand.[140] Although parasympathetic stimulation appears to dilate small coronary arteries,[14] the extent of cholinergic regulation of large coronary arteries is also controversial.[141]

Intravenous use of norepinephrine induces a brief fall, followed by a sustained rise, in coronary vascular resistance, accompanied by a decline in coronary sinus pO_2.[142] The early vasodilatation can be eliminated by beta-adrenoceptor blockade and presumably results from the augmented myocardial oxygen consumption consequent to stimulation of myocardial beta receptors. The later increase in coronary vascular resistance can be prevented by alpha-adrenoceptor blockade and is caused by the stimulation of alpha receptors in the coronary vascular bed by norepinephrine. Blockade of $alpha_1$ receptors in patients with coronary artery disease attenuates the coronary vasoconstrictor response to the cold pressor test[143] and to cigarette smoking,[144] indicating that both responses are mediated by stimulation of these receptors.

REFLEX CONTROL. Baroreceptor activity affects coronary vascular resistance reflexly. With carotid occlusion, baroreceptor hypotension leads to reflex adrenergic stimulation, increased metabolic activity, and secondary coronary dilatation. When this augmentation of myocardial beta receptor–mediated activity is prevented by beta blockade, reflex coronary vasoconstriction secondary to carotid hypotension is unmasked.[145] Stimulation of the distal ends of the vagi produces coronary vasodilatation,[145,146] an effect

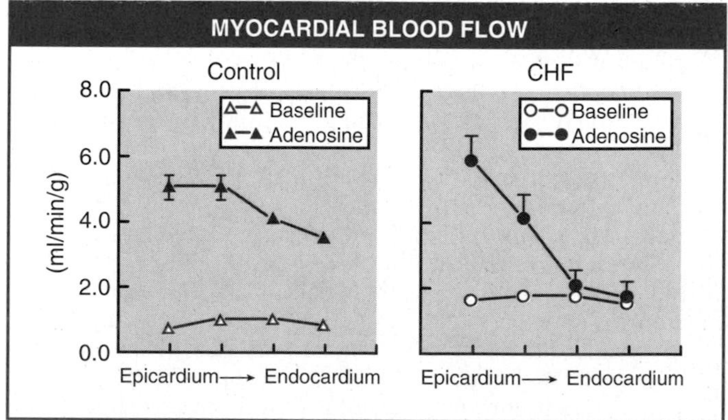

FIGURE 36–15. The reduction in subendocardial reserve as reflected by diminished responses of endocardial blood flow to near maximal vasodilation with adenosine. There was near exhaustion of subendocardial reserve in the dogs with left ventricular failure (CHF). (Reproduced with permission from Vatner, S. F., Shannon, R., and Hitinger, L.: Reduced subendocardial coronary reserve, a potential mechanism for impaired diastolic function in the hypertrophied and failing heart. Circulation *81*(Suppl. III):III–8, 1990. Copyright American Heart Association.)

mediated by the release of acetylcholine from vagal nerve endings that can be blocked by atropine.[111]

Stimulation of the carotid sinus nerves results in a substantial reduction in coronary vascular resistance,[147] an effect that can be prevented by alpha-receptor blockade. This finding indicates that adrenergic coronary constrictor tone is present in the resting conscious dog and the coronary vasodilation attendant upon stimulation of the carotid sinus nerves results from a reduction in this tone. Alpha receptor–mediated constrictor tone appears to persist in the coronary vascular bed during exercise, despite the coexisting metabolic vasodilation.[148] $Alpha_1$ adrenoceptor stimulation is capable of causing epicardial vasoconstriction in ischemic myocardium, thereby influencing favorably the transmural distribution of blood flow to the subendocardium[149,150] during exercise.

Efferent neural influences on the coronary vascular bed may also be activated reflexly by cardiopulmonary parasympathetic receptors. Stimulation of these receptors leads to reflex systemic and coronary vasodilation,[151] while stimulation of somatic afferent fibers increases coronary resistance through alpha-adrenergically mediated vasoconstriction.[152] Activation of chemoreceptors initially causes coronary dilation, a reflex that is mediated by the vagi and can be abolished by atropine.[111] Intracoronary injection of veratrum alkaloids, as well as other metabolically active substances, induces reflex bradycardia and hypotension (the Bezold-Jarisch reflex),[153] both the afferent and efferent limbs of which involve the vagus nerves.[151] Neurally controlled and alpha-adrenoceptor mediated constriction of stenotic lesions of the coronary vascular bed in humans has been observed on coronary arteriograms[150] during the handgrip test.[154]

TONIC CORONARY VASOCONSTRICTION. There is evidence for tonic coronary constriction mediated by adrenergic nerves.[147] Acute surgical denervation of the heart reduces coronary vascular resistance and lowers arteriovenous oxygen extraction and raises coronary venous O_2 content (primary vasodilation).[155] Coronary vascular resistance in dogs as well as patients with innervated hearts declines by almost 25 per cent in response to alpha-adrenoceptor blockade and the resultant release of basal coronary constrictor mediated by alpha receptors.[156] However, coronary vascular resistance does *not* diminish when patients with transplanted hearts are subjected to alpha-adrenoceptor blockade because in these patients, cardiac denervation, an element of transplantation, had already abolished the coronary constrictor tone.

An increase in adrenergic outflow does *not* appear to be responsible for the episodes of coronary spasm in most patients with Prinzmetal's (variant) angina[157] or in the genesis of ischemia in syndrome X (see p. 1343).[158] However, it has been reported that alpha-adrenoceptor stimulation can induce coronary spasm that can be prevented by phenoxybenzamine or prazosin in some patients with variant angina.[150] The finding in some patients with chronic stable angina that administration of alpha-receptor blockers can reduce exercise-induced ST-segment depression and angina[150,159,160] indicates that alpha receptor–mediated coronary vasoconstriction may play a contributory role in the development of myocardial ischemia resulting in these patients. It has also been reported that cocaine is a potent coronary vasoconstrictor both in dogs and humans,[161] and because this effect can be prevented by an alpha-receptor blocker, phentolamine, it appears to be mediated, at least in part, by alpha-adrenergic stimulation.[162]

Effects of Coronary Stenoses

Limitation of coronary blood flow by atherosclerotic plaques is related principally to their geometric features, including the severity and length of narrowings, their stiffness or partial distensibility, and the presence of superimposed platelet aggregation and thrombosis.[163]

As blood traverses a stenosis, pressure (energy) is lost. To estimate this pressure loss, principles of fluid dynamics have been applied and tested in animal models as well as in patients.[164–166] Although the formulas are complex, they have been simplified as follows:[163]

$$\Delta P = \frac{1.8 \cdot Q}{d^4_{sten}} + \frac{6.1 \cdot Q^2}{d^4_{sten}}$$

where ΔP is the pressure drop across a stenosis in millimeters of mercury, Q is the flow across the stenosis in milliliters per second, and d_{sten} is the minimal stenosis lumen diameter in millimeters. The first term accounts for viscous friction between layers of fluid in the stenotic segment leading to frictional energy losses. The second term reflects energy losses occurring when the "pressure energy" of normal arterial flow is transferred first to the kinetic energy of high velocity flow and then, at the exit from the stenosis, to the turbulent energy of distal flow eddies (separation losses).

CORONARY BLOOD FLOW. At normal levels of arterial flow, both frictional and separation losses contribute to the stenosis resistance and to the presence of a pressure gradient. As flow increases, separation losses, which increase with the square of the flow, become increasingly prominent and viscous losses become negligible. Thus, increases in blood flow and pressure drops across the stenosis are related in an exponential manner (Fig. 36–16). Augmentation of coronary blood flow is associated with elevations in pressure gradients across the stenotic orifice and reductions in poststenotic perfusion pressure.

Brown et al.[163] have pointed out three common clinical situations in which the transstenotic pressure gradient elevations due to flow increases may be important in the pathogenesis of myocardial ischemia: (1) Pharmacological dilators of coronary resistance arterioles, such as dipyrida-

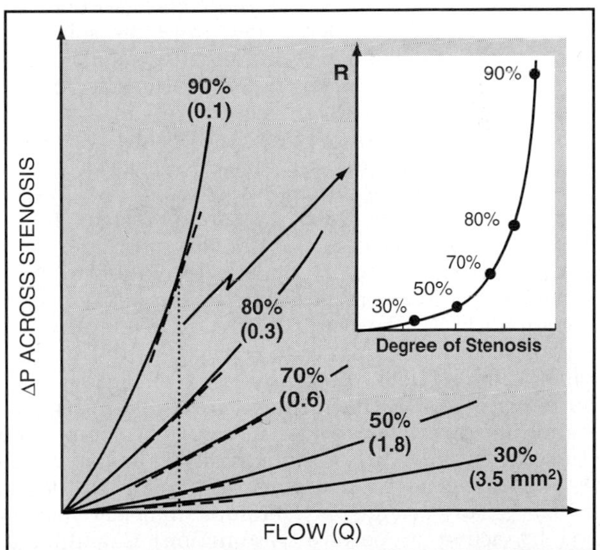

FIGURE 36–16. Relation between pressure reduction across a stenosis (ΔP) and flow through the stenosis (Q̇). Relations are shown for concentric stenoses of 30, 50, 70, 80, and 90 per cent internal diameter. The numbers in parentheses below each per cent diameter stenosis represent residual luminal cross-sectional area, calculated on the basis of a normal internal diameter of 3 mm and cross-sectional area of 7.1 mm². The level of flow corresponding to basal metabolic needs is represented by the vertical dotted line; stenosis resistances for this level of flow are shown as the dashed tangent lines to the individual pressure-flow relations. In the inset on the right, stenosis resistance (R) is plotted as a function of degree of stenosis. (From Klocke, F. J.: Measurements of coronary blood flow and degree of stenosis: Current clinical implications and continuing uncertainties. Newsletter of the Council on Clinical Cardiology of the American Heart Association. Vol 7, No. 3, July 1982.)

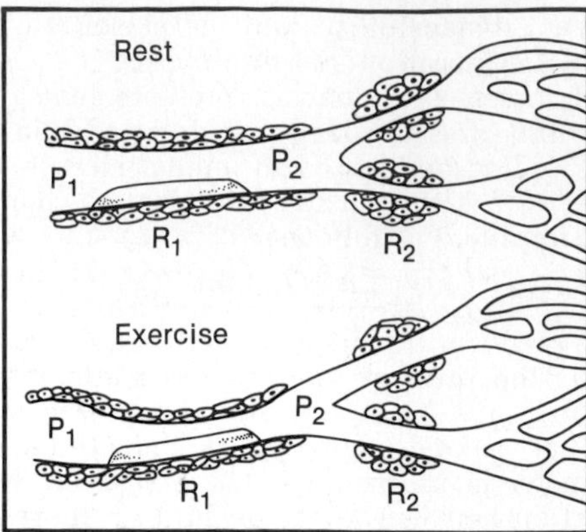

FIGURE 36–17. Diagrammatic representation of vessel collapse when myocardial flow increases. Under baseline conditions (Rest, *top*), flow across the stenosis (R_1) is modest and a large pressure gradient (P_1-P_2) does not develop. With a vasodilator intervention such as exercise *(bottom)*, the pressure gradient across the stenosis (P_1-P_2) increases. The resulting fall in intraluminal pressure may lead to collapse of the vessel at the level of the obstruction, thereby increasing the degree of stenosis. This leads to dilatation of the distal vessels (R_2). (From Epstein, S. E., Cannon, R. O., III, and Talbot, T. L.: Hemodynamic principles in the control of coronary blood flow. Am. J. Cardiol. *56:*9E, 1985.)

mole and adenosine, increase the transstenotic flow and pressure gradient. When subendocardial resistance vessels become fully dilated, their perfusion becomes perfusion pressure dependent. Redistribution of flow from the subendocardium to the subepicardium develops as the transstenotic pressure gradient increases and pressure distal to the stenosis falls. This is one mechanism of "coronary steal." A fall in aortic perfusion pressure reduces subendocardial flow further. (2) During physical activity, coronary blood flow rises to meet the increase in myocardial oxygen demand,[167,168] leading to an increase in transstenotic pressure gradient and a fall in the distal perfusion pressure, resulting in redistribution of blood flow from the subendocardium toward the subepicardium, an effect similar to that observed with the administration of pharmacological vasodilators (Fig. 36–17). Furthermore, the fall in intraluminal pressure may lead to collapse of the vessel at the level of the obstruction, thereby increasing the degree of stenosis. (3) The reduced oxygen-carrying capacity of anemia is compensated for by increases in coronary blood flow because the myocardium cannot sufficiently increase its oxygen extraction significantly. The augmentation of flow is associated with a marked increase in the transstenotic pressure gradient.[163,169] Not surprisingly, therefore, anemia is poorly tolerated in patients with coronary artery disease.

SEVERITY OF STENOSIS. At any level of blood flow, the single most important determinant of stenosis resistance is the minimum diameter of the stenosis. The transstenotic pressure drop is inversely proportional to the *fourth* power of the minimum luminal diameter. As a consequence, a relatively small change in luminal diameter (such as caused by active or passive vasomotion) is amplified to produce marked hemodynamic effects in the presence of severe stenoses.[163,170] For example, when the diameter stenosis is increased from 80 to 90 per cent, the resistance of a stenosis rises nearly threefold.[165]

ENTRANCE AND EXIT EFFECTS. Blood flow velocity (kinetic energy) increase and pressure (static energy) decreases in a narrowed arterial segment. The conversion of static to kinetic energy would occur with little loss of energy if the flow remained laminar, according to the Bernoulli principle.[163,166] Laminar flow can be preserved if the entrance and the exit of the stenotic segment are tapered gradually. However, most stenoses have abrupt transitions where energy losses associated with separation of laminar flow into eddy currents (vortices) occurs. The separation energy losses are particularly pronounced at the exits of stenoses.

LENGTH OF STENOSES. For most stenoses, the length of the narrowed segment has only a modest effect on the physiological significance of the obstruction. However, in very long narrowed segments, significant turbulence occurs along the wall of the stenotic segment, and energy is dissipated as heat when eddies impact on the wall; stenosis length may become important under these conditions.[171]

DYNAMIC CHANGES IN STENOSIS SEVERITY. Examination of the morphology of pressure-fixed human coronary arteries has revealed eccentricity of atherosclerotic plaques which involve only a portion of the arterial wall while the remaining arc of the wall is relatively normal and often compliant.[172] This provides a mechanism by which changes in distending pressure or vascular tone may alter luminal caliber and stenosis resistance. For example, most atherosclerotic stenosis in patients can dilate actively in response to nitroglycerin or constrict in response to ergonovine or alpha-adrenergic stimuli.[173]

Dynamic changes in stenosis severity and resistance due to alterations in intraluminal distending pressure have been demonstrated in compliant stenoses, both in experimental models and in patients with coronary artery disease.[163,174,175] As blood flow velocity rises in the stenotic segment, distending pressure falls, leading to passive collapse of a pliable segment. Passive collapse of a stenosis associated with the use of vasodilators occurs with agents that selectively dilate distal resistance vessels. The administration of dipyridamole to patients with coronary artery disease causes narrowing of severely stenotic pliable segments as well as of the normal arterial segments distal to the stenoses.[176] Passive collapse of pliable stenosis may also occur when aortic pressure is lowered.

EFFECTS OF CORONARY STENOSIS IN THE INTACT CORONARY BED. The effect of a coronary stenosis depends on the degree to which the resistance to flow caused by the stenosis can be compensated for by dilation of arterioles distal to the stenosis.[177] Gould and Lipscomb[178] concluded that in normal dogs, resting coronary flow is not altered until the constriction reaches at least 85 per cent of the diameter. Therefore, resting coronary flow is little affected by mild or

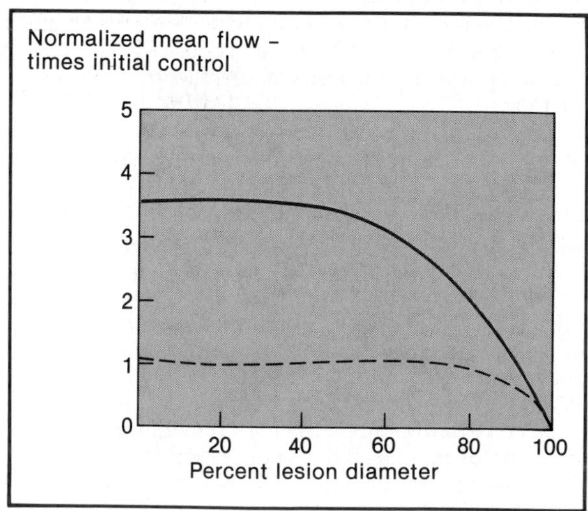

FIGURE 36–18. Relationship between resting *(dashed line)* and maximal coronary blood flow *(solid line)* and percentage of diameter stenosis in a dog. Progressive coronary stenosis was achieved by progressively narrowing a short segment of a proximal coronary artery. Resting coronary blood flow did not change until coronary diameter stenosis exceeded 80 per cent. Maximal coronary blood flow began to decrease when per cent diameter stenosis exceeded 50 per cent. (From Marcus, M. L.: The Coronary Circulation in Health and Disease. New York, McGraw-Hill, 1983, and modified from Gould, K. L., and Lipscomb, L.: Effects of coronary stenoses on coronary flow reserve and resistance. Am. J. Cardiol. *34:*50, 1974.)

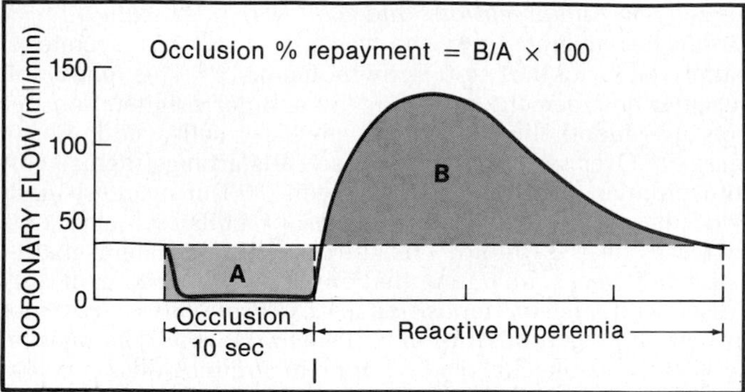

FIGURE 36–19. Mean coronary flow prior to, during, and following coronary occlusion. Arrow indicates the release of occlusion. Area A represents the flow debt, and area B its repayment. (From Gould, K. L.: Coronary Artery Stenosis. New York, Elsevier, 1991, p. 13.)

moderate stenoses and is an insensitive measure for evaluating coronary artery disease. *Maximal* coronary blood flow, however, begins to decline when diameter stenosis exceeds 30 to 45 per cent (Fig. 36–18). The capacity to increase coronary blood flow in response to increased oxygen demand is abolished when diameter stenosis exceeds 90 per cent.

Insights derived from such animal studies need to be applied cautiously in clinical practice. The simple use of relative per cent diameter stenosis determined by coronary arteriography has important limitations, because it does not account for other geometric characteristics of the stenosis such as its absolute diameter, length, exit angle, or eccentricity. The determination of relative per cent diameter narrowing may be misleading in the setting of diffuse disease where segments adjacent to the stenosis are also reduced in caliber. The hemodynamic effects of serial stenoses are also difficult to assess from arteriograms.[170] It is not surprising, then, that the correlation between per cent diameter stenosis and the physiological significance of a given obstruction in patients is poor, especially for lesions of moderate severity.[179,180]

Coronary Flow Reserve and Hyperemia

Ischemia caused by transient coronary arterial occlusion is followed by an increase in blood flow above control levels, a response called reactive hyperemia (Fig. 36–19). The marked vasodilation that characterizes reactive hyperemia is probably related to the accumulation of metabolites, especially adenosine (see p. 1163). The difference between basal coronary blood flow and peak flow during reactive hyperemia represents the *coronary flow reserve.*

Because of the limitations inherent in coronary angiography, attention has been directed to physiological approaches for assessing the severity of coronary stenoses. As noted earlier, maximal blood flow is a more sensitive index of stenosis severity than resting blood flow. Because methods for measuring maximal coronary flow in absolute terms are not readily available, the concept of *coronary flow reserve,* defined as the ratio of maximal flow to resting flow, has been developed and refined into an accepted functional measure of resistance to coronary blood flow. Abnormal resistance may be caused by stenosis and/or microcirculatory disorders.[170,179,181]

Three types of stimuli have been used to elicit maximal coronary blood flow: metabolic stress, pharmacological coronary dilation, and transient coronary occlusion. Intense treadmill or bicycle exercise yields near maximal four- to six-fold flow increases[182] and is thereby a widely accepted stimulus for assessing flow responses. Maximal increases in coronary blood flow can also be produced by pharmacological coronary vasodilators. Adenosine and papaverine (Fig. 36–20) have a rapid onset and brief duration of action, can be administered directly into the coronary artery, and are therefore particularly well-suited for studies in the catheterization laboratory.[183] Transient occlusion of a coronary artery by an angioplasty balloon with the measurement of reactive hyperemia is the third stimulus.

INVASIVE MEASUREMENT OF FLOW RESERVE. Several techniques for determining coronary flow reserve have been developed for use during cardiac catheterization. Catheter- or guidewire-based Doppler systems allow continuous measurement of phasic and mean coronary blood flow velocity.[184,185] Miniaturized Doppler crystals have been placed at the tip of angioplasty guidewires, permitting measurements of coronary blood flow velocity[186,187] (Fig. 36–20). The thermodilution method measures flow in the coronary venous system, either in the great cardiac vein (which drains the left anterior descending artery territory) or in the coronary sinus (which drains the left anterior descending and circumflex artery territories).[189] These approaches have demonstrated only a weak inverse correlation between angiographic estimates of per cent diameter stenosis and

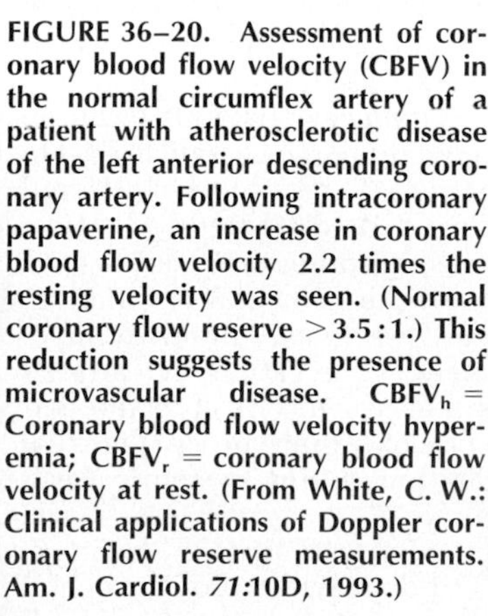
FIGURE 36–20. Assessment of coronary blood flow velocity (CBFV) in the normal circumflex artery of a patient with atherosclerotic disease of the left anterior descending coronary artery. Following intracoronary papaverine, an increase in coronary blood flow velocity 2.2 times the resting velocity was seen. (Normal coronary flow reserve >3.5 : 1.) This reduction suggests the presence of microvascular disease. $CBFV_h$ = Coronary blood flow velocity hyperemia; $CBFV_r$ = coronary blood flow velocity at rest. (From White, C. W.: Clinical applications of Doppler coronary flow reserve measurements. Am. J. Cardiol. *71*:10D, 1993.)

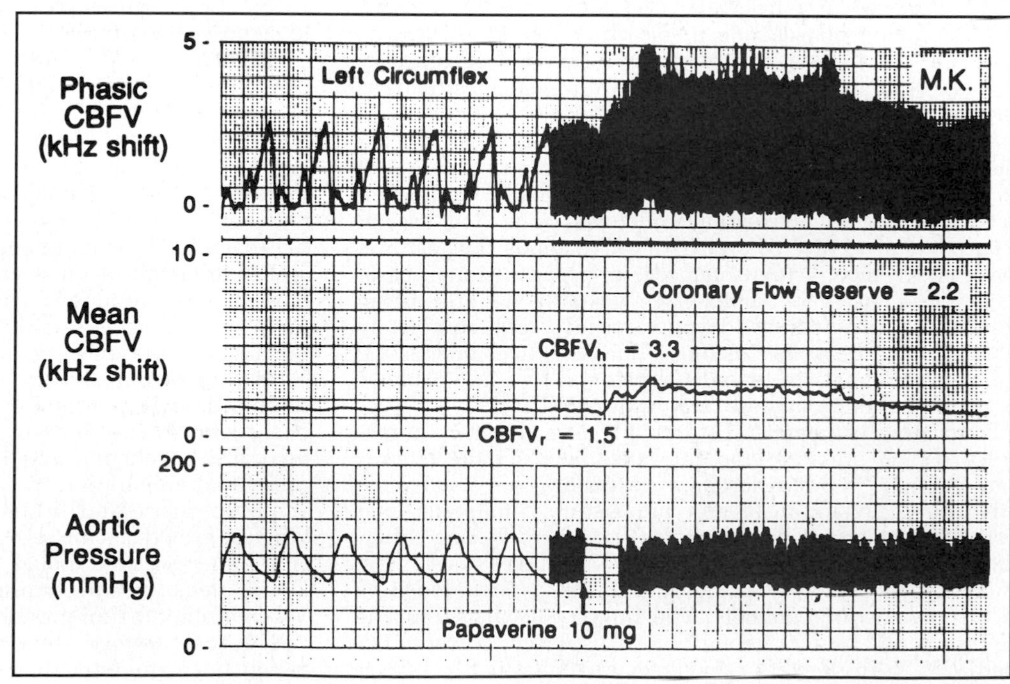

coronary reserve, particularly for stenoses of moderate (intermediate) severity.[180]

NONINVASIVE MEASUREMENT OF FLOW RESERVE. Digital subtraction angiography can also be used to estimate regional coronary blood flow in a downstream area by measuring the time of arrival and/or the rapidity of clearance of injected x-ray contrast medium.[188] Radionuclide stress myocardial perfusion imaging (thallium-201, sestamibi) is used widely to quantify coronary flow reserve (see p. 288). Some laboratories are investigating the use of positron-emission tomography, ultrafast computed tomography, and nuclear magnetic resonance imaging for the same purpose.[190] Flow reserve is typically assessed by these techniques during exercise or with pharmacological vasodilators. In contrast to catheterization-based techniques that measure an *absolute* coronary flow reserve index (the quotient of maximal and basal flow), cardiac imaging techniques assess *relative* coronary flow reserve by comparing the perfusion of ischemic regions of the left ventricle with presumably normally perfused reference regions.[191]

Imaging techniques yield a less quantitative index of flow reserve than catheter-based techniques. In addition, results can be misleading in the setting of diffuse coronary disease when a normal reference region is not available. Together, absolute and relative coronary flow reserves provide a more complete description of physiological stenosis severity than does either alone.[191]

There is a poor correlation between the severity of stenoses and their propensity to cause myocardial infarction, sudden ischemic death, or unstable angina. Most atherosclerotic lesions responsible for these complications are either not appreciated on angiograms obtained shortly before the event or are mild stenoses of inconsequential hemodynamic significance.[192–194] Pathological studies have revealed that myocardial infarctions are usually caused by ruptures of plaques that are not necessarily severe, with formation of a superimposed occlusive thrombus.[195] These findings suggest that although measurements of coronary flow reserve may be useful in the assessment of the severity of stenoses and in the identification of severe lesions responsible for exertional angina, they are *not* likely to identify the more dangerous plaques responsible for unstable angina, acute myocardial infarction, and ischemic sudden death.

Coronary Collateral Circulation

Following total or near-total occlusion of a coronary artery, perfusion of ischemic myocardium occurs by way of collaterals—vascular channels that interconnect ordinary arteries.[190] Preexisting collaterals are thin-walled structures ranging in diameter from 20 to 200 μm.[196,197] The density of preexisting collaterals varies greatly among different species.[197] Acute coronary occlusion produces no infarction at all in guinea pigs because of an exceptionally well-developed network of preexisting collaterals. The dog has an intermediate density of preexisting collaterals that can deliver, on average, 5 to 10 per cent of preocclusional, basal flow. Pigs, rats, and rabbits have virtually no preexisting collaterals, and infarcts develop rapidly and completely with acute coronary occlusion.[197] The density of preexisting collateral channels in humans appears to be comparable to or somewhat more modest than in dogs.[198]

Preexisting collaterals are normally closed and nonfunctional, as no pressure gradient exists between the arteries they connect.[199] After coronary occlusion, the distal pressure drops precipitously and preexisting collaterals open virtually instantly. The transformation of preexisting collaterals into mature collaterals occurs in three stages. The initial stage (the first 24 hours) involves *passive widening* of the preexisting channels. The internal elastic lamina is ruptured and its fragments are displaced toward the media.[196,197] The second stage (1 day to 3 weeks) is characterized by *inflammation and cellular proliferation*.[196,197] Monocytes migrate into the vascular wall and secrete a variety of cytokines and growth factors.[201] This phase of vascular enlargement is marked by cellular proliferation involving endothelium, smooth muscle cells, and fibroblasts.[202] Over several weeks, these cells arrange themselves into circular and longitudinal layers.[198] During these first two phases, the luminal diameter of collateral channels increases nearly 10-fold. The third stage of collateral maturation (3 weeks to 6 months) involves thickening of the vessel wall due to *deposition of extracellular matrix* and further cellular proliferation.[203] In its final state, the mature collateral vessel may reach 1 mm in luminal diameter. Its three-layer structure is nearly indistinguishable from a normal coronary artery of the same size.[204]

Factors Promoting Collateral Growth

Mechanical forces determine the size of collateral channels in the early minutes and hours after coronary occlusion. Pressure gradients across preexisting collaterals augment blood flow and create shear stresses,[201] which in turn lead to activation of endothelial cells with expression of leukocyte adhesion molecules and secretion of growth factors.[205] Ischemia or hypoxia may initiate the process of vascular transformation by causing intense dilation of native coronary collateral channels, but these stimuli probably have only a limited role in further collateral angiogenesis.[201] Other chemical stimuli likely contribute to growth of collateral channels, including a variety of growth factors and proto-oncogenes. These are rapidly expressed following coronary occlusion, in part due to enhanced transcriptional activity.[206]

HEREDITARY FACTORS. These play an important role in determining the density of preexisting collaterals. For example, coronary occlusion in Black Russian rabbits results in a large infarct, as preexisting collaterals are virtually absent. New Zealand White rabbits, on the other hand, have a greater number of preexisting collaterals and are more resistant to the ischemic effects of a coronary occlusion.[197]

SEVERITY OF OBSTRUCTION. The severity of coronary obstruction is a critical determinant of the development of coronary collateral channels. In dogs, the growth of collaterals is not stimulated until a coronary stenosis reduces the luminal cross-sectional area by at least 80 per cent.[200] In patients, coronary collaterals do not develop until a stenosis of at least 70 per cent is present. Beyond this threshold value, the growth of collateral channels is directly related to stenosis severity.[207]

EXERCISE. This stimulus has no effect on the preexisting coronary collaterals in the absence of coronary occlusions or stenoses.[200] Even in the presence of severe coronary stenoses, the effects of exercise training have been inconsistent and overall quite small in animals.[208]

PHARMACOLOGICAL AGENTS. Coronary collaterals dilate in response to nitrates[200] and beta-adrenergic agonists.[204] On the other hand, calcium antagonists,[209] beta blockers,[210] and alpha-adrenergic agonists have no detectable direct effect on collateral function, whereas vasopressin[204] and serotonin[211] are potent constrictors of the collateral circulation. Such a constriction of collateral vessels may intensify myocardial ischemia during platelet aggregation or arterial thrombosis when serotonin is released locally into the coronary circulation, and it may contribute to episodes of myocardial ischemia and infarction during systemic vasopressin administration.[204]

Intracoronary and systemic administration of basic fibroblast growth factor (b-FGF) to dogs with coronary occlusion enhances endothelial cell proliferation, increases collateral density, and improves collateral blood flow.[212,213] Vascular endothelial growth factor (VEGF) is an endothelial cell–specific mitogen that markedly enhances collateral development following femoral artery occlusion in rabbits[214,215] and coronary occlusion in dogs.[216] Both b-FGF and VEGF are members of the family of heparin-binding growth factors, and some of their actions may be potentiated by the addition of heparin. Some[217,218] but not all[219] investigators have found that the administration of heparin can enhance or accelerate collateral development.

ENDOGENOUS VASODILATORS. The release of endogenous vasodilators such as prostacyclin and nitric oxide maintains collaterals in a dilated state.[219a] Inhibition of prostaglandin synthesis with indomethacin[220] or aspirin[221] results in marked reductions in collateral blood flow. Inhibition of nitric oxide synthesis with N^G-nitro-L-arginine methyl ester (L-NAME) also leads to marked reductions in collateral blood flow.[222] Thus, these two endothelium-derived factors play a central role in the maintenance of collateral flow.

FUNCTIONAL CAPACITY OF COLLATERALS. Mature collaterals can provide normal levels of perfusion to collateral-dependent regions at rest or during moderate exercise in dogs with chronic coronary occlusion.[200] However, during maximal exercise or maximal pharmacologically induced vasodilation, flow to regions perfused by collaterals may be less than normal, especially in subendocardial regions.[197] Relief of coronary occlusion leads to a rapid disappearance of functional and angiographic evidence of coronary collaterals. However, when a previously occluded vessel is reoccluded months later, the collateral circulation functions fully within 60 minutes.[200]

CORONARY COLLATERALS IN HUMANS. Controversy has existed in the past regarding the importance of coronary collaterals in humans.[197,200] However, it is now clear that coronary collaterals can mitigate the severity of myocardial ischemia and myocardial necrosis. Some patients with total occlusion of a major coronary artery may demonstrate no evidence of myocardial infarction and have normal ventricular function at rest.[200] Myocardium in the distribution of occluded coronary arteries with angiographically apparent collaterals has been shown to have better contractile function and less fibrosis than regions in the distribution of noncollateralized occluded vessels.[223]

Percutaneous transluminal coronary angioplasty (PTCA) has served as a model of controlled coronary artery occlusion in humans. During PTCA, collateral filling to the artery being dilated can be visualized by contrast injection into the contralateral coronary artery using a second angiographic catheter.[224] Filling through the collateral artery has been shown to increase significantly during balloon inflation,[225] with the opening of preformed collaterals. These recruitable collaterals afford protection from myocardial ischemia during balloon inflation as judged from the extent and severity of electrocardiographic ST-segment elevation, the appearance of wall-motion abnormalities,[225] and metabolic studies of transmyocardial lactate extraction.[226]

Coronary collaterals also limit the size of myocardial infarction and the clinical sequelae of coronary occlusion. Patients with acute myocardial infarction in whom thrombolytic therapy was unsuccessful may show subsequent improvement in regional and global wall motion if residual flow was improved by extensive collaterals.[218,227] Total occlusion of the left anterior descending coronary artery in association with poor collateral blood supply predisposes to left ventricular aneurysm formation after anterior myocardial infarction. However, coronary collaterals may prevent left ventricular aneurysm formation in such patients by limiting the progression of the wavefront of necrosis from the subendocardial to subepicardial layers and leaving a viable rim of myocardium or by improving the process of healing of the infarcted tissue.[218]

Recently, successful restoration of antegrade coronary blood flow several days or weeks after myocardial infarction has been shown to improve regional wall motion. The use of myocardial contrast echocardiography demonstrated an association between collateral blood flow and myocardial viability.[228] It may be presumed that low levels of collateral blood flow, not detectable by angiography, maintained the myocardium in a viable although "hibernating" state (see p. 1176).

ENHANCING COLLATERAL FORMATION. There has been much interest in finding ways to enhance collateral function in patients with coronary stenoses. In experimental animals with coronary occlusion, exercise has no influence on collateral development.[197,208,229,230] In the few available clinical studies that utilized repeat coronary angiography, an increase in collaterals occurred only with progression in the severity of coronary artery stenoses, but not with long-term exercise programs.[231,232] The reduction of myocardial ischemia observed after an exercise program is most likely the result of exercise conditioning rather than collateral

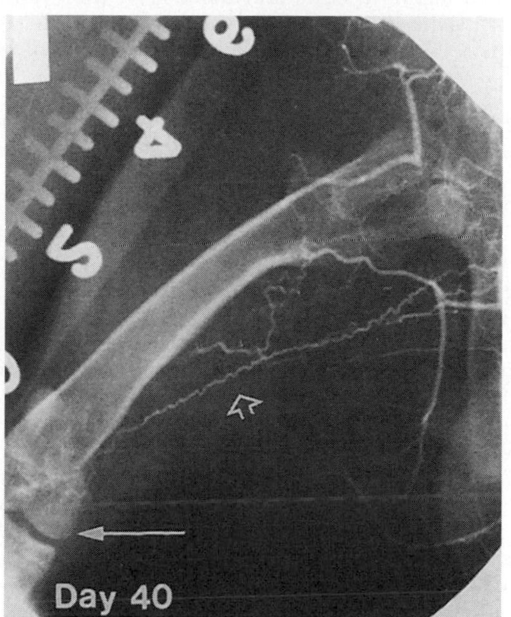

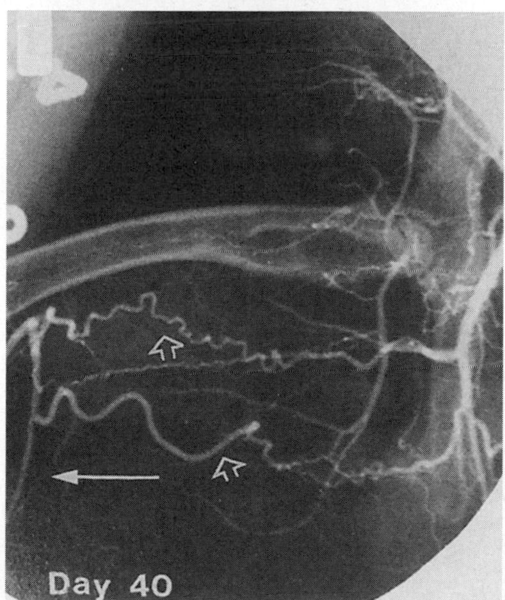

FIGURE 36–21. Selective internal iliac angiography of control rabbit performed at day 40 (control, untreated, *top*) and of VEGF-treated rabbit at day 40 (*bottom*). VEGF was administered as a single intraarterial bolus into the internal iliac artery of rabbits with severe ipsilateral ischemia. The angiogram shown here has yielded angiographic scores of 0.17 and 0.41. Distal reconstitution, barely apparent in the control group (arrows), was evident in the VEGF-treated group (arrows). Direct and linear extension of internal iliac artery to popliteal and/or saphenous arteries was also more evident in VEGF-treated group (open arrows). (From Takeshita, S., et al.: Therapeutic angiogenesis. J. Clin. Invest. *93*:662, 1994, by copyright permission of the American Society for Clinical Investigation.)

expansion. Preliminary studies have suggested that repeat exercise stress combined with injections of heparin may raise the ischemia threshold and improve collateral blood flow[218,233] and that heparin may improve collateral blood flow after myocardial infarction.[234]

Advances in molecular biology are bringing to clinical testing gene therapy for arterial disease.[235,236] After encouraging animal experiments (Fig. 36–21), a clinical trial has been initiated to evaluate whether local delivery of a gene encoding for vascular endothelial growth factor (VEGF) can enhance collateral development in patients with obstructive atherosclerosis involving the lower extremities. An improved understanding of the molecular and cellular mechanisms of angiogenesis should lead to other innovative approaches to augment collateral blood flow more effectively in patients with atherosclerotic stenoses in a variety of vascular beds.

CONSEQUENCES OF MYOCARDIAL ISCHEMIA

Myocardial Stunning and Hibernation

(See also pp. 89 and 388)

For four decades following Tennant and Wiggers' classic observation on the effects of coronary occlusion on myocardial contraction,[237] it was believed that transient severe ischemia caused either irreversible cardiac injury—that is, infarction, or prompt recovery. However, in the 1970's it became clear that after a brief episode of severe ischemia, prolonged myocardial dysfunction with gradual return of contractile activity occurred, a condition termed myocardial stunning[238–240] (Fig. 36–22). Stunning may occur following exercise-induced ischemia[241] and coronary spasm.[242] It affects both systolic and diastolic function[240,243] and can occur in the globally as well as the regionally ischemic heart. Clinically, myocardial stunning probably occurs most frequently in patients who have undergone ischemic cardiac arrest during cardiopulmonary bypass[244]; such hearts may not recover normal function for days. In patients with a myocardial infarction (both with and without the administration of reperfusion thrombolytic therapy), reversibly injured, functionally stunned myocardium lies adjacent to infarcted myocardium.[245,246] Myocardial stunning is an important feature of unstable angina (see p. 1332).

DETERMINANTS OF STUNNING. The severity of the ischemic stress is an important influence in the genesis of myocardial stunning. Bolli et al.[247] found a close relationship

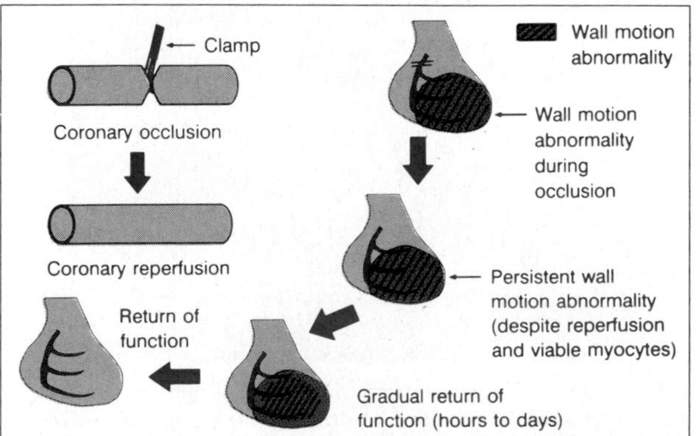

FIGURE 36–22. Schematic diagram of stunned myocardium. During coronary occlusion, a wall motion abnormality of the left ventricle is present in the region supplied by the occluded artery. With relief of ischemia and re-establishment of coronary blood flow, there is a persistent wall motion abnormality despite reperfusion and viable myocytes. There is then gradual improvement in function that requires hours to days for recovery. (From Kloner, R. A., Przyklenk, K., and Patel, B.: Altered myocardial states: The stunned and hibernating myocardium. Am. J. Med. *86*(Suppl. 1A):14, 1986.)

TABLE 36–3 THE PROPOSED MECHANISMS OF MYOCARDIAL STUNNING

1. Insufficient energy production by mitochondria
2. Impaired energy use by myofibrils
3. Impaired sympathetic neuronal responsiveness
4. Impaired myocardial perfusion
5. Damage to the extracellular collagen matrix
6. Decreased sensitivity of myofilaments to calcium
7. Calcium overload
8. Excitation-contraction uncoupling due to dysfunction of sarcoplasmic reticulum
9. Generation of damaging oxygen free radicals

Modified from Bolli, R.: Postischemic myocardial stunning. *In* Yellon, D. M., and Jennings, R. B. (eds.): Myocardial Protection: The Pathophysiology of Reperfusion and Reperfusion Injury. New York, Raven Press, Ltd., 1992.

between the magnitude of blood flow reduction during 15-minute periods of coronary artery occlusion and the degree of myocardial dysfunction after reperfusion. The severity of stunning is always greater in the subendocardial layers of the left ventricular wall which are more ischemic than the subepicardial layers.[247,248] The duration of ischemia is a second important factor.[248]

MECHANISMS OF STUNNING. The sequence of biochemical events whereby transient myocardial ischemia leads to protracted depression of myocardial contractility has not been elucidated definitively.[249] The proposed mechanisms are listed in Table 36-3. Insufficient energy production, impaired energy use by myofibrils, and impaired myocardial perfusion[250] are unlikely mechanisms because the contractility of the stunned myocardium can be transiently but rapidly restored by inotropic stimulation.[251–253] More likely mechanisms include a transient calcium overload of myocytes immediately after reperfusion,[254,255] excitation-contraction uncoupling due to ischemia-induced dysfunction of the sarcoplasmic reticulum,[256] and generation of oxygen free radicals.[257–260] Despite evidence that reperfusion-induced cellular changes are at least in part responsible for myocardial stunning, it is unlikely that reperfusion alone accounts for all of the postischemic damage. More likely, ischemia of the myocardium is associated with multiple and severe metabolic derangements, and recovery of function cannot be expected instantaneously even if no additional injury occurs upon reperfusion.[261,262]

MYOCARDIAL HIBERNATION. Chronic hypoperfusion of the myocardium ("hibernation") is a reversible cause of left ventricular dysfunction. Radionuclide imaging techniques, positron emission tomography, and stress (dobutamine) echocardiography are capable of assessing myocardial perfusion and viability and are helpful in determining whether myocardial dysfunction is due to necrosis or hibernation.

ISCHEMIC PRECONDITIONING. (See p. 1214)

Hemodynamic Consequences of Ischemia

Because the heart has virtually no stores of oxygen, within seconds of coronary occlusion its relatively high rate of energy expenditure results in a sudden, striking decline of myocardial oxygen tension and loss of contractility. If sufficiently widespread, regional impairment of myocardial contractile activity depresses global left ventricular function, causing reductions of stroke volume, stroke work, cardiac output, and ejection fraction while elevating ventricular end-diastolic volume and pressure. Clinical evidence of heart failure occurs when regional asynergy is so severe and extensive that the uninvolved myocardium cannot sustain the normal hemodynamic burden. Left ventricular failure usually develops when contraction ceases in 20 to 25 per cent of the left ventricle. With loss of 40 per cent

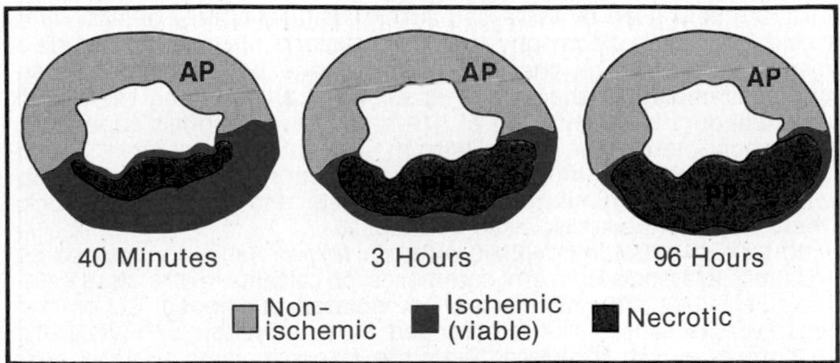

FIGURE 36–23. Progression of cell death versus time after circumflex coronary occlusion in dogs. Necrosis occurs first in the subendocardial myocardium. With longer occlusions, a wavefront of cell death moves from the subendocardial zone across the wall to involve progressively more of the transmural thickness of the ischemic zone. In contrast, the lateral margins in the subendocardial region of the infarct are established as early as 40 minutes after occlusion and are sharply defined by the anatomic boundaries of the ischemic bed. AP = anterior papillary muscle; PP = posterior papillary muscle. (From Reimer, K. A., Hill, M. L., and Jennings, R. B.: Prolonged depletion of ATP and of the adenine nucleotide pool due to delayed resynthesis of adenine nucleotides following reversible myocardial ischemic injury in dogs. J. Mol. Cell. Cardiol. *13:*229, 1981.)

or more of the left ventricular myocardium, severe pump failure ensues, and, if this loss is acute, cardiogenic shock develops.

Myocardial ischemia and infarction alter not only the contractile (systolic) properties of the heart but also its diastolic properties (see pp. 1194 and 1195). Ischemia causes both a leftward shift and an increase in the slope of the left ventricular end-diastolic pressure-volume relation so that ventricular pressure is higher at any volume[263] (Fig. 13–14, p. 403). Myocardial ischemia also impairs ventricular relaxation,[264] as evidenced by a decreased rate of the ventricular pressure decline (negative dP/dt) and ventricular wall thinning, and it prolongs the isovolumetric relaxation period.[264,265] With regional ischemia, the reduction of compliance is limited to the ischemic region, whereas the nonischemic region operates on a higher and steeper portion of its (normal) pressure-volume curve. Thus, the ischemia-induced changes in diastolic properties increase the resistance to ventricular filling.

Thus, ischemia causes impairment of cardiac contraction and incomplete ventricular emptying (systolic failure). In addition, it impairs ventricular relaxation and shifts the diastolic pressure-volume curve leftward (diastolic failure). The combination of systolic and diastolic failure leads to elevated ventricular filling pressures, causing symptoms of pulmonary congestion.

The "Wavefront" of Ischemic Necrosis

As already noted (see p. 1174), within seconds of a coronary artery occlusion, blood begins to flow through preexisting collateral channels to the artery distal to the site of occlusion. Collateral flow is lowest and myocardial oxygen consumption highest in the subendocardium, and therefore ischemia is most severe in this region. In the normal myocardium, thickening and shortening are greater in the subendocardium, as is wall stress, accounting for the higher subendocardial energy requirements.[266,267] Consistent with these findings, higher rates of metabolic activity, lower tissue oxygen tension,[268] and greater oxygen extraction have been found in this region.[269] As a consequence, ischemia becomes most severe and myocardial cells undergo necrosis first in the subendocardium, commencing as early as 15 to 20 minutes after coronary artery occlusion. Necrosis progresses toward the epicardium, gradually involving the less severely ischemic outer layers (Fig. 36–23). The progression of the wavefront of necrosis[269a] is slowed by the presence of residual blood flow when the coronary occlusion is incomplete or when well-developed collaterals are present at the time of occlusion.[270] The progression of the wavefront is accelerated when myocardial ischemia is unusually severe, when collateral blood flow is low, in the presence of marked arterial hypotension (e.g., in patients in cardiogenic shock), and in the presence of elevated myocardial

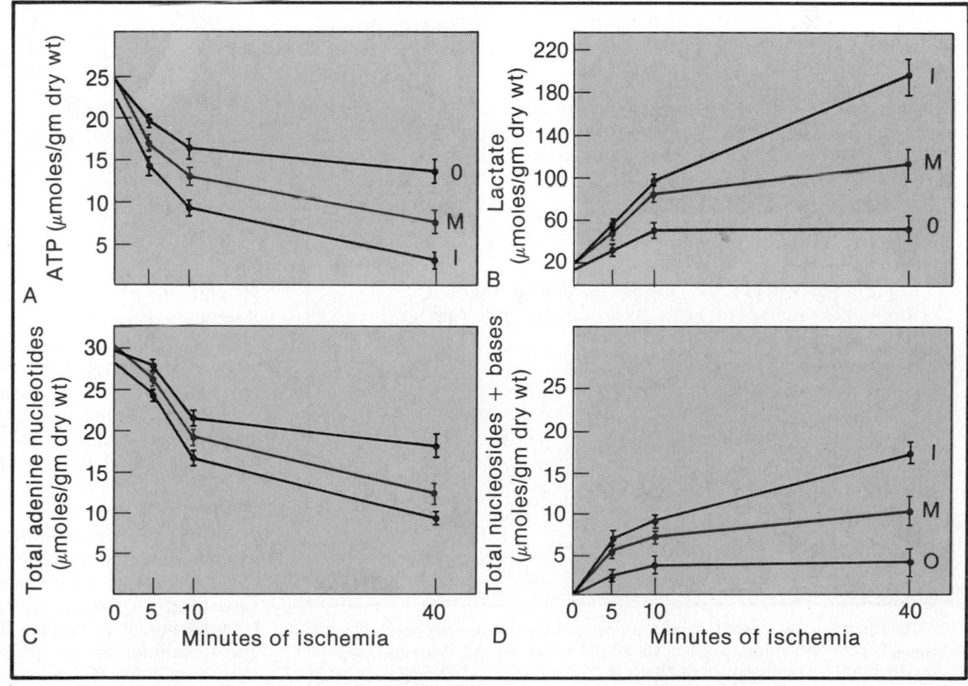

FIGURE 36–24. Time course of metabolic changes during myocardial ischemia plotted by transmural layer (I = inner, subendocardial; M = middle; O = outer, subepicardial). Ischemia was induced by circumflex occlusion in anesthetized dogs. Data for different times are based on different groups of dogs; *N* = 4 to 6; brackets indicate plus or minus one standard error of the mean. *A,* More rapid depletion of ATP in the inner layer, highly significant after 5 min of ischemia ($P < 0.01$). *B,* Tissue lactate accumulation, with the most rapid accumulation in the subendocardium. For all layers there was a progressive increase in lactate content during the first 10 min of ischemia. Between 10 and 40 min there was continued lactate accumulation in the inner and middle layers, but not in the outer layer. *C,* Total adenine nucleotide content (ATP + ADP + AMP). Adenine nucleotide degradation was most rapid in the subendocardium. Note the time lag between ATP depletion (graph A) and adenine nucleotide breakdown. *D,* Total nucleosides and bases, which are the products of adenine nucleotide degradation. Accumulation was fastest in the subendocardium. As with lactate (graph B), nucleoside and base content in the outer layer was maximal by 10 minutes and was not further increased at 40 minutes, even though adenine nucleotide breakdown in this layer continued (graph C). (From Reimer, K. A., and Jennings, R. B.: Myocardial ischemia, hypoxia, and infarction. *In* Fozzard, H. A., Jennings, R. B., Haber, E., Katz, A. M., and Morgan, H. E. [eds.]: The Heart and Cardiovascular System. 2nd ed. New York, Raven Press, 1991, p. 1888. From the studies of Murry, C. E., et al.: Collateral blood flow and transmural location: Independent determinants of ATP in ischemic canine myocardium. Fed. Proc. *44:*823, 1985.)

oxygen demand, as may be caused by inotropic stimulation (tachycardia or fever).

The transmural progression of necrosis has been demonstrated in dogs with a variable duration of coronary occlusion prior to reperfusion,[271] and in humans.[272] The recognition of the time-dependent progression of necrosis is the basis of interventions designed to arrest the progression of necrosis as rapidly as possible by reperfusion of occluded coronary arteries, using thrombolytic therapy or angioplasty.

Effects of Ischemia on Myocardial Metabolism

HIGH-ENERGY PHOSPHATE METABOLISM. During the first minutes of severe ischemia, the production of high-energy phosphates (the sum of ATP and creatine phosphate [CP]) declines and is greatly exceeded by their utilization. Therefore, tissue stores of high-energy phosphates decline progressively, with CP stores falling more rapidly than ATP stores. CP is depleted by transfer of high-energy phosphate to ADP as oxidative synthesis of ATP declines. In the absence of normal oxidative phosphorylation, ADP is converted to AMP (in the myokinase reaction), which in turn is broken down to adenosine and ultimately to inosine, hypoxanthine, and xanthine.[273] These changes are more striking in the subendocardium (Fig. 36–24). When tissue is only reversibly injured by ischemia (i.e., when its viability can still be maintained by reperfusion), ATP stores are usually greater than 60 per cent of control, and electron microscopy may reveal only glycogen loss, nuclear chromatin clumping, intermyofibrillar edema, and mitochondrial swelling but no sarcolemmal damage or accumulation of amorphous dense bodies in the mitochondria. When ATP content is reduced below 20 per cent of control values, cells become unable to regenerate high-energy phosphate or to maintain physiological ionic gradients and cell volume. The combination of reduced myocardial high-energy phosphate stores, cell swelling, and sarcolemmal damage (potentially attributable to oxygen-derived free radicals, causing lipid peroxidation) appears to play a key role in cell death with ischemia or reperfusion (Table 36–4).

OXIDATIVE PHOSPHORYLATION. The importance of oxidative phosphorylation—that is, the coupling of ATP synthesis to aerobic respiration—for the metabolic integrity of myocardium is underscored by some simple considerations. Complete oxidation of 1 mole of glucose gives rise to the net production of 36 moles of ATP. In contrast, only 2 moles of ATP are produced from anaerobic metabolism of 1 mole of glucose. Thus, even if the profound derangements in intermediary metabolism associated with increased production of reducing equivalents accompanying anaerobic glycolysis could be corrected, an 18-fold increase in glycolytic flux would be required for myocardium to synthesize comparable quantities of ATP via anaerobic compared with aerobic metabolism. The failure of energy production to keep pace with demand in ischemic cells is manifested by a prompt decline in the concentration of CP, a major constituent of myocardial high-energy phosphate stores.

ALTERATIONS IN CELLULAR ELECTROPHYSIOLOGY. The effects of ischemia on the electrophysiological properties of cardiac muscle are numerous and complex. Ischemia-induced ventricular tachyarrhythmias can be caused by increased automaticity, triggered activity, and reentry. The early electrophysiological hallmarks of ischemia include a marked diminution in the resting membrane potential, the action potential amplitude, the rate of upstroke of phase 0, and the action potential duration. Activation of ATP-sensitive K^+ channels appears to be responsible for the latter. Within 10 minutes of ischemia, action potential alterations in amplitude and duration become prominent, with subsequent diminution of excitability and conduction block. These alterations are discussed in Chap. 20.

ROLE OF CALCIUM IN ISCHEMIC INJURY. Myocardial injury induced by ischemia is associated with complexes of calcium in the tissue detectable by electron microscopy. As pointed out above, ischemia—whatever its cause—is characterized by a reduction of myocardial ATP stores, which interferes with the transsarcolemmal Na^+-K^+ exchange, which in turn elevates intracellular $[Na^+]$, raising intracellular $[Ca^{++}]$ through an enhanced Na^+-Ca^{++} exchange (see p. 386). Lowered ATP stores also reduce Ca^{++} uptake by the sarcoplasmic reticulum and reduce extrusion of Ca^{++} from cells. The resultant augmented intracellular $[Ca^{++}]$[274] causes mitochondrial Ca^{++} overload, which decreases ATP production further. Activation of intracellular Ca^{++} ATPases augments ATP usage and activates sarcolemmal phospholipases, which release membrane phospholipid degradation products whose detergent properties impair the integrity of the cell membrane.[275]

Calcium antagonists interfere with Ca^{++} influx through voltage-dependent channels. Beta-adrenoreceptor agonists recruit additional receptor-operated channels, and beta-adrenoreceptor blockers reduce Ca^{++} influx by interfering with this recruitment of receptor-operated channels. Thus, one would expect beta blockers and Ca^{++}

TABLE 36–4 POTENTIAL CAUSES OF IRREVERSIBILITY

High-energy phosphate depletion/cessation of anaerobic glycolysis
- Catabolism without resynthesis of macromolecules
- Reduced transsarcolemmal gradients of Na^+ and K^+
  - Cell swelling
- Calcium overload
  - Activation of phospholipases/proteases
  - Impaired mitochondrial function
  - Activation of ATPases

Catabolite accumulation (lactate, H^+ (acidosis), fatty acid derivatives, free radicals, ammonia, inorganic phosphate, etc.)
- Enzyme denaturation
- Membrane damage
- Increased intracellular osmolarity
  - Cell swelling

Cell death may be related to the consequences of one or both general features of ischemic injury shown above. Some effects of ischemia may be related to both high-energy phosphate depletion and catabolite accumulation. For example, cell swelling may be due both to loss of ATP-dependent ion transport and to intracellular production of small-molecular-weight catabolites.

From Reimer, K. A., and Jennings, R. B.: Myocardial ischemia, hypoxia and infarction. *In* Fozzard, H. A., Haber, E., Jennings, R. B., et al. (eds.): The Heart and Cardiovascular System. 2nd ed. New York, Raven Press, 1991, pp. 1875–1974.

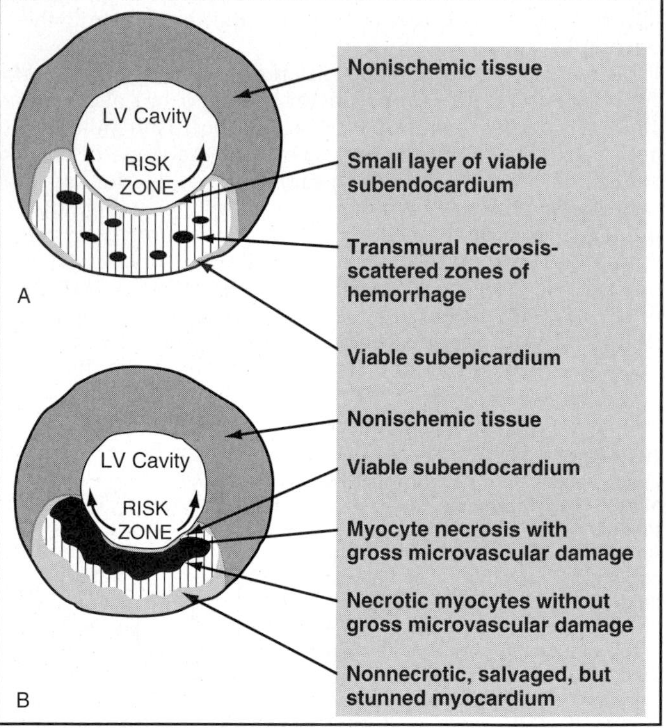

FIGURE 36–25. *A,* Schematic diagram showing a transverse section through a canine left ventricle subjected to a permanent coronary occlusion without reperfusion. The white area represents nonischemic myocardium supplied by the nonoccluded vessel. The infarct (hatched area) is transmural or near-transmural. There are scattered zones of hemorrhage (solid black). A small layer of viable subendocardium is present, which derives its oxygen directly from the ventricular cavity. Where collateral flow is high, there may be a small rim of surviving subepicardium (shaded areas). *B,* Schematic diagram showing a transverse section through a canine left ventricle subjected to coronary occlusion followed within 1 or 2 hours by coronary reperfusion. The hatched and solid black areas represent the infarct that is confined to the inner half of the myocardium. The solid black areas represent the zone of gross microvascular damage including zones of no-reflow and hemorrhage. It is smaller than and contained within the total infarct. The remainder of the infarct without severe microvascular damage is represented by the hatched area and is located in the midmyocardium. The epicardial portion of the ischemic zone (stippled area) has been salvaged by coronary reperfusion. It is nonnecrotic but stunned (postischemic ventricular dysfunction) for hours to days following coronary reperfusion. (From Braunwald, E., and Kloner, R. A.: Myocardial reperfusion: A double-edged sword? J. Clin. Invest. *76:*1715, 1985, by copyright permission of the American Society for Clinical Investigation.)

antagonists to have similar effects in the treatment of ischemia. Indeed, both groups of compounds delay ischemia-induced necrosis and, particularly when combined with reperfusion, reduce the extent of myocardial necrosis.[276–280]

REPERFUSION INJURY

Despite the unequivocal utility of reperfusion in limiting cell death in the presence of severe ischemia, reperfusion can elicit a number of adverse reactions that may limit its beneficial actions[281,282] (Fig. 36–25).

ACCELERATION OF MYOCYTE NECROSIS. After reperfusion, ischemic cells often suddenly develop ultrastructural changes indicative of cell death, including "explosive swelling"[283] and widespread architectural disruption. Nevertheless, it is likely that most—perhaps all—of the myocytes in which necrosis is accelerated by reperfusion were already irreversibly injured by the time reperfusion occurred and that reperfusion merely hastened the death of cells already destined not to recover. If reperfusion does cause necrosis of reversibly injured myocardium, the quantity of tissue so affected is likely small.

THE "NO-REFLOW" PHENOMENON. This refers to the failure to achieve sustained reperfusion after a prolonged period of ischemia. The areas of reduced or absent reflow often appear to result from ischemia-induced microvascular damage and myocardial contracture. However, the no-reflow phenomenon does not appear to augment myocyte death, because the zone of reflow is contained within areas in which myocytes were already necrotic at the time of the onset of reperfusion (Fig. 36–25).

REPERFUSION-INDUCED HEMORRHAGE. Reperfused infarcts frequently contain hemorrhagic areas.[284] Reperfusion-induced hemorrhage, like the "no-reflow" phenomenon, is caused largely by microvascular damage. It is generally contained within areas of myocardium already necrotic at the time of reperfusion.[285]

Thus, it appears that reperfusion can be detrimental by causing arrhythmias and can contribute to myocardial stunning, although it is not clear that this process causes necrosis of many *reversibly* injured ischemic cells.[286]

REFERENCES

DETERMINANTS OF MYOCARDIAL OXYGEN CONSUMPTION

1. Reimer, K. A., and Jennings, R. B.: Myocardial ischemia, hypoxia and infarction. *In* Fozzard, H. A., Haber, E., Jennings, R. B., et al. (eds.): The Heart and Cardiovascular System. 2nd ed. New York, Raven Press, 1991, pp. 1875–1974.
2. Braunwald, E.: Control of myocardial oxygen consumption: Physiologic and clinical considerations. Am. J. Cardiol. *27:*416, 1971.
3. Klocke, F. J., Braunwald, E., and Ross, J., Jr.: Oxygen cost of electrical activation of the heart. Circ. Res. *18:*357, 1966.
4. Loiselle, D. S.: Cardiac basal and activation metabolism. *In* Jacob, R., Just, H. J., and Holubarsch, D. H. (eds.): Cardiac Energetics: Basic Mechanisms and Clinical Implications. New York, Springer-Verlag, 1987, pp. 37–50.
5. Evans, C. L., and Matsuoka, Y.: The effect of various mechanical conditions on the gaseous metabolism and efficiency of the mammalian heart. J. Physiol. *49:*378, 1915.
6. Sarnoff, S. J., Braunwald, E., Welch, G. H., Jr., et al.: Hemodynamic determinants of oxygen consumption of the heart with special reference to the tension-time index. Am. J. Physiol. *192:*148, 1958.
7. Braunwald, E., Sarnoff, S. J., Case, R. B., et al.: Hemodynamic determinants of coronary flow: Effect of changes in aortic pressure and cardiac output on the relationship between myocardial oxygen consumption and coronary blood flow. Am. J. Physiol. *192:*157, 1958.
8. Boerth, R. C., Covell, J. W., Pool, P. E., and Ross, J., Jr.: Increased myocardial oxygen consumption and contractile state associated with increased heart rate in dogs. Circ. Res. *24:*725, 1969.
9. Rooke, G. A., and Feigl, E. O.: Work as a correlate of canine left ventricular oxygen consumption, and the problem of catecholamine oxygen wasting. Circ. Res. *50:*273, 1982.
10. Suga, H.: Ventricular energetics. Physiol. Rev. *70:*247, 1990.
10a. Kameyama, T., Asanoi, H., Ishizaka, S., et al.: Energy conversion efficiency in human left ventricle. Circulation *85:*988, 1992.
11. Takaoka, H., Takeuchi, M., Odake, M., et al.: Comparison of hemodynamic determinants for myocardial oxygen consumption under different contractile states in human ventricle. Circulation *87:*59, 1993.
12. Graham, T. P., Jr., Covell, J. W., Sonnenblick, E. H., et al.: Control of myocardial oxygen consumption: Relative influence of contractile state and tension development. J. Clin. Invest. *47:*375, 1968.
13. Vik-Mo, H., and Mjos, O. D.: Influence of free fatty acids on myocardial oxygen consumption and ischemic injury. Am. J. Cardiol. *48:*361, 1981.

REGULATION OF CORONARY BLOOD FLOW

14. Young, M. A., and Vatner, S. F.: Regulation of large coronary arteries. Circ. Res. *59:*579, 1986.
15. Provenza, D. V., and Scherlis, S.: Coronary circulation in dog's heart: Demonstration of muscle sphincters in capillaries. Circ. Res. *7:*318, 1959.
16. Olsson, R. A., and Bugni, W. J.: Coronary circulation. *In* Fozzard, H. A., Jennings, R. B., Haber, E., et al. (eds.): The Heart and Cardiovascular System. New York, Raven Press, 1986, pp. 987–1038.
17. Bache, R. J., and Hess, D. S.: Reactive hyperemia following one-beat coronary occlusions in the awake dog. Am. J. Physiol. *250:*H474, 1986.
18. Sadick, N., Dube, G. P., McHale, P. A., and Greenfield, J. C., Jr.: Metabolic mediation of single brief diastolic occlusion reactive hyperemic responses. Am. J. Physiol. *253:*H25, 1987.
19. Dube, G. P., Bemis, K. G., and Greenfield, J. C., Jr.: Distinction between metabolic and myogenic mechanisms of coronary hyperemic response to brief diastolic occlusion. Circ. Res. *68:*1313, 1991.
20. Marcus, M. L.: The coronary circulation. *In* Marcus, M. L. (ed.): The Coronary Circulation in Health and Disease. New York, McGraw-Hill Book Co., 1983, pp. 65–92.
21. Sparks, H. V., Jr., and Bardenheuer, H.: Regulation of adenosine formation by the heart. Circ. Res. *58:*193, 1986.
22. Berne, R. M.: The role of adenosine in the regulation of coronary blood flow. Circ. Res. *47:*807, 1980.
23. Belardinelli, L., Linden, J., and Berne, R. M.: The cardiac effects of adenosine. Prog. Cardiovasc. Dis. *32:*73, 1989.
24. Headrick, J. P., Ely, S. W., Matherne, G. P., and Berne, R. M.: Myocardial adenosine, flow, and metabolism during adenosine antagonism and adrenergic stimulation. Am. J. Physiol. *264:*H61, 1993.
25. Radford, M. J., McHale, P. A., Sadick, N., et al.: Effect of aminophylline on coronary reactive and functional hyperaemic response in conscious dogs. Cardiovasc. Res. *18:*377, 1984.
26. Sawmiller, D. R., Linden, J., and Berne, R. M.: Effects of xanthine amine congener on hypoxic coronary resistance and venous and epicardial adenosine concentrations. Cardiovasc. Res. *28:*604, 1994.
27. Ely, S. W., Matherne, G. P., Coleman, S. D., and Berne, R. M.: Inhibition of adenosine metabolism increases myocardial interstitial adenosine concentrations and coronary flow. J. Mol. Cell. Cardiol. *24:*1321, 1992.
28. Martin, S. E., Lenhard, S. D., Schmarkey, L. S., et al.: Adenosine regulates coronary blood flow during increased work and decreased supply. Am. J. Physiol. *264:*H1438, 1993.
29. Billman, G. E.: Effects of aminophylline on behaviorally induced coronary blood flow increases. Am. J. Physiol. *253:*H548, 1987.
30. Jones, C. E., Hurst, T. W., and Randall, J. R.: Effect of aminophylline on coronary functional hyperemia and myocardial adenosine. Am. J. Physiol. *243:*H480, 1982.
31. Rossen, J. D., Oskarsson, H., Minor, R. L., et al.: Effect of adenosine antagonism on metabolically mediated coronary vasodilation in humans. J. Am. Coll. Cardiol. *23:*1421, 1994.
32. Yamabe, H., Okumura, K., Ishizaka, H., et al.: Role of endothelium-derived nitric oxide in myocardial reactive hyperemia. Am. J. Physiol. *263:*H8, 1992.
32a. DiCarleto, P. E., and Gimbrone, M. A. Jr.: Vascular endothelium. *In* Fuster, V., Ross, R., and Topol, E. J. (eds.): Atherosclerosis and Coronary Artery Disease. Philadelphia, Lippincott-Raven, 1996, pp. 387–400.
33. Furchgott, R. F., and Zawadzki, J. V.: The obligatory role of endothelial cells in the relaxation of arterial smooth muscle by acetylcholine. Nature *288:*373, 1980.
34. Needleman, P., and Kaley, S.: Cardiac and coronary prostaglandin synthesis and function. N. Engl. J. Med. *298:*1122, 1978.
35. Vanhoutte, P. M.: Endothelium-derived relaxing and contracting factors. Adv. Nephrol. *19:*3, 1990.
36. Palmer, R. M., Ferrige, A. G., and Moncada, S.: Nitric oxide release accounts for the biological activity of endothelium-derived relaxing factor. Nature *327:*524, 1987.
37. Ignarro, L. J., Byrns, R. E., Buga, G. M., and Wood, K. S.: Endothelium-derived relaxing factor from pulmonary artery and vein possesses pharmacological and chemical properties identical to those of nitric oxide radical. Circ. Res. *61:*866, 1987.
38. Myers, P. R., Minor, R. L., Jr., Guerra, R., Bates, J. N., and Harrison, D. G.: The vasorelaxant properties of the endothelium-derived relaxing factor more closely resemble S-nitrosocysteine than nitric oxide. Nature *345:*161, 1990.
39. Palmer, R. M., Ashton, D. S., and Moncada, S.: Vascular endothelial cells synthesize nitric oxide from L-arginine. Nature *333:*664, 1988.
40. Lamas, S., Marsden, P. A., Li, G. K., et al.: Endothelial nitric oxide synthase: Molecular cloning and characterization of a distinct constitutive enzyme isoform. Proc. Natl. Acad. Sci. U.S.A. *89:*6348, 1992.
41. Vanhoutte, P. M., and Shimokawa, H.: Endothelium-derived relaxing factor and coronary vasospasm. Circulation *80:*1, 1989.
42. Martin, W., Furchgott, R. F., Villani, D., and Jothianandan, D.: Depression of contractile responses in rat aorta by spontaneously released endothelium-derived relaxing factor. J. Pharmacol. Exp. Ther. *237:*529, 1986.
43. Vane, J. R., Anggard, E. E., and Botting, R. M.: Regulatory functions of the vascular endothelium. N. Engl. J. Med. *323:*27, 1990.
44. Furchgott, R. F.: The 1989 Ulf von Euler lecture: Studies on endothelium-dependent vasodilation and the endothelium-derived relaxing factor. Acta. Physiol. Scand. *139:*257, 1990.
45. Lüscher, T. F., and Tanner, F. C.: Endothelial regulation of vascular tone and growth. Am. J. Hypertens. *6:*283S, 1993.
46. Ludmer, P. L., Selwyn, A. P., Shook, T. L., et al.: Paradoxical vasoconstriction induced by acetylcholine in atherosclerotic coronary arteries. N. Engl. J. Med. *315:*1046, 1986.
47. Lefroy, D. C., Crake, T., Uren, N. G., et al.: Effect of inhibition of nitric oxide synthesis on epicardial coronary artery caliber and coronary blood flow in humans. Circulation *88:*43, 1993.
47a. Quyyumi, A. A., Dakak, N., Andrews, N. P., et al.: Nitric oxide activity

in the human coronary circulation. Impact of risk factors for coronary atherosclerosis. J. Clin. Invest. *95:*1747, 1995.

48. Golino, P., Piscione, F., Willerson, J. T., et al.: Divergent effects of serotonin on coronary artery dimensions and blood flow in patients with coronary atherosclerosis and control patients. N. Engl. J. Med. *324:*641, 1991.
49. Matsuyama, K., Yasue, H., Okumura, K., et al.: Effects of H_1-receptor stimulation on coronary arterial diameter and coronary hemodynamics in humans. Circulation *81:*65, 1990.
50. Nabel, E. G., Selwyn, A. P., and Ganz, P.: Large coronary arteries in humans are responsive to changes in blood flow: An endothelium-dependent mechanism that fails in patients with atherosclerosis. J. Am. Coll. Cardiol. *16:*349, 1990.
51. Drexler, H., Zeiher, A. M., Wollschläger, H., et al.: Flow-dependent coronary artery dilatation in humans. Circulation *80:*466, 1989.
52. Weidinger, F. F., McLenachan, J. M., Cybulsky, M. I., et al.: Hypercholesterolemia enhances macrophage recruitment and dysfunction of regenerated endothelium after balloon injury of the rabbit iliac artery. Circulation *84:*755, 1991.
53. Shimokawa, H., Aarhus, L. L., and Vanhoutte, P. M.: Porcine coronary arteries with regenerated endothelium have a reduced endothelium-dependent responsiveness to aggregating platelets and serotonin. Circ. Res. *61:*256, 1987.
54. Fish, R. D., Nabel, E. G., Selwyn, A. P., et al.: Responses of coronary arteries of cardiac transplant patients to acetylcholine. J. Clin. Invest. *81:*21, 1988.
55. Zeiher, A. M., Drexler, H., Wollschläger, H., and Just, H.: Modulation of coronary vasomotor tone in humans: Progressive endothelial dysfunction with different early stages of coronary atherosclerosis. Circulation *83:*391, 1991.
56. McFadden, E. P., Clarke, J. G., Davies, G. J., et al.: Effect of intracoronary serotonin on coronary vessels in patients with stable angina and patients with variant angina. N. Engl. J. Med. *324:*648, 1991.
57. Cox, D. A., Vita, J. A., Treasure, C. B., et al.: Atherosclerosis impairs flow-mediated dilation of coronary arteries in humans. Circulation *80:*458, 1989.
58. Furchgott, R. F., Carvalho, M. H., Khan, M. T., and Matsunaga, K.: Evidence for endothelium-dependent vasodilation of resistance vessels by acetylcholine. Blood Vessels *24:*145, 1987.
59. Aalkjaer, C., Heagerty, A. M., Swales, J. D., and Thurston, H.: Endothelium-dependent relaxation in human subcutaneous resistance vessels. Blood Vessels *24:*85, 1987.
60. Vallance, P., Collier, J., and Moncada, S.: Effects of endothelium-derived nitric oxide on peripheral arteriolar tone in man. Lancet *2:*997, 1989.
61. Creager, M. A., Cooke, J. P., Mendelsohn, M. E., et al.: Impaired vasodilation of forearm resistance vessels in hypercholesterolemic humans. J. Clin. Invest. *86:*228, 1990.
62. Treasure, C. B., Vita, J. A., Cox, D. A., et al.: Endothelium-dependent dilation of the coronary microvasculature is impaired in dilated cardiomyopathy. Circulation *81:*772, 1990.
63. Sellke, F. W., Armstrong, M. L., and Harrison, D. G.: Endothelium-dependent vascular relaxation is abnormal in the coronary microcirculation of atherosclerotic primates. Circulation *81:*1586, 1990.
64. Zeiher, A. M., Drexler, H., Wollschläger, H., and Just, H.: Endothelial dysfunction of the coronary microvasculature is associated with impaired coronary blood flow regulation in patients with early atherosclerosis. Circulation *84:*1984, 1991.
64a. Quyyumi, A., Dakak, N., Andrews, N. P., et al.: Contribution of nitric oxide to metabolic coronary vasodilation in the human heart. Circulation *92:*320, 1995.
65. Yeung, A. C., Vekshtein, V. I., Krantz, D. S., et al.: The effect of atherosclerosis on the vasomotor response of coronary arteries to mental stress. N. Engl. J. Med. *325:*1551, 1989.
66. Gordon, J. B., Ganz, P., Nabel, E. G., et al.: Atherosclerosis influences the vasomotor response of epicardial coronary arteries to exercise. J. Clin. Invest. *83:*1946, 1989.
67. Nabel, E. G., Selwyn, A. P., and Ganz, P.: Paradoxical narrowing of atherosclerotic coronary arteries induced by increases in heart rate. Circulation *81:*850, 1990.
68. Meredith, I. T., Yeung, A. C., Weidinger, F. F., et al.: Role of impaired endothelium-dependent vasodilation in ischemic manifestations of coronary artery disease. Circulation *87:*V–56, 1993.
69. Vita, J. A., Treasure, C. B., Yeung, A. C., et al.: Patients with evidence of coronary endothelial dysfunction as assessed by acetylcholine infusion demonstrate marked increase in sensitivity to constrictor effects of catecholamines. Circulation *85:*1390, 1992.
70. Zeiher, A. M., Drexler, H., Wollschläger, H., et al.: Coronary vasomotion in response to sympathetic stimulation in humans: Importance of the functional integrity of the endothelium. J. Am. Coll. Cardiol. *14:*1181, 1989.
71. Levine, G. N., Keaney, J. F., Jr., and Vita, J. A.: Cholesterol reduction in cardiovascular disease. N. Engl. J. Med. *332:*512, 1995.
72. Fuster, V., Stein, B., Ambrose, J. A., et al.: Atherosclerotic plaque rupture and thrombosis: Evolving concepts. Circulation *82*(Suppl. II):II–47, 1990.
72a. Stary, H. C., Chandler, A. B., Dinsmore, R. E., et al.: A definition of advanced types of atherosclerotic lesions and a histological classification of atherosclerosis. Circulation *92:*1355, 1995.
73. Maseri, A., Severi, S., DeNes, D. M., et al.: "Variant" angina: One aspect of a continuous spectrum of vasospastic myocardial ischemia: Pathogenetic mechanisms, estimated incidence and clinical and coronary angiographic findings in 138 patients. Am. J. Cardiol. *42:*1019, 1978.
74. Van den Berg, E. K., Schmitz, J. M., Benedict, C. R., et al.: Transcardiac serotonin concentration is increased in selected patients with limiting angina and complex coronary lesion morphology. Circulation *79:*116, 1989.
75. Zeiher, A. M., Krause, T., Schächinger, V., et al.: Impaired endothelium-dependent vasodilatation of coronary resistance vessels is associated with exercise-induced myocardial ischemia. Circulation *91:*2345, 1995.
76. Zeiher, A. M., Goebel, H., Schächinger, V., and Ihling, C.: Tissue endothelin-1 immunoreactivity in the active coronary atherosclerotic plaque. Circulation *91:*941–947, 1995.
77. Motz, W., Vogt, M., Rabenau, O., et al.: Evidence of endothelial dysfunction in coronary resistance vessels in patients with angina pectoris and normal coronary angiograms. Am. J. Cardiol. *68:*996, 1991.
78. Quyyumi, A. A., Cannon, R. O., III, Panza, J. A., et al.: Endothelial dysfunction in patients with chest pain and normal coronary arteries. Circulation *86:*1864, 1992.
79. Egashira, K., Inour, T., Hirooka, Y., et al.: Evidence of impaired endothelium-dependent coronary vasodilatation in patients with angina pectoris and normal coronary angiograms. N. Engl. J. Med. *328:*1659, 1993.
80. Vita, J. A., Treasure, C. B., Nabel, E. G., et al.: The coronary vasomotor response to acetylcholine relates to risk factors for coronary artery disease. Circulation *81:*491, 1990.
81. Egashira, K., Inou, T., Hirooka, Y., et al.: Impaired coronary blood flow response to acetylcholine in patients with coronary risk factors and proximal atherosclerotic lesions. J. Clin. Invest. *91:*29, 1993.
81a. Zeiher, A. M., Schächinger, V., and Minners, J.: Long-term cigarette smoking impairs endothelium-dependent coronary arterial vasodilator function. Circulation *92:*1094, 1995.
82. Anderson, T. J., Meredith, I. T., Yeung, A. C., et al.: The effect of cholesterol-lowering and antioxidant therapy on endothelium-dependent coronary vasomotion. N. Engl. J. Med. *332:*488, 1995.
83. Treasure, C. B., Klein, J. L., Weintraub, W. S., et al.: Beneficial effects of cholesterol-lowering therapy on the coronary endothelium in patients with coronary artery disease. N. Engl. J. Med. *332:*481, 1995.
84. Egashira, K., Hirooka, Y., Kai, H., et al.: Reduction in serum cholesterol with pravastatin improves endothelium-dependent coronary vasomotion in patients with hypercholesterolemia. Circulation *89:*2519, 1994.
84a. Leung, W. H., Lau, C. P., and Wong, C. K.: Beneficial effect of cholesterol-lowering therapy on coronary endothelium-dependent relaxation in hypercholesterolemic patients. Lancet *341:*1496, 1993.
85. Yanagisawa, M., Kurihara, H., Kimura, S., et al.: A novel potent vasoconstrictor peptide produced by vascular endothelial cells. Nature *332:*411, 1988.
86. Seo, B., Oemar, B. S., Siebenmann, R., et al.: Both ET_A and ET_B receptors mediate contraction to endothelin-1 in human blood vessels. Circulation *89:*1203, 1994.
87. Lüscher, T. F.: Endothelin: Systemic arterial and pulmonary effects of a new peptide with potent biological properties. Am. Rev. Respir. Dis. *146:*S56, 1992.
88. Lerman, A., Edwards, B. S., Hallett, J. W., et al.: Circulating and tissue endothelin immunoreactivity in advanced atherosclerosis. N. Engl. J. Med. *325:*997, 1991.
89. Stewart, D. J., Kubac, G., Costello, K. B., and Cernacek, P.: Increased plasma endothelin-1 in the early hours of acute myocardial infarction. J. Am. Coll. Cardiol. *18:*38, 1991.
90. Wei, C. M., Lerman, A., Rodeheffer, R. J., et al.: Endothelin in human congestive heart failure. Circulation *89:*1580, 1994.
91. Lüscher, T. F., Boulanger, C. M., Dohi, Y., and Yang, Z.: Endothelium-derived contracting factors. Hypertension *19:*117, 1992.
92. Ehrenreich, H., Anderson, R. W., Fox, C. H., et al.: Endothelins, peptides with potent vasoactive properties, are produced by human macrophages. J. Exp. Med. *172:*1741, 1990.
93. Moreno, P. R., Falk, E., Palacios, I. F., et al.: Macrophage infiltration in acute coronary syndromes: Implications for plaque rupture. Circulation *90:*775, 1994.
94. Van der Wal, A. C., Becker, A. E., Van der Loos, C. M., and Das, P. K.: Site of intimal rupture or erosion of thrombosed coronary atherosclerotic plaques is characterized by an inflammatory process irrespective of the dominant plaque morphology. Circulation *89:*36, 1994.
95. Lüscher, T. F.: Endothelin, endothelin receptors, and endothelin antagonists. Curr. Opin. Nephrol. Hypertens. *3:*92, 1994.
96. Scandinavian Simvastatin Survival Study Group: Randomised trial of cholesterol lowering in 4444 patients with coronary heart disease: The Scandinavian Simvastatin Survival Study (4S). Lancet *344:*1383, 1994.
97. Johnson, P. C.: Autoregulation of blood flow. Circ. Res. *59:*483, 1986.
98. Olsson, R. A., Bunger, R., and Spaan, J. A. E.: Coronary circulation. *In* Fozzard, H. A., Haber, E., Jennings, R. B., et al. (eds.): The Heart and Cardiovascular System. 2nd ed. New York, Raven Press, 1991, pp. 1392–1426.
99. Harrison, D. G., Florentine, M. S., Brooks, L. A., et al.: The effect of hypertension and left ventricular hypertrophy on the lower range of coronary autoregulation. Circulation *77:*1108, 1988.
100. Rouleau, J., Boerboom, L. E., Surjadhana, A., and Hoffman, J. I. E.: The role of autoregulation and tissue diastolic pressures in the transmural distribution of left ventricular blood flow in anesthetized dogs. Circ. Res. *45:*804, 1979.

101. Hoffman, J. I. E.: Maximal coronary flow and the concept of coronary vascular reserve. Circulation *70:*153, 1984.
102. Marcus, M. L.: The coronary circulation. *In* Marcus, M. L. (ed.): The Coronary Circulation in Health and Disease. New York, McGraw-Hill Book Co., 1983, pp. 93–112.
103. Smith, T. P., Jr., and Canty, J. M., Jr.: Modulation of coronary autoregulatory responses by nitric oxide: Evidence for flow-dependent resistance adjustments in conscious dogs. Circ. Res. *73:*232, 1993.
104. Ueeda, M., Silvia, S. K., and Olsson, R. A.: Nitric oxide modulates coronary autoregulation in the guinea pig. Circ. Res. *70:*1296, 1992.
105. Lansman, J. B., Hallam, T. J., and Rink, T. J.: Single stretch-activated ion channels in vascular endothelial cells as mechanotransducers? Nature *325:*811, 1987.
106. Oien, A. H., and Aukland, K.: A mathematical analysis of the myogenic hypothesis with special reference to autoregulation of renal blood flow. Circ. Res. *52:*241, 1983.
107. Bayliss, W. M.: On the local reaction of the arterial wall to changes of internal pressure. J. Physiol. (Lond.) *28:*220, 1902.
108. Rajagopalan, S., Dube, S., and Canty, J. M., Jr.: Regulation of coronary diameter by myogenic mechanisms in arterial microvessels greater than 100 microns in diameter. Am. J. Physiol. *268:*H788, 1995.
109. Chilian, W. M., and Marcus, M. L.: Effects of coronary and extravascular pressure on intramyocardial and epicardial blood velocity. Am. J. Physiol. *248:*H170, 1985.
110. Marcus, M. L., and Harrison, D. G.: Physiologic basis for myocardial perfusion imaging. *In* Schelbert, H. R., Skorton, D. J., and Wolf, G. L. (eds.): Cardiac Imaging, A Companion to Braunwald's Heart Disease. Philadelphia, W.B. Saunders Co., 1991, pp. 8–23.
111. Berne, R. M., and Rubio, R.: Coronary circulation. *In* Berne, R. M., Speralakis, N., and Geiger, S. R. (eds.): Handbook of Physiology: Section 2, The Cardiovascular System. Bethesda, American Physiologic Society, 1979, p. 897.
111a. Zhang, J., Duncker, D. J., Ya, X., et al.: Effect of left ventricular hypertrophy secondary to chronic pressure overload on transmural myocardial 2-deoxyglucose uptake. Circulation *92:*1274, 1995.
112. Braunwald, E., Ross, J., Jr., and Sonnenblick, E. H.: Regulation of coronary blood flow. *In* Mechanisms of Contraction of the Normal and Failing Heart, 2nd ed. Boston, Little, Brown, and Co., 1976, p. 200.
113. Austin, R. E., Jr., Smedira, N. G., Squiers, T. M., and Hoffman, J. I.: Influence of cardiac contraction and coronary vasomotor tone on regional myocardial blood flow. Am. J. Physiol. *266:*H2542, 1994.
114. Farhi, E. R., Klocke, F. J., Mates, R. E., et al.: Tone-dependent waterfall behavior during venous pressure elevation in isolated canine hearts. Circ. Res. *68:*392, 1991.
115. Hoffman, J. I., and Spaan, J. A.: Pressure-flow relations in coronary circulation. Physiol. Rev. *70:*331, 1990.
116. Chilian, W. M.: Microvascular pressures and resistances in the left ventricular subepicardium and subendocardium. Circ. Res. *69:*561, 1991.
117. Klocke, F. J.: Coronary blood flow in man. Prog. Cardiovasc. Dis. *19:*117, 1976.
118. Weiss, H. R., Neubauer, J. A., Lipp, J. A., and Sinha, A. K.: Quantitative determination of regional oxygen consumption in the dog heart. Circ. Res. *42:*394, 1978.
119. Hoffman, J. I.: Transmural myocardial perfusion. Prog. Cardiovasc. Dis. *29:*429, 1987.
120. Gallagher, K. P., Osakada, G., Matsuzaki, M., et al.: Myocardial blood flow and function with critical coronary stenosis in exercising dogs. Am. J. Physiol. *243:*H698, 1982.
121. Bache, R. J., McHale, P. A., and Greenfield, J. C., Jr.: Transmural myocardial perfusion during restricted coronary inflow in the awake dog. Am. J. Physiol. *232:*H645, 1977.
122. Ball, R. M., and Bache, R. J.: Distribution of myocardial blood flow in the exercising dog with restricted coronary artery inflow. Circ. Res. *38:*60, 1976.
123. Rembert, J. C., Boyd, L. M., Watkinson, W. P., and Greenfield, J. C., Jr.: Effect of adenosine on transmural myocardial blood flow distribution in the awake dog. Am. J. Physiol. *239:*H7, 1980.
124. Gewirtz, H., Williams, D. O., Ohley, W. H., and Most, A. S.: Influence of coronary vasodilation on the transmural distribution of myocardial blood flow distal to a severe fixed coronary artery stenosis. Am. Heart J. *106:*674, 1983.
125. O'Keefe, D. D., Hoffman, J. I., Cheitlin, R., et al.: Coronary blood flow in experimental canine left ventricular hypertrophy. Circ. Res. *43:*43, 1978.
126. Hittinger, L., Shannon, R. P., Bishop, S. P., et al.: Subendocardial exhaustion of blood flow reserve and increased fibrosis in conscious dogs with heart failure. Circ. Res. *65:*971, 1989.
127. Shannon, R. P., Komamura, K., Shen, Y. T., et al.: Impaired regional subendocardial coronary flow reserve in conscious dogs with pacing-induced heart failure. Am. J. Physiol. *265:*H801, 1993.
128. Nathan, H. J., and Feigl, E. O.: Adrenergic vasoconstriction lessens transmural steal during coronary hypoperfusion. Am. J. Physiol. *250:*H645, 1986.
129. Heller, G. V., Barbour, M. M., Dweik, R. B., et al.: Effects of intravenous theophylline on exercise-induced myocardial ischemia. I. Impact on the ischemic threshold. J. Am. Coll. Cardiol. *21:*1075, 1993.
130. Kumada, T., Gallagher, K. P., Shirato, K., et al.: Reduction of exercise-induced regional myocardial dysfunction by propranolol. Circ. Res. *46:*190, 1980.
131. Vatner, S. F., Baig, H., Manders, W. T., et al.: Effects of propranolol on regional myocardial function, electrograms, and blood flow in conscious dogs with myocardial ischemia. J. Clin. Invest. *60:*353, 1977.
132. Vatner, S. F.: Alpha-adrenergic tone in the coronary circulation of the concious dog. Fed. Proc. *43:*2867, 1984.
133. Woodman, O. L., and Vatner, S. F.: Coronary vasoconstriction mediated by $alpha_1$ and $alpha_2$ adrenoceptors in conscious dogs. Am. J. Physiol. *253:*H388, 1987.
134. Young, M. A., Vatner, D. E., Knight, D. R., et al.: Alpha-adrenergic vasoconstriction and receptor subtypes in large coronary arteries of calves. Am. J. Physiol. *255:*H1452, 1988.
135. Morgan, K. G., Papageorgiou, P., and Jiang, M. J.: Pathophysiologic role of calcium in the development of vascular smooth muscle tone. Am. J. Cardiol. *64:*35F, 1989.
136. Johns, A., Leitjen, P., Yamamoto, H., et al.: Calcium regulation in vascular smooth muscle contractility. Am. J. Cardiol. *59:*18A, 1987.
137. Rinkema, L. E., Thomas, J. X., Jr., and Randall, W. C.: Regional coronary vasoconstriction in response to stimulation of stellate ganglia. Am. J. Physiol. *243:*H410, 1982.
138. Murray, P. A., Lavallee, M., and Vatner, S. F.: Alpha-adrenergic–mediated reduction in coronary blood flow secondary to carotid chemoreceptor reflex activation in conscious dogs. Circ. Res. *54:*96, 1984.
139. Feldman, R. D., Christy, J. P., Paul, S. T., and Harrison, D. G.: Beta-adrenergic receptors on canine coronary collateral vessels: Characterization and function. Am. J. Physiol. *257:*H1634, 1989.
140. Vatner, S. F., and Hintze, T. H.: Mechanism of constriction of large coronary arteries by beta-adrenergic receptor blockade. Circ. Res. *53:*389, 1983.
141. Cox, D. A., Hintze, T. H., and Vatner, S. F.: Effects of acetylcholine on large and small coronary arteries in conscious dogs. J. Pharmacol. Exp. Ther. *225:*764, 1983.
142. Vatner, S. F., Higgins, C. B., and Braunwald, E.: Effects of norepinephrine on coronary circulation and left ventricular dynamics in the conscious dog. Circ. Res. *34:*812, 1974.
143. Kern, M. J., Horowitz, J. D., Ganz, P., et al.: Attenuation of coronary vascular resistance by selective $alpha_1$-adrenergic blockade in patients with coronary artery disease. J. Am. Coll. Cardiol. *5:*840, 1985.
144. Winniford, M. D., Jansen, D. E., Reynolds, G. A., et al.: Cigarette smoking–induced coronary vasoconstriction in atherosclerotic coronary artery disease and its prevention by calcium antagonists and nitroglycerin. Am. J. Cardiol. *59:*203, 1987.
145. Hackett, J. G., Abboud, F. M., Mark, A. L., et al.: Coronary vascular responses to stimulation of chemoreceptors and baroreceptors. Circ. Res. *31:*8, 1972.
146. Higgins, C. B., Vatner, S. F., and Braunwald, E.: Parasympathetic control of the heart. Pharmacol. Rev. *25:*119, 1973.
147. Vatner, S. F., Franklin, D., Van Citters, R. L., and Braunwald, E.: Effects of carotid sinus nerve stimulation on the coronary circulation of conscious dogs. Circ. Res. *27:*11, 1970.
148. Heyndrickx, G. R., Muylaert, P., and Pannier, J. L.: Alpha-adrenergic control of oxygen delivery to myocardium during exercise in conscious dog. Am. J. Physiol. *242:*H805, 1982.
149. Laxson, D. D., Dai, X. Z., Homans, D. C., and Bache, R. J.: The role of $alpha_1$- and $alpha_2$-adrenergic receptors in mediation of coronary vasoconstriction in hypoperfused ischemic myocardium during exercise. Circ. Res. *65:*1688, 1989.
150. Heusch, G.: Alpha-adrenergic mechanisms in myocardial ischemia. Circulation *81:*1, 1990.
151. Feigl, E. O.: Reflex parasympathetic coronary vasodilation elicited from cardiac receptors in the dog. Circ. Res. *37:*175, 1975.
152. Pitetti, K. H., Iwamoto, G. A., Mitchell, J. H., and Ordway, G. A.: Stimulating somatic afferent fibers alters coronary arterial resistance. Am. J. Physiol. *256:*R1331, 1989.
153. Jarisch, A., and Zotterman, Y.: Depressor reflexes from the heart. Acta Physiol. Scand. *16:*31, 1948.
154. Brown, B. G., Lee, A. B., Bolson, E. L., and Dodge, H. T.: Reflex constriction of significant coronary stenosis as a mechanism contributing to ischemic left ventricular dysfunction during isometric exercise. Circulation *70:*18, 1984.
155. Brachfeld, N., Monroe, R. G., and Gorlin, R.: Effects of pericoronary denervation on coronary hemodynamics. Am. J. Physiol. *199:*174, 1960.
156. Macho, P., and Vatner, S. F.: Effects of prazosin on coronary and left ventricular dynamics in conscious dogs. Circulation *65:*1186, 1982.
157. Chierchia, S., Davies, G., Berkenboom, G., et al.: Alpha-adrenergic receptors and coronary spasm: An elusive link. Circulation *69:*8, 1984.
158. Galassi, A. R., Kaski, J. C., Pupita, G., et al.: Lack of evidence for alpha-adrenergic receptor mediated mechanisms in the genesis of ischemia in syndrome X. Am. J. Cardiol. *64:*264, 1989.
159. Gould, L., Reddy, C. V., and Gombrecht, R. F.: Oral phentolamine in angina pectoris. Jpn. Heart J. *14:*393, 1973.
160. Berkenboom, G. M., Abramowicz, M., Vandermoten, P., and Degre, S. G.: Role of alpha adrenergic coronary tone in exercise-induced angina pectoris. Am. J. Cardiol. *57:*195, 1986.
161. Hayes, S. N., Moyer, T. P., Morley, D., and Bove, A. A.: Intravenous cocaine causes epicardial coronary vasoconstriction in the intact dog. Am. Heart J. *121:*1639, 1991.
162. Lange, R. A., Cigarroa, R. G., Yancy, C. W., et al.: Cocaine-induced coronary-artery vasoconstriction. N. Engl. J. Med. *321:*1557, 1989.
163. Brown, B. G., Bolson, E. L., and Dodge, H. T.: Dynamic mechanisms in human coronary stenosis. Circulation *70:*917, 1984.
164. Young, D. F., Cholvin, N. R., and Roth, A. C.: Pressure drop across artificially induced stenoses in the femoral arteries of dogs. Circ. Res. *36:*735, 1975.
165. Klocke, F. J.: Measurements of coronary blood flow and degree of ste-

nosis: Current clinical implications and continuing uncertainties. J. Am. Coll. Cardiol. *1*:31, 1983.
166. Gould, K. L.: Dynamic coronary stenosis. Am. J. Cardiol. *45*:286, 1980.
167. Ball, R. M., Bache, R. J., Cobb, F. R., and Greenfield, J. C., Jr.: Regional myocardial blood flow during graded treadmill exercise in the dog. J. Clin. Invest. *55*:43, 1975.
168. Bache, R. J., Vrobel, T. R., Ring, W. S., et al.: Regional myocardial blood flow during exercise in dogs with chronic left ventricular hypertrophy. Circ. Res. *48*:76, 1981.
169. Geha, A. S., and Baue, A. E.: Graded coronary stenosis and coronary flow during acute normovolemic anemia. World J. Surg. *2*:645, 1978.
170. Gould, K. L.: Pressure-flow characteristics of coronary stenoses in unsedated dogs at rest and during coronary vasodilation. Circ. Res. *43*:242–253, 1978.
171. Goldberg, S. J.: The principles of pressure drop in long segment stenosis. Herz *11*:291, 1986.
172. Freudenberg, H., and Lichtlen, P. R.: The normal wall segment in coronary stenosis—a postmortem study. Z. Kardiol. *70*:863, 1981.
173. Brown, B. G., Bolson, E. L., Petersen, R. B., et al.: The mechanisms of nitroglycerin action: Stenosis vasodilation as a major component of the drug response. Circulation *64*:1089, 1981.
174. Schwartz, J. S., Bache, R. J.: Effect of arteriolar dilation on coronary artery diameter distal to coronary stenoses. Am. J. Physiol. *249*:H981, 1985.
175. Santamore, W. P., and Walinsky, P.: Altered coronary flow response to vasoactive drugs in the presence of coronary arterial stenosis in the dog. Am. J. Cardiol. *45*:276, 1980.
176. Brown, B. G., Josephson, M. A., Petersen, R. B., et al.: Intravenous dipyridamole combined with isometric handgrip for near maximal acute increases in coronary flow in patients with coronary artery disease. Am. J. Cardiol. *48*:1077, 1981.
177. Klocke, F. J.: Measurements of coronary flow reserve: Defining pathophysiology versus making decisions about patient care. Circulation *76*:1183, 1987.
178. Gould, K. L., and Lipscomb, K.: Effects of coronary stenoses on coronary flow reserve and resistance. Am. J. Cardiol. *34*:48, 1974.
179. Wilson, R. F., Marcus, M. L., and White, C. W.: Prediction of the physiologic significance of coronary arterial lesions by quantitative lesion geometry in patients with limited coronary artery disease. Circulation *75*:723, 1987.
180. Donohue, T. J., Kern, M. J., Aguirre, F. V., et al.: Assessing the hemodynamic significance of coronary artery stenoses: Analysis of translesional pressure-flow velocity relationships in patients. J. Am. Coll. Cardiol. *22*:449, 1993.
181. Marcus, M., Wright, C., Doty, D., et al.: Measurements of coronary velocity and reactive hyperemia in the coronary circulation of humans. Circ. Res. *49*:877, 1981.
182. Vatner, S. F., Higgins, C. B., Franklin, D., and Braunwald, E.: Role of tachycardia in mediating the coronary hemodynamic response to severe exercise. J. Appl. Physiol. *32*:380, 1972.
183. Nahser, P. J., Brown, R. E., Oskarsson, H., et al.: Maximal coronary flow reserve and metabolic coronary vasodilation in patients with diabetes mellitus. Circulation *91*:635, 1995.
184. Doucette, J. W., Corl, P. D., Payne, H. M., et al.: Validation of a Doppler guide wire for intravascular measurement of coronary artery flow velocity. Circulation *85*:1899, 1992.
185. DiMario, C., Gil, R., and Serruys, P. W.: Long-term reproducibility of coronary flow velocity measurements in patients with coronary artery disease. Am. J. Cardiol. *75*:1177, 1995.
186. Kern, M. J., and Anderson, H. V. (eds.): A symposium: The clinical applications of the intracoronary Doppler guidewire flow velocity in patients: Understanding blood flow beyond the coronary stenosis. Am. J. Cardiol. *71*:1D–86D, 1993.
187. White, C. W., Wright, C. B., Doty, D. B., et al.: Does visual interpretation of the coronary arteriogram predict the physiological importance of a coronary stenosis? N. Engl. J. Med. *310*:819, 1984.
188. Reiber, J. H. C., Koning, G., Van der Zwet, P. M. J., et al.: Assessment of myocardial flow reserve with the DCI. Medica Mundi *38*:81, 1993.
189. Ganz, W., Tamura, K., Marcus, H. S., et al.: Measurement of coronary sinus blood flow by continuous thermodilution in man. Circulation *44*:181, 1971.
190. Marcus, M. L., Schelbert, H. R., Skorton, D. J., and Wolf, G. I. (eds.): Cardiac Imaging. Philadelphia, W. B. Saunders Co., 1991.
191. Gould, K. L., Kirkeeide, R. L., and Buchi, M.: Coronary flow reserve as a physiologic measure of stenosis severity. J. Am. Coll. Cardiol. *15*:459, 1990.
192. Little, W. C., Constantinescu, M., Applegate, R. J., et al.: Can coronary angiography predict the site of a subsequent myocardial infarction in patients with mild to moderate coronary artery disease? Circulation *78*:1157–1166, 1988.
193. Ambrose, J. A., Tannenbaum, M. A., Alexopoulos, D., et al.: Angiographic progression of coronary artery disease and the development of myocardial infarction. J. Am. Coll. Cardiol. *12*:56, 1988.
194. Giroud, D., Li, J. M., Urban, P., et al.: Relation of the site of acute myocardial infarction to the most severe coronary arterial stenosis at prior angiography. Am. J. Cardiol. *69*:729, 1992.
195. Davies, M. J., and Thomas, A. C.: Plaque fissuring: The cause of acute myocardial infarction, sudden ischaemic death and crescendo angina. Br. Heart J. *53*:363, 1985.
196. Kanazawa, T.: Coronary collateral circulation. Jpn. Circ. J. *58*:151, 1994.
197. Schaper, W., Gorge, G., Winkler, B., and Schaper, J.: The collateral circulation of the heart. Prog. Cardiovasc. Dis. *31*:57, 1988.
198. Goldstein, R. E., Michaelis, L. L., Morrow, A. G., and Epstein, S. E.: Coronary collateral function in patients without occlusive coronary artery disease. Circulation *51*:118, 1975.
199. Marcus, M. L., and Harrison, D. G.: Physiologic basis for myocardial perfusion imaging. *In* Schelbert, H. R., Skorton, D. J., and Wolf, G. L. (eds.): Cardiac Imaging, A Companion to Braunwald's Heart Disease. Philadelphia, W. B. Saunders Co., 1991, pp. 8–23.
200. Marcus, M. L.: The coronary circulation. *In* Marcus, M. L. (ed.): The Coronary Circulation in Health and Disease. New York, McGraw-Hill Book Co., 1983, pp. 221–241.
201. Schaper, W.: New paradigms for collateral vessel growth. Basic Res. Cardiol. *88*:193–198, 1993.
202. Pasyk, S., Schaper, W., Schaper, J., et al.: DNA synthesis in coronary collaterals after coronary artery occlusion in conscious dog. Am. J. Physiol. *242*:H1031, 1982.
203. Schaper, W., and Pasyk, S.: Influence of collateral flow on the ischemic tolerance of the heart following acute and subacute coronary occlusion. Circulation *53*(Suppl. 1):57, 1976.
204. Harrison, D. G., and Simonetti, I.: Neurohumoral regulation of collateral perfusion. Circulation *83*(Suppl. 3):62, 1991.
205. Nagel, T., Resnick, N., Atkinson, W. J., et al.: Shear stress selectively upregulates intercellular adhesion molecule-1 expression in cultured human vascular endothelial cells. J. Clin. Invest. *94*:885, 1994.
206. Knoll, R., Arras, M., Zimmermann, R., et al.: Changes in gene expression following short coronary occlusions studied in porcine hearts with run-on assays. Cardiovasc. Res. *28*:1062, 1994.
207. Rentrop, K. P., Thornton, J. C., Feit, F., and Van Buskirk, M.: Determinants and protective potential of coronary arterial collaterals as assessed by an angioplasty model. Am. J. Cardiol. *61*:677, 1988.
208. Schaper, W.: Influence of physical exercise on coronary collateral blood flow in chronic experimental two-vessel occlusion. Circulation *65*:905–912, 1982.
209. Pupita, G., Mazzara, D., Centanni, M., et al.: Ischemia in collateral-dependent myocardium: Effects of nifedipine and diltiazem in man. Am. Heart J. *126*:86, 1993.
210. Cohen, M. V.: Lack of effect of propranolol on canine coronary collateral development during progressive coronary stenosis and occlusion. Cardiovasc. Res. *27*:249–254, 1993.
211. Hollenberg, N.: Serotonin, atherosclerosis, and collateral vessel spasm. Am. J. Hypertens. *1*:312S–316S, 1988.
212. Unger, E. F., Banai, S., Shou, M., et al.: Basic fibroblast growth factor enhances myocardial collateral flow in a canine model. Am. J. Physiol. *266*:H1588, 1994.
213. Lazarous, D. F., Scheinowitz, M., Shou, M., et al.: Effects of chronic systemic administration of basic fibroblast growth factor on collateral development in the canine heart. Circulation *91*:145, 1995.
214. Bauters, C., Asahara, T., Zheng, L. P., et al.: Physiological assessment of augmented vascularity induced by VEGF in ischemic rabbit hindlimb. Am. J. Physiol. *267*:H1263, 1994.
215. Takeshita, S., Pu, L. Q., Stein, L. A., et al.: Intramuscular administration of vascular endothelial growth factor induces dose-dependent collateral augmentation in a rabbit model of chronic limb ischemia. Circulation *90*(Suppl. II):228, 1994.
216. Banai, S., Jaklitsch, M. T., Shou, M., et al.: Angiogenic-induced enhancement of collateral blood flow to ischemic myocardium by vascular endothelial growth factor in dogs. Circulation *89*:2183, 1994.
217. Carroll, S. M., White, F. C., Roth, D. M., and Bloor, C. M.: Heparin accelerates coronary collateral development in a porcine model of coronary artery occlusion. Circulation *88*:198, 1993.
218. Sasayama, S., and Fujita, M.: Recent insights into coronary collateral circulation. Circulation *85*:1197, 1992.
219. Cohen, M. V., Chukwuogo, N., and Yarlagadda, A.: Heparin does not stimulate coronary-collateral growth in a canine model of progressive coronary-artery narrowing and occlusion. Am. J. Med. Sci. *306*:75, 1993.
219a. Frank, M. W., Harris, K. R., Ahlin, K. A., and Klocke, F. J.: Endothelium-derived relaxing factor (nitric oxide) has a tonic vasodilating action on coronary collateral vessels. J. Am. Coll. Cardiol. *27*:658, 1996.
220. Altman, J. D., Dulas, D., Pavek, T., et al.: Endothelial function in well-developed canine coronary collateral vessels. Am. J. Physiol. *264*:H567, 1993.
221. Altman, J. D., Dulas, D., Pavek, T., and Bache, R. J.: Effect of aspirin on coronary collateral blood flow. Circulation *87*:583, 1993.
222. Randall, M. D., and Griffith, T. M.: EDRF plays central role in collateral flow after arterial occlusion in rabbit ear. Am. J. Physiol. *263*:H752, 1992.
223. Schwarz, F., Flameng, W., Ensslen, R., et al.: Effect of collaterals on left ventricular function at rest and during stress. Am. Heart J. *95*:570, 1978.
224. Rentrop, K. P., Cohen, M., Blanke, H., and Phillips, R. A.: Changes in collateral channel filling immediately after controlled coronary artery occlusion by an angioplasty balloon in human subjects. J. Am. Coll. Cardiol. *5*:587, 1985.
225. Cohen, M., and Rentrop, K. P.: Limitation of myocardial ischemia by collateral circulation during sudden controlled coronary artery occlusion in human subjects: A prospective study. Circulation *74*:469, 1986.
226. Mizuno, K., Horiuchi, K., Matui, H., et al.: Role of coronary collateral vessels during transient coronary occlusion during angioplasty assessed by hemodynamic, electrocardiographic and metabolic changes. J. Am. Coll. Cardiol. *12*:624, 1988.
227. Schwartz, H., Leiboff, R. L., Katz, R. J., et al.: Arteriographic predictors of spontaneous improvement in left ventricular function after myocardial infarction. Circulation *71*:466, 1985.

228. Sabia, P. J., Powers, E. R., Ragosta, M., et al.: An association between collateral blood flow and myocardial viability in patients with recent myocardial infarction. N. Engl. J. Med. *327*:1825–1831, 1992.
229. Franklin, B. A.: Exercise training and coronary collateral circulation. Med. Sci. Sports Exerc. *23*:648–653, 1991.
230. McKirnan, M. D., and Bloor, C. M.: Clinical significance of coronary vascular adaptations to exercise training. Med. Sci. Sports Exerc. *26*:1262, 1994.
231. Hellerstein, H. K.: Acceleration of collaterals due to physical activity—dogma or fact. Bibl. Cardiol. *36*:125, 1977.
232. Ferguson, R. J., Petitclerc, R., Choquette, G., et al.: Effect of physical training on treadmill exercise capacity, collateral circulation and progression of coronary disease. Am. J. Cardiol. *34*:764, 1974.
233. Fujita, M., Sasayama, S., Asanoi, H., et al.: Improvement of treadmill capacity and collateral circulation as a result of exercise with heparin pretreatment in patients with effort angina. Circulation *77*:1022, 1988.
234. Ejiri, M., Fujita, M., Miwa, K., et al.: Effects of heparin treatment on collateral development and regional myocardial function in acute myocardial infarction. Am. Heart J. *119*:248, 1990.
235. Isner, J. M., and Feldman, L. J.: Gene therapy for arterial disease. Lancet *344*:1653, 1994.
236. Isner, J. M., Walsh, K., Symes, J., et al.: Arterial gene therapy for therapeutic angiogenesis in patients with peripheral artery disease. Circulation *91*:2687, 1995.

CONSEQUENCES OF MYOCARDIAL ISCHEMIA

237. Tennant, R., and Wiggers, C. J.: The effect of coronary occlusion on myocardial contractions. Am. J. Physiol. *112*:351, 1935.
238. Heyndrickx, G. R., Millard, R. W., McRitchie, R. J., et al.: Regional myocardial functional and electrophysiological alterations after brief coronary occlusion in conscious dogs. J. Clin. Invest. *56*:978, 1975.
239. Braunwald, E., and Kloner, R. A.: The stunned myocardium: Prolonged, postischemic ventricular dysfunction. Circulation *66*:1146, 1982.
240. Ellis, S. G., Henschke, C. I., Sandor, T., et al.: Time course of functional and biochemical recovery of myocardium salvaged by reperfusion. J. Am. Coll. Cardiol. *1*:1047, 1983.
241. Thaulow, E., Guth, B. D., Heusch, G., et al.: Characteristics of regional myocardial stunning after exercise in dogs with chronic coronary stenosis. Am. J. Physiol. *257*:H113, 1989.
242. Fournier, C., Boujon, B., Hebert, J., et al.: Stunned myocardium following coronary spasm. Am. Heart J. *121*:593, 1991.
243. Charlat, M. L., O'Neill, P. G., Hartley, C. J., et al.: Prolonged abnormalities of left ventricular diastolic wall thinning in the "stunned" myocardium in conscious dogs: Time course and relation to systolic function. J. Am. Coll. Cardiol. *13*:185, 1989.
244. Braunwald, E.: The stunned myocardium: Newer insights into mechanisms and clinical implications. J. Thorac. Cardiovasc. Surg. *100*:310, 1990.
245. Patel, B., Kloner, R. A., Przyklenk, K., and Braunwald, E.: Postischemic myocardial "stunning": A clinically relevant phenomenon. Ann. Intern. Med. *108*:626, 1988.
246. Zimmermann, R., Mall, G., Rauch, B., et al.: Residual ^{201}Tl activity in irreversible defects as a marker of myocardial viability: Clinicopathological study. Circulation *91*:1016, 1995.
247. Bolli, R., Patel, B. S., Hartley, C. J., et al.: Nonuniform transmural recovery of contractile function in the "stunned" myocardium. Am. J. Physiol. *257*:H375, 1989.
248. Preuss, K. C., Gross, G. J., Brooks, H. L., and Warltier, D. C.: Time course of recovery of "stunned" myocardium following variable periods of ischemia in conscious and anesthetized dogs. Am. Heart J. *114*:696, 1987.
249. Marban, E.: Myocardial stunning and hibernation: The physiology behind the colloquialisms. Circulation *83*:681, 1991.
250. Bolli, R., Triana, J. F., and Jeroudi, M. O.: Prolonged impairment of coronary vasodilation after reversible ischemia: Evidence for microvascular "stunning." Circ. Res. *67*:332, 1990.
251. Ellis, S. G., Wynne, J., Braunwald, E., et al.: Response of reperfusion-salvaged stunned myocardium to inotropic stimulation. Am. Heart J. *107*:13, 1984.
252. Arnold, J. M. O., Braunwald, E., Sandor, T., and Kloner, R. A.: Inotropic stimulation of reperfused myocardium with dopamine: Effects on infarct size and myocardial function. J. Am. Coll. Cardiol. *6*:1026, 1985.
253. Heusch, G., Schafer, S., and Kroger, K.: Recruitment of inotropic reserve in "stunned" myocardium by the cardiotonic agent AR-L 57. Basic Res. Cardiol. *83*:602, 1988.
254. Lazdunski, M., Frelin, C., and Frelin, P.: The sodium/hydrogen exchange system in cardiac cells: Its biochemical and pharmacological properties and its role in regulating internal concentrations of sodium and internal pH. J. Mol. Cell. Cardiol. *17*:1029, 1985.
255. Tani, M., and Neely, J. R.: Role of intracellular Na^+ in Ca^{2+} overload and depressed recovery of ventricular function of reperfused ischemic rat hearts: Possible involvement of H^+-Na^+ and Na^+-Ca^{2+} exchange. Circ. Res. *65*:1045, 1989.
256. Krause, S. M., Jacobus, W. E., and Becker, L. C.: Alterations in cardiac sarcoplasmic reticulum calcium transport in the postischemic "stunned" myocardium. Circ. Res. *65*:526, 1989.
257. Przyklenk, K., and Kloner, R. A.: Superoxide dismutase plus catalase improve contractile function in the canine model of the "stunned" myocardium. Circ. Res. *58*:148, 1986.
258. Bolli, R., Patel, B. S., Jeroudi, M. O., et al.: Iron-mediated radical reactions upon reperfusion contribute to myocardial "stunning." Am. J. Physiol. *259*:H1901, 1990.
259. Koerner, J. E., Anderson, B. A., and Dage, R. C.: Protection against postischemic myocardial dysfunction in anesthetized rabbits with scavengers of oxygen-derived free radicals: Superoxide dismutase plus catalase, N-2-mercaptopropionyl glycine and captopril. J. Cardiovasc. Pharmacol. *17*:185, 1991.
260. Dage, R. C., Anderson, B. A., Mao, S. J. T., and Koerner, J. E.: Probucol reduces myocardial dysfunction during reperfusion after short-term ischemia in rabbit heart. J. Cardiovasc. Pharmacol. *17*:158, 1991.
261. Bolli, R.: Postischemic myocardial stunning. *In* Yellon, D. M., and Jennings, R. B. (eds.): Myocardial Protection: The Pathophysiology of Reperfusion and Reperfusion Injury. New York, Raven Press, 1992.
262. Hearse, D. J.: Stunning: A radical re-view. Cardiovasc. Drugs Ther. *5*:853, 1991.
263. Jennings, R. B., and Reimer, K. A.: Factors involved in salvaging ischemic myocardium: Effects of reperfusion of arterial blood. Circulation *68*(Suppl. I):I-25, 1983.
264. Visner, M. S., Arentzen, C. E., Parrish, D. G., et al.: Effects of global ischemia on the diastolic properties of the left ventricle in the conscious dog. Circulation *71*:610, 1985.
265. Momomura, S. I., Ferguson, J. J., Miller, M. J., et al.: Regional myocardial blood flow and left ventricular diastolic properties in pacing-induced ischemia. J. Am. Coll. Cardiol. *17*:781, 1991.
266. Yin, F. C. P.: Ventricular wall stress. Circ. Res. *49*:829, 1981.
267. Dunn, R. B., and Griggs, D. M.: Transmural gradients in ventricular tissue metabolites produced by stopping coronary blood flow in the dog. Circ. Res. *37*:438, 1975.
268. Moss, A. J.: Intramyocardial oxygen tension. Cardiovasc. Res. *2*:314, 1968.
269. Weiss, H. R., and Sinha, A. K.: Regional oxygen saturation of small arteries and veins in the canine myocardium. Circ. Res. *42*:119, 1978.
269a. Reimer, K. A., and Jennings, R. B.: The "wavefront phenomenon" of myocardial ischemic cell death. II. Transmural progression of necrosis within the framework of ischemic bed size (myocardium at risk) and collateral flow. Lab. Invest. *40*:633, 1979.
270. Naka, Y., Stern, D. M., and Pinsky, D. J.: The pathophysiology of myocardial ischemia, necrosis, and reperfusion. *In* Fuster, V., Ross, R., and Topol, E. J. (eds.): Atherosclerosis and Coronary Artery Disease. Philadelphia, Lippincott-Raven, 1996, pp. 807–818.
271. Ganz, W., Watanabe, I., Kanamasa, K., et al.: Does reperfusion extend necrosis? A study in a single territory of myocardial ischemia—half reperfused and half not reperfused. Circulation *82*:1020, 1990.
272. Lee, J. T., Ideker, R. E., and Reimer, K. A.: Myocardial infarct size and location in relation to the coronary vascular bed at risk in man. Circulation *64*:526, 1981.

EFFECTS OF ISCHEMIA ON MYOCARDIAL METABOLISM

273. Jennings, R. B., Reimer, K. A., Hill, M. L., and Mayer, S. E.: Total ischemia in dog hearts in vitro. I. Comparison of high energy phosphate production, utilization and depletion, and of adenine nucleotide catabolism in total ischemia in vitro vs. severe ischemia in vivo. Circ. Res. *49*:892, 1981.
274. Marban, E., Koretsune, Y, Corretti, M., et al.: Calcium and its role in myocardial cell injury during ischemia and reperfusion. Circulation *80*(Suppl. IV):80, 1989.
275. Sedlis, S. P., Corr, P. B., Sobel, B. E., and Ahumada, G. G.: Lysophosphatidyl choline potentiates Ca^{++} accumulation in rat cardiac myocytes. Am. J. Physiol. *244*:H32, 1983.
276. Kloner, R. A., DeBoer, L. W. V., Carlson, N., and Braunwald, E.: The effect of verapamil on myocardial ultrastructure during and following release of coronary artery occlusion. Exp. Mol. Pathol. *36*:277, 1982.
277. Braunwald, E., Muller, J. E., Kloner, R. A., and Maroko, P. R.: Role of beta-adrenergic blockade in the therapy of patients with myocardial infarction. Am. J. Med. *74*:113, 1983.
278. Hammerman, H., Kloner, R. A., Briggs, L. L., and Braunwald, E.: Enhancement of salvage of reperfused myocardium by early beta-adrenergic blockade (timolol). J. Am. Coll. Cardiol. *3*:1438, 1984.
279. Lo, H. M., Kloner, R. A., and Braunwald, E.: Effect of intracoronary verapamil on infarct size in the ischemic, reperfused canine heart: Critical importance of the timing of treatment. Am. J. Cardiol. *56*:672, 1985.
280. Campbell, C. A., Kloner, R. A., Alker, K. J., and Braunwald, E.: Effect of verapamil on infarct size in dogs subjected to coronary artery occlusion with transient reperfusion. J. Am. Coll. Cardiol. *8*:1169, 1986.
281. Forman, M. B., Virmani, R., and Puett, D. W.: Mechanisms and therapy of myocardial reperfusion injury. Circulation *81*(Suppl. IV):69, 1990.
282. Lefer, A. M., Tsao, P. S., Lefer, D. J., and Ma, X-L.: Role of endothelial dysfunction in the pathogenesis of reperfusion injury after myocardial ischemia. FASEB, J. *5*:2029, 1991.
283. Jennings, R. B., Schaper, J., Hill, M. L., et al.: Effect of reperfusion late in the phase of reversible ischemic injury: Changes in cell volume, electrolytes, metabolites, and ultrastructure. Circ. Res. *56*:262, 1985.
284. Kloner, R. A., Ellis, S. G., Lange, R., and Braunwald, E.: Studies of experimental coronary artery reperfusion: Effects on infarct size, myocardial function, biochemistry, ultrastructure, and microvascular damage. Circulation *68*(Suppl. I):8, 1983.
285. Kloner, R. A., Ellis, S. G., Carlson, N. V., and Braunwald, E.: Coronary reperfusion for the treatment of acute myocardial infarction: Postischemic ventricular dysfunction. Cardiology *70*:233, 1983.
286. Hearse, D. J., and Bolli, R.: Reperfusion-induced injury: Manifestations, mechanisms and clinical relevance. Cardiovasc. Res. *26*:101, 1992.

Chapter 37
Acute Myocardial Infarction

ELLIOTT M. ANTMAN, EUGENE BRAUNWALD

Changing Patterns in Clinical Care of Patients with Acute Myocardial Infarction 1184
PATHOLOGY 1185
Role of Acute Plaque Change 1186
Gross Pathological Changes 1189
PATHOPHYSIOLOGY 1194
Left Ventricular Function 1194
Circulatory Regulation 1195
Ventricular Remodeling 1195
Pathophysiology of Other Organ Systems . 1196
CLINICAL FEATURES 1198
Predisposing Factors 1198
History 1198
Physical Examination 1199
Laboratory Examinations 1202
MANAGEMENT 1207
Prehospital Care 1207
Management in the Emergency Department 1208
Reperfusion of Myocardial Infarction 1213
Coronary Thrombolysis 1215
Coronary Angioplasty 1221
Surgical Reperfusion 1223
Antithrombotic and Antiplatelet Therapy . . 1223
Hospital Management 1226
Pharmacological Therapy 1228
HEMODYNAMIC DISTURBANCES IN ACUTE MYOCARDIAL INFARCTION 1233
Hemodynamic Assessment 1233
Hemodynamic Abnormalities 1234
Left Ventricular Failure 1235
Cardiogenic Shock 1238
Right Ventricular Infarction 1240
Mechanical Causes of Heart Failure 1241
ARRHYTHMIAS IN ACUTE MYOCARDIAL INFARCTION 1245
Ventricular Arrhythmias 1246
Bradyarrhythmias 1249
Conduction Disturbances 1250
Supraventricular Tachyarrhythmias 1253
Other Complications 1254
CONVALESCENCE, DISCHARGE, AND POST-MYOCARDIAL INFARCTION CARE 1257
Risk Stratification 1258
Secondary Prevention 1263
REFERENCES 1266

CHANGING PATTERNS IN CLINICAL CARE OF PATIENTS WITH ACUTE MYOCARDIAL INFARCTION

Despite impressive strides in diagnosis and management over the last three decades, acute myocardial infarction (AMI) continues to be a major public health problem in the industrialized world. In the United States nearly 1.5 million patients annually suffer from AMI (about one patient every 20 seconds).[1] More than 1 million patients with suspected AMI are admitted yearly to coronary care units in the United States; in only 30 to 50 per cent of patients is the diagnosis confirmed.[2] Although the death rate from AMI has declined by about 30 per cent over the last decade, its development is still a fatal event in approximately one-third of patients.[1] About 50 per cent of the deaths associated with AMI occur within 1 hour of the event and are attributable to arrhythmias, most often ventricular fibrillation (Chap. 24). Because AMI may strike an individual during the most productive years, it can have profound deleterious psychosocial and economic ramifications. In the United States, the yearly economic burden of coronary artery disease is in excess of $60 billion.[1] Perhaps as much as half of this cost is related to AMI and its prevention and treatment. Utilizing national statistics and a previously validated Coronary Heart Disease Policy Model,[3] investigators at the Harvard School of Public Health estimate that the average annual cost of caring for a patient with AMI in 1996 is $12,000.

Driven in large part by the need for cost-saving measures,[4] contemporary care of patients with AMI is becoming increasingly influenced by managed care systems[5] and guidelines for clinical practice (Table 63–14, p. 1972).[2,5a] Coronary care practice is better equipped than other fields of cardiovascular medicine to face this transition from pathophysiologically based decision-making to evidence-based decision-making, given the rich data base of over 500,000 patients with suspected AMI studied in clinical trials and efforts at summarizing a vast amount of data using meta-analysis.[6–10] Valuable and often complementary insights are also available from observational registries and outcomes research projects using medical claims data bases.[11–13] New therapies for AMI are being evaluated not only for evidence of safety and efficacy but also for their cost-effectiveness in caring for patients and their impact on quality of life.[14–16] However, despite an abundance of cost-effectiveness information analyzed from a societal perspective using data from clinical trials, clinicians weighing the risk-benefit ratio at the bedside of an individual patient with AMI may have difficulty applying the findings for several reasons: uncertainty whether the benefits observed in a strictly defined trial population are applicable to a wider selection of patients,[17] limited data on specific subgroups, variations in the absolute level of baseline risk,[18,19] and variations in patient preferences.[20,21] The information in this chapter on various treatment strategies should therefore be used as a guide and not a substitute for carefully reasoned clinical decision-making on a case-by-case basis.

IMPROVEMENTS IN OUTCOME. A steady decline in the mortality rate from AMI has been observed across several population groups since 1960.[22–24a] This drop in mortality appears to be caused by a fall in the incidence of AMI (replaced in part by an increase in the rate of unstable angina[25,26]) and a fall in the case fatality rate once a myocardial infarction has occurred[27] (Fig. 37–1). In addition, clinicians are now more astute at identifying those patients who are at increased risk of AMI[28] and benefit from more aggressive prophylactic cardiovascular treatments to prevent it from occurring when they undergo noncardiac surgery (e.g., intravenous nitroglycerin perioperatively[29]).

Several landmarks in the management of patients have contributed to the decline in mortality from AMI.[30] In the mid-1960's the concept of coronary care units was introduced. The first decade of coronary care was notable for detailed analysis and vigorous management of cardiac arrhythmias. Subsequently, introduction of the pulmonary artery balloon flotation catheter set the stage for bedside hemodynamic monitoring and more precise management of heart failure and cardiogenic shock associated with AMI. The modern reperfusion era of coronary care was ushered in by intracoronary and then intravenous thrombolysis, increased use of aspirin, and development of primary percutaneous transluminal coronary angioplasty (PTCA) for AMI.[31] Drug therapy continues to be an integral aspect of the treatment of patients with AMI, with noteworthy advances in the use of beta-adrenoceptor blockers, antithrombotic regimens, nitrates, and angiotensin-converting enzyme (ACE) inhibitors.[7,32]

LIMITATIONS OF CURRENT THERAPY. Despite the gratifying success of medical therapy for AMI, several observations indicate that considerable room for improvement exists. The short-term mortality of patients with AMI who receive aggressive reperfusion therapy as part of a randomized trial is in the range of 6.5 per cent,[33] whereas observational data

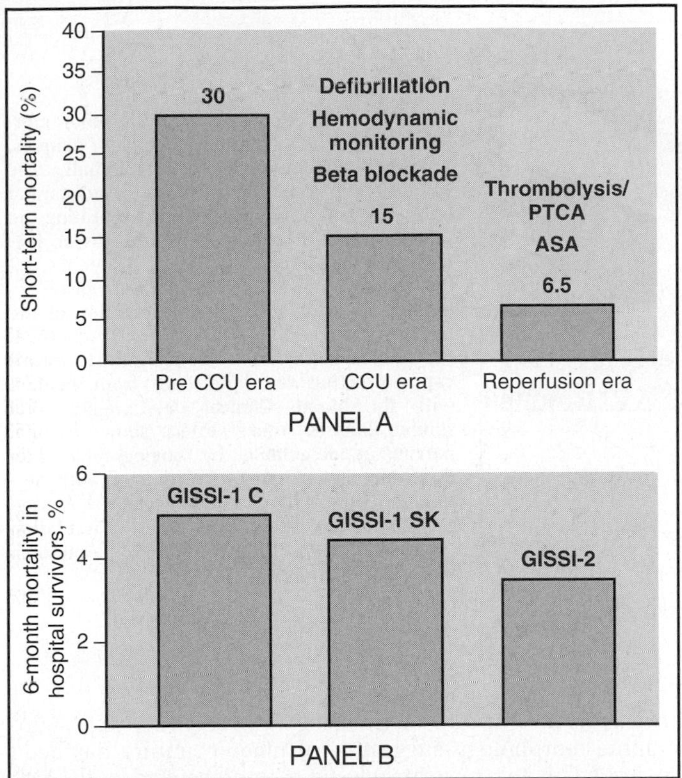

FIGURE 37–1. A, The impact of medical therapy for acute MI on short-term mortality. In the pre-CCU era acute MI short-term mortality (30-day) was estimated to be 30 per cent. Implementation of the CCU concept with defibrillation, sophisticated hemodynamic monitoring, and beta blockade reduced this to 15 per cent. A further mortality reduction was ushered in by the reperfusion era; combinations of thrombolysis, primary PTCA, and aspirin are now employed. (Modified from Antman, E. M.: General hospital management. *In* Julian, D., and Braunwald, E. (eds.): Management of Acute Myocardial Infarction. London, W. B. Saunders Company. Ltd., 1994, p. 31.) B, Six-month mortality for patients who survived the hospital phase of acute MI in the control (placebo) arm of the GISSI (GISSI-1 C) Study is compared with that in the GISSI-1 streptokinase arm (GISSI-1 SK). These results document the long-term benefits of thrombolytic therapy in reducing mortality. Further evidence that long-term use of aspirin and beta blockers contributes to a reduction in mortality can be seen in the third bar, which indicates 6-month mortality in GISSI-2. Compared with the GISSI-1 trial, at 6 months following infarction, greater proportions of patients in GISSI-2 were receiving aspirin (76 per cent versus 46 per cent, $P < 0.001$) and beta blockers (24 per cent versus 11 per cent, $P < 0.001$). (From Volpi, A., De Vita, C., Franzosi, M. G., et al.: Determinants of 6-month mortality in survivors of myocardial infarction after thrombolysis: Results of the GISSI-2 data base. Circulation *88*:416, 1993. Copyright 1993 American Heart Association.)

bases such as The National Registry of Myocardial Infarction suggest that the mortality rate in AMI patients not receiving reperfusion therapy is about 13 per cent.[12] In addition, the mortality rate from AMI in patients enrolled in randomized trials is considerably lower than that observed in patients who are excluded from such trials. For example, the 18-month mortality in the 2180 patients *excluded* from the Danish Verapamil Infarction Trial II (DAVIT II) was 25.6 per cent, whereas it was only 13.9 per cent in the placebo group enrolled in the trial.[34]

Although the survival of elderly patients (>age 65) following AMI has improved significantly,[35] advanced age consistently emerges as one of the principal determinants of mortality in AMI.[36–38] The 30-day and 1-year mortality rates for Medicare patients with AMI treated in 1990 were 23 per cent and 36 per cent, respectively.[35] Despite reluctance to use potentially life-saving drug therapies in the elderly, cardiac catheterization and other invasive procedures are being performed more commonly at some point during hospitalization in elderly AMI patients. Nevertheless, evidence suggests that the greatest reductions in mortality for elderly patients are derived from those strategies employed during the first 24 hours[39]—a time frame in which prompt and appropriate use of life-saving pharmacotherapy is of paramount importance, emphasizing the need to extend advances in drug therapy for AMI to the elderly.

Despite trends toward greater use of mortality-reducing therapies such as thrombolytics, aspirin, and beta-adrenoceptor blockers in patients with AMI,[40,41] these drugs still appear to be underutilized[42,43] (especially in the elderly[44,44a]), whereas calcium antagonists appear to be overutilized.[45,46] Considerable variation exists in practice patterns for management of patients with AMI.[47–50] This variation is seen not only on an international level[47,51] but also regionally within countries[49,50] and across medical specialties[52]; such variations in practice are correlated with differences in outcome after AMI.[52a]

Variation has also been observed in the treatment patterns of certain population subgroups with AMI—notably women and blacks. Although the unadjusted rates of thrombolytic use and referral for cardiac catheterization and angioplasty are lower[53,54] and mortality rates are higher in women with AMI,[10,55,56] gender differences are less apparent (but may not disappear entirely) once adjustment is made for baseline variables such as comorbidities and age[55–57] (Chap. 51). Although black patients with AMI in Veterans Administration Hospitals in the United States undergo fewer cardiac procedures such as cardiac catheterization than their white counterparts (even after adjustment for patient and hospital characteristics), they experience equivalent survival rates.[58]

PATHOLOGY

Almost all myocardial infarctions result from coronary atherosclerosis, generally with superimposed coronary thrombosis[58a]. Nonatherogenic forms of coronary artery disease are discussed on p. 1349 and causes of AMI without coronary atherosclerosis are shown in Table 37–1, p. 1193.

Prior to the thrombolytic era, clinicians typically divided AMI patients into those suffering a Q-wave or non-Q-wave infarct, based on the evolution of the pattern on the electrocardiogram (ECG) over several days following AMI. The term "Q-wave infarction" was frequently considered to be virtually synonymous with "transmural infarction," whereas "non-Q-wave infarctions" were often referred to as "subendocardial infarctions." Important advances have occurred in our understanding of the pathophysiology of AMI, leading to a reorganization of clinical presentations into what is now referred to as the *acute coronary syndromes,* the spectrum of which includes unstable angina, non-Q-wave infarction, and Q-wave infarction (Figs. 37–2 to 37–5).

ROLE OF ACUTE PLAQUE CHANGE

Slowly accruing high-grade stenoses of epicardial coronaries may progress to complete occlusion but do not usually precipitate AMI, probably because of the development of a rich collateral network (see p. 1174) over time. However, during the natural evolution of atherosclerotic plaques, especially those that are lipid-laden, an abrupt and catastrophic transition may occur, characterized by plaque rupture and exposure of substances that promote platelet activation and thrombin generation[59–65] (Figs. 37–2

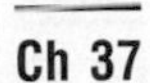

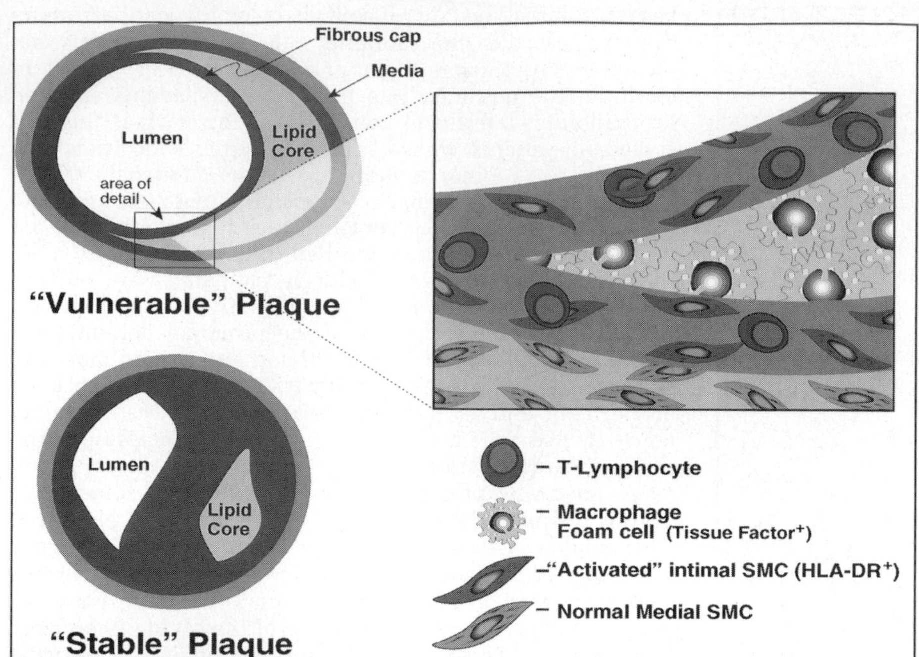

FIGURE 37–2. Comparison of the characteristics of "vulnerable" and "stable" plaques. Vulnerable plaques grow outward initially. The vulnerable plaque typically has a substantial lipid core and a thin fibrous cap separating the thrombogenic macrophages bearing tissue factor from the blood. At sites of lesion disruption, smooth muscle cells (SMCs) are often activated, as detected by their expression of the transplantation antigen HLA-DR. In contrast, the stable plaque has a relatively thick fibrous cap protecting the lipid core from contact with the blood. Clinical data suggest that stable plaques more often show luminal narrowing detectable by angiography than do vulnerable plaques. (Reproduced with permission from Libby, P.: Molecular bases of the acute coronary syndromes. Circulation *91*:2844, 1995. Copyright 1995 American Heart Association.)

to 37–4). The resultant thrombus interrupts blood flow and leads to an imbalance between oxygen supply and demand and, if this imbalance is severe and persistent, to myocardial necrosis (Fig. 36–23, p. 1177).

COMPOSITION OF PLAQUES. At autopsy, the atherosclerotic plaque of patients who died of MI is composed primarily of fibrous tissue of varying density and cellularity with superimposed thrombus.[66–67a] Calcium, lipid-laden foam cells, and extracellular lipid each constitute 5 to 10 per cent of the remaining area.[66] The atherosclerotic plaques that are associated with thrombosis and a total occlusion, located in infarct-related vessels, are generally more complex and irregular than those in vessels not associated with MI.[68] Histological studies of these lesions often reveal plaque rupture or fissuring[60,68,69] (Fig. 37–6). Angiographic morphology suggestive of plaque rupture has been identified in the majority of stenoses associated with AMI or abrupt onset of unstable angina.[70] This finding is rare in the noninfarct-related vessels of AMI patients and in the vessels of patients with chronic stable angina.[70]

Platelet-rich thrombi are often associated with the surface of the most advanced atherosclerotic lesions, called complicated plaques, which are characterized by fibrocalcific degeneration, deposition of lipid, calcium, fibrous tissue, necrotic debris, extravasated blood, and a fibrous cap (Figs. 37–2 and 37–3). Impaired endothelial cell function may contribute to atherogenesis through release of growth factors.[68] Luminal narrowing may potentiate platelet activation

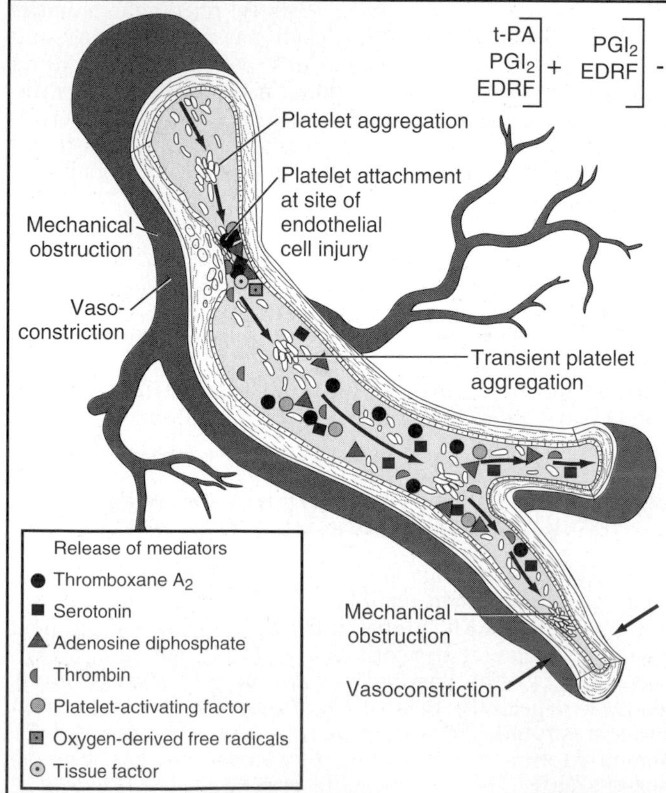

FIGURE 37–3. Schematic diagram suggesting probable mechanisms responsible for the conversion from chronic coronary heart disease to acute coronary artery disease syndromes. In this scheme, endothelial injury, usually at sites of atherosclerotic plaques and usually plaque ulceration or fissuring, is associated with platelet adhesion and aggregation and the release or activation of selected mediators, including thromboxane A_2, serotonin (5HT), adenosine diphosphate (ADP), platelet-activating factor (PAF), thrombin, tissue factor, and oxygen-derived free radicals. The accumulation of these mediators promotes platelet aggregation and mechanical obstruction of the narrowed artery. Thromboxane A_2, 5HT, thrombin, and PAF are vasoconstrictors at sites of endothelial injury. ADP, 5HT, and tissue factor have mitogenic influences and promote the development of neointimal proliferation. Therefore, the conversion from chronic stable to acute unstable coronary heart disease syndromes is most likely associated with endothelial injury, platelet aggregation, accumulation of platelet and other cell-derived mediators, further platelet aggregation, and vasoconstriction, with consequent dynamic narrowing of the coronary artery lumen. The relative absence of prostacyclin (PGI_2), t-PA (tissue plasminogen activator), and EDRF (nitrous oxide) at sites of endothelial injury contributes to the development of thrombosis, vasoconstriction, and neointimal proliferation. There are many different reasons for endothelial injury in addition to atherosclerotic plaque fissuring or ulceration, including flow shear stress, hypertension, immune complex deposition with complement activation, and mechanical injury to the endothelium as it occurs with coronary artery angioplasty, atherectomy, and stent placement and following heart transplantation. (From Willerson, J. T., Cohen, L. S., and Maseri, A.: Pathophysiology and clinical recognition. *In* Willerson, J. T., and Cohen, J. N. [eds.]: Cardiovascular Medicine. New York, Churchill Livingstone, 1995, p. 335.)

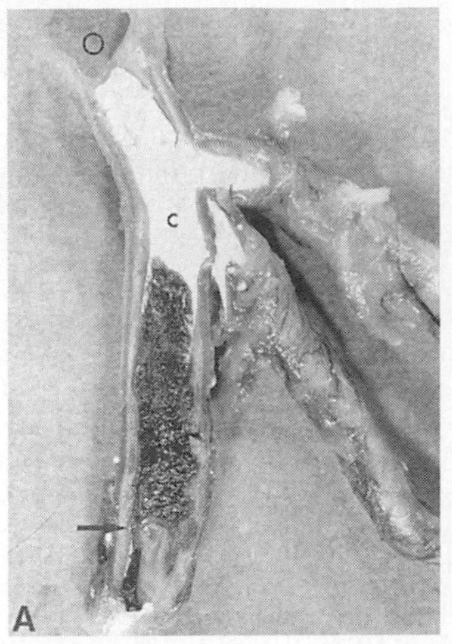

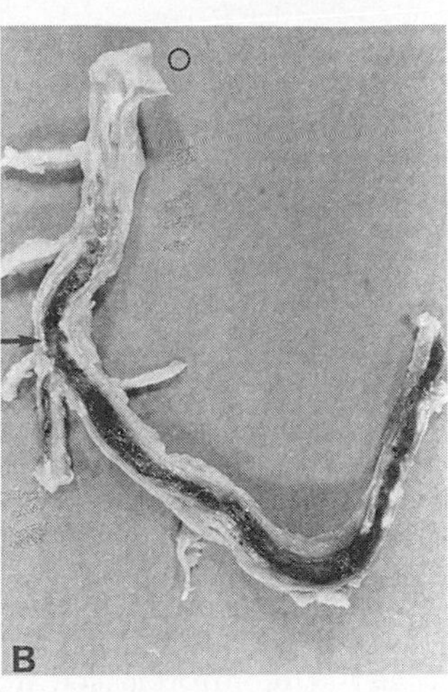

FIGURE 37–4. Thrombus propagation. ***A,*** **Left anterior descending coronary artery cut open longitudinally, showing a dark (red) stagnation thrombosis propagating upstream from the initiating rupture/platelet-rich thrombus at the arrow. In this case, the thrombus has propagated proximally up to the nearest major side branch (the first diagonal branch).** ***B,*** **The right coronary artery cut open longitudinally, showing a huge stagnation thrombosis propagating downstream from the initiating rupture/platelet-rich thrombus at the arrow. Unlike upstream thrombus propagation, downstream propagation may, as in this case, occlude major side branches. O = coronary ostium; c = contrast medium injected postmortem. (From Falk, E.: Coronary thrombosis: Pathogenesis and clinical manifestations. Am. J. Cardiol.** ***68*****:28B, 1991.)**

through augmentation of shear forces. Young persons with coronary thrombotic events have been described as having a genetic polymorphism in glycoprotein IIb/IIIa, possibly altering platelet-fibrinogen interactions.[71] This observation raises the possibility of screening for patients at increased risk of coronary thrombosis in the event of plaque rupture.

In patients with MI, coronary thrombi are usually superimposed on or adjacent to atherosclerotic plaques (Figs. 37–3 and 37–4).[65] These coronary arterial thrombi, which are approximately 1 cm in length in most cases, adhere to the luminal surface of an artery and are composed of platelets, fibrin, erythrocytes, and leukocytes.[72] The composition of the thrombus may vary at different levels: A white thrombus is composed of platelets, fibrin, or both, and a red thrombus is composed of erythrocytes, fibrin, platelets, and leukocytes. Early thrombi are usually small and nonocclusive and are composed almost exclusively of platelets.

PLAQUE FISSURING AND RUPTURE. The process of plaque fissuring is an area of intense investigation and is likely to be multifactorial in nature[64] (Figs. 37–2 and 37–3). Libby has summarized the evidence suggesting that T lymphocytes in human atheroma elaborate the cytokine interferon-gamma (IFN-γ) that markedly inhibits the ability of vascular smooth muscle cells to form interstitial collagen in vulnerable regions of the fibrous cap over an atherosclerotic plaque.[68] Furthermore, in atherosclerotic plaques prone to rupture there is an increased rate of formation of metalloproteinase enzymes such as collagenase, gelatinase, and stromelysin that degrade components of the protective interstitial matrix.[65,68,73] These proteinases may be elaborated by activated macrophages and mast cells that have been shown to accumulate in high concentration at the site of atheromatous erosions and plaque rupture in patients who died of AMI.[63,74,75] Examination of specimens from directional atherectomy reveals a much higher content of macrophages in patients with unstable angina or AMI compared with patients with chronic stable angina.[64] In addition to these structural aspects of vulnerable plaques, stresses induced by intraluminal pressure, coronary vasomotor tone, tachycardia (cyclic stretching and compression),[65] and disruption of nutrient vessels[76] combine to produce plaque rupture at the margin of the fibrous cap near an adjacent plaque-free segment of the coronary artery wall (shoulder region of plaque).[65,77] A number of key physiological parameters such as systolic blood pressure, heart rate, blood viscosity, endogenous tissue plasminogen activator (t-PA) activity, plasminogen activator inhibitor-1 (PAI-1) levels, plasma cortisol levels, and plasma epinephrine levels that exhibit circadian variations act in concert to produce a heightened propensity to plaque rupture and coronary thrombosis between 6 and 11 A.M., yielding the circadian clustering of AMI and relative resistance to thrombolytic therapy in the early morning hours.[78,79]

ACUTE CORONARY SYNDROMES. If, when plaque rupture occurs, a sufficient quantity of thrombogenic substances is exposed, the coronary artery lumen may become obstructed

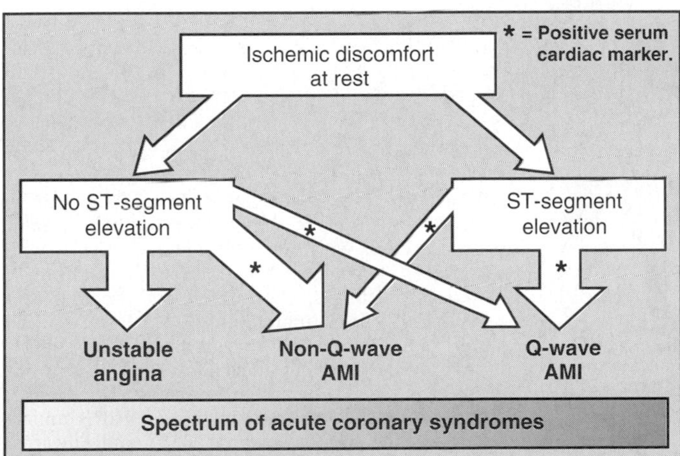

FIGURE 37–5. Acute coronary syndromes. Patients with ischemic discomfort may present with or without ST-segment elevation on the electrocardiogram. The majority (large arrow) of patients with ST-segment elevation ultimately develop a Q-wave acute myocardial infarction (AMI), whereas a minority (small arrow) develop a non-Q-wave AMI. Of the patients who present without ST-segment elevation, the majority (large arrows) are ultimately diagnosed with either unstable angina or non-Q-wave AMI based on the presence or absence of a cardiac marker such as CK-MB detected in the serum; a minority of such patients ultimately develop a Q-wave AMI. The spectrum of clinical conditions ranging from unstable angina to non-Q-wave AMI and Q-wave AMI is referred to as the acute coronary syndromes.

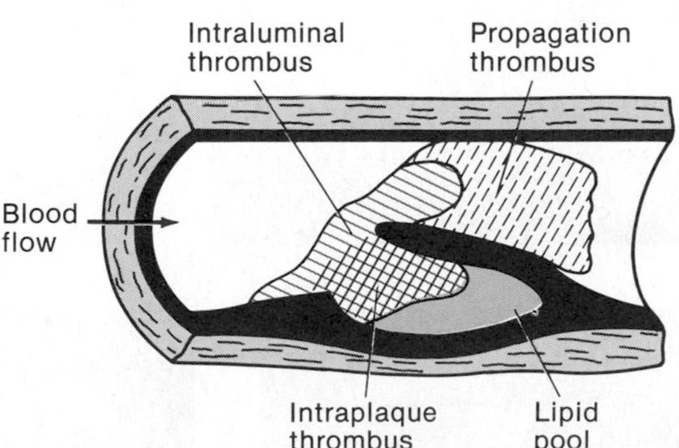

FIGURE 37–6. Representation of a longitudinal reconstruction of a coronary artery showing the histological components of an occluding thrombus. Much of the thrombus at the site of occlusion is contained within the plaque and compresses the lumen from outside. Intraluminal thrombus develops adjacent to a plaque fissure and then propagates downstream. A plug of lipid has extruded into the lumen. (Reproduced with permission from Davies, M. J.: A macro and micro view of coronary vascular insult in ischemic heart disease. Circulation ***82*****[Suppl. II]:38, 1990. Copyright 1990 American Heart Association.)**

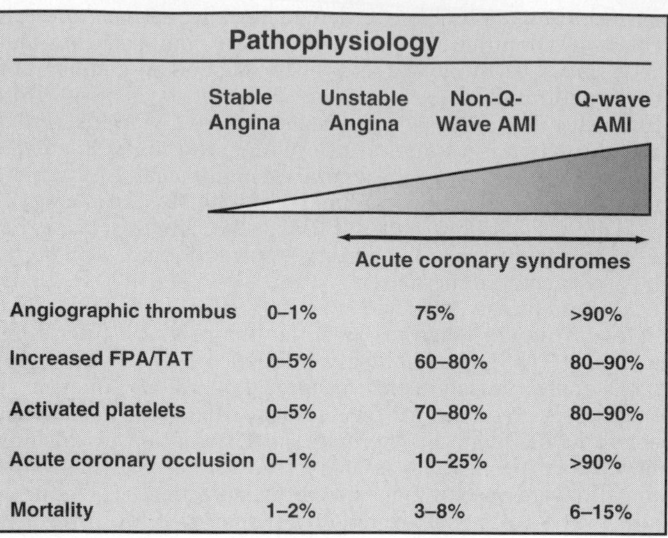

	Stable Angina	Unstable Angina / Non-Q-Wave AMI	Q-wave AMI
Angiographic thrombus	0–1%	75%	>90%
Increased FPA/TAT	0–5%	60–80%	80–90%
Activated platelets	0–5%	70–80%	80–90%
Acute coronary occlusion	0–1%	10–25%	>90%
Mortality	1–2%	3–8%	6–15%

FIGURE 37–7. Comparison of pathophysiological findings in patients with acute coronary syndromes. Progression from unstable angina to Q-wave AMI across the acute coronary syndrome spectrum is associated with a progressively increasing incidence of detection of thrombus at angiography, evidence of activation of the coagulation cascade (release of fibrinopeptide A [FPA] and generation of thrombin-antithrombin [TAT] complexes), activation and aggregation of platelets, and ultimately complete occlusion of the culprit coronary artery. The greater diminution in regional coronary blood flow and the larger amount of myocardium that progresses to necrosis with Q-wave AMI result in higher mortality rates than occurs in patients with unstable angina or non-Q-wave AMI. (From Cannon, C. P., and Rutherford, J. D.: The clinical spectrum of ischemic heart disease. *In* Antman, E. M., and Rutherford, J. D. [eds.]: Coronary Care Medicine: A Practical Approach. Boston, Marinus Nijhoff, 1996.)

by a combination of fibrin, platelet aggregates, and red blood cells[65] (Figs. 37–3, 37–4, and 37–6). An adequate collateral network that prevents necrosis from occurring can result in clinically silent episodes of coronary occlusion.[80] The rupture of plaques is now considered to be the common pathophysiological substrate of the *acute coronary syndromes* that range from unstable angina through non-Q-wave AMI and Q-wave AMI (Figs. 37–5 and 37–7). The dynamic process of plaque rupture may evolve to a completely occlusive thrombus, typically producing ST elevation on the electrocardiogram and ultimately necrosis involving the full or nearly full thickness of the ventricular wall in a zone subtended by the affected coronary artery (i.e., transmural myocardial infarction, often with *Q wave* development on the ECG). Less obstructive thrombi and/or those that are constituted by less robust fibrin formation and a greater proportion of platelet aggregates produce the syndromes of *unstable angina* (see p. 1331) and *non-Q-wave AMI,* typically presenting as ST-segment depression and/or T-wave inversion on the ECG (Figs. 37–5 and 37–7). Relief of transient vasospasm (induced by thromboxane A_2 and serotonin released from activated platelets) or spontaneous lysis and restoration of antegrade flow in the culprit coronary vessel in less than 20 minutes usually does not result in histological evidence of necrosis, the release of biochemical markers of necrosis, or persistent changes on the electrocardiogram; the resulting condition is unstable angina (Figs. 37–5 and 37–7). Episodes of plaque rupture more prolonged and more severe than those producing unstable angina typically result in release of a biochemical marker of necrosis but a less extensive pattern of necrosis than is found in patients with ST-elevation MI. When clinical evidence of necrosis is detected (now possible in a greater number of patients with sensitive markers such as cardiac-specific troponin T or I) (see p. 1203) and no pathological Q waves evolve on the ECG, a diagnosis of non-Q-wave AMI is made, a condition midway between Q-wave infarction and unstable angina (Figs. 37–5 and 37–7). Often, patients with non-Q-wave MI have a pattern of myocardial necrosis that is less confluent in nature and more concentrated in the inner third of the ventricular wall because restoration of blood flow prevented the wavefront of necrosis from extending across the thickness of the ventricular wall.

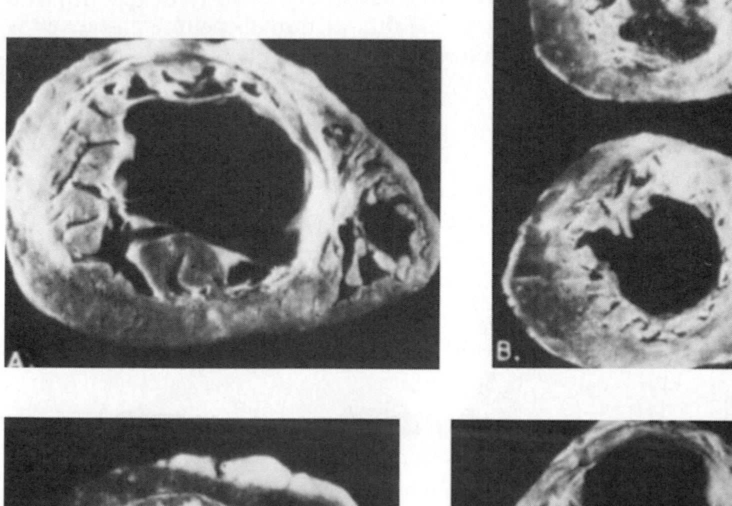

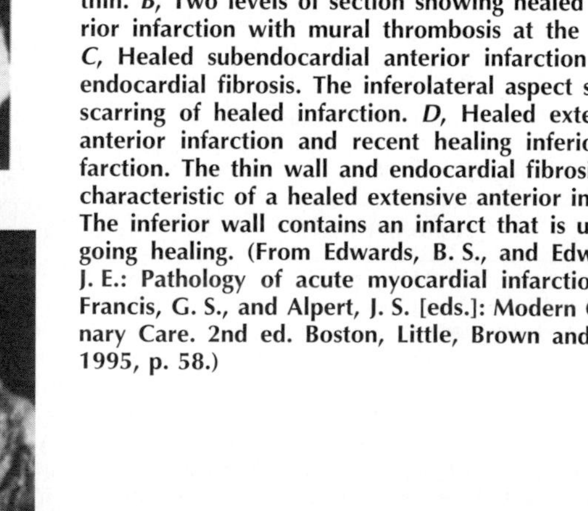

FIGURE 37–8. Examples of gross appearance of heart with healed MI. *A,* Healed extensive anteroseptal infarction. The involved part of the wall is thin. *B,* Two levels of section showing healed anterior infarction with mural thrombosis at the apex. *C,* Healed subendocardial anterior infarction with endocardial fibrosis. The inferolateral aspect shows scarring of healed infarction. *D,* Healed extensive anterior infarction and recent healing inferior infarction. The thin wall and endocardial fibrosis are characteristic of a healed extensive anterior infarct. The inferior wall contains an infarct that is undergoing healing. (From Edwards, B. S., and Edwards, J. E.: Pathology of acute myocardial infarction. *In* Francis, G. S., and Alpert, J. S. [eds.]: Modern Coronary Care. 2nd ed. Boston, Little, Brown and Co., 1995, p. 58.)

Some patients with stenotic atherosclerotic lesions experience AMI without evidence of plaque rupture or superimposed thrombosis. AMI occurs in clinical circumstances that produce a marked reduction in myocardial oxygen supply (e.g., prolonged severe vasospasm, as in Prinzmetal's variant angina (see p. 1340), or associated with a marked increase in myocardial oxygen demand (see below). These infarcts are located along the least well perfused inner one-third to one-half of the ventricular wall and often extend beyond the target territory perfused by a single coronary vessel. The ECG in such patients may show deep T-wave inversions or diffuse ST-segment depression.

Correlation with Evolutionary Changes on ECG

Autopsy data have shown that the ECG lacks sufficient sensitivity and specificity to permit reliable distinction of transmural from subendocardial infarcts because patients with transmural infarcts may not develop Q waves and Q waves may be seen in patients with autopsy evidence of a subendocardial (nontransmural) AMI.[81] These remarks notwithstanding, a crude categorization of patients into Q-wave and non-Q-wave patterns based on the ECG is useful because Q-wave AMIs are usually associated with greater ventricular damage, a greater tendency to infarct expansion and remodeling, and a higher mortality rate.[82–84]

GROSS PATHOLOGICAL CHANGES

On gross inspection, AMI may be divided into two major types: transmural infarcts, in which myocardial necrosis involves the full thickness (or nearly full thickness) of the ventricular wall, and subendocardial (nontransmural) infarcts, in which the necrosis involves the subendocardium, the intramural myocardium, or both without extending all the way through the ventricular wall to the epicardium (Fig. 37–8).[58a]

An occlusive coronary thrombosis appears to be far more common when the infarction is transmural and localized to

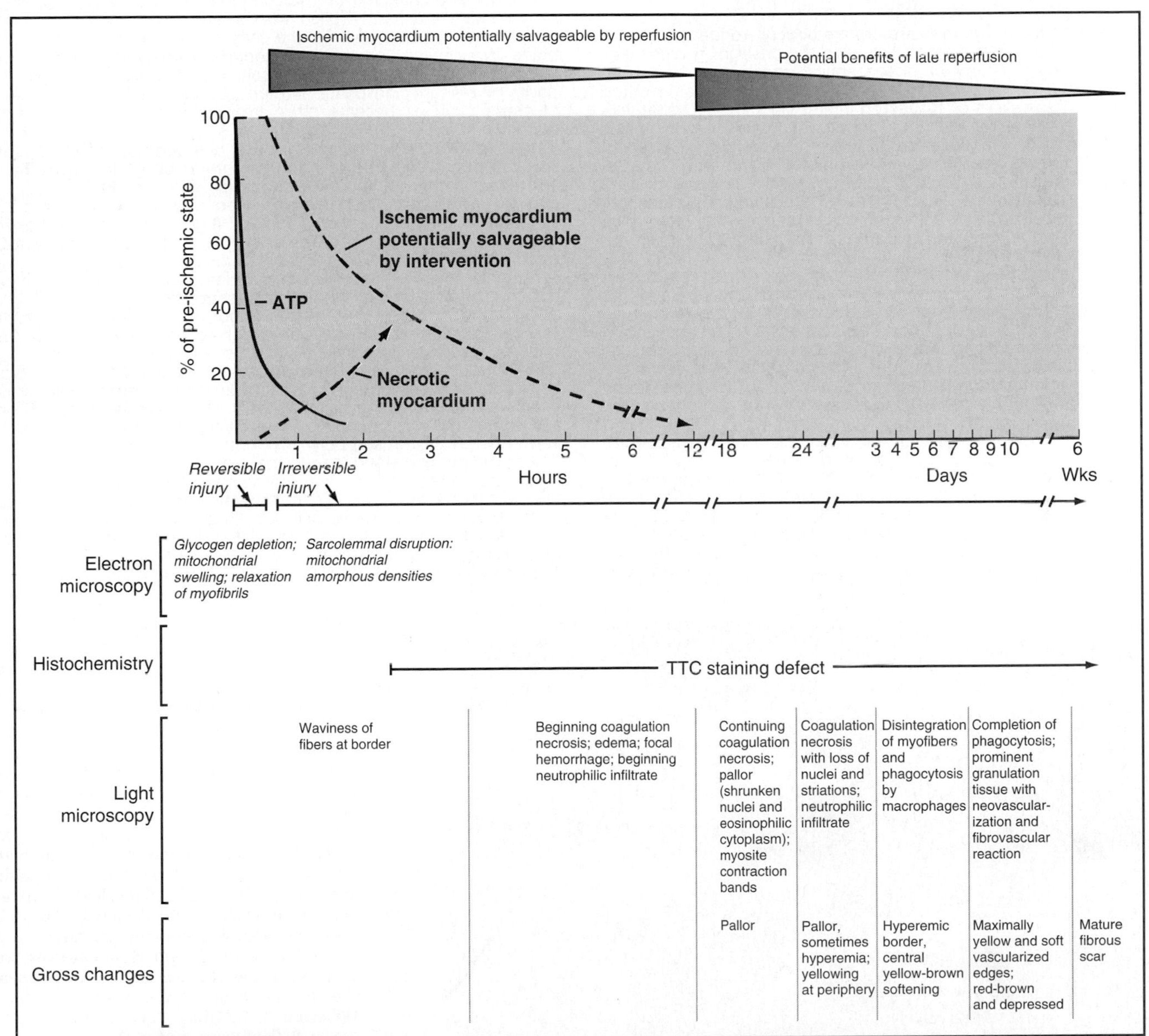

FIGURE 37–9. Temporal sequence of early biochemical, ultrastructural, histochemical, and histological findings after onset of MI. At the top of the figure are schematically shown the time frames for early and late reperfusion of the myocardium supplied by an occluded coronary artery. For approximately one-half hour following the onset of even the most severe ischemia, myocardial injury is potentially reversible; after that there is progressive loss of viability that is complete by 6 to 12 hours. The benefits of reperfusion (both early and late) are greatest when it is achieved early, with progressively smaller benefits occurring as reperfusion is delayed. (Figure developed in collaboration with Dr. Frederick J. Schoen.)

the distribution of a single coronary artery[85] (Figs. 37–4 and 37–7). Nontransmural infarctions, however, frequently occur in the presence of severely narrowed but still patent coronary arteries. Patchy nontransmural infarction may arise from thrombolysis or PTCA of an originally occlusive thrombus with restoration of blood flow *before* the wavefront of necrosis has extended from the subendocardium across the full thickness of the ventricular wall (Fig. 36–23, p. 1177). The histological pattern of necrosis may differ, with contraction band injury (see below) occurring almost twice as often in nontransmural as in transmural infarction.[85] Paradoxically, before their infarction, patients with nontransmural infarcts have, on average, a more severe stenosis in the infarct-related coronary artery than do patients suffering from transmural infarcts.[86] This finding suggests that a more severe obstruction occurring before infarction protects against the development of transmural infarction, perhaps by fostering the development of collateral circulation. It also accords with the concept that less severely stenotic but lipid-laden plaques with a fragile cap are responsible for the abrupt presentation of ST-segment elevation that may evolve to transmural infarctions.

Gross alterations of the myocardium are difficult to identify until at least 6 to 12 hours have elapsed following the onset of necrosis (Fig. 37–9). However, a variety of histochemical approaches have been used to identify zones of necrosis that can be discerned after only 2 to 3 hours. Tissue slices of suspected infarct sites are immersed in a solution of triphenyltetrazolium chloride (TTC), which stains viable myocardium brick red (because of preserved dehydrogenase enzymes that form a red formazen precipitate[87]) and leaves the infarcted region pale as a result of failure of uptake of the vital dye[88] (Fig. 37–9). The nitroblue tetrazolium (NBT) staining technique can similarly distinguish viable zones of myocardium, which stain dark blue, from necrotic areas of myocardium that therefore remain uncolored and identifiable.[89]

Initially, the myocardium in the affected region may appear pale and slightly swollen. Eighteen to 36 hours after the onset of the infarct, the myocardium is tan or reddish purple (due to trapped erythrocytes), with a serofibrinous exudate evident on the epicardium in transmural infarcts. These changes persist for approximately 48 hours; the infarct then turns gray, and fine yellow lines, secondary to neutrophilic infiltration, appear at its periphery. This zone gradually widens and during the next few days extends throughout the infarct.

Eight to 10 days following infarction, the thickness of the cardiac wall in the area of the infarct is reduced as necrotic muscle is removed by mononuclear cells. The cut surface of an infarct of this age is yellow, surrounded by a reddish purple band of granulation tissue that extends through the necrotic tissue by 3 to 4 weeks. Commencing at this time and extending over the next 2 to 3 months, the infarcted area gradually acquires a gelatinous, ground-glass, gray appearance, eventually converting into a shrunken, thin, firm scar, which whitens and firms progressively with time[81] (Fig. 37–9). This process begins at the periphery of the infarct and gradually moves centrally. The endocardium below the infarct increases in thickness and becomes gray and opaque.

Histological and Ultrastructural Changes

ELECTRON MICROSCOPY. In experimental infarction, the earliest ultrastructural changes in cardiac muscle following ligation of a coronary artery, noted within 20 minutes, consist of reduction in the size and number of glycogen granules, intracellular edema, and swelling and distortion of the transverse tubular system, the sarcoplasmic reticulum, and the mitochondria (Figs. 37–9 and 37–10).[81,90] These early changes are reversible. Changes after 60 minutes of occlusion include myocardial cell swelling, mitochondrial abnormalities such as swelling and internal disruption, and development of amorphous, flocculent aggregation and margination of nuclear chromatin, and relaxation of myofibrils. After 20 minutes to 2 hours of ischemia, changes in some cells become irreversible, and there is progression of these alterations; additional changes include indistinct tight junctions at the intercalated discs, swollen sacs of the sarcoplasmic reticulum at the level of the A band, greatly enlarged mitochondria with few cristae, thinning and fractionation of myofilaments, disappearance of the heterochromatin, rarefaction of the euchromatin and peripheral aggregation of chromatin in the nucleus, disorientation of myofibrils, and clumping of mitochondria. Cells irreversibly damaged by ischemia are usually swollen, with an enlarged sarcoplasmic space; the sarcolemma may peel off the cells, defects in the plasma membrane may appear, and the mitochondria are fragmented. The swollen mitochondria obtained from ischemic myocardium contain deposits of calcium phosphate and amorphous matrix densities. Many of these changes become more intense when blood flow is restored.[81,90]

LIGHT MICROSCOPY. It was previously believed that no light microscopic changes could be seen in infarcted myocardium until 8 hours after interruption of blood flow. However, in some infarcts a pattern of wavy myocardial fibers may be seen 1 to 3 hours after onset, especially at the periphery of the infarct (Fig. 37–9). It is hypothesized that wavy fibers result from the stretching and buckling of noncontractile fibers as forces are transmitted to them from adjacent viable contractile fibers.[81,84] After 8 hours, edema of the interstitium becomes evident, as do increased fatty deposits in the muscle fibers, along with infiltration of neutrophilic polymorphonuclear leukocytes and red blood cells. Muscle cell nuclei become pyknotic and then undergo karyolysis, and small blood vessels undergo necrosis.

By 24 hours there is clumping of the cytoplasm and loss of cross striations, with appearance of focal hyalinization and irregular crossbands in the involved myocardial fibers. The nuclei become pyknotic and sometimes even disappear. The myocardial capillaries in the involved region dilate, and polymorphonuclear leukocytes accumulate, first at the periphery and then in the center of the infarct. During the first 3 days, the interstitial tissue becomes edematous and red blood cells may extravasate (Fig. 37–9). Generally, on about the fourth day after infarction, removal of necrotic fibers by macrophages begins, again commencing at the periphery (Fig. 37–9). Later, lymphocytes, macrophages, and fibroblasts infiltrate between myocytes, which become fragmented. At 8 days the necrotic muscle fibers have become

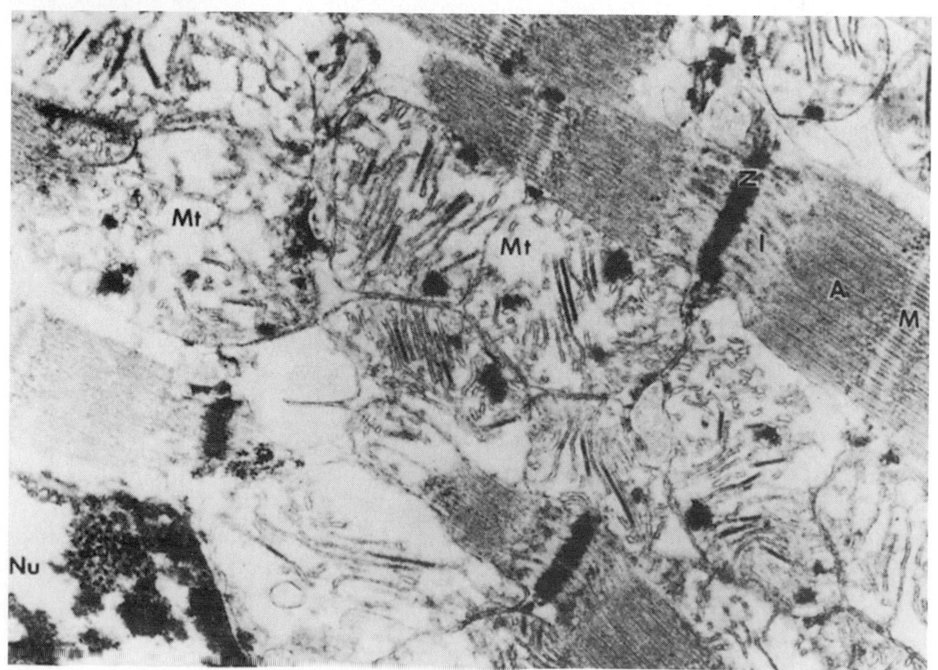

FIGURE 37–10. Electron micrograph of a muscle cell from the center of an infarct produced by permanent coronary occlusion in the dog. The myofibrils are fixed in a relaxed state and exhibit I, A, M, and Z bands. There is slight edema and no glycogen. (The clusters of granules resembling glycogen probably are ribosomes.) The mitochondria (Mt) are swollen and have linear densities and amorphous matrix (flocculent) densities. The nucleus (Nu) has clumped chromatin along the nuclear membrane and large lucent areas. (Tissue fixed with glutaraldehyde and osmium. Epoxy section stained with uranyl acetate and lead citrate, ×19,500.) (From Willerson, J. T., Hillis, L. D., and Buja, L. D. (eds.): Pathogenesis and pathology of ischemic heart disease. *In* Ischemic Heart Disease. Clinical and Pathophysiological Aspects. New York, Raven Press, 1982, p. 47.)

dissolved; by about 10 days the number of polymorphonuclear leukocytes is reduced, and granulation tissue first appears at the periphery. Ingrowth of blood vessels and fibroblasts continues, along with removal of necrotic muscle cells, until the fourth to sixth week following infarction, by which time much of the necrotic myocardium has been removed. This process continues along with increasing collagenization of the infarcted area. By the sixth week, the infarcted area has usually been converted into a firm connective tissue scar with interspersed intact muscle fibers (Fig. 37–9).

Patterns of Myocardial Necrosis

COAGULATION NECROSIS. This results from severe, persistent ischemia and is usually present in the central region of infarcts, which results in the arrest of muscle cells[91] in the relaxed state and the passive stretching of ischemic muscle cells. On light microscopy the myofibrils are stretched, many with nuclear pyknosis, vascular congestion, and healing by phagocytosis of necrotic muscle cells (Fig. 37–9). There is evidence of mitochondrial damage with prominent amorphous (flocculent) densities but no calcification.

NECROSIS WITH CONTRACTION BANDS. This form of myocardial necrosis, also termed *contraction band necrosis* or *coagulative myocytolysis*, results primarily from severe ischemia followed by reflow.[81] It is caused by increased Ca^{++} influx into dying cells, resulting in the arrest of cells in the contracted state. It is seen in the periphery of large infarcts and is present to a greater extent in nontransmural than in transmural infarcts.[85] The entire infarct may show this form of necrosis when reperfusion occurs experimentally or by surgery[91] (Fig. 37–11). Although patches of contraction band necrosis are found after successful reperfusion by thrombolytic therapy,[92] their presence in a large segment of the infarcts of patients who did not receive such therapy suggests that reperfusion through spontaneous thrombolysis or the release of spasm or both have occurred. It is characterized by hypercontracted myofibrils with contraction bands and mitochondrial damage, frequently with calcification, marked vascular congestion, and healing by lysis of muscle cells.

MYOCYTOLYSIS. Ischemia without necrosis generally causes no acute changes that are visible by light microscopy. However, severe prolonged ischemia can cause myocyte vacuolization, often termed myocytolysis. Prolonged severe ischemia, which is potentially reversible, causes cloudy swelling, as well as hydropic, vascular, and fatty degeneration.[93] Frequently seen at the borders of an infarct as well as in patchy areas of infarction in patients with chronic ischemic heart disease, myocytolysis is characterized by edema and cell swelling, lysis of myofibrils and nuclei, no neutrophilic response, and healing by lysis and phagocytosis of necrotic myocytes and ultimately scar formation.[94]

MODIFICATION OF PATHOLOGICAL CHANGES BY REPERFUSION

Early after the onset of ischemia, contractile dysfunction is observed that is believed to be due in part to shortening of the action potential duration, reduced cytosolic free calcium levels, and intracellular acidosis.[95] When reperfusion of myocardium undergoing the evolutionary changes from ischemia to infarction occurs sufficiently early (i.e., within 15 to 20 minutes), it may successfully prevent necro-

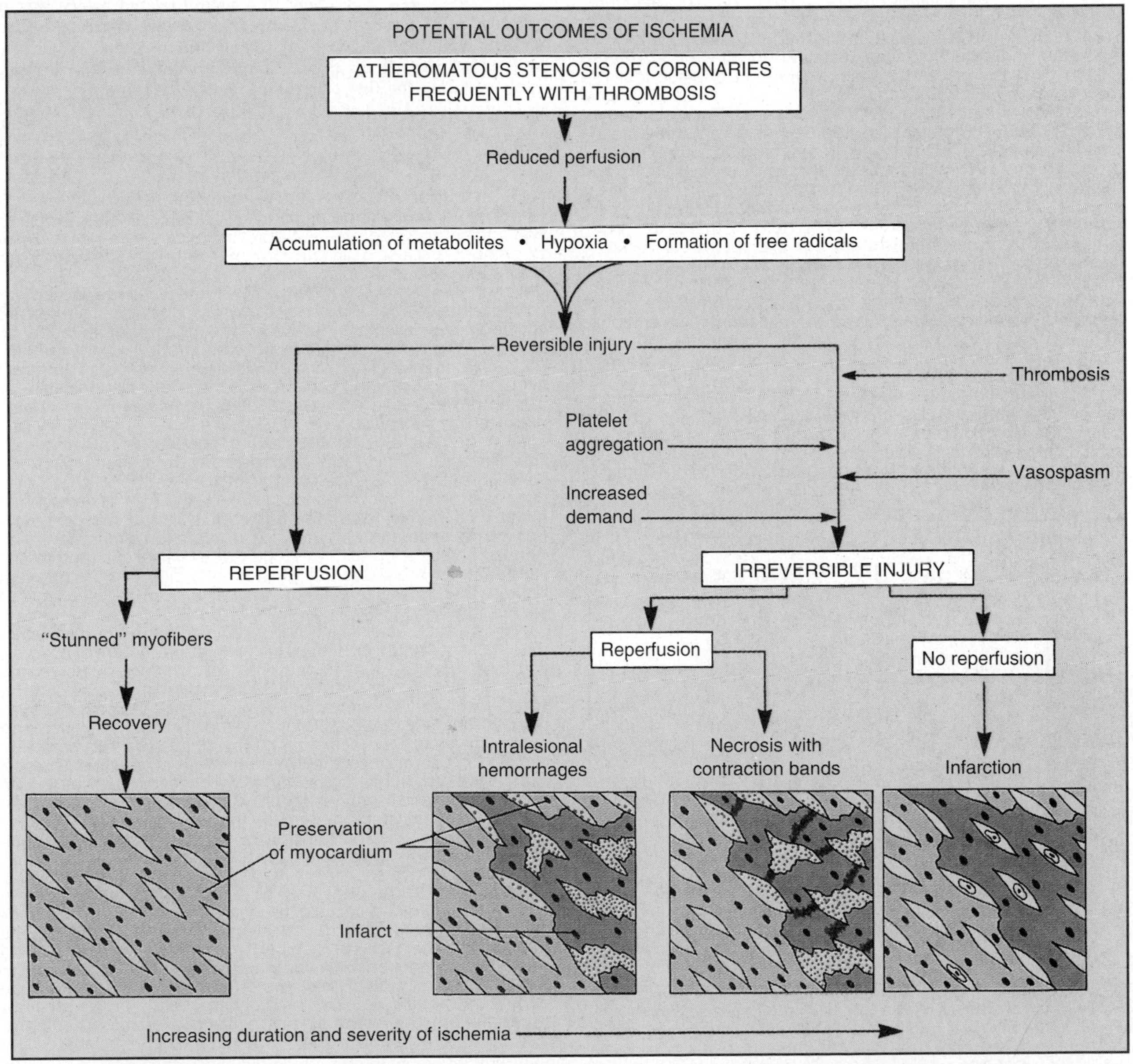

FIGURE 37–11. Several potential outcomes of reversible and irreversible ischemic injury to the myocardium. (From Schoen, F. J.: The heart. *In* Cotran, R. S., Kumar, V., and Robbins, S. L. (eds.): Pathologic Basis of Disease. 5th ed. Philadelphia, W. B. Saunders Company, 1994, p. 538.)

sis from developing. Beyond such a very early stage, the number of salvaged myocytes and therefore the amount of salvaged myocardial tissue (area of necrosis/area at risk) is directly related to the length of time the coronary artery has been totally occluded,[88] the level of myocardial oxygen consumption, and the collateral blood flow (Fig. 37–11). Typical pathological findings of reperfused infarcts include a histological mixture of necrosis, hemorrhage within zones of irreversibly injured myocytes,[96] coagulative myocytolysis with contraction bands, and distorted architecture of the cells in the reperfused zone[81] (Fig. 37–11). Following reperfusion, mitochondria in nonviable myocytes develop deposits of calcium phosphate and ultimately a large fraction of the cells may calcify. Reperfusion of infarcted myocardium also accelerates the washout of intracellular proteins ("serum cardiac markers"), producing an exaggerated and early peak value of substances such as CK-MB and cardiac-specific troponin T and I.[97]

CORONARY ANATOMY AND LOCATION OF INFARCTION

In over 75 per cent of patients with MI who come to autopsy, more than one coronary artery is severely narrowed.[94,98] One-third to two-thirds of patients with AMI have critical obstruction (to less than 25 per cent of luminal area) of all three coronary arteries, whereas the remainder are equally divided between those having one-vessel disease and those having two-vessel disease.[98,99] Coronary arteriographic studies in surviving patients show that a higher percentage have one-vessel disease. Angiographic studies performed in the earliest hours of AMI in patients presenting with ST-segment elevation have revealed approximately a 90 per cent incidence of total occlusion of the infarct-related vessel.[100,101] Recanalization from spontaneous thrombolysis[101,102] as well as attrition due to some mortality among those patients with total occlusion results in a diminishing incidence of angiographically totally occluded vessels in the period following myocardial infarction (Fig. 37–12).[99] In contrast to patients with a Q-wave infarction, those patients who sustain a non-Q-wave infarction have a much lower incidence of complete occlusion of the infarct-related coronary artery (Figs. 37–7 and 37–13).

Thus, transmural infarcts occur distal to an acutely totally occluded coronary artery with thrombus superimposed on a ruptured plaque. However, the converse is not the case, in that chronic total occlusion of a coronary artery is not always associated with myocardial infarction. Collateral blood flow and other factors—such as the level of myocardial metabolism, the presence and location of stenoses in other coronary arteries, the rate of development of the obstruction, and the quantity of myocardium supplied by the obstructed vessel—all influence the viability of myocardial cells distal to the occlusion. In many series of patients studied at necropsy or by coronary arteriography, a small number (<5 per cent) of patients with AMI are found to have normal coronary vessels.[94,99] In these patients, an embolus that has lysed, a transiently occlusive platelet aggregate, or a prolonged episode of severe coronary spasm may have been responsible for the reduction in coronary flow.

Studies of patients who ultimately develop AMI after having undergone coronary angiography at some time before its occurrence have been helpful in clarifying coronary anatomy before infarction. Although high-grade stenoses, when present,[103] more frequently lead to AMI than do less severe lesions, the majority of occlusions actually

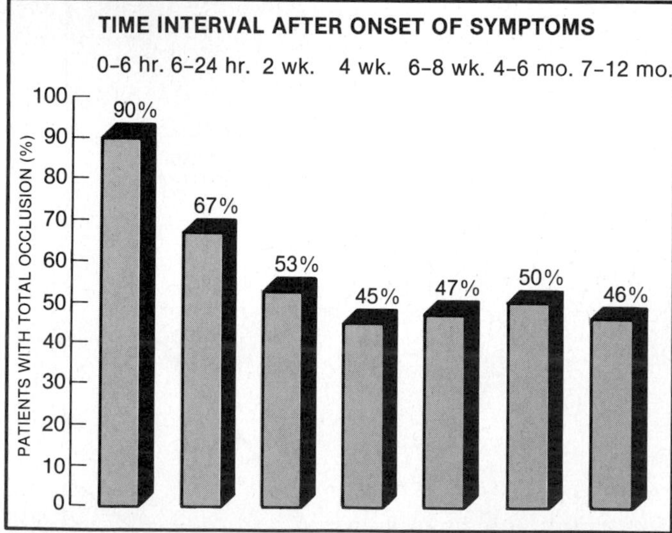

FIGURE 37–12. Percentage of patients with total coronary occlusion at different time intervals after the onset of symptoms of AMI. (Adapted from deFeyter, P. J., van den Brand, M., Serruys, P. W., and Wijns, W.: Early angiography after myocardial infarction: What have we learned? Am. Heart J. *109*:194, 1985.)

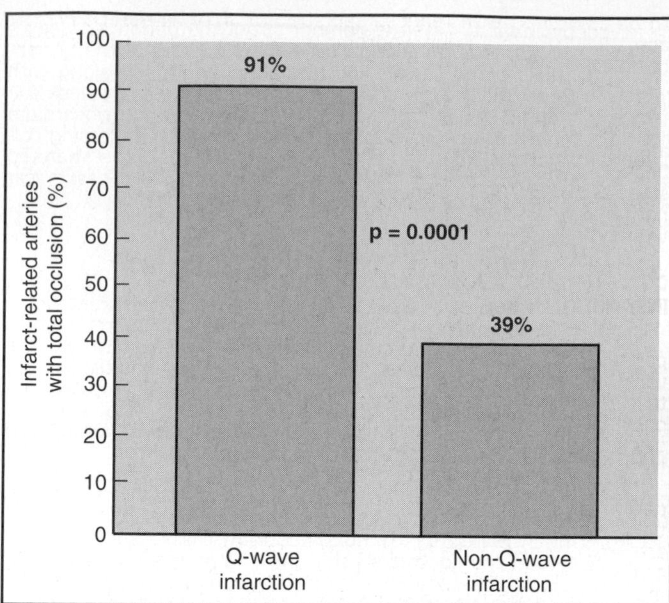

FIGURE 37–13. Prevalence of total occlusion of infarct-related artery in patients during the first 6 hours of acute Q-wave infarction versus non-Q-wave infarction. The infarct-related artery was totally occluded in 91 per cent of patients with Q-wave versus 39 per cent of patients with non-Q-wave infarction. (From Keen, W. D., Savage, M. P., Fischman, D. L., et al.: Comparison of coronary angiographic findings during the first 6 hours of non-Q-wave and Q-wave myocardial infarction. Am. J. Cardiol. *74*:324, 1994. Copyright 1994 by excerpta Medica Inc.)

occur in vessels with a previously identified stenosis of less than 50 per cent on angiograms performed months to years earlier.[104] This finding supports the concept that AMI occurs as a result of sudden thrombotic occlusion at the site of rupture of previously nonobstructive but lipid-rich plaques.[103]

Rather frequently, when an area of the ventricle is perfused by collateral vessels, an infarct occurs at a distance from a coronary occlusion. For example, following the gradual obliteration of the lumen of the right coronary artery, the inferior wall of the left ventricle may be maintained viable by collateral vessels arising from the left anterior descending coronary artery. In this circumstance, an occlusion of the left anterior descending artery may cause an infarct of the diaphragmatic wall.

RIGHT VENTRICULAR INFARCTION. Depending on the criteria used, approximately 50 per cent of patients with inferior infarction have some involvement of the right ventricle.[105] Among these patients, right ventricular infarction occurs exclusively in those with transmural infarction of the inferoposterior wall and the posterior portion of the septum. Right ventricular infarction almost invariably develops in association with infarction of the adjacent septum and left ventricular myocardium, but isolated infarction of the right ventricle is seen in 3 to 5 per cent of autopsy-proven cases of myocardial infarction.[106]

Regardless of whether or not it is combined with involvement of the left ventricle, right ventricular infarction is generally associated with obstructive lesions of the right coronary artery. However, right ventricular infarction occurs less commonly than would be anticipated from the frequency of atherosclerotic lesions involving the right coronary artery.[107] This discrepancy probably can be explained by the lower oxygen demands of the right ventricle, because right ventricular infarcts occur more commonly in conditions associated with increased right ventricular oxygen needs such as pulmonary hypertension and right ventricular hypertrophy.[105,108] Moreover, the intercoronary collateral system of the right ventricle is richer than that of the left, and the thinness of the right ventricular wall allows the chamber to derive some nutrition from the blood within the right ventricular cavity.

ATRIAL INFARCTION. This may be seen in up to 10 per cent of patients with AMI if PR segment displacement is used as the criterion for atrial infarction.[109] Although isolated atrial infarction may be observed in 3.5 per cent of autopsies of patients with AMI,[110] it often occurs in conjunction with ventricular infarction and can cause rupture of the atrial wall.[111] This type of infarct is more common on the right than the left side, occurs more frequently in the atrial appendages than in the lateral or posterior walls of the atrium, and can result in thrombus formation.[112] The difference in incidence between right and left atrial infarction might be explained by the considerably higher oxygen content of left atrial blood. Atrial infarction is frequently accompanied by atrial arrhythmias. It has also been reported to be associated with reduced secretion of atrial natriuretic peptide and a low cardiac output syndrome when right ventricular infarction coexists.[113]

CORONARY ARTERY SPASM (see also p. 1341). In addition to causing AMI in patients with Prinzmetal's angina (p. 1340), coronary artery spasm may also cause intimal damage that can initiate formation of an atherosclerotic plaque.[114] Epicardial coronary artery spasm has been identified in patients with fixed atherosclerotic coronary artery stenosis before, during, and after AMI. An association between coronary artery spasm and coronary artery thrombosis has also been documented clinically.[115]

COLLATERAL CIRCULATION IN ACUTE MYOCARDIAL INFARCTION (see also p. 1174)

The coronary collateral circulation is particularly well developed in patients with (1) coronary occlusive disease, especially when it is severe, with the reduction of the luminal cross-sectional area by more than 75 per cent in one or more major vessels; (2) chronic hypoxia, as occurs in severe anemia, chronic obstructive pulmonary disease, and cyanotic congenital heart disease; and (3) left ventricular hypertrophy, which intensifies coronary collaterals.

The magnitude of coronary collateral flow is one of the principal determinants of infarct size.[116] Indeed, it is rather common for patients with abundant collaterals to have totally occluded coronary arteries without evidence of infarction in the distribution of that artery; thus, the survival of the myocardium distal to such occlusions must depend on collateral blood flow. Even if collateral perfusion existing at the time of coronary occlusion is not successful in improving contractile function, it may still exert a beneficial effect by preventing the formation of a left ventricular aneurysm.[117] Some collaterals are seen in nearly 40 per cent of patients with an acute total occlusion,[118] and more begin to appear soon after the total occlusion occurs.[100] It is likely that the presence of a high-grade stenosis (>90 per cent), possibly with periods of intermittent total occlusion, permits the development of collaterals that remain only as potential conduits until a total occlusion occurs or recurs. The latter event then brings these channels into full operation.

The incidence of collaterals 1 to 2 weeks following AMI varies considerably and may be as high as 75 to 100 per cent in patients with persistent occlusion of the infarct vessel, or as low as 17 to 42 per cent in patients with subtotal occlusion.[119]

NONATHEROSCLEROTIC CAUSES OF ACUTE MYOCARDIAL INFARCTION

Numerous pathological processes other than atherosclerosis can involve the coronary arteries (see p. 1349) and result in myocardial infarction (Table 37–1).[90,119a] For example, coronary arterial occlusions can be the result of embolization of a coronary artery. Emboli most frequently lodge in the distribution of the left anterior descending coronary artery, commonly in the distal epicardial and intramural branches. The causes of coronary embolism are numerous: infective endocarditis and nonbacterial thrombotic endocarditis (see Chap. 33), mural thrombi, prosthetic valves,[120] neoplasms,[121] air that is introduced at the time of cardiac surgery,[122] and calcium deposits from manipulation of calcified valves at operation. In situ thrombosis of coronary arteries can occur secondary to chest wall trauma (see Chap. 44).

A variety of inflammatory processes can be responsible for coronary artery abnormalities, some of which mimic atherosclerotic disease and may predispose to true atherosclerosis.[123] Epidemiological evidence suggests that viral infections, particularly with coxsackie B, may be an uncommon cause of AMI.[124] Viral illnesses precede AMI occasionally in young persons who are later shown to have normal coronary arteries.[125]

Syphilitic aortitis may produce marked narrowing or occlusion of one or both coronary ostia,[126] whereas Takayasu's arteritis may result in obstruction of the coronary arteries (see Chap. 45).[127] Necrotizing arteritis, polyarteritis nodosa,[128] mucocutaneous lymph node syndrome (Kawasaki disease) (see p. 994),[129] systemic lupus erythematosus (see p. 1778) and giant cell arteritis[130] (see Chap. 56) can cause coronary occlusion. Therapeutic levels of mediastinal radiation can cause thickening and hyalinization of the walls of coronary arteries, with subsequent infarction.[131] AMI may also be the result of coronary arterial involvement in amyloidosis (see p. 1797), Hurler syndrome, pseudoxanthoma elasticum,[132] and homocystinuria (see Chap. 49).

As cocaine abuse has become more common, reports of AMI following the use of cocaine have appeared with increasing frequency. Cocaine may cause AMI in patients with normal coronary arteries, preexisting MI, documented coronary artery disease, or coronary artery spasm.[133–135] AMI associated with cocaine has also been reported following its topical use in nasal septoplasty[136] and in neonates whose mothers used the drug.[137] Recurrent MI after further cocaine abuse has been reported as well.

Cocaine may cause AMI by at least three mechanisms: (1) increasing myocardial oxygen demand through increases in heart rate and blood pressure, (2) diminishing coronary artery flow resulting from either coronary vasospasm and/or thrombosis, and (3) active myocarditis (either hypersensitivity or toxic).[134,135,138,139] In very high doses, cocaine appears to have a direct toxic effect on heart muscle which may produce cardiac failure and sudden death with extensive myocyte necrosis.[133,134]

TABLE 37–1 CAUSES OF MYOCARDIAL INFARCTION WITHOUT CORONARY ATHEROSCLEROSIS

CORONARY ARTERY DISEASE OTHER THAN ATHEROSCLEROSIS
Arteritis
Luetic
Granulomatous (Takayasu disease)
Polyarteritis nodosa
Mucocutaneous lymph node (Kawasaki) syndrome
Disseminated lupus erythematosus
Rheumatoid arthritis
Ankylosing spondylitis
Trauma to coronary arteries
Laceration
Thrombosis
Iatrogenic
Radiation (radiotherapy for neoplasia)
Coronary mural thickening with metabolic disease or intimal proliferative disease
Mucopolysaccharidoses (Hurler disease)
Homocystinuria
Fabry disease
Amyloidosis
Juvenile intimal sclerosis (idiopathic arterial calcification of infancy)
Intimal hyperplasia associated with contraceptive steroids or with the postpartum period
Pseudoxanthoma elasticum
Coronary fibrosis caused by radiation therapy
Luminal narrowing by other mechanisms
Spasm of coronary arteries (Prinzmetal's angina with normal coronary arteries)
Spasm after nitroglycerin withdrawal
Dissection of the aorta
Dissection of the coronary artery
EMBOLI TO CORONARY ARTERIES
Infective endocarditis
Nonbacterial thrombotic endocarditis
Prolapse of mitral valve
Mural thrombus from left atrium, left ventricle, or pulmonary veins
Prosthetic valve emboli
Cardiac myxoma
Associated with cardiopulmonary bypass surgery and coronary arteriography
Paradoxical emboli
Papillary fibroelastoma of the aortic valve ("fixed embolus")
Thrombi from intracardiac catheters or guidewires
CONGENITAL CORONARY ARTERY ANOMALIES
Anomalous origin of left coronary from pulmonary artery
Left coronary artery from anterior sinus of Valsalva
Coronary arteriovenous and arteriocameral fistulas
Coronary artery aneurysms
MYOCARDIAL OXYGEN DEMAND-SUPPLY DISPROPORTION
Aortic stenosis, all forms
Incomplete differentiation of the aortic valve
Aortic insufficiency
Carbon monoxide poisoning
Thyrotoxicosis
Prolonged hypotension
HEMATOLOGICAL (IN SITU THROMBOSIS)
Polycythemia vera
Thrombocytosis
Disseminated intravascular coagulation
Hypercoagulability, thrombosis, thrombocytopenic purpura
MISCELLANEOUS
Cocaine abuse
Myocardial contusion
Myocardial infarction with normal coronary arteries
Complication of cardiac catheterization

Modified from Cheitlin, M., et al.: Myocardial infarction without atherosclerosis. JAMA *231*:951, 1975. Copyright 1975, American Medical Association.

MYOCARDIAL INFARCTION WITH ANGIOGRAPHICALLY NORMAL CORONARY VESSELS

Approximately 6 per cent of all patients with AMI and perhaps four times that percentage of patients with this diagnosis under the age of 35 years do not have coronary atherosclerosis demonstrated by coronary arteriography or at autopsy.[99,100,140] Perhaps half of the patients of this group, in turn, have a variety of other lesions involving the coronary vessels or myocardium (Table 37-1), whereas the others have no detectable coronary obstructive lesions.[141,142] Patients with AMI and normal coronary arteries tend to be young and to have relatively few coronary risk factors, except that they often have a history of cigarette smoking.[140] Usually they have no history of angina pectoris prior to the infarction.[140] The infarction in these patients is usually not preceded by any prodrome, but the clinical, laboratory, and ECG features of AMI are otherwise indistinguishable from those present in the overwhelming majority of patients with AMI who have classic obstructive atherosclerotic coronary artery disease. In patients who recover, areas of localized dyskinesis and hypokinesis can often be demonstrated by left ventricular angiography. Many of these cases are caused by coronary artery spasm and/or thrombosis, perhaps with underlying endothelial dysfunction or small plaques that are not apparent on coronary angiography.[143] Additional suggested causes include (1) coronary emboli (perhaps from a small mural thrombus, a prolapsed mitral valve,[144] or a myxoma); (2) coronary artery disease in vessels too small to be visualized by coronary arteriography or coronary arterial thrombosis with subsequent recanalization (Table 37-1); (3) a variety of hematological disorders causing in situ thrombosis in the presence of normal coronary arteries (polycythemia vera, cyanotic heart disease with polycythemia,[145] sickle cell anemia,[146] disseminated intravascular coagulation, thrombocytosis, and thrombotic thrombocytopenic purpura); augmented oxygen demand (thyrotoxicosis,[147] amphetamine use[148]); (5) hypotension secondary to sepsis, blood loss, or pharmacological agents; and (6) anatomical variations such as anomalous origin of a coronary artery (see p. 909), coronary arteriovenous fistula (see p. 908), or a myocardial bridge (see p. 258).

PROGNOSIS. The long-term outlook for patients who have survived an AMI with angiographically normal coronary vessels on arteriography appears to be substantially better than for patients with MI and obstructive coronary artery disease.[149] Following recovery from the initial infarct, recurrent infarction, heart failure, and death are unusual in patients with normal coronary arteries.[150] Indeed, most of these patients have normal exercise electrocardiograms and only a minority develop angina pectoris.

PATHOPHYSIOLOGY

LEFT VENTRICULAR FUNCTION

Systolic Function

Upon interruption of antegrade flow in an epicardial coronary artery, the zone of myocardium supplied by that vessel immediately loses its ability to shorten and perform contractile work.[151,152] Four abnormal contraction patterns develop in sequence[153]: (1) dyssynchrony, i.e., dissociation in the time course of contraction of adjacent segments; (2) hypokinesis, reduction in the extent of shortening; (3) akinesis, cessation of shortening; and (4) dyskinesis, paradoxical expansion, systolic bulging.[154,155] Accompanying dysfunction of the infarcting segment initially is hyperkinesis of the remaining normal myocardium. The early hyperkinesis of the noninfarcted zones is thought to be the result of acute compensatory mechanisms, including increased activity of the sympathetic nervous system and the Frank-Starling mechanism.[84] A portion of this compensatory hyperkinesis is ineffective work because contraction of the noninfarcted segments of myocardium causes dyskinesis of the infarct zone.[156] Increased motion of the noninfarcted region subsides within 2 weeks of infarction, during which time some degree of recovery can be seen in the infarct region as well, particularly if reperfusion (see p. 1213) of the infarcted area occurs and myocardial stunning diminishes.[157]

Patients with AMI often also show reduced myocardial contractile function in noninfarcted zones. This may result from previous obstruction of the coronary artery supplying the noninfarcted region of the ventricle and loss of collaterals from the freshly occluded infarct related vessel, a condition that has been termed "ischemia at a distance."[158] Conversely, the presence of collaterals developing before MI may allow for greater preservation of regional systolic function in an area of distribution of the occluded artery and improvement in left ventricular ejection fraction early after infarction.[159]

If a sufficient quantity of myocardium undergoes ischemic injury, left ventricular pump function becomes depressed; cardiac output, stroke volume, blood pressure, and peak dP/dt are reduced[155]; and end-systolic volume is increased. In fact, the degree to which end-systolic volume increases is perhaps the most powerful predictor of mortality following AMI.[160] Paradoxical systolic expansion of an area of ventricular myocardium further decreases the left ventricular stroke volume. As necrotic myocytes slip past each other, the infarct zone thins and elongates, especially in patients with large anterior infarcts, leading to infarct expansion (see p. 1195). As the ventricle dilates during the first few hours to days following infarction, regional and global wall stress increases according to Laplace's law. In some patients a vicious circle of dilatation begetting further dilatation is initiated.[83,161] The degree of ventricular dilatation, which depends closely on infarct size, patency of the infarct-related artery,[162] and activation of the local renin-angiotensin system in the noninfarcted portion of the ventricle, can be favorably modified by ACE inhibition therapy even in the absence of symptomatic left ventricular dysfunction.[163-165]

With the passage of time, edema and cellular infiltration and ultimately fibrosis increase the stiffness of the infarcted myocardium back to and beyond control values. Increasing stiffness in the infarcted zone of myocardium improves left ventricular function because it prevents paradoxical systolic wall motion.

Rackley and collaborators have demonstrated a linear relationship between specific parameters of left ventricular function and the likelihood of developing clinical symptoms such as dyspnea and ultimately a shocklike state.[166] The earliest abnormality is a reduction in diastolic compliance (see below), which can be observed with infarcts that involve only 8 per cent of the total left ventricle on angiographic examination. When the abnormally contracting segment exceeds 15 per cent, the ejection fraction may be reduced and elevations of left ventricular end-diastolic pressure and volume occur. The risk of developing physical signs and symptoms of left ventricular failure also increase proportionally to increasing areas of abnormal left ventricular wall motion.[155] Clinical heart failure accompanies areas of abnormal contraction exceeding 25 per cent, and cardiogenic shock, often fatal, accompanies loss of more than 40 per cent of the left ventricular myocardium.[166]

Unless infarct extension occurs, some improvement in wall motion takes place during the healing phase, as recovery of function occurs in initially reversibly injured (stunned) myocardium (Fig. 37-11). Regardless of the age of the infarct, patients who continue to demonstrate abnormal wall motion of 20 to 25 per cent of the left ventricle are likely to manifest hemodynamic signs of left ventricular failure.

Diastolic Function

Left ventricular diastolic properties are altered in infarcted and ischemic myocardium, leading initially to an increase but later to a reduction in left ventricular compliance. These changes are associated with a decrease in the peak rate of decline in left ventricular pressure (peak (−) dP/dt), an increase in the time constant of left ventricular pressure fall (τ), and an initial rise in left ventricular end-diastolic pressure.[167] Over a period of several weeks, end-diastolic volume increases and diastolic pressure begins to fall toward normal.[84] As with impairment of systolic function, the magnitude of the diastolic abnormality appears to be related to the size of the infarct.

CIRCULATORY REGULATION

The abnormality in circulatory regulation that is present in AMI is diagrammed in Figure 37–14. The process begins with an anatomical or functional obstruction in the coronary vascular bed, which results in regional myocardial ischemia and, if the ischemia persists, in infarction. If the infarct is of sufficient size, it depresses overall left ventricular function so that left ventricular stroke volume falls and filling pressures rise. A marked depression of left ventricular stroke volume ultimately lowers aortic pressure and reduces coronary perfusion pressure; this condition may intensify myocardial ischemia and thereby initiate a vicious circle (Fig. 37–14). The inability of the left ventricle to empty also leads to an increased preload—that is, it dilates the well-perfused, normally functioning portion of the left ventricle. This compensatory mechanism tends to restore stroke volume to normal levels, but at the expense of a reduced ejection fraction. However, the dilatation of the left ventricle also elevates ventricular afterload, because Laplace's law (see p. 379) dictates that at any given arterial pressure the dilated ventricle must develop a higher wall tension. This increased afterload not only depresses left ventricular stroke volume but also elevates myocardial oxygen consumption, which in turn intensifies myocardial ischemia. When regional myocardial dysfunction is limited and the function of the remainder of the left ventricle is normal, compensatory mechanisms sustain overall left ventricular function. If a large portion of the left ventricle becomes necrotic, pump failure occurs; i.e., overall left ventricular function becomes so depressed that the circulation cannot be sustained despite the dilatation of the remaining viable portion of the ventricle.

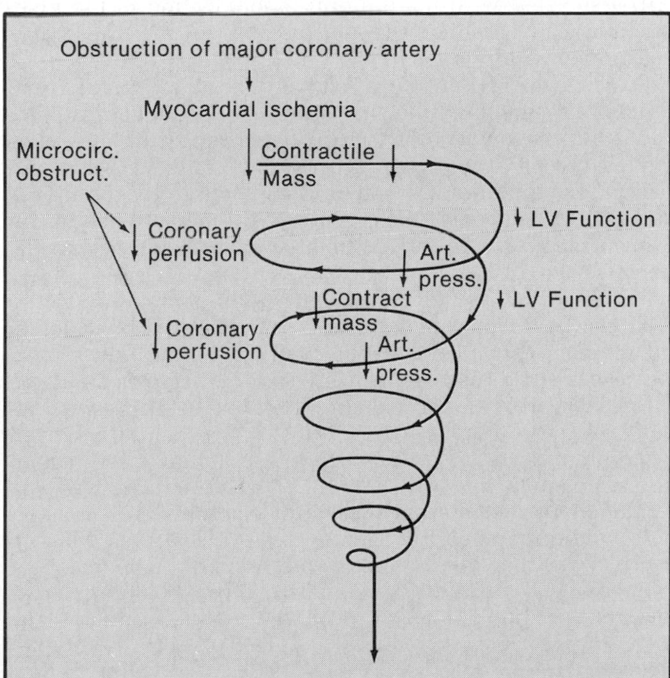

FIGURE 37–14. The sequence of events in the vicious circle in which coronary artery obstruction leads to cardiogenic shock and progressive circulatory deterioration. (From Pasternak, R. C., and Braunwald, E.: Acute myocardial infarction. *In* Isselbacher, K. J., et al. (eds.): Harrison's Principles of Internal Medicine. New York, McGraw-Hill Book Co., 1994.)

VENTRICULAR REMODELING

As a consequence of MI, the changes in left ventricular size, shape, and thickness involving both the infarcted and the noninfarcted segments of the ventricle described above occur and are collectively referred to as *ventricular remodeling.* This process, in turn, can influence ventricular function and prognosis.[83,84] A combination of changes in left ventricular dilation and hypertrophy of residual noninfarcted myocardium is responsible for remodeling. After the size of infarction, the two most important factors driving the process of left ventricular dilatation are ventricular loading conditions and infarct artery patency[83,162,168] (Fig. 37–15). Elevated ventricular pressure contributes to increased wall stress and the risk of infarct expansion, and a patent infarct artery accelerates myocardial scar formation and increases tissue turgor in the infarct zone, reducing the risk of infarct expansion and ventricular dilatation.

INFARCT EXPANSION. An increase in the size of the infarcted segment, known as infarct expansion, is defined as "acute dilatation and thinning of the area of infarction not explained by additional myocardial necrosis."[169] Infarct expansion appears to be caused by (1) a combination of slippage between muscle bundles, reducing the number of myocytes across the infarct wall; (2) disruption of the normal myocardial cells; and (3) tissue loss within the necrotic zone.[169] It is characterized by disproportionate thinning and dilation of the infarct zone prior to formation of a firm, fibrotic scar. The degree of infarct expansion appears to be related to the preinfarction wall thickness, with existing hypertrophy possibly protecting against infarct thinning.[170] The apex is the thinnest region of the ventricle and an area of the heart that is particularly vulnerable to infarct expansion.[171] Wall stress $(\sigma) = \frac{PR}{2h}$, where P = pressure, R = radius of curvature, and h = wall thickness.[171] Infarction of the apex secondary to occlusion of the left anterior descending coronary artery causes the radius of curvature at the apex to increase, exposing this normally thin region to a marked elevation in wall stress. This concept was reported by Picard et al., who observed greater infarct segment lengthening at the apex in dogs subjected to left anterior descending coronary artery occlusion than in the posterior zone of the left ventricle in dogs subjected to left circumflex coronary artery occlusion.[172]

When it is present, infarct expansion is associated with both a higher mortality and a higher incidence of nonfatal complications, such as heart failure and ventricular aneurysm.[84,173] Infarct expansion has been noted in more than three-fourths of the hearts of patients succumbing to AMI and one-third to one-half of all patients with anterior Q-wave infarctions.[173] Infarct expansion is best recognized echocardiographically as elongation of the noncontractile region of the ventricle.[174] When expansion is severe enough to cause symptoms, the most characteristic clinical finding is deterioration of systolic function associated with new or louder gallop sounds and new or worsening pulmonary congestion. Rupture of the ventricle may be considered to be a consequence of extreme infarct expansion.[175]

VENTRICULAR DILATATION. Although infarct expansion plays an important role in the ventricular remodeling that occurs early following myocardial infarction, remodeling is also caused by dilatation of the viable portion of the ventricle, commencing immediately following AMI, and progressing for months or years thereafter[176] (Fig. 37–15). As opposed to distention, dilatation may be accompanied by a shift of the pressure-volume curve of the left ventricle to

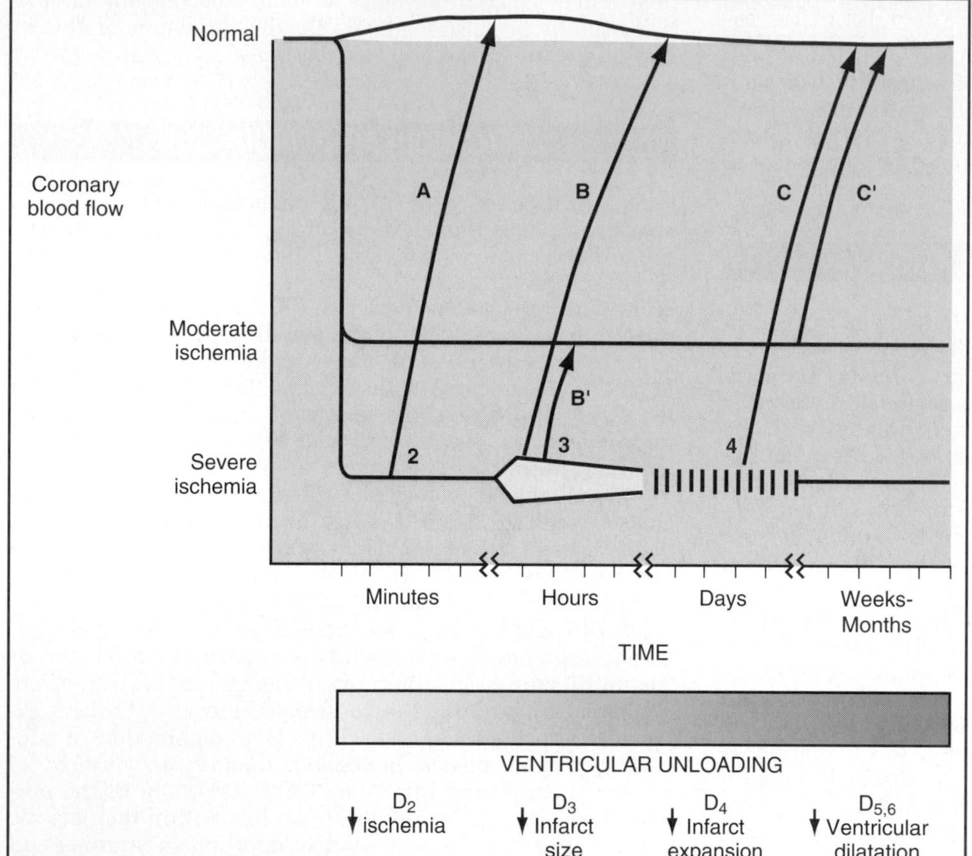

FIGURE 37–15. Therapeutic maneuvers in various stages of ischemia and infarction. Severely ischemic tissue (2) may be reperfused, thereby averting MI (A). Infarcting tissue (3) may be reperfused, leading to sparing of myocardial tissue (B). If blood flow is restored only in part (B′), the myocardium may remain noncontractile although viable, i.e., hibernating. After completion of the infarct (4), late reperfusion (C) may still be useful. Mechanical reperfusion of moderately ischemic myocardium (C′) may restore contractility of hibernating myocardium to normal. Ventricular unloading may be useful throughout the pre- and post-infarct periods. Unloading may reduce ischemia (D_2), infarct size (D_3), infarct expansion (D_4), and ventricular dilation ($D_{5,6}$). (From Braunwald, E., and Pfeffer, M. A.: Ventricular enlargement and remodeling following acute myocardial infarction: Mechanisms and management. Am. J. Cardiol. *68*:4D, 1991.)

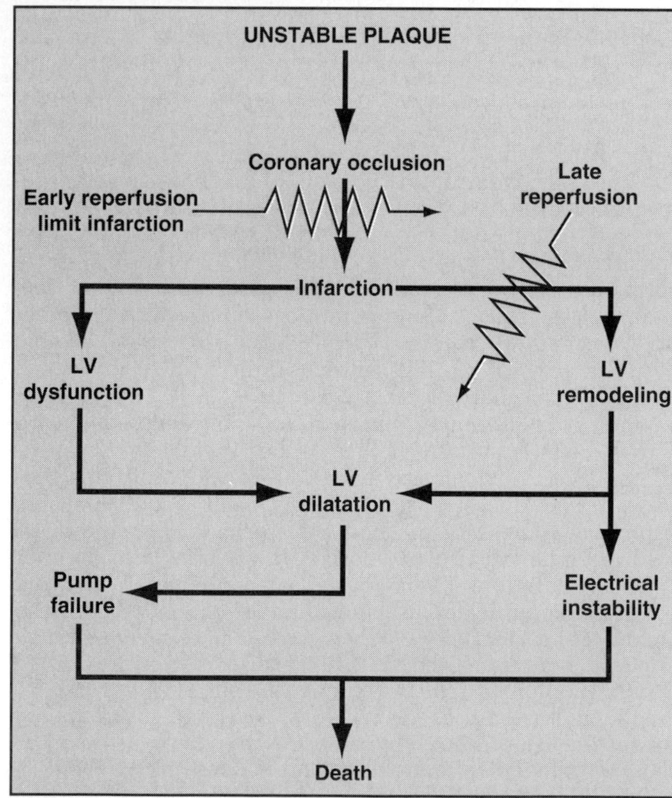

FIGURE 37–16. Flow chart showing postulated sequence of events from an unstable atherosclerotic plaque to death. The original paradigm emphasizing early reperfusion is shown at the left; the expanded paradigm illustrating the benefits of late reperfusion is shown at the right. (Reproduced with permission from Kim, C. B., and Braunwald, E.: Potential benefits of late reperfusion of infarcted myocardium: The open artery hypothesis. Circulation *88*:2426, 1993. Copyright 1993 American Heart Association.)

the right, resulting in a larger left ventricular volume at any given diastolic pressure (see p. 1194).[177] This global dilatation of the noninfarct zone may be viewed as a compensatory mechanism that maintains stroke volume in the face of a large infarction. However, ventricular dilatation is also associated with nonuniform repolarization of the myocardium that predisposes the patient to life-threatening ventricular arrhythmias.[178]

Following AMI, an extra load is placed on the residual functioning myocardium,[84] a load that presumably is responsible for the compensatory hypertrophy of the uninfarcted myocardium. This hypertrophy could help to compensate for the functional impairment caused by the infarct and may be responsible for some of the hemodynamic improvement seen in the months after infarction in some patients.[179]

EFFECTS OF TREATMENT. Ventricular remodeling after AMI can be affected by several factors, the first of which is infarct size (Fig. 37–15). Acute reperfusion and other measures to restrict the extent of myocardial necrosis limit the increase in ventricular volume following AMI,[180] and evidence suggests that an open infarct artery per se achieved even late after coronary occlusion also attenuates ventricular enlargement[162,181] (Fig. 37–16). The second factor is scar formation in the infarct. Glucocorticosteroids and nonsteroidal anti-inflammatory agents given early after MI can cause scar thinning and greater infarct expansion,[182] whereas ACE inhibitors[83,84] attenuate ventricular enlargement (see p. 1229) (Figs. 37–15 and 37–16).

PATHOPHYSIOLOGY OF OTHER ORGAN SYSTEMS

PULMONARY

Changes in pulmonary gas exchange, ventilation, and distribution of perfusion all occur with AMI.[187] Hypoxemia is a frequent conco quence, with a severity, in general, proportional to that of left ventricular failure. There is an inverse relation between pulmonary artery diastolic pressure and arterial oxygen tension in patients with AMI. This suggests that increased pulmonary capillary hydrostatic pressure leads to interstitial edema, which results in arteriolar and bronchiolar compression that ultimately causes perfusion of poorly ventilated alveoli with resultant hypoxemia.[184,185] In addition to hypoxemia, there is a fall in diffusing capacity.[185] Hyperventilation often occurs in patients with AMI and may cause hypocapnia and respiratory alkalosis, particularly in restless, anxious patients with pain. With reversal of heart failure, hypoxemia and intrapulmonary shunting diminish.

INCREASE IN INTERSTITIAL WATER. A positive correlation has been demonstrated between pulmonary extravascular (interstitial) water content, left ventricular filling pressure, and the clinical signs and symptoms of left ventricular failure.[185] The increase in pulmonary extravascular water may be responsible for the alterations in pulmonary mechanics observed in patients with AMI, i.e., reduction of airway conductance, pulmonary compliance, forced expiratory volume and midexpiratory flow rate, and an increase in closing volume—the last presumably related to the widespread closure of small, dependent airways during the first 3 days following AMI.[186] Ultimately, severe increases in extravascular water may lead to pulmonary edema. Recovery of left ventricular function or diuresis reduces abnormally elevated values for closing volumes—i.e., the lung volume at which airway closure commences—to normal.

The "closing volume" can encroach on and sometimes exceed functional residual volume. This can lead to arterial hypoxemia by the shunting of blood through alveoli that are not well ventilated.

REDUCTION OF VITAL CAPACITY. Virtually all lung volume indices—total lung capacity, functional residual capacity, and residual volume, as well as vital capacity—fall in the presence of AMI.[187] These reductions correlate with the elevations of left-sided filling pressures and are most probably due to increases in pulmonary extravascular water. Lung volumes, oxygenation, and airway resistance all return toward normal by the time of hospital discharge for most patients.[187] Increased pulmonary venous pressure also results in redistribution of pulmonary blood flow from the bases to the apices of the lung in patients with AMI,[188] altering the relationship between ventilation and perfusion. However, at follow-up examination 3 to 25 weeks after MI, the ventilation-perfusion relationship has usually returned to normal or almost so.

REDUCTION OF AFFINITY OF HEMOGLOBIN FOR OXYGEN. In patients with MI, particularly when complicated by left ventricular failure or cardiogenic shock, the affinity of hemoglobin for oxygen is reduced, i.e., the P_{50} is increased.[189] The increase in P_{50} results from increased levels of erythrocyte 2,3-diphosphoglycerate (2,3-DPG), which constitutes an important compensatory mechanism, responsible for an estimated 18 per cent increase in oxygen release from oxyhemoglobin in patients with cardiogenic shock.[189]

ENDOCRINE

PANCREAS. Hyperglycemia and impaired glucose tolerance are common in patients with AMI. Although the absolute levels of blood insulin are often in the normal range, they are usually inappropriately low for the level of blood sugar, and there may be relative insulin resistance as well. Patients with cardiogenic shock often demonstrate marked hyperglycemia and depressed levels of circulating insulin, often with complete suppression of insulin secretion in response to tolbutamide.[190] These abnormalities in insulin secretion and the resultant impaired glucose tolerance appear to be secondary to a reduction in pancreatic blood flow as a consequence of splanchnic vasoconstriction accompanying severe left ventricular failure. In addition, increased activity of the sympathetic nervous system with augmented circulating catecholamines inhibits insulin secretion and augments glycogenolysis, also contributing to the elevation of blood sugar.[191]

Glucose appears to be a more favorable energy source than free fatty acids for the ischemic myocardium by more efficiently replenishing Krebs cycle and stimulating contractile performance.[192,193] Because hypoxic heart muscle derives a considerable portion of its energy from the metabolism of glucose (see Chap. 36) and because insulin is essential for the uptake of glucose by the myocardium as well as for myocardial protein synthesis and inhibition of lysosomal activity, the deleterious effects of insulin deficiency are clear. These metabolic considerations, combined with epidemiological observations that diabetic patients have a markedly worse prognosis,[194] have served as the foundation for efforts to more aggressively administer insulin-glucose infusions to diabetics with AMI (see p. 1901).

ADRENAL MEDULLA. Excessive secretion of catecholamines produces many of the characteristic signs and symptoms of AMI. The plasma and urinary catecholamine levels are highest during the first 24 hours after the onset of chest pain,[191] with the greatest rise in plasma catecholamine secretion occurring during the first hour after the onset of MI.[195] These high levels of circulating catecholamines in patients with AMI correlate with the occurrence of serious arrhythmias and result in an increase in myocardial oxygen consumption, both directly and indirectly, as a consequence of catecholamine-induced elevation of circulating free fatty acids.[193] As might be anticipated, the concentration of circulating catecholamines correlates with the extent of myocardial damage and incidence of cardiogenic shock, as well as both early and late mortality rates.[196]

Circulating catecholamines enhance platelet aggregation; when this occurs in the coronary microcirculation, the release of the potent vasoconstrictor thromboxane A_2 may further impair cardiac perfusion. The marked increase in sympathetic activity associated with AMI serves as the foundation for beta-adrenoceptor blocker regimens in the acute phase (see p. 1211).

LOCAL MYOCARDIAL AND SYSTEMIC RENIN-ANGIOTENSIN SYSTEM. Noninfarcted regions of the myocardium appear to exhibit activation of the tissue renin-angiotensin system with increased angiotensin II production.[84,165] Both locally and systemically generated angiotensin II may stimulate the production of various growth factors such as platelet-derived growth factor and transforming growth factor-β that promote compensatory hypertrophy in the noninfarcted myocardium as well as control the structure and tone of the infarct-related coronary and other myocardial vessels.[84,197,198] Additional potential actions of angiotensin II that have a more negative impact on the infarction process include release of endothelin, PAI-1, and aldosterone, which may cause vasoconstriction, impaired fibrinolysis, and increased sodium retention, respectively.[84,197,198] Inhibition of generation of circulating and tissue angiotensin II is one of the proposed mechanisms of benefit from ACE inhibitors in AMI.[84]

NATRIURETIC PEPTIDES. The peptides atrial natriuretic factor (ANF) and N-terminal pro-ANF are released from cardiac atria in response to elevation of atrial pressure. In a case-control study from the TIMI II trial, Hall and colleagues have shown that elevated N-terminal pro-ANF levels within the first 12 hours of AMI are highly predictive of an increased mortality risk in the year following infarction.[199] A novel protein, brain natriuretic peptide (BNP), originally isolated from porcine brain, has been shown to be secreted by human ventricular myocardium. It appears to be released early after AMI, peaking at about 16 hours.[200] Patients with anterior infarction, lower cardiac index, and more significant congestive heart failure after AMI have higher levels of BNP and also show a second peak of BNP release about 5 days after infarction.[200] These intriguing observations suggest that BNP levels may be a marker of the degree of left ventricular dysfunction in AMI and that markedly elevated levels of BNP correlate with a worse prognosis.

ADRENAL CORTEX. Plasma and urinary 17-hydroxycorticosteroids and ketosteroids, as well as aldosterone, are also markedly elevated in patients with AMI.[191] Their concentrations correlate directly with the peak level of serum creatine kinase,[196] implying that the stress imposed by larger infarcts is associated with greater secretion of adrenal steroids. The magnitude of the elevation of cortisol correlates with infarct size and mortality.[201] Glucocorticosteroids also contribute to the impairment of glucose tolerance.

THYROID GLAND. Although patients with AMI are generally euthyroid, evidence indicates a significant transient decrease in serum triiodothyronine (T_3), levels, a fall that is most marked on about the third day after the infarct.[202] This fall in T_3 is usually accompanied by a rise in reverse T_3, with variable changes or no change in thyroxine (T_4) and thyroid-stimulating hormone (TSH) levels. The alteration in peripheral T_4 metabolism appears to correlate with infarct size and may be mediated by the rise in endogenous levels of cortisol which accompanies AMI.[203]

RENAL FUNCTION

Both prerenal azotemia and acute renal failure can complicate the marked reduction of cardiac output that occurs in cardiogenic shock. On the other hand, an increase in circulating atrial natriuretic peptide (see p. 405) occurs following AMI, an increase that is correlated with the severity of left ventricular failure.[204] An increase in atrial natriuretic peptide is also found when right ventricular infarction accompanies inferior wall infarction, suggesting that this hormone may play a role in the hemodynamic disturbances that accompany right ventricular infarction (see p. 1240).[205]

HEMATOLOGICAL FUNCTION

PLATELETS. AMI generally occurs in the presence of extensive coronary and systemic atherosclerotic plaques, which may serve as the site for the formation of platelet aggregates, a sequence that has been suggested as the initial step in the process of coronary thrombosis, coronary occlusion, and subsequent MI. Circulating platelets are hyperaggregable in patients with AMI.[62,206] Findings suggestive of a hypercoagulable state as a risk factor for AMI are discussed on page 1153, and the role of platelets in AMI is discussed on page 1333. Platelets from AMI patients have an increased propensity for aggregation locally in the area of a disrupted plaque and also release vasoactive substances such as thromboxane A_2[62,207] (Figs. 37–2, 37–3, and 37–7).

COAGULATION TESTS. Elevated levels of serum fibrinogen degradation products, an end-product of thrombosis—as well as release of distinctive proteins when platelets are activated,[208] i.e., platelet factor 4 and beta-thromboglobulin—have been reported in some patients with AMI.[209,210] Fibrinopeptide A, a protein released from fibrin by thrombin, is a marker of ongoing thrombosis and is elevated during the early hours of AMI[211] (see Chap. 58 and Fig. 37–7, p. 1188). The interpretation of the coagulation tests in patients with AMI may be complicated by elevated blood levels of catecholamines, concomitant shock, and/or pulmonary embolism, conditions that are all capable of altering various tests of platelet and coagulation function. Thus, it is not yet clear whether the aforementioned changes are the causes or consequences of AMI.

LEUKOCYTES. AMI is usually accompanied by leukocytosis, which is related to the necrotic process and its magnitude and to elevated glucocorticoid levels. Activation of neutrophils may produce important intermediates, such as leukotriene B_4 and oxygen free radicals, that have important microcirculatory effects.[212]

BLOOD VISCOSITY. Clinical and epidemiological studies suggest that several hemostatic and hemorheological factors (e.g., fibrinogen, Factor VII, plasma viscosity, hematocrit, red blood cell aggregation, total white cell count) are involved in the pathophysiology of atherosclerosis and also play an integral role in acute thrombotic events.[213] An increase in blood viscosity also occurs in patients with AMI. During the first few days after infarction, this is mainly attributable to hemoconcentration, but later the increases in plasma viscosity and red cell aggregation correlate with elevated serum concentrations of $alpha_2$ globulin and fibrinogen, which are nonspecific reactions to tissue necrosis and are also responsible for the elevated sedimentation rate characteristic of AMI.[214] The high values of blood viscosity indices are observed most frequently in patients with complications such as left ventricular failure, cardiogenic shock, and thromboembolism.

CLINICAL FEATURES

PREDISPOSING FACTORS

In as many one-half of patients with AMI, a precipitating factor or prodromal symptoms can be identified.[214a] Although adequate control studies have not been carried out, evidence suggests that unusually heavy exercise (particularly in fatigued or emotionally stressed patients) may play a role in precipitating AMI. Such infarctions could be the result of marked increases in myocardial oxygen consumption in the presence of severe coronary arterial narrowing. It has been suggested that unusually heavy exertion or mental stress such as that caused by anger[215,215a] may trigger plaque disruption, leading to AMI.[78] A number of reports have documented that upsetting life events occur commonly in patients who subsequently suffer an MI.[216,216a] Such events have been quantified and scored as "Life Change Units." Rahe and coworkers noted, on retrospective analysis, a significant buildup of Life Change Units in patients who subsequently suffered myocardial infarction or died suddenly.[216] Patients with known coronary disease who have been hospitalized for treatment of an acute coronary syndrome–related event and who subsequently report a high level of stress in their life have an increased risk of rehospitalization for cardiovascular reasons and also for "hard" events such as death and myocardial infarction.[217,218] Of interest, however, one study has provided evidence that in a multivariate analysis adjusting for other cardiac risk factors, job strain did not affect the outcome (including nonfatal AMI) in patients with angiographically proven coronary artery disease.[219]

Accelerating angina and rest angina, two patterns of unstable angina, may culminate as AMI (Fig. 37–7). Surgical procedures associated with acute blood loss have also been noted as precursors of AMI (see p. 1759). Reduced myocardial perfusion secondary to hypotension (e.g., hemorrhagic or septic shock) and increased myocardial oxygen demands secondary to aortic stenosis, fever, tachycardia, and agitation can also be responsible for myocardial necrosis. Other factors reported as predisposing to AMI include respiratory infections, hypoxemia of any cause, pulmonary embolism, hypoglycemia, administration of ergot preparations, use of cocaine, sympathomimetics, serum sickness, allergy, and on rare occasion wasp stings may all be triggers of AMI. In patients with Prinzmetal's angina (see p. 1340), AMI may develop in the territory of the coronary artery that repeatedly undergoes spasm.[220] Rarely, munition workers exposed to high concentrations of nitroglycerin may develop MI when they are withdrawn from this exposure, suggesting that it is caused by vasospasm.[221]

Trauma may precipitate an AMI in one of two ways. Myocardial contusion and hemorrhage into the myocardium may actually cause cell necrosis, or the injury may involve a coronary artery, causing occlusion of that vessel with resultant AMI (see Chap. 44). Neurological disturbances (transient ischemic attacks or strokes) may also precipitate AMI. Concern has been raised on the basis of a case-control study that patients with hypertension who are receiving short-acting calcium antagonists, particularly in high doses, are at increased risk of developing AMI.[222] Because of possible selection bias in the patients who received calcium antagonists, these results must be viewed cautiously and clinicians should await the results of ongoing multicenter trials (e.g., ALLHAT) before withdrawing calcium antagonists from patients who might be benefiting from their antihypertensive effect (reduction of stroke).[223,224]

CIRCADIAN PERIODICITY. An analysis of a large number of patients hospitalized with MI, studied as a part of the Multicenter Investigation of Limitation of Infarct Size (MILIS), revealed a pronounced circadian periodicity for the time of onset of AMI, with peak incidence of events between 6 A.M. and 12 noon.[225] Circadian rhythms affect many physiological and biochemical parameters; the early morning hours are associated with rises in plasma catecholamines and cortisol and increases in platelet aggregability. Interestingly, the characteristic circadian peak was *absent* in patients receiving beta blocker or aspirin therapy before their presentation with AMI.[226,227]

HISTORY

PRODROMAL SYMPTOMS. Despite recent advances in the laboratory detection of AMI, the history remains of substantial value in establishing a diagnosis.[228,228a] The prodrome is usually characterized by chest discomfort, resembling classic angina pectoris (described on p. 1291), but it occurs at rest or with less activity than usual and can therefore be classified as unstable angina. However, the latter is often not disturbing enough to induce patients to seek medical attention, and if they do, they may not be hospitalized. Among patients who are hospitalized for unstable angina, fewer than 10 per cent develop AMI (see p. 1336). Of the patients with AMI presenting with prodromal symptoms of unstable angina, approximately one-third have had symptoms from 1 to 4 weeks before hospitalization; in the remaining two-thirds, symptoms predated admission by 1 week or less, with one-third of these patients (20 per cent of all with prodromes) having had symptoms for 24 hours or less.[229] A feeling of general malaise or frank exhaustion often accompanies other symptoms preceding AMI.

NATURE OF THE PAIN (see also p. 1291). The pain of AMI is variable in intensity; in most patients it is severe and in some instances intolerable. The pain is prolonged, usually lasting for more than 30 minutes and frequently for a number of hours. The discomfort is described as constricting, crushing, oppressing, or compressing; often the patient complains of a sensation of a heavy weight or a squeezing in the chest. Although the discomfort is typically described as a choking, viselike, or heavy pain, it may also be characterized as a stabbing, knifelike, boring, or burning discomfort. The pain is usually retrosternal in location, spreading frequently to both sides of the anterior chest, with predilection for the left side. Often the pain radiates down the ulnar aspect of the left arm, producing a tingling sensation in the left wrist, hand, and fingers. Some patients note only a dull ache or numbness of the wrists in association with severe substernal or precordial discomfort. In some instances, the pain of AMI may begin in the epigastrium and simulate a variety of abdominal disorders, a fact that often causes MI to be misdiagnosed as "indigestion." In other patients the discomfort of AMI radiates to the shoulders, upper extremities, neck, jaw, and interscapular region, again usually favoring the left side. In patients with preexisting angina pectoris, the pain of infarction usually resembles that of angina with respect to location. However, it is generally much more severe, lasts longer, and is not relieved by rest and nitroglycerin.

In some patients, particularly the elderly, AMI is manifested clinically not by chest pain but rather by symptoms of acute left ventricular failure and chest tightness or by marked weakness or frank syncope. These symptoms may be accompanied by diaphoresis, nausea, and vomiting.[230] The pain of AMI may have disappeared by the time the physician first encounters the patient (or the patient reaches the hospital), or it may persist for many hours. Opiates—in particular, morphine—usually relieve the pain. Both angina pectoris and the pain of AMI are thought to arise from nerve endings in ischemic or injured, but not necrotic, myocardium.[231] Thus, in MI, stimulation of nerve fibers in an ischemic zone of myocardium surrounding the necrotic central area of infarction probably gives rise to the pain.

Pain often disappears suddenly and completely when blood flow to the infarct territory is restored. In patients in whom reocclusion occurs after thrombolysis, pain recurs if the initial reperfusion has left viable myocardium. Thus, what has previously been thought of as the "pain of infarction," sometimes lasting for many hours, probably represents pain caused by ongoing ischemia. The recognition that pain implies ischemia and not infarction heightens the importance of seeking ways to relieve the ischemia, for which the pain is a marker. This finding suggests that the clinician should not be complacent about ongoing cardiac pain under any circumstances.

OTHER SYMPTOMS. Nausea and vomiting occur in more than 50 per cent of patients with transmural MI and severe chest pain,[232] presumably owing to activation of the vagal reflex or to stimulation of left ventricular receptors as part of the Bezold-Jarisch reflex (see p. 1171). These symptoms occur more commonly in patients with inferior MI than in those with anterior MI. Moreover, nausea and vomiting are common side effects of opiates. When the pain of AMI is epigastric in location and is associated with nausea and vomiting, the clinical picture may easily be confused with that of acute cholecystitis, gastritis, or peptic ulcer. Occasionally a patient complains of diarrhea or a violent urge to evacuate the bowels during the acute phase of MI. Other symptoms include feelings of profound weakness, dizziness, palpitations, cold perspiration, and a sense of impending doom. On occasion, symptoms arising from an episode of cerebral embolism or other systemic arterial embolism are the first signs of AMI. The aforementioned symptoms may or may not be accompanied by chest pain.

Differential Diagnosis

The pain of AMI may stimulate the pain of acute pericarditis (see p. 1481), which is usually associated with some pleuritic features; i.e., it is aggravated by respiratory movements and coughing and often involves the shoulder, ridge of the trapezius, and neck. An important feature that distinguishes pericardial pain from ischemic discomfort is that ischemic discomfort never radiates to the trapezius ridge, a characteristic site of radiation of pericardial pain.[233] Pleural pain is usually sharp, knife-like, and aggravated in a cyclical fashion by each breath, which distinguishes it from the deep, dull, steady pain of AMI. Pulmonary embolism (see Chap. 46) generally produces pain laterally in the chest, is often pleuritic in nature, and may be associated with hemoptysis. The pain due to acute dissection of the aorta (see p. 1556) is usually localized in the center of the chest, is extremely severe and described by the patient as a "ripping" or "tearing" sensation, is at its maximal intensity shortly after onset, persists for many hours, and often radiates to the back or the lower extremities. Often one or more major arterial pulses are absent. Pain arising from the costochondral and chondrosternal articulations may be associated with localized swelling and redness; it is usually sharp and "darting" and is characterized by marked localized tenderness.

SILENT MI AND ATYPICAL PRESENTATION. Population studies suggest that between 20 and 60 per cent of nonfatal MIs are unrecognized by the patient and are discovered only on subsequent routine electrocardiographic[234,235] or postmortem examinations. Of these unrecognized infarctions, approximately half are truly silent, with the patients unable to recall any symptoms whatsoever. The other half of patients with so-called silent infarction can recall an event characterized by symptoms compatible with acute infarction when leading questions are posed after the electrocardiographic abnormalities are discovered. Unrecognized or silent infarction occurs more commonly in patients without antecedent angina pectoris[235] and in patients with diabetes and hypertension. Silent MI is often followed by silent ischemia (see p. 1344). The prognosis of patients with silent and symptomatic presentations of AMI appears similar.[235]

In an analysis of atypical presentations of AMI, Bean[236] lists the following: (1) congestive heart failure—beginning de novo or worsening of established failure; (2) classic angina pectoris without a particularly severe or prolonged attack; (3) atypical location of the pain; (4) central nervous system manifestations, resembling those of stroke, secondary to a sharp reduction in cardiac output in a patient with cerebral arteriosclerosis; (5) apprehension and nervousness; (6) sudden mania or psychosis; (7) syncope; (8) overwhelming weakness; (9) acute indigestion; and (10) peripheral embolization.

PHYSICAL EXAMINATION

GENERAL APPEARANCE. Patients suffering an AMI often appear anxious and in considerable distress.[228a] An anguished facial expression is common, and—in contrast to patients with severe angina pectoris, who often lie, sit, or stand still, recognizing that all forms of activity increase the discomfort—some patients suffering an AMI may be restless and move about in an effort to find a comfortable position. They often massage or clutch their chests and frequently describe their pain with a clenched fist held against the sternum (the "Levine" sign, named after Dr. Samuel A. Levine). In patients with left ventricular failure and sympathetic stimulation, cold perspiration and skin pallor may be evident; they typically sit or are propped up in bed, gasping for breath. Between breaths, they may complain of chest discomfort or a feeling of suffocation. Cough productive of frothy, pink, or blood-streaked sputum is common.

Patients in cardiogenic shock often lie listlessly, making few if any spontaneous movements. The skin is cool and clammy, with a bluish or mottled color over the extremities, and there is marked facial pallor with severe cyanosis of the lips and nailbeds. Depending on the degree of cerebral perfusion, the patient in shock may converse normally or may evidence confusion and disorientation.

HEART RATE. The heart rate may vary from a marked bradycardia to a rapid regular or irregular tachycardia, depending on the underlying rhythm and the degree of left ventricular failure. Most commonly, the pulse is rapid and regular initially (sinus tachycardia at 100 to 110 beats/

min), slowing as the patient's pain and anxiety are relieved; premature ventricular beats are common, occurring in more than 95 per cent of patients evaluated within the first 4 hours after the onset of symptoms.[237]

BLOOD PRESSURE. The majority of patients with uncomplicated AMI are normotensive, although the reduced stroke volume accompanying the tachycardia may cause declines in systolic and pulse pressures and elevation of diastolic pressure. Among previously normotensive patients, a hypertensive response occasionally is seen during the first few hours, with the arterial pressure exceeding 160/90 mm Hg, presumably as a consequence of adrenergic discharge secondary to pain and agitation. It is common for previously hypertensive patients to become normotensive without treatment following AMI, although many of these previously hypertensive patients eventually regain their elevated levels of blood pressure, generally 3 to 6 months after infarction. In patients with massive infarction, arterial pressure falls acutely, owing to left ventricular dysfunction and venous pooling secondary to administration of morphine or nitrates or both; as recovery occurs, the arterial pressure tends to return to preinfarction levels.

Patients in cardiogenic shock (see p. 1238), by definition, have systolic pressures below 90 mm Hg and evidence of end-organ hypoperfusion. However, hypotension alone does not necessarily signify cardiogenic shock because some patients with inferior infarction in whom the Bezold-Jarisch reflex is activated may also transiently have systolic blood pressure below 90 mm Hg.[238] Their hypotension eventually resolves spontaneously, although the process can be accelerated by intravenous atropine (0.5 to 1.0 mg) and assumption of the Trendelenburg position. Other patients who are initially only slightly hypotensive may demonstrate gradually falling blood pressures with progressive reduction in cardiac output over several hours or days as they develop cardiogenic shock as a consequence of increasing ischemia and extension of infarction (Fig. 37–14). Evidence of autonomic hyperactivity is common, varying in type with the location of the infarction. At some time in their initial presentation, more than half of patients with inferior MI have evidence of excess parasympathetic stimulation, with hypotension, bradycardia, or both, whereas about half of patients with anterior MI show signs of sympathetic excess, having hypertension, tachycardia, or both.[239]

TEMPERATURE AND RESPIRATION. Most patients with extensive AMI develop fever, a nonspecific response to tissue necrosis, within 24 to 48 hours of the onset of infarction. Body temperature often begins to rise within 4 to 8 hours after the onset of infarction, and rectal temperature may reach 101° to 102°F. Fever usually resolves by the fifth or sixth day following infarction.

The respiratory rate may be slightly elevated soon after the development of an AMI; in patients without heart failure, it results from anxiety and pain because it returns to normal with treatment of physical and psychological discomfort. In patients with left ventricular failure, the respiratory rate correlates with the severity of failure; patients with pulmonary edema may have respiratory rates exceeding 40 per minute. However, the respiratory rate is not necessarily elevated in patients with cardiogenic shock. Cheyne-Stokes (periodic) respiration (see p. 455) may occur in elderly individuals with cardiogenic shock and heart failure, particularly after opiate therapy and in the presence of cerebrovascular disease.

JUGULAR VENOUS PULSE. The height and contour of the jugular venous pulse reflect right atrial and right ventricular diastolic pressures (see p. 18). Because these pressures are usually normal or only slightly elevated in patients with AMI (even in the presence of mild to moderate left ventricular failure), it is not surprising that usually the jugular venous pulse fails to show any abnormalities. The *a* wave may be prominent in patients with pulmonary hypertension secondary to left ventricular failure or reduced compliance. In contrast, right ventricular infarction (whether or not it accompanies left ventricular infarction) often results in marked jugular venous distention and, when it is complicated by necrosis or ischemia of right ventricular papillary muscles, tall *c-v* waves of tricuspid regurgitation are evident. In patients with AMI and cardiogenic shock, the jugular venous pressure is usually elevated. In patients with AMI, hypotension, and hypoperfusion (findings that may resemble those of patients with cardiogenic shock) but who have flat neck veins, it is likely that the depression of left ventricular performance may be related, at least in part, to hypovolemia. The differentiation can be made only by assessing left ventricular performance using echocardiography or by measuring left ventricular filling pressure with a pulmonary artery flotation catheter.

CAROTID PULSE. Palpation of the carotid arterial pulse provides a clue to the left ventricular stroke volume; a small pulse suggests a reduced stroke volume, whereas a sharp, brief upstroke is often observed in patients with mitral regurgitation or ruptured ventricular septum with a left-to-right shunt. Pulsus alternans reflects severe left ventricular dysfunction.

THE CHEST. Moist rales are audible in patients who develop left ventricular failure and/or a reduction of left ventricular compliance with AMI. Diffuse wheezing may be present in patients with severe left ventricular failure. Cough with hemoptysis, suggesting pulmonary embolism with infarction, may also occur. In 1967 Killip proposed a prognostic classification scheme based on the presence and severity of rales detected in patients presenting with AMI.[240] Class I patients are free of rales and a third heart sound. Class II patients have rales but to only a mild-moderate degree (<50 per cent of lung fields) and may or may not have an S_3. Patients in Class III have rales in more than half of each lung field and frequently have pulmonary edema. Finally, Class IV patients are in cardiogenic shock. Despite overall improvement in mortality in each class, compared with data observed during the original development of the classification scheme, the latter remains useful today as evidenced by data from recent large MI trials.[10]

Cardiac Examination

PALPATION. Despite severe symptoms and extensive myocardial damage, the findings on examination of the heart may be quite unremarkable in patients with AMI.[241] Palpation of the precordium may yield normal findings, but in patients with transmural AMI it more commonly reveals a presystolic pulsation, synchronous with an audible fourth heart sound, reflecting a vigorous left atrial contraction filling a ventricle with reduced compliance. In the presence of left ventricular systolic dysfunction, an outward movement of the left ventricle may be palpated in early diastole, coincident with a third heart sound. When the anterior or lateral portion of the ventricle is dyskinetic, an abnormal systolic pulsation is present in the third, fourth, or fifth interspace to the left of the sternum. In some patients, this paradoxical precordial impulse is clearly separable from the point of maximal impulse, which is more lateral and to the left. In other patients, the abnormal impulse is a diffuse, rippling, precordial movement, approximately 5 to 10 cm in diameter, not clearly separable from the point of maximal impulse and can be appreciated near the left anterior axillary line. Patients with longstanding hypertension or previous infarction with left ventricular hypertrophy often demonstrate a laterally displaced, sustained apical impulse.

AUSCULTATION. The heart sounds, particularly the first sound, are frequently muffled and occasionally inaudible immediately after the infarct, and their intensity increases during convalescence. A soft first heart sound may also reflect prolongation of the P-R interval. Patients with marked ventricular dysfunction and/or left bundle branch block may have paradoxical splitting of the second heart sound (see p. 33). Patients with postinfarction angina may also develop a transient, paradoxically split second heart sound during anginal episodes.

A *fourth heart sound* is almost universally present in patients in sinus rhythm with AMI and is usually best heard between the left sternal border and the apex. This sound reflects the atrial contribution to ventricular filling and is particularly prominent in AMI patients due to a reduction in left ventricular compliance (see p. 1235) and elevation of left ventricular end-diastolic pressure, even in the absence of left ventricular systolic dysfunction. This finding is of limited diagnostic value because it is commonly audible in most patients with chronic ischemic heart disease and is recordable, although not often audible, in many normal subjects older than 45 years.

A *third heart sound* in AMI usually reflects severe left ventricular dysfunction with elevated ventricular filling pressure. It is caused by rapid deceleration of transmitral blood flow during protodiastolic filling of the left ventricle with resultant oscillations of the cardiohemic system (i.e., myocardium and stream of blood flowing from left atrium to left ventricle)[242] and is usually heard in patients with large infarctions. This sound is detected best at the apex, with the patient in the left lateral recumbent position, and is more common in patients with transmural anterior infarctions than in those with inferior or nontransmural infarctions. The mortality of patients who manifest a third heart sound during the acute phase of MI is higher than that of patients without such a sound.[243] A third heart sound may be caused not only by left ventricular failure but also by increased inflow into the left ventricle, as occurs when mitral regurgitation or ventricular septal defect complicates AMI. Third and fourth heart sounds emanating from the left ventricle are heard best at the apex; in patients with right ventricular infarcts, these sounds may be heard along the left sternal border and are intensified by inspiration.

Systolic murmurs, transient or persistent, are commonly audible in patients with AMI and generally result from mitral regurgitation secondary to dysfunction of the mitral valve apparatus (papillary muscle dysfunction, left ventricular dilatation). A new, prominent apical holosystolic murmur, accompanied by a thrill, may represent rupture of a head of a papillary muscle (see p. 1243). The findings in rupture of the interventricular septum are similar, although the murmur and thrill are usually most prominent along the left sternal border and may be audible at the right sternal border as well. The systolic murmur of tricuspid regurgitation (caused by right ventricular failure due to pulmonary hypertension and/or right ventricular infarction or by infarction of a right ventricular papillary muscle) is also heard along the left sternal border. It is characteristically intensified by inspiration and is accompanied by a prominent *c-v* wave in the jugular venous pulse and a right ventricular fourth sound.

Pericardial friction rubs are audible in 6 to 30 per cent of all patients with AMI and in a higher percentage of patients with transmural infarctions.[233] Rubs are notorious for their evanescence and, hence, are probably even more common than reported; frequent auscultation in patients with transmural infarction often results in the discovery of a rub that might otherwise have gone unnoticed. Although friction rubs may be heard within 24 hours or as late as 2 weeks after the onset of infarction, most commonly they are noted on the second or third day.[233] Occasionally, in patients with extensive infarction, a loud rub may be heard for many days. About 40 per cent of patients with AMI and a pericardial friction rub have a pericardial effusion on echocardiographic study,[244] but only rarely are the classic electrocardiographic changes of pericarditis (see p. 1483) seen.[233] Delayed onset of the rub and the associated discomfort of pericarditis (as late as 3 months postinfarction) are characteristic of the post–myocardial infarction (Dressler) syndrome (see p. 1256).

Pericardial rubs are most readily audible along the left sternal border or just inside the point of maximal impulse. Loud rubs may be audible over the entire precordium and even over the back. Occasionally, only the systolic portion of a rub is heard; it may be confused with a systolic murmur, and the diagnosis of rupture of the ventricular septum or mitral regurgitation may be incorrectly considered.

Other Findings

FUNDI. Hypertension, diabetes, and generalized atherosclerosis commonly accompany AMI, and because these conditions may produce characteristic changes in the fundus, a careful funduscopic examination may provide information concerning the underlying vascular status; this is particularly useful in patients unable to provide a detailed history.

ABDOMEN. As already noted, in patients with AMI, particularly in an inferior location with diaphragmatic irritation, the pain may be localized to the epigastrium or the right upper quadrant. Pain in the abdomen associated with nausea, vomiting, restlessness, and even abdominal distention is often interpreted by patients as a sign of "indigestion,"[236] resulting in self-medication with antacids, and it may suggest an acute abdominal process to the physician. Right heart failure, characterized by hepatomegaly and a positive abdominojugular reflux, is unusual in patients with acute left ventricular infarction but does occur in patients with severe and prolonged left ventricular failure or right ventricular infarction.

EXTREMITIES. Coronary atherosclerosis is often associated with systemic atherosclerosis, and it is therefore common for patients with AMI to have a history of intermittent claudication and to demonstrate physical findings of peripheral vascular disease. Thus, diminished peripheral arterial pulses, loss of hair, and atrophic skin in the lower extremities are noted frequently in patients with coronary artery disease. Peripheral edema is a manifestation of right ventricular failure and, like congestive hepatomegaly, is unusual in patients with acute left ventricular infarction. Cyanosis of the nailbeds is common in patients with severe left ventricular failure and is particularly striking in patients with cardiogenic shock.

NEUROPSYCHIATRIC FINDINGS (see also p. 1880). Except for the altered mental status that occurs in patients with AMI who have a markedly reduced cardiac output and cerebral hypoperfusion, the neurological examination is normal unless the patient has suffered cerebral embolism secondary to a mural thrombus. Indeed, an underlying MI is common in patients with cerebral embolic stroke.[245] In patients with cerebrovascular accidents, 13 per cent have an associated AMI (see p. 1879); in contrast, in a series of patients with AMI, only 2 per cent suffered a stroke. The relationship between stroke and AMI was confined to patients with large myocardial infarctions, as reflected in markedly elevated serum creatine kinase concentrations.[245] The coincidence between these two conditions may be explained by systemic hypotension due to MI precipitating a cerebral infarction and the converse, as well as by mural emboli from the left ventricle causing cerebral emboli.

Patients with AMI often exhibit alterations of the emotional state, including intense anxiety, denial, and depression. Medical staff caring for AMI patients must be sensitive to changes in the patient's emotional state—a calm, professional atmosphere, with thorough explanations of equipment and prognosis, can help alleviate the distress associated with AMI.[246]

Serum Markers of Cardiac Damage

The World Health Organization (WHO) criteria for the diagnosis of AMI require that at least two of the following three elements be present: a history of ischemic-type chest discomfort, evolutionary changes on serially obtained ECG tracings, and a rise and fall in serum cardiac markers.[247] There is considerable variability in the pattern of presentation of AMI with respect to these three elements, as exemplified by the following statistics. ST-segment elevation and Q waves on the ECG, two features that are highly indicative of AMI, are seen in only about half of AMI cases on presentation.[248] Approximately one-fourth of patients with AMI do not present with classic chest pain, and the event would go unrecognized unless an ECG were recorded fortuitously in temporal proximity to the infarction or permanent pathological Q waves are seen on later tracings.[249,250] Nondiagnostic ECGs are recorded in approximately half of patients presenting to emergency departments with chest pain suspicious for MI who ultimately are shown to have an AMI.[251] Among patients admitted to the hospital with a chest pain syndrome, fewer than 20 per cent are subsequently diagnosed as having had an AMI.[252,253] Therefore, in the majority of patients, clinicians must obtain serum cardiac marker measurements at periodic intervals to either establish or exclude the diagnosis of AMI[254]; such measurements may also be useful for a rough quantitation of the size of infarction.[255]

As myocytes become necrotic, the integrity of the sarcolemmal membrane is compromised and intracellular macromolecules (serum cardiac markers) begin to diffuse into the cardiac interstitium and ultimately into the microvasculature and lymphatics in the region of the infarct[97,256] (Fig. 37–17 and Table 37–2). The rate of appearance of these macromolecules in the peripheral circulation depends on several factors, including intracellular location, molecular weight, local blood and lymphatic flow, and the rate of elimination from the blood.[97,256,257]

Given the accelerated pace of decision-making in patients with acute coronary syndromes and emphasis on reduction of length of hospital stay,[258] there is considerable interest in evaluating new serum cardiac markers,[97] shortening assay time in the central chemistry laboratory,[259] and designing rapid whole blood bedside assays.[260] For optimal specificity, a serum marker of MI should be present in high concentration in the myocardium and be absent from nonmyocardial tissue and serum.[97,256] For optimal sensitivity it should be rapidly released into the blood after myocardial injury, and there should be a stoichiometric relationship between the plasma level of the marker and the extent of myocardial injury.[254] For ease of clinical use, the marker should persist in blood for an appropriate length of time to provide a convenient diagnostic time window (Table 37–2). Finally, the assay methodology should be inexpensive and easy to perform.

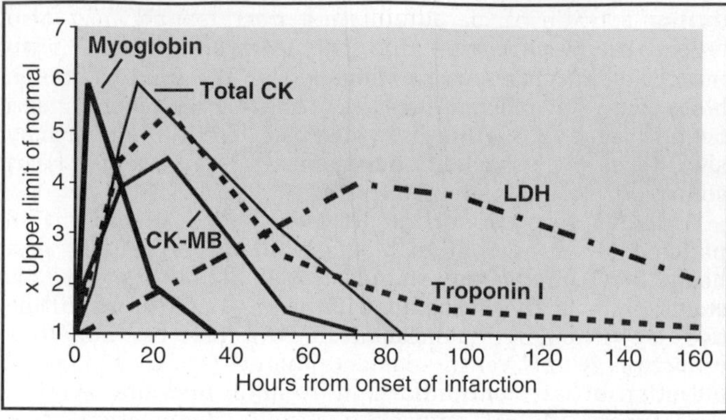

FIGURE 37–17. Time course of elevations of serum markers after AMI. This figure summarizes the relative timing, rate of rise, peak values, and duration of elevation above the upper limit of normal for multiple serum markers following AMI. Although traditionally total CK, CK-MB, and lactic dehydrogenase (LDH [with isoenzymes]) are measured, the relatively slow rate of rise above normal for CK and the potential confusion with noncardiac sources of enzyme release for both total CK and LDH have inspired the search for additional serum markers. The smaller molecule myoglobin is released quickly from infarcted myocardium but is not cardiac specific. Therefore, elevations of myoglobin that may be detected quite early after the onset of infarction require confirmation with a more cardiac-specific marker such as CK-MB or troponin I. Troponin I (and troponin T; not shown) rises more slowly than myoglobin and may be useful for diagnosis of infarction even up to 3 to 4 days after the event. Assays for cardiac-specific troponin I and troponin T using monoclonal antibodies are now available. (From Antman, E. M.: General hospital management. *In* Julian, D. G., and Braunwald, E. (eds.): Management of Acute Myocardial Infarction. London, W.B. Saunders Ltd., 1994, p. 63.)

CREATINE KINASE (CK). Serum CK activity exceeds the normal range within 4 to 8 hours following the onset of AMI and declines to normal within 2 to 3 days (Fig. 37–7). Although the peak CK occurs on average at about 24 hours, peak levels occur earlier in patients who have had reperfu-

TABLE 37–2 MOLECULAR MARKERS USED OR PROPOSED FOR USE IN THE DIAGNOSIS OF ACUTE MYOCARDIAL INFARCTION

MARKER	MW (D)	RANGE OF TIMES TO INITIAL ELEVATION (h)	MEAN TIME TO PEAK ELEVATIONS (NONTHROMBOLYSIS)	TIME TO RETURN TO NORMAL RANGE	MOST COMMON SAMPLING SCHEDULE
hFABP	14,000–15,000	1.5	5–10 h	24 h	On presentation, then 4 h later
Myoglobin	17,800	1–4	6–7 h	24 h	Frequent; 1–2 h after CP
MLC	19,000–27,000	6–12	2–4 d	6–12 d	Once at least 12 h after CP
cTnI	23,500	3–12	24 h	5–10 d	Once at least 12 h after CP
cTnT	33,000	3–12	12 h–2 d	5–14 d	Once at least 12 h after CP
MB-CK	86,000	3–12	24 h	48–72 h	Every 12 h × 3*
MM-CK tissue isoform	86,000	1–6	12 h	38 h	60–90 min after CP
MB-CK tissue isoform	86,000	2–6	18 h	Unknown	60–90 min after CP
Enolase	90,000	6–10	24 h	48 h	Every 12 h × 3
LD	135,000	10	24–48 h	10–14 d	Once at least 24 h after CP
MHC	400,000	48	5–6 d	14 d	Once at least >2 d after CP

hFABP = heart fatty acid binding proteins; MLC = myosin light chain; cTnI = cardiac troponin I; cTnT = cardiac troponin T; MB-CK = MB isoenzyme of creatine kinase (CK); MM-CK = MM isoenzyme of CK; LD = lactate dehydrogenase; MHC = myosin heavy chain; CP = chest pain.

* Increased sensitivity can be achieved with sampling every 6 or 8 h.

Modified from Adams, J., III, Abendschein, D., and Jaffe, A.: Biochemical markers of myocardial injury. Is MB creatine kinase the choice for the 1990s? Circulation *88:*750, 1993. Copyright 1993 American Heart Association.

sion as a result of the administration of thrombolytic therapy or mechanical recanalization (as well as in patients with early spontaneous thrombolysis). Because the time-activity curve of serum CK is influenced by reperfusion, and because reperfusion itself influences infarct size, reperfusion interferes with estimation of infarct size by enzyme analysis.[97,261]

Although elevation of the serum CK is a sensitive enzymatic detector of AMI that is routinely available in most hospitals,[97,262] important drawbacks include false-positive results in patients with muscle disease, alcohol intoxication, diabetes mellitus, skeletal muscle trauma, vigorous exercise, convulsions, intramuscular injections, thoracic outlet syndrome, and pulmonary embolism.[97,257,263]

CK ISOENZYMES. Three isoenzymes of CK (MM, BB, and MB) have been identified by electrophoresis. Extracts of brain and kidney contain predominantly the BB isoenzyme, skeletal muscle contains principally MM but does contain some MB (1 to 3 per cent),[264] and both MM and MB isoenzymes are present in cardiac muscle. The MB isoenzymes of CK may also be present in minor quantities in the small intestine, tongue, diaphragm, uterus, and prostate.[265] Strenuous exercise, particularly in trained long-distance runners or professional athletes, may cause elevation of both total CK and CK-MB.[97,266,267] Despite the fact that small quantities of CK-MB isoenzyme are found in tissues other than the heart, elevated serum activity of CK-MB may be considered, for practical purposes, to be the result of AMI (except in the case of trauma or surgery on the aforementioned organs, which contain small quantities of the enzyme). Earlier CK-MB assay methods that were in common use included radioimmunoassay and agarose gel electrophoresis techniques; these have now been largely supplanted by highly sensitive and specific enzyme immunoassays that utilize monoclonal antibodies directed against CK-MB.[268] Mass assays report results in nanograms per milliliter rather than units per milliliter and have been confirmed to be more accurate than CK-MB activity assays, especially in patients presenting within 4 hours of the onset of AMI.[269] It has been proposed that a ratio (relative index) of $\frac{\text{CK-MB mass}}{\text{CK activity}}$ of about 2.5 per cent is indicative of a myocardial rather than skeletal source of the CK-MB elevation.[270] Although this ratio may be satisfied by many patients with AMI, it is inaccurate in several circumstances: (1) When high levels of total CK are present because of skeletal muscle injury (a large quantity of CK-MB must be released from the myocardium to satisfy criteria); (2) Chronic skeletal muscle injury releases large amounts of CK-MB; (3) Total CK measurements are within the normal reference range for the laboratory and CK-MB is elevated (possibly indicating that a microinfarction has occurred).[97] Patients with minimally elevated CK-MB and normal CK have a prognosis that is generally worse than that for patients with suspected MI but no CK-MB elevation.[271] Thus, whether or not such elevations represent true "microinfarctions" may be less important than the prognostic connotations of this isolated elevation.

Clinicians should not rely on measurements of CK and CK-MB at a single point in time but instead should evaluate the temporal rise and fall of serially obtained values; skeletal muscle release of CK-MB generally remains elevated for a longer time than myocardial release of CK-MB and produces a "plateau" pattern of CK-MB values over several days, in contrast to the shorter time course of skeletal muscle CK-MB elevation, as depicted in Figure 37–17. Furthermore, the availability of new serum markers such as cardiac-specific troponin I and T (cTnI and cTnT) (Fig. 37–17 and Table 37–2) may help distinguish skeletal from cardiac muscle damage.

In addition to AMI secondary to coronary obstruction, other forms of injury to cardiac muscle—such as those resulting from myocarditis, trauma, cardiac catheterization, shock, and cardiac surgery—may also produce elevated serum CK-MB levels.[97] These latter causes of elevation of serum CK-MB values can usually be readily distinguished from AMI by the clinical setting.

CK ISOFORMS. Isoforms of the MM and MB isoenzymes have been identified.[272] These are subtypes of the individual isoenzymes and are formed in the circulation when an enzyme known as carboxypeptidase cleaves lysine residues from the carboxy terminus of the myocardial form of the enzyme (CK-MM3 and CK-MB2), producing isoforms with a different electrophoretic mobility (CK-MM2, CK-MM1, and CK-MB1). Certain isoforms appear to be released into the blood quite rapidly—perhaps as soon as 1 hour—after the onset of infarction. In one study an absolute level of the CK-MB2 isoform > 1.0 U/L or ratio of $\frac{\text{CK-MB2}}{\text{CK-MB1}} > 1.5$ had a sensitivity for diagnosing AMI of 59 per cent at 2 to 4 hours and of 92 per cent at 4 to 6 hours.[273] A rapid high-voltage electrophoretic assay for these isoforms has been developed and preliminary results in experienced research laboratories suggest it may permit early identification of patients with AMI and early detection of successful reperfusion (peak $\frac{\text{CK-MB2}}{\text{CK-MB1}} > 3.8$ at 2 hours).[259,274]

MYOGLOBIN. This protein is released into the circulation from injured myocardial cells and can be demonstrated within a few hours after the onset of infarction[275,276] (Fig. 37–17 and Table 37–2). Peak levels of serum myoglobin are reached considerably earlier (1 to 4 hours) than peak values of serum CK.[97] In contrast to CK, myoglobin (which has a molecular weight of only 17,800) is readily excreted into the urine. A more rapid rise in serum myoglobin has been observed following reperfusion, and its measurement has been suggested as a useful index of successful reperfusion[97,277] and even infarct size.[278] However, the clinical value of serial determinations of myoglobin in AMI is limited by the brief duration of its elevation (< 24 hours) and by the lack of specificity. The latter results from the fact that myoglobin is a constituent of skeletal muscle. Because of its lack of cardiac specificity, an isolated measurement of myoglobin within the first 4 to 8 hours following onset of chest discomfort in patients with a nondiagnostic ECG should not be relied upon to make the diagnosis of AMI but should be supplemented by a more cardiac-specific marker such as CK-MB, cTnI, or cTnT (Table 37–2).

CARDIAC-SPECIFIC TROPONINS. The troponin complex consists of three subunits that regulate the calcium-mediated contractile process of striated muscle.[279] These are troponin C, which binds Ca^{++}; troponin I (TnI), which binds to actin and inhibits actin-myosin interactions; and troponin T (TnT), which binds to tropomyosin, thereby attaching the troponin complex to the thin filament (see Fig. 12–4, p. 364). Although the majority of TnT is incorporated in the troponin complex, approximately 6 per cent is dissolved in the cytosol[280]; about 2 to 3 per cent of TnI is found in a cytosolic pool.[281]

Although both TnT and TnI are present in cardiac and skeletal muscle, they are encoded by different genes and the amino acid sequence differs.[282] This permits the production of antibodies that are specific for the cardiac form (cTnT and cTnI) and has led to the development of quantitative assays for cTnT and cTnI that have been approved by the FDA for clinical use[281,283–286] (Fig. 37–17 and Table 37–2). Several studies have confirmed the reliability of these new quantitative assays for detecting myocardial injury, and measurement of cTnT or cTnI has been proposed as a new diagnostic criterion for MI.[97,257,263,281,286–288] A qualitative, rapid, bedside assay for cTnT has also been approved for diagnosing AMI.[288a]

Because CK-MB is found in skeletal muscle, the cut-off value for an elevated CK-MB is typically set a few units above the upper end of the reference range. However, because cTnT or cTnI is not detected in the peripheral circulation under normal circumstances, the cut-off value for these analytes may be set only slightly above the "noise" level of the assay.[257,285] Furthermore, whereas CK-MB usually increases 10- to 20-fold above the upper limit of the reference range, cTnT and cTnI typically increase more than 20 times above the reference range. These features of the cardiac-specific troponin assays provide an improved signal-to-noise ratio, enabling the detection of even minor degrees of myocardial necrosis.[260,289–291] In patients with AMI, cTnT and cTnI first begin to rise above the upper reference limit by 3 hours from the onset of chest pain.[287] Elevations of cTnI may persist for 7 to 10 days following AMI; elevations of cTnT may persist for up to 10 to 14 days.

The kinetics of release of cTnT are similar for patients with Q-wave and non-Q-wave AMI.[257,292] Patients with AMI who undergo successful recanalization of the infarct-related artery have a rapid release of cTnT that may be useful as an indicator of reperfusion.[97,293,294] In theory the same should hold true for cTnI, but criteria for reperfusion have not been established yet. Also, although CK-MB measurements return to the normal range by 72 hours following infarction, the degeneration of the contractile apparatus produces a continuous release of cTnI from the complex for 5 to 10 days and cTnT for 10 to 14 days after AMI, permitting late diagnosis of infarction.[97,257]

When comparing the diagnostic efficiency of cTnT versus CK-MB for AMI, it is important to bear in mind that the cTnT assay is probably capable of detecting episodes of myocardial necrosis that are below the detection limit of the current CK-MB assays. The somewhat vague term of "minor myocardial damage" has been used to describe the pathological process in patients who have a chest pain syndrome and elevated cTnT but in whom CK-MB is in the normal range.[282,289] At the present time it remains unclear whether such patients have release of cTnT from a cytosolic pool in response to reversible ischemia or they have actually sustained "microinfarctions." However, it has been established that patients with a chest pain syndrome suspicious for AMI who have a normal CK-MB and elevated cTnT have an increased risk for adverse clinical outcome, including death, recurrent nonfatal infarction, and need for revascularization with PTCA or CABG.[260,282,289,295]

The independent diagnostic and prognostic value of measurement of cTnT or cTnI versus CK-MB or other serum cardiac markers is currently under investigation.[296–299] Until sufficient information in a large enough sample of patients is available, no definitive recommendations regarding the prognostic implications of these markers can be made.

LACTIC DEHYDROGENASE (LDH). The activity of this enzyme exceeds the normal range by 24 to 48 hours after the onset of AMI, reaches a peak 3 to 6 days after the onset of pain, and returns to normal levels 8 to 14 days after the infarction[97] (Fig. 37–17). Total LDH, although sensitive, is not specific; false-positive elevations occur in patients with hemolysis, megaloblastic anemia, leukemia, liver disease, hepatic congestion, renal disease, a variety of neoplasms, pulmonary embolism, myocarditis, skeletal muscle disease, and shock.[300]

LDH comprises five isoenzymes, which are numbered in the order of the rapidity of their migration toward the anode of an electrophoretic field. LDH_1 moves most rapidly, whereas LDH_5 is the slowest. Fractionation of the serum LDH into its five isoenzymes increases diagnostic accuracy because the heart contains principally LDH_1. Most conditions causing elevated serum total LDH activity, such as liver or skeletal muscle disease or injury, are readily distinguished from AMI by analysis of LDH isoenzymes. Increased serum LDH_1 activity precedes elevation of serum total LDH and usually occurs within 8 to 24 hours after infarction.[97] Because hemolysis also raises serum LDH_1 activity, particular care must be taken in the withdrawal and handling of the blood specimens.

Many laboratories report a ratio of LDH_1/LDH_2 greater than 1.0 as a cut-off defining abnormality. However, even a ratio as low as 0.76 has been reported to be more than 90 per cent sensitive and specific for the diagnosis of AMI.[97] Although LDH isoenzyme testing may be useful, it is likely that LDH isoenzyme analysis for the diagnosis of AMI will be superseded by newer, more cardiac-specific late markers such as cTnT or cTnI (Table 37–2).

OTHER SERUM CARDIAC MARKERS. For many years the activity of serum glutamic oxaloacetic acid transferase (SGOT)—now generally referred to as aspartate aminotransferase (AST)—was monitored for diagnosis of AMI. However, because false-positive elevations occur frequently (with most hepatic or skeletal muscle diseases, following intramuscular injections or pulmonary embolism, with shock) and because the time course of elevation offers no advantage relative to other serum markers, its incremental benefit for the diagnosis of AMI is negligible, and it is no longer routinely used.

Other promising serum cardiac markers that are under development include heart fatty acid binding proteins (hFABP), myosin light chains (MLC), myosin heavy chains (MHC), and glycogen phosphorylase isoenzyme BB (GPBB).[97,301,302] These markers offer the potential for earlier diagnosis (hFABP, GPBB) and a longer diagnostic window (MLC, MHC), but their relative roles compared with traditional markers such as CK-MB and newer markers such as CK-MB isoforms, cTnT, or cTnI remain to be defined. Carbonic anhydrase III is a protein found only in skeletal muscle and not cardiac muscle.[303] With injury to skeletal muscle it is released in a fixed relationship to myoglobin, and therefore the ratio of myoglobin to carbonic anhydrase III may be a useful means of excluding a cardiac source of myoglobin elevation.[304]

RECOMMENDATIONS FOR MEASUREMENT OF SERUM MARKERS. Although most hospitals obtain CK and CK-MB measurements when evaluating patients with suspected AMI, this practice may change in the near future as assays for more rapidly released markers such as myoglobin and more cardiac-specific markers such as troponin T and troponin I become available clinically.[287]

It seems reasonable for clinicians to measure either cTnT or cTnI in patients with suspected AMI. From a cost-effectiveness perspective, it is unnecessary to measure both a cardiac-specific troponin and CK-MB at all time points. Routine diagnosis of AMI can be accomplished within 12 hours using CK-MB, cTnT, or cTnI by obtaining measurements approximately every 8 to 12 hours. Retrospective diagnosis or diagnosis of AMI in the presence of skeletal muscle injury is more readily accomplished with cTnT or cTnI. Future directions for research with the cardiac troponins involve evaluating their ability to aid in the diagnosis of AMI that occurs following cardiac[305] and noncardiac surgery[286] and interventional catheterization procedures and in identifying myocardial injury from conditions other than AMI, such as myocarditis.[306]

Other Laboratory Measurements

Numerous nonspecific manifestations may be recognized in patients with AMI. Although they are not generally employed in establishing the diagnosis, awareness of their coexistence with infarction is important in order to avoid misinterpretation or erroneous diagnosis of other disorders.

SERUM LIPIDS. These are often determined in patients with AMI. However, the results may be misleading because numerous factors that can alter the values are operating at the time of the patient's admission to the hospital. Serum triglycerides are affected by caloric intake, intravenous glucose, and recumbency.

During the first 24 to 48 hours after admission, total cholesterol and HDL cholesterol remain at or near baseline values but generally fall precipitously after that.[307,308] The fall in HDL cholesterol after AMI is greater than the fall in total cholesterol; thus, the ratio of total cholesterol to HDL cholesterol is no longer useful for risk assessment early after MI.[309] In review of the revised, more aggressive guidelines for management of hyperlipidemia in patients with clinical manifestations of coronary artery disease,[310] a lipid profile should be obtained on all AMI patients who are admitted within 24 to 48 hours of symptoms. For patients admitted beyond 24 to 48 hours, it is best to defer determinations of serum lipid levels until at least 8 weeks after the infarction has occurred.

HEMATOLOGICAL MANIFESTATIONS. The elevation of the white blood count usually develops within 2 hours after the onset of chest pain, reaches a peak 2 to 4 days following infarction, and returns to normal in 1 week; the peak white blood cell count usually ranges between 12 and 15×10^3 per cubic millimeter but occasionally rises to as high as 20 × 10^3 per cubic millimeter in patients with large transmural AMI. Often there is an increase in the percentage of polymorphonuclear leukocytes and a shift of the differential count to band forms. Using a combination of abnormal leukocyte differential count and CK-MB was found to be especially helpful in the recognition of AMI when the initial ECG tracing was nondiagnostic.[311]

The erythrocyte sedimentation rate (ESR) is usually normal during the first day or two after infarction, even though fever and leukocytosis may be present. It then rises to a peak on the fourth or fifth day and may remain elevated for several weeks. The increase in the ESR is secondary to elevated plasma alpha$_2$ globulin fibrinogen,[312] but the peak does not correlate well with the size of the infarction or with the prognosis. The hematocrit often increases during the first few days following infarction as a consequence of hemoconcentration.[214]

Electrocardiographic Findings

(See also p. 127)

In the majority of patients with AMI, some change can be documented when serial electrocardiograms (ECGs) are compared.[312a] However, many factors limit the ability of the ECG to diagnose and localize MI: the extent of myocardial injury, the age of the infarct, its location (e.g., the 12-lead ECG is relatively insensitive to infarction in the posterolateral region of the left ventricle), the presence of conduction defects, the presence of previous infarcts or acute pericarditis, changes in electrolyte concentrations, and the administration of cardioactive drugs. Nevertheless, serial standard 12-lead ECGs remain a clinically useful method for the detection and localization of MI.[255] Even when left bundle branch block is present on the ECG, MI can be diagnosed when striking ST-segment deviation is present beyond that which can be explained by the conduction defect.[312b]

Although general agreement exists on electrocardiographic and vectorcardiographic criteria for the recognition of infarction of the anterior and inferior myocardial walls (Table 4–3, p. 129), less agreement is found on criteria for lateral and posterior infarcts[313]; here even the terminology may be confusing. It has been reported that patients with an abnormal R wave in V_1 (0.04 sec in duration and/or R/S ratio ≥ 1 in the absence of preexcitation or right ventricular hypertrophy) with inferior or lateral Q waves have an increased incidence of isolated occlusion of a dominant left circumflex coronary artery without collateral circulation; such patients have a lower ejection fraction, increased end-systolic volume, and higher complication rate than patients with inferior infarction due to isolated occlusion of the right coronary artery.[314]

More sophisticated forms of ECG recordings including high-resolution electrocardiography, body surface potential mapping of ST segments, and continuous vectorcardiography have all been reported in small series of patients to augment the 12-lead ECG in diagnosing AMI, but the lack of ready availability of equipment and the special expertise required limits the use of these techniques.[315–317] Of potentially more widespread clinical applicability is a clinical and ECG algorithm for predicting the presence of AMI that provides a computerized reading of the tracing along with a statement of the patient's risk of adverse cardiovascular events with and without reperfusion therapy.[318]

Although most patients continue to demonstrate the ECG changes from an infarction for the rest of their lives, particularly if they evolve Q waves, in a substantial minority the typical changes disappear, Q waves can regress,[319] and the ECG can even return to normal after a number of years. Under many circumstances Q-wave patterns may simulate MI. Conditions that may mimic the electrocardiographic features of MI by producing a pattern of "pseudoinfarction" include ventricular hypertrophy, conduction disturbances, preexcitation, primary myocardial disease, pneumothorax, pulmonary embolus, amyloid heart disease, primary and metastatic tumors of the heart, traumatic heart disease, intracranial hemorrhage, hyperkalemia, pericarditis, early repolarization, and cardiac involvement with sarcoidosis.[320]

Q-WAVE AND NON-Q-WAVE INFARCTION. As noted earlier (see p. 1189), the presence or absence of Q waves on the surface ECG does not reliably predict the distinction between transmural and nontransmural (subendocardial) AMI.[82,321] Q waves on the ECG signify abnormal electrical activity but are not synonymous with irreversible myocardial damage. Also, the absence of Q waves may simply reflect the insensitivity of the standard 12-lead ECG, especially in the posterior zones of the left ventricle.[82] True pathological subendocardial AMI, as recognized at autopsy, is seen with ST-segment depression and/or T-wave changes only about 50 per cent of the time.[322] Angiographic studies in AMI patients without ST-segment elevation show a higher incidence of subtotal occlusion of the culprit coronary vessel and greater collateral flow to the infarct zone[323,324] (Fig. 37–7). Observational data suggest that AMI without ST-segment elevation is seen more commonly in elderly patients and patients with a prior MI.[325,326]

Nevertheless, for the prognostic importance of identifying two different populations, a distinction should be made between AMI with and without Q waves, recognizing that the latter constitutes a heterogeneous group of abnormalities.[82,327,328] Changes in the ST segment and T wave are quite nonspecific and may occur in a variety of conditions, including stable and unstable angina pectoris, ventricular hypertrophy, acute and chronic pericarditis, myocarditis, early repolarization, electrolyte imbalance, shock, and metabolic disorders and following the administration of digitalis (see Chap. 4). Serial ECGs may be of considerable aid in differentiating these conditions from non-Q-wave infarction.[82,329] Transient changes favor angina or electrolyte disturbances, whereas persistent changes argue for infarction if other causes such as shock, administration of digitalis, and persistent metabolic disorders can be eliminated. In the final analysis, the diagnosis of nontransmural infarction rests more on the combination of clinical findings and the elevation of serum enzymes than on the ECG.

ISCHEMIA AT A DISTANCE. Patients with new Q waves and ST-segment elevation diagnostic for AMI in one territory often have ST-segment depression in other territories. These additional ST-segment changes may be caused by ischemia in a territory other than the area of infarction, termed "ischemia at a distance," or by reciprocal electrical phenomena.[330,331] A good deal of attention has been directed to associated ST-segment depression in the anterior leads, when it occurs in patients with acute inferior MI.[332,333] However, despite the clinical importance of differentiation among causes of anterior ST-segment depression in such patients—including anterior ischemia, posterior wall infarction, and true reciprocal changes—such a differentiation cannot be made reliably by electrocardiographic or even vectrocardiographic techniques. Although precordial ST-segment depression is more commonly associated with extensive infarction of the posterior, lateral, or inferior septal segments—rather than anterior wall subendocardial ischemia—imaging techniques such as two-dimensional echocardiography are necessary to ascertain whether an anterior wall motion abnormality is present. Regardless of whether the anterior ST-segment changes reflect anterior wall ischemia or are reciprocal to changes elsewhere, this finding, as with ischemia at a distance, implies a poorer prognosis than if such changes are not present.[330,331,333,334]

RIGHT VENTRICULAR INFARCTION. ST-segment elevation in right precordial leads (V_1, V_3R–V_6R) is a relatively sensitive and specific sign of right ventricular infarction.[335,336] Occasionally ST-segment elevation in leads V_2 and V_3 may be due to acute right ventricular infarction; this appears to occur only when the injury to the left inferior wall is minimal.[337] Usually, the concurrent inferior wall injury suppresses this anterior ST-segment elevation resulting from right ventricular injury. Likewise, right ventricular infarction appears to reduce the anterior ST-segment depression often observed with inferior wall myocardial infarction.[338] A QS or QR pattern in leads V_3R and/or V_4R also suggest right ventricular myocardial necrosis but has less predictive accuracy than ST-segment elevation in these leads.[339]

ATRIAL INFARCTION. The most common electrocardiographic patterns are depression or elevation of the PR segment, alterations in the contour of the P wave, and abnormal atrial rhythms, including atrial flutter, atrial fibrillation, wandering atrial pacemaker, and AV nodal rhythm.[340]

Imaging

ROENTGENOGRAPHY. The initial chest roentgenogram in patients with AMI is almost invariably a portable film obtained in the emergency room or the coronary care unit. Two findings are common: signs of left ventricular failure and cardiomegaly. Although the pulmonary vascular markings on the roentgenogram reflect left ventricular end-diastolic pressure, significant temporal discrepancies may occur because of what have been termed diagnostic lags and post-therapeutic lags. Up to 12 hours may elapse before pulmonary edema accumulates after ventricular filling pressure has become elevated. The post-therapeutic phase lag represents a longer time interval; up to 2 days are required for pulmonary edema to resorb and the radiographic signs of pulmonary congestion to clear after ventricular filling pressure has returned toward normal. The degree of congestion and the size of the left side of the heart on the chest film are useful for defining groups of patients with AMI who are at increased risk of dying after the acute event.[341]

Echocardiography

(See also pp. 87 to 90 and Fig. 3–87, p. 86)

TWO-DIMENSIONAL ECHOCARDIOGRAPHY. The relative portability of echocardiographic equipment makes this technique ideal for the assessment of patients with AMI hospitalized in the coronary care unit or even in the emergency department before admission.[342,342a] In patients with chest pain compatible with AMI but with a nondiagnostic ECG (Fig. 37–18), the finding on echocardiography of a distinct region of disordered contraction can be helpful diagnostically because it supports the diagnosis of myocardial ischemia.[343–345] Echocardiography is also useful in evaluating patients with chest pain and a nondiagnostic ECG who are suspected of having an aortic dissection. The identification of an intimal flap consistent with an aortic dissection is a crucial observation because it represents a major contraindication to thrombolytic therapy (see p. 1554).

Areas of abnormal regional wall motion are observed almost universally in patients with AMI, and the degree of wall motion abnormality can be categorized with a semiquantitative wall motion score index.[346] Abnormal wall motion is less often noted echocardiographically when the infarction is nontransmural; however, abnormalities are still present in more than two-thirds of these patients. Left ventricular function estimated from two-dimensional echocardiograms correlates well with measurements from angiography and is useful in establishing prognosis following AMI.[347] Furthermore, the early use of echocardiography can aid in the early detection of potentially viable but stunned myocardium (contractile reserve),[348,349] residual provocable ischemia,[350] patients at risk for the development of congestive heart failure following AMI,[351] and mechanical complications of AMI.[352]

Whereas transthoracic imaging is adequate in most patients, occasional patients have poor echo windows, especially if they are undergoing mechanical ventilation. In such patients transesophageal echocardiography can be safely performed[353] and can be useful in evaluating ventricular septal defects and papillary muscle dysfunction.[352]

DOPPLER ECHOCARDIOGRAPHY. This technique (see p. 56) allows for assessment of blood flow in the cardiac chambers and across cardiac valves. Used in conjunction with two-dimensional echocardiography, it is helpful in detecting and assessing the severity of mitral or tricuspid regurgitation following AMI.[354] Identification of the site of acute ventricular septal rupture, as well as quantification of shunt flow across the resulting defect, is also possible.[355]

Other Imaging Modalities

COMPUTED TOMOGRAPHY (CT) (see p. 337). This technique can provide useful cross-sectional information in patients with MI. In addition to the assessment of cavity di-

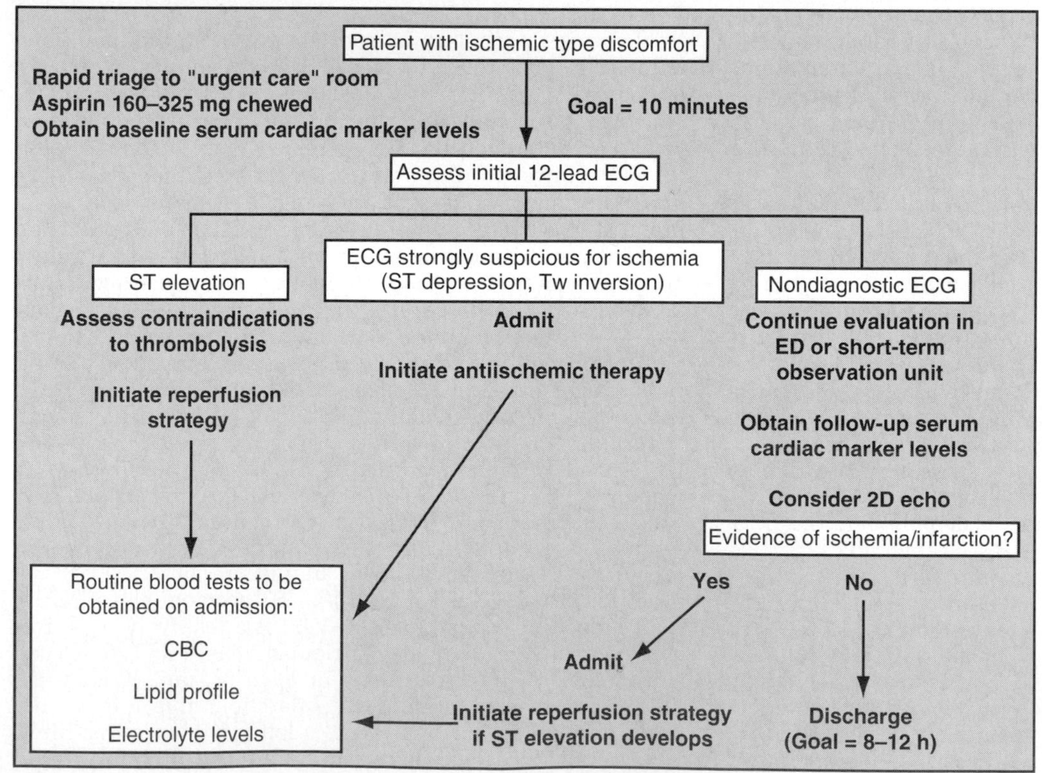

FIGURE 37–18. Algorithm for management of patients with suspected AMI in emergency department. All patients with ischemic-type discomfort should be rapidly evaluated and receive aspirin. The initial 12-lead electrocardiogram (ECG) is used to define the acute management strategy. Patients with ST-segment elevation should be considered candidates for reperfusion, whereas those without ST-segment elevation whose ECG and clinical history are strongly suspicious for ischemia should be admitted for initiation of antiischemic therapy. Patients with a nondiagnostic ECG should undergo further evaluation in the emergency department or short-term observation unit with ultimate disposition based on the results of serial serum cardiac marker levels and echocardiographic findings. Routine blood tests that should be obtained in all patients admitted include a complete blood count (CBC), lipid profile, and electrolyte levels.

mensions and wall thickness,[356] left ventricular aneurysms may be detected, and, of particular importance in AMI, intracardiac thrombi can be identified. Although cardiac CT is a less convenient technique, it probably is more sensitive for thrombus detection than is echocardiography.[357]

MAGNETIC RESONANCE IMAGING (MRI) (see Figs. 10–3, p. 320 and 10–4, p. 321). In addition to localizing and sizing the area of infarction, MRI techniques are capable of early recognition of MI and of providing an assessment of the severity of the ischemic insult.[358–360a] Although imaging with this technique presents practical problems for routine studies in coronary care unit patients because patients must be transported to the MRI facility, this modality holds much promise because of its ability to assess perfusion of infarcted and noninfarcted tissue as well as of reperfused myocardium; to identify areas of jeopardized but not infarcted myocardium; to identify myocardial edema, fibrosis, wall thinning, and hypertrophy; to assess ventricular chamber size and segmental wall motion; and to identify the temporal transition between ischemia and infarction.[358,361]

NUCLEAR IMAGING. Radionuclide angiography, perfusion imaging, infarct-avid scintigraphy, and positron-emission tomography have been used to evaluate patients with AMI. Nuclear cardiac imaging techniques (Fig. 9–21, p. 287, Figs. 9–30 and 9–31, p. 296) can be useful for detecting AMI[362]; assessing infarct size,[363] collateral flow,[116] and jeopardized myocardium; determining the effects of the infarct on ventricular function; and establishing prognosis of patients with AMI.[363,363a] However, the necessity of moving a critically ill patient from the coronary care unit (CCU) to the nuclear medicine department limits their practical application unless a portable gamma camera is available. The ACC/AHA Task Force Committee on Cardiac Radionuclide Imaging has *not* recommended the *routine* use of any radionuclide imaging technique for the purpose of diagnosing AMI, but considered rest radionuclide angiography for assessment of right and left ventricular function and stress myocardial perfusion imaging for detection of ischemia as usually appropriate and potentially useful (Class I).[362] The committee further emphasized that before ordering cardiac radionuclide imaging in individual patients, the quality of the laboratory, the expertise of the staff performing and evaluating the test results, and the potential impact of positive and negative results on subsequent clinical decision-making all be carefully considered.[362]

Estimation of Infarct Size

ELECTROCARDIOGRAPHY. Interest in limiting infarct size, in large part because of the recognition that the quantity of myocardium infarcted has important prognostic implications, has focused attention on the accurate determination of MI size. The sum of ST-segment elevations measured from multiple precordial leads correlates with the extent of myocardial injury in patients with anterior MI.[364] QRS scoring systems and planar or vectorcardiographic techniques to estimate infarct size have also been developed. Although they demonstrate good correlations with infarct size at autopsy and with enzymatic estimates, formal sizing of infarcts by ECG technique is not necessary in most patients. Of note, however, there is a relationship between the number of ECG leads showing ST elevation and mortality—patients with 8 or 9 of 12 leads with ST elevation have three to four times the mortality of those with only 2 or 3 leads with ST elevation.[365] The duration of ischemia time as estimated from continuous ST segment monitoring is correlated with infarct size, the ratio of infarct size to area at risk, and the extent of regional wall motion abnormality observed at 7 days and 30 days after AMI.[364]

SERUM CARDIAC MARKER METHODS. In order to estimate infarct size by analysis of serum cardiac marker levels, it is necessary to account for the quantity of the marker lost from the myocardium, its volume of distribution, and its release ratio.[97] Serial measurements of proteins released by necrotic myocardium, particularly CK and its MB isoenzyme, are helpful in determining AMI size. Clinically, the peak CK or CK-MB provides an approximate estimate of infarct size and is widely used prognostically. In the prethrombotic era, quantification of the cumulative release of CK or CK-MB correlated with other techniques for estimating infarct size in vivo as well as with the area of necrosis at autopsy. However, coronary artery reperfusion dramatically changes the wash-out kinetics of CK from myocardium, resulting in early and exaggerated peak enzyme levels and limiting the usefulness of CK curves as a measure of infarct size.[261] Whether structural proteins such as the troponins, whose release ratios are less affected by rapid changes in coronary flow, offer an advantage in this regard requires further investigation.[97]

NONINVASIVE IMAGING TECHNIQUES. Echocardiography (see Chap. 3), radionuclide scintigraphy[363] (see Chap. 9), CT scanning (see Chap. 10), and MRI[360] (see Chap. 10) have all been utilized for the clinical and experimental assessment of infarct size. Infarct-avid scintigraphy and myocardial perfusion imaging have been used to quantify infarct size. Estimation of infarct size by quantitative tomographic ^{99m}Tc-sestamibi imaging appears to be less limited by ventricular geometry and can distinguish small infarcts and ischemia from infarcted myocardium more readily than other noninvasive methods.[363] Tomography has improved on planar techniques employing technetium-99m pyrophosphate to image AMI (see p. 285).[366] Imaging of radiolabeled myosin-specific antibodies, which bind to myosin exposed by the loss of plasma membrane in early myocardial necrosis, holds promise for highly accurate quantification of infarct size.[87,367,368] Contrast-enhanced MRI imaging has been helpful in demonstrating the regional heterogeneity of infarction patterns in patients with persistently occluded infarct arteries versus those with successfully reperfused vessels.[369]

MANAGEMENT

Physician practices have changed dramatically as newer approaches to the care of the AMI patient have become available.[35,36,45] Almost all physicians in the United States have access to intensive care facilities for their patients with AMI. The current average hospital length of stay is 5 to 6 days, less than half of what it was in 1970. The National Registry of Myocardial Infarction, an observational data base of practice patterns reflecting treatment of 240,989 patients with AMI at 1073 hospitals between 1990 and 1993, reported that nearly 80 per cent of patients with AMI received aspirin.[12] Invasive and/or noninvasive procedures to evaluate prognosis and the need for further therapy are now used in most post-MI patients, whereas only a small percentage of patients had such procedures performed 25 years ago.[35,36,45] Finally, thrombolytic therapy and angioplasty are now the standard of care in appropriately selected patients.[370–374] The combination of these measures has led to a decline in the short-term mortality from AMI.[22]

PREHOSPITAL CARE

The prehospital care of patients with suspected acute myocardial infarction is a crucial element bearing directly on the likelihood of survival. Most deaths associated with AMI occur within the first hour of its onset and are usually due to ventricular fibrillation[375] (see also Chap. 24). Accordingly, the importance of the immediate implementation of definitive resuscitative efforts and of rapidly transporting the patient to a hospital cannot be overemphasized.[376] Major components of the delay from the onset of symptoms consistent with AMI to treatment include the following[375]: (1) the time for the patient to recognize the seriousness of the problem and seek medical attention; (2) prehospital evaluation, treatment, and transportation; (3) the time for diagnostic measures and initiation of treatment in the hospital.

Patients must be educated to seek immediate medical

attention should they develop manifestations of AMI. The GISSI investigators have analyzed the epidemiology of avoidable delays in the care of patients with AMI in Italy since 1990 and reported that the decision time by the patient played a more significant role than home-to-hospital time and in-hospital time in delay to treatment of AMI.[377] Patient-related factors that were correlated with longer decision to seek medical attention included advanced age, living alone, low intensity of initial symptoms, history of diabetes, occurrence of symptoms at night, and involvement of a general practitioner before arrival in the emergency department.[377]

Health care professionals should heighten the level of awareness of patients at risk for AMI (e.g., those with hypertension, diabetes, history of angina pectoris). They should review and reinforce with patients and their families the need for seeking urgent medical attention for a pattern of symptoms including chest discomfort, extreme fatigue, and dyspnea, especially if accompanied by diaphoresis, lightheadedness, palpitations, or a sense of impending doom.[378] Although many patients shun such discussions and tend to minimize the likelihood of ever needing emergency cardiac treatment, emphasis should be placed on the prevention and treatment of potentially fatal arrhythmias as well as salvage of the jeopardized myocardium by reperfusion, for which time is crucial.[379] Patients should also be instructed in the proper use of sublingual nitroglycerin that should be taken as one tablet at the onset of ischemic-type discomfort and repeated at 5-minute intervals for a total of three doses. If the symptoms have not dissipated within 15 minutes, the patient should be rapidly transported to a medical facility that has the capability of recording and interpreting an electrocardiogram, providing advanced cardiac life support and cardiac monitoring, and initiating reperfusion therapy with either thrombolysis or angioplasty if indicated.[2] Primary care physicians need to take a larger role in helping implement strategies to facilitate early treatment.[378]

Well-equipped ambulances and helicopters staffed by personnel trained in the acute care of the infarction victim (mobile CCUs) allow definitive therapy to commence while the patient is being transported to the hospital.[380] To be used effectively, they must be placed strategically within a community, and excellent radio communication systems must be available. These units should be equipped with battery-operated monitoring equipment, a DC defibrillator, oxygen, endotracheal tubes and suction apparatus, and commonly used cardiovascular drugs. A radiotelemetry system that allows transmission of the ECG signal to the hospital is desirable but not essential. The effectiveness of such a system depends upon the competency of paramedics, transmission distances, and the availability of expert consultation on the receiving end.[381] Observations of simple variables such as heart rate and blood pressure permit initial classification of patients into high- or low-risk subgroups[382] because those patients initially presenting with hypotension have a mortality in excess of 30 per cent, whereas young patients with isolated sinus bradycardia and a normal or elevated blood pressure appear to have a mortality that is under 5 per cent.[10]

In addition to prompt defibrillation, the efficacy of prehospital care appears to depend on several factors, including early relief of pain with its deleterious physiological sequelae, reduction of excessive activity of the autonomic nervous system, and abolition of prelethal arrhythmias, such as ventricular tachycardia. However, these efforts must not inhibit rapid transfer to the hospital, which might possibly diminish the benefit of the patient's early entry into the health care system.

PREHOSPITAL THROMBOLYSIS. The potential benefits of prehospital thrombolysis have been evaluated in five randomized trials that collectively randomized 6318 patients.[382–386] Although none of the individual trials showed a significant reduction in mortality with prehospital initiated thrombolytic therapy, there was a generally consistent observation of benefit from earlier treatment, and a meta-analysis of all the available trials demonstrated a 17 per cent reduction in mortality (95 per cent CI: 2 per cent to 29 per cent).[386]

Several factors must be weighed when communities consider whether their ambulances and emergency transport vehicles should have capabilities of initiating thrombolytic therapy. The greatest reduction in mortality is observed when reperfusion can be initiated within 60 to 90 minutes of the onset of symptoms.[10,375] It has been suggested that the streamlining of emergency department triage practices so that treatment can be started within 30 minutes, when coupled with the 15 to 30 minute transport time that is common in most urban centers, may be more cost effective than equipping all ambulances to administer prehospital thrombolytic therapy.[387] The latter would require extensive training of personnel, installation of computer-assisted electrocardiographs or systems for radio transmission of the ECG signal to a central station, and stocking of medicine kits with the necessary drug supplies.[381,388–390] However, in selected communities where transport delays may be 90 minutes or longer and experienced personnel or physicians are available on ambulances, prehospital thrombolytic therapy is probably beneficial.[390]

MANAGEMENT IN THE EMERGENCY DEPARTMENT

Physicians evaluating patients in the emergency department must confront the difficult task of rapidly identifying patients who require urgent reperfusion therapy, triaging lower risk patients to the appropriate facility within the hospital, and not discharging patients home inappropriately while avoiding unnecessary admissions.[375,391,392] As emphasized in Figure 37–18, a history of ischemic-type discomfort and the initial 12-lead electrocardiogram (Fig. 37–19) are the primary tools for screening patients with acute coronary syndromes in the emergency department.[376,393] ST-segment elevation on the electrocardiogram of a patient with a history compatible with AMI (see p. 1205) is highly suggestive of thrombotic occlusion of an epicardial coronary artery,[100,323,324] and its presence should serve as the trigger for a well-rehearsed sequence of rapid assessment of the patient for contraindications to thrombolysis and initiation of a reperfusion strategy[375,391] (Fig. 37–20).

Because lethal arrhythmias can occur suddenly in patients with an acute coronary syndrome, all patients should rapidly have a 12-lead ECG performed while a brief targeted history is taken[375,391] (Fig. 37–18). Patients should then be attached to a bedside ECG monitor and intravenous access obtained for infusion of 5 per cent dextrose in water. If the initial ECG shows ST-segment elevation of 1 mm or more in at least two contiguous leads (Fig. 37–19) or a new or presumably new left bundle branch block, the patient should be screened immediately for any contraindications to thrombolysis (Table 37–3) to help facilitate expeditious initiation of reperfusion therapy (see p. 1215). The National Heart Attack Alert Program recommends that emergency departments strive for a goal of treating eligible AMI patients with thrombolytic therapy within 30 minutes[375,391] (Fig. 37–21).

Patients with an initial ECG that reveals new or presumably new ST-segment depression and/or T-wave inversion, while not considered candidates for thrombolytic therapy, should be treated as though they are suffering from AMI without ST elevation or unstable angina (a distinction to be made subsequently after scrutiny of serial ECGs and serum cardiac marker measurements) (Fig. 37–5).

The available data fail to show a benefit of thrombolysis

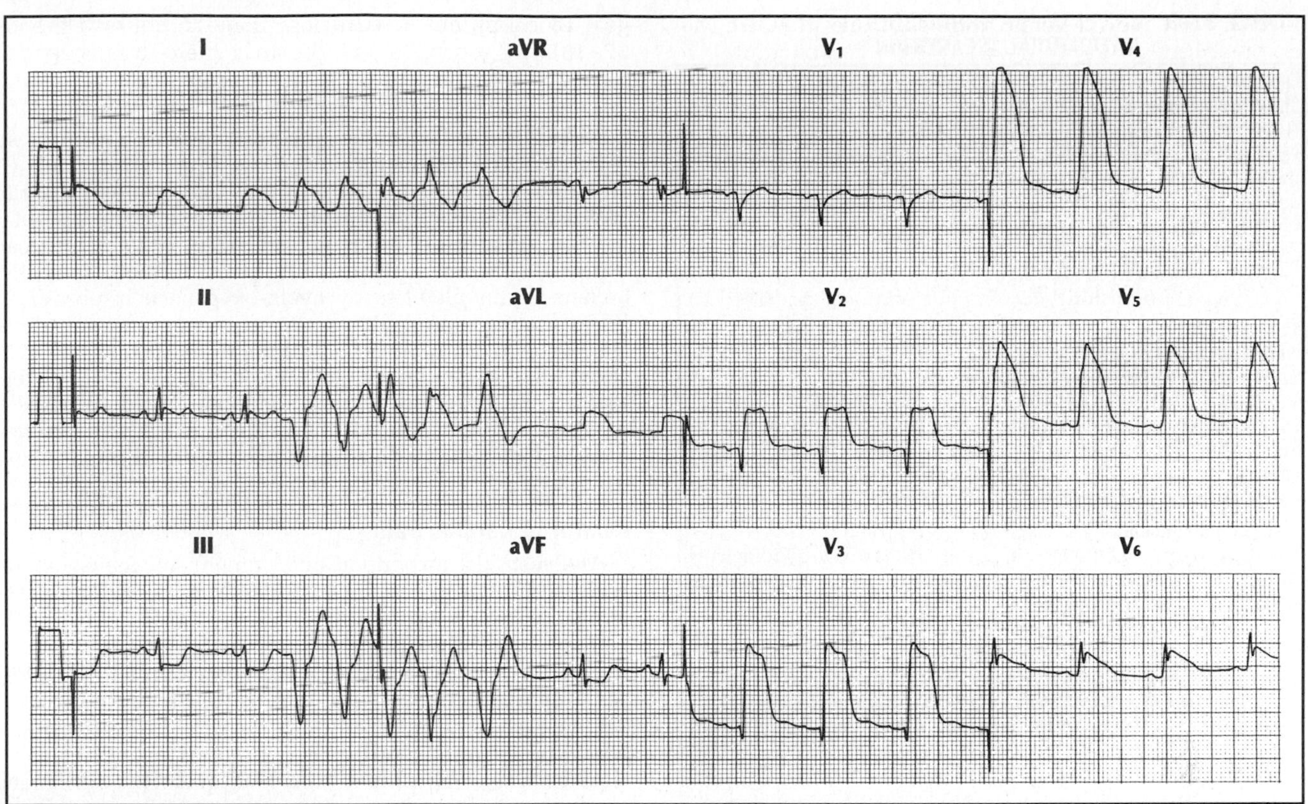

FIGURE 37–19. This 12-lead ECG was obtained from a middle-aged man admitted with an extensive anterior AMI. (Note pathological Q waves in the precordial leads and marked repolarization abnormalities in the anterior and lateral leads.) A five-beat salvo of nonsustained ventricular tachycardia is seen extending over the transition between leads III and aV_f. (From Antman, E. M., and Rutherford, J. D.: Coronary Care Medicine. Boston, Martinus Nijhoff Publishing, 1986, p. 81.)

in AMI patients who do not present with ST-segment elevation[10,394,395] (Fig. 37–18). Management of the AMI patient without ST-segment elevation is an important problem[396] because about 40 to 50 per cent of patients with AMI are not considered candidates for thrombolysis on the basis of an initial ECG that does not show ST-segment elevation.[397,398] Some patients without ST-segment elevation on the initial ECG may subsequently experience a worsening of ischemic discomfort, develop ST-segment elevation (presumably when a subtotal occlusion of the culprit coronary artery progresses to total occlusion), and become candidates for reperfusion therapy (Table 37–3). Therefore, pa-

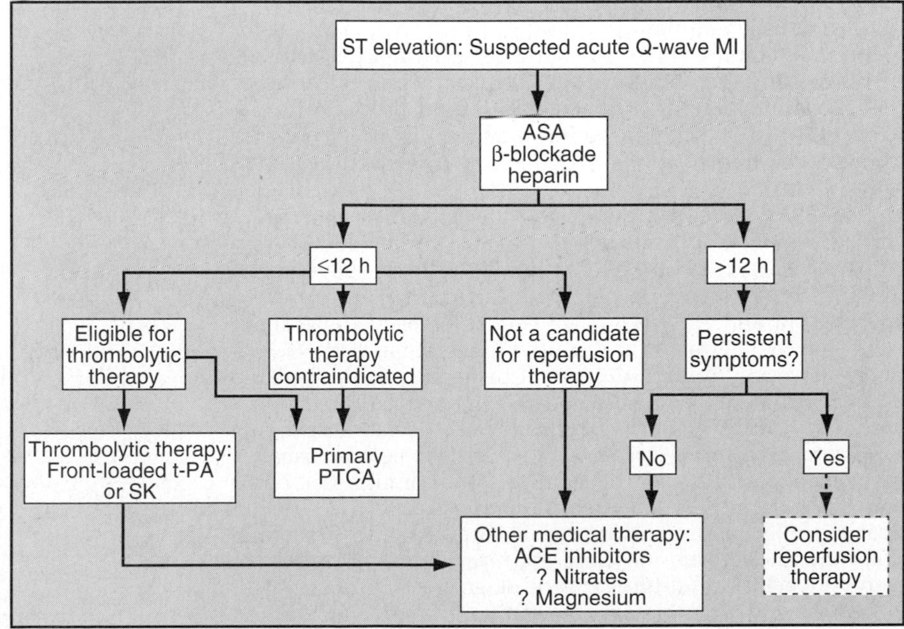

FIGURE 37–20. Recommendations for management of patients with an acute Q-wave MI. All patients suspected of having a Q-wave MI (i.e., ST-segment elevation on electrocardiogram [ECG]) should receive aspirin (ASA), beta blockers (in the absence of contraindications), and an antithrombin (particularly if tissue-type plasminogen activator [t-PA] is used for thrombolytic therapy). Whether heparin is required in patients receiving streptokinase (SK) remains a matter of controversy; the small additional risk for intracranial hemorrhage may not be offset by the survival benefit afforded by adding heparin to SK therapy. Patients treated within 12 hours who are eligible for thrombolytics should expeditiously receive either front-loaded t-PA or SK or be considered for primary percutaneous transluminal coronary angioplasty (PTCA). Primary PTCA is also to be considered when lytic therapy is contraindicated. Individuals treated after 12 hours should receive the initial medical therapy noted above and, on an individual basis, may be candidates for angiotensin-converting enzyme (ACE) inhibitors (particularly if left ventricular function is impaired). Further information is required to place the role of magnesium in proper perspective. After discharge, all patients should receive aspirin and a beta blocker (in the absence of contraindications). Dietary modifications and, if needed, treatment to reduce LDL-cholesterol and elevate HDL-cholesterol are strongly encouraged, as is life style modification (including regular physical exercise and cessation of cigarette smoking). (Modified from Antman, E. M.: Medical therapy for acute coronary syndromes: An overview. *In* Califf, R. M. [ed.]: Acute Myocardial Infarction and Other Acute Ischemic Syndromes, vol. 8. Braunwald, E. (ed.): Atlas of Heart Diseases. Philadelphia, Current Science, 1996 [pp. 10–10.25].)

TABLE 37–3 CRITERIA FOR THROMBOLYSIS IN ACUTE MYOCARDIAL INFARCTION

Indications
1. Chest pain consistent with AMI
2. Electrocardiographic changes
   ST-segment elevation >0.1 mV in at least two contiguous leads
   New or presumably new left bundle branch block
3. Time from onset of symptoms
   <6 hours: most beneficial
   6–12 hours: lesser but still important benefits
   >12 hours: diminishing benefits but may still be useful in selected patients

Absolute Contraindications
1. Active internal bleeding (excluding menses)
2. Suspected aortic dissection
3. Recent head trauma or known intracranial neoplasm
4. History of cerebrovascular accident known to be hemorrhagic
5. Major surgery or trauma <2 wks

Relative Contraindications*
1. Blood pressure >180/110 mm Hg on at least two readings
2. History of chronic, severe hypertension with or without drug therapy
3. Active peptic ulcer
4. History of cerebrovascular accident
5. Known bleeding diathesis or current use of anticoagulants
6. Prolonged or traumatic cardiopulmonary resuscitation
7. Diabetic hemorrhagic retinopathy or other hemorrhagic ophthalmic condition
8. Pregnancy
9. Prior exposure to streptokinase or APSAC (This contraindication is particularly important in the initial 6- to 9-month period after streptokinase or APSAC administration and applies to reuse of any streptokinase-containing agent but does not apply to t-PA or urokinase.)

* These should be considered on a case-by-case analysis or risk versus benefit. In instances in which these contraindications (particularly 1 to 5) have paramount importance, such as more active peptic ulcer with history of bleeding, they become absolute contraindications when weighed against a less than life-threatening, evolving AMI.

Adapted from AHA Medical/Scientific Statement Special Report (1990): ACC/AHA guidelines for the early management of patients with acute myocardial infarction. Circulation *82*:707; Anderson, H. V., and Willerson, J. T.: Thrombolyis in acute myocardial infarction. N. Engl. J. Med. *329*:703, 1993. Copyright 1993 Massachusetts Medical Society.

tients whose ECG is highly suggestive of myocardial ischemia should be admitted to a hospital unit with facilities for continuous monitoring of the ECG (either the CCU or intermediate care unit) that will alert the staff if arrhythmias or ST elevation occurs. Arrangements should be made for 12-lead ECGs to be obtained approximately every 8 hours for the first 24 hours, or more frequently if ischemic discomfort recurs.

Patients with a history suggestive of AMI (see p. 1198) and an initial nondiagnostic ECG (i.e., no obvious ST-segment deviation or T-wave inversion) should have serial tracings obtained while being evaluated in the emergency department for AMI (Fig. 37–18). Emergency department staff may be alerted to the sudden development of ST segment elevation by periodic visual inspection of the bedside ECG monitor, by continuous ST-segment recording, or by auditory alarms when the ST-segment deviation exceeds programmed limits. Decision aids such as computer-based diagnostic algorithms,[399,399a] identification of high-risk clinical indicators,[400] rapid determination of cardiac serum markers,[260] two-dimensional echocardiographic screening for regional wall motion abnormalities,[343,344,401,402] and myocardial perfusion imaging[403] are of greatest clinical utility when the ECG is nondiagnostic. In an effort to improve the cost effectiveness of care of patients with a chest pain syndrome, nondiagnostic ECG, and low suspicion of AMI but in whom the diagnosis has not been entirely excluded, many medical centers have developed critical pathways[404,405] that involve a coronary observation unit with a goal of ruling out AMI in less than 12 hours[392,406,407] (Fig. 37–18).

General Treatment Measures

ASPIRIN. This agent is effective across the entire spectrum of acute coronary syndromes (Figs. 37–5 and 37–7) and now forms part of the initial management strategy of patients with suspected AMI (Fig. 37–18). The pharmacology of aspirin is presented on page 1819. The goal of aspirin treatment is to quickly block formation of thromboxane A_2 in platelets by cyclo-oxygenase inhibition.[408,409] Because low doses (40 to 80 mg) take several days to achieve full antiplatelet effect,[410] at least 160 to 325 mg should be administered acutely in the emergency department.[411] In order to achieve therapeutic blood levels rapidly, the patient should chew the tablet, thus promoting buccal absorption rather than absorption through the gastric mucosa.

Control of Cardiac Pain

Analgesia is an important element of management of AMI patients in the emergency department. Often there is a tendency to underdose the patient for fear of obscuring response to anti-ischemic or reperfusion therapy. This should be avoided because pain contributes to the heightened sympathetic activity that is particularly prominent during the early phase of AMI. Control of cardiac pain is typically accomplished with a combination of nitrates, analgesics (e.g., morphine), oxygen, and beta-adrenoceptor blockers. Similar pharmacological principles apply in the coronary care unit, where many of the therapies discussed below are continued after initial dosing in the emergency department.[412] Because the pain associated with MI is related to ongoing ischemia (see p. 1198), many interventions that act to improve the oxygen supply-demand relationship (by either increasing supply or decreasing demand) may lessen the pain associated with AMI.

ANALGESICS. Although a wide variety of analgesic agents has been used to treat the pain associated with AMI, including meperidine, pentazocine, and morphine, the latter remains the drug of choice, except in patients with well-documented morphine hypersensitivity. Four to 8 mg should be administered intravenously and doses of 2 to

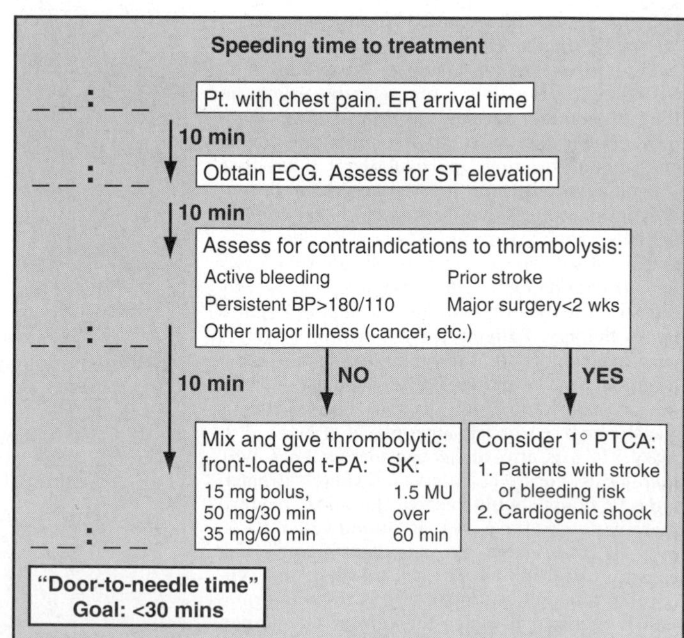

FIGURE 37–21. Algorithm for rapid triage of patients in the emergency room (ER) to provide thrombolysis with the shortest possible "door-to-needle" time. (From Cannon, C. P., Antman, E. M., Walls, R., and Braunwald, E.: Time as an adjunctive agent to thrombolytic therapy. J. Thromb. Thrombolysis *1*:31, 1994.)

8 mg repeated at intervals of 5 to 15 minutes until the pain is relieved or evident toxicity—i.e., hypotension, depression of respiration, or severe vomiting—precludes further administration of the drug. In some patients, remarkably large cumulative doses of morphine (2 to 3 mg/kg) may be required and are usually tolerated.[30]

The reduction of anxiety resulting from morphine diminishes the patient's restlessness and the activity of the autonomic nervous system, with a consequent reduction of the heart's metabolic demands. The beneficial effect of morphine in patients with pulmonary edema is unequivocal and may relate to several factors, including peripheral arterial and venous dilatation (particularly among patients with excessive sympathoadrenal activity), reduction of the work of breathing, and slowing of heart rate secondary to combined withdrawal of sympathetic tone and augmentation of vagal tone.[30]

Hypotension following the administration of nitroglycerin (Fig. 37–22) and morphine can be minimized by maintaining the patient in a supine position and elevating the lower extremities if systolic arterial pressure declines below 100 mm Hg. Obviously, such positioning is undesirable in the presence of pulmonary edema, but morphine rarely produces hypotension under these circumstances. The concomitant administration of atropine in doses of 0.5 to 1.5 mg intravenously may be helpful in reducing the excessive vagomimetic effects of morphine, particularly when hypotension and bradycardia are present before it is administered. Respiratory depression is an unusual complication of morphine in the presence of severe pain or pulmonary edema, but as the patient's cardiovascular status improves, impairment of ventilation may supervene and should be watched for. It can be treated with naloxone, in doses of 0.1 to 0.2 mg intravenously initially, repeated after 15 minutes if necessary. Nausea and vomiting may be troublesome side effects of large doses of morphine and may be treated with a phenothiazine.

Other analgesics such as meperidine are less effective than is morphine but are equally likely to produce side effects and are prone to augment ventricular rate. Preliminary reports of treatment of AMI patients with the synthetic and semisynthetic narcotics fentanyl and sufentanil, patient controlled analgesia, and thoracic epidural anesthesia are encouraging, but the experience is too limited to recommend the use of these agents and modalities in routine practice.[413]

NITRATES. By virtue of their ability to enhance coronary blood flow by coronary vasodilation and to decrease ventricular preload by increasing venous capacitance, sublingual nitrates are indicated for most patients with an acute coronary syndrome. At present, the only groups of patients with AMI in whom sublingual nitroglycerin should *not* be given are those with inferior MI and suspected right ventricular infarction[105] or marked hypotension (systolic pressure <90 mm Hg), especially if accompanied by bradycardia.

Once it is ascertained that hypotension is not present, a sublingual nitroglycerin tablet should be administered and the patient observed carefully for improvement in symptoms or change in hemodynamics. If an initial dose is well tolerated and appears to be of benefit, further nitrates should be administered, with careful monitoring of the vital signs. Even small doses may produce sudden hypotension and bradycardia, a reaction that can be life-threatening but can usually be easily reversed with intravenous atropine if it is recognized quickly (Fig. 37–22). Long-acting oral nitrate preparations should be avoided in the very early course of AMI because of the frequently changing hemodynamic status of the patient. In patients with a prolonged period of waxing and waning chest pain, intravenous nitroglycerin may be of benefit in controlling symptoms and correcting ischemia, but frequent monitoring of blood pressure is required.[30]

BETA-ADRENOCEPTOR BLOCKERS. These drugs have been used in the early hours of AMI in attempts to limit the size of the infarct (see p. 1212). In the course of these studies, it has been recognized that beta blockers relieve pain and reduce the need for analgesics in many patients, presumably by reducing ischemia.[414] Patients most suited for the use of beta blockers early in the course of AMI are those who also have sinus tachycardia and hypertension because beta blockers lower both the heart rate and arterial blood pressure, thereby lowering myocardial oxygen demand. A popular and relatively safe protocol for the use of a beta blocker in this situation is as follows: (1) Patients with heart failure (rales > 10 cm up from diaphragm), hypotension (BP < 90 mm Hg), bradycardia (heart rate < 60 bpm), or heart block (PR > 0.24 sec) are first excluded.[415] (2) Metoprolol is given in three 5-mg boluses. (3) Patients are observed for 2 to 5 minutes after each bolus, and if heart rate falls below 60 beats/min or systolic blood pressure falls below 100 mm Hg, no further drug is given; a total of three intravenous doses (15 mg) is administered. (4) If hemodynamic stability continues, 15 minutes after the last intravenous dose, the patient is begun on oral metoprolol, 50 mg every 6 hours for 2 days, then switched to 100 mg twice daily. An infusion of an extremely short-acting beta blocker, esmolol (50 to 250 μg/kg/min), may be useful in patients with relative contraindications to beta blockade in whom heart rate slowing is considered highly desirable.[416]

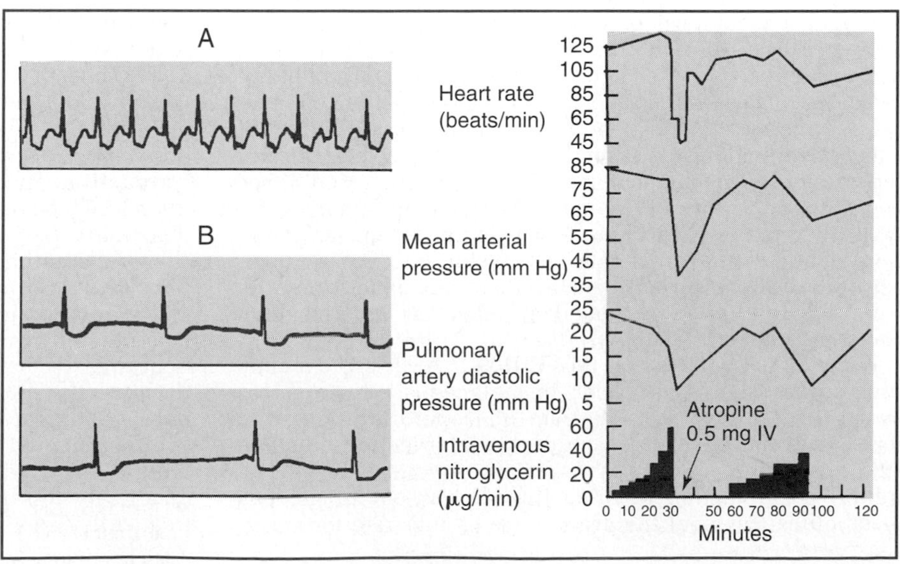

FIGURE 37–22. Sinus bradycardia and hypotension provoked by intravenous nitroglycerin in a patient with AMI. Intravenous nitroglycerin at a dose of 20 to 40 μg/min in a patient with anteroseptal AMI and sinus tachycardia (*A*) provoked profound sinus bradycardia (*B*) and hypotension. This was quickly reversed with intravenous atropine, 0.5 mg, but recurred after reinstitution of intravenous nitroglycerin. (From Come, P. C., and Pitt, B.: Nitroglycerin-induced severe hypotension and bradycardia in patients with acute myocardial infarction. Circulation *54*:624, 1976. Copyright 1976 American Heart Association.)

Unlike beta blockers, calcium antagonists are of little if any acute value in AMI and may, in fact, be hazardous.[414,417,418]

OXYGEN. Hypoxemia may occur in patients with AMI and is usually secondary to ventilation-perfusion abnormalities that are sequelae of left ventricular failure; pneumonia and intrinsic pulmonary disease are additional causes of hypoxemia. It is common practice to treat all patients hospitalized with AMI with oxygen for at least 24 to 48 hours, based on the empirical assumption of hypoxia and evidence that increased oxygen in the inspired air may protect ischemic myocardium.[419,420] However, this practice may not be cost effective. Augmentation of the fraction of oxygen in the inspired air does not elevate oxygen delivery significantly in patients who are not hypoxemic. Furthermore, it may increase systemic vascular resistance and arterial pressure and thereby lower cardiac output slightly.

In view of these considerations, arterial oxygen saturation may be estimated by pulse oximetry (an increasingly available technology), and oxygen therapy may be omitted if it is normal. On the other hand, oxygen should be administered to patients with AMI when arterial hypoxemia is clinically evident or can be documented by measurement. In these patients, serial arterial blood gas measurements may be employed to follow the efficacy of oxygen therapy. Although patients with AMI may exhibit a reduction in precordial ST-segment elevation during 100 per cent oxygen breathing, no long-term effect on survival or on the development of complications has been documented.[420]

In general, the delivery of 2 to 4 liters/min of 100 per cent oxygen by mask or nasal prongs for 6 to 12 hours is satisfactory for most patients with mild hypoxemia. If arterial oxygenation is still depressed on this regimen, the flow rate may have to be increased, and other causes for hypoxemia should be sought. In patients with pulmonary edema, endotracheal intubation and positive-pressure controlled ventilation may be necessary.

Limitation of Infarct Size

Infarct size is an important determinant of prognosis in patients with AMI.[421] Patients who succumb from cardiogenic shock generally exhibit either a single massive infarct or a small to moderate-sized infarct superimposed on multiple prior infarctions.[422,423] Survivors with large infarcts frequently exhibit late impairment of ventricular function,[356,424] and the long-term mortality rate is higher than for survivors with small infarcts, who tend not to develop cardiac decompensation.[84,171,425]

In view of the prognostic importance of infarct size, the concept that modification of infarct size is possible has attracted a great deal of experimental and clinical attention.[426] Efforts to limit the size of the infarct have been divided among three different (sometimes overlapping) approaches: (1) early reperfusion,[421,427] (2) reduction of myocardial energy demands, and (3) manipulation of sources of energy production in the myocardium.[193,428] Although early reperfusion ("time-dependent effect of reperfusion") has been the major focus of modern management strategies for AMI, it is important to note that in addition to the limitation of infarct size, even late reperfusion of ischemic myocardium conveys several benefits that contribute to mortality reduction ("time-independent effect of reperfusion,") (see p. 1213)[162,421,429] (Fig. 37–16).

THE DYNAMIC NATURE OF INFARCTION. AMI is a dynamic process that does not occur instantaneously but evolves over hours (Fig. 37–9). The fate of jeopardized, ischemic tissue may be affected favorably by interventions that restore perfusion, reduce myocardial oxygen requirements, inhibit accumulation of or facilitate wash-out of noxious metabolites, augment the availability of substrate for anaerobic metabolism,[192,193,421,430–433] or blunt the effects of mediators of injury (such as calcium overload or oxygen free radicals)[192,193,433–439] that compromise the structure and function of intracellular organelles and constituents of cell membranes. Strong evidence in experimental animals and suggestive evidence in patients indicate that ischemic preconditioning (see p. 1214) prior to sustained coronary occlusion decreases infarct size and is associated with a more favorable outcome, with decreased risk of extension of infarction and recurrent ischemic events.[440–444] Brief episodes of ischemia in one coronary vascular bed may precondition myocardium in a remote zone, attenuating the size of infarction in the latter when sustained coronary occlusion occurs.[441]

The perfusion of the myocardium in the infarct zone appears to be reduced maximally immediately following coronary occlusion. Up to one-third of patients may develop spontaneous recanalization of an occluded infarct-related artery beginning at 12 to 24 hours. This delayed spontaneous reperfusion has been associated with improvement of left ventricular function because it improves healing of infarcted tissue, prevents ventricular remodeling, and reperfuses hibernating myocardium. However, in order to *maximize* the amount of salvaged myocardium by *accelerating* the process of reperfusion and also implementing it in those patients who would otherwise have an occluded infarct-related artery, the strategies of pharmacologically induced thrombolysis and primary PTCA of the infarct vessel have been developed (see pp. 1215 and 1221).

Additional factors that may contribute to limitation of infarct size in association with reperfusion include relief of coronary spasm, improved systemic hemodynamics (augmentation of coronary perfusion pressure and reduced left ventricular end-diastolic pressure), and development of collateral circulation.[432] The prompt implementation of measures designed to protect ischemic myocardium and support myocardial perfusion may provide sufficient time for the development of anatomical and physiological compensatory mechanisms that limit the ultimate extent of infarction (Figs. 37–18 and 37–21).

AMI in hospitalized patients may be complicated by extension of infarction or early reinfarction (Fig. 37–23). Depending on the criteria utilized for detection, the incidence of these complications ranges from 8 to 30 per cent.[173] It is possible that interventions designed to protect ischemic myocardium during the initial event may also reduce the incidence of extension of infarction or early reinfarction.

ROUTINE MEASURES FOR INFARCT SIZE LIMITATION. Whereas reperfusion of ischemic myocardium is the most important technique for limiting infarct size, several routine measures to accomplish this goal are applicable to all patients with AMI, whether or not a reperfusion therapy is prescribed. The treatment strategies discussed in this section may be initiated in the emergency department (Fig. 37–18) and then continued in the coronary care unit.

It is important to maintain an optimal balance between myocardial oxygen supply and demand so that as much as possible of the jeopardized zone of the myocardium surrounding the most profoundly ischemic zones of the infarct can be salvaged. During the period before irreversible injury has occurred, myocardial oxygen consumption should be minimized by maintaining the patient at rest, physically and emotionally, and by utilizing mild sedation and a quiet atmosphere that may lower heart rate, a major determinant of myocardial oxygen consumption. If the patient was receiving a beta-adrenoceptor blocking agent at the time the clinical manifestations of the infarction commenced, the drug should be continued unless a specific contraindication develops, such as left ventricular systolic failure or bradyarrhythmia. Marked sinus bradycardia (heart rate less than approximately 50 beats/min) and the frequently coexisting hypotension should be treated with

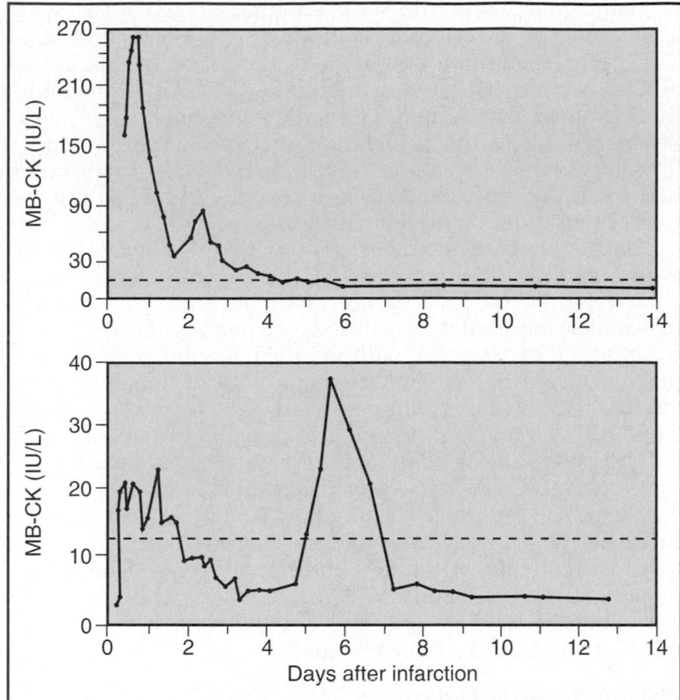

FIGURE 37–23. MB creatine kinase (MB-CK) time-activity curves for a patient in whom myocardial extension developed prior to return of plasma MB-CK to baseline (top) and a patient in whom extension occurred after return of MB-CK to baseline (bottom). (From Muller, J. E., Rude, R. E., Braunwald, E., et al.: Myocardial infarct extension: Occurrence, outcome, and risk factors in the MILIS. Ann. Intern. Med. *108*:1, 1988.)

postural maneuvers (the Trendelenburg position) to increase central blood volume and atropine and electrical pacing, but not with isoproterenol. On the other hand, the routine administration of atropine, with the resultant increase in heart rate, to patients without serious bradycardia is contraindicated. All forms of tachyarrhythmias require prompt treatment because they increase myocardial oxygen needs.

Congestive heart failure should be treated promptly. Given their multiple beneficial actions in AMI patients, ACE inhibitors are the first line of drugs indicated in the treatment of congestive heart failure associated with AMI unless the patient is hypotensive (see p. 495). Drugs such as isoproterenol that increase myocardial oxygen consumption should be avoided.

As discussed above, arterial oxygenation should be restored to normal in patients with hypoxemia, such as occurs in patients with chronic pulmonary disease, pneumonia, or left ventricular failure. Oxygen-enriched air should be administered to patients with hypoxemia, and bronchodilators and expectorants should be used when indicated. Severe anemia, which can also extend the area of ischemic injury, should be corrected by the cautious administration of packed red cells, accompanied by a diuretic if there is any evidence of left ventricular failure. Associated conditions, particularly infections and the accompanying tachycardia, fever, and elevated myocardial oxygen needs, require immediate attention.

Systolic arterial pressure should not be allowed to deviate by more than approximately 25 to 30 mm Hg from the patient's usual level unless marked hypertension had been present before the AMI. It is likely that each patient has an optimal range of arterial pressure; as coronary perfusion pressure deviates from this level, the unfavorable balance between oxygen supply (which is related to coronary perfusion pressure) and myocardial oxygen demand (which is related to ventricular wall tension) that ensues increases the extent of ischemic injury.

REPERFUSION OF MYOCARDIAL INFARCTION

GENERAL CONCEPTS. Although reperfusion occurs spontaneously in some patients, persistent thrombotic occlusion is present in the majority of patients with AMI while the myocardium is undergoing necrosis.[100] Timely reperfusion of jeopardized myocardium represents the most effective way of restoring the balance between myocardial oxygen supply and demand. The extent of protection appears to be related directly to the rapidity with which reperfusion is implemented after the onset of coronary occlusion[382,427,445–449] (Fig. 37–9). Preliminary data exist suggesting that following thrombolytic therapy more rapid reperfusion (and smaller infarcts) occurs in patients with AMI preceded by unstable angina compared with those without preinfarction angina.[449a]

In some patients, particularly those with cardiogenic shock, tissue damage occurs in a "stuttering" manner rather than abruptly, a condition that might more properly be termed subacute infarction. This concept of the nature of the infarction process, as well as the observation that the incidence of complications of AMI in both the early and late postinfarction periods is a function of infarct size,[450] underscores the need for careful history-taking to ascertain whether the patient appears to have had repetitive cycles of spontaneous reperfusion and reocclusion. "Fixing" the time of onset of the infarction process in such patients can be difficult. In such patients with waxing and waning ischemic discomfort, a rigid time interval from the first episode of pain should not be used when determining whether a patient is "outside the window" for benefit from acute reperfusion therapy.

PATHOPHYSIOLOGY OF MYOCARDIAL REPERFUSION. Prevention of cell death by the restoration of blood flow depends on the severity and duration of pre-existing ischemia. Substantial experimental and clinical evidence exists indicating that recovery of left ventricular systolic function, improvement in diastolic function, and reduction in overall mortality are more favorably influenced, the earlier that blood flow is restored[10,421,427] (Fig. 37–16). Collateral coronary vessels also appear to play a role in the successful left ventricular function following reperfusion.[432,451] They provide sufficient perfusion of myocardium to retard cell death and are probably of greater importance in patients having reperfusion later rather than 1 to 2 hours after coronary occlusion.

Reperfusion Injury

(See p. 1179)

The process of reperfusion, although beneficial in terms of myocardial salvage, may come at a cost due to a process known as *reperfusion injury*[452,453] (Fig. 37–11) (see also Fig. 36–25, p. 1178). Kloner has summarized the data on the four types of reperfusion injury that have been observed in experimental animals.[454] These consist of (1) lethal reperfusion injury—a term referring to reperfusion-induced death of cells that were still viable at the time of restoration of coronary blood flow, (2) vascular reperfusion injury—progressive damage to the microvasculature such that there is an expanding area of no reflow and loss of coronary vasodilatory reserve,[455] (3) stunned myocardium—salvaged myocytes display a prolonged period of contractile dysfunction following restoration of blood flow owing to abnormalities of intracellular biochemistry leading to reduced energy production[88,436] (see pp. 388 and 1176) (Fig. 37–11), and (4) reperfusion arrhythmias—bursts of ventricular tachycardia and on occasion ventricular fibrillation that occur within seconds of reperfusion.[237] The available evidence suggests that vascular reperfusion injury, stunning, and reperfusion arrhythmias can all occur in patients with AMI. The concept of lethal reperfusion injury of potentially salvageable myocardium remains controversial, both in experimental animals and in patients.[81,454,456–459]

Reperfusion does increase the cell swelling that occurs with ischemia.[460,461] Reperfusion of the myocardium in which the microvasculature is damaged leads to the creation of a hemorrhagic infarct[462] (Fig. 37–11). Thrombolytic therapy appears more likely to produce hemorrhagic infarction than reperfusion by mechanical means. Although concern has been raised that this hemorrhage may lead to extension of the infarct, this does not appear to be the case.[463] Histological study of patients not surviving in spite of successful reperfusion has revealed hemorrhagic infarcts, but this hemorrhage usually does not extend beyond the area of necrosis.[96,464]

The loss of magnesium with ischemia, followed during reperfusion by the sudden exposure of severely ischemic cells to both calcium and oxygen upon restoration of flow, has been observed to affect the severity of ischemic damage in several animal species.[435–437,440,465,466] Toxicity from oxygen-derived free radicals mediated at least in part by stimulated leukocytes has attracted considerable attention for its possible role in extending myocardial injury and contributing to calcium overload and inability to regulate cell volume.[467,468] Observations in reperfused patients with AMI indicate that cardiac inflammatory responses are mediated by the cytokines IL-8 and IL-6, opening new options for reducing reperfusion injury by developing pharmacological interventions specifically targeted against specific cytokines.[469] Experimental models of AMI have revealed a consistent message—interventions that attenuate reperfusion injury exert their maximal beneficial effect if blood levels (and presumably myocardial tissue concentrations) are elevated at the time reperfusion occurs.[457–459,468,470,471] The effectiveness of agents such as superoxide dismutase and magnesium rapidly declines the later they are administered after reperfusion; eventually no beneficial effect is detectable in animal models after 45 to 60 minutes of reperfusion has elapsed.[459] This concept is strengthened further by investigations with novel agents such as liposomal PGE_1[472] and inhibitors of Na^+-H^+ exchange[473] that substantially reduce the amount of myocardial injury that occurs with reperfusion when they are administered prior to restoration of coronary blood flow. Drugs such as beta-adrenoceptor blockers, which delay the death of ischemic cells, may, if administered prophylactically to patients at high risk of occlusion (or reocclusion) or in the earliest phases of the development of an AMI, enhance the quantity of myocardium salvaged by early reperfusion.[474,475]

Ischemic Preconditioning

The intriguing observation that brief periods of experimental coronary occlusion and reperfusion prior to a more sustained period of occlusion lasting less than 1.5 to 3 hours result in marked reduction in the amount of necrosis that develops has led to the concept of *ischemic preconditioning*.[440,453,476] Recent data suggest that during the period of brief coronary occlusion adenosine receptors are activated which initiate a cascade of intracellular events culminating in phosphorylation of a membrane protein that is responsible for the protective effect. The leading candidate membrane protein is the ATP-dependent potassium channel that, when activated, causes a shortening of the action potential duration, a decrease in calcium influx, a reduction in contractile force generation, and thereby an energy-sparing effect.[477] The implications of ischemic preconditioning, including a possible modification of the severity of myocardial infarction, are profound and have stimulated interest in ATP-dependent potassium channel openers such as nicorandil, bimakalim, and other "preconditioning-mimetic" agents for potential use in patients with AMI.[440,478,479]

Another potential mechanism for the acute response to ischemic preconditioning is a slowing of glycolysis with attenuation of intracellular acidosis.[480–480b] A "second window" of preconditioning has been described by Marber et al. that appears 24 hours or more after the initial preconditioning episodes and may be mediated by molecular adaptation leading to the production of heat shock protein.[481] Preconditioning appears to be associated with a more oxidized cellular redox state, which may contribute to protection against subsequent bouts of ischemia.[482]

Clinical observations consistent with the concept of ischemic preconditioning include the "warm-up phenomenon" reported by many angina patients (i.e., angina early in exercise necessitating a brief rest period followed by a resumption of exercise without angina) and a lower in-hospital death rate in AMI patients who have a history of angina within the 48-hour period that precedes infarction.[440,442] A history of preinfarction angina in patients with a first Q-wave MI has been reported to be associated with a lower peak CK activity, lower in-hospital incidence of sustained ventricular tachycardia and fibrillation, and a lower incidence of pump failure and cardiac mortality.[444] Of interest, in patients with a first anterior Q-wave MI, a history of preinfarction angina was associated with a higher ejection fraction, smaller end-diastolic volume, and a lower incidence of aneurysm formation.[444]

Reperfusion Arrhythmias

Transient sinus bradycardia occurs in many patients with inferior infarcts at the time of acute reperfusion; it is most often accompanied by some degree of hypotension. This combination of hypotension and bradycardia with a sudden increase in coronary flow has been ascribed to the activation of the Bezold-Jarisch reflex.[483] Premature ventricular contractions, accelerated idioventricular rhythm, and nonsustained ventricular tachycardia are also seen commonly following successful reperfusion. In experimental animals with AMI, ventricular fibrillation occurs shortly after reperfusion, but this arrhythmia is not as frequent in patients as in the experimental setting. Although some investigators have postulated that early afterdepolarizations participate in the genesis of reperfusion ventricular arrhythmias, Vera et al. have shown that early afterdepolarizations are present both during ischemia and during reperfusion and are therefore unlikely to be involved in the development of reperfusion ventricular tachycardia or fibrillation.[484]

When present, rhythm disturbances may actually be a marker of successful restoration of coronary flow.[485] However, although reperfusion arrhythmias have a high sensitivity for detecting successful reperfusion, the high incidence of identical rhythm disturbances in patients without successful coronary artery reperfusion limits their specificity for detection of restoration of coronary blood flow. In general, clinical features are poor markers of reperfusion, with no single clinical finding or constellation of findings being reliably predictive of angiographically demonstrated coronary artery patency.[486]

In an overview of randomized trials in which thrombolytic therapy was compared with placebo, Solomon et al. reported *no* increase in the risk of ventricular tachycardia or ventricular fibrillation in patients receiving thrombolytic therapy.[487] Thus, although reperfusion arrhythmias may show a temporal clustering at the time of restoration of coronary blood flow in patients with successful thrombolysis, the overall incidence of such arrhythmias appears to be similar in patients not receiving a thrombolytic agent who may develop these arrhythmias as a consequence of spontaneous coronary artery reperfusion or the evolution of the infarct process itself. These considerations, as well as the fact that the brief "electrical storm" occurring at the time of reperfusion is generally innocuous, indicate that no prophylactic antiarrhythmic therapy is necessary when thrombolytics are prescribed.[487]

Late Establishment of Patency of the Infarct Vessel

It has been suggested that improved survival and ventricular function after successful reperfusion are not due entirely to limitation of infarct size[162,421,488] (Fig. 37–16). Both experimental and clinical evidence indicate that the benefits of a patent artery include a favorable effect on ventricular remodeling (improved healing of infarcted tissue and prevention of infarct expansion),[83,171,425,489,489a] enhancement of collateral flow,[490] improvement in diastolic and systolic function,[491–495] increased electrical stability,[496–498] and reduced long-term mortality.[499,500] Late reperfusion of the artery perfusing an infarction provides a vascular scaffolding in the infarct zone[501] and increases the influx of inflammatory cells that participate in the formation of a mature fibrous scar.[502] The vascular scaffold and firmer myocardial scar prevent infarct segment lengthening and decrease the tendency to infarct expansion and aneurysm formation.[488] Poorly contracting or noncontracting myocardium in a zone that is supplied by a stenosed infarct-related artery with slow antegrade perfusion may still contain viable myocytes. This situation is referred to as *hibernating* myocardium[453] (see p. 1176), and its function can be improved by percutaneous transluminal coronary angioplasty (PTCA) to augment flow in the infarct-related artery.[503] Late reperfusion of the infarct-related artery by thrombolysis or late restoration of flow via PTCA[504] enhances the electrical stability of the infarcted zone and is probably related to the reduced incidence of ventricular fibrillation and automatic firing of implantable cardioverter-defibrillator devices.[505,506] The beneficial effect of late (within 16 days) reperfusion of the infarct-related artery is independent of left ventricular function and other mortality-reducing therapies such as ACE inhibitors[499] (see p. 1229).

Summary of Effects of Myocardial Reperfusion

As illustrated in Figure 37–16, rupture of an unstable plaque in the culprit vessel produces complete occlusion of the infarct-related coronary artery. AMI occurs with the ensuing development of left ventricular dilatation and ultimate death through a combination of pump failure and electrical instability. Early reperfusion (i.e., thrombolysis, primary PTCA) shortens the duration of coronary occlusion, minimizes the degree of ultimate left ventricular dysfunction and dilatation, and reduces the probability that the AMI patient will develop pump failure or malignant ventricular tachyarrhythmias. Late reperfusion (after approximately 4 to 6 hours have elapsed since the onset of coronary artery occlusion) appears to affect favorably the process of infarct healing and minimizes left ventricular remodeling and the ultimate development of pump dysfunction and electrical instability.

CORONARY THROMBOLYSIS

Many years elapsed between the first report of intracoronary clot lysis in an experimental animal and the widespread use of thrombolytic agents in AMI.[31,507] With publication of the first GISSI trial of over 11,000 patients in 1986,[508] in which intravenous streptokinase was shown to result in a significant reduction in mortality in patients treated within 6 hours of the onset of symptoms, the routine use of thrombolytic therapy in AMI was established. It is now clear that thrombolysis recanalizes thrombotic occlusion associated with AMI (Fig. 37–24), and restoration of coronary flow reduces infarct size and improves myocardial function and survival.[10,421]

INTRACORONARY THROMBOLYSIS. Clinical investigation in the area of pharmacological reperfusion of ischemic myocardium initially focused on the use of intracoronary thrombolysis in the early hours of AMI.[31,427,509,510] The fact that viability could be maintained in a portion of the successfully reperfused myocardium was reflected in studies showing the restoration of contractile activity.[511,512] Most reported experience with intracoronary thrombolysis has not been in randomized controlled trials, largely because it has been thought difficult to withhold thrombolytic therapy once a thrombotic coronary artery occlusion has been visualized angiographically, and it has not been considered ethical to catheterize patients if randomization to no thrombolytic therapy were possible for a portion of the patients. Because of the delay involved in catheterizing patients with AMI, current consensus is that intracoronary administration of thrombolytic therapy should be reserved for patients who develop coronary thrombosis during the course of an angiographic procedure and in whom either a coronary catheter is already in place or such placement is easily and rapidly achieved.

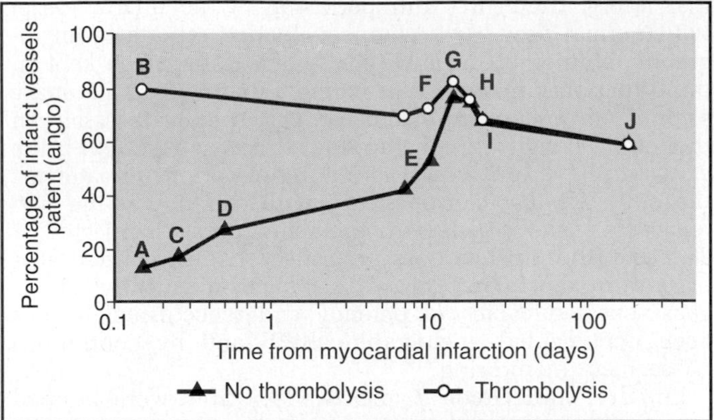

FIGURE 37–24. Comparison of angiographically documented infarct-related coronary artery patency rates in 10 separate clinical studies and time from MI as modulated by early administration of a thrombolytic agent versus nonthrombolytic (conventional) therapy. The x-axis is a semilogarithmic scale of time in days from myocardial infarction. Note that the difference in patency rates becomes diminishingly small within the first 2 to 3 weeks after infarction. (From Rumberg, J. A., and Gersh, B. J.: Coronary artery patency and left ventricular remodeling after myocardial infarction: mechanisms and mechanics. *In* Califf, R. M., Mark, D. B., and Wagner, G. S. [eds.]: Acute Coronary Care. St. Louis, Mosby-Year Book, 1995, p. 122.)

INTRAVENOUS THROMBOLYSIS. This form of thrombolytic therapy has several important advantages over intracoronary use. Because only the placement of a peripheral intravenous line is required, therapy may be initiated early, in a variety of locations (home, ambulance, helicopter, emergency department) and at relatively low cost. The subject of intravenous thrombolysis has perhaps been one of the most rapidly evolving areas in the management of patients with AMI, especially over the last decade.[512a]

PATENCY OF THE INFARCT-RELATED ARTERY. In the 1980's more than 20 trials were conducted that collectively enrolled over 8000 patients and established the patency rates of the infarct-related artery at 60 minutes, 90 minutes, 180 minutes, and 1 to 21 days following thrombolysis with a variety of regimens: conventional dose t-PA (alteplase), accelerated-dose t-PA, streptokinase, urokinase, anisoylated plasminogen streptokinase activator complex (APSAC) given alone or in combination (e.g., t-PA plus urokinase or streptokinase). The results of these trials have been summarized in several recent reviews.[427,513,514]

In order to provide a level of standardization for comparison of the various regimens, most investigators focus on the status of the infarct vessel at 90 minutes and describe the flow according to the TIMI grading system: Grade 0 = complete occlusion of the infarct related artery; Grade 1 = some penetration of the contrast material beyond the point of obstruction but without perfusion of the distal coronary bed; Grade 2 = perfusion of the entire infarct vessel into the distal bed but with delayed flow compared with a normal artery; Grade 3 = full perfusion of the infarct vessel with normal flow.[515,516] When evaluating reports of angiographic studies of thrombolytic agents, it must be kept in mind that only in studies in which a pretreatment coronary arteriogram documents occlusion of the culprit vessel can the term *recanalization* be applied if flow is restored. If the status of the culprit vessel is not known prior to treatment, the only fact that can be stated with certainty is the *patency rate* of the vessel at the moment contrast is injected.[513] This snapshot in time does not reflect the fluctuating status of flow in the infarct vessel that characteristically undergoes repeated cycles of patency and reocclusion, as has been documented angiographically[517] and by continuous ST-segment monitoring.[518]

Initially TIMI Grade 2 and Grade 3 flow were lumped into the favorable category of coronary patency that was compared with a combined TIMI Grade 0 and Grade 1 flow into an unfavorable category of persistent occlusion. However, TIMI Grade 2 flow should not be lumped with Grade 3 flow because it has been recognized that TIMI Grade 3 flow is far superior to Grade 2 in terms of infarct size reduction and both short-term[519] and long-term[520] mortality benefit. Therefore, TIMI Grade 3 flow should be considered to be the goal of reperfusion therapy.[521–523] However, Ito et al. have shown that even some patients with TIMI Grade 3 flow do not necessarily achieve adequate myocardial perfusion at the tissue level, as demonstrated on contrast echocardiography.[455] In an effort to provide a more quantitative statement of the briskness of coronary blood flow in the infarct artery and also to account for differences in the size and length of vessels (e.g., LAD versus RCA) and interobserver variability, Gibson and coworkers have developed the *TIMI frame count*—a simple count of the number of angiographic frames elapsed until the contrast arrives in the distal bed of the vessel of interest.[524] The TIMI frame count for patients with Grade 3 flow is in the range of 35 ± 13 frames, compared with 88 ± 31 frames for Grade 2 flow—this difference in frame counts correlates with CK release, left ventricular function, and clinical outcome.[524]

Despite the obvious mortality benefit afforded patients who rapidly achieve and maintain TIMI Grade 3 flow, the problems of "no reflow" at the myocardial level,[369] intermittent patency after successful clot lysis, and the risk of reocclusion has led Lincoff and Topol to pose the intriguing notion that there is an "illusion of reperfusion" because probably only one-quarter to one-third of patients treated with thrombolytics truly receive optimal reperfusion.[525] This has stimulated interest in development of alternative thrombolytic regimens (see p. 1220), evaluation of the benefits and risks of adjunctive therapies (see p. 1826), and evaluation of conjunctive therapies that help minimize myocardial damage (see p. 1221). Novel approaches to maintaining coronary artery patency after thrombolysis using tissue factor pathway inhibitor[526] and enhancing the concentration of nitric oxide in the coronary circulation[527] are being explored in experimental animals.

Effect on Mortality

There is no doubt that early intravenous therapy and thrombolytic drugs improve survival in patients with AMI[10,511] (Fig. 37–25). Mortality varies considerably depending on patients included for study and adjunctive therapies employed. The benefit of thrombolytic therapy appears to be greatest when agents are administered as early as possible, with the most dramatic results when the drug is given less than 1 to 2 hours after symptoms begin.[382,528] The impact of early treatment was first clearly shown in the initial GISSI trial[508] and confirmed in ISIS-2.[529] The GISSI-1 and ISIS-2 trials taken together with the ISAM[530] (streptokinase), AIMS[531] (APSAC), and ASSEST[532] (t-PA) trials are the critical elements of the portfolio of scientific evidence that thrombolytic therapy reduces mortality.[513]

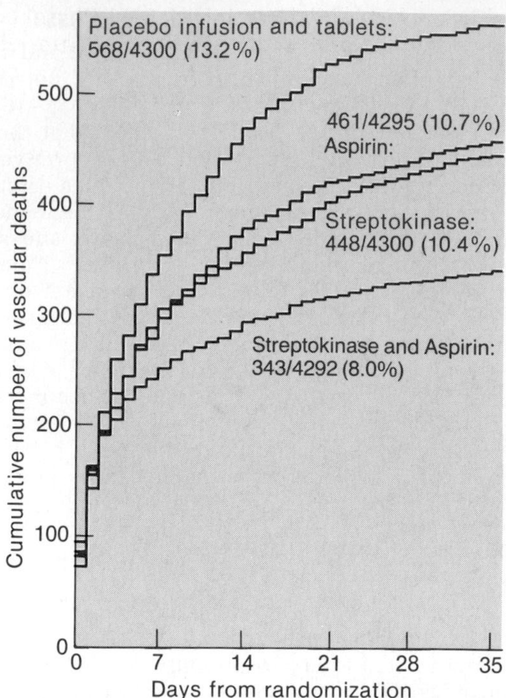

FIGURE 37–25. Cumulative vascular mortality (deaths from cardiac, cerebral, hemorrhagic, or other known vascular disease, or unknown causes) in days 0 to 35 of the Second International Study of Infarct Survival (ISIS-2). The four curves describe mortality for patients allocated (i) active streptokinase only, (ii) active aspirin only, (iii) both active treatments, and (iv) neither. Note that individually aspirin and streptokinase have a favorable effect of similar magnitudes and together the benefits appear additive. (From ISIS-2 [Second International Study of Infarct Survival] Collaborative Group: Randomized trial of intravenous streptokinase, oral aspirin, both, or neither among 17,187 cases of suspected acute myocardial infarction: ISIS-2. Lancet *2*:349, 1988. © by The Lancet Ltd.)

The Fibrinolytic Therapy Trialists' (FTT) Collaborative Group has performed a comprehensive overview of nine trials of thrombolytic therapy, each of which enrolled more than 1000 patients[10] (Fig. 37–26). The data base for the FTT overview consisted of a total of 58,600 patients, including 6177 (10.5 per cent) who died, 564 (1.0 per cent) who sustained a stroke, and 436 (0.7 per cent) who sustained major noncerebral bleeds. A time-dependent effect[421] of thrombolytic therapy on mortality was evident in that the number of lives saved per 1000 patients treated in relation to the time from symptom onset to initiation of thrombolysis was as follows: 0 to 1 hour—35 per 1000; 2 to 3 hours—25 per 1000; 4 to 6 hours—19 per 1000; 7 to 12 hours—16 per 1000. The absolute mortality rates for the control and fibrinolytic groups stratified by presenting features are shown in Figure 37–26. The overall results indicated an 18 per cent reduction in short-term mortality, but as much as a 25 per cent reduction in mortality for the subset of 45,000 patients with ST-segment elevation or bundle branch block. There was a mortality reduction of 22 per cent in those patients with anterior ST-segment elevation and 11 per cent in those with inferior ST elevation. The patients presenting with ST-segment depression had an excess mortality of 11 per cent that serves as part of the foundaton for the observation that thrombolytic therapy does not benefit patients presenting with ST-segment depression. Two trials, LATE and EMERAS, viewed together provide evidence that a mortality reduction may still be observed in patients treated with thrombolytics between 6 and 12 hours from the onset of ischemic symptoms.[533,534] The data from LATE and EMERAS and the FTT overview form the basis for extending the "window" of treatment with thrombolytics up to 12 hours from the onset of symptoms.

The mortality effect of thrombolytic therapy in elderly patients is of considerable interest. Whereas patients greater than the age of 75 were initially excluded from randomized trials of thrombolytic therapy, they now constitute about 15 per cent of the patients studied in recent megatrials of thrombolysis.[33,535] Barriers to initiation of therapy in older patients with AMI include a protracted period of delay in seeking medical care, a lower incidence of ischemic discomfort and greater incidence of atypical symptoms and concomitant illnesses, and an increased incidence of nondiagnostic ECGs.[35,230,536,537] Younger patients with AMI achieve a slightly greater relative reduction in mortality compared with elderly patients, but the higher absolute mortality in the elderly results in similar absolute mortality reductions. Thus, as seen in Figure 37–26, there was a 26 per cent decrease in mortality in patients who were less than 55 years of age (11 lives saved per 1000 with thrombolytic therapy) and a 4 per cent reduction in mortality in patients older than age 75 (10 lives saved per 1000 treated).

Other important baseline characteristics that impact on the mortality effect of thrombolytic therapy include the vital signs at presentation and the presence of diabetes mellitus (Fig. 37–26). For example, there was an 18 per cent decrease in mortality for patients presenting with a systolic pressure less than 100 mm Hg (62 lives saved per 1000 treated), compared with a 12 per cent reduction in mortality for patients with a systolic pressure of 175 mm Hg or more (10 lives saved per 1000 treated). Patients with a history of diabetes mellitus experienced a mortality reduction of 21 per cent (37 lives saved per 1000 treated), compared with a mortality reduction of 15 per cent (15 lives saved per 1000 treated) in patients without a history of diabetes.

A number of models have been developed to integrate the many clinical variables that affect a patient's mortality risk prior to administration of thrombolytic therapy. In the TIMI II trial, patients were classified as low risk if they *lacked* any of the following: age of 70 years or more,

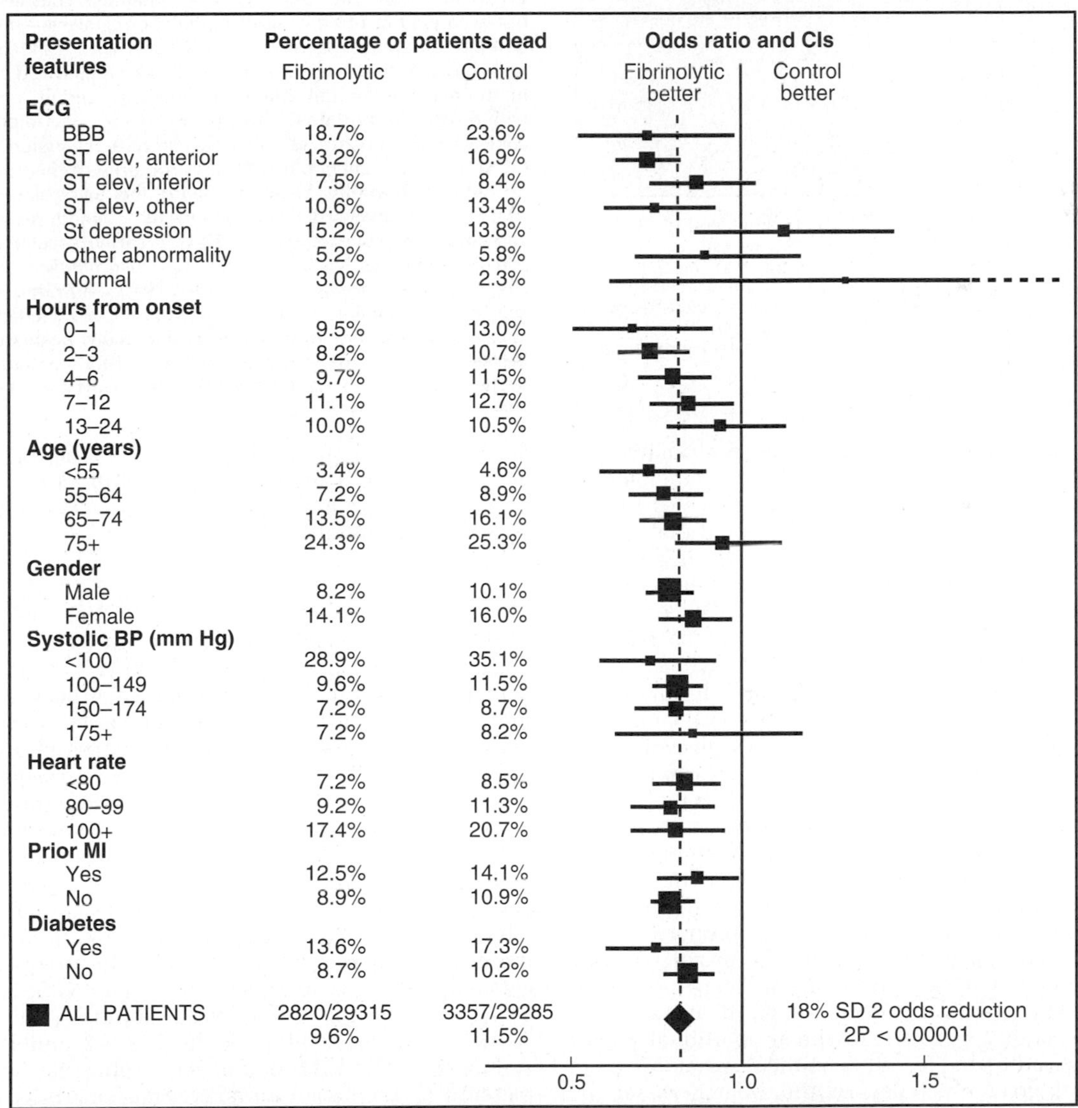

FIGURE 37–26. Mortality differences during days 0 to 35 subdivided by presentation features in a collaborative overview of results from nine trials of thrombolytic therapy. The absolute mortality rates are shown for fibrinolytic and control groups in the center portion of the figure for each of the clinical features at presentation listed on the left side of the figure. The ratio of the odds of death in the fibrinolytic group to that in the control group is shown for each subdivision (colored square), along with its 99 per cent confidence interval (horizontal line). The summary odds ratio at the bottom of the figure corresponds to an 18 per cent proportional reduction in 35-day mortality and is highly statistically significant. This translates to a reduction of 18 deaths per 1000 patients treated with thrombolytic agents. (From Fibrinolytic Therapy Trialists' [FTT] Collaborative Group: Indications for fibrinolytic therapy in suspected acute myocardial infarction: Collaborative overview of mortality and major morbidity results from all randomized trials of more than 1000 patients. Lancet *343*:311, 1994. © by The Lancet Ltd.)

TABLE 37–4 A) MORTALITY 6 WEEKS FOLLOWING THROMBOLYTIC THERAPY FOR EACH OF EIGHT RISK FACTORS IN 3261 PATIENTS*

RISK FACTOR	DEATHS BY 6 WEEKS (%)
None	1.5
Age ≥70 years	11.2
Previous infarction	7.9
Anterior infarction	5.6
Atrial fibrillation	10.6
Rales in more than one-third of lung fields	12.4
Hypotension and sinus tachycardia	10.1
Female gender	7.1
Diabetes mellitus	8.5

B) MORTALITY 6 WEEKS FOLLOWING THROMBOLYTIC THERAPY ACCORDING TO NUMBER OF RISK FACTORS† PRESENT INITIALLY

NO. OF RISK FACTORS	NO. OF PATIENTS	NO. OF DEATHS WITHIN 6 WEEKS	MORTALITY RATE (%)
0	864	13	1.5
1	1384	32	2.3
2	689	48	7.0
3	231	30	13.0
≥4	93	16	17.2

* Seventy-eight patients with cardiogenic shock or pulmonary edema were excluded.

† Possible risk factors listed in A.

Data from analysis of patients enrolled in Phase II of the Thrombolysis in Myocardial Infarction (TIMI) trial. Hillis, L. D., Foreman, S., and Braunwald, E.: Risk stratification before thrombolytic therapy in patients with acute myocardial infarction. Reprinted by permission of the American College of Cardiology. J. Am. Coll. Cardiol. *16*:313, 1990.

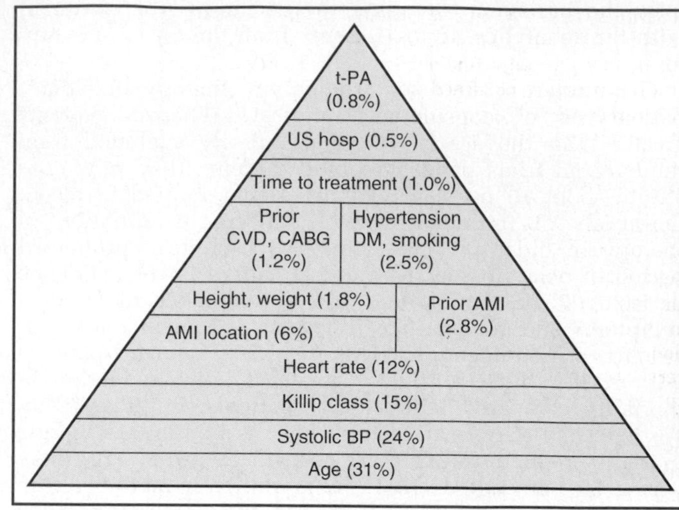

FIGURE 37–27. Influence of clinical characteristics on 30-day mortality after MI in patients treated with thrombolytic agents based on experience from the GUSTO Trial. Although considerable attention has been paid to optimizing thrombolytic regimens—indeed, the small absolute differences in mortality observed with different thrombolytic regimens are controversial—it should be emphasized that the choice of the agent is far less important than are certain clinical variables with respect to mortality. This pyramid depicts the importance of such clinical characteristics as calculated from a regression analysis in the GUSTO Trial. Numbers in parentheses represent the proportion of risk for 30-day mortality associated with the particular characteristics. AMI = acute myocardial infarction; BP = blood pressure; CABG = coronary artery bypass grating; CVD = cardiovascular disease; DM = diabetes mellitus; t-PA = tissue-type plasminogen activators; US Hosp = patients treated in a United States hospital. (Adapted from Lee, K. L., Woodlief, L. H., Topol, E. J., et al.: Predictors of 30-day mortality in the era of reperfusion for acute myocardial infarction: Results from an international trial of 41,021 patients. Circulation *91*:1659, 1995. Copyright 1995 American Heart Association.)

previous infarction, atrial fibrillation, anterior infarction, rales in more than one-third of the lung fields, hypotension and sinus tachycardia, female gender, and diabetes mellitus[538] (Table 37–4). However, it should be noted that statistical modeling of mortality risk such as that cited above cannot cover all clinical scenarios and should not substitute for clinical judgment in individual cases. For example, patients with inferior MI who might otherwise be considered to have a low risk of mortality and for whom many physicians have questioned the benefits of thrombolytic therapy might be in a much higher mortality risk subgroup if their inferior infarction is associated with right ventricular infarction,[539] precordial ST-segment depression,[540] or ST-segment elevation in the lateral precordial leads.[541] The GUSTO I investigators developed a regression model to illustrate the relative importance of clinical characteristics on 30-day mortality in contemporary thrombolytic-treated patients.[542] The mortality "pyramid" shown in Figure 37–27 clearly demonstrates that much greater proportions of the risk of mortality are contributed by the systolic blood pressure and heart rate at presentation than precisely which thrombolytic agent was selected (e.g., the use of t-PA contributed less than 1 per cent to the proportional effect on mortality after adjusting for other clinical variables).

As a result of greater patency of the infarct vessel in patients treated with thrombolytic agents,[513] the clinical benefits that appear to accrue and contribute to the reduction in mortality include reductions in left ventricular failure,[543] malignant arrhythmias,[532,544] and serious complications of AMI such as septal rupture and cardiogenic shock.[530,532,544] The short-term survival benefit enjoyed by patients who receive thrombolytic therapy is maintained over the 1- to 5-year follow-up that has been reported in a number of studies.[545] However, room for improvement remains given reports of reocclusion rates of the infarct related artery as high as 10 per cent in hospital[513] and up to 30 per cent by 3 months,[546] and reinfarction rates as high as 5 per cent in hospital[513] and 7 per cent within the first year[547] in thrombolytic-treated patients.

Comparison of Thrombolytic Agents

There has been considerable controversy regarding the efficacy of various thrombolytic agents.[547a] Three megatrials comparing thrombolytic regimens have been reported. The first was GISSI-2,[548] which compared t-PA (alteplase, 100 mg over 3 hours) with streptokinase (1.5 MU over 30 to 60 minutes). All patients received oral aspirin; one-half received subcutaneous heparin. There was no difference in mortality in the group that received conventional dose t-PA (8.9 per cent) versus the group who received streptokinase (8.5 per cent). The ISIS-3 investigators reported no differences in mortality in a three-arm trial comparing streptokinase, 1.5 million units over 1 hour (10.6 per cent), t-PA (in the double-chain form as duteplase in contrast to the single-chain form as alteplase studied in GISSI-2) (10.3 per cent), and APSAC, 30 mg over 3 minutes (10.5 per cent).[535] A meta-analysis combining the GISSI-2 and ISIS-3 results summarized the information on a collective total of 48,294 patients.[535] Identical mortality rates of 10 per cent at 35 days were seen in the t-PA– and streptokinase-treated patients.

In the GUSTO I trial (Fig. 37–28), 41,021 patients were randomized into one of four treatment arms: streptokinase, 1.5 MU over 60 minutes with immediate intravenous heparin to a target APTT of 60 to 85 seconds; accelerated t-PA with immediate intravenous heparin; a combination arm of intravenous t-PA (1 mg/kg over 60 minutes) and streptokinase (1.0 MU over 60 minutes); and streptokinase, 1.5 MU over 60 minutes with subcutaneous heparin. The 30-day

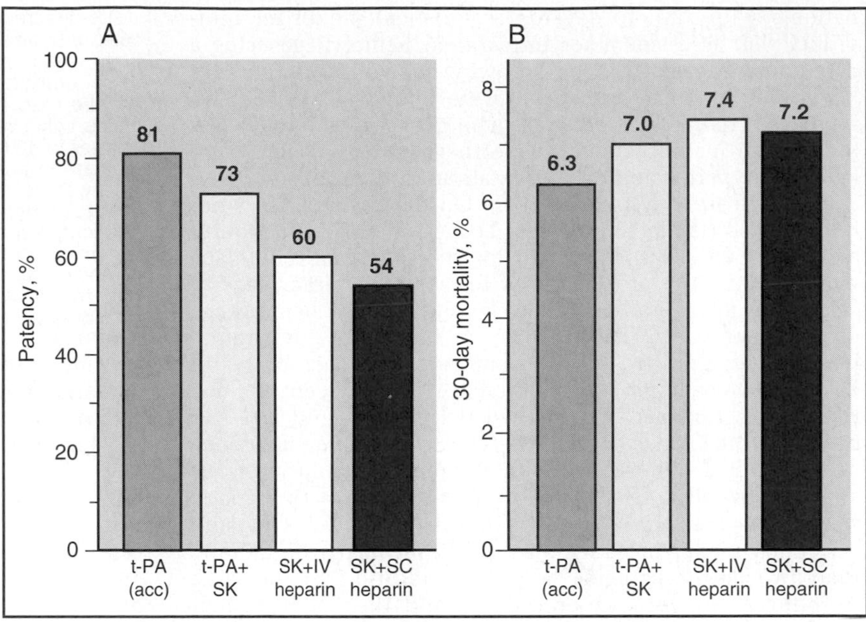

FIGURE 37–28. *A* and *B*, Results of the Angiographic Substudy of the GUSTO Trial along with the 30-day mortality findings from the main study. The regimen that consisted of accelerated t-PA and intravenous (IV) heparin achieved the highest level of infarct-related artery patency (flow ≥ TIMI Grade II) by 90 minutes. Although the other regimens shown eventually "caught up" in terms of patency, it was apparently too late to provide the maximum reduction in mortality seen with the accelerated t-PA regimen. One drawback of regimens that achieve such early and sustained infarct-related patency is the associated small but definite increase in the risk for bleeding, the most serious complication being intracranial hemorrhage that results in a cerebrovascular accident (CVA). SC = subcutaneous; SK = streptokinase. (Adapted from The GUSTO Angiographic Investigators: The effects of tissue plasminogen activator, streptokinase, or both on coronary-artery patency, ventricular function, and survival after acute myocardial infarction. N. Engl. J. Med. *329:*1615, 1993; and The GUSTO Investigators: An international randomized trial comparing four thrombolytic strategies for acute myocardial infarction. N. Engl. J. Med. *329:*673, 1993. Copyright Massachusetts Medical Society.)

mortality for the accelerated t-PA group was 6.3 per cent, streptokinase plus subcutaneous heparin 7.2 per cent, streptokinase plus intravenous heparin 7.4 per cent, and streptokinase plus t-PA combination plus intravenous heparin 7.0 per cent (Fig. 37–28).

In the GUSTO Angiographic Substudy involving 2431 patients, those with TIMI Grade 0 or 1 flow had a 30-day mortality of 9.8 per cent that was reduced to 7.9 per cent in patients with TIMI Grade 2 flow and 4.3 per cent in those with TIMI Grade 3 flow.[519] The 90-minute patency rates for the infarct-related artery in the four treatment arms were as follows (Fig. 37–28): accelerated t-PA 81 per cent (54 per cent Grade 3 flow), combination t-PA plus streptokinase 73 per cent (38 per cent Grade 3 flow), streptokinase plus intravenous heparin 60 per cent (32 per cent Grade 3 flow), and streptokinase plus subcutaneous heparin 54 per cent (29 per cent Grade 3 flow). This early gradient in patency rates favoring t-PA was no longer apparent beyond 180 minutes, presumably because of a "catch-up" phenomenon whereby late patency rates with streptokinase approach those of front-loaded t-PA, albeit beyond a time when as much myocardial salvage is possible as with t-PA. A related observation on early arterial patency was made in the TIMI 4 trial that randomized patients with AMI presenting within 6 hours to receive either front-loaded t-PA, APSAC, or a combination of a reduced dose of both t-PA and APSAC.[549] The 90-minute patency rate for front-loaded t-PA was 84 per cent (60 per cent Grade 3), APSAC 73 per cent (43 per cent Grade 3), and the combination 68 per cent (45 per cent Grade 3). A mortality trend favoring t-PA compared with both of the other treatment regimens was seen at 1 year.[549]

EFFECT ON LEFT VENTRICULAR FUNCTION. Although precise measurements of infarct size would be an ideal endpoint for clinical reperfusion studies, such measures have been found to be impractical.[550] Attempts to use left ventricular ejection fraction as a surrogate for infarct size have not been productive because little difference is seen in ejection fraction between treatment groups that show a significant difference in mortality.[421,513] Alternative methods of assessing left ventricular function, such as end-systolic volume[551] or quantitative echocardiography,[552] are more revealing because patients with smaller volumes and better-preserved ventricular shape have an improved survival.

As with survival, improvement in global left ventricular function is related to the time of thrombolytic treatment, with greatest improvement occurring with earliest therapy.[513,553,554] Greater improvement in left ventricular function has been reported with anterior than with inferior infarcts.[421] Earlier trials failed to demonstrate any difference in global left ventricular function when streptokinase and t-PA were compared.[555,556] The angiographic substudy in GUSTO I reported detailed regional wall motion analyses stratified by thrombolytic regimen.[519] Patients who received the accelerated t-PA regimen had significantly less depression of regional wall motion in the ischemic zone, as evidenced by fewer abnormal chords when their ventricular silhouettes were subjected to segmental wall motion analysis. In addition, this patient group tended to have a slightly higher global ejection fraction and slightly reduced end-systolic volume index at 90 minutes following initiation of thrombolytic therapy. The totality of the data presented in the GUSTO angiographic substudy[519] is consistent with the hypothesis that more rapid and complete restoration of normal coronary blood flow in the infarct-related artery with t-PA was associated with an improvement in regional and global left ventricular function (presumably through greater myocardial salvage in the ischemic zone) and that this difference in function compared to that obtained with streptokinase may have contributed to the mortality differences observed at 30 days and beyond (Fig. 37–28).[372]

Complications of Thrombolytic Therapy

Recent (<1 year) exposure to streptococci or streptokinase produces some degree of antibody-mediated resistance to streptokinase (and APSAC) in most patients. Although this is of clinical consequence only rarely, it is recommended that patients not receive streptokinase for AMI if they have been treated with a streptokinase product within the last year. In the International t-PA/SK Mortality Trial, allergic reactions were seen in 1.7 per cent of patients given streptokinase. Hypotension can be expected in up to 10 per cent.[529] Bleeding complications are, of course, most common and potentially the most serious.[513,557] Most bleeding is relatively minor with all agents, with more serious episodes occurring in patients requiring invasive procedures.[558,559] Overall, 70 per cent of bleeding episodes occur at the site of vascular punctures.[558–560] Intracranial hemorrhage is the most serious complication of thrombolytic therapy[513,561–563]; its frequency varies with the clinical characteristics of the patient and the thrombolytic prescribed.[562,564]

Collaborators from the European Cooperative Society Group (ECSG) and GISSI, TAMI, TIMI, and ISAM groups pooled their respective data bases on thrombolytic-treated patients with AMI to develop a statistical model for individual risk assessment for intracranial hemorrhage using a case-control format.[564] The following four clinical variables known at hospital admission were shown to predict an increased risk of intracranial hemorrhage: age > 65 years (odds ratio for intracranial hemorrhage = 2.2), weight < 70 kg (2.1), hypertension on presentation (2.0), and use of t-PA as opposed to streptokinase (1.6). On the basis of the number of these risk factors present at the time of evaluation of a patient who is a candidate for thrombolysis, clinicians may estimate the probability of intracranial hemorrhage.[564] Assuming an overall incidence of intracranial hemorrhage of 0.75 per cent, the expected incidence of intracranial hemorrhage stratified by the number of risk factors would be 0.26 per cent for no risk factors, 0.96 per cent for one risk factor, 1.32 per cent for two risk factors, and 2.17 per cent for three risk factors.[544,565] The incremental incidence of intracranial hemorrhage with thrombolysis appears to be at least partially offset by a lower frequency of thrombotic strokes, so that the overall incidence of stroke is usually not much higher in patients receiving thrombolytic therapy than in control patients.[508,529,561] In addition to the risks introduced by invasive procedures and the features cited above, fibrinogen depletion and a prolonged activated partial thromboplastin time (aPTT) level (>90 sec) during therapy confer an increased risk of bleeding in patients receiving thrombolytic therapy.[535,548,556,558,559]

There have been reports of an "early hazard" with thrombolytic therapy,[566,567] i.e., an excess of deaths in the first 24 hours in thrombolytic-treated patients compared with controls (especially in elderly patients treated > 12 hours).[10,568,569] However, this excess early mortality is more than offset by the deaths prevented beyond the first day, culminating in an 18 per cent (13 to 23 per cent) reduction in mortality by 35 days.[10] The mechanisms responsible for this early hazard are not clear but probably are multiple, including an increased risk of myocardial rupture[570] (particularly in the elderly),[567,571] fatal intracranial hemorrhage,[561] inadequate myocardial reperfusion resulting in pump failure and cardiogenic shock,[571,572] and possible reperfusion injury of reperfused myocardium.[454] Reports of more unusual complications such as splenic rupture,[573] aortic dissection,[574] and cholesterol embolization[575] have also appeared.

OTHER THROMBOLYTIC AGENTS

In addition to accelerated t-PA (alteplase) and streptokinase, two other thrombolytic agents—urokinase and anisoylated streptokinase plasminogen activator complex (APSAC, anistreplase)—have been approved by the United States Food and Drug Administration for the treatment of AMI. Urokinase (see p. 1821), a naturally occurring plasminogen activator, has been undergoing evaluation for treatment of AMI for at least three decades. Although it offers the potential advantage of less antigenicity than with streptokinase, infarct artery patency rates are about the same as those achieved with streptokinase.[513,514,576] Although it is prescribed in an intravenous regimen for AMI in some countries, given its high cost and lack of advantage over streptokinase, its use in the United States is almost exclusively for intracoronary infusion (6000 IU/minute to an average cumulative dose of 500,000 IU[577]) to lyse intracoronary thrombi that are believed to be responsible for an evolving AMI. APSAC, usually administered in a dose of 30 mg over 2 to 5 minutes intravenously, has a side-effect profile similar to that of streptokinase, a patency profile similar to that of conventional-dose t-PA, and a mortality benefit similar to that of streptokinase or t-PA (double-chain form, duteplase).[513,535,549,578,579] The lack of any compelling advantages (other than bolus administration) and costs higher than streptokinase have relegated APSAC to an extremely infrequently prescribed drug for AMI in the United States.

Recombinant human single-chain urokinase-type plasminogen activator (see p. 1821) (scuPA or pro-urokinase) has been produced both in nonglycosylated (e.g., saruplase) and glycosylated (e.g., Abbott-74187) forms. Pro-urokinase preparations have been studied alone[580] and in combination with urokinase[581] and t-PA.[582] Synergism has been suggested for these combinations, allowing for lower drug doses with higher clot specificity without an increase in bleeding complications. Combinations of urokinase and t-PA,[583,584] streptokinase and t-PA,[33,585] and APSAC and t-PA[579] have also been tested to take advantage of synergistic effects of multiple plasminogen activators. As yet, none of these combinations has proved clearly to be of additional benefit and none is recommended for routine use in AMI patients.

Site-directed mutagenesis has been used to produce t-PA molecules with altered pharmacokinetic and functional properties.[586] Reteplase (r-PA), a t-PA mutant that retains only the kringle-2 and protease domains and lacks glycosylated side chains, has a longer half-life than alteplase, permitting bolus administration.[587] Following encouraging results from phase 2 angiographic trials,[588,589] r-PA (two boluses of 10 MU separated by 30 minutes) was compared with streptokinase in a large phase 3 trial (INJECT).[590] The INJECT trial reported 35-day mortality rates of 9.02 per cent for r-PA and 9.53 per cent for streptokinase; at 6 months these rates were 11.0 per cent and 12.1 per cent, respectively (P = NS). Bleeding rates were similar in the two treatment arms. Given its demonstrated equivalence to streptokinase and advantage of ease of administration, r-PA may be a useful addition to the list of available thrombolytic agents; it is now being tested against accelerated t-PA in a large phase 3 mortality trial (GUSTO-3).

Another promising mutant of t-PA is TNK-tPA, which contains a new glycosylation site on kringle 1 (decreases rate of clearance), lacks another glycosylation on kringle 1 (decreases rate of clearance and increases fibrin specificity), and contains a 4-amino acid substitution in the protease domain (increases fibrin specificity and resistance to PAI-1).[591] Initial experience in patients (TIMI 10 Pilot) suggests that TNK-tPA has sufficiently slowed plasma clearance to permit single-bolus administration and greater fibrin specificity than alteplase t-PA and achieves a 90-minute patency rate that is at least comparable to that of alteplase t-PA.[592] Additional trials are under way.

Other approaches to development of new thrombolytic agents have included using recombinant DNA technology to produce staphylokinase[593] and vampire bat t-PA,[594] potent thrombolytics with fibrin specificity. It remains to be determined how immunogenic these molecules are and whether they will be useful clinically.

Recommendations for Thrombolytic Therapy

NET CLINICAL BENEFIT OF THROMBOLYSIS. Perhaps one of the most important messages from all of the available evidence is that thrombolytic therapy is underutilized in patients with AMI. Fendrick and colleagues have calculated that if every patient with AMI for whom thrombolytic therapy is recommended under current guidelines were treated with aspirin and a thrombolytic agent, more than 4000 additional lives would be saved annually in the United States.[595] Of all the currently approved regimens, accelerated t-PA is the most effective at recanalization of the infarct-related artery and restoration of normal coronary blood flow in the ischemic zone.[596] It is also the most expensive of the available treatment regimens, and this has engendered considerable discussion of the relative benefits of t-PA versus streptokinase, the intracranial hemorrhage risk difference in patients treated with t-PA versus streptokinase, and the cost effectiveness of substitution of t-PA for streptokinase in the treatment of AMI.[597–603]

Against the mortality benefits associated with administration of t-PA versus streptokinase must be weighed the excess risk of stroke that is estimated to be 2 to 3 per 1000 patients treated. When the entire cohort of patients enrolled in the GUSTO I trial was analyzed for the net clinical benefit of the various thrombolytic regimens (e.g., composite endpoint of 30 days' mortality or nonfatal stroke), a small but statistically significant benefit was still seen for the accelerated t-PA regimen (7.2 per cent) versus the streptokinase plus subcutaneous heparin regimen (7.9 per cent) and streptokinase plus intravenous heparin regimen (8.2 per cent).[33] However, this net clinical advantage of accelerated-dose t-PA regimen does not apply equally to all patients with AMI.[15,427] Patients with a higher baseline risk of mortality experience a greater mortality benefit with the accelerated t-PA regimen compared with streptokinase.[15,387] On average, the use of t-PA in place of streptokinase costs an additional $33,000 per year of life saved; t-PA is less cost effective in younger patients and more cost effective in older patients who are at higher risk of mortality.[15]

CHOICE OF AGENT. Analysis of the net clinical benefit and cost effectiveness of t-PA versus streptokinase does not easily yield recommendations for treatment because clinicians must weigh the risk of mortality and risk of intracranial hemorrhage when confronting a thrombolytic-eligible patient with AMI; additional considerations may be the constraints placed on physicians' therapeutic decision-making by the health care system in which they are practicing.[603] We are in agreement with the general recommendations by Martin and Kennedy[427] and Simoons and Arnold[604] that categorize patients into those that are at high risk of death (advanced age, female gender, depressed left ventricular function, anterior MI, bundle branch block, total magnitude of ST-segment elevation, diabetes, heart rate greater than 100 beats/min, systolic pressure less than 100 mm Hg, long delay since onset of ischemic discomfort),[427,604] and high risk of intracranial hemorrhage (age greater than 65 years). In the subgroup of patients presenting within 4 hours of symptom onset, the speed of reperfusion of the infarct vessel is of paramount importance and a high-intensity thrombolytic regimen such as accelerated t-PA is the preferred treatment, except in those individuals in whom the risk of death is low (e.g., a young patient with a small inferior MI) and the risk of intracranial hemorrhage is increased (e.g., acute hypertension), in whom streptokinase and accelerated t-PA are approximately equivalent choices. For those patients presenting between 4 and 12 hours after the onset of chest discomfort, the speed of reperfusion of the infarct vessel is of lesser importance, and therefore streptokinase and accelerated t-PA are generally equivalent options, given the difference in costs. Of note, for those patients presenting between 4 and 12 hours from symptom onset with a low mortality risk but an increased risk of intracranial hemorrhage (e.g., elderly patients with inferior MI, blood pressure greater than 100 mm Hg, and heart rate less than 100 beats/min), streptokinase is probably preferable to t-PA because of cost considerations if thrombolytic therapy is prescribed at all in such a patient.

LATE THERAPY. No mortality benefit was demonstrated in the LATE and EMERAS trials when thrombolytics were routinely administered to patients between 12 and 24 hours,[533,534] although we believe it is still reasonable to consider thrombolytic therapy in appropriately selected patients with persistent symptoms and ST elevation on ECG beyond 12 hours (Fig. 37–20). Persistent chest pain late after the onset of symptoms correlates with a higher incidence of collateral or antegrade flow in the infarct zone and is therefore a marker for patients with viable myocardium that might be salvaged.[605] Because elderly patients treated with thrombolytics more than 12 hours after the onset of symptoms are at increased risk of cardiac rupture,[567] it is our practice to restrict late thrombolytic administration to younger patients (<65 years) with ongoing ischemia, especially those with large anterior infarctions. The elderly patient with ongoing ischemic symptoms but presenting late (>12 hours) is probably better managed with direct (primary) PTCA (see below) than with thrombolytic therapy.

Before the institution of thrombolytic therapy, consideration should be given to the patient's need for intravascular catheterization, as would be required for the placement of an arterial pressure monitoring line, a pulmonary artery catheter for hemodynamic monitoring, or a temporary transvenous pacemaker. If any of these are required, ideally they should be placed as expeditiously as possible *before* infusion of the thrombolytic agent. If such procedures require an additional delay of more than 30 minutes, they should be deferred as long as possible after thrombolytic therapy is begun. In the early hours after institution of thrombolytic therapy, such catheterization should be performed only if crucial to survival, and then sites where excessive bleeding can be controlled should be chosen (e.g., subclavian vein catheterization should be avoided).

As noted above, all patients with suspected AMI should receive aspirin (160 to 325 mg) regardless of the thrombolytic agent prescribed. Aspirin should be continued indefinitely (see p.1264). The issues surrounding antithrombin therapy as an adjunct to thrombolysis are complex and are discussed in detail in a subsequent section (see p. 1224).

CORONARY ANGIOPLASTY

(See also p. 1313)

It is now established that reperfusion can be achieved by emergency PTCA.[606–610] Using a guidewire and balloon catheter, it is technically easier to cross a total occlusion consisting of a fresh thrombus than to cross a longstanding occlusion of a coronary artery. Thus, wire-guided balloon angioplasty can be useful to achieve reperfusion in two quite different circumstances[611]: (1) in lieu of thrombolytic therapy where it is referred to as *direct* or *primary angioplasty*,[612] and (2) as adjunctive therapy with thrombolysis or as a management strategy in the subacute phase of AMI (days 2 to 7) in patients who do not receive thrombolysis. Several clinical scenarios have been described that represent different categories of use of PTCA when it is not selected as the primary reperfusion strategy (see Chap. 39).[370,611,613] When thrombolysis has failed to reperfuse the infarct vessel or a severe stenosis is present in the infarct vessel, a *rescue PTCA* may be performed as soon as possible. Alternatively, strategies of empirical *immediate* (i.e., performed urgently within a few hours) or *deferred* (i.e., performed within the first week) PTCA have been proposed for all patients with residual critical stenosis (>70 per cent of lumen diameter) who receive thrombolysis. Finally, a more conservative approach of *elective* PTCA may be used to manage AMI patients only when spontaneous or exercise-provoked ischemia occurs whether or not they have received a previous course of thrombolytic therapy.

Primary Angioplasty

An important advantage of primary PTCA in AMI is the ability to achieve reperfusion of the infarct vessel without the risk of bleeding associated with thrombolytic therapy.[370,610,613–615a] In addition, primary PTCA (performed predominantly in experienced centers) as compared with thrombolytic therapy has been shown in several randomized trials and registries to yield higher patency rates of the infarct vessel both at 90 minutes (about 90 per cent for PTCA versus 65 per cent for thrombolysis).[519,546,606,610,616,617] In a randomized trial of primary PTCA versus intravenous streptokinase for AMI in patients presenting an average of 3 hours after symptom onset, de Boer et al.[617] found that infarct size measured by enzyme release was reduced by 23 per cent and global and regional left ventricular function was improved in the group undergoing PTCA. Systematic overviews[618,619] of seven trials of primary PTCA versus thrombolysis[606–608,620–623] collectively enrolling just under 1200 patients revealed a 40 per cent reduction in short-term mortality in patients treated with primary PTCA versus thrombolysis (Fig. 37–29); a similar reduction in the composite endpoint of death or nonfatal AMI by 6 weeks was also observed. When primary PTCA is performed in experienced centers with a well-staffed invasive angiography team, hospital length of stay and follow-up costs are less than for the patients with AMI who are treated by thrombolytic therapy.[16,608,609,624]

Why have these dramatic differences favoring primary PTCA over thrombolytic therapy been observed? In addition to the high level of technical expertise in the dedicated centers that have reported promising results with primary PTCA, differences in the adequacy of reperfusion and responses of ischemic myocardium to restoration of flow by thrombolysis and mechanical means should be considered.[617] Early patency of the infarct-related artery is higher

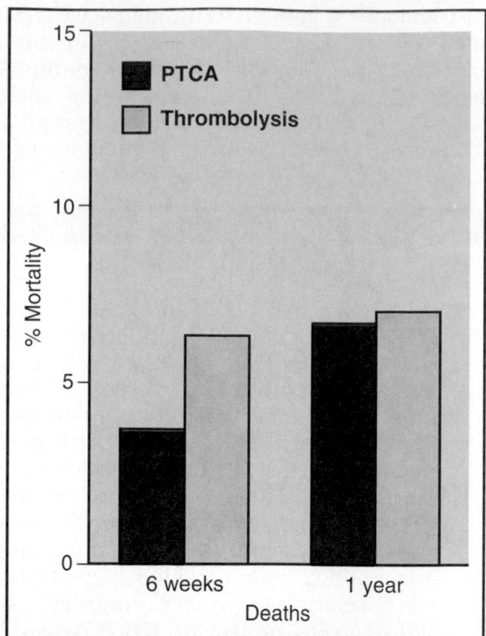

FIGURE 37–29. Comparison of mortality in AMI patients treated with primary PTCA versus thrombolysis. Pooled data from seven randomized trials reveal a significantly lower mortality at 6 weeks in the patients treated with PTCA. A nonsignificant trend favoring PTCA was present at 1 year. (Adapted from Michels, K. B., and Yusuf, S.: Does PTCA in acute myocardial infarction affect mortality and reinfarction rates?: A quantitative overview (meta-analysis) of the randomized clinical trials. Circulation *91*:476, 1995; Copyright 1995 American Heart Association.)

with direct PTCA, full reperfusion (TIMI Grade 3 flow) is higher, the degree of residual stenosis is less,[617] reocclusion rates are lower,[546,616,625–627] and collateral flow to noninfarct-related myocardial zones is probably increased[607]—all features that promote better healing in the infarct zone, less left ventricular dilatation,[628] and reduced morbidity and mortality. Ohnishi and coworkers have reported in a canine model of AMI that pharmacological lysis of coronary thrombi associated with production of a systemic lytic state is associated with nonspecific protease activity, activation of neutrophils, complement activation, and platelet activation with release of vasoactive substances that appear to cause delayed recovery of contractile function due to reperfusion injury.[463] In contrast, mechanical recanalization of the infarct vessel does not produce the interstitial edema, contraction band necrosis, and microvascular hemorrhage seen with thrombolytic therapy[462] (Fig. 37–11).

The clinical trial results and intriguing experimental observations cited above must be placed in perspective when one considers implementing primary PTCA as a treatment strategy for the majority of patients with AMI. Fewer than 20 per cent of hospitals in the United States[609,629] and less than 10 per cent of hospitals in Europe[630] can perform primary PTCA, and an even smaller proportion are capable of performing it on an emergency basis 24 hours a day, 7 days a week. It remains to be determined whether lower-volume PTCA centers with less experienced investigators can replicate the encouraging results reported to date.[630,631] In addition, it is unclear whether on-site cardiac surgical backup is a necessary component of a primary PTCA strategy for AMI.[632] The potential cost implications of offering primary PTCA to all eligible patients with AMI are staggering and have been the subject of considerable ongoing debate in several countries.[614,633]

Angioplasty as an Adjunct to Thrombolysis

Ellis et al. have summarized the heterogeneous outcomes reported in observational series of *rescue* PTCA after failed thrombolysis.[634] Although procedural success was obtained in about 80 per cent of patients, the average rate of reocclusion was 18 per cent, and the average mortality was 10.6 per cent. Two randomized trials subsequently compared rescue PTCA versus conservative therapy in patients with an occluded infarct vessel despite thrombolysis.[635,636] The RESCUE trial focused on the subset of AMI patients with an anterior infarction and reported a reduction in the composite endpoint of death or congestive heart failure by 30 days in the PTCA group.[636] When combined with the trial by Belenkie et al.,[635] a mortality rate of 5.4 per cent was seen in the rescue PTCA group versus 12.9 per cent in the conservative group, which was not statistically significant.[618]

Following thrombolytic therapy in patients who clinically appear to have reperfused, PTCA, whether applied immediately or deferred, has the theoretical benefit of further opening of a stenosed coronary artery to increase flow, perhaps enhancing myocardial recovery and diminishing the possibility of reocclusion. Several trials have compared immediate, early (within several hours to a few days), or deferred (delayed for 4 days) PTCA versus no PTCA, whereas others have compared immediate versus deferred PTCA or immediate versus deferred versus no PTCA; a summary of the design features and main findings of 16 trials that collectively enrolled about 6200 patients in these categories has been published along with meta-analysis of the mortality results.[618] Although none of the individual comparisons of strategies achieved conventional statistical significance, a consistent theme was observed—the *routine empirical* use of PTCA (either immediate or delayed) following thrombolysis was associated with a trend toward *increased* mortality.[370,613,618] In addition, there were higher rates of abrupt reclosure of the infarct-related coronary artery and complications, including reinfarction and the need for urgent coronary artery bypass surgery, while providing no benefit in terms of recovery of ventricular function.[565,637–639] Possible explanations for the increased hazard associated with PTCA soon after thrombolysis include exacerbation of platelet activation and thrombosis at the site of plaque rupture and increased bleeding, including hemorrhagic dissections of the target vessel.[637,640–643] There is also no evidence to support empirical deferred PTCA in patients without evidence of recurrent or provocable ischemia. The TOPS trial randomized patients with a negative exercise test several days following thrombolysis to either medical therapy or medical therapy plus PTCA.[644] There was no benefit in terms of rest or exercise ejection fraction, but there were disturbing trends toward a higher rate of abrupt vessel closure and non-Q-wave MI acutely and a lower rate of infarct-free survival at 1 year follow-up in the PTCA-treated patients.[644]

Recommendations for Use of PTCA in AMI

Although this field is evolving rapidly, at the time of this writing it appears that primary PTCA, when carried out by experienced interventional cardiologists in high-volume angiography laboratories, is at least as effective as and may actually be superior to thrombolytic therapy.[610a] It is our practice to refer thrombolytic-ineligible patients to primary PTCA and also to select primary PTCA as the reperfusion method of choice if the patient is at relatively high risk of intracerebral hemorrhage consequent to thrombolytic therapy (see p. 1220), or if the anticipated time to placement of angioplasty catheters is less than 1 hour from the patient's presentation to the emergency department. In the special circumstances of cardiogenic shock, a serious problem that affects about 5 to 7 per cent of patients with AMI,[422,645] the observational data to date appear to be more favorable with primary PTCA than thrombolysis[646–648] (see p. 1239) and in the absence of other life-threatening comorbidities (e.g., advanced cancer), we therefore refer cardiogenic shock patients for primary PTCA. Nonrandomized observational data from the GUSTO trial support the use of PTCA for management of shock both in patients who arrive in shock and in those who develop it during hospitalization (30-day mortality was 33 to 40 per cent in PTCA-treated patients, compared with 75 per cent in medically treated patients). An ongoing randomized study of PTCA versus medical therapy (SHOCK trial) will provide important, definitive data on the relative benefit of PTCA for cardiogenic shock.[646]

Patients in whom thrombolytic therapy fails to achieve reperfusion represent candidates for PTCA (rescue angioplasty), and in such patients PTCA can usually be safe and effective (greater than 80 per cent success rates).[649] Until there are better ways to recognize patients who might benefit from "rescue angioplasty," the question of optimal treatment of thrombolytic failure remains unresolved.[650] However, patients with evolving chest pain and ST-segment elevations that persist for 90 minutes following the onset of administration of a thrombolytic agent are candidates for emergency catheterization and, if the infarct-related vessel is occluded, for rescue angioplasty. Elective PTCA can be considered for most patients receiving thrombolytic therapy in whom ischemia develops at rest, during ambulation in the hospital, or during a prehospital discharge exercise test.[613,639,641,651] We do not consider it necessary to carry out routine coronary arteriography on asymptomatic patients with negative prehospital discharge exercise tests to identify patients who have severe obstruction in whom PTCA can be performed.

Evidence exists from observational studies, retrospective reviews of multicenter trials, as well as a recent randomized trial that routine prophylactic use of intra-aortic balloon counterpulsation following PTCA for AMI reduces the risk of reocclusion.[652–654] Whether or not thrombolysis was used, prophylactic intra-aortic balloon counterpulsation may be useful for 24 to 48 hours as an adjunct to maintain vessel patency following PTCA of the infarct vessel in those patients in whom it is judged that a sudden reocclusion of the target vessel would be associated with severe hemodynamic compromise.

SURGICAL REPERFUSION

There have been extensive improvements in intraoperative myocardial preservation with cardioplegia and hypothermia and in surgical techniques. These have allowed surgical reperfusion in patients with AMI to be carried out at quite low short- and long-term mortality rates—approximately 2 per cent in-hospital and 25 per cent 10-year mortality rates in selected centers. This has kept alive the concept of emergency coronary revascularization as a possible measure to protect jeopardized myocardium in patients suffering AMI.[655–657] As appears to be the case for all methods designed to limit infarct size, salvage of myocardium is most successful if surgery is performed within the first 4 to 6 hours of the onset of the acute event.[658] In the usual patient who develops an AMI outside of the hospital, it is logistically almost impossible to bring the patient to the hospital, carry out a clinical evaluation, outline the coronary anatomy by arteriography, assemble the surgical team, commence operation, and place the patient on cardiopulmonary bypass in less than 4 to 6 hours after the onset of the event. It is therefore unlikely that surgical reperfusion can or will be applied in the *routine* treatment of AMI. Indeed, the operation is contraindicated in patients with uncomplicated transmural infarcts more than 6 hours after the onset of the event. When carried out at this time, surgical reperfusion appears to produce marked hemorrhage into the area of infarction.[659] In some patients with AMI, including some with cardiogenic shock, infarction appears to occur in a stuttering manner over an interval of several days.[660] Revascularization carried out more than 6 hours after the onset of the event might be of benefit in this group, but this has yet to be rigorously established.

About 10 to 20 per cent of AMI patients are currently referred for coronary bypass grafting for one of the following indications: persistent or recurrent chest pain despite thrombolysis or PTCA,[661] high-risk coronary anatomy (e.g., left main stenosis) discovered at catheterization, or a complication of AMI such as ventricular septal rupture or severe mitral regurgitation due to papillary muscle dysfunction. Patients with AMI with continued severe ischemic and hemodynamic instability are likely to benefit from emergency revascularization. PTCA is the preferable technique when revascularization is needed in the first 48 to 72 hours following AMI; surgery should be reserved for those in whom PTCA has been unsuccessful or whose anatomy dictates the need for coronary artery bypass grafting, such as patients with left main or extensive multivessel coronary artery disease.

Patients undergoing successful thrombolysis but with important residual stenoses, who on anatomical grounds are more suitable for surgical revascularization than for PTCA, have undergone coronary artery bypass surgery with quite low mortality (about 4 per cent) and morbidity *provided* that they are operated on more than 24 hours from AMI; those patients requiring urgent or emergency CABG within 24 to 48 hours of AMI have mortality rates between 15 and 20 per cent.[657,661,662] When surgery is performed under urgent conditions with active and ongoing ischemia or cardiogenic shock, operative mortality rises steeply.[663,664] At autopsy, such patients have extensive myocardial necrosis that is often hemorrhagic.[665] Patients who are referred urgently for CABG within 6 to 12 hours of receiving a thrombolytic should receive aprotinin and fresh-frozen plasma to correct their coagulation system deficit and minimize the requirements for blood transfusion. Although postoperative chest tube drainage with relatively minor bleeding occurs more commonly than after elective bypass surgery, this problem is not of major concern.[666]

ANTITHROMBOTIC AND ANTIPLATELET THERAPY

Antithrombotic Therapy

Despite 30 years of active clinical investigation, the use of antithrombotic agents after AMI remains controversial. The rationale for administering heparin (see p. 1978) acutely in AMI includes prevention of deep venous thrombosis, pulmonary embolism, ventricular thrombus formation, and cerebral embolization. In addition, establishing and maintaining patency of the infarct-related artery, whether or not a patient receives thrombolytic therapy, is another common rationale for heparin therapy in AMI.

Randomized trials in AMI conducted in the prethrombolytic era (between 1969 and 1973) showed that the risks of pulmonary embolism, stroke, and reinfarction were reduced in patients who received intravenous heparin.[667–669] Relative mortality was reduced by approximately 10 to 30 per cent, but hemorrhagic complications increased by a factor of 2- to 4-fold. A meta-analysis reported in 1977 indicated a significant reduction of mortality favoring the use of anticoagulation in the hospital phase of AMI[670]; some of the mortality reduction effects in this meta-analysis may have been due to long-term oral anticoagulant therapy superimposed on acute intravenous heparin initiated during the hospital phase.[671,672] With the introduction of the thrombolytic era and importantly after the publication of ISIS-2,[529] the situation became more complicated because of strong evidence of a substantial mortality reduction with aspirin alone and confusing and conflicting data regarding the risk-benefit ratio of heparin used as an adjunct to aspirin or in combination with aspirin and a thrombolytic agent. Several reviews have summarized the available information.[672–674]

EFFECT ON MORTALITY. In the SCATI trial of streptokinase for AMI, in which patients were randomized to receive either delayed subcutaneous heparin or placebo as the *sole* adjunctive therapy (i.e., no aspirin), there was a trend toward lower mortality in the heparin group.[675] No randomized trial data are available comparing aspirin alone versus aspirin plus heparin in patients not receiving thrombolytic therapy. In the combined data set of GISSI-2 and ISIS-3 (totaling over 62,000 patients), the 35-day mortality was 10.0 per cent in the patients receiving subcutaneous heparin versus 10.2 per cent in the patients not receiving any subcutaneous heparin.[672,674] In addition, in the GUSTO study, no difference was seen in the 35-day mortality rate in patients receiving streptokinase plus subcutaneous heparin (7.2 per cent) or intravenous heparin (7.4 per cent).[33] Nonrandomized subgroup analyses from the LATE trial of 2821 patients who received t-PA showed a 35-day mortality of 7.6 per cent when intravenous heparin was administered, compared with 10.4 per cent when no heparin was given.[533,672] Thus, the available information suggests that intravenous heparin is probably of no benefit in patients receiving streptokinase but may be helpful in patients receiving t-PA.

EFFECT ON PATENCY OF INFARCT ARTERY

A number of angiographic studies have examined the role of heparin therapy in establishing and maintaining patency of the infarct-related artery in patients with AMI. Comparison of these trials is difficult because of potentially important differences in study design, including whether aspirin was administered along with heparin, the thrombolytic agent that was administered, and variations in the time of diagnostic coronary arteriography. The Bleich[676] and HART[677] studies showed a higher infarct-related artery patency rate in AMI patients treated with t-PA plus heparin than t-PA plus placebo (71 to 82 per cent versus 43 to 52 per cent infarct-related artery patency at 7 to 72 hours). The European Cooperative Study Group performed angiograms relatively late, i.e., 48 to 120 hours following t-PA, and still showed a somewhat greater patency rate of the infarct-related artery in the heparin-treated patients.[678] The LIMITS (Liquemin in Myocardial Infarction During Thrombolysis with Saruplase) study investigators reported that AMI patients who are treated with unglycosylated single-chain urokinase-type plasminogen activator (saruplase) and are also treated with intravenous heparin (but no aspirin) achieve a higher patency rate of the infarct-related artery at 6 to 12 hours (79 per cent) than those in the control group (57 per cent).[580] The TAMI-3 study suggested that in patients receiving aspirin plus t-PA, no patency benefit was achieved by the immediate intravenous administration of heparin and that it could therefore be delayed for at least 60 to 90 minutes after thrombolysis.[679]

Although a slightly better 90-minute infarct-related artery patency rate was observed in the OSIRIS (streptokinase plus aspirin) study[680] in patients who received heparin versus placebo (82 per cent patency versus 72 per cent), the GUSTO angiographic substudy[519] showed no benefit of intravenous heparin versus subcutaneous heparin in patients who received streptokinase plus aspirin with respect to 90-minute infarct-related artery patency (60 per cent versus 54 per cent). Heparin afforded no benefit in terms of late patency (5-day) of the infarct-related artery in the DUCCS-1 study of patients receiving APSAC plus aspirin.[681]

In a randomized double-blind trial (APSIM) of APSAC versus conventional-dose heparin (500 IU/kg/24 hours), the patency rate of the infarct-related artery was 77 per cent in the thrombolytic group versus only 37 per cent in the heparin group.[682] However, the HEAP (Heparin in Early Patency) investigators have presented intriguing data that a large single intravenous bolus of 300 units per kilogram of heparin to AMI patients presenting in less than 6 hours with ST-segment elevation results in a 90-minute patency rate of the infarct-related artery of 60 per cent with 36 per cent TIMI Grade 3 flow.[683]

EFFECT ON LEFT VENTRICULAR THROMBUS. Anticoagulant therapy significantly reduces the incidence of echocardiographically documented left ventricular thrombi.[671] These benefits are observed most prominently in patients with anterior myocardial infarction, particularly those with a large area of wall motion abnormality. In the thrombolytic era, the incidence of left ventricular thrombi is reduced.[684,685] Although co-administration of heparin does not appear to affect the incidence of left ventricular thrombus formation in patients who receive thrombolytic therapy, the thrombi protrude less into the ventricular cavity when heparin is administered.[686]

COMPLICATIONS OF ANTITHROMBOTIC THERAPY

Although heparin may induce thrombocytopenia through an immunological mechanism, this is seen only rarely, probably occurring in only 2 to 3 per cent of patients.[687,687a] The most serious complication of antithrombotic therapy is bleeding—especially intracranial hemorrhage—when thrombolytic agents are prescribed (see p. 1219). Major hemorrhagic events occur more frequently in patients of low body weight, advanced age, and marked prolongation of the aPTT (greater than 90 to 100 seconds).[558,559] Frequent monitoring of the aPTT (facilitated by use of a bedside testing device) reduces the risk of major hemorrhagic complications in patients treated with heparin.[688] A standardized nomogram, adopted from treatment regimens for patients with pulmonary embolism, is commonly used to adjust heparin infusions in patients with AMI.[689] It should be noted, however, that during the first 12 hours following thrombolytic therapy, the aPTT may be elevated from the thrombolytic agent alone (particularly if streptokinase is administered), making it difficult to accurately interpret the effects of a heparin infusion on the patient's coagulation status.

NEW ANTITHROMBOTIC AGENTS

(See also p. 1821)

Potential disadvantages of infusions of unfractionated heparin include dependency on antithrombin III for inhibition of thrombin activity, sensitivity to platelet factor 4, inability to inhibit clot-bound thrombin, marked interpatient varability in therapeutic response, and the need for frequent aPTT monitoring. In an effort to circumvent these disadvantages of unfractionated heparin, there has been interest in the development of novel antithrombotic compounds.[690] The prototypical direct antithrombin is hirudin, which has been made available for clinical investigation using recombinant technology (see p. 1820). The TIMI-9 trial compared intravenous unfractionated heparin with intravenous hirudin in AMI patients receiving thrombolytic therapy (accelerated-dose t-PA or streptokinase). Hirudin was equal to heparin in effectiveness but was not superior when analyzed using a composite primary endpoint of the sum of death, nonfatal AMI, or congestive heart failure/cardiogenic shock, or the harder composite endpoint of the sum of death or nonfatal MI.[691] The GUSTO IIB study showed no statistically significant reduction in the incidence of death or nonfatal recurrent infarction by 30 days with hirudin versus heparin in MI patients with ST-segment elevation as well as those without.[691a]

The potential beneficial effects of low molecular weight heparin preparations, particularly those that have a high anti-X_a:anti-II_a ratio, are now being examined in AMI patients in both the presence and the absence of thrombolytic therapy.

Recommendations for Antithrombotic Therapy

Given the pivotal role thrombin plays in the pathogenesis of AMI, antithrombotic therapy remains an important therapeutic intervention. As reviewed on page 1225, all patients with an acute coronary syndrome should receive antiplatelet therapy (aspirin remains the recommended agent at this time). Until the results of ongoing studies are available, we believe that the recommendations below are a reasonable approach.

For patients who do *not* receive thrombolytic therapy, overviews of the available data indicate that heparin reduces mortality and morbidity from serious complications such as reinfarction and thromboembolism.[692,693] Therefore, in the absence of contraindications to anticoagulation we routinely use heparin in *all* AMI patients presenting with ST elevation who are not candidates for thrombolysis and also prescribe it for AMI patients presenting without ST elevation. Minimum therapy should consist of 7500 IU subcutaneously every 12 hours; however, it is the practice of many clinicians to administer intravenous heparin at full therapeutic dosage to such patients.[671] Dosing regimens that are based on weight (bolus 70 U/kg and infusion of 15 U/kg/hr) may more rapidly and safely establish a therapeutic level of heparin (target aPTT about 1.5 to 2 times control)[694,695]; in the average-sized patient this corresponds to an intravenous bolus of 5000 U and infusion of 1000 U/hr. The heparin infusion is continued for at least 48 hours, and then a decision is made about the patient's ongoing need for intravenous antithrombotic therapy based on factors such as the presence or absence of recurrent ischemia and plans for catheterization. Patients with a large anterior infarction with or without an echocardiographically demonstrated thrombus are at increased risk of cerebral embolism and should receive oral anticoagulant therapy (target INR 2.0 to 3.0) for at least 3 months following AMI.[684,685] Additional recommendations on long-term oral anticoagulant therapy after AMI are given on page 1265.

For patients receiving thrombolytic therapy with either streptokinase or APSAC, there is no apparent mortality benefit of immediate intravenous heparin, and we do not recommend its use if those thrombolytics are prescribed. The only exception to this are patients who have another compelling indication for anticoagulation such as a large anterior infarction with a significant wall motion abnormality[671] or atrial fibrillation (see p. 1253)—in this case we generally use intravenous heparin administered to a target aPTT of 60 to 70 seconds. The relative benefits of routine use of delayed (4 to 12 hours), high-dose (12,500 IU twice daily) subcutaneous heparin in patients receiving streptokinase remain unresolved.[695a]

On the basis of the principle that t-PA is a more fibrin-specific lytic agent and the evidence that infarct-related artery patency rates are higher in patients receiving intravenous heparin adjunctively with t-PA, it is commonly recommended that with t-PA, intravenous heparin should be administered.[671] A bolus of 5000 IU followed by an initial infusion of 1000 IU/hr or a bolus of 70 IU/kg followed by an initial infusion of 15 IU/kg/hr is appropriate.[696] In current practice the target aPTT range is 50 to 70 seconds.[2] Patients should be monitored for any signs of bleeding and frequent measurements of the aPTT (at least once every 12 to 24 hours) are recommended, because the incidence of hemorrhage increases with marked prolongation of the aPTT.[558,559] The infusion should be maintained for at least 24 to 48 hours following administration of t-PA.

Because of concern about the possibility of a rebound increase in thrombin generation and recurrent ischemia following cessation of heparin therapy[697,698] (see p. 1823), some clinicians have suggested a tapering of heparin infusions rather than abrupt discontinuation.

Antiplatelet Therapy

As discussed earlier (see p. 1110), platelets play a major role in the thrombotic response to rupture of a coronary artery plaque.[65,699] Aggregates of platelets are integrally involved in the development of AMI, both with and without ST-segment elevation.[207,699a] Platelet-rich thrombi are also more resistant to thrombolysis than are fibrin and erythrocyte-rich thrombi.[700,701] Thus, there is a sound scientific basis for inhibiting platelet aggregation in *all* AMI patients, regardless of whether a thrombolytic is prescribed. Comprehensive overviews of randomized trials of antiplatelet therapy have summarized the overwhelming evidence of benefit of antiplatelet therapy for a wide range of vascular disorders[9,702,703] (Fig. 37–30). In patients at risk for AMI, patients with a documented prior AMI, and patients in the acute phase of an AMI, dramatic reductions (between 25 to 50 per cent) in mortality, nonfatal reduction of recurrent infarction, and nonfatal stroke are achieved by antiplatelet therapy.[9] Not unexpectedly, the absolute benefits are greatest in those patients at highest baseline risk.[9] Although several antiplatelet regimens have been evaluated, the agent most extensively tested has been aspirin and this also is the drug for which the most compelling evidence of benefit exists.[411,704]

The ISIS-2 study was the largest trial of aspirin in AMI and provides the single strongest piece of evidence that aspirin reduces mortality in AMI[529] (Fig. 37–25). Of interest, in contrast to the observations of a time-dependent mortality effect of thrombolytic therapy (see p. 1220), the mortality reduction with aspirin was similar in patients treated within 4 hours (25 per cent reduction in mortality), between 5 and 12 hours (21 per cent reduction), and between 13 and 24 hours (21 per cent reduction). There was an overall 23 per cent reduction in mortality from aspirin in ISIS-2 that was largely additive to the 25 per cent reduction in mortality from streptokinase, so that patients receiving both therapies experienced a 42 per cent reduction in mortality.[529] The mortality reduction was as high as 53 per cent in those patients who received both aspirin and streptokinase within 6 hours of symptoms. Of particular interest was the fact that the combination of streptokinase and aspirin reduced mortality from 23.8 per cent to 15.8 per cent (34 per cent reduction) *without* increasing the risk of stroke or hemorrhage.[671]

Recommendations for Antiplatelet Therapy

Some uncertainty about the optimal dose of aspirin for acute treatment of AMI remains.[705] In general, high doses of aspirin are not more effective than lower doses but are more likely to provoke gastrointestinal side effects.[411] However, adequate cyclo-oxygenase inhibition (and reduction in thromboxane A_2 production) takes several days to accomplish with less than 75 mg of aspirin, and loading doses of 160 to 325 mg (preferably chewed) are therefore recommended for all AMI patients without a history of aspirin allergy whether they present with ST elevation or not and whether they undergo reperfusion with thrombolytics or PTCA or are treated with a more conservative medical regimen (Fig. 37–18). Active peptic ulcer disease is a relative contraindication to antiplatelet therapy.[2] For patients with severe nausea and vomiting, aspirin suppositories (325 mg) can be used. Aspirin should be continued indefinitely in patients with AMI.

NEW ANTIPLATELET REGIMENS. Alternative regimens for inhibiting platelet function are under active development (see Chap. 58). Although thromboxane synthase inhibitors,[706] thromboxane and serotonin receptor antagonists,[707] and agents with combined actions on thromboxane synthesis and the thromboxane receptor have been explored,[708,709] the most promising class of agents are the glycoprotein IIb/IIIa receptor antagonists, which interfere with the final common pathway for platelet aggregation.[207,710] When combined with accelerated-dose t-PA and aspirin in patients with ST-elevation AMI, integrelin, a cyclic peptide antagonist of the IIb/IIIa receptor, achieves patency rates of the infarct-related artery between 70 and 80 per cent[711] and reduces the amount of ST-segment deviation observed over time with a continuous ECG monitor.[712]

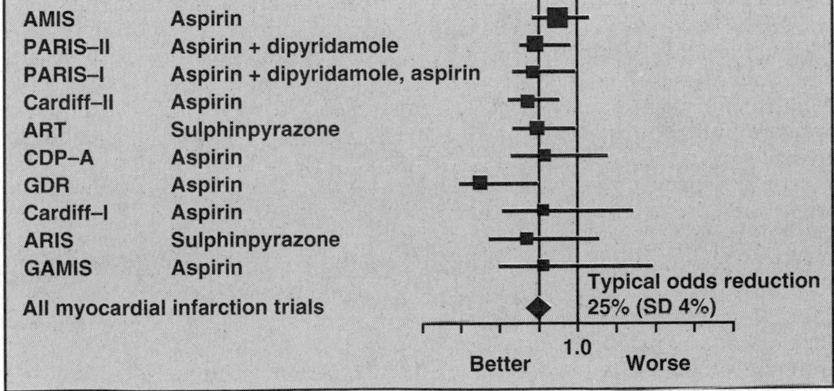

FIGURE 37–30. Results of aspirin therapy after MI. Meta-analysis of several placebo-controlled trials of antiplatelet therapy after MI (predominantly aspirin), indicating a 25 per cent reduction in the odds for mortality in patients receiving the active therapy. (Adapted from Antiplatelet Trialists' Collaboration: Secondary prevention of vascular disease by prolonged antiplatelet treatment. BMJ *296*:320, 1988.)

Coronary Care Units

Deaths from primary ventricular fibrillation in AMI have been prevented because the coronary care unit (CCU) allows continuous monitoring of cardiac rhythm by highly trained nurses with the authority to initiate immediate treatment of arrhythmias in the absence of physicians, and because of the specialized equipment (defibrillators, pacemakers) and drugs available. Although all of these benefits can be achieved for patients scattered throughout the hospital, the clustering of patients with AMI in the CCU has greatly improved the efficient use of the trained personnel, facilities, and equipment. In recent years, with increasing emphasis on hemodynamic monitoring and treatment of the serious complications of AMI with such modalities as thrombolytic therapy, afterload reduction, and intraaortic balloon counterpulsation, the CCU has assumed even greater importance.[30,713] As interventional strategies including thrombolytic therapy and acute coronary angioplasty are used more routinely in AMI patients, facilities in which patients may undergo diagnostic and therapeutic angiographic procedures are being integrated into the CCU structure.

At the same time, the value of CCUs for patients with uncomplicated AMI has been questioned and restudied.[30,714] With increasing attention directed to the limitation of resources and to the economic impact of intensive care, there have been efforts to select patients for whom hospitalization in a CCU would likely be of benefit (see p. 1749).[713] The ECG, on presentation, particularly in conjunction with previous tracings[715] and an immediate general clinical assessment, can be useful both for predicting which patients will have the diagnosis of AMI confirmed and identifying low-risk patients who may require less intensive care.[393,716,717] Of patients with a history of typical chest pain but with a normal ECG in the emergency department, less than 20 per cent ultimately have an AMI on that admission, and less than 1 per cent develop any significant complication.[718] Thus, a patient with a normal ECG may not require admission to a full-fledged CCU. Careful analysis of the quality of pain may help identify such low-risk patients as well. Patients without a history of angina pectoris or MI presenting with pain that is sharp or stabbing and pleuritic, positional, or reproduced by palpation of the chest wall are extremely unlikely to have an AMI.[719] Computer-guided decision protocols are being developed to aid clinicians in identifying those AMI patients who require admission to the CCU as opposed to a less intensive hospital ward.[720]

Contemporary CCUs typically have equipment available for noninvasive monitoring of single or multiple ECG leads, cardiac rhythm, ST-segment deviation, arterial pressure, and arterial oxygen saturation.[721] Computer algorithms for detection and analysis of arrhythmias are superior to visual surveillance by skilled CCU staff.[722] However, even the most sophisticated ECG monitoring systems are susceptible to artifacts due to patient movement or noise on the signal from poor skin preparation when monitoring electrodes are applied.[30] Noninvasive monitoring of arterial blood pressure using a sphygmomanometric cuff that undergoes cycles of inflation and deflation at programmed intervals is suitable for the majority of patients admitted to a CCU. Invasive arterial monitoring is preferred in patients with a low output syndrome under circumstances in which inotropic therapy is initiated for severe left ventricular failure (see p. 1194).[30]

The CCU remains the appropriate hospital unit for patients with complicated infarctions (e.g., hemodynamic instability, recurrent arrhythmias) and those patients requiring intensive nursing care for devices such as an intra-aortic balloon pump (see p. 1221). For patients with a low risk of mortality from AMI (see p. 1235), the clinician should consider admission to an intermediate care facility (see below) equipped with simple ECG monitoring and resuscitation equipment. This strategy has been shown to be cost effective[723] and may reduce CCU utilization by one-third, shorten hospital stays, and have no deleterious effect on patients' recovery. Intermediate care units for low-risk AMI patients may also be appealing to patients who stand to gain little benefit from the high staffing, intense activity, and elaborate technology available in current CCUs (with their attendant high costs) and who may be disturbed by that activity and equipment.

RECOMMENDATIONS FOR ADMISSION TO THE CCU. (1) Patients with clear-cut AMI, presenting within 12 to 24 hours of symptoms, should, in most instances, be admitted to an intensive CCU. (2) Most patients with severe unstable angina should also be admitted to the CCU, particularly if episodes of chest pain occur at rest, high doses of intravenous nitroglycerin (e.g., $\geq 300\ \mu g/min$) are required to relieve chest pain, or frequent adjustments of intravenous nitroglycerin infusions are required because of fluctuating symptoms and hemodynamic status. (3) Once an AMI is ruled out (ideally by 12 hours) and symptoms are controlled with oral or topical pharmacological agents, discharge from the CCU should be considered. (4) AMI patients with an uncomplicated status, such as those without a history of previous infarction, persistent ischemic-type discomfort, congestive heart failure, hypotension, heart block, or hemodynamically compromising ventricular arrhythmias, may be safely transferred out of the CCU within 24 to 36 hours. (5) In patients with a complicated AMI, the duration of the CCU stay should be dictated by the need for "intensive" care—that is, hemodynamic monitoring, close nursing supervision, intravenous vasoactive drugs, and frequent changes in the medical regimen.

General Measures for Management of AMI

The CCU staff must be sensitive to patient concerns about mortality, prognosis, and future productivity. A calm, quiet atmosphere and the "laying on of hands" with a gentle but confident touch helps allay anxiety and reduce sympathetic tone, ultimately leading to a reduction in hypertension, tachycardia, and arrhythmias.[30] To reduce the risk of nausea and vomiting early after infarction and to reduce the risk of aspiration, during the first 4 to 12 hours after admission patients should receive either nothing by mouth or a clear liquid diet. Subsequently a diet with 50 to 55 per cent of calories from complex carbohydrates and up to 30 per cent from mono- and unsaturated fats should be given. The diet should be enriched in foods that are high in potassium, magnesium, and fiber but low in sodium (Table 37–5).

The results of laboratory tests obtained in the CCU should be scrutinized for any derangements potentially contributing to arrhythmias, such as hypoxemia, hypovolemia, disturbances of acid-based balance or of electrolytes, and drug toxicity. Oxazepam, 15 to 30 mg orally four times a day, is useful to allay the anxiety that is common in the first 24 to 48 hours.[724] Delirium may be provoked by medications frequently used in the CCU, including antiarrhythmic drugs, H_2 blockers, narcotics, and beta blockers. Potentially offending agents should be discontinued in patients with an abnormal mental status. Haloperidol, a butyrophenone, may be used safely in patients with AMI beginning with a dose of 2 mg intravenously for mildly agitated patients and 5 to 10 mg for progressively more agitated patients.[724] Hypnotics, such as temazepam, 15 to 30 mg or an equivalent, should be provided as needed for sleep. Dioctyl sodium sulfosuccinate, 200 mg daily, or another stool softener should be used to prevent constipation and straining.

"Coronary precautions" that do *not* appear to be supported by evidence from clinical research[2] include the

TABLE 37–5 GUIDELINES FOR DIET THERAPY IN THE CARDIAC CARE UNIT

1. NPO prior to evaluation by physician
2. *Kilocalories and protein:* the diet should initially be planned to provide adequate kilocalories and protein to maintain the patient's initial weight. Caloric restrictions may subsequently be initiated for weight loss if needed
3. *Fats:* the diet should be limited to $\leq$30% of total calories from fat. Foods high in cholesterol and saturated fats should be avoided. One or two eggs per week may be given if requested and/or to ensure adequate protein intake; egg substitutes should also be available and encouraged
4. *Carbohydrates:* complex carbohydrates should constitute 50–55% of total calories
5. *Fiber:* the diet should contain fiber consistent with a balanced mixed diet, including fresh fruit and vegetables, whole-grain bread, and cereals. Foods that may cause gastrointestinal intolerance should be eliminated on an individual basis.
6. *Sodium:* a "no added salt" (NAS) diet (3–4 g Na^+) is recommended, with adjustment as indicated by clinical status. The NAS diet order excludes a salt shaker as well as foods high in sodium (greater than 300 mg per serving)
7. *Potassium:* foods high in potassium should be encouraged except for patients with renal insufficiency
8. *Quantity:* small, frequent feedings may be recommended on an individual basis
9. *Fluids:* use of regular coffee should not be restricted. Decaffeinated beverages and weak tea may be offered as substitutes if desired by the patient
10. *Education:* the principal goal of patient education and long-term planning is to achieve and maintain ideal body weight and to adhere to dietary adjustments as ordered by the physician

Modified from Antman, E. M.: General hospital management. *In* Julian, D., and Braunwald, E. (eds.): Management of Acute Myocardial Infarction. London, W. B. Saunders Ltd., 1994, p. 35.

avoidance of iced fluids,[725,726] hot beverages,[727] caffeinated beverages,[728] rectal examinations,[729] back rubs,[730] and assistance with eating.[30]

PHYSICAL ACTIVITY. In the absence of complications, patients with AMI need not be confined to bed for more than 12 hours and, unless they are hemodynamically compromised, they may use a bedside commode shortly after admission.[731] Progression of activity should be individualized depending upon the patient's clinical status, age, and physical capacity; a suggested schedule for activity progression is shown in Table 37–6.

In patients without hemodynamic compromise, early ambulation—including dangling feet on the side of the bed, sitting in a chair, standing, and walking around the bed—does not cause important changes in heart rate, blood pressure, or pulmonary wedge pressure.[731] Although heart rate increases slightly (usually by less than 10 per cent), pulmonary wedge pressures fall slightly as the patient assumes the upright posture for activities. Early ambulatory activities are rarely associated with any symptoms, and when symptoms do occur, they generally are related to hypotension. Thus, when Levine and Lown proposed the "armchair" treatment of AMI in the 1950's, they were undoubtedly correct that stress to the myocardium is less in the upright position.[732] As long as blood pressure and heart rate are monitored carefully, early ambulation offers considerable psychological and physical benefit without any clear medical risk.

The Intermediate Coronary Care Unit

AMI patients are at risk for late in-hospital mortality from recurrent ischemia or infarction, hemodynamically significant ventricular arrhythmias, and severe congestive heart failure after discharge from the CCU. Therefore, continued surveillance in intermediate CCUs (also called step-down units) is justifiable. Risk factors for mortality in the hospital after discharge from the coronary care unit include significant congestive heart failure evidenced by persistent sinus tachycardia for more than 2 days and rales greater than one-third of the lung fields; recurrent ventricular tachycardia and ventricular fibrillation; atrial fibrillation or flutter while in the CCU; intraventricular conduction delays or heart block; anterior location of infarction; and recurrent episodes of angina with marked electrocardiographic ST-segment abnormalities at low activity levels.[538,733] Although it has not been shown rigorously,[734] it is likely that a reduction in late hospital mortality can be achieved with the use of intermediate CCUs, which permit prolonged continuous monitoring of the electrocardiogram and prompt, effective treatment of ventricular fibrillation and other serious arrhythmias.

The availability of intermediate care units may also be helpful in identifying those patients who remain free of complications and are suitable candidates for early discharge from the hospital. Several reports suggest that aggressive reperfusion protocols with angioplasty or thrombolytics can reduce length of hospital stay.[735,736] In patients who are believed to have undergone successful reperfusion, the *absence* of early sustained ventricular tachyarrhythmias, hypotension, or heart failure, coupled with a well-preserved left ventricular ejection fraction, predicts a low risk of late complications in-hospital. Such patients are suitable candidates for discharge from the hospital in less than 5 days from the onset of symptoms.

Following AMI, patients are often eager for information, in need of reassurance, confused by misinformation and prior impressions, capable of counterproductive denial, and

TABLE 37–6 ACTIVITY PROGRESSION FOLLOWING MYOCARDIAL INFARCTION

GENERAL GUIDELINES

When progressing through the stages noted below, specific activities should be stopped for increasing shortness of breath or the patient's perception of fatigue or detection of an increase in the heart rate of >20–30 beats/min^{-1}. Vital signs should be monitored before and following progression from one stage to the next and also from one level to the next within each stage. Energy-conserving techniques should be emphasized and the use of prophylactic nitroglycerin should be reviewed with the patient

STAGE I (DAY 1–2)

Use a bedpan/commode. Feed self-prepared tray with arm and back support. Complete assistance with bathing. Passive range of motion (ROM) to all extremities. Active ankle motion (with footboard if available). Emphasis on relaxation and deep breathing

Partially bathe upper body with back support. Bed to chair transfers for 1–2 hours per day. Active ROM to all extremities 5–10 times (sitting or supine)

STAGE II (DAY 3–4)

Bathe, groom, self-dress sitting on bed or chair. Bed to chair transfers ad lib. Ambulate in room with gradual increase in duration and frequency

May shower or stand at sink to bathe. May dress in own clothes. Supervised ambulation outside of room (100–600 feet several times per day) (33–200 meters)

Partially bathe upper body with back support. Bed to chair 20–30 min daily. Active assisted to active ROM all extremities: 5–10 times (sitting or supine)

STAGE III (DAY 5–7)

Ambulate 600 feet (200 meters) three times per day. May shampoo hair (e.g., activity with arms over head)

Supervised stair walking

Predischarge exercise tolerance test

From Antman, E. M.: General hospital management. *In* Julian, D., and Braunwald, E. (eds.): Management of Acute Myocardial Infarction. London, W. B. Saunders Ltd., 1994, p. 34.

simply frightened. Intermediate care facilities provide ideal settings and ample opportunities to begin the rehabilitation process. The capacity for the early detection of problems following AMI and the social and educational benefits of grouping such patients together strongly argue for continued utilization of intermediate CCUs. Furthermore, the economic advantage of grouping such patients together for sharing of skilled personnel and resources outweighs any questions raised by the lack of a clear consensus regarding reduced mortality. An additional potential advantage is the facilitation of patient education in a group setting with lectures and audiovisual programs.

PHARMACOLOGICAL THERAPY

The rationale and recommendations for initiation of several pharmacological measures to treat AMI in the emergency department have been reviewed previously (see p. 1210) (Fig. 37–18). The early use of beta blockers, ACE inhibitors, calcium antagonists, and magnesium and nitrates is discussed in this section. Secondary prevention with some of these agents is discussed subsequently (see p. 1263).

Beta Blockers

(See also p. 1978)

The effects of beta blockers on AMI can be divided into those that are immediate (when the drug is given very early in the course of infarction) and long-term (secondary prevention), when the drug is initiated sometime after infarction (see p. 1211).[736a] The immediate intravenous administration of beta-adrenoceptor blockers reduces cardiac index, heart rate, and blood pressure.[414] The net effect is a reduction in myocardial oxygen consumption per minute and per beat. Favorable effects of acute intravenous administration of beta-adrenoceptor blockers on the balance of myocardial oxygen supply and demand are reflected in reductions in chest pain,[737] in the proportion of patients with threatened infarction who actually evolve AMI,[738] and in the development of ventricular arrhythmias.[739,740] Because beta-adrenoceptor blockade diminishes circulating levels of free fatty acids by antagonizing the lipolytic effects of catecholamines and because elevated levels of fatty acids augment myocardial oxygen consumption and probably increase the incidence of arrhythmias, these metabolic actions of beta-blocking agents may also be beneficial to the ischemic heart.[739]

Objective evidence of beneficial effects of beta blockers in acute myocardial ischemia has been reported using the precordial ST-segment mapping technique.[741] Acute beta blockade probably reduces infarct size in AMI. Reduction in release of cardiac enzymes with beta blockade[742] is suggestive of a smaller infarct, as is the preservation of R waves and reduction in the development of Q waves.[743]

RESULTS OF MULTICENTER TRIALS. At least 27 randomized beta blocker trials involving more than 27,000 patients have been undertaken.[32,744] Several trials have been performed to test the effects of early beta blockade in myocardial infarction. The largest of these, ISIS-1, involving more than 16,000 patients, reported a significant reduction in mortality among the patients randomized to intravenous atenolol compared with placebo-treated patients.[745] The findings of a meta-analysis of data from the 27 early beta blocker trials (in the prethrombolytic era) are summarized in Figure 37–31. Intravenous followed by oral beta blocker therapy is associated with about a 15 per cent relative reduction in mortality, nonfatal reinfarction, and nonfatal cardiac arrest.[746] Although antagonism of sympathetic stimulation to the heart might be expected to exacerbate pulmonary edema in patients with occult heart failure, usually only small changes in pulmonary capillary wedge pressure occur when the drug is used in patients with AMI.[739] Thus, in appropriately selected patients the benefits noted above occur at a cost of about a 3 per cent incidence of provocation of congestive heart failure or complete heart block and a 2 per cent incidence of the development of cardiogenic shock[746] (Fig. 37–31).

Because reduction of infarct size in AMI patients treated with beta blockers is likely to occur only with early treatment (≤4 hours from the onset of pain), investigators have sought other explanations for the reduction in the mortality in the acute phase which has been observed.[745] Intriguing observations from the ISIS-1 trial raise the possibility that a reduction in the development of cardiac rupture or electromechanical dissociation during the first day is achieved with early beta blockade.[747]

In the TIMI-II trial the addition of a beta blocker (metoprolol) to thrombolytic therapy was studied.[641] Although recurrent ischemia and reinfarction were reduced by immediate intravenous versus delayed use of metoprolol, mortality was not reduced nor was ventricular function improved. Thus, immediate intravenous beta blockade, although clinically beneficial, may not enhance salvage of myocardium in the setting of early reperfusion but may confer clinical benefit by means of its antiischemic effect.[475]

RECOMMENDATIONS. Given the overall favorable effects of beta blockade in the aforementioned clinical trials, patients in a hyperdynamic state (sinus tachycardia, hypertension, no evidence of heart failure or bronchospasm) as well as patients seen in the first 4 hours appear to be good candidates for this therapy, regardless of whether or not thrombolytic therapy is employed. Unless there are contraindications (see p. 1978), beta blockade probably should be continued in patients who develop AMI. In addition, beta blockers are indicated in patients in whom infarction is complicated by persistent or recurrent ischemic pain, progressive or repetitive serum enzyme elevations suggestive of infarct extension, or tachyarrhythmias early after the onset of infarction. If adverse effects of beta blockers develop or if patients present with complications of infarction that are contraindications to beta blockade such as heart failure or heart block, the beta blocker should be withheld.

SELECTION OF BETA BLOCKER. Favorable effects have been reported with atenolol, timolol, and alprenolol; these benefits probably occur with propranolol and with esmolol, an

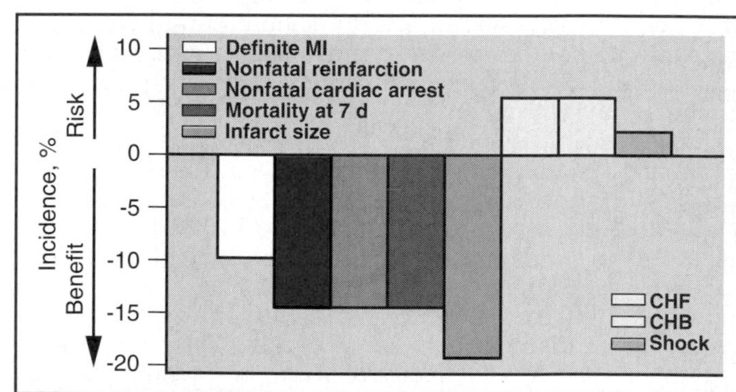

FIGURE 37–31. Results of intravenous beta blockade in acute MI: Acute phase of treatment. The benefits of beta blockers given intravenously followed by oral administration for 1 week in patients with suspected AMI include reductions in the rate of development of definite MI, in the incidence of nonfatal reinfarction and cardiac arrest, mortality at 7 days, and infarct size. In appropriately selected patients — i.e., those with a heart rate 60 beats/min or higher, systolic blood pressure 100 mm Hg or more, P-R interval less than 0.24 sec, rales in less than one-third of the lung field, and no history of bronchospastic lung disease—the risks for congestive heart failure (CHF), complete heart block (CHB), and cardiogenic shock are acceptably low. (Adapted from data in Yusuf, S.: The use of beta-blockers in the acute phase of myocardial infarction. *In* Califf, R. M., and Wagner, C. S. [eds.]: Acute Coronary Care 1986. Boston, Martinus Nijhoff, 1985, pp. 73–88.)

ultrashort-acting agent, as well. In the absence of any favorable evidence supporting the benefit of agents with intrinsic sympathomimetic activity (ISA), such as pindolol and oxprenolol, and with some unfavorable evidence for these agents in secondary prevention,[748] beta blockers with ISA probably should not be chosen for treatment of AMI. Occasionally the clinician may wish to proceed with beta blocker therapy even in the presence of relative contraindications, such as a history of mild asthma, mild bradycardia, mild heart failure, or first-degree heart block. In this situation, a trial of esmolol may help determine whether the patient can tolerate beta blockade.[416,748] Because the hemodynamic effects of this drug, with a half-life of 9 minutes, disappear in less than 30 minutes, it offers considerable advantage over longer-acting agents when the risk of a beta blocker complication is relatively high.

ACE Inhibitors

In 1992, with the publication of the SAVE trial,[749] ACE inhibitors were established as an important addition to the list of treatments for AMI. The rationale for their use includes experimental and clinical evidence of a favorable impact on ventricular remodeling, improvement in hemodynamics, and reductions in congestive heart failure.[84,171,425,750] There is now unequivocal evidence from eight randomized, placebo-controlled mortality trials collectively enrolling over 100,000 patients, that ACE inhibitors reduce death from AMI.[751] These eight trials may be grouped into two categories. The first *selected* AMI patients for randomization, based on features indicative of increased mortality such as left ventricular ejection fraction less than 40 per cent,[749] clinical signs and symptoms of congestive heart failure,[752] anterior location of infarction,[753] and abnormal wall motion score index[754] (Fig. 37–32). The second group were *unselective* trials that randomized all patients with AMI provided they had a minimum systolic pressure of approximately 100 mm Hg (ISIS-4 and GISSI-3 as shown in Figure 37–33; CONSENSUS II[755] and Chinese Captopril Study[756]). With the exception of the SMILE trial,[753] all of the selective trials initiated ACE inhibitor therapy between 3 and 16 days after AMI and maintained it for 1 to 4 years, whereas the unselective trials all initiated treatment within the first 24 to 36 hours and maintained it for only 4 to 6 weeks.

A consistent survival benefit was observed in all of the trials already noted, except for CONSENSUS II, the one study that utilized an intravenous preparation early in the course of AMI.[755] Estimates of the mortality benefit of ACE inhibitors in the unselective, short duration of therapy trials was 5 per 1000 patients treated. Recent analysis of these unselective short-term trials indicates that approximately one-third of the lives saved occurred within the first 1 to 2 days.[751] Not unexpectedly, greater survival benefits of 42 to 76 lives saved per 1000 patients treated were obtained in the selective, long duration of therapy trials. Of note, there was generally a 20 per cent reduction in the risk of death attributable to ACE inhibitor treatment in the selective trials. The mortality reduction with ACE inhibitors is accompanied by significant reductions in the development of congestive heart failure, supporting the underlying pathophysiological rationale for administering this class of drugs in AMI.[749,752,754,757] In addition, some data suggest that ischemic events, including recurrent infarction and the need for coronary revascularization, can also be reduced by chronic administration of ACE inhibitors after an AMI.[758]

The mortality benefits of ACE inhibitors are additive to those achieved with aspirin and beta blockers.[749,757] Thus, ACE inhibitors should not be considered a substitute for these other therapies with proven benefit in AMI patients. The benefits of ACE inhibition appear to be a class effect because mortality and morbidity have been reduced by several agents. However, to replicate these benefits in clinical practice, physicians should select a specific agent and prescribe the drug according to the protocols utilized in the successful clinical trials reported to date.

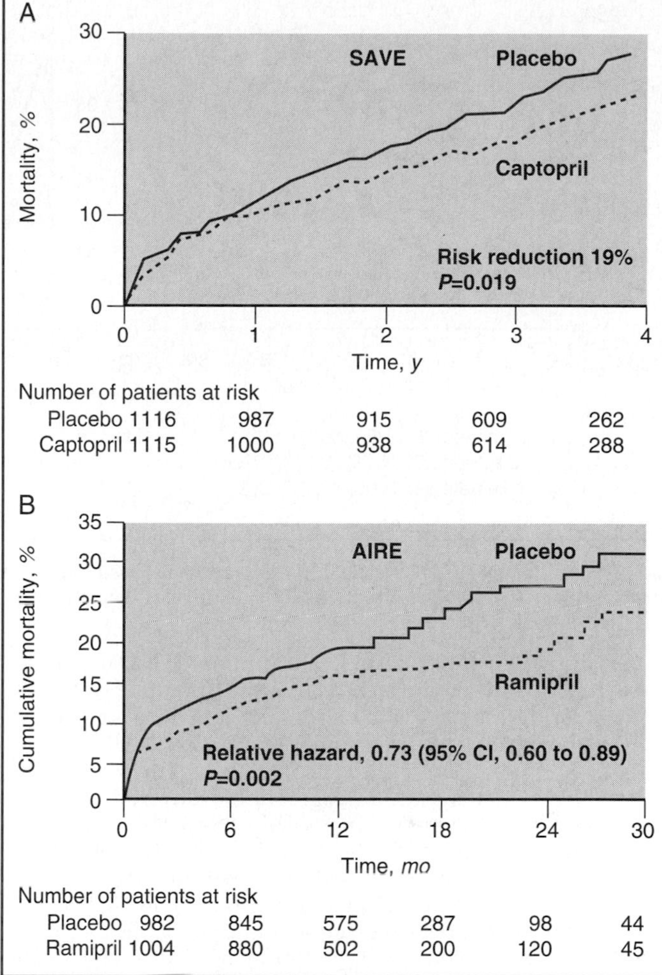

FIGURE 37–32. Benefits of long-term administration of angiotensin-converting enzyme (ACE) inhibitors to patients with AMI who have clinical evidence of left ventricular dysfunction. Among patients given active therapy (either captopril or ramipril) in the SAVE (Survival and Ventricular Enlargement) Trial (*A*) and the AIRE (Acute Infarction Ramipril Efficacy) Study (*B*), long-term mortality was reduced approximately 25 per cent. Additional benefits of ACE inhibitor therapy included reductions in recurrent hospitalizations for congestive heart failure and recurrent MI (not shown). (*A* adapted from Pfeffer, M. A., Braunwald, E., Moye, L. A., et al., on behalf of the SAVE Investigators: Effect of captopril on mortality and morbidity in patients with left ventricular dysfunction after myocardial infarction: Results of the Survival and Ventricular Enlargement Trial. N. Engl. J. Med. *327*:669, 1992; *B* adapted from The Acute Ramipril Efficacy [AIRE] Study Investigators: Effect of ramipril on mortality and morbidity of survivors of acute myocardial infarction with clinical evidence of heart failure. Lancet *342*:821, 1993. © by The Lancet Ltd.)

The major *contraindications* to the use of ACE inhibitors in AMI include hypotension in the setting of adequate preload, known hypersensitivity, and pregnancy. Adverse reactions include hypotension, especially after the first dose, and intolerable cough with chronic dosing; much less commonly angioedema can occur (see p. 474).

RECOMMENDATIONS FOR USE OF ACE INHIBITORS. After administration of aspirin, initiating reperfusion strategies and where appropriate beta blockade (see p. 1228), *all* AMI patients should be considered for ACE inhibition therapy. Although there is little disagreement that high-risk AMI patients (elderly, anterior infarction, prior infarction, Killip class II or greater, and asymptomatic patients with evidence of depressed global ventricular function on an imaging study) should receive life-long treatment with ACE inhibitors,[425,759] short term (4 to 6 weeks) therapy to a broader

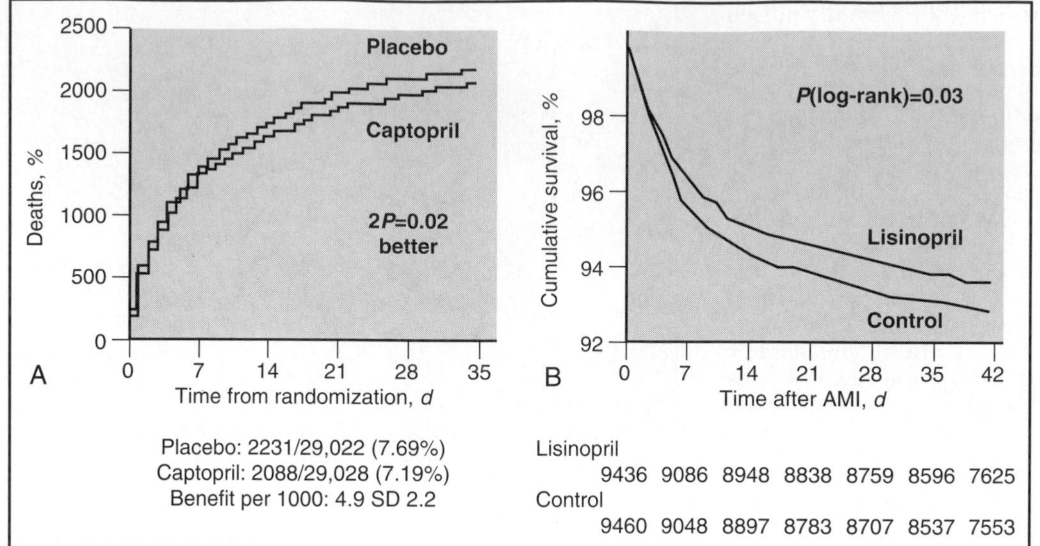

FIGURE 37–33. Results of treatment with angiotensin-converting enzyme (ACE) inhibitors after MI. Two trials of acute therapy in unselected patients (i.e., both with and without evidence of left ventricular dysfunction) have shown that ACE inhibitors reduce mortality at 4 to 6 weeks. This effect was seen in two different patient populations and with two different ACE inhibitors, captopril (*A*) and lisinopril (*B*), attesting to the consistency and general applicability of the observations. (Adapted from ISIS-4 [Fourth International Study of Infarct Survival] Collaborative Group: A randomized factorial trial assessing early oral captopril, oral mononitrate, and intravenous magnesium sulphate in 5850 patients with suspected acute myocardial infarction. Lancet *345*:669, 1995; and Gruppo Italiano per lo Studio della Sopravvivenza nell'Infarto Miocardico: GISSI-3: Effects of lisinopril and transdermal glyceryl trinitrate singly and together on 6-week mortality and ventricular function after acute myocardial infarction. Lancet *343*:1115, 1994. © by The Lancet Ltd.)

group of patients has also been proposed based on the pooled results of the unselective mortality trials.[18,760,761]

Considering all the available data, we favor a strategy of an initial trial of oral ACE inhibitors in all AMI patients with congestive heart failure as well as in hemodynamically stable patients with ST-segment elevation or left bundle branch block, commencing within the first 24 hours. In the absence of congestive heart failure, we do *not* recommend their use in AMI patients without ST-segment changes or only ST segment depression on ECG. Prior to hospital discharge, left ventricular function should be evaluated. ACE inhibition therapy should be continued indefinitely in patients with congestive heart failure, evidence of a reduction in global function, or a large regional wall motion abnormality. In patients without these findings at discharge, ACE inhibitors may be discontinued.

Nitrates

(See also p. 1211)

Sublingual nitroglycerin very rarely opens occluded coronary arteries. However, in patients with AMI the potential for reductions in ventricular filling pressures, wall tension, and cardiac work coupled with improvement in coronary blood flow, especially in ischemic zones,[762] and antiplatelet effects[763] make nitrates a logical and attractive pharmacological intervention in AMI.[764–766]

In patients with AMI, the administration of nitroglycerin and other nitrates such as isosorbide dinitrate reduces pulmonary capillary wedge pressure and systemic arterial pressure, left ventricular chamber volume, infarct size,[767,768] and the incidence of mechanical complications.[768] As with other interventions to spare ischemic myocardium in AMI, intravenous nitroglycerin appears to be of greatest benefit in patients treated earliest.[768]

CLINICAL TRIAL RESULTS. In the prethrombolytic era, 10 randomized trials of acute administration of intravenous nitroglycerin (or nitroprusside, another nitric oxide donor) collectively enrolled 2042 patients. A meta-analysis of these trial results showed a reduction in mortality of 35 per cent associated with nitrate therapy.[769]

In the thrombolytic era two megatrials of nitrate therapy have been conducted—GISSI-3[757] and ISIS-4.[761] In GISSI-3, there was no independent effect of nitrates on short-term mortality.[757] Similarly, in ISIS-4, no effect of a mononitrate on 35-day mortality was observed. A pooled analysis of over 80,000 patients treated with nitrate-like preparations intravenously or orally in 22 trials revealed a mortality rate of 7.7 per cent in the control group, which was reduced to 7.4 per cent in the nitrate group. These data are consistent with a small treatment effect of nitrates on mortality such that 3 to 4 fewer deaths would occur for every 1000 patients treated.[761]

NITRATE PREPARATIONS AND MODE OF ADMINISTRATION. Intravenous nitroglycerin can be administered safely to patients with evolving MI as long as the dose is titrated carefully to avoid induction of reflex tachycardia or systemic arterial hypotension.[770] Patients with inferior wall infarction are particularly sensitive to an excessive fall in preload, particularly if concurrent right ventricular infarction is present.[771] In such cases nitrate-induced venodilatation could impair cardiac output and reduce coronary block flow, thus worsening myocardial oxygenation rather than improving it.[772]

A useful regimen employs an initial infusion rate of 5 to 10 μg/min with increases of 5 to 20 μg/min until the mean arterial blood pressure is reduced by 10 per cent of its baseline level in normotensive patients and by 30 per cent for hypertensive patients, but in no case below a systolic pressure of 90 mm Hg.[764,768] Alternatively, nitroglycerin may be administered as a sustained-release oral preparation (30 to 60 mg/day) or as an ointment (1 to 3 inches every 6 to 8 hours for patients with a systolic pressure greater than 120 mm Hg). Nitroglycerin can also be given sublingually at doses of 0.3 to 0.6 mg. This route may be more hazardous because the rate of absorption is difficult to control and arterial pressure may decline precipitously.

ADVERSE EFFECTS. Clinically significant methemoglobinemia has been reported to occur during administration of intravenous nitroglycerin.[773] Although uncommon, this problem is seen when unusually large doses of nitrates are administered. It is important not only for its potential to cause symptoms of lethargy and headache but also because elevated methemoglobin levels can impair the oxygen-carrying capacity of blood, potentially exacerbating ischemia. Dilatation of the pulmonary vasculature supplying poorly ventilated lung segments may produce a ventilation-perfusion mismatch.

Tolerance to intravenous nitroglycerin (as manifested by increasing nitrate requirements) develops in many patients, often as soon as 12 hours after the infusion is started.[774] Despite the theoretical and demonstrated benefit of sulfhydryl agents in diminishing tolerance, their use has not become widespread.[775]

RECOMMENDATIONS FOR NITRATES IN AMI. Nitroglycerin is indicated for the relief of persistent pain and as a vasodilator in patients with infarction associated with left ventricular failure. In the absence of recurrent angina or congestive heart failure, we do not routinely prescribe them in AMI patients. Higher-risk patients such as those with large transmural infarctions, especially of the anterior wall, have the most to gain from nitrates in terms of reduction of ventricular remodeling, and we therefore routinely use intravenous nitrates for 24 to 48 hours in such patients. There is no clear benefit to empirical long-term cutaneous or oral nitrates in the asymptomatic patient, and we therefore do not prescribe nitrates beyond the first 48 hours unless angina or ventricular failure is present.

Calcium Antagonists

(See also p. 1978)

Despite sound experimental and clinical evidence of an antiischemic effect,[776] calcium antagonists have *not* been found to be helpful in the acute phase of AMI, and concern has been raised in several systematic overviews about an increased risk of mortality when they are prescribed on a routine basis to AMI patients.[414,417,418] Perhaps in response to the lack of compelling data showing a beneficial effect and concerns about the risk of excess mortality coupled with more convincing evidence of benefit from aspirin and beta blockers, many clinicians have decreased their use of calcium antagonists in the setting of AMI.[12,40,41,45] A distinction should be made between the dihydropyridine type of calcium antagonists (e.g., nifedipine) and the nondihydropyridine calcium antagonists (e.g., verapamil and diltiazem).[417,777,777a]

NIFEDIPINE. In multiple trials involving a total of over 5000 patients, the immediate-release preparation of nifedipine has not shown any reduction in infarct size,[778–781] prevention of progression to infarction,[778,780] control of recurrent ischemia,[780] or lowering of mortality.[782] When trials of the immediate-release form of nifedipine are pooled in a meta-analysis, evidence suggests a dose-related increased risk of in-hospital mortality (especially above 80 mg of nifedipine),[418,783] although posthospital mortality does not appear to be increased in nifedipine-treated patients.[784,785] Nifedipine does not appear to be helpful in conjunction with either thrombolytic therapy[786] or beta blockade.[779,787] A potential mechanism by which the immediate release form of nifedipine may be harmful in AMI is coronary hypoperfusion due to an abrupt fall in systolic pressure from peripheral vasodilatation. The abrupt fall in arterial pressure may also provoke a reflex action of the renin-angiotensin system and sympathetic discharge that produces tachycardia.[776] Thus, we do not recommend use of immediate-release nifedipine early in the treatment of AMI. No trials of the sustained-release preparations of nifedipine in AMI have been reported to date.

VERAPAMIL AND DILTIAZEM. When administered during the acute phase of AMI, these drugs have not had any demonstrated favorable effect on infarct size or other important endpoints in patients with AMI, with the exception of control of supraventricular arrhythmias.[782,788] Although the possibility has been raised that verapamil and diltiazem in the first few days following AMI may be helpful in preventing reinfarction in patients with non-Q-wave infarction,[788–791] the data supporting this contention are not statistically robust and require further evaluation in future studies. Subgroup analyses of MDPIT and DAVIT-II trials with both diltiazem and verapamil have suggested that mortality is reduced in patients free of heart failure in the CCU.[792,793] These subgroup analyses must be interpreted with caution because in the MDPIT study about 50 per cent of patients in the placebo and diltiazem groups were also receiving beta blockers that may have contributed to the observed mortality reduction[792]; and in the DAVIT-II study patients with an indication for beta blockers were excluded from the trial.[793] Furthermore, both the MDPIT and DAVIT-II studies were conducted in an era when aspirin, ACE inhibitors, and early use of coronary angiography for recurrent ischemia were not as common as they are now. Thus, based on the available data, we do *not* recommend the routine use of either verapamil or diltiazem in AMI regardless of whether it is believed that the patient is suffering from a Q-wave or non-Q-wave infarction. Their use should be avoided in patients with Killip class II or greater hemodynamic findings.

Magnesium

Patients with AMI may have a total body deficit of magnesium because of a low dietary intake, advanced age, or prior diuretic use. They may also acquire a functional deficit of available magnesium due to trapping of free magnesium in adipocytes, as soaps are formed when free fatty acids are released by catecholamine-induced lipolysis with the onset of infarction.[794–796] Myocardial and urinary losses of magnesium that occur during AMI may increase a patient's magnesium requirement. The magnesium cation serves as a critical cofactor in over 300 intracellular enzymatic processes, including several that are integrally involved in mitochondrial function, energy production, maintenance of trans-sarcolemmal ionic gradients, cell volume control, and resting membrane potential.[794,797,798] Experimental models of AMI in at least four different animal species have shown that supplemental administration of magnesium before coronary occlusion, during occlusion, coincident with reperfusion, or for a short time interval (15 to 45 minutes) after reperfusion reduces infarct size and prevents myocardial stunning due to reperfusion injury.[459] However, delayed administration of magnesium beyond a very short interval (15 to 60 minutes) following reperfusion is no longer effective in reducing myocardial damage.[459]

Since 1984, several trials of routine supplemental administration of intravenous magnesium in patients with suspected AMI have been conducted. By 1992 about 1300 patients had been randomized, and meta-analyses of the seven trials conducted to that point suggested that patients who received magnesium had a 45 per cent lower risk of mortality.[7,799] In 1992, the LIMIT-2 trial reported a 24 per cent reduction in mortality at 28 days in patients treated with magnesium compared with placebo (Fig. 37–34). This mortality reduction appeared to be mediated through a re-

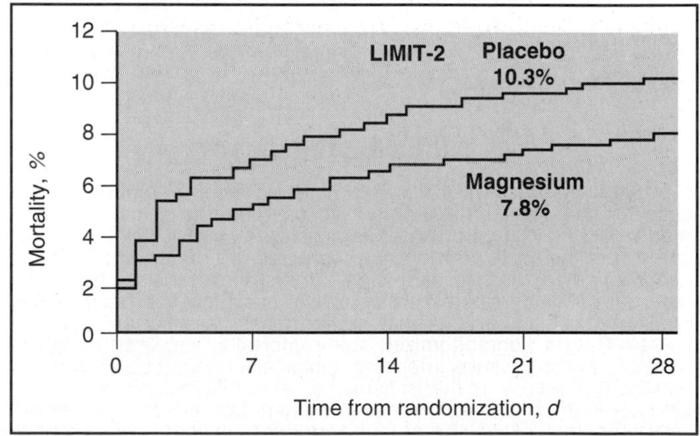

FIGURE 37–34. Results of intravenous (IV) magnesium therapy in acute MI. Two trials of magnesium conducted in the thrombolytic era. In LIMIT-2 (Second Leicester Intravenous Magnesium Intervention Trial), magnesium was administered relatively early and concurrently with thrombolytic agents in the 36 per cent of patients who received thrombolytic therapy. A 24 per cent reduction in mortality was seen at 28 days in patients treated with magnesium. (Adapted from Woods, K. L., Fletcher, S., Roffe, C., et al.: Intravenous magnesium sulphate in suspected acute myocardial infarction: results of the Second Leicester Intravenous Magnesium Intervention Trial [LIMIT 2]. Lancet *339*:1553, 1992. © by The Lancet Ltd.)

duction in congestive heart failure. Long-term follow-up of LIMIT-2 revealed a 20 per cent reduction in ischemic heart disease–related mortality over an average of 4.5 years.[800,801]

Unexpectedly, the ISIS-4 trial reported no effect of magnesium on 35-day mortality.[761] However, concern about interpretation has been raised over the low overall mortality of the control group in ISIS-4 (due to widespread use of aspirin and administration of thrombolytics to 75 per cent of patients) and the late administration of magnesium after pharmacological reperfusion and markedly delayed treatment (median of 12 hours) in patients who did not receive thrombolytic therapy.[459,800–802] Thus, despite the 58,050 patients randomized in ISIS-4, it is not clear that serum magnesium levels were elevated at the time of reperfusion in the cohort of patients randomized to magnesium or in any subgroup of them. Because of the trivial cost of magnesium, its ease of administration, its widespread availability, and the fact that it has the potential to reduce mortality in high-risk AMI patients (e.g., elderly patients who are not candidates for thrombolysis), another large-scale, randomized, multicenter trial (MAGIC)[459] is planned to define more explicitly the role of magnesium in AMI.

RECOMMENDATIONS. Because of the risk of cardiac arrhythmias when electrolyte deficits are present in the early phase of infarction, all patients with AMI should have a serum magnesium measurement on admission. We advocate repleting magnesium deficits to maintain a serum magnesium level of 2.0 mEq/liter or more. In the presence of hypokalemia (<4.0 mEq/liter) during the course of treatment of AMI, the serum magnesium should be rechecked and repleted if necessary because it is often difficult to correct a potassium deficit in the presence of a concurrent magnesium deficit. Episodes of torsades de pointes (see p. 684) should be treated with 1 to 2 gm of magnesium delivered as a bolus over about 5 minutes. Although routine early (ideally <6 hours from the onset of chest pain) supplemental magnesium administration may be helpful in certain high-risk patients such as the elderly or those for whom reperfusion therapy is contraindicated,[803] additional data are needed before definite recommendations regarding patient selection and dosing can be made. There does not appear to be any benefit to routine late (>6 hours) administration of magnesium to patients with uncomplicated AMI who do not have electrolyte deficits.

Because it may cause vasodilation and hypotension, magnesium infusions should not be administered in patients with a systolic pressure less than 80 to 90 mm Hg. Patients with renal failure may not excrete magnesium normally and should not be considered candidates for supplemental magnesium infusions.

Other Approaches

GLUCOSE-INSULIN-POTASSIUM. Administration of a solution of glucose-insulin-potassium (300 gm of glucose, 50 units of insulin, and 80 mEq of KCl in 1000 ml of water administered at a rate of 1.5 ml/kg/hr) lowers the concentration of plasma free fatty acids and improves ventricular performance, as reflected in systolic arterial pressure, cardiac output, and stroke work at any level of left ventricular filling pressure[804]; also the frequency of ventricular premature beats decreases.[805] In a nonrandomized study, mortality appeared to be reduced,[806] hemodynamics improved, global ejection fraction increased, and both asynergy in the ischemic zone and pulmonary artery diastolic pressure reduced.[805] However, no definitive effect on enzymatically estimated infarct size or long-term mortality has been described in a prospective, controlled, randomized trial.[805]

The DIGAMI (Diabetes Mellitus Insulin-Glucose Infusion in Acute Myocardial Infarction) Study reported a significant 30 per cent relative

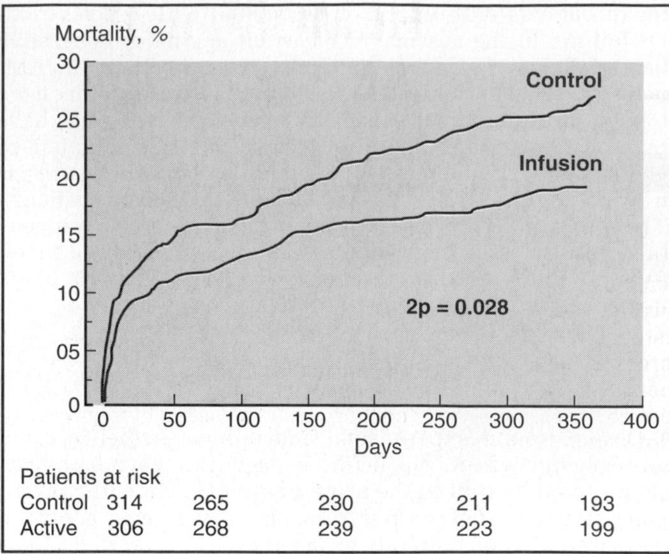

FIGURE 37–35. Actuarial mortality curves in patients receiving insulin-glucose infusion and in controls of the Diabetes Mellitus Insulin-Glucose Infusion in Acute Myocardial Infarction (DIGAMI) study during 1 year of follow-up. Numbers below graph indicate the number of patients at different times of observation. Active = patients receiving infusion. (From Malmberg, K., Ryden, L., Efendic, S., et al.: Randomized trial of insulin-glucose infusion followed by subcutaneous insulin treatment in diabetic patients with acute myocardial infarction (DIGAMI Study): Effects on mortality at 1 year. Reprinted with permission from the American College of Cardiology. J. Am. Coll. Cardiol. *26*:57, 1995.)

decrease in mortality at 1 year in diabetics with AMI who received a strict regimen of an insulin-glucose infusion for 24 hours, followed by 3 months of subcutaneous injections of insulin four times daily as compared with standard therapy[807] (Fig. 37–35). Thus, "infusions of glucose-insulin-potassium (GIK) may provide necessary metabolic support for the ischemic myocardium; this may be particularly important in patients with large anterior infarcts and cardiogenic shock."[192,193]

INTRAAORTIC BALLOON COUNTERPULSATION (see also p. 1239). From a theoretical standpoint, intraaortic balloon counterpulsation might be expected to limit infarct size for several reasons. In experimental animals, intraaortic balloon counterpulsation decreases preload, increases coronary blood flow, and improves cardiac performance. No definitive information is available indicating that intraaortic balloon counterpulsation alters the prognosis in patients with relatively uncomplicated infarction. Leinbach et al., however, have reported an immediate, persistent fall in ST-segment elevation. This occurred in patients with anterior MI who had preservation of precordial R waves and good ventricular function,[808] in whom the left anterior descending coronary artery was not totally occluded and who underwent intraaortic balloon pumping within 6 hours.

Given the relatively frequent rate of complications[809] after intraaortic balloon insertion and the absence of convincing data for infarct size reduction, intraaortic balloon pumping should be reserved for hemodynamically compromised patients and for those with refractory ischemia. Although noninvasive external forms of counterpulsation have been developed, these approaches have not been rigorously studied in patients with AMI.

OTHER AGENTS. Oxygen-derived free radicals are abundant in ischemic tissue and may contribute to myocardial injury, particularly following reperfusion (see p. 1214). Although evidence from studies in animals suggested that the extent of myocardial necrosis and postischemic dysfunction can be affected favorably by treatment with oxygen free radical scavengers such as superoxide dismutase,[435,467] initial results in patients have not been encouraging.[468] Alternative forms of antioxidant therapy including vitamins E and C are being studied in experimental animals, but there is uncertainty about their potential role in patients.[810–812] Given the important role that nitric oxide (NO) plays in regulating platelet activation, interest has arisen in developing techniques for increasing NO production or providing exogenous NO donors in the setting of AMI other than the nitrates discussed above.[527,813]

HEMODYNAMIC DISTURBANCES IN ACUTE MYOCARDIAL INFARCTION

HEMODYNAMIC ASSESSMENT

In patients with clinically uncomplicated AMI, invasive hemodynamic monitoring is not necessary because the status of the circulation can be assessed by careful clinical evaluation. This ordinarily consists of monitoring of heart rate and rhythm, repeated measurement of systemic arterial pressure by cuff, obtaining chest roentgenograms to detect heart failure, careful and repeated auscultation of the lung fields for pulmonary congestion, measurement of urine flow, examination of the skin and mucous membranes for evidence of the adequacy of perfusion, and arterial sampling for pO_2, PCO_2, and pH when hypoxemia or metabolic acidosis is suspected.

In contrast, in patients with AMI whose ventricular contractile performance is not normal, it is important to assess the degree of hemodynamic compromise in order to initiate therapy with drugs such as vasodilators and diuretics. In the past, central venous or right atrial pressure was used to gauge the degree of left ventricular failure in patients with AMI. However, this technique is fraught with error because central venous pressure actually reflects right rather than left ventricular function. Right ventricular function and therefore systemic venous pressure may be normal or nearly so in patients with significant left ventricular failure.[814] Conversely, patients with right ventricular failure due to right ventricular infarction or pulmonary embolism may exhibit elevated right atrial and central venous pressures despite normal left ventricular function.[813] Low values for right atrial and central venous pressures imply hypovolemia, whereas elevated right atrial pressures usually result from right ventricular failure secondary to left ventricular failure, pulmonary hypertension, or right ventricular infarction, or less commonly from tricuspid regurgitation or pericardial tamponade.

Major advances in the management of AMI have resulted from the hemodynamic monitoring that has become widespread in CCUs[816–818a] (Table 37–7). This often consists of both an intraarterial catheter and a pulmonary artery catheter for measurement of pulmonary artery, pulmonary artery occlusive (equivalent to pulmonary wedge), and right atrial pressures, and cardiac output by thermodilution. In patients with hypotension, a Foley catheter provides accurate and continuous measurement of urine output.

TABLE 37–7 INDICATIONS FOR HEMODYNAMIC MONITORING OF ACUTE MYOCARDIAL INFARCTION

Management of complicated AMI
Hypovolemia vs. cardiogenic shock
Ventricular septal rupture vs. acute mitral regurgitation
Severe left ventricular failure
Right ventricular failure
Refractory ventricular tachycardia
Differentiating severe pulmonary disease from left ventricular failure
Assessment of cardiac tamponade
Assessment of therapy in *selected* individuals
Afterload reduction in patients with severe left ventricular failure
Inotropic agent therapy
Beta blocker therapy
Temporary pacing (ventricular vs. atrioventricular)
Intraaortic balloon counterpulsation
Mechanical ventilation

From Gore, J. M., and Zwernet, P. L.: Hemodynamic monitoring of acute myocardial infarction. *In* Francis, G. S., and Alpert, J. S. (eds.): Modern Coronary Care. Boston, Little, Brown & Co., 1990, p. 138.

NEED FOR INVASIVE MONITORING. The use of invasive hemodynamic monitoring[814] is based on the following principal factors:

1. Difficulty of interpreting clinical and radiographic findings of pulmonary congestion because of phase lags, such as those occurring after diuretic therapy. Severe depression of cardiac index and/or elevation of left ventricular filling pressure may be unsuspected in as many as 15 per cent of patients when estimates are based exclusively on clinical criteria.[814]
2. Need for identifying noncardiac causes of arterial hypotension, particularly hypovolemia.
3. Possible contribution of reduced ventricular compliance to impaired hemodynamics, requiring judicious adjustment of intravascular volume to optimize left ventricular filling pressure.
4. Difficulty in assessing the severity and somctimes even determining the presence of lesions such as mitral regurgitation and ventricular septal defect when the cardiac output or the systemic pressures are depressed.
5. Establishing a baseline of hemodynamic measurements and guiding therapy in patients with clinically apparent pulmonary edema or cardiogenic shock.
6. Underestimation of systemic arterial pressure by the cuff method in patients with intense vasoconstriction.

The prognosis and the clinical status are related to both the cardiac output and the pulmonary artery wedge pressure. Patients with normal cardiac output after AMI have an extremely low expected mortality; prognosis worsens as cardiac output declines. Patients with intraventricular conduction defects, atrioventricular (AV) block, or both after anterior infarction have lower cardiac indices and higher pulmonary capillary wedge pressures than do patients without these conduction disturbances. On the other hand, patients with these conduction defects and inferior MI usually do not demonstrate such hemodynamic abnormalities.

PULMONARY ARTERY PRESSURE MONITORING. Patients most likely to benefit from pulmonary artery catheter monitoring include those whose AMI is complicated by (1) hypotension that is not easily corrected by fluid administration; (2) hypotension in the presence of congestive heart failure; (3) hemodynamic compromise severe enough to require intravenous vasopressors or vasodilators or intraaortic balloon counterpulsation; (4) mechanical lesions (or suspected ones) such as cardiac tamponade, severe mitral regurgitation, and a ruptured ventricular septum[819]; and (5) right ventricular infarction.[105] Other indications for hemodynamic monitoring include assessment of the effects of mechanical ventilation, differentiating pulmonary disease from left ventricular failure as the cause of hypoxemia, and management of septic shock[30] (Table 37–7).

Before inserting a pulmonary artery catheter into a patient with an AMI, the physician must decide that the potential benefit of the information to be obtained outweighs any potential risks. Major complications from pulmonary artery catheters are relatively rare (about 3 to 5 per cent of cases),[818] but severe problems can occur, including sepsis, pulmonary infarction, and pulmonary artery rupture. By minimizing the duration of catheterization and by strict adherence to aseptic techniques, risk can be diminished.[819]

Accurate determination of hemodynamics by clinical assessment is difficult in critically ill patients. The use of a pulmonary artery catheter often leads to important changes in therapy which would not have occurred if the hemodynamic information had not been available.[820] Some believe, however, that the pulmonary artery catheter is often overused. It has been suggested that until clinical trials assess-

TABLE 37–8 HEMODYNAMIC CLASSIFICATIONS OF PATIENTS WITH ACUTE MYOCARDIAL INFARCTION

A. BASED ON CLINICAL EXAMINATION[a]		B. BASED ON INVASIVE MONITORING[b]	
Class	Definition	Subset	Definition
I	Rales and S3 absent	I	Normal hemodynamics PCWP <18, CI >2.2
II	Rales over <50% of lung	II	Pulmonary congestion PCWP >18, CI <2.2
III	Rales over >50% of lung fields (pulmonary edema)	III	Peripheral hypoperfusion PCWP <18, CI >2.2
IV	Shock	IV	Pulmonary congestion and peripheral hypoperfusion PCWP >18, CI <2.2

Modified from (a) Killip, T. and Kimball, J.: Treatment of myocardial infarction in a coronary care unit. A two year experience with 250 patients. Am. J. Cardiol. *20:*457, 1967; and (b) Forrester, J., Diamond, G., Chatterjee, K., et al.: Medical therapy of acute myocardial infarction by the application of hemodynamic subsets. N. Engl. J. Med. *295:*1356, 1976.

PCWP = pulmonary capillary wedge pressure; CI = cardiac index.

ing its benefit are performed, the use of this technique should be curbed.[821,822] (At least one such trial has suggested that complications and mortality are actually higher in patients who received pulmonary artery catheterization,[823] although such patients might have been at higher risk initially.) These observations emphasize the importance of patient selection, meticulous technique, and correct interpretation of the data obtained.

Hemodynamic Abnormalities

In 1976, Swan, Forrester, and their associates measured the cardiac output and wedge pressure simultaneously in a large series of patients with AMI and identified four major hemodynamic subsets of patients (Table 37–8): (1) patients with normal perfusion and without pulmonary congestion (normal cardiac output and normal wedge pressure); (2) patients with normal perfusion and pulmonary congestion (normal cardiac output and elevated wedge pressure); (3) patients with decreased perfusion but without pulmonary congestion (reduced cardiac output and normal wedge pressure); and (4) patients with decreased perfusion and pulmonary congestion (reduced cardiac output and elevated wedge pressure).[817] This classification, which overlaps with a crude clinical classification proposed earlier by Killip and Kimball (Table 37–8), has proved to be quite useful, but it should be noted that patients frequently pass from one category to another with therapy and sometimes apparently even spontaneously.

HEMODYNAMIC SUBSETS. These are usually reflected in the patient's clinical status. Hypoperfusion usually becomes evident clinically when the cardiac index falls below approximately 2.2 liters/min/m^2, whereas pulmonary congestion is noted when the wedge pressure exceeds approximately 20 mm Hg. However, approximately 25 per cent of patients with cardiac indices less than 2.2 liters/min/m^2 and 15 per cent of patients with elevated pulmonary capillary wedge pressures are not recognized clinically. Discrepancies in hemodynamic and clinical classification of patients with AMI arise for a variety of reasons. Patients may exhibit "phase lags" as clinical pulmonary congestion develops or resolves, symptoms secondary to chronic obstructive pulmonary disease may be confused with those resulting from pulmonary congestion, or longstanding left ventricular dysfunction may mask signs of hypoperfusion secondary to compensatory vasoconstriction.[817]

The hemodynamic findings shown in Tables 37–8 and 37–9 allow for rational approaches to therapy. The goals of hemodynamic therapy are to maintain ventricular performance, support blood pressure, and protect jeopardized myocardium. Because these goals occasionally may be at cross purposes, recognition of the hemodynamic profile, as assessed clinically or as available from hemodynamic monitoring, is required before optimal therapeutic interventions can be designed along the lines discussed below.

Hypotension in the Prehospital Phase

During the prehospital phase of AMI, invasive hemodynamic monitoring is not feasible, and during this period, therapy should be guided by frequent clinical assessment and measurement of arterial pressure by cuff, with the recognition that intense vasoconstriction can provide a falsely low pressure measured by this method. Hypotension associated with bradycardia often reflects excessive vagotonia. Relative or absolute hypovolemia is often present when hypotension occurs with a normal or rapid heart rate, particularly among patients receiving diuretics just prior to the occurrence of infarction. Marked diaphoresis, reduction of fluid intake, or vomiting during the period preceding and accompanying the onset of AMI may all contribute to the development of hypovolemia. Even if the effective vascular volume is normal, relative hypovolemia may be present because ventricular compliance is reduced in AMI and a

TABLE 37–9 HEMODYNAMIC PATTERNS FOR COMMON CLINICAL CONDITIONS

	CHAMBER PRESSURES (mmHg)				
CARDIAC CONDITION	RA	RV	PA	PCW	CI
Normal	0–6	25/0–6	25/0–12	6–12	≥2.5
AMI without LVF	0–6	25/0–6	30/12–18	≤18	≥2.5
AMI with LVF	0–6	30–40/0–6	30–40/18–25	>18	>2.0
Biventricular failure	>6	50–60/>6	50–60/25	18–25	>2.0
RVMI	12–20	30/12–20	30/12	≤12	<2.0
Cardiac tamponade	12–16	25/12–16	25/12–16	12–16	<2.0
Pulmonary embolism	12–20	50–60/12–20	50–60/12	<12	<2.0

From Gore, J. M. and Zwerner, P. L. Hemodynamic monitoring of acute myocardial infarction. In: Francis, G. S. and Alpert, J. S. (eds.) Modern Coronary Care, pp. 139–164, 1990. Boston, Little, Brown and Co.

AMI = acute myocardial infarction; CI = cardiac index; LVF = left ventricular failure; PA = pulmonary artery; PCW = pulmonary capillary wedge; RA = right atrium; RV = right ventricle; RVMI = right ventricular myocardial infarction.

left ventricular filling pressure as high as 20 mm Hg may be needed to provide an optimal preload.

MANAGEMENT. In the absence of rales involving more than one-third of the lung fields, the patient should be put in the reverse Trendelenburg position, and in those with sinus bradycardia and hypotension, atropine should be administered (0.3 to 0.6 mg intravenously repeated at 3- to 10-minute intervals up to 2.0 mg). If these measures do not correct the hypotension, normal saline should be administered intravenously, beginning with a bolus of 100 ml followed by 50-ml increments every 5 minutes. The patient should be carefully observed and the infusion stopped when the systolic pressure returns to approximately 100 mm Hg, if the patient becomes dyspneic, or if pulmonary rales develop or increase. Because of the poor correlation between left ventricular filling pressure and mean right atrial pressure, assessment of systemic (even central) venous pressure is of limited value as a guide to fluid therapy.

Administration of cardiotonic agents is indicated during the prehospital phase if systemic hypotension persists despite correction of hypovolemia and excessive vagotonia. In the absence of invasive hemodynamic monitoring, assessment of peripheral vascular resistance must be based on clinical observations. If cutaneous vasoconstriction is present, therapy with dobutamine, which stimulates cardiac contractility without unduly accelerating heart rate and which does not increase the impedance to ventricular outflow, may be helpful (see p. 1237). In hypotensive patients with AMI with clinical evidence of vasodilatation, an uncommon circumstance, phenylephrine hydrochloride is preferable, although this agent, which increases coronary as well as peripheral vascular tone, should be used with caution.

Hypovolemic Hypotension

Recognition of hypovolemia is of particular importance in hypotensive patients with AMI because of the hazard it poses and because of the improvement in circulatory dynamics that can be achieved so readily and safely by augmentation of vascular volume. Because hypovolemia is often occult, it is frequently overlooked in the absence of invasive hemodynamic monitoring. Hypovolemia may be absolute, with low left ventricular filling pressure (< 8 mm Hg), or relative, with normal (8 to 12 mm Hg) or even modestly increased (13 to 18 mm Hg) left ventricular filling pressures. Because of the reduction of left ventricular compliance that occurs with acute ischemia and infarction (see p. 1194), left ventricular filling pressures between 13 and 18 mm Hg, although above the upper limits of normal, may actually be suboptimal.

Exclusion of hypovolemia as the cause of hypotension requires the documentation of a reduced cardiac output despite left ventricular filling pressure exceeding 18 mm Hg. If, in a hypotensive patient, the pulmonary capillary wedge pressure (ordinarily measured as the pulmonary artery occlusive pressure) is below this level, fluid challenge should be carried out as described above. If hypovolemia is documented or suspected, the fluid replaced should resemble the fluid lost. Thus, when a low hematocrit complicates AMI, infusion of packed red blood cells or whole blood is the treatment of choice. On the other hand, crystalloid or colloid solutions should be administered when the hematocrit is normal or elevated.

Hypotension caused by right ventricular infarction may be confused with that caused by hypovolemia because both are associated with a low, normal, or minimally elevated left ventricular filling pressure. The findings and management of right ventricular infarction are discussed on page 1240.

The Hyperdynamic State

When infarction is not complicated by hemodynamic impairment, no therapy other than general supportive measures and treatment of arrhythmias is necessary. However, if the hemodynamic profile is of the hyperdynamic state, i.e., elevation of sinus rate, arterial pressure, and cardiac index, occurring singly or together in the presence of a normal or low left ventricular filling pressure, and if other causes of tachycardia such as fever, infection, and pericarditis can be excluded, treatment with beta-adrenoceptor blockers is indicated (see p. 1211). Presumably, the increased heart rate and blood pressure are the result of inappropriate activation of the sympathetic nervous system, possibly secondary to augmented release of catecholamines, pain and anxiety, or some combination of these.

LEFT VENTRICULAR FAILURE

Even in the thrombolytic era, left ventricular dysfunction remains the single most important predictor of mortality following AMI (Fig. 37–36). In patients with AMI, heart failure is characterized either by systolic dysfunction alone or by both systolic and diastolic dysfunction.[824] Left ventricular diastolic dysfunction leads to pulmonary venous hypertension and pulmonary congestion, whereas systolic dysfunction is principally responsible for a depression of cardiac output and of the ejection fraction. Clinical manifestations of left ventricular failure become more common

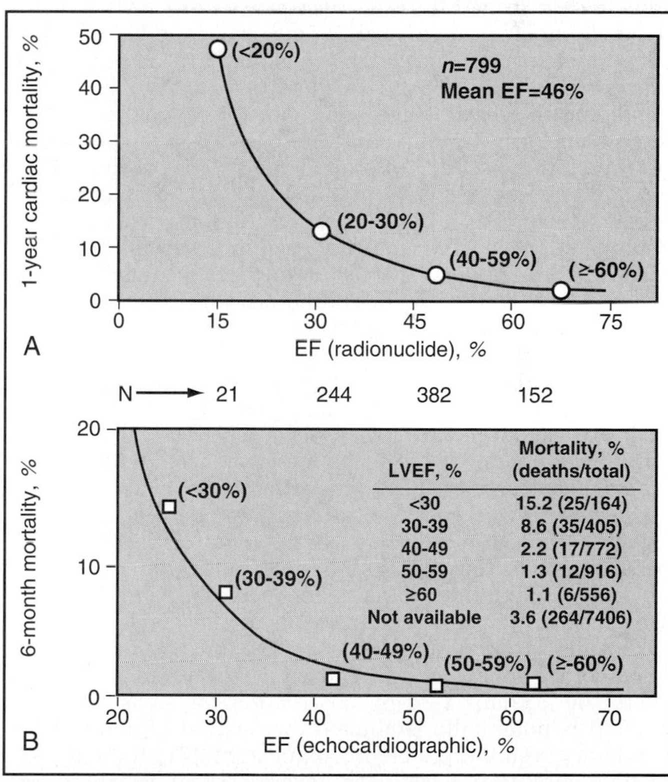

FIGURE 37–36. Impact of left ventricular (LV) function on survival following MI. The curvilinear relationship between LV ejection fraction (LVEF) is quite reproducible, whether EF is determined by the radionuclide method (*A*), as in the prethrombolytic era, or by the echocardiographic method (*B*), as in the thrombolytic era. Among patients with an LVEF below 40 per cent, mortality is markedly increased at 6 months and 1 year. Thus, interventions such as thrombolysis, aspirin, and angiotensin-converting enzyme (ACE) inhibitors should be of considerable benefit in patients with AMI to minimize the amount of LV damage and interrupt the neurohumoral activation seen with congestive heart failure. (*A* adapted from Multicenter Postinfarction Research Group: Risk stratification and survival after myocardial infarction. N. Engl. J. Med. *309*:331, 1983; *B* adapted from Volpi, A., De Vita, C., Franzosi, M. G., et al.: Determinants of 6-month mortality in survivors of myocardial infarction after thrombolysis: Results of the GISSI-2 data base. Circulation *88*:416, 1993. Copyright 1993 American Heart Association.)

as the extent of the injury to the left ventricle increases. Mortality increases in association with the severity of the hemodynamic deficit.[817]

THERAPEUTIC IMPLICATIONS. Classification of patients with AMI by hemodynamic subsets has therapeutic relevance. As already noted, patients with normal wedge pressures and hypoperfusion often benefit from infusion of fluids, because the peak value of stroke volume is usually not attained until left ventricular filling pressure reaches 18 to 24 mm Hg.[814] However, a low level of left ventricular filling pressure does not imply that left ventricular damage is necessarily slight. Such patients may be relatively hypovolemic and/or may have suffered a right ventricular infarct with or without severe left ventricular damage.[825]

The relation between ventricular filling pressure and cardiac index when preload is increased by an infusion of saline or dextran can provide valuable hemodynamic information, in addition to that obtained from baseline measurements. For example, the ventricular function curve rises steeply (marked increase in cardiac index, small increase in filling pressure) in patients with normal left ventricular function and hypovolemia, whereas the curve rises gradually or remains flat in those patients with a combination of hypovolemia and depressed cardiac function.

Invasive hemodynamic monitoring is essential to guide therapy of patients with severe left ventricular failure (pulmonary capillary wedge pressure > 18 mm Hg *and* cardiac index < 2.5 liters/min/m^2).

AVOIDANCE OF HYPOXEMIA. Patients whose AMI is complicated by congestive heart failure characteristically develop hypoxemia due to a combination of pulmonary vascular engorgement (and in some cases pulmonary interstitial edema), diminished vital capacity, and respiratory depression from narcotic analgesics. Hypoxemia can impair the function of ischemic tissue at the margin of the infarct and thereby contribute to establishing or perpetuating the vicious circle (Fig. 37–14). The ventilation-perfusion mismatch that results in hypoxemia requires careful attention to ventilatory support. Increasing fractions of inspired oxygen (FIO_2) via face mask should be used initially, but if the oxygen saturation of the patient's blood cannot be maintained above 85 to 90 per cent on 100 per cent FIO_2, strong consideration should be given to endotracheal intubation with positive-pressure ventilation. The improvement of arterial oxygenation and hence myocardial oxygen supply may help to restore ventricular performance. Positive end-expiratory pressure (PEEP) may diminish systemic venous return and reduce effective left ventricular filling pressure. This may require reduction in the amount of PEEP, normal saline infusions to maintain left ventricular filling pressure, adjustment of the rate of infusion of vasodilators such as nitroglycerin, or some combination of the above. Because myocardial ischemia frequently occurs during the return to unsupported spontaneous breathing,[826] the weaning process should be accompanied by observation for signs of ischemia and is potentially facilitated by a period of intermittent mandatory ventilation before extubation. Continuous ST-segment monitoring has been recommended for these patients.[826]

When wheezing complicates pulmonary congestion, bronchodilators that act primarily on beta$_2$-adrenoceptors, such as isoetharine or metaproterenol, given as aerosols, or terbutaline, are more desirable than conventional bronchodilators, such as isoproterenol or epinephrine. The latter act primarily on beta$_1$-receptors, which, by increasing myocardial oxygen consumption, can increase ischemia.

Although positive inotropic agents may be useful, they do not represent the initial therapy of choice in patients with AMI. Instead, heart failure is managed most effectively first by reduction of ventricular preload, and then, if possible, by lowering afterload. Arrhythmias may contribute to hemodynamic compromise as discussed on page 1246 and should be treated promptly in patients with left ventricular failure.

DIURETICS (see also p. 498). Mild heart failure in patients with AMI frequently responds well to diuretics such as furosemide, administered intravenously in doses of 10 to 40 mg, repeated at 3- to 4-hour intervals if necessary. The resultant reduction of pulmonary capillary pressure reduces dyspnea, and the lowering of left ventricular wall tension that accompanies the reduction of left ventricular diastolic volume diminishes myocardial oxygen requirements and may lead to improvement of contractility and augmentation of the ejection fraction, stroke volume, and cardiac output. The reduction of elevated left ventricular filling pressure may also enhance myocardial oxygen delivery by diminishing the impedance to coronary perfusion attributable to elevated ventricular wall tension. It may also improve arterial oxygenation by reducing pulmonary vascular congestion.

The intravenous administration of furosemide reduces pulmonary vascular congestion and pulmonary venous pressure within 15 minutes, before renal excretion of sodium and water has occurred; presumably this action results from a direct dilating effect of this drug on the systemic arterial bed. It is important not to reduce left ventricular filling pressure much below 18 mm Hg, the lower range associated with optimal left ventricular performance in AMI, because this may reduce cardiac output further and cause arterial hypotension. Excessive diuresis may also result in hypokalemia, with its attendant risk of digitalis intoxication.

AFTERLOAD REDUCTION (see also p. 494). Myocardial oxygen requirements depend on left ventricular wall stress, which in turn is proportional to the product of peak developed left ventricular pressure, volume, and wall thickness. Vasodilator therapy is recommended in patients with AMI complicated by (1) heart failure unresponsive to treatment with diuretics, (2) hypertension, (3) mitral regurgitation, or (4) ventricular septal defect. In these patients, treatment with vasodilator agents increases stroke volume and may reduce myocardial oxygen requirements and thereby lessen ischemia. Hemodynamic monitoring of systemic arterial and, in many cases, pulmonary capillary wedge (or at least pulmonary artery) pressure and cardiac output in patients treated with these agents is important. Improvement of cardiac performance and energetics requires three simultaneous effects: (1) reduction of left ventricular afterload, (2) avoidance of excessive systemic arterial hypotension in order to maintain effective coronary perfusion pressure, and (3) avoidance of excessive reduction of ventricular filling pressure with consequent diminution of cardiac output. In general, pulmonary capillary wedge pressure should be maintained at approximately 20 mm Hg and arterial pressure above 90/60 mm Hg in patients who were normotensive before developing the AMI.

Vasodilator therapy is particularly useful when AMI is complicated by mitral regurgitation or rupture of the ventricular septum. In such patients, vasodilators alone or in combination with intraaortic balloon counterpulsation can sometimes serve as a "holding maneuver" and provide hemodynamic stabilization to permit definitive catheterization and angiographic studies to be carried out and to prepare the patient for early surgical intervention. Because of the precarious state of patients with complicated infarction and the need for meticulous adjustment of dosage, therapy is best initiated with agents that can be administered intravenously and that have a short duration of action, such as nitroprusside,[827,828] nitroglycerin,[829,830] or isosorbide dinitrate.[831] After initial stabilization, the medication of choice is generally an ACE inhibitor,[832] but long-acting nitrates given by mouth, sublingually, or by ointment[833] may also be useful.

Nitroglycerin. This drug has been shown in animal experiments to be less likely than nitroprusside to produce a "coronary steal," i.e., to divert blood flow from the ischemic to the nonischemic zone.[834] Therefore, apart from consideration of its routine use in AMI patients discussed earlier (see p. 1230), it may be a particularly useful vasodilator in patients with AMI complicated by left ventricular failure.[767,768,835] Ten to 15 μg/min is infused and the dose is increased by 10 μg/min every 5 minutes until (1) the desired effect (improvement of hemodynamics or relief of ischemic chest pain) is achieved or (2) a decline in systolic arterial pressure to 90 mm Hg, or by more than 15 mm Hg, has occurred. Although both nitroglycerin and nitroprusside lower systemic arterial pressure, systemic vascular resistance, and the heart rate–systolic blood pressure product, the reduction of left ventricular filling pressure is more prominent with nitroglycerin because of its relatively greater effect than nitroprusside on venous capacitance vessels. Nevertheless, in patients with severe left ventricular failure, cardiac output often increases despite the reduction in left ventricular filling pressure produced by nitroglycerin.

Oral Vasodilators. The use of oral vasodilators in the treatment of chronic congestive heart failure is discussed on page 474. In patients with AMI and persistent heart failure, long-term treatment with a converting enzyme inhibitor should be carried out. As noted on page 1229, this reduced ventricular load decreases the remodeling of the left ventricle that occurs commonly in the period after MI and thereby reduces the development of heart failure and risk of death.[83,84]

DIGITALIS (see also p. 480). Although digitalis increases the contractility and the oxygen consumption of normal hearts, when heart failure is present the diminution of heart size and wall tension frequently results in a net reduction of myocardial oxygen requirements.[836] In animal experiments it fails to improve ventricular performance immediately following experimental coronary occlusion, but salutary effects are elicited when it is administered several days later.[837] The absence of early beneficial effects may be due to the inability of ischemic tissue to respond to digitalis or the already maximal stimulation of contractility of the normal heart by circulating and neuronally released catecholamines.

Although the issue is still controversial, arrhythmias may be increased by digitalis glycosides when they are given to patients in the first few hours after the onset of MI, particularly in the absence of hypokalemia. Also, undesirable peripheral systemic and coronary vasoconstriction may result from the rapid intravenous administration of rapidly acting glycosides such as ouabain.[837]

Administration of digitalis to patients with AMI in the hospital phase should generally be reserved for the management of supraventricular tachyarrhythmias such as atrial flutter and fibrillation and of heart failure that persists despite treatment with diuretics, vasodilators, and beta-adrenoceptor agonists. There is no indication for its use as an inotropic agent in patients without clinical evidence of left ventricular dysfunction, and it is too weak an inotropic agent to be relied upon as the principal cardiac stimulant in patients with overt pulmonary edema or cardiogenic shock. It may, however, be useful as a supplement to vasodilator agents and in the treatment of persistent or recurrent left ventricular failure.[838]

Cardiac glycosides appear to become progressively more effective in the treatment of heart failure as the interval from onset of infarction lengthens; i.e., they are more effective in the treatment of chronic than of acute heart failure secondary to ischemic heart disease. Of note, in a direct comparison of captopril versus digoxin for prevention of left ventricular remodeling and dysfunction following AMI, Bonaduce and colleagues found that patients in whom captopril therapy was initiated 7 to 10 days after onset of infarction had less left ventricular remodeling and better-preserved global left ventricular function than patients receiving digitalis.[839] In addition, the possibility that continued administration of digitalis might contribute to late mortality in the 2 years following AMI has been raised[840–844] and debated.[845,846] Although it is clear that mortality is greater in patients treated with digoxin after AMI, it is not clear that this increase in mortality is due to digoxin itself or to confounding variables that correlate with use of digoxin.[846,847] At this time, digoxin appears to be indicated in AMI patients only if they exhibit supraventricular tachyarrhythmias or overt heart failure that is not adequately controlled by ACE inhibitors and diuretics.

BETA-ADRENOCEPTOR AGONISTS. When left ventricular failure is severe, as manifested by marked reduction of cardiac index (<2 liters/min/m^2), and pulmonary capillary wedge pressure is at optimal (18 to 24 mm Hg) or excessive (>24 mm Hg) levels despite therapy with diuretics, beta-adrenoceptor agonists are indicated. Although isoproterenol is a potent cardiac stimulant and improves ventricular performance, it should be avoided in AMI patients. It also causes tachycardia and augments myocardial oxygen consumption and lactate production[848]; in addition, it reduces coronary perfusion pressure by causing systemic vasodilation and in animal experiments it increases the extent of experimentally induced infarction.[849] Norepinephrine also increases myocardial oxygen consumption because of its peripheral vasoconstrictor as well as positive inotropic actions.

Dopamine and dobutamine (see p. 502) may be particularly useful in patients with AMI and reduced cardiac output, increased left ventricular filling pressure, pulmonary vascular congestion, and hypotension.[850] Fortunately, the potentially deleterious alpha-adrenergic vasoconstrictor effects exerted by dopamine occur only at higher doses than those required to increase contractility. Its vasodilating actions on renal and splanchnic vessels and its positive inotropic effects generally improve hemodynamics and renal function.[851] In patients with AMI and severe left ventricular failure, this drug should be administered at a dose of 3 μg/kg/min while monitoring pulmonary capillary wedge and systemic arterial pressures as well as cardiac output. The dose may be increased stepwise to 20 μg/kg/min, in order to reduce pulmonary capillary wedge pressure to approximately 20 mm Hg and elevate cardiac index to exceed 2 liters/min/m^2. However, it must be recognized that doses exceeding 5 μg/kg/min activate peripheral alpha receptors and cause vasoconstriction.

Dobutamine has a positive inotropic action comparable to that of dopamine but a slightly less positive chronotropic effect[852] and less vasoconstrictor activity. In patients with AMI, dobutamine improves left ventricular performance without augmenting enzymatically estimated infarct size.[853] It may be administered in a starting dose of 2.5 μg/kg/min and increased stepwise to a maximum of 30 μg/kg/min. Both dopamine and dobutamine must be given carefully and with constant monitoring of the ECG, systemic arterial pressure, and pulmonary artery or pulmonary artery occlusive pressure and, if possible, with frequent measurements of cardiac output. The dose must be reduced if the heart rate exceeds 100 to 110 beats/min, if supraventricular or ventricular tachyarrhythmias are precipitated, or if ST-segment changes increase.

OTHER POSITIVE INOTROPIC AGENTS. Amrinone and milrinone are noncatecholamine, nonglycoside, phosphodiesterase inhibitors with inotropic and vasodilating action[854] (see p. 502). Although these drugs have been used in patients undergoing cardiac surgery,[855,856] reported experience with them in the setting of AMI is limited.[857] In patients with left ventricular failure following AMI, amrinone increases cardiac output while reducing pulmonary wedge pressure and systemic vascular resistance[858,859]; heart rate increases only at relatively high doses.[859] In AMI patients studied, no exacerbation of angina or increased incidence of arrhythmias has been reported.[858] Thus, these phosphodiesterase inhibitors appear to be useful in selected patients whose heart failure persists despite treatment with diuretics, who are not hypotensive, and who are likely to benefit from both an enhancement in contractility and afterload reduction. The initial intravenous dosage of amrinone is 0.75 mg/kg infused slowly over several minutes. This is then followed by a maintenance infusion started at 5 to 10 μg/kg/min and titrated to the patient's hemodynamic response. The total daily dose should not exceed 10 mg/kg.[860] Milrinone should be given as a loading dose of 50 μg/kg over 10 minutes, followed by a maintenance infusion of 0.375 to 0.75 μg/kg/min.

CARDIOGENIC SHOCK

This severest clinical expression of left ventricular failure is associated with extensive damage to the left ventricular myocardium in more than 80 per cent of AMI patients in whom it occurs[860a]; the remainder have a mechanical defect such as ventricular septal or papillary muscle rupture or predominant right ventricular infarction.[646] In the past cardiogenic shock has been reported to occur in up to 20 per cent of patients with AMI,[861] but estimates from recent large randomized trials of thrombolytic therapy and observational data bases report an incidence rate in the range of 7 per cent.[422,423,645,862] About 10 per cent of patients with cardiogenic shock present with this condition at the time of admission, whereas 90 per cent develop it during hospitalization.[645] This low-output state is characterized by elevated ventricular filling pressures, low cardiac output, systemic hypotension, and evidence of vital organ hypoperfusion (e.g., clouded sensorium, cool extremities, oliguria, acidosis).[422,423,863] Patients with cardiogenic shock due to AMI are more likely to be older, to have a history of a prior MI or congestive heart failure, and to have sustained an anterior infarction at the time of development of shock.[422] When shock develops in the course of AMI, it usually is due to infarct extension[864] (Fig. 37–23). The prognosis of patients with cardiogenic shock is poor, with fatality rates of about 70 per cent.[422,646,862]

PATHOLOGICAL FINDINGS. At autopsy, more than two-thirds of patients with cardiogenic shock demonstrate stenosis of 75 per cent or more of the luminal diameter of all three major coronary vessels, usually including the left anterior descending coronary artery.[865] Almost all patients with cardiogenic shock are found to have thrombotic occlusion of the artery supplying the major region of recent infarction.[866,867] Page et al., who studied 20 cardiogenic shock patients at autopsy, found that all exhibited necrosis of at least 40 per cent of the left ventricle.[866] In contrast, 35 per cent or less of the left ventricle had been destroyed in all but 1 of 14 patients who succumbed without having been in cardiogenic shock.[866] Similar findings were reported by Alonso et al.[867] Patients with cardiogenic shock had lost an average of 51 per cent of the left ventricular myocardium (range: 35 to 68 per cent), whereas in a group of patients with AMI who died suddenly of arrhythmias and who had never been in cardiogenic shock, necrosis averaged 23 per cent (range: 14 to 31 per cent) of the left ventricle.[867]

Patients who die as a consequence of cardiogenic shock often have "piecemeal" necrosis, i.e., progressive myocardial necrosis from marginal extension of their infarct into an ischemic zone bordering on the infarction. This is generally associated with persistent elevation of CK-MB. Early deterioration in left ventricular function secondary to apparent extension of infarction may, in some cases, result from expansion of the necrotic zone of myocardium without actual extension of the necrotic process (Fig. 37–37). Shear forces that develop during ventricular systole can disrupt necrotic myocardial muscle bundles, with resultant expansion and thinning of the akinetic zone of myocardium, which in turn results in deterioration of overall left ventricular function.

At autopsy, patients with cardiogenic shock consistently demonstrate marginal extension of recent areas of infarction (see p. 1194).[866,867] Additionally, focal areas of necrosis are frequently found in regions of the left and right ventricles that are not adjacent to the major area of recent infarction.[866] Such extensions and focal lesions are probably in part the result of the shock state itself because they can also be found in the hearts of patients dying of noncardiogenic shock. Infarction of the ischemic periinfarction zone can be precipitated by a number of factors that adversely affect the supply of oxygen or the metabolic demand in this zone of myocardium. These include a reduction of coronary perfusion pressure causing impaired myocardial perfusion in the presence of atherosclerotic obstructions of the nonculprit artery. An augmentation of myocardial oxygen demand resulting from the local release of catecholamines from ischemic adrenergic nerve endings in the heart as well as from circulating endogenous or infused catecholamines may also play a role. Patients with rupture of the ventricular septum or of a papillary muscle can also exhibit cardiogenic shock. These patients often have smaller infarcts than do those with cardiogenic shock secondary to ventricular failure without a mechanical lesion. The prognosis is better in such patients because the smaller infarct

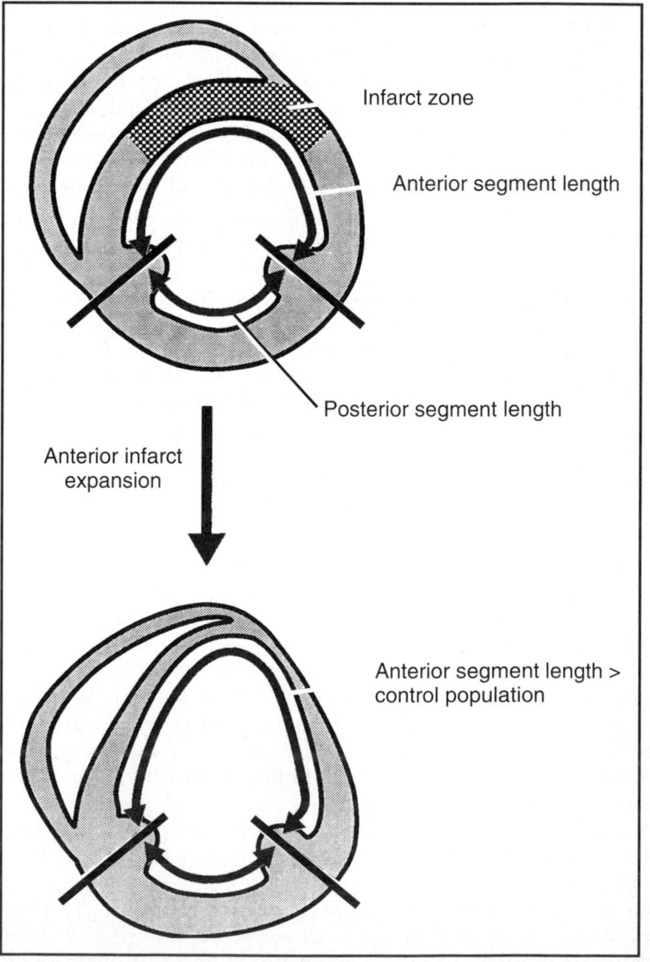

FIGURE 37–37. Infarct expansion after transmural anterior myocardial infarction. (From Tice, F. D., and Kisslo, J.: Echocardiographic assessment and monitoring of the patient with AMI: Prospects for the thrombolytic era. *In* Califf, R. M., Mark, D. B., and Wagner, G. S. (eds.): Acute Coronary Care. St. Louis, Mosby-Year Book, 1995, p. 496.)

allows their left ventricle to support the circulation if the mechanical defect has been corrected surgically.

PATHOPHYSIOLOGY. The shock state in patients with AMI appears to be the result of a vicious circle, demonstrated in Figure 37–14 (see p. 1195).[422,423,863] According to this formulation, coronary obstruction leads to myocardial ischemia, which impairs myocardial contractility and ventricular performance. This, in turn, reduces arterial pressure and therefore coronary perfusion pressure, leading to further ischemia and extension of necrosis until the left ventricle has insufficient contracting myocardium to sustain life. The progressive nature of the myocardial insult in this syndrome is reflected in the stuttering and progressive evolution of elevations in the plasma enzyme–time activity curves of markers specific for myocardial injury. Consideration of the vicious circle also points to the hazard of hypovolemic hypotension in patients with AMI but without cardiogenic shock. Hypotension, whatever its cause, reduces coronary perfusion, especially of myocardium in the territory of obstructive arteries, and thereby may enhance necrosis.

DIAGNOSIS. Cardiogenic shock is characterized by marked and persistent (>30 min) hypotension with systolic arterial pressure less than 80 mm Hg and a marked reduction of cardiac index (generally < 1.8 liters/mm/m^2) in the face of elevated left ventricular filling pressure (pulmonary capillary wedge pressure > 18 mm Hg). Spurious estimates of left ventricular filling pressure based on measurements of the pulmonary artery wedge pressure can occur in the presence of marked mitral regurgitation, in which the tall *v* wave in the left atrial (and pulmonary artery wedge) pressure tracing elevates the mean pressure above left ventricular end-diastolic pressure. Accordingly, mitral regurgitation and other mechanical lesions such as ventricular septal defect, ventricular aneurysm, and pseudoaneurysm must be excluded before the diagnosis of cardiogenic shock due to impairment of left ventricular function can be established. Mechanical complications should be suspected in any patient with AMI in whom circulatory collapse occurs.[422,423,863] Immediate hemodynamic, angiographic, and echocardiographic evaluations are necessary in patients with cardiogenic shock. It is important to exclude mechanical complications because primary therapy of such lesions usually requires immediate operative treatment with intervening support of the circulation by intraaortic balloon counterpulsation.

Medical Management

When the aforementioned mechanical complications are not present, cardiogenic shock is due to impairment of left ventricular function. Although dopamine or dobutamine usually improves the hemodynamics in these patients, unfortunately neither appears to improve hospital survival significantly. Similarly, vasodilators have been utilized in an effort to elevate cardiac output and to reduce left ventricular filling pressure. However, by lowering the already markedly reduced coronary perfusion pressure, myocardial perfusion can be compromised further, accelerating the vicious circle illustrated in Figure 37–14 (see p. 1195). Vasodilators may nonetheless be used in conjunction with intraaortic balloon counterpulsation and inotropic agents in an effort to increase cardiac output while sustaining or elevating coronary perfusion pressure.[422,423,863]

The systemic vascular resistance is usually elevated in patients with cardiogenic shock, but occasionally resistance is normal and in a few cases vasodilation actually predominates. When systemic vascular resistance is not elevated (i.e., <1800 dynes/sec/cm^5) in patients with cardiogenic shock, norepinephrine, which has both alpha- and beta-adrenoceptor agonist properties (in doses ranging from 2 to 10 μg/min), may be employed to increase diastolic arterial pressure, maintain coronary perfusion, and improve contractility. However, there is no definitive evidence that ultimate outcome is affected by this drug.[868] Norepinephrine should be used only when other means, including balloon counterpulsation, fail to maintain arterial diastolic pressure above 50 to 60 mm Hg in a previously normotensive patient. The use of alpha-adrenoceptor agents such as phenylephrine and methoxamine is contraindicated in patients with cardiogenic shock (unless systemic vascular resistance is inordinately low).

Intraaortic Balloon Counterpulsation

(See also p. 535)

Intraaortic balloon counterpulsation may be useful in patients with cardiogenic shock due to mechanical defects following AMI (see pp. 1241 to 1245) or to severe left ventricular dysfunction when other medical measures fail.[869–872] The balloon is inserted percutaneously[873] or, rarely, via an arterial cutdown in the femoral artery and advanced into the thoracic aorta via the femoral artery. Phased pulsations, electrocardiographically synchronized, allow for inflation at the time of closure of the aortic valve and deflation just before the onset of systole. The augmented coronary perfusion pressure during diastole enhances coronary blood flow because coronary vascular resistance is minimal during this portion of the cardiac cycle. Because the balloon is deflated throughout systole, the left ventricle ejects against a lower impedance. Hemodynamic changes generally include a 10 to 20 per cent increase in cardiac output, a reduction in systolic and increase in diastolic arterial pressure with little change in mean pressure, a diminution of heart rate, and an increase in urine output.[869,872] The reduction in left ventricular afterload reduces myocardial oxygen consumption, and, as a consequence, anaerobic metabolism and myocardial ischemia are diminished.[869] Favorable effects are sometimes reflected in prompt resolution of electrocardiographic signs of ischemia.

INDICATIONS. Intraaortic balloon counterpulsation is utilized in the treatment of AMI in three groups of patients: (1) those whose conditions are hemodynamically unstable and in whom support of the circulation is required for the performance of cardiac catheterization and angiography carried out to assess lesions that are potentially correctable surgically or by angioplasty; (2) those with cardiogenic shock that is unresponsive to medical management; and (3) rarely, those with persistent ischemic pain that is unresponsive to treatment with inhalation of 100 per cent oxygen, beta-adrenoceptor blockade, and nitrates. Unfortunately, among patients with cardiogenic shock, improvement is often only temporary, and "balloon dependence" commonly develops.[870,872] Patients with cardiogenic shock treated with this modality can be successfully weaned from the supporting system only occasionally. Counterpulsation alone does not improve overall survival in patients either with or without a surgically remediable mechanical lesion.[870,871]

COMPLICATIONS. These occur infrequently but include damage to or perforation of the aortic wall, ischemia distal to the site of insertion of the balloon in the femoral artery, thrombocytopenia, hemolysis, renal emboli, and mechanical failure such as rupture of the balloon.[809,874] Those at highest risk include patients with peripheral vascular disease, the elderly, and women, particularly if they are small. These factors should be taken into consideration before an attempt is made to institute intraaortic balloon counterpulsation. Because of the potential for vascular bleeding complications, there has been reluctance to use intraaortic pumps in patients who have undergone thrombolytic therapy. However, despite the increased bleeding risk, because of the poor outcome among patients with shock following thrombolysis (usually ineffective thrombolysis), this modality should be considered in selected patients who are candidates for an aggressive approach to revascularization.

Reperfusion

Reversal of cardiogenic shock by acute reperfusion has been reported, usually with thrombolytic therapy, emergency PTCA, or a combination of these measures.[422,423,863] In several uncontrolled series of patients, the mortality of cardiogenic shock appears to have been reduced to about 35 per cent by early angioplasty or coronary artery bypass surgery.[875] Encouraging evidence favoring early angiography and revascularization has been reported in a cardiogenic shock registry.[646] Another small retrospective series reported that patients with cardiogenic shock who underwent a successful angioplasty had a better 1-year survival than either those who did not undergo a successful angioplasty or those who received only medical therapy.[876] These promising results must be interpreted cautiously because selection bias due to exclusion of elderly and moribund patients may have inflated the estimate of the beneficial effect of angioplasty.

Of the five therapies frequently used to treat patients with cardiogenic shock (vasopressors, intraaortic balloon counterpulsation, thrombolysis, angioplasty, and coronary artery bypass surgery), the first two are useful temporizing maneuvers, but only early revascularization appears to reduce mortality.[646] Because this conclusion is based on uncontrolled data, an international randomized trial (SHOCK) is underway to define whether revascularization with either angioplasty or bypass surgery is superior to conventional medical therapy. The results of randomized trials will also provide information on the overall costs to the health care system of implementing an aggressive treatment program.

We recommend assessment of patients on an individualized basis to determine their desire for aggressive care[877] and overall candidacy for further treatment (e.g., age, mental status, comorbidities). Patients who are potential candidates for revascularization should then rapidly receive intraaortic balloon counterpulsation and be referred for coronary arteriography. Those with suitable anatomy should be revascularized with angioplasty or coronary artery bypass surgery. In appropriately selected patients, emergency cardiac transplantation has also been used successfully to manage cardiogenic shock.[878]

SURGERY. Surgical treatment in cardiogenic shock (aside from correcting mechanical abnormalities) may involve bypassing occluded as well as severely obstructed nonoccluded vessels. Occlusion of one major vessel may cause left ventricular dysfunction and hypotension, which can then lead to hypoperfusion and ischemia of myocardium subserved by the other diseased vessels. Left ventricular function may be improved by relief of this ischemia with revascularization. It is possible that left ventricular bypass, a technique that reduces left ventricular oxygen demands more drastically, may ultimately prove to be more effective in improving survival in patients with cardiogenic shock than intraaortic balloon counterpulsation[879]; however, it is still experimental. Emergency percutaneous cardiopulmonary bypass has been used in a small series of patients before catheterization.[880] Although relatively successful in pilot studies, this complex strategy cannot be widely recommended until tested further.

RIGHT VENTRICULAR INFARCTION

A characteristic hemodynamic pattern (Table 37–10) has been observed in patients with right ventricular infarction,[881,882] which frequently accompanies inferior left ventricular infarction[541] or rarely occurs in isolated form.[883,884] Right-heart filling pressures (central venous, right atrial, and right ventricular end-diastolic pressures) are elevated whereas left ventricular filling pressure is normal or only slightly raised[825]; right ventricular systolic and pulse pressures are decreased, and cardiac output is often markedly depressed. Rarely, this disproportionate elevation of right-sided filling pressure causes right-to-left shunting through a patent foramen ovale.[885] This possibility should be considered in patients with right ventricular infarction who have unexplained systemic hypoxemia. The finding of an elevation in atrial natriuretic factor in this condition has led to the suggestion that abnormally high levels of this peptide might be in part responsible for the hypotension seen in right ventricular infarction.[205]

TABLE 37–10 FEATURES OF RIGHT VENTRICULAR INFARCTION

Inferior-posterior myocardial infarction
Clinical findings may include:
Normal or depressed right ventricular function
Shock
Tricuspid regurgitation
Ruptured ventricular septum
Hemodynamic measurements
Abnormally elevated right atrial pressure
Normal right ventricular and pulmonary artery systolic pressures
Increased ratio of right ventricular to left ventricular filling pressure
Depressed right ventricular function curve
Scintigraphy
Uptake in right ventricular free wall
Increased right ventricular dimensions and decreased wall motion
Echocardiography
Increased right ventricular dimension
Absence of pericardial effusion
Cardiac enzymes
Increased magnitude of enzyme values relative to degree of left ventricular dysfunction
Cardiac catheterization
Involvement of right (usually) or left (rarely) circumflex coronary arteries
Right ventricular akinesis
Differential diagnosis
Hypotension with acute myocardial infarction
Pericardial tamponade
Constrictive pericarditis
Pulmonary embolus

Modified from Rackley, C. E., Russell, R. O., Jr., Mantle, J. A., et al.: Right ventricular infarction and function. Am. Heart J. *101*:215, 1981.

Diagnosis

Many patients with the combination of normal left ventricular filling pressure and depressed cardiac index have right ventricular infarcts (with accompanying inferior left ventricular infarcts). The hemodynamic picture may superficially resemble that seen in patients with pericardial disease (see Chap. 45).[825] It includes elevated right ventricular filling pressure; steep, right atrial *y* descent; and an early diastolic drop and plateau (square root sign) in the right ventricular pressure tracing. Moreover, Kussmaul's sign (an increase in jugular venous pressure with inspiration, p. 453) and pulsus paradoxus (a fall in systolic pressure of greater than 10 mm Hg with inspiration, p. 1488) may be present in patients with right ventricular infarction. In fact, Kussmaul's sign in the setting of inferior wall AMI is highly predictive of right ventricular involvement.

The ECG may provide the first clue that right ventricular involvement is present in the patient with inferior wall MI. Most patients with right ventricular infarction have ST-segment elevation in lead V_4R (right precordial lead in V_4 position)[339,886] (Fig. 4–39, p. 134). Transient elevation of the ST segment in any of the right precordial leads may occur with right ventricular MI, and the presence of ST-segment elevation of 0.1 mV or more in any one or combination of leads V_4R, V_5R, and V_6R in patients with the clinical picture of acute MI is highly sensitive and specific for the diagnosis of right ventricular MI.[339,887]

ECHOCARDIOGRAPHY AND RADIONUCLIDE ANGIOGRAPHY. Echocardiography is helpful in the differential diagnosis[888] because in right ventricular infarction, in contrast to pericardial tamponade, no significant quantities of pericardial fluid are seen. On two-dimensional echocardiography, abnormal wall motion of the right ventricle as well as right ventricular dilatation and depression of right ventricular ejection fraction are noted.[888,889] Gated equilibrium radionuclide angiography is also useful for recognizing right ventricular MI.[881,890] Serial studies have shown that some degree of recovery of an initially depressed right ventricular ejection fraction is the rule with right ventricular MI,[754,881,891] whereas this is less apparent in left ventricular ejection fraction.

HEMODYNAMICS. Loss of atrial transport in patients with right ventricular infarction can result in marked reductions in stroke volume and arterial blood pressure.[891] As already noted, disproportionate elevation of the right-sided filling pressure is the hemodynamic hallmark of right ventricular infarction. Therefore, ventricular pacing may fail to increase cardiac output, and atrioventricular sequential pacing may be required.[129,892] In general, the hemodynamic importance of right ventricular infarction in patients with inferior infarction is reflected in the observations of Marmor et al. They noted that although infarct sizes (reflected in CK release curves) were similar in patients with anterior and inferior infarcts, the former had severe depression of the left ventricular ejection fraction and the latter had more severe depression of the right ventricular ejection fraction.[893]

Treatment

In patients with hypotension due to right ventricular MI, hemodynamics may be improved by a combination of expanding plasma volume to augment right ventricular preload and cardiac output and, when left ventricular failure is present, arterial vasodilators. The initial therapy for hypotension in patients with right ventricular infarction should almost always be volume expansion. However, if hypotension has not been corrected after one or more liters of fluid have been administered briskly, consideration should be given to hemodynamic monitoring with a pulmonary artery catheter, because further volume infusion may be of little use and may produce pulmonary congestion.[815] Vasodilators reduce the impedance to left ventricular outflow and in turn left ventricular diastolic, left atrial, and pulmonary (arterial) pressures, thereby lowering the impedance to right ventricular outflow and enhancing right ventricular output. A remarkably high survival rate of 60 per cent, albeit in a small series of patients with right ventricular infarction and serious and prolonged hypotension, emphasizes the importance of recognition and vigorous medical therapy of this cause of serious hypotension in MI.[894]

Right ventricular infarction is common among patients with inferior left ventricular infarction. Therefore, otherwise unexplained systemic arterial hypotension or diminished cardiac output, or marked hypotension in response to small doses of nitroglycerin[771] in patients with inferior infarction, should lead to the prompt consideration of this diagnosis. In view of the importance of atrial transport, patients requiring pacing should have atrial or atrioventricular sequential pacing.[892] Replacement of the tricuspid valve and repair of the valve with annuloplasty rings have been carried out in the treatment of severe tricuspid regurgitation secondary to right ventricular infarction.

MECHANICAL CAUSES OF HEART FAILURE

Free Wall Rupture

The most dramatic complications of AMI are those that involve tearing or rupture of acutely infarcted tissue.[895,895a] The clinical characteristics of these lesions vary considerably and depend on the site of rupture, which may involve the papillary muscles, the interventricular septum, or the free wall of either ventricle. The overall incidence of these complications is hard to assess because clinical and autopsy series differ considerably.[896,897] However, as a group they are probably responsible for about 15 per cent of all deaths from AMI.[895,898] The comparative clinical profile of these complications, as gathered from different studies, is shown in Table 37–11. A large autopsy study in 1989 suggests that the incidence of myocardial rupture has increased since the late 1960's, with a rate of 31 per cent among necropsied cases.[897] The prior use of corticosteroids or nonsteroidal antiinflammatory agents has been implicated as predisposing to rupture as a result of impaired healing. Controversy remains about the actual relationship between the use of such agents and the frequency of rupture, with several series suggesting a correlation of rupture with their use[899,900] and others not.[896,901] Conversely, the early use of thrombolytic therapy appears to reduce the incidence of cardiac rupture,[464,567] an effect that is responsible in part for improved survival with effective thromboly-

TABLE 37–11 CLINICAL PROFILE OF MECHANICAL COMPLICATIONS OF MYOCARDIAL INFARCTION

VARIABLE	VENTRICULAR SEPTAL DEFECT	FREE WALL RUPTURE	PAPILLARY MUSCLE RUPTURE
Age (mean, years)	63	69	65
Days post-MI	3–5	3–6	3–5
Anterior MI	66%	50%	25%
New murmur	90%	25%	50%
Palpable thrill	Yes	No	Rare
Previous MI	25%	25%	30%
Echocardiographic findings			
Two-dimensional	Visualize defect	May have pericardial effusion	Flail or prolapsing leaflet
Doppler	Detect shunt	—	Regurgitant jet in LA
PA catheterization	Oxygen step-up in RV	Equalization of diastolic pressure	Prominent *V* wave in PCW tracing
Mortality			
Medical	90%	90%	90%
Surgical	50%	Case reports	40–90%

MI = myocardial infarction; LA = left atrium; PA = pulmonary artery; RV = right ventricle; PCW = pulmonary capillary wedge.
Modified from Labovitz, A. J., et al.: Mechanical complications of acute myocardial infarction. Cardiovasc. Rev. Rep. *5*:948, 1984.

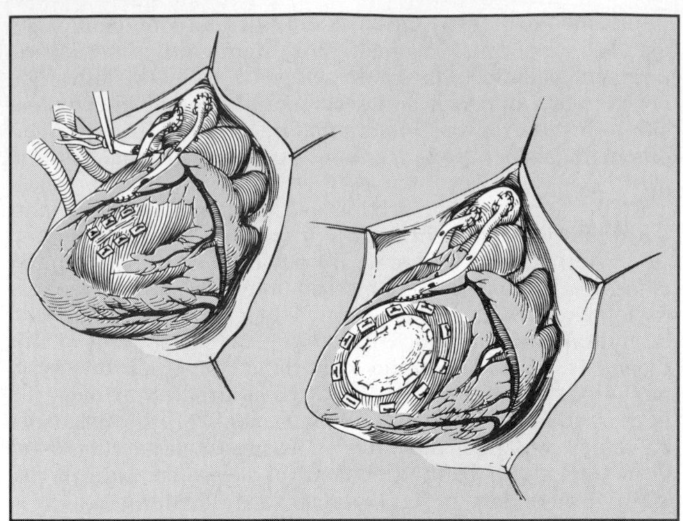

FIGURE 37–38. Free-wall perforation of the left ventricle. On the left is a direct suture repair of a small rupture. On the right is a Dacron patch closure of a larger rupture. Note the coronary artery bypass grafting which was also done at the time of surgery. (From Canacho, M. T., Muehrcke, D. D., and Loop. F. D.: Mechanical complications. *In* Julian, D. G., and Braunwald, E. [eds.]: Management of Acute Myocardial Infarction. London, W. B. Saunders Ltd., 1994, p. 310.)

sis. Late thrombolytic therapy may actually *increase* the risk of cardiac rupture despite improving overall survival.[567,902]

Rupture of the free wall of the infarcted ventricle (Fig. 37–38) occurs in up to 10 per cent of patients dying in the hospital of AMI.[895] Thinness of the apical wall, marked intensity of necrosis at the terminal end of the blood supply, poor collateral flow, the shearing effect of muscular contraction against an inert and stiffened necrotic area, and aging of the myocardium with laceration of the myocardial microstructure have all been proposed as the local factors that lead to rupture.[903–905]

CLINICAL CHARACTERISTICS. The following are some features that characterize this serious complication of AMI:

1. Occurs more frequently in the elderly and possibly more frequently in women than in men with infarction.[901]
2. Appears to be more common in hypertensive than in normotensive patients.[901,903]
3. Occurs approximately seven times more frequently in the left than the right ventricle and seldom occurs in the atria.
4. Usually involves the anterior or lateral walls[895,896] of the ventricle in the area of the terminal distribution of the left anterior descending coronary artery.
5. Is usually associated with a relatively large transmural infarction involving at least 20 per cent of the left ventricle.[896]
6. Occurs between 1 day and 3 weeks, but most commonly 1 to 4 days, following infarction.
7. Is usually preceded by infarct expansion, i.e., thinning and a disproportionate dilatation within the softened necrotic zone.[907]
8. Most commonly results from a distinct tear in the myocardial wall or a dissecting hematoma that perforates a necrotic area of myocardium (Fig. 37–38).
9. Usually occurs near the junction of the infarct and the normal muscle.
10. Occurs less frequently in the center of the infarct, but when rupture occurs here, it is usually during the second rather than the first week following the infarct.
11. Rarely occurs in a greatly thickened ventricle or in an area of extensive collateral vessels.[904]
12. Most often occurs in patients *without* previous infarction.[896,906]

Rupture of the free wall of the left ventricle usually leads to hemopericardium and death from cardiac tamponade. Occasionally, rupture of the free wall of the ventricle occurs as the first clinical manifestation in patients with undetected or silent myocardial infarction, and then it may be considered a form of "sudden cardiac death" (see Chap. 24).

The course of rupture varies from catastrophic, with an acute tear leading to immediate death, to subacute with nausea, hypotension, and pericardial type of discomfort being the major clinical clues to its presence.[895,908] Survival depends on the recognition of this complication, hemodynamic stabilization of the patient—usually with inotropic agents and/or intraaortic balloon pump—and most importantly on prompt surgical repair.[908]

PSEUDOANEURYSM. Incomplete rupture of the heart may occur when organizing thrombus and hematoma, together with pericardium, seal a rupture of the left ventricle and thus prevent the development of hemopericardium (Fig. 37–39). With time, this area of organized thrombus and pericardium can become a pseudoaneurysm (false aneurysm) that maintains communication with the cavity of the left ventricle.[909] In contrast to true aneurysms, which always contain some myocardial elements in their walls, the walls of pseudoaneurysms are composed of organized hematoma and pericardium and lack any elements of the original myocardial wall. Pseudoaneurysms can become quite large, even equaling the true ventricular cavity in size, and they communicate with the left ventricular cavity through a narrow neck. Frequently, pseudoaneurysms contain significant quantities of old and recent thrombus, superficial portions of which can cause arterial emboli. Pseudoaneurysms can drain off a portion of each ventricular stroke volume exactly as do true aneurysms. The diagnosis

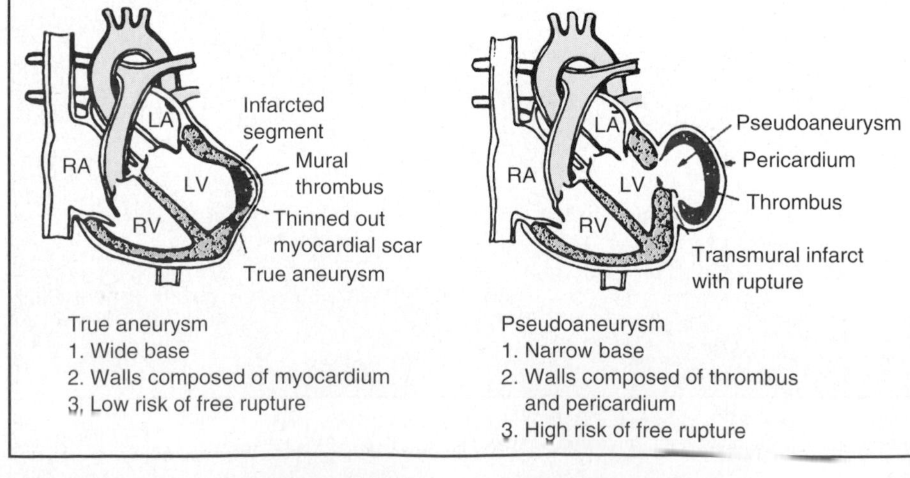

FIGURE 37–39. Differences between a pseudoaneurysm and a true aneurysm. (From Shah, P. K.: Complications of acute myocardial infarction. *In* Parmley, W., and Chatterjee, K. [eds.]: Cardiology. Philadelphia, J. B. Lippincott, 1987.)

of pseudoaneurysm can usually be made by two-dimensional echocardiography (Fig. 3–91, p. 87) and contrast angiography, although at times differentiation between true aneurysm and pseudoaneurysm may be difficult by any imaging technique.[910]

DIAGNOSIS. The rupture usually is first suggested by the development of sudden profound shock, often rapidly leading to electromechanical dissociation due to pericardial tamponade. Immediate pericardiocentesis confirms the diagnosis and relieves the pericardial tamponade, at least momentarily. If the patient's condition is relatively stable, echocardiography may help in establishing the diagnosis of tamponade. Under the most favorable conditions, cardiac catheterization can be carried out, not necessarily to confirm the diagnosis of rupture but to delineate the coronary anatomy. This is helpful so that, in addition to ventricular repair, coronary artery bypass surgery can be performed in patients in whom high-grade obstructive lesions are present. In patients in whom hemodynamics are critically compromised, establishment of the diagnosis should be followed immediately by surgical resection of the necrotic and ruptured myocardium with primary reconstruction (Fig. 37–38). When rupture is subacute and a pseudoaneurysm is suspected or present, prompt elective surgery is indicated because rupture of the pseudoaneurysm occurs relatively frequently.[908]

Rupture of the Interventricular Septum

Although rupture of the interventricular septum previously was reported in up to 11 per cent of autopsied cases,[911] clinical experience suggests that its incidence is probably in the range of 2 per cent of AMI patients,[895,912,913] perhaps because death usually is not immediate, and patients frequently can reach a referral center where this complication is treated. Clinical features associated with an increased risk of rupture of the interventricular septum include lack of development of a collateral network, advanced age, hypertension, and possibly thrombolysis.[894,912–914]

The perforation may range in length from one to several centimeters. It may be a direct through-and-through opening, or it may be more irregular and serpiginous.[915,916] The size of the defect determines the magnitude of the left-to-right shunt and the extent of hemodynamic deterioration, which in turn affects the likelihood of survival.[895,917] As in rupture of the free wall of the ventricle, transmural infarction underlies rupture of the ventricular septum. Rupture of the septum with an anterior infarction tends to be apical in location, whereas inferior infarctions are associated with perforation of the basal septum and with a worse prognosis than those in an anterior location.[918] Virtually all patients have multivessel coronary artery disease, with the majority exhibiting lesions in all of the major vessels. The likelihood of survival depends on the degree of impairment of ventricular function and the size of the defect.[918–920]

A ruptured interventricular septum is characterized by the appearance of a new harsh, loud holosystolic murmur that is heard best at the lower left sternal border and that is usually accompanied by a thrill. Biventricular failure generally ensues within hours to days. The defect can also be recognized by two-dimensional echocardiography with color flow Doppler imaging[921–923] or insertion of a pulmonary artery balloon catheter to document the left-to-right shunt.

Catheter placement of an umbrella-shaped device within the ruptured septum has been reported to stabilize the conditions of critically ill patients with acute septal rupture following AMI.[924]

Rupture of a Papillary Muscle

Partial or total rupture of a papillary muscle is a rare but often fatal complication of transmural MI[895,913,925] (Fig. 37–40). Inferior wall infarction can lead to rupture of the posteromedial papillary muscle,[926] which occurs more commonly than rupture of the anterolateral muscle, a consequence of anterolateral MI.[927,928] Rupture of a right ventricular papillary muscle is rare but can cause massive tricuspid regurgitation and right ventricular failure. Complete transection of a left ventricular papillary muscle is incompatible with life because the sudden massive mitral regurgitation that develops cannot be tolerated. Rupture of a portion of a papillary muscle, usually the tip or head of the muscle, resulting in severe, although not necessarily overwhelming, mitral regurgitation is much more frequent and is not immediately fatal. Unlike rupture of the ventricular septum, which occurs with large infarcts, papillary muscle rupture occurs with a relatively small infarction in approximately one-half of the cases seen.[929] The extent of coronary artery disease in these patients sometimes is modest as well.

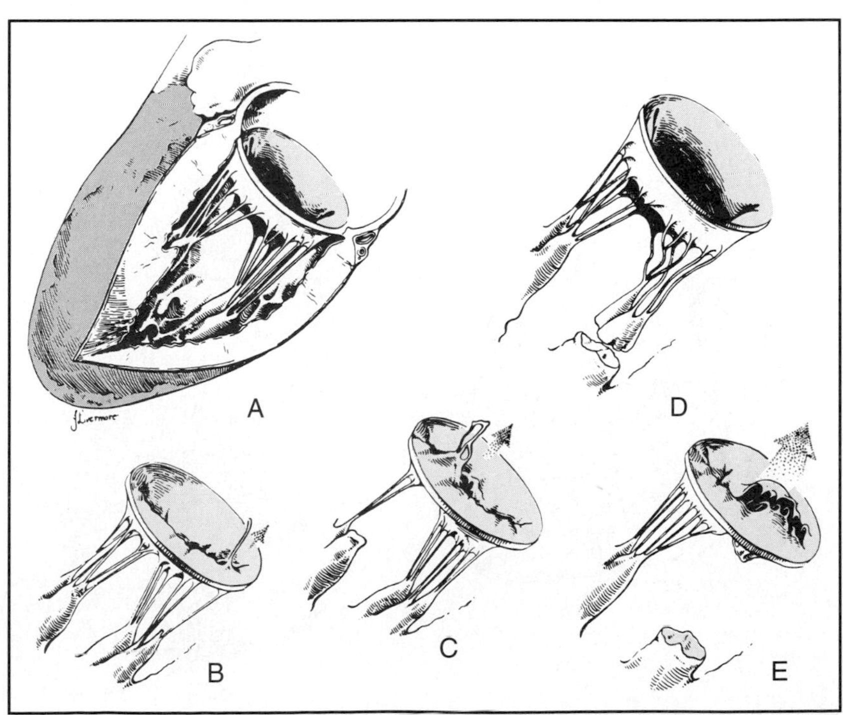

FIGURE 37–40. Mitral regurgitation after MI due to papillary head rupture. *A*, Normal annulus, chordae leaflets, and papillary structures. *B*, Ruptured posterolateral chordae with mild posterolateral regurgitant jet at the commissure. *C*, Partial papillary head rupture of the anterolateral papillary muscle with moderate mitral regurgitation of the anterolateral commissure. *D*, Complete rupture of the posteromedial papillary muscle. *E*, Severe regurgitation with anterior and posterior mitral leaflet flail segments due to the loss of the posterolateral papillary muscle. (From Camacho, M. T., Muehrcke, D. D., and Loop, F. D.: Mechanical complications. *In* Julian, D. G., and Braunwald, E. [eds.]: Management of Acute Myocardial Infarction. London, W. B. Saunders, Ltd., 1994, p. 305.)

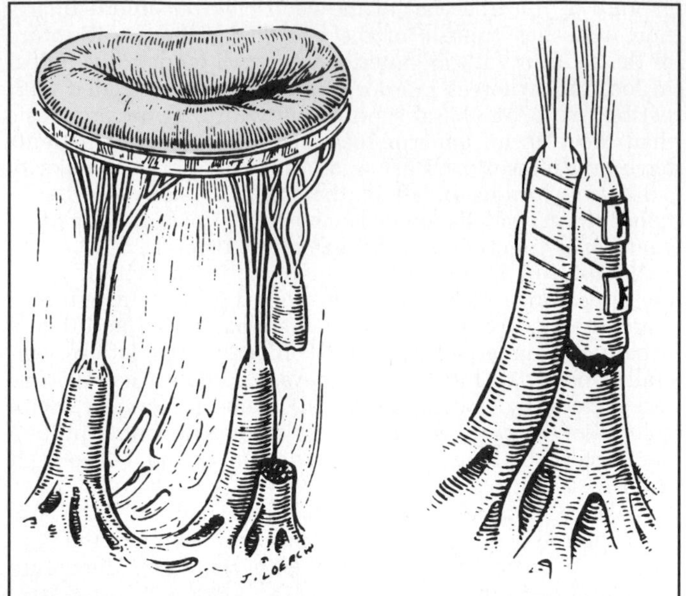

FIGURE 37–41. Repair of a totally ruptured papillary muscle head. On the left are the findings at surgery of a ruptured papillary head. On the right is a repair technique in which the ruptured papillary head is sutured to an adjacent papillary head for competence of the posterior medial papillary support structure. (From Camacho, M. T., Muehrcke, D. D., and Loop, F. D.: Mechanical complications. *In* Julian, D. G., and Braunwald, E. [eds.]: Management of Acute Myocardial Infarction. London, W. B. Saunders Ltd., 1994, p. 307.)

In a small number of patients, rupture of more than one cardiac structure is noted clinically[930] or at postmortem examination; all possible combinations of rupture of the free left ventricular wall, the interventricular septum, and papillary muscles have been described.[915]

As with patients who have a ruptured ventricular septal defect, those with papillary muscle rupture manifest a new holosystolic murmur and develop increasingly severe heart failure. In both conditions the murmur may become softer or disappear as arterial pressure falls. Mitral regurgitation due to partial or complete rupture of a papillary muscle may be promptly recognized echocardiographically.[931] Color flow Doppler imaging is particularly helpful in distinguishing acute mitral regurgitation from a ventricular septal defect in the setting of AMI[932] (Table 37–11). Therefore, an echocardiogram should be obtained immediately on any patient in whom the diagnosis is suspected, because hemodynamic deterioration can ensue rapidly. Echocardiography also often permits differentiation of papillary muscle rupture from other, generally less severe forms of mitral regurgitation that occur with AMI.[933]

Differentiation Between Ventricular Septal Rupture and Mitral Regurgitation

It may be difficult, on clinical grounds, to distinguish between acute mitral regurgitation and rupture of the ventricular septum in patients with AMI who suddenly develop a loud systolic murmur.[934] This differentiation can be made most readily by color flow Doppler echocardiography.[932,935] In addition, a right-heart catheterization with a balloon-tipped catheter can readily distinguish between these two complications.[933] As already noted, patients with ventricular septal rupture demonstrate a "step-up" in oxygen saturation in blood samples from the right ventricle and pulmonary artery compared with those from the right atrium. Patients with acute mitral regurgitation lack this step-up; they may demonstrate tall *c-v* waves in both the pulmonary capillary and pulmonary arterial pressure tracings.

Invasive monitoring, which is essential in these patients, also allows for the critically important assessment of ventricular function. Right and left ventricular filling pressures (right atrial pressure and pulmonary capillary wedge pressure) dictate fluid administration or the use of diuretics, whereas measurements of cardiac output and mean arterial pressure are obtained for calculation of systemic vascular resistance as a guide for vasodilator therapy. Unless systolic pressure is below 90 mm Hg, this therapy, generally using nitroglycerin or nitroprusside, should be instituted as soon as possible once hemodynamic monitoring is available. This may be critically important for stabilizing the patient's condition in preparation for further diagnostic studies and surgical repair. If vasodilator therapy is not tolerated or if it fails to achieve hemodynamic stability, intraaortic balloon counterpulsation should be rapidly instituted.

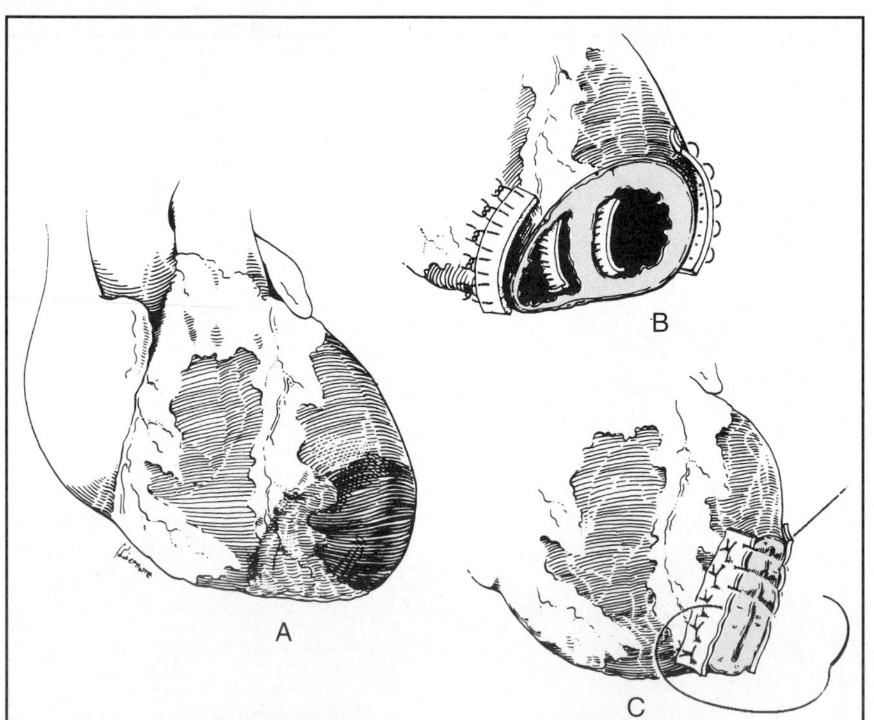

FIGURE 37–42. Repair of an apical ventricular septal defect. *A*, Large apical aneurysm with underlying ventricular septal defect. *B*, Interrupted suture repair is performed by excising the apex of the right and left ventricles, including the ventricular septal defect, with reapproximation of the left and right ventricular free walls along with the septum using Teflon felt strips for hemostasis. *C*, Over-and-over suture reinforcement of the repair for further hemostasis. (From Camacho, M. T., Muehrcke, D. D., and Loop, F. D.: Mechanical complications. *In* Julian, D. G., and Braunwald, E. [eds.]: Management of Acute Myocardial Infarction. London, W. B. Saunders Ltd., 1994, p. 296.)

Surgical Treatment

Operative intervention is most successful in patients with AMI and circulatory collapse when a surgically correctable mechanical lesion such as ventricular septal defect or mitral regurgitation can be identified and repaired.[913,936] In such patients the circulation should at first be supported by intraaortic balloon pulsation and a positive inotropic agent such as dopamine or dobutamine in combination with a vasodilator, unless the patient is hypotensive. Operation should not be delayed in patients with a correctable lesion who agree to an aggressive management strategy and require pharmacological and/or mechanical (counterpulsation) support.[912,936,937] Such patients frequently develop a serious complication—infection, adult respiratory distress syndrome, extension of the infarct, or renal failure—if operation is delayed. Surgical survival is predicted by early operation, short duration of shock, and mild degrees of right and left ventricular impairment.[912,934,936] When the hemodynamic status of a patient with one of these mechanical lesions complicating an AMI remains stable after the patient has been weaned from pharmacological and/or mechanical support, it may be possible to postpone operation for 2 to 4 weeks to allow some healing of the infarct to occur. Surgical repair may involve either correction of mitral regurgitation, insertion of a prosthetic mitral valve repair, or closure of a ventricular septal defect, usually accompanied by coronary revascularization[913] (Figs. 37–40 to 37–42).

ARRHYTHMIAS IN ACUTE MYOCARDIAL INFARCTION

The genesis and diagnosis of arrhythmias are presented in Chapters 20 and 22 and their treatment in Chapters 21 and 23. The role of arrhythmias in complicating the course of patients with AMI and the prevention and treatment of these arrhythmias in this setting are discussed here and summarized in Table 37–12.

The incidence of arrhythmias is higher in those patients seen earlier after the onset of symptoms. Many serious arrhythmias develop before hospitalization, even before the patient is monitored.[938] Some abnormality of cardiac rhythm also occurs in the majority of patients with AMI treated in CCUs.[939,940] When patients are seen very early during the course of MI, they almost invariably exhibit evidence of increased activity of the autonomic nervous system. Thus, sinus bradycardia, sometimes associated with AV block, and hypotension reflect augmented vagal activity.

TABLE 37–12 CARDIAC ARRHYTHMIAS AND THEIR MANAGEMENT DURING ACUTE MYOCARDIAL INFARCTION

CATEGORY	ARRHYTHMIA	OBJECTIVE OF TREATMENT	THERAPEUTIC OPTIONS
1. Electrical instability	Ventricular premature beats	Correction of electrolyte deficits and increased sympathetic tone	Potassium and magnesium solutions, beta blocker
	Ventricular tachycardia	Prophylaxis against ventricular fibrillation, restoration of hemodynamic stability	Antiarrhythmic agents; cardioversion/defibrillation
	Ventricular fibrillation	Urgent reversion to sinus rhythm	Defibrillation; bretylium tosylate
	Accelerated idioventricular rhythm	Observation unless hemodynamic function is compromised	Increase sinus rate (atropine, atrial pacing); antiarrhythmic agents
	Nonparoxysmal AV junctional tachycardia	Search for precipitating causes (e.g., digitalis intoxication); suppress arrhythmia only if hemodynamic function is compromised	Atrial overdrive pacing; antiarrhythmic agents; cardioversion relatively contraindicated if digitalis intoxication present
2. Pump failure/ Excessive sympathetic stimulation	Sinus tachycardia	Reduce heart rate to diminish myocardial oxygen demands	Antipyretics; analgesics; consider beta blocker unless CHF present; treat latter if present with anticongestive measures (diuretics, afterload reduction)
	Atrial fibrillation and/or atrial flutter	Reduce ventricular rate; restore sinus rhythm	Verapamil, digitalis glycosides; anticongestive measures (diuretics, afterload reduction); cardioversion; rapid atrial pacing (for atrial flutter)
	Paroxysmal supraventricular tachycardia	Reduce ventricular rate; restore sinus rhythm	Vagal maneuvers; verapamil, cardiac glycosides, beta-adrenergic blockers; cardioversion; rapid atrial pacing
3. Bradyarrhythmias and conduction disturbances	Sinus bradycardia	Acceleration of heart rate only if hemodynamic function is compromised	Atropine; atrial pacing
	Junctional escape rhythm	Acceleration of sinus rate only if loss of atrial "kick" causes hemodynamic compromise	Atropine; atrial pacing
	Atrioventricular block and intraventricular block		Insertion of pacemaker

Modified from Antman, E. M., and Rutherford, J. D. (eds): Coronary Care Medicine: A Practical Approach. Boston, Martinus Nijhoff Publishing, 1986, p. 78.

MECHANISM OF ARRHYTHMIAS. Activation of receptors within atrial and ventricular myocardium by ischemic or necrotic tissue may cause enhanced efferent sympathetic activity, increased concentrations of circulating catecholamines, and local release of catecholamines from nerve endings within the heart. The last phenomenon may also result from direct ischemic damage of adrenergic neurons.[940a] In addition, ischemic myocardium may be hyperreactive to the arrhythmogenic effects of norepinephrine,[941] which may vary strikingly in concentration in different portions of the ischemic heart.[942] Sympathetic stimulation of the heart may also enhance the automaticity of ischemic Purkinje fibers. Furthermore, catecholamines facilitate propagation of slow current responses mediated by calcium, and stimulation of ischemic myocardium by catecholamines may exacerbate arrhythmias dependent on such currents.[941] Finally, it has been demonstrated that transmural infarction can interrupt both afferent and efferent limbs of the sympathetic nervous system innervating myocardium distal to the area of infarction (but still viable)[942] (see p. 1192). In addition to the potential for modifying a variety of cardiovascular reflexes, this creation of autonomic imbalance may promote the development of arrhythmias.[942] This explains why beta-adrenoceptor blocking agents may also be helpful in the treatment of ventricular arrhythmias, particularly when the latter are associated with other signs of heightened adrenergic activity.

Experimental and clinical studies have suggested that electrolyte disturbances (e.g., hypokalemia, hypomagnesemia, acidosis), elevated free fatty acid levels, and oxygen-derived free radicals also contribute to the development of arrhythmias. The severity of these abnormalities, with the size of infarction and the perfusion status of the infarct-related coronary artery, appears to determine a patient's risk for developing the most serious rhythm disturbance—primary ventricular fibrillation (i.e., ventricular fibrillation occurring in the absence of congestive heart failure or cardiogenic shock).

The treatment of tachyarrhythmias involves not only the use of antiarrhythmic drugs but also correction of abnormalities of plasma electrolyte concentrations, acid-base balance disturbances, hypoxemia, anemia, and digitalis intoxication. In addition, it is essential to treat pericarditis, pulmonary emboli, and pneumonia or other infections, which may give rise to sinus tachycardia or other supraventricular tachyarrhythmias.

Arrhythmias occurring in patients with AMI require aggressive treatment when they (1) impair hemodynamics; (2) compromise myocardial viability by augmenting myocardial oxygen requirements; or (3) predispose to malignant ventricular arrhythmias, i.e., ventricular tachycardia, ventricular fibrillation, or asystole. Evidence indicates that both the diminished threshold to ventricular fibrillation[943] and the incidence of malignant ventricular arrhythmias associated with infarction[944] are affected by the extent of the underlying infarction.[945]

HEMODYNAMIC CONSEQUENCES. Patients with significant left ventricular dysfunction have a relatively fixed stroke volume and depend on changes in heart rate to alter cardiac output. However, there is a narrow range of heart rate over which the cardiac output is maximal, with significant reductions occurring at both faster and slower rates. Thus, all forms of bradycardia and tachycardia may depress the cardiac output in patients with AMI. Although the optimal rate insofar as cardiac output is concerned may exceed 100 per minute, it is important to consider that heart rate is one of the major determinants of myocardial oxygen consumption and that at more rapid heart rates myocardial energy needs can be elevated to levels that adversely affect ischemic myocardium. Therefore, in patients with AMI, the optimal rate is usually lower, in the range of 60 to 80 beats/min.

A second factor to consider in assessing the hemodynamic consequences of a particular arrhythmia is the loss of the atrial contribution to ventricular preload.[946] Studies in patients without AMI have demonstrated that loss of atrial transport decreases left ventricular output by 15 to 20 per cent.[947] However, in patients with reduced diastolic left ventricular compliance of any cause (including AMI), atrial systole is of greater importance for left ventricular filling. In patients with AMI, atrial systole boosts end-diastolic volume by 15 per cent, end-diastolic pressure by 29 per cent, and stroke volume by 35 per cent.[948]

VENTRICULAR ARRHYTHMIAS

Ventricular Premature Beats (VPBs)

(See also p. 675)

Prior to the widespread use of reperfusion therapy, aspirin, beta blockers, and intravenous nitrates in the management of AMI, it was believed that frequent VPBs (more than five per minute), VPBs with multiform configuration, early coupling (the "R-on-T" phenomenon), and repetitive patterns in the form of couples or salvos (Fig. 37–19) presaged ventricular fibrillation. However, it is now clear that such "warning arrhythmias" are present in as many patients who do not develop fibrillation as those who do.[237] Several reports have shown that primary ventricular fibrillation (see below) occurs without antecedent warning arrhythmias and may even develop in spite of suppression of warning arrhythmias.[949,950] On the other hand, frequent and complex VPBs and R-on-T beats are commonly observed in patients with AMI who never develop ventricular fibrillation.[949,951,952] Campbell et al. have analyzed these observations by pointing out that both primary ventricular fibrillation and VPBs, especially R-on-T beats, all occur during the early phase of AMI when considerable heterogeneity of electrical activity is present.[237,953,954] Although R-on-T beats expose this heterogeneity and can precipitate ventricular fibrillation in a small minority of patients, the ubiquitous nature of VPBs in AMI and the extremely infrequent nature of ventricular fibrillation in the current era of AMI management produces unacceptably low sensitivity and specificity of ECG patterns observed on monitoring systems for identifying patients at risk of ventricular fibrillation.[237]

MANAGEMENT. Given the declining incidence of ventricular fibrillation in AMI seen in CCUs over the last three decades (Fig. 37–43*A*), the prior practice of prophylactic suppression of VPBs with antiarrhythmic drugs no longer is necessary and may actually be associated with an increased risk of fatal bradycardic and asystolic events[955,956] (Fig. 37–44). Therefore, we pursue a conservative course when VPBs are observed in AMI and do not routinely prescribe antiarrhythmic drugs but instead determine whether recurrent ischemia or electrolyte (Fig. 37–43*B*) or metabolic disturbances are present.

When, at the very inception of an infarction, VPBs are encountered in the presence of sinus tachycardia, augmented sympathoadrenal stimulation is often a contributing factor and may be treated by beta-adrenoceptor blockade. In fact, early administration of an intravenous beta blocker is effective in reducing the incidence of ventricular fibrillation in evolving MI[957–959] (see p. 1228).

Accelerated Idioventricular Rhythm

(See p. 683)

Commonly defined as a ventricular rhythm with a rate of 60 to 125 beats/min, and frequently called "slow ventricular tachycardia," this arrhythmia is seen in up to 20 per cent of patients with AMI. It occurs frequently during the first 2 days, with about equal frequency in anterior and inferior infarctions, and probably results from enhanced automaticity of Purkinje fibers. Most episodes are of short duration, and the arrhythmia may terminate abruptly, slow

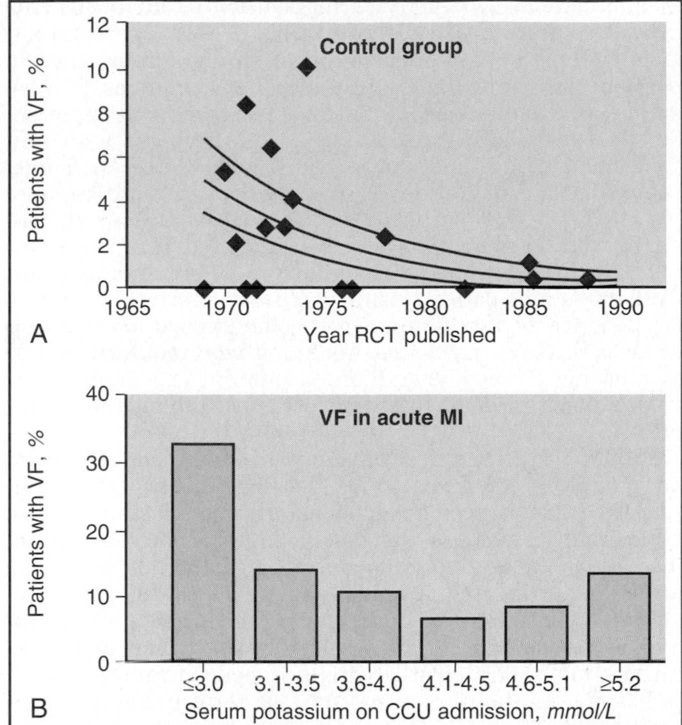

FIGURE 37–43. *A*, Temporal changes in primary ventricular fibrillation (VF), as shown in this regression analysis of the results of 18 randomized controlled trials (RCTs) in which lidocaine was administered prophylactically to patients with AMI. In 1970, the estimated risk for primary VF in the control group (heavy line) was 4.5 per cent (lighter lines represent 95 per cent confidence intervals). By 1990, this risk was substantially below 1 per cent, probably owing to such factors as the increased use of beta blockers, more aggressive repletion of electrolyte deficits, more effective therapies for left ventricular dysfunction, the decreased use of diuretics, and more effective sedation and anxiolytic therapy. *B*, Importance of electrolyte deficits, as shown in this study in which the risk for VF was strikingly increased in patients who presented to the critical care unit (CCU) with hypokalemia. (*A* adapted from Antman, E. M., and Berlin, J. A.: Declining incidence of ventricular fibrillation in myocardial infarction: Implications for the prophylactic use of lidocaine. Circulation *86:*764, 1992; *B* adapted from Nordrehaug, J. E., and van der Lippe, G.: Hypokalemia and ventricular fibrillation in acute myocardial infarction. Br. Heart J. *50:*525, 1983.)

gradually before termination, or be overdriven by acceleration of the basic cardiac rhythm. Variation of the rate is common.

Accelerated idioventricular rhythm is often observed shortly after successful reperfusion has been established.[960,961] However, the frequent occurrence of these rhythms in patients without reperfusion limits their reliability as markers of restoration of patency of the infarct-related coronary artery.[962,963] In contrast to rapid ventricular tachycardia, accelerated idioventricular rhythms are thought not to affect prognosis. There is no definitive evidence that this arrhythmia, when left untreated, increases the incidence of either ventricular fibrillation or death.[964] Therefore we do not routinely treat accelerated idioventricular rhythms. In the rare patient with clear-cut hemodynamic compromise or recurrent angina related to accelerated idioventricular rhythms, we attempt to accelerate the sinus rate with atropine or atrial pacing; suppressive antiarrhythmic therapy with lidocaine or procainamide is usually not used unless there is unequivocal precipitation of more serious ventricular tachyarrhythmias.

Ventricular Tachycardia

(See also p. 677)

Nonsustained ventricular tachycardia is usually defined as three or more consecutive ventricular ectopic beats (at a rate > 100 beats/min and lasting < 30 sec; Fig. 37–19); sustained ventricular tachycardia refers to similar rhythms that last longer than 30 seconds or cause hemodynamic compromise *that requires intervention.* (Although most brief runs of ventricular tachycardia cause some reduction in blood pressure that is observed on arterial line pressure tracings, the majority of such episodes are not recognized by the patient[237]). Additional descriptive features of note for sustained ventricular tachycardia are whether the ECG appearance is monomorphic or polymorphic.[965,966] This may be of importance because the former is more likely to be due to a myocardial scar and require aggressive strategies to prevent its recurrence and the latter may be more responsive to measures directed against ischemia. When continuous ECG recordings during the first 12 hours of AMI are analyzed, nonsustained paroxysms of monomorphic or polymorphic ventricular tachycardia may be seen in up to 67 per cent of patients.[954] These *nonsustained* runs of ventricular tachycardia do not appear to be associated with an increased mortality risk, either during hospitalization or over the first year.[966] Episodes of *sustained* ventricular tachycardia during the first 48 hours following AMI are often polymorphic and are associated with a hospital mortality of about 20 per cent.[966] However, the 1-year mortality in patients with sustained ventricular tachycardia who survive to hospital discharge is not increased over that of patients who had only nonsustained runs of ventricular tachycardia or no episodes of ventricular tachycardia during the first 48 hours.[966]

Ventricular tachycardia occurring late in the course of AMI is more common in patients with transmural infarction and left ventricular dysfunction, is likely to be sustained, usually induces marked hemodynamic deterioration, and is associated with both an increased hospital mortality and long-term mortality.[939,967]

MANAGEMENT. Since hypokalemia may increase the risk of developing ventricular tachycardia,[968] low serum potassium should be identified quickly after a patient's admission for AMI and should be treated promptly. The serum

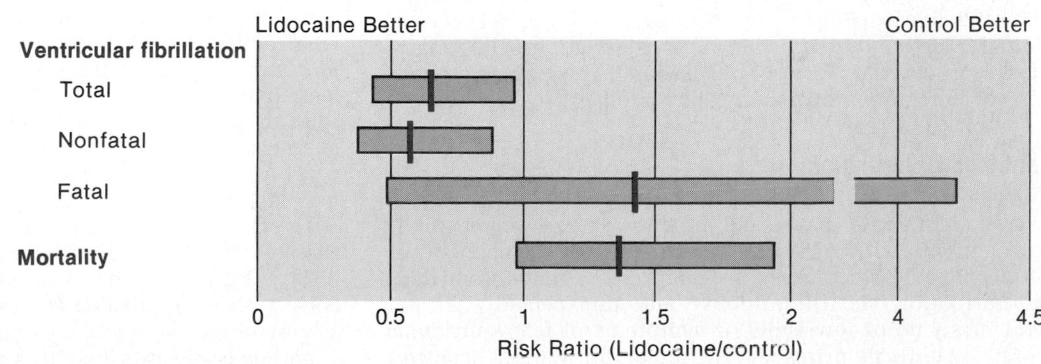

FIGURE 37–44. Pooled results of 14 randomized controlled trials of lidocaine in patients with suspected AMI suggest that the drug increases mortality despite reducing the risk of ventricular fibrillation. Patients received the drug intravenously (nine trials) or by intramuscular injection (five trials) and were followed for roughly the length of treatment (24 to 48 hours of IV administration, a few hours for IM). The narrow vertical bars represent the risk ratio derived from the pooled data, and the broad horizontal bars show the 95 per cent confidence limits for these ratios. (Adapted from Antman, E. M., and Braunwald, E.: Acute MI: Management in the 1990s. Hosp. Pract. July 15, 1990, p. 73.)

potassium level should be maintained above 4.5 mEq/liter and serum magnesium above 2 mEq/liter.[30]

Rapid abolition of sustained ventricular tachycardia in patients with AMI is mandatory because of its deleterious effect on pump function and because it frequently deteriorates into ventricular fibrillation. When the ventricular rate is rapid (>150/min) and/or there is a decline in arterial pressure, a single attempt at "thumpversion," i.e., striking a sharp blow to the precordium, is indicated (see p. 680). Rapid polymorphic ventricular tachycardia should be managed similar to ventricular fibrillation, with an unsynchronized discharge of 200 joules, whereas monomorphic ventricular tachycardia should be treated with a synchronized discharge of 100 joules.[969] Occasionally lower energy (10 to 20 joules) synchronized discharges can terminate monomorphic ventricular tachycardia.

When the ventricular rate is slower than approximately 150/min and the arrhythmia is well tolerated hemodynamically, antiarrhythmic therapy with one of the following regimens should be attempted[2]:

1. *Lidocaine*—initial bolus of 1.0 to 1.5 mg/kg followed by supplemental boluses of 0.5 to 0.75 mg/kg every 5 to 10 min as needed to a maximum of 3 mg/kg. A maintenance infusion of 20 to 50 μg/kg/min (1 to 4 mg/min) may then be started. It should be recognized that the metabolism of lidocaine is slowed not only in patients with heart failure or hypotension but also in those with diminution of hepatic blood flow due to effects of pharmacological agents such as propranolol.[970] The rate of infusion should be lower in patients with renal failure. Therefore, careful titration is needed to avoid toxicity, manifested primarily by central nervous system hyperactivity, as well as by depression of intraventricular and atrioventricular conduction and cardiac contractility. Saturation of an extravascular pool normally occurs after a continuous infusion of approximately 3 hours, at which time blood levels increase despite maintenance of a constant infusion rate.[971] At this time, it may be desirable to reduce the rate of administration by about 25 per cent (see also p. 605).
2. *Procainamide*—loading infusion of 12 to 17 mg/kg over about 20 to 30 minutes, followed by a maintenance infusion of 1 to 4 mg/min (see also p. 603).
3. *Amiodarone*—loading infusion of 150 mg, followed by a constant infusion of 1.0 mg/min for up to 6 hours and then a maintenance infusion at 0.5 mg/min (see also p. 613).

After reversion to sinus rhythm, every effort should be made to correct underlying abnormalities such as hypoxia, hypotension, acid-base or electrolyte disturbances, and digitalis excess. Although no definitive data are available, it is a common clinical practice to continue maintenance infusions of antiarrhythmic drugs for several days following an index episode of ventricular tachycardia and to discontinue the drug and either observe the patient for recurrence or perform a diagnostic electrophysiology study. Patients with recurrent or refractory ventricular tachycardia should be considered for specialized procedures such as implantation of antitachycardia devices or surgery (see p. 621). Occasionally, urgent attempts at revascularization with angioplasty or coronary artery bypass graft surgery may help control refractory ventricular tachycardia.[965,972]

Ventricular Fibrillation

(See also p. 686)

This arrhythmia may occur in three settings in hospitalized patients with AMI. (Its occurrence as a mechanism of sudden death is discussed in Chap. 24.) *Primary* ventricular fibrillation occurs suddenly and unexpectedly in patients with no or few signs or symptoms of left ventricular failure. Although primary ventricular fibrillation occurred in up to 10 per cent of patients hospitalized with AMI several decades ago, analyses suggest that its incidence has declined dramatically[955,973,974] (Fig. 37–43*A*). Approximately 60 per cent of episodes occur within 4 hours and 80 per cent within 12 hours of the onset of symptoms.[954] *Secondary* ventricular fibrillation, on the other hand, is often the final event of a progressive downhill course with left ventricular failure and cardiogenic shock.[237] So-called *late* ventricular fibrillation develops more than 48 hours following AMI and frequently but not exclusively occurs in patients with large infarcts and ventricular dysfunction. Patients with intraventricular conduction defects and anterior wall infarction, patients with persistent sinus tachycardia, atrial flutter, or fibrillation early in the clinical course, and those with right ventricular infarction who require ventricular pacing are at higher risk for suffering late in-hospital ventricular fibrillation than are patients without these features.

PROGNOSIS. The effect of primary ventricular fibrillation on prognosis continues to be debated. The MILIS study suggested that it does not have an adverse effect on hospital mortality, whereas the first GISSI trial suggested that there is an excess mortality due to primary ventricular fibrillation during the hospital phase but not thereafter.[975] On the other hand, secondary ventricular fibrillation occurring in association with marked left ventricular failure or cardiogenic shock clearly entails a poor prognosis, with in-hospital mortality rates of 40 to 60 per cent.[976] With the availability of amiodarone and new antitachycardia devices, the prognosis of late ventricular fibrillation is improving and is probably driven more by residual ventricular function and recurrent ischemia than the arrhythmic risk per se.[977]

PROPHYLAXIS. In the early years of MI care in CCUs, concern about the risk of primary ventricular fibrillation led to aggressive monitoring for warning ventricular arrhythmias (see p.1226) and the initiation of antiarrhythmic therapy when they appeared. Later, when it was shown that warning arrhythmias could not be relied upon to predict the risk of ventricular fibrillation, arrhythmia prophylaxis became routine.[978,979] Lidocaine has been studied most extensively in this regard and has been shown to reduce the incidence of ventricular fibrillation,[980] leading to its widespread routine use in CCUs in patients with known or suspected AMI. However, we no longer endorse that CCU practice for the following reasons:

1. As already noted, the incidence of ventricular fibrillation in patients hospitalized for AMI is decreasing so that the risk for the arrhythmia is now much lower than it was several decades ago (probably under 5 per cent) (Fig. 37–43*A*). The reasons for this reduction in ventricular fibrillation are not clear but probably include general improvements in the care of AMI patients, greater use of beta blockers, aggressive repletion of electrolytes, prompt treatment of ischemia and congestive heart failure, and reduction in infarct size from reperfusion strategies.[955]
2. There is no evidence that prophylaxis with lidocaine actually reduces mortality in hospitalized patients with AMI because they can almost always be promptly defibrillated. Furthermore, there appear to be trends to excess mortality risk when lidocaine is used on a routine prophylactic basis[956,980] (Fig. 37–44).
3. Beta-adrenoceptor blockers, which should be administered promptly to the majority of patients with AMI (see p. 1211), have been shown to reduce not only ventricular fibrillation[959] but also mortality from AMI.[745]
4. There is an association between hypokalemia and the risk of ventricular fibrillation in the CCU[981,982] (Fig. 37–43*B*). Although it has not been conclusively shown that correction of hypokalemia to a level of 4.5 mEq/liter actually reduces the incidence of ventricular fibrillation, our experience suggests that this probably is protective and of little risk. The data on magnesium and the risk of ventricu-

lar fibrillation are incomplete at present. Despite the fact that no consistent relationship between hypomagnesemia and ventricular fibrillation has been observed,[982] magnesium deficits may still be involved in the risk of ventricular fibrillation because intracellular magnesium levels are reduced in AMI and are not adequately reflected by serum measurements.[983] For these reasons, plus the fact that it is often difficult to repair a potassium deficit without administering supplemental magnesium, we routinely replete magnesium to a level of 2 mEq/liter.

The only situation in which we might consider prophylactic lidocaine (bolus of 1.5 mg/kg followed by 20 to 50 μg/kg/min) would be the unusual circumstance in which a patient within the first 12 hours of an AMI must be managed in a facility where cardiac monitoring is not available and equipment for prompt defibrillation is not readily accessible.

MANAGEMENT (see also p. 687). The likelihood of successful restoration of an effective cardiac rhythm declines rapidly with time after the onset of uncorrected ventricular fibrillation. Irreversible brain damage may occur within 1 to 2 minutes, particularly in elderly patients. The treatment of ventricular fibrillation is an unsynchronized electrical countershock with at least 200 to 300 joules, implemented as rapidly as possible. This interrupts fibrillation and restores an effective cardiac rhythm in patients under direct medical observation in the CCU. When ventricular fibrillation occurs outside an intensive care unit, resuscitative efforts are much less likely to be successful, primarily because the time interval between the onset of the episode and institution of definitive therapy tends to be prolonged. Because closed-chest cardiopulmonary resuscitation with external cardiac compression provides only a marginal cardiac output even under optimal circumstances, countershock could be implemented as soon as possible after the detection of ventricular fibrillation rather than deferred under the mistaken impression that adequate circulatory and respiratory support can be maintained in the interim. Failure of electrical countershock to restore an effective cardiac rhythm is due almost always to rapidly recurrent ventricular tachycardia or ventricular fibrillation, to electromechanical dissociation, or, very rarely, to electrical asystole.

Ventricular fibrillation often recurs rapidly and repeatedly when the metabolic milieu of the heart has been compromised by severe or prolonged hypoxemia, acidosis, electrolyte abnormalities, or digitalis intoxication. Under these conditions, continued cardiopulmonary resuscitation, prompt implementation of pharmacological and ventilatory maneuvers designed to correct these abnormalities, and rapidly repeated attempts with electrical countershock may be effective. Even though repeated shocks with excessive energy may damage the myocardium and elicit arrhythmias, speed is essential and prompt efforts with high-intensity shocks (generally 300 to 400 watt-seconds) are justified. When ventricular fibrillation persists without documented interruption by electrical countershock, administration of epinephrine either by the intracardiac route (up to 10 ml of a 1:10,000 concentration) or intravenous route (1 mg initially) may facilitate a subsequent defibrillation attempt.

Successful interruption of ventricular fibrillation or prevention of refractory recurrent episodes may also be facilitated by administration of bretylium tosylate, 5 mg/kg intravenously, repeated 5 to 20 minutes later if necessary (see p. 615), or amiodarone (75 to 150 mg bolus). When synchronous cardiac electrical activity is restored by countershock but contraction is ineffective—i.e., during electromechanical dissociation—the usual underlying cause is very extensive myocardial ischemia or necrosis or rupture of the ventricular free wall or septum.[984,985] If rupture has not occurred, intracardiac administration of calcium gluconate or epinephrine may promote restoration of an effective heartbeat. We do *not* usually administer bicarbonate injections to correct acidosis because of the high osmotic load they impose and the fact that hyperventilation of the patient is probably a more suitable means of clearing the acidosis.

BRADYARRHYTHMIAS

Sinus Bradycardia

(See also p. 645)

Sinus bradycardia is a common arrhythmia occurring during the early phases of AMI, and it is particularly frequent in patients with inferior and posterior infarction.[986] Observations in mobile CCUs indicate that 25 to 40 per cent of patients with AMI have electrocardiographic evidence of sinus bradycardia within the first hour after the onset of symptoms; however, 4 hours after infarction commences, the incidence of sinus bradycardia has declined to 15 to 20 per cent.[938] Stimulation of cardiac vagal afferent receptors (which are more common in the inferoposterior than the anterior or lateral portions of the left ventricle), with resulting efferent cholinergic stimulation of the heart, produces vagotonia with resultant bradycardia and hypotension. This is a manifestation of the Bezold-Jarisch reflex[987] that is mediated by the vagus nerves and occurs during reperfusion, particularly of the right coronary artery.[483,529,530,988] Often sinus bradycardia is a component of vasovagal or vasodepressor response, which may be intensified by severe pain as well as by morphine, and may be related to vasovagal syncope (see p. 863).[989]

On the basis of data obtained in experimental infarction and from some clinical observations, it appears that the increased vagal tone that produces sinus bradycardia during the early phase of AMI may actually be protective, perhaps because it reduces myocardial oxygen demands.[986] Thus, the acute mortality rate appears to be as low in patients with sinus bradycardia as in patients without this arrhythmia.

MANAGEMENT. Isolated sinus bradycardia, unaccompanied by hypotension or ventricular ectopy, should be observed rather than treated initially. In the first 4 to 6 hours following infarction, if the sinus rate is extremely slow (under 40 to 50 bpm), administration of intravenous atropine in aliquots of 0.3 to 0.6 mg every 3 to 10 minutes (with a total dose not exceeding 2 mg) to bring heart rate up to approximately 60 beats/min often abolishes the VBPs commonly associated with this degree of sinus bradycardia. Atropine often contributes to restoration of arterial pressure and hence coronary perfusion and should be employed if hypotension accompanying any degree of sinus bradycardia is present. The favorable effects of atropine may be accompanied by regression of ST-segment elevation. Elevation of the lower extremities also often elevates arterial pressure by redistributing blood from the systemic venous bed to the thorax, thereby augmenting ventricular preload, cardiac output, and arterial pressure.

Sinus bradycardia occurring more than 6 hours after the onset of the AMI is often transitory, is caused by sinus node dysfunction or atrial ischemia rather than vagal hyperactivity, is usually not accompanied by hypotension, and does not usually predispose to ventricular arrhythmias. Treatment is not required unless ventricular performance is compromised or the administration of a beta-adrenoceptor blocker or high doses of antiarrhythmic drugs (which may slow the sinus rate further) is planned. When atropine is ineffective and the patient is symptomatic and/or hypotensive, electrical pacing is indicated (see Chap. 23). In patients with depressed ventricular performance, who require the atrial contribution to ventricular filling, atrial pacing or atrioventricular sequential pacing is superior to simple ventricular pacing.[892]

ATRIOVENTRICULAR AND INTRAVENTRICULAR BLOCK

Ischemic injury can produce conduction block at any level of the AV or intraventricular conduction system. Such blocks may occur in the atrioventricular node and the bundle of His, producing various grades of AV block; in either main bundle branch, producing right or left bundle branch block; and in the anterior and posterior divisions of the left bundle, producing left anterior or left posterior (fascicular) divisional blocks. Disturbances of conduction can, of course, occur in various combinations. The mechanisms and recognition of intraventricular and atrioventricular conduction disturbances are discussed in Chapter 22.

First-Degree AV Block (see also p. 688)

First-degree AV block (Fig. 22–49, p. 688) occurs in less than 15 per cent of patients with AMI admitted to CCUs. His bundle electrocardiographic studies have shown that almost all patients with first-degree AV block have disturbances in conduction above the bundle of His, i.e., intranodal. The localization of the site of block is important because development of complete heart block and ventricular asystole is restricted almost exclusively to those patients with first-degree block in whom the conduction disturbance is *below* the bundle of His; this occurs more commonly in patients with anterior infarction and those with associated bifascicular block.[990]

First-degree AV block generally does not require specific treatment. However, if digitalis intoxication is suspected as the cause, this drug should be discontinued. Beta blockers and calcium antagonists (other than nifedipine) prolong AV conduction and may be responsible for first-degree AV block as well. However, discontinuation of these drugs in the setting of AMI has the potential of increasing ischemia and ischemic injury. Therefore, it is our practice not to decrease the dosage of these drugs unless the PR interval is greater than 0.24 sec. Only if higher-degree block or hemodynamic impairment occurs should these agents be stopped. If the block is a manifestation of excessive vagotonia and is associated with sinus bradycardia and hypotension, administration of atropine, as already outlined, may be helpful. Continued electrocardiographic monitoring is important in such patients in view of the possibility of progression to higher degrees of block.[991]

Second-Degree AV Block

MOBITZ TYPE I OR WENCKEBACH (Fig. 22–51, p. 689). Mobitz type I block occurs in up to 10 per cent of patients with AMI admitted to CCUs and accounts for about 90 per cent of all patients with AMI and second-degree AV block. This type of block (1) generally occurs within the AV node, (2) is usually associated with narrow QRS complexes, (3) is presumably secondary to ischemic injury, (4) occurs more commonly in patients with inferior than anterior myocardial infarction, (5) is usually transient and does not persist for more than 72 hours after infarction, (6) may be intermittent, and (7) rarely progresses to complete AV block (Table 37–13). First-degree and type I second-degree AV blocks do not appear to affect survival, are most commonly associated with occlusion of the right coronary artery, and are caused by ischemia of the AV node.

Specific therapy is not required in patients with second-degree AV block of the Mobitz type I variety when the ventricular rate exceeds 50 beats/min and ventricular irritability, heart failure, and bundle branch block are absent. However, if these complications develop or if the heart rate falls below approximately 50 beats/min and the patient is symptomatic, immediate treatment with atropine (0.3 to 0.6 mg) is indicated; temporary pacing systems are almost never needed in the management of this arrhythmia.

MOBITZ TYPE II (Fig. 22–52, p. 689). This is a rare conduction defect following AMI, occurring in only 10 per cent of all cases of second-degree block.[992] Thus, the overall incidence of Mobitz type II block after infarction is less than 1 per cent. In contrast to Mobitz type I block, type II second-degree block (1) usually originates from a lesion in the conduction system below the bundle of His, (2) is associated with a wide QRS complex, (3) often but not invariably reflects trifascicular block with impaired conduction distal to the bundle of His, (4) often progresses suddenly to complete AV block, and (5) is almost always associated with anterior rather than inferior infarction (Table 37–13).

Because of its potential for progression to complete heart block, Mobitz type II second-degree AV block should be treated with a temporary external or transvenous demand pacemaker with the rate set at approximately 60 beats/min.

Complete (Third-Degree) AV Block (see also p. 691)

The AV conduction system has a dual blood supply, the AV branch of the right coronary artery and the septal perforating branch from the left anterior descending coronary artery.[993] Therefore, complete AV block can occur in patients with either anterior or inferior infarction. Complete AV block develops in 5 to 15 per cent of patients with AMI[994,995]; the incidence may be even higher in patients with right ventricular infarction.[105] As with other forms of AV block, the prognosis depends on the anatomical location of the block in the conduction system and the size of the infarction.[996]

Complete heart block in patients with inferior infarction usually results from an intranodal or supranodal lesion[997] and develops gradually, often progressing from first-degree or type I second-degree block (Table 37–13). The escape rhythm is usually stable without asystole and often junctional, with a rate exceeding 40 beats/min and a narrow QRS complex in 70 per cent of cases and a slower rate and wide QRS in the others. This form of complete AV block is often transient, may be responsive to pharmacological antagonism of adenosine with methylxanthines,[998] and resolves in the majority of patients within a few days.[999] The mortality may approach 15 per cent unless right ventricular infarction is present, in which case the mortality associated with complete AV block may be more than doubled.[1000]

In patients with anterior infarction, third-degree AV block often occurs suddenly, 12 to 24 hours after the onset of infarction, although it is usually preceded by intraventricular block and often Mobitz type II (not first-degree or Mobitz type I) AV block (Table 37–13). Such patients have unstable escape rhythms with wide QRS complexes and rates less than 40 beats/min; ventricular systole may occur quite suddenly. The mortality in this group of patients is extremely high, approximately 70 to 80 per cent.[1001]

PROGNOSIS. This depends on the extent and secondarily on the anatomical site of the myocardial injury.[999,1002] Patients with inferior infarction often have concomitant ischemia or infarction of the AV node secondary to hypoperfusion of the AV node artery. However, the His-Purkinje system usually escapes injury in such individuals. Patients with inferior MI who develop AV block usually have lesions in both the right and left anterior descending coronary arteries.[1003] Likewise, patients with inferior MI and AV block have larger infarcts and more depressed right ventricular and left ventricular function than do patients with inferior infarct and no AV block. As already noted, junctional escape rhythms with narrow QRS complexes occur commonly in this setting. In patients with anterior infarction, AV block usually develops as a result of extensive septal necrosis that involves the bundle branches. The high mortality in this group of patients with slow idioventricular rhythm and wide QRS complexes is the consequence of extensive myocardial necrosis resulting in severe left ventricular failure and often shock.

Although data suggest that complete AV block is *not* an

TABLE 37–13 ATRIOVENTRICULAR (AV) CONDUCTION DISTURBANCES IN ACUTE MYOCARDIAL INFARCTION

	LOCATION OF AV CONDUCTION DISTURBANCE	
	Proximal	Distal
Site of block	Intranodal	Intranodal
Site of infarction	Inferoposterior	Anteroseptal
Compromised arterial supply	RCA (90%), LCX (10%)	Septal perforators of LAD
Pathogenesis	Ischemia, necrosis, hydropic cell swelling, excess parasympathetic activity	Ischemia, necrosis, hydropic cell swelling
Predominant type of AV nodal block	First-degree (PR > 200 ms) Mobitz type I second-degree	Mobitz type II second-degree Third-degree
Common premonitory features of third-degree AV block	(a) First–second-degree AV block (b) Mobitz I pattern	(a) Intraventricular conduction block (b) Mobitz II pattern
Features of escape rhythm following third-degree block		
(a) Location	(a) Proximal conduction system (His bundle)	(a) Distal conduction system (bundle branches)
(b) QRS width	(b) <0.12/sec*	(b) >0.12/sec
(c) Rate	(c) 45–60/min but may be as low as 30/min	(c) Often <30/min
(d) Stability of escape rhythm	(d) Rate usually stable; asystole uncommon	(d) Rate often unstable with moderate to high risk of ventricular asystole
Duration of high-grade AV block	Usually transient (2–3 days)	Usually transient but some form of AV conduction disturbance and/or intraventricular defect may persist
Associated mortality rate	Low unless associated with hypotension and/or congestive heart failure	High because of extensive infarction associated with power failure or ventricular arrhythmias
Pacemaker therapy		
(a) Temporary	(a) Rarely required; may be considered for bradycardia associated with left ventricular power failure, syncope, or angina	(a) Should be considered in patients with anteroseptal infarction and acute bifascicular block
(b) Permanent	(b) Almost never indicated because conduction defect is usually transient	(b) Indicated for patients with high-grade AV block with block in His–Purkinje system and those with transient advanced AV block and associated bundle branch block

Modified from Antman, E. M. and Rutherford, J. D.: Coronary Care Medicine: A Practical Approach. Boston: Martinus Nijhoff, 1986; Dreifus, L. S., et al.: Guidelines for implantation of cardiac pacemakers and antiarrhythmia devices. Reprinted with permission from the American College of Cardiology. J. Am. Coll. Cardiol. *18*:1, 1991.

* Some studies suggest that a wide QRS escape rhythm (>0.12 sec) following high-grade AV block in inferior infarction is associated with a worse prognosis.

RCA = right coronary artery; LCX = left circumflex coronary artery; LAD = left anterior descending coronary artery.

independent risk factor for mortality,[1004] whether temporary transvenous pacing per se improves survival of patients with anterior AMI remains controversial. Some investigators contend that ventricular pacing is useless when employed to correct complete AV block in patients with anterior infarction in view of the poor prognosis in this group regardless of therapy. We agree with others,[993,1005] however, that ventricular or AV sequential pacing is indicated in essentially all patients with AMI with complete AV block. Pacing is likely to protect against transient hypotension with its attendant risks of extending infarction and precipitating malignant ventricular tachyarrhythmias. Also pacing protects against asystole, a particular hazard in patients with anterior infarction and infranodal block. Improved survival with pacing probably occurs in only a small fraction of patients with complete AV block and anterior wall infarcts because the extensive destruction of the myocardium that almost invariably accompanies this condition results in a very high mortality rate, even in paced patients.

Given these considerations, an extremely large series of patients would be required to demonstrate the small reduction of mortality that might be achieved by pacing. The absence of data supporting such an effect, however, by no means excludes the possibility that it may be present. Although it is generally agreed that pacing is indicated in patients with inferior wall infarction and complete AV block, it is of particular importance if the ventricular rate is very slow (<40 to 50 beats/min), if ventricular irritability or hypotension is present, or if pump failure develops; atropine is only rarely of value in these patients. Only when complete heart block develops in less than 6 hours after the onset of symptoms is atropine likely to abolish the AV block or cause acceleration of the escape rhythm.[1006] In such cases the AV block is more likely to be transient and related to increases in vagal tone rather than the more persistent block seen later in the course of MI, which generally requires cardiac pacing.

Intraventricular Block

In the prethrombolytic era studies of intraventricular conduction disturbances, i.e., block within one or more of the three subdivisions (fascicles) of the His-Purkinje system (the anterior and posterior divisions of the left bundle and the right bundle, p. 121), had been reported to occur in 5 to 10 per cent of patients with AMI.[1005,1007–1009] The right bundle branch and the left posterior division have a dual blood supply from the left anterior descending and right coronary arteries, whereas the left anterior division is supplied by septal perforators originating from the left anterior descending coronary artery. Not all conduction blocks observed in patients with AMI can be considered to be complications of infarcts because almost half are already present at the time the first ECG is recorded, and they may represent antecedent disease of the conduction system.[1007]

ISOLATED LEFT ANTERIOR DIVISIONAL BLOCK (see p. 121). This occurs in 3 to 5 per cent of patients with AMI[1010] and in an additional 5 per cent of patients with associated right bundle branch block. Isolated left anterior divisional block is unlikely to progress to complete AV block.[1005,1009,1011] Mortality is increased in these patients, although not as much as in patients with other forms of conduction block.

LEFT POSTERIOR DIVISIONAL BLOCK. This occurs in only 1 to 2 per cent of patients with AMI admitted to coronary care units. The posterior fascicle is larger than the anterior fascicle, and, in general, a larger infarct is required to block it. As a consequence, mortality is markedly increased.[1012] Complete AV block is not a frequent complication of either form of isolated divisional block.[1005,1009,1011,1012]

RIGHT BUNDLE BRANCH BLOCK. This defect alone occurs in approximately 2 per cent of patients with AMI and frequently leads to AV block because it is often a new lesion, associated with anteroseptal infarction.[1007,1012] Isolated right bundle branch block is associated with an increased mortality risk in patients with anterior MI even if complete AV block does not occur, but this appears to be the case only if it is accompanied by congestive heart failure.[1007,1009,1010,1012–1015]

BIFASCICULAR BLOCK. The combination of right bundle branch block with either left anterior or posterior divisional block or the combination of left anterior and posterior divisional blocks (i.e., left bundle branch block) is known as bidivisional or bifascicular block (see p. 123). If new block occurs in two of the three divisions of the conduction system, the risk of developing complete AV block is quite high. Mortality is also high because of the occurrence of severe pump failure secondary to the extensive myocardial necrosis required to produce such an extensive intraventricular block.[1011] Left bundle branch block occurs in approximately 5 per cent of patients with AMI. Although the latter defect progresses to complete AV block only half as frequently as does right bundle branch block, it is associated with as high a mortality as right bundle branch block and the other two forms of bifascicular block[939,1009,1012,1013] and with a high late mortality. Patients with intraventricular conduction defects, particularly right bundle branch block,[1016] account for the majority of patients who develop ventricular fibrillation late in their hospital stay. However, the high mortality in these patients occurs even in the absence of high-grade AV block and appears to be related to cardiac failure and massive infarction rather than to the conduction disturbance.

Preexisting bundle branch block or divisional block is less often associated with the development of complete heart block in patients with AMI than are conduction defects acquired during the course of the infarct.[1009] Bidivisional block in the presence of prolongation of the P-R interval (first-degree AV block) may indicate disease of the third subdivision rather than of the AV node. In such cases, termed trifascicular block, nearly 40 per cent progress to complete heart block, a risk that is considerably greater than the risk of complete heart block without first-degree AV block.[1005]

Complete bundle branch block (either left or right), the combination of right bundle branch block and left anterior divisional (fascicular) block, and any of the various forms of trifascicular block are all more often associated with anterior than inferoposterior infarction. All these forms are more frequent with large infarcts and in older patients and have a higher incidence of other accompanying arrhythmias than is seen in patients without bundle branch block.[1013]

Use of Pacemakers in AMI

(See also p. 1964)

TEMPORARY PACING. Just as is the case for complete AV block, transvenous ventricular pacing has not resulted in statistically demonstrable improvement in prognosis among patients with AMI who develop intraventricular conductions defects. However, temporary pacing is advisable in some of these patients because of the high risk of developing complete AV block. This includes patients with new bilateral (bifascicular) bundle branch block, i.e., right bundle branch block with left anterior or posterior divisional block and alternating right and left bundle branch block; first-degree AV block adds to this risk. Isolated new block in only one of the three fascicles even with P-R prolongation and preexisting bifascicular block and normal P-R interval poses somewhat less risk; these patients should be monitored closely, with insertion of a temporary pacemaker deferred unless higher-degree AV block occurs.

It has been proposed on the basis of results of an analysis of several large series of well-characterized patients that the risk of developing complete heart block following AMI can be predicted.[1011] The presence (new or preexisting) of any of the following conduction disturbances is considered a risk factor: first-degree AV block, Mobitz type I second-degree AV block, Mobitz type II second-degree AV block, left anterior hemiblock, left posterior hemiblock, right bundle branch block, and left bundle branch block. Each risk factor was assigned a score of 1, and the risk score was calculated as the sum of these electrocardiographic risk factors. The incidence of complete heart block occurred as follows: risk score 0, 1.2 to 6.8 per cent incidence; risk score 1, 7.8 to 10.4 per cent incidence; risk score 2, 25.0 to 30.1 per cent incidence; and risk score 3, 36 per cent or greater incidence.[1011] Some authorities have pointed out deficiencies in this scoring system in that Mobitz type II AV block is assigned a score of only 1 point but appears to carry more significance; also there is no differentiation between preexisting and newly appearing bundle branch block.[1017]

We believe that failure to demonstrate improved prognosis statistically does not belie the potential value of pacemaker therapy; it probably reflects the overriding impact on mortality of the extensive infarction responsible for the development of the conduction abnormality and the large number of patients required to permit statistical documentation of reduction of mortality.

In assessing the need for temporary pacing (Table 37–13), the clinician must keep in mind that between 10 and 20 per cent of patients develop pacemaker-related complications.[1018] A pericardial friction rub develops in approximately 5 per cent of patients but does not necessarily indicate cardiac perforation, nor is such a finding an indication for withdrawal of the pacemaker electrode. Arrhythmias requiring cardioversion, right ventricular perforation, and local infectious complications occur in 1 to 3 per cent of cases.[1018] Pacemaker malfunction also occurs rather frequently and is, in part, related to the experience of the clinical team in managing the device and its insertion.

Although external temporary cardiac pacing was introduced in 1952,[1019] its widespread clinical use did not occur until relatively recently owing to technical refinements making the technique safe, quickly applicable, and relatively well tolerated. Noninvasive external temporary cardiac pacing is now possible routinely in conscious patients and is acceptable to many but not all patients because of the discomfort.[1020] Used in a standby mode, it is virtually free of complications and contraindications and provides an important alternative to transvenous endocardial pacing. Once it is clinically evident that continuous pacing is required, external pacing, which is generally not well tolerated for more than minutes to hours, should be replaced by a temporary transvenous pacemaker (Table 37–13).

PERMANENT PACING. The question of permanent pacing in survivors of AMI associated with conduction defects is still controversial (Table 37–13). Patients with inferior infarction with transient type II second-degree block or complete AV block without an associated intraventricular conduction defect do not appear to require permanent pacing. Some contend that prophylactic pacing makes little difference in the long-term survival of patients with AMI and bundle branch block complicated by transient high-degree block.[1021] On the other hand, in a retrospective multicenter study, survivors of AMI and bundle branch block who experienced transient high-degree (Mobitz type II second-degree, or third-degree) block had a high incidence of recurrent high-degree AV block and sudden death, and this incidence was reduced by insertion of a permanent demand pacemaker.[1005,1009] Thus, these findings suggest a role for prophylactic permanent pacing in patients with AMI and bundle branch block with transient high-degree AV block.

The question of the advisability of permanent pacemaker insertion is complicated by the fact that not all sudden deaths in this population are due to recurrent high-degree block. A high incidence of late in-hospital ventricular fibrillation occurs in CCU survivors with anteroseptal MI complicated by either right or left bundle branch block.[1016] If the propensity for this arrhythmia continued, ventricular fibrillation rather than asystole due to failure of AV conduction and of the infranodal pacemaker could be responsible for late sudden death.

Long-term pacing is often helpful when complete heart block persists throughout the hospital phase in a patient with AMI, when sinus node function is markedly impaired, or when Mobitz II second- or third-degree block occurs intermittently. When high-grade AV block is associated with newly acquired bundle branch block or other criteria of impairment of conduction system function, prophylactic long-term pacing may be justified as well. Thus, despite the difficulty of proving that long-term pacing improves survival after MI because of the high mortality associated with extensive infarction frequently responsible for high degrees of heart block, prophylactic long-term pacing is prudent.

ASYSTOLE. This arrhythmia has been reported to occur in 1 to 14 per cent of patients with AMI admitted to CCUs,[939] This wide variation in incidence reflects differences in the definition of this event. The lower incidence rates include only patients who develop asystole either as a primary event or following abnormalities of AV or intraventricular conduction, whereas the higher rates include patients who develop asystole as a terminal complication. In either event, the mortality is very high.

The presence of apparent ventricular asystole on monitor displays of continuously recorded electrocardiograms may be misleading, because the mechanism may in fact be fine ventricular fibrillation. Because of the predominance of ventricular fibrillation as the cause of cardiac arrest in this setting, initial therapy should include electrical countershock, even if definitive electrocardiographic documentation of this arrhythmia is not available. In the rare instance in which asystole can be documented to be the responsible electrophysiological disturbance, immediate transcutaneous pacing (or stimulation with a transvenous pacemaker if one is already in place) is indicated.[1020]

SUPRAVENTRICULAR TACHYARRHYTHMIAS

SINUS TACHYCARDIA (see also p. 645). This arrhythmia is typically associated with augmented sympathetic activity and may provoke transient hypertension or hypotension. Common causes are anxiety, persistent pain, left ventricular failure, fever, pericarditis, hypovolemia, pulmonary embolism, and the administration of cardioaccelerator drugs such as atropine, epinephrine, or dopamine; rarely it occurs in patients with atrial infarction. Sinus tachycardia is particularly common in patients with anterior infarction, expecially if there is significant accompanying left ventricular dysfunction.[1022] It is an undesirable rhythm in patients with AMI because it results in an augmentation of myocardial oxygen consumption, as well as a reduction in the time available for coronary perfusion, thereby intensifying myocardial ischemia and/or external myocardial necrosis. Persistent sinus tachycardia may signify persistent heart failure and under these circumstances is a poor prognostic sign associated with an excess mortality. An underlying cause should be sought and appropriate treatment instituted, e.g., analgesics for pain, diuretics for heart failure, oxygen, beta blockers and nitroglycerin for ischemia, and aspirin for fever or pericarditis.

Administration of beta-adrenoceptor blocking agents, in the dosage and manner described on page 612, may be helpful in the treatment of sinus tachycardia, particularly when this arrhythmia is a manifestation of a hyperdynamic circulation, which is seen particularly in young patients with an initial MI without extensive cardiac damage. However, beta blockade is contraindicated in patients in whom the sinus tachycardia is a manifestation of hypovolemia or of pump failure, the latter reflected by a systolic arterial pressure below 100 mm Hg, rales involving more than one-third of the lung fields, a pulmonary capillary wedge pressure exceeding 20 to 25 mm Hg, or a cardiac index below approximately 2.2 liters/min/m^2. A possible exception to this is a patient in whom persistent ischemia is believed to be the cause or the result of tachycardia—cautious administration of an ultrashort-acting beta-adrenoceptor blocker such as esmolol (25 to 200 μg/kg/min) may be tried to ascertain the patient's response to slowing of the heart rate.[416]

ATRIAL PREMATURE CONTRACTIONS (see also p. 650). Atrial premature contractions, and the atrial tachyarrhythmias (paroxysmal supraventricular tachycardia, atrial flutter, and atrial fibrillation) that they often herald, may be caused by atrial distention secondary to increases in left ventricular diastolic pressure, by pericarditis with its associated atrial epicarditis, or, less commonly, by ischemic injury to the atria[1023] and sinus node. Atrial premature beats per se are not associated with an increase in mortality,[1023] and cardiac output is unaffected. No specific therapy is needed, but it should be kept in mind that these beats may indicate excessive autonomic stimulation or the presence of overt or occult heart failure—conditions that may be assessed by physical examination, chest roentgenography, and echocardiography.

PAROXYSMAL SUPRAVENTRICULAR TACHYCARDIA (see also p. 677). This arrhythmia occurs in less than 10 per cent of patients with AMI but requires aggressive management because of the rapid ventricular rate.[1024,1025] Augmentation of vagal tone by manual carotid sinus stimulation may restore sinus rhythm. The drug of choice for paroxysmal supraventricular tachycardia in the non-AMI patient is adenosine (6 to 12 mg).[1025] Few data exist to guide therapy with adenosine in the AMI patient, but we believe that it can be used safely provided that hypotension (systolic pressure $<$100 mm Hg) is not present prior to its administration. Intravenous verapamil (5 to 10 mg), diltiazem (15 to 20 mg), or metoprolol (5 to 15 mg) are suitable alternatives in patients without significant left ventricular dysfunction. In the presence of congestive heart failure or hypotension, DC countershock or rapid atrial stimulation via a transvenous intraatrial electrode should be utilized. Although digitalis glycosides may be useful in augmenting vagal tone, thereby terminating the arrhythmia, their effect is often delayed.

ATRIAL FLUTTER AND FIBRILLATION (see also pp. 652 and 654). Atrial flutter is the least common major atrial arrhythmia associated with AMI, occurring in less than 5 per cent of patients.[1023] Atrial flutter is usually transient, and in AMI it is typically a consequence of augmented sympathetic stimulation of the atria, often occurring in patients with left ventricular failure or pulmonary emboli in whom the arrhythmia intensifies hemodynamic deterioration.[938,939,1026]

Atrial fibrillation is far more common than flutter, occurring in 10 to 15 per cent of patients with AMI.[1027,1027a] As with atrial premature contractions and atrial flutter, fibrillation is usually transient and tends to occur in patients with left ventricular failure but is also observed in patients with pericarditis and ischemic injury to the atria and right ventricular infarction.[105,1028] The increased ventricular rate and the loss of the atrial contribution to left ventricular filling result in a significant reduction in cardiac output. Atrial fibrillation during AMI is associated with increased mortality and stroke, particularly in patients with anterior wall infarction.[1024,1027,1029] However, because it is more common in patients with clinical and hemodynamic manifestations of extensive infarction and a poor prognosis, atrial fibrillation is probably a marker of poor prognosis, with only a small independent contribution to increased mortality.[1023]

Management. Atrial flutter and fibrillation in patients with AMI are treated in a manner similar to these conditions in other settings (see pp. 654 and 656). Because of the possibility that the rapid ventricular rate and hypotension associated with these arrhythmias can increase infarct size and because of the important role played by atrial contraction in the support of cardiac output in patients with AMI, treatment must be prompt, especially when the ventricular rate exceeds 100 beats/min. When hemodynamic decompensation is prominent, electrical cardioversion is indicated, beginning with 25 to 50 joules for atrial flutter and 50 to 100 joules for atrial fibrillation, with gradual increase if the initial shock is not successful. For patients without hemodynamic compromise, the first maneuver should be to slow the ventricular rate. Ideally, a beta-adrenoceptor blocker (e.g., metoprolol in 5-mg intravenous boluses every 5 to 10 minutes to a total dose of 15 to 20 mg, followed by 25 to 50 mg orally every 6 hours) should be used because of the combined effects of ischemia and sympathetic tone that are usually present in patients with atrial fibrillation. If there is concern about the patient's ability to tolerate beta blockade, esmolol may be used (see p. 610). Intravenous doses of verapamil or diltiazem (see p. 616) are attractive alternatives because of their ability to slow the ventricular rate promptly, but they should be used with caution if at all in patients with pulmonary congestion. In patients with congestive heart failure, digitalis is the principal agent used to slow the ventricular response, although the onset of its effect may be delayed for several hours. Digitalis may be supplemented by small intravenous doses of a beta blocker, which also prolongs the AV nodal refractory period: 1 to 4 mg of propranolol in divided doses is often quite effective in reducing the ventricular rate and is well tolerated, even in patients with mild heart failure and a rapid ventricular rate. An additional important option for the treatment of atrial flutter is the use of rapid atrial stimulation via a transvenous intraatrial electrode (see p. 624).[1030] Because of the increased risk of embolism in atrial fibrillation, intravenous anticoagulation with heparin should be instituted in the absence of any contraindications.

Attention should be directed to the management of the underlying cause, usually heart failure, and then a decision must be made about the advisability of antiarrhythmic therapy to restore and maintain sinus rhythm. In patients who have acute atrial flutter or fibrillation without a history of atrial fibrillation and in whom congestive symptoms are either absent or easily controlled, we usually administer intravenous procainamide (2 to 4 mg/min) for 24 to 48 hours. The goal is to achieve pharmacological cardioversion or secondarily to establish a therapeutic concentration of the drug in preparation for DC cardioversion.[1031]

In view of the mounting evidence of an increased risk of proarrhythmia from antiarrhythymic drugs prescribed for atrial fibrillation, as well as an adverse interaction between recurrent ischemia and antiarrhythmic drugs, we are reluctant to prescribe type I antiarrhythmic agents over the intermediate or long term in patients with AMI.[1032–1035] Amiodarone appears to be an increasingly attractive antiarrhythmic drug for suppression of recurrences of atrial fibrillation.[1036,1037] This drug is also useful for prevention of ventricular arrhythmias and can block the AV node should atrial fibrillation recur—all desirable features following AMI. It may be prescribed in a low dose (200 mg/day), thereby reducing the risk of toxicity. Although experience is limited, we agree with the suggestion that amiodarone is probably the most logical choice of drugs for suppression of atrial fibrillation following AMI[387,1036,1037]; often only a short course of treatment (6 weeks) is needed because the risk of atrial fibrillation decreases as time passes following infarction.

Patients with recurrent episodes of atrial fibrillation should be treated with oral anticoagulants (to reduce the risk of stroke), even if sinus rhythm is present at the time of hospital discharge, because no antiarrhythmic regimen can be relied upon to be completely effective in suppressing atrial fibrillation. In the absence of contraindications, the majority of patients should receive a beta blocker after AMI; in addition to their several other beneficial effects in MI and post-MI patients, these agents are helpful in slowing the ventricular rate should atrial fibrillation recur.

JUNCTIONAL RHYTHMS (see also p. 659). These arrhythmias are often transient, occur during the first 48 hours of the infarction, typically develop and terminate gradually, and are characterized by QRS complexes that resemble those of normally conducted beats. Retrograde P waves may be evident, or AV dissociation may occur, with the junctional rate slightly in excess of the underlying sinus rate. Junctional rhythms fall into two categories:

1. AV junctional rhythm at a rate of 35 to 60 beats/min in which the AV junctional tissue simply assumes the role of the dominant pacemaker when the sinus node is depressed. This arrhythmia is generally a benign protective escape rhythm that is commonly seen among patients with a slow sinus rate in the presence of inferior myocardial infarction. When there is hemodynamic impairment, transvenous sequential AV pacing may be required to facilitate ventricular performance and maintain adequate peripheral perfusion.

2. Accelerated junctional rhythm (nonparoxysmal junctional tachycardia) is less common and occurs when there is increased automaticity of the junctional tissue, which usurps the role of pacemaker, usually appearing at a rate of 70 to 130 beats/min. This arrhythmia is seen more commonly with inferior than anterior AMI and may also appear in patients with digitalis intoxication. In studies conducted during the prethrombolytic era, the appearance of accelerated junctional rhythm in the setting of anterior infarction was associated with a poor prognosis, but this was not observed when it occurred in patients with inferior infarction.[1038]

OTHER COMPLICATIONS

Recurrent Chest Discomfort

Evaluation of postinfarction chest discomfort may be complicated by previous abnormalities on the ECG and a vague description of the discomfort by the patient who either may be exquisitely sensitive to fleeting discomfort or may deny a potential recrudescence of symptoms. The critical task for clinicians is to distinguish recurrent angina or infarction from nonischemic causes of discomfort that might be caused by infarct expansion (see p. 1195), pericarditis, pulmonary embolism, and noncardiac conditions. Important diagnostic maneuvers include a repeat physical examination, repeat ECG, and assessment of the response to sublingual nitroglycerin, 0.4 mg. (The use of noninvasive diagnostic evaluation for recurrent ischemia in patients whose symptoms only appear with moderate levels of exertion is discussed on page 1295.)

RECURRENT ISCHEMIA AND INFARCTION. The incidence of postinfarction angina without reinfarction is between 20 and 30 per cent.[641] It does not appear to be reduced by the use of thrombolytic therapy as the management strategy during the acute phase,[33,1039] but has been reported to be lower in patients who undergo primary PTCA for AMI.[606] When accompanied by ST and T-wave changes in the same leads where Q waves have appeared, it may be due to occlusion of an initially patent vessel, reocclusion of an initially recanalized vessel,[626] or coronary spasm.[1040]

Extension of the original zone of necrosis or *reinfarction* in a separate myocardial zone can be a difficult diagnosis, especially within the first 24 hours after the index event.[173] It is more convenient to refer to both extension and reinfarction collectively under the more general term *recurrent infarction*.[387] Serum cardiac markers may still be elevated from the initial infarction, and it may not be possible to distinguish the ECG changes that are part of the normal evolution after the index infarction (see p. 1205) from those due to recurrent infarction. Because the cardiac-specific troponins (see p. 1203) remain elevated for more than 1 week following the index event, they are of less value for diagnosing recurrent infarction than are more rapidly rising and falling markers such as CK-MB. Within the first 18 to 24 hours following the initial infarction, when serum cardiac markers may not have returned to the normal range, recurrent infarction should be strongly considered when there is repeat ST-segment elevation on the ECG. Although pericarditis remains a possibility in such patients, the two can usually be distinguished by the presence of a rub and lack of responsiveness to nitroglycerin in patients with pericardial discomfort.

Beyond the first 24 hours, when serum cardiac markers such as CK-MB have usually returned to the normal range (see p. 1203), recurrent infarction may be diagnosed either by re-elevation of the CK-MB above the upper limit of normal and increased by at least 50 per cent of the previous value or the appearance of new Q waves on the ECG.[641,1041] Because of variations in patient populations and definitions of recurrent infarction, estimates of the incidence of this complication of AMI range from about 5 per cent to as high as 20 per cent within the first 6 weeks and may be somewhat higher in patients who have received thrombolytic therapy.[33,641,1042–1044] Marmor reported that recurrent infarction occurred frequently in obese females and was most common in patients with nontransmural infarction.[1045] It is apparently more common in patients with diabetes mellitus, those with a previous MI, and those with an early peaking CK-MB curve (<15 hours), but it is not predictable from the angiographic appearance of the coronary artery early after infarction—at least when thrombolytic therapy has been given.[1043]

Regardless of whether postinfarction angina is persistent or limited, its presence is important because short-term morbidity is higher among such patients; mortality may be increased if the recurrent ischemia is accompanied by ECG changes and hemodynamic compromise.[1046–1050] Recurrent infarction (due in many cases to reocclusion of the infarct-related coronary artery) carries serious adverse prognostic information because it is associated with a two to fourfold higher rate of in-hospital complications (congestive heart failure, heart block) and mortality.[626,1044,1051,1052] The mortality rate at 1 to 3 years following the initial infarction is higher in those patients who suffered from recurrent infarction during their index hospitalization.[1053,1054] Presumably, the higher mortality is related to the larger mass of myocardium whose function becomes compromised.

Of the standard therapies that are routinely prescribed during the acute phase of AMI, aspirin and beta blockers have been associated with a reduction in the incidence of recurrent infarction.[641,746,1055] The data on heparin are less convincing.[2]

Management. As with the acute phase of treatment of AMI, algorithms for management of patients with recurrent ischemic discomfort at rest center on the 12-lead ECG[387,1056] (Fig. 37–45). Those patients with ST-segment reelevation should either receive repeat thrombolysis[1057–1059] or be referred for urgent catheterization and PTCA.[1060] Insertion of an intraaortic balloon pump (see p. 1232) may help stabilize the patient while other procedures are being arranged. For patients believed to have recurrent ischemia who do not have evidence of hemodynamic compromise, an attempt should be made to control symptoms with sublingual or intravenous nitroglycerin and intravenous beta blockade to slow the heart rate to 60 beats/min.[387] When hypotension, congestive heart failure, or ventricular arrhythmias develop during recurrent ischemia, urgent catheterization and revascularization are indicated.

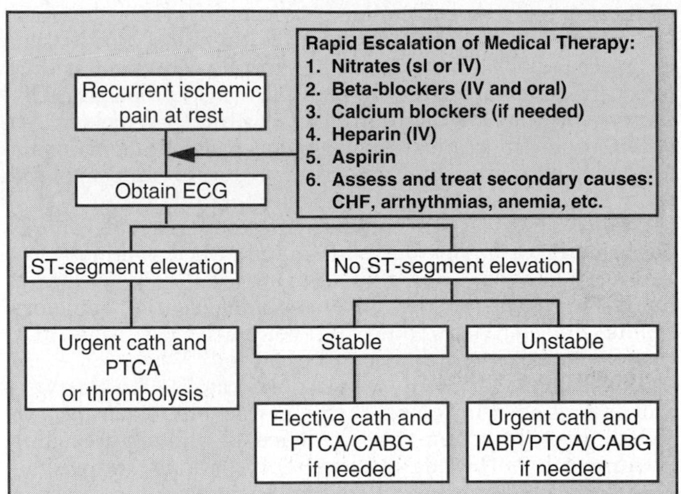

FIGURE 37–45. **Treatment of recurrent ischemic events. (From Cannon, C. P., Ganz, L. I., and Stone, P. H.: Complicated myocardial infarction. *In* Rippe, J. M., Irwin, R. S., Fink, M. P., and Cerra, F. B. [eds.]: Intensive Care Medicine. 3rd ed. Boston, Little, Brown & Company, 1995.)**

Pericardial Effusion and Pericarditis

(See also pp. 1481 and 1485)

PERICARDIAL EFFUSION. Effusions are generally detected echocardiographically, and their incidence varies with technique, criteria, and laboratory expertise. They occur in approximately 25 per cent of patients after MI.[244] Effusions are more common in patients with anterior MI and with larger infarcts and when congestive failure is present.[1061] The majority of pericardial effusions that are seen following AMI do not cause hemodynamic compromise; when tamponade occurs, it is usually due to ventricular rupture or hemorrhagic pericarditis.[233,1062]

The reabsorption rate of a postinfarction pericardial effusion is slow, with resolution often taking several months. The presence of an effusion does not indicate that pericarditis is present; although they may occur together, the majority of effusions occur without other evidence of pericarditis.[1063]

PERICARDITIS. When secondary to transmural AMI, pericarditis may produce pain as early as the first day and as late as 6 weeks after MI. The pain of pericarditis may be confused with that resulting from postinfarction angina, recurrent infarction, or both. An important distinguishing feature is the radiation of the pain to either trapezius ridge, a finding that is nearly pathognomonic of pericarditis and rarely seen with ischemic discomfort.[233] Transmural myocardial infarction, by definition, extends to the epicardial surface and is responsible for local pericardial inflammation. An acute fibrinous pericarditis (pericarditis epistenocardica) occurs commonly after transmural infarction,[1064] but the majority of patients do not report any symptoms from this process.[233] Although transient pericardial friction rubs are relatively common among patients with transmural infarction within the first 48 hours, pain or electrocardiographic changes occur much less often.[1065] However, the development of a pericardial rub appears to be correlated with a larger infarct and greater hemodynamic compromise.[1066] The discomfort of pericarditis usually becomes worse during a deep inspiration, but it may be relieved or diminished when the patient sits up and leans forward (see Chap. 43).

Although anticoagulation clearly increases the risk for hemorrhagic pericarditis early after MI, this complication has not been reported with sufficient frequency during heparinization or following thrombolytic therapy to warrant absolute prohibition of such agents when a rub is present, but the detection of a pericardial effusion on echocardiogram is usually an indication for discontinuation of anticoagulation.[233] In patients in whom continuation or initiation of anticoagulant therapy is strongly indicated (such as during cardiac catheterization or following coronary angioplasty), heightened monitoring of clotting parameters and observation for clinical signs of possible tamponade are needed. Late pericardial constriction due to anticoagulant-induced hemopericardium has been reported.[1067]

Treatment of pericardial discomfort consists of aspirin, but usually in higher doses than prescribed routinely following infarction—doses of 650 mg orally every 4 to 6 hours may be needed. Nonsteroidal antiinflammatory agents and steroids should be avoided because they may interfere with myocardial scar formation.[1068]

DRESSLER SYNDROME. Also known as the postmyocardial infarction syndrome,[1069–1071] this usually occurs 1 to 8 weeks after infarction. Its incidence is difficult to define because it often blends imperceptibly with the more common early post–myocardial infarction pericarditis. Dressler cited an incidence of 3 to 4 per cent of all AMI patients in 1957,[1072] but the incidence has decreased dramatically since that time.[1070,1073] Clinically, patients with Dressler's syndrome present with malaise, fever, pericardial discomfort, leukocytosis, an elevated sedimentation rate, and a pericardial effusion. At autopsy, patients with this syndrome usually demonstrate localized fibrinous pericarditis[1074] containing polymorphonuclear leukocytes.[1069] The cause of this syndrome is not clearly established, although the detection of antibodies to cardiac tissue has raised the notion of an immunopathological process.[1075] Treatment is with aspirin, 650 mg, as often as every 4 hours. Glucocorticosteroids or nonsteroidal antiinflammatory agents are best avoided in patients with Dressler syndrome within 4 weeks of AMI because of their potential to impair infarct healing,[1076] to cause ventricular rupture,[900] and to increase coronary vascular resistance. Aspirin in large doses is effective. Four weeks after AMI, nonsteroidal antiinflammatory agents and in occasional patients corticosteroids are necessary to control what may be severe, recurrent symptoms.

Venous Thrombosis and Pulmonary Embolism

Almost all pulmonary emboli originate from thrombi in the veins of the lower extremities (see Chap. 46); much less commonly, they originate from mural thrombi overlying an area of right ventricular infarction. Bed rest and heart failure predispose to venous thrombosis and subsequent pulmonary embolism, and both of these factors occur commonly in patients with AMI, particularly those with large infarcts. Several decades ago, at a time when patients with AMI were routinely subjected to prolonged periods of bed rest, significant pulmonary embolism was found in more than 20 per cent of patients with MI coming to autopsy,[1077] and massive pulmonary embolism accounted for 10 per cent of deaths from AMI.[1078] In recent years, with early mobilization and the widespread use of low-dose anticoagulant prophylaxis, pulmonary embolism has become an uncommon cause of death in this condition. When pulmonary embolism does occur in patients with AMI, management is generally along the lines described for noninfarction patients (see Chap. 46).

Left Ventricular Aneurysm

The term *left ventricular aneurysm* (often termed *true aneurysm*) is generally reserved for a discrete, dyskinetic area of the left ventricular wall with a broad neck (to differentiate it from pseudoaneurysm due to a contained myocardial rupture).[1079,1080] True left ventricular aneurysms probably develop in less than 5 to 10 per cent of all patients with AMI and perhaps somewhat more frequently in patients with transmural infarction (especially anterior).[1081] The wall of the true aneurysm is thinner than the rest of the left ventricle (Fig. 37–39), and it is usually composed of fibrous tissue as well as necrotic muscle, occasionally mixed with viable myocardium. Aneurysm formation presumably occurs when intraventricular tension stretches the noncontracting infarcted heart muscle, thus producing infarct expansion,[907] a relatively weak, thin layer of necrotic muscle, and fibrous tissue that bulges with each cardiac contraction. With the passage of time, the wall of the aneurysm becomes more densely fibrotic, but it continues to bulge with systole, causing some of the left ventricular stroke volume during each systole to be ineffective.

When an aneurysm is present after anterior MI, there is generally a total occlusion of a poorly collateralized left anterior descending coronary artery.[1082] An aneurysm is rarely seen with multivessel disease when there are either extensive collaterals or a nonoccluded left anterior descending artery.[1082,1083] Aneurysms usually range from 1 to 8 cm in diameter.[1084] They occur approximately four times more often at the apex and in the anterior wall than in the inferoposterior wall.[1084] The overlying pericardium is usually densely adherent to the wall of the aneurysm, which may even become partially calcified after several years. True left ventricular aneurysms (in contrast to pseudoaneurysms) rarely rupture soon after development. Late rupture, when the true aneurysm has become stabilized by the formation of dense fibrous tissue in its wall, almost never occurs.[909]

Mortality in patients with a left ventricular aneurysm is up to six times higher than in patients without aneurysms, even when compared with that in patients with comparable left ventricular ejection fraction.[1085] Death in these patients is often sudden and presumably related to the high incidence of ventricular tachyarrhythmias that occur with aneurysms.

The presence of persistent ST-segment elevation in an electrocardiographic area of infarction, classically thought to suggest aneurysm formation, actually indicates a large infarct but does not necessarily imply an aneurysm.[1086] The diagnosis of aneurysm is best made noninvasively by an echocardiographic study by radionuclide ventriculography, or at the time of cardiac catheterization by left ventriculography. With the loss of shortening from the area of the aneurysm, the remainder of the ventricle must be hyperkinetic in order to compensate. With relatively large aneurysms, complete compensation is impossible. The stroke volume falls or, if maintained, it is at the expense of an increase in end-diastolic volume, which in turn leads to increased wall tension and myocardial oxygen demand. Heart failure may ensue, and angina may appear or worsen.

TREATMENT. Aggressive management of AMI, including coronary thrombolysis, may diminish the incidence of ventricular aneurysms. Surgical aneurysmectomy generally is successful only if there is relative preservation of contractile performance in the nonaneurysmal portion of the left ventricle.[1087] In such circumstances, when the operation is performed for worsening heart failure or angina, operative mortality is relatively low and clinical improvement can be expected.[1087] Aneurysmectomy (Fig. 38–32, p. 1348) and special procedures carried out to control ventricular tachyarrhythmias occurring with left ventricular aneurysms are described on page 1348.

Left Ventricular Thrombus and Arterial Embolism

Mural thrombi (Fig. 37–46) occur in approximately 20 per cent of patients with AMI who do not receive anticoagulant therapy; the incidence rises to 40 per cent with anterior infarction and to as high as 60 per cent in patients with large anterior infarcts that involve the apex of the left ventricle.[1088–1090] The most convenient and accurate method for diagnosing left ventricular thrombosis is two-dimensional echocardiography[1090] (Fig. 3–93, p. 88). It is hypothesized that endocardial inflammation during the acute phase of infarction provides a thrombogenic surface for clots to form in the left ventricle.[1090] With extensive transmural infarction of the septum, however, mural thrombi

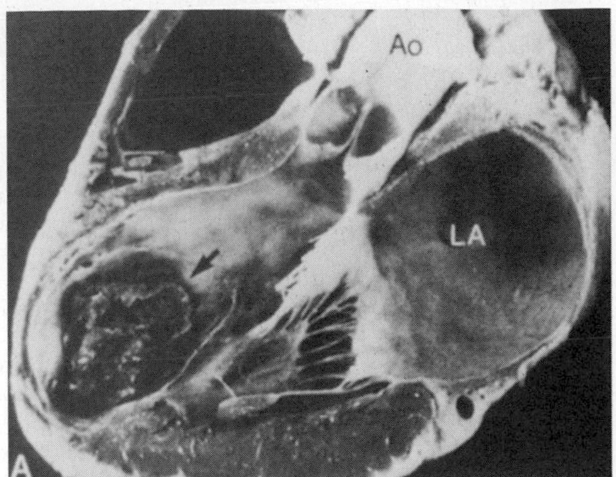

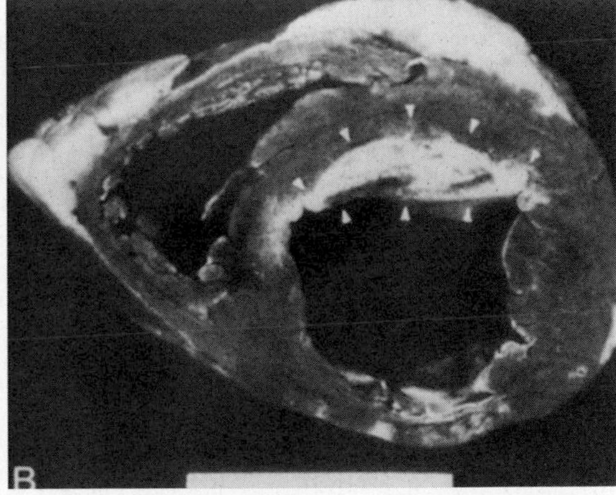

FIGURE 37–46. Postinfarction left ventricular mural thrombus. *A*, Recent thrombus (arrow) with central ulceration. Systemic embolization occurred in this patient. *B*, Old organized thrombus (arrowheads) adjacent to area of infarction. (From Edwards, W. D.: Pathology of myocardial infarction and reperfusion. *In* Gersh, B. J., and Rahimtoola, S. H. [eds.]: Acute Myocardial Infarction. New York, Chapman & Hall, 1991, p. 29.)

may overlie infarcted myocardium in both ventricles. Prospective studies have suggested that patients who develop a mural thrombus early (within 48 to 72 hours of infarction) have an extremely poor early prognosis,[912,1091] with a high mortality from the complications of a large infarction (shock, reinfarction, rupture, and ventricular tachyarrhythmia), rather than emboli from the left ventricular thrombus.[1092]

Although a mural thrombus adheres to the endocardium overlying the infarcted myocardium, superficial portions of it can become detached and produce systemic arterial emboli. Although estimates vary based on patient selection, about 10 per cent of mural thrombi result in systemic embolization.[1088,1093,1094] Echocardiographically detectable features that suggest a given thrombus is more likely to embolize include increased mobility and protrusion into the ventricular chamber, visualization in multiple views, and contiguous zones of akinesis and hyperkinesis.[1090,1095,1096]

MANAGEMENT. About two decades ago three trials involving 3500 patients showed a reduction in the incidence of *systemic embolism* in AMI from 3 per cent to 1 per cent.[668,669,1097] Over the past decade six randomized trials involving only 560 patients tested whether anticoagulant therapy reduced the incidence of *left ventricular thrombus formation*.[675,1093,1098–1101] Collectively these smaller trials showed that anticoagulation (intravenous heparin or high-dose subcutaneous heparin) reduced the development of *thrombi* by 50 per cent, but, because of the low event rate, it was not possible to demonstrate a reduction in the incidence of *systemic embolism*. Additional data from thrombolytic trials suggest that thrombolysis reduces the rate of thrombus formation and the character of the thrombi so that they are less protuberant.[675,686,1102] Of note, however, the data from thrombolytic trials are difficult to interpret because of the confounding effect of antithrombotic therapy with heparin.[1093,1098,1101] Recommendations for anticoagulation vary considerably,[1103–1106] and thrombolysis has precipitated fatal embolization.[1107] Nevertheless, anticoagulation for 3 to 6 months with warfarin is advocated for many patients with demonstrable mural thrombi[1089,1106] (see p. 1265)

Based on the available data, it is our practice to recommend anticoagulation (intravenous heparin to elevate the aPTT to 1.5 to 2.0 times control, followed by a minimum of 3 to 6 months of warfarin) in the following clinical situations: (1) an embolic event has already occurred or (2) the patient has a large anterior infarction whether or not a thrombus is visualized echocardiographically. We are also inclined to follow the same anticoagulation practice in patients with infarctions other than in the anterior distribution if a thrombus or large wall motion abnormality is detected.

Aspirin, although probably not capable of affecting thrombus size in most patients, may prevent further platelet deposition on existing thrombi[1108] and also is protective against recurrent ischemic events (see p. 1264). It should be prescribed in conjunction with warfarin to patients who are candidates for long-term anticoagulation therapy based on the indications discussed above.

CONVALESCENCE, DISCHARGE, AND POST–MYOCARDIAL INFARCTION CARE

Prolonged hospitalization and enforced bed rest for any illness may lead to complications (particularly in elderly patients) such as constipation, decubitus ulcers, excessive resorption of bone with formation of renal calculi, atelectasis, thrombophlebitis, pulmonary emboli, urinary retention, mild anemia due to repetitive blood sampling for diagnostic tests, impaired oral intake of fluids, bleeding from the gastrointestinal tract due to stress ulcers, and deconditioning of cardiovascular reflex responses to postural changes. Because of the precarious status of the heart recovering from AMI, avoidance of such complications is of primary importance. For example, constipation may lead to straining, transitory reduction of venous return and diminution of cardiac output, impaired coronary perfusion, and ventricular arrhythmias, occasionally culminating in ventricular fibrillation. Early use of a bedside commode, stool softeners, and a bed-chair regimen appear to be useful in avoiding many of the difficulties encountered previously among patients with AMI confined to bed for several weeks.

Although concern has been raised from studies in animals[1109] that early physical activity might unfavorably influence ventricular remodeling, perhaps by causing infarct extension, no evidence indicates that this concern is relevant to patients, and early mobilization appears to be warranted in most stable AMI patients. For the patient with an uncomplicated AMI, washing and personal care may begin within the first 24 hours. If the convalescence continues uneventfully, limited ambulation within the room can be begun on the second or third day (Table 37–6). Once early ambulatory activities are begun, advancement in the activity should depend on the patient's condition. A shower may be allowed some time after the third day.

TIMING OF HOSPITAL DISCHARGE. The time of discharge from the hospital is variable. As noted earlier (see p. 1227), patients who have undergone aggressive reperfusion protocols and have no significant ventricular arrhythmias, recurrent ischemia, or congestive heart failure have been safely discharged in less than 5 days. More commonly discharge occurs 5 or 6 days after admission for patients who experience no complications, who can be followed readily at home, and whose family setting is conducive to convalescence. Most complications that would preclude early discharge occur within the first day or two of admission; therefore, patients suitable for early discharge can be identified early during the hospitalization.[733,1110–1112] Several controlled trials and many uncontrolled trials of early discharge after AMI have failed to show any increase in risk in patients appropriately selected for early discharge.[736,1113]

For patients who have experienced a complication, discharge is deferred until their condition has been stable for several days and it is clear that they are responding appropriately to necessary medications such as antiarrhythmic agents, vasodilators, or positive inotropic agents or that they have undergone the appropriate work-up for recurrent ischemia.

COUNSELING. Before discharge from the hospital, all patients should receive detailed instruction concerning physical activity. Initially, this should consist of ambulation at home but avoidance of isometric exercise such as lifting; several rest periods should be taken daily. In addition, the patient should be given fresh nitroglycerin tablets and instructed in their use and should receive careful instructions about the use of any other medications prescribed. As convalescence progresses, graded resumption of activity should be encouraged. Many approaches have been utilized, ranging from formal rigid guidelines to general advice advocating moderation and avoidance of any activity that evokes symptoms. Sexual counseling is often overlooked during recovery from MI and should also be included as part of the educational process.[1114] Such counseling should begin early after AMI and should include the recommendation that sexual activity be resumed after successful completion of either early submaximal or later symptom-limited exercise stress testing.[1115]

Some evidence indicates that behavioral alteration is possible after recovery from MI and that this may improve prognosis.[1116] A cardiac rehabilitation program with supervised physical exercise and an educational component has been recommended for most MI patients following discharge.[1117] Although the overall clinical benefit of such programs continues to be debated,[1118] there is little question that most people derive considerable knowledge and psychological security from such interventions and they continue to be endorsed by experienced clinicians.[1081,1119] Meta-analyses of randomized trials of medically supervised rehabilitation programs versus usual care that were conducted in an era before widespread use of beta-adrenoceptor blockers and thrombolytics have shown a reduction in cardiovascular death but no change in the incidence of nonfatal reinfarction.[1118–1120] The physical and psychological aspects of rehabilitation of patients convalescing from AMI are discussed in Chapter 40.

RISK STRATIFICATION

The process of risk stratification following AMI occurs in three stages—initial presentation, in-hospital course (CCU, intermediate care unit), and at the time of hospital discharge. The tools used to form an integrated assessment of the patient consist of baseline demographic information, serial electrocardiograms and serum cardiac marker measurements, hemodynamic monitoring data, a variety of noninvasive tests, and, if performed, the findings at cardiac catheterization.

INITIAL PRESENTATION. Certain demographic and historical factors are associated with a poor prognosis in patients with AMI, including female gender,[56,1121] age greater than 70 years,[10,1122,1123] a history of diabetes mellitus,[1124] prior angina pectoris, and previous MI[1125–1127] (Fig. 37–47). Diabetes mellitus, in particular, appears to confer a three- to fourfold increase in risk.[1128,1129] Whether this is due to accelerated atherosclerosis or some other characteristic induced by the diabetic state (such as a larger infarct size[1130]) is unclear.[1131] (Surviving diabetic patients also experience a more complicated post–myocardial infarction course, including a greater incidence of postinfarction angina, infarct extension, and heart failure.[1124])

In addition to playing a central role in the decision pathway for management of patients with AMI based on the presence or absence of ST-segment elevation (see p. 1205), the 12-lead electrocardiogram carries important prognostic information. Mortality is greater in patients experiencing anterior wall MI than after inferior MI, even when corrected for infarct size.[1132,1133] Patients with right ventricular infarction complicating inferior infarction, as suggested by ST-segment elevation in V_4R, have a greater mortality rate than patients sustaining an inferior infarction without right ventricular involvement.[541] Patients with multiple leads showing ST elevation and a high sum of ST-segment elevation have an increased mortality, especially if their infarct is anterior in location.[10,365,1134] Patients whose ECG demonstrates persistent advanced heart block (e.g., Mobitz type II, second-degree, or third-degree AV block) or new intraventricular conduction abnormalities (bifascicular or trifascicular) in the course of an AMI have a worse prognosis than do patients without these abnormalities. The influence of high degrees of heart block is particularly important in patients with right ventricular infarction, for such patients have a markedly increased mortality.[1000] Other electrocardiographic findings that augur poorly are persistent horizontal or downsloping ST-segment depression,[1135] Q waves in multiple leads, evidence of right ventricular infarction accompanying inferior infarction,[105] ST-segment depressions in anterior leads in patients with inferior infarction,[332,540,1136] and atrial arrhythmias (especially atrial fibrillation).[538,1137]

Data from the thrombolytic era have confirmed that important determinants of short- and long-term prognosis appear to be similar in patients who have received thrombolytic therapy compared with those who did not.[538,542,1138] A constellation of clinical factors can be detected at the time of presentation to help select patients at particularly high risk of death in the first 4 to 6 weeks following AMI[538,542] (Table 37–4).

HOSPITAL COURSE. Recurrent ischemia and infarction following AMI, either in the same location as the index infarction or "at a distance" (see p. 1205), influence prognosis adversely.[330] Poor prognosis comes from the loss of viable myocardium, with the resulting larger area of infarction creating a greater compromise in ventricular function. Postinfarction angina generally connotes a less favorable prognosis because it indicates the presence of jeopardized myocardium.[1139] In the current era of aggressive revascularization, early postinfarction angina often

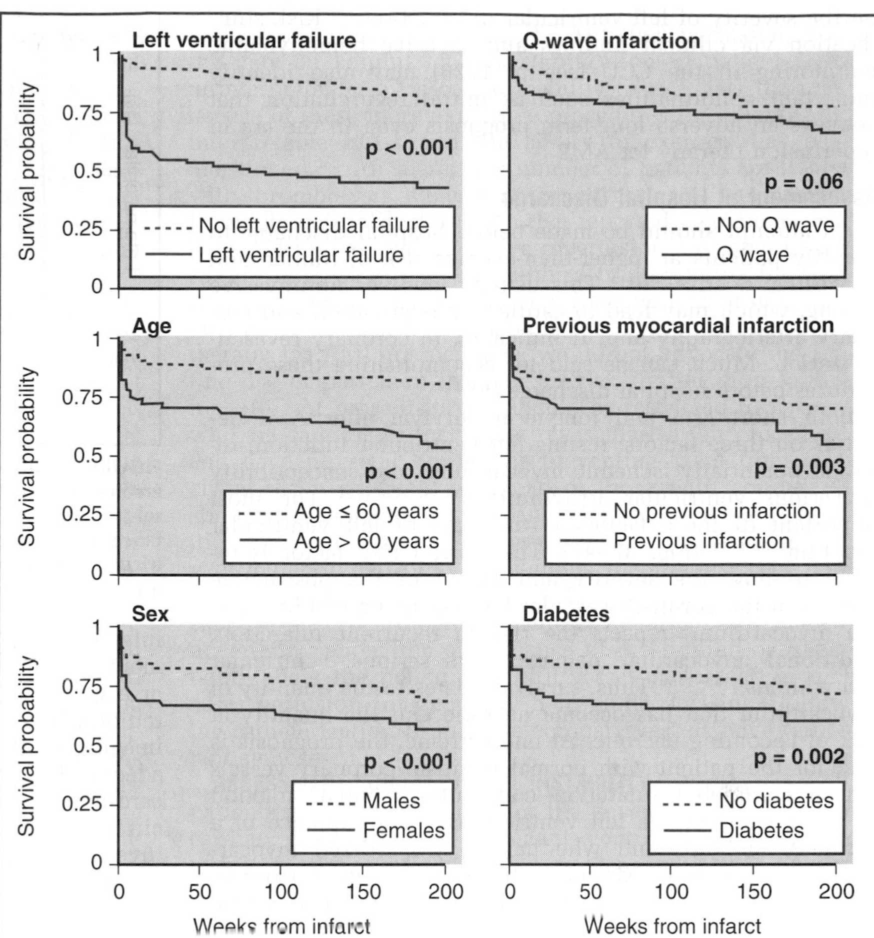

FIGURE 37–47. Kaplan-Meier survival curves illustrating the effects on prognosis after infarction or left ventricular failure, Q-wave infarction, age, gender, diabetes, and history of myocardial infarction. (From Stevenson, R., Ranjadayalan, K., Wilkinson, P., et al.: Short and long term prognosis of acute myocardial infarction since introduction of thrombolysis. BMJ *307*:349, 1993.)

leads to early interventions that tend to improve outcome, diminishing the long-term impact and significance of angina early after AMI. Silent postinfarction ischemia detected by ambulatory monitoring is associated with the same unfavorable prognosis as asymptomatic ischemia after AMI.[1140]

Patients with non-Q-wave AMI are a heterogeneous group presenting with a variety of ECG abnormalities, including ST-segment depression, T-wave inversion, or even no clear abnormality on the standard 12-lead tracing. Nevertheless, non-Q-wave AMI can be viewed as a distinct clinical entity that is due in most patients to a subtotal occlusion of the culprit coronary vessel.[1141] It appears to be increasing in frequency,[329] probably owing to a combination of factors, including more widespread use of antiischemic therapies in the population (e.g., aspirin), the increasing age of the population,[1142,1143] and more sensitive assays for serum markers that may detect smaller infarctions, altering a patient's diagnosis from unstable angina to non-Q-wave MI.[282,289] Following thrombolysis, the classification of infarcts into Q-wave and non-Q-wave categories should be deferred to the period of convalescence because of the tendency of Q waves to both appear and regress after the first 24 hours.[1141a]

Patients with non-Q-wave infarction tend to have smaller infarcts initially and a lower incidence of heart failure early after infarction.[82,1144] However, the higher incidence of subtotal occlusion of the infarct-related artery results in more frequent angina (related to the presence of preserved myocardium with marginal blood supply),[82,1144] leading to the notion that non-Q-wave AMI is an "incomplete" infarction.[1144] The hospital mortality in patients with non-Q-wave infarcts is lower than that in patients with Q-wave infarct,[82,1144] but an increased risk of reinfarction results in long-term mortality similar to that seen in patients with Q-wave AMI[1145] (Fig. 37–47). In addition to recurrent infarction, other factors associated with a higher risk of morbidity and mortality in patients with non-Q-wave infarction include advanced age, pulmonary congestion associated with infarction, persistent ST-segment depression, and easily provoked ischemic changes on a predischarge exercise test or ambulatory ECG monitor.[82,1146,1147]

The recognition of differences between the early natural histories of these two forms of infarction suggests the need for a more aggressive diagnostic approach, including a careful noninvasive search for ischemia. Often coronary arteriography followed by early coronary angioplasty or coronary bypass surgery is advised in patients who have sustained an acute non-Q-wave infarction.[82,1144]

Despite the logic inherent in this approach, no firm evidence indicates that an early invasive strategy decreases the risk of death or nonfatal infarction compared with a more conservative approach, as reported by the TIMI-IIIB investigators.[395] However, those patients in TIMI-IIIB who were randomized to early diagnostic catheterization and revascularization had lower rates of rehospitalization and a reduced need for antiischemic medications. The majority of patients in the conservative arm ultimately crossed over to a revascularization strategy within the next 12 months. These observations led us to recommend early use of angiography and, if the coronary anatomy is appropriate, either angioplasty or coronary bypass surgery in non-Q-wave AMI patients who have no contraindications to these procedures and who have access to a high-quality tertiary care center capable of performing revascularization with a low risk of complications.

Soon after CCUs were instituted, it became apparent that left ventricular function is an important early determinant of survival. Hospital mortality from AMI depends directly

bution of intervals between normal beats) less than 15 are used.[1161,1190] The ATRAMI (Autonomic Tone and Reflexes After Myocardial Infarction) study has reported that among 1284 postinfarction patients, the finding of a depressed baroreflex sensitivity value (<3.0 msec/mm Hg) was associated with about a threefold increase in the risk of mortality.[1160]

Despite the increased risk of arrhythmic events following AMI in patients who are found to have abnormal results on one or more of the noninvasive tests described above, several points should be emphasized. The low positive predictive value (<30 per cent) for the noninvasive screening tests limits their usefulness when viewed in isolation. Although the predictive value of screening tests can be improved by combining several of them together, the therapeutic implications of an increased risk profile for arrhythmic events have not been established. In the face of mortality reductions achievable with the general use of beta blockers, ACE inhibitors, aspirin, and revascularization when appropriate following infarction, it is unclear whether interventions such as amiodarone or implantable defibrillators targeted for high-risk asymptomatic patients reduce mortality.[1193] Until the results of ongoing randomized trials evaluating therapy with amiodarone following

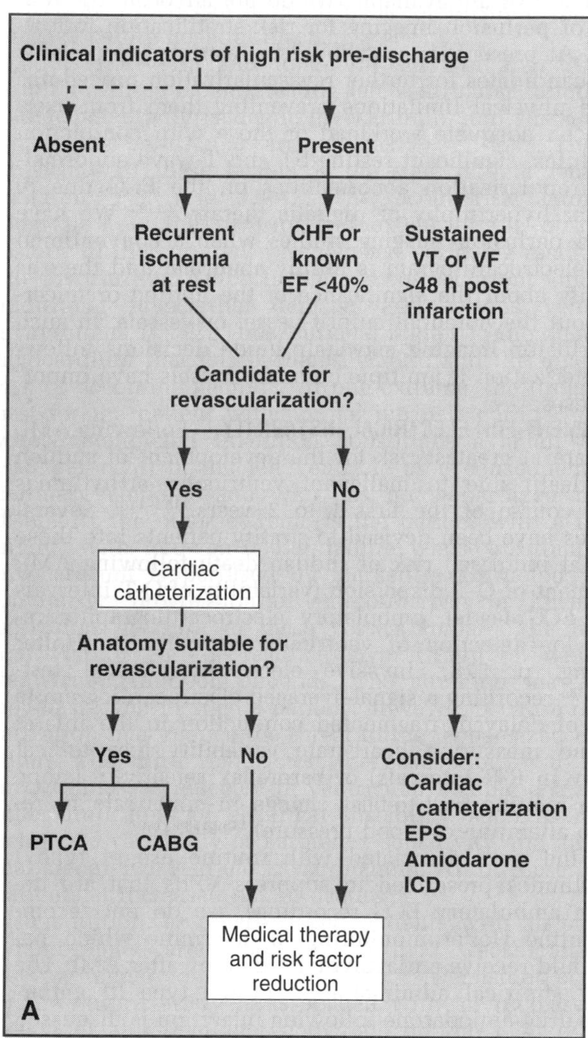

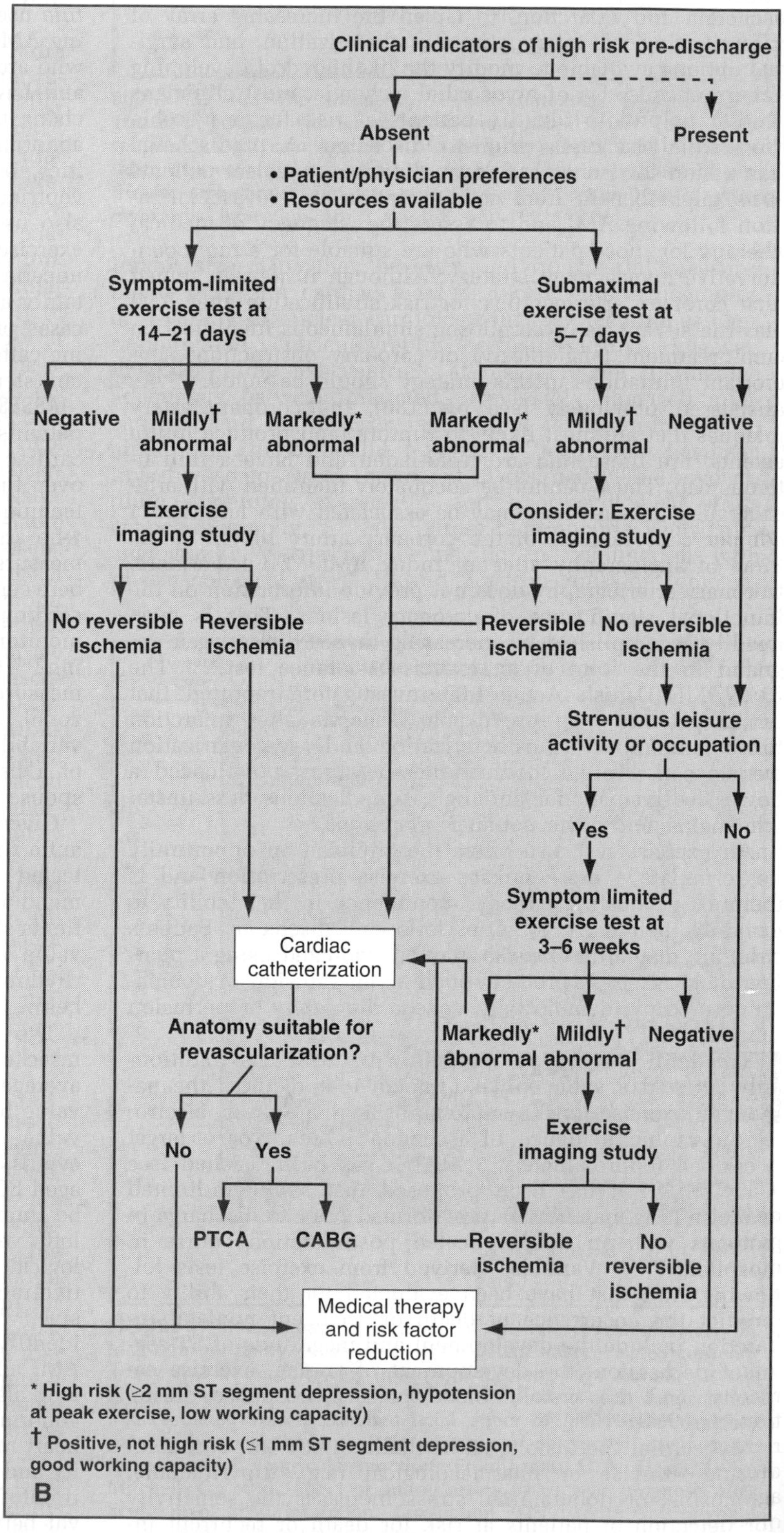

FIGURE 37–50. Management algorithm for risk stratification following acute myocardial infarction. *A*, Patients with clinical indicators of high risk at hospital discharge such as recurrent ischemia at rest or depressed left ventricular function should be considered candidates for revascularization and referral to cardiac catheterization for ultimate triage to either angioplasty/coronary artery bypass graft surgery or medical therapy and risk factor reduction. Patients with life-threatening arrhythmias such as sustained ventricular tachycardia (VT) or ventricular fibrillation (VF) should be considered for diagnostic cardiac catheterization, electrophysiology study (EPS), and management with either amiodarone or an implantable cardioconverter-defibrillator (ICD) or both. *B*, Patients without indicators of high risk at hospital discharge can be evaluated either with a submaximal exercise test prior to discharge (at 5 to 7 days) or with a symptom-limited exercise test at 14 to 21 days. Patients with either a markedly abnormal exercise test or evidence of reversible ischemia on an exercise imaging study should be referred for cardiac catheterization. Patients with a negative exercise test or no evidence of reversible ischemia on an exercise imaging study can be managed with medical therapy and risk factor reduction.

AMI (EMIAT, CAMIAT) and management strategies for patients at risk for sudden death (CABG-PATCH, MUSTT, MADIT) are available, we do not recommend the routine use of noninvasive screening measures for electrical instability. At present such tests should be considered research tools that require additional data on patient outcomes when clinicians act on the results of an abnormal finding.[2,1194]

Recommendations for Predischarge Management

An algorithm for predischarge management of patients at varying levels of risk following infarction is outlined in Figure 37-50. Initially, a judgment is made as to the presence of clinical variables indicative of high risk for future cardiac events. Patients with spontaneous episodes of ischemia or depressed left ventricular function who are considered suitable candidates for revascularization based on their overall medical condition should be referred for cardiac catheterization (Fig. 37–50*A*). The former group of patients is at increased risk of recurrent infarction (and subsequent increased mortality risk[1054]), whereas the latter group may benefit from revascularization surgery if multivessel coronary artery disease is identified at catheterization (see Chap. 38). Patients with sustained ventricular tachycardia or ventricular fibrillation that occurs more than 48 hours after the acute event (Fig. 37–50*A*) are at increased risk of sudden cardiac death and should be considered for diagnostic electrophysiology study and treatment as outlined in Chapter 22.

In the absence of high-risk clinical indicators, two management strategies are possible, and the choice between them may be influenced by patient and physician preferences and the availability of resources in the patient's local community for the necessary follow-up procedures (Fig. 37–50*B*). Initial exercise testing can use conventional electrocardiography with supplementation by a perfusion imaging study for patients with uninterpretable resting ECGs or an equivocal (i.e., mildly abnormal) initial electrocardiographic result. Submaximal exercise testing can be performed before discharge to triage patients to an early catheterization strategy or medical therapy strategy. Plans for a follow-up symptom-limited exercise test in patients without clear indications for catheterization are formulated based on the patient's life style and occupation. Patients who undergo aggressive reperfusion therapy and have an uncomplicated course in the CCU may be suitable candidates for early hospital discharge with plans for a symptom-limited exercise test 2 to 3 weeks later. Subsequent decisions about continued medical therapy or referral for cardiac catheterization can then be made as outlined in Figure 37–50*B*.

SECONDARY PREVENTION OF ACUTE MYOCARDIAL INFARCTION

(See also p. 1184)

The concept of secondary prevention of reinfarction and death after recovery from an AMI has been investigated actively for several decades. Problems in proving the efficacy of various interventions have been related both to the ineffectiveness of certain strategies and to the difficulty in proving a benefit as mortality and morbidity have improved following AMI. Nevertheless, patients who survive the initial course of AMI are at increased risk because of coronary artery disease and its complications; therefore, it is imperative that efforts be made to reduce this risk.[7,1195–1197] Although secondary prevention drug trials generally have tested one form of therapy against placebo in an attempt to demonstrate a benefit of that therapy, the physician must remember that disciplined clinical care of the individual patient is far more important than rote use of an agent found beneficial in the latest drug trial.[17]

LIFE STYLE MODIFICATION. Efforts to improve survival and the quality of life after MI that relate to life style modification of known risk factors are considered in Chapter 35. Of these, cessation of smoking and control of hypertension are probably most important. It has been shown that within 2 years of quitting smoking, the risk of a nonfatal MI in these former smokers falls to a level similar to that in patients who never smoked.[1198] Being hospitalized for an AMI is a powerful motivation for patients to cease cigarette smoking, and this is an ideal time to encourage that clearly beneficial and highly cost-effective life style change.[1199,1200] It is also an ideal time to begin to treat hypertension, to counsel patients to achieve optimal body weight, and to consider various strategies to improve the patient's lipid profile (see below).

Physicians caring for patients following an AMI need to be sensitive to the fact that some patients experience major depression following infarction, and the development of this problem is an independent risk factor for mortality.[1201] In addition, lack of an emotionally supportive network in the patient's environment following discharge is associated with an increased risk of mortality and recurrent cardiac events.[1202,1203] The precise mechanisms relating depression and lack of social support to worse prognosis after AMI are not clear, but one possibility is lack of adherence to prescribed treatments, a behavior that has been shown to be associated with increased risk of mortality following infarction.[1204] Evidence exists that a comprehensive rehabilitation program utilizing primary health care personnel who counsel patients and make home visits favorably impacts the clinical course of patients following infarction and reduces the rate of rehospitalization for recurrent ischemia and infarction.[1205] A supportive physician attitude can also have a positive impact on the rate of return to work after AMI.[1206]

MODIFICATION OF LIPID PROFILE. Compelling evidence now exists that an increased cholesterol level, and most importantly an increased LDL cholesterol level, is associated with an increased risk of coronary heart disease.[310,1207] Based on this observation and the finding in the CARE trial that lowering cholesterol reduces the risk of coronary heart disease,[1208] the Adult Treatment Panel II Guidelines recommend a target LDL cholesterol of less than 100 mg/dl in patients with clinically evident coronary heart disease.[310] This recommendation clearly applies to patients with AMI, and it is therefore important to obtain a lipid profile on admission in all patients admitted with acute infarction.[2] (It should be recalled that cholesterol levels may fall 24 to 48 hours following infarction.[307,308])

Surveys of physician practice in the past have revealed a disappointingly low rate of treatment of hypercholesterolemia in patients with proven coronary artery disease, indicating considerable room for improvement in this aspect of secondary prevention following AMI.[1209] Perhaps the most dramatic evidence favoring reduction of cholesterol in patients with clinically overt coronary heart disease is the 30 per cent reduction in total mortality and 42 per cent reduction in coronary heart disease–related deaths over 5.4 years in patients receiving simvastatin for an elevated cholesterol in the Scandinavian Simvastatin Survival Study(4S).[1210] Of particular interest was the relatively constant 35 per cent reduction in coronary death and nonfatal infarction with simvastatin across a wide range of baseline cholesterol levels.[1211]

Recommendations. All patients recovering from AMI should be considered potential candidates for modification of their lipid profile. Initial therapy should consist of an AHA Step II diet (<7 per cent of total calories as saturated fat and cholesterol <200 mg/day). We strongly advise adherence to a target LDL cholesterol of less than 125 mg/dl. This requires drug therapy in the majority of patients, and our preference at present is to prescribe an HMG CoA reductase inhibitor prior to hospital discharge (see Chap. 35) in patients with an LDL cholesterol greater than 130 on admission (Fig. 37–18).

ANTIPLATELET AGENTS. On the basis of 11 randomized trials in 20,000 patients with a prior infarction, the Antiplatelet Trialists' Collaboration reported a 25 per cent reduction in the risk of recurrent infarction, stroke, or vascular death in patients receiving prolonged antiplatelet therapy (36 fewer events for every 1000 patients treated).[9] No antiplatelet therapy proved superior to aspirin, and daily doses of aspirin between 80 and 325 mg appear to be effective.[2] Data from the Worcester Heart Attack Study suggest that when an AMI occurs in chronic users of aspirin, it is likely to be smaller and non-Q-wave in nature.[1212] Experimental data on late reperfusion in a rat model of coronary occlusion suggest that aspirin treatment following AMI increases the patency of the microvasculature in the infarcted area, resulting in less infarct expansion and thicker myocardial walls in the infarct zone.[1213] The compelling arguments cited above serve as the basis for the recommendation that all patients recovering from AMI should, in the absence of contraindications, remain on aspirin for an indefinite period.[2,17] Patients with true aspirin allergy should be treated with sulfinpyrazone (400 mg twice daily) or ticlopidine (250 mg twice daily),[9] although the data indicating that these agents reduce mortality following AMI are not nearly as robust as those for aspirin, and some recommend treating aspirin-intolerant patients with warfarin.[671]

ACE INHIBITORS. The rationale for the acute use of ACE inhibitors following AMI has been discussed earlier (see p. 1229). To prevent late remodeling of the left ventricle and also to decrease the likelihood of recurrent ischemic events,[749,758] we advocate indefinite therapy with an ACE inhibitor to all patients with clinically evident congestive heart failure, a moderate decrease in global ejection fraction, or a large regional wall motion abnormality, even in the face of a normal global ejection fraction. A decision-analytic model that tested strategy of prescription of ACE inhibitors to hypothetical 50- to 80-year-old patients with an ejection fraction of 40 per cent or less following AMI reported incremental cost-effectiveness ratios of $4,000 to $10,000 per quality-adjusted life-year (QALY).[1214] These calculations compare quite favorably with the costs of other commonly accepted medical procedures such as angioplasty for one- or two-vessel coronary artery disease ($8,000 to $111,000 per QALY).[1214]

BETA-ADRENOCEPTOR BLOCKERS. Meta-analyses of trials from the prethrombolytic era involving over 20,000 patients who received beta-adrenoceptor blockers in the convalescent phase of AMI have shown a 20 per cent reduction in long-term mortality.[7,744,748] When beta blockade is initiated early (<6 hours) in the acute phase of infarction and continued in the chronic phase of treatment, some of the benefit may result from a reduction in infarct size.[748,1215] However, in the majority of patients who have beta blockade initiated during the convalescent phase of AMI, reduction in long-term mortality is probably due to a combination of an antiarrhythmic effect (prevention of sudden death) and prevention of reinfarction.[414,745,748,1186,1216,1217]

Overviews of the results of trials of beta-adrenoceptor blockers with agonist activity have not shown a beneficial effect on mortality compared with more convincing evidence of a beneficial effect and little evidence of harm for trials of beta blockers without agonist activity (odds ratio 0.69[0.61–0.79]).[414] No differences are seen when cardioselective and noncardioselective agents are compared. The greatest mortality benefit from chronic beta blockade following AMI is seen in patients with the greatest baseline risk—those with compromised ventricular function and ventricular arrhythmias.[1186,1218] The results of the Beta-Blocker Pooling Project, in which data were examined from nine separate studies involving more than 10,000 patients, suggest a highly significant reduction in overall mortality among treated patients with pump failure.[1219]

Recommendations. Although some controversy exists regarding their utility in patients with a non-Q-wave infarction,[1219a] we remain persuaded of the benefits of immediate intravenous beta-adrenoceptor blockade (to reduce infarct size and cardiac rupture—see p. 1211) and long-term therapy with beta blockers, including patients who undergo thrombolysis or angioplasty (see below). Therefore, we begin therapy as early as possible (see p. 1228), continue treatment during hospitalization, and prescribe beta blockers at discharge, as long as contraindications (see p. 1978) are not present. Patients with a relative contraindication to beta blockade (moderate heart failure, bradyarrhythmias) undergo a monitored trial of therapy in the hospital. The dosage should be sufficient to blunt the heart rate response to stress or exercise. Much of the impact of beta blockers in preventing mortality occurs in the first weeks; treatment should commence as soon as possible.[748]

Some controversy exists as to how long patients should be treated.[1220,1221] The collective data from five trials providing information on long-term follow-up of beta-adrenoceptor blockers following infarction suggest that therapy should be continued for at least 2 to 3 years[32,1222,1223] (Fig. 37–51). At that time, if the beta blocker is well tolerated and if there is no reason to discontinue therapy, such therapy probably should be continued in most patients.

Not all patients derive the same benefit from beta blocker therapy. The cost-effectiveness of treatment in medium- or high-risk persons compares very favorably with that of many other accepted interventions such as coronary bypass surgery, angioplasty, and lipid-lowering therapy.[1221] In patients with an extremely good prognosis (first AMI, good ventricular function, no angina, negative stress test, and no complex ventricular ectopy) in whom a mortality rate of approximately 1 per cent per year can be anticipated, beta blockers would have a smaller impact on survival. However, it is our preference to prescribe beta blockers to such patients for whatever postinfarction benefit is achieved and also to have them as part of the patient's usual regimen should AMI recur at an unpredictable time in the future.

NITRATES. Although these agents are suitable for management of specific conditions following AMI such as recurrent angina or as part of a treatment regimen for congestive heart failure, little evidence indicates that they reduce mortality when prescribed on a routine basis to all patients with infarction.[757,761]

ANTICOAGULANTS (see also p. 1828). At least three theoretical reasons exist for anticipating that anticoagulants might be beneficial in the long-term management of pa-

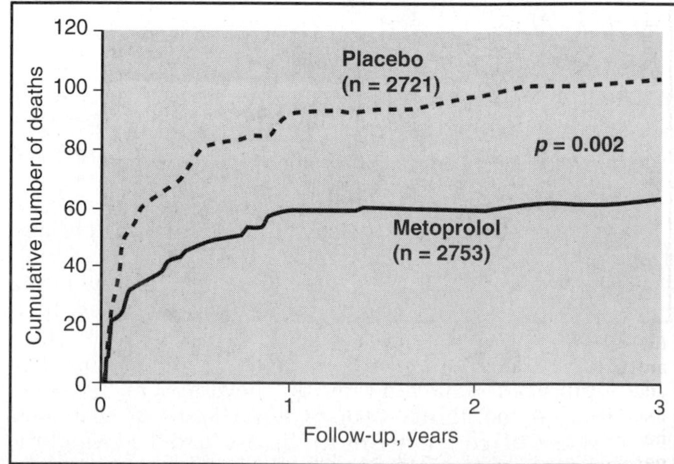

FIGURE 37–51. Prevention of sudden death with long-term beta blockade following MI. Analysis of pooled data from 5 trials in which long-term metoprolol therapy was used after MI revealed a 40 per cent reduction in incidence of sudden cardiac death in both men and women. (From Olsson, G., Wikstrand, J., Warnold, I., et al.: Metoprolol-induced reduction in postinfarction mortality: Pooled results from five double-blind randomized trials. Eur. Heart J. *13*:28, 1992.)

tients after AMI: (1) Because the coronary occlusion responsible for the AMI is often due to a thrombus, anticoagulants might be expected to halt, slow progression, or prevent the development of new thrombi elsewhere in the coronary arterial tree. (2) Anticoagulants might be expected to diminish the formation of mural thrombi and resultant systemic embolization (see p. 1256). (3) Anticoagulants might be expected to reduce the incidence of venous thrombosis and pulmonary embolization.

After several decades of evaluation, the weight of evidence now suggests that anticoagulants have a favorable effect on late mortality, stroke, and reinfarction among patients hospitalized with AMI[7,1224–1226] (Fig. 37–52). Long-term anticoagulant therapy has also been shown to be a cost-effective intervention following AMI, with the major cost savings coming from reductions in the rate of recurrent infarction and related interventions.[1227]

Previous small trials of aspirin versus oral anticoagulation have led to conflicting results, with no clear consensus regarding superiority of either antithrombotic strategy.[1228,1229] The APRICOT Investigators reported that after initially successful thrombolysis, aspirin-treated patients had lower rates of reinfarction, need for revascularization, and mortality than did coumadin-treated patients.[546] As expected, cost-effectiveness calculations show that aspirin is associated with a very favorable economic profile, but its true efficacy compared with or combined with oral anticoagulation remains unknown.[1230] The Coumadin Aspirin Reinfarction Study (CARS) was discontinued prematurely due to lack of evidence of benefit of reduced-dose aspirin (80 mg daily) with either 1 or 3 mg of warfarin daily compared with aspirin 160 mg alone daily. Data on the relative benefits of aspirin versus a combination of aspirin plus warfarin will be forthcoming from the ongoing Combination Hemotherapy and Mortality Prevention (CHAMP) Study.[1230]

Therefore, at present we recommend routine use of aspirin in all AMI patients without contraindications and add warfarin to patients with clear indications for anticoagulation such as deep vein thrombosis, pulmonary embolism, mural thrombus seen at echocardiography, a large regional wall motion abnormality (especially anterior) seen at echocardiography even in the absence of a visualized thrombus, atrial fibrillation, and a history of embolic cerebrovascular accident.

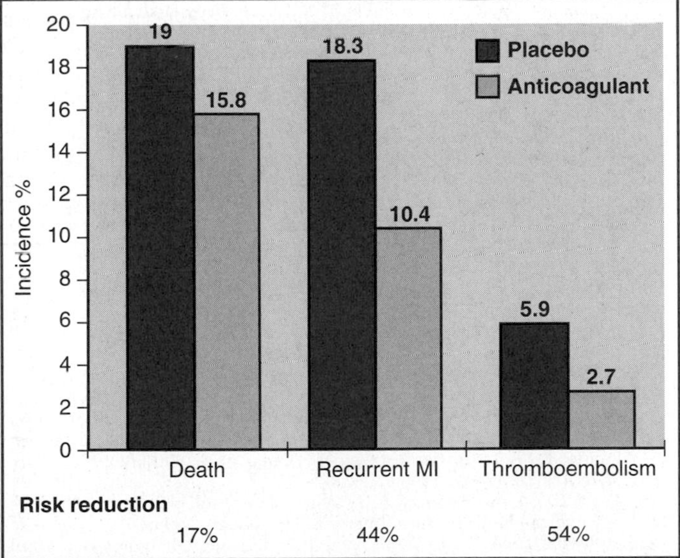

FIGURE 37–52. Meta-analysis of trials of patients who received oral anticoagulant therapy compared with control subjects. These results add to the evidence that long-term warfarin therapy reduces the risks for death, recurrent MI, and thromboembolism. In WARIS, the risk for hemorrhage was 0.6 per cent per year for major hemorrhage and 3.3 per cent for minor hemorrhage; however, it will be of considerable interest to see whether lower levels of anticoagulation (Coumadin, 1 to 3 mg) in conjunction with small amounts of aspirin (80 to 160 mg/d) is safe and effective. This possibility is being tested in the CARS and CHAMP studies. (Adapted from Devine, N., Azarnia, N., Nelson, K., et al.: Long-term anticoagulants in post myocardial infarction patients: A meta-analysis. Circulation *86*:I-259, 1992. Copyright 1992 American Heart Association.)

CALCIUM ANTAGONISTS (see also p. 1231). At present we do not recommend the routine use of calcium antagonists for secondary prevention of infarction. A possible exception is a patient who cannot tolerate a beta-adrenoceptor blocker because of adverse effects on bronchospastic lung disease but who has well-preserved left ventricular function; such patients may be candidates for a rate-slowing calcium antagonist such as diltiazem or verapamil.

ANTIARRHYTHMICS. Although it has been recognized for decades that antiarrhythmic therapy can control atrial and ventricular arrhythmias effectively in many patients, careful reviews of clinical trials following AMI have reported an increased risk of mortality with type I drugs.[1231,1232] The most notable postinfarction trial in this area was the Cardiac Arrhythmia Suppression Trial (CAST), which tested whether encainide, flecainide, or moricizine for suppression of ventricular arrhythmias detected on ambulatory electrocardiographic monitoring would reduce the risk of cardiac arrest and death over the long term. Both the first phase of the trial (encainide or flecainide versus placebo) and the second phase of the trial (moricizine versus placebo) were stopped prematurely because of increased mortality in the active treatment groups.[1232–1234] The mechanism of the increased risk following AMI remains a subject of investigation, but one hypothesis that has been put forth is an adverse interaction between recurrent ischemia and the presence of an antiarrhythmic drug because the risk of death or cardiac arrest was greater in patients with a non-Q-wave AMI than with Q-wave AMI.[1034] Sodium channel blockade by antiarrhythmics may exacerbate electrophysiological differences between subepicardial and subendocardial zones of myocardium, rendering the latter more susceptible to ischemic injury.[1234a]

Subsequent to CAST, another postinfarction prophylactic antiarrhythmic drug trial was undertaken with oral D-sotalol (Survival With ORal D-sotalol = SWORD). This trial was designed to test the hypothesis that prophylactic administration of D-sotalol to patients with depressed left ventricular function (ejection fraction $\leq$ 40 per cent) and either a recent (6 to 42 days) or remote (>42 days) AMI would reduce total mortality. SWORD also was stopped prematurely after enrollment of only 3121 of a planned 6400 patients because statistical evidence of increased mortality emerged in the active treatment group.[1235]

Four prospective, randomized, placebo-controlled trials compared the empirical prophylactic use of amiodarone versus placebo following AMI (Fig. 37–53). A meta-analysis of these trials revealed an encouraging 55 per cent reduction in sudden death and 46 per cent reduction in total mortality.[1236] The Canadian Amiodarone Myocardial Infarction Trial (CAMIAT) showed that amiodarone reduced VPD frequency in patients with recent MI; this correlated with a reduction in arrhythmic death or resuscitation from ventricular fibrillation. However, 42 per cent of patients discontinued amiodarone during maintenance therapy in CAMIAT because of intolerable side effects. The European Amiodarone Myocardial Infarction Trial (EMIAT) showed a reduction in arrhythmic death following MI in patients with depressed left ventricular function, but there was no reduction in total mortality or other cardiovascular-related mortality.

At the present time, the *routine* use of antiarrhythmic agents (including amiodarone) cannot be recommended. Given the data cited earlier on the protective effects of beta-adrenoceptor blockers against sudden death (see p. 1228) and the ability of aspirin to reduce the risk of reinfarction (see p. 1827), it is unclear that additional mortality reductions would be achieved by the empirical addition of amiodarone in the patient who is convalescing from an AMI and is free of symptomatic sustained ventricular arrhythmias. Whether subgroups of patients with indicators

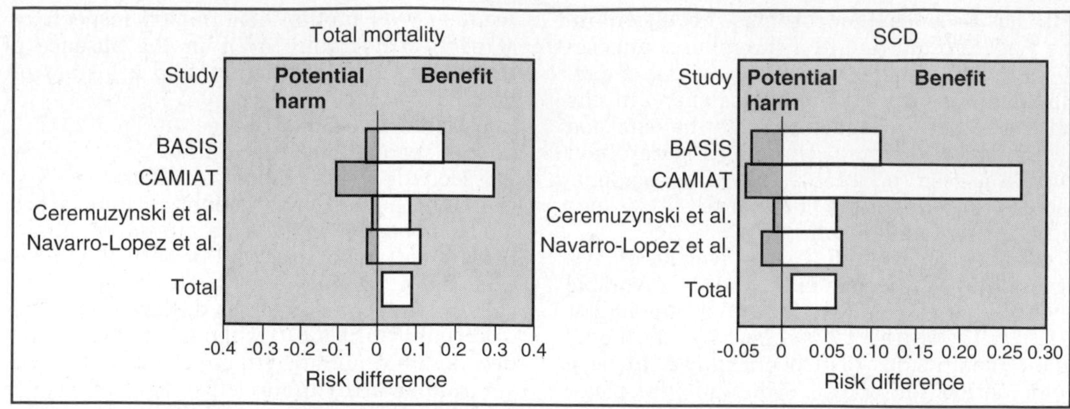

FIGURE 37–53. Amiodarone trials after infarction. Four prospective, randomized, placebo-controlled trials have investigated the benefits of empiric long-term amiodarone prophylaxis following MI. Data from the individual studies are plotted along with the pooled estimate using meta-analytic techniques. The two plots depict the 95 per cent confidence intervals for the risk differences describing the effects of amiodarone on total mortality and sudden cardiac death. Plots of this nature depict benefits from the active therapy (amiodarone) to the right of the vertical line and potential harm to the left. Total mortality in the placebo-treated group was 11.2 per cent, compared with 6.1 per cent in the amiodarone-treated group. This indicates a relative reduction in total mortality of nearly 46 per cent and an absolute reduction ranging from 1.3 per cent to 8.2 per cent, explained almost entirely by the reduction in sudden death from 6.9 per cent in the placebo group to 3.1 per cent in the amiodarone group. (From Zarembski, D. G., Nolan, P. E., Jr., Slack, M. K., et al.: Empiric long-term amiodarone prophylaxis following myocardial infarction: A meta-analysis. Arch. Intern. Med. *153*:2661, 1993.)

of high risk of sudden death, such as abnormal heart rate variability or reduced baroreflex sensitivity, should be treated and if so by what strategy remains to be determined.

HORMONE REPLACEMENT THERAPY (see also p. 1708). Estrogen replacement therapy has been reported to be helpful in the primary prevention of coronary heart disease,[1237] improves the coronary artery disease risk factor profile in postmenopausal women,[1238,1238a] and appears to reduce mortality in women with moderate coronary heart disease.[1239] However, the decision to prescribe hormone replacement therapy is often a complex one that involves weighing risks of breast cancer versus modification of a coronary artery disease risk factor profile.[1240] At present we recommend consideration of hormone replacement therapy in postmenopausal women who have suffered an AMI.

Acknowledgment

Drs. Richard Pasternak and Burton Sobel co-authored this chapter with one of the present authors in the third and fourth editions of this textbook. Portions of the chapter appearing in the fourth edition have been retained. The important influence of Drs. Pasternak and Sobel on this chapter is gratefully acknowledged.

REFERENCES

CHANGING PATTERNS IN CLINICAL CARE

1. American Heart Association: Heart and Stroke Facts: 1996Statistical Supplement. Dallas, American Heart Association, 1996, pp. 1-23.
2. Committee to Develop Guidelines for the Management of Patients with Acute Myocardial Infarction: Guidelines for the management of patients with acute myocardial infarction: A report of the American College of Cardiology/American Heart Association Task Force on Practice Guidelines. J. Am. Coll. Cardiol. *(in press).*
3. Weinstein, M. C., Coxson, P. G., and Wilman, L.: Forecasting coronary heart disease incidence, mortality, and cost: The Coronary Heart Disease Policy Model. Am. J. Public Health *77*:1417, 1987.
4. Goldman, L.: Cost-awareness in medicine. *In* Isselbacher, K. H., Braunwald, E., Wilson, J. D., et al. (eds.): Harrison's Principles of Internal Medicine. New York, McGraw-Hill Book Co., 1994, p. 38.
5. Every, N. R., Fihn, S. D., Maynard, C., et al.: Resource utilization in treatment of acute myocardial infarction: Staff-model health maintenance organization versus fee-for-service hospitals. J. Am. Coll. Cardiol. *26*:401,1995.
5a. The Task Force on the Management of Acute Myocardial Infarction of the European Society of Cardiology: Acute myocardial infarction: prehospital and in-hospital management. Eur. Heart J. *17*:43, 1996.
6. Yusuf, S., Sleight, P., Held, P., et al.: Routine medical management of acute myocardial infarction: Lessons from overviews of recent randomized controlled trials. Circulation *82*(Suppl. II):117, 1990.
7. Antman, E., Lau, J., Kupelnick, B., et al.: A comparison of results of meta-analyses of randomized control trials and recommendations of clinical experts. JAMA *268*:240, 1992.
8. Lau, J., Antman, E. M., Jimenez-Silva, J., et al.: Cumulative meta-analysis of therapeutic trials for myocardial infarction. N. Engl. J. Med. *327*:248, 1992.
9. Antiplatelet Trialists' Collaboration: Collaborative overview of randomized trials of antiplatelet therapy. I. Prevention of death, myocardial infarction, and stroke by prolonged antiplatelet therapy in various categories of patients. BMJ *308*:81, 1994.
10. Fibrinolytic Therapy Trialists (FTT) Collaborative Group: Indications for fibrinolytic therapy in suspected acute myocardial infarction: Collaborative overview of early mortality and major morbidity results from all randomised trials of more than 1000 patients. Lancet *343*:311, 1994.
11. Rogers, W. J.: What is the optimal tool to define appropriate therapy: The randomized clinical trial, meta-analysis, or outcomes research? Commentary. Cur. Opin. Cardiol. *9*:401, 1994.
12. Rogers, W., Bowlby, L., Chandra, N., et al.: Treatment of myocardial infarction in the United States (1990 to 1993): Observations from the National Registry of Myocardial Infarction. Circulation *90*:2103, 1994.
13. Hlatky, M.: Observational databases. *In* Califf, R. M., Mark, D. B., and Wagner, G. S. (eds.): Acute Coronary Care. 2nd ed. St. Louis, Mosby-Year Book, 1995, p. 145.
14. Kupersmith, J., Holmes-Rovner, M., Hogan, A., et al.: Cost-effectiveness analysis in heart disease. Part I. General principles. Prog. Cardiovasc. Dis. *37*:161, 1994.
15. Mark, D. B., Hlatky, M. A., Califf, R. M., et al.: Cost effectiveness of thrombolytic therapy with tissue plasminogen activator as compared with streptokinase for acute myocardial infarction. N. Engl. J. Med. *332*:1418, 1995.
16. Goldman, L.: Cost and quality of life: Thrombolysis and primary angioplasty. J. Am. Coll. Cardiol. *25*:38S, 1995.
17. Julian, D.: The practical implications of clinical trials: Putting it all together. *In* Julian, D., and Braunwald, E. (eds.): Management of Acute Myocardial Infarction. London, W. B. Saunders Company, 1994, p. 407.
18. Walsh, J. T., Gray, D., Keating, N. A., et al.: ACE for whom? Implications for clinical practice of post-infarct trials. Br. Heart J. *73*:470, 1995.
19. Antman, E. M., and Califf, R. M.: Clinical trials and meta-analysis. *In* Smith, T. W. (ed.): Cardiovascular Therapeutics. Philadelphia, W. B. Saunders Company, 1996.
20. Asch, D. A., and Hershey, J. C.: Why some health policies don't make sense at the bedside. Ann. Intern. Med. *122*:846, 1995.
21. Rothwell, P. M.: Can overall results of clinical trials be applied to all patients? Lancet *345*:1616, 1995.
22. de Vreede, J. J. M., Gorgels, A. P. M., Verstraaten, G. M. P., et al.: Did prognosis after acute myocardial infarction change during the past 30 years? A meta-analysis. J. Am. Coll. Cardiol. *18*:698, 1991.
23. Naylor, C. D., and Chen, E.: Population-wide mortality trends among patients hospitalized for acute myocardial infarction: The Ontario experience, 1981 to 1991. J. Am. Coll. Cardiol. *24*:1431, 1994.
24. Behar, S., Goldbourt, U., Barbash, G., et al.: Twenty-five-year mortality rate decrease in patients in Israel with a first episode of acute myocardial infarction. Am. Heart J. *130*:453, 1995.
24a. Gheorghiade, M., Razumma, P., Borzak, S., et al.: Decline in the rate of hospital mortality from acute myocardial infarction: Impact of changing management strategies. Am. Heart J. *131*:250, 1996.
25. Whitney, E. J., Shear, C. L., Mantell, G., et al.: The case for unstable

angina pectoris as a primary endpoint in primary prevention studies. Am. J. Cardiol. *70*:738, 1992.

26. Davidson, C.: Cardiac rehabilitation in the district hospital. *In* Jones, D., and West, R. (eds.): Cardiac Rehabilitation. London, BMJ Publishing Group, 1995, p. 144.
27. Pell, S., and Fayerweather, W. E.: Trends in the incidence of myocardial infarction and in associated mortality and morbidity in a large employed population, 1957–1983. N. Engl. J. Med. *312*:1005, 1985.
28. Younis, L. T., Miller, D. D., and Chaitman, B. R.: Preoperative strategies to assess cardiac risk before noncardiac surgery. Clin. Cardiol. *18*:447, 1995.
29. Mason, J. J., Owens, D. K., Harris, R. A., et al.: The role of coronary angiography and coronary revascularization before noncardiac vascular surgery. JAMA *273*:1919, 1995.
30. Antman, E. M.: General hospital management. *In* Julian, D. G., and Braunwald, E. (eds.): Management of Acute Myocardial Infarction. Philadelphia, W. B. Saunders Company, 1994, p. 29.
31. Rentrop, K. P.: Restoration of anterograde flow in acute myocardial infarction: The first 15 years. J. Am. Coll. Cardiol. *25*:1S, 1995.
32. Yusuf, S., Wittes, J., and Friedman, L.: Overview of results of randomized clinical trials in heart disease. I. Treatments following myocardial infarction. JAMA *260*:2088, 1988.
33. The GUSTO Investigators: An international randomized trial comparing four thrombolytic strategies for acute myocardial infarction. N. Engl. J. Med. *329*:673, 1993.
34. Madsen, J. K., and Hansen, J. F.: Mortality of patients excluded from the Danish Verapamil Infarction Trial II: The DAVIT-II Study Group. Eur. Heart J. *14*:377, 1993.
35. Pashos, C. L., Newhouse, J. P., and McNeil, B. J.: Temporal changes in the care and outcomes of elderly patients with acute myocardial infarction, 1987 through 1990. JAMA *270*:1832, 1993.
36. Udvarhelyi, I. S., Gatsonis, C., Epstein, A. M., et al.: Acute myocardial infarction in the Medicare population: Process of care and clinical outcomes. JAMA *268*:2530, 1992.
37. Maggioni, A., Maseri, A., Fresco, C., et al.: Age-related increase in mortality among patients with first myocardial infarctions treated with thrombolysis. N. Engl. J. Med. *329*:1442, 1993.
38. White, H. D., Granger, C., Gore, J., et al.: Older age is associated with a large increase in mortality and total stroke, but not non-fatal disabling stroke: Results of the GUSTO trial. Circulation *90*(Suppl. I):563, 1994.
39. McClellan, M., McNeil, B. J., and Newhouse, J. P.: Does more intensive treatment of acute myocardial infarction in the elderly reduce mortality? Analysis using instrumental variables. JAMA *272*:859, 1994.
40. Latini, R., Avanzini, F., Zuanetti, G., et al.: Changing patterns of pharmacological treatment after myocardial infarction: The GISSI experience. J. Am. Coll. Cardiol. *23*:210A, 1994.
41. Antman, E. M., Cannon, C. P., Mueller, J., et al.: Do clinical trial results influence physician drug use in myocardial infarction? Circulation *90*(Suppl. I):167, 1994.
42. Sial, S. H., Malone, M., Freeman, J. L., et al.: Beta blocker use in the treatment of community hospital patients discharged after myocardial infarction. J. Gen. Intern. Med. *9*:599, 1994.
43. Kennedy, H. L., and Rosenson, R. S.: Physician use of beta-adrenergic blocking therapy: A changing perspective. J. Am. Coll. Cardiol. *26*:547, 1995.
44. Meehan, T. P., Hennen, J., Radford, M. J., et al.: Process and outcome of care for acute myocardial infarction among Medicare beneficiaries in Connecticut: A quality improvement demonstration project. Ann. Intern. Med. *122*:928, 1995.
44a. Krumholz, H. M., Radford, M. J., Ellerbeck, E. F., et al.: Aspirin in the treatment of acute myocardial infarction in elderly Medicare beneficiaries. Patterns of use and outcomes. Circulation *92*:2841, 1995.
45. Pashos, C. L., Normand, S. T., Garfinkle, J. B., et al.: Trends in the use of drug therapies in patients with acute myocardial infarction: 1988 to 1992. J. Am. Coll. Cardiol. *23*:1023, 1994.
46. Ellerbeck, E. F., Jencks, S. F., Radford, M. J., et al.: Quality of care for Medicare patients with acute myocardial infarction: A four-state pilot study from the Cooperative Cardiovascular Project. JAMA *273*:1509, 1995.
47. Rouleau, J. L., Moye, L. A., Pfeffer, M. A., et al.: A comparison of management patterns after acute myocardial infarction in Canada and the United States. N. Engl. J. Med. *328*:779, 1993.
48. Pilote, L., Racine, N., and Hlatky, M. A.: Differences in the treatment of myocardial infarction in the United States and Canada. Arch. Intern. Med. *154*:1090, 1994.
49. Pilote, L., Califf, R. M., Sapp, S., et al.: Regional variation across the United States in the management of acute myocardial infarction. N. Engl. J. Med. *333*:565, 1995.
50. Guadagnoli, E., Hauptman, P. J., Ayanian, J. Z., et al.: Variation in the use of cardiac procedures after acute myocardial infarction. N. Engl. J. Med. *333*:573, 1995.
51. Ketley, D., and Woods, K. L.: Impact of clinical trials on clinical practice: Example of thrombolysis for acute myocardial infarction. Lancet *342*:891, 1993.
52. Ayanian, J., Hauptman, P., Guadagnoli, E., et al.: Knowledge and practices of generalist and specialist physicians regarding drug therapy for acute myocardial infarction. N. Engl. J. Med. *331*:1136, 1994.
52a. Mark, D. B., Naylor, C. D., Hlatky, M. A., et al.: Use of medical resources and quality of life after acute myocardial infarction in Canada and the United States. N. Engl. J. Med. *331*:1130, 1994.
53. Lincoff, A. M., Califf, R. M., Ellis, S. G., et al.: Thrombolytic therapy for women with myocardial infarction: Is there a gender gap? J. Am. Coll. Cardiol. *22*:1780, 1993.
54. Krumholz, H. M., Douglas, P. S., Lauer, M. S., et al.: Selection of patients for coronary angiography and coronary revascularization early after myocardial infarction: Is there evidence for a gender bias? Ann. Intern. Med. *116*:785, 1992.
55. Becker, R. C., Terrin, M., Ross, R., et al.: Comparison of clinical outcomes for women and men after acute myocardial infarction. Ann. Intern. Med. *120*:638, 1994.
56. Bueno, H., Almazan, A., Lopez-Sendon, J. L., et al.: Influence of sex on the short-term outcome of elderly patients with a first acute myocardial infarction. Circulation *92*:1133, 1995.
57. White, H. D., Barbash, G. I., Modan, M., et al.: After correcting for worse baseline characteristics, women treated with thrombolytic therapy for acute myocardial infarction have the same mortality and morbidity as men except for a high incidence of hemorrhagic stroke. Circulation *88*:2097, 1993.
58. Peterson, E. D., Wright, S. M., Daley, J., et al.: Racial variation in cardiac procedure use and survival following acute myocardial infarction in the Department of Veterans Affairs. JAMA *271*:1175, 1994.

PATHOLOGY OF ACUTE MYOCARDIAL INFARCTION

58a. Fallon, J. T.: Pathology of myocardial infarction and reperfusion. *In* Fuster, V., Ross, R., and Topol, E. J. (eds.): Atherosclerosis and Coronary Artery Disease. Philadelphia, Lippincott-Raven, 1996, pp. 791–796.
59. Constantinides, P.: Plaque fissures in human coronary thrombosis. J. Athero. Res. *6*:1, 1966.
60. Davies, M. J., and Thomas, A. C.: Plaque fissuring—the cause of acute myocardial infarction, sudden ischemic death, and crescendo angina. Br. Heart J. *53*:363, 1985.
61. Falk, E.: Coronary thrombosis: Pathogenesis and clinical manifestations. Am. J. Cardiol. *68*:28B, 1991.
62. Willerson, J. T.: Conversion from chronic to acute coronary heart disease syndromes: Role of platelets and platelet products. Tex. Heart Inst. J. *22*:13, 1995.
63. Davies, M. J., Richardson, P. D., Woolf, N., et al.: Risk of thrombosis in human atherosclerotic plaques: Role of extracellular lipid, macrophage, and smooth muscle cell content. Br. Heart J. *69*:377, 1993.
64. Falk, E., Shah, P. K., and Fuster, V.: Pathogenesis of plaque disruption. *In* Fuster, V., Ross, R., and Topol, E. J. (eds.): Atherosclerosis and Coronary Artery Disease. Philadelphia, Lippincott-Raven, 1996, pp. 492–510.
65. Falk, E., Shah, P. K., and Fuster, V.: Coronary plaque disruption. Circulation *92*:657, 1995.
66. Kragel, A. H., Reddy, S. G., Wittes, J. T., et al.: Morphometric analysis of the composition of atherosclerotic plaques in the four major epicardial coronary arteries in acute myocardial infarction and in sudden coronary death. Circulation *80*:1747, 1989.
67. Roberts, W. C.: Preventing and arresting coronary atherosclerosis. Am. Heart J. *130*:580, 1995.
67a. Stary, H. C.: The histological classification of atherosclerotic lesions in human coronary arteries. *In* Fuster, V., Ross, R., and Topol, E. J. (eds.): Atherosclerosis and Coronary Artery Disease. Philadelphia, Lippincott-Raven, 1996, pp. 463–474.
68. Libby, P.: Molecular basis of the acute coronary syndromes. Circulation *91*:2844, 1995.
69. Falk, E.: Plaque rupture with severe pre-existing stenosis precipitating thrombosis: Characteristics of coronary atherosclerotic plaque underlying fatal occlusion thrombi. Br. Heart J. *50*:127, 1983.
70. Wilson, R. F., Holida, M. D., and White, C. W.: Quantitative angiographic morphology of coronary stenoses leading to myocardial infarction or unstable angina. Circulation *73*:286, 1986.
71. Weiss, E. J., Bray, P. F., Schulman, S. P., et al.: Fibrinogen receptor polymorphism Pl^{A2}: An inherited platelet risk factor for early coronary thrombotic events. Circulation *92*(Suppl.):I-30, 1995.
72. Falk, E.: Morphologic features of unstable atherothrombotic plaques underlying acute coronary syndrome. Am. J. Cardiol. *63*:114E, 1989.
73. Galis, Z., Sukhova, G., Lark, M., et al.: Increased expression of matrix metalloproteinases and matrix degrading activity in vulnerable regions of human atherosclerotic plaques. J. Clin. Invest. *94*:2493, 1994.
74. Kovanen, P. T., Kaartinen, J., and Paavonen, T.: Infiltrates of activated mast cells at the site of coronary atheromatous erosion or rupture in myocardial infarction. Circulation *92*:1084, 1995.
75. Constantinides, P.: Infiltrates of activated mast cells at the site of coronary atheromatous erosion or rupture in myocardial infarction. Circulation *92*:1083, 1995.
76. Barger, A., Beeuwkes, I. R., Lainey, L., et al.: Hypothesis: Vasa vasorum and neovascularization of human coronary arteries. N. Engl. J. Med. *310*:175, 1984.
77. Cheng, G. C., Loree, H. M., Kamm, R. D., et al.: Distribution of circumferential stress in ruptured and stable atherosclerotic lesions: A structural analysis with histopathologic correlation. Circulation *87*:1179, 1993.
78. Waxman, S., and Muller, J. E.: Risk factors for an acute ischemic event. *In* Califf, R. (ed.): Acute Myocardial Infarction and Other Acute Ischemic Syndromes. Vol 8 of Braunwald, E. (series ed.): Atlas of Heart Diseases. Philadelphia, Current Science, 1996, pp. 2–2.14.

79. Braunwald, E.: Morning resistance to thrombolytic therapy. Circulation *91*:1604, 1995.
80. Danchin, N.: Is myocardial revascularization for tight coronary stenoses always necessary? Viewpoint. Lancet *342*:224, 1993.
81. Schoen, F. J.: The heart. *In* Cotran, R. S., Kumar, V., and Robbins, S. L. (eds.): Pathologic Basis of Disease. Philadelphia, W. B. Saunders Company, 1994, p. 517.
82. Piérard, L. A.: Non-Q-wave, incomplete infarction. *In* Julian, D., and Braunwald, E. (eds.): Management of Acute Myocardial Infarction. London, W. B. Saunders Ltd., 1994, p. 315.
83. Pfeffer, M. A., and Braunwald, E.: Ventricular remodeling after myocardial infarction: Experimental observations and clinical implications. Circulation *81*:1161, 1990.
84. Vaughan, D. E., and Pfeffer, M. A.: Ventricular remodeling following myocardial infarction and angiotensin-converting enzyme and ACE inhibitors. *In* Fuster, V., Ross, R., and Topol, E. J. (eds.): Atherosclerosis and Coronary Artery Disease. Philadelphia, Lippincott-Raven, 1996, pp. 1193–1205.
85. Freifeld, A. G., Schuster, E. H., and Bulkley, B. H.: Nontransmural versus transmural myocardial infarction. Am. J. Med. *75*:423, 1983.
86. Ambrose, J. A., Tannenbaum, M. A., Alexopoulos, D., et al.: Angiographic progression of coronary artery disease and the development of myocardial infarction. J. Am. Coll. Cardiol. *12*:56, 1988.
87. Jain, D., Crawley, J. C., Lahiri, A., et al.: Indium-111 antimyosin images compared with triphenyl tetrazolium chloride staining in a patient six days after myocardial infarction. J. Nucl. Med. *31*:231, 1990.
88. Ytrehus, K., and Downey, J. M.: Experimental models assessing the physiology of myocardial ischemia. Curr. Opin. Cardiol. *8*:581, 1993.
89. Vivaldi, M. T., Kloner, R. A., and Schoen, F. J.: Triphenyltetrazolium staining of irreversible ischemic injury following coronary artery occlusion in rats. Am. J. Pathol. *121*:522, 1985.
90. Buja, L. M., and McAllister, H. A., Jr.: Coronary artery disease: Anatomic abnormalities. *In* Willerson, J. T., and Cohn, J. N. (eds.): Cardiovascular Medicine. New York, Churchill Livingstone, 1995, p. 316.
91. Kloner, R. A., Ellis, S. G., Lange, R., et al.: Studies of experimental coronary artery reperfusion: Effects on infarct size, myocardial function, biochemistry, ultrastructure and microvascular damage. Circulation *68*:1, 1983.
92. Matsuda, M., Fujiwara, J., Onodera, T., et al.: Quantitative analysis of infarct size, contraction band necrosis, and coagulation necrosis in human autopsied hearts with acute myocardial infarction after treatment with selective intracoronary thrombolysis. Circulation *76*:981, 1987.
93. Schlesinger, M. J., and Reiner, L.: Focal myocytolysis of the heart. Am. J. Physiol. *31*:443, 1955.
94. Buja, L. M., and Willerson, J. T.: Clinicopathologic correlates of acute ischemic heart disease syndromes. Am. J. Cardiol. *47*:343, 1981.
95. Gasser, R. N. A., and Klein, W.: Contractile failure in early myocardial ischemia: Models and mechanisms. Cardiovasc. Drugs Ther. *8*:813, 1994.
96. Gertz, S. D., Kalan, J. M., Kragel, A. N., et al.: Cardiac morphologic findings in patients with acute myocardial infarction treated with tissue plasminogen activator. Am. J. Cardiol. *65*:953, 1990.
97. Adams, J., III, Abendschein, D., and Jaffe, A.: Biochemical markers of myocardial injury: Is MB creatine kinase the choice for the 1990s? Circulation *88*:750, 1993.
98. Roberts, W. C., Potkin, B. N., Solus, D. E., et al.: Mode of death, frequency of healed and acute myocardial infarction, number of major epicardial coronary arteries severely narrowed by atherosclerotic plaque, and heart weight in fatal atherosclerotic coronary artery disease: Analysis of 889 patients studied at necropsy. J. Am. Coll. Cardiol. *15*:196, 1990.
99. Betriu, A., Castaner, A., Sanz, G. A., et al.: Angiographic finding 1 month after myocardial infarction: A prospective study of 259 survivors. Circulation *65*:1099, 1982.
100. DeWood, M. A., Spores, J., Notske, R. N., et al.: Prevalence of total coronary artery occlusion during the early hours of transmural myocardial infarction. N. Engl. J. Med. *303*:897, 1980.
101. Ong, L., Reiser, P., Coromilas, J., et al.: Left ventricular function and rapid release of creatine kinase MB in acute myocardial infarction: Evidence for spontaneous reperfusion. N. Engl. J. Med. *309*:1, 1983.
102. DeWood, M. A., Notske, R. N., Simpson, C. S., et al.: Prevalence and significance of spontaneous thrombolysis in transmural myocardial infarction. Eur. Heart J. *6*:33, 1985.
103. Ellis, S., Alderman, E. L., Cain, K., et al.: Morphology of left anterior descending coronary territory lesions as a predictor of anterior myocardial infarction: A CASS registry study. J. Am. Coll. Cardiol. *13*:1481, 1989.
104. Little, W. C., Constantinescu, M., Applegate, R. J., et al.: Can coronary angiography predict the site of a subsequent myocardial infarction in patients with mild-to-moderate coronary artery disease? Circulation *78*:1157, 1988.
105. Kinch, J. W., and Ryan, T. J.: Right ventricular infarction. N. Engl. J. Med. *330*:1211, 1994.
106. Mittal, S. R.: Isolated right ventricular infarction. Int. J. Cardiol. *46*:53, 1994.
107. Rackley, C. E., Russell, R. O., Jr., Mantle, J. A., et al.: Right ventricular infarction and function. Am. Heart J. *101*:215, 1981.
108. Setaro, J. F., and Cabin, H. S.: Right ventricular infarction. Cardiol. Clin. *10*:69, 1992.
109. Nielsen, F. E., Andersen, H. H., Gram-Hansen, P., et al.: The relationship between ECG signs of atrial infarction and the development of supraventricular arrhythmias in patients with acute myocardial infarction. Am. Heart J. *123*:69, 1992.
110. Ventura, T., Colantonio, D., Leocata, P., et al.: Isolated atrial myocardial infarction: Pathological and clinical features in 10 cases. Cardiologia *36*:345, 1991.
111. Alonso-Orcajo, N., Izquierdo-Garcia, F., and Simarro, E.: Atrial rupture and sudden death following atrial infarction. Int. J. Cardiol. *46*:82, 1994.
112. Iga, K., Konishi, T., and Kusukawa, R.: Intracardiac thrombi in both the right atrium and right ventricle after acute inferior-wall myocardial infarction. Int. J. Cardiol. *46*:169, 1994.
113. Yasuda, S., Nonogi, H., Miyazaki, S., et al.: Hyposecretion of atrial natriuretic peptide due to associated right atrial infarction in a patient with acute right ventricular infarction? Eur. Heart J. *15*:718, 1994.
114. Conti, C. R.: Myocardial infarction: Thoughts about pathogenesis and the role of coronary artery spasm. Am. Heart J. *110*:187, 1985.
115. Vincent, G. M., Anderson, J. L., and Marshall, H. W.: Coronary spasm producing coronary thrombosis and myocardial infarction. N. Engl. J. Med. *309*:220, 1983.
116. Christian, T. F., Gibbons, R. J., Clements, I. P., et al.: Estimates of myocardium at risk and collateral flow in acute myocardial infarction using electrocardiographic indexes with comparison to radionuclide and angiographic measures. J. Am. Coll. Cardiol. *26*:388, 1995.
117. Hirai, T., Fujita, M., Nakajima, H., et al.: Importance of collateral circulation for prevention of left ventricular aneurysm formation in acute myocardial infarction. Circulation *79*:791, 1989.
118. Markis, J. E., Brewer, C. C., Alderman, J., et al.: Myocardial infarction without early coronary angiographic evidence of occlusion: The NHLBI thrombolysis in myocardial infarction trial (TIMI). Circulation *72*(Suppl. III):56S, 1985.
119. Schwartz, H., Leiboff, R. H., Bren, G. B., et al.: Temporal evolution of the human coronary collateral circulation after myocardial infarction. J. Am. Coll. Cardiol. *4*:1088, 1984.
119a. Harrison, D. C.: Nonatherosclerotic coronary disease. *In* Fuster, V., Ross, R., and Topol, E. J. (eds.): Atherosclerosis and Coronary Artery Disease. Philadelphia, Lippincott-Raven, 1996, pp. 757–772.
120. Dollar, A. L., Pierre-Louis, M. L., McIntosh, C. L., et al.: Extensive multifocal myocardial infarcts from cloth emboli after replacement of mitral and aortic valves with cloth-covered caged-ball prostheses. Am. J. Cardiol. *64*:410, 1989.
121. Ackermann, D. M., Hyma, B. A., and Edwards, W. D.: Malignant neoplastic emboli to the coronary arteries. Hum. Pathol. *18*:955, 1987.
122. Obarski, T. P., Loop, F. D., Cosgrove, D. M., et al.: Frequency of acute myocardial infarction in valve repairs versus valve replacement for pure mitral regurgitation. Am. J. Cardiol. *65*:887, 1990.
123. Parrillo, J. E., and Fauci, A. S.: Necrotizing vasculitis, coronary angiitis, and the cardiologist. Am. Heart J. *99*:547, 1980.
124. Spodick, D. H.: Inflammation and the onset of myocardial infarction. Ann. Intern. Med. *99*:547, 1985.
125. Miklozek, C. L., Crumpacker, C. S., Royal, H. D., et al.: Myocarditis presenting as acute myocardial infarction. Am. Heart J. *115*:768, 1988.
126. Connolley, J. E., Eldridge, F. L., Calvin, J. W., et al.: Proximal coronary artery obstruction. N. Engl. J. Med. *271*:213, 1964.
127. Roberts, W. C., MacGregor, R. R., DeBlanc, H. J., et al.: The prepulseless phase of pulseless disease, or pulseless disease with pulses. Am. J. Med. *46*:313, 1969.
128. Pick, R. A., Glover, M. U., and Vieweg, W. V. R.: Myocardial infarction in a young woman with isolated coronary arteritis. Chest *82*:378, 1982.
129. van Camp, G., Deschamps, P., Mestrez, F., et al.: Adult onset Kawasaki disease diagnosed by the echocardiographic demonstration of coronary aneurysms. Eur. Heart J. *16*:1155, 1995.
130. Lie, J. L., Failoni, D. D., and Davis, D. C. J.: Temporal arteritis with giant cell aortitis, coronary arteritis, and myocardial infarction. Arch. Pathol. Lab. Med. *110*:857, 1986.
131. Joensuu, H.: Acute myocardial infarction after heart irradiation in young patients with Hodgkin's disease. Chest *95*:388, 1989.
132. Huang, S., Kumar, G., Steele, H. D., et al.: Cardiac involvement in pseudoxanthoma elasticum. Am. Heart J. *74*:680, 1967.
133. Isner, J. M., and Chokshi, S. K.: Cardiac complications of cocaine abuse. Annu. Rev. Med. *42*:133, 1991.
134. Kloner, R. A., Hale, S., Alker, K., et al.: The effects of acute and chronic cocaine use on the heart. Circulation *85*:407, 1992.
135. Chakko, S., and Myerburg, R. J.: Cardiac complications of cocaine abuse. Clin. Cardiol. *18*:67, 1995.
136. Ashchi, M., Wiedemann, H. P., and James, K. B.: Cardiac complication from use of cocaine and phenylephrine in nasal septoplasty. Arch. Otolaryngol. Head Neck Surg. *121*:681, 1995.
137. Bulbul, Z. R., Rosenthal, D. N., and Kleinman, C. S.: Myocardial infarction in the perinatal period secondary to maternal cocaine abuse: A case report and literature review. Arch. Pediatr. Adoles. Med. *148*:1092, 1994.
138. Lange, R. A., and Willard, J. E.: The cardiovascular effects of cocaine. Heart Dis. Stroke *2*:136, 1993.
139. Killam, A. L.: Cardiovascular and thrombosis pathology associated with cocaine use. Hematol. Oncol. Clin. North Am. *7*:1143, 1993.
140. Alpert, J. S.: Myocardial infarction with angiographically normal coronary arteries. Arch. Intern. Med. *154*:265, 1994.
141. Glover, M. V., Kuber, M. T., Warren, S. E., et al.: Myocardial infarction before age 36: Risk factor and arteriographic analysis. Am. J. Cardiol. *49*:1600, 1982.

142. Ciraulo, D. A., Bresnahan, G. F., Frankel, P. S., et al.: Transmural myocardial infarction with normal coronary angiograms and with single vessel coronary obstruction: Clinical-angiographic features and five-year follow-up. Chest *83*:196, 1983.
143. Braunwald, E.: Coronary spasm and acute myocardial infarction—New possibility for treatment and prevention. N. Engl. J. Med. *299*:1301, 1978.
144. Makino, H., and Al-Saidr, H.: Myocardial infarction in patients with mitral valve prolapse and normal coronary arteries. J. Am. Coll. Cardiol. *1*:661, 1983.
145. Yeager, S. B., and Freed, M. D.: Myocardial infarction as a manifestation of polycythemia in cyanotic heart disease. Am. J. Cardiol. *53*:952, 1984.
146. Martin, C. R., Cobb, C., Tatter, D., et al.: Acute myocardial infarction in sickle cell anemia. Arch. Intern. Med. *143*:830, 1983.
147. Bergeron, G. A., Goldsmith, R., and Schiller, N. B.: Myocardial infarction, severe, reversible ischemia, and shock following excess thyroid administration in a woman with normal coronary arteries. Arch. Intern. Med. *148*:1450, 1988.
148. Carson, P., Oldroyd, K., and Phadke, K.: Myocardial infarction due to amphetamine. BMJ *294*:1525, 1987.
149. Pecora, M. J., Roubin, G. S., Cobbs, B. W., et al.: Presentation and late outcome of myocardial infarction in the absence of angiographically significant coronary artery disease. Am. J. Cardiol. *62*:363, 1988.
150. Raymond, R., Lynch, J., Underwood, D., et al.: Myocardial infarction and normal coronary aortography: A 10 year clinical and risk analysis of 74 patients. J. Am. Coll. Cardiol. *11*:471, 1988.

PATHOPHYSIOLOGY OF ACUTE MYOCARDIAL INFARCTION

151. Tennant, R., and Wiggins, C. J.: The effect of coronary occlusion on myocardial contraction. Am. J. Physiol. *112*:351, 1935.
152. Theroux, P., Franklin, D., Ross, J., Jr., et al.: Regional myocardial function during acute coronary artery occlusion and its modification by pharmacologic agents in the dog. Circ. Res. *35*:896, 1974.
153. Herman, M. V., Heinle, R. A., Klein, M. D., et al.: Localized disorders in myocardial contraction. N. Engl. J. Med. *227*:222, 1967.
154. Swan, H. J. C., Forrester, J. S., Diamond, G., et al.: Hemodynamic spectrum of myocardial infarction and cardiogenic shock. Circulation *45*:1097, 1972.
155. Forrester, J. S., Wyatt, H. L., Daluz, P. L., et al.: Functional significance of regional ischemic contraction abnormalities. Circulation *54*:64, 1976.
156. Low, W. Y., Chen, Z., Guth, B., et al.: Mechanisms of augmented segment shortening in nonischemic areas during acute ischemia of the canine left ventricle. Circ. Res. *56*:351, 1985.
157. Bourdillon, P. D. V., Broderick, T. M., Williams, E. S., et al.: Early recovery of regional left ventricular function after reperfusion in acute myocardial infarction assessed by serial two-dimensional echocardiography. Am. J. Cardiol. *63*:641, 1989.
158. Schuster, E. H., and Bulkley, B. H.: Ischemia at a distance after acute myocardial infarction: A cause of early postinfarction angina. Circulation *62*:509, 1980.
159. Cortina, A., Ambrose, J. A., Prieto-Granada, J., et al.: Left ventricular function after myocardial infarction: Clinical and angiographic correlations. J. Am. Coll. Cardiol. *5*:619, 1985.
160. White, H. D., Norris, R. M., Brown, M. A., et al.: Left ventricular end-systolic volume as the major determinant of survival after recovery from myocardial infarction. Circulation *76*:44, 1987.
161. Braunwald, E., and Pfeffer, M. A.: Ventricular enlargement and remodeling following acute myocardial infarction: Mechanisms and management. Am. J. Cardiol. *68*:1D, 1991.
162. Braunwald, E., and Kim, C. B.: Late establishment of patency of the infarct-related artery. *In* Julian, D., and Braunwald, E. (eds.): Acute Myocardial Infarction. London, W. B. Saunders Ltd., 1994, p. 147.
163. Pfeffer, M. A., Lamas, G. A., Vaughan, D. E., et al.: Effect of captopril on progressive ventricular dilatation after anterior myocardial infarction. N. Engl. J. Med. *319*:80, 1988.
164. Jeremy, R. W., Hackworthy, R. A., Bautovich, G., et al.: Infarct artery perfusion and changes in left ventricular volume in the month after acute myocardial infarction. J. Am. Coll. Cardiol. *9*:989, 1987.
165. Hirsch, A. T., Talsnecs, C. E., Schunkert, H., et al.: Tissue specific activation of cardiac angiotensin converting enzyme in experimental heart failure. Circ. Res. *69*:475, 1991.
166. Rackley, C. E., Russell, R. O., Jr., et al.: Modern approach to the patient with acute myocardial infarction. Curr. Probl. Cardiol. *1*:49, 1977.
167. Waters, D. D., DaLuz, P., Wyatt, H. L., et al.: Early changes in regional and global left ventricular function induced by graded reduction in regional coronary perfusion. Am. J. Cardiol. *39*:537, 1977.
168. Pfeffer, J. M., Pfeffer, M. A., Fletcher, P. J., et al.: Progressive ventricular remodeling in rat with myocardial infarction. Am. J. Physiol. *260*:H1406, 1991.
169. Weisman, H. F., Bush, D. E., Mannisi, J. A., et al.: Cellular mechanisms of myocardial infarct expansion. Circulation *78*:186, 1988.
170. Pirolo, J. S., Hutchins, G. M., and Moore, G. W.: Infarct expansion: Pathologic analysis of 204 patients with a single myocardial infarct. J. Am. Coll. Cardiol. *7*:349, 1986.
171. Pfeffer, M. A.: Left ventricular remodeling after acute myocardial infarction. Annu. Rev. Med. *46*:455, 1995.
172. Picard, M. H., Wilkins, G. T., Gillam, L. D., et al.: Immediate regional endocardial surface expansion following coronary occlusion in the canine left ventricle: Disproportionate effects of anterior versus inferior ischemia. Am. Heart J. *121*:753, 1991.
173. Weisman, H. F., and Healy, B.: Myocardial infarct expansion, infarct extension, and reinfarction: Pathophysiologic concepts. Prog. Cardiovasc. Dis. *30*:73, 1987.
174. Jugdutt, B. I., and Michorowski, B. L.: Role of infarct expansion in rupture of the ventricular septum after acute myocardial infarction: A two-dimensional echocardiographic study. Clin. Cardiol. *10*:641, 1987.
175. Schuster, E. H., and Bulkley, B. H.: Expansion of transmural myocardial infarction: A pathophysiologic feature in cardiac rupture. Circulation *60*:1532, 1979.
176. Abernathy, M., Sharpe, N., Smith, H., et al.: Echocardiographic prediction of left ventricular volume after myocardial infarction. J. Am. Coll. Cardiol. *17*:1527, 1991.
177. McKay, R. G., Pfeffer, M. A., Pasternak, R. C., et al.: Left ventricular remodeling after myocardial infarction: A corollary. Circulation *74*:693, 1986.
178. Dambrink, J.-H. E., Sippens Groenewegen, A., van Gilst, W. H., et al.: Association of left ventricular remodeling and nonuniform electrical recovery expressed by nondipolar QRST integral map patterns in survivors of a first anterior myocardial infarction. Circulation *92*:300, 1995.
179. Ginzton, L. E., Conant, R., Rodrigues, D. M., et al.: Functional significance of hypertrophy of the noninfarcted myocardium after myocardial infarction in humans. Circulation *80*:816, 1989.
180. Lavie, C. J., O'Keefe, J. H., Jr., Chesebro, J. H., et al.: Prevention of late ventricular dilatation after acute myocardial infarction by successful thrombolytic reperfusion. Am. J. Cardiol. *66*:31, 1990.
181. Braunwald, E.: The open-artery theory is alive and well—again. N. Engl. J. Med. *329*:1650, 1993.
182. Hammerman, H., Kloner, R. A., Hale, S., et al.: Dose-dependent effects of short-term methylprednisone on myocardial infarct extent, scar formation, and ventricular function. Circulation *68*:446, 1983.
183. Cortese, D., and Viggiano, R. W.: The lungs in acute myocardial infarction. *In* Gersh, B. J., and Rahimtoola, S. H. (eds.): Acute Myocardial Infarction. New York, Elsevier, 1991, p. 398.
184. Biddle, T. L., Yu, P. N., Hodges, M., et al.: Hypoxemia and lung water in acute myocardial infarction. Am. Heart J. *92*:692, 1976.
185. Hales, C. A., and Kazemi, H.: Clinical significance of pulmonary function tests: Pulmonary function after uncomplicated myocardial infarction. Chest *72*:350, 1977.
186. Hales, C. A., and Kazemi, H.: Small-airways function in myocardial infarction. N. Engl. J. Med. *290*:761, 1974.
187. Gray, B. A., Hyde, R. W., Hodges, M., et al.: Alterations in lung volume and pulmonary function in relation to hemodynamic changes in acute myocardial infarction. Circulation *59*:551, 1979.
188. Kazemi, H., Parsons, E. F., Valenca, L. M., et al.: Distribution of pulmonary blood flow after myocardial ischemia and infarction. Circulation *41*:1025, 1970.
189. DaLuz, P. L., Cavanilles, J. M., Michaels, S., et al.: Oxygen delivery, anoxic metabolism and hemoglobin-oxygen affinity (P50) in patients with acute myocardial infarction and shock. Am. J. Cardiol. *36*:148, 1975.
190. Vetter, N. J., Adams, W., Strange, R. C., et al.: Initial metabolic and hormonal response to acute myocardial infarction. Lancet *1*:284, 1974.
191. Ceremuzynski, L.: Hormonal and metabolic reactions evoked by acute myocardial infarction. Circ. Res. *48*:767, 1981.
192. Taegtmeyer, H.: Metabolic support of the postischaemic heart. Lancet *345*:1552, 1995.
193. Opie, L. H.: Glucose and the metabolism of ischaemic myocardium. Lancet *345*:1520, 1995.
194. Zuanetti, G., Latini, R., Maggioni, A. P., et al.: Influence of diabetes on mortality in acute myocardial infarction: Data from the GISSI-2 study. J. Am. Coll. Cardiol. *22*:1788, 1993.
195. Rouleau, J. J., Dagerais, G.-R., Packer, M., et al.: Selective activation of neurohormonal systems in post-infarction left ventricular dysfunction. J. Am. Coll. Cardiol. *17*:21A, 1991.
196. Karlsberg, R. P., Cryer, P. E., and Roberts, R.: Serial plasma catecholamine response early in the course of clinical acute myocardial infarction: Relationship to infarct extent and mortality. Am. Heart J. *102*:24, 1981.
197. Dzau, V. J., Gibbons, G. H., Cooke, J. P., et al.: Vascular biology and medicine in the 1990s: Scope, concepts, potentials, and perspectives. Circulation *87*:705, 1993.
198. Pitt, B.: The role of angiotensin-converting enzyme inhibitors during the early phase. *In* Julian, D., and Braunwald, E. (eds.): Management of Acute Myocardial Infarction. London, W. B. Saunders Ltd., 1994, p. 253.
199. Hall, C., Cannon, C. P., Forman, S., et al.: Prognostic value of N-terminal proatrial natriuretic factor plasma levels measured within the first 12 hours after myocardial infarction. J. Am. Coll. Cardiol. *26*:1452, 1995.
200. Morita, E., Yause, H., Yoshimura, M., et al.: Increased plasma levels of brain natriuretic peptide in patients with acute myocardial infarction. Circulation *88*:82, 1993.
201. Bain, R. J., Fox, J. P., Jagger, J., et al.: Serum cortisol levels predict infarct size and patient mortality. Int. J. Cardiol. *37*:145, 1992.
202. Wiersinga, W. M., Lie, K. I., and Touber, J. L.: Thyroid hormones in acute myocardial infarction. Clin. Endocrinol. *14*:367, 1981.

203. Kahana, L., Keidar, S., Sheinfeld, M., et al.: Endogenous cortisol and thyroid hormone levels in patients with acute myocardial infarction. Clin. Endocrinol. *19:*131, 1983.
204. Tomoda, H.: Atrial natriuretic peptide in acute myocardial infarction. Am. J. Cardiol. *62:*1122, 1988.
205. Robalino, B. D., Petrella, R. W., Jubran, F. Y., et al.: Atrial natriuretic factor in patients with right ventricular infarction. J. Am. Coll. Cardiol. *15:*546, 1990.
206. Willerson, J. T., Golino, P., Eidt, J., et al.: Platelet mediators and unstable coronary artery disease. Circulation *80:*198, 1989.
207. Frishman, W. H., Burns, B., Atac, B., et al.: Novel antiplatelet therapies for treatment of patients with ischemic heart disease: Inhibitors of the platelet glycoprotein IIb/IIIa integrin receptor. Am. Heart J. *130:*877, 1995.
208. Fitzgerald, D. J., Roy, L., Catella, F., et al.: Platelet activation in unstable coronary disease. N. Engl. J. Med. *315:*983, 1986.
209. Fuster, V.: Lewis A. Conner Memorial Lecture: Mechanisms leading to myocardial infarction: Insights from studies of vascular biology. Circulation *90:*2126, 1994.
210. Tracey, R. P., and Bovill, E. G.: The coagulation system. *In* Califf, R. M. (ed.): Acute Myocardial Infarction and Other Acute Ischemic Syndromes. Philadelphia, Current Medicine, 1996.
211. Freudenberger, R., and Fuster, V.: Acute coronary syndromes: Thrombosis and thrombolysis. *In* Smith, T. W. (ed.): Cardiovascular Therapeutics. Philadelphia, W. B. Saunders Company, 1996.
212. Engler, R. L., Dahlgren, M. D., Morris, D. D., et al.: Role of leukocytes in response to acute myocardial ischemia and reflow in dogs. Am. J. Physiol. *251:*H314, 1986.
213. Koenig, W., and Erns, E.: The possible role of hemorheology in atherothrombogenesis. Atherosclerosis *94:*93, 1992.
214. Hershberg, P. I., Wells, R. E., and McGandy, R. B.: Hematocrit and prognosis in patients with acute myocardial infarction. JAMA *219:*855, 1972.

CLINICAL FEATURES

214a. Braunwald, E.: Acute myocardial infarction—the value of being prepared. N. Engl. J. Med. *334:*51, 1996.
215. Mittleman, M. A., Maclure, M., Sherwood, J. B., et al.: Triggering of acute myocardial infarction onset by episodes of anger. Circulation *92:*1720, 1995.
215a. Muller, J. E., Tofler, G. H., and Mittleman, M.: Triggering of onset of myocardial infarction and sudden cardiac death. *In* Fuster, V., Ross, R., and Topol, E. J. (eds.): Atherosclerosis and Coronary Artery Disease. Philadelphia, Lippincott-Raven, 1996, pp. 819–834.
216. Rahe, R. H., Romo, M., Bennett, L., et al.: Recent life changes, myocardial infarction, and abrupt coronary death. Arch. Intern. Med. *133:*221, 1974.
216a. Muller, J. E., Tofler, G. H., and Mittleman, M.: Triggering of onset of myocardial infarction and sudden cardiac death. *In* Fuster, V., Ross, R., and Topol, E. J. (eds.): Atherosclerosis and Coronary Artery Disease. Philadelphia, Lippincott-Raven, 1996, pp. 819–834.
217. Allison, T. G., Williams, D. E., Miller, T. D., et al.: Medical and economic costs of psychologic distress in patients with coronary artery disease. Mayo Clin. Proc. *70:*734, 1995.
218. Pasternak, R. C.: Psychologic factors and course after myocardial infarction: Maturing of a risk factor. Mayo Clin. Proc. *70:*809, 1995.
219. Hlatkly, M. A., Lam, L. C., Lee, K. L., et al.: Job strain and the prevalence and outcome of coronary artery disease. Circulation *92:*327, 1995.
220. Maseri, A., L'Abbate, A., Baroldi, G., et al.: Coronary vasospasm as a possible cause of myocardial infarction. N. Engl. J. Med. *299:*1271, 1978.
221. Lange, R. L., Reid, M. S., Tresch, D. D., et al.: Nonatheromatous ischemic heart disease following withdrawal from chronic industrial nitroglycerin exposure. Circulation *46:*666, 1972.
222. Psaty, B. M., Heckbert, S. R., Koepsell, T. D., et al.: The risk of myocardial infarction associated with antihypertensive drug therapies. JAMA *274:*620, 1995.
223. Lenfant, C.: The calcium channel blocker scare: Lessons for the future. Circulation *91:*2855, 1995.
224. Buring, J. E., Glynn, R. J., and Hennekens, C. H.: Calcium channel blockers and myocardial infarction: A hypothesis formulated but not yet tested. JAMA *274:*654, 1995.
225. Muller, J. E., Stone, P. H., Turi, Z. G., et al.: Circadian variation in the frequency of onset of acute myocardial infarction. N. Engl. J. Med. *313:*1315, 1985.
226. Willich, S. N., Linderer, T., Wegscheider, K., et al.: Increasing morning incidence of myocardial infarction in the ISAM study: Absence with prior β-adrenergic blockade. Circulation *80:*853, 1989.
227. Ridker, P. M., Manson, J. E., Buring, J. E., et al.: Circadian variation of acute myocardial infarction and the effect of low-dose aspirin in a randomized trial of physicians. Circulation *82:*897, 1990.
228. Willerson, J. T., Cohen, L. S., and Maseri, A.: Coronary artery disease: Pathophysiology and clinical recognition. *In* Willerson, J. T., and Cohn, J. N. (eds.): Cardiovascular Medicine. New York, Churchill Livingstone, 1995, p. 333.
228a. Huggins, G. S., and O'Gara, P. T.: Clinical presentation and diagnostic evaluation. *In* Fuster, V., Ross, R., and Topol, E. J. (eds.): Atherosclerosis and Coronary Artery Disease. Philadelphia, Lippincott-Raven, 1996.
229. Harper, R. W., Kennedy, G., DeSanctis, R. W., et al.: The incidence and pattern of angina prior to acute myocardial infarction: A study of 577 cases. Am. Heart J. *97:*178, 1979.
230. Muller, R., Gould, L., Betu, R., et al.: Painless myocardial infarction in the elderly. Am. Heart J. *119:*202, 1990.
231. Malliani, A., and Lombardi, F.: Consideration of the fundamental mechanisms eliciting cardiac pain. Am. Heart J. *103:*575, 1982.
232. Ingram, D. A., Fulton, R. A., Portal, R. W., et al.: Vomiting as a diagnostic aid in acute ischemic cardiac pain. BMJ *281:*636, 1980.
233. Spodick, D. H.: Pericardial complications of myocardial infarction. *In* Francis, G. S., and Alpert, J. S. (eds.): Coronary Care. Boston, Little, Brown and Co., 1995, p. 333.
234. Yano, K., and MacLean, C. J.: The incidence and prognosis of unrecognized myocardial infarction in Honolulu, Hawaii, Heart Program. Arch. Intern. Med. *149:*1528, 1989.
235. Sigurdsson, E., Thorgeirsson, G., Sigvaldason, H., et al.: Unrecognized myocardial infarction: Epidemiology, clinical characteristics, and the prognostic role of angina pectoris: The Reykjavik study. Ann. Intern. Med. *122:*96, 1995.
236. Bean, W. B.: Masquerade of myocardial infarction. Lancet *1:*1044, 1977.
237. Campbell, R. W. F.: Arrhythmias. *In* Julian, D., and Braunwald, E. (eds.): Management of Acute Myocardial Infarction. London, W.B. Saunders Ltd., 1994, p. 223.
238. Chadda, K. D., Lichstein, E., Gupta, P. K., et al.: Bradycardia-hypotension syndrome in acute myocardial infarction: Reappraisal of the overdrive effects of atropine. Am. J. Med. *59:*158, 1975.
239. Webb, S. W., Adgey, A. A., and Pantridge, J. F.: Autonomic disturbance at onset of acute myocardial infarction. BMJ *818:*89, 1982.
240. Killip, T., and Kimball, J. T.: Treatment of myocardial infarction in a coronary care unit: A two year experience with 250 patients. Am. J. Cardiol. *20:*457, 1967.
241. Gadsboll, N., Hoilund-Carlsen, P. F., et al.: Symptoms and signs of heart failure in patients with myocardial infarction: Reproducibility and relationship to chest x-ray, radionuclide venticulography and right heart catheterization. Eur. Heart J. *10:*1017, 1989.
242. Manson, A. L., Nudelman, S. P., Hagley, M. T., et al.: Relationship of the third heart sound to transmitral flow velocity deceleration. Circulation *92:*388, 1995.
243. Riley, C. P., Russell, R. O. J., and Rackley, C. E.: Left ventricular gallop sound and acute myocardial infarction. Am. Heart J. *86:*598, 1973.
244. Galve, E., Garcia Del Castillo, H., Evangelista, A., et al.: Pericardial effusion in the course of myocardial infarction: Incidence, natural history, and clinical relevance. Circulation *73:*294, 1986.
245. Thompson, P. L., and Robinson, J. S.: Stroke after acute myocardial infarction: Relation to infarct size. BMJ *2:*457, 1978.
246. Duryee, R.: The efficacy of inpatient education after myocardial infarction. Heart Lung *21:*217, 1992.

LABORATORY EXAMINATIONS

247. Pedoe-Tunstall, H., Kuulasmaa, K., Amouyel, P., et al.: Myocardial infarction and coronary deaths in the World Health Organization MONICA Project. Circulation *90:*583, 1994.
248. Goldberg, R., Gore, J., Alpert, J., et al.: Incidence and case fatality rates of acute myocardial infarction (1975–1984): The Worcester Heart Attack Study. Am. Heart J. *115:*761, 1988.
249. Kannel, W.: Prevalence and clinical aspects of unrecognized myocardial infarction and sudden unexpected death. Circulation *75*(Suppl. II):II, 1987.
250. Grimm, R., Tillingshast, S., Daniels, K., et al.: Unrecognized myocardial infarction: Experience in the multiple risk factor intervention trial (MRFIT). Circulation *75*(Suppl. II):6, 1987.
251. Gibler, W., Lewis, L., Erb, R., et al.: Early detection of acute myocardial infarction in patients presenting with chest pain and nondiagnostic ECGs: Serial CKMB sampling in the emergency department. Ann. Emerg. Med. *19:*1359, 1990.
252. Hedges, J. R., Young, G. P., Henkel, G. F., et al.: Serial ECGs are less accurate than serial CK-MB results for emergency department diagnosis of myocardial infarction. Ann. Emerg. Med. *21:*1445, 1992.
253. Gibler, W. B., Young, G. P., Hedges, J. R., et al.: Acute myocardial infarction in chest pain patients with nondiagnostic ECGs: Serial CK-MB sampling in the emergency department: The Emergency Medicine Cardiac Research Group. Ann. Emerg. Med. *21:*504, 1992.
254. Sacks, D. B.: Troponin T: A cardiac specific-marker. *In* Goldman, L., and Katus, H. A. (eds.): Cardiac Troponin T for the Diagnosis of Myocardial Injury. Deerfield, IL, Discovery International, 1994, p. 3.
255. Murray, C., and Alpert, J. S.: Diagnosis of acute myocardial infarction. Curr. Opin. Cardiol. *9:*465, 1994.
256. Ellis, A. K.: Serum protein measurements and the diagnosis of acute myocardial infarction. Circulation *83:*1107, 1991.
257. Mair, J., Dienstl, F., and Puschendorf, B.: Cardiac troponin T in the diagnosis of myocardial injury. Crit. Rev. Clin. Lab. Sci. *29:*31, 1992.
258. Collinson, P. O., Ramhamadamy, E. M., Stubbs, P. J., et al.: Rapid enzyme diagnosis of patients with acute chest pain reduces patient stay in the coronary care unit. Ann. Clin. Biochem. *30:*17, 1993.
259. Puleo, P. R., Meyer, D., Wathen, C., et al.: Use of a rapid assay of subforms of creatine kinase MB to diagnose or rule out acute myocardial infarction. N. Engl. J. Med. *331:*561, 1994.
260. Antman, E. M., Grudzien, C., and Sacks, D.: Evaluation of a rapid bedside assay for detection of serum cardiac troponin T. JAMA *273:*1279, 1995.

261. Roberts, R.: Enzymatic estimation of infarct size: Thrombolysis induced its demise: Will it now rekindle its renaissance? Circulation *81*:707, 1990.
262. Lee, T. H., and Goldman, L.: Serum enzyme assays in the diagnosis of acute myocardial infarction. Ann. Intern. Med. *105*:221, 1986.
263. Adams, J. E., Bodor, G. S., Davila-Roman, V. G., et al.: Cardiac troponin I: A marker with high specificity for cardiac injury. Circulation *88*:101, 1993.
264. Tsung, J. S., and Tsung, S. S.: Creatine kinase isoenzymes in extracts of various human skeletal muscles. Clin. Chem. *32*:1568, 1986.
265. Roberts, R., and Sobel, B. E.: Isoenzymes of creatine phosphokinase and diagnosis of myocardial infarction. Ann. Intern. Med. *79*:741, 1973.
266. Jaffe, A. S., Garfinkel, B. T., Ritter, C. S., et al.: Plasma MB creatine kinase after vigorous exercise in professional athletes. Am. J. Cardiol. *53*:856, 1984.
267. Apple, F.: Creatine kinase-MB. Lab. Med. *23*:298, 1992.
268. Vaidya, H. C., Maynard, Y., Dietzler, D. N., et al.: Direct measurement of creatine-kinase MB activity in serum after extraction with a monoclonal antibody specific to the MB isoenzyme. Clin. Chem. *32*:657, 1986.
269. Bakker, A. J., Gorgels, J. P. M. C., van Vlies, B., et al.: Contribution of creatine kinase MB mass concentration at admission to early diagnosis of myocardial infarction. Br. Heart J. *72*:112, 1994.
270. El Allaf, M., Chapelle, J., El Allaf, D., et al.: Differentiating muscle damage from myocardial injury by means of the serum creatine kinase (CK) isoenzyme MB mass measure/total CK activity ratio. Clin. Chem. *32*:291, 1986.
271. Yusuf, S., Collins, R., Lin, L., et al.: Significance of elevated MB isoenzyme with normal creatine kinase in acute myocardial infarction. Am. J. Cardiol. *59*:245, 1987.
272. Roberts, R., and Kleiman, N.: Earlier diagnosis and treatment of acute myocardial infarction necessitates the need for a "new diagnostic mind-set." Circulation *89*:872, 1994.
273. Puleo, P. R., Guadagno, P. A., Roberts, R., et al.: Early diagnosis of acute myocardial infarction based on assay for subforms of creatine kinase-MB. Circulation *82*:759, 1990.
274. Puleo, P. R., and Perryman, B.: Noninvasive detection of reperfusion in acute myocardial infarction based on plasma activity of creatine kinase MB subfractions. J. Am. Coll. Cardiol. *17*:1047, 1991.
275. Ohman, E. M., Casey, C., Bengston, J. R., et al.: Early detection of acute myocardial infarction: Additional diagnostic information from serum concentrations of myoglobin in patients without ST elevation. Br. Heart J. *63*:335, 1990.
276. Zabel, M., Hohnloser, S. H., Koster, W., et al.: Analysis of creatine kinase, CK-MB, myoglobin, and troponin T time-activity curves for early assessment of coronary artery reperfusion after intravenous thrombolysis. Circulation *87*:1542, 1993.
277. Abendschein, D. R., Ellis, A. K., Eisenberg, P. R., et al.: Prompt detection of coronary recanalization by analysis rates of change of concentrations of macromolecular markers in plasma. Coron. Artery Dis. *2*:201, 1991.
278. Yamashita, T., Abe, S., Arima, S., et al.: Myocardial infarct size can be estimated from serial plasma myoglobin measurements within 4 hours of reperfusion. Circulation *87*:1840, 1993.
279. Katus, H., Scheffold, T., Remppis, A., et al.: Proteins of the troponin complex. Lab. Med. *23*:311, 1992.
280. Katus, H. A., Remppis, A., Scheffold, T., et al.: Intracellular compartmentation of cardiac troponin T and its release kinetics in patients with reperfused and nonreperfused myocardial infarction. Am. J. Cardiol. *67*:1360, 1991.
281. Adams, J. E., Schechtman, K. B., Landt, Y., et al.: Comparable detection of acute myocardial infarction by creatine kinase MB isoenzyme and cardiac troponin I. Clin. Chem. *40*:1291, 1994.
282. Hamm, C. W.: New serum markers for acute myocardial infarction. N. Engl. J. Med. *331*:607, 1994.
283. Katus, H. A., Looser, S., Hallermayer, K., et al.: Development and in vitro characterization of a new immunoassay of cardiac troponin T. Clin. Chem. *38*:386, 1992.
284. Wu, A. H. B., Valdes, R., Jr., Apple, F. S., et al.: Cardiac troponin-T immunoassay for diagnosis of acute myocardial infarction. Clin. Chem. *40*:900, 1994.
285. Bodor, G. S., Porter, S., Landt, Y., et al.: Development of monoclonal antibodies for an assay of cardiac troponin-I and preliminary results in suspected cases of myocardial infarction. Clin. Chem. *38*:2203, 1992.
286. Adams, J. E., Sicard, G. A., Allen, B. T., et al.: Diagnosis of perioperative myocardial infarction with measurement of cardiac troponin I. N. Engl. J. Med. *330*:670, 1994.
287. Mair, J., Morandell, D., Genser, N., et al.: Equivalent early sensitivities of myoglobin, creatine kinase MB mass, creatine kinase isoform ratios, and cardiac troponins I and T for acute myocardial infarction. Clin. Chem. *41*:1266, 1995.
288. Newby, L. K., Gibler, W. B., Ohman, W. M., et al.: Biochemical markers in suspected acute myocardial infarction: The need for early assessment. Clin. Chem. *41*:1263, 1995.
288a. Müller-Bardorff, M., Freitag, H., Scheffold, T., et al.: Development and characterization of a rapid assay for bedside determinations of cardiac troponin T. Circulation *92*:2869, 1995.
289. Hamm, C., Ravkilde, J., Gerhardt, W., et al.: The prognostic value of serum troponin T in unstable angina. N. Engl. J. Med. *327*:146, 1992.
290. Guest, T. M., Ramanathan, A. V., Tuteur, P. G., et al.: Myocardial injury in critically ill patients: A frequently unrecognized complication. JAMA *273*:1945, 1995.
291. Larue, C., Calzolari, C., Bertinchant, J. P., et al.: Cardiac-specific immunoenzymometric assay of troponin I in the early phase of acute myocardial infarction. Clin. Chem. *39*:972, 1993.
292. Katus, H. A., Remppis, A., Neumann, F. J., et al.: Diagnostic efficiency of troponin T measurements in acute myocardial infarction. Circulation *83*:902, 1991.
293. Remppis, A., Scheffold, T., Karrer, O., et al.: Assessment of reperfusion of the infarct zone after acute myocardial infarction by serial cardiac troponin T measurements in serum. Br. Heart J. *71*:242, 1994.
294. Abe, S., Arima, S., Yamashita, T., et al.: Early assessment of reperfusion therapy using cardiac troponin T. J. Am. Coll. Cardiol. *23*:1382, 1994.
295. Ravkilde, J., Horder, M., Gerhardt, W., et al.: Diagnostic performance and prognostic value of serum troponin T in suspected acute myocardial infarction. Scand. J. Clin. Lab. Invest. *53*:677, 1993.
296. Ravkilde, J., Nissen, H., Horder, M., et al.: Independent prognostic value of serum creatine kinase isoenzyme MB mass, cardiac troponin T and myosin light chain levels in suspected acute myocardial infarction: Analysis of 28 months of follow-up in 196 patients. J. Am. Coll. Cardiol. *25*:574, 1995.
297. Hamm, C. W., and Katus, H. A.: New biochemical markers for myocardial cell injury. Curr. Opin. Cardiol. *10*:355, 1995.
298. Ohman, E. M., Armstrong, P., Califf, R. M., et al.: Risk stratification in acute ischemic syndromes using serum troponin T. J. Am. Coll. Cardiol. (Special Issue):148A, 1995.
299. Antman, E. M., Tanasijevic, M. J., Cannon, C. P., et al.: Cardiac troponin I on admission predicts death by 42 days in unstable angina and improved survival with an early invasive strategy: Results from TIMI IIIB. Circulation *92*(Suppl.): I-663, 1995.
300. Marshall, T., Williams, J., and Williams, K. M.: Electrophoresis of serum enzymes and proteins following acute myocardial infarction. J. Chromatogr. *569*:323, 1991.
301. Rabitzsch, G., Mair, J., Lechleitner, P., et al.: Immunoenzymometric assay of human glycogen phosphorylate isoenzyme BB in diagnosis of ischemic myocardial injury. Clin. Chem. *41*:966, 1995.
302. Apple, F. S.: Glycogen phosphorylase BB and other cardiac proteins: Challenges to creatine kinase MB as the marker for detecting myocardial injury. Clin. Chem. *41*:963, 1995.
303. Vaananen, H. K., Syrjala, H., Rahkila, P., et al.: Serum carbonic anhydrase III and myoglobin concentrations in acute myocardial infarction. Clin. Chem. *36*:635, 1990.
304. Vuori, J., Rasi, S., Takala, T., et al.: Dual-label time-resolved fluoroimmunoassay for simultaneous detection of myoglobin and carbonic anhydrase III in serum. Clin. Chem. *37*:2087, 1991.
305. Eikvar, L., Pillgram-Larsen, J., Skjaeggestad, Ø., et al.: Serum cardiospecific troponin T after open heart surgery in patients with and without perioperative myocardial infarction. Scand. J. Clin. Lab. Invest. *54*:329, 1994.
306. Franz, W. M., Remppis, A., Scheffold, T., et al.: Serum troponin T: A diagnostic marker for acute myocarditis? Circulation *90*(Suppl. I):67, 1994.
307. Gore, J. M., Goldberg, R. J., Matsumoto, A. S., et al.: Validity of serum total cholesterol level obtained within 24 hours of acute myocardial infarction. Am. J. Cardiol. *54*:722, 1984.
308. Ryder, R., Hayes, T., Mulligan, I., et al.: How soon after myocardial infarction should plasma lipid values be assessed? BMJ *289*:1651, 1984.
309. Ronnemaa, T., Viikari, J., Irjala, K., et al.: Marked decrease in serum HDL cholesterol level during acute myocardial infarction. Acta Med. Scand. *207*:161, 1980.
310. Expert Panel on Detection, Evaluation and Treatment of High Blood Cholesterol in Adults: Summary of the second report of the National Cholesterol Education Program (NCEP) Expert Panel on Detection, Evaluation, and Treatment of High Blood Cholesterol in Adults (Adult Treatment Panel II). JAMA *269*:3015, 1993.
311. Thomson, S. P., Gibbons, R. J., Smars, P. A., et al.: Incremental value of the leukocyte differential and the rapid creatine kinase-MB isoenzyme for the early diagnosis of myocardial infarction. Ann. Intern. Med. *122*:335, 1995.
312. Eastham, R. D., and Morgan, E. H.: Plasma-fibrinogen levels in coronary-artery disease. Lancet *2*:1196, 1963.
312a. Parker, A. B. III., Waller, B. F., and Gering, L. E.: Usefulness of the 12-lead electrocardiogram in detection of myocardial infarction: Electrocardiographic-anatomic correlations—Part I. Clin. Cardiol. *19*:55, 1996.
312b. Sgarbossa, E. B., Pinski, S. L., Barbagelata, A., et al.: Electrocardiographic diagnosis of evolving acute myocardial infarction in the presence of left bundle-branch block. N. Engl. J. Med. *334*:481, 1996.
313. Cooksey, J. D., Dunn, M., and Massie, E.: Clinical Vectorcardiography and Electrocardiography. 2nd ed. Chicago, Year Book Medical Publishers, 1977, p. 361.
314. Shen, W. F., Tribouilloy, C., Mirode, A., et al.: Isolated circumflex coronary artery occlusion as a cause of myocardial infarction. Am. J. Noninvas. Cardiol. *7*:204, 1993.
315. Ben-Haim, S. A., Gil, A., and Edoute, Y.: Beat-to-beat morphologic variability of the electrocardiogram for the evaluation of chest pain in the emergency room. Am. J. Cardiol. *70*:1139, 1992.
316. Kornreich, F., Montague, T. J., and Rautaharju, P. M.: Body surface potential mapping of ST segment changes in acute myocardial infarction. Circulation *87*:773, 1993.
317. Lundin, P., Eriksson, S. V., Erhardt, L., et al.: Continuous vectorcar-

diography in patients with chest pain indicative of acute ischemic heart disease. Cardiology *81*:145, 1992.

318. Selker, H. P., Griffith, J. L., and Beshansky, J. R.: The Acute Cardiac Ischemia Time-Insensitive Predictive Instrument (ACI-TIPI): A Decision Aid for Emergency Department Triage and a Measure of Appropriateness of Coronary Care Unit Use. *In* Califf, R. M., Mark, D. B., and Wagner, G. S. (eds.): Acute Coronary Care. St. Louis, Mosby, 1995, p. 201.
319. Coll, S., Betriu, A., De Flores, T., et al.: Significance of Q-wave regression after transmural acute myocardial infarction. Am. J. Cardiol. *61*:739, 1988.
320. Taussig, A. S., et al.: Misleading ECGs: Patterns of infarction. J. Cardiovasc. Med. *9*:1147, 1983.
321. Phibbs, B.: "Transmural" versus "subendocardial" myocardial infarction: An electrocardiographic myth. J. Am. Coll. Cardiol. *1*:561, 1983.
322. Levine, H. D.: Subendocardial infarction in retrospect: Pathologic, cardiographic, and ancillary features. Circulation *72*:790, 1985.
323. Dacanay, S., Kennedy, H. L., Uretz, E., et al.: Morphological and quantitative angiographic analyses of progression of coronary stenoses: A comparison of Q-wave and non-Q-wave myocardial infarction. Circulation *90*:1739, 1994.
324. Keen, W. D., Savage, M. P., Fischman, D. L., et al.: Comparison of coronary angiographic findings during the first six hours of non-Q-wave and Q-wave myocardial infarction. Am. J. Cardiol. *74*:324, 1994.
325. Kudenchuk, P. J., Ho, M. T., Weaver, W. D., et al.: Accuracy of computer-interpreted electrocardiography in selecting patients for thrombolytic therapy: MITI Project Investigators. J. Am. Coll. Cardiol. *17*:1486, 1991.
326. Weaver, W. D., Litwin, P. E., Martin, J. S., et al.: Effect of age on use of thrombolytic therapy and mortality in acute myocardial infarction: The MITI Project Group. J. Am. Coll. Cardiol. *18*:657, 1991.
327. Spodick, D. H.: Q-wave infarction versus S-T infarction: Non-specificity of electrocardiographic criteria for differentiating transmural and non-transmural lesions. Am. J. Cardiol. *51*:913, 1983.
328. Zema, M. J.: Q wave, S-T segment, and T wave myocardial infarction. Am. J. Med. *78*:391, 1985.
329. Goldberg, R. J., Gore, J. M., Alpert, J. S., et al.: Non-Q wave myocardial infarction: Recent changes in occurrence and prognosis—a community-wide perspective. Am. Heart J. *113*:273, 1987.
330. Schuster, E. H., and Bulkley, B. H.: Early post-infarction angina: Ischemia at a distance and ischemia in the infarct zone. N. Engl. J. Med. *305*:1101, 1981.
331. Ferguson, D. W., Pandian, N., Kioschos, J. M., et al.: Angiographic evidence that reciprocal ST-segment depression during acute myocardial infarction does not indicate remote ischemia: Analysis of 23 patients. Am. J. Cardiol. *53*:55, 1984.
332. Mukharji, J., Murray, S., Lewis, S. E., et al.: Is anterior ST depression with acute transmural inferior infarction due to posterior infarction? J. Am. Coll. Cardiol. *4*:28, 1984.
333. Mirvis, D. M.: Physiologic bases for anterior ST segment depression in patients with acute inferior wall myocardial infarction. Am. Heart J. *116*:1308, 1988.
334. Muller, D. W. M., Topol, E. J., Califf, R. M., et al.: Relationship between antecedent angina pectoris and short-term prognosis after thrombolytic therapy for acute myocardial infarction. Am. Heart J. *119*:224, 1990.
335. Lopez-Sendon, J., Coma-Canella, I., Alcasena, S., et al.: Electrocardiographic findings in acute right ventricular infarction: Sensitivity and specificity of electrocardiographic alterations in right precordial leads V4R, V3R, V1, V2, and V3. J. Am. Coll. Cardiol. *6*:1273, 1985.
336. Kulbertus, H. E.: Right ventricular infarction. *In* Julian, D., and Braunwald, E. (eds.): Management of Acute Myocardial Infarction. London, W. B. Saunders Ltd., 1994, p. 331.
337. Geft, I. L., Shah, P. K., Rodriguez, L., et al.: ST elevations in leads V1 to V5 may be caused by right coronary artery occlusion and acute right ventricular infarction. Am. J. Cardiol. *53*:991, 1984.
338. Lew, A. S., Maddahi, J., Shah, P. K., et al.: Factors that determine the direction and magnitude of precordial ST-segment deviations during inferior wall acute myocardial infarction. Am. J. Cardiol. *55*:883, 1985.
339. Robalino, B. D., Whitlow, P. L., Underwood, D. A., et al.: Electrocardiographic manifestations of right ventricular infarction. Am. Heart J. *118*:138, 1989.
340. Silvertssen, E., Hoel, B., Bay, G., et al.: Electrocardiographic atrial complex and acute atrial myocardial infarction. Am. J. Cardiol. *31*:450, 1973.
341. Brattler, A., Karliner, J. S., Higgins, C. B., et al.: The initial chest x-ray in acute myocardial infarction: Prediction of early and late mortality and survival. Circulation *61*:1004, 1980.
342. Katz, A. S., Harrigan, P., and Parisi, A. F.: The value and promise of echocardiography in acute myocardial infarction and coronary artery disease. Clin. Cardiol. *15*:401, 1992.
342a. Nishimura, R. A.: Acute myocardial infarction: The role of echocardiography. *In* Fuster, V., Ross, R., and Topol, E. J. (eds.): Atherosclerosis and Coronary Artery Disease. Philadelphia, Lippincott-Raven, 1996, pp. 855–876.
343. Berning, J., and Steensgard-Hansen, F.: Early estimation of risk by echocardiographic determination of wall motion index in an unselected population with acute myocardial infarction. Am. J. Cardiol. *65*:567, 1990.
344. Sabia, P., Abbott, R. D., Afrookteh, A., et al.: Importance of two-dimensional echocardiographic assessment of left ventricular function in patients presenting to the emergency room with cardiac-related symptoms. Circulation *84*:1615, 1991.
345. Hepner, A. M., and Armstrong, W. F.: Echocardiography in acute myocardial infarction. *In* Francis, G. S., and Alpert, J. S. (eds.): Coronary Care. Boston, Little, Brown and Co., 1995, p. 473.
346. Segar, D. S., Brown, S. E., Sawada, S. G., et al.: Dobutamine stress echocardiography: Correlation with coronary lesion severity as determined by quantitative angiography. J. Am. Coll. Cardiol. *19*:1197, 1992.
347. Kuhn, M. B., Egeblad, H., Hojberg, S., et al.: Prognostic value of echocardiography compared to other clinical findings: Multivariate analysis based on long-term survival in 456 patients. Cardiology *86*:157, 1995.
348. Salustri, A., Elhendy, A., Garyfallydis, P., et al.: Prediction of improvement of ventricular function after first acute myocardial infarction using low-dose dobutamine stress echocardiography. Am. J. Cardiol. *74*:853, 1994.
349. Camarano, G., Ragosta, M., Gimple, L. W., et al.: Identification of viable myocardium with contrast echocardiography in patients with poor left ventricular systolic function caused by recent or remote myocardial infarction. Am. J. Cardiol. *75*:215, 1995.
350. Takeuchi, M., Araki, M., Nakashima, Y., et al.: The detection of residual ischemia and stenosis in patients with acute myocardial infarction with dobutamine stress echocardiography. J. Am. Soc. Echocardiogr. *7*:242, 1994.
351. Finkelhor, R. S., Sun, J. P., Castellanos, M., et al.: Predicting left heart failure after a myocardial infarction: A preliminary study of the value of echocardiographic measures of left ventricular filling and wall motion. J. Am. Soc. Echocardiogr. *4*:215, 1991.
352. Tice, F. D., and Kisslo, J.: Echocardiographic assessment and monitoring of the patient with acute myocardial infarction: Prospects for the thrombolytic era. *In* Califf, R. M., Mark, D. B., and Wagner, G. S. (eds.): Acute Coronary Care. St. Louis, Mosby-Year Book, 1994, p. 489.
353. Pearson, A. C., Castello, R., and Labovitz, A. J.: Safety and utility of transesophageal echocardiography in the critically ill patient. Am. Heart J. *119*:1083, 1990.
354. Harrison, J. K., and Bashore, T. M.: Assessment and management of the critically ill patient with valvular heart disease. *In* Califf, R. M., Mark, D. B., and Wagner, G. S. (eds.): Acute Coronary Care. St. Louis, Mosby-Year Book, 1995, p. 719.
355. Smyllie, J. H., Sutherland, G. R., Geuskens, R., et al.: Doppler color flow mapping in the diagnosis of ventricular septal rupture and acute mitral regurgitation after myocardial infarction. J. Am. Coll. Cardiol. *15*:1449, 1990.
356. Hirose, K., Reed, J. E., and Rumberger, J. A.: Serial changes in regional right ventricular free wall and left ventricular septal wall lengths during the first 4 to 5 years after index anterior wall myocardial infarction. J. Am. Coll. Cardiol. *26*:394, 1995.
357. Foster, C. J., Sekiya, T., Love, H. G., et al.: Identification of intracardiac thrombus: Comparison of computed tomography and cross-sectional echocardiography. Br. J. Radiol. *60*:327, 1987.
358. Baer, F. M., Theissen, P., Voth, E., et al.: Morphologic correlate of pathologic Q waves as assessed by gradient-echo magnetic resonance imaging. Am. J. Cardiol. *74*:430, 1994.
359. Johnston, D. L., Gupta, V. K., Wendt, R. E., et al.: Detection of viable myocardium in segments with fixed defects on thallium-201 scintigraphy: Usefulness of magnetic resonance imaging early after acute myocardial infarction. Magn. Reson. Imaging *11*:949, 1993.
360. Holman, E. R., van Jonbergen, H. P., van Dijkman, P. R., et al.: Comparison of magnetic resonance imaging studies with enzymatic indexes of myocardial necrosis for quantification of myocardial infarct size. Am. J. Cardiol. *71*:1036, 1993.
360a. Kantor, H. L., and Toussaint, J. F.: Acute myocardial infarction: The role of magnetic resonance. *In* Fuster, V., Ross, R., and Topol, E. J. (eds.): Atherosclerosis and Coronary Artery Disease. Philadelphia, Lippincott-Raven, 1996, pp. 905–920.
361. Yokota, C., Nonogi, H., Miyazaki, S., et al.: Gadolinium-enhanced magnetic resonance imaging in acute myocardial infarction. Am. J. Cardiol. *75*:577, 1995.
362. Committee on Radionuclide Imaging: ACC/AHA Task Force Report: Guidelines for clinical use of cardiac radionuclide imaging. J. Am. Coll. Cardiol. *25*:521, 1995.
363. Miller, T. D., Christian, T. F., Hopfenspirger, M. R., et al.: Infarct size after acute myocardial infarction measured by quantitative tomographic ^{99m}Tc sestamibi imaging predicts subsequent mortality. Circulation *92*:334, 1995.
363a. Beller, G. A.: Acute myocardial infarction: The role of radionuclide imaging. *In* Fuster, V., Ross, R., and Topol, E. J. (eds.): Atherosclerosis and Coronary Artery Disease. Philadelphia, Lippincott-Raven, 1996, pp. 877–894.
364. Hasche, E. T., Fernandes, C., Freedman, S. B., et al.: Relation between ischemia time, infarct size, and left ventricular function in humans. Circulation *92*:710, 1995.
365. Mauri, F., Gasparini, M., Barbonaglia, L., et al.: Prognostic significance of the extent of myocardial injury in acute myocardial infarction treated by streptokinase (the GISSI trial). Am. J. Cardiol. *63*:1291, 1989.
366. Zaret, B. L., and Wackers, F. J.: Nuclear cardiology. N. Engl. J. Med. *329*:775, 1993.
367. Antunes, M. L., Tresgallo, M. E., Seldin, D. W., et al.: Effect of infarct size measured from antimyosin single-photon emission computed tomographic scans on left ventricular remodeling. J. Am. Coll. Cardiol. *18*:1263, 1991.

368. Johnson, L. L., Seldin, D. W., Keller, A. M., et al.: Dual isotope thallium and indium antimyosin SPECT imaging to identify acute infarct patients at further ischemic risk. Circulation *81*:37, 1990.
369. Lima, J. A. C., Judd, R. M., Bazille, A., et al.: Regional heterogeneity of human myocardial infarcts demonstrated by contrast-enhanced MRI: Potential mechanisms. Circulation *92*:1117, 1995.

MANAGEMENT OF ACUTE MYOCARDIAL INFARCTION

370. Topol, E. J.: Mechanical interventions for acute myocardial infarction. *In* Topol, E. J. (ed.): Textbook of Interventional Cardiology. Philadelphia, W. B. Saunders Company, 1994, p. 292.
371. Zahger, D., and Gotsman, M. S.: Thrombolysis in the era of randomized trials. Curr. Opin. Cardiol. *10*:372, 1995.
372. Holmes, D. R., Califf, R. M., and Topol, E. J.: Lessons we have learned from the GUSTO trial. J. Am. Coll. Cardiol. *25*:10S, 1995.
373. Smith, S. M.: Current management of acute myocardial infarction. Dis. Mon. *41*:363, 1995.
374. van de Werf, F., Califf, R. M., Armstrong, P. W., et al.: Clinical perspective: Progress culminating from ten years of clinical trials on thrombolysis for acute myocardial infarction. Eur. Heart J. *16*:1024, 1995.

PREHOSPITAL CARE

375. National Heart Attack Alert Program Coordinating Committee—60 Minutes to Treatment Working Group: Emergency department: Rapid identification and treatment of patients with acute myocardial infarction. Ann. Emerg. Med. *23*:311, 1994.
376. Gibler, W. B., Kereiakes, D. J., Dean, E. N., et al.: Prehospital diagnosis and treatment of acute myocardial infarction: A north-south perspective: The Cincinnati Heart Project and the Nashville Prehospital TPA Trial. Am. Heart J. *121*:1, 1991.
377. GISSI-Avoidable Delay Study Group: Epidemiology of avoidable delay in the care of patients with acute myocardial infarction in Italy. Arch. Intern. Med. *155*:1481, 1995.
378. National Heart Attack Alert Program: Patient/bystander recognition and action: Rapid identification and treatment of acute myocardial infarction (NIH Publication 93-3303). Bethesda, MD, National Heart, Lung, and Blood Institute, 1994, p. 1.
379. Reilly, A., Dracup, K., and Dattolo, J.: Factors influencing prehospital delay in patients experiencing chest pain. Am. J. Crit. Care. *3*:300, 1994.
380. Lombardi, G., Gallagher, J., and Gennis, P.: Outcome of out-of-hospital cardiac arrest in New York City: The Pre-Hospital Arrest Survival Evaluation (PHASE) Study. JAMA *271*:678, 1994.
381. National Heart Attack Alert Program: 9-1-1: Rapid identification and treatment of acute myocardial infarction (NIH Publication 94-3302). Bethesda, MD, National Heart, Lung, and Blood Institute, 1994, p. 1.
382. Weaver, W. D., Cerqueira, M., Hallstrom, A. P., et al.: Prehospital-initiated vs. hospital-initiated thrombolytic therapy: The Myocardial Infarction Triage and Intervention Trial. JAMA *270*:1211, 1993.
383. Castaigne, A., Herve, C., Duval-Moulin, A., et al.: Prehospital use of APSAC: Results of a placebo-controlled study. Am. J. Cardiol. *64*:30A, 1989.
384. Schofer, J., Buttner, J., Geng, G., et al.: Prehospital thrombolysis in acute myocardial infarction. Am. J. Cardiol. *66*:1429, 1990.
385. GREAT Group: Feasibility, safety, and efficacy of domicillary thrombolysis by general practitioners: Grampian region early anistreplase trial. BMJ *305*:548, 1992.
386. The European Myocardial Infarction Project Group: Prehospital thrombolytic therapy in patients with suspected acute myocardial infarction. N. Engl. J. Med. *329*:383, 1993.
387. Califf, R. M.: Acute myocardial infarction. *In* Smith, T. W. (ed.): Cardiovascular Therapeutics. Philadelphia, W. B. Saunders Company, 1996.
388. National Heart Attack Alert Program: Emergency medical dispatching: Rapid identification and treatment of acute myocardial infarction (NIH Publication 94-3287). Bethesda, MD, National Heart, Lung, and Blood Institute, 1994, p. 1.
389. National Heart Attack Alert Program: Staffing and equipping emergency medical services systems: Rapid identification and treatment of acute myocardial infarction (NIH Publication 93-3304). Bethesda, MD, National Heart, Lung, and Blood Institute, 1994, p. 1.
390. Vincent, R.: Pre-hospital management. *In* Julian, D., and Braunwald, E. (eds.): Management of Acute Myocardial Infarction. London, W. B. Saunders Ltd., 1994, p. 3.

MANAGEMENT IN THE EMERGENCY DEPARTMENT

391. National Heart Attack Alert Program: Emergency Department: Rapid identification and treatment of patients with acute myocardial infarction (NIH Publication 93-3278). Bethesda, MD, National Heart, Lung, and Blood Institute, 1993.
392. Kaul, S., and Abbott, R. D.: Evaluation of chest pain in the Emergency Department. Ann. Intern. Med. *121*:976, 1994.
393. Karlson, B. W., Herlitz, J., Wiklund, O., et al.: Early prediction of acute myocardial infarction from clinical history, examination, and electrocardiogram in the emergency room. Am. J. Cardiol. *68*:171, 1991.
394. Karlsson, J. E., Berglund, U., Bjorkholm, A., et al.: Thrombolysis with recombinant human tissue-type plasminogen activator during instability in coronary artery disease: Effect on myocardial ischemia and need for coronary revascularization: TRIC Study Group. Am. Heart J. *124*:1419, 1992.
395. The TIMI IIIB Investigators: Effects of tissue plasminogen activator and a comparison of early invasive and conservative strategies in unstable angina and non-Q-wave myocardial infarction: Results of the TIMI IIIB Trial. Circulation *89*:1545, 1994.
396. Granger, C. B.: Early management of acute coronary syndromes: Need for better understanding and treatment strategies. Clinician *13*:44, 1995.
397. Cragg, D., Friedman, H., Bonema, J., et al.: Outcome of patients with acute myocardial infarction who are ineligible for thrombolytic therapy. Ann. Intern. Med. *115*:173, 1991.
398. Granger, C., Christopher, D., Stebbins, A., et al.: Thrombolytic therapy treats the tip of the MI iceberg: Results from the GUSTO MI registry. Circulation *90*(Suppl. I):663, 1994.
399. Goldman, L., Cook, E., Brand, D., et al.: A computer protocol to predict myocardial infarction in emergency department patients with chest pain. N. Engl. J. Med. *318*:797, 1988.
399a. Baxt, W. G., and Skora, J.: Prospective validation of artificial neural network trained to identify acute myocardial infarction. Lancet *347*:12, 1996.
400. Fuchs, R., and Scheidt, S.: Improved criteria for admission to cardiac care units. JAMA *246*:2037, 1985.
401. Peels, C. H., Visser, C. A., Funke Kupper, A. J., et al.: Usefulness of two-dimensional echocardiography for immediate detection of myocardial ischemia in the emergency room. Am. J. Cardiol. *65*:687, 1990.
402. Armstrong, W.: Echocardiography in acute myocardial infarction. *In* Francis, G., and Alpert, J. (eds.): Modern Coronary Care. Boston, Little, Brown and Co., 1990, p. 455.
403. Wackers, F., Kie, K., Liem, K., et al.: Potential value of thallium-201 scintigraphy as a means of selecting patients for the coronary care unit. Br. Heart J. *41*:111, 1979.
404. Nelson, M.: Critical pathways in the emergency department. J. Emerg. Nurs. *19*:110, 1993.
405. Lyle, K.: Enhancing early cardiac care: Critical pathways and practice guidelines in the ED and CPED. Clinician *13*:60, 1995.
406. Gaspoz, J. M., Lee, T. H., Weinstein, M. C., et al.: Cost-effectiveness of a new short-stay unit to "rule out" acute myocardial infarction in low risk patients. J. Am. Coll. Cardiol. *24*:1249, 1994.
407. Barish, R. A., and Doherty, R. J.: Establishing a chest pain center in an academic medical center: The University of Maryland experience. Clinician *13*:39, 1995.
408. Stein, B., and Fuster, V.: Clinical pharmacology of platelet inhibitors. *In* Fuster, V., and Verstraete, M. (eds.): Thrombosis in Cardiovascular Disorders. Philadelphia, W. B. Saunders Company, 1992, p. 99.
409. Meyer, B. J., and Chesebro, J. H.: Aspirin and anticoagulants. *In* Julian, D., and Braunwald, E. (eds.): Management of Acute Myocardial Infarction. London, W. B. Saunders Ltd., 1994, p. 163.
410. Reilly, I. A. G., and Fitzgerald, G. A.: Inhibition of thromboxane formation *in vivo* and *ex vivo*: Implications for therapy with platelet inhibitory drugs. Blood *69*:180, 1987.
411. Fuster, V., Dyken, M. L., Voonas, P. S., et al.: Aspirin as a therapeutic agent in cardiovascular disease: Special Writing Group. Circulation *87*:659, 1993.
412. Herlitz, J.: Analgesia in myocardial infarction. Drugs *37*:939, 1989.
413. Kock, M., Blomberg, S., Emanuelsson, H., et al.: Thoracic epidural anesthesia improves global and regional left ventricular function during stress-induced myocardial ischemia in patients with coronary artery disease. Anesth. Analg. *71*:625, 1990.
414. Chamberlain, D.: β-Blockers and calcium antagonists. *In* Julian, D., and Braunwald, E. (eds.): Management of Acute Myocardial Infarction. London, W. B. Saunders Ltd., 1994, p. 193.
415. Hjalmarson, A., Elmfeldt, D., Herlitz, J., et al.: Effect on mortality of metoprolol in acute myocardial infarction, a double-blind randomized trial. Lancet *2*:823, 1981.
416. Kirshenbaum, J. M., Kloner, R. F., McGowan, N., et al.: Use of an ultrashort-acting beta receptor blocker (esmolol) in patients with acute myocardial ischemia and relative contraindications to beta-blockade therapy. J. Am. Coll. Cardiol. *12*:773, 1988.
417. Yusuf, S., Held, P., and Furberg, C.: Update of effects of calcium antagonists in myocardial infarction or angina in light of the second Danish Verapamil Infarction Trial (DAVIT-II) and other recent studies. Am. J. Cardiol. *67*:1295, 1991.
418. Furberg, C. D., Psaty, B. M., and Meyer, J. V.: Nifedipine: Dose-related increase in mortality in patients with coronary heart disease. Circulation *92*:1236, 1995.
419. Maroko, P., Radvany, P., Braunwald, E., et al.: Reduction of infarct size by oxygen inhalation following acute coronary occlusion. Circulation *52*:360, 1975.
420. Madias, J. E., and Hood, W. B., Jr.: Reduction of precordial ST-segment elevation in patients with anterior myocardial infarction by oxygen breathing. Circulation *53*:198, 1976.
421. Gersh, B. J., and Anderson, J. L.: Thrombolysis and myocardial salvage: Results of clinical trials and the animal paradigm—paradoxic or predictable? Circulation *88*:296, 1993.
422. Califf, R. M., and Bengtson, J. R.: Cardiogenic shock. N. Engl. J. Med. *330*:1724, 1994.
423. O'Gara, P. T.: Primary pump failure. *In* Fuster, V., Ross, R., and Topol, E. (eds.): Atherosclerosis and Coronary Artery Disease. New York, Raven Press, 1995, p. 1051.
424. Gaudron, P., Eilles, C., Kugler, I., et al.: Progressive left ventricular dysfunction and remodeling after myocardial infarction. Circulation *87*:755, 1993.
425. Pfeffer, M.: ACE inhibition in acute myocardial infarction. N. Engl. J. Med. *332*:118, 1995.

426. Maroko, P. R., and Braunwald, E.: Modification of myocardial infarct size after coronary occlusion. Ann. Intern. Med. *79:*720, 1973.
427. Martin, G. V., and Kennedy, J. W.: Choice of thrombolytic agent. *In* Julian, D., and Braunwald, E. (eds.): Management of Acute Myocardial Infarction. London, W. B. Saunders Ltd., 1994, p. 71.
428. Iliceto, S., Scrutinio, D., Bruzzi, P., et al.: Effects of L-carnitine administration on left ventricular remodeling after acute anterior myocardial infarction: The L-Carnitine Ecocardiografia Digitalizzata Infarto Miocardico (CEDIM) Trial. J. Am. Coll. Cardiol. *26:*380, 1995.
429. Hahn, R., Wond, S. C., Brown, E., et al.: Early benefits of late coronary reperfusion on reducing myocardial infarct expansion: Echo findings and ultrastructural basis. J. Am. Coll. Cardiol. *21:*301A, 1993.
430. Rude, R. E., Muller, J. E., and Braunwald, E.: Efforts to limit the size of myocardial infarcts. Ann. Intern. Med. *95:*736, 1981.
431. Kubler, W., and Doorey, A.: Reduction of infarct size: An attractive concept: Useful or possible in human? Br. Heart J. *53:*5, 1985.
432. Christian, T. F., Schwartz, R. S., and Gibbons, R. J.: Determinants of infarct size in reperfusion therapy for acute myocardial infarction. Circulation *86:*81, 1992.
433. Taegtmeyer, H.: Energy metabolism of the heart: From basic concepts to clinical applications. Curr. Probl. Cardiol. *19:*57, 1994.
434. Kusuoka, H., and Marban, E.: Role of altered calcium homeostasis in stunned myocardium. *In* Kloner, R. A., and Przyklenk, K. (eds.): Stunned Myocardium. New York, Marcel Dekker, 1993, p. 197.
435. Bolli, R.: Oxygen-derived free radicals and postischemic myocardial dysfunction ("stunned myocardium"). J. Am. Coll. Cardiol. *12:*239, 1988.
436. Bolli, R.: Myocardial "stunning" in man. Circulation *86:*1671, 1992.
437. Weglicki, W. B., Phillips, T. M., Mak, I. T., et al.: Cytokines, neuropeptides, and reperfusion injury during magnesium deficiency. Ann. N. Y. Acad. Sci. *723:*246, 1994.
438. Airaghi, L., Lettino, M., Manfredi, M. G., et al.: Endogenous cytokine antagonists during myocardial ischemia and thrombolytic therapy. Am. Heart J. *130:*204, 1995.
439. Przyklenk, K., and Kloner, R. A.: Oxygen radical scavenging agents as adjuvant therapy with tissue plasminogen activator in a canine model of coronary thrombolysis. Cardiovasc. Res. *27:*925, 1993.
440. Kloner, R. A., and Yellon, D.: Does ischemic preconditioning occur in patients? J. Am. Coll. Cardiol. *24:*1133, 1994.
441. Przyklenk, K., Bauer, B., Ovize, M., et al.: Regional ischemic "preconditioning" protects remote virgin myocardium from subsequent sustained coronary occlusion. Circulation *87:*893, 1993.
442. Kloner, R. A., Shook, T., Przyklenk, K., et al.: Previous angina alters in-hospital outcome in TIMI 4: A clinical correlate to preconditioning? Circulation *91:*37, 1995.
443. Kloner, R. A., Muller, J., and Davis, V.: Effects of previous angina pectoris in patients with first acute myocardial infarction not receiving thrombolytics: MILIS Study Group: Multicenter Investigation of the Limitation of Infarct Size. Am. J. Cardiol. *75:*615, 1995.
444. Anzai, T., Yoshikawa, T., Asakura, Y., et al.: Preinfarction angina as a major predictor of left ventricular function and long-term prognosis after a first Q wave myocardial infarction. J. Am. Coll. Cardiol. *26:*319, 1995.

REPERFUSION OF MYOCARDIAL INFARCTION

445. Morgan, C. D., Roberts, R. S., Haq, A., et al.: Coronary patency, infarct size and left ventricular function after thrombolytic therapy for acute myocardial infarction: Results from the tissue plasminogen activator: Toronto (TPAT) placebo-controlled trial: TPAT Study Group. J. Am. Coll. Cardiol. *17:*1451, 1991.
446. Cerqueira, M. D., Maynard, C., and Ritchie, J. L.: Radionuclide assessment of infarct size and left ventricular function in clinical trials of thrombolysis. Circulation *84:*100, 1991.
447. Bassand, J. P., Machecourt, J., Cassagnes, J., et al.: Multicenter trial of intravenous anisoylated plasminogen streptokinase activator complex (APSAC) in acute myocardial infarction: Effects on infarct size and left ventricular function. J. Am. Coll. Cardiol. *13:*988, 1989.
448. Ritchie, J. L., Cerqueira, M., Maynard, C., et al.: Ventricular function and infarct size: The Western Washington Intravenous Streptokinase in Myocardial Infarction Trial. J. Am. Coll. Cardiol. *11:*689, 1988.
449. Althouse, R., Maynard, C., Cerqueira, M. D., et al.: The Western Washington Myocardial Infarction Registry and Emergency Department Tissue Plasminogen Activator Treatment Trial. Am. J. Cardiol. *66:*1289, 1990.
449a. Andreotti, F., Pasceri, V., Hackett, D. R., et al.: Preinfarction angina as a predictor of more rapid coronary thrombolysis in patients with acute myocardial infarction. N. Engl. J. Med. *334:*7, 1995.
450. van der Laarse, A., van Leeuwen, F. T., Krul, R., et al.: The size of infarction as judged enzymatically in 1974 patients with acute myocardial infarction: Relation with symptomatology, infarct localization and type of infarction. Int. J. Cardiol. *19:*191, 1988.
451. Topol, E. J., and Ellis, S. G.: Coronary collaterals revisited: Accessory pathway to myocardial preservation during infarction. Circulation *83:*1084, 1991.
452. Virmani, R., et al.: Reperfusion injury in the ischemic myocardium. Cardiovasc. Pathol. *1:*117, 1992.
453. Kloner, R. A., and Przylenk, K.: Understanding the jargon: A glossary of terms used (and misused) in the study of ischaemia and reperfusion. Cardiovasc. Res. *27:*162, 1993.
454. Kloner, R. A.: Does reperfusion injury exist in humans? J. Am. Coll. Cardiol. *21:*537, 1993.
455. Ito, H., Tomooka, T., Sakai, N., et al.: Lack of myocardial perfusion immediately after successful thrombolysis: A predictor of poor recovery of left ventricular function in anterior myocardial infarction. Circulation *85:*1699, 1992.
456. Gottleib, R. A., Burleson, K. O., Kloner, R. A., et al.: Reperfusion injury induces apoptosis in rabbit cardiomyocytes. J. Clin. Invest. *94:*1621, 1994.
457. Herzog, W. R., Schlossberg, M. L., MacMurdy, K. S., et al.: Timing of magnesium therapy affects experimental infarct size. Circulation *92:*2622, 1995.
458. Christensen, C. W., Rieder, M. A., Silverstein, E. L., et al.: Magnesium sulfate reduces myocardial infarct size when administered prior to but not after coronary reperfusion in a canine model. Circulation *92:*2617, 1995.
459. Antman, E. M.: Magnesium in acute MI: Timing is critical. Circulation *92:*2367, 1995.
460. Kloner, R. A., Ganote, C. E., and Jennings, R. B.: The "no-reflow" phenomenon after temporary coronary occlusion in the dog. J. Clin. Invest. *54:*1496, 1974.
461. Entman, M. L., Michael, L., Rossen, R. D., et al.: Inflammation in the course of early myocardial ischemia. FASEB J. *5:*2529, 1991.
462. Waller, B. F., Rothbaum, D. A., Pinkerton, C. A., et al.: Status of the myocardium and infarct-related coronary artery in 19 necropsy patients with acute recanalization using pharmacologic (streptokinase, r-tissue plasminogen activator), mechanical (percutaneous transluminal coronary angioplasty) or combined types of reperfusion therapy. J. Am. Coll. Cardiol. *9:*785, 1987.
463. Ohnishi, Y., Butterfield, M. C., Saffitz, J. E., et al.: Deleterious effects of a systemic lytic state on reperfused myocardium: Minimization of reperfusion injury and enhanced recovery of myocardial function by direct angioplasty. Circulation *92:*500, 1995.
464. Gertz, S. D., Kragel, A. H., Kalan, J. M., et al.: Comparison of coronary and myocardial morphologic findings in patients with and without thrombolytic therapy during fatal first acute myocardial infarction. Am. J. Cardiol. *66:*904, 1990.
465. Ferrari, R., Albertini, A., Curello, S., et al.: Myocardial recovery during post-ischaemic reperfusion: Effects of nifedipine, calcium, and magnesium. J. Mol. Cell. Cardiol. *18:*487, 1986.
466. Steenbergen, C., Murphy, E., Levy, L., et al.: Elevation in cytosolic free calcium concentration early in myocardial ischemia in perfused rat heart. Circ. Res. *60:*700, 1987.
467. Werns, S. W., Shea, M. J., Driscoll, E. M., et al.: The independent effects of oxygen radical scavengers on canine infarct size reduction by superoxide dismutase but not catalase. Circ. Res. *56:*895, 1985.
468. Flaherty, J. T., Pitt, B., Gruber, J. W., et al.: Recombinant human superoxide dismutase (h-SOD) fails to improve recovery of ventricular function in patients undergoing coronary angioplasty for acute myocardial infarction. Circulation *89:*1982, 1991.
469. Neumann, F.-J., Ott, I., Gawaz, M., et al.: Cardiac release of cytokines and inflammatory responses in acute myocardial infarction. Circulation *92:*748, 1995.
470. du Toit, E. F., and Opie, L. H.: Modulation of severity of reperfusion stunning in the isolated rat heart by agents altering calcium flux at reperfusion. Circ. Res. *70:*960, 1992.
471. Silver, M. J., Sutton, J. M., Hook, S., et al.: Adjunctive selectin blockade successfully reduces infarct size beyond thrombolysis in the electrolytic canine coronary artery model. Circulation *92:*492, 1995.
472. Smalling, R. W., Feld, S., Ramanna, N., et al.: Infarct salvage with liposomal prostaglandin E_1 administered by intravenous bolus immediately before reperfusion in a canine infarction-reperfusion model. Circulation *92:*935, 1995.
473. Klein, H. H., Pich, S., Bohle, R. M., et al.: Myocardial protection by Na^+-H^+ exchange inhibition in ischemic, reperfused porcine hearts. Circulation *92:*912, 1995.
474. TIMI Study Group: Comparison of invasive and conservative strategies after treatment with intravenous tissue plasminogen activator in acute myocardial infarction: Results of the Thrombolysis in Myocardial Infarction (TIMI) Phase II Trial. N. Engl. J. Med. *302:*618, 1989.
475. Roberts, R., Rogers, W. J., Mueller, H. S., et al.: Immediate versus deferred beta-blockade following thrombolytic therapy in patients with acute myocardial infarction: Results of the Thrombolysis in Myocardial Infarction (TIMI) II-B Study. Circulation *83:*422, 1991.
476. Murry, C. E., Jennings, R. B., and Reimer, K. A.: What is ischemic preconditioning? *In* Przylenk, K., Kloner, R. A., and Yellon, D. M. (eds.): Ischemic Preconditioning: The Concept of Endogenous Cardioprotection. Norwell, MA, Kluwer Academic, 1994, p. 3.
477. Gross, G. J., and Auchampach, J. A.: Blockade of ATP-sensitive potassium channels prevents myocardial preconditioning in dogs. Circ. Res. *70:*222, 1992.
478. Mizumura, T., Nithipatikom, K., and Gross, G. J.: Bimakalim, an ATP-sensitive potassium channel opener, mimics the effects of ischemic preconditioning to reduce infarct size, adenosine release, and neutrophil function in dogs. Circulation *92:*1236, 1995.
479. Hearse, D. J.: Activation of ATP-sensitive potassium channels: A novel pharmacological approach to myocardial protection? Cardiovasc. Res. *30:*1, 1995.
480. Wolfe, C. L., Stevens, R. E., Vissern, F. L. J., et al.: Loss of myocardial protection after preconditioning correlates with the time course of

glycogen recovery within the preconditioned segment. Circulation *87*:881, 1993.

480a. Barbosa, V., Sievers, R. E., Zaugg, C. E., and Wolfe, C. L.: Preconditioning ischemia time determines the degree of glycogen depletion and infarct size reduction in rat hearts. Am. Heart J. *131*:224, 1996.

480b. Sandhu, R., Thomas, U., Diaz, R. J., and Wilson, G. J.: Effect of ischemic preconditioning of the myocardium on cAMP. Circ Res. *78*:137, 1996.

481. Marber, M. S., Latchman, D. S., Walker, M., et al.: Cardiac stress protein elevation 24 hours after brief ischemia or heat stress is associated with resistance to myocardial infarction. Circulation *88*:1264, 1993.

482. Chen, W., Gabel, S., Steenbergen, C., et al.: A redox-based mechanism for cardioprotection induced by ischemic preconditioning in perfused rat heart. Circ. Res. *77*:424, 1995.

483. Wei, J. Y., Markis, J. E., Malagold, M., et al.: Cardiovascular reflexes stimulated by reperfusion of ischemic myocardium in acute myocardial infarction. Circulation *67*:796, 1983.

484. Vera, Z., Pride, H. P., and Zipes, D. P.: Reperfusion arrhythmias: Role of early afterdepolarizations studied by monophasic action potential recordings in the intact canine heart during autonomically denervated and stimulated sites. J. Cardiovasc. Electrophysiol. *6*:532, 1995.

485. Goldberg, S., Greenspon, A. J., Urban, P. L., et al.: Reperfusion of arrhythmia: A marker of restoration of antegrade flow during intracoronary thrombolysis for acute myocardial infarction. Am. Heart J. *105*:26, 1983.

486. Califf, R. M., O'Neill, W., Stack, R. S., et al.: Failure of simple clinical characteristics to predict perfusion status after intravenous thrombolysis. Ann. Intern. Med. *108*:658, 1988.

487. Solomon, S. D., Ridker, P. M., and Antman, E. M.: Ventricular arrhythmias in trials of thrombolytic therapy for acute myocardial infarction: A meta-analysis. Circulation *88*:2575, 1993.

488. Kim, C., and Braunwald, E.: Potential benefits of late reperfusion of infarcted myocardium: The open artery hypothesis. Circulation *88*:2426, 1993.

489. Hochman, J. S., and Choo, H.: Limitation of myocardial infarct expansion by reperfusion independent of myocardial salvage. Circulation *75*:299, 1987.

489a. Alhaddad, A. I., Kloner, R. A., Hakim, I., et al.: Benefits of late coronary artery reperfusion on infarct expansion progressively diminish over time: Relation to viable islets of myocytes within the scar. Am. Heart J. *131*:451, 1996.

490. Braunwald, E.: Coronary artery patency in patients with myocardial infarction. J. Am. Coll. Cardiol. *16*:1550, 1990.

491. Schröder, R., Neuhaus, K. L., Linderer, T., et al.: Impact of late coronary artery reperfusion on left ventricular function one month after acute myocardial infarction (results from the ISAM study). Am. J. Cardiol. *64*:878, 1989.

492. Lavie, C. J., O'Keefe, J. H., Chesebro, J. H., et al.: Prevention of late ventricular dilatation after acute myocardial infarction by successful thrombolytic reperfusion. Am. J. Cardiol. *66*:31, 1990.

493. Topol, E. J., Califf, R. M., Vandormael, M., et al.: A randomized trial of late reperfusion therapy for acute myocardial infarction: Thrombolysis and Angioplasty in Myocardial Infarction-6 Study Group. Circulation *85*:2090, 1992.

494. Golia, G., Marino, P., Rametta, F., et al.: Reperfusion reduces left ventricular dilatation without infarct size limitation by late reperfusion in the acute and chronic phases after myocardial infarction. Am. Heart J. *127*:499, 1994.

495. Nidorf, S. M., Siu, S. C., Galambos, G., et al.: Benefit of late coronary reperfusion on ventricular morphology and function after myocardial infarction. J. Am. Coll. Cardiol. *21*:683, 1993.

496. Zaman, A. G., Morris, J. L., Smylie, J. H., et al.: Late potentials and ventricular enlargement after myocardial infarction. Circulation *88*:905, 1993.

497. Hii, J. T. Y., Traboulsi, M., Mitchell, L. B., et al.: Infarct artery patency predicts outcome of serial electropharmacological studies in patients with malignant ventricular arrhythmias. Circulation *87*:764, 1993.

498. Steinberg, J. S., Hochman, J. S., Morgan, C. D., et al.: The effects of thrombolytic therapy administered 6–24 hours after myocardial infarction on the signal-averaged ECG: Results of a multicenter randomized trial. J. Am. Coll. Cardiol. *21*:225A, 1993.

499. Lamas, G. V., Flaker, G. C., Mitchell, G., et al.: Effects of infarct artery patency on prognosis after acute myocardial infarction. Circulation *92*:1101, 1995.

500. White, H. D., Cross, D. B., Elliott, J. M., et al.: Long-term prognostic importance of patency of the infarct-related coronary artery after thrombolytic therapy for acute myocardial infarction. Circulation *89*:61, 1994.

501. Pirzada, F. A., Weiner, J. M., and Hood, W. B. J.: Experimental myocardial infarction: Accelerated myocardial stiffening related to coronary reperfusion following ischemia. Chest *74*:190, 1978.

502. Richard, V., Murry, C. E., and Reimer, K. A.: Healing of myocardial infarcts in dogs: Effects of late reperfusion. Circulation *92*:1891, 1995.

503. Montalescot, G., Faraggi, M., Drobinski, G., et al.: Myocardial viability in patients with Q wave myocardial infarction and no residual ischemia. Circulation *86*:47, 1992.

504. Boehrer, J. D., Glamann, D. B., Lange, R. A., et al.: Effect of coronary angioplasty on late potentials one to two weeks after acute myocardial infarction. Am. J. Cardiol. *70*:1515, 1992.

505. Gang, E. S., Lew, A. S., Hong, M., et al.: Decreased incidence of ventricular late potentials after successful thrombolytic therapy for acute myocardial infarction. N. Engl. J. Med. *321*:712, 1989.

506. Horvitz, L. L., Pietrolungo, J. F., Suri, R. S., et al.: An open infarct-related artery is associated with a lower risk of lethal arrhythmias in patients with a left ventricular aneurysm. Circulation *86*:I, 1992.

CORONARY THROMBOLYSIS

507. Fletcher, A. P., Alkjaersig, N., Smyrniotis, F. E., et al.: The treatment of patients suffering from early myocardial infarction with massive and prolonged streptokinase therapy. Trans. Assoc. Am. Physicians *71*:287, 1958.

508. Gruppo Italiano Per Lo Studio Della Streptochinasi Nell'Infarct Miocardico (GISSI): Effectiveness of intravenous thrombolytic treatment in acute myocardial infarction. Lancet *1*:397, 1986.

509. van de Werf, F., Ludbrook, P. A., Bergmann, S. R., et al.: Coronary thrombolysis with tissue-type plasminogen activator in patients with evolving myocardial infarction. N. Engl. J. Med. *310*:609, 1984.

510. Kennedy, J., Ritchie, J., Davis, K., et al.: The Western Washington randomized trial of intracoronary streptokinase in acute myocardial infarction: A 12-month follow-up report. N. Engl. J. Med. *312*:1073, 1985.

511. Tiefenbrunn, A. J., and Sobel, B. E.: Thrombolysis and myocardial infarction. Fibrinolysis *5*:1, 1991.

512. Tiefenbrunn, A. J.: Clinical benefits of thrombolytic therapy in acute myocardial infarction. Am. J. Cardiol. *69*:3, 1992.

512a. Lincoff, A. M., and Topol, E. J.: Acute myocardial infarction: Acute management: thrombolytic therapy. *In* Fuster, V., Ross, R., and Topol, E. J. (eds.): Atherosclerosis and Coronary Artery Disease. Philadelphia, Lippincott-Raven, 1996, pp. 955–978.

513. Granger, C. B., Califf, R. M., and Topol, E. J.: Thrombolytic therapy for acute myocardial infarction: A review. Drugs *44*:293, 1992.

514. Topol, E.: Thrombolytic intervention. *In* Topol, E. (ed.): Textbook of Interventional Cardiology. 2nd ed. Philadelphia, W. B. Saunders Company, 1994, p. 68.

515. TIMI Study Group: The Thrombolysis in Myocardial Infarction (TIMI) Trial: Phase I findings. N. Engl. J. Med. *312*:932, 1985.

516. Chesebro, J. H., Knatterud, G., Roberts, R., et al.: Thrombolysis in Myocardial Infarction (TIMI) Trial, Phase 1: A comparison between intravenous tissue plasminogen activator and intravenous streptokinase. Circulation *76*:142, 1987.

517. Gold, H. K., Leinbach, R. C., Garabedian, H. D., et al.: Acute coronary reocclusion after thrombolysis with recombinant human tissue-type plasminogen activator: Prevention by a maintenance infusion. Circulation *73*:347, 1986.

518. Langer, A., Krucoff, M. W., Klootwijk, P., et al.: Noninvasive assessment of speed and stability of infarct-related artery reperfusion: Results of the GUSTO ST segment monitoring study: Global Utilization of Streptokinase and Tissue Plasminogen Activator for Occluded Coronary Arteries. J. Am. Coll. Cardiol. *25*:1552, 1995.

519. The GUSTO Angiographic Investigators: The comparative effects of tissue plasminogen activator, streptokinase, or both on coronary artery patency, ventricular function and survival after acute myocardial infarction. N. Engl. J. Med. *329*:1615, 1993.

520. Lenderink, T., Simoons, M. L., Van Es, G.-A., et al.: Benefits of thrombolytic therapy is sustained throughout five years and is related to TIMI perfusion grade 3 but not grade 2 flow at discharge. Circulation *92*:1110, 1995.

521. Karagounis, L., Sorensen, S. G., Menlove, R. L., et al.: Does Thrombolysis in Myocardial Infarction (TIMI) perfusion grade 2 represent a mostly patent artery or a mostly occluded artery? Enzymatic and electrocardiographic evidence from the TEAM-2 study. J. Am. Coll. Cardiol. *19*:1, 1992.

522. Clemmensen, P., Ohman, E. M., Sevilla, D. C., et al.: Impact of infarct artery patency on the relationship between electrocardiographic and ventriculographic evidence of acute myocardial ischaemia. Eur. Heart J. *15*:1356, 1994.

523. Vogt, A., von Essen, R., Tebbe, U., et al.: Impact of early perfusion status of the infarct-related artery on short-term mortality after thrombolysis for acute myocardial infarction: Retrospective analysis of four German multicenter studies. J. Am. Coll. Cardiol. *21*:1391, 1993.

524. Gibson, C. M., Cannon, C. P., Baim, D. S., et al.: TIMI frame count: A new standardization of infarct-related artery flow grade, and its relationship to clinical outcomes in the TIMI-4 trial. Circulation *90*(Suppl I):220, 1994.

525. Lincoff, A. M., and Topol, E. J.: Illusion of reperfusion: Does anyone achieve optimal reperfusion during acute myocardial infarction? Circulation *87*:1792, 1993.

526. Abendschein, D. R., Meng, Y. Y., Torr-Brown, S., et al.: Maintenance of coronary patency after fibrinolysis with tissue factor pathway inhibitor. Circulation *92*:944, 1995.

527. Yao, S.-K., Akhtar, S., Scott-Burden, T., et al.: Endogenous and exogenous nitric oxide protect against intracoronary thrombosis and reocclusion after thrombolysis. Circulation *92*:1005, 1995.

528. Weaver, W. D.: Time to thrombolytic treatment: Factors affecting delay and their influence on outcome. J. Am. Coll. Cardiol. *25*:3S, 1995.

529. ISIS-2 (Second International Study of Infarct Survival) Collaborative Group: Randomised trial of intravenous streptokinase, oral aspirin, both, or neither among 17,187 cases of suspected acute myocardial infarction: ISIS-2. Lancet *2*:349, 1988.

530. ISAM (Intravenous Streptokinase in Acute Myocardial Infarction)

Study Group: A prospective trial of intravenous streptokinase in acute myocardial infarction (ISAM). N. Engl. J. Med. *314*:1465, 1986.
531. AIMS Trial Study Group: Effect of intravenous APSAC on mortality after acute myocardial infarction: Preliminary report of a placebo-controlled clinical trial. Lancet *1*:545, 1988.
532. Wilcox, R. G., von der Lippe, G., Olsson, C. G., et al.: Trial of tissue plasminogen activator for mortality reduction in acute myocardial infarction: Anglo-Scandinavian Study of Early Thrombolysis (ASSET). Lancet *1*:525, 1988.
533. LATE (Late Assessment of Thrombolytic Efficacy) Study Group: Late Assessment of Thrombolytic Efficacy (LATE) study with alteplase 6–24 hours after onset of acute myocardial infarction. Lancet *342*:759, 1993.
534. EMERAS (Estudio Multicentrico Estreptoquinasa Republicas de America del Sur) Collaborative Group: Randomized trial of late thrombolysis in acute myocardial infarction. Lancet *342*:767, 1993.
535. ISIS-3 (Third International Study of Infarct Survival) Collaborative Group: ISIS-3: A randomized trial of streptokinase vs tissue plasminogen activator vs anistreplase and of aspirin plus heparin vs aspirin alone among 41,299 cases of suspected acute myocardial infarction. Lancet *339*:753, 1992.
536. Krumholz, H. M., Pasternak, R. C., Weinstein, M. C., et al.: Efficacy and cost-effectiveness of thrombolytic therapy in elderly patients with suspected acute myocardial infarction. N. Engl. J. Med. *327*:7, 1992.
537. Topol, E. J., and Califf, R. M.: Thrombolytic therapy for elderly patients. N. Engl. J. Med. *327*:45, 1992.
538. Hillis, L. D., Forman, S., Braunwald, E., et al.: Risk stratification before thrombolytic therapy in patients with acute myocardial infarction. J. Am. Coll. Cardiol. *16*:313, 1990.
539. Zehender, M., Kasper, W., Kauder, E., et al.: Right ventricular infarction as an independent predictor of prognosis after acute inferior myocardial infarction. N. Engl. J. Med. *328*:981, 1993.
540. Peterson, E. G., Hathaway, W. R., Zabel, K. M., et al.: The prognostic importance of anterior ST-segment depression in inferior myocardial infarctions: Results in 16,185 patients. J. Am. Coll. Cardiol. *25*:342A, 1995.
541. Berger, P. B., and Ryan, T. J.: Inferior myocardial infarction: High-risk subgroups. Circulation *81*:401, 1990.
542. Lee, K. L., Woodlief, L. H., Topol, E. J., et al.: Predictors of 30-day mortality in the era of reperfusion for acute myocardial infarction: Results from an international trial of 41,021 patients. Circulation *91*:1659, 1995.
543. Serruys, P. W., Simoons, M. L., Suryapranata, H., et al.: Preservation of global and regional left ventricular function after early thrombolysis in acute myocardial infarction. J. Am. Coll. Cardiol. *7*:729, 1986.
544. Van de Werf, F., Arnold, A. E. R., and for the European Cooperative Study Group for Recombinant Tissue Type Plasminogen Activator: Intravenous tissue plasminogen activator and size of infarct, left ventricular function, and survival in acute myocardial infarction. BMJ *297*:1374, 1988.
545. Gruppo Italiano Per Lo Studio Della Streochi and Nasi Nell'Infarto Miocardico: Long-term effects of intravenous thrombolysis in acute myocardial infarction: Final report of the GISSI study. Lancet *2*:871, 1987.
546. Meijer, A., Verheugt, F. W. A., Werter, C. J. P. J., et al.: Aspirin versus coumadin in the prevention of reocclusion and recurrent ischemia after successful thrombolysis: a prospective placebo-controlled angiographic study: Results of the APRICOT Study. Circulation *87*:1524, 1993.
547. Schroder, R., Neuhaus, K. L., Leizorovicz, A., et al.: A prospective placebo-controlled double-blind multicenter trial of intravenous streptokinase in acute myocardial infarction (ISAM): Long-term mortality and morbidity. J. Am. Coll. Cardiol. *9*:197, 1987.
547a. Collen, D.: Fibrin-selective thrombolytic therapy for acute myocardial infarction. Circulation *93*:857, 1996.
548. The International Study Group: In-hospital mortality and clinical course of 20,891 patients with suspected acute myocardial infarction randomised between alteplase and streptokinase with or without heparin. Lancet *2*:71, 1990.
549. Cannon, C. P., McCabe, C. H., Diver, D. J., et al.: Comparison of front-loaded recombinant tissue-type plasminogen activator, anistreplase and combination thrombolytic therapy for acute myocardial infarction: Results of the Thrombolysis in Myocardial Infarction (TIMI) 4 trial. J. Am. Coll. Cardiol. *24*:1602, 1994.
550. Califf, R. M., Harrelson-Woodlief, L., and Topol, E. J.: Left-ventricular ejection fraction may not be useful as an end point of thrombolytic therapy comparative trials. Circulation *82*:1847, 1990.
551. White, H. D., Norris, R. M., Brown, M. A., et al.: Effect of intravenous streptokinase on left ventricular function and early survival after acute myocardial infarction. N. Engl. J. Med. *317*:850, 1987.
552. St. John Sutton, M., Pfeffer, M. A., Plappert, T., et al.: Quantitative two-dimensional echocardiographic measurements are major predictors of adverse cardiovascular events after acute myocardial infarction: The protective effects of captopril. Circulation *89*:68, 1994.
553. Sheehan, F. H.: Measurement of left ventricular function as an end-point in trials of thrombolytic therapy. Coronary Art. Dis. *1*:13, 1990.
554. Lavie, C. J., Gersh, B. J., and Chesebro, J. H.: Reperfusion in acute myocardial infarction. Mayo Clin. Proc. *65*:549, 1990.
555. Wackers, F. J. T., Terrin, M. L., Kayden, D. S., et al.: Quantitative radionuclide assessment of regional ventricular function after thrombolytic therapy for acute myocardial infarction: Results of Phase I Thrombolysis in Myocardial Infarction (TIMI) Trial. J. Am. Coll. Cardiol. *13*:998, 1989.
556. Gruppo Italiano per lo Studio della Sopravvivenza nell'Infarto Miocardico: GISSI-2: A factorial randomised trial of alteplase versus streptokinase and heparin versus no heparin among 12,490 patients with acute myocardial infarction. Lancet *336*:65, 1990.
557. Califf, R. M., Fortin, D. F., Tenaglia, A. N., et al.: Clinical risks of thrombolytic therapy. Am. J. Cardiol. *69*:3, 1992.
558. Antman, E. M., for the TIMI 9A Investigators: Hirudin in acute myocardial infarction: Safety report from the Thrombolysis and Thrombin Inhibition in Myocardial Infarction (TIMI) 9A trial. Circulation *90*:1624, 1994.
559. The Global Use of Strategies to Open Occluded Coronary Arteries (GUSTO) IIa Investigators: A randomized trial of intravenous heparin versus recombinant hirudin for acute coronary syndromes. Circulation *90*:1631, 1994.
560. Sane, D. C., Califf, R. M., Topol, E. J., et al.: Bleeding during thrombolytic therapy for acute myocardial infarction: Mechanisms and management. Ann. Intern. Med. *111*:1010, 1989.
561. Gore, J. M., Granger, C. B., Simoons, M. L., et al.: Stroke after thrombolysis: Mortality and functional outcomes in the GUSTO-I Trial. Circulation *92*:2811, 1995.
562. Maggioni, A. P., Franzosi, M. G., Santoro, E., et al.: The risk of stroke in patients with acute myocardial infarction after thrombolytic and antithrombotic treatment. N. Engl. J. Med. *327*:1, 1992.
563. De Jaegere, P. P., Arnold, A. A., Balk, A. H., et al.: Intracranial hemorrhage in association with thrombolytic therapy: Incidence and clinical predictive factors. J. Am. Coll. Cardiol. *19*:289, 1992.
564. Simoons, M., Maggioni, A., Knatterud, G., et al.: Individual risk assessment for intracranial hemorrhage during thrombolytic therapy. Lancet *342*:1523, 1993.
565. Simoons, M. L., Arnold, A. E. R., Betriu, A., et al.: Thrombolysis with tissue plasminogen activator in acute myocardial infarction: No additional benefit from immediate percutaneous coronary angioplasty. Lancet *1*:197, 1988.
566. Mauri, F., DeBiase, A. M., Franzosi, M. G., et al.: In-hospital causes of death in the patients admitted to the GISSI study. G. Ital. Cardiol. *17*:37, 1987.
567. Honan, M. B., Harrell, F. E., Reimer, K. A., et al.: Cardiac rupture, mortality and the timing of thrombolytic therapy: A meta-analysis. J. Am. Coll. Cardiol. *16*:359, 1990.
568. Maynard, C., Weaver, D., Litwin, P. E., et al.: Hospital mortality in acute myocardial infarction in the era of reperfusion therapy (the Myocardial Infarction Triage and Intervention Project). Am. J. Cardiol. *72*:877, 1993.
569. Ohman, E. M., Topol, E. J., Califf, R. M., et al.: An analysis of the cause of early mortality after administration of thrombolytic therapy: The Thrombolysis Angioplasty in Myocardial Infarction Study Group. Coronary Art. Dis. *4*:957, 1993.
570. Becker, R. C., Charlesworth, A., Wilcox, R. G., et al.: Cardiac rupture associated with thrombolytic therapy: Impact of time to treatment in the late assessment of thrombolytic efficacy (LATE) study. J. Am. Coll. Cardiol. *25*:1063, 1995.
571. Kleiman, N., White, H., Ohman, E., et al.: Mortality within 24 hours of thrombolysis for myocardial infarction: The importance of early reperfusion. Circulation *90*:2658, 1994.
572. Kleiman, N. S., Terrin, M., Mueller, H., et al.: Mechanisms of early death despite thrombolytic therapy: Experience from the Thrombolysis in Myocardial Infarction Investigation Phase II (TIMI II) Study. J. Am. Coll. Cardiol. *19*:1129, 1992.
573. Weiner, M. D., and Ong, L. S.: Streptokinase and splenic rupture. Am. J. Med. *86*:249, 1989.
574. Blankenship, J. C., and Almquist, A. K.: Cardiovascular complications of thrombolytic therapy in patients with a mistaken diagnosis of acute myocardial infarction. J. Am. Coll. Cardiol. *14*:1579, 1989.
575. Queen, M., Biem, J., Moe, G. W., et al.: Development of cholesterol embolization syndrome after intravenous streptokinase for acute myocardial infarction. Am. J. Cardiol. *65*:1042, 1990.
576. Wall, T. C., Phillips, H. R., Stack, R. S., et al.: Results of high dose intravenous urokinase for acute myocardial infarction. Am. J. Cardiol. *65*:124, 1990.
577. Tennant, S. N., Dixon, J., Venable, T. C., et al.: Intracoronary thrombolysis in patients with acute myocardial infarction: Comparison of the efficacy of urokinase with streptokinase. Circulation *69*:756, 1984.
578. Neuhaus, K.-L., Von Essen, R., Tebbe, U., et al.: Improved thrombolysis in acute myocardial infarction with front-loaded administration of alteplase: Results of the rt-PA-APSAC Patency Study (TAPS). J. Am. Coll. Cardiol. *19*:885, 1992.
579. Anderson, J. L.: Review of anistreplase (APSAC) for acute myocardial infarction. *In* Anderson, J. L. (ed.): Modern Management of Acute Myocardial Infarction in the Community Hospital. New York, Marcel Dekker, 1991, p. 149.
580. Tebbe, U., Windeler, J., Boesl, I., et al.: Thrombolysis with recombinant unglycosylated single-chain urokinase-type plasminogen activator (saruplase) in acute myocardial infarction: Influence of heparin on early patency rate (LIMITS Study). J. Am. Coll. Cardiol. *26*:365, 1995.
581. Weaver, W. D., Hartmann, J. R., Anderson, J. L., et al.: New recombinant glycosylated prourokinase for treatment of patients with acute myocardial infarction: Prourokinase Study Group. J. Am. Coll. Cardiol. *24*:1242, 1994.
582. Zarich, S. W., Kowalchuk, G. J., Weaver, W. D., et al.: Sequential combination thrombolytic therapy for acute myocardial infarction: Re-

sults of the pro-urokinase and t-PA enhancement of thrombolysis (PATENT) trial. J. Am. Coll. Cardiol. *16*:374, 1995.

583. Califf, R. M., Topol, E. J., Stack, R. S., et al.: Evaluation of combination thrombolytic therapy and timing of cardiac catheterization in acute myocardial infarction: Results of Thrombolysis and Angioplasty in Myocardial Infarction—Phase 5 randomized trial. Circulation *83*:1543, 1991.
584. Urokinase and Alteplase in Myocardial Infarction Collaborative Group: Combination of urokinase and alteplase in the treatment of myocardial infarction. Coronary Art. Dis. *2*:225, 1991.
585. Grines, C. L., Nissen, S. E., Booth, D. C., et al.: A prospective, randomized trial comparing combination half-dose tissue-type plasminogen activator and streptokinase with full-dose tissue-type plasminogen activator: Kentucky Acute Myocardial Infarction Trial (KAMIT) Group. Circulation *84*:540, 1991.
586. Verstraete, M., and Lijnen, H. R.: Novel thrombolytic agents. Cardiovasc. Drugs Ther. *8*:801, 1994.
587. Neuhaus, K. L., von Essen, R., Vogt, A., et al.: Dose finding with a novel recombinant plasminogen activator (BM 06.022) in patients with acute myocardial infarction: Results of the German Recombinant Plasminogen Activator Study: A study of the Arbeitsgemeinschaft Leitender Kardiologischer Krankenhausarzte (ALKK). J. Am. Coll. Cardiol. *24*:55, 1994.
588. Bode, C., Smalling, R. W., Sen, S., et al.: Recombinant plasminogen activator angiographic phase II international dose finding study (RAPID): Patency analysis and mortality endpoints. Circulation *88*(Suppl. I):292, 1993.
589. Weaver, W. D., Bode, C., Burnett, C., et al.: Reteplase vs. Alteplase Patency Investigation During Myocardial Infarction Trial (RAPID 2). J. Am. Coll. Cardiol. (Special Issue):87A, 1995.
590. International Joint Efficacy Comparison of Thrombolytics: Randomised, double-blind comparison of reteplase double-bolus administration with streptokinase in acute myocardial infarction (INJECT): Trial to investigate equivalence. Lancet *346*:329, 1995.
591. Keyt, B. A., Paoni, N. F., Refino, C. J., et al.: A faster-acting and more potent form of tissue plasminogen activator. Proc. Natl. Acad. Sci. U.S.A. *91*:3670, 1994.
592. Meeting Highlights: AHA 68th Scientific Sessions, "TIMI 10A: TNK for acute myocardial infarction." Circulation *93*:843, 1996.
593. Collen, D., and Lijnen, H. R.: Staphylokinase, a fibrin-specific plasminogen activator with therapeutic potential? Blood *84*:680, 1994.
594. Montoney, M., Gardell, S. J., and Marder, V. J.: Comparison of the bleeding potential of vampire bat salivary plasminogen activator versus tissue plasminogen activator in an experimental rabbit model. Circulation *91*:1540, 1995.
595. Fendrick, A., Ridker, P., and Bloom, B.: Improved health care benefits of increased use of thrombolytic therapy. Arch. Intern. Med. *154*:1605, 1994.
596. Simoons, M. L.: Another coronary reperfusion regimen. Lancet *346*:324, 1995.
597. Ridker, P. M., O'Donnell, C., Marder, V. J., et al.: Large-scale trials of thrombolytic therapy for acute myocardial infarction: GISSI-2, ISIS-3, and GUSTO 1. Ann. Intern. Med. *119*:530, 1993.
598. Lee, K. L., Califf, R. M., Simes, J., et al.: Holding GUSTO up to the light. Ann. Intern. Med. *120*:876, 1994.
599. Ridker, P. M., O'Donnell, C. J., Marder, V. J., et al.: A response to "Holding GUSTO up to the light." Ann. Intern. Med. *120*:882, 1994.
600. Ridker, P. M., O'Donnell, C. J., Marder, V. J., et al.: More on the GUSTO trial. Ann. Intern. Med. *121*:818, 1994.
601. Lee, K. L., Califf, R. M., and Topol, E. J.: The last word on GUSTO, for now. Ann. Intern. Med. *120*:970, 1994.
602. Hennekens, C. H., O'Donnell, C. J., Ridker, P. M., et al.: Current issues concerning thrombolytic therapy for acute myocardial infarction. J. Am. Coll. Cardiol. *25*:18S, 1995.
603. Lee, T. H.: Cost effectiveness of tissue plasminogen activator. N. Engl. J. Med. *332*:1443, 1995.
604. Simoons, M. L., and Arnold, A. E.: Tailored thrombolytic therapy: A perspective. Circulation *88*:2556, 1993.
605. Brodie, B. R., Stuckey, T. D., Hansen, C., et al.: Benefit of late coronary reperfusion in patients with acute myocardial infarction and persistent ischemic chest pain. Am. J. Cardiol. *74*:538, 1994.

CORONARY ANGIOPLASTY IN ACUTE MYOCARDIAL INFARCTION

606. Grines, C. L., Browne, K. F., Marco, J., et al.: A comparison of immediate angioplasty with thrombolytic therapy for acute myocardial infarction. N. Engl. J. Med. *328*:673, 1993.
607. Zijlstra, F., de Boer, M. J., Hoorntje, J. C. A., et al.: A comparison of immediate coronary angioplasty with intravenous streptokinase in acute myocardial infarction. N. Engl. J. Med. *328*:680, 1993.
608. Gibbons, R. J., Holmes, D. R., Reeder, G. S., et al.: Immediate angioplasty compared with the administration of a thrombolytic agent followed by conservative treatment for myocardial infarction: The Mayo Coronary Care Unit and Catheterization Laboratory Groups. N. Engl. J. Med. *328*:685, 1993.
609. Lange, R. A., and Hillis, L. D.: Immediate angioplasty for acute myocardial infarction. N. Engl. J. Med. *328*:726, 1993.
610. Stewart, R. E., and O'Neill, W. W.: Direct angioplasty for acute myocardial infarction. Curr. Opin. Cardiol. *10*:367, 1995.
610a. King, S. B. III., and Holmes, D. R. III: Coronary angioplasty for acute myocardial infarction. *In* Fuster, V., Ross, R., and Topol, E. J. (eds.): Atherosclerosis and Coronary Artery Disease. Philadelphia, Lippincott-Raven, 1996, pp. 1143–1156.
611. Topol, E. J.: Coronary angioplasty for acute myocardial infarction. Ann. Intern. Med. *109*:970, 1988.
612. Eckman, M. H., Wong, J. B., Salem, D. N., et al.: Direct angioplasty for acute myocardial infarction: A review of outcomes in clinical subsets. Ann. Intern. Med. *117*:667, 1992.
613. De Franco, A. C., and Topol, E. J.: Angiography and angioplasty. *In* Julian, D., and Braunwald, E. (eds.): Management of Acute Myocardial Infarction. London, W. B. Saunders Ltd., 1994, p. 107.
614. Grines, C. L., and O'Neill, W. W.: Primary angioplasty: The optimal reperfusion strategy in the United States. Br. Heart J. *73*:405, 1995.
615. O'Neill, W. W., Brodie, B. R., Ivanhoe, R., et al.: Primary coronary angioplasty for acute myocardial infarction (the Primary Angioplasty Registry). Am. J. Cardiol. *73*:627, 1994.
616. Brodie, B. R., Grines, C. L., Ivanhoe, R., et al.: Six-month clinical and angiographic follow-up after direct angioplasty for acute myocardial infarction: Final results from the Primary Angioplasty Registry. Circulation *90*:156, 1994.
617. de Boer, M. J., Hoorntje, J. C. A., Ottervanger, J. P., et al.: Immediate coronary angioplasty versus intravenous streptokinase in acute myocardial infarction: Left ventricular ejection fraction, hospital mortality and reinfarction. J. Am. Coll. Cardiol. *23*:1004, 1994.
618. Michels, K. B., and Yusuf, S.: Does PTCA in acute myocardial infarction affect mortality and reinfarction rates? A quantitative overview (meta-analysis) of the randomized clinical trials. Circulation *91*:476, 1995.
619. Vaitkus, P. T.: Percutaneous transluminal coronary angioplasty versus thrombolysis in acute myocardial infarction: A meta-analysis. Clin. Cardiol. *18*:35, 1995.
620. O'Neill, W., Timmis, G. C., Bourdillon, P. D., et al.: A prospective randomized clinical trial of intracoronary streptokinase versus coronary angioplasty for acute myocardial infarction. N. Engl. J. Med. *314*:812, 1986.
621. DeWood, M. A., Fisher, M. J., and for the Spokane Heart Research Group: Direct PTCA versus intravenous rtPA in acute myocardial infarction: Preliminary results from a prospective randomized trial. Circulation *80*(Suppl. II):418, 1989.
622. Ribeiro, E. E., Silva, L. A., Carneiro, R., et al.: Randomized trial of direct coronary angioplasty versus intravenous streptokinase in acute myocardial infarction. J. Am. Coll. Cardiol. *22*:376, 1993.
623. Elizaga, J., Garcia, E. J., Delcan, J. L., et al.: Primary coronary angioplasty versus systemic thrombolysis in acute anterior myocardial infarction: In-hospital results from a prospective randomized trial. Circulation *88*(Suppl. I):411, 1993.
624. Zijlstra, F.: Primary angioplasty is the most effective treatment for an acute myocardial infarction. Br. Heart J. *73*:403, 1995.
625. Himbert, D., Juliard, J. M., Steg, P. G., et al.: Primary coronary angioplasty for acute myocardial infarction with contraindication to thrombolysis. Am. J. Cardiol. *71*:377, 1993.
626. Ohman, E. M., Califf, R. M., Topol, E. J., et al.: Consequences of reocclusion after successful reperfusion therapy in acute myocardial infarction. Circulation *82*:781, 1990.
627. Stone, G. W., Grines, C. L., Browne, K. F., et al.: Implications of recurrent ischemia after reperfusion therapy in acute myocardial infarction: A comparison of thrombolytic therapy and primary angioplasty. J. Am. Coll. Cardiol. *26*:66, 1995.
628. Leung, W. H., and Lau, C. P.: Effects of severity of the residual stenosis of the infarct-related coronary artery on left ventricular dilation and function after acute myocardial infarction. J. Am. Coll. Cardiol. *20*:307, 1992.
629. American Heart Association: Facilities and services in the United States, In hospital statistics 1992–1993. Chicago, AHA, 1992, p. 208.
630. de Jaegere, P. P., and Simoons, M. L.: Immediate angioplasty: A conservative view from Europe: Cost effectiveness needs to be considered. Br. Heart J. *73*:407, 1995.
631. Bedotto, J. B., Kahn, J. K., Rutherford, B. D., et al.: Failed direct coronary angioplasty for acute myocardial infarction: In-hospital outcome and predictors of death. J. Am. Coll. Cardiol. *22*:690, 1993.
632. Vaitkus, P. T.: Limitations of primary angioplasty in acute myocardial infarction: Effectiveness depends on the clinical and operational context. Br. Heart J. *73*:409, 1995.
633. Boyle, R. M.: Immediate angioplasty in the United Kingdom. Br. Heart J. *73*:413, 1995.
634. Ellis, S. G., van de Werf, F., Ribeiro-da Silva, E., et al.: Present status of rescue coronary angioplasty: Current polarization of opinion and randomized trials. J. Am. Coll. Cardiol. *19*:681, 1992.
635. Belenkie, I., Traboulsi, M., Hall, C. A., et al.: Rescue angioplasty during myocardial infarction has a beneficial effect on mortality: A tenable hypothesis. Can. J. Cardiol. *8*:357, 1992.
636. Ellis, S. G., da Silva, E. R., Heyndrickx, G., et al.: Randomized comparison of rescue angioplasty with conservative management of patients with early failure of thrombolysis for acute anterior myocardial infarction. Circulation *90*:2280, 1994.
637. Topol, E. J., Califf, R. M., George, B. S., et al.: A randomized trial of immediate versus delayed elective angioplasty after intravenous tissue plasminogen activator in acute myocardial infarction. N. Engl. J. Med. *317*:581, 1987.
638. Rogers, W. J., Baim, D. S., Gore, J. M., et al.: Comparison of immediate invasive, delayed invasive, and conservative strategies after tissue-type plasminogen activator: Results of the Thrombolysis in Myocardial Infarction (TIMI) Phase II-A Trial. Circulation *81*:1457, 1990.

639. Holmes, D., and Topol, E. J.: Reperfusion momentum: Lessons from the randomization trials of immediate coronary angioplasty for myocardial infarction. J. Am. Coll. Cardiol. *14*:1572, 1989.
640. The TIMI Research Group: Immediate vs delayed catheterization and angioplasty following thrombolytic therapy for acute myocardial infarction: TIMI II A results. JAMA *260*:2849, 1988.
641. The TIMI Study Group: Comparison of invasive and conservative strategies after treatment with intravenous tissue plasminogen activator in acute myocardial infarction: Results of the Thrombolysis in Myocardial Infarction (TIMI) Phase II Trial. N. Engl. J. Med. *320*:618, 1989.
642. SWIFT (Should We Intervene Following Thrombolysis?) Trial Study Group: SWIFT trial of delayed elective intervention v. conservative treatment after thrombolysis with anistreplase in acute myocardial infarction. BMJ *302*:555, 1991.
643. Özbeck, C., Dyckmans, J., Sen, S., et al.: Comparison of invasive and conservative strategies after treatment with streptokinase in acute myocardial infarction: Results of a randomized trial (SIAM). J. Am. Coll. Cardiol. *15*:63A, 1990.
644. Ellis, S. G., Mooney, M. R., George, B. S., et al.: Randomized trial of late elective angioplasty versus conservative management for patients with residual stenoses after thrombolytic treatment of myocardial infarction: Treatment of Post-Thrombolytic Stenoses (TOPS) study group. Circulation *86*:1400, 1992.
645. Holmes, D. R., Bates, E. R., Kleiman, N. S., et al.: Contemporary reperfusion therapy for cardiogenic shock: The GUSTO-1 trial experience. J. Am. Coll. Cardiol. *26*:668, 1995.
646. Hochman, J. S., Boland, J., Sleeper, L. A., et al.: Current spectrum of cardiogenic shock and effect of early revascularization on mortality: Results of an International Registry: SHOCK Registry Investigators. Circulation *91*:873, 1995.
647. Aguirre, F. V., Meritt, R. F., and Carollo, S. C.: The role of coronary angiography after thrombolysis. Curr. Opin. Cardiol. *10*:381, 1995.
648. Vaitkus, P. T.: The continuing evolution of percutaneous transluminal coronary angioplasty in the treatment of coronary artery disease. Coronary Art. Dis. *6*:429, 1995.
649. Ellis, S. G., da Silva, E. R., Heyndrickx, G., et al.: Randomized comparison of rescue angioplasty with conservative management of patients with early failure of thrombolysis for acute anterior myocardial infarction. Circulation *90*:2280, 1994.
650. Erbel, R., Pop, T., Diefenbach, C., et al.: Long-term results of thrombolytic therapy with and without percutaneous transluminal coronary angioplasty. J. Am. Coll. Cardiol. *14*:276, 1989.
651. Guerci, A. D., and Ross, R. S.: TIMI II and the role of angioplasty in acute myocardial infarction. N. Engl. J. Med. *320*:663, 1989.
652. Ishihara, M., Sato, H., Tateishi, H., et al.: Intraaortic balloon pumping as the postangioplasty strategy in acute myocardial infarction. Am. Heart J. *122*:385, 1991.
653. Ohman, E. M., Califf, R. M., George, B. S., et al.: The use of intraaortic balloon pumping as an adjunct to reperfusion therapy in acute myocardial infarction: The Thrombolysis and Angioplasty in Myocardial Infarction (TAMI) study group. Am. Heart J. *121*:895, 1991.
654. Ohman, E. M., George, B. S., White, C. J., et al.: Use of aortic counterpulsation to improve sustained coronary artery patency during acute myocardial infarction: Results of a randomized trial: The Randomized IABP study group. Circulation *90*:792, 1994.
655. DeWood, M. A., Notske, R. N., Berg, R., et al.: Medical and surgical management of early Q wave myocardial infarction. I. Effects of surgical reperfusion on survival, recurrent myocardial infarction, sudden death and functional class at 10 or more years of follow-up. J. Am. Coll. Cardiol. *14*:65, 1989.
656. Schaff, H. V.: Myocardial infarction: The role of bypass surgery. *In* Fuster, V., Ross, R., and Topol, E. J. (eds.): Atherosclerosis and Coronary Artery Disease. Philadelphia, Lippincott-Raven, 1996, pp. 1157–1166.
656a. Verstraete, M., Chesebro, J., and Fuster, V.: Acute myocardial infarction: Antithrombotic therapy. *In* Fuster, V., Ross, R., and Topol, E. J. (eds.): Atherosclerosis and Coronary Artery Disease. Philadelphia, Lippincott-Raven, 1996, pp. 979–994.
657. Kereiakes, D. J., Topol, E. J., George, B. S., et al.: Favorable early and long-term prognosis following coronary bypass surgery therapy for myocardial infarction: Results of a multicenter trial: TAMI Study Group. Am. Heart J. *118*:199, 1989.
658. Schaff, H. V.: The role of bypass surgery in acute myocardial infarction. *In* Gersh, B. J., and Rahimtoola, S. H. (eds.): Acute Myocardial Infarction. New York, Elsevier, 1991, p. 386.
659. Montoya, A., Mulet, J., Pifarre, R., et al.: Hemorrhagic infarct following myocardial revascularization. J. Thorac. Cardiovasc. Surg. *75*:206, 1978.
660. Kagen, L., Scheidt, S., and Butt, A.: Serum myoglobin in myocardial infarction: The "staccato phenomenon": Is acute myocardial infarction in man an intermittent event? Am. J. Med. *62*:86, 1977.
661. Gersh, B. J., Chesebro, J. H., Braunwald, E., et al.: Coronary artery bypass surgery after thrombolytic therapy in the Thrombolysis in Myocardial Infarction Trial, Phase II (TIMI II). J. Am. Coll. Cardiol. *25*:395, 1995.
662. Tardiff, B. E., Califf, R. M., Morris, D., et al.: Coronary revascularization surgery following myocardial infarction: Effect of bypass surgery on survival following thrombolysis. *(In press).*
663. Naunheim, K. S., Kesler, K. A., Kanter, K. R., et al.: Coronary artery bypass for recent infarction: Predictors of mortality. Circulation *78*(Suppl. I):122, 1988.
664. Kennedy, J. W., Ivey, T. D., Misbach, G., et al.: Coronary artery bypass graft surgery early after acute myocardial infarction. Circulation *79*(Suppl. I):73, 1989.
665. Kalan, J. M., and Roberts, W. C.: Morphologic findings in patients undergoing coronary artery bypass grafting for acute myocardial infarction. Am. J. Cardiol. *62*:144, 1988.
666. Kay, P., Ahmad, A., Floten, S., et al.: Emergency coronary artery bypass surgery after intracoronary thrombolysis for evolving myocardial infarction. Int. J. Cardiol. *7*:281, 1985.

ANTITHROMBOTIC AND ANTIPLATELET THERAPY

667. Report of the Working Party on Anticoagulant Therapy in Coronary Thrombosis to the Medical Research Council: Assessment of short-term anticoagulant administration after cardiac infarction. BMJ *1*:335, 1969.
668. Drapkin, A., and Merskey, C.: Anticoagulant therapy after acute myocardial infarction: Relation of therapeutic benefit to patient's age, sex, and severity of infarction. JAMA *222*:541, 1972.
669. Veterans Administration Cooperative Study: Anticoagulants in acute myocardial infarction. Results of a cooperative clinical trial. JAMA *225*:724, 1973.
670. Chalmers, T. C., Matta, R. J., Smith, H., et al.: Evidence favoring the use of anticoagulants in the hospital phase of acute myocardial infarction. N. Engl. J. Med. *297*:1091, 1977.
671. Cairns, J. A., Hirsh, J., Lewis, H. D., et al.: Antithrombotic agents in coronary artery disease. Chest *108*(Suppl.):3805, 1995.
672. O'Donnell, C. J., Ridker, P. M., Hebert, P. R., et al.: Antithrombotic therapy for acute myocardial infarction. J. Am. Coll. Cardiol. *25*:23S, 1995.
673. Ridker, P. M., Hebert, P. R., Fuster, V., et al.: Are both aspirin and heparin justified as adjuncts to thrombolytic therapy for acute myocardial infarction? Lancet *341*:1574, 1993.
674. Hennekens, C. H., O'Donnell, C. J., and Ridker, P. M.: Current and future perspectives on antithrombotic therapy of acute myocardial infarction. Eur. Heart J. *16*(Suppl.):2, 1995.
675. The SCATI Group: Randomised controlled trial of subcutaneous calcium-heparin in acute myocardial infarction. Lancet *1*:182, 1989.
676. Bleich, S. D., Nichols, T., Schumacher, R. R., et al.: Effect of heparin on coronary patency after thrombolysis with tissue plasminogen activator in acute myocardial infarction. Am. J. Cardiol. *66*:1412, 1990.
677. Hsia, J., Hamilton, W. P., Kleiman, N., et al.: A comparison between heparin and low-dose aspirin as adjunctive therapy with tissue plasminogen activator for acute myocardial infarction. N. Engl. J. Med. *323*:1433, 1990.
678. de Bono, D. P., Simoons, M. I., Tijssen, J., et al.: Effect of early intravenous heparin on coronary patency, infarct size, and bleeding complications after alteplase thrombolysis: Results of a randomized double blind European Cooperative Study Group trial. Br. Heart J. *67*:122, 1992.
679. Topol, E. J., George, B. S., Kereiakes, D. J., et al.: A randomized controlled trial of intravenous tissue plasminogen activator and early intravenous heparin in acute myocardial infarction. Circulation *79*:281, 1989.
680. Col, J., Decoster, O., Hanique, G., et al.: Infusion of heparin conjunct to streptokinase accelerates reperfusion of acute myocardial infarction: Results of a double blind randomized study (OSIRIS). Circulation *86*(Suppl. I):259, 1992.
681. O'Connor, C. M., Meese, R., Carney, R., et al.: A randomized trial of intravenous heparin in conjunction with anistreplase (anisoylated plasminogen streptokinase activator complex) in acute myocardial infarction: The Duke University Clinical Cardiology Study (DUCCS). J. Am. Coll. Cardiol. *23*:11, 1994.
682. Bassand, J. P., Machecourt, J., Cassagnes, J., et al.: A multicenter double-blind trial of intravenous APSAC versus heparin in acute myocardial infarction: Final report of the APSIM study. J. Am. Coll. Cardiol. *11*:232A, 1988.
683. Verheugt, F. W. A., Marsh, R. C., Veen, G., et al.: Megadose bolus heparin as primary reperfusion therapy for acute myocardial infarction: The HEAP pilot study. Eur. Heart J. *16*(Suppl.):176, 1995.
684. Vaitkus, P. T., and Barnathan, E. S.: Usefulness of echocardiography in managing left ventricular thrombi after acute myocardial infarction. Am. J. Cardiol. *66*:387, 1990.
685. Vaitkus, P., and Barnathan, E.: Embolic potential, prevention and management of mural thrombus complicating anterior myocardial infarction: A meta-analysis. J. Am. Coll. Cardiol. *22*:1004, 1993.
686. Vecchio, C., Chiarella, F., Lupi, G., et al.: Left ventricular thrombus in anterior acute myocardial infarction after thrombolysis: A GISSI-2 connected study. Circulation *84*:512, 1991.
687. Warkentin, T. E.: Heparin-induced thrombocytopenia. Annu. Rev. Med. *40*:31, 1989.
687a. Warkentin, T. E., Levine, M. N., Hirsh, J., et al.: Heparin-induced thrombocytopenia in patients treated with low-molecular-weight heparin or unfractionated heparin. N. Engl. J. Med. *332*:1330, 1995.
688. Becker, R. C., Cyr, J., Corrao, J. M., et al.: Bedside coagulation monitoring in heparin-treated patients with active thromboembolic disease: A coronary care unit experience. Am. Heart J. *128*:719, 1994.
689. Cruikshank, M. K., Levine, M. N., Hirsh, J., et al.: A standard nomogram for the management of heparin therapy. Arch. Intern. Med. *151*:333, 1991.
690. Verstraete, M., and Zoldhelyi, P.: Novel antithrombotic drugs in development. Drugs *49*:856, 1995.
691. Meeting Highlights: AHA 68th Scientific Sessions, "TIMI 9B: Heparin

versus hirudin as adjunctive therapy for thrombolysis in acute myocardial infarction." Circulation *93*:843, 1996.
691a. Topol, E. The GUSTO IIB Trial. Presentation, Am. Coll. Cardiol., 1996.
692. MacMahon, S., Collins, R., Knight, C., et al.: Reduction in major morbidity and mortality by heparin in acute myocardial infarction. Circulation *78*(Suppl. II):98, 1988.
693. Vaitkus, P. T., Berlin, J. A., Schwartz, J. S., et al.: Stroke complicating acute myocardial infarction: A meta-analysis of risk modification by anticoagulation and thrombolytic therapy. Arch. Intern. Med. *152*:2020, 1992.
694. Granger, C. B., Hirsch, J., Califf, R. M., et al.: Activated partial thromboplastin time and outcome after thrombolytic therapy for acute myocardial infarction. Circulation *93*:870, 1996.
695. Hassan, W. M., Flaker, G. C., Feutz, C., et al.: Improved anticoagulation with a weight adjusted heparin nomogram in patients with acute coronary syndromes: A randomized trial. J. Thromb. Thrombol. *2*:245, 1996.
695a. White, H. D., and Yusuf, S.: Issues regarding the use of heparin following streptokinase therapy. J. Thromb. Thrombol. *2*:5, 1995.
696. Ward, S. R., and Topol, E. J.: How best to use heparin in MI patients given thrombolysis. J. Crit. Illness *10*:385, 1995.
697. Theroux, P., Waters, D., Lam, J., et al.: Reactivation of unstable angina after the discontinuation of heparin. N. Engl. J. Med. *327*:141, 1992.
698. Granger, C. B., Miller, J. M., Bovill, E. G., et al.: Rebound increase in thrombin generation and activity after cessation of intravenous heparin in patients with acute coronary syndromes. Circulation *91*:1929, 1995.
699. Fuster, V., Badimon, L., Badimon, J. J., et al.: The pathophysiology of coronary artery disease and the acute coronary syndromes. N. Engl. J. Med. *326*:242, 1992.
699a. Weitz, J. I., Califf, R. M., Ginsberg, J.S., et al.: New antithrombotics. Chest *108*(Suppl.):471S, 1995.
700. Jang, I. K., Gold, H. K., Ziskind, A. A., et al.: Differential sensitivity of erythrocyte-rich and platelet-rich arterial thrombi to lysis with recombinant tissue-type plasminogen activator: A possible explanation for resistance to coronary thrombolysis. Circulation *79*:920, 1989.
701. Coller, B. S.: Platelets and thrombolytic therapy. N. Engl. J. Med. *322*:33, 1990.
702. Antiplatelet Trialists' Collaboration: Collaborative overview of randomised trials of antiplatelet therapy. II. Maintenance of vascular graft or arterial patency by antiplatelet therapy. BMJ *308*:159, 1994.
703. Antiplatelet Trialists' Collaboration: Collaborative overview of randomised trials of antiplatelet therapy. III. Reduction in venous thrombosis and pulmonary embolism by antiplatelet prophylaxis among surgical and medical patients. BMJ *308*:235, 1994.
704. Patrono, C.: Aspirin as an antiplatelet drug. N. Engl. J. Med. *330*:1287, 1994.
705. Buerke, M., Pittroff, W., Melyer, J., et al.: Aspirin therapy: Optimized platelet inhibition with different loading and maintenance doses. Am. Heart J. *130*:465, 1995.
706. Yao, S.-K., Ober, J. C., Ferguson, J. J., et al.: Combination of inhibition of thrombin and blockade of thromboxane A_2 synthetase and receptors enhances thrombolysis and delays reocclusion in canine coronary arteries. Circulation *86*:1993, 1992.
707. Golino, P., Buja, M., Ashton, J. H., et al.: Effect of thromboxane and serotonin receptor antagonists on intracoronary platelet deposition in dogs with experimental stenosed coronary arteries. Circulation *78*:701, 1988.
708. Yasuda, T., Gold, H. K., Yaotia, H., et al.: Antithrombotic effects of ridogrel, a combined thromboxane A_2 synthetase inhibitor and prostaglandin endoperoxide-receptor antagonist, in a platelet-mediated coronary artery occlusion preparation in the dog. Coronary Art. Dis. *2*:1103, 1991.
709. The RAPT Investigators: Randomized trial of ridogrel, a combined thromboxane A_2 synthase inhibitor and thromboxane A_2/prostaglandin endoperoxide receptor antagonist, versus aspirin as adjunction to thrombolysis in patients with acute myocardial infarction: The Ridogrel Aspirin Patency Trial (RAPT). Circulation *89*:588, 1994.
710. Lefkovits, J., Plow, E. F., and Topol, E. J.: Platelet glycoprotein IIb/IIIa receptors in cardiovascular medicine. N. Engl. J. Med. *332*:1553, 1995.
711. Ohman, E. M., Kleiman, N. S., Talley, J. D., et al.: Simultaneous platelet glycoprotein IIb/IIIa integrin blockade with accelerated tissue plasminogen activator in acute myocardial infarction. Circulation *90*(Suppl. I):564, 1994.
712. Krucoff, M. W., Ohman, E. M., Trollinger, K. M., et al.: Beneficial impact of a platelet inhibitor, integrelin, on parameters of continuous 12-lead ST-segment recovery from myocardial infarction. Circulation 92(Suppl.):I-416, 1995.
713. Lee, T. H., and Goldman, L.: The coronary care unit turns 25: Historical trends and future directions. Ann. Intern. Med. *108*:887, 1988.
714. Davison, G., Suchman, A. L., and Goldstein, B. J.: Reducing unnecessary coronary care unit admissions: A comparison of three decision aids. J. Gen. Intern. Med. *5*:474, 1990.
715. Lee, T. H., Cook, E. F., Weisberg, M. C., et al.: Impact of the availability of a prior electrocardiogram on the triage of the patient with acute chest pain. J. Gen. Intern. Med. *5*:381, 1990.
716. Lee, T. H.: Chest pain in the emergency department: Uncertainty and the test of time. Mayo Clin. Proc. *66*:963, 1991.
717. Bell, M. R., Montarello, J. K., and Steele, P. M.: Does the emergency room electrocardiogram identify patients with suspected acute myocardial infarction who are at low risk of acute complications? Aust. N. Z. J. Med. *20*:564, 1990.
718. Brush, J. E., Brand, D. A., Acampora, D., et al.: Use of the initial electrocardiogram to predict in-hospital complications of acute myocardial infarction. N. Engl. J. Med. *312*:1137, 1985.
719. Lee, T. L., Cook, E. F., Weisberg, M., et al.: Acute chest pain in the emergency ward: Identification and evaluation of low risk patients. Arch. Intern. Med. *145*:65, 1985.
720. Aase, O., Jonsbu, J., Liestøl, K., et al.: Decision support by computer analysis of selected case history variables in the emergency room among patients with acute chest pain. Eur. Heart J. *14*:441, 1993.
721. Mirvis, D., Berson, A., Goldberger, A., et al.: Instrumentation and practice standards for electrocardiographic monitoring in special care units. Circulation *79*:464, 1989.
722. Romhilt, D., Bloomfield, S., Chou, T., et al.: Unreliability of conventional electrocardiographic monitoring for arrhythmia detection in coronary care units. Am. J. Cardiol. *31*:457, 1973.
723. Fineberg, H., Scadden, D., and Goldman, L.: Management of patients with a low probability of acute myocardial infarction: Cost-effectiveness of alternatives to coronary care unit admission. N. Engl. J. Med. *310*:1301, 1984.
724. Stern, T. A.: Psychiatric management of acute myocardial infarction in the coronary care unit. Am. J. Cardiol. *60*:59J, 1987.
725. Kirchhoff, K. T., Holm, K., Foreman, M. D., et al.: Electrocardiographic response to ice water ingestion. Heart Lung *19*:41, 1990.
726. Sortur, S. V., and Khadilkar, S. V.: Worsening of cardiac arrhythmia following drinking chilled water in a patient of acute myocardial infarction. J. Assoc. Phys. India *35*:311, 1987.
727. Gross, L., and Malaya, R.: Extrinsically induced arrhythmia in acute myocardial infarction. JAMA *228*:1021, 1974.
728. Lynn, L. A., and Kissinger, J. F.: Coronary precautions: Should caffeine be restricted after myocardial infarction? Heart Lung *21*:365, 1992.
729. Kirchhoff, K. T.: An examination of the physiologic basis for coronary precautions. Heart Lung *10*:874, 1981.
730. Bauer, W. C., and Dracup, K. A.: Physiologic effects of back massage in patients with acute myocardial infarction. Focus Crit. Care. *14*:42, 1987.
731. Winslow, E. H., Lane, L., and Gaffney, A.: Oxygen uptake and cardiovascular response in patients with acute myocardial infarction. J. Cardiopul. Rehabil. *4*:348, 1984.
732. Levine, S. A., and Lown, B.: "Armchair" treatment of acute coronary thrombosis. JAMA *148*:1365, 1952.
733. Krone, R.: The role of risk stratification in the early management of a myocardial infarction. Ann. Intern. Med. *116*:223, 1992.
734. Weinberg, S. L.: Intermediate coronary care—observations on the validity of the concept. Chest *73*:154, 1978.
735. Topol, E. J., Burek, K., O'Neill, W. W., et al.: A randomized controlled trial of early hospital discharge three days after myocardial infarction in the era of reperfusion. N. Engl. J. Med. *318*:1083, 1988.
736. Mark, D. B., Sigmon, K., Topol, E. J., et al.: Identification of acute myocardial infarction patients suitable for early hospital discharge after aggressive interventional therapy: Results from the Thrombolysis and Angioplasty in Acute Myocardial Infarction Registry. Circulation *83*:1186, 1991.
736a. Frishman, W. H.: Acute myocardial infarction: Role of β-adrenergic blockers. *In* Fuster, V., Ross, R., and Topol, E. J. (eds.): Atherosclerosis and Coronary Artery Disease. Philadelphia, Lippincott-Raven, 1996, pp. 1205–1214.

PHARMACOLOGICAL THERAPY

737. Waagstein, F., and Hjalmaarson, A. C.: Double-blind study of the effect of cardioselective beta-blockade on chest pain in acute myocardial infarction. Acta Med. Scand. *587*(Suppl.):201, 1975.
738. Norris, R. M., Clarke, E. D., Sammel, N. L., et al.: Protective effect of propranolol in threatened myocardial infarction. Lancet *2*:907, 1978.
739. Mueller, H. S., and Ayres, S. M.: The role of propranolol in the treatment of acute myocardial infarction. Prog. Cardiovasc. Dis. *19*:405, 1977.
740. The MIAMI Trial Research Group: Metoprolol in acute myocardial infarction: Arrhythmias. Am. J. Cardiol. *56*:35G, 1985.
741. Gold, H. K., Leinbach, C., and Maroko, P. R.: Propranolol-induced reduction of signs of ischemic injury during acute myocardial infarction. Am. J. Cardiol. *38*:689, 1976.
742. The MIAMI Trial Research Group: Metoprolol in acute myocardial infarction: Enzymatic estimation of infarct size. Am. J. Cardiol. *56*:27G, 1985.
743. The International Collaborative Study Group: Reduction of infarct size with the early use of timolol in acute myocardial infarction. N. Engl. J. Med. *310*:9, 1984.
744. Held, P. H., and Yusuf, S.: Effects of beta-blockers and calcium channel blockers in acute myocardial infarction. Eur. Heart J. *14*:18, 1993.
745. ISIS-1 (First International Study of Infarct Survival) Collaborative Group: Randomized trial of intravenous atenolol among 16,027 cases of suspected acute myocardial infarction. Lancet *2*:57, 1986.
746. Yusuf, S.: The use of beta-blockers in the acute phase of myocardial infarction. *In* Califf, R. M., and Wagner, G. S. (eds.): Acute Coronary Care 1986. Boston, Martinus Nijhoff, 1985, p. 73.
747. ISIS-1 (First International Study of Infarct Survival) Collaborative Group: Mechanisms for the early mortality reduction produced by beta-blockade started early in acute myocardial infarction: ISIS-1. Lancet *1*:921, 1988.
748. Yusuf, S., Peto, R., Lewis, J., et al.: Beta blockade during and after myocardial infarction: An overview of the randomized trials. Prog. Cardiovasc. Dis. *27*:335, 1985.

749. Pfeffer, M. A., Braunwald, E., Moye, L. A., et al.: Effect of captopril on mortality and morbidity in patients with left ventricular dysfunction after myocardial infarction. N. Engl. J. Med. *327*:669, 1992.
750. Pfeffer, J. M., Pfeffer, M. A., and Braunwald, E.: Influence of chronic captopril therapy on the infarcted left ventricle of the rat. Circ. Res. *57*:84, 1985.
751. Latini, R., Maggioni, A. P., Flather, M., et al.: "ACE-inhibitor use in patients with myocardial infarction": Summary of evidence from clinical trials. Circulation *32*:3132, 1995.
752. The Acute Infarction Ramipril Efficacy (AIRE) Study Investigators: Effect of ramipril on mortality and morbidity of survivors of acute myocardial infarction with clinical evidence of heart failure. Lancet *342*:821, 1993.
753. Ambrosioni, E., Borghi, C., Magnani, B., et al.: Effects of the early administration of zofenopril on mortality and morbidity in patients with anterior myocardial infarction: Results of the Survival of Myocardial Infarction Long-Term Evaluation Trial. N. Engl. J. Med. *332*:280, 1995.
754. Køber, L., Torp-Pedersen, C., Carlsen, J. E., et al.: A clinical trial of the angiotensin-converting-enzyme inhibitor trandolapril in patients with left ventricular dysfunction after myocardial infarction. N. Engl. J. Med. *333*:1670, 1995.
755. Swedberg, K., Held, P., Kjekshus, J., et al.: Effects of early administration of enalapril on mortality in patients with acute myocardial infarction: Results of the Cooperative North Scandinavian Enalapril Survival Study II (CONSENSUS II). N. Engl. J. Med. *327*:678, 1992.
756. Chinese Cardiac Study Collaborative Group: Oral captopril versus placebo among 13,634 patients with suspected myocardial infarction: Interim report from the Chinese Cardiac Study (CCS-1). Lancet *345*:686, 1995.
757. Gruppo Italiano per lo Studio della Sopravvivenza nell'Infarto Miocardico: GISSI-3: Effects of lisinopril and transdermal glyceryl trinitrate singly and together on 6-week mortality and ventricular function after acute myocardial infarction. Lancet *343*:1115, 1994.
758. Rutherford, J. D., Pfeffer, M. A., Moye, L. A., et al.: Effects of captopril on ischemic events after myocardial infarction: Results of the Survival and Ventricular Enlargement Trial. Circulation *90*:1731, 1994.
759. Lindsay, H. S. J., Zaman, A. G., and Cowan, J. C.: ACE inhibitors after myocardial infarction: Patient selection or treatment for all? Br. Heart J. *73*:397, 1995.
760. Coats, A. J. S.: ACE inhibitors after myocardial infarction: Selection and treatment for all. Br. Heart J. *73*:395, 1995.
761. ISIS-4 Collaborative Group: ISIS-4: A randomized factorial trial assessing early oral captopril, oral mononitrate, and intravenous magnesium sulphate in 58,050 patients with suspected acute myocardial infarction. Lancet *345*:669, 1995.
762. Horowitz, L. D., Gorlin, R., Taylor, W. J., et al.: Effects of nitroglycerin in regional myocardial blood flow in coronary artery disease. J. Clin. Invest. *50*:1578, 1971.
763. Loscalzo, J.: Antiplatelet and antithrombotic effects of organic nitrates. Am. J. Cardiol. *70*:18B, 1992.
764. Wilhelmsen, L.: Nitrates. *In* Julian D., and Braunwald, E. (eds.): Management of Acute Myocardial Infarction. London, W. B. Saunders Ltd., 1994, p. 241.
765. Jugdutt, B. I.: Nitrates in myocardial infarction. Cardiovasc. Drugs Ther. *8*:635, 1994.
766. Abrams, J.: The role of nitrates in coronary heart disease. Arch. Intern. Med. *155*:357, 1995.
767. Bussmann, W. D., Passek, D., Seidel, W., et al.: Reduction of CK and CK-MB indexes of infarct size by intravenous nitroglycerin. Circulation *63*:615, 1981.
768. Jugdutt, B. I., and Warnica, J. W.: Intravenous nitroglycerin therapy to limit myocardial infarct size, expansion, and complications: Effect of timing, dosage, and infarct location. Circulation *78*:906, 1988.
769. Yusuf, S., Collins, R., MacMahon, S., et al.: Effect of intravenous nitrates on mortality in acute myocardial infarction: An overview of the randomized trials. Lancet *1*:1088, 1988.
770. Chatterjee, K., and Parmley, W. W.: Vasodilator therapy for acute myocardial infarction and chronic congestive heart failure. J. Am. Coll. Cardiol. *1*:133, 1983.
771. Ferguson, J. J., Diver, D. J., Boldt, M., et al.: Significance of nitroglycerin-induced hypotension with inferior wall acute myocardial infarction. Am. J. Cardiol. *64*:311, 1989.
772. Osuna, P. B., Moreno, M. G., Jimenez, A. A., et al.: Isosorbide dinitrate sublingual therapy for inferior myocardial infarction: Randomized trial to assess infarct size limitation. Am. J. Cardiol. *55*:330, 1985.
773. Kaplan, K. J., Taber, M., Teagarden, J. R., et al.: Association of methemoglobinemia and intravenous nitroglycerin administration. Am. J. Cardiol. *55*:181, 1985.
774. Jugdutt, B. I., and Warnica, J. W.: Tolerance with low dose intravenous nitroglycerin therapy in acute myocardial infarction. Am. J. Cardiol. *64*:581, 1989.
775. Levy, W. E., Katz, R. J., Ruffalo, R. L., et al.: Potentiation of the hemodynamic effects of acutely administered nitroglycerin by methionine. Circulation *78*:640, 1988.
776. Opie, L. H., Frishman, W. H., and Thandani, U.: Calcium channel antagonists (Calcium entry blockers). *In* Opie, L. H. (ed.): Drugs for the Heart. Philadelphia, W. B. Saunders Co., 1995, p. 50.
777. Messerli, F. H.: "Cardioprotection"—Not all calcium antagonists are created equal. Am. J. Cardiol. *66*:855, 1990.
777a. Moss, A. J.: Acute myocardial infarction: Role of calcium channel blockers. *In* Fuster, V., Ross, R., and Topol, E. J. (eds.): Atherosclerosis and Coronary Artery Disease. Philadelphia, Lippincott-Raven, 1996, pp. 1215–1222.
778. Muller, J., Morrison, J., Stone, P. H., et al.: Nifedipine therapy for patients with threatened and acute myocardial infarction: A randomized, double-blind, placebo-controlled comparison. Circulation *69*:740, 1984.
779. Sirnes, P. A., Overskeid, K., Pederson, T. R., et al.: Evolution of infarct size during the early use of nifedipine in patients with acute myocardial infarction: The Norwegian Nifedipine Multicenter Trial. Circulation *70*:738, 1984.
780. Branagan, J. P., Walsh, K., Kelly, P., et al.: Effect of early treatment with nifedipine in suspected acute myocardial infarction. Eur. Heart J. *7*:859, 1986.
781. Gottlieb, S. O., Becker, L. C., Weiss, J. L., et al.: Nifedipine in acute myocardial infarction: An assessment of left ventricular function, infarct size, and infarct expansion: A double blind, randomised, placebo controlled trial. Br. Heart J. *59*:411, 1988.
782. Skolnick, A. E., and Frishman, W. H.: Calcium channel blockers in myocardial infarction. Arch. Intern. Med. *149*:1669, 1989.
783. Yusuf, S.: Calcium antagonists in coronary artery disease and hypertension: Time for reevaluation? Circulation *92*:1079, 1995.
784. Opie, L. H., and Messerli, R. H.: Nifedipine and mortality: Grave defects in the dossier. Circulation *92*:1068, 1995.
785. Kloner, R. A.: Nifedipine in ischemic heart disease. Circulation *92*:1074, 1995.
786. Erbel, R., Pop, T., Meinertz, T., et al.: Combination of calcium channel blocker and thrombolytic therapy in acute myocardial infarction. Am. Heart J. *115*:529, 1988.
787. Report of the Holland Interuniversity Nifedipine/Metoprolol Trial Research Group: Early treatment of unstable angina in the coronary care unit: A randomised, double-blind, placebo-controlled comparison of recurrent ischaemia and thrombolytic therapy in patients treated with nifedipine or metoprolol or both. Br. Heart J. *56*:400, 1986.
788. The Danish Study Group on Verapamil in Myocardial Infarction: Verapamil in acute myocardial infarction. Eur. Heart J. *54*:516, 1984.
789. Gibson, R. S., Boden, W. E., Theroux, P., et al.: Diltiazem and reinfarction in patients with non-Q wave myocardial infarction: Results of a double-blind, randomized, multicenter trial. N. Engl. J. Med. *315*:423, 1986.
790. Hansen, J. F.: Treatment with verapamil after an acute myocardial infarction: Review of the Danish studies on verapamil in myocardial infarction (DAVIT I and II). Drugs *2*:43, 1991.
791. Hansen, J. F.: Calcium antagonists and myocardial infarction. Cardiovasc. Drugs Ther. *5*:665, 1991.
792. The Multicenter Diltiazem Postinfarction Trial Research Group: The effect of diltiazem on mortality and reinfarction after myocardial infarction. N. Engl. J. Med. *319*:385, 1988.
793. The Danish Study Group on Verapamil in Myocardial Infarction: Effect of verapamil on mortality and major events after acute infarction (the Danish Verapamil Infarction Trial II-DAVIT II). Am. J. Cardiol. *66*:779, 1990.
794. Arsenian, M. A.: Magnesium and cardiovascular disease. Prog. Cardiovasc. Dis. *35*:271, 1993.
795. Flink, E. B., Brick, J. E., and Shane, S. R.: Alterations of long-chain free fatty acid and magnesium concentrations in acute myocardial infarction. Arch. Intern. Med. *141*:441, 1981.
796. Antman, E.: Randomized trials of magnesium for acute myocardial infarction: Big numbers do not tell the whole story. Am. J. Cardiol. *75*:391, 1995.
797. Woods, K. L.: Possible pharmacological actions of magnesium in acute myocardial infarction. Br. J. Clin. Pharmacol. *32*:3, 1991.
798. Shechter, M., Kaplinsky, E., and Rabinowitz, B.: The rationale of magnesium supplementation in acute myocardial infarction: A review of the literature. Arch. Intern. Med. *152*:2189, 1992.
799. Teo, K. K., and Yusuf, S.: Role of magnesium in reducing mortality in acute myocardial infarction: A review of the evidence. Drugs *46*:347, 1993.
800. Woods, K. L., and Fletcher, S.: Long-term outcome after intravenous magnesium sulphate in suspected acute myocardial infarction: The second Leicester Intravenous Magnesium Intervention Trial (LIMIT-2). Lancet *343*:816, 1994.
801. Woods, K. L.: Mega-trials and management of acute myocardial infarction. Lancet *346*:611, 1995.
802. Antman, E., Lau, J., Berkey, C., et al.: Large versus small trials of magnesium for acute myocardial infarction: Big numbers do not tell the whole story. Circulation *90*(Suppl. I):325, 1994.
803. Shechter, M., Hod, H., Kaplinsky, E., et al.: Magnesium therapy in acute myocardial infarction when patients are not candidates for thrombolytic therapy. Am. J. Cardiol. *75*:321, 1995.
804. Mantle, J. A., Rogers, W. J., McDaniel, H. G., et al.: Metabolic support of mechanical performance in myocardial infarction in man—a randomized clinical trial of glucose-insulin-potassium. Am. J. Cardiol. *43*:395, 1979.
805. Rogers, W. J., Segall, P. H., McDaniel, H. G., et al.: Prospective randomized trial of glucose-insulin-potassium in acute myocardial infarction. Am. J. Cardiol. *43*:801, 1979.
806. Heng, M. K., Norris, R. M., Singh, B. N., et al.: Effects of glucose and glucose-insulin-potassium on haemodynamics and enzyme release after acute myocardial infarction. Br. Heart J. *39*:748, 1977.
807. Malmberg, K., Ryden, L., Efendic, S., et al.: Randomized trial of insu-

lin-glucose infusion followed by subcutaneous insulin treatment in diabetic patients with acute myocardial infarction (DIGAMI Study): Effects on mortality at 1 year. J. Am. Coll. Cardiol. *26*:57, 1995.
808. Leinbach, R. C., Gold, H. K., Harper, R. W., et al.: Early intraaortic balloon pumping for anterior myocardial infarction without shock. Circulation *58*:204, 1978.
809. Alderman, J. D., Gabliani, G. I., McCabe, C. H., et al.: Incidence and management of limb ischemia with percutaneous wire-guided intraaortic balloon catheters. J. Am. Coll. Cardiol. *9*:524, 1987.
810. Herbaczynska-Cedro, K., Klosiewicz-Wasek, B., Cedro, K., et al.: Supplementation with vitamins C and E suppresses leukocyte oxygen free radical production in patients with myocardial infarction. Eur. Heart J. *16*:1044, 1995.
811. Guarnieri, C., Giordano, E., Muscari, C., et al.: Vitamin E can protect myocardium against oxidative damage. Cardiovasc. Res. *30*:153, 1995.
812. Klein, H. H.: Vitamin E cannot protect myocardium against oxidative damage. Cardiovasc. Res. *30*:156, 1995.
813. Williams, M. W., Taft, C. S., Ramnauth, S., et al.: Endogenous nitric oxide (NO) protects against ischaemia-reperfusion injury in the rabbit. Cardiovasc. Res. *30*:79, 1995.

HEMODYNAMIC DISTURBANCES

814. Rackley, C. E., Satler, L. F., Pearle, D. L., et al.: Use of hemodynamic measurements for management of acute myocardial infarction. *In* Rackley, C. E. (ed.): Advances in Critical Care Cardiology. Philadelphia, F. A. Davis Co., 1986, p. 3.
815. Gewirtz, H., Gold, H. K., Fallon, J. T., et al.: Role of right ventricular infarction in cardiogenic shock associated with inferior myocardial infarction. Br. Heart J. *42*:719, 1979.
816. Swan, H. J. C., Ganz, W., Forrester, J. S., et al.: Catheterization of the heart in man with use of a flow-directed balloon-tipped catheter. N. Engl. J. Med. *283*:447, 1970.
817. Forrester, J. S., Diamond, G., Chatterjee, K., et al.: Medical therapy of acute myocardial infarction by application of hemodynamic subsets. N. Engl. J. Med. *295*:1356, 1976.
818. Paglairello, G.: The Pulmonary Artery (Swan-Ganz) Catheter. Int. J. Technol. Assess. Health Care *9*:202, 1993.
818a. Ganz, W., Shah, P. K., and Forrester, J. S.: Acute myocardial infarction: The role of hemodynamic assessment. *In* Fuster, V., Ross, R., and Topol, E. J. (eds.): Atherosclerosis and Coronary Artery Disease. Philadelphia, Lippincott-Raven, 1996, pp. 895–904.
819. Goldenheim, P. D., and Kazemi, H.: Cardiopulmonary monitoring of critically ill patients. N. Engl. J. Med. *311*:776, 1984.
820. Eisenberg, P. R., Jaffe, A. S., and Schuster, D. P.: Clinical evaluation compared to pulmonary artery catheterization in the hemodynamic assessment of critically ill patients. Crit. Care Med. *12*:549, 1984.
821. Robin, E. D.: The cult of the Swan-Ganz catheter. Ann. Intern. Med. *103*:445, 1985.
822. Robin, E. D.: Death by pulmonary artery flow-directed catheter: Time for a moratorium? Chest *92*:727, 1987.
823. Gore, J. M., Goldberg, R. J., Spodick, D. H., et al.: A community-wide assessment of the use of pulmonary artery catheters in patients with acute myocardial infarction. Chest *92*:721, 1987.
824. Noble, R. J.: Myocardial infarction with hypotension. Chest *99*:1012, 1991.
825. Coma-Canella, I. L.-S. J., and Gamallo, C.: Low output syndrome in right ventricular infarction. Am. Heart J. *98*:613, 1979.
826. Rasanen, J., Nikki, O. P., and Heikkila, J.: Acute myocardial infarction complicated by respiratory failure: The effects of mechanical ventilation. Chest *85*:21, 1984.
827. Cohn, J. N., Franciosa, J. A., Francis, G. S., et al.: Effect of short term infusion on sodium nitroprusside in mortality rate in acute myocardial infarction complicated by left ventricular failure: Results of a Veterans Administration Cooperative Study. N. Engl. J. Med. *306*:1129, 1982.
828. Passamani, E. R.: Nitroprusside in myocardial infarction. N. Engl. J. Med. *306*:1168, 1982.
829. Chiariello, M., Gold, H. K., Leinbach, R. C., et al.: Comparison between the effects of nitroprusside and nitroglycerin on ischemic injury during acute myocardial infarction. Circulation *54*:766, 1976.
830. Flaherty, J. T.: Intravenous nitroglycerin. Johns Hopkins Med. J. *151*:36, 1982.
831. Rabinowitz, B., Tamari, I., Elazar, E., et al.: Intravenous isosorbide dinitrate in patients with refractory pump failure and acute myocardial infarction. Circulation *65*:771, 1982.
832. Cohn, J. N.: Editorial—Progress in vasodilator therapy for heart failure. N. Engl. J. Med. *302*:1414, 1980.
833. Franciosa, J. A., Mikulic, E., Cohn, J. N., et al.: Hemodynamic effects of orally administered isosorbide dinitrate in patients with congestive heart failure. Circulation *50*:1020, 1974.
834. Chiariello, M., Gold, H. K., Leinbach, R. C., et al.: Comparison between the effects of nitroprusside and nitroglycerin on ischemic injury during acute myocardial infarction. Circulation *54*:766, 1976.
835. Derrida, J. P., Sal, R., and Chiche, P.: Favorable effects of prolonged nitroglycerin infusion in patients with acute myocardial infarction. Am. Heart J. *96*:833, 1978.
836. Covell, J. W., Braunwald, E., Ross, J., et al.: Studies on digitalis XVI: Effects on myocardial oxygen consumption. J. Clin. Invest. *45*:1535, 1966.
837. Ross, J. J., Waldhausen, J. S., and Braunwald, E.: Studies on digitalis. I. Direct effects on peripheral vascular resistance. J. Clin. Invest. *39*:930, 1960.
838. Marchionni, N., Pini, R., Vanucci, A., et al.: Hemodynamic effects of digoxin in acute myocardial infarction in man: A randomized controlled trial. Am. Heart J. *109*:63, 1985.
839. Bonaduce, D., Petretta, M., Arrichiello, P., et al.: Effects of captopril treatment on left ventricular remodeling and function after anterior myocardial infarction: Comparison with digitalis. J. Am. Coll. Cardiol. *19*:858, 1992.
840. Moss, A. J., Davis, H. T., Conard, D. L., et al.: Digitalis-associated cardiac mortality after myocardial infarction. Circulation *64*:1150, 1981.
841. Ryan, T. J., Bailey, K. R., McCabe, C. H., et al.: The effects of digitalis on survival in high-risk patients with coronary artery disease. Circulation *67*:735, 1983.
842. Digitalis Subcommittee of the Multicenter Post-Infarction Research Group: The mortality risk associated with digitalis treatment after myocardial infarction. Cardiovasc. Drugs Ther. *1*:125, 1987.
843. Mølstad, P., and Abdelnoor, M.: Digitoxin-associated mortality in acute myocardial infarction. Eur. Heart J. *12*:65, 1991.
844. Køber, L., Torp-Pedersen, C., Hildebrandt, C., et al.: Digoxin is an independent risk factor for long term mortality after acute myocardial infarction. Eur. Heart J. *13*(Suppl.):1897, 1992.
845. Bigger, J. T., Fleiss, J. L., Rolnitzky, L. M., et al.: Effect of digitalis treatment on survival after acute myocardial infarction. Am. J. Cardiol. *55*:623, 1985.
846. Muller, J. E., Turi, Z. G., Stone, P. H., et al.: Digoxin therapy and mortality after myocardial infarction: Experience in the MILIS Study. N. Engl. J. Med. *314*:265, 1986.
847. Mølstad, P.: Digitalis in patients after myocardial infarction. Herz *18*:118, 1993.
848. Mueller, H., Ayres, S. M., Giannelli, S., et al.: Effect of isoproterenol, 1-norepinephrine, and intra-aortic counterpulsation on hemodynamics and myocardial metabolism in shock following acute myocardial infarction. Circulation *45*:335, 1972.
849. Shell, W. E., and Sobel, B. E.: Deleterious effects of increased heart rate on infarct size in the conscious dog. Am. J. Cardiol. *31*:474, 1973.
850. Ichard, C., Ricome, J. L., Rimailho, A., et al.: Combined hemodynamic effects of dopamine and dobutamine in cardiogenic shock. Circulation *67*:620, 1983.
851. Holzer, J., Karliner, J. S., O'Rourke, R. A., et al.: Effectiveness of dopamine in patients with cardiogenic shock. Am. J. Cardiol. *32*:79, 1973.
852. Tuttle, R. R., and Mills, J.: Development of a new catecholamine to selectively increase cardiac contractility. Circ. Res. *36*:185, 1975.
853. Maekawa, K., Liang, C. S., Hood, W. B. J., et al.: Comparison of dobutamine and dopamine in acute myocardial infarction: Effects of systemic hemodynamics, plasma catecholamines, blood flows and infarct size. Circulation *67*:750, 1983.
854. DiBianco, R.: Acute positive inotropic intervention: The phosphodiesterase inhibitors. Am. Heart J. *121*:1871, 1991.
855. Sherry, K. M., and Locke, T. J.: Use of milrinone in cardiac surgical patients. Cardiovasc. Drugs Ther. *7*:671, 1993.
856. Wynands, J. E.: The role of amrinone in treating heart failure during and after coronary artery surgery supported by cardiopulmonary bypass. J. Cardiac Surg. *9*:453, 1994.
857. Verma, S. P., Silke, B., Reynolds, G. W., et al.: Modulation of inotropic therapy by venodilation in acute heart failure: A randomised comparison of four inotropic agents, alone and combined with isosorbide dinitrate. J. Cardiovasc. Pharmacol. *19*:24, 1992.
858. Taylor, S. H., Verma, S. P., Hussain, M., et al.: Intravenous amrinone in left ventricular failure complicated by acute myocardial infarction. Am. J. Cardiol. *56*:29B, 1985.
859. Verma, S. P. S. B., and Taylor, S. H.: Hemodynamic dose-response effects of amrinone in left ventricular failure complicating myocardial infarction. Br. J. Clin. Pharmacol. *19*:540P, 1985.
860. Colucci, W. S., Wright, R. F., and Braunwald, E.: New positive inotropic agents in the treatment of congestive heart failure. N. Engl. J. Med. *314*:349, 1986.
860a. O'Gara, P. T.: Acute myocardial infarction: Primary pump failure. *In* Fuster, V., Ross, R., and Topol, E. J. (eds.): Atherosclerosis and Coronary Artery Disease. Philadelphia, Lippincott-Raven, 1996, pp. 1051–1064.

CARDIOGENIC SHOCK

861. Scheidt, S., Ascheim, R., and Killip, T.: Shock after acute myocardial infarction: A clinical and hemodynamic profile. Am. J. Cardiol. *26*:556, 1970.
862. Goldberg, R. J., Gore, J. M., Alpert, J. S., et al.: Cardiogenic shock after acute myocardial infarction: Incidence and mortality from a community-wide perspective, 1975 to 1988. N. Engl. J. Med. *325*:1117, 1991.
863. Hochman, J. S., and LeJemetel, T.: Management of cardiogenic shock. *In* Julian, D. G., and Braunwald, E. (eds.): Management of Acute Myocardial Infarction. London, W. B. Saunders Ltd., 1994, p. 267.
864. Hands, M. E., Rutherford, J. D., Muller, J. E., et al.: The in-hospital development of cardiogenic shock after myocardial infarction: Incidence, predictors of occurrence, outcome and prognostic factors. J. Am. Coll. Cardiol. *14*:40, 1989.
865. Wackers, F. J., Lie, K. I., Becker, A. E., et al.: Coronary artery disease in patients dying from cardiogenic shock or congestive heart failure in the setting of acute myocardial infarction. Br. Heart J. *38*:906, 1976.
866. Page, D. L., Caulfield, J. B., Kastor, J. A., et al.: Myocardial changes associated with cardiogenic shock. N. Engl. J. Med. *285*:133, 1971.

867. Alonso, D. R., Scheidt, S., Post, M., et al.: Pathophysiology of cardiogenic shock: Quantification of myocardial necrosis, clinical, pathologic and electrocardiographic correlation. Circulation *48*:588, 1973.
868. Mueller, H., Ayres, S. M., Gregory, J. J., et al.: Hemodynamics, coronary blood flow, and myocardial metabolism in coronary shock: Response to L-norepinephrine and isoproterenol. J. Clin. Invest. *49*:1885, 1970.
869. Mueller, H., Ayres, S. M., Conklin, E. F., et al.: The effects of intraaortic counterpulsation on cardiac performance and metabolism in shock associated with acute myocardial infarction. J. Clin. Invest. *50*:1885, 1971.
870. Johnson, S. A., Scanlon, P. J., Loeb, H. S., et al.: Treatment of cardiogenic shock in myocardial infarction by intraaortic balloon counterpulsation and surgery. Am. J. Med. *62*:687, 1977.
871. O'Rourke, M. F., Norris, R. M., Campbell, T. J., et al.: Randomized controlled trial of intraaortic balloon counterpulsation in early myocardial infarction with acute heart failure. Am. J. Cardiol. *47*:815, 1981.
872. Corral, C. H., and Vaughn, C. C.: Intraaortic balloon counterpulsation: An eleven-year review and analysis of determinants of survival. Texas Heart Inst. J. *13*:39, 1986.
873. Goldberg, M. J., Rubenfire, M., Kantrowitz, A., et al.: Intraaortic balloon pump insertion: A randomized study comparing percutaneous and surgical techniques. J. Am. Coll. Cardiol. *9*:515, 1987.
874. Isner, J. M., Cohen, S. J., Viruari, R., et al.: Complications of the intraaortic balloon counterpulsation device: Clinical and morphologic observations in 45 necropsy patients. Am. J. Cardiol. *45*:250, 1980.
875. Bates, E. R., and Topol, E. J.: Limitations of thrombolytic therapy for acute myocardial infarction complicated by congestive heart failure and cardiogenic shock. J. Am. Coll. Cardiol. *18*:1077, 1991.
876. Eltchaninoff, H., Simpfendorfer, C., Franco, I., et al.: Early and 1-year survival rates in acute myocardial infarction complicated by cardiogenic shock: A retrospective study comparing coronary angioplasty with medical treatment. Am. Heart J. *130*:459, 1995.
877. Danis, M., Patrick, D. L., Southerland, L. I., et al.: Patients' and families' preferences for medical intensive care. JAMA *260*:797, 1988.
878. Champagnac, D., Claudel, J. P., Chevalier, P., et al.: Primary cardiogenic shock during acute myocardial infarction: Results of emergency cardiac transplantation. Eur. Heart J. *14*:925, 1993.
879. Pae, W. E., Jr., and Pierce, W. S.: Temporary left ventricular assistance in acute myocardial infarction and cardiogenic shock: Rationale and criteria for utilization. Chest *79*:692, 1981.
880. Shawl, F. A., Domanski, M. J., Hernandez, T. J., et al.: Emergency percutaneous cardiopulmonary bypass support in cardiogenic shock from acute myocardial infarction. Am. J. Cardiol. *64*:967, 1989.

RIGHT VENTRICULAR INFARCTION

881. Shah, P. K., Maddahi, J., Berman, D. S., et al.: Scintigraphically detected predominant right ventricular dysfunction in acute myocardial infarction: Clinical and hemodynamic correlates and implications for therapy and prognosis. J. Am. Coll. Cardiol. *6*:1264, 1985.
882. O'Rourke, R. A., and Dell'Italia, L. J.: Right ventricular myocardial infarction. *In* Fuster, V., Ross, R., and Topol, E. J. (eds.): Atherosclerosis and Coronary Artery Disease. Philadelphia, Lippincott-Raven, 1996, pp. 1079–1096.
883. Forman, M. B., Goodin, J., Phelan, B., et al.: Electrocardiographic changes associated with isolated right ventricular infarction. J. Am. Coll. Cardiol. *4*:640, 1984.
884. Roberts, N., Harrison, D. G., Reimer, K. A., et al.: Right ventricular infarction with shock but without significant left ventricular infarction: A new clinical syndrome. Am. Heart J. *110*:1047, 1985.
885. Bansal, R. C., Marsa, R. J., Holland, D., et al.: Severe hypoxemia due to shunting through a patent foramen ovale: A correctable complication of right ventricular infarction. J. Am. Coll. Cardiol. *5*:188, 1985.
886. Candell-Riera, J., Figueras, J., Valle, V., et al.: Right ventricular infarction: Relationships between ST segment elevation in $V4_R$ and hemodynamic, scintigraphic, and echocardiographic findings in patients with acute inferior myocardial infarction. Am. Heart J. *101*:281, 1981.
887. Braat, S. H., Brugada, P., De Zwaan, C., et al.: Value of electrocardiogram in diagnosing right ventricular involvement in patients with an acute inferior wall myocardial infarction. Br. Heart J. *49*:368, 1983.
888. Lopez-Sendon, J., Garcia-Fernandez, M. A., Coma-Canella, I., et al.: Segmental right ventricular function after acute myocardial infarction: Two-dimensional echocardiographic study in 63 patients. Am. J. Cardiol. *51*:390, 1983.
889. Arditti, A., Lewin, R. F., Hellman, C., et al.: Right ventricular dysfunction in acute inferoposterior myocardial infarction: An echocardiographic isotopic study. Chest *87*:307, 1985.
890. Starling, M. R., Dell'Italia, L. J., Chaudhuri, T. K., et al.: First transit and equilibrium radionuclide angiography in patients with inferior transmural myocardial infarction: Criteria for the diagnosis of associated hemodynamically significant right ventricular infarction. J. Am. Coll. Cardiol. *4*:923, 1984.
891. Dell'Italia, L. J., Starling, M. R., Crawford, M. H., et al.: Right ventricular infarction: Identification by hemodynamic measurements before and after volume loading and correlation with noninvasive techniques. J. Am. Coll. Cardiol. *4*:931, 1984.
892. Topol, E. J., Goldshlager, N., Ports, T. A., et al.: Hemodynamic benefit of atrial pacing in right ventricular myocardial infarction. Ann. Intern. Med. *96*:594, 1982.
893. Marmor, A., Geltman, E. M., Biello, D. R., et al.: Functional response of the right ventricle to myocardial infarction: Dependence on the site of left ventricular infarction. Circulation *64*:1005, 1981.
894. Lorell, B., Leinbach, R. C., Pohost, G. M., et al.: Right ventricular infarction: Clinical diagnosis and differentiation from cardiac tamponade and pericardial constriction. Am. J. Cardiol. *43*:465, 1979.

MECHANICAL CAUSES OF HEART FAILURE

895. Reeder, G. S.: Identification and treatment of complications of myocardial infarction. Lancet *70*:880, 1995.
895a. Kuhn, F. E., and Gersh, B. J.: Acute myocardial infarction: Mechanical complications. *In* Fuster, V., Ross, R., and Topol, E. J. (eds.): Atherosclerosis and Coronary Artery Disease. Philadelphia, Lippincott-Raven, 1996, pp. 1065–1079.
896. Pohjola-Sintonen, S., Muller, J. E., Stone, P. H., et al.: Ventricular septal and free wall rupture complicating acute myocardial infarction: Experience in the Multicenter Limitation of Infarct Size. Am. Heart J. *117*:809, 1989.
897. Reddy, S. G., and Roberts, W. C.: Frequency of rupture of the left ventricular free wall or ventricular septum among necropsy cases of fatal acute myocardial infarction since introduction of coronary care units. Am. J. Cardiol. *63*:906, 1989.
898. Pappas, P. J., Cernaianu, A. C., Baldino, W. A., et al.: Ventricular free-wall rupture after myocardial infarction. Chest *99*:892, 1991.
899. Bulkley, B. H., and Roberts, W. C.: Steroid therapy during acute myocardial infarction: A cause of delayed healing and of ventricular aneurysm. Am. J. Med. *56*:244, 1974.
900. Silverman, H. W., and Pfeifer, M. P.: Relation between use of anti-inflammatory agents and left ventricular free wall rupture during acute myocardial infarction. Am. J. Cardiol. *59*:363, 1987.
901. Shapira, I., Isakov, A., Burke, M., et al.: Cardiac rupture in patients with acute myocardial infarction. Chest *92*:219, 1987.
902. Becker, R., Charlesworth, A., Wilcox, R., et al.: Late thrombolysis accelerates the onset of cardiac rupture. Circulation *90*(Suppl. I):563, 1994.
903. Edmondson, H. A., and Hoxie, H. J.: Hypertension and cardiac rupture: Clinical and pathological study of 72 cases, in 13 of which rupture of the interventricular septum occurred. Am. Heart J. *24*:719, 1942.
904. London, R. E., and London, S. B.: Rupture of the heart: A critical analysis of 47 consecutive autopsy cases. Circulation *31*:202, 1965.
905. Kassis, E., Vogelsang, M., and Lyngoborg, K.: Cardiac rupture complicating myocardial infarction: A study concerning early diagnosis and possible management. Dan. Med. Bull. *48*:164, 1981.
906. Mann, J. M., and Roberts, W. C.: Rupture of the left ventricular free wall during acute myocardial infarction: Analysis of 138 necropsy patients and comparison with 50 necropsy patients with acute myocardial infarction without rupture. Am. J. Cardiol. *62*:847, 1988.
907. Schuster, E. H., and Bulkley, B. H.: Expansion of transmural myocardial infarction: A pathophysiologic factor in cardiac rupture. Circulation *60*:1532, 1979.
908. Oliva, P. B., Hammill, S. C., and Edwards, W. D.: Cardiac rupture, a clinically predictable complication of acute myocardial infarction: Report of 70 cases with clinicopathologic correlations. J. Am. Coll. Cardiol. *22*:720, 1993.
909. Vlodaver, Z., Coe, J. L., and Edwards, J. E.: True and false left ventricular aneurysms. Circulation *51*:567, 1975.
910. Lascault, G., Reeves, F., and Drobinski, G.: Evidence of the inaccuracy of standard echocardiographic and angiographic criteria used for the recognition of true and "false" left ventricular inferior aneurysms. Br. Heart J. *60*:125, 1988.
911. Lundberg, S., and Soderstrom, J.: Perforation of the interventricular septum in myocardial infarction. Acta Med. Scand. *172*:413, 1962.
912. Held, A. C., Cole, P. L., Lipton, B., et al.: Rupture of the interventricular septum complicating acute myocardial infarction: A multicenter analysis of clinical findings and outcome. Am. Heart J. *116*:1330, 1988.
913. Camacho, M. T., Muehrcke, D. D., and Loop, F. D.: Mechanical complications. *In* Julian, D., and Braunwald, E. (eds.): Management of Acute Myocardial Infarction. London, W. B. Saunders Ltd., 1994, p. 291.
914. Westaby, S., Parry, A., Ormerod, O., et al.: Thrombolysis and postinfarction ventricular septal rupture. J. Thorac. Cardiovasc. Surg. *104*:1506, 1992.
915. Edwards, B. S., Edwards, W. D., and Edwards, J. E.: Ventricular septal rupture complicating acute myocardial infarction: Identification of simple and complex types in 53 autopsied hearts. Am. J. Cardiol. *54*:1201, 1984.
916. Mann, J. M., and Roberts, W. C.: Acquired ventricular septal defect during acute myocardial infarction: Analysis of 38 unoperated necropsy patients and comparison with 50 unoperated necropsy patients without rupture. Am. J. Cardiol. *62*:8, 1988.
917. Lemery, R., Smith, H. C., Giuliani, E. R., et al.: Prognosis in rupture of the ventricular septum after acute myocardial infarction and role of early surgical intervention. Am. J. Cardiol. *70*:147, 1992.
918. Cummings, R. G., Reimer, K. A., Califf, R., et al.: Quantitative analysis of right and left ventricular infarction in the presence of postinfarction ventricular septal defect. Circulation *77*:33, 1988.
919. Radford, M. J., Johnson, R. A., Daggett, W. M., Jr., et al.: Ventricular septal rupture: A review of clinical and physiologic features and an analysis of survival. Circulation *64*:545, 1981.
920. Moore, C. A., Nygaard, T. W., Kaiser, D. L., et al.: Postinfarction ventricular septal rupture: The importance of location of infarction and

right ventricular function in determining survival. Circulation *74:*45, 1986.
921. Bansal, R. C., Eng, A. K., and Shakudo, M.: Role of two-dimensional echocardiography, pulsed, continuous wave and color flow Doppler techniques in the assessment of ventricular septal rupture after myocardial infarction. Am. J. Cardiol. *65:*852, 1990.
922. Helmcke, F., Mahan, E. F., Nanda, N. C., et al.: Two-dimensional echocardiography and Doppler color flow mapping in the diagnosis and prognosis of ventricular septal rupture. Circulation *81:*1775, 1990.
923. Fortin, D. G., Sheikh, K.H., and Kisslo, J.: The utility of echocardiography in the diagnostic strategy of postinfarction ventricular septal rupture: A comparison of two-dimensional echocardiography versus Doppler color flow imaging. Am. Heart J. *121:*25, 1991.
924. Lock, J. E., Block, P. C, McKay, R. G., et al.: Transcatheterization closure of ventricular septal defects. Circulation *78:*361, 1988.
925. Chwa, E., Gonzalez, A., Bahr, R. D., et al.: Papillary muscle rupture: A reversible cause of cardiogenic shock. Maryland Med. J. *41:*893, 1992.
926. Manning, W. J., Waksmonski, C. A., and Boyle, N. G.: Papillary muscle rupture complicating inferior myocardial infarction: Identification with transesophageal echocardiography. Am. Heart J. *129:*191, 1995.
927. Barbour, D. J., and Roberts, W. C.: Rupture of a left ventricular papillary muscle during acute myocardial infarction: Analysis of 22 necropsy patients. J. Am. Coll. Cardiol. *8:*588, 1986.
928. Coma-Canella, I., Gamallo, C., Onsurve, P. M., et al.: Anatomic findings in acute papillary muscle necrosis. Am. Heart J. *118:*1188, 1989.
929. Nishimura, R. A., Schaff, H. V., Shub, C., et al.: Papillary muscle rupture complicating acute myocardial infarction. Am. J. Cardiol. *51:*373, 1983.
930. Lader, E., Colvin, S., and Tunick, P.: Myocardial infarction complicated by rupture of both ventricular septum and right ventricular papillary muscle. Am. J. Cardiol. *52:*424, 1983.
931. Come, P. C., Riley, M. F., Weintraub, R., et al.: Echocardiographic detection of complete and partial papillary muscle rupture during acute myocardial infarction. Am. J. Cardiol. *56:*787, 1985.
932. Buda, A. J.: The role of echocardiography in the evaluation of mechanical complications of acute myocardial infarction. Circulation *84:*1109, 1991.
933. Sharma, S. K., Seckler, J., Israel, D. H., et al.: Clinical, angiographic and anatomic findings in acute severe ischemic mitral regurgitation. Am. J. Cardiol. *70:*277, 1992.
934. Shah, P. K., and Francis, G. S.: Pump failure, shock, and cardiac rupture in acute myocardial infarction. *In* Francis, G. S., and Alpert, J. S. (eds.): Coronary Care. Boston, Little, Brown and Company, 1995, p. 289.
935. Goldman, A. P., Glover, M. U., Mick, W., et al.: Role of echocardiography/Doppler in cardiogenic shock: Silent mitral regurgitation. Ann. Thorac. Surg. *52:*296, 1991.
936. Jones, M. T., Schofield, P. M., Dark, J. F., et al.: Surgical repair of acquired ventricular septal defects: Determinants of early and late outcome. J. Thorac. Cardiovasc. Surg. *93:*680, 1987.
937. Dresdale, A. R., and Paone, G.: Surgical treatment of acute myocardial infarction. Henry Ford Hosp. Med. J. *39:*245, 1991.

VENTRICULAR ARRHYTHMIAS

938. Pantridge, J. F., and Adgey, A. A. J.: Pre-hospital coronary care: The mobile coronary care unit. Am. J. Cardiol. *24:*666, 1969.
939. Meltzer, L. E., and Cohen, H. E.: The incidence of arrhythmias associated with acute myocardial infarction. *In* Meltzer, L. E., and Dunning, A. J. (eds.): Textbook of Coronary Care. Philadelphia, Charles Press, 1972.
940. Norris, N. M.: Myocardial Infarction. New York, Churchill-Livingstone, 1982, p. 322.
940a. Kidwell, G. A., and Chung, M. K.: Ischemic ventricular arrhythmias. *In* Fuster, V., Ross, R., and Topol, E. J. (eds.): Atherosclerosis and Coronary Artery Disease. Philadelphia, Lippincott-Raven, 1996, pp. 995–1012.
941. Corr, P. B., and Gillis, R. A.: Autonomic neural influences on the dysrhythmias resulting from myocardial infarction. Circ. Res. *43:*1, 1978.
942. Barber, M. J., Mueller, T. M., Davies, B. G., et al.: Interruption of sympathetic and vagal-mediated afferent responses by transmural myocardial infarction. Circulation *72:*623, 1985.
943. Bloor, C. M., Ehsani, A., White, F. C., et al.: Ventricular fibrillation threshold in acute myocardial infarction and its relation to myocardial infarct size. Cardiovasc. Res. *9:*468, 1975.
944. Geltman, E. M., Ehsani, A. A., Campbell, M. K., et al.: The influence of location and extent of myocardial infarction on long-term ventricular dysrhythmia and mortality. Circulation *60:*805, 1979.
945. Roque, F., Amuchastegui, L. M., Lopez Morillos, M. A., et al.: Beneficial effects of timolol on infarct size and late ventricular tachycardia in patients with myocardial infarction. Circulation *76:*610, 1987.
946. Lassers, B. E., Anderton, J. L., George, M., et al.: Hemodynamic effects of artificial pacing in complete heart block complicating acute myocardial infarction. Circulation *38:*308, 1968.
947. Ruskin, J., McHale, P. A., Harley, A., et al.: Pressure-flow studies in man: Effects of atrial systole on left ventricular function. J. Clin. Invest. *49:*472, 1970.
948. Rahimtoola, S. H., Ehsani, A., Sinno, M. Z., et al.: Left atrial transport function in myocardial infarction: Importance of its booster function. Am. J. Med. *59:*686, 1975.
949. El-Sherif, N., Myerburg, R. J., Scherlag, B. J., et al.: Electrocardiographic antecedents of primary ventricular fibrillation: Value of the R-on-T phenomenon in myocardial infarction. Br. Heart J. *38:*415, 1976.
950. Weinberg, B., and Zipes, D.: Strategies to manage the post-MI patient with ventricular arrhythmias. Clin. Cardiol. *12:*86, 1989.
951. Lee, K. J., Wellens, H. J. J., Dorsnar, E., et al.: Observations on patients with primary ventricular fibrillation complicating acute myocardial infarction. Circulation *52:*755, 1975.
952. Surawicz, B.: R on T phenomenon: Dangerous and harmless. J. Appl. Cardiol. *1:*39, 1986.
953. Campbell, R. W. F., Murray, A., and Julian, D. G.: Relation of ventricular arrhythmias to ventricular fibrillation. Br. Heart J. *43:*109, 1980.
954. Campbell, R. W. F., Murray, A., and Julian, D. G.: Ventricular arrhythmias in first 12 hours of acute myocardial infarction: Natural history study. Br. Heart J. *46:*351, 1981.
955. Antman, E. M., and Berlin, J. A.: Declining incidence of ventricular fibrillation in myocardial infarction: Implications for the use of lidocaine. Circulation *84:*764, 1992.
956. Hine, L. K., Laird, N., Hewitt, P., et al.: Meta-analytic evidence against prophylactic use of lidocaine in acute myocardial infarction. Arch. Intern. Med. *149:*2694, 1989.
957. Hjalmarson, A., Herlitz, J., Holmberg, S., et al.: The Goteborg metoprolol trial: Effects on mortality and morbidity in acute myocardial infarction. Circulation *67:*26, 1983.
958. Yusuf, S., Sleight, P., Rossi, P., et al.: Reduction in infarct size, arrhythmias and chest pain by early intravenous beta blockade in suspected acute myocardial infarction. Circulation *67:*12, 1983.
959. Norris, R. M., Barnaby, P. F., Brown, M. A., et al.: Prevention of ventricular fibrillation during acute myocardial infarction by intravenous propranolol. Lancet *2:*883, 1984.
960. Gressin, V., Gorgels, A., Louvard, Y., et al.: ST-segment normalization time and ventricular arrhythmias as electrocardiographic markers of reperfusion during intravenous thrombolysis for acute myocardial infarction. Am. J. Cardiol. *71:*1436, 1993.
961. Gressin, V., Gorgels, A. P., Louvard, Y., et al.: Is arrhythmogenicity related to the speed of reperfusion during thrombolysis for myocardial infarction? Eur. Heart J. *14:*516, 1993.
962. Six, A. J., Louwerenburg, J. H., Kingma, J. H., et al.: Predictive value of ventricular arrhythmias for patency of the infarct-related coronary artery after thrombolytic therapy. Br. Heart J. *66:*143, 1991.
963. Maggioni, A. P., Zuanetti, G., Franzosi, M. G., et al.: Prevalence and prognostic significance of ventricular arrhythmias after acute myocardial infarction in the fibrinolytic era: GISSI-2 results. Circulation *87:*312, 1993.
964. Bigger, J. T., Jr., Dresdale, R. J., Heissenbuttel, R. H., et al.: Ventricular arrhythmias in ischemic heart disease: Mechanism, prevalence, significance, and management. Prog. Cardiovasc. Dis. *19:*255, 1977.
965. Wolfe, C. L., Nibley, C., Bhandari, A., et al.: Polymorphous ventricular tachycardia associated with acute myocardial infarction. Circulation *84:*1543, 1991.
966. Eldar, M., Sievner, Z., Goldbourt, U., et al.: Primary ventricular tachycardia in acute myocardial infarction: Clinical characteristics and mortality: The SPRINT Study Group. Ann. Intern. Med. *117:*31, 1992.
967. Kleiman, R. B., Miller, J. M., Buxton, A. E., et al.: Prognosis following sustained ventricular tachycardia occurring early after myocardial infarction. Am. J. Cardiol. *62:*528, 1988.
968. Nordrehaug, J. E., Johannessen, K. A., and von der Lippe, G.: Serum potassium concentration as a risk factor of ventricular arrhythmias early in acute myocardial infarction. Circulation *71:*654, 1985.
969. Emergency Cardiac Care Committee and Subcommittees, American Heart Association: Guidelines for cardiopulmonary resuscitation and emergency cardiac care. III. Adult advanced cardiac life support. JAMA *268:*2172, 1992.
970. Feely, J., Wade, D., McAllister, C. B., et al.: Effect of hypotension on liver blood flow and lidocaine disposition. N. Engl. J. Med. *307:*866, 1982.
971. LeLorier, J., Grenon, D., Latour, Y., et al.: Pharmacokinetics of lidocaine after prolonged intravenous infusions in uncomplicated myocardial infarction. Ann. Intern. Med. *87:*700, 1977.
972. Bhaskaran, A., Seth, A., Kumar, A., et al.: Coronary angioplasty for the control of intractable ventricular arrhythmia. Clin. Cardiol. *18:*480, 1995.
973. Volpi, A., Maggioni, A., Franzosi, M. G., et al.: In-hospital prognosis of patients with acute myocardial infarction complicated by primary ventricular fibrillation. N. Engl. J. Med. *317:*257, 1987.
974. Chiriboga, D., Yarzebski, J., Goldberg, R. J., et al.: Temporal trends (1975 through 1990) in the incidence and case-fatality rate of primary fibrillation complicating acute myocardial infarction: A community wide perspective. Circulation *89:*998, 1994.
975. Volpi, A., Cavalli, A., Franzosi, M. G., et al.: One-year prognosis of primary ventricular fibrillation complicating acute myocardial infarction. Am. J. Cardiol. *63:*1174, 1989.
976. Behar, S., Reicher Ress, H., Schechter, M., et al.: Frequency and prognostic significance of secondary ventricular fibrillation complicating acute myocardial infarction. Am. J. Cardiol. *71:*152, 1993.
977. Jensen, G. V. H., Torp-Pedersen, C., Kober, L., et al.: Prognosis of late versus early ventricular fibrillation in acute myocardial infarction. Am. J. Cardiol. *66:*10, 1990.
978. Lown, B., Fakhro, A. M., Hood, W. B., et al.: The coronary care unit: New perspectives and directions. JAMA *199:*188, 1967.
979. Harrison, D. C.: Should lidocaine be administered routinely to all patients after acute myocardial infarction? Circulation *58:*581, 1978.

980. MacMahon, S., Collins, R., Peto, R., et al.: Effects of prophylactic lidocaine in suspected acute myocardial infarction: An overview of results from the randomized, controlled trials. JAMA *260:*1910, 1988.
981. Nordrehaug, J. E., and Lippe, G. V. D.: Hypokalemia and ventricular fibrillation in acute myocardial infarction. Br. Heart J. *50:*525, 1983.
982. Higham, P. D., Adams, P. C., Murray, A., et al.: Plasma potassium, serum magnesium and ventricular fibrillation: A prospective study. Q. J. Med. *86:*609, 1993.
983. Haigney, M. C. P., Silver, B., Tanglao, E., et al.: Noninvasive measurement of tissue magnesium and correlation with cardiac levels. Circulation *92:*2190, 1995.
984. Bellotto, F., Forman, R., and Buja, G.: Electromechanical dissociation in the acute myocardial infarction: A review of the literature shows the need for a codified definition. J. Electrophysiol. *2:*517, 1988.
985. Charlap, S., Kahlam, S., Lichstein, E., et al.: Electromechanical dissociation: Diagnosis, pathophysiology, and management. Am. Heart J. *118:355,* 1989.

BRADYARRHYTHMIAS

986. Graner, L. E., Gershen, B. J., Orlando, M. M., et al.: Bradycardia and its complications in the pre-hospital phase of acute myocardial infarction. Am. J. Cardiol. *32:*607, 1973.
987. Mark, A. L.: The Bezold-Jarisch reflex revisited: Clinical implications of inhibitory reflexes originating in the heart. J. Am. Coll. Cardiol. *1:*90, 1983.
988. Koren, G., Weiss, A. T., Ben-David, J., et al.: Bradycardia and hypotension following reperfusion with streptokinase (Bezold-Jarish reflex): A sign of coronary thrombolysis and myocardial salvage. Am. Heart J. *112:*468, 1986.
989. Come, P. C., and Pitt, B.: Nitroglycerin-induced severe hypotension and bradycardia in patients with acute myocardial infarction. Circulation *54:*624, 1976.
990. Rotman, M., Wagner, G. S., and Wallace, A. G. P.: Bradyarrhythmias in acute myocardial infarction. Circulation *45:*703, 1972.
991. Norris, R. M., and Mercer, C. J.: Significance of idioventricular rhythms in acute myocardial infarction. Prog. Cardiovasc. Dis. *16:*455, 1974.
992. Bhandari, A. K., and Sager, P. T.: Management of peri-infarctional ventricular arrhythmias and conduction disturbances. *In* Naccarelli, G. V. (ed.): Cardiac Arrhythmias: A Practical Approach. Mt. Kisco, NY, Futura Publishing, 1991, p. 283.
993. Fisch, J. R., Zipes, D. P., and Fisch, C.: Bundle branch block in sudden death. Prog. Cardiovasc. Dis. *23:*187, 1980.
994. Berger, P. B., Ruocco, N. A., Jr., Ryan, T. J., et al.: Incidence and prognostic implications of heart block complicating inferior myocardial infarction treated with thrombolytic therapy: Results from TIMI II. J. Am. Coll. Cardiol. *20:*533, 1992.
995. McDonald, K., O'Sullivan, J. J., Conroy, R. M., et al.: Heart block as a predictor of in-hospital death in both acute inferior and acute anterior myocardial infarction. Q. J. Med. *74:*277, 1990.
996. Goldberg, R. J., Zevallos, J. C., Yarzebski, J., et al.: Prognosis of acute myocardial infarction complicated by complete heart block (the Worcester Heart Attack Study). Am. J. Cardiol. *69:*1135, 1992.
997. Bilbao, F. J., Zabalza, I. E., Vilanova, J. R., et al.: Atrioventricular block in posterior acute myocardial infarction: A clinicopathologic correlation. Circulation *75:*733, 1987.
998. Bertolet, B. D., McMurtrie, E. B., Hill, J. A., et al.: Theophylline for the treatment of atrioventricular block after myocardial infarction. Ann. Intern. Med. *123:*509, 1995.
999. Clemmensen, P., Bates, E. R., Califf, R. M., et al.: Complete atrioventricular block complicating inferior wall acute myocardial infarction treated with reperfusion therapy: TAMI Study Group. Am. J. Cardiol. *67:*225, 1991.
1000. Mavric, Z., Zaputovic, L., Matana, A., et al.: Prognostic significance of complete atrioventricular block in patients with acute inferior myocardial infarction with and without right ventricular involvement. Am. Heart J. *119:*823, 1990.
1001. Kostuk, W. J., and Beanlands, D. S.: Complete heart block associated with acute myocardial infarction. Am. J. Cardiol. *26:*380, 1970.
1002. Lilavie, C. J., and Gersh, P. J.: Mechanical and electrical complication of acute myocardial infarction. Mayo Clin. Proc. *65:*709, 1990.
1003. Bassan, R., Maia, I. G., Bozza, A., et al.: Atrioventricular block in acute inferior wall myocardial infarction: Harbinger of associated obstruction of the left anterior descending coronary artery. J. Am. Coll. Cardiol. *8:*773, 1986.
1004. Nicod, P., Gilpin, E., Dittrich, H., et al.: Long-term outcome in patients with inferior myocardial infarction and complete atrioventricular block. J. Am. Coll. Cardiol. *12:*589, 1988.
1005. Hindman, M. C., Wagner, G. S., Jaro, M., et al.: The clinical significance of bundle branch block complicating acute myocardial infarction. 2. Indications for temporary and permanent pacemaker insertion. Circulation *58:*689, 1978.
1006. Feigl, D., Ashkenazy, J., and Kishon, Y.: Early and late atrioventricular block in acute inferior myocardial infarction. J. Am. Coll. Cardiol. *4:*35, 1984.
1007. Klein, R. C., Vera, Z., and Mason, D. T.: Intraventricular conduction defects in acute myocardial infarction: Incidence, prognosis and therapy. Am. Heart J. *108:*1007, 1984.
1008. Hollander, G., Nadiminti, V., Lichstein, E., et al.: Bundle branch block in acute myocardial infarction. Am. Heart J. *105:*738, 1983.
1009. Hindman, M. C., Wagner, G. S., Jaro, M., et al.: The clinical significance of bundle branch block complicating acute myocardial infarction. 1. Clinical characteristics, hospital mortality, and one-year follow-up. Circulation *58:*679, 1978.
1010. Scheinman, M. M., and Gonzalez, R. P.: Fascicular block and acute myocardial infarction. JAMA *244:*2646, 1980.
1011. Lamas, G. A., Mueller, J. E., Turi, A. G., et al.: A simplified method to predict occurrence of complete heart block during acute myocardial infarction. Am. J. Cardiol. *57:*1213, 1986.
1012. Mullins, C. B., and Atkins, J. M.: Prognoses and management of ventricular conduction blocks in acute myocardial infarction. Mod. Concepts Cardiovasc. Dis. *45:*129, 1976.
1013. Dubois, C., Pierard, L. A., Smeets, J.-P., et al.: Short- and long-term prognostic importance of complete bundle-branch complicating acute myocardial infarction. Clin. Cardiol. *11:*292, 1988.
1014. Ricou, F., Nicod, P., Gilpin, E., et al.: Influence of right bundle branch block on short- and long-term survival after acute anterior myocardial infarction. J. Am. Coll. Cardiol. *17:*858, 1991.
1015. Ricou, F., Nicod, P., Gilpin, E., et al.: Influence of right bundle branch block on short- and long-term survival after inferior Q-wave myocardial infarction. Am. J. Cardiol. *67:*1143, 1991.
1016. Lie, K. I., Liem, K. L., Schuilenburg, R. M., et al.: Early identification of patients developing late in-hospital ventricular fibrillation after discharge from the coronary care unit. Am. J. Cardiol. *41:*674, 1978.
1017. DeGuzman, M., Cawanish, D. T., and Rahimtoola, S. H.: AV node–His Purkinje system disease: AV block (acute). *In* Bogan, E., and Wilcoff, K. (eds.): Clinical Cardiac Pacing. Philadelphia, W. B. Saunders Company, 1995, p. 321.
1018. Hynes, J. K., Holmes, D. R., Jr., and Harrison, C. E.: Five-year experience with temporary pacemaker therapy in the coronary care unit. Mayo Clin. Proc. *58:*122, 1983.
1019. Zoll, P.: Resuscitation of the heart in ventricular standstill by external electrical stimulation. N. Engl. J. Med. *247:*768, 1952.
1020. Zoll, P. M., Zoll, R. H., Falk, R. H., et al.: External non-invasive temporary cardiac pacing: Clinical trials. Circulation *71:*937, 1985.
1021. Ginks, W. R., Sutton, R., Oh, W., et al.: Long-term prognosis after acute inferior infarction with atrioventricular block. Br. Heart J. *39:*186, 1977.

SUPRAVENTRICULAR TACHYARRHYTHMIAS

1022. Crimm, A., Severance, H. W., Coffey, K., et al.: Prognostic significance of isolated sinus tachycardia during the first three days of acute myocardial infarction. Am. J. Med. *76:*983, 1984.
1023. Berisso, M. Z., Carratino, L., Ferroni, A., et al.: Frequency, characteristics and significance of supraventricular tachyarrhythmias detected by 24-hour electrocardiographic recording in the late hospital phase of acute myocardial infarction. Am. J. Cardiol. *65:*1064, 1990.
1024. Serrano, C. V., Ramires, J. A. F., Mansur, A. P., et al.: Importance of the time of onset of supraventricular tachyarrhythymias on prognosis of patients with acute myocardial infarction. Clin. Cardiol. *18:*84, 1995.
1025. Ganz, L. I., and Friedman, P. L.: Supraventricular tachycardia. N. Engl. J. Med. *332:*162, 1995.
1026. DeSanctis, R. W., Block, P., and Hutter, A. M.: Tachyarrhythmias in myocardial infarction. Circulation *45:*681, 1972.
1027. Behar, S., Zahavi, Z., Goldbourt, U., et al.: Long-term prognosis of patients with paroxysmal atrial fibrillation complicating acute myocardial infarction. Eur. Heart J. *13:*45, 1992.
1027a. Madias, J. E., Patel, D. C., and Singh, D.: Atrial fibrillation in acute myocardial infarction. A prospective study based on data from a consecutive series of patients admitted to the coronary care unit. Clin. Cardiol. *19:*180, 1996.
1028. Hod, H., Lew, A. S., Heltai, M., et al.: Early atrial fibrillation during evolving myocardial infarction: A consequence of impaired left atrial perfusion. Circulation *75:*146, 1987.
1029. Crenshaw, B. S., Ward, S. R., Stebbins, A. L., et al.: Risk factors and outcomes in patients with atrial fibrillation following acute myocardial infarction. Circulation *92*(Suppl.):I-777, 1995.
1030. Kirkorian, G., Moncada, E., Chevalier, P., et al.: Radiofrequency ablation of atrial flutter: Efficacy of an anatomically guided approach. Circulation *90:*2804, 1994.
1031. Suttorp, M. J., Kingma, J. H., Jessurun, E. R., et al.: The value of class IC antiarrhythmic drugs for acute conversion of paroxysmal atrial fibrillation or flutter to sinus rhythm. J. Am. Coll. Cardiol. *16:*1722, 1990.
1032. Hine, L., Laird, N., Hewitt, P., et al.: Meta-analysis of empirical long-term antiarrhythmic therapy after myocardial infarction. JAMA *262:*3037, 1989.
1033. Coplen, S., Antman, E., Berlin, J., et al.: Efficacy and safety of quinidine therapy for maintenance of sinus rhythm after cardioversion: A meta-analysis of randomized control trials. Circulation *82:*1106, 1990.
1034. Akiyama, T., Pawitan, Y., Greenberg, H., et al.: Increased risk of death and cardiac arrest from encainide and flecainide in patients after non-Q-wave acute myocardial infarction in the Cardiac Arrhythmia Suppression Trial: CAST Investigators. Am. J. Cardiol. *68:*1551, 1991.
1035. Cowan, J. C.: Antiarrhythmic drugs in the management of atrial fibrillation. Br. Heart J. *70:*304, 1993.
1036. Middlekauff, H. R., Wiener, I., and Stevenson, W. G.: Low-dose amiodarone for atrial fibrillation. Am. J. Cardiol. *72:*26, 1993.
1037. Podrid, P. J.: Amiodarone: Reevaluation of an old drug. Ann. Intern. Med. *122:*689, 1995.
1038. Fishenfeld, J., Desser, K. B., and Benchimol, A.: Non-paroxysmal A-V

junctional tachycardia associated with acute myocardial infarction. Am. Heart J. *86*:754, 1973.

OTHER COMPLICATIONS

1039. Simoons, M. L., Brand, M., de Zwaan, C., et al.: Improved survival after early thrombolysis in acute myocardial infarction. Lancet *2*:578, 1985.
1040. Koiwaya, Y., Torii, S., Takeshita, A., et al.: Postinfarction angina caused by coronary arterial spasm. Circulation *65*:275, 1982.
1041. Cannon, C. P., McCabe, C. H., Henry, T. D., et al.: A pilot trial of recombinant desulfatohirudin compared with heparin in conjunction with tissue-type plasminogen activator and aspirin for acute myocardial infarction: Results of the Thrombolysis in Myocardial Infarction (TIMI) 5 trial. J. Am. Coll. Cardiol. *23*:993, 1994.
1042. Cohen, L. S.: Managing patients after myocardial infarction. Hosp. Prac. *25*:49, 1990.
1043. Ellis, S. G., Topol, E. J., George, B. S., et al.: Recurrent ischemia without warning: Analysis of risk factors for in-hospital ischemic events following successful thrombolysis with intravenous tissue plasminogen activator. Circulation *80*:1159, 1989.
1044. Ohman, E. M., Armstrong, P. M., Guerci, A. D., et al.: Reinfarction after thrombolytic therapy: Experience from the GUSTO trial. Circulation *88*(Suppl. I):490, 1993.
1045. Marmor, A., Sobel, B. E., and Roberts, E.: Factors presaging early recurrent myocardial infarction ("extension"). Am. J. Cardiol. *48*:603, 1981.
1046. Benhorin, J., Andrews, M. L., Carleen, E. D., et al.: Occurrence, characteristics, and prognostic significance of early postacute myocardial infarction angina pectoris. Am. J. Cardiol. *62*:679, 1988.
1047. Mueller, H. S., Cohen, L. S., Braunwald, E., et al.: Predictors of early morbidity and mortality after thrombolytic therapy of acute myocardial infarction: Analyses of patient subgroups in the Thrombolysis in Myocardial Infarction (TIMI) trial, phase II. Circulation *85*:1254, 1992.
1048. Silva, P., Galli, M., Campolo, L., et al.: Prognostic significance of early ischemia after acute myocardial infarction in low-risk patients. Am. J. Cardiol. *71*:1142, 1993.
1049. Barbagelata, A., Granger, C. B., Topol, E. J., et al.: Isolated recurrent ischemia after thrombolytic therapy: Incidence, importance, and cost. Am. J. Cardiol. *76*:1007, 1995.
1050. Betriu, A., Califf, R. M., Granger, C., et al.: Importance of clinical findings during post-infarction angina in determining prognosis: Results from the GUSTO trial. J. Am. Coll. Cardiol. *23*:27A, 1994.
1051. Muller, J. E., Rude, R. E., Braunwald, E., et al.: Myocardial infarct extension: Occurrence, outcome, and risk factors in the Multicenter Investigation of Limitation of Infarct Size. Ann. Intern. Med. *108*:1, 1988.
1052. Maisel, A. S., Ahnve, S., Gilpin, E., et al.: Prognosis after extension of myocardial infarct: The role of Q wave or non-Q wave infarction. Circulation *71*:211, 1985.
1053. Cannon, C. P., McCabe, C. H., Schweiger, M. J., et al.: Prospective validation of a composite end point for evaluation of new thrombolytic regimens for acute MI: Results from the TIMI 4 trial. Circulation *88*(Suppl. I):60, 1993.
1054. Mueller, H. S., Forman, S. A., Menegus, M. A., et al.: Prognostic significance of nonfatal reinfarction during 3-year follow-up: Results of the Thrombolysis in Myocardial Infarction (TIMI) Phase II Clinical Trial. J. Am. Coll. Cardiol. *26*:900, 1995.
1055. Roux, S., Christeller, S., and Ludin, E.: Effects of aspirin on coronary reocclusion and recurrent ischemia after thrombolysis: A meta-analysis. J. Am. Coll. Cardiol. *19*:671, 1992.
1056. Cannon, C. P., Ganz, L. I., and Stone, P. H.: Complicated myocardial infarction. *In* Rippe, J. M., Irwin, R. S., Fink, M. P., et al. (eds.): Intensive Care Medicine. Boston, Little, Brown and Company, 1995, p. 477.
1057. Barbash, G. I., Hod, H., Roth, A., et al.: Repeat infusions of recombinant tissue-type plasminogen activator in patients with acute myocardial infarction and early recurrent myocardial ischemia. J. Am. Coll. Cardiol. *16*:779, 1990.
1058. Purvis, J. A., McNeil, A. J., Roberts, M. J. D., et al.: First-year follow-up after repeat thrombolytic therapy with recombinant-tissue plasminogen activator for myocardial reinfarction. Coronary Artery Dis. *3*:713, 1992.
1059. Simoons, M. L., Arnout, J., van den Brand, M., et al.: Retreatment with alteplase for early signs of reocclusion after thrombolysis: The European Cooperative Study Group. Am. J. Cardiol. *71*:524, 1993.
1060. Topol, E. J., Holmes, D. R., and Rogers, W. J.: Coronary angiography after thrombolytic therapy for acute myocardial infarction. Ann. Intern. Med. *114*:877, 1991.
1061. Sugiura, T., Iwasaka, T., Takayama, Y., et al.: Factors associated with pericardial effusion in acute Q wave myocardial infarction. Circulation *81*:477, 1990.
1062. Barrington, W., Smith, J. E., and Himmelstein, S. I.: Cardiac tamponade following treatment with tissue plasminogen activator: An atypical hemodynamic response to pericardiocentesis. Am. Heart J. *121*:1227, 1991.
1063. Clemmensen, P., Grande, P., Saunamäki, K., et al.: Evolution of electrocardiographic and echocardiographic abnormalities during the 4 years following first myocardial infarction. Eur. Heart J. *16*:1063, 1995.
1064. Erhardt, L.: Clinical and pathological observations in different types of acute myocardial infarction: A study of 84 patients deceased after treatment in a coronary care unit. Acta Med. Scand. *560*(Suppl.):1, 1974.
1065. Krainin, F. M., Flessas, A. P., and Spodick, D. H.: Infarction-associated pericarditis: Rarity of diagnostic electrocardiogram. N. Engl. J. Med. *311*:1211, 1984.
1066. Wall, T. C., Califf, R. M., Harrelson-Woodlief, L., et al.: Usefulness of a pericardial friction rub after thrombolytic therapy during acute myocardial infarction in predicting amount of myocardial damage. Am. J. Cardiol. *66*:1418, 1990.
1067. Karim, A. H., and Salomon, J.: Constrictive pericarditis after myocardial infarction: Sequela of anticoagulant-induced hemopericardium. Am. J. Med. *79*:389, 1985.
1068. Kloner, R., Fishbein, M., Lew, H., et al.: Mummification of the infarcted myocardium by high dose corticosteroids. Circulation *57*:56, 1978.
1069. Dressler, W.: The post-myocardial infarction syndrome: A report of forty-four cases. Arch. Intern. Med. *103*:28, 1959.
1070. Lichtstein, E., Arsura, E., Hollander, G., et al.: Current incidence of postmyocardial infarction (Dressler's) syndrome. Am. J. Cardiol. *50*:1269, 1982.
1071. Khan, A. H.: The postcardiac injury syndromes. Clin. Cardiol. *15*:67, 1992.
1072. Dressler, W., Yurkovsky, J., and Starr, M. C.: Hemorrhagic pericarditis, pleurisy, and pneumonia complicating recent myocardial infarction. Am. Heart J. *54*:42, 1957.
1073. Northcote, R. J., Hutchinson, S. J., and McGuinness, J. B.: Evidence for the continued existence of the postmyocardial infarction (Dressler's syndrome). Am. J. Cardiol. *53*:1201, 1984.
1074. Lichstein, E., Liu, H. M., and Gupta, P.: Pericarditis complicating acute myocardial infarction: Incidence of complications and significance of electrocardiogram on admission. Am. Heart J. *87*:246, 1974.
1075. Uuskiula, M. M., Lamp, K. M., and Martin, S. I.: Relationship between the clinical course of acute myocardial infarction and specific sensitization of lymphocytes and lymphotoxin production. Kardiologiia *26*:57, 1987.
1076. Brown, E. J., Jr., Kloner, R. A., Schoen, F. J., et al.: Scar thinning due to ibuprofen administration after experimental myocardial infarction. Am. J. Cardiol. *51*:877, 1983.
1077. Eppinger, E. C., and Kennedy, J. A.: The cause of death in coronary thrombosis, with special reference to pulmonary embolism. Am. J. Med. Sci. *195*:104, 1938.
1078. Hellerstein, H. K., and Martin, J. W.: Incidence of thromboembolic lesions accompanying myocardial infarction. Am. Heart J. *33*:443, 1947.
1079. Gueron, M., Wanderman, K. L., Hirsch, M., et al.: Pseudoaneurysm of the left ventricle after myocardial infarction: A curable form of myocardial rupture. J. Thorac. Cardiovasc. Surg. *69*:736, 1975.
1080. Kahn, J., and Fisher, M. R.: MRI of cardiac pseudoaneurysm and other complications of myocardial infarction. Magn. Reson. Imaging. *9*:159, 1991.
1081. Schoen, F. J.: Ischemic heart disease. *In* Schoen, F. J. (ed.): Interventional and Surgical Cardiovascular Pathology. Clinical Correlations and Basic Principles. Philadelphia, W. B. Saunders Company, 1989, p. 58.
1082. Forman, M. B., Collins, H. W., Kopelman, H. A., et al.: Determinants of left ventricular aneurysm formation after acute anterior myocardial infarction: A clinical and angiographic study. J. Am. Coll. Cardiol. *8*:1256, 1986.
1083. Hirai, T., Fujita, M., Nakajima, H., et al.: Importance of collateral circulation for prevention of left ventricular aneurysm formation in acute myocardial infarction. Circulation *79*:791, 1989.
1084. Abrams, D. L., Edelist, A., Luria, M. H., et al.: Ventricular aneurysm: A reappraisal based on a study of 65 consecutive autopsied cases. Circulation *27*:164, 1963.
1085. Meizlish, J. L., Berger, H. J., Plankey, M., et al.: Functional left ventricular aneurysm formation after acute anterior transmural myocardial infarction: Incidence, natural history, and prognostic implications. N. Engl. J. Med. *311*:1001, 1984.
1086. Lindsay, J., Jr., Dewey, D. C., Talesnick, B. S., et al.: Relation of ST-segment elevation after healing of acute myocardial infarction to the presence of left ventricular aneurysm. Am. J. Cardiol. *54*:84, 1984.
1087. Brawley, R. K., Magovern, G. J., Jr., Gott, V. L., et al.: Left ventricular aneurysmectomy: Factors influencing postoperative results. J. Thorac. Cardiovasc. Surg. *85*:712, 1983.
1088. Keeley, E. C., and Hillis, L. D.: Left ventricular mural thrombus after acute myocardial infarction. Clin. Cardiol. *19*:83, 1996.
1089. Halperin, J. L., and Fuster, V.: Left ventricular thrombi and cerebral embolism. N. Engl. J. Med. *320*:392, 1989.
1090. Halperin, J. L., and Petersen, P.: Thrombosis in the cardiac chambers: Ventricular dysfunction and atrial fibrillation. *In* Fuster, V., and Verstraete, M. (eds.): Thrombosis in Cardiovascular Disorders. Philadelphia, W. B. Saunders Company, 1992, p. 215.
1091. Funke Kupper, A. J., Verheugt, F. W. A., Peels, C. H., et al.: Left ventricular thrombus incidence and behavior studied by serial two-dimensional echocardiography in acute anterior myocardial infarction: Left ventricular wall motion, systemic wall motion, systemic embolism and oral anticoagulation. J. Am. Coll. Cardiol. *13*:1514, 1989.
1092. Stein, B., Halperin, J. L., and Fuster, V.: Prevention of left ventricular mural thrombosis and arterial embolism during and after myocardial infarction. Coronary Artery Dis. *1*:180, 1990.
1093. Gueret, P., Dubourg, O., Ferrier, A., et al.: Effects of full-dose heparin anticoagulation on the development of left ventricular thrombosis in acute myocardial infarction. J. Am. Coll. Cardiol. *8*:419, 1986.
1094. Fernandez-Ortiz, A., Jand, I.-K., and Fuster, V.: Anticoagulant and platelet inhibitory agents for myocardial infarction. *In* Francis, G. S.,

and Alpert, J. S. (eds.): Coronary Care. Boston, Little, Brown and Company, 1995, p. 569.
1095. Stratton, J. R., and Resnick, A. D.: Increased embolic risk in patients with left ventricular thrombi. Circulation *75*:1004, 1987.
1096. Jugdutt, B. I., Sivaram, C. A., Wortman, C., et al.: Prospective two-dimensional echocardiographic evaluation of left ventricular thrombus and embolism after myocardial infarction. J. Am. Coll. Cardiol. *13*:554, 1989.
1097. Working Party on Anticoagulant Therapy in Coronary Thrombosis to the Medical Research Council: An assessment of long-term anticoagulant administration after cardiac infarction: BMJ *2*:837, 1964.
1098. Nordrehaug, J. E., Johannessen, K. A., and von der Lippe, G.: Usefulness of high-dose anticoagulants in preventing left ventricular thrombus in acute myocardial infarction. Am. J. Cardiol. *55*:1941, 1985.
1099. Davis, M. J. E., and Ireland, M. A.: Effect of early anticoagulation on the frequency of left ventricular thrombi after anterior wall acute myocardial infarction. Am. J. Cardiol. *57*:1244, 1986.
1100. Arvan, S., and Boscha, K.: Prophylactic anticoagulation for left ventricular thrombi after acute myocardial infarction: A prospective randomized trial. Am. Heart J. *113*:688, 1987.
1101. Turpie, A. G. G., Robinson, J. G., Doyle, D. J., et al.: Comparison of high-dose with low-dose subcutaneous heparin to prevent left ventricular mural thrombosis in patients with acute transmural anterior myocardial infarction. N. Engl. J. Med. *320*:352, 1989.
1102. Held, A. C., Gore, J. M., Paraskos, J., et al.: Impact of thrombolytic therapy on left ventricular mural thrombi in acute myocardial infarction. Am. J. Cardiol. *62*:310, 1988.
1103. Halperin, J. L., and Fuster, V.: Left ventricular thrombus and stroke after myocardial infarction: Toward prevention or perplexity? J. Am. Coll. Cardiol. *14*:912, 1989.
1104. Nihoyannopoulos, P., Smith, G. C., Maseri, A., et al.: The natural history of left ventricular thrombus in myocardial infarction: A rationale in support of masterly inactivity. J. Am. Coll. Cardiol. *14*:903, 1989.
1105. Stein, B., Fuster, V., Halperin, J. L., et al.: Antithrombitic therapy in cardiac disease: An emerging approach based on pathogenesis and risk. Circulation *80*:1501, 1989.
1106. Kouvaras, G., Chronopoulos, G., Soufras, G., et al.: The effects of long-term antithrombotic treatment on left ventricular thrombi in patients after an acute myocardial infarction. Am. Heart J. *119*:73, 1990.
1107. Keren, A., Goldberg, S., Gottlieb, S., et al.: Natural history of left ventricular thrombi: Their appearance and resolution in the posthospitalization period of acute myocardial infarction. J. Am. Coll. Cardiol. *15*:790, 1990.
1108. Stratton, J. R., and Ritchie, J. L.: The effects of antithrombotic drugs in patients with left ventricular thrombi: Assessment with indium-111 platelet imaging and two-dimensional echocardiography. Circulation *69*:561, 1984.

CONVALESCENCE, DISCHARGE, AND POST–MYOCARDIAL INFARCTION CARE

1109. Hammerman, H., Kloner, R. A., Alker, K. J., et al.: Effects of transient increased afterload during experimentally induced acute myocardial infarction in dogs. Am. J. Cardiol. *55*:566, 1985.
1110. Gheorghiade, M., Anderson, J., Rosman, H., et al.: Risk identification at the time of admission to coronary care unit in patients with suspected myocardial infarction. Am. Heart J. *116*:1212, 1988.
1111. Parsons, R. W., Jamrozik, K. D., Hobbs, M. S., et al.: Early identification of patients at low risk of death after myocardial infarction and potentially suitable for early hospital discharge. BMJ *308*:1006, 1994.
1112. Newby, L. K., Califf, R. M., Guerci, A., et al.: Early discharge in the thrombolytic era: An analysis of criteria for uncomplicated infarction from the Global Utilization for Streptokinase and t-PA for Occluded Coronary Arteries (GUSTO) trial. J. Am. Coll. Cardiol. 1996 *(in press).*
1113. Pryor, D. B., Hindman, M. C., Wagner, G. S., et al.: Early discharge after acute myocardial infarction. Ann. Intern. Med. *99*:528, 1983.
1114. Ockene, I. S., Clemow, L. P., and Ockene, J. K.: Psychosocial and behavioral factors during recovery from myocardial infarction. *In* Francis, G. S., and Alpert, J. S. (eds.): Coronary Care. Boston, Little, Brown and Company, 1995, p. 595.
1115. Tardif, G. S.: Sexual activity after a myocardial infarction. Arch. Phys. Med. Rehabil. *70*:763, 1989.
1116. Mendes de Leon, C. F., Powell, L. H., and Kaplan, B. H.: Changes in coronary-prone behaviors in the Recurrent Coronary Prevention Project. Psychosom. Med. *53*:407, 1991.
1117. Squires, R. W., Gau, G. T., Miller, T. D., et al.: Cardiovascular rehabilitation: Status, 1990. Mayo Clin. Proc. *65*:731, 1990.
1118. O'Connor, G. T., Buring, J. E., Yusuf, S., et al.: An overview of randomized trials of rehabilitation with exercise after myocardial infarction. Circulation *80*:234, 1989.
1119. Dennis, C. A.: Rehabilitation following acute myocardial infarction. *In* Francis, G. S., and Alpert, J. S. (eds.): Coronary Care. Boston, Little, Brown and Company, 1995, p. 629.
1120. Balady, G. J., Fletcher, B. J., Froelicher, E.S., et al.: Cardiac rehabilitation programs: A statement for healthcare professionals from the American Heart Association. Circulation *90*:1602, 1994.
1121. Tofler, G. H., Stone, P. H., Muller, J. E., et al.: Effects of gender and race on prognosis after myocardial infarction: Adverse prognosis for women, particularly black women. J. Am. Coll. Cardiol. *9*:473, 1987.
1122. Tofler, G. H., Muller, J. E., Stone, P. H., et al.: Factors leading to shorter survival after acute myocardial infarction in patients aging 65 to 75 years compared with younger patients. Am. J. Cardiol. *62*:860, 1988.
1123. Marcus, F. I., Friday, K., McCans, J., et al.: Age-related prognosis after acute myocardial infarction (the Multicenter Diltiazem Postinfarction Trial). Am. J. Cardiol. *65*:559, 1990.
1124. Stone, P. H., Muller, J. E., Hartwell, T., et al.: The effect of diabetes mellitus on prognosis and serial left ventricular function after acute myocardial infarction: Contribution of both coronary disease and diastolic left ventricular dysfunction to the adverse prognosis. J. Am. Coll. Cardiol. *14*:49, 1989.
1125. DeBusk, R. F., Kraemer, H. C., and Nash, E.: Stepwise risk stratification soon after acute myocardial infarction. Am. J. Cardiol. *52*:1161, 1983.
1126. Merrilees, M. A., Scott, P. J., and Norris, R. M.: Prognosis after myocardial infarction: Results of 15 year follow-up. BMJ *288*:356, 1984.
1127. Benhorin, J., Moss, A. J., Oakes, D., et al.: Prognostic significance of nonfatal myocardial reinfarction. J. Am. Coll. Cardiol. *15*:253, 1990.
1128. Smith, J. W., Marcus, F. I., Serokman, R., et al.: Prognosis of patients with diabetes mellitus after acute myocardial infarction. Am. J. Cardiol. *54*:718, 1984.
1129. Abbott, R. D., Donaue, R. P., Kannel, W. B., et al.: The impact of diabetes on survival following myocardial infarction in men vs women: The Framingham Study. JAMA *260*:3456, 1988.
1130. Rennert, G., Saltz-Rennerts, H., Wanderman, K., et al.: Size of acute myocardial infarcts in patients with diabetes mellitus. Am. J. Cardiol. *55*:1629, 1985.
1131. Gwilt, D. J. G., Petri, M., Lewis, P. W., et al.: Myocardial infarct size and mortality in diabetic patients. Br. Heart J. *54*:466, 1985.
1132. Maisel, A. S., Gilpin, E., Holt, B., et al.: Survival after hospital discharge in matched populations with inferior or anterior myocardial infarction. J. Am. Coll. Cardiol. *6*:731, 1985.
1133. Hands, M. E., Lloyd, B. L., Robinson, J. S., et al.: Prognostic significance of electrocardiographic site of infarction after correction for enzymatic size of infarction. Circulation *73*:885, 1986.
1134. Zabel, K. M., Hathaway, W. R., Peterson, E. D., et al.: Baseline electrocardiogram predicts 30-day mortality among 32,182 patients with acute myocardial infarction treated with thrombolysis. J. Am. Coll. Cardiol. *25*:342A, 1995.
1135. Bates, E. R., Clemmensen, P. M., Califf, R. M., et al.: Precordial ST segment depression predicts a worse prognosis in inferior infarction despite reperfusion therapy: The Thrombolysis and Angioplasty in Myocardial Infarction (TAMI) Study Group. J. Am. Coll. Cardiol. *16*:1538, 1990.
1136. Wong, C. K., Freedman, S. B., Bautovich, G., et al.: Mechanism and significance of precordial ST-segment depression during inferior wall acute myocardial infarction associated with severe narrowing of the dominant right coronary artery. Am. J. Cardiol. *71*:1025, 1993.
1137. Goldberg, R. J., Seeley, D., Becker, R. C., et al.: Impact of atrial fibrillation on the in-hospital and long-term survival of patients with acute myocardial infarction: A community-wide perspective. Am. Heart J. *119*:996, 1990.
1138. Chaitman, B. R., Thompson, B. W., Kern, M. J., et al.: Tissue plasminogen activator followed by percutaneous transluminal coronary angioplasty: One year TIMI phase II pilot results. Am. Heart J. *119*:213, 1990.
1139. Bosch, X., Théroux, P., Walters, D., et al.: Early postinfarction ischemia: Clinical, angiographic, and prognostic significance. Circulation *75*:988, 1987.
1140. Tzivoni, D., Gavish, A., Zin, D., et al.: Prognostic significance of ischemic episodes in patients with previous myocardial infarction. Am. J. Cardiol. *62*:661, 1988.
1141. DeWood, M. A., Stifter, W. F., Simpson, C. S., et al.: Coronary arteriographic findings soon after non-Q wave myocardial infarction. N. Engl. J. Med. *315*:417, 1986.
1141a. Matetzky, S., Barabash, G. I., Rabinowitz, B., et al.: Q wave and non-Q wave myocardial infarction after thrombolysis. J. Am. Coll. Cardiol. *26*:1445, 1995.
1142. Devlin, W., Cragg, D., Jacks, M., et al.: Comparison of outcome in patients with acute myocardial infarction aged > 75 years with that in younger patients. Am. J. Cardiol. *75*:573, 1995.
1143. Krikorian, R. K., and Vacek, J. J.: Non-Q-wave myocardial infarction in the elderly: Clinical characteristics and management. Am. J. Ger. Cardiol. *4*:41, 1995.
1144. Gibson, R. S.: Non-Q-wave myocardial infarction. *In* Fuster, V., Ross, R., and Topol, E. J. (eds.): Atherosclerosis and Coronary Artery Disease. Philadelphia, Lippincott-Raven, 1996, pp. 1097–1124.
1145. Berger, C. J., Murabito, J. M., Evans, J. C., et al.: Prognosis after first myocardial infarction: Comparison of Q wave and non-Q wave myocardial infarction in the Framingham Heart Study. JAMA *268*:1545, 1992.
1146. Krone, R. J., Greenberg, J., Dwyer, E. M., et al.: Long-term prognostic significance of ST segment depression during acute myocardial infarction. J. Am. Coll. Cardiol. *22*:361, 1993.
1147. Mickley, H., Pless, P., Nielsen, J. R., et al.: Residual myocardial ischemia in first non-Q versus Q wave infarction: Maximal exercise testing and ambulatory ST segment monitoring. Eur. Heart J. *14*:18, 1993.
1148. Johnston, T. S., and Wenger, N. K.: Risk stratification after myocardial infarction. Curr. Opin. Cardiol. *8*:621, 1993.
1149. Pitt, B.: Evaluation of the postinfarct patient. Circulation *91*:1855, 1995.

1150. Figueredo, V., and Cheitlin, M. D.: Risk stratification. *In* Julian, D., and Braunwald, E. (eds.): Management of Acute Myocardial Infarction. London, W. B. Saunders Ltd., 1994, p. 361.
1151. Wolff, A. A., and Karliner, J. S.: Overall risk stratification and management strategies for patients with acute myocardial infarction. *In* Francis, G. S., and Alpert, J. S. (eds.): Coronary Care. Boston, Little, Brown and Company, 1995, p. 741.
1152. Multicenter Postinfarction Research Group: Risk stratification and survival after myocardial infarction. N. Engl. J. Med. *309:*331, 1983.
1153. Volpi, A., De Vita, C., Franzosi, M. G., et al.: Determinants of 6-month mortality in survivors of myocardial infarction after thrombolysis: Results of the GISSI-2 data base: The Ad Hoc Working Group of the Gruppo Italiano per lo Studio della Sopravvivenza nell'Infarto Miocardico (GISSI)-2 Data Base. Circulation *88:*416, 1993.
1154. Stevenson, R., Ranjadayalan, K., Wilkinson, P., et al.: Short and long term prognosis of acute myocardial infarction since introduction of thrombolysis. BMJ *307:*349, 1993.
1155. Jereczek, M., Andresen, D., Schroder, J., et al.: Prognostic value of ischemia during Holter monitoring and exercise testing after acute myocardial infarction. Am. J. Cardiol. *72:*8, 1993.
1156. Myers, M. G., Baigrie, R. S., Charlat, M. L., et al.: Are routine non-invasive tests useful in prediction of outcome after myocardial infarction in elderly people? Lancet *342:*1069, 1993.
1157. Ruberman, W., Weinblatt, E., Goldberg, J. D., et al.: Ventricular premature complexes and sudden death after myocardial infarction. Circulation *64:*297, 1981.
1158. Gomes, J. A., Winters, S. L., Ip, J.: Post myocardial infarction stratification and signal-averaged electrocardiogram. Prog. Cardiovasc. Dis. *35:*263, 1993.
1159. McClements, B. M., Adgey, A. A.: Value of signal-averaged electrocardiography, radionuclide ventriculography, Holter monitoring and clinical variables for prediction of arrhythmic events in survivors of acute myocardial infarction in the thrombolytic era. J. Am. Coll. Cardiol. *21:*1419, 1993.
1160. La Rovere, M. T., Bigger, J. T., Marcus, F. I., et al.: Prognostic value of depressed baroreflex sensitivity: The ATRAMI Study. Circulation *92*(Suppl.):I-777, 1995.
1161. Task Force of the European Society of Cardiology and The North American Society of Pacing and Electrophysiology: Heart rate variability—standards of measurement, physiological interpretation, and clinical use. Circulation *93:*1043, 1996.
1162. Aguirre, F. V., Kern, M. J., Hsia, J., et al.: Importance of myocardial infarct artery patency on the prevalence of ventricular arrhythmia and late potentials after thrombolysis in acute myocardial infarction. Am. J. Cardiol. *68:*1410, 1991.
1163. Morris, K. G.: Use of radionuclide angiography following acute myocardial infarction. *In* Califf, R. M., Mark, D. B., and Wagner, G. S. (eds.): Acute Coronary Care. St. Louis, Mosby, 1995, p. 797.
1164. Fletcher, G. F., Balady, G., Froelicher, V. F., et al.: Exercise standards: A statement for healthcare professionals from the American Heart Association. Circulation *91:*580, 1995.
1165. Pilote, L., Silberberg, J., Lisbona, R., et al.: Prognosis in patients with low left ventricular ejection fraction after myocardial infarction. Circulation *80:*1636, 1989.
1166. Dilsizian, V., and Bonow, R. O.: Current diagnostic techniques of assessing myocardial viability in patients with hibernating and stunned myocardium. Circulation *87:*1, 1993.
1167. Crawford, M. H.: Risk stratification after myocardial infarction with exercise and Doppler echocardiography. Circulation *84*(Suppl. I):163, 1991.
1168. Bach, D. S., and Armstrong, W. F.: Dobutamine stress echocardiography. Am. J. Cardiol. *69:*18, 1992.
1169. Previtali, M., Poli, A., Lanzarini, L., et al.: Dobutamine stress echocardiography for assessment of myocardial viability and ischemia in acute myocardial infarction treated with thrombolysis. Am. J. Cardiol. *72:*16, 1993.
1170. Watada, H., Ito, H., Oh, H., et al.: Dobutamine stress echocardiography predicts reversible dysfunction and quantitates the extent of irreversibly damaged myocardium after reperfusion of anterior myocardial infarction. J. Am. Coll. Cardiol. *24:*624, 1994.
1171. Pellikka, P. A., Roger, V. L., Oh, J. K., et al.: Stress echocardiography. Part II. Dobutamine stress echocardiography: Techniques, implementation, clinical applications, and correlations. Mayo Clin. Proc. *70:*16, 1995.
1172. Picano, E., Pingitore, A., Sicari, R., et al.: Stress echocardiographic results predict risk reinfarction early after uncomplicated acute myocardial infarction: Large-scale multicenter study. J. Am. Coll. Cardiol. *26:*908, 1995.
1173. Coma-Canella, I., del Val Gomez Martinez, M., Rodigro, F., et al.: The dobutamine stress test with thallium-201 single-photon emission computed tomography and radionuclide angiography: Postinfarction study. J. Am. Coll. Cardiol. *22:*399, 1993.
1174. Sansoy, V., Glover, D. K., Watson, D. D., et al.: Comparison of thallium-201 resting redistribution with technetium-99m sestamibi uptake and functional response to dobutamine for assessment of myocardial viability. Circulation *92:*994, 1995.
1175. Yoshida, K., and Gould, K. L.: Quantitative relation of myocardial infarct size and myocardial viability by positron emission tomography to left ventricular ejection fraction and 3-year mortality with and without revascularization. J. Am. Coll. Cardiol. *22:*984, 1993.
1176. Mark, W. I., Webster, M. B., Chesebro, J. H., et al.: Myocardial infarction and coronary artery occlusion: A prospective 5-year angiographic study. J. Am. Coll. Cardiol. *15:*218A, 1990.
1176a. Meeting Highlights: AHA 68th Scientific Sessions, "Invasive Versus Medical Treatment of Postinfarction Ischemia" (DANAMI Study). Circulation *93:*846, 1996.
1177. Juneau, M., Colles, P., Theroux, P., et al.: Symptom-limited versus low level exercise testing before hospital discharge after myocardial infarction. J. Am. Coll. Cardiol. *20:*927, 1992.
1178. Jain, A., Myers, G. H., Sapin, P. M., et al.: Comparison of symptom-limited and low level exercise tolerance tests early after myocardial infarction. J. Am. Coll. Cardiol. *22:*1816, 1993.
1179. Stevenson, R., Umachandran, V., Ranjadayalan, K., et al.: Reassessment of treadmill stress testing for risk stratification in patients with acute myocardial infarction treated by thrombolysis. Br. Heart J. *70:*415, 1993.
1180. Gibson, R. S., and Beller, G. A.: Value of predischarge myocardial perfusion scintigraphy. *In* Fuster, V., Ross, R., and Topol, E. J. (eds.): Atherosclerosis and Coronary Artery Disease. Philadelphia, Lippincott-Raven, 1996, pp. 1167–1192.
1181. Lavie, C. J., Gibbons, R. J., Zinsmeister, A. R., et al.: Interpreting results of exercise studies after acute myocardial infarction altered by thrombolytic therapy, coronary angioplasty or bypass. Am. J. Cardiol. *67:*116, 1991.
1182. Moss, A. J., Goldstein, R. E., Hall, W. J., et al.: Detection and significance of myocardial ischemia in stable patients after recovery from an acute coronary event. JAMA *269:*2379, 1993.
1183. Moss, A. J., Davis, H. T., DeCamilla, J., et al.: Ventricular ectopic beats and their relation to sudden and nonsudden cardiac death after myocardial infarction. Circulation *60:*998, 1979.
1184. Bigger, J. T., Fleiss, J. L., Kleiger, R., et al.: The relationships between ventricular arrhythmias, left ventricular dysfunction, and mortality in the 2 years after myocardial infarction. Circulation *69:*250, 1984.
1185. Mukharji, J., and MILIS Study Group: Risk factors for sudden death after acute myocardial infarction. Am. J. Cardiol. *54:*31, 1984.
1186. Kostis, J. B., Byington, R., Friedman, L. M., et al.: Prognostic significance of ventricular ectopic activity in survivors of acute myocardial infarction. J. Am. Coll. Cardiol. *10:*231, 1987.
1187. Morganroth, J., and Bigger, J. T., Jr.: Pharmacologic management of ventricular arrhythmias after the Cardiac Arrhythmia Suppression Trial. Am. J. Cardiol. *65:*1497, 1990.
1188. Richards, D. A., Byth, K., Ross, D. L., et al.: What is the best predictor of spontaneous ventricular tachycardia and sudden death after myocardial infarction? Circulation *83:*756, 1991.
1188a. Prystowsky, E. N.: Acute myocardial infarction: Role of electrophysiologic testing prior to hospital discharge. *In* Fuster, V., Ross, R., and Topol, E. J. (eds.): Atherosclerosis and Coronary Artery Disease. Philadelphia, Lippincott-Raven, 1996, pp. 1257–1266.
1189. Hohnloser, S. H., Franck, P., Klingenheben, T., et al.: Open infarct artery, late potentials, and other prognostic factors in patients after acute myocardial infarction in the thrombolytic era: A prospective trial. Circulation *90:*1747, 1994.
1190. Farrell, T. G., Bashir, Y., Cripps, T., et al.: Risk stratification for arrhythmic events in postinfarction patients based on heart rate variability, ambulatory electrocardiographic variables and the signal-averaged electrocardiogram. J. Am. Coll. Cardiol. *18:*687, 1991.
1190a. Gomes, J. A.: Acute myocardial infarction: Role of signal averaging. *In* Fuster, V., Ross, R., and Topol, E. J. (eds.): Atherosclerosis and Coronary Artery Disease. Philadelphia, Lippincott-Raven, 1996, pp. 1245–1256.
1191. Bourke, J. P., Richards, D. A. B., Ross, D. L., et al.: Routine programmed electrical stimulation in survivors of acute myocardial infarction for prediction of spontaneous ventricular tachyarrhythmias during follow-up: Results, optimal stimulation protocol, and cost-effective screening. J. Am. Coll. Cardiol. *18:*780, 1991.
1192. Pedretti, R., Etro, M. D., Laporta, A., et al.: Prediction of late arrhythmic events after acute myocardial infarction from combined use of noninvasive prognostic variables and inducibility of sustained monomorphic ventricular tachycardia. Am. J. Cardiol. *71:*1131, 1993.
1193. Gilman, J. K., Jalal, S., and Naccarelli, G. V.: Predicting and preventing sudden death from cardiac causes. Circulation *90:*1083, 1994.
1194. Pieper, S. J., and Hammil, S. C.: Heart rate variability: Technique and investigational application in cardiovascular medicine. Mayo Clin. Proc. *70:*955, 1995.
1195. Moss, A. J., and Benhorin, J.: Prognosis and management after a first myocardial infarction. N. Engl. J. Med. *322:*743, 1990.
1196. Schoenberger, J. A.: Advances in the primary and secondary prevention of coronary heart disease. Curr. Opin. Cardiol. *8:*557, 1993.
1197. Hinstridge, V., and Speight, T. M.: An overview of therapeutic interventions in myocardial infarction: Emphasis on secondary prevention. Drugs *2:*8, 1991.
1198. Rosenberg, L., Kaufman, D. W., Helmrich, S. P., et al.: The risk of myocardial infarction after quitting smoking in men under 55 years of age. N. Engl. J. Med. *313:*1511, 1985.
1199. Rigotti, N. A., Singer, D. E., Mulley, A. G., Jr., et al.: Smoking cessation following admission to a coronary care unit. J. Gen. Intern. Med. *6:*305, 1991.
1200. Krumholz, H. M., Cohen, B. J., Tsevat, J., et al.: Cost-effectiveness of a smoking cessation program after myocardial infarction. J. Am. Coll. Cardiol. *22:*1697, 1993.
1201. Frasure-Smith, N., Lesperance, F., and Talajic, M.: Depression follow-

ing myocardial infarction: Impact on 6-month survival. JAMA *270*:1819, 1993.
1202. Berkman, L. F., Leo-Summers, L., and Horwitz, R. I.: Emotional support and survival after myocardial infarction. Ann. Intern. Med. *117*:1003, 1992.
1203. Bucher, H. C.: Social support and prognosis following first myocardial infarction. J. Gen. Intern. Med. *9*:409, 1994.
1204. Gallagher, E. J., Viscoli, C. M., and Horwitz, R. I.: The relationship of treatment adherence to the risk of death after myocardial infarction in women. JAMA *270*:742, 1993.
1205. Bondestam, E., Breikss, A., and Hartford, M.: Effects of early rehabilitation on consumption of medical care during the first year after acute myocardial infarction in patients > or = 65 years of age. Am. J. Cardiol. *75*:767, 1995.
1206. Dennis, C., Houston-Miller, N., Schwartz, R. G., et al.: Early return to work after uncomplicated myocardial infarction: Results of a randomized trial. JAMA *260*:214, 1988.
1207. Wong, N. D., Wilson, P. W. F., and Kannel, W. B.: Serum cholesterol as a prognostic factor after myocardial infarction: The Framingham Study. Ann. Intern. Med. *115*:687, 1991.
1208. Braunwald, E., Pfeffer, M., and Sacks, F.: The CARE Trial: Presented at American College of Cardiology, 1996.
1209. Cohen, M., Byrne, M., Levine, B., et al.: Low rate of treatment of hypercholesterolemia by cardiologists in patients with suspected and proven coronary artery disease. Circulation *83*:1294, 1991.
1210. Scandinavian Simvistatin Survival Study Group: Randomised trial of cholesterol lowering in 4444 patients with coronary heart disease: The Scandinavian Simvastatin Survival Study (4S). Lancet *344*:1383, 1994.
1211. Scandinavian Simvistatin Survival Study Group: Baseline serum cholesterol and treatment effect in the Scandinavian Simvastatin Survival Study (4S). Lancet *345*:1274, 1995.
1212. Col, N. F., Yarzebski, J., Gore, J. M., et al.: Does aspirin consumption affect the presentation or severity of acute myocardial infarction? Arch. Intern. Med. *155*:1386, 1995.
1213. Alhaddad, I. A., Tkaczevski, L., Siddiqui, F., et al.: Aspirin enhances the benefits of late reperfusion on infarct shape: A possible mechanism of the beneficial effects of aspirin on survival after acute myocardial infarction. Circulation *91*:2819, 1995.
1214. Tsevat, J., Duke, D., Goldman, L., et al.: Cost-effectiveness of captopril therapy after myocardial infarction. J. Am. Coll. Cardiol. *26*:914, 1995.
1215. Herlitz, J., Elmfeldt, D., Holmberg, S., et al.: Goteborg metoprolol trial: Mortality and causes of death. Am. J. Cardiol. *53*:9D, 1984.
1216. Olsson, G., Rehnqvist, N., Sjögren, A., et al.: Long-term treatment with metoprolol in acute myocardial infarction: Effect on 3 year mortality and morbidity. J. Am. Coll. Cardiol. *5*:1428, 1985.
1217. The Norwegian Multicenter Study Group: Timolol-induced reduction in mortality and reinfarction in patients surviving acute myocardial infarction. N. Engl. J. Med. *304*:801, 1981.
1218. Chadda, K., Goldstein, S., Byington, R., et al.: Effect of propranolol after acute myocardial infarction in patients with congestive heart failure. Circulation *73*:503, 1986.
1219. Beta-Blocker Pooling Project Research Group: The Beta-Blocker Pooling Project (BBPP): Subgroup findings from randomized trials in postinfarction patients. Eur. Heart J. *9*:8, 1988.
1219a. O'Rourke, R. A.: Are beta-blockers really underutilized in postinfarction patients? J. Am. Coll. Cardiol. *26*:1437, 1995.
1220. Olsson, G., Levin, L.-A., and Rehnqvist, N.: Economic consequences of postinfarction prophylaxis with β blockers: Cost effectiveness of metoprolol. Br. Heart J. *294*:339, 1987.
1221. Goldman, L., Sia, S. T. B., Cook, E. F., et al.: Costs and effectiveness of routine therapy with long-term beta-adrenergic antagonists after acute myocardial infarction. N. Engl. J. Med. *319*:152, 1988.
1222. Brand, D. A., Newcomer, L. N., Freiburger, A., et al.: Cardiologists' practices compared with practice guidelines: use of beta-blockade after myocardial infarction. J. Am. Coll. Cardiol. *26*:1432, 1995.
1223. Goldstein, S.: Review of beta blocker myocardial infarction trials. Clin. Cardiol. *12*:54, 1989.
1224. Smith, P., Arnesen, H., and Holme, I.: The effect of warfarin on mortality and reinfarction after myocardial infarction. N. Engl. J. Med. *323*:147, 1990.
1225. Devine, N., Azarnia, N., Nelson, K., et al.: Long-term anticoagulants in post myocardial infarction patients: A meta-analysis. Circulation *86*(Suppl. I):259, 1992.
1226. Anticoagulants in the Secondary Prevention of Events in Coronary Thrombosis (ASPECT) Research Group: Effect of long-term oral anticoagulant treatment on mortality and cardiovascular morbidity after myocardial infarction. Lancet *343*:499, 1994.
1227. van Bergen, P. F. M. M., Jonker, J. J. C., van Hout, B. A., et al.: Costs and effects of long-term oral anticoagulant treatment after myocardial infarction. JAMA *273*:925, 1995.
1228. Breddin, K., Loew, D., Lechner, K., et al.: The German-Austrian aspirin trial: A comparison of acetylsalicylic acid, placebo, and phenprocoumon in secondary prevention of myocardial infarction. Circulation *62*(Suppl. V):V63, 1980.
1229. The EPSIM Research Group: A controlled comparison of aspirin and oral anticoagulants in prevention of death after myocardial infarction. N. Engl. J. Med. *307*:701, 1982.
1230. Cairns, J. A., and Markham, B. A.: Economics and efficacy in choosing oral anticoagulants or aspirin after myocardial infarction. JAMA *273*:965, 1995.
1231. Teo, K. K., Yusuf, S., and Furberg, C. D.: Effects of prophylactic antiarrhythmic drug therapy in acute myocardial infarction. JAMA *270*:1589, 1993.
1232. Epstein, A. E., Hallstrom, A. P., Rogers, W. J., et al.: Mortality following ventricular arrhythmia suppression by encainide, flecainide, and moricizine after myocardial infarction: The original design concept of the Cardiac Arrhythmia Suppression Trial (CAST). JAMA *270*:2451, 1993.
1233. Echt, D. S., Liebson, P. R., Mitchell, L. B., et al.: Mortality and morbidity in patients receiving encainide, flecainide, or placebo: The Cardiac Arrhythmia Suppression Trial. N. Engl. J. Med. *324*:781, 1991.
1234. The Cardiac Arrhythmia Suppression Trial II Investigators: Effects of the antiarrhythmic agent moricizine on survival after myocardial infarction. N. Engl. J. Med. *327*:227, 1992.
1234a. Krishnan, S. C., Shivkumar, K., Garan, H., et al.: Increased vulnerability of the subendocardium to ischaemic injury: An electrophysiological explanation. Lancet *346*:1612, 1995.
1235. Waldo, A. L., Camm, A. J., de Ruyter, H., et al.: Preliminary mortality results from the Survival with Oral D-Sotalol (SWORD) Trial. J. Am. Coll. Cardiol. *25*(Special Issue):15A, 1995.
1236. Zarembski, D. G., Nolan, P. E., Slack, M. K., et al.: Empiric long-term amiodarone prophylaxis following myocardial infarction: A meta-analysis. Arch. Intern. Med. *153*:2661, 1993.
1237. Stevenson, J. C., Crook, D., Godsland, I. F., et al.: Hormone replacement therapy and the cardiovascular system: Nonlipid effects. Drugs *47*(Suppl. 2):35, 1994.
1238. The Writing Group for the PEPI Trial: Effects of estrogen or estrogen/progestin regimens on heart disease risk factors in postmenopausal women: The postmenopausal estrogen/progestin interventions (PEPI) trial. JAMA *273*:199, 1995.
1238a. Samaan, S. A., and Crawford, M.H.: Estrogen and cardiovascular function after menopause. J. Am. Coll. Cardiol. *26*:1403, 1995.
1239. Lobo, R. A., and Speroff, L.: International consensus conference on postmenopausal hormone therapy and the cardiovascular system. Fertil. Steril. *61*:592, 1994.
1240. Colditz, G. A., Hankinson, S. E., Hunter, D. J., et al.: The use of estrogens and progestins and the risk of breast cancer in postmenopausal women. N. Engl. J. Med. *332*:1589, 1995.

Chapter 38
Chronic Coronary Artery Disease

BERNARD J. GERSH, EUGENE BRAUNWALD, JOHN D. RUTHERFORD

STABLE ANGINA PECTORIS 1290
Clinical Manifestations 1290
Pathophysiology 1293
Noninvasive Testing 1295
Catheterization, Angiography, and Coronary Arteriography 1298
Medical Management 1299
PERCUTANEOUS TRANSLUMINAL CORONARY ANGIOPLASTY AND RELATED CATHETER-BASED TECHNIQUES 1313
CORONARY ARTERY BYPASS SURGERY . . .1316
Technical Considerations 1316
Outcome of Surgery 1319
Selection of Patients for Coronary Bypass Surgery 1321
Results 1323
Comparisons Between PTCA and CABG . . .1329
Coronary Bypass Surgery in Patients with Associated Vascular Disease 1331
UNSTABLE ANGINA 1331
PRINZMETAL'S VARIANT ANGINA 1340
OTHER MANIFESTATIONS OF CORONARY ARTERY DISEASE 1343
Chest Pain with Normal Coronary Arteriogram .1343
Silent Myocardial Ischemia 1344
Heart Failure .1346
Cardiac Arrhythmias 1349
Nonatheromatous Coronary Artery Disease 1349
REFERENCES .1349

Chronic coronary artery disease (CAD) is most commonly due to obstruction of the coronary arteries by atheromatous plaques[1]; the pathogenesis of atherosclerosis is described in Chap. 34. Factors that predispose to this condition are discussed in Chap. 35, the control of coronary blood flow in Chap. 36, and acute myocardial infarction in Chap. 37; sudden cardiac death, another significant consequence of CAD is presented in Chap. 24.

The importance of CAD in contemporary society is attested to by the almost epidemic number of persons afflicted[2–3a]—especially when this number is compared with the anecdotal reports of its occurrence in the medical literature before this century. More than 11 million Americans have CAD, which causes more deaths, disability, and economic loss in industrialized nations than any other group of diseases. About 6.3 million persons in the United

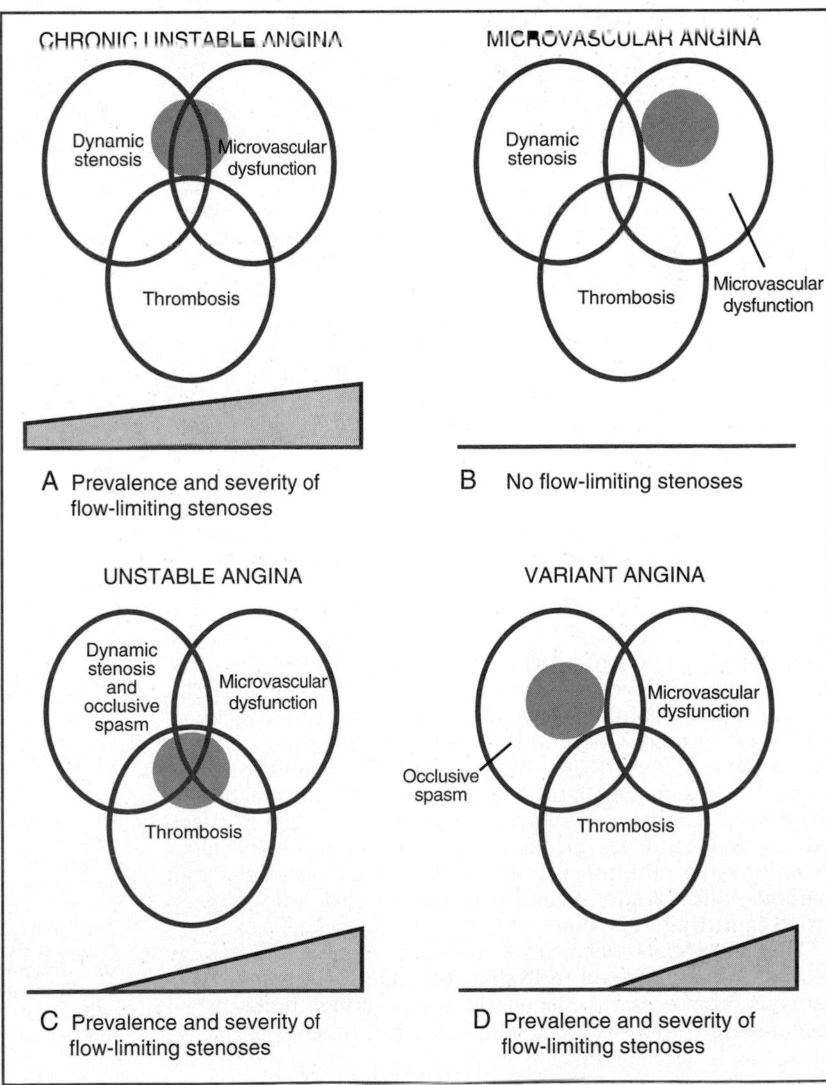

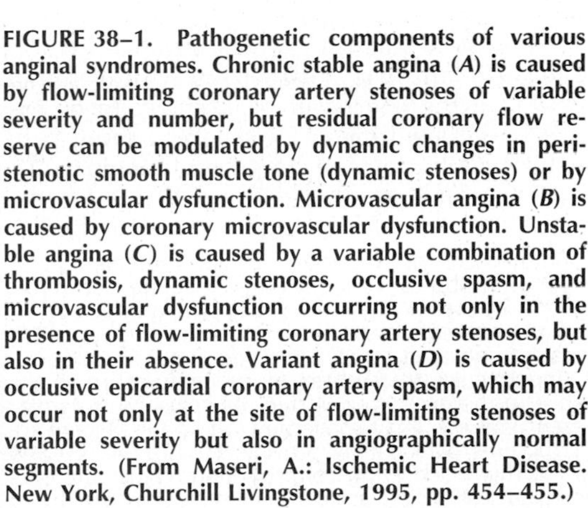
FIGURE 38–1. Pathogenetic components of various anginal syndromes. Chronic stable angina (*A*) is caused by flow-limiting coronary artery stenoses of variable severity and number, but residual coronary flow reserve can be modulated by dynamic changes in peristenotic smooth muscle tone (dynamic stenoses) or by microvascular dysfunction. Microvascular angina (*B*) is caused by coronary microvascular dysfunction. Unstable angina (*C*) is caused by a variable combination of thrombosis, dynamic stenoses, occlusive spasm, and microvascular dysfunction occurring not only in the presence of flow-limiting coronary artery stenoses, but also in their absence. Variant angina (*D*) is caused by occlusive epicardial coronary artery spasm, which may occur not only at the site of flow-limiting stenoses of variable severity but also in angiographically normal segments. (From Maseri, A.: Ischemic Heart Disease. New York, Churchill Livingstone, 1995, pp. 454–455.)

States have a history of CAD, and the estimated cost for the treatment of heart disease is $56 billion annually. The direct and indirect costs have been estimated at $14 billion per year. Given the current magnitude of the problem and the increasing prevalence of CAD which is anticipated because of the aging of the population, the recognition, management, and prevention of CAD are of major public health importance.[2] However, in the past three decades, encouraging reductions in the consequences of CAD have been noted (see p. 1126).[4] For example, between 1961 and 1991, the age-adjusted death rate for CAD declined by 52 per cent, more so in men than in women.[1] Similar trends have been observed in many industrialized nations with different health care systems. Multiple causes may have contributed to this favorable trend. These include the impact of reduction of risk factors (Chap. 35), improvements in socioeconomic circumstances including enhanced access to care, and new methods of diagnosis and treatment.

There is no uniform presenting syndrome for CAD. Chest discomfort is usually the predominant symptom in chronic (stable) angina (see p. 1291), unstable angina (p. 1334), Prinzmetal's (variant) angina (p. 1340), microvascular angina (p. 1343) (Fig. 38–1), and acute myocardial infarction (p. 1198). However, syndromes of CAD also occur in which ischemic chest discomfort is absent or not prominent. These include asymptomatic (silent) myocardial ischemia (p. 1344), congestive heart failure, cardiac arrhythmias, and sudden death (p. 747). There are also nonatherosclerotic causes of obstructive CAD[6] (p. 1349). Myocardial ischemia may also occur in the *absence* of obstructive CAD, as in the case of aortic valve disease, hypertrophic cardiomyopathy, idiopathic dilated cardiomyopathy, and luetic aortitis. Moreover, CAD may coexist with these other forms of heart disease. It may also be present in patients with noncardiac disease, e.g., esophageal disorders (p. 1291), confusing the differential diagnosis of chest discomfort.

STABLE ANGINA PECTORIS

CLINICAL MANIFESTATIONS

CHARACTERISTICS OF ANGINA (see also p. 4). Angina pectoris is a discomfort in the chest or adjacent areas caused by myocardial ischemia brought on by exertion and associated with a disturbance of myocardial function but without myocardial necrosis.[7] Heberden's initial description of the chest discomfort as conveying a sense of "strangling and anxiety" is still remarkably pertinent, although adjectives frequently used to describe this distress include "vise-like," "constricting," "suffocating," "crushing," "heavy," and "squeezing." In other patients, the quality of the sensation is more vague and is described as a mild pressure-like discomfort or an uncomfortable numb sensation. The site of the discomfort is usually retrosternal, but radiation is common and usually occurs down the ulnar surface of the left arm; the right arm and the outer surfaces of both arms may also be involved[7–9] (Fig. 1-1, p. 6). Anginal discomfort above the mandible or below the epigastrium is rare. Anginal "equivalents" (i.e., symptoms of myocardial ischemia other than angina), such as dyspnea, faintness, fatigue, and eructations, are common, particularly in the elderly. A history of abnormal exertional dyspnea may be an early indicator of CAD even when angina is absent or when there is no electrocardiographic evidence of ischemic heart disease.[10] Dyspnea at rest or with exertion may be a manifestation of very severe ischemia leading to elevation of the left ventricular filling pressure.

A careful clinical history is the key to the correct diagnosis and is particularly important in this era of cost-conscious practice of medicine, when it may obviate the need for more expensive testing. If the quality of the pain, its duration, precipitating factors, and associated symptoms are taken into consideration, it is usually possible to arrive at a correct diagnosis (Table 1–3, p. 5). The typical episode of angina pectoris usually begins gradually and reaches its maximum intensity over a period of minutes before dissipating. It is unusual for angina pectoris to reach its maximum severity within seconds, and it is characteristic that patients with angina usually prefer to rest, sit, or stop walking during episodes.[7]

Typical angina pectoris is relieved within minutes by rest or by the use of nitroglycerin. The response to the latter is often a useful diagnostic tool, although it should be remembered that esophageal pain and other syndromes may also respond to nitroglycerin.[11] A delay of more than 5 to 10 minutes before relief is obtained suggests that the symptoms are either not due to ischemia or, alternatively, due to severe ischemia. The phenomenon of "first effort" or "warm-up" angina is used to describe the ability of some patients who develop angina with exertion to subsequently continue at the same level of exertion without symptoms after an intervening period of rest. It has been postulated that this may be due to ischemic preconditioning.[12]

The fact that the anginal discomfort varies considerably among patients and that other entities can mimic it often makes the differential diagnosis of chest pain difficult.[7,8,13] (Table 1–1, p. 3). Characteristics that are *not* suggestive of angina are fleeting, momentary chest pains described as "needle jabs" or "sticking pains," discomfort that is aggravated or precipitated by breathing or by a single movement of the trunk or arm, pain that is relieved within a few seconds of lying horizontally, discomfort relieved within a few seconds by one or two swallows of food or water and that is localized to a very small area (e.g., an area the size of the tip of a finger). Pain that is associated with or reproduced by pressure on the chest wall is unlikely to be angina pectoris, as is the syndrome of constant, aching pain that is present for hours at a time. In general, anginal discomfort does not last for more than 30 minutes unless the patient is having a myocardial infarction or an arrhythmia.

MECHANISM. The mechanisms of cardiac pain and the neural pathways remain poorly understood.[14] It is presumed that the discomfort arises from sensory endplates of the intracardiac sympathetic nerves. The afferent fibers traverse the nerves that connect to the upper five thoracic sympathetic ganglia and upper five distal thoracic roots of the spinal cord. Impulses are transmitted by the spinal cord to the thalamus and hence to the neocortex. Within the spinal cord, cardiac sympathetic afferent impulses may converge with impulses from somatic thoracic structures, which may provide a basis for referred cardiac pain (e.g., to the chest).[15] The contribution of vagal afferents to ischemic pain is unclear. Using positron emission tomography to examine changes in regional cerebral blood flow associated with angina pectoris, it was proposed that cortical activation is necessary for the sensation of pain, but that the thalamus may act as a gate to afferent pain signals.[16]

Triggers. The specific substances or triggers that stimulate the sensory nerve endings and begin the series of interactions that culminate in chest discomfort have not been identified. Attention has been paid to a variety of substances, including peptides that are released from cells as a result of transient ischemia, such as adenosine, bradykinin, histamine, and serotonin.[17] In one study, adenosine administered intravenously reproduced the symptom in over 90 per cent of patients with angina. Another hypothesis has suggested that mechanical stretching of a coronary artery may be the cause of pain.[17] Thus, the link between ischemic events at a tissue level and the perception of pain remains a subject of investigation.[17]

Differential Diagnosis of Chest Pain

(see Table 1–2, p. 3 and Fig. 1–2, p. 6)

The differentiation of various disorders from CAD is challenging because the severity of the chest pain and the seriousness of the underlying disorder are not necessarily related. Compounding the difficulty in differential diagnosis is the common myth that pain in the left arm or left side of the chest is an ominous sign signifying the presence of CAD. However, a host of disorders can cause discomfort in these locations.

ESOPHAGEAL DISORDERS. The common painful esophageal disorders that may simulate or coexist with angina pectoris are gastroesophageal reflux and disorders of esophageal motility, including diffuse spasm as well as "nutcracker" esophagus characterized by high-amplitude peristaltic contractions and vigorous achalasia.[19] Symptomatic esophageal reflux is common and is estimated to occur in 7 to 14 per cent of an otherwise "healthy" United States population. The typical characteristics of esophageal and cardiac pain are shown in Table 38–1. The classic presentation of esophageal pain is "heartburn," particularly in relationship to changes in posture and meals and in association with dysphagia. Esophageal spasm also may cause constant retrosternal discomfort of uniform intensity or severe spasmodic pain during or after swallowing.

There is no simple way to diagnose esophageal disease as the cause of chest pain, and the predictive value of each of the standard tests is poor. In one series of 200 patients with esophageal pain, heartburn was the presenting feature in 85 per cent, 21 per cent described pain radiating to the arms, and 5 per cent to the fingers, and 22 per cent experienced pain initiated by exertion.[20] To further compound the difficulty in distinguishing between angina and esophageal pain, both may be relieved by nitroglycerin.[21] However, esophageal pain is often relieved by milk, antacids, foods, or occasionally warm liquids.

GASTROESOPHAGEAL REFLUX. The esophageal acid perfusion, or Bernstein test, may be helpful in its use of alternate infusions of dilute acid and normal saline by a nasal gastric catheter, placing the tip at the level of the midesophagus.[22] Infusion of acid produces pain in over 90 per cent of patients with subjective and objective evidence of gastroesophageal acid reflux, but it is particularly useful if the patient's symptoms are reproduced.[23] Acid reflux into the esophagus can also be recognized by recording the pH from an electrode at the tip of a catheter inserted into the distal esophagus.

ESOPHAGEAL MOTILITY DISORDERS. These are not uncommon in patients with retrosternal chest pain of unclear cause and should be specifically excluded or confirmed, if possible. In addition to chest pain, the majority of such patients have dysphagia. Although barium studies may reveal motility problems, esophageal manometry may show diffuse esophageal spasm, increased pressure at the lower esophageal sphincter, and other motility disorders. Provocative pharmacological agents such as methacholine may provoke esophageal pain and manometric signs of spasm. Surgical or medical therapy of esophageal reflux improves symptoms in patients whose chest pain coincides with documented episodes of reflux.[24]

CHEST PAIN AND NORMAL CORONARY ARTERIES. It is important to distinguish between chest pain due to esophageal disease and chest pain secondary to ischemia with normal coronary arteries. This condition, also known as *syndrome X,* is discussed later in this chapter (see p. 1343). The incidence of esophageal disease is substantial among patients with nonischemic chest pain and normal coronary arteries. In one study of patients with "angina-like pain" believed to be noncardiac in origin (most of whom had undergone coronary angiography), the combination of esophageal motility and distal esophageal pH monitoring showed evidence of symptomatic esophageal disease in 24 per cent.[25] A more complex problem is determining if part or all of the symptoms in patients with *known* CAD is due to esophageal disease. Both CAD and esophageal disease are common clinical entities that may coexist. A diagnostic evaluation for an esophageal disorder may be indicated in patients with CAD who have a poor symptomatic response to antianginal therapy in the absence of documentation of severe ischemia or in patients with persistent symptoms despite adequate coronary revascularization.

BILIARY COLIC. This symptom is sometimes confused with angina pectoris. It is usually caused by a rapid rise in biliary pressure due to obstruction of the cystic or bile duct. The pain is steady, usually lasts 2 to 4 hours, and subsides spontaneously without any symptoms between attacks. It is generally most intense in the right upper abdomen but may also be felt in the epigastrium or precordium. This discomfort is often referred to the scapula, may radiate around the costal margin to the back, or rarely may be felt in the shoulder, suggesting diaphragmatic irritation. Although nausea and vomiting are common, the relationship of the pain to meals is variable. Although a history of dyspepsia, flatulence, fatty food intolerance, and indigestion may be associated with cholelithiasis, these symptoms are also commonly experienced by the general population. Ultrasonography is accurate in diagnosing gallstones and allows determination of gallbladder size, thickness, and whether or not the bile ducts are dilated. Failure to opacify the gallbladder on oral cholecystography may indicate nonfunction due to disease.

COSTOSTERNAL SYNDROME. In 1921, Tietze first described a syndrome of local pain and tenderness, usually limited to the anterior chest wall, associated with swelling of the costal cartilages. This condition causes pain that can resemble angina pectoris. The full-blown Tietze syndrome, i.e., pain associated with tender swelling of the costochondral junctions, is uncommon, whereas costochondritis causing tenderness of the costochondral junctions (without swelling) is relatively common.[26] Pain on palpation of these joints is a useful clinical sign. Local pressure should be applied routinely to the anterior chest wall during the examination of the patient. Treatment of costochondritis usually consists of reassurance and anti-inflammatory agents.

CERVICAL RADICULITIS. This may occur as a constant ache, sometimes resulting in a sensory deficit. The pain may be related to motion of the neck, just as motion of the shoulder triggers attacks of pain due to bursitis. A hyperalgesic area of skin, noted by running the finger down the back and exerting pressure, may lead to the suspicion of thoracic root pain. Occasionally, pain mimicking angina can be due to compression of the brachial plexus via cervical ribs. Physical examination may also detect pain brought about by movement of an arthritic shoulder, a calcified shoulder tendon, and the like. The musculoskeletal disorders that can mimic angina include subacromial bursitis and costochondritis.

OTHER CAUSES OF ANGINA-LIKE PAIN. *Acute myocardial infarction* is usually associated with prolonged (>30 min-

TABLE 38–1 SIMILARITIES AND DIFFERENCES BETWEEN ESOPHAGEAL AND CARDIAC PAIN

	SIMILARITIES OF CARDIAC AND ESOPHAGEAL PAIN	DISTINGUISHING FEATURES OF ESOPHAGEAL PAIN
Location	Mid or lower retrosternal. May be a severe epigastric pain with radiation up to neck.	High epigastric, behind xiphoid process or in low retrosternal area.
Nature	Heaviness, squeezing, tightness, or burning. Can be associated with weakness, diaphoresis, and anxiety.	Often burning or perceived as spasm. Heartburn is frequent association. Can be associated with increased salivation. Dysphagia occurs.
Radiation	Upward toward throat. May radiate to left neck, shoulder, or arm.	Tends to ascend but not radiate to left side. Radiation to both shoulders and/or arms is less frequent. When pain begins in lower retrosternal area it often radiates down to epigastrium.
Precipitants	After eating. Angina is more likely with physical activity after eating.	After eating certain foods—alcohol, coffee, spices. Less likely to be brought on by exertion. Can be precipitated by change in posture, e.g., by lying down.
Duration	Can last a short duration (2 to 10 min).	May last hours; may wax and wane.
Relieving factors	May be relieved or released by nitroglycerin, standing, and relaxing.	

Modified from Miller, A. J.: Diagnosis of Chest Pain. New York, Raven Press, 1988, pp. 74–76.

utes), severe pain that, apart from duration and intensity, may be similar to angina pectoris (see p. 1198). It is associated with characteristic electrocardiographic and enzyme findings.

Severe pulmonary hypertension may be associated with exertional chest pain with the characteristics of angina pectoris, and, indeed, this pain is thought to be due to right ventricular ischemia which develops during exertion (see p. 788). Other associated symptoms include exertional dyspnea, dizziness, and syncope. Associated findings on physical examination, such as a parasternal lift, palpable and loud pulmonary component of the second sound, and right ventricular hypertrophy on the electrocardiogram usually are readily recognized.

Pulmonary embolism presents with dyspnea as the cardinal symptom, but chest pain may be associated (see p. 1587). Pleuritic pain suggests pulmonary infarction, and a history of exacerbation of the pain with inspiration, along with a pleural friction rub, usually helps to distinguish it from angina pectoris.

The pain of *acute pericarditis* (see p. 1481) at times may be difficult to distinguish from angina pectoris. However, pericarditis tends to occur in younger patients than does angina, and the diagnosis depends on chest pain, a pericardial friction rub, and electrocardiographic changes. The chest pain usually is sudden in onset, severe and persistent and is intensified by coughing, swallowing, and inspiration. Relief may be obtained by sitting up and leaning forward; palpation of the trapezius ridge often causes discomfort. A pericardial friction rub can be detected in most patients if listened for carefully, at different times, and with the patient in different positions. Early, widespread ST-segment elevations may be present. Some patients with pericardial disease describe a vague retrosternal discomfort without the characteristics of pleuropericarditis, but a relationship to exertion is not present. Pain due to hepatic congestion may complicate the clinical history.

In many of the disorders just mentioned, angina pectoris can usually be excluded by a careful history and physical examination. It must be emphasized, however, that chronic CAD can and frequently does coexist with any of these other disorders and that noncardiac disease can trigger a true angina attack in a patient with CAD. For example, among patients with severe, disabling angina, obstructive sleep apnea may be a common precipitant of nocturnal angina, which may respond dramatically to the initiation of continuous positive airway pressure.[27]

Physical Examination

GENERAL EXAMINATION. The physical examination has often been considered relatively unhelpful in patients with chronic CAD and stable angina, and, indeed, it is often entirely normal. Nonetheless, a diligently performed physical examination can provide useful clues to the diagnosis and in the identification of patients with risk factors for CAD. The value of the examination is enhanced when performed during and soon after an episode of angina pectoris. Not only should the examination be directed at the cardiovascular system, but particular attention should be directed to the presence of comorbid conditions that exert a major impact on prognosis and on the risks and expectations of coronary revascularization procedures.

Inspection of the eyes may reveal a *corneal arcus,* and examination of the skin may show xanthomas (Fig. 2–2, p. 17). The size of the corneal arcus appears to correlate positively with age and levels of cholesterol and low-density lipoproteins.[28] *Xanthelasma,* in which lipid deposits are intracellular, appear to be promoted by increased levels of triglycerides and a relative deficiency of high-density lipoproteins. In the Lipid Research Clinic study,[29] the incidence of both xanthelasma and corneal arcus increased with age and was highest in patients with type II hyperlipoproteinemia and usually low in those with the type IV phenotype. Retinal arteriolar changes (see p. 15) are common in patients with CAD and diabetes mellitus or hypertension.

There appears to be some correlation between CAD and *diagonal earlobe crease* (except in native American Indians and Asians). There is often a unilateral diagonal earlobe crease in younger persons with CAD that becomes bilateral with advancing age.[30]

The *blood pressure* may be chronically elevated or may rise acutely (along with heart rate) during an angina attack. Changes in blood pressure may precede (and precipitate) or follow (and be caused by) angina.

Other important features of the general physical examination are abnormalities of the arterial pulses and of the venous system. The association between peripheral vascular disease and CAD is strong and well documented.[31,32] This is not confined to patients with symptomatic or clinically overt peripheral vascular or carotid artery disease but is seen also in asymptomatic subjects with a reduced ankle-brachial blood pressure index or evidence of early carotid disease on ultrasonography.[33] The presence of carotid and peripheral arterial disease on palpation and auscultation increases the likelihood that chest discomfort of unclear origin is caused by CAD. Evaluation of the patient's venous system, particularly in the legs, may have an important bearing on the type of grafting procedure employed in subsequent coronary bypass surgery.

CARDIAC EXAMINATION. The presence of murmurs of hypertrophic cardiomyopathy or aortic valve disease suggests that angina may be due to conditions other than (or in addition to) CAD. It is often helpful to examine the heart *during* an episode of pain because ischemia may produce transient left ventricular dysfunction with a third heart sound and pulmonary rales detectable on physical examination. A softening of the mitral component of the first heart sound due to ischemic left ventricular dysfunction may also be demonstrated during angina. Paradoxical splitting of the second heart sound (see p. 33) may occur transiently during an angina attack and appears to be related to asynergy and prolongation of left ventricular contraction, resulting in delayed closure of the aortic valve. If other obvious cardiac diseases are absent, a third or loud fourth heart sound suggests ischemia as the basis for the chest pain. These sounds are common in patients with angina at rest, and their frequency is increased during handgrip exercise[34] even if the latter does not precipitate angina pectoris. A sustained apical cardiac impulse is common in patients with moderate or severe left ventricular dysfunction.

When patients with CAD lie in the left lateral recumbent position, dyskinetic bulges at the apex may be palpable. These bulges correspond to dyskinetic areas and often complement the auscultatory findings of diastolic filling sounds.[35,36] Transient apical systolic murmurs are quite common in CAD and have been attributed to reversible papillary muscle dysfunction secondary to transient myocardial ischemia. When persistent, such murmurs may be due to papillary muscle fibrosis, often a manifestation of subendocardial infarction or a regional wall motion abnormality altering the alignment of the papillary muscles in relation to other components of the mitral valve apparatus. These murmurs are more prevalent in patients with extensive CAD, especially those with prior myocardial infarction and left ventricular dysfunction. The systolic murmurs may assume a variety of configurations (early, late, or holosystolic) and may be accentuated by exertion or during angina. A midsystolic click, often followed by a late systolic murmur produced by mitral valve prolapse (see p. 1032), also occurs in patients with CAD. A diastolic murmur or a continuous murmur is a rare finding in CAD and has been attributed to turbulent flow across a proximal coronary artery stenosis.[37]

PATHOPHYSIOLOGY

Angina pectoris results from myocardial ischemia, which is caused by an imbalance between myocardial oxygen requirements (MVO_2) and oxygen supply.[37a] The former may be elevated by increases in heart rate, left ventricular wall stress, and contractility (see p. 1161); the latter is determined by coronary blood flow and the coronary arterial oxygen content (Figs. 38–1 and 38–2).

ANGINA DUE TO INCREASED MYOCARDIAL OXYGEN DEMAND. In this condition, sometimes termed "demand angina," MVO_2 increases in the face of a constant oxygen supply. The increased MVO_2 commonly stems from norepinephrine release by adrenergic nerve endings, a physiological response to exertion, emotion, or mental stress. Of great importance to MVO_2 is the *rate* at which any task is carried out. Hurrying is particularly likely to precipitate angina, as are efforts involving motion of the hands over the head. The effects of emotion on the ratio of oxygen supply and demand are complex. Mental stress may increase adrenergic tone, reduce vagal activity, and increase blood pressure.[38] Anger may produce constriction in coronary arteries with preexisting narrowing without necessarily affecting oxygen demand.[39] Other factors causing angina due to an increase in MVO_2 in patients with obstructive CAD include exercise after eating and the excessive metabolic demands imposed by chills, fever, thyrotoxicosis, tachycardia from any cause, and hypoglycemia. Among patients with stable, fixed obstructive CAD, several studies using ambulatory electrocardiographic monitoring have documented the importance of increases in MVO_2 and, in particular, heart rate as a precipitant of ischemia. In these patients, in contrast to those with unstable angina (see p. 1331), ischemic episodes are preceded by significant increases in heart rate, and the likelihood of developing ischemia is proportional to both the magnitude and the duration of the heart rate increase.[11,40]

In all of these conditions, underlying fixed coronary artery obstruction is usually present, and the other factors (e.g., exertion, emotion, or fever) precipitate ischemia and chest discomfort by stimulating myocardial oxygen needs in the presence of a fixed and limited myocardial oxygen supply.

ANGINA DUE TO TRANSIENT DECREASED OXYGEN SUPPLY. There is increasing evidence that not only unstable angina but chronic stable angina may also be caused by transient reductions of oxygen supply as a consequence of coronary vasoconstriction,[1,41,42] a condition sometimes termed "supply angina." The coronary arterial bed is well innervated, and a variety of stimuli alter coronary tone (see p. 1163). Nonocclusive intracoronary thrombi are another cause of reduced oxygen supply and myocardial ischemia, usually causing angina at rest (unstable angina, p. 1331) rather than chronic stable angina.

Patients with angina precipitated by a transient reduction in myocardial oxygen supply comprise a spectrum based upon the severity of the underlying fixed defect and the degree of the dynamic change in coronary arterial tone. In the typical patient with stable angina, the degree of fixed obstruction is sufficient to result in an inadequate coronary flow rate to cope with the increased oxygen demands of exercise. However, superimposed upon this, episodes of transient coronary vasoconstriction may cause additional limitations to coronary flow reserve in many patients.[43]

In rare patients without organic obstructing lesions, severe dynamic obstruction alone can cause myocardial ischemia and resultant angina (Prinzmetal's angina, p. 1340). On the other hand, in patients with severe fixed obstruction to coronary flow, only a minor increase in dynamic obstruction is necessary for blood flow to fall below a critical level and cause myocardial ischemia (Fig. 38–3).

FIXED COMPARED WITH VARIABLE-THRESHOLD ANGINA. The variability of the threshold for angina differs widely among patients with chronic angina. In patients with fixed-threshold angina precipitated by increased oxygen demands, with few if any dynamic (vasoconstrictor) components, the level of physical activity required to precipitate angina is relatively constant. Characteristically, these patients can predict the amount of physical activity that will precipitate angina, e.g., walking up exactly two flights of stairs at a customary pace. When these patients are tested on a treadmill or bicycle, the pressure-rate product that elicits angina and/or electrocardiographic evidence of ischemia is constant or almost so.

Changes in the blood pressure–heart rate product (the double product) provide an approximation of alterations of myocardial oxygen requirements. In patients with fixed-threshold, demand angina,

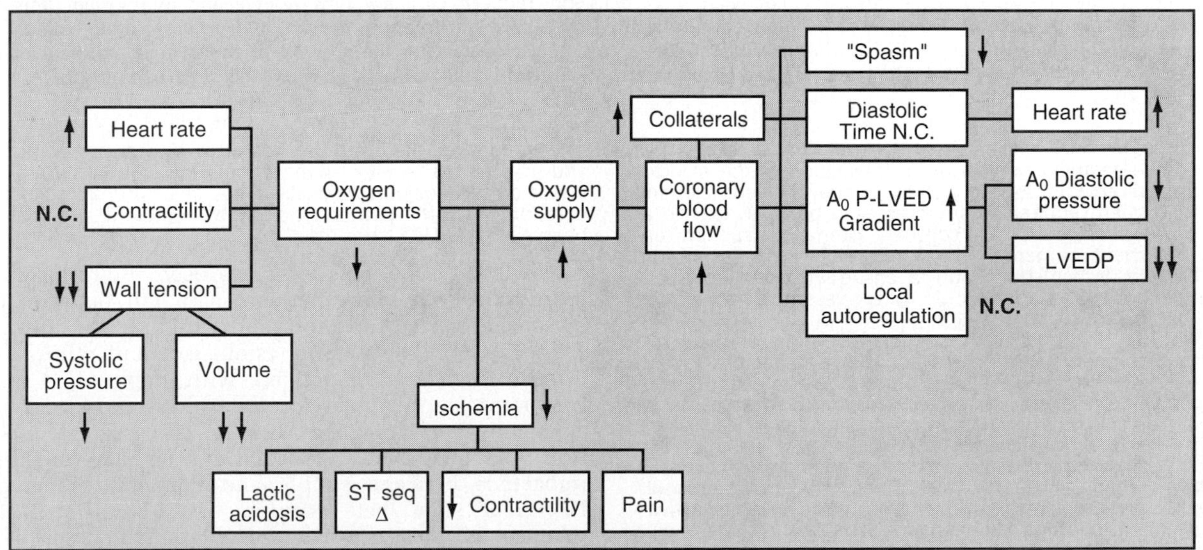

FIGURE 38–2. Factors influencing balance between myocardial oxygen requirements *(left)* and supply *(right)*. Arrows indicate effects of nitrates. In relieving angina pectoris, nitrates exert favorable effects by reducing oxygen requirements and increasing supply. Although a reflex increase in heart rate would tend to reduce the time for coronary flow, dilation of collaterals and enhancement of the pressure gradient for flow to occur as the LVEDP falls tend to increase coronary flow. A_0P = aortic pressure; LVEDP = left ventricular end-diastolic pressure; NC = no change. (From Frishman, W. H.: Pharmacology of the nitrates in angina pectoris. Am. J. Cardiol. *56*:81, 1985.)

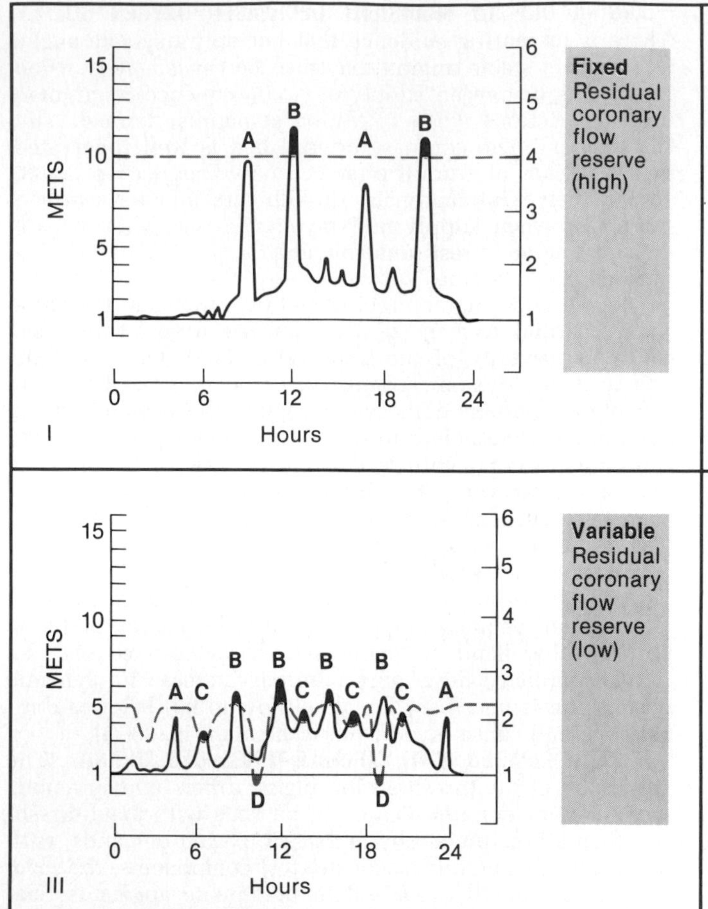

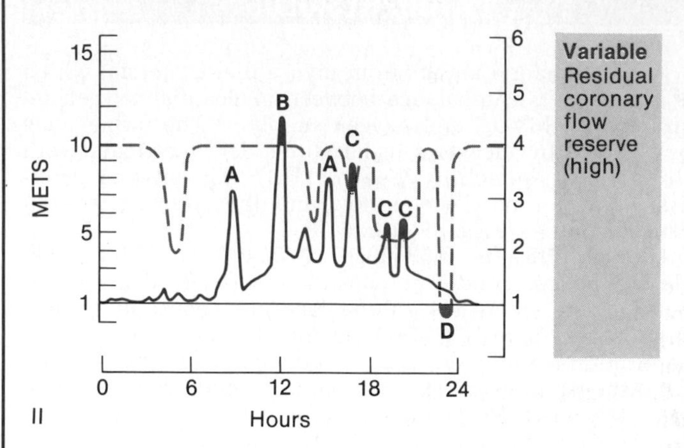

FIGURE 38–3. Schematic illustration of the relation between physical activity (during 24 hours) expressed as METS (multiple of basal metabolic oxygen consumption) and coronary flow reserve. Normally, during resting conditions, coronary flow reserve exactly matches the metabolic demand. However, when metabolic demands increase to a maximum of 16 METS, coronary flow reserve increases up to six times the resting value to match the increased demand for flow by the myocardium so that no ischemia occurs.

I. In this situation, a patient has a moderately severe fixed coronary artery obstruction that reduces coronary flow reserve to four times the resting value. *A,* The patient can exercise up to approximately 10 METS without developing ischemia; *B,* however, exercise above approximately 10 METS triggers ischemia.

II. In this situation, the patient has a moderately severe stenosis that fixes the coronary reserve at four times resting levels as in I. In addition, there is a variable stenosis. Therefore, residual coronary flow reserve has an upper limit that is fixed but that can decrease because of the presence of the mechanisms that transiently interfere with coronary blood flow. Thus, the residual coronary flow reserve can vary throughout the day. Under these conditions, if the patient exercises beyond the maximal residual coronary flow reserve, ischemia will always develop (*B*). However, the patient may also develop ischemia on other occasions after smaller degrees of exercise, when residual coronary flow reserve is decreased by these functional factors (*C*). Occasionally, coronary flow reserve decreases so that resting flow is impaired and ischemia occurs at rest (*D*). At other times of the day, this patient can exercise below the level of his maximal residual coronary flow reserve without experiencing ischemia (*A*).

III. In this situation, the patient has a very severe fixed stenosis and also variable stenosis. Maximal residual coronary flow reserve is reduced to little more than two times the resting value of coronary flow, thus allowing the patient to exercise up to a level of about 5 METS in the absence of any transient impairment of coronary flow. The combination of markedly reduced coronary flow reserve and of transient impairment of coronary flow results in frequent occurrences of ischemic episodes caused by excessive increase of demand above the maximal residual coronary flow (*B*) or by transient impairment of flow during exertion (*C*) or at rest (*D*). However, in the absence of transient impairment of flow, the patient can tolerate activities below 5 METS (*A*). (Modified from Maseri, A., Chierchia, S., and Kaski, J. C.: Mixed angina pectoris. Am. J. Cardiol., *56:*31E and 32E, 1985.)

the specific threshold at which ischemia develops (as reflected in angina and/or ST-segment depression) is a function of the myocardial oxygen requirements. As the activity of the left ventricle (and therefore its oxygen requirements) increases, a point is reached at which perfusion distal to a critical coronary arterial obstruction cannot supply sufficient oxygen to the myocardium perfused by the obstructed artery; ischemia and angina ensue. This relationship is, however, modified by the effects of coronary vasomotor tone upon myocardial oxygen supply (Fig. 38–3).[44]

The majority of patients with variable-threshold angina have atherosclerotic coronary arterial narrowing, but dynamic obstruction caused by vasoconstriction plays an important role in causing myocardial ischemia.[45] These patients typically have "good days," when they are capable of substantial physical activity, and "bad days," when even minimal activity can cause clinical and/or electrocardiographic evidence of myocardial ischemia or when angina occurs even at rest. Often, even in the course of a single day, they may be capable of substantial physical activity at one time, while minimal activity results in angina at another. Patients with variable-threshold angina often complain of a circadian variation of angina which is more common in the morning. Angina on exertion and sometimes even at rest may be precipitated by cold temperatures,[46,47] emotion, and mental stress. A cold environment has been shown to increase peripheral resistance, both at rest and during exercise.[48–51] The rise in arterial pressure, by augmenting myocardial oxygen requirements, lowers the threshold for the development of angina. An alternative or additional explanation is the development of cold-induced coronary vasoconstriction.

Worsening of exercise tolerance after a meal is well documented and may be the result of a more rapid increase in $M\dot{V}O_2$ when exercise is carried out postprandially. A dynamic coronary vasoconstrictor component to the pathophysiology of postprandial angina has also been suggested.[58]

MIXED ANGINA. This term has been proposed by Maseri to describe the many patients who fall between the two extremes of fixed-threshold and variable-threshold angina[53] (Fig. 38–3II). The pathophysiological and clinical correlations of ischemia in patients with stable CAD may have important implications for the selection of anti-ischemic agents, as well as for their timing. The greater the contribution from increased myocardial oxygen requirements to the imbalance between supply and demand, the greater the likelihood that beta-blocking agents will be effective, whereas nitrates and calcium channel blocking agents, at least on theoretical grounds, are likely to be especially effective in episodes due primarily to vasoconstriction. The finding that in most patients with chronic stable angina an increase in $M\dot{V}O_2$ precedes episodes of ischemia, i.e., that they have demand angina, argues in favor of beta-blockers as essential therapeutic agents.[54]

GRADING OF ANGINA PECTORIS. A system of grading the

severity of angina pectoris proposed by the Canadian Cardiovascular Society has gained widespread acceptance.[55] The system is a modification of the New York Heart Association functional classification but allows patients to be categorized in more specific terms. Other grading systems include the specific activity scale developed by Goldman[56] and an anginal "score" developed by Califf et al.[57] The latter integrates the clinical features and "tempo" of angina together with electrocardiographic ST- and T-wave changes and offers independent prognostic information above that provided by age, gender, left ventricular function, and the coronary angiographic anatomy. A limitation of all of these grading systems is their dependence on accurate patient observation and patients' widely varying tolerance for symptoms.[58]

CORRELATION BETWEEN HISTORICAL FEATURES AND CORONARY ANGIOGRAPHY. Diamond and Forrester estimated the presence of angiographic CAD to be 90 per cent, 50 per cent, and 15 per cent, respectively, in middle-aged adults with histories of typical angina, atypical angina, or nonanginal chest pain, respectively, but only 3 to 4 per cent among asymptomatic middle-aged adults.[59] Although the clinical manifestations of CAD, including rest angina and nocturnal and postprandial angina, tend to be more severe among patients with multivessel than with single-vessel disease, neither the severity, duration, nature of the pain, nor its precipitating factors correlate with the extent of disease at angiography. Perhaps the most striking example of the lack of historical-arteriographic correlations is in two subgroups of patients—those with advanced obstructive CAD who are asymptomatic with "silent ischemia" (see p. 1344) and those with Prinzmetal's or variant angina who may have episodes of very severe anginal discomfort, yet with minimal or no underlying coronary atherosclerosis (see p. 1341).

The presentation of CAD and angina differs in men and women. These differences are discussed in Chap. 51.

NONINVASIVE TESTING

Resting Electrocardiogram

This is normal in approximately one-half of patients with chronic stable angina pectoris (Chap. 4). Patients with normal tracings at rest may have severe angina, but they usually have not previously suffered extensive infarction. The most common electrocardiographic abnormalities are nonspecific ST-T changes with or without evidence of prior transmural infarction. There are numerous pitfalls in the use of the *resting* electrocardiogram in the diagnosis of myocardial ischemia. ST-T wave abnormalities are common in the general population, with an overall prevalence of 8.5 per cent for men and 7.7 per cent for women in the Framingham Heart Study.[60] The prevalence increases with increasing age and in subjects with hypertension or diabetes mellitus, in cigarette smokers, and in women.[61] In addition to myocardial ischemia, other conditions that can produce ST-T wave abnormalities include left ventricular hypertrophy and dilatation, electrolyte abnormalities, neurogenic effects, and antiarrhythmic drugs.[61] In patients with CAD, however, the occurrence of ST-T wave abnormalities in the resting electrocardiogram may correlate with the severity of the underlying heart disease, including the number of vessels involved and the presence of left ventricular dysfunction.[62] This may explain the adverse impact of ST-T wave changes upon prognosis in these patients. In contrast, a normal resting electrocardiogram is a more favorable long-term prognostic sign in patients with suspected or definite CAD.[63] However, both the sensitivity and specificity of such electrocardiographic changes in patients with chronic stable angina are low.

A variety of conduction disturbances, most frequently left bundle branch block and left anterior fascicular block, occur in patients with chronic stable angina, and they are often associated with marked impairment in left ventricular function,[64] reflecting multivessel disease and previous myocardial damage. In patients with chronic stable angina, abnormal Q waves are relatively specific but insensitive indicators of prior myocardial infarction. A variety of arrhythmias, especially ventricular premature beats, may be present on the electrocardiogram, but they too have low sensitivity and specificity for CAD.

Interval electrocardiograms may reveal the development of Q-wave infarctions that have gone unrecognized clinically. The increasing use of ambulatory electrocardiographic monitoring has shown that many patients with symptomatic myocardial ischemia also have episodes of silent ischemia that would otherwise go unrecognized during normal daily activities (see p. 1344).

Left ventricular hypertrophy on the electrocardiogram in patients with chronic stable angina should suggest the presence of underlying hypertension, aortic stenosis, or hypertrophic obstructive cardiomyopathy. This finding is a poor prognostic factor in patients with angina.[65]

Noninvasive Stress Testing

Noninvasive stress testing can provide useful and often indispensable information required to establish the diagnosis and estimate the prognosis in patients with chronic stable angina.[65] However, several studies have emphasized that the indiscriminate use of such tests may provide limited *incremental* information provided by noninvasive testing in patients with stable CAD, over and above that provided by the physicians' detailed and thoughtful clinical assessment.[66–69b] The appropriate application of noninvasive tests requires consideration of Bayesian principles (Fig. 5–11, p. 162). These state that the reliability of any test is defined by its sensitivity and specificity, and its predictive accuracy depends upon the prevalence of disease in the population under study. In an era of emphasis on cost-effectiveness, optimal utilization requires an assessment of the *incremental* amount of information provided by a test, over and above that which can be obtained from the standard clinical variables alone (Chap. 53).

Prior to undertaking noninvasive testing, it is appropriate to ask the question: What will be the response to the test if it is positive or if it is negative? If the answer is the same, the need for the test should be reconsidered.

Exercise Electrocardiography

(See also Chap. 5)

DIAGNOSIS OF CORONARY ARTERY DISEASE. As a screening test for CAD, the exercise electrocardiogram is useful in that it is relatively simple and inexpensive. It is particularly helpful in patients with chest pain syndromes who are considered to have moderate probability of CAD, and in whom the resting electrocardiogram is normal, provided that they are capable of achieving an adequate workload.[69a,70] Although the incremental value of exercise testing in diagnosing CAD is limited to patients in whom the estimated prevalence of CAD is either high or low, the test provides useful, additional information about the severity of ischemia, and the degree of functional limitation as well as the prognosis.[66,69a,71,72]

Certain symptomatic, electrocardiographic, and hemodynamic responses to treadmill exercise testing suggest the presence of significant obstruction in one or more coronary arteries. The most useful exercise electrocardiographic variable for the detection of CAD, and in particular multivessel disease, is the ST-segment shift during exercise and recovery (see p. 157).[73] The predictive value for the detection of CAD is 90 per cent, if typical chest discomfort occurs during exercise with ST horizontal or downward sloping depression of 1 mm or more. ST-segment depression of 2 mm or more accompanied by typical chest discomfort is virtually diagnostic of significant CAD.[72,73] In the absence of typical angina pectoris, downsloping or horizontal ST-segment depression of 1 mm or more has a predictive value of 70 per cent for the detection of significant coronary stenosis, but this increases to 90 per cent with ST-segment depression of 2 mm or more. The early onset of ST-segment depression during exercise, its long persistence following discontinuation of exercise, a downsloping or horizontal depression, and a low work capacity or exercise duration are all strongly associated with multivessel disease. Exercise-induced QRS prolongation also appears to be a function of exercise-induced ischemia[74] and is related to the extent of exercise-induced segmental contraction abnormalities.

In view of the relatively low overall sensitivity (approximately 75 per cent) of exercise stress electrocardiography in CAD, a negative result does not exclude this diagnosis. However, the likelihood of three-vessel or left main disease is markedly reduced by a negative test.

A major limitation of the sensitivity of the end exercise electrocardiogram is that it cannot be interpreted in many patients. This includes patients who are incapable of reaching the level of exercise required for near maximal effort (85 per cent or more of maximal predicted heart rate), particularly those receiving beta-adrenergic blockers, or those who develop fatigue, leg cramps, or dyspnea, and patients with abnormalities in the baseline electrocardiogram including those taking digitalis. In these patients, noninvasive imaging with exercise or pharmacological stress testing or diagnostic coronary angiography may be indicated.

INFLUENCE OF ANTIANGINAL THERAPY. Antianginal pharmacological therapy reduces the sensitivity of exercise testing as a screening tool. Beta blockade increases the exercise duration and suppresses, diminishes, or delays the appearance of ST-segment depression and thus obscures the diagnostic interpretation of exercise testing.[75] Because beta blockade reduces the sensitivity of the test, a negative exercise test in patients receiving antianginal drugs does *not* exclude significant and possibly life-threatening myocardial ischemia. Therefore, if the purpose of the exercise test is to *diagnose* ischemia, it should be performed, if possible, in the absence of antianginal medications. The advisability of withdrawing medications in an individual patient before exercise testing is a matter of judgment. Two or 3 days are required for patients receiving long-acting beta blockers. Unless the patient has severe angina, sublingual nitroglycerin for 1 or 2 days is likely to be sufficient to control symptoms if other therapy is withdrawn. For long-acting nitrates, calcium antagonists, and short-acting beta blockers, discontinuing the medications the day before testing usually suffices. If the purpose of the exercise test is to identify safe levels of daily activity or the extent of functional disability, the test should be carried out while the patient is taking the usual medications.

Nuclear Cardiology Techniques

(See Chap. 9)

STRESS MYOCARDIAL PERFUSION IMAGING (see also p. 288). In this technique, the radionuclide is injected at peak exercise or at symptom-limited endpoints, such as angina pectoris or dyspnea; the patient is encouraged to exercise for another 30 to 45 seconds to ensure that the initial myocardial uptake of the tracer reflects a perfusion pattern at peak stress[76,77] and the images are obtained several minutes later when the patient is at rest. Important advances in the assessment of myocardial viability and ischemia include both 24-hour delayed redistribution imaging and rest thallium-201 reinjection protocols[78–80] as well as the use of technetium-99m (Tc-99m)–labeled perfusion agents (isonitriles).

Exercise thallium (or isonitrile) scintigraphy, simultaneous with electrocardiography, is superior to exercise electrocardiography alone in the detection of CAD, in the identification of multivessel disease, in localizing diseased vessels, and in the detection of myocardial viability in regions of abnormal wall motion with or without Q-waves,[81] both in patients with and without normal resting electrocardiograms.[82] The published results using visual analysis of exercise-redistribution images include more than 4000 patients with angiographic documentation of the presence or absence of coronary disease. In these studies, the sensitivity averaged 82 per cent and the specificity 88 per cent. In these same patients, conventional ECG exercise stress testing had a sensitivity ranging from 50 to 80 per cent.[83]

Stress myocardial scintigraphy is particularly helpful in the diagnosis of CAD in patients with abnormal resting electrocardiograms, such as those with left ventricular hypertrophy and strain and left bundle branch block. Among homogeneous populations of symptomatic patients, the magnitude of ST-segment depression on symptom-limited exercise testing correlates well with the extent of ischemia as assessed by quantitative thallium-201 scintigraphy. In *mixed* populations in which the proportion of false-positive ST-segment responses increases, greater reliance is placed upon thallium scintigraphy to assess the presence and magnitude of ischemia.[84] Thallium-201 scintigraphy provides important information in regard to prognosis (p. 274).[85–88]

Because stress myocardial scintigraphy is a relatively expensive test (three to four times the cost of an exercise electrocardiogram), certain issues should be considered: (1) a regular exercise electrocardiogram should always be obtained first in patients with chest pain and a normal resting electrocardiogram for screening and detection of CAD; (2) stress myocardial perfusion scintigraphy should *not* be used as a screening test in patients in whom the prevalence of coronary disease is low or moderate; (3) stress myocardial perfusion scintigraphy is more sensitive in detecting CAD, especially in patients with single-vessel coronary artery disease, than exercise electrocardiography.[89]

Pharmacological Nuclear Stress Testing (see also p. 289). For patients unable to exercise adequately, especially the elderly and patients with peripheral vascular disease and those limited by dyspnea, pharmacological stimulation with dipyridamole and adenosine prior to scintigraphic imaging may be employed.[90–95a] In a comparison of 2000 patients undergoing adenosine and dipyridamole pharmacological stress testing, adenosine was shown to cause a slightly greater degree of systemic vasodilation than dipyridamole. Although adverse effects occurred less often with dipyridamole than with adenosine, these were more difficult to manage and necessitated more monitoring time as well as the fairly frequent intravenous use of aminophylline for reversal.[90] In patients with asthma, dobutamine thallium scintigraphy is a useful and safe alternative to dipyridamole and adenosine.[92] A promising new pharmacological stress agent still under investigation is arbutamine, a sympathomimetic agent designed to simulate exercise, that is delivered via a closed-loop delivery device controlled by hemodynamic feedback. It is potentially superior to dobutamine, dipyridamole, and adenosine, but further studies are needed.[95b,95c]

EXERCISE RADIONUCLIDE ANGIOGRAPHY. The use of exercise radionuclide angiography in the detection and estimation of prognosis in CAD has fallen out of favor. Failure to increase the ejection fraction by 5 per cent or more was proposed as a diagnostic test for CAD.[77] However, this is a nonspecific finding that may occur in other conditions that compromise left ventricular function as well as in some healthy women. Although a combination of clinical and exercise variables, including peak ejection fraction, has been shown to be helpful in the identification of patients with severe CAD, the addition of radionuclide ventriculography in patients with normal electrocardiograms at rest adds little to the diagnostic information provided by clinical and other exercise variables.[85]

Echocardiography

(See also p. 89)

Two-dimensional echocardiography is useful in the evaluation of patients with chronic CAD, by assessing global and regional left ventricular function in the absence and presence of ischemia, as well as in establishing left ventricular hypertrophy and associated valve disease. Echocardiography is relatively inexpensive and safe. Rarely, coronary artery occlusion can be diagnosed by transesophageal echocardiography.[96] Stress echocardiography, in which imaging is carried out immediately after exercise, allows the detection of regional ischemia by identifying new areas of wall motion disorders. Adequate images can be obtained in more than 85 per cent of patients, and the test is highly reproducible. The inability to image at peak exercise is only a minor disadvantage because most wall motion abnormalities do not normalize immediately upon cessation of exercise. Several studies have shown that exercise echocardiography can *detect* the presence of CAD with an accuracy similar to that of stress thallium scintigraphic imaging and is superior to exercise electrocardiography alone.[97–99a]

PHARMACOLOGICAL STRESS ECHOCARDIOGRAPHY (see also p. 86). Among patients unable to exercise or those in whom the quality of the echocardiographic images during or immediately after exercise is poor, alternative echocardiographic approaches are available. These include transesophageal pacing with transesophageal echocardiography,[100] high-dose dipyridamole infusion, adenosine infusion, or dobutamine stress echocardiography. Arbutamine is a promising alternative agent.[100a] Whereas exercise echocardiography is the stress test of choice in patients able to achieve an adequate level, pacing and dobutamine stress echocardiography are more sensitive than dipyridamole.[101,102] Atropine increases the accuracy of dobutamine echocardiography, especially in patients taking beta blockers.[103] In one of the few direct comparisons in the same patients of exercise echocardiography, dobutamine echocardiography, and dipyridamole echocardiography, the sensitivity of exercise or dobutamine echocardiography was similar and was significantly higher than that of dipyridamole echocardiography. Specificity did not differ significantly among the tests. Moreover, in patients with known CAD, exercise and dobutamine echocardiography were superior to dipyridamole echocardiography in the assessment of the extent of disease.[101]

Several reports attest to the accuracy of dobutamine stress echocardiography in the detection of significant CAD.[104,105] Transesophageal dobutamine stress echocardiography has been shown to be feasible, safe, and accurate for the detection of myocardial ischemia. This may allow extension of dobutamine stress testing to patients with inadequate transthoracic echocardiographic imaging.[106] Although it has been shown that dobutamine stress echocardiography and exercise echocardiography are superior to exercise electrocardiographic testing alone and that these techniques are an excellent alternative to scintigraphic imaging, it has not been established that stress echocardiography is preferable or necessary in all patients who are otherwise suitable for exercise electrocardiographic testing. It is usually not cost-effective to utilize both techniques, and the choice of which stress to use and when is determined in part by the characteristics of the patients and the level of expertise and experience in any particular laboratory in addition to direct costs.

Clinical Application of Noninvasive Testing

GENDER DIFFERENCES IN THE DIAGNOSIS OF CAD (see also Chap. 51). Based upon earlier studies that documented a very high frequency of false-positive stress tests in women compared to men,[107] it is now generally accepted that electrocardiographic stress testing is not as reliable in women as it is in men. However, the prevalence of CAD among women in the patient populations under study was low, and the major explanation for the lower positive predictive value of exercise electrocardiography in women can be accounted for on the basis of Bayesian principles.[108,109] Once men and women are stratified appropriately according to the pretest prevalence of disease, the results of stress testing are similar.[110]

Soft tissue attenuation artifacts, especially those caused by breast tissue in women, may reduce the diagnostic accuracy of myocardial perfusion scintigraphy in women.[111] Exercise radionuclide ventriculography has little if any place in the *diagnosis* of CAD in women, because a fall or no increase in ejection fraction at higher rates of exercise has been noted to occur in healthy women. However, among women without a prior history of myocardial infarction, exercise echocardiography was superior to exercise electrocardiography in the detection of CAD.[111a]

IDENTIFICATION OF PATIENTS AT HIGH RISK. When applying noninvasive tests to the diagnosis and management of CAD, it is useful to grade the results as negative, indeterminate, positive—not high risk, and positive—high risk. The criteria for high-risk positivity are shown in Table 38–2.

Regardless of the severity of symptoms, patients with high-risk noninvasive tests have a very high likelihood of CAD and, if they have no obvious contraindications to revascularization, should undergo coronary arteriography. Such patients, even if asymptomatic, are at risk of having left main or three-vessel CAD with impaired left ventricular function. They are at high risk of experiencing coronary events, and their prognosis may often be improved by coronary bypass surgery. In contrast, patients with clearly negative exercise tests, regardless of symptoms, have an excellent prognosis which cannot usually be improved by revascularization. If they do not have serious symptoms, they usually do not require coronary arteriography.

ASYMPTOMATIC PERSONS. In asymptomatic persons or in those with chest pain not likely to be angina, who are being screened for CAD, i.e., patients in whom the pretest likelihood of coronary disease is low (less than 15 per cent), a negative exercise electrocardiogram excludes, for practical purposes, ischemic heart disease. However, if in such a patient there is an abnormal exercise electrocardiographic test, several alternatives exist. If the test is positive but not high risk and the patient demonstrates excellent exercise capacity (i.e., to stage IV of a Bruce protocol or the equivalent), the likelihood of left main coronary disease or multivessel CAD is low, the prognosis is excellent, and the

TABLE 38–2 CRITERIA FOR HIGH RISK ON NONINVASIVE TESTING

HIGH-RISK EXERCISE ELECTROCARDIOGRAPHIC VARIABLES
≥2.0 mm ST-segment depression
≥1 mm ST-segment depression in stage I
ST-segment depression in multiple leads
ST-segment depression for greater than 5 minutes during the recovery period
Achievement of a workload of less than 4 METS or a low exercise maximal heart rate
Abnormal blood pressure response
Ventricular arrhythmias
HIGH-RISK THALLIUM-201 SCINTIGRAPHIC VARIABLES
Multiple perfusion defects (total plus reversible defects) in more than one vascular supply region (e.g., defects in coronary supply regions of the left anterior descending and left circumflex vessels)
Increased lung thallium-201 uptake reflecting exercise-induced left ventricular dysfunction
Postexercise transient left ventricular cavity dilation

From Beller, G. A.: Current status of nuclear cardiology techniques. Curr. Probl. Cardiol. *16*:463, 1991.

patient may usually be observed without further testing. If, on the other hand, such a patient has a high-risk positive exercise electrocardiogram (see p. 1295), coronary angiography is usually indicated to determine whether or not left main CAD or severe multivessel disease with left ventricular dysfunction is present. If the patient falls into an intermediate category (a positive but not high-risk exercise test), then a stress imaging study (echocardiography or perfusion scintigraphy) may provide further information. If both studies are abnormal but not high risk, the likelihood of CAD approaches 90 per cent.

PATIENTS WITH ATYPICAL ANGINA. In these patients, the pretest probability of CAD is approximately 50 per cent. If two noninvasive tests are abnormal, the likelihood of CAD exceeds 95 per cent; if both tests are normal, it falls below 5 per cent. When test results are discordant, they should be evaluated in the light of the exercise level achieved, the presence of accompanying symptoms, and whether or not one of the tests is positive with high risk. Thus, for example, a patient with atypical angina and a normal exercise electrocardiogram who develops multiple large perfusion defects on a stress thallium-201 scintigram at a heart rate of 130 beats/min has a much greater likelihood of having CAD than one who has a normal exercise electrocardiogram and develops a single small perfusion defect without chest pain at a heart rate of 185 beats/min.

PATIENTS WITH TYPICAL ANGINA. In patients with high pretest likelihood of disease of approximately 90 per cent, noninvasive testing is most valuable for estimating the extent and severity of CAD and thereby the prognosis. The development of a high-risk positive stress test points to multivessel disease and a high risk of subsequent coronary events, and unless there are contraindications to revascularization, coronary angiography is indicated.

OTHER TESTS

BIOCHEMICAL TESTS. Serum levels of cardiac enzymes are normal in patients with chronic stable angina, which serves to differentiate them from patients with acute myocardial infarction. There are more relevant discriminators in patients with unstable angina (see p. 1332), in whom elevations in serum creatine phosphokinase (CPK) and a newer marker, serum troponin T (see p. 1335), may be a useful prognostic indicator.[111]

In younger patients (<45 years) with chronic stable angina, metabolic abnormalities that are risk factors for the development of CAD are frequently detected. These include hypercholesterolemia and other dyslipidemias (Chap. 35), carbohydrate intolerance, and insulin resistance.[112,113] All patients with established or suspected CAD warrant biochemical evaluation of total cholesterol, low-density lipoprotein cholesterol, high-density lipoprotein cholesterol, triglycerides, and fasting blood sugar.

CHEST ROENTGENOGRAM. This is usually within normal limits in patients with chronic stable angina, particularly if they have a normal resting electrocardiogram and have not experienced a myocardial infarction. If cardiomegaly is present, it is indicative of either severe CAD with prior myocardial infarction, preexisting hypertension, concomitant valvular heart disease, or an associated nonischemic condition such as cardiomyopathy. The presence of coronary calcification on fluoroscopy is indicative of underlying CAD (see p. 223). In patients with CAD who are scheduled to undergo an invasive procedure, the additional benefit of chest radiography is in the identification of other conditions that could alter or complicate therapy, e.g., chronic obstructive lung disease, chest infections, or neoplasms.[114]

ELECTRON BEAM OR ULTRAFAST COMPUTED TOMOGRAPHY (CT) (see also p. 336). Noninvasive detection of CAD has long been possible through detecting calcification associated with plaques by fluoroscopy. Such calcific deposits are diagnostic of coronary atherosclerosis.[115] Electron beam cardiac CT as a screening technique for coronary atherosclerosis is now available in a number of centers.[115a] However, the relationship of a positive test to subsequent cardiac events in asymptomatic patients has not been established.[116,117] The *absence* of calcium on CT is strongly predictive of the absence of significant atherosclerotic disease.[118] An analysis by a committee of the American Heart Association on the potential value of electron beam CT or ultrafast CT concluded that, while the technique is highly predictive for the *presence* of atherosclerosis, the *degree* of atherosclerosis cannot be predicted and the prognostic importance has not yet been established. Although this modality was considered to have great potential, it was *not* recommended for routine screening of patients.[119,120]

CATHETERIZATION, ANGIOGRAPHY, AND CORONARY ARTERIOGRAPHY

The clinical examination and noninvasive techniques described above are extremely valuable in establishing the diagnosis of CAD and are indispensable to an overall assessment of patients with this condition. However, the definitive diagnosis of CAD and a precise assessment of its anatomical severity and its effects upon cardiac performance require cardiac catheterization, coronary arteriography, and left ventricular angiography[120a] (Chaps. 7 and 9). Among patients with chronic stable angina pectoris referred for coronary arteriography, approximately 25 per cent of patients each have one-, two-, or three-vessel disease (i.e., >70 per cent luminal diameter narrowing). Five to 10 per cent have obstruction of the left main coronary artery, and in approximately 15 per cent no critical obstruction is detectable. Coronary angiographic findings differ between patients whose first presentation is acute myocardial infarction and chronic stable angina. Patients with unheralded myocardial infarction have fewer diseased vessels, fewer stenoses and chronic occlusions, and less diffuse disease than do chronic stable angina patients, suggesting that the pathophysiological substrate and the propensity to thrombosis differ between the two groups of patients.[121] In patients with chronic angina who have a history of prior infarction, total occlusion of at least one major coronary artery is more common than in those without such a history.

Coronary artery ectasia, i.e., patulous, aneurysmal dilatation involving most of the length of a major epicardial coronary artery, is present in approximately 1 to 3 per cent of patients with obstructive CAD at autopsy or angiography. This angiographic lesion does not appear to affect symptoms, survival, or the incidence of myocardial infarction.[122,123] Coronary ectasia should be distinguished from discrete *coronary artery aneurysms,* which are almost never found in arteries without severe stenoses, are most common in the left anterior descending coronary artery, and are usually associated with extensive CAD.[124] These discrete atherosclerotic coronary artery aneurysms do not appear to rupture, and their resection is not warranted.

Coronary collateral vessels (see p. 1174) may protect against myocardial infarction when total occlusion occurs, provided that they are of adequate size.[125] In patients with abundant collateral vessels, myocardial infarct size is smaller than in patients without collaterals and total occlusion of a major epicardial artery may not lead to left ventricular dysfunction.[126] In patients with chronic occlusion of a major coronary artery but without infarction, collateral-dependent myocardial segments show nearly normal baseline blood flow and oxygen consumption but severely limited flow reserve. This provides an explanation for the ability of collaterals to protect against resting ischemia but not exercise-induced angina.[127]

Myocardial bridging of coronary arteries (Fig. 8–23, p. 258) is observed in angiographically normal coronary arteries and normally does not constitute a hazard. Occasionally, compression of a portion of a coronary artery by a myocardial bridge can be associated with clinical manifestations of myocardial ischemia during strenuous physical activity and may even initiate malignant ventricular arrhythmias.[128,129]

LEFT VENTRICULAR FUNCTION. *Ventricular relaxation,* as reflected in the early diastolic ventricular filling rate, may be impaired at rest in patients with chronic CAD. Diastolic filling becomes even more abnormal (slowed) during exercise, when ischemia intensifies. In patients with chronic stable angina, the frequency of elevation of left ventricular end-diastolic pressure and reduced cardiac output at rest, generally attributed to abnormal left ventricular dynamics, increases with the number of vessels exhibiting critical narrowing and with the number of prior infarctions.[130] However, there is a great deal of overlap among individual patients so that the severity of coronary arterial disease cannot be predicted from these two measurements. The left ventricular end-diastolic pressure may be elevated secondary to reduced ventricular compliance, left ventricular systolic failure, or a combination of these two processes.[131] Both impaired systolic and diastolic function may occur as a consequence of acute, reversible ischemia and/or chronic scar formation. In many patients with normal hemodynamics in the resting state, abnormalities of left ventricular function can be elicited by dynamic or isometric exercise. Elevations of left ventricular end-diastolic pressure usually occur *before* the patient develops angina and before there is electrocardiographic ST-segment depression.

Left ventricular function can be assessed by means of biplane contrast ventriculography. Global abnormalities of left ventricular function are reflected in elevations of left ventricular end-diastolic and end-systolic volumes and depression of the ejection fraction (see p. 425). These changes, are, however, quite nonspecific. Abnormalities of *regional* wall motion (hypokinesis, akinesia, or dyskinesia) are more characteristic of CAD because the latter is usually regional in distribution. Also, hyperkinetic contraction of nonischemic myocardium, detected by left ventriculography, may compensate for hypokinetic or akinetic ischemic or necrotic myocardium, thereby maintaining normal or nearly normal global left ventricular function, despite marked depression of function in one region of the ventricle.[133]

Left ventricular function (global or regional) may be normal at rest in patients with chronic CAD without previous myocardial infarction but may become abnormal during or after stress. Abnormalities of left ventricular function detected angiographically may signify irreversible damage, i.e., prior infarction, or it may indicate acute ischemia or chronic hypoperfusion sufficient to maintain the viability but not the contractility of the myocardium, i.e., "myocardial hibernation"[133–135] (see pp. 388 and 1176). Reversibility of this form of left ventricular dysfunction in patients with CAD and chronic stable angina is reflected in improved contraction assessed angiographically by an inotropic stimulus (postextrasystolic potentiation[136] or the infusion of a sympathomimetic amine[137]) or in long-term improvement after myocardial revascularization.

In addition to demonstrating areas of asynergy, left ventriculography may also show mitral valve prolapse, which occurs in approximately 20 per cent of patients with obstructive CAD[138] and probably results from impaired contractility of the ventricular myocardium and papillary muscles. Mitral regurgitation secondary to left ventricular dilatation may be observed in patients with chronic stable angina and ischemic cardiomyopathy.

CORONARY BLOOD FLOW AND MYOCARDIAL METABOLISM. Cardiac catheterization can also document abnormal myocardial metabolism in patients with chronic stable angina. With a catheter in the coronary sinus, arterial and coronary venous lactate measurements are obtained at rest and after suitable stresses, such as the infusion of isoproterenol[139] or pacing-induced tachycardia.[140] Because lactate is a byproduct of anaerobic glycolysis, its production by the heart and subsequent appearance in coronary sinus blood is a reliable sign of myocardial ischemia (see p. 1204). When combined with coronary arteriography, this technique may be helpful in localizing significant coronary obstructive lesions and mycoardial ischemia.[141]

Studies of coronary flow reserve (maximum flow divided by resting flow) and of endothelial function are frequently abnormal in patients with CAD and chronic stable angina. They are discussed on pp. 200 and 1166.

MEDICAL MANAGEMENT

There are five aspects to the comprehensive management of chronic, stable angina: (1) identification and treatment of associated diseases, which can precipitate or worsen angina; (2) reduction of coronary risk factors; (3) general and nonpharmacological methods, with particular attention toward adjustments of lifestyle; (4) pharmacological management; and (5) revascularization by percutaneous transluminal angioplasty (or other catheter-based techniques) or by coronary bypass surgery.[141a] Although discussed individually, all five of these approaches must be considered, often simultaneously, in each patient. Among the medical therapies only two—aspirin and effective lipid lowering—have been convincingly shown to reduce mortality and morbidity in patients with chronic stable angina. Other therapies such as nitrates, beta blockers, and calcium antagonists have been shown to improve symptomatology and exercise performance, but their effect, if any, on survival has not been demonstrated.

TREATMENT OF ASSOCIATED DISEASES

A number of common medical conditions that can increase myocardial oxygen demands or reduce oxygen delivery may present with new angina pectoris or the exacerbation of previously stable angina. These include anemia, marked weight gain, occult thyrotoxicosis, fever, infections, and tachycardia. Drugs such as amphetamines and isoproterenol all increase myocardial oxygen demands, as do other agents that stimulate the sympathetic nervous system. Cocaine, which can cause acute coronary spasm and myocardial infarction, is discussed on p. 1340. Congestive heart failure, by causing cardiac dilatation and tachyarrythmias including sinus tachycardia, can increase myocardial oxygen needs with an increase in the frequency and severity of angina. Identification and treatment of these conditions is critical to the management of chronic stable angina.

Reduction of Coronary Risk Factors

HYPERTENSION (see also Chaps. 26 and 27). The epidemiological links between an elevated blood pressure and CAD mortality and severity are well established.[142,143] Hypertension increases myocardial oxygen demands and intensifies ischemia in patients with preexisting obstructive coronary vascular disease. Increased left ventricular mass due to left ventricular hypertrophy is a stronger predictor of myocardial infarction and coronary heart disease death than is the actual degree of blood pressure elevation.[144] A meta-analysis of clinical trials of treatment for mild to moderate hypertension showed a statistically significant 16 per cent reduction of CAD events and mortality in patients receiving antihypertensive therapy.[145] It is logical to extend these observations on the benefits of antihypertensive therapy to patients with established CAD. Therefore, blood pressure control is an essential aspect of management of patients with chronic stable angina.

In conjunction with antihypertensive therapy, attainment of an ideal body weight is particularly important in obese patients in whom weight reduction, in addition to aiding blood pressure control, raises the threshold for and may even abolish angina pectoris.

CIGARETTE SMOKING. This is one of the most powerful risk factors for the development of CAD in all age groups (see p. 1147), and cardiac events occur at a younger age in smokers. In a study of Australian men and women with premature CAD, smoking and lipid abnormalities were the two variables most relevant to the *severity* of CAD.[143] Among patients with angiographically documented CAD, cigarette smokers have a higher 5-year mortality and relative risk of infarction or sudden death than those who have stopped smoking,[146] and smoking cessation lessens the risks of adverse coronary events in patients with established CAD.[147] In patients who have undergone coronary bypass surgery, the cessation of cigarette smoking has been shown to decrease substantially both morbidity and mortality.[148,149]

Cigarette smoking may be responsible for aggravating angina pectoris other than through the progression of atherosclerosis. It may increase myocardial oxygen demands and reduce coronary blood flow[150,150a] by means of an alpha-adrenergically mediated increase in coronary artery tone and thereby cause acute ischemia.[151] Cigarette smoking also appears to interfere with the efficacy of antianginal drugs; improvements in exercise tolerance and a reduction in angina pectoris occur when cigarette smoking is discontinued in patients with angina receiving a beta blocker or calcium antagonist.[152] Smoking cessation is one of the most effective and certainly the least expensive approaches to the prevention of disease progression in native vessels and bypass grafts. Techniques for smoking cessation are discussed on p. 1148.

Passive cigarette smoking,[153] the inhalation of smog and carbon monoxide, and ascent to high altitude all lower the threshold for angina, and their avoidance represents an important aspect of therapy. Symptoms may also be aggravated or exercise performance impaired in patients with chronic stable angina who encounter some specific environmental situations (traffic tunnels, houses with defective gas furnaces, and closed automobiles during heavy highway traffic).[154] The mechanism is probably decreased oxygen delivery to the myocardium. Every effort must be made to avoid these aggravating stimuli.[155]

MANAGEMENT OF DYSLIPIDEMIA (see also Chap. 35). Cholesterol lowering by diet and drugs has been shown to reduce the incidence of CAD in primary prevention trials. Among men with moderate hypercholesterolemia in the West of Scotland trial, treatment with pravastatin significantly reduced the incidence of myocardial infarction and death without adversely affecting the risk of death from non-cardiovascular causes.[155a] In patients with *established* CAD, lipid-lowering therapy has demonstrated a significant reduction in disease progression and in subsequent cardiovascular events.[156–159,159b] Angiographic trials of cholesterol lowering in patients with chronic CAD, many of whom had chronic stable angina, have shown that the effects on coronary obstruction are modest whereas the reduction in cardiovascular events is quite impressive. Two studies have shown that aggressive lipid-lowering drugs significantly improve endothelium-mediated responses in the coronary arteries of patients with atherosclerosis.[160,161] These findings may explain the disproportionate reduction in coronary events in patients treated with cholesterol-lowering therapy, despite very small degrees of anatomical regression of atherosclerotic stenoses. The results from the Scandinavian Simvastatin Survival Study (4S) of patients with a history of angina or prior myocardial infarction provide convincing evidence that lipid-lowering therapy significantly improves overall survival and reduces cardiovascular mortality in patients with coronary heart disease.[159]

The revised National Cholesterol Education Program Guidelines (see p. 1990) advocate cholesterol-lowering therapy in *all* patients with coronary heart disease or extracardiac atherosclerosis to LDL levels below 100 mg/dl.

ESTROGEN REPLACEMENT THERAPY (see also p. 1707). The male gender and, in women, the postmenopausal state, are risk factors for the development and progression of CAD. Epidemiological studies have shown that the favorable cardiovascular risk profile in premenopausal women changes after the menopause, in that the levels of total cholesterol, low-density lipoprotein cholesterol (LDL-C), apolipoprotein B, and triglycerides all increase while high-density lipoprotein cholesterol (HDL-C) decreases slightly or remains unchanged.[162,163] Several long-term studies have identified reduced HDL-C and increased triglyceride levels as powerful predictors of CAD risk among postmenopausal women.[164,165] Moreover, numerous, large cross-sectional studies and a randomized trial[166] strongly suggest that postmenopausal hormone replacement therapy with estrogens, alone or in combination with medroxyprogesterone acetate, has a favorable effect upon the cardiovascular risk factor lipid profile (by increasing HDL-C and lowering LDL-C and triglyceride levels[167,168]) and upon the incidence of cardiovascular events[169,170] and the extent of atherosclerosis as determined by carotid ultrasonography.[171]

The beneficial effect of estrogen replacement therapy is probably not limited to altering favorably the lipid profile. It may also involve the interaction between estrogen and estrogen receptors in blood vessels, the maintenance of normal endothelial function (see p. 1166) and their direct modulating effects upon vascular tone. Estrogen replacement therapy may reduce LDL oxidation and uptake by the arterial wall and alter favorably the hemostatic profile.[172,172a] One study of estrogen replacement therapy suggested that the greatest benefit was in women with established CAD and least in those with normal coronary vessels.[173] Thus, the case for estrogen replacement therapy as secondary prevention of CAD is strong[174] (as it is in the primary prevention in women with multiple risk factors for CAD). The National Cholesterol Education Program (NCEP) has tentatively endorsed estrogen therapy as a method of lowering lipid levels in postmenopausal women with *established* CAD.[175]

ANTIOXIDANTS. Oxidized LDL particles are strongly linked to the pathophysiology of atherogenesis (see p. 1116), and epidemiological data support an association between low levels of beta-carotene and myocardial infarction, at least among smokers.[176–178] Other studies imply that a high dietary intake of antioxidants, including flavonoids (polyphenolic antioxidants) naturally present in vegetables, fruits, tea, and wine and vitamin E, is associated with a decline in coronary heart disease events.[177–179] Large randomized trials evaluating the effects of antioxidant supplementation, as well as probucol, a lipid-lowering agent with additional antioxidant properties, are under way. Until the results are available, no firm recommendations can be made regarding antioxidant intake in patients with chronic stable angina. Nonetheless, in a subgroup analysis of patients who had undergone previous coronary bypass surgery, coronary artery lesion progression was less in subjects with a supplementary vitamin E intake of 100 IU per day or more compared with patients with a lower intake.[178]

EXERCISE (see also Chap. 40). The conditioning effect of exercise on skeletal muscles allows a greater workload at any level of total body oxygen consumption. By decreasing the heart rate at any level of exertion, a higher cardiac output can be achieved at any level of myocardial oxygen consumption. The combination of these two effects of exercise conditioning permits the patient with chronic stable angina to increase physical performance substantially following institution of a continuing exercise program.[180]

Most of the information about the physiological effects of exercise and their effect on prognosis in patients with CAD is derived from studies in patients entered into cardiac rehabilitation programs,[181,182] many of whom have sustained a prior myocardial infarction. There is less information on the benefits of exercise in patients with chronic stable CAD, but one study has confirmed a striking and direct relationship between the intensity of exercise and favorable changes in the morphology of obstructive lesions on angiography.[183]

Other studies in patients with known coronary heart disease have demonstrated the beneficial effects of prolonged exercise training on cardiac performance, effort tolerance, quality of life, and stress-induced myocardial ischemia.[184,185] The question of whether or not exercise accelerates the development of collateral vessels in patients with chronic CAD remains unsettled.

Thus, the available evidence suggests that regular, supervised physical exercise should be recommended for most patients with documented CAD and chronic stable angina. It is safe if begun under supervision[186] and, if survivors of a myocardial infarction can be used as a yardstick, it is probably cost-effective.[187] The psychological benefits of exercise are difficult to evaluate. However, exercise conditioning programs may be quite helpful in increasing the self-confidence of patients with chronic CAD (as they are in patients recovering from acute myocardial infarction). Patients who are involved in exercise programs usually are also more likely to be health conscious, to pay attention to diet and weight, and to discontinue cigarette smoking. Thus, in addition to a conditioning effect on skeletal and cardiac muscle, regular dynamic exercise provides the patient with a feeling of well-being, an important consideration in the management of any chronic disease.

For all of the aforementioned reasons, patients should be urged to participate in regular exercise programs—usually walking (see below)—in conjunction with their drug therapy.

ASPIRIN (see also p. 1827). Although platelet hyperaggregability is not considered to be a risk factor for myocardial infarction, reduction of platelet aggregability with aspirin reduces the risk of development of this complication. Moreover, in patients with stable CAD, enhanced thrombin-induced platelet aggregation is strongly associated with angiographic progression of the disease, and a higher incidence of clinical events. The platelet abnormalities may be a marker of increased risk in addition to playing a causative role in the development of coronary events.[188] A meta-analysis on 140,000 patients comprising 300 studies confirmed the prophylactic benefit of aspirin in both male and female patients with angina pectoris, prior myocardial infarction, or prior stroke and after bypass surgery.[189] In a Swedish trial of both men and women with chronic stable angina, 75 mg of aspirin, in conjunction with the beta blocker sotalol, caused a 34 per cent reduction in acute myocardial infarction and sudden death.[190] In a smaller study confined to men with chronic stable angina but without a history of myocardial infarction, 325 mg aspirin on alternate days reduced the risk of myocardial infarction during 5 years of follow-up by 87 per cent.[191] Therefore, 75 to 325 mg of aspirin daily is advisable in patients with chronic stable angina without contraindications to this drug.

Although coumadin has proven beneficial in postinfarct patients, no data support the use of chronic anticoagulation in patients with stable angina.

BETA BLOCKERS. The value of beta blockers in reducing death and recurrent myocardial infarction in patients who have experienced a myocardial infarction is well established[192,193] (see p. 1228), as is their usefulness in the treatment of angina (see p. 1304). Whether these drugs are also of value in preventing infarction and sudden death in patients with chronic stable angina is not clear. However, there is no reason to assume that the favorable effects of beta blockers on ischemia and perhaps upon arrhythmias should not apply to patients with chronic stable angina pectoris. Therefore, it is sensible to use these drugs when angina or hypertension or both are present in patients with chronic CAD and when these drugs are well tolerated.

ANGIOTENSIN-CONVERTING ENZYME (ACE) INHIBITORS. Several small studies that evaluated the effect of ACE inhibitors on the severity of angina pectoris and ischemia have provided conflicting results but were limited by small sample size and brief duration of therapy.[194–198]

A surprising and perhaps far-reaching finding from recent randomized trials of ACE inhibitors in postinfarct and other patients with ischemic and nonischemic causes of left ventricular dysfunction was a striking reduction in the subsequent incidence of ischemic events such as myocardial infarction, unstable angina, and the need for coronary revascularization procedures.[199–203] Data from four trials including approximately 11,000 patients showed a statistically significant risk reduction in myocardial infarction of 21 per cent and in subsequent unstable angina of 15 per cent.[203] The potentially beneficial effects of ACE inhibitors include a reduction in left ventricular hypertrophy, vascular hypertrophy, progression of atherosclerosis, plaque rupture, and thrombosis, in addition to a potentially favorable influence on myocardial oxygen supply/demand relationships, cardiac hemodynamics, and a reduction of sympathetic activity.[203]

Despite these intriguing observations, prospective randomized trials showing the effects of these drugs in patients with chronic stable angina without left ventricular dysfunction have not been completed. Therefore, as of this writing, ACE inhibitors are *not* recommended in patients with chronic stable angina pectoris in the absence of other conditions that would warrant treatment with this class of drugs, i.e., hypertension, heart failure, or asymptomatic left ventricular dysfunction.

Counseling and Changes in Life Style

The psychosocial issues faced by the patient who develops chronic stable angina for the first time are similar to, although usually less intense, than those experienced by the patient with an acute myocardial infarction. Many patients have an unrealistically gloomy perception of their prognosis; they should be offered a realistic appraisal, together with an understandable explanation of the pertinent clinical features of the disease.

An important aspect of the physician's role is to counsel patients in the kinds of work they can do and in their leisure activities, eating habits, vacation plans, and the like. Certain changes in life style may be helpful, such as modifying strenuous activities if they constantly and repeatedly produce angina. These changes may be minor in many instances. For example, golfing could be modified to include use of a golf cart instead of walking. A history of CAD and stable angina is not inconsistent with the ability to continue to perform vigorous exertion. This is important not only in regard to recreational activities and life style but also for patients in whom physical exertion is required in their employment. Isometric activities such as weight lifting[204] and other activities such as snow shoveling, which involves an energy expenditure between 60 and 65 per cent of peak oxygen consumption,[205] and cross-country or downhill skiing[206] are undesirable. In addition, some activities expose the individual to the detrimental effects of cold on the oxygen demand/supply relationship,[48,49,207] and these too should be avoided if possible.

Thoughtful counseling, which may include supervised exercise sessions simulating the particular activity in question, can play a vital role in maintaining a productive and enjoyable life style in patients with chronic stable angina. Many activities, such as shopping or climbing stairs, need not be discontinued by the patient with chronic angina; often it is necessary merely to perform them more slowly or to pause for brief periods of rest. The patient with chronic stable angina should avoid excessive fatigue and exhaustion. Although it is desirable to minimize the number of bouts of angina, an occasional episode is not to be feared. Indeed, unless patients occasionally reach their angina threshold, they may not appreciate the extent of their exercise capacity. The vast majority of patients with chronic stable angina should not be treated as invalids. Often the propensity for angina actually declines, perhaps as a result of the development of collaterals and/or because of training effects.

Eliminating or reducing the factors that precipitate anginal episodes is of obvious importance. Patients learn their usual threshold by trial and error. Because many anginal episodes are precipitated by increases in the mechanical activity of the heart (owing to increases in myocardial oxygen consumption), patients should avoid sudden bursts of activity, particularly after long periods of rest or after meals and in cold weather. Chronic and unstable angina exhibit a circadian rhythm characterized by a lower angina threshold shortly after arising.[208,208a] Therefore, morning activities such as showering, shaving, and dressing should be done at a slower pace, and if necessary with use of prophylactic nitroglycerin. The stress of sexual intercourse is approximately equal to that of climbing one flight of stairs at a normal pace or to any activity that induces a heart rate of approximately 120 beats/min. With proper precautions, i.e., commencing more than 2 hours postprandially and taking an additional dose of a short-acting beta blocker 1 hour before and nitroglycerin 15 minutes before, the majority of patients with chronic stable angina are able to continue satisfactory sexual activity.

Just as there is a role for exercise in the management of CAD, so is there a role for rest, especially in situations in which angina has become frequent or severe. Marked restriction of activity or even complete bed rest, in addition to drug therapy, may be necessary to control symptoms. In less critical situations, merely reducing the amount of time spent working or increasing the rest periods has a beneficial effect. For example, a long lunch break including a short nap may be beneficial. It may be helpful for the patient to use a face mask or scarf to cover the mouth or nose in cold weather. A hot, humid environment may also precipitate angina, and air conditioning may be a necessity rather than a luxury for patients with chronic angina. Large meals can have a similar effect if they are followed by exertion. An effort should be made to minimize emotional outbursts because they too increase myocardial oxygen requirements and sometimes induce coronary vasoconstriction. Occasionally, antianxiety drugs and sedatives or relaxation techniques using biofeedback mechanisms may be useful. Hostility is an adverse risk factor in CAD.

Nitrates

(See also pp. 1336 and 1342)

Mechanism of Action

Although the clinical effectiveness of amyl nitrite in angina pectoris was first described in 1867 by Brunton, organic nitrates are still the drugs most commonly used in the treatment of patients with this condition. The action of these agents is to relax vascular smooth muscle.[208b] The vasodilator effects of nitrates are evident in both systemic (including coronary) arteries and veins in normal subjects and in patients with ischemic heart disease, but they appear to be predominant in the venous circulation. The venodilator effect reduces ventricular preload,[209] which in turn reduces myocardial wall tension and oxygen requirements. The actions of nitrates to reduce both preload and afterload make them useful in the treatment of heart failure (Fig. 38–2) as well as angina pectoris.

Posture is important in evaluating the hemodynamic effects of nitrates. In a patient in the supine position, venous return is normally greater but exercise tolerance and the angina threshold are lower than in the upright position. The hemodynamic and angina-relieving effects of nitrates are most marked when patients are sitting or standing, i.e., when the preload-reducing effects of these drugs are most prominent. By reducing the heart's mechanical activity, volume, and oxygen consumption, nitrates increase exercise capacity in patients with ischemic heart disease, thereby allowing a greater total body workload to be achieved before the angina threshold is reached.

EFFECTS ON THE CORONARY CIRCULATION. Conductance Vessels (see Table 38–6, p. 1306). There is evidence, obtained from quantitative, computer-assisted measurements of coronary arterial diameter, that nitroglycerin causes dilatation of epicardial stenoses. These are often eccentric lesions, and nitroglycerin causes relaxation of smooth muscle in the wall of the coronary artery that is not encompassed by the plaque. Even a small increase in the narrowed arterial lumen can produce a significant reduction in resistance to blood flow across obstructed regions (Fig. 36–7, p. 1165).[210] Nitrates may also exert a beneficial effect in patients with an impaired coronary flow reserve by alleviating vasoconstriction due to endothelial dysfunction.[211]

REDISTRIBUTION OF BLOOD FLOW. Studies in experimental animals with coronary obstruction have shown that nitroglycerin causes redistribution of blood flow from normally perfused to ischemic areas, particularly in the subendocardium.[212] This may be mediated in part by an increase in collateral blood flow and in part by a lowering of ventricular diastolic pressure, thereby reducing subendocardial compression. In patients with chronic stable angina responsive to nitroglycerin, topical nitroglycerin under resting conditions alters myocardial perfusion by preferentially increasing flow to areas of reduced perfusion with little or no change in global myocardial perfusion.[213]

The results of studies of nitroglycerin on coronary blood flow in patients have been conflicting. Some studies have reported increased blood flow after sublingual or intravenous nitroglycerin,[213,214] but most report no change or reduced flow.[215] However, because myocardial oxygen demand fell, the net effect on oxygen balance became favorable in the latter studies. Using intracoronary injection of xenon-133 (as well as in retrograde perfusion studies performed during coronary bypass surgery), it was shown that blood flow in regions of myocardium perfused by stenotic coronary arteries rose after administration of nitroglycerin when well-developed collaterals supplying those regions were present.[216] In patients with chronic stable angina, topical nitroglycerin alters myocardial perfusion by preferentially increasing flow to areas of reduced perfusion with little or no change in global myocardial perfusion.[213]

The presence of well-developed collaterals may be an important determinant of a good therapeutic response to nitrates.[216–218] After systemic nitroglycerin, the heart can be paced to higher rates before angina occurs. But this is not the case after intracoronary administration, implying that the systemic effects of nitrates may predominate in patients with pure effort angina.[215] The nitrates have also been shown to improve ventricular wall motion in patients with CAD, as demonstrated by contrast ventriculography,[219] echocardiography, and radionuclide ventriculography, both at rest and during exercise. They also reduce the extent of myocardial ischemia, as reflected in exercise-thallium tomographic perfusion defect therapy.[220]

ANTITHROMBOTIC EFFECTS. The stimulation of guanylate cyclase by nitric oxide (NO) results in inhibitory actions on platelets in addition to vasodilation. Although the antithrombotic effects of intravenous nitroglycerin have been demonstrated both in patients with unstable angina and those with chronic stable angina,[221–223] the clinical significance of these actions is not clear.

CELLULAR MECHANISM OF ACTION. Nitrates have the ability to cause vasodilation whether or not the endothelium is intact.[224] After entering the vascular smooth muscle cell, nitrates are converted to reactive (NO) or S-nitrosothiols, which activate intracellular guanylate cyclase to produce cyclic guanosine monophosphate (GMP),[224,225] which in turn triggers smooth muscle relaxation and antiplatelet aggregatory effects (Fig. 38–4). Sulfhydryl (SH) groups are required for both the formation of NO and the stimulation of guanylate cyclase, and nitroglycerin-induced vasodilation can be enhanced by prior administration of *N*-acetylcysteine, an agent that increases the availability of SH groups.[226] This action of *N*-acetylcysteine potentiates the peripheral hemodynamic responses[226] and the coronary vasodilator effect of nitroglycerin[216] and reverses the partial tolerance to the coronary vasodilator effect of nitroglycerin.

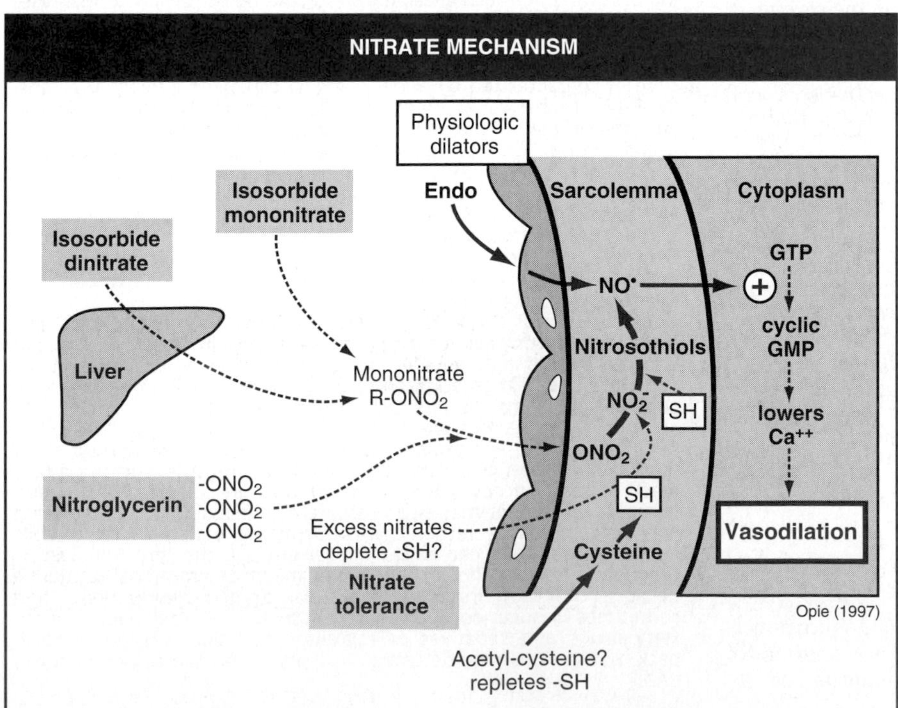

FIGURE 38–4. Mechanisms of the effects of nitrates in the generation of nitric oxide (NO) and the stimulation of guanylate cyclase cyclic GMP, which mediates vasodilation. Sulfhydryl (SH) groups are required for the formation of NO and the stimulation of guanylate cyclase. Isosorbide dinitrate is metabolized by the liver, whereas this is bypassed by the mononitrates. Abbreviations are as follows: SH = sulfhydryl; GTP = guanosine triphosphate; GMP = guanosine monophosphate. (Redrawn from Opie, L. H.: Drugs for the Heart. 4th ed. Philadelphia, W. B. Saunders Company, 1995, p. 33. Figure copyright L. H. Opie.)

TABLE 38–3 RECOMMENDED DOSING REGIMENS FOR LONG-TERM NITRATE THERAPY

PREPARATION OF AGENT	DOSE	SCHEDULE
Nitroglycerin		
Ointment	0.5–2 inches	2–3 times/d
Buccal or transmucosal	1–3 mg	3 times/d
Transdermal patch	0.4–1.2 mg/h for 12 to 14 hours, after which patch is removed	
Oral sustained release	9.0–13.5 mg	2–3 times/d*
Isosorbide dinitrate		
Oral	10–60 mg	2–3 times/d
Oral sustained release	80–120 mg	Once daily
Isosorbide-5-mononitrate		
Oral	20–30 mg	Twice daily given 7–8 h apart
Oral sustained release	60–240 mg	Once daily

* Very limited data available on efficacy.

From Abrams, J.: Medical therapy of stable angina pectoris. *In* Beller, G.: Chronic Ischemic Heart Disease. Atlas of Heart Diseases, vol. 5. Braunwald, E. (ed.). Philadelphia, Current Medicine, 1995, p. 7.18.

Types of Preparations and Routes of Administration

(Table 38–3)

Nitroglycerin administered sublingually remains the drug of choice for the treatment of acute angina episodes and for the prevention of angina. Because sublingual administration avoids first-pass hepatic metabolism, a transient but effective concentration of the drug rapidly appears in the circulation. The half-life of nitroglycerin itself is brief, and it is rapidly converted to two inactive metabolites, both of which are found in the urine after nitroglycerin administration. The liver possesses large amounts of hepatic glutathione organic nitrate reductase, the enzyme that breaks down nitroglycerin, but there is also evidence that blood vessels (veins and arteries) may metabolize nitrates directly. Within 30 to 60 minutes, hepatic breakdown has abolished the hemodynamic and clinical effects.

The usual sublingual dose is 0.3 to 0.6 mg, and most patients respond within 5 minutes to one or two 0.3-mg tablets. If symptoms are not relieved by a single dose, additional doses of 0.3 mg may be taken at 5-minute intervals, but no more than 1.2 mg should be used within a 15-minute period. The development of tolerance (see below) is rarely a problem with intermittent usage. Sublingual nitroglycerin is especially useful when it is taken *prophylactically* shortly before physical activities that are likely to cause angina are undertaken. Used for this purpose, it may prevent angina for up to 40 minutes.

ADVERSE REACTIONS. These are common and include headache, flushing, and hypotension (Table 38–4). The latter is rarely severe, but in some patients, particularly in the face of an unstable ischemic syndrome, volume depletion, and the upright posture, nitrate-induced hypotension is accompanied by a paradoxical bradycardia, consistent with a vasovagal or vasodepressor response. This reaction is more common in the elderly, who are less able to tolerate hypovolemia. The administration of nitrates before a meal, particularly in patients with a tendency toward postprandial hypotension, may enhance venous pooling, preload reduction, and the extent of the fall in blood pressure after the meal.[228] In addition, the partial pressure of oxygen in arterial blood may fall after large doses of nitroglycerin because of a *ventilation-perfusion imbalance* caused by inability of the pulmonary vascular bed to constrict in areas of alveolar hypoxia, thereby leading to perfusion of less hypoxic tissues.[229] *Methemoglobinemia* is a rare complication of very large doses of nitrates; commonly used doses of nitrates cause small elevations of methemoglobin that probably are not of clinical significance.

PREPARATIONS (Table 38–3). **Nitroglycerin Tablets.** These tend to lose their potency, especially if exposed to light, and should be kept in dark containers. Other nitrate preparations are available in sublingual, buccal, oral, spray, and ointment form. An oral nitroglycerin spray that dispenses metered, aerosolized doses of 0.4 mg may be better absorbed than the sublingual form in patients with dry mucosal membranes.[230] It can also be quickly sprayed onto, or under, the tongue. For prophylaxis, the spray should be used 5 to 10 minutes before angina-provoking activities.

Isosorbide Dinitrate. This is an effective antianginal agent but with low bioavailability after oral administration. It undergoes rapid hepatic metabolism, and there are marked variations in plasma concentrations after oral administration. It has two metabolites (one has a potent vasodilator action) that are cleared less rapidly than the parent drug and are excreted unchanged in the urine. It is available in tablets for sublingual use, in chewable form, in tablets for oral use, and in sustained-release capsules.

Partial or complete nitrate tolerance (see below) develops with regimens of isosorbide dinitrate when it is administered as 30 mg three or four times daily.[231] A dosage schedule should be adopted that allows a 10- to 12-hour nitrate-free interval. If the drug is administered on a three-times-daily schedule (e.g., at 8:00 A.M., 1 P.M., and 6 P.M.), the antianginal benefit lasts for approximately 6 hours, and the magnitude of the antianginal benefit decreases with each successive dose.[231]

Isosorbide-5-Mononitrate. This active metabolite of the dinitrate is completely bioavailable with oral administration, because it does not undergo first-pass hepatic metabolism[232] and is efficacious in the treatment of chronic stable angina.[233] Plasma levels of isosorbide-5-mononitrate reach their peak between 30 minutes and 2 hours after ingestion, and the drug has a plasma half-life of 4 to 6 hours. A single

TABLE 38–4 SIDE EFFECTS OF ANTIANGINAL DRUGS*

	HYPOTENSION FLUSHING, HEADACHE	LEFT VENTRICULAR DYSFUNCTION	DECREASED HEART RATE ATRIOVENTRICULAR BLOCK†	GASTROINTESTINAL SYMPTOMS	BRONCHOCONSTRICTION‡	EDEMA
Beta blockers	0	++	+++	+	+++	0
Nitrates	+++	0	0	0	0	0
Diltiazem	+	+	+	0	0	+
Nifedipine	+++	0	0	0	0	+++
Verapamil	+	+	++	++	0	+
Amlodipine	+	0	0	0	0	+++
Bepridil	+	+	+	0	0	0

* 0 = absent; + = mild; ++ = moderate; +++ = sometimes severe.

† In patients with sick sinus node syndrome or conduction system disease.

‡ In patients with obstructive lung disease.

Reprinted by permission from Braunwald, E.: Mechanism of action of calcium channel blocking agents. N. Engl. J. Med. *307*:1618, 1982. Copyright Massachusetts Medical Society.

20-mg tablet still exhibits activity 8 hours after administration. Tolerance has not been demonstrated using once-a-day or eccentric dosing intervals but does occur with a twice-daily dosing regimen at 12-hour intervals. The only sustained-release preparation of isosorbide-5-mononitrate is *Imdur,* which is given once daily in a dose of 30 to 240 mg. Presumably this preparation provides a sufficiently low level of nitrates for a long enough period of time to avoid tolerance, because the duration of activity is estimated to be 12 hours or less.

Topical Nitroglycerin. OINTMENT. Nitroglycerin ointment (15 mg/inch) is efficacious when applied (most commonly to the chest) in strips of 0.5 to 2.0 inches. Delay in the onset of action is approximately 30 minutes. Because it is effective for 4 to 6 hours, this form of the drug is particularly useful in patients with severe angina or unstable angina who are confined to bed and chair. Nitroglycerin ointment also may be used prophylactically after retiring by patients with nocturnal angina. Skin permeability increases with increased hydration, and absorption is also enhanced if the paste is covered with plastic whose edges are taped to the skin.

TRANSDERMAL PATCHES. A silicone gel or polymer matrix impregnated with nitroglycerin results in absorption for 24 to 48 hours at a rate determined by various methods of preparation of the patch, including a semipermeable membrane placed between the drug reservoir and the skin. The release rate of the patches varies from 2.5 to 15 mg per 24 hours. Relatively low doses (2.5 mg to 5 mg per 24 hours) may not produce sufficient plasma and tissue concentrations to sustain consistent, effective antianginal effects. Transdermal nitroglycerin therapy has been shown to increase exercise duration and maintains anti-ischemic effects for 12 hours after patch application throughout 30 days of therapy, without significant evidence of nitrate tolerance or rebound phenomenon,[234] provided that the patch is not applied for more than 12 out of 24 hours.

NITRATE TOLERANCE

This phenomenon has been demonstrated with all forms of nitrate administration which maintain continuous blood levels of the drug.[231,234–236] Although nitrate tolerance is rapid in onset, renewed responsiveness is easily established after a short nitrate-free interval. The problem of tolerance applies to all nitrate preparations and is particularly important in patients with chronic stable angina pectoris, as opposed to those receiving short-acting courses of nitrates (e.g., unstable angina and myocardial infarction).[237,238] Nitrate tolerance appears to be limited to the capacitance and resistance vessels in that it has not been noted in the large conductance vessels, including the epicardial coronary arteries and radial arteries, despite continuous administration of nitroglycerin for 48 hours.[239]

A meta-analysis of randomized clinical trials of nitroglycerin patches suggested that in doses of 5 to 10 mg, exercise duration was improved early after administration but by 24 hours the effect of nitroglycerin on exercise performance was attenuated by the development of nitrate tolerance.[235] However, a regimen in which transdermal nitroglycerin was applied for 12 hours and removed for 12 hours improved exercise performance for 8 to 12 hours after application of the patch. After 1 month of such therapy, responsiveness to transdermal nitroglycerin remained virtually unchanged. Therefore, after application of a transdermal nitroglycerin patch one can expect therapeutic efficacy (improved exercise performance) for 8 to 12 hours. Provided a substantial nitrate-free interval (of 10 to 12 hours) exists every 24-hour period, sustained improvement in exercise performance may be maintained. If a state of tolerance is induced, a nitrate-free interval restores responsiveness. If large intermittent doses of transdermal or oral nitrates are employed (equivalent to 20 mg per 24 hours of a transdermal patch), it is possible that rebound angina may occur during the nitrate-free period.

MECHANISMS. Several mechanisms of nitrate tolerance have been proposed.[219] Their relative importance has not been defined.

Depletion of Sulfhydryl (SH) Groups. Perhaps the most widely accepted explanation of nitrate tolerance is that a depletion of intracellular SH cofactors occurs and that these are a crucial component of the metabolic conversion of nitroglycerin to nitric oxide or S-nitrosothiols, a conversion necessary for the activation of guanylate cyclase.[240]

Neurohormonal Activation. There may be nonspecific activation of neurohormonal mechanisms in response to the hypotensive effects of nitrates with a resultant increase in plasma catecholamines, plasma renin activity, and arginine vasopressin causing sodium retention and weight gain.[241] It has been suggested that angiotensin-converting enzyme inhibitors modify nitrate tolerance by blunting the neurohormonal responses to nitrate therapy.[242]

Plasma Volume Expansion. Plasma volume expansion occurs during continuous nitrate administration,[241] even in the absence of neurohormonally mediated sodium retention.[242] It may be the result of a fluid shift from the extravascular to the intravascular space in response to the vasodilating or hemodynamic actions of nitrates.[243]

Downregulation of Nitrate Receptors. It has been proposed that high-affinity receptors, which respond to low concentrations of nitrates, are downregulated during the development of tolerance. The activity of low-affinity receptors is maintained and these continue to respond but to increasing concentrations of nitrate.[244]

MANAGEMENT. The only practical strategy is to provide a "nitrate-free" interval. The optimal interval is unknown, but with patches or ointment of nitroglycerin or preparations of isosorbide dinitrate or isosorbide-5-mononitrate, *a 12-hour off period is recommended.*[244–248] The timing of administration should be adapted to the pattern of symptoms, e.g., whether angina is predominantly exercise-related during the day or nocturnal.

NITRATE WITHDRAWAL. A common form of nitrate withdrawal (rebound) is observed in patients whose angina is intensified after discontinuation of large doses of long-acting nitrates.[249] The potential for rebound can be modified by adjusting the dose and timing of administration in addition to the use of other antianginal drugs. Moreover, nitroglycerin administered by the sublingual route does not result in tolerance, and even after 2 weeks of therapy there is no reduction in efficacy when sublingual nitroglycerin is administered two or three times daily.[250]

Because of the possibility of nitrate dependence, nitrate therapy should be withdrawn carefully. In individuals exposed to industrial doses of nitroglycerin, nitrate tolerance, nitrate dependence, and withdrawal symptoms may cause serious problems. During the manufacture of dynamite, substantial levels of nitrates are often present in the atmosphere and can be absorbed through the skin and lungs. After an acute response of headache, hypotension, palpitations, and gastrointestinal disturbances, adaptation occurs.[251] Withdrawal from this environment may result in angina unrelated to exertion or emotion. In fact, spontaneous coronary vasospasm and acute myocardial infarction have been documented during a period of withdrawal.

Beta-Adrenoceptor Blocking Agents

(See also p. 853)

Four beta-adrenoceptor blocking drugs have been approved for the treatment of angina in the United States, and this class of agents constitutes a cornerstone of therapy of this condition. In addition to their anti-ischemic properties, beta blockers are effective antihypertensives (see p. 854) and antiarrhythmics (p. 610). Also, they have been shown to reduce mortality and reinfarction in post–myocardial infarct patients (p. 1264). This combination of actions makes them extremely useful in the management of chronic stable angina. A number of studies have shown that beta-adrenoceptor blockers, in doses that are generally well tolerated, reduce the frequency of anginal episodes and raise the anginal threshold, both when given alone and when added to other antianginal agents.

The salutary action of these drugs (which have a chemical structure resembling that of beta-adrenoceptor agonists) depends on their ability to cause competitive inhibition of the effects of neuronally released and circulating catecholamines on beta adrenoceptors[252–254] (Table 38–5). Beta blockade reduces myocardial oxygen consumption primarily by slowing heart rate; the slower heart rate in turn increases the fraction of the cardiac cycle occupied by diastole with a corresponding increase in the time available for coronary perfusion (Fig. 38–5; Table 38–6). These drugs also reduce exercise-induced rises in blood pressure and limit exercise-induced increases in contractility. Thus, beta blockers reduce myocardial oxygen demands primarily during activity or excitement when surges of increased sympathetic activity occur.[255] Thus, in the face of impaired myocardial perfusion, the effects of beta blockers on myocardial oxygen demands may critically and favorably alter the imbalance between supply and demand, resulting in the elimination of ischemia.

Beta blockers reduce blood flow to most organs by means of the combination of unopposed alpha-adrenergic vasoconstriction and blockade of the $beta_2$ receptors. Complications are relatively minor, but in patients with peripheral

TABLE 38–5 PHYSIOLOGICAL ACTIONS OF β-ADRENERGIC RECEPTORS

ORGAN	RECEPTOR TYPE	RESPONSE TO STIMULUS
Heart		
SA node	β_1	Increased heart rate
Atria	β_1	Increased contractility and conduction velocity
AV node	β_1	Increased automaticity and conduction velocity
His-Purkinje system	β_1	Increased automaticity and conduction velocity
Ventricles	β_1	Automaticity, contractility, and conduction velocity
Arteries		
Peripheral	β_2	Dilatation
Coronary	β_2	Dilatation
Carotid	β_2	Dilatation
Other	β_1	Increased insulin release
		Increased liver and muscle glycogenolysis
Lungs	β_2	Dilatation of bronchi
Uterus	β_2	Smooth muscle relaxation

From Abrams, J.: Medical therapy of stable angina pectoris. *In* Beller, G.: Chronic Ischemic Heart Disease. Atlas of Heart Diseases, vol. 5. Braunwald, E. (ed.). Philadelphia, Current Medicine, 1995, p. 7.19.

vascular disease, the reduction in blood flow to skeletal muscles with the use of the nonselective beta blockers may reduce maximal exercise capacity. In patients with preexisting left ventricular dysfunction, beta blockade may increase ventricular volume and thereby enhance oxygen demands.

Characteristics of Different Beta Blockers

(Table 38–7)

SELECTIVITY. Two major subtypes of beta receptors, designated $beta_1$ and $beta_2$, are present in different proportions in different tissues. $Beta_1$ receptors predominate in the heart, and their stimulation leads to an increase in heart rate, AV conduction and contractility, the release of renin from juxtaglomerular cells in the kidneys, and lipolysis in adipocytes. $Beta_2$ stimulation causes bronchodilation, vasodilation, and glycogenolysis. *Nonselective* beta-blocking drugs (propranolol, nadolol, penbutolol, pindolol, sotalol, timolol, carteolol) block both $beta_1$ and $beta_2$ receptors, whereas *cardioselective* beta blockers (acebutolol, atenolol, betaxolol, bisoprolol, esmolol, and metoprolol) block $beta_1$ receptors while having lesser effects on $beta_2$ receptors. Thus, cardioselective beta blockers reduce myocardial oxygen demands while tending not to block bronchodilation, vasodilation, or glycogenolysis. However, as the doses of these drops are increased, this cardioselectivity diminishes. Because cardioselectivity is only relative, the use of cardioselective beta blockers in doses sufficient to control angina may still cause bronchoconstriction in some susceptible patients.

Some beta blockers also cause vasodilatation. These include labetalol (an alpha-adrenergic blocking agent and $beta_2$ agonist, p. 487), and two investigational drugs, carvedilol (with alpha- and $beta_1$-blocking activity) and bucindolol (a nonselective beta blocker that causes direct [non–alpha-adrenergic mediated] vasodilation).[256,257]

ANTIARRHYTHMIC ACTIONS (see also p. 610). Beta blockers have antiarrhythmic properties as a direct effect of their ability to block sympathoadrenal myocardial stimulation, which in certain situations may be arrhythmogenic.[258] Sotalol (see p. 615) has combined class II (beta-blocking) and class III antiarrhythmic activities; it is an attractive drug when it is desired to treat angina and suppress ventricular tachyarrhythmias.[259,260]

INTRINSIC SYMPATHOMIMETIC ACTIVITY (ISA). Beta blockers with ISA (acebutolol, carteolol, celiprolol, penbutolol, pindolol) are partial beta agonists that also produce blockade by shielding beta receptors from more potent beta agonists. Pindolol and acebutolol produce low-grade beta stimulation when sympathetic activity is low (at rest), whereas these partial agonists behave more like conventional beta blockers when sympathetic activity is high. Agents with ISA may not be as effective as those without this property at reducing heart rate or the frequency, duration, and magnitude of ambulatory ST-segment changes or increasing the duration of exercise in patients with severe angina.[261–263]

POTENCY. This can be measured by the ability of beta blockers to inhibit the tachycardia produced by isoproterenol. All drugs are considered in reference to propranolol, which is given a value of 1.0 (Table 38–7). Timolol and pindolol are the most potent agents, and acebutolol and labetalol are the least.

LIPID SOLUBILITY. The hydrophilicity or lipid solubility of beta blockers is a major determination of their absorption and metabolism. The lipid-soluble (lipophilic) beta blockers, propranolol, metoprolol, and pindolol, are readily absorbed from the gastrointestinal tract, are metabolized predominantly by the liver, have a relatively short half-life, and usually require administration twice or more daily to achieve continuing pharmacological effects. The water-soluble (hydrophilic) beta blockers (atenolol, sotalol, and nadolol) are not as

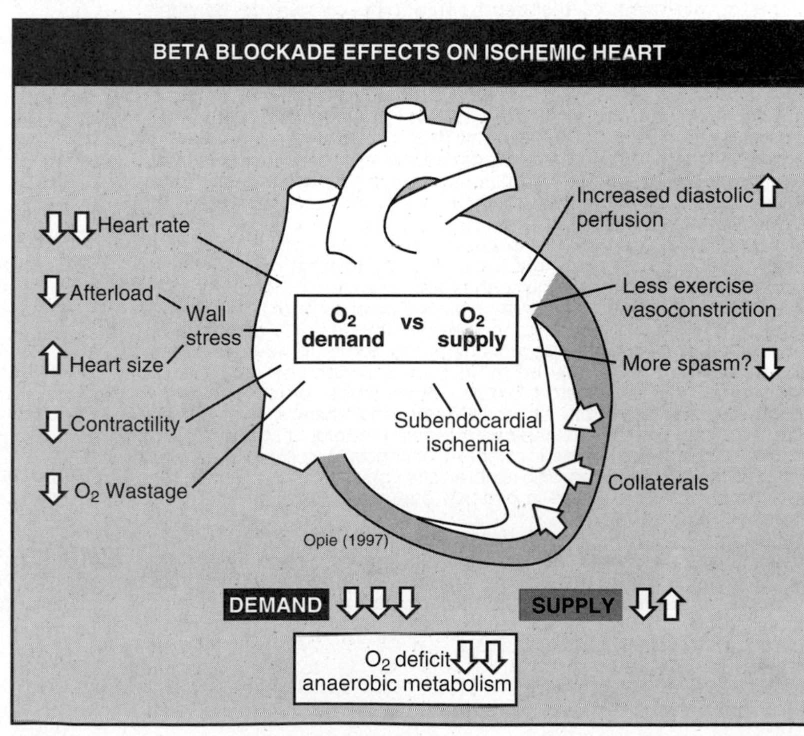

FIGURE 38–5. Effects of beta blockade on the ischemic heart. Beta blockade has a beneficial effect on the ischemic myocardium, unless (1) the preload rises substantially as in left heart failure or (2) there is vasospastic angina when spasm may be promoted in some patients. Note recent proposal that beta blockade diminishes exercise-induced vasoconstriction. (Redrawn from Opie, L. H.: Drugs for the Heart. 4th ed. Philadelphia, W. B. Saunders Company, 1995. Figure copyright L. H. Opie.)

TABLE 38–6 EFFECTS OF ANTIANGINAL AGENTS ON INDICES OF MYOCARDIAL OXYGEN SUPPLY AND DEMAND*

		BETA-ADRENOCEPTOR BLOCKERS				CALCIUM ANTAGONISTS		
		ISA†		Cardio-Selective				
INDEX	NITRATES	*No*	*Yes*	*No*	*Yes*	Nifedipine	Verapamil	Diltiazem
Supply								
Coronary resistance								
Vascular tone	↓↓	↑	0	↑	0↑	↓↓↓	↓↓↓	↓↓↓
Intramyocardial diastolic tension	↓↓↓	↑	0	↑	↑	↓↓	0↑	0
Coronary collateral circulation	↑	0	0	0	0	↑	0	↑
Duration of diastole	0(↓)	↑↑↑	0↓	↑↑↑	↑↑↑	0↑(↓↓)	↑↑↑(↓)	↑↑(↓)
Demand								
Intramyocardial systolic tension								
Preload	↓↓↓	↑	0	↑	↑	↓0	↑0↓	0↓
Afterload (peripheral vascular resistance)	↓	↑	↑	↑↑	↑	↓↓	↓	↓
Contractility	0(↑)	↓↓↓	↓	↓↓↓	↓↓↓	↓(↑↑)‡	↓↓(↑)‡	↓(↑)‡
Heart rate	0(↑)	↓↓↓	0↓	↓↓↓	↓↓↓	0(↑↑)	↓↓(↑)	↓↓(↑)

* ↑ = increase, ↓ = decrease, 0 = little or no definite effect. Number of arrows represents relative intensity of effect. Symbols in parentheses indicate reflex-mediated effects.

† ISA = intrinsic sympathomimetic activity.

‡ Effect of calcium entry on left ventricular *contractility,* as assessed in the intact animal model. The net effect on *left ventricular performance* is variable, being influenced by alterations in afterload, reflex cardiac stimulation, and the underlying state of the myocardium.

From Shub, C., et al.: Selection of optimal drug therapy for the patient with angina pectoris. Mayo Clin. Proc. *60*:539, 1985.

readily absorbed from the gastrointestinal tract, are not as extensively metabolized, have relatively long plasma half-lives, and can be administered once daily. If either metoprolol or propranolol is administered intravenously, a much higher concentration reaches the bloodstream, and therefore intravenous dosing has much greater potency than oral dosing.

ALPHA-ADRENOCEPTOR BLOCKING ACTIVITY. The alpha-blocking potency of labetalol is approximately 20 per cent of its beta-blocking potency, and it is also one of the weaker beta blockers compared with propranolol,[264] although it possesses significant ISA (Table 38–7). Its combined alpha- and beta-blocking effects make it a particularly useful antihypertensive agent (see p. 487), and it is especially so in patients with hypertension and angina. The major side effects of labetalol are postural hypotension and retrograde ejaculation.[254]

OXIDATION PHENOTYPE. Metoprolol and propranolol are lipid-soluble beta blockers noted for the variability of their pharmacokinetics, drug metabolism, and pharmacodynamics. The oxidative metabolism of metoprolol exhibits the debrisoquin type of genetic polymorphism; poor hydroxylators, or metabolizers (up to 10 per cent of Caucasians), have significant prolongation of the elimination half-life of the drug compared with extensive hydroxylators or metabolizers. Thus, angina might be controlled by a single daily dose of metoprolol in poor metabolizers, whereas extensive metabolizers require the same dose two or three times a day.[265] If a patient exhibits an exaggerated clinical response (e.g., extreme bradycardia) following administration of metoprolol, propranolol, or other lipid-soluble beta blockers, it may be the result of prolongation of the elimination half-life due to slow oxidative metabolism.

EFFECTS ON SERUM LIPIDS. Beta-blocker therapy (with agents lacking ISA) usually cause no significant changes in total or LDL cholesterol but they increase triglycerides and reduce HDL cholesterol.[266] The most commonly studied drug has been propranolol, which can increase plasma triglyceride concentrations by up to 50 per cent and reduce HDL cholesterol by approximately 15 per cent. Adverse effects upon the lipid profile may be more frequent with the nonselective than with $beta_1$-selective blockers. Two drugs possessing ISA—acebutolol and pindolol—do not significantly change total cholesterol, triglyerides, or LDL cholesterol, and pindolol *increases* serum HDL cholesterol. The effects of these changes in serum lipids after long-term administration of beta blockers for either hypertension or angina must be considered in patients begun and maintained on this therapy.[267]

MEMBRANE-STABILIZING ACTIVITY. This property refers to the "quinidine-like" effect of certain beta blockers that reduces the rate of rise of the cardiac action potential (see p. 612). The clinical relevance of this effect is negligible (except perhaps in cases of overdose) because it is observed only at concentrations far exceeding therapeutic levels.[268]

DOSAGE. For optimal results, the dosage of beta blocker should be carefully adjusted. In the case of propranolol, it is useful to start with 80 mg of propranolol daily (20 mg four times a day) or comparable doses of other blockers. Twenty-four to 48 hours are required for the drug to achieve an antianginal effect. Efficacy is determined by drug effects on heart rate and symptoms, and, when these are unclear, their effect on exercise performance on a stress test can be evaluated. Resting heart rate should be reduced to between 50 and 60 beats/min, and an increase of less than 20 beats/min should be seen with modest exercise (e.g., climbing one flight of stairs).[269] The usual dosage of propranolol ranges from 80 to 320 mg/day, but some patients require (and tolerate) much higher doses. Therapy needs to be individualized and requires repeated checking of the patient during the initial period of drug administration.

ADVERSE EFFECTS AND CONTRAINDICATIONS. Most of the adverse reactions are a consequence of their beta-blocking properties and include cardiac effects (severe sinus bradycardia, sinus arrest, AV block, reduced left ventricular contractility), bronchoconstriction, fatigue, mental depression, nightmares, gastrointestinal upset, sexual dysfunction, intensification of insulin-induced hypoglycemia, and cutaneous reactions (Tables 38–4 and 38–8). Lethargy, weakness, and fatigue may be caused by reduced cardiac output or may arise from a direct effect on the central nervous system. Bronchoconstriction results from a blockade of $beta_2$ receptors in the tracheobronchial tree. As a consequence, asthma and chronic obstructive lung disease are contraindications to beta blockers, even to $beta_1$-selective agents.[270]

In patients who already have impaired left ventricular function, congestive heart failure may be intensified, an effect that can be counteracted, in part, by the use of digitalis or diuretics. Beginning therapy with a very low dose (e.g., metoprolol 10 mg daily for the first week and then gradually raising it has been shown to be beneficial in selected patients with idiopathic dilated cardiomyopathy and, to a lesser extent, in patients with heart failure due to ischemic heart disease) (see p. 1264).[271]

Beta blockers should be used with *great caution* in patients with cardiac conduction disease involving either the sinus node or the AV conduction system. In patients with

TABLE 38–7 PHARMACOKINETICS AND PHARMACOLOGY OF SOME BETA-ADRENOCEPTOR BLOCKERS

	ATENOLOL	METOPROLOL	NADOLOL	PINDOLOL	PROPRANOLOL	TIMOLOL	PROPRANOLOL HCl	ACEBUTOLOL	LABETALOL	BISOPROLOL	BETAXOLOL	CARTEOLOL	PENBUTOLOL
Extent of absorption (%)	≃50	>95	≃30	>90	90	>90	>90	≃70	>90	>90	>90	>90	100
Extent of bioavailability (% of dose)	≃40	≃50	≃30	≃90	≃30	75	≃30	≃50	≃25	80	90	85	100
Beta-blocking plasma concentration	0.2–0.5 μg ml	50–100 ng ml	50–100 ng ml	50–100 ng ml	50–100 ng ml	50–100 ng ml	50–100 ng ml	0.2–2.0 μg ml	0.7–3.0 μg ml	16–70	20–50		
Protein binding (%)	<5	12	≃30	57	93	≃10	93	30–40	≃50	30	50–60	23–30	80–98
Lipophilicity*	Low	Moderate	Low	Moderate	High	Low	High	Low	Low	Moderate	Moderate	Low	High
Elimination half-life (hr)	6 to 9	3 to 4	14 to 25	3 to 4	3.5 to 6.0	3 to 4	3–4	3–4‡	≃6	7–15	12–22	5–7	
Drug accumulation in renal disease	Yes	No	Yes	No	No	No	No	Yes§	No	Yes	Yes	Yes	Yes
Predominant route of elimination†	RE (mostly unchanged)	HM	RE	RE (≃40% unchanged) and HM	HM	RE (≃20% unchanged) and HM	HM	HM§	HM	HM 50% RE 50%	HM	RE	HM
β_1-blocker potency ratio (propranolol = 1)	1.0	1.0	1.0	6.0	1.0	6.0	1.0	0.3	0.3	10	4	10	1
Relative β_1 sensitivity	+	+	0	0	0	0	0	Yes	0	+	+	0	0
Intrinsic sympathetic activity	0	0	0	+	0	0	0	+	0	0	0	+	+
Membrane-stabilizing activity	0	0	0	+	++	0	++	+	0	0	0	0	0
Usual maintenance dose	50–100 mg qd	50–100 mg qid	40–80 mg qd	5–20 mg tid	60 mg qid	20 mg bid	60 mg qid	200–600 mg bid	100–600 mg/day	5–20 mg qd	5–20 mg qd	2.5–10 mg qd	20 mg qd
FDA-approved indications													
Hypertension	Yes	Yes	Yes	Yes	Yes	Yes	—	Yes	Yes	Yes	Yes	Yes	Yes
Angina	Yes	Yes	Yes	No	Yes	No	—	No	No	No	No	No	No
Post myocardial infarction	Yes	Yes	No	No	Yes	Yes	—	No	No	No	No	No	No

* Determined by the distribution ratio between octanol and water.

† RE = renal excretion; HM = hepatic metabolism.

‡ Half-life of the active metabolite, diacetolol, is 12 to 15 hours.

§ Acebutolol is mainly eliminated by the liver, but its major metabolite, diacetolol, is excreted by the kidney.

Modified from Frishman, W. H., et al.: Antianginal agents, Part 2: β-Blockers. Hosp. Formul. *21*:62, 1986.

TABLE 38–8 CANDIDATES FOR USE OF β-BLOCKING AGENTS FOR ANGINA

Ideal Candidates
Prominent relationship of physical activity to attacks of angina
Coexistent hypertension
History of supraventricular or ventricular arrhythmia
Postmyocardial infarction angina
Prominent anxiety state
Poor Candidates
Asthma or reversible airway component in chronic lung patients
Diabetes
Severe left ventricular dysfunction
Congestive heart failure resulting from systolic impairment
History of depression
Raynaud's phenomenon
Peripheral vascular disease
Bradyarrhythmia

From Abrams, J.: Medical therapy of stable angina pectoris. *In* Beller, G.: Chronic Ischemic Heart Disease. Atlas of Heart Diseases, vol. 5, Braunwald, E. (ed.). Philadelphia, Current Medicine, 1995, p. 7.14.

symptomatic conduction disease, beta blockers are contraindicated unless a pacemaker is in place. In patients with asymptomatic sinus node dysfunction or first degree AV block, beta blockers may be tolerated, but their administration requires careful observation. Pindolol, because of its ISA activity, may be preferable in this situation. Blockade of noncardiac $beta_2$ receptors inhibits catecholamine-induced glycogenolysis so that noncardioselective beta blockers can impair the defense to insulin-induced hypoglycemia.[272] Blockade of $beta_2$ receptors also inhibits the vasodilating effects of catecholamines in peripheral blood vessels and leaves the constrictor (alpha-adrenergic) receptors unopposed and thereby enhances vasoconstriction. Noncardioselective beta blockers may precipitate episodes of Raynaud's phenomenon in patients with this condition and may cause uncomfortable coldness of the distal extremities. Reduced flow to the limbs may occur in patients with peripheral vascular disease.[273]

Abrupt withdrawal of beta-adrenoceptor blocking agents after prolonged administration can result in increased total ischemic activity in patients with chronic stable angina. This may be caused by a return to the previously high levels of myocardial oxygen demand while the underlying atherosclerotic process has progressed.[274] Occasionally such withdrawal can precipitate unstable angina and rarely even provoke myocardial infarction. If abrupt withdrawal of beta blockers is required, patients should be instructed to reduce exertion, manage angina episodes with sublingual nitroglycerin, and/or substitute a calcium antagonist.

Calcium Antagonists

(See also p. 855)

The critical role played by calcium ions in the normal contraction of cardiac and vascular smooth muscle is discussed on p. 366. Calcium antagonists are a heterogeneous group of compounds that inhibit calcium ion movement through slow channels in cardiac and smooth muscle membranes by noncompetitive blockade of voltage-sensitive L-type calcium channels (Fig. 12–10, p. 367).[275–278] There are three major classes of calcium antagonists—the dihydropyridines (of which nifedipine is the prototype), the phenylalkylamines (of which verapamil is the prototype), and the modified benzothiazepines (of which diltiazem is the prototype). The two predominant effects of calcium antagonists result from blocking entry of calcium ions and slowing the recovery of the channel.[275,276] The phenylalkylamines have a marked effect upon the recovery of the channel and thereby exert depressant effects on cardiac pacemakers and conduction, whereas the dihydropyridines, which do not impair channel recovery, have little effect on the conduction system.

The efficacy of calcium antagonists in patients with angina pectoris is related to the reduction in myocardial oxygen demand, together with an increase in oxygen supply which they induce (Table 38–6)[208a]; the latter is particularly important in patients in whom a prominent vasospastic or vasoconstrictor component may be present (i.e., Prinzmetal's variant angina [see p. 1340], patients with variable threshold angina [p. 1293], and patients with abnormal small coronary arteries and impaired vasodilator reserve[279]). Calcium antagonists may be effective on their own in combination with beta-adrenoceptor blockers and nitrates in patients with chronic stable angina.[280–282a]

Six calcium antagonists—verapamil, nifedipine, diltiazem, nicardipine, amlodipine, and bepridil—have been approved by the Food and Drug Administration (FDA) in the United States for the treatment of angina pectoris (Table 38–9). All of these agents are effective in causing relaxation of vascular smooth muscle in both the systemic arterial and coronary arterial beds. In addition, blockade of the entry of calcium into myocytes results in a negative inotropic effect, which is counteracted to some extent by peripheral vascular dilation and by activation of the sympathetic nervous system in response to drug-induced hypotension.[283] However, the negative inotropic effect must be considered in patients with significant left ventricular dysfunction.

Calcium antagonists have a rapid onset of action and are metabolized by the liver, resulting in a limited bioavailability of between 13 and 52 per cent and a half-life of between 3 and 12 hours. Amlodipine and bepridil are exceptions in that both drugs have long half-lives and may be administered once daily. In the case of some of the other calcium antagonists, sustained-release preparations have been shown to be effective.

ANTIATHEROGENIC ACTION. Studies in experimental animals, both primates and nonprimates, have suggested that calcium antagonists might have an antiatherogenic effect, and human studies support this.[284–286] In multicenter, randomized trials utilizing quantitative coronary arteriography, patients showing mild coronary artery disease developed significantly fewer new lesions taking nifedipine than did patients taking placebo. However, preexisting lesions did not appear to be affected. Prolonged follow-up is necessary to determine whether these angiographic observations are accompanied by clinical benefits. In patients undergoing cardiac transplantation, diltiazem has been reported to be beneficial in reducing the frequency and severity of coronary arteriopathy in the transplanted heart[287] (see p. 526).

NIFEDIPINE. This dihydropyridine is a particularly effective dilator of vascular smooth muscle and is a more potent vasodilator than either diltiazem or verapamil. Although its in vitro actions on myocardium and specialized cardiac tissue are similar to those of other agents, the concentration required to reproduce effects on these tissues is not reached in vivo because of the early appearance of its powerful vasodilating effects. Thus, in clinical practice the potential negative chronotropic, inotropic, and dromotropic (on AV conduction) effects of nifedipine are seldom a problem, although even nifedipine can worsen heart failure in patients with preexisting chronic congestive heart failure.[288]

In contrast to beta blockers, which reduce heart rate and the rate pressure product at rest and during exercise, nifedipine reduces only systolic pressure.[289,290] Thus, the beneficial effects of nifedipine in the treatment of angina result from its capacity to reduce myocardial oxygen needs resulting from its afterload-reducing effect and to increase myocardial oxygen delivery consequent to its dilating action on the coronary vascular bed (Table 38–6). In patients without heart failure, nifedipine causes modest reflex increases in ejection fraction, velocity of circumferential fiber

TABLE 38–9 PHARMACOKINETICS OF CALCIUM ANTAGONISTS USED COMMONLY FOR ANGINA PECTORIS*

	DILTIAZEM	NICARDIPINE	NIFEDIPINE	NIFEDIPINE GITS	VERAPAMIL	AMLODIPINE	FELODIPINE	ISRADIPINE	BEPRIDIL
Usual adult dose	IV: 0.25 mg/kg bolus then 0.15 mg/kg/hr Oral: 30–90 mg tid or qid	IV: 10–15 mg/hr for 30 min then 3–5 mg/hr Oral: 20–30 mg tid	SL: 10–30 mg tid or qid Oral: 10–30 mg tid or qid	Oral: 30–60 mg daily	IV: 0.075 to 0.015 mg/kg Oral: 80–120 mg tid or qid	2.5–10 mg qd	5–20 mg qd	2.5–5.0 mg bid	200–400 mg qd
Extent of absorption (%)	80–90	-100	90	>90	90	>90	>90	>90	>90
Extent of bioavailability (% of dose)	40–70	30	65–75	45–75	20–35	60–65	20	15–24	>80
Onset of action	Oral: <15 min	<20 min	SL: <3 min Oral: <20 min	Approximately 6 hr	IV: 2 min Oral: 2 hr	1–2 hr	2 hr	20 min	2–3 hr
Peak effect	Oral: 30 min	1 hr	Oral: 1–2 hr	After 6 hr	IV 3–5 min Oral 3–4 hr	6–12 hr	2–5 hr	1.5 hr	8 h
Therapeutic serum levels (ng/ml)	50–200	30–50	25–100	25–100	80–300	5–20	1–5	2–10	500–2000
Elimination half-life (hr)	3.5–6.0	2.0–4.0	2.0–5.0	2.0–5.0	3.0–7.0†	30–50	9	8	26–64
Elimination	60% metabolized by liver; remainder excreted by kidneys	High first-pass hepatic metabolism	High first-pass hepatic metabolism	High first-pass hepatic metabolism	85% eliminated by first-pass hepatic metabolism	Hepatic	High first-pass hepatic metabolism	High first-pass hepatic metabolism	Hepatic
Heart rate	↓	↑	↑↑	↑	↓	0	↑	0	↓
Peripheral vasc. resistance	↓	↓	↓↓↓	↓↓	↓	↓↓↓	↓↓↓	↓↓↓	↓
FDA approved indications									
Hypertension	Yes	Yes	Yes	Yes	Yes	Yes	Yes	Yes	Yes
Angina	Yes	Yes	Yes	Yes	Yes	Yes	No	No	Yes
Coronary spasm	Yes	No	Yes	Yes	Yes	Yes	No	No	No

* All agents approved by FDA for treatment of angina pectoris.
† 4.5–12 hr with multiple dosing.
GITS, gastrointestinal therapeutic system; IV, intravenous; SL, sublingual.

shortening, heart rate, and cardiac index; these increases can be blocked by beta-adrenoceptor blockade.

The dose is 10 mg orally every 8 hours, increased stepwise to 20 mg every 6 hours, guided by the blood pressure response to a minimal dose of 160 mg. An extended-release formulation utilizing the gastrointestinal therapeutic system (GITS) of drug delivery (Table 38–9) is designed to deliver 30, 60, or 90 mg of nifedipine in a single daily dose at a relatively constant rate over a 24-hour period and is useful for the treatment of chronic stable angina, Prinzmetal's angina, and hypertension.[291] The efficacy of the extended-release preparation, either alone or in conjunction with beta blockers, in reducing episodes of angina and of ischemia on ambulatory monitoring has been documented.[292]

Adverse Effects. These occur in 15 to 20 per cent of patients and require discontinuation of medication in about 5 per cent. Most adverse effects are related to the systemic vasodilation and include headache, dizziness, palpitations, flushing, hypotension, and leg edema (unrelated to heart failure). Gastrointestinal side effects, including nausea, epigastric pressure, and vomiting, are noted in approximately 5 per cent of patients. Rarely, in patients with extremely severe, fixed coronary obstructions, nifedipine aggravates angina, presumably by lowering arterial pressure excessively with subsequent reflex tachycardia. For this reason, combined therapy of angina with nifedipine and a beta blocker is particularly effective and superior to nifedipine alone.[281,282] Most of the adverse effects are reduced by the use of the extended-release preparations. Review of multiple clinical trials has revealed that short-acting nifedipine may cause an increase in mortality.[292a] There are no firm data that this risk applies to extended-release nifedipine or to other calcium antagonists.[292b,292c] Clearly, insufficient data are available to assess the long-term risks (if any) of calcium antagonists in chronic CAD. As of this writing it is recommended that patients with CAD—especially those with acute coronary syndromes—not receive short-acting nifedipine. Instead, they may be placed on extended-release nifedipine or on another calcium antagonist.

A comparison of the side effects of nifedipine with those of other calcium antagonists is shown in Table 38–4. Because of its potent vasodilator effects, nifedipine is *contraindicated* in patients who are hypotensive or who have severe aortic valve stenosis and in patients with unstable angina who are *not* simultaneously receiving a beta blocker and in whom reflex-mediated increases in heart rate may be harmful. Nifedipine (or one of the second-generation dihydropyridines) is the calcium antagonist of choice in patients with mild left ventricular dysfunction, sinus bradycardia, sick sinus syndrome, and AV block (particularly if a beta-adrenoceptor blocking agent is concurrently administered and additional drug therapy of angina is indicated).[281] This is because in the dosages used clinically these agents have fewer negative effects on myocardial contractility or on the specialized automatic and conduction systems than does verapamil or diltiazem. Nonetheless, in patients with more serious left ventricular dysfunction, all calcium antagonists—even nifedipine—can precipitate heart failure.[288]

Nifedipine interacts significantly with prazosin (resulting in excessive hypotension), cimetidine, and phenytoin (resulting in increased bioavailability of nifedipine and increased quinidine clearance). Nifedipine increases blood levels of propranolol and when the two drugs are used together there is a risk of an added negative inotropic and hypotensive effect.[290] In patients with Prinzmetal's variant angina, abrupt cessation of nifedipine therapy may result in a rebound increase in the frequency and duration of attacks (see p. 1343).

VERAPAMIL (see also p. 616). Verapamil dilates systemic and coronary resistance vessels and large coronary conductance vessels. It slows heart rate and reduces myocardial contractility. This combination of actions results in a reduction of the myocardial oxygen demands, the basis for the drug's efficacy in the management of chronic stable angina. Thrombus formation and whole blood platelet aggregation levels in response to thrombin are decreased by verapamil (as well as to transdermal nitroglycerin). To what extent the clinical benefits of verapamil and nitrates are related to their effects on platelet aggregation and thrombus formation is uncertain.[293]

Verapamil accelerates left ventricular diastolic filling at rest and during exercise in patients with chronic stable angina, whereas beta blockade does not have this effect.[294] Despite the marked negative inotropic effects of verapamil in isolated cardiac muscle preparations, changes in contractility are modest in patients with normal cardiac function. However, in patients with cardiac dysfunction, verapamil, like beta blockers, may reduce cardiac output, elevate left ventricular filling pressure, and cause clinical heart failure. In clinically useful doses, verapamil inhibits calcium influx into specialized cardiac cells, sometimes causing slowing of heart rate and AV conduction. Therefore, it is contraindicated in patients with preexisting atrioventricular nodal disease or sick sinus syndrome, congestive heart failure, and suspected digitalis or quinidine toxicity. In the treatment of effort-related angina, verapamil is comparable to propranolol, causing dose-dependent reductions in the frequency of anginal episodes, although the combination results in better exercise capacity than either alone.[294]

The usual starting dose of verapamil for oral administration is 40 to 80 mg three times daily to a maximum dose of 480 mg/day (Table 38–9). Sustained-release capsules of verapamil are available (60 mg, 90 mg, and 120 mg), and starting doses are 60 to 120 mg twice daily with a usual optimal dose range of 240 to 360 mg/day.

Verapamil interacts significantly with a number of other drugs. *Intravenous* verapamil should not be used together with a beta blocker (given intravenously *or* orally), nor should a beta blocker be administered intravenously in patients receiving oral verapamil. The bioavailability of verapamil is increased by cimetidine and carbamazepine, whereas verapamil may increase plasma levels of cyclosporine and digoxin and may be associated with excessive hypotension in patients receiving quinidine or prazosin. Hepatic enzyme inducers such as phenobarbital may reduce the effects of verapamil.

Adverse effects of verapamil are noted in approximately 10 per cent of patients and relate to systemic dilation (hypotension and facial flushing), gastrointestinal symptoms (constipation and nausea), and central nervous system reactions such as headache and dizziness. A rare side effect is gingival hyperplasia appearing after 1 to 9 months of therapy.[283]

DILTIAZEM. Diltiazem's actions are intermediate between those of nifedipine and verapamil. In clinically useful doses its vasodilator effects are less profound than nifedipine's, and its cardiac depressant action (on the sinoatrial and AV nodes and myocardium) less than those of verapamil. This profile may explain the remarkably low incidence of adverse effects of diltiazem. This drug is a systemic vasodilator, lowering arterial pressure at rest and during exertion and increasing the workload required to produce myocardial ischemia, but it may also increase myocardial oxygen delivery. Although diltiazem causes little vasodilation of epicardial coronary arteries under basal conditions, it may enhance perfusion of the subendocardium distal to a flow-limiting coronary stenosis[295]; it also blocks exercise-induced coronary vasoconstriction.[291] In patients with ischemic heart disease, diltiazem reduces afterload and depresses myocardial systolic function but improves left ventricular relaxation.[296] In patients with chronic stable angina receiving maximally tolerated doses of diltiazem there is a significant reduction in heart rate at rest, but there is no effect on peak blood pressure achieved during exercise, and the duration of symptom-limited treadmill exercise is prolonged.

The dose of diltiazem is 30 to 60 mg four times daily, although higher doses are sometimes needed. A sustained-release formulation (Diltiazem CD) has been approved for the once-daily treatment of systemic hypertension and angina pectoris and is available in capsules of 120 mg, 180 mg, 240 mg, and 300 mg.[297]

Diltiazem is a highly effective antianginal agent. Both atenolol and diltiazem are of similar efficacy in increasing nonischemic exercise duration in patients with variable-threshold angina and act primarily by slowing the resting heart rate.[298] High doses (mean dose 340 mg) have been shown to be a relatively safe addition to maximally tolerated doses of isosorbide dinitrate and a beta blocker, causing increases in exercise tolerance and resting and exercise left ventricular ejection fraction.[297] Major side effects are similar to those of the other calcium channel blockers and related to vasodilatation, but these are relatively infrequent, particularly if the dose does not exceed 240 mg/day.[283] As is the case with verapamil, diltiazem should be used with caution in patients with sick sinus syndrome and AV block. In patients with preexisting left ventricular dysfunction, diltiazem may exacerbate or precipitate heart failure.[283]

Diltiazem interacts with other drugs, including beta-adrenergic blocking agents (causing enhanced negative inotropic, chronotropic, and dromotropic effects), flecainide, and cimetidine (which increases the bioavailability of diltiazem), and diltiazem has been associated with increased plasma levels of cyclosporine, carbamazepine, and lithium carbonate. Diltiazem may cause excess sinus node depression if administered with disopyramide and reduce digoxin clearance, especially in patients with renal failure.[299]

Second-Generation Calcium Antagonists

The "second-generation" calcium antagonists (nicardipine, isradipine, amlodipine, and felodipine) are mainly dihydropyridine derivatives, with nifedipine, the prototypical agent. There is also considerable experience with nimodipine, hisoldipine, and nitrendipine, which, however, are not licensed in the United States. These agents differ in potency, tissue specificity, and pharmacokinetics and in general are potent vasodilators due to greater vascular selectivity than with the "first generation" antagonists, i.e., verapamil, nifedipine, and diltiazem.

AMLODIPINE. This agent, which is less lipid soluble than nifedipine, has a slow, smooth onset and ultralong duration of action (plasma half-life = 36 hours). It causes marked coronary and peripheral dilatation and may be useful in the treatment of patients with angina accompanied by hypertension. It may be used as a once-daily hypotensive or antianginal agent.[300] In a series of randomized placebo-controlled studies in patients with stable exercise-induced angina pectoris, amlodipine has been shown to be effective and well tolerated.[301] It has little, if any, negative inotropic action and may be especially useful in patients with chronic angina and left ventricular dysfunction. It has been suggested that amlodipine may be useful in the treatment of heart failure, but definitive proof awaits the outcome of current ongoing trials.[302,303] Preliminary data from the placebo-controlled Prospective Randomized Amlodipine Survival Evaluation (PRAISE) study demonstrated no increase in mortality or hospitalization for life-threatening cardiovascular events in patients with New York Heart Class III-IV failure and a mean ejection fraction of 21 per cent when amlodipine was added to a full regimen of digoxin, diuretic, and ACE inhibitor therapy. In patients with nonischemic dilated cardiomyopathy, all-cause mortality was 21.5 per cent in those assigned to amlodipine versus 34.5 per cent in those assigned to placebo; a 45 per cent reduction in relative risk ($P = 0.001$). No significant difference in survival was observed in patients with ischemic cardiomyopathy. These data *suggest* that in patients with congestive heart failure due to ischemic heart disease, who need a calcium channel antagonist for hypertension or angina, survival is not adversely affected by amlodipine.[302]

NICARDIPINE. This drug has a similar half-life to nifedipine (2 to 4 hours), but intravenous administration is easier because it is water soluble without associated light sensitivity.[283] It also appears to have greater vascular selectivity. Nicardipine may be used as an antianginal and antihypertensive agent requiring thrice-daily administration, although a sustained-release formulation is available for twice-daily dosing in hypertension. For chronic stable angina pectoris, it appears to be as effective as verapamil or diltiazem, and its efficacy is enhanced when combined with a beta blocker.

FELODIPINE AND ISRADIPINE. In the United States, both drugs are approved by the FDA for the treatment of hypertension but not angina pectoris.[283] A recent study documented similar efficacy between felodipine and nifedipine in patients with chronic stable angina.[304] *Felodipine* has also been reported to be more vascular selective than nifedipine and to have a mild *positive* inotropic effect due to calcium channel agonist properties. *Isradipine* has a longer half-life than nifedipine and demonstrates greater vascular sensitivity.

BEPRIDIL. This calcium antagonist interacts with the dihydropyridine binding site and has a sodium channel blocking effect.[283] It markedly prolongs the atrial refractory period and may be useful in the treatment of patients with angina and arrhythmias, although it is also arrhythmogenic and causes Q-T prolongation and *torsades de pointes*.[305] Although chemically unrelated to the other calcium channel blockers, bepridil has been shown to be an effective antianginal agent. Nonetheless, because of its potential to prolong the Q-T interval and cause torsades de pointes, the drug should be reserved for patients in whom other antianginal drugs have failed.[283] Interactions with antiarrhythmic agents, tricyclic antidepressants, and cardiac glycosides are potentially hazardous.

Medical Management of Angina Pectoris

RELATIVE ADVANTAGES OF BETA BLOCKERS AND CALCIUM ANTAGONISTS. The choice between a beta blocker and a calcium channel antagonist as initial therapy in patients with chronic stable angina is controversial because both classes of agents are effective in relieving symptoms and reducing ischemia.[141a,283a,283b] Because long-term administration of beta blockers has been found to prolong life in patients after acute myocardial infarction and in the treatment of hypertension, many have extrapolated these findings to patients with angina and prefer these agents to calcium antagonists. The authors of this chapter consider this extrapolation to be a reasonable one. In addition, a possible risk of short-acting nifedipine in CAD has been raised (see p. 1310), although this possibility is unresolved. However, it must be recognized that beta blockers (without intrinsic sympathomimetic activity) increase serum triglycerides and decrease HDL cholesterol with uncertain long-term consequences.[266,267] In contrast, the long-term administration of calcium antagonists has *not* been shown to improve long-term survival following acute myocardial infarction, although diltiazem apparently is effective in preventing severe angina and early reinfarction after non-Q-wave infarction[306] and verapamil reduces reinfarction rates,[307] while nifedipine has been associated with the development of fewer new coronary artery lesions[284,285] in patients with established CAD.

The choice of the drug with which to initiate therapy is influenced by a number of clinical factors (Table 38–10).

1. Calcium antagonists are the preferable agents in patients with a history of asthma or chronic obstructive lung disease and/or with wheezing on clinical examination, in whom beta blockers, even relatively selective agents, are contraindicated.

TABLE 38–10 RECOMMENDED DRUG THERAPY (CALCIUM ANTAGONIST VS BETA BLOCKER) IN PATIENTS WHO HAVE ANGINA IN CONJUNCTION WITH OTHER MEDICAL CONDITIONS*

CLINICAL CONDITION	RECOMMENDED DRUG (ALTERNATIVE DRUG)
Cardiac arrhythmias and conduction abnormalities	
Sinus bradycardia	Nifedipine**
Sinus tachycardia (not due to cardiac failure)	Beta blocker
Supraventricular tachycardia	Verapamil or beta blocker
Atrioventricular block	Nifedipine**
Rapid atrial fibrillation (with digitalis)	Verapamil or beta blocker
Ventricular arrhythmias	Beta blocker (± group 1 antiarrhythmic agent)
Left ventricular dysfunction	
Congestive heart failure	
Mild (LVEF ≥ 40%)	Nifedipine** (verapamil, diltiazem, or beta blockers cautiously)
Moderate to severe (LVEF < 40%)	Nifedipine** (cautiously, in combination with other therapy)
Left-sided valvular heart disease†	
Aortic stenosis (mild)‡	Beta blocker
Aortic insufficiency	Nifedipine**
Mitral regurgitation	Nifedipine**
Mitral stenosis§	Beta blocker
Miscellaneous medical conditions	
Systemic hypertension	Beta blocker (calcium antagonists)
Severe preexisting headaches	Beta blockers (verapamil or diltiazem)
COPD with bronchospasm or asthma	Nifedipine,** verapamil, or diltiazem
Hyperthyroidism	Beta blocker
Raynaud's syndrome	Nifedipine**
Claudication	Nifedipine,** verapamil, or diltiazem (low-dose $beta_1$ blocker or beta-ISA)
Depression	Nifedipine,** verapamil, or diltiazem
Neurasthenia or fatigue states	Nifedipine,** verapamil, or diltiazem
Insulin-dependent diabetes mellitus	Nifedipine,** verapamil, or diltiazem (low-dose $beta_1$ blocker or beta-ISA)

* From Shub, C., et al.: Selection of optimal drug therapy for the patient with angina pectoris. Mayo Clin. Proc. *60*:539, 1985.

Beta-ISA = beta blocker with intrinsic sympathomimetic activity such as pindolol or acebutolol; COPD = chronic obstructive pulmonary disease; LVEF = left ventricular ejection fraction.

† Surgical therapy should be considered for patients with severe valvular heart disease; beta blockers are not routinely used in patients with valvular heart disease and left ventricular failure.

‡ Vasodilators may increase aortic valve gradient, and beta blockers can cause left ventricular failure. Any of these drugs should be used with extreme caution in patients with severe aortic stenosis.

§ If congestive heart failure (associated with normal left ventricular function) occurs in a patient with angina, severe mitral stenosis, and rapid atrial fibrillation, a beta blocker (in combination with digitalis) may be used to decrease the heart rate.

** Long-acting slow-release nifedipine.

2. Nifedipine (long-acting) or nicardipine is the calcium antagonist of choice in patients with sick sinus syndrome, sinus bradycardia, or significant AV conduction disturbances, whereas beta blockers and verapamil should be used only with great caution in such patients. In patients with symptomatic conduction disease, neither a beta blocker nor a calcium blocker should be used unless a pacemaker is in place. If a beta blocker is required in patients with asymptomatic evidence of conduction disease, pindolol, which has the greatest intrinsic sympathomimetic activity, is useful. In the case of calcium channel blockers, nifedipine or nicardipine is preferable to verapamil and diltiazem, but careful observation for deterioration of conduction is mandatory.

3. Calcium antagonists are clearly preferred in patients suspected of having Prinzmetal's variant angina; beta blockers may even aggravate angina under these circumstances.

4. Calcium antagonists may be preferred over beta blockers in patients with significant, symptomatic peripheral arterial disease because the latter may cause peripheral vasoconstriction.

5. Beta blockers should usually be avoided in patients with histories of significant depressive illness, sexual dysfunction, sleep disturbance, nightmares, fatigue, or lethargy.

6. The presence of moderate to severe left ventricular dysfunction in patients with angina limits the therapeutic options. Obviously, cardiac failure may be controlled with diuretics, digitalis, and angiotensin-converting enzyme inhibitors, and nitrates can be used for the management of angina. However, when cardiac failure is treated and angina persists, other agents may be required. Verapamil and beta blockers are more likely to be associated with adverse effects under these circumstances. Nifedipine and diltiazem are reasonable choices if the left ventricular ejection fraction is greater than 30 per cent and overt cardiac failure does not exist.[308] Whether amlodipine or a highly vascular-selective calcium antagonist, such as felodipine, will prove to be superior in such patients remains to be seen, but initial results with amlodipine are encouraging.[302].

7. Nifedipine should *not* be used as the initial and only agent in patients with unstable angina (see p. 1337), but treatment should be initiated with nitrates and beta blockers to avoid the reflex-mediated tachycardia associated with nifedipine alone that may aggravate unstable angina.[309] However, long-acting nifedipine may be helpful when added to a beta blocker.

8. Hypertensive patients with angina pectoris do well with either beta blockers or calcium antagonists because both agents have antihypertensive effects.

9. Patients with ischemia (symptomatic and asymptomatic) detected by ambulatory electroardiography are improved by both classes of agents. A combination is more effective than either alone.[310]

10. A beta blocker is usually considered first when there is a relatively fixed anginal threshold and myocardial ischemia is caused primarily by an increase in myocardial oxygen demand in the face of a fixed supply. Conversely, in patients with variable-threshold angina in whom reductions of myocardial blood supply may be caused by alterations in coronary vasomotor tone, a calcium antagonist has been presumed to be preferable to a beta blocker. However, although this is a logical approach, its validity remains to be proven.

COMBINATION THERAPY. The combination of a beta-adrenoreceptor blocker, calcium antagonist, and long-acting nitrate is widely used in the management of chronic stable angina. When adrenergic blockers and calcium antagonists are used together in the treatment of angina pectoris, a number of issues should be considered:

1. The addition of a beta blocker enhances the clinical effect of nifedipine and other dihydropyridines.
2. In patients with moderate or severe left ventricular dysfunction, sinus bradycardia, or AV conduction disturbances, combination therapy with calcium antagonists and beta blockers either should be avoided or should be initiated with caution.[311] In patients with AV conduction system disease, the preferred combination is long-acting nifedipine or another dihydropyridine and a beta blocker. The negative inotropic effects of calcium antagonists are not usually a problem in combined therapy with low doses of beta blockers but can become significant with higher doses. With such doses, nifedipine and nicardipine are the calcium antagonists of choice, but they should be used cautiously.
3. The combination of a dihydropyridine and a long-acting nitrate (without a beta blocker) is not an optimal combination because both are vasodilators.

Approach to the Patient with Chronic Stable Angina

1. Identify and treat precipitating factors, such as anemia, uncontrolled hypertension, thyrotoxicosis, tachyarrhythmias, uncontrolled congestive heart failure, and concomitant valvular heart disease.
2. Initiate risk factor modification, physical exercise, and life style counseling.
3. Initiate pharmacotherapy with aspirin and sublingual nitroglycerin. Employ the latter for the alleviation of symptoms and prophylactically (see p. 1302).
4. In many patients, sublingual nitroglycerin is the only anti-ischemic agent required, but if episodes occur more than two or three times per week, the next step is the addition of *either* a beta blocker or a calcium antagonist; the choice is discussed above. The decision to add a beta blocker or calcium antagonist to a nitrate is not based entirely on the frequency and severity of symptoms. The need to treat concomitant hypertension or the presence of a prior myocardial infarction may indicate the use of one of these agents even in patients in whom episodes of symptomatic angina are infrequent.
5. If angina persists, add a long-acting nitrate using eccentric dosing schedules to prevent nitrate tolerance. An assessment of the pattern and the timing of angina often helps govern the timing of drug administration.
6. If angina persists despite two antianginal agents (a long-acting nitrate preparation with either a beta blocker *or* calcium antagonist), add the third antianginal agent.
7. Coronary angiography, with a view to considering coronary revascularization, is indicated in patients with refractory symptoms or ischemia despite optimal medical therapy; it should also be carried out in patients with "high-risk" noninvasive tests (see p. 165) and in those with occupations or life styles that indicate a more aggressive approach.

PERCUTANEOUS TRANSLUMINAL CORONARY ANGIOPLASTY AND RELATED CATHETER-BASED TECHNIQUES

(See also Chap. 39)

Percutaneous transluminal coronary angioplasty (PTCA) and other catheter-based techniques represent a major therapeutic advance in the management of chronic stable angina.[312,313] Their importance to the management of CAD in the United States is reflected by a performance of approximately 360,000 procedures in 1993, a more than 10-fold increase during the last decade.[314] This increase has not been accompanied by a reduction in the number of patients undergoing coronary bypass surgery.[315]

PATIENT SELECTION (Table 63–8, p. 1955). Improved technology and increasing operator experience have expanded the pool of patients with both single and multivessel disease who are candidates for PTCA (and other catheter-based techniques for revascularization). Factors that need to be taken into account in patient selection include the following:

1. The need for revascularization (surgical or catheter-based) as opposed to medical therapy
2. The likelihood of a successful catheter-based revascularization based upon angiographic characteristics of the lesion—type A, B, or C lesions,[316] which characterize complexity as mild, moderate, or severe, respectively (Table 39–3, p. 1370)
3. The risk and potential consequences of acute PTCA failure
4. The likelihood of restenosis
5. The need for complete revascularization
6. The presence of comorbid conditions and the suitability of the patient for surgery
7. Patient preference

The patient with chronic stable angina who is ideal for PTCA, i.e., who is at low risk for complications and in whom the likelihood of technical success is high, is a male with chronic stable angina less than 70 years of age, with single-vessel and single-lesion CAD, the anatomical characteristics of a type A lesion with less than 90 per cent stenosis, no history of congestive heart failure, and an ejection fraction greater than 40 per cent.

Features associated with increased risk for PTCA include advanced age, female gender, a history of congestive heart failure, the presence of left ventricular dysfunction,[317–319] left main coronary artery equivalent disease, unstable angina, recent thrombolytic therapy, and type B or C lesions. However, it has been suggested that the classification of type A, B, and C lesions may be simplistic in the light of increasing operative experience and new technologies.[320] The presence of the aforementioned features does not necessarily contraindicate PTCA but should raise the threshold for performing the procedure. Lower procedural volumes in individual laboratories have also been shown to correlate with increased complications.[320a]

ACUTE OUTCOME. Continued improvements in the technical aspects of PTCA as well as increasing operator experience have had a favorable impact on the rate of primary success (usually defined as an increase of diameter narrowing >20 per cent and a final diameter obstruction <50 per cent) and a reduction in complications. This has occurred despite a broadening of the selection criteria for PTCA to include older and sicker patients with more complex anatomy.[312,319,321] Current expectations for angioplasty are an overall success rate in excess of 90 per cent with an acute complication rate of under 5 per cent, particularly in patients with single-vessel disease.

ABRUPT CLOSURE. This refers to a sustained and significate reduction in flow in the target vessel, which is usually recognized prior to leaving the laboratory.[322] In addition to clinical signs and symptoms of ischemia, the angiographic appearance of extensive dissection or thrombus is strongly associated with subsequent total occlusion. The incidence of abrupt closure ranges from 2 to 11 per cent, depending, in part, upon the definitions used; subsequent morbidity and mortality are high. Clinical risk factors for acute closure include advanced age, female gender, unstable angina pectoris, diabetes, chronic hemodialysis, and recent thrombolytic therapy.[323–325] Angiographic correlates of abrupt closure include proximity of the lesion to a branch vessel, lesion length greater than 10 mm, the presence of thrombus, diffuse disease, angulated lesions, diameter stenosis of 80 to 90 per cent, and calcified lesions.[326,327]

Management. The treatment objectives of abrupt closure are to establish adequate coronary perfusion as a bridge to coronary bypass surgery, or, in some patients, as a definitive strategy. Newer therapeutic options have reduced the morbidity of acute vessel closure and include prolonged balloon inflations, stent placement (Fig. 39–10, p. 1380); the use of autoperfusion catheters (Fig. 39–2, p. 1367), adjunctive hemodynamic support, and in some patients the administration of a thrombolytic agent.[312,321,328–331] A reduction in distal flow without apparent dissection or distal embolization occurs in about 2 per cent of patients undergoing PTCA and is frequently reversed by intracoronary verapamil or diltiazem, suggesting that microvascular spasm is responsible.[332,333]

A randomized trial of a monoclonal antibody to the platelet glycoprotein IIb/IIIa receptor in patients considered at "high risk" of complications after coronary angioplasty has documented a reduction in periprocedural adverse outcome[334] (Table 39–2, p. 1370), but with increased bleeding complications.[335]

Long-Term Results. For the majority of patients undergoing PTCA, the intermediate and late outcomes can be characterized by a low mortality or nonfatal myocardial infarction rate. Long-term prognosis after an initially successful PTCA is similar between men and women.[336]

COMPARISON BETWEEN PTCA AND MEDICAL THERAPY. The first major randomized trial involving PTCA was the Veterans Administration Comparison of Angioplasty with Medical Therapy in the treatment of single-vessel coronary artery disease.[337] Eighty-six per cent of the patients had stable angina, all were male, and the duration of follow-up was 6 months. PTCA was distinctly superior to medical therapy in the relief of angina and in the improvement in exercise tolerance, although repeat PTCA or CABG was required in 15 per cent of patients by 6 months (Fig. 38–6). A conclusion that can be drawn from this study is that a trial of medical therapy followed by PTCA in the event of treatment failure is a reasonable initial strategy for patients with stable angina and single-vessel disease. Nonetheless, indices of quality of life, including functional capacity and the patient's perception of well-being, were significantly better among patients treated with PTCA.[337a] In a small randomized trial of PTCA, medical therapy and coronary bypass surgery in patients with a proximal stenosis of the left anterior descending coronary artery, there was no difference in the combined endpoint of cardiac death, myocardial infarction, or refractory angina requiring revascularization between PTCA and medical therapy. Coronary bypass surgery, however, was superior to the other two therapeutic modalities.[337b]

The Duke University data base provides important information on the relative benefits of bypass surgery, PTCA, and medical therapy upon survival in 9263 patients referred for cardiac catheterization between 1984 and 1990.[338] Adjusted 5-year survival for patients with single-vessel disease was similar—95 per cent with PTCA and 94 per cent with medical therapy; in patients with two-vessel disease, this was 91 per cent versus 86 per cent, respectively; and in patients with three-vessel disease, it was 81 per cent versus 72 per cent. These trends suggest that PTCA is superior to medical management in patients with multivessel disease (Fig. 38–7). The 10-year follow-up of the first series of patients who underwent PTCA performed by Gruentzig is encouraging, with a survival rate of 95 per cent in patients with single-vessel disease and 81 per cent in patients with multivessel disease.[339] In the NHLBI Registry, 5-year survival was 93.2 per cent in patients with single-vessel disease, 88.8 per cent in patients with two-vessel disease, and 86 per cent with three-vessel disease. Both early and late outcomes appear to be improving.[340] Restenosis, the Achilles heel of angioplasty (see below), continues to exert the major influence upon long-term outcome.[321] The recurrence of angina is frequent,[341–350] leading to the need for coronary bypass surgery in approximately 20 per cent of patients after 1 to 3 years and of repeat PTCA in approximately 40 per cent by 3 years.[351]

PTCA IN PATIENTS WITH LEFT VENTRICULAR DYSFUNCTION. Several studies of PTCA in patients with left ventricular dysfunction have documented a high initial procedural success rate with successful dilatation of one lesion in 88 per cent and of 76 per cent for all lesions. However, long-term results were less favorable. Two-year survival among

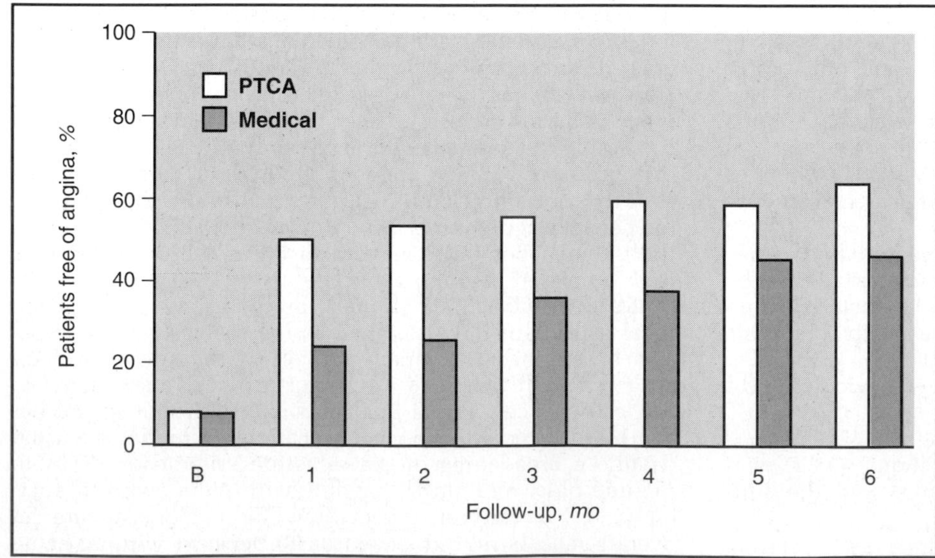

FIGURE 38–6. The percentage of patients free of angina at 1-month intervals after randomization in the Veterans Administration ACME trial. The horizontal axis shows the month after randomization (baseline B) in clinic visits at months 1 through 6 for each treatment group. PTCA = percutaneous transluminal coronary angioplasty. (From Gersh, B. J.: Natural history of chronic coronary artery disease. *In* Beller, G. A. [ed.]: Chronic Ischemic Heart Disease. Atlas of Heart Diseases, vol. 5. Philadelphia, Current Medicine, 1995, p. 1.21. Adapted from Parisi, A. F., et al.: A comparison of angioplasty with medical therapy in the treatment of single-vessel coronary artery disease. N. Engl. J. Med. *326*:10, 1992. Copyright Massachusetts Medical Society.)

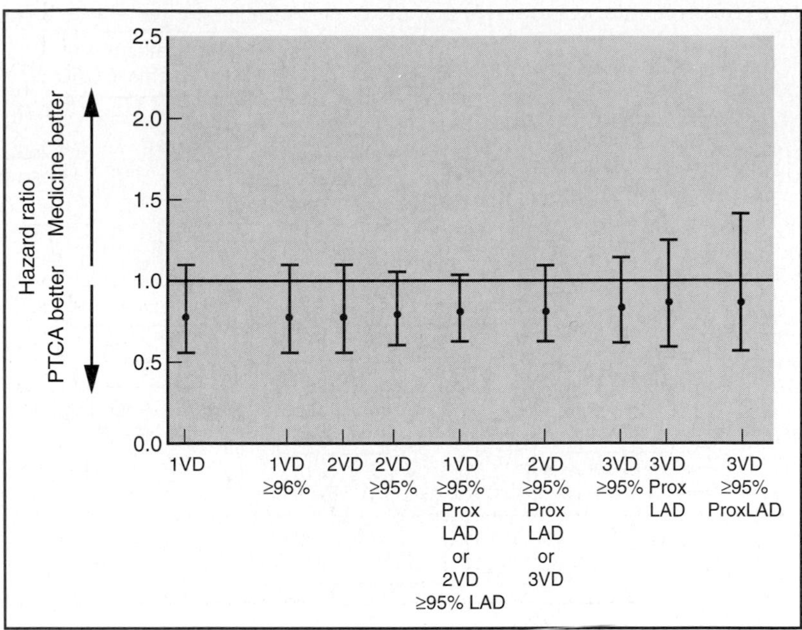

FIGURE 38–7. Hazard ratios for percutaneous transluminal coronary angioplasty (PTCA) versus medicine, calculated from the Cox regression model to evaluate relative survival differences. Points indicate hazard ratios for each level of the coronary artery disease index; bars indicate 99 per cent confidence intervals. Horizontal line at ratio 1.0 indicates point of prognostic equivalence between treatments. Hazard ratios below the line favor PTCA; those above the line favor medicine. VD = vessel disease; Prox LAD = proximal left anterior descending coronary artery. (Reproduced with permission from Mark, D. B., Nelson, C. L., Califf, R. M., et al.: Continuing evaluation of therapy for coronary artery disease: Initial results from the era of coronary angioplasty. Circulation *89:*2015, 1994. Copyright American Heart Association.)

patients with an ejection fraction of 0.40 or less and multivessel disease was only approximately 75 per cent.[352] In another series, 23 per cent of patients with an ejection fraction of 0.35 or less died during a 21-month mean follow-up.[353] In a recent report from the National Heart, Lung and Blood Institute registry, the 4-year survival in patients with very poor left ventricular function in whom the ejection fraction was less than 0.25 was only 45 per cent.[341] Another recent study demonstrated similar results with a 3-year survival of 83 per cent and 92 per cent in patients with ejection fractions of 0.31 to 0.35 and 0.36 to 0.40, respectively, but only 69 per cent in patients with an ejection fraction of 0.30 or less.[341,354] To achieve a good outcome in patients with multivessel disease and left ventricular dysfunction, particularly if angina or ischemia is severe, revascularization should be complete.[342] This is often difficult to achieve with PTCA and other catheter-based revascularization techniques, particularly in the presence of chronic total occlusions. This limitation of angioplasty in the achievement of complete revascularization is an important factor contributing to the relatively disappointing results of this procedure in patients with significant left ventricular dysfunction and multivessel disease.[317]

RESTENOSIS. Although a striking improvement has occurred in the initial results of PTCA during the past 15 years, restenosis continued to dominate late events. The most frequently used definition is a greater than 50 per cent diameter stenosis and/or greater than 50 per cent late loss of the acute luminal gain,[344,347] but there is no clear consensus regarding the optimal angiographic definition.[355] The incidence is approximately 30 to 40 per cent, occurs within 6 months of the procedure, and depends on the patient population, the complexity of the lesion, and the definition of restenosis,[344] but it does not appear to have declined despite a plethora of therapeutic approaches directed toward its prevention. The use of stenting has been found, however, to reduce this complication (Table 39–10, p. 1380). Neither the development of symptoms[355a] nor an abnormal exercise stress electrocardiogram is particularly reliable in the recognition of restenosis, but both are helpful in guiding subsequent therapy.[344]

MECHANISMS OF AND RISK FACTORS FOR RESTENOSIS. The pathogenesis of restenosis in response to mechanical injury is incompletely understood and multifactorial. Traditionally, restenosis has been considered to be due to the development of neointimal thickening as a result of migration and stimulation of smooth muscle by growth factors (see p. 1372). The elastic properties of the vessel undergoing PTCA and its recoil in the development of restenosis have also received attention. Clinical variables that appear to be associated with increased rates of restenosis include diabetes, severe angina, male sex, smoking, and older age.[347] *Anatomical* factors include total occlusion, left anterior descending coronary artery location, saphenous vein graft lesions, long lesions, and multivessel or multilesion PTCA.[349,350] *Procedural* variables include a greater residual stenosis, following PTCA, severe dissection, the absence of an intimal tear, the use of inappropriately sized balloons, and the presence of thrombus.

PREVENTION OF RESTENOSIS. A plethora of pharmacological agents of different categories has been evaluated for the prevention of restenosis after coronary angioplasty, with generally disappointing results. None has shown unequivocal success. The EPIC trial of a monoclonal blocking antibody to the platelet glycoprotein IIb/IIIa receptor documented a reduction in clinical endpoints at 6 months, which may, in part, be related to a decline in the incidence of restenosis.[34,355a]

The frequency of restenosis after PTCA and the desire to expand the pool of patients with chronic CAD amenable to transcatheter techniques have spawned the development of a variety of other devices, described in Chap. 39. Two randomized trials of directional coronary atherectomy versus standard balloon angioplasty, however, have failed to document any clinically relevant superiority of one form of therapy over the other,[356,357] but these trials have been criticized on the basis that the optimal results with directional coronary atherectomy were not attained.[358] Two randomized trials demonstrated a reduction in the rate of restenosis and in clinical events in patients receiving balloon-expandable stents compared with patients undergoing standard balloon angioplasty (Table 39–8, p. 1374).[358a] However, this benefit was achieved at a cost of a significantly higher risk of vascular complications and a longer hospital stay and costs.[359-360a] Although rapidly gaining in popularity, the long-term effects of stents have not yet been well defined, and their exact place remains to be defined.

MANAGEMENT OF RESTENOSIS. Restenosis is amenable to repeat PTCA, but it is not entirely clear whether lesions that have developed restenosis are more likely to develop restenosis after a subsequent percutaneous intervention.[361] Among patients with stable or unstable angina and restenosis, a 93 per cent anatomical success rate after repeat angioplasty has been reported, and most patients experienced significant long-term clinical improvement. However, the likelihood of recurrent angina requiring subsequent bypass surgery was greater than in patients undergoing PTCA for the first time.[362] In patients undergoing a third PTCA for restenosis at the same site, an interval of less than 3 months between the second and third procedures was strongly associated with further restenosis, suggesting that such patients should be considered for coronary bypass surgery.[363]

CHRONIC TOTAL OCCLUSION. This poses a formidable obstacle to PTCA success, particularly in the presence of bridging collaterals, an estimated duration of occlusion of more than 3 months, and a vessel diameter of 3 mm.[364-366,366a] After initially successful elective coronary angioplasty of total occlusions, the restenosis rate was 45 per cent in vessels with total occlusions, compared with 34 per cent in those with subtotal obstruction ($P < 0.001$). This is due primarily to an increased number of total occlusions at follow-up angiography (19.2 per cent compared with 5.0 per cent for stenoses, $P < 0.001$).[365] The role of stents is under evaluation.[365a] Explanations for the higher reocclusion rate are speculative, but a major potential contributor could be an increased collateral circulation around previously occluded arteries, a higher incidence of previous myocardial infarction, and more myocardial fibrosis in the distribution of the totally occluded arteries, leading to a reduction in total demand for flow to

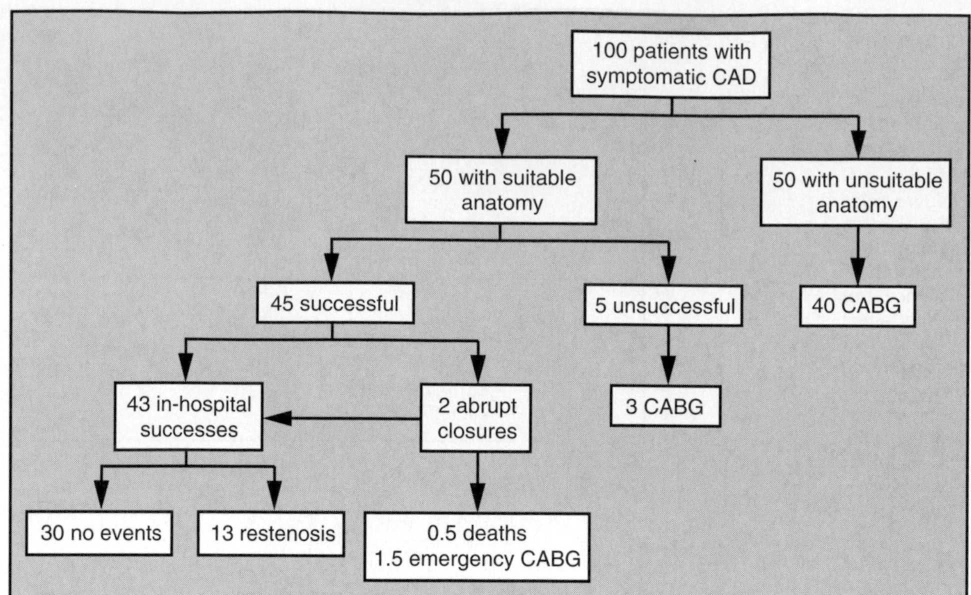

FIGURE 38–8. The limitations of balloon PTCA. Approximately one-half of patients who present with symptomatic coronary artery disease (CAD) and are in need of revascularization are candidates for PTCA. The remaining patients are ineligible because of unfavorable coronary anatomy, which most commonly results from chronic total occlusion more than 3 months in duration. Of the suitable candidates, a small percentage have an unsuccessful procedure and subsequently require CABG. A small percentage of patients who have a successful procedure develop abrupt vessel closure, and 20 to 30 per cent of patients develop restenosis that necessitates a repeat procedure. Thus, approximately 30 per cent of all patients who need myocardial revascularization are successfully treated and free of complications after PTCA. (From Faxon, D. P.: Coronary angioplasty for stable angina pectoris. *In* Beller, G. A. and Braunwald, E. [eds.]: Chronic Ischemic Heart Disease. Atlas of Heart Diseases, vol. 5. Philadelphia, Current Medicine, 1995, p. 9.16.)

the distal bed. Slow flow across the previously occluded lesion is likely to cause reocclusion consequent to thrombosis rather than fibrointimal hyperplasia or vascular recoil.

PTCA IN WOMEN (see p. 1704).

PTCA IN THE ELDERLY. The mortality and rate of periprocedural complications is increased in elderly patients undergoing PTCA.[367,368] Among hospital survivors, the late recurrence of angina appears to be higher in the elderly than in younger patients. On the other hand, PTCA may be more appropriate than coronary bypass surgery for the frail elderly with comorbid conditions who require revascularization but in whom the risks of surgery are higher.[368a]

PTCA IN CORONARY BYPASS GRAFTS. Coronary artery bypass surgery and PTCA are often considered to be competitive procedures, but it is more appropriate to view them as complementary. Patients who have undergone prior coronary bypass surgery, in whom repeat revascularization is under consideration, may be amenable to PTCA of native vessels or of bypass grafts.[369–372] This application of angioplasty and other transcatheter techniques is increasing rapidly and is particularly helpful in elderly patients, who would otherwise be facing a second or third coronary bypass operation. However, the initial and late success rates of PTCA in bypass grafts, particularly in saphenous vein conduits, are lower than in native vessels.[369] Results are better with dilatation of distal graft lesions; angiographic success rates approach 90 per cent at the distal site of the graft insertion, 70 per cent in the mid portion, and 55 per cent proximally.

Multiple factors increase the likelihood of *unfavorable* results of PTCA of vein grafts[370]; these include a graft age of 4 to 6 years, diffuse graft disease, chronic total occlusions, vein graft thrombus, and the site of the stenosis (i.e., proximal, mid, or distal). Until new techniques for maintaining long-term vein graft patency after PTCA are shown to be effective, balloon angioplasty should be considered only as a palliative procedure for patients with severe symptoms.[370]

COMPARISON OF PTCA AND CORONARY ARTERY BYPASS SURGERY (see p. 1374).

CONCLUSION. PTCA represents a major advance in the management of chronic stable angina. However, its limitations must be recognized. Only approximately half of all patients with symptomatic CAD are suitable candidates for this procedure, and of this half, only about 60 per cent have successful procedures *and* escape restenosis (Fig. 38–8).

OTHER CATHETER-BASED TECHNIQUES. Lasers, stents, rotablaters and atherectomy[372] are discussed in Chap. 39.

CORONARY ARTERY BYPASS SURGERY

In 1964 Garrett, Dennis, and DeBakey first used coronary artery bypass grafting (CABG) as a "bailout" procedure.[373] This was followed by the widespread use of the technique by Favoloro and Johnson and their respective collaborators in the late 1960s.[374,375] The use of the internal mammary artery (IMA) graft was pioneered by Kolesov in 1966 and Green in 1968.[376,377]

The number of coronary bypass operations in the United States has increased substantially from 180,000 in 1983 to approximately 300,000 in 1993.[314] The advent of PTCA may have blunted the growth of coronary artery bypass surgery somewhat. Nevertheless, CABG remains one of the most frequently performed operations in the United States; approximately 1 in every 1000 persons undergoes CABG on an annual basis, and this procedure results in the expenditure of almost $50 billion annually.[378]

The appropriate use of invasive cardiovascular procedures is undergoing increasing scrutiny. It is, therefore, reassuring to note that in studies of coronary angiography and bypass surgery in New York State and Canada, only 6 per cent and 4 per cent of bypass procedures, respectively, were considered inappropriate.[379] Patients with chronic stable angina represented 48 per cent of those undergoing bypass surgery in the United States and 61 per cent of those in Canada.

Technical Considerations

When the decision has been reached to proceed with coronary bypass surgery, administration of beta-adrenoreceptor blockers, nitrates, and calcium antagonists is continued until operation. It is crucial to minimize perioperative damage and to protect the myocardium. The most commonly used method involves a single period of aortic cross-clamping with intermittent infusion of cold cardioplegia.[380] Continued low-flow normothermic cardioplegic infusion may be equally effective in maintaining cardiac arrest and minimizing cardiac damage.[315] Cardioplegic solutions may be sanguinous, involving high concentrations of potassium with or without added substances, such as oxygen, buffers, and free radical scavengers.[381] Retrograde cardioplegia through the coronary sinus facilitates a more uniform distribution of cardioplegic solution. Many surgeons now use a combination of antegrade and retrograde perfusion[382] as well as topical hypothermia with cold saline or ice slush as an adjunct. Renewed interest in coronary bypass surgery without cardiopulmonary bypass has been stimulated by the desire to avoid blood transfusions, by economic issues, and by the wish to avoid the damaging effects of bypass, particularly in the elderly and in patients with heavily calcified aortas.[383]

VENOUS CONDUITS. The saphenous vein is used mainly for distal branches of the right and circumflex coronary arteries and for sequential grafts to these vessels and diagonal branches (Figs. 38–9 and 38–10). In emergency situations, many surgeons prefer the saphenous vein, which can be harvested and grafted more rapidly, to the internal mammary artery. Arm vein grafts are not as effective as either saphenous veins or internal mammary artery grafts.

Eight to 12 per cent of saphenous vein grafts become occluded during the early perioperative period. Trauma to the vein during surgical preparation can denude the endothelium, impair the intrinsic fibrinolytic activity of saphenous vein, and damage the vessel wall, predisposing to early thrombosis.[384] Careful harvesting of the graft, with particular attention to the avoidance of overdistention and the use of modified storage solutions, has been shown to improve patency and preserve the integrity of the graft in both animal models and the clinical setting.[380]

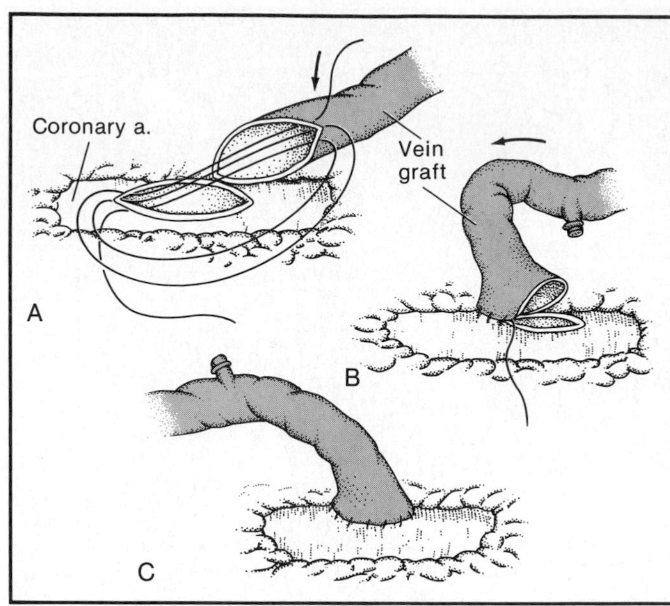

FIGURE 38–10. The venocoronary anastomosis to the proximal portion of the arteriotomy. (From Cohn, L. H.: Surgical techniques of emergency coronary revascularization. *In* Cohn, L. H. [ed.]: The Treatment of Acute Myocardial Ischemia: An Integrated Medical-Surgical Approach. Mt. Kisco, N.Y., Futura Publishing Co., 1979, p. 87.)

INTERNAL MAMMARY ARTERY BYPASS GRAFTS. The internal mammary artery (IMA), also known as the internal thoracic artery, usually is remarkably free of atheroma, especially in patients under the age of 65 years. When it is grafted to a coronary artery (Figs. 38–11 and 38–12), it appears to be virtually immune to the development of intimal hyperplasia, which is almost universally seen in aortocoronary vein grafts.[384a] Atherosclerotic changes in the IMA develop in only a small percentage of patients after coronary bypass surgery. The IMA is delicate, and great care has to

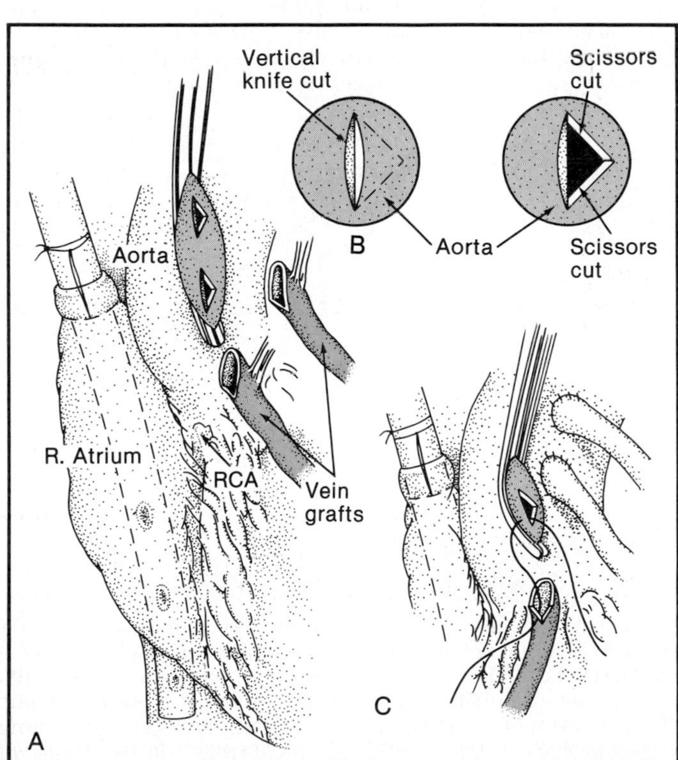

FIGURE 38–9. The aorticovenous anastomosis in a coronary arterial–saphenous vein bypass graft. *A* shows the direction of the anastomotic site for left-sided grafts; *B* shows details of aortic orifices; *C* shows the direction of right coronary artery (RCA) grafts. (From Cohn, L. H.: Surgical techniques of emergency coronary revascularization. *In* Cohn, L. H. [ed.]: The Treatment of Acute Myocardial Ischemia: An Integrated Medical-Surgical Approach. Mt. Kisco, N.Y., Futura Publishing Co., 1979, p. 87.)

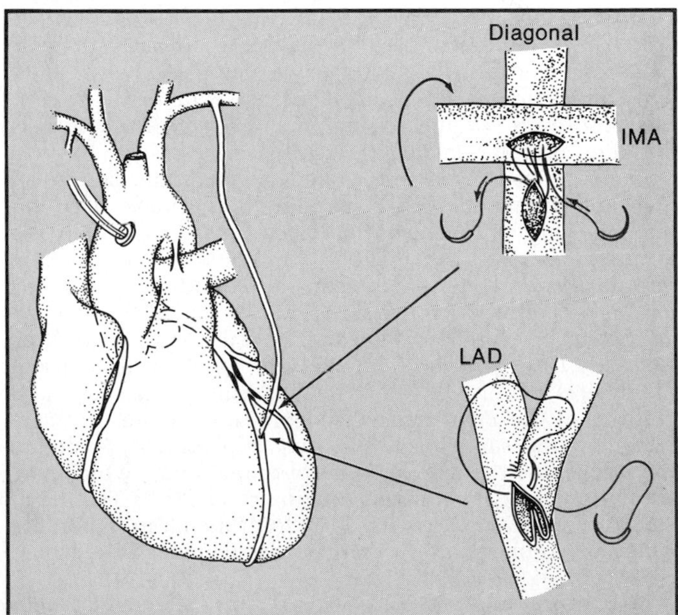

FIGURE 38–11. Internal mammary grafting: In situ left internal mammary artery (IMA) graft to the left anterior descending artery (end-to-side) and diagonal branch (side-to-side) employing the diamond anastomotic technique to the latter. The details show the IMA pedicle rolled up over the diagonal coronary artery to facilitate exposure and use of continuous suture. (From Jones, E. L.: Extended use of the internal mammary coronary artery bypass. J. Cardiac Surg. *1*:13, 1986.)

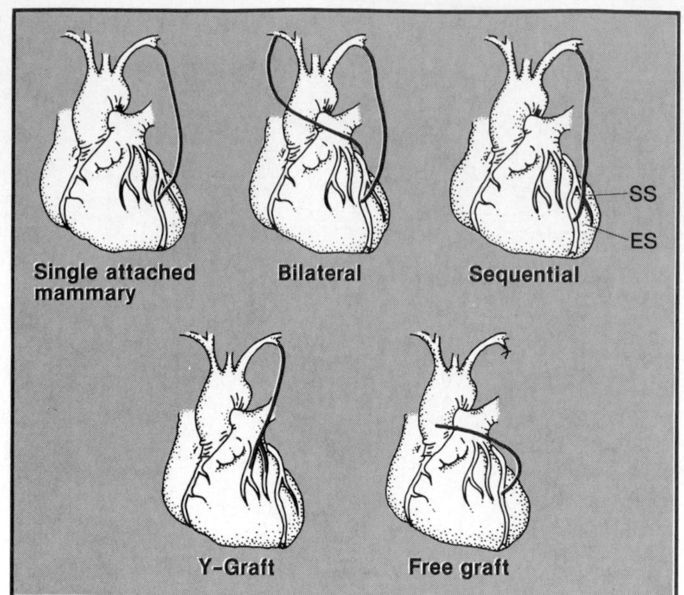

FIGURE 38–12. Different types of internal mammary artery grafts. A single attached internal mammary artery graft (either the right or left) remains attached proximally to the subclavian artery and is connected to the coronary arteries. Bilateral internal mammary artery grafts (right and left) are joined end to side to coronary arteries. Sequential internal mammary artery grafts consist of an attached or free internal mammary artery with one or more side-to-side anastomoses and one end-to-side anastomosis. The internal mammary artery Y graft has two terminal branches of either the attached or free internal mammary artery sutured to two coronary arteries. A free internal mammary graft is placed by transecting the right or left internal mammary artery near its origin in the subclavian artery, and the proximal artery is anastomosed to the aorta with the distal end to the coronary artery. (From Tector, A. J., et al.: Expanding the use of the internal mammary artery to improve patency in coronary artery bypass grafting. J. Thorac. Cardiovasc. Surg. *91*:9, 1986.)

be taken to mobilize the vessel without traumatizing it.[385] This prolongs the operative time and often requires entry into the pleural space. The "skeletonization" technique of IMA dissection, in which the artery is taken down with a strip of endothoracic fascia containing internal thoracic veins and endolymphatic tissue, achieves high flow rates and the pleural space is not usually opened.[380] However, this procedure is time consuming and the IMA therefore is not often used for emergency surgery.

Comparative morphological and angiographic studies of IMA and saphenous vein bypass grafts that have been implanted long term show that accelerated atherosclerosis occurs commonly in saphenous vein grafts but is extremely rare in IMA grafts. There are several potential explanations for the superiority of the IMA graft.[380] The media of the artery may derive nourishment from the lumen as well as from the vasa vasorum, and the internal elastic lamina of the IMA is uniform.[386] Moreover, the finding that the endothelium of the IMA produces significantly more prostacyclin than the saphenous vein may explain why endothelium-dependent relaxation is more pronounced, which may allow flow-dependent autoregulation to occur.[387] The diameter of the IMA graft usually is a closer match to that of the recipient coronary artery than is the diameter of a saphenous vein.

In contrast to the 40 to 60 per cent patency for vein grafts at 10 to 12 years following coronary surgery, that of IMA grafts exceeds 90 per cent.[315] Long-term patency rates were 95 per cent to the left anterior descending coronary artery, 88 per cent to the left circumflex, and 76 per cent to the right coronary artery and were higher for left than for right IMA grafts, and higher for in situ than for free IMA grafts. However, fibrointimal proliferation may occasionally develop in IMA grafts and cause narrowing and may be a factor in late graft closure.[380]

Loop et al. described improved 10-year survival in patients who received an IMA graft to the anterior descending coronary artery alone, or combined with one or more saphenous vein grafts, compared with survival in patients who had only saphenous vein bypass grafts (Fig. 38–13).[388,389a,389b] This important observation has been confirmed.[389] Patients receiving the IMA graft have a decreased risk of late death, myocardial infarction, cardiac events, and reoperations, and this clinical advantage persists for up to 20 years.[388,390,391] Most surgeons now believe that whenever it is technically feasible, IMA grafting is the preferable treatment, at least for lesions of the anterior descending coronary artery.

Although the benefits of the single IMA graft over the saphenous vein graft alone are not in dispute, it is unclear whether bilateral IMA grafts are superior to a single IMA graft to the left anterior descending coronary artery.[389] The use of bilateral grafts is technically more demanding, but late reoperation rates are reduced in patients receiving bilateral IMA grafts.

Complications of Arterial Conduits. Inadequate flow rates with evidence of myocardial ischemia in the perioperative period are rare after IMA grafts to the left anterior descending coronary artery or its diagonal branches.[380] Perioperative spasm is the presumed cause and can be managed by the administration of sodium nitroprusside or a combination of glyceryl trinitrate and verapamil.[392] Other complications include an increased incidence of sternal wound infections, which is more frequent in obese patients and in diabetics and after bilateral IMA implants.[390]

Other Conduits. The right gastroepiploic artery is increasingly used as a conduit in patients in whom the IMA and saphenous veins have been exhausted and in younger patients, particularly among those with hyperlipidemia.[315,380] The graft is most frequently placed to the right coronary artery.[391] Initial results suggested that patency rates were inferior to those for the IMA, but this may have been part of a "learning curve," with recent data suggesting

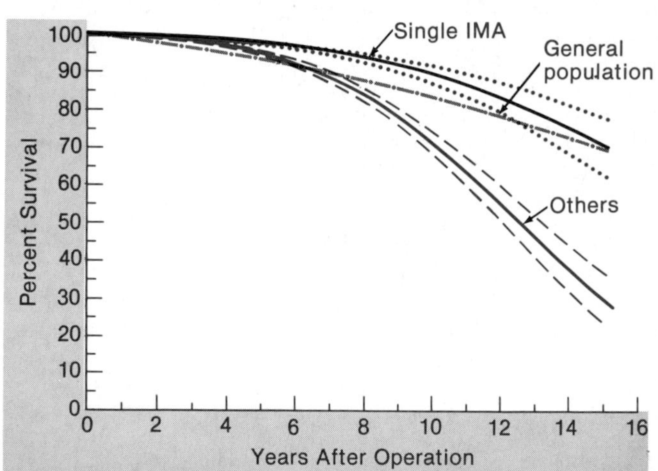

FIGURE 38–13. Survival of patients with extensive three-vessel disease according to whether or not a single internal mammary artery graft (IMA) to the left anterior descending coronary artery was used as a conduit in addition to whatever vein grafts were necessary. "General population" refers to an age, race, and gender-matched general population from government statistics and "Others" refers to patients revascularized without a single IMA graft applied to the left anterior descending coronary artery. These data strongly suggest that having a single IMA graft applied to the left anterior descending coronary artery is beneficial to survival in patients with extensive three-vessel coronary artery disease. (Modified from Kirklin, J. W., et al.: Summary of a consensus concerning death and ischemic events after coronary artery bypass grafting. Circulation *79*[Suppl. I]:81, 1989, copyright American Heart Association.)

that patency rates are equal. Other conduits that have been employed include the radial artery and the inferior epigastric artery.[393]

MILD NATIVE VESSEL OBSTRUCTION. Intraoperative studies have shown that native arteries with less than 50 per cent luminal diameter obstruction often have minimal, if any, pressure gradients across the lesions and little difference in blood flow through the artery distal to the graft when the bypass graft is opened. Patients with higher grade obstructions usually have greater pressure gradients across the lesions. Patency rates of IMA grafts to vessels with less than 50 per cent stenosis are lower than to vessels with more significant lesions.

THE DISTAL VASCULATURE. The state of the distal coronary vasculature is important for the fate of bypass grafts. Late patency of grafts is related to coronary arterial runoff as determined by the diameter of the coronary artery into which the graft is inserted, the size of the distal vascular bed, and the severity of coronary atherosclerosis distal to the site of insertion of the graft. The highest graft patency rates are found when the lumina of the vessels distal to the graft insertion are greater than 1.5 mm in diameter, perfuse a large vascular bed, and are free of atheroma obstructing more than 25 per cent of the vessel lumen.

FLOW RATES. When measured at the time of operation, flow rates through saphenous vein grafts average nearly 70 ml/min. Those in which the flow is less than 45 ml/min—and especially less than 25 ml/min—are more frequently associated with graft closure than those with flow rates exceeding 45 ml/min.[394] The possible causes for reduced flow include (1) subcritical obstruction of the coronary artery, (2) a technically poor anastomosis, with narrowing of the lumen due to kinking of the vessel or pinching at the site of anastomosis, (3) a small myocardial mass perfused by the graft, and (4) a diseased distal vascular bed.

OTHER SURGICAL PROCEDURES FOR ISCHEMIC HEART DISEASE. Coronary bypass surgery may be combined with surgical procedures aimed at correction of atherosclerotic disease elsewhere in the cardiovascular system, with correction of mechanical complications of myocardial infarction (mitral regurgitation at ventricular septal defect), left ventricular aneurysmectomy, and concomitant valvular heart disease.[395,396] Not unexpectedly, morbidity and mortality are correspondingly increased owing to the added complexity of the procedure and, in many patients who require these other procedures, the presence of underlying left ventricular dysfunction.

Outcome of Surgery

OPERATIVE MORTALITY. As Kirklin et al. have pointed out, risk factors for death following coronary artery surgery may be considered in five categories: (1) preoperative factors related to CAD, including recent acute myocardial infarction, hemodynamic instability, left ventricular dysfunction, extensive CAD, the presence of left main coronary artery disease, and severe or unstable angina; (2) preoperative factors related to the aggressiveness of the arteriosclerotic process, as reflected in associated carotid peripheral vascular disease; (3) preoperative biological factors (older age at operation, diabetes mellitus, and perhaps female gender); (4) intraoperative factors (intraoperative ischemic damage and failure to use IMA grafts)[397]; and (5) environmental or institutional factors, including the specific surgeon and treatment protocols used.[398]

The patient population undergoing coronary bypass surgery has been changing over time, particularly with the wider use of PTCA and other catheter-based procedures. In comparison with the 1970's, patients undergoing coronary bypass surgery today are older, include a higher percentage of women, are "sicker," in that a greater proportion have unstable angina, three-vessel disease, prior coronary revascularization with either coronary bypass surgery or PTCA, left ventricular dysfunction, and comorbid conditions, including hypertension, diabetes, and peripheral vascular disease.[399]

In-hospital mortality after isolated coronary bypass surgery was characterized by a steady decline from 1967 to the early 1980's. Overall mortality for elective first bypass procedures in the United States from 1980 to 1990 was 2.2 per cent in 58,384 patients in the Society of Thoracic Surgeons data base. It was 2.6 per cent in elective patients without IMA grafts and 1.3 per cent in patients receiving such an implant.[399] More recently there has been a stabilization or even a slight overall increase in morbidity and mortality, which reflects the changing characteristics toward an older and sicker population of patients undergoing operation.[400,400a]

Changing Late Results of Coronary Bypass Surgery. Two competing influences warrant a reevaluation of the late results of coronary bypass surgery in the contemporary era. Improved surgical and perioperative techniques, including the use of IMA grafts, improve long-term outcome. On the other hand, the survival to discharge of high-risk patients, who may have died during the perioperative period during an earlier era, may have an opposite effect upon late outcome. In addition, as already noted, the patient population undergoing CABG has shifted toward a greater proportion of older, higher risk patients with a worse prognosis. This trend may substantially alter downward the expectations of late outcome.

PERIOPERATIVE COMPLICATIONS. Perioperative morbidity (see also Chap. 52) has also increased because of a larger fraction of higher risk patients.

PERIOPERATIVE MYOCARDIAL INFARCTION. The diagnosis of perioperative myocardial infarction is hampered by the lack of specificity of repolarization abnormalities and enzyme changes during the perioperative period. Predictors of perioperative myocardial infarction in the Coronary Artery Surgery Study (CASS) were female gender, severe perioperative angina pectoris, severe stenosis of the left main coronary artery, and three-vessel disease.[401] Unstable angina and prolonged cardiopulmonary bypass times are also risk factors.[402] Perioperative myocardial infarction, particularly if it is associated with hemodynamic or arrhythmic complications or preexisting left ventricular dysfunction, has a major adverse effect upon early and late prognosis.[403]

RESPIRATORY COMPLICATIONS. Postoperative changes in pulmonary function after coronary bypass surgery are frequent and troublesome, but rarely serious, except in patients with preexisting chronic lung disease or the elderly.

BLEEDING. Impaired hemostasis and bleeding complications are an inherent risk of coronary bypass surgery. Reoperation for bleeding is required in 2 to 5 per cent of patients.[404] Cardiopulmonary bypass causes derangements of the intrinsic coagulation and fibrinolytic systems in addition to platelet function. The risk of bleeding is increased with age, a smaller surface area, reoperation, bilateral internal thoracic artery grafts, and the preoperative use of heparin, aspirin, and thrombolytic agents. The prophylactic use of epsilon-aminocaproic acid (aprotinin), which may prevent degradation of platelet function, is associated with a significant reduction in both blood loss and transfusion requirements.[405]

WOUND INFECTIONS. Major perioperative wound complications, especially mediastinitis and/or wound dehiscence, occur in approximately 1 per cent of patients.[406] These are associated with a markedly increased in-hospital mortality, morbidity, and length of stay. This risk is substantially increased by the use of double IMA grafts, particularly in diabetics.[406]

POSTOPERATIVE HYPERTENSION. This complication can occur in up to one-third of all patients after coronary bypass surgery (see p. 830). The mechanism is unclear, but it may be related to increased levels of circulating catecholamines and renin. It is important to control postoperative hypertension to prevent myocardial ischemia, cardiac failure, and excessive perioperative bleeding. Postoperative hypertension rarely presents a problem with the use of drugs such as calcium antagonists[407] or nitrates.[408] Esmolol, a short-acting beta-blocking agent (see p. 487), appears to be equally effective in reducing arterial pressure and also slows heart rate.[409]

CEREBROVASCULAR COMPLICATIONS. These include stroke, the incidence of which is 1 to 5 per cent and is age related.[410] Delayed returns of a normal level of consciousness occurs in approximately 3 per cent of patients,[411] and intellectual dysfunction in the early postoperative period, as assessed by a battery of neurocognitive tests, has been noted in approximately 75 per cent of patients.[412] Transient mild visual deficits are common.[410] Fortunately, major long-term sequelae are uncommon. Mild degrees of confusion, agitation, and delusional behavior are frequent and usually transient. The elderly are particularly vulnerable.

ATRIAL FIBRILLATION. This is one of the most frequent complications of coronary bypass surgery. It occurs in up to 40 per cent of patients, primarily within 2 to 3 days.[413,414] In the early postoperative period, rapid ventricular rates and loss of atrial transport may compromise systemic hemodynamics and increase the risk of embolization. Beta blockers are useful in the treatment of the condition once established, and trials have suggested a benefit for the prophylactic value of these drugs.[413]

CONDUCTION DISTURBANCES AND BRADYARRHYTHMIAS. The incidence of postoperative bradyarrhythmias requiring permanent pacemaker implantation was 0.8 per cent in a series of 1614 consecutive patients discharged from the hospital after coronary bypass surgery.[415] Predictive factors were preoperative left bundle branch block, concomitant left ventricular aneurysmectomy, and older age. The majority of patients continued to require permanent pacemaker support during follow-up.[415] Patients with CAD who develop fascicular conduction disturbances often have diffuse myocardial disease and an unfavorable prognosis. The causes of death are ventricular arrhythmias and cardiac failure.

COMPLICATION IN THE OBESE. While obesity per se does not appear to increase significantly the operative mortality,[416] it is associated with a higher incidence of complications, including sternotomy dehiscence, impaired leg wound healing following saphenous vein excision,[417] postoperative hypertension, and bronchoconstriction.

SYMPTOMATIC RESULTS. Major relief of angina pectoris occurs in more than 90 per cent of appropriately selected patients after coronary bypass surgery.[416a] Approximately three-quarters of patients are free from ischemic events, sudden death, occurrence of a myocardial infarction, or return of angina for 5 years after coronary artery surgery and nearly half for at least 10 years.[398] However, by 15 years only about 15 per cent of patients can be expected to be alive and free of an ischemic event.

In the bypass surgery arms of recent randomized trials of PTCA and CABG (see p. 1375), recurrent angina pectoris was reported in 21.5 per cent to 34 per cent of patients at a follow-up ranging from 2 to 3 years, but (Canadian Classification) grade III or IV angina was present in only 6 per cent at 2.5 years in the RITA trial.[418] Only 12 per cent of patients in the Emory Angioplasty Surgery Study (EAST) reported class II, III, or IV angina after 3 years of follow-up (see p. 1375).[351]

RETURN TO EMPLOYMENT. Return to full employment has been disappointing in some series. Among participants in the surgical arm of EAST, whose mean age was 61 years at entry, only 38.5 per cent were gainfully employed at 3 years.[351] In contrast, in a study of patients under the age of 65 years who were employed at the time of revascularization, 79 per cent of patients who had bypass surgery were working at 1 year, and, after adjustment for baseline characteristics, the 1-year employment rates were the same among patients treated with surgery, angioplasty, or medical therapy.[419] Factors that affect adversely the prospects of patients returning to work include advanced age, postoperative angina, and a period of either unemployment or disability before surgery.[420,421] Forty-seven per cent of patients undergoing bypass surgery in the EAST trial were able to engage in moderate or strenuous activity 3 years after the procedure.[351] However, with time there is a fall off in symptomatic benefit, and there is a suggestion that by 10 years after coronary vein graft surgery the relief of symptoms and improved exercise performance noted at 5 years have decreased to levels seen in medically treated patients.[422]

GRAFT PATENCY. Experimental studies and observations in patients suggest that there are several phases of disease development in venous aortocoronary artery bypass grafts. The occlusion rate, which is high in the first year, decreases substantially between the first and sixth years. Between 6 and 10 years after operation the attrition rate for grafts increases again. Early occlusion (prior to hospital discharge) occurs in 8 to 12 per cent of venous grafts, and by 1 year 15 to 30 per cent of vein grafts have become occluded.[423,424] After the first year, the annual occlusion rate is 2 per cent per year and rises to approximately 4 per cent per year between years 6 and 10. At 10 years, approximately one-third of vein grafts which are patent at 1 year have become occluded, one-third demonstrate significant atherosclerosis, and one-third appear to be unchanged.[423] Moreover, 20 to 40 per cent of grafts that are patent at 10 years after surgery are stenotic.[315,380]

Early Phase (First Month). Technical factors that may cause thrombotic closure at the proximal or distal anastomoses include kinking due to excessive length, tension due to insufficient length, poor graft flow, and inadequate distal runoff. Atheroma at the arteriotomy site may predispose to early thrombotic occlusion. Surgical manipulation of the saphenous vein during harvesting and preparation prior to grafting play key roles in initiating the sequence of endothelial damage with subsequent platelet and fibrin deposition, leading to thrombosis.[384,424,425] Interruption of the nutrient blood flow to the vein wall may also be involved.[423]

Intermediate Phase (1 Month to 1 Year). In vein grafts that have been implanted in the arterial circulation for 1 month to 1 year, there is substantial endothelial denudation and proliferation and migration of medial cells to the intima. Even in the face of endothelial continuity, progressive migration of vascular smooth muscle cells through the internal elastic lamina into the intima may occur.[384,426] The initial phase of rapid proliferation is followed after several months by a marked increase in the connective tissue matrix, which further increases intimal and medial thickness. These events are promoted by aggregation of platelets and secretion of growth factors. This accelerated process of intimal hyperplasia and thickening is an early stage of atherosclerotic plaque formation and is believed to occur because of interaction between platelets and macrophages and endothelial damage. If the proliferation is severe and localized, as may occur at the site of the anastomosis between the grafts and the recipient artery, total occlusion can occur within 1 year. Histological studies of grafts that occlude within 1 year often show either substantial thrombosis with minimal intima-medial changes or marked intimal hyperplasia or superimposed thrombus.[427]

Late Phase (Beyond 1 Year). Some investigators believe that the development of atherosclerosis in vein grafts, as in native arteries, is a continuum starting from platelet deposition and advancing to smooth muscle cell proliferation and finally to lipid incorporation into the plaque. By 10 years, nearly one-half of venous grafts patent at 5 years have become occluded.[428] Beyond the first year, particularly after 3 to 5 years, the histological appearance of occluded or obstructed coronary bypass grafts is consistent with atherosclerosis. There is clear evidence of mature lipid-laden plaques, foam cells, cholesterol clefts, ulceration, and areas of calcification with disruption of the medial layer.[429] Although there are similarities to the atherosclerotic lesions of arterial disease, vein graft atherosclerosis is more diffuse circumferentially.[430] Marked friability of the atherosclerotic lesions may cause intermittent coronary embolization,[431] which complicates revascularization procedures, such as reoperation or PTCA of vein grafts.

DETERMINATION OF GRAFT PATENCY. Although determination of graft patency usually involves postoperative angiography, radionuclide techniques, which assess myocardial perfusion, may also indicate graft patency.[432] Contrast-enhanced computed tomography has been used to assess patency of saphenous vein grafts (Fig. 10–36, p. 338).

PROGRESSION OF DISEASE IN NONGRAFTED ARTERIES. Disease progression, defined as a worsening of a preexisting lesion or appearance of a new diameter narrowing of 50 per cent or greater, can occur at a rate of 20 to 40 per cent over 5 to 10 years in nongrafted native vessels.[433] The rate of disease progression appears highest in arterial segments already showing evidence of disease,[434] and it is between three and six times higher in grafted native coronary arteries than in ungrafted native vessels. Disease progression is also greater in arteries with patent grafts than in arteries with occluded grafts[435] and usually occurs proximal to the site of graft insertion.[433,434] These data suggest that bypassing an artery with minimal disease, even if initially successful, may ultimately be harmful to the patient who incurs both the risk of graft closure and the increased risk of accelerated obstruction of the native vessels.

EFFECTS OF THERAPY ON VEIN GRAFT OCCLUSION AND NATIVE VESSEL PROGRESSION. A meta-analysis of clinical trials suggests that antiplatelet or anticoagulant therapy after coronary artery bypass surgery may prevent graft occlusion.[436]

ANTIPLATELET THERAPY (see also p. 1225). In a prospective randomized double-blind trial, dipyridamole (started 48 hours before operation) plus aspirin (started 7 hours after operation) was compared with placebo treatment. Within 1 month of operation 3 per cent of vein-graft distal anastomoses were occluded in the treated patients, compared with 10 per cent in the placebo group.[437] At angiography performed 1 year after operation, 11 per cent of vein-graft distal anastomoses were occluded in the treated group and 25 per cent in the placebo group.[438] There was no significant increase in blood loss, transfusions, or reoperations in the treated group during the perioperative period. Subsequent studies suggested that dipyridamole is *not* an essential component and that low doses of aspirin (40 to 80 mg/day) may be sufficient.[439]

A Veterans Administration Cooperative Study Group has also examined the effect of specific antiplatelet therapy on vein graft after coronary artery bypass grafting.[440] Early graft patency rates were 92 per cent for aspirin (with or without dipyridamole) compared with 85 per cent for placebo. At 1 year the graft occlusion rate in all of the aspirin groups combined was 16 per cent compared with 23 per cent for the placebo group.[440] Aspirin started 6 hours after surgery appears to be as effective in preventing vein graft complications as is aspirin begun 12 hours preoperatively, but the former has the added benefit of reducing bleeding complications.[441] A meta-analysis of 17 trials of prevention of vein graft occlusion suggested that 100 mg to 325 mg of daily aspirin was more effective than a high dosage (975 mg).[439] Aspirin should be continued indefinitely following coronary bypass surgery. However, aspirin does not affect patency of an internal mammary artery graft.[442]

THERAPY OF HYPERLIPIDEMIA AND OTHER RISK FACTORS. Several studies have drawn attention to the relationship between vein graft atherosclerosis and elevated levels of LDL cholesterol, Lp(a), and reduced HDL cholesterol levels.[424,443–447] The randomized Cholesterol Lowering Atherosclerosis Study (CLAS) of hyperlipidemic men who had undergone coronary bypass surgery demonstrated a significant reduction in disease progression in native vessels and in bypass grafts with lipid-lowering pharmacotherapy.[444] It is essential to maintain ideal body weight, reduce total and LDL cholesterol levels, and permanently cease smoking following coronary artery surgery.[446] In patients randomized to bypass surgery in the Coronary Artery Surgery Study (CASS), mortality and morbidity were lower among men who quit smoking than those who continued to smoke after entry.[148]

Selection of Patients for Coronary Bypass Surgery

The indications for coronary bypass surgery consist of the need for improvement of the quality or quantity of life. Patients whose angina is not controlled by medical management or who have unacceptable side effects with such management should be considered for coronary revascularization. If, on the basis of the coronary anatomy, the patient is a suitable candidate for PTCA and is not in a subgroup that requires operation (such as three-vessel disease with left ventricular dysfunction), angioplasty is ordinarily the procedure of choice.[447a] If the patient is a failure of medical therapy and is not a good candidate for PTCA, then coronary bypass surgery should be considered. This procedure is also indicated in patients with CAD, regardless of symptoms, in whom survival is likely to be prolonged.[448]

In making the critical decision regarding revascularization, it is important to assess the patient's prognosis (Table 38–11) and how it may be affected by operation. The key initial step is to stratify patients into categories of risk with continued medical therapy, based upon an analysis of clinical, noninvasive, and, in some patients, angiographic variables. This process defines the *indications* for revascularization over medical therapy; more recent randomized trial data are helpful in defining which *modality* of revascularization (PTCA or surgery) is preferable (see p. 1374).

TABLE 38–11 DETERMINANTS OF ADVERSE PROGNOSIS IN CORONARY ARTERY DISEASE

Cardiac Determinants
Left ventricular dysfunction
Extent of myocardial jeopardy—extent of ischemia at rest and on exercise and number of large vessels diseased
Extent of myocardium in jeopardy
Abnormal arrhythmic substrate
Clinical and Electrocardiographic Modifying Factors
Advanced age
History of congestive heart failure
Diabetes
Rapidly accelerating angina
Resting electrocardiographic abnormalities
Left ventricular hypertrophy and hypertension
Peripheral vascular disease
Hyperlipidemia

Natural History of Angina Pectoris

CLINICAL AND ELECTROCARDIOGRAPHIC CRITERIA. Data from the Framingham Study, obtained prior to the widespread use of aspirin, beta blockers, and aggressive modification of risk factors, showed that the average annual mortality rate of patients with chronic stable angina was 4 per cent.[449] The combination of these treatments has improved prognosis. Remission of angina may occur in up to one-third of patients with angina of recent onset, but this is unusual if the condition has been present for several years. Numerous studies attest to the adverse prognostic impact of congestive heart failure (based upon a clinical history of cardiomegaly on chest radiography), prior myocardial infarction, hypertension, and advanced age in patients with stable angina pectoris.[449–451] A third heart sound is a useful clinical predictor of an abnormal left ventricular ejection fraction and an adverse prognosis in patients with CAD. The severity of angina, especially the tempo of intensification, is also an important predictor of outcome.

On the other hand, a normal resting electrocardiogram in patients with stable angina pectoris speaks in favor of well-preserved left ventricular function and a favorable long-term prognosis (see p. 1295).[351,452] Left ventricular hypertrophy, as determined on the electrocardiogram or echocardiogram, is associated with an increased mortality secondary to the effects of hypertension and left ventricular dysfunction.[453]

ANGIOGRAPHIC CRITERIA. The independent impact of multivessel disease and left ventricular dysfunction, and their interaction upon the prognosis of patients with CAD, has been well documented[454–456] (Fig. 38–14). These two risk factors are synergistic in that the adverse effects on prognosis of impaired ventricular function are more pronounced as the number of stenotic vessels increases.[455] When all of the other factors are held constant, the number of coronary arteries with significant stenoses is one of the most powerful prognostic factors. More elaborate classifications of the extent of disease have not provided much additional information, other than the greater the extent of jeopardized myocardium, the worse the prognosis. Among medically treated patients in CASS, 12-year survival was 91 per cent in patients with chronic angina and angiographically normal vessels. In the presence of single-vessel disease, it was 86 per cent in patients with at least one obstruction of 30 to 50 per cent; 79 per cent in patients with at least one stenosis of 50 to 70 per cent, and 74 per

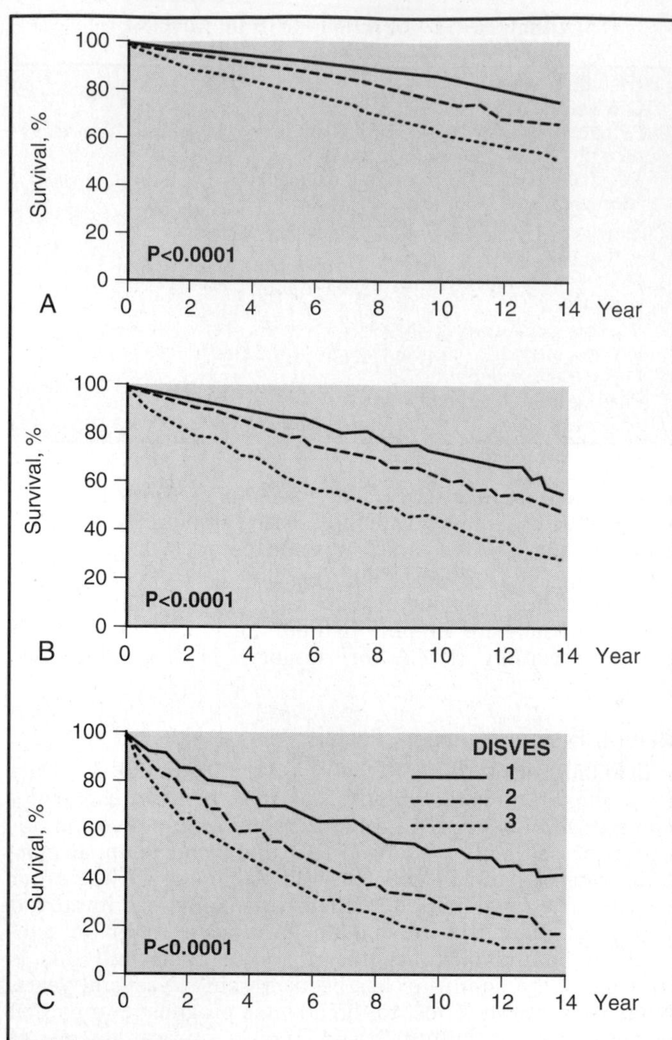

FIGURE 38–14. Graphs showing survival for medically treated CASS patients. *A*, Patients with one-, two-, or three-vessel disease and ejection fraction 50 to 100 per cent by number of diseased vessels (DISVES). *B*, Patients with one-, two-, or three-vessel disease and ejection fraction 35 to 49 per cent by number of diseased vessels. *C*, Patients with one-, two-, or three-vessel disease and ejection fraction 0 to 34 per cent by number of diseased vessels. (Reproduced with permission from Emond, M., et al.: Long-term survival of medically treated patients in the Coronary Artery Surgery Study [CASS] registry. Circulation *90:*2645, 1994. Copyright American Heart Association.)

cent in patients with single-vessel disease and a stenosis of 70 per cent or more.[455]

Studies in symptomatic patients have revealed that if only one of the three major coronary arteries has more than 50 per cent stenosis, the annual mortality rate is approximately 2 per cent.[457] The importance to survival of the quantity of myocardium that is jeopardized is reflected in the observation that an obstructive lesion proximal to the first septal perforating branch of the left anterior descending coronary artery was associated with a 5-year survival of 90 per cent, compared with 98 per cent in patients with more distal lesions.[457] The survival rate of patients with isolated right CAD at 5 years appeared to be higher (96 per cent) than in patients with disease of the left anterior descending coronary artery (92 per cent). The overall survival of medically treated patients with left anterior descending and left circumflex CAD was not significantly different, but both were less than the survival of patients with isolated right CAD.[457]

In symptomatic patients (or in asymptomatic survivors of myocardial infarction, if two of the major arteries exhibit severe stenosis, the 5-year mortality is approximately 9 per cent, and if all three vessels are stenotic it rises to approximately 15 per cent.[458,459] In an observational study of patients with obstructive CAD who initially were treated medically, 15-year survival rates were 48, 28, 18, and 9 per cent for patients with single-, double-, triple-, and left main vessel disease, respectively.[454] In addition to the number of vessels involved, the severity of obstruction is also important. Prognosis in patients with 50 to 75 per cent narrowing is better than in those with more than 75 per cent narrowing.[460]

High-grade lesions of the left main coronary artery or its "equivalents" are particularly life threatening (Fig. 38–15).[461] Mortality among medically treated patients has been reported as 29 per cent at 18 months, 39 per cent at 2 years, and 43 per cent at 5 years.[462,463] Survival is better for patients having a 50 to 70 per cent stenosis (1- and 3-year survivals of 91 per cent and 66 per cent, respectively) than for patients with a greater than 70 per cent left main coronary artery stenosis (1- and 3-year survivals of 72 and 41 per cent).[464] Furthermore, a number of characteristics found at catheterization or on noninvasive examination are predictors of an adverse prognosis in patients with 70 per cent or greater left main coronary artery stenosis; these include chest pain at rest, ST-T wave changes on the resting electrocardiogram, cardiomegaly on the chest roentgenogram, a history of congestive heart failure, findings of left ventricular dysfunction at catheterization, and elevation of the arterial–mixed venous oxygen difference.[464]

The severity of symptoms is a useful prognostic factor in conjunction with arteriographic findings and left ventricular function. In asymptomatic or mildly symptomatic patients who have one- or two-vessel disease, the prognosis is excellent, and the annual mortality is approximately 1.5 per cent. Even in patients with three-vessel disease who have good exercise capacity (achievement of 85 per cent predicted heart rate or workload of 100 watts or more), the annual mortality rate also is relatively low, 4 per cent.[465]

LIMITATIONS OF ANGIOGRAPHY. The pathophysiological significance of coronary stenoses lies in their impact upon resting and exercise-induced blood flow, in addition to their potential for plaque rupture with superimposed thrombotic occlusion. It is generally accepted that a stenosis of greater than 60 per cent of the luminal diameter is hemodynamically significant, in that it may be responsible for a reduction in exercise-induced myocardial blood flow causing angina and ischemia[466] (see p. 1293). The functional significance of obstruction of "intermediate" severity (approximately 50 per cent diameter stenosis)[467] is less well established.

Another limitation to the routine use of coronary angiography for prognosis in patients with chronic stable angina is its inability to identify which coronary lesions can be considered to be at high risk for future events, such as myocardial infarction or sudden death. Although it is widely accepted that myocardial infarction is the result of thrombotic occlusion at the site of a plaque rupture[468] (see p. 1188), a growing body of evidence suggests that it is not necessarily the plaque causing the most severe stenosis which subsequently ruptures. Several studies of patients undergoing serial coronary angiograms indicate that myocardial infarction often arises from rupture of the plaque which did *not* cause critical obstruction (see p. 1192). Mild lesions can rupture, thrombose, and occlude, leading to myocardial infarction and sudden death.[469–472] In contrast, arteries with severe preexisting stenoses may proceed to clinically silent complete occlusion, often without infarction, presumably due to the formation of collaterals.

In summary, angiographic documentation of the extent of CAD is an indispensable step in the selection of patients for coronary revascularization, particularly if the interaction between the anatomical extent of disease, left ventricular function, and the severity of ischemia is taken into account. However, angiography is not helpful in predicting the site of subsequent occlusions which could cause myo-

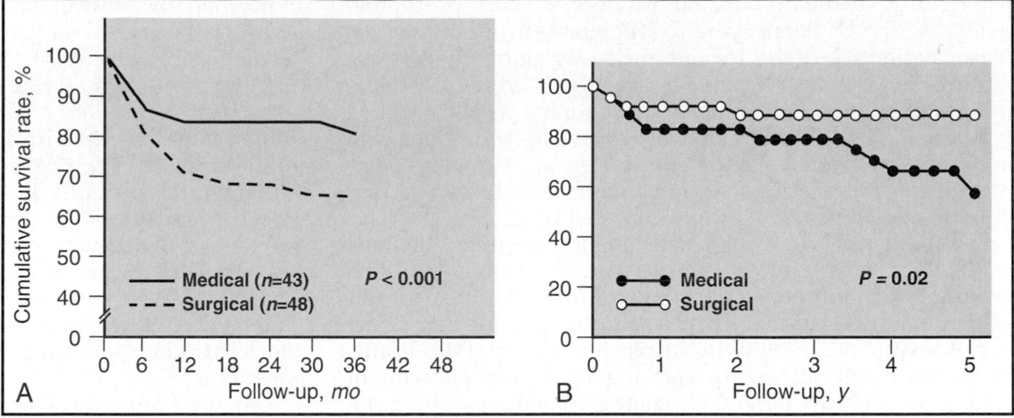

FIGURE 38–15. Cumulative survival with medical and surgical therapy in patients with symptomatic left main coronary disease greater than 50% from the Veterans Administration Cooperative Study (A) and the Coronary Artery Surgery Study patients with left main coronary artery disease (B). (From Gersh, B. J.: Natural history of chronic coronary artery disease. *In* Beller, G. A., and Braunwald, E. [eds.]: Chronic Ischemic Heart Disease. Atlas of Heart Diseases. Philadelphia, Current Medicine, 1995. Adapted from Takaro, T., Hultgren, H. N., Lipton, M. J., et al.: The VA cooperative randomized study of surgery for coronary arterial occlusive disease. II. Subgroup with significant left main lesions. Circulation 51[Suppl. III]: 107, 1976. Copyright American Heart Association.)

cardial infarction or sudden cardiac death, particularly in the individual patient.

NONINVASIVE TESTING (see p. 1295). In the estimation of prognosis in patients with chronic stable angina pectoris, stress testing with or without imaging may provide useful information (Table 38–2)[71,451] (Chaps. 3, 5, and 9). Depending upon the nature of the study, the patient's functioning status, the severity of ischemia, the extent of "jeopardized" myocardium, and ventricular function can all be assessed by these tests. In patients in whom left ventricular function and coronary anatomy have already been defined, stress testing may provide additional prognostic information regarding the functional significance of specific angiographic lesions.

From a clinical standpoint, the initial approach to a patient with chronic stable angina and a normal resting electrocardiogram is to perform a standard exercise electrocardiogram. In patients with major electrocardiographic conduction abnormalities (left or right bundle branch block) or in patients with resting ST-segment changes, in whom the response to exercise may be difficult to interpret, it is reasonable to proceed directly to a stress imaging study. The latter can be determined by nuclear techniques or echocardiography. The choice depends on the expertise available to any individual institution.

One of the most important prognosticators derived from exercise stress testing is exercise duration or capacity.[473] In an 8-year follow-up of medically treated patients with angiographically confirmed CAD and a positive exercise test, the duration of exercise correlated significantly with survival.[71] Patients reaching stage 4 of a Bruce protocol had a survival rate of 93 per cent, compared to only 45 per cent in patients who terminated exercise in stage 1.[71] This relationship between exercise duration and long-term survival was independent of whether the exercise was terminated because of dyspnea, fatigue, or angina. In a 16-year follow-up study from the CASS registry, exercise capacity was shown to be an extremely powerful predictor of survival, particularly among men, and to be helpful in the identification of patients likely to benefit from coronary revascularization.[474] Other factors identified with a poor prognosis in individual series of patients with chronic stable angina are described in Table 38–2.

Prognostic Scores. Mark et al. have incorporated exercise test results into a prognostic score, which stratified patients with stable CAD into three risk groups with 5-year mortality rates of 3 per cent, 9 per cent, and 28 per cent, respectively, and then showed that this score contained information beyond that provided by clinical and catheterization data.[475] Similar studies at the Long Beach Veterans Administration Medical Center considered both clinical and exercise predictors of cardiovascular mortality. A simple score based upon a history of congestive heart failure, ST-segment depression on the resting electrocardiogram, and a fall in systolic blood pressure below rest during exercise identified three categories of risk with annual cardiac mortality rates of 1 per cent, 7 per cent, and 12 per cent, respectively.[476]

Stress Thallium-201 Myocardial Perfusion Imaging. The value of thallium scintigraphy in the stratification of patients with stable CAD is based upon the documentation of scintigraphic variables, indicative of patients at high risk (see p. 1296) (Table 38–2). Among patients presenting with chest pain, and including patients with angiographically proven CAD, a normal stress perfusion study was associated with a cardiac event rate of less than 1 per cent per year.[477,478]

Pharmacological Perfusion Imaging. Pharmacological stress perfusion imaging techniques with dipyridamole, adenosine, or dobutamine have an established place as an alternative to exercise perfusion imaging in establishing prognosis in patients with stable CAD.[69a,69b,91,93,479,480,480a] These techniques have been particularly useful in patients with peripheral vascular disease and in the elderly.[95,481,482]

Pharmacological (Stress) Echocardiography. There is increasing evidence that echocardiography with exercise[483a] or pharmacological stress (dobutamine, arbutamine, or dipyridamole) can also be useful for risk stratification.[483a,484,485]

Results

Relief of Angina Pectoris

As early as 1972, a committee of the American Heart Association indicated that the most widely accepted indication for surgical revascularization was "significant disability from moderate to severe angina pectoris, unresponsive to optimal medical care."[486] Two and a half decades later, angina pectoris despite medical management remains the principal indication. However, coronary bypass surgery is now being carried out in increasing numbers of patients with multivessel coronary disease and either mild to moderate symptoms, left ventricular dysfunction, or poor exercise tolerance, because of the improved survival in these groups. Patients with unstable angina and left ventricular dysfunction as well as survivors of acute myocardial infarction are also undergoing revascularization with increasing frequency.

Relief of angina pectoris occurs in up to 95 per cent of patients with chronic stable angina following coronary artery bypass surgery. More than half of the patients become totally asymptomatic, at least initially. Most of the others experience substantial symptomatic relief. The major randomized trials have all demonstrated greater relief of angina, better exercise performance, and a lower requirement for antianginal medications for surgically compared with medically treated patients 5 years postoperatively.[448,487,488,498] After 5 years, differences in symptoms between patients initially treated medically and surgically are diminished, owing in part to the high "cross-over" rate from medical to surgical therapy in patients with continued symptoms, and a progression of disease in vein grafts and non-bypassed vessels in the surgical group.[487,488] The reoperation rate for recurrence of symptoms has been reported to be in the range of 6 to 8 per cent per year.[489]

For patients with persistent angina despite adequate medical therapy and for those who cannot tolerate the usual antianginal medications and who are not ideal candidates for PTCA, coronary bypass surgery provides excellent symptomatic relief.[490] With increasing use of IMA grafts, long-term relief of angina and freedom from subsequent cardiac events are improved, compared with previous patient populations who have received coronary artery vein grafts alone.

In summary, after 5 years, approximately three fourths of surgically treated patients can be predicted to be free from an ischemic event, sudden death, occurrence of myocardial infarction, or return of angina; about half remain free for approximately 10 years, and about 15 per cent for 15 or more years.[398,491,492] Symptomatic improvement is best maintained in patients with the most complete revascularization.[420]

Effects of Surgery on Survival in Patients with Chronic Stable Angina

Current clinical practice has been shaped by three major randomized trials into which patients were enrolled between 1972 and 1979, The Veterans Administration (VA), European Cardiac Society Study (ECSS), and the NIH-supported CASS.[493–499] These trials antedated the widespread use of the IMA for revascularization, as well as of aspirin and coronary angioplasty. Only CASS included women and only the VA trial included patients over the age of 65 years. High-risk patients, defined in terms of symptoms, severity of ischemia, age, extent of CAD, and left ventricular dysfunction, were generally excluded from the ECCS and CASS, even though such patients benefit the most from revascularization. The VA trial included a larger number of high-risk patients, and in the ECSS 42 per cent of patients had class III angina (Canadian Cardiovascular Society Criteria). In contrast, in CASS, all patients had either mild angina (Class I-II) or were asymptomatic after myocardial infarction.

In the VA study, there was no significant difference in overall survival between the groups initially assigned to medical and surgical treatment after 11 years of follow-up. However, higher risk subsets, including patients with left main coronary disease and patients who had three-vessel disease with impaired left ventricular function, initially had a significant survival advantage with surgery, although the magnitude of the difference decreased between 7 and 11 years. On retrospective analysis, a higher risk subset, with two or more of the following risk factors —New York Heart Association class III or IV angina; a history of hypertension; a history of prior myocardial infarction; and ST-segment depression on the resting electrocardiogram—experienced a survival benefit from operation.[497]

Patients randomized to an initial surgical approach also experienced an overall survival advantage in the ECSS[498] (Fig. 38–16). The benefits of surgery were greater in patients at higher risk, including patients with multivessel disease, which included the proximal left anterior descending coronary artery, older patients, those with evidence of ischemia or infarction on the resting electrocardiogram, patients with peripheral vascular disease, and those with a markedly positive stress test. There was no significant difference in survival between medical and surgical treatment in patients with one-vessel disease and those with two-vessel disease without critical stenosis of the proximal left anterior descending coronary artery. In the CASS randomized trial, there was no difference in overall survival between the medically and surgically treated groups.[493,499] However, survival of patients at higher risk, with a left ventricular ejection fraction between 35 and 50 per cent was improved by surgery.[493]

The results of the ECCS suggest that in patients with moderately severe angina pectoris and normal ventricular function, if several risk factors, such as age greater than 50 years, an abnormal electrocardiogram at rest, ST-segment depression greater than 1.5 mm during exercise, and peripheral arterial disease are present, coronary angiography should be performed. If three-vessel disease (coronary artery diameter stenoses > 75 per cent) or obstruction of the proximal left anterior descending coronary artery and one other major vessel is present, surgery appears to be superior to medical therapy.[448] Other clinical risk factors in patients with three-vessel disease and normal ventricular function that might lead to surgical rather than medical therapy include severe angina pectoris (class III or IV), a

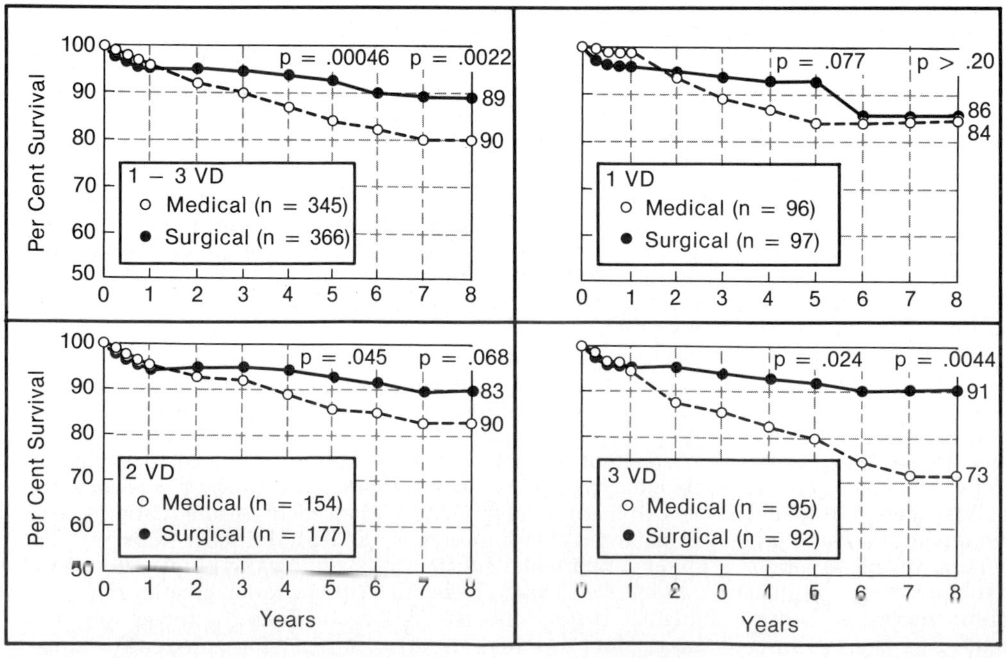

FIGURE 38–16. Cumulative survival curves for patients in the European Coronary Surgery Study. To compare the European prospective randomized coronary surgery study with other studies, a cohort of 711 patients was identified as having greater than 75 per cent obstruction in one, two, or three vessels. A significant improvement in survival with surgery was found in the total cohort and in the subgroup with three-vessel disease; however, there was no significant difference in survival between the two treatments in patients with one-vessel disease and those with two-vessel disease without proximal left anterior descending stenosis. (Reproduced with permission from Varnauskas, E., and the European Coronary Surgery Study Group: Survival, myocardial infarction, and employment status in a prospective, randomized study of coronary bypass surgery. Circulation 72(Suppl. V):90, 1985. Copyright American Heart Association.)

history of myocardial infarction, and resulting ST-segment depression.

LEFT MAIN CORONARY ARTERY STENOSIS. There is general agreement that surgical treatment improves survival in patients with left main coronary artery obstruction[500] or its "equivalent" (Fig. 38–15). The CASS registry demonstrated that the superiority of revascularization was equivalent in both symptomatic and asymptomatic patients with disease affecting the left main coronary artery.[462] Although coronary bypass surgery appears to confer the most benefit on patients with severe degrees of left main coronary artery disease and/or those patients with impaired left ventricular function, it is still beneficial in *all* patients with left main coronary stenoses greater than 60 per cent, which has recently been confirmed in a 16-year follow-up study from the CASS registry.[463]

There is continuing debate about whether there is a "left main equivalent" anatomy, which has a natural history similar to that of left main coronary disease. The condition in question may consist of disease in the proximal portions of both the left anterior descending and left circumflex coronary arteries. We believe that the ominous nature of significant left main coronary disease exists because a single event (rupture of a single plaque) can cause infarction of a very large quantity of myocardium. While combined disease of the proximal left anterior descending and circumflex coronary arteries does identify a subgroup of high-risk patients, the prognosis is not as poor as it is for patients with left main coronary artery disease.[502] Nevertheless, patients with combined stenoses of 70 per cent or greater in the left anterior descending coronary artery, before the first septal perforating branch, and in the proximal circumflex coronary artery before the first obtuse marginal branch, who have impaired ventricular function, also have improved survival and less angina following surgical revascularization than if they are treated medically, particularly in the face of left ventricular dysfunction.[503]

OVERVIEW OF THE RANDOMIZED TRIALS. A systematic overview of the seven randomized trials (the three aforementioned large trials and four smaller trials) which compared coronary bypass surgery with medical therapy between 1972 and 1984 yielded 2649 patients (Table 38–12).[448] Patients undergoing coronary bypass surgery had a significantly lower mortality at 5, 7, and 10 years, but by 10 years 41 per cent of the patients initially randomized to medical treatment had undergone CABG. The advantage for surgery was greatest in patients with left main coronary artery disease. An improvement in survival was also noted with surgical treatment in patients with one- or two-vessel disease and stenosis of the proximal left anterior descending coronary artery. In this published meta-analysis, the results for single- versus double-vessel disease in patients with left anterior descending coronary artery disease were not presented separately but it is likely that the majority of the benefit was in the patients with double-vessel disease.[448] Among patients without obstruction of the proximal left anterior descending coronary artery, the reduction in mortality was confined to those with left main coronary artery or three-vessel disease. Patients were further stratified into high-, moderate-, and low-risk subgroups using criteria developed by the Veterans Administration Cooperative Study.[495] These were based upon clinical criteria, including the severity of angina, history of hypertension, prior myocardial infarction, and ST-segment depression at rest. Low-risk patients had none of the four risk factors aside from ST-segment depression, whereas those with two or three risk factors were considered to be at high risk. In patients at high risk, the mortality reduction was 29 per cent at 10 years versus 10 per cent in patients at moderate risk. In low-risk patients, there was a nonsignificant trend toward a greater mortality with bypass surgery.

The results of all the trials and registries[496] taken together indicate that the "sicker" the patient (based upon the severity of symptoms or ischemia, age, the number of vessels diseased, and the presence of left ventricular dysfunction), the greater the benefit of surgical over medical therapy on survival (Table 38–12; Fig. 38–17).[338] Among low-risk patients and patients with single-vessel disease, no trial has demonstrated any benefit upon survival.

TABLE 38–12 EFFECTS OF CORONARY ARTERY BYPASS GRAFT SURGERY ON SURVIVAL*

SUBGROUP	MEDICAL TREATMENT MORTALITY RATE (%)	p FOR CABG SURGERY VS MEDICAL TREATMENT
Vessel disease		
One vessel	9.9	0.18
Two vessels	11.7	0.45
Three vessels	17.6	<0.001
Left main artery	36.5	0.004
No LAD disease		
One or two vessels	8.3	0.88
Three vessels	14.5	0.02
Left main artery	45.8	0.03
Overall	12.3	0.05
LAD disease present		
One or two vessels	14.6	0.05
Three vessels	19.1	0.009
Left main artery	32.7	0.02
Overall	18.3	0.001
LV function		
Normal	13.3	<0.001
Abnormal	25.2	0.02
Exercise test status		
Missing	17.4	0.10
Normal	11.6	0.38
Abnormal	16.8	<0.001
Severity of angina		
Class O, I, II	12.5	0.005
Class III, IV	22.4	0.001

* Systematic overview of coronary artery bypass graft surgery upon survival in comparison with medical therapy based on data from the 7 randomized trials comparing a strategy of initial coronary artery bypass graft surgery with one of initial medical therapy; illustrates subgroup results at 5 years.

From Yusuf, S., Zucker, D., Peduzzi, P., et al.: Effect of coronary artery bypass graft surgery on survival. Overview of 10 year results from randomized trials by the Coronary Artery Bypass Graft Surgery Trialists Collaboration, Lancet *344*:563, 1994.

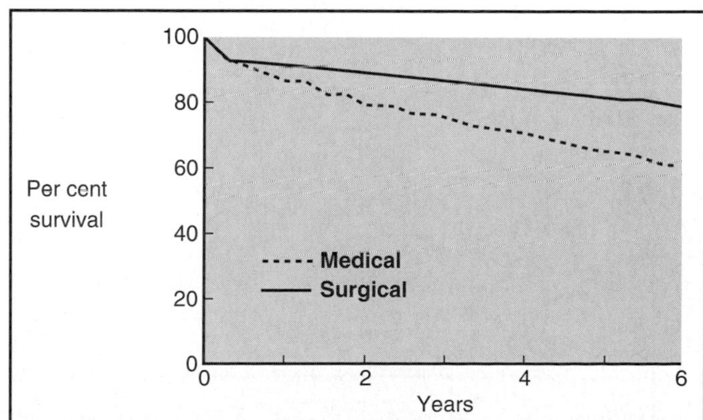

FIGURE 38–17. Cumulative 6-year survival rates in surgical and medical groups in the coronary artery surgery study (CASS) registry of 1491 patients 65 years or older. In addition to improved survival, at 5 years chest pain was absent in 62 per cent of the surgical group and 29 per cent of the medical group ($P < 0.0001$). Benefit of surgical treatment was greatest in the "high-risk" patients and was not observed in a subgroup at "low risk" who had mild angina, good ventricular function, and absence of left main CAD. (From Gersh, B. J., Kronmal, R. A., and Schaff, H. V.: Comparison of coronary artery bypass surgery and medical therapy in patients 65 years of age or older. N. Engl. J. Med. *313*:217, 1985. Copyright Massachusetts Medical Society.)

Thus, coronary bypass surgery prolongs survival in patients with significant left main coronary artery disease irrespective of symptoms, in patients with multivessel disease and impaired left ventricular function, and in patients with three-vessel disease that includes the proximal left anterior descending coronary artery (irrespective of left ventricular function).[448,490] Surgical therapy also has been demonstrated to prolong life in patients with *two-vessel disease* and left ventricular dysfunction, particularly in those with a critical stenosis of the proximal left anterior descending coronary artery. Although no study has documented a survival benefit with surgical treatment in patients with *single-vessel disease,* there is some evidence that such patients who have impaired left ventricular function have a poor long-term survival.[504] Such patients with angina and/or evidence of ischemia at a low or moderate level of exercise, especially those with obstruction of the proximal left anterior descending coronary artery, may benefit from coronary revascularization by either angioplasty or bypass surgery.

EFFECT OF SURGERY ON SUBSEQUENT MYOCARDIAL INFARCTION. The major randomized trials of patients with mild to moderate angina suggested that the likelihood of occurrence of myocardial infarction after 5 to 10 years of follow-up was similar in medically and surgically treated patients.[495–498,505,506] In the CASS, the reported annual risk of nonfatal Q wave myocardial infarction was 2.2 per cent per year with medical treatment compared with 2.8 per cent per year with surgical treatment.[506] However, in an observational study carried out in patients at higher risk for ischemic events (i.e., those with severe angina and three-vessel disease), a benefit of surgical treatment on the incidence of infarction was demonstrated.[507,508]

Patients with Depressed Left Ventricular Function

Over the last two decades, left ventricular dysfunction has changed from a relative contraindication to a strong indication for coronary revascularization.[509,510] Patients with impaired left ventricular function may demonstrate enhancement of left ventricular function and an improved long-term survival after coronary revascularization compared with medical treatment (Fig. 38–18).[511–514] Indeed, the most striking survival advantage as well as symptomatic and functional improvement is displayed by patients with the most impaired ventricular function in whom the prognosis with medical therapy is poor. In patients with a history of heart failure and three-vessel coronary artery disease, coronary bypass surgery may also reduce the incidence of sudden death.[514]

In one study which examined the late results of surgical and medical therapy for patients with CAD and resting left ventricular ejection fraction of 35 per cent or less, 7-year survival and freedom from nonfatal infarction were greater in the surgically than in the medically treated patients.[515] In other studies surgical treatment was shown to prolong survival in patients with ejection fractions of 25 per cent or less.[451] When these observations are taken together with the results of the Duke data base, it appears that if operative mortality is lower than approximately 7 per cent, surgery is likely to offer an advantage over medical therapy in patients with viable ischemic myocardium and severely depressed left ventricular function.[516]

However, congestive heart failure remains a powerful predictor of perioperative mortality and a poorer long-term outcome.[510,511] In the CASS registry, there was an increasing operative mortality with more severe degrees of left ventricular dysfunction[517] (Fig. 38–14). Patients with nor-

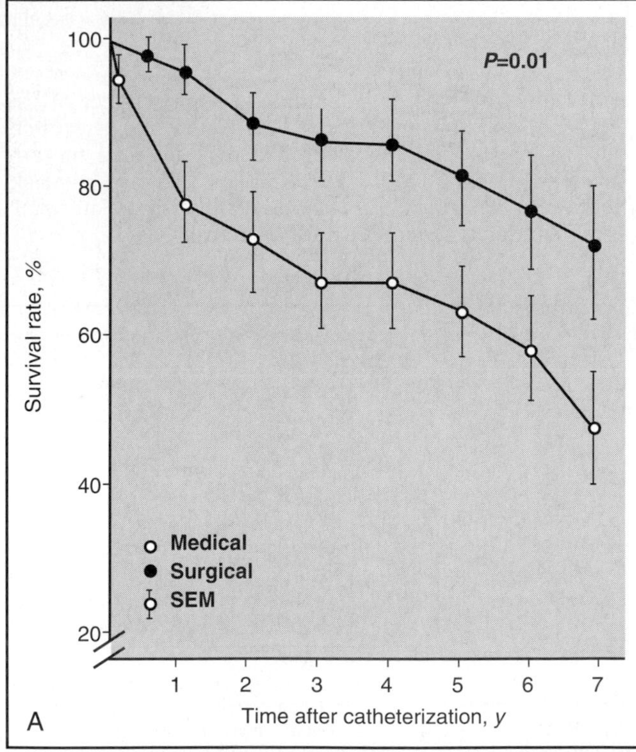

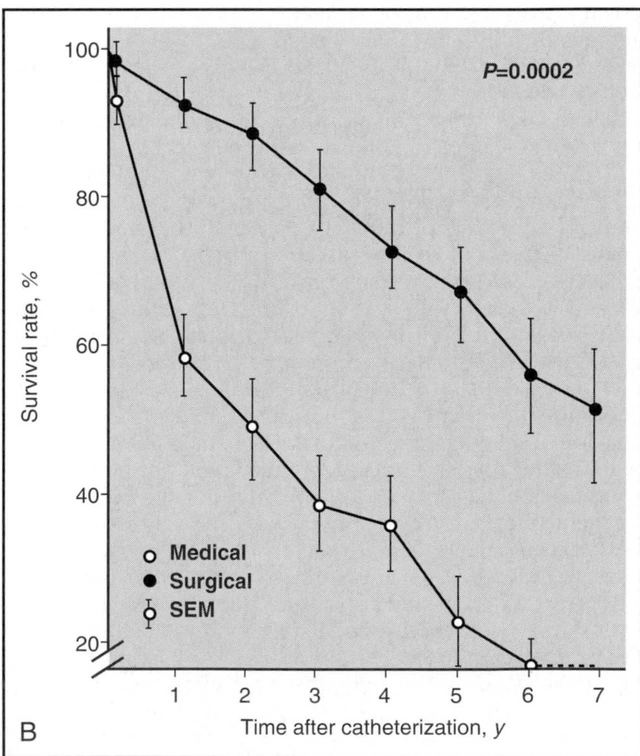

FIGURE 38–18. *A,* Cumulative survival of 47 patients treated surgically and 62 treated medically. All patients had an ejection fraction between 26 and 35 per cent. Seven-year survival rates were 73 and 50 per cent, respectively. *B,* Cumulative survival of 30 patients treated surgically and 53 treated medically. All patients had an ejection fraction of 25 per cent or less. Seven-year survival rates were 46 per cent and 15 per cent, respectively. (From Gersh, B. J.: Natural history of chronic coronary artery disease. *In* Beller, G. A. and Braunwald, E. [eds.]: Chronic Ischemic Heart Disease. Atlas of Heart Diseases, vol. 5. Philadelphia, Current Medicine, 1995, p. 1.16. Adapted from Piggott, J. D., et al.: Late results of surgical and medical therapy for patients with coronary artery disease and depressed left ventricular function. J. Am. Coll. Cardiol. *5:*1036, 1985.)

mal or nearly normal left ventricular function had an operative mortality rate of 2 per cent and a 5-year survival of 92 per cent. Patients with moderate impairment (ejection fraction 0.35 to 0.49) had an operative mortality of 4.2 per cent and a 5-year survival of 80 per cent, and in those with poor ventricular function (ejection fraction <0.35) the operative mortality was 6.2 per cent and 5-year survival 65 per cent. More recent data on patients with an ejection fraction of 30 per cent or less demonstrated an in-hospital surgical mortality rate of 8.4 per cent.[511]

MYOCARDIAL HIBERNATION. Improvement in survival and left ventricular function following CABG depends on successful reperfusion of viable but noncontractile or poorly contracting "hibernating" myocardium (see p. 388 and 1215). Two related pathophysiological conditions, myocardial *stunning* (prolonged but temporary postischemic ventricular dysfunction without myocardial necrosis) and myocardial *hibernation* (persistent left ventricular dysfunction when myocardial perfusion is chronically reduced but sufficient to maintain the viability of tissue) have been described. The reduction in myocardial contractility in hibernating myocardium conserves metabolic demands and may be protective.

Hibernating myocardium can cause abnormal systolic and/or diastolic ventricular function.[518,519] The predominant clinical feature of myocardial ischemia in these patients may not be angina, but dyspnea secondary to elevation of left ventricular diastolic pressure. Symptoms resulting from chronic left ventricular dysfunction may be inappropriately ascribed to myocardial necrosis and scarring when the symptoms may, in fact, be reversed when the chronic ischemia is relieved by coronary revascularization.

DETECTION OF HIBERNATING MYOCARDIUM. A reduction in *diastolic* wall thickness of dysfunctional left ventricular segments is indicative of scarring. On the other hand, akinetic or dyskinetic segments with preserved diastolic wall thickness may represent a mixture of scarred and viable myocardium. Diastolic wall thickness and segmental function can be assessed by echocardiography, magnetic resonance imaging, fast computed tomography, and angiocardiography. A useful strategy for the assessment of dysfunctional segments has been developed by Maseri (Fig. 38–19).

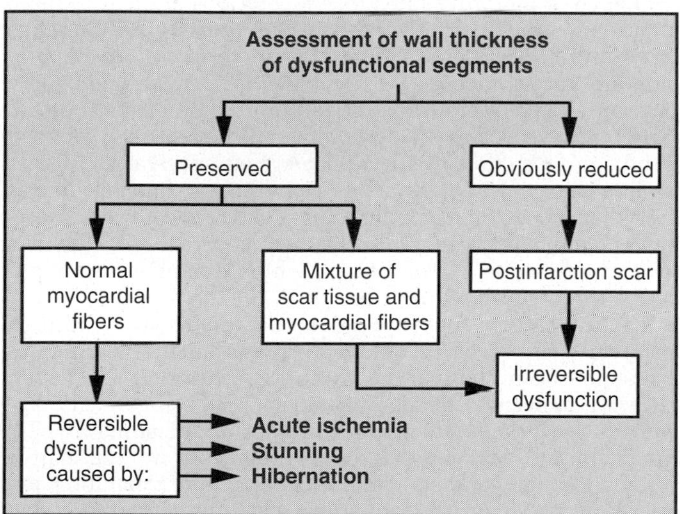

FIGURE 38–19. Flow diagram for the practical assessment of noncontractile segments of myocardial wall potentially recoverable by revascularization procedures. An obviously reduced wall thickness is indicative of postinfarction scar. The absence of contractile function in segments of the ventricular wall with preserved wall thickness may be caused by different mechanisms. An acute ischemic cause can be excluded by administration of sublingual nitrates. Stunning can be excluded by repeating the ventricular wall motion study several days after the last ischemic episode. Hibernating myocardium should be distinguished from a mixture of scar tissue and viable myocardial cells. (From Maseri, A.: Ischemic Heart Disease. New York, Churchill Livingstone, 1995, p. 642.)

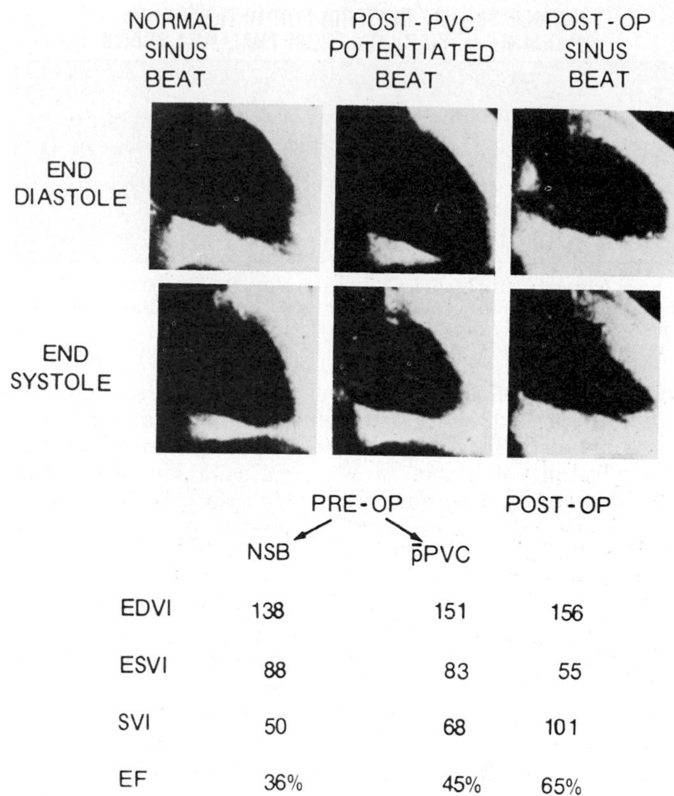

FIGURE 38–20. Examples of the ventriculographic analysis performed to evaluate the effects of an inotropic stimulus, including some of the calculations made. p̄PVC = premature ventricular contraction; PRE-OP = preoperative; POST-OP = postoperative; NSB = normal sinus beat; p̄PVC = after premature ventricular contraction; EDVI = end-diastolic volume index (ml/m²); ESVI = end-systolic volume index (ml/m²); SVI = stroke volume index (ml/m²); EF = ejection fraction. (From Popio, K. A., et al.: Post extrasystolic potentiation as a predictor of potential myocardial viability. Am. J. Cardiol. *39*:944, 1977.)

The term *contractile reserve* is used to describe the ability of wall segments of hibernating myocardium to exhibit augmented contractility, often causing an improvement in global ejection fraction in response to a suitable stimulus (Fig. 38–20). The demonstration of contractile reserve and of improvement in contractility after revascularization results from the fact that many hypokinetic (and even akinetic) areas of the ventricular wall are composed entirely or in part of viable, hibernating myocardium or of a mixture of the latter and fibrous scar. The viable muscle is capable of responding to a sympathomimetic agent or postextrasystolic potentiation and its contractile state may also respond to improved perfusion after operation. In contrast, necrotic tissue obviously cannot be stimulated to contract by any pharmacological or hemodynamic intervention or by improved perfusion. In patients with poor left ventricular function and poor contractile reserve (<10 per cent increase in ejection fraction with inotropic stimulation), perioperative mortality is high and long-term survival is poorer than in patients with equally depressed left ventricular function but normal contractile reserve.[137]

Positron emission tomography (PET) has evolved as the noninvasive "gold standard" for assessing viability, with a positive predictive value of 78 to 85 per cent and a negative predictive value of 78 to 92 per cent[520–522a] (Fig. 9–40, color plate 7). The high cost, technical difficulty, and need for a cyclotron limit this technique's widespread applicability. In 1991, a committee of the American Heart Association indicated that "201-thallium imaging may provide

TABLE 38–13 CRITERIA FOR DETERMINING MYOCARDIAL VIABILITY FROM THALLIUM SCANS

1. Normal thallium uptake on early scan
2. Complete thallium redistribution on delayed images
3. Defect fill-in following thallium reinjection
4. Partial redistribution of an initial defect on delayed images if defect cts > 50% peak counts
5. Mild fixed defect with defect cts > 50% peak cts

From Johnson, L. L.: Thallium-201 to assess myocardial viability. *In* Iskandrian, A. S., and van der Wall, E. E. (eds.): Myocardial Viability. Dordrecht, The Netherlands, Kluwer, 1994, pp. 19–37. cts = counts.

most of the clinical relevant data regarding viable myocardium in patients with left ventricular dysfunction" and recommended that PET be used in patients in whom the identification of viable myocardium is a key issue that would change patient management in respect to revascularization. This was considered particularly appropriate if the results from thallium-201 scintigraphy performed were equivocal.[523]

In the last 5 years, there have been further refinements to thallium scintigraphic techniques, including reinjection, rest-redistribution imaging, and quantitative analysis.[524–526] (Fig. 9–1, p. 275; Table 38–13). These new developments have enhanced considerably the sensitivity and specificity for thallium in the prediction of viability in apparently "fixed" defects. New tracers, such as the radiolabeled long-chain fatty acid, 123-iodine-iodophenylpentadecanoic acid (IPPA), in conjunction with thallium SPECT and sestamibi imaging appear to be promising in the assessment of viability as well.[527]

Dobutamine echocardiography may also be useful in the detection of myocardial ischemia. Increasing doses of dobutamine, up to a maximum of 40 μg/kg/min, are used (see p. 1297). On the other hand, low-dose dobutamine (5 to 20 μg/kg/min)[528,528a] can provide information regarding *reversibility* of segmental dysfunction. In patients with chronic CAD, this has been shown to be a promising, easily accessible, and less costly alternative to PET in the prediction of recovery of left ventricular function after revascularization.[528,528a] Myocardial contrast echocardiography during cardiac catheterization is also a promising investigation technique for defining myocardial segments with poor left ventricular function, which are viable and amenable to improvement following revascularization.[529]

Surgical Treatment in Special Groups

WOMEN (see also Ch. 51). It is clear that there are marked differences in the utilization rates of coronary bypass surgery between men and women.[530,531] However, it is unclear whether these differences represent an overutilization in men or underutilization in women or both. Compared with men, women who undergo coronary bypass surgery are "sicker" as defined by age, comorbidity, the severity of angina, and history of congestive heart failure.[531]

Many series have demonstrated a higher morbidity and mortality in coronary surgery in women. The Society of Thoracic Surgeons data base provides a broad perspective of outcomes in the United States.[399] Mortality was almost double in women compared with men, 4.6 per cent and 2.8 per cent, respectively. Perioperative morbidity, including myocardial infarction, respiratory failure, and stroke, was also significantly higher in women. Most of these differences can be accounted for by the "sicker" preoperative status of women, the higher rate of nonelective procedures, and perhaps by the smaller coronary arteries. However, a small independent detrimental effect of female gender persists in most multivarate analyses.[532, 533] Despite the increased perioperative mortality and morbidity in women, late survival is similar in men and women,[531,534,535] but the relief of anginal symptoms appears to be less in women.[536]

YOUNGER PATIENTS. Patients aged 35 or younger usually have hyperlipidemia and other major risk factors for CAD.[537] Despite the severity of the underlying disease and the rapidity of the atherosclerotic process, coronary bypass surgery is associated with excellent actuarial survival rates of 94 per cent at 5 years and 85 per cent at 10 years in these patients.[537] However, during longer follow-up, atherosclerosis of the venous grafts becomes an increasingly important problem in these patients,[538] which underlies the current trend to use bilateral IMA grafts and other arterial conduits in younger patients.

THE ELDERLY. The presence of CAD increases strikingly among the elderly, as does morbidity and mortality. In the United States, the utilization of noninvasive cardiovascular procedures in the elderly is extensive, and approximately half of all such procedures are performed in patients over the age of 65 years. Even though hospital mortality with CABG in the elderly has declined steadily,[538–540] age remains an important risk factor for mortality and morbidity and costs, although relief of angina is similar.[541,541a] The increase in perioperative mortality and morbidity in the elderly is, in part, due to diffuse atherosclerotic emboli (see p. 1696).[541b] Predictors of an adverse outcome include the presence and number of comorbid conditions and the presence of noncardiac vascular disease.

Evaluation of the elderly for coronary bypass surgery should take into account other less tangible factors related to quality of life and the potential ability to benefit from the operation. These include not only the chronological age of the patient, but also the estimated physiological age, comorbid conditions, the patient's attitude, including his/her understanding of the risks and expectations of the procedure, as well as an assessment of the patient's level of activity and current life style.

PATIENTS REQUIRING REOPERATION. At least 10 per cent of coronary artery procedures are now reoperations. This percentage is rising rapidly,[399,489,542] and in some centers exceeds 20 per cent. The indications for reoperation include progression of atherosclerosis in native vessels, incomplete revascularization at the time of the first operation, and both early and late graft failure.

Operative mortality rates for reoperations are two to three times higher than that of the initial procedure and range from 2 to 10 per cent.[543] The clinical results after reoperation are not as good as those after a primary procedure. By 5 years after reoperation surgery, approximately half of the patients have recurrent symptoms. However, late survival results are excellent, with a 90 per cent survival at 5 years and 75 per cent at 10 years.[544] Nonetheless, late survival is less than for patients undergoing a first procedure. This is understandable given the older age, severe CAD, and frequency of comorbid conditions, which comprise the population undergoing reoperation.[545]

The indications for reoperation compared with continued medical therapy or percutaneous transcatheter techniques have not been defined in a randomized trial. Moreover, they are subject to change given the increasingly wide application of percutaneous techniques to diseased bypass grafts and to lesions that have progressed in the native circulation. In general, the indications for reoperation are based upon the same principles that apply to initial disease, although the higher risk and poorer late outcome of reoperation than for initial operation need to be taken into account.

OTHER HIGH-RISK SUBGROUPS. Patients with *familial hyperlipidemia* have long been considered to be at particular risk for an adverse late outcome after coronary bypass surgery. More encouraging results have been reported after the use of an IMA or other arterial conduit, in conjunction with aggressive lipid-lowering therapy.[546] The risks of cardiac surgery in patients with *end-stage renal disease* are markedly increased. Nonetheless, the reported results (63 per cent cumulative survival over 5 years in patients with

NYHA class II-III symptoms) justify treating symptomatic patients on dialysis, but before the onset of severe congestive heart failure.[547] Elderly *diabetics* with angiographically proven coronary artery disease are more likely to be female, with evidence of peripheral vascular disease and a higher number of coronary occlusions compared with age-matched nondiabetic patients.[548] In a cohort of CASS registry patients, diabetes was an independent predictor of mortality. However, the relative survival benefit of coronary bypass surgery versus medical therapy was comparable in diabetic and nondiabetic patients, with a significant reduction in mortality of 44 per cent provided by surgery over medical therapy in the former.[548]

Summary of Indications for Coronary Revascularization

1. Certain anatomical subsets of patients are candidates for coronary bypass surgery, irrespective of the severity of symptoms or left ventricular dysfunction. These include patients with significant left main coronary artery disease and most patients with three-vessel disease, which includes the proximal left anterior descending coronary artery, especially those with left ventricular dysfunction.

2. The benefits of coronary bypass surgery are well documented in patients with left ventricular dysfunction and multivessel disease, irrespective of symptoms. In patients whose dominant symptom is heart failure without severe angina, the benefits of coronary revascularization are less well defined, but this approach should be considered in patients with evidence of significant contractile reserve.

3. The primary objective of coronary revascularization in patients with one-vessel disease is the relief of significant symptoms or objective evidence of severe ischemia. For the majority of these, PTCA is the revascularization modality of choice.

4. In patients with angina who are *not* considered to be at high risk, survival is similar in surgically and medically treated patients.

5. All of the indications discussed above relate to the potential benefits of surgery over medical therapy on *survival*. Coronary revascularization using angioplasty or bypass surgery is highly efficacious in relieving symptoms and may be considered for patients with moderate to severe ischemic symptoms who are dissatisfied with medical therapy, even if they are not in a high-risk subset. In such patients the optimal method of revascularization is selected on the basis of arteriographic findings.

Comparisons Between PTCA and CABG

OBSERVATIONAL STUDIES. Comparisons between angioplasty and coronary bypass surgery in patients with multivessel disease indicate that mortality and nonfatal myocardial infarction rates are similar between the two groups. The relief of angina is greater and the need for repeat revascularization is substantially lower after surgery. Among patients with left ventricular dysfunction, survival after surgery appears to be better than after angioplasty, probably because of the ability to achieve more complete revascularization with the former.[549] Indeed, complete revascularization is achieved by PTCA in only 25 to 50 percent of patients with two-vessel disease and in 10 to 25 per cent of patients with three-vessel disease.[342,343] In the future, improvements in transcatheter techniques, particularly in the ability to treat chronic total occlusions, may improve the results of this approach in patients with left ventricular dysfunction.

Outcome data 1 year after PTCA in patients (most of whom had single-vessel disease) indicate that approximately 20 per cent of patients undergo CABG; recurrence of symptoms and/or the need for repeat revascularization procedures is high (approximately 40 per cent). Bypass surgery provided a clear survival benefit over angioplasty in the Duke University data base in patients with severe two-vessel disease which included 95 per cent or greater obstruction of the proximal left anterior descending coronary artery and in all forms of three-vessel disease[338] (Fig. 38–21). On the other hand, the effect on survival of the methods of revascularization was equal in patients with two-vessel disease, without proximal left anterior descending coronary artery obstruction.

RANDOMIZED TRIALS. Four randomized trials comparing PTCA with coronary bypass surgery in patients with multivessel disease have been published[314,351,418,550–551c] and are described in Table 39–7, p. 1374. Two randomized trials have compared PTCA with CABG in patients confined to those with single-vessel disease, and the RITA trial included patients with single as well as multivessel disease.[337b,418,551b] An appreciation of the baseline characteristics of the patients entered into these trials is critical to the placement of these trials into a clinical context. Approximately two-thirds of the patients who were eligible clinically were excluded on angiographic grounds, including the presence of chronic total occlusions, complex stenoses, left main coronary artery disease, and the inability to achieve functionally adequate revascularization with angioplasty as well as by recent myocardial infarction and

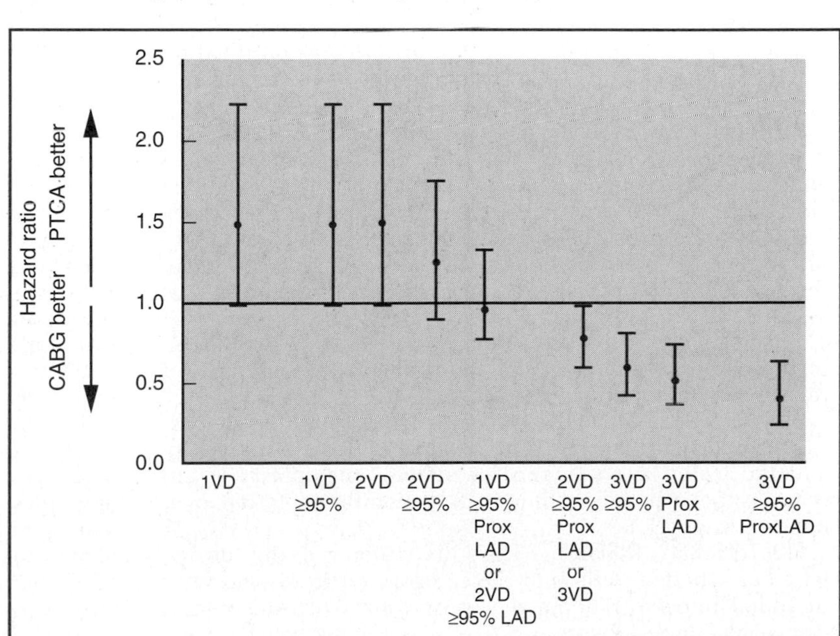

FIGURE 38–21. Hazard ratios for coronary artery bypass graft surgery (CABG) versus percutaneous transluminal coronary angioplasty (PTCA). Points below 1.0 favor CABG. VD = vessel disease; Prox LAD = proximal left anterior descending coronary artery. (Reproduced with permission from Mark, D. B., Nelson, C. L., Califf, R. M., et al.: Continuing evaluation of therapy for coronary artery disease: Initial results from the era of coronary angioplasty. Circulation *89:*2015, 1994. Copyright American Heart Association.)

previous revascularization. In the RITA and ERACI trials, the ability to achieve "equivalent" degrees of revascularization in the two groups was an inclusion criterion.[351,418] Moreover, the majority of patients entered into the trials had well-preserved left ventricular function with a mean ejection fraction exceeding 50 per cent. Patients with significant left ventricular dysfunction and multivessel disease were underrepresented in these trials.

The BARI trial (Bypass Angioplasty Revascularization Investigation), which was carried out in North America in patients with multivessel disease, is the largest of the randomized trials of coronary bypass surgery and PTCA and the only trial with sufficient statistical power to detect differences in mortality. Preliminary data demonstrate a significant difference in 5-year survival in favor of coronary bypass surgery in the approximately 300 diabetic patients receiving therapy for diabetes; no difference in mortality was noted among the remaining approximately 1500 patients (nondiabetics or diabetics not receiving treatment). It should be emphasized that these data are preliminary, but a recent meta-analysis of the randomized trials of CABG and PTCA in patients with multivessel disease (excluding the BARI data) demonstrated a trend toward an overall adverse outcome after hospital discharge in patients treated with PTCA.[314a]

Given the differences between the studies, it is reassuring that the results are remarkably consistent among the trials and with observational data.[551a] In this highly selected group of patients, after 1 to 3 years of follow-up, there were no significant differences in mortality or in the rate of myocardial infarction between patients treated with angioplasty and coronary bypass surgery.[551a] Moreover, as anticipated from observational data, the rate of subsequent revascularization procedures as well as the recurrence of angina were considerably higher in the angioplasty group.[551a] For example, in the EAST study, at 3 years only 13 per cent of patients in the CABG group required additional revascularization (surgery or angioplasty), compared with 54 per cent of the patients in the PTCA group.[351] Another consistent but predictable finding was the lower in-hospital cost in patients undergoing angioplasty. However, the need for recurrent hospitalizations and repeat revascularization procedures over the subsequent period of follow-up contributed to an increase in postdischarge costs in the angioplasty group[552,552a] and almost equal expenditures over a 3-year time span.

The Choice Between Coronary Angioplasty and Bypass Surgery

(Table 38–14)

The medical management of chronic CAD as outlined on pp. 1299 to 1313 involves the reduction of reversible risk factors, life style alterations counseling, the treatment of conditions that intensify angina, and the pharmacological management of ischemia. When an unacceptable level of angina persists, and/or the patient experiences troubling side effects from the anti-ischemic drugs, the coronary anatomy should be defined to allow selection of the appropriate technique for revascularization. In patients in whom the angina is controlled, noninvasive testing is carried out and coronary arteriography is carried out in those having a "high-risk" result (see p. 1297). Following the elucidation of the coronary anatomy, the selection of the technique of revascularization is made as follows:

SINGLE-VESSEL DISEASE. Among patients with single-vessel disease in whom revascularization is deemed necessary and the lesion is anatomically suitable, angioplasty or another catheter-based technique is generally preferred over bypass surgery.

MULTIVESSEL DISEASE. The first step is to decide whether a patient falls into the category of those who were included into the randomized trials comparing angioplasty and bypass surgery. Patients were included in the trials only if it was believed that equivalent degrees of revascularization were achieved by both techniques and most patients with occluded coronary arteries were excluded. The majority of patients had double-vessel disease and well-preserved left ventricular function.[551a] The lack of any difference in late mortality and in myocardial infarction between the two groups in such patients indicates that angioplasty is a reasonable *initial* strategy, provided that the patient accepts the distinct possibility of symptom recurrence and need for a repeat revascularization procedure. Patients with a single, localized lesion in each affected vessel and preserved left ventricular function fare best with angioplasty. The BARI trial results in diabetics raise additional questions in this subgroup of patients, but further analyses are needed before definitive conclusions can be drawn.[314a]

TABLE 38–14 COMPARISON OF REVASCULARIZATION STRATEGIES IN MULTIVESSEL DISEASE

	ADVANTAGES	DISADVANTAGES
PTCA	Less invasive	Restenosis
	Shorter hospital stay	High incidence of incomplete revascularization
	Lower initial cost	Relative inefficacy in patients with severe LV dysfunction
	Easily repeated	Uncertain long-term outcome (>10 y)
	Effective in relieving symptoms	Limited to specific anatomic subsets
CABG	Effective in relieving symptoms	Cost
	Improved survival in certain subsets	Increased risk of a repeat procedure due to late graft closure
	Ability to achieve complete revascularization	
	Wider applicability	Morbidity

Modified from Faxon, D. P.: Coronary angioplasty for stable angina pectoris. *In* Beller, G. and Braunwald, E. (eds.): Chronic Ischemic Heart Disease. Atlas of Heart Diseases, vol. 5. Philadelphia, Current Medicine, 1995.

NEED FOR COMPLETE REVASCULARIZATION. Complete revascularization is an important goal in patients with left ventricular dysfunction and/or multivessel disease. The major advantage of bypass surgery over PTCA is the ability to achieve complete revascularization, particularly in patients with three-vessel disease. In the majority of such patients, particularly those with chronic total coronary occlusion, left ventricular dysfunction, or left main coronary artery disease, coronary bypass surgery is the procedure of choice.[312] Among patients with borderline left ventricular function (ejection fraction between 45 per cent and 50 per cent) and milder degrees of ischemia, PTCA may provide adequate revascularization, even if it is not anatomically complete.

Many patients fall into a gray zone in which either method of revascularization is suitable. Other factors that come into consideration include (1) access to a high quality team and operator with an excellent record of success; (2) patient preference; some patients are made anxious by the idea that following angioplasty they are at high risk of symptom recurrence and may require reintervention. Such patients are better candidates for surgical treatment; (3) patient's age and comorbidity; frail, very elderly patients and those with comorbid conditions, such as cancer or serious hepatic disease with a limited life span, who have disabling angina are often better candidates for angioplasty; (4) angioplasty is often preferable in younger patients (<50 years) with the expectation that they may require surgery some time in the future and that angioplasty will postpone the need for operation; this sequence may be preferable to two operations.

Coronary Bypass Surgery in Patients with Associated Vascular Disease

The management of patients with combined CAD and peripheral vascular disease, involving the carotid arteries, the abdominal aorta, or the vessels of the lower extremities, presents many challenges.[553] Combined disease is becoming increasingly important as the population of patients under consideration for CABG ages and as technical improvements allow the application of coronary revascularization to ever more complex cases.

IMPACT OF CAD IN PATIENTS WITH PERIPHERAL VASCULAR DISEASE. Clinically apparent CAD occurs frequently in patients with peripheral vascular disease.[31] The prevalence of clinically unrecognized CAD, as documented by angiographic studies, is even higher.[553] Among patients undergoing peripheral vascular surgery, the late outcomes are dominated by cardiac causes of morbidity and mortality.[553–555] Conversely, in patients with CAD the presence of peripheral vascular disease, even if it is asymptomatic, is associated with an adverse prognosis.[556]

If coronary revascularization is performed prior to the vascular surgery in patients with combined peripheral vascular and CAD, the perioperative mortality of the vascular procedure is reduced.[31,557] In seven series totaling 1237 patients undergoing vascular surgical procedures, the mean operative mortality was 1.5 per cent among patients with prior coronary bypass surgery, similar to the 1.3 per cent mortality rate in patients without clinically apparent CAD, and substantially lower than the 6.8 per cent mortality rate in patients with clinically suspected but uncorrected CAD.[31] Late mortality in patients with peripheral vascular disease is also reduced among those who have undergone prior coronary bypass surgery.[558,559] However, because patients with CAD with peripheral atherosclerosis tend to be older and to have more widespread vascular disease and end-organ damage than patients without peripheral atherosclerosis, the perioperative mortality and morbidity consequent to CABG are high and the late outcome not as favorable.[31,540,541,560] Diffuse *atheroembolism* (see p. 1320) is a particularly serious complication of coronary bypass surgery in patients with peripheral vascular disease and aortic atherosclerosis.[541] It is a major cause of perioperative death, stroke, neurocognitive dysfunction, and multiple organ dysfunction after bypass surgery.

It is important to identify CAD and to estimate its severity in patients who are candidates for peripheral vascular surgery. The diagnostic problem is intensified by the fact that these patients often have limited walking capacity and therefore may not develop effort angina. Pharmacological stress myocardial perfusion scintigraphy or echocardiography can be employed. The identification of "high risk" patients using these techniques (see p. 1297) should lead to coronary angiography and, depending on the anatomic findings, to coronary revascularization, often prior to peripheral vascular surgery.

Thus, the presence of peripheral vascular disease suggests that the patient may also have high-risk CAD, with potential benefit from bypass surgery in the long term. In the ECSS, patients with CAD and peripheral vascular disease treated surgically had a much better survival than did medically treated patients.[498] In the CASS registry, patients with peripheral vascular disease and three-vessel CAD who received surgical treatment also exhibited a major reduction in late mortality and morbidity compared with those who managed medically.[31] Observations such as these argue for consideration of coronary revascularization in patients with peripheral vascular disease who have significant CAD. The major indication for coronary revascularization prior to vascular surgery in patients with known chronic coronary artery disease is the intention of improving *long-term* prognosis as opposed to perioperative outcomes alone, because the latter have markedly improved in the current era of sophisticated pre- and perioperative care.[31]

CAROTID ARTERY DISEASE (see also p. 1879). In patients with stable CAD and *carotid artery disease* in whom endarterectomy is planned, exercise stress testing and consideration of coronary revascularization can ordinarily be performed postoperatively.[31] Although the presence of asymptomatic carotid bruits increases the risk of stroke after coronary bypass surgery,[561] there is little to suggest that prophylactic carotid endarterectomy reduces the risk of perioperative stroke in such patients.[562,563]

MANAGEMENT. Patients with severe or unstable coronary disease can be categorized into two groups according to the severity and instability of the accompanying vascular disease.[31] When the noncoronary vascular procedures are elective, they can generally be postponed until the cardiac symptoms have stabilized, either by intensive medical therapy or by revascularization. A combined procedure is necessary in patients with both unstable CAD and an unstable vascular condition, e.g., frequent recurrent transient ischemic attacks or a rapidly expanding abdominal aortic aneurysm.[562,564,565] In some patients in this category, PTCA offers the potential for stabilizing the patient from a cardiac standpoint, prior to proceeding with a definitive vascular repair.[566]

UNSTABLE ANGINA

Coronary artery disease represents a spectrum of conditions, with acute transmural infarction at one end of the spectrum, ranging successively through nontransmural infarction, unstable angina, and chronic stable angina, to silent ischemia at the other. Unstable angina (previously also known as preinfarction angina, crescendo angina, acute coronary insufficiency, and intermediate coronary syndrome) is at the center of this spectrum. This condition is frightening and disabling in nature and may herald acute myocardial infarction. In 1991, the US National Center for Health Statistics reported 570,000 hospitalizations carrying a diagnosis of unstable angina, resulting in 3.1 million hospital days, making it one of the most common serious cardiovascular disorders.[567]

DEFINITION. In addition to the absence of clear-cut electrocardiographic and cardiac enzyme changes diagnostic of a myocardial infarction, the currently used definition of unstable angina pectoris depends on the presence of one or more of the following three historical features: (1) crescendo angina (more severe, prolonged, or frequent) superimposed on a preexisting pattern or relatively stable, exertion-related angina pectoris; (2) angina pectoris of new onset (usually within 1 month), which is brought on by minimal exertion; or (3) angina pectoris at rest as well as with minimal exertion. In some patients, the ischemic episode of unstable angina pectoris can be related to obvious precipitating factors, such as anemia, infection, thyrotoxicosis, or cardiac arrhythmias, and the condition is then called *secondary unstable angina*.[568] Prinzmetal's ("variant") angina is also characterized by angina at rest and may be considered to be a form of unstable angina, but it is pathogenetically distinct and is discussed on p. 1340.

CLASSIFICATION. The syndrome of unstable angina describes a broad population of patients.[568a] They may be patients with single-vessel or multivessel coronary artery disease; a minority have no critically severe obstruction on coronary arteriography. They may or may not have a history of prior myocardial infarction or chronic angina, may have unstable angina while receiving no medical therapy, or may be suffering severe, transient episodes of ischemia despite a combination of medications including full doses of nitrates, calcium antagonists, beta blockers, aspirin, and intravenous heparin.

To categorize this heterogeneous population, one of the authors of this chapter proposed a classification that focuses on three important issues[568] (Table 38–15): (1) the severity of the clinical manifestations, (2) the clinical circumstances in which the unstable angina occurs, and (3) whether or not the symptomatic ischemic episodes are accompanied by transient electrocardiographic changes. This classification notes whether or not rest pain is present, whether rest pain has occurred within the preceding 48 hours, and whether the unstable angina is provoked by conditions such as anemia, fever, infection, and tachyarrhythmias. It is also proposed that the amount of therapy administered be taken into account.[568a]

Severity of Unstable Angina. The severity is graded according to whether or not rest pain has occurred and, if so, its timing. Class I is defined as the onset of severe, accelerated angina, occurring within 2 months of presentation, *without* rest pain. Also included in this class are patients with chronic stable angina who have developed angina that is distinctly more frequent, severe, longer in duration, or precipitated by substantially less exertion than previously. Class II refers to patients with a history of rest angina during the preceding 2 months, but not the preceding 48 hours. Class III refers to patients who have experienced one or more episodes of angina at rest within the preceding 48 hours.

In contrast to unstable angina, Class I, chronic exertional angina is by definition stable, and although it may have developed recently, it is not severe or frequent, as defined above. Angina that is severe and/or frequent and remains unchanged for more than 2 months is also *not* considered to be unstable. Patients with prolonged (>30 min) chest discomfort accompanied by ST-segment *elevation* are *not* considered to have unstable angina.

Clinical Circumstances in Which Unstable Angina Occurs. Unstable angina is also classified according to the clinical circumstances in which it occurs. Class A (secondary unstable angina) refers to patients, usually with underlying obstructive CAD, in whom the imbalance between myocardial oxygen supply and demand causing the instability results from conditions that are *extrinsic* to the coronary vascular bed. This includes patients in whom reductions of myocardial oxygen supply result from anemia or hypoxemia, while increases in myocardial oxygen demand which precipitate unstable angina may be caused by such conditions as fever, infection, uncontrolled hypertension, aortic stenosis, tachyarrhythmia, unusual emotional stress, and thyrotoxicosis. Class B (primary unstable angina) occurs in the *absence* of an identifiable extracoronary condition responsible for intensifying ischemia and in patients who have not suffered a myocardial infarction within the preceding 2 weeks. This is the most common form of unstable angina and includes a large majority of patients with underlying coronary atherosclerosis and an unstable plaque that has caused subtotal coronary occlusion. Class C (postinfarction unstable angina) is present in patients who develop unstable angina within 2 weeks of a documented acute myocardial infarction; it occurs in approximately 20 per cent of patients following infarction.

This is a clinical classification, which can be related to underlying disease. For example, Class III patients (with recent rest angina) are more likely to have intracoronary thrombus, and heparin may be of greater value in such patients than in patients in Classes I and II. A clinical score based upon this classification is an important predictor of intracoronary thrombus and lesion complexity.[569] Two prospective studies of patients admitted for suspected unstable angina demonstrated that this classification is an appropriate instrument to predict survival, infarct-free survival, and infarct free-survival without intervention.[570,571]

TABLE 38–15 CLASSIFICATION OF UNSTABLE ANGINA

SEVERITY	
Class I	**New-onset, severe, or accelerated angina.** **Patients with angina of less than 2 months' duration, severe or occurring three or more times per day, or angina that is distinctly more frequent and precipitated by distinctly less exertion. No rest pain in the last 2 months.**
Class II	**Angina at rest. Subacute.** **Patients with one or more episodes of angina at rest during the preceding month but not within the preceding 48 hours.**
Class III	**Angina at rest. Acute.** **Patients with one or more episodes at rest within the preceding 48 hours.**
CLINICAL CIRCUMSTANCES	
Class A	**Secondary unstable angina.** **A clearly identified condition extrinsic to the coronary vascular bed that has intensified myocardial ischemia, e.g., anemia, infection, fever, hypotension, tachyarrhythmia, thyrotoxicosis, hypoxemia secondary to respiratory failure.**
Class B	**Primary unstable angina.**
Class C	**Postinfarction unstable angina (within 2 weeks of documented myocardial infarction).**
INTENSITY OF TREATMENT	
1.	**Absence of treatment or minimal treatment.**
2.	**Occurring in presence of standard therapy for chronic stable angina (conventional doses of oral beta blockers, nitrates, and calcium antagonists).**
3.	**Occurring despite maximally tolerated doses of all three categories of oral therapy, including intravenous nitroglycerin.**

From Braunwald, E.: Unstable angina: A classification. Circulation *80*:410, 1989. Copyright 1989 American Heart Association.

Pathophysiology

As already pointed out, the majority of patients with unstable angina have severe obstructive CAD, and episodes of myocardial ischemia can be precipitated by either an increase in myocardial oxygen demands and/or a reduction in supply.[572] Episodes of spontaneous (rest) angina can be preceded by a reduction of myocardial oxygen supply due to a further reduction in lumen diameter consequent to transient vasoconstrictor influences, and/or platelet thrombi (Fig 38–1*C*). Elevations of arterial pressure and/or tachycardia, which lead to increases in myocardial oxygen requirements, can also provoke episodes of unstable angina.

In many patients with unstable angina and episodes of rest pain who are continuously monitored, an interesting sequence of events has been demonstrated. First, there is a reduction of coronary sinus oxygen saturation (which, in the presence of constant myocardial oxygen needs, signifies a reduction of coronary blood flow). This is followed by ST-segment depression, and only then does chest discomfort appear. Blood pressure and/or heart rate may rise secondary to the latter.[573] Thus, in many patients with unstable angina, ischemia appears to be precipitated by a reduction in oxygen supply, rather than an increase in oxygen demand, the latter being the most common precipitant of chronic stable angina. It is also likely that in some episodes of unstable angina an increase in myocardial oxygen demand and a reduction in supply occur simultaneously. In a patient with critical coronary obstruction, a mild increase in myocardial oxygen demand and a small reduction in supply could act in concert to produce critical ischemia and unstable angina. Such a sequence could explain the circadian variation in the distribution of ischemic events in patients with unstable angina in which patients with a low coronary reserve exhibited a higher incidence of severe ischemia in the morning.[208a,574]

Evidence indicates that the development of unstable angina may be preceded by marked recent progression in the extent and severity of CAD.[575,575a] Other important mechanisms contributing to the reduction of oxygen supply, and therefore to the precipitation of ischemic episodes in patients with unstable angina with severe underlying obstructive CAD, include the platelet aggregation, thrombosis, and coronary vasoconstriction, which are discussed below.

PLATELET AGGREGATION. There is substantial evidence to support the role of platelet aggregation either as a primary phenomenon or secondary to plaque rupture or fissure in the precipitation of ischemic episodes in patients with unstable angina as well as myocardial infarction (Fig. 37–7, p. 1188). It is likely that other factors may also be operative, such as increases in sympathetic vascular tone, elevated circulating catecholamine levels, hypercholesterolemia, leukocyte activation,[575b] and impaired fibrinolysis. These may be manifested by increased serum concentrations of plasminogen activator inhibitor type-I, (PAI-1) in addition to the activation of alpha$_2$-adrenergic and serotonergic platelet receptors, which may promote platelet aggregation.[576–578]

Platelets and the coronary vascular endothelium interact in a complex manner; platelets produce thromboxane A_2, a proaggregatory and vasoconstrictor substance (see p. 1165), whereas the normal endothelium produces the antiaggregatory vasodilator prostacyclin (prostaglandin I_2), as well as tissue plasminogen activator (t-PA) and endothelium-derived relaxing factor (see p. 1164). It has been speculated that the abrupt conversion from chronic stable angina to unstable angina may result from the more intense myocardial ischemia initiated by platelet aggregation,[578] from coronary vasoconstriction resulting from the local accumulation of thromboxane A_2 and serotonin, and also from reductions in the local concentrations of endothelially derived vasodilators and inhibitors of platelet aggregation.[579]

In patients with unstable angina who have had pain within the preceding 24 hours, the finding of elevated metabolites of thromboxane A_2 derived from aggregating platelets in plasma and urine suggests that local release of thromboxane may be associated with the episodes of unstable angina.[578] The reductions in coronary blood flow in canine preparations with marked coronary obstruction appear to be abolished by platelet inhibitors, including aspirin, sulfinpyrazone, prostacyclin, ibuprofen, and indomethacin but *not* by heparin, nitroglycerin, or papaverine.[580] This finding suggests that these reductions are mediated by platelet aggregation rather than by vasospasm or fibrin deposition. Furthermore, four separate clinical trials have now shown that aspirin can protect against death and nonfatal acute myocardial infarction in patients with unstable angina[581–584] (p. 1829). The beneficial impact of a GP-IIb/IIIa platelet receptor blocker (see p. 1629), which is a potent inhibitor of platelet aggregation, upon recurrent ischemic events in patients with unstable angina, provides further evidence in support of a major role of platelet aggregation in the pathophysiology of unstable angina.[585,586] Finally, in patients with unstable angina who suffer sudden death, aggregates of platelet emboli have been found in small intramyocardial vessels in segments of myocardium immediately downstream from a major epicardial coronary artery containing an atheromatous plaque that has undergone fissuring and on which mural thrombus had developed.[587]

THROMBOSIS. In addition to platelet aggregation, the presence of an active thrombotic process in patients with unstable angina is suggested by increased serum concentrations of fibrin-related antigen and D-dimer (the principal breakdown fragment of fibrin), tissue plasminogen activator and tissue plasminogen activator inhibitor-I,[588,589] prothrombin fragment 1+2, and fibrinopeptide-A.[590,591] These changes do not occur in patients with chronic stable angina and suggest that a hypercoagulable state is not just a marker of the acute thrombotic episode, but persists after clinical stabilization.[590] In patients with unstable angina pectoris, intracoronary thrombus formation is associated with a hypercoagulable state in association with diminished fibrinolytic activity.[592] Several studies in patients with unstable angina have shown intracoronary filling defects having the appearance of thrombi at angiography[593,594] (Fig. 38–22), and this finding has been confirmed by coronary angioscopy.[595,596] Furthermore, when thrombolytic therapy is administered to patients with unstable angina and recent pain, dissolution of intracoronary filling defects has been observed.[593,594,597] Finally, postmortem observations in many patients with unstable angina have suggested an ongoing thrombotic process in a major coronary artery. This process may accumulate in total occlusion, which is responsible for infarction and/or sudden death.[598]

CORONARY CONSTRICTION. Quantitative angiography has shown vasomotor hyperreactivity localized to regions of preexisting coronary atheroma in patients with unstable angina.[599] Postmortem studies have shown that in the majority of significantly diseased coronary arteries a portion of the circumference is circumscribed by normal arterial walls.[600] Therefore, it is likely that a normal pliable muscular elastic arc of vessel wall provides a mechanism whereby normal (vasoconstriction) or abnormally intense (vasospasm) increases in vasomotor tone may narrow lumen caliber and thus flow resistance.[601]

Endothelial dysfunction may lead to vasoconstriction by promoting the release of physiological mediators of vasoconstriction such as endothelin-I, or by inhibiting the release of vasodilator substances, such as prostacyclin and endothelium-derived relaxing factor (see p. 1164).[602,603] Endothelial dysfunction may also impair fibrinolysis in the acute ischemic syndromes because functioning endothe-

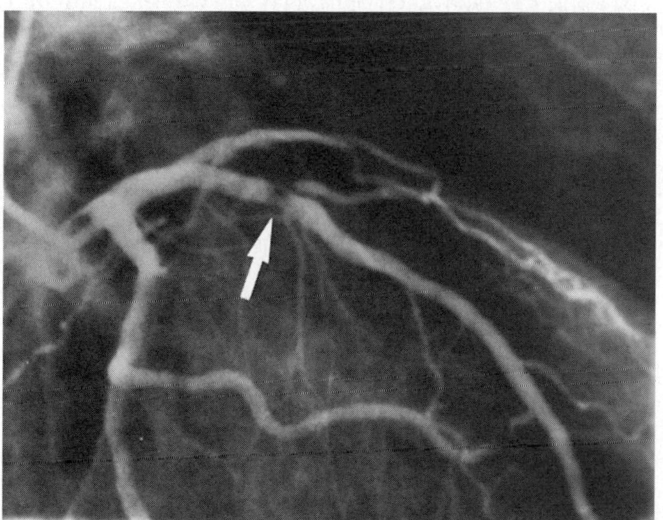

FIGURE 38–22. Coronary artery thrombus in a patient with unstable angina. A 60-year-old man was admitted to the hospital with a history of crescendo angina and prolonged rest pain. He had electrocardiographic T-wave inversions in leads V_2-V_5, I, aV_L and no abnormalities of serial cardiac enzymes. After 72 hours of hospital treatment with aspirin, heparin, and beta blocker therapy he had a further episode of rest pain associated with 5- to 8-mm anterior ST-segment elevations. Coronary angiography was performed, and the left coronary artery (right anterior oblique caudal projection) is shown. In the left anterior descending coronary artery, at the level of the second diagonal branch, an irregular hazy filling defect is present (arrow). It is surrounded by angiographic contrast medium and extends into the diagonal branch itself. After 4 further days of heparin and antianginal therapy, a repeat coronary angiogram was obtained, and the size of the intracoronary filling defect had decreased, confirming that it was a coronary thrombus.

lium is required to secrete and bind tissue plasminogen activator and plasminogen. Thromboxane A_2, which is released and synthesized by aggregating platelets, is a powerful local vasoconstrictor.[604]

It is likely that progression of atherosclerosis, platelet aggregation, thrombus formation, and changes in vasomotor tone may operate either alone or together at different times in individual patients to produce unstable angina. Alterations in coronary artery tone at the site of plaques may initiate and/or be exacerbated by local formation of platelet thrombi with resulting ischemia. In addition, growth factors, in particular fibroblast growth factor, may be involved in the transformation from stable to unstable angina by causing enhanced smooth muscle proliferation in preexisting atherosclerotic lesions.[605] Thus, unstable angina is a complex, dynamic syndrome that perhaps is often a precursor of myocardial infarction; both conditions share a common patholophysiological link.

Clinical and Laboratory Findings

SYMPTOMS. The chest discomfort in unstable angina is similar in *quality* to that of classic effort-induced angina, although it is often more intense, is usually described as pain, may persist for as long as 30 minutes, and occasionally awakens the patient from sleep.[606] Several clues should alert the physician to a changing pattern of angina and the development of unstable angina. These include an abrupt and persistent reduction in the threshold of physical activity that provokes angina; an increase in the frequency, severity, and duration of angina; the development of rest angina or nocturnal angina, radiation of the discomfort to an additional or new site; and the onset of new associated features such as diaphoresis, nausea, vomiting, palpitation, or dyspnea. The usual regimen of rest and sublingual nitroglycerin administration which controls chronic stable angina, often provides only temporary or incomplete relief in unstable angina.

PHYSICAL EXAMINATION. This may reveal transient diastolic (third and fourth) heart sounds and a dyskinetic apical impulse suggesting left ventricular dysfunction, or a transient systolic murmur of mitral regurgitation during or immediately after an ischemic episode. These findings are nonspecific, because they may also be present in patients with chronic stable angina or acute myocardial infarction. Nonetheless, physical examination may provide important clues to adverse prognosis based upon evidence of acute congestive heart failure or systemic hypotension during an episode of pain.

ELECTROCARDIOGRAM. Transient ST-segment deviations (depression or elevation) and/or T-wave inversions occur commonly, but not universally, in unstable angina. Dynamic shifts in the ST-segment (≥1 mm of ST-depression or elevation) or T-wave inversions that resolve at least partially when symptoms are relieved, are important markers of an adverse prognosis, i.e., subsequent acute myocardial infarction or death.[606,607] An unusual, subtle electrocardiographic manifestation of unstable angina is the presence of transient, inverted U waves.[608] Patients with ST changes in the anteroseptal leads, often associated with significant stenosis of the left anterior descending coronary artery, appear to be a particularly high-risk group (Fig. 38–23).[609] The diagnostic accuracy of an abnormal electrocardiogram is enhanced if a prior tracing is available for comparison.[610]

Usually these electrocardiographic changes clear completely or partially with the relief of pain. Persistence for more than 12 hours may suggest that a non–Q-wave infarction has occurred.

If patients have a typical history of chronic stable angina pectoris or established CAD (previous myocardial infarction, abnormal coronary arteriogram, or a history of a positive noninvasive stress test), the diagnosis of unstable angina may be based on clinical symptoms even in the absence of electrocardiographic changes. It is in the subgroup of patients without evidence of previous CAD and no electrocardiographic changes associated with pain that the diagnosis may be inaccurate.

CONTINUOUS ELECTROCARDIOGRAPHIC MONITORING. Ischemic chest pain is not a reliable or sensitive marker of transient acute myocardial ischemia. Episodes of primary reduction in coronary blood flow may be associated with variable and minor electrocardiographic changes that precede symptoms of pain or discomfort.[573] Investigations using continuous electrocardiographic monitoring, which were conducted before the widespread use of aspirin and heparin, documented that up to 60 per cent of patients with unstable angina experienced asymptomatic episodes of ST-segment depression.[611] More recent studies on patients treated with aspirin and heparin have demonstrated that the incidence of transient ST-segment deviation has decreased to between 5 and 20 per cent. More than 85 to 90 per cent of the ischemic episodes detected by Holter monitoring techniques are not associated with chest pain.[612] Furthermore, the presence of ischemia, detected by Holter monitoring, serves as a predictor of unfavorable outcome during hospital admission[613] and follow-up.[561,612] Asymptomatic ischemic electrocardiographic changes are frequently accompanied by transient reductions in myocar-

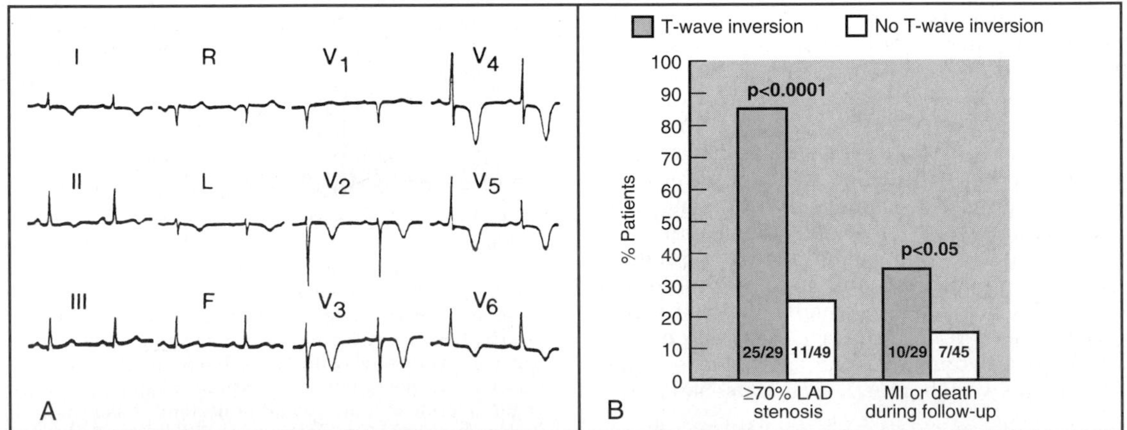

FIGURE 38–23. Unstable angina. *A,* Symmetrical anterior T-wave inversion with isoelectric ST segment frequently associated with critical stenosis of the left anterior descending coronary artery. *B,* Prevalence of significant stenosis of the left anterior descending coronary artery (LAD) and the incidence of cardiac events in patients with and without new T-wave inversion. MI = myocardial infarction. (From Haines, D. E., Raabe, D. S., Gundel, W., and Wackers, F. J.: Anatomic and prognostic significance of new T-wave inversion in unstable angina. Am. J. Cardiol. *52*:14, 1983.)

dial perfusion and abnormalities of ventricular function.[614] More evidence is needed to determine the prognostic significance not only of silent ischemia but of the "total ischemic burden" based upon ambulatory or continuous electrocardiographic monitoring in patients with unstable angina pectoris.[615]

OTHER LABORATORY TESTS. Findings on chest roentgenogram, serum cholesterol level, and carbohydrate tolerance are similar to those observed in patients with chronic stable angina (see p. 1295). Unlike acute myocardial infarction, nonspecific indicators of tissue necrosis, such as leukocytosis and fever, are usually absent. Cardiac enzymes are not abnormally elevated; when cardiac specific enzymes are elevated, by definition the diagnosis is acute myocardial infarction and not unstable angina.

Cardiac troponin-T is a regulatory protein that is a specific marker of myocardial cell injury (see p. 407). In patients with unstable angina, it appears to be a more sensitive indicator of myocardial cell injury than is serum creatine kinase MB activity.[117] Recent evidence suggests a relationship between unstable angina (and other acute ischemic syndromes) and markers of an active inflammatory response. Two circulating acute-phase reactants, C-reactive protein and serum amyloid-A protein, which are sensitive indicators of inflammation, have been shown to be elevated in patients with unstable angina even when creatine kinase and cardiac troponin-T levels were normal, and these proteins are markers of an adverse prognosis.[616]

Coronary Anatomy

CORONARY ARTERIOGRAPHIC FINDINGS. These vary according to the population under study and are dependent upon the patient's history and mode of presentation.[617,618,618a] Patients in whom unstable angina is superimposed on longstanding, stable angina often have multivessel disease, whereas patients with new onset of rest pain may have disease involving only a single coronary artery. Among all patients with unstable angina, three-vessel disease is found in approximately 40 per cent, two-vessel disease in 20 per cent, left main coronary artery disease in approximately 20 per cent, single-vessel disease in about 10 per cent, and no critical obstruction in the remaining 10 per cent. In contrast, in patients in whom unstable angina is the *initial* presentation of CAD (approximately half of all patients with unstable angina), the distribution of CAD is different in that approximately 50 per cent have single-vessel disease (the majority with left anterior descending coronary artery involvement), and less than 20 per cent have three-vessel disease.[619,620]

Among the subset of patients with unstable angina with normal coronary arteriograms or nonobstructive disease are some in whom the diagnosis of angina pectoris is probably incorrect. In the remainder, coronary spasm, the spontaneous lysis of a coronary thrombus, abnormalities of the microvascular circulation, or the presence of a lesion overlooked on coronary arteriography may be responsible. Fourteen per cent of patients with unstable angina enrolled into the TIMI IIIA trial had no luminal diameter stenosis of a major coronary artery of 60 per cent or greater on the baseline arteriogram. In half of these, no visually detectable coronary stenosis was noted. Nearly one-third of the patients without critical coronary stenoses had impaired angiographic filling, suggesting a pathophysiological role for coronary microvascular dysfunction.[621] The short-term prognosis in patients with unstable angina and no critical obstruction of an epicardial coronary artery is excellent.

Postmortem angiograms, histological examinations, and coronary arteriograms typically display eccentric stenoses with scalloped or overhanging edges more frequently in patients with unstable angina than in patients with chronic stable angina (see p. 256).[622] In contrast, lesions with concentric, symmetrical narrowing or asymmetrical narrowing with smooth borders and a broad neck are more common in patients with stable angina. Acute progression had occurred from a previously insignificant lesion in many patients with known coronary anatomy and stable angina pectoris who were restudied after an episode of acute unstable angina.[622] Eccentric lesions with a narrow neck due to one or more overhanging edges or irregular, scalloped borders, or both are the most common morphological feature of disease progression. This finding may represent either a disrupted atherosclerotic plaque, a partially lysed thrombus, or the combination.[623]

When comparing the angiographic findings in patients with chronic stable angina with those having unstable angina, the latter exhibited a higher frequency of complex lesions and thrombus (Fig. 38–22).[569,575a] Coronary arteriography has shown a 40 per cent incidence of coronary thrombi in patients presenting early after the onset of rest angina.[624] Cardiac events (death, myocardial infarction, and the need for urgent revascularization) were more frequent in patients with coronary thrombus (73 per cent), complex coronary morphology (55 per cent), or multivessel disease (58 per cent) than in patients without these angiographic features (17 per cent, 31 per cent, and 7 per cent, respectively). Similarly, intracoronary thrombi were present in 75 per cent of patients requiring urgent coronary arteriography for persistent angina later during admission.[624]

AUTOPSY STUDIES. These suggest that patients with unstable angina have more severe and extensive coronary obstruction than other patients with CAD.[623] Such studies also have shown that about 70 per cent of specimens of diseased arterial segments with significant narrowings (greater than or equal to 50 per cent diameter) have an eccentric, residual arterial lumen that is partially circumscribed by an arc of at least 00 degrees of normal arterial wall which could be responsible for vasoconstriction.[600]

Plaque fissuring has been implicated in acute coronary syndromes, including acute myocardial infarction (Fig. 37–7, p. 1187) and unstable angina.[625] The type of plaque most likely to undergo fissuring is one with an eccentrically situated pool of extracellular lipid contained within the intima. This pool is separated from the blood in the lumen of the artery by a cap of fibrous tissue covered by endothelium. The cap seems most likely to tear at its lateral margin where it is attached to more normal intima. Blood enters the lipid cavity from the lumen, and because of the thrombogenicity of the subendothelial tissues that are exposed, thrombus develops within the plaque itself. This thrombus can expand the volume of the plaque, but subsequently the tear may reseal, restabilize, and heal. Pathological as well as coronary arteriographic studies have suggested the presence of subtotally occlusive coronary arterial thrombi in patients with unstable angina.[626] Plaque fissures heal by the proliferation of smooth muscle, which can contribute to an increase in the severity of chronic obstruction. Some episodes of plaque fissuring are followed by the development of thrombus within the coronary arterial lumen.

CORONARY ANGIOSCOPY. This technique has also revealed complex plaques or thrombi that may not be detected by coronary angiography in patients with unstable angina.[595] The frequency and characteristics of coronary artery thrombi have been evaluated using percutaneous transluminal coronary angioscopy by Mizuno and associates.[596] Patients with unstable angina were frequently observed to have grayish-white (platelet) thrombi, whereas reddish (fibrin) thrombi were more commonly observed in patients with acute myocardial infarction. Moreover, occlusive thrombi occurred frequently in patients with acute myocardial infarction but were not present in patients with unstable angina.

VENTRICULAR FUNCTION. This is usually well preserved in patients with unstable angina, except in those who have had prior myocardial infarction. However, during and following episodes of acute ischemia, localized areas of asynergy are present and stroke volume and ejection fraction decline, whereas left ventricular end-systolic and end-diastolic volumes rise, as does left ventricular filling pressure. Nitroglycerin may restore both global and regional left ventricular function in patients with unstable angina. More recent data demonstrate that angina at rest may be followed by prolonged depression of contractile function in the territory supplied by the "culprit lesion"; this may persist for up to 24 hours or longer[627,628] and represents myocardial stunning (see p. 1176).

Natural History

Unstable angina and acute myocardial infarction are closely related pathogenetically and clinically. Whereas approximately half of patients with acute myocardial infarction report a prodrome of unstable angina shortly before infarction, the opposite is not the case; i.e., only a minority of patients with unstable angina pectoris develop early infarction. Although patients with unstable angina may present difficult management problems, approximately 95 per cent do not in fact develop myocardial infarction over the short term, although recurrent unstable ischemic events are common.[575a] Among patients presenting with unstable angina, who stabilized on standard medical therapy and who were on a waiting list for elective coronary angiography, 57 per cent developed an adverse event (acute coronary syndrome or angiographic total coronary occlusion) during an average follow-up of 8 months.[629] Documentation of all cardiac admissions to coronary and intensive care units in Hamilton, Ontario, over the 1-year period 1979–1980 revealed that in 811 patients admitted with unstable angina, hospital mortality was 1.5 per cent (compared with 17 per cent for acute myocardial infarction), 1-year mortality was 9.2 per cent (compared with 27 per cent for acute myocardial infarction), and only 16 per cent of the patients who died with unstable angina did so during the initial hospitalization. Repeat hospital admission occurred in 28 per cent of patients with unstable angina.[630] In the TIMI III registry of 3318 patients with unstable angina, 21 per cent "ruled in" for a non-Q-wave myocardial infarction on the initial hospitalization; 62 per cent underwent coronary angiography, 22 per cent angioplasty, and 13 per cent coronary bypass surgery. In the subsequent 42 days, 2.4 per cent died and 2.9 per cent experienced a new myocardial infarction.[631]

EXERCISE TESTING. After stabilization of symptoms and before discharge from the hospital, exercise testing can be performed safely in patients admitted with unstable angina who have become asymptomatic.[567,632,633] A normal resting electrocardiogram and an exercise test negative for ischemia in such patients is associated with a 5-year survival greater than 95 per cent. On the other hand, a high-risk exercise stress test (Table 38–2) identifies patients at high risk for subsequent morbid and fatal events.

Exercise thallium scintigraphy after clinical stabilization of unstable angina has demonstrated that the size of the myocardial perfusion defect is a useful predictor of the extent of coronary artery disease[634] and of patients at higher risk for subsequent fatal and morbid events.[635] Exercise electrocardiography, exercise thallium scintigraphy, and dipyridamole thallium scintigraphy showed a similar accuracy in dichotomizing patients with unstable angina into low- and high-risk subgroups for future cardiac events.[567] Two-dimensional echocardiography often reveals transient abnormalities of ventricular wall motion. When persistent, these too are associated with an adverse prognosis.[636]

Data from the Duke Cardiovascular Data Bank demonstrate that the diagnosis of unstable angina at the time of hospital admission carries a risk of death which is intermediate between that of stable angina and that of acute myocardial infarction. The mortality risk in the acute ischemic syndromes is time-dependent, and by 2 months mortality rates were similar in all three populations. Patients with unstable angina who appear to have a worse prognosis and to be at high risk for adverse events while in the hospital are older,[631] have continuing rest pain despite medical therapy, and demonstrate thrombi, complex coronary morphology, or multivessel disease at coronary arteriography. Ischemia detected by Holter monitoring and significant ST-T wave changes on the electrocardiogram at presentation also suggest an unfavorable outcome.[611–613]

Management

Medical Management

APPROACH. Unstable angina pectoris is a serious, potentially dangerous condition, and its management must be approached with this in mind. The pivotal first step in the management of suspected unstable angina is a prompt evaluation and triage in the emergency room and the immediate initiation of anti-ischemic therapy.[636a] In patients in whom the diagnosis is uncertain and in those considered to be at low-risk (see below), outpatient management may be appropriate. In selected low-risk patients (Table 63–17, p. 1982), an exercise test after a period of observation in the emergency department, which is positive but not "high risk," may identify those who can be discharged on medical therapy.[567] However, the majority of patients with unstable angina should be admitted to the hospital, generally to a coronary care unit or a monitored step-down bed depending upon severity and acuity of the clinical presentation.

The patient should be immediately placed at bed rest. Removal from an emotionally taxing situation, the presence of a quiet atmosphere, physical and emotional rest, the physician's reassurance, mild sedation, and antianxiety drugs are all helpful and by themselves diminish or relieve episodes of rest pain in perhaps half of all patients. Placing the bed into the reverse Trendelenburg position (feet down) is a simple measure that may be helpful, as may the inhalation of 100 per cent oxygen during periods of pain. A vigorous effort must be undertaken immediately to diagnose and treat conditions that may be responsible for transient increases in myocardial oxygen demands, such as infection, fever, thyrotoxicosis, anemia, arrhythmias, exacerbation of preexisting heart failure, concurrent illness (particularly of the pulmonary tract, leading to coughing and hypoxemia, and acute gastrointestinal disturbances, causing vomiting, retching, or diarrhea), tachyarrhythmias (which increase myocardial oxygen demand), and severe bradyarrhythmias (which reduce myocardial perfusion). Control of these aggravating factors is helpful in an additional 10 to 15 per cent of patients.

The electrocardiogram should be monitored continuously; diagnostic tests to rule out a myocardial infarction should include serial CK-MB enzymes. The routine use of other laboratory measurements such as serum troponin-T is under investigation.[117] Invasive monitoring is usually not necessary unless the patient exhibits hemodynamic instability.

NITRATES (see p. 1302). These are a mainstay of therapy. In addition to frequently relieving and preventing recurrence of ischemic pain, nitrates have been shown to improve global and regional left ventricular function. Nitrates may be given sublingually, orally, topically, or intravenously, and they may be of the short- or long-acting variety (Table 38–3). Intravenous nitroglycerin offers the advantage of more consistent control of ischemic episodes during the first 24 hours of treatment. An additional advantage of intravenous nitroglycerin in patients already receiving standard therapy of oral or topical nitrates and beta-blocking drugs is that it reduces the number of anginal episodes, and the need for sublingual nitroglycerin and analgesics. Intravenous nitroglycerin should be started in a dose of 5 to 10 μg/min by continuous infusion and increased by 10 μg/min every 5 to 10 minutes until relief of symptoms or limiting side effects (headache or hypotension with a systolic blood pressure of 90 mm Hg, or more than 30 per cent below starting mean arterial pressure).[408,567] It is recommended that patients on intravenous nitroglycerin be switched to an oral or topical nitrate once they have been symptom-free for 24 hours. Tolerance to continuous intravenous nitroglycerin therapy develops within 24 to 48 hours (p. 1304).

BETA-ADRENOCEPTOR BLOCKERS (see p. 1304). Beta blockers should be administered to all patients with unstable angina, without contraindications to these drugs (Table 38–4).[567] In patients who have not previously received these drugs, the addition of a beta blocker[637,638] or the combination of a beta blocker and nitrates[639] reduces episodes of recurrent ischemia and the occurrence of myocardial infarction.[633,639] In patients already receiving nitrates and/or calcium antagonists who develop unstable angina, the addition of beta blockers reduces the frequency and duration of both symptomatic and silent ischemic episodes. When rapid beta blockade is desired, intravenous esmolol is efficacious and safe, even in patients with compromised left ventricular function.[640] Resolution of drug effect occurs within 20 minutes of discontinuing this drug.

In patients who are already taking a beta blocker at the time unstable angina develops, the drug should be continued unless contraindications are present. The dosage of beta blockers should be adjusted so that the resting heart rate is reduced to between 50 and 60 beats/min. Beta blockade may improve pulmonary congestion if the elevated pulmonary venous pressure is due to an ischemia-induced reduction of left ventricular compliance or left ventricular systolic failure. Rarely, heart failure may be precipitated by beta blockade in patients with previous infarction.

CALCIUM ANTAGONISTS (see also p. 1308). These drugs are as effective as beta blockers in relieving symptoms.[633,637–639] However, an overview of all randomized trials of calcium antagonists in unstable angina suggests that they do *not* prevent the development of acute myocardial infarction or reduce mortality.[641] One randomized, double-blind comparison of recurrent ischemia in patients with unstable angina treated with nifedipine or metoprolol, or both, was terminated prematurely because it appeared that nifedipine therapy alone might have been associated with more nonfatal myocardial infarctions within the first 48 hours of treatment than therapy with metoprolol alone or with a combination of nifedipine and metoprolol.[639] Studies of patients with unstable angina have suggested that the addition of nifedipine to beta blocker therapy or to a combination of nitrates and beta blockers is useful in relieving angina and reducing the subsequent short-term risk of death, myocardial infarction, or the need for urgent coronary artery surgery.[639,642] The possible risks of short-acting nifedipine are discussed on p. 1310. It is therefore recommended that calcium antagonists be used as *second-line* therapy in patients with continued ischemia, despite nitrates and beta blockers. Particular caution should be used in adding a calcium antagonist to a beta blocker in patients with left ventricular dysfunction.

ASPIRIN AND TICLOPIDINE. The potential importance of platelet activation and thrombus formation in the pathogenesis of unstable angina (see p. 1333) has established an important role for aspirin in the management of these patients. Indeed, several randomized trials of aspirin have shown that aspirin reduces the incidence of myocardial infarction and death from cardiac causes by approximately 50 per cent.[581–584,643] Therefore, there is now widespread agreement that aspirin should be started as soon as the diagnosis of unstable angina is established and should then be continued indefinitely (Fig. 38–24). The recommended doses are 160 to 325 mg/day, although lower doses have

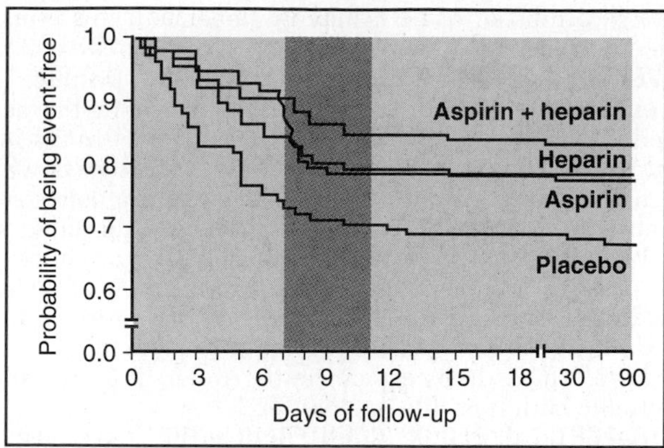

FIGURE 38–24. Kaplan-Meier event-free curves for patients in the four study groups. The curves cover the study period of 7 days, which included the double-blind administration of the study drugs; a 96-hour period early after drug discontinuation, from day 7 to day 11 (indicated by the rectangle); and a follow-up period extending through 3 months. The time of drug discontinuation was adjusted to day 7 for all patients for comparability. The rate of attrition in the heparin group after the discontinuation of the study drug was important, but not when aspirin was administered concomitantly with heparin. (Modified from Theroux, P., Waters, O., Lam, J., et al.: Reactivation of unstable angina after the discontinuation of heparin. N. Engl. J. Med. *327*:141, 1992. Copyright Massachusetts Medical Society.)

proven beneficial. The only contraindications are ongoing major hemorrhage, a recent history of life-threatening bleeding, or a clear-cut history of hypersensitivity to aspirin.[567,644,677]

For the minority of patients with unstable angina with these contraindications, *ticlopidine* in a dose of 250 mg twice daily is a suitable alternative. A multicenter randomized trial of ticlopidine in unstable angina reported a 47% reduction in cardiovascular death and a 46% reduction in nonfatal myocardial infarction at 6 months.[644,645,677]

HEPARIN (see also p. 1823). Intravenous heparin is effective in patients with unstable angina.[583,584] Several trials have suggested that intravenous heparin may be superior to aspirin[646] or that the combination is superior to either drug alone (Fig. 38–24).[584,647] The case for using the combination is strengthened further by the demonstration that rebound angina may be precipitated by discontinuation of heparin in patients who are not taking aspirin.[647–649] There is evidence that this is due to a true "rebound" phenomenon secondary to an increase in thrombin activity after a cessation of heparin.[649a] The more gradual discontinuation of heparin might attenuate this response, and has been recommended in recently published guidelines,[567] but remains unproven. The recommended initial dose of heparin is an 80 units/kg intravenous bolus followed by a constant intravenous infusion of 18 units/kg/hour. An activated partial thromboplastin time (aPTT) is obtained 6 hours after beginning the infusion or 6 hours after any dosage change, and the heparin infusion is adjusted to an aPTT of between 45 and 70 seconds, using a nomogram[650,651] both in patients treated with thrombolytics alone or in combination with PTCA.[655a]

THROMBOLYTIC THERAPY. The initial promise of thrombolytic therapy in acute myocardial infarction raised expectations that this would also be a useful form of therapy in unstable angina, a closely related condition pathogenetically. Despite strong evidence implicating platelet aggregation and thrombosis in unstable angina, these expectations have not been met. Thrombolytic agents have *not* been beneficial, and there is a trend toward a detrimental effect.[567,652–655] The combination of aspirin plus a high dose of low molecular weight heparin has been shown in one trial to be associated with fewer recurrent ischemic events than aspirin alone or aspirin plus unfractionated heparin.[651a] There is some evidence, however, that low-dose, prolonged infusion of t-PA may be beneficial; this remains to be confirmed.[656]

INVESTIGATIVE ANTITHROMBOTIC AGENTS. Despite the proven benefits of both aspirin and heparin in the acute ischemic syndromes, both drugs have their limitations. Aspirin interferes with only one of several pathways which lead to platelet aggregation. Heparin requires a cofactor for its action; it is ineffective against clot-bound thrombin and may be inactivated by a number of substances, which are generated by platelet aggregation and thrombosis. Given these limitations, the attraction of the newer antithrombotic (see p. 1817) and antiplatelet agents (see p. 1818) is understandable. These drugs are currently under intensive study in patients with unstable angina.[585,657]

INTRAAORTIC BALLOON COUNTERPULSATION (see also p. 1232). The large majority of patients with unstable angina respond to therapy with heparin, aspirin, nitrates, calcium antagonists, and beta blockers, and true refractory unstable angina is uncommon. In a series of patients referred to a tertiary care center for "refractory" unstable angina, almost all were rendered chest pain–free with a more aggressive medical regimen, and only 9 per cent were considered to be truly refractory.[658] Intraaortic balloon counterpulsation is considered when medical therapy has failed, and it is usually effective in stabilizing the patient's condition, both symptomatically and hemodynamically. Intraaortic balloon counterpulsation is usually initiated either before or during coronary arteriography with a view to continuing it through revascularization.[659] This technique is useful primarily because it allows the safe performance of coronary arteriography and ensures that the patient goes to coronary bypass surgery or PTCA under optimal conditions. Although there has never been a randomized trial of the efficacy of intraaortic balloon counterpulsation in patients with unstable angina, it is an extremely effective method for the control of ischemia in this setting. However, local complications related to intraaortic balloon placement are common in the elderly, women, and diabetics.[660]

INDICATIONS FOR CATHETERIZATION AND ANGIOGRAPHY. After initial therapy with bed rest, oxygen, analgesics, aspirin, heparin, nitrates, beta-adrenoreceptor blocking drugs, and/or calcium antagonists, more than 80 per cent of patients who are hospitalized with unstable angina become asymptomatic within 48 hours, and their electrocardiographic signs of transient ischemia disappear. During this period, serial electrocardiographic and enzyme evaluations confirm that no infarction has taken place, thereby differentiating them from patients with acute myocardial infarction.

In patients in whom medical therapy fails with recurrent angina or electrocardiographic changes of recurrent ischemia, the initial diagnostic approach may be to proceed with cardiac catheterization in order to evaluate them for revascularization.[660a] In such patients, noninvasive testing is unlikely to provide sufficient incremental information so as to alter the proposed treatment strategy. In patients who respond to initial medical therapy and those in whom the indications for intervention are less clear-cut, noninvasive evaluation is indicated for further risk stratification.[567]

The approach to patients who have stabilized on medical therapy was comprehensively addressed by the AHCPR Clinical Practice Guidelines (Table 63–17, p. 1983) and is based, in part, on the results of the TIMI-IIIB trial.[567,652] This trial suggested that early coronary arteriography followed by revascularization may be the most appropriate approach for patients admitted to a center with facilities for high-quality PTCA and bypass surgery, provided that there are no contraindications to revascularization and the coronary anatomy is suitable. An initially more conservative strategy of continuing medical therapy at home in patients who have stabilized on intensive medical management in the hospital is appropriate for patients with unstable angina who do not have access to a tertiary care center, those with contraindications to revascularization, those who refuse it, and those who are considered to be at extremely low risk for cardiac events on continued medical therapy. The latter includes patients with unstable angina who have not experienced rest pain, patients with new-onset angina with an onset more than 2 weeks earlier, and those with a normal or unchanged electrocardiogram during pain. If such patients become asymptomatic on medical management and do *not* exhibit a "high-risk" stress test (see p. 1297), they may be followed *without* angiography with a very low incidence of an adverse cardiac outcome, i.e., death or myocardial infarction.

Catheterization and arteriography are helpful in the majority of patients with unstable angina in that they identify several subgroups of patients and can thus be used to guide therapy: (1) patients with left main coronary artery disease—the most life-threatening form of disease—in whom urgent surgery is indicated; (2) patients with multivessel obstructive disease without a clear "culprit" lesion who are not suitable for PTCA; unless there are contraindications, we recommend that in such patients coronary artery bypass surgery be planned on a semiurgent basis (within 10 days) after the patient's hemodynamic condition has stabilized; (3) patients with multivessel disease and left ventricular dysfunction who should also be revascularized; (4) patients with single-vessel or double-vessel disease with normal left ventricular function and a discrete narrow proximal lesion (i.e., "culprit" lesion) amenable to PTCA or other catheter-based revascularization (see p. 1313); (5) a small number of patients (about 10 per cent of all patients with unstable angina) with no demonstrable CAD, in whom the prognosis appears to be excellent with medical management and in whom revascularization is obviously not necessary. In some of these patients, coronary spasm is responsible for the angina, and this can be established by provocative testing at the time of coronary arteriography (see p. 264); intensification of therapy with nitrates and calcium antagonists would then be indicated; and (6) patients with diffuse distal CAD unsuitable for angioplasty or bypass grafting.

Maximal medical therapy and heparinization should be maintained up to and continued through the time of cardiac catheterization. The risks of coronary arteriography are slightly greater in patients with unstable than in those with chronic stable angina.[661] This risk is increased further in patients who continue to have symptoms despite optimal medical management.

Revascularization

PERCUTANEOUS TRANSLUMINAL CORONARY ANGIOPLASTY (PTCA). In patients with unstable angina, successful PTCA results in the immediate cessation of ischemic episodes as well as in improvement in both regional and global ischemic left ventricular dysfunction.[662] The initial success rate of dilation of significant stenoses is 83 to 93 per cent.[663–666] Although the acute complications of PTCA are slightly higher in patients with unstable as opposed to stable angina,[663–667] late outcomes are similar.[668,669] Patients with unstable angina appear to be at a somewhat higher risk of developing a myocardial infarction at the time of PTCA than patients with chronic stable angina.[663] The risk factors for a procedure-related complication include very severe degrees of stenosis, the presence of thrombus, ST-segment elevations, or persistent T-wave inversions and the number of lesions attempted.[664] The incidence of ischemic complications in patients with unstable angina undergoing PTCA was reduced by treatment with the chimeric monoclonal anti-IIb/IIIa antibody 7E3 in the randomized EPIC trial[670] (see p. 1369).

If angioplasty is performed immediately after the onset of unstable angina, the complication rate is higher and the success rate is lower. Some have therefore advocated deferring angioplasty for 4 to 7 days in patients with an intraluminal filling defect with the appearance of thrombus, thus allowing time for continued therapy with aspirin and intravenous heparin to be effective. It appears that delayed angioplasty in such patients is safe and effective, although it does increase the length of hospitalization.[671]

The incidence of restenosis following PTCA is generally similar in patients with unstable angina and chronic stable angina, although in some analyses the presence of unstable angina emerges as an independent predictor of a higher rate of restenosis.[664,666] The risk factors for restenosis in patients with unstable angina appear to be multifactorial and include poor perfusion beyond the "culprit" lesion, multiple irregularities in the vessel being dilated, the presence of intraluminal thrombus, involvement of the left anterior descending coronary artery, and the presence of collateral vessels. In patients with medically refractory rest angina who are also considered at high risk for coronary bypass surgery, the 2-year mortality after PTCA was comparable to that in a similar group of "high-risk" patients undergoing coronary bypass surgery at the same institution.[671]

Despite the aforementioned problems, angioplasty and related catheter-based techniques[672] are now a cornerstone in the treatment of unstable angina. The 5-year survival rate exceeds 90 per cent, and approximately three-fourths of patients remain free of angina following successful angioplasty.[663–666,673] The incidence of myocardial infarction during long-term follow-up does not differ substantially from that following PTCA for chronic stable angina.[673]

CORONARY BYPASS SURGERY. In patients with *refractory* unstable angina who have not suffered recent myocardial infarction, the operative mortality for coronary artery surgery is 3.7 per cent, approximately twice that observed in patients with chronic stable angina pectoris, and the incidence of perioperative myocardial infarction is 10 per cent. The later mortality rate is approximately 2 per cent per year, and the rate of nonfatal infarction is 3 to 4 per cent per year.

The Veterans Administration Cooperative Study compared medical with surgical management in 468 patients with unstable angina. No difference in two-year mortality was observed overall, although in patients with left ventricular dysfunction surgical therapy conferred a survival advantage that was sustained for 5 years[676,677] (Fig. 38–25). Subsequent follow-up has demonstrated that the survival advantage of surgery after 5 and 8 years of follow-up did not reach statistical significance at 10 years when patients were analyzed according to the "intention to treat" principle. But if patients who "crossed over" to surgical therapy were censored, there remained a highly significant advantage to surgical treatments.[677] In addition, the cumulative rate of repeat hospitalizations was lower in patients treated with surgery, and the quality of their life appeared to be better.[678] Rahimtoola et al. assessed the late results of bypass surgery performed for unstable angina in more than 1000 patients between 1970 and 1982. The actuarial 5- and 10-year survival rates were 92 per cent and 83 per cent, respectively.[679]

The results of coronary bypass surgery compared with medical therapy in patients with unstable angina are consistent with the findings in patients with chronic stable angina (see p. 1959) in that the major benefit of surgical over medical therapy is in the "sickest" patients, characterized by the presence of multivessel disease, severe symptoms, and left ventricular dysfunction.[679a] Thus, operation appears to be the treatment of choice for patients with unstable angina pectoris, abnormal left ventricular function, and extensive CAD.[677] Risk factors for increased operative mortality in patients undergoing coronary artery bypass grafting for unstable angina are also similar to those for chronic stable angina and include advanced age, clinical and laboratory evidence of left ventricular dysfunction, and the need for an intraaortic balloon for preoperative control of angina.[680] In patients who have postinfarction unstable angina, the independent predictors of perioperative mortality include the presence of an anterior transmural myocardial infarction and the need for preoperative intraaortic balloon pumping for either continuing angina or congestive heart failure.[674] In patients who have undergone coronary bypass grafting and later develop unstable angina, the risk of subsequent death and myocardial infarction is higher because they are less suitable candidates for further revascularization.[601]

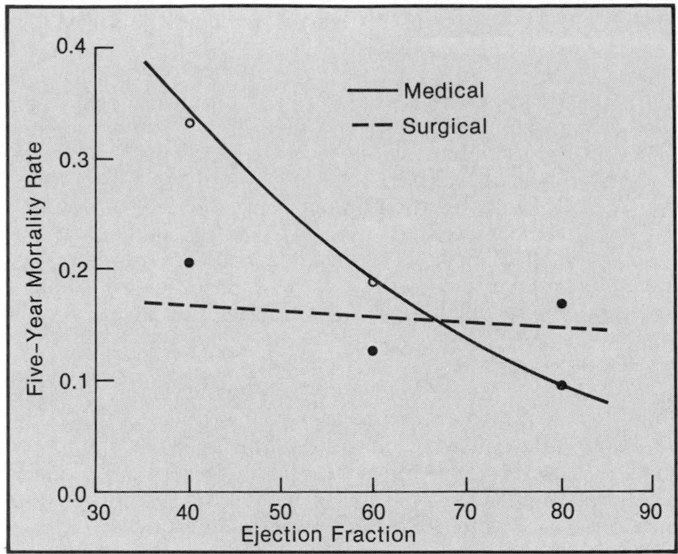

FIGURE 38–25. Mortality following medical and surgical treatment of unstable angina using ejection fraction as a continuous variable. Curves computed by logistic regression analysis based on 5-year mortality of 468 patients with unstable angina randomized to medical (open circles) and surgical (closed circles) therapy. The mean observed per cent mortality is illustrated for ejection fraction intervals 0.30–0.49, 0.50–0.69, and >0.70. The worse the ejection fraction, the poorer the survival in medically treated patients; thus, surgery should be recommended for patients with unstable angina and reduced ejection fraction for three-vessel coronary artery disease suitable for surgical revascularization because it offers improved 5-year survival. (Reproduced with permission from Parisi, A. F., et al.: Medical compared with surgical management of unstable angina: 5-year mortality and morbidity in the Veterans Administration Study. Circulation *80:*1176, 1989. Copyright American Heart Association.)

Management: A Summary

The role of coronary arteriography and reperfusion and the timing of such therapy remain controversial in patients with unstable angina. Patients with unstable angina who respond to intensive medical therapy may be managed by either an aggressive approach with early angiography or more conservatively based upon the results of the TIMI-IIIB trial.[652] One can make a strong case, however, for routine coronary angiography in all patients with unstable angina and evidence of left ventricular dysfunction and in patients with adverse prognostic features, such as a recent myocardial infarction, persistent T-wave inversion in the anterior leads, or significant ST-segment depression during episodes of angina.[682] In patients with unstable angina and multivessel disease, the approach to PTCA, other catheter-based techniques, or coronary bypass surgery must be individualized, as in patients with chronic stable angina (see p. 1298).

If a patient has received intensive medical therapy for a 48-hour period and there is persistent evidence of continuing ischemia, it is our policy to proceed with catheterization and coronary arteriography. Intraaortic balloon counterpulsation is often instituted either before or during cardiac catheterization if the patient exhibits hemodynamic instability or continued rest pain. If the patient has single-vessel disease and well-maintained left ventricular function, then PTCA is performed, if technically feasible. On the other hand, in patients in whom there is evidence of left main coronary disease, ventricular dysfunction, or multivessel disease and the anatomy is suitable for bypass grafting, operation is performed immediately.

PRINZMETAL'S VARIANT ANGINA

In 1959, Prinzmetal et al. described an unusual syndrome of cardiac pain secondary to myocardial ischemia that occurs almost exclusively at rest, is usually not precipitated by physical exertion or emotional stress, and is associated with electrocardiographic ST-segment elevations.[683] This syndrome, now known as *Prinzmetal's* or *variant angina,* may be associated with acute myocardial infarction and severe cardiac arrhythmias, including ventricular tachycardia and fibrillation, as well as sudden death.

Mechanisms

Variant angina pectoris has been demonstrated convincingly to be due to coronary artery spasm.[1,684,684a] (Fig. 38–11). The latter causes a transient, abrupt, marked reduction in the diameter of an epicardial (or large septal) coronary artery resulting in myocardial ischemia. This occurs in the absence of any preceding increases in myocardial oxygen demand, as reflected in elevations of heart rate or blood pressure. The reduction in diameter can usually be reversed by nitroglycerin, sometimes requiring large doses, and can occur in either normal or diseased coronary arteries. The striking reduction in luminal diameter is usually focal and involves a single site. Measurements of great cardiac vein flow and left anterior descending coronary artery diameters in patients with vasospastic angina suggest that not only epicardial but also the resistance coronary arteries are affected by the coronary vasomotion disorder.[685] This focal, severe vasospasm should not be confused with vasoconstriction of both the large and small coronary vessels, a *normal* response to stimuli such as cold exposure. The latter response is much less intense and occurs diffusely throughout the coronary vascular bed.

In patients with Prinzmetal's angina, basal coronary artery tone may be increased. Although responses to ergonovine, acetylcholine, and nitrates are greater in spastic segments of the coronary arteries, there is also hypersensitivity to vasoconstrictor stimuli throughout the entire coronary artery tree.[686] Sites of spasm in Prinzmetal's angina may be adjacent to atheromatous plaques. It has been suggested that in this subgroup of patients the basic abnormality may be hypercontractility of the arterial wall associated with the atherosclerotic process itself. Other suggested mechanisms include endothelial injury (which reverses the dilator response to a variety of stimuli, e.g., acetylcholine [see p. 1342]) and hypercontractility of vascular smooth muscle due to vasoconstrictor mitogens, leukotrienes, serotonin,[687] and higher local concentrations of blood-borne vasoconstriction in areas adjacent to neovascularized atherosclerotic plaques.

Iodine-123 metaiodobenzylguanidine (^{123}I MIBG) positron emission–computed tomography (PET) (see p. 307) has been carried out in patients with Prinzmetal's angina in whom coronary vasospasm has been provoked by the intracoronary administration of acetylcholine. This technique has demonstrated regional myocardial sympathetic dysinnervation, which was not observed in patients with significant obstructive CAD disease and in subjects with normal coronary arteries. The region of myocardial sympathetic dysinnervation was usually located in the area of distribution of the vessel developing vasospasm.[688]

Coronary spasm in patients with variant angina may induce stasis and result in the conversion of fibrinogen to fibrin in the coronary vessels, with elevated levels of plasma fibrinopeptide A, an index of fibrin formation.[689] The latter displays significant circadian variation in plasma concentration, with the peak levels occurring from midnight to early morning, in parallel with the frequency of the ischemic attacks in these patients.[690] In addition, these patients also demonstrate a morning peak in the values of plasminogen activator antigen and free plasminogen activator inhibitor activity.[691] The possibility that vasospasm may induce leukocyte adhesion in the coronary circulation in the initiation of an inflammatory process has been suggested.[691a]

Cigarette smoking is an important risk factor for Prinzmetal's angina.[692,693] *Magnesium sulfate* has been shown to terminate cold pressor–induced anginal attacks, to prevent induction of further attacks,[694] and to suppress attacks induced by hyperventilation[695] and exercise in these patients.[696]

Cocaine, which blocks the presynaptic uptake of the neurotransmitters norepinephrine and dopamine, causes alpha-adrenergically mediated coronary constriction when taken intranasally.[697] There is a high incidence of spontaneous, silent myocardial ischemia detected by Holter monitoring in cocaine abusers during the early stages of withdrawal.[698] The possibility that coronary vasoconstriction may be mediated by therapeutic or illicit cocaine use in patients with suspected coronary artery spasm should always be considered. Spasm causing total occlusion of a coronary vessel, in response to intracoronary ergonovine, has been demonstrated after blunt thoracic trauma.[699] Both *hyperinsulinemia* and *insulin resistance* may be risk factors for variant angina, in the causation of early atheromatous lesions and the subsequent development of occlusive lesions.[699a]

Clinical Manifestations

Patients with variant angina tend to be younger than patients with chronic stable angina or unstable angina, and many do not exhibit classic coronary risk factors except that they are often heavy cigarette smokers.[693] The anginal discomfort is often extremely severe, is generally referred to as "pain," and may be accompanied by syncope, the latter presumably caused by arrhythmias. Attacks of Prinzmetal's angina tend to be clustered between midnight and 8 A.M.[690] Patients studied by means of ambulatory electrocardiography, even those without clinically apparent angina pectoris, show more frequent abnormalities in the morning. In contrast to the situation in patients with unstable angina, the rest pain in patients with Prinzmetal's angina has usually not progressed from a period of chronic stable angina. Although exercise capacity is usually well preserved in patients with Prinzmetal's angina, some patients experience typical pain and ST-segment elevations not only at rest but during or after exertion as well.

Clinical features do not reliably differentiate patients with Prinzmetal's angina with normal or mildly abnormal coronary arteriograms from those with this syndrome and severe coronary obstruction.[699b] However, the latter may have a combination of fixed-threshold, exertion-induced angina with ST-segment depression, as well as episodes of rest angina with ST-segment elevation. Rarely, Prinzmetal's angina develops following coronary artery bypass surgery,[700] and occasionally it appears to be a manifestation of a generalized vasospastic disorder associated with attacks of migraine and Raynaud's phenomenon; it has also been reported in association with aspirin-induced asthma.[701] Some patients appear to demonstrate a distinct relationship between emotional distress and episodes of coronary vasospasm. Alcohol withdrawal may precipitate variant angina,[702] and alcohol ingestion may prevent coronary spasm.[703] Variant angina has been reported to be provoked by 5-fluorouracil[704] and by cyclophosphamide (see p. 1803).[705]

Cardiac examination is usually normal in the absence of ischemia (unless the patient has suffered a previous myocardial infarction) but often reveals signs of dyskinesis and impaired left ventricular function during episodes of myocardial ischemia.

ELECTROCARDIOGRAM. The key to the diagnosis of variant angina lies in the detection of ST-segment elevation with pain (Fig. 38–26). In some patients, episodes of ST-segment depression follow episodes of ST-segment elevation and are associated with T-wave changes. ST-segment and T-wave alternans[706] is the result of ischemic conduction delay and may be associated with potentially lethal ventricular arrhythmias.[707] R-wave "growth" may also be associated with the occurrence of ventricular arrhythmias.[708] Many patients exhibit multiple episodes of asymptomatic ST-segment elevation (silent ischemia). The ST-segment deviations may be present in any leads; the concurrent presence of ST-segment elevations in both the inferior and anterior leads (reflecting extensive ischemia) is associated with an increased risk of sudden death.[709]

Transient conduction disturbances may occur during episodes of ischemia.[710] Ventricular ectopic activity is more frequent during longer episodes of ischemia, is often associated with ST-segment T-wave alternans,[708] and is of ominous prognostic import.

In survivors of out-of-hospital cardiac arrest without flow-limiting coronary stenoses, spontaneous or induced focal coronary spasm has been found to be associated with life-threatening ventricular arrhythmias. In some patients, reperfusion rather than ischemia itself correlates with the onset of ventricular arrhythmias (Fig. 38–27).[711] Myocardial cell damage, as reflected by the release of small quantities of CK-MB, may occur in the absence of persistent electrocardiographic changes in patients with prolonged attacks of variant angina; transient Q waves have been observed.[712] Transmural myocardial infarction due to coronary artery spasm in the absence of angiographically demonstrable obstructive coronary artery disease has been described.[713]

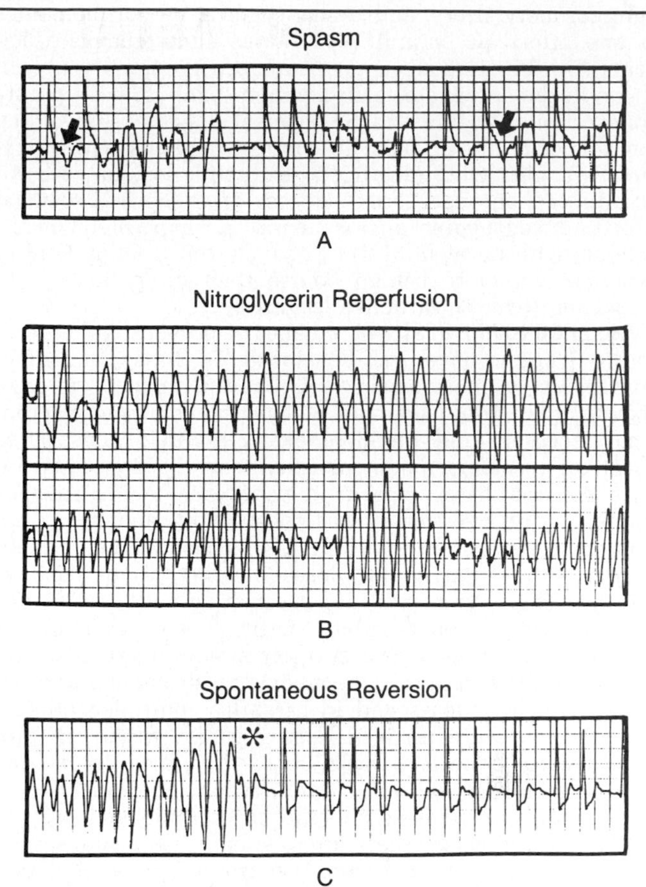

FIGURE 38–27. Arrhythmia during silent ischemia and reperfusion. Selected strips from a 2.5-minute continuous recording (lead II) in Patient 2 during an angiographically documented spasm of the right coronary artery are shown. Tracing A began 24 seconds after the onset of ST-segment elevations (arrows) and demonstrates premature ventricular contractions and salvos. The top strip of tracing B was recorded 70 seconds after onset, immediately after the sublingual administration of nitroglycerin (1/150 grain); the bottom strip of tracing B was recorded 36 seconds later. Tracing C was recorded 130 seconds after onset and shows spontaneous reversion (asterisk) and atrial fibrillation. (From Myerburg, R. J., Kessler, K. M., Mallon, S. M., et al.: Life-threatening ventricular arrhythmias in patients with silent myocardial ischemia due to coronary artery spasm. N. Engl. J. Med. *326:*1451, 1992. Copyright Massachusetts Medical Society.)

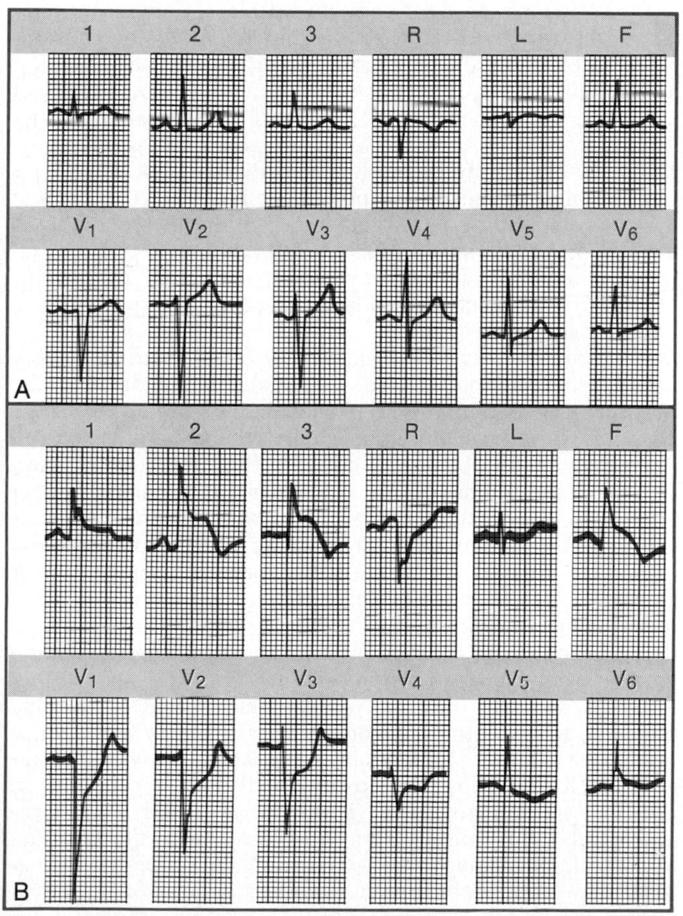

FIGURE 38–26. ECG (*A*) prior to an episode of Prinzmetal's angina and (*B*) during an episode of Prinzmetal's angina. ST segments are now markedly elevated in the inferior leads, with reciprocal depression in the anterior leads. After nitroglycerin was given, the electrocardiogram returned to baseline. (From Berman, N. D., et al.: Prinzmetal's angina with coronary artery spasm. Angiographic, pharmacologic, metabolic and radionuclide perfusion studies. Am. J. Med. *60:*727, 1976.)

Exercise testing in patients with variant angina is of limited value because the response is so variable. Approximately equal numbers of patients show ST-segment depression, no change in ST segments during exercise, or ST-segment elevation, reflecting the presence of underlying fixed CAD in some patients, the absence of significant lesions in others, and the provocation of spasm by exercise in the remainder.

Hemodynamic and Arteriographic Studies

Spasm of a proximal coronary artery with resultant transmural ischemia has been convincingly documented arteriographically and is the diagnostic hallmark of Prinzmetal's angina.[714] Echocardiographic studies performed during episodes of spontaneous variant angina have demonstrated abnormalities in ventricular function that precede the onset of symptoms of angina and electrocardiographic changes.[715]

Significant fixed proximal coronary obstruction of at least one major vessel occurs in the majority of patients, and in them spasm usually occurs within 1 cm of the obstruction. The remainder have normal coronary arteries in the absence of ischemia. Spasm is most common in the right coronary artery, and it may occur at one or more sites in one artery or in multiple arteries simultaneously. Patients with Prinzmetal's angina and normal coronary arteriograms in the absence of pain are more likely to have purely nonexertional angina and ST-segment elevations involving inferior leads during pain. In contrast, patients with Prinzmetal's angina who have fixed obstructive lesions with superimposed coronary artery spasm often have associated effort-induced angina and ischemia in anterolateral leads. Patients with no or mild fixed coronary obstruction tend to experience a more benign course than do patients with associated severe obstructive lesions.

THE ERGONOVINE TEST. A number of provocative tests for coronary spasm have been developed. Of these, the ergonovine test is the most sensitive. Ergonovine maleate, an ergot alkaloid that stimulates both alpha-adrenergic and serotonergic receptors and therefore exerts a direct constrictive effect on vascular smooth muscle,[716] has been used to induce coronary artery spasm in patients with Prinzmetal's angina. Coronary arteries that constrict spontaneously appear to be abnormally sensitive to this agent. When administered intravenously in doses ranging from 0.05 to 0.40 mg, ergonovine provides a sensitive and specific test for provoking coronary artery spasm. There is an inverse correlation between the dose of ergonovine required to induce a positive test and the frequency of spontaneous attacks.[717] In low doses and in carefully controlled clinical situations, ergonovine is a relatively safe drug, but prolonged coronary artery spasm precipitated by ergonovine may cause myocardial infarction. Because of this hazard, it is recommended that ergonovine be administered only to patients in whom coronary arteriography has demonstrated normal or nearly normal coronary arteries and in gradually increasing doses, beginning with a very low dose.

The ergonovine test should be carried out only in a setting where appropriate resuscitative equipment, drugs, and personnel are readily available, usually in the cardiac catheterization laboratory, and with a catheter poised to enter the coronary arteries, so that the angiographic diagnosis of spasm can be made and intracoronary nitroglycerin administered to abolish the spasm.

The response of the *normal* coronary arterial bed to larger doses ($\geq$0.40 mg) of ergonovine is a diffuse reduction in arterial caliber. In patients with atypical chest pain who do not have Prinzmetal's angina, sequential intravenous bolus injections of ergonovine maleate result in progressive diffuse reductions in coronary dimensions. These vasoconstrictor responses appear to be accentuated in women and in patients with intimal coronary arteriographic irregularities, suggesting the existence of minor atherosclerotic disease. This dose-dependent phenomenon differs from the abnormal response in Prinzmetal's angina, which is characterized by severe focal spasm, usually at much lower doses of the agent. The sensitivity of the ergonovine test is high in patients with active disease (who have at least one attack daily) and lower in patients with sporadic episodes of variant angina.[718]

HYPERVENTILATION. This stimulus has also been demonstrated to provoke some episodes of intense angina,[719] electrocardiographic ST-segment elevations, angiographic evidence of coronary artery spasm, and ventricular arrhythmias.[718] In patients with active disease who have at least one daily attack of Prinzmetal's angina, the sensitivity of hyperventilation was 95 per cent, compared with 100 per cent for ergonovine. However, in patients with less frequent attacks of angina, hyperventilation has a lower sensitivity than ergonovine and, therefore, is of more limited diagnostic value.[718]

ACETYLCHOLINE. Intracoronary injections of acetylcholine have been shown to induce severe coronary spasm in patients with variant angina. This spasm should not be confused with the mild diffuse constriction that acetylcholine induces in patients with abnormal coronary endothelium. Because this method allows induction of spasm separately in the left and right coronary arteries, it is useful in patients with known multivessel disease or spasm. In such patients, the use of intracoronary acetylcholine has been shown to be sensitive, reliable, and safe.[720] Indeed, the sensitivity (95 per cent) and the specificity (99 per cent) of acetylcholine for induction of coronary spasm[720,721] are comparable to those of ergonovine.

Methacholine, a parasympathomimetic drug, histamine,[712] and dopamine[722] also can induce coronary artery spasm. Like ergonovine and acetylcholine, these agents are capable of causing marked coronary artery spasm in patients with variant angina who have severe underlying arteriosclerotic coronary artery narrowing and in those without such fixed stenoses. Exercise, the cold pressor test, and induced alkalosis all can cause coronary spasm in patients with variant angina, but none of these tests is as sensitive as ergonovine or acetylcholine.

MYOCARDIAL PERFUSION SCINTIGRAPHY. Localization of the myocardial perfusion defect to an area perfused by a coronary artery in which spasm can be demonstrated by arteriography has been reported using thallium-201 scintigraphy,[723] and a reduction in coronary sinus flow during episodes of spasm has also been noted. These studies support the relationship between coronary spasm and the resultant myocardial perfusion and ischemia.

Management

There are several important differences between the optimal management of Prinzmetal's variant angina and classic (stable and unstable) angina.

1. Patients with both variant and classic angina usually respond well to nitrates; sublingual or intravenous nitroglycerin often abolishes attacks of variant angina promptly, and long-acting nitrates are useful in preventing attacks.[724] However, the mechanism of action of the drugs may differ in the two types of angina. As already discussed (see p. 1302), in chronic (effort-induced) stable angina, as well as in unstable angina, one important action of the nitrates is to reduce myocardial oxygen needs and the second is to cause coronary vasodilation. In Prinzmetal's angina, nitrates abolish or prevent myocardial ischemia *exclusively* by exerting a direct vasodilating effect on the spastic coronary arteries.

2. In patients with classic angina (stable and unstable), beta-adrenoreceptor blockade is usually beneficial, but the response in patients with Prinzmetal's angina to these agents is variable. Some, particularly those with associated fixed lesions, exhibit a reduction in the frequency of exertion-induced angina caused primarily by augmentation of myocardial oxygen requirements. In others, however, nonselective beta-adrenoreceptor blockers may actually be detrimental, because blockade of the $beta_2$ receptors, which subserve coronary dilation, allows unopposed alpha receptor–mediated coronary vasoconstriction to occur; in these patients, the duration of episodes of vasotonic angina may be prolonged by propranolol.[725]

3. In contrast to the variable effectiveness of beta blockers, the calcium antagonists are extremely effective in preventing the coronary artery spasm of variant angina,[726,727] and they should ordinarily be prescribed in maximally tolerated doses. These drugs, along with long- and short-acting nitrates, are the mainstay of therapy. Because calcium antagonists act through a different mechanism than do nitrates, the vasodilatory actions of these two classes of drugs may be additive. Similar efficacy rates have been noted for nifedipine, diltiazem, and verapamil. Rarely, a patient responds to only one of these three agents, and even less commonly simultaneous administration of two or even three antagonists is required.[728] Slow-release nifedipine has been shown to be highly effective in suppressing not only symptomatic but also asymptomatic myocardial ischemia in patients with variant angina.[729] Once-

daily felodipine has also been shown to be highly effective in preventing ergonovine-induced myocardial ischemia in patients with variant angina.[730] Reports have suggested a rebound of symptoms when calcium antagonists are discontinued.[731]

4. Prazosin, a selective alpha-adrenoreceptor blocker (see p. 852), has also been found to be of value in patients with Prinzmetal's angina.[732] Aspirin, helpful in unstable angina (see p. 1337), may actually *increase* the severity of ischemic episodes in patients with Prinzmetal's angina because it inhibits biosynthesis of the naturally occurring coronary vasodilator prostacyclin.[733]

5. Coronary angioplasty and occasionally coronary artery bypass surgery may be helpful in patients with variant angina with discrete, proximal fixed obstructive lesions.[734] Calcium antagonists should be continued for at least 6 months following successful revascularization. PTCA and coronary artery bypass surgery are *contraindicated* in patients with isolated coronary artery spasm without accompanying obstructive disease.

Prognosis

Many patients with Prinzmetal's angina pass through an acute, active phase, with frequent episodes of angina and cardiac events during the first 6 months after presentation. Long-term survival at 5 years is excellent (89 to 97 per cent).[735] The extent and severity of CAD and the activity of the disease have an adverse influence on long-term survival free of myocardial infarction. Nonfatal myocardial infarction occurs in up to 20 per cent of patients and death in up to 10 per cent during this period. Patients with variant angina who develop serious arrhythmias (ventricular tachycardia, ventricular fibrillation, high-degree atrioventricular block, or asystole) during spontaneous episodes of pain are at a higher risk for sudden death.[736] Patients with Prinzmetal's angina and severe obstructive coronary artery lesions are at greater risk for persistent anginal symptoms, acute myocardial infarction, and death.[737] In most patients who survive an infarction or the initial 3- to 6-month period of frequent episodes, the condition stabilizes and there is a tendency for symptoms and cardiac events to diminish with time. In patients who experience such remissions, cautious tapering of calcium antagonists may be attempted. For reasons that are not clear, some patients, after a relatively quiescent period of months or even years, experience a recrudescence of vasospastic activity with frequent and severe episodes of ischemia.[738] Fortunately, these patients respond to re-treatment with calcium antagonists and nitrates. Most patients in whom symptoms recur after a pain-free period demonstrate spasm on provocative testing at the same location as previously demonstrated and respond once more to treatment with nitrates and calcium antagonists.

OTHER MANIFESTATIONS OF CORONARY ARTERY DISEASE

CHEST PAIN WITH NORMAL CORONARY ARTERIOGRAM

The syndrome of angina or angina-like chest pain with a normal coronary arteriogram, often referred to as *syndrome X,* is an important clinical entity that should be differentiated from classic ischemic heart disease caused by CAD. In this condition the prognosis is usually excellent,[739–741] in contrast to the variable outcome in patients with angina caused by coronary atherosclerosis. Patients with chest pain with normal coronary arteriograms may constitute as many as 10 to 20 per cent of those undergoing coronary arteriography because of the clinical suspicion of angina. The cause(s) of the syndrome is unclear. True myocardial ischemia, reflected in the production of lactate by the myocardium during exercise or pacing, is present in some of these patients.[742]

It is postulated that the syndrome of angina pectoris with normal coronary arteries reflects a number of conditions. Included in syndrome X are patients with microvascular dysfunction in whom angina may be the result of ischemia.[743] This condition is frequently referred to as *microvascular angina* (Fig. 38–1*B*). In others, chest discomfort without ischemia may be due to abnormal pain perception or sensitivity. This may result in an awareness of chest pain in response to stimuli such as arterial stretch or changes in heart rate, rhythm, or contractility.[744] A sympathovagal imbalance with sympathetic predominance in some of these patients has also been postulated. At the time of cardiac catheterization, some patients with syndrome X are unusually sensitive to intracardiac instrumentation, with typical chest pain being consistently produced by direct right atrial stimulation and saline infusion.[744] Other patients appear to have a combination of microvascular dysfunction and abnormal pain sensitivity (Fig. 38–23*B*). Studies with intravascular ultrasound have demonstrated the anatomical and physiological heterogeneity of syndrome X, with a spectrum ranging from normal coronary arteries to vessels with intimal thickening and atheromatous plaque.[744a]

MICROVASCULAR DYSFUNCTION OR INADEQUATE VASODILATOR RESERVE (see also p. 1173). Patients with chest pain and angiographically normal coronary arteries and no evidence of large vessel spasm even after an acetylcholine challenge may demonstrate an abnormally reduced capacity to reduce coronary resistance and increase coronary flow in response to stimuli such as exercise, dipyridamole, and atrial pacing. These patients also have an exaggerated response of small coronary vessels to vasoconstrictor stimuli and an impaired response to intracoronary papavarine[745] (Fig. 36–20, p. 1173). This abnormality appears to affect the smaller resistance vessels that are not visible angiographically, while the large proximal conductance vessels are normal.[745a] The reduced vasodilator reserve in the microcirculation may be associated with exercise-induced regional wall-motion abnormalities as well as abnormalities of diastolic function.[746] The reduced coronary flow reserve may cause abnormalities of myocardial perfusion which are detectable by means of positron emission tomography.[747] It has been reported that these patients also have an impairment of vasodilator reserve in forearm vessels[748] and airway hyperresponsiveness,[749] suggesting that, in addition to their coronary circulation, smooth muscle in their systemic arteries and other organs may be affected.

A link between coronary microvascular dysfunction and ischemia in response to exercise is an attractive concept that could explain abnormal left ventricular function resulting from exercise in some patients with chest pain and normal coronary arteries.[747,750,751] Abnormal endothelial function and increased sympathetic drive or responsiveness have been reported.[752,753]

EVIDENCE FOR ISCHEMIA. Despite general acceptance that microvascular and/or endothelial dysfunction is present in many patients with syndrome X, whether ischemia is in fact the putative cause of the symptoms in these patients is not at all clear.[750,751] The development of left ventricular dysfunction and of electrocardiographic or scintigraphic abnormalities during exercise in some of these patients supports an ischemic etiology. On the other hand, support for a noncardiac cause for the pain is provided by several reports of behavioral or psychiatric disorders in patients with chest pain and normal coronary angiograms.[754,755]

The absence of definitive evidence of ischemia in some patients with syndrome X has focused attention upon alternative nonischemic causes of cardiac-related pain, including a reduced threshold for pain perception—the so-called sensitive heart syndrome.[744,751,756] Esophageal dysmotility and the reproduction of pain with the infusion of hydrochloric acid into the esophagus (Bernstein test) or intraesophageal balloon distention have been reported in some of these patients.[757] These observations suggest that some patients with this syndrome may not have cardiac disease at all.

CLINICAL FEATURES. The syndrome of angina or angina-like chest pain with normal epicardial arteries occurs more frequently in women,[758] many of whom are premenopausal, whereas obstructive CAD is found more commonly in men and postmenopausal women. Fewer than half of the patients with syndrome X have typical angina pectoris; the majority have a variety of forms of atypical chest pain. Although the features are frequently atypical, the chest pain may nonetheless be severe and disabling.[758] The condition may be benign in regard to survival, but it may have adverse effects on the quality of life, employment, and increased use of health care resources.

In some patients with minimal or no coronary disease, an exaggerated preoccupation with personal health is associated with the chest pain, and panic disorder may be responsible in a proportion of such patients.[754] Potts and Bass found that two-thirds of patients with chest pain and normal coronary arteries have predominantly psychiatric disorders.[758a] Others have reported that the incidence of obstructive CAD is extremely low in patients with atypical chest pain who are anxious and/or depressed.[759,760] The association between syndrome X and insulin resistance warrants further study.

FINDINGS ON PHYSICAL AND LABORATORY EXAMINATION. Abnormal physical findings reflecting ischemia, such as a precordial bulge, gallop sound, and the murmur of mitral regurgitation, are uncommon in syndrome X. The resting electrocardiogram may be normal, but nonspecific ST-T wave abnormalities are often observed, sometimes occurring in association with the chest pain. Approximately 20 per cent of patients with chest pain and normal coronary arteriograms have positive exercise tests. However, many of the patients with this syndrome fail to complete the exercise test, discontinuing because of fatigue or mild chest discomfort. Left ventricular function is usually normal at rest and during stress,[746] unlike the situation in obstructive CAD in which function often becomes impaired during stress. A small percentage of patients with syndrome X exhibit lactate production and ST-segment depression during exercise, signifying significant ischemia. Some patients show abnormal myocardial perfusion reserve, but there is no consistent pattern of abnormal myocardial blood flow.

PROGNOSIS. Important prognostic information on patients with angina and either normal or nearly normal coronary arteriograms has been obtained from the CASS registry.[761] In patients with an ejection fraction of 50 per cent or more, the 7-year survival rate was 96 per cent for patients with a normal arteriogram and 92 per cent for those whose arteriographic study revealed mild disease (<50 per cent luminal stenosis). In such patients, an ischemic response to exercise was not associated with increased mortality, although a history of smoking or hypertension was. Thus, long-term survival of patients with anginal chest pain and normal coronary angiograms is excellent, markedly better than in patients with obstructive CAD and no different from that in an age-matched general population.[750,751,762,763] Nonetheless, the symptoms are persistent, and most patients continue to experience chest pain leading to repeated cardiac catheterizations and hospital admissions.[750,764]

MANAGEMENT. In patients with angina-like chest pain syndrome and normal epicardial coronary arteries, esophageal abnormalities should be considered (see p. 1291). Such patients may show either motility disorders of the esophagus or abnormal reflux. Exercise electrocardiography and/or myocardial perfusion scintigraphy are often helpful in excluding obstructive CAD. When a noninvasive stress test is positive, or even in patients with serious disability and multiple hospital admissions in whom it is negative, the documentation of normal coronary arteries by coronary angiography provides an objective basis for firm reassurance.

In patients with the syndrome in whom ischemia can be demonstrated by noninvasive stress testing, a trial of anti-ischemic therapy with nitrates and beta blockers is logical, but the response to this therapy is often poor.[751] In contrast to patients with organic coronary artery disease, sublingual nitrates are ineffective in improving exercise tolerance in patients with syndrome X, and, in some, exercise tolerance may further deteriorate.[765] Calcium antagonists are effective in reducing the frequency and severity of angina and improving exercise tolerance in some patients. When these conditions are present, the treatment of esophageal reflux and dysmotility may be effective.

Estrogen has been shown to attenuate normal coronary vasomotor responses to acetylcholine, to increase coronary blood flow, and to potentiate endothelium-dependent vasodilation in postmenopausal women.[766,767] Although estrogen would therefore seem to be a logical treatment for postmenopausal women with syndrome X, its clinical effectiveness in these patients has yet to be documented. Imipramine (50 mg) has been reported to be helpful in some patients.[755]

SILENT MYOCARDIAL ISCHEMIA

Two forms of silent myocardial ischemia are recognized. The first and less common form, designated type I silent ischemia, occurs in patients with obstructive CAD, sometimes severe, who *do not experience angina at any time;* some type I patients do not even experience pain in the course of myocardial infarction. Epidemiological studies of sudden death (Chap. 24), as well as clinical and postmortem studies of patients with silent myocardial infarction, and studies of patients with chronic angina pectoris suggest that many patients with extensive coronary artery obstruction never experience angina pectoris in any of its recognized forms (stable, unstable, or variant).[768] These patients with type I silent ischemia may be considered to have a defective anginal warning system. Both the patient and physician may be unaware of the presence of ischemic heart disease until a fatal event ensues or an infarction is detected on routine electrocardiogram.

In the Framingham Study, one-quarter of patients who developed myocardial infarction had unrecognized infarctions, detected only by pathological Q waves on routine 2-year electrocardiogram, and of these approximately half were truly silent.[769] This important observation has been confirmed.[770] In other patients, symptomatic myocardial infarction is the first clinical manifestation of CAD, although postmortem or angiographic studies indicate that severe coronary artherosclerosis must have existed prior to the infarction yet the patient had never complained of angina. Such patients with silent ischemia may be identified prior to such an event by an abnormal electrocardiogram (occasionally at rest, more commonly during exercise), by the presence of arrhythmias, or by means of coronary arteriography performed as a result of a positive exercise test.

The second and much more frequent form, designated type II silent ischemia, occurs in patients with the usual forms of chronic stable angina, unstable angina, and Prinzmetal's angina. When monitored, patients with this form of silent ischemia exhibit some episodes of ischemia that are associated with chest discomfort and other episodes that are not—i.e., episodes of silent (asymptomatic) ischemia. The "total ischemic burden" in these patients refers to the total period of ischemia, both symptomatic and asymptomatic.

AMBULATORY ELECTROCARDIOGRAPHY. The extensive use of ambulatory electrocardiographic monitoring has led to a greater appreciation of the high frequency of type II "silent" ischemia (Fig. 38–28).[768] It has become apparent that anginal pain is a poor indicator and an underestimator of the frequency of significant cardiac ischemia.[771–773] Exercise-induced hemodynamic changes indicative of myocardial ischemia (increasing left ventricular end-diastolic pressure and decreasing left ventricular ejection fraction) occur in patients with CAD, irrespective of the development of ischemic discomfort.[774] Ambulatory studies in patients with type II silent ischemia have demonstrated that, although increases in myocardial oxygen demand often lead to ischemia, many episodes of ischemia, both symptomatic and asymptomatic, are not preceded by an acceleration of heart rate or a rise in arterial pressure. This suggests that reductions in myocardial oxygen supply make an important contribution to the initiation of both symptomatic and asymptomatic ischemic episodes in these patients.[775]

Transient ST-segment depression of 0.1 mV or more that lasts for more than 30 seconds is a very rare finding in normal subjects.[776] Patients with known CAD show a strong correlation between such transient ST-segment depression and independent measurements of impaired regional myocardial perfusion and ischemia using rubidium-82 uptake measured by positron-emission tomography.[777,778] In patients with type II silent ischemia, perfusion defects occur in the same myocardial regions during symptomatic and asymptomatic episodes of ST-segment depression.

Type II silent ischemia is extremely common. Thus, analyses of ambulatory electrocardiograms in patients with exertion-induced angina suggest that the majority of ischemic episodes occurring during normal daily activities are, in fact, asymptomatic. Their frequency is such that it has been suggested that overt angina pectoris is merely the "tip of the ischemic iceberg." Episodes of silent ischemia have been estimated to be present in approximately half of all patients with angina, although a higher prevalence has been reported in diabetics.[768–770] Episodes of ST-segment depression, both symptomatic and asymptomatic, exhibit a circadian rhythm and are more common in the morning.[773] Asymptomatic nocturnal ST-segment changes are almost invariably an indicator of two- or three-vessel CAD or left main coronary artery stenosis.

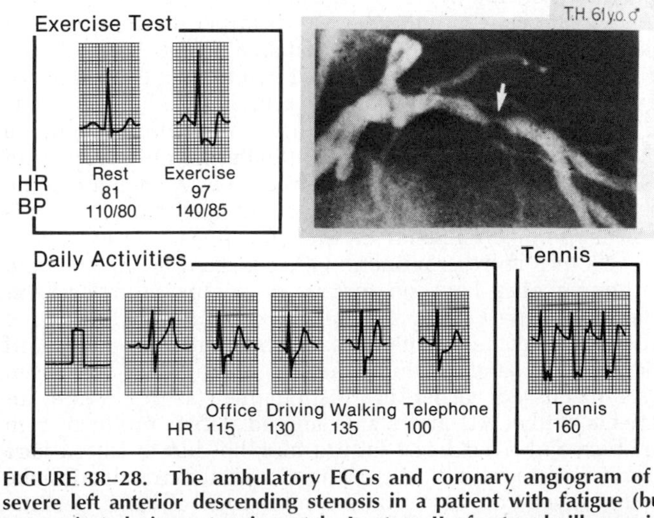

FIGURE 38–28. The ambulatory ECGs and coronary angiogram of a severe left anterior descending stenosis in a patient with fatigue (but not angina) during a tennis match. In stage II of a treadmill exercise test (Bruce protocol), 4 mm of ST-segment depression were seen in lead V_5. Ambulatory Holter monitoring of lead V_5 demonstrates ischemic ST-segment depressions during a number of ordinary activities, e.g., walking, telephoning. During a game of tennis, marked ST-segment depression was recorded when the patient was asymptomatic. (Reproduced with permission from Nabel, E. G., et al.: Characteristics and significance of ischemia detected by ambulatory electrocardiographic monitoring. Circulation *75*[Suppl. II]:74, 1987. Copyright American Heart Association.)

Pharmacological agents that reduce or abolish episodes of symptomatic ischemia, i.e., nitrates, beta blockers, and calcium antagonists, also reduce or abolish episodes of silent ischemia.[771,779]

MECHANISMS OF SILENT ISCHEMIA. It is not clear why some patients with unequivocal evidence of ischemia do not experience chest pain whereas others are symptomatic. Maseri has proposed that silent ischemia results from a variable combination of an increased sensitivity to painful stimuli and coronary microvascular dysfunction[1] (Fig. 38–29). Investigation into the causes of silent ischemia has focused primarily upon four areas: (1) The association between diabetes and both silent ischemia and "painless infarctions" has been attributed to an autonomic neuropathy.[781–784] (2) Patients with silent ischemia have been shown to have a high threshold for other forms of pain such as that resulting from electrical shocks or limb ischemia.[785,786] (3) These patients produce an excessive quantity of endogenous opioids (endorphins), which raise the pain threshold.[787,788] (4) In patients with type II silent ischemia, the asymptomatic episodes may result from a less severe ischemia than the symptomatic episodes. In some of these patients, shorter periods of ischemia on Holter electrocardiography tend to be asymptomatic, whereas longer periods are accompanied by angina.[788–790a] It is not clear which of these four possibilities or a combination plays a dominant role in the production of silent ischemia.

PROGNOSIS. Irrespective of the mechanism(s) responsible, ample evidence supports the view that myocardial ischemia, regardless of whether it is symptomatic or asymptomatic, is of prognostic importance in patients with CAD. The presence of frequent and accelerating episodes of ST-segment depression on ambulatory electrocardiography, whether silent or symptomatic, identifies a group of patients with CAD at higher risk of subsequent events than patients with fewer or no such episodes.[779,791] In asymptomatic patients, the presence of exercise-induced ST-segment depression has been shown to predict a four- to five-fold increase in cardiac mortality compared with those without this finding.[792] It has been reported that multiple episodes of asymptomatic ischemia detected by ambulatory electrocardiography are a predictor of an adverse outcome,[793] but it is not clear that the detection of such episodes contributes *independent* prognostic information.[780,780a]

Whereas the adverse prognosis of asymptomatic but electrocardiographically abnormal stress tests is clear, the clinical value of the detection of silent ischemia by ambulatory electrocardiographic monitoring has not been established. Exercise electrocardiography can identify the majority of patients likely to have significant ischemia during their daily activities[791] and remains the most important screening test for significant CAD. Many patients with type I silent ischemia have been identified because of an asymptomatic positive exercise electrocardiogram obtained following a myocardial infarction. In such patients with a defective anginal warning system, it is reasonable to assume that asymptomatic ischemia has a significance similar to symptomatic ischemia and that their management with respect to coronary angiography and revascularization should be similar.

MANAGEMENT. Drugs that are effective in preventing episodes of symptomatic ischemia (nitrates, calcium antagonists, and beta blockers) are effective in reducing or eliminating episodes of silent ischemia as well[794,795] (Fig. 38–

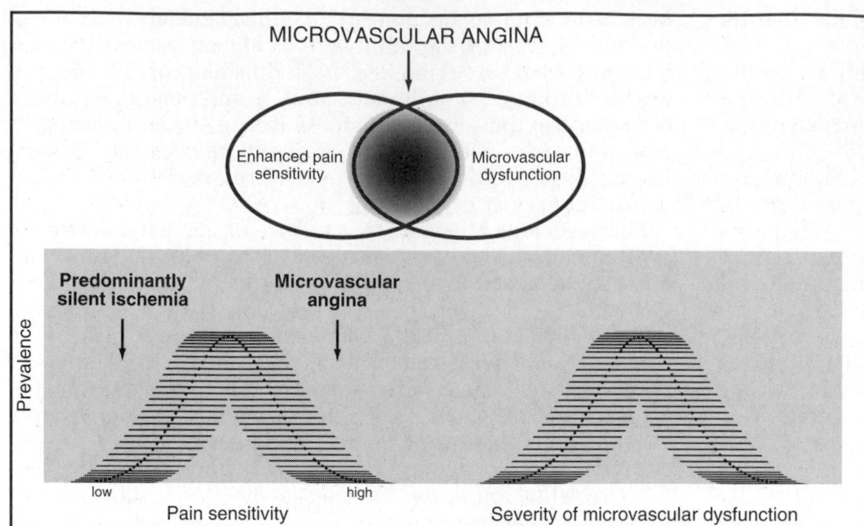

FIGURE 38–29. Proposed pathogenetic mechanisms of microvascular angina. The syndrome results from a variable combination of two components: an increased sensitivity to painful stimuli associated with a coronary microvascular dysfunction (indicated by recurring ST-segment depression), both of which have a bell-shaped prevalence in the population. Furthermore, within any individual, either component may vary in time (indicated by the horizontal lines). In patients with a markedly enhanced sensitivity to pain, even a minimal microvascular dysfunction can cause angina. Conversely, some patients with severe microvascular dysfunction (indicated by recurring ST-segment depression) may not come to medical attention if they have a normal or a low sensitivity to pain. (From Maseri, A.: Ischemic Heart Disease. New York, Churchill Livingstone, 1995, p. 522.)

30). In one randomized study, metoprolol was superior to diltiazem in reducing the mean number of ischemic episodes and mean duration of ischemia.[796] Nitrates are helpful. A combination of a beta blocker and a calcium antagonist is superior to either class of drug alone in suppressing ischemia detected by ambulatory electrocardiography. Although the suppression of ischemia in patients with asymptomatic ischemia is a worthwhile objective, whether treatment should be guided by symptoms or by ischemia as reflected in ambulatory electrocardiography has not been established. The Asymptomatic Cardiac Ischemia Pilot (ACIP) study demonstrated that cardiac ischemia can be suppressed in 40 to 55 per cent of patients with either medication or revascularization, but the outcomes were similar between patients assigned to an "ischemia-guided" strategy as opposed to an "angina-guided" strategy.[797–797d] These data have provided the foundation for a prospective, large randomized trial, including coronary revascularization as one of the therapeutic modalities.

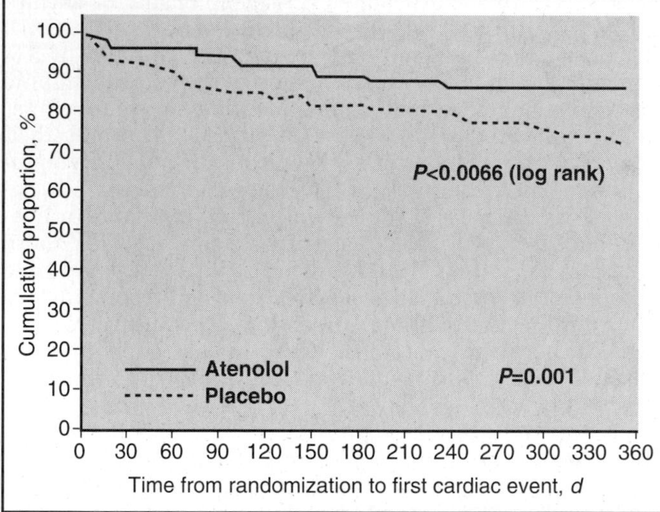

FIGURE 38–30. Atenolol in silent ischemia trial (ASIST). The recently reported ASIST is the first controlled trial to demonstrate modification of cardiac risk through treatment of silent myocardial ischemia (SMI). A total of 306 asymptomatic or minimally symptomatic patients with coronary artery disease, positive exercise tests, and ambulatory electrocardiographic (ECG episodes) of SMI were randomized to receive atenolol or placebo. Ambulatory ECG monitoring was repeated at 4 weeks, and outcome was assessed after 1 year. At 4 weeks, atenolol was associated with a significant reduction in SMI. After 1 year, a significant (56 per cent) relative reduction in adverse events (death, resuscitated ventricular tachycardia and fibrillation, nonfatal myocardial infarction, and unstable or worsening angina) was found when patients given atenolol were compared with those given placebo. The presence of ischemia at 4 weeks was the most important independent factor associated with adverse outcomes after 1 year. (From Bertolet, B. D., and Pepine, C. J.: Silent Myocardial Ischemia. *In* Beller, G. A. and Braunwald, E. [eds.]: Chronic Ischemic Heart Disease. Atlas of Heart Diseases, vol. 5. Philadelphia, Current Medicine, 1995, p. 8.9.)

HEART FAILURE

Manifestations of congestive heart failure are common in patients with chronic CAD. Heart failure may be the dominant clinical feature in some patients, especially those who have sustained prior myocardial infarction(s), in whom ischemic areas have become replaced with a fibrous scar, leading to disappearance or reduction of the angina. The three most common causes of congestive heart failure are (1) an inadequate quantity of normally contracting myocardium, (2) left ventricular aneurysm, and (3) mitral regurgitation due to papillary muscle dysfunction. The first is the most common of the three.

Ischemic Cardiomyopathy

In 1970 Burch and colleagues first used the term *ischemic cardiomyopathy* to describe the condition in which CAD results in severe myocardial dysfunction, with clinical manifestations often indistinguishable from those of primary dilated cardiomyopathy (see p. 1407).[798] Symptoms of heart failure, caused by ischemic myocardial dysfunction (hibernation), diffuse fibrosis, and multiple infarctions, alone or in combination, may dominate the clinical picture of CAD. In some patients with chronic CAD, angina may be the principal clinical manifestation at one time, but later this symptom diminishes or even disappears as heart failure becomes more prominent. Other patients with ischemic cardiomyopathy have no history of angina or myocardial infarction (type I silent ischemia, see p. 1344), and it is in this subgroup that ischemic cardiomyopathy is often confused with dilated cardiomyopathy.

As discussed earlier in this chapter (see p. 1293), in patients with CAD and stable angina, left ventricular dysfunction and overt heart failure may be due to a localized infarct, scattered fibrosis, ischemic noncontractile (hibernating) myocardium, or some combination of these. A similar situation exists in patients without angina who present with heart failure and little or no angina as their primary manifestation of CAD. It is important to recognize hibernating myocardium in patients with ischemic cardiomyopathy because symptoms resulting from chronic left ventricular dysfunction may be incorrectly thought to result from necrotic and scarred myocardium rather than from a reversible ischemic process. Hibernating myocardium may be present in patients with known or suspected CAD with a degree of cardiac dysfunction or heart failure not readily accounted for by prior myocardial infarctions.

The outlook for patients with ischemic cardiomyopathy treated medically is quite poor, and revascularization or cardiac transplantation may be considered.[799] The prognosis is particularly poor in patients in whom the ischemic cardiomyopathy is secondary to multiple myocardial infarctions and in those with associated ventricular arrhythmias. On the other hand, patients whose heart failure, even if severe, is secondary to large segments of reversibly injured but viable (hibernating) myocardium have a better prognosis following revascularization. Thus, the key to the management of patients with ischemic cardiomyopathy is to assess the extent of residual viable myocardium with a view to coronary revascularization. Techniques for detecting hibernating myocardium are described on p. 1327.

Left Ventricular Aneurysm

This is usually defined as a segment of the ventricular wall that exhibits paradoxical (dyskinetic) systolic expansion. Chronic fibrous aneurysms interfere with ventricular performance principally through loss of contractile tissue. Aneurysms made up largely of a mixture of scar tissue and viable myocardium or of thin scar tissue also cause a mechanical disadvantage by a combination of paradoxical expansion and loss of effective contraction. *False aneurysms* (pseudoaneurysms) represent localized myocardial rupture, in which the hemorrhage is limited by pericardial adhesions, and have a mouth that is considerably smaller than the maximal diameter (Fig. 38–31).

The frequency of ventricular aneurysms depends on the incidence of transmural myocardial infarction and congestive heart failure in the population studied. Left ventricular aneurysm can also result from myocardial infarction secondary to blunt chest trauma.[800] More than 80 per cent of left ventricular aneurysms are located anterolaterally near the apex. They are often associated with total occlusion of the left anterior descending coronary artery and a poor collateral blood supply.[801] Approximately 5 to 10 per cent of aneurysms are located posteriorly. Three-quarters of patients with aneurysms have multivessel CAD.[802]

Almost half of the patients with moderate or large aneurysms have symptoms of heart failure (with or without associated angina), a third have severe angina alone, and approximately 15 per cent have symptomatic ventricular arrhythmias, which may be intractable and life threatening.[803] Mural thrombi are found in almost half of patients with chronic left ventricular aneurysms and can be detected by angiography and two-dimensional echocardiography (Fig. 3–93, p. 88). Systemic embolic events in patients with thrombi in left ventricular aneurysms tend to occur within the initial 4 to 6 months after infarction.

DETECTION. Clues to the presence of aneurysm include persistent ST-segment elevations on the resting electrocardiogram (in the absence of chest pain) and a characteristic bulge of the silhouette of the left ventricle on a chest roentgenogram (see p. 228). These findings, when clear-cut, are relatively specific, but they have limited sensitivity. Radionuclide ventriculography and two-dimensional echocardiography can demonstrate ventricular aneurysm more readily; the latter is also helpful in distinguishing between true and false aneurysms, based upon the demonstration of a narrow neck in relationship to cavity size in the latter.[804] Color-flow echocardiographic imaging is useful in establishing the diagnosis because flow "in and out" of the aneurysm as well as abnormal flow within the aneurysm can be detected, and subsequent pulsed Doppler imaging can reveal a "to-and-fro" pattern with characteristic respiratory variation of the peak systolic velocity.[804] Computed

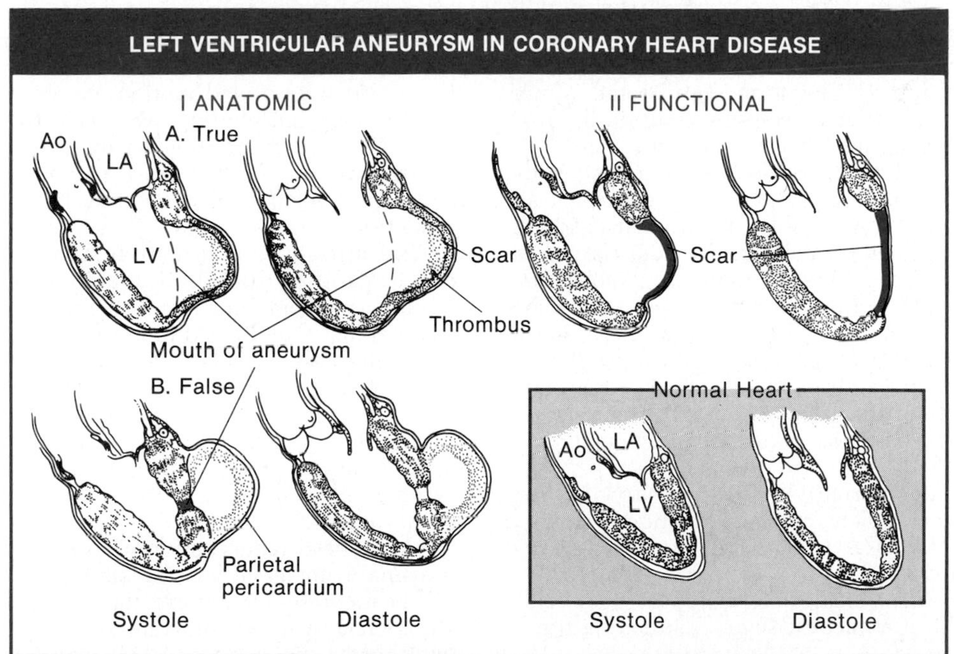

FIGURE 38–31. Hearts in systole and diastole with true and false anatomical and functional left ventricular aneurysms and healed myocardial infarction. A normal heart in systole and diastole is shown for comparison. The true anatomical left ventricular aneurysm protrudes during both systole and diastole, has a mouth that is as wide as or wider than the maximal diameter, has a wall that was formerly the wall of the left ventricle, and is composed of fibrous tissue with or without residual myocardial fibers. A true aneurysm may or may not contain thrombus and almost never ruptures once the wall is healed. The false anatomical left ventricular aneurysm protrudes during both systole and diastole, has a mouth that is considerably smaller than the maximal diameter of the aneurysm and represents a myocardial rupture site, has a wall made up of parietal pericardium, virtually always contains thrombus, and often ruptures. The functional left ventricular aneurysm protrudes during ventricular systole but not during diastole and consists of fibrous tissue with or without myocardial fibers. (From Cabin, H. S., and Roberts, W. C.: Left ventricular aneurysm, intraaneurysmal thrombus and systemic embolus in coronary heart disease. Chest *77*:586, 1980.)

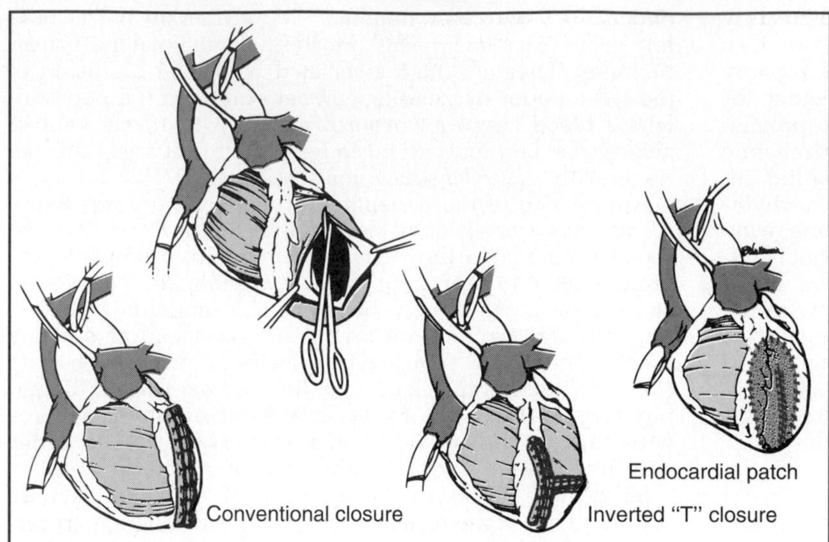

FIGURE 38–32. Operative techniques used in left ventricular aneurysm repair. The figure depicts resection of the ventricular aneurysm enclosure by one of three methods. The conventional closure is illustrated on the left. The "T" closure and the endocardial patch techniques were developed in an attempt to restore normal left ventricular geometry. (From Komeda, M., David, T. E., Malik, A., et al.: Operative risks and long-term results of operation for left ventricular aneurysm. Ann. Thorac. Surg. *53*:22, 1992.)

tomography and magnetic resonance imaging are reliable noninvasive techniques for the identification of left ventricular aneurysms (Fig. 10–34, p. 337) and screening for resectability.[805] However, biplane left ventriculography remains the most precise method available for outlining a true left ventricular aneurysm, assessing septal motion, and determining the quantity of functioning residual myocardium.

LEFT VENTRICULAR ANEURYSMECTOMY. True ventricular aneurysms do not rupture, and operative excision is carried out to improve the clinical manifestations, most often heart failure, but sometimes also angina, embolization, and life-threatening tachyarrhythmias.[803,806] Coronary revascularization is frequently carried out along with aneurysmectomy, especially in patients in whom angina accompanies heart failure.

A large left ventricular aneurysm in a patient with symptoms of heart failure, particularly if angina pectoris is also present, is an indication for operation. The operative mortality rate for left ventricular aneurysmectomy is approximately 10 per cent (ranging from 2 to 19 per cent).[806,807] Risk factors for early death include poor left ventricular function, recent myocardial infarction, the presence of mitral regurgitation, and intractable ventricular arrhythmias.[807–809] Operation carries a particularly high risk in patients with severe heart failure, a low-output state, and akinesis of the interventricular septum, as assessed echocardiographically.[810] Akinesis or dyskinesia of the posterior basal segment of the left ventricle and significant right coronary artery stenoses are additional risk factors.[810] Pseudoaneurysms rupture frequently and should therefore be resected on an urgent basis as soon as the diagnosis is established.[811]

Risk factors for late mortality following survival from operation include incomplete revascularization, impaired systolic function of the basal segments of the ventricle and of the septum not involved by the aneurysm, the presence of a large aneurysm with a small quantity of residual viable myocardium, and the presence of severe cardiac failure as the presenting feature.

Improvement in left ventricular function has been reported in survivors of resection of left ventricular aneurysms complicated by cardiac failure.[808,809] A concomitant improvement in exercise performance may also occur, particularly in patients who have undergone complete revascularization. In patients carefully selected for surgical treatment, 70 to 80 per cent of survivors are in NYHA Class I or II after 5 years, with a 10-year actuarial survival of 69 per cent in patients undergoing left ventricular aneurysmectomy and revascularization, compared with 57 per cent in those undergoing left ventricular aneurysmectomy alone.[812]

New surgical approaches to the repair of left ventricular aneurysms are designed to restore normal left ventricular geometry by using an alternative method of epicardial closure and/or an endocardial patch to divide the area of the aneurysm from the remainder of the ventricular cavity (Fig. 38–32).[813–815]

Mitral Regurgitation Secondary to Coronary Artery Disease

Mitral regurgitation is an important cause of heart failure in some patients with CAD. Rupture of a papillary muscle, or of the head of a papillary muscle, usually causes severe acute mitral regurgitation in the course of acute myocardial infarction (Fig. 37–40, p. 1243). Chronic mitral regurgitation in patients with CAD is most commonly caused by papillary muscle dysfunction due to ischemia or fibrosis[816] in concert with a wall motion abnormality in the region of the papillary muscle (Fig. 32–10, p. 1019) and/or by dilatation of the mitral annulus; many of the latter patients have ventricular aneurysms. Most patients with chronic CAD and mitral regurgitation have suffered a prior myocardial infarction.

Clinical features that help to identify mitral regurgitation due to papillary muscle dysfunction as the cause of acute pulmonary edema or of milder symptoms of left-sided failure include a loud systolic murmur and demonstration of a flail mitral valve leaflet on echocardiography. The latter is the preferred diagnostic technique because the timing and duration of the murmur are variable. Instead of being only mid to late systolic, as was originally thought, murmurs may be holosystolic or early systolic. Doppler echocardiography is helpful in assessing the severity of the regurgitation (see p. 72).

As in mitral regurgitation of other causes, the left atrium is usually not greatly enlarged unless mitral regurgitation has been present for more than 6 months (Fig. 32–14, p. 1021). The electrocardiogram is nonspecific, and most patients have angiographic evidence of multivessel CAD. In patients with ischemic mitral regurgitation, in addition to the severity of regurgitation, advanced age, comorbid disorders (renal failure or pulmonary dysfunction), ventricular dysfunction, the need for intensive care management, and the extent of CAD all influence long-term survival adversely.[316]

In patients with posterior papillary muscle dysfunction resulting from acute myocardial infarction, reperfusion therapy with thrombolysis or PTCA may be attempted initially because urgent surgery is often accompanied by a very high hospital mortality. In patients with rupture of a papillary muscle, or, more frequently, one or more heads of a papillary muscle, immediate surgery is required provided that there is a chance of satisfactory outcome.[817] The procedure of choice, when possible, is mitral valve repair rather than replacement. The decision is based upon the anatomical characteristics of the structures comprising the mitral valve apparatus, the urgency of the need for surgery, and individual expertise.

Ischemic mitral regurgitation secondary to dilatation of the mitral annulus is common in patients with ischemic cardiomyopathy and can intensify the severity of the left ventricular failure. Improvement of left ventricular function by medical therapy with reduction of left ventricular volume and the annular diameter reduces the severity of mitral regurgitation (see p. 1026). Direct surgical treatment of the mitral valve is not indicated in these patients, although if other indications are present multivessel myocardial revascularization may be helpful.

CARDIAC ARRHYTHMIAS

Various degrees and forms of ventricular ectopic activity are the most common arrhythmias in patients with chronic CAD. In some patients with CAD, cardiac arrhythmias are the dominant clinical manifestation of the disease. That there is a substantial subgroup of patients with CAD and occult arrhythmias is suggested by the frequency with which sudden death is the first manifestation of this condition. The frequency and severity of ventricular arrhythmias induced during exercise tests and ambulatory monitoring correlate, in general, with the degree of arteriographically documented CAD. Patients with severe left ventricular dysfunction associated with multivessel disease have more high-grade ectopic activity than do those with normal ventricular function and single-vessel disease.

The recognition and management of patients with malignant ventricular arrhythmias and/or sudden cardiac death due to chronic CAD are discussed in detail in Chap. 24.

NONATHEROMATOUS CORONARY ARTERY DISEASE

Although atherosclerosis is, by far, the most important cause of CAD, a number of other conditions may also be responsible.[818,818a] The most common causes of nonatheromatous CAD resulting in myocardial ischemia are the syndrome of angina-like pain with normal coronary arteriograms, i.e., so-called syndrome X, and Prinzmetal's angina, both of which have been discussed earlier in this chapter (see pp. 1343 and 1340).

Nonatheromatous CAD may also result from diverse abnormalities. These include congenital abnormalities in the origin or distribution of the coronary arteries (see pp. 908 and 967). The most important of these are anomalous origin of a coronary artery (usually the left) from the pulmonary artery, origin of both coronary arteries from either the right or left sinus of Valsalva, and coronary arteriovenous fistula. Anomalous origin of either the left main coronary artery or right coronary artery from the aorta with subsequent coursing between the aorta and pulmonary trunk is a rare and sometimes fatal coronary arterial anomaly.[819]

In an autopsy study of 150 cases of sudden death in persons 35 years or younger, death was attributed to CAD in 48. In 16 of these, the disease was not atherosclerosis but attributable to abnormalities in the origin and course of the coronary arteries, including a deep intramyocardial course, ostial obstruction, an abnormal origin of the right or left coronary artery, or spontaneous dissection of a coronary artery. In one patient, effort-induced acute myocardial infarction was noted in the presence of an intramural coronary arterial trunk.[820]

A number of inherited connective tissue disorders are associated with myocardial ischemia. These include the Marfan syndrome (causing aortic and coronary artery dissection; p. 1671), Hurler syndrome (causing coronary obstruction), homocystinuria (causing coronary artery thrombosis; p. 1673), Ehlers-Danlos syndrome (coronary artery dissection; p. 1672), and pseudoxanthoma elasticum (causing accelerated CAD; p. 1673). Kawasaki disease (the mucocutaneous lymph node syndrome) may cause coronary artery aneurysms and ischemic heart disease in children (p. 994).

Spontaneous dissection of a coronary artery can cause unheralded myocardial infarction and sudden death and is often discovered first at postmortem examination. Two-thirds of the described cases have occurred in women, and one-half of these were associated with the postpartum state.[821] In patients who survive spontaneous coronary artery dissection, there is a 20 per cent mortality over the subsequent 3 years. In general, coronary revascularization is recommended, particularly in patients who have ongoing ischemia.

Coronary vasculitis due to connective tissue diseases or autoimmune forms of vasculitis, including polyarteritis nodosum,[822] giant-cell [temporal] arteritis,[823] and scleroderma,[824] is well described (Chap. 56). Coronary arteritis is seen at autopsy in about 20 per cent of patients with rheumatoid arthritis but is rarely associated with clinical manifestations.[825] The incidence of CAD is increased in women with systemic lupus erythematosus.[826] In patients with systemic lupus erythematosus CAD has been attributed to a vasculitis, immune complex–mediated endothelial damage, and coronary thrombosis due to antiphospholipid antibodies,[826–828] as well as to accelerated atherosclerosis (see p. 1779). The antiphospholipid syndrome, which presents with arterial and venous thrombosis and is associated with the presence of antiphospholipid antibodies, may be associated with myocardial infarction, angina, and diffuse left ventricular dysfunction.[828]

Rarely, *Takayasu's arteritis* (see p. 1572) is associated with angina, myocardial infarction, and cardiac failure in patients under the age of 40 years.[829] Coronary blood flow may be decreased by involvement of the ostia or proximal segments of the coronary arteries, but disease of distal coronary segments is rare.[830,831] The average age of onset of symptoms is 24 years, and event-free survival at 10 years after diagnosis is approximately 60 percent.[829] Luetic aortitis may also produce myocardial ischemia by causing obstruction of coronary ostia (see p. 1441).

An unusual cause of nonatherosclerotic coronary artery disease, but one that is well described, is radiation-induced coronary stenosis following radiation therapy[832] (see p. 1799). Radiation injury may be latent and may not be manifest clinically for many years after therapy, and it has been suggested that hypercholesterolemia may exacerbate the process.[833]

Myocardial ischemia not caused by coronary atherosclerosis can also result from embolism, infective endocarditis (Chap. 33), implanted prosthetic cardiac valves (Chap. 32), calcified aortic valves, mural thrombi, and primary cardiac tumors (Chap. 42).

An interesting nonatherosclerotic myocardial ischemic syndrome has been described in workers in the nitrate industry who apparently experience nitrate withdrawal symptoms on weekends. It is presumed to be secondary to coronary spasm when there is no counterstimulation to the vasoconstriction that they undergo as an adaptation to the vasodilating actions of the high concentrations of nitrates to which they have been exposed (see p. 1302).[834]

Cocaine use is a well-documented cause of chest pain and in particular acute myocardial infarction.[834a]

CARDIAC TRANSPLANT–ASSOCIATED CORONARY ARTERIOPATHY (see p. 525). This condition is frequently observed in cardiac transplant survivors. It is a rapidly evolving, diffuse, concentric arteriosclerosis involving epicardial and intramural coronary vessels.[835,836] It is presumed to be caused by chronic immune injury to the coronary endothelium of the donor heart, but the precise mechanism and risk factors have not been clarified. Other suggested etiologic factors include opportunistic infections (cytomegalovirus infection), immunosuppressive therapy, cyclosporine-induced endothelial injury, and elevated lipid levels. Acute myocardial infarction can result, and this complication is usually not accompanied by chest pain or typical electrocardiographic changes. Infarction in these patients is associated with a high mortality rate, and, at anatomical examination, there is diffuse disease of the coronary arteries and multiple foci of nontransmural cardiac infarction. The management of this form of CAD is difficult, usually requires a second cardiac transplantation, and is discussed on p. 526.

REFERENCES

1. Maseri, A.: Ischemic Heart Disease. New York, Churchill Livingstone, 1995, 713 pp.
2. Centers for Disease Control and Prevention: National Center for Health Statistics, National Vital Statistics and The United States Bureau of the Census. Health, United States 1993, p. 31.
3. AHA: Heart and Stroke Facts: 1995 Statistical Supplement. Dallas, American Heart Association, 1995.

3a. Kannel, W. B.: Incidence, prevalence, and mortality of coronary artery disease. *In* Fuster, V., Ross, R., and Topol, E. J. (eds.): Atherosclerosis and Coronary Artery Disease. Philadelphia, Lippincott, 1996, pp. 13–24.

4. Goldberg, R. J., Gorak, E. J., Yarzebski, J., et al.: A community-wide perspective of sex differences and temporal trends in the incidence and survival rates after acute myocardial infarction out-of-hospital deaths caused by coronary heart disease. Circulation *87*:1947, 1993.
5. Davis, D. L., Dinse, G. E., and Hoeld, G.: Decreasing cardiovascular disease and increasing cancer among whites in the U.S.A. from 1972 through 1987. JAMA *271*:431, 1994.
6. Virmani, R., and Forman, M. B.: Nonatherosclerotic Ischemic Heart Disease. 1st ed. New York, Raven Press, 1989.

STABLE ANGINA PECTORIS

7. Matthews, M. B., and Julian, D. G.: Angina pectoris: Definition and description. *In* Julian, D. G. (ed.): Angina Pectoris, 2nd ed. New York, Churchill Livingstone, 1985, p. 2.
8. Christie, L. G., Jr., and Conti, C. R.: Systematic approach to evaluation of angina-like chest pain: Pathophysiology and clinical testing with emphasis on objective documentation of myocardial ischemia. Am. Heart J. *102*:897, 1981.

8a. DeServi, S., Arbustini, E., Marsico, F., et al.: Correlation between clinical and morphologic findings in unstable angina. Am. J. Cardiol. *77*:128, 1996.

9. Angina pectoris. *In* Fowler, N. O. (ed.): Diagnosis of Heart Disease. New York, Springer-Verlag, 1991, pp. 187–206.
10. Cook, D. G., and Shaper, A. G.: Breathlessness, angina pectoris, and coronary artery disease. Am. J. Cardiol. *63*:921, 1989.

11. Andrews, T. C., Fenton, T., Toyosaki, N., et al.: Subsets of ambulatory myocardial ischemia based on heart rate activity: Circadian distribution and response to anti-ischemic medication. Circulation *88*:92, 1993.
12. Marber, M. S., Joy, M. D., and Yellond, M.: Is warm-up in angina ischemic preconditioning? Br. Heart J. *72*(Edit.):213, 1994.
13. Constant, J.: The clinical diagnosis of nonanginal chest pain: The differentiation of angina from nonanginal chest pain by history. Clin. Cardiol. *6*:11, 1983.
14. Maseri, A., Crea, F., Kaski, J. C., and Davies, G.: Mechanisms and significance of cardiac ischemic pain. Prog. Cardiovasc. Dis. *35*:1, 1992.
15. Janes, R. D., Brandys, J. C., Hopkins, D. A., et al.: Anatomy of human extrinsic cardiac nerves and ganglia. Am. J. Cardiol. *57*:299, 1986.
16. Rosen, S. D., Paulesu, E., and Frith, C. D.: Central nervous pathways mediating angina pectoris. Lancet *344*:147, 1994.
17. Crea, F., Pupita, G., Galassi, A. R., et al.: Role of adenosine in pathogenesis of anginal pain. Circulation *81*:164, 1990.
18. Lam, H. G., Dekker, W., Kan, G., et al.: Esophageal dysfunction as a cause of angina pectoris ("linked angina"): Does it exist? Am. J. Med. *96*:359, 1994.
19. Davies, H. A., Jones, D. B., Rhodes, J., and Newcombe, R. G.: Angina-like esophageal pain: Differentiation from cardiac pain by history. J. Clin. Gastroenterol. *7*:477, 1985.
20. Henderson, R. D., Wigle, E. D., Sample, K., and Marryatt, G.: Atypical chest pain of cardiac and esophageal origin. Chest *73*:24, 1978.
21. Brand, D. L., Ilves, R., and Pope, C. E.: Evaluation of esophageal function in patients with central chest pain. Acta Med. Scand. *644*(Suppl.):53, 1981.
22. Bernstein, L. M., Fruin, R. C., and Pacini, R.: Differentiation of esophageal pain from angina pectoris: Role of the esophageal acid perfusion test. Medicine *41*:143, 1962.
23. Henderson, R. D., and Maryatt, G.: Characteristics of esophageal pain. Acta Med. Scand. *544*(Suppl.):49, 1981.
24. DeMeester, T. R., O'Sullivan, G. C., Bermudez, G., et al.: Esophageal function in patients with angina-type chest pain and normal coronary angiograms. Ann. Surg. *196*:488, 1982.
25. Brand, D. L., Martin, D., and Pope, C. E.: Esophageal manometrics in patients with angina-like chest pain. Am. J. Dig. Dis. *22*:300, 1977.
26. Epstein, S. E., Gerber, L. H., and Borer, J. S.: Chest wall syndrome: A common cause of unexplained cardiac pain. JAMA *241*:2793, 1979.
27. Franklin, K. A., et al.: Sleep apnea and nocturnal angina. Lancet *345*:1085, 1995.
28. Winder, A. F.: Relationship between corneal arcus and hyperlipidemia is clarified by studies in familial hypercholesterolaemia. Br. J. Ophthalmol. *67*:789, 1983.
29. Segal, P., Insull, W., Chambless, L. E., et al.: The association of dyslipoproteinemia with corneal arcus and xanthelasma: The Lipid Research Clinic's Program Prevalence Study. Circulation *73*:108, 1986.
30. Tranchesi, B., Jr., Barbosa, V., de Albuquerque, C. P., et al.: Diagonal earlobe crease as a marker of the presence and extent of coronary atherosclerosis. Am. J. Cardiol. *70*:1417, 1992.
31. Gersh, B. J., Rihal, C. S., Rooke, T. W., and Ballard, D. J.: Evaluation and management of patients with both peripheral vascular and coronary artery disease. J. Am. Coll. Cardiol. *18*:203, 1991.
32. Eagle, K. A., Rihal, C. S., Foster, E. D., et al.: Long-term survival in patients with coronary artery disease: Importance of peripheral vascular disease. J. Am. Coll. Cardiol. *23*:1091, 1994.
33. Ogren, M., Hedblad, B., Isacsson, S. O., et al.: Non-invasively detected carotid stenosis and coronary heart disease in men with leg arteriosclerosis. Lancet *342*:1138, 1993.
34. Cohn, P. F., Thompson, S., Strauss, W., et al.: Diastolic heart sounds during static (handgrip) exercise in patients with chest pain. Circulation *47*:1217, 1973.
35. Heckerling, P. S., Weiner, S. L., Wolfkiel, C. J., et al.: Accuracy and reproducibility of precordial percussion and palpation for detecting increased left ventricular end-diastolic volume and mass: A comparison of physical findings and ultrafast computed tomography of the heart. JAMA *270*:1943, 1993.
36. Ranganathan, N., Juma, Z., and Sivaciyan, V.: The apical impulse in coronary heart disease. Clin. Cardiol. *8*:20, 1985.
37. Sangster, J. F., and Oakley, C. M.: Diastolic murmur of coronary artery stenosis. Br. Heart J. *35*:840, 1973.
37a. Schwartz, G. G., and Karliner, J. S.: Pathophysiology of chronic stable angina. *In* Fuster, V., Ross, R., and Topol, E. J. (eds.): Atherosclerosis and Coronary Artery Disease. Philadelphia, J. B. Lippincott, 1996, pp. 1389–1400.
38. Jiang, W., Hayano, J., Coleman, E. R., et al.: Relation of cardiovascular responses to mental stress and cardiac vagal activity in coronary artery disease. Am. J. Cardiol. *72*:551, 1993.
39. Boltwood, M. D., Taylor, C. B., Burke, M. B., et al.: Anger report predicts coronary artery vasomotor response to mental stress and atherosclerotic segments. Am. J. Cardiol. *72*:1361, 1993.
40. Panza, J. A., Diodati, J. G., Callahan, T. S., et al.: Role of increase in heart rate in determining the occurrence and frequency of myocardial ischemia during daily life in patients with stable coronary artery disease. J. Am. Coll. Cardiol. *20*:1092, 1992.
41. Hillis, L. D., and Braunwald, E.: Coronary artery spasm. N. Engl. J. Med. *299*:695, 1978.
42. Ganz, P., Abben, R. P., and Barry, W. H.: Dynamic variations in resistance of coronary arterial narrowings in angina pectoris at rest. Am. J. Cardiol. *59*:66, 1987.
43. Tousoulis, D., Davies, G., McFadden, E., et al.: Coronary vasomotor effects of serotonin in patients with angina. Circulation *88*:1518, 1993.
44. Epstein, S. E., and Talbot, T. L.: Dynamic coronary tone in precipitation, exacerbation and relief of angina pectoris. Am. J. Cardiol. *48*:797, 1981.
45. Maseri, A.: Medical therapy of chronic stable angina pectoris. Circulation *82*:2258, 1990.
46. Benhorin, J., Banai, S., Moriel, M., et al.: Circadian variations in ischemic threshold and their relation to occurrence of ischemic episodes. Circulation *87*:808, 1993.
47. Juneau, M., Johnstone, M., Dempsey, E., and Waters, D. D.: Exercise-induced myocardial ischemia in a cold environment: Effect of antianginal medications. Circulation *79*:1015, 1989.
48. Epstein, S. E., Stampfer, M., Beiser, G. D., et al.: Effects of a reduction in environmental temperature on the circulatory response to exercise in man: Implications concerning angina pectoris. N. Engl. J. Med. *280*:7, 1969.
49. Marchant, B., Donaldson, G., Mridha, K., et al.: Mechanisms of cold intolerance in patients with angina. J. Am. Coll. Cardiol. *23*:630, 1994.
50. Gottdiener, J. S., Krantz, D. S., Howell, R. H., et al.: Induction of silent myocardial ischemia with mental stress testing: Relation to the triggers of ischemia during daily life activities and to ischemia's functional severity. J. Am. Coll. Cardiol. *24*:1645, 1994.
51. Dodds, P. A., Bellamy, C. M., Muirhead, R. A., and Perry, R. A.: Vasoconstrictor peptides and cold intolerance in patients with stable angina pectoris. Br. Heart J. *73*:25, 1995.
52. Colles, P., Juneau, M., Gregoire, J., et al.: Effect of a standardized meal on the threshold of exercise-induced myocardial ischemia in patients with stable angina. J. Am. Coll. Cardiol. *21*:1052, 1993.
53. Maseri, A., Chierchia, S., and Keski, J. C.: Mixed angina pectoris. Am. J. Cardiol. *56*:30E, 1985.
54. Parker, J. D., Testa, M. A., Jimenez, A. H., et al.: Morning increase and ambulatory ischemia in patients with stable coronary artery disease: Importance of physical activity in increased cardiac demand. Circulation *89*:604, 1994.
55. Campeau, L.: Grading of angina pectoris. Circulation *54*:522, 1976.
56. Goldman, L., Hashimoto, B., Cook, E. F., and Loscalzo, A.: Comparative reproducibility and validity of systems for assessing cardiovascular functional class: Advantages of a new specific activity scale. Circulation *64*:1227, 1981.
57. Califf, R. M., Mark, D. B., Harrell, F. E., et al.: Importance of clinical measures of ischemia in the prognosis of patients with documented coronary artery disease. J. Am. Coll. Cardiol. *11*:20, 1988.
58. Cox, J. L., Naylor, D., Johnstone, D. E., et al.: Limitations of Canadian Cardiovascular Society classification of angina pectoris. Am. J. Cardiol. *74*:276, 1994.
59. Diamond, G. A., and Forrester, J. S.: Analysis of probability as an aid in the clincial diagnosis of coronary artery disease. N. Engl. J. Med. *300*:1350, 1979.
60. Kannel, W. B., Anderson, K., and McGee, D. L.: Nonspecific electrocardiographic abnormality as a predictor of coronary heart disease: The Framingham Study. Am. Heart J. *113*:370, 1987.
61. Mirvis, D. M., El-Zeky, F., Vander Zwaag, R., et al.: Clinical and pathophysiologic correlates of ST-T wave abnormalities in coronary artery disease. Am. J. Cardiol. *66*:699, 1990.
62. Miranda, C. P., Lehmann, K. G., and Froehlicher, V. F.: Correlation between resting ST segment depression, exercise testing, coronary angiography, and long-term prognosis. Am. Heart J. *122*:1617, 1991.
63. Crenshaw, J. H., Mirvis, D. M., El-Zeky, F., et al.: Interactive effects of ST-T wave abnormalities on survival of patients with coronary artery disease. J. Am. Coll. Cardiol. *18*:1413, 1991.
64. Hamby, R. I., Weissman, R. H., Prakash, M. N., and Hoffman, L.: Left bundle branch block: A predictor of poor left ventricular function in coronary artery disease. Am. Heart J. *106*:471, 1983.
65. Hammermeister, K. E., DeRouen, T. A., and Dodge, H. T.: Variables predictive of survival in patients with coronary disease: Selection by univariate and multivariate analyses from the clinical, electrocardiographic, exercise, arteriographic, and quantitative angiographic evaluations. Circulation *59*:421, 1979.
65a. Pattillo, R. W., Fuchs, S., Johnson, J., et al.: Predictors of prognosis by quantitative assessment of coronary angiography, single photon emission computed tomography thallium imaging, and treadmill exercise testing. Am. Heart J. *131*:582, 1996.
66. Chang, J. A., and Froelicher, V. F.: Clinical and exercise test markers of prognosis in patients with stable coronary artery disease. Curr. Probl. Cardiol. *19*:533, 1994.
67. Peterson, M. C., Holbrook, J. H., Hales, D., et al.: Contributions of the history, physical examination and laboratory investigation in making medical diagnoses. West. J. Med. *156*:163, 1992.
68. Marantz, P. R., Tobin, J. N., Wassertheil-Smoller, S., et al.: Prognosis in ischemic heart disease: Can you tell as much at the bedside as in the nuclear laboratory? Arch. Intern. Med. *152*:2433, 1992.
69. Pryor, D. B., Shore, L., McCants, C. B., et al.: Value of the history and physical in identifying patients at increased risk for coronary artery disease. Ann. Intern. Med. *118*:81, 1993.
69a. Christian, T. F., Miller, T. D., Bailey, K.R., and Gibbons, R.J.: Exercise tomographic thallium-201 imaging in patients with severe coronary artery disease and normal electrocardiograms. Ann. Intern. Med. *121*:825, 1994.
69b. Berman, D.S., Hachamovitch, R., Kiat, H., et al.: Incremental value of prognostic testing in patients with known or suspected ischemic heart disease: A basis for optimal utilization of exercise technetium-99m Sestamibi myocardial perfusion single-photon emission computed tomography. J. Am. Coll. Cardiol. 26:639, 1995.

70. Wilson, R. F., Marcus, M. L., Christensen, B. V., et al.: Accuracy of exercise electrocardiography in detecting physiologically significant coronary arterial lesions. Circulation *83:*412, 1991.
71. Bogaty, P., Dagenais, G. R., Cantin, B., et al.: Prognosis in patients with a strongly positive exercise electrocardiograph. Am. J. Cardiol. *64:*1284, 1989.
72. Weiner, D. A., McCabe, C., Hueter, D. C., et al.: The predictive value of anginal chest pain as an indicator of coronary disease during exercise testing. Am. Heart J. *96:*458, 1978.
73. Ribisl, P. M., Morris, C. K., Kawaguchi, T., et al.: Angiographic patterns and severe coronary artery disease: Exercise test correlates. Arch. Intern. Med. *152:*1618, 1992.
74. Michaelides, A., Ryan, J. M., VanFossen, D., et al.: Exercise-induced QRS prolongation in patients with coronary artery disease: A marker of myocardial ischemia. Am. Heart J. *126:*1320, 1993.
75. Ho, S. W., McComish, M. J., and Taylor, R. R.: Effect of beta adrenergic blockade on the results of exercise testing related to the extent of coronary artery disease. Am. J. Cardiol. *55:*258, 1985.
76. Coyne, E. P., Belvedere, D. A., Vande Streek, P. R., et al.: Thallium-201 scintigraphy after intravenous infusion of adenosine compared with exercise thallium testing in the diagnosis of coronary artery disease. J. Am. Coll. Cardiol. *17:*1289, 1991.
77. Gibbons, R. J., Fyke, F. E., Clements, I. P., et al.: Noninvasive identification of severe coronary artery disease using exercise radionuclide angiography. J. Am. Coll. Cardiol. *11:*28, 1988.
78. Dilsizian, V., Smeltzer, W. R., Freedman, N. M., et al.: Thallium reinjection after stress-redistribution imaging: Does 24-hour delayed imaging after reinjection enhance detection of viable myocardium? Circulation *83:*1247, 1991.
79. Bonow, R. O., Dilsizian, V., Cuocolo, A., and Bacharach, S. L.: Identification of viable myocardium in patients with chronic coronary artery disease and left ventricular dysfunction: Comparison of thallium scintigraphy with reinjection and PET imaging with ^{18}F-fluorodeoxyglucose. Circulation *83:*26, 1991.
80. Dilsizian, V., Perone-Filardi, P., Arrighi, J. A., et al.: Concordance and discordance between stress-redistribution-reinjection and rest-redistribution thallium imaging for assessing viable myocardium: Comparison with metabolic activity by PET. Circulation *88:*941, 1993.
81. Brown, K. A.: Prognostic value of thallium-201 myocardial perfusion imaging: A diagnostic tool comes of age. Circulation *83:*363, 1991.
82. European Coronary Surgery Study Group (ECSSG): Long-term results of prospective randomized study of coronary artery bypass surgery and stable angina pectoris. Lancet *2:*1173, 1982.
83. Assessment of myocardial perfusion and viability. *In* Cerqueira, M. D. (ed.): Nuclear Cardiology. Cambridge, MA, Blackwell Scientific Publications, 1994, p. 160.
84. Taylor, A. J., Sackett, M. C., and Beller, G. A.: The degree of ST-segment depression on symptom-limited exercise testing: Relation to the myocardial ischemia burden as determined by thallium-201 scintigraphy. Am. J. Cardiol. *75:*228, 1995.
85. Beller, G. A.: Current status of nuclear cardiology techniques: Curr. Probl. Cardiol. *16:*451, 1991.
86. Kotler, T. S., and Diamond, G. A.: Exercise thallium-201 scintigraphy in the diagnosis and prognosis of coronary artery disease. Ann. Intern. Med. *113:*684, 1990.
87. Christian, T. F., Miller, T. D., Bailey, K. R., and Gibbons, R. J.: Noninvasive identification of severe coronary artery disease using exercise tomographic thallium-201 imaging. Am. J. Cardiol. *70:*14, 1992.
88. Kaul, S., Lilly, D. R., Gascho, J. A., et al.: Prognostic utility of the exercise thallium-201 test in ambulatory patients with chest pain: Comparison with cardiac catheterization. Circulation *77:*745, 1988.
89. Port, S. C., Oshima, M., Ray, G., et al.: Assessment of single-vessel coronary artery disease: Results of exercise electrocardiography, thallium-201 myocardial perfusion imaging and radionuclide angiography. J. Am. Coll. Cardiol. *6:*75, 1985.
90. Johnston, D. L., Daley, J. R., Hodge, D. O., et al.: Hemodynamic responses and adverse effects associated with adenosine and dipyridamole pharmacological stress testing: A comparison of 2,000 patients. Mayo Clin. Proc. *70:*331, 1995.
91. Iskandrian, A. S., Heo, J., Lemek, J., et al.: Identification of high risk patients with left main and three vessel coronary artery disease by adenosine-single photon emission computed tomographic thallium imaging. Am. Heart J. *125:*1130, 1993.
92. Pennell, D. J., Underwood, S. R., and Ell, P. J.: Safety of dobutamine stress for thallium-201 myocardial perfusion tomography in patients with asthma. Am. J. Cardiol. *71:*1346, 1993.
93. Gupta, N. C., Esterbrooks, D. J., Hilleman, B. E., and Mohiuddin, S. M.: Multicenter Adenosine Study Group: Comparison of adenosine in exercise thallium-201 single-photon emission computed tomography (SPECT) myocardial perfusion imaging. J. Am. Coll. Cardiol. *19:*248, 1992.
94. Nishimura, S., Mahmarian, J. J., Boyce, T. M., and Verani, M. S.: Equivalence between adenosine and exercise thallium-201 myocardial tomography: A multicenter, prospective, crossover trial. J. Am. Coll. Cardiol. *20:*265, 1992.
95. Shaw, L., Chaitman, B. R., Hilton, T. C., et al.: Prognostic value of dipyridamole thallium-201 imaging in elderly patients. J. Am. Coll. Cardiol. *19:*1390, 1992.
95a. Dagianti, A., Penco, M., Agati, L., et al.: Stress echocardiography: Comparison of exercise, dipyridamole and dobutamine in detecting and predicting the extent of coronary artery disease. J. Am. Coll. Cardiol. *26:*1180, 1995.
95b. Kiat, H., Iskandrian, A. S., Villegas, B.J., et al.: Arbutamine stress thallium-201 single-photon emission computed tomography using a computerized closed-loop delivery center system multicenter trial for evaluation and safety of diagnosis accuracy. J. Am. Coll. Cardiol. *26:*1159, 1995.
95c. Dennis, C. A., Poole, P. E., Perrins, E.J., et al.: Stress testing with closed-loop arbutamine as an alternative to exercise. J. Am. Coll. Cardiol. *26:*1151, 1995.
96. Decker, P. J., Scott, C. H., and Fishman, L. S.: A rare case of coronary artery occlusion diagnosed by echocardiography. Am. J. Cardiol. *75:*104, 1995.
97. Marwick, T. H., Nemec, J. J., Pashkow, F. J., et al.: Accuracy and limitations of exercise echocardiography in a routine clinical setting. J. Am. Coll. Cardiol. *19:*74, 1992.
98. Quinones, M. A., Verani, M. S., Haichin, R. M., et al.: Exercise echocardiography versus 201 Tl single-photon emission computed tomography in evaluation of coronary artery disease: Analysis of 292 patients. Circulation *85:*1026, 1992.
99. Roger, V. L., Pellikka, P. A., Oh, J. K., et al.: Identification of multivessel coronary artery disease by exercise echocardiography. J. Am. Coll. Cardiol. *24:*109, 1994.
99a. Marwick, T. H., Torelli, J., Harka, K., et al.: Influence of left ventricular hypertrophy and detection of coronary artery disease using exercise echocardiography. J. Am. Coll. Cardiol. *26:*1180, 1995.
100. Iliceto, S., Galiuto, L., Marangelli, V., and Rizzon, P.: Clinical use of stress echocardiography: Factors affecting diagnostic accuracy. Eur. Heart J. *15:*672, 1994.
100a. Cohen, J. L., Chan, K. L., Jaarsman, W., et al.: Arbutamine echocardiography: Efficacy and safety of a new pharmacologic stress agent to induce myocardial ischemia and to detect coronary artery disease. J. Am. Coll. Cardiol. *26:*1168, 1995.
101. Dagianti, A., Penco, N., Agati, L., et al.: Stress echocardiography: Comparison of exercise dipyridamole and dobutamine in detecting and predicting the extent of coronary artery disease. J. Am. Coll. Cardiol. *26:*18, 1995.
102. Marangelli, V., Iliceto, S., Piccinni, G., et al.: Detection of coronary artery disease by digital stress echocardiography: Comparison of exercise, transesophageal atrial pacing and dipyridamole echocardiography. J. Am. Coll. Cardiol. *24:*117, 1994.
103. Fioretti, P. M., Poldermans, D., Salustri, A., et al.: Atropine increases the accuracy of dobutamine stress echocardiography in patients taking beta-blockers. Eur. Heart J. *15:*355, 1994.
104. Marwick, T., Willemart, B., D'Hondt, A. M., et al.: Selection of the optimal nonexercise stress for the evaluation of ischemic regional myocardial dysfunction and malperfusion. Circulation *87:*345, 1993.
105. Beleslin, B. D., Ostojic, M., Stepanovic, J., et al.: Stress echocardiography in the detection of myocardial ischemia: Head-to-head comparison of exercise, dobutamine and dipyridamole tests. Circulation *90:*1168, 1994.
106. Frohwein, S., Klein, L., Lane, A., et al.: Transesophageal dobutamine stress echocardiography in the evaluation of coronary artery disease. J. Am. Coll. Cardiol. *25:*823, 1995.
107. Sketch, M. H., Mohiuddin, S. M., Lynch, J. D., et al.: Significant sex differences in the correlation of electrocardiographic exercise testing in coronary arteriograms. Am. J. Cardiol. *36:*169, 1975.
108. Proceedings of an N.H.L.B.I. Conference: Exercise ECG testing with and without radionuclide studies. *In* Cardiovascular Health and Disease in Women. Greenwich, CT, Le Jacq Communications, Inc., 1993, p. 74.
109. Pryor, D. B., Shaw, L., and Harrell, F. E.: Estimating the likelihood of severe coronary artery disease. Am. J. Med. *90:*553, 1991.
110. Shaw, L. J., Miller, D. D., Romeis, J. C., et al.: Gender differences in the noninvasive evaluation and management of patients with suspected coronary artery disease. Ann. Intern. Med. *120:*559, 1994.
111. Hamm, C. W., Ravkilde, J., Gerhardt, W., et al.: The prognostic value of serum troponin T in unstable angina. N. Engl. J. Med. *327:*146, 1992.
111a. Marwick, T. H., Anderson, T., Williams, J., et al.: Exercise electrocardiography is an accurate and cost-efficient technique for detection of coronary artery disease in women. J. Am. Coll. Cardiol *26:*335, 1995.
112. French, J. K., Elliott, J. M., Williams, B. F., et al.: Association of angiographically detected coronary artery disease with low levels of high-density lipoprotein cholesterol and systemic hypertension. Am. J. Cardiol. *71:*505, 1993.
113. NIH Consensus Development Panel: Triglyceride, high-density lipoprotein, and coronary heart disease. JAMA *269:*505, 1993.
114. Pearson, M., and Layton, C.: Value of the chest radiograph before cardiac catheterization in adults. Br. Heart J. *72:*505, 1994.
115. Chae, S. C., Heo, J., Iskandrian, A. S., et al.: Identification of extensive coronary artery disease in women by exercise single-photon emission computed tomographic (SPECT) thallium imaging. J. Am. Coll. Cardiol. *21:*1305, 1993.
115a. Kajinami, K., Seki, H., Takekoshi, N., et al.: Noninvasive prediction of coronary atherosclerosis by quantification of coronary artery calcification using electron beam computed tomography. Comparison with electrocardiographic and thallium exercise stress test results. J. Am. Coll. Cardiol. *26:*1209, 1995.
116. Loecker, T. H., Schwartz, R. S., Cottac, W., et al.: Fluoroscopic coronary artery calcification and associated coronary disease in asymptomatic young men. J. Am. Coll. Cardiol. *19:*1167, 1992.
117. Rumberger, J. A., Sheedy, P. F., III, Breen, J. F., et al.: Coronary calcium as determined by electron beam computer tomography and coronary disease on arteriograms: Effects of patients' sex on diagnosis. Circulation *91:*1363, 1995.

118. Detrano, R., Wong, N., Tang, W., et al.: Prognostic significance of cardiac cinefluoroscopy for coronary calcific deposits in asymptomatic, high risk subjects. J. Am. Coll. Cardiol. *24*:354, 1994.
119. Simons, D. B., Schwartz, R. S., Edwards, W. D., et al.: Noninvasive definition of anatomic coronary artery disease by ultrafast computed tomographic scanning: A quantitative pathological comparison study. J. Am. Coll. Cardiol. *20*:1118, 1992.
120. Committee on Advanced Cardiac Imaging and Technology, Council on Clinical Cardiology, American Heart Association: Potential value of ultrafast computed tomography to screen for coronary artery disease. Circulation *87*:2071, 1993.
120a. Ellis, S. G.: Chronic stable angina: Role of coronary angiography. *In* Fuster, V., Ross, R., and Topol, E. J. (eds): Atherosclerosis and Coronary Artery Disease. Philadelphia, J. B. Lippincott, 1996, pp. 1433–1450.
121. Bogaty, P., Brecker, S. J., White, S. E., et al.: Comparison of coronary angiographic findings in acute and chronic first presentation of ischemic heart disease. Circulation *87*:1938, 1993.
122. Stajduhar, K. C., Laird, J. R., Rogan, K. M., and Wortham, D. C.: Coronary arterial ectasia: Increased prevalence in patients with abdominal aortic aneurysm as compared to occlusive atherosclerotic peripheral vascular disease. Am. Heart J. *125*:86, 1993.
123. Hartnell, G. G., Parnell, B. M., and Pridie, R. B.: Coronary artery ectasia: Its prevalence and clinical significance in 4993 patients. Br. Heart J. *54*:392, 1985.
124. Tunick, P. A., Slater, J., Kronzon, I., and Glassman, E.: Discrete atherosclerotic coronary artery aneurysms: A study of 20 patients. J. Am. Coll. Cardiol. *15*:279, 1990.
125. Agarwal, J. B., and Helfant, R. H.: Functional importance of coronary collateral circulation. Int. J. Cardiol. *4*:94, 1983.
126. Newman, P. E.: The coronary collateral circulation: Determinants and functional significance in ischemic heart disease. Am. Heart J. *102*:431, 1981.
127. Vanoverschelde, J. L., Winjns, W., Depre, C., et al.: Mechanisms of chronic regional postischemic dysfunction in humans: New insights from the study of noninfarcted collateral-dependent myocardium. Circulation *87*:1513, 1993.
128. Kracoff, O. G., Ovsyshcher, I., and Gueron, M.: Malignant course of a benign anomaly: Myocardial bridging. Chest *92*:1113, 1987.
129. Bestetti, R. B., Costa, R. S., Kazava, D. K., and Oliviera, J. S.: Can isolated myocardial bridging of the left anterior descending coronary artery be associated with sudden death during exercise? Acta Cardiol. *46*:27, 1991.
130. Moraski, R. E., Russell, R. O., Jr., Smith, M., and Rackley, C. E.: Left ventricular function in patients with and without myocardial infarction and one, two or three-vessel coronary artery disease. Am. J. Cardiol. *35*:1, 1975.
131. Mann, T., Brodie, B. R., Grossman, W., and McLaurin, L. P.: Effect of angina on the left ventricular diastolic pressure-volume relationship. Circulation *35*:761, 1977.
132. Stack, R. S., Phillips, H. R., 3d., Grierson, D. S., et al.: Functional improvement of jeopardized myocardium following intracoronary streptokinase infusion in acute myocardial infarction. J. Clin. Invest. *72*:84, 1983.
133. Rahimtoola, S. H.: The hibernating myocardium. Am. Heart J. *117*:211, 1989.
134. Braunwald, E., and Rutherford, J. D.: Reversible ischemic left ventricular dysfunction: Evidence for the "hibernating myocardium." J. Am. Coll. Cardiol. *8*:1467, 1986.
135. Marban, E.: Myocardial stunning and hibernation: The physiology behind the colloquialisms. Circulation *83*:681, 1991.
136. Popio, K. A., Gorlin, R., Bechtel, D., and Levine, J. A.: Postextrasystolic potentiation as a predictor of potential myocardial viability: Preoperative analyses compared with studies after coronary bypass surgery. Am. J. Cardiol. *39*:944, 1977.
137. Nesto, R. W., Cohn, L. H., Collins, J. J., Jr., et al.: Inotropic contractile reserve: A useful predictor of increased 5-year survival and improved postoperative left ventricular function in patients with coronary artery disease and reduced ejection fraction. Am. J. Cardiol. *50*:39, 1982.
138. Verani, M. S., Carroll, R. J., and Falsetti, H. L.: Mitral valve prolapse in coronary artery disease. Am. J. Cardiol. *37*:1, 1976.
139. Herman, M. V., Elliott, W. C., and Gorlin, R.: An electrocardiographic, anatomic, and metabolic study of zonal myocardial ischemia in coronary heart disease. Circulation *35*:834, 1967.
140. Gertz, E. W., Wisneski, J. A., Neese, R., et al.: Myocardial lactate metabolism: Evidence of lactate release during net chemical extraction in man. Circulation *63*:1273, 1981.
141. Cannon, P. J., Weiss, M. B., and Sciacca, R. R.: Myocardial blood flow in coronary artery disease: Studies at rest and during stress with inert gas washout techniques. Prog. Cardiovasc. Dis. *20*:95, 1977.
141a. Rutherford, J. D.: Chronic stable angina: Medical management. *In* Fuster, V., Ross, R., and Topol, E. J. (eds): Atherosclerosis and Coronary Artery Disease. Philadelphia, J. B. Lippincott, 1996, pp. 1419–1432.
142. Stamler, J., Stamler, R., and Neaton, J. D.: Blood pressure, systolic and diastolic, and cardiovascular risks. Arch. Intern. Med. *153*:598, 1993.
143. Wang, X. L., Tam, C., McCredie, R. M., and Wilcken, D. E.: Determinants of severity of coronary artery disease in Australian men and women. Circulation *89*:1974, 1994.
144. Devereux, R. B., and Roman, M. J.: Inter-relationships between hypertension, left ventricular hypertrophy and coronary heart disease. J. Hypertens. *11*(Suppl. 4):S3, 1993.
145. Hebert, P. R., Moser, M., Mayer, J., et al.: Recent evidence on drug therapy of mild to moderate hypertension and decreased risk of coronary heart disease. Arch. Intern. Med. *153*:578, 1993.
146. Vliestra, R. E., Kronmal, R. E., Oberman, A., et al.: Effect of cigarette smoking on survival of patients with angiographically documented coronary artery disease: Report from CASS Registry. JAMA *255*:1023, 1986.
147. Hermanson, B., Omenn, G. S., Kronmal, R. A., and Gersch, B. J.: Beneficial six-year outcome of smoking cessation in older men and women with coronary artery disease: Results from the CASS Registry. N. Engl. J. Med. *319*:1365, 1988.
148. Cavender, J. B., Rogers, W. J., Fisher, L. D., et al.: Effects of smoking on survival and morbidity in patients randomized to medical or surgical therapy in the Coronary Artery Surgery Study (CASS): Ten-year follow-up. J. Am. Coll. Cardiol. *20*:287, 1992.
149. Pearson, T., Rapaport, E., Criqui, M., et al.: Optimal risk factor management in the patient after coronary revascularization: A statement for healthcare professionals from an American Heart Association Writing Group. Circulation *90*:3125, 1994.
150. Nicod, P., Rehr, R., Winniford, M. D., et al.: Acute systemic and coronary hemodynamic and serologic responses to cigarette smoking in long-term smokers with atherosclerotic coronary artery disease. J. Am. Coll. Cardiol. *4*:964, 1984.
150a. Czernin, J., Sun, K., Bruken, R., et al.: Effect of acute and long-term smoking on myocardial blood flow and flow reserve. Circulation *91*:2891, 1995.
151. Winniford, M. D., Wheelan, K. R., Kremers, M. S., et al.: Smoking-induced coronary vasoconstriction in patients with atherosclerotic coronary artery disease: Evidence for adrenergically mediated alterations in coronary artery tone. Circulation *73*:662, 1986.
152. Deanfield, J., Wright, C., Kirkler, S., et al.: Cigarette smoking and the treatment of angina with propranolol, atenolol, and nifedipine. N. Engl. J. Med. *310*:951, 1984.
153. Aronow, W. S.: Effect of passive smoking on angina pectoris. N. Engl. J. Med. *299*:21, 1978.
154. Allred, E. N., Bleecker, E. R., Chaitman, B. R., et al.: Short-term effects of carbon monoxide exposure on the exercise performance of subjects with coronary artery disease. N. Engl. J. Med. *321*:1426, 1989.
155. Adams, K. F., Koch, G., Chatterjee, B., et al.: Acute elevation of blood carboxyhemoglobin to 6% impairs exercise performance and aggravates symptoms in patients with ischemic heart disease. J. Am. Coll. Cardiol. *12*:900, 1988.
155a. Shepherd, J., Cobbe, S. W., Ford, I., et al.: Prevention of coronary heart disease with pravastatin in men with hypercholesterolemia. N. Engl. J. Med. *16*:333, 1995.
156. Pitt, B., Mancini, G. B. J., Ellis, S. G., et al.: Pravastatin limitation of atherosclerosis in the coronary arteries (PLACI): Reduction of atherosclerosis progression in clinical events. J. Am. Coll. Cardiol. *26*:1133, 1995.
157. Rubins, H. B., Robins, S. J., Collins, D., et al.: Distribution of lipids in 8500 men with coronary artery disease. Am. J. Cardiol. *175*:1196, 1995.
158. Blankenhorn, D. H., Azen, S. P., Kramsch, D. M., et al.: Coronary angiographic changes with lovastatin therapy: The Monitored Atherosclerosis Regression Study (MARS). Ann. Intern. Med. *119*:969, 1993.
159. Scandinavian Simvastatin Survival Study Group: Randomised trial of cholesterol lowering in 4444 patients with coronary heart disease: the Scandinavian Simvastatin Survival Study (4S). Lancet *344*:1383, 1994.
160. Anderson, T. J., Meredith, I. T., Yeung, A. C., et al.: The effect of cholesterol-lowering and antioxidant therapy on endothelium-dependent coronary vasomotion. N. Engl. J. Med. *332*:488, 1995.
161. Treasure, C. B., Klein, J. L., Weintraub, W. S., et al.: Beneficial effects of cholesterol-lowering therapy on the coronary endothelium in patients with coronary artery disease. N. Engl. J. Med. *332*:481, 1995.
162. Bonithon-Kopp, C., Scarabin, P. Y., Darne, B., et al.: Menopause-related changes in lipoproteins and some other cardiovascular risk factors. Int. J. Epidemiol. *19*:42, 1990.
163. van Beresteijn, E. C., Korevaar, J. C., Huijbregts, P. C., et al.: Perimenopausal increase in serum cholesterol: A 10-year longitudinal study. Am. J. Epidemiol. *137*:383, 1993.
164. Bass, K. M., Newschaffer, C. J., Klage, M. J., and Bush, T. L.: Plasma lipoprotein levels as predictors of cardiovascular death in women. Arch. Intern. Med. *153*:2209, 1993.
165. Stensvold, I., Tverdal, A., Urdal, P., and Graff-Iversen, S.: Non-fasting serum triglyceride concentration and mortality from coronary heart disease and any cause in middle aged Norwegian women. Br. Med. J. *307*:1318, 1993.
166. The Post Menopausal Estrogen/Progestin Interventions (PEPI) Trial, the writing group for the PEPI trial: Effects of estrogen or estrogen/progestin regimens on heart disease, risk factors in post menopausal women. JAMA *273*:199, 1995.
167. Vaziri, S. M., Evans, J. C., Larson, M. J., and Wilson, P. W.: The impact of female hormone usage on the lipid profile. Arch. Intern. Med. *153*:2200, 1993.
168. Nabulsi, A. A., Folsom, A. R., White, A., et al.: Association of hormone-replacement therapy with various cardiovascular risk factors in post-menopausal women. N. Engl. J. Med. *328*:1069, 1993.
169. Grady, D., Rubin, S. M., Petitti, D. B., et al.: Hormone therapy to prevent disease and prolong life in postmenopausal women. Ann. Intern. Med. *117*:1016, 1992.

170. Rosenberg, L., Palmer, J. R., and Shapiro, S.: A case-control study of myocardial infarction in relation to use of estrogen supplements. Am. J. Epidemiol. *137*:54, 1993.

171. Manolio, T. A., Furberg, C. D., Shemanski, L., et al.: Associations of post-menopausal estrogen use with cardiovascular disease and its risk factors in older women. Circulation *88*:2163, 1993.

172. LaRosa, J. C.: Estrogen: Risk versus benefit for the prevention of cardiovascular disease. Cor. Art. Dis. *4*:588, 1993.

172a. Gebara, O. C. E., Mittleman, M. A., Sutherland, P., et al.: Association between increased estrogen status and increased fibrinolytic potential in the Framingham offspring study. Circulation *91*:1952, 1995.

173. Sullivan, J. M.: Hormone replacement in the secondary prevention of cardiovascular disease. *In* Wenger, N. K., Speroff, T., and Packad, B. (eds.): Proceedings of a NHLBI Conference: Cardiovascular Health and Disease in Women. Greenwich, CT, Le Jacq Communications, Inc., 1993, p. 189.

174. Sullivan, J. M., Vander Zwaag, R., Hughes, J. P., et al.: Estrogen replacement and coronary artery disease: Effect on survival in postmenopausal women. Arch. Intern. Med. *150*:2557, 1990.

175. Expert Panel on Detection, Evaluation and Treatment of High Blood Cholesterol in Adults: Summary of the second report of the National Cholesterol Education Program (NCEP): Expert panel on detection, evaluation and treatment of high blood cholesterol in adults (adult treatment panel II). JAMA *269*:3015, 1993.

176. Kardinaal, A. F., Kok, F. J., Ringstad, J., et al.: Antioxidants in adipose tissue and risk of myocardial infarction: The EURAMIC study. Lancet *342*:1379, 1993.

177. Jha, P., Flather, M., Lonn, E., et al.: The antioxidant vitamins and cardiovascular disease: a critical review of epidemiologic and clinical trial data. Ann. Intern. Med. *123*:816, 1995.

178. Hodis, H. N., Mack, W. G., LaBree, L., et al.: Serial coronary angiographic evidence that antioxidant vitamin intake reduces progression of coronary artery atherosclerosis. JAMA *273*:1849, 1995.

179. Stampfer, M. J., Hennekens, C. H., Manson, J. E., et al.: Vitamin E consumption and the risk of coronary disease in women. N. Engl. J. Med. *328*:1444, 1993.

180. Ferguson, R. J., Taylor, A. W., Cote, P., et al.: Skeletal muscle and cardiac changes with training in patients with angina pectoris. Am. J. Physiol. *243*:H830, 1982.

181. Bittner, V., and Oberman, A.: Efficacy studies in coronary rehabilitation. Cardiol. Clin. *11*:333, 1993.

182. Hedback, B., Perk, J., and Wodlin, P.: A long-term reduction of cardiac mortality after myocardial infarction: 10-Year results of a comprehensive rehabilitation program. Eur. Heart J. *14*:831, 1993.

183. Hambrecht, R., Niebauer, J., Marburger, C., et al.: Various intensities of leisure time physical activity in patients with coronary artery disease: Effects of coronary respiratory fitness and progression of coronary atherosclerotic lesions. J. Am. Coll. Cardiol. *22*:468, 1993.

184. Shuler, G., Hambrecht, R., Schlierf, G., et al.: Myocardial perfusion and regression of coronary artery disease in patients on a regimen of intensive physical exercise and low-fat diet. J. Am. Coll. Cardiol. *19*:34, 1992.

185. Ades, P. A., Waldmann, M. L., Poehlman, E. T., et al.: Exercise conditioning in older coronary patients: Submaximal lactate response and endurance capacity. Circulation *88*:572, 1993.

186. Stratton, J. R., Levy, W. C., Cerqueira, M. D., et al.: Cardiovascular responses to exercise: Effects of aging and exercise training in healthy men. Circulation *89*:1648, 1994.

187. Oldridge, N., Furlong, W., Feeny, D., et al.: Economic evaluation of cardiac rehabilitation soon after acute myocardial infarction. Am. J. Cardiol. *72*:154, 1993.

188. Lam, J. Y. T., Latour, J., Lesperance, J., et al.: Platelet aggregation, coronary artery disease, progression in future coronary events. Am. J. Cardiol. *73*:333, 1994.

189. Antiplatelet Trialists' Collaboration: Collaborative overview of randomized trial of antiplatelet therapy. I. Prevention of death, myocardial infarction and stroke by prolonged antiplatelet therapy in various categories of patients. Br. Med. J. *308*:81, 1994.

190. SAPAT (Swedish Angina Pectoris Aspirin Trial) Group, Juul-Moller, S., Edvardsson, N., Jahnmatz, B., et al.: Double-blind trial of aspirin in primary prevention of myocardial infarction in patients with stable chronic angina pectoris. Lancet *340*:1421, 1992.

191. Ridker, P. M., Manson, J. E., Gaziano, J. M., et al.: Low-dose aspirin therapy for chronic stable angina: A randomized, placebo-controlled clinical trial. Ann. Intern. Med. *114*:835, 1991.

192. The Beta-Blocker Pooling Project Research Group: The Beta-blocker Pooling Project (BBPP): Subgroup findings from randomized trials in post-infarction patients. Eur. Heart J. *9*:8, 1988.

193. Goldman, L., Sia, S. T., Cook, E. F., et al.: Costs and effectiveness of routine therapy with long-term beta-adrenergic antagonists after acute myocardial infarction. N. Engl. J. Med. *319*:152, 1988.

194. Daly, P., Mettauer, B., Rouleau, J. L., et al.: Lack of reflex increase in myocardial sympathetic tone after captopril: Potential anti-anginal effect. Circulation *71*:317, 1985.

195. Strozzi, C., Portaluppi, F., Cocco, G., and Urso, L.: Ergometric evaluation of the effects of enalapril maleate in normotensive patients with stable angina. Clin. Cardiol. *11*:246, 1988.

196. Simon, J., Gibbs, R., Crean, P. A., et al.: The variable effects of angiotensin converting enzyme inhibition on myocardial ischemia in chronic stable angina. Br. Heart J. *62*:112, 1989.

197. Cleland, J. G., Henderson, E., McLenachan, J., et al.: Effect of captopril, an angiotensin-converting enzyme inhibitor, in patients with angina pectoris and heart failure. J. Am. Coll. Cardiol. *17*:733, 1991.

198. Sogaard, P., Gotzsche, C. O., Ravkilde, J., and Thygesen, K.: Effects of captopril on ischemia and dysfunction of the left ventricle after myocardial infarction. Circulation *87*:1093, 1993.

199. Pfeffer, M. A., Braunwald, E., Moye, L. A., et al.: Effect of captopril on mortality and morbidity in patients with left ventricular dysfunction after myocardial infarction. N. Engl. J. Med. *327*:669, 1992.

200. SOLVD Investigators: Effects of enalapril on survival in patients with reduced left ventricular ejection fractions and congestive heart failure. N. Engl. J. Med. *325*:293, 1991.

201. SOLVD Investigators: Effect of enalapril on mortality and the development of heart failure in asymptomatic patients with reduced left ventricular ejection fractions. N. Engl. J. Med. *327*:685, 1992.

202. The Acute Infarction Ramipril Efficacy (AIRE) Study Investigators: Effect of ramipril on mortality and morbidity of survivors of acute myocardial infarction with clinical evidence of heart failure. Lancet *342*:821, 1993.

203. Lonn, E. M., Yusuf, S., Jha, P., et al.: Emerging role of angiotensin-converting enzyme inhibitors in cardiac and vascular protection. Circulation *90*:2056, 1994.

204. Featherstone, J. F., Holly, R. G., and Amsterdam, E. A.: Physiologic responses to weight lifting in coronary artery disease. Am. J. Cardiol. *71*:287, 1993.

205. Franklin, B. A., Hogan, P., Bonzheim, K., et al.: Cardiac demands on heavy snow shoveling. JAMA *273*:880, 1995.

206. Kahn, J. F., Jouanin, J. C., Espirito-Santo, J., and Monod, H.: Cardiovascular responses to leisure alpine skiing in habitually sedentary middle-aged men. J. Sports Sci. *11*:31, 1993.

207. Luurila, O. J., Karjalainen, J., Viitasalo, N., and Toivonen, L.: Arrhythmias and ST segment deviation during prolonged exhaustive exercise (ski marathon) in healthy, middle-aged men. Eur. Heart J. *15*:507, 1994.

208. Rocco, M. B., Barry, J., Campbell, S., et al.: Circadian variation of transient myocardial ischemia in patients with coronary artery disease. Circulation *75*:395, 1987.

208a. Figueras, J., and Lidon, R. M.: Early morning reduction in ischemic threshold in patients with unstable angina and significant coronary disease. Circulation *92*:1737, 1995.

208b. Robertson, R. M., and Robertson, D.: Drugs used for the treatment of myocardial ischemia. *In* Hardman, J. G., et al. (eds): Goodman & Gilman's The Pharmacological Basis of Therapeutics. 9th ed. New York, McGraw-Hill, 1996, pp. 759–780.

209. Williams, J. F., Jr., Glick, G., and Braunwald, E.: Studies on cardiac dimensions in intact unanesthetized man. V. Effects of nitroglycerin. Circulation *32*:767, 1965.

210. Brown, B. G., Bolson, E., Petersen, R. B., et al.: The mechanisms of nitroglycerin action: Stenosis vasodilatation as a major component of the drug response. Circulation *64*:1089, 1981.

211. Parker, J. O.: Nitrates and angina pectoris. Am. J. Cardiol. *72*:3C, 1993.

212. Bache, R. J., Ball, R. M., Cobb, F. R., et al.: Effects of nitroglyerin on transmural myocardial blood flow in the unanesthetized dog. J. Clin. Invest. *55*:1219, 1975.

213. Fallen, E. L., Nahmias, C., Scheffel, A., et al.: Redistribution of myocardial blood flow with topical nitroglycerin in patients with coronary artery disease. Circulation *91*:1381, 1995.

214. Sudhir, K., MacGregor, J. S., Barbant, S. D., et al.: Assessment of coronary conductance and resistive vessel reactivity in response to nitroglycerine, ergonovine and adenosine: In vivo studies with simultaneous intravascular two-dimensional and Doppler ultrasound. J. Am. Coll. Cardiol. *21*:1261, 1993.

215. Ganz, W., and Marcus, H. S.: Failure of intracoronary nitroglycerin to alleviate pacing-induced angina. Circulation *46*:880, 1972.

216. Dove, J. T., Shah, P. M., and Schreiner, B. F.: Effect of sublingually administered nitroglycerin on left ventricular wall motion in coronary artery disease. Circulation *49*:682, 1974.

217. Ohno, A., Fujita, M., Miwa, K., et al.: Importance of coronary collateral circulation for increased treadmill exercise capacity by nitrates in patients with stable effort angina pectoris. Cardiology *78*:323, 1991.

218. Cohen, M. V., Downey, J. M., Sonnenblick, E. H., and Kirk, E. S.: The effects of nitroglycerin on coronary collaterals and myocardial contractility. J. Clin. Invest. *52*:2836, 1973.

219. Dove, J. T., Shah, P. M., Schreiner, B. F.: Effects of nitroglycerin on left ventricular wall motion in coronary artery disease. Circulation *49*:662, 1974.

220. Mahmarian, J. J., Fenimore, N. L., Marks, G. F., et al.: Transdermal nitroglycerin patch therapy reduces the extent of exercise-induced myocardial ischemia: Results of a double-blind, placebo-controlled trial using quantitative thallium-201 tomography. J. Am. Coll. Cardiol. *24*:25, 1994.

221. Chirkov, Y. Y., Naukalis, J. I., Sage, E., and Horowitz, J. D.: Antiplatelet effects of nitroglycerin in healthy subjects and in patients with stable angina pectoris. J. Cardiovasc. Pharmacol. *21*:384, 1993.

222. Lacoste, L. L., Theroux, P., Lidon, R. M., et al.: Antithrombotic properties of transdermal nitroglycerin in stable angina pectoris. Am. J. Cardiol. *73*:1058, 1994.

223. Andrews, R., May, J. A., Vickers, J., and Heptinstall, S.: Inhibition of platelet aggregation by transdermal glyceryl trinitrate. Br. Heart J. *72*:575, 1994.

224. Murad, F.: Cyclic guanosine monophosphate as a mediator of vasodilation. J. Clin. Invest. *78*:1, 1986.

225. Anderson, T. J., Meredith, I. T., Ganz, P., et al.: Nitric oxide and nitro-

vasodilators: Similarities, differences and potential interactions. J. Am. Coll. Cardiol. *24*:555, 1994.

226. Horowitz, J. D., Antman, E. M., Lorell, B. H., et al.: Potentiation of the cardiovascular effects of nitroglycerin by N-acetylcysteine. Circulation *68*:1247, 1983.

227. Winniford, M. D., Kennedy, P. L., Wells, P. J., and Hillis, L. D.: Potentiation of nitroglycerin-induced coronary dilatation by N-acetylcysteine. Circulation *73*:138, 1986.

228. Jansen, R. W., and Lipsitz, L. A.: Postprandial hypotension: Epidemiology, pathophysiology and clinical management. Ann. Intern. Med. *122*:286, 1995.

229. Hales, C. A., and Westphal, D.: Hypoxemia following the administration of sublingual nitroglycerin. Am. J. Med. *65*:911, 1978.

230. Parker, J. O., Vankoughnett, K. A., and Farrell, B.: Nitroglycerin lingual spray: Clinical efficacy and dose-response relation. Am. J. Cardiol. *57*:1, 1986.

231. Bassan, M. M.: The daylong pattern of the antianginal effect of long-term three times daily administered isosorbide dinitrate. J. Am. Coll. Cardiol. *16*:936, 1990.

232. de Belder, M. A., Schneeweiss, A., and Camm, A. J.: Evaluation of the efficacy and duration of action of isosorbide mononitrate in angina pectoris. Am. J. Cardiol. *65*:6J, 1990.

233. Nordlander, R., and Walter, M.: Once- versus twice-daily administration of controlled-release isosorbide-5-mononitrate 60 mg in the treatment of stable angina pectoris: A randomized, double-blind, cross-over study: The Swedish Multicenter Group. Eur. Heart J. *15*:108, 1994.

234. Parker, J. O., Amies, M. H., Hawkinson, R. W., et al.: Intermittent transdermal nitroglycerin therapy in angina pectoris: Clinically effective without tolerance or rebound. Circulation *91*:1368, 1995.

235. Munzel, T., Heitzer, T., Kurz, S., et al.: Dissociation of coronary vascular tolerance and neurohormonal adjustments during long-term nitroglycerin therapy in patients with stable coronary artery disease. J. Am. Coll. Cardiol. *27*:297, 1996.

236. Mangione, N. J., and Glasser, S. P.: Phenomenon of nitrate tolerance. Am. Heart J. *128*:137, 1994.

237. Demots, H., and Glasser, S. P.: Intermittent transdermal nitroglycerin therapy in the treatment of chronic stable angina. J. Am. Coll. Cardiol. *13*:786, 1989.

238. Abrams, J.: Clinical aspects of nitrate tolerance. Eur. Heart J. *12*:42, 1991.

239. Jeserich, M., Munzel, T., Pape, L., et al.: Absence of vascular tolerance in conductance vessels after 48 hours of intravenous nitroglycerin in patients with coronary artery disease. J. Am. Coll. Cardiol. *26*:50, 1995.

240. Packer, M.: What causes tolerance to nitroglycerin? The 100 year old mystery continues. J. Am. Coll. Cardiol. *16*:932, 1990.

241. Parker, J. D., Farrell, B., Fenton, T., et al.: Counter-regulatory responses to continuous and intermittent therapy with nitroglycerin. Circulation *84*:2336, 1991.

242. Parker, J. D., and Parker, J. O.: Effect of therapy with an angiotensin-converting enzyme inhibitor of hemodynamic and counter-regulatory responses during continuous therapy with nitroglycerin. J. Am. Coll. Cardiol. *21*:1445, 1993.

243. Dupuis, J., Lalonde, G., Lemieux, R., and Rouleau, J. L.: Tolerance to intravenous nitroglyerin in patients with congestive heart failure: Rate of increased intravascular volume, neurohumoral activation and task of prevention with N-acetylcysteine. J. Am. Coll. Cardiol. *16*:923, 1990.

244. Watanabe, H., Kakihana, M., Ohtsuka, S., et al.: Platelet cyclic GNP: A potentially useful indicator to evaluate the effects of nitroglycerin on nitrate tolerance. Circulation *88*:29, 1993.

245. Schaer, D. F., Buff, L. A., and Katz, R. J.: Sustained antianginal efficacy of transdermal nitroglycerin patches using an overnight 10-hour nitrate-free interval. Am. J. Cardiol. *61*:46, 1988.

246. Fox, K. M., Dargie, H. J., Deanfield, J., and Maseri, A., on behalf of the Transdermal Nitrate Investigators: Avoidance of tolerance and lack of rebound with intermittent dose titrated transdermal glyceral trinitrate. Br. Heart J. *66*:151, 1991.

247. DeMots, H., and Glasser, S. P.: Intermittent transdermal nitroglycerin therapy in the treatment of chronic stable angina. J. Am. Coll. Cardiol. *13*:786, 1989.

248. de Belder, M. A., Schneeweiss, A., and Camm, A. J.: Evaluation of the efficacy and duration of action of isosorbide mononitrate in angina pectoris. Am. J. Cardiol. *65*:6J, 1990.

249. Przybojewski, J. Z., and Heyns, M. H.: Acute coronary vasospasm secondary to industrial nitroglycerin withdrawal. S. Afr. Med. J. *63*:158, 1983.

250. May, D. C., Popma, J. J., Black, W. H., et al.: In vivo induction and reversal of nitroglycerin tolerance in human coronary arteries. N. Engl. J. Med. *317*:805, 1987.

251. Schwartz, A.: The cause, relief, and prevention of headaches arising from contact with dynamite. N. Engl. J. Med. *235*:541, 1948.

252. Hoffman, B. B., and Lefkowitz, R. J.: Catecholamines, sympathomimetic drugs, and adrenergic receptor antagonists. *In* Hardman, J. G., et al. (eds.): Goodman & Gilman's The Pharmacological Basis of Therapeutics. 9th ed. New York, McGraw-Hill, 1996, pp. 199–248.

253. Lefkowitz, R. J., and Caron, M. G.: Adrenergic receptors: Models for the study of receptors coupled to guanine nucleotide regulatory proteins. J. Biol. Chem. *263*:4993, 1988.

254. Opie, L. H., Sonnenblick, E. H., Kaplan, N. M., et al.: Beta-blocking agents. *In* Opie, L. H. (ed.): Drugs for the Heart. 4th ed. Philadelphia, W. B. Saunders Company, 1995, pp. 1–3.

255. Parker, J. D., Testama, A., Jimenez, A. H., et al.: Morning increase in ambulatory ischemia in patients with stable coronary artery disease: Importance of physical activity in increased cardiac demand. Circulation *89*:604, 1994.

256. Bristow, M. R., O'Connell, J. B., Gilbert, E. M., et al.: Dose-response of chronic beta-blocker treatment in heart failure from either idiopathic dilated or ischemic cardiomyopathy. Circulation *89*:1632, 1994.

257. Olse, S. L., Gilbert, E. M., Renlund, D. G., et al.: Carvedilol improves left ventricular function and symptoms in chronic heart failure: A double-blind randomized study. J. Am. Coll. Cardiol. *25*:1225, 1995.

258. Steinbeck, G., Andresen, D., Bach, P., et al.: A comparison of electrophysiologically guided anti-arrhythmic drug therapy with beta-blocker therapy in patients with symptomatic, sustained ventricular tachyarrhythmias. N. Engl. J. Med. *327*:987, 1992.

259. Anastasiou-Nana, M. I., Gilbert, E. M., Miller, R. H., et al.: Usefulness of d,l Sotalol for suppression of chronic ventricular arrhythmias. Am. J. Cardiol. *67*:511, 1991.

260. Singh, B. N., Deedwania, P., Nademanee, K., et al.: Sotalol: A review of its pharmacodynamic and pharmacokinetic properties and therapeutic use. Drugs *34*:311, 1987.

261. Frishman, W. H.: Pindolol: A new β-adrenoceptor antagonist with partial agonist activity. N. Engl. J. Med. *308*:940, 1983.

262. Kostis, J. B., Frishman, W., Hosler, M. H., et al.: Treatment of angina pectoris with pindolol: The significance of intrinsic sympathomimetic activity of beta blockers. Am. Heart J. *104*:496, 1982.

263. Quyyumi, A. A., Wright, C., Mockus, L., and Fox, K. M.: Effect of partial agonist activity in beta blockers in severe angina pectoris: A double-blind comparison of pindolol and atenolol. Br. Med. J. *289*:951, 1984.

264. Frishman, W., and Halprin, S.: Clincial pharmacology of the new beta-adrenergic blocking drugs. VII. New horizons in beta-adrenoceptor blockade therapy—labetolol. Am. Heart J. *98*:660, 1979.

265. Lennard, M. S.: The polymorphic oxidation of beta-adrenoceptor antagonists. Pharmacol. Ther. *41*:461, 1989.

266. Lehtonen, A.: Effect of beta blockers and blood lipid profile. Am. Heart J. *109*:1192, 1985.

267. Northcote, R. J., Todd, I. C., and Ballantyne, D.: Beta blockers and lipoproteins: A review of current knowledge. Scott. Med. J. *31*:220, 1986.

268. Henry, J. A., and Cassidy, S. L.: Membrane stabilizing activity: A major cause of fatal poisoning. Lancet *1*:1414, 1986.

269. Borzak, S., Fenton, T., Glasser, S. P., et al. for the Angina and Silent Ischemia Study Group (ASISG): Discordance between effects of anti-ischemic therapy on ambulatory ischemia, exercise performance and anginal symptoms in patients with stable angina pectoris. J. Am. Coll. Cardiol. *21*:1605, 1993.

270. Opie, L. H., Sonnenblick, E. H., Kaplan, N. M., et al.: Beta-agents. *In* Opie, L. H. (ed.): Drugs for the Heart. 4th ed. Philadelphia, W. B. Saunders Company, 1995, pp. 20–23.

271. Waagstein, F., Bristow, M. R., Swidberg, K., et al.: Beneficial effects of metoprolol in idiopathic dilated cardiomyopathy. Lancet *342*:1441, 1993.

272. Deacon, S. P., Karunanayake, A., and Barnett, D.: Acebutolol, atenolol and propranolol and metabolic responses to acute hypoglycemia in diabetes. Br. Med. J. *2*:1255, 1977.

273. Hiatt, W. R., Stoll, S., and Nies, A. S.: Effect of beta-adrenergic blockers on the peripheral circulation in patients with peripheral vascular disease. Circulation *72*:1226, 1985.

274. Miller, R. R., Olsen, H. G., Amsterdam, E. A., and Mason, D. T.: Propranolol withdrawal rebound phenomenon: Exacerbation of coronary events after abrupt cessation of antianginal therapy. N. Engl. J. Med. *293*:416, 1975.

275. Katz, A. M.: Cardiac ion channels. N. Engl. J. Med. *328*:1244, 1993.

276. Hurwitz, L., Partridge, L. D., and Leach, J. D. (eds.): Calcium Channels: Their Properties, Functions, Regulation and Clinical Relevance. Boca Raton, FL, CRC Press, 1991.

277. Opie, L. H.: Calcium channel antagonists. Part I. Fundamental properties: Mechanisms, classification, sites of action. Cardiovasc. Drugs Ther. *1*:411, 1987.

278. Wood, A. J.: Calcium antagonists: Pharmacologic differences and similarities. Circulation *80*(Suppl. IV):184, 1989.

279. Cannon, R. O., Watson, R. M., Rosing, D. R., and Epstein, S. E.: Efficacy of calcium channel blocker therapy for angina pectoris resulting from small-vessel coronary artery disease and abnormal vasodilator reserve. Am. J. Cardiol. *56*:242, 1985.

280. Braunwald, E.: Mechanisms of action of calcium-channel blocking agents. N. Engl. J. Med. *307*:1618, 1982.

281. Strauss, W. E., and Parisi, S. F.: Combined use of calcium-channel and beta-adrenergic blockers for the treatment of chronic stable angina. Ann. Intern. Med. *109*:570, 1988.

282. Packer, M.: Combined beta-adrenergic and calcium-entry blockade in angina pectoris. N. Engl. J. Med. *320*:709, 1989.

282a. Opie, L. H.: Calcium channel antagonists in the treatment of coronary artery disease: Fundamental pharmacological properties relevant to clinical use. Prog. Cardiovasc. Dis. *38*:273, 1996.

283. Frishman, W. H.: Current Cardiovascular Drugs. 2nd ed. Philadelphia, Current Medicine, 1995, pp. 129–148.

283a. Ryden, L., and Malmberg, K.: Calcium channel blockers or beta receptor antagonists for patients with ischaemic heart disease. What is the best choice? Eur. Heart J. *17*:1, 1996.

283b. Fox, K. M., Mulcahy, D., Findlay, I., et al.: The Total Ischaemic Burden European Trial (TIBET): Effects of atenolol, nifedipine SR and their combination on the exercise test and the total ischaemic burden in 608 patients with stable angina. Eur. Heart J. *17*:96, 1996.

284. Lichtlen, P. R., Hugenholtz, P. G., Raffenbeul, W., et al.: Retardation of angiographic progression of coronary artery disease by nifedipine: Results of the International Nifedipine Trial on Antiatherosclerotic Therapy (INTACT). Lancet *335*:1109, 1990.
285. Loaldi, A., Polese, A., Montorsi, P., et al.: Comparison of nifedipine, propranolol and isosorbide dinitrate on angiographic progression and regression of coronary arterial narrowings in angina pectoris. Am. J. Cardiol. *64*:433, 1989.
286. Waters, D., and Lesperance, J.: Interventions that beneficially influence the evolution of coronary atherosclerosis: The case for calcium channel blockers. Circulation *86*(Suppl. III):111, 1992.
287. Schroeder, J. S., Gao, S. Z., Alderman, E. L., et al.: A preliminary study of diltiazem in the prevention of coronary artery disease in heart transplant recipients. N. Engl. J. Med. *328*:164, 1993.
288. Elkayam, U., Amin, J., Mehra, A., et al.: A prospective, randomized, double-blind, crossover study to compare the efficacy and safety of chronic nifedipine therapy with that of isosorbide dinitrate and their combination in the treatment of chronic congestive heart failure. Circulation *82*:1954, 1990.
289. Vetrovec, G. W.: Hemodynamic and electrophysiologic effects of first- and second-generation calcium antagonists. Am. J. Cardiol. *73*:34a, 1994.
290. Opie, L. H., Frishman, W. H., and Thadani, U.: Calcium channel antagonists (calcium entry blockers). *In* Opie, L. H. (ed.): Drugs for the Heart. 4th ed. Philadelphia, W. B. Saunders Company, 1995, p. 53.
291. Wallace, W. A., Willington, K. L., Chess, M. A., et al.: Comparison of nifedipine gastrointestinal therapeutic system and atenolol on anti-anginal efficacies and exercise hemodynamic responses in stable angina pectoris. Am. J. Cardiol. *73*:23, 1994.
292. Parmley, W. W., Nestor, W., Singh, B. N., et al.: Attenuation of the circadian patterns of myocardial ischemia with nifedipine GITS in patients with chronic stable angina. J. Am. Coll. Cardiol. *19*:1380, 1992.
292a. Furberg, C. D., Psaty, B. M., and Meyer, J. V.: Nifedipine: Dose related increase in mortality in patients with coronary heart disease. Circulation *92*:1737, 1995.
292b. Opie, L. H., and Messerli, F. H.: Nifedipine and mortality: Grave defects in the dossier. Circulation *92*:1068, 1995.
292c. Yusuf, S.: Calcium antagonists in coronary artery disease and hypertension. Time for reevaluation. Circulation *92*:1079, 1995.
293. LaCoste, L., Lamb, J. Y. T., Hung, J., et al.: Oral verapamil inhibits platelet thrombus formation in humans. Circulation *89*:630, 1994.
294. Leon, M. B., Rosing, D. R., Bonow, R. O., et al.: Clinical efficacy of verapamil alone and combined with propranolol in treating patients with chronic stable angina pectoris. Am. J. Cardiol. *48*:131, 1981.
295. Bache, R. J.: Effects of calcium entry blockade on myocardial blood flow. Circulation *80*(Suppl. IV):40, 1989.
296. Murakami, T., Hess, O. M., and Krayenbuehl, H. P.: Left ventricular function before and after diltiazem in patients with coronary artery disease. J. Am. Coll. Cardiol. *5*:723, 1985.
297. Klinke, W., Baird, M., Juneau, M., et al.: Anti-anginal efficacy and safety of control-delivery diltiazem QD versus an equivalent dose of immediate-release diltiazem. Cardiovasc. Drugs Ther. *9*:319, 1995.
298. Nadazin, A., and Davies, G. J.: Investigation of therapeutic mechanisms of atenolol and diltiazem in patients with variable-threshold angina. Am. Heart J. *127*:312, 1994.
299. Piepho, R. W., Culbertson, V. L., and Rhodes, R. S.: Drug interactions with the calcium-entry blockers. Circulation *75*(Suppl. V):V181, 1987.
300. Abernethy, D. R.: An overview of the pharmacokinetics and pharmacodynamics of amlodipine in elderly persons with systemic hypertension. Am. J. Cardiol. *73*:10A, 1994.
301. Ezekowitz, M. D., Hossack, K., Metta, J. L., et al.: Amlodipine in chronic stable angina: Results of a multicenter double-blind crossover trial. Am. Heart J. *129*:527, 1995.
302. Packer, M., For the Prospective Randomized Amlodipine Survival Evaluation [PRAISE] Investigators: Presented at the Annual Scientific Sessions of the American College of Cardiology, New Orleans, LA, March 1995.
303. Landau, A. G., Gentilucci, M., Cavusoglu, E., and Frishman, W. H.: Calcium antagonists for the treatment of congestive heart failure. Cor. Art. Dis. *5*:37, 1994.
304. Ekelund, L. G., Ulvenstam, G., Walldius, G., and Aberg, A.: Effects of felodipine versus nifedipine on exercise tolerance in stable angina pectoris. Am. J. Cardiol. *73*:658, 1994.
305. Frishman, W. H.: Comparative efficacy and concomitant use of bepridil and beta-blockers in the management of angina pectoris. Am. J. Cardiol. *69*:50D, 1992.
306. Multicentre Diltiazem Postinfarction Trial Research Group: The effect of diltiazem on mortality and reinfarction after myocardial infarction. N. Engl. J. Med. *319*:385, 1988.
307. The Danish Study Group on Verapamil in Myocardial Infarction: Effect of verapamil on mortality and major events after acute myocardial infarction: The Danish Verapamil Infarction Trial II-DAVIT II. Am. J. Cardiol. *66*:779, 1990.
308. Boden, W. E., Bough, E. W., Reichman, M. J., et al.: Beneficial effects of high-dose diltiazem in patients with persistent effort angina on beta blockers and nitrates: A randomized, double-blind, placebo-controlled cross-over study. Circulation *71*:1197, 1985.
309. HINT Research Group: Early treatment of unstable angina in the coronary care unit: A randomised, double-blind, placebo-controlled comparison of recurrent ischaemia in patients treated with nifedipine or metoprolol or both: Report of the Holland Interuniversity Nifedipine/Metoprolol Trial (HINT). Br. Heart J. *56*:400, 1986.
310. White, H. D., Polak, J. F., Wynne, J., et al.: Addition of nifedipine to maximal nitrate and beta-adrenoreceptor blocker therapy in coronary artery disease. Am. J. Cardiol. *55*:1303, 1985.
311. Packer, M., Meller, J., Medina, N., et al.: Hemodynamic consequences of combined beta-adrenergic and slow calcium channel blockade in men. Circulation *65*:660, 1982.

PERCUTANEOUS TRANSLUMINAL CORONARY ANGIOPLASTY

312. Gersh, B. J.: Coronary revascularization in the 1990's: A cardiologist's perspective. Can. J. Cardiol. *10*:661, 1994.
313. King, S. B. III., and Holmes, D. J., Jr.: Chronic stable angina: Role of coronary intervention. *In* Fuster, V., Ross, R., and Topol, E. J. (eds): Atherosclerosis and Coronary Artery Disease. Philadelphia, J. B. Lippincott, 1996, pp. 1485–1504.
314. National Heart, Lung and Blood Institute Alert, No. 21, 1995.
315. Lytle, B. W., and Cosgrove, D. M.: Coronary artery bypass surgery. Curr. Probl. Surg. *29*:756, 1992.
316. Ryan, T. J., Bauman, W. B., Kennedy, J. W., et al.: ACC/AHA Task Force Report: Guidelines for percutaneous transluminal coronary angioplasty: A report of the American College of Cardiology/American Heart Association Task Force on assessment of diagnostic and therapeutic cardiovascular procedures [Committee on Percutaneous Transluminal Angioplasty]. J. Am. Coll. Cardiol. *22*:2033, 1993.
317. Kimmel, S. C., Berlin, J. A., Strom, B. L., et al.: Development and validation of a simplified predictive index for major complications in contemporary percutaneous transluminal coronary angioplasty practice. J. Am. Coll. Cardiol. *26*:931, 1995.
318. Serota, H., Deligonul, U., Lee, W-H., et al.: Predictors of cardiac survival after percutaneous transluminal coronary angioplasty in patients with severe left ventricular dysfunction. Am. J. Cardiol. *67*:367, 1991.
319. Holmes, D. R., Holubkov, R., Vlietstra, R. E., and the coinvestigators of the NHLBI Transluminal Coronary Angioplasty Registry: Comparison of complications during percutaneous transluminal coronary angioplasty from 1977 to 1981 and from 1985 to 1986. J. Am. Coll. Cardiol. *12*:1149, 1988.
320. Faxon, D. P., Holmes, D. R., Hartzler, G., et al.: ABCs of coronary angioplasty: Have we simplified it too much? Cathet. Cardiovasc. Diagn. *25*:1, 1992.
320a. Jollis, J. G., Peterson, E. D., DeLong, E. R., et al.: The relation between the volume of coronary angioplasty procedures in hospitals treating Medicare beneficiaries and short-term mortality. N. Engl. J. Med. *331*:1625, 1994.
321. Landau, C., Lange, R. A., and Hillis, L. D.: Percutaneous transluminal coronary angioplasty (review). N. Engl. J. Med. *330*:981, 1994.
322. Lincoff, A. M.: Patients at high risk for ischemic complications. J. Invest. Cardiol. *6*(Suppl. A):13A, 1994.
323. Kuntz, R. E., Piana, R., Pomerantz, R. M., et al.: Changing incidence and management of abrupt closure following coronary intervention in the new device era. Cathet. Cardiovasc. Diagn. *27*:183, 1992.
324. Lincoff, A. M., Popma, J. J., Ellis, S. G., et al.: Abrupt vessel closure complicating coronary angioplasty: Clinical, angiographic and therapeutic profile. J. Am. Coll. Cardiol. *19*:926, 1992.
325. deFeyter, P. J., deJaegere, P. P., and Serruys, P. W.: Incidence, predictors and management of acute coronary occlusion after coronary angioplasty. Am. Heart J. *127*:643, 1994.
326. Reeder, G. S., Bryant, S. C., Suman, V. J., et al.: Intracoronary thrombus: Still a risk factor for PTCA failure? Cathet. Cardiovasc. Diagn. *34*:191, 1995.
327. Tan, K., Sulke, N., Taub, N., and Sowton, E.: Clinical and lesion morphologic determinants of coronary angioplasty success and complications: Current experience. J. Am. Coll. Cardiol. *24*:855, 1995.
328. Lincoff, A. M., Topol, E. J., Chapekis, A. T., et al.: Intracoronary stenting compared with conventional therapy for abrupt vessel closure complicating coronary angioplasty: A matched case-control study. J. Am. Coll. Cardiol. *21*:866, 1993.
329. Sutton, J. M., Ellis, S. G., Roubin, G. S., et al.: Major clinical events after coronary stenting: The multicentre registry of acute and elective Gianturco-Roubin stent placement: Gianturco-Roubin Intracoronary Stent Investigator Group. Circulation *89*:1126, 1994.
330. Gibbs, J. S., Sigwart, U., and Buller, N. P.: Temporary stent as a bail-out device during percutaneous transluminal coronary angioplasty: Preliminary clinical experience. Br. Heart J. *71*:372, 1994.
331. Schomig, A., Kastrati, A., Dietz, R., et al.: Emergency coronary setting for dissection during percutaneous transluminal coronary angioplasty: Angiographic follow-up after stenting and after repeat angioplasty of the stent segment. J. Am. Coll. Cardiol. *23*:1053, 1994.
332. Piana, R. N., Paik, G. Y., Moscucci, M., et al.: Incidence and treatment of "no-reflow" after percutaneous coronary intervention. Circulation *89*:2514, 1994.
333. Weyrens, F. J., Mooney, J., Lesser, J., and Mooney, M. R.: Intracoronary diltiazem for microvascular spasm after interventional therapy. Am. J. Cardiol. *75*:849, 1995.
334. The EPIC Investigators: Use of a monoclonal antibody directed against the platelet glycoprotein IIb/IIIa receptor in high-risk coronary angioplasty. N. Engl. J. Med. *330*:956, 1994.
335. Aguirre, F. V., Topol, E. J., Ferguson, J. J., et al.: Bleeding complications with a chimeric antibody to platelet glycoprotein IIb/IIIa integrin in patients undergoing percutaneous coronary intervention. Circulation *91*:282, 1995.
336. Detre, K., Yeh, W., Kelsey, S., et al.: Has improvement in PTCA inter-

angina and non–Q-wave myocardial infarction: Results of the TIMI-IIIB trial. Circulation *89:*1545, 1994.

653. Schreiber, T. L., Rizik, D., White, C., et al.: Randomized trial of thrombolysis versus heparin in unstable angina. Circulation *86:*1407, 1992.
654. Bar, F. W., Verheugt, F. W., Cohl, J., et al.: Thrombolysis in patients with unstable angina improves the angiographic, but not the clinical outcome: Results of UNASEM, a multicenter, randomized, placebo-controlled clinical trial with anistreplase. Circulation *86:*150, 1992.
655. Freeman, M. R., Langer, A., Wilson, R. F., et al.: Thrombolysis in unstable angina: Randomized double-blind trial of t-PA and placebo. Circulation *85:*150, 1992.
655a. Mehran, R., Ambrose, J. A., Bongu, R. M., et al.: Angioplasty of complex lesions and ischemic rest angina. Results of the thrombolysis and angioplasty in unstable angina (TAUSA) trial. J. Am. Coll. Cardiol. *26:*961, 1995.
656. Romeo, F., Rosano, G. M., Martuscelli, E., et al.: Effectiveness of prolonged low dose recombinant tissue-type plasminogen activator for refractory unstable angina. J. Am. Coll. Cardiol. *25:*1295, 1995.
657. Fuchs, J., Cannon, C. P., and the TIMI VII Investigators: Hirulog in the treatment of unstable angina. Results of the thrombin inhibition in myocardial ischemia (TIMI) VII trial. Circulation *92:*727, 1995.
658. Grambow, D. W., and Topol, E. J.: Effect of maximal medical therapy on refractoriness of unstable angina pectoris. Am. J. Cardiol. *70:*577, 1992.
659. Szatmary, L. J., Marco, J., Fajadet, J., and Caster, L.: The combined use of diastolic counterpulsation and coronary dilation in unstable angina due to multivessel disease under unstable hemodynamic conditions. Int. J. Cardiol. *19:*59, 1988.
660. Makhoul, R. G., Cole, C. W., and McCann, R. L.: Vascular complications of the intra-aortic balloon pump: An analysis of 436 patients. Am. Surg. *59:*564, 1993.
660a. Willerson, J. T.: Management of the patient with unstable angina after the initial therapy. *In* Fuster, V., Ross, R., and Topol, E. J. (eds.): Atherosclerosis and Coronary Artery Disease. Philadelphia, J. B. Lippincott, 1996, pp. 1327–1338.
661. Kennedy, J. W.: Complications associated with cardiac catheterization and angiography. Cathet. Cardiovasc. Diagn. *8:*5, 1982.
662. DeFeyter, P. J., Suryapranata, H., Serruys, P. W., et al.: Effects of successful percutaneous transluminal coronary angioplasty on global and regional left ventricular function in unstable angina pectoris. Am. J. Cardiol. *60:*993, 1987.
663. Kamp, O., Beatt, K. J., deFeyter, P. J., et al.: Short-, medium-, and long-term follow-up after percutaneous transluminal coronary angioplasty for stable and unstable angina pectoris. Am. Heart J. *117:*991, 1989.
664. DeFeyter, P. J., and Serruys, P. W.: Unstable angina. Role of coronary interventions. *In* Fuster, V., Ross, R., and Topol, E. J. (eds.): Atherosclerosis and Coronary Artery Disease. Philadelphia, Lippincott-Raven, 1996, pp. 1351–1358.
665. Grassman, E. D., Leya, F., Johnson, S. A., et al.: Percutaneous transluminal coronary angioplasty for unstable angina: Predictors of outcome in a multicenter study. J. Thrombosis Thrombolysis *1:*73, 1994.
666. Halon, D. A., Merdler, A., Shefer, A., et al.: Identifying patients at high risk for restenosis after percutaneous transluminal coronary angioplasty for unstable angina pectoris. Am. J. Cardiol. *64:*289, 1989.
667. Tenaglia, A. N., and Stack, R. S.: Angioplasty for acute coronary syndromes. Annu. Rev. Med. *44:*465, 1993.
668. Stammen, F., DeScheerder, I., Glazier, J. J., et al.: Immediate and follow-up results of the conservative coronary angioplasty strategy for unstable angina pectoris. Am. J. Cardiol. *69:*1533, 1992.
669. Ruygrok, P., deJaegere, P., Van Domburg, R., et al.: Unstable angina patients fare no worse than stable patients 10 years after balloon angioplasty. J. Am. Coll. Cardiol. *25*(Abs.):249-A, 1995.
670. The EPIC Investigators: Use of a monoclonal antibody directed against the platelet glycoprotein IIb/IIIa receptor in high-risk coronary angioplasty. N. Engl. J. Med. *330:*956, 1994.
671. Morrison, D. A., Sacks, J., Grover, F., et al.: Effectiveness of percutaneous transluminal coronary angioplasty for patients with medically refractory rest angina pectoris and high risk of adverse outcomes with coronary artery bypass grafting. Am. J. Cardiol. *75:*237, 1995.
672. Abdelmeguid, A. E., Ellis, S. G., Sapp, S. K., et al.: Directional coronary atherectomy in unstable angina. J. Am. Coll. Cardiol. *24:*46, 1994.
673. Talley, J. D., Hurst, J. W., King, S. B., III, et al.: Clinical outcome 5 years after attempted percutaneous transluminal coronary angioplasty in 427 patients. Circulation *77:*820, 1988.
674. Gardner, T. J., Stuart, R. S., Greene, P. S., and Baumgartner, W. A.: The risk of coronary bypass surgery for patients with postinfarction angina. Circulation *79*(Suppl., I):I79, 1989.
675. Kaiser, G. C., Schaff, H. V., and Killip, T.: Myocardial revascularization for unstable angina pectoris. Circulation *79*(Suppl. I):I60, 1989.
676. Luchi, R. J., Scott, S. M., and Deupree, R. H.: Comparison of medical and surgical treatment for unstable angina pectoris: Results of a Veterans Administration Cooperative Study. N. Engl. J. Med. *316:*977, 1987.
677. Scott, S. N., Deupree, R. H., Sharma, G. V., et al.: VA study of unstable angina: 10-year results show duration of surgical advantage for patients with impaired ejection fraction. Circulation *90*(Suppl.):II-120, 1994.
678. Booth, D. C., Deupree, R. H., Hultgren, H. N., et al.: Quality of life after bypass surgery for unstable angina: 5-year follow-up results of a Veterans Affairs Cooperative Study. Circulation *83:*87, 1991.
679. Rahimtoola, S. H., Nunley, D., Grunkemeier, G., et al.: Ten-year survival after coronary bypass surgery for unstable angina. N. Engl. J. Med. *308:*676, 1983.
679a. Schoff, H. V.: Unstable angina. Role of bypass surgery. *In* Fuster, V., Ross, R., and Topol, E. J. (eds.): Atherosclerosis and Coronary Artery Disease. Philadelphia, J. B. Lippincott, 1996, pp. 1359–1366.
680. Naunheim, K. S., Fiore, A. C., Arango, D. C., et al.: Coronary artery bypass grafting for unstable angina pectoris: Risk analysis. Ann. Thorac. Surg. *47:*569, 1989.
681. Waters, D. D., Walling, A., Roy, D., and Theroux, P.: Previous coronary artery bypass grafting as an adverse prognostic factor in unstable angina pectoris. Am. J. Cardiol. *58:*465, 1986.
682. Murphy, J. G., and Gersh, B. J.: Pros and cons of revascularization versus a conservative approach. *In* Rutherford, J. D. (ed.): Unstable Angina. New York, Marcel Dekker, 1992, p. 247.

PRINZMETAL'S VARIANT ANGINA

683. Prinzmetal, M., Kennamer, R., Merliss, R., et al.: A variant form of angina pectoris. Am. J. Med. *27:*375, 1959.
684. Cohen, M.: Variant angina pectoris. *In* Fuster, V., Ross, R., and Topol, E. J. (eds.): Atherosclerosis and Coronary Artery Disease. Philadelphia, J. B. Lippincott, 1996, pp. 1367–1376.
684a. Crea, F., Kaski, J. C., Masori, A., et al.: Key references on coronary artery spasm. Circulation *89:*2442, 1994.
685. Nakamura, Y., Yamaguro, T., Inoki, I., et al.: Vasomotor response to ergonovine of epicardial and resistance coronary arteries in the nonspastic vascular bed in patients with vasospastic angina. Am. J. Cardiol. *74:*1006, 1994.
686. Hoshio, A., Kotake, H., and Mashiba, H.: Significance of coronary artery tone in patients with vasospastic angina. J. Am. Coll. Cardiol. *14:*604, 1989.
687. McFadden, E. P., Clarke, J. G., Davies, G. J., et al.: Effect of intracoronary serotonin on coronary vessels in patients with stable angina and patients with variant angina. N. Engl. J. Med. *324:*648, 1991.
688. Takano, H., Nakamura, T., Satou, T., et al.: Regional myocardial sympathetic dysinnervation in patients with coronary vasospasm. Am. J. Cardiol. *75:*324, 1995.
689. Irie, T., Imaizumi, T., Matuguchi, T., et al.: Increased fibrinopeptide A during anginal attacks in patients with variant angina. J. Am. Coll. Cardiol. *14:*589, 1989.
690. Ogawa, H., Yasue, H., Oshima, S., et al.: Circadian variation of plasma fibrinopeptide A level in patients with variant angina. Circulation *80:*1617, 1989.
691. Masuda, T., Ogawa, H., Miyao, Y., et al.: Circadian variation in fibrinolytic activity in patients with variant angina. Br. Heart J. *71:*156, 1994.
692. Nobuyoshi, M., Abe, M., Nosaka, H., et al.: Statistical analysis of clinical risk factors for coronary artery spasm: Identification of the most important determinant. Am. Heart J. *124:*32, 1992.
693. Sugiishi, M., and Takatsu, F.: Cigarette smoking is a major risk factor for coronary spasm. Circulation *87:*76, 1993.
694. Cohen, L., and Kitzes, R.: Prompt termination and/or prevention of cold-pressor-stimulus–induced vasoconstriction of different vascular beds by magnesium sulfate in patients with Prinzmetal's angina. Magnes. Trace Elem. *5:*144, 1986.
695. Miyagi, H., Yasue, H., Okumura, K., et al.: Effect of magnesium on anginal attack induced by hyperventilation in patients with variant angina. Circulation *79:*597, 1989.
696. Kugiyama, K., Yasue, H., Okumura, K., et al.: Suppression of exercise-induced angina by magnesium sulfate in patients with variant angina. J. Am. Coll. Cardiol. *12:*1177, 1988.
697. Lange, R. A., Cigarroa, R. G., and Yancy, C. W., Jr.: Cocaine-induced coronary-artery vasoconstriction. N. Engl. J. Med. *321:*1557, 1989.
698. Nademanee, K., Gorelick, D. A., Josephson, M. A., et al.: Myocardial ischemia during cocaine withdrawal. Ann. Intern. Med. *111:*876, 1989.
699. Fourneir, J. A., Sanchez, A. F., and Cortacero, J.-A. P.: Selective ergonovine induced coronary artery spasm and ST-segment alternans after blunt thoracic trauma. Int. J. Cardiol. *47:*290, 1995.
699a. Shinozaki, K., Suzuki, M., Ikebuchi, I., et al.: Insulin resistance associated with compensatory hyperinsulinemia as an independent risk factor for vasospastic angina. Circulation *92:*1749, 1995.
699b. Onaka, H., Yasue, H., Shimada, S., et al.: Clinical observation of spontaneous anginal attacks and multivessel spasm in variant angina pectoris with normal coronary arteries: Evaluation by 24-hour 12-lead electrocardiography with computer analysis. J. Am. Coll. Cardiol. *27:*38, 1996.
700. Waters, D. D., Theroux, P., Crittin, J., et al.: Previously undiagnosed variant angina as a cause of chest pain after coronary artery bypass surgery. Circulation *61:*1159, 1980.
701. Habbab, M. A., Szwed, S. A., and Haft, I.: Is coronary arterial spasm part of the aspirin-induced asthma syndrome? Chest *90:*141, 1986.
702. Pijls, N. H., and van der Werf, T.: Prinzmetal's angina associated with alcohol withdrawal. Cardiology *75:*226, 1988.
703. Matsuguchi, T., Araki, H., Nakamura, N., et al.: Prevention of vasospastic angina by alcohol ingestion: Report of 2 cases. Angiology *39:*394, 1988.
704. Kleiman, N. S., Lehane, D. E., Geyer, C. E., Jr., et al.: Prinzmetal's angina during 5-fluorouracil chemotherapy. Am. J. Med. *82:*566, 1987.
705. Stefenelli, T., Zielinski, C. C., Mayr, H., and Scoheithauer, W.: Prinzmetal's angina during cyclophosphamide therapy. Eur. Heart J. *9:*1155, 1988.
706. Chockalingam, V., Jagnathan, V., Chandrasekar, P. V., et al.: A case of ST-segment and T-wave alternans. Arch. Intern. Med. *143:*1792, 1983.
707. Salerno, J. A., Previtali, M., Panciroli, C., et al.: Ventricular arrhythmias during acute myocardial ischaemia in man: The role and significance of R-ST-T alternans and the prevention of ischaemic sudden death by medical treatment. Eur. Heart J. *7*(Suppl. A):63, 1986.

708. Bayes de Luna, A., Carreras, F., Cladellias, M., et al.: Holter ECG study of the electrocardiographic phenomena in Prinzmetal angina attacks with emphasis on the study of ventricular arrhythmias. J. Electrocardiol. *18*:267, 1985.
709. Yasue, H., Takizawa, A., Nagao, M., et al.: Long-term prognosis for patients with variant angina and influential factors. Circulation *78*:1, 1988.
710. Ortega-Carnicer, J., Garcia-Nieto, F., Malillos, M., and Sanchez-Fernandez, A.: Transient left posterior hemiblock during Prinzmetal's angina culminating in acute myocardial infarction. Chest *84*:638, 1983.
711. Myerburg, R. J., Kessler, K. M., Mallon, S. M., et al.: Life threatening ventricular arrhythmias in patients with silent myocardial ischemia due to coronary artery spasm. N. Engl. J. Med. *326*:1451, 1992.
712. Meller, J., Conde, C. A., Donoso, E., and Dack, S.: Transient Q waves in Prinzmetal's angina. Am. J. Cardiol. *35*:691, 1975.
713. Gersh, B. J., Bassendine, M., Forman, R., et al.: Coronary artery spasm and myocardial infarction in the absence of angiographically demonstrable coronary artery disease. Mayo Clin. Proc. *56*:700, 1981.
714. Masuda, Y., Ozaki, M., Ogawa, H., et al.: Coronary arteriography and left ventriculography during spontaneous and exercise-induced ST-segment elevation in patients with variant angina. Am. Heart J. *106*:509, 1983.
715. Distante, A., Rovai, D., Picano, E., et al.: Transient changes in left ventricular mechanics during attacks of Prinzmetal's angina: An M-mode echocardiographic study. Am. Heart J. *107*:465, 1984.
716. Yokoyama, M., Akita, H., Hirata, K., et al.: Supersensitivity of isolated coronary artery to ergonovine in a patient with variant angina. Am. J. Med. *89*:507, 1990.
717. Harding, M. B., Leithe, M. E., Mark, D. B., et al.: Ergonovine maleate testing during cardiac catheterization: A 10 year perspective in 3,447 patients without significant coronary artery disease or Prinzmetal's variant angina. (erratum J. Am. Coll. Cardiol. *21*:848, 1993). J. Am. Coll. Cardiol. *20*:107, 1992.
718. Previtali, M., Ardissino, D., Barberis, P., et al.: Hyperventilation and ergonovine tests in Prinzmetal's variant angina pectoris in men. Am. J. Cardiol. *63*:17, 1989.
719. Minoda, K., Yasue, H., Kugiyama, K., et al.: Comparison of the distribution of myocardial blood flow between exercise-induced and hyperventilation-induced attacks of coronary spasm: A study with thallium-201 myocardial scintigraphy. Am. Heart J. *127*:1474, 1994.
720. Okumura, K., Yasue, H., Matsuyama, K., et al.: Sensitivity and specificity of intracoronary injection of acetylcholine for the induction of coronary artery spasm. J. Am. Coll. Cardiol. *12*:883, 1988.
721. Okumura, K., Yasue, H., Matsuyama, K., et al.: Effect of H1 receptor stimulation on coronary artery diameter in patients with variant angina: Comparison with effect of acetylcholine. J. Am. Coll. Cardiol. *17*:338, 1991.
722. Crea, F., Chierchia, S., Kaski, J. C., et al.: Provocation of coronary spasm by dopamine in patients with active variant angina pectoris. Circulation *74*:262, 1986.
723. Maseri, A., Parodi, O., Severi, S., and Pesola, A.: Transient transmural reduction of myocardial blood flow, demonstrated by thallium-201 scintigraphy, as a cause of variant angina. Circulation *54*:280, 1976.
724. Ginsburg, R., Lamb, I. H., Schroeder, J. S., et al.: Randomized-blind comparison of nifedipine and isosorbide dinitrate therapy in variant angina pectoris due to coronary artery spasm. Am. Heart J. *103*:44, 1982.
725. Robertson, R. M., Wood, A. J. J., Vaughn, W. K., et al.: Exacerbation of vasotonic angina pectoris by propranolol. Circulation *6*:281, 1982.
726. Antman, E., Muller, J., Goldberg, S., et al.: Nifedipine therapy for coronary-artery spasm: Experience in 127 patients. N. Engl. J. Med. *302*:1269, 1980.
727. Ginsburg, R., Lamb, I. H., Schroeder, J. S., et al.: Randomized double-blind comparison of nifedipine and isosorbide dinitrate therapy in variant angina pectoris due to coronary artery spasm. Am. Heart J. *103*:44, 1982.
728. Prida, X. E., Gelman, J. S., Feldman, R. L., et al.: Comparison of diltiazem and nifedipine alone and in combination in patients with coronary artery spasm. J. Am. Coll. Cardiol. *9*:412, 1987.
729. Morikami, Y., and Yasue, H.: Efficacy of slow-release nifedipine on myocardial ischemic episodes in variant angina pectoris. Am. J. Cardiol. *68*:580, 1991.
730. Chimienti, M., Negroni, M. S., Pusineri, E., et al.: Once daily felodipine in preventing ergonovine-induced myocardial ischemia in Prinzmetal's variant angina. Eur. Heart J. *15*:389, 1994.
731. Pesola, A., Lauro, A., Gallo, R., et al.: Efficacy of diltiazem in variant angina: Results of a double-blind crossover study in CCU by Holter monitoring: The possible occurrence of a withdrawal syndrome. G. Ital. Cardiol. *17*:329, 1987.
732. Tzivoni, D., Keren, A., Benhorin, J., et al.: Prazosin therapy for refractory variant angina. Am. Heart J. *105*:262, 1983.
733. Miwa, K., Kambara, H., and Kawai, C.: Effect of aspirin in large doses on attacks of variant angina. Am. Heart J. *105*:351, 1983.
734. Corcos, T., David, P. R., Bourassa, M. G., et al.: Percutaneous transluminal coronary angioplasty for the treatment of variant angina. J. Am. Coll. Cardiol. *5*:1046, 1985.
735. Yasue, H., Takizawa, D., Nagao, M., et al.: Long-term prognosis of patients with variant angina and influential factors. Circulation *78*:1, 1988.
736. Shimokawa, H., Nagasaw, A. K., Irie, T., et al.: Clinical characteristics and long-term prognosis of patients with variant angina: A comparative study between Western and Japanese populations. Int. J. Cardiol. *18*:331, 1988.
737. Mark, D. B., Califf, R. M., Morris, K. G., et al.: Clinical characteristics and long-term survival of patients with variant angina. Circulation *69*:880, 1984.
738. Ozaki, Y., Takatsu, F., Osugi, J., et al.: Long term study of recurrent vasospastic angina using coronary angiograms during ergonovine provocation tests. Am. Heart J. *123*:1191, 1992.

CHEST PAIN WITH NORMAL CORONARY ARTERIOGRAM

739. Kemp, H. G., Kronmal, R. A., Vlietstra, R. E., and Frye, R. L.: Seven-year survival of patients with normal and near normal coronary arteriograms: A CASS registry study. J. Am. Coll. Cardiol. *7*:479, 1986.
740. Papanicolaou, M. N., Califf, R. M., Hlatky, M. A., et al.: Prognostic implications of angiographically normal and insignificantly narrowed coronary arteries. Am. J. Cardiol. *58*:1181, 1986.
741. Maseri, A., Crea, F., Kaski, C., and Crake, T.: Mechanisms of angina pectoris in syndrome X. J. Am. Coll. Cardiol. *17*:499, 1991.
742. Camici, P. G., Marraccini, P., Lorenzoni, R., et al.: Coronary hemodynamics and myocardial metabolism in patients with syndrome X: Response to pacing stress. J. Am. Coll. Cardiol. *17*:1461, 1991.
743. Bortone, A. S., Hess, O. M., Eberli, F. R., et al.: Abnormal coronary vasomotion during exercise in patients with normal coronary arteries and reduced coronary flow reserve. Circulation *79*:516, 1989.
744. Shapiro, L. M., Crake, T., and Poole-Wilson, P. A.: Is altered cardiac sensation responsible for chest pain in patients with normal coronary arteries? Clinical observation during cardiac catheterization. Br. Med. J. *296*:170, 1988.
744a. Wiederman, J. G., Schwartz, A., Apfelbaum, M., et al.: Anatomic and physiologic heterogeneity in patients with syndrome X. An intravascular ultrasound study. J. Am. Coll. Cardiol. *25*:131, 1995.
745. Chauhan, A., Mullens, P. A., Petch, M. C., et al.: Is coronary flow reserve in response to papaverine really normal in syndrome X? Circulation *89*:1998, 1994.
745a. Cannon, R. O.: The microcirculation in atherosclerotic coronary artery. *In* Fuster, V., Ross, R., and Topol, E. J. (eds.): Atherosclerosis and Coronary Artery Disease. Philadelphia, Lippincott-Raven, 1996, pp. 773–790.
746. Cannon, R. O., Bonow, R. O., Bacharach, S. L., et al.: Left ventricular dysfunction in patients with angina pectoris, normal epicardial coronary arteries, and abnormal vasodilator reserve. Circulation *71*:218, 1985.
747. Geltman, E. M., Henes, C. G., Senneff, M. J., et al.: Increased myocardial perfusion at rest and diminished perfusion reserve in patients with angina and angiographically normal coronary arteries. J. Am. Coll. Cardiol. *16*:586, 1990.
748. Sax, F. L., Cannon, R. O., Hanson, C., and Epstein, S. E.: Impaired forearm vasodilator reserve in patients with microvascular angina. N. Engl. J. Med. *317*:1366, 1987.
749. Cannon, R. O., III, Peden, D. B., Berkebile, C., et al.: Airway hyperresponsiveness in patients with microvascular angina: Evidence for a diffuse disorder of smooth muscle responsiveness. Circulation *82*:2011, 1990.
750. Cannon, R. O.: Chest pain with normal coronary angiograms. *In* Fuster, V., Ross, R., and Topol, E. J. (eds.): Atherosclerosis and Coronary Artery Disease. Philadelphia, J. B. Lippincott, 1996, pp. 1577–1590.
751. Cannon, R. O., III: The sensitive heart: A syndrome of abnormal cardiac pain perception. JAMA *273*:883, 1995.
752. Vrints, C. J., Bult, H., Hitter, E., et al.: Impaired endothelium-dependent cholinergic coronary vasodilation in patients with angina and normal coronary arteriograms. J. Am. Coll. Cardiol. *19*:21, 1992.
753. Bugiardin, R., Pozzati, A., Ottani, F., et al.: A spectrum of ischemic syndromes involving functional abnormalities of the epicardial and microvascular coronary circulation. J. Am. Coll. Cardiol. *22*:417, 1993.
754. Carter, C., Maddock, R., and Amsterdam, E.: Panic disorder and chest pain in the coronary care unit. Psychosomatica *23*:302, 1992.
755. Cannon, R. O., Quyyumi, A. A., Mincemoyer, R., et al.: Imipramine in patients with chest pain despite normal coronary angiograms. N. Engl. J. Med. *330*:1411, 1994.
756. Lagerqvist, R., Sylven, C., and Waldenstrom, A.: Lower threshold for adenosine-induced chest pain in patients with angina and normal coronary angiograms. Br. Heart J. *68*:282, 1992.
757. DeMeester, T. R., O'Sullivan, G. C., Bermudez, G., et al.: Esophageal function in patients with angina-type chest pain and normal coronary angiograms. Ann. Surg. *196*:488, 1982.
758. Rosen, S. D., Uren, N. G., Kaski, J. C., et al.: Coronary vasodilator reserve, pain perception and sex in patients with syndrome X. Circulation *90*:50, 1994.
758a. Potts, S. G., Bass, C. M., et al.: Psychological morbidity in patients with chest pain and normal or near-normal coronary arteries. A long-term follow-up study. Psychol. Med. *25*:339, 1995.
759. Kaski, J. C., Rosano, G. M., Collins, P., et al.: Cardiac syndrome X: Clinical characteristics and left ventricular function. J. Am. Coll. Cardiol. *25*:807, 1995.
760. Channer, K. S., James, M. A., Papouchado, M., et al.: Anxiety and depression in patients with chest pain referred for exercise testing. Lancet *2*:820, 1985.
761. Kemp, H. G., Kronmal, R. A., Vlietstra, R. E., et al.: Seven-year survival of patients with normal or near normal coronary arteriograms: A CASS registry study. J. Am. Coll. Cardiol. *7*:479, 1986.
762. Ockene, I. S., Shay, M. J., Alpert, J. S., et al.: Unexplained chest pain in patients with normal coronary arteriograms: A follow-up study of functional status. N. Engl. J. Med. *303*:1249, 1980.
763. Pupita, G., Kaski, J. C., Galassi, A. R., et al.: Long-term variability of

angina pectoris and electrocardiographic signs of ischemia in syndrome X. Am. J. Cardiol. *64*:139, 1989.
764. Romeo, J., Rosano, G. M., Martuscelli, E., et al.: Long-term follow-up of patients initially diagnosed with syndrome X. Am. J. Cardiol. *71*:669, 1993.
765. Lanza, G. A., Manzoli, A., Bia, E., et al.: Acute effects of nitrates in exercise testing in patients with syndrome X: Clinical and pathophysiological implications. Circulation *90*:2695, 1994.
766. Gilligan, D. M., Quyyumi, A. A., Cannon, R. O., 3d, et al.: Effects of physiological levels of estrogen on coronary vasomotor function in postmenopausal women. Circulation *89*:2545, 1994.
767. Reis, E., Gloth, S. T., Blumenthal, R. S., et al.: Ethinyl estradiol acutely attenuates abnormal coronary vasomotor responses to acetylcholine in postmenopausal women. Circulation *89*:52, 1994.

SILENT MYOCARDIAL ISCHEMIA

768. Kellermann, J. J., and Braunwald, E. (eds.): Silent Myocardial Ischemia: A Critical Appraisal. Basel, Karger, 1990.
769. Kannel, W. B., and Abbott, R. D.: Incidence and prognosis of unrecognized myocardial infarction. N. Engl. J. Med. *3*:1144, 1984.
769a. Cohn, P. F.: Silent ischemia. *In* Fuster, V., Ross, R., and Topol, E. J. (eds.): Atherosclerosis and Coronary Artery Disease. Philadelphia, J. B. Lippincott, 1996, pp. 1561–1576.
770. Sigurdsson, E., Thorgeirsson, G., Sigvaldason, H., and Sigfussen, N.: Unrecognized myocardial infarction: Epidemiology, clinical characteristics, and the prognostic role of angina pectoris: The Reykjavik study. Ann. Intern. Med. *122*:96, 1995.
771. Mulcahy, D., Keegan, J., Crean, P., et al.: Silent ischemia in chronic stable angina: A study of its frequency and characteristics in 150 patients. Br. Heart J. *60*:417, 1988.
772. Epstein, S. E., Quyyumi, A. A., and Bonow, R. A.: Myocardial ischemia: Silent or symptomatic. N. Engl. J. Med. *318*:1038, 1988.
773. Rocco, M. B., Barry, J., Campbell, S., et al.: Circadian variation of transient myocardial ischemia in patients with coronary artery disease. Circulation *75*:395, 1987.
774. Hirzel, H. O., Leutwyler, R., and Kralyenbuehl, H. P.: Silent myocardial ischemia: Hemodynamic changes during dynamic exercise in patients with proven coronary artery disease despite absence of angina pectoris. J. Am. Coll. Cardiol. *6*:275, 1985.
775. Chierchia, S., Gallino, A., Smith, G., et al.: Role of heart rate in pathophysiology of chronic stable angina. Lancet *2*:1353, 1984.
776. Deanfield, J. E., Ribiero, P., Oakley, K., et al.: Analysis of ST-segment changes in normal subjects: Implications for ambulatory monitoring in angina pectoris. Am. J. Cardiol. *54*:1321, 1984.
777. Deanfield, J., Shea, M., Ribeiro, P., et al.: Transient ST-segment depression as a marker of myocardial ischemia during daily life. Am. J. Cardiol. *54*:1195, 1984.
778. Quyyumi, A. A., Mockus, L., Wright, C., and Fox, K. M.: Morphology of ambulatory ST-segment changes in patients with varying severity of coronary artery disease. Br. Heart J. *53*:186, 1985.
779. Cohn, P. F.: Silent Myocardial Ischemia and Infarction. 3rd ed. New York, Marcel Dekker, Inc., 1993, p. 73.
780. Mulcahy, D., Purcell, H., Patel, D., and Fox, K.: Asymptomatic ischaemia during daily life in stable coronary artery disease: Relevant or redundant? Br. Heart J. *72*:5, 1994.
780a. Quyyumi, A. A., Panza, J. A., Diodati, J. G., et al.: Prognostic implications of myocardial ischemia during daily life in low risk patients with coronary artery disease. J. Am. Coll. Cardiol. *21*:700, 1993.
781. Aronow, W. S., Mercando, A. D., and Epstein, S.: Prevalence of silent myocardial ischemia detected by 24-hour ambulatory electrocardiography, and its association with new coronary events at 40 month follow-up in elderly diabetic and nondiabetic patients with coronary artery disease. Am. J. Cardiol. *69*:555, 1992.
782. Ranjadayalan, K., Umachandran, V., Ambepityia, G., et al.: Prolonged anginal perceptual threshold in diabetes: Effects of exercise capacity and myocardial ischemia. J. Am. Coll. Cardiol. *16*:1120, 1990.
783. Nesto, R. W., Philips, R. T., Kett, K. G., et al.: Angina and exertional myocardial ischemia in diabetic and non-diabetic patients: Assessment by exercise thallium scintigraphy. Ann. Intern. Med. *108*:170, 1988.
784. Naka, M., Haramatsu, K., Aizawa, T., et al.: Silent myocardial ischemia in patients with non–insulin dependent diabetes mellitus as judged by treadmill exercise testing and coronary arteriography. Am. Heart J. *123*:46, 1992.
785. Glazier, J. J., Chierchia, S., Brown, M. J., and Maseri, A.: Importance of generalized defective perception of painful stimuli as a cause of silent myocardial ischemia in chronic stable angina pectoris. Am. J. Cardiol. *58*:667, 1986.
786. Droste, C., and Roskamm, H.: Experimental pain measurement in patients with asymptomatic myocardial ischemia. J. Am. Coll. Cardiol. *1*:940, 1983.
787. Sheps, D. S., Ballenger, M. N., DeGent, G. E., et al.: Psychophysical responses to a speech stressor: Correlation of plasma-beta endorphin levels at rest and after psychological stress with thermally measured pain threshold in patients with coronary artery disease. J. Am. Coll. Cardiol. *25*:1499, 1995.
788. Hikita, H., Kurita, A., Takase, B., et al.: Usefulness of plasma beta-endorphin levels, pain threshold and autonomic function in assessing silent myocardial ischemia in patients with and without diabetes mellitus. Am. J. Cardiol. *72*:140, 1993.
789. Marwick, T. H.: Is silent ischemia painless because it is mild? J. Am. Coll. Cardiol. *25*:1513, 1995.
790. Nihoyannapoulos, P., Marsonis, A., Joshi, J., et al.: Magnitude of myocardial dysfunction is greater in painful than in painless myocardial ischemia: An exercise echocardiographic study. J. Am. Coll. Cardiol. *25*:1507, 1995.
790a. Klein, J., Chaors, Y., Burman, D. S., et al.: Is "silent" myocardial ischemia really as severe as symptomatic ischemia? The analytical effect of patient selection biases. Circulation *89*:1958, 1994.
791. Petretta, M., Bonaduce, D., Bianchi, V., et al.: Characteristics and prognostic significance of silent myocardial ischemia or predischarge electrocardiographic monitoring in unselected patients with myocardial infarction. Am. J. Cardiol. *69*:579, 1992.
792. Ekelund, L. G., Suchindran, C. M., McMahon, R. P., et al.: Coronary heart disease morbidity and mortality in hypercholesterolemic men predicted from an exercise test: The Lipid Research Clinics Coronary Primary Prevention Trial. J. Am. Coll. Cardiol. *14*:556, 1989.
793. Deedwania, P. C.: Comparison of the prognostic values of ischemia during daily life and ischemia induced by treadmill exercise testing. Am. J. Cardiol. *74*:15B, 1994.
794. Stern, S., Cohn, P. F., and Pepine, C. J.: Silent myocardial ischemia. Curr. Probl. Cardiol. *18*:301, 1993.
795. TIBET Study Group, Total Ischemia Burden European Trial (TIBET): Effective treatment on exercise and Holter ECG and angina. Circulation *86*(Suppl. I):I-713, 1992.
796. Portegies, M. C. M., Sijbring, P., Gobel, E. J. A. N., et al.: Efficacy of metoprolol and diltiazem in treating silent myocardial ischemia. Am. J. Cardiol. *74*:1095, 1994.
797. Knatterud, G. L., Bourassa, B. M. J., Papine, C. J., et al.: Effective treatment strategies to suppress ischemia in patients with coronary artery disease: Twelve-week results of the Asymptomatic Cardiac Ischemia Pilot (ACIP) study. J. Am. Coll. Cardiol. *24*:11, 1994.
797a. Chaitman, B. R., Stone, P. H., Knatterud, G. L., et al.: Asymptomatic Cardiac Ischemia Pilot (ACIP) study: Impact of anti-ischemia therapy and 12-week rest electrocardiogram and exercise test outcomes. J. Am. Coll. Cardiol. *26*:585, 1995.
797b. Roberts, W. J., Bourassa, M. G., Andrews, T. C., et al.: Asymptomatic Cardiac Ischemia Pilot (ACIP) study. Outcome at 1-year for patients with asymptomatic cardiac ischemia randomized to medical therapy or revascularization. J. Am. Coll. Cardiol. *26*:594, 1995.
797c. Bourassa, M. G., Pepine, C. J., Foreman, S. A., et al.: Asymptomatic Cardiac Ischemia Pilot (ACIP) study. Effects of coronary angioplasty and coronary artery bypass graft surgery on recurrent angina and ischemia. J. Am. Coll. Cardiol. *26*:606, 1995.

HEART FAILURE

798. Burch, G. E., Giles, T. D., and Colcolough, H. L.: Ischemic cardiomyopathy. Am. Heart J. *79*:291, 1970.
799. Kron, I. L., Flanagan, T. L., Blackbourne, L. H., et al.: Coronary revascularization rather than cardiac transplantation for chronic ischemic cardiomyopathy. Ann. Surg. *210*:348, 1989.
800. Grieco, J. G., Montoya, A., Sullivan, H. J., et al.: Ventricular aneurysm due to blunt chest injury. Ann. Thorac. Surg. *47*:322, 1989.
801. Hirai, T., Fujita, M., Nakajima, H., et al.: Importance of collateral circulation for prevention of left ventricular aneurysm formation in acute myocardial infarction. Circulation *79*:791, 1989.
802. Barratt-Boyes, B. G., White, H. D., Agnew, T. M., et al.: The results of surgical treatment of left ventricular aneurysms: An assessment of the risk factors affecting early and late mortality. J. Thorac. Cardiovasc. Surg. *87*:87, 1984.
803. Stephenson, L. W., Hargrove, W. C., Ratcliffe, M. B., et al.: Surgery for left ventricular aneurysm: Early survival with and without endocardial resection. Circulation *79*(Suppl. X):1, 1989.
804. Sutherland, G. R., Smyllie, J. H., and Roelandt, J. R.: Advantages of colour flow imaging in the diagnosis of left ventricular pseudoaneurysm. Br. Heart J. *61*:59, 1989.
805. Marcus, M. L., Stanford, W., Hajduczok, Z. D., and Weiss, R. M.: Ultrafast computed tomography in the diagnosis of cardiac diseases. Am. J. Cardiol. *64*:54E, 1989.
806. Couper, G. S., Bunton, R. W., Birjiniuk, V., et al.: Relative risks of left ventricular aneurysmectomy in patients with akinetic scars versus true dyskinetic aneurysms. Circulation *82*(Suppl. IV):248, 1990.
807. Cosgrove, D. M., Lytle, B. W., Taylor, P. C., et al.: Ventricular aneurysm resection. Circulation *79*(Suppl. I):97, 1989.
808. Mangschau, A., Forfang, K., Rootwelt, K., and Frysaker, T.: Improvement in cardiac performance and exercise tolerance after left ventricular aneurysm surgery: A prospective study. Thorac. Cardiovasc. Surg. *36*:320, 1988.
809. Louagie, Y., Alouini, T., Lesperance, J., and Pelletier, L. C.: Left ventricular aneurysm complicated by congestive heart failure: An analysis of long-term results and risk factors of surgical treatment. J. Cardiovasc. Surg. *30*:648, 1989.
810. Barratt-Boyes, B. G., White, H. D., Agnew, T. M., et al.: Results of surgical treatment of left ventricular aneurysm: An assessment of the risk factors affecting early and late mortality. J. Thorac. Cardiovasc. Surg. *87*:87, 1984.
811. Ivert, T., Almdahl, S. M., Lunde, P., and Lindblom, D.: Post infarction left ventricular pseudoaneurysm—echocardiographic diagnosis and surgical repair. Cardiovasc. Surg. *2*:463, 1994.

812. Olearchyk, A. S., Lemole, G. M., and Spagna, P. M.: Left ventricular aneurysm: Ten years' experience in surgical treatment of 244 cases: Improved clinical status, hemodynamics and long-term longevity. J. Thorac. Cardiovasc. Surg. *88*:544, 1984.
813. Prates, P. R., Vitola, D., Sant'anna, J. R., et al.: Surgical repair of ventricular aneurysms: Early results with Cooley's technique. Texas Heart Inst. J. *20*:19, 1993.
814. Dor, V., Montiglio, F., Sabatier, M., et al.: Left ventricular shape changes induced by aneurysmectomy with endoventricular circular patch plasty reconstruction. Eur. Heart J. *15*:1063, 1994.
815. Komeda, M., David, T. E., Malik, A., et al.: Operative risks and long-term results of operation for left ventricular aneurysm. Ann. Thorac. Surg. *53*:22, 1992.
816. Rankin, J. S., Hickey, M. S., Smith, L. R., et al.: Ischemic mitral regurgitation. Circulation *79*(Suppl. I):I-116, 1989.
817. Replogle, R. L., and Campbell, C. D.: Surgery for mitral regurgitation associated with ischemic heart disease. Circulation *79*(Suppl. I):122, 1989.
818. Drexler, H., and Schroeder, J. S.: Unusual forms of ischemic heart disease. Curr. Opin. Cardiol. *9*:457, 1994.
818a. Harrison, D. C.: Nonatherosclerotic coronary disease. *In* Fuster, V., Ross, R., and Topol, E. J. (eds.): Atherosclerosis and Coronary Artery Disease. Philadelphia, Lippincott-Raven, 1996, pp. 757–772.
819. Kragel, A. H., and Roberts, W. C.: Anomalous origin of either the right or left main coronary artery from the aorta with subsequent coursing between aorta and pulmonary trunk· Analysis of 32 necroscopy cases. Am. J. Cardiol. *62*:771, 1988.
820. Corrado, D., Thiene, E. G., Cocco, P., and Frescura, C.: Non-atherosclerotic coronary artery disease and sudden death in the young. Br. Heart J. *68*:601, 1992.
821. DeMaio, S. J., Jr., Kinsella, S. H., and Silverman, M. E.: Clinical course and long-term prognosis of spontaneous coronary artery dissection. Am. J. Cardiol. *64*:471, 1989.
822. Schrader, M. L., Hochman, J. S., and Bulkley, B. A.: The heart and polyarteritis nodosa: A clinicopathologic study. Am. Heart J. *109*:1353, 1985.
823. Saito, S., Arai, H., Kim, K., and Aoki, N.: Acute myocardial infarction in a young adult due to solitary giant cell arteritis of the coronary artery diagnosed antemortemly by primary directional coronary atherectomy. Cathet. Cardiovasc. Diagn. *33*:245, 1994.
824. LeRoy, E. C.: The heart in systemic sclerosis. N. Engl. J. Med. *310*:188, 1984.
825. Morris, P. B., Imber, M. J., Heinsimer, J. A., et al.: Rheumatoid arthritis and coronary arteritis. Am. J. Cardiol. *57*:689, 1986.
826. Bidani, A. K., Roberts, J. L., Schwartz, M. N., and Lewis, E. J.: Immunopathology of cardiac lesions in fatal sytemic lupus erythematosus. Am. J. Med. *69*:849, 1980.
827. Korbet, S. M., Schwartz, M. M., and Lewis, E. J.: Immune complex deposition and coronary vasculitis in systemic lupus erythematosus: Report of two cases. Am. J. Med. *77*:141, 1984.
828. Leung, W. H., Wong, K. L., Lau, C. P., et al.: Association between antiphospholipid antibodies and cardiac abnormalities in patients with systemic lupus erythematosus. Am. J. Med. *89*:411, 1990.
829. Subramanyan, R., Joy, J., and Balakrishnan, K. G.: Natural history of aortoarteritis (Takayasu's disease). Circulation *80*:429, 1989.
830. Kihara, M., Kimura, K., Yakuwa, H., et al.: Isolated left coronary ostial stenosis as the sole arterial involvement in Takayasu's disease. J. Intern. Med. *232*:353, 1992.
831. Case records of the Massachusetts General Hospital Case 4-1995: A 26-year-old woman with recurrent angina after a triple-coronary-artery bypass graft. N. Engl. J. Med. *332*:380, 1995.
832. Scholz, K. H., Herrmann, C., Tebbe, U., et al.: Myocardial infarction in young patients with Hodgkin's disease: Potential pathogenic role of radiotherapy, chemotherapy and splenectomy. Clin. Invest. *71*:57, 1993.
833. Wan, S. K., and Babb, J. D.: Radiation-induced stenosis of the left main coronary artery. Cathet. Cardiovasc. Diagn. *28*:225, 1993.
834. Lange, R. L., Reid, M. S., Tresch, D. D., et al.: Nonatheromatous ischemic heart disease following withdrawal from chronic industrial nitroglycerin exposure. Circulation *46*:666, 1972.
834a. Hollander, J. E.: The management of cocaine-associated myocardial ischemia. N. Engl. J. Med. *333*:1267, 1995.
835. Paavonen, T., Mennander, A., Lautenschlager, I., et al.: Endothelialitis and accelerated arteriosclerosis in human heart transplant coronaries. J. Heart Lung Transpl. *12*:117, 1993.
836. Schuler, S., Matschke, K., Loebe, M., et al.: Coronary artery disease in patients with hearts from older donors: Morphologic features and therapeutic implications. J. Heart Lung Transpl. *12*:100, 1993.

Chapter 39
Interventional Catheterization Techniques

A. MICHAEL LINCOFF, ERIC J. TOPOL

HISTORY 1366
PERCUTANEOUS TRANSLUMINAL CORONARY ANGIOPLASTY 1366
Procedural Outcome and Complications ... 1368
Long-Term Outcome 1371
NEW DEVICES FOR PERCUTANEOUS CORONARY REVASCULARIZATION 1376
Coronary Atherectomy 1376
Intracoronary Stents 1378
Lasers and Other Ablative Energy 1382
INTRAVASCULAR IMAGING TECHNIQUES .. 1383
NONCORONARY ARTERIAL REVASCULARIZATION 1384
PERCUTANEOUS BALLOON VALVULOPLASTY 1385
INTERVENTIONS FOR CONGENITAL HEART DISEASE 1386
QUALITY OF CARE AND CREDENTIALING .. 1386
FUTURE DIRECTIONS 1387
REFERENCES 1387

HISTORY

Interventional cardiology, the application of catheter-based techniques to the treatment of coronary artery, valvular, or congenital cardiac diseases, arose as the culmination of the use of catheters as instruments for the *diagnosis* of heart disease. Cournand and Ranges[1] and others first reported the potential utility of the right-heart catheter in 1941, ushering in a period during which cardiac catheterization was used to evaluate congenital and rheumatic defects and leading ultimately to the development in the late 1950's and 1960's of selective coronary arteriography by Sones and Judkins. The earliest percutaneous *treatment* of a cardiovascular disorder was the Rashkind balloon septostomy to create interatrial defects in patients with transposition of the great vessels.[2]

Dotter and Judkins introduced the therapeutic application of percutaneous "angioplasty" of atherosclerotic peripheral vascular stenoses in 1964,[3] although their cumbersome system of multiple coaxial catheters failed to gain widespread acceptance because of the frequent occurrence of traumatic, hemorrhagic, or embolic vascular complications. The modern era of cardiovascular intervention began as an outgrowth of these ideas, however, with the development by Andreas Gruentzig of a double-lumen balloon catheter, with which dilatation of arterial lesions in the iliac and femoral vessels could be safely achieved with a high rate of procedural success. Miniaturization of this balloon catheter system led to the first percutaneous transluminal coronary angioplasty (PTCA) procedure performed by Gruentzig in September, 1977 in Zurich, where a high-grade narrowing in the proximal left anterior descending coronary artery of a 37-year-old man was successfully dilated,[4] leading to sustained resolution of the stenosis at 1-month angiographic follow-up.

Since the initial application of balloon angioplasty to the treatment of coronary artery disease in humans in 1977, there has been explosive growth in the field of interventional cardiology. While percutaneous revascularization was initially restricted to relatively young patients with stable angina, normal left ventricular function, and proximal, discrete, subtotal, noncalcified concentric stenoses of a single coronary artery, current indications for this procedure have expanded to include unstable angina and acute myocardial infarction, elderly patients and those with depressed left ventricular function, multivessel coronary artery disease, and stenoses with complex morphology or in coronary artery bypass grafts.

A variety of "new devices" for coronary intervention have been developed which allow atherosclerotic plaque to be excised, pulverized, aspirated, ablated by laser or other energy, or supported by metal prosthetic scaffolds, each of which has been advocated to overcome some of the limitations of balloon angioplasty in treating lesions with high-risk characteristics or in reversing the complications of balloon dilatation. The role of adjunctive pharmacological therapy in preventing ischemic complications has been established, with ongoing evaluation of several promising new agents. Novel imaging techniques, including intravascular ultrasonography, fiberoptic angioscopy, and Doppler flow assessment, provide information regarding plaque morphology and physiological function which is complementary to data derived from conventional contrast angiography, facilitating the selection of optimal means of revascularization and assessment of outcome.

Several randomized trials are under way or have been completed to evaluate the efficacy of percutaneous revascularization relative to that of coronary artery bypass surgery in the management of advanced coronary artery disease. Finally, there has been parallel development of new methods for nonsurgical treatment of peripheral vascular and cardiac valve stenoses, as well as transcatheter therapies of congenital cardiac defects.

PERCUTANEOUS TRANSLUMINAL CORONARY ANGIOPLASTY

Since the introduction of coronary balloon angioplasty into clinical practice in 1977,[5] improvements in equipment design and operator experience have permitted this procedure to be applied to the treatment of a broad spectrum of coronary artery disease. More than 400,000 percutaneous revascularization procedures are carried out each year by balloon angioplasty or related "new device" technologies in the United States,[6,7] now exceeding the number of coronary artery bypass surgeries.

ANGIOPLASTY EQUIPMENT. Equipment used during the earliest period of balloon angioplasty was comparatively primitive. Guide catheters were composed of solid Teflon, a material that did not allow adequate retention of shape or torque control. Balloon catheters were bulky and difficult to pass across tight coronary stenoses, with initial designs using no guidewire. Balloon angioplasty was thus confined primarily to proximal lesions in nontortuous vessels.

Wall construction of contemporary guide catheters has evolved into a composite of different layers, conferring improved stability, shape retention, and torque control to catheters with less traumatic distal tips, smaller external diameters, and larger inner lumen dimensions. A variety of preformed shapes are now available, thus optimizing coaxial coronary ostial engagement and support for passage of dilatation catheters. "Over-the-wire" balloon catheter systems have been developed, wherein a freely movable guidewire is passed through the entire length of the central lumen of the angioplasty catheter (Fig. 39–1); such steerable guidewires, with diameters of only 0.009 to 0.018 inch and specialized tips of varying degrees of stiffness, can be precisely shaped, allowing even distal coronary lesions beyond tortuosity to be routinely accessed. Perhaps most remarkable has been the evolution of the balloon angioplasty catheter, with current deflated profiles as small as 1 mm and shaft constructions that optimize trackability and transmission of "push" force. Different polymers are used as balloon materials, permitting accurate sizing, conformability to angulated lesions, and dilatation of rigid lesions with pressures as high as 18 to 20 atmospheres. Specialized catheter designs now include those with the capability of providing distal coronary perfusion during balloon inflation or after abrupt vessel closure (Fig. 39–2) and those with balloons as long as 80 mm intended for diffuse coronary lesions.

Finally, there have been substantial improvements in the quality of radiographic imaging in the cardiac catheterization laboratory. The development of high-resolution fluoroscopy, digital image reconstruction, and on-line com-

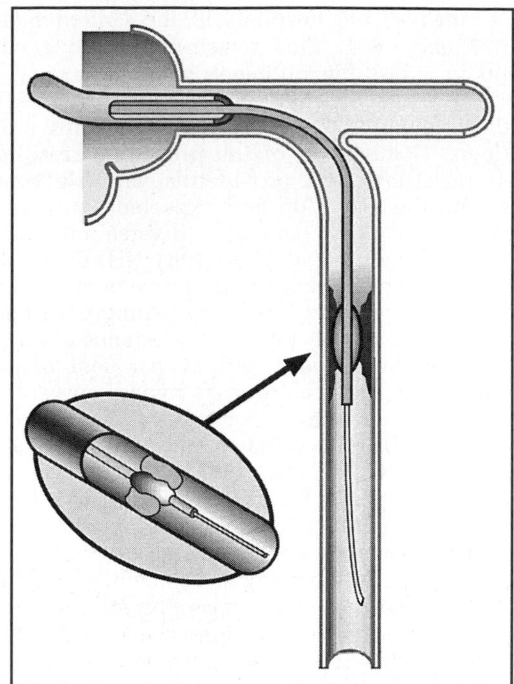

FIGURE 39–1. Diagram of balloon angioplasty catheter with movable guidewire.

puterized quantitative analysis has permitted clear visualization of small-diameter guidewires and catheters within the vasculature, the use of high-definition frozen frames as coronary "road maps," accurate assessment of luminal dimensions before and after revascularization, and improved detection of adverse outcomes such as vascular wall dissection or thrombus formation.

TECHNIQUE. Patients receive antiplatelet therapy with aspirin, 80 to 325 mg daily, ideally beginning at least 1 day prior to the coronary angioplasty procedure. Following local anesthesia, vascular access is achieved by percutaneous femoral puncture or, less frequently, brachial puncture or cutdown. At some institutions or in some high-risk patients, a catheter is placed in the pulmonary artery for monitoring of right heart pressures. The coronary vessel is intubated with a No. 7 to 9 French (2.3 to 3.0 mm diameter) guide catheter, and arteriography performed in orthogonal radiographic projections demonstrating unforeshortened views of the target stenosis. Stable coaxial orientation of the guide catheter within the coronary ostium without damping of the pressure waveform must be assured. Systemic heparinization is universally employed, as an initial bolus followed by a continuous infusion or additional periodic boluses, with most laboratories monitoring the adequacy of anticoagulation during the procedure by measurement of activated clotting times (target ≥300 seconds). A steerable coronary guidewire, the tip of which has been shaped into a curve appropriate for the specific coronary anatomy, is advanced through the guide catheter into the coronary vessel and manipulated under fluoroscopic guidance across the stenosis by rotation of its distal tip using a manual torquing handle.

A balloon angioplasty catheter of suitable inflated diameter (usually ≤110 per cent of the estimated "normal" vessel diameter) is advanced across the guidewire to the stenosis and inflated over a period of seconds or minutes to a pressure at which the balloon appears fully expanded under fluoroscopy (typically at 4 to 8 atmospheres). The duration of balloon inflation may vary from 15 seconds to 2 to 3 minutes or more at the operator's discretion. Some evidence indicates that acute angiographic outcome may be improved by prolongation of balloon inflation time,[8] although the duration of inflation is usually limited primarily by the development of ischemic signs or symptoms due to interruption of distal coronary blood flow. Inadequate improvement in the degree of stenosis may be treated by repeat balloon inflations, exchange over the guidewire for a balloon catheter of larger inflated diameter, or exchange for another percutaneous revascularization device.

After the angioplasty procedure, patients are observed at least overnight in an inpatient cardiology unit for the infrequent development of recurrent myocardial ischemia or hemorrhagic complications; postprocedural ischemia, particularly if prolonged and associated with electrocardiographic changes, usually necessitates urgent repeat angiography and revascularization. If a suboptimal angiographic result is obtained during the angioplasty procedure, particularly if coronary dissection or thrombus is present, heparin anticoagulation is usually continued by infusion for at least several hours. Patients are maintained indefinitely on daily aspirin therapy. Routine long-term follow-up is not uniform but often includes risk factor modification and surveillance for recurrent ischemia by stress testing 3 to 6 months following revascularization.

PATHOPHYSIOLOGY. The mechanisms by which coronary balloon angioplasty may improve vessel luminal dimensions have been characterized by studies in animal models, cadaveric human arterial models, and specimens obtained from patients who died following successful or complicated coronary angioplasty; the recent development of intravascular ultrasound imaging has provided a powerful means of studying the in vivo arterial response during and following percutaneous revascularization[9] (Figs. 3–15, p. 58, and 39–7, p. 1377). The radial force exerted by balloon dilatation within a coronary artery universally produces endothelial denudation with variable degrees of fracture and separation of plaque from the underlying media, stretching of the medial and adventitial layers, and fracture or dissection of the media. Based on these findings, Waller[10] has postulated five different mechanisms for the hemodynamic benefit derived from balloon angio-

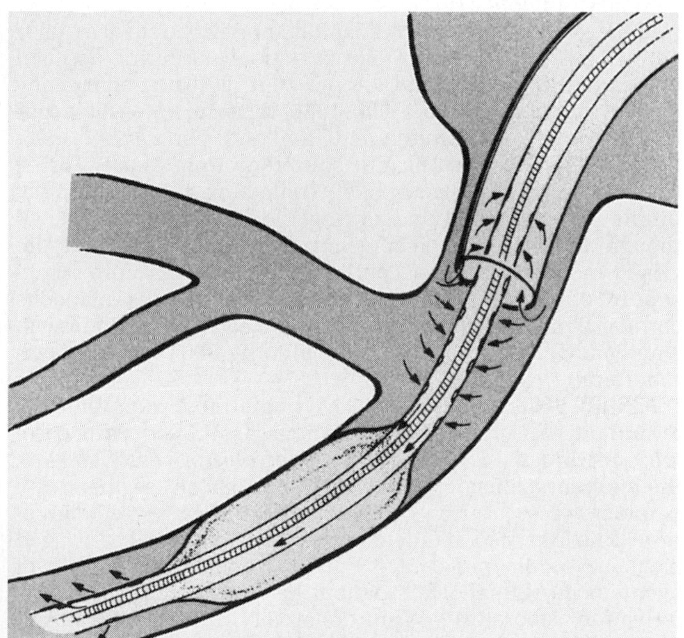

FIGURE 39–2. Schematic diagram of an autoperfusion balloon catheter. Distal coronary perfusion can be maintained during balloon angioplasty using this catheter design (Advanced Cardiovascular Systems, Inc., Mountain View, CA). Once an autoperfusion catheter is inflated across the stenosis, blood enters sideholes proximal to the balloon, flows passively through the central lumen, and exits the catheter via sideholes distal to the coronary occlusion. Flow rates are proportional to proximal arterial perfusion pressure. (From Folland, E. D.: Balloon angioplasty. *In* Topol, E. J., and Serruys, P. [eds.]: Current Review of Interventional Cardiology. Philadelphia, Current Medicine, 1994, p. 1.8.)

plasty (Fig. 39–3); for any particular lesion, one or more of these mechanisms may be operative. *Plaque compression* appears to play only a minor role in the improvement of the dense fibrocalcific stenoses typically present in advanced coronary artery disease. A major mechanism of balloon angioplasty appears to be *plaque fracture,* with immediate formation of fissures within the atherosclerotic lesion which provide channels for blood flow; the ultimate luminal geometry and extent of enlargement are influenced by subsequent plaque healing and remodeling. An important degree of additional expansion in cross-sectional area is obtained when more extensive arterial injury results in localized *medial dissection* accompanying plaque fracture. *Stretching* with minimal compression of concentric dense fibrocollagenous plaques may also occur, providing an immediate improvement of luminal diameter, which may be partially or completely attenuated, however, by elastic recoil. Similarly, vessels in which an eccentric plaque is dilated may be enlarged simply as a result of *stretching of plaque-free arterial segments* with little or no fracture or compression of plaque, with a propensity for early loss of luminal dimensions due to gradual relaxation of the overstretched segment.

Procedural Outcome and Complications

Gruentzig et al. reported the short-term results among the first 50 patients to undergo balloon angioplasty in 1979.[5] Procedural success was achieved in only 32 of these 50 patients (64 per cent), with the majority of failures due to inability to reach or cross the coronary stenoses using the equipment available at the time.

The National Heart, Lung, and Blood Institute (NHLBI) established a voluntary registry of 3248 consecutive PTCA cases performed at 105 hospitals in the United States between 1977 and 1981. This registry was reopened from 1985–1986 to assess the influence of technological developments and greater operator experience, with 15 of the sites in the original 1977–1981 registry enrolling a total of 2094 patients. Comparison of the procedural results from these two registries[11] has provided a valuable source of data regarding the evolution and expected short-term outcomes of this technique among a diverse population of patients. During the original 1977–1981 NHLBI registry experience, angiographic success (improvement in luminal stenosis by ≥20 per cent), as in Gruentzig's first cohort, was achieved in only 67 per cent of stenoses for which angioplasty was attempted,[11] and 21 per cent of patients required urgent or elective coronary bypass surgery during the hospitalization period; 22 per cent of lesions could not be passed by the balloon catheter and an additional 7 per cent could not be dilated. By 1985–1986, however, despite an increased proportion of patients with advanced age, impaired left ventricular function, unstable angina, multivessel coronary disease, total occlusions, and complex stenosis morphology, angiographic success was achieved in 88 per cent of lesions,[11] with elective bypass surgery performed in only 2.2 per cent. More recent reports of data derived during 1989 and 1990–1991 have corroborated the NHLBI findings, with procedural failure rates of only 3.7 per cent and 7.7 per cent, respectively.[12,13]

The majority of patients treated with coronary angioplasty experience substantial immediate relief of symptoms of myocardial ischemia. The procedure has been estimated to be effective in decreasing or eliminating angina in 88 per cent and 76 per cent of patients,[14] respectively, with improvement or resolution of ischemic signs on exercise stress testing following successful balloon dilatation.[15] The extent of improvement in symptom status is better among patients with single-vessel coronary artery disease than among those with multivessel involvement.[16,17]

Major ischemic complications occur infrequently during coronary angioplasty. Even during the early 1977–1981 NHLBI experience, the in-hospital mortality rate was only 1.2 per cent, with 4.9 per cent of patients suffering nonfatal myocardial infarction and 5.8 per cent requiring emergency bypass surgery. In the 1985–1986 registry, rates of death and myocardial infarction (1.0 and 4.3 per cent, respectively) were not significantly different from those during the earlier study period, likely reflecting the greater risk profile of patients treated during the later time period, although the need for emergency bypass surgery had declined modestly (3.4 per cent). Among an even more recent cohort of patients undergoing multivessel percutaneous coronary intervention at five experienced clinical sites, an emergency bypass surgery rate of only 0.9 per cent was reported.[18]

ABRUPT VESSEL CLOSURE. The single most important determinant of ischemic complications associated with coronary angioplasty is the occurrence of *abrupt vessel closure,* the sudden occlusion of the target or adjacent segment of a coronary vessel during or after percutaneous revascularization. The reported incidence of abrupt closure has ranged from 4.2 to 8.3 per cent,[19–22] with roughly one-quarter of events occurring after the patient has left the cardiac catheterization laboratory. While relatively infrequent, abrupt vessel closure has important clinical sequelae (Table 39–1).

The pathophysiological mechanisms of abrupt coronary occlusion are similar to those that produce the therapeutic benefit derived from balloon dilatation. Although plaque and medial fissuring induced by balloon angioplasty usually remains localized, extensive disruption of the medial layer can occur, leading to obstructive dissection flaps or intramural hematoma (Fig. 39–4). Exposure of subendothelial vascular wall components results in platelet deposition and activation with formation of thrombin; occlusive thrombosis may occur, often in association with blood

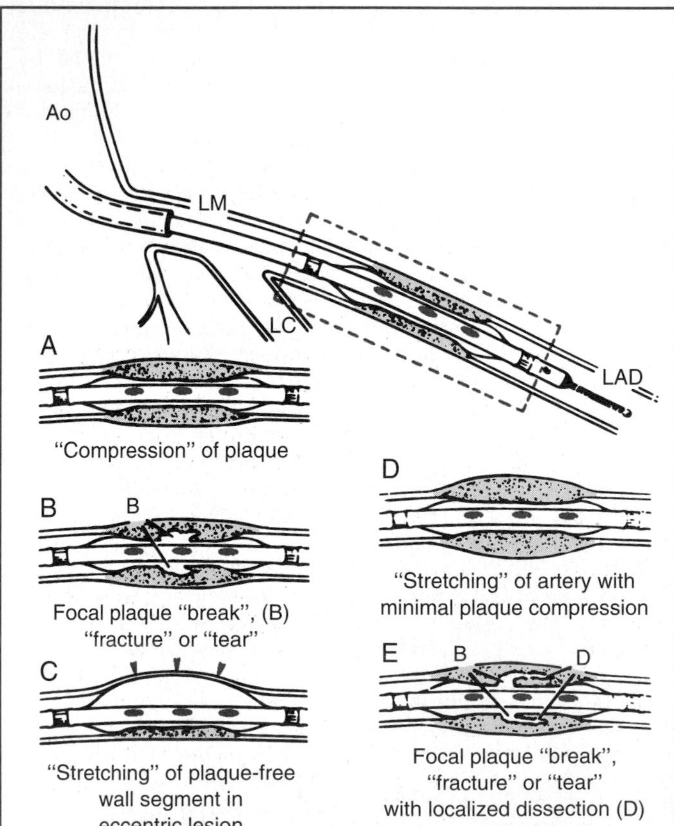

FIGURE 39–3. Diagram of five possible mechanisms of coronary balloon angioplasty. Ao = aorta; LAD = left anterior descending artery; LC = left circumflex artery; LM = left main artery. (From Waller, B. F.: Coronary luminal shape and the arc of disease free wall: Morphologic observations and clinical relevance. J. Am. Coll. Cardiol. *6*:1100, 1985.)

TABLE 39–1 REPORTED CLINICAL SEQUELAE OF ABRUPT VESSEL CLOSURE

SERIES	YEARS	DEATH (%)	MI (%)	CABG (%)
NHLBI Registry I	1979–81	4.9	4.1	7.2
Beth Israel Hospital	1981–86	2.0	3.5	3.3
Emory University	1982–86	2.0	5.4	5.5
Cleveland Clinic	1983–85	0	4.3	4.1
NHLBI Registry II	1985–86	4.9	4.0	4.0
Thoraxcenter	1986–88	6.0	3.6	3.0
University of Michigan	1988–90	8.0	2.0	2.0
Beth Israel Hospital	1989–91	2.5	3.1	2.3

CABG = coronary artery bypass graft surgery; MI = myocardial infarction; NHLBI = National Heart, Lung, and Blood Institute.

From Lincoff, A. M., and Topol, E. J.: Abrupt vessel closure. *In* Topol, E. J. (ed.): Textbook of Interventional Cardiology. 2nd ed. Philadelphia, W. B. Saunders Company, 1994, p. 207.

stasis produced by medial dissection flaps. In some patients, particularly those with unstable ischemic syndromes, propagation of pre-existent mural thrombus present at the treatment site may be the predominant mechanism of coronary obstruction.

A number of preventive measures may limit the occurrence of abrupt vessel closure during coronary angioplasty. Pharmacological approaches have focused on suppression of both platelet aggregation and thrombus formation at the site of balloon dilatation or on preprocedural resolution of pre-existent mural thrombus. Aspirin, an irreversible inactivator of thromboxane A_2 synthesis and inhibitor of platelet activation, has been demonstrated to reduce the incidence of periprocedural myocardial infarction or occlusive coronary thrombosis.[23]

Although no controlled trials have assessed the efficacy of heparin in the prevention of abrupt closure, observational data suggest that this agent may be useful prior to, during, or after the angioplasty procedure. Among patients with unstable angina or angiographically visible intracoronary thrombus, treatment with aspirin and continuous heparin infusion for 3 to 7 days before percutaneous revascularization has been associated with improved procedural success, diminished risk of periprocedural vessel occlusion, and angiographic regression of thrombus.[24,25] Although the necessary or target dose for heparin therapy during coronary intervention has never been definitively evaluated, the probability of abrupt vessel closure or ischemic complications appears to be inversely related to the level of anticoagulation[26]; administration of sufficient heparin to achieve an activated coagulation time of 300 to 350 seconds or more prior to initiating coronary angioplasty is thus routinely recommended.[27,28] Finally, although randomized trials have failed to demonstrate a benefit derived from therapy with heparin after uncomplicated angioplasty,[29,30] the temporal relationship noted between discontinuation or inadequate doses of postprocedural heparin suggests that this agent may be useful in preventing closure in selected patients with suboptimal angiographic results following balloon angioplasty.[31]

In contrast to heparin and aspirin, however, adjunctive therapy with thrombolytic agents before balloon angioplasty has *not* been shown to confer clinical benefit, may in fact be detrimental among patients with unstable angina, and is clearly associated with an increased risk of hemorrhagic complications.[32,33] Procedural mechanical factors that may reduce the risk of abrupt closure include selection of appropriately sized balloons to avoid excessive overdilation relative to the normal coronary diameter,[34,35] the use of long (30 to 40 mm) balloons for angulated or diffuse lesions, and gradual and prolonged inflations.[8,36]

A recent large-scale clinical trial, the EPIC trial, demonstrated the efficacy of c7E3Fab (Abciximab, Centocor, Inc., Malvern, PA), a novel monoclonal antibody fragment directed against the platelet membrane glycoprotein IIb/IIIa receptor which binds circulating fibrinogen and cross-links adjacent platelets as the final common pathway to platelet aggregation.[37] Administration of c7E3Fab for 12 hours during and following high-risk coronary angioplasty or atherectomy, in addition to conventional therapy with heparin and aspirin, reduced the incidence of death, myocardial infarction, or urgent repeat revascularization by 35 per cent over the subsequent 30 days[38] (Table 39–2, see also p. 1820).

If abrupt closure occurs, initial management typically consists of repeat prolonged balloon dilatation to induce adhesion of obstructive dissection flaps to the arterial wall or compression of intraluminal thrombus.[22] A number of "new device" technologies, most prominently intracoronary

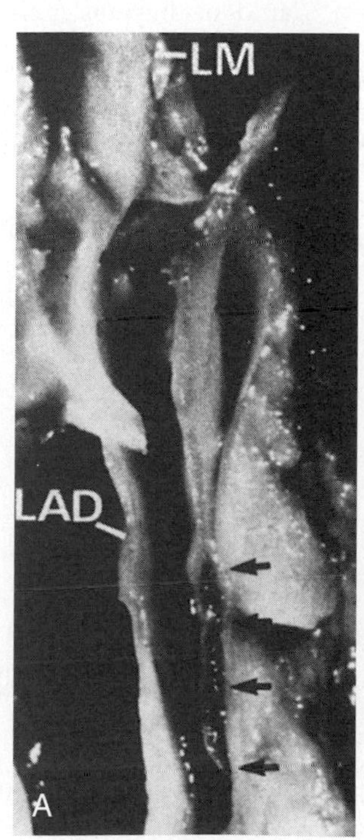

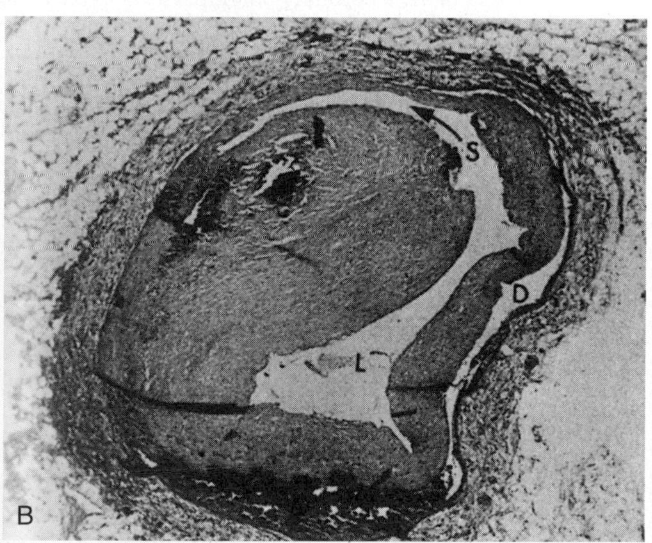

FIGURE 39–4. Pathological findings of coronary dissection following balloon angioplasty. *A,* Localized coronary artery dissection *(arrows)* is present at angioplasty site in left anterior descending artery (LAD). LM = left main coronary artery. (From Waller, B. F.: Early and late morphologic changes in human coronary arteries after PTCA. Clin. Cardiol. *6:*363, 1983.) *B,* Section of left anterior descending artery at site of angioplasty, revealing splitting (S, *arrow*) of the atherosclerotic plaque and dissecting hematoma of the outer media (D). The split has enlarged the original lumen (L). (From Block, P. C., Myler, R. K., Stertzer, S., and Fallon, J. T.: Morphology after transluminal angioplasty in human beings. N. Engl. J. Med. *305:*383, 1981. Copyright 1981, Massachusetts Medical Society.)

TABLE 39–2 OUTCOME IN EPIC TRIAL TESTING AT 30 DAYS AND 6 MONTHS

	PLACEBO (N = 696)	c7E3 FAb BOLUS (N = 695)	c7E3 FAb BOLUS + INFUSION (N = 708)	P VALUE
	% of Patients			
30-day events				
Composite*	12.8	11.4	8.3	0.009
Death	1.7	1.3	1.7	0.96
Nonfatal MI	8.6	6.2	5.2	0.013
Emergency PTCA	4.5	3.6	0.8	<0.001
Emergency CABG	3.6	2.3	2.4	0.177
6-month events				
Composite†	35.1	32.6	27.0	0.001
Death	3.4	2.6	3.1	0.832
Nonfatal MI	10.5	8.0	6.9	0.016
PTCA	20.9	19.9	14.4	0.001
CABG	10.9	9.9	9.4	0.343
Target vessel revascularization (PTCA or CABG)	22.3	21.0	16.5	0.007

CABG = coronary artery bypass graft surgery; MI = myocardial infarction; PTCA = coronary angioplasty.

* 30-day composite endpoint = death, myocardial infarction, or emergency PTCA, CABG, stent, or intra-aortic balloon pump placement.

† 6-month composite endpoint = death, myocardial infarction, any PTCA, or any CABG.

Data from EPIC Investigators: Use of a monoclonal antibody directed against the platelet glycoprotein IIb/IIIa receptor in high-risk coronary angioplasty. N. Engl. J. Med. *330*:956, 1994; and Topol, E. J., Califf, R. M., Weisman, H. S., et al.: Reduction of clinical restenosis following coronary intervention with early administration of platelet IIb/IIIa integrin blocking antibody. Lancet *343*:881, 1994.

stents that "scaffold" the disrupted angioplasty site (see p. 1378), also hold promise as means of successfully managing abrupt closure, even in settings where prolonged balloon dilatation has failed. Intracoronary administration of thrombolytic agents has been used successfully in selected patients with thrombotic coronary occlusion,[39] although the preponderance of published data suggest that this strategy is of limited usefulness.[21,22,32]

Notwithstanding the expansion of catheterization laboratory strategies for management of abrupt closure, emergency coronary artery bypass surgery is required in a proportion of patients (Table 39–1) because of failure to achieve stable vessel recanalization. The autoperfusion catheter (Fig. 39–2) can be used to protect jeopardized myocardium while the patient is prepared for operation. Current guidelines issued by the American College of Cardiology and the American Heart Association thus mandate the presence of on-site cardiac surgical facilities for the performance of elective coronary angioplasty.[7] Even at experienced, high-volume surgical centers, however, emergency surgical revascularization performed in this setting does not yield results equivalent to more elective procedures. Perioperative death and myocardial infarction occur more frequently than would be expected for comparable patients managed by primary elective surgery, with published mortality rates ranging from 1.4 to 19 per cent and perioperative Q wave infarction rates from 20 to 57 per cent.[40]

RISK FACTORS FOR ISCHEMIC COMPLICATIONS. Clinical, angiographic, and procedural parameters have been identified which are associated with mortality or morbidity during percutaneous coronary revascularization. Unstable angina has been associated with elevated risks for mortality (up to 5.4 per cent), myocardial infarction (up to 12 per cent), and emergency surgery (up to 12 per cent).[41–43] Interventions performed within 1 to 2 weeks after the onset of unstable ischemic symptoms appear to be associated with a particular hazard,[41,42,44,45] while the complication profile among patients with unstable angina in whom revascularization could be delayed for 2 to 4 weeks may be the same as in patients with stable angina.[44] Other clinical variables associated with ischemic risk include acute myocardial infarction, diabetes mellitus,[46] and possibly female gender[47,48] and advanced age.[49,50]

Multivariate analyses have demonstrated that coronary angiographic assessment provides a powerful means of preprocedural risk stratification. A number of angiographic risk factors have been identified and formally incorporated

TABLE 39–3 AMERICAN COLLEGE OF CARDIOLOGY/AMERICAN HEART ASSOCIATION CLASSIFICATION OF LESION TYPE

Type A Lesions (high success, >85%; low risk)	
Discrete (<10 mm length)	Little or no calcification
Concentric	Less than totally occlusive
Readily accessible	Not ostial in location
Nonangulated segment <45°	No major branch involvement
Smooth contour	Absence of thrombus
Type B Lesions (moderate success, 60–85%; moderate risk)	
Tubular (10–20 mm length)	Moderate to heavy calcification
Eccentric	Total occlusion <3 months old
Moderate tortuosity of proximal segment	Ostial in location
Moderately angulated segment, 45–90°	Bifurcation lesions requiring double guidewires
Irregular contour	Some thrombus present
Type C Lesions (low success, <60%; high risk)	
Diffuse (>2 cm length)	Total occlusion >3 months old
Excessive tortuosity of proximal segment	Inability to protect major sidebranches
Extremely angulated segments >90°	Degenerated vein grafts with friable lesions

From Ryan, T. J., Faxon, D. P., Gunnar, R. M., et al.: Guidelines for percutaneous transluminal coronary angioplasty. A report of the American College of Cardiology/American Heart Association Task Force on assessment of diagnostic and therapeutic cardiovascular procedures (subcommittee on percutaneous transluminal coronary angioplasty). J. Am. Coll. Cardiol. *12*:529, 1988.

TABLE 39–4 CORRELATES OF MORTALITY AFTER ABRUPT CLOSURE

Female gender
Age >65–70 years
History of congestive heart failure
Left ventricular ejection fraction ≤30%
Unstable angina
Multivessel or left main coronary disease
Collaterals arising from target vessel
Proximal right coronary artery dilation
Jeopardy score
New-onset angina

into a coronary lesion classification by an American College of Cardiology and American Heart Association task force[51] (Table 39–3); this schema defines characteristics of so-called Type A, B, and C lesions based on expected procedural success rates and risks of complications. This scoring system has been independently validated by Ellis and colleagues,[46] among others, who demonstrated that procedural success rates declined from 92 per cent to 61 per cent for Type A versus C lesions, respectively, with an increase in the complication rate from 2 to 21 per cent. Importantly, however, individual angiographic analyses have had inadequate statistical power to accurately estimate the magnitude of risk associated with the various angiographic risk factors,[52] and abrupt closure thus often remains unforeseeable. Nevertheless, in the absence of identifiable angiographic risk factors, procedural success in the hands of skilled operators should exceed 90 to 92 per cent.[12,13,46]

A suboptimal angiographic result following angioplasty may also portend an increased risk of subsequent abrupt closure. The most important procedural correlate of abrupt closure is the occurrence of coronary dissection (Fig. 39–4) during balloon angioplasty. Dissections detectable by angiography likely represent the most extreme of the spectrum of intimal/medial disruptions which occur during all balloon angioplasty procedures. Ischemic risk following dissection is related to the length of the dissection, residual stenosis and luminal diameter.[20,48,53,54]

If abrupt closure occurs during coronary angioplasty, the risk of mortality is influenced by several clinical and angiographic factors (Table 39–4). Most of the clinical predictors likely portend an inadequate myocardial or systemic reserve to compensate for an acute ischemic insult, whereas the angiographic parameters reflect the amount of myocardium in jeopardy for ischemia or infarction.[55–59]

Long-Term Outcome

Among patients who have undergone initially successful coronary angioplasty, outcome over the first 6 to 12 months is influenced primarily by the development of recurrent stenoses at treated sites ("restenosis"), while events over the longer term appear to depend on progression of atherosclerotic disease. Several groups have obtained outcome data for up to 10 years following percutaneous revascularization. Reported rates of survival have been excellent by 1, 5, and 10 years of follow-up, at 97 per cent,[60,61] 88 to 97 per cent,[60–63] and 78 to 90 per cent,[64,65] respectively. Survival free from myocardial infarction or coronary bypass surgery has been somewhat less favorable, however, ranging from 81 to 90 per cent at 1 year,[60,61] 79 per cent at 5 years,[63] and 65 per cent at 10 years.[64]

Recurrence of ischemic signs or symptoms among patients treated with coronary angioplasty appears to occur primarily over the first year following the procedure. The 1985–1986 NHLBI Registry reported that 72 per cent of treated patients were alive and free of anginal symptoms by 1 year follow-up,[60] although intercurrent coronary artery bypass surgery or repeat percutaneous revascularization had been performed during that time period in 6.4 per cent and 20.7 per cent of patients in that Registry, respectively. By 5-year follow-up, clinical status was essentially the same, with 73 per cent of patients reported alive and free of symptoms in the NHLBI series[66] and 85 per cent in the Emory report.[63] Of the 119 patients surviving for 10 years in the original cohort of 133 successfully treated by Gruentzig in Zurich, 75 per cent were symptom-free, with repeat angioplasty or coronary bypass surgery each carried out in 31 per cent of patients.[64]

Long-term outcome following percutaneous revascularization is clearly inferior among patients with multivessel rather than single-vessel coronary disease.[60,62,64,65] Rates of mortality, myocardial infarction, coronary bypass surgery, and repeat percutaneous intervention were all significantly worse among patients with multivessel disease than those with single-vessel disease at 1-, 5-, or 10-year follow-up in reports of the Emory,[65] NHLBI,[60] or Zurich[64] experience. Signs and symptoms of myocardial ischemia have also been more frequent among patients with multivessel disease in several reports.[16,17,64] The apparently less favorable long-term prognosis for patients with multivessel disease treated by balloon angioplasty may be related in part to the completeness of revascularization. Patients undergoing coronary artery bypass surgery usually achieve complete revascularization. In contrast, complete revascularization is achieved in only a minority of patients with multivessel disease undergoing coronary angioplasty.

In a report of the 1985–1986 NHLBI Registry experience,[67] complete revascularization was attempted in only 33 per cent and 15 per cent of patients with two-vessel and three-vessel disease, respectively, and was successful in 23 per cent and 9 per cent. Similarly in the Mayo Clinic series, complete revascularization was accomplished in 41 per cent.[68] The reason for failure to attempt or accomplish complete revascularization by percutaneous techniques was the presence, most commonly, of a chronic total occlusion, but also of complex or diffuse atherosclerosis or a stenosis of only intermediate severity (50 to 69 per cent diameter stenosis).[67,68] Moreover, particularly among patients with unstable angina, a strategy of dilatation of only the "culprit lesion" has been advocated and demonstrated to provide symptomatic relief in many patients.[69]

The impact of complete revascularization on clinical outcome among patients with multivessel coronary disease treated percutaneously, however, remains unresolved. Although the extent of revascularization appears to influence prognosis among patients undergoing coronary bypass surgery,[70] the relative ease with which repeat procedures may be carried out by percutaneous methods and the risk of restenosis following dilatation of even those lesions of intermediate severity may diminish the importance of complete revascularization among patients undergoing balloon angioplasty. In fact, results of different published studies have varied considerably regarding the outcome among patients with complete versus incomplete revascularization. Although some series have suggested that patients with incomplete revascularization are more symptomatic and more likely to require subsequent coronary bypass surgery,[71] others have failed to demonstrate a significant difference in long-term outcome between the groups of patients defined by the extent of revascularization.[68,72,73] In the Mayo Clinic series,[68] for example, differences in baseline clinical and angiographic features appeared to account entirely for the apparent excess risk for mortality, coronary bypass surgery, or the development of severe angina among patients with incomplete revascularization. Faxon and colleagues have suggested that patients with incomplete revascularization that is nevertheless *functionally adequate* (defined as successful dilatation of all stenoses in bypassable vessels subserving viable myocardium) have a prognosis at 1 year that is equivalent to those with complete revascularization.[72]

Restenosis

The principal factor limiting the long-term benefit of coronary angioplasty is restenosis, the angiographic renarrowing of the vessel lumen following successful balloon dilatation of a vascular lesion. The incidence of restenosis has remained largely unchanged since the introduction of coronary angioplasty, with reported rates ranging from 30 to 50 per cent or more depending upon the method of follow-up and the criteria used to define restenosis. A recent analysis using a private insurance claims data base of 2101 patients treated with coronary angioplasty has provided an estimate of the economic cost of restenosis; surgery or PTCA was required in 30 per cent of these patients within the subsequent 1 year, at a projected total of 1.6 billion dollars in charges within the United States.[6]

Restenosis has traditionally been an angiographic diagnosis, defined most commonly as greater than 50 per cent diameter stenosis at follow-up angiography.[74,75] The most common clinical manifestation of restenosis is recurrence of anginal chest pain.[34,76] Myocardial infarction as the first indication of restenosis is extremely rare, and it has been speculated that the fibroproliferative restenotic lesion is less likely than the lipid-laden native atherosclerotic plaque to undergo plaque rupture.[77] The presence of angiographic restenosis has only limited predictive value for the occurrence of clinical events, however, with up to 30 per cent of patients with restenosis found to be asymptomatic.[76,78,79] Hillegass and colleagues have estimated that the positive predictive value of symptoms for the occurrence of angiographic restenosis is approximately 60 per cent, whereas the likelihood that asymptomatic patients are free from angiographic restenosis (negative predictive value) is approximately 85 per cent.[80] The apparent discordance between clinical outcome and angiographic restenosis is likely related to the influence of collateral vessels,[78] incomplete revascularization, or progression of atherosclerotic disease in other arteries, as well as to the limitations of a dichotomous definition of restenosis, in which intermediate narrowings of 50 to 70 per cent are classified together with more severe lesions as restenotic but are unlikely to produce ischemic symptoms. Moreover, estimation of the true *functional* severity of stenoses by angiography may be problematic, as has been suggested by intravascular ultrasound and Doppler flow studies.

The time course of angiographic restenosis has been elucidated by important serial angiographic studies performed by Serruys and colleagues[81] and Nobuyoshi and associates.[82] Taken together, these two studies suggested an immediate loss of luminal diameter over the first 24 hours after angioplasty, stabilization or slight improvement in the lesion appearance during the first month, progressive loss of luminal diameter over the period between 1 and 4 months, and a relative plateau after 4 months. Restenosis rates were 12.7 per cent, 43.0 per cent, 49.4 per cent, and 52.5 per cent at 1, 3, 6, and 12 months, respectively, in the Nobuyoshi report.[82] At any given time following percutaneous revascularization, changes in luminal diameter appear to occur in nearly all patients, but with the extent of renarrowing normally distributed and only a proportion of patients satisfying dichotomous criteria for restenosis.[83] Typically, ischemic symptoms due to restenosis develop within 6 months of the coronary angioplasty procedure[76,83a]; patients presenting with angina after 6 months more frequently have progression of coronary disease in other vessels than restenosis.[84]

The pathogenesis of restenosis is complex (see p. 1315) and likely multifactorial. Pathological studies of the limited numbers of patients undergoing necropsy following successful balloon angioplasty have suggested that there may be two important subgroups of restenosis lesions: those exhibiting "atherosclerotic plaque only" without morphological evidence of previous balloon angioplasty (approximately 30 per cent of patients), and those with intimal fibrous hyperplasia superimposed upon previous intimal-medial fractures and dissections.[85,86] Restenosis within lesions that do not show evidence of prior balloon injury or intimal hyperplasia likely results from stretching of disease-free arterial wall (in eccentric lesions) or of atherosclerotic plaque (in concentric stenoses) during initial balloon dilatation, followed by "chronic elastic recoil" of the stretched arterial segments.[85] Recent studies have also suggested that shrinkage or remodeling of arterial cross-sectional area may occur following balloon dilatation, with pathological findings in animal models demonstrating structural changes extending throughout the arterial wall.[87,88] Serial intravascular ultrasound studies in humans have also supported the concept that remodeling may be an important mechanism of restenosis following coronary intervention.[89]

In lesions exhibiting intimal fibrous hyperplasia following balloon angioplasty, restenosis appears to be the result of an excessive arterial response to injury.[89a] The magnitude

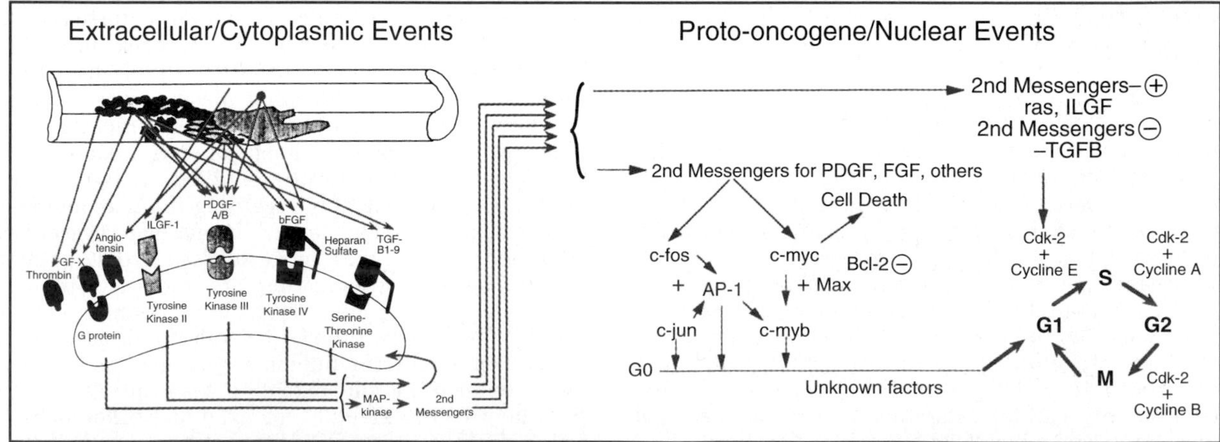

FIGURE 39–5. Possible pathways leading to neointimal hyperplasia component of restenosis. Fundamental pathways have been demonstrated, but not all are known to exist in arterial smooth muscle cells. ILGF = insulin-like growth factor; PDGF = platelet-derived growth factor; bFGF = basic fibroblast growth factor; TGFβ = transforming growth factor β; GFX = growth factor "X" (unknown growth factors); MAPkinase = mitogen activated kinase. (From Lincoff, A. M., Topol, E. J., and Ellis, S. G.: Local drug delivery for the prevention of restenosis. Fact, fancy, and future. Circulation *90:*2070, 1994. Copyright American Heart Association.)

of this response, and hence the amount of proliferative tissue, has been noted in animal models and human pathological studies to be proportional to the degree of arterial injury during percutaneous revascularization.[85,90] The cascade of events leading to the formation of the neointimal proliferative lesion in response to arterial injury is not completely understood but has been characterized to some extent in animal models and in vitro systems[91–97] (Fig. 39–5). Balloon angioplasty produces endothelial denudation, plaque disruption, and exposure of subendothelial components, leading to platelet deposition and activation, thrombus formation, and release of mitogens from activated platelets and endothelium. Circulating monocytes, macrophages, and polymorphonuclear leukocytes are recruited by endothelial and platelet migratory factors to the site of arterial injury. Growth and chemotactic factors released from platelets, inflammatory cells, endothelium, and smooth muscle cells induce proliferation and migration of vascular smooth muscle cells from the arterial media to intima and synthesis of extracellular collagen and proteoglycan matrix. Excessive fibrocellular accumulation results in luminal narrowing and restenosis.

Several retrospective studies have identified clinical, anatomical, and procedural factors that may influence the risk of restenosis following coronary angioplasty (Table 39–5). Owing to differences in definitions, angiographic follow-up, and patient populations in these studies, however, the associations between many of these features and restenosis have been variable. Among the clinical factors, only the presence of unstable angina (new or recent onset, accelerating, occurring at rest),[74–76,98–100] variant angina,[101–103] and diabetes mellitus[75,76,99,104] has consistently predicted an elevated incidence of restenosis. The anatomical factors listed in Table 39–5 may predict elevated restenosis risk due to excessive plaque burden or excessive dilatation forces required to achieve an acceptable angiographic result. Similarly, procedural variables associated with restenosis tend to be related to inadequacy of the initial procedural result, with quantitative angiographic studies demonstrating that the extent of postprocedural enlargement in luminal diameter is a potent predictor of angiographic outcome.[105]

Research into means of diminishing or preventing restenosis following coronary angioplasty has thus far been largely unsuccessful. A number of pharmacological agents have been tested which, by virtue of their effects in vitro or in animal models, might be expected to favorably influence different components of the arterial response to injury (Table 39–6).[105a] Unfortunately, clinical trials have failed to demonstrate an unequivocal reduction in the incidence of angiographic restenosis with any of these agents.[80] Although many of these negative clinical studies have accurately reflected the failure of the pharmacological therapy under evaluation to control the restenotic response, some of the trials have been flawed by overly restrictive entry criteria, inadequate sample sizes, or poor rates of angiographic follow-up.[80,106] One promising agent may be the c7E3 Fab antibody fragment against the platelet membrane glycoprotein IIb/IIIa receptor, which reduced the need for repeat coronary revascularization by 28 per cent over 6 months in a large-scale clinical trial (Table 39–2), although systematic angiographic follow-up was not performed to determine the mechanism of this benefit.[107] One of the "new device" technologies for percutaneous revascularization, intracoronary stenting (see p. 1378), has been demonstrated in randomized controlled angiographic trials to be useful in the prevention of restenosis (Table 39–10, p. 1380), albeit in a relatively select group of patients and with a significant risk of hemorrhagic or thrombotic complications.[108,109]

TABLE 39–5 CLINICAL, ANATOMICAL, AND PROCEDURAL CORRELATES OF RESTENOSIS

Clinical Factors
Unstable angina
Variant angina
Diabetes mellitus
Male gender
Cigarette smoking
Hypercholesterolemia
End-stage renal disease
Anatomical Factors
Severe preangioplasty stenosis
Proximal stenosis
Left anterior descending artery stenosis
Long stenosis
Saphenous vein graft stenosis
Chronic total occlusion
Lesion calcification
Bend stenosis
Bifurcation stenosis
Ostial stenosis
Presence of collaterals
Procedural Factors
Postangioplasty stenosis > 30%
Use of undersized balloon
Small residual minimal luminal diameter

Adapted from Popma, J. J., and Topol, E. J.: Factors influencing restenosis after coronary angioplasty. Am. J. Med. *88*:1, 1990; with permission.

TABLE 39–6 PHARMACOLOGICAL AGENTS TESTED IN CLINICAL TRIALS FOR PREVENTION OF RESTENOSIS

Antiplatelet Agents
Aspirin (± dipyridamole)
Ticlopidine
Thromboxane A_2 inhibitors
Serotonin receptor antagonist
Prostacyclin analogs
Anticoagulants
Warfarin
Heparin
Enoxaparin (low molecular weight heparin)
Hirudin
Calcium Channel Antagonists
Diltiazem
Nifedipine
Verapamil
Antiproliferative Agents
Colchicine
Trapidil
Corticosteroids
Angiotensin-converting Enzyme Inhibitor
Cilazapril
Lipid-lowering Agents
Lovastatin
Fish oil

Adapted from Hillegass, W. B., Ohman, E. M., and Califf, R. M.: Restenosis: The clinical issues. *In* Topol, E. J. (ed.): Textbook of Interventional Cardiology. 2nd ed. Philadelphia, W. B. Saunders Company, 1994, p. 415.

Repeat revascularization of patients with angiographic restenosis is generally reserved for those with clinical symptoms or demonstrable ischemia, as the prognosis in asymptomatic patients is quite favorable.[78,110] Although restenosis may recur following subsequent dilatations, sustained patency can ultimately be achieved in most patients by repeat angioplasty procedures.[111,112]

Comparative Trials of Coronary Angioplasty

Only one randomized trial has been performed evaluating the efficacy of PTCA relative to medical therapy, the Angioplasty Compared to Medicine (ACME) study carried out within the Veterans Administration.[113] Among 212 patients with single-vessel coronary disease and stable angina, an abnormal stress test, or recent myocardial infarction, treatment with coronary angioplasty resulted in a greater likelihood of freedom from angina and better performance during treadmill testing than did intensification of medical therapy over 6 months follow-up; patients

TABLE 39–7 RANDOMIZED TRIALS OF BYPASS SURGERY VERSUS CORONARY ANGIOPLASTY IN PATIENTS WITH MULTIVESSEL CORONARY DISEASE

		STUDY ENDPOINTS		ENTRY CRITERIA		
TRIAL	NUMBER	Primary	Secondary	Clinical	Angiographic	FOLLOW-UP PERIOD
RITA[115]	1011	Death + MI	Repeat revascularization, angina severity, exercise tolerance, employment status	Revascularization appropriate by PTCA or CABG	1, 2, 3 vessels >50% stenosis, equivalent revascularization feasible by CABG or PTCA	5 years
GABI[117]	359	Freedom from angina	Death, MI, repeat revascularization	Revascularization appropriate by PTCA or CABG, Class III angina	2 or 3 vessels >70% stenosis, no total occlusions	1 year
EAST[118]	392	Death + QMI + large ischemic burden on thallium	Repeat revascularization, angina severity, angiographic status	Revascularization appropriate by PTCA or CABG	2 or 3 vessels >50% stenosis	3 years
ERACI[116]	127	Death + MI + repeat revascularization + angina	In-hospital complications, completeness of revascularization	Revascularization appropriate by PTCA or CABG	2 or 3 vessel disease, complete revascularization feasible	5 years
CABRI	1054	Angina, functional capacity	Death, MI, repeat revascularization, angiography, L function	Revascularization appropriate by PTCA or CABG	2 or 3 vessels >50% stenosis	5 years
BARI	1829	Death	MI, angina, repeat revascularization, treadmill performance, angiography, L function	Revascularization appropriate by PTCA or CABG	2 or 3 vessels >50% stenosis	5 years

CABG = Coronary artery bypass graft surgery; L = left ventricle; MI = myocardial infarction; N = number of enrolled patients; PTCA = coronary angioplasty; BARI = Bypass Angioplasty Revascularization Investigation; CABRI = Coronary Angioplasty Bypass Revascularization Investigation; EAST = Emory Angioplasty versus Surgery Trial; ERACI = Argentine Randomized Trial of Percutaneous Transluminal Coronary Angioplasty Versus Coronary Artery Bypass Surgery in Multivessel Disease; GABI = German Angioplasty Bypass Surgery Investigation; RITA = Randomized Intervention Treatment of Angina; QMI = Q-wave MI.

Adapted from Gersh, B. J.: Efficacy of percutaneous transluminal coronary angioplasty (PTCA) in coronary artery disease: Why we need randomized trials. *In* Topol, E. J. (ed.): Textbook of Interventional Cardiology. 2nd ed. Philadelphia, W. B. Saunders Company, 1994, p. 251.

within the angioplasty group more frequently required coronary artery bypass surgery than those randomized to medicine (6.7 versus 0 per cent, $P < 0.01$), however, and 15 per cent underwent repeat PTCA. Among 101 patients with double-vessel disease in the same trial, the benefit of angioplasty compared with medical therapy appeared to be less marked than for those with single-vessel disease.[114] A large-scale prospective nonrandomized analysis of more than 9000 patients treated at Duke University over a 7-year period observed a trend toward a 20 per cent reduction in long-term mortality by PTCA relative to medicine for patients with single-vessel coronary disease or less severe forms of double-vessel disease, although for double-vessel disease with proximal left anterior descending artery involvement or for triple-vessel disease, the effects of PTCA and medical therapy on survival appeared to be equivalent.[62]

Six randomized clinical trials have been performed or are under way comparing coronary angioplasty with bypass surgery in patients with multivessel coronary disease (Table 39–7), and interim or final results have been reported for five[115–118] (Table 39–8, see also p. 1330). At one year follow-up, the ERACI,[116] GABI,[117] and CABRI[119] trials reported no difference between angioplasty and surgery with respect to in-hospital or 1-year mortality. Myocardial infarction rates were equivalent between the two therapies in the ERACI and CABRI studies, although in-hospital infarction rates were higher among surgically treated patients in GABI (8.1 versus 2.3 per cent, $P = 0.022$).

In all three studies, substantially more patients required repeat coronary revascularization following initial PTCA (44 per cent versus 6 per cent in GABI and 40 per cent versus 8.6 per cent in CABRI). The RITA[115] and EAST[118] trials have reported outcome among patients followed for

TABLE 39–8 PTCA VERSUS CABG TRIALS: CLINICAL OUTCOME

	RITA		ERACI		GABI		CABRI		EAST	
	PTCA	CABG	PTCA	CABG	PTCA	CABG	PTCA	CABG	PTCA	CABG
Randomized	510	501	63	64	182	177	541	513	198	194
Early Outcome	In-hospital		In-hospital		In-hospital		30 days		In-hospital	
Death (%)	0.8	1.2	1.5	4.6	1.1	2.3	1.7	0.9	1.0	1.0
MI (%)	3.5	2.4	6.3	6.2	2.3*	8.1*	3.1	2.9	2.0	10.3*
Reintervention (%)	6.7	NA	1.5	1.5	11.0	1.7*	10.1	1.6*	10.1	0*
Late Outcome	2–2.5 years		1 year		1 year		1 year		3 years	
Death (%)	3.1	3.6	4.8	4.6	2.2	5.1	3.9	2.1	7.1	6.2
MI (%)	6.7	5.2	9.5	7.8	3.8	7.3	2.9	3.3	14.6	19.6
PTCA (%)	18.2	0.8	14.2	3.3	27.5	1.1	20.1	7.2	40	13
CABG (%)	18.8	3.2†	17.5	0†	22.5	4.0†	20.2	1.4†	21.2	0.5†
Angina-free (%)	69*	7	62	86	71	74	85	91	80	88
Event-free survival (%)	62*	8	64	84	56	94	60	85*	46	70*

* Statistically significant difference
† Statistically significant difference for all reinterventions (CABG + PTCA)
CABG = Coronary artery bypass graft surgery; MI = myocardial infarction; NA = not available; PTCA = coronary angioplasty.
Trials: RITA = Randomized Intervention Treatment of Angina; ERACI = Argentine Randomized Trial of Percutaneous Transluminal Coronary Angioplasty versus Coronary Bypass Surgery in Multivessel Disease; GABI = German Angioplasty versus Bypass Surgery Investigation; CABRI = Coronary Angioplasty versus Bypass Revascularization Investigation; EAST = Emory Angioplasty Surgery Trial.
From Moliterno, D. J., Elliott, J. M., and Topol, E. J.: Randomized trials of myocardial revascularization. Curr. Probl. Cardiol. *20*:171, 1995, with permission.

2.5 and 3 years, respectively. Both studies found no differences between patients treated with surgery or PTCA in the incidence of death or myocardial infarction over this follow-up period, nor was there a difference between treatment groups with regard to the prevalence of large ischemic defects on thallium scanning in EAST. As with ERACI and GABI, however, RITA and EAST observed a 3- to 4-fold higher rate of repeat coronary revascularization among patients who were initially treated with balloon angioplasty. Similar results were reported for 134 patients with isolated proximal left anterior descending artery disease followed for 2.5 years after randomization to PTCA or internal mammary artery bypass grafting.[120] The results of the large-scale BARI trial, with primary endpoints at 5 years follow-up, have yet to be reported.

The existing randomized data can be summarized as demonstrating equivalent clinical outcome with regard to "hard" endpoints of death and myocardial infarction among patients managed with initial strategies of either coronary angioplasty or bypass surgery, although with a somewhat greater periprocedural morbidity following treatment with surgery and a greater need for repeat revascularization in patients undergoing angioplasty. It is important to recognize, however, that only a minor proportion of patients screened at the institutions participating in these trials were actually randomized (4 per cent in GABI and 8 per cent in EAST), with many patients excluded from enrollment due to clinical or anatomical factors that were thought to render them unsuitable for PTCA (such as left main disease or chronically occluded vessels). Thus, the results of these randomized trials must be interpreted within the context of the patient populations examined and cannot necessarily be extrapolated to the patients with more complex or severe coronary disease. Moreover, these trials were carried out prior to the widespread use of new device technologies for coronary intervention, and thus, particularly in view of the impact of coronary stenting, may not accurately reflect the current state of the art of percutaneous coronary revascularization.

Indications for Coronary Angioplasty

(See also pp. 1313 and 1954)

Despite the growing body of data regarding the risk factors for acute and long-term complications and the efficacy of coronary angioplasty compared with medical therapy or surgical revascularization, a consensus on firm indications for the procedure has not been established. Coronary angioplasty is effective in relieving symptoms in patients with single-vessel and multivessel coronary disease, even when applied to stenoses with relative high-risk characteristics; although the need for repeat revascularization is the most common adverse outcome, repeat procedures can usually be performed without significant morbidity. Selection of patients for PTCA involves careful consideration of the extent of symptoms or ischemic myocardium, the response to medical therapy, the risk of abrupt vessel closure, the likelihood of fatal or serious morbid outcomes in the event of abrupt closure, the prospects for complete or "functionally complete" revascularization, the expected incidence of restenosis, and the suitability of the patient for coronary artery bypass surgery.

The only "absolute contraindications" to angioplasty are the absence of a hemodynamically significant coronary stenosis, significant (>50 per cent stenosis) left main coronary disease unprotected by at least one patent bypass graft, and (in the United States, at least) absence of on-site cardiac surgical support.[7] In general, angioplasty is considered the revascularization procedure of choice for patients with angina or an ischemic response on exercise testing who have single-vessel or double-vessel coronary disease without proximal left anterior descending artery involvement,[121] although the usefulness of medical therapy in this setting must not be disregarded. Among patients who are candidates for surgical revascularization, the benefits of coronary artery bypass appear clear in the setting of severe symptoms and multivessel coronary disease that either cannot be completely revascularized or that is poorly amenable to angioplasty due to the presence of diffuse coronary involvement, a severely degenerated saphenous vein graft target, or a single remaining conduit for myocardial circulation.[7,14,62]

CORONARY ANGIOPLASTY FOR ACUTE MYOCARDIAL INFARCTION (see also p. 1221). Several randomized trials have examined the role of coronary angioplasty as primary or adjunctive therapy for patients with acute myocardial infarction. Given the known limitations of thrombolytic therapy in this setting, including delayed reperfusion, failed or incomplete reperfusion, and reocclusion, balloon angioplasty has intuitive appeal as a means of restoring infarct vessel patency or treating residual stenoses following thrombolysis to prevent recurrent ischemia or reocclusion. Five different strategies for percutaneous revascularization for acute infarction have thus been advocated: (1) *primary angioplasty* to achieve acute infarct vessel reperfusion without prior administration of thrombolytic agents, (2) *urgent adjunctive coronary angioplasty* performed routinely within a few hours after successful thrombolytic reperfusion to treat an underlying stenosis, (3) *deferred adjunctive coronary angioplasty* of the infarct-related artery carried out routinely within the first week of thrombolysis to prevent recurrent ischemia, (4) *conservative adjunctive coronary angioplasty* applied selectively to patients who demonstrate spontaneous recurrent or inducible ischemia following thrombolysis for myocardial infarction, and (5) *rescue coronary angioplasty* performed immediately in patients for whom thrombolytic agents have failed to achieve infarct vessel reperfusion.

Several observational reports have suggested that primary PTCA may be as effective as thrombolytic therapy in reducing mortality and salvaging left ventricular function during acute myocardial infarction.[122,123] Importantly, many of the patients treated with angioplasty in these series would have been considered ineligible for thrombolytic therapy because of excessive risk for hemorrhage or other exclusionary criteria. Four small-scale randomized trials have compared direct angioplasty to intravenous thrombolytic therapy for acute infarction,[124–127] the largest of which, the Primary Angioplasty in Myocardial Infarction (PAMI) study,[124] randomized 395 patients to PTCA or tissue plasminogen activator (t-PA). PAMI demonstrated a lower incidence of death or reinfarction by hospital discharge and during 6 months follow-up among patients treated with PTCA compared with thrombolysis. Although the data regarding the use of acute angioplasty as primary therapy for acute infarction appear quite promising, the limitations of these studies, including the small numbers of patients tested and the failure to compare with accelerated t-PA, must be surmounted before the efficacy of direct balloon angioplasty relative to optimal thrombolytic therapy can be firmly established.

Three large randomized trials have examined the strategy of immediate adjunctive coronary angioplasty following successful thrombolysis with t-PA.[128–130] Despite differences in design, the findings of these studies were concordant: urgent PTCA in this setting offers no clinical benefit, with a trend toward greater mortality, reocclusion, and recurrent ischemia in the immediate angioplasty arm of each trial and no differences in ventricular function. The failure of angioplasty to improve outcome following successful thrombolysis may be due to a diminished likelihood of procedural success and increased risk of thrombotic occlusion when balloon dilatation is performed within recently lysed clot. Similarly, two major trials examining the strategy of "deferred" routine percutaneous revascularization in the days following successful thrombolysis also failed to detect a clinical benefit from the more aggressive approach,[131,132] again with a slight trend toward more frequent death or reinfarction among patients undergoing PTCA. Thus, the conservative approach of reserving percutaneous revascularization for situations of spontaneous or demonstrable ischemia appears to be most suitable for the majority of stable patients following apparently successful thrombolysis for acute infarction. In contrast to the routine adjunctive strategy, however, the application of PTCA as a mode of "rescue" for failed thrombolysis may offer significant benefit, at least for patients with large myocardial infarctions. In a controlled trial of 150 patients with anterior infarction and persistently occluded infarct arteries after thrombolysis,[133] randomization to rescue PTCA resulted in a substantial reduction in the endpoints of death or severe congestive heart failure (16.6 versus 6.4 per cent for PTCA and conservative therapy, respectively, $P = 0.05$).

NEW DEVICES FOR PERCUTANEOUS CORONARY REVASCULARIZATION

The development of new devices for percutaneous revascularization has been motivated by the recognition that despite improvements in equipment design and operator experience, balloon angioplasty remains substantially limited by the risk of procedural complications, difficulties in achieving an adequate angiographic result, and the persistently high incidence of restenosis when this technique is applied to certain patient or coronary lesion subsets. Stenoses that are complex, calcified, long, bulky, eccentric, totally occluded, within saphenous vein grafts, or associated with thrombus are particularly challenging to treat with conventional methods of balloon dilatation. In part, the limitations of coronary angioplasty in this regard are thought to be related to the uncontrolled plaque disruption and vessel stretching induced by balloon dilatation, leading unpredictably to coronary dissection and excessive vascular trauma (Fig. 39–4) and the resultant sequelae of acute ischemic events or late restenotic "response to injury." The potential efficacy of new devices relative to PTCA may be twofold. First, these techniques have been purported to produce a more predictable degree of arterial trauma, thereby reducing the risk of abrupt coronary closure; additionally, the mechanical support of the arterial wall afforded by one class of devices, stents, appears to successfully reverse vascular disruption induced by other methods of revascularization and to prevent ischemic complications. Second, in that plaque is actually removed or elastic recoil eliminated by new devices interventions, these techniques may achieve a better improvement in luminal dimensions than does PTCA, thereby potentially leading to a larger residual lumen at long-term follow-up and less restenosis ("bigger is better").[105]

Following the introduction into investigational use of directional atherectomy for the treatment of coronary stenoses in 1986, six new devices have been approved by the Food and Drug Administration (FDA) since 1990 and a number of others are in various stages of review. Interventional cardiologists have embraced these techniques with great enthusiasm, yet few of these methods have been compared in controlled clinical trials to balloon angioplasty. Observational data, in the form of single-center or multicenter registries, are useful in assessing safety and efficacy during the early stages of clinical testing of new devices but are limited by selection bias and the frequent requirement for adjunctive balloon angioplasty to obtain an acceptable final angiographic result. Thus, the most appropriate indications and limitations of most new devices remain to be defined. Table 39–9 summarizes the potential "niches" for new devices for percutaneous coronary interventions.[133a]

TABLE 39–9 POTENTIAL "NICHES" FOR NEW DEVICES FOR PERCUTANEOUS CORONARY INTERVENTION: EFFICACY RELATIVE TO BALLOON ANGIOPLASTY SUGGESTED BY PUBLISHED OBSERVATIONAL AND RANDOMIZED TRIAL DATA

INDICATION	STENT	ROTO	TEC	LASER	DCA
Acute Outcome					
Treat abrupt vessel closure	++	NA	NA	NA	+
Complex lesion morphology					
Calcification	−	++	−−	+	−−
Thrombus	−−	−	+	+	+
Saphenous vein graft	++	−	+	+	+
Degenerated saphenous vein graft	0	−−	++	+	0
Eccentric	+	+	−	−	++
Ostial	+	++	−	+	+
Long	+	++	0	+	−
"Undilatable" (rigid) stenosis	−	++	−	+	−−
Long-term Outcome					
Reduce restenosis	++	0	0	0	0

DCA = directional coronary atherectomy; Roto = rotational atherectomy (Rotablator); TEC = transluminal extraction catheter.

Assessment of efficacy is for use of new device alone or in combination with balloon angioplasty only. Some devices may be more effective than balloon angioplasty when used in combination with other devices, such as rotational atherectomy followed by stenting for undilatable or calcified stenoses.

NA Data regarding efficacy relative to balloon angioplasty not available.
++ Appears to be substantially more effective than balloon angioplasty
\+ Possibly more effective than balloon angioplasty
0 Appears equivalent to balloon angioplasty
− Possibly less effective (or associated with higher complication risk) than balloon angioplasty
−− Appears to be substantially less effective (or associated with higher complication risk) than balloon angioplasty

Coronary Atherectomy

Three different devices that remove atheromatous material from coronary lesions have been approved for clinical use. Two of these, the directional and extraction atherectomy catheters, operate on the principle of physically cutting the stenosis using a spinning blade, while rotational atherectomy abrades and pulverizes the plaque. Each technique has been extensively evaluated in patients and advocated for particular coronary lesion subsets.

DIRECTIONAL CORONARY ATHERECTOMY. The directional coronary atherectomy catheter (Simpson Coronary Atherocath, Devices for Vascular Intervention, Inc., Redwood City, CA) consists of a metal cylinder at its distal end, which houses a coaxial rotating cup-shaped blade (Fig. 39–6*A*).

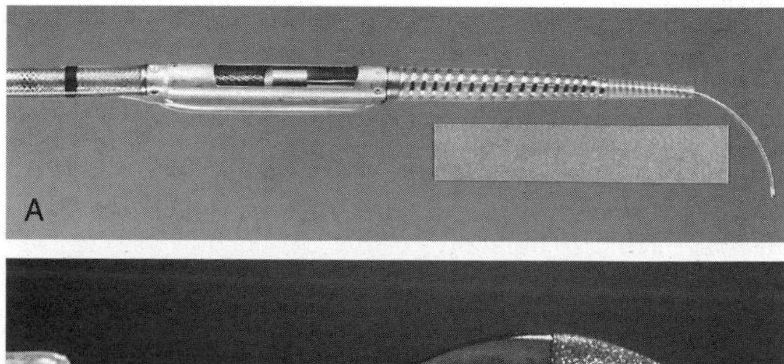

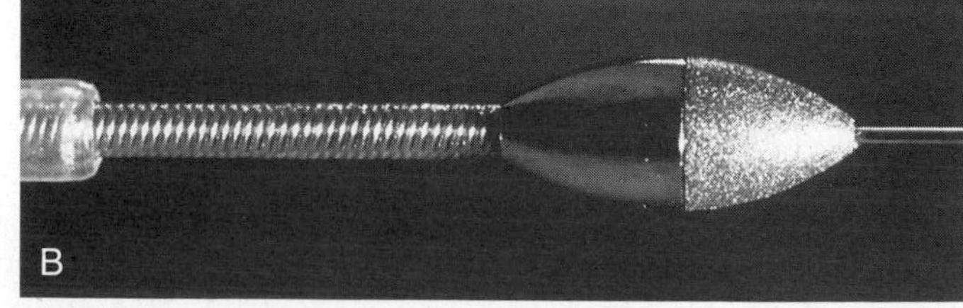

FIGURE 39–6. Atherectomy devices. *A*, Directional atherectomy. (Courtesy of Devices for Vascular Interventions, Redwood City, CA.) *B*, Rotational atherectomy. (Courtesy of Heart Technology, Seattle, WA.)

One side of the cylindrical housing contains a window 9 mm in length over a 120-degree arc, with a noncompliant balloon attached to the metal housing opposite the window. A flexible conical nosecone at the distal tip of the housing serves as a collecting chamber for excised atheromatous tissue. Once passed over a guidewire to the coronary stenosis, the eccentric balloon is inflated to low pressure (1 to 2 atmospheres), pressing the window against the plaque and invaginating the atherosclerotic tissue into the cutting chamber. The cutter within the housing, connected by a drive cable through the shaft of the catheter to an external drive unit, is activated and slowly pushed forward through the housing as it spins at approximately 2000 rpm; tissue prolapsing into the catheter is excised and pushed forward into the hollow nosecone collecting chamber. The balloon is deflated and the catheter torqued to reorient the window to other diseased quadrants. Following multiple cuts, some of which may be performed with the balloon inflated to higher pressures (2 to 4 atmospheres), the catheter is withdrawn and fragments of excised plaque are retrieved from the distal nosecone. Many patients require adjunctive balloon angioplasty following atherectomy to achieve an optimal angiographic result.

The mechanism of enlargement of luminal diameter by directional atherectomy appears to be twofold. Clearly, plaque excision reduces the obstructive bulk of atheroma (Fig. 39–7), but intravascular ultrasound studies and geometric calculations suggest that the majority of improvement in luminal dimensions is a result of dilatation by the atherectomy catheter balloon.[134,135] Atherectomy into the plaque, arterial media, and even adventitia may change the compliance of the artery and allow selective and sustained stretching of the arterial wall.

Observational registry experience demonstrated directional atherectomy to be effective and safe for treating a wide variety of coronary stenoses,[136] with an overall procedural success rate of 85 per cent following atherectomy, increasing to 92 per cent with adjunctive balloon angioplasty. Rates of in-hospital death, nonfatal Q wave myocardial infarction, and emergency coronary bypass surgery were similar to those associated with PTCA: 0.5 per cent, 0.9 per cent, and 4.0 per cent, respectively. Plaque removal by directional atherectomy may produce an angiographic result superior to that obtainable by balloon angioplasty, particularly for lesions that are eccentric, ostial, restenotic, or associated with intraluminal thrombus.[137,138] Failures of atherectomy are most frequently due to inability to pass the bulky catheter to or across the coronary stenosis, although other complications include coronary occlusion, embolization, and perforation. As with balloon angioplasty, outcome using this technique is influenced by clinical and coronary morphological features.

Three multicenter randomized trials have evaluated the hypothesis that directional atherectomy can reduce restenosis rates relative to balloon angioplasty.[139–141] In the Coronary Angioplasty Versus Excisional Atherectomy Trial[139] (CAVEAT-1), immediate angiographic success rates and postprocedural luminal diameters were greater among the 512 patients with de novo native coronary artery stenoses allocated to directional atherectomy than the 500 undergoing balloon angioplasty, although only a nonsignificant trend toward reduced restenosis rates in the atherectomy group was observed (50 versus 57 per cent, $P = 0.06$). Importantly, however, acute procedural ischemic complications (death, myocardial infarction, emergency bypass surgery, and abrupt closure) occurred significantly more frequently among patients randomized to atherectomy than to PTCA (11 versus 5 per cent, $P < 0.001$), as did the actuarial incidence of death or myocardial infarction by 6 months follow-up (9.4 versus 3.6 per cent, $P = 0.0002$). Moreover, atherectomy resulted in higher hospital costs, longer procedure times, and longer fluoroscopy times than balloon angioplasty. Notably, 1-year follow-up of the CAVEAT-1 cohort demonstrated a higher mortality for patients treated with atherectomy than with angioplasty (2.2 versus 0.6 per cent, $P = 0.035$), although the explanation for this observation is thus far elusive.[142]

The Canadian Coronary Atherectomy Trial (CCAT)[140] focused on patients undergoing revascularization of de novo proximal left anterior descending artery stenoses, an anatomical location believed to be particularly well suited for atherectomy owing to its large luminal diameter and the relatively high risk for restenosis following balloon angioplasty. As with CAVEAT-1, acute procedural success rates and luminal dimensions were superior following atherectomy, but no difference in restenosis rates was observed (46 versus 43 per cent for atherectomy and angioplasty, respectively, $P = 0.71$). Finally, CAVEAT-2[141] compared the two techniques among patients with saphenous vein graft stenoses, with no significant difference in the rates of 6-month restenosis (45.6 per cent and 50.5 per cent following atherectomy and angioplasty, respectively, $P = 0.49$), although there was a trend toward fewer repeat target vessel revascularization procedures in atherectomy-treated patients (18.6 versus 26.2 per cent, $P = 0.09$).

Some authors,[143] citing the thesis of "bigger is better," have attributed the absence of demonstrable long-term advantage of atherectomy over angioplasty in these three trials to the failure of the interventional operators to perform atherectomy to obtain a residual stenosis close to 0

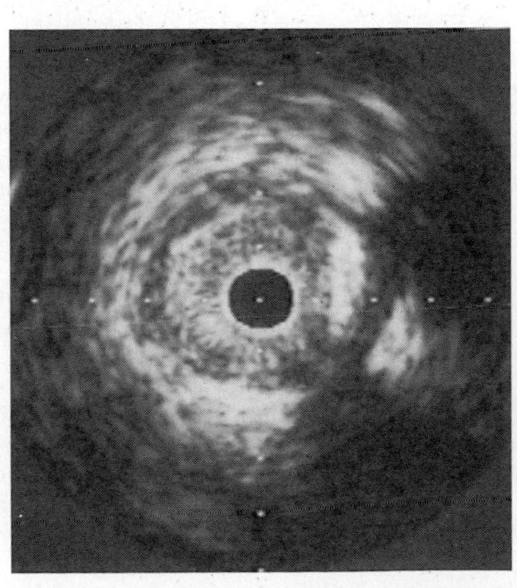

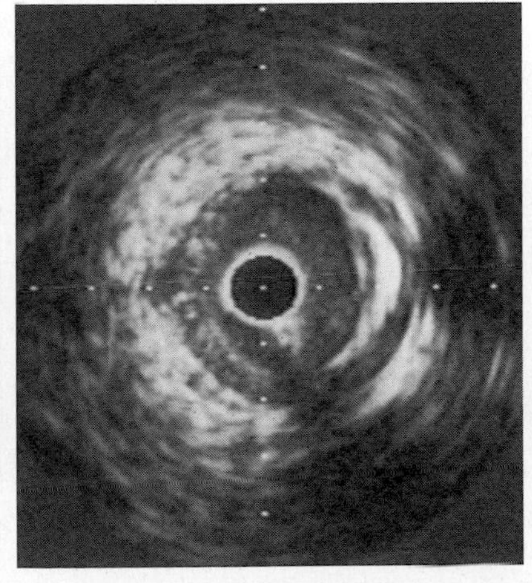

FIGURE 39–7. Intravascular ultrasound images before and after directional coronary atherectomy. *Left,* Circumferential atheromatous plaque with severe luminal compromise prior to atherectomy. Arc of calcification with ultrasound shadowing is visible between 1 and 4 o'clock. *Right,* Following directional atherectomy, there is nearly complete removal of atherosclerotic plaque material with an excellent residual lumen. The arc of calcium is still present. (From Nissen, S. E., Tuzcu, E. M., and DeFranco, A. C.: Coronary intravascular ultrasound: Diagnostic and interventional applications. *In* Topol, E. J. [ed.]: Textbook of Interventional Cardiology. Update 14. Philadelphia, W. B. Saunders Company, 1994, p. 219.)

per cent.[144] Whether such an approach of "aggressive" atherectomy will reduce the incidence of restenosis compared to angioplasty, without an unacceptably high incidence of acute ischemic complications, is being tested in an ongoing randomized trial. Until results of this trial become available, the settings in which directional atherectomy may lead to a convincingly better clinical or long-term angiographic outcome remain unclear.

ROTATIONAL ATHERECTOMY. The rotational atherectomy catheter (Rotablator, Heart Technology, Inc., Bellevue, WA) uses a rapidly spinning abrasive tip welded to the end of a flexible metal drive shaft to grind or "polish" the internal lumen of an atherosclerotic plaque. The distal end of the catheter consists of an elliptical burr coated with 10- to 40-μm diamond chips (Fig. 39–6*B*) which rotates at 170,000 to 200,000 rpm while slowly advanced across the atherosclerotic plaque. Rotational atherectomy produces abraded atheromatous particles of less than 10 to 12 μm in diameter which typically pass downstream without obstruction of the microcirculation,[145] although larger debris may be formed by rotablation of heavily calcified stenoses. Multiple passes of the Rotablator are typically performed until no resistance is encountered; progressively larger burrs ranging in size from 1.25 to 2.5 mm may be used.

Rotational atherectomy theoretically operates on the principle of "differential cutting," where rigid material such as calcium or fibrotic plaque is preferentially pulverized rather than the elastic components of the arterial wall.[146] As such, this technique has been particularly advocated for heavily calcified, inelastic or "nondilatable," eccentric, and diffuse coronary lesions (Fig. 39–8). Intravascular ultrasound studies of heavily calcified lesions treated with rotational atherectomy appear to confirm that the primary mechanism of improvement of luminal dimension is selective removal of calcified plaque, with little or no stretching of the vessel itself.[147] Adjunctive balloon angioplasty, however, required in most cases because of the relatively small diameters of available Rotablator burrs,[148] further increases the luminal area by vessel stretching and plaque fracture.

A recent report from the multicenter rotational atherectomy registry of 709 patients treated at 17 institutions with the Rotablator demonstrated a high rate of procedural success (94.7 per cent), which appeared unrelated to traditional high-risk characteristics.[149] Rates of death, Q-wave myocardial infarction, non-Q-wave infarction, and emergency bypass surgery were 0.8 per cent, 0.9 per cent, 5.2 per cent, and 1.7 per cent, respectively; restenosis at 6 months was documented in 37.7 per cent of patients who returned for angiographic follow-up. Other analyses have generally confirmed these findings,[148,150] also identifying delayed coronary runoff ("slow reflow"), possibly resulting from distal embolization of microparticulate debris or microcavitation bubbles, as an important contributor to the incidence of periprocedural myocardial infarction. Although observational data thus suggest that rotational atherectomy may be useful in treating certain lesion subsets that appear poorly suited for balloon angioplasty, randomized trials comparing this technique with other forms of percutaneous coronary revascularization have yet to be performed.

TRANSLUMINAL EXTRACTION ATHERECTOMY. The transluminal extraction catheter (TEC, InterVentional Technologies, Inc., San Diego, CA) was designed to excise and extract atheromatous material and has been applied primarily to diffusely degenerated saphenous vein grafts and to thrombus-containing lesions. It consists of a flexible, hollow torque tube, the distal end of which consists of two blades oriented in a conical configuration. Once activated within the coronary vasculature, the torque tube spins at 750 rpm with vacuum applied through its lumen; this design is intended to aspirate plaque and thrombus cut by the rotating blades through the hollow tube into an external vacuum bottle.

The multicenter observational TEC registry experience reported a procedural success rate of 88 per cent,[151] with major complications occurring in 5.7 per cent of patients, including death, myocardial infarction following occlusion or embolization, emergency bypass surgery, and vessel perforation in 2.2 per cent, 1.3 per cent, 2.3 per cent, and 1 per cent, respectively.[152] The relatively high rate of complications observed in this registry may be related in part to the prevalence of high-risk characteristics among patients treated with this device, such as degenerated saphenous vein grafts or acute myocardial infarction.[151] In contrast to balloon angioplasty, in which vein graft age has been associated with the risk of ischemic complications,[153] procedural success with TEC in bypass grafts appears to be unrelated to graft age[151]; distal embolization may occur in up to 23 per cent of patients nonetheless,[154] particularly from diffusely degenerated grafts and following adjunctive balloon angioplasty. Restenosis rates among different subsets of patients treated with the TEC catheter have not been better than those obtained with PTCA, ranging from 45 to 51 per cent in native coronary arteries and 46 to 53 per cent in vein grafts.[151]

Intracoronary Stents

As an alternative to the removal of plaque material by atherectomy, intravascular stents may be used to support and maintain stretch of a diseased segment of artery, thus eliminating acute or chronic recoil, scaffolding disrupted or friable atherosclerotic tissue, minimizing contact between blood and thrombogenic subintimal arterial wall components, and optimizing coronary blood flow dynamics. There has been a broad observational experience with the use of stents as a means of treating abrupt closure or im-

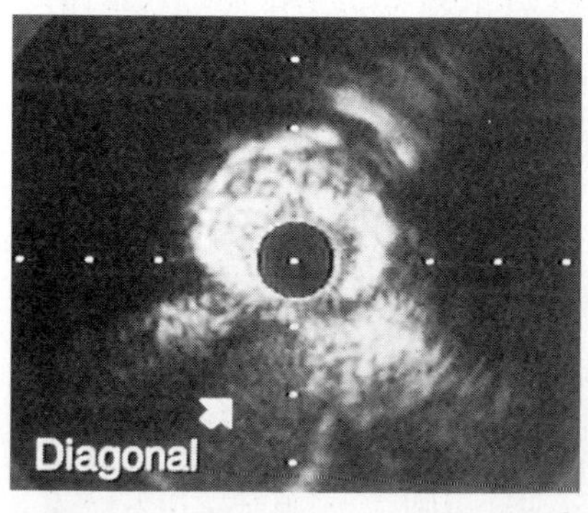

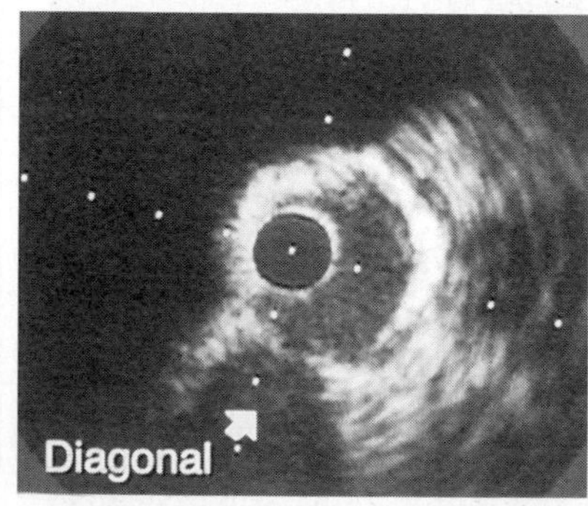

FIGURE 39–8. Intravascular ultrasound images before and after rotational atherectomy (Rotablator). Presence of a visible diagonal branch of the left anterior descending artery in both images documents matching of location and orientation within the artery. *Left,* Densely calcified atherosclerotic plaque with severe compromise of vessel lumen prior to rotational atherectomy; deep vascular structures are obscured by nearly complete shadowing of ultrasound beam by calcification. *Right,* Following rotational atherectomy, there is significant removal of calcified plaque with marked improvement in vascular lumen. More deep wall structures are visible after removal of calcium. (From DeFranco, A. C., Tuzcu, E. M., and Nissen, S. E.: Diagnostic and interventional applications of coronary intravascular ultrasound. *In* Topol, E. J., and Serruys, P. [eds.]: Current Review of Interventional Cardiology. Philadelphia, Current Medicine, 1995, pp. 174–191.)

proving an inadequate angiographic result during percutaneous revascularization, and two randomized trials have demonstrated efficacy in reducing the incidence of restenosis.

Stents currently in clinical use are composed of various metals that have been demonstrated to possess adequate radial hoop strength and to be biocompatible without degradation. The major disadvantage of metallic stents is their potential for thrombogenicity at the blood-tissue interface, with the resultant risk of acute thrombotic closure or distal embolization. Stents have thus been designed with various mesh or coil configurations to minimize the surface area of exposed metal; nevertheless, early experience with most of these designs indicated that intensive anticoagulation was required for the 2 to 3 months following stent placement before re-endothelialization occurs. Such vigorous anticoagulation regimens, consisting of aspirin, heparin, warfarin, and often dipyridamole and dextran, are associated with a substantial risk of hemorrhagic complications, particularly from vascular access sites. Recent data, however, suggest that *optimal* stent implantation with enhanced antiplatelet therapy may obviate the need for long-term warfarin in many patients.

WALLSTENT. The Wallstent (Medinvent, Schneider Europe, Zurich, Switzerland) was the first stent to be used in humans and is the only self-expanding stent design in clinical use. It consists of a flexible woven stainless steel mesh tube available in a number of lengths, which is delivered to the stenosis site on a catheter in a constrained form and deployed by withdrawal of an overlying membrane (Fig. 39–9*A*). By virtue of its self-expanding properties, the Wallstent does not require balloon dilatation for implantation and maintains a residual radial expansion force on the arterial wall.

The outcome of the initial clinical experience with the Wallstent by a group of European investigators (antedating all other stent projects) highlighted both the promise and risks associated with the use of stents in coronary arteries.[155,156] A total of 265 patients, many of whom had relatively complex pathology including saphenous vein graft stenoses, were treated with the Wallstent at different institutions with widely varying anticoagulation regimens. A limited number of stents were subsequently retrieved from patients undergoing coronary artery bypass surgery, demonstrating deposition of platelets, fibrin, and leukocytes during the first 3 to 7 days following implantation, with subsequent ingrowth of varying degrees of neointima by 3 to 10 months. Although the restenosis rate following placement of the Wallstent in this series was an encouraging 27 per cent (18 per cent in native coronary vessels, 39 per cent in saphenous vein grafts), enthusiasm for this device was dampened by the prohibitively high subacute thrombotic occlusion rate of 15 per cent. Eleven of the 265 patients (4.1 per cent) died during the hospitalization period, the majority due either to myocardial infarction sustained during thrombotic stent closure (seven patients) or to intracranial hemorrhage (three patients) related to the intensive anticoagulation regimen. Other hemorrhagic complications, including femoral hematomas or gastrointestinal and genitourinary bleeding, were observed more frequently than in balloon angioplasty series. It is likely that the high incidence of adverse events in this first stenting experience was related to the "learning curve" for proper patient and lesion selection and the management of anticoagulation; after withdrawal of the coronary Wallstent from the market in 1990, this device is undergoing renewed clinical investigation in the United States and is commonly used in Europe.

GIANTURCO-ROUBIN STENT. The Gianturco-Roubin Flexstent (Cook, Inc., Bloomington, IN) was the first coronary stent approved by the FDA for the indication of abrupt or threatened closure. It consists of a single 0.006-inch diameter stainless steel wire wrapped into an interdigitating serpentine coil and mounted on a balloon catheter (Fig. 39–9*B*); this flexible, low-profile system is placed across a coronary lesion and the stent deployed by balloon inflation. During preclinical animal studies, placement of the Gianturco-Roubin stent was followed by early nonocclusive thrombus deposition, with subsequent reconstitution of an endothelial layer by 2 weeks that appeared morphologically normal by 6 months.[157]

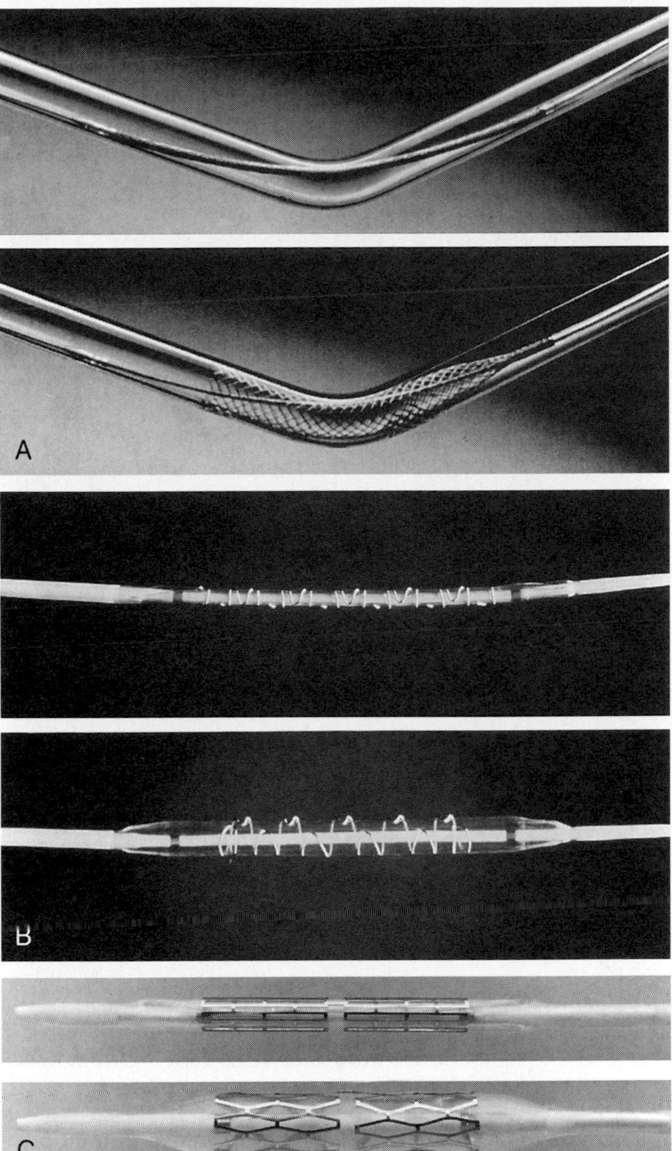

FIGURE 39–9. Intracoronary stents. *A*, Self-expanding Wallstent. *Top*, Prior to deployment. *Bottom*, Nearly completely deployed by withdrawal of constraining membrane. (Courtesy of Schneider, USA, Minneapolis, MN.) *B*, Gianturco-Roubin balloon-expandable coil stent. *Top*, Undeployed, wrapped around delivery balloon. *Bottom*, Deployed by expansion of delivery balloon. (Courtesy of Cook, Inc., Bloomington, IN.) *C*, Palmaz-Schatz balloon-expandable slotted tube stent. *Top*, Undeployed, wrapped around delivery balloon. *Bottom*, Deployed by expansion of delivery balloon. (Courtesy of Johnson and Johnson Interventional Systems, Warren, NJ.)

An extensive registry experience has demonstrated the effectiveness of the Gianturco-Roubin stent in reversing abrupt or threatened coronary closure (Fig. 39–10), although randomized controlled trials have not been reported. In the largest single-center series,[158] 115 patients had the stent placed as either primary or bailout therapy for severe dissection or vessel closure with a 93 per cent rate of angiographic resolution. Among this group of patients who would have been expected to be at very high risk for ischemic events with conventional therapy (Table

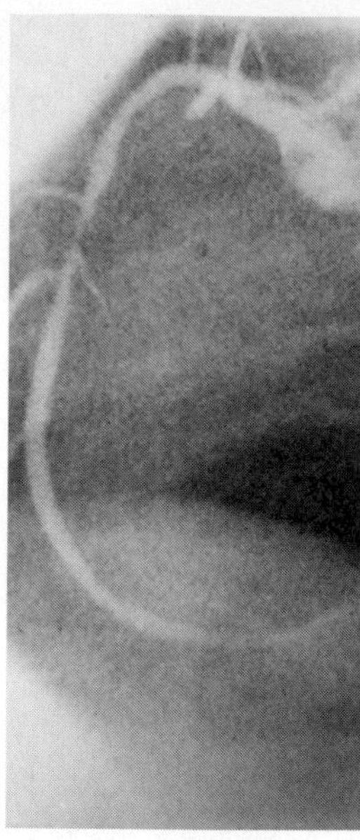
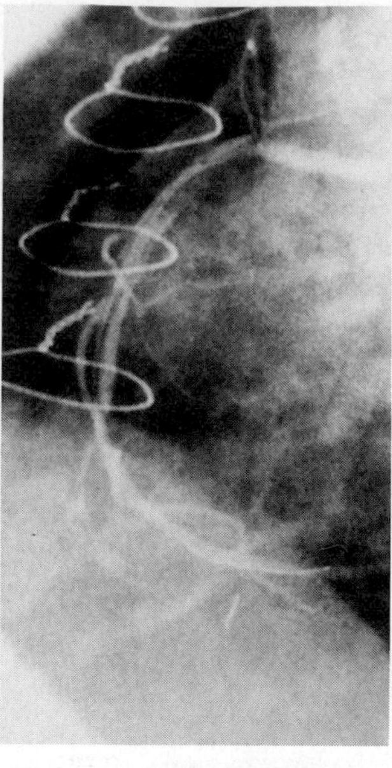
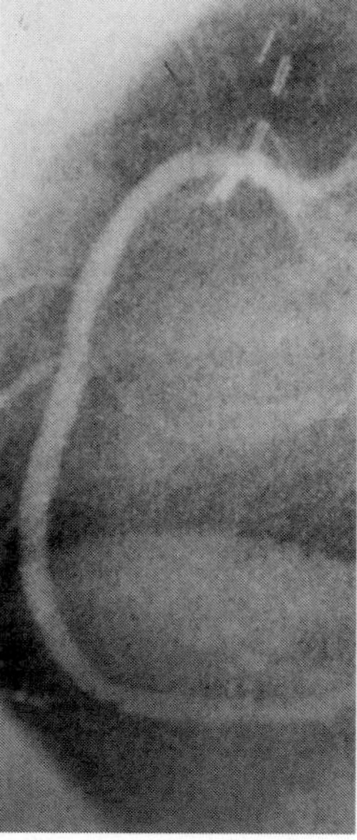

FIGURE 39–10. Angiographic efficacy of stenting for treating coronary dissection. *Left,* Stenosis in mid-right coronary artery prior to intervention. *Middle,* Extensive spiral dissection extending from the tip of the guide catheter to the acute margin of the vessel. *Right,* Final appearance of the vessel after the insertion of three overlapping Gianturco-Roubin stents. The vessel is widely patent with brisk distal flow. (From Muller, D. W. M., and Ellis, S. G.: Advances in coronary angioplasty: Endovascular stents. Coron. Artery Dis. *1*:438, 1990.)

39–1), complications following stent implantation were infrequent; death occurred in 1.7 per cent, emergency bypass surgery in 4.2 per cent, and Q-wave and non-Q-wave infarction in 7 per cent and 9 per cent, respectively. Similarly, in a larger multicenter registry experience of 415 patients treated for abrupt closure, rates of death, myocardial infarction, and coronary bypass surgery were 3 per cent, 5 per cent, and 12 per cent, respectively.[152] Despite anticoagulation with aspirin, dipyridamole, heparin, dextran, warfarin, and occasionally urokinase, however, stent thrombosis has been reported to occur in 6 to 12 per cent of these patients[158–160]; bleeding complications associated with anticoagulation have ranged from 11 to 25 per cent.[158,159] Placement of the Gianturco-Roubin stent has not yet been documented to appreciably affect restenosis risk, with angiographic restenosis rates within 6 months ranging from 40 to 45 per cent.[158,159]

PALMAZ-SCHATZ STENT. The Palmaz-Schatz stainless steel slotted tube stent (Johnson and Johnson Interventional Systems, Warren, NJ) is deployed by balloon expansion within a coronary lesion, assuming a meshwork of adjacent parallelograms (Fig. 39–9*C*). The advantage of this design over wire coil stents appears to be its greater radial support strength; longitudinal flexibility of this somewhat stiff stent was improved by incorporation of a single filament articulation point at its center. As with the Gianturco-Roubin stent, preclinical studies with this device documented early thrombus deposition (usually nonocclusive), followed by endothelialization within 3 weeks.[161]

During the initial clinical experience with the Palmaz-Schatz stent, with only aspirin and dipyridamole administered during the posthospitalization period, a subacute thrombosis rate of 18 per cent was observed.[162] This thrombosis risk was reduced to 4 to 5 per cent following elective implantation by the addition of warfarin therapy for 1 to 3 months.[162,163] Noncomparative reports suggested that use of this stent might lead to a reduced incidence of restenosis.[164a] Among 206 patients in whom Palmaz-Schatz stents were placed in native coronary arteries, restenosis occurred in only 16.3 per cent of de novo and 35 per cent of restenotic lesions.[164] Similarly, among 200 focal saphenous vein graft lesions, for which restenosis rates following balloon angioplasty approaching 70 per cent have been reported,[165] treatment with the Palmaz-Schatz stent was associated with angiographic restenosis in only 17 per cent of patients.[166]

Two randomized trials comparing Palmaz-Schatz stent placement to conventional balloon angioplasty have confirmed that this device can reduce the frequency of restenosis following percutaneous revascularization in patients with de novo native coronary stenoses.[108,109] In the Belgium and Netherlands Stent Study[109,109a] (BENESTENT), angiographic restenosis at 6 months follow-up was present in 22 per cent and 32 per cent of patients in the stent and PTCA groups, respectively, while in the Stent Restenosis Study[108] (STRESS), restenosis rates were 31 per cent and 42 per cent among lesions treated with stents or balloon angioplasty (Table 39–10). The mechanism by which stents reduced the incidence of restenosis in these trials was acute improvement in the immediate angiographic result relative to balloon angioplasty, not a reduction in neointimal hyperplasia. Postprocedural luminal diameters were substantially greater following stenting than after PTCA, which, despite *significantly more loss* in luminal diameter over the subsequent 6 months, translated to greater luminal

TABLE 39–10 OUTCOME IN BENESTENT AND STRESS TRIALS OF STENTING VERSUS CORONARY ANGIOPLASTY

	BENESTENT		STRESS	
	Stent (N = 259)	PTCA (N = 257)	Stent (N = 205)	PTCA (N = 202)
Early Events	In-hospital		14 days	
Death (%)	0	0	0	1.5
Myocardial infarction (%)	3.4	3.1	5.4	5.0
CABG (%)	3.1	1.6	2.4	4.0
Repeat PTCA (%)	0.4	1.2	2.0	1.0
Late Events	7 months		240 days	
Death (%)	0.8	0.4	1.5	1.5
Myocardial infarction (%)	4.2	4.6	6.3	6.9
CABG (%)	6.2	4.4	4.9	8.4
Repeat PTCA (%)	13.5*	23.3	11.2	12.4
Target vessel revascularization (%)	NR	NR	10.2	15.4
Restenosis Rate† (%)	22*	32	32*	42

* Statistically significant difference
† >50% diameter stenosis on follow-up angiography
CABG = coronary artery bypass graft surgery; NR = not reported; PTCA = coronary angioplasty.
Data from Serruys, P. W., de Jaegere, P., Kiemeneij, F., et al.: A comparison of balloon-expandable-stent implantation with balloon angioplasty in patients with coronary artery disease. N. Engl. J. Med. *331*:489, 1994; and Fischman, D. L., Leon, M. B., Baim, D. S., et al.: A randomized comparison of coronary-stent placement and balloon angioplasty in the treatment of coronary artery disease. N. Engl. J. Med. *331*:496, 1994. Copyright Massachusetts Medical Society.

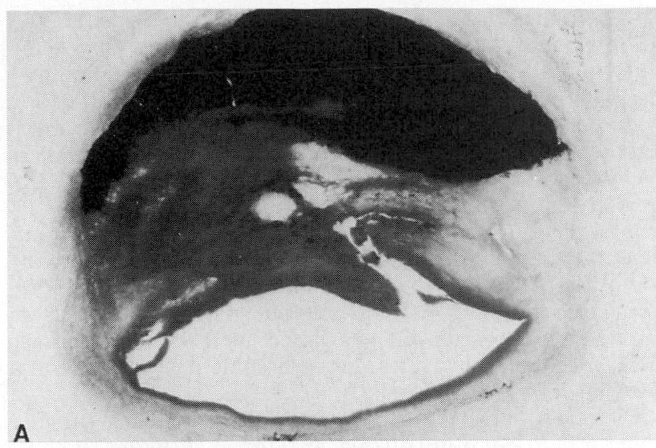

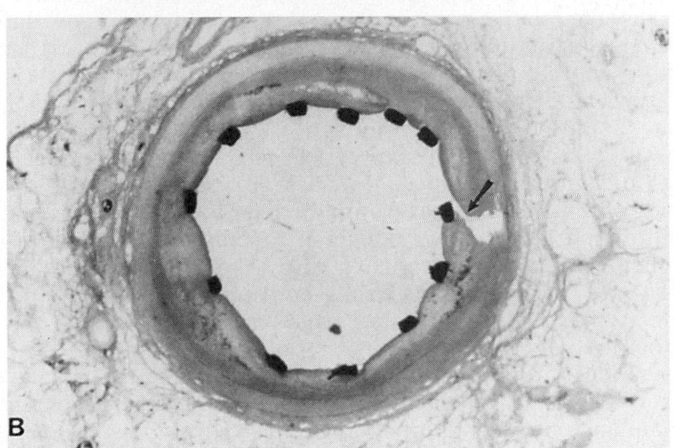

FIGURE 39–11. Pathological efficacy of stenting for treating coronary dissection. *A,* Micrograph of dilated but not stented human cadaver coronary artery with a typical intimal and medial dissection and luminal collapse. *B,* Dilated and stented human cadaver coronary artery with a large intimal and medial tear "tacked up" by the stent struts *(arrow).* (Reproduced with permission from Schatz, R. A.: A view of vascular stents. Circulation *79:*445, 1989. Copyright American Heart Association.)

diameters at follow-up. The decrease in angiographic restenosis documented in these two trials was accompanied by clinical benefit as well, with significant reductions in the need for repeat target vessel revascularization (13.5 per cent versus 23.3 per cent in BENESTENT, 10.2 per cent versus 15.4 per cent in STRESS). Bleeding and vascular complications, however, developed more frequently among patients treated with stents who had received heparin, aspirin, dextran, dipyridamole, and warfarin (13.5 per cent versus 3.1 per cent in BENESTENT and 7.3 per cent versus 4.0 per cent in STRESS), although subacute stent closure occurred in only 3.4 to 3.5 per cent. The findings of these two trials led to approval of the Palmaz-Schatz stent by the FDA in 1994 for the prevention of restenosis in de novo atherosclerotic lesions.

The Palmaz-Schatz stent has also been successfully employed as a "bailout" procedure following abrupt or threatened vessel closure or for suboptimal results following other forms of percutaneous revascularization (Fig. 39–11). Preliminary results of a small randomized trial have confirmed that stent placement for failed angioplasty results in more frequent resolution and fewer ischemic complications than do other forms of therapy such as prolonged repeat balloon inflations.[167]

OTHER STENT DESIGNS. Various other balloon-expandable stent designs are currently under clinical investigation. The Wiktor sinusoidal coil[168] (Medtronic Interventional Vascular, Minneapolis, MN) and Strecker wire mesh[169] (Boston Scientific, Watertown, MA) stents are composed of tantalum, a radiopaque metal that renders these stents particularly simple to position precisely within coronary vessels. Early results derived from human implantations appear to be similar to those obtained with earlier stent designs. A nickel-titanium alloy (nitinol) with "thermal memory" properties has been used to construct a balloon-expandable stent that can be removed within several days of implantation; heated fluid administered through a specialized intracoronary catheter causes the stent to collapse around the catheter into its predeployment configuration.[170] This and other temporary stent designs may be useful in situations where only transient mechanical support is required. Various coatings, including polymers, pharmacological agents, and endothelial cells, have been applied to stent surfaces and tested in animal models with the intent of reducing thrombosis or limiting neointimal hyperplasia. A heparin-coated Palmaz-Schatz stent is currently under pilot-phase clinical investigation, with early results suggesting that systemic anticoagulation can be markedly diminished without an increased risk for thrombotic complications.

OPTIMAL STENT IMPLANTATION AND REDUCED ANTICOAGULATION. Intravascular ultrasound studies performed after implantation of the Palmaz-Schatz and other stents have demonstrated that despite the angiographic appearance of complete stent expansion, most stents are in fact inadequately deployed by traditional balloon inflation pressures (6 to 8 atmospheres) with poor apposition of stent struts to the arterial wall.[171] Repeat balloon inflations within the stents using larger balloons or higher pressures (up to 16 atmospheres) result in improved luminal dimensions with complete implantation of the stent struts within the plaque material (Fig. 39–12). Based upon these findings and the hypothesis that stent thrombosis may arise primarily at sites of poorly supported arterial plaque or stent struts protruding into the arterial lumen, several groups of investigators have recently evaluated outcome *without* warfarin

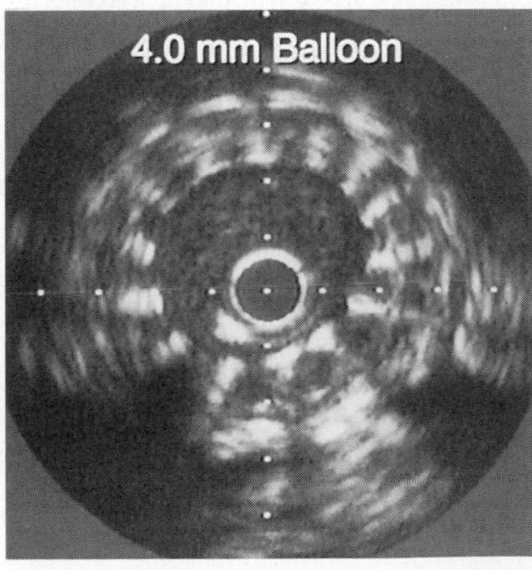

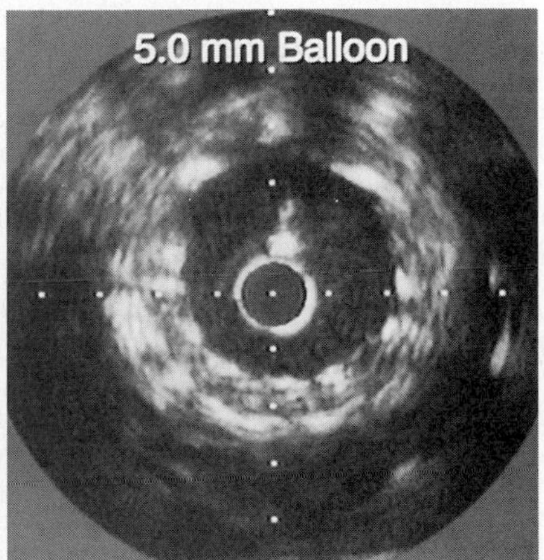

FIGURE 39–12. Intravascular ultrasound images after intracoronary stent placement. *Left,* Following deployment of a Palmaz-Schatz intracoronary stent using a 4.0-mm-diameter balloon, echogenic stent struts between 3 and 7 o'clock can be seen to be incompletely apposed to the underlying vascular wall. *Right,* Following inflations of a 5.0-mm balloon within the stent, complete apposition of all stent struts against the arterial wall is visible. (From Defranco, A. C., Tuzcu, E. M., and Nissen, S. E.: Diagnostic and interventional applications of coronary intravascular ultrasound. *In* Topol, E. J., and Serruys, P. [eds.]: Current Review of Interventional Cardiology. Philadelphia, Current Medicine, 1995, pp. 174–191.)

therapy following "optimal" stent implantation.[164a,172,173] Initial series uniformly employed intravascular ultrasonography to demonstrate that stent struts were completely expanded following high-pressure balloon inflations, although subsequent reports have suggested that ultrasonography may not routinely be necessary.[174] Enhanced antiplatelet therapy with ticlopidine in addition to aspirin for several weeks has usually been considered a key component of this reduced anticoagulation regimen, with some groups using low molecular weight heparin as well. The incidence of subacute thrombosis during antiplatelet therapy without warfarin following optimal stent implantation has been surprisingly low, usually less than 2 to 3 per cent, with rates of vascular and hemorrhagic complications equivalent to those for coronary balloon angioplasty.[174a] Observational reports have suggested that this method of stenting may also result in lower rates of late restenosis than traditional stenting techniques, by virtue of the improved postprocedural angiographic result.[175]

If the strategy of optimal stent implantation by high-pressure balloon inflations, with or without intravascular ultrasound guidance, proves to eliminate the need for intensive anticoagulation while preserving or enhancing the benefits of stenting in reducing the incidence of restenosis and treating abrupt or threatened coronary closure, a major transformation in the practice of interventional cardiology may follow. Without the thrombotic or hemorrhagic risks traditionally associated with stent placement, this technique may be applied to a wide variety of coronary lesions that would otherwise be considered at "high risk" for acute complications or subsequent restenosis, with a consequent broadening of the indications for percutaneous coronary revascularization. Importantly, however, widespread acceptance of stenting should await the acquisition of long-term follow-up (5 years or more) experience in patients with this prosthesis.

Lasers and Other Ablative Energy

Other new devices for percutaneous coronary intervention have been developed with mechanisms of action similar to those of atherectomy catheters or stents. Instead of mechanical excision of atherosclerotic material, thermal, photochemical, or acoustic energy is used to ablate coronary plaque. Additionally, compliance and other physical properties of the arterial wall may be modified by these devices, resulting in decreased elastic recoil and sealing of disrupted dissection flaps. Although several types of ablative techniques are currently under investigation, only the excimer laser has been approved by the FDA for coronary revascularization.

THERMAL BALLOON ANGIOPLASTY. Laser, radiofrequency, and microwave energy have all been used to deliver heat to coronary stenoses during balloon inflations. Heating of the vascular wall occurs either by direct radiation (laser and microwave) or conduction of heat from the fluid within the balloon (radiofrequency). Preclinical studies in animal models have indicated that each of these devices may reduce elastic recoil, weld disrupted tissue planes, desiccate intraluminal thrombus, and produce a better postprocedural luminal enlargement than conventional balloon angioplasty, with varying degrees of necrosis of the arterial wall, medial thinning, straightening of the elastic laminae, and protein coagulation.

A laser balloon catheter employs an Nd:YAG near-infrared laser source that is transmitted through a fiberoptic to a diffusing silica fiber within the angioplasty balloon. Although experience with laser balloon angioplasty following conventional PTCA demonstrated this technique to be effective in improving the angiographic result in many patients with relatively high-risk coronary lesions and reversing severe dissections or acute or threatened closure,[176,177] this device was withdrawn from clinical use because of the high incidence of restenosis and major clinical events.[177] A radiofrequency balloon catheter has been used in a technique of physiologically controlled low stress angioplasty (PLOSA), based on the concept that thermal modification of the arterial wall at moderate temperatures (approximately 60°C) during balloon inflations with pressures as low as 2 atmospheres may allow vascular distention without disruption, thus minimizing elastic recoil and the restenotic healing response. In pilot-phase clinical experience, immediate clinical and angiographic results following PLOSA were similar to those that would be expected following conventional balloon angioplasty[178]; an intravascular ultrasound evaluation has failed to detect a difference in the mechanisms of luminal enlargement by PLOSA and PTCA.[179]

LASER ANGIOPLASTY. Laser angioplasty devices directly ablate atherosclerotic plaque by three different mechanisms, the relative contributions of which depend upon the wavelength and intensity of laser energy, the mode of operation (continuous or pulsed), the lasing media (blood, saline, or radiographic contrast), the degree of tissue contact, and the absorption characteristics of different components of vascular tissue. *Thermal* effects melt or vaporize tissue and denature proteins. The precision or selectivity of thermal plaque ablation may be optimized by use of ultraviolet or infrared laser energy delivered in pulses of short duration, operating characteristics that minimize diffusion of heat away from the target zone and injury of adjacent tissue. *Acoustic* pressure transients arise from plasma or vapor bubble formation during pulsed, high-energy laser operation, producing plaque and tissue disruption and likely playing a major role in the development of ischemic complications during laser angioplasty. *Photodissociation* occurs when absorption of laser energy leads to direct rupture of intramolecular bonds within a tissue without appreciable heating, an effect that is highly specific to the absorption characteristics of individual tissue components. Although photodissociation is thus the ideal objective of laser angioplasty, thermal and acoustic mechanisms appear to predominate under clinical conditions.

Pulsed lasers currently used for vascular applications operate with wavelengths in the ultraviolet (excimer), mid-infrared (holmium), or visible (dye) range. Despite the initial excitement surrounding the use of "high technology" lasers for coronary revascularization, clinical expectations of exceptional efficacy, selectivity, and safety have been inadequately fulfilled. Immediate results of laser angioplasty have proven to be unpredictable and not clearly different from those obtained by conventional balloon dilatation, even for complex lesion subsets thought to be most suited for laser ablation. Moreover, laser angioplasty has been associated with an increased risk for procedural complications, including dissection, abrupt closure, and perforation. Registry studies have thus far failed to detect a reduction in the incidence of restenosis using this technique.

Excimer Laser. This has been the most extensively evaluated coronary laser system. High-intensity, short-duration (100 to 200 nsec) pulses of 308-nm ultraviolet light are transmitted through a fiberoptic bundle catheter to the coronary stenosis, where the laser energy is absorbed by proteins within the plaque. Histopathological changes resulting from excimer laser ablation in animal models have included focal crater formation without charring and localized intimal disruption. In two large clinical series[180,181] of over 3500 patients undergoing excimer laser coronary angioplasty, immediate procedural success was achieved in approximately 90 per cent, despite the high prevalence of complex morphological features, with adjunctive balloon angioplasty required in up to 95 per cent of patients to improve the narrow lumen achieved by laser ablation alone. Although rates of in-hospital death, myocardial infarction, and emergency bypass surgery were similar to those expected for balloon angioplasty, coronary dissection and perforation appeared to occur more frequently, in 16 to 22 per cent and 1.6 to 2.4 per cent of treated lesions, respectively. Angiographic restenosis occurred in 46 per cent of patients following successful excimer laser angioplasty.[182] Two recent randomized trials comparing excimer laser to conventional balloon angioplasty for the treatment of long[183] or totally occluded[184] lesions failed to demonstrate a difference between these two techniques in long-term clinical or angiographic outcome. The development of directional laser catheters may improve the safety and outcome of excimer laser angioplasty in certain lesion subsets.

Other lasers under clinical investigation include the *holmium* and *pulsed dye* lasers. The holmium infrared laser energy is absorbed by water within atherosclerotic and vascular tissue. Early clinical results using this device have been similar to those obtained with excimer, with no apparent reduction in restenosis. The visible light produced by the pulsed dye laser is absorbed primarily by hemoglobin, and the energy threshold for ablation of thrombus is 100-fold lower than that for arterial tissue. This device may thus find a "niche" as a means of thrombolysis during myocardial infarction or acute ischemic syndromes.

THERAPEUTIC ULTRASOUND. The ablative effects of high-intensity, low-frequency ultrasound have been attributed primarily to mechanical vibration and cavitation. Tissues containing a heavy matrix of collagen or elastin, such as arterial wall, are resistant to ultrasound, while those without elastic support, such as thrombus or atherosclerotic plaque, are disrupted by ultrasonic energy. Ultrasound ablation of atherosclerotic plaque or thrombi may thus be accomplished at energy levels below that required to damage normal arterial wall structures. Preclinical studies have demonstrated the potential efficacy of catheter-based ultrasound devices in recanalizing resistant, totally or subtotally occluded arterial segments or dissolving intravascular thrombus.[185] Pilot-phase human investigation is currently under way.

INTRAVASCULAR IMAGING TECHNIQUES

Despite improvements in the resolution of coronary radiographic imaging and the development of computerized angiographic digital reconstruction, several inherent limitations remain to the use of angiography as a means of assessing coronary lesion morphology and the results of percutaneous revascularization. Coronary angiography visualizes only the opacified lumen of the artery, rendering this technique inadequate to evaluate pathological structures within the vascular wall. Substantial atherosclerosis may develop before reduction in luminal dimensions,[186] a process that cannot be discerned by angiographic assessment. The two-dimensional view provided by the coronary angiogram is often inadequate to appreciate the severity of eccentric or complex lesions and underestimates the degree of stenosis in the presence of diffuse coronary disease extending into adjacent "normal" segments. Three new modalities have thus been applied clinically in the setting of percutaneous coronary intervention to more precisely visualize the arterial wall and vascular lumen or assess the functional significance of a coronary stenosis.

INTRAVASCULAR ULTRASONOGRAPHY (see also Fig. 3–15, p. 58). There has been rapid evolution of technology for miniaturization of high-frequency transducers to permit ultrasound imaging from within the coronary vasculature. Ultrasound energy emitted from an intraluminal probe penetrates into the vascular wall, with reflections formed at the interfaces between tissue components with different acoustic properties. Intravascular ultrasonography (IVUS) thus produces high-resolution cross-sectional images that not only delineate absolute luminal dimensions, but also the extent and structure of the atherosclerotic plaque and the arterial wall (Fig. 39–5). Images produced by this technique correlate well with histological findings.[187,188]

Two types of intravascular ultrasound catheters have been developed. *Solid state* designs consist of multiple transducers located circumferentially around the tip of the catheter, which are electronically activated in sequence to produce a 360-degree image; *mechanical scanners* employ a rotating transducer (or a rotating reflector with a fixed transducer) at the tip of the catheter. Cross-sectional images are formed by computerized analysis of ultrasound energy reflected from the tissue to the transducer. Serial cross-sectional images obtained throughout a vessel segment may be integrated to form a three-dimensional computerized reconstruction.[189] Current ultrasound catheters used for coronary arteries have distal tips ranging in diameter from 0.9 to 1.7 mm, allowing interrogation of distal coronary segments.

Intravascular ultrasonography has been employed clinically to identify angiographically inapparent atherosclerotic plaque, quantify luminal dimensions, and characterize the composition of stenotic lesions ("soft" plaque, "hard" plaque, calcification [Figs. 39–7, 39–8, 39–12, and 39–13], thrombus). Several groups have demonstrated that diffuse atherosclerotic disease is frequently detectable by IVUS in arteries that appear to be angiographically normal, particularly in segments adjacent to stenotic lesions,[190] due in part to the Glagov phenomenon of arterial remodeling[186]; the true plaque burden within a coronary vessel is thus often much more extensive than would be expected from its an-

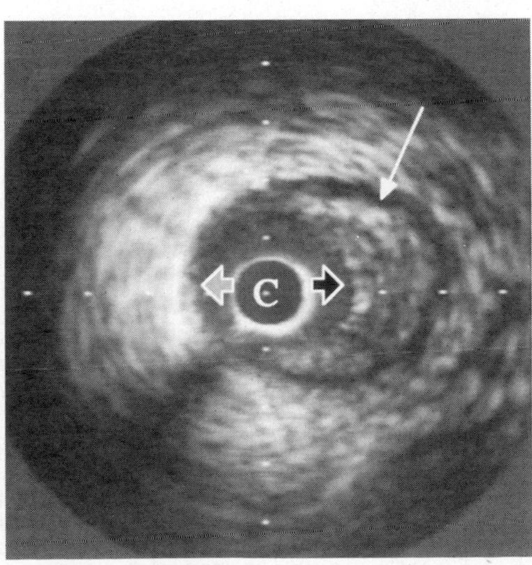

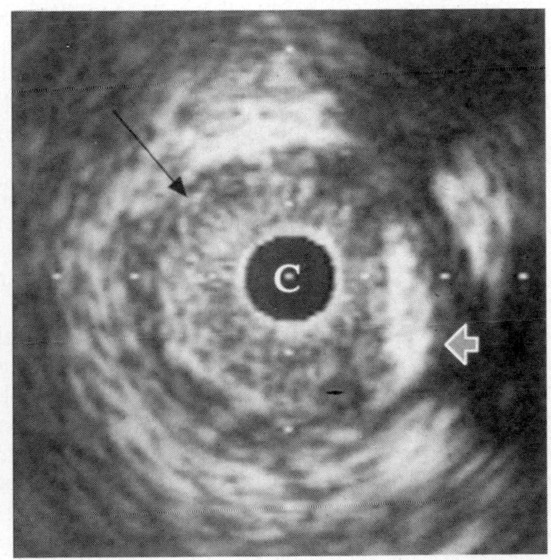

FIGURE 39–13. Examples of intracoronary ultrasound images. C designates ultrasound transducer catheter (1.3 mm diameter) in center of each vessel. Tick marks represent 1 mm distance. *Left,* Eccentric atheromatous lesion. Wide gray arrow denotes undiseased arterial intima, wide black arrow denotes soft crescentic atherosclerotic plaque, narrow white arrow indicates hypoechoic arterial media. *Right,* Circumferential atheromatous lesion with severe compromise of arterial lumen. Wide gray arrow denotes arc of calcification, with dropout of structural features located deep to calcium due to shadowing of ultrasound beam. Narrow black arrow indicates arterial media. (Courtesy of S. Nissen, M.D., Cleveland Clinic Foundation.)

giographic appearance. Similarly, ultrasonography has been useful in assessing the degree of luminal compromise in lesions that appear to be equivocal or indeterminate by angiography due to tortuosity, foreshortening, or vessel overlap, such as in the left main coronary artery.[191,192] IVUS has been shown to be significantly more sensitive than angiography in detecting the presence of calcium within an atherosclerotic lesion,[193] and some investigators have also suggested this modality may be useful in differentiating thrombus from other plaque components.[194]

Intravascular ultrasound studies have contributed markedly to our understanding of the mechanisms of balloon angioplasty[9] and new device interventions[134,147,195] (Figs. 39–7, 39–8, and 39–12); this technique has been employed clinically to guide the application and assess the results of percutaneous revascularization techniques. Identification of certain morphological features by ultrasonography may predict the outcome of percutaneous intervention[196] and aid selection of the best device to obtain an optimal angiographic result.[197] For example, localized deposits of calcium may predispose to medial dissection during balloon angioplasty.[198] Superficial calcium may be considered an indication for the use of rotational atherectomy, bulky eccentric noncalcified lesions for directional atherectomy, intraluminal thrombus for extraction atherectomy or thrombolysis, and fibrotic plaque for stenting or balloon angioplasty.[197] Serial IVUS examinations may also be performed during the revascularization procedure to assess interim results and guide further interventional therapy (Fig. 39–12). Prototype devices have been developed in which an ultrasound transducer is integrated into a balloon angioplasty catheter or directional atherectomy device, optimizing the coronary intervention by concurrent IVUS imaging. Following percutaneous revascularization, intravascular ultrasonography provides a more accurate estimation of luminal dimensions than does angiography,[199] owing to the irregular luminal contour produced by most interventional techniques. IVUS also appears to be the most sensitive method for evaluating the completeness of lesion dilatation, plaque removal, or stent deployment and for detecting plaque disruption or medial dissection, observations that may be correlated with subsequent ischemic complications or restenosis.

CORONARY ANGIOSCOPY. Direct visualization of the lumen of a coronary artery in living patients was made practical by the development of low-profile, flexible, fiberoptic imaging catheters with sufficient fiber density to provide high-resolution images. The most advanced angioscope design currently in clinical use (Baxter Edwards, Irvine, CA) is passed into the coronary artery over a standard angioplasty guidewire, a soft latex occlusion balloon is inflated proximal to the area of interest, and warm Ringer's lactate is infused to create a blood-free field for imaging. The movable imaging bundle containing 5000 fibers (pixels) can be advanced distally as much as 5 cm beyond the occlusion balloon to visualize the arterial segment under high-intensity illumination, with images transmitted through the fiberoptic to a video camera and monitor.

Coronary angioscopy can be performed safely during diagnostic cardiac catheterization or percutaneous revascularization procedures. Pathological structures in the lumen and on the surface of the vascular wall can often be more clearly delineated by angioscopy than by angiography or even intravascular ultrasonography. Stable atheromatous lesions appear as white fibrotic or yellow lipid-laden plaques within the arterial wall with smooth or slightly irregular surfaces.[200] Saphenous vein graft stenoses often appear more complex, with friable plaque components and diffuse disease.[201] In the setting of unstable ischemic syndromes, however, most "culprit lesion" plaques are found by angioscopy to have visible clefts or dissections, with up to 94 per cent associated with white (platelet-rich) or red (erythrocyte- and fibrin-rich) thrombi.[202,203] In the setting of coronary intervention, angioscopy appears to be valuable as a more sensitive means than angiography of identifying intraluminal thrombus, elucidating the mechanism of abrupt or threatened closure, or assessing the completeness of stent deployment[204] or plaque removal by atherectomy.[205]

INTRACORONARY DOPPLER. Measurement of blood flow velocity using the Doppler principle was until recently a complex procedure reserved largely for research applications. The development of piezoelectric crystals that may be mounted at the distal tip of a coronary guidewire has enabled intracoronary Doppler to be used routinely in the clinical evaluation of stenosis severity and the results of coronary intervention. As intracoronary Doppler allows assessment of the *physiological* significance of a coronary lesion, this technique provides data that are complementary to the structural and geometric information derived from other forms of imaging in the catheterization laboratory.

The Doppler guidewire currently in widespread use has the dimensions, flexibility, and handling characteristics of a typical 0.018-inch-diameter angioplasty guidewire. The small cross-sectional area of this wire produces minimal disturbance of the flow profile across a vascular stenosis, thus enabling accurate measurement of blood flow velocities beyond tight coronary lesions. Three alterations in the normal intracoronary velocity patterns have been identified by the Doppler technique which are associated with hemodynamically significant coronary lesions: reduced diastolic/systolic velocity ratio, reduced distal/proximal flow velocity ratio, and blunted hyperemic response.[206]

Clinical applications of intracoronary Doppler include evaluation of the functional significance of intermediate lesions (50 to 70 per cent stenosis) by coronary angiography, diagnosis of abnormalities in coronary vasodilatory reserve, and the assessment of outcome, complications, collateral flow, and additional lesions during percutaneous coronary revascularization. The extent to which continuous Doppler flow measurements in the distal vessel normalize during coronary intervention provides an immediate indication of the adequacy of luminal enlargement, while deterioration in flow parameters appears to be an early signal of impending coronary closure. Cyclical variations in intracoronary Doppler flow velocities may signal the presence of platelet aggregation and intraluminal thrombus formation in an artery with a satisfactory angiographic result following percutaneous intervention, with the potential for late thrombotic coronary occlusion.

NONCORONARY ARTERIAL REVASCULARIZATION

Techniques for percutaneous noncoronary arterial revascularization have been developed in parallel with those for coronary intervention, with increasing application to lesions that would previously have been treated by reconstructive vascular surgery. Although balloon angioplasty has been the traditional mainstay of peripheral arterial revascularization, the role of new device technologies, particularly stents, as a means of improving procedural results and decreasing restenosis has expanded.

PERIPHERAL BALLOON ANGIOPLASTY. Percutaneous transluminal angioplasty (PTA) has proven highly effective in treating claudication, rest pain, ischemic ulcers, and poor wound healing due to ileofemoral and runoff vessel disease. Percutaneous revascularization techniques are associated with less morbidity and shorter recovery periods than surgery and allow preservation of venous conduits in patients who may require future surgery for coronary, cerebrovascular, or peripheral vascular disease. Alternatively, PTA may be used as an adjunct to surgical revascularization, to improve in-flow or outflow to a graft, or to treat anastomotic stenoses arising from prior surgery. Initial success rates for balloon angioplasty of aortic bifurcation occlusive disease have been reported as high as 92 per cent, with 81 per cent and 72 per cent patency rates at 3 and 5 years.[207]

A randomized trial comparing surgery to angioplasty among patients with lower extremity arterial disease demonstrated no difference in long-term outcome following initially successful results by either of the two treatment techniques[208]; initial procedural failure occurred more frequently in patients treated with balloon angioplasty but did not increase the risk of limb loss or subsequent surgical failure. Femoropopliteal disease more commonly presents as diffuse or occluded lesions than does iliac atherosclerosis, yet outcome following treatment of femoropopliteal disease in recent series has largely been favorable, with initial success rates of approximately 90 per cent[209] and 5-year patency rates of nearly 60 per cent.[210] The infrapopliteal and distal tibial circulation are also approached with improving technical success.

Balloon angioplasty has become the preferred procedure for revascularization of renal artery stenoses due to fibromuscular dysplasia, with acute success rates in excess of 90 per cent.[207,211] Atherosclerotic disease of the renal arteries is somewhat more difficult to treat percutaneously, particularly if diffuse or ostial. Balloon dilatation has also been successfully applied in recent years to aortic and mesenteric vessels. Early work using balloon angioplasty to treat stenoses of the subclavian or extracranial carotid and vertebral arteries has proceeded cautiously owing to major concern regarding the risk of distal embolization from these vessels.[207,212] Despite the effectiveness of surgical carotid endarterectomy, however, percutaneous revascularization may prove to be preferable for patients with severe medical comorbidities or lesions within the intrathoracic or distal carotid vessels which are not easily accessible by surgery.

NEW DEVICES FOR PERIPHERAL REVASCULARIZATION. Directional atherectomy, rotational atherectomy, transluminal extraction atherectomy, and excimer laser have all been evaluated for peripheral arterial revascularization. These devices may be particularly useful for debulking total occlusions or eccentric lesions but in general are associated with acute success and restenosis rates similar to those of balloon angioplasty. Intraluminal stenting, however, may prove to be a substantial advance over balloon angioplasty in many situations. When implanted in large vessels, such as ileofemoral arteries, chronic anticoagulation is not required. Stents appear to limit the restenosis risk in nonrandomized reports[213] and are useful in lesions that are less amenable to balloon angioplasty, such as ostial renal stenoses[214] or total occlusions. Early experience has suggested that stents may also limit the embolic risk during treatment of ulcerated carotid or vertebral artery lesions. Recently, repair of abdominal aortic aneurysms has been reported using percutaneously deployed prosthetic grafts anchored to the arterial wall by proximal and distal metallic stents.[215] Endovascular stent grafts have also been used in carotid and other peripheral arteries and represent a promising alternative to surgical revascularization.

PERCUTANEOUS BALLOON VALVULOPLASTY

AORTIC VALVULOPLASTY (see also p. 1044). Although surgical valve replacement has proven to be highly effective treatment for aortic valve stenosis, surgical mortality and morbidity may be elevated in some patients, particularly the elderly or those with other comorbidities. Percutaneous balloon valvuloplasty has thus been proposed as a less invasive means of treating aortic stenosis. Although early experience with this procedure demonstrated encouraging acute procedural results, short-lived hemodynamic benefit and high rates of restenosis were subsequently documented. Percutaneous treatment of aortic stenosis is now reserved primarily for patients who are either (1) not candidates for surgical valve replacement, but in whom balloon valvuloplasty would be expected to palliate severe symptoms or stabilize cardiogenic shock, or (2) potentially suitable for definitive surgical treatment in the future but first require stabilization of aortic stenosis for urgent noncardiac surgery.

Both anterograde and retrograde approaches have been described, the latter performed via puncture of the interatrial septum. The aortic valve is crossed with an extra stiff guidewire, over which a dilation balloon measuring 15 to 23 mm in diameter is passed; correct sizing of the balloon is accomplished by either echocardiographic or radiographic measurements or by increasing balloon sizes until inflation produces transient hypotension. Multiple inflations are performed until the properly sized balloon is fully inflated. If results of dilatation are suboptimal (aortic valve area less than 0.5 cm^2) despite full inflation, a double balloon technique may be employed. Balloon dilatation improves the valvular cross-sectional area primarily by fracture of calcific deposits, although to a lesser extent, splitting of fused commissures or stretching of the valvular annulus also occurs. Acute complications of aortic valvuloplasty include aortic regurgitation, leaflet avulsion or aortic rupture, ventricular perforation, systemic embolization or stroke, and peripheral vascular injury from the large-bore catheters and sheaths.

Acutely following aortic balloon valvuloplasty, the aortic valve area is typically doubled and the transvalvular gradient halved.[216,217] Most patients experience an improvement in functional status,[216,217] and subsequent mortality risk is likely reduced if the valve area has been increased to greater than 0.7 cm^2. Long-term outcome appears to be best among patients with preserved left ventricular function[219] and those in whom echocardiography performed several days after the procedure demonstrates sustained improvement in valve area and gradient (thus, minimal annular recoil).[218] Overall, however, more than half of patients develop recurrence of symptoms during the first 6 months and the vast majority within 1 year following successful aortic valvuloplasty, although symptomatic improvement may persist despite evidence of valvular restenosis by cardiac catheterization.[216,217]

MITRAL VALVULOPLASTY (see also p. 1016). In contrast to aortic valvuloplasty, percutaneous mitral balloon valvuloplasty has been shown to provide substantial and sustained clinical benefit in selected patients with rheumatic mitral stenosis. Immediate hemodynamic results are usually excellent and procedural complications uncommon, with long-term outcome among suitable patients similar to that among patients treated with open surgical commissurotomy.[220]

There is no one standard technique of balloon mitral valvuloplasty. The valve is usually approached in an anterograde direction via an interatrial septal puncture, although a retrograde technique has been reported. One or two tubular balloons or a specialized nylon-rubber (Inoue) balloon is advanced across the mitral valve and repetitive inflations performed until the balloons have fully expanded (Fig. 39–14). The Inoue technique is less cumbersome and as effective as valvuloplasty performed using single or double tubular balloons, and generally results in a smaller atrial septal puncture. The mechanism of improvement in the valve area is via splitting of fused commissures. Acute complications include leaflet tears or chordal or papillary rupture leading to mitral regurgitation, ventricular perforation, tamponade resulting from transseptal puncture, and systemic embolization.

Hemodynamic improvement following mitral valvuloplasty occurs immediately, with valve area increasing on average by 1.0 cm^2, with a prompt drop in pulmonary pres-

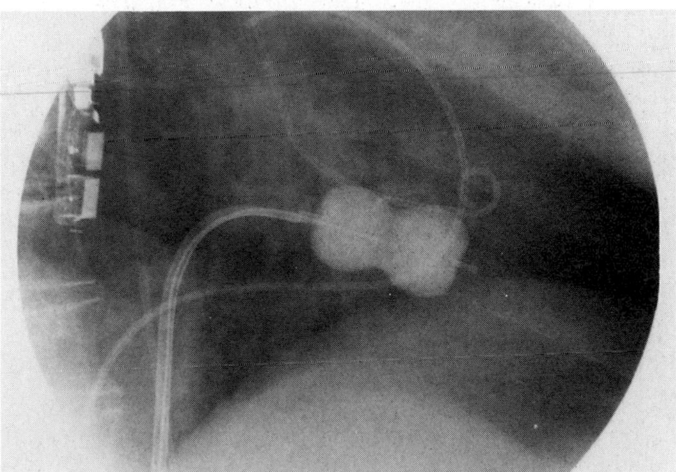

FIGURE 39–14. Cineangiogram frame during mitral valvuloplasty using Inoue balloon. The "waist" of the inflating balloon is within the stenotic mitral valve. A pigtail catheter within the left ventricle and a pulmonary artery catheter are also visible.

sures (Fig. 32–8, p. 1016).[221] Echocardiographic criteria have been developed to identify which patients with symptomatic mitral stenosis are most likely to derive benefit from this procedure[222]; these criteria have been shown to be the most important predictors of procedural outcome. The valve is assessed on the basis of four characteristics, each of which is graded on a scale of 0 to 4 (favorable to unfavorable): leaflet mobility, valvular thickening, subvalvular thickening, and valvular calcification. A good procedural result (valve area >1.5 cm^2) was obtained in 91 per cent of patients with a cumulative score of 8 or less but only 33 per cent of those with echocardiographic scores greater than 12 in a large single center experience.[221] Outcome by 4 years follow-up was generally good, with 91 per cent of patients alive and 67 per cent free from mitral valve replacement or severe (NYHA Class III–IV) heart failure.[221] Long-term outcome in this cohort was best among patients with lower echocardiographic scores, no mitral calcification on fluoroscopy, no atrial fibrillation, good functional class prior to valvuloplasty, and a large immediate postprocedural valve area. A randomized trial comparing mitral balloon valvuloplasty to open surgical commissurotomy among patients with favorable valvular anatomy demonstrated comparable initial hemodynamic results and clinical outcome among patients treated with either technique, although hemodynamic findings at 3 years were more favorable in the balloon valvuloplasty group.[220]

INTERVENTIONS FOR CONGENITAL HEART DISEASE

(See also Chap. 29)

Since the origin of the field of interventional cardiology in 1966 with balloon atrial septostomy,[2] a procedure directed at congenital heart disease, pediatric interventional cardiologists have developed percutaneous techniques for relieving congenital valvular and great vessel stenoses and transcatheter closure of aberrant vascular channels. Some of these methods, such as pulmonary balloon valvuloplasty, have gained widespread acceptance, whereas others are in early stages of clinical investigation.

BALLOON VALVULOPLASTY. Percutaneous balloon dilation of isolated congenital semilunar valvular stenoses has proven to be highly effective in providing long-term hemodynamic and symptomatic benefit in neonatal, pediatric, and adult patients. The pathology of congenital pulmonic and aortic stenosis consists of variable degrees of valvular deformity and commissural fusion, but, in contrast to acquired forms of valvular heart disease, severe thickening and calcification are less frequently present. Balloon valvuloplasty in these patients thus substantially reduces the extent of ventricular outflow obstruction, primarily through splitting along the lines of commissural fusion, although tearing of the valve leaflets may occur as well.

Kan and associates described the first clinical application of balloon valvuloplasty[223] in 1982, in which excellent acute improvement in transvalvular gradient was achieved in five children with *pulmonary valve stenosis.* In the report of the Pediatric Valvuloplasty Registry[224] in which 784 children underwent this procedure, mean gradient decreased acutely from 71 to 28 mm Hg, with the least benefit observed among patients with pulmonary valve dysplasia. Procedural mortality was only 0.2 per cent. Pulmonary valvuloplasty may be particularly challenging in neonates with severe stenosis or pulmonary atresia, in whom catheterization of the pulmonary artery may be difficult and require graded dilatation (see p. 926). Among the limited number of patients for whom long-term (2 to 5 years) follow-up is available, late results of pulmonic valvuloplasty appear to be excellent.[225,226] Valve gradients have on average been even lower than those immediately following valvuloplasty,[225,226] with less frequent development of pulmonic regurgitation or ventricular arrhythmias than in matched patients treated surgically.[226] Balloon pulmonary valvuloplasty may therefore be curative for patients with pulmonary stenosis and is considered the procedure of choice.

Unlike pulmonary valve stenosis, *congenital aortic stenosis* tends to be progressive over time, with a substantial rate of restenosis over 5 to 20 years following surgical valvotomy. Balloon aortic valvuloplasty can be performed in this group of patients with a satisfactory acute outcome (see p. 918); among 204 patients in the Pediatric Valvuloplasty Registry,[224] mean transvalvular gradient decreased from 77 to 30 mm Hg. Mortality risk was 2.4 per cent, confined entirely to patients 3 months old or less, with 10.2 per cent of patients exhibiting some increase in aortic regurgitation. Although long-term follow-up data are not yet available, no restenosis was observed in one series by a mean of 1.7 years after aortic valvuloplasty.[227]

OTHER PERCUTANEOUS INTERVENTIONS FOR CONGENITAL HEART DISEASE. Pulmonary artery stenosis or hypoplasia may be effectively treated by catheter-based technologies (see p. 924). Success rates following balloon dilatation of these vessels have ranged from 50 to 60 per cent, with failures due primarily to elastic recoil.[228] The use of balloon-expandable intraluminal stents is under investigation, with very encouraging immediate and short-term results in the limited number of patients studied thus far.[229] Long-term effectiveness and management strategies following stent placement in growing children must be evaluated. There has also been a limited experience with balloon angioplasty or stent placement for management of aortic coarctation, venous obstruction, or stenoses of Fontan shunts.

A variety of devices for transcatheter closure of the atrial septal defect, patent ductus arteriosus (PDA), or anomalous systemic-pulmonary collateral vessels are under preclinical or clinical evaluation. Current implants for closure of atrial septal defects are based on a double-disc design, in which part of the device lies in the right and left atria on either side of the defect. Small to moderate-size atrial septal defects have been effectively closed using clamshell or buttoned occluder devices in early clinical trials, although deployment failures, residual interatrial shunting, or late embolic events or device failures have been reported in a sizeable proportion of patients.[230,231] The Rashkind PDA Occluder, another double-disc design, has been investigated for closure of the persistently patent ductus arteriosus in over 650 patients, with low mortality risk and a 5 to 10 per cent rate of residual ductus murmur.[232] Embolization coils and a modified buttoned occluder are also under evaluation for patent ductus arteriosus closure.

QUALITY OF CARE AND CREDENTIALING

Advances in the technology for percutaneous coronary revascularization have been accompanied by a dramatic increase in the number of procedures carried out in the United States as well as a proliferation in the number of operators and sites performing these interventions. In a survey by the American College of Cardiology, fully 43 per cent of members stated that they performed coronary angioplasty.[233] Several studies have highlighted considerable variability in practice patterns and outcome associated with percutaneous revascularization procedures. An examination of a private insurance data base, for example, demonstrated substantial differences between geographical regions and types of hospitals with respect to per capita rates of coronary angioplasty, utilization of preprocedural functional testing, hospital charges and length of stay, and crossover to bypass surgery.[6] Indications for coronary revascularization in studies conducted in New York state were found to be much more frequently "uncertain" or "inappropriate" for angioplasty[234] than for coronary bypass surgery.[235]

Operator and institutional experience and caseload appear to substantially influence angioplasty practice and outcome. The number of cases per interventional operator per year in the United States has been estimated to range widely from 1 to 700, but with a median of only 22 to 35.[236] Similarly, a recent Medicare data base analysis revealed that the annual volume of angioplasty procedures per hospital carried out in Medicare beneficiaries ranged from 1 to 987, with half of patients treated at centers that performed 54 or fewer angioplasties in this patient population per year.[237] Two large-scale studies have demonstrated that mortality and complications occur more frequently among patients treated at low-volume centers. In a statewide survey of angioplasty procedures performed among nearly 25,000 patients in California,[238] the risk of death or emergency coronary bypass surgery was 43 to 49 per cent higher at centers performing less than 200 cases per year than at centers with annual institutional volumes of more than 400 cases. A larger analysis of more than 217,000 Medicare patients treated throughout the United States confirmed the association between outcome and institutional volume, noting a fall in 30-day mortality from 4.2 per cent among patients treated at lowest volume sites to 2.7 per cent at high-volume centers.[237]

Based upon recognition of the consistent association between operator skill and experience and efficacy of percutaneous revascularization, the American College of Cardiology and American Heart Association have promulgated guidelines for minimal levels of training and experience.[7] The American Board of Internal Medicine is considering a Certificate of Added Qualification for interventional cardiology equivalent to that for cardiac electrophysiology. For the time being, however, credentialing in interventional cardiology is at the discretion of individual institutions. Nevertheless, it is recommended that interventional operators have undergone a formal angioplasty training program, during which a minimum of 125 procedures, including 75 as the primary operator, were performed. It should be noted that these guidelines for operator volume were derived empirically without prospective validation.[7] Further, in order to maintain privileges to carry out coronary angioplasty, a minimum of 75 procedures should be performed each year as primary operator. Finally, it is recommended that an institutional minimum of 200 cases annually is "essential for maintenance of quality and safe care."[7] The issue of institutional and operator procedural volume is even more problematic when new devices for percutaneous revascularization are considered; assessment of competence is complex owing to the steep "learning curves" associated with many of these devices, their relatively infrequent use at many centers, and the absence of validated mechanisms of teaching operators who are not part of training programs.

FUTURE DIRECTIONS

The remarkable development of new and enhanced techniques for percutaneous coronary revascularization over the last 15 years has led to considerable expansion in the list of candidates for the procedure and improvements in immediate and long-term outcome. Continued progress is certain. While the technology for balloon angioplasty may remain relatively stable, the development of new devices for percutaneous revascularization will continue, with somewhat more enlightened and realistic expectations of the biological responses within the coronary artery. Indications and methods for existing modalities will be refined, with randomized trials playing a key role in defining the specific settings for their use. Novel technologies will be introduced and developed, directed at the efficient removal or modification of arterial plaque with minimal arterial trauma or at site-specific drug delivery to inhibit thrombosis and restenosis. Concurrently, as intravascular ultrasound and angioscopy will be further refined and integrated into revascularization devices, allowing precise guidance and optimization of plaque ablation or remodeling while limiting associated coronary injury. Finally, understanding of the vascular biology of percutaneous revascularization, thrombosis, and restenosis will improve, leading to pharmacological therapies designed to ameliorate adverse thrombotic, proliferative, and remodeling responses. It is realistic to expect that both acute-phase results and long-term outcome of percutaneous revascularization can be markedly improved, with further extension of these techniques in the management of obstructive coronary artery disease.

REFERENCES

HISTORY

1. Cournand, A. F., and Ranges, H. S.: Catheterization of the right auricle in man. Proc. Soc. Exp. Biol. Med. *46*:462, 1941.
2. Rashkind, W. J., and Miller, W. W.: Creation of an atrial septal defect without thoracotomy: Palliative approach to complete transposition of the great vessels. JAMA *196*:991, 1966.
3. Dotter, C. T., and Judkins, M. P.: Transluminal treatment of arteriosclerotic obstruction: Description of a new technique and preliminary report of its application. Circulation *30*:654, 1964.
4. Gruentzig, A. R.: Transluminal dilatation of coronary artery stenosis (letter). Lancet *1*:263, 1978.

PERCUTANEOUS TRANSLUMINAL CORONARY ANGIOPLASTY

5. Gruentzig, A. R., Senning, A., and Siegenthaler, W. E.: Nonoperative dilatation of coronary-artery stenosis. Percutaneous transluminal coronary angioplasty. N. Engl. J. Med. *301*:61, 1979.
6. Topol, E. J., Ellis, S. G., Cosgrove, D. M., et al.: Analysis of coronary angioplasty practice in the United States with an insurance-claims data base. Circulation *87*:1489, 1993.
7. Ryan, T. J., Bauman, W. B., Kennedy, J. W., et al.: Guidelines for percutaneous transluminal coronary angioplasty. A report of the American College of Cardiology/American Heart Association Task Force on Assessment of Diagnostic and Therapeutic Cardiovascular Procedures (Committee on Percutaneous Transluminal Coronary Angioplasty). J. Am. Coll. Cardiol. *22*:2033, 1993.
8. Ohman, E. M., Marquis, J. F., Ricci, D. R., et al.: A randomized comparison of the effects of gradual prolonged versus standard primary balloon inflation on early and late outcome. Results of a multicenter clinical trial. Circulation *89*:1118, 1994.
9. Honye, J., Mahon, D. J., Jain, A., et al.: Morphological effects of coronary balloon angioplasty in vivo assessed by intravascular ultrasound imaging. Circulation *85*:1012, 1992.
10. Waller, B. F.: Coronary luminal shape and the arc of disease free wall: Morphologic observations and clinical relevance. J. Am. Coll. Cardiol. *6*:1100, 1985.
11. Detre, K., Holubkov, R., Kelsey, S., et al.: Percutaneous transluminal coronary angioplasty in 1985–1986 and 1977–1981. The National Heart, Lung, and Blood Registry. N. Engl. J. Med. *318*:265, 1988.
12. Kahn, J. K., and Hartzler, G. O.: Frequency and causes of failure with contemporary balloon coronary angioplasty and implications for new technologies. Am. J. Cardiol. *66*:858, 1990.
13. Myler, R. K., Shaw, R. E., Stertzer, S. H., et al.: Lesion morphology and coronary angioplasty: Current experience and analysis. J. Am. Coll. Cardiol. *19*:1641, 1992.
14. Wong, J. B., Sonnenberg, F. A., Salem, D. N., and Pauker, S. G.: Myocardial revascularization for chronic stable angina. Analysis of the role of percutaneous transluminal coronary angioplasty based on data available in 1989. Ann. Intern. Med. *113*:852, 1990.
15. Rosing, D. R., Cannon, R. D., Watson, R. M., et al.: Three year anatomic, functional, and clinical follow-up after successful percutaneous transluminal coronary angioplasty. J. Am. Coll. Cardiol. *9*:1, 1987.
16. Faxon, D. P., Ruocco, N., and Jacobs, A. K.: Long-term outcome of patients after percutaneous transluminal coronary angioplasty. Circulation *81*:IV-9, 1990.
17. Gruentzig, A. R., King, S. B., Schlumpf, M., and Siegenthaler, W.: Long-term follow-up after percutaneous transluminal coronary angioplasty. The early Zurich experience. N. Engl. J. Med. *316*:1127, 1987.
18. Ellis, S. G., Cowley, M. J., Whitlow, P. L., et al.: Prospective case-control comparison of percutaneous transluminal coronary revascularization in patients with multivessel disease treated in 1986–1987 versus 1991: Improved in-hospital and 12-month results. Multivessel Angioplasty Prognosis Study (MAPS) Group. J. Am. Coll. Cardiol. *25*:1137, 1995.
19. Kuntz, R. E., Piana, R., Pomerantz, R. M., et al.: Changing incidence and management of abrupt closure following coronary intervention in the new device era. Cathet. Cardiovasc. Diagn. *27*:189, 1992.

20. Detre, K. M., Holmes, D. R., Holubkov, R., et al.: Incidence and consequences of periprocedural occlusion. The 1985–1986 National Heart, Lung, and Blood Institute percutaneous transluminal coronary angioplasty registry. Circulation *82:*739, 1990.
21. de Feyter, P. J., van den Brand, M., Jaarman, G. J., et al.: Acute coronary artery occlusion during and after percutaneous transluminal coronary angioplasty. Frequency, prediction, clinical course, management, and follow-up. Circulation *83:*927, 1991.
22. Lincoff, A. M., Popma, J. J., Ellis, S. G., et al.: Abrupt vessel closure complicating coronary angioplasty: Clinical, angiographic, and therapeutic profile. J. Am. Coll. Cardiol. *19:*926, 1992.
23. Schwartz, L., Bourassa, M. G., Lesperance, J., et al.: Aspirin and dipyridamole in the prevention of restenosis after percutaneous transluminal coronary angioplasty. N. Engl. J. Med. *318:*1714, 1988.
24. Laskey, M. A., Deutsch, E., Barnathan, E., et al.: Influence of heparin therapy on percutaneous transluminal coronary angioplasty outcome in unstable angina pectoris. Am. J. Cardiol. *65:*1425, 1990.
25. Laskey, M. A., Deutsch, E., Hirshfeld, J. W. J., et al.: Influence of heparin therapy on percutaneous transluminal coronary angioplasty outcome in patients with coronary arterial thrombus. Am. J. Cardiol. *65:*179, 1990.
26. McGarry, T. F., Gottlieb, R. S., Morganroth, J., et al.: The relationship of anticoagulation level and complications after successful percutaneous transluminal coronary angioplasty. Am. Heart J. *123:*1445, 1992.
27. Dougherty, K. G., Gaos, C. M., Bush, H. S., et al.: Activated clotting times and activated partial thromboplastin times in patients undergoing coronary angioplasty who receive bolus doses of heparin. Cathet. Cardiovasc. Diagn. *26:*260, 1992.
28. Bowers, J., and Ferguson, J. J.: The use of activated clotting times to monitor heparin therapy during and after interventional procedures. Clin. Cardiol. *17:*357, 1994.
29. Ellis, S. G., Roubin, G. S., Wilentz, J., et al.: Effect of 18- to 24-hour heparin administration for prevention of restenosis after uncomplicated coronary angioplasty. Am. Heart J. *117:*777, 1989.
30. Friedman, H. Z., Cragg, D. R., Glazier, S. M., et al.: Randomized prospective evaluation of prolonged versus abbreviated intravenous heparin therapy after coronary angioplasty. J. Am. Coll. Cardiol. *24:*1214, 1994.
31. Gabliani, G., Deligonul, U., Kern, M. J., and Vandormael, M.: Acute coronary occlusion occurring after successful percutaneous transluminal coronary angioplasty: Temporal relationship to discontinuation of anticoagulation. Am. Heart J. *116:*696, 1988.
32. Vaitkus, P. T., and Laskey, W. K.: Efficacy of adjunctive thrombolytic therapy in percutaneous transluminal coronary angioplasty. J. Am. Coll. Cardiol. *24:*1415, 1994.
33. Ambrose, J. A., Almeida, O. D., Sharma, S. K., et al.: Adjunctive thrombolytic therapy during angioplasty for ischemic rest angina. Results of the TAUSA Trial. Circulation *90:*69, 1994.
34. Roubin, G. S., Douglas, J. S., King, S. B., et al.: Influence of balloon size on initial success, acute complications, and restenosis after percutaneous transluminal coronary angioplasty. A prospective randomized study. Circulation *78:*557, 1988.
35. Nichols, A. B., Smith, R., Berke, A. D., et al.: Importance of balloon size in coronary angioplasty. J. Am. Coll. Cardiol. *13:*1094, 1989.
36. Tenaglia, A. N., Quigley, P. J., Kereiakes, D. J., et al.: Coronary angioplasty performed with gradual and prolonged inflation using a perfusion balloon catheter: Procedural success and restenosis rate. Am. Heart J. *124:*585, 1992.
37. Phillips, D. R., Charo, I. F., Parise, L. V., and Fitzgerald, L. A.: The platelet membrane glycoprotein IIb/IIIa complex. Blood *71:*831, 1988.
38. EPIC Investigators: Use of a monoclonal antibody directed against the platelet glycoprotein IIb/IIIa receptor in high-risk coronary angioplasty. N. Engl. J. Med. *330:*956, 1994.
39. Schieman, G., Cohen, B. M., Kozina, J., et al.: Intracoronary urokinase for intracoronary thrombus accumulation complicating percutaneous transluminal coronary angioplasty in acute ischemic syndromes. Circulation *82:*2052, 1990.
40. Lincoff, A. M., and Topol, E. J.: Abrupt vessel closure. *In* Topol, E. J. (ed.): Textbook of Interventional Cardiology. 2nd ed. Philadelphia, W. B. Saunders Company, 1994, p. 207.
41. de Feyter, P. J., Serruys, P. W., Soward, A., et al.: Coronary angioplasty for early postinfarction unstable angina. Circulation *74:*1365, 1986.
42. de Feyter, P. J., Suryapranata, H., Serruys, P. W., et al.: Coronary angioplasty for unstable angina: Immediate and late results in 200 consecutive patients with identification of risk factors for unfavorable early and late outcome. J. Am. Coll. Cardiol. *12:*324, 1988.
43. de Feyter, P. J.: Coronary angioplasty in unstable angina. Am. Heart J. *118:*860, 1989.
44. Myler, R. K., Shaw, R. E., Stertzer, S. H., et al.: Unstable angina and coronary angioplasty. Circulation *82:*II-88, 1990.
45. Stammen, F., De Scheerder, I., Glazier, J. J., et al.: Immediate and follow-up results of the conservative coronary angioplasty strategy for unstable angina pectoris. Am. J. Cardiol. *69:*1533, 1995.
46. Ellis, S. G., Vandormael, M. G., Cowley, M. J., et al.: Coronary morphologic and clinical determinants of procedural outcome with angioplasty for multivessel coronary disease. Implications for patient selection. Circulation *82:*1193, 1990.
47. Cowley, M. J., Dorros, G., [illegible], et al.: Acute coronary events associated with percutaneous transluminal coronary angioplasty. Am. J. Cardiol. *53:*12, 1984.
48. Ellis, S. G., Roubin, G. S., King, S. B., et al.: Angiographic and clinical predictors of acute closure after native vessel coronary angioplasty. Circulation *77:*372, 1988.
49. Kern, M. J., Deligonul, U., Galan, K., et al.: Percutaneous transluminal coronary angioplasty in octogenarians. Am. J. Cardiol. *61:*457, 1988.
50. Kelsey, S. F., Miller, D. P., Holubkov, R., et al.: Results of percutaneous transluminal coronary angioplasty in patients ≥ 65 years of age (from the 1985 to 1986 National Heart, Lung, and Blood Institute's coronary angioplasty registry). Am. J. Cardiol. *66:*1033, 1990.
51. Ryan, T. J., Faxon, D. P., Gunnar, R. M., et al.: Guidelines for percutaneous transluminal coronary angioplasty. A report of the American College of Cardiology/American Heart Association Task Force on assessment of diagnostic and therapeutic cardiovascular procedures (subcommittee on percutaneous transluminal coronary angioplasty). J. Am. Coll. Cardiol. *12:*529, 1988.
52. Tenaglia, A. N., Fortin, D. F., Frid, D. J., et al.: A simple scoring system to predict PTCA abrupt closure. J. Am. Coll. Cardiol. *19*(Abs.):139, 1992.
53. Black, A. J. R., Namay, D. L., Niederman, A. L., et al.: Tear of dissection after coronary angioplasty—morphologic correlates of an ischemic complication. Circulation *79:*1035, 1989.
54. Huber, M. S., Mooney, J. F., Madison, J., and Mooney, M. R.: Use of a morphologic classification to predict clinical outcome after dissection from coronary angioplasty. Am. J. Cardiol. *68:*467, 1991.
55. Ellis, S. G., Myler, R. K., King, S. B., et al.: Causes and correlates of death after unsupported coronary angioplasty: Implications for use of angioplasty and advanced support techniques in high-risk settings. Am. J. Cardiol. *68:*1447, 1991.
56. Ellis, S. G., Roubin, G. S., King, S. B., et al.: In-hospital cardiac mortality after acute closure after coronary angioplasty: Analysis of risk factors from 8,207 procedures. J. Am. Coll. Cardiol. *11:*211, 1988.
57. Califf, R. M., Phillips, H. R., Hindman, M. C., et al.: Prognostic value of a coronary artery jeopardy score. J. Am. Coll. Cardiol. *5:*1055, 1985.
58. Holmes, D. R. J., Holubkov, R., Vlietstra, R. E., et al.: Comparison of complications during percutaneous transluminal coronary angioplasty from 1977 to 1981 and from 1985 to 1986: The National Heart Lung, and Blood Institute Percutaneous Transluminal Coronary Angioplasty Registry. J. Am. Coll. Cardiol. *12:*1149, 1988.
59. Bergelson, B. A., Jacobs, A. K., Cupples, L. A., et al.: Prediction of risk for hemodynamic compromise during percutaneous transluminal coronary angioplasty. Am. J. Cardiol. *70:*1540, 1992.
60. Detre, K., Holubkov, R., Kelsey, S., et al.: One-year follow up results of the 1985–1986 National Heart, Lung, and Blood Institute's percutaneous transluminal coronary angioplasty registry. Circulation *80:*421, 1989.
61. O'Keefe, J. H. Jr., Rutherford, B. D., McConahay, D. R., et al.: Multivessel coronary angioplasty from 1980 to 1989: Procedural results and long-term outcome. J. Am. Coll. Cardiol. *16:*1097, 1990.
62. Mark, D. B., Nelson, C. L., Califf, R. M., et al.: Continuing evolution of therapy for coronary artery disease. Initial results from the era of coronary angioplasty. Circulation *89:*2015, 1994.
63. Talley, J. D., Hurst, J. W., King, S. B., et al.: Clinical outcome 5 years after attempted percutaneous transluminal coronary angioplasty in 427 patients. Circulation *77:*820, 1988.
64. King, S. B. I., and Schlumpf, M.: Ten-year completed follow-up of percutaneous transluminal coronary angioplasty: The early Zurich experience. J. Am. Coll. Cardiol. *22:*353, 1993.
65. Weintraub, W. S., Douglas, J. S., Morris, D. C., et al.: Long term follow-up after PTCA in patients with single and multivessel coronary artery disease. J. Am. Coll. Cardiol. *23*(Abs.):352, 1994.
66. Kent, K., Cowley, M., Detre, K., et al.: Report of five-year outcome for 1977–81 and 1985–86 cohorts of the NHLBI PTCA registry. J. Am. Coll. Cardiol. *86*(Abs.):I-55, 1992.
67. Bourassa, M. G., Holubkov, R., Yeh, W., et al.: Strategy of complete revascularization in patients with multivessel coronary artery disease (a report from the 1985–1986 NHLBI PTCA Registry). Am. J. Cardiol. *70:*174, 1992.
68. Bell, M. R., Bailey, K. R., Reeder, G. S., et al.: Percutaneous transluminal angioplasty in patients with multivessel coronary disease: How important is complete revascularization for cardiac event-free survival? J. Am. Coll. Cardiol. *16:*553, 1990.
69. Wohlgelernter, D., Cleman, M., Highman, H. A., and Zaret, B. L.: Percutaneous transluminal coronary angioplasty of the "culprit lesion" for management of unstable angina pectoris in patients with multivessel coronary disease. Am. J. Cardiol. *56:*460, 1986.
70. Jones, E. L., Craver, J. M., Guyton, R. A., et al.: Importance of complete revascularization in performance of the coronary bypass operation. Am. J. Cardiol. *51:*7, 1983.
71. Deligonul, U., Vandormael, M. G., Kern, M. J., et al.: Coronary angioplasty: A therapeutic option for symptomatic patients with two and three vessel coronary disease. J. Am. Coll. Cardiol. *11:*1173, 1988.
72. Faxon, D. P., Ghalilli, K., Jacobs, A. K., et al.: The degree of revascularization and outcome after multivessel coronary angioplasty. Am. Heart J. *123:*854, 1992.
73. Reeder, G. S., Holmes, D. R. J., Detre, K., et al.: Degree of revascularization in patients with multivessel coronary disease: A report from the National Heart, Lung, and Blood Institute percutaneous transluminal coronary angioplasty registry. Circulation *77:*638, 1988.
74. Leimgruber, P., Roubin, G. S., Hollman, J., et al.: Restenosis after successful coronary angioplasty in patients with single-vessel disease. Circulation [illegible]
75. Ellis, S. G., Roubin, G. S., King, S. B., et al.: Importance of stenosis morphology in the estimation of restenosis risk after elective per-

cutaneous transluminal coronary angioplasty. Am. J. Cardiol. *63*:30, 1989.
76. Holmes, D. R., Vlietstra, R. E., Smith, H. C., et al.: Restenosis after percutaneous transluminal coronary angioplasty: A report of the PTCA Registry of the National Heart, Lung, and Blood Institute. Am. J. Cardiol. *53*:77, 1984.
77. Nobuyoshi, M., Kimura, T., Ohishi, H., et al.: Restenosis after percutaneous transluminal coronary angioplasty: Pathologic observations in 20 patients. J. Am. Coll. Cardiol. *17*:433, 1991.
78. Popma, J. J., VanDenBerg, E. K., and Dehmer, G.: Long-term outcome of patients with asymptomatic restenosis after percutaneous transluminal coronary angioplasty. Am. J. Cardiol. *62*:1298, 1988.
79. Bengtson, J. R., Mark, D. B., Honan, M. B., et al.: Detection of restenosis after elective percutaneous transluminal coronary angioplasty using the exercise treadmill test. Am. J. Cardiol. *65*:28, 1990.
80. Hillegass, W. B., Ohman, E. M., and Califf, R. M.: Restenosis: the clinical issues. *In* Topol, E. J. (ed.): Textbook of Interventional Cardiology. 2nd ed. Philadelphia, W. B. Saunders Company, 1993, p. 415.
81. Serruys, P. W., Liujten, H. E., Beatt, K. J., et al.: Incidence of restenosis after successful coornary angioplasty: A time-related phenomenon. A quantitative angiographic study in 342 consecutive patients at 1, 2, 3, and 4 months. Circulation *77*:361, 1988.
82. Nobuyoshi, M., Kimura, T., Nosaka, H., et al.: Restenosis after successful percutaneous transluminal coronary angioplasty: Serial angiographic follow-up of 229 patients. J. Am. Coll. Cardiol. *12*:616, 1988.
83. Rensing, B. J., Hermans, W. R. M., Deckers, J. W., et al.: Lumen narrowing after percutaneous transluminal coronary balloon angioplasty follows a near gaussian distribution: A quantitative angiographic study in 1445 successfully dilated lesions. J. Am. Coll. Cardiol. *19*:939, 1992.
83a. Moliterno, D. J., and Topol, E. J.: Clinical evaluation of restenosis. *In* Fuster, V., Ross, R., and Topol, E. J. (eds.): Atherosclerosis and Coronary Artery Disease. Philadelphia, Lippincott-Raven, 1996, pp. 1505–1526.
84. Joelson, J. M., Most, A. S., and Williams, D. O.: Angiographic findings when chest pain recurs after successful percutaneous transluminal coronary angioplasty. Am. J. Cardiol. *60*:792, 1987.
85. Waller, B. F., Pinkerton, C. A., Orr, C. M., et al.: Restenosis 1 to 24 months after clinically successful coronary balloon angioplasty: A necropsy study of 20 patients. J. Am. Coll. Cardiol. *17*:58, 1991.
86. Waller, B. F., Pinkerton, C. A., Orr, C. M., et al.: Morphologic observations late (>30 days) after clinically successful coronary balloon angioplasty: An analysis of 20 necropsy patients and review of 41 necropsy patients with coronary angioplasty restenosis. Circulation *83*:I-90, 1991.
87. Post, M. J., Borst, C., and Kuntz, R. E.: The relative importance of arterial remodeling compared with intimal hyperplasia in lumen renarrowing after balloon angioplasty. A study in the normal rabbit and the hypercholesterolemic Yucatan micropig. Circulation *89*:2816, 1994.
88. Kakuta, T., Currier, J. W., Haudenschild, C. C., et al.: Differences in compensatory vessel enlargement, not intimal formation, account for restenosis after angioplasty in the hypercholesterolemic rabbit model. Circulation *89*:2809, 1994.
89. Mintz, G. S., Kovach, J. A., Javier, S. P., et al.: Geometric remodeling is the predominant mechanism of late lumen loss after coronary angioplasty. Circulation *88*(Abs.):I-654, 1993.
89a. Falk, E., and Nobuyoshi, M.: Differences between atherosclerosis and restenosis. Harrison, D.C.: Nonatherosclerotic coronary disease. *In* Fuster, V., Ross, R., and Topol, E. J. (eds.): Atherosclerosis and Coronary Artery Disease. Philadelphia, Lippincott-Raven, 1996, pp. 683–700.
90. Schwartz, R. S., Huber, K. C., Murphy, J. G., et al.: Restenosis and the proportional neointimal response to coronary artery injury: Results in a porcine model. J. Am. Coll. Cardiol. *19*:267, 1992.
91. Ip, J. H., Fuster, V., Badimon, L., et al.: Syndromes of accelerated atherosclerosis: Role of vascular injury and smooth muscle cell proliferation. J. Am. Coll. Cardiol. *15*:1667, 1990.
92. Clowes, A. W., Reidy, M. A., and Clowes, M. M.: Mechanisms of stenosis after arterial injury. Lab. Invest. *49*:208, 1983.
93. Clowes, A. W., and Schwartz, S. M.: Significance of quiescent smooth muscle migration in the injured rat carotid artery. Circ. Res. *56*:139, 1985.
94. Forrester, J. S., Fishbein, M., Helfant, R., and Fagin, J.: A paradigm for restenosis based on cell biology: Clues for the development of new preventive therapies. J. Am. Coll. Cardiol. *17*:758, 1991.
95. Glagov, S.: Intimal hyperplasia, vascular modeling, and the restenosis problem. Circulation *89*:2888, 1994.
96. Schwartz, R. S., Holmes, D. R., and Topol, E. J.: The restenosis paradigm revisited: An alternative proposal for cellular mechanisms. J. Am. Coll. Cardiol. *20*:1284, 1992.
97. Lindner, V., Lappi, D. A., Baird, A., et al.: Role of basic fibroblast growth factor in vascular lesion formation. Circ. Res. *68*:106, 1991.
98. Hirshfeld, J. W., Schwartz, J. S., Jugo, R., et al.: Restenosis after coronary angioplasty: A multivariate statistical model to relate lesion and procedure variables to restenosis. J. Am. Coll. Cardiol. *18*:647, 1991.
99. Lambert, M., Bonan, R., Cote, G., et al.: Multiple coronary angioplasty: A model to discriminate systemic and procedural factors related to restenosis. J. Am. Coll. Cardiol. *12*:310, 1988.
100. Guiteras, V. P., Bourassa, M. G., David, P. R., et al.: Restenosis after successful percutaneous transluminal coronary angioplasty: The Montreal Heart Institute experience. Am. J. Cardiol. *60*:50, 1987.
101. Bertrand, M. E., Lablanche, J. M., Fourrier, J. L., et al.: Relation to restenosis after percutaneous transluminal coronary angioplasty to vasomotion of the dilated coronary arterial segment. Am. J. Cardiol. *63*:277, 1989.
102. Bertrand, M. E., LaBlanche, J. M., Thieuleux, F. A., et al.: Comparative results of percutaneous transluminal coronary angioplasty in patients with dynamic versus fixed coronary stenosis. J. Am. Coll. Cardiol. *8*:504, 1986.
103. Corcos, T., David, P. R., Bourassa, M. G., et al.: Percutaneous transluminal coronary angioplasty for the treatment of variant angina. J. Am. Coll. Cardiol. *5*:1046, 1985.
104. Austin, G. E., Lynn, M., and Hollman, J.: Laboratory test results as predictors of recurrent coronary artery stenosis following angioplasty. Arch. Pathol. Lab. Med. *111*:1158, 1987.
105. Kuntz, R. E., Gibson, C. M., Nobuyoshi, M., and Baim, D. S.: Generalized model of restenosis after conventional balloon angioplasty, stenting, and directional atherectomy. J. Am. Coll. Cardiol. *21*:15, 1993.
105a. Pratt, R. E., and Dzau, V. J.: Pharmacological strategies to prevent restenosis. Lessons learned from blockade of the renin-angiotensin system. Circulation *93*:848, 1996.
106. Popma, J. J., Califf, R. M., and Topol, E. J.: Clinical trials of restenosis after coronary angioplasty. Circulation *84*:1426, 1991.
107. Topol, E. J., Califf, R. M., Weisman, H. S., et al.: Reduction of clinical restenosis following coronary intervention with early administration of platelet IIb/IIIa integrin blocking antibody. Lancet *343*:881, 1994.
108. Fischman, D. L., Leon, M. B., Baim, D. S., et al.: A randomized comparison of coronary-stent placement and balloon angioplasty in the treatment of coronary artery disease. N. Engl. J. Med. *331*:496, 1994.
109. Serruys, P. W., de Jaegere, P., Kiemeneij, F., et al.: A comparison of balloon-expandable-stent implantation with balloon angioplasty in patients with coronary artery disease. N. Engl. J. Med. *331*:489, 1994.
109a. Macaya, C., Serruys, P. W., Ruygrok, P., et al.: Continued benefit of coronary stenting versus balloon angioplasty: One-year clinical follow-up of Benestent trial. J. Am. Coll. Cardiol. *27*:255, 1996.
110. Hernandez, R. A., Macaya, C., Iniguez, A., et al.: Midterm outcome of patients with asymptomatic restenosis after coronary balloon angioplasty. J. Am. Coll. Cardiol. *19*:1402, 1992.
111. Teirstein, P. S., Hoover, C. A., Ligon, R. W., et al.: Repeat coronary angioplasty: Efficacy of a third angioplasty for a second restenosis. J. Am. Coll. Cardiol. *13*:291, 1989.
112. Black, A. J. R., Anderson, V., Roubin, G. S., et al.: Repeat coronary angioplasty: Correlates of a second restenosis. J. Am. Coll. Cardiol. *11*:714, 1988.
113. Parisi, A. F., Folland, E. D., Hartigan, P., and Veterans Affairs ACME Investigators: A comparison of angioplasty with medical therapy in the treatment of single-vessel coronary artery disease. N. Engl. J. Med. *326*:10, 1992.
114. Folland, E. D., Parisi, A. F., Hartigan, P., for the VA ACME Investigators: PTCA vs medicine for double vessel disease: Initial results of the randomzied VA ACME trial. Circulation *84*(Abs.):II-252, 1991.
115. RITA Trial Participants: Coronary angioplasty versus coronary artery bypass surgery: The Randomized Intervention Treatment of Angina (RITA) trial. Lancet *335*:1315, 1993.
116. Rodriguez, A., Boullon, F., Perez-Balino, N., et al.: Argentine randomized trial of percutaneous transluminal coronary angioplasty versus coronary artery bypass surgery in multivessel disease (ERACI): In-hospital results and 1-year follow up. J. Am. Coll. Cardiol. *22*:1060, 1993.
117. Hamm, C. W., Reimers, J., Ischinger, T., et al.: A randomized study of coronary angioplasty compared with bypass surgery in patients with symptomatic multivessel coronary disease. N. Engl. J. Med. *331*:1037, 1994.
118. King, S. B., Lembo, N. J., Weintraub, W. S., et al.: A randomized trial comparing coronary angioplasty with coronary bypass surgery. N. Engl. J. Med. *331*:1044, 1994.
119. Moliterno, D. J., Elliott, J. M., and Topol, E. J.: Randomized trials of myocardial revascularization. *In* O'Rourke, R. A. (ed.): Current Problems in Cardiology. Vol. XX. Linn, MO, C. V. Mosby, 1995, p. 121.
120. Goy, J. J., Eeckhout, E., Burnand, B., et al.: Coronary angioplasty versus left internal mammary artery grafting for isolated proximal left anterior descending artery stenosis. Lancet *343*:1449, 1994.
121. Mark, D. B., Lam, L. C., Lee, K. L., et al.: Effects of coronary angioplasty, coronary bypass surgery, and medical therapy on employment in patients with coronary artery disease. A prospective comparison study. Ann. Intern. Med. *120*:111, 1994.
122. Eckman, M. H., Wong, J. B., Salem, D. N., and Pauker, S. G.: Direct angioplasty for acute myocardial infarction. A review of outcomes in clinical subsets. Ann. Intern. Med. *117*:667, 1992.
123. O'Keefe, J. H., Rutherford, B. D., McConahay, D. D. R., et al.: Early and late results of coronary angioplasty without antecedent thrombolytic therapy for acute myocardial infarction. Am. J. Cardiol. *64*:1221, 1989.
124. Grines, C. L., Browne, K. F., Marco, J., et al.: A comparison of immediate angioplasty with thrombolytic therapy for acute myocardial infarction. N. Engl. J. Med. *328*:673, 1993.
125. de Boer, M. J., Hoorntje, J. C. A., Ottervanger, J. P., et al.: Immediate coronary angioplasty versus intravenous streptokinase in acute myocardial infarction: Left ventricular ejection fraction, hospital mortality and reinfarction. J. Am. Coll. Cardiol. *23*:1004, 1994.
126. Gibbons, R. J., Holmes, D. R., Reeder, G. S., et al.: Immediate angioplasty compared with the administration of a thrombolytic agent followed by conservative treatment for myocardial infarction. N. Engl. J. Med. *328*:685, 1993.
127. Ribeiro, E. E., Silva, L. A., Carneiro, R., et al.: A randomized trial of direct PTCA vs intravenous streptokinase in acute myocardial infarction. J. Am. Coll. Cardiol. *17*:152, 1991.
128. TIMI Research Group: Immediate vs. delayed catheterization and angio-

dial perfusion even in the absence of formal exercise training.[19,20]

OTHER FACTORS. Concomitant illnesses, such as chronic obstructive pulmonary disease and peripheral vascular disease, can limit the capacity for exercise before the effects of ischemia or left ventricular dysfunction are manifested. The common cardiovascular drugs, including nitrates, beta blockers, and calcium channel blockers, increase the exercise capacity by increasing coronary blood flow, decreasing myocardial oxygen demand, or improving hemodynamics during exercise.[21–23] Angiotensin-converting enzyme inhibitors appear to be particularly beneficial for increasing capacity for exercise in patients with congestive heart failure, probably because of their effects on peripheral circulation.[24–26]

Effects of Exercise Training

SKELETAL MUSCLE. The primary physiological improvements from exercise training are on skeletal muscle performance and are directly related to increases in capillary density, oxidative enzyme content, myoglobin concentration,[6,14] and increased numbers and size of mitochondria.[27] These changes increase skeletal muscle perfusion and the efficiency of extraction of oxygen.

MYOCARDIAL PERFORMANCE. Current evidence suggests that myocardial performance may improve in patients with coronary disease subjected to training programs that are either of a higher intensity, greater frequency, or longer duration than those traditionally provided in cardiac rehabilitation.[28,29] In contrast to low- and moderate-intensity programs, patients in high-intensity programs have shown improvements in myocardial oxygenation using electrocardiographic and perfusion measures.[29,30] The minimal intensity, frequency, and duration required for such effects have not been established.

Exercise training lowers heart rate and blood pressure at rest and, at submaximal exercise, increases peak MET capacity and increases both endurance and strength. The lower the initial MET capacity, the greater the benefit in most patients.[31,32] Patients with a combination of myocardial ischemia and resting left ventricular dysfunction are less likely to benefit from short-term exercise training.[33] Treatment with beta blockers does not prevent a training effect in patients with coronary heart disease although the training effect may be blunted.[22] Other benefits of exercise, include reduction of weight, improved glucose tolerance in patients with diabetes, raised high-density lipoprotein (HDL) cholesterol levels, and psychological benefits including a greater confidence to resume customary activities more quickly.[31,34]

MORBIDITY AND MORTALITY. Exercise training has not been definitively shown to improve morbidity and mortality in patients with coronary heart disease. Only one of 22 randomized trials of cardiac rehabilitation with exercise training demonstrated a statistically significant cardiovascular mortality benefit.[35] However, all other studies were limited by inadequate sample size, short follow-up or crossovers after randomization. Two meta-analyses showed that overall mortality and cardiovascular mortality, defined as fatal reinfarction or sudden death, were reduced by 20 per cent to 25 per cent in patients randomized to exercise training. Rates of nonfatal reinfarction were similar in exercise and control groups[36,37] (Fig. 40–2). The magnitude of benefit is similar to that seen in the randomized trials of prophylactic beta blockade after myocardial infarction,[38] suggesting that exercise training may be equally beneficial.

Selection of Patients for Exercise Testing and Training

PATIENTS ELIGIBLE FOR EXERCISE TRAINING. The indications for exercise training have been expanded to include higher-risk patients in recent years. The safety and efficacy of training in patients previously considered to be at high risk, particularly those with congestive heart failure, has

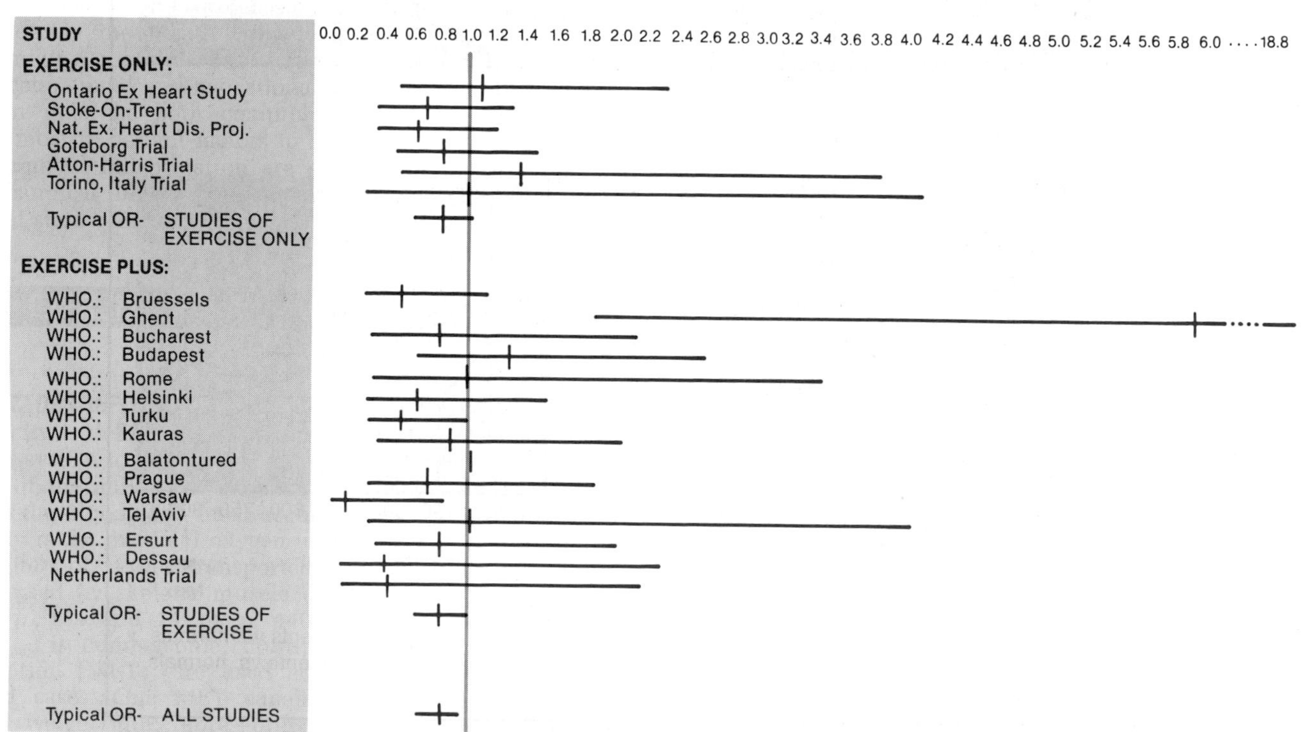

FIGURE 40–2. Chart of effects of pooling from randomized trials of cardiac rehabilitation on the estimate of mortality 3 years after randomization. Short vertical lines indicate the point estimates; horizontal lines depict the 95 per cent confidence intervals. "Exercise Plus" usually refers to life style and dietary modifications in both the exercise and control groups. (Reproduced with permission from O'Connor, G. T., Buring, J. E., Yusuf, S., et al.: An overview of randomized trials of rehabilitation with exercise after myocardial infarction. Circulation *80*:234, 1989. Copyright American Heart Association.)

been demonstrated. Exercise training benefits patients recovering from myocardial infarction, coronary artery bypass graft surgery, coronary angioplasty, valve surgery and cardiac transplantation, and those with stable angina and compensated congestive heart failure.[31,34,39,40] Prescription for exercise should be based upon the results of exercise tests. Cardiopulmonary stress testing may provide additional information helpful for prescribing exercise training in patients with congestive heart failure.[27,41] Patients ineligible for exercise testing because of severe angina, uncompensated congestive heart failure, and uncontrolled arrhythmias are not candidates for exercise training. Other limiting noncardiac illnesses such as chronic obstructive pulmonary disease, peripheral vascular disease, stroke, and orthopedic disease do not necessarily obviate exercise testing and training because specialized techniques, such as arm-crank ergometry, can be used.[42]

EXERCISE TESTING. Exercise testing to a symptom or sign limit should be performed as soon after a cardiac event as the patient's condition permits. In uncomplicated cases, testing can be performed 7 to 21 days after myocardial infarction,[43] 3 to 10 days following coronary angioplasty,[44] and 14 to 28 days following cardiac surgery. Exercise testing is performed later in patients who have undergone cardiac surgery to minimize the detrimental effects of wound healing and pulmonary dysfunction on performance of exercise.

Submaximal exercise testing is commonly used prior to or soon after discharge from hospital because of the perceived safety of such testing compared with maximal testing (see also Chap. 5). Maximal testing is then performed at 6 to 8 weeks following discharge from hospital. However, there is no evidence that submaximal testing is safer than symptom-limited testing in properly selected patients,[43] and there are disadvantages to submaximal testing. Prognostically important signs of myocardial ischemia, left ventricular dysfunction and arrhythmias, may not be elicited by submaximal testing. Patients may be inappropriately limited in their customary activities and in exercise training if submaximal testing is used to evaluate physical capacity.[45,46] Return to work may be significantly delayed.[47,48]

Because capacity for exercise is reduced in patients recovering from a cardiac event, a modified treadmill protocol should be used. Table 40-1 compares the standard Bruce protocol with a modified Naughton protocol. The Bruce protocol increases by 2 to 3 METs at each stage and quickly surpasses the average capacity of patients recovering from a cardiac event. The modified Naughton protocol starts at a lower MET workload and increases at 1-MET increments. This gradual progression is better tolerated and provides a more accurate assessment of MET capacity. The usual symptomatic endpoints are dyspnea and fatigue, whereas moderate angina, dizziness, and claudication occur less commonly. Signs that are important endpoints include high-grade ventricular arrhythmias (such as triplets), a fall in systolic blood pressure of 20 mm Hg compared with the previous stage, and marked ischemia.

Although the exercise test is the basis of the prescription for exercise, certain test results contraindicate exercise training. Severe exercise-induced ischemia, arrhythmias, or left ventricular dysfunction must be corrected before patients can be allowed to exercise. Exercise testing should be repeated after treatment to confirm that the abnormalities, in fact, have resolved. Less severe abnormalities that occur at high heart rates and workloads are not necessarily contraindications to exercise training, especially if patients are being given maximal medical therapy, and no other treatment options are available. In some instances, the exercise prescription is modified as discussed below, and more intensive surveillance is used during exercise training. The advisability of early testing and training after anterior myocardial infarction has been questioned because of experimental and clinical evidence showing formation of abnormal myocardial scars.[49,50] However, evaluation of patients recovering from anterior myocardial infarction found that moderate exercise training was not associated with worsening left ventricular topography or function.[51]

TABLE 40-1 COMPARISON OF THE MODIFIED NAUGHTON AND BRUCE PROTOCOLS FOR TREADMILL EXERCISE TESTING

		MODIFIED NAUGHTON			BRUCE		
Min	METs	Stage	Speed (mph)	Grade (%)	Stage	Speed (mph)	Grade (%)
3	3	1	2.0	3.5			
3	4	2	2.0	7.0			
3	5	3	2.0	10.5	1	1.7	10.0
3	6	4	2.0	14.0			
3	7	5	2.0	17.5	2	2.5	12.0
3	8	6	3.0	12.5			
3	9	7	3.0	15.0			
3	10	8	3.0	17.0	3	3.4	14.0

The prognostic value of exercise testing after myocardial infarction has been questioned.[45,52] For purposes of rehabilitation, the absence of exercise-induced ischemic abnormalities with preserved exercise capability identifies a group of patients at very low risk for a recurrent cardiac event, irrespective of the use of a thrombolytic agent at the time of infarction.[53,54] Issues related to exercise testing are more completely developed in Chapter 5.

Exercise Prescription

INDIVIDUALIZED PRESCRIPTION IN UNCOMPLICATED CASES. The exercise prescription is individualized, based on the results of the symptom-limited exercise test. The components of the prescription are summarized by the acronym *FIT*: *f*requency, *i*ntensity, and *t*ime. The minimum frequency needed to improve cardiovascular fitness is three times weekly. Intensity is most easily prescribed as a target heart rate. The time or duration of exercise is usually 30 to 60 minutes for each session but is also individually determined. Thresholds for frequency, intensity, and duration have not been established, and the guidelines suggested reflect recommendations of national organizations.[31,32,34,39,55] Modifications of the prescription for complicated cases are described below.

The conditioning effect is a balance between the intensity and duration of exercise. The intensity of exercise is based upon the peak heart rate achieved during exercise testing. A low intensity is prescribed initially to allow the patient to complete 1-hour sessions without excessive fatigue. A target heart rate of 65 per cent of peak heart rate is a common starting point. In some instances, especially after cardiac surgery, the resting pulse is high, and 65 per cent of the peak heart rate places the target rate near the resting pulse. In those cases, a slightly higher initial target of 75 per cent may be used. Alternatively, 40 to 50 per cent of the difference between the peak and the resting heart rate may be calculated and added to the resting pulse to determine the target. For convenience, the target is given as a 10-second count.

COMPONENTS OF EXERCISE SESSIONS. Exercise sessions, whether performed individually or in a group, should last 1 hour. Each session includes a warm-up period, a period of aerobic and muscular conditioning, and a cool-down period. A 10-minute warm-up includes stretching and light calisthenics to prevent musculoskeletal injury and gradually increase the heart rate. A 40-minute conditioning period is best spent in aerobic exercise, such as walking, jogging, and bicycling, during the first several weeks of training. Swimming is excellent aerobic exercise but creates problems with surveillance, pulse monitoring, and response in the event of a cardiovascular emergency. The exercise session is concluded with a 10-minute cool-down using stretching exercises similar to those in the warm-up period. This is especially important for coronary patients in whom ventricular arrhythmias are commonly precipitated by the abrupt cessation of moderate or high-intensity exercise.[56,57]

Aerobic conditioning, rather than strength training, is emphasized in the first several weeks of exercise training. Arm training, especially isometric exercise, is usually proscribed in the early training period because it causes a disproportionate increase in blood pressure compared with heart rate[58] and may compromise sternal wound healing in the first 4 to 6 weeks after cardiac surgery. Standard exercise programs emphasizing dynamic leg training by walking, jogging, and bicycling also increase arm strength and endurance even without specific arm training.[59] If arm and shoulder strength training is important, patients can begin using light hand weights during walk-jog exercises early in the exercise program. Circuit and strength training emphasizing muscular conditioning in both upper and lower extremities may be advantageous to some patients later in their training program.[60–63] This is especially true of patients who perform a significant amount of upper extremity work in their jobs.

ADVANCING THE PRESCRIPTION. The Borg scale of rate of perceived exertion (RPE)[64] is a useful tool for advancing the exercise prescription during training. As shown in Table 40-2, the RPE scale gives a numeric value to a perceived level of exertion. Patients should exercise at an RPE of 13 to 15. As patients become more fit, the RPE will fall, and the intensity of exercise may then be increased. The target is usually increased by 5 per cent to 10 per cent of the peak heart rate. Ultimately, patients should be able to exercise at 85 per cent of their peak heart rate for the entire session, and most patients reach this intensity within eight to 12 sessions.

Follow-up treadmill testing should be performed 4 to 8 weeks after beginning training. Many patients will achieve significantly higher heart rates on subsequent testing. Higher achieved heart rates are related to improvements in chronotropic competence in some patients and the ability to achieve a maximal cardiovascular effort in others previously limited by severe skeletal muscle deconditioning.[13] The follow-up treadmill test can be used to advance the exercise prescription for most patients and to allow some to graduate to lower levels of surveillance during exercise.

PATIENTS WITH MYOCARDIAL ISCHEMIA. Patients with exercise-induced myocardial ischemia should receive optimal therapy to eliminate or ameliorate the problem. Some patients will still show evidence of ischemia. Assuming that ischemia does not occur at extremely low workloads, these patients may still exercise safely as long as their target heart rate remains well below that at which ischemia occurs.[65] Limiting the maximal target heart rate to 10 beats/min below that at which ischemic abnormalities occur is clinically useful. Increased surveillance during exercise, such as with continuous electrocardiographic monitoring, is also recommended in the initial stages of exercise training.[31,34,39]

TABLE 40–2 BORG SCALE OF RATE OF PERCEIVED EXERTION (RPE)

	6
Very, very light	7
	8
Very light	9
	10
Light	11
	12
Somewhat hard	13
	14
Hard	15
	16
Very hard	17
	18
Very, very hard	19
	20

From Borg, G.: Perceived exertion as an indicator of somatic stress. Scand. J. Rehabil. Med. *2*:92, 1970.

PATIENTS WITH HEART FAILURE. These patients are at higher risk for complications related to exercise but also tend to have the most significant improvements from exercise training. Supervised exercise training has been shown to be safe in patients with heart failure.[3,27,66,67] The exercise prescription often must be modified for patients with heart failure because of their limited endurance. Shorter periods of aerobic training, lower target heart rates, and intermittent rest periods can all be used to limit the degree of fatigue felt by these patients.[27] The ultimate target heart rate should also be kept 10 beats/min below that at which significant symptoms of dyspnea and fatigue occur on exercise testing.

In patients with heart failure, the presence of inducible ischemia generally predicts a poor response to exercise training. These patients are less likely to show a training effect with the usual duration of training[19,65] and are more likely to have complications related to coronary disease during follow-up.[4,65]

PATIENTS WITH ARRHYTHMIAS. These patients present a significant challenge to the clinician because of controversies regarding therapy and the uncertainty of the safety of exercise. No definitive data are available regarding the safety of exercise in patients with arrhythmias. Patients with exercise-induced ventricular arrhythmias and coronary disease are at high risk for both fatal events and nonfatal ischemic complications.[56] The usual clinical approach in cardiac rehabilitation is to exclude patients with severe exercise-induced arrhythmias from exercise training until suppression of the arrhythmia has been achieved. Higher levels of surveillance are recommended during exercise using continuous electrocardiographic monitoring. It is unknown whether exercise training affects arrhythmias.[68] One study has shown a reduction in ventricular arrhythmia frequency with training, perhaps due to modulation of sympathetic response during exercise.[69] Stable patterns of arrhythmia during electrocardiogram-monitored exercise training are often used as evidence to allow patients to begin supervised, unmonitored exercise. However, the safety of this approach has not been documented.

Risks of Exercise Training

Exercise training is not without risks. The greatest risk lies in patients with untreated or unrecognized left ventricular dysfunction, myocardial ischemia, and ventricular arrhythmias. In patients receiving optimal therapy, the greatest risk lies in exercising at or above the level at which the abnormalities can be elicited by exercise testing.[70] For this reason, the maximum target heart rate used in exercise training must be lower than the heart rate at which abnormalities become evident on testing.

PATIENT SELECTION AND SURVEILLANCE. Safe exercise training is best assured by proper selection of patients and adequate surveillance during exercise. Guidelines to stratify risk of exercise training have been published by several professional organizations.[31,39,40,55] Patients at high risk for cardiovascular complications during exercise have one or more of the characteristics listed in Table 40-3.[39,71] Every attempt should be made to ameliorate or correct high-risk conditions before recommending exercise. If the abnormality cannot be corrected, the risks and benefits of exercise training should be carefully considered and the highest level of surveillance during exercise recommended. Patients in whom the risks of exercise outweigh the benefits despite optimal medical therapy should be informed of the risks and counseled not to exercise. Because the natural history of conditions such as congestive heart failure limits

TABLE 40–3 INDICATIONS FOR CONTINUOUS ELECTROCARDIOGRAPHIC MONITORING DURING EXERCISE TRAINING

CLINICAL INDICATION	OBJECTIVE SIGNS
Severe left ventricular dysfunction Congestive heart failure History of cardiogenic shock	Ejection fraction <30%
Severe exercise-induced ischemia	ST-segment depression ≥ 0.2 mV Angina at a workload ≤ 5 METs Multiple perfusion defects (Exercise nuclear study) Multiple dyskinetic segments (Exercise echocardiography study)
Complex ventricular arrhythmia (at rest or exercise-induced) Previous cardiac arrest	Nonsustained ventricular tachycardia
Hypotensive response to exercise	Systolic drop of 20 mm Hg or more at increasing load
Low functional capacity	Peak workload ≤ 5 METs
Inability to self-monitor heart rate	

prognosis, patients and physicians should be aware of the need for close medical follow-up beyond that available in supervised exercise programs.

The highest level of surveillance is supervised group exercise with continuous electrocardiographic monitoring. Approximately 15 per cent to 25 per cent of patients eligible for exercise training have one or more of the characteristics in Table 40–3 and require continuous electrocardiographic monitoring.[31,34,39] The next level of surveillance is unmonitored group exercise training supervised by health professionals with advanced cardiac life-support certification. Patients without high-risk characteristics, and those who improve during electrocardiogram-monitored training can participate in supervised, unmonitored group training.[72] Very low-risk patients can safely exercise independently after learning the principles of pulse monitoring and recognition of symptoms. In general, low-risk patients have an exercise capacity of eight METs or more without symptoms or signs of left ventricular dysfunction, myocardial ischemia, or ventricular arrhythmias. These criteria may be used to graduate patients from supervised programs.[73]

All patients should be taught to monitor their pulse and recognize symptoms during exercise. The concepts of the target heart rate and RPE are conveyed and reinforced during group exercise sessions. These principles and concepts guide patients in independent, safe, and effective exercise after completion of a formal exercise program. Patients who are unable or unwilling to follow the exercise prescription should receive higher levels of surveillance.

SAFETY OF SUPERVISED PROGRAMS. Despite the potential for cardiovascular complications during exercise, supervised programs have an extremely good safety record. In a survey of 167 programs, the incidence rate per million patient hours of exercise for fatal events was 1.3, for myocardial infarction 3.4, and for resuscitated cardiac arrests 8.9. There were no significant differences in rates for continuous electrocardiogram-monitored compared with intermittently monitored programs.[71] The event rates in this study were significantly lower than in a survey performed a decade earlier[74] and were reconfirmed in a more recent study.[75] The reasons for improvement are speculative. Improved risk stratification, improved revascularization and medical therapies, more rigorous standards for cardiac rehabilitation programs, and increased awareness of the necessity of monitoring high-risk patients may have contributed to the improved safety record.

SECONDARY PREVENTION

Comprehensive cardiac rehabilitation includes an aggressive approach to treatment of risk factors. Lipid lowering is discussed in Chapter 35, treatment of hypertension in Chapter 27, and control of diabetes mellitus in Chapter 61. In this chapter, attention is directed on cessation of cigarette smoking in secondary prevention.

RISKS. Cigarette smoking is an established risk factor for the development of angina and myocardial infarction[76] and increases the risk for recurrent infarction and death.[77] Survivors of myocardial infarction who continue to smoke have twice the rate of recurrent infarction and cardiac death compared with patients who quit smoking. The risk of a second cardiac event declines rapidly after cessation of smoking. Within 3 years of myocardial infarction, former smokers have approximately the same risk for reinfarction as survivors of myocardial infarction who never smoked.[78,79] Patients who continue to smoke after coronary bypass surgery have two to six times the expected mortality compared with nonsmokers or those who quit smoking after surgery.[80,81]

PATHOPHYSIOLOGY. The pathophysiology underlying the increased risk for death and reinfarction is uncertain. Platelet aggregation, thrombosis, coronary spasm, and diminished coronary and collateral flow reserve have all been implicated.[76,82,83] Fibrinogen levels are significantly higher in smokers than nonsmokers and increase the primary risk of myocardial infarction.[77] Although the degree of coronary atherosclerosis is not closely correlated with smoking habits, the risk for myocardial infarction in smokers is strongly correlated with the extent of coronary artery disease and plasma cholesterol levels.[84]

ETIOLOGY OF TOBACCO DEPENDENCE. Smoking is a complex behavior with physiological, psychological, and sociological roots. There are several theories regarding the etiology, although no single theory is adequate to explain all aspects of smoking behavior. Physiological dependence on nicotine causes acute craving for cigarettes with abrupt cessation of smoking. Smoking is a habit that appears to minimize negative emotions such as distress, anger, and fear and counteracts feelings of insecurity. It may also be used as a coping mechanism to transfer such negative emotions into a socially acceptable behavior. Finally, a smoking habit may have deep sociological origins such as modeling behavior after parents and peers.[85]

PROGRAMS FOR CESSATION OF SMOKING. Demographic and psychological factors identify patients who are more likely to continue smoking after a cardiac event. Lower occupational and educational levels, smoking of a larger number of cigarettes, increasing age, and higher rates of consumption of alcohol are demographic factors associated with continued smoking.[86] Psychological factors, such as a less negative attitude regarding smoking, higher anxiety levels, and a low sense of personal control over life events, identify those smokers who are less likely to quit smoking after a cardiac event.[76]

Myocardial infarction, coronary surgery, and coronary angioplasty are sufficient impetus to stop smoking in 20 per cent to 60 per cent of patients.[87,88] Patients who receive strong advice to stop smoking from health professionals are more likely to quit and remain abstinent compared with those who do not receive such advice.[89–91] This is particularly true of patients who believe that they are at personal risk if they continue smoking. Unfortunately, high acute rates of cessation are associated with high rates of recidivism in the absence of interventions to maintain abstinence.

Cessation of smoking is facilitated by treating both the physiological and psychological aspects of the habit. Hospital confinement for myocardial infarction or coronary surgery usually provides sufficient time for the physiological manifestations of nicotine withdrawal, such as irritability, emotionality, inability to concentrate, nausea, and headache, to resolve. In patients who continue to crave cigarettes, nicotine dependence is strong, and more gradual nicotine withdrawal may be necessary.[76]

Nicotine withdrawal can be managed by tapering cigarette smoking, gradually changing to lower-nicotine cigarettes, or using nicotine-replacement therapy. Transdermal nicotine patches and oral nicotine polacrilex raise serum nicotine levels to 30 per cent to 60 per cent of the level obtained with cigarette smoking[92,93] which is sufficient to significantly blunt the craving for cigarettes.[94,95] Smokers using nicotine replacement therapy are twice as likely to be abstinent from cigarettes 1 year following treatment compared with those not using nicotine replacement therapy.[96,97] Although prescription of nicotine polacrilex alone does not decrease the long-term rate of abstinence,[98] there is evidence that transdermal nicotine patches increase rates of abstinence, even in the absence of adjuvant behavioral therapy.[97]

Behavioral therapy, with or without nicotine replacement, increases long-term rates of abstinence. Such therapy can be provided by physicians, nurses, or other trained personnel.[94] Using techniques of self-control or substitution of healthful behaviors for smoking assist the patient in abstinence. Role-playing cigarette refusal and enlisting social support of family, friends, and coworkers reinforces nonsmoking behavior. Long-term rates of abstinence up to 70 per cent have been achieved with formal programs, particularly with patients who have recently diagnosed coronary disease.[99] Behavioral interventions are best targeted to the period immediately after cessation of smoking, as relapse in the first 2 to 3 weeks is highly predictive of continued smoking.[93,99]

PSYCHOLOGICAL FACTORS

COMMON PSYCHIATRIC PROBLEMS. Severe psychological stress or major depression complicate myocardial infarction in approximately 15 per cent of cases and have been associated with significantly higher rates of morbidity and mortality.[100,101] Although most professionals providing cardiac rehabilitation believe that exercise training and related services provide significant psychological benefits, severe stress or major depression require specific therapy. There is evidence that specific therapy for severe stress can influence outcome positively, although comparable data for major depression are lacking.[102] The more common and less disabling problems of delirium in the acute care setting and anxiety and minor depression during early recovery are generally transient and easily treated.[103,104]

SELF-EFFICACY. Acute cardiac illnesses have many psychosocial sequelae including medical restrictions on even the most routine of activities. These restrictions are reinforced by family, friends, and coworkers who perceive a poor prognosis and are concerned that physical and emotional stress can further damage the heart. If patients have a poor understanding of their illness, fear of recurrent cardiac problems leads to a sense of loss of control and a lack of confidence to resume customary activities. This lack of confidence can be a significant impediment to the resumption of a full and active life.

Self-efficacy is a psychological term describing how a person's judgment regarding the capacity for performance of a task or action is an important determinant of whether that person will attempt the task or action.[105] Self-efficacy reflects confidence and is highly predictive of action. Self-efficacy for specific tasks can be rated on 0 to 100 per cent confidence scales. For example, self-efficacy scales have been validated for physical activity that predicts whether a coronary patient will be successful with a regular exercise program.[106–108] The most common areas of low self-efficacy for coronary patients are physical exertion, emotional stress, and sexual activity.[105]

Self-efficacy can be increased in coronary patients by four methods: persuasion, information, vicarious experience, and enactive techniques. Using exercise as an example, physicians can persuade patients that they are capable of exercising. Patients can be informed about what sensations to expect with exercise, so they do not misread normal physiological responses, such as tachycardia, as grave symptoms. Vicarious experiences can be shared by other patients who have successfully undertaken exercise programs. The most powerful method for increasing exercise self-efficacy is the performance of a supervised exercise test.[105,108]

Self-efficacy is a useful measure for predicting potential success for other important behavioral changes such as cessation of smoking and dietary modification.[108,109] In circumstances of low self-efficacy, informative, persuasive, vicarious and enactive techniques to raise self-efficacy are helpful for increasing the rate of success for behavioral change. Spousal perceptions are equally important. Self-efficacy scales that rate spouses' perceptions of the patients' potential for success with a particular task are also highly predictive of success or failure. Support and encouragement by the spouse in change of behavior are extremely important for success. Spousal self-efficacy can be raised using similar techniques as for patients.[110]

TYPE A BEHAVIOR. Although Type A behavior is recognized as a risk factor for the development of coronary artery disease,[111] its effect on prognosis is unknown. Conflicting results are reported in several studies, although there are limitations in each. The major limitations are the populations studied, the instruments used to classify behavior, the duration of follow-up, and the endpoints studied. One of the most important concepts that has emerged from the Type A controversy is recognition that the construct probably reflects a collection of behaviors, not all of which are related to either the development or prognosis of coronary disease. Of the three primary characteristics of Type A behavior—competitive striving for achievement, time urgency, and hostility–only the latter appears to be independently related to outcomes of coronary disease, but there is continued controversy in this area.[112–114] There is limited evidence that modification of Type A behavior can change prognosis of coronary disease.[115] Further investigation is needed before such therapy can be recommended.

VOCATIONAL REHABILITATION

The cost of cardiovascular disability is high. The direct costs of care for patients with heart disease are estimated at $85 billion annually in the United States.[116] Indirect costs, due to goods and services not provided because of cardiovascular illness, are several times greater. Indirect costs can be significantly reduced by increasing the numbers of patients who return to work and shortening the interval between a cardiac event and return to work.

FACTORS RELATED TO EMPLOYMENT. Employment after a cardiac event is related to demographic, medical, and psychosocial factors. Patients unemployed at the time of a cardiac event, those over the age of 60, and those with blue-collar jobs are significantly less likely to work after the event.[117] Retirement and disability benefits are more easily obtained after age 60, encouraging patients to leave the work force. Blue-collar workers, especially those who are unskilled, are easily replaced in the work force and consequently lose their jobs more commonly after a cardiac event.[118]

After a cardiac event, the medical condition of the patient and the advice provided by the physician regarding return to work are the most important factors influencing the rate of reemployment in previously employed patients.[47,48] In the absence of demographic and psychosocial impediments, the physician must first ensure that the risk of a cardiovascular complication is low and will not be increased by returning to work. The physician must then determine if the patient has the physical capacity to perform occupational work. Finally, the physician must provide explicit advice regarding the timing of return to work and any work restrictions that the patient and employer must follow.

FACILITATING REEMPLOYMENT. In the majority of patients recovering from cardiac surgery and myocardial infarction, a careful clinical evaluation and a symptom-limited treadmill test are sufficient to guide the physician in the return-to-work decision. Accurate methods to stratify the risk of recurrent coronary events rely on clinical information obtained during hospitalization and specialized testing performed during or shortly after hospitalization.[46] More than half of patients surviving myocardial infarction have no symptoms or signs of congestive heart failure or myocardial ischemia. Their risk of cardiac death, myocardial infarction, or unstable angina in the year following the primary event is less than 10 per cent. A symptom-limited exercise capacity on treadmill testing of 7 METs or more without ischemia lowers the risk to under 3 per cent.[119]

The treadmill test also establishes peak physical capacity that can be related to the patient's occupational work. Individuals can sustain 6 to 8 hours of continuous effort at 40 per cent of their peak MET capacity. Continuous tolerance for work declines at higher levels, averaging 4 hours at 60 per cent of peak capacity and 2 hours above 60 per cent of peak capacity.[120] The average job has an energy requirement well under 5 METs, which means that a peak capacity of 7 to 10 METs is sufficient for most individuals to perform their occupational work.[120] There is evidence that with increasing levels of automation, current guidelines overestimate the work requirements for household and occupational activities.[121,122] Only 16 per cent of Americans perform jobs requiring manual labor, and that percentage declines rapidly with age.[123] Most manual labor jobs require only intermittent high-energy expenditure, which significantly prolongs tolerance for work.

Intensive physical reconditioning is not necessary for the average patient to return to work. In patients with very low functional capacity and those with higher occupational physical requirements, an exercise training program can hasten their return to work. Unless the patient's job requires lifting and carrying of moderate to heavy loads, the standard aerobic training previously described is sufficient to expedite return to work. In specialized circumstances, exercise programs that include upper extremity isometric training can be provided. Work simulation and specialized training programs may be helpful in unusual circumstances. In the particular circumstance of jobs affecting public safety, such as with pilots, police, and fire fighters, more stringent requirements regarding return to work are legislated.[124]

The average interval between uncomplicated myocardial infarction and return to work is 70 to 90 days; it averages 15 to 30 days after coronary angioplasty and 50 to 100 days after uncomplicated coronary surgery.[47,117,120] These intervals can be shortened substantially with a coordinated approach using risk stratification, treadmill testing, and explicit physician advice regarding the timing of return to work. In employed patients without high-risk clinical characteristics or severe treadmill ischemia, the time from myocardial infarction was shortened from 75 to 51 days in a randomized trial of an early return-to-work intervention. Recurrent cardiac events averaged 3.5 per cent in the 6 months after infarction and were no higher in patients returning to work earlier compared with those returning to work later.[47] Similar results were obtained in a subsequent study that also demonstrated very low-risk patients without evidence of ischemia on treadmill testing could return to work safely approximately 1 month after myocardial infarction.[48] Although these studies did not include a special program for patients performing manual labor, the intervention was as successful in the 11 to 17 per cent of the population performing manual labor as it was in the sedentary workers. Higher-risk patients with evidence of congestive heart failure or myocardial ischemia accounted for 23 per cent of all employed patients under the age of 60 and were specifically excluded from study. Return-to-work decisions in such patients must be individualized.[47,48]

BENEFITS OF REEMPLOYMENT. The benefits of an early return to work are financial and psychological. In the trial discussed above,[47] patients randomized to the return to work intervention earned $2100 more than patients randomized to usual care in the 6 months following myocardial infarction. Although not specifically examined, financial benefits to employers probably accrued including increased productivity and reduced costs of temporary employees and disability insurance payments.[125] Interventions that increase the numbers of patients returning to work and shorten the interval between the illness and reemployment will have the greatest impact on reducing the economic burden of cardiovascular disability.

ORGANIZATION OF CARDIAC REHABILITATION SERVICES

For most patients, cardiac rehabilitation begins in the hospital following a cardiac event and continues for several months thereafter. Traditionally, cardiac rehabilitation has been provided in phases with activity guidelines based upon the time from the cardiac event. Although phased rehabilitation provides a framework, individual patients will progress more slowly or quickly depending upon their age, condition prior to their cardiac event, the severity of illness, and motivation. The rehabilitation program should be individualized to facilitate a rate of recovery commensurate with the patient's status.[39]

Inpatient Rehabilitation

Hospitalization has been significantly shortened for patients recovering from myocardial infarction and cardiac surgery. Therefore, inpatient rehabilitation must make patients self-sufficient in the activities of daily living in a short period of time. The behavioral changes required for secondary prevention may be introduced in the hospital but are mainly deferred until patients are at home.

EARLY MOBILIZATION. Early mobilization reduces the detrimental effects of bed rest as discussed previously[7–9] and maximizes the rate at which customary activities can be resumed. In the coronary care unit, assisted range of motion exercises can be initiated in the first 24 to 48 hours for most patients. Patients in stable condition should be encouraged to sit in a chair for increasing periods each day to minimize depletion of intravascular volume, deconditioning of skeletal muscle, and orthopedic impairment. Self-care activities, such as shaving, oral hygiene, and sponge bathing, should be encouraged as soon as the patient's condition is stable.

GRADUATED PHYSICAL ACTIVITY. On transfer of the patient from the intensive care unit, a graduated program of physical and self-care activities can begin. Upright posture should be encouraged as much as tolerated. Patients should walk with assistance at least twice daily. Although some inpatient programs suggest walking specific distances each day, ambulation can be based on the patient's tolerance. In that way, patients are neither pushed beyond their tolerance nor held back in their recovery. The target heart rate and RPE scale can be used to individualize the intensity and time of activity. For each session, standing heart rate and blood pressure are obtained, followed by 5 minutes of range of motion and flexibility exercises. Patients are then assisted with walking at a rate that keeps the pulse within the range of resting pulse plus 20 beats per minute and the RPE less than 14. Most patients will tolerate a minimum of 5 minutes of walking the first day. As long as the pulse and RPE remain within prescribed limits, walking time can be increased until patients are walking at least 30 minutes twice daily. At that point, the walking sessions should include stair climbing to ensure that patients can perform that task at home. Patients able to walk unassisted for 30 minutes and climb stairs have sufficient strength and endurance for most activities of daily living.

EDUCATION AND COUNSELING. During the periods of assisted ambulation, the nurse or physical therapist teaches patients how to count their pulse, use the RPE scale, and recognize important symptoms. Before discharge from the hospital, patients are taught how to access emergency medical care; learn the names, dosages, effects, and side-effects of their medications; and have specific questions regarding their cardiac status answered. During these or other times, basic information regarding the risk factors for coronary disease should be presented with emphasis on those that affect the patient.

At the time of hospital discharge, patients should receive very specific advice about resumption of activities at home. Even common-sense knowledge should not be presumed by the health professionals caring for the patient. The spouse should receive the advice with the patient because the retention of information by hospitalized patients is limited, and most disagreements between patient and spouse in the early recovery period are related to perceptions of medical advice given.[126–129] A simple approach to providing guidelines for physical activities is to treat them as forms of exercise. Patients can use the resting pulse plus 20 beats-per-minute rule for most household activities. The patient quickly will learn the heart rate response to each activity and be confident in undertaking such activities at home. Patients should be told what restrictions are placed on common activities such as climbing stairs, lifting, driving, socializing with visitors, shopping, and walking outdoors.

Activities that involve more mental than physical stress, such as driving, socializing, and shopping, concern patients and family at the time of discharge from the hospital. Mental stress has been shown to affect cardiac performance negatively.[130–133] However, in studies directly comparing the physiological stress of exercise with formal methods of psychological stress, the hemodynamic response was always significantly greater with exercise than mental stress.[134–137] The pathophysiology of mental stress and its influence on prognosis are incompletely understood.[135,136,138,139] It appears unlikely that mental stress, unless severe, will precipitate a cardiac event soon after myocardial infarction or in the setting of stable coronary disease.

Early Postdischarge Exercise Testing and Rehabilitation

ACTIVITIES BEFORE EXERCISE TESTING. The interval between hospital discharge and formal cardiac rehabilitation should be as brief as possible. During this period, patients can continue their walking program as prescribed in the hospital. They should walk a minimum of 30 minutes twice daily at a target heart rate within the resting pulse plus 20 beats/min range at an RPE of less than 14. Patients able to tolerate the duration of walking should be encouraged to add a third session or increase the two sessions to 45 minutes each. Secondary prevention efforts can begin as patients are motivated and have time to begin behavioral changes. Initial visits with a dietitian may be scheduled if weight loss or reduction of cholesterol is necessary.[140] A smoking abstinence program may begin during this period.[99] Patients should be provided with resources to teach them about coronary disease and risk-factor management.[141]

RECOMMENDATIONS FOLLOWING EXERCISE TESTING. A postdischarge exercise test is a good focal point for the subsequent rehabilitation effort. The formal exercise prescription may then be given. Goals for weight loss, reduction of serum cholesterol, cessation of smoking, and return to work may be established. In the absence of significant abnormalities on the treadmill test, patients may begin most customary activities such as driving, sexual activity, and light lifting. Although lifting is often proscribed for 6 to 8 weeks after myocardial infarction and cardiac surgery, studies suggest that lifting and carrying of moderate loads is not dangerous after uncomplicated myocardial infarction and cardiac surgery. In patients with coronary disease, including those recovering from myocardial infarction, static lifting and combined static lifting and dynamic treadmill walking were associated with similar or lower double products compared with dynamic treadmill walking alone. In these studies, there was no evidence of myocardial ischemia induced by static lifting alone.[142–144]

SEXUAL ACTIVITY. The most common sexual problems of coronary patients are reduced or absent libido, avoidance of sexual activity even if libido has recovered, impotence, and premature or delayed ejaculation in men. The causes of sexual dysfunction include preexisting conditions, fear of precipitating a cardiac event, depression, and medications, especially beta blockers and diuretics. In addition, the sexual partner may believe that sexual activity could precipitate a cardiac event and therefore may avoid sexual activity. Because patients are reluctant to discuss sexual dysfunction, the physician should address issues of sexuality and consider the effects of medications on sexual drive.[129,145–148]

The hemodynamic response to sexual intercourse has been evaluated in patients recovering from myocardial infarction. The maximal heart rate during sexual intercourse averages 120 beats/min, which approximates maximal heart rates attained in the performance of other customary activities.[147] The hemodynamic response to sexual activity is far greater with an unfamiliar compared with a familiar partner, in unfamiliar settings, and after excessive eating and consumption of alcohol.[145] The exercise test can be used to gauge the potential cardiac stress of sexual activity. Patients without significant treadmill abnormalities can be advised to resume sexual activity gradually. Cardiac work associated with sexual intercourse can be minimized by adopting relaxed positions such as side-to-side rather than top-to-bottom postures that increase the isometric work.[145,147] Patients should be told to report symptoms such as angina, prolonged dyspnea, excessive fatigue, or tachycardia lasting more than 10 minutes after intercourse. In sedentary individuals, such symptoms may be the only manifestation of exercise-induced ischemia or left ventricular dysfunction.

Outpatient Rehabilitation Programs

Formal cardiac rehabilitation programs typically have both medical and program directors. The medical director is a physician, whereas the program director may be trained in a variety of disciplines. The rehabilitation team is multidisciplinary and includes nurses, physical therapists, exercise physiologists, dietitians, vocational counselors, and psychologists. When smaller programs cannot support the broad range of services, a referral network that includes all the disciplines is necessary. Adequate facilities for outpatient exercise training are needed. If high-risk patients are included, continuous electrocardiographic monitoring must be available. Equipment and training for cardiopulmonary resuscitation is mandatory.

EXERCISE TRAINING. Exercise training guidelines have

been presented earlier. Most patients can benefit from group exercise programs. The standard group training program provides three sessions weekly for 8 to 12 weeks. Some patients require more prolonged training, whereas others may progress to independent exercise more quickly. In such groups, proper techniques of exercise training can be reinforced, and patients can learn how to perform safe and effective exercise independently. The group setting is also an opportunity for patients to receive reliable information from health professionals regarding coronary disease and risk-factor modification. Although difficult to quantitate, there is an obvious benefit of the social support provided by interactions with other patients in various stages of recovery from coronary illness. Group exercise sessions are often the focal point for the development of educational programs and support groups.

RISK FACTOR MODIFICATION. A comprehensive program of cardiac rehabilitation should combine exercise training with risk factor modification (Chap. 35). Smoking abstinence programs and dietary counseling are the two most important additional services a program should provide. Continued reinforcement of the principles of risk-factor modification improves compliance with behavioral programs.[89,106,108,149]

Current evidence suggests that cardiac rehabilitation programs offering exercise training, smoking abstinence, and cholesterol treatment programs can improve the rates of morbidity and mortality of patients with coronary artery disease.[36,37] Cardiac rehabilitation programs can also facilitate functional recovery.[150–152] Early risk stratification, including treadmill testing, can identify patients requiring further treatment and hasten the resumption of customary activities of low-risk patients. Education and counseling can improve psychosocial outcomes. Significant economic benefits can be realized when vocational rehabilitation is included in a cardiac rehabilitation program.[47,48] Participation in a cardiac rehabilitation program may decrease subsequent costs of care through reductions in numbers of rehospitalizations and use of other medical services.[107,125,153–155] As the principles of cardiac rehabilitation become more broadly applied, larger numbers of patients with coronary disease will benefit medically, socially, and psychologically.

REFERENCES

EXERCISE IN CARDIAC REHABILITATION

1. DeBusk, R. F.: Why is cardiac rehabilitation not widely used? (Editorial). West. J. Med. *156*:206, 1992.
2. Roberts, J. M., Sullivan, M., Froelicher, V. F., et al.: Predicting oxygen uptake from treadmill testing in normal subjects and coronary artery disease patients. Am. Heart J. *108*:1454, 1984.
3. Coats, A. J.: Exercise rehabilitation in chronic heart failure. J. Am. Coll. Cardiol. *22*:172A–177A, 1993.
4. Sullivan, M. J., Higginbotham, M. B., and Cobb, F. R.: Exercise training in patients with severe left ventricular dysfunction. Circulation *78*:506, 1988.
5. Sullivan, M. J., Higginbotham, M. B., and Cobb, F. R. Exercise training in patients with chronic heart failure delays ventilatory anaerobic threshold and improves submaximal exercise performance. Circulation *79*:324, 1989.
6. Adamopoulos, S., Coats, A. J., Brunotte, F., et al.: Physical training improves skeletal muscle metabolism in patients with chronic heart failure. J. Am. Coll. Cardiol. *21*:1101, 1993.
7. Teasell, R., and Dittmer, D. K.: Complications of immobilization and bed rest. Part 2: Other complications. Can. Fam. Physician *39*:1440, 1445, 1993.
8. Dittmer, D. K., and Teasell, R.: Complications of immobilization and bed rest. Part 1: Musculoskeletal and cardiovascular complications. Can. Fam. Physician *39*:1428, 1435, 1993.
9. Hughson, R. L., Yamamoto, Y., Blabler, A. P., et al.: Effect of 28-day head-down bed rest with countermeasures on heart rate variability during LBNP. Aviat. Space Environ. Med. *65*:293, 1994.
10. Weins, R. D., Lafia, P., Marder, C. M., et al.: Chronotropic incompetence in clinical exercise testing. Am. J. Cardiol. *54*:74, 1984.
11. Thoren, P. N.: Activation of left ventricular receptors with non-medulated vagal afferent fibers during occlusion of a coronary artery in the cat. Am. J. Cardiol. *37*:146, 1976.
12. Wetherbee, S., Franklin, B. A., Hollingsworth, V., et al.: Relationship between arm and leg training work loads in men with heart disease: Implications for exercise prescription. Chest *99*:1271, 1991.
13. Haskell, W. L., and DeBusk, R. F.: Cardiovascular responses to repeated treadmill testing soon after myocardial infarction. Circulation *60*:1247, 1979.
14. Sullivan, M. J., Green, H. J., and Cobb, F. R.: Skeletal muscle biochemistry and histology in ambulatory patients with long-term heart failure. Circulation *81*:518, 1990.
15. Sullivan, M. J., Knight, D. J., Higginbotham, M. B., and Cobb, F. R.: Relation between central and peripheral hemodynamics during exercise in patients with chronic heart failure: Muscle blood flow is reduced with maintenance of arterial perfusion pressure. Circulation *80*:769, 1989.
16. McKelvie, R. S., Teo, K. K., McCartney, N., et al.: Effects of exercise training in patients with congestive heart failure: A critical review. J. Am. Coll. Cardiol. *25*:789, 1995.
17. Smith, R. F., Johnson, G., Ziesche, S., et al.: Functional capacity in heart failure. Comparison of methods for assessment and their relation to other indexes of heart failure. The V-HeFT VA Cooperative Studies Group. Circulation *87*(Suppl. 6):VI88, 1993.
18. Sullivan, M. J., and Cobb, F. R.: Central hemodynamic response to exercise in patients with chronic heart failure. Chest *101*:340S, 1992.
19. Ades, P. A., Grunvald, M. H., and Weiss, R. M.: Usefulness of myocardial ischemia as a predictor of training effect in cardiac rehabilitation after acute myocardial infarction or coronary artery bypass grafting. Am. J. Cardiol. *63*:1032, 1989.
20. Rice, K. R., Gervino, E., Jarisch, W. R., and Stone P. H.: Effects of nifedipine on myocardial perfusion during exercise in chronic stable angina pectoris. Am. J. Cardiol. *65*(16):1097, 1990.
21. Stone, P. H., Gibson, R. S., Glasser, S. P., et al.: Comparison of propranolol, diltiazem, and nifedipine in the treatment of ambulatory ischemia in patients with stable angina: Differential effects on ambulatory ischemia, exercise performance, and anginal symptoms. The ASIS Study Group. Circulation *82*:1962, 1990.
22. Gordon, N. F., and Duncan J. J.: Effect of beta-blockers on exercise physiology: implications for exercise training. Med. Sci. Sports Exerc. *23*:668, 1991.
23. MacGowan, G. A., O'Callaghan, D., Webb, H., and Horgan, J. H.: The effects of verapamil on training in patients with ischemic heart disease. Chest *101*:141, 1992.
24. Mancini, D. M., Davis, L., Wexler, J. P., et al.: Dependence of enhanced maximal exercise performance on increased peak skeletal muscle perfusion during long-term captopril therapy in heart failure. J. Am. Coll. Cardiol. *10*:845, 1987.
25. Drexler, H., Banhardt, U., Meinertz, T., et al. Contrasting peripheral short-term effects of converting enzyme inhibition in patients with congestive heart failure: A double blind, placebo-controlled trial. Circulation *79*:491, 1989.
26. Dickstein, K., and Aarsland, T.: Effect on exercise performance of enalapril therapy initiated early after myocardial infarction. Nordic Enalapril Exercise Trial. J. Am. Coll. Cardiol. *22*:975, 1993.
27. Hanson, P.: Exercise testing and training in patients with chronic heart failure. Med. Sci. Sports Exerc. *26*:527, 1994.
28. Hagberg, J. M.: Physiologic adaptations to prolonged high-intensity exercise training in patients with coronary artery disease. Med. Sci. Sports Exerc. *23*:661, 1991.
29. Rogers, M. A., Yamamotao, C., Hagberg, J. M., et al.: The effect of 7 years of intense training in patients with coronary artery disease. J. Am. Coll. Cardiol. *10*:321, 1987.
30. Laslett, L. J., Paumer, L., and Amsterdam, E. A.: Increase in myocardial oxygen consumption indexes by exercise training at onset of ischemia in patients with coronary artery disease. Circulation *71*:958, 1985.
31. American College of Sports Medicine. Position stand. Exercise for patients with coronary artery disease. Med. Sci. Sports Exerc. *26*:1, 1994.
32. Cox, M. H.: Exercise training programs and cardiorespiratory adaptation. Clin. Sports Med. *10*:19, 1991.
33. Squires, R. W., Lavie, C. J., Brandt, T. R. et al.: Cardiac rehabilitation in patients with severe ischemic left ventricular dysfunction. Mayo Clin. Proc. *62*:997, 1987.
34. Statement on exercise: A position statement for health professionals by the Committee on Exercise and Cardiac Rehabilitation of the Council on Clinical Cardiology, American Heart Association. Circulation *81*:396, 1990.
35. Kallio,V., Hamalainen, H., Hakkila, J., et al.: Reduction in sudden deaths by a multifactorial intervention programme after acute myocardial infarction. Lancet *2*:1091, 1979.
36. O'Connor, G. T., Buring, J. E., Yusuf, S., et al.: An overview of randomized trials of rehabilitation with exercise after myocardial infarction. Circulation *80*:234, 1989.
37. Oldridge, N. B., Guyatt, G. H., Fischer, M. E., et al.: Cardiac rehabilitation after myocardial infarction: Combined experience of randomized clinical trials. JAMA *260*:945, 1988.
38. Yusuf, S., Peto, R., Lewis, J., et al.: Beta blockade during and after myocardial infarction: An overview of randomized trials. Prog. Cardiovasc. Dis. *27*:335, 1985.
39. American Association for Cardiovascular and Pulmonary Rehabilitation. Guidelines for Cardiac Rehabilitation Programs. Ed. 2 Champaign, Ill., Human Kinetics, 1995.
40. Fletcher, G. F., Froelicher, V. F., Hartley, L. H., et al.: Exercise standards: A statement for health professionals from the American Heart Association. Circulation *82*:228, 1990.

41. Weber, K. T., and Janicki, J. S.: Cardiopulmonary exercise testing for the evaluation of heart failure. Am. J. Cardiol. *55:*22A, 1985.
42. Levandoski, S. G., Sheldahl, L. M., Wilke, N. A., et al.: Cardiopulmonary responses of coronary artery disease patients to arm and leg cycle ergometry. J. Cardiopulm. Rehabil. *10:*39, 1990.
43. Juneau, M., Colles, P., Theroux, P., et al.: Symptom-limited versus low level exercise testing before hospital discharge after myocardial infarction. J. Am. Coll. Cardiol. *20:*927, 1992.
44. Ben-Ari, E., and Rothbaum, D. Clinical and exercise considerations for the percutaneous transluminal coronary angioplasty patient. J. Cardiopulm. Rehabil. *11:*145, 1991.
45. Lavie, C. J., Gibbons, R. J., Zinsmeister, A. R., and Gersh, B. J.: Interpreting results of exercise studies after acute myocardial infarction altered by thrombolytic therapy, coronary angioplasty or bypass. Am. J. Cardiol. *67:*116, 1991.
46. Krone, R. J.: The role of risk stratification in the early management of a myocardial infarction. Ann. Intern. Med. *116:*223, 1992.
47. Dennis, C., Houston-Miller, N., Schwartz, R. G., et al.: Early return to work after uncomplicated myocardial infarction: Results of a randomized trial. JAMA *260:*214, 1988.
48. Pilote, L., Thomas, R. J., Dennis, C., et al.: Return to work after uncomplicated myocardial infarction: A trial of practice guidelines in the community. Ann. Intern. Med. *117:*383, 1992.
49. Gaudron, P., Hu, K., Schamberger, R., et al.: Effect of endurance training early or late after coronary artery occlusion on left ventricular remodeling, hemodynamics, and survival in rats with chronic transmural myocardial infarction. Circulation *89:*402, 1994.
50. Jugdutt, B. S., Michorowski, B. L., Kappagoda, C. T., et al.: Exercise training after anterior Q-wave myocardial infarction: Importance of regional left ventricular function or topography. J. Am. Coll. Cardiol. *12:*362, 1988.
51. Giannuzzi, P., Tavazzi, L., Temporelli, P. L., et al.: Long-term physical training and left ventricular remodeling after anterior myocardial infarction: Results of the Exercise in Anterior Myocardial Infarction (EAMI) trial. EAMI Study Group. J. Am. Coll. Cardiol. *22:*1821, 1993.
52. Moss, A. J., Goldstein, R. E., Hall, W. J., et al.: Detection and significance of myocardial ischemia in stable patients after recovery from an acute coronary event. Multicenter Myocardial Ischemia Research Group. JAMA *269:*2379, 1993.
53. Sacknoff, D. M., and Coplan, N. L.: Exercise testing for stratifying cardiac risk following thrombolytic therapy for acute myocardial infarction [Editorial]. Am. Heart J. *124:*1400, 1992.
54. Piccalo, G., Pirelli, S., Massa, D., et al.: Value of negative predischarge exercise testing in identifying patients at low risk after acute myocardial infarction treated by systemic thrombolysis. Am. J. Cardiol. *70:*31, 1992.
55. American College of Sports Medicine: Position Stand. Physical activity, physical fitness, and hypertension. Med. Sci. Sports Exerc. *25:*1, 1993.
56. Marieb, M. A., Beller, G. A., Gibson, R. S., et al.: Clinical relevance of exercise-induced ventricular arrhythmias in suspected coronary artery disease. Am. J. Cardiol. *66:*172, 1990.
57. Sparks, K. E., Shaw, D. K., Eddy, D., et al.: Alternatives for cardiac rehabilitation patients unable to return to a hospital-based program. Heart Lung *22:*298, 1993.
58. Bertagnoli, K., Hanson, P., and Ward, A.: Attenuation of exercise-induced ST depression during combined isometric and dynamic exercise in coronary artery disease. Am. J. Cardiol. *65:*314, 1990.
59. Ben-Ari, E., Kellermann, J. J., Rothbaum, D. A., et al.: Effects of prolonged intensive versus moderate leg training on the untrained arm exercise response in angina pectoris. Am. J. Cardiol. *59:*231, 1987.
60. Haennel, R. G., Quinney, H. A., and Kappagoda, C. T.: Effects of hydraulic circuit training following coronary artery bypass surgery. Med. Sci. Sports Exerc. *23:*158, 1991.
61. Sparling, P. B., Cantwell, J. D., Dolan, C. M., and Niederman, R. K.: Strength training in a cardiac rehabilitation program: A six-month follow-up. Arch. Phys. Med. Rehabil. *71:*148, 1990.
62. Faigenbaum, A. D., Skrinar, G. S., Cesare, W. F., et al.: Physiologic and symptomatic responses of cardiac patients to resistance exercise. Arch. Phys. Med. Rehabil. *71:*395, 1990.
63. McCartney, N., McKelvie, R. S., Haslam, D. R., and Jones, N. L.: Usefulness of weightlifting training in improving strength and maximal power output in coronary artery disease. Am. J. Cardiol. *67:*939, 1991.
64. Borg, G.: Perceived exertion as an indicator of somatic stress. Scand. J. Rehabil. Med. *2:*92, 1970.
65. Arvan, S.: Exercise performance of the high-risk acute myocardial infarction patient after cardiac rehabilitation. Am. J. Cardiol. *62:*197, 1988.
66. Coats, A. J., Adamopoulos, S., Radaelli, A., et al.: Controlled trial of physical training in chronic heart failure: Exercise performance, hemodynamics, ventilation, and autonomic function. Circulation *85:*2119, 1992.
67. Rossi, P.: Physical training in patients with congestive heart failure. Chest *101:*350S, 1992.
68. O'Hara, G. E., Brugada, P., Rodriguez, L. M., et al.: Incidence, pathophysiology and prognosis of exercise-induced sustained ventricular tachycardia associated with healed myocardial infarction. Am. J. Cardiol. *70:*875, 1992.
69. Hertzeanu, H. L., Shemesh, J., Aron, L. A., et al.: Ventricular arrhythmias in rehabilitated and nonrehabilitated post-myocardial infarction patients with left ventricular dysfunction. Am. J. Cardiol. *71:*24, 1993.
70. Van Camp, S. P., and Peterson, R. A.: Identification of the high-risk cardiac rehabilitation patient. J. Cardiopulm. Rehabil. *9:*103, 1989.
71. Van Camp, S. P., and Peterson, R. A.: Cardiovascular complications of outpatient cardiac rehabilitation programs. JAMA *256:*1160, 1986.
72. Greenland, P., and Chu, J. S.: Efficacy of cardiac rehabilitation services: With emphasis on patients after myocardial infarction. Ann. Intern. Med. *109:*650, 1988.
73. DeBusk, R. F., Haskell, W. L., Miller, N. H., et al.: Medically directed at-home rehabilitation soon after clinically uncomplicated acute myocardial infarction. Am. J. Cardiol. *55:*251, 1985.
74. Haskell, W. L.: Cardiovascular complications during exercise training of cardiac patients. Circulation *57:*920, 1978.
75. Hossack, J. M., and Hartwig, R.: Cardiac arrest associated with supervised cardiac rehabilitation. J. Cardiac Rehabil. *2:*402, 1992.

SECONDARY PREVENTION

76. Lakier, J. B.: Smoking and cardiovascular disease. Am. J. Med. *93:*8S, 1992.
77. Dobson, A. J., Alexander, H. M., Heller, R. F., and Lloyd D. M. How soon after quitting smoking does risk of heart attack decline? J. Clin. Epidemiol. *44:*1247, 1991.
78. Kawachi, I., Colditz, G. A., Stampfer, M. J., et al.: Smoking cessation in relation to total mortality rates in women: A prospective cohort study. Ann. Intern. Med. *119:*992, 1993.
79. Kawachi, I., Colditz, G. A., Stampfer, M. J., et al.: Smoking cessation and time course of decreased risks of coronary heart disease in middle-aged women. Arch. Intern Med *154:*169, 1994.
80. Cavender, J. B., Rogers, W. J., Fisher, L. D., et al.: Effects of smoking on survival and morbidity in patients randomized to medical or surgical therapy in the Coronary Artery Surgery Study (CASS): 10-year follow-up. CASS Investigators. J. Am. Coll. Cardiol. *20:*287, 1992.
81. Ramanathan, K. B., Vander Zwaag, R., Maddock, V., et al.: Interactive effects of age and other risk factors on long-term survival after coronary artery surgery. J. Am. Coll. Cardiol. *15:*1493, 1990.
82. Caralis, D. G., Deligonul, U., Kern, M. J., and Cohen, J. D.: Smoking is a risk factor for coronary spasm in young women. Circulation *85:*905, 1992.
83. Terres, W., Weber, K., Kupper, W., and Bleifield, W.: Age, cardiovascular risk factors and coronary heart disease as determinants of platelet function in men: A multivariate approach. Thromb. Res. *62:*649, 1991.
84. Robinson, J. G., and Leon, A. S.: The prevention of cardiovascular disease: Emphasis on secondary prevention. Med. Clin. North Am. *78:*69, 1994.
85. Sherman, C. B.: Health effects of cigarette smoking. Clin. Chest Med. *12:*643, 1991.
86. Freund, K. M., D'Agostino, R. B., Belanger, A. J., et al.: Predictors of smoking cessation: The Framingham Study. Am. J. Epidemiol. *135:*957, 1992.
87. Crouse, J. D., and Hagaman, A. P.: Smoking cessation in relation to cardiac procedures. Am. J. Epidemiol. *134:*699, 1991.
88. Rigotti, N. A., McKool, K. M., and Shiffman, S.: Predictors of smoking cessation after coronary artery bypass graft surgery: Results of a randomized trial with 5-year follow-up. Ann. Intern. Med. *120:*287, 1994.
89. Schwartz, J. L.: Methods of smoking cessation. Med. Clin. North Am. *76:*451, 1992.
90. Rigotti, N. A., Singer, D. E., Mulley, A. G., Jr., and Thibault, G. E.: Smoking cessation following admission to a coronary care unit. J. Gen. Intern. Med. *6:*305, 1991.
91. Frank, E., Winkleby, M. A., Altman, D. G., et al.: Predictors of physician's smoking cessation advice. JAMA *266:*3139, 1991.
92. Hurt, R. D., Dale, L. C., Offord, K. P., et al.: Serum nicotine and cotinine levels during nicotine-patch therapy. Clin. Pharmacol. Ther. *54:*98, 1993.
93. Kenford, S. L., Fiore, M. C., Jorenby, D. E., et al.: Predicting smoking cessation: Who will quit with and without the nicotine patch. JAMA *271:*589, 1994.
94. Hurt, R. D., Dale, L. C., Fredrickson, P. A., et al.: Nicotine patch therapy for smoking cessation combined with physician advice and nurse follow-up: One-year outcome and percentage of nicotine replacement. JAMA *271:*595, 1994.
95. Tonnesen, P., Norregaard, J., Simonsen, K., and Sawe U. A double-blind trial of a 16-hour transdermal nicotine patch in smoking cessation. N. Engl. J. Med. *325:*311, 1991.
96. Silagy, C., Mant, D., Fowler, G., and Lodge, M.: Meta-analysis on efficacy of nicotine replacement therapies in smoking cessation. Lancet *343:*139, 1994.
97. Fiore, M. C., Smith, S. S., Jorenby, D. E., and Baker, T. B.: The effectiveness of the nicotine patch for smoking cessation: A meta-analysis. JAMA *271:*1940, 1994.
98. Tsevat, J.: Impact and cost-effectiveness of smoking interventions. Am. J. Med. *93:*43S, 1992.
99. Taylor, C. B., Houston-Miller, N., Killen, J. D., and DeBusk, R. F.: Smoking cessation after acute myocardial infarction: Effects of a nurse-managed intervention. Ann. Intern. Med *113:*118, 1990.

PSYCHOLOGICAL FACTORS

100. Frasure-Smith, N.: In-hospital symptoms of psychological stress as predictors of long-term outcome after acute myocardial infarction in men. Am. J. Cardiol. *67:*121, 1991.
101. Frasure-Smith, N., Lesperance, F., and Talajic, M.: Depression following myocardial infarction. Impact on 6-month survival. JAMA *270:*1819, 1993.

102. Brown, M. A., Munford, A. M., and Munford, P. R.: Behavior therapy of psychological distress in patients after myocardial infarction or coronary bypass. J. Cardiopulm. Rehabil. *13:*201, 1993.
103. Kavan, M. G., Elsasser, G. N., and Hurd, R. H.: Depression after acute myocardial infarction: The role of primary care physicians in rehabilitation. Postgrad. Med. *89:*83, 1991.
104. Ladwig, K. H., Roll, G., Breithardt, G., et al.: Post-infarction depression and incomplete recovery 6 months after acute myocardial infarction. Lancet *343:*20, 1994.
105. Bandura, A.: Self-efficacy mechanism in human agency. Am. Psychol. *37:*122, 1982.
106. Damrosch, S.: General strategies for motivating people to change their behavior. Nurs. Clin. North Am. *26:*833, 1991.
107. Oldridge, N. B., and Rogowski, B. L.: Self-efficacy and in-patient cardiac rehabilitation. Am. J. Cardiol. *66:*362, 1990.
108. Robertson, D., and Keller, C.: Relationships among health beliefs, self-efficacy, and exercise adherence in patients with coronary artery disease. Heart Lung *21:*56, 1992.
109. Vidmar, P. M., and Rubinson, L.: The relationship between self-efficacy and exercise compliance in a cardiac population. J. Cardiopulm. Rehabil. *14:*246, 1994.
110. Ewart, C. K., Taylor, B., Reese, L. B., et al.: Exercise testing to enhance wives' confidence in their husbands' cardiac capability soon after uncomplicated acute myocardial infarction. Am. J. Cardiol. *55:*635, 1985.
111. The review panel on coronary-prone behavior and coronary heart disease. Coronary-prone behavior and coronary heart disease: A critical review. Circulation *63:*1199, 1981.
112. Dembroski, T., MacDougall, J., Costa, P., and Grandits, C.: Components of hostility as predictors of sudden death and myocardial infarction in the multiple risk factor intervention trial. Psychosom. Med. *51:*514, 1989.
113. Helmer, D. C., Ragland, D. R., and Syme, S. L.: Hostility and coronary artery disease. Am. J. Epidemiol. *133:*112, 1991.
114. Maruta, T., Hamburgen, M. E., Jennings, C. A., et al.: Keeping hostility in perspective: Coronary heart disease and the Hostility Scale on the Minnesota Multiphasic Personality Inventory. Mayo Clin. Proc. *68:*109, 1993.
115. Friedman, M., Thoreson, C. E., Gill, J. J., et al.: Alteration of Type A behavior and its effect on cardiac recurrences in post myocardial infarction patients: Summary results of the recurrent coronary prevention project. Am. Heart J. *112:*653, 1986.

VOCATIONAL REHABILITATION

116. Wittels, E. H., Hay, J. W., and Gotto, A. M.: Medical costs of coronary artery disease in the United States. Am. J. Cardiol. *65:*432, 1990.
117. Mark, D. B., Lam, L. C., Lee, K. L., et al.: Identification of patients with coronary disease at high risk for loss of employment: A prospective validation study. Circulation *86:*1485, 1992.
118. Guillette, W., Judge, R. D., Koehn, E., et al.: Committee report on economic, administrative, and legal factors influencing the insurability and employability of patients with ischemic heart disease: 20th Bethesda conference. J. Am. Coll. Cardiol. *14:*1010, 1989.
119. Pryor, D. B., Bruce, R. A., Chaitman, B. R., et al.: Task force I: Determination of prognosis in patients with ischemic heart disease: 20th Bethesda conference. J. Am. Coll. Cardiol. *14:*1016, 1989.
120. Haskell, W. L., Brachfeld, N., Bruce, R. A., et al.: Task force II: Determination of occupational working capacity in patients with ischemic heart disease: 20th Bethesda conference. J. Am. Coll. Cardiol. *14:*1025, 1989.
121. Wilke, N. A., Sheldahl, L. M., Dougherty, S. M., et al.: Baltimore Therapeutic Equipment work simulator: Energy expenditure of work activities in cardiac patients. Arch. Phys. Med. Rehabil. *74:*419, 1993.
122. Wilke, N. A., Sheldahl, L. M., Dougherty, S. M., et al.: Energy costs of household tasks in women with coronary artery disease. Am. J. Cardiol. *75:*670, 1995.
123. Bureau of Labor Statistics. Handbook of Labor Statistics. Washington, D.C.: U.S. Department of Labor, 1993.
124. DeBusk, R. F.: Determination of cardiac impairment and disability: 20th Bethesda conference. J. Am. Coll. Cardiol. *14:*1043, 1989.
125. Picard, M. H., Dennis, C., Schwartz, R. G., et al.: Cost-benefit of early return to work after uncomplicated myocardial infarction. Am. J. Cardiol. *63:*1308, 1989.
126. Cupples, S. A.: Effects of timing and reinforcement of preoperative education on knowledge and recovery of patients having coronary artery bypass graft surgery. Heart Lung *20:*654, 1991.
127. Duryee, R.: The efficacy of inpatient education after myocardial infarction. Heart Lung *21:*217, 1992.
128. Nyamathi, A., Jacoby, A., Constancia, P., and Ruvevich, S.: Coping and adjustment of spouses of critically ill patients with cardiac disease. Heart Lung *21:*160, 1992.
129. Beach, E. K., Maloney, B. H., Plocica, A. R., et al.: The spouse: A factor in recovery after acute myocardial infarction. Heart Lung *21:*30, 1992.
130. Burg, M. M., Jain, D., Soufer, R., et al.: Role of behavioral and psychological factors in mental stress-induced silent left ventricular dysfunction in coronary artery disease. J. Am. Coll. Cardiol. *22:*440, 1993.
131. Coumel, P., and Leenhardt, A. Mental activity, adrenergic modulation, and cardiac arrhythmias in patients with heart disease. Circulation *83:*1158, 1991.
132. Follick, M. J., Ahern, D. K., Gorkin, L., et al.: Relation of psychosocial and stress reactivity variables to ventricular arrhythmias in the Cardiac Arrhythmia Pilot Study (CAPS). Am. J. Cardiol. *66:*63, 1990.
133. Ironson, G., Taylor, C. B., Boltwood, M., et al.: Effects of anger on left ventricular ejection fraction in coronary artery disease. Am. J. Cardiol. *70:*281, 1992.

ORGANIZATION OF CARDIAC REHABILITATION SERVICES

134. Specchia, G., Falcone, C., Traversi, E., et al.: Mental stress as a provocative test in patients with various clinical syndromes of coronary heart disease. Circulation *83*(Suppl. 4):II108, 1991.
135. Specchia, G., Falcone, C., Traversi, E., et al.: Mental stress as provocative test in patients with various clinical syndromes of coronary heart disease. Circulation *83:*108, 1991.
136. Rozanski, A., Krantz, D. S., and Bairey, C. N.: Ventricular responses to mental stress testing in patients with coronary artery disease: Pathophysiological implications. Circulation *83:*137, 1991.
137. Gottdiener, J. S., Krantz, D. S., Howell, R. H., et al.: Induction of silent myocardial ischemia with mental stress testing: Relation to the triggers of ischemia during daily life activities and to ischemic functional severity. J. Am. Coll. Cardiol. *24:*1645, 1994.
138. L'Abbate, A., Simonetti, I., Carpeggiani, C., and Michelassi, C.: Coronary dynamics and mental arithmetic stress in humans. Circulation *83:*94, 1991.
139. Grignani, G., Soffiantino, F., Zucchella, M., et al.: Platelet activation by emotional stress in patients with coronary artery disease. Circulation *83:*128, 1991.
140. Montgomery, D. A., and Amos, R. J.: Nutritional information needs during cardiac rehabilitation: Perceptions of the cardiac patient and spouse. J. Am. Diet Assoc. *91:*1078, 1991.
141. Squires, R. W., Gau, G. T., Miller, T. D., et al.: Cardiovascular rehabilitation: Status, 1990. Mayo Clin. Proc. *65:*731, 1990.
142. DeBusk, R. F., Valdez, R., Houston, N., and Haskell, W.: Cardiovascular responses to dynamic and static effort soon after myocardial infarction. Circulation *58:*368, 1978.
143. Wilke, N. A., Sheldahl, S. G., Levandoski, S. G., et al.: Weight carrying versus handgrip exercise testing in men with coronary artery disease. Am. J. Cardiol. *64:*736, 1989.
144. Featherstone, J. F., Holly, R. G., and Amsterdam, E. A.: Physiologic responses to weight lifting in coronary artery disease. Am. J. Cardiol. *71:*287, 1993.
145. Cooper, A. J.: Myocardial infarction and advice on sexual activity. Practitioner *229:*575, 1985.
146. Hamilton, G. A., and Seidman, R. N.: A comparison of the recovery period for women and men after an acute myocardial infarction. Heart Lung *22:*308, 1993.
147. Tardif, G. S.: Sexual activity after a myocardial infarction. Arch. Phys. Med. Rehabil. *70:*763, 1989.
148. Froelicher, E. S., Kee, L. L., Newton, K. M., et al.: Return to work, sexual activity and other activities after acute myocardial infarction. Heart Lung *23:*423, 1994.
149. van Dixhoorn, J., Duivenvoorden, H. J., and Pool J.: Success and failure of exercise training after myocardial infarction: Is the outcome predictable? J. Am. Coll. Cardiol. *15:*974, 1990.
150. Allen, J. K.: Physical and psychosocial outcomes after coronary artery bypass graft surgery: Review of the literature. Heart Lung *19:*49, 1990.
151. Bethell, H. J., and Mullee, M. A.: A controlled trial of community-based coronary rehabilitation. Br. Heart J. *64:*370, 1990.
152. Juneau, M., Geneau, S., Marchand, C., and Brosseau, R.: Cardiac rehabilitation after coronary bypass surgery. Cardiovasc. Clin. *21:*25, 1991.
153. Ades, P. A., Huang, D., and Weaver, S. O.: Cardiac rehabilitation participation predicts lower rehospitalization costs. Am. Heart J. *123:*916, 1992.
154. Levin, L. A., Perk, J., and Hedback, B.: Cardiac rehabilitation: A cost analysis. J. Intern. Med. *230:*427, 1991.
155. Oldridge, N. B.: Cardiac rehabilitation services: What are they and are they worth it? Compr. Ther. *17:*59, 1991.

Chapter 41
The Cardiomyopathies and Myocarditides

JOSHUA WYNNE and EUGENE BRAUNWALD

Endomyocardial Biopsy 1404
DILATED CARDIOMYOPATHY 1407
Idiopathic Dilated Cardiomyopathy 1407
Alcoholic Cardiomyopathy 1412
HYPERTROPHIC CARDIOMYOPATHY 1414
RESTRICTIVE AND INFILTRATIVE CARDIOMYOPATHIES 1426
Amyloidosis. 1427
Inherited Infiltrative Disorders Causing Cardiomyopathy. 1430
Sarcoidosis 1431
Endomyocardial Disease 1431
MYOCARDITIS. 1435
Viral Myocarditis 1437
Rickettsial Myocarditis 1439
Bacterial Myocarditis 1439
Whipple Disease 1440
Spirochetal Infections 1440
Fungal Infections of the Heart 1441
Protozoal Myocarditis 1442
Metazoal Myocardial Disease 1444
TOXIC, CHEMICAL, IMMUNE, AND PHYSICAL DAMAGE TO THE HEART. 1445
Hypersensitivity. 1448
Giant Cell Myocarditis 1449
Physical Agents 1449
REFERENCES .1449

The cardiomyopathies constitute a group of diseases, outlined in Table 41–1, in which the dominant feature is involvement of the heart muscle itself. They are distinctive because they are not the result of pericardial, hypertensive, congenital, valvular, or ischemic diseases. The term *ischemic cardiomyopathy* (see p. 1346) refers to the condition in which coronary artery disease causes multiple infarctions or diffuse fibrosis and leads to left ventricular dilatation with congestive heart failure; it may or may not be associated with angina pectoris.[1,2] Although the diagnosis of cardiomyopathy requires the exclusion of these etiological factors, the features of cardiomyopathy are often sufficiently distinctive—both clinically and hemodynamically—to allow a positive diagnosis to be made.[3] With increasing awareness of this condition, along with improvements in diagnostic techniques, cardiomyopathy is being recognized as a significant cause of morbidity and mortality.[4] Whether the result of improved recognition or of other factors, the incidence and prevalence of cardiomyopathy appear to be increasing.[4,5]

A variety of schemes has been proposed for classifying the cardiomyopathies. The most widely recognized classification is that promulgated by the World Health Organization (WHO) (Fig. 41–1),[5a] although there have been objections to this scheme[6–8] (Tables 41–1 and 41–2). In the WHO classification, the term *cardiomyopathy* is restricted to diseases solely involving the heart muscle that are of unknown cause; other diseases that affect the myocardium but are of known cause or are part of a generalized systemic disorder are termed *specific heart muscle diseases.* Although conceptually sound, this classification system may be overly rigid for the clinician, because the *clinical* features of a given cardiomyopathy are often identical to those of one of the specific heart muscle diseases. We prefer to use the term *secondary cardiomyopathy* to identify those patients with a specific heart muscle disease that clinically closely simulates an idiopathic or *primary* cardiomyopathy.

Three basic types of functional impairment have been described (Table 41–2): (1) *dilated* (formerly called congestive), the most common form, characterized by ventricular dilatation, contractile dysfunction, and often symptoms of congestive heart failure; (2) *hypertrophic,* recognized by inappropriate left ventricular hypertrophy, often with asymmetrical involvement of the interventricular septum, usually with preserved or enhanced contractile function; and (3) *restrictive,* the most common form in western countries, marked by impaired diastolic filling, in some cases with endocardial scarring of the ventricle. Most forms of secondary cardiomyopathy are characterized by the dilated cardiomyopathy pattern. The distinction between these three functional categories is not absolute, and often there is overlap[6]; in particular, patients with hypertrophic cardiomyopathy also have increased wall stiffness (as a consequence of the myocardial hypertrophy) and thus present some of the features of a restrictive cardiomyopathy. It is difficult to fit a few conditions (such as arrhythmogenic right ventricular dysplasia, early or "latent" cardiomyopathy, and the entity of mildly dilated cardiomyopathy) neatly into the traditional functional classification scheme.[6–9]

Endomyocardial Biopsy

Evaluation of some patients suspected of suffering from a cardiomyopathy has been facilitated by the use of endo-

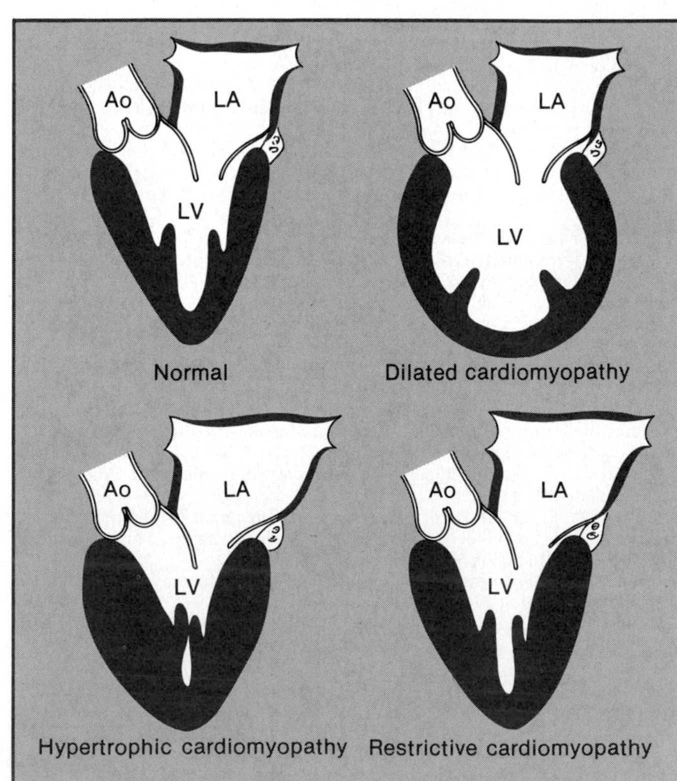

FIGURE 41–1. Diagram comparing three morphologic types of cardiomyopathies of unknown cause. Ao = Aorta, LA = left atrium, LV = left ventricle. (From Waller, B. F.: Pathology of the cardiomyopathies. J. Am. Soc. Echocardiog. *1*:4, 1988.)

TABLE 41–1 IMPORTANT CAUSES OF CARDIOMYOPATHY AND MYOCARDITIS

1. **Inflammatory**
   - a. Infective
     - Viral
     - Rickettsial
     - Bacterial
     - Mycobacterial
     - Spirochetal
     - Fungal
     - Parasitic
   - b. Noninfective
     - Collagen diseases
     - Granulomatous
     - Kawasaki
2. **Metabolic**
   - a. Nutritional
     - Thiamine
     - Kwashiorkor
     - Pellagra
     - Scurvy
     - Hypervitaminosis D
     - Obesity
     - Selenium deficiency
     - Carnitine deficiency
   - b. Endocrine
     - Acromegaly
     - Thyrotoxicosis
     - Myxedema
     - Uremia
     - Cushing's disease
     - Pheochromocytoma
     - Diabetes mellitus
   - c. Altered metabolism
     - Gout
     - Oxalosis
     - Porphyria
   - d. Electrolyte imbalance
3. **Toxic**
   - a. Cobalt
   - b. Alcohol
   - c. Bleomycin
   - d. Adriamycin
   - e. Phenothiazines and antidepressants
   - f. Antimony compounds
   - g. Carbon monoxide
   - h. Lead
   - i. Emetine and dehydroemetine
   - j. Chloroquine
   - k. Lithium
   - l. Cyclophosphamide
   - m. Hydrocarbons
   - n. Catecholamines
   - o. Phosphorus
   - p. Mercury
   - q. Insect stings
   - r. Snake bites
   - s. Paracetamol
   - t. Reserpine
   - u. Corticosteroids
   - v. Cocaine
   - w. Methysergide
4. **Infiltrative**
   - a. Amyloidosis
   - b. Hemochromatosis
   - c. Neoplastic
   - d. Glycogen storage disorders
   - e. Sarcoidosis
   - f. Mucopolysaccharidosis
   - g. Fabry disease
   - h. Whipple disease
   - i. Gaucher disease
   - j. Sphingolipidoses
5. **Fibroplastic**
   - a. Endomyocardial fibrosis
   - b. Endocardial fibroelastosis
   - c. Löffler's fibroplastic endocarditis
   - d. Carcinoid
6. **Hematological**
   - a. Sickle cell anemia
   - b. Polycythemia vera
   - c. Thrombotic thrombocytopenic purpura
   - d. Leukemia
7. **Hypersensitivity**
   - a. Methyldopa
   - b. Penicillin
   - c. Sulfonamides
   - d. Tetracycline
   - e. Phenindione
   - f. Phenylbutazone
   - g. Antituberculous drugs
   - h. Giant cell myocarditis
   - i. Cardiac transplant rejection
8. **Genetic**
   - a. Hypertrophic cardiomyopathy
     - With gradient
     - Without gradient
   - b. Neuromuscular
     - Duchenne muscular dystrophy
     - Facioscapulohumeral muscular dystrophy
     - Limb-girdle dystrophy of Erb
     - Myotonia dystrophica
     - Friedreich's ataxia
     - Kearns-Sayre syndrome
     - Nemaline cardiomyopathy
     - Multicore cardiomyopathy
9. **Miscellaneous acquired**
   - a. Postpartum cardiomyopathy
   - b. Obesity
10. **Idiopathic**
    - a. Idiopathic dilated cardiomyopathy
    - b. Idiopathic restrictive cardiomyopathy
    - c. Idiopathic hypertrophic cardiomyopathy
    - d. Idiopathic arrhythmogenic right ventricular dysplasia
11. **Physical agents**
    - a. Heat stroke
    - b. Hypothermia
    - c. Radiation
    - d. Tachycardia

myocardial biopsy (see p. 186).[10,11] Using a flexible bioptome, the clinician easily and safely may obtain tissue samples from the right (and occasionally left) ventricle via a transvenous (or transarterial) approach (Fig. 41–2). The availability of disposable transfemoral bioptomes has further facilitated endomyocardial biopsy. Two-dimensional echocardiography may help guide the placement of the bioptome and reduce or eliminate radiation exposure.[12–15] Endomyocardial biopsy results in a small tissue sample (average size 1 to 2 mm), and multiple samples (usually four or more) are required because pronounced topographic variations may be found within the myocardium. Which

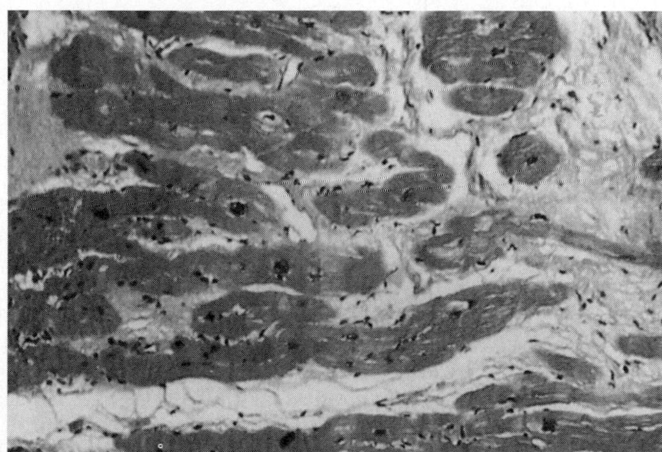
A

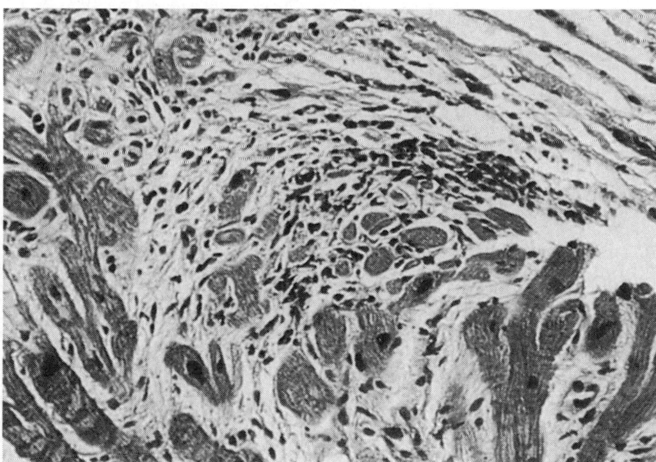
B

FIGURE 41–2. Histological specimens obtained by right ventricular endomyocardial biopsy. *A,* Idiopathic dilated cardiomyopathy with varying degrees of interstitial fibrosis and myocyte hypertrophy (trichrome stain, ×210). *B,* Myocarditis with dense focal area of mononuclear cell infiltrate adjacent to necrotic and degenerating myocytes, with irregular myocytic hypertrophy and dense interstitial fibrosis (hematoxylin and eosin, ×210). (From Dec, G. W., and Fuster, V.: Idiopathic dilated cardiomyopathy. N. Engl. J. Med. *331*:1564, 1994. Copyright Massachusetts Medical Society.)

TABLE 41–2 FUNCTIONAL CLASSIFICATION OF THE CARDIOMYOPATHIES

	DILATED	RESTRICTIVE	HYPERTROPHIC
Symptoms	Congestive heart failure, particularly left-sided Fatigue and weakness Systemic or pulmonary emboli	Dyspnea, fatigue Right-sided congestive heart failure Signs and symptoms of systemic disease: amyloidosis, iron storage disease, etc.	Dyspnea, angina pectoris Fatigue, syncope, palpitations
Physical Examination	Moderate to severe cardiomegaly; S_3 and S_4 Atrioventricular valve regurgitation, especially mitral	Mild to moderate cardiomegaly: S_3 or S_4 Atrioventricular valve regurgitation; inspiratory increase in venous pressure (Kussmaul's sign)	Mild cardiomegaly Apical systolic thrill and heave; brisk carotid upstroke S_4 common Systolic murmur that increases with Valsalva maneuver
Chest Roentgenogram	Moderate to marked cardiac enlargement, especially left ventricular Pulmonary venous hypertension	Mild cardiac enlargement Pulmonary venous hypertension	Mild to moderate cardiac enlargement Left atrial enlargement
Electrocardiogram	Sinus tachycardia Atrial and ventricular arrhythmias ST-segment and T-wave abnormalities Intraventricular conduction defects	Low voltage Intraventricular conduction defects AV conduction defects	Left ventricular hypertrophy ST-segment and T-wave abnormalities Abnormal Q waves Atrial and ventricular arrhythmias
Echocardiogram	Left ventricular dilatation and dysfunction Abnormal diastolic mitral valve motion secondary to abnormal compliance and filling pressures	Increased left ventricular wall thickness and mass Small or normal-sized left ventricular cavity Normal systolic function Pericardial effusion	Asymmetrical septal hypertrophy (ASH) Narrow left ventricular outflow tract Systolic anterior motion (SAM) of the mitral valve Small or normal-sized left ventricle
Radionuclide Studies	Left ventricular dilatation and dysfunction (RVG)	Infiltration of myocardium (^{201}Tl) Small or normal-sized left ventricle (RVG) Normal systolic function (RVG)	Small or normal-sized left ventricle (RVG) Vigorous systolic function (RVG) Asymmetrical septal hypertrophy (RVG or ^{201}Tl)
Cardiac Catheterization	Left ventricular enlargement and dysfunction Mitral and/or tricuspid regurgitation Elevated left- and often right-sided filling pressures Diminished cardiac output	Diminished left ventricular compliance "Square root sign" in ventricular pressure recordings Preserved systolic function Elevated left- and right-sided filling pressures	Diminished left ventricular compliance Mitral regurgitation Vigorous systolic function Dynamic left ventricular outflow gradient

RVG = Radionuclide ventriculogram; ^{201}Tl = thallium-201.

patients should be subjected to biopsy remains controversial, but there is general agreement that biopsy may be of benefit in certain specific situations; there is little debate as to its clinical utility in detecting infiltrative disorders of the myocardium and in monitoring for anthracycline cardiotoxicity and cardiac transplant rejection (Table 41–3).[10,11]

TABLE 41–3 CLINICAL INDICATIONS FOR ENDOMYOCARDIAL BIOPSY

DEFINITE
Monitoring of cardiac allograft rejection Monitoring of anthracycline cardiotoxicity
POSSIBLE
Detection and monitoring of myocarditis Diagnosis of secondary cardiomyopathies Differentiation between restrictive and constrictive heart disease
UNCERTAIN
Unexplained, life-threatening ventricular tachyarrhythmias AIDS Formulation of prognosis in idiopathic dilated cardiomyopathy

From Mason, J. W., and O'Connell, J. B.: Clinical merit of endomyocardial biopsy. Circulation *79*:971, 1989. Copyright American Heart Association.

Although on occasion endomyocardial biopsy may identify a specific etiological agent in an individual patient with cardiac disease of uncertain cause (Table 41–4), the clinical utility of routine biopsy in cardiomyopathy is limited (particularly because no definitive pattern has been found in dilated cardiomyopathy) (Table 41–5).[5] It has been estimated that a specific etiologic diagnosis is obtained by biopsy in less than 10 per cent of patients with cardiomyopathy, and a treatable disease is found in only about 2 per cent.[10,11]

Dallas Criteria. Interpretation of biopsy specimens had been plagued by a high degree of interobserver variability; the adoption of a generally accepted set of histological definitions,[16] the *Dallas criteria,* appears to have substantially improved agreement. It is hoped that newer immunohistochemical and molecular biological techniques (such as the polymerase chain reaction or in situ hybridization techniques to detect viral infection of the heart) may expand further the diagnostic utility of endomyocardial biopsy.[16–21]

TABLE 41–4 SPECIFIC DIAGNOSES THAT CAN BE CONFIRMED BY MYOCARDIAL BIOPSY

Cardiac allograft rejection	Fabry disease of the heart	Henoch-Schönlein purpura
Myocarditis	Carcinoid disease	Rheumatic carditis
Giant cell myocarditis	Irradiation injury	Chagasic cardiomyopathy
Doxorubicin cardiotoxicity	Glycogen storage disease	Chloroquine cardiomyopathy
Cardiac amyloidosis	Cardiac tumors of cardiac origin	Lyme carditis
Cardiac sarcoidosis	Cardiac tumors of noncardiac origin	Carnitine deficiency cardiomyopathy
Cardiac hemochromatosis	Kearns-Sayre syndrome	Right ventricular lipomatosis
Endocardial fibrosis	Cytomegalovirus infection	Hypereosinophilic syndrome
Endocardial fibroelastosis	Toxoplasmosis	

From Mason, J. W., and O'Connell, J. B.: Clinical merit of endomyocardial biopsy. Circulation *79*:971, 1989, reprinted by permission of the American Heart Association, Inc.

TABLE 41–5 ENDOMYOCARDIAL BIOPSY CHARACTERISTICS

DILATED CARDIOMYOPATHY	HYPERTROPHIC CARDIOMYOPATHY
Light Microscopy	**Light Microscopy**
Increase in myofiber size	Endocardial thickening and fibrosis
Attenuation of cells	Marked myocardial hypertrophy
Hyperchromatic, irregular shaped nuclei	Large, bizarre nuclei
Interstitial, focal, perivascular fibrosis	Myofiber disorganization
	Interstitial fibrosis
Electron Microscopy	**Electron Microscopy**
Hypertrophic changes	Myofibrillar disarray
Increased number of sarcomeres and mitochondria	Increased side-to-side junctions
Large, lobulated nuclei	Increased cell branching
Z-band abnormalities	Increased glycogen
Irregular invaginations of sarcolemma	
Widened, convoluted, intercalated discs	**MYOCARDITIS**
Degenerative Changes	**Light and Electron Microscopy**
Myofilament loss	Inflammatory infiltrate, usually lymphocytic
Aggregation of glycogen and mitochondria	Necrosis or degeneration of adjacent myocytes
Pleomorphic mitochondria	Uninvolved, normal myocardium
Myelin figures, lipid vacuoles	Absence of severe chronic myocardial changes

From Leatherbury, L., Chandra, R. S., Chapiro, S. R., and Perry, L. W.: Value of endomyocardial biopsy in infants, children, and adolescents with dilated or hypertrophic cardiomyopathy and myocarditis. Reprinted from the American College of Cardiology. J. Am. Coll. Cardiol. *12*:1547, 1988.

DILATED CARDIOMYOPATHY

IDIOPATHIC DILATED CARDIOMYOPATHY

Dilated cardiomyopathy (DCM) is a syndrome characterized by cardiac enlargement and impaired systolic function of one or both ventricles (Fig. 41–3). Although it was formerly called congestive cardiomyopathy, the term *dilated cardiomyopathy* is now preferred because the earliest abnormality usually is ventricular enlargement and systolic contractile dysfunction, with congestive heart failure often (but not invariably) developing later. In an occasional patient, the predominant finding is that of contractile dysfunction with only a mildly dilated left ventricle.[22,23]

The incidence of DCM is reported to be about 5 to 8 cases per 100,000 population per year and appears to be increasing, although the true figure likely is higher as a consequence of underreporting of mild or asymptomatic cases.[5,24] It occurs almost three times more frequently in blacks and males than in whites and females, and this difference does not appear to be related solely to differing degrees of hypertension, cigarette smoking, or alcohol use[4,5,25–27]; furthermore, survival in blacks appears to be worse than in whites.[23,28]

Although the cause is not definable in many cases, more than 75 specific diseases of heart muscle can produce the clinical manifestations of DCM. It is likely that this condition represents a final common pathway that is the end result of myocardial damage produced by a variety of cytotoxic, metabolic, immunological, familial, and infectious mechanisms.[24] Alcohol, for example, may lead to severe cardiac dysfunction and may produce clinical, hemodynamic, and pathological findings identical to those present in idiopathic dilated cardiomyopathy (see p. 1412).

The natural history of DCM is not well established. Many

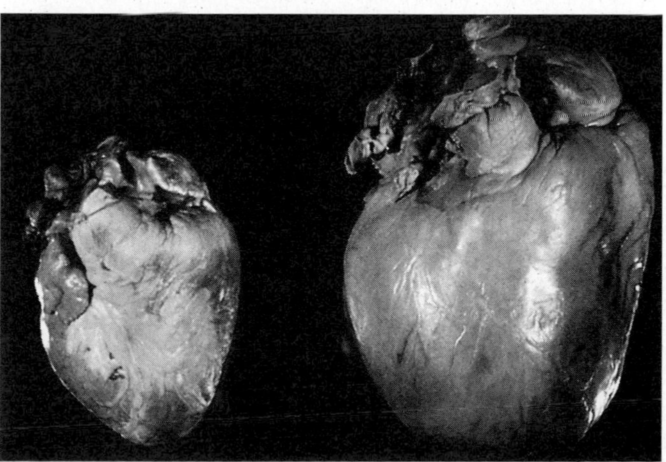

FIGURE 41–3. Gross pathology of normal heart *(left)* and heart in idiopathic dilated cardiomyopathy *(right),* characterized by biventricular hypertrophy and four-chamber enlargement. (From Kasper, E. K., Hruban, R. H., and Baughman, K. L.: Idiopathic dilated cardiomyopathy. *In* Abelmann, W. H., and Braunwald, E., [eds.]: Cardiomyopathies, Myocarditis, and Pericardial Disease. Atlas of Heart Diseases. Vol. 2. Philadelphia, Current Medicine, 1995, pp. 3.1–3.18.)

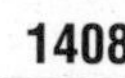

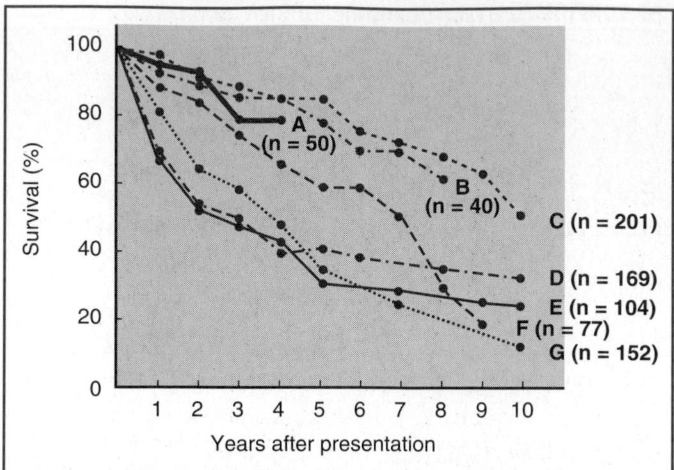

FIGURE 41–4. Survival of patients with idiopathic dilated cardiomyopathy in seven published series (A to G). n = number of patients studied. To identify each specific series, see article by Dec and Fuster. (From Dec, G. W., and Fuster, V.: Idiopathic dilated cardiomyopathy. N. Engl. J. Med. *331*:1564, 1994. Copyright Massachusetts Medical Society.)

patients have minimal or no symptoms and the progression of the disease in these patients is unclear, although there is some evidence that the long-term prognosis is not good.[29] Nevertheless, in symptomatic patients the course usually is one of progressive deterioration, with a quarter of newly diagnosed patients referred to major medical centers dying within a year, and half dying within 5 years, although a minority improve, with a reduction in cardiac size and longer survival (Fig. 41–4).[22,24] Recent data suggest that in patients with mild dilatation not referred to a medical center the prognosis may be more favorable, reflecting earlier diagnosis and better treatment (Fig. 41–5).[3,5,24] About a quarter of patients with recent onset DCM improve spontaneously, even some sick enough initially to be considered for cardiac transplantation.[30,31] In some patients clinical and functional improvements may occur years after initial presentation. A variety of clinical predictors of patients at enhanced risk of death in DCM have been identified (Table 41–6).[32] However, the predictive reliability of any single feature is not high.[33] It may be difficult to predict with any accuracy the clinical course and outcome in an individual

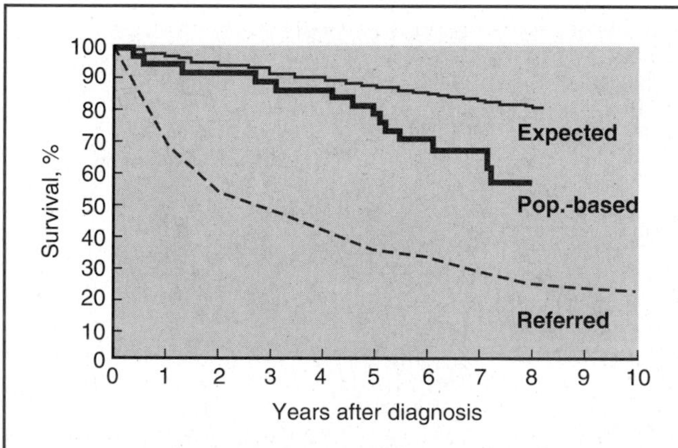

FIGURE 41–5. Survival of patients with idiopathic dilated cardiomyopathy, contrasting the poor survival in the cohort referred to a major medical center (Referred) with the much better survival in the nonreferred population-based cohort (Pop.-based). Both survival curves are compared with the expected survival of a 1980 Minnesota white cohort (Expected). (From Sugrue, D. D., Rodeheffer, R. J., Codd, M. B., et al.: The clinical course of idiopathic dilated cardiomyopathy. A population-based study. Ann. Intern. Med. *117*:117, 1992.)

TABLE 41–6 FACTORS ASSOCIATED WITH REDUCED SURVIVAL IN DILATED CARDIOMYOPATHY

S_3
Left ventricular conduction delay
Elevation of filling pressures
Absence of left ventricular thickening
Age > 55 years
Cardiac enlargement
Depressed cardiac output
Depressed ejection fraction
Depressed serum sodium levels
Elevated serum norepinephrine levels
Functional class
Ventricular arrhythmias
Large thallium defects
Myocardial biopsy findings
Ventricular shape (more spherical)

patient.[5,24] Nevertheless, greater ventricular enlargement and worse dysfunction tend to correlate with poorer prognosis.[24,32,34–36] Cardiopulmonary exercise testing also can provide prognostic information (see p. 153). Marked limitation of exercise capacity manifested by reduced maximal systemic oxygen uptake (especially when below 10 to 12 ml/kg/min) is a reliable predictor of mortality and is used widely as an indicator for consideration of cardiac transplantation.[24] It has been suggested that specific endomyocardial biopsy morphological findings (such as loss of intracellular myofilaments) may offer some predictive information regarding prognosis[24,37,38] (Table 41–5).

Pathology

POSTMORTEM EXAMINATION. This reveals enlargement and dilatation of all four chambers; the ventricles are more dilated than the atria (Fig. 41–3). Although the thickness of the ventricular wall is increased in some cases, the degree of hypertrophy often is less than might be expected given the severe dilatation present.[24] The development of left ventricular hypertrophy appears to have a protective or beneficial role in dilated cardiomyopathy, presumably because it reduces systolic wall stress and thus protects against further cavity dilatation.[39,40] The cardiac valves are intrinsically normal, and intracavitary thrombi, particularly in the ventricular apex, are common.[24,41] The coronary arteries usually are normal. The right ventricle is preferentially involved in some cases of dilated cardiomyopathy, sometimes on a familial basis.

HISTOLOGICAL EXAMINATION. Microscopic study reveals extensive areas of interstitial and perivascular fibrosis, particularly involving the left ventricular subendocardium (Fig. 41–2). Small areas of necrosis and cellular infiltrate are seen on occasion, but these typically are not prominent features.[41] There is marked variation in myocyte size; some myocardial cells are hypertrophied and others are atrophied.[41] Cardiac biopsy specimens obtained during life demonstrate a variety of similar abnormalities, including interstitial fibrosis, cellular infiltrates, myocyte hypertrophy, and myocardial cell degeneration.[42] No viruses or other etiological agents have been identified with any regularity in tissue from patients with DCM. Particularly disappointing has been the failure to identify any immunological, histochemical, morphological, ultrastructural, or microbiological marker that might be used to establish the diagnosis of idiopathic dilated cardiomyopathy or to clarify its cause.

Etiology

It is likely that idiopathic DCM represents a common expression of myocardial damage that has been produced by a variety of as yet unestablished myocardial insults. Although the cause(s) remain unclear,[43] interest has centered on three possible basic mechanisms of damage: familial and genetic factors; viral myocarditis and other cytotoxic insults; and immunological abnormalities (Fig. 41–6).[23,24,44]

Familial linkage of DCM occurs more commonly than often appreciated. In 20 per cent of patients, a first-degree relative also shows evidence of DCM, suggesting that familial transmission is relatively frequent.[5,23,45–48,48a] Most familial cases demonstrate autosomal dominant transmission[23,48] (see p. 1665), but the disease is genetically quite heterogeneous, and autosomal recessive[49] and X-linked inheritance[46,50,51] has been found. One form of familial X-linked dilated cardiomyopathy is due to a deletion in the promotor region and the first exon of the gene that codes for the protein dystrophin, a component of the cytoskeleton of myocytes.[50] This has fueled speculation that a resulting deficiency of cardiac dystrophin is the cause of the dilated cardiomyopathy.[46] Mutations involving mitochondrial DNA have been reported as well.[52–55] Whether any of the patients without apparent familial linkage have a genetic predisposition to DCM remains unknown.[46] There is great interest in using molecular genetic techniques to identify markers of disease susceptibility in asymptomatic carriers at risk for the eventual development of overt clinical DCM.[51,56,56a] An example of such a marker may be the angiotensin-converting enzyme DD genotype that is found with increased frequency in DCM patients.[57] One intriguing familial metabolic deficiency is that of carnitine, with improvement occurring in the myopathy with carnitine repletion.[58,59]

There has been wide speculation that an episode of subclinical viral myocarditis initiates an autoimmune reaction that culminates in the development of full-blown DCM.[60–62] Although this hypothesis is inviting, it remains largely unsupported[63]; it has been estimated that only 15 per cent of patients with myocarditis progress to DCM.[64] In some patients who exhibit the clinical features of DCM, endomyocardial biopsy reveals evidence of an inflammatory myocarditis. The reported frequency of finding evidence of an inflammatory infiltrate in DCM varies widely and undoubtedly depends largely on patient selection and the criteria used for diagnosis; using rigorous criteria, only about 10 per cent (or less) of patients with DCM have biopsy evidence of myocarditis.[10,11] Other evidence favoring the concept that DCM is a postviral disorder includes the presence of high antibody viral titers,[60,65] viral-specific RNA sequences,[66,67] and apparent viral particles[64] in patients with "idiopathic" dilated cardiomyopathy. On the other hand, the more rigorous technique of polymerase chain reaction generally has not confirmed the presence of viral remnants in the myocardium of most cardiomyopathy patients,[68–71] although data are conflicting.[72–74]

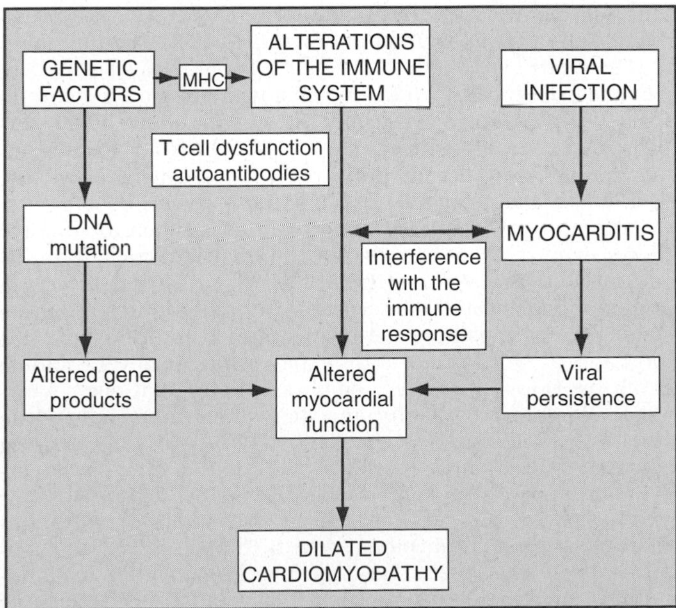

FIGURE 41–6. Hypotheses to explain the pathogenesis of dilated cardiomyopathy. (From Mestroni, L., Krajinovic, M., Severini, G. M., et al.: Familial dilated cardiomyopathy. Br. Heart J. *72*:S35, 1994.)

Abnormalities of both humoral and cellular immunity have been found in patients with DCM,[23,44,75–77] although the findings have not been completely reproducible. There is speculation that antibodies might be the *result* of myocardial damage, rather than the cause.[78] There appears to be an association with specific HLA Class II antigens (such as DR4 and DQw4), suggesting that abnormalities of immunoregulation may play a role in DCM.[56,79] Circulating antimyocardial antibodies to a variety of antigens (including the myosin heavy chain, the beta-adrenoreceptor, the muscarinic receptor, laminin, and mitochondria) have been identified.[44,45,76,80–84] Abnormalities of various T cells, including cytotoxic T cells, suppressor T lymphocytes, and natural killer cells have been found in some but not all studies.[24,85] It has been suggested that these putative immunological abnormalities may be the consequence of prior viral myocarditis.[85] It is thought that viral components may be incorporated into the cardiac sarcolemma, only to serve as an antigenic source that directs the immune response to attack the myocardium. Nevertheless, the precise role of either humoral or cellular immunomodulation in the pathogenesis of DCM remains unestablished.[24]

A variety of other possible causes has been proposed, although none is accepted as *the* cause of DCM. Thus, endocrine abnormalities as well as the effects of chemicals or toxins have been suggested as possible etiological factors. It has been suggested that microvascular hyperreactivity (spasm) may lead to myocellular necrosis and scarring, with resultant heart failure, although this remains speculative.[1,39] From a clinical standpoint, the more important causes of secondary DCM include alcohol and cocaine abuse, human immunodeficiency virus,[86] metabolic abnormalities, and the cardiotoxicity of anticancer drugs (especially doxorubicin).

ABNORMALITIES OF THE SYMPATHETIC NERVOUS SYSTEM. Several abnormalities of the sympathetic nervous system have been demonstrated in DCM, but they appear to be more the result than the cause of the disease.[24,87] A reduction in density of membrane-associated beta-adrenoceptors[88–90] is believed to be a consequence of the development of anti–beta-adrenoceptor autoantibodies.[76,82] An alteration in the signal transmission pathway by which the beta-receptors stimulate the contractile apparatus (the G-protein system) has been found as well. Inhibition of this system is enhanced in DCM patients, perhaps accounting for their depressed contractile function. An increase of the α subunits of the inhibitory guanine nucleotide–binding protein ($G_{i\alpha}$) has been reported to occur in the membranes of myocytes from failing hearts.[91–93] This abnormality has been shown to be more profound in myocardial membranes from hearts with dilated than in those with ischemic cardiomyopathy.[94] This increase in $G_{i\alpha}$ is associated with a striking reduction of basal adenylate cyclase activity and of the positive inotropic effects of isoproterenol and of the phosphodiesterase inhibitor milrinone (see p. 484). These findings suggest that the increase of $G_{i\alpha}$ might contribute to the reduced effects of endogenous catecholamines in DCM. The precise cause of contractile dysfunction at the cellular level in patients with DCM remains unclear. Although there are demonstrable abnormalities of cellular metabolism and calcium handling by cardiomyopathic tissue,[1,95–99] the significance of these findings is not yet clear.

Clinical Manifestations

(Fig. 41–7)

HISTORY. Symptoms usually develop gradually in patients with DCM. Some patients are asymptomatic and yet have left ventricular dilatation for months or even years which is clinically recognized only later when symptoms develop or when routine chest roentgenography demonstrates cardiomegaly.[100] Other patients, after recovery from what appears to be a systemic viral infection, develop symptoms of heart failure for the first time. In still others, severe heart failure develops acutely during an episode of myocarditis; although some recovery occurs, chronic manifestations of diminished cardiac reserve persist and heart failure reappears months or years later. It is important to carefully question the patient and family about alcohol consumption, because excessive alcohol consumption is a major cause of secondary DCM, and its cessation may result in substantial clinical improvement.[24] Although patients of any age may be affected, the disease is most common in middle age and is more frequent in men than in women.

The most striking symptoms are those of left ventricular failure. Fatigue and weakness due to diminished cardiac output are common. Exercise intolerance is common and

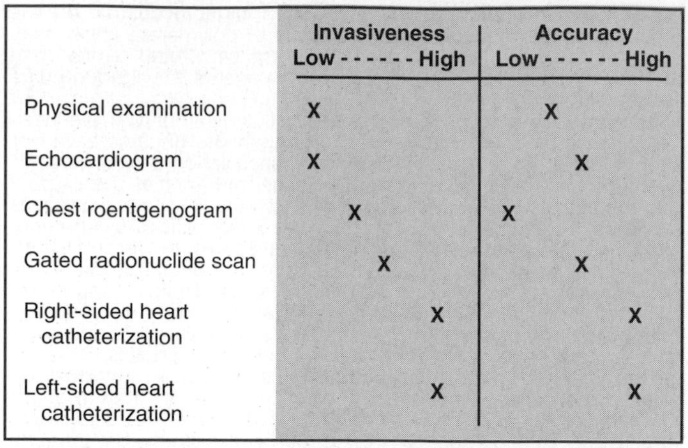

	Invasiveness Low ------ High				Accuracy Low ------ High			
Physical examination	X					X		
Echocardiogram	X						X	
Chest roentgenogram		X			X			
Gated radionuclide scan			X				X	
Right-sided heart catheterization				X				X
Left-sided heart catheterization				X				X

FIGURE 41–7. Assessment of utility of diagnostic techniques in idiopathic dilated cardiomyopathy. (From Manolio, T. A., Baughman, K. L., Rodeheffer, R., et al.: Prevalence and etiology of idiopathic dilated cardiomyopathy [summary of a National Heart, Lung, and Blood Institute workshop]. Am. J. Cardiol. *69*:1458, 1992.)

relates, at least in part, to reduced skeletal muscle perfusion as well as histological and biochemical alterations in the exercising muscle groups.[101] Right heart failure is a late and ominous sign and is associated with a particularly poor prognosis. Chest pain occurs in about one-third of patients and may suggest concomitant ischemic heart disease.[3,24,102] A reduction in the vasodilator reserve of the coronary microvasculature in DCM suggests that subendocardial ischemia may play a role in the genesis of chest pain despite angiographically normal coronary arteries.[103] Chest pain secondary to pulmonary embolism and abdominal pain secondary to congestive hepatomegaly are frequent in the late stages of illness.

PHYSICAL EXAMINATION. This usually reveals variable degrees of cardiac enlargement and findings of congestive heart failure. The systolic blood pressure is usually normal or low, and the pulse pressure is narrow, reflecting a diminished stroke volume. *Pulsus alternans* (see p. 22) is common when severe left ventricular failure is present. The jugular veins are distended when right heart failure appears, but on initial presentation most patients do not have evidence of this.[24] Prominent *a* and *v* waves are visible, the latter a late manifestation of the presence of tricuspid valvular regurgitation. The liver may be engorged and pulsatile. Peripheral edema and ascites are present when right heart failure is advanced. Wheezing resulting from bronchospasm may be found, apparently as a consequence of bronchial hyperresponsiveness.[104]

The precordium usually reveals left and, occasionally, right ventricular impulses, but the heaves are not sustained, as they are in patients with ventricular hypertrophy. The apical impulse is usually displaced laterally, reflecting left ventricular dilatation. A presystolic *a* wave may be palpable. The second heart sound is usually normally split, although paradoxical splitting (see p. 33) may be detected in the presence of left bundle branch block, an electrocardiographic finding that is not unusual in dilated cardiomyopathy. If pulmonary hypertension is present, the pulmonary component of the second heart sound may be accentuated, and the splitting may be narrow. Presystolic gallop sounds (S_4) are almost universally present and often precede the development of overt congestive heart failure.[24] Ventricular gallops (S_3) are the rule once cardiac decompensation occurs, and a summation gallop is heard when there is concomitant tachycardia. Systolic murmurs are common and are usually due to mitral or, less commonly, tricuspid valvular regurgitation.[24] Mitral regurgitation results from enlargement and abnormal motion of the mitral annulus; ventricular dilatation with resultant distortion of the geometry of the subvalvular apparatus ("papillary muscle dysfunction") plays a lesser role.[105] Gallop sounds and regurgitant murmurs can often be elicited or intensified by isometric handgrip exercise with its attendant enhancement of systemic vascular resistance and impedance to left ventricular outflow (see p. 48). Systemic emboli resulting from dislodgment of intracardiac thrombi from the left atrium and ventricle and pulmonary emboli that originate in the venous system of the legs are common late complications.

NONINVASIVE LABORATORY EXAMINATIONS. To identify potentially reversible secondary causes of dilated cardiomyopathy, several basic screening biochemical tests are indicated, including determination of serum phosphorus (hypophosphatemia), serum calcium (hypocalcemia), serum creatinine and urea nitrogen (uremia), thyroid function studies (hypo- and hyperthyroidism), and iron studies (hemochromatosis). It is prudent to test for the human immunodeficiency virus (HIV) as well, as this infection is an important and often unrecognized cause of congestive heart failure.[86] The *chest roentgenogram* usually reveals generalized cardiomegaly and pulmonary vascular redistribution; interstitial and alveolar edema are less common on initial presentation.[24] Pleural effusions may be present, and the azygos vein and superior vena cava may be dilated when right heart failure supervenes.

Electrocardiography. The electrocardiogram often shows sinus tachycardia when heart failure is present. The entire spectrum of atrial and ventricular tachyarrhythmias may be seen. Poor R-wave progression and intraventricular conduction abnormalities, especially left bundle branch block, are common.[24] Anterior Q waves may be present when there is extensive left ventricular fibrosis, even without a discrete myocardial scar.[24,106] ST-segment and T-wave abnormalities are common, as are P-wave changes, especially left atrial abnormality.[106] Ambulatory monitoring demonstrates the ubiquity of ventricular arrhythmias, with about half of monitored patients with DCM exhibiting nonsustained ventricular tachycardia.[24] There is no consensus that complex or frequent ventricular arrhythmias predict sudden (presumably arrhythmic) death, although they do appear to predict total mortality.[106–108] Perhaps ventricular arrhythmias as detected on ambulatory monitoring are a marker for the extent of myocardial damage in DCM and therefore are *associated* with sudden death without necessarily being its *cause.* In occasional cases, particularly in children, recurrent and/or incessant supraventricular or ventricular tachyarrhythmias may actually be the *cause* (rather than the result) of ventricular dysfunction.[109–112] In those cases, restoration of sinus rhythm or slowing of the heart rate may be therapeutic.

Echocardiography. Two-dimensional and Doppler forms of echocardiography are useful in assessing the degree of impairment of left ventricular function and for excluding concomitant valvular or pericardial disease (Chap. 3).[5] In addition to examining all four cardiac valves for evidence of structural or functional abnormalities, echocardiography allows evaluation of the size of the ventricular cavity and thickness of the ventricular walls. A pericardial effusion may be demonstrated on occasion. Doppler studies are useful in delineating the severity of mitral (and tricuspid) regurgitation.[76,82] Patients with a pattern of left ventricular filling on Doppler studies which simulates that seen with restrictive cardiomyopathy appear to have more advanced disease.[113] Combining echocardiography with dobutamine infusion may identify patients with left ventricular dysfunction due to coronary artery disease by demonstrating provocable regional differences in wall motion and thus distinguish them from patients with idiopathic DCM.[114,114a] It has been suggested that *thallium-201* imaging may be helpful in distinguishing left ventricular enlargement caused by DCM from that caused by coronary artery disease,[115,116] although there is not complete agreement on this point.[24,117] Scanning with *gallium* or *antimyosin antibody* (see p. 296) may help to identify patients more likely to have evidence of myocarditis on biopsy, although whether this finding is useful clinically is not yet established.[24,118–120]

Radionuclide Ventriculography. Like echocardiography, radionuclide ventriculography reveals increased end-diastolic and end-systolic left ventricular volumes, reduced ejection fractions in both ventricles, and wall-motion abnormalities; it is used most commonly when echocardiography is technically suboptimal.[24] Like echocardiography, it may demonstrate segmental wall motion abnormalities in DCM even in the absence of coronary artery disease, the disease process that most commonly produces regional dysfunction. In most patients it is not necessary to carry out serial studies or batteries of noninvasive tests in order to follow patients with DCM and evaluate their response to treatment.

CARDIAC CATHETERIZATION AND ANGIOCARDIOGRAPHY. Only select patients with DCM require cardiac catheterization[24] (particularly those with chest pain and a suspicion of ischemic disease, or patients thought to have a treatable systemic disease such as sarcoidosis or hemochromatosis). When cardiac catheterization is done, the left ventricular end-diastolic, left atrial, and pulmonary artery wedge pressures are usually elevated. Modest degrees of pulmonary arterial hypertension are common. Advanced cases may demonstrate right ventricular dilatation and failure as well, with resultant elevation of the right ventricular end-diastolic, right atrial, and central venous pressures.

Left ventriculography demonstrates enlargement of this chamber, typically with diffuse reduction in wall motion. Segmental wall motion abnormalities are not uncommon and may simulate the angiographic findings in ischemic heart disease.[121] However, prominent localized wall disorders are more characteristic of ischemic heart disease, whereas diffuse global dysfunction is more typical of DCM. The ejection fraction is reduced and the end-systolic volume is increased as a result of the impairment of left ventricular contractility. Sometimes left ventricular thrombi may be visualized within the left ventricle as intracavitary filling defects. Mild mitral regurgitation is often present. On occasion, it may be difficult to distinguish left ventricular dilatation secondary to severe mitral regurgitation due to intrinsic mitral valve disease from DCM with secondary mitral regurgitation.

Coronary arteriography usually reveals normal vessels, although coronary vasodilatory capacity may be impaired[103,122,123]; in some cases this may relate to marked elevation of the left ventricular filling pressures.[124] This examination may be of particular value in excluding coronary artery disease in patients with abnormal Q waves on the electrocardiogram or regional left ventricular wall motion abnormalities on noninvasive testing. Coronary arteriography thus helps to distinguish between myocardial infarction as a result of obstructive coronary artery disease, and extensive localized myocardial fibrosis secondary to severe DCM in the absence of coronary artery obstruction.

Management

Because the cause of idiopathic dilated cardiomyopathy is unknown, specific therapy is not possible. Treatment, therefore, is for heart failure, as discussed in Chapter 17.[125] Physical, dietary, and pharmacological interventions may help to control symptoms; only cardiac transplantation[125a] (Chap. 18) and specific pharmacological therapy (the vasodilators enalapril or hydralazine plus nitrates, and the beta-adrenoceptor blocker carvedilol) have been shown to prolong life (Table 41–7).[24,125–128,128a] Although the demonstrated benefits of vasodilator therapy are more equivocal in asymptomatic patients, we favor their use when not contraindicated in hopes of limiting progressive ventricular dilatation and preventing or delaying symptomatic deterioration.

Because of evidence that activation of the sympathetic nervous system may have deleterious cardiac effects (rather

TABLE 41–7 APPROACH TO MANAGEMENT OF DILATED CARDIOMYOPATHY

Initiate conventional management with digoxin, diuretics, and angiotensin-converting enzyme inhibitors or hydralazine/isosorbide dinitrate.
Consider beta-adrenergic blockade if symptoms persist.
Add anticoagulation for ejection fraction less than 0.30, history of thromboembolic phenomena, or detection of mural thrombi.
If symptomatic at rest despite above measures, add intravenous dobutamine and/or phosphodiesterase inhibitor and consider cardiac transplantation.

Adapted from O'Connell, J. B., Moore, C. K., and Waterer, H. C.: Treatment of end stage dilated cardiomyopathy. Br. Heart J. *72:*S52, 1994.

than being an important compensatory mechanism as traditionally thought), beta-adrenoceptor blockade (usually with metoprolol) has been suggested as treatment for DCM[24] (see p. 487). Results to date generally have been favorable, with evidence of improved symptoms, exercise capacity, and left ventricular function, and a suggestion that survival has been improved.[24,129–136] Beta-adrenoceptor blockade has been surprisingly well tolerated, with infrequent aggravation of heart failure (which, on occasion, may be profound). The mechanism of beneficial action of beta-adrenoceptorblockers is unknown[125] but may relate to: (1) negative chronotropic effect with reduced myocardial oxygen demand, (2) reduced myocardial damage due to catecholamines, (3) improved diastolic relaxation, (4) inhibition of sympathetically mediated vasoconstriction, (5) increase ("upregulation") in myocardial beta-adrenoceptor density,[137] or (6) improved calcium handling at slower rates.[88,138–141] Despite the encouraging data, the use of beta-adrenoceptor blockade in DCM still is considered investigational. Recent data indicate that carvedilol (a beta-adrenoceptor blocker with alpha-adrenoceptor blocking and antioxidant effects) substantially reduces mortality in DCM.[128a]

Because of the possible link between DCM, microvascular circulatory abnormalities, and abnormal myocardial calcium handling, there has been interest in the use of calcium antagonists. Diltiazem in particular appears to be safe and preliminary results regarding clinical utility are encouraging, although myocardial depression is an important potential side effect of the calcium antagonists as a group. Combining a calcium antagonist with a vasodilator does not appear to have any additional beneficial effects on reducing mortality in DCM.[141a] At present, the use of calcium antagonists in DCM is considered investigational and not yet first-line therapy.[125,142]

Although there is no definitive evidence that antiarrhythmic agents prolong life or prevent sudden death in DCM,[24,125,142a] it may be appropriate to use them in the treatment of symptomatic arrhythmias. Because of the adverse effects of most available agents, many of which depress myocardial contractility and have a proarrhythmic effect (see Chap. 21), treatment should be individualized, with both efficacy and toxicity carefully monitored. Unfortunately, electrophysiological testing is of limited utility in DCM because it is positive in a minority of patients at risk[24,143]; the lack of inducibility of ventricular tachyarrhythmias does not identify a low-risk group, and pharmacological suppression of provoked arrhythmias does not necessarily predict freedom from recurrences.[144] The recording of late potentials by the signal-averaged electrocardiogram appears to be of benefit in assessing the risk of death,[145–147] although this has not been a universal finding and awaits further confirmation.[148,149] Implantation of the internal defibrillator (see p. 732) should be considered in appropriate candidates with symptomatic ventricular tachyarrhythmias.[125,143,150,151]

Even in the absence of controlled clinical trials demonstrating their efficacy,[152,153] anticoagulants are recommended in patients with DCM and heart failure (particularly in the presence of atrial fibrillation or a prior stroke) (see p. 509).[24] Anticoagulants should be used even without direct clinical or echocardiographic evidence of thrombus formation if there are no specific contraindications to these agents with a target prolongation of the prothrombin time to 2.0 to 3.0 (international normalized ratio [INR]).[24] In those patients with chronic heart failure secondary to DCM and lymphocytic infiltrate on myocardial biopsy, treatment with corticosteroids and immunosuppressive agents has been advocated. Prednisone therapy does not appear to have a clinically important effect on symptoms, exercise performance, or ejection fraction (in more than just the short term) and is associated with significant complications in half the patients so treated.[154,155] Routine clinical use of immunosuppressive therapy thus cannot be recommended at present.[24,125]

Surgical treatment (such as with mitral annuloplasty) or replacement of regurgitant valves has been attempted in some patients with prominent atrioventricular valvular regurgitation. The results of operation are usually less than satisfactory because of the degree of pre-existing cardiac dysfunction and damage. In appropriate patients, cardiac transplantation may be an alternative (Chap. 18), with a 5-year survival rate of over 70 per cent.[24] Surgical translocation of the latissimus dorsi muscle to wrap around the heart and augment cardiac performance (dynamic cardiomyoplasty) appears to have benefited some patients who are not otherwise suitable candidates for cardiac transplantation.[156–162]

ALCOHOLIC CARDIOMYOPATHY

Chronic excessive consumption of alcohol may be associated with congestive heart failure, hypertension, cerebrovascular accidents, arrhythmias, and sudden death; it is the major cause of secondary, nonischemic dilated cardiomyopathy in the Western world and accounts for upwards of one-third of all cases of DCM.[163–165] It is estimated that two-thirds of the adult population use alcohol to some extent, and more than 10 per cent are heavy users.[166] Therefore, it is not surprising that alcoholic cardiomyopathy is a major problem. Ceasing alcohol consumption early in the course of alcoholic cardiomyopathy may halt the progression or even reverse left ventricular contractile dysfunction, unlike nonalcoholic cardiomyopathy that often is marked by progressive clinical deterioration.[39]

The consumption of alcohol may result in myocardial damage by three basic mechanisms: (1) a presumed direct toxic effect of alcohol or its metabolites; (2) nutritional effects, most commonly in association with thiamine deficiency that leads to beriberi heart disease (see p. 461); and (3) rarely, toxic effects due to additives in the alcoholic beverage (cobalt)[167] (see p. 1413). There had been speculation that alcohol caused myocardial damage only through dietary deficiencies, but it is now clear that alcoholic cardiomyopathy occurs in the absence of nutritional deficiencies.[163,166,168]

Typical Oriental beriberi may coexist with alcoholic cardiomyopathy, although it is no longer seen with any frequency.[169] The distinguishing features of each include peripheral vasodilatation and high-output heart failure, often right-sided, in the former and reduced contractility with typically left-sided low-output failure in the latter.[163,169]

Alcohol results in acute as well as chronic depression of myocardial contractility and may produce reversible cardiac dysfunction even when ingested by normal nonalcoholic individuals.[170] What is responsible for the transition from the reversible acute effects to permanent myocardial damage remains unclear.[171]

The precise mechanisms of cardiac depression produced by alcohol is undetermined,[172] but a direct toxic effect on striated muscle is likely (particularly because alcoholics often demonstrate concomitant skeletal myopathy and cardiomyopathy).[163,166] In acute studies, alcohol and its metabolite acetaldehyde have been shown to interfere with a number of membrane and cellular functions that involve the transport and binding of calcium, mitochondrial respiration, myocardial lipid metabolism, myocardial protein synthesis, and signal transduction.[166,170,171] Studies in isolated ferret papillary muscles have shown that ethanol in concentrations similar to those occurring in intoxicated humans depresses myocardial contractility by interfering with excitation-contraction coupling through inhibition of the interaction between calcium and the myofilaments.[170] The accumulation of metabolites of ethanol in the myocardium may interfere with normal myocardial lipid metabolism and may play a role in the pathogenesis of alcohol-induced myocardial damage.[171] The role that other associated electrolyte imbalances (hypokalemia, hypophosphatemia, hypomagnesemia) may play in alcohol-mediated damage has not been settled.[168]

PATHOLOGY. The gross and microscopic pathological findings are nonspecific and similar to those observed in idiopathic DCM, with interstitial fibrosis, myocytolysis, evidence of small vessel coronary artery disease, and myocyte hypertrophy.[163,173,174] Electron microscopy shows enlarged and disorganized mitochondria, with large glycogen-containing vacuoles.[168]

Clinical Manifestations

Alcoholic cardiomyopathy most commonly occurs in men 30 to 55 years of age who have been heavy consumers of whisky, wine, or beer, usually for more than 10 years.[164,174] Although alcoholic cardiomyopathy may be observed in the homeless, malnourished, "skid row" alcoholic man, many patients are well-nourished individuals of middle and even upper socioeconomic status without liver disease or peripheral neuropathy. Accordingly, unless a high index of suspicion is maintained, it may be easy to miss a history of alcohol abuse. Persistent questioning of the patient and particularly the relatives of patients with unexplained cardiomegaly or cardiomyopathy is often required to elicit a history of alcoholism.

It is frequently possible to demonstrate mild depression of cardiac function in chronic alcoholics even before cardiac dysfunction becomes clinically manifest.[164,175] Abnormalities of both systolic function (reduced ejection fraction) and diastolic function (increased myocardial wall stiffness) have been demonstrated in alcoholic patients without cardiac symptoms by a variety of invasive and noninvasive techniques.[176] Although overt alcoholic liver disease and cardiac involvement usually do not occur together, even cirrhotic patients without signs or symptoms of heart disease have demonstrable evidence of asymptomatic myocardial disease.[164]

The development of symptoms may be insidious, although some patients have acute and florid left-sided congestive heart failure. A paroxysm of atrial fibrillation is a relatively frequent initial presenting finding.[164] More advanced cases demonstrate findings of biventricular failure, with left ventricular dysfunction usually dominating. Dyspnea, orthopnea, and paroxysmal nocturnal dyspnea frequently are observed. Palpitations and syncope due to tachyarrhythmias, usually supraventricular, occasionally are present. Angina pectoris does not occur unless there is concomitant coronary artery disease or aortic stenosis, although atypical chest pain may be seen.

PHYSICAL EXAMINATION. The cardiac findings resemble those seen in idiopathic dilated cardiomyopathy. Examination usually reveals a narrow pulse pressure, often with an elevated diastolic pressure secondary to excessive peripheral vasoconstriction. There is cardiomegaly, and protodiastolic (S_3) and presystolic (S_4) gallop sounds are common.[164] An apical systolic murmur of mitral regurgitation often is found. The severity of right heart failure varies, but jugular venous distention and peripheral edema are common. A concomitant skeletal muscle myopathy involving the shoulder and pelvic girdle is a frequent finding, and the degree of muscle weakness and histological abnormality in the skeletal muscles parallels that in the heart.[163,168]

LABORATORY EXAMINATION. The *chest roentgenogram* in the advanced case demonstrates considerable cardiac enlargement, pulmonary congestion, and pulmonary venous hypertension (see p. 219). Pleural effusions often are seen. *Electrocardiographic abnormalities* are common and frequently are the only indication of alcoholic heart disease during the preclinical phase. Alcoholic patients without other evidence of heart disease often are seen after developing palpitations, chest discomfort, or syncope, typically following a binge of alcohol consumption on a weekend, particularly during the year-end holiday season. This is dubbed the "holiday heart syndrome." The most common arrhythmia observed is atrial fibrillation, followed by atrial flutter and frequent ventricular premature contractions.[164] Alcohol consumption may predispose to atrial flutter or fibrillation, even in nonalcoholics.[168] Hypokalemia may play a role in the genesis of some of these arrhythmias. Supraventricular arrhythmias are also frequently observed in patients with overt alcoholic cardiomyopathy. Sudden, unexpected death is not uncommon in young adult alcoholics, and it is likely that ventricular fibrillation is responsible.[164]

Atrioventricular conduction disturbances (most commonly first-degree heart block), bundle branch block, left ventricular hypertrophy, poor R-wave progression across the precordium, and repolarization abnormalities are common electrocardiographic findings.[164] Prolongation of the Q-T interval is noted frequently. ST-segment and T-wave changes are often restored to normal within several days after cessation of alcohol consumption.

The hemodynamic findings observed at cardiac catheterization and the assessment of left ventricular function by noninvasive methods (echocardiography and isotope angiography) resemble those found in idiopathic DCM.

MANAGEMENT. The *natural history* of alcoholic cardiomyopathy depends on the drinking habits of the patient. Total abstinence in the early stages of the disease may lead to resolution of the manifestations of congestive heart failure and a return of heart size toward normal, although patients with severe heart failure may show no improvement in function or prognosis.[164] Continued alcohol consumption leads to further myocardial damage and fibrosis, with the development of refractory congestive heart failure. Death may also be due to arrhythmia, heart block, and systemic or pulmonary embolism.

The key to the long-term treatment of alcoholic cardiomyopathy is *immediate and total abstinence* as early in the course of the disease as possible.[164] This may be quite effective in improving the signs and symptoms of congestive heart failure.[177,177a] The reversibility of alcoholic myocardial depression is supported by the demonstration of a reduction of myocardial uptake of labeled monoclonal antimyosin antibodies (a marker of myocyte damage) in alcoholics who stop drinking.[120] The prognosis in patients who continue to drink, particularly if they have been symptomatic for a long time, is poor. In the overall population of patients with alcoholic cardiomyopathy, between 40 and 50 per cent succumb within a 3- to 6-year period, especially if they continue to drink.[164] Prolonged bed rest is thought to result in functional improvement, although its major benefit may simply be the decreased alcohol consumption.[164]

The management of acute episodes of congestive heart failure is similar to that of idiopathic DCM (see p. 1411 and Table 41–7). For patients with severe congestive heart failure, it is prudent to administer thiamine on the chance that beriberi may be contributing to the heart failure.[169] Whether to use chronic anticoagulation (as is usually recommended for idiopathic DCM) is a difficult question; we usually do not prescribe warfarin because of the risk of bleeding due to noncompliance, trauma, and overanticoagulation due to hepatic dysfunction.

COBALT CARDIOMYOPATHY

A previously unrecognized syndrome of severe congestive heart failure appeared in the mid-1960s, first in Canada and subsequently in the United States and Europe.[167] The disease was found in people who drank a particular brand of beer to which cobalt sulfate had been added as a foam stabilizer. Since cobalt was removed from the process, no more cases of the disease have been reported. On very rare occasions occupational exposure to cobalt may result in myocardial damage and attendant congestive heart failure.[167,178]

ARRHYTHMOGENIC RIGHT VENTRICULAR DYSPLASIA

(See also p. 324)

This unique cardiomyopathy (which is also called right ventricular cardiomyopathy) is marked by partial or total replacement of right ventricular muscle by adipose and fibrous tissue (Fig. 41–8) and may be associated with reentrant ventricular tachyarrhythmias of right ventricular origin (left bundle branch block configuration of the QRS complex).[179–182] The cause of the myocardial changes is unclear, but in about one-third of the cases there is autosomal dominant inheritance of the disease.[182–184] It appears to be distinct from Uhl's disease, which is marked by extreme thinning of the ventricular wall. The diagnosis is based on a constellation of clinical, electrocardiographic, histological, and echocardiographic findings.[182,185] Typical clinical features include male predominance, normal physical examination, inverted T waves in the right precordial electrocardiographic leads, symptoms of palpitations and syncope, and a risk of sudden

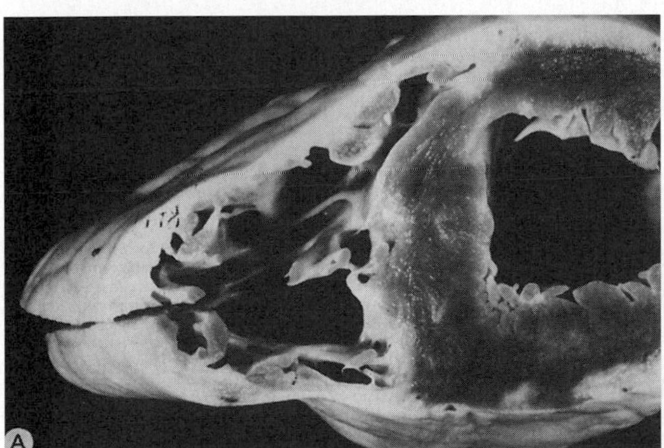

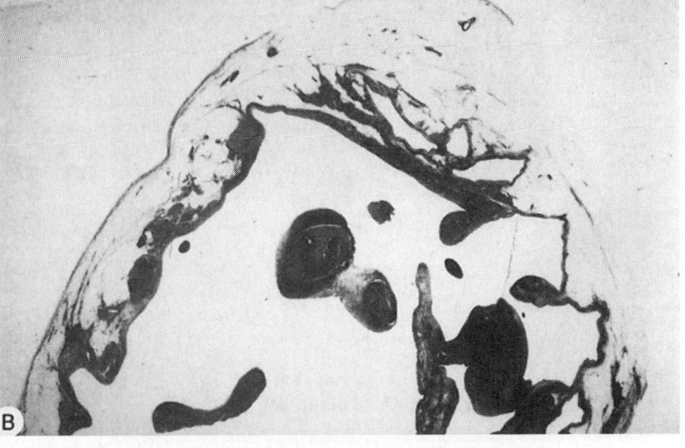

FIGURE 41–8. Pathological findings in a 39-year-old man with arrhythmogenic right ventricular dysplasia and a family history of sudden death. *A,* Cross-section of the heart showing pronounced adipose infiltration of the right ventricular free wall and nearly normal left ventricle and ventricular septum. *B,* Histological view of the right ventricular free wall showing myocardial atrophy and massive fibrofatty replacement. (Azan, ×1). (From McKenna, W. J., Thiene, G., Nava, A., et al.: Diagnosis of arrhythmogenic right ventricular dysplasia/cardiomyopathy. Task Force of the Working Group Myocardial and Pericardial Disease of the European Society of Cardiology and of the Scientific Council on Cardiomyopathies of the International Society and Federation of Cardiology. Br. Heart J. *71:*215, 1994.)

death.[182,184,186–188] In some patients with ventricular arrhythmias of no evident cause, clinically subtle right ventricular dysplasia may be etiologic.[189–192]

Noninvasive and invasive evaluation demonstrate a dilated, poorly contractile right ventricle, usually with a normal left ventricle, although some degree of left ventricular dysfunction has been seen.[193,194] Magnetic resonance imaging (MRI) shows promise for identifying patients with this condition.[195] Antiarrhythmic therapy, especially with beta-adrenoceptor blockers, often is effective in controlling the arrhythmias.[190,192] The arrhythmias appear to be related to abnormalities of regional right ventricular sympathetic innervation, as demonstrated by noninvasive scintigraphy.[180] Cryoablation of the presumed arrhythmogenic focus has been successful in resolving the ventricular arrhythmia in some patients.[196]

HYPERTROPHIC CARDIOMYOPATHY

Although first described about a century ago, the unique features of hypertrophic cardiomyopathy (HCM) were not studied systematically until the late 1950s.[197,198] The characteristic finding was inappropriate myocardial hypertrophy that occurred in the absence of an obvious cause for the hypertrophy (such as aortic stenosis or systemic hypertension), often predominantly involving the interventricular septum of a nondilated left ventricle that showed hyperdynamic ventricular function (Fig. 41–9).[198] A distinctive clinical feature was soon recognized in some patients with HCM—a dynamic pressure gradient in the subaortic area that divided the left ventricle into a high-pressure apical region and a lower-pressure subaortic region (Fig. 41–10). Although subsequent studies have shown that only a minority of patients (perhaps a quarter)[199] demonstrate this outflow gradient, its unique features attracted much attention and led to a myriad of terms (more than 75) used to describe the disease (among the more popular terms were *idiopathic hypertrophic subaortic stenosis (IHSS)* and *muscular subaortic stenosis*). The term *hypertrophic cardiomyopathy* is now preferred because most patients do not have an outflow gradient or "stenosis" of the left ventricular outflow tract. Because hypertrophy typically occurs in the absence of a pressure gradient, the characteristic distinguishing feature of HCM is myocardial hypertrophy that is out of proportion to the hemodynamic load.

The physiological characteristics of HCM differ substantially from those of DCM (Table 41–8). The most characteristic pathophysiological abnormality in HCM is *diastolic*

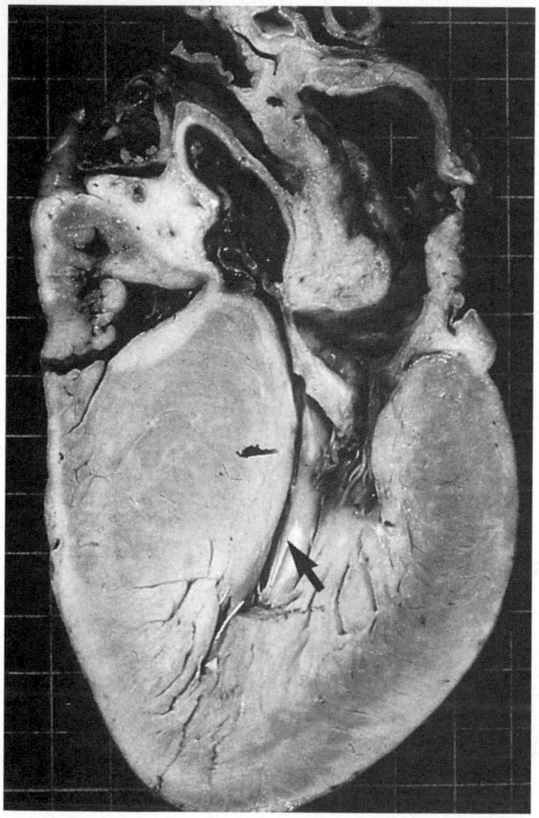

FIGURE 41–9. Pathological findings in a patient with hypertrophic cardiomyopathy with a left ventricular outflow tract gradient during life. The heart is opened in the longitudinal plane. This patient had mitral regurgitation that was partially due to abnormal insertion of an anomalous papillary muscle (arrow) onto the ventricular surface of the anterior mitral leaflet. (Modified from Wigle, E. D., Sasson, Z., Henderson, M. A., et al.: Hypertrophic cardiomyopathy. The importance of the site and the extent of hypertrophy: A review. Prog. Cardiovasc. Dis. 28:1, 1985.)

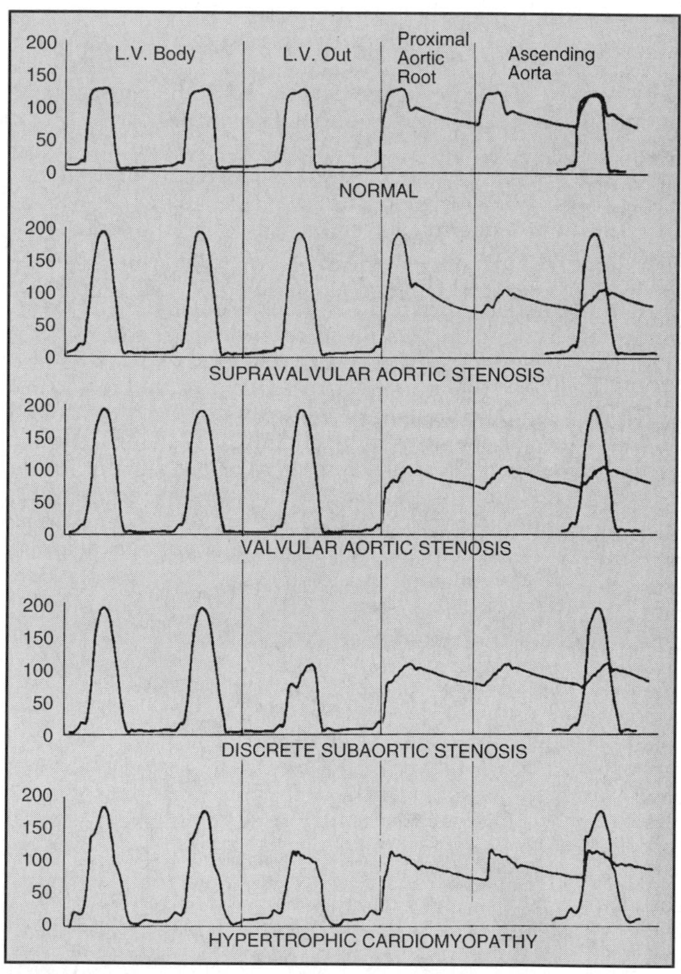

FIGURE 41–10. Left heart pressures in various conditions. In each horizontal panel there is an idealized depiction of the pressure tracing that would be obtained as a catheter is withdrawn from the left ventricular body through the left ventricular outflow tract into the proximal aortic root. On the far right is a superimposition of the pressures in the left ventricular body and in the aorta. The vertical lines bound the regional catheter position within the heart during withdrawal. All forms of discrete stenosis (supravalvular, valvular, and subvalvular) have delayed aortic upstroke rates downstream from the stenosis. Only in hypertrophic cardiomyopathy is the aortic upstroke rate rapid and parallel to the left ventricular pressure. LV = Left ventricular, Out = outflow tract. (From Criley, J. M., and Siegel, R. J.: Subaortic stenosis revisited: The importance of the dynamic pressure gradient. Medicine [Baltimore] *72*:412, 1993.)

TABLE 41–8 DIFFERENCES IN SYSTOLIC AND DIASTOLIC FUNCTION IN DILATED (CONGESTIVE) AND HYPERTROPHIC CARDIOMYOPATHY

	DILATED CARDIOMYOPATHY	HYPERTROPHIC CARDIOMYOPATHY
Left ventricular volume		
End-diastolic	Increased	Normal
End-systolic	Markedly increased	Decreased
Left ventricular mass	Increased	Markedly increased
Mass/volume ratio	Decreased	Increased
Systolic function		
Ejection fraction	Decreased	Normal or increased
Myocardial shortening	Decreased	Increased
Wall stress	Increased	Decreased
Diastolic function		
Chamber stiffness	Decreased	Increased
Myocardial stiffness	Increased	Increased

From Chatterjee, K.: Pathophysiology of cardiomyopathy. *In* Giles, T. D., and Sander, G. E. (eds.): Cardiomyopathy. Middleton, MA, PSG Publishing Co., 1988, p. 65.

rather than systolic dysfunction (see also pp. 402 and 447).[197] Thus, HCM is characterized by abnormal stiffness of the left ventricle with resultant impaired ventricular filling. This abnormality in diastolic relaxation produces increased left ventricular end-diastolic pressure with resulting pulmonary congestion and dyspnea, the most common symptoms in HCM, despite typically hyperdynamic left ventricular systolic function. The disease appears to be genetically transmitted in about half the patients as an autosomal dominant trait with disease loci on one of at least four different chromosomes (chromosomes 1, 11, 14, and 15).[200,201] The cause of HCM (see p. 1417) in the remainder of patients is unknown. Morphological evidence of the disease is found in about one-fourth of the first-degree relatives of a patient with HCM; in many of the relatives the disease is milder than in the propositus, the degree of hypertrophy is less and is more localized, and outflow gradients usually are lacking. Symptoms often are absent or minimal, and the disease is detected only by echocardiography. The overall prevalence of HCM is low and has been estimated to occur in 0.02 to 0.2 per cent of the population.[202,202a] It is found in 0.5 per cent of unselected patients referred for an echocardiographic examination.[203]

Pathology

MACROSCOPIC EXAMINATION. This typically discloses a marked increase in myocardial mass, and the ventricular cavities are small (Fig. 41–9).[198] The left ventricle is usually more involved with the hypertrophic process than is the right.[204] The atria are dilated and often hypertrophied, reflecting the high resistance to filling of the ventricles caused by diastolic dysfunction and the effects of atrioventricular valve regurgitation. The pattern and extent of left ventricular hypertrophy in HCM vary greatly from patient to patient, and a characteristic feature is heterogeneity in the amount of hypertrophy evident in different regions of the left ventricle.[198] A typical feature found in most patients with HCM is disproportionate involvement of the interventricular septum and anterolateral wall compared with the posterior segment of the free wall of the left ventricle.[198] When hypertrophy is largely localized to the septum, the process has been called asymmetrical septal hypertrophy (ASH). Other patterns of hypertrophy may be seen on occasion, including concentric left ventricular hypertrophy, with symmetrical thickening of the left ventricle involving the septum and free wall equally. This variant may occasionally be seen in patients with the genetically transmitted as well as the sporadic forms of HCM. The differentiation of the "physiological" hypertrophy that occurs in some highly trained male athletes from that seen in HCM may be difficult; athletes may demonstrate left ventricular wall thicknesses up to 16 mm in the absence of HCM (normal < 12 mm) (Fig. 41–11).[205–207] Some patients with HCM have substantial hypertrophy in unusual locations, such as the posterior portion of the septum, the posterobasal free wall, and the midventricular level.[198] One unusual variant demonstrates marked posterior wall hypertrophy and virtually no septal hypertrophy; patients with this form of HCM tend to be young and severely symptomatic.[208]

An inverse relationship exists between the extent of hypertrophy and age. Whether this is due to premature death of younger patients with greater hypertrophy or progressive reduction in the extent of hypertrophy is unknown.[198]

Apical HCM. A variant with predominant involvement of the apex is common in Japan and is estimated to represent a quarter of Japanese HCM patients.[209] In other parts of the world, apical HCM is much less common. Typical features include a characteristic spade-like configuration of the left ventricle during angiographic study (although some patients with this variant do not demonstrate this abnormality),[210] giant negative T waves in the precordial electrocardiographic leads, the absence of an intraventricular pressure gradient, mild symptoms, and a generally benign course.[198,211,212]

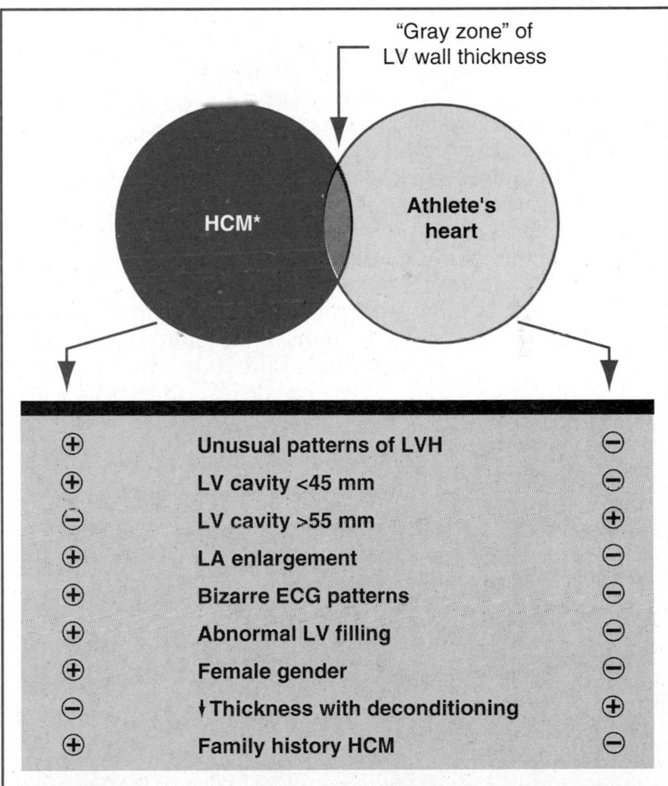

FIGURE 41–11. Criteria used to distinguish hypertrophic cardiomyopathy from athlete's heart. The shaded area (gray zone) indicates that there can be overlap between the two diagnoses, and the criteria listed below indicate which diagnosis would be favored (+) or less likely (−) for each criterion. ↓ = Decreased, HCM = hypertrophic cardiomyopathy, LA = left atrial, LV = left ventricular, LVH = left ventricular hypertrophy. * = Assumes that systolic anterior motion of the mitral valve is absent because its presence would indicate the presence of hypertrophic cardiomyopathy even in an athlete. (Reproduced by permission from Maron, B. J., Pelliccia, A., and Spirito, P.: Cardiac disease in young trained athletes. Insights into methods for distinguishing athlete's heart from structural heart disease, with particular emphasis on hypertrophic cardiomyopathy. Circulation *91:* 1596, 1995. Copyright 1995 American Heart Association.)

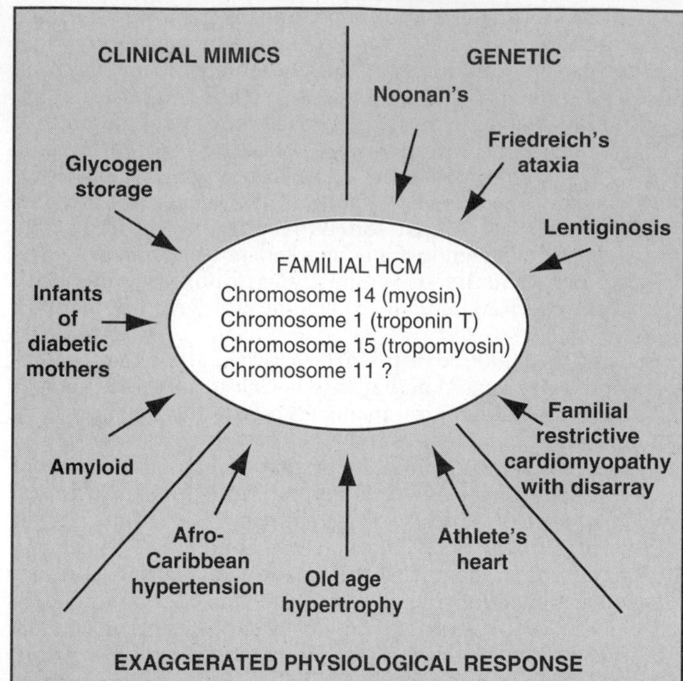

FIGURE 41–12. Classification of the causes of myocardial hypertrophy that can be confused with or may be related to familial hypertrophic cardiomyopathy. (From Davies, M. J., and McKenna, W. J.: Hypertrophic cardiomyopathy: An introduction to pathology and pathogenesis. Br. Heart J. *72*:S2, 1994.)

Two variants of HCM are seen particularly in elderly women. The first, termed *hypertensive hypertrophic cardiomyopathy of the elderly,* is characterized by severe concentric left ventricular hypertrophy and small left ventricular cavity size, and is associated with hypertension.[213,214] The second presentation also is marked by an especially small left ventricular cavity but with relatively mild hypertrophy; other findings include marked anterior displacement of the mitral valve, extensive submitral (annular) calcification, a left ventricular outflow gradient, and the late appearance of severe and progressive symptoms.[215] In contrast to young patients with HCM, the elderly patient is more likely to show a localized septal bulge just below the aortic valve and is less likely to have marked abnormalities in the orientation and curvature of the septum.[216]

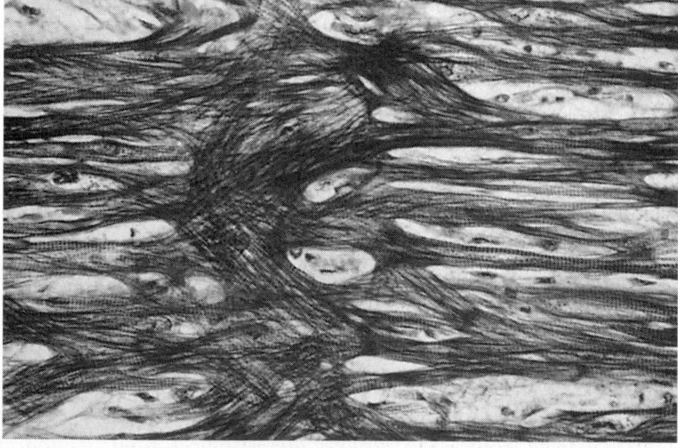

FIGURE 41–13. Histological specimen of a patient with hypertrophic cardiomyopathy showing myofibrillar disarray. In the central area the myofibrils cross each other in a disorganized manner, but in adjacent areas on each side the appearance is more normal, with parallel arrays of myofibrils. (PTHA stain, ×240). (From Davies, M. J., and McKenna, W. J.: Hypertrophic cardiomyopathy: An introduction to pathology and pathogenesis. Br. Heart J. *72*:S2, 1994.)

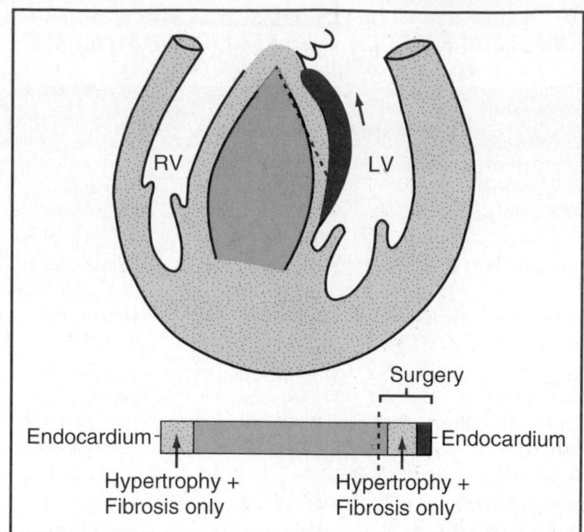

FIGURE 41–14. Diagrammatic representation showing usual location of myocyte disarray in interventricular septum in hypertrophic cardiomyopathy. This explains why disarray is usually deep or absent in septectomy specimen, and why endomyocardial biopsy (3-mm maximum dimension) is also unlikely to sample zone of disarray. RV = Right ventricle, LV = left ventricle. (From Tazelaar, H. D., and Billingham, M. E.: The surgical pathology of hypertrophic cardiomyopathy. Arch. Pathol. Lab. Med. *111*:257, 1987.)

A variety of disparate conditions may present similar gross morphological features as HCM, including hyperparathyroidism, infants of diabetic mothers, neurofibromatosis, generalized lipodystrophy, lentiginosis, pheochromocytoma, Friedreich's ataxia, and Noonan syndrome (Fig. 41–12).[217,218] Rarely, the findings may be simulated by amyloid, glycogen storage disease, or tumor involvement of the septum.[219,220]

HISTOLOGY. Microscopic findings in HCM are distinctive, with myocardial hypertrophy and gross disorganization of the muscle bundles resulting in a characteristic whorled pattern; abnormalities are found in the cell-to-cell arrangement (disarray) and disorganization of the myofibrillar architecture within a given cell (Fig. 41–13).[198] Fibrosis is usually prominent[221] and may be extensive enough to produce grossly visible scars. Foci of disorganized cells are often interspersed between areas of hypertrophied but otherwise normal-appearing muscle cells. Interstitial (matrix) connective tissue elements are increased.[198] Disarray in HCM patients is found in grossly hypertrophied myocardial segments as well as relatively normal segments.[222] Although abnormally arranged cardiac muscle cells initially were considered specific for HCM, it is now recognized that they may be found in a variety of acquired and congenital heart conditions.[198] What is unique about the disarray in HCM is its ubiquity and frequency. Findings in almost all HCM patients have some degree of disarray, and most have involvement of 5 per cent or more of the myocardium; in contrast, disarray findings in non-HCM patients (when they occur) usually involve only about 1 per cent of the myocardium[198] (Fig. 41–14).

Abnormal intramural coronary arteries, with a reduction in the size of the lumen and thickening of the vessel wall, are common in HCM, occurring in more than 80 per cent of patients.[198,199] This abnormality occurs most frequently in the ventricular septum; it also has been observed in infants who died of this condition and could represent a congenital component of the condition. The prominence of abnormal intramural coronary arteries in areas of extensive myocardial fibrosis is consistent with the hypothesis that these abnormalities may be responsible for the development of myocardial ischemia.[198]

Etiology

The cause of the myocardial hypertrophy in HCM remains unknown.[223] Suggestive data link abnormal myocardial calcium kinetics[224] and specific features of HCM, particularly the abnormalities of diastolic function.[197] Abnormal calcium fluxes with a resultant increase in intracellular calcium concentration appear to occur as a consequence of an increase in the number of calcium channels.[225,226] This in turn may produce (in an as yet undefined process) hypertrophy and cellular disarray.

Other suggested causes of HCM include (1) abnormal sympathetic stimulation because of heightened responsiveness of the heart to or excessive production of circulating catecholamines[227] or reduced neuronal uptake of cardiac norepinephrine[228]; (2) abnormally thickened intramural coronary arteries that do not dilate normally and lead to myocardial ischemia, with resultant fibrosis and abnormal compensatory hypertrophy; (3) subendocardial ischemia, possibly related to abnormalities of the microcirculation, that depletes the energy stores essential for the sequestration of calcium during diastole, resulting in persistent interaction of the contractile elements during diastole and attendant increased diastolic stiffness; and (4) structural abnormalities, including a catenoid configuration of the septum, that lead to myocardial cell hypertrophy and disarray.

GENETICS OF HYPERTROPHIC CARDIOMYOPATHY (see also pp. 1664 to 1665). Familial HCM occurs as an autosomal dominant mendelian-inherited disease about 50 per cent of the time.[200,229] It is thought that some if not all of the sporadic forms of the disease may be due to spontaneous mutations.[229,230] At least five different genes on at least four chromosomes are associated with HCM, with over three dozen different mutations discovered thus far (Fig. 41–15).[200,223] The proteins encoded by three of the genes have been identified. Familial HCM thus is a genetically heterogeneous disease (i.e., it can be caused by genetic defects at more than one locus).[231,232] However, the genetic heterogeneity does *not* appear to explain the clinical variability. The genetic basis of HCM was first reported in 1989 by Seidman and her collaborators, who reported the existence of a disease gene located on 14 q1 (i.e., the long arm of the 14th chromosome in the band closest to the centromere) and termed it *FHC-1* (for familial hypertrophic cardiomyopathy).[233,234] Subsequently they found this to be the gene encoding for beta cardiac myosin heavy chain (βMHC); it is now known as CMH1 (cardiomyopathy, hypertrophic, 1).[200] Sequencing of this gene in one family with HCM revealed that the abnormality was caused by a gene duplication in which the alpha and beta MHC genes were fused and present in an extra copy. In the second family, there was a point mutation in the beta MHC sequence that alters the myosin's arginine to glutamine. Both of these mutations affect the polypeptides crucial to the structure of myofibrils and might be responsible for the myocyte and myofibrillar disarray characteristic of familial HCM. Other disease loci that have been identified include CMH2 on chromosome 1 g3 (encoding for troponin T); CMH3 on chromosome 15 q2 (encoding for α tropomyosin); CMH4 on chromosome 11, and an additional gene that is not yet localized.[200,201,235] It is estimated that about 30 per cent of familial HCM is due to mutations of the cardiac myosin heavy chain gene, 15 per cent is caused by mutations of the cardiac troponin T gene, less than 3 per cent is due to mutations of the α tropomyosin gene, and the remainder to mutations of other unidentified genes.[235a]

There is wide variation in the phenotypic expression of a given mutation of a given gene, with variability in clinical symptoms and degree of hypertrophy expressed.[200,236–238] Of particular interest are mutations of the troponin T gene that typically result in only modest hypertrophy but indicate a poor prognosis and a high risk of sudden death.[235a] Conversely, certain genes and mutations are associated with more favorable prognoses (Fig. 41–16).[239,240] It is possible to detect the CMH1 gene in DNA extracted from blood lymphocytes, so the disease can be detected in childhood even before it becomes clinically evident.[241] It is likely that soon it may be possible to screen for all or most of the genes associated with HCM.[200,201] In some patients with an abnormal gene and no echocardiographic evidence of HCM, the electrocardiogram is abnormal.[242] Therefore, otherwise unexplained abnormalities of the electrocardiogram in first-degree relatives of patients with HCM may be indicative of a carrier or preclinical state.[242]

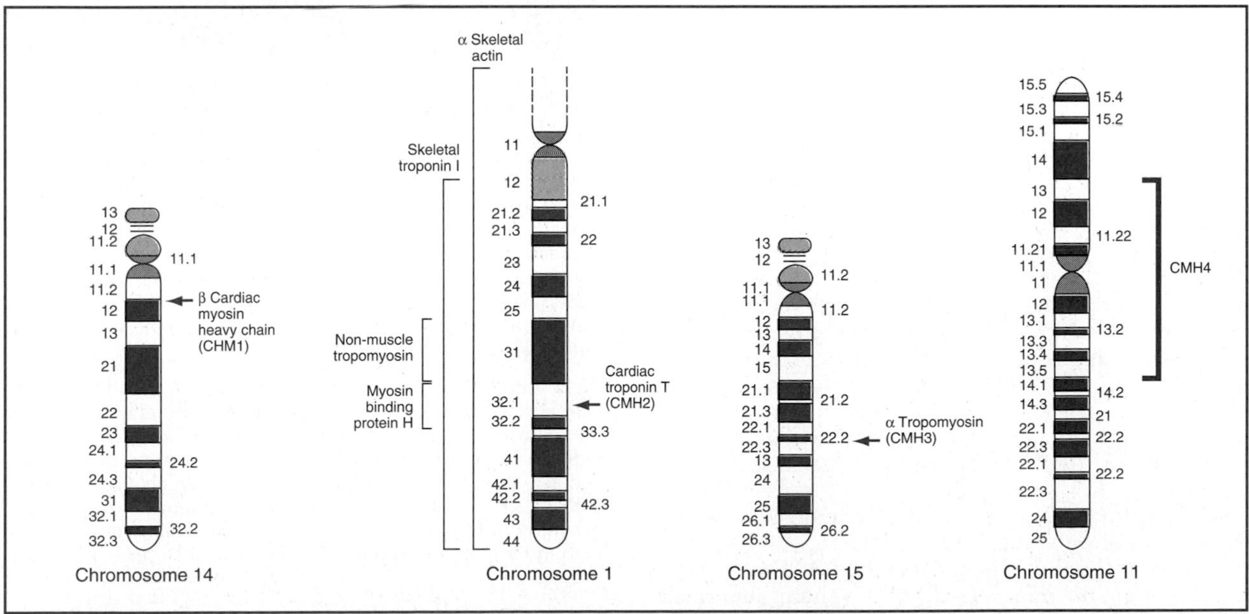

FIGURE 41–15. Diagrammatic depiction of the four chromosomes containing known disease gene loci for hypertrophic cardiomyopathy. The disease loci (designated CMH1-4) and relevant genes are identified by arrows (where the gene itself is known) or by square brackets showing the range of possible map locations. The positions of four other contractile protein genes, previously considered gene candidates for CMH2 on chromosome 1, are also shown by square brackets. (From Watkins, H.: Multiple disease genes cause hypertrophic cardiomyopathy. Br. Heart J. *72*:S4, 1994.)

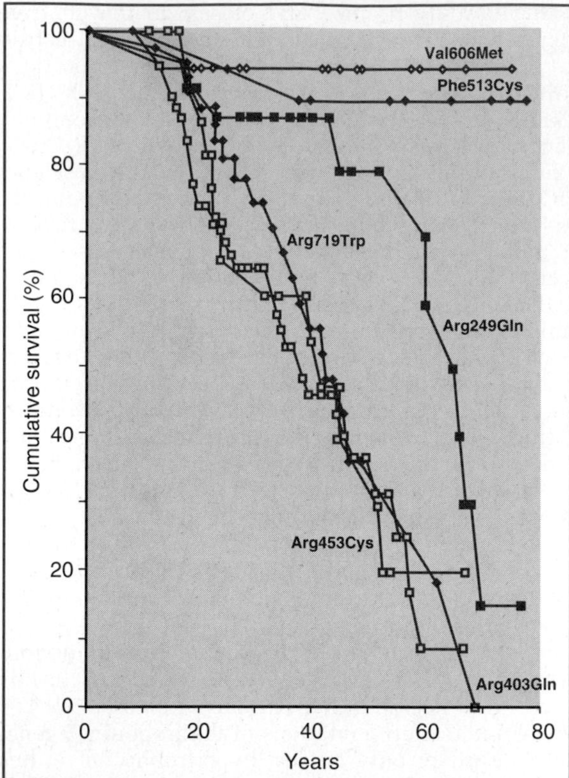

FIGURE 41–16. Kaplan-Meier curves showing the survival of affected individuals with different mutations for hypertrophic cardiomyopathy. (From Watkins, H.: Multiple disease genes cause hypertrophic cardiomyopathy. Br. Heart J. *72*:S4, 1994.)

Pathophysiology

SYSTOLE. Since the initial descriptions of HCM, the feature that has attracted the greatest attention is the dynamic pressure gradient (Fig. 41–10). Although this pressure gradient was initially thought to be due to a muscular sphincter action in the subaortic region or was an artifact, it appears to be related to further narrowing of an already small outflow tract (narrowed by the prominent septal hypertrophy and possibly abnormal location of the mitral valve) by systolic anterior motion (SAM) of the mitral valve against the hypertrophied septum.[198]

There continues to be considerable controversy about the cause and significance of the outflow gradient.[243,244] Central to the disagreement is whether there is true obstruction to left ventricular ejection or whether the pressure gradient is simply the consequence of vigorous ventricular emptying.[243] Most now favor the view that a true mechanical impediment to left ventricular ejection occurs when outflow gradients are present and is the result of distal portions of the mitral valve apparatus moving anteriorly across the outflow tract and contacting the ventricular septum in midsystole. It is likely that the mitral valve is displaced anteriorly because of Venturi effects and as a result of the increased ejection velocities produced by the abnormal left ventricular outflow tract orientation and geometry[245] (Fig. 41–17).

DIASTOLE. Most patients with HCM demonstrate abnormalities of diastolic function (see pp. 402 and 447) whether or not a pressure gradient is present and whether or not they are symptomatic (Fig. 41–18).[246,247] These abnormalities of global diastolic filling are largely independent of the extent and distribution of myocardial hypertrophy; patients with mild and apparently localized hypertrophy may demonstrate prominent diastolic dysfunction, suggesting that the myopathic process occurs in ventricular regions that are not macroscopically hypertrophied.[248] Others have found that diastolic filling varies in different regions of the left ventricle and is influenced by the thickness of the septum.[249] Diastolic dysfunction in turn leads to increased filling pressure despite a normal or small left ventricular cavity and appears to result from abnormalities of left ventricular relaxation and distensibility.[250] Early diastolic filling is impaired when relaxation is prolonged, perhaps related to abnormal calcium kinetics, subendocardial ischemia, or the abnormal loading conditions found in HCM.[225,251] Late diastolic filling is altered when left ventricular distensibility is impaired; as a consequence, filling pressures rise. HCM may cause abnormal distensibility of the ventricle because of fibrosis or cellular disorganization.[221,225]

MYOCARDIAL ISCHEMIA. Myocardial ischemia is common and multifactorial in HCM (Table 41–9). Major causes include impaired vasodilator reserve (perhaps related to the thickened and narrowed small intramural coronary arteries found in HCM)[252–254]; increased oxygen demand, especially in patients with outflow gradients; and elevated filling pressures with resultant subendocardial ischemia.[198]

Clinical Manifestations

SYMPTOMS. The majority of patients with HCM are asymptomatic or only mildly symptomatic[255] and often are

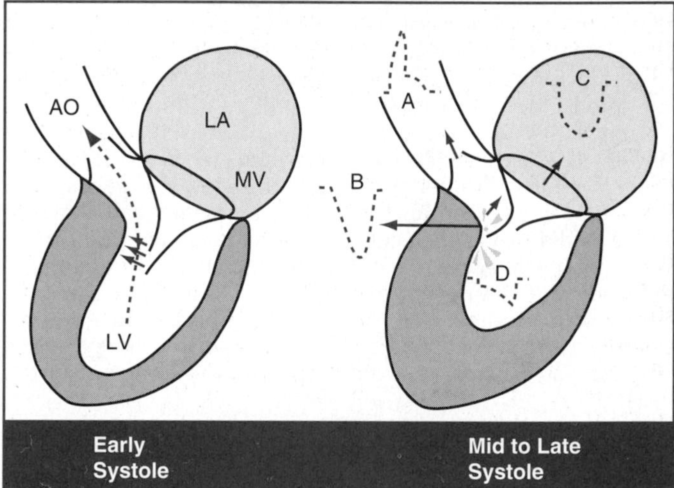

FIGURE 41–17. ***Left,*** **Proposed mechanism of mitral leaflet systolic anterior motion (SAM) in early systole in hypertrophic cardiomyopathy (HCM). Ventricular septal hypertrophy causes narrowed outflow tract, as result of which ejection velocity is rapid and path of ejection *(dashed line)* is closer to mitral leaflets (MV) than is normal. This results in Venturi forces (three short oblique arrows in outflow tract) drawing anterior and/or posterior mitral leaflets toward septum. Subsequent mitral leaflet-septal contact results in obstruction to left ventricular (LV) outflow and concomitant mitral regurgitation as seen on right panel. By midsystole, SAM-septal contact is well established, causing marked narrowing of LV outflow tract with obstruction to outflow. LA = Left atrium.**

Right, **Proximal to level of SAM-septal contact, converging lines indicate acceleration of jet just proximal to obstruction and narrowing of jet width that occurs. Distal to obstruction, arrow and diverging lines indicate high-velocity flow that emanates from site of SAM-septal contact, directed posterolaterally at considerable angle from normal path of aortic outflow. In late systole, although forward flow continues into outflow tract and aorta (AO), the volume of flow is much less than in early nonobstructed systole. Typical Doppler flow patterns are shown.**

A, **Integrated Doppler flow signal in ascending aorta; *B,* high outflow tract velocity recorded by continuous wave (CW) Doppler at site of SAM-septal contact; *C,* presence of mitral regurgitation recorded by CW Doppler; *D,* late systolic velocity peak that can be recorded in apical region of LV. (Reproduced with permission from Wigle, E. D.: Hypertrophic cardiomyopathy: A 1987 viewpoint. Circulation *75*:312, 1987. Copyright 1987 American Heart Association.)**

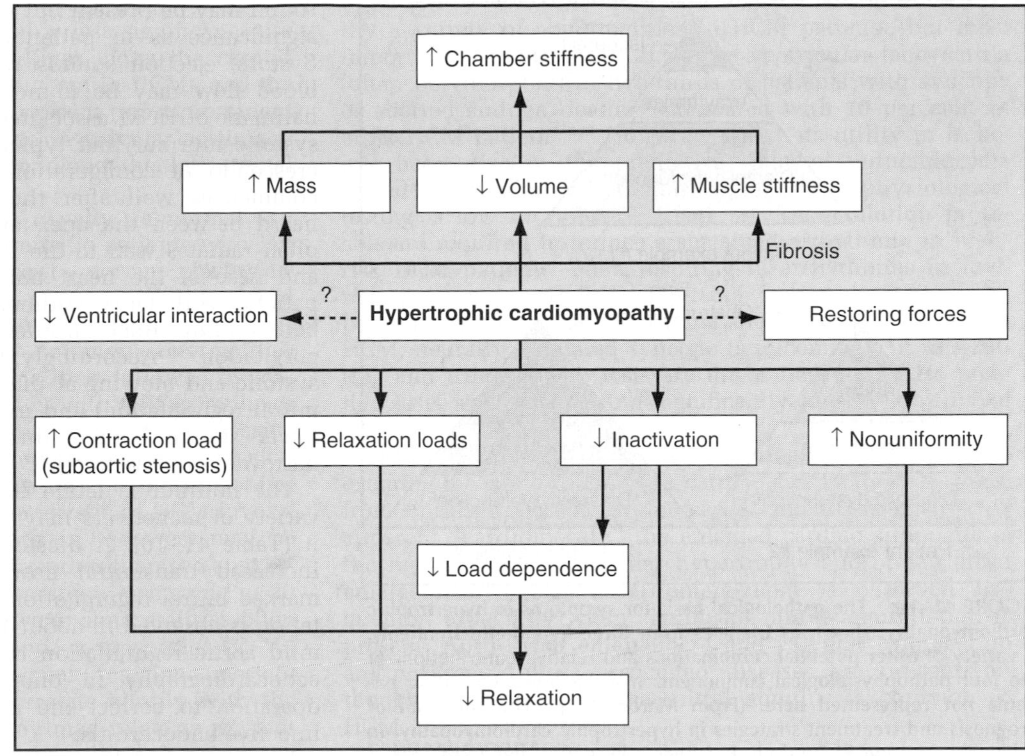

FIGURE 41–18. Diastolic dysfunction in HCM. There is increased chamber stiffness or decreased compliance as a result of increased muscle mass and the resulting decreased ventricular volume. Increased muscle stiffness from myocardial fibrosis also occurs. Thus, all three factors that affect the stiffness or compliance of the ventricle are altered in a way that increases chamber stiffness. Left ventricular relaxation in HCM is impaired because of changes in loading conditions, decreased inactivation, and increased nonuniformity. The subaortic stenosis in obstructive HCM represents a contraction load on the ventricle, which delays and impairs relaxation. Coronary and ventricular filling loads, which aid in relaxation, are reduced in HCM because of the degree of hypertrophy and other reasons. High myoplasmic calcium results in decreased inactivation, which impairs relaxation both directly and indirectly by reducing the load dependence of the relaxation process. Finally, much nonuniformity exists in HCM, which also impairs relaxation. Thus all three factors controlling relaxation are altered to impair it in HCM. (From Wigle, E. D., Kitching, A. D., Rakowski, H.: Hypertrophic cardiomyopathy. *In* Abelmann, W. H., and Braunwald, E. [eds.]: Cardiomyopathies, Myocarditis, and Pericardial Disease. Atlas of Heart Diseases. Vol. 2. Philadelphia, Current Medicine, 1995.)

identified during screening of relatives of a patient with HCM. Unfortunately, the first clinical manifestation of the disease in such individuals may be sudden death. The disease is identified most often in adults in their 30s and 40s; it occurs more often than commonly suspected in elderly patients. The condition has been observed at necropsy in stillborns and both clinically and pathologically in octogenarians. The importance of recognizing this disorder in children at the earliest possible time is highlighted by the higher mortality rate in younger patients; death is often sudden and unexpected. When HCM is first diagnosed in older patients, several features are distinctive and are in contrast to findings in younger patients: generally mild degrees of left ventricular hypertrophy; frequent demonstration of outflow gradients; and appearance of marked symptoms only after age 55.[256] A particularly high index of suspicion of this condition must be maintained to make the clinical diagnosis in the elderly because their symptoms may easily be confused with those of coronary artery or aortic valve disease. Because syncope and sudden death have been associated with competitive sports and severe exertion in patients with HCM, it is important to diagnose this condition so that these activities may be proscribed. The disease is slightly more common in men, although women may be more likely to be severely disabled and may initially present at a younger age than men.[257]

The clinical picture varies considerably, ranging from the asymptomatic relative of a patient with recognized HCM who has a slightly abnormal echocardiogram but no other manifestation of the illness to the patient with incapacitating symptoms. A general relationship exists between the extent of hypertrophy and the severity of symptoms, but the relationship is not absolute, and some patients have severe symptoms with only mild and apparently localized hypertrophy, and vice versa.[190] A complex interaction occurs between left ventricular hypertrophy, the left ventricular pressure gradient, diastolic dysfunction, and myocardial ischemia, which accounts for the great variability in symptoms from patient to patient (Fig. 41–19).

The most common symptom is *dyspnea*, occurring in up to 90 per cent of symptomatic patients, which is largely a consequence of the elevated left ventricular diastolic (and therefore left atrial and pulmonary venous) pressure, which results principally from impaired ventricular filling owing to diastolic dysfunction.[198] Angina pectoris (found in about three-fourths of symptomatic patients), fatigue, and presyncope and syncope are also common. Palpitations, paroxysmal nocturnal dyspnea, overt congestive heart failure, and dizziness are found less frequently, although severe congestive heart failure culminating in death may be seen. Exertion tends to exacerbate many of the symptoms.[258] A variety of mechanisms may contribute to the production of angina pectoris (Table 41–9). It is at least in part the result of an imbalance between oxygen supply and demand as a consequence of the greatly increased myocardial mass. Transmural infarction may occur in the absence of narrowing of the extramural coronary arteries.[198] Abnormalities of the small coronary arteries may contribute to myocardial ischemia, particularly during exertion, and perhaps 20 per cent of older patients with hypertrophic cardiomyopathy may have concurrent atheromatous obstructive coronary artery disease. Impaired diastolic relaxation may produce subendocardial ischemia as a result of prolonged maintenance of wall tension with a concomitant slower-than-normal decrease in the impedance to coronary blood flow. Syncope may result from inadequate cardiac output with exertion or from cardiac arrhythmias. It occurs

TABLE 41–9 PROPOSED CAUSES OF ISCHEMIA IN HCM DESPITE NORMAL EPICARDIAL CORONARY ARTERIES

Increased muscle mass
Inadequate capillary density
Elevated diastolic filling pressures
Abnormal intramural coronary arteries
Impaired vasodilatory reserve
Systolic compression of arteries
Enhanced myocardial oxygen demand (increased wall stress)

ited, particularly in asymptomatic patients and those without outflow gradients.

Beta-adrenoceptor blockers, calcium antagonists, and the conventional antiarrhythmic agents do not appear to suppress serious ventricular arrhythmias or reduce the frequency of supraventricular arrhythmias. However, *amiodarone* is effective in the treatment of both supraventricular and ventricular tachyarrhythmias in HCM.[314] Although there is some belief that amiodarone improves prognosis in HCM,[340] only limited and inconclusive data are available. Amiodarone may also improve symptoms and exercise capacity, although its putative beneficial effects on diastolic ventricular function are controversial.[199,271] Experience with *sotalol,* although limited, has been generally favorable; in addition to its antiarrhythmic effects on supraventricular and ventricular arrhythmias, its beta-adrenoceptor blocking effects are beneficial.[341] We do not favor empirical use of amiodarone (or other antiarrhythmic agents for that matter) and share the concern about possible proarrhythmic effects and potential toxicity, including sudden death.[229,268,271,342]

Strenuous exercise should be avoided because of the risk of sudden death; although more deaths in HCM occur during rest or mild activity, almost half the deaths occur during or just after strenuous physical activity.[281] Even though many individuals with subclinical HCM exercise vigorously, the threat of sudden death is sufficiently real that competitive sports are proscribed in patients with marked hypertrophy or other factors believed to be associated with increased risk (Table 41–11).[205] Atrial fibrillation should usually be pharmacologically or electrically converted because of the hemodynamic consequences of the loss of the atrial contribution to ventricular filling in this disorder. Anticoagulants should be given to patients with chronic atrial fibrillation when no contraindication exists. Infective endocarditis may occur in about 5 per cent of patients, and antibiotic prophylaxis is indicated.[198] The infection usually occurs on the aortic valve or mitral apparatus, on the endocardium, or at the site of the contact lesion on the septum; thus, chronic endocardial trauma may provide a nidus for subsequent infection.

DDD PACING. Insertion of a dual-chamber DDD pacemaker may be useful in some patients with an outflow gradient and severe symptoms,[343–348,348a] but it is likely that no more than 10 per cent of HCM patients are candidates. Symptoms generally are improved, and the gradient is reduced by an average of about 50 per cent.[198] Benefits have been described even after termination of pacing, suggesting a modification of myocardial properties.[345,347] The long-term utility of pacing, however, is not known at present.[349,349a,349b] The benefit of its use in patients without a resting outflow gradient is even more equivocal; it usually improves symptoms and exercise capacity, but there is no improvement or even worsening of various hemodynamic variables and pharmacological therapy usually needs to be reinstituted.[350] Therefore, its use in this setting generally is not recommended at present. In high-risk patients or those surviving a cardiac arrest, insertion of an implantable cardioverter-defibrillator should be considered.[273] A few patients have benefited from intentional infarction of a portion of the interventricular septum by the infusion of alcohol into a selectively catheterized septal artery.[350a]

SURGICAL TREATMENT. A variety of surgical procedures aimed at reducing the outflow gradient have been developed and are most commonly used in the markedly symptomatic patient with a gradient above 50 mm Hg who has not responded well to medical management.[198,261,351,352,352a] The most popular operation for HCM consists of excising a portion of the hypertrophied septum. A transaortic approach with septal myotomy-myectomy is the most widely used procedure, although left transventricular as well as combined transaortic and left ventricular approaches have also been used successfully. Operative management is facilitated by intraoperative echocardiography, and operative mortality is now less than 5 per cent[268,352–354]; large centers have reported series of patients with mortalities under 3 per cent.[198,261] Operation often relieves the obstruction as well as the mitral regurgitation. The reduction in left ventricular systolic pressure produced by the operation leads to reduced evidence of postoperative myocardial ischemia on thallium stress testing.[355] Patients over the age of 65 as well as under the age of 10 years have undergone successful operations; the operative risk is higher in older patients.[349]

Surgery results in long-term improvement in symptoms and exercise capacity in most patients.[356,357] Occasional patients experience myocardial damage and fibrosis as a consequence of the procedure.[355] Significant aortic regurgitation is an uncommon complication of the transaortic valve approach, occurring in less than 4 per cent of patients.[261] Myotomy-myectomy may be combined with other necessary operative procedures (particularly coronary artery bypass grafting), although the risk is increased.[354] There has been recent enthusiasm for combining septal myotomy-myectomy with plication of the anterior leaflet of the mitral valve.[358] Although mitral valve replacement or repair is performed in fewer centers than myotomy-myectomy, the long-term results also have been favorable, with symptomatic benefit and an improvement in hemodynamics.[359] The rationale for this operation is that it abolishes obstruction by preventing SAM of the mitral valve (see p. 91). It appears to be of particular value in patients with less than severe (<18 mm) hypertrophy of the upper septum or other atypical septal morphology, in those with previous myotomy-myectomy with persistent severe symptoms and obstruction, and in patients with intrinsic mitral valve disease.[360] In appropriate candidates not responding to maximal standard medical and surgical therapy, cardiac transplantation may be an option; this usually is required only for patients who have entered the dilated phase of HCM and have intractable symptoms of congestive heart failure.[361]

RESTRICTIVE AND INFILTRATIVE CARDIOMYOPATHIES

Of the three major functional categories of the cardiomyopathies (dilated, hypertrophic, and restrictive), the restrictive are the least common in Western countries, although secondary forms of restrictive cardiomyopathy such as endomyocardial disease (see p. 1431) are common in specific geographical regions.[362,363] The hallmark of the restrictive cardiomyopathies is abnormal diastolic function; the ventricular walls are excessively rigid and impede ventricular filling. Contractile function, on the other hand, often is unimpaired, even in many cases of extensive infiltration of the myocardium.[6,364] Thus, restrictive cardiomyopathy bears some functional resemblance to constrictive pericarditis, which is also characterized by normal or nearly normal systolic function but abnormal ventricular filling.[365,366] Differentiation of the two conditions is mandatory because of the potential for successful surgical treatment of constriction (Table 43–8, p. 1503).[219,363,363a]

A variety of specific pathological processes may result in restrictive cardiomyopathy, although the cause often remains unknown. Myocardial fibrosis, infiltration, or endomyocardial scarring is usually responsible for the abnormal diastolic behavior; there often is histological evidence of

TABLE 41–13 CLASSIFICATION OF THE RESTRICTIVE CARDIOMYOPATHIES

MYOCARDIAL
Noninfiltrative
Idiopathic
Scleroderma
Infiltrative
Amyloid
Sarcoid
Gaucher disease
Hurler disease
Storage Diseases
Hemochromatosis
Fabry disease
Glycogen storage diseases
ENDOMYOCARDIAL
Endomyocardial fibrosis
Hypereosinophilic syndrome
Carcinoid
Metastatic malignancies
Radiation
Anthracycline toxicity

myocyte hypertrophy.[366,367] Myocardial involvement with amyloid is a common cause of secondary restrictive cardiomyopathy, although it can be caused by a variety of other conditions (Table 41–13).[363]

Some patients may manifest the clinical features of a restrictive cardiomyopathy and yet exhibit the pathological findings of left ventricular hypertrophy and fibrosis[6]; certainly ventricular hypertrophy, especially HCM, can cause diminished ventricular compliance, but not restrictive cardiomyopathy per se. Restrictive cardiomyopathy on occasion is inherited; in those cases there may be an associated skeletal muscle myopathy.[367,368]

HEMODYNAMICS. The clinical and hemodynamic features of restrictive heart disease simulate those of chronic constrictive pericarditis; endomyocardial biopsy, CT scanning (Fig. 10–40, p. 340), MRI (Fig. 10–14, p. 325) and radionuclide angiography (Fig. 43–28, p. 1504) may be particularly useful in differentiating the two diseases by demonstrating myocardial scarring or infiltration (biopsy) or thickening of the pericardium (CT and MRI).[362,363,369,370] With the use of these modalities, exploratory thoracotomy should rarely be required; nevertheless, if the differentiation between constriction and restrictive cardiomyopathy cannot be established with certainty, surgical exploration is in order.[219] The characteristic hemodynamic feature in both conditions is a deep and rapid early decline in ventricular pressure at the onset of diastole, with a rapid rise to a plateau in early diastole (although this finding is absent in some patients with restrictive cardiomyopathy).[365,367] This dip and plateau has been termed the "square root" sign (Fig. 43–19, p. 1502) and is manifested in the atrial pressure tracing as a prominent *y* descent followed by a rapid rise and plateau.[219] The *x* descent may also be rapid, and the combination results in the characteristic M or W waveform in the atrial pressure tracing. The *a* wave is prominent and often is of the same amplitude as the *v* wave. Both systemic and pulmonary venous pressures are elevated, although patients with restrictive heart disease typically have left ventricular filling pressures that exceed right ventricular filling pressure by more than 5 mm Hg[366]; this difference is accentuated by exercise, fluid challenge, and Valsalva maneuver (although not all patients demonstrate this finding).[219,371] In this respect they differ from patients with constrictive pericarditis, in whom diastolic pressures are similar in both ventricles, usually differing by no more than 5 mm Hg.[365] The pulmonary artery systolic pressure is often greater than 50 mm Hg in patients with restrictive cardiomyopathy but is lower in constrictive pericarditis.[362,365] Furthermore, the plateau of the right ventricular diastolic pressure is usually at least one-thrd of the peak right ventricular systolic pressure in patients with constrictive pericarditis, whereas it is frequently less in restrictive cardiomyopathy.[365] Patients who demonstrate all three typical hemodynamic features (difference of biventricular diastolic pressures, pulmonary artery systolic pressure, ratio of right ventricular diastolic to systolic pressure) can be classified correctly, although in one-fourth the differentiation between constriction and restriction cannot be made on hemodynamic grounds.[365]

CLINICAL MANIFESTATIONS. Exercise intolerance is frequent because of the inability of patients with restrictive cardiomyopathy to increase their cardiac output by tachycardia without further compromising ventricular filling. Weakness and dyspnea are often prominent. Exertional chest pain may be prominent in some patients but is usually absent. Particularly in advanced cases, the central venous pressure is elevated, with attendant peripheral edema, enlarged liver, ascites, and anasarca. *Physical examination* may reveal jugular venous distention, and an S_3, S_4, or both. An inspiratory increase in venous pressure (Kussmaul sign, p. 1497) may be seen. However, in contrast to constrictive pericarditis, the apex impulse is usually palpable in restrictive cardiomyopathy.

Various ancillary laboratory findings in addition to endomyocardial biopsy, CT scanning, and MRI[369] may be useful in distinguishing between constrictive and restrictive disease. While pericardial calcification is neither absolutely sensitive nor specific for constrictive pericarditis (see p. 1499), its presence in a patient in whom the differential diagnosis rests between restrictive cardiomyopathy and constrictive pericarditis lends strong support to the latter diagnosis.[219] The *echocardiogram* may demonstrate thickening of the left ventricular wall and an increase of left ventricular mass in patients with infiltrative disease causing restrictive cardiomyopathy (Fig. 41–21).[362] The pattern of filling of the left ventricle differs in the two conditions, as can be demonstrated by digitized echocardiograms,[372] transthoracic[373–375] and transesophageal[376,377] Doppler ultrasonography, and radionuclide ventriculography.[378,379] In patients with constrictive pericarditis, respiratory variations in left ventricular isovolumic relaxation time and peak mitral valve velocity in early diastole are prominent; however, this finding is not present in patients with restrictive cardiomyopathy (nor in normal subjects).[375]

The prognosis in restrictive cardiomyopathy is quite variable; usually it is one of relentless symptomatic progression and high mortality.[219] No specific therapy (other than symptomatic) is available (excepting the secondary restrictive cardiomyopathy due to iron overload which is improved by removal of the iron), although there is speculation that calcium antagonists may be of some value.[362]

AMYLOIDOSIS

ETIOLOGY AND TYPES. Amyloidosis is a disease complex that results from deposition of unique twisted B-pleated sheet fibrils formed from various proteins by several different pathogenic mechanisms.[363,380,381] Amyloid may be found in almost any organ, but clinically evident disease does not appear unless infiltration is extensive. Several classification systems have been used to characterize the different clinical presentations of amyloidosis. The condition with the traditional designation of primary amyloidosis is now known to be caused by the production of an amyloid protein composed of portions of immunoglobulin light chain (designated AL) by a monoclonal population of plasma cells, often as a consequence of multiple myeloma.[382] Secondary amyloidosis is due to the production of a nonimmunoglobulin protein termed AA.[380]

Familial amyloidosis, inherited as an autosomal dominant trait, results from the production of a variant prealbumin protein termed transthyretin; more than 50 different point mutations have been described so far.[383–385] It generally occurs in one of three clinical presentations: progressive neuropathy, cardiomyopathy, or nephropathy.[381] Senile systemic amyloidosis is due to the production of either an atrial natriuretic-like protein or transthyretin[380,386] and is becoming

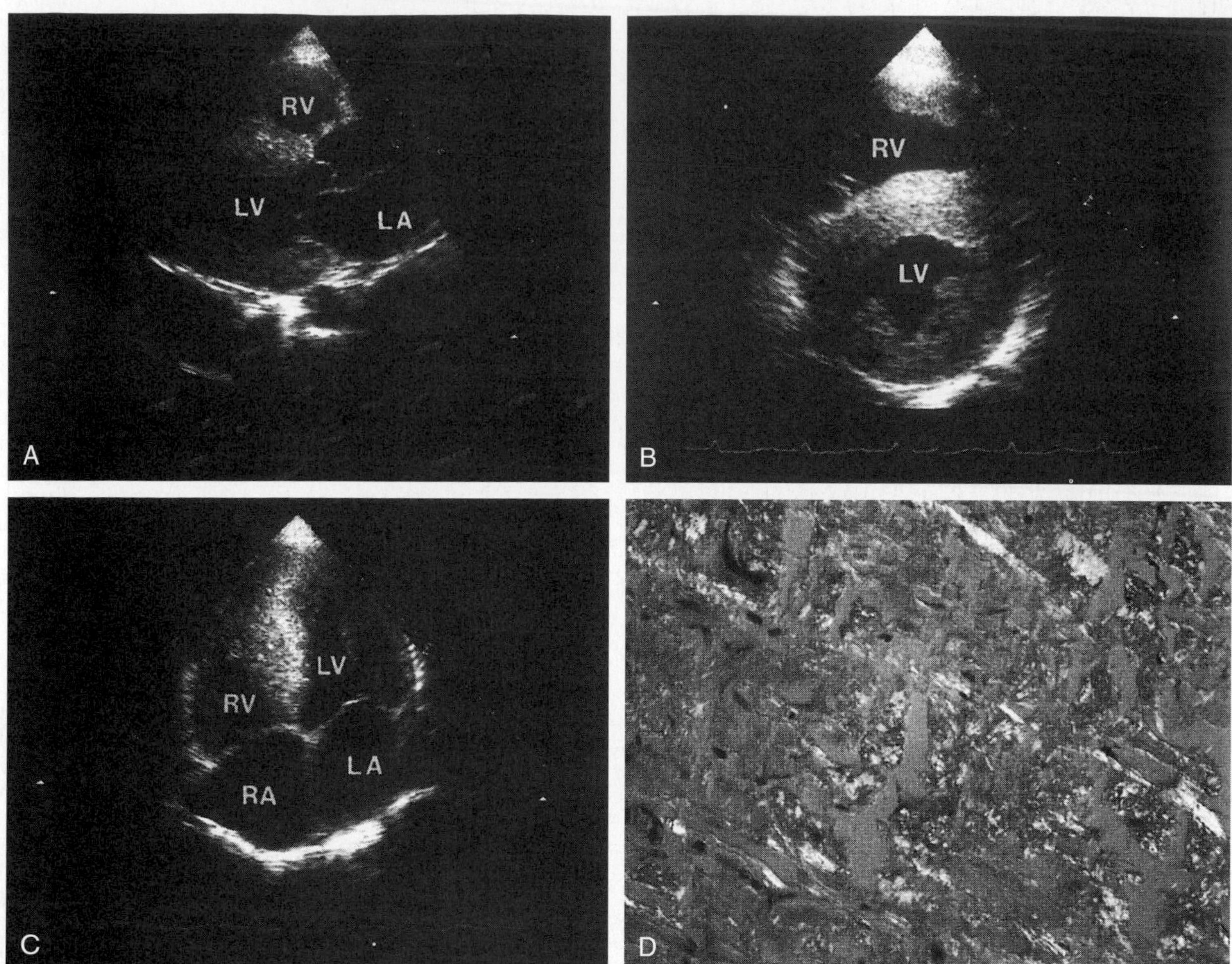

FIGURE 41–21. Two-dimensional echocardiogram in various orientations (*A* to *C*) and cardiac biopsy specimen *(D)* of a 68-year-old man with cardiac amyloidosis. *A,* Parasternal long-axis view shows marked increase of wall thickness of the left ventricle and thickening of both the mitral and aortic valves. *B,* Parasternal short-axis view of the left ventricle shows an increase in wall thickness and a prominent speckled pattern of the myocardium that is characteristic of infiltrative cardiomyopathy. *C,* Apical four-chamber view shows hypertrophy of both ventricles and thickening of both the mitral and tricuspid valves and the interatrial septum. *D,* Endomyocardial biopsy specimen demonstrates amyloid protein showing apple-green birefringence when viewed under polarized light (Congo red stain, ×3). LA = Left atrium; LV = left ventricle; RA = right atrium; RV = right ventricle. (From Douglas, P. S.: Images in clinical medicine. N. Engl. J. Med. *327:*1574, 1992. Copyright Massachusetts Medical Society.)

increasingly common as the average age of the population increases. Scattered deposits of amyloid localized to the aorta or atria are virtually ubiquitous in individuals over the age of 80.[363,380] Small deposits of amyloid may often be found in the pulmonary vessels or the vessels of other organs as well.

Cardiac Amyloidosis

Involvement of the heart is a common finding and is the most frequent cause of death in amyloidosis associated with an immunocyte dyscrasia.[387] Clinically apparent heart disease is present in one-third of patients, although the heart is virtually always involved when studied pathologically.[381] In secondary amyloidosis, on the other hand, clinically significant cardiac involvement is uncommon[388]; the myocardial deposits are typically small and perivascular and usually do not result in significant myocardial dysfunction.[380] Familial amyloidosis is associated with overt cardiac involvement in about one-quarter of the afflicted patients, usually late in the course of the disease.[389] The clinical course is usually dominated by neurological or renal dysfunction, although death is due to heart failure or arrhythmia about half the time.[389] Cardiac involvement in senile amyloidosis varies from small atrial deposits that do not result in functional impairment to extensive ventricular involvement with resultant cardiac failure.[385]

Cardiac amyloidosis occurs more commonly in men than in women, and it is rare before the age of 30 years.[381] Even in the familial form, the onset of clinical cardiac disease usually does not occur before the age of 35 years and generally occurs much later in life.[388]

PATHOLOGY. The pathological findings often include mild atrial enlargement, usually without significant ventricular dilatation. The walls of both ventricles are typically firm, rubbery, noncompliant, and thickened. Amyloid is present between the myocardial fibers (Fig. 41–21*D*), with extensive deposition in the papillary muscles occurring commonly. Endocardial involvement of the atria[382] and ventricles is frequent. Amyloidosis often results in focal thickening of or deposits on the cardiac valves, but these abnormalities do not appear to interfere with valvular function other than to produce murmurs. The intramural coronary arteries and veins frequently contain amyloid deposits in the media and adventitia, occasionally compromising the lumina of the vessels.[364,384]

CLINICAL MANIFESTATIONS. Involvement of the cardiovascular system by amyloidosis occurs in four general forms:

1. The most common presentation of cardiac amyloidosis is that of *restrictive cardiomyopathy.*[219] Right-sided findings dominate the clinical presentation; peripheral

edema is a prominent finding, whereas paroxysmal nocturnal dyspnea and orthopnea are absent.[363] Amyloid infiltration of the myocardium results in increased stiffness of the myocardium, producing the characteristic diastolic dip and plateau (square root sign) in the ventricular pressure pulse that may simulate constrictive pericarditis. In contrast to the accelerated early left ventricular diastolic filling found in constrictive pericarditis, cardiac amyloidosis is marked by an impaired rate of early diastolic filling.

2. A second common presentation is congestive heart failure due to systolic dysfunction.[219,385] Hemodynamic evidence of restriction of ventricular filling may not be prominent in these patients. In some patients amyloid deposition in the atrium may be responsible for loss of atrial transport function despite the maintenance of electrical "sinus" rhythm and the precipitation of congestive heart failure.[382] The course of this form of the disease is often relentless progression, usually poorly responsive to treatment. Angina pectoris occurs on occasion despite angiographically normal coronary arteries.[364]

3. Orthostatic hypotension is the third mode of presentation, occurring in about 10 per cent of cases. Although most likely due to amyloid infiltration of the autonomic nervous system or of blood vessels, amyloid deposition in the heart and adrenals may contribute to this manifestation. Hypovolemia as a result of the nephrotic syndrome secondary to renal amyloidosis may aggravate the postural hypotension.[389]

4. An abnormality of cardiac impulse formation and conduction is the fourth and least common mode of presentation and may result in arrhythmias and conduction disturbances.[380] Sudden death, presumably arrhythmic in origin, is relatively common.[389]

Physical Examination. This often reveals congestive heart failure, especially right-sided[363]; a systolic murmur due to atrioventricular valvular regurgitation may be present. Jugular venous distention, a protodiastolic gallop, hepatomegaly, peripheral edema, and a narrow pulse pressure are found in patients presenting with restrictive cardiomyopathy. A fourth heart sound is uncommon, presumably due to amyloid infiltration of the atrium. Patients typically are normotensive or hypotensive; even previously hypertensive individuals usually have a fall in blood pressure as the disease progresses.

Noninvasive Testing. The *chest roentgenogram* usually shows cardiomegaly in patients with systolic dysfunction, although heart size may be normal in patients with the restrictive form.[363] Pulmonary congestion may be prominent in patients with congestive heart failure. The *electrocardiogram* is often abnormal; the most characteristic feature (but often absent) is diffusely diminished voltage.[363] Myocardial infarction is often simulated because of small or absent R waves in right precordial leads or, less frequently, by Q waves in the inferior leads.[380] Arrhythmias, particularly atrial fibrillation, are common, although they rarely are the presenting feature of cardiac amyloidosis. Complex ventricular arrhythmias are found frequently in patients with cardiac amyloidosis, and in some may be a harbinger of sudden death.[384] Various forms of AV conduction defects are often seen.[389] Abnormalities of AV conduction appear to be particularly common in familial amyloidosis with polyneuropathy.[389] Sinus node involvement is common, and the clinical and electrocardiographic features of the sick sinus syndrome may be present (see p. 648).

Echocardiography (Fig. 3–102, p. 92) in advanced cases most commonly reveals increased thickness of the walls of the ventricles, small ventricular chambers, dilated atria, and thickening of the interatrial septum,[380] although the findings are more prominent in the familial than in the primary (AL) form (Fig. 41–21).[364] Left ventricular dysfunction may be seen, especially in advanced cases, but systolic function often is surprisingly normal.[364] Early preclinical unsuspected cardiac involvement may be detectable only by echocardiography or Doppler ultrasonography.[390] Although the cardiac valves may be thickened, they usually move normally.[385] A pericardial effusion is common but rarely results in tamponade. The appearance of the thickened cardiac walls is often distinctive on two-dimensional echocardiography, demonstrating a granular sparkling texture, presumably due to the amyloid deposit.[219,391] In some cases the pattern of increased wall thickness is nonuniform and may resemble HCM.[219] Echocardiographic demonstration of thick left ventricular walls with concomitant low voltage on the electrocardiogram appears to distinguish cardiac amyloidosis from pericardial disease or left ventricular hypertrophy, and this distinctive voltage/mass ratio is characteristic of myocardial infiltration by amyloid.[391] Doppler ultrasonography[392] and radionuclide ventriculography[393] routinely demonstrate abnormalities of diastolic function, and by estimating the degree of cardiac involvement by amyloid, provide prognostic information.[394]

Scintigraphy with technetium-99m pyrophosphate is often strongly positive with prominent amyloid involvement,[395] although in a minority of cases it is falsely negative.[219,391] Positive scans tend to correlate with extensive cardiac involvement. Scanning with indium-labeled antimyosin antibody may also detect cardiac amyloid involvement.[396]

DIAGNOSIS. Whereas two or three decades ago the clinical diagnosis of systemic amyloidosis was made correctly antemortem only 25 per cent of the time, with more recent clinical awareness of the disease and the utilization of *biopsy techniques,* the diagnosis is now made before death in the majority of cases. An abdominal fat aspirate has been the single most useful diagnostic procedure, combining the attributes of ease of performance, sensitivity, and safety.[363] Biopsy of rectum, gingiva, bone marrow, liver, kidney, and various other tissues has also been used. Endomyocardial biopsy of the right or left ventricles may be helpful in establishing the diagnosis of cardiac amyloidosis if the abdominal fat aspirate is negative.[363]

MANAGEMENT. The treatment of cardiac amyloidosis is generally unsatisfactory and ineffective, although it is speculated that alkylating agents may have some role in primary (AL) amyloidosis.[363,385,397] Digitalis glycosides should be used with caution because patients with cardiac amyloidosis appear to be particularly sensitive to digitalis preparations, and the use of ordinary doses may lead to serious arrhythmias; this may relate to selective binding of digoxin to amyloid fibrils in the myocardium.[363] Similarly, nifedipine binds to amyloid fibrils; its use and that of the other calcium antagonists may lead to exacerbation of congestive heart failure symptoms due to an enhanced negative inotropic effect.[363,398] Insertion of a permanent pacemaker may be beneficial in the short term in patients with symptomatic conducting system disease. Careful use of low doses of diuretics and vasodilators may afford some symptomatic benefit,[381] but there is a real risk of hypotension with use of these agents. In patients with atrial standstill due to amyloid infiltration, anticoagulation may be appropriate even in the absence of atrial arrhythmias, as there is some risk of thrombus formation, presumably as a consequence of stasis in the atrium.[382] A few patients have undergone cardiac transplantation, with inferior long-term results (39 per cent survival at 4 years in one study) due to progressive amyloidosis in other organs; accordingly, cardiac transplantation is not recommended in these patients.[399] An heroic alternative approach for the familial form of cardiac amyloidosis is simultaneous heart and liver transplantation because the circulating transthyretin in these patients is produced in the liver and can be corrected with liver transplantation.[384,385] No therapy is effective for the senile form.[385]

INHERITED INFILTRATIVE DISORDERS CAUSING CARDIOMYOPATHY

The intramyocardial accumulation or infiltration of an abnormal metabolic product typically produces a restrictive picture with impaired diastolic ventricular filling. Systolic impairment may be seen as well but is not invariably found. A variety of infiltrative diseases, often inherited, may result in this hemodynamic picture, including the glycogenoses, the mucopolysaccharidoses, Fabry disease, and Gaucher disease.

FABRY DISEASE

Fabry disease (angiokeratoma corporis diffusum universale) is an X-linked recessive disorder of glycosphingolipid metabolism due to a deficiency of the lysosomal enzyme α-galactosidase A as a consequence of one of more than four dozen mutations.[400–402] Some mutations result in no detectable α-galactosidase A activity and widespread manifestations throughout the body, whereas others produce some degree of enzyme activity with attendant atypical variants of Fabry disease with involvement limited solely to the myocardium.[403,404,404a] The disease is characterized by an intracellular accumulation of a neutral glycolipid, with prominent involvement of the skin and kidneys as well as the myocardium in the classic form. *Histological examination* often reveals widespread involvement of the myocardium, vascular endothelium, conducting tissues, and valves, particularly the mitral valve (Fig. 41–22).[403] The major clinical manifestations of the disease result from the accumulation of the glycolipid substrate in endothelial cells, with eventual occlusion of small arterioles. The accumulation of the glycolipid occurs in the lysosomes of the cardiac tissues and is responsible for the multiple cardiovascular manifestations of Fabry disease.

CARDIAC FINDINGS. These typically include angina and myocardial infarction despite angiographically normal coronary arteries (due to accumulation of lipid moieties in coronary endothelial cells), increased left ventricular wall thickness simulating HCM (due to accumulation in myocytes), left ventricular dysfunction and failure, and mitral regurgitation (due to deposition in valvular fibroblasts).[403] Symptomatic cardiovascular involvement occurs eventually in most affected males, whereas female carriers usually are asymptomatic or only minimally symptomatic. Systemic hypertension, mitral valve prolapse, and congestive heart failure are common clinical manifestations. *Electrocardiographic* abnormalities include AV block or a short P-R interval, and ST-segment and T-wave abnormalities.[405] The *echocardiogram* usually reveals increased left ventricular wall thickness as a result of glycolipid deposition, which may simulate HCM.[403] Differentiation from other hypertrophic or restrictive processes (such as cardiac amyloidosis) may not be possible on echocardiographic grounds but may be possible with nuclear MRI. *Endomyocardial biopsy* may be of considerable value in making a definitive diagnosis, as is low plasma α-galactosidase A activity.[403]

GAUCHER DISEASE

Gaucher disease is an uncommon inherited disorder of glycosyl ceramide metabolism. It is secondary to a deficiency of the enzyme β-glucosidase and results in accumulation of cerebrosides in the spleen, liver, bone marrow, lymph nodes, brain, and myocardium. Diffuse interstitial infiltration of the left ventricle by cells laden with cerebroside occurs, with attendant reduced left ventricular compliance and cardiac output. Clinical evidence of cardiac involvement is uncommon, but when present it is characterized by left ventricular dysfunction, hemorrhagic pericardial effusion, increased left ventricular wall mass, and thickening of the left-sided valves.[406–408] Liver transplantation may produce a reduction in tissue infiltration by cerebrosides.[409]

HEMOCHROMATOSIS

(See also p. 1674)

Hemochromatosis is characterized by excessive deposition of iron in a variety of parenchymal tissues (heart, liver, gonads, and pancreas). It may occur (1) as a familial (autosomal recessive)[410] or idiopathic disorder, (2) in association with a defect in hemoglobin synthesis resulting in ineffective erythropoiesis, (3) in chronic liver disease, and (4) with excessive oral or parenteral intake of iron (or blood transfusions) over many years.[411–413] Although patients who have iron deposits in the myocardium almost always have deposits in other organs (e.g., liver, spleen, pancreas, bone marrow), the severity of myocardial involvement varies widely and only roughly parallels that in other organs. Cardiac involvement leads to a mixed dilated/restrictive cardiomyopathic presentation with both systolic and diastolic dysfunction, often with associated arrhythmias.[411,414,415] Myocardial damage is thought to be due to direct tissue toxicity of the free iron moiety rather than simply to tissue infiltration.[411] Although cirrhosis and hepatocellular carcinoma are the most common causes of death, cardiac mortality is an important additional concern (especially in the group of patients—usually men—who present at a young age).[413,416]

PATHOLOGICAL FINDINGS. These consist of a dilated heart with thickened ventricular walls.[417] Myocardial iron deposits are found within the sarcoplasmic reticulum and are most common in the subepicardial region, followed by the subendocardial region, and are least common in the midmyocardial wall.[418] They are more extensive in ventricular than in atrial myocardium. Involvement of the cardiac conducting system is common. Myocardial degeneration and fibrosis may also occur (Fig. 57–5, p. 1791).

The severity of myocardial dysfunction is proportional to the quantity of iron present in the myocardium.[417] Extensive deposits of cardiac iron (particularly those grossly visible at postmortem examination) are invariably associated with cardiac dysfunction.

CLINICAL MANIFESTATIONS. These vary widely, depending on the extent of myocardial involvement. Some patients remain asymptomatic despite echocardiographic evidence of myocardial involvement, which is expressed initially as increased left ventricular wall thickness and later as chamber enlargement and contractile dysfunction.[417] In such cases, a variety of noninvasive techniques (CT and especially MRI) may demonstrate early subclinical myocardial involvement in which treatment is most effective.[411,419] Symptomatic cardiac involvement is usually associated with electrocardiographic abnormalities, including ST-segment and T-wave abnormalities, as well as supraventricular arrhythmias[417,420]; these electrocardiographic changes correlate with the degree of iron deposit in the heart.

Cardiac involvement usually is evident from the clinical and echocardiographic features; endomyocardial biopsy may be useful to confirm (but not exclude) the diagnosis.[413] The diagnosis is aided by finding an elevated plasma iron level, a normal or low total iron-binding capacity, and markedly elevated values for serum ferritin, urinary iron, liver iron, and especially saturation of transferrin.[413] Repeated phlebotomies or the use of the chelating agent desferrioxamine may be clinically beneficial[410,411] (see p. 1791).

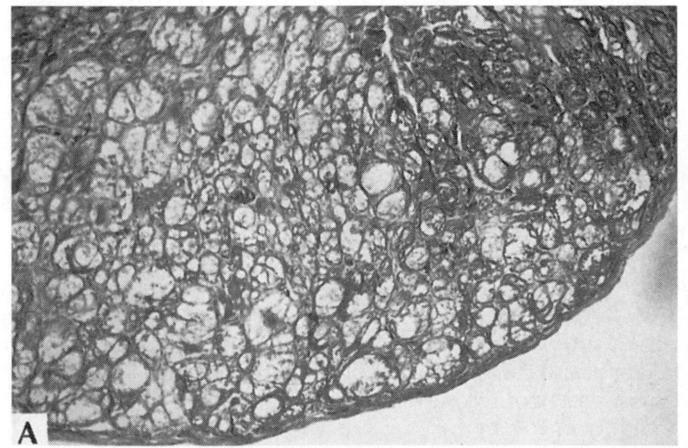

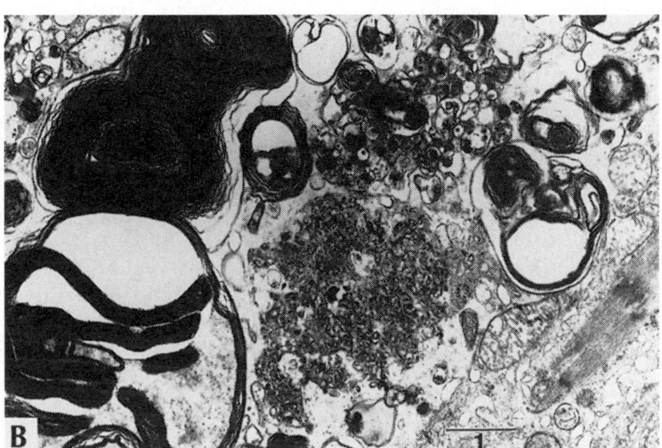

FIGURE 41–22. Histological findings in Fabry disease. *A,* Endomyocardial biopsy showing markedly vacuolated myocytes. *B,* Transmission electron microscopic appearance of the characteristic intracellular deposits of whorled membrane-bound glycoproteins. Bar = 1 μm. (From Butany, J., and Schoen, F. J.: Endomyocardial biopsy. *In* Abelmann, W. H., and Braunwald, E. [eds.]: Cardiomyopathies, Myocarditis, and Pericardial Disease. Atlas of Heart Diseases. Vol. 2. Philadelphia, Current Medicine, 1995, pp. 12.1–12.17.)

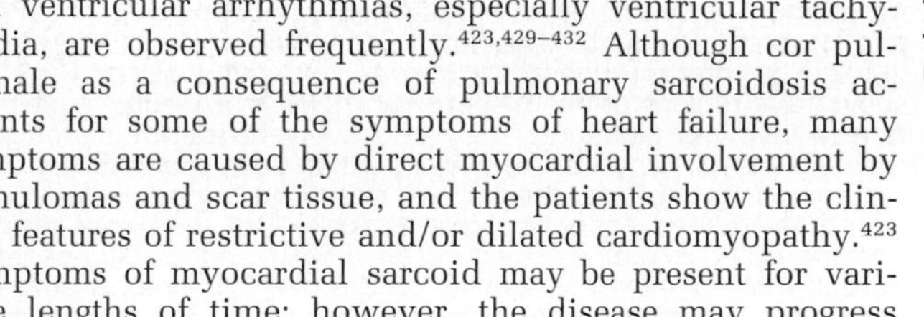

FIGURE 41–23. Endomyocardial biopsy specimen from a patient with glycogen storage disease. The intracytoplasmic lucency is caused by accumulation of glycogen. (From Kasper, E. K., Hruban, R. H., and Baughman, K. L.: Idiopathic dilated cardiomyopathy. *In* Abelmann, W. H., and Braunwald, E. [eds.]: Cardiomyopathies, Myocarditis, and Pericardial Disease. Atlas of Heart Diseases. Vol. 2. Philadelphia, Current Medicine, 1995, pp. 3.1–3.18.)

GLYCOGEN STORAGE DISEASES

Adult patients may demonstrate cardiac involvement in these diseases (Fig. 41–23); in Type III (glycogen debranching enzyme deficiency), cardiac involvement is found only in patients with deficient enzyme in muscle tissue.[421] Cardiac involvement is marked most commonly by apparent left ventricular hypertrophy on the electrocardiogram and echocardiogram.[220,421]

SARCOIDOSIS

Sarcoidosis is a granulomatous disorder of unknown cause, characterized by multisystem involvement. Infiltration of the lungs, reticuloendothelial system, and skin usually dominates the clinical picture, but virtually any tissue may be affected. The most important manifestation results from pulmonary involvement. This often leads to diffuse fibrosis that may result in fatal right heart failure. Primary cardiac involvement is not often recognized clinically, although it may be demonstrated at autopsy in 20 to 30 per cent of cases, most of which demonstrate generalized sarcoidosis.[422–426]

Clinical manifestations of sarcoid heart disease are present in less than 5 per cent of patients, although myocardial involvement may result in heart block, congestive heart failure, ventricular arrhythmias, and sudden death.[423] Myocardial sarcoidosis may have restrictive as well as congestive features because cardiac infiltration by sarcoid granulomas results not only in increased stiffness of the ventricular wall but in diminished systolic contractile function as well. Myocardial sarcoidosis typically affects young or middle-aged adults of either gender; there usually is evidence of generalized sarcoidosis.[422–424,427]

PATHOLOGY. The typical pathological feature of sarcoidosis is the presence of noncaseating granulomas, which occur in many organs. They infiltrate the myocardium and may eventually become fibrotic scars.[423] The granulomas may involve any region of the heart, although the left ventricular free wall and the interventricular septum are the most common sites, and extensive granulomas and scar tissue in the cephalad portion of the interventricular septum is a constant finding in patients with abnormalities of the conduction system.[428] Cardiac infiltration may range from a few scattered lesions to extensive involvement.[423] Because of the variable cardiac involvement, myocardial biopsy may be positive in only about half of the patients, and therefore a negative biopsy by no means excludes the diagnosis.[423] Transmural involvement is common, and large portions of the ventricular wall may be replaced by scar tissue, which may lead to aneurysm formation. Although involvement of small coronary artery branches may be found in sarcoidosis, the larger conductance vessels are uninvolved.[423]

CLINICAL MANIFESTATIONS. Sudden death is the most feared and unfortunately one of the more common manifestations of cardiac sarcoidosis.[423,429–432] Conduction disturbances and congestive heart failure are common manifestations of symptomatic involvement in nonfatal cases, but many patients are asymptomatic despite extensive cardiac involvement.[425] Syncope is common and may reflect paroxysmal arrhythmias or conduction disturbances.[423] Atrial and ventricular arrhythmias, especially ventricular tachycardia, are observed frequently.[423,429–432] Although cor pulmonale as a consequence of pulmonary sarcoidosis accounts for some of the symptoms of heart failure, many symptoms are caused by direct myocardial involvement by granulomas and scar tissue, and the patients show the clinical features of restrictive and/or dilated cardiomyopathy.[423] Symptoms of myocardial sarcoid may be present for variable lengths of time; however, the disease may progress rapidly to death, and in some patients the interval from the onset of the cardiac symptoms to death is measured in months. Survival may be considerably longer, however.[423]

Cardiac dysfunction is often severe and progressive. Occasionally, patients with extensive involvement develop overt left ventricular aneurysms.[423] Pericardial effusions are not uncommon in patients with sarcoidosis.[433]

The *physical examination* may reveal findings of extracardiac sarcoid or may be totally normal. A systolic murmur reflecting mitral regurgitation is common. This appears to be more the result of left ventricular dilatation than of direct sarcoid involvement of the papillary muscles.

The *electrocardiogram* frequently is abnormal in patients with known sarcoid and most commonly demonstrates T-wave abnormalities. Sarcoidosis appears to have an affinity for involvement of the AV junction and bundle of His, and thus varying degrees of intraventricular or AV block are common.[423] With extensive myocardial involvement, pathological Q waves may appear and simulate myocardial infarction. Characteristic features of *echocardiography* include left ventricular dilatation and dysfunction, often with regional wall motion abnormalities suggestive of ischemic heart disease[423,434]; a small to moderate-sized pericardial effusion is seen in about 20 per cent.[433]

DIAGNOSIS. In many cases the diagnosis may be suspected in patients with bilateral hilar lymphadenopathy on chest roentgenogram in whom there is clinical or electrocardiographic evidence of myocardial disease. *Endomyocardial biopsy* may be useful in establishing the diagnosis, although the nonuniform involvement of the heart by sarcoidosis means that a negative biopsy does not exclude the diagnosis.[426] The *echocardiogram* demonstrates diffuse and often regional left ventricular wall motion abnormalities in patients with clinical cardiac involvement.[435] *Myocardial imaging* with *thallium-201* may be helpful in demonstrating segmental perfusion defects that result from sarcoid infiltration of the myocardium.[436–440] Imaging may also indicate the presence of right ventricular hypertrophy in patients with right ventricular overload due to pulmonary fibrosis and pulmonary hypertension. Uptake of technetium pyrophosphate, gallium, and labeled antimyosin antibody may aid in the diagnosis, as may nuclear MRI.[423,437,438,441–443]

MANAGEMENT. The treatment of myocardial sarcoidosis is difficult. Arrhythmias are often refractory to antiarrhythmic drugs.[430] Permanent pacing may be helpful in patients with conducting system involvement.[426] Although the matter is not settled, corticosteroids may be of some benefit in treating the conduction disturbances, arrhythmias, and myocardial dysfunction of sarcoidosis.[422,423,426,444–448] Because the risk of sudden death appears to be greatest in patients with extensive myocardial involvement, it may be reasonable to attempt to halt the progression of the disease with steroids before irreversible fibrosis occurs. Insertion of an implantable cardioverter-defibrillator may be considered in appropriate patients at high risk of sudden death.[430,449] Heart or heart-lung transplantation has been used in selected patients with intractable heart failure.[426,450]

ENDOMYOCARDIAL DISEASE

DEFINITION AND PATHOGENESIS. Endomyocardial disease (EMD) is a common form of secondary restrictive cardiomyopathy in equatorial

Africa and is encountered with less frequency in South America, Asia, and nontropical countries, including the United States.[362,451,452] It is marked by intense endocardial fibrotic thickening of the apex and subvalvular regions of one or both ventricles that results in obstruction to inflow of blood into the respective ventricle, thus producing restrictive physiology. For many years it had been thought that there are two variants of the disease, one occurring principally in tropical countries (termed endomyocardial fibrosis, EMF, or Davies disease) and the other in temperate countries (Löffler endocarditis parietalis fibroplastica, or hypereosinophilic syndrome).[363] This conclusion was reached in part because the pathological findings in advanced cases are identical.[453,454] Despite the pathological similarities, differences occur in clinical presentation. In addition to the geographical differences, the temperate form of the disease (Löffler endocarditis) acts as a more aggressive and rapidly progressive disorder, affecting principally males, and is associated with hypereosinophilia, thromboembolic phenomena, and generalized arteritis.[363] EMF, conversely, shows no gender predilection, occurs in younger patients, and is not associated with an intense eosinophilia.[363,455]

It has also been postulated that Löffler endocarditis and EMF are different phases in a single disease that results from the toxic effect of eosinophils on the heart.[454,456–458] Under this formulation, an initial hypereosinophilia of whatever cause results in damage to the myocardium that produces the first phase of EMD: a necrotic phase, marked by an intense myocarditis, rich in eosinophils, and with an associated arteritis (i.e., Löffler endocarditis).[457,459] This initial phase occurs within the first few months of illness. It appears to be followed by a thrombotic stage, occurring about a year after initial presentation, during which the myocarditis has receded, nonspecific thickening of the myocardium is beginning, and there is a variable degree of superimposed thrombus formation.[457] The last stage is one of fibrosis, presenting all of the features of EMF.[454] The three stages —necrotic, thrombotic, and fibrotic—have been defined on the basis of postmortem material, and it is not suggested that each patient with advanced disease (manifested by EMF) has necessarily passed through the earlier phases.

There is now, however, increasing speculation that this continuum occurs only in the temperate countries, and the endemic EMF found in tropical countries is a distinct and separate disease, as a link with eosinophilia has been virtually impossible to document.[363,460,461] The fibrosis of tropical EMF has been linked to the higher levels of cerium and lower concentrations of magnesium that apparently are found in endemic areas.[460,461]

The possible role of *eosinophils* in the production of the cardiac abnormalities has intrigued investigators for years.[454,457,462] Eosinophils may damage tissues by direct invasion or by the release of toxic substances.[456] The presence of degranulated peripheral eosinophils in patients with Löffler endocarditis suggests that the protein constituents of the eosinophil's granule may be cardiotoxic,[463] first producing the necrotic phase of EMD, followed by the thrombotic and fibrotic phases after the disappearance of the initial eosinophilia.[454]

Because the clinical manifestations of EMD demonstrate geographical and clinical differences, Löffler endocarditis and EMF are discussed separately, even though they could be part of the same disease continuum.

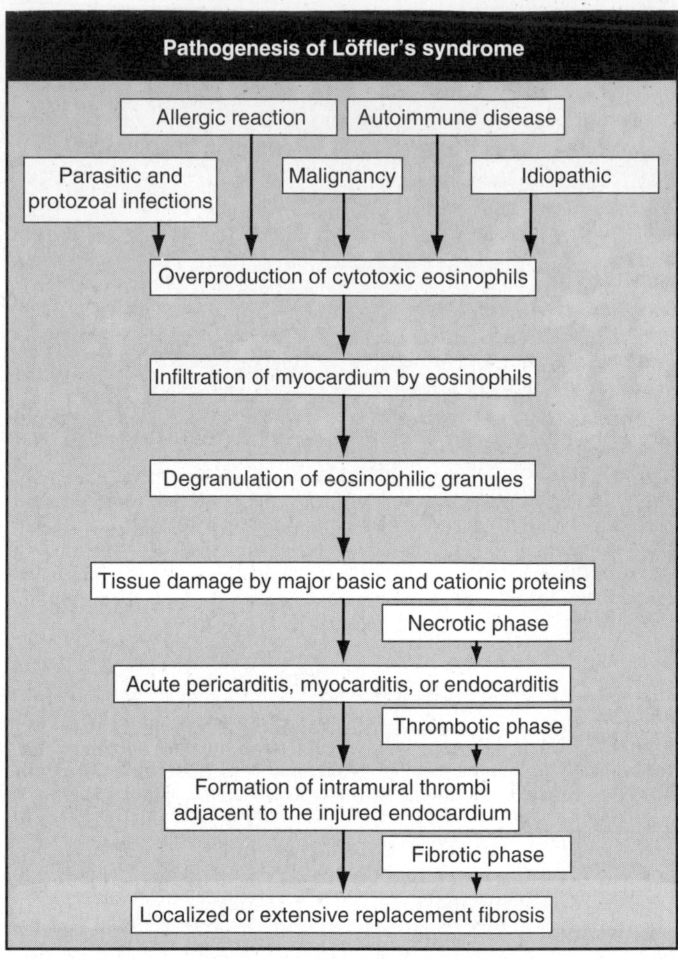

FIGURE 41–24. The pathogenesis of Löffler's syndrome. Tissue damage is caused by major basic and cationic proteins derived from cytotoxic eosinophils. These cytotoxic proteins may stay in the myocardium for a prolonged period and produce continuous tissue damage. In the fibrotic phase, various types of heart diseases, such as endomyocardial fibrosis, dilated cardiomyopathy, AV block, or valvular regurgitation can be seen according to the difference of the most dominantly involved site. (From Hirota, Y.: Restrictive cardiomyopathy, cardiac amyloidosis, and hypereosinophilic heart disease. *In* Abelmann, W. H., and Braunwald, E. [eds.]: Cardiomyopathies, Myocarditis and Pericardial Disease. Atlas of Heart Diseases. Vol. 2. Philadelphia, Current Medicine, 1995.)

Löffler Endocarditis: The Hypereosinophilic Syndrome

Marked eosinophilia of any cause may be associated with endomyocardial disease (Fig. 41–24). The typical patient who presents with Löffler endocarditis is a man in his fourth decade who lives in a temperate climate and has the hypereosinophilic syndrome (i.e., persistent eosinophilia with ≥1500 eosinophils/mm^3 for at least 6 months or until death, with evidence of organ involvement).[362,363,457,464] Cardiac involvement in the hypereosinophilic syndrome is the rule, occurring in more than three-fourths of patients.[454,465] Hypereosinophilia and cardiac involvement are also seen in the Churg-Strauss syndrome, which is differentiated by asthma or allergic rhinitis and a necrotizing vasculitis.[363,466] The cause of the eosinophilia in most patients with Löffler endocarditis is unknown, although in some it may be the result of leukemia, or it may be reactive (i.e., secondary to various parasitic, allergic, granulomatous, hypersensitivity, or neoplastic disorders).[459,462,465]

PATHOLOGY. In the hypereosinophilic syndrome, a variety of organs are usually involved besides the heart, including the lungs, bone marrow, and brain.[362,454,457] Cardiac involvement is often biventricular, with mural endocardial thickening of the inflow portions and apex of the ventricles.[363] Histological findings include variable degrees of (1) an acute inflammatory eosinophilic myocarditis involving the myocardium and endocardium; (2) thrombosis, fibrinoid change, and inflammatory reaction involving small intramural coronary vessels; (3) mural thrombosis, often containing eosinophils; and (4) fibrotic thickening of up to several millimeters.[363,457]

CLINICAL MANIFESTATIONS. The principal clinical features include weight loss, fever, cough, skin rash, and congestive heart failure. Although early cardiac involvement may be asymptomatic, overt cardiac dysfunction occurs in more than half the patients and may be right- and/or left-sided.[454] Cardiomegaly, often without overt symptoms of congestive heart failure, may be present, and the murmur of mitral regurgitation is common.[457] Systemic embolism is frequent and may lead to neurological and renal dysfunction. Death is usually due to congestive heart failure, often with associated renal, hepatic, or respiratory dysfunction.[363]

LABORATORY EXAMINATION. The *chest roentgenogram* may reveal cardiomegaly and pulmonary congestion or, less commonly, pulmonary infiltrates. The *electrocardiogram* most commonly shows nonspecific ST-segment and T-wave abnormalities.[363,465] Arrhythmias, especially atrial fibrillation, and conduction defects, particularly right bundle branch block, may also be present.

The *echocardiogram* commonly demonstrates localized thickening of the posterobasal left ventricular wall, with absent or markedly limited motion of the posterior leaflet of the mitral valve.[362,363] There may be obliteration of the apex by thrombus. Enlargement of the atria may be seen, along with Doppler ultrasound evidence of atrioventricular valve regurgitation.[363] Systolic function often is well preserved, in keeping with the restrictive picture seen in this condition.[454]

The *hemodynamic* consequences of the dense endocardial scarring seen in Löffler endocarditis are those of a restrictive cardiomyopathy, with abnormal diastolic filling due to increased stiffness of the ventricles and a reduction in the size of the ventricular cavity by organized thrombus.[454,457] Atrioventricular valvular regurgitation may occur because of involvement of the supporting apparatus of the mitral or tricuspid valves.[454] *Cardiac catheterization* reveals markedly elevated ventricular filling pressures, and there may be evidence of tricuspid or mitral regurgitation. A characteristic feature on angiocardiography is largely preserved systolic function with obliteration of the apex of the ventricles.[457] The diagnosis is often confirmed by percutaneous endomyocardial biopsy,[457] but the biopsy is not invariably positive.[462]

MANAGEMENT. Medical therapy during the course of early Löffler endocarditis and surgical therapy during the later phases of fibrosis may have a positive effect on symptoms and survival. Corticosteroids appear to have a beneficial effect on acute myocarditis,[459] and together with cytotoxic drugs (hydroxyurea in particular), may improve survival substantially.[454,457,465] A limited number of patients not responding to standard therapy have responded to treatment with interferon.[462,464] Routine cardiac therapy with digitalis, diuretics, afterload reduction, and anticoagulation as indicated are adjuncts in the management of these patients.[454,457] Surgical therapy (see Management of EMF, p. 1434) appears to offer significant palliation of symptoms once the fibrotic stage has been reached.[363,457,465]

Endomyocardial Fibrosis

EMF occurs most commonly in tropical and subtropical Africa, particularly Uganda and Nigeria.[461] It is typified by fibrous endocardial lesions of the inflow portion of the right or left ventricle or both and often involves the AV valves, resulting in regurgitation.[452,460] It is a relatively frequent cause of heart failure and death in equatorial Africa, accounting for 10 to 20 per cent of deaths due to heart disease.[362,363]

Although most prominent in Africa, it is also found in tropical and subtropical regions in the rest of the world, including India,[452] Brazil, Colombia, and Sri Lanka. EMF is most common in specific ethnic groups, notably the Rwanda tribe in Uganda, and in people of low socioeconomic status.[461] The disease is equally frequent in both genders, and, although most common in children and young adults, its reported age range is 4 to 70 years.[362,455] It is most common in blacks, but cases have been reported occasionally in whites in temperate climates, rarely in the absence of prior residence in tropical areas.

PATHOLOGY

A pericardial effusion, which may be quite large, may be present.[461] The heart is normal in size or slightly enlarged, but massive cardiomegaly does not occur. The right atrium is often dilated, and in patients with severe right ventricular involvement there may be massive enlargement of this chamber. Indentation of the right border of the heart above the apex as a result of apical scarring may occur.[461]

Combined right and left ventricular disease occurs in about half the cases, with pure left ventricular involvement occurring in 40 per cent and pure right ventricular involvement in the remaining 10 per cent of patients who are examined post mortem.[362,453] When affected, the right ventricle exhibits extensive, dense, fibrous thickening of the inflow tract and apex, with involvement of the papillary muscles and chordae tendineae. Involvement of the right ventricle may lead to obliteration of the apex, with a mass of thrombus and fibrous tissue filling the cavity.[453] The tricuspid valve is often pulled down and distorted by the fibrous process involving the supporting structures. Right atrial thrombi occur commonly. Left ventricular involvement is similar, with fibrosis extending from the apex up the inflow portion of the left ventricle to the posterior mitral valve leaflet. The anterior leaflet of the mitral valve and the outflow portion of the left ventricle are usually spared. Thrombi often overlie the endocardial lesions, and widely distributed endocardial calcific deposits may occur. The coronary arteries are uninvolved, as is the remainder of the body.[362]

HISTOLOGIC FINDINGS. Microscopically, the involved endocardium demonstrates a thick layer of collagen tissue on top of a layer of loosely arranged connective tissue.[467] Septa composed of fibrous and granulation tissue extend for variable distances into the myocardium.[362,467] Interstitial edema is often present, but there is no prominent cellular infiltration. Small patches of fibroelastosis may occur in both ventricular outflow tracts beneath the semilunar valves but are thought to be a secondary phenomenon due to local trauma rather than a result of the basic pathological process.

CLINICAL MANIFESTATIONS

As already noted, EMF may involve both ventricles or either ventricle selectively; left-sided involvement results in symptoms of pulmonary congestion, whereas predominant right-sided disease may present features of a restrictive cardiomyopathy and therefore simulate constrictive pericarditis. There is often regurgitation of one or both AV valves. The onset of the disease is usually insidious, but it is sometimes ushered in by an acute febrile illness. Rarely, the disease appears to stabilize; although survival for up to 12 years has been observed, EMF is usually relentlessly progressive.[363] Death is due to progressive myocardial failure, often associated with pulmonary congestion, infection, or infarction, or sudden, unexpected cardiovascular collapse, presumably arrhythmic in origin.[362] Survival appears to be unrelated to site of predominant involvement (right or left ventricle), although patients presenting in advanced right-sided failure have a worse prognosis than other patients.[363,455]

RIGHT VENTRICULAR EMF. Pure or predominant right ventricular involvement is characterized by fibrous obliteration of the right ventricular apex that diminishes the capacity of this chamber.[453] The fibrosis often extends to the supporting apparatus of the tricuspid valve,[468,469] resulting in tricuspid regurgitation.[470] Clinical manifestations in patients with right-sided involvement include an elevated jugular venous pressure, a prominent *v* wave, and a rapid *y* descent. A protodiastolic gallop sound may be heard along the lower sternal border, reflecting right ventricular dysfunction.[453] The liver is usually large and pulsatile, and ascites, splenomegaly, and peripheral edema are common. Pulmonary congestion is not present in the absence of left-sided involvement, and the pulmonary artery and pulmonary capillary wedge pressures are normal. A pericardial effusion, which is sometimes quite large, may be present. The right atrium is often enlarged, sometimes massively so.

Laboratory Findings. The *electrocardiogram* is usually abnormal, with diminished QRS voltage (probably resulting from the presence of a pericardial effusion), ST-segment and T-wave abnormalities, and findings of right atrial enlargement, especially a qR pattern in lead V_1.[471] The *chest roentgenogram* demonstrates cardiac enlargement, usually with gross prominence of the right atrium and a pericardial effusion. Calcification in the walls of the right or, less commonly, the left ventricle may be seen.[452] *Echocardiography* may demonstrate right ventricular thickening, obliteration of the apex, dilated atrium, strong echoes emanating from the endocardial surface, and abnormal septal motion in patients with tricuspid regurgitation.[453,461,472] At *angiography* the right ventricular apex is characteristically not visualized because of obliteration by the fibrous endocardium, but tricuspid regurgitation, right atrial enlargement, and filling defects in the right atrium due to intraatrial thrombi are sometimes seen.[362] Early angiographic changes that may be present before advanced disease develops include a change in the endocardial appearance, small apical filling defects, and mild tricuspid regurgitation.

LEFT VENTRICULAR EMF. With predominant *left-sided* involvement, the endomyocardial fibrosis invades the apex of the ventricle and usually the chordae tendineae or the posterior mitral valve leaflet as well, leading to mitral regurgitation.[473] The murmur may be confined to late systole, as is characteristic of the papillary muscle dysfunction type of murmur, or it may be pansystolic. Findings of pulmonary hypertension may be prominent. A protodiastolic gallop is commonly heard.

Laboratory Findings. The *electrocardiogram* usually shows T-wave abnormalities and diminished QRS voltage in the presence of a pericardial effusion, although left ventricular hypertrophy may be present.[362,363] There may be findings of left atrial abnormality. As with right-sided involvement, atrial fibrillation often is present. *Echocardiographic* features include thickening and reduced motion of the posterobasal wall and posterior mitral leaflet, increased echoreflectivity of the endocardium, preserved systolic wall motion in the presence of apical obliteration, dilated atrium, and Doppler ultrasound evidence of mitral regurgitation.[363] *Cardiac catheterization* often reveals pulmonary hypertension, with elevated left ventricular filling pressures and a reduced cardiac index.[473] The left ventriculogram usually shows mitral regurgitation, and a filling defect due to an intracavitary thrombus within the ventricle may be seen on occasion.[362] Coronary arteriography does not reveal obstructive disease.

BIVENTRICULAR EMF. This form of EMF occurs more frequently than either isolated right- or left-sided disease.[474] If there is more than minimal right ventricular involvement, severe pulmonary hypertension does not occur, and the right-sided findings dominate the clinical presentation. Typical patients with biventricular involvement may have the features of right ventricular EMF, with only a mitral regurgitant murmur to suggest left ventricular involvement. Systemic embolization may occur in up to 15 per cent of patients; infective endocarditis is even less frequent and is found in less than 2 per cent.

DIAGNOSIS

This is based on the presence in an individual of the typical clinical and laboratory features, particularly angiography, from the appropriate geographical area. Eosinophilia is usually not a prominent feature and when present may reflect associated parasitic infestation. *Endomyocardial biopsy* may occasionally be helpful in establishing the diagnosis. However, this risks dislodging a mural thrombus, with resultant embolization, and left-sided biopsy is *not* recommended. In addition, because the disease is often focal, the biopsy may miss the pathological process, particularly if a right ventricular biopsy is performed in a patient with isolated left-sided disease.[461]

MANAGEMENT

The medical treatment of EMF is often difficult and not particularly effective.[473] In patients with advanced disease, the outlook is poor, with a 35 to 50 per cent 2-year mortality.[455,474] Substantially better survival may be seen in less symptomatic patients who have milder forms of the disease.[474,475] Digitalis glycosides may be helpful in controlling the ventricular rate in patients with atrial fibrillation,[363] but the response of congestive symptoms is disappointing. Diuretics are not particularly helpful in the treatment of ascites.[363] Once endomyocardial disease has reached the fibrotic stage, surgery offers the possibility of symptomatic improvement and is the treatment of choice.[362] Operative excision of the fibrotic endocardium and replacement of the mitral and/or tricuspid valves have led to substantial symptomatic improvement, especially with predominant left-sided involvement.[461,475,476] Mitral valve repair, rather than replacement, can be accomplished in some patients.[477] Postoperative catheterization has provided objective evidence of hemodynamic improvement with a reduction in ventricular filling pressures, an increase in cardiac output, and normalization of the angiographic appearance.[476] Operative mortality has been high, running between 15 and 25 per cent in the larger series,[363,461,471,475] although it appears to be lower if replacement of valves can be avoided.[476,477]

Endocardial Fibroelastosis

(See p. 991)

Carcinoid Heart Disease

ETIOLOGY AND PATHOLOGY. The carcinoid syndrome is caused by a metastasizing carcinoid tumor and is characterized by cutaneous flushing, diarrhea, bronchoconstriction, and endocardial plaques composed of a unique type of fibrous tissue. The vasomotor, bronchoconstrictor, and cardiac manifestations are undoubtedly related to circulating humoral substances secreted by the tumor,[478,479] although the precise substance(s) responsible remains to be elucidated.[480,481] Virtually all patients develop diarrhea and flushing, and cardiac abnormalities are found on echocardiography in more than half; clinically apparent and severe right-sided disease is seen in a quarter of patients.[478,479]

Sixty to 90 per cent of tumors arise in the small bowel and appendix, and the rest originate in other areas of the gastrointestinal tract and bronchus.[478] Carcinoid tumors of the ileum are the most likely to metastasize, with involvement of the regional lymph nodes and liver. Usually only carcinoid tumors that invade the liver result in carcinoid heart disease.[478] The cardiac lesions may be related to large circulating quantities of serotonin, bradykinin, or other substances secreted by the tumor, which usually are inactivated by the liver, lungs, and brain.[481a] Hepatic metastases apparently allow large quantities of tumor products to reach the heart without being inactivated by the liver. The preferential right-sided involvement presumably is related to inactivation of the offending humoral substance(s) by the lungs. In 5 to 10 per cent of cases, significant left-sided valvular disease develops,[482] related in most to passage of blood directly from the right to the left side of the heart through a patent foramen ovale, or less commonly by tumor involvement of the lungs.[478]

The characteristic *pathological* findings are fibrous plaques that involve the "downstream" aspect of the tricuspid and pulmonic valves, the endocardium of the cardiac chambers, and the intima of the venae cavae, pulmonary artery, and coronary sinus. The fibrous tissue in the plaques results in distortion of the valves, leading to both stenosis and regurgitation.[478] Histologically, the plaques consist of deposits of fibrous tissue located superficially on the endocardium, often with extension into the underlying layers.[479,481] Ultrastructural and immunohistochemical studies have demonstrated that the plaques are composed of smooth muscle cells embedded in a stroma rich in acid mucopolysaccharides and collagen.[481] Metastatic involvement of the myocardium itself is rare.[478]

CLINICAL MANIFESTATIONS. *Physical examination* usually reveals a systolic murmur along the left sternal border, produced by tricuspid regurgitation; in some cases, there may be a concomitant murmur of pulmonic stenosis and/or regurgitation.[478]

The *chest roentgenogram* is normal in half the patients, but may reveal enlargement of the heart, and pleural effusions or nodules[478]; the pulmonary artery trunk is typically of normal size, without evidence of post-stenotic dilatation as occurs in congenital pulmonic stenosis. No specific *electrocardiographic pattern* is diagnostic of carcinoid heart disease.[478] Right atrial enlargement may be seen on occasion, but electrocardiographic evidence of right ventricular hypertrophy usually is lacking. Nonspecific ST-segment and T-wave abnormalities and sinus tachycardia are the most common findings,[478] although severely symptomatic patients usually have low QRS voltage.[483] *Echocardiography* may reveal evidence of tricuspid and/or pulmonary valve thickening, along with right atrial and right ventricular dilatation; small pericardial effusions are present in a minority.[478,479,484]

The *hemodynamic findings* most commonly encountered are those of tricuspid regurgitation (see p. 1058) and occasionally pulmonic stenosis. A rare patient with the carcinoid syndrome demonstrates a hyperkinetic state (which may lead to high-output heart failure) but without the typical cardiac lesions; in one patient this was caused by profound vasodilatation by substance P.[485]

MANAGEMENT. In patients with mild congestive heart failure this consists of digitalis and diuretics. Symptomatic improvement and improved survival have been noted with the use of somatostatin analogs.[483] Balloon valvuloplasty of the right-sided valves has produced symptomatic improvement in a few patients with stenotic tricuspid or pulmonary valves,[486] although others have developed recurrent symptoms despite "successful" valvuloplasty.[487] Surgical replacement of the tricuspid valve and pulmonic valvotomy or valvectomy may result in symptomatic improvement in severely symptomatic patients with serious valvular dysfunction, although the operative mortality is high (35 per cent in one series).[483] Surgery may improve the functional status and survival of patients with carcinoid heart disease, but patients over the age of 60 years have a very high surgical mortality (reportedly over 50 per cent).[482] The long-term mortality remains high regardless of treatment modality, with half the patients dead within 1 to 2 years.[478,483]

Obesity and Heart Disease

(See p. 1152)

Diabetic Cardiomyopathy

(See p. 1150)

Myocarditis is said to be present when the heart is involved in an inflammatory process, often caused by an infectious agent. The inflammation may involve the myocytes, interstitium, vascular elements, and/or pericardium; involvement of the latter structure is discussed in Chapter 43.

Myocarditis has been described during and following a wide variety of viral, rickettsial, bacterial, protozoal, and metazoal diseases; indeed, virtually any infectious agent may produce cardiac inflammation (Table 41–14).[488] Infectious agents cause myocardial damage by three basic mechanisms: (1) invasion of the myocardium; (2) production of a myocardial toxin, e.g., diphtheria; and (3) immunologically mediated myocardial damage.[489–491] The principal mechanism of heart involvement in viral myocarditis is believed to be a cell-mediated immunological reaction to new cell surface changes or a new antigen related to the virus, and not merely the result of cell damage caused by viral replication.[492–494] Additional evidence for an immune-mediated mechanism is the demonstration of a marked increase in major histocompatibility complex antigen expression in the biopsy specimens from patients with myocarditis.[495] Antibodies against intracellular components may also play a role.[496] Patients with ongoing myocarditis (unlike those with resolved myocarditis) have myocytes that express the intercellular adhesion molecule termed ICAM-1, and it is speculated that the persistent expression of ICAM-1 may play a role in continued myocardial inflammation.[494] Although often mistakenly limited to inflammation due to an infective agent, myocarditis may also be caused by allergic reactions and pharmacological agents, as well as occurring during the course of some systemic diseases such as vasculitis.

TABLE 41–14 PRINCIPAL INFECTIOUS ETIOLOGICAL AGENTS ASSOCIATED WITH MYOCARDITIS

BACTERIAL INFECTIONS	
Streptococcal	Brucellosis
Staphylococcal	Diphtheria
Pneumococcal	Salmonellosis
Meningococcal	Tuberculosis
Haemophilus	Tularemia
Gonococcal	
SPIROCHETAL INFECTIONS	
Leptospirosis	Relapsing fever
Lyme disease	Syphilis
FUNGAL INFECTIONS	
Aspergillosis	Coccidiodomycosis
Actinomycosis	Cryptococcosis
Blastomycosis	Histoplasmosis
Candidiasis	
PARASITIC INFECTIONS	
Cysticercosis	Trichinosis
Schistosomiasis	Trypanosomiasis
Toxoplasmosis	Visceral larva migrans
RICKETTSIAL INFECTIONS	
Rocky Mountain spotted fever	Scrub typhus
Q fever	Typhus
VIRAL INFECTIONS	
Adenovirus	*Mycoplasma pneumoniae*
Arbovirus	Poliomyelitis
Coxsackievirus	Psittacosis
Cytomegalovirus	Respiratory syncytial virus
Echovirus	Rabies
Encephalomyocarditis virus	Rubella
Hepatitis	Rubeola
Human immunodeficiency virus	Vaccina
Infectious mononucleosis	Varicella
Influenza	Variola
Mumps	Yellow fever

Adapted from Marboe, C. C., and Fenoglio, J. J.: Pathology and natural history of human myocarditis. Pathol. Immunopathol. Res. *7*:226, 1988.

Myocarditis may be an acute or a chronic process and may occur during the peripartum period (see p. 1851). In North America, viruses (especially enteroviruses) are presumed to be the most common agents producing myocarditis,[497,498] whereas in South America, Chagas' disease (produced by *Trypanosoma cruzi*) is far more common.[499] The identification of the specific etiological agent responsible for infectious myocarditis usually rests on the associated extracardiac findings because the cardiovascular signs and symptoms are often nonspecific.[490] The histological findings vary, depending on the stage of the disease, the mechanism of myocardial damage, and the specific etiological agent. Myocardial involvement may be focal or diffuse, but the myocardial lesions are generally randomly distributed in the heart, and thus the clinical consequences depend to a large extent on the size and number of the lesions. However, a single small lesion may have profound consequences if it is located within the cardiac conducting system. The histological findings are usually nonspecific (except for some parasitic and granulomatous forms of myocarditis), and with certain exceptions (Table 41–4), myocardial biopsy seldom elucidates the specific etiological agent.

The natural history of myocarditis is varied, as shown in Figure 41–25.

CLINICAL MANIFESTATIONS. The clinical expression of myocarditis ranges from the asymptomatic state secondary to focal inflammation to fulminant fatal congestive heart failure due to diffuse myocarditis.[488] An initial episode of viral myocarditis, perhaps unrecognized and forgotten, may be the initial event that eventually culminates in an "idiopathic" DCM.[16] In experimental animals, the structural and functional myocardial alterations that follow viral myocarditis may persist well beyond the stage of viral replication and myocardial inflammatory response, and the late changes resemble those of DCM.[500]

The outcome after viral myocarditis is quite variable,[488] perhaps related to differing genetic susceptibility of individual patients. In most patients, the event is entirely self-limited and often unrecognized.[498,501] More overt myocarditis may result in acute congestive heart failure.[488,502] In others, unrecognized myocarditis may be the cause of arrhythmias in what appears to be a structurally normal heart.[503] Some patients with chest pain and angiographically normal coronary arteries may have had subclinical myocarditis at some point in the past. Most intriguing is the possibility that viral myocarditis may culminate in DCM, presumably as a consequence of viral-mediated immunological cardiac damage.[501]

Although transient electrocardiographic abnormalities suggesting myocardial involvement are noted in many patients with infectious disease, most patients do not have other clinical manifestations of myocarditis.[504,505] It is postulated that these electrocardiographic changes reflect subclinical myocardial involvement. That unrecognized myocardial involvement occurs with systemic infections is supported by histological evidence of unsuspected myocarditis during routine postmortem examinations; this occurs about 1 per cent of the time.[506] Some degree of myocardial involvement, often subepicardial in location, also frequently occurs in patients with acute pericarditis.

Because myocardial involvement is subclinical in most acute infectious diseases, the majority of patients have no specific complaints referable to the cardiovascular system[504]; the presence of myocarditis is often inferred from ST-segment and T-wave abnormalities on the electrocardiogram.[488] From a clinical viewpoint, myocardial involvement

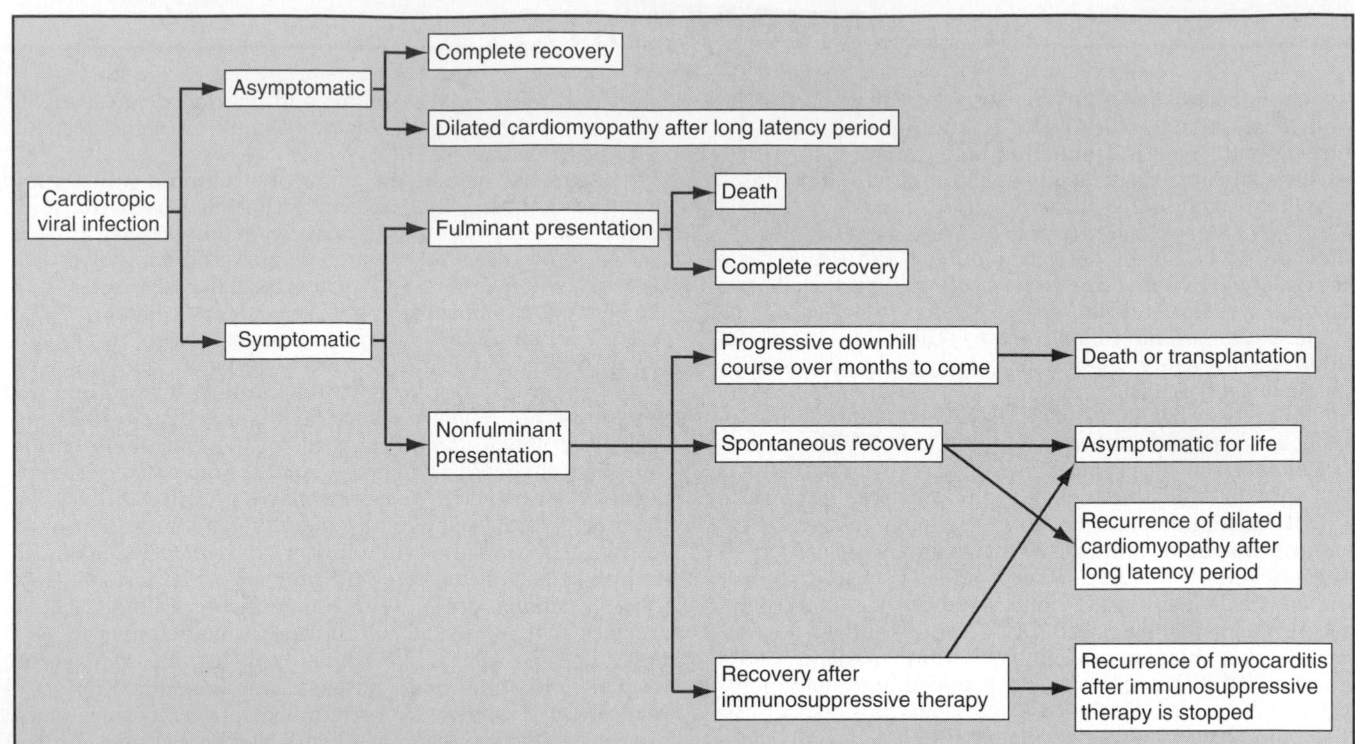

FIGURE 41–25. The natural history of human myocarditis. Most patients with mild symptoms of acute myocarditis are not seen by cardiologists and most of these patients appear to recover fully. Of the patients with symptomatic heart disease typically seen by cardiologists, a small number have fulminant presentations and either die in the acute stage or appear to recover fully. Of the remaining patients with myocarditis, a few are characterized by a progressive downhill course over a period of months to years that ends in death from heart failure or intractable arrhythmias. Some spontaneously recover and remain asymptomatic for life, and others have an asymptomatic period followed by development of dilated cardiomyopathy. (From Herskowitz, A., and Ansari, A. A.: Myocarditis. *In* Abelmann, W. H., and Braunwald, E. [eds.]: Cardiomyopathies, Myocarditis, and Pericardial Disease. Atlas of Heart Diseases. Vol. 2. Philadelphia, Current Medicine, 1995.)

is associated with nonspecific symptoms, including fatigue, dyspnea, palpitations, and precordial discomfort.[119,488] Chest pain usually reflects associated pericarditis, but precordial discomfort suggestive of myocardial ischemia is occasionally observed.[119] In some cases, the clinical presentation (with chest pain, electrocardiographic abnormalities, increased muscle enzyme levels, and regional wall motion abnormalities) may simulate an acute myocardial infarction.[507,508]

Physical Examination. Tachycardia is usual and may be out of proportion to the temperature elevation.[488] The first heart sound is often muffled, and a protodiastolic gallop may be present. A transient apical systolic murmur may appear,[488] but diastolic murmurs are rare. Clinical evidence of congestive heart failure occurs only in the more severe cases.[488] The heart is usually normal in size in the clinically silent cases, but it may be dilated in patients with congestive heart failure. Pulmonary and systemic emboli may occur.

Laboratory Findings. *Electrocardiographic* abnormalities are usually transient and occur far more frequently than does clinical myocardial involvement. The most common changes are abnormalities of the ST segment and T wave, but atrial and in particular ventricular arrhythmias, AV and intraventricular conduction defects, and, rarely, Q waves may be seen.[488] Complete AV block is usually transient and resolves without sequelae, but it is occasionally a cause of sudden death in patients with myocarditis.[509] Intraventricular conduction abnormalities are associated with more severe myocardial damage and a worse prognosis.[509,510] On *radiological examination,* heart size may range from normal to markedly enlarged, and pulmonary congestion may be present in patients with fulminant disease.[488] *Echocardiography* demonstrates some degree of left ventricular dysfunction (surprisingly often regional in nature) in many patients with clinical myocarditis, although wall motion may be normal. Often findings may include increased wall thickness, left ventricular thrombi, and abnormal diastolic filling despite normal systolic function.[511] *Radionuclide scanning* after the administration of gallium-67, indium-111 antimyosin antibody, or technetium-99m pyrophosphate may identify inflammatory and necrotic changes characteristic of myocarditis, as may nuclear MRI.[119,488,512–514]

DIAGNOSIS. This is often predicated on the identification of the associated systemic illness and its characteristic features.[16] The diagnosis of viral myocarditis is supported by the identification of the virus in stool, throat washings, blood, myocardium, or pericardial fluid, or by a distinct (usually fourfold) increase in virus-neutralizing antibody, complement-fixation, or hemagglutination inhibition titers, but cultures usually are negative and serological tests nondiagnostic.[490,498] Even in fatal cases, isolation of virus from the myocardium at necropsy is unusual.[488,515] *Endomyocardial biopsy* frequently is used to confirm the diagnosis of myocarditis (Fig. 41–2).[16] A borderline or negative biopsy does not exclude the diagnosis,[516,517] and, if clinically indicated, a repeat biopsy may be appropriate and diagnostic.[518] Molecular biological techniques (using tissue obtained by endomyocardial biopsy) offer promise as a way of rapidly and confidently diagnosing acute myocarditis.[20]

PATHOLOGY. Patients with myocarditis demonstrate a wide spectrum of gross and histological changes, reflecting the range of disease seen clinically. Grossly, the hearts in acute cases are flabby, with focal hemorrhages; in chronic cases, the heart is enlarged and hypertrophied.[500] The histological hallmark of myocarditis is an inflammatory myocardial infiltrate, with associated evidence of myocyte damage (Fig. 41–2).[488,500] The inflammatory infiltrate may be composed of a variety of cell types, including polymorphonuclear cells, lymphocytes, macrophages, plasma cells, eosinophils, and/or giant cells.[500] In bacterial myocarditis, polymorphonuclear cells predominate; in viral infections, lymphocytes predominate; and in hypersensitivity myocarditis, eosinophils are seen in abundance.[500] Routine histological examination of the heart rarely provides a specific diagnosis, although in some instances electron microscopic and immunofluorescent techniques may allow elucidation of a specific cause.

MANAGEMENT. Therapy is often supportive and is usually directed at the more prominent systemic manifestations of the disease.[488] The demonstration of a particular predilection for involvement of the AV conducting system in some forms of myocarditis suggests that patients with suspected myocarditis should be observed closely for any evidence of conduction abnormality. Bed rest (or at least restricted activity) is advisable[488,505] because exercise in experimental animals with myocarditis is deleterious.[490,500] Because myocarditis often occurs in young adults, it is important to limit their athletic activities; it is recommended that athletes abstain from sports for a 6-month convalescent period, and until heart size and function have returned to normal.[205] Congestive heart failure responds to routine management,[488] including digitalization and diuresis, although patients with myocarditis appear to be particularly sensitive to digitalis, and toxicity should be watched for. Significant symptomatic arrhythmias should be treated with antiarrhythmic agents, although beta-adrenoceptor blockers are probably best avoided in view of their negative inotropic action[519]; participation in athletic and sporting activities should be proscribed until arrhythmias have resolved.[205]

The use of corticosteroids is controversial.[491,520–522] Although these agents were previously thought to be proscribed in acute viral myocarditis (because increased tissue necrosis and viral replication have been demonstrated following their use in experimental myocarditis), their use in a small number of patients has not been associated with similar dire short-term consequences.[500,501] A randomized trial of immunosuppression in myocarditis found no improvement in left ventricular ejection fraction or survival.[522a] Nonsteroidal anti-inflammatory agents—indomethacin, salicylates, and ibuprofen,[523] along with cyclosporine[524,525]—are contraindicated during the acute phase of viral myocarditis (the first 2 weeks) because they increase myocardial damage.[488,491,505] On the other hand, nonsteroidal anti-inflammatory agents appear to be safe in the late phase of myocarditis.[523] At least in children, high-dose intravenous gamma globulin appears to be associated with more rapid resolution of left ventricular dysfunction, and perhaps improved survival.[526] In experimental models of myocarditis, the converting enzyme inhibitor captopril has beneficial effects in the acute phase of myocarditis; human data are not yet available.[527,528]

It is hoped that effective antiviral agents,[522,529] immunosuppressive agents,[490] or antilymphocyte monoclonal antibodies for treating viral myocarditis will be available soon for clinical use.[488,505,530] It may also be possible, in the future, to treat patients with myocarditis with agents that stimulate production of interferon because this substance affords protection against the effects of viral myocarditis, at least in experimental animals.[490,531] Antibiotics may also be employed with benefit in infections caused by atypical pneumonia and psittacosis.

VIRAL MYOCARDITIS

Approximately two dozen viruses may be associated with clinical evidence of myocarditis (Table 41–14).[500] The myocarditis characteristically develops after a lag period of several weeks following the initial systemic infection, suggesting involvement of an immunological mechanism. In animals, a variety of factors appears to enhance susceptibility to myocardial damage, including radiation, malnutrition, steroids, exercise, and previous myocardial injury. Viral myocarditis may be particularly virulent in infants[498] and in pregnant women.

COXSACKIEVIRUS. Both Coxsackie viruses A and B may produce myocarditis, although infection with Coxsackie B is more common; this agent is the most frequent cause of viral myocarditis, causing more than half the cases.[490,532–534] The myocardium appears to be particularly susceptible to the effects of this virus because of the apparent affinity of myocardial membrane receptors for the viral particles. Necropsy often demonstrates a pericardial effusion, pericarditis, cardiac enlargement, and a predominantly mononuclear inflammatory infiltrate, with necrosis of the atrial and ventricular myocardium. In some cases, focal myocardial necrosis simulating myocardial infarction is seen, despite normal coronary arteries.[535]

Although most infections are benign, self-limited, and subclinical, Coxsackie myocarditis appears to be particularly virulent in the neonate and child.[502,536] In most infections in adults, the other clinical manifestations of viral involvement, such as pleurodynia, myalgia, upper respiratory tract symptoms, and arthralgias, predominate.[532] Severe cases in the adult are characterized by myopericardial involvement with pleuritic or pericarditic chest pain, palpitations, and fever. Many patients with overt myocardial involvement develop congestive heart failure with cardiomegaly and pulmonary edema.[502,537]

The *electrocardiogram* is virtually always abnormal, with ST-segment and T-wave abnormalities and arrhythmias, often ventricular in origin; AV conduction disturbances are common.[536,537] Blood levels of myocardial enzymes (serum transaminases, creatine kinase) may be normal or elevated, reflecting the absence or presence of variable degrees of clinically detectable myocardial necrosis.[502] *Echocardiography* may reveal diffuse and regional left ventricular wall motion abnormalities that usually improve or disappear over time.[533,538]

Most patients recover completely within weeks,[502] although the electrocardiogram and ventricular function may require months to return to normal. Rarely, Coxsackie myocarditis is fatal in adults.[537] Some patients become symptomatic following resolution of the infection, and they may present years later with dilated cardiomyopathy.[533]

Treatment is symptomatic, and despite occasional postmortem evidence of intracardiac thrombi, anticoagulation should probably be avoided because of the risk of a hemorrhagic pericardial effusion. Bed rest is indicated during the acute course of myocarditis, but no convincing evidence exists that a period of prolonged rest after apparent resolution of the acute process is useful. Heart failure and cardiac arrhythmias are treated in the usual fashion.

CYTOMEGALOVIRUS. Unrecognized infection with cytomegalovirus (CMV) is extremely common in childhood, and the majority of the adult population have antibodies to CMV.[539] Primary infection after the age of 35 years is uncommon, and generalized infection usually occurs only in immunosuppressed patients with neoplastic disease, after transplantation, and with HIV infection.[540–542] The cardiovascular manifestations in adults are generally limited to asymptomatic and transient electrocardiographic abnormalities. Symptomatic cardiac involvement is rare, although a hemorrhagic pericardial effusion or myocarditis with left ventricular dysfunction and attendant congestive heart failure may occur.[541–543] The diagnosis of CMV myocarditis may be suggested by the presence of viral inclusions in myocardial biopsy specimens and confirmed by the detection of viral DNA in the myocardium.[540,544] Although fatalities are unusual, when they do occur, histological examination of the heart may reveal focal lymphocytic infiltration and fibrosis.

DENGUE. Although previous dengue epidemics often were associated with symptomatic cardiac involvement, more recent outbreaks have been associated with fewer apparent cardiac complications.[545] Nonspecific electrocardiographic repolarization abnormalities are common but typically benign and transient.[545,546] Transient ventricular arrhythmias may be seen on occasion.

HEPATITIS. Clinical cardiac involvement in hepatitis is rare; an occasional patient may develop fulminant myocarditis with congestive heart failure, hypotension, and death.[547,548] The characteristic *pathological changes* in the myocardium associated with viral hepatitis are minute foci of necrosis of isolated muscle bundles, often surrounded by lymphocytes and a diffuse serous inflammation.[548] The ventricles may be dilated, with petechial hemorrhages. Hemorrhage into the myocardium may be a conspicuous finding.[548] Myocardial damage may be produced indirectly through an immune-mediated mechanism or directly by viral invasion of the heart.[548]

Symptomatic myocarditis is generally observed in the first to third week of illness. Patients may have dyspnea, palpitations, and anginal chest pain; fatalities have been reported.[548,549] *Electrocardiographic changes,* including bradycardia, ventricular premature beats, and ST-segment and T-wave abnormalities, may be seen during the course of hepatitis.[548] These abnormalities are usually transient and asymptomatic, although congestive heart failure, cardiomegaly, and sudden death have been reported.[547,548]

Heart involvement in the acquired immunodeficiency syndrome (AIDS) may consist of metastatic involvement from Kaposi's sarcoma, a wide variety of infective and nonspecific forms of myocarditis, pericarditis with or without an effusion, endocarditis (especially nonbacterial thrombotic endocarditis), and dilated cardiomyopathy (Table 41–15).[550–552] Cardiac involvement occurs in about one-quarter to one-half of patients (on the basis of echocardiographic, endomyocardial biopsy, and autopsy findings) (Fig. 41–26 and 41–27)[552–554]; however, it leads to clinically apparent heart disease in only approximately 10 per cent.[555–560] When there are clinical manifestations, congestive heart failure is the most common finding and is due to left ventricular dilatation and dysfunction, simulating a dilated cardiomyopathy.[86,550] Because of the frequency of opportunistic pulmonary infections, dyspnea may be attributed incorrectly to lung disease rather than congestive heart failure; echocardiography may be useful in identifying left ventricular dysfunction as the cause of the dyspnea.[550,551] Particular surveillance for cardiac toxoplasmosis in HIV infection should be maintained, as it may be the precipitant for symptomatic congestive heart failure and is potentially treatable.[561] Other common clinical and echocardiographic findings that result in symptoms in a minority of patients include pericardial effusion (usually but not invariably without cardiac tamponade), ventricular arrhythmias, repolarization changes on the electrocardiogram, marantic endocarditis, and right ventricular dilatation and hypertrophy.[551,552,555,559,560]

TABLE 41–15 CARDIAC LESIONS IN AIDS

- **MYOCARDITIS**
  - Opportunistic infections
    - *Pneumocystis carinii*
    - *Mycobacterium tuberculosis*
    - *Mycobacterium avium-intracellulare*
    - *Cryptococcus neoformans*
    - *Aspergillus fumigatus*
    - *Candida albicans*
    - *Histoplasma capsulatum*
    - *Coccidioides immitis*
    - *Toxoplasma gondii*
    - Herpes simplex
  - Viral agents
    - Cytomegalovirus
    - Human immunodeficiency virus (HIV)
    - Herpes simplex
  - Lymphocytic myocarditis
  - Noninflammatory myocardial necrosis
    - Microvascular spasm?
- **ENDOCARDITIS**
  - Marantic endocarditis (nonbacterial thrombotic endocarditis)
  - Bacterial endocarditis
  - Aspergillus endocarditis
- **PERICARDITIS**
  - Infectious
    - Tuberculous
    - Herpes simplex
    - Histoplasmosis
    - *Cryptococcus*
  - Noninfectious
  - Pericardial effusion
- **CARDIOMEGALY**
  - Right ventricular hypertrophy or dilation
  - Biventricular dilation (dilated cardiomyopathy)
- **VASCULAR LESIONS**
  - Arteriopathy
  - Myocardial infarction
- **MALIGNANCY**
  - Kaposi's sarcoma
  - Malignant lymphoma
- **TOXIC LESIONS**
  - Drug-induced
    - Drugs used in combating opportunistic infections
    - Anti-HIV drugs

Modified from Acierno, L. J.: Cardiac complications in acquired immunodeficiency syndrome (AIDS): A review. Reprinted by permission of the American College of Cardiology. J. Am. Coll. Cardiol. *13*:1144, 1989.

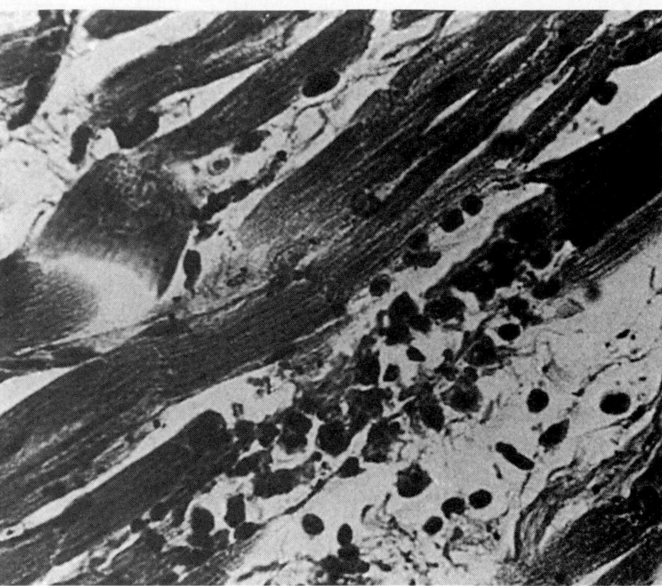

FIGURE 41–26. Example of lymphocytic myocarditis showing myocyte necrosis in AIDS patient (×400, reduced by 5 per cent). (From Baroldi, G., Corallo, S., Moroni, M., et al.: Focal lymphocytic myocarditis in acquired immunodeficiency syndrome (AIDS): A correlative morphologic and clinical study in 26 consecutive fatal cases. Reprinted by permission from the American College of Cardiology. J. Am. Coll. Cardiol. *12*:463, 1988.)

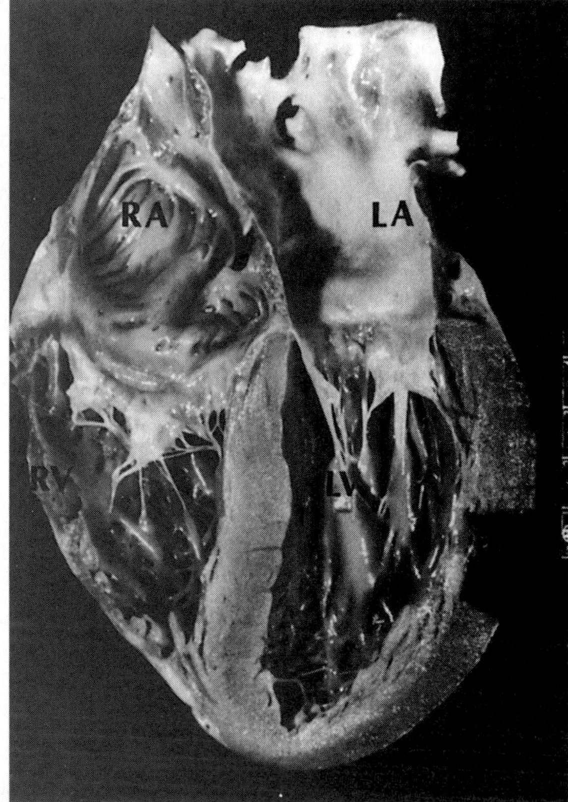

FIGURE 41–27. Marked dilatation of all four chambers of the heart in a patient with AIDS. LA = Left atrium, RA = right atrium. (Reproduced by permission from Cohen, I. S., Anderson, D. W., Virmani, R., et al.: Congestive cardiomyopathy in association with the acquired immunodeficiency syndrome. N. Engl. J. Med. *315*:628, 1986. Copyright Massachusetts Medical Society.)

The cause of myocardial damage in HIV infection is not clearly established and likely is multifactorial.[562] Although some of the cardiac effects are due to the commonly associated opportunistic infections, damage as a consequence of the HIV virus itself and/or through activation of the immune system is thought to be likely.[550,555,556,563,564] Whether agents used to treat AIDS (such as zidovudine [AZT]) may be cardiotoxic themselves has not been resolved.[564a]

Pathological cardiac findings in AIDS patients are common, with myocarditis the most frequent.[552] Although opportunistic infections caused by a wide variety of viral, fungal (Fig. 41–28, p. 1441), parasitic, and bacterial pathogens account for some cases of myocarditis, most are unexplained but are suspected to be related to the HIV itself.[552,556,565] Isolation of HIV from the myocardium has added further credence to this speculation.[556] It has been speculated that the HIV-related myocarditis may result in the dilated cardiomyopathy found in some patients.[550] Other important postmortem findings include pericardial effusions, right and/or left ventricular dilatation, and nonbacterial thrombotic endocarditis.[552,555]

Treatment of AIDS-associated heart disease may afford some degree of symptomatic improvement.[552,566] Relief of cardiac tamponade, therapy for infective myocarditis, and treatment of congestive heart failure have resulted in at least short-term palliation.[552,567]

INFECTIOUS MONONUCLEOSIS. Evident cardiac involvement in infectious mononucleosis is extremely rare, although nonspecific ST-segment and T-wave abnormalities may be seen. In rare cases, pericarditis and myocarditis (even simulating a myocardial infarction) may be present.[568]

INFLUENZA. Although clinically apparent myocarditis is rare in influenza, the presence of preexisting cardiovascular disease greatly increases the risk of morbidity and mortality.[569] During epidemics, 5 to 10 per cent of infected patients may experience cardiac symptoms.[16] Postmortem findings in fatal cases include biventricular dilatation,[522] with evidence of a mononuclear infiltrate,[570] especially in perivascular areas.

Cardiac involvement typically occurs within 1 to 2 weeks of the onset of the illness and may be severe, sometimes contributing to mortality.[522] The *clinical manifestations* include dyspnea, palpitations, anginal chest pain, arrhythmia, and heart failure; there may be concomitant involvement of the pericardium.[522] Sinus tachycardia or, less commonly, sinus bradycardia may be seen. The *electrocardiogram* may show transient ST-segment and T-wave abnormalities, conduction defects, and even complete AV block; death may be associated with massive hemorrhagic pulmonary edema due to viral or bacterial involvement of the lungs.[571]

LASSA FEVER. Lassa fever, a major cause of death in West Africa that is caused by an arenavirus, often is associated with electrocardiographic abnormalities[572] that may represent subclinical myocardial involvement. More than half the patients demonstrate nonspecific repolarization changes and low voltage.[572] Pericardial involvement may occur.[573] *Pathological findings* include myocardial congestion, edema, and a mononuclear cellular infiltrate. In most cases, however, the putative cardiac involvement does not appear to play a major clinical role.[572]

MUMPS. Myocardial involvement during the course of mumps is rarely recognized.[574,575] The hearts of only a few patients with mumps have come to postmortem examination, and they have been found to be both dilated and hypertrophied. Histologically, there is diffuse interstitial fibrosis, with infiltration of mononuclear cells and areas of focal necrosis.[574]

Cardiac involvement is usually unrecognized clinically, and the diagnosis of myocarditis is based on nonspecific electrocardiographic changes.[574] Transient ST-segment and T-wave abnormalities are most common, but extrasystoles and atrioventricular conduction block may occur.[574–576] Tachycardia, a transient apical systolic murmur, and protodiastolic gallop may be present.[574–576]

POLIOMYELITIS. Myocarditis occurs about 5 to 10 per cent of the time during epidemics and is a frequent finding in fatal cases of poliomyelitis, occurring in half or more of all patients dying with this disease; death may be sudden.[16] Although myocardial involvement is usually focal and minimal in extent, some patients with bulbar disease succumb early in the course of the illness, often with cardiovascular collapse.[577,578] These patients all have viral infection of the medulla and severe systemic vasoconstriction that leads to pulmonary edema. Myocarditis appears to contribute to the heart failure.[577] The *electrocardiogram* is frequently abnormal, with ST-segment and T-wave abnormalities, prolongation of the P-R and Q-T intervals,[579] premature contractions, tachycardia, and atrial fibrillation. *Treatment* is symptomatic, with aggressive support of pulmonary function; tracheostomy and prolonged mechanical ventilatory support may be required. Fortunately, this disease has been largely eliminated by immunization.

RESPIRATORY SYNCYTIAL VIRUS. Although respiratory syncytial virus is an important cause of respiratory disease, particularly in children, it rarely results in cardiac involvement.[580] Congestive heart failure and complete heart block have been seen on occasion.[581]

RUBELLA AND RUBEOLA. Congenital cardiovascular lesions may develop in the offspring when *rubella* is contracted by the mother during the first trimester of pregnancy, with persistent ductus arteriosus and pulmonary artery maldevelopment as prominent anomalies.[498] Rare cases of postgestational myocarditis occur, with attendant conduction defects and heart failure.[582,583]

Overt myocarditis is quite rare in *rubeola*,[534] although transient electrocardiographic abnormalities, including prolongation of the P-R interval, ST-segment and T-wave changes, AV conduction abnormalities, and ventricular tachycardia, have been reported.[584] Congestive heart failure occurs on rare occasions, and its appearance is a poor prognostic sign, often indicating a fatal outcome.[585] Histological examination of the heart in fatal cases has revealed evidence of myocarditis characterized predominantly by a perivascular lymphocytic infiltrate.[584]

VARICELLA. Clinical myocarditis is a rare finding in varicella, although unsuspected myocarditis is common in fatal varicella.[586] Occasionally a patient may develop overt clinical evidence of myocarditis with congestive heart failure.[586–588] Histological findings include rare but characteristic intranuclear inclusion bodies within the myocardial cells, along with interstitial edema, cellular infiltrates, and myonecrosis.[587] The electrocardiogram may show conduction abnormalities, including complete heart block; sudden death occurs rarely.[589]

VARIOLA AND VACCINIA. Cardiac involvement following smallpox is rare, although several cases of myocarditis associated with acute cardiac failure and death have been reported. Myocarditis with pericardial effusion and congestive heart failure has also been observed as a complication of smallpox vaccination[590]; an immunological mechanism has been suggested, and dramatic responses to steroids have been reported. The histological changes include a mixed mononuclear infiltrate, with interstitial edema and occasional degenerating or necrotic muscle bundles.[591]

RICKETTSIAL MYOCARDITIS

The rickettsial diseases frequently are associated with evidence of myocardial involvement, but usually it is subclinical. Transient ST-segment and T-wave alterations in particular are observed commonly. The circulatory collapse that may accompany these diseases is largely a manifestation of abnormalities of the peripheral vascular bed, but a myocardial component may also be present. The basic histopathological process is a vasculitis, with a periarterial interstitial infiltrate.

Q FEVER. Endocarditis is the most common cardiac manifestation of infection with *R. burnettii* (Q fever).[592] Myocarditis is not a prominent feature,[593] although dyspnea and chest pain, perhaps reflecting associated pericarditis, occur frequently. The electrocardiogram may demonstrate transient ST-segment and T-wave changes as well as paroxysmal ventricular arrhythmias. Abnormalities of the immune system have been implicated in the pathogenesis of the disease.[594]

ROCKY MOUNTAIN SPOTTED FEVER. Clinical evidence of myocarditis is more common than often appreciated in Rocky Mountain spotted fever (caused by *R. rickettsii*), and the heart is often involved in the multisystem damage that occurs as the result of a widespread vasculitis.[595–597] Unsuspected left ventricular dysfunction is common, and echocardiographic evidence of dysfunction may persist in some patients.[595]

SCRUB TYPHUS. Myocarditis is common during the course of scrub typhus (tsutsugamushi disease, caused by *R. tsutsugamushi*), especially in fatal cases.[598,599] The histological findings are those of a focal panvasculitis involving the small blood vessels. Myocardial necrosis is unusual, but hemorrhage into the heart and subepicardial petechiae may occur.[599] Clinical evidence of myocardial involvement typically is not severe and is usually not associated with residual cardiac damage.[598] The electrocardiogram may show nonspecific ST-segment and T-wave abnormalities, as well as first-degree AV block.[599] A protodiastolic gallop and apical systolic murmur suggestive of mitral regurgitation are occasionally found.[598]

BACTERIAL MYOCARDITIS

BRUCELLOSIS. Cardiac involvement in the course of brucellosis is uncommon, usually consisting of endocarditis. Myocardial involvement, when it occurs, is manifested by T-wave abnormalities and prolongation of AV conduction.[600] An occasional patient develops fulminant myocarditis, with a lymphocytic and polymorphonuclear infiltrate.[600]

CLOSTRIDIA. Cardiac involvement is common in patients with clostridial infections with multiple organ involvement.[601] The myocardial damage results from the toxin elaborated by the bacteria, but the precise actions of the toxin remain to be elucidated.[602] The *pathological findings* are distinctive, with gas bubbles usually present in the myocardium. Areas of degenerated muscle fibers are apparent, but an inflammatory infiltrate is usually absent.[601] *C. perfringens* may cause myocardial abscess formation, with myocardial perforation and resultant purulent pericarditis.[603]

DIPHTHERIA. Myocardial involvement is one of the more serious complications of diphtheria and occurs in up to one-quarter of cases.[604,605] Indeed, myocardial involvement is the most common cause of death in this infection, and half of the fatal cases demonstrate cardiac involvement.[605] Cardiac damage is due to the liberation by the diphtheria bacillus of a toxin that inhibits protein synthesis by interfering with the transfer of amino acids from soluble RNA to polypeptide chains under construction. The toxin has a particular affinity for the cardiac conducting system.[604]

Pathological findings include a flabby and dilated heart with a myocardium that has a "streaky" appearance. Microscopic examination reveals characteristic fatty infiltration of the myocytes,[605] often with an interstitial inflammatory infiltrate, myocytolysis, and hyaline necrosis of muscle fibers. With time, fibrosis and hypertrophy of the remaining myocardial cells develop. The conduction system is often involved.

Clinical signs of cardiac dysfunction typically appear at the end of the first week of the illness. Cardiomegaly and severe congestive heart failure are often present. A protodiastolic gallop and pulmonary congestion may be prominent features. Elevation of the serum transaminase levels may be seen; a high level is associated with a poor prognosis. Sudden circulatory failure and death may occur. Many patients develop ST-segment and T-wave abnormalities, but atrial and ventricular arrhythmias and conduction defects may also occur.[605] Persistently abnormal electrocardiograms are common following diphtheritic myocarditis, as are cardiomegaly and symptoms of reduced cardiac reserve. Some patients recover fully.

Because of the serious effects of the toxin on the myocardium, antitoxin should be administered as rapidly as possible.[605] Antibiotic therapy is of less urgency. Overt congestive heart failure may be resistant to therapy with cardiac glycosides. The development of complete AV block is an ominous complication, and mortality is high despite insertion of a transvenous pacemaker.[604]

LEGIONNAIRES' DISEASE. Although pneumonia, rhabdomyolysis, renal failure, and hepatic as well as central nervous system involvement are common with *Legionella pneumophila*, overt cardiac involvement is not.[606] Occasional electrocardiographic changes may be noted, consisting primarily of ST-segment and T-wave abnormalities; ventricular arrhythmias may be seen. Rarely, pericardial effusion, myocarditis with evidence of myocardial necrosis, or congestive heart failure may be seen.[606,607]

MENINGOCOCCUS. Myocardial involvement is common during the course of fatal meningococcal infections but is less commonly recognized in the usual case.[608,609] *Pathological findings* include hemorrhagic myocardial lesions, occasionally associated with intracellular organisms.[608] An interstitial myocarditis composed of lymphocytes, plasma cells, and polymorphonuclear leukocytes may be observed, occasionally with myonecrosis.[608]

Meningococcal myocarditis may result in congestive heart failure as well as in pericardial effusion with tamponade.[609] Death may occur suddenly and be associated with involvement of the atrioventricular node.[608]

MYCOPLASMA PNEUMONIAE. Electrocardiographic abnormalities are common during the course of atypical pneumonia, although clinically apparent myocarditis is not.[534] When carditis occurs, it may be serious, and, rarely, fatal.[610] Nonspecific ST-segment and T-wave abnormalities are the most common manifestations of cardiac involvement; a rare patient may develop complete heart block.[610] The electrocardiographic findings usually resolve within 1 to 2 weeks. A cell-mediated autoimmune myocarditis has been postulated as the cause of the changes.[534] Pericarditis may be a prominent finding, and congestive heart failure is occasionally seen.[611] A protodiastolic gallop[612] and pericardial friction rub may be noted in occasional cases. Complete recovery is the rule in most patients,[612] although occasional patients may have persistent sequelae, including arrhythmias.[611]

PSITTACOSIS. Myocarditis complicating psittacosis is a relatively common occurrence and is characterized by congestive heart failure and acute pericarditis.[613,614] *Pathological changes* include fibrinous pericarditis as well as endocarditis and myocarditis. Fever, chest pain, electrocardiographic changes, cardiomegaly, systemic emboli, tachycardia, and hypotension may occur. Although most patients recover completely, fatalities have been reported.[613] The systemic infection may be treated effectively with tetracycline, but the effect of the antibiotic on the myocardium is unknown.

SALMONELLA. Symptomatic myocardial involvement during salmonella infections is rare,[615–617] although electrocardiographic abnormalities are often seen, suggesting subclinical myocarditis.[618] Other cardiovascular complications include infected mural thrombi, occasionally resulting in pulmonary and systemic emboli, and mycotic aneurysms.[619] Myocardial abscesses may rupture, producing fatal cardiac tamponade. Myocarditis with congestive heart failure occurs most commonly in children who are severely ill with salmonellosis, and it is associated with a high mortality.[620] When myocarditis occurs, it often develops rapidly, with evidence of biventricular failure, tachycardia, a protodiastolic gallop, an apical systolic murmur of mitral regurgitation, and peripheral edema.[620]

Electrocardiographic abnormalities include ST-segment and T-wave changes, prolonged P-R or Q-T intervals, and low QRS voltage.[618,621]

STREPTOCOCCUS. The most commonly detected cardiac finding following beta-hemolytic streptococcal infection is acute rheumatic fever, which is discussed in detail in Chapter 55.

Involvement of the heart by the streptococcus may produce a myocarditis that is distinct from acute rheumatic carditis.[622,623] It is characterized by an interstitial infiltrate composed of mononuclear cells with occasional polymorphonuclear leukocytes[624]; the infiltrate may be focal or diffuse and may be localized to the subendocardial or perivascular region. There may be small areas of myocardial necrosis.[624] *Electrocardiographic abnormalities,* including prolongation of the P-R and Q-T intervals, occur frequently. Although these abnormalities are rarely associated with other clinical manifestations of myocardial involvement, sudden death, conduction disturbances, and arrhythmias may occur.[622,624]

TUBERCULOSIS. Tuberculous involvement of the myocardium (not as a complication of tuberculous pericarditis) is extremely rare, particularly since the introduction of drugs effective against tuberculosis.[625,626] Most cases of myocardial tuberculosis are clinically silent and are diagnosed only at autopsy.[625] Tuberculous involvement of the myocardium occurs via hematogenous or lymphatic spread, or directly from contiguous structures; it may lead to arrhythmias, including atrial fibrillation and ventricular tachycardia, complete atrioventricular block, congestive heart failure, left ventricular aneurysms, and sudden death.[625–627]

WHIPPLE DISEASE

Intestinal lipodystrophy, or Whipple disease, may be associated with myocardial involvement, and PAS-positive macrophages may be found in the myocardium, pericardium, and heart valves of patients with this disorder.[628,629] Coronary artery lesions, with smooth muscle necrosis, panarteritis, and medial scarring, are not rare.[630] Electron microscopy has demonstrated rod-shaped structures in the myocardium similar to those found in the small intestine, and it has been suggested that they are the causative agent of the myocardial abnormalities. There may be an associated inflammatory infiltrate and foci of fibrosis.[628] The valvular fibrosis may be severe enough to result in aortic regurgitation and mitral stenosis.[630] Although asymptomatic, nonspecific electrocardiographic changes are most common; systolic murmurs, pericarditis, and even overt congestive heart failure may occur.[629] Antibiotic therapy appears to be effective in treating the basic disease; however, relapses can occur, often more than 2 years after initial diagnosis.[631,632]

SPIROCHETAL INFECTIONS

LEPTOSPIROSIS (WEIL DISEASE). Most patients with leptospiral infections have mild or subclinical disease and little evidence of heart involvement. Cardiac involvement in severe or fatal leptospirosis is common, however, with 50 to 100 per cent of fatal cases demonstrating evidence of myocarditis.[633] Many patients with severe systemic disease demonstrate first-degree heart block and transient ST-segment and T-wave abnormalities, presumably reflecting myocarditis.[633,634] Bradycardia despite fever, ventricular premature depolarizations, congestive heart failure, and pericarditis may be seen as well.[633,634] The *pathological findings* in the occasional fatal case include petechiae or large foci of hemorrhage (often located in the epicardium), an interstitial myocardial infiltration (often subendocardial in location), aortitis, and coronary arteritis.[633]

LYME CARDITIS. Lyme disease is caused by a tickborne spirochete *(Borrelia burgdorferi)*.[635] It usually begins during the summer months with a characteristic skin rash (erythema chronicum migrans), followed in weeks to months by neurologic, joint, or cardiac involvement; some clinical manifestations may persist for years.[636]

About 10 per cent of patients with Lyme disease develop evidence of transient cardiac involvement, the most common manifestation being variable degrees of AV block.[636–639] The location of the block appears to be at the level of the AV node.[635] Syncope due to complete heart block is frequent with cardiac involvement because often there is an associated depression of ventricular escape rhythms.[635,640] Ventricular tachycardia occurs uncommonly.[638] Diffuse ST-segment and T-wave abnormalities and transient, usually asymptomatic, left ventricular dysfunction may be found in some patients, although cardiomegaly or symptoms of congestive heart failure are rare.[639,641] A positive gallium or indium antimyosin antibody scan may point to suspected cardiac involvement in this disease.[635,642,643] The demonstration of spirochetes in myocardial biopsies of some patients with Lyme carditis suggests that the cardiac manifestations are due to a direct toxic effect, although there is speculation that immune-mediated mechanisms may be involved as well.[635]

The value of specific therapy in Lyme carditis remains uncertain,[644] and even without therapy the disease usually is self-limited with complete recovery the rule; nevertheless, it is thought that treating the early manifestations of the disease may prevent development of late complications.[645] Patients with second-degree or complete heart block should be hospitalized and undergo continuous electrocardiographic monitoring.[644] Temporary transvenous pacing may be required for up to a week or longer in patients with high-grade block.[635] Although the efficacy of antibiotics is not established, they are utilized routinely in Lyme carditis. Intravenous antibiotics (ceftriaxone, 2 gm, or penicillin G, 20 million units daily for 14 days) are suggested, although oral antibiotics (doxycycline, 100 mg twice daily, or amoxicillin, 500 mg three times daily for 14 to 21 days) may be used when there is only mild cardiac involvement (first-degree AV block of less than 40 msec duration).[645] Whether anti-inflammatory agents (salicylates, corticosteroids) can ameliorate heart block is not clear.[640]

RELAPSING FEVER. Many infections are currently observed in Ethiopia. During pandemics, mortality may be particularly high, reaching 70 per cent, although sporadic cases are often more benign.[646] Cardiac involvement is said to be a common complication and is often implicated as a cause of death, although one report involving 63 children did not find evidence of cardiac involvement.[647] AV conduction defects occur frequently and may be responsible for sudden death, although tachyarrhythmias have also been implicated.[646] Numerous petechiae are observed with a diffuse histiocytic interstitial infiltrate, particularly around small arterioles in the left ventricle.

SYPHILIS. Aortitis is the most common manifestation of luetic involvement of the cardiovascular system.[648] Aortic regurgitation and coronary ostial narrowing are associated findings. Syphilitic involvement of the myocardium itself in the form of gumma formation is uncommon and usually unsuspected clinically.[648] Involvement of the base of the interventricular septum may result in damage to the conduction system and AV block.[648] In one case a ruptured left ventricular aneurysm was found as a result of syphilitic endarteritis.[649]

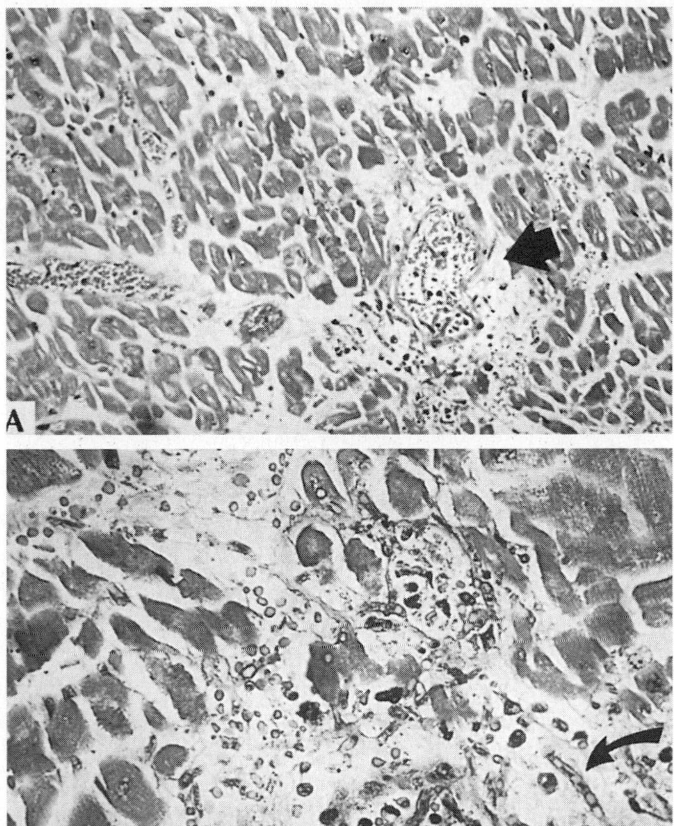

FIGURE 41–28 Aspergillus myocarditis in a patient with AIDS. *A,* Section of heart with blood vessel and mild inflammation (arrow) (× 330). *B,* High-powered examination of this area reveals fungal hyphae invading through a blood vessel wall and into the myocardium (arrow) (× 825). (Courtesy of G. K. Haines, Northwestern University, Chicago, IL.)

FUNGAL INFECTIONS OF THE HEART

Cardiac fungal infections occur most frequently in patients with malignant disease and/or those receiving chemotherapy, steroids, radiation, or immunosuppressive therapy. Cardiac surgery, intravenous drug abuse, and infection with HIV are also predisposing factors for fungal cardiac involvement.

ACTINOMYCOSIS. Myocarditis is a rare complication of actinomycotic infection, occurring in less than 2 per cent of patients.[650] However, cardiac involvement is quite serious when it does occur. Involvement of the heart most commonly is the result of direct extension of disease within the thorax.[650,651] Initially the pericardium is invaded, with eventual obliteration of the pericardial space. The myocardium may be involved by extension of the pericardial process. Myocardial seeding is less common.[650] The myocardial lesion is a suppurative, necrotizing abscess containing the organism, surrounded by granulation tissue. Both right- and left-sided failure are common manifestations. A pericardial rub may be heard, sometimes associated with clinical evidence of a pericardial effusion or constriction.[650,651]

ASPERGILLOSIS. Myocardial involvement is not uncommon in generalized aspergillosis, and when it occurs it is usually fatal.[652] It is being encountered increasingly in the immunocompromised patient.[653–655] On pathologic examination, myocardial necrosis and infarction caused by thrombosis of vessels that contain fungal mycelia are commonly seen, along with myocardial abscesses and pericardial involvement (Fig. 41–28).[654,656] The electrocardiogram may be normal in the face of significant myocardial damage, but T-wave changes may be present. The *diagnosis* of aspergillus infection is often difficult.[655] Identification of aspergillus through open lung biopsy, aspiration lung biopsy, transtracheal aspiration, or bronchial brush technique may be successful.[654,657] Treatment is difficult and usually unsuccessful.[654]

BLASTOMYCOSIS. Involvement of the heart by the fungus is quite uncommon, even in the immunocompromised heart. When involvement occurs, it is most often by direct extension from the pericardium.

CANDIDIASIS. Disseminated monilial infections are common opportunistic infections, particularly in the compromised host.[658] Endocarditis is the most frequent manifestation of cardiac involvement (see p. 1082), occurring most commonly in cardiac surgical patients or drug addicts, although multiple abscesses of the myocardium may occur as associated or independent findings.[659] Complete heart block may be caused by microabscesses of the conduction system.[658]

COCCIDIOIDOMYCOSIS. Involvement of the heart is rare in patients with generalized coccidioidomycosis.[660] The hearts may be grossly normal, although epicardial lesions with resultant pericarditis are common, and progression to constrictive pericarditis may occur (p. 1498). A nonspecific, focal interstitial, and perivascular cellular infiltrate with associated muscle fiber degeneration and interstitial edema is commonly found, although granulomas containing fungi are also seen sometimes.

CRYPTOCOCCOSIS. Cryptococcal infection of the myocardium occurs most commonly in immunocompromised patients with disseminated malignancy or HIV infection.[661] *Pathological examination* may show cardiac dilatation, with epithelial granulomas, giant cells, and an inflammatory infiltrate.[661] When congestive heart failure occurs, pulmonary congestion and muffled heart sounds may be found on physical examination, and cardiomegaly on the chest roentgenogram.[661] The *electrocardiogram* may show first-degree AV block and T-wave inversions; ventricular arrhythmias have been observed.

HISTOPLASMOSIS. Cardiac involvement in histoplasmosis is rare and usually is related to mediastinal fibrosis, the most serious complication of histoplasmosis.[662,663] Pericarditis with effusion may occur (see p. 1510), and superior vena caval obstruction has been observed.[663]

Myocardial involvement is uncommon, although atrial arrhythmias and T-wave abnormalities have been reported.

MUCORMYCOSIS. Cardiac involvement in the setting of disseminated mucormycosis occurs in about 20 per cent of patients and is characterized by fungal invasion of the coronary arteries with resultant areas of myocardial infarction.[664] Valvular and pericardial involvement may be seen as well. Clinical manifestations are nonspecific, and cardiac involvement often is not suspected but may include congestive heart failure, arrhythmias, conduction defects, and endocarditis.[664]

PROTOZOAL MYOCARDITIS

Trypanosomiasis (Chagas' Disease)

Chagas' disease is caused by the protozoan *Trypanosoma cruzi.* The major cardiovascular manifestation is an extensive myocarditis that typically becomes evident years after the initial infection. The disease is prevalent in Central and South America, particularly in Brazil, Argentina, and Chile, where it is a major public health problem (Fig. 41–29). Upwards of 20 million people are thought to be infected with the parasite, and an estimated 100 million are at risk of infection.[499,665,666] In rare cases, the disease may be found in nonendemic areas as a consequence of transfusion with contaminated blood products[667]; somewhat more common is that patients with the disease emigrate to nonendemic areas.[499]

The natural history of Chagas' disease is characterized by three phases: acute, latent, and chronic. During the *acute phase,* the disease is transmitted to humans (usually below the age of 20 years)[668,669] through the bite of a reduviid bug (subfamily Triatominae), which harbors the parasite in its gastrointestinal tract.[670] This insect acquires the disease from feeding on infected animals, including the armadillo, raccoon, opossum, and skunk as well as domestic dogs and cats. The reduviid bug, popularly known in Argentina as "vinchuca," meaning "to let oneself drop," lives in the walls and roofs of houses and, during nocturnal feedings, drops from the ceiling onto the sleeping person below. The bug then often bites the person around the eyes, and infection of the human host occurs when the trypanosomes in the animal's feces gain entry through abraded skin or through the conjunctivae. Occasionally, this results in unilateral periorbital edema and swelling of the eyelid, termed *Romaña's sign,*[499] while entry through the skin may result in a lesion called a *chagoma.* Transmission may occur through blood transfusions as well as congenitally, although this appears to be uncommon.[668]

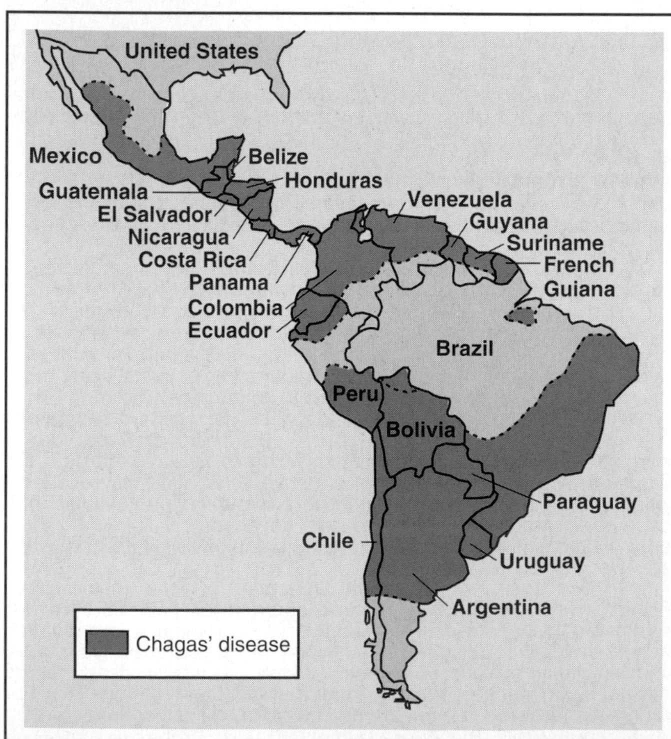

FIGURE 41–29. Distribution of Chagas' disease in the Americas. (From Acquatella, H.: Chagas' disease. *In* Abelmann, W. H., and Braunwald, E. [eds.]: Cardiomyopathies, Myocarditis, and Pericardial Disease. Atlas of Heart Diseases. Vol. 2. Philadelphia, Current Medicine, 1995, pp. 8.1–8.18.)

ACUTE TRYPANOSOMIASIS. Following inoculation, the protozoa multiply and then migrate widely throughout the body. In less than 10 per cent of cases an acute illness occurs[666,669]; the latter is fatal in about 10 per cent of patients.[499]

Pathological examination during the acute phase often reveals parasites in the cardiac fibers with a marked cellular infiltrate, particularly around cardiac cells that have ruptured and released the parasites.[671] Involvement may extend into the endocardium, resulting in thrombus formation, and into the epicardium, resulting in pericardial effusion. The pathogenesis of the myocardial lesions of acute Chagas' disease appears to relate in large part to immune lysis by antibody and cell-mediated immunity directed against antigens released from *T. cruzi*–infected cells, which become adsorbed onto the surface of infected and noninfected host cells.[670]

Clinical Manifestations. These include fever, muscle pains, sweating, hepatosplenomegaly, myocarditis with congestive heart failure, and, occasionally, meningoencephalitis.[666] Most patients recover, and their symptoms resolve over several months. Young children most commonly develop clinical acute disease and generally are more seriously ill than adults.

CHRONIC TRYPANOSOMIASIS. The disease then enters a *latent phase* without clinical symptoms; however, there is evidence of early and progressive subclinical cardiomyopathy. Electrocardiographic changes often appear at this stage and are a marker for the eventual clinical heart disease and increased mortality to become evident later. At an average of 20 years after the initial (and usually unrecognized) infestation, approximately 30 per cent of infected individuals develop findings of *chronic Chagas' disease,* the manifestations of which cover a wide spectrum from asymptomatic but seropositive patients through those with electrocardiographic abnormalities to those with advanced disease characterized by cardiomegaly, congestive heart failure, arrhythmias, thromboembolic phenomena, atypical chest pain, right bundle branch block, and sudden death.[672–675] In the advanced stage, cardiac dilatation typically involves all the cardiac chambers, although right-sided enlargement may predominate.[676]

The central paradox in the pathogenesis of this disorder is the negative correlation between the severity of disease and the level of parasitemia. It is not unusual to be unable to detect parasites in patients dying of Chagas' disease.[665,677] An autoimmune mechanism has been proposed.[499,678–680] It appears (at least in an animal model) that self-reactive cytotoxic T lymphocytes develop following the initial infection, and these lymphocytes are able to lyse normal host cells, perhaps related to cross-reacting antigens of *T. cruzi* and striated muscle.[39] A variety of antibodies against myocyte sarcoplasmic reticulum, laminin, and other constituents have also been implicated in the pathogenesis of Chagas' myocarditis.[679] It is thought that the acute phase results in the release from parasite-modified host cells of self-components that are immunogenic.[670] Another hypothesis suggests that cardiac parasympathetic denervation leads to eventual chronic Chagas' disease.[499,665]

Pathology. Nerves and autonomic ganglia are frequently abnormal, and megaesophagus and megacolon may occur; less commonly, there is dilatation of the stomach, duodenum, ureter, and bronchi. Different strains of *T. cruzi* may account for the geographical differences in the expression of Chagas' disease; in Brazil, megaesophagus and megacolon are common, but these conditions are unusual in Venezuela.[681] Lesions of the cardiac nerves are routinely found in patients with chronic Chagas' disease, with evidence of cardiac parasympathetic denervation.[666] Pathological cardiac findings include cardiac enlargement, with dilatation and hypertrophy of all cardiac chambers. In more than half the patients, the left (and occasionally right) ventricular apex is thin and bulging, resembling an aneurysm (Fig. 41–30).[499,665,672] Thrombus formation is frequent and may fill much of the apex; the right atrium also frequently contains thrombus. It has been suggested that this characteristic apical aneurysm may be the result of intravascular platelet aggregation leading to focal myocardial necrosis.[682]

The microscopic findings are principally those of extensive fibrosis, particularly of the left ventricle.[668] A chronic cellular infiltrate composed of lymphocytes, plasma cells, and macrophages often is present.[666] Preferential involvement of the right bundle branch and the anterior fascicle of the left bundle branch by inflammatory and fibrotic changes explains the frequent occurrence of right bundle branch and left anterior fascicular block.[499] The basement membranes of capillaries, vascular smooth muscle cells, and myocytes are thickened.[670] It is unusual to be able to find parasites in the myofibers of autopsied patients.[665]

Clinical Manifestations. These include anginal chest pain, symptomatic conducting system disease, and sudden death[499]; chronic progressive heart failure, often predominantly right-sided, is the rule in advanced cases. Thus, although pulmonary congestion is occasionally noted, the usual findings include fatigue due to diminished cardiac output, peripheral edema, ascites, and hepatic congestion.[672] Tricuspid regurgitation is often present, particularly in patients with severe right-sided heart failure, although mitral regurgitation is frequently present as well. The second heart sound is widely split, often with an accentuated pulmonic component, reflecting the combined effects of right bundle branch block and pulmonary hypertension. Autonomic dysfunction is common, with marked abnormalities in the expected reflex changes in heart rate produced by various maneuvers.

The *chest roentgenogram* often demonstrates severe cardiomegaly, with or without pulmonary venous hypertension.[672] *Electrocardiographic abnormalities* are the rule late in the course of the disease,[674] particularly in patients who are seroreactive to *T. cruzi* antigen. Right bundle branch block, left anterior hemiblock, atrial fibrillation, and ventricular premature depolarizations are the most common findings in patients with chronic Chagas' disease.[499,666,672,683,684] ST-segment and T-wave abnormalities also are common,[683] as are Q waves; P-wave abnormalities and AV block are seen less frequently.[499] Early in the disease, the electrocardiogram may be normal or nearly so.[674,676] Administration of the antiarrhythmic agent ajmaline may precipitate the appearance of electrocardiographic abnormalities and thus identify patients with as yet clinically silent cardiac involvement. Furthermore, electrophysiological testing of asymptomatic patients, even those with normal electrocardiograms, may demonstrate abnormalities of the conducting system in many.

Ventricular arrhythmias are a prominent feature of chronic Chagas' disease.[666] Frequent ventricular premature depolarizations, often with multiple morphologies, are seen frequently, and bouts of ventricular tachycardia may occur.[673,683] Ventricular arrhythmias are particularly common during and following exercise,[666] occurring in the majority of patients subjected to stress electrocardiographic testing (including some without any clinical evidence of cardiac involvement). Ventricular tachycardia induced by electrophysiological testing[685] is most common in patients with evidence of conduction abnormalities on the electrocardiogram, low ejection fraction, and apical left ventricular aneurysm.[670] Syncope and sudden death due to ventricular fibrillation are constant threats and may develop even before cardiomegaly or heart failure.[499,666,686,687] Sinus bradycardia may also be seen, even in patients with severe heart failure when a tachycardia would be expected, presumably related to cardiac autonomic dysfunction.[666] Atrial arrhythmias, including atrial fibrillation (often with a slow ventricular response), also may occur.[666] Thromboembolic phenomena are a frequent complication, occurring in more than 50 per cent of the patients.

The *echocardiographic findings* in advanced cases are those of a dilated cardiomyopathy with increased end-diastolic and end-systolic volumes and reduced ejection fraction, often with enlargement of the left atrium and right ventricle.[666] Diastolic filling of the left ventricle is frequently abnormal, even in those without other clinical or echocardiographic evidence of cardiac involvement. In the majority of advanced cases, the echocardiographic appearance is distinctive, with left ventricular posterior wall hypokinesis and relatively preserved interventricular septal motion; an apical aneurysm is often seen on two-dimensional echocardiography. Ten to 15 per cent of asymptomatic patients demonstrate apical dyskinesis.

Radionuclide ventriculography may, like echocardiography, demonstrate right or left ventricular wall motion abnormalities in the absence of an overall depression of global ventricular function.[688] Perfusion scanning with thallium-201 may show fixed defects (corresponding to areas of fibrosis) as well as evidence of reversible ischemia.[499,689]

Left ventricular cineangiography in advanced cases shows a dilated, hypokinetic left ventricle with a large api-

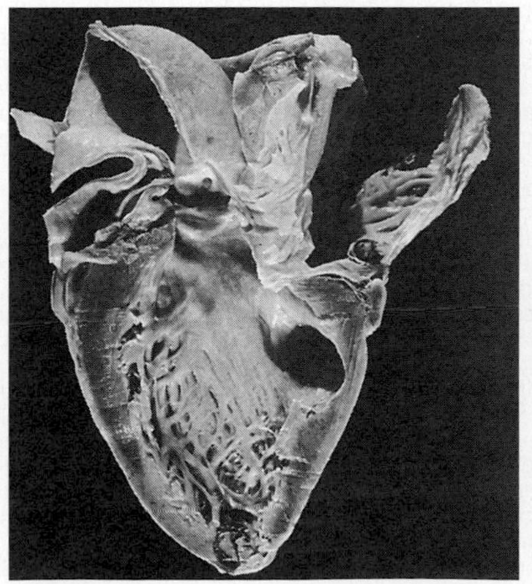

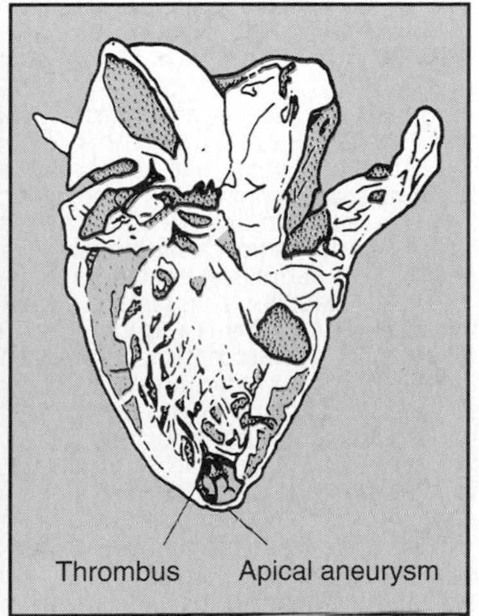

FIGURE 41–30. The heart from a patient who died suddenly with Chagas' disease. The narrow-necked left ventricular apical aneurysm is typical of Chagas' disease. (From Acquatella, H.: Chagas' disease. *In* Abelmann, W. H., and Braunwald, E. [eds.]: Cardiomyopathies, Myocarditis, and Pericardial Disease. Atlas of Heart Diseases. Vol. 2. Philadelphia, Current Medicine, 1995, pp. 8.1–8.18.)

cal aneurysm[499] containing intracavitary thrombus, often with evidence of mitral regurgitation. *Coronary angiography* is usually normal,[499] although abnormalities of the coronary microcirculation have been suggested as a cause of the clinical manifestations of Chagas' disease.

The *complement-fixation test* (Machado-Guerreiro test) is useful in diagnosis; it has high sensitivity and specificity for the identification of chronic Chagas' disease.[499] Also used in diagnosis are the indirect immunofluorescent antibody, the enzyme-linked immunosorbent assay (ELISA), and the hemagglutination tests.[499,690] Another test that is occasionally useful is the detection of parasites in the blood of patients with chronic Chagas' disease (which occurs in 30 to 40 per cent of cases) by means of *xenodiagnosis*.[669] The patient is bitten by reduviid bugs bred in the laboratory; the subsequent identification of parasites in the intestine of the insect is proof of infection in the human host.

MANAGEMENT. The treatment of Chagas' disease remains difficult; although slowly progressive at first, once cardiac decompensation develops there is usually a rapid and inexorable progression to death, which is usually due to arrhythmia, although congestive failure and systemic thromboembolism account for additional mortality.[499,691] Patients at greatest risk of mortality are those with left ventricular enlargement and especially those with impaired left ventricular function.[684,686] Major efforts are aimed at interrupting transmission of the parasite to humans; such vector control methods have been generally successful.[499,667,668] They may prevent not only the initial infection but also reinfection that may play a role in determining the severity of the resulting cardiomyopathy. *Amiodarone* appears to be particularly effective in controlling the ubiquitous ventricular arrhythmias seen in Chagas' disease, although whether this translates into improved survival remains to be established.[669] Anticoagulation may be of some benefit in preventing recurrent thromboembolic episodes. Although antiparasitic agents such as nifurtimox and benzimidazole are effective in reducing parasitemia, no evidence indicates that they are efficacious in curing the disease.[499,690] A promising avenue of approach appears to be immunoprophylaxis, although a clinically useful vaccine is not yet available. Insertion of an implantable cardioverter-defibrillator,[692] use of the latissimus dorsi muscle wrap around the heart (dynamic cardiomyoplasty),[693,694] and heart transplantation have been performed in a few patients[695] but are not practical options for the vast majority of patients.

AFRICAN TRYPANOSOMIASIS. African sleeping sickness, caused by *Trypanosoma gambiense* or *T. rhodesiense,* may be associated with myocardial abnormalities, although they are usually of less functional significance than in Chagas' disease.[696] *T. rhodesiense,* in particular, may lead to cardiac failure,[696] although the central nervous system findings (excessive somnolence) usually dominate the clinical picture.

Pathological examination often reveals pericardial fluid.[696] The heart is not as greatly dilated and hypertrophied as it is in Chagas' disease and may appear grossly to be normal. There is often epicardial thickening with a cellular exudate composed of lymphocytes, plasma cells, and histiocytes. The myocardium typically displays a diffuse interstitial infiltrate, often with zones of patchy fibrosis and interstitial edema.[697]

Nonspecific *electrocardiographic* changes, commonly ST-segment and T-wave abnormalities and prolongation of the Q-T interval, are observed in at least half the patients.[696] Unlike Chagas' disease, arrhythmias and conduction disturbances are usually not prominent features, and the arterial pressure is usually normal. Some patients have asymptomatic cardiomegaly,[696] although both pulmonary congestion and peripheral edema have been reported.

TOXOPLASMOSIS. *Toxoplasma* infections are caused by an obligate intracellular parasite *(T. gondii);* both congenital and acquired forms may occur. Symptomatic acquired toxoplasmic infections involving the heart are uncommon. They occur most commonly in immunosuppressed patients with malignant diseases and occasionally in patients with AIDS and following cardiac or bone marrow transplantation.[561,698] An inflammatory infiltrate, often with eosinophils and variable degrees of edema and degeneration of the muscle bundles, and pericardial effusion are often present.[698]

Most adult cases are asymptomatic, but *Toxoplasma* infections may produce a severe, fatal disease with multisystem involvement.[561] Toxoplasmic myocarditis, often with pericarditis, may occur as an isolated disease process or as part of a multisystem disseminated disease.[561] Manifestations may include arrhythmias (atrial and ventricular), sudden death, AV block, pericarditis, and heart failure.[561] Large pericardial effusions may be seen on occasion.[698] Diagnosis may be aided by endomyocardial biopsy.[567]

Treatment is with a combination of pyrimethamine and triple sulfonamides, but the response to therapy is variable[567]; it appears to have no effect on the cyst form.[561]

MALARIA. Although myocardial changes may be demonstrated during the course of malaria, particularly with *Plasmodium falciparum,* clinical findings to indicate cardiac involvement are rare.[699,700] The heart generally demonstrates few gross abnormalities. The principal findings are histological. The capillaries are often filled and even distended with an accumulation of parasites, sometimes totally occluding the lumen of the vessels. Thrombosis of the capillaries and ischemic myocardial changes may be seen.[700] Focal myocardial damage may be present, along with an interstitial infiltrate composed of lymphocytes, plasma cells, and macrophages.[700] In rare cases, cardiac failure may contribute to or even cause death.[700] ST-segment and T-wave changes on the electrocardiogram may be the only clinical indications of myocardial involvement.[699]

METAZOAL MYOCARDIAL DISEASE

ECHINOCOCCUS (HYDATID CYST). *Echinococcus* is endemic in many sheep-raising areas of the world, particularly Argentina, Uruguay, New Zealand, Greece, North Africa, and Iceland, but cardiac involvement in hydatid disease is uncommon, occurring in less than 2 per cent of cases.[701–703] The usual host of *Echinococcus granulosus* is the dog, but human beings may serve as intermediate hosts (rather than the sheep, the usual intermediate host) if they accidentally ingest ova from contaminated dog feces.

When cardiac involvement is present, the cysts usually are intramyocardial in the interventricular septum or left ventricular free wall; involvement of the right ventricle or atrium may occur.[702–704] Involvement of the tricuspid valve may be seen on occasion,[702] and pericardial involvement with compression of the heart is not uncommon.[702,704] In most cases, a single cardiac cyst is present.[701,702]

A myocardial cyst may degenerate and calcify, develop daughter cysts, or rupture. Rupture of the cyst is the most dreaded complication; rupture into the pericardium may result in acute pericarditis, which may progress to chronic constrictive pericarditis. Rupture into the cardiac chambers may result in systemic or pulmonary emboli.[705,706] Rapidly progressive pulmonary hypertension may occur with rupture of right-sided cysts, with subsequent embolization of hundreds of scolices into the pulmonary circulation.[702] The liberation of hydatid fluid into the circulation may produce profound, fatal circulatory collapse due to an anaphylactic reaction to the protein constituents of the fluid.[702]

Symptoms depend on the location, size, and integrity of the cyst; patients may be asymptomatic or in profound circulatory collapse.[701,702] The *electrocardiogram* may reflect the location of the cyst; T-wave changes and loss of QRS voltage may occur with left ventricular involvement, while AV conduction defects or right bundle branch block may be seen with involvement of the interventricular septum. Chest pain is usually due to rupture of the cyst into the pericardial space with resultant pericarditis. Large cystic masses may sometimes produce right-sided obstruction.[701,702]

Diagnosis. Recognition of an echinococcal cyst of the heart is a relatively simple matter if there is evidence of cysts in other organs, particularly the liver and lung. However, a cardiac cyst may be an isolated, solitary finding. The *chest roentgenogram* frequently shows an abnormal cardiac silhouette or a calcified lobular mass adjacent to the left ventricle. Although CT and nuclear MRI may aid in the detection and localization of heart cysts, two-dimensional echocardiography is thought to be the best choice.[702,704,707] *Eosinophilia,* present in some patients, is a useful adjunctive finding. The *Casoni skin test* is not very helpful because both false-positive and false-negative results occur. Serological tests, including hemagglutination and complement fixation, are more useful.

Management. Until recently, treatment for hydatid disease was limited to surgical excision.[704,708] Because of the significant risk of rupture of the cyst and its attendant serious and sometimes fatal consequences, surgical excision is generally recommended, even for asymptomatic patients. The surgical results have been generally favorable. Experience suggests that the benzimidazole derivative mebendazole may be somewhat useful in the medical management of this disease.[709]

VISCERAL LARVA MIGRANS. People are occasional accidental hosts of the roundworm infestations of dogs due to *Toxocara canis,* but cardiac involvement is rare. Most cases occur in children 1 to 3 years of age.[710] Myocarditis may occur in association with invasion of the myocardium by larvae.[710] The myocardial lesions include granulomas or extensive inflammatory infiltrates (often with eosinophils) with foci of muscle necrosis.[710] Congestive heart failure and death may occur, although asymptomatic cardiac involvement may be seen as well.[710]

SCHISTOSOMIASIS AND RELATED DISEASE. Direct cardiac involvement in schistosomiasis, heterophyiasis, and cysticercosis is distinctly unusual. The principal cardiovascular manifestation of schistosomiasis is right heart overload as a consequence of embolization of the ova to the pulmonary vasculature, with attendant pulmonary hypertension.

TRICHINOSIS. Infestation with *Trichinella spiralis* is a common human finding. Mild myocarditis is frequent, but symptomatic involvement is uncommon and may be responsible for the majority of fatalities.[711,712] Less frequently, death is due to pulmonary embolism secondary to venous thrombosis, or encephalitis.[712]

Although the parasite may invade the heart, it does not usually encyst there, and it is rare to find larvae or larval fragments in the myocardium. Nonetheless, *pathological findings* at autopsy may be impressive. The heart may be dilated and flabby and a pericardial effusion may be present. A prominent focal infiltrate composed of lymphocytes and eosinophils is commonly found, with occasional microthrombi in the intramural arterioles.[712] Areas of muscle degeneration and necrosis are present. The actual cause of the myocardial lesions is debated; whether they bear any relationship to the ubiquitous eosinophilia is uncertain.[712]

Clinical Manifestations. Myocarditis usually is mild and goes unnoticed, but in occasional cases it is manifested by congestive heart failure and chest pain, usually appearing around the third week of the disease, when the general constitutional symptoms are abating.[713] Physical examination may be normal, or there may be gross cardiomegaly with severe congestive heart failure. Sudden death may occur, usually in the fourth to eighth week of the illness.

Electrocardiographic abnormalities may be detected in one-fourth of patients with trichinosis and parallel the time course of clinical cardiac involvement, initially appearing in the second or third week and usually resolving by the seventh week of the illness.[714] The most common electrocardiographic abnormalities are repolarization abnormalities and conduction defects.[714] The electrocardiographic changes usually resolve completely.

The definitive *diagnosis* is based on the demonstration of larval forms in tissue biopsy samples, usually of the gastrocnemius muscle.[714] Eosinophilia, when present, is a supportive finding. The skin test is usually but not invariably positive. Treatment is with corticosteroids; dramatic improvement in cardiac function has been reported following their use.[714]

TOXIC, CHEMICAL, IMMUNE, AND PHYSICAL DAMAGE TO THE HEART

A wide variety of substances other than infectious agents may act on the heart and damage the myocardium. In some cases, the damage is acute, transient, and associated with evidence of an inflammatory infiltrate with myocyte necrosis (such as with arsenicals and lithium); in other cases, a hypersensitivity reaction occurs, without evidence of necrosis (as with sulfonamides). Other agents that damage the myocardium may lead to chronic changes with resulting histological evidence of fibrosis and a clinical picture of a dilated cardiomyopathy. Furthermore, many offending stimuli may be associated with both acute and chronic phases (e.g., alcohol, doxorubicin). The response often is related to the dose and rate of exposure.

Numerous chemicals and drugs (both industrial and therapeutic) may lead to cardiac damage and dysfunction. Several physical agents (e.g., radiation and excessive heat) may also result in myocardial damage. Furthermore, myocardial involvement may be evident in a variety of systemic disease, which are described in Part V of this book.

COCAINE. The illicit use of this drug has increased dramatically recently. It has been associated with a variety of cardiovascular complications, including myocardial ischemia and infarction (unassociated with obstructive coronary artery disease in about one-third), accelerated atherosclerosis, arrhythmias and sudden death, electrophysiological effects, coronary vasoconstriction, myocarditis, dilated cardiomyopathy, rupture of the aorta, cerebrovascular events, increased platelet aggregation, arterial thrombosis, and an apparent predisposition to the development of endocarditis[715–733] (Fig. 41–31). The actual frequency of these complications is in some dispute[734]; the number of adverse events reported in the literature is far less than the casual impression of medical caregivers in inner-city hospitals would suggest.[735] In one study of cocaine abusers who presented to the hospital with chest pain, the frequency of documented myocardial infarction was low.[736] The effects of cocaine on the myocardium itself include transient depression of ventricular function whether the drug is taken acutely or chronically (Fig. 41–32),[720,737,738] scattered areas of myocardial necrosis and myocarditis unrelated to coronary artery disease (which in some cases include contraction band necrosis), and fibrosis.[739,740] In a few cases there has been evidence of dilated cardiomyopathy.[723,737] Even asymptomatic cocaine abusers may have clinically silent myocardial depression.[738]

The cardiovascular effects of cocaine likely are related to its principal pharmacological effects: blocking the reuptake of catecholamines in the presynaptic neurons; blocking sodium channels, leading to local anesthetic, membrane-stabilizing effects; and reducing spontaneous sympathetic activity as a result of effects on the brain stem.[729,739] It has been speculated that the myocardial damage seen with cocaine relates to excess catecholamines damaging myocytes because their reuptake is blocked; this may lead to calcium overload of the cells, or perhaps to local vasoconstriction with subsequent ischemic damage.[724] Vasoconstriction has also been shown as a direct effect of cocaine itself.[741] The monocellular infiltrate (myocarditis) that has been found may merely be a reaction to the associated myocyte death or could be a hypersensitivity reaction to the cocaine, a metabolite,[724] or a contaminant.

Treatment is empirical; nitrates, alpha-adrenoceptor blockers, calcium antagonists, and thrombolytic therapy (for acute myocardial infarctions) have been advocated but without any definite demonstration of their efficacy.[723,742] Beta-adrenoceptor blockers probably should be avoided, as they have been shown to further reduce coronary blood flow and increase coronary vascular resistance during cocaine use, and may predispose to cocaine-mediated cardiac conduction defects.[719,723,739,743]

DAUNORUBICIN AND DOXORUBICIN (See pp. 1800 to 1803)

INTERFERON-ALPHA. Interferon-alpha is a leukocyte-derived protein used therapeutically to treat malignancies and HIV infections.

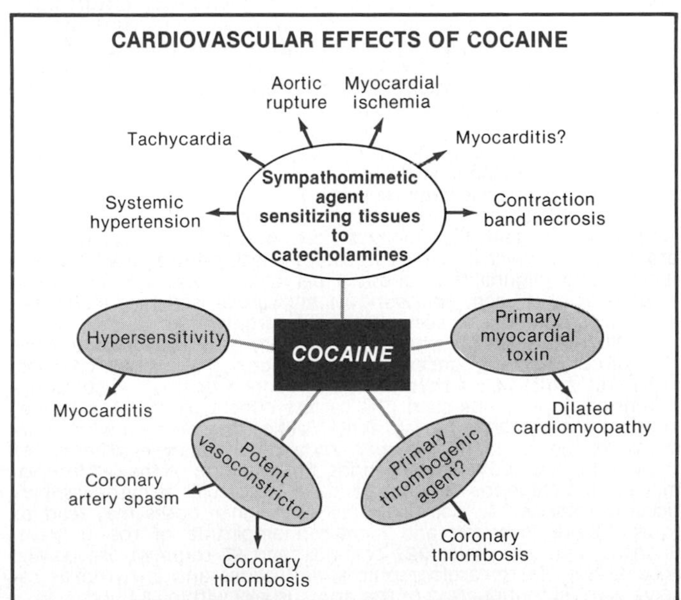

FIGURE 41–31. Diagram showing the effects of cocaine on the heart. (From Waller, B. F.: Cocaine and the heart. Indiana Med. *81*:956, 1988.)

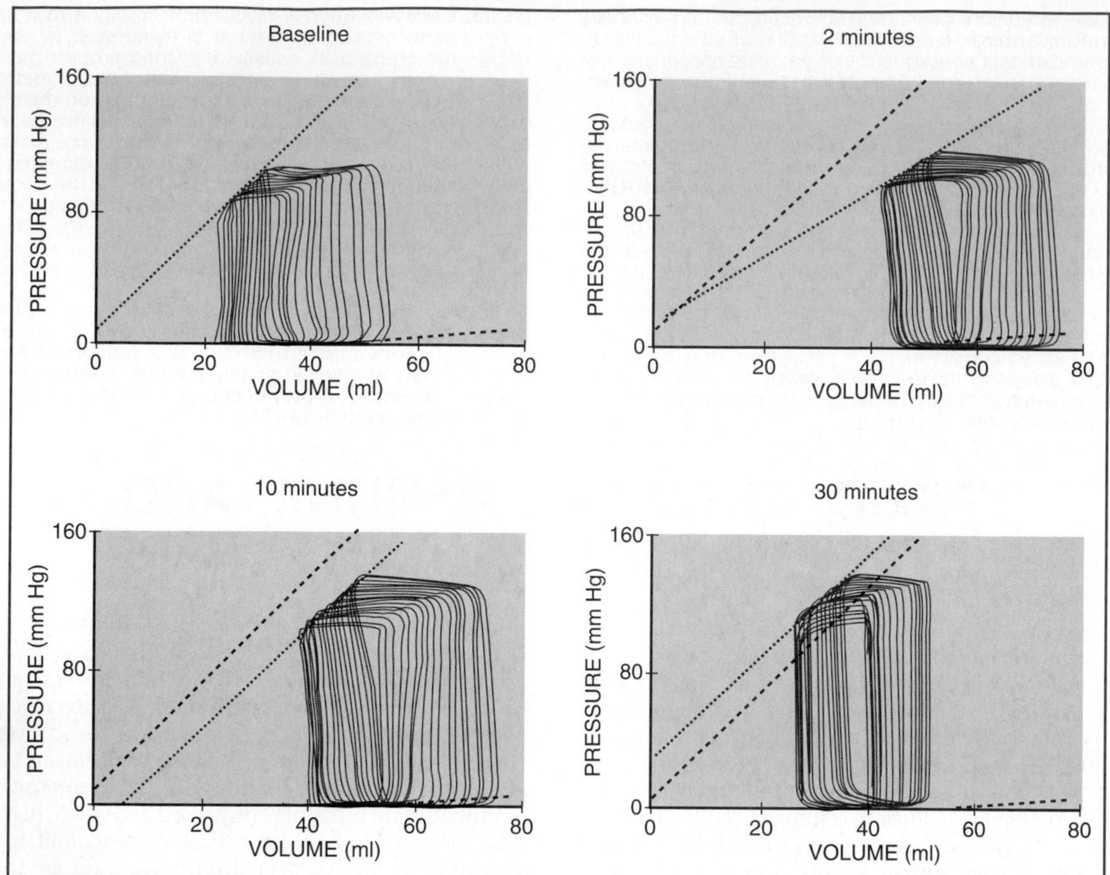

FIGURE 41–32. Left ventricular pressure-volume loops in canine subjected to injection of cocaine. The dashed line at the left upper boundary is the end-systolic pressure-volume relationship that defines the contractile state of the ventricle. There is evidence of contractile depression *(dotted line)* at 2 minutes, with partial resolution at 10 minutes. By 30 minutes there has been complete recovery of the transient myocardial depression. (From Liu, C. P., Tunin, C., and Kass, D. A.: Transient time course of cocaine-induced cardiac depression versus sustained peripheral vasoconstriction. Reprinted by permission of the American College of Cardiology. J. Am. Coll. Cardiol. *21*:260, 1993.)

Cardiotoxicity, usually consisting of hypotension, tachycardia, and transient arrhythmias, occurs in a minority of patients (perhaps up to 10 per cent).[744,745] Several patients have developed congestive heart failure and the clinical picture of a dilated cardiomyopathy during interferon-alpha therapy; in at least some patients, cardiomyopathy resolves rapidly with discontinuation of interferon.[745]

TRICYCLIC ANTIDEPRESSANTS. Although sudden death, disturbances in rhythm, and abnormalities of atrioventricular conduction may be seen with the tricyclic antidepressants, particularly when taken as an overdose,[746] important depression of left ventricular function is usually not seen, even in patients with pre-existing heart disease. Particular caution is indicated when using tricyclic antidepressants in patients with prior myocardial infarction and/or pre-existing ventricular arrhythmias, as these agents have a class I antiarrhythmic effect and might be proarrhythmic in these settings.[746] A rare case of hypersensitivity myocarditis has been reported.[747]

INTERLEUKIN-2 (see also p. 1803). The lymphokine interleukin-2, an antineoplastic agent, has significant cardiovascular toxicity, the most prominent of which is a diffuse capillary leak syndrome with hypotension and oliguria.[748] In about 5 per cent of patients, additional cardiotoxicity is seen, consisting of myocardial ischemia, infarction, injury, arrhythmias, and eosinophilic myocarditis.[748–750]

PHENOTHIAZINES. The phenothiazines may be associated with a variety of cardiac disturbances, including electrocardiographic changes, atrial and ventricular arrhythmias, and sudden death.[751] Postural hypotension may also be seen. The cardiac effects are largely dose-dependent. Electrocardiographic abnormalities may be seen with as little as 200 mg of thioridazine per day and consist of lengthening of the Q-T interval and T-wave changes. Prolongation of the Q-T interval may set the stage for the emergence of ventricular arrhythmias, particularly torsades de pointes (p. 685).[751] Higher doses may lead to frank T-wave inversion and increased amplitude of the U wave. Changes in the P wave, QRS complex, and ST segment are usually absent. The electrocardiographic abnormalities and arrhythmias resolve with discontinuation of the drug, usually within 48 hours.

Pathological changes in the hearts of patients who have received psychotropic drugs and who have died suddenly include the deposition of acid mucopolysaccharide between muscle bundles in periarteriolar regions as well as the conduction system, with myofibrillar degeneration, and endothelial proliferation in the smaller blood vessels, although a direct causal relationship between drug administration and cardiomyopathic changes is only inferential.[752] A variety of explanations have been invoked for the apparent cardiac damage, including direct toxic effects of the phenothiazines on the myocardium, stimulation of higher autonomic centers, and changes in circulating or myocardial levels of catecholamines.

EMETINE. Cardiovascular changes are said to be common with the chronic use of emetine, a drug often employed in the treatment of amebiasis and schistosomiasis as well as the active ingredient in ipecac syrup (used for childhood poisoning).[753] Myocardial lesions may be observed in some but not all patients at autopsy, and similar cardiac damage is noted in experimental animals given emetine.[753,754] The myocardial lesions consist of myofibrillar degeneration and necrosis,[754] with an interstitial infiltrate of mononuclear cells and histiocytes.

The *electrocardiogram,* which may be abnormal in 50 per cent of treated patients, most commonly shows reduced T-wave amplitude or inversion. Prolongation of the Q-T interval and ST-segment shifts may also be seen, although abnormalities of the P wave, P-R segment, and QRS complex are infrequent. The electrocardiographic changes usually resolve within weeks or months after cessation of treatment. Sinus tachycardia and hypotension may also be seen, although clinical evidence of myocardial toxicity is usually lacking. Only rare fatalities have been reported.[755] *Dehydroemetine* results in electrocardiographic abnormalities similar to those of emetine, but they are less prominent and of shorter duration.

METHYSERGIDE. The widespread fibrotic reactions seen with this drug can also involve the heart. Up to 1 per cent of patients treated long term may develop typically left-sided valvular lesions, resulting in stenosis and regurgitation.[752] Fibrotic endocardial and pericardial lesions are also seen on occasion, producing a hemodynamic picture of restrictive and constrictive disease.[756]

CHLOROQUINE. This drug has been widely used in the prophylaxis and treatment of a variety of parasitic and other diseases, including collagen and dermatologic disorders.[757] Electrocardiographic changes may be seen with its use, along with conduction disturbances and features of a restrictive cardiomyopathy.[757] In toxic doses, chloroquine may result in depressed cardiac output, bradycardia, arrhythmias, heart block, and death. Characteristic histological changes are found by electron microscopy (Fig. 41–33).[757]

ANTIMONY COMPOUNDS. Various antimony compounds, such as stibophen and tartar emetic, have been widely used in the treatment of schistosomiasis; less toxic agents are now becoming available. The antimony compounds are associated with electrocardiographic changes in almost all patients.[758] Typical *electrocardiographic changes* include prolongation of the Q-T interval with flattening or inversion of T waves.[758] ST-segment shifts and P-wave changes may be seen, although the QRS complex usually demonstrates no abnormality. The majority of patients do not demonstrate cardiac findings, although chest pain, bradycardia, hypotension, ventricular arrhythmias (including paroxysmal ventricular tachycardia), and sudden death may occur.[758]

LITHIUM. Lithium carbonate, used in the treatment of bipolar disorders, is associated with T-wave changes in one-fourth or more of patients who receive the drug.[759] Clinical evidence of myocardial involvement is usually lacking, although intoxication with lithium may be associated with ventricular arrhythmias, symptomatic sinus node abnormalities, AV conduction disturbances, congestive heart failure, and in rare cases, death.[759] In fatal lithium toxicity, the heart is said to be dilated, with evidence of myofibrillar degeneration associated with a lymphocytic interstitial infiltrate and fibrosis, although no definite proof is available that these changes are due to lithium.[759]

HYDROCARBONS. Ingestion of hydrocarbons may result in fragmentation and vacuolization of the muscle fibers with loss of cross-striations.[760] Electrocardiographic changes, arrhythmias, and cardiomegaly may occur. Involvement of the central nervous, renal, hepatic, and pulmonary systems may dominate the clinical presentation and obscure the myocardial damage, which may well contribute to the mortality of hydrocarbon ingestion.[760]

The *fluorinated hydrocarbons,* commonly used as aerosol propellants, appear to be cardiac toxins, contrary to their reputation of being inert. In animal preparations at least, the aerosol propellants cause ventricular tachyarrhythmias, depress myocardial contractility, and lower systemic vascular resistance and arterial pressure.[761] These cardiovascular effects may be involved in the sudden deaths seen in individuals who abuse aerosols for their psychotropic effect.[761]

CATECHOLAMINES. A severe reversible dilated cardiomyopathy has been observed in conjunction with pheochromocytoma, and the myocardial damage has been attributed to high levels of circulating catecholamines (see p. 829).[762–764] Similar changes have been demonstrated in experimental animals treated with prolonged infusions of L-norepinephrine.[763,764] Catecholamines also may produce acute myocarditis, with focal myocardial necrosis, inflammation, epicardial hemorrhages, tachycardia, and arrhythmias.[765] Similar findings have been described with excessive use of beta-adrenoceptor agonist inhalants and methylxanthines in the treatment of decompensated pulmonary disease.[766] The cardiomyopathy associated with pheochromocytoma is one of the conditions that should be considered when heart failure suddenly appears without other obvious explanation.[763,764]

A variety of mechanisms of myocardial damage have been suggested.[767] A direct toxic effect may be involved, or the damage may be secondary to relative tissue hypoxia because of heightened metabolic demands. Alternatively, the damage may result from changes in autonomic tone, enhanced lipid mobility, calcium overload, damaging effects of catecholamine oxidation products (free radicals), or increased sarcolemmal permeability.[765,767,768] Catecholamine-induced vasospasm also may play a role.[764]

LEAD. The prominent features in lead poisoning generally center on the gastrointestinal and central nervous systems. However, myocardial involvement may contribute to or be the principal cause of death in some cases.[769] Electrocardiographic changes, atrioventricular conduction defects, and overt congestive heart failure may occur.[769] The electrocardiographic and myocardial changes appear to be reversible with chelation therapy.[769]

CARBON MONOXIDE. Both acute and chronic carbon monoxide toxicity can occur. Although central nervous system findings usually dominate the clinical presentation, significant and occasionally fatal cardiac abnormalities may be present.[770] Because carbon monoxide has a higher affinity for hemoglobin than does oxygen, reduced amounts of oxygen are delivered to the tissues. Thus, the cardiac toxicity may be partially caused by myocardial hypoxia, but a direct toxic effect of the gas on myocardial mitochondria may play an even more important role.[771,772] The *histological features* include focal areas of necrosis, most marked in the subendocardium. Focal perivascular infiltrates and punctate hemorrhages are also seen.[772]

Cardiac involvement may appear promptly after exposure, or it may be delayed for up to several days. Palpitations, sinus tachycardia, and various arrhythmias, including ventricular extrasystoles and atrial fibrillation, are common.[773] Bradycardia and AV block may occur in more severe cases.[773] In patients with ischemic heart disease, angina pectoris and myocardial infarction may be precipitated. Electrocardiographic ST-segment and T-wave abnormalities are quite common. Transient right and/or left ventricular wall motion abnormalities may be present.[772] Administration of 100 per cent oxygen, bed rest, and surveillance for serious rhythm or conduction abnormalities usually permit rapid recovery.

HYPOCALCEMIA. In rare patients with chronic hypocalcemia (often due to hypoparathyroidism), congestive heart failure may occur and resolve only when the serum calcium level is raised.[774] Rapid transfusion of citrated blood can produce hypocalcemia and reversible myocardial depression, as can ambulatory peritoneal dialysis in patients with chronic renal failure.[775]

HYPOPHOSPHATEMIA. A form of reversible left ventricular dysfunction may be seen with severe hypophosphatemia. Restoration of the serum phosphate level to normal results in hemodynamic recovery.

HYPOMAGNESEMIA. Focal cardiac necrosis is found in experimental magnesium deficiency and may account for the supraventricular and ventricular arrhythmias and electrocardiographic changes that are seen clinically. In addition to arrhythmias, coronary spasm and acute myocardial infarction may be seen.[776] A rare case of fatal cardiomyopathy has been reported.[776,777]

TAURINE DEFICIENCY. A deficiency of taurine, an amino acid found in high concentration in cardiac and retinal tissue, produces a dilated cardiomyopathy in cats that is reversible with oral taurine supplementation.[778] Whether a similar condition exists in humans is not known; this has been the subject of speculation.[779]

CARNITINE DEFICIENCY. Carnitine, an essential cofactor for the oxidation of fatty acids, produces a hypertrophic or dilated cardiomyopathy in children when deficient.[780–783] Carnitine supplementation can lead to symptomatic and functional improvement[700,703–785]; determination of carnitine levels therfore is important in children with unexplained cardiomyopathy.[780] Myocardial carnitine levels are reduced in the hearts of patients with dilated cardiomyopathy, but the significance of this observation is not known at present.[781]

SELENIUM DEFICIENCY. Dietary deficiency of the trace element selenium appears to be one of the principal factors responsible for a form of dilated cardiomyopathy endemic to certain rural areas in China,[786] although the etiological role played by selenium has been

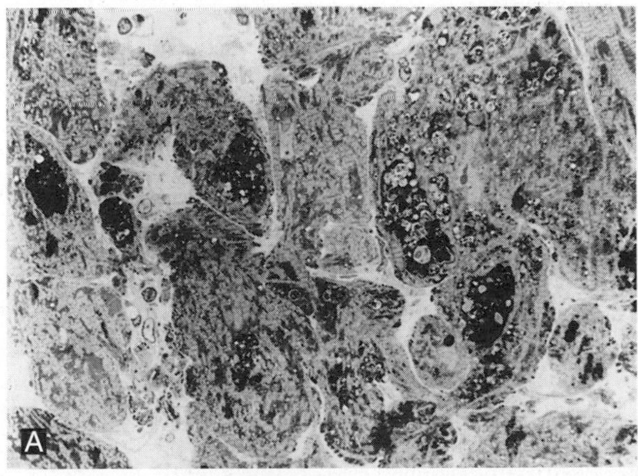

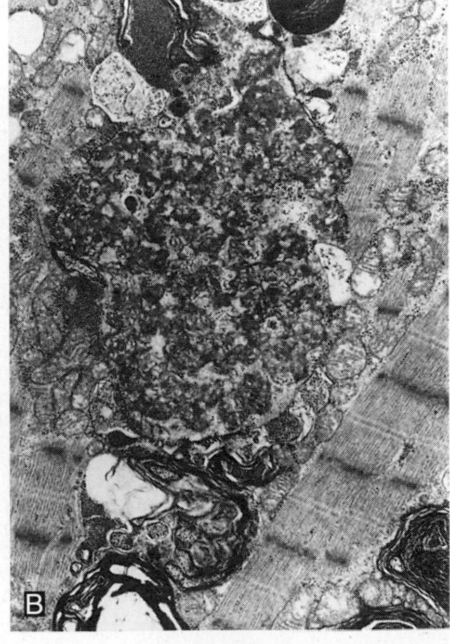

FIGURE 41–33. Endomyocardial biopsy specimen from a patient with chloroquine cardiomyopathy. *A,* 1-μm-thick section demonstrating numerous cytoplasmic inclusions that occupy the central area of myocytes (alkaline toluidine blue stain, ×700). *B,* Electron micrograph demonstrating that the cytoplasmic inclusions are composed of irregularly arranged electron-dense concentric lamellae and curvilinear bodies (×30,000). (Reproduced by permission from Ferrans, V. J., Hall, R. J., and McAllister, H. A. Jr.: Chloroquine-induced cardiomyopathy. Circulation *88:*785, 1993; copyright, 1993 American Heart Association.)

questioned.[787,788] Termed *Keshan disease*, it affects mainly children and young women and apparently is prevented by the prophylactic administration of sodium selenite tablets.[787,789] A similar cardiomyopathy may be found in Occidentals subjected to prolonged parenteral hyperalimentation; supplementation with oral selenium may reverse the cardiomyopathy.[788,790,791]

SCORPION STING. The venom of the scorpion is mainly neurotoxic, but cardiac findings may be prominent and even fatal, particularly in children.[792–795] Electrocardiographic changes and myocardial damage with elevated serum cardiac enzyme levels are common findings.[795] Hearts are normal on gross examination, with prominent microscopic changes usually but not invariably present, particularly in the subendocardial region and papillary muscles. Degeneration and necrosis of muscle fibers are noted, with interstitial edema and a mononuclear infiltrate.[795] The histological features of scorpion sting suggest high levels of circulating catecholamines and are similar to those seen with experimental catecholamine infusion and in pheochromocytoma.[792] The parasympathetic system appears to be stimulated as well.[792]

The *electrocardiogram* often initially shows tall, peaked T waves that progress to inversions and ST-segment shifts. Q waves may appear, and the Q-T interval is usually prolonged.[796] Atrial, junctional, and ventricular arrhythmias may occur. Tachycardia, hypertension, anxiety, diaphoresis, and pulmonary edema—findings resembling those of a massive catecholamine effect—are striking in many patients.[796] A smaller number of patients are seen in shock with peripheral vascular collapse. Most deaths are due to pulmonary edema, presumably the result of left ventricular dysfunction.[797] Occasionally, sudden and unexpected deaths occur in a smaller percentage of patients, presumably as a consequence of arrhythmias. Adrenergic blocking agents and the use of specific antivenom appear to be useful in the management of the cardiovascular manifestation of scorpion stings.[794]

WASP AND SPIDER STINGS. Stings by the vespine wasps may lead to anaphylaxis, with hypotension, circulatory collapse, and cyanosis.[798] Occasional patients may have chest pain and clinical findings compatible with acute myocardial infarction.[798] The mechanism of myocardial damage is unclear; perhaps it merely reflects necrosis from profound hypotension, although a direct toxic effect on the myocardium or an indirect effect on the coronary arteries may be involved.[798]

SNAKE BITE. Cardiac complications are not prominent features of snake bites, and the clinical picture is usually dominated by the neurological, hematological, and vascular damage produced by the snakebite toxin.[799,800] Myocardial involvement is seen on occasion and may rarely contribute to morbidity and mortality. T-wave abnormalities are the most common manifestation of myocardial involvement, although ST-segment depression, QRS prolongation, and AV conduction defects may also be seen.[751] The electrocardiographic changes are usually transient, but when persistent they are attributed to direct myocardial damage due to the toxin. Death may occur from circulatory collapse, myocardial depression, or myocardial infarction due to hypotension and coronary artery thrombosis. Coronary artery vasospasm may also be involved.[801,802]

ARSENIC. Myocardial involvement may be seen in both acute and chronic arsenical poisoning, usually from pesticides; the heart may be dilated, with accumulation of pericardial fluid.[803] Multiple local and confluent areas of subepicardial and subendocardial hemorrhage are characteristic findings. The myocardium is usually abnormal, with evidence of a perivascular mononuclear infiltrate.[803]

Clinically unrecognized interstitial myocarditis is manifested by T-wave inversions and ST-segment depressions, along with prolongation of the Q-T interval.[803] The electrocardiographic changes usually revert to normal within 2 to 4 weeks. The electrocardiographic abnormalities appear to resolve more rapidly when BAL (British antilewisite, dimercaprol) is used in therapy.[803]

CYCLOPHOSPHAMIDE (see also p. 1803). High doses of cyclophosphamide have been associated with electrocardiographic changes, congestive heart failure, and death from hemorrhagic myocarditis.[804] In the majority of patients treated, a reversible decrease of QRS voltage and systolic function is seen, often asymptomatic, although more than 20 per cent may succumb as a consequence of myopericarditis.[805] The myocardial damage appears to result from direct endothelial damage and resultant fibrin microthrombi in the capillaries.

AZIDE. Sodium azide, a chemical preservative that interferes with oxidative phosphorylation, may produce fatal acute cardiotoxicity when accidentally ingested.[806,807] Pathological findings include marked interstitial edema and myofibrillar degeneration. Clinical features include arrhythmias, myocardial ischemia, left ventricular dysfunction, and hypotension.[806]

PARACETAMOL. Paracetamol, a phenacetin metabolite, may result in massive liver necrosis. On occasion it also results in fatty degeneration and focal necrosis of the myocardium after an overdose.[808]

5-FLUOROURACIL. This antineoplastic agent has been associated with cardiotoxicity manifested by chest pain, electrocardiographic changes, and arrhythmia.[809,810] Swelling of myocardial fibers without an inflammatory infiltrate has been found at necropsy.[811]

PACLITAXEL. The most common cardiac effect of paclitaxel is sinus bradycardia, usually asymptomatic, which occurs in about one-fourth of patients.[812] A variety of other findings (ischemia, arrhythmias, conduction defects) have been noted on occasion, but usually in patients with pre-existing cardiac pathology; the etiologic role of paclitaxel is not established.[812]

HYPERSENSITIVITY

Hypersensitivity to a variety of agents may result in allergic reactions that involve the myocardium. A variety of drugs (most commonly the sulfonamides, the penicillins, and methyldopa) or other sensitizers may lead to an allergic myocarditis (Table 41–16),[813] characterized by peripheral eosinophilia and a perivascular infiltration of the myocardium by eosinophils, lymphocytes, and histiocytes; necrosis is seen on occasion.[814,815] Hypersensitivity myocarditis is rarely recognized clinically and is often first discovered at postmortem examination, although it is occasionally diagnosed on endomyocardial biopsy.[815,816] Most patients who have hypersensitivity myocarditis are not critically ill, but die suddenly, presumably the consequence of an arrhythmia. An occasional patient has intense eosinophilic infiltration of the myocardium of no obvious cause, with prominent necrosis evident and findings of hemodynamic collapse; some of these patients may have undiagnosed hypersensitivity myocarditis.[463,814,816] Because of the potential for significant deleterious effects, a high index of suspicion for this condition should be maintained; in one unusual case, penicillin residue in pet food led to hypersensitivity myocarditis in a young child.[817] Therapy includes discontinuation of the offending agent and corticosteroids and/or immunosuppression therapy in severe cases.[814,816]

METHYLDOPA. Although hepatitis is the most frequently encountered serious adverse reaction to methyldopa, sudden and unexpected death has been reported in a number of patients found at necropsy to have had an unsuspected myocarditis.[815,816] The *histological findings* have the characteristics of an allergic myocarditis, showing an interstitial inflammatory infiltrate with abundant eosinophils,[815] a vasculitis, and focal myocardial necrosis. Electrocardiographic changes include sinus bradycardia, sinus pauses, and first- and second-degree AV block.[818]

PENICILLIN. Allergic reactions to penicillin are fairly common, but myocardial involvement is rare.[819] *Histological findings* consist of a perivascular and interstitial infiltrate composed of eosinophils and mononuclear cells.[815] Both myocardial infarction and pericarditis may occur and account for some of the electrocardiographic changes.[817,820] Transient electrocardiographic changes may be the only manifestation of cardiac involvement, with sinus tachycardia, ST-segment elevation, and T-wave inversion.[817]

SULFONAMIDES. Sulfonamides may result in myocardial damage owing to a hypersensitivity vasculitis as well as a myocarditis.[820] In fatal cases eosinophilic myocarditis,[815] sometimes with granulomas, usually can be demonstrated. Although usually clinically silent, myocardial involvement may produce severe and even fatal congestive heart failure.[816] Electrocardiographic changes are usually absent, but nonspecific ST-segment and T-wave abnormalities may be seen.

TETRACYCLINE. Allergic reactions to antibiotics of the tetracycline class include fever, tachycardia, and first-degree AV block. Postmortem findings include cardiac dilatation, fibrinoid muscle cell degeneration, and a diffuse interstitial and perivascular infiltrate.[815]

TABLE 41–16 PRINCIPAL DRUGS CAPABLE OF CAUSING HYPERSENSITIVITY MYOCARDITIS

Antibiotics	**Anti-inflammatory**
Amphotericin B	Indomethacin
Ampicillin	Oxyphenbutazone
Chloramphenicol	Phenylbutazone
Penicillin	
Tetracycline	**Diuretics**
Streptomycin	Acetazolamide
	Chlorthalidone
Sulfonamides	Hydrochlorothiazide
Sulfadiazine	Spironolactone
Sulfisoxazole	
	Others
Anticonvulsants	Amitriptyline
Phenindione	Methyldopa
Phenytoin	Sulfonylureas
Carbamazepine	Tetanus toxoid
Antituberculous	
Isoniazid	
Paraaminosalicylic acid	

From Kounis, N. G., Zavras, G. M., Soufras, G. D., and Kitrou, M. P.: Hypersensitivity myocarditis. Ann. Allergy *62*:71, 1989.

ANTITUBERCULOUS DRUGS. Most reactions to antituberculous drugs consist of a fever, rash, or both, but serious and fatal cardiac reactions may occur on rare occasions. *Paraaminosalicylic acid* may lead to the development of interstitial edema, acute inflammatory infiltrate, refractory congestive heart failure, hypotension, and ventricular irritability.[821]

Streptomycin has been implicated as an unusual cause of myocarditis. Pathological findings may include cardiac dilatation, myocarditis with necrosis, hemorrhage, and a fibrinous pericardial effusion.[821] Clinically, it may be associated with chest pain, dyspnea, fever, and rash, followed by collapse and death.

GIANT CELL MYOCARDITIS

Giant cell myocarditis is a rare disease of unknown cause characterized by the presence of multinucleated giant cells in the myocardium. (It is included here because of the possibility that it may be of immune or autoimmune origin.) Also called granulomatous myocarditis, this condition is typically a rapidly fatal disease, often of young to middle-aged adults.[822] *Pathological findings* are usually impressive. The ventricles are dilated, and mural thrombi may be present. A serpiginous area of myocardial necrosis may be seen involving the right as well as the left ventricle.[822] Multinucleated giant cells are found, particularly at the margins of the areas of myocardial necrosis; the giant cells appear to be of macrophage rather than myocyte origin.[823]

Giant cell myocarditis occurs on occasion in association with systemic diseases such as sarcoidosis, systemic lupus erythematosus, drug hypersensitivity, infections (especially syphilis and tuberculosis), and thyrotoxicosis, but the cause of the disease remains obscure.[822] In many ways the clinical features suggest a viral myocarditis except for the rapid and virulent course. However, despite careful investigation there has been no serological or bacteriological evidence of an infectious cause.[822,823] It has been suggested that the cause is an autoimmune reaction, although little evidence aside from the histological findings supports this view.[822,823]

Both genders are equally affected; the onset typically is rapid, with dyspnea, chest pain, orthopnea, and hypotension. Fever is usually present, with electrocardiographic evidence of widespread myocardial involvement. Conduction defects, ventricular arrhythmias, and AV block are common.[822] Overt congestive heart failure and sudden death may occur.[824] Therapy (other than cardiac transplantation[825,826]) often is unsuccessful, although corticosteroids and immunosuppressive agents appear to have benefited some patients. Because the prognosis in general is poor, empirical immunosuppressive therapy probably is warranted.[822,823,827–829] Occasional patients have had long-term survival.[825]

PHYSICAL AGENTS

HEAT STROKE. This condition results from failure of the thermoregulatory center following exposure to high ambient temperature and is manifested principally by hyperpyrexia and central nervous system dysfunction. However, cardiovascular abnormalities (usually electrocardiographic) appear to be common; pulmonary edema and right ventricular dysfunction may occur,[830] along with hypotension and circulatory collapse. *Pathological changes* include dilatation of the right side of the heart, particularly the right atrium. Hemorrhages of the subendocardium and the subepicardium are frequently seen at necropsy and often involve the interventricular septum and posterior wall of the left ventricle.[830] Histological findings include degeneration and necrosis of muscle fibers as well as interstitial edema.[830] Possible factors responsible for myocardial damage include direct thermal injury, myocardial hypoxia secondary to circulatory collapse, decreased coronary blood flow, and metabolic abnormalities resulting from widespread injury to other organs.

Sinus tachycardia is invariably present, whereas atrial and ventricular arrhythmias are usually absent. Transient prolongation of the Q-T interval may be seen, along with ST-segment and T-wave abnormalities. It may take up to several months for these repolarization abnormalities to resolve. Serum enzyme levels may be elevated and may reflect myocardial damage, at least in part.[830]

HYPOTHERMIA. Low temperature may also result in myocardial damage. Cardiac dilatation may occur with epicardial petechiae and subendocardial hemorrhages. Microinfarcts are found in the ventricular myocardium, presumably related to abnormalities in the microcirculation.[831] The lesions are not due to the low temperature per se but appear to be the result of the circulatory collapse, hemoconcentration, capillary slugging, and depressed cellular metabolism that accompany hypothermia. Clinical manifestations of hypothermia include sinus bradycardia, conduction disturbances, atrial (and occasionally ventricular) fibrillation, hypotension, a fall in cardiac output, reversible myocardial depression, and a characteristic deflection of the terminal portion of the QRS pattern (Osborn wave).[831,832] Treatment includes core warming, cardiopulmonary resuscitation, and management of pulmonary, hematological, and renal complications.[832]

RADIATION. The use of ionizing radiation during radiation therapy (or less commonly after radiation accidents) may result in a variety of occasionally acute but usually chronic cardiac complications, including pericarditis with effusion, tamponade, or constriction; coronary artery fibrosis and myocardial infarction; valvular abnormalities; myocardial fibrosis; and conduction disturbances.[833–835] Although the heart has been regarded as one of the organs more resistant to the effects of radiation, the clinical significance of radiation-induced heart disease is greater than usually thought.[834] Although radiation probably results in some degree of tissue damage in all patients, clinically significant cardiac involvement occurs in the minority of patients, usually long after the radiation treatment has ended.[834] Radiation-induced cardiac damage is related to the dose of radiation, the mass of heart irradiated, and the dose schedule of the radiation.

The late cardiac damage that may follow irradiation appears to result from a long-lasting injury of the capillary endothelial cells, which leads to cell death, capillary rupture, and microthrombi.[834] Because of this damage to the microvasculature, ischemia results and is followed by myocardial fibrosis. In addition to microvascular damage, the major epicardial coronary arteries may become narrowed, especially at the ostia.[835,836]

Only an occasional patient manifests acute cardiac abnormality clinically with radiation therapy; typically this consists of acute pericarditis. A mild, transient, asymptomatic depression of left ventricular function may be seen early after radiation therapy.[837] The more common clinical expressions of radiation heart disease occur months or years after the exposure. The pericardium is the most common site of clinical involvement, with findings of chronic pericardial effusion or pericardial constriction.[834] Myocardial damage occurs less frequently and is characterized by myocardial fibrosis with or without endocardial fibrosis or fibroelastosis. Left and/or right ventricular dysfunction at rest or with exercise appears to be a common, albeit usually asymptomatic, finding 5 to 20 years after radiation therapy, especially in those in whom the now-outmoded technique of a single anteroposterior port was used.[834,838,839] Occasional patients may develop usually asymptomatic left-sided (and rarely right-sided) valvular regurgitation (or on occasion stenosis) that rarely requires valve replacement; often there is a latent period of a decade or more between the radiation exposure and the development of valvular deformity.[833,839–842] Electrocardiographic abnormalities, heart block, and a variety of arrhythmias may be seen months or years after therapeutic radiation, although usually they are of limited clinical significance.[840,843,844]

REFERENCES

1. Siu, S. C., and Sole, M. J.: Dilated cardiomyopathy. Curr. Opin. Cardiol. *9*:337, 1994.
2. Hare, J. M., Walford, G. D., Hruban, R. H., et al.: Ischemic cardiomyopathy: Endomyocardial biopsy and ventriculographic evaluation of patients with congestive heart failure, dilated cardiomyopathy and coronary artery disease. J. Am. Coll. Cardiol. *20*:1318, 1992.
3. Sugrue, D. D., Rodeheffer, R. J., Codd, M. B., et al.: The clinical course of idiopathic dilated cardiomyopathy. A population-based study. Ann. Intern. Med. *117*:117, 1992.

4. Coughlin, S. S., Comstock, G. W., and Baughman, K. L.: Descriptive epidemiology of idiopathic dilated cardiomyopathy in Washington County, Maryland, 1975–1991. J. Clin. Epidemiol. *46:*1003, 1993.
5. Manolio, T. A., Baughman, K. L., Rodeheffer, R., et al.: Prevalence and etiology of idiopathic dilated cardiomyopathy (summary of a National Heart, Lung, and Blood Institute workshop). Am. J. Cardiol. *69:*1458, 1992.
5a. Richarrdson, P., McKenna, W., Bristow, M., et al.: Report of the 1995 World Health Organization/International Society and Federation of Cardiology Task Force on the Definition and Classification of Cardiomyopathies. Circulation *93:*841, 1996.
6. Keren, A., and Popp, R. L.: Assignment of patients into the classification of cardiomyopathies. Circulation *86:*1622, 1992.
7. Boffa, G. M., Thiene, G., Nava, A., and Dalla Volta, S.: Cardiomyopathy: A necessary revision of the WHO classification. Int. J. Cardiol. *30:*1, 1991.
8. Abelmann, W. H.: Introduction. *In* Abelmann W. H. (ed.): Cardiomyopathies, Myocarditis, and Pericardial Disease. Current Medicine *1:*2, 1995.
9. Goodwin, J. F.: Cardiomyopathies and specific heart muscle diseases. Definitions, terminology, classifications and new and old approaches. Postgrad. Med. J. *68*(Suppl. 1):S3, 1992.
10. Kasper, E. K., Agema, W. R., Hutchins, G. M., et al.: The causes of dilated cardiomyopathy: A clinicopathologic review of 673 consecutive patients. J. Am. Coll. Cardiol. *23:*586, 1994.
11. Mason, J. W.: Endomyocardial biopsy and the causes of dilated cardiomyopathy. J. Am. Coll. Cardiol. *23:*591, 1994.
12. Pytlewski, G., Georgeson, S., Burke, J., et al.: Endomyocardial biopsy under transesophageal echocardiographic guidance can be safely performed in the critically ill cardiac transplant recipient. Am. J. Cardiol. *73:*1019, 1994.
13. Balzer, D., Moorhead, S., Saffitz, J. E., et al.: Pediatric endomyocardial biopsy performed solely with echocardiographic guidance. J. Am. Soc. Echocardiogr. *6:*510, 1993.
14. Blomstrom-Lundqvist, C., Noor, A. M., Eskilsson, J., and Persson, S.: Safety of transvenous right ventricular endomyocardial biopsy guided by two-dimensional echocardiography. Clin. Cardiol. *16:*487, 1993.
15. Bell, C. A., Kern, M. J., Aguirre, F. V., et al.: Superior accuracy of anatomic positioning with echocardiographic-over fluoroscopic-guided endomyocardial biopsy. Cathet. Cardiovasc. Diagn. *28:*291, 1993.
16. Herskowitz, A., Campbell, S., Deckers, J., et al.: Demographic features and prevalence of idiopathic myocarditis in patients undergoing endomyocardial biopsy. Am. J. Cardiol. *71:*982, 1993.
17. Kyu, B., Matsumori, A., Sato, Y., et al.: Cardiac persistence of cardioviral RNA detected by polymerase chain reaction in a murine model of dilated cardiomyopathy. Circulation *86:*522, 1992.
18. Archard, L. C., Bowles, N. E., Cunningham, L., et al.: Molecular probes for detection of persisting enterovirus infection of human heart and their prognostic value. Eur. Heart J. *12*(Suppl. D):56, 1991.
19. Jin, O., Sole, M. J., Butany, J. W., et al.: Detection of enterovirus RNA in myocardial biopsies from patients with myocarditis and cardiomyopathy using gene amplification by polymerase chain reaction. Circulation *82:*8, 1990.
20. Martin, A. B., Webber, S., Fricker, F. J., et al.: Acute myocarditis. Rapid diagnosis by PCR in children. Circulation *90:*330, 1994.
21. Okada, I., Matsumori, A., and Kyu, B.: Detection of viral RNA in experimental coxsackievirus B3 myocarditis of mice using the polymerase chain reaction. Int. J. Exp. Pathol. *73:*721, 1992.

DILATED CARDIOMYOPATHY

22. Keren, A., Gottlieb, S., Tzivoni, D., et al.: Mildly dilated congestive cardiomyopathy. Use of prospective diagnostic criteria and description of the clinical course without heart transplantation. Circulation *81:*506, 1990.
23. Mestroni, L., Krajinovic, M., Severini, G. M., et al.: Familial dilated cardiomyopathy. Br. Heart J. *72:*S35, 1994.
24. Dec, G. W., and Fuster, V.: Medical progress: Idiopathic dilated cardiomyopathy. N. Engl. J. Med. *331:*1564, 1994.
25. Coughlin, S. S., Neaton, J. D., Sengupta, A., and Kuller, L. H.: Predictors of mortality from idiopathic dilated cardiomyopathy in 356,222 men screened for the Multiple Risk Factor Intervention Trial. Am. J. Epidemiol. *139:*166, 1994.
26. Coughlin, S. S., Labenberg, J. R., and Tefft, M. C.: Black-white differences in idiopathic dilated cardiomyopathy: The Washington DC Dilated Cardiomyopathy Study. Epidemiology *4:*165, 1993.
27. Coughlin, S. S., Szklo, M., Baughman, K., and Pearson, T. A.: The epidemiology of idiopathic dilated cardiomyopathy in a biracial community. Am. J. Epidemiol. *131:*48, 1990.
28. Coughlin, S. S., Gottdiener, J. S., Baughman, K. L., et al.: Black-white differences in mortality in idiopathic dilated cardiomyopathy: The Washington DC Dilated Cardiomyopathy Study. J. Natl. Med. Assoc. *86:*583, 1994.
29. Redfield, M. M., Gersh, B. J., Bailey, K. R., and Rodeheffer, R. J.: Natural history of incidentally discovered, asymptomatic idiopathic dilated cardiomyopathy. Am. J. Cardiol. *74:*737, 1994.
30. Steimle, A. E., Stevenson, L. W., Fonarow, G. C., et al.: Prediction of improvement in recent onset cardiomyopathy after referral for heart transplantation. J. Am. Coll. Cardiol. *23:*553, 1994.
31. Semigran, M. J., Thaik, C. M., Fifer, M. A., et al.: Exercise capacity and systolic and diastolic ventricular function after recovery from acute dilated cardiomyopathy. J. Am. Coll. Cardiol. [illegible], 1994.
32. Fruhwald, F. M., Dusleag, J., Eber, B., et al.: Long-term outcome and prognostic factors in dilated cardiomyopathy. Preliminary results. Angiology *45:*763, 1994.
33. Anguita, M., Arizon, J. M., Bueno, G., et al.: Clinical and hemodynamic predictors of survival in patients aged <65 years with severe congestive heart failure secondary to ischemic or nonischemic dilated cardiomyopathy. Am. J. Cardiol. *72:*413, 1993.
34. Borggrefe, M., Block, M., and Breithardt, G.: Identification and management of the high risk patient with dilated cardiomyopathy. Br. Heart J. *72:*S42, 1994.
35. De Maria, R., Gavazzi, A., Recalcati, F., et al.: Comparison of clinical findings in idiopathic dilated cardiomyopathy in women versus men. The Italian Multicenter Cardiomyopathy Study Group (SPIC). Am. J. Cardiol. *72:*580, 1993.
36. Saxon, L. A., Stevenson, W. G., Middlekauff, H. R., et al.: Predicting death from progressive heart failure secondary to ischemic or idiopathic dilated cardiomyopathy. Am. J. Cardiol. *72:*62, 1993.
37. Pelliccia, F., d'Amati, G., Cianfrocca, C., et al.: Histomorphometric features predict 1-year outcome of patients with idiopathic dilated cardiomyopathy considered to be at low priority for cardiac transplantation. Am. Heart J. *128:*316, 1994.
38. Yamada, T., Fukunami, M., Ohmori, M., et al.: Which subgroup of patients with dilated cardiomyopathy would benefit from long-term beta-blocker therapy? A histologic viewpoint. J. Am. Coll. Cardiol. *21:*628, 1993.
39. Abelmann, W. H., and Lorell, B. H.: The challenge of cardiomyopathy. J. Am. Coll. Cardiol. *13:*1219, 1989.
40. Kuroda, T., Shiina, A., Suzuki, O., et al.: Prediction of prognosis of patients with idiopathic dilated cardiomyopathy: A comparison of echocardiography with cardiac catheterization. Jpn. J. Med. *28:*180, 1989.
41. Ferrans, V. J.: Pathologic anatomy of the dilated cardiomyopathies. Am. J. Cardiol. *64:*9C, 1989.
42. Schaper, J., Froede, R., Hein, S., et al.: Impairment of the myocardial ultrastructure and changes of the cytoskeleton in dilated cardiomyopathy. Circulation *83:*504, 1991.
43. Bender, J. R.: Idiopathic dilated cardiomyopathy. An immunologic, genetic, or infectious disease, or all of the above? Circulation *83:*704, 1991.
44. Neumann, D. A.: Autoimmunity and idiopathic dilated cardiomyopathy. Mayo Clin. Proc. *69:*193, 1994.
45. Michels, V. V., Moll, P. P., Rodeheffer, R. J., et al.: Circulating heart autoantibodies in familial as compared with nonfamilial idiopathic dilated cardiomyopathy. Mayo Clin. Proc. *69:*24, 1994.
46. Michels, V. V.: Progress in defining the causes of idiopathic dilated cardiomyopathy. N. Engl. J. Med. *329:*960, 1993.
47. Zachara, E., Caforio, A. L., Carboni, G. P., et al.: Familial aggregation of idiopathic dilated cardiomyopathy: Clinical features and pedigree analysis in 14 families. Br. Heart J. *69:*129, 1993.
48. Michels, V. V., Moll, P. P., Miller, F. A., et al.: The frequency of familial dilated cardiomyopathy in a series of patients with idiopathic dilated cardiomyopathy. N. Engl. J. Med. *326:*77, 1992.
48a. Goerss, J. B., Michels, V. V., Burnett, J., et al.: Frequency of familial dilated cardiomyopathy. Eur. Heart J. *16* (Suppl O):2, 1996.
49. Kelly, D. P., and Strauss, A. W.: Inherited cardiomyopathies. N. Engl. J. Med. *330:*913, 1994.
50. Muntoni, F., Cau, M., Ganau, A., et al.: Brief report: Deletion of the dystrophin muscle-promoter region associated with X-linked dilated cardiomyopathy. N. Engl. J. Med. *329:*921, 1993.
51. Towbin, J. A., Hejtmancik, J. F., Brink, P., et al.: X-linked dilated cardiomyopathy. Molecular genetic evidence of linkage to the Duchenne muscular dystrophy (dystrophin) gene at the Xp21 locus. Circulation *87:*1854, 1993.
52. Remes, A. M., Hassinen, I. E., Ikaheimo, M. J., et al.: Mitochondrial DNA deletions in dilated cardiomyopathy: A clinical study employing endomyocardial sampling. J. Am. Coll. Cardiol. *23:*935, 1994.
53. Silvestri, G., Santorelli, F. M., Shanske, S., et al.: A new mtDNA mutation in the tRNA(Leu(UUR)) gene associated with maternally inherited cardiomyopathy. Hum. Mutat. *3:*37, 1994.
54. Tranchant, C., Mousson, B., Mohr, M., et al.: Cardiac transplantation in an incomplete Kearns-Sayre syndrome with mitochondrial DNA deletion. Neuromuscul. Disord. *3:*561, 1993.
55. Anan, R., Nakagawa, M., Miyata, M., et al.: Cardiac involvement in mitochondrial diseases. A study on 17 patients with documented mitochondrial DNA defects. Circulation *91:*955, 1995.
56. Carlquist, J. F., Menlove, R. L., Murray, M. B., et al.: HLA class II (DR and DQ) antigen associations in idiopathic dilated cardiomyopathy. Validation study and meta-analysis of published HLA association studies. Circulation *83:*515, 1991.
56a. Mestroni, L., Krajinovic, M., Severini, G. M., et al.: Molecular genetics of dilated cardiomyopathies. Eur. Heart J. *16* (Suppl O):5, 1996.
57. Raynolds, M. V., Bristow, M. R., Bush, E. W., et al.: Angiotensin-converting enzyme DD genotype in patients with ischaemic or idiopathic dilated cardiomyopathy. Lancet *342:*1073, 1993.
58. Bakker, H. D., Scholte, H. R., Luyt-Houwen, I. E., et al.: Neonatal cardiomyopathy and lactic acidosis responsive to thiamine. J. Inherit. Metab. Dis. *14:*75, 1991.
59. Bratton, S. L., Garden, A. L., Bohan, T. P., et al.: A child with valproic acid–associated carnitine deficiency and carnitine-responsive cardiac dysfunction. J. Child Neurol. *7:*413, 1992.
60. Muir, P., Nicholson, F., Tilzey, A. J., et al.: Chronic relapsing pericarditis and dilated cardiomyopathy: Serological evidence of persistent enterovirus infection. Lancet *1:*804, 1989.
61. Shabetai, R.: Myocarditis and dilated cardiomyopathy: [illegible] distant relatives? Cardiology *76:*332, 1989.
62. Sole, M. J., and Liu, P.: Viral myocarditis: A paradigm for understand-

ing the pathogenesis and treatment of dilated cardiomyopathy. J. Am. Coll. Cardiol. *22*:99A, 1993.
63. Keeling, P. J., Lukaszyk, A., Poloniecki, J., et al.: A prospective case-control study of antibodies to coxsackie B virus in idiopathic dilated cardiomyopathy. J. Am. Coll. Cardiol. *23*:593, 1994.
64. O'Connell, J. B.: Immunosuppression for dilated cardiomyopathy. N. Engl. J. Med. *321*:1119, 1989.
65. Tracy, S., Chapman, N. M., McManus, B. M., et al.: A molecular and serologic evaluation of enteroviral involvement in human myocarditis. J. Mol. Cell Cardiol. *22*:403, 1990.
66. Why, H. J., Meany, B. T., Richardson, P. J., et al.: Clinical and prognostic significance of detection of enteroviral RNA in the myocardium of patients with myocarditis or dilated cardiomyopathy. Circulation *89*:2582, 1994.
67. Bowles, N. E., Rose, M. L., Taylor, P., et al.: End-stage dilated cardiomyopathy. Persistence of enterovirus RNA in myocardium at cardiac transplantation and lack of immune response. Circulation *80*:1128, 1989.
68. Grasso, M., Arbustini, E., Silini, E., et al.: Search for Coxsackievirus B3 RNA in idiopathic dilated cardiomyopathy using gene amplification by polymerase chain reaction. Am. J. Cardiol. *69*:658, 1992.
69. Keeling, P. J., Jeffery, S., Caforio, A. L., et al.: Similar prevalence of enteroviral genome within the myocardium from patients with idiopathic dilated cardiomyopathy and controls by the polymerase chain reaction. Br. Heart J. *68*:554, 1992.
70. Weiss, L. M., Liu, X. F., Chang, K. L., and Billingham, M. E.: Detection of enteroviral RNA in idiopathic dilated cardiomyopathy and other human cardiac tissues. J. Clin. Invest. *90*:156, 1992.
71. Giacca, M., Severini, G. M., Mestroni, L., et al.: Low frequency of detection by nested polymerase chain reaction of enterovirus ribonucleic acid in endomyocardial tissue of patients with idiopathic dilated cardiomyopathy. J. Am. Coll. Cardiol. *24*:1033, 1994.
72. Martino, T. A., Liu, P., and Sole, M. J.: Viral infection and the pathogenesis of dilated cardiomyopathy. Circ. Res. *74*:182, 1994.
73. Schwaiger, A., Umlauft, F., Weyrer, K., et al.: Detection of enteroviral ribonucleic acid in myocardial biopsies from patients with idiopathic dilated cardiomyopathy by polymerase chain reaction. Am. Heart J. *126*:406, 1993.
74. Satoh, M., Tamura, G., Segawa, I., et al.: Enteroviral RNA in dilated cardiomyopathy. Eur. Heart J. *15*:934, 1994.
75. Caforio, A. L., Keeling, P. J., Zachara, E., et al.: Evidence from family studies for autoimmunity in dilated cardiomyopathy. Lancet *344*:773, 1994.
76. Limas, C., Limas, C. J., Boudoulas, H., et al.: Anti-beta-receptor antibodies in familial cardiomyopathy: Correlation with HLA-DR and HLA-DQ gene polymorphisms. Am. Heart J. *127*:382, 1994.
77. Carlquist, J. F., Ward, R. H., Husebye, D., et al.: Major histocompatibility complex class II gene frequencies by serologic and deoxyribonucleic acid genomic typing in idiopathic dilated cardiomyopathy. Am. J. Cardiol. *74*:918, 1994.
78. Barry, W. H.: Mechanisms of immune-mediated myocyte injury. Circulation *89*:2421, 1994.
79. Limas, C., Limas, C. J., Boudoulas, H., et al.: HLA-DQA1 and DQB1 gene haplotypes in familial cardiomyopathy. Am. J. Cardiol. *74*:510, 1994.
80. Neumann, D. A., Burek, C. L., Baughman, K. L., et al.: Circulating heart-reactive antibodies in patients with myocarditis or cardiomyopathy. J. Am. Coll. Cardiol. *16*:839, 1990.
81. Limas, C. J., and Limas, C.: Immune-mediated modulation of sarcoplasmic reticulum function in human dilated cardiomyopathy. Basic Res. Cardiol. *87*(Suppl. 1):269, 1992.
82. Magnusson, Y., Wallukat, G., Waagstein, F., et al.: Autoimmunity in idiopathic dilated cardiomyopathy. Characterization of antibodies against the beta 1-adrenoceptor with positive chronotropic effect. Circulation *89*:2760, 1994.
83. Fu, L. X., Magnusson, Y., Bergh, C. H., et al.: Localization of a functional autoimmune epitope on the muscarinic acetylcholine receptor-2 in patients with idiopathic dilated cardiomyopathy. J. Clin. Invest. *91*:1964, 1993.
84. Caforio, A. L., Grazzini, M., Mann, J. M., et al.: Identification of alpha- and beta-cardiac myosin heavy chain isoforms as major autoantigens in dilated cardiomyopathy. Circulation *85*:1734, 1992.
85. Caforio, A. L. P.: Role of autoimmunity in dilated cardiomyopathy. Br. Heart J. *72*:S30, 1994.
86. Herskowitz, A., Vlahov, D., Willoughby, S., et al.: Prevalence and incidence of left ventricular dysfunction in patients with human immunodeficiency virus infection. Am. J. Cardiol. *71*:955, 1993.
87. Tomita, T., Murakami, T., Iwase, T., et al.: Chronic dynamic exercise improves a functional abnormality of the G stimulatory protein in cardiomyopathic BIO 53.58 Syrian hamsters. Circulation *89*:836, 1994.
88. Gilbert, E. M., Olsen, S. L., Renlund, D. G., and Bristow, M. R.: Beta-adrenergic receptor regulation and left ventricular function in idiopathic dilated cardiomyopathy. Am. J. Cardiol. *71*:23C, 1993.
89. Merlet, P., Delforge, J., Syrota, A., et al.: Positron emission tomography with 11C CGP-12177 to assess beta-adrenergic receptor concentration in idiopathic dilated cardiomyopathy. Circulation *87*:1169, 1993.
90. Bristow, M. R., Anderson, F. L., Port, J. D., et al.: Differences in beta-adrenergic neuroeffector mechanisms in ischemic versus idiopathic dilated cardiomyopathy. Circulation *84*:1024, 1991.
91. Feldman, A. M., Jackson, D. G., Bristow, M. R., et al.: Immunodetectable levels of the inhibitory guanine nucleotide-binding regulatory proteins in failing human heart: Discordance with measurements of adenylate cyclase activity and levels of pertussis toxin substrate. J. Mol. Cell Cardiol. *23*:439, 1991.
92. Bristow, M. R., and Feldman, A. M.: Changes in the receptor-G protein-adenylyl cyclase system in heart failure from various types of heart muscle disease. Basic Res. Cardiol. *87*(Suppl. 1):15, 1992.
93. Feldman, A. M., Tena, R. G., Kessler, P. D., et al.: Diminished beta-adrenergic receptor responsiveness and cardiac dilation in hearts of myopathic Syrian hamsters (BIO 53.58) are associated with a functional abnormality of the G stimulatory protein. Circulation *81*:1341, 1990.
94. Bohm, M., Gierschik, P., Jakobs, K. H., et al.: Increase of Gi alpha in human hearts with dilated but not ischemic cardiomyopathy. Circulation *82*:1249, 1990.
95. Wikman-Coffelt, J., Stefenelli, T., Wu, S. T., et al.: $[Ca^{2+}]i$ transients in the cardiomyopathic hamster heart. Circ. Res. *68*:45, 1991.
96. Hasenfuss, G., Reinecke, H., Studer, R., et al.: Relation between myocardial function and expression of sarcoplasmic reticulum $Ca^{(2+)}$-ATPase in failing and nonfailing human myocardium. Circ. Res. *75*:434, 1994.
97. Studer, R., Reinecke, H., Bilger, J., et al.: Gene expression of the cardiac $Na^{(+)}$-Ca^{2+} exchanger in end-stage human heart failure. Circ. Res. *75*:443, 1994.
98. Jeck, C. D., Zimmermann, R., Schaper, J., and Schaper, W.: Decreased expression of calmodulin mRNA in human end-stage heart failure. J. Mol. Cell Cardiol. *26*:99, 1994.
99. Go, L. O., Moschella, M. C., Watras, J., et al.: Differential regulation of two types of intracellular calcium release channels during end-stage heart failure. J. Clin. Invest. *95*:888, 1995.
100. Stewart, R. A., McKenna, W. J., and Oakley, C. M.: Good prognosis for dilated cardiomyopathy without severe heart failure or arrhythmia. Q. J. Med. *74*:309, 1990.
101. Caforio, A. L., Rossi, B., Risaliti, R., et al.: Type 1 fiber abnormalities in skeletal muscle of patients with hypertrophic and dilated cardiomyopathy: Evidence of subclinical myogenic myopathy. J. Am. Coll. Cardiol. *14*:1464, 1989.
102. Komajda, M., Jais, J. P., Reeves, F., et al.: Factors predicting mortality in idiopathic dilated cardiomyopathy. Eur. Heart J. *11*:824, 1990.
103. Treasure, C. B., Vita, J. A., Cox, D. A., et al.: Endothelium-dependent dilation of the coronary microvasculature is impaired in dilated cardiomyopathy. Circulation *81*:772, 1990.
104. Cabanes, L. R., Weber, S. N., Matran, R., et al.: Bronchial hyperresponsiveness to methacholine in patients with impaired left ventricular function. N. Engl. J. Med. *320*:1317, 1989.
105. Feldman, M. D., and Beller, G. A.: Is secondary mitral regurgitation in congestive heart failure a marker of clinical importance? J. Am. Coll. Cardiol. *15*:181, 1990.
106. Wilensky, R. L., Yudelman, P., Cohen, A. I., et al.: Serial electrocardiographic changes in idiopathic dilated cardiomyopathy confirmed at necropsy. Am. J. Cardiol. *62*:276, 1988.
107. Keogh, A. M., Baron, D. W., and Hickie, J. B.: Prognostic guides in patients with idiopathic or ischemic dilated cardiomyopathy assessed for cardiac transplantation. Am. J. Cardiol. *65*:903, 1990.
108. De Maria, R., Gavazzi, A., Caroli, A., et al.: Ventricular arrhythmias in dilated cardiomyopathy as an independent prognostic hallmark. Italian Multicenter Cardiomyopathy Study (SPIC) Group. Am. J. Cardiol. *69*:1451, 1992.
109. Corey, W. A., Markel, M. L., Hoit, B. D., and Walsh, R. A.: Regression of a dilated cardiomyopathy after radiofrequency ablation of incessant supraventricular tachycardia. Am. Heart J. *126*:1469, 1993.
110. Cruz, F. E., Cheriex, E. C., Smeets, J. L., et al.: Reversibility of tachycardia-induced cardiomyopathy after cure of incessant supraventricular tachycardia. J. Am. Coll. Cardiol. *16*:739, 1990.
111. Yoshimura, H., Ishikawa, T., Kuji, N., et al.: Two cases of dilated cardiomyopathy associated with incessant supraventricular tachycardia who showed a favorable response to beta-blockade. Heart Vessels *5*(Suppl.):88, 1990.
112. Katritsis, D., Leatham, E., Pumphrey, C., et al.: Low-energy DC catheter ablation of left atrial ectopic tachycardia that had resulted in reversible cardiomyopathy. PACE Pacing Clin. Electrophysiol. *16*:1345, 1993.
113. Pinamonti, B., Di Lenarda, A., Sinagra, G., and Camerini, F.: Restrictive left ventricular filling pattern in dilated cardiomyopathy assessed by Doppler echocardiography: Clinical, echocardiographic and hemodynamic correlations and prognostic implications. Heart Muscle Disease Study Group. J. Am. Coll. Cardiol. *22*:808, 1993.
114. Sharp, S. M., Sawada, S. G., Segar, D. S., et al.: Dobutamine stress echocardiography: Detection of coronary artery disease in patients with dilated cardiomyopathy. J. Am. Coll. Cardiol. *24*:934, 1994.
114a. Vigna, C., Russo, A., De Rito, V., et al.: Regional wall motion analysis by dobutamine stress echocardiography to distinguish between ischemic and nonischemic dilated cardiomyopathy. Am. Heart J. *131*:537, 1996.
115. Tauberg, S. G., Orie, J. E., Bartlett, B. E., et al.: Usefulness of thallium-201 for distinction of ischemic from idiopathic dilated cardiomyopathy. Am. J. Cardiol. *71*:674, 1993.
116. Doi, Y. L., Chikamori, T., Tukata, J., et al.: Prognostic value of thallium-201 perfusion defects in idiopathic dilated cardiomyopathy. Am. J. Cardiol. *67*:188, 1991.
117. Glamann, D. B., Lange, R. A., Corbett, J. R., and Hillis, L. D.: Utility of various radionuclide techniques for distinguishing ischemic from nonischemic dilated cardiomyopathy. Arch. Intern. Med. *152*:769, 1992.
118. Werner, G. S., Figulla, H. R., Munz, D. L., et al.: Myocardial indium-111 antimyosin uptake in patients with idiopathic dilated cardiomyopathy: Its relation to haemodynamics, histomorphometry, myocardial enteroviral infection, and clinical course. Eur. Heart J. *14*:175, 1993.
119. Dec, G. W., Palacios, I., Yasuda, T., et al.: Antimyosin antibody cardiac

475. Mady, C., Pereira Barretto, A. C., de Oliveira, S. A., et al.: Effectiveness of operative and nonoperative therapy in endomyocardial fibrosis. Am. J. Cardiol. *63*:1281, 1989.
476. de Oliveira, S. A., Pereira Barreto, A. C., Mady, C., et al.: Surgical treatment of endomyocardial fibrosis: A new approach. J. Am. Coll. Cardiol. *16*:1246, 1990.
477. Uva, M. S., Jebara, V. A., Acar, C., et al.: Mitral valve repair in patients with endomyocardial fibrosis. Ann. Thorac. Surg. *54*:89, 1992.
477a. La Vecchia, L., Bedogni, F., Bozzola, L., et al.: Prediction of recovery after abstinence in alcoholic cardiomyopathy: Role of hemodynamic and morphometric parameters. Clin. Cardiol. *19*:45, 1996.
478. Pellikka, P. A., Tajik, A. J., Khandheria, B. K., et al.: Carcinoid heart disease. Clinical and echocardiographic spectrum in 74 patients. Circulation *87*:1188, 1993.
479. Lundin, L.: Carcinoid heart disease. A cardiologist's viewpoint. Acta Oncol. *30*:499, 1991.
480. Waltenberger, J., Lundin, L., Oberg, K., et al.: Involvement of transforming growth factor-beta in the formation of fibrotic lesions in carcinoid heart disease. Am. J. Pathol. *142*:71, 1993.
481. Lundin, L., Funa, K., Hansson, H. E., et al.: Histochemical and immunohistochemical morphology of carcinoid heart disease. Pathol. Res. Pract. *187*:73, 1991.
481a. Robiolio, P. A., Rigolin, V. H., Wilson, J. S., et al.: Carcinoid heart disease. Correlation of high serotonin levels with valvular abnormalities detected by cardiac catheterization and echocardiography. Circulation *92*:790, 1995.
482. Robiolio, P. A., Rigolin, V. H., Harrison, J. K., et al.: Predictors of outcome of tricuspid valve replacement in carcinoid heart disease. Am. J. Cardiol. *75*:485, 1995.
483. Connolly, H. M., Nishimura, R. A., Smith, H. C., et al.: Outcome of cardiac surgery for carcinoid heart disease. J. Am. Coll. Cardiol. *25*:410, 1995.
484. Lundin, L., Landelius, J., Andren, B., and Oberg, K.: Transoesophageal echocardiography improves the diagnostic value of cardiac ultrasound in patients with carcinoid heart disease. Br. Heart J. *64*:190, 1990.
485. Yun, D., and Heywood, J. T.: Metastatic carcinoid disease presenting solely as high-output heart failure. Ann. Intern. Med. *120*:45, 1994.
486. Onate, A., Alcibar, J., Inguanzo, R., et al.: Balloon dilation of tricuspid and pulmonary valves in carcinoid heart disease. Tex. Heart Inst. J. *20*:115, 1993.
487. Grant, S. C., Scarffe, J. H., Levy, R. D., and Brooks, N. H.: Failure of balloon dilatation of the pulmonary valve in carcinoid pulmonary stenosis. Br. Heart J. *67*:450, 1992.

MYOCARDITIS

488. Peters, N. S., and Poole-Wilson, P. A.: Myocarditis—continuing clinical and pathologic confusion. Am. Heart J. *121*:942, 1991.
489. Herzum, M., and Maisch, B.: Humoral and cellular immune reactions to the myocardium in myocarditis. Herz *17*:91, 1992.
490. See, D. M., and Tilles, J. G.: Viral myocarditis. Rev. Infect. Dis. *13*:951, 1991.
491. Olinde, K. D., and O'Connell, J. B.: Inflammatory heart disease: Pathogenesis, clinical manifestations, and treatment of myocarditis. Annu. Rev. Med. *45*:481, 1994.
492. Leslie, K. O., Schwarz, J., Simpson, K., and Huber, S. A.: Progressive interstitial collagen deposition in Coxsackievirus B3-induced murine myocarditis. Am. J. Pathol. *136*:683, 1990.
493. Seko, Y., Matsuda, H., Kato, K., et al.: Expression of intercellular adhesion molecule-1 in murine hearts with acute myocarditis caused by coxsackievirus B3. J. Clin. Invest. *91*:1327, 1993.
494. Toyozaki, T., Saito, T., Takano, H., et al.: Expression of intercellular adhesion molecule-1 on cardiac myocytes for myocarditis before and during immunosuppressive therapy. Am. J. Cardiol. *72*:441, 1993.
495. Herskowitz, A., Ahmed-Ansari, A., Neumann, D. A., et al.: Induction of major histocompatibility complex antigens within the myocardium of patients with active myocarditis: A nonhistologic marker of myocarditis. J. Am. Coll. Cardiol. *15*:624, 1990.
496. Rose, N. R., Neumann, D. A., and Herskowitz, A.: Coxsackievirus myocarditis. Adv. Intern. Med. *37*:411, 1992.
497. McNulty, C. M.: Active viral myocarditis: Application of current knowledge to clinical practice. Heart Dis. Stroke *1*:135, 1992.
498. Hyypia, T.: Etiological diagnosis of viral heart disease. Scand. J. Infect. Dis. *88*(Suppl.):25, 1993.
499. Hagar, J. M., and Rahimtoola, S. H.: Chagas' heart disease in the United States. N. Engl. J. Med. *325*:763, 1991.
500. Marboe, C. C., and Fenoglio, J. J. Jr.: Pathology and natural history of human myocarditis. Pathol. Immunopathol. Res. *7*:226, 1988.
501. Davies, M. J., and Ward, D. E.: How can myocarditis be diagnosed and should it be treated? Br. Heart J. *68*:346, 1992.
502. Gowrishankar, K., and Rajajee, S.: Varied manifestations of viral myocarditis. Indian J. Pediatr. *61*:75, 1994.
503. Friedman, R. A., Kearney, D. L., Moak, J. P., et al.: Persistence of ventricular arrhythmia after resolution of occult myocarditis in children and young adults. J. Am. Coll. Cardiol. *24*:780, 1994.
504. Abelmann, W. H.: Myocarditis and dilated cardiomyopathy. West. J. Med. *150*:458, 1989.
505. Peters, N. S., and Poole-Wilson, P. A.: Myocarditis—a controversial disease. J. R. Soc. Med. *84*:1, 1991.
506. Gravanis, M. B., and Sternby, N. H.: Incidence of myocarditis. A 10-year autopsy study from Malmo, Sweden. Arch. Pathol. Lab. Med. *115*:390, 1991.
507. Narula, J., Khaw, B. A., Dec, G. W. Jr., et al.: Brief report: Recognition of acute myocarditis masquerading as acute myocardial infarction. N. Engl. J. Med. *328*:100, 1993.
508. Dec, G. W. Jr., Waldman, H., Southern, J., et al.: Viral myocarditis mimicking acute myocardial infarction. J. Am. Coll. Cardiol. *20*:85, 1992.
509. Morgera, T., Di Lenarda, A., Dreas, L., et al.: Electrocardiography of myocarditis revisited: Clinical and prognostic significance of electrocardiographic changes. Am. Heart J. *124*:455, 1992.
510. Matsuura, H., Palacios, I. F., Dec, G. W., et al.: Intraventricular conduction abnormalities in patients with clinically suspected myocarditis are associated with myocardial necrosis. Am. Heart J. *127*:1290, 1994.
511. James, K. B., Lee, K., Thomas, J. D., et al.: Left ventricular diastolic dysfunction in lymphocytic myocarditis as assessed by Doppler echocardiography. Am. J. Cardiol. *73*:282, 1994.
512. Memel, D. S., DeRogatis, A. J., and William, D. C.: Ga-67 citrate myocardial uptake in a patient with AIDS, toxoplasmosis, and myocarditis. Clin. Nucl. Med. *16*:315, 1991.
513. Matsumori, A., Yamada, T., Tamaki, N., et al.: ^{111}In monoclonal antimyosin antibody imaging: Imaging of myocardial infarction and myocarditis. Jpn. Circ. J. *54*:333, 1990.
514. Matsouka, H., Hamada, M., Honda, T., et al.: Evaluation of acute myocarditis and pericarditis by Gd-DTPA enhanced magnetic resonance imaging. Eur. Heart J. *15*:283, 1994.
515. Huber, S. A.: Viral myocarditis—a tale of two diseases. Lab. Invest. *66*:1, 1992.
516. Hauck, A. J., Kearney, D. L., and Edwards, W. D.: Evaluation of postmortem endomyocardial biopsy specimens from 38 patients with lymphocytic myocarditis: Implications for role of sampling error. Mayo Clin. Proc. *64*:1235, 1989.
517. Chow, L. H., Radio, S. J., Sears, T. D., and McManus, B. M.: Insensitivity of right ventricular endomyocardial biopsy in the diagnosis of myocarditis. J. Am. Coll. Cardiol. *14*:915, 1989.
518. Dec, G. W., Fallon, J. T., Southern, J. F., and Palacios, I.: "Borderline" myocarditis: An indication for repeat endomyocardial biopsy. J. Am. Coll. Cardiol. *15*:283, 1990.
519. Rezkalla, S., Kloner, R. A., Khatib, G., et al.: Effect of metoprolol in acute coxsackievirus B3 murine myocarditis. J. Am. Coll. Cardiol. *12*:412, 1988.
520. Maisch, B., Schonian, U., Crombach, M., et al.: Cytomegalovirus associated inflammatory heart muscle disease. Scand. J. Infect. Dis. *88*(Suppl.):135, 1993.
521. Jones, S. R., Herskowitz, A., Hutchins, G. M., and Baughman, K. L.: Effects of immunosuppressive therapy in biopsy-proved myocarditis and borderline myocarditis on left ventricular function. Am. J. Cardiol. *68*:370, 1991.
522. Chan, K. Y., Iwahara, M., Benson, L. N., et al.: Immunosuppressive therapy in the management of acute myocarditis in children: A clinical trial. J. Am. Coll. Cardiol. *17*:458, 1991.
522a. Mason, J. W., O'Connell, J. B., Herskowitz, A., et al.: A clinical trial of immunosuppressive therapy for myocarditis. N. Engl. J. Med. *333*:269, 1995.
523. Rezkalla, S. H., and Kloner, R. A.: Management strategies in viral myocarditis. Am. Heart J. *117*:706, 1989.
524. Kishimoto, C., and Abelmann, W. H.: Absence of effects of cyclosporine on myocardial lymphocyte subsets in Coxsackievirus B3 myocarditis in the aviremic stage. Circ. Res. *65*:934, 1989.
525. Kishimoto, C., Thorp, K. A., and Abelmann, W. H.: Immunosuppression with high doses of cyclophosphamide reduces the severity of myocarditis but increases the mortality in murine Coxsackievirus B3 myocarditis. Circulation *82*:982, 1990.
526. Drucker, N. A., Colan, S. D., Lewis, A. B., et al.: Gamma-globulin treatment of acute myocarditis in the pediatric population. Circulation *89*:252, 1994.
527. Rezkalla, S., Kloner, R. A., Khatib, G., and Khatib, R.: Beneficial effects of captopril in acute coxsackievirus B3 murine myocarditis. Circulation *81*:1039, 1990.
528. Rezkalla, S., Kloner, R. A., Khatib, G., and Khatib, R.: Effect of delayed captopril therapy on left ventricular mass and myonecrosis during acute coxsackievirus murine myocarditis. Am. Heart J. *120*:1377, 1990.
529. Ray, C. G., Icenogle, T. B., Minnich, L. L., et al.: The use of intravenous ribavirin to treat influenza virus-associated acute myocarditis. J. Infect. Dis. *159*:829, 1989.
530. Kishimoto, C., and Abelmann, W. H.: Monoclonal antibody therapy for prevention of acute coxsackievirus B3 myocarditis in mice. Circulation *79*:1300, 1989.
531. Kishimoto, C., Crumpacker, C. S., and Abelmann, W. H.: Prevention of murine coxsackie B3 viral myocarditis and associated lymphoid organ atrophy with recombinant human leucocyte interferon alpha A/D. Cardiovasc. Res. *22*:732, 1988.
532. Hingorani, A. D.: Postinfectious myocarditis. BMJ *304*:1676, 1992.
533. Remes, J., Helin, M., Vaino, P., and Rautio, P.: Clinical outcome and left ventricular function 23 years after acute coxsackie virus myopericarditis. Eur. Heart J. *11*:182, 1990.
534. Saiman, L., and Prince, A.: Infections of the heart. Adv. Pediatr. Infect. Dis. *4*:139, 1989.
535. Frustaci, A., and Maseri, A.: Localized left ventricular aneurysms with normal global function caused by myocarditis. Am. J. Cardiol. *70*:1221, 1992.
536. Wolfgram, L. J., and Rose, N. R.: Coxsackievirus infection as a trigger of cardiac autoimmunity. Immunol. Res. *8*:61, 1989.
537. Joy, J., Rao, Y. Y., Raveendranath, M., et al.: Coxsackie viral myocarditis: A clinical and echocardiographic study. Indian Heart J. *42*:441, 1990.
538. Pinamonti, B., Alberti, E., Cigalotto, A., et al.: Echocardiographic findings in myocarditis. Am. J. Cardiol. *62*:285, 1988.

539. Lowry, R. W., Adam, E., Hu, C., et al.: What are the implications of cardiac infection with cytomegalovirus before heart transplantation? J. Heart Lung Transplant. *13:*122, 1994.
540. Partanen, J., Nieminen, M. S., Krogerus, L., et al.: Cytomegalovirus myocarditis in transplanted heart verified by endomyocardial biopsy. Clin. Cardiol. *14:*847, 1991.
541. Gonwa, T. A., Capehart, J. E., Pilcher, J. W., and Alivizatos, P. A.: Cytomegalovirus myocarditis as a cause of cardiac dysfunction in a heart transplant recipient. Transplantation *47:*197, 1989.
542. Shabtai, M., Luft, B., Waltzer, W. C., et al.: Massive cytomegalovirus pneumonia and myocarditis in a renal transplant recipient: Successful treatment with DHPG. Transplant. Proc. *20:*562, 1988.
543. Schindler, J. M., and Neftel, K. A.: Simultaneous primary infection with HIV and CMV leading to severe pancytopenia, hepatitis, nephritis, perimyocarditis, myositis, and alopecia totalis. Klin. Wochenschr. *68:*237, 1990.
544. Powell, K. F., Bellamy, A. R., Catton, M. G., et al.: Cytomegalovirus myocarditis in a heart transplant recipient: Sensitive monitoring of viral DNA by the polymerase chain reaction. J. Heart Lung Transplant. *8:*465, 1989.
545. George, R.: Dengue haemorrhagic fever in Malaysia: A review. Southeast Asian J. Trop. Med. Public Health *18:*278, 1987.
546. Songco, R. S., Hayes, C. G., Leus, C. D., and Manaloto, C. O. R.: Dengue fever/dengue haemorrhagic fever in Filipino children: Clinical experience during the 1983–1984 epidemic. Southeast Asian J. Trop. Med. Public Health *18:*284, 1987.
547. Singh, D. S., Gupta, P. R., Gupta, S. S., et al.: Cardiac changes in acute viral hepatitis in Varanasi (India): Case reports. J. Trop. Med. Hyg. *92:*243, 1989.
548. Ursell, P. C., Habib, A., Sharma, P., et al.: Hepatitis B virus and myocarditis. Hum. Pathol. *15:*481, 1984.
549. Mahapatra, R. K., and Ellis, G. H.: Myocarditis and hepatitis B virus. Angiology *36:*116, 1985.
550. Jacob, A. J., and Boon, N. A.: HIV cardiomyopathy: A dark cloud with a silver lining? Br. Heart J. *66:*1, 1991.
551. Francis, C. K.: Cardiac involvement in AIDS. Curr. Probl. Cardiol. *15:*569, 1990.
552. Kaul, S., Fishbein, M. C., and Siegel, R. J.: Cardiac manifestations of acquired immune deficiency syndrome: A 1991 update. Am. Heart J. *122:*535, 1991.
553. Anderson, D. W., Virmani, R., Reilly, J. M., et al.: Prevalent myocarditis at necropsy in the acquired immunodeficiency syndrome. J. Am. Coll. Cardiol. *11:*792, 1988.
554. Baroldi, G., Corallo, S., Moroni, M., et al.: Focal lymphocytic myocarditis in acquired immunodeficiency syndrome (AIDS): A correlative morphologic and clinical study in 26 consecutive fatal cases. J. Am. Coll. Cardiol. *12:*463, 1988.
555. Akhras, F.: HIV and opportunistic infections: which makes the heart vulnerable? Br. J. Clin. Pract. *47:*232, 1993.
556. Grody, W. W., Cheng, L., and Lewis, W.: Infection of the heart by the human immunodeficiency virus. Am. J. Cardiol. *66:*203, 1990.
557. Acierno, L.: Cardiac complications in acquired immunodeficiency syndrome (AIDS): A review. J. Am. Coll. Cardiol. *13:*1144, 1989.
558. Blanchard, D. G., Hagenhoff, C., Chow, L. C., et al.: Reversibility of cardiac abnormalities in human immunodeficiency virus (HIV)-infected individuals: A serial echocardiographic study. J. Am. Coll. Cardiol. *17:*1270, 1991.
559. Levy, W. S., Simon, G. L., Rios, J. C., and Ross, A. M.: Prevalence of cardiac abnormalities in human immunodeficiency virus infection. Am. J. Cardiol. *63:*86, 1989.
560. Himelman, R. B., Chung, W. S., Chernoff, D. N., et al.: Cardiac manifestations of human immunodeficiency virus infection: A two-dimensional echocardiographic study. J. Am. Coll. Cardiol. *13:*1030, 1989.
561. Hofman, P., Drici, M. D., Gibelin, P., et al.: Prevalence of toxoplasma myocarditis in patients with the acquired immunodeficiency syndrome. Br. Heart J. *70:*376, 1993.
562. Herskowitz, A., Willoughby, S., Wu, T. C., et al.: Immunopathogenesis of HIV-1-associated cardiomyopathy. Clin. Immunol. Immunopathol. *68:*234, 1993.
563. Beschorner, W. E., Baughman, K., Turnicky, R. P., et al.: HIV-associated myocarditis. Pathology and immunopathology. Am. J. Pathol. *137:*1365, 1990.
564. Herskowitz, A., Wu, T. C., Willoughby, S. B., et al.: Myocarditis and cardiotropic viral infection associated with severe left ventricular dysfunction in late-stage infection with human immunodeficiency virus. J. Am. Coll. Cardiol. *24:*1025, 1994.
564a. Lipshultz, S. E., Orav, E. J., Sanders, S. P., et al.: Cardiac structure and function in children with human immunodeficiency virus infection treated with zidovudine. N. Engl. J. Med. *327:*1260, 1992.
565. Cox, J. N., di Dio, F., Pizzolato, G. P., et al.: Aspergillus endocarditis and myocarditis in a patient with the acquired immunodeficiency syndrome (AIDS). A review of the literature. Virchows Arch. A. Pathol. Anat. Histopathol. *417:*255, 1990.
566. Grange, F., Kinney, E. L., Monsuez, J. J., et al.: Successful therapy for *Toxoplasma gondii* myocarditis in acquired immunodeficiency syndrome. Am. Heart J. *120:*443, 1990.
567. Albrecht, H., Stellbrink, H. J., Fenske, S., et al.: Successful treatment of *Toxoplasma gondii* myocarditis in an AIDS patient. Eur. J. Clin. Microbiol. Infect. Dis. *13:*500, 1994.
568. Tyson, A. A. Jr., Hackshaw, B. T., and Kutcher, M. A.: Acute Epstein-Barr virus myocarditis simulating myocardial infarction with cardiogenic shock. South. Me d. J. *82:*1184, 1989.
569. Sprenger, M. J., Van Naelten, M. A., Mulder, P. G., and Masurel, N.: Influenza mortality and excess deaths in the elderly, 1967–1982. Epidemiol. Infect. *103:*633, 1989.
570. Agnholt, J., Sorensen, H. T., Rasmussen, S. N., et al.: Cardiac hypersensitivity to 5-aminosalicylic acid. Lancet *1:*1135, 1989.
571. Ruben, F. L., and Cate, T. R.: Influenza pneumonia. Semin. Respir. Infect. *2:*122, 1987.
572. Cummins, D., Bennett, D., Fisher-Hoch, S. P., et al.: Electrocardiographic abnormalities in patients with Lassa fever. J. Trop. Med. Hyg. *92:*350, 1989.
573. McCormick, J. B., King, I. J., Webb, P. A., et al.: Lassa fever: A case-control study of the clinical diagnosis and course of Lassa fever. J. Infect. Dis. *155:*445, 1987.
574. Ozkutlu, S., Soylemezoglu, O., Calikoglu, A. S., et al.: Fatal mumps myocarditis. Jpn. Heart J. *30:*109, 1989.
575. Ward, S. C., Wiselka, M. J., and Nicholson, K. G.: Still's disease and myocarditis associated with recent mumps infection. Postgrad. Med. J. *64:*693, 1988.
576. Chaudary, S., and Jaski, B. E.: Fulminant mumps myocarditis. Ann. Intern. Med. *110:*569, 1989.
577. Hildes, J. A., Schaberg, A., and Alcock, A. U. W.: Cardiovascular collapse in acute poliomyelitis. Circulation *12:*986, 1955.
578. Teloh, H. A.: Myocarditis in poliomyelitis. Arch. Pathol. *55:*408, 1953.
579. Weinstein, L., and Shelokov, A.: Cardiovascular manifestations of acute poliomyelitis. N. Engl. J. Med. *244:*281, 1951.
580. Pahl, E., and Gidding, S. S.: Echocardiographic assessment of cardiac function during respiratory syncytial virus infection. Pediatrics *81:*830, 1988.
581. Martin, J. T., Kugler, J. D., Gumbiner, C. H., et al.: Refractory congestive heart failure after ribavirin in infants with heart disease and respiratory syncytial virus. Nebr. Med. J. *75:*23, 1990.
582. Hoyer, S., Berglin, E., Pettersson, G., et al.: Cardiac transplantation in patients with active myocarditis. Transplant. Proc. *22:*1450, 1990.
583. Frustaci, A., Abdulla, A. K., Caldarulo, M., and Buffon, A.: Fatal measles myocarditis. Cardiologia *35:*347, 1990.
584. Degen, J. A. Jr.: Visceral pathology in measles: A clinicopathologic study of 100 fatal cases. Am. J. Med. Sci. *194:*104, 1937.
585. Weinstein, L.: Cardiovascular manifestations in some of the common infectious diseases. Mod. Concepts Cardiovasc. Dis. *23:*229, 1954.
586. Lorber, A., Zonis, Z., Maisuls, E., et al.: The scale of myocardial involvement in varicella myocarditis. Int. J. Cardiol. *20:*257, 1988.
587. Tsintsof, A., Delprado, W. J., and Keogh, A. M.: Varicella zoster myocarditis progressing to cardiomyopathy and cardiac transplantation. Br. Heart J. *70:*93, 1993.
588. Waagner, D. C., and Murphy, T. V.: Varicella myocarditis. Pediatr. Infect. Dis. J. *9:*360, 1990.
589. Rich, R., and McErlean, M.: Complete heart block in a child with varicella. Am. J. Emerg. Med. *11:*602, 1993.
590. Matthews, A. W., and Griffiths, I. D.: Post-vaccinal pericarditis and myocarditis. Br. Heart J. *36:*1043, 1974.
591. Finlay-Jones, L. R.: Fatal myocarditis after vaccinations for smallpox. N. Engl. J. Med. *270:*41, 1964.
592. Chevalier, P., Moncada, E., Kirkorian, G., et al.: Q fever-induced EMF. Am. Heart J. *125:*1818, 1993.
593. Gur, H., Gefel, D., and Tur-Kaspa, R.: Transient electrocardiographic changes during two episodes of relapsing brucellosis. Postgrad. Med. J. *60:*544, 1984.
594. Maisch, B.: Rickettsial perimyocarditis—a follow-up study. Heart Vessels *2:*55, 1986.
595. Marin-Garcia, J., and Barrett, F. F.: Myocardial function in Rocky Mountain spotted fever: Echocardiographic assessment. Am. J. Cardiol. *51:*341, 1983.
596. Marin-Garcia, J., and Mirvis, D. M.: Myocardial disease in Rocky Mountain spotted fever: Clinical, functional, and pathologic findings. Pediatr. Cardiol. *5:*149, 1984.
597. Marin-Garcia, J.: Left ventricular dysfunction in Rocky Mountain spotted fever. Clin. Cardiol. *6:*501, 1983.
598. Ganjoo, R. K., Sharma, S. N., and Roy, A. K.: Typhus myocarditis. J. Assoc. Physicians India *37:*357, 1989.
599. Yotsukura, M., Aoki, N., Fukuzumi, N., and Ishikawa, K.: Review of a case of tsutsugamushi disease showing myocarditis and confirmation of Rickettsia by endomyocardial biopsy. Jpn. Circ. J. *55:*149, 1991.
600. Jubber, A. S., Gunawardana, D. R., and Lulu, A. R.: Acute pulmonary edema in Brucella myocarditis and interstitial pneumonitis. Chest *97:*1008, 1990.
601. Roberts, W. C., and Beard, G. W.: Gas gangrene of the heart in clostridial septicemia. Am. Heart J. *74:*482, 1967.
602. Stevens, D. L., Troyer, B. E., Merrick, D. T., et al.: Lethal effects and cardiovascular effects of purified alpha- and theta-toxins from *Clostridium perfringens.* J. Infect. Dis. *157:*272, 1988.
603. Guneratne, P.: Gas gangrene (abscess) of heart. N. Y. State J. Med. *75:*1766, 1975.
604. Stockins, B. A., Lanas, F. T., Saavedra, J. G., and Opazo, J. A.: Prognosis in patients with diphtheric myocarditis and bradyarrhythmias: Assessment of results of ventricular pacing. Br. Heart J. *72:*190, 1994.
605. Havaldar, P. V., Patil, V. D., Siddibhavi, B. M., et al.: Fulminant diphtheritic myocarditis. Indian Heart J. *41:*265, 1989.
606. Armengol, S., Domingo, C., and Mesalles, E.: Myocarditis: A rare complication during Legionella infection. Int. J. Cardiol. *37:*418, 1992.
607. Devriendt, J., Staroukine, M., Schils, E., et al.: Legionellosis and "torsades de pointes." Acta Cardiol. *45:*329, 1990.

608. Sandler, M. A., Pincus, P. S., Weltman, M. D., et al.: Meningococcaemia complicated by myocarditis. A report of 2 cases. S. Afr. Med. J. *75*:391, 1989.
609. Ejlertsen, T., Vesterlund, T., and Schmidt, E. B.: Myopericarditis with cardiac tamponade caused by *Neisseria meningitidis* serogroup W135. Eur. J. Clin. Microbiol. Infect. Dis. *7*:403, 1988.
610. Agarwala, B. N., and Ruschhaupt, D. G.: Complete heart block from mycoplasma pneumoniae infection. Pediatr. Cardiol. *12*:233, 1991.
611. Murray, B. J.: Nonrespiratory complications of *M. pneumoniae* infection. Am. Fam. Physician *37*:127, 1988.
612. Karjalainen, J.: A loud third heart sound and asymptomatic myocarditis during *Mycoplasma pneumoniae* infection. Eur. Heart J. *11*:960, 1990.
613. Page, S. R., Stewart, J. T., and Bernstein, J. J.: A progressive pericardial effusion caused by psittacosis. Br. Heart J. *60*:87, 1988.
614. Odeh, M., and Oliven, A.: Chlamydial infections of the heart. Eur. J. Clin. Microbiol. Infect. Dis. *11*:885, 1992.
615. Lerner, A. M.: A new continuing fatigue syndrome following mild viral illness. A proscription to exercise. Chest *94*:901, 1988.
616. Delapenha, R. A., Greaves, W. L., Mani, V., and Frederick, W. R.: Typhoid fever with unusual clinical features. South. Med. J. *81*:417, 1988.
617. Burt, C. R., Proudfoot, J. C., Roberts, M., and Horowitz, R. H.: Fatal myocarditis secondary to Salmonella septicemia in a young adult. J. Emerg. Med. *8*:295, 1990.
618. Wander, G. S., Khurana, S. B., and Puri, S.: Salmonella myopericarditis presenting with acute pulmonary oedema. Indian Heart J. *44*:55, 1992.
619. Utley, J. R., Story, J. R., and Dandilides, P. C.: Resection of infected ventricular aneurysm *(Salmonella)* following saddle embolus. J. Card. Surg. *8*:143, 1993.
620. Singh, S., and Singhi, S.: Cardiovascular complications of enteric fever. Indian Pediatr. *29*:1319, 1992.
621. Kovoor, P., Mathew, M., Abraham, T., and Taneja, P. K.: Enteric fever complicated by myocarditis, hepatitis and shock. J. Assoc. Physicians India *36*:353, 1988.
622. Putterman, C., Caraco, Y., and Shalit, M.: Acute nonrheumatic perimyocarditis complicating streptococcal tonsillitis. Cardiology *78*:156, 1991.
623. Maher, D., and Ostrowski, J.: Highly virulent *Streptococcus pyogenes* rheumatic pancarditis and fatal septicaemia with septic shock. J. Infect. *26*:195, 1993.
624. Karjalainen, J.: Streptococcal tonsillitis and acute nonrheumatic myopericarditis. Chest *95*:359, 1989.
625. Bali, H. K., Wahi, S., Sharma, B. K., et al.: Myocardial tuberculosis presenting as restrictive cardiomyopathy. Am. Heart J. *120*:703, 1990.
626. O'Neill, R. G., Rokey, R., Greenberg, S., and Pacifico, A.: Resolution of ventricular tachycardia and endocardial tuberculoma following antituberculous therapy. Chest *100*:1467, 1991.
627. Chan, A. C., and Dickens, P.: Tuberculous myocarditis presenting as sudden cardiac death. Forensic Sci. Int. *57*:45, 1992.
628. Southern, J. F., Moscicki, R. A., Magro, C., et al.: Lymphedema, lymphocytic myocarditis, and sarcoidlike granulomatosis. Manifestations of Whipple's disease. JAMA *261*:1467, 1989.
629. Sossai, P., DeBoni, M., and Cielo, R.: The heart and Whipple's disease. Int. J. Cardiol. *23*:275, 1989.
630. James, T. N., and Bulkley, B. H.: Abnormalities of the coronary arteries in Whipple's disease. Am. Heart J. *105*:481, 1983.
631. Keinath, R. D., Merrell, D. E., Vlietstra, R., and Dobbins, W. O. III: Antibiotic treatment and relapse in Whipple's disease. Long-term follow-up of 88 patients. Gastroenterology *88*:1867, 1985.
632. Feldman, M.: Whipple's disease. Am. J. Med. Sci. *291*:56, 1986.
633. Dixon, A. C.: The cardiovascular manifestations of leptospirosis. West. J. Med. *154*:331, 1991.
634. Watt, G., Padre, L. P., Tuazon, M., and Calubaquib, C.: Skeletal and cardiac muscle involvement in severe, late leptospirosis. J. Infect. Dis. *162*:266, 1990.
635. McAlister, H. F., Klementowicz, P. T., Andrews, C., et al.: Lyme carditis: An important cause of reversible heart block. Ann. Intern. Med. *110*:339, 1989.
636. van der Linde, M. R., Crijns, H. J., De Koning, J., et al.: Range of atrioventricular conduction disturbances in Lyme borreliosis: A report of four cases and review of other published reports. Br. Heart J. *63*:162, 1990.
637. van der Linde, M. R.: Lyme carditis: Clinical characteristics of 105 cases. Scand. J. Infect. Dis. (Suppl.)*77*:81, 1991.
638. Haywood, G. A., O'Connell, S., and Gray, H. H.: Lyme carditis: A United Kingdom perspective. Br. Heart J. *70*:15, 1993.
639. Asch, E. S., Bujak, D. I., Weiss, M., et al.: Lyme disease: an infectious and postinfectious syndrome. J. Rheumatol. *21*:454, 1994.
640. Vlay, S. C., Dervan, J. P., Elias, J., et al.: Ventricular tachycardia associated with Lyme carditis. Am. Heart J. *121*:1558, 1991.
641. Rees, D. H., Keeling, P. J., McKenna, W. J., and Axford, J. S.: No evidence to implicate *Borrelia burgdorferi* in the pathogenesis of dilated cardiomyopathy in the United Kingdom. Br. Heart J. *71*:459, 1994.
642. Stanek, G., Klein, J., Bittner, R., and Glogar, D.: Isolation of *Borrelia burgdorferi* from the myocardium of a patient with longstanding cardiomyopathy. N. Engl. J. Med. *322*:249, 1990.
643. Kimball, S. A., Janson, P. A., and LaRaia, P. J.: Complete heart block as the sole presentation of Lyme disease. Arch. Intern. Med. *149*:1897, 1989.
644. Cox, J., and Krajden, M.: Cardiovascular manifestations of Lyme disease. Am. Heart J. *122*:1449, 1991.
645. Rahn, D. W., and Malawista, S. E.: Lyme disease: Recommendations for diagnosis and treatment. Ann. Intern. Med. *114*:472, 1991.
646. Wengrower, D., Knobler, H., Gillis, S., and Chajek-Shaul, T.: Myocarditis in tick-borne relapsing fever. J. Infect. Dis. *149*:1033, 1984.
647. Mekasha, A.: Louse-borne relapsing fever in children. J. Trop. Med. Hyg. *95*:206, 1992.
648. Jackman, J. D. Jr., and Radolf, J. D.: Cardiovascular syphilis. Am. J. Med. *87*:425, 1989.
649. Chino, M., Minami, T., and Nishikawa, K.: Ruptured ventricular aneurysm in secondary syphilis. Lancet *342*:935, 1993.
650. Nahass, R. G., Scholz, P., Mackenzie, J. W., and Gocke, D. J.: Chronic constrictive pericarditis. A case report and review of the literature. Arch. Intern. Med. *149*:1202, 1989.
651. Slutzker, A. D., and Claypool, W. D.: Pericardial actinomycosis with cardiac tamponade from a contiguous thoracic lesion. Thorax *44*:442, 1989.
652. Berarducci, L., Ford, K., Olenick, S., and Devries, S.: Invasive intracardiac aspergillosis with widespread embolization. J. Am. Soc. Echocardiogr. *6*:539, 1993.
653. Russack, V.: *Aspergillus terreus* myocarditis: Report of a case and review of the literature. Am. J. Cardiovasc. Pathol. *3*:275, 1990.
654. Hori, M. K., Knight, L. L., Carvalho, P. G., and Stevens, D. L.: Aspergillar myocarditis and acute coronary artery occlusion in an immunocompromised patient. West. J. Med. *155*:525, 1991.
655. Massin, E. K., Zeluff, B. J., Carrol, C. L., et al.: Cardiac transplantation and aspergillosis. Circulation *90*:1552, 1994.
656. Rogers, J. G., Windle, J. R., McManus, B. M., and Easley, A. R. Jr.: Aspergillus myocarditis presenting as myocardial infarction with complete heart block. Am. Heart J. *120*:430, 1990.
657. McCalmont, T. H., Silverman, J. F., and Geisinger, K. R.: Cytologic diagnosis of aspergillosis in cardiac transplantation. Arch. Surg. *126*:394, 1991.
658. Hall, J. C., and Giltman, L. I.: Candida myocarditis in a patient with chronic active hepatitis and macronodular cirrhosis. J. Tenn. Med. Assoc. *79*:473, 1986.
659. Atkinson, J. B., Connor, D. H., Robinowitz, M., et al.: Cardiac fungal infections: Review of autopsy findings in 60 patients. Hum. Pathol. *15*:935, 1984.
660. Vartivarian, S. E., Coudron, P. E., and Markowitz, S. M.: Disseminated coccidioidomycosis. Unusual manifestations in a cardiac transplantation patient. Am. J. Med. *83*:949, 1987.
661. Lafont, A., Wolff, M., Marche, C., et al.: Overwhelming myocarditis due to *Cryptococcus neoformans* in an AIDS patient. Lancet *2*:1145, 1987.
662. Garrett, H. E. Jr., and Roper, C. L.: Surgical intervention in histoplasmosis. Ann. Thorac. Surg. *42*:711, 1986.
663. Loyd, J. E., Tillman, B. F., Atkinson, J. B., and Des Prez, R. M.: Mediastinal fibrosis complicating histoplasmosis. Medicine (Baltimore) *67*:295, 1988.
664. Jackman, J. D. Jr., and Simonsen, R. L.: The clinical manifestations of cardiac mucormycosis. Chest *101*:1733, 1992.
665. Rossi, M. A.: Comparison of Chagas' heart disease to arrhythmogenic right ventricular cardiomyopathy. Am. Heart J. *129*:626, 1995.
666. Hagar, J. M., and Rahimtoola, S. H.: Chagas' heart disease. Curr. Probl. Cardiol. *20*:825, 1995.
667. Grant, I. H., Gold, J. W. M., Wittner, M., et al.: Transfusion-associated acute Chagas' disease acquired in the United States. Ann. Intern. Med. *111*:849, 1989.
668. Mota, E. A., Guimaraes, A. C., Santana, O. O., et al.: A nine year prospective study of Chagas' disease in a defined rural population in northeast Brazil. Am. J. Trop. Med. Hyg. *42*:429, 1990.
669. Morris, S. A., Tanowitz, H. B., Wittner, M., and Bilezikian, J. P.: Pathophysiological insights into the cardiomyopathy of Chagas' disease. Circulation *82*:1900, 1990.
670. Sadigursky, M., von Kreuter, B. F., Ling, P. Y., and Santos-Buch, C. A.: Association of elevated anti-sarcolemma, anti-idiotype antibody levels with the clinical and pathologic expression of chronic Chagas myocarditis. Circulation *80*:1269, 1989.
671. Palacios-Pru, E., Carrasco, H., Scorza, C., and Espinoza, R.: Ultrastructural characteristics of different stages of human chagasic myocarditis. Am. J. Trop. Med. Hyg. *41*:29, 1989.
672. Bestetti, R. B., Freitas, O. C., Muccillo, G., and Oliveira, J. S.: Clinical and morphological characteristics associated with sudden cardiac death in patients with Chagas' disease. Eur. Heart J. *14*:1610, 1993.
673. Carrasco, H. A., Guerrero, L., Parada, H., et al.: Ventricular arrhythmias and left ventricular myocardial function in chronic chagasic patients. Int. J. Cardiol. *28*:35, 1990.
674. Casado, J., Davila, D. F., Donis, J. H., et al.: Electrocardiographic abnormalities and left ventricular systolic function in Chagas' heart disease. Int. J. Cardiol. *27*:55, 1990.
675. Rossi, M. A.: Microvascular changes as a cause of chronic cardiomyopathy in Chagas' disease. Am. Heart J. *120*:233, 1990.
676. Espinosa, R. A., Pericchi, L. R., Carrasco, H. A., et al.: Prognostic indicators of chronic chagasic cardiopathy. Int. J. Cardiol. *30*:195, 1991.
677. Jones, E. M., Colley, D. G., Tostes, S., et al.: Amplification of a *Trypanosoma cruzi* DNA sequence from inflammatory lesions in human chagasic cardiomyopathy. Am. J. Trop. Med. Hyg. *48*:348, 1993.
678. Reis, D. D., Jones, E. M., Tostes, S., et al.: Expression of major histocompatibility complex antigens and adhesion molecules in hearts of patients with chronic Chagas' disease. Am. J. Trop. Med. Hyg. *49*:192, 1993.

679. Sanchez, J. A., Milei, J., Yu, Z. X., et al.: Immunohistochemical localization of laminin in the hearts of patients with chronic chagasic cardiomyopathy: Relationship to thickening of basement membranes. Am. Heart J. *126:*1392, 1993.
680. Mengel, J. O., and Rossi, M. A.: Chronic chagasic myocarditis pathogenesis: Dependence on autoimmune and microvascular factors. Am. Heart J. *124:*1052, 1992.
681. Oliveira, J. S. M., and Marin-Neto, J. A.: Parasympathetic impairment in Chagas' heart disease: Cause or consequence? Int. J. Cardiol. *21:*153, 1988.
682. Abelmann, W. H.: The dilated cardiomyopathies: Experimental aspects. Cardiol. Clin. *6:*219, 1988.
683. Bestetti, R. B., Santos, C. R., Machado-Junior, O. B., et al.: Clinical profile of patients with Chagas' disease before and during sustained ventricular tachycardia. Int. J. Cardiol. *29:*39, 1990.
684. Bestetti, R. B., Dalbo, C. M., Freitas, O. C., et al.: Noninvasive predictors of mortality for patients with Chagas' heart disease: A multivariate stepwise logistic regression study. Cardiology *84:*261, 1994.
685. Giniger, A. G., Retyk, E. O., Laino, R. A., et al.: Ventricular tachycardia in Chagas' disease. Am. J. Cardiol. *70:*459, 1992.
686. Carrasco, H. A., Parada, H., Guerrero, L., et al.: Prognostic implications of clinical, electrocardiographic and hemodynamic findings in chronic Chagas' disease. Int. J. Cardiol. *43:*27, 1994.
687. de Paola, A. A. V., Gomes, J. A., Miyamoto, M. H., and Fo, E. E.: Transcoronary chemical ablation of ventricular tachycardia in chronic chagasic myocarditis. J. Am. Coll. Cardiol. *20:*480, 1992.
688. Marin-Neto, J. A., Marzullo, P., Sousa, A. C., et al.: Radionuclide angiographic evidence for early predominant right ventricular involvement in patients with Chagas' disease. Can. J. Cardiol. *4:*231, 1988.
689. Marin-Neto, J. A., Marzullo, P., Marcassa, C., et al.: Myocardial perfusion abnormalities in chronic Chagas' disease as detected by thallium-201 scintigraphy. Am. J. Cardiol. *69:*780, 1992.
690. Kirchhoff, L. V.: Is *Trypanosoma cruzi* a new threat to our blood supply? Ann. Intern. Med. *111:*773, 1989.
691. de Paola, A. A. V., Horowitz, L. N., Miyamoto, M. H., et al.: Angiographic and electrophysiologic substrates of ventricular tachycardia in chronic chagasic myocarditis. Am. J. Cardiol. *65:*360, 1990.
692. de Paola, A. A. V., Horowitz, L. N., Miyamoto, M. H., et al.: Automatic implantable defibrillator with VVI pacemaker in a patient with chronic Chagas myocarditis and total atrioventricular block. Am. Heart J. *118:*415, 1989.
693. Bocchi, E. A., Moreira, L. F., Bellotti, G., et al.: Hemodynamic study during upright isotonic exercise before and six months after dynamic cardiomyoplasty for idiopathic dilated cardiomyopathy or Chagas' disease. Am. J. Cardiol. *67:*213, 1991.
694. Jatene, A. D., Moreira, L. F., Stolf, N. A., et al.: Left ventricular function changes after cardiomyoplasty in patients with dilated cardiomyopathy. J. Thorac. Cardiovasc. Surg. *102:*132, 1991.
695. Bocchi, E. A., Bellotti, C., Uip, D., et al.: Long-term follow-up after heart transplantation in Chagas' disease. Transplant. Proc. 25:1329, 1993.
696. Tsala Mbala, P., Blackett, K., and Mbonifor, C. L.: Functional and immunologic involvement in human African trypanosomiasis caused by *Trypanosoma gambiense.* Bull. Soc. Pathol. Exot. Filiales *81:*490, 1988.
697. Holmes, P. H.: Pathophysiology of parasitic infections. Parasitology *94:*S29, 1987.
698. Adair, O. V., Randive, N., and Krasnow, N.: Isolated toxoplasma myocarditis in acquired immune deficiency syndrome. Am. Heart J. *118:*856, 1989.
699. Franzen, D., Curtius, J. M., Heitz, W., et al.: Cardiac involvement during and after malaria. Clin. Investig. *70:*670, 1992.
700. Sharma, S. N., Mohapatra, A. K., and Machave, Y. V.: Chronic falciparum cardiomyopathy. J. Assoc. Physicians India *35:*251, 1987.
701. Russo, G., Tamburino, C., Cuscuna, S., et al.: Cardiac hydatid cyst with clinical features resembling subaortic stenosis. Am. Heart J. *117:*1385, 1989.
702. Oliver, J. M., Sotillo, J. F., Dominguez, F. J., et al.: Two-dimensional echocardiographic features of echinococcosis of the heart and great blood vessels. Clinical and surgical implications. Circulation *78:*327, 1988.
703. Akhtar, M. J.: Hydatid disease of the right ventricle and role of tomographic scanning in its diagnosis. Int. J. Cardiol. *33:*432, 1991.
704. Abid, A., Khayati, A., and Zargouni, N.: Hydatid cyst of the heart and pericardium. Int. J. Cardiol. *32:*108, 1991.
705. Bayezid, O., Ocal, A., Isik, O., et al.: A case of cardiac hydatid cyst localized on the interventricular septum and causing pulmonary emboli. J. Cardiovasc. Surg. (Torino) *32:*324, 1991.
706. Benomar, A., Yahyaoui, M., Birouk, N., et al.: Middle cerebral artery occlusion due to hydatid cysts of myocardial and intraventricular cavity cardiac origin. Two cases. Stroke *25:*886, 1994.
707. Cantoni, S., Frola, C., Gatto, R., et al.: Hydatid cyst of the interventricular septum of the heart: MR findings. A.J.R. *161:*753, 1993.
708. Miralles, A., Bracamonte, L., Pavie, A., et al.: Cardiac echinococcosis. Surgical treatment and results. J. Thorac. Cardiovasc. Surg. *107:*184, 1994.
709. Urbanyi, B., Rieckmann, C., Hellberg, K., et al.: Myocardial echinococcosis with perforation into the pericardium. J. Cardiovasc. Surg. (Torino) *32:*534, 1991.
710. Dao, A. H., and Virmani, R.: Visceral larva migrans involving the myocardium: Report of two cases and review of literature. Pediatr. Pathol. *6:*449, 1986.
711. Compton, S. J., Celum, C. L., Lee, C., et al.: Trichinosis with ventilatory failure and persistent myocarditis. Clin. Infect. Dis. *16:*500, 1993.
712. Fourestie, V., Douceron, H., Brugieres, P., et al.: Neurotrichinosis. A cerebrovascular disease associated with myocardial injury and hypereosinophilia. Brain *116:*603, 1993.
713. Ursell, P. C., Habib, A., Babchick, O., et al.: Myocarditis caused by *Trichinella spiralis.* Arch. Pathol. Lab. Med. *108:*4, 1984.
714. Lopez-Lozano, J. J., Garcia Merino, J. A., and Liano, H.: Bilateral facial paralysis secondary to trichinosis. Acta Neurol. Scand. *78:*194, 1988.

TOXIC, CHEMICAL, IMMUNE AND PHYSICAL DAMAGE TO THE HEART

715. Sauer, C. M.: Recurrent embolic stroke and cocaine-related cardiomyopathy. Stroke *22:*1203, 1991.
716. Henzlova, M. J., Smith, S. H., Prchal, V. M., and Helmcke, F. R.: Apparent reversibility of cocaine-induced congestive cardiomyopathy. Am. Heart J. *122:*577, 1991.
717. Eisenberg, M. J., Mendelson, J., Evans, G. T. Jr., et al.: Left ventricular function immediately after intravenous cocaine: A quantitative two-dimensional echocardiographic study. J. Am. Coll. Cardiol. *22:*1581, 1993.
718. Pilati, C. F., Espinal, A. R., and Pukys, T. F.: Persistent left ventricular dysfunction after cocaine treatment in rabbits. Proc. Soc. Exp. Biol. Med. *203:*100, 1993.
719. Clarkson, C. W., Chang, C., Stolfi, A., et al.: Electrophysiological effects of high cocaine concentrations on intact canine heart. Evidence for modulation by both heart rate and autonomic nervous system. Circulation *87:*950, 1993.
720. Liu, C. P., Tunin, C., and Kass, D. A.: Transient time course of cocaine-induced cardiac depression versus sustained peripheral vasoconstriction. J. Am. Coll. Cardiol. *21:*260, 1993.
721. Om, A.: Cardiovascular complications of cocaine. Am. J. Med. Sci. *303:*333, 1992.
722. Kimura, S., Bassett, A. L., Xi, H., and Myerburg, R. J.: Early afterdepolarizations and triggered activity induced by cocaine. A possible mechanism of cocaine arrhythmogenesis. Circulation *85:*2227, 1992.
723. Kloner, R. A., Hale, S., Alker, K., and Rezkalla, S.: The effects of acute and chronic cocaine use on the heart. Circulation *85:*407, 1992.
724. Brogan, W. C. 3rd, Lange, R. A., Glamann, D. B., and Hillis, L. D.: Recurrent coronary vasoconstriction caused by intranasal cocaine: Possible role for metabolites. Ann. Intern. Med. *116:*556, 1992.
725. Minor, R. L. Jr., Scott, B. D., Brown, D. D., and Winniford, M. D.: Cocaine-induced myocardial infarction in patients with normal coronary arteries. Ann. Intern. Med. *115:*797, 1991.
726. Tracy, C. M., Bachenheimer, L., Solomon, A., et al.: Evidence that cocaine slows cardiac conduction by an action on both AV nodal and His-Purkinje tissue in the dog. J. Electrocardiol. *24:*257, 1991.
727. Moliterno, D. J., Lange, R. A., Gerard, R. D., et al.: Influence of intranasal cocaine on plasma constituents associated with endogenous thrombosis and thrombolysis. Am. J. Med. *96:*492, 1994.
728. Jennings, L. K., White, M. M., Sauer, C. M., et al.: Cocaine-induced platelet defects. Stroke *24:*1352, 1993.
729. Hageman, G. R., and Simor, T.: Attenuation of the cardiac effects of cocaine by dizocilpine. Am. J. Physiol. *264:*H1890, 1993.
730. Stewart, G., Rubin, E., and Thomas, A. P.: Inhibition by cocaine of excitation-contraction coupling in isolated cardiomyocytes. Am. J. Physiol. *260:*H50, 1991.
731. Isner, J. M., and Chokshi, S. K.: Cardiac complications of cocaine abuse. Annu. Rev. Med. *42:*133, 1991.
732. Petty, G. W., Brust, J. C., Tatemichi, T. K., and Barr, M. L.: Embolic stroke after smoking "crack" cocaine. Stroke *21:*1632, 1990.
733. Majid, P. A., Patel, B., Kim, H. S., et al.: An angiographic and histologic study of cocaine-induced chest pain. Am. J. Cardiol. *65:*812, 1990.
734. Lange, R. A., and Willard, J. E.: The cardiovascular effects of cocaine. Heart Dis. Stroke *2:*136, 1993.
735. Chakko, S., and Myerburg, R. J.: Cardiac complications of cocaine abuse. Clin. Cardiol. *18:*67, 1995.
736. Gitter, M. J., Goldsmith, S. R., Dunbar, D. N., and Sharkey, S. W.: Cocaine and chest pain: clinical features and outcome of patients hospitalized to rule out myocardial infarction. Ann. Intern. Med. *115:*277, 1991.
737. Chokshi, S. K., Moore, R., Pandian, N. G., and Isner, J. M.: Reversible cardiomyopathy associated with cocaine intoxication. Ann. Intern. Med. *111:*1039, 1989.
738. Chakko, S., Fernandez, A., Mellman, T. A., et al.: Cardiac manifestations of cocaine abuse: A cross-sectional study of asymptomatic men with a history of long-term abuse of "crack" cocaine. J. Am. Coll. Cardiol. *20:*1168, 1992.
739. Kloner, R. A., and Hale, S.: Unraveling the complex effects of cocaine on the heart. Circulation *87:*1046, 1993.
740. Virmani, R., Robinowitz, M., Smialek, J. E., and Smyth, D. F.: Cardiovascular effects of cocaine: an autopsy study of 40 patients. Am. Heart J. *115:*1068, 1988.
741. Egashira, K., Morgan, K. G., and Morgan, J. P.: Effects of cocaine on excitation contraction coupling of aortic smooth muscle from the feret. J. Clin. Invest. *87:*1322, 1991.
742. Hale, S. L., Alker, K. J., Rezkalla, S. H., et al.: Nifedipine protects the

pletely normal perfusion of the opposite lung, a pattern unusual with typical pulmonary emboli.

Cardiac Manifestations

The specific signs and symptoms produced by tumors are more closely related to their precise anatomical location than to their histological types.[34] Thus, it is useful to consider the constellation of findings typical of each location. The presentation of *pericardial tumors* is considered on page 1522 and will not be discussed here except to point out that primary tumors of the myocardium and endocardium may extend into the pericardial space and produce many of the clinical manifestations of pericardial tumors, including hemorrhagic pericardial effusion and compression of the heart by the effusion or the tumor itself.

MYOCARDIAL TUMORS. When clinically apparent, myocardial tumors most commonly result in disturbances of conduction or rhythm,[35–38] the precise nature of which is determined by the location of the tumor. Thus, tumors in the area of the atrioventricular node, typically angiomas and mesotheliomas, may produce atrioventricular (AV) conduction disturbances, including complete heart block and asystole, and can lead to sudden death.[35–38] A wide variety of arrhythmias may be produced, including atrial fibrillation or flutter, paroxysmal atrial tachycardia with or without block, nodal rhythm, ventricular premature beats, ventricular tachycardia, and ventricular fibrillation.[34,38] Intramural tumors may also produce symptoms by virtue of their size and location. Impairment of ventricular performance may simulate congestive, restrictive, or hypertrophic cardiomyopathy (Chap. 41). Tumor infiltration of the myocardial wall occasionally causes myocardial rupture.[39]

LEFT ATRIAL TUMORS. Mobile, pedunculated, left atrial tumors may prolapse to variable degrees into the mitral valve orifice, resulting in obstruction to atrioventricular blood flow and, frequently, mitral regurgitation. The resultant signs and symptoms often mimic those of mitral valve disease[1,5,39] (Table 42–2), especially mitral stenosis (see p. 1011)[40] and include dyspnea, orthopnea, paroxysmal nocturnal dyspnea, pulmonary edema, cough, hemoptysis, chest pain, peripheral edema, and fatigue. However, weight loss, pallor, syncope, and sudden death—manifestations that are uncommon with mitral valve disease—also occur. It is not unusual for the symptoms to be sudden in onset, intermittent, and related to the patient's body position.[5,34] Although the majority of symptoms produced by left atrial tumors are nonspecific, the occurrence of paroxysmal symptoms that arise characteristically in a particular body position and are out of proportion to the clinical findings should raise suspicion of a left atrial tumor. The most common primary cardiac tumor presenting in the left atrium is the benign myxoma, which, in the large majority of cases, is solitary (see p. 1467).

Physical Examination. This may disclose signs of pulmonary congestion, an S_4, a loud S_1 which is often widely split, a holosystolic murmur which is loudest at the apex and resembles mitral regurgitation, and a diastolic murmur resulting from obstruction to flow through the mitral orifice produced by the tumor. The loud S_1 that occurs in patients with left atrial myxoma may be due to the late onset of mitral valve closure resulting from prolapse of the tumor through the mitral valve orifice.[41] Consequently the left ventricular–left atrial pressure crossover occurs at a higher pressure, as in patients with mitral stenosis or a short P-R interval. It has been suggested that the finding of a loud S_1 in the absence of a short P-R interval or a mitral diastolic murmur should raise the suspicion of a left atrial tumor.[41] In many cases an early diastolic sound, termed a tumor plop, can be identified. It is thought to be produced as the tumor strikes the endocardial wall or as its excursion is abruptly halted. Although in most cases the tumor plop occurs later than the opening snap of the mitral valve and earlier than the S_3, it is not surprising that this sound is frequently confused with the opening snap or the S_3.

RIGHT ATRIAL TUMORS. Right atrial tumors frequently produce symptoms of right heart failure, including fatigue, peripheral edema, ascites, hepatomegaly, and prominent *a* waves in the jugular venous pulse.[34,42–44a] The average time interval from the symptomatic presentation to the correct diagnosis of right atrial tumor may be years. The development of right heart failure may be rapidly progressive and is often associated with new systolic or diastolic murmurs or both. The murmurs are generally the result of tumor obstruction to tricuspid valve flow or of tricuspid regurgitation caused by tumor interference with valve closure or valve destruction caused directly or indirectly by the tumor.[45] It is not surprising that right atrial tumors have been misdiagnosed as Ebstein's anomaly of the tricuspid valve, constrictive pericarditis, tricuspid stenosis, carcinoid syndrome, superior vena caval syndrome, and cardiomyopathy (Table 42–2). Pulmonary embolism and pulmonary hypertension occur and may simulate classic thromboembolic disease.[43] Right atrial hypertension may cause right-to-left shunting through a patent foramen ovale, with systemic hypoxia, cyanosis, clubbing, and polycythemia.[44a] Whereas myxomas occur much more commonly in the left atrium than in the right atrium, sarcomas occur more commonly in the right atrium.

Physical Examination. This may reveal peripheral edema, evidence of superior vena caval obstruction, hepatomegaly, and ascites. An early diastolic rumbling murmur, alone or in combination with a holosystolic murmur secondary to tricuspid regurgitation, may demonstrate respiratory or positional variation. Because of the rarity of *isolated* rheumatic tricuspid valvular disease, the lack of other valvular findings should raise the question of a right atrial tumor. A protodiastolic tumor plop has been described and is thought to be similar in etiology to that produced by left atrial tumors.[46] The jugular venous pressure may be elevated, and a prominent *a* wave and steep *y* descent may be present.

RIGHT VENTRICULAR TUMORS. Right ventricular tumors often present with right heart failure as a result of obstruction to right ventricular filling or outflow. Clinical manifestations include peripheral edema, hepatomegaly, ascites, shortness of breath, syncope, and sudden death.

A systolic ejection murmur at the left sternal border is usually found on physical examination. A presystolic murmur and a diastolic rumble[34] have been noted and are thought to be due to obstruction of the tricuspid valve. An S_3 may be audible, and a low-pitched diastolic sound that coincides with the maximal anterior excursion of the tumor has been ascribed either to tumor or to late closure of the pulmonary valve.[47] P_2 is often delayed, and its intensity may be normal, decreased, or increased. Tumor emboli to the pulmonary arteries may result in pulmonary hypertension, and the presence of tumor in the pulmonic valve orifice may lead to pulmonary regurgitation. The jugular veins are frequently distended with a prominent *a* wave and may demonstrate Kussmaul's sign (see p. 19).

The cardiac findings often lead to a diagnosis of pulmonic stenosis, restrictive cardiomyopathy, or tricuspid regurgitation. Whereas pulmonic stenosis is often asymptomatic and slowly progressive, the symptoms of right ventricular tumors are often rapidly progressive, and there is no poststenotic dilatation or systolic ejection click.

LEFT VENTRICULAR TUMORS. When left ventricular tumors are predominantly intramural in location, they are often asymptomatic, or they may present as conduction disturbances or arrhythmias, or they may interfere with ventricular function. However, when the tumor also has a significant intracavitary component, there may be obstruction to left ventricular outflow, resulting in syncope and findings consistent with left ventricular failure. Atypical chest pain has also been reported and, in some cases, may

TABLE 42–3 RELATIVE INCIDENCE OF BENIGN TUMORS OF THE HEART

BENIGN TUMOR	% OF GROUP Adults	Children	Infants
Myxoma	46	15	0
Lipoma	21	0	0
Papillary fibroelastoma	16	0	0
Rhabdomyoma	2	46	65
Fibroma	3	15	12
Hemangioma	5	5	4
Teratoma	1	13	18
Mesothelioma of the AV node	3	4	2
Granular cell tumor	1	0	0
Neurofibroma	1	1	0
Lymphangioma	1	0	0
Hamartoma	0	1	0

Data representing the extensive investigations of the Armed Forces Institute of Pathology as well as the cumulative experience of other researchers. A total of 265, 82, and 49 benign tumors were found in adults (aged >16 years), children (aged 1 to 16 years), and infants (aged <1 year), respectively. Myxomas were the most common reported benign tumors in adults, whereas rhabdomyomas were the most common benign tumors in both children and infants; benign teratomas also occurred frequently in children and infants.

From Allard, M. F. et al.: Primary cardiac tumors. *In* Goldhaber, S., and Braunwald, E. (eds): Atlas of Heart Diseases. Philadelphia, Current Medicine, 1995, pp. 15.1–15.22.

reflect obstruction of a coronary artery either directly by tumor involvement or as a result of a tumor embolus to the coronary artery.

Physical Examination. This reveals a systolic murmur, and both the murmur and the blood pressure may vary with position. Left ventricular tumors may simulate the findings of aortic stenosis, subaortic stenosis, hypertrophic cardiomyopathy, endocardial fibroelastosis, and coronary artery disease.

Benign Versus Malignant Tumors

The types of benign and malignant mesenchymal tumors that may develop in the heart are typical of those occurring in any mass of striated muscle and connective tissue. Although the exact incidence of each specific tumor type cannot be stated, about 75 per cent of all cardiac tumors are benign histologically and the remainder are malignant.[1] The majority of benign cardiac tumors are myxomas, followed in frequency by a wide variety of other tumors (Table 42–3). Almost all malignant cardiac tumors are sarcomas, and of these the angiosarcoma and rhabdomyosarcoma are the most common forms (Table 42–4).

TABLE 42–4 RELATIVE INCIDENCE OF PRIMARY MALIGNANT TUMORS OF THE HEART

TUMOR TYPE	% OF GROUP Adults	Children	Infants
Angiosarcoma	33	0	0
Rhabdomyosarcoma	21	33	66
Mesothelioma	16	0	0
Fibrosarcoma	11	11	33
Malignant lymphoma	6	0	0
Extraskeletal osteosarcoma	4	0	0
Thymoma	3	0	0
Neurogeic sarcoma	3	11	0
Leiomyosarcoma	1	0	0
Liposarcoma	1	0	0
Synovial sarcoma	1	0	0
Malignant teratoma	0	44	0

A total of 117, nine, and three malignant tumors were found in adults (aged >16 years), children (aged 1 to 16 years), and infants (aged <1 year), respectively. Angiosarcomas were the most commonly reported malignant tumors in adults, but rhabdomyosarcomas and mesotheliomas were also relatively common. Malignant teratomas were the most common tumors in children. Rhabdomyosarcomas were the most frequently reported malignant tumors in infants, with fibrosarcomas the second most common.

From Allard, M. F., et al.: Primary cardiac tumors. *In* Goldhaber, S., and Braunwald, E. (eds): Atlas of Heart Diseases, Philadelphia, Current Medicine, 1995, pp. 15.1–15.22.

Although it is often difficult or impossible to differentiate histologically benign from malignant tumors prior to operation, certain findings may be helpful. Characteristics suggestive of malignancy include the presence of distant metastases, local mediastinal invasion, evidence of rapid growth in tumor size, hemorrhagic pericardial effusion, precordial pain, location of the tumor on the right side of the heart or on the atrial free wall, evidence of combined intramural and intracavitary location, and extension into the pulmonary veins. Benign tumors are more likely to occur on the left side of the interatrial septum and to grow slowly. Although benign tumors do not metastasize, distant tumor emboli may mimic peripheral or pulmonary metastases.[48] The preoperative differentiation between benign and malignant tumors may occasionally be made by examination of peripheral tumor emboli recovered by arteriotomy or by biopsy of skin or muscle.[5,27,29,30]

SPECIFIC CARDIAC TUMORS

Benign Tumors

Myxomas

As already pointed out, myxomas are the most common type of primary cardiac tumor, comprising 30 to 50 per cent of the total in most pathological series.[1–6] The mean age of patients with sporadic myxoma is 56 years, and 70 per cent are females. However, myxomas have been described in patients ranging in age from 3 to 83 years and are now not infrequently diagnosed in elderly patients in whom the symptoms and signs of cardiac tumor may have been attributed to other causes for a substantial time. Approximately 86 per cent of myxomas occur in the left atrium, and over 90 per cent are solitary[5,6] (Fig. 42–1). In the left atrium, the usual site of attachment is in the area of the fossa ovalis. Myxomas also may occur in the right atrium and, less often, in the right or left ventricle. Multiple tumors may occur in the same chamber or in a combination of chambers. Although myxomas may occasionally be found on the posterior left atrial wall, tumors presenting in this location should raise the suspicion of malignancy. Myxomas of the mitral and tricuspid valves have been reported.[44,48]

The clinical signs and symptoms produced by cardiac myxomas include nonspecific manifestations as already discussed, embolization, and mechanical interference with cardiac function (Table 42–1). Not surprisingly, the symptoms produced by cardiac myxomas may simulate a wide variety of other cardiac and noncardiac conditions (Table 42–2).

FAMILIAL MYXOMAS. Familial cardiac myxomas constitute approximately 10 per cent or less of all myxomas and appear to have an autosomal dominant transmission.[1,49,50,50a] Some patients with cardiac myxoma have a syndrome, frequently called "syndrome myxoma" or "Carney syndrome," that also consists of: (1) myxomas in other locations (breast or skin), (2) spotty pigmentation (lentigines, pigmented nevi, or both) (Fig. 42–2), and (3) endocrine overactivity (pituitary adenoma, primary pigmented nodular adrenocortical disease, or testicular tumors involving the endocrine components).[51–53] Patients with the Carney syndrome tend to be younger (mean age, 20's), are more likely to have myxomas in locations other than the left atrium, sometimes have bilateral tumors, and are more likely to develop recurrences (Table 42–5).

Although the etiology of the syndrome myxoma is unknown, it has been proposed to result from a widespread abnormality resulting in excessive proliferation of certain mesenchymal cells, and excessive glycosaminoglycans

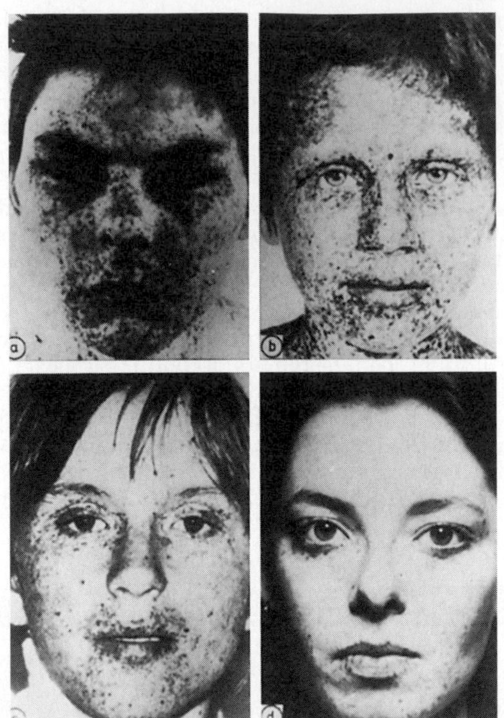

FIGURE 42–2. Four patients with extensive facial freckling, a finding that is associated with "syndrome myxoma." Patients with this syndrome tend to be younger than patients with sporadic myxoma and have a substantially higher incidence of ventricular, multiple, biatrial, recurrent, and familial myxomas of the heart. In addition, these patients, in contrast to patients with sporadic myxoma, may have noncardiac myxomas and endocrine neoplasms. (From Vidaillet, H. J., Jr., et al.: "Syndrome myxoma": a subset of patients with cardiac myxoma associated with pigmented skin lesions and peripheral and endocrine neoplasms. Br. Heart J. *57:* 247, 1987.)

(GAG) production by them, possibly analogous to the neural masses in von Recklinghausen's neurofibromatosis.[54] Patients may have two or more components of this complex, and generally the first component is diagnosed at a relatively young age (mean age, 18 years). Some patients have been said to have the NAME syndrome (*n*evi, *a*trial myxoma, *m*yxoid neurofibroma, *e*phelides)[50a,55] or the LAMB syndrome (*l*entigines, *a*trial *m*yxoma, and *b*lue nevi).[56]

Because cardiac myxomas may be familial, routine echocardiographic screening of first-degree relatives is appropriate, particularly if the patient is young or has multiple tumors. In one recent study, screening of families of six patients with familial myxoma yielded four close relatives with cardiac myxoma.[57] Moreover, in patients with a familial history or other components of the syndrome described above who are undergoing resection, a careful search should be made preoperatively for multiple cardiac myxomas. Postoperatively, these patients should be observed closely for the development of other tumors; this occurs in 12 to 22 per cent of such patients.[58] The pathological features of familial myxomas do not differ from those occurring sporadically (see below).[59]

TABLE 42–5 COMPARISON OF THE CLINICAL FEATURES OF SPORADIC MYXOMA AND SYNDROME MYXOMA

FEATURE	SPORADIC	SYNDROME
Age (yr) (range)	56 (39–82)	25 (10–56)
Female/male ratio	2.7:1	1.8:1
Patients (No.)	70	44
Cardiac myxomas (No.)	72	103
Distributions of myxomas (%)		
Atrial/ventricular	100/0	87/13
Single/multiple	99/1	50/50
Biatrial	0	23
Recurrent	0	18
Familial	0	27
Freckling (%)	0	68
Noncardiac tumors (%)	0	57
Endocrine neoplasm (%)	0	30

Vidaillet, H. J., Jr., et al.: "Syndrome myxoma": A subset of patients with cardiac myxoma associated with pigmented skin lesions and peripheral and endocrine neoplasms. Br. Heart J. *57*:247, 1987.

PATHOLOGY. Most cardiac myxomas are received by the pathologist as surgically excised specimens that have been removed for clinical symptomatology. Rarely, cardiac myxomas are encountered incidentally at autopsy. The pathological characteristics of myxomas are well described and are independent of location.[1,48,60–62]

Gross Pathology. Myxomas are gelatinous (often termed myxoid), smooth and round with a glistening surface, or variably friable, and either irregular or polypoid (Fig. 42–2). They are either sessile or pedunculated with a distinct stalk, which may be narrow or broad. In approximately 90 per cent of cases arising in the atria, the base of attachment is the atrial septum, usually in the region of the limbus of the fossa ovalis. In approximately 10 per cent of cases, the point of origin is the posterior or anterior atrial wall or atrial appendage; valvular myxomas are rare. Cardiac myxomas can be multicentric. Areas of hemorrhage are frequent. The tumors average 4 to 8 cm in diameter but range from less than 1 cm to 15 cm or greater.

Histology. The diagnosis of myxoma is made by the observation of characteristic patterns of cells (often called "lipidic" cells) embedded in a myxoid stroma rich in glycosaminoglycans (GAGs) (Fig. 42–3).[60–62] Myxoma cells have a round, elongated or polyhedral shape, scant pink cytoplasm, and an ovoid nucleus with an open chromatin pattern; they are occasionally multinuclear. Although they may be present individually, myxoma cells are typically present as cords, rings, or florets, sometimes as multiple layers surrounding vascular structures. Diagnosis of myxoma requires the presence of characteristic isolated or clustered collections of myxoma cells. Hemorrhages, macrophages, often containing iron pigment, and lymphocytes and plasma cells are variably present. Calcification is present in approximately 10 to 20 per cent of cardiac myxomas. Extramedullary hematopoiesis, glandular structures lined by mucin-filled goblet cells,[63] and cellular atypia may be present in a minority of cases; these features may simulate malignancy. Since emboli from myxomas usually derive from the most superficial portions, they may have less definitive histologic features than the intracardiac lesion from which they originated.

Ultrastructural and Immunohistochemical Findings. Myxoma cells have abundant fine cytoplasmic filaments similar to those of smooth muscle cells.[62] The cells most resemble embryonic mesenchymal cells with multipotential capabilities for cellular differentiation, including vasoformative activity, and are especially similar to embryonic endocardial cushion tissue.[64] *Immunohistochemical studies* demonstrate variable positivity for the endothelial cell markers Factor VIII–related antigen and *Ulex europaeus*. More consistent positivity is obtained when myxomas are stained for *vimentin,* indicative of the mesenchymal derivation of the cells, as well as some neuroendocrine markers and smooth muscle cell antigens. Analysis by immunohistochemistry has not been useful for either diagnostic purposes or elucidation of histogenesis.

Embolization. Although myxomas or other benign cardiac tumors can cause death from coronary or cerebral embolization,[65] metastatic tumor implantation with wasting is rare. Occasional reports suggest that myxomas may have a malignant counterpart, with local invasion of the interatrial septum, recurrence, or metastasis. However, some cases of purported malignancy probably represent malignant tumors of other types with extensive areas of myxoid degeneration or of multicentricity that was not appreciated, inadequate excision, or embolization of benign lesions.

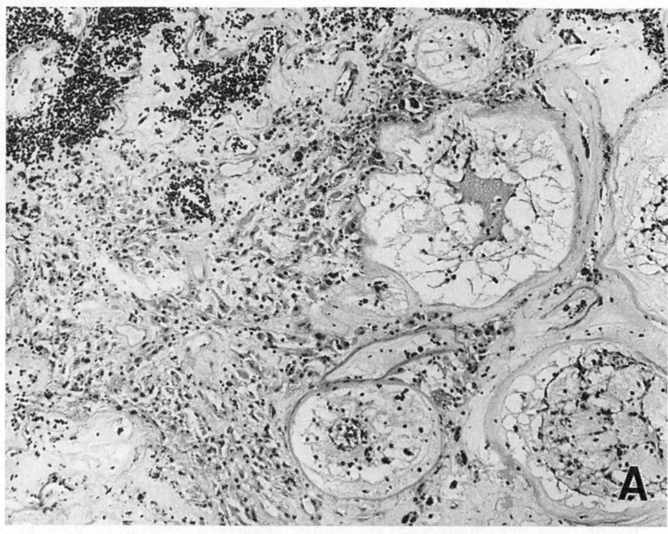

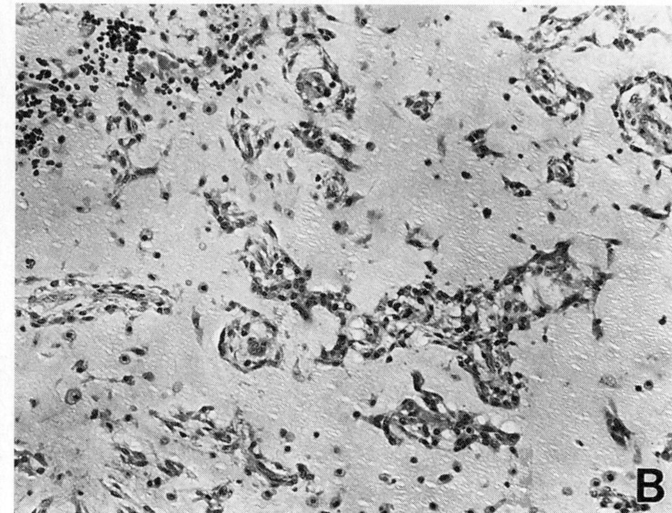

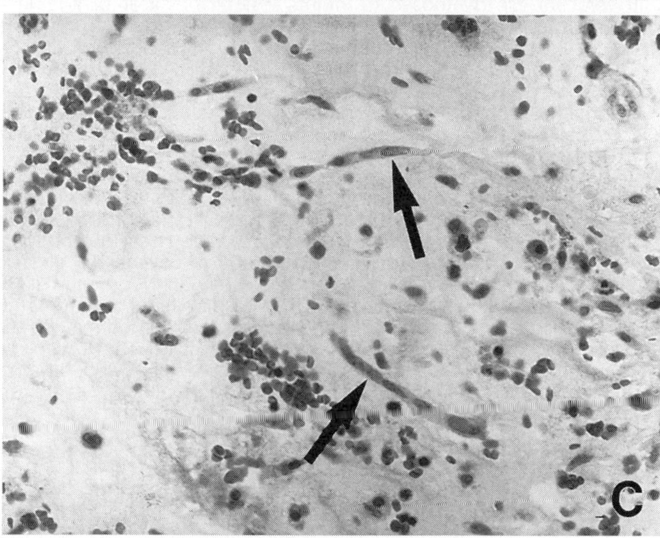

FIGURE 42–3. Characteristic histological features of myxoma. *A,* Low-power view demonstrating individual tumor cells, clusters, and islands scattered throughout the characteristic pale-staining granular extracellular matrix. Hemorrhage is present at upper left. Scattered inflammatory cells are also present. *B,* Medium-power view, demonstrating groups of polygonal myxoma cells. *C,* High-magnification view, showing individual variably rounded to elongated myxoma cells, some arranged in cords (arrows). *A,* 50×; *B,* 175×; *C,* 400×; all stained with hematoxylin and eosin.

Many of the morphological features of organizing mural thrombi resemble those of myxoma, including abundant loose amorphous extracellular matrix, connective tissue cells, and small vascular channels. It is difficult to distinguish between some myxomas and mural thrombi in various stages of organization; indeed, cellular intracardiac thrombi and peripheral thromboemboli occasionally erroneously receive a diagnosis of myxoma. The resemblance to organizing/organized thrombi has been put forth as evidence that myxomas have a thrombotic origin,[66] but most investigators currently find this notion untenable.[60,64]

Histogenesis. The histogenesis of cardiac myxomas is uncertain, but the weight of evidence favors benign neoplasia, with the tumor probably originating from subendocardial nests of primitive mesenchymal cells that may differentiate into several cell types, including endothelial and lipidic cells. Cytogenetic analyses demonstrating clonal chromosomal abnormalities provide the best support for this concept. One study of the cytogenetics of eight cases[67] yielded three with telomeric associations involving chromosome 2 (one with Carney's syndrome); in the same study, four other cases had nonclonal rearrangements involving the short arm of chromosome 12. In an additional recently reported myxoma from a patient with Carney's syndrome, clonal telomeric associations between chromosomes 13 and 15 were demonstrated, and similar nonclonal associations between chromosomes 12 and 17 and others were observed.[68] Nevertheless, the most convincing case of clonal structural aberrations was recently reported by Dijkhuizen,[69] in which a cardiac myxoma from a 48-year-old man had normal chromosome number but a complex clonal rearrangement, which included a breakpoint at 12p12, the location of the *Ki-ras* oncogene. The authors speculated that *Ki-ras* might play a role in the origin of cardiac myxoma. The presence of aneuploidy in some cardiac myxomas provides additional support for the concept of a neoplastic origin.[70]

Before the discussion of nonmyxomatous cardiac tumors is continued below, it should be noted that peculiar microscopic-sized cellular cardiac lesions have been noted incidentally as part of endomyocardial biopsy or surgically removed tissue specimens or at cardiac surgery, free-floating or loosely attached to a valvular or endocardial mass.[71,72] Not neoplastic, they have been termed *M*esothelial/monocytic *I*ncidental *C*ardiac *E*xcrescences ("MICE"). Histologically, such lesions are composed largely of clusters and ribbons of mesothelial cells and entrapped erythrocytes and leukocytes, embedded within a fibrin mesh. Previously considered to be a reactive mesothelial and/or monocytic (histiocytic) hyperplasia, they are now considered to be common artefacts—formed by compaction of mesothelial strips (likely from the pericardium) or other tissue debris and fibrin which are transported via catheters or around an operative site on a cardiotomy suction tip.[73] Such tissue fragments are of importance only in that they should not be confused with metastatic carcinoma.

PAPILLARY TUMORS OF HEART VALVES (PAPILLARY FIBROELASTOMA). The most common tumors of the cardiac valves, papillary fibroelastomas of the cardiac valves and adjacent endocardium, are found not uncommonly postmortem and may be identified during life by two-dimensional echocardiography.[74,75] Although many are clinically insignificant, they have the potential to embolize to vital structures or cause valvular dysfunction, and those on the aortic valve can partially obstruct a coronary arterial orifice.[76] These lesions have a characteristic frond-like appearance resembling a sea anemone, may be single or multiple up to 3 or 4 cm in diameter, and may occur on any valve or on papillary muscle, chordae tendineae, or endocardium, usually attached by a short pedicle (Fig. 42–4). Most often, the ventricular surface of semilunar valves and the atrial surface of atrioventricular valves are affected. The tricuspid valve is most commonly involved in children and the mitral and aortic valves in adults. Histologically, the tumor is covered by endothelium that surrounds a core of loose connective tissue rich in GAGs, collagen, and elastic fibers and containing smooth muscle cells (often as a fine meshwork surrounding a central collagen or dense elastic fiber core).

Pathogenesis. The pathogenesis of these lesions is unsettled, but it appears that they may originate secondary to endocardial trauma and/or the organization of mural thrombi.[66] Papillary tumors are generally distinguished from Lambl's excrescences, which are acellular deposits of thrombus and connective tissue covered by a single layer of endothelium and are found on heart valves at the site of endothelial damage in many adults, particularly along the closure margins of the aortic valve cusps. In contrast, papillary fibroelastomas are unusually found at valvular contact areas.

RHABDOMYOMAS. These are the most common cardiac tumors of infants and children; approximately three-fourths occur in patients younger than 1 year.[77,78] They occur with equal frequency in the left and right ventricular and septal myocardium; nearly all are multiple. Approximately one-third also involve either one or both atria. In approximately half of affected patients, at least one of the tumors is intracavitary and obstructive. Nonspecific clinical manifestations, including cardiomegaly, right or left ventricular failure or both, an S_3, S_4, and systolic or diastolic murmurs, may mimic mitral stenosis, mitral atresia, aortic stenosis, subaortic stenosis, or infundibular pulmonic stenosis.

Association with Tuberous Sclerosis. Rhabdomyomas are strongly associated with tuberous sclerosis, a familial syndrome characterized by hamartomas in several organs, epilepsy, mental deficiency, and adenoma sebaceum.[79–81] A recent study indicated that at least 80 per cent of patients with cardiac rhabdomyomas have tuberous sclerosis, and 60 per cent of patients with tuberous sclerosis less than 18 years old have cardiac rhabdomyomas.[81] Conversely, approximately 50 per cent or more of patients having tuberous sclerosis but no signs or symptoms of cardiac disease have been shown to have findings on echocardiography that are consistent with one or more rhabdomyomas. Rhabdomyomas causing significant intracavity obstruction may result in death within the first 24 hours of life, whereas patients with less severe involvement may either remain asymptomatic or have difficulty during infancy or early childhood.

Pathology. Rhabdomyomas are yellow-gray and range from 1 mm to several centimeters in diameter. They are circumscribed but not encapsulated; microscopically, they are easily distinguished from the surrounding myocardium as clusters of abnormal cells. The microscopic hallmark, termed the "spider cell," is a large (up to 80 mm diameter) cell containing a central cytoplasmic mass that is suspended by fine fibrillar processes radiating to the periphery, thus giving the appearance of a spider hanging in a net. Such cells are sufficiently characteristic that the tumor may be diagnosed by fine-needle aspiration.[82] The cytoplasm is rich in glycogen and stains positively with periodic acid–Schiff reagent. Electron microscopy demonstrates myofibrils, cytoplasmic and mitrochondrial glycogen, and apparent intercellular junctions similar to intercalated discs. Immunohistochemistry reveals diffuse positivity for myoglobin, actin, desmin and vimentin, and the absence of neuroendocrine markers, similar to the staining pattern of the adjacent cardiac muscle. Evidence suggests that rhabdomyomas are actually myocardial hamartomas or malformations rather than true neoplasms. In support of this concept is their multiple occurrence and preponderance in children, especially in those with tuberous sclerosis.

FIBROMAS. Fibromas are benign connective tissue tumors that occur predominantly in children and constitute the second most common type of primary cardiac tumor occurring in the pediatric age group.[83] The majority occur before the age of 10 years, and about 40 per cent are diagnosed in infants less than 1 year of age. Males and females appear to be equally affected. Derived from fibroblasts and considered low-grade connective tissue tumors, cardiac fibromas resemble and have the same biological behavior as soft tissue fibromatoses at other sites.

Pathology. Almost all cardiac fibromas occur within the ventricular myocardium, most frequently within the anterior free wall of the left ventricle or the interventricular septum and much less often in the posterior left ventricular wall or right ventricle. Typically, they are gray, firm, circumscribed, not encapsulated, and range in size from 3 to 10 cm. Grossly, they exhibit a whorled appearance on cut sections. Microscopically, cardiac fibromas consist of elongated fibroblasts admixed with fibrous tissue consisting mostly of collagen. Their cellularity is variable, and mitotic figures are rarely, if ever, seen. Fibrous tissue is intermingled with adjacent myocardial fibers at the margins of the lesion. Calcification and islands of bone formation may be seen microscopically and occasionally radiographically. The *Corlin syndrome,* the main features of which are multiple nevoid basal cell carcinomas, cysts of the jaw, and skeletal abnormalities, may be associated in some cases with cardiac tumors, either fibromas or fibrous histiocytomas.[84]

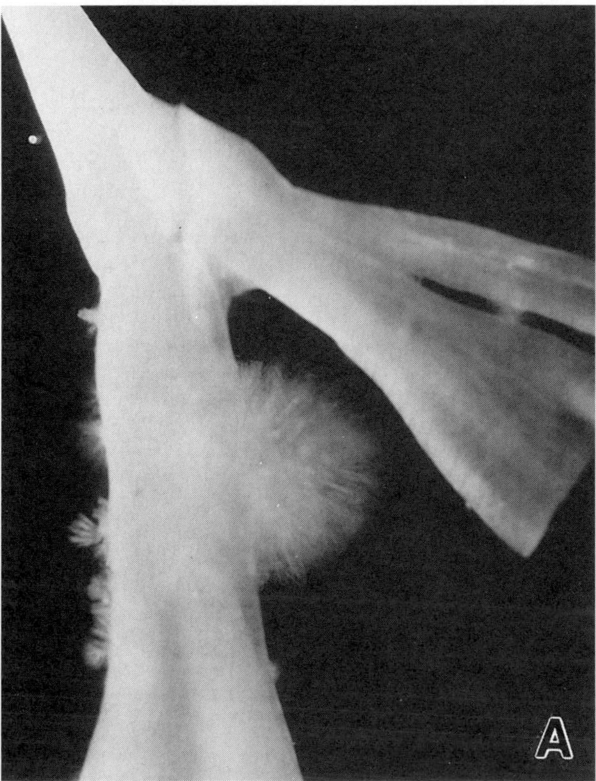

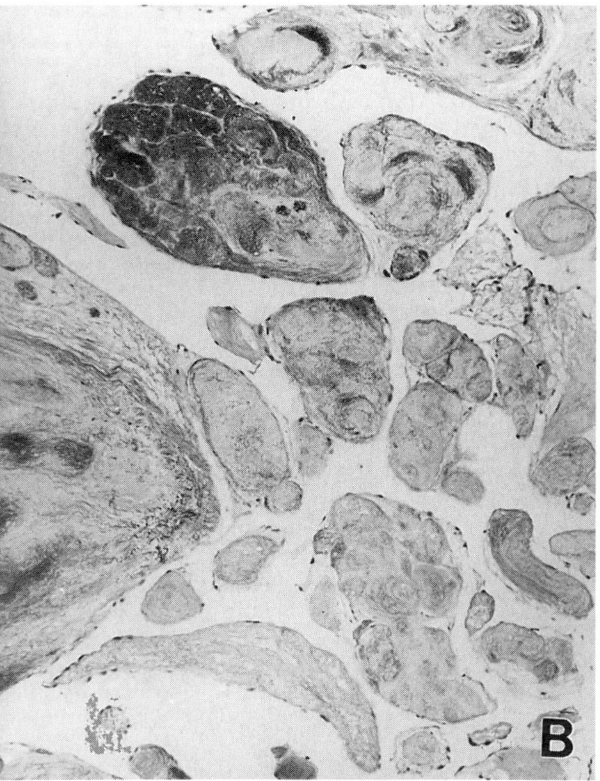

FIGURE 42–4. Papillary fibroelastoma. *A,* Gross photograph demonstrating resemblance of this lesion to a sea anemone, with myriad papillary fronds, arising from the chordae tendineae near the mitral leaflet. In this case, multiple lesions were present, all associated with the mitral valve apparatus. *B,* Histological appearance of papillary fibroelastoma, demonstrating the multiple papillary fronds consisting of a collagen core surrounded by elastic fibers and loose connective tissue, all covered by endocardial endothelium. 100×; stained with elastica van Gieson stain (elastin black).

Clinical Manifestations. Although fibromas may be incidental findings at postmortem examination, approximately 70 per cent at some time cause mechanical interference with intracardiac flow, ventricular contraction abnormalities, or conduction disturbances. Clinical manifestations are protean and include murmurs, atypical chest pain, congestive heart failure and signs of subaortic stenosis, valvular or infundibular pulmonic stenosis with right ventricular hypertrophy, tricuspid stenosis, conduction disturbances, ventricular tachycardia, and sudden death. As in the case of rhabdomyomas, the increased usage of echocardiography has rarely resulted in the detection of cardiac fibromas in patients without cardiac signs or symptoms. Surgical excision of cardiac fibromas may be possible.[85,86]

LIPOMAS AND LIPOMATOUS HYPERTROPHY OF THE ATRIAL SEPTUM. Lipomas occur at all ages and with equal frequency in both sexes. Most range in diameter from 1 to 15 cm, although some have been reported to weigh more than 2 kg. Most tumors are sessile or polypoid and occur in the subendocardium or subpericardium, although about one-fourth are completely intramuscular. Subendocardial tumors with intracavity extension produce symptoms that are characteristic of their location, whereas subepicardial tumors may cause compression of the heart and pericardial effusion. The most common chambers affected are the left ventricle, right atrium, and interatrial septum. Intramural tumors may be asymptomatic or result in arrhythmias, AV or intraventricular conduction disturbances, or mechanical interference. However, many tumors are clinically silent and are found only at autopsy or become apparent on a routine chest roentgenogram.

Microscopically, the lesions are usually well encapsulated, composed of typical mature fat cells, and occasionally contain fibrous connective tissue (fibrolipoma), muscular tissue (myolipoma), or vacuolated brown (fetal) fat resembling a hibernoma.

Whereas lipomas are true neoplasms, a condition termed *lipomatous hypertrophy of the interatrial septum* represents the occurrence of a nonencapsulated hyperplastic accumulation of mature and fetal adipose tissue within the interatrial septum. These lesions range from 1 to 7 cm in dimension, most often protrude into the right atrium, and are more common in obese, elderly, or female patients.[87] A variety of atrial arrhythmias have been attributed to these lesions, but a cause-and-effect relationship has been difficult to establish.[87] Since this lesion may occasionally be detected by cineangiography, echocardiography, computed tomography, or other diagnostic techniques, the major clinical dilemma is the differential diagnosis and treatment of an intraatrial filling defect.

ANGIOMAS. Composed of benign proliferations of endothelial cells, hemangiomas and lymphangiomas are extremely rare.[88] Anatomically, they may occur in any part of the heart, but usually they are intramural, often in the interventricular septum or AV node, where they may cause complete heart block and sudden death. Cardiac tamponade due to hemopericardium may be the presenting clinical syndrome. More commonly found in the right heart chambers, hemangiomas are red, hemorrhagic, generally sessile or polypoid subendocardial nodules, ranging from 2 to 4 cm in diameter. Histologically, the tumors consist of endothelium-lined spaces which may contain blood, lymph, or thrombi; they are classified according to the predominant type of proliferating vascular channel. Dilated, often thrombosed, subendocardial blood vessels (varices) are frequently mistaken for hemangiomas; they are usually found incidentally.

TERATOMAS. These tumors, which contain elements of all three germ cell layers, occur within the heart less frequently than in the anterior mediastinum.[89] Teratomas are generally observed in children, and when located within the heart, they occur predominantly within the right atrium, right ventricle, or the interatrial or interventricular septum.

CYSTIC TUMOR ("MESOTHELIOMA") OF THE ATRIOVENTRICULAR NODE. Of controversial histogenesis, these small tumors (usually less than 15 mm in largest dimension) frequently cause death by complete heart block, ventricular fibrillation,[36] or cardiac tamponade.[90] They occur in patients of virtually any age as poorly circumscribed, often multicystic nodules in the atrial septum, immediately cephalad to the commissure of the septal and anterior leaflets of the tricuspid valve, in the region of the AV node. These lesions are characterized by tubules and cysts lined by flat or cuboidal cells that are devoid of mitotic activity, but may have secretory function. Although often considered to be derived from mesothelial rests, similar to the adenomatoid tumors of the ovary and testis that they resemble histologically, recent studies have suggested an endodermal rather than mesothelial origin.[91,92]

ENDOCRINE TUMORS OF THE HEART. Approximately 2 per cent of *paragangliomas* are intrathoracic, and of these, most are located in the posterior mediastinum. However, these tumors can also occur in close association with the left atrial or left ventricular epicardium, where they are thought to have arisen from sympathetic fibers to the heart or from ectopic chromaffin cells. More rarely still, paragangliomas may arise within the interatrial septum. Tumors in any of these locations may secrete catecholamines and therefore can be associated with signs and symptoms characteristic of pheochromocytoma.[93]

Rarely, benign *thyroid tumors* arise within the heart, presumably from ectopic rests of thyroid tissue. These tumors most often arise from the interventricular septum and present, not infrequently, as obstruction to right ventricular outflow.

Malignant Cardiac Tumors

About one-fourth of all cardiac tumors exhibit malignant histological characteristics and invasive or metastatic behavior. Nearly all of these are sarcomas, thus making these tumors second only to myxomas in overall frequency. Sarcomas may occur at any age but are most common between the third and fifth decades, are distinctly unusual in infant and children, and show no sex preference. In decreasing order of frequency the sites involved are the right atrium, left atrium, right ventricle, left ventricle, and interventricular septum.

Sarcomas derive from mesenchyme and therefore may display a wide variety of morphological types, including angiosarcoma, rhabdomyosarcoma, fibrosarcoma, osteosarcoma, and others.[94–96]

From a clinical viewpoint, sarcomas characteristically display a rapid downhill course. Death most often occurs from a few weeks to 2 years after the onset of symptoms. These tumors proliferate rapidly and generally cause death through widespread infiltration of the myocardium, obstruction of flow within the heart, or distant metastases. About 75 per cent of all patients with cardiac sarcomas have pathological evidence of distant metastases at the time of death.[1,97,98] The most frequent sites are the lungs, thoracic lymph nodes, mediastinum, and vertebral column; less often the liver, kidneys, adrenals, pancreas, bone, spleen, and bowel are involved.

The cardiac findings are determined primarily by the location of the tumor and by the extent of intracavitary obstruction. Typical presentations include progressive, unexplained, congestive heart failure, particularly of the right side; precordial pain; pericardial effusion; tamponade; arrhythmias; conduction disturbances; obstruction of the venae cavae; and sudden death. Tumors limited to the myocardium without intracavitary extension may produce no cardiac symptoms or may cause arrhythmias and conduction disturbances. Because of the rapid growth potential of sarcomas, they commonly extend into the cardiac chambers, the pericardial space, or both. In about 20 per cent of cases, the tumor is sessile or polypoid. When there is extension into the pericardial space, hemorrhagic pericardial effusion is common and tamponade may occur. Because the right side of the heart is most commonly affected, sarcomas frequently cause signs of right heart failure as a result of obstruction of the right atrium, right ventricle, or tricuspid or pulmonic valves. In addition, obstruction of the superior vena cava may result in swelling of the face and upper extremities, whereas obstruction of the inferior vena cava may result in visceral congestion.

ANGIOSARCOMAS. Included within this category are angiosarcomas and Kaposi's sarcomas.[99,100] All 40 patients in one series were adults. In distinction to most other cardiac sarcomas, in which the sex distribution is equal, there appears to be a 2:1 male-to-female ratio among patients with angiosarcomas. These tumors have a striking predilection for the right atrium (Fig. 42–5) and may be infiltrative or polypoid in nature. Microscopically, angiosarcomas are characterized by ill-defined but variable anastomotic vascular channels lined with atypical, often heaped-up, endothelial cells. By electron microscopy, immature endothelial cells, primitive pericytes, and undifferentiated mesenchymal cells may be identified.[101]

RHABDOMYOSARCOMAS. These are tumors of striated muscle which often diffusely infiltrate the myocardium but which may also, on occasion, form a polypoid extension into the cardiac chambers and therefore have been clinically mistaken for myxoma.[102] Rhabdomyoblasts (cross-striations by light microscopy; thick and thin filaments and Z-band material by electron microscopy) are the histological hallmark of this tumor, and 20 to 30 per cent of the tumors have cross-striations.

FIBROSARCOMAS AND MALIGNANT FIBROUS HISTIOCYTOMAS. Fibrosarcomas of the heart have a whitish, soft "fish flesh" consistency characteristic of these tumor types elsewhere in the body.[101a] Fibroblastic in differentiation, they are composed of spindle-shaped cells with elongated blunt-ended nuclei, and frequent mitoses. They may contain areas of hemorrhage and necrosis and extensively infiltrate the heart, often involving more than one cardiac chamber. A thrombus may form in an obstructed pulmonary vein, in the vena cava, or over the mural surface of the tumor.

LYMPHOMAS. Although cardiac involvement of a systemic lym-

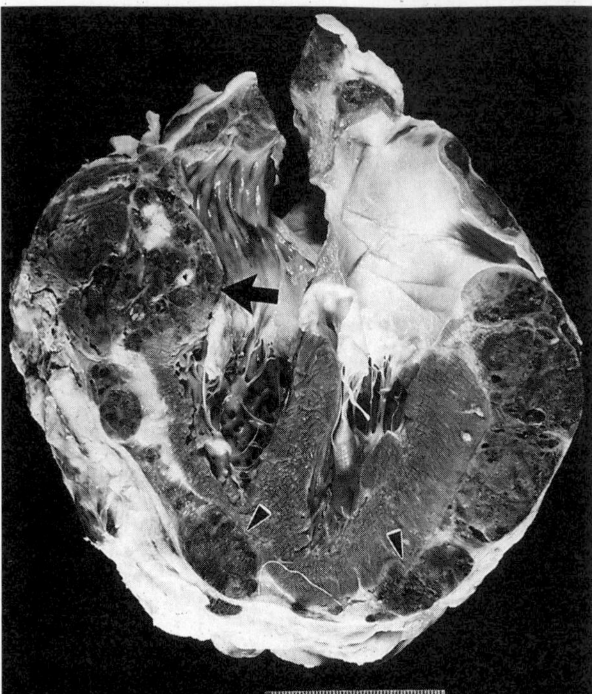

FIGURE 42–5. Massive pericardial angiosarcoma, with deep myocardial invasion at multiple sites (arrowheads), particularly at right atrium (arrow). (From Schoen, F. J.: Interventional and Surgical Cardiovascular Pathology: Clinical Correlations and Basic Principles. Philadelphia, W. B. Saunders Company, 1989.)

phoma has been reported in 25 to 36 per cent of cases, primary lymphoma involving only the heart or pericardium is much less common.[102,103] Myocardial infiltration by lymphoma may be nodular or diffuse, and the clinical syndrome of hypertrophic cardiomyopathy has been mimicked. Some of these tumors are predominantly intracavitary.

PULMONARY ARTERY SARCOMAS. Sarcomas of the pulmonary artery trunk, main branches, or pulmonic valves may present as tumor emboli to the lungs or as right ventricular outflow obstruction.[104] These tumors usually present after the fourth decade, show a 2:1 female predominance, and may originate from undifferentiated tissue of the bulbis cordis. Typical symptoms include dyspnea, chest pain, cough, and hemoptysis and may be associated with radiographic findings of a pulmonary hilar mass or cardiomegaly. Right ventricular injection of contrast material helps to delineate the tumor. Although most reported cases were previously diagnosed at autopsy, it is likely that early diagnosis, surgical resection, and possibly chemotherapy may have an impact on survival of future patients with this tumor.[105]

DIAGNOSTIC TECHNIQUES

Although certain clinical manifestations may be suggestive of a cardiac tumor, no clinical finding or set of findings is pathognomonic. Furthermore, the majority of cardiac tumors produce signs and symptoms typical of the common forms of heart disease. The development of modern diagnostic methods has had a major impact on the diagnosis and hence the natural history of cardiac tumors. It is not unusual for cardiac tumors to be diagnosed and cured in patients who are totally asymptomatic or without signs of cardiovascular disease.[106] Although cardiac catheterization made possible the definitive preoperative diagnosis of cardiac tumors, it was not until the advent of echocardiography that it was feasible to evaluate all patients suspected of this diagnosis. Both M-mode and two-dimensional echocardiography are effective screening techniques. However, two-dimensional echocardiography, and particularly transesophageal imaging (Fig. 42–6), is more sensitive and provides considerably more information regarding the site of tumor attachment, pattern of tumor movement, and size. In many centers, the information provided by two-dimensional echocardiography, computed tomography (CT), or magnetic resonance imaging (MRI) (Fig. 42–7) is considered sufficient to proceed directly to surgery without cardiac catheterization and angiography. However, catheterization and angiography should not be omitted in the absence of a technically adequate two-dimensional echocardiographic study, CT, or MRI that has visualized all four cardiac chambers.

It is imperative that noninvasive evaluation, preferably by two-dimensional echocardiography (or CT or MRI), be performed before cardiac catheterization whenever the diagnosis of cardiac tumor is considered. When left atrial myxoma is suspected, it is safest to visualize the left atrium by injecting the contrast agent into the pulmonary artery and film during the levophase. It is particularly important to avoid the transseptal approach, since this risks dislodgment of fragments of tumor that may be attached in the region of the fossa ovalis. Furthermore, since cardiac tumors may be multiple and present in more than one chamber, all four chambers should be visualized noninvasively prior to cardiac catheterization whenever possible.

Clinical and Noninvasive Methods

CLINICAL EXAMINATION. When valvular or myocardial disease is suspected on clinical grounds, certain atypical

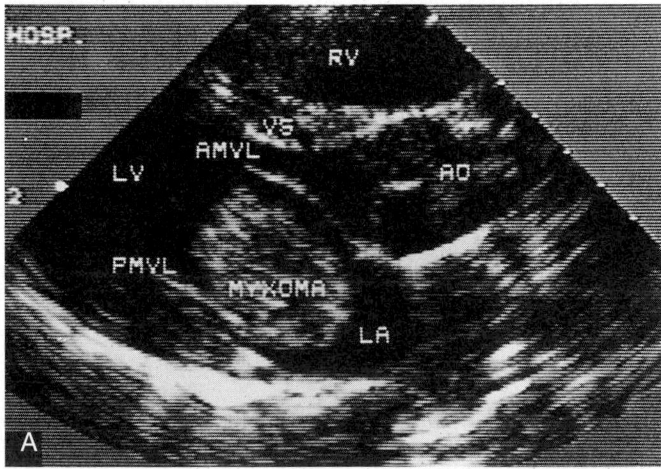

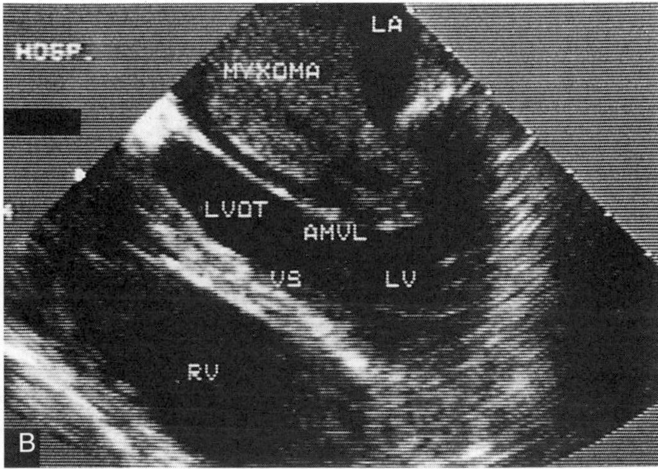

FIGURE 42–6. Transthoracic two-dimensional echocardiogram (*A*) and transesophageal two-dimensional echocardiogram (*B*) showing a left atrial (LA) mass prolapsing into and obstructing the mitral valve orifice. Note the superior resolution of the transesophageal echocardiogram. Although not visible here, the myxoma was attached to the mid-portion of the atrial septum. (From Allard, M. F., et al.: Primary cardiac tumors. *In* Goldhaber, S. Z., and Braunwald, E. (eds.): Cardiopulmonary Diseases and Cardiac Tumors. Atlas of Heart Diseases. Vol. 3. Philadelphia, Current Medicine, 1995, pp. 15.1–15.22.)

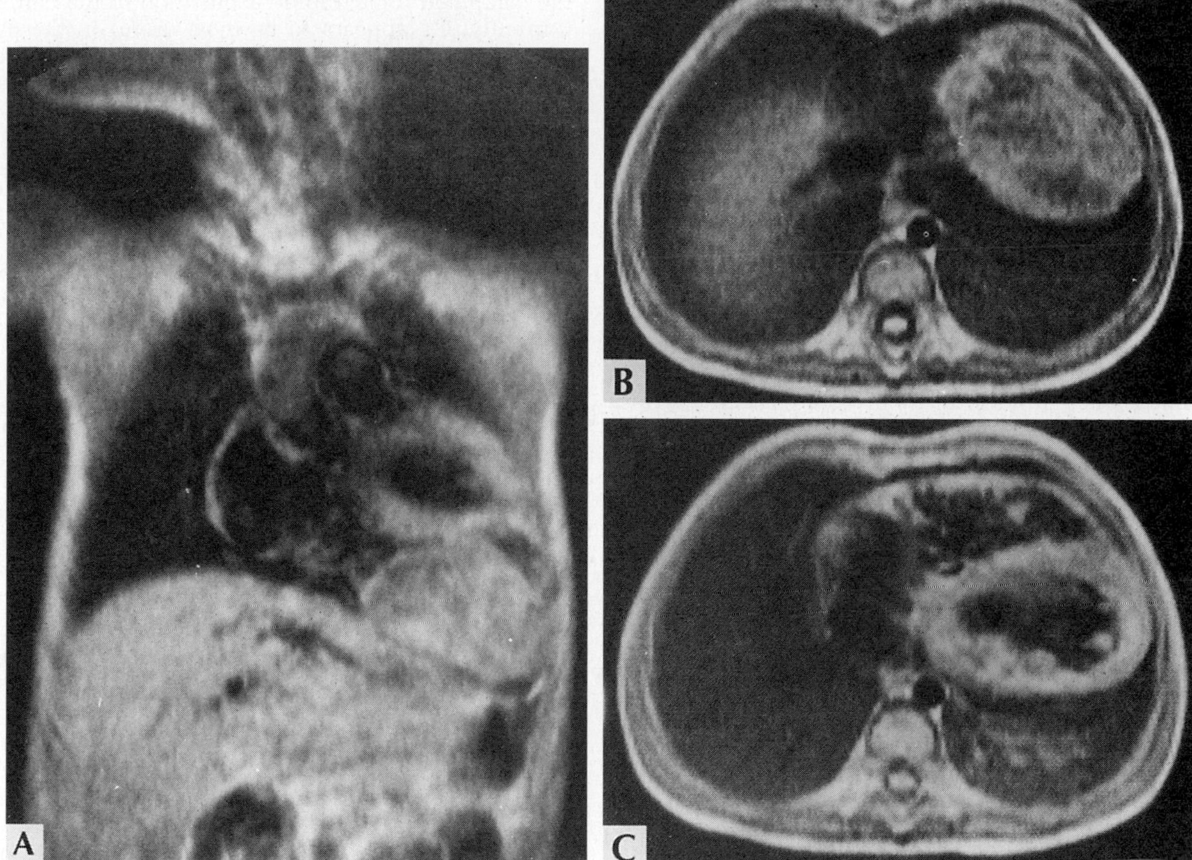

FIGURE 42–7. Magnetic resonance images illustrating a large tumor in the right ventricular apex, impinging on the apical septum. In the coronal view, the prominent mass indents the septum *(A)*. In the axial views, the tumor shows areas of tissue inhomogeneity *(B)* and indents the ventricular septum *(C)*. (From Allard, M. F., et al.: Primary cardiac tumors. *In* Goldhaber, S. Z., and Braunwald, E. (eds.): Cardiopulmonary Diseases and Cardiac Tumors. Atlas of Heart Disease. Vol. 3. Philadelphia, Current Medicine, 1995, pp. 15.1–15.22.)

findings may raise the question of cardiac tumor. The intensity of the systolic or diastolic murmur caused by a left atrial myxoma is often exquisitely sensitive to positional change, a finding atypical of valvular heart disease. S_1 may be delayed as a consequence of an elevated left atrial pressure, as in mitral stenosis. It is often intense and widely split, and an early systolic sound may occur, representing tumor movement toward the atrium during systole. In addition, a tumor "plop" may be present about 100 msec after S_2, which appears to result from the sudden tension of the tumor stalk as it prolapses into the left ventricle during diastole or from the tumor striking the myocardium. The tumor plop *precedes* the end of the rapid filling wave of the apexcardiogram and can thereby be differentiated from an S_3; as noted, it usually occurs later than an opening snap. Systolic time intervals are usually consistent with a reduced stroke volume. Apexcardiography often shows a deep notch on the upstroke, which occurs at the time of extrusion of the tumor through the mitral valve in early systole.

Right atrial tumors may also result in a widely split S_1 and an early systolic sound. The S_2 may be paradoxically split as a result of early pulmonic valve closure. A tumor plop and systolic and diastolic murmurs, which are increased by inspiration, may also occur with right atrial tumors. The jugular venous pulse tracing may reflect obstruction of the tricuspid orifice, demonstrating an accentuated *a* wave, attenuation of the *x* descent, or an early, broad *v* wave.

RADIOLOGICAL EXAMINATION

Cardiac tumors may display several findings on plain chest roentgenograms. These include alterations in cardiac contour, changes in overall cardiac size, specific chamber enlargement, alterations in pulmonary vascularity, and intracardiac calcification (Chap. 7). The cardiac contour may be normal, may display generalized or specific chamber enlargement that mimics virtually any type of valvular heart disease, or may demonstrate a bizarre appearance. Pericardial effusions are rather common and generally indicate invasion of the pericardial space by a malignant tumor. Mediastinal widening, due to hilar and paramediastinal adenopathy, may indicate spread of a malignant cardiac tumor. A bumpy, irregular, or fuzzy cardiac border may be seen when the pericardium is involved. Cardiac enlargement may reflect rapid tumor growth, particularly in the case of sarcomas, whereas specific chamber enlargement is frequently due to intracavitary obstruction, particularly by pedunculated tumors such as myxomas. Thus, left atrial myxoma may produce the radiological pattern characteristic of mitral stenosis. Occasionally a large tumor mass displaces the heart and may simulate enlargement of a specific chamber.

Calcification visible by roentgenographic methods may occur with several types of cardiac tumor, including rhabdomyomas, fibromas, hamartomas, teratomas, myxomas, and angiomas. Visualization of intracardiac calcium in an infant or a child is unusual and should immediately raise the question of an intracardiac tumor. Cardiac fluoroscopy and laminography may be helpful in differentiating calcification of cardiac tumor from that of other structures, such as cardiac valves, coronary arteries, pericardium, and mural thrombus. Occasionally, calcified atrial polypoid tumors may be seen to prolapse into the ventricle during diastole. Fluoroscopy is also useful in differentiating cardiac tumor from ventricular aneurysm, both of which may result in a localized protrusion on plain chest roentgenograms. However, on fluoroscopic examination, cardiac tumors do not display the paradoxical motion during ventricular contraction that is characteristic of ventricular aneurysm.

ECHOCARDIOGRAPHY (see Fig. 3–105, p. 94). Two-dimensional echocardiography provides substantial advantages over conventional M-mode echocardiography for the diagnosis and preoperative evaluation of intracardiac tumors.[5] In the majority of cases of cardiac tumors, the information provided by two-dimensional echocardiography provides adequate information regarding tumor size, attachment, and mobility to allow operative resection without preoperative angiography. This technique is sensitive for detection of small tumors and is especially useful for detection of left ventricular tumors and tumors that do not prolapse through the mitral or tricuspid valve orifices.

Left atrial myxomas have been classified by their echocardiographic appearance as follows: Class I tumors are small and prolapse through the mitral valve; Class II tumors are small and nonprolapsing; Class III tumors are large and prolapse; and Class IV tumors are large and nonprolapsing.[107] The increased sensitivity of two-dimensional echocardiography makes possible the diagnosis of cardiac tumors in neonates and in utero.[108] The improved diagnostic power and widespread use of two-dimensional echocardiography have resulted in an increase in the detection of primary cardiac tumors,[106] in many cases prior to the onset of clinical signs or symptoms.

Two-dimensional echocardiography may facilitate the differentiation between left atrial thrombus and myxoma, because the former typically produces a layered appearance and is generally situated in the posterior portion of the atrium, whereas the latter is often mottled in appearance and rarely occurs in the posterior portion of the atrium. In some atrial myxomas, areas of echolucency may be seen within the tumor mass, corresponding to areas of hemorrhage within the tumor. Since these areas of echolucency are not found in thrombotic or infective lesions, this finding may be of value in the differential diagnosis of an intraatrial mass. Continuous-mode Doppler ultrasonography may be useful for evaluating the hemodynamic consequences of valvular obstruction or incompetence caused by cardiac tumors.[109]

Transesophageal Echocardiography (see Fig. 3–106, p. 95). This approach provides an unimpeded view of both atria and the atrial septum, and appears to be superior to transthoracic echocardiography in many patients.[110] The potential advantages of transesophageal echocardiography include improved resolution of the tumor and its attachment (Fig. 42–6), the ability to detect some masses not visualized by transthoracic echocardiography, and improved visualization of right atrial tumors. In 17 patients suspected of having a cardiac tumor, transthoracic echocardiography yielded four false-positives and two false-negatives, whereas transesophageal echocardiography resulted in only one false-positive and no false-negatives.[111] In the same series, transesophageal echocardiography proved to be superior for visualizing anatomic details such as tumor contour, cysts, and calcification, and identified a stalk in 10 or 11 tumors subsequently shown to have a stalk at surgery, whereas transthoracic echocardiography identified a stalk in only 5 of the 11 tumors. Transesophageal echocardiography has been used to guide the percutaneous biopsy of a right atrial myxoma.[112] Although transesophageal echocardiography does not appear warranted on a routine basis, it should be considered when the transthoracic study is suboptimal or confusing.

RADIONUCLIDE IMAGING. Gated blood pool scanning has been used to identify atrial, ventricular, and intramural tumors.[113] Radionuclide ventriculography generally has a lower rate of resolution than does echocardiography or contrast injection angiography and therefore may be less sensitive for the detection of small filling defects. In some cases in which the cardiac tumor was not evident by routine static or dynamic radionuclide imaging, it has been possible to delineate the tumor and its movement during a cardiac cycle by use of a computer-generated composite functional image.[113]

COMPUTED TOMOGRAPHY. CT of the heart has been used to demonstrate cardiac tumors.[114] Although more experience will be necessary to establish its role, certain advantages are apparent. These include a high degree of tissue discrimination, which may allow definition of the degree of intramural tumor extension; evaluation of the extracardiac structures; and the ability to construct images in any plane. Resolution appears to be improved substantially by gating the computed tomographic acquisition to the cardiac cycle. Currently, CT appears to be most useful in the evaluation of suspected tumors of the heart to determine the degree of myocardial invasion and the involvement of pericardial and extracardiac structures. Ultrafast CT, a technique that uses electron beam technology, has a short scanning acquisition time that eliminates the motion artifacts occurring with conventional CT and appears to be useful for assessment of intracardiac masses.[114]

MAGNETIC RESONANCE IMAGING. MRI may be of considerable value in the detection and delineation of cardiac tumors and in some cases may depict the size, shape, and surface characteristics of the tumor more clearly than two-dimensional echocardiography[115] (Fig. 10–18, p. 326). The larger field of view with MRI (Fig. 42–7) provides better definition of tumor prolapse, secondary valve obstruction, and cardiac chamber size than does two-dimensional echocardiography. Contrast enhancement with Gd-DTPA and multislice imaging in the transaxial, sagittal, and long axes can provide precise three-dimensional information. MRI can also provide information regarding tissue composition that can help to differentiate tumors from thrombi.[116]

Angiography

Cardiac catheterization and selective angiocardiography are not necessary in all cases of cardiac tumors, since, as already discussed, in many cases adequate preoperative information may be obtained by echocardiography, CT, or MRI. However, several circumstances exist in which the risk and expense of cardiac catheterization are outweighed by the supplemental information it may provide. These situations include cases in which (1) noninvasive evaluation has not been adequate in defining fully tumor location or attachment; (2) all four cardiac chambers have not been adequately visualized noninvasively; (3) a malignant cardiac tumor is considered likely; or (4) other cardiac lesions may coexist with a cardiac tumor and possibly dictate a different surgical approach. For instance, when a malignant cardiac tumor is suspected, cardiac angiography may provide valuable information regarding the degree of myocardial, vascular, and/or pericardial invasion. Likewise, in certain cases, such as the presence of pulmonary hypertension or the coexistence of significant valvular or coronary artery lesions, cardiac catheterization and angiography may provide information that significantly affects the surgical approach.[117]

The major angiographic findings in patients with cardiac tumors include (1) compression or displacement of cardiac chambers or large vessels, (2) deformity of cardiac chambers, (3) intracavitary filling defects, (4) marked variations in myocardial thickness, (5) pericardial effusion, and (6) local alterations in wall motion. Displacement of the cardiac chambers or the great vessels without deformation of the internal contour may be observed in both benign and malignant tumors, whereas deformation of a cardiac chamber usually indicates an infiltrating malignant lesion. The most frequent angiographic findings are intracavitary filling defects, which may be either fixed or mobile. Fixed defects may be lobulated or appear as a coarse nodularity of the myocardium often difficult to distinguish from a mural thrombus. Such defects may reflect endocardial tumors with broad attachments or intramural tumors with intracavitary extension. Mobile intracavitary defects are usually pedunculated tumors, typically myxomas, although the stalk may be difficult to visualize. Such tumors may prolapse into the AV valve orifice during diastole or, in the case of ventricular tumors, into the left ventricular outflow tract during systole. An atrial ball thrombus may mimic a pedunculated tumor, but is more likely to be associated with clot in the atrial appendage.

A localized increase in myocardial wall thickness, especially when accompanied by a pericardial effusion, suggests an infiltrating malignant tumor. It is often difficult to differentiate myocardial thickening from pericardial effusion, but this may be aided by observation of the thickness of the right atrial wall. Since the right atrial wall is seldom infiltrated by tumor, the finding of right atrial thickening to greater than 5 mm suggests a pericardial effusion.[117] In myocardial infiltration, localized areas of disordered wall motion may also be noted by cineangiography. Coronary arteriography may in some cases allow visualization of the vascular supply of the tumor, thus demarcating the extent of tumor invasion, the source of its blood supply, and its relation to the coronary arteries.[118,119] However, the vascular pattern of cardiac tumors has not proved to be a useful sign of malignancy.

False-negative angiographic studies generally occur when the diagnosis is not suspected prior to catheterization. False-positive studies are most often the result of thrombus, but may also be produced by many entities, such as streaming of nonopaque venous blood, a hematoma in the atrial septum, an aneurysm of the muscular or membranous ventricular septum, Bernheim syndrome, congenital septal dysplasia, and hydatid cysts of the interventricular septum.

The major risk of angiography is peripheral embolization due to dislodgement of a fragment of tumor or of an associated thrombus. Therefore, the thorough evaluation of all cardiac chambers by noninvasive methods prior to catheterization is recommended in patients suspected of having cardiac tumors so that contrast material can be injected into the chamber proximal (upstream) to the location of the tumor. The transseptal approach to the left atrium (see p. 186) is particularly hazardous because of the frequent occurrence of left atrial myxomas in the region of the fossa ovalis.[120]

TREATMENT AND PROGNOSIS

Benign Tumors

Operative excision is the treatment of choice for most benign cardiac tumors and in many cases results in a complete cure.[5,121–123] Although many tumors are histologically benign, all cardiac tumors are potentially lethal as a result of intracavitary or valvular obstruction, peripheral embolization, and disturbances of rhythm or conduction. Unfortunately, it is not unusual for patients to die or experience a major complication while awaiting operation, and therefore it is mandatory to carry out the operation promptly after the diagnosis has been established.

Although some epicardial tumors may be removed without the aid of extracorporeal circulation, most intramural and intracavitary tumors must be excised under direct vision, requiring use of the heart-lung machine. Closed approaches are not now recommended because of increased risk of dislodging tumor fragments. In addition, excision cannot be as complete, and adequate inspection of the other cardiac chambers for additional tumors is not possible.

The dislodgment of tumor fragments constitutes a major risk of operation and may result in peripheral emboli or the dispersion of micrometastases, which may seed peripherally. To reduce this risk, manipulation of the heart prior to cardiopulmonary bypass should be minimized. Some surgeons recommend that venous cannulation for cardiopulmonary bypass be performed via the femoral or azygos vein rather than through the right atrium to avoid dislodging an unsuspected right atrial tumor. In addition, the tumor should be removed en bloc when possible, and the chamber then irrigated well with saline.

ATRIAL MYXOMAS. Numerous reports document complete cure of left and right atrial myxomas with follow-up periods of 10 to 15 years.[124,125] In about 1 to 5 per cent of cases a recurrence or second cardiac myxoma has been reported following resection of the initial myxoma.[126,127] Possible causes of the second tumor include incomplete excision of the original tumor with regrowth, growth from a second "pretumorous" focus, i.e., metasynchronous, or intracardiac implantation from the original tumor. Because of the first two possibilities, some surgeons have advocated excision of the entire region of the fossa ovalis and repair of the resultant atrial septal defect to remove presumably high concentrations of "pretumor" cells thought to be located in that region. In one case, the large size of a myxoma, together with its location on the posterior left atrial wall, necessitated complete removal of the heart, followed by autotransplantation, i.e., reimplantation of the patient's excised heart.[127a] Laser photocoagulation of a 1-cm area around the stalk attachment site has also been suggested as a way of eradicating pretumorous cells without the necessity of creating an atrial septal defect.[128] Other surgeons have reported equally successful long-term recurrence-free periods with simple excision of the tumor and a small rim at the base. It now appears that in approximately 7 per cent of patients with (1) a familial history of cardiac myxoma, (2) features of the complex of lentigines and other abnormalities described on page 1467, or (3) synchronous tumor appearance (i.e., multiple tumors at the time of presentation), the incidence of a second tumor occurring at some time in the future is in the range of 12 to 22 per cent, as compared to approximately 1 per cent for patients with sporadic atrial myxoma.[127] It is believed that tumor recurrence in these cases is from a second pretumorous focus of cells. In these high-risk patients, a careful search for multiple tumors preoperatively and more extensive resection of the underlying endocardium, atrial septum, or both is recommended. Careful echocardiographic follow-up for detection of metasynchronous tumors is recommended[127] in all patients following resection of a myxoma.

OTHER BENIGN TUMORS. Successful excision has also been reported for ventricular myxomas, as well as most other types of benign cardiac tumor, including rhabdomyoma, hamartoma, fibroma, lipoma, hemangioma, and papillary fibroelastoma.[129–131] The major surgical considerations in excision of ventricular tumors include preservation of adequate ventricular myocardium, maintenance of proper atrioventricular valve function, and preservation of as much of the conduction system as possible. Often, however, papillary muscles, chordae tendineae, or the AV conduction system must be sacrificed during the resection of a tumor, thereby necessitating replacement of the atrioventricular valve, implantation of a pacemaker, or both.

Malignant Tumors

Operation is not an effective treatment for the great majority of primary malignant tumors of the heart because of the large mass of cardiac tissue involved or the presence of metastases. The major role for surgery in such cases is to establish a diagnosis in order to exclude the possibility of a curable benign tumor. Nevertheless, in some cases palliation of hemodynamics and/or constitutional symptoms and extension of life may be achieved by aggressive therapy. Survivals of 1 to 3 years have been reported following partial resection, chemotherapy, radiation therapy, orthotopic cardiac transplantation or various combinations of these modalities.[132–136] In some instances, localized recurrences have been eliminated by multiple operations. Some success in palliation of symptoms has been reported following the combination of chemotherapy and radiation therapy[137] and radiation therapy alone.[136] Lymphosarcoma of the heart frequently responds to chemotherapy, radiation therapy, or both.[138,139] Unfortunately, many other reports indicate a failure to alter the course of cardiac sarcomas despite various combinations of surgery, chemotherapy, and radiation therapy.

REFERENCES

CLINICAL PRESENTATION

1. Allard, M. F., Taylor, G. P., Wilson, J. E., and McManus, B. M.: Primary cardiac tumors. *In* Goldhaber, S. Z. and Braunwald, E. (eds.): Cardiopulmonary Diseases and Cardiac Tumors. Atlas of Heart Diseases. vol. 3. Philadelphia, Current Medicine, 1995, pp. 15.1–15.22.
2. Reynan, K.: Frequency of primary tumors of the heart. Am. J. Cardiol. *77*:107, 1996.
3. Lam, K. Y. L., Dickens, P., and Chan, A. C. L.: Tumors of the heart. Arch. Pathol. Lab. Med. *117*:1027, 1993.
4. Tazelaar, H. D., Locke, T. J., and McGregir, C. G. A.: Pathology of surgically excised primary cardiac tumors. Mayo Clin. Proc. *67*:957, 1992.
5. Salcedo, E. E., Cohen, G. I., White, R. D., and Davison, M. B.: Cardiac tumors: Diagnosis and treatment. Curr. Probl. Cardiol. *17*:73, 1992.
6. Hanson, E. C.: Cardiac tumors: A current perspective. N. Y. State J. Med. *92*:41, 1992.
7. Goodwin, J. F.: Symposium on cardiac tumors. The spectrum of cardiac tumors. Am. J. Cardiol. *21*:307, 1968.
8. St. John Sutton, M. G., Mercier, L., Guliani, E. R., and Lie, J. T.: Atrial myxomas: A review of clinical experience in 40 patients. Mayo Clin. Proc. *55*:371, 1980.
9. Hirano, T., Taga, T., and Yasukawa, K.: Human B-cell differentiation

factor defined by an anti-peptide antibody and its possible role in autoantibody production. Proc. Natl. Acad. Sci. USA *84*:228, 1987.
10. Borden, E. C., and Chin, P.: Interleukin-6: A cytokine with potential diagnostic and therapeutic roles. J. Lab. Clin. Med. *123*:824, 1994.
11. Wada, A., Kanda, T., Hayashi, R., et al.: Cardiac myxoma metastasized to the brain: Potential role of endogenous interleukin-6. Cardiology *83*:208, 1993.
12. Takahara, H., Mori, A., Tabata, R., et al.: Left atrial myxoma with production of interleukin-6. J. Jpn. Assoc. Thorac. Surg. *40*:326, 1992.
13. Seino, Y., Ikeda, U., and Shimada, K.: Increased expression of interleukin-6 mRNA in cardiac myxomas. Br. Hoart J. *69*:565, 1993.
14. Seguin, J. R., Beigbeder, J.-Y., Hvass, U., et al.: Interleukin-6 production by cardiac myxomas may explain constitutional symptoms. J. Thorac. Cardiovasc. Surg. *103*:599, 1992.
15. Jourdan, M., Bataille, R., Sequin, J., et al.: Constitutive production of interleukin-6 and immunologic features in cardiac myxomas. Arthritis Rheum. *33*:398, 1990.
16. Curry, H. L. F., Matthews, J. A., and Robinson, J.: Right atrial myxoma mimicking a rheumatic disorder. Br. Med. J. *1*:542, 1967.
17. Savige, J. A., Yeung, S. P., Davis, D. J., et al.: Anti-neutrophil cytoplasmic antibodies associated with atrial myxoma. Am. J. Med. *85*:755, 1988.
18. Graham, S. L., and Sellers, A. L.: Atrial myxoma with multiple myeloma. Arch. Intern. Med. *139*:116, 1979.
19. Leonhardt, E. T. G., and Kullenberg, K. P. G.: Bilateral atrial myxomas with multiple arterial aneurysms. A syndrome mimicking polyarteritis nodosa. Am. J. Med. *62*:792, 1977.
20. Byrd, W. E., Matthews, O. P., and Hunt, R. E.: Left atrial myxoma presenting as a systemic vasculitis. Arthritis Rheum. *23*:240, 1980.
21. Feldman, A. R., and Keeling, J. H.: Cutaneous manifestation of atrial myxoma. J. Am. Acad. Dermatol. *21*:1080, 1989.
22. Quinn, T. J., Condini, M. A., and Harris, A. A.: Infected cardiac myxoma. Am. J. Cardiol. *53*:381, 1984.
23. Whitman, M. S., Rovito, M. A., Klions, D., and Tunkel, A. R.: Infected atrial myxoma: Case report and review. Clin. Infect. Dis. *18*:657, 1994.
24. Hashimoto, H., Takahashi, H., Fujiwara, Y., et al.: Acute myocardial infarction due to coronary embolization from left atrial myxoma. Jpn. Circ. J. *57*:1016, 1993.
25. De Carli, S., Sechi, L. A., Ciani, R., et al.: Right atrial myxoma with pulmonary embolism. Cardiology *84*:368, 1994.
26. Miyauchi, Y., Endo, T., Kuroki, S., and Hayakawa, H.: Right atrial myxoma presenting with recurrent episodes of pulmonary embolism. Cardiology *81*:178, 1992.
27. Eriksen, U. H., Baandrup, U., and Jensen, B. S.: Total disruption of left atrial myxoma causing a cerebral attack and a saddle embolus in the iliac bifurcation. Int. J. Cardiol. *35*:127, 1992.
28. Boussen, K., Moalla, M., Blondeau, P., et al.: Embolization of cardiac myxomas masquerading as polyarteritis nodosa. J. Rheumatol. *18*:283, 1991.
29. Weerasena, N. A., Groome, D., Pollock, J. G., and Pollock, J. C.: Atrial myxoma as the cause of acute lower limb ischemia in a teenager. Scott. Med. J. *34*:440, 1989.
30. Reed, R. J., Utz, M. P., and Terezakis, N.: Embolic and metastatic cardiac myxoma. Am. J. Dermatopathol. *11*:157, 1989.
31. Michael, A. S., Mikhael, M. A., and Christ, M.: Myxoma of the heart presenting with recurrent episodes of hemorrhagic cerebral infarction: MR findings. J. Comput. Assist. Tomogr. *13*:123, 1989.
32. Knepper, L. E., Biller, J., Adams, H. P., Jr., and Bruno, A.: Neurologic manifestations of atrial myxoma. A 12-year experience and review. Stroke *19*:1435, 1988.
33. Heath, D., and Mackinnon, J.: Pulmonary hypertension due to myxoma of the right atrium. With special reference to the behavior of emboli of myxoma in the lung. Am. Heart J. *68*:227, 1964.
34. Harvey, W. P.: Clinical aspects of cardiac tumors. Am. J. Cardiol. *21*:328, 1968.
35. Kawano, H., Okada, R., Kawano, Y., et al.: Mesothelioma in the atrioventricular node. Case report. Jpn. Heart J. *35*:255, 1994.
36. Balasundaram, S., Halees, S. A., and Duran, C.: Mesothelioma of the atrioventricular node: First successful follow-up after excision. Eur. Heart J. *13*:718, 1992.
37. James, T. N., and Galakhov, I.: De subitaneis mortibus XXVI. Fatal electrical instability of the heart associated with benign congenital polycystic tumor of the atrioventricular node. Circulation *56*:667, 1977.
38. Strauss, W. E., Asinger, R. W., and Hodges, M.: Mesothelioma of the AV node: Potential utility of pacing. PACE *11*:1296, 1988.
39. Lantz, D. A., Dougherty, T. H., and Lucca, M. J.: Primary angiosarcoma of the heart causing cardiac rupture. Am. Heart J. *118*:186, 1989.
40. Mitral stenosis and left atrial myxoma. *In* Fowler, N. O.: Diagnosis of Heart Disease. New York, Springer-Verlag, 1991, pp. 146–159.
41. Gershlick, A. H., Leech, G., Mills, P. G., and Leatham, A.: The loud first heart sound in left atrial myxoma. Br. Heart J. *52*:403, 1984.
42. Teoh, K. H., Mulji, A., Tomlinson, C. W., and Lobo, F. V.: Right atrial myxoma originating from the eustachian tube. Can. J. Cardiol. *9*:441, 1993.
43. Heck, H. A., Jr., Gross, C. M., and Houghton, J. L.: Long-term severe pulmonary hypertension associated with right atrial myxoma. Chest *102*:301, 1992.
44. Pessotto, R., Santini, F., Piccin, C., et al.: Cardiac myxoma of the tricuspid valve: Description of a case and review of the literature. J. Heart Valve Dis. *3*:344, 1994.
44a. Savino, J. S., and Weiss, S. J.: Right atrial tumor. N. Engl. J. Med. *333*:1608, 1995.
45. Waxler, E. B., Kawai, N., and Kasparian, H.: Right atrial myxoma: Echocardiographic, phonocardiographic and hemodynamic signs. Am. Heart J. *82*:251, 1972.
46. Keren, A., Chenzbruna, A., Schuger, L., et al.: The etiology of tumor plop in a patient with huge right atrial myxoma. Chest *95*:1147, 1989.
47. Hada, Y., Wolfe, C., Murry, C. F., and Craige, E.: Right ventricular myxoma. Case report and review of phonocardiographic auscultatory manifestations. Am. Heart J. *100*:871, 1980.
48. Gosse, P., Herpin, D., Roudant, R., et al.: Myxoma of the mitral valve diagnosed by echocardiography. Am. Heart J. *111*:803, 1986.

SPECIFIC CARDIAC TUMORS

49. Carney, J. A., Hruska, L. S., Beauchamp, G. D., and Gordon, H.: Dominant inheritance of the complex of myxomas, spotty pigmentation and endocrine overactivity. Mayo Clin. Proc. *61*:165, 1986.
50. Van Gelder, H. M., O'Brien, D. J., Staples, E. D., and Alexander, J. A.: Familial cardiac myxoma. Ann. Thorac. Surg. *53*:419, 1992.
50a. Koopman, R. J., and Happle, R.: Autosomal dominant transmission of the NAME syndrome (nevi, atrial myxoma, mucinosis of the skin and endocrine overactivity). Hum. Genet. *86*:300, 1991.
51. Carney, J. A., Gordon, J., Carpenter, P. C., et al.: The complex of myxomas, spotty pigmentation and endocrine overactivity. Medicine *64*:270, 1985.
52. Vidaillet, H. J., Jr., Seward, J. B., Fyke, F. E., et al.: "Syndrome myxoma": A subset of patients with cardiac myxoma associated with pigmented skin lesions and peripheral and endocrine neoplasms. Br. Heart J. *57*:247, 1987.
53. Bennett, W. S., Skelton, T. N., and Lehan, P. H.: The complex of myxomas, pigmentation and endocrine overactivity. Am. J. Cardiol. *65*:399, 1990.
54. Carney, J. A., and Behnaz, C. T.: Myxoid fibroadenoma and allied conditions (myxomatosis) of the breast. Am. J. Surg. Pathol. *15*:713, 1991.
55. Vidaillet, H. J., Jr., Seward, J. B., Fyke, E., and Tajik, A. J.: NAME syndrome (nevi, atrial myxoma, myxoid neurofibroma, ephelides): A new and unrecognized subset of patients with cardiac myxoma. Minn. Med. *67*:695, 1984.
56. Rhodes, A. R., Silverman, R. A., Harrist, T. J., and Perez-Atayde, A. R.: Mucocutaneous lentigines, cardiomucocutaneous myxoma, and multiple blue nevi: The "LAMB" syndrome. Am. Acad. Dermatol. *10*:72, 1984.
57. Farah, M. G.: Familial cardiac myxoma. A study of relatives of patients with myxoma. Chest *105*:65, 1994.
58. McCarthy, P. M., Piehler, J. M., Schaff, H. V., et al.: The significance of multiple, recurrent, and "complex" cardiac myxomas. Thorac. Cardiovasc. Surg. *91*:389, 1986.
59. Carney, J. A.: Differences between nonfamilial and familial cardiac myxoma. Am. J. Surg. Pathol. *9*:53, 1985.
60. McAllister, H. A., Jr.: Tumors of the heart and pericardium. *In* Silver, M. D. (ed.): Cardiovascular Pathology. 2nd ed. New York, Churchill Livingstone, 1991, p. 1297.
61. Burke, A. P., and Virmani, R.: Cardiac myxoma. A clinicopathologic study. Am. J. Clin. Pathol. *100*:671, 1993.
62. Ferrans, V. J., and Roberts, W. L.: Structural features of cardiac myxomas. Histology, histochemistry and electron microscopy. Hum. Pathol. *4*:111, 1973.
63. Goldman, B. I., Frydman, C., Harpaz, N., et al.: Glandular cardiac myxomas. Cancer *59*:1767, 1987.
64. Lie, J. T.: The identity and histogenesis of cardiac myxomas: A controversy put to rest. Arch. Pathol. Lab. Med. *113*:724, 1989.
65. Hashimoto, H., Takahashi, H., Fujiwara, Y., et al.: Acute myocardial infarction due to coronary embolization from left atrial myxoma. Jpn. Circ. J. *57*:1016, 1993.
66. Salyer, W. R., Page, D. L., and Hutchins, G. M.: The development of cardiac myxomas and papillary endocardial lesions from mural thrombus. Am. Heart J. *89*:4, 1975.
67. Dewald, G. W., Dahl, R. J., Spurbeck, B. S., et al.: Chromosomally abnormal clones and non-random telomeric translocations in cardiac myxomas. Mayo Clin. Proc. *62*:558, 1987.
68. Richkind, K. E., Wason, D., and Vidaillet, H.: Cardiac myxoma characterization by clonal telomeric association. Genes Chrom. Cancer *9*:68, 1994.
69. Dijkhuizen, T., van den Berg, E., and Molenaar, W. M.: Cytogenetics of a case of cardiac myxoma. Cancer Genet. Cytogenet. *73*:73, 1992.
70. Seidman, J. D., Berman, J. J., Hitchcock, C. L., et al.: DNA analysis of cardiac myxomas: Flow cytometry and image analysis. Hum. Pathol. *22*:494, 1991.
71. Luthringer, D. J., Virmani, R., Weiss, S. W., and Rosai, J.: A distinctive cardiovascular lesion resembling histiocytoid (epithelioid) hemangioma. Am. J. Surg. Pathol. *14*:993, 1990.
72. Veinot, J. P., Tazelaar, H. D., Edwards, W. D., and Colby, T. V.: Mesothelial/monocytic incidental cardiac excrescences: Cardiac MICE. Mod. Pathol. *7*:9, 1994.
73. Courtice, R. W., Stinson, W.A., and Walley, V. M.: Tissue fragments recovered at cardiac surgery masquerading as tumoral proliferations. Am. J. Surg. Pathol. *18*:167, 1994.

PAPILLARY TUMORS OF HEART VALVES

74. Shahian, D. W., Labib, S. B., and Chang, G.: Cardiac papillary fibroelastoma. Ann. Thorac. Surg. *59*:538, 1995.

75. LiMandri, G., Homma, S., Di Tullio, M. R., et al.: Detection of multiple papillary fibroelastomas of the tricuspid valve by transesophageal echocardiography. J. Am. Soc. Echo. *7*:315, 1994.
76. Pomerance, A.: Papillary "tumours" of the heart valves. J. Pathol. Bacteriol. *87*:135, 1981.
77. Fenoglio, J. J., McAllister, H. A., and Ferrans, V. J.: Cardiac rhabdomyoma: A clinicopathologic and electron microscopic study. Am. J. Cardiol. *38*:241, 1976.
78. Burke, A. P., and Virmani, R.: Cardiac rhabdomyoma: A clinicopathologic study. Mod. Pathol. *4*:70, 1991.
79. Bass, J. L., Breningstall, G. N., and Swaiman, K. F.: Echocardiographic incidence of cardiac rhabdomyoma in tuberous sclerosis. Am. J. Cardiol. *55*:137, 1985.
80. Gibbs, J. L.: The heart and tuberous sclerosis. An echocardiographic and electrocardiographic study. Br. Heart J. *54*:596, 1985.
81. Webb, D. W., Thomas, R. D., and Osborne, J. P.: Cardiac rhabdomyomas and their association with tuberous sclerosis. Arch. Dis. Child. *68*:367, 1993.
82. Moriarty, A. T., Nelson, W. A., and McGahey, B.: Fine-needle aspiration of rhabdomyosarcoma of the heart. Acta Cytologica. *34*:74, 1990.
83. Van der Hauwaert, L. G.: Cardiac tumours in infancy and childhood. Br. Heart J. *33*:125, 1971.
84. Jones, K. L., Wolf, P. L., Jensen, P., et al.: The Gorlin syndrome: A genetically determined disorder associated with cardiac tumor. Am. Heart J. *111*:1013, 1986.
85. Miralles, A., Bracamonte, L., Soncul, H., et al.: Cardiac tumors: Clinical experience and surgical results in 74 patients. Ann. Thorac. Surg. *52*:886, 1991.
86. Tazelaar, H. D., Locke, T. J., and McGregor, C. G. A.: Pathology of surgically excised primary cardiac tumors. Mayo Clin. Proc. *67*:957, 1992.
87. Prior, J. T.: Lipomatous hypertrophy of cardiac interatrial septum. Arch Pathol. *78*:11, 1964.
88. Chao, J. C., Reyes, C. V., and Hwang, M. H.: Cardiac hemangioma. South. Med. J. *83*:44, 1990.
89. Cox, J. N., Friedli, B., Mechmeche, M., et al.: Teratoma of the heart. Virchows Arch. (A) *402*:163, 1983.
90. Meysman, M., Noppen, M., Demeyer, G., and Vincken, W.: Malignant epithelial mesothelioma presenting as cardiac tamponade. Eur. Heart J. *14*:1576, 1993.
91. Monma, N., Satodate, R., Tashiro, A., and Segawa, I.: Origin of so-called mesothelioma of the atrioventricular node. Arch. Pathol. Lab. Med. *115*:1026, 1991.
92. Burke, M. A. P., Anderson, P. G., Virmani, R., et al.: Tumor of the atrioventricular nodal region. Arch. Pathol. Lab. Med. *114*:1057, 1990.
93. David, T. E., Lenkei, S. C., Marquez-Julio, A., et al.: Pheochromocytoma of the heart. Ann. Thorac. Surg. *41*:98, 1986.

MALIGNANT CARDIAC TUMORS

94. Putnam, J. B., Sweeney, M. S., Colon, R., et al.: Primary cardiac sarcomas. Ann. Thorac. Surg. *51*:906, 1991.
95. Burke, A. P., Cowan, D., and Virmani, R.: Primary sarcoma of the heart. Cancer *69*:387, 1992.
96. Thomas, C. R., Johnson, G. W., Stoddard, M. F., and Clifford, S.: Primary malignant cardiac tumors: Update 1992. Med. Pediatr. Oncol. *20*:519, 1992.
97. Whorton, C. M.: Primary malignant tumor of the heart. Cancer *2*:245, 1949.
98. Burke, A. P., and Virmani, R.: Osteosarcomas of the heart. Am. J. Surg. Pathol. *15*:289, 1991.
99. Klima, U., Wimmer-Greinecker, G., Harringer, W., et al.: Cardiac angiosarcoma—a diagnostic dilemma. Cardiovasc. Surg. *1*:674, 1993.
100. Herrmann, M. A., Shankerman, R. A., Edwards, W. D., et al.: Primary cardiac angiosarcoma: A clinicopathologic study of six cases. J. Thorac. Cardiovasc. Surg. *103*:655, 1992.
101. Keohane, M. E., Lazzam, C., Halperin, J. L., et al.: Angiosarcoma of the left atrium mimicking myxoma. Case report. Hum. Pathol. *20*:599, 1989.
101a. Basso, C., Stefani, A., Calabrese, F., et al.: Primary right atrial fibrosarcoma diagnosed by endocardial biopsy. Am. Heart J. *131*:399, 1996.
102. Proctor, M. S., Tracy, G. P., and Von Koch, L.: Primary cardiac B-cell lymphoma. Am. Heart J. *118*:179, 1989.
103. Kasai, K., Kuwao, S., Sato, Y., et al.: Case report of primary cardiac lymphoma. The applications of PCR to the diagnosis of primary cardiac lymphoma. Acta Pathol. Jpn. *42*:667, 1992.
104. Marvasti, M. A., Obeid, A. I., Potts, J. L., and Parker, F. B.: Approach in the management of atrial myxoma with long-term follow-up. Ann. Thorac. Surg. *38*:53, 1984.
105. Bleisch, N., Kraus, F.: Polypoid sarcoma of the pulmonary trunk. Cancer *46*:314, 1980.

DIAGNOSIS, TREATMENT, PROGNOSIS

106. Lane, G. E., Kapples, E. J., Thompson, R. C., et al.: Quiescent left atrial myxoma. Am. Heart J. *127*:1629, 1994.
107. Charuzi, Y., Bolger, A., Beeder, C., and Lew, A. S.: A new echocardiographic classification of left atrial myxoma. Am. J. Cardiol. *55*:614, 1985.
108. Dennis, M. A., Appareti, K., Manco-Johnson, M. L., et al.: The echocardiographic diagnosis of multiple fetal cardiac tumors. Ultrasound Med. *4*:327, 1985.
109. Panidis, I. P., Mimtz, G. S., and McAllisterm M.: Hemodynamic consequences of the left atrial myxomas as assessed by Doppler ultrasound. Am. Heart J. *111*:927, 1986.
110. Edwards, L. C. III, and Louie, E. K.: Transthoracic and transesophageal echocardiography for the evaluation of cardiac tumors, thrombi, and valvular vegetations. Am. J. Card. Imag. *8*:45, 1994.
111. Shyu, K-G., Chen, J-J., Cheng, J-J., et al.: Comparison of transthoracic and transesophageal echocardiography in the diagnosis of intracardiac tumors in adults. J. Clin. Ultrasound *22*:381, 1994.
112. Azuma, T., Ohira, A., Akagi, H., et al.: Transvenous biopsy of a right atrial tumor under transesophageal echocardiographic guidance. Am. Heart J. *131*:402, 1996.
113. Bough, E., Bodem, W., Gandsman, E., et al.: Radionuclide diagnosis of left atrial myxoma with computer-generated functional images. Am. J. Cardiol. *52*:1365, 1986.
114. Bleiweis, M. S., Georgiou, D., and Brundage, B. H.: Detection of intracardiac masses by ultrafast computed tomography. Am. J. Card. Imag. *8*:63, 1994.
115. Fujita, N., Caputo, G. R., and Higgins, C. B.: Diagnosis and characterization of intracardiac masses by magnetic resonance imaging. Am. J. Card. Imag. *8*:69, 1994.
116. Reddy, D. B., Jena, Col. A., and Venugopal, P.: Magnetic resonance imaging (MRI) in evaluation of left atrial masses: An in vitro and in vivo study. J. Cardiovasc. Surg. *35*:289, 1994.
117. Fueredi, G. A., Knetchtges, T. E., and Czarnecki, D. J.: Coronary angiography in atrial myxoma: Findings in nine cases. Am. J. Roentgenol. *152*:737, 1989.
118. Singh, R. N., Burkholder, J. A., and Magovern, G. J.: Coronary arteriography as an aid in left atrial myxoma diagnosis. Cardiovasc. Intervent. Radiol. *7*:40, 1984.
119. Weyne, A. E., Heyndrickx, G. R., Cavelier, C. C., et al.: Cardiac imaging techniques in the diagnosis of angiosarcoma of the heart: Report of two cases. Postgrad. Med. J. *61*:271, 1985.
120. Pendyck, F., Pierce, E. C., Baron, M. G., and Lukban, S. B.: Embolization of left atrial myxoma after transseptal cardiac catheterization. Am. J. Cardiol. *30*:569, 1972.
121. Wiatrowska, B. A., Walley, V. M., Masters, R. G., et al.: Surgery for cardiac tumors: The University of Ottawa Heart Institute experience (1980–1991). Can. J. Cardiol. *9*:65, 1993.
122. MacGowan, S. W., Sidhu, P., Aherne, T., et al.: Atrial myxoma: National incidence, diagnosis and surgical management. Ir. J. Med. Sci. *162*:223, 1993.
123. Aru, G. M., Falchi, S., Cardu, G., et al.: The role of transesophageal echocardiography in the monitoring of cardiac mass removal: A review of 17 cases. J. Card. Surg. *8*:554, 1993.
124. Larsson, S., Lopore, V., and Kennergren, C.: Atrial myxomas: Results of 25 years' experience and review of the literature. Surgery *105*:695, 1989.
125. Bortolotti, U., Maraglino, G., Rubino, M., et al.: Surgical excision of intracardiac myxomas: A 20-year follow-up. Ann. Thorac. Surg. *49*:449, 1990.
126. Waller, D. A., Ettles, D. F., Saunders, N. R., and Williams, G.: Recurrent cardiac myxoma: The surgical implications of two distinct groups of patients. Thorac. Cardiovasc. Surg. *37*:226, 1989.
127. McCarthy, P. M., Piehler, J. M., Schaff, H. V., et al.: The significance of multiple, recurrent, and "complex" cardiac myxomas. Thorac. Cardiovasc. Surg. *91*:389, 1986.
127a Scheid, H. H., Nestle, H. W., Kling, D., et al.: Resection of a heart tumor using autotransplantation. Thorac. Cardiovasc. Surg. *36*:40, 1988.
128. Mesnildrey, P., Bloch, G., Cachera, J. P., and Piwicna, A.: Atrial myxoma: A new surgical approach using neodynium:yttrium-aluminum-garnet laser photocoagulation. J. Thorac. Cardiovasc. Surg. *98*:313, 1989.
129. Goldman, S., Lortscher, R., and Pappas, G.: Surgical treatment for rhabdomyoma of the right atrium causing arrhythmias. J. Thorac. Cardiovasc. Surg. *89*:802, 1985.
130. Corno, A., deSimone, G., Catena, G., and Marcelletti, C.: Cardiac rhabdomyoma: Surgical treatment in the neonate. Thorac. Cardiovasc. Surg. *87*:725, 1984.
131. Orringer, M. B., Sisson, J. C., Glazer, G., et al.: Surgical treatment of cardiac pheochromocytomas. J. Thorac. Cardiovasc. Surg. *89*:753, 1985.
132. Aufiero, T. X., Pae, W. E. Jr., Clemson, B. S., et al.: Heart transplantation for tumor. Ann. Thorac. Surg. *56*:1174, 1993.
133. Yuh, D. D., Kubo, S. H., Francis, G. S., et al.: Primary cardiac lymphoma treated with orthotopic heart transplantation: A case report. J. Heart Lung Transplant. *13*:538, 1994.
134. Baay, P., Karawande, S. V., Kushner, J. P., et al.: Successful treatment of a cardiac angiosarcoma with combined modality therapy. J. Heart Lung Transplant. *13*:923, 1994.
135. Crespo, M. G., Pulpon, L. A., Pradas, G., et al.: Heart transplantation for cardiac angiosarcoma: Should its indication be questioned? J. Heart Lung Transplant. *12*:527, 1993.
136. Baay, P., Karwande, S. V., Kushner, J. P., et al.: Successful treatment of a cardiac angiosarcoma with combined modality therapy. J. Heart Lung Transplant. *13*:923, 1994.
137. Hollingworth, J. H., and Sturgill, B. C.: Treatment of primary angiosarcoma of the heart. Am. Heart J. *78*:254, 1969.
138. Terry, L. N., and Kilgerman, M. M.: Pericardial and myocardial involvement by lymphomas and leukemias. The role of radiotherapy. Cancer *25*:1003, 1970.
139. Gerfein, O. B.: Lymphosarcoma of the right atrium. Angiographic and hemodynamic documentation of response to chemotherapy. Arch. Intern. Med. *135*:325, 1975.

Chapter 43
Pericardial Diseases

BEVERLY H. LORELL

Anatomy 1478
Functions of the Pericardium 1478
Limitations of Cardiac Distention 1480

ACUTE PERICARDITIS 1481

PERICARDIAL EFFUSION 1485
Pericardial Effusion Without Cardiac Compression 1485
Cardiac Tamponade 1486
Pathophysiology 1486
Clinical Manifestations 1489
Laboratory Studies 1490
Cardiac Catheterization 1492
Pericardiocentesis 1493
Pericardiotomy and Pericardiectomy 1495

CONSTRICTIVE PERICARDITIS 1496
Pathophysiology 1496
Etiology 1498
Clinical Features 1498
Cardiac Catheterization and Angiography . . . 1502
Hemodynamic Differentiation Among Constrictive Pericarditis, Cardiac Tamponade, and Restrictive Cardiomyopathy 1503
Management 1504
Effusive-Constrictive Pericarditis 1505

SPECIFIC FORMS OF PERICARDITIS 1505
Viral Pericarditis 1505
Tuberculous Pericarditis 1507
Bacterial (Purulent) Pericarditis 1508
Fungal Pericarditis 1510
Other Infectious Pericarditis 1511
Pericarditis Following Acute Myocardial Infarction 1511
Uremic Pericarditis 1512
Neoplastic Pericarditis 1513
Radiation Pericarditis 1516
Pericarditis Related to Hypersensitivity or Autoimmunity 1517
Acute Rheumatic Fever 1517
Systemic Lupus Erythematosus 1518
Rheumatoid Arthritis 1518
Progressive Systemic Sclerosis 1518
Pericarditis in Other Connective Tissue Disorders 1519
Drug- and Toxin-Related Pericarditis 1519
Post-Surgical Constrictive Pericarditis 1521
Other Forms of Pericardial Disease 1521
Myxedema Pericardial Disease 1521
Cholesterol Pericarditis 1522
Chylopericardium 1522
Traumatic Pericarditis 1522
Pericardial Cysts 1522
Congenital Absence and Defects of the Pericardium 1522

REFERENCES 1524

ANATOMY

The pericardium forms a strong flask-shaped sac with short tubelike extensions that enclose the origins of the aorta and its junction with the aortic arch, the pulmonary artery where it branches, the proximal pulmonary veins, and venae cavae. Fibrous tissue of the pericardium actually blends with adventitia of the great arteries to form very strong attachments. In addition, the pericardium has firm ligamentous attachments anteriorly to the sternum and xiphoid process, posteriorly to the vertebral column, and inferiorly to the diaphragm.[1,2] The human pericardium receives its arterial blood supply from small branches of the aorta and internal mammary and musculophrenic arteries. The pericardium is innervated by the vagus, left recurrent laryngeal nerve, and esophageal plexus and also has rich sympathetic innervation from the stellate and first dorsal ganglia and the cardiac, aortic, and diaphragmatic plexuses. The phrenic nerves course over the pericardium en route to the diaphragm. The afferent nerves responsible for pain perception appear to be transmitted via the phrenic nerve entering the spinal cord at C4–C5.[2] Peripheral sensory fibers that enter the dorsal root ganglia at C8–T2 supply both the brachial plexus and the pericardium, which provides a possible morphological explanation for referred pericardial pain.[3]

THE TWO LAYERS OF THE PERICARDIUM. The pericardium is composed of a fibrous outer layer and an inner serous membrane composed of a single layer of mesothelial cells. The inner serous layer is intimately attached to the surface of the heart and epicardial fat to form the visceral pericardium, and this inner serous membrane reflects back on itself to line the outer fibrous layer to form the parietal pericardium.

The pericardium has two major serosal tunnels: the transverse sinus, which lies posterior to the great arteries and anterior to the atria and superior vena cava, and the oblique sinus, which lies posterior to the left atrium so that the posterior left atrial wall is actually separated from the pericardial space. The serous visceral pericardium is attached to the parietal pericardium by delicate connective tissue with elastin fibers. The parietal pericardium is composed of collagen fibers interlaced with extensive elastic fibers, which are wavy during childhood and become progressively straighter with age, suggesting that young pericardia are more compliant than those of the elderly.

ELECTRON MICROSCOPY. This reveals that exuberant microvilli and long, single cilia project from the serous mesothelium composing the visceral pericardium and the inner lining of the parietal pericardium,[4] which increase markedly the surface area available for fluid transport. Both microvilli and cilia provide a specialized surface to permit movement of the pericardial membranes over each other during each cardiac cycle and to permit the pericardium to accommodate changes in cardiac shape during contraction. In addition, numerous small fenestrations or pores less than 50 μ in diameter provide direct communication between the pericardial and pleural cavities in mammals.[5]

PERICARDIAL FLUID. The human pericardium normally contains up to 50 ml of clear fluid. The visceral pericardium is believed to be the source of normal pericardial fluid and excessive fluid in disease states. Normal pericardial fluid appears to be an ultrafiltrate of plasma because electrolytes are present in pericardial fluid in concentrations compatible with such an ultrafiltrate; protein concentrations are about one-third those of the plasma, and albumin is present in a higher ratio in pericardial fluid, reflecting its lower molecular weight. Current data suggest that drainage of the pericardial space occurs both by the thoracic duct via the parietal pericardium and by the right lymphatic duct via the right pleural space.

Pericardial fluid also contains phospholipids that serve as a lubricant to reduce friction between the surfaces of the parietal pericardium and the visceral pericardium.[6] The pericardium appears to produce prostaglandins in response to physiological stimuli that may modulate efferent cardiac sympathetic stimulation and alter cardiac electrophysiological properties.[7] The clinical implications of this potential regulatory effect of the pericardium on electrical conduction of the heart are not yet known.

FUNCTIONS OF THE PERICARDIUM

The pericardium's ligamentous attachments help to fix the heart anatomically and prevent excessive motion with changes in body position. The pericardium also reduces friction between the heart and surrounding organs and provides a barrier against the extension of infection and malignancy from contiguous organs to the heart itself. The role of the pericardium in the regulation of the circulation is controversial because congenital absence of the pericardium is not associated with overt disturbances of cardiac function. However, observations in both dogs and humans indicate that the pericardium may play a role in (1) the distribution of hydrostatic forces on the heart, (2) the prevention of acute cardiac dilatation, and (3) diastolic coupling of the two ventricles.

The normal pericardium is relatively stiff, and the relationship between pressure within the pericardium and total intrapericardial volume, which is the sum of the volume of the heart itself and the reserve volume of the surrounding pericardial sac, appears as a steep curve when plotted on a graph.[1] Once the pericardium is filled, intrapericardial pressure rises sharply as volume is increased (Fig. 43–1). Thus, the stiffness of the pericardium increases when the load is increased, and then it becomes almost inextensible. Although much of our knowledge regarding the physiological role of the pericardium has been derived from experimental studies in dogs, it is important to recognize that the human pericardium is about three times as thick and much less distensible than canine pericardium.[8] Usually, the pericardial sac is filled with a thin film of fluid distributed throughout the pericardial space in such a way that the pericardial reserve volume is not exceeded. This permits respiratory and postural changes in cardiac volume and total intrapericardial volume to occur without significant changes in intrapericardial pressure. When measured with a fluid-filled or micromanometer-tipped catheter, pericardial pressure is nearly equal to intrapleural pressure and varies from −5 to +5 cm H_2O during the respiratory cycle.[9]

INTRAPERICARDIAL PRESSURE. Normal intrapericardial pressure is zero or negative. This has major implications for our understanding of the influence of pericardial pressure on the transmural distending pressure of the cardiac chambers and the operation of the Frank-Starling mechanism in the beat-to-beat regulation of stroke volume.[10] The transmural distending pressure of either vehicle is the difference between intracardiac and intrapericardial pressures and is independent of gravity. When intrapericardial pressure is assumed to be negative, normally a substantial transmural distending pressure would be expected to exist across both ventricles. For example, when left ventricular end-diastolic pressure is +8 mm Hg and intrapericardial pressure is −2 mm Hg relative to atmosphere, the actual left ventricular distending pressure would be $8 - (-2) =$ 10 mm Hg, and when right ventricular end-diastolic pressure is 4 mm Hg and intrapericardial pressure is −2 mm Hg relative to the atmosphere, the actual right ventricular distending pressure would be $4 - (-2) = 6$ mm Hg.

Studies using micromanometer pressure measurements support the view that pericardial pressure is usually very low and thus exerts only a small influence on the average transmural distending pressure of the heart as long as pericardial reserve volume is not exceeded by volume loading.[9] Under normal conditions, it is clear that the pericardium does influence the pattern of venous return and ventricular filling that occurs in every cardiac cycle. Ventricular ejection is accompanied by abrupt descent of the atrioventricular junction (the "base" of the heart) and a reduction in right atrial pressure, manifest by the *x* descent* in the right atrial pressure pulse as well as by a decline in intrapericardial pressure. These changes result in a surge of venous return during systole, particularly when ventricular and pericardial pressures are increased. This acceleration of venous return during systolic ejection is diminished by opening of the pericardium.

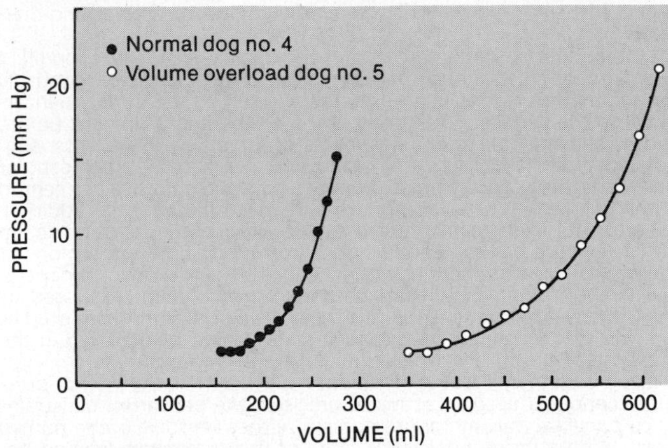

FIGURE 43–1. Pericardial pressure-volume curves from a normal dog *(left)* and from a dog with chronic volume overload *(right)*. Note that the normal pressure-volume curve *(right)* is initially flat but becomes extremely steep as total volume within the pericardium increases. In response to chronic cardiac dilatation, the pericardium enlarges in size and mass such that the pericardium can accommodate a large volume of low pressure *(right curve)*. (Reproduced by permission from Freeman, G. L., and LeWinter, M. M.: Pericardial adaptations during chronic dilation in dogs. Circ. Res. *54*:294, 1984. Copyright American Heart Association.)

When the volume of the heart or other contents of the pericardial sac increase and exceed the elastic limits of the pericardium during diastole, the heart operates on the steep portion of the curve relating intrapericardial pressure and volume, resulting in marked increases in intrapericardial and intracardiac pressures. However, the difference between the two pressures, i.e., the transmural pressure, usually declines. In the extreme case of cardiac tamponade, in which both intrapericardial and intracardiac pressures are markedly increased, the transmural pressure distending the ventricles may fall precipitously toward zero, resulting in decreased ventricular diastolic volumes and preload. These findings, taken together, support the classic view that the pericardium is a distensible "loosely fitting" sac that modestly affects stroke volume by changes in intrapericardial pressure and transmural pressure and exerts a substantial influence only at higher ventricular and pericardial pressures.

CHALLENGES TO THE "CLASSIC VIEW." This classic view has been seriously challenged by Smiseth and coworkers,[11] who contend that the use of either fluid-filled or micromanometer catheters underestimates pericardial pressure and its influence on transmural distending pressures in normal hearts. They have shown in dogs that the measurement of the *surface contact pressure* of the pericardium against the heart using a flat balloon is more accurate than a fluid-filled catheter in estimating the actual pericardial pressure (the fall in left ventricular pressure observed immediately after opening the pericardium in the absence of any change in chamber volume). Observations from dogs and from humans indicate that when the amount of fluid in the pericardial sac is small, pericardial pressure measured in this way is much higher than intrathoracic pressure or pericardial pressure measured with a fluid-filled or micromanometer catheter, whereas pericardial pressures measured by either a balloon or fluid-filled catheter are similar when a substantial volume of pericardial fluid (40 to 50 ml) is present.[12,13] Thus the controversy regarding the concept of pericardial surface contact pressure does not detract from the accuracy or the clinical utility of measuring intrapericardial pressure with a catheter in patients with large pericardial effusions and cardiac tamponade.

However, these arguments profoundly challenge classic views regarding the normal physiology of the heart and the accurate measurement of the transmural pressure of each ventricle. These studies have emphasized that intrapericardial surface contact pressure is not zero or negative and, to the contrary, is virtually equal to right atrial pressure.[11,12] A further assumption is that differences in pericardial surface contact pressure do not exist over different chambers of the heart. This analysis indicates that left ventricular transmural pressure in normal hearts should be estimated by subtracting right atrial pressure rather than intrathoracic pressure. It also carries the remarkable implication that the transmural distending pressure of the normal

*It is recognized that the descent in venous pressure after the *a* wave is usually termed the *x* descent and, after the *c* wave, the *x′* descent. In this chapter, the major systolic venous pressure descent after the *a* and *c* waves is termed the *x* descent.

right ventricle is extremely small, and negligible or zero at end-diastole.

Experiments by Santamore et al.[14] and Slinker et al.[15] have modified this concept and indicate that closed flat-balloon catheters probably exaggerate the constraining pressure exerted by the normal pericardium on the surface of the heart. Recent experiments in dogs before and after pericardiectomy, as well as observations in patients, suggest that pericardial constraint accounts for about 96 per cent of right atrial intracavitary pressure in the dog, and about 90 per cent in humans when central venous pressure is 10 mm Hg.[16] In addition, experiments indicate that the pressure exerted by the pericardium on the surface of the heart is not uniform over different regions of the heart.[17] Measurements by Chew et al.[18] of in situ regional pericardial strain in dogs show that the normal pericardium is strained by the underlying heart, even during vena caval occlusion. These studies indicate that a completely unloaded state cannot be achieved in the presence of an intact pericardium.

Taken together, these experiments suggest that right atrial pressure cannot be used to estimate precisely the pericardial constraint or to calculate transmural pressures of either ventricle in the normal heart. Furthermore, pericardial catheter measurements tend to underestimate while pericardial balloons tend to overestimate pericardial pressure, which appears to be within the range of 0.2 to 3 mm Hg under normal physiological conditions. Finally, these experiments confirm that the pericardium modifies the filling and intracavitary pressures of both ventricles, particularly when cardiac distention occurs.

LIMITATIONS OF CARDIAC DISTENTION

The relatively nondistensible pericardium may help to limit acute distention of the heart. This was appreciated as early as 1898 by Bernard, who used a pump to increase pressure in excised hearts with and without the pericardium and noted that hearts unsupported by the pericardium ruptured at lower pressures than did hearts with intact pericardia.[19] Subsequent studies in dogs demonstrated that the pericardium restrains right and left ventricular filling, so that ventricular volume is greater at any given ventricular pressure with the pericardium removed than with the pericardium intact. Thus, acute changes in intracardiac and total intrapericardial volume result in an upward shift of both the left and right ventricular pressure-volume relationships, which is in part mediated by the restraining effect of the pericardium and an increase in intrapericardial pressure.[15,20,21] As ventricular volumes increase, the proportional contribution of the pericardium to end-diastolic pressure of the thin-walled right ventricle increases relative to that of the left ventricle.[15] Thus, as the heart is distended, the pericardium makes a greater contribution to right ventricular end-diastolic pressure than to left ventricular end-diastolic pressure.

EFFECTS OF ACUTE VOLUME LOADING. The hemodynamic effects of acute volume loading and vasodilators are in part mediated by pericardial constraint. Shirato et al.[22] demonstrated that acute volume loading with dextran in dogs with intact pericardia resulted in an upward shift in the left ventricular pressure–segment length relation; i.e., left ventricular pressure was higher at any given segment length, whereas the reduction of venous return and cardiac volume by means of nitroprusside administration shifted the curves downward toward control levels. This occurred because nitroprusside and other vasodilators that decrease right heart filling reduce the total volume occupied by the heart within the pericardial space and thus reduce the restraining of the left ventricle by the pericardium; in turn, this causes a downward shift of the left ventricular pressure-volume relation so that a given left ventricular volume is associated with lower left ventricular diastolic pressure.

After pericardiectomy, volume loading results in a rightward shift in the pressure-segment length relation and, after nitroprusside, a leftward shift along a single curve.[22] When the effect of the pericardium is eliminated by plotting left ventricular transmural pressure versus segment length, the points during all interventions fall along a single curve. Smiseth et al.[23] have extended these findings and have shown that the opposite effects of angiotensin (upward shift) and nitroprusside (downward shift) of the left ventricle pressure-volume relation depend on changes in intrapericardial pressure mediated by shifts in blood volume from the heart to systemic vascular beds.

EFFECTS OF CHRONIC VOLUME LOADING. A restraining effect of the pericardium has been observed early in the course of chronic volume overloading induced by formation of arteriovenous shunts in dogs prior to enlargement of the pericardium by stretch or hypertrophy. However, this restraining effect was not apparent in dogs studied late during the course of chronic volume overload.[24] This occurs because chronic left ventricular enlargement and hypertrophy are accompanied by an increase in the compliance of the pericardial chamber and an increase in total pericardial volume due to the addition of new pericardial tissue.[25] In addition to its effects on ventricular filling, pericardial pressure also appears to influence indices of isovolumic relaxation of the left ventricle. Frais et al.[26] showed that alterations in the asymptote and time constant of left ventricular pressure decay (tau) in dogs subjected to volume loading vary with changes in intrapericardial pressure.

These observations suggest that shifts in the left and right ventricular diastolic pressure-volume relations following volume loading or vasodilator administration are largely due to changes in intrapericardial pressure. However, the pericardium does not affect *intrinsic* myocardial compliance; neither does it account for changes in the left ventricular diastolic pressure-volume relationship observed during ischemia.[27]

VENTRICULAR INTERDEPENDENCE. The pericardium also contributes to diastolic coupling between the two ventricles. The distention of one ventricle alters the distensibility of the other, even in the absence of the pericardium.[28] This effect appears to be mediated in part by shared encircling muscle bands and by the interventricular septum, which tends to bulge into the left ventricle, causing a change in the shape of the left ventricle when the right ventricle is distended.[29] In the absence of the pericardium, large increases in right ventricular volume and pressure are required to cause an appreciable increase in left ventricular filling pressure.[30] In contrast, the presence of an intact pericardium markedly accentuates the coupling between ventricular diastolic pressures.[31] When right ventricular volume and pressure are increased with the normal pericardium intact, right and left ventricular filling pressures are closely correlated, and left ventricular volume is smaller than in the absence of the pericardium. In the absence of the pericardium, cardiac distensibility is primarily related to properties of the myocardium. This effect of the pericardium on the interaction between the two ventricles is accentuated in experimental constrictive pericarditis when the distensibility of the pericardium is decreased.[32] This effect of the pericardium on diastolic ventricular interaction is present at normal filling pressures and becomes of increasing importance at high right ventricular filling pressures. During volume loading in normal conscious dogs, it has been shown that pericardial pressure exerts a disproportionately greater effect on the thin-walled right ventricle, which suggests that the pericardium couples diastolic function of the two ventricles via its influence on right ventricular filling and geometry.[9,15]

Although normal pericardium does not appear to contribute importantly to the interaction of the ventricles during systole at normal filling pressures,[33] it does influence global and regional systolic function during conditions of acute distention of the heart.[34,35] Kanazawa et al.[34] showed that removal of the pericardium in dogs caused insignificant changes in stroke volume, whereas removal of the pericardium during volume loading caused a substantial increase in stroke volume associated with an increase in end-diastolic segment length and systolic excursion. Although pericardial pressure was not measured, it is likely that this increase in stroke volume was due to the Frank-Starling mechanism via an increase of the transmural distending pressure of the ventricle following removal of the pericardium. Furthermore, during volume overload, the pericardium caused an upward shift in the left ventricular end-systolic pressure-volume relationship in the absence of a change in inotropic state. Pericardial constraint also appears to modify regional systolic function during acute right ventricular pressure overload and distention. Goto et al.[35] found that acute right ventricular loading in dogs results in nonuniform decreases in regional left ventricular shortening, an effect that is enhanced by the presence of the pericardium.

The pericardium also appears to limit maximal body oxygen consumption by limiting stroke volume and cardiac output during maximal exercise in conscious dogs.[36] These observations suggest that the normal pericardium exerts a restraining effect and modifies ventricular interaction during systole at high ventricular filling pressures.

In *summary*, there is experimental evidence from canine studies that the pericardium limits acute distention of the heart, enhances the effect that distention of one ventricle has on the diastolic pressure-volume relations and systolic function of the contralateral ventricle, and modifies cardiac growth.

FUNCTIONS OF THE PERICARDIUM IN HUMANS. There is substantial evidence that the restraining effects of the pericardium are clinically relevant. For example, in humans after pericardiotomy, there is a downward shift of the left ventricular pressure-volume curve that is increasingly prominent as left ventricular volume increases.[37] Similarly, routine pericardial closure after open-heart surgery has been shown to result in an increase in right heart filling pressure associated with a reduction in left ventricular diastolic cavity dimension and cardiac output, whereas open-

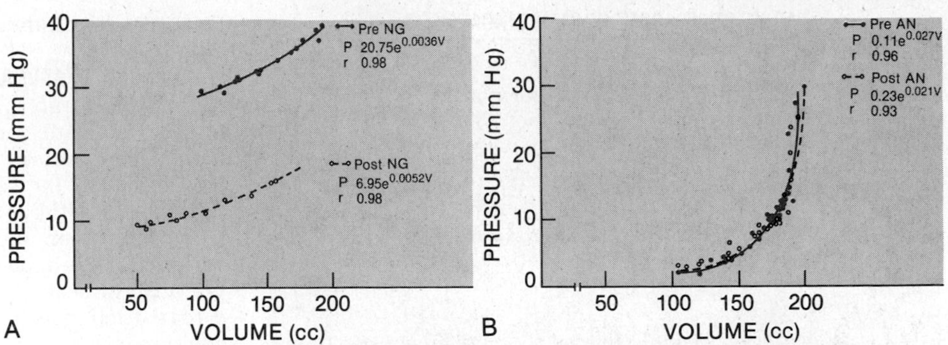

FIGURE 43–2. Left ventricular pressure-volume curves in man *(A)* before and after nitroglycerin (NG) and *(B)* before and after amyl nitrite (AN). Nitroglycerin, which causes venodilation and reduces total intrapericardial volume, shifts the curve downward and leftward. In contrast, the curves before and after amyl nitrite, which causes arterial dilation, can be superimposed. (Reproduced by permission from Ludbrook, P. A., et al.: Influence of right ventricular hemodynamics on left ventricular diastolic pressure-volume relations in man. Circulation *59:*21, 1979. Copyright American Heart Association.)

ing of the pericardium causes the opposite effects.[38] In addition, angiotensin, nitroprusside, and nitroglycerin infusions, which alter intracardiac volume, cause acute shifts in the left ventricular diastolic pressure-volume relation in humans,[39] an effect that has been shown in animal studies to depend on the presence of the constraint of the pericardium.[23] Ludbrook demonstrated in humans that the downward shift in the left ventricular pressure-volume curve that occurs during nitroglycerin administration is not observed with amyl nitrite, which alters aortic pressure but has little acute effect on intrapericardial volumes (Fig. 43–2).[39,40] After pericardiotomy and loss of the restraining effect of the pericardium, the human left ventricular pressure-volume curve is not altered by nitroprusside administration.[41] These observations indicate that the beneficial effects of interventions such as nitroprusside infusion, in which an augmentation of stroke volume may be observed at a lower ventricular filling pressure, are in part due to an alteration of apparent cardiac distensibility mediated by reducing the restraining effect of the pericardium.[42]

The pericardium may also provide a significant restraining effect on acute cardiac dilatation during acute volume loading in humans.[43] Extrapolating the findings of dog experiments may underestimate the restraining effect of the human pericardium during acute volume loading because normal human pericardium is thicker and shows much greater viscous responses than canine pericardium.[8] In patients, volume overload due to acute mitral regurgitation is sometimes associated with striking elevation and equilibration of diastolic pressures in all four cardiac chambers similar to that observed in constrictive pericardial disease (see p. 1501), but these findings do not appear to be present in patients with chronic volume overload.[44] Similarly, acute right ventricular infarction is sometimes associated with elevation and equilibration of diastolic right and left ventricular pressures[45] that have been shown experimentally to be related to the elevation of intrapericardial pressure.[46]

EFFECTS ON MYOCARDIAL GROWTH. The restraining effect of the pericardium also appears to modulate chronic changes in cardiac volume and physiological growth of the human heart. Because animal studies have suggested that left ventricular mass increases after pericardiectomy, Tischler et al.[47] used quantitative two-dimensional echocardiography to examine changes in left ventricular volume and mass in 25 patients with normal left ventricular ejection fraction 1 day before and 6 weeks and 7 months after elective bypass surgery with the pericardium left widely open. Both left ventricular end-diastolic volume and left ventricular mass were significantly increased by 6 weeks after surgery, and by 7 months after surgery, left ventricular end-diastolic volume had increased by 29 per cent and left ventricular mass had increased by 20 per cent in the absence of changes in systemic arterial blood pressure, left ventricular end-systolic wall stress, or end-systolic volume. It is likely that these effects on left ventricular mass were mediated by an increase in the transmural distending pressure following opening of the pericardium. These observations support the notion that the relief of pericardial constraint in humans results in a stimulus for myocardial growth and an increase in left ventricular mass.

ROLE IN HEART FAILURE. The role of the pericardium in the pathogenesis of chronic heart failure in patients is controversial and not yet well understood. Although compensatory enlargement and increased capacitance of the pericardium are likely to occur in humans with chronic cardiac enlargement, it is feasible that acute increases in venous return in patients with heart failure could accentuate the effects of the pericardium on ventricular diastolic and systolic function. Consistent with this hypothesis, Janicki studied the effects of the augmentation of venous return by exercise in 61 patients with chronic heart failure and deduced that pericardial constraint became evident when stroke volume abruptly became invariant and a similar increment in right and left heart filling pressures occurred during progressive exercise.[48] In this study, pericardial constraint became evident during exercise in half of the patients. Thus, it appears that the pericardium can be an important determinant of the limits of systolic pump function and result in the coupling of right and left ventricular diastolic pressures in patients with heart failure.

ACUTE PERICARDITIS

Acute pericarditis is a syndrome due to inflammation of the pericardium characterized by chest pain, a pericardial friction rub, and serial electrocardiographic abnormalities. The incidence of pericardial inflammation detected in several autopsy series ranges from 2 to 6 per cent, whereas pericarditis is diagnosed clinically in only about 1 of 1000 hospital admissions. This suggests that pericarditis is frequently inapparent clinically, although it may occur in the presence of a vast number of medical and surgical disorders (Table 43–1). The most common causes of the syndrome of acute pericarditis include idiopathic or viral pericarditis, uremia, bacterial infection, acute myocardial infarction, pericardiotomy associated with cardiac surgery, tuberculosis, neoplasm, and trauma. All types of pericarditis are more common in men than in women, and in adults compared with young children. The relative frequency of causes of pericarditis depend on the clinical setting. Presumed viral or idiopathic pericarditis is common in an outpatient setting, whereas pericarditis related to trauma, neoplasm, and uremia is seen more frequently in tertiary hospitals.

The *pathological changes* of acute pericarditis are those of acute inflammation, including the presence of polymorphonuclear leukocytes, increased pericardial vascularity, and deposition of fibrin. Inflammation may also involve the superficial myocardium, and fibrinous adhesions may form between the pericardium and epicardium and between the pericardium and adjacent sternum and pleura. The visceral pericardium may also react to acute injury by exudation of fluid. The pathological and clinical features of specific causes of pericarditis are discussed later in this chapter. This section focuses on clinical features common to acute pericarditis of many causes.

HISTORY. *Chest pain* is frequently the chief complaint of patients with acute pericarditis; its quality and location are variable. Pain is often localized to retrosternal and left precordial regions and frequently radiates to the trapezius ridge and neck (Table 43–2). Occasionally it may be local-

TABLE 43–1 CAUSES OF PERICARDITIS

1. **Idiopathic** (nonspecific)
2. **Viral Infections:** Coxsackie A virus, Coxsackie B virus, echovirus, adenovirus, mumps virus, infectious mononucleosis, varicella, hepatitis B, AIDS (acquired immunodeficiency syndrome)
3. **Tuberculosis**
4. **Acute Bacterial Infection:** pneumococcus, staphylococcus, streptococcus, gram-negative septicemia, *Neisseria meningitidis, Neisseria gonorrhoeae,* tularemia, *Legionella pneumophila*
5. **Fungal Infections:** histoplasmosis, coccidioidomycosis, *Candida,* blastomycosis
6. **Other Infections:** toxoplasmosis, amebiasis, mycoplasma, *Nocardia,* actinomycosis, echinococcosis, Lyme disease
7. **Acute Myocardial Infarction**
8. **Uremia:** untreated uremia; in association with hemodialysis
9. **Neoplastic Disease:** lung cancer, breast cancer, leukemia, Hodgkin's disease, lymphoma
10. **Radiation**
11. **Autoimmune Disorders:** acute rheumatic fever, systemic lupus erythematosus, rheumatoid arthritis, scleroderma, mixed connective tissue disease, Wegener's granulomatosis, polyarteritis nodosa
12. **Other Inflammatory Disorders:** sarcoidosis, amyloidosis, inflammatory bowel disease, Whipple disease, temporal arteritis, Behçet disease
13. **Drugs:** hydralazine, procainamide, phenytoin, isoniazid, phenylbutazone, dantrolene, doxorubicin, methysergide, penicillin (with hypereosinophilia)
14. **Trauma:** including chest trauma; hemopericardium following thoracic surgery; pacemaker insertion; cardiac diagnostic procedures; esophageal rupture; pancreatic-pericardial fistula
15. **Delayed Postmyocardial-Pericardial Injury Syndromes:**
    a. Postmyocardial infarction (Dressler) syndrome
    b. Postpericardiotomy syndrome
16. **Dissecting Aortic Aneurysm**
17. **Myxedema**
18. **Chylopericardium**

ized to the epigastrium, mimicking an "acute abdomen," or have a dull or oppressive quality, with radiation to the left arm similar to the ischemic pain of myocardial infarction. The pain is often aggravated by lying supine, coughing, deep inspiration, and swallowing and is eased by sitting up and leaning forward. Sometimes it is noted with each heartbeat. The pain associated with pericarditis may arise from inflammation of both the pericardium and the adjacent pleura, accounting for the pleuritic nature of the discomfort. Pericardial pain may also be provoked by stretch of the pericardial sac due to the presence of intrapericardial fluid. The inspiratory and positional aggravation of pericardial pain may be confused with chest pain caused by acute pulmonary embolism. It is important also to recognize that acute pericarditis may develop in about 4 per cent of patients a few days after acute pulmonary embolism.[49]

Acute pericarditis may also cause *dyspnea.* This symptom is related in part to the need to breathe shallowly to avoid pericardiopleuritic chest pain. Dyspnea may be aggravated by the presence of fever or by the development of a large pericardial effusion that compresses adjacent bronchi and pulmonary parenchyma. Additional symptoms such as cough, sputum production, or weight loss may be due to an underlying systemic disease such as tuberculosis or uremia. The classic clinical features of chest pain and dyspnea are more subtle in elderly patients with pericarditis and are easily confused with other causes of chest pain.[50]

PHYSICAL EXAMINATION: THE FRICTION RUB. The *pericardial friction rub* (p. 45) is the pathognomonic physical finding of acute pericarditis. It is a scratching, grating, high-pitched sound, described by Laennec's associate Victor Collin as "the squeak of leather of a new saddle under the rider." Although the sound is believed to arise from friction between the roughened pericardial and epicardial surfaces, a loud pericardial rub may also be heard in the presence of scant or large pericardial effusions.[51] The pericardial friction rub is classically described as having three components that are related to cardiac motion during atrial systole (presystole), ventricular systole, and rapid ventricular filling in early diastole. Spodick's prospective analysis of the pericardial friction rub revealed that the presystolic component is present in about 70 per cent of cases, while a ventricular systolic component is the loudest and most easily heard component, present in almost all cases.[52] The rapid diastolic filling component is detected less frequently and may be slurred into that of atrial contraction, resulting in a biphasic "to-and-fro" rub. In this series, a true three-component rub was detected about half the time and at the lower left sternal border. The single-component rub is the least common but is likely to be the auscultatory finding in patients with atrial fibrillation.

An important feature of the pericardial friction rub is that it is often evanescent and may change in quality from one examination to the next. Detection of the rub is aided by listening with the stethoscope diaphragm applied firmly to the chest at the lower left sternal border during inspiration and full expiration with the patient sitting up and leaning forward. Occasionally, rubs may be detected with the patient lying supine with arms extended above the head during inspiration or suspended respiration. The single-component pericardial friction rub may be mistaken for a systolic murmur or tricuspid or mitral regurgitation. A pericardial rub may also be confused with the crunch of air in the mediastinum or the artifact of skin scratching against the stethoscope. Pericardial friction rubs may be differentiated from murmurs by (1) the use of exercise to permit detection of a classic three-component rub, (2) the failure of a rub to radiate widely or to vary in timing and duration with inspiration or a change in posture in a manner characteristic of regurgitant murmurs, and (3) by the confirmatory finding of typical electrocardiographic and echocardiographic changes of pericarditis.

TABLE 43–2 PERICARDIAL VERSUS ISCHEMIC PAIN

	ISCHEMIA	PERICARDITIS
Location	Retrosternal; left shoulder, arm	Precordium; left trapezius ridge
Quality	Pressure, burning, buildup	Sharp, pleuritic; or dull, oppressive
Thoracic motion	No effect	Increased by breathing, rotating thorax
Duration	Angina; 1 or 2 to 15 min Unstable angina: ½ hr to hours	Hours or days
Effort	Stable angina: usually Unstable angina or infarction: usually not	No relation
Posture	No effect; may sit, belch, use Valsalva or knee-chest position for relief	Leaning forward for relief; aggravated by recumbency

From Fowler, N. O.: Acute pericarditis. *In* Fowler, N. O. (ed.): The Pericardium in Health and Disease. Mt. Kisco, NY, Futura Publishing Co., 1985, p. 158.

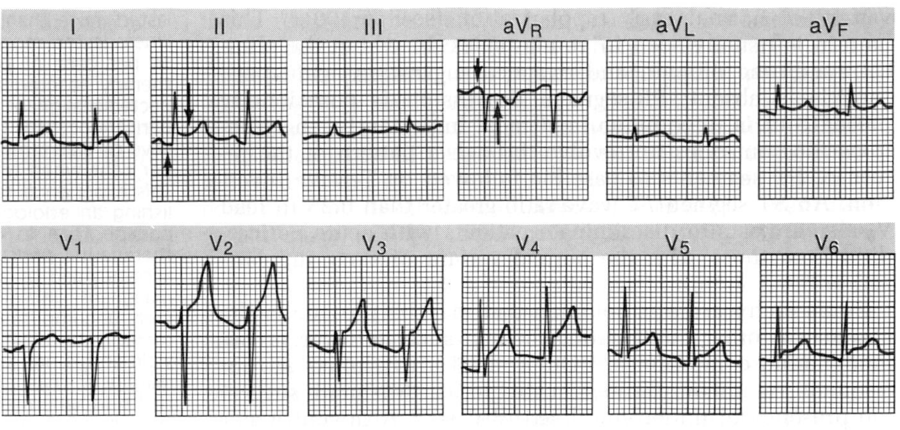

FIGURE 43–3. Stage I electrocardiographic changes from a patient with acute pericarditis. Diffuse ST-segment elevation, which is concave upward, is present in all leads except aV_R and V_1. (A short P-R interval unrelated to acute pericarditis is also present.) Depression of the PR segment, an electrocardiographic abnormality that is common in patients with acute pericarditis, is not evident because of the short P-R interval.

ELECTROCARDIOGRAM. Serial electrocardiograms are extremely helpful in confirming the diagnosis of acute pericarditis. Electrocardiographic changes can occur a few hours or days after the onset of pericardial pain, and the electrocardiographic diagnosis of acute pericarditis is made by detecting the serial appearance of four stages of abnormalities of the ST segments and T waves (Fig. 43–3).[53] These changes are believed to be related to an actual current of injury caused by superficial myocardial inflammation or epicardial injury. There are four stages in the evolution of acute pericarditis (Table 43–3). Stage I electrocardiographic changes accompany the onset of chest pain and are virtually diagnostic of acute pericarditis. These comprise ST-segment elevation, which, unlike the pattern of ST-segment elevation in acute myocardial infarction, is concave upward and usually present in all leads except aVr and V1. The T waves are usually upright in the leads with ST-segment elevation. The ST-segment axis in the frontal plane also differs in these two conditions and is reported to range from 30 to 60 degrees in acute pericarditis, unlike acute anterior myocardial infarction in which the ST-segment axis varies from 100 to 120 degrees.[54]

Recent studies of body surface potential mapping in patients with acute pericarditis suggest that the mechanism of ST elevation is a current flowing from the epicardial surface out into the thorax and back into the heart through the atria and great vessels.[55] Stage II occurs several days later and represents the return of ST segments to baseline, accompanied by T-wave flattening. This change in the ST segments usually occurs prior to the appearance of T-wave inversion. In contrast, T waves in acute myocardial infarction often become inverted before the ST segments return to baseline. Stage III is characterized by inversion of the T waves so that the T-wave vector becomes directed opposite to the ST-segment vector. T-wave inversion is generally present in most leads and is not associated with the loss of R-wave voltage or the appearance of Q waves. These features help to differentiate this stage of nonspecific T-wave inversion from changes associated with the evolution of transmural or subendocardial myocardial infarction. Stage IV represents the reversion of T-wave changes to normal, which may occur up to weeks or months later. T-wave inversion may occasionally persist indefinitely in patients with chronic pericardial inflammation due to tuberculosis, uremia, or neoplastic pericardial disease.

Electrocardiographic abnormalities appear in about 90 per cent of cases of acute pericarditis,[53,56] and the finding of typical Stage I changes or a classic evolution of all four stages can be diagnostic even when other clinical features of pericarditis are misleading. All four stages are detected in about 50 per cent of patients with acute pericarditis. In addition, depression of the PR segment occurs in about 80 per cent of patients with acute pericarditis.[53] Depression of the PR segment occurs during the early stages of ST-segment elevation or T-wave inversion, is usually present in both limb and precordial leads, and may reflect abnormal atrial repolarization due to atrial inflammation.

Variations of the patterns already described are present in slightly less than 50 per cent of patients with pericarditis and include (1) isolated PR-segment depression, (2) the absence of one or more stages of the ST-segment and T-wave changes, (3) evolution of Stage I (ST-segment elevation) directly to Stage IV (reversion of T waves to normal), (4) persistence of T-wave inversion, (5) appearance of ST-segment changes in only a few leads, (6) the appearance of marked T-wave inversion before the ST segments returned to baseline, and (7) the absence of any serial electrocardiographic changes whatsoever.[57]

Regional ST-segment deviation may be confused with electrocardiographic changes of regional myocardial ischemia. ST-segment elevation in the right precordial leads has been described in acute pericarditis.[58] The frequency of acute right precordial ST-segment elevation in acute pericarditis has not been systematically studied, and this finding could cause confusion with acute right ventricular infarction.

In addition to the features already described that help to distinguish the ST-segment changes of pericarditis from those of acute myocardial infarction, the changes of Stage I must also be differentiated from the electrocardiographic

TABLE 43–3 FOUR-STAGE ("TYPICAL") ECG EVOLUTION OF ACUTE PERICARDITIS

SEQUENCE	LEADS OF "EPICARDIAL" DERIVATION (I, II, aV_L, aV_F, V_{3-6})			LEADS REFLECTING "ENDOCARDIAL" POTENTIAL aV_R, OFTEN V_1, SOMETIMES V_2		
Stage	J-ST*	T Waves	PR Segment	ST Segment	T Waves	PR Segment
I	Elevated	Upright	Depressed or isoelectric	Depressed	Inverted	Elevated or isoelectric
II early	Isoelectric	Upright	Isoelectric or depressed	Isoelectric	Inverted	Isoelectric or elevated
II late	Isoelectric	Low to flat to inverted	Isoelectric or depressed	Isoelectric	Shallow to flat to upright	Isoelectric or elevated
III	Isoelectric	Inverted	Isoelectric	Isoelectric	Upright	Isoelectric
IV	Isoelectric	Upright	Isoelectric	Isoelectric	Inverted	Isoelectric

* J-ST = junction of S (or T) wave with the end of the QRS complex.
Modified from Spodick, D. H.: Electrocardiographic changes in acute pericarditis. Am. J. Cardiol. *33*:470, 1974.

paradoxical pulse can be accurately quantified by means of an intraarterial catheter but may be estimated by cuff sphygmomanometry. The cuff should be inflated 20 mm Hg above systolic pressure and slowly deflated until the Korotkoff sounds are heard only during expiration. The cuff should then be deflated to the point at which Korotkoff sounds are heard equally well in inspiration and expiration. The difference between these pressures is the estimated magnitude of pulsus paradoxus.

Other disorders with systemic venous distention, pulsus paradoxus, and clear lungs that can be confused with cardiac tamponade include obstructive pulmonary disease, constrictive pericarditis, restrictive cardiomyopathy, and massive pulmonary embolism. Pulsus paradoxus is occasionally noted during severe hypovolemia due to hemorrhagic shock, but jugular venous distention is usually absent. Cardiac tamponade may be confused with shock due to right ventricular infarction with jugular venous distention and clear lungs.[45] However, the hemodynamics of right ventricular infarction are more like those of pericardial constriction than of tamponade (see p. 1496).

LOW-PRESSURE TAMPONADE. The clinical findings may be further modified in patients with so-called *low-pressure cardiac tamponade* in whom jugular venous distention is absent and the right atrial pressure is low. This syndrome, which occurs in the setting of hypovolemia, represents an early stage in the development of cardiac tamponade in which accumulation of a pericardial effusion causes intrapericardial pressure to rise and equilibrate with low right heart diastolic filling pressures.[116] Pericardiocentesis reduces intrapericardial pressure and causes the separation of right atrial and intrapericardial pressures. Low-pressure cardiac tamponade tends to occur in patients with tuberculosis and neoplastic pericarditis complicated by severe dehydration.

TENSION PNEUMOPERICARDIUM. This condition causes hemodynamic changes similar to those of acute hemorrhagic cardiac tamponade. It is being increasingly recognized as a cause of cardiac tamponade with high mortality in infants during mechanical ventilation and in adults as a result of penetrating chest trauma, gastric and esophageal rupture, carcinomatous bronchopericardial fistula, gas production from contiguous infection, and diagnostic procedures such as sternal bone marrow aspiration.[117] Characteristic clinical findings include muffled heart sounds, bradycardia, and shifting tympany over the precordium. Unique auscultatory findings can be detected, including a metallic cracking sound, and the bruit de moulin, which was described in the first report of pneumopericardium in 1844 by Bricheteau as "the noise made by floats of a mill wheel as they strike the water,"[118] and which indicates the presence of both air and fluid in the pericardial space.

Laboratory Studies

CHEST ROENTGENOGRAM. There are no roentgenographic features diagnostic of cardiac tamponade. The heart may appear completely normal in size in cardiac tamponade that develops from acute hemopericardium due to cardiac rupture or laceration. On the other hand, if an effusion that accumulates more slowly to more than approximately 250 ml is responsible, the cardiac silhouette may be enlarged with a water bottle configuration (Fig. 7–47, p. 234). This finding suggests the presence of a large pericardial effusion but supplies no information about its hemodynamic significance. In patients with cardiac tamponade due to tension pneumopericardium, the chest roentgenogram usually shows that the heart is surrounded by air delineated by a strip of soft tissue extending up the aorta consisting of the pericardium.

ELECTROCARDIOGRAM. The electrocardiographic abnormalities seen in acute cardiac tamponade include those of acute pericarditis and pericardial effusion per se. The development of electrical alternans is a more specific indicator of pericardial tamponade and reflects pendular swinging of the heart within the pericardial space (Fig. 43–8).[119] Electrical alternans may also be related to a beat-to-beat alteration of right and left ventricular filling.

Electrical alternans may also occur in constrictive pericarditis, in tension pneumothorax, after myocardial infarction, and with severe cardiac muscle dysfunction. However, the appearance of electrical alternans in a patient with a known pericardial effusion is highly suggestive of cardiac tamponade—a finding that has been confirmed in experimental cardiac tamponade.[120] Electrical alternans of the QRS complex may occur in a 2:1 or 3:1 pattern. Alternans is usually limited to the QRS complex, but alternans of the P wave, QRS complex, and T wave may rarely occur in extreme cardiac tamponade. Both the abnormal heart motion within the pericardial sac and electrical alternans disappear when pericardial fluid is aspirated.

ECHOCARDIOGRAM (see also p. 93). In patients with jugular venous distention and the possibility of cardiac tamponade, echocardiography is extremely useful and should be performed prior to consideration of pericardiocentesis (Table 43–6). In a rare patient who is in extremis from the

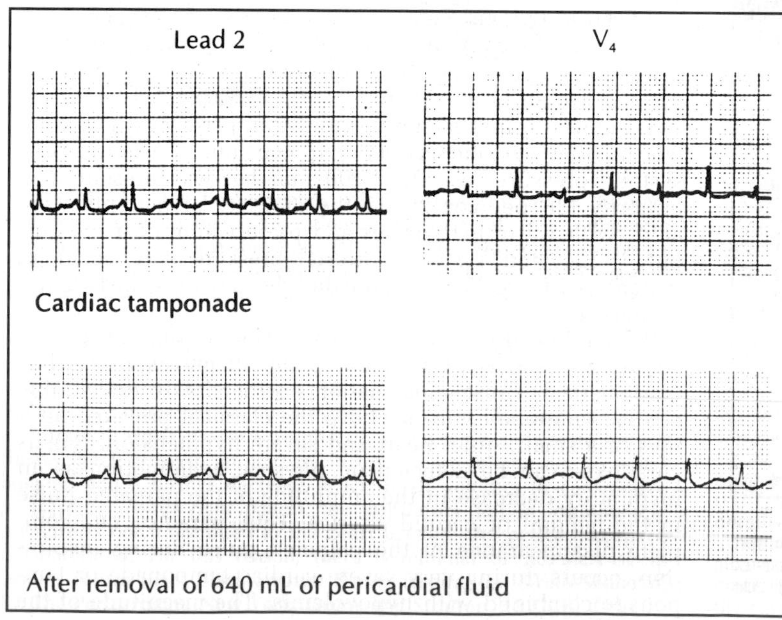

FIGURE 43–8. Electrical alternans of the QRS complex in a patient with cardiac tamponade. Electrical alternans of the QRS complex may also occur with pericarditis without tamponade, with supraventricular or ventricular tachycardia, and with coronary artery disease. Total alternans, involving P, QRS, and T complexes, is almost diagnostic of cardiac tamponade. (From Fowler, N.: Pericardial disease. *In* Abelmann, W. H. [ed.]: Cardiomyopathies, Myocarditis, and Pericardial Disease, in Braunwald, E. (series ed.): Atlas of Heart Diseases. Philadelphia, Current Medicine, 1995.)

TABLE 43–6 ECHOCARDIOGRAPHIC FINDINGS IN CARDIAC TAMPONADE

Right atrial diastolic collapse
Right ventricular early diastolic collapse
Left atrial collapse
Abnormal inspiratory increase in tricuspid valve flow and >15% inspiratory decrease of mitral valve flow
Abnormal inspiratory increase of right ventricular dimension with abnormal inspiratory decrease of left ventricular dimension
Inspiratory decrease of mitral valve DE excursion and EF slope
Inferior vena caval plethora (failure to decrease proximal diameter by ≥50% on sniff or deep inspiration)
Left ventricular pseudohypertrophy
Swinging heart

extremely rapid development of cardiac tamponade, the physician may have to rely on the history and physical findings to make a judgment about the need for pericardiocentesis. If echocardiography is readily available and the patient with suspected cardiac tamponade is not moribund, obtaining an echocardiogram increases the likelihood of diagnosing cardiac tamponade correctly and prevents inappropriate and potentially lethal attempts at pericardiocentesis or pericardiotomy. First, the echocardiogram helps to document the presence and magnitude of pericardial effusion (Fig. 3–104, p. 93). The absence of echocardiographic evidence of pericardial effusion virtually excludes the diagnosis of cardiac tamponade, *with the exception of the postoperative cardiac surgery patient in whom loculated fluid or thrombus may cause cardiac compression.* Second, the echocardiogram can rapidly differentiate cardiac tamponade from other causes of systemic venous hypertension and arterial hypotension, including constrictive pericarditis, cardiac muscle dysfunction, and right ventricular infarction. The appearance of dense echoes in the pericardial space or extrinsic to the pericardium suggests the presence of compression by material other than free fluid. Echocardiograms can often detect both massive extracardiac hematoma and extrinsic compression of the heart by tumor, which can cause cardiac compression with the physiology of cardiac constriction or cardiac tamponade.

Two-dimensional and Doppler echocardiography can provide additional clues that pericardial effusion is associated with cardiac tamponade. The presence of pulsus paradoxus is associated with sudden leftward motion of the septum during inspiration and an exaggerated increase in right ventricular size.[108,121] This characteristic respiratory variation in ventricular preload can also be detected by the Doppler ultrasound findings of exaggerated tricuspid and pulmonic flow velocities and reduction of peak mitral flow velocity with the onset of inspiration and the opposite changes after the onset of expiration (Fig. 43–7).[122,123] When the inspiratory reduction in left ventricular filling is extreme, the aortic valve may close prematurely or fail to open[124] and mitral valve opening may be delayed until atrial systole. Recent combined hemodynamic and echocardiographic-Doppler studies in patients with tamponade before and during pericardiocentesis show that the presence and magnitude of respiratory variation in mitral flow velocity are *not* predictive of the magnitude of hemodynamic compromise.[125] Cardiac tamponade is also associated with "pseudohypertrophy" (an increase in left ventricular diastolic wall thickness), which correlates inversely with the decrease in cavity volume, but the independent prognostic value of this sign is not known.[126] Diastolic right atrial and right ventricular compression or collapse occur early during the development of cardiac tamponade[101,102,103] (Fig. 43–9). Left atrial and left ventricular diastolic collapse can occur when regional left heart compression is present.[100,127]

Right ventricular diastolic collapse appears to be more predictive of cardiac tamponade than pulsus paradoxus, particularly during hypovolemia, and these echocardiographic signs may be reversed by volume expansion.[128,129] Right ventricular diastolic collapse may be absent in the presence of right ventricular hypertrophy and can occur when a large pleural effusion causes elevation of intrapericardial pressure by external compression.[130] Thus, the echocardiographic findings of pericardial effusion, an inspiratory increase in right ventricular dimensions, and right atrial and ventricular diastolic collapse strongly suggest the diagnosis of cardiac tamponade, but these changes are not 100 per cent sensitive or specific. Experimental studies confirm that a single echocardiogram cannot always predict the presence or severity of cardiac tamponade.[131]

Furthermore, hemodynamic observations at our institution in a consecutive series of 50 patients with suspected cardiac tamponade and echocardiographic evidence of right atrial and ventricular diastolic collapse showed that these echocardiographic findings were uniformly associated with elevation of pericardial pressure and the near equilibration of right atrial and right ventricular pressures.[132] However,

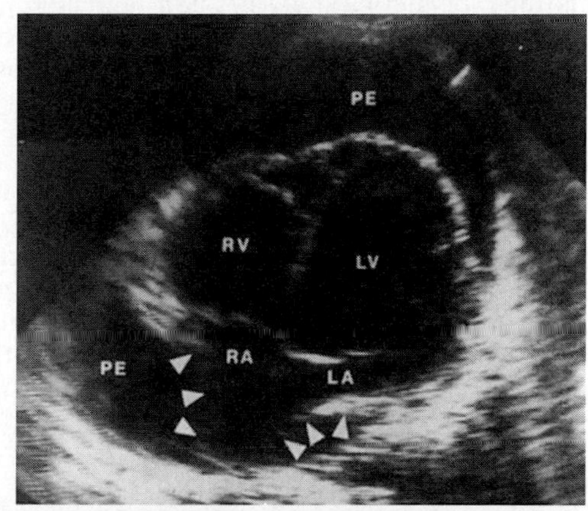

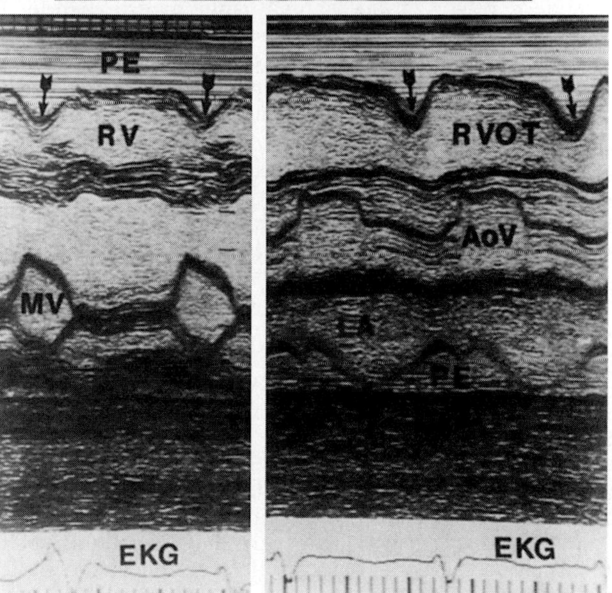

FIGURE 43–9. Two-dimensional *(upper panel)* and M-mode *(lower panels)* echocardiograms from a patient with a malignant pericardial effusion and cardiac tamponade. The two-dimensional image shows a large pericardial effusion (PE) adjacent to the borders of the right ventricle (RV), right atrium (RA), and left ventricle (LV). The effusion is sufficiently large that fluid is also present behind the left atrium (LA). Diastolic compression (white arrowheads) of both the right and left atria is present. The M-mode images also show striking diastolic compression (dark arrows) of the right ventricle during diastole when the mitral valve (MV) is open and compression of the right ventricular outflow tract (RVOT) in early to mid diastole after aortic valve (AoV) closure.

right heart diastolic collapse was associated with a wide spectrum of hemodynamic derangement, including a subset of patients with minimal elevation of right atrial pressure and the preservation of a normal cardiac output and systemic arterial pressure. Eisenberg et al. have examined the prognostic value of echocardiography in 187 hospitalized patients with pericardial effusion, of whom 16 (9 per cent) subsequently required pericardiocentesis or surgical drainage.[133] This study concluded that the size of the pericardial effusion was the most powerful predictor of outcome, whereas right heart diastolic collapse, distention of the superior vena cava, and altered response to respiration added little prognostic information. Thus, the recognition of patients with cardiac tamponade by echocardiography requires complementary clinical and hemodynamic assessment to distinguish patients with milder degrees of cardiac compression from those with hemodynamic decompensation who require urgent drainage of pericardial fluid.

We agree with Fowler's recent suggestion that in most patients, cardiac tamponade requiring pericardial drainage should be diagnosed by a clinical examination showing elevated systemic venous pressure, tachycardia, dyspnea, and pulsus paradoxus.[87] Many patients with echocardiographic findings of pericardial effusion and right heart compression who do not have these clinical findings may be observed closely, and pericardial drainage may not be necessary. In contrast, in patients with suspected cardiac perforation or rupture who have echocardiographic signs of pericardial effusion and right heart compression, urgent pericardial drainage by pericardiocentesis or surgery is almost always needed. Cardiac tamponade is a *clinical,* not an echocardiographic or a radionuclide, diagnosis that is established definitively by documentation of the elevation and equilibration of intrapericardial and right atrial pressures and the reversal of these findings by evacuation of pericardial fluid.

Cardiac Catheterization

Cardiac catheterization is invaluable in establishing the hemodynamic importance of pericardial effusion. Except in extreme emergencies, such as when the patient is moribund, we prefer to catheterize the right heart and pericardial space in conjunction with pericardiocentesis. Cardiac catheterization (1) provides absolute confirmation of the diagnosis of cardiac tamponade; (2) quantitates the hemodynamic compromise; (3) guides pericardiocentesis by documenting that pericardial aspiration is associated with hemodynamic improvement; and (4) permits the detection of coexisting hemodynamic problems, including left ventricular failure, effusive-constrictive pericarditis (see p. 1505), and unsuspected pulmonary hypertension in patients with malignant effusions.

Cardiac catheterization typically demonstrates elevation of right atrial pressure with a characteristic preserved systolic x descent and absence of or a diminutive diastolic y descent. When intrapericardial and right atrial pressures are recorded simultaneously, both are elevated and virtually identical (Fig. 43–10); both pressures fall during inspiration, and intrapericardial pressure may fall slightly below right atrial pressure during systolic ejection at the time of the x descent. If intrapericardial pressure is not elevated, and if right atrial and intrapericardial pressures are not virtually identical, the diagnosis of cardiac tamponade must be reconsidered.

Right ventricular mid-diastolic pressure is elevated and equal to right atrial and intrapericardial pressures and lacks the dip-and-plateau configuration characteristic of constrictive pericarditis. Because right ventricular and pulmonary artery systolic pressures are equal to the sum of the pressure developed by the right ventricle plus the intrapericardial pressure, right ventricular and pulmonary artery systolic pressures are usually moderately elevated, in the range of 35 to 50 mm Hg. In the case of severe cardiac compression, right ventricular systolic pressure may be reduced and only slightly higher than right ventricular diastolic pressure.

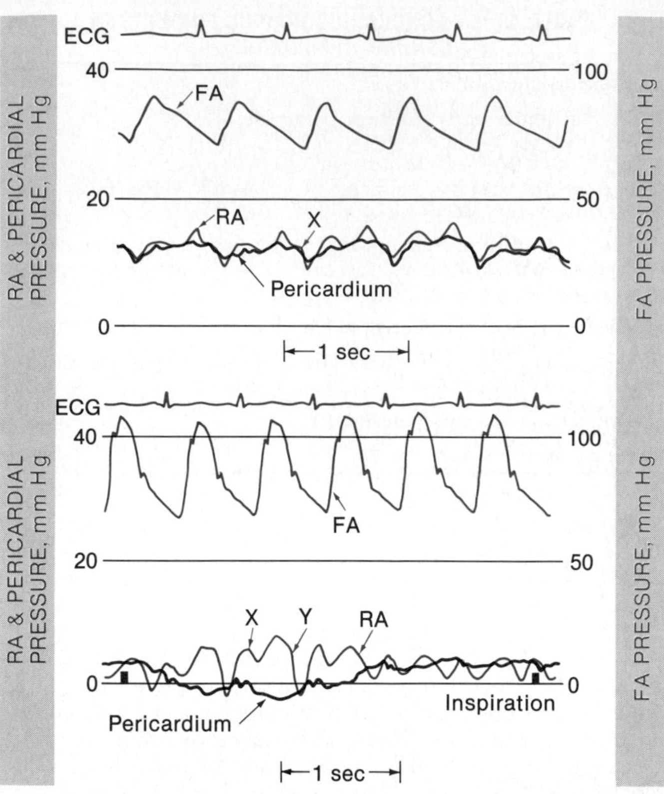

FIGURE 43–10. Simultaneous right atrial (RA) and intrapericardial pressures (scale 0 to 40 mm Hg) and femoral artery pressure (scale 0 to 100 mm Hg) from a patient with decompensated cardiac tamponade. Before pericardiocentesis *(upper panel),* systemic hypotension is present, and there is elevation and equalization of right atrial and intrapericardial pressures. Note that a systolic x descent is present, but the diastolic y descent is absent, suggesting that right atrial emptying is impeded by compression of the right ventricle in early diastole. After aspiration of about 300 ml of pericardial fluid *(lower panel),* cardiac tamponade is relieved, as shown by the restoration of intrapericardial pressure to zero, the restoration of right atrial pressure to a normal level, and the improvement in systemic arterial pressure. The right atrial tracing shows the appearance of a diastolic y descent, which indicates the relief of cardiac compression and restoration of normal right atrial emptying in early diastole. Although this degree of fluid aspiration relieved tamponade physiology, an additional 1500 ml of fluid was subsequently aspirated from the pericardial space. (Modified from Lorell, B. H., and Grossman, W.: Profiles in constrictive pericarditis, restrictive cardiomyopathy, and cardiac tamponade. *In* Grossman, W., and Baim, D. S. [eds.]: Cardiac Catheterization, Angiography and Intervention. Philadelphia, Lea and Febiger, 1991, p. 644.)

Usually the pulmonary capillary wedge pressure and left ventricular diastolic pressure are elevated and equal to intrapericardial pressure when recorded simultaneously. During expiration, the pulmonary capillary wedge pressure is usually slightly higher than intrapericardial pressure, resulting in a pressure gradient that promotes left-heart filling. During inspiration, the pulmonary capillary wedge pressure may transiently decrease more than intrapericardial pressure such that the pressure gradient between the pulmonary venous circulation and the left heart is reduced or absent. In patients with severe underlying left ventricular dysfunction or hypertrophy and elevation of the left ventricular diastolic pressure, cardiac tamponade can be present when intrapericardial and right atrial pressures are equal but lower than left ventricular diastolic pressure. Depending on the severity of cardiac compression, left ventricular systolic and aortic pressures may be normal or reduced.

Pulsus paradoxus can be easily documented by intraarterial catheterization and pressure measurement. Simultaneous recording of systemic arterial and right ventricular pressures shows that the inspiratory pressure variation is out of phase. Stroke volume is usually markedly depressed. Cardiac output may be normal, owing to the compensatory effect of tachycardia, or it may be markedly reduced when cardiac tamponade is severe; systemic vascular resistance is usually elevated.

Angiographic studies add no additional information if echocardiographic findings suggestive of cardiographic tamponade were obtained prior to cardiac catheterization. In an otherwise normal heart, right and left ventricular end-diastolic volumes are usually reduced with normal or increased ejection fractions.

Aspiration of pericardial fluid results initially in the lowering of the identical intrapericardial, right atrial, right ventricular, and left ventricular diastolic pressures, followed by a fall of intrapericardial pressure below right atrial pressure and reappearance of the *y* descent in the right atrial waveform (Fig. 43–10). Further aspiration causes intrapericardial pressure to fall to a mean level of zero and to fluctuate with changes in intrathoracic pressure. Because the pressure-volume curve of the pericardium is steep, the initial aspiration of 50 to 100 ml of pericardial fluid usually leads to striking reduction in intrapericardial pressure, marked improvement in systemic arterial pressure and cardiac output, and abolition of pulsus paradoxus. The reduction of intrapericardial pressure is often followed by diuresis, related both to the augmentation of cardiac output and the release of atrial natriuretic factor.[93–95]

If intrapericardial pressure falls to zero or becomes negative and right atrial pressure remains elevated, *effusive-constrictive pericarditis* (see p. 1505) should be strongly considered, especially in patients with underlying neoplasm or prior radiation. Other causes of continued elevation of right atrial pressure after successful pericardiocentesis include the coexistence of cardiac tamponade and preexisting left ventricular dysfunction, causing, in turn, pulmonary hypertension and right atrial hypertension, tricuspid valve disease, and restrictive cardiomyopathy. In patients with suspected malignant disease, pulmonary hypertension due to pulmonary microvascular tumor is an important cause of persistent elevation of right atrial pressure and the failure to relieve dyspnea after complete drainage of the pericardial space.[132]

The distinction between cardiac tamponade and the superior vena cava syndrome must always be made in patients with neoplastic disease in whom these lesions may occur singly or together. In patients with obstruction of the superior vena cava, cardiac tamponade may be suspected from the presence of elevated jugular venous pressure and pulsus paradoxus due to respiratory distress. In this condition (without accompanying cardiac tamponade), pressure in the superior vena cava is markedly elevated, with dampened pulsations, and exceeds right atrial and inferior vena cava pressures. Two-dimensional and Doppler echocardiography may not be successful in distinguishing between these conditions because cardiac tamponade as well as other causes of elevated central venous pressure may modify the appearance and respiratory fluctuation of flow in the venae cavae.[123,133] If elevation of jugular venous pressure persists after relief of cardiac tamponade in patients with neoplastic disease, obstruction of the superior vena cava, as reflected in a pressure gradient between the superior vena cava and right atrium, should be sought. Superior vena caval obstruction may be amenable to radiation therapy.

Pericardiocentesis

Hemodynamic support during preparation of the patient for pericardiocentesis or pericardiotomy should include administration of intravenous fluid, blood, plasma, or saline. The rationale for volume expansion is that it has been shown to delay the appearance of right ventricular diastolic collapse and hemodynamic deterioration.[102] In experimental cardiac tamponade, administration of norepinephrine and dobutamine has produced an increase in cardiac output, whereas dobutamine appears to delay the onset of tissue hypoxia by promoting a greater augmentation of cardiac output and oxygen delivery at any level of intrapericardial pressure.[134] The vasodilators hydralazine and nitroprusside have also been employed in experimental cardiac tamponade to promote an increase in cardiac output secondary to the reduction of elevated systemic resistance.[135] The administration of vasodilators in conjunction with volume expansion must be done with extreme caution in patients with cardiac tamponade, because it may be hazardous in patients with borderline or frank hypotension. Beta-adrenergic blockade should be avoided because increased adrenergic activity helps to maintain cardiac output. Positive-pressure ventilation should be avoided whenever possible because it has been shown to depress cardiac output further in patients with cardiac tamponade.[136]

Pericardial fluid under pressure causing tamponade can be evacuated by (1) percutaneous pericardiocentesis using a needle or catheter, (2) pericardiotomy via a subxiphoid incision, or (3) partial or extensive surgical pericardiectomy. Considerable controversy exists regarding the exact indications for pericardiocentesis, although the procedure has been performed extensively since its initial demonstration in 1840 by the Viennese physician Franz Schuh. The benefits of pericardiocentesis include the rapid relief of cardiac tamponade and the opportunity to obtain accurate hemodynamic measurements before and after pericardial aspiration. The major risk of percutaneous pericardiocentesis is laceration of the heart, coronary arteries, or lung. Prior to the 1970s, pericardiocentesis was usually performed blindly at the bedside using a sharp needle without hemodynamic or echocardiographic monitoring, and the risk of death or life-threatening complications appeared to be as high as 20 per cent.[137]

TECHNIQUE. The modern approach is exemplified by the Stanford experience in 123 patients.[138] In the majority of patients, pericardiocentesis was performed by a cardiologist in the cardiac catheterization laboratory using a subxiphoid approach under fluoroscopic guidance with hemodynamic and electrocardiographic monitoring. In this experience, five deaths occurred in association with pericardiocentesis; nonfatal hemopericardium developed in an additional five patients. Pericardiocentesis in this study was successful in obtaining pericardial fluid in 106 of 123 patients. Importantly, the probability of success in safely obtaining fluid was directly related to the size of the pericardial effusion because fluid was obtained in 93 per cent of patients with large effusions located both anteriorly and posteriorly on echocardiogram but in only 58 per cent with a small posterior pericardial effusion. In 23 patients a specific etiological diagnosis was possible from analysis of the pericardial fluid. Cardiac tamponade was successfully relieved by pericardiocentesis in 61 per cent, whereas the remainder required subsequent surgical drainage owing either to failure to relieve tamponade or to recurrence after pericardiocentesis. Surgery was most frequently required in patients with acute traumatic hemopericardium (see p. 1536). An unsuspected physiological cause of increased systemic venous pressure other than simple cardiac tamponade was documented in 40 per cent of the patients studied, including effusive-constrictive pericarditis in 17 per cent, congestive heart failure in 16 per cent, and coexisting neoplastic superior vena caval obstruction in 5 per cent. Similar experiences regarding the efficacy and safety of pericardiocentesis have been reported by ourselves in a consecutive series of 50 patients[132] and others.[139,140]

Two-dimensional echocardiography is useful in guiding

pericardiocentesis. Callahan et al.[141] have reported their experience in 132 consecutive pericardiocenteses guided by two-dimensional echocardiography. Pericardiocentesis was successful in obtaining pericardial fluid in 95 per cent of the procedures. There were no deaths, one pneumothorax, and three minor complications. Partial or complete surgical pericardiectomy was subsequently required in 25 per cent of patients for recurrent effusion, chronic relapsing pericarditis, or effusive-constrictive disease. Two-dimensional echocardiographic guidance is particularly helpful in percutaneous pericardiocentesis in patients with loculated pericardial effusion after cardiac surgery.

RISKS AND COMPLICATIONS. Thus, pericardiocentesis is now safer than it was a decade ago, and when the procedure is performed by an experienced operator, the risk of developing a life-threatening complication is generally less than 5 per cent.[132,138–142] The procedure is most likely to be successful and uncomplicated when performed in patients with clear-cut echocardiographic evidence of a large effusion with an anterior clear space of 10 mm or more. These recent experiences with pericardiocentesis indicate that the procedure should usually be performed in conjunction with hemodynamic measurements, including right heart and intrapericardial pressures, to (1) document the presence of the physiological changes of cardiac tamponade prior to attempted pericardiocentesis and (2) exclude other important coexisting causes of elevated jugular venous pressure, such as effusive-constrictive disease, superior vena caval obstruction, and left ventricular failure. There is rarely justification for performing blind needle pericardiocentesis at the bedside in the absence of optimal hemodynamic monitoring or of a prior echocardiogram documenting the presence of a large anterior and posterior effusion.

Pericardiocentesis is likely to be either complicated or unsuccessful in improving hemodynamics in patients with (1) acute traumatic hemopericardium in which blood enters the pericardial space as rapidly as it can be aspirated, (2) a small pericardial effusion judged to be less than 200 ml in size, (3) absence of an anterior effusion based on echocardiogram, (4) a loculated effusion, or (5) clot and fibrin as well as fluid filling the mediastinal or pericardial space postoperatively. Acute hemopericardium secondary to laceration, puncture of the heart, or leaking left ventricular or aortic aneurysm is likely to recur rapidly after pericardiocentesis. This procedure should be used only as an emergency temporizing measure prior to surgical pericardial exploration in which repair of the heart or aorta may be necessary. Surgical drainage is also usually preferred in patients with tamponade caused by purulent pericarditis to permit extensive drainage and in patients with suspected or known tuberculous pericarditis to permit bacteriological and histological examination of pericardial biopsy specimens. A rare but important complication that may occur after the relief of cardiac tamponade is the development of sudden ventricular dilatation and acute pulmonary edema.[143,144] The mechanism is probably a sudden increase in pulmonary venous blood flow following the relief of pericardial compression in the presence of underlying ventricular dysfunction.

COMBINED CATHETERIZATION AND PERICARDIOCENTESIS

We prefer the following method of combined catheterization and pericardiocentesis, which allows documentation of increased intrapericardial pressure and assessment of hemodynamic improvement after pericardiocentesis.[145] In contrast to traditional bedside sharp-needle pericardiocentesis, this method utilizes a soft catheter for pericardial aspiration and eliminates the prolonged presence of a sharp needle in the pericardial sac, thereby minimizing the risk of cardiac laceration. If possible, pericardiocentesis should be performed in a cardiac procedure laboratory where radiographic and hemodynamic monitoring facilities are optimal and by cardiologists experienced with hemodynamic measurements and the procedure itself. Before the procedure, the patient's blood should be typed and crossmatched and the cardiac surgery team alerted.

Pericardiocentesis is performed after the recording of baseline right atrial, right ventricular, pulmonary artery, and pulmonary capillary wedge pressures using a balloon-tipped catheter and cardiac output. Before pericardiocentesis, the transducer system that will be used to record intrapericardial pressure should be leveled with the other transducers, calibrated, and connected to a short length of fluid-filled tubing and a stopcock. Care should be taken to use equisensitive transducers and to avoid an underdamped catheter-transducer system.

PATIENT POSITION AND ROUTE. Pericardiocentesis is carried out with the patient's thorax and head tilted up, which enhances the pooling of the effusion anteriorly and inferiorly. Although multiple sites have been advocated for pericardiocentesis, we strongly prefer the subxiphoid route because it is extrapleural and avoids the coronary, pericardial, and internal mammary arteries. The skin is shaved, cleansed, and prepared in aseptic fashion, and the skin and subcutaneous tissue are anesthetized with 1 per cent lidocaine. The skin is pierced with a No. 11 blade, 0.5 cm below and to the left of the xiphoid process, and the subcutaneous tissues are spread with a small curved clamp.

NEEDLE INSERTION. A long, 8-inch, thin-walled No. 18-gauge pointed needle (pericardiocentesis kit, Mansfield Scientific, Inc., Mansfield, MA) is attached via a stopcock to a hand-held syringe containing 1 per cent lidocaine. One port of the stopcock is connected to the short length of fluid-filled tubing and the transducer that will be used to measure pericardial pressure (Fig. 43–11). The thin-walled needle commonly used for lumbar puncture is not adequate because its long sharp bevel poses some hazard. The metal hub of the needle may be attached by a sterile connector to the V lead of an electrocardiographic machine, and the electrocardiogram should be continuously recorded. *It is essential that the electrocardiographic apparatus have equipotential grounding with no chance of a current wave that could induce ventricular fibrillation.* If this condition cannot be assured, it is safer to omit electrocardiographic monitoring from the needle.

The needle is directed posteriorly until the tip passes posterior to the bony cage. The hub of the needle is then pressed toward the diaphragm, and the needle is advanced with a 15-degree posterior tilt, either directly toward the patient's head or toward the right or left shoulder. As the needle is smoothly and slowly advanced, the operator periodically attempts to aspirate fluid and then injects a small amount of lidocaine to clear the needle and to provide anesthesia of the deep tissues. The needle is advanced until the pericardial membrane is felt to "give" and pericardial fluid is aspirated or until ST-segment elevation and ventricular premature beats appear on the electrocardiogram, indicating that the needle has reached the

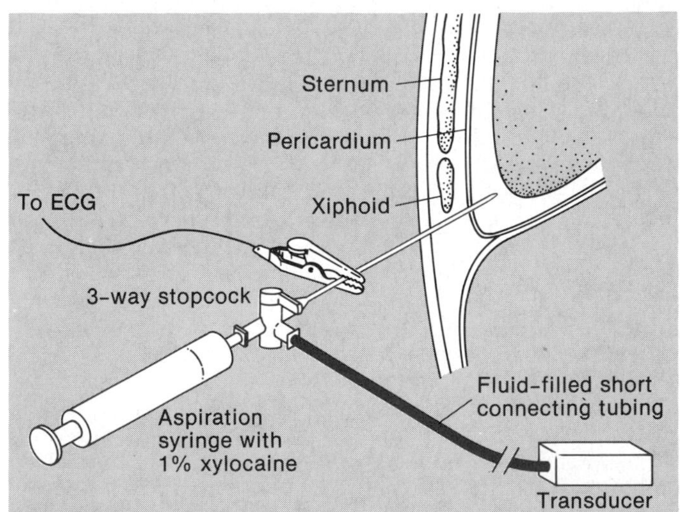

FIGURE 43–11. Pericardiocentesis using the subxiphoid approach, which avoids the major epicardial vessels. A hollow needle, which is attached via a stopcock to an aspiration syringe and to a short length of connecting tubing to a transducer, is used to enter the pericardial space. When fluid is initially aspirated, the pressure waveform at the needle tip should be briefly examined to confirm that the needle tip is in the pericardial space. A floppy-tipped guidewire is then passed through the hollow needle, the needle is exchanged for a soft flexible catheter with end and side holes to facilitate safe and thorough drainage of the pericardial sac. (Modified from Lorell, B. H., and Grossman, W.: Profiles in constrictive pericarditis, restrictive cardiomyopathy, and cardiac tamponade. *In* Grossman, W., and Baim, D. S. [eds.]: Cardiac Catheterization, Angiography and Intervention. Philadelphia, Lea and Febiger, 1991, p. 643.)

epicardium. In the latter case, the needle is promptly and smoothly withdrawn while the operator attempts to aspirate pericardial fluid until the needle lies within the fluid-filled pericardial space and the ECG changes disappear. If fluid cannot be freely aspirated, the needle is slowly withdrawn out of the body, avoiding lateral motion; the needle is flushed and the procedure repeated.

If hemorrhagic fluid is freely aspirated and it is not clear whether the needle is in the ventricle, atrium, or pericardial space, a few milliliters of contrast medium may be injected under fluoroscopic observation. If the contrast medium instantly swirls and disappears, the needle is within a cardiac chamber; in contrast, the appearance of sluggish layering of contrast medium inferiorly indicates that the needle is correctly positioned. When fluid can be freely aspirated, the stopcock is turned into its transducer and needle tip, and phasic right atrial pressures are simultaneously displayed. If the needle tip is in the pericardial space, pericardial and right atrial pressures should be equal with identical waveforms. A soft floppy-tip 0.038-inch guidewire is then passed through the hollow needle so that its tip lies within the pericardial space, as confirmed by fluoroscopy. A soft tampered large-bore lumen No. 6 French or 7 French catheter with multiple sideholes and an end hole is advanced over the guidewire, the guidewire is removed, and a few milliliters of fluid are aspirated. The catheter is then promptly connected to the prepared transducer, and intrapericardial pressure is recorded simultaneously with right atrial and systemic arterial pressure to document the presence of cardiac tamponade.

THE PERICARDIAL FLUID. Fluid samples are then aspirated from the catheter and sent for analysis of protein, amylase, glucose, and cholesterol content; hematocrit and white blood cell count; and bacteriological culture for aerobic and anaerobic bacteria, tuberculosis, and fungi. In most cases, a generous sample of fluid should also be sent in a heparinized container for cytological examination. Right atrial, systemic arterial, and intrapericardial pressures should then be recorded periodically as aliquots of fluid are removed—not only until intrapericardial pressure falls to zero but until no further fluid can be aspirated; intrapericardial pressure may return to normal levels after removal of only 50 to 100 ml of fluid in the presence of an effusion of 1 to 2 liters. *In our experience, extremely thorough drainage can be accomplished by connecting the intrapericardial catheter via sterile noncollapsible tubing to a stoppered sterile glass bottle with a vacuum.* This should be done only when a soft catheter is in the pericardial space because vacuum suction would be hazardous with sharp needle drainage. When no further fluid can be aspirated or drained, cardiac output and systemic arterial pressure as well as right atrial, right ventricular, and pulmonary capillary wedge pressures should be recorded, the last three simultaneously. The jugular veins should also be examined.

COMPLETION OF DRAINAGE. Successful relief of cardiac tamponade is documented by (1) the fall of intrapericardial pressure to levels of −3 and +3 mm Hg, (2) the fall of elevated right atrial pressure and separation between right- and left-heart filling pressures, (3) augmentation of cardiac output, and (4) disappearance of pulsus paradoxus. The presence of continued elevation and equilibration of right and left ventricular diastolic pressures with the appearance of a prominent *y* descent in the right atrial pressure tracing strongly suggests the presence of constricting pericardium due to effusive-constrictive pericarditis (see p. 1505). Jugular venous distention despite a fall in right atrial pressure should raise the question of coexisting superior vena caval obstruction, particularly in patients with known or suspected malignant disease.

Some cardiologists advocate the routine injection of a small volume of CO_2 or air into the pericardial space to outline the pericardium at the end of the procedure. This procedure has not been shown to be of aid in identifying unsuspected tumor masses,[138] and we do not advocate it. When the pericardial space is nearly obliterated, there is also the risk of injecting gas into a pleural cavity or cardiac chamber or the production of air tamponade.

POSTASPIRATION MANAGEMENT. It is often desirable to leave the intrapericardial catheter in place for several hours to permit repeated aspiration of fluid if cardiac tamponade recurs or to allow instillation of a nonabsorbable corticosteroid or antineoplastic agent in special cases. The catheter may be sutured securely to the skin and attached via a three-way stopcock to a closed drainage system. If the fluid is hemorrhagic or rich in fibrin, the catheter must be cleared frequently with a few millimeters of fluid. Dilute heparin may be instilled into the catheter to prevent clotting. The catheter should usually be removed after 24 to 48 hours because of the risk of introducing infection and producing iatrogenic purulent pericarditis. However, in some patients, continuous catheter drainage for several days has been reported to be necessary and effective in relieving cardiac tamponade.[141,146]

Percutaneous pericardial drainage in infants and children can be done without complications using a modification of this approach in which a catheter is inserted over a curved guidewire into the pericardial space under fluoroscopic control.[146]

Following pericardiocentesis, the majority of patients should be observed for about 24 hours in an intensive care setting for recurrence of cardiac tamponade. It is frequently helpful to obtain an echocardiogram soon after pericardiocentesis to establish the appearance of the heart and pericardium following aspiration.

PERCUTANEOUS BALLOON PERICARDIOTOMY. The technique of percutaneous balloon pericardiotomy was proposed by Palacios et al.,[147] and the experience of the first 50 patients with either larger pericardial effusions or tamponade undergoing this procedure as part of a multicenter registry has been recently reported.[148] In this series, the majority (88 per cent) had large pericardial effusions and a history of malignancy. Balloon pericardiotomy is performed as part of percutaneous pericardiocentesis with measurement of pericardial fluid and sampling of fluid for cytology and other studies. Approximately 200 ml of fluid is then left within the pericardial sac. After further dilation of the pericardial tract, a 20-mm diameter, 3-cm-long dilating balloon (Mansfield) is advanced over a guidewire to straddle the parietal pericardium, and the balloon is manually inflated to create a tear ("window") in the pericardium (Fig. 43–12). Sometimes additional punctures and balloon-induced rents in the pericardium are performed. After the pericardiotomy, the pericardial catheter is reinserted over a guidewire and all remaining fluid is drained. Postprocedure echocardiography and chest radiography (to monitor accumulation of left pleural effusion) should be done 24 hours later and at monthly follow-up.

This procedure was successful in 46 patients (92 per cent) in relieving tamponade with a short follow-up of 3 months, whereas two patients required early operation and

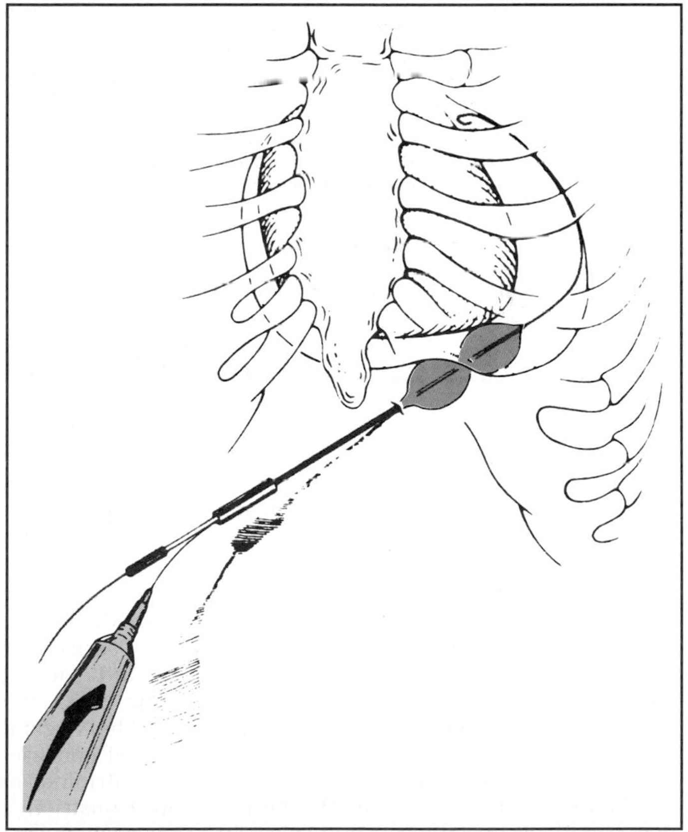

FIGURE 43–12. Illustration of the percutaneous balloon pericardiotomy technique. After partial drainage of the pericardium using a pericardial catheter, an 0.038-inch stiff J-tip wire is introduced into the pericardial space. A 3-cm-long dilating balloon is then advanced over the guidewire to "straddle" the parietal pericardial membrane and manually inflated to create a rent in the pericardium. (Modified from Ziskind, A. A., et al.: Percutaneous balloon pericardiotomy for the treatment of cardiac tamponade and large pericardial effusions: Description of technique and report of the first 50 cases. J. Am. Coll. Cardiol. *21*:1, 1993; reprinted by permission of the American College of Cardiology.)

TABLE 43–7 CLINICAL AND HEMODYNAMIC COMPRESSIVE PERICARDIAL DISEASE

	CARDIAC TAMPONADE	SUBACUTE "ELASTIC" CONSTRICTION	CHRONIC "RIGID" CONSTRICTION
Duration of symptoms	Hours to days	Weeks to months	Months to years
Chest pain, friction rub	Usual	Recent past	Remote
Pulsus paradoxus	Prominent	Usually prominent	Slight or absent
Kussmaul's sign	Absent	Usually absent	Often present
Early diastolic knock	Absent	Usually absent	Often present
Heart size on chest roentgenogram	Usually enlarged	Usually enlarged	Usually normal, sometimes enlarged
Pericardial calcification	Absent	Rare	Often present
Abnormal P waves or atrial fibrillation	Absent	Absent	Often present
Venous (right atrial) waveform	X or Xy	Xy or XY	XY or xY
Pericardial effusion	Always present	Often present	Absent

X and Y = prominent *x* and *y* descents, respectively; *x* and *y* = inconspicuous *x* and *y* descents.
Modified from Hancock, E. W.: On the elastic and rigid forms of constrictive pericarditis. Am. Heart J. *100*:917, 1980.

throughout the cardiac cycle, and respiratory changes in intrathoracic pressure usually are transmitted to the cardiac chambers.[165] Thus, patterns of ventricular filling and waveforms in the subacute form of fibroelastic compression tend to resemble those of cardiac tamponade rather than of constrictive pericarditis and include a systemic venous waveform with a predominant *x* descent or equal *x* and *y* descents, an inconspicuous early diastolic dip in the ventricular waveform, an inspiratory fall in systemic venous and right atrial pressures, and the presence of pulsus paradoxus (Table 43–7).

Etiology

Tuberculosis was formerly the leading cause of constrictive pericarditis in Western nations as reported in the classic series of Paul[166] and Andrews[167] and their coworkers. In disadvantaged nations, this is still true, whereas with the advent of antituberculosis therapy this disease now accounts for 15 per cent or less of cases in developed nations.[168,169] The largest number of cases of constrictive pericarditis today are of unknown cause (42 per cent) and are attributed to earlier clinically inapparent viral pericarditis.[169] In the past decade, constrictive pericarditis after cardiac surgery has emerged as an important cause (see p. 1734). In a series of 84 consecutive patients with constrictive pericarditis seen from 1979 to 1989, the largest numbers of cases were of unknown and presumed viral origin (55 per cent).[170] Postsurgical pericarditis accounted for 4 per cent of all cases, tuberculosis accounted for 12 per cent, and prior mediastinal radiation therapy accounted for 5 per cent of cases.[170] Other nontubercular causes include chronic renal failure treated with hemodialysis (see p. 1935); connective tissue disorders, including rheumatoid arthritis and systemic lupus erythematosus (p. 1776); and neoplastic pericardial infiltration or encasement of the heart due most commonly to lung cancer, breast cancer, Hodgkin's disease, and lymphoma. Constrictive pericarditis can develop after incomplete drainage of purulent pericarditis (p. 1509) and as a complication of fungal infections (p. 1510) and parasitic infections (p. 1511). It may occasionally follow pericarditis associated with acute myocardial infarction and the postpericardiotomy syndrome, (p. 1520), and in association with pulmonary asbestosis.[171]

CONSTRICTIVE PERICARDITIS IN CHILDREN (see also p. 1509). Constrictive pericarditis is far less common in children than in adults and may rarely occur following a viral syndrome in a child mistakenly thought to have hepatitis or a protein-losing enteropathy. When constrictive pericarditis occurs in young children, tuberculosis should be strongly considered because it was a proved or highly likely cause of 56 per cent of 84 children with constrictive pericarditis reported in the literature.[172] Nontraumatic hemopericardium has been reported in children and young adults with congenital bleeding disorders complicated by a second process such as endocarditis or viral syndrome, and constrictive pericarditis has occurred following pericardial bleeding due to congenital afibrinogenemia.[173] The newly described familial syndrome of pericarditis, arthritis, and camptodactyly (flexion contractures) is a rare cause of constrictive pericarditis in children and young adults.[174] A rare congenital cause of constrictive pericarditis is *mulibrey nanism,* an autosomal recessive disorder characterized by dwarfism, constrictive pericarditis, abnormal fundi, and fibrous dysplasia of the long bones.[175]

Clinical Features

In patients in whom systemic venous and right atrial pressures are modestly elevated (10 to 15 mm Hg), left ventricular filling pressure is also usually only modestly elevated. In this setting, symptoms secondary to systemic venous congestion such as edema, abdominal swelling, and discomfort due to ascites and passive hepatic congestion may predominate. Vague abdominal symptoms such as postprandial fullness, dyspepsia, flatulence, and anorexia may also be present. When both right and left heart filling pressures are elevated to the level of 15 to 30 mm Hg, symptoms of pulmonary venous congestion, such as exertional dyspnea, cough, and orthopnea, are present. Pleural effusions and elevation of the diaphragm due to ascites may also contribute to dyspnea. Severe platypnea, the symptom of dyspnea in the upright position, whose mechanism is not understood, is noted occasionally in chronic constrictive pericarditis.[176] Severe fatigue, weight loss, and muscle wasting suggest the presence of fixed or reduced cardiac output. Chest pain typical of angina may be related to underperfusion of the coronary arteries or compression of an epicardial coronary artery by the thickened pericardium.[164]

PHYSICAL EXAMINATION. The single most important finding is elevation of jugular venous pressure. If the neck is examined casually, or if the patient is examined supine so that jugular venous pressure is measured above the angle of the jaw, this important clue to the presence of constrictive pericarditis may be missed. A prominent feature of the elevated jugular venous pressure is the rapidly collapsing negative wave of the diastolic *y* descent. In patients in sinus rhythm, both *x* and *y* descents can be distinguished; the *x* descent is synchronous with the carotid pulse while the diastolic *y* descent is out of phase with the carotid pulse. These features may be difficult to detect in patients with tachycardia, tachypnea, or arrhythmia. It may also be difficult to distinguish between right heart failure due to tricuspid regurgitation and chronic constrictive pericarditis by neck vein examination at the bedside. The finding of

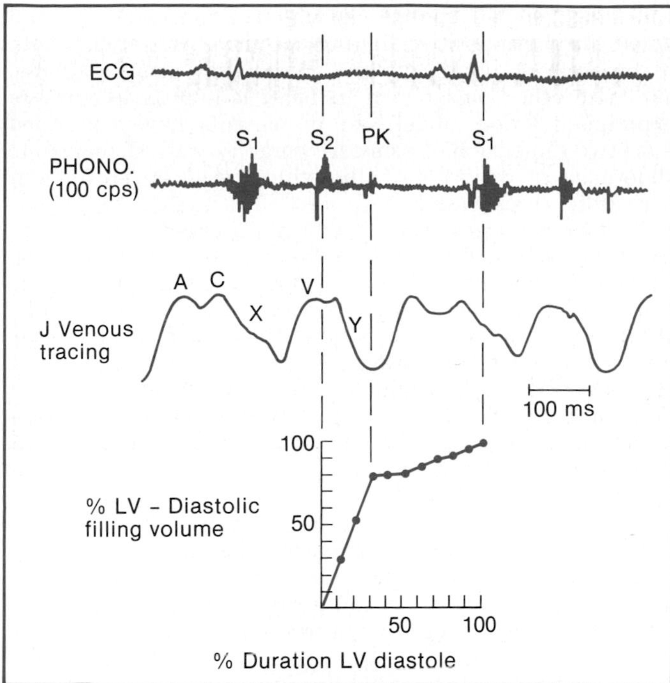

FIGURE 43–14. The electrocardiogram (ECG), phonocardiogram (PHONO), jugular venous pulse tracing, and left ventricular (LV) diastolic filling curve in a patient with constrictive pericarditis and pericardial knock (PK). The pericardial knock (PK) occurs simultaneously with the nadir of the diastolic *y* descent and sudden plateau of the LV filling curve. (From Tyberg, T. I., et al.: Genesis of pericardial knock in constrictive pericarditis. Am. J. Cardiol. *46*:570, 1980.)

Kussmaul's sign (an inspiratory increase in systemic venous pressure) is difficult to appreciate at the bedside and may be confused with exaggerated amplitude of the venous waves during inspiration.

The arterial pulse may be normal or show diminished pulse pressure. Severe pulsus paradoxus is uncommon in rigid constrictive pericarditis and rarely exceeds 10 mm Hg unless pericardial fluid under pressure is also present. Systolic retraction of the apical impulse occurs in the majority of patients and usually consists of an unobtrusive diffuse precordial movement. The most impressive abnormality during auscultation is the diastolic pericardial knock, an early diastolic sound that is often heard along the left sternal border in rigid constrictive pericarditis, infrequently heard in subacute constrictive pericarditis of the fibroelastic variety, and not heard in pure cardiac tamponade. The pericardial knock usually occurs 0.09 to 0.12 second after A_2 and corresponds in timing to the sudden cessation of ventricular filling and the premature diastolic plateau of the diastolic ventricular volume curve[177] (Fig. 43–14). The pericardial knock tends to occur earlier and to have a higher acoustic frequency than the typical S_3 gallop sound, and therefore it may be confused with the opening snap of mitral stenosis. Widening of the split between the aortic and pulmonic components of the second heart sound may occur in constrictive pericarditis. This is attributed to (1) a fixed right ventricular stroke volume during inspiration due to pericardial compression and (2) premature aortic valve closure due to a transitory inspiratory decrease in left ventricular stroke volume.

Hepatomegaly is usually present, and prominant hepatic pulsations that conform to the jugular venous pulse can be detected in 70 per cent of patients.[178] Other evidence of hepatic dysfunction secondary to passive liver congestion and diminished cardiac output may include ascites, icterus, spider angiomas, and palmar erythema. Constrictive pericarditis may rarely have the presenting feature of hepatic coma.[179] In young patients with competent venous valves, edema of the extremities may be noticeably absent in the presence of marked abdominal distention. Older patients with long-standing constrictive pericarditis may have enormous ascites and massive edema of the scrotum, thighs, and calves.[180] In contrast, the upper torso and arms may show evidence of marked muscle wasting and cachexia. The volume overload of pregnancy can occasionally promote the development of symptoms and signs of severe constriction in women who were asymptomatic with pericardial disease prior to pregnancy.[181]

CHEST ROENTGENOGRAM (see also p. 235). The cardiac silhouette may be small, normal, or enlarged. Cardiac enlargement may be apparent because of coexisting pericardial effusion, the contribution of an enormously thickened pericardium, or preexisting cardiac chamber enlargement or hypertrophy. The right superior mediastinum may be prominent as a result of engorgement of the superior vena cava, and left atrial enlargement is common.[182] Extensive calcification of the pericardium is present in approximately half the patients and raises the possibility of a tubercular etiology. The location of calcification is helpful in distinguishing between pericardial and myocardial aneurysm calcium because pericardial calcification is predominantly located over the right heart chambers and in the atrioventricular grooves, whereas isolated calcification of the left ventricular apex or posterior wall suggests left ventricular aneurysm. However, this finding is not specific for constrictive pericarditis in that *a calcified pericardium is not necessarily a constricted one.* The lateral chest film is particularly useful for the detection of pericardial calcium in the atrioventricular groove or along the anterior and diaphragmatic surfaces of the right ventricle (Fig. 43–15). Fluoroscopy may be helpful in distinguishing pericardial calcification from calcium within the wall of a myocardial aneurysm or thrombus or within the mitral or aortic valves, mitral annulus, or coronary arteries. Pleural effusions are present in about 60 per cent of patients, and unexplained persistent pleural effusion can be the presenting manifesta-

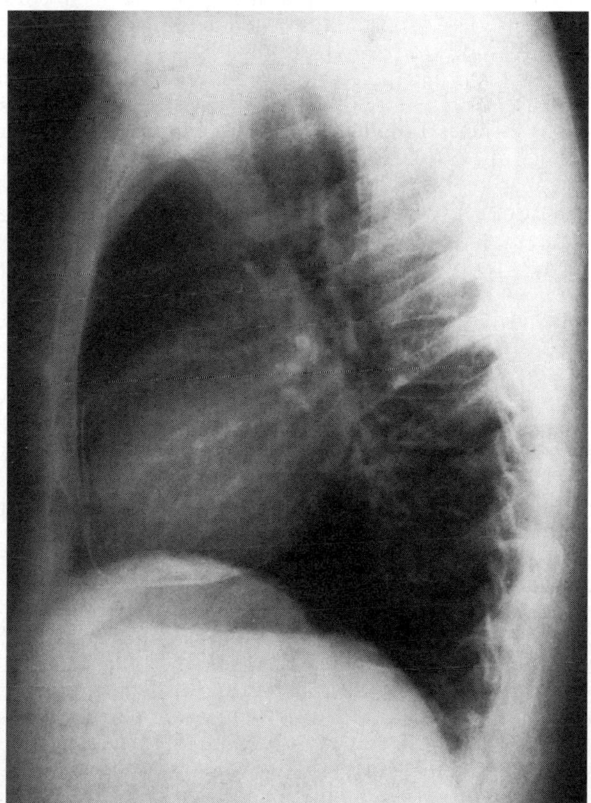

FIGURE 43–15. Lateral chest roentgenogram showing calcification of the pericardium in a patient with chronic constrictive pericarditis of idiopathic (postviral) etiology. The eggshell rim of pericardial calcification is often best appreciated in the lateral projection.

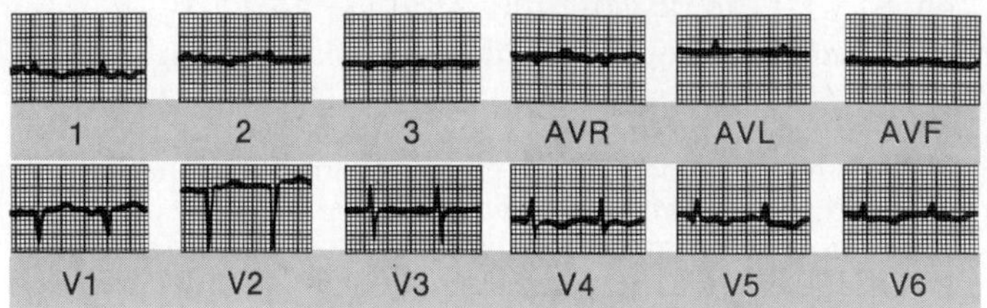

FIGURE 43–16. Electrocardiogram from a patient with surgically proven constrictive pericarditis and normal coronary arteries who had symptoms of chronic fatigue, dyspnea, and chest pain. The electrocardiogram is notable for the presence of a wide, notched P wave and diffuse T-wave inversion. These changes were initially mistakenly thought to be related to coronary insufficiency.

tion.[183] Because left atrial pressure is commonly elevated to 15 to 30 mm Hg, there may be evidence of redistribution of blood flow, but Kerley's B lines or infiltrates suggestive of frank pulmonary edema are rare.

ELECTROCARDIOGRAM. Electrocardiographic findings include low QRS voltage, generalized T-wave inversion or flattening, and left atrial abnormalities suggestive of P mitrale (Fig. 43–16). Atrial fibrillation occurs in less than half the patients with constrictive pericarditis and is thought to be related to longstanding elevation of atrial pressures and atrial enlargement. In a postmortem study of constrictive pericarditis, Levine noted that atrioventricular block, intraventricular conduction defects, and pseudoinfarction patterns with deep wide Q waves seemed to be related to an extension of calcification into the myocardium and around the coronary arteries, compromising coronary blood flow.[163] An unusual pattern that simulates right ventricular hypertrophy with right-axis deviation may be present in about 5 per cent of patients and due to dense pericardial scar overlying the right ventricle in association with compensatory dilation and hyperkinesis of the outflow tract.[184]

ECHOCARDIOGRAM. One distinct M-mode echocardiographic pattern of pericardial thickening in constrictive pericarditis consists of two parallel lines representing the visceral and parietal pericardia separated by a clear space of at least 1 mm; another consists of multiple dense echoes.[185] Other M-mode echocardiographic abnormalities include abrupt posterior motion of the interventricular septum in early diastole, coinciding with the pericardial knock, abrupt posterior motion during atrial systole, reduced amplitude of left ventricular posterior wall motion, and premature pulmonic valve opening secondary to a high right ventricular early diastolic pressure. These changes are also seen in other disorders with high right ventricular early diastolic pressure, such as tricuspid and pulmonic regurgitation. Engle et al.[186] reviewed M-mode echocardiograms from 40 patients with proven constrictive pericarditis and 40 normal subjects. They observed that normal left ventricular size, left atrial enlargement, flattened diastolic ventricular wall motion, and abnormal septal motion were found in most patients, but no single feature was diagnostic of constrictive pericarditis. Left atrial dilatation as well as abnormalities of wall motion tend to normalize after successful pericardiectomy.[187]

Two-dimensional echocardiography in constrictive pericarditis shows an immobile and dense appearance of the pericardium, abrupt displacement of the interventricular septum during early diastolic filling ("septal bounce"), prominent early diastolic filling, and an abnormal contour of the junction of the left ventricle and left atrial posterior wall.[188] Dilatation of the hepatic veins and inferior vena cava, intense and spontaneous contrast in the inferior vena cava, and distention of the inferior vena cava with blunted respiratory fluctuations in diameter ("plethora") are also observed in patients with constrictive pericarditis. Himelman et al.[189] reviewed the diagnostic value of pericardial adhesions, septal bounce, and vena cava plethora and noted that false-positive findings occurred in patients with pacemakers or bundle branch block after pericardiotomy, and with other causes of right heart failure. Studies in an experimental dog model and in patients have confirmed that two-dimensional echocardiography can demonstrate abnormal early diastolic filling but greatly overestimates pericardial thickness.[190]

Doppler echocardiography of the engorged hepatic vein has been reported to show a *W*-wave pattern that corresponds to the characteristic pattern of right atrial filling and consists of rapid forward flow during early diastole, abrupt deceleration and subsequent reverse flow before the *a* wave, and a second wave of rapid forward flow during early systolic ejection with reverse flow in late systole.[191] Constrictive pericarditis is also associated with characteristic Doppler patterns of transvalvular and central venous flow velocities during respiration.[192,193] In constrictive pericarditis, the pericardial shell isolates the heart from changes in intrathoracic pressure. Because the thickened pericardium isolates the heart from the lungs, inspiration causes a decrease in the pressure gradient between the pulmonary capillaries and the left heart, resulting in an inspiratory decrease in diastolic mitral inflow and pulmonary venous flow velocities. This decrease in left ventricular filling results in a leftward shift of the interventricular septum, allowing augmented diastolic inspiratory inflow into the right ventricle manifest as increased early diastolic tricuspid inflow and hepatic vein flow velocities during inspiration. Opposite changes occur during early expiration (Fig. 43–17). The marked limitation of right heart filling during expiration also causes exaggeration of the normal pattern of expiratory reversal of hepatic vein flow during diastole.

In a study of 28 patients who underwent exploratory thoracotomy, 22 of 23 patients with Doppler findings of constrictive pericarditis were found to have this diagnosis at operation, whereas Doppler features consistent with restriction were found in four patients, three of whom were found to have constriction and one a restrictive myopathy.[193] In two patients with a normal pericardium, one patient had a normal Doppler study whereas one patient had

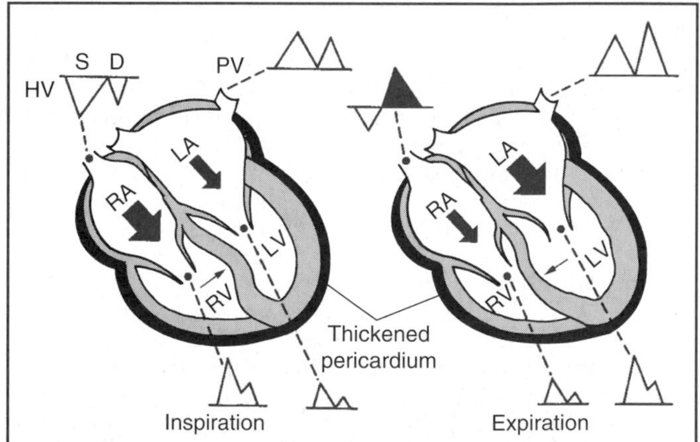

FIGURE 43–17. The effects of respiration on transvalvular flow in constrictive pericarditis. Because the pericardial shell isolates the heart from inspiratory pressure changes in the lungs, early inspiration causes a reduction in the driving pressure gradient between the pulmonary capillaries and the left atrium (LA), which leads to a decrease in pulmonary venous (PV) and mitral valve velocities. This reduction in left ventricular (LV) filling causes a slight leftward bowing of the septum associated with an inspiratory increase in right heart filling manifest as increased tricuspid inflow and diastolic hepatic venous (HV) flow velocities *(left panel)*. The opposite changes are seen during expiration. (Adapted from Oh, J. K., et al.: Diagnostic role of Doppler echocardiography in constrictive pericarditis. J. Am. Coll. Cardiol. *23*:154, 1994; reprinted by permission of the American College of Cardiology.)

Doppler findings of constriction related to chronic pulmonary disease with a normal pericardium. These observations illustrate that respiratory Doppler flow patterns suggestive of constriction are highly sensitive but also occur in conditions in which a dilated right ventricle is constrained by the normal pericardium, such as chronic lung disease, pulmonary embolism, and right ventricular infarction. Transient findings of "constrictive" respiratory changes in Doppler flow velocities have also been observed during the resolution of acute pericarditis with pericardial effusion, presumably related to transient stiffening and thickening of the inflamed pericardium.[194]

CT AND MRI. CT has also emerged as a valuable tool in the evaluation of suspected constrictive pericarditis. The technique is especially useful in identifying pericardial thickening and in identifying other findings compatible with constrictive pericarditis, including dilation of the venae cavae and deformation of the right ventricle, and increased filling fraction of the ventricles in early diastole.[195,196] Nonvisualization of the left ventricular posterolateral wall by CT suggests coexisting myocardial fibrosis or atrophy and may predict a poor outcome following pericardiectomy.[197]

Experience with MRI in patients with constrictive pericarditis suggests that it can also detect pericardial thickening, dilation of the venae cavae and hepatic veins, narrowing of the right ventricle, and dilatation of the right atrium[198,199] (Figs. 43–18 and Fig. 16–14, p. 325). MRI is probably the most sensitive imaging technique currently available for delineating the thickness of the pericardium, the morphology of regional or annular thickening or calcification, and the relationship of extracardiac masses to the pericardium and surface of the heart.[198,199] Both CT scanning and MRI have the potential to identify patients with a thickened pericardium and associated myocardial atrophy and fibrosis. Although the number of patients reported to date is relatively small, the identification of myocardial atrophy and/or fibrosis may have prognostic value in patients subjected to pericardial exploration. In a series of 7 patients with severe atrophy or fibrosis and pericardial thickening who underwent pericardiectomy, 100 per cent died of acute heart failure, whereas 4 (9 per cent) of 43 patients without myocardial atrophy died following pericardiectomy.[199] In assessing the role of these expensive imaging technologies, it must be emphasized that severe constrictive physiology can occur in the presence of a diseased but minimally thickened pericardium, whereas *pericardial thickening or calcification alone is not diagnostic of hemodynamically significant constrictive pericarditis.*[196]

The use of noninvasive imaging techniques, especially two-dimensional echocardiography, to assist in discrimination between constrictive pericarditis and restrictive cardiomyopathy is discussed below.

OTHER LABORATORY FINDINGS. Other abnormal laboratory findings may be present as a result of chronic elevation of right atrial pressure causing passive congestion of the liver, kidneys, and gastrointestinal tract. These include depressed serum albumin, elevated serum globulin, elevated conjugated and unconjugated serum bilirubin, and abnormal hepatocellular function tests. In patients with hepatomegaly and ascites, liver biopsy may show histological features similar to the Budd-Chiari syndrome, including hepatic venule thrombi and ductular proliferation.[200] Chylous ascites may occur because of impedance of lymphatic drainage due to central venous hypertension.[201] Protein-losing enteropathy may be evident from the presence of albumin in the stool and lymphangiectasis on small-bowel biopsy.[202] Elevated systemic venous pressure may also produce variable degrees of albuminuria as well as pronounced protein loss consistent with the nephrotic syndrome.[203] Nonspecific evidence of the presence of chronic disease such as normocytic and normochromic anemia may be found.

DIFFERENTIAL DIAGNOSIS. Constrictive pericarditis should be suspected in patients with jugular venous distention, unexplained pleural effusion, hepatomegaly, systemic edema, or ascites. It must be distinguished from superior vena caval obstruction, nephrotic syndrome, hepatic and intra-abdominal disease due to malignancy, and other cardiac causes of right atrial hypertension, including restrictive cardiomyopathy, tricuspid stenosis, tricuspid regurgitation, hypertrophic cardiomyopathy, and right atrial myxoma. It may be extremely difficult to distinguish patients with constrictive pericarditis from those with restrictive physiology due to amyloidosis, sarcoidosis, radiation injury, hemochromatosis, and the hypereosinophilic syndrome, which may involve pericardium as well as the myocardium.[204–207] Both constrictive pericarditis and restrictive cardiomyopathy may show the electrocardiographic changes of atrial fibrillation, left atrial abnormalities, and diffuse low QRS voltage with T-wave flattening. The presence of atrioventricular block and conduction disturbances simulating myocardial infarction favors the diagnosis of restrictive cardiomyopathy. Echocardiography in some patients with restrictive cardiomyopathy may show abnormal thickening of the ventricular myocardium or a peculiar "sparkling" appearance when amyloidosis is present. The simultaneous use of electrocardiography and echocardiography to demonstrate a reduction of the voltage/mass ratio has been described in patients with amyloid

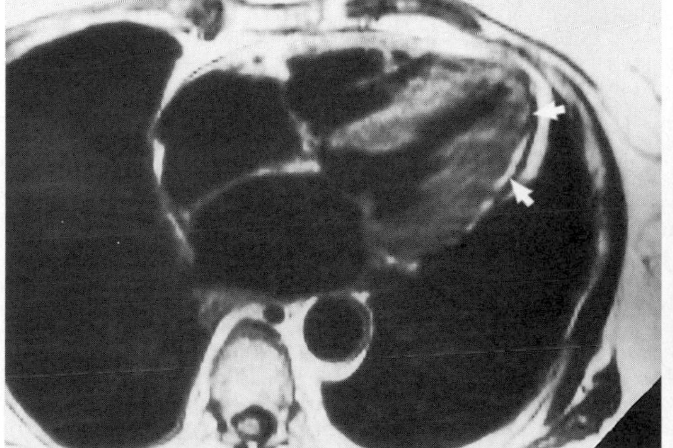

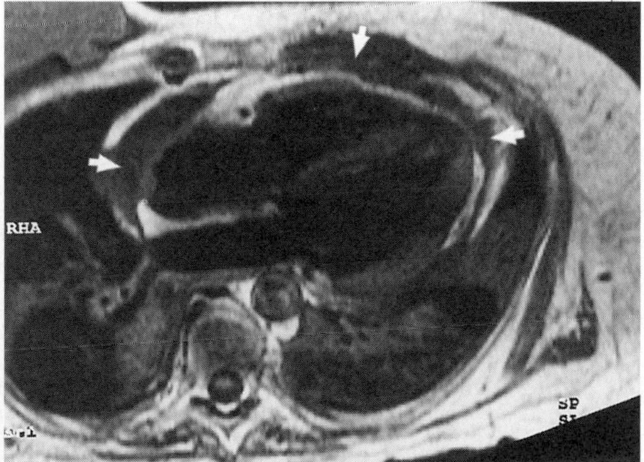

FIGURE 43–18. *Left,* Spin-echo magnetic resonance image in the transverse plane of a normal heart and thin pericardium (≤3 mm) of a normal adult. *Right,* Spin-echo magnetic resonance image (transverse plane) of the heart of a patient with a thickened pericardium (white arrows) and hemodynamic documentation of constrictive pericarditis at cardiac catheterization.

restrictive cardiomyopathy in whom diffuse low QRS voltage is associated with increased thickness of the left ventricular wall due to amyloid deposition.[208]

In the presence of findings suggestive of constrictive pericarditis, right- and left-heart catheterization should be performed to document the presence of constrictive physiology and to exclude other causes of right atrial hypertension. Diuresis should be avoided prior to catheterization because hypovolemia may obscure the characteristic hemodynamic findings. MRI, cardiac catheterization, and angiography, often with endomyocardial biopsy, are usually decisive in discriminating between constrictive pericarditis and restrictive cardiomyopathy in many patients, but in a small minority exploratory thoracotomy may be required.

Cardiac Catheterization and Angiography

Cardiac catheterization is useful in the assessment of patients suspected of having constrictive pericarditis to (1) document the presence of elevation and equilibration of diastolic filling pressures, (2) assess the effect of constrictive pericarditis on stroke volume and cardiac output, (3) evaluate myocardial systolic function, (4) assist in the difficult discrimination between constrictive pericarditis and restrictive cardiomyopathy, and (5) exclude compression of the coronary arteries or regional outflow tract compression by the fibrotic pericardium.

Catheterization of both the right and left ventricles should be performed to permit simultaneous recording of right and left heart filling pressures. Typical findings include the elevation and virtual identity (within 5 mm Hg) of right atrial, right ventricular diastolic, left atrial (pulmonary capillary wedge), and left ventricular diastolic pressures before the *a* wave. Right atrial pressure is characterized by a preserved systolic *x* descent, a prominent early diastolic *y* descent, and *a* and *v* waves that are small and equal in height and result in the typical M or W configurations (Fig. 43–19). Both the right and left ventricular diastolic pressures show an early diastolic dip followed by a plateau. This sign may be obscured by the presence of tachycardia, although the equilibration of diastolic pressures persists during exercise (Fig. 43–20), and by the damping effect of connecting tubes or bubbles within the catheters and transducers. Right ventricular and pulmonary artery systolic pressures are usually modestly elevated, in the range of 35 to 40 mm Hg, and rarely exceed 60 mm Hg. When hemodynamics in the baseline state are unremarkable, the rapid infusion of about 1000 ml of warmed saline over 6 to 8 minutes may unmask these findings in the rare patient with occult constrictive pericarditis.[209]

Careful recordings during respiration show that mean right atrial pressure fails to decrease normally or actually rises during inspiration. Because inspiration is associated with transient pooling of blood within the pulmonary bed and reduction in right ventricular afterload, inspiration causes a fall in pulmonary artery and right ventricular systolic pressures, pulmonary capillary wedge pressure, and left ventricular diastolic pressure. Because constrictive pericarditis is associated with inspiratory swings in right ventricular filling which are less marked than those observed in cardiac tamponade, pulsus paradoxus is usually absent or less prominent than that observed in cardiac tamponade. Both cardiac output and stroke volume are low-normal or depressed. When they are depressed, compensatory tachy-

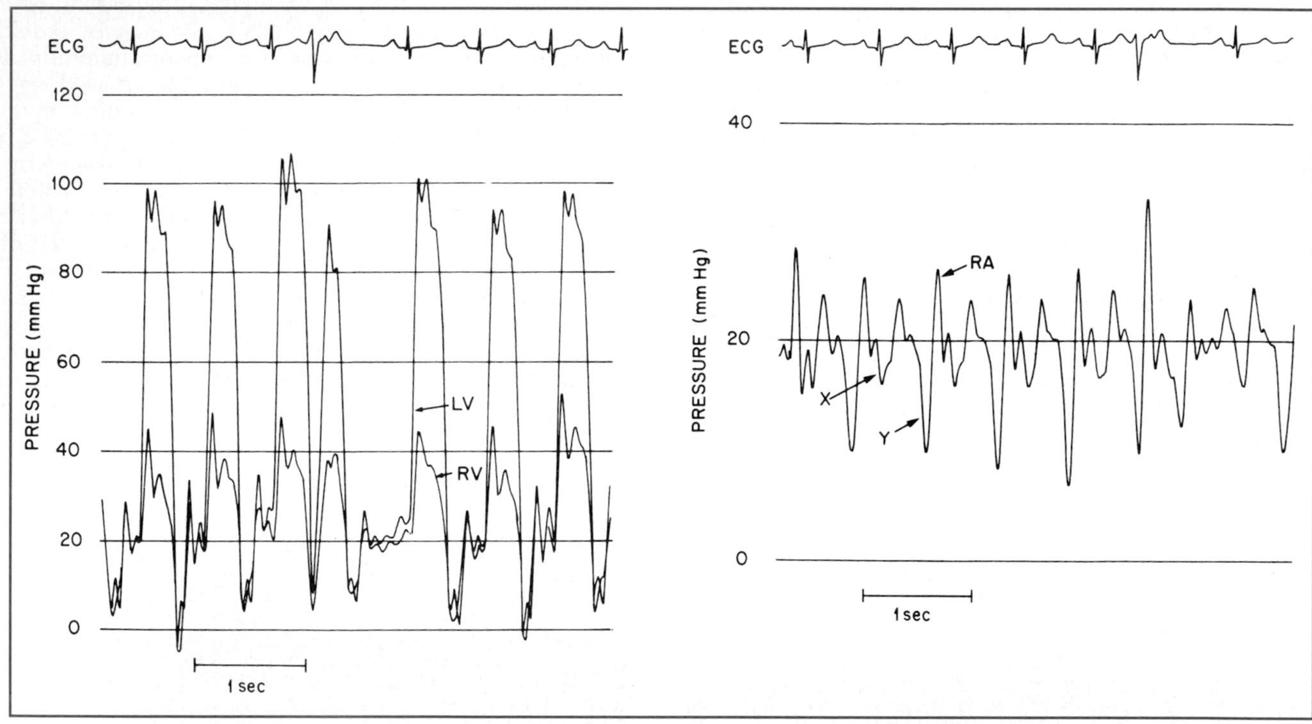

FIGURE 43–19. *Left,* Left (LV) and right (RV) ventricular pressures recorded simultaneously in the same patient with constrictive pericarditis illustrate that the presence of resting tachycardia partially obscures evaluation of the diastolic waveforms, and underdamping of the left ventricular pressure-transducer system accentuates an undershoot of left ventricular pressure in early diastole and an overshoot during atrial contraction. A long diastole following a premature beat permits the recognition of equilibrium of left and right ventricular diastolic pressures and the appreciation of a dip-and-plateau component of the ventricular waveform. *Right,* Right atrial (RA) pressure recording from a patient with constrictive pericarditis, illustrating that the pressure is elevated and equal throughout diastole. Note the prominent Y descent in the right atrial waveform, which indicates that the right atrial emptying is rapid and unimpeded in early diastole. The nadir of the Y descent corresponds with the abrupt cessation of early diastolic ventricular filling. The prominent X and Y descents give the right atrial waveform its characteristic M- or W-shaped appearance in constrictive pericarditis. (From Lorell, B. H., and Grossman, W.: Profiles in constrictive pericarditis, restrictive cardiomyopathy, and cardiac tamponade. *In* Grossman, W., and Baim, D. S. [eds.]: Cardiac Catheterization and Angiography. Philadelphia, Lea and Febiger, 1995).

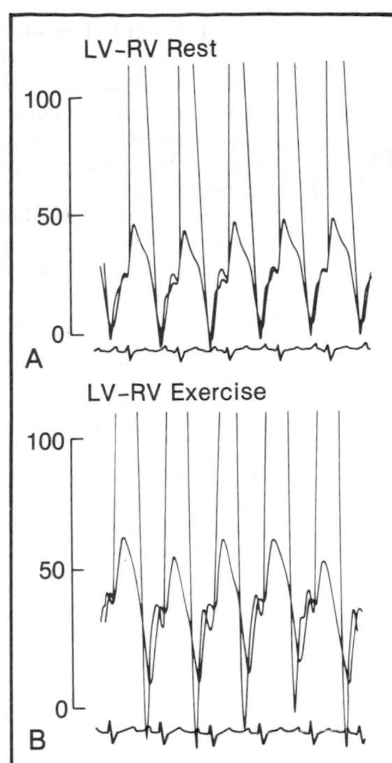

FIGURE 43-20. **Representative left (LV) and right ventricular (RV) pressure tracings obtained at rest *(A)* and during exercise *(B)* from a patient with constrictive pericarditis. The diastolic equalization of pressures that is present at rest persists during exercise when the diastolic pressure of both ventricles is substantially higher. (From Robbins, M. A., et al.: Resting and exercise hemodynamics in constrictive pericarditis and a case of cardiac amyloidosis mimicking constriction. Cathet. Cardiovasc. Diagn. 9:463, 1983.)**

cardia and an elevation of systemic vascular resistance may be found.

The left ventricular angiogram usually demonstrates that left ventricular end-systolic and end-diastolic volumes are normal or decreased. In the absence of myocardial fibrosis or inflammation, both isovolumic and ejection phase indices of systolic function are normal. Venous angiography or simple fluoroscopy may demonstrate dilatation of the superior vena cava and straightening of the right heart border; pericardial thickening may be detectable. These findings contrast with those of cardiac tamponade in which diastolic compression of the superior vena cava and right atrium is present. Coronary angiography may demonstrate that the coronary arteries are within the coronary silhouette rather than on the surface of the heart, and rarely, diastolic pinching or external compression of the coronary arteries may be detected.[164,210] In rare patients, careful hemodynamic measurements may demonstrate the presence of regional pericardial constriction causing pulmonary outflow tract obstruction, which can be confirmed by right ventricular angiography or noninvasive echocardiography or CT imaging.

HEMODYNAMIC DIFFERENTIATION AMONG CONSTRICTIVE PERICARDITIS, CARDIAC TAMPONADE, AND RESTRICTIVE CARDIOMYOPATHY

Although both constrictive pericarditis and tamponade are characterized by elevation and equilibrium of right and left ventricular diastolic pressures, several hemodynamic features differ. In contrast with patients with constrictive pericarditis, patients with cardiac tamponade demonstrate (1) marked pulsus paradoxus, (2) a fall in right atrial pressure during inspiration, (3) elevation of intrapericardial pressure, (4) a right atrial pressure tracing with a predominant *x* descent and absence of or an attenuated *y* descent, and (5) lack of a prominent dip-and-plateau pattern in the right and left ventricular pressure pulses.

The findings of cardiac catheterization help to differentiate some but not all patients with constrictive pericarditis from those with restrictive cardiomyopathy (Table 43-8) due to amyloidosis, radiation injury, hemochromatosis, or other causes. In both conditions, right

TABLE 43-8 CONSTRICTIVE PERICARDITIS VERSUS RESTRICTIVE CARDIOMYOPATHY

	CONSTRICTIVE PERICARDITIS	RESTRICTIVE CARDIOMYOPATHY
S_3 gallop	Absent	May be present
Pericardial knock	May be present	Absent
Palpable systolic apical impulse	Absent	May be present
Pericardial calcification	Present 50%	Absent
Pulsus paradoxus	May be present	May be present
Equal RV and LV diastolic pressures	Usually present	LV > RV
Rate of LV filling	80% in first half of diastole	40% in first half of diastole
PEP/LVET	Av. 0.31	Av. 0.48 (congestive failure)
CAT scan, echo, MRI	Thickened pericardium	Normal pericardium

Modified from Fowler, N. O.: Constrictive pericarditis. *In* Fowler, N. O. (ed.): The Pericardium in Health and Disease. Mt. Kisco, NY, Futura Publishing Co., 1985, p. 319.

and left ventricular diastolic pressures are elevated, stroke volume and cardiac output are depressed, left ventricular end-diastolic volume is normal or decreased, and diastolic filling is impaired. A diagnosis of restrictive cardiomyopathy is more likely when marked right ventricular systolic hypertension is present (pressure > 60 mm Hg) and left ventricular diastolic pressure exceeds right ventricular diastolic pressure at rest or during exercise by more than 5 mm Hg.[211] However, in some patients with restrictive cardiomyopathy, hemodynamics at rest and during exercise may be indistinguishable from constrictive pericarditis, with equilibration of right and left ventricular diastolic pressures and a predominant dip-and-plateau pattern in the ventricular waveforms.[145,212-214]

Angiographically, straightening of the right heart border may be present in both conditions, and thickening of the heart border may be detected as a result of either pericardial or myocardial thickening. The finding of a depressed left ventricular ejection fraction in the presence of a small heart has been suggested as a discriminating feature of restrictive cardiomyopathy. However, the left ventricular ejection fraction may be normal in some patients with restrictive cardiomyopathy and, conversely, is occasionally reduced in patients with constrictive pericarditis.[212,213]

ANALYSIS OF VENTRICULAR FILLING. Frame-by-frame analysis of left ventricular filling using left ventricular angiograms has been suggested as a method for distinguishing between constrictive pericarditis and restrictive cardiomyopathy.[215] In constrictive pericarditis, early diastolic filling tends to be excessively rapid in contrast to restrictive cardiomyopathy, in which early diastolic filling is slower than normal with greater dependence on the atrial contribution to filling. The discrimination between these patterns of left ventricular filling in constrictive pericarditis versus restrictive cardiomyopathy has also been accomplished using noninvasive methods, including the assessment of diastolic filling by radionuclide angiography[216] (Fig. 43-21), and Doppler echocardiography.[192,217]

ANALYSIS OF FLOW VELOCITIES. The use of transthoracic Doppler echocardiography for the analysis of respiratory changes in transvalvular flow velocities and the use of transesophageal Doppler echocardiography to analyze patterns of pulmonary venous flow velocity during respiration have been proposed to distinguish between these conditions.[192,217,218]

Recent clinical studies suggest that the marked respiratory variations in transvalvular, hepatic, and pulmonary flow velocities which are characteristic of constrictive pericarditis can correctly identify about 85 per cent of patients with constrictive pericarditis.[193,219,220] False-positive patterns of constrictive respiratory variations in flow velocities can occur in patients with chronic pulmonary disease and pulmonary embolism, and these respiratory flow velocity patterns can be more difficult to distinguish in patients with constrictive pericarditis and atrial fibrillation. This marked respiratory variation in Doppler flow velocities is not usually observed in restrictive cardiomyopathy (Fig. 43-22). In contrast, restrictive cardiomyopathy, including amyloid heart disease, is characterized by a spectrum of echo-Doppler abnormalities, including slowed left ventricular relaxation associated with a reduced transmitral early diastolic pressure gradient which is evident as a reduced peak velocity of early transmitral diastolic flow (E wave) and enhanced flow velocity during atrial contraction (A wave). More severe restrictive myopathy may progress to "pseudonormalization" of Doppler flow velocity patterns and to the advanced stage of "restrictive" flow patterns characterized by a short isovolumic relaxation time, increase in E wave peak velocity clear-cut evidence of tuberculosis.[277,281] Furthermore, the finding of granulomas and caseous material without viable bacilli is also not diagnostic of tuberculous pericarditis because these findings can be present in chronic pericardial disease due to rheumatoid arthritis and sarcoidosis. The measurement of a high level of adenosine deaminase activity (>40 units/liter) in pleural or pericardial fluid, although not diagnostic, is supportive of a diagnosis of tuberculous pericarditis.[282] In a prospective study of 26 patients with large pericardial effusion who underwent therapeutic pericardioscopy with drainage and biopsy, a level of adenosine deaminase activity of 40 units/liter or higher in pericardial fluid had a sensitivity of 93 per cent and specificity of 97 per cent for the diagnosis of tuberculous pericarditis.[282] Furthermore, the combined measurement of adenosine deaminase and carcinoembryonic antigen in pericardial effusion discriminated patients with tuberculous pericarditis from those with malignant effusion. Tuberculous pericarditis has also been presumptively diagnosed by PCR in pericardial biopsy specimen.[283]

It may be necessary to make a presumptive clinical diagnosis of tuberculous pericarditis in severely ill patients with a large hemorrhagic pericardial effusion, a positive tuberculin skin test, and systemic symptoms such as weight loss and anorexia, even when examinations of the pericardial fluid and biopsy do not reveal tuberculosis. In such patients, clinical improvement may occur after initiation of antituberculosis chemotherapy. It should be emphasized that the tuberculin skin test alone is not a reliable indicator of tuberculous pericarditis because it may be negative in as many as 30 per cent of patients with documented tuberculosis due to anergy, and is positive in about 30 to 40 per cent of patients with acute idiopathic pericarditis and benign natural history.[69,168] Making a presumptive clinical diagnosis of tuberculous pericarditis requires careful judgment because; on the one hand, treatment should not be withheld from seriously ill patients, while, on the other, it is not prudent to commit patients with nontuberculous effusions to a prolonged course of multiple-drug antituberculosis therapy. The systematic approach suggested by Permanyer-Miralda et al. (see p. 1484) appears to have a high likelihood of identifying patients with tuberculous pericarditis with very low risk of either missing active tuberculosis or inappropriately applying blind antituberculous therapy.[69] This strategy remains to be validated in other populations, such as patients at high risk for HIV infection.

MANAGEMENT. In the era before antituberculosis chemotherapy, tuberculous pericarditis was rapidly fatal, with an early mortality rate greater than 80 per cent; the remaining patients had a protracted course of months to years with frequently fatal outcome due to miliary tuberculosis or constrictive pericarditis. Since the introduction of early chemotherapy, mortality from acute tuberculous pericarditis has fallen to less than 50 per cent, but the effectiveness of antituberculosis chemotherapy in preventing the development of constrictive pericarditis is controversial.[273,274] In a recent series of 294 consecutive patients with acute pericarditis, 13 patients were shown to have tuberculous pericarditis and 7 of these (54 per cent) developed constrictive pericarditis requiring pericardiectomy.[277]

Treatment of tuberculous pericarditis includes hospitalization with bedrest and particular attention to findings of physical examination, electrocardiography, and echocardiography that suggest the development of an enlarging pericardial effusion and tamponade or constrictive pericarditis. Initial chemotherapy should usually consist of a three-drug regimen, such as oral isoniazid, oral ethambutol, and intramuscular streptomycin. The use of corticosteroids has been advocated to reduce pericardial inflammation and enhance resorption of pericardial effusion.

In a controlled trial in South Africa, 143 patients with tuberculous pericarditis and clinical signs of constrictive physiology were randomized to receive antitubercular drug therapy with prednisolone or placebo added during the first 11 weeks of treatment.[284] In this trial, clinical improvement occurred more rapidly, and there was a lower mortality at 24 months (4 versus 11 per cent) and a lower requirement for pericardiectomy (21 versus 30 per cent) in the prednisolone versus placebo-treated cohort. The use of steroids earlier in the course of tuberculous pericarditis before the development of constrictive physiology has not been studied in a clinical trial. We believe that corticosteroids should be reserved for critically ill patients with recurrent large effusion who do not respond to pericardial drainage and antituberculosis drugs alone.

In patients with documented cardiac tamponade or with a large pericardial effusion seen on the echocardiogram, the effusion should be drained initially by percutaneous pericardiocentesis with continued catheter drainage. Pericardiectomy should be performed after 4 to 6 weeks of antituberculosis drug therapy if patients develop large recurrent effusions or cardiac compression due to effusive-constrictive disease or early constrictive pericarditis.[273,284] Pericardiectomy should be performed early in the course in patients with clinical and hemodynamic evidence of chronic cardiac compression with anticipation of a good outcome. In a South African study of 113 patients with severe constrictive tuberculous pericarditis who underwent pericardiectomy, 97 per cent were discharged from the hospital; in the majority, hepatomegaly and edema promptly resolved, whereas resolution of venous congestion required 2 to 3 months in some patients.[285] Mortality is higher among patients who undergo pericardiectomy at the late stage of calcific pericardial constriction.[265,285]

BACTERIAL (PURULENT) PERICARDITIS

Although the clinical spectrum of bacterial purulent pericarditis has changed over the past five decades, mortality remains high. Since the introduction of antibiotics in the 1940's, the overall incidence as well as the incidence of bacterial pericarditis detected at autopsy have decreased.[286,287] Purulent pericarditis continues to occur primarily as a complication of pneumonia or empyema due to staphylococci, pneumococci, and streptococci.[287,288] Acute self-limited pericarditis has also been observed in young adults with acute streptococcal tonsillitis in the absence of rheumatic fever.[289] The incidence of hospital-acquired penicillin-resistant staphylococcal pericarditis in post-thoracotomy patients has increased, and there is a widened spectrum of organisms responsible for bacterial pericarditis, including non-group A streptococcus[290] the gram-negative bacilli (*Proteus, Escherichia coli, Pseudomonas, Klebsiella*),[286] *Brucella melitensis*,[291] *Salmonella* species,[292,293] *Neisseria gonorrhoeae*,[294] *Haemophilus influenzae*,[295] *Francisella tularensis*,[296] and other unusual pathogens.[297-301]

Purulent pericarditis is rarely caused by anaerobic bacteria, and a recent review of 30 cases showed that isolated anaerobic bacteria were identified in 57 per cent and with a mixture of facultative or aerobic bacteria in 43 per cent of cases.[302] Infection usually occurs from a contiguous source of infection or via hematogenous seeding related to subdiaphragmatic or intrapulmonary abscess, gastrointestinal malignancy or rupture, and rarely in association with gas gangrene due to *Clostridium septicemia*.[297,302-305] It is now established that *Neisseria meningitidis*, particularly from serogroup C and W, can cause either a primary infection of the pericardium in the absence of meningitis, or secondary pericarditis complicating meningitis and sepsis.[306] *Legionella pneumophila*, the causative organism in legionnaire's disease, has been reported as a cause of purulent pericarditis associated with pneumonia and as a primary infection.[307] Important predisposing factors for the development of purulent pericarditis include a preexisting pericardial effusion as in uremic pericarditis, as well as immunosuppression due to burns, immunotherapy, lymphoma, leukemia, or AIDS (see p. 1506).

The routes of pericardial infection have also changed. Direct pulmonary extension of bacterial pneumonia or empyema now accounts for between 20 and 50 per cent of cases of purulent pericarditis.[287,297] Today, purulent pericarditis tends to occur in adults via (1) contiguous spread from an early postoperative infection after thoracic surgery or trauma, (2) infection related to infective endocarditis, (3) extension from a subdiaphragmatic suppurative source, and (4) hematogenous spread during bacteremia.

In patients with endocarditis, bacterial pericarditis is a life-threatening complication that is detected ante mortem in about 1 of 25 patients with endocarditis,[308] in about 1 of 8 patients with endocarditis studied at autopsy, and in a higher percentage of those with staphylococcal endocarditis.[286] In such patients, bacterial pericarditis may develop (1) by extension from a valve ring abscess, (2) by rupture of an aneurysm, (3) by extension from a myocardial abscess, or (4) from a septic coronary embolus.[309] An infected myocardial infarction or aortic aneurysm may also be a source for the development of purulent bacterial pericarditis. In patients with AIDS, the high rate of skin and nasal colonization and use of intravenous catheters contribute to the development of *Staphylococcus aureus* pericarditis.[310] Extension of a subdiaphragmatic abscess into the pericardial space is a rare source of purulent pericarditis.[302,305]

BACTERIAL PERICARDITIS IN CHILDREN. In children, the most common organisms include *Staphylococcus aureus* followed by *Haemophilus influenzae* and *Neisseria meningitis*.[311,312] *H. influenzae* pericarditis has been increasingly recognized in young children and is usually characterized by a mild prodromal illness followed by the rapid development of cardiac compression and death due to pericardial effusion.[313,314] Pediatric illnesses associated with the development of bacterial pericarditis include pharyngitis, pneumonia, meningitis, otitis media, impetigo, endocarditis, and bacterial arthritis. The development of bacterial pericarditis in infants and children carries a high mortality—approaching 70 per cent, depending on the organism, and the risk of extremely rapid early development of constrictive pericarditis, if it is not diagnosed early.[311,315] The high mortality in children appears to be reduced by early diagnosis and combined treatment with parenteral antibiotics and open surgical pericardial drainage, if effusion recurs after initial pericardiocentesis. Following this contemporary approach for parenteral antibiotics and early drainage of purulent fluid, a recent series of purulent pericarditis in children reported a mortality of 2 per cent without late development of constriction.[311]

PATHOLOGY. Bacterial pericarditis is usually frankly suppurative by the time it is detected clinically. The inflammation may result in organization and dense adhesions with a loculated pericardial effusion followed by obliteration of the pericardial space, thickening, and eventual calcification of the pericardium. In some patients, the inflammation may involve the adjacent sternum, pleura, and diaphragm with formation of dense adhesions between the parietal pericardium and contiguous structures. The evolution of this inflammatory process has been studied in an animal model of pericarditis caused by the injection of heat-killed staphylococci into the pericardial space.[316]

CLINICAL FEATURES. Bacterial pericarditis is usually an acute fulminant illness of only a few days' duration. In one series,[297] the mean duration of symptoms prior to hospitalization was only 3 days. High fevers, shaking chills, night sweats, and dyspnea are common. In most patients the symptom of typical pericardial chest pain is absent. Tachycardia is present in nearly all patients, but a pericardial friction rub is present in less than half. In many cases the pericarditis remains unsuspected because of the dominant presence of symptoms and signs related to an underlying known infection, such as pneumonia or mediastinitis following complicated thoracic surgery or trauma. The appearance of new jugular venous distention and pulsus paradoxus may be the first evidence of pericardial involvement, and these ominous signs reflect the development of cardiac tamponade due to the acute accumulation of suppurative fluid under pressure. In one series, cardiac tamponade developed acutely in 38 per cent of patients with previously unsuspected purulent pericarditis and contributed to death in the majority.[297]

LABORATORY FINDINGS. These usually include a leukocytosis with a marked leftward shift. The chest roentgenogram usually shows enlargement of the cardiac shadow and, less commonly, widening of the mediastinitis. In the majority of cases the roentgenogram shows evidence of underlying pneumonia, empyema, or mediastinitis. Electrocardiographic changes typically include ST-segment and T-wave changes characteristic of pericarditis in the majority of patients. The appearance of electrical alternans suggests the possibility of cardiac tamponade. In patients with suspected infective endocarditis, the appearance of a prolonged P-R interval, atrioventricular dissociation, or bundle branch block is strong evidence of extension of infection from the valve ring into the adjacent myocardium. The latter is an important predisposing factor for the development of pericarditis, especially in patients with staphylococcal endocarditis.[297]

PERICARDIAL FLUID. This usually shows polymorphonuclear leukocytosis and sometimes frank pus. Pericardial-glucose levels are usually depressed, and the protein content is increased; lactate dehydrogenase values may also be markedly elevated.

Purulent bacterial pericarditis should be suspected in a debilitated patient with unexplained high spiking fevers, dyspnea, markedly elevated white blood cell count, and an increase in the size of the cardiac silhouette on chest roentgenogram. The key to the diagnosis, which unfortunately is frequently not made before death, is a high index of suspicion. An echocardiogram should be promptly obtained to look for evidence of a new pericardial effusion and/or loculation of fluid with adhesions. Spontaneous contrast echoes in a patient with suspected purulent pericarditis raise the possibility of a gas-producing bacterial infection.[317] Both indium and gallium scintigraphy have been reported to show a "halo sign" of increased pericardial tracer uptake in bacterial pericarditis, but this finding can also be seen in viral, tuberculous, and other forms of pericarditis.[279,318,319]

NATURAL HISTORY. Despite the lower incidence of purulent bacterial pericarditis in the antibiotic era, overall survival continues to be extremely poor, averaging about 30 per cent in modern series.[297,320] The poor prognosis stems in large part from failure of clinical diagnosis before death. In patients treated only with antibiotics without pericardial drainage, the rapid unsuspected development of a large pericardial effusion may result in sudden cardiovascular collapse and death due to cardiac tamponade. The high mortality from purulent pericarditis can be reduced substantially through the institution of both appropriate parenteral antibiotic therapy and early complete surgical drainage.[287,297,320,321] Early surgical drainage of the pericardium may help to prevent the complication of constrictive pericarditis. In a recent surgical series of pericardiectomy with antibiotic treatment, the surgical mortality was 8 per cent, with a 5-year survival of 91 per cent and no late cases of pericardial constriction.[321] Successful treatment of bacterial endocarditis with long-term simple catheter drainage of the pericardial space has been reported, but experience with this approach is limited.[322,323] The instillation of intrapericardial urokinase in three patients with purulent fibrinous pericarditis has also been reported.[323]

Meningococcal Pericarditis. The pericardium may become infected early during meningococcal sepsis (in the presence or absence of meningitis), causing purulent pericarditis with cardiac tamponade, as described earlier. In these cases the pericardial fluid is frankly purulent, and viable organisms can usually be isolated. In addition, sterile pericarditis may occur late in the convalescent period in association with arthritis, pleuritis, and ophthalmitis. This syndrome appears to have an immunological cause, does not require further antibiotic therapy if the primary infection has been adequately treated, and responds to antiinflammatory agents. Febrile, self-limited polyserositis with pericarditis has also been reported after effective treatment of sepsis due to *Staphylococcus aureus*,[324] and in young adults with acute streptococcal tonsillitis in the absence of rheumatic fever.[289]

MANAGEMENT. Suspicion of the presence of purulent pericardial fluid is an indication to explore the pericardial space. This may be done by percutaneous pericardiocentesis only if there is echocardiographic evidence of a large anterior and posterior pericardial effusion that may be safely tapped or, preferably, by a generous subxiphoid pericardiotomy with thorough pericardial drainage. Both pericardial fluid and pericardial tissue should be immediately studied by means of Gram-stained, acid-fast, and fungal smears by an experienced examiner. The fluid should then be cultured for aerobic and anaerobic bacteria with appropriate antibiotic sensitivity testing and for fungi and tuberculosis. Pericardial fluid should also be examined; the number of white blood cells, the differential count, hematocrit, and glucose and protein content should be determined. Cultures of blood, sputum, and recent surgical wounds should also be obtained.

Results of Gram staining of the pericardial fluid should be used in the selection of antibiotic therapy. If the effusion is purulent but no organisms can be easily identified and tuberculosis is not considered likely, therapy should be initiated with both a semisynthetic antistaphylococcal antibiotic and an aminoglycoside. Depending on the results of the cultures of the pericardial fluid and blood, antibiotic therapy may then be modified. High concentrations of antibiotics can be achieved in pericardial fluid, so that instillation of antibiotics into the pericardial space is not warranted.[325] However, systemic antibiotics alone are inadequate treatment, and prompt and thorough surgical drainage of the pericardium is essential in almost all patients with bacterial pericarditis.[297,313,321] Percutaneous aspiration of a large effusion may be extremely helpful in making an initial bacteriological diagnosis and initiating therapy, and percutaneous aspiration followed by catheter drainage is sometimes effective in preventing recurrent effusion.[322,323,326] However, purulent pericardial effusions are likely to recur, and more extensive surgical drainage may be needed in some patients after antibiotic therapy has been initiated. Open drainage, through creation of a subxiphoid pericardiotomy, is usually adequate when the diagnosis is made early and when the pericardial fluid is thin and the pericardium minimally thickened. This procedure is also the preferred route of drainage in severely disabled patients because it can be performed under local anesthesia and avoids the pleural cavities. In a patient with a thick purulent effusion and dense adhesions with loculation, extensive pericardiectomy is needed to achieve adequate drainage and to prevent development of constrictive pericarditis,[286,297,315,321] which can occur very early after presentation.[327]

FUNGAL PERICARDITIS

ETIOLOGY AND PATHOPHYSIOLOGY. Histoplasmosis is the most common cause of fungal pericarditis. This diagnosis should be considered in young and otherwise healthy patients suspected of having acute viral or tuberculous pericarditis who live in the Ohio or Mississippi River Valley or the Western Appalachians, where the fungus is endemic.[328] In these areas, histoplasmosis is acquired by inhalation of spores during small rural outbreaks from bird or bat droppings and during major urban outbreaks related to excavation and building demolition. Coccidioidomycosis pericarditis occurs in patients who have inhaled chlamydospores from soil or dust in areas of the American Southwest, particularly the San Joaquin Valley, and Argentina, where it is endemic.[329,330] Other fungal infections responsible for pericarditis include aspergillosis, blastomycosis, and those caused by *Candida albicans* and *Candida tropicalis*.[331–334] Groups at increased risk for the development of fungal pericarditis consequent to disseminated infection include drug addicts, patients who are immunosuppressed or who have received potent broad-spectrum antibiotics, and patients recovering from complicated open-heart surgery.

Histoplasmosis pericarditis most commonly develops as a noninfectious inflammatory response to infection confined to adjacent mediastinal lymph nodes and rarely by direct or hematogenous infection in patients with disseminated infection.[328,335] The isolation of organisms from pericardial fluid is unusual, and its predilection for young immunocompetent males suggests that self-limited histoplasmosis pericarditis usually represents a sterile immune reaction. Pericarditis due to fungi other than histoplasmosis may occur as a complication of open-heart surgery in adults and children as a result of spread from contiguous infected lymph nodes or pulmonary lesions or hematogenous dissemination in immunosuppressed patients with fungal sepsis.

PATHOLOGY. Pericardial fluid may accumulate extremely rapidly and to massive quantities in patients with histoplasmosis. The fluid can be serous or hemorrhagic with increased protein content and polymorphonuclear leukocytosis. In cases of fungal pericarditis due to agents other than *Histoplasma*, exudative pericardial effusions may accumulate more slowly, so that an effusion may be present for months. Histoplasmosis and other fungal pericardial effusions occasionally become organized, with pericardial thickening, the appearance of granulomas and multinucleated giant cells, and the development of a constricting, calcified pericardium.[328,335]

Histoplasmosis in patients with disseminated infection may rarely cause infection of the myocardium and endocardium as well as of the pericardium.[335] Similarly, aspergillosis, candidiasis, and coccidioidomycosis may cause pericarditis in the context of pulmonary infection, endocarditis, and myocardial abscess.[329–332] Therefore, cardiac decompensation in patients with fungal pericarditis may be due either to the presence of cardiac compression from a pericardial effusion or a constricting pericardium or to an underlying myocardial infection.

CLINICAL FEATURES. The clinical course of histoplasmosis pericarditis is now better understood from two large urban outbreaks in which 6.3 per cent of 712 patients with clinically recognized histoplasmosis had acute pericarditis.[328] Almost all of the patients had a preceding respiratory illness, and pericardial pain and typical electrocardiographic changes at presentation. The chest roentgenogram was always abnormal, an enlarged cardiac silhouette was present in 95 per cent, and pleural effusions and intrathoracic adenopathy were present in two-thirds of the patients. Notably, the "classic" manifestations of histoplasmosis—acute self-limited disseminated infection or severe cavitary pulmonary infection—were absent. However, more than 40 per cent of patients had hemodynamic compromise or frank cardiac tamponade consistent with other reports.[328,335] Histoplasmosis pericarditis can rarely occur in the less common setting of severe prolonged disseminated infection evident by fever, anemia, leukopenia, and the syndrome of pneumonitis progressing to pulmonary cavitation, massive hepatomegaly, meningitis, myocarditis, or endocarditis. Severe disseminated infections are especially likely to occur in young infants, elderly males, and immunosuppressed patients.

Coccidioidomycosis Pericarditis. This condition does not occur in the brief self-limited influenza-like form of the infection but is instead a complication of the progressive disseminated form of coccidioidomycosis.[329,330] Blacks, Filipinos, and Chicanos appear to be especially vulnerable to the development of disseminated coccidioidomycosis. These patients are usually chronically ill and debilitated, with fever, weight loss, and the complications of pulmonary cavitations with lymphadenopathy, osteomyelitis, and meningitis. In immunocompromised patients, the insidious appearance of symptoms of fungal pericarditis and underlying myocardial infection may initially be overlooked because attention is focused on symptoms related to underlying lymphoma, leukemia, or known valvular endocarditis. Physical findings suggestive of cardiac compression (jugular venous distention, hypotension, pulsus paradoxus) may be the first clues to the diagnosis of fungal pericarditis.

DIAGNOSIS. Histoplasmosis Pericarditis. In young and otherwise healthy adults with evidence of pericarditis, a presumptive clinical diagnosis of histoplasmosis pericarditis can be made on the basis of (1) residence or travel in an endemic area, (2) an elevated complement fixation titer of at least 1:32, and (3) a positive immunodiffusion test.[328] Most patients do not show a progressive rise in titer, because pericarditis usually occurs after initial mild or asymptomatic pneumonitis such that titers are high when first measured. Histoplasmin skin tests are not helpful, and their use may falsely elevate antibody titers.[328] *Histoplasma* may be isolated from specimens from invasive biopsies of mediastinal nodes, but cultures or methenamine silver stains rarely identify the organism in extrapulmonary sites such as the liver, bone marrow, and pericardium in patients with benign, self-limited forms of pericarditis. Histoplasmosis pericarditis that occurs in the setting of severe disseminated infection must be differentiated from sarcoidosis, tuberculosis, Hodgkin's disease, and brucellosis. Histological tissue examination and culture are important in disseminated progressive histoplasmosis, and in this setting the organism may be isolated from extrapericardial sites such as the bone marrow, exudate from ulcers, or sputum by inoculation on Sabouraud's medium or by guinea pig inoculation with subsequent subculture of the spleen.

Coccidioidomycosis Pericarditis. A presumptive diagnosis of coccidioidomycosis pericarditis is made in a patient with pericarditis who has (1) a history of dust exposure in an endemic area in the American Southwest, California Central Valley, or South America, (2) a characteristic clinical picture of disseminated coccidioidomycosis involving the lungs and other organs, (3) the appearance of a positive serum precipitin test early in the infection followed by a rising positive complement-fixation antibody titer, and (4) microscopic evidence of the characteristic spherule in biopsy material. A definitive diagnosis is made by culture identification of the organism on Sabouraud's medium. Coccidioidin skin tests are often negative in the presence of progressive disseminated disease.

Other Fungal Pericarditis. If pericarditis due to other fungal organisms is suspected, appropriate complement-fixing antibody titers should be measured. Serology and precipitin tests for *Candida* are not sensitive or specific, and the diagnosis of candida pericarditis depends on growth of the fungus from several sites other than superficially contaminated catheters in association with immunosuppression or complicated cardiac surgery.[332] Depending on the clinical setting, it may be important to obtain pericardial fluid and a pericardial biopsy specimen. It must be emphasized that the microscopic finding of granulomas alone is nonspecific and may occur in tuberculosis, fungal and parasitic infections, and sarcoid involvement of the pericardium. Therefore, histological documentation of the characteristic appearance of the fungus and subsequent culture identification are important.

MANAGEMENT. *Histoplasmosis pericarditis* is generally a benign illness that resolves within 2 weeks and does not require treatment with amphotericin.[328] Nonsteroidal anti-inflammatory drugs or steroids appear to shorten the duration of chest pain, fever, pericardial friction rub, and effusion.[328] Patients should always be hospitalized because histoplasmosis may cause the rapid development of massive effusions with acute cardiac tamponade that require emergency pericardiocentesis or pericardiectomy.[328,335] Although pericardial calcification and pericardial constriction have been reported in histoplasmosis pericarditis, these complications are uncommon. Intravenous amphotericin B is required only for patients with histoplasmosis pericarditis and severe disseminated systemic disease.

In *nonhistoplasmosis fungal pericarditis* the diagnosis is rarely made before death. Spontaneous remissions do not occur; infection progresses until the patient dies either of the underlying disease or of fungal pericardial and myocardial involvement. Survival from nonhistoplasmosis fungal pericarditis has been reported in occasional patients treated with parenteral antifungal therapy and surgical drainage by pericardiectomy.[332,336] Drug therapy for pericarditis associated with disseminated coccidioidomycosis, aspergillosis, and blastomycosis consists of prolonged intravenous therapy with amphotericin B. The South American form of blastomycosis may require the addition of a sulfonamide. Candida pericarditis associated with fungal sepsis and disseminated infection is treated with amphotericin B, in addition to pericardiectomy.[332] Candida pericarditis has been successfully treated with antifungal therapy and drainage of pericardiocentesis, but there is little experience with this approach.[333] In many cases of nonhistoplasmosis fungal pericarditis, chronic pericardial fungal infection progresses to severe pericardial constriction or, less commonly, cardiac tamponade. Therefore, depending on the patient's underlying medical condition, pericardiectomy is usually indicated. Intrapericardial instillation of antifungal agents has not proved helpful in these diseases. The serious toxicity associated with prolonged amphotericin B administration underscores the importance of making a definitive diagnosis after histological examination or culture.

Pericarditis complicated by the development of cardiac tamponade and chronic constrictive pericarditis may also be caused by *Actinomyces israelii* and *Nocardia asteroides,* which are intermediate forms between fungi and bacteria.[337–339] These organisms may cause indolent infections and invasion of the pericardium from thoracic, abdominal, or cervicofascial abscesses.

OTHER INFECTIOUS PERICARDITIS

The mycoplasmas, fastidious organisms that cause pulmonary and urogenital disease, are newly recognized as pathogens that can cause pericarditis in association with large pericardial effusions.[340] Mycoplasma pericarditis appears to occur in patients who are immunocompromised or have undergone cardiac surgery. The parasite *Toxoplasma gondii,* which is usually acquired by accidental cyst ingestion in endemic areas, is a cause of myocarditis, acute pericarditis with tamponade, and chronic pericardial effusion.[341–343] The prevalence of *Toxoplasma* as a cause of acute pericarditis of unknown origin may be underestimated.[69] Toxoplasmosis pericarditis can occur in the setting of fever of unknown origin with lymphadenopathy in both normal and immunosuppressed patients.[342–344] It is presumptively diagnosed by documenting high IgM or rising IgG antibodies, and definitively diagnosed by inoculation of infected pericardial fluid into mice, and it is usually treated with sulfadiazine and pyrimethamine antibiotic therapy in addition to drainage of pericardial fluid.

Other parasitic causes include amebiasis,[345–347] schistosomiasis,[348] and echinococcosis.[349,350] The diagnosis of amebic pericarditis is facilitated by the demonstration of multiple cystic lesions in the region of the pericardium by chest roentgenography and two-dimensional echocardiography.[347] Uncommon causes of parasitic pericarditis include dracunculosis,[351] cysticercosis, and filariasis.[352] These unusual infections rarely cause acute cardiac tamponade but may cause chronic constrictive pericarditis. The spirochetes *Borrelia burgdorferi* and *Babesia microti* are increasingly recognized as causes of pericarditis with tamponade and myocarditis in association with tick-borne Lyme disease.[353,354] The diagnosis can be made by the demonstration of IgM and IgG antibodies in pericardial fluid by indirect immunofluorescence and identification of spirochetes in pericardial or myocardial biopsies or synovial biopsies. Lyme pericarditis is usually treated by a 14-day course of intravenous ceftriaxone, and pericardial drainage if needed. The psittacosis agent, *Chlamydia psittaci,* an obligate intracellular parasite-like bacterium that causes a febrile pneumonitis via bird-to-human transmission; and the recently discovered respiratory pathogen *Chlamydia pneumoniae* are also rare causes of effusive pericarditis.[355,356]

PERICARDITIS FOLLOWING ACUTE MYOCARDIAL INFARCTION

(See also p. 1255)

Pericarditis is a common occurrence during the first few days after acute myocardial infarction.[357,358] The incidence of early postmyocardial infarction pericarditis varies from 28 to 40 per cent of fatal transmural infarctions studied at autopsy.[359] In a review by Oliva et al. of 14 reports of postinfarction pericarditis, the mean incidence of postinfarction pericarditis detected by a friction rub alone was 14 per cent, whereas the mean incidence was 25 per cent if the symptom of classic positional chest pain or a rub or both were used as diagnostic criteria.[359] The recent use of thrombolytic therapy in acute myocardial infarction appears to have caused about a 50 per cent reduction in the incidence of early postinfarction pericarditis.[359–363] Furthermore, observations from the GISSI trial have shown that the earlier the thrombolytic treatment is initiated, the lower is the incidence of pericarditis, and that pericardial involvement is strongly associated with several indices of infarct size.[362] The late development of Dressler syndrome is now exceedingly rare in patients who have received thrombolytic therapy with successful reperfusion.[364] In a prospective study of 703 patients with acute myocardial infarction, pericarditis, defined by the detection of a pericardial friction rub, occurred in 25 per cent of patients with transmural infarction and in 9 per cent of patients with non-Q-wave infarction.[365]

Fibrinous pericarditis is detected in about 10 per cent of patients with non-Q-wave infarction at autopsy.[366] Pericarditis is more prevalent in anterior than in inferior infarction[365] and also occurs following lateral and predominant right ventricular infarction. Other forms of pericardial involvement after myocardial infarction include acute pericardial hemorrhage secondary to cardiac rupture and the late occurrence of Dressler syndrome (see p. 1256).

CLINICAL FEATURES. Pericarditis is recognized clinically by the appearance of a pericardial friction rub within 12 hours to 10 days after acute myocardial infarction. In most patients with postinfarction pericarditis, a pericardial friction rub appears on the first, second, or third day after infarction.[358,359,365] In about 70 per cent of patients, the presence of a pericardial rub is accompanied by pleuritic or positional chest pain.[365] There is usually a slight temperature elevation, but pneumonitis is uncommon. Appearance of a new friction rub more than 10 days after acute infarction probably represents the onset of Dressler syndrome or pericarditis complicating a second infarction. Because pericardial friction rubs are notoriously evanescent, serial auscultatory evaluation of the patient in various positions in a quiet room is important for detection. Pericardial rubs with a single systolic component heard near the apex may be confused with a new murmur of mitral regurgitation due to papillary muscle dysfunction or rupture. Postinfarction pericarditis does not directly cause hemodynamic deterioration unless pericardial effusion under pressure develops, causing cardiac tamponade.

In a series of patients with acute infarction and pericardial effusion,[367] the use of heparin did not appear to be associated with increased risk. However, hemorrhagic cardiac tamponade related to the use of anticoagulants has been reported as a rare complication in patients with postinfarction pericarditis.[368] Constrictive pericarditis has been reported as a sequel of hemopericardium after infarction.[369]

The typical diagnostic electrocardiographic changes of acute pericarditis are extremely rare in early postinfarction pericarditis.[358] Two types of atypical T-wave evolution have been observed in patients with regional postinfarction pericarditis preceding myocardial rupture. These two patterns of T-wave evolution consist of T waves that remain

TABLE 43–10 CAUSES OF TUMORS METASTATIC TO THE PERICARDIUM

PRIMARY MALIGNANT NEOPLASM	FREQUENCY (%)
Lung carcinoma	40
Breast carcinoma	22
Gastrointestinal carcinoma	3
Other carcinomas	6
Leukemia and lymphoma	15
Melanoma	3
Sarcoma	4
Other (including malignant mesothelioma, germ cell tumors)	7

Relative frequency of neoplasms metastatic to the pericardium in 1315 patients.

Data from Goodie, R. B.: Secondary tumors of the heart and pericardium. Br. Heart J. *17*:183, 1955; and Scott, R. W., and Garvin, C. F.: Tumors of the heart and pericardium. Am. Heart J. *17*:431, 1939.

pericardial teratomas are a rare cause of hydrops fetalis in utero and in neonates.[418]

PRIMARY PERICARDIAL TUMORS. Primary malignant neoplasms of the pericardium are rare and are predominantly due to mesothelioma, including that arising after asbestos and fiber glass exposure,[419,420] and, less frequently, to benign localized fibrous mesothelioma, malignant fibrosarcoma, angiosarcoma, lipomas and liposarcomas, and benign and primary malignant teratomas.[421–424] Rare primary neoplasms of the pericardium occasionally have been reported in association with congenital developmental disorders such as tuberous sclerosis.[425] Cathecholamine-secreting pheochromocytoma is a rare primary neoplasm of the pericardium.[426] In patients with AIDS, an increasing number of patients have been reported with malignant involvement of the pericardium and heart due to Kaposi's sarcoma and cardiac lymphoma.[258,259,427,428] Pericardial tamponade can be an early presentation of HIV infection, and purulent pericarditis as well as malignancy must always be excluded in these patients.[258,259]

PERICARDIAL METASTASES. These may involve the heart in several ways: (1) extension and attachment to the pericardium of a malignant mediastinal mass, (2) nodular tumor deposits from hematogenous or lymphatic spread (Fig. 43–23), (3) diffuse pericardial thickening and infiltration with tumor, and (4) local infiltration of the pericardium.[408]

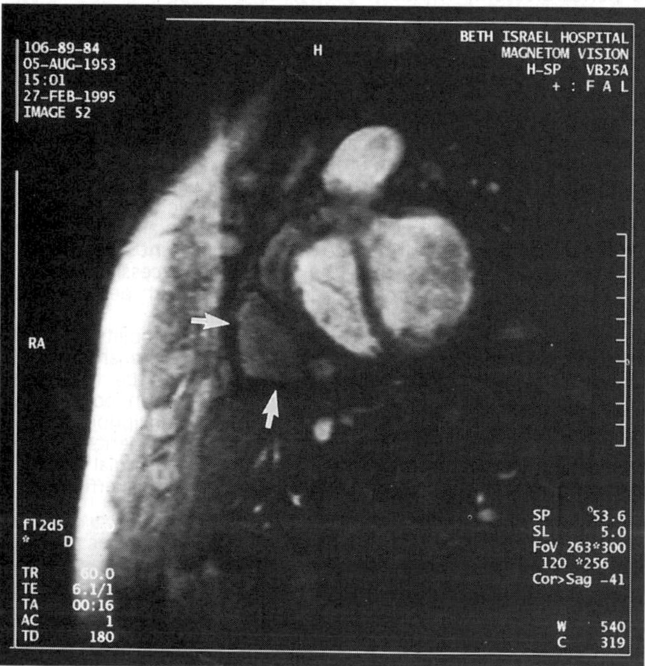

FIGURE 43–23. Spin-echo magnetic resonance image of the heart and pericardium from a patient with non-Hodgkin's lymphoma and elevation of right atrial and right ventricular diastolic pressures. The scan showed a discrete large mass (white arrows) within the pericardial sac which overlaid and compressed the right ventricle. Biopsy of the mass confirmed the presence of intrapericardial lymphoma. (Courtesy of W. Manning, M.D.)

In the majority of cases, the epicardium and myocardium are *not* involved.

EFFUSION IN NEOPLASTIC PERICARDITIS. Neoplastic pericarditis may cause several syndromes of cardiac compression. Neoplastic involvement of the pericardium may result in serosanguineous or hemorrhagic effusions, which may develop extremely rapidly, causing acute or subacute cardiac tamponade.[428a] Pericardial involvement by tumors such as sarcomas, mesotheliomas, and melanomas can also erode the cardiac chamber or intrapericardial blood vessels, causing acute pericardial distention and abrupt fatal cardiac tamponade. A rare cause of hemorrhagic effusion and cardiac tamponade is intrapericardial extramedullary hematopoiesis associated with preleukemic conditions and during blast crisis with Philadelphia chromosome–positive chronic myeloid leukemia and chronic myelomonocytic leukemia.[429,430] Cardiac compression may also occur as a consequence of the development of both thickened pericardium and pericardial effusion under pressure (effusive-constrictive pericarditis), or it may be caused by thickening of the pericardium produced by tumor encasement of the heart, causing the physiology of constrictive pericarditis.

Not all pericardial effusions associated with mediastinal cancer are malignant. Asymptomatic pericardial effusions are common in patients with mediastinal lymphoma and Hodgkin's disease.[431] These evanescent effusions are frequently detected during staging procedures and presumably develop as a result of impaired lymphatic drainage. Transient effusions may also occur in association with mediastinal thymoma and primary cardiac tumors.[432,433] Fracp et al. have observed that small, clinically unsuspected pericardial effusions detectable by echocardiography are common in women with metastatic breast cancer.[434] In a prospective study of 38 women with metastatic breast cancer in whom echocardiography was done on a routine basis, 53 per cent were found to have small pericardial effusions that did not progress to cause hemodynamic embarrassment in any patient. It is uncertain whether small pericardial effusions in asymptomatic women with metastatic breast cancer are due to indolent malignant pericardial involvement or impaired lymphatic drainage.

CLINICAL FEATURES. Neoplastic pericarditis is often totally asymptomatic and detected only as an incidental finding at autopsy. However, it is the most common specific cause of acute pericarditis in developed countries. In a prospective series of patients with acute pericarditis of unknown cause, a diagnostic protocol revealed an unsuspected malignant etiology in 5 per cent of patients.[68] In patients with undiagnosed cancer, leukemia, or primary pericardial tumors, cardiac tamponade can be the initial manifestation.[408,415,421] In patients with known malignancy, symptoms resulting from pericardial involvement may be incorrectly attributed to the underlying neoplasm, so that malignant pericarditis is not suspected until symptoms and signs of severe cardiac compression appear.

In patients with malignant pericarditis, dyspnea is by far the most common symptom.[408,410,435] Other frequent symptoms and physical findings include chest pain, cough, orthopnea, and hepatomegaly. Distant heart sounds and a pericardial friction rub are rarely detected, which is in part probably due to a low index of suspicion.[408,435] In the majority of patients the diagnosis is made only when there is evidence of cardiac compression or frank cardiac tamponade, manifest as jugular venous distention, pulsus paradoxus, and hypotension.[436]

The *chest roentgenogram* is abnormal in more than 90 per cent of patients with malignant pericarditis and may show pleural effusion, cardiac enlargement, mediastinal widening, a hilar mass, or, less commonly, an irregular nodular contour of the cardiac silhouette. The *electrocardiogram* is usually abnormal but nonspecific, showing tachycardia, ST- and T-wave changes, low QRS voltage, and occasionally atrial fibrillation. In occasional patients, persistent tachycardia or electrocardiographic changes are the initial findings that lead to the diagnosis. Electrocardiographic findings that are rarely seen in pericarditis, such as atrioventricular conduction disturbances, suggest malignant invasion of the myocardium and conduction system.

DIAGNOSIS. Patients with cancer and pericarditis benefit from a systematic evaluation, and these patients should not be summarily assumed to have a preterminal condition. The diagnosis of malignant pericarditis depends on both documentation of pericardial inflammation and substantiation that pericarditis is due to neoplasm. It is often not appreciated that in approximately half the patients with symptomatic pericarditis and neoplastic disease there is a nonmalignant cause; most commonly the condition is due to prior radiation or to idiopathic causes.[138,408] Many patients with advanced neoplastic disease are immunosuppressed as a consequence of their malignant disease and/or therapy and are therefore also at risk for tuberculous and fungal pericarditis. Acute pericarditis has also been rarely reported as a complication of intravenous administration of the chemotherapeutic agents doxorubicin and daunorubicin. Sudden tamponade during chemotherapy for bone marrow transplantation for malignancy and thalassaemia has been described. This complication accounted for 29 per cent of all deaths within 1 month of treatment in a series of 400 consecutive transplant patients.[437] The mechanism is not yet understood but may be related to the drug-conditioning regimen.

Neoplastic pericarditis with cardiac compression must be differentiated from other causes of jugular venous distention, hepatomegaly, and peripheral edema in cancer patients. The most important of these are (1) underlying left ventricular dysfunction secondary to prior cardiac disease or doxorubicin cardiac toxicity, (2) superior vena caval obstruction, (3) malignant hepatic involvement with portal hypertension, and (4) microvascular tumor spread in the lungs with secondary pulmonary hypertension.

Echocardiography often provides critical information about the presence and size of a pericardial effusion and the thickness and motion of the pericardium and may suggest the presence of abnormal diastolic filling of the heart due to cardiac compression. Two-dimensional echocardiography may be helpful in the detection of irregular undulating masses that protrude into the pericardial space and define the presence of pericardial space-occupying lesions.[438] *CT* and *MRI* (Fig. 43–23) can also detect the presence of pericardial effusions and, in some instances, may give added information regarding the presence and location of space-occupying masses within the pericardium and adjacent mediastinum and lungs.[423,439]

PERICARDIOCENTESIS AND CARDIAC CATHETERIZATION. We recommend that pericardiocentesis using the catheter drainage technique (see p. 1493) be performed in conjunction with cardiac catheterization in cancer patients with suspected cardiac tamponade in whom a large pericardial effusion is documented by echocardiography. Two additional diagnoses should always be systematically evaluated during cardiac catheterization in these patients: (1) Superior vena caval obstruction may coexist with malignant cardiac tamponade and contribute to the development of facial edema and jugular venous distention and should be systematically excluded at cardiac catheterization in cancer patients. (2) Cyanosis, hypoxemia, and elevation of the pulmonary vascular resistance are not features of cardiac tamponade, and pulmonary microvascular tumor (lymphangitic tumor) should be strongly suspected in a patient with these findings, hypoxemia, or persistent dyspnea following pericardiocentesis. Support for this diagnosis can be obtained at the same setting as pericardiocentesis and right-heart catheterization by obtaining a sample of blood from the pulmonary capillary wedge position for cytological analysis using the right-heart catheter.[440]

The appearance of the pericardial fluid does not differentiate among neoplastic, radiation, or idiopathic causes. Because treatment strategies differ, it is necessary to carry out a meticulous cytological examination of pericardial fluid in an attempt to differentiate malignant pericarditis from radiation-induced or idiopathic pericarditis. Cytological examination of pericardial fluid is diagnostic of a malignant neoplasm in about 85 per cent of the cases of malignant pericarditis.[138,408,441] False-negative cytological diagnoses are uncommon in carcinomatous pericarditis but occur more commonly with involvement by lymphoma or mesothelioma.[441] The measurement of carcinoembryonic antigen (CEA) may add to the diagnostic yield of the examination of pericardial fluid in patients with suspected neoplastic pericarditis[282]; open pericardial biopsy may be required if the results of cytological examination of pericardial fluid are normal. If a sufficiently large biopsy specimen is obtained, open pericardial biopsy should provide a histological diagnosis in up to 90 per cent of cases. However, false-negative diagnoses may occur if only a small tissue sample is obtained, and in critically ill patients open pericardial biopsy is not without risk. Optically guided percutaneous pericardioscopy with biopsy is a new and alternative approach for the diagnosis of suspected neoplastic pericardial involvement.[155,156]

In patients with echocardiographic evidence of a thickened pericardium and the physical findings of cardiac compression (jugular venous distention, edema, ascites, and hepatomegaly), cardiac catheterization is useful for documenting the presence of constrictive physiology before a decision is made to proceed with aggressive surgical intervention, i.e., extensive pericardiectomy.

NATURAL HISTORY. If cardiac tamponade can be avoided or successfully treated, the mere presence of neoplastic pericarditis does not imply that death is imminent. Because lung cancer and breast cancer are by far the most common causes of malignant pericarditis with cardiac tamponade, both the management strategy and subsequent natural history usually depend on the type of underlying malignant disease. The natural history of neoplastic pericarditis in patients treated for cardiac tamponade was studied using a Kaplan-Meier analysis in two series.[150,408] In both series, the mean survival was 4 months with 25 per cent surviving 1 year. We studied the outcome of a consecutive series of 29 patients with malignant pericardial effusion and tamponade managed with pericardiocentesis in whom the 1-year survival rate was 17 per cent compared with 91 per cent for 21 patients with nonmalignant effusion.[132] These series indicate that a subset of about 25 per cent of patients with cardiac tamponade due to malignant pericarditis who are managed surgically or with pericardiocentesis survive 1 year or longer.

The outcome in patients with malignant pericarditis due to breast cancer is strikingly better than that in patients with lung cancer or other metastatic carcinomas. Following surgical treatment of cardiac tamponade in lung cancer patients, Piehler et al. reported that the mean survival was only 3.5 months, in contrast with breast cancer patients in whom mean survival was 9 months with survivorship extending to more than 5 years.[150] Similarly, Stewart et al. reported that the median survival following surgical treatment of malignant effusion in lung cancer patients was 2 months, compared with a survival of 8.4 months for breast cancer.[406] In one series of breast cancer patients with malignant pericarditis managed with pericardiectomy or pericardiotomy, the overall median survival was 17 months.[434] A similar prolonged survival in patients with malignant effusion due to breast cancer has been reported by others.[408,441,442]

MANAGEMENT. Decisions about the management of neoplastic pericardial effusion depend on the underlying condition of the patient, the presence or absence of clinical manifestations related to cardiac compression, and the prognosis and treatment options available for the specific histology and stage of the underlying malignant disease. At one end of the spectrum are debilitated patients with end-stage malignant disease for whom there is no promising treatment option for the underlying malignant disease and for whom the prognosis is bleak. In this setting, diagnostic procedures should be as brief and painless as possible, and intervention should be directed toward alleviation of symptoms with a goal of improving the quality of the remaining roidism should always be considered as the cause of pericardial effusion in patients following mediastinal radiation therapy, in whom 25 per cent develop radiation-induced thyroid dysfunction.[452] The *ECG* often shows nonspecific abnormalities, including low QRS voltage and flattened or inverted T waves, due to either myxedematous heart disease or pericardial effusion. In myxedematous patients with cardiac compression from a pericardial effusion, the expected compensatory tachycardia may be absent. Massive macroglossia has been reported as a feature of hypothyroidism and pericardial effusion with elevated venous pressure.[602]

Myxedematous pericardial effusions tend to regress slowly and ultimately disappear over a period of months after patients have been treated with thyroid replacement and have returned to the euthyroid state.[598,601] Cardiac tamponade has been reported, but it is a rare complication.[601,603,604]

CHOLESTEROL PERICARDITIS

Cholesterol pericarditis results from pericardial injury associated with deposition of cholesterol crystals and a mononuclear cell inflammatory reaction consisting of foam cells, macrophages, and giant cells. The presence of cholesterol crystals in the pericardial space is believed to provoke a chronic inflammatory response that results in effusion and may ultimately lead to the development of constrictive pericarditis. A pericardial effusion that contains microscopic cholesterol crystals typically has a glittering "gold" appearance. The similarities in the lipid and cholesterol contents of pericardial fluid and serum in some patients with cholesterol pericarditis suggest that simple transudation may explain the high cholesterol content in the pericardial space.

MANAGEMENT. The management of patients with cholesterol pericarditis includes detection and treatment of an underlying predisposing condition associated with the development of cholesterol pericarditis, such as tuberculous, rheumatoid, or myxedematous pericarditis or hypercholesterolemia. However, in the majority of cases, cholesterol pericarditis occurs in the absence of a clear underlying disease.[605] Cholesterol pericardial effusions are usually large, but because they develop slowly, cardiac tamponade is an unusual complication.[606] Pericardiectomy is indicated in the unlikely event of cardiac tamponade as well as in the treatment of massive cholesterol pericardial effusion, which may cause dyspnea and chest pain.[607] The development of constrictive pericarditis requiring pericardiectomy has been reported but is extremely rare.[608]

CHYLOPERICARDIUM

Idiopathic chylopericardium is rare, and chylopericardium is usually associated with mechanical obstruction of the thoracic duct or its drainage into the left subclavian vein resulting from (1) surgical or traumatic rupture of the thoracic duct or (2) lymphatic blockage by neoplasms, tuberculosis, or congenital lymphangiomatosis.[609,610] Thoracic duct obstruction with failure of adequate collateral drainage then results in the reflux of chyle through lymphatics draining the pericardium. Most patients with chylopericardium are asymptomatic and come to clinical attention when a large, slowly accumulating pericardial effusion is detected on chest roentgenogram or echocardiogram.

The presence of a connection between a damaged thoracic duct and the pericardial space can be established by lymphangiography and radionuclide lymphangiography with technetium-99m antimony sulfur colloid, as well as by the recovery of ingested Sudan III, a lipophilic dye, from pericardial aspirate.[609,610] CT may demonstrate density compatible with fat in the pericardial space.[611] The pericardial fluid is usually milky white in a high cholesterol and triglyceride content, protein content greater than 3.5 gm/dl, and microscopic fat droplets demonstrated with a Sudan III stain.[610] Lymphopericardium, which is due to pericardial angiomas as part of generalized lymphangiectasis, is characterized by clear pericardial fluid.

Cardiac tamponade and constrictive pericarditis are rare complications.[610,611] Chylopericardium has been reported as a rare cause of cardiac tamponade after cardiac surgery.[612,613] The management of symptomatic chylopericardium consists of efforts to reduce the likelihood of recurrence. These include ingestion of a diet rich in medium-chain triglycerides or, if this is unsuccessful, in ligation of the thoracic duct and parietal pericardiectomy to evacuate chylous fluid and prevent reaccumulation.[610,613]

TRAUMATIC PERICARDITIS

(See also p. 1536)

In addition to penetrating or nonpenetrating cardiac trauma (Chap. 44), other important causes of traumatic pericarditis include rupture of the esophagus into the pericardial space, which may occur from esophageal erosion secondary to esophageal carcinoma or sudden rupture of the esophageal contents into the pericardial space in Boerhaave's syndrome, or as a complication of esophagogastrectomy. Pericarditis with tamponade and late constriction has also followed esophageal perforation by accidental ingestion of tooth picks and fish bones.[614,615] Traumatic pericarditis due to esophageal rupture is usually followed by intense erosive pericardial inflammation and infection. Esophageal rupture or perforation may also be followed by the development of an esophagopericardial fistula.[616] These disorders usually require immediate surgical intervention and are associated with a high mortality, although medical management with spontaneous fistula closure has been reported.[616] Pericarditis may also occur secondary to pancreatitis associated with a pericardial effusion with high amylase content and, rarely, the development of cardiac tamponade or a pancreatic-pericardial fistula.[617] The incidence of occult pericardial effusion in patients with acute alcoholic pancreatitis is significantly higher (47 per cent) than in control subjects (11 per cent).[617] The development of fistulas to the pericardium in response to ulcer formation, malignant disease, or surgery may occur from other sites, including the stomach,[618] biliary tract,[619] colon,[620] and bronchi.[621]

Pericardial trauma may also give rise to unusual traumatic syndromes, including cardiovascular collapse following herniation of the heart through a rent in the pericardium caused by trauma, or prior pericardiotomy mimicking congenital partial absence of the pericardium with cardiac subluxation,[622] and intrapericardial diaphragmatic hernia.[623] Diagnosis of cardiac herniation can be made by CT and MRI.[624] Life-threatening cardiac herniation may also occur following radical left pneumonectomy with partial pericardial resection.[625] Intrapericardial herniation of loops of bowel following manual reduction of an umbilical hernia is a rare complication that can be diagnosed by echocardiography.[626]

PERICARDIAL CYSTS

Pericardial cysts are rare developmental anomalies and are typically located at the right costophrenic angle.[627] Unusual locations include the left costophrenic angle, hilum, and superior mediastinum at the level of the aortic arch. They are usually unilocular and filled with clear liquid, giving rise to the term *springwater cysts*.

Pericardial cysts usually do not cause symptoms or unusual physical findings. Rarely, chest pain may occur owing to torsion of the cyst. These lesions typically come to medical attention as an unsuspected finding of a round, sharply defined mass along the right cardiac border on a chest roentgenogram. The size of the cyst in asymptomatic patients may vary over time.[627,628] In most cases, a cyst can be differentiated from solid tumor or aneurysm by two-dimensional echocardiography or CT (Fig. 43–25).[628] When a suspected pericardial cyst is in an unusual location, angiography may occasionally be needed to discriminate a cyst from an aneurysm or pseudoaneurysm. Pericardial cysts located at the right costophrenic angle can be accurately diagnosed and treated by percutaneous aspiration under fluoroscopic guidance.[629] Because long-term follow-up studies have shown that most asymptomatic patients do not develop symptoms, most patients should be managed conservatively, without surgical exploration.[630]

Other benign developmental abnormalities of the pericardium include benign intrapericardial teratomas and intrapericardial bronchial cysts, which can be identified by CT.[631]

CONGENITAL ABSENCE AND DEFECTS OF THE PERICARDIUM

Congenital absence of the pericardium was first described anatomically by Realdus Columbus in 1559, but its antemortem detection did not occur until 1959.[632] In patients with pericardial agenesis, the anomaly usually involves a partial defect of the left-sided pericardium, which is potentially lethal, in 70 per cent; total absence in 9 per cent; partial absence of the right-sided pericardium, and absence of the inferior pericardium, in 17 per cent.[633] There is a 3:1 male/female predominance among patients with pericardial defects, and about 30 per cent have other congenital anomalies, including atrial septal defect, bicuspid aortic valve, bronchogenic cysts, or pulmonic sequestration. A familial occurrence of congenital absence of the pericardium has been reported.[634]

Total absence of the pericardium is not usually associated with symptoms. Occasionally the patient may complain of chest discomfort and palpitations. The cause of these symptoms is unknown, but they may be related to torsion of the great vessels due to excess mobility of the heart. Most asymptomatic patients come to attention because of an unexplained heart murmur or abnormal chest roentgenogram. The extremely rare complication of acute chest pain due to strangulation of the heart between the diaphragm and the pulmonary ligament has been reported.[635]

TOTAL ABSENCE OF THE LEFT PERICARDIUM. Patients with total absence of the left pericardium often have widened splitting of the second heart sound, a hyperdynamic precordial impulse, leftward displacement of the apical impulse, and a systolic murmur at the upper left sternal border that may be related to turbulent blood flow in an unusually mobile heart. ECG abnormalities include right-axis deviation due to levoposition of the heart, incomplete right bundle branch block, clockwise displacement of the QRS transition zone of the precordial leads, and tall and peaked P waves in the right precordial leads.[636]

The standard posteroanterior view of the chest roentgenogram re-

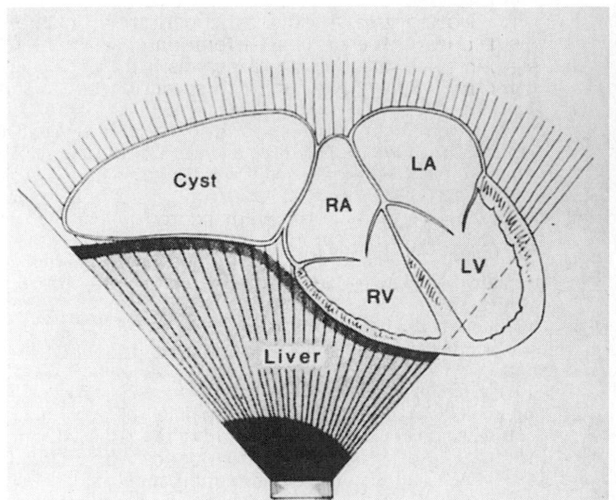

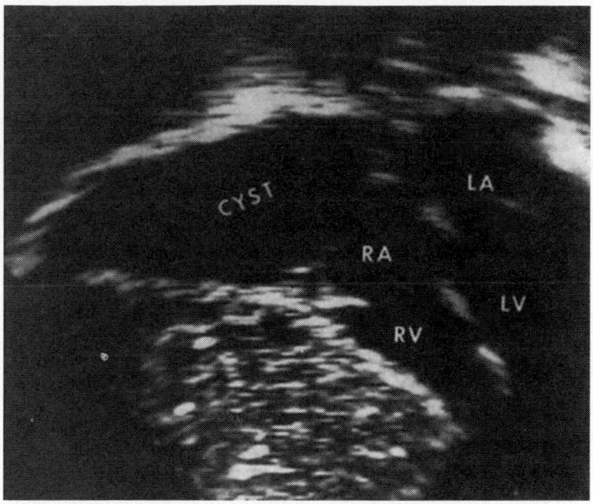

FIGURE 43–25. Two-dimensional subcostal echocardiographic appearance of a well-demarcated benign pericardial cyst adjacent to the right atrial (RA) wall. (From Hynes, J. K., et al.: Two-dimensional echocardiographic diagnosis of pericardial cyst. Mayo Clin. Proc. *58*:60, 1983.)

veals marked leftward displacement of the cardiac silhouette, prominence of the main pulmonary artery, and interposition of radiolucent lung tissue between the aorta and main pulmonary artery or between the left hemidiaphragm and inferior cardiac border. This anomaly must be differentiated from other conditions that cause prominence of the left hilum or pulmonary artery on the standard chest film, including pulmonic valve stenosis, atrial septal defect, idiopathic dilatation of the pulmonary artery, and hilar adenopathy.

M-mode *echocardiographic findings* simulate those seen in right ventricular volume overload, including dilatation of the right ventricle and paradoxical anterior motion of the septum in systole, which is an artifact related to exaggerated cardiac rotation. Two-dimensional echocardiography can demonstrate localized bulging of the left ventricular contour and the drop off of pericardial echoes.[637] Radionuclide perfusion imaging can be used to confirm the diagnosis by demonstration of a wedge of lung tissue between the heart and left hemidiaphragm[638]; CT and MRI can also be used to detect absence of the left pericardium by demonstrating visibility of the right pericardium and absence of the left pericardium, absence of the preaortic recess, and the abnormal presence of a wedge of lung between the aorta and pulmonary artery.[639]

Findings at catheterization are usually normal. Cardiac catheterization with angiography is indicated only if there is a strong suspicion of associated congenital anomalies requiring surgical correction. Usually no specific therapy is required for management of complete absence of the left-sided pericardium.

PARTIAL ABSENCE OF THE PERICARDIUM. Partial left-sided pericardial defects may be complicated by herniation of the left atrial appendage, atrium, or left ventricle through the defect, associated with chest pain, syncope, and sudden death from cardiac strangulation.[640–642] The chest roentgenogram usually shows the nonspecific finding of prominence of the second arch of the left heart border, which must be distinguished from pulmonary artery dilation or aneurysm of the left atrial appendage.[643] Two-dimensional echocardiography and MRI are helpful in demonstrating dilation of the left atrial appendage that extends beyond the pulmonary artery[643,644] (Fig. 43–26). Pulmonary artery angiography with follow-through of contrast opacification to the left heart is the standard method of definitively demonstrating herniation of the left atrium or left atrial appendage beyond the left heart border.[643,644] Partial herniation of the heart and diastolic collapse and compression of the coronary arteries through the defect is a complication of this anomaly that uncommonly may contribute to the development of chest pain and coronary artery strictures.[642,645]

The even rarer anomaly of partially right-sided pericardial defect may be associated with inspiratory right-sided chest pain secondary to herniation of the right atrium and right ventricle through the defect or herniation of lung into the pericardial cavity. The chest roentgenogram may show an unusual protuberance of the right heart border, and technetium-99m cardiac blood pool imaging may demonstrate that the abnormal contour of the right heart border fills simultaneously with the right atrium.[646] Right atrial angiography in the left anterior oblique projection is helpful in documenting herniation of the right atrium and right ventricle through the pericardial defect. Surgical treatment of partial left- or right-sided pericardial defects is usually indicated to relieve symptoms and prevent cardiac strangulation. The defect may be approached by excision of the atrial appendage, pericardioplasty, or pericardiotomy.[647]

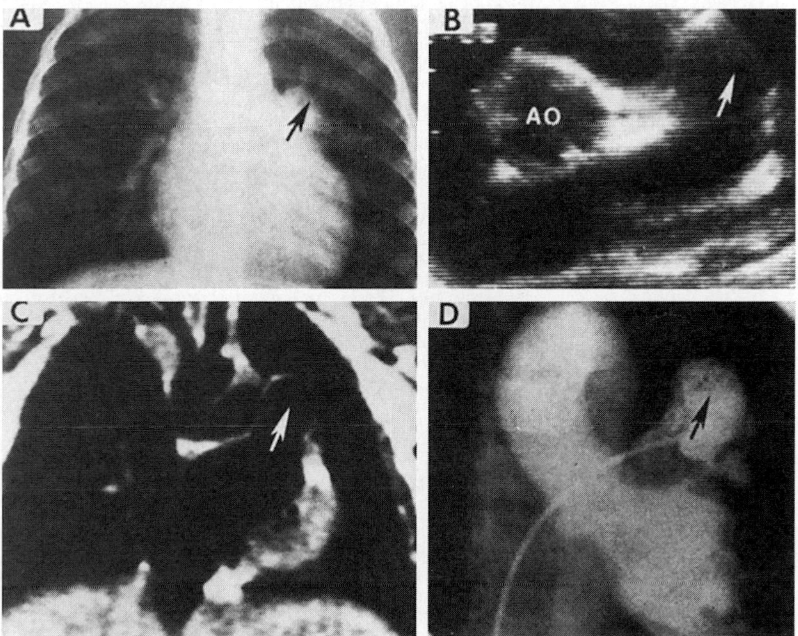

FIGURE 43–26. Noninvasive diagnostic features of partial absence of the left pericardium. The chest roentgenogram *(A)* shows knoblike prominence of the left atrial appendage (arrow). The short-axis cross-sectional two-dimensional echocardiogram *(B)* shows an enlarged left atrial appendage (arrow) extending beyond the pulmonary artery. The frontal plane magnetic resonance image *(C)* shows enlargement and lateral protuberance of the left atrial appendage (arrow). A contrast cineangiogram *(D)* with the catheter positioned across a patent foramen ovale in the left atrial appendage shows a characteristic wedge of lung between the aorta and pulmonary artery and confirms the herniation of the left atrial appendage (arrow). (From Altman, C. A., et al.: Noninvasive diagnostic features of partial absence of the pericardium. Am. J. Cardiol. *63*:1536, 1989.)

REFERENCES

ANATOMY AND FUNCTIONS

1. Fowler, N. O.: Pericardial diseases. *In* Diagnosis of Heart Disease. New York, Springer-Verlag, 1991, pp. 292–313.
2. Holt, J. P.: The normal pericardium. Am. J. Cardiol. *26*:455, 1970.
3. Alles, A., and Dom, R. M.: Peripheral sensory nerve fibers that dichotomize to supply the brachium and the pericardium in the rat. Brain Res. *342*:382, 1970.
4. Ishihara, T., Ferrans, V. J., Jones, M., et al.: Histologic and ultrastructural features of a normal human parietal pericardium. Am. J. Cardiol. *46*:744, 1980.
5. Fukuo, Y., Nakatani, T., Shinohara, H., and Matsuda, T.: Pericardium of rodents: Pores connect the pericardial and pleural cavities. Anat. Res. *220*:132, 1988.
6. Hills, B. A., and Butler, B. D.: Phospholipids identified on the pericardium and their ability to impart boundary lubrication. Ann. Biomed. Eng. *13*:573, 1985.
7. Miyazaki, T., Pride, H. P., and Zipes, D. P.: Prostaglandins in the pericardial fluid modulate neural regulation of cardiac electrophysiological properties. Circ. Res. *66*:163, 1990.
8. Lee, M. D., Fung, Y. C., Shabetai, R., and LeWinter, M. M.: Biaxial mechanical properties of human pericardium and canine comparisons. Am. J. Physiol. *253*:H75, 1987.
9. Tyson, G. S., Jr., Maier, G. W., Olsen, C. O., et al.: Pericardial influences on ventricular filling in the conscious dog. Circ. Res. *54*:173, 1984.
10. Shabetai, R.: Pericardial and cardiac pressure. Circulation *77*:1, 1988.
11. Smiseth, O. A., Frais, M. A., Kingma, I., et al.: Assessment of pericardial constraint in dogs. Circulation *71*:158, 1985.
12. Smiseth, O. A., Frais, M. A., Kingma, I., et al.: Assessment of pericardial constraint: The relation between right ventricular filling pressure and pericardial pressure measured after pericardiocentesis. J. Am. Coll. Cardiol. *7*:307, 1986.
13. Boltwood, C. M., Jr.: Ventricular performance related to transmural filling pressure in clinical tamponade. Circulation *73*:428, 1987.
14. Santamore, W. P., Constantinesco, M., and Little, W. C.: Direct assessment of right ventricular transmural pressure. Circulation *75*:744, 1987.
15. Slinker, B. K., Ditchey, R. V., Bell, S. P., and LeWinter, M. M.: Right heart pressure does not equal pericardial pressure in the potassium chloride arrested canine heart in situ. Circulation *7G*:357, 1987.
16. Hamilton, D. R., Dani, R. S., Semlacher, R. A., et al: Right atrial and right ventricular transmural pressures in dogs and humans. Effects of the pericardium. Circulation *90*:2492, 1994.
17. Hoit, B. D., Lew, W. Y., and LeWinter, M.: Regional variation in pericardial contact pressure in the canine ventricle. Am. J. Physiol. *255*:H1370, 1988.
18. Chew, P. H., Humphrey, J. D., and Yin, F. C.: Regional finite deformations of the in situ canine pericardium. Am. J. Physiol. *264*:H97, 1993.
19. Bernard, H. L.: The functions of the pericardium. J. Physiol. *22*:43, 1898.
20. Junemann, M., Smiseth, O. A., Refsum, H., et al.: Quantification of effect of pericardium on LV diastolic PV relation in dogs. Am. J. Physiol. *252*:H963, 1987.
21. Gilbert, J. C., and Glantz, S. A.: Determinants of ventricular filling and of the diastolic pressure-volume relation. Circ. Res. *64*:827, 1989.
22. Shirato, K., Shabetai, R., Bhargave, V., et al.: Alteration of the left ventricular diastolic pressure-segment length relation produced by the pericardium. Circulation *57*:1191, 1978.
23. Smiseth, O. A., Manyari, D. E., Lima, J. A., et al.: Modulation of vascular capacitance by angiotensin and nitroprusside: A mechanism of changes in pericardial pressure. Circulation *76*:875, 1987.
24. LeWinter, M. M., and Pavelec, R.: Influence of the pericardium on left ventricular end-diastolic pressure-segment relations during early and later stages of experimental chronic volume overload in dogs. Circ. Res. *50*:501, 1982.
25. Freeman, G. L., and LeWinter, M. M.: Pericardial adaptations during chronic cardiac dilation in dogs. Circ. Res. *54*:294, 1984.
26. Frais, M. A., Bergman, D. W., Kingma, I., et al.: The dependence of the time constant of left ventricular isovolumic relaxation (tau) on pericardial pressure. Circulation *81*:1071, 1990.
27. Serizawa, T., Carabello, B. A., and Grossman, W.: Effect of pacing induced ischemia on left ventricular diastolic pressure-volume relations in dog with coronary stenosis. Circ. Res. *46*:430, 1980.
28. Armoore, J. N., Santamore, W. P., Coring, W. J., and George, D. T.: Computer simulation of the effects of ventricular interdependence on indices of left ventricular systolic function. J. Biomed. Eng. *14*:257, 1992.
29. Brinker, J. A., Weiss, J. L., Lappe, D. L., et al.: Leftward septal displacement during right ventricular loading in man. Circulation *61*:626, 1980.
30. Lorell, B. H., Palacios, I., Daggett, W. M., et al.: Right ventricular distention and left ventricular compliance. Am. J. Physiol. *240*:H87, 1981.
31. Hoit, B. D., Dalton, N., Bhargava, V., and Shabetai, R.: Pericardial influences on right and left ventricular filling dynamics. Circ. Res. *68*:197, 1991.
32. Santamore, W. P., Bartlett, R., Van Buren, S. J., et al.: Ventricular coupling in constrictive pericarditis. Circulation *74*:597, 1986.
33. Mangano, D. T.: The effect of the pericardium on ventricular systolic function in man. Circulation *61*:352, 1980.
34. Kanazawa, M., Shirato, K., Ishikawa, K., et al.: The effect of pericardium on the end-systolic pressure-segment length relationship in canine left ventricle in acute volume overload. Circulation *68*:1290, 1983.
35. Goto, Y., Slinker, B. K., and LeWinter, M. M.: Nonhomogeneous left ventricular regional shortening during acute right ventricular pressure overload. Circ. Res. *65*:43, 1989.
36. Stray-Gendersen, J., Musch, T. I., Haidet, G. C., et al.: The effect of pericardiectomy on maximal oxygen consumption and maximal cardiac output in untrained dogs. Circ. Res. *58*:523, 1986.
37. Ringertz, H. G., Misbach, G. A., and Tyberg, J. V.: Effect of the normal pericardium on the left ventricular diastolic pressure-volume relationship. Acta Radiol. *22*:529, 1981.
38. Jarvinen, A., Peltola, K., Rasanen, J., and Heikkila, J.: Immediate hemodynamic effects of pericardial closure after open-heart surgery. Scand. J. Thorac. Cardiovasc. Surg. *21*:131, 1987.
39. Ludbrook, P. A., Byrne, J. D., Kurnik, P. B., and McKnight, R. C.: Influence of reduction of preload and afterload by nitroglycerin on left ventricular diastolic pressure-volume relations and relaxation in man. Circulation *56*:937, 1977.
40. Ludbrook, P. A., Byrne, J. D., and McKnight, R. C.: Influence of right ventricular hemodynamics on left ventricular diastolic pressure-overload relations in man. Circulation *59*:21, 1979.
41. Wong, C. Y., and Spotnitz, H. M.: Effect of nitroprusside on end-diastolic pressure-diameter relations of the human left ventricle after pericardiectomy. J. Thorac. Cardiovasc. Surg. *82*:350, 1981.
42. Ross, J., Jr.: Acute displacement of the diastolic pressure-volume curve of the left ventricle: Role of the pericardium and the right ventricle. Circulation *59*:32, 1979.
43. Lee, M. J., and Boughner, D. R.: Mechanical properties of human pericardium. Circ. Res. *57*:475, 1985.
44. Bartle, S. H., and Hermann, H. J.: Acute mitral regurgitation in man. Hemodynamic evidence and observations indicating an early role for the pericardium. Circulation *36*:839, 1967.
45. Lorell, B. H., Leinbach, R. C., Pohost, G. M., et al.: Right ventricular infarction. Am. J. Cardiol. *43*:465, 1979.
46. Goldstein, J. A., Vlahakes, G. H., Verrier, E. D., et al.: The role of right ventricular systolic dysfunction and elevated intrapericardial pressure in the genesis of low output in experimental right ventricular infarction. Circulation *65*:513, 1982.
47. Tischler, M. D., Rowan, M., and LeWinter, M. M.: Increased left ventricular mass after thoracotomy and pericardiectomy. A role for the relief of pericardial constraint? Circulation *87*:1921, 1993.
48. Janicki, J. S.: Influence of the pericardium and ventricular interdependence of left ventricular diastolic and systolic function in patients with heart failure. Circulation *81*(Suppl. II):15, 1990.

ACUTE PERICARDITIS

49. Garty, I., Mader, R., and Schonfeld, S.: Post pulmonary embolism pericarditis. Clin. Nucl. Med. *19*:519, 1994.
50. Wenger, N. K.: Pericardial disease in the elderly. Cardiovasc. Clin. *22*:97, 1992.
51. Markiewicz, W., Brik, A., Brook, G., et al.: Pericardial rub in pericardial effusion: Lack of correlation with amount of fluid. Chest *77*:643, 1980.
52. Spodick, D. H.: Pericardial rub: Prospective, multiple observer investigation of pericardial friction rub in 100 patients. Am. J. Cardiol. *35*:357, 1975.
53. Spodick, D. H.: Diagnostic electrocardiographic sequences in acute pericarditis: Significance of PR segment and PR vector changes. Circulation *48*:575, 1973.
54. Kouvaras, G., Soufras, G., Chronopoulos, G., et al.: The ST segment as a different diagnostic feature between acute pericarditis and acute inferior myocardial infarction. Angiology *41*:207, 1990.
55. Teh, B. S., Walsh, J., Bell, A. J., et al.: Electrical current paths in acute pericarditis. J. Electrocardiol. *26*:291, 1993.
56. Toriya Martinez, R. N., and Gonzalez Hermosillo, J. A.: Acute nonspecific pericarditis. Arch. Inst. Cardiol. Mex. *57*:307, 1987.
57. Bruce, M. A., and Spodick, D. H.: Atypical electrocardiogram in acute pericarditis: Characteristics and prevalence. J. Electrocardiol. *13*:61, 1980.
58. Carson, W.: Maximal spatial ST vector of ST segment elevation in the right praecordial leads on electrocardiogram due to acute pericarditis. Eur. Heart. J. *9*:665, 1988.
59. Wanner, W. R., Schaal, S. F., Bashore, T. M., et al.: Repolarization variant vs. acute pericarditis. A prospective electrocardiographic and echocardiographic evaluation. Chest *83*:180, 1983.
60. Ginzton, L. E., and Laks, M. M.: The differential diagnosis of acute pericarditis. Circulation *65*:1004, 1982.
61. Dressler, N.: Sinus tachycardia complicating and outlasting pericarditis. Am. Heart J. *72*:422, 1966.
62. Spodick, D. H.: Frequency of arrhythmias in acute pericarditis determined by Holter monitoring. Am. J. Cardiol. *53*:842, 1984.
63. Weiss, J. M., and Spodick, D. H.: Association of left pleural effusion with pericardial disease. N. Engl. J. Med. *308*:696, 1983.
64. Olson, H. G., Lyons, K. P., Aronow, W. S., et al.: Technetium-99m stannous pyrophosphate myocardial scintigrams in pericardial disease. Am. Heart J. *99*:459, 1980.
65. Kodama, K., Igase, M., Funada, J., et al.: Gallium-67 citrate scintigraphy in idiopathic pericarditis: Report of a case. Jpn. Circ. J. *58*:298, 1994.

66. Matsouka, H., Hamada, M., Honda, T., et al.: Evaluation of acute myocarditis and pericarditis by Gd-DTPA enhanced magnetic resonance imaging. Eur. Heart J. *15*:283, 1994.
67. Karjalainen, J., and Heikkila, J.: Acute pericarditis: Myocardial enzyme release as evidence for myocarditis. Am. Heart J. *111*:546, 1986.
68. Saner, H. E., Gobel, F. L., Nicoloff, D. M., and Edwairds, J. E.: Aortic dissection presenting as pericarditis. Chest *91*:71, 1987.
69. Permanyer-Miralda, G., Sagrista-Sauleda, J., and Soler-Soler, J.: Primary acute pericardial disease: A prospective series of 231 consecutive patients. Am. J. Cardiol. *56*:623, 1985.
70. Arunsalam, S., and Siegel, R. J.: Rapid resolution of symptomatic acute pericarditis with ketorolac tromethamine: A parenteral nonsteroidal anti-inflammatory agent. Am. Heart J. *125*:1455, 1993.
71. Sagrista-Sauleda, J., Permanyer-Miralda, G., Candell-Riera, J., et al.: Transient cardiac constriction: An unrecognized pattern of evolution in effusive acute idiopathic pericarditis. Am. J. Cardiol. *59*:961, 1987.
72. Fowler, N. O., and Harbin, A. D.: Recurrent pericarditis: Follow-up of 31 patients. J. Am. Coll. Cardiol. *7*:300, 1986.
73. Melchior, T. M., Ringsdal, V., Hildebrandt, P., and Torp-Pedersen, C.: Recurrent acute idiopathic pericarditis treated with intravenous methylprednisone given as pulse therapy. Am. Heart J. *123*:1086, 1992.
74. Hatcher, C. R., Logue, R. B., Logan, W. D., et al.: Pericardiectomy for recurrent pericarditis. J. Thorac. Cardiovasc. Surg. *62*:371, 1971.
75. Permanyer-Miralda, G., Sagrista-Sauleda, J., Shabetai, R., et al.: Acute pericardial disease: An approach to etiologic diagnosis and treatment. *In* Soler-Soler, J., Permanyer-Miralda, G., and Sagrista-Sauleda, J. (eds.): Pericardial Disease: New Insights and Old Dilemmas. Dordrecht, The Netherlands, Kluwer Academic Publishers, 1990, pp. 193–214.
76. Millaire, A., deGroote, P., Decoulx, E., et al.: Treatment of recurrent pericarditis with colchicine. Eur. Heart J. *15*:120, 1994.
77. Adler, Y., Zandman-Goddard, G., Ravid, M., et al.: Usefulness of colchicine in preventing recurrences of pericarditis. Am. J. Cardiol. *73*:916, 1994.
78. Guindo, J., Rodriguez de la Serna, A., Ramio, J., et al.: Recurrent pericarditis. Relief with colchicine. Circulation *82*:1117, 1990.

PERICARDIAL EFFUSION

79. Carsky, E. W., Mauceri, R. A., and Azimi, F.: The epicardial fat pad sign: Analysis of frontal and lateral chest radiographs in patients with pericardial effusion. Radiology *137*:303, 1980.
80. Miller, S. W.: Imaging pericardial disease. Radiol. Clin. North Am. *27*:1113, 1989.
81. Horowitz, M. S., Schultz, C. S., and Stinson, E. B.: Sensitivity and specificity of echocardiographic diagnosis of pericardial effusion. Circulation *50*:239, 1974.
82. Berger, M., Bobak, K., Jelveh, M., and Goldberg, E.: Pericardial effusion diagnosed by echocardiography. Clinical and electrocardiographic findings. Chest *74*:174, 1978.
83. Enein, M., Zina, A. A., Kassem, M., and el-Tabbakh, G.: Echocardiography of the pericardium in pregnancy. Obstet. Gynecol. *69*:851, 1987.
84. Friedman, M. J., Sahn, D. J., and Haber, K.: Two-dimensional echocardiography and B-mode ultrasonography for the diagnosis of loculated pericardial effusion. Circulation *60*:1644, 1979.
85. Soler-Soler, J.: Massive chronic idiopathic pericardial effusion. *In* Soler-Soler, J., Permanyer-Miralda, G., and Sagrista-Sauleda, J. (eds.): Pericardial Disease: New Insights and Old Dilemmas. Dordrecht, The Netherlands, Kluwer Academic Publishers, 1990, pp. 153–165.
86. Reddy, P. S., Curtiss, E. I., O'Toole, J. D., and Shaver, J. A.: Cardiac tamponade: Hemodynamic observations in man. Circulation *58*:265, 1978.
87. Fowler, N. O.: Cardiac tamponade. A clinical or an echocardiographic diagnosis? Circulation *87*:1738, 1993.
88. Harasawa, H., Li, K. S., Nakamoto, T., et al.: Ventricular coupling via the pericardium: Normal versus tamponade. Cardiovasc. Res. *27*:1470, 1993.
89. Nakamoto, T., Li, K. S., Johnston, W. E., and Santamore, W. P.: Differential effects of positive end expiratory pressure and cardiac tamponade on left-right ventricular mechanical function in the dog. Cardiovasc. Res. *26*:148, 1992.
90. Shibamoto, T., Hayashi, T., Jr., Saeki, Y., et al.: Differential control of sympathetic outflow to kidney, heart, adrenal gland, and liver during systemic hypotension produced by cardiac tamponade in anesthetized dogs. Circ. Shock *39*:114, 1993.
91. Nishikawa, Y., Roberts, J. P., Talcott, M. R., et al.: Accelerated myocardial relaxation in conscious dogs during acute tamponade. Am. J. Physiol. *266*:H1953, 1994.
92. Pegram, B. L., Kardon, M. B., and Bishop, V. S.: Changes in left ventricular internal diameter with increasing pericardial pressure. Cardiovasc. Res. *9*:707, 1975.
93. Mancini, G. B. J., McGillem, M. J., Bates, E. R., et al.: Hormonal responses to cardiac tamponade: Inhibition of release of atrial natriuretic factor despite elevation of atrial pressures. Circulation *76*:884, 1987.
94. Stokhof, A. A., Overduin, L. M., Mol, J. A., and Rijnbek, A.: Effects of pericardiocentesis on circulating concentrations of atrial natriuretic hormone and arginine vasopressin in dogs with spontaneous pericardial effusion. Eur. J. Endocrinol. *130*:357, 1994.
95. Casale, P. N., Fifer, M. A., Graham, R. M., and Palacios, I. F.: Relation of atrial pressure and plasma levels of atrial natriuretic factor in cardiac tamponade. Am. J. Cardiol. *73*:610, 1994.
96. Wechsler, A. S., Auerbach, B. J., Graham, T. C., and Sabiston, D. C.: Distribution of intramyocardial blood flow during pericardial tamponade: Correlation with microscopic anatomy and intrinsic myocardial contractility. J. Thorac. Cardiovasc. Surg. *68*:847, 1974.
97. Kostreva, D. R., Castaner, A., Pedersen, D. H., and Kampine, J. P.: Nonvagally mediated bradycardia during tamponade or severe hemorrhage. Cardiology *68*:65, 1981.
98. Fowler, N. O., and Gabel, M.: The hemodynamic effects of cardiac tamponade: Mainly the result of atrial, not ventricular, compression. Circulation *71*:154, 1985.
99. Fowler, N. O., Gabel, M., and Buncher, C. R.: Cardiac tamponade: A comparison of right versus left heart compression. J. Am. Coll. Cardiol. *12*:187, 1988.
100. Schwartz, S. L., Pandian, N. G., Cao, Q. L., et al.: Left ventricular diastolic collapse in regional left heart cardiac tamponade. An experimental echocardiographic and hemodynamic study. J. Am. Coll. Cardiol. *22*:907, 1993.
101. Leimgruber, P. P., Klopfenstein, H. S., Wann, L. S., and Brooks, H. L.: The hemodynamic derangement associated with right ventricular diastolic collapse in cardiac tamponade: An experimental echocardiographic study. Circulation *68*:612, 1983.
102. Klopfenstein, H. S., Cogswell, T. L., Bernath, G. A., et al.: Alternations in intravascular volume affect the relation between right ventricular diastolic collapse and the hemodynamic severity of cardiac tamponade. J. Am. Coll. Cardiol. *6*:1057, 1985.
103. Singh, S., Wann, L. S., Schuchard, G. H., et al.: Right ventricular and right atrial collapse in patients with cardiac tamponade—a combined echocardiographic and hemodynamic study. Circulation *70*:966, 1984.
104. Ruskin, J., Bache, R. J., Rembert, J. C., and Greenfield, J. C., Jr.: Pressure-flow studies in man: Effect of respiration on left ventricular stroke volume. Circulation *48*:79, 1973.
105. Shabetai, R., Fowler, N. O., Fenton, J. C., and Masangkay, M.: Pulsus paradoxus. J. Clin. Invest. *44*:1882, 1965.
106. Shabetai, R., Fowler, N. O., and Gueron, M.: The effects of respiration on aortic pressure and flow. Am. Heart J. *65*:525, 1963.
107. Savitt, M. A., Tyson, G. S., Elbeery, J. R., et al.: Physiology of cardiac tamponade and paradoxical pulse in conscious dogs. Am. J. Physiol. *265*:H1996, 1993.
108. Gonzales, M. S., Basnight, M. A., Appleton, C. P., et al.: Experimental pericardial effusion: Relation of abnormal respiratory variation in mitral flow velocity to hemodynamics and diastolic right heart collapse. J. Am. Coll. Cardiol. *17*:239, 1991.
109. Settle, H. P., Jr., Engel, P. J., Fowler, N. O., et al.: Echocardiographic study of the paradoxical arterial pulse in chronic obstructive lung disease. Circulation *62*:1297, 1980.
110. Winer, H. E., and Krozon, I.: Absence of paradoxical pulse in patients with cardiac tamponade and atrial septal defects. Am. J. Cardiol. *44*:378, 1979.
111. Cunningham, M. J., Safian, R. D., Come, P. C., and Lorell, B. H.: Absence of pulsus paradoxus in a patient with cardiac tamponade and coexisting pulmonary artery obstruction. Am. J. Med. *83*:973, 1987.
112. Guberman, B. A., Fowler, N. O., Engel, P. J., et al.: Cardiac tamponade in medical patients. Circulation *64*:633, 1981.
113. Beck, C. S.: Two cardiac compression triads. JAMA *104*:714, 1935.
114. Sznajder, J. I., Evander, E., Pollak, E. R., et al.: Pericardial effusion causes interstitial pulmonary edema in dogs. Circulation *76*:843, 1987.
115. Brown, J., MacKinnon, D., King, A., and Vanderbush, E.: Elevated arterial blood pressure in cardiac tamponade. N. Engl. J. Med. *327*:463, 1992.
116. Labib, S. B., Udelson, J. E., and Pandian, N. G.: Echocardiography in low pressure cardiac tamponade. Am. J. Cardiol. *63*:1156, 1989.
117. Katzir, D., Klinovsky, E., Kent, V., et al.: Spontaneous pneumopericardium: Case report and review of the literature. Cardiology *76*:305, 1989.
118. Bricheteau: Observat d'hydropneumopercarde accompane d'un fluctuation perceptible a l'orielle. Arch. Gen. Med. *4*:334, 1844.
119. Usher, B. W., and Popp, R. L.: Electrical alternans: Mechanism in pericardial effusion. Am. Heart J. *83*:459, 1972.
120. Friedman, H. S., Lajam, F., Calderon, J., et al.: Electrocardiographic features of experimental cardiac tamponade in closed-chest dogs. Eur. J. Cardiol. *6*:311, 1977.
121. D'Cruz, I. A., Cohen, H. C., Prabhus, R., and Glick, G.: Diagnosis of cardiac tamponade by echocardiography (changes in mitral valve motion and ventricular dimensions with special reference to paradoxical pulse). Circulation *52*:460, 1975.
122. Appleton, C. P., Hatle, L. K., and Popp, R. L.: Cardiac tamponade and pericardial effusion: Respiratory variation in transvalvular flow velocities studied by Doppler echocardiography. J. Am. Coll. Cardiol. *11*:1020, 1988.
123. Burstow, D. J., Jae, K. O., Baileys, K. R., et al.: Cardiac tamponade: Characteristic Doppler observations. Mayo Clin. Proc. *64*:312, 1989.
124. Shindler, D. M., Reddy, K., Shindler, O. I., and Kostis, J. B.: Failure of the aortic valve to open during inspiration in cardiac tamponade. Chest *82*:797, 1982.
125. Simeonidou, E., Hamouratidis, N., Tzimas, K., et al.: Respiratory variation in mitral flow velocity in pericardial effusion and cardiac tamponade. Angiology *45*:213, 1994.
126. DiSegni, E., Feinberg, M. S., Sheinowitz, M., et al.: Left ventricular

503. Grant, S. C., Levy, R. D., Venning, M. C., et al.: Wegener's granulomatosis and the heart. Br. Heart J. *71*:82, 1994.
504. Csonka, G. W., and Oates, J. K.: Pericarditis and electrocardiographic changes in Reiter's syndrome. Br. Med. J. *1*:866, 1957.
505. Goldman, M. J., and Lau, F. Y. K.: Acute pericarditis associated with serum sickness. N. Engl. J. Med. *250*:278, 1954.
506. Shapiro, L., and Buckingham, R. B.: Septic rheumatoid pericarditis complicating Felty's syndrome. Arthritis Rheum. *24*:1435, 1981.
507. Sonnenblick, M., Nesher, G., and Rosin, A.: Nonclassical organ involvement in temporal arteritis. Semin. Arthritis Rheum. *19*:183, 1989.
508. Sarrouj, B. J., Zampino, D. J., and Cilurso, A. M.: Pericarditis as the initial manifestation of inflammatory bowel disease. Chest *106*:1911, 1994.
509. Cullen, S., Duff, D. F., Denham, B., and Ward, O. C.: Cardiovascular manifestations in Kawasaki disease. Ir. J. Med. Sci. *158*:253, 1989.
510. Zimand, S., Tauber, T., Hegesch, T., and Aladjem, M.: Familial Mediterranean fever presenting with massive cardiac tamponade. Clin. Exp. Rheumatol. *12*:67, 1994.
511. Crake, T., Sandie, G. I., Crisp, A. J., and Record, C. O.: Constrictive pericarditis and intestinal hemorrhage due to Whipple's disease. Postgrad. Med. J. *59*:194, 1983.
512. Dawes, P. T., and Atherton, S. T.: Coeliac disease presenting as recurrent pericarditis. Lancet *1*:1021, 1981.
513. Naschitz, J. E., Yeshurun, D. Miselevich, I., and Boss, J. H.: Colitis and pericarditis in a patient with eosinophilic fasciitis. A contribution to the multisystem nature of eosinophilic fasciitis. J. Rheumatol. *16*:688, 1989.
514. Nicolosi, A. C., Almassi, G. H., and Komorowski, R.: Cardiac tamponade secondary to giant lymph node hyperplasia (Castleman's disease). Chest *105*:637, 1994.
515. Wanner, W. R., Williams, T. E., Fulkerson, P. K., et al.: Postoperative pericarditis following thymectomy for myasthenia gravis. A prospective study. Chest *83*:647, 1983.
516. King, D. L.: Rhabdomyolysis with pericardial tamponade. Ann. Emerg. Med. *23*:583, 1994.
517. Silverman, K. J., Hutchins, G. M., and Bulkley, B. H.: Cardiac sarcoid: A clinicopathologic study of 84 unselected patients with systemic sarcoidosis. Circulation *58*:1204, 1978.
518. Garrett, J., O'Neill, H., and Blake, S.: Constrictive pericarditis associated with sarcoidosis. Am. Heart J. *107*:394, 1984.
519. Diderholm, E., Eklund, A., Orinius, E., and Widstrom, O.: Exudative pericarditis in sarcoidosis. Sarcoidosis *6*:60, 1989.
520. Alarcon-Segovia, D.: Drug-induced lupus syndromes. Mayo Clin. Proc. *44*:664, 1969.
521. Browning, C. A., Bishop, R. L., Heilpern, R. J., et al.: Accelerated constrictive pericarditis in procainamide-induced systemic lupus erythematosus. Am. J. Cardiol. *53*:376, 1984.
522. Harrington, T. M., and Davis, D. E.: Systemic lupus–like syndrome induced by methyldopa therapy. Chest *79*:696, 1981.
523. Lim, A. G., and Hine, K. R.: Fever, vasculitic rash, arthritis, pericarditis, and pericardial effusion after mesalazine. Br. Med. J. *308*:113, 1994.
524. Pent, M. T., Ganapathy, S., Holdsworth, C. D., and Channer, K. C.: Mesalazine induced lupus-like syndrome. Br. Med. J. *308*:113, 1994.
525. Schoenwetter, A. H., and Silber, E. N.: Penicillin hypersensitivity, acute pericarditis and eosinophilia. JAMA *191*:136, 1965.
526. Slater, E. E.: Cardiac tamponade and peripheral eosinophilia in a patient receiving cromolyn sodium. Chest *73*:878, 1978.
527. Dell-Isola, B, Rezgui, N., Thiollieres, J. M., et al.: Acute pericarditis with eosinophilia after ingestion of tryptophan. Rev. Prat. *43*:2563, 1993.
528. Yates, R. C., and Olson, K. B.: Drug-induced pericarditis. Report of three cases due to 6-amino-9-D-psicofuranosylpurine. N. Engl. J. Med. *265*:274, 1961.
529. Krehlik, J. M., Hindson, D. A., Crowley, J. J., Jr., and Knight, L. L.: Minoxidil-associated pericarditis and fatal cardiac tamponade. West. J. Med. *143*:527, 1985.
530. Miller, D. H., and Haas, L. F.: Pneumonitis, pleural effusion and pericarditis following treatment with dantrolene. J. Neurol. Neurosurg. Psych. *47*:553, 1984.
531. Lipworth, B. J., and Oakley, D. G.: Surgical treatment of constrictive pericarditis due to practolol. A case report. J. Cardiovasc. Surg. *29*:408, 1988.
532. Haugtomt, H., and Haerem, J.: Pulmonary edema and pericarditis after inhalation of Teflon fumes. Tidsskr. Nor. Laegeforen *109*:584, 1989.
533. Harbin, A. D., Gerson, M. C., and O'Connell, J. B.: Simulation of acute myopericarditis by constrictive pericardial disease with endomyocardial fibrosis to methysergide therapy. J. Am. Coll. Cardiol. *4*:196, 1984.
534. Bristow, M. R., Thompson, P. D., Martin, R. P., et al.: Early anthracycline toxicity. Am. J. Med. *65*:823, 1978.
535. Cazin, B., Gorin, N. C., Laporte, J. P., et al.: Cardiac complications after bone marrow transplantation. Cancer *57*:2061, 1986.
536. Ratliff, N. B., McMahon, J. T., Shirey, E. K., and Groves, L. K.: Silicone pericarditis. Cleve. Clin. Q. *51*:185, 1984.
537. Fraker, T. D., Jr., Walsh, T. E., Morgan, R. J., and Kim, K.: Constrictive pericarditis after the Beck operation. Am. J. Cardiol. *54*:931, 1984.
538. Sonakul, D., Thakerngpol, K., and Pocaree, P.: Cardiac pathology in 76 thalassemic patients. Birth Defects *23*:177, 1988.
539. Cordioli, E., Tondini, C., Pizzi, C., and Bugiardini, R.: Exudative pericarditis with pleural plaques caused by exposure to asbestos, resolved with steroidal treatment. Minerva Med. *85*:555, 1994.
540. Abdun Nur, D., Marcus, C. S., and Russell, F. E.: Pericarditis associated with scorpionfish (Scorpaena buttata) sting. Toxicon *19*:579, 1981.
541. Dressler, W.: A postmyocardial infarction syndrome. Preliminary report of a complication resembling idiopathic recurrent benign pericarditis. JAMA *160*:1379, 1956.
542. Lichstein, E., Arsura, E., Hollander, G., et al.: Current incidence of postmyocardial infarction (Dressler's) syndrome. Am. J. Cardiol. *50*:1269, 1982.
543. Jerjes-Sanchez, C., Ibarra-Perez, C., Ramirez-Rivera, A., et al.: Dressler-like syndrome after pulmonary embolism and infarction. Chest *92*:115, 1987.
544. Dressler, W.: The post-myocardial infarction syndrome. A report of forty-four cases. Arch. Intern. Med. *103*:28, 1959.
545. Van der Geld, H.: Anti-heart antibodies in the post-pericardiotomy and the post-myocardial infarction syndrome. Lancet *2*:617, 1964.
546. Liem, K. L., ten Veen, J. H., Lie, K. I., et al.: Incidence and significance of heart muscle antibodies in patients with acute myocardial infarction and unstable angina. Acta Med. Scand. *206*:473, 1971.
547. Khan, A. H.: The postcardiac delayed injury syndromes. Clin. Cardiol. *15*:67, 1992.
548. Hutchison, S. J., McKillop, J. H., and Hutton, I.: Failure of gallium-67 citrate imaging to diagnose post-myocardial infarction (Dressler's) syndrome. Eur. J. Nucl. Med. *13*:52, 1987.
549. Madsen, S. M., and Jakobsen, T. J.: Colchicine treatment of recurrent steroid-dependent pericarditis in a patient with post-myocardial-infarction syndrome (Dressler's syndrome). Ugeskr. Laeger *154*:3427, 1992.
550. Goldhaber, S. Z., Lorell, B. H., and Green, L. H.: Constrictive pericarditis. A case requiring pericardiectomy following Dressler's postmyocardial infarction syndrome. J. Thorac. Cardiovasc. Surg. *81*:793, 1981.
551. Kanawaty, D. S., Burggraf, G. W., and Abdollah, H.: Constrictive pericarditis and anemia post myocardial infarction. Can. J. Cardiol. *5*:147, 1989.
552. Soloff, L. A., Zatuchni, J., Janton, D. H., et al.: Reactivation of rheumatic fever following mitral commisurotomy. Circulation *8*:481, 1953.
553. Engle, M. A., and Ito, T.: The postpericardiotomy syndrome. Am. J. Cardiol. *7*:73, 1961.
554. Peters, R. W., Scheinman, M. M., Raskin, S., and Thomas, A. N.: Unusual complications of epicardial pacemakers. Am. J. Cardiol. *45*:1088, 1980.
555. Escaned, J., Ahmad, R. A., and Shiu, M. F.: Pleural effusion following coronary perforation during balloon angioplasty: An unusual presentation of the postpericardiotomy syndrome. Eur. Heart J. *13*:716, 1992.
556. Livelli, F. D., Jr., Johnson, R. A., McEnany, M. T., et al.: Unexplained in-hospital fever following cardiac surgery: Natural history, relationship to postpericardiotomy syndrome and a prospective study of therapy with indomethacin versus placebo. Circulation *57*:968, 1978.
557. Engle, M. A., Gay, W. A., Jr., Zabriskie, J. B., and Senterfit, L. B.: The postpericardiotomy syndrome: 25 years' experience. J. Cardiovasc. Med. *4*:321, 1984.
558. Kaminsky, M. E., Rodan, B. A., Osborne, D. R., et al.: Postpericardiotomy syndrome. Am. J. Radiol. *138*:503, 1982.
559. DeSaulniers, D., Gervais, N., and Rouleau, J.: Does pericardial drainage decrease the frequency of the postpericardiotomy syndrome? Can. J. Surg. *24*:265, 1981.
560. Nkere, U. U., Whawell, S. A., Thompson, J. N., and Taylor, E. M.: Changes in pericardial morphology and fibrinolytic activity during cardiopulmonary bypass. J. Thorac. Cardiovasc. Surg. *106*:339, 1993.
561. Ofori-Krakye, S. K., Tyberg, T. I., Geha, A. S., et al.: Late cardiac tamponade after open heart surgery: Incidence, role of anticoagulants in its pathogenesis and its relationship to the postpericardiotomy syndrome. Circulation *63*:1323, 1981.
562. Kassanoff, A. H., and Martirossian, M. G.: Postpericardiotomy and post-myocardial infarction syndrome presenting as noncardiac pulmonary edema. Chest *99*:1410, 1991.
563. Weitzman, L. B., Tinkler, W. P., Kronzon, I., et al.: The incidence and natural history of pericardial effusion after cardiac surgery—an echocardiographic study. Circulation *69*:506, 1984.
564. King, T. E., Jr., Stelzner, T. J., and Sahn, S. A.: Cardiac tamponade complicating the postpericardiotomy syndrome. Chest *83*:500, 1983.
565. Russo, A. M., O'Connor, W. H., and Waxman, H. L.: Atypical presentations and echocardiographic findings in patients with cardiac tamponade occurring early and later after cardiac surgery. Chest *104*:71, 1993.
566. Terada, Y., Saitoh, T., Shimoyama, Y., et al.: Late cardiac tamponade after open heart surgery. Kyobu Geka *47*:128, 1994.
567. Carrel, T., Jennl, R., Ritter, M., and Turina, M.: Late pericardial tamponade: A dangerous complication of postoperative anticoagulation following heart surgery. Schweiz. Med. Wochenschr. *123*:2401, 1993.
568. D'Cruz, I. A., Overton, D. H., and Pai, G. M.: Pericardial complications of cardiac surgery: Emphasis on the diagnostic role of echocardiography. J. Card. Surg. *7*:257, 1992.
569. Malour, J. F., Alam, S., Gharzeddine, W., and Stefadouros, M. A.: The role of anticoagulation in the development of pericardial effusion and late tamponade after cardiac surgery. Eur. Heart J. *15*:583, 1994.
570. Reichert, C. L., Visser, C. A., Koolen, J. J., et al.: Transesophageal echocardiography in hypotensive patients after cardiac operations. Comparison with hemodynamic parameters. J. Thorac. Cardiovasc. Surg. *104*:321, 1992.
571. Rex, D. K., Rogers, D. W., Mohammed, Y., and Williams, E. S.: Post-cardiac surgery tamponade mimicking acute hepatitis. J. Clin Gastroenterol. *14*:136, 1992.
572. Battle, R. W., and Tischler, M. D.: Late postoperative cardiac tamponade presenting as a pulsatile epigastric mass. Scand. J. Thorac. Cardiovasc. Surg. *27*:183, 1993.

573. Maggiano, H. J., Higgins, T. L., Lobo, W., et al.: Superior vena cava syndrome after open heart surgery. Cleve. Clin. J. Med. *59:*93, 1992.
574. Berge, K. H., Lanier, W. L., and Reeder, G. S.: Occult cardiac tamponade detected by transesophageal echocardiography. Mayo Clin. Proc. *67:*667, 1992.
575. Chuttani, K., Tischler, M. D., Pandian, N. G., et al.: Diagnosis of cardiac tamponade after cardiac surgery: Relative value of clinical, echocardiographic, and hemodynamic signs. Am. Heart J. *127:*913, 1994.
576. Susini, G, Pepi, M., Sisillo, E., et al.: Percutaneous pericardiocentesis versus subxiphoid pericardiotomy in cardiac tamponade due to postoperative pericardial effusion. J. Cardiothorac. Vasc. Anesthesia *7:*178, 1993.
577. Friedrich, S. P., Berman, A. D., Baim, D. S., and Diver, D. J.: Myocardial perforation in the cardiac catheterization laboratory: Incidence, presentation, diagnosis, and management. Cathet. Cardiovasc. Diagn. *32:*99, 1994.
578. Deckers, J. W., Hare, J. M., and Baughman, K. L.: Complications of transvenous right ventricular endomyocardial biopsy in adult patients with cardiomyopathy: A seven-year survey of 546 consecutive diagnostic procedures in a tertiary referral center. J. Am. Coll. Cardiol. *19:*43, 1992.
579. B-Lundqvist, C., Olsson, S. B., and Varnauskas, E.: Transseptal left heart catheterization: A review of 278 studies. Clin. Cardiol. *9:*21, 1986.
580. Goldbaum, T. S., Jacob, A. S., Smith, D. F., et al.: Cardiac tamponade following percutaneous transluminal coronary angioplasty. Cath. Cardiovasc. Diag. *11:*413, 1985.
581. Seggewiss, H., Schmidt, H. K., Mellwig, K. P., et al.: Acute pericardial tamponade after percutaneous transluminal coronary angioplasty (PTCA). Z. Kardiol. *82:*721, 1993.
582. Gunther, H. V., Strupp, G., Volmar, J., et al.: Coronary stent implantation: Infarction and abscess with fatal outcome. Z. Kardiol. *82:*521, 1993.
583. Rosenthal, E., Qureshi, S. A., Sakadekar, A. P., et al.: Technique of percutaneous laser-assisted valve dilatation for valvar atresia in congenital heart disease. Br. Heart J. *69:*556, 1993.
584. Bichel, J.: Serious complications of sternal puncture. Ugeskr. Laeger *151:*442, 1989.
585. Mellon, J. K., Galvin, J. F., Bowe, P. C., et al.: Oesophago-pericardial fistula and cardiac tamponade after oesophagoscopy. Eur. J. Cardiothorac. Surg. *2:*282, 1988.
586. Puhakka, H. J.: Complications of mediastinoscopy. J. Laryngol. Otol. *103:*312, 1989.
587. Brown, D. L., and Luchi, R. J.: Cardiac tamponade and constrictive pericarditis complicating endoscopic sclerotherapy. Arch. Intern. Med. *147:*2169, 1987.
588. Greene, T. O., Portnow, A. S., and Huang, S. K.: Acute pericarditis resulting from an endocardial active fixation screw-in atrial lead. Pacing Clin. Electrophysiol. *17:*21, 1994.
589. Isselbacher, E. M., Cigarroa, J. E., and Eagle, K. A.: Cardiac tamponade complicating proximal aortic dissection. Is pericardiocentesis harmful? Circulation *90:*2375, 1994.
590. Ng, A. S. H., Dorosti, K., and Sheldon, W. C.: Constrictive pericarditis following cardiac surgery—Cleveland Clinic Experience: Report of 12 cases and review. Cleve. Clin. Q. *50:*39, 1984.
591. Cimino, J. J., and Kogan, A. D.: Constrictive pericarditis after cardiac surgery: Report of three cases and review of the literature. Am. Heart J. *118:*1292, 1989.
592. Carrier, M., Hudson, G., Paquet, E., et al.: Mediastinal and pericardial complications after transplantation. Not-so-unusual postoperative problems? Cardiovasc. Surg. *2:*395, 1994.
593. Hinkamp, T. J., Sullivan, H. J., Montoya, A., et al.: Chronic cardiac rejection masking as constrictive pericarditis. Ann. Thorac. Surg. *57:*1579, 1994.
594. Killian, D. M., Furiasse, J. G., Scanlon, P. J., et al.: Constrictive pericarditis after cardiac surgery. Am. Heart J. *118:*563, 1989.
595. Kabbani, S. S., Bashour, T., Ellertson, D. G., et al.: Constrictive pericarditis following myocardial revascularization: A possible cause of graft occlusion. Am. Heart J. *110:*493, 1985.
596. Almassi, G. H., Chapman, R. D., Troup, P. J., et al.: Constrictive pericarditis associated with patch electrodes of the automatic implantable cardioverter-defibrillator. Chest *92:*369, 1987.
597. Kassanoff, A. H., Levin, C. B., Wyndham, C. R., and Mills, L. J.: Implantable cardioverter defibrillator infection causing constrictive pericarditis. Chest *102:*960, 1992.

OTHER FORMS OF PERICARDIAL DISEASE

598. Kerber, R. E., and Sherman, B.: Echocardiographic evaluation of pericardial effusion in myxedema. Incidence and biochemical and clinical correlations. Circulation *52:*823, 1975.
599. Hardisty, C. A., Naik, D. R., and Munro, D. S.: Pericardial effusion in hypothyroidism. Clin. Endocrinol. *13:*349, 1980.
600. Parving, H., Hansen, J. M., Nielsen, S. V., et al.: Mechanisms of edema formation in myxedema-increased protein extravasation and relatively slow lymphatic drainage. N. Engl. J. Med. *301:*460, 1981.
601. Zimmerman, J., Yahalom, J., and Bar-On, H.: Clinical spectrum of pericardial effusion as the presenting feature of hypothyroidism. Am. Heart J. *106:*770, 1983.
602. Meares, N., Brande, S., and Burgess, K.: Massive macroglossia as a presenting feature of hypothyroid-associated pericardial effusion. Chest *104:*1632, 1993.
603. Manolis, A. S., Varriale, P., and Ostrowski, R. M.: Hypothyroid cardiac tamponade. Arch. Intern. Med. *147:*1167, 1987.
604. Rubillon, J. F., Sanchez, B., Vuolo-Figaud, A. M., et al.: Cardiac tamponade in severe hypothyroidism. A rare cause. Presse Med. *22:*1221, 1993.
605. Rosenbau, D. L., and Yu, P. N.: Idiopathic cholesterol pericarditis with effusion. Am. Heart J. *70:*515, 1965.
606. Van Buren, P. C., and Roberts, W. C.: Cholesterol pericarditis and cardiac tamponade with congenital hypothyroidism in adulthood. Am. Heart J. *119:*697, 1990.
607. Ridenhouse, C. E., and Kiphart, R. J.: Idiopathic cholesterol pericarditis treatment with pericardiectomy. Ann. Thorac. Surg. *4:*360, 1967.
608. Stanley, R. J., Subramanian, R., and Lie, J. T.: Cholesterol pericarditis terminating as constrictive calcific pericarditis. Follow-up study of patient with 40-year history of disease. Am. J. Cardiol. *46:*511, 1980.
609. Bhatti, M. A., Ferrante, J. W., Gielchinsky, I., and Norman, J. C.: Pleuropulmonary and skeletal lymphangiomatosis with chylothorax and chylopericardium. Ann. Thorac. Surg. *40:*398, 1985.
610. Rose, D. M., Colvin, S. B., Danilowicz, D., and Isom, O. W.: Cardiac tamponade secondary to chylopericardium following cardiac surgery: Case report and review of the literature. Ann. Thorac. Surg. *34:*333, 1982.
611. Morishita, Y., Taira, A., Furoi, A., et al.: Constrictive pericarditis secondary to primary chylopericardium. Am. Heart J. *109:*373, 1985.
612. Pereira, W. M., Kalil, R. A., Prates, P. R, and Nesralla, I. A.: Cardiac tamponade due to chylopericardium after cardiac surgery. Ann. Thorac. Surg. *46:*572, 1988.
613. Bar-El, Y., Smolinsky, A., and Yellin, A.: Chylopericardium as a complication of mitral valve replacement. Thorax *44:*74, 1989.
614. Meyns, B. P., Faveere, B. C., Van de Werf, F. J., et al.: Constrictive pericarditis due to ingestion of a toothpick. Ann. Thorac. Surg. *57:*489, 1994.
615. Sharland, M. G., and McCaughan, B. C.: Perforation of the esophagus by a fish bone leading to cardiac tamponade. Ann. Thorac. Surg. *56:*969, 1993.
616. Naggar, C. Z., Daly, P. A., Burke, M. J., and Swartz, M. R.: Successful medical management of esophagopericardial fistula. Heart Lung *16:*47, 1987.
617. Variyam, E. P., and Shah, A.: Pericardial effusion and left ventricular function in patients with acute alcoholic pancreatitis. Arch. Intern. Med. *147:*923, 1987.
618. Letoquart, J. P., Fasquel, J. L., L'Huillier, J. P., et al.: Gastropericardial fistula. Review of the literature apropos of an original case. J. Chir. (Paris) *127:*6, 1990.
619. Song, Z. L.: Cholangiothoracic fistulae. Chung Hua Wai Ko Tsa Chih *27:*269, 1989.
620. Isolauri, J., and Markkula, H.: Recurrent ulceration and colopericardial fistula as late complications of colon interposition. Ann. Thorac. Surg. *44:*84, 1987.
621. Ali, I., and Beg, M. H.: Traumatic bronchopericardial fistula presenting as cardiac tamponade. J. Thorac. Cardiovasc. Surg. *95:*740, 1988.
622. Aho, A. J., Vanttinen, E. A., and Nelimarkka, O. I.: Rupture of the pericardium with luxation of the heart after blunt trauma. J. Trauma *27:*560, 1987.
623. Callejas, M. A., Mestres, C. A., Catalan, M., and Sanchez-Lloret, J.: Traumatic intrapericardial diaphragmatic rupture. Thorac. Cardiovasc. Surg. *32:*376, 1984.
624. Kirsch, J. D., and Escarous, A.: CT diagnosis of traumatic pericardium rupture. J. Comput. Assist. Tomogr. *13:*523, 1989.
625. Cassorla, L., and Katz, J. A.: Management of cardiac herniation after intrapericardial pneumonectomy. Anesthesiology *60:*362, 1984.
626. DuBroft, R. J., and Hoffman, I.: Intestinal tamponade: Cardiac compression by intestinal contents. J. Am. Soc. Echocardiogr. *7:*89, 1994.
627. Feigin, D. S., Fenoglio, J. J., McAllister, H. A., and Madewell, J. E.: Pericardial cysts: A radiologic-pathologic correlation and review. Radiology *125:*15, 1977.
628. Hynes, J. K., Tajik, A. J., Osborn, M. J., et al.: Two-dimensional echocardiographic diagnosis of pericardial cyst. Mayo Clin. Proc. *58:*60, 1983.
629. Klatte, E. C., and Yune, H. Y.: Diagnosis and treatment of pericardial cysts. Radiology *104:*541, 1972.
630. Unverferth, D. V., and Wooley, C. F.: The different diagnosis of paracardiac lesions: Pericardial cysts. Cath. Cardiovasc. Diag. *5:*31, 1979.
631. Moncada, R., Baglia, K., Moguillansky, S. J., et al.: CT diagnosis of congenital intrapericardial masses. J. Comput. Assist. Tomogr. *9:*56, 1985.
632. Ellis, K., Leeds, N. E., and Himmelstein, A.: Congenital deficiencies in partial pericardium: Review of two new cases including successful diagnosis by plain roentgenography. Am. J. Roentgenol. *82:*125, 1959.
633. Letanche, G., Gayet, C., Souguet, P. J., et al.: Agenesis of the pericardium: Clinical, echocardiographic and MRI aspects. Rev. Pneumol. Clin. *44:*105, 1988.
634. Taysi, K., Hartmann, A. F., Shackelford, G. D., and Sundarum, V.: Congenital absence of the pericardium in a family. Am. J. Med. Genet. *21:*77, 1985.
635. Cohlmann, H. R., and van Ingen, G. J.: Symptomatic congenital complete absence of the left pericardium. Case report and review of the literature. Eur. Heart J. *10:*670, 1989.

636. Inoue, H., Fujii, J., Mashima, S., and Marao, S.: Pseudo right atrial overloading pattern in complete defect of the left pericardium. J. Electrocardiol. *14*:413, 1981.
637. Candan, I., Erol, C., and Sonel, A.: Cross sectional echocardiographic appearance in presumed congenital absence of the left pericardium. Br. Heart J. *55*:405, 1986.
638. D'Altoria, R. A., and Caro, J. Y.: Congenital absence of the left pericardium detected by imaging of the lung: Case report. J. Nucl. Med. *18*:267, 1977.
639. Gutierrez, F. R., Shackelford, G. D., McKnight, R. C., et al.: Diagnosis of congenital absence of left pericardium by MR imaging. J. Comput. Assist. Tomogr. *9*:551, 1985.
640. Saito, R., and Hotta, F.: Congenital pericardial defect associated with cardiac incarceration: Case Report. Am. Heart J. *100*:866, 1980.
641. Jones, J. W., and McManus, B. M.: Fatal cardiac strangulation by congenital partial pericardial defect. Am. Heart J. *107*:183, 1984.
642. Auch-Schweik, W., Bonzel, T., Krause, T., et al.: Differential diagnosis of chest pain and diagnostic findings in pericardial defects combined with coronary artery disease. Clin. Cardiol. *11*:650, 1988.
643. Altman, C. A., Ettedgui, J. A., Wozney, P., and Beerman, L. B.: Noninvasive diagnostic features of partial absence of the pericardium. Am. J. Cardiol. *63*:1536, 1989.
644. Ruys, F., Paulus, W., Stevens, C., and Brutsaert, D.: Expansion of the left atrial appendage is a distinctive cross-sectional echocardiographic feature of congenital defect of the pericardium. Eur. Heart J. *4*:738, 1983.
645. Wolff, F., Fritz, A., Dumeny, P., and Eisenmann, B.: Diastolic coronary prolapse in partial left pericardial agenesis. Arch. Mal. Coeur. *80*:206, 1987.
646. Minocha, G. K., Falicov, R. E., and Nijensohn, E.: Partial right-sided congenital pericardial defect with herniation of the right atrium and right ventricle. Chest *76*:484, 1979.
647. Bernal, J. M., Lepiedra, J. O., Gonzalez, I., et al.: Angiocardiographic demonstration of partial defect of the pericardium with herniation of the left atrium and ventricle. J. Cardiovasc. Surg. *27*:344, 1986.

Chapter 44
Traumatic Heart Disease

PETER F. COHN, EUGENE BRAUNWALD

NONPENETRATING CARDIAC INJURY 1535
Pericardium .1536
Myocardium .1536
Complications of Cardiac Resuscitation . . .1539
PENETRATING CARDIAC INJURY 1539
INJURIES TO CARDIAC VALVES, PAPILLARY MUSCLES, AND CHORDAE TENDINEAE . . .1541
INJURIES TO THE CORONARY ARTERIES AND GREAT VESSELS 1542
REFERENCES .1544

Violent injury accounts for the majority of deaths in persons under 40 years of age in the United States, and among these victims cardiac trauma is one of the leading causes of death.[1,2] For example, chest injuries are directly responsible for more than 25 per cent of the 50,000 to 60,000 deaths that result annually from automobile accidents and contribute significantly to another 25 per cent of these deaths.[3] The increasing frequency of physical violence has also resulted in a corresponding increase in the incidence of traumatic heart disease, especially in *young adult males.* These are the most frequent victims, because they are more likely to have automobile and motorcycle accidents, to incur injuries while performing heavy labor, and, as the daily headlines attest, to be involved in or victims of acts of physical violence.

The frequency of these mishaps is increasing. In Houston,[4] a 30-year analysis of 4459 patients with cardiovascular injuries (86 per cent of whom were males) showed a steady rise between 1958 (averaging 27 patients/yr) and 1988 (213 patients/yr) (Table 44–1). In addition, the incidence of medically-related cardiac trauma is also rising, such as increased use of intravascular and intracardiac catheters leading to penetrating injuries of the heart and great vessels, and resuscitative cardiac massage causing a variety of nonpenetrating injuries of these organs.

The two principal, immediate consequences of cardiac injury are *exsanguinating hemorrhage* and *cardiac tamponade.* Effective treatment has resulted in an increasing number of immediate survivors, and later sequelae— including myocardial infarction, ventricular aneurysm and pseudoaneurysm, ventricular septal defect, valvular damage, recurrent pericarditis, and constrictive pericarditis—are becoming far more common. Serious cardiac trauma is frequently overlooked in patients with nonpenetrating injury, particularly when other structures such as the thoracic cage and lungs are obviously damaged. Such oversight can be tragic, because the lethal consequences of cardiac injury may suddenly emerge after the superficial injuries have been attended to. Clearly, a much higher index of suspicion of this possibility is necessary if the increasing magnitude of this problem is to be halted and reversed.

NONPENETRATING CARDIAC INJURY

Nonpenetrating injuries result from the effects of external physical forces, but it is important to recognize that these forces need not necessarily be applied directly to the chest, because injuries to the heart and great vessels may also occur with trauma to other parts of the body.

The most common cause of nonpenetrating injury in civilian life is probably that directly related to *vehicular impact,*[5] either by direct compression, usually with the steering wheel squeezing the heart between the sternum and the spine, or by indirect compression. Causes of nonpenetrating injuries other than automobile and motorcycle accidents include direct blows to the chest by any kind of blunt object or missile, such as a clenched fist and various kinds of sporting equipment, as well as by the kicks of animals, falls, and cardiac resuscitative procedures. Fractures of the bony structures of the chest wall *are not* necessary accompaniments of cardiac injury in any of these situations. This point is of crucial importance, because *the absence of such obvious injuries following trauma should by no means exclude the possibility of nonpenetrating injury to the heart.* The clinical manifestations may not be apparent for days or even weeks after the accident.

Pathological findings following nonpenetrating cardiac injury usually include some degree of *pericarditis,* which may be associated with the late development of *pericardial constriction.* Changes in the heart itself range from minute ecchymotic areas in the subepicardium or subendocardium to transmural contusions with edematous, fragmented, or necrotic muscle fibers, surrounded at first by red blood cells and invaded soon thereafter by polymorphonuclear leukocytes. The external appearance of the heart may be misleading in the case of nonpenetrating injury, as large areas of intramural contusion, including involvement of the interventricular septum, may not be apparent.[6] In patients who survive the injury, healing is by scar formation resembling that following acute myocardial infarction, and post-traumatic aneurysms resembling postinfarction aneurysms may develop.[7] The types of cardiac injury resulting from blunt (nonpenetrating) trauma are listed in Table 44–2, the

TABLE 44–1 ETIOLOGY OF PATIENT CARDIOVASCULAR INJURIES: 1958–1988

ETIOLOGY	1958–63	1964–69	1970–73	1974–78	1979–83	1984–88	TOTAL
Gunshot wound	42	236	436	501	625	456	2296
Stab/laceration	64	110	161	229	362	463	1389
Blunt trauma	1	17	58	90	62	76	304
Shotgun wound	1	15	45	55	61	37	214
Iatrogenic	1	1	0	0	4	25	31
Other/unknown	54	20	111	25	3	12	225
Total	163	399	811	900	1117	1069	4459

From Mattox, K. L., et al.: Five thousand seven hundred sixty cardiovascular injuries in 4459 patients: Epidemiologic evaluation 1958 to 1988. Ann. Surg. *209*:698, 1989.

TABLE 44–2 TYPES OF CARDIAC INJURY FROM BLUNT TRAUMA

A. MYOCARDIUM
1. Contusion
2. Laceration
3. Rupture
4. Septal perforation
5. Aneurysm, pseudoaneurysm
6. Hemopericardium, tamponade
7. Thrombosis, systemic embolism

B. PERICARDIUM
1. Pericarditis
2. Postpericardiotomy syndrome
3. Constrictive pericarditis
4. Pericardial laceration
5. Hemorrhage
6. Cardiac herniation

C. ENDOCARDIAL STRUCTURES
1. Rupture of papillary muscle
2. Rupture of chordae tendineae
3. Rupture of atrioventricular and semilunar valves

D. CORONARY ARTERY
1. Thrombosis
2. Laceration
3. Fistula

From Jackson, D. H., and Murphy, G. W.: Nonpenetrating cardiac trauma. Mod. Conc. Cardiovasc. Dis. *45*:123, 1976. Copyright 1976 American Heart Association.

most severe forms being rupture of the aortic or mitral valve and rupture of the interventricular septum or even of the free wall of a cardiac chamber. The relative incidences of the various consequences of nonpenetrating cardiac trauma are shown in Table 44–3.

TABLE 44–3 NONPENETRATING CARDIAC TRAUMA

TYPE AND/OR SITE OF INJURY	NO. OF CASES	CASES COMBINED WITH AORTIC RUPTURE	TOTAL
Rupture	273	80	353
Right ventricle	56	10	66
Left ventricle	46	13	59
Right atrium	35	6	41
Left atrium	24	2	26
IV septum	25(20*)	7(4*)	32(24*)
IA septum	18(10*)	5(3*)	23(13*)
Multiple chamber ruptures	69	37	106
Contusion/laceration	105	24	129
Pericardial laceration	18	18	36
Hemopericardium	13	12	25
Valvular laceration/rupture	1(2†)	0(4†)	1(6†)
Aortic valve	1(1†)	0(2†)	1(3†)
Pulmonic valve	0(4†)	0	0(4†)
Tricuspid valve	0(8†)	0	0(8†)
Mitral valve	0(8†)	0(1†)	0(9†)
Mitral and tricuspid valves	0(1†)	0(1†)	0(2†)
Coronary artery laceration/rupture	0(7†)	1(2†)	1(9†)
Papillary muscle laceration/rupture	1(23†)	0	1(23†)
TOTAL	411	135	546

Numbers in parentheses indicate more significant associated cardiac injuries (tabulated in another column).
* Associated with other sites of cardiac rupture.
† Combined with cardiac rupture or other cardiac injury.
From Parmley, L. F., et al.: Nonpenetrating traumatic injury of the heart. Circulation *18*:371, 1958. Copyright 1958 American Heart Association.

Pericardium

Injury to the pericardium in blunt trauma may range from contusion to laceration or rupture. Whether the pericardium tears or not, some degree of traumatic pericarditis is found at autopsy or operation in most patients sustaining severe blunt trauma of the chest, especially of the precordial area. In their classic study Parmley et al. reported pericardial laceration or rupture in 249 of 546 autopsy cases of nonpenetrating trauma to the heart[8]; however, it should be noted that this rarely occurs as an isolated lesion (Table 44–3) and is usually associated with cardiac contusion and even more serious cardiac injury. On the basis of a series of landmark experiments in a canine model, in which 14 of 18 dogs receiving sublethal blunt chest trauma developed pericardial rents, DeMuth et al. suggested that a higher frequency of pericardial tears than is generally appreciated occurs in survivors of chest trauma.[9] Clinically, a tear in the pericardium can occur as a consequence of blunt trauma, and delayed herniation of the heart through the rent may then compromise circulatory function acutely.

CLINICAL FEATURES AND DIAGNOSIS. Traumatic pericarditis is manifested by the development of a typical pericardial friction rub and ST–T-wave changes on the electrocardiogram characteristic of pericarditis (see p. 1482). During and immediately following the acute episode, the major problem is not the pericarditis itself but its most common complications, i.e., hemopericardium and resultant tamponade, discussed on page 1486. Commonly, the patient is restless, with hypotension, oliguria or anuria, distant heart sounds, and pulsus paradoxus. There is usually diffuse low voltage on the electrocardiogram. Pericardial fluid on the echocardiogram (see p. 1486) is a key finding.[10]

TREATMENT AND PROGNOSIS. As a rule, uncomplicated pericarditis secondary to cardiac trauma simply resolves. Tamponade, however, requires emergency operative treatment, as discussed below. Recurrent pericardial effusions sometimes associated with chest pain and fever, i.e., the so-called postpericardiotomy syndrome, occur in a small number of patients. The cause of this syndrome is not clear (see p. 1520). Although patients with recurrent effusion usually respond to aspirin or nonsteroidal antiinflammatory agents, occasionally glucocorticosteroids are necessary. *Constrictive pericarditis* (see p. 1496) occurs as a rare complication of traumatic pericarditis, with or without recurrent effusions.

Myocardium

CONTUSION. Myocardial contusion usually produces no significant symptoms and often goes unrecognized. At times, manifestations of the injury are masked by injury to the chest wall or other organs.[6,11,12] This is important because as many as 75 per cent of patients with myocardial contusion can have signs of external chest injury.[13] Thus there is a higher frequency of diagnosis of cardiac contusion associated with increasing awareness of the lesion.

Clinical Features and Diagnosis. The most common symptom of myocardial contusion is precordial pain resembling that of myocardial infarction, but the pain from other sites of chest trauma can confuse the clinical picture.[12,13] As with myocardial infarction, nitroglycerin and related drugs have little effect in relieving the pain. The *electrocardiogram* probably represents one of the most helpful tools for recognizing contusion of the left ventricle. Either nonspecific ST–T abnormalities or the classic findings of pericarditis are the most common changes noted. Initially, electrocardiographic signs of deeper injury to the myocardium, i.e., pathological Q waves, may be dwarfed by pericardial inflammation; only as the latter subsides does injury to the myocardium become more evident. However, because the possibility of cardiac trauma is often not considered in trauma victims, an electrocardiogram is often not recorded immediately on patients with chest injuries and

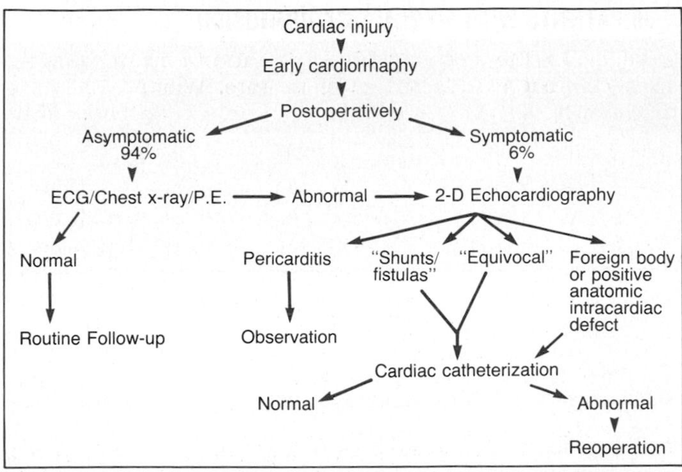

FIGURE 44–1. A recommended decision schema for post-traumatic cardiac evaluation. Following cardiac injury, repair is generally carried out by simple cardiorrhaphy. This algorithm shows a suggested approach to detect residual damage following emergency cardiorrhaphy. (From Mattox, K. L., et al.: Cardiac evaluation following heart injury. J. Trauma *25*:758, © by Williams and Wilkins, 1985.)

the diagnosis may be missed. Just as in acute myocardial infarction, serial findings, i.e., the evolution of Q waves and the subsidence of the ST-segment and T-wave abnormalities, are crucial. The sensitivity and specificity of electrocardiographic findings are less than 100 per cent, however; hence the need for additional tests.

A recommended decision schema for evaluating cardiac injury immediately after early cardiorrhaphy (suturing of the heart) is depicted in Figure 44–1.

SERUM ENZYMES. Because *enzyme levels* may be elevated by trauma to noncardiac as well as to cardiac tissue, they too are of limited diagnostic value. With the widespread availability of reliable measurements of the MB band of creatine kinase (CK), the presence or absence of cardiac necrosis can be better documented in patients with blunt trauma. Indeed, with the electrocardiogram and CK-MB as screening tests, the detection of myocardial contusion has increased from 7 to 17 per cent in patients with blunt chest trauma entering the Henry Ford Hospital.[14] Similarly, at the Mayo Clinic 58 of 291 such patients (20 per cent) had elevations of CK-MB.[15] However, false-positive elevations of the CK-MB isoenzyme can also be seen if the total CK is greater than 20,000 units; this can occur after massive injury to skeletal muscle.

RADIONUCLIDE IMAGING (see Chap. 9). Myocardial perfusion is reduced in areas of myocardial contusion. Contused myocardium concentrates ^{99m}Tc-pyrophosphate in amounts comparable to those observed in ischemic injury. Scanning following injection of radioactive thallium to detect areas of reduced perfusion and of labeled pyrophosphate to locate areas of recent necrosis may be expected to identify patients with myocardial damage following blunt trauma, to localize this damage, and to indicate the extent of the damage. Radionuclide ventriculography often shows a reduced ventricular ejection fraction in such patients. These tests show changes similar to those observed in patients with acute myocardial infarction (Chap. 37). Sutherland et al.[16] used radionuclide ventriculography to define focal defects in ventricular wall motion. They subgrouped the 43 patients whom they studied into those with right ventricular abnormalities (18), left ventricular abnormalities (4), biventricular abnormalities (6), and neither kind (15). They described the state of right ventricular pump function using modified ventricular function curves and found it to be surprisingly well preserved. Schamp et al. also found a high (83 per cent) frequency of right ventricular abnormalities in the 40 patients they studied.[17]

ECHOCARDIOGRAPHY. In addition to identifying pericardial effusion, *two-dimensional echocardiography* is also useful in evaluating cardiac injuries, including myocardial contusion. Such findings as abnormal wall motion and chamber enlargement can be detected with this technique. Echocardiography is useful when the patient with suspected cardiac injury first undergoes testing, as well as after emergency thoracotomy and cardiac repair in an effort to detect residual cardiac damage. When confirmed with pulsed-Doppler echocardiography, intracardiac shunts and regurgitant lesions can be demonstrated.

Because patients with severe chest wall injuries often have suboptimal transthoracic echocardiographic results, the development of the transesophageal approach has significantly added to the value of echocardiography in diagnosing cardiac injury. For example, Karalis et al.[10] reported that 20 of 105 patients whose transthoracic echocardiographic results were nondiagnostic had wall motion abnormalities on transesophageal echocardiography. The spectrum of myocardial injury detected by the combined techniques in their study is depicted in Figure 44–2.

ARRHYTHMIAS. A wide variety of arrhythmias is common with areas of extensive contusion, and ventricular tachycardia that degenerates into ventricular fibrillation represents a frequent cause of death in these patients, although atrial fibrillation is also commonly associated with a poor outcome.[6] The precise mechanism responsible for these arrhythmias has not been defined. In addition, both atrioventricular and intraventricular conduction defects, as well as sinus node dysfunction, are seen.[19,20] Blunt impact to the chest can also lead to cardiac arrest *without* obvious signs of structural injury.[20a] In contrast to acute myocardial infarction, cardiac contusion rarely leads to severe *heart failure* unless massive damage to a valve or rupture of the interventricular septum has occurred.[21,22] However, some impairment of right and/or left ventricular function, as reflected in depressed ejection fractions and ventricular function (myocardial performance) curves, may be found.[16] In the animal model, alcohol ingestion potentiates the effect of blunt trauma on the myocardium.[23] This gives added strength to the warning not to mix drinking and driving.

Treatment and Prognosis. In this era of progressively earlier ambulation of patients with acute myocardial infarction, a similar approach appears to be reasonable after several days of close observation for myocardial contusion. Several groups have concluded that in trauma patients in stable condition, contusion neither increases the complication rate nor necessitates intensive care unit monitoring.[24,25] In a study from the Boston City Hospital, Cachecho et al.[11] prospectively divided 336 patients admitted to the surgical intensive care unit with possible myocardial contusion into three groups: (1) those with a normal electrocardiogram, (2) those with an abnormal one, and (3) those with either normal or abnormal electrocardiograms but with many associated thoracic or extrathoracic injuries. Noninvasive studies were most abnormal in the latter group (Table 44–4), who were also the oldest (mean age 40). Cardiac complications were absent in Groups 1 and 2 as opposed to 19/138 in Group 3. The authors concluded that young patients with minor blunt trauma and a normal or slightly abnormal electrocardiogram do not benefit from cardiac monitoring. From the point of view of physical activity, we recommend treating these patients in a manner similar to that for those with acute myocardial infarction with comparable extent of myocardial damage (Chap. 37). However, treatment with *anticoagulants and obviously with thrombolytics* is con-

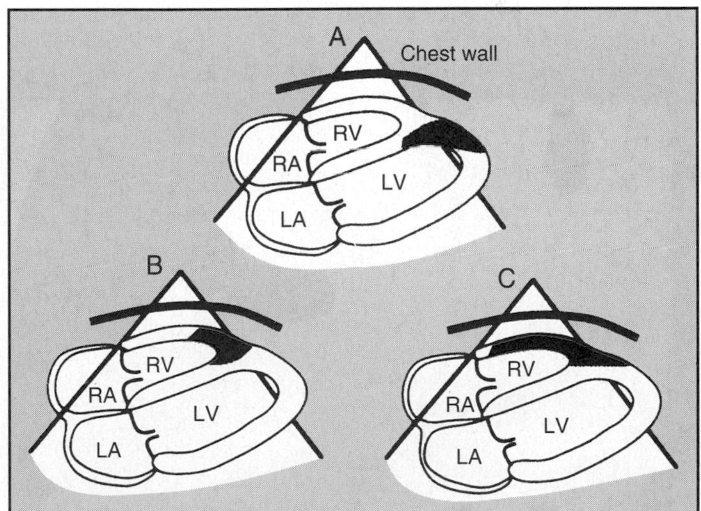

FIGURE 44–2. Spectrum of myocardial injury detected by echocardiography among 105 patients. When the left ventricle (LV) was injured, the myocardial contusion was limited to a small area of the LV spectrum and apex (A). When the right ventricle (RV) was injured, the myocardial contusion in 72 per cent of patients (B) was limited to a small area of the RV anteroapical wall; however, in the other 28 per cent (C) the myocardial contusion was extensive, involving most of the anterior RV wall and apex. LA = left atrium, RA = right atrium. (From Karalis, D. G., et al.: The role of echocardiography in blunt chest trauma: A transthoracic and transesophageal echocardiographic study. J. Trauma *36*:53, © by Williams and Wilkins, 1994.)

TABLE 44–4 RESULTS OF NONINVASIVE STUDIES IN 36 PATIENTS WITH MYOCARDIAL CONTUSION

	GROUP 1		GROUP 2		GROUP 3	
	NO. OF STUDIES	NO. POSITIVE (%)	NO. OF STUDIES	NO. POSITIVE (%)	NO. OF STUDIES	NO. POSITIVE (%)
CPK-MB*	155	1 (0.6)	43	0 (0)	138	2 (1.4)
2D-Echo†	56	0 (0)	28	0 (0)	56	3 (5.3)
GBP‡	65	3 (4.6)	30	2 (6.6)	66	10 (15)
ECG§	155	0 (0)	43	43 (100)	138	44 (32)

All group 2 patients had an abnormal trauma floor ECG; % positive in parentheses.
* CPK-MB = Creatine phosphokinase myocardial band.
† Echo = two-dimensional echocardiography.
‡ GBP = gated blood pool scan.
§ ECG = serial electrocardiograms.
From Cachecho, R., et al.: The clinical significance of myocardial contusion. J. Trauma *33*:68–73, 1992. © by Williams and Wilkins, 1992.

traindicated, because intramyocardial or intrapericardial hemorrhage may be precipitated or exacerbated. Atrial fibrillation, when present, usually reverts to sinus rhythm spontaneously. If it does not, digitalis glycosides may be used to slow the ventricular rate and may also cause reversion to sinus rhythm. Chest pain is best treated with analgesics; nonsteroidal antiinflammatory agents are not advised because they might interfere with myocardial healing (see p. 1210). When the postcardiac injury syndrome occurs, corticosteroids have proved helpful.[26]

As already noted, the prognosis for complete or partial recovery is generally excellent, but these patients require careful follow-up to observe for late complications, ranging from ventricular arrhythmias to cardiac rupture. Coronary occlusion,[27–29] aorto–right atrial fistula,[30] and ventricular aneurysms (Fig. 44–3)[7] are occasional sequelae, and there is no agreement about whether or not surgical resection of the last-named is required. It is our policy to use the presence of heart failure as an indication for operation of aneurysms analogous to that in patients with postinfarct aneurysms (see p. 1256). Pseudoaneurysms, however, require immediate repair (see p. 1242).

Although many analogies can be drawn between the cardiac necrosis caused by trauma and that caused by ischemic heart disease, a number of crucial differences must be emphasized. Patients with acute myocardial infarction secondary to coronary artery disease generally have diffuse, obstructive, gradually progressive coronary atherosclerosis, are frequently middle-aged or elderly, and may have underlying heart disease such as that secondary to prolonged hypertension or diabetes mellitus; patients with traumatic myocardial contusion generally have normal coronary vessels and only a discrete area of myocardial damage; most often, they are young and without underlying cardiovascular illness. Hence, the long-term prognosis in surviving patients with myocardial necrosis secondary to trauma tends to be far better than in patients with myocardial infarction secondary to atherosclerotic coronary artery disease.

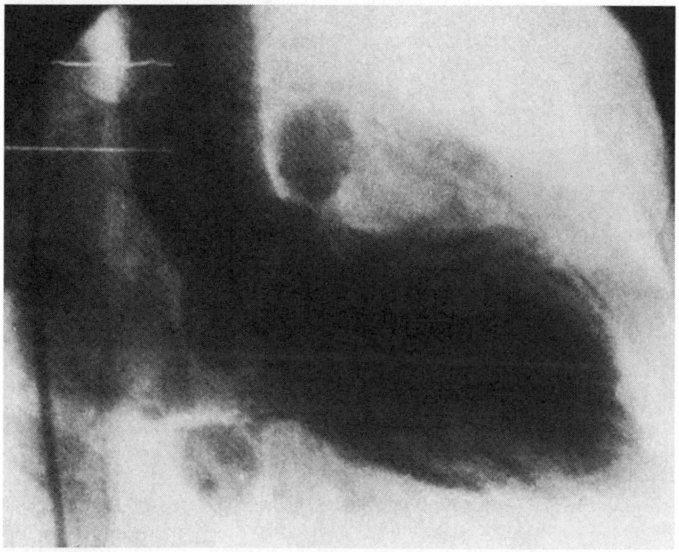

FIGURE 44–3. Right anterior oblique left ventriculogram. Submitral aneurysms appear as saccular narrow-necked structures at superior and inferior portions of mitral annulus during diastole. Top of inferior aneurysm is compressed by left atrium. (From Matthews, R. V., et al.: Chest trauma and subvalvular left ventricular aneurysms. Chest *95*:474, 1989.)

CARDIAC RUPTURE. There appear to be two mechanisms of cardiac rupture: (1) acute laceration due to compression of the heart by direct force, and (2) contusion and hemorrhage leading to necrosis, softening, and rupture several days following the trauma.[31] Rupture of a cardiac chamber usually, but not always, results in immediate death. It is this minority of patients who survive the initial trauma that must be assessed and treated immediately in the emergency department setting.[32]

Clinical Features and Diagnosis. In the patient who survives the first few minutes of cardiac rupture, the clinical picture of cardiac tamponade described above is common. Although ventricular rupture is far more common than is atrial rupture, the latter occurs particularly following automobile accidents, as detailed in a series of 63 patients reported from Tokyo (Fig. 44–4).[33] Wearing a seatbelt does not necessarily prevent this complication of motor vehicle accidents, as noted in a large series from Helsinki.[34] Rupture of the interventricular septum should be suspected in patients who develop severe congestive heart failure immediately or within several days of the trauma, together with a new holosystolic murmur along the left sternal border; however, trauma to the mitral valve apparatus, which may be manifested with a similar picture clinically, must be excluded. On the basis of a series of 546 autopsy cases of nonpenetrating injury to the heart, the incidence of rupture of the ventricular septum has been estimated by Parmley et al. to be almost 10 per cent, with a similar number of patients experiencing rupture of the atrial septum (Table 44–3).[8] These lesions may occur without other serious cardiac injuries, but occasionally other abnormalities are present, including valve cusp perforations and a variety of intracardiac shunts. Although the predilection for perforation of the ventricular septum is highest at the apex, any portion of the muscular septum may be involved, and multiple perforations are not uncommon. The diagnosis of ventricular septal defect and of damage to the mitral valve apparatus can be confirmed by means of catheterization, demonstration of an oxygen step-up in the right ventricle, left ventricular angiography, as well as by color-flow Doppler echocardiography[10,18] (see p. 1541).

Treatment and Prognosis. Patients with external rupture of the heart obviously require emergency surgery if they are to have any chance of survival. Although operation should not be postponed, pericardiocentesis and expansion of the intravascular volume can be carried out while the most rapid preparations possible for operation are undertaken. Successful surgical treatment of external

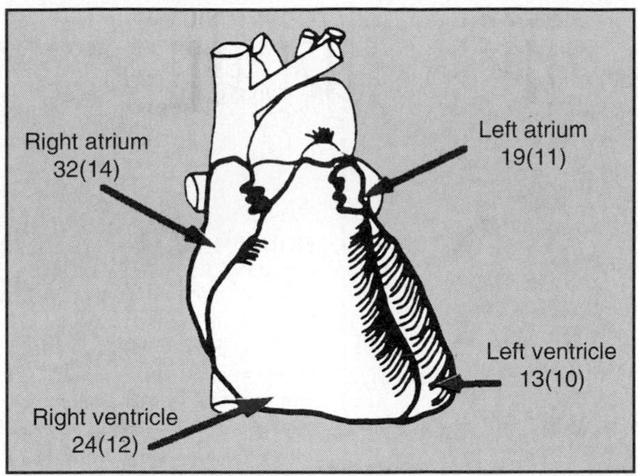

FIGURE 44–4. Location of cardiac rupture. There were 20 cases with multiple chamber injuries. Fourteen had two chambers ruptured, five had three chambers ruptured, and one had four chambers ruptured. In parentheses are numbers of multiple chamber injuries. (From Kato, K., et al.: Blunt traumatic rupture of the heart: An experience in Tokyo. J. Trauma *36*:859, © by Williams and Wilkins, 1994.)

cadiac rupture has been reported in a small number of cases.[33–35] In contrast, patients with rupture of the interventricular septum do not always require emergency operation. Indeed, many defects are small, with minimal left-to-right shunts, and may even heal spontaneously. If heart failure develops subsequently, as occurs in many patients, surgical correction should be carried out promptly and is often successful.[36]

Complications of Cardiac Resuscitation

Closed-chest (external) cardiac massage (see p. 763) is generally thought to be safe and simple—so much so that it is included as part of the cardiopulmonary resuscitation technique taught to lay persons. What is not sufficiently appreciated is that the procedure itself can result in serious complications, which may go unrecognized because many of the patients succumb to the cardiac arrest itself.[37] Even at postmortem examination, the complications may be improperly attributed to the underlying cardiac disease.

Rupture of the left ventricle is a more common complication of cardiac massage than is rupture of the right ventricle. However, rupture of either chamber may occur and may be life-threatening if the patient survives the arrhythmia that necessitated massage in the first place. Because in most instances external resuscitation is performed for patients with myocardial infarction, it may not always be clear whether the left ventricular rupture preceded the massage or occurred as a consequence of it.

Rupture of right ventricular papillary muscles with acute tricuspid regurgitation has also been reported as a complication of closed-chest cardiac massage, as has rupture of the atria and aorta and dissecting hematoma of a coronary artery.[38] A variety of noncardiovascular traumatic lesions, such as fracture of the sternum, hemothorax, pneumothorax, and laceration of abdominal organs may occur. Because of the efficacy of cardiopulmonary resuscitation and its increasing use by paramedical personnel and lay people, an increasing number of such complications may be anticipated in the future. This increased incidence will be stemmed only by educational programs for all individuals likely to employ this technique.

PENETRATING CARDIAC INJURY

Penetrating cardiac injuries occurring in civilian life are due to a variety of objects, such as bullets, knives, ice picks, and the like. The demographics of penetrating cardiac trauma in Jefferson County, Alabama were reviewed by Naughton, et al.[39] As with blunt trauma, male victims predominated and gunshot wounds were the major mechanism of injury. Penetrating injuries may also be due to the inward displacement of ribs or sternal fragments accompanying chest injuries. The chamber most commonly involved in this type of injury is the right ventricle because of its anterior position, followed, in descending order of frequency, by the left ventricle, the right atrium, and the left atrium. However, penetrating wounds of the precordium are not the only types of wounds that may result in cardiac injury. Occasionally, wounds of other areas of the chest, as well as of the neck and upper abdomen, are associated with penetration of the heart. In addition, intravenous or intracardiac catheters may fracture and become impaled within the walls of a great vessel or cardiac chamber (Chap. 6). Migration of an indwelling venous catheter into the pulmonary artery, which may ultimately lead to perforation of this vessel, is another complication that has increased in frequency with its widespread use in intensive care units. Formerly, thoracotomy was necessary to remove these catheter fragments, but catheters with snares and other devices are now available for this purpose.[40,44]

Perforation of the right ventricle with a transvenous pacing electrode is not uncommon, but tamponade is rare. During cardiac catheterization, perforation of the thin-walled right atrium or outflow tract of the right ventricle has been reported. Such patients usually require only careful observation, but when tamponade occurs, immediate drainage is mandatory. Coronary angioplasty[42] and endomyocardial biopsy[43,44] can also result in tamponade. Dissection of the aorta or arch vessels has been reported as a complication of retrograde arterial catheterization and occasionally is also severe enough to require operative intervention.

Penetrating wounds of the heart often result in laceration of the pericardium, sometimes occurring alone but usually associated with laceration of the myocardium itself. One or more chambers but also the cardiac valves and their accessory structures, as well as the interventricular and interatrial septa, may be perforated. Occasionally, low-velocity missiles may penetrate the cardiac chambers but may be retained within the myocardium.

The most common penetrating injuries resulting from physical violence are stab and gunshot wounds.[2,39,45] The former do not necessarily cause extensive cellular destruction adjacent to the wound; they resemble surgical incisions, and transmural wounds in the thick-walled left ventricle may actually seal quickly without disastrous consequences. In contrast, bullet wounds are associated with bleeding that is not usually self-limited and extensive cellular destruction in and adjacent to the path of the bullet. When a coronary artery is lacerated or perforated, myocardial infarction may ensue.

CLINICAL FEATURES AND DIAGNOSIS. The clinical picture of a penetrating wound of the heart depends on several factors, including the object responsible for the injury (e.g., bullet, knife, ice pick), the size of the wound, and the precise location of the structures injured. Pericardial laceration occurring by itself is uncommon and of relatively little significance unless infection supervenes. Rather, the injuries to underlying cardiac structures usually determine the clinical presentation, course, and choice of treatment. However, the nature of the pericardial wound is important, i.e., whether or not the wound is open and allows free drainage of intrapericardial blood. If the pericardium remains open and extravasated blood can pass freely into the pleural cavities or mediastinum, cardiac tamponade will not develop, at least initially, and the presenting signs and symptoms will be those of hemorrhage and hemothorax. On the other hand, if the pericardium does *not* permit free drainage because its opening has been obliterated by a blood clot, adjacent lung tissue, or other structures, or because a flap develops in the pericardial rent, immediate exsanguination may be averted, but tamponade may occur

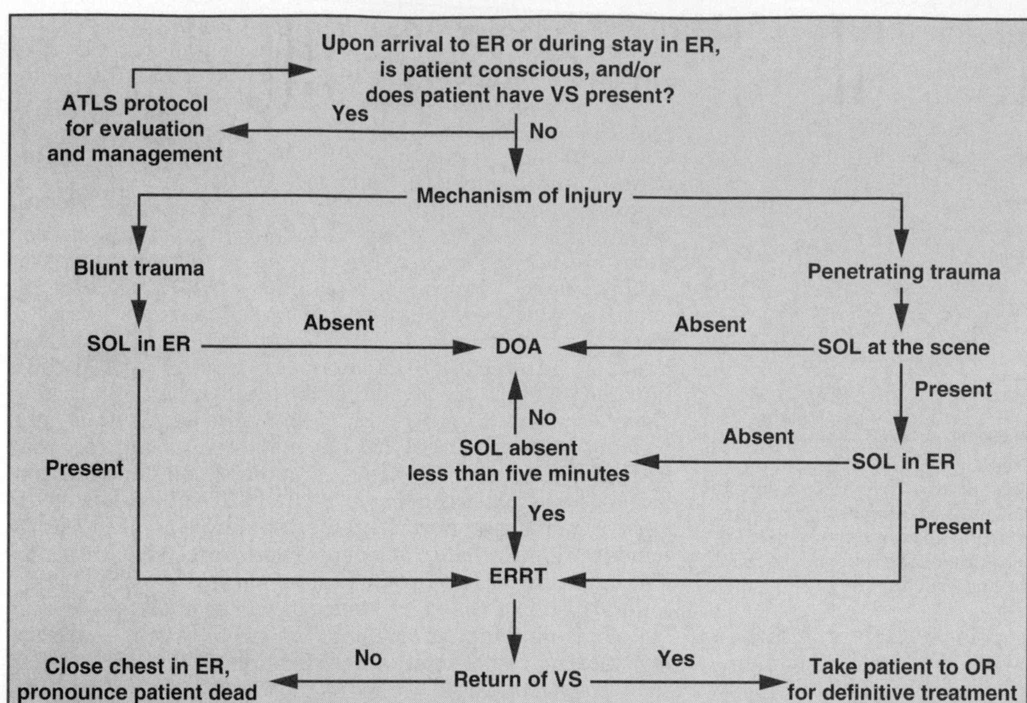

FIGURE 44–5. Emergency room resuscitative thoracotomy algorithm. ER = emergency room, ATLS = advanced trauma life support, SOL = signs of life, DOA = dead on arrival, ERRT = emergency room resuscitative thoracotomy, VS = vital signs. (From Boyd, M., et al.: Emergency room resuscitative thoracotomy: When is it indicated? J. Trauma *33:*714, © by Williams and Wilkins, 1994.)

minutes or hours later. In some instances, blood accumulates both intra- and extrapericardially.

Whether the hemorrhage is intra- or extrapericardial, its severity can often be surmised from the clinical picture. Traumatic penetrating lesions of the heart are usually associated with injuries to the lungs and other organs, which may predominate at first; a high index of suspicion of cardiac penetration is necessary when patients are evaluated following thoracic or upper abdominal trauma. Although extensive injuries to the pericardium and underlying heart are usually immediately fatal or result in shock, delayed clinical manifestations of cardiac injury as a result of hemorrhage, infection, retained foreign bodies, or arrhythmias may become apparent after the other bodily injuries have been attended to. Failure to give serious consideration to the possibility that *cardiac* damage has occurred in a patient with obvious noncardiac trauma may lead to an unanticipated catastrophe.

Although echocardiography is extremely valuable in the recognition of pericardial effusion[10,18,20,46] (see p. 93), foreign bodies in the heart,[47] and intracardiac shunts,[10,18,48,49] it is not always readily available in an emergency setting. When agitation, cool and clammy skin, neck vein distention, pulsus paradoxus, and other classic findings of tamponade (considered earlier) are present, the diagnosis can be relatively simple; in patients without such typical findings, the clinical picture may be attributed to blood loss, especially since volume expansion can improve the hemodynamic state, at least temporarily. Whether or not pericardiocentesis should be performed as a diagnostic test is controversial. If nonclotting blood is obtained, the diagnosis of hemopericardium is confirmed, and the accompanying decompression may constitute effective, albeit temporary, initial treatment. If the pericardiocentesis is negative, however, cardiac tamponade cannot be ruled out. Because, as discussed later, the primary management in any event is thoracotomy, it seems pointless to waste valuable time with pericardial aspiration unless there is doubt regarding the diagnosis.

MANAGEMENT. The definitive treatment of cardiac wounds *accompanied by severe hemorrhage* is immediate thoracotomy and cardiorrhaphy.[50] Although multiple pericardiocenteses are no longer considered a substitute for thoracotomy in the treatment of cardiac wounds associated with cardiac tamponade, there may still be a role for pericardial aspiration *while the patient is being prepared for operation*. The availability in many hospitals of surgical teams and equipment for cardiopulmonary bypass has permitted the safe and effective repair of many penetrating injuries of the heart.

Emergency department resuscitative thoracotomy has also been advocated in selected instances. (Figure 44–5 illustrates one proposed algorithm).[51,52] The best survival rate is in those patients with penetrating wounds and signs of life present in the emergency department. It is therefore not surprising that successful prehospital resuscitative measures can increase the success of a hospital emergency procedure.[53] A novel approach to hospital emergency thoracotomy cardiac stapling was successfully used in 28 patients with penetrating cardiac injuries at the San Francisco General Hospital[54] between 1987 and 1992. This technique also prevents the surgeon from exposure to contaminated needle sticks while suturing the heart. Operative treatment includes repair of the pericardium, myocardium, aorta, and valves as well as of any lacerations of the coronary arteries. At operation, the heart and great vessels should be thoroughly examined for the presence of multiple wounds. When the bullet has penetrated the anterior wall of the heart, the posterior wall should always be inspected for an exit wound before the chest is closed. Many victims of penetrating cardiac injury, young and other-

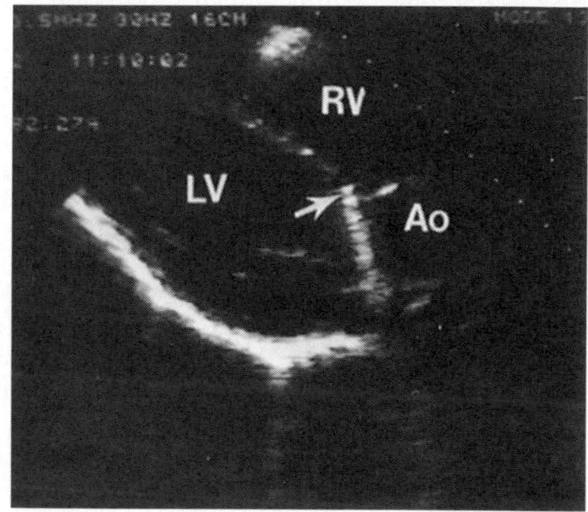

FIGURE 44–6. Two-dimensional echocardiographic image in the left parasternal long-axis view. A bullet fragment (arrow) is located high in the interventricular septum and has the typical appearance of such missiles with dense trailing reverberations. Ao = aortic root; LV = left ventricle; RV = right ventricle. (From Hassett, A., et al.: Utility of echocardiography in the management of patients with penetrating missile wounds of the heart. Reprinted with permission of the American College of Cardiology. J. Am. Coll. Cardiol. *7:*1151, 1986.)

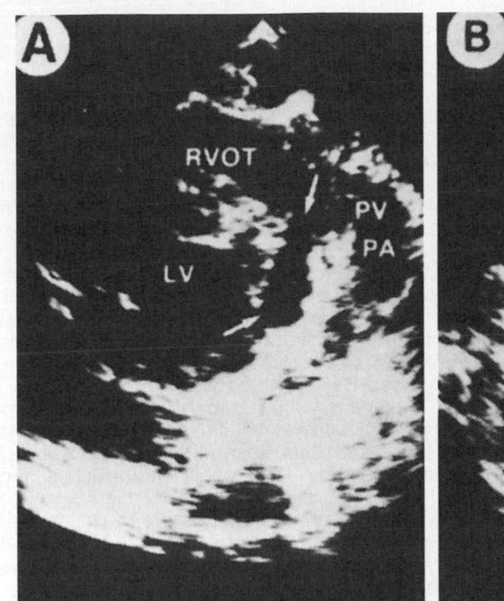

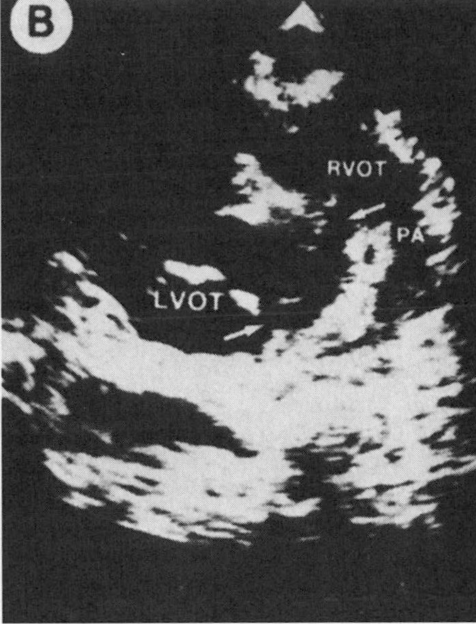

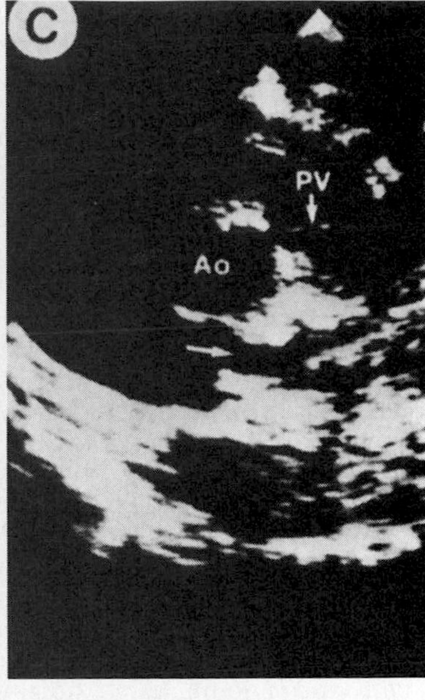

FIGURE 44–7. Two-dimensional echocardiogram from the parasternal short-axis position in a patient with a ventricular septal defect caused by knife stabbing. *A,* A defect is seen in the interventricular septum (arrows) between the left ventricle (LV) and the right ventricular outflow tract (RVOT) just proximal to the pulmonary valve (PV). *B,* At a slightly higher level the defect originates in the left ventricular outflow tract (LVOT) and exits in the distal right ventricular outflow tract. *C,* At an even higher level, but just below the aorta (Ao) and left atrium, a portion of the defect is seen (arrow). PA = pulmonary artery. (From Goldfarb, M. S., et al.: Two-dimensional Doppler echocardiographic diagnosis of a traumatic intracardiac shunt. Am. J. Cardiol. *57*:494, 1986.)

wise in good health, can withstand relatively long periods of hypoperfusion without irreversible brain, renal, or cardiac damage. Therefore, one should err on the side of aggressive attempts at resuscitation in patients who arrive moribund in the operating room. Retained foreign bodies in the heart are less of a problem in civilian than in military injuries, because shootings in civilian life usually occur at short range and thus result in through-and-through wounds.

There is disagreement concerning whether or not retained foreign bodies should be removed. Certainly, if the projectile is accessible, it should be removed; echocardiography (Fig. 44–6) can be helpful in locating foreign bodies.[47,55] If deemed not dangerous, they can probably be left in place (as has been done in the pulmonary arteries[56]), although there is some risk of later infection, pain, aneurysm formation, or migration of the foreign body.[55] In addition, dealing with a patient who is preoccupied with the knowledge that he or she has a foreign body retained in or close to the heart may present some difficulty; indeed, anxiety can become excessive, impairing the patient's function more than the physical damage and, occasionally, becoming an indication for reoperation and extraction of the object. The serious consequences of a foreign body embolus from the left ventricle also encourage a more aggressive surgical policy toward foreign bodies lodged in that chamber than in the right ventricle. Foreign bodies embedded at strategic points in great vessels may erode the vessel and cause potentially severe hemorrhage or may embolize[55] and should, if possible, be removed.

Late complications of penetrating wounds of the heart are quite common and include post-traumatic pericarditis and infection as well as arrhythmias, ventricular septal defect, and ventricular aneurysm.

PROGNOSIS. The outlook following a penetrating wound depends, first and foremost, on the extent of the injury. Gunshot wounds of the heart are more often fatal than are stab wounds, while among the latter, knife wounds are more serious than are ice pick wounds. Salvage rates are lower in patients with extrapericardial hemorrhage compared with tamponade and also with penetrating wounds involving thin-walled structures such as the atria or the pulmonary artery, since they rarely seal off spontaneously, whereas injury to the ventricles is associated with distinctly higher survival.

The state of consciousness and the extent of damage, if any, to the central nervous system at the time the patient is brought to the hospital also affect prognosis. It is clear that delay in performing the initial thoracotomy also adversely influences the chances for survival.

Rupture of the interventricular septum (Fig. 44–7) is often a late complication of penetrating injury as it is with blunt injury. Asfaw et al. described 12 patients with stab wounds who presented with cardiac tamponade and who had epicardial and pericardial wounds that were repaired at thoracotomy.[57] Days to years later, septal defects were diagnosed, but only four patients were symptomatic enough to warrant subsequent reoperation for closure of the defect. Residual injuries requiring reoperation can often be detected with color-flow Doppler echocardiography.[10,18]

INJURIES TO CARDIAC VALVES, PAPILLARY MUSCLES, AND CHORDAE TENDINEAE

Patients with preexisting valvular heart disease may be at higher risk than those with normal valves for the development of valvular injury following blunt trauma. Parmley et al. cited a 9 per cent incidence of valvular injury in their report of 546 cases of nonpenetrating chest trauma (Table 44–3).[8] In most series (although not in Parmley's) damage to the aortic valve is by far the most common of these lesions (Fig. 44–8). Indeed, sustained damage of the aortic

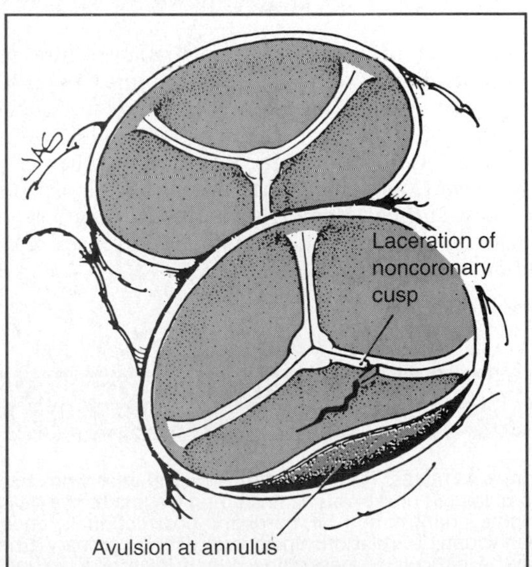

FIGURE 44–8. Diagram showing laceration of noncoronary cusp and avulsion at annulus of aortic valve following blunt trauma. (From German, D. S., et al.: Acute aortic valvular incompetence following blunt thoracic deceleration injury: Case report. J. Trauma *30*:1411, © by Williams and Wilkins, 1990.)

valve should be suspected in any patient without a history of heart disease who has a heart murmur after severe blunt trauma to the chest. Damage to cardiac valves may also occur as a consequence of penetrating wounds of the heart, but, in contrast to the damage caused by nonpenetrating injury, these are rarely solitary lesions.[58,59] Blunt chest trauma has also been reported to cause bioprosthetic valve dysfunction.[60]

CLINICAL FEATURES AND DIAGNOSIS. New, loud, musical murmurs are characteristic of injury to the valves and their supporting structures. The combination of a high-pitched diastolic blowing murmur with a widened pulse pressure following blunt trauma to the chest suggests rupture of the *aortic valve.* The murmur and the hemodynamic consequences of the rupture may not appear for several days following the trauma. Aortic regurgitation may also occur transiently owing to perivalvular edema or hemorrhage.

Rupture of the *mitral valve* or of a papillary muscle appears to occur as a consequence of sudden obstruction of left ventricular outflow due to blunt injury in early diastole.[61] It is usually associated with the development of precordial pain and a loud, harsh holosystolic murmur that radiates to the apex. Fulminant pulmonary edema quickly develops; compensation in those patients with lesser degrees of regurgitation due to torn leaflets or chordae tendineae may remain for longer periods of time, although they may eventually show signs of decompensation.

Rupture of the *tricuspid valve* is not as rare as previously thought[62] and is more benign than mitral valve rupture, with symptoms ranging from fatigue to ascites and edema. Physical findings can be striking, with prominent systolic venous pulsations, hepatic pulsations, and a typical holosystolic murmur with inspiratory accentuation.

TREATMENT AND PROGNOSIS. The prognosis depends largely on the severity of the regurgitation. Because the lesion usually develops suddenly, the ventricle does not have the opportunity to adapt to this burden, as it does in most forms of chronic valvular regurgitation. Obviously, the baseline condition of the ventricle prior to the trauma, the presence of other injuries occurring simultaneously, and the severity of the regurgitation affect the heart's ability to tolerate the insult. When effective surgical treatment is not possible, survival without the need for operation is not uncommon in patients with mild or moderate regurgitation. With severe left ventricular failure due to a ruptured mitral valve or papillary muscle, however, early surgery is mandatory.

The diagnosis of acute left ventricular failure may be difficult immediately after serious trauma, because fractured ribs and pulmonary contusions may be blamed for the shortness of breath and dyspnea. When left ventricular failure develops slowly or the lesion is not hemodynamically significant, as with lesser degrees of injury, medical therapy may suffice. Hemorrhage into a papillary muscle may cause late necrosis and delayed rupture, and these patients must be observed carefully.

INJURIES TO THE CORONARY ARTERIES AND GREAT VESSELS

CORONARY ARTERIES. Transmural myocardial infarctions have been reported following blunt trauma (including trauma to the head),[63] but angiographic confirmation of coronary obstruction is uncommon, and, when found, its relationship to preexisting coronary atherosclerosis may be difficult to determine. When infarction occurs, it may not be clear whether it results directly from myocardial contusion, from trauma to a coronary artery, or from some combination of these two processes. In many cases of myocardial infarction, preexisting coronary artery disease has been present, and it is reasonable to postulate that the injury dislodges a plaque, which then obstructs the vessel completely. However, it is also possible that a normal coronary artery becomes occluded, by either a traumatically induced intimal tear or hemorrhage.[64] Indeed, coronary arteriography has provided strong evidence that myocardial infarction follows blunt chest trauma in previously asymptomatic persons with normal vessels except for complete obstruction of the vessel supplying the infarcted area.[29] The complications of myocardial infarction—arrhythmias, pump failure, and late development of aneurysms—are similar when the lesion has an atherosclerotic basis, and treatment is similar as well. However, it may be anticipated that *following survival from the initial episode, the long-term prognosis will be more favorable in patients with traumatic damage of a coronary artery,* because the remaining vessels are usually normal. There are exceptions, however.[65]

ANEURYSM. Left ventricular *aneurysm and pseudoaneurysm* following injury to the coronary arteries can lead to ventricular rupture, cardiac failure, embolism, or arrhythmia. Operative intervention is indicated in the presence of a pseudoaneurysm, in which the myocardium has actually ruptured but in which a thrombus, fibrous tissue, and/or pericardium prevent exsanguination, because external rupture—an event that is usually fatal—is likely to occur ultimately if the condition is left untreated. Pseudoaneurysm can often be differentiated from true aneurysm by contrast or radionuclide angiography (see p. 1347).

FISTULA. Formation of an *arteriovenous fistula* is an unusual complication of traumatic damage of a coronary artery.[66] Injury to the right coronary artery is more commonly followed by an arteriovenous fistula than is injury to the left. The venous side of the fistula may be the coronary sinus, the great cardiac vein, the right atrium, or the right ventricle; in the last instance, the fistula should be termed an "arteriocameral fistula." The murmur in traumatic coronary arteriovenous or arteriocameral fistula is usually loud, widely radiating, and continuous; the electrocardiogram frequently shows transmural myocardial infarction, and the roentgenogram exhibits cardiomegaly with increased pulmonary vascularity. In patients who do not undergo surgical repair, symptoms of congestive heart failure and chest pain are frequent unless the shunt is minimal.

The left anterior descending coronary artery is the vessel most commonly involved, and at operation, the treatment of choice is suture-ligation of the cut vessel with coronary artery bypass grafting if the lacerated vessel is large and the lesion is a proximal one. Not all patients will require cardiopulmonary bypass during surgery.[67] Angiography is not advised in the emergency setting, as it is with nonpenetrating trauma. However, postoperative angiography is useful in

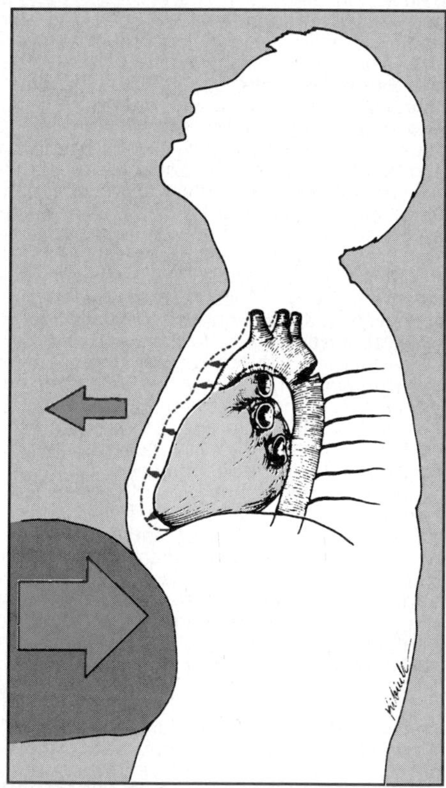

FIGURE 44–9. When the body is suddenly arrested against an obstacle, the heart and horizontal portion of the aortic arch continue their forward movement, while the descending aorta is fixed to the spine by the intercostal arteries ("deceleration" mechanism of injury). The aortic tear is posterior in this example, but it can also be anteromedial if there is upward displacement of the heart. (From Maggisano, R., and Cina, C.: Traumatic rupture of the thoracic aorta. *In* McMurtry, R. Y. and McLellan, B. A. [eds.]: *Management of Blunt Trauma.* Baltimore, Williams and Wilkins, 1990, pp. 206–226.)

localizing the presence of possible residual injuries such as a coronary arteriocameral fistula.

GREAT VESSELS. Rupture of the aorta is one of the most common traumatic lesions involving the heart or great vessels. It is most common after automobile accidents[68-70] but can also occur after falls from heights or other types of crushing injuries.[71] In automobile accidents, most commonly rupture occurs at the isthmus (Fig. 44–9), whether the collisions are head-on or broadside.[68]

It has been estimated that 10 to 20 per cent of patients with ruptured aortas live long enough to be treated successfully under ideal circumstances, which include a high level of awareness of the possibility of aortic rupture in victims of automobile accidents as well as a well-coordinated team approach.[70] As with cardiac injury, rupture of the aorta may be overshadowed by injuries to other organs, and the diagnosis may be overlooked.[71] Common clinical and radiological findings are listed in Table 44–5. Patients with aortic rupture often complain of pain in the back in addition to the chest, as do patients with aortic dissection (see p. 1556). If the expanding mediastinal hematoma or false aneurysm narrows the aortic lumen, or if the torn intima and media cause partial aortic obstruction, ischemia of the spinal cord and kidneys may ensue. A systolic murmur may be heard in the midscapular region, and widening of the superior mediastinum is visible on the chest roentgenogram (Fig. 45–9, p. 1558) along with other findings.[72,73]

A diagnostic triad that occurs in well over half the cases of ruptured aorta was initially reported by Symbas et al.[74] It consists of (1) increased arterial pressure and pulse amplitude in the upper extremities, (2) decreased pressure and pulse amplitude in the lower extremities, and (3) radiological evidence of widening of the superior mediastinum. CT scanning is *not* a useful screening procedure,[75] but transesophageal echocardiography has become increasingly useful in documenting aortic lacerations (Fig. 44–10).[76-79] Despite these advances the procedure is not infallible,[80,81] and Vlahakes and Warren[82] recommend that "at each institution results of transesophageal echocardiography be calibrated against the existing gold standard of aortography." When equivocal echocardiography results are obtained—or a negative study is obtained in patients strongly suspected of aortic rupture—an aortogram should be obtained. The entire thoracic aorta and its branches should be visualized so as not to overlook a rupture occurring at an unusual site or multiple sites of rupture.

TABLE 44–5 CLINICAL AND RADIOGRAPHIC CHARACTERISTICS OF 93 PATIENTS EVALUATED FOR AORTIC TRAUMA

CHARACTERISTIC	RUPTURE (N = 11)	NO RUPTURE (N = 82)
Age—yr		
Mean ± SD	42.9 ± 15.1	44.5 ± 19.2
Range	17–66	13–87
Sex—M/F	7/4	62/20
Mechanism of injury—no. (%)		
Motor vehicle accident (unrestrained)	7 (63.6)	48 (58.5)
Motor vehicle accident (restrained)	2 (18.2)	12 (14.6)
Pedestrian hit by car	0	8 (9.8)
Motorcycle accident	1 (9.1)	6 (7.3)
Fall	1 (9.1)	5 (6.1)
Gunshot	0	1 (1.2)
Crushed by car	0	2 (2.4)
External chest trauma—no. (%)	2 (18.2)	16 (19.5)
Intubation—no. (%)	5 (45.5)	30 (36.6)
Systolic blood pressure—mm Hg		
Mean ± SD	118.8 ± 33.4	130.6 ±26.5
Range	70–170	76–198
Heart rate—beats/min		
Mean ± SD	115.7 ± 30.3	103.8 ± 22.9
Range	62–167	60–178
Glasgow coma score		
Mean ± SD	12.1 ±3.8	12.3 ± 3.8
Range	6–15	3–15
Injury-severity score*		
Mean ± SD	51.1 ± 15.2	26.7 ± 13.3
Range	25–75	5–75
Chest-film findings		
No. of signs/patient		
Mean	2.70	2.48
Range	0–6	1–6
Wide mediastinum—no. (%)	10 (90.9)	74 (90.2)
Normal—no (%)	1 (9.1)	0
Death—no. (%)	4 (36.4)	9 (11.0)

* $P < 0.001$ for the comparison between the groups.
None of the deaths were due to aortic injury.
From Smith, M. D., et al.: Transesophageal echocardiography in the diagnosis of traumatic rupture of the aorta. N. Engl. J. Med. *332*:356, 1995.

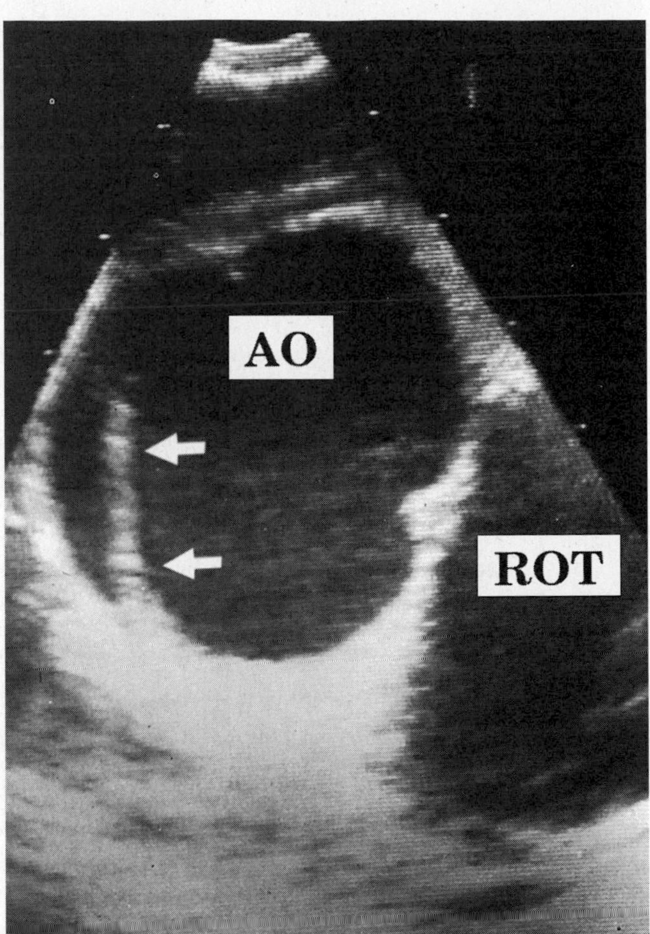

FIGURE 44–10. Transesophageal echocardiographic view of the aortic root (AO) just above the origin of the right coronary artery. White arrows indicate an intimal flap on the right aortic wall. ROT, right outflow tract. (From Catoire, P., et al.: Traumatic laceration of the ascending aorta detected by transesophageal echocardiography. Ann. Emerg. Med. *23*:356, 1994.)

PENETRATING TRAUMA TO THE GREAT VESSELS. This is usually the result of bullet or stab wounds and occurs most commonly in conjunction with cardiac wounds. Cardiac tamponade is a frequent complication of injury to the intrapericardial segment of one of the great vessels, but when it is extrapericardial, massive hemothorax is usually the presenting finding. The superior vena cava, trachea, or esophagus or some combination of these structures may be compressed if a large mediastinal hematoma forms as a result of bleeding. Injury to the innominate or carotid arteries may compress these vessels, with resultant neurological signs. An arteriovenous fistula may develop with symptoms of congestive heart failure accompanied by a systolic or, more commonly, a continuous murmur. These fistulous connections may also involve the systemic and pulmonary vessel. Blunt trauma has also been reported to cause transection of the inferior vena cava.[83]

Penetrating injury to the great vessels should be suspected in any patient in whom a projectile traverses the mediastinum and is suggested by radiological evidence of a widened mediastinum. Aortography should be performed immediately, provided that emergency thoracotomy for shock or tamponade can be deferred briefly. Immediate operation, sometimes using a heparinized shunt between the ascending and descending aorta, should be carried out as soon as the diagnosis of thoracic aortic disruption has been established whether by blunt or penetrating injury.[84] Camp et al.[70] described their experience with 75 patients with lacerations of the descending thoracic aorta secondary to blunt trauma who reached the hospital alive. There was a significantly higher mortality rate in patients over 55 than in younger patients, 82.4 vs. 12 per cent $p < 0.001$. The authors concluded that elderly patients may be better candidates for *nonsurgical* management.

Antiadrenergic agents such as guanethidine, reserpine, and propranolol, which have been utilized in the treatment of spontaneous dissection of the aorta (see p. 1565), may also have a role in treatment of patients with aortic rupture if, for logistical reasons, operation must be deferred.

REFERENCES

1. Cheitlin, M. D.: Cardiovascular trauma. Circulation *65*:1529; *66*:244, 1982.
2. Henderson, V. J., Smith, R. S., Fry, W. R., et al.: Cardiac injuries: Analysis of an unselected series of 251 cases. J. Trauma *36*:341, 1994.
3. Sherman, M. M., Saini, U. K., Yarnoz, M. D., et al.: Management of penetrating heart wounds. Am. J. Surg. *135*:553, 1978.
4. Mattox, K. L., Feliciano, D. V., Burch, J., et al.: Five thousand seven hundred sixty cardiovascular injuries in 4459 patients: Epidemiologic evolution 1958 to 1987. Ann. Surg. *209*:698, 1989.

NONPENETRATING CARDIAC INJURY

5. Glock, Y., Massabuau, P., and Puel, P.: Cardiac damage in nonpenetrating chest injuries. J. Cardiovasc. Surg. *30*:27, 1989.
6. McLean, R. F., Devitt, J. H., McLellan, B. A., et al.: Significance of myocardial contusion following blunt chest trauma. J. Trauma *33*:240, 1992.
7. Matthews, R. V., French, W. J., and Criley, J. M.: Chest trauma and subvalvular left ventricular aneurysms. Chest *95*:474, 1989.
8. Parmley, L. F., Manion, W. C., and Mattingly, T. W.: Nonpenetrating traumatic injury of the heart. Circulation *18*:371, 1958.
9. DeMuth, W. E., Lerner, E. H., and Liedtke, A. J.: Nonpenetrating injury of the heart: An experimental model. J. Trauma *13*:639, 1973.
10. Karalis, D. G., Victor, M. F., Davis, G. A., et al.: The role of echocardiography in blunt chest trauma: A transthoracic and transesophageal echocardiographic study. J. Trauma *36*:53, 1994.
11. Cachecho, R., Grindlinger, G. A., and Lee, V. W.: The clinical significance of myocardial contusion. J. Trauma *33*:68, 1992.
12. Tenzer, M. L.: The spectrum of myocardial contusion: A review. J. Trauma *25*:620, 1985.
13. Snow, N., Richardson, J. D., and Flint, L. M., Jr.: Myocardial contusion: Implications for patients with multiple traumatic injuries. Surgery *92*:744, 1982.
14. Torres-Mirabal, P., Gruenberg, J. C., Brown, R. S., and Obeid, F. N.: Spectrum of myocardial contusion. Am. Surg. *48*:383, 1982.
15. Frazee, R. C., Mucha, P., Jr., Farnell, M. B., and Miller, F. A., Jr.: Objective evaluation of blunt cardiac trauma. J. Trauma *26*:510, 1986.
16. Sutherland, G. R., Cheung, H. W., Holliday, R. L., et al.: Hemodynamic adaptation to acute myocardial contusion complicating blunt chest injury. Am. J. Cardiol. *57*:291, 1986.
17. Schamp, D. J., Plotnick, G. D., Croteau, D., et al.: Clinical significance of radionuclide angiographically-determined abnormalities following acute blunt chest trauma. Am. Heart J. *116*:500, 1988.
18. Mattox, K. L., Limacher, M. C., Feliciano, D. V., et al.: Cardiac evaluation following heart injury. J. Trauma *25*:758, 1985.
19. Cooperman, Y., Low, S., and Laniado, S.: Traumatic heart block. PACE *12*:25, 1989.
20. Bognolo, D. A., Rabow, F. I., Vijayanagar, R. R., and Eckstein, P. F.: Traumatic sinus node dysfunction. Ann. Emerg. Med. *11*:319, 1982.

20a. Maron, B. J., Poliac, L. C., Kaplan, J. A. and Mueller, F. O.: Blunt impact to the chest leading to sudden death from cardiac arrest during sports activities. N. Engl. J. Med. *333*:337, 1995.

21. Évora, P. R. B., Ribeiro, P. J. F., Brasil, J. C. F., et al.: Late surgical repair of ventricular septal defect due to nonpenetrating chest trauma: Review and report of two contrasting cases. J. Trauma *25*:1007, 1985.
22. German, D. S., Shapiro, M. I., and Willman, V. L.: Acute aortic valvular incompetence following blunt thoracic deceleration injury: Case report. J. Trauma *30*:1411, 1990.
23. Desiderio, M. A.: The potentiation of the response to blunt cardiac trauma by ethanol in dogs. J. Trauma *26*:467, 1986.
24. Dubrow, T. J., Mihalka, J., Eisenhauer, D. M., et al.: Myocardial contusion in the stable patient: What level of care is appropriate? Surgery *106*:267, 1989.
25. Soliman, M. H., and Waxman, K.: Value of a conventional approach to the diagnosis of traumatic cardiac contusion after chest injury. Crit. Care Med. *15*:218, 1987.
26. Wiegand, L., and Zwillich, C. W.: The post-cardiac injury syndrome following blunt chest trauma: Case report. J. Trauma *34*:445, 1993.
27. Watt, A. H., and Stephens, M. R.: Myocardial infarction after blunt chest trauma incurred during rugby football that later required cardiac transplantation. Br. Heart J. *55*:408, 1986.
28. Espinosa, R., Badui, E., Castaño, R., and Madrid, R.: Acute posterior wall myocardial infarction secondary to football chest trauma. Chest *88*:928, 1985.
29. Unterberg, C., Buchwald, A., and Viegand, V.: Traumatic thrombosis of the left main coronary artery and myocardial infarction caused by blunt chest trauma. Clin. Cardiol. *12*:672, 1989.
30. Chang, H., Chu, S-H., and Lee, Y-T.: Traumatic aorto-right atrial fistula after blunt chest injury. Ann. Thorac. Surg. *45*:778, 1989.
31. Getz, B. S., Davies, E., Steinberg, S. M., et al.: Blunt cardiac trauma resulting in right atrial rupture. J. A. M. A. *255*:761, 1986.
32. Brathwaite, C. E. M., Rodriguez, A., Turney, S. Z., et al.: Blunt traumatic cardiac rupture: A 5-year experience. Ann. Surg. *212*:701, 1990.
33. Kato, K., Kushimoto, S., Mashiko, K., et al.: Blunt traumatic rupture of the heart: An experience in Tokyo. J. Trauma *36*:859, 1994.
34. Santavirta, S., and Arajarvi, E.: Ruptures of the heart in seatbelt wearers. J. Trauma *32*:275, 1992.
35. Leavitt, B. J., Meyer, J. A., Morton, J. R., et al.: Survival following nonpenetrating traumatic rupture of cardiac chambers. Ann. Thorac. Surg. *44*:532, 1987.
36. End, A., Rodler, S., Oturanlar, D., et al.: Elective surgery for blunt cardiac trauma. J. Trauma *37*:798, 1994.
37. Eisenberg, M. S., Horwood, B. T., Cummins, R. O., et al.: Cardiac arrest and resuscitation: A tale of 29 cities. Ann. Emerg. Med. *19*:179, 1990.
38. Baker, P. B., Keyhani-Rofagha, S., Graham, R. L., and Sharma, H. M.: Dissecting hematoma (aneurysm) of coronary arteries. Am. J. Med. *80*:317, 1986.

PENETRATING CARDIAC INJURY

39. Naughton, M. J., Brissie, R. M., Bessey, P. Q., et al.: Demography of penetrating cardiac trauma. Ann. Surg. *209*:676, 1989.
40. Auge, J. M., Oriol, A., Serra, C., and Crexells, C.: The use of pigtail catheters for retrieval of foreign bodies from the cardiovascular system. Cathet. Cardiovasc. Diagn. *10*:625, 1984.
41. McIvor, M. E., Kaufman, S. L., Satre, R., et al.: Search and retrieval of a radiolucent foreign object. Cath. Cardiovasc. Diagn. *16*:19, 1989.
42. Goldbaum, T. S., Jacob, A. S., Smith, D. F., et al.: Cardiac tamponade following percutaneous transluminal coronary angioplasty: Four case reports. Cathet. Cardiovasc. Diagn. *11*:413, 1985.
43. Przybojewski, J. Z.: Endomyocardial biopsy: A review of the literature. Cathet. Cardiovasc. Diagn. *11*:287, 1985.
44. Anastasious-Nana, M. I., O'Connell, J. B., Nanas, J. N., et al.: Relative efficiency and risk of endomyocardial biopsy: Comparisons in heart transplant and nontransplant patients. Cath. Cardiovasc. Diagn. *16*:7, 1989.
45. Shirani, J., Zafari, A. M., Hill, V. E., et al.: Long asymptomatic survival with a bullet adjacent to the left main coronary artery, the only site of atherosclerotic plaque in the coronary tree. Am. Heart J. *128*:1043, 1994.
46. Nagy, K. K., Lohmann, C., Kim, D. O., and Barrett, J.: Role of echocardiography in the diagnosis of occult penetrating cardiac injury. J. Trauma *38*:859, 1995.
47. Hassett, A., Moran, J., Sabiston, D. C., and Kisslo, J.: Utility of echocardiography in the management of patients with penetrating missile wounds of the heart. J. Am. Coll. Cardiol. *7*:1151, 1986.
48. Miller, J. T., Richards, K. L., Miller, J. F., and Crawford, M. H.: Doppler echocardiographic determination of the cause of a systolic murmur following penetrating chest trauma. Am. Heart J. *111*:988, 1986.
49. Goldfarb, M. S., Walpole, H. T., Jr., Landolt, C. C., et al.: Two-dimensional Doppler echocardiographic diagnosis of a traumatic intracardiac shunt. Am. J. Cardiol. *57*:494, 1986.
50. Martin, L. F., Mavroudis, C., Dyess, D. L., et al.: The first 70 years' experience managing cardiac disruption due to penetrating and blunt injuries at the University of Louisville. Am. Surg. *52*:14, 1986.
51. Lorenz, H. P., Steinmetz, B., Lieberman, J., et al.: Emergency thoracotomy: Survival correlates with physiologic status. J. Trauma *32*:780, 1992.
52. Boyd, M., Vanek, V. W., and Bourguet, C. C.: Emergency room resuscitative thoracotomy: When is it indicated? J. Trauma *33*:714, 1992.
53. Durham, A. A., Richardson, R. J., Wall, M. J., Jr., et al.: Emergency center thoracotomy: Impact of prehospital resuscitation. J. Trauma *32*:775, 1992.
54. Macho, J. R., Markison, R. E., and Schecter, W. P.: Cardiac stapling in the management of penetrating injuries of the heart: Rapid control of hemorrhage and decreased risk of personal contamination. J. Trauma *34*:711, 1993.
55. Bergin, P. J.: Aortic thrombosis and peripheral embolization after thoracic gunshot wound diagnosed by transesophageal echocardiography. Am. Heart J. *119*:688, 1990.
56. Kortbeek, J. B., Clark, J. A., and Carraway, R. C.: Conservative management of a pulmonary artery bullet embolism: Case report and review of the literature. J. Trauma *33*:906, 1992.
57. Asfaw, I., Thoms, N. W., and Arfulu, A.: Interventricular septal defects from penetrating injuries of the heart: A report of 12 cases and review of the literature. J. Thorac. Cardiovasc. Surg. *69*:450, 1975.
58. Rustad, D. G., Hopeman, A. R., Murr, P. C., and VanWay, C. W., III: Aorta-cardiac fistula with aortic valve injury from penetrating trauma. J. Trauma *26*:266, 1986.
59. Werne, C., Sagraves, S. G., and Costa, C.: Mitral and tricuspid valve rupture from blunt trauma sustained during a motor vehicle collision. J. Trauma *29*:15, 1989.
60. Rumisek, J. D., Robonowitz, M., Virmani, R., et al.: Bioprosthetic heart valve rupture associated with trauma. J. Trauma *26*:276, 1986.
61. Cho, M-C., Kim, D-W., Hong, J-M., et al.: Left ventricular and papillary muscle rupture following blunt chest trauma. Am. J. Cardiol. *76*:424, 1995.
62. Gayet, C., Pierre, B., Delahaye, J-P., et al.: Traumatic tricuspid insufficiency: An underdiagnosed disease. Chest *92*:429, 1987.
63. Bashour, T. T., Morelli, R. L., Cunningham, T., and Budge, W. R.: Acute

coronary thrombosis following head trauma in a young man. Am. Heart J. *119*:676, 1990.
64. Sabbah, H. N., Mohyi, J., and Stein, P. D.: Coronary arteriography in dogs following blunt cardiac trauma: A longitudinal assessment. Cath. Cardiovasc. Diagn. *15*:155, 1988.
65. Watt, A. H., and Stephens, M. R.: Myocardial infarction after blunt chest trauma incurred during rugby football that later required cardiac transplantation. Br. Heart J. *55*:408, 1986.
66. Martin, R., Mitchell, A., and Dhalla, N.: Late pericardial tamponade and coronary arteriovenous fistula after trauma. Br. Heart J. *55*:216, 1986.
67. Reissman, P., Rivkind, A., Jurim, O., et al.: Simon D: Case Report: The management of penetrating cardiac trauma with major coronary artery injury—is cardiopulmonary bypass essential? J. Trauma *33*:773, 1992.
68. Feczko, J. D., Lynch, L., Pless, J. E., et al.: An autopsy case review of 142 nonpenetrating (blunt) injuries of the aorta. J. Trauma *33*:846, 1992.
69. Ben-Menachem, Y.: Rupture of the thoracic aorta by broadside impacts in road traffic and other collisions: Further angiographic observations and preliminary autopsy findings. J. Trauma *35*:363, 1993.
70. Camp, P. C., Jr., Rogers, F. B., Shackford, S. R., et al.: Blunt traumatic thoracic aortic lacerations in the elderly: An analysis of outcome. J. Trauma *37*:418, 1994.
71. Shaikh, K. A., Schwab, C. W., and Camishion, R. C.: Aortic rupture in blunt trauma. Am. Surg. *52*:47, 1986.
72. Gundry, S. R., Burney, R. E., Mackenzie, J. R., et al.: Assessment of mediastinal widening associated with traumatic rupture of the aorta. J. Trauma *23*:293, 1983.
73. Heystraten, F. M., Rosenbusch, G., Kingma, L. M., et al.: Chest radiography in acute traumatic rupture of the thoracic aorta. Acta Radiol. *29*:411, 1988.
74. Symbas, P. N., Tyras, D. H., Ware, R. E., and Hatcher, C. R., Jr.: Rupture of the aorta: A diagnostic triad. Ann. Thorac. Surg *15*:405, 1973.
75. Miller, F. B., Richardson, J. D., Thomas, H. A., et al.: Role of CT in diagnosis of major arterial injury after blunt thoracic trauma. Surgery *106*:596, 1989.
76. Catoire, P., Bonnet, F., Delaunay, L., et al.: Traumatic laceration of the ascending aorta detecting by transesophageal echocardiography. Ann. Emerg. Med. *23*:356, 1994.
77. Smith, M. K., Cassidy, J. M., Souther, S., et al.: Transesophageal echocardiography in the diagnosis of traumatic rupture of the aorta. N. Engl. J. Med. *332*:356, 1995.
78. Catoire, P., Orliaguet, G., Liu, N., et al.: Systematic transesophageal echocardiography for detection of mediasternal lesions in patients with multiple injuries. J. Trauma *38*:96, 1995.
79. Vignon, P., Gueret, P., Vedrinne, J-M., et al.: Role of transesophageal echocardiography in the diagnosis and management of traumatic aortic disruption. Circulation *92*:2959, 1995.
80. Oxorn, D., and Towers, M.: Traumatic aortic disruption: False positive diagnosis on transesophageal echocardiography. J. Trauma *39*:386, 1995.
81. Saletta, S., Lederman, E., Fein, S., et al.: Transesophageal echocardiography for the initial evaluation of the widened mediastinum in trauma patients. J. Trauma *39*:137, 1995.
82. Vlahakes, G. J., and Warren, R. L.: Traumatic rupture of the aorta. N. Engl. J. Med. *332*(Edit.):356, 1995.
83. Peitzman, A. B., Udekwu, A. O., Pevec, W., and Albrink, M.: Transection of the inferior vena cava from blunt thoracic trauma: Case reports. J. Trauma *29*:534, 1989.
84. Akins, C. W., Buckley, M. J., Daggett, W., et al.: Acute traumatic disruption of the thoracic aorta: A ten-year experience. Ann. Thorac. Surg. *31*:305, 1981.

Chapter 45
Diseases of the Aorta

ERIC M. ISSELBACHER, KIM A. EAGLE, ROMAN W. DESANCTIS

THE NORMAL AORTA 1546
EXAMINATION OF THE AORTA 1546
AORTIC ANEURYSMS 1547
Abdominal Aortic Aneurysms 1547
Thoracic Aortic Aneurysms 1550
AORTIC DISSECTION 1554
Clinical Manifestations 1556
Diagnostic Techniques 1558
Management 1564
Atypical Aortic Dissection 1568
Aortic Trauma 1570
AORTIC ATHEROMATOUS EMBOLI 1570
ACUTE AORTIC OCCLUSION 1571
AORTOARTERITIS SYNDROMES 1572
Takayasu's Arteritis 1572
Giant Cell Arteritis 1573
REFERENCES 1576

THE NORMAL AORTA

FUNCTION

Appropriately called "the greatest artery" by the ancients, the aorta is admirably suited for its task. In an average lifetime, this thin but large and remarkably tough vessel must absorb the impact of 2.3 to 3 billion heartbeats while carrying roughly 200 million liters of blood through the body. Arteries can be categorized as either *conductance* or *resistance* vessels. Conductance vessels are the conduits for blood, and the aorta is the ultimate conductance vessel.

The aorta is composed of three layers: the thin inner layer, or *intima;* a thick middle layer, or *media;* and a rather thin outer layer, the *adventitia.* The strength of the aorta lies in the media, which is composed of laminated but intertwining sheets of elastic tissue arranged in a spiral manner that affords maximum tensile strength. Indeed, as thin as it is, the aortic wall can withstand the experimental pressure of thousands of millimeters of mercury without bursting. In contrast to the peripheral arteries, the aortic media contains relatively little smooth muscle and collagen between the elastic layers. It is this tremendous accretion of elastic tissue that gives the aorta not only tensile strength but also distensibility and elasticity, which serve a vital circulatory role. The aortic intima is a thin and delicate layer that is lined by endothelium and easily traumatized. The adventitia contains mainly collagen and carries the important vasa vasorum, which nourish the outer half of the aortic wall, including much of the media.

During ventricular systole, the aorta is distended by the force of the blood ejected into it by the left ventricle, and in this manner part of the kinetic energy generated by the contracting left ventricle is converted into potential energy stored in the aortic wall. Then, during diastole, this potential energy is transformed back into kinetic energy as the aortic walls recoil, propelling the blood in the aortic lumen distally into the arterial bed. Thus, the aorta plays an essential role in maintaining forward circulation of the blood in diastole after it is delivered into the aorta by the left ventricle during systole. The pulse wave itself, with its milking effect, is transmitted along the aorta to the periphery at a speed of about 5 m/sec. This is much faster than the velocity of the intraluminal blood itself, which travels at only 40 to 50 cm/sec.

The systolic pressure developing within the aorta is a function of the volume of blood ejected into the aorta, the compliance or distensibility of the aorta, and the resistance to blood flow. This resistance is determined primarily by the tone of the peripheral muscular arteries and arterioles, and to a slight extent by the inertia of the column of blood in the aorta when systole commences.

In addition to its conductance and pumping functions, the aorta also plays a role in indirectly controlling systemic vascular resistance and heart rate. Pressure-responsive receptors, analogous to those in the carotid sinus, lie in the ascending aorta and aortic arch and send afferent signals to the vasomotor center in the brain stem by way of the vagus nerves. Raising the intra-aortic pressure causes reflex bradycardia and reduction of systemic vascular resistance, whereas lowering the pressure increases the heart rate and vascular resistance.

ANATOMICAL CONSIDERATIONS

The aorta is divided anatomically into its thoracic and abdominal components. The thoracic aorta is further divided into the *ascending, arch,* and *descending* segments, while the abdominal aorta consists of *suprarenal* and *infrarenal* segments.

The ascending aorta is 5 cm long and has two distinct segments. The lower segment is the *aortic root,* beginning at the level of the aortic valve and extending to the sinotubular junction. This is the widest portion of the ascending aorta, measuring about 3.3 cm in width. The bases of the aortic leaflets are supported by the aortic root from which the three sinuses of Valsalva bulge outward to allow for the full excursion of aortic valve leaflets during systole. In addition, the two coronary arteries arise from these sinuses of Valsalva. The upper tubular segment of the ascending aorta rises to join the aortic arch. Normally the ascending aorta sits just to the right of midline, with its proximal portion lying within the pericardial cavity. Nearby structures include the pulmonary artery anteriorly and leftward, the left atrium, right pulmonary artery, and right mainstem bronchus posteriorly, and the right atrium and superior vena cava to the right.

The *arch of the aorta* gives rise to all of the brachiocephalic arteries. From the ascending aorta it courses slightly leftward in front of the trachea and then proceeds posteriorly to the left of the trachea and esophagus. The pulmonary artery bifurcation and right pulmonary artery lie inferior to the arch, as does the left lung. The recurrent laryngeal nerve loops underneath the arch distally, and the phrenic and vagus nerves lie to the left.

The *descending thoracic aorta* begins in the posterior mediastinum to the left of the vertebral column and gradually courses in front of the vertebral column as it descends, occupying a position immediately behind the esophagus. Distally it passes through the diaphragm, usually at the level of the twelfth thoracic vertebra.

The point at which the aortic arch joins the descending aorta is called the *aortic isthmus.* The aorta is especially vulnerable to trauma at this site because it is here that the relatively mobile portion of the aorta—the ascending aorta and arch—becomes relatively fixed to the thoracic cage by the pleural reflections, the paired intercostal arteries, and the left subclavian artery. This is also where coarctations of the aorta are located.

The abdominal aorta continues from the thoracic aorta, giving off the important splanchnic arteries and ending at its bifurcation at the level of the fourth lumbar vertebra.

AGING OF THE AORTA

As discussed above, the elastic properties of the aorta are crucial to its normal function. However, it has been well demonstrated that the elasticity and distensibility of the aorta decline with age. Such changes are seen even in normal healthy adults, and for unknown reasons these changes occur earlier and are more progressive among men than women.[1] The loss of elasticity and aortic compliance likely accounts for the increase in pulse pressure commonly seen in the elderly. This progressive loss of aortic elasticity with aging is accelerated among those with hypertension compared with age-matched normotensive controls.[2] Similarly, those with hypercholesterolemia[3] or coronary artery disease show a greater loss of elasticity than do controls.[4] Conversely, among healthy athletes elasticity is higher than among their age-matched controls.[4]

Histologically, the aging aortic wall exhibits fragmentation of elastin with a concomitant increase in collagen, resulting in an increased collagen-to-elastin ratio that contributes to the loss of aortic distensibility observed physiologically.[5] Recent experimental animal data suggest that impairment of vasa vasorum flow to the aortic wall results in stiffening of the aorta with similar histological changes and may therefore be one cause of the degenerative changes seen with age.[6]

In animal models it has been demonstrated that a loss of aortic distensibility directly affects the mechanical performance of the left ventricle, producing increases in left ventricular systolic pressure and wall tension and in end-diastolic pressure and volume.[7] Furthermore, reduced aortic compliance causes a 20 to 40 per cent increase in myocardial oxygen consumption in order to maintain a given stroke volume.[8] It is therefore likely that, over time, the changes in aortic compliance seen with age may cause clinically important alterations in cardiac function.[7]

EXAMINATION OF THE AORTA

Unless the aorta is abnormally enlarged, the only location in which it can be palpated is the abdomen. The ease with which it can be felt depends largely on the body habitus and the pulse pressure: It is readily felt in thin individuals. It may be quite sensitive to palpation. Auscultation usually is unrevealing in aortic diseases, except for occasional bruits at the sites of narrowing of the aorta or its arterial branches. Diseases of the aortic root and proximal ascending aorta sometimes involve the aortic valve, with resultant aortic regurgitation that may be detectable on auscultation. Regurgitant murmurs secondary to root dilatation, rather than primary valvular disease, are often loudest along the right sternal border.

Chest roentgenography and fluoroscopy are valuable and simple procedures for assessing the aorta. Normally, the ascending aorta is not visible on the direct anteroposterior chest roentgenogram. The aorta is seen as a "knob" in the superior mediastinum just to the left of the vertebral column. The lateral border of the descending thoracic aorta can often be distinguished to the left of the spine. On the lateral chest roentgenogram, the aortic root and proximal ascending aorta are visible as an indistinct shadow in the middle of the mediastinum arising from the base of the heart. The ascending aorta and arch are best demonstrated in a left anterior oblique projection—a view that should always be included when disease of the thoracic aorta is suspected (Fig. 7–17, p. 216).

A number of imaging modalities are available for diagnostic examination of the aorta. These include aortography, computed tomographic scanning, magnetic resonance imaging, and both transthoracic and transesophageal echocardiography. The use of intravascular ultrasonography for the diagnosis of aortic pathology is under investigation. The respective utility of these imaging modalities is discussed below in the context of specific aortic diseases.

AORTIC ANEURYSMS

The term *aortic aneurysm* refers to a pathological dilatation of the normal aortic lumen involving one or several segments. Although there is perhaps no universally accepted definition, an aortic aneurysm is best described as a permanent localized dilatation of the aorta having a diameter at least 1.5 times that of the expected normal diameter of that given aortic segment.[9] Aneurysms are usually described in terms of their location, size, morphology, and etiology. The morphology of an aortic aneurysm is typically either *fusiform,* which is the more common shape, or *saccular.* A fusiform aneurysm is fairly uniform in shape, with symmetrical dilatation that involves the full circumference of the aortic wall. The dilatation seen in saccular aneurysms, on the other hand, is more localized, appearing as an outpouching of only a portion of the aortic wall. In addition, there may be a *pseudoaneurysm* or *false aneurysm* of the aorta, which is not actually an aneurysm at all but rather a well-defined collection of blood and connective tissue outside the vessel wall. This may be a consequence of a contained rupture of the aortic wall.

The presence of an aortic aneurysm may be a marker of more diffuse aortic disease. Overall, up to 13 per cent of all patients diagnosed with an aortic aneurysm are found to have multiple aneurysms,[10] with up to 25 to 28 per cent of those with thoracic aortic aneurysms having concomitant abdominal aortic aneurysms.[11,12] For this reason, Crawford and Cohen have recommended that a patient in whom an aortic aneurysm is discovered undergo examination of the entire aorta for the possible presence of other aneurysms.[10]

Abdominal Aortic Aneurysms

Abdominal aortic aneurysms are much more common than are thoracic aortic aneurysms. Age is an important risk factor, as the incidence rises rapidly after 55 years of age in men and 70 years of age in women,[13] and abdominal aortic aneurysms occur four to five times more frequently in men than in women. The incidence of abdominal aneurysms has increased threefold in recent decades, from 8.7 per 100,000 person-years in 1951 to 1960 to 36.5 per 100,000 person-years in 1971 to 1980.[14] Because the incidence of abdominal aneurysms of all sizes has increased, it is believed that these data at least in part reflect a true increase in the disease incidence. Other factors that may have contributed to the marked rise in the incidence of such aneurysms include the increasing mean age of the population, a greater awareness of the association of aneurysmal disease with other prevalent cardiovascular conditions, and improvements in diagnostic evaluation. The prevalence of abdominal aortic aneurysms in the population 50 years of age and older is at least 3 per cent.[15]

ETIOLOGY AND PATHOGENESIS. Although it is now evident that abdominal aortic aneurysms arise as a consequence of multiple interacting factors, classically atherosclerosis has been considered the common underlying etiology. The infrarenal abdominal aorta is most affected by the atherosclerotic process and is similarly the most common site of abdominal aneurysm formation; only a fraction of abdominal aortic aneurysms are suprarenal, with these tending to arise only as an extension of a thoracic (thoracoabdominal) aneurysm. The atherosclerotic process less often involves the descending thoracic aorta, and involvement of the ascending aorta is distinctly uncommon.

Atherosclerotic disease of the aorta may produce either stenotic obstruction, a process that tends to be confined to the infrarenal abdominal aorta, or aneurysmal dilatation; why one process should predominate over the other in any given individual is unknown.[15] Although the mechanism by which atherosclerosis results in aortic aneurysms is obscure, a recent hypothesis may account for the disease's predilection for the infrarenal abdominal aorta over other segments.[16] The media of the infrarenal aorta in humans has no vasa vasorum, and as a consequence at least the inner media must receive oxygen and nutrients by diffusion from the aortic lumen. Atherosclerotic disease causes thickening of the intima and may thereby compromise the diffusion of such oxygen and nutrients to the medial layer. Exacerbated by increases in aortic wall stress from hypertension, this hypoxemia may lead to ischemic injury of the media, thus initiating a process of degeneration of the media and its elastic elements.[16] The damage produces a weakening of the aortic wall which over time allows the formation of fusiform or, less commonly, saccular dilatation of the aorta. As the aorta then widens, tension in the vessel wall rises in accordance with Laplace's law, which states that tension is proportional to the product of pressure and radius. Further widening results in even greater wall tension, which in turn leads to acceleration of aneurysm enlargement. A vicious circle is thus established in which the dilatation is often rapidly progressive.

Although atherosclerosis certainly contributes to the pathogenesis of abdominal aortic aneurysms, genetic and cellular factors play important roles as well. A genetic predisposition to the development of abdominal aortic aneurysms has been repeatedly suggested by studies of familial incidence, with up to 28 per cent of patients who have an abdominal aortic aneurysm having a first-degree relative similarly affected.[17] A recent report analyzing 313 pedigrees has confirmed the importance of familial factors in the pathogenesis of abdominal aortic aneurysms and supports the hypothesis that abdominal aortic aneurysm might be a predominantly genetic disease.[18] At present, however, no genetic marker has been shown to be definitively related to aneurysm formation, and it appears likely that the genetic factors involved may be heterogeneous.

An area of expanding investigation is the role of the cellular mechanisms in the pathogenesis of aortic aneurysms. Destruction of the media and its elastic tissue is the striking histological feature of aortic aneurysms when compared with the normal aorta. Experimental evidence indicates excessive activity of proteolytic enzymes in the aortas of affected patients which may lead to the deterioration of structural matrix proteins such as elastin and collagen in the aortic media, and thereby promote or perpetuate the formation of aneurysms. Studies have shown that aneurysmal aortas contain elastolytic activity with an active elastase not present in the normal aorta[19] and that other active proteolytic enzymes are present as well. An active inflammatory process may also contribute, given that an abnormal presence of macrophages[20] and elevated levels of cytokines[21] have been demonstrated in aneurysmal aortic tissue.

As a result of flow turbulence through the aneurysmal aortic segment, blood may stagnate along the walls and thus allow the formation of mural thrombus. Such thrombus, as well as atherosclerotic debris, may embolize distally and compromise the circulation of tributary arteries. However, the major risk posed by abdominal aortic aneurysms is that of aneurysm rupture. When rupture does occur, 80 per cent rupture into the left retroperitoneum, which may contain the rupture, whereas most of the remainder rupture into the peritoneal cavity, causing uncontrolled hemorrhage and rapid circulatory collapse.[22] Rarely, an aneurysm may rupture into the inferior vena cava, iliac vein, or renal vein.[23,24]

addition, routine coronary arteriography in those undergoing aneurysm repair revealed severe correctable coronary artery disease in 31 per cent of all patients, including an 18 per cent incidence in patients without prior clinical manifestations of coronary disease.[57] Moreover, among those with angiographically significant coronary artery disease, multivessel disease was seen in the majority.[57]

Studies by Boucher et al.[58] and Eagle et al.[59] have suggested that dipyridamole-thallium cardiac scanning (see p. 288) is an effective means of identifying patients at highest risk for perioperative ischemic events. Patients with reversible thallium defects in multiple segments of myocardium are at highest risk,[60] and it is in this subgroup that coronary angiography is likely to be most helpful. The safety of dipyridamole-thallium studies in such patients has been well established. Although exercise thallium scintigraphy is also a useful screening method,[61] many patients with vascular disease fail to achieve an adequate heart rate owing to limited exercise capacity. Other techniques shown to be effective for preoperative evaluation of myocardial ischemia include dobutamine stress echocardiography[62] and electrocardiogram exercise testing in patients with a normal baseline electrocardiogram and adequate exercise tolerance.

Selective preoperative evaluation to identify the presence and severity of coronary artery disease among patients with clinical markers of coronary artery disease has been widely advocated,[63] and some further suggest screening those with strong cardiac risk factors despite the absence of clinical evidence of coronary artery disease.[64,65] Although patients found to have significant correctable coronary artery disease are presumed to benefit from preoperative coronary revascularization with selective coronary artery bypass surgery or angioplasty, at present this conclusion remains unproved.[64] The data available from nonrandomized studies of patients with significant coronary artery disease undergoing vascular surgery do demonstrate a lower mortality for those who have undergone coronary bypass surgery.[66] Furthermore, a recent randomized study demonstrates that the long-term outcome of patients having combined peripheral vascular disease and high-risk coronary artery disease is improved by coronary artery revascularization in those with three-vessel coronary disease.[67] As is the case for coronary artery bypass surgery, there are as yet no available data to confirm that preoperative coronary angioplasty for significant coronary stenoses decreases the risk from major vascular surgery.

In addition to such preoperative screening and potential coronary revascularization, operative risk secondary to cardiac ischemic events may be further reduced through the use of perioperative invasive hemodynamic monitoring and careful perioperative surveillance for evidence of ischemia.[68,69] Furthermore, myocardial ischemia and perhaps myocardial infarction may be prevented by using beta-adrenergic blockers perioperatively.[70]

Late Survival. A review by Kiell and Ernst of late survival following abdominal aortic aneurysm repair among almost 2500 patients revealed 1-, 5-, and 10-year survival rates of 93, 63, and 40 per cent, respectively.[26] The long-term survival of those with concomitant coronary artery disease has been found to be approximately 10 per cent lower than for those without coronary disease.[71]

MEDICAL MANAGEMENT. Risk factor modification is fundamental in the medical management of abdominal aortic aneurysms. Hypercholesterolemia and hypertension should be carefully controlled. Most patients with abdominal aortic aneurysms are cigarette smokers, and smoking must be discontinued. Beta blockers have long been considered an important therapy for reducing the risk of aneurysm expansion and rupture, and both animal and human studies support such a role. Brophy et al.[72] demonstrated that propranolol delays the development of aneurysms in a mouse model prone to develop spontaneous aortic aneurysms. Interestingly, it appears that the drug's efficacy in this model may have been independent of reductions of blood pressure or dP/dt but rather may have been the result of changes in connective tissue metabolism and the structure of the aortic wall. In humans, a recent study has shown that the mean rate of abdominal aortic aneurysm expansion was slower among patients treated with beta blockers than among those not treated with beta blockers, with the effect most marked among large aneurysms.[49]

Should one elect to observe an abdominal aortic aneurysm of 4.0 cm in size or larger, careful routine follow-up is indicated in order to detect either rapid expansion ($\geq$0.5 cm/year) or an increase in size to 5.0 cm or larger, either of which is an indication for surgery.[73] CT scanning every 6 months, and perhaps as frequently as every 3 months for those at higher risk, has been advocated as an effective method of following such patients.[32]

Thoracic Aortic Aneurysms

Thoracic aortic aneurysms are much less common than are aneurysms of the abdominal aorta, and their incidence did not increase over the same 30-year period that saw a marked increase in the incidence of abdominal aortic aneurysms (as noted above).[12] Thoracic aneurysms are classified by the portion of aorta involved, i.e., the ascending, arch, or descending thoracic aorta. This anatomical distinction is important because the etiology, natural history, and therapy of thoracic aneurysms differ for each of these segments. Aneurysms of the descending aorta occur most commonly, followed by aneurysms of the ascending aorta, whereas arch aneurysms occur much less often.[11] In addition, descending thoracic aneurysms may extend distally to involve the abdominal aorta, creating what is known as a *thoracoabdominal aortic aneurysm*. Sometimes the entire aorta may be ectatic, with localized aneurysms seen at sites in both the thoracic and abdominal aorta.

ETIOLOGY AND PATHOGENESIS. Aneurysms of the ascending thoracic aorta most often result from the process of *cystic medial degeneration* (or *cystic medial necrosis*). Histologically cystic medial degeneration has the appearance of smooth muscle cell necrosis and elastic fiber degeneration, with the appearance in the media of cystic spaces filled with mucoid material. Although these changes occur most frequently in the ascending aorta, in some cases the entire aorta may be similarly affected. The histological changes lead to weakening of the aortic wall, which in turn results in the formation of a fusiform aneurysm. Such aneurysms often involve the aortic root and may consequently result in aortic regurgitation. The term *annuloaortic ectasia* is often used to describe this condition (see below).

Cystic medial degeneration is found in virtually all cases of the Marfan syndrome[74] and may be associated with other connective tissue disorders as well, such as Ehlers-Danlos syndrome. The Marfan syndrome (see p. 1669) is an autosomal dominant heritable disorder of connective tissue that has recently been discovered to be due to mutations of one of the genes for fibrillin, a structural protein that helps to direct and orient elastin in the developing aorta.[75] These mutations result in a decrease in the amount of elastin in the aortic wall,[76] together with a loss of the elastin's normally highly organized structure. As a consequence, from an early age the marfanoid aorta exhibits markedly abnormal elastic properties and increased systemic pulse wave velocities, and over time the aorta exhibits progressively increasing degrees of stiffness and dilatation.[77]

In those patients without the Marfan syndrome, however, it is not possible to recognize the histological diagnosis of cystic medial degeneration prospectively (i.e., without surgery or necropsy).[78] This fact has significantly limited our understanding of medial degeneration and its natural history, and it remains unclear to what extent this syndrome may represent an independent disease process versus a manifestation of another disease state. It has long been suspected that some patients who have annuloaortic ectasia and proven cystic medial degeneration without the classic phenotypic manifestations of the Marfan syndrome may, in fact, have a variation or forme fruste of the Marfan syndrome,[79] although this remains unproved. On the contrary, many patients with ascending thoracic aortic aneurysms appear to have nothing more than idiopathic cystic medial degeneration.

ATHEROSCLEROSIS. Atherosclerotic aneurysms infrequently occur in the ascending aorta and, when they do, tend to be associated with diffuse aortic atherosclerosis.

Aneurysms in the aortic arch are often contiguous with aneurysms of the ascending or descending aorta. They may be due to atherosclerotic disease, cystic medial degeneration, syphilis, or other infections. The predominant cause of aneurysms of the descending thoracic aorta is atherosclerosis.[81] These aneurysms tend to originate just distal to the origin of the left subclavian artery and may be either fusiform or saccular.[82] The pathogenesis of such atherosclerotic aneurysms in the thoracic aorta may be similar to that of abdominal aneurysms but has not been extensively examined.

SYPHILIS. This was once a common cause of ascending thoracic aortic aneurysm, but today it has become a rarity in most major medical centers[12,80] as a result of aggressive antibiotic treatment of the disease in its early stages. The latent period from initial spirochetal infection to aortic complications may range from 5 to 40 years but is most commonly 10 to 25 years. During the secondary phase of the disease there is direct spirochetal infection of the aortic media, most commonly involving the ascending aorta. The muscular and elastic medial elements are destroyed by the infection and inflammatory response and replaced by fibrous tissue that frequently calcifies. Weakening of the aortic wall from medial destruction results in progressive aneurysmal dilatation. In addition, the infection may spread into the aortic root, and the subsequent root dilatation may result in aortic regurgitation.

INFECTIOUS AORTITIS. This rare cause of aortic aneurysm may result from a primary infection of the aortic wall, causing aortic dilatation with the formation of fusiform or saccular aneurysms (see p. 1547). More commonly, infected or *mycotic* aneurysms may arise secondarily from an infection occurring in a preexisting aneurysm of another etiology. When an infected aneurysm involves the ascending aorta, it is often the consequence of direct spread from aortic bacterial endocarditis.

Several other causes of thoracic aortic aneurysms are discussed in detail elsewhere in this chapter, including aortic infection (see p. 1575), giant cell arteritis (p. 1573), aortic trauma (p. 1543), and aortic dissection (p. 1554). Note that the clinical presentation, natural history, and therapy of thoracic aneurysms discussed below apply specifically to *nondissecting thoracic aortic aneurysms.*

Clinical Manifestations

Forty per cent of patients with thoracic aortic aneurysms are asymptomatic at the time of diagnosis,[11] with such aneurysms typically discovered as incidental findings on a routine physical examination or chest roentgenogram. When patients do experience symptoms, the symptoms tend to reflect either a vascular consequence of the aneurysm or a local mass effect. Vascular consequences include aortic regurgitation due to dilatation of the aortic root, often associated with secondary congestive heart failure; myocardial ischemia or infarction due to local compression of the coronary arteries by enlarged sinuses of Valsalva; sinus of Valsalva aneurysms that may rupture into the right side of the heart to cause a continuous murmur and congestive heart failure; and thromboembolism causing stroke, lower extremity ischemia, renal infarction, or mesenteric ischemia.

Local mass effect from an ascending or arch aneurysm may cause superior vena cava syndrome due to obstruction of venous return via compression of the superior vena cava or innominate veins. Aneurysms of the arch or descending aorta may compress the trachea (Fig. 45–2) or mainstem bronchus, producing tracheal deviation, wheezing, cough, dyspnea (with symptoms that may be positional), hemoptysis, or recurrent pneumonitis. Compression of the esophagus may produce dysphagia, and compression of the recurrent laryngeal nerve may cause hoarseness. Chest pain and back pain occur in 37 per cent and 21 per cent, respectively, of nondissecting aneurysms[11] and result from direct compression of other intrathoracic structures or from erosion into adjacent bone. Typically such pain is steady, deep, boring, and at times extremely severe.

As with abdominal aortic aneurysms, the most worrisome consequence of thoracic aneurysms is leakage or rupture. Rupture is accompanied by the dramatic onset of excruciating pain, usually in the region where less severe pain had previously existed. Rupture occurs most commonly into the left intrapleural space or the intrapericardial space, presenting as hypotension. The third most common site of rupture is from the descending thoracic aorta into the adjacent esophagus (an aortoesophageal fistula), presenting as life-threatening hematemesis.[83] Acute aneurysm expansion, which may herald rupture, can cause similar pain. Thoracic aneurysms may also develop aortic dissection, which is discussed in detail later in this chapter.

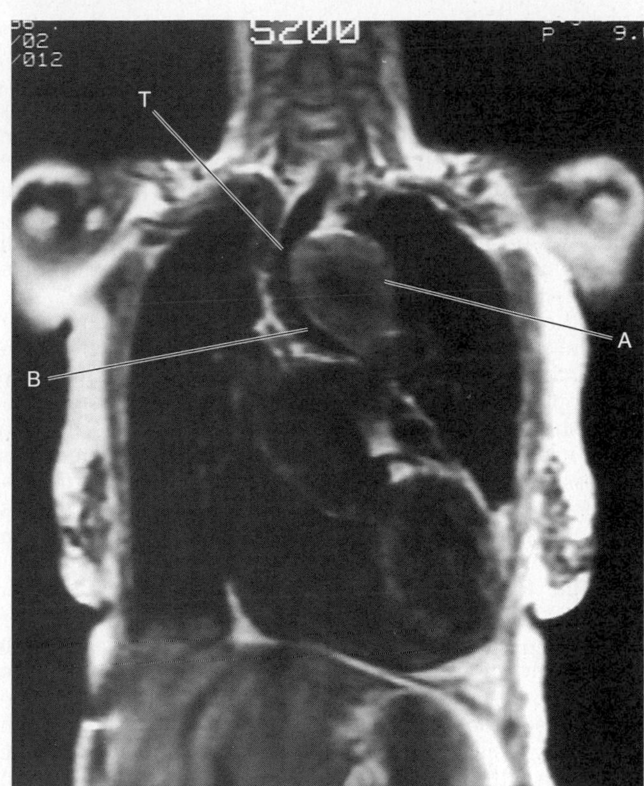

FIGURE 45–2. MRI in the coronal projection of a large thoracic aortic aneurysm in an elderly woman presenting with a complaint of dyspnea and cough. In this view the markedly dilated aortic arch (A) compresses the trachea (T), causing rightward tracheal deviation. The aneurysm also compresses the left mainstem bronchus (B). In addition, all four cardiac chambers are dilated, consistent with the patient's known idiopathic dilated cardiomyopathy.

DIAGNOSIS AND SIZING. Many thoracic aneurysms are readily visible on chest roentgenogram (Fig. 45–3), presenting as widening of the mediastinal silhouette, enlargement of the aortic knob, or displacement of the trachea from midline. Unfortunately, smaller aneurysms, especially saccular ones, may not be evident on chest roentgenogram; therefore, this technique cannot exclude the diagnosis of aortic aneurysm.

Aortography is still the preferred modality for the preoperative evaluation of thoracic aortic aneurysms and precise

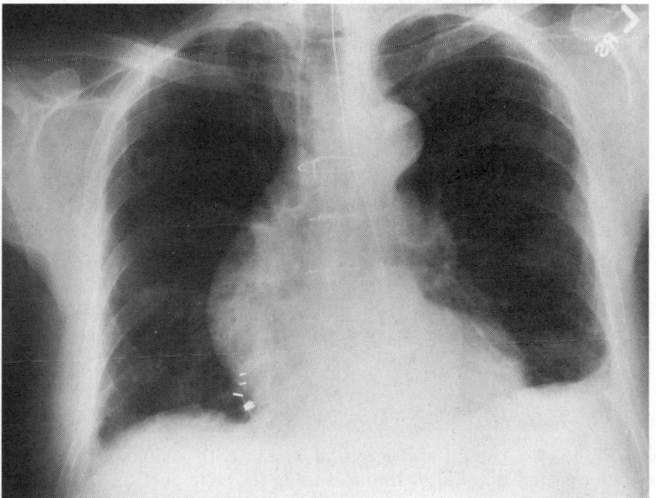

FIGURE 45–3. Chest roentgenogram of a patient with a very large aneurysm of the ascending thoracic aorta. Evident are both marked widening of the mediastinum and an abnormal aortic contour.

definition of the anatomy of the aneurysm and great vessels (Fig. 45–4). As is the case for abdominal aortic aneurysms, contrast-enhanced CT scanning is very accurate in detecting and sizing thoracic aortic aneurysms[84] and is useful as a method to follow aneurysm size. MRI is also useful in defining thoracic aortic anatomy and detecting aneurysms[85] (Fig. 45–2) and is of particular utility in patients with preexisting aortic disease. MR angiography may prove especially useful in defining the anatomy of the aortic branch vessels, but its utility in evaluating thoracic aortic aneurysms has not yet been extensively studied.

Transthoracic echocardiography is not very accurate for diagnosing thoracic aneurysms and is particularly limited in its ability to examine the descending thoracic aorta. Transesophageal echocardiography (TEE), a far more accurate method for assessing the thoracic aorta, has become widely used for detection of aortic dissection. There has been less experience with TEE in evaluation of nondissecting thoracic aneurysms. (The advantages and disadvantages of each imaging modality are discussed in greater detail on p. 356.)

NATURAL HISTORY. Defining the natural history of thoracic aortic aneurysms is complex, given the numerous contributing factors. The cause of an aneurysm may affect both its rate of growth and propensity for rupture. The presence or absence of aneurysm symptoms is another important predictor, as symptomatic patients have a much poorer prognosis than those without symptoms,[81] in large part because the onset of new symptoms is frequently a harbinger of rupture or death. Moreover, the high prevalence of additional cardiovascular diseases in these patients may have a dramatic impact on mortality; in fact, second to aneurysm rupture, the most common causes of death in this population are other cardiovascular diseases.[82,86]

Several small studies of the natural history of thoracic aortic aneurysms have been reported, but the data are far more limited than those available regarding abdominal aortic aneurysms. In the largest modern series, the 1-, 3-, and 5-year survival rates for patients with thoracic aortic aneurysms not undergoing surgical repair were approximately 65, 36, and 20 per cent, respectively.[12,86,87] Aneurysm rupture occurs in 32 to 68 per cent of patients not treated surgically, with rupture accounting for 32 to 47 per cent of all patient deaths.[81,86,87] Fewer than half of the patients with rupture may arrive at the hospital alive,[80] as mortality at 6 hours is 54 per cent and at 24 hours reaches 76 per cent.[80] There is no apparent association between thoracic aneurysm location and the risk of death due to rupture.[86]

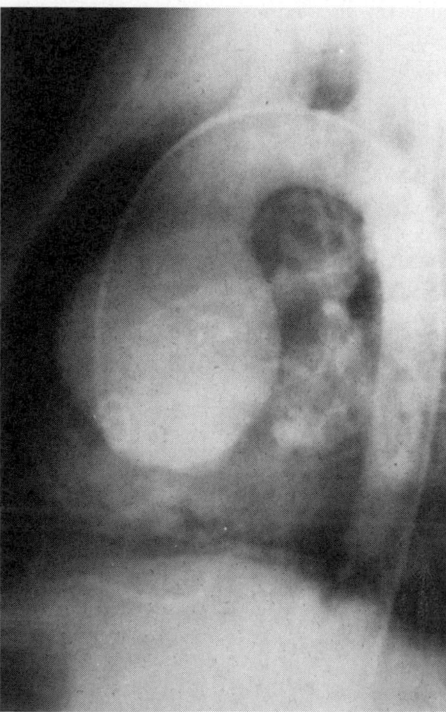

FIGURE 45–4. Lateral aortogram in a man with annuloaortic ectasia and aneurysmal dilation of the ascending thoracic aorta. The bulbous, pear-shaped aortic root can easily be seen. The left ventricle is partially opacified consequent to aortic regurgitation. (Courtesy of Christos Athanasoulis, M.D., and Arthur Waltman, M.D., Section of Vascular Radiology, Massachusetts General Hospital, Boston.)

Because size is an important predictor of the risk of aneurysm rupture, several studies have examined the rate of expansion of thoracic aortic aneurysms. As with abdominal aneurysms, initial size is the only independent predictor of the rate of thoracic aneurysm growth,[84] although some data also suggest that descending thoracic aneurysms may expand more slowly than others.[88] In a recent report, Dapunt et al. followed 67 patients with thoracic aortic aneurysm using serial CT scanning and found a mean rate of expansion of 0.43 cm/year.[89] The only independent predictor of a rapid expansion (greater than 0.5 cm/year) was an initial aortic diameter larger than 5.0 cm: Those aneurysms that were 5.0 cm or smaller showed mean growth rates of 0.17 cm/year, whereas those larger than 5.0 cm grew by 0.79 cm/year. Unfortunately, even when controlling for initial aneurysm size, there was still substantial variation in individual aneurysm growth rates, making such mean growth rates of little value in predicting aneurysm growth for a given patient. More helpful, however, was the finding that growth rates among small aneurysms were more consistent, with only 1 of 25 aneurysms 4.0 cm or less at baseline showing rapid growth. Two additional findings in this series were that no aneurysm smaller than 5.0 cm ruptured during the follow-up period, and that the only variable predictor of survival was initial aneurysm size.

Management

SURGICAL TREATMENT. The optimal timing of surgical repair of thoracic aortic aneurysms remains uncertain for several reasons. First, as noted above, the available data on the natural history of thoracic aneurysms are limited, especially with respect to the outcomes of surgical intervention. Second, with the high incidence of coexisting cardiovascular disease in this population, many patients die of other cardiovascular causes before their aneurysms ever rupture. Finally, significant risks are associated with thoracic aortic surgery, particularly in the arch and descending aorta, which in many cases may outweigh the potential benefits of aortic repair.

We currently recommend surgery when thoracic aortic aneurysms reach 6.0 cm or larger, or often 7.0 cm or larger in patients at high operative risk. Indications for surgery in smaller aneurysms include rapid rate of expansion, associated significant aortic regurgitation, or the presence of aneurysm-related symptoms. In patients with the Marfan syndrome, given their higher risk of dissection and rupture, we recommend repair of thoracic aneurysms when they reach only 5.5 cm in size.[90] Surgery should be considered even sooner in Marfan patients at especially high risk, such as those with rapid and progressive aortic dilatation, those with a family history of the Marfan syndrome plus aortic dissection, or women planning pregnancy. Of course, the aggressiveness with which surgical repair is undertaken in any case should be appropriately influenced by the general condition of the individual patient.

Thoracic aortic aneurysms are generally resected and replaced with a prosthetic sleeve of appropriate size (Fig. 45–5). Cardiopulmonary bypass is necessary for the removal of ascending aortic aneurysms, and partial bypass to support the circulation distal to the aneurysm is often advisable in resection of descending thoracic aortic aneurysms. A temporary Gott shunt may be used from the proximal aorta to the aorta beyond the aneurysm in order to perfuse the distal circulation while the aortic site being

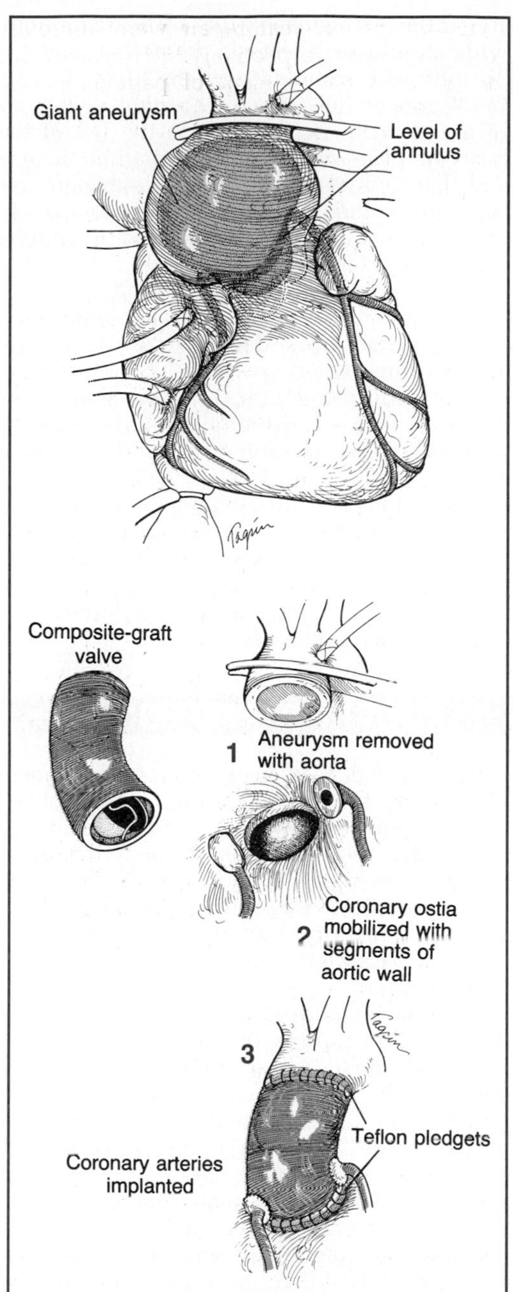

FIGURE 45–5. Technique for the composite graft replacement of an aneurysm of the ascending aorta. *Top,* The aneurysm is shown, involving the sinuses of Valsalva. The patient is on total cardiopulmonary bypass. *Bottom,* The composite graft is shown, with a low-profile, tilting-disc aortic prosthesis attached to its inferior end. (1) The aneurysm is resected with the native aortic valve. (2) The coronary ostia have been excised and mobilized with a button of aortic wall. (3) The composite graft has been secured in place using Teflon felt reinforcement for the suture line. The coronary artery ostia are then reimplanted directly to the graft.

repaired is cross-clamped.[91] The use of such adjuncts is less important, however, than the nature and extent of the aneurysm in determining the incidence of postoperative complications.[92]

The use of a composite graft consisting of a Dacron tube with a prosthetic aortic valve sewn into one end (Bentall procedure) is generally the method of choice in treating ascending thoracic aneurysms involving the root which are associated with significant aortic regurgitation.[93] The valve and graft are sewn directly into the aortic annulus, and the coronary arteries then reimplanted into the Dacron aortic graft (Fig. 45–5). The operative risk for mortality is about 5 per cent.[93] For those patients with structurally normal aortic valve leaflets whose aortic regurgitation is secondary to dilatation of the root, David et al. have successfully repaired the native valve by either reimplanting it in a Dacron graft or reconstructing the aortic root. In a recent series, 41 of 45 patients had mild or no aortic regurgitation after this method of aortic valve repair and were stable at a mean of 18 months.[94]

Aneurysms of the aortic arch may be successfully excised surgically, but the procedure may be particularly challenging. The brachiocephalic vessels must be removed from the aortic arch prior to its resection. Then, after interposition of the prosthetic tube graft, the island of native aortic tissue containing the brachiocephalic vessels is reimplanted into the graft and normal cerebral perfusion restored. There is, however, a significantly increased risk of stroke secondary to variable periods of cerebral ischemia. The incidence of stroke in recent series is 3 to 7 per cent.[95,96] The standard method for carrying out this operation today is with the use of profound hypothermic circulatory arrest, as introduced by Griepp et al. in 1974.[97] Some have attempted to add selective cerebral perfusion during aneurysmectomy, but cannulation techniques are difficult. In fact, the incidence of stroke may actually be as high or higher with this method, possibly due to cannulation-induced cerebral emboli.[96,99] A more recent adjunct for cerebral protection during hypothermic arrest is the use of retrograde cerebral perfusion via a superior vena cava cannula.[95] Not only does this technique provide nutrients and oxygen to the brain,[100] but it may also serve to flush out both air and particulate matter from the cerebral and carotid arteries that would otherwise embolize. The results of retrograde cerebral perfusion have thus far been quite encouraging, with trends toward lower stroke rates in recent reports.[95,99]

More than half of the patients undergoing surgical repair of a thoracic aortic aneurysm in Crawford's series had multiple aortic segments involved, and almost three-quarters of those with descending thoracic aneurysms had multiple involvement.[98] Such widespread aneurysmal dilatation of the aorta presents a particular challenge to the surgeon and often precludes operation. However, Crawford et al. have demonstrated that it is possible to successfully replace virtually the entire diseased thoracic and abdominal aorta.[98] A method known as the "elephant trunk" technique, carried out in sequential stages of aortic replacement, has been shown to facilitate such extensive surgical procedures and reduce the associated risks.[101]

Elective surgical repair of ascending and descending thoracic aortic aneurysms has a 90 to 95 per cent early survival rate in most centers.[102,103] Major complications are technical, especially hemorrhage from tearing of the diseased aorta. A catastrophic complication of resection of descending thoracic aortic aneurysms is postoperative paraplegia secondary to interruption of the blood supply to the spinal cord. The incidence of paraplegia ranges from 0 to 17 per cent,[91,92] although most series show an incidence of about 5 to 6 per cent.[92,104] A number of methods have been proposed to reduce the likelihood of paraplegia, although none has proved to be consistently safe and effective. One of the more promising techniques involves maintaining distal aortic perfusion during surgery with the use of the heparinless Gott shunt (aorto-aorta bypass).[91] Although some groups have achieved good success with such techniques,[91] others have had mixed results. Controlled trials might better clarify the efficacy of these techniques.

An alternative approach to the surgical management of descending thoracic aneurysms, as recently reported by Dake et al., is the use of a transluminally placed endovascular stent-graft. This technique has the advantage of being far less invasive than surgery and has the potential of reducing the incidence of paraplegia from surgically induced spinal cord ischemia. The authors report successful device deployment in all 14 of their patients, with documented thrombosis of the residual aneurysm lumen surrounding the stent-graft in 12.[105] Although still experimental at present, such a device may in the future have an important role in the management of patients who are at risk for aortic rupture but are otherwise poor surgical candidates. Unfortunately, the curvilinear nature of the ascending aorta and arch makes application of similar techniques to aneurysms of these proximal aortic segments far more problematic.

Complications of associated atherosclerosis, such as myocardial infarction, cerebrovascular accidents, and renal failure, often become manifested under the massive physiological stress of aortic surgery. The most frequent causes of early postoperative death are myocardial infarction, congestive heart failure, stroke, renal failure, hemorrhage, respiratory failure, and sepsis. Advanced age, emergency operation, prolonged aortic cross-clamp time, extent of the aneurysm, diabetes, prior aortic surgery, aneurysm symptoms, and intraoperative hypotension are the most important factors determining perioperative morbidity and mortality.[106] Many patients with atherosclerotic aneurysms are heavy smokers, and pulmonary complications following surgery are common. The left lung may be severely traumatized by compression during resection of large aneurysms of the descending thoracic aorta, a complication that may seriously jeopardize the patient's survival, particularly in the setting of underlying pulmonary disease.

Late deaths are usually associated with cardiac complications, aneurysm rupture, respiratory failure, or stroke.[102] Aneurysm rupture may be due to aneurysm formation at the graft margins or the appearance of new aneurysms at other aortic sites.[11]

MEDICAL MANAGEMENT. The long-term impact of medical therapy on aneurysm growth and survival in patients with typical atherosclerotic thoracic aneurysms has not been examined. However, in a recent report, Shores et al. examined the efficacy of beta blockers in adult patients with the Marfan syndrome.[107] They randomized 70 patients to treatment with propranolol versus no beta blocker therapy and followed them over a 10-year period. The treated group showed a significantly slower rate of aortic dilatation, fewer adverse clinical endpoints (death, aortic dissection, aortic regurgitation, aortic root >6 cm), and significantly lower mortality from the 4-year point onward.[107] Although this study examined only the effect of beta blockade in the Marfan syndrome, it follows logically that medical therapy to reduce dP/dt and control blood pressure is essential to the treatment of thoracic aortic aneurysm, both for those with smaller aneurysms being followed serially and for patients having undergone aortic aneurysm repair.

Annuloaortic Ectasia

The term *annuloaortic ectasia* was first used by Ellis et al. in 1961 to describe a clinicopathological condition seen in a subset of patients with thoracic aortic aneurysms in whom idiopathic dilatation of the proximal aorta and the aortic annulus leads to pure aortic regurgitation.[108] The entity has subsequently been recognized with increasing frequency and makes up about 5 to 10 per cent of the population undergoing aortic valve replacement for pure aortic regurgitation. Annuloaortic ectasia is more common in men than in women, typically presenting in the fourth, fifth, and sixth decades with progressively more severe aortic regurgitation. Sudden onset of symptoms followed by rapid progression is occasionally seen.

The common pathological feature shared by patients with annuloaortic ectasia is that of cystic medial degeneration of the afflicted aortic wall, leading to progressive dilatation. With widening of the aortic root, the valve annulus dilates and the aortic leaflets are pulled apart, resulting in aortic regurgitation, despite the fact that the aortic valve leaflets themselves are structurally normal. The weakened aortic walls are also prone to dissection. When aortic dissection does occur, the dissection tends to be small, circumscribed, and confined to the ascending aorta.

Clinically, little distinguishes the aortic regurgitation in patients with annuloaortic ectasia from that due to other causes. On physical examination, the diastolic murmur tends to be of greater intensity to the right of the sternum in cases of annuloaortic ectasia and to the left of the sternum in cases of primary aortic regurgitation. Lemon and White found that two features—acute or subacute development of symptoms and the presence of associated chest pain—were more common in patients with annuloaortic ectasia than primary aortic regurgitation.[109]

The chest roentgenogram usually shows a grossly dilated aortic root and ascending aorta with left ventricular enlargement proportional to the degree of aortic regurgitation. Aortographically, annuloaortic ectasia has one of three typical appearances. Most common is a pear-shaped enlargement of the ascending aorta (Fig. 45–4). Also seen are diffuse symmetrical dilatation and dilatation limited to the aortic root.[109]

Surgical correction is usually undertaken for relief of aortic regurgitation when it is severe and responsible for symptoms of left ventricular failure or when the left ventricle or ascending aorta is increasing in size. In such cases, the aortic valve together with the proximal ascending aorta is usually replaced with a composite graft.

AORTIC DISSECTION

Acute aortic dissection is an uncommon but potentially catastrophic illness that occurs with an incidence of at least 2000 cases per year in the United States.[110,111] Early mortality is as high as 1 per cent per hour if untreated,[112] but survival may be significantly improved by the timely institution of appropriate medical and/or surgical therapy. Prompt clinical recognition and definitive diagnostic testing are therefore essential in the management of patients with aortic dissection.

Aortic dissection is believed to begin with the formation of a tear in the aortic intima that directly exposes an underlying diseased medial layer to the driving force (or pulse pressure) of the intraluminal blood (Fig. 45–6*A*). This blood penetrates the diseased medial layer and cleaves the laminar plane of the media in two, thus dissecting the aortic wall. Driven by persistent intraluminal pressure, the dissection process extends a variable length along the aortic wall, typically antegrade (driven by the forward force of aortic blood flow) but sometimes retrograde from the site of intimal tear. The blood-filled space between the dissected layers of the aortic wall becomes the *false lumen.* Shear forces may lead to further tears in the *intimal flap* (the inner portion of the dissected aortic wall), producing exit sites or additional entry sites for blood flow in the false lumen. The false lumen may become distended with blood, causing the intimal flap to bow into the *true lumen,* thereby narrowing its caliber and distorting its shape.

It has also been suggested that aortic dissection may begin instead with the rupture of the vasa vasorum within the aortic media, i.e., with the development of an intramural hematoma (Fig. 45–6*B*). Local hemorrhage then secondarily ruptures through the intimal layer, creating the intimal tear and aortic dissection. The fact that in autopsy series as many as 13 per cent of aortic dissections do not have an identifiable intimal tear[113] argues that, at least in this minority of cases, independent medial hemorrhage is the primary cause of dissection. On the other hand, one might argue that the lack of an intimal tear in these patients indicates that they do not, in fact, have classic aortic dissection, but rather suffer intramural hematoma of the aorta, a closely related condition (see below).

CLASSIFICATION. Most classification schemes for aortic dissection are based on the fact that the vast majority of aortic dissections originate in one of two locations: (1) the ascending aorta, within several centimeters of the aortic

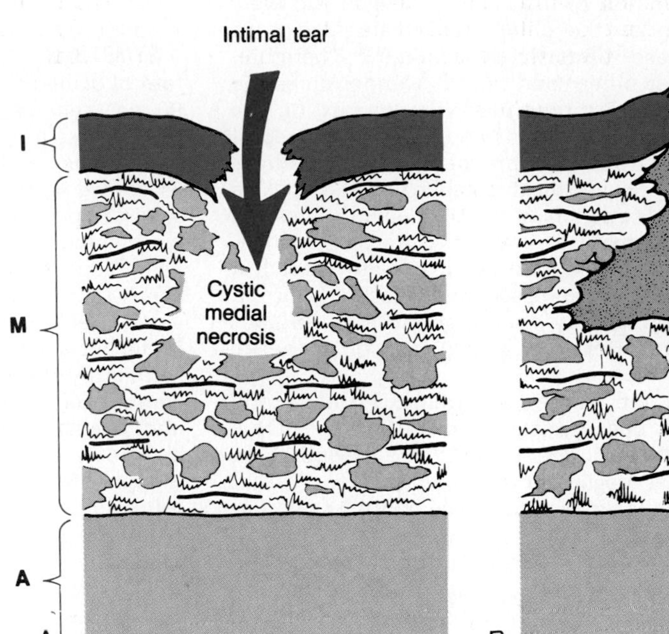

FIGURE 45–6. Proposed mechanisms of initiation of aortic dissection. In both cases, cystic medial necrosis is present. In *A*, an intimal tear is the initial event, allowing aortic blood to enter the media. In *B*, the primary event is hemorrhage into the media, with secondary rupture of the overlying intima. I = intima; M = media; A = adventitia.

valve, and (2) the descending aorta, just distal to the origin of the left subclavian artery at the site of the ligamentum arteriosum.[111] Sixty-five per cent of intimal tears occur in the ascending aorta, 20 per cent in the descending aorta, 10 per cent in the aortic arch, and 5 per cent in the abdominal aorta.[98]

There are three major classification systems to define the location and extent of aortic involvement, as defined in Table 45–1 and depicted in Figure 45–7: (1) DeBakey types I, II, and III[114]; (2) Stanford types A and B[115]; and (3) anatomical categories "proximal" and "distal." All three schemes share the same basic principle of distinguishing those aortic dissections with and without ascending aortic involvement for prognostic and therapeutic reasons; in general, surgery is indicated for dissections involving the ascending aorta, whereas medical management is reserved for those dissections without ascending aortic involvement. Accordingly, because both DeBakey types I and II involve the ascending aorta, they are grouped together for simplicity in the Stanford (type A) and anatomical (proximal) classification systems. Aortic dissections confined to the abdominal aorta,[116] although quite uncommon, are best categorized as type B or distal dissections. Proximal or type A dissections occur in about two-thirds of cases, with distal dissections composing the remaining one-third.

In addition to its location, aortic dissection is also classified according to its duration, defined as the length of time from symptom onset to medical evaluation. The mortality from dissection and its risk of progression decrease progressively over time, making therapeutic strategies for long-standing aortic dissections quite different from those for dissections presenting acutely. A dissection present less than 2 weeks is defined as "acute," whereas those present 2 weeks or more are defined as "chronic" because the mortality curve for untreated aortic dissections begins to level off at 75 to 80 per cent at this time.[112] At diagnosis, about two-thirds of aortic dissections are acute and the remaining third are chronic.[117]

ETIOLOGY AND PATHOGENESIS. Medial degeneration, as

TABLE 45–1 COMMONLY USED CLASSIFICATION SYSTEMS TO DESCRIBE AORTIC DISSECTION

TYPE	SITE OF ORIGIN AND EXTENT OF AORTIC INVOLVEMENT
DeBakey	
Type I	Originates in the ascending aorta, propagates at least to the aortic arch and often beyond it distally
Type II	Originates in and is confined to the ascending aorta
Type III	Originates in the descending aorta and extends distally down the aorta or, rarely, retrograde into the aortic arch and ascending aorta
Stanford	
Type A	All dissections involving the ascending aorta, regardless of the site of origin
Type B	All dissections not involving the ascending aorta
Descriptive	
Proximal	Includes DeBakey types I and II or Stanford type A
Distal	Includes DeBakey type III or Stanford type B

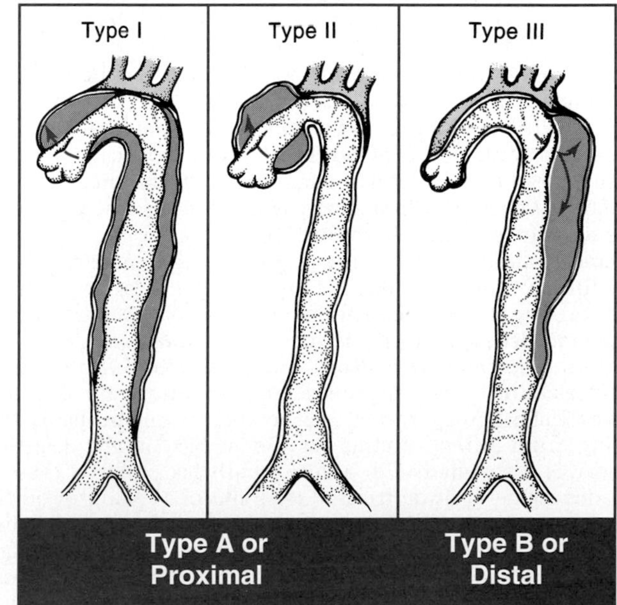

FIGURE 45–7. Commonly used classification systems for aortic dissection. (Refer to Table 45–1 for definitions.)

evidenced by deterioration of the medial collagen and elastin, is considered to be the chief predisposing factor in most nontraumatic cases of aortic dissection.[78,95] Therefore, any disease process or other condition that undermines the integrity of the elastic or muscular components of the media predisposes the aorta to dissection. Cystic medial degeneration is an intrinsic feature of several hereditary defects of connective tissue, most notably the Marfan (see p. 1671) and Ehlers-Danlos (see p. 1672) syndromes. In addition to their propensity to develop thoracic aortic aneurysms, patients with the Marfan syndrome are indeed at high risk of developing aortic dissection—especially proximal dissection—at a relatively young age. In fact, the Marfan syndrome accounts for 6 to 9 per cent of all aortic dissections.[117,118]

In the absence of the Marfan syndrome, histologically classic cystic medial degeneration is identified in only a minority of cases of aortic dissection.[117,118] Nevertheless, the degree of medial degeneration found in most other cases of aortic dissection still tends to be qualitatively and quantitatively much greater than that expected as part of the aging process. Although the cause of such medial degeneration remains unclear, advanced age and hypertension appear to be two of the most important factors.

The peak incidence of aortic dissection is in the sixth and seventh decades of life, with men affected twice as often as women.[117] A coexisting history of hypertension is found in almost 80 per cent of cases in a recent series of 236 cases of aortic dissection from Spittell et al.[117] Bicuspid aortic valve is a well-established risk factor for proximal aortic dissection and historically has been found in 7 to 14 per cent of all aortic dissections.[117,118] Interestingly, the risk of aortic dissection appears to be independent of the severity of the bicuspid valve stenosis.[118] Certain other congenital cardiovascular abnormalities predispose the aorta to dissection, including unicuspid aortic valve and possibly coarctation of the aorta.[118] Aortic dissection has also been reported to occur in association with the Noonan[119] and the Turner syndromes.[117,120] Rarely, aortic dissection complicates arteritis involving the aorta (see p. 1574), particularly giant cell arteritis.[117] A number of reports describe aortic dissection in association with cocaine abuse among younger men,[121] but no direct causal relationship has yet been established.

An unexplained relationship exists between pregnancy and aortic dissection (see p. 1855). About half of all aortic dissections in women under 40 years of age occur during pregnancy, typically in the third trimester[122] and also occasionally in the early postpartum period.[123] Increases in blood volume, cardiac output, and blood pressure seen in late pregnancy may contribute to the risk,[124] although this explanation cannot account for postpartum occurrence. Women with the Marfan syndrome and a dilated aortic root are at particular risk of suffering acute aortic dissection during pregnancy,[125] and in some cases the diagnosis of the Marfan syndrome is first made when such women present with a peripartum aortic dissection.

Direct trauma to the aorta may also cause aortic dissection. Blunt trauma tends to cause localized tears, hematomas, or frank aortic disruption rather than classic aortic dissection (see p. 1543). Iatrogenic trauma, on the other hand, is associated with true aortic dissection. Intraarterial catheterization and the insertion of intraaortic balloon pumps[126] both may induce aortic dissection, probably resulting from direct trauma to the aortic intima. Cardiac surgery is associated with a very small risk of aortic dissection occurring at an aortic incision site or the site of aortic cross-clamping.[127] The majority of these dissections are discovered intraoperatively and repaired at that time, although 20 per cent are detected only after a delay.[128] A distinct group of cardiac surgical patients undergoing aortic valve replacement suffer aortic dissection as a late complication, usually not until several years after the procedure.[129]

Clinical Manifestations

SYMPTOMS. By far the most common presenting symptom of acute aortic dissection is severe pain, found in 74 to 90 per cent of cases,[117,130] whereas the large majority of those presenting without pain are found to have chronic dissections.[117] The pain is typically of sudden onset, and is as severe at its inception as it ever becomes, contrasting with the pain of myocardial infarction, which usually has a crescendo-like onset. In fact, the pain may be all but unbearable in some instances, forcing the patient to writhe in agony, fall to the ground, or pace restlessly in an attempt to gain relief. Several features of the pain should arouse suspicion of aortic dissection. The quality of the pain as described by the patient is often morbidly appropriate to the actual event, with adjectives such as "tearing," "ripping," and "stabbing" frequently used. Another important characteristic of the pain of aortic dissection is its tendency to migrate from its point of origin to other sites, generally following the path of the dissection as it extends through the aorta. Such migratory pain was noted in 70 per cent of our cases.[130]

The location of pain may be quite helpful in suggesting the location of the aortic dissection, because localized symptoms tend to reflect involvement of the underlying aorta. In the series by Spittell et al.,[117] when the location of chest pain was anterior only (or if the most severe pain was anterior), more than 90 per cent had involvement of the ascending aorta. Conversely, when the chest pain was interscapular only (or when the most severe pain was interscapular), more than 90 per cent had involvement of the descending thoracic aorta (i.e., DeBakey type I or III). The presence of any pain in the neck, throat, jaw, or face strongly predicted involvement of the ascending aorta, whereas pain anywhere in the back, abdomen, or lower extremities strongly predicted involvement of the descending aorta.

Less common symptoms at presentation, occurring with or without associated chest pain, include congestive heart failure, syncope, cerebrovascular accident, ischemic peripheral neuropathy, paraplegia, and cardiac arrest or sudden death. The presence of acute congestive heart failure in this setting is almost invariably due to severe aortic regurgitation induced by a proximal aortic dissection (discussed below). The occurrence of syncope without focal neurological signs, in 4 to 5 per cent of aortic dissections,[117,130] may be an ominous sign suggesting a surgical emergency. It is associated most often with a rupture of a proximal aortic dissection into the pericardial cavity with resultant cardiac tamponade, and less often with rupture of the descending thoracic aorta into the intrapleural space.[117]

PHYSICAL FINDINGS. Although extremely variable, the findings on physical examination generally reflect the location of the aortic dissection and extent of associated cardiovascular involvement. In some cases physical findings alone may be sufficient to suggest the diagnosis, whereas in other cases such pertinent findings may be subtle or absent, even in the presence of extensive aortic dissection. Hypertension is seen in more than 80 to 90 per cent of those with distal aortic dissection but is less common in proximal dissection. Hypotension, on the other hand, occurs much more commonly among those with proximal than distal aortic dissection.[130] True hypotension usually is the result of cardiac tamponade, intrapleural rupture, or intraperitoneal rupture. Dissection involving the brachiocephalic vessels may result in "pseudohypotension," an inaccurate measurement of blood pressure due to compromise or occlusion of the brachial arteries.

The physical findings most typically associated with aortic dissection—pulse deficits, the murmur of aortic regurgitation, and neurological manifestations—are more characteristic of proximal than of distal dissection. The presence of *pulse deficits* (diminution or absence) in patients with

PLATE 10

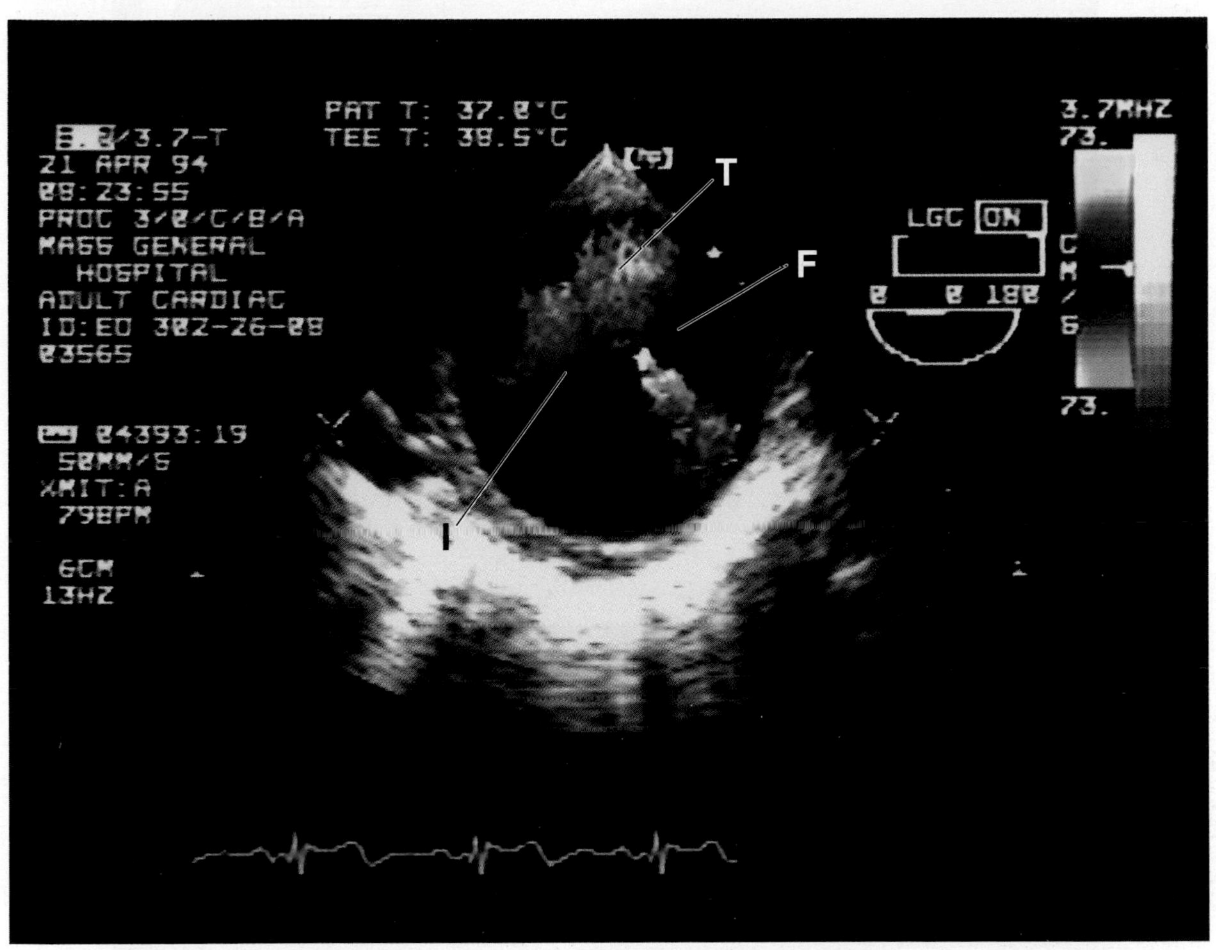

FIGURE 45–16. A cross-sectional transesophageal echocardiogram of a descending aortic dissection demonstrating a site of intimal tear. Blood flow (in orange) is evident in the true lumen (T) during systole, while a narrow jet of high-velocity blood (in blue) crosses into the false lumen (F) through a tear in the intimal flap (I).

PLATE 11

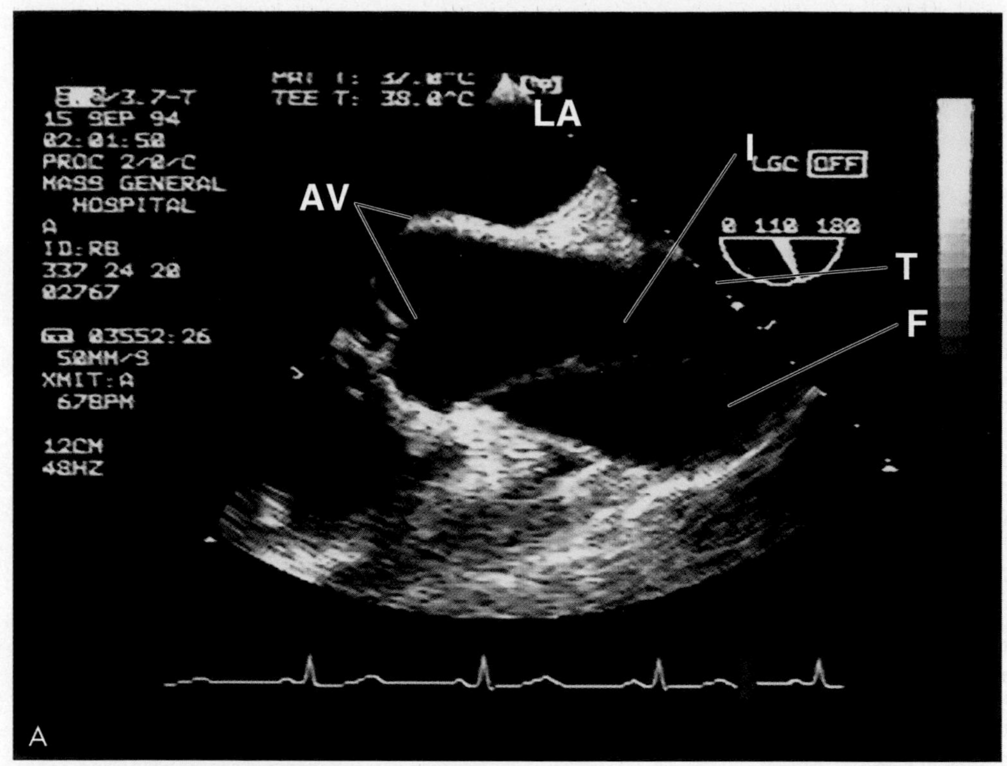

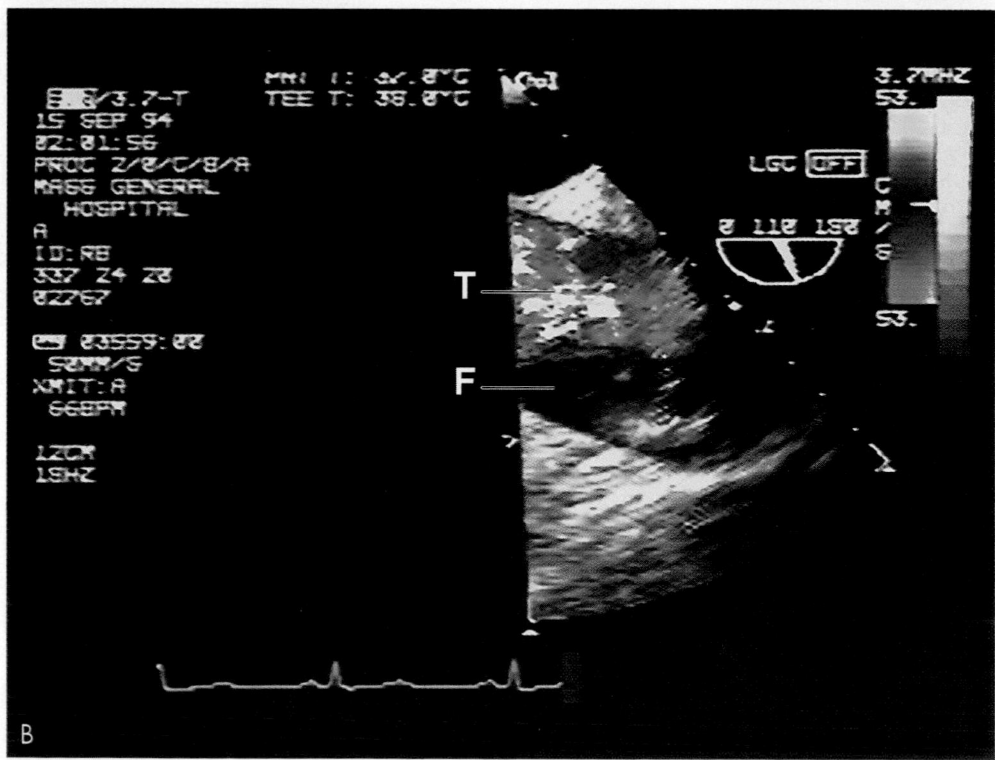

FIGURE 45–17. A transesophageal echocardiogram of the proximal ascending aorta in long axis in a patient with a proximal aortic dissection. *A*, The left atrium (LA) is closest to the transducer. The aortic valve (AV) is seen on the left in this view, with the ascending aorta extending to the right. Within the proximal aorta is an intimal flap (I), which originates just at the level of the sinotubular junction above the right sinus of Valsalva. The true lumen (T) and the false lumen (F) are separated by the intimal flap. *B*, The addition of color flow Doppler in the same view confirms the presence of two distinct lumens. The true lumen (T) fills completely with brisk blood flow (bright blue color), while at the same time there is minimal retrograde flow (dark orange) in the false lumen (F).

acute chest pain strongly suggests the presence of aortic dissection. Pulse deficits are present in about 50 per cent of proximal aortic dissection and occur throughout the arterial tree but are seen in only 15 per cent of distal dissections, where they usually involve the femoral or left subclavian arteries. Such pulse deficits result from extension of the dissection flap into an artery with compression of the true lumen by the false channel, or from proximal obstruction of flow due to a mobile portion of the intimal flap overlying the vessel's orifice. Whichever the cause, the pulse deficits in aortic dissection may be transient, secondary to decompression of the false lumen by distal reentry into the true lumen or to movement of the intimal flap away from the occluded orifice.

Aortic regurgitation is an important feature of proximal aortic dissection, with the murmur of aortic regurgitation detected in anywhere from 16 to 67 per cent of cases.[117,130] When aortic regurgitation is present in patients with distal dissection, it generally antedates the dissection and may be the result of preexisting dilatation of the aortic root due to the underlying aortic pathology, such as cystic medial degeneration. The murmur of aortic regurgitation associated with proximal dissection often has a musical quality and may be heard better along the right than the left sternal border. It may wax and wane, the intensity varying directly with the height of the arterial blood pressure. Depending on the severity of the regurgitation, other peripheral signs of aortic incompetence may be present, such as collapsing pulses and a wide pulse pressure. However, in some cases congestive heart failure secondary to severe acute aortic regurgitation may occur with little or no murmur and no peripheral signs of aortic runoff.

The aortic regurgitation associated with proximal aortic dissection, occurring in one-half to two-thirds of cases,[131] may result from any of several mechanisms, as depicted in Figure 45–8. First, the dissection may dilate the aortic root, widening the annulus so that the aortic leaflets are unable to coapt properly in diastole. Second, in an asymmetrical dissection, pressure from the dissecting hematoma may depress one leaflet below the coaptation line of the others so as to render the valve incompetent. Third, the annular support of the leaflets or the leaflets themselves may be torn, causing leaflet flail. Lastly, in the setting of an extensive or circumferential intimal tear, the unsupported intimal flap may prolapse into the left ventricular outflow tract,[132] occasionally appearing as frank intimal intussusception,[133] producing severe aortic regurgitation.

Neurological manifestations occur in as many as 6 to 19 per cent of all aortic dissections[117,130,134] but are more common with proximal dissection. Cerebrovascular accidents may occur in 3 to 6 per cent when there is direct involvement of the innominate or left common carotid arteries.[134] Less frequently, patients may present with altered consciousness or even coma. When spinal artery perfusion is compromised (more common in distal dissection[117]), ischemic spinal cord damage may produce paraparesis or paraplegia.[135]

In a small minority, about 1 to 2 per cent of cases,[117,136] a proximal dissection flap may involve the ostium of a coronary artery and cause acute myocardial infarction. The dissection more often affects the right coronary artery than the left, explaining why these myocardial infarctions tend to be inferior in location.[117] Unfortunately, when secondary myocardial infarction does occur, its symptoms may complicate the clinical picture by obscuring the symptoms of the primary aortic dissection. Most worrisome is the possibility that, in the setting of electrocardiographic evidence of myocardial infarction, the underlying aortic dissection may go unrecognized. Moreover, the consequences of such a misdiagnosis in the era of thrombolytic therapy can be catastrophic. In a recent review of the literature, Kamp et al. described an early mortality of 71 per cent (many from cardiac tamponade) among 21 cases of aortic dissection treated with thrombolysis.[137] It thus remains essential that when evaluating patients with acute myocardial infarction—particularly inferior infarctions—one carefully consider the possibility of an underlying aortic dissection before thrombolytic or anticoagulant therapy is instituted. Although some physicians feel reassured that performing a chest roentgenogram prior to the institution of thrombolysis is adequate to exclude the diagnosis of dissection, a blinded study of roentgenogram interpretation in this setting suggests that this is not sufficient.[138]

Extension of aortic dissection into the abdominal aorta may cause other vascular complications. Compromise of one or both renal arteries occurs in about 5 to 8 per cent[134,139] and may lead to renal ischemia or frank infarction, resulting in severe hypertension and acute renal failure. Mesenteric ischemia and infarction are also occasional complications of abdominal dissection, seen in 3 to 5 per cent of cases.[134,139] In addition, aortic dissection may extend into the iliac arteries, causing femoral pulse deficits (12 per cent[134]) and acute lower extremity ischemia. If in such cases the associated chest pain is minimal or absent, the pulse deficit and ischemic peripheral neuropathy may be mistaken for a peripheral embolic event.

Additional clinical manifestations of aortic dissection include the presence of pleural effusions, seen more commonly on the left side. The effusion typically arises secondary to an exudative inflammatory reaction around the involved aorta, but in some cases may result from a hemothorax due to a transient rupture or leak from a descending dissection. Several rarely encountered clinical manifestations of aortic dissection include hoarseness,[117] upper airway obstruction,[140] rupture into the tracheobronchial tree with hemoptysis,[117] dysphagia,[117] hematemesis due to rupture into the esophagus,[141] superior vena cava syndrome,[117] pulsation of the sternoclavicular joint,[142] pulsating neck masses, Horner syndrome, and unexplained fever.[143] Other rare presentations associated with the presence of a continuous murmur include rupture of the aortic dissection into the right atrium,[144] into the right ventricle,[145] or into the left atrium with secondary congestive heart failure.[146]

A variety of conditions may mimic aortic dissection. These include myocardial infarction or ischemia, acute aortic regurgitation without dissection, nondissecting thoracic or abdominal aortic aneurysms, pericarditis, musculoskeletal pain, or mediastinal tumors. Diagnostic confusion may be particularly likely when a patient with chest pain presents coincidentally with another clinical symptom, physical finding, or chest roentgenographic finding typically associated with aortic dissection.[147]

LABORATORY FINDINGS. Chest roentgenography is included in the discussion of clinical manifestations of aortic dissection rather than in the discussion of diagnostic techniques because an abnormal incidental finding on a routine

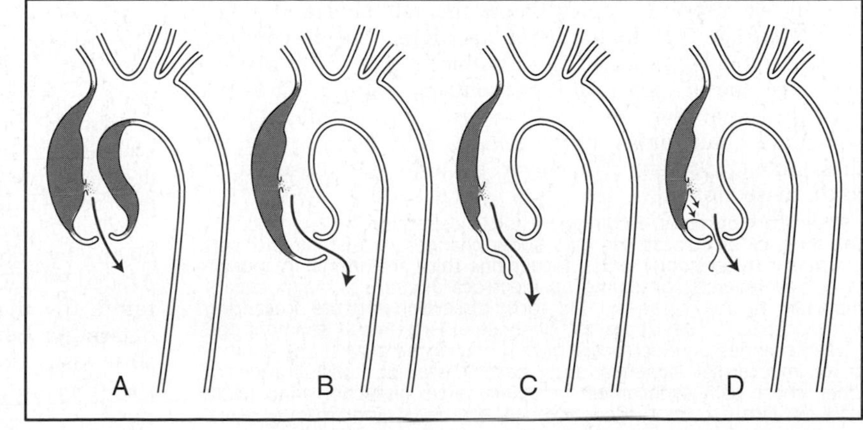

FIGURE 45–8. Mechanisms of aortic regurgitation in proximal aortic dissection. *A,* An extensive or circumferential tear dilates the aortic root and annulus, preventing the aortic valve leaflets from coapting. *B,* With asymmetrical dissection, pressure from the false lumen depresses one aortic leaflet below the coaptation line of the other leaflets. *C,* The annular support is disrupted, resulting in a flail aortic leaflet. *D,* Prolapse of a mobile intimal flap through the aortic valve during diastole prevents leaflet coaptation.

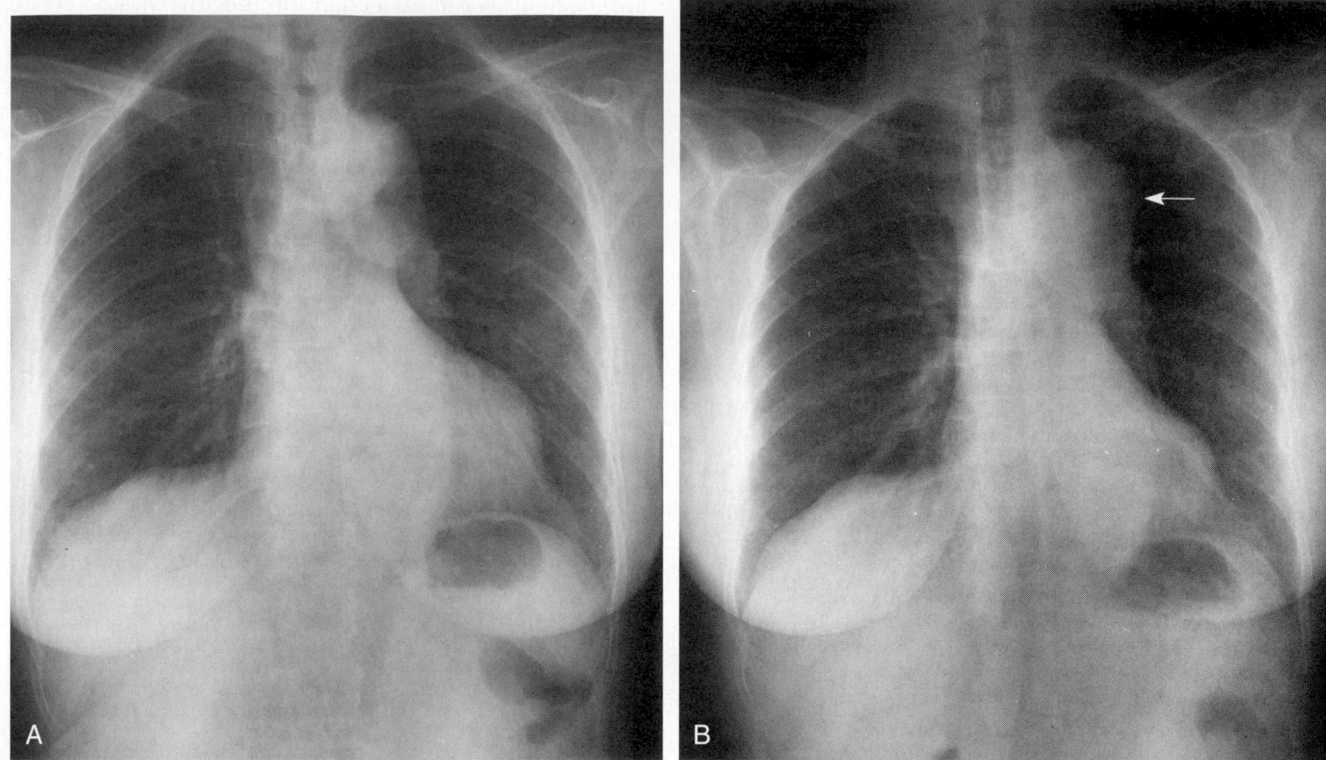

FIGURE 45–9. Chest roentgenogram of a patient with aortic dissection. *A,* The patient's baseline study from 3 years prior to admission, with a normal appearing aorta. *B,* The chest roentgenogram upon admission, which is remarkable for the interval enlargement of the aortic knob (arrow). The patient was found to have a proximal aortic dissection. (From Isselbacher, E. M., Cigarroa, J. E., and Eagle, K. A.: Aortic dissection. *In* Creager, M. (ed.): Vascular Disease. Braunwald, E. [series ed.]: Atlas of Heart Diseases, vol. 7. Philadelphia, Current Medicine, 1996.)

chest roentgenogram may first raise clinical suspicion of aortic dissection. Moreover, although chest roentgenography may help support a diagnosis of suspected aortic dissection, the findings are nonspecific and rarely diagnostic. The findings of chest roentgenography, therefore, add to the other available clinical data used in deciding if suspicion of aortic dissection warrants proceeding to a more definitive diagnostic study.

The most common abnormality seen on chest roentgenogram in aortic dissection is a widening of the aortic silhouette, appearing in 81 to 90 per cent of cases[117,130] and sometimes with a localized bulge overlying the site of origin. Less often, nonspecific widening of the superior mediastinum is seen. If calcification of the aortic knob is present, separation of the intimal calcification from the outer aortic soft tissue border by more than 1.0 cm—the "calcium sign"—is suggestive, although not diagnostic, of aortic dissection (Fig. 45–9). Comparison of the current chest roentgenogram with a previous study may reveal acute changes in the aortic or mediastinal silhouettes that would otherwise have gone unrecognized. Pleural effusions may occasionally be present, typically on the left side and more often associated with dissection involving the descending aorta. Although the majority of patients with aortic dissection have one or more of these roentgenographic abnormalities, the remainder, up to 12 per cent,[117] have chest roentgenograms that appear unremarkable. Therefore, a normal chest roentgenogram can never exclude the presence of aortic dissection.

Electrocardiographic findings in aortic dissection are nonspecific. One-third of electrocardiograms show changes consistent with left ventricular hypertrophy, and another one-third are normal in appearance. Nevertheless, obtaining an electrocardiogram is diagnostically important for two reasons: (1) in aortic dissection patients presenting with nonspecific chest pain, the absence of ischemic ST-segment and T-wave changes on electrocardiogram may argue against the diagnosis of myocardial ischemia and thereby prompt consideration of other chest pain syndromes including aortic dissection; and (2) in patients with proximal dissection, the electrocardiogram may reveal acute myocardial infarction when the dissection flap has involved a coronary artery.

Because of the variable extent of aortic, branch vessel, and cardiac involvement occurring with aortic dissection, the signs and symptoms associated with the condition occur sporadically. Consequently, the presence or absence of aortic dissection cannot be diagnosed accurately in most cases on the basis of symptoms and clinical findings alone. In the series from Spittell et al., of all aortic dissections (presenting without a known diagnosis) the initial clinical diagnosis was aortic dissection in only 62 per cent,[117] and the other 38 per cent were thought initially to have myocardial ischemia, congestive heart failure, nondissecting aneurysms of the thoracic or abdominal aorta, symptomatic aortic stenosis, pulmonary embolism, and so forth. Among this 38 per cent in whom aortic dissection went undiagnosed at presentation, nearly two-thirds had their aortic dissection detected incidentally while undergoing a diagnostic procedure for other clinical questions, and in nearly one-third the aortic dissection remained undiagnosed until necropsy.[117] Given the clinical challenge that detection of aortic dissection presents, physicians should remain vigilant for any risk factors, symptoms, and signs consistent with aortic dissection if a timely diagnosis is to be made.

Diagnostic Techniques

Once the diagnosis of aortic dissection is suspected on clinical grounds, it is essential to confirm the diagnosis both promptly and accurately.[147a] The diagnostic modalities currently available for this purpose include aortography, contrast-enhanced CT, MRI, and transthoracic or transesophageal echocardiography. Each modality has certain advantages and disadvantages with respect to diagnostic accuracy, speed, convenience, risk, and cost, but none is appropriate in all situations.

When comparing the four imaging modalities, one must begin by considering what diagnostic information is needed.[148] First and foremost, the study must confirm or refute the diagnosis of aortic dissection. Second, it must determine whether the dissection involves the ascending aorta (i.e., proximal or type A) or is confined to the descending aorta or arch (i.e., distal or type B). Third, if possible, it should identify a number of the anatomical features of the dissection, including its extent, the sites of entry and reentry, the presence of thrombus in the false lumen, branch vessel involvement by the dissection, the presence and severity of aortic regurgitation, the presence or absence of pericardial effusion, and any coronary artery involvement by the intimal flap. Unfortunately, no single imaging modality provides all of this anatomical detail. Choice of diagnostic modalities should therefore be guided by the clinical scenario and by targeting information that will best assist patient management.

AORTOGRAPHY. Retrograde aortography was the first accurate diagnostic technique for evaluating suspected aortic dissection. The diagnosis of aortic dissection is based on direct angiographic signs, including visualization of two lumens or an intimal flap (considered diagnostic), as in Figure 45–10, or indirect signs (considered suggestive), such as deformity of the aortic lumen, thickening of the aortic walls, branch vessel abnormalities, and aortic regurgitation.[149,150] Earnest et al. showed that the false lumen was visualized in 87 per cent, the intimal flap in 70 per cent, and the site of intimal tear in 56 per cent of dissections.[151]

Aortography had long been considered the diagnostic standard for the evaluation of aortic dissection because for several decades it was the only accurate method for diagnosing aortic dissection ante mortem, although its true sensitivity could not be defined. However, the recent introduction of alternative diagnostic modalities has indicated that aortography is not as sensitive as previously thought. A prospective study by Erbel et al. in 1989 found that for the diagnosis of aortic dissection the sensitivity and specificity of aortography were 88 and 95 per cent, respectively.[152] Furthermore, a recent series by Bansal et al. found that the sensitivity of aortography was only 77 per cent when the definition of aortic dissection included intramural hematoma with noncommunicating dissection[153] (see p. 1568). False-negative aortograms occur because of thrombosis of the false lumen, equal and simultaneous opacification of both the true and false lumens,[154] or the presence of an intramural hematoma.

Important advantages of aortography include its ability to delineate the extent of the aortic dissection, including branch vessel involvement (Figs. 45–11 and 45–12). It is also useful in detecting some of the major complications of aortic dissection, such as thrombus in the false lumen or the presence of aortic regurgitation (Fig. 45–11), and often in revealing the patency of the coronary arteries (Fig. 45–10). Moreover, aortography is widely available and surgeons are very comfortable with its use. In addition to the limited sensitivity of aortography, other disadvantages are the inherent risks of the invasive procedure, the risks associated with the use of contrast material, and the time in completing the study, both in assembling an angiography team and because of the procedure's long duration. Lastly, it requires that potentially unstable patients travel to the angiography suite.

COMPUTED TOMOGRAPHY. In contrast-enhanced CT scanning, aortic dissection is diagnosed by the presence of two distinct aortic lumens, either visibly separated by an inti-

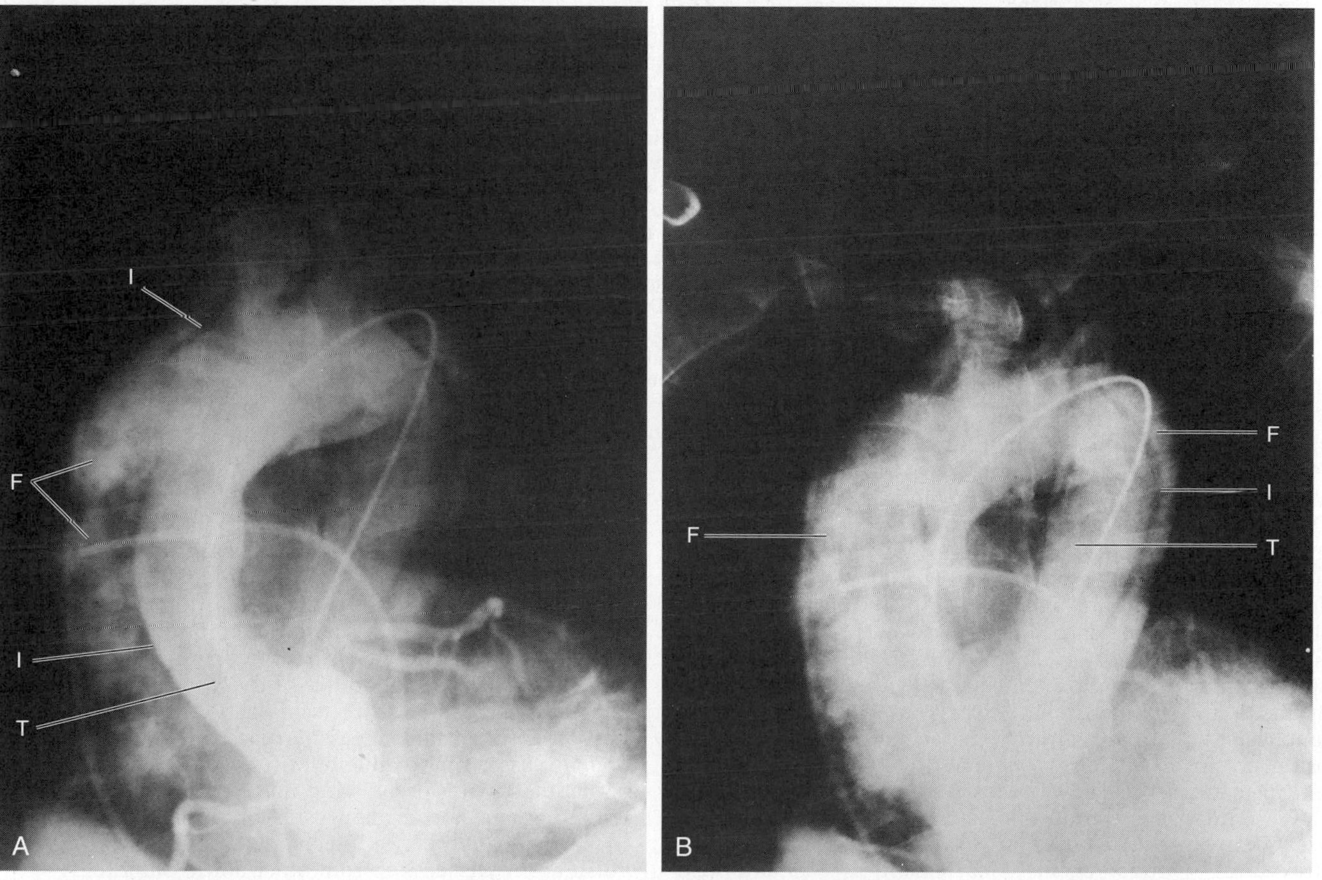

FIGURE 45–10. Thoracic aortogram in the anteroposterior view demonstrating the presence of a proximal aortic dissection. *A*, The well-opacified true lumen (T) and the poorly opacified false lumen (F) are separated by an intimal flap (I), which is visible in the ascending aorta as a thin radiolucent line within the aorta. Additionally, the proximal portions of both coronary arteries are well visualized. *B*, In a subsequent aortographic exposure, the false lumen has filled-in late and the intimal flap is now clearly visible as it courses distally down the descending aorta. (*A* from Cigarroa, J. E., Isselbacher, E. M., DeSanctis, R. W., and Eagle, K. A.: Diagnostic imaging in the evaluation of suspected aortic dissection: Old standards and new directions. N. Engl. J. Med. *328*:35, 1993. *B* from Isselbacher, E. M., Cigarroa, J. F., and Eagle, K. A.: Aortic dissection. *In* Creager, M. (ed.): Vascular Disease. Braunwald, E. [series ed.]: Atlas of Heart Diseases, vol. 7. Philadelphia, Current Medicine, 1996.)

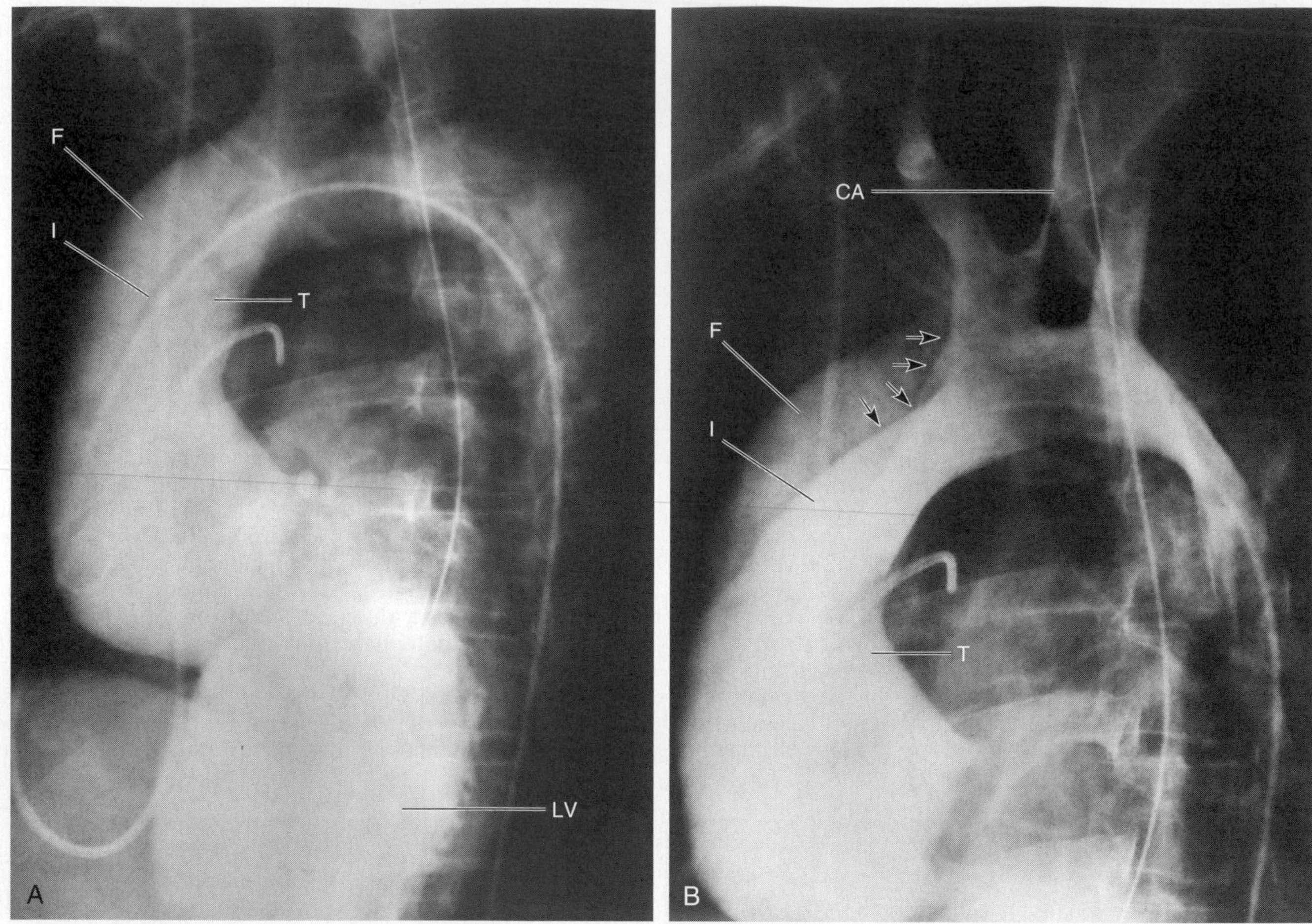

FIGURE 45–11. Aortogram in the left oblique view demonstrating a proximal aortic dissection and its associated cardiovascular complications. *A*, The aortic root is dilated. The true lumen (T) and false lumen (F) are separated by the intimal flap (I), which is faintly visible as a radiolucent line following the contour of the pigtail catheter. The abundance of contrast in the left ventricle (LV) is indicative of significant aortic insufficiency (see Fig. 45–8). *B*, The true lumen is better opacified than the false lumen and two planes of the intimal flap can now be distinguished (arrows). The branch vessels are opacified and there is marked narrowing of the right carotid artery (CA), suggesting that its lumen is compromised by the dissection. (*A* from Cigarroa, J. E., Isselbacher, E. M., DeSanctis, R. W., and Eagle, K. A.: Diagnostic imaging in the evaluation of suspected aortic dissection: Old standards and new directions. N. Engl. J. Med. *328*:35, 1993. *B* from Isselbacher, E. M., Cigarroa, J. E., and Eagle, K. A.: Aortic dissection. *In* Creager, M. (ed.): Vascular Disease. Braunwald, E. [series ed.]: Atlas of Heart Diseases, vol. 7. Philadelphia, Current Medicine, 1996.)

mal flap (Fig. 45–13) or distinguished by a differential rate of contrast opacification. Indirect signs of aortic dissection may also be evident.[148] In two large prospective series of patients with suspected aortic dissection, Erbel et al.[152] found contrast-enhanced CT scanning to have a sensitivity of 83 per cent with a specificity of 100 per cent, while Nienaber et al.[155] found a sensitivity of 94 per cent with a specificity of 87 per cent. Recent advances, such as ultrafast CT scanning with an electron beam,[156] which provides superior image resolution, and helical CT scanning, which permits a three-dimensional display of the aorta and its branches,[38] will likely improve the accuracy of CT in diagnosing aortic dissection as well as in better defining anatomical features.[157]

CT scanning has the advantage that, unlike aortography, it is noninvasive. However, it does require the use of an intravenous contrast agent. Most hospitals are equipped with a readily accessible CT scanner, available on an emergency basis. CT is also helpful in identifying the presence of thrombus in the false lumen and detecting the presence of a pericardial effusion. A disadvantage of CT scanning is that its sensitivity for aortic dissection is lower than that for other available modalities. Moreover, an intimal flap is identified in only two-thirds of cases, and the site of intimal tear is rarely identified.[158] CT scanning also cannot reliably detect the presence of aortic regurgitation or involvement of the branch vessels.

MAGNETIC RESONANCE IMAGING. The use of MRI has particular appeal for diagnosing aortic dissection in that it is entirely noninvasive and does not require the use of intravenous contrast material or ionizing radiation. Furthermore, MRI produces high-quality images in the transverse, sagittal, and coronal planes, as well as in a left anterior oblique view that displays the entire thoracic aorta in one plane (Fig. 45–14). The availability of these multiple views facilitates the diagnosis of aortic dissection and the determination of its extent and in many cases reveals the presence of branch vessel involvement. MRI is ideal for the evaluation of patients with preexisting aortic disease, such as those with thoracic aortic aneurysms or prior aortic-graft repair because it provides sufficient anatomical detail to distinguish aortic dissection from other aortic pathology.[139]

In the series by Nienaber et al.,[155] MRI was used to evaluate 105 patients with suspected aortic dissection and was found to have both a sensitivity and specificity of 98 per cent, consistent with previous findings.[159,160] MRI had a sensitivity of 88 per cent for identifying the site of intimal tear, 98 per cent for the presence of thrombus, and 100 per cent for the presence of a pericardial effusion. Furthermore, the use of the cine-MRI technique in a subset of these

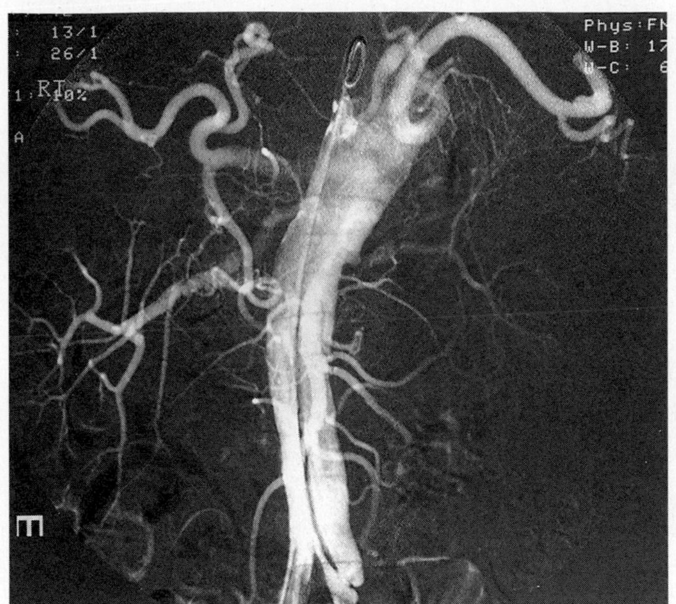

FIGURE 45–12. Digital subtraction angiogram of the abdominal aorta to assess the status of renal perfusion in a patient with a distal thoracic aortic dissection. This study confirmed the presence of an intimal flap extending down into the left common iliac artery. The celiac axis, superior mesenteric artery, and right renal artery are widely patent and fill from the true lumen. The left renal artery fills from the false lumen, with the intimal flap involving the ostium of the artery and impairing distal flow. As a consequence there is minimal contrast excretion by the left kidney compared with the right.

patients showed an 85 per cent sensitivity for detecting aortic regurgitation.

The remarkably high accuracy of MRI has made it the current gold standard for diagnosing the presence or absence of aortic dissection. Still, MRI does have a number of disadvantages. It is contraindicated in patients with pacemakers, certain types of vascular clips, and certain older types of metallic prosthetic heart valves.[161] MRI provides only limited images of the branch vessels and does not consistently identify the presence of aortic regurgitation. MR scanners are not available in many hospitals and, when present, may not be readily available on an emergency basis. Many patients with aortic dissection are hemodynamically unstable, often intubated or receiving intravenous antihypertensive medications with arterial pressure monitoring, but the MR scanners limit the presence of many monitoring and support devices in the imaging suite and also limit patient accessibility during the lengthy study. Understandably, concern for the safety of unstable patients has led many physicians to conclude that the use of MRI is relatively contraindicated for unstable patients. Notably, despite such concerns, in the studies by Nienaber et al.[155,159] no complications occurred among their unstable aortic dissection patients during the performance of MRI.

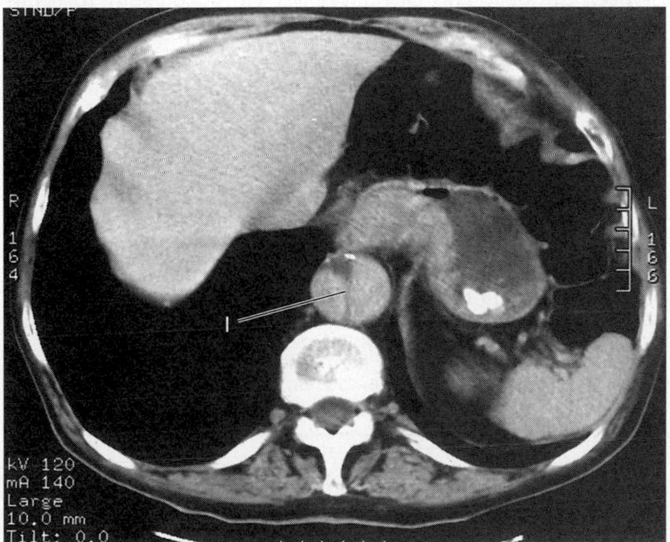

FIGURE 45–13. Contrast-enhanced CT scan of the chest at the level of the diaphragm showing an intimal flap (I) separating the two lumens of an aortic dissection of the descending thoracic aorta.

ECHOCARDIOGRAPHY. Echocardiography is well suited for the evaluation of patients with suspected aortic dissection because it is readily available in most hospitals and is noninvasive and quick to perform, and the full examination can be completed at the bedside. The echocardiographic finding considered diagnostic of an aortic dissection is the presence of an undulating intimal flap within the aortic lumen separating true and false channels. Reverberations and other artifacts can cause linear echodensities within the aortic lumen that mimic aortic dissection; to definitively distinguish an intimal flap from such artifacts, the flap should be identified in more than one view, it should have a motion independent of that of the aortic walls or other cardiac structures, and there should be a differential in color Doppler flow patterns between the two lumens. In cases in which the false lumen is thrombosed, displacement of intimal calcification[152] or thickening of the aortic wall may suggest aortic dissection.

Transthoracic Echocardiography. This technique has a sensitivity of 59 to 85 per cent and specificity of 63 to 96 per cent for the diagnosis of aortic dissection. Its sensitivity is as high as 78 to 100 per cent for dissections involving the ascending aorta but drops to only 31 to 55 per cent for dissections of the descending aorta.[148] Such poor sensitivity, especially in the case of distal dissections, significantly limits the general utility of this technique. Furthermore, image quality is often adversely affected by obesity, emphysema, mechanical ventilation, or small intercostal spaces.

Transesophageal Echocardiography. The proximity of the esophagus to the aorta enables TEE to overcome many of the limitations of transthoracic imaging and permits the use of higher frequency ultrasonography, which provides better anatomical detail (Fig. 45–15). The examination is generally performed at the bedside with the patient under sedation or light general anesthesia and typically requires 10 to 15 minutes to complete.[162,163] The procedure is relatively noninvasive and requires no intravenous contrast or ionizing radiation. Relative contraindications include known esophageal disease (strictures, tumors, and varices), and the required esophageal intubation may not be tolerated in up to 3 per cent of patients. The incidence of important side effects (such as hypertension, bradycardia, bronchospasm, or, rarely, esophageal perforation) is much less than 1 per cent.[163] One important disadvantage of TEE is its limited ability to visualize the distal ascending aorta and proximal arch owing to the interposition of the air-filled trachea and left mainstem bronchus. Although the use of biplane and multiplane probes has helped reduce this problem, a blind spot persists in the proximal aortic arch.[164]

The results of large prospective studies by Erbel et al.[152] and Nienaber et al.[155] demonstrated that the sensitivity of TEE for aortic dissection is 98 to 99 per cent. The sensitivity for detecting an intimal tear was 73 per cent (Fig. 45–16) and for the presence of thrombus in the false lumen, 68 per cent.[155] Furthermore, TEE detected both aortic regurgitation and pericardial effusion in 100 per cent.[155] The specificity of TEE for the diagnosis of aortic dissection is less well defined. Although Erbel et al. found the specificity to be as high as 97 per cent,[152] Nienaber et al. found it to be 77 per cent.[155] However, in the latter study the early inexperience of those performing the examinations and the use of monoplane transducers may have contributed to the incidence of false positives.

Several methods have been suggested to reduce the possibility of false-positive diagnosis by TEE,[148] including the use of biplane or mul-

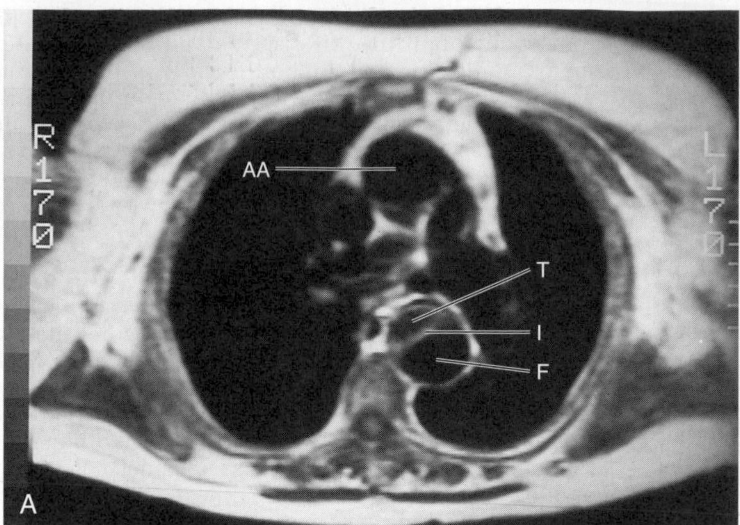

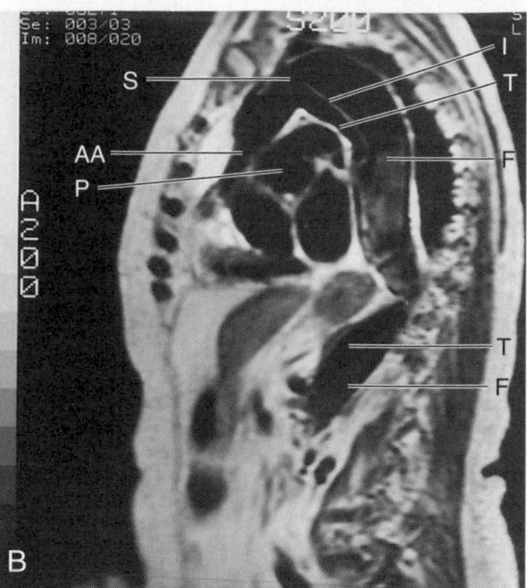

FIGURE 45–14. Magnetic resonance images in two planes in a patient with a distal aortic dissection. *A,* This image in the transverse plane through the upper thorax at the level of the pulmonary artery shows an intact ascending aorta (AA), but in the descending aorta reveals an intimal flap (I) separating the true (T) and false (F) lumens. *B,* This image in the sagittal plane of the aorta shows the site of intimal tear (S) together with the intimal flap (I), which begins just distal to the take-off of the left subclavian artery and spirals distally along the descending aorta. The true (T) and false (F) lumens are identified in both the descending thoracic aorta above as well as in the abdominal aorta below. The ascending aorta (AA) is uninvolved by the dissection. Also seen here is the pulmonary artery (P) at its bifurcation. Notice that in both views the false lumen originates posteriorly and is wider than the true lumen. This pattern is quite typical in distal aortic dissections. (From Isselbacher, E. M., Cigarroa, J. E., and Eagle, K. A.: Aortic dissection. *In* Creager, M. (ed.): Vascular Disease. Braunwald, E. [series ed.]: Atlas of Heart Diseases. Philadelphia, Current Medicine, 1996.)

tiplane ultrasound transducers and confirmation of two lumens by the demonstration of differential color flow patterns (Fig. 45–17). We have proposed[148] that if, in addition to an intimal flap, confirmatory evidence of at least one other echocardiographic feature of aortic dissection is identified, the aortic dissection may be called "definite." If an intimal flap alone is seen (i.e., one that is not considered an artifact) with no other supporting evidence, the diagnosis of dissection should not be considered definitive, and examination with another imaging modality should be sought to exclude the possibility of a false positive. If this conservative approach were applied to the echocardiographic interpretations in the study by Nienaber et al.,[155] the specificity of "definite" aortic dissection would have been 100 per cent.[148]

In addition to its high sensitivity for detecting aortic dissection, TEE may provide other important information useful to the surgeon. Some surgeons wish to know preoperatively if the intimal flap involves the ostia of the coronary arteries, but this determination has traditionally required the performance of coronary angiography.[165]

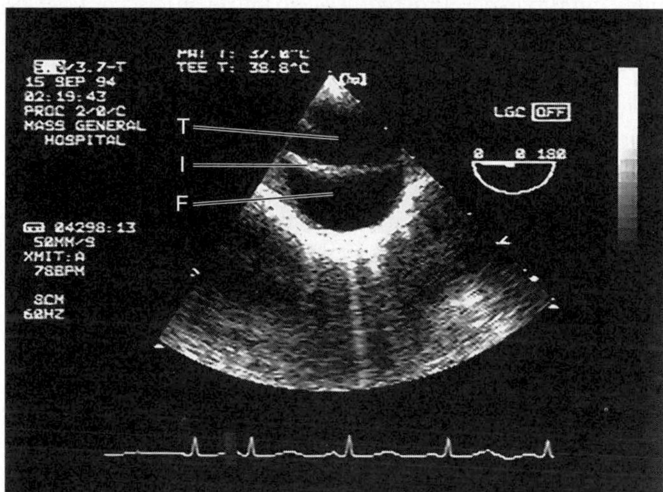

FIGURE 45–15. A cross-sectional transesophageal echocardiogram of the descending thoracic aorta demonstrating an aortic dissection. The aorta is dilated. Evident is an intimal flap (I) dividing the true lumen (T) anteriorly and the false lumen (F) posteriorly. The true lumen fills during systole and therefore is seen bowing slightly into the false lumen in this systolic image.

Ballal et al.[166] performed TEE on 34 patients with aortic dissection, seven of whom had coronary artery involvement confirmed at surgery. In six of these seven patients, TEE identified the intimal flap extending into the coronary ostia. However, TEE delineates only the very proximal portions of the coronary arteries so when the assessment of coronary atherosclerosis is necessary, coronary angiography is still required (see below).

Among patients presenting with suspected aortic dissection, the diagnosis is excluded in 42 to 68 per cent,[159,167,168] yielding a group of patients with a chest pain syndrome of unknown etiology. Granato et al.[168] found that transthoracic echocardiography was helpful in establishing an alternative cause of chest pain in 42 per cent of these cases, by identifying cardiac abnormalities such as left ventricular wall motion abnormalities, aortic stenosis, the presence of pericardial effusion or cardiac tamponade. More recently, Chan[169] found that among patients found not to have dissection, TEE detected other aortic abnormalities in 73 per cent and evidence of acute myocardial infarction or ischemia in 23 per cent.

INTRAVASCULAR ULTRASONOGRAPHY. One of the most recent developments in the echocardiographic evaluation of aortic dissection has been the utilization of intravascular ultrasonography to define the detailed anatomy of the involved aorta and determine the extent of dissection. The intravascular ultrasound catheter is inserted through an introducer in the femoral artery and positioned within the aortic lumen under fluoroscopic guidance. The aorta is then imaged in a transverse plane through its short axis, allowing visualization of the two lumens and the intimal flap.

The most extensive assessment of this technique to date was reported by Yamada et al.,[170] who studied 15 patients with previously known chronic aortic dissection and compared the findings of intravascular ultrasonography with those of other established imaging modalities. Intravascular ultrasonography accurately detected the intimal flap in all segments of the aorta, although it was poor at detecting the sites of intimal tear in the thoracic aorta, probably due to vessel curvature. However, intravascular ultrasonography was quite useful in the evaluation of the abdominal aorta: It demonstrated the origins of the renal arteries and the distal extent of dissection in all cases and identified the site of intimal tear of the abdominal aorta in 78 per cent of cases. Accurate assessment of the abdominal aorta

FIGURE 45–16. See color plate 10.

FIGURE 45–17. See color plate 11.

with this technique may have particular relevance given the inability of TEE to image this portion of the aorta. Furthermore, intravascular ultrasonography may play an important role in the positioning and deployment of endovascular stenting devices[171] (see below). Nevertheless, the potential future role of intravascular ultrasonography in both the evaluation and management of patients with aortic dissection requires further study.

Selecting an Imaging Modality

Each of the four imaging modalities has particular advantages and disadvantages. In selecting among them, one must consider the accuracy as well as the safety and availability of each test. MRI and TEE are the most sensitive of the four studies, but given its unsurpassed specificity, MRI is considered by most to be the present gold standard for evaluating aortic dissection. The four modalities differ in their ability to detect the complications associated with dissection, so the specific diagnostic information sought by the treating physician and/or surgeon should bear upon the procedure chosen. A summary of the diagnostic performance of each of the four imaging modalities is presented in Table 45–2.

Both the accessibility of imaging studies and the time required to complete them are key considerations given the high early mortality of unoperated proximal aortic dissection. Aortography can rarely be performed on an emergency basis, requiring the assembly of an angiography team at night, and carries the risks of an invasive procedure and the use of a contrast agent. MRI, although optimal in its accuracy, is also generally unavailable on an emergency basis and poses the risks of limited patient monitoring and accessibility during the lengthy procedure. CT scanning is more readily available in most emergency rooms and is quickly completed. TEE is also readily available in most larger centers and can be completed quickly at the bedside, making it ideal for evaluating unstable patients. The practical assessment of the four imaging modalities is summarized in Table 45–3.

In the setting in which all of these imaging modalities are available, we believe that TEE should be considered first in the evaluation of suspected aortic dissection, in light of its accuracy, safety, speed, and convenience. In many institutions TEE has indeed become the procedure of choice,[172] with surgeons taking patients to the operating room on the basis of the echocardiographic findings alone.[173,174] In institutions where TEE is not readily available, CT scanning instead serves as an effective screening test for aortic dissection. However, if the diagnosis of aortic dissection is confirmed by CT, after patient transfer to a tertiary care center an additional diagnostic study may be required to more completely define the aortic anatomy prior to surgery. However, in such instances, the patient may be taken directly to the operating room, where a TEE can then be performed to confirm the diagnosis and better define the dissection anatomy without unduly delaying surgery.[173]

Although MRI is less practical than other modalities for the assessment of suspected acute aortic dissection, it is nonetheless well suited for stable or chronic dissections. Given its extraordinary accuracy and its high-quality detailed images, we recommend the use of MRI for following patients with aortic dissection, whether treated medically or surgically, as a means of identifying subsequent aneurysm formation, extension of the dissection, or other complications.

Despite its relative disadvantages, aortography still plays an important role when clear definition of the anatomy of the branch vessels is essential for management. The performance of aortography should also be considered when a definitive diagnosis is not made by one or more of the other imaging modalities.

In the final analysis, each institution must determine its own best diagnostic approach in the evaluation of suspected aortic dissection based on available human and material resources and the speed with which such resources can be mobilized. It must be emphasized that regardless of which of the four imaging modalities are available at a given institution, the levels of skill and experience of those who carry out each diagnostic procedure must, with good reason, also be considerations in deciding the study of choice.

TABLE 45–2 DIAGNOSTIC PERFORMANCE OF IMAGING MODALITIES IN THE EVALUATION OF SUSPECTED AORTIC DISSECTION

DIAGNOSTIC PERFORMANCE	ANGIO	CT	MRI	TEE
Sensitivity	++	++	+++	+++
Specificity	+++	+++	+++	++/+++
Site of intimal tear	++	+	+++	++
Presence of thrombus	+++	++	+++	+
Presence of aortic insufficiency	+++	−	+	+++
Pericardial effusion	−	++	+++	+++
Branch vessel involvement	+++	+	++	+
Coronary artery involvement	++	−	−	++

Key: +++ excellent, ++ good, + fair, − not detected. Angio = angiography; CT = computed tomography; MRI = magnetic resonance imaging; TEE = transesophageal echocardiography.

Modified from Cigarroa, J.E., Isselbacher, E.M., DeSanctis, R.W., and Eagle, K.A.: Diagnostic imaging in the evaluation of suspected aortic dissection: Old standards and new directions. N. Engl. J. Med. *328*:35, 1993. Copyright by the Massachusetts Medical Society.

TABLE 45–3 PRACTICAL ASSESSMENT OF IMAGING MODALITIES IN THE EVALUATION OF SUSPECTED AORTIC DISSECTION

ADVANTAGES OF STUDY	ANGIO	CT	MRI	TEE
Readily available	Fairly	Quite	Fairly	Very
Quickly performed	Fairly	Quite	Fairly	Very
Performed at bedside	No	No	No	Yes
Noninvasive	No	Yes	Yes	Yes
IV contrast	Yes	Yes	No	No
Cost	High	Reasonable	Moderate	Reasonable

Angio = angiography; CT = computed tomography; MRI = magnetic resonance imaging; TEE = transesophageal echocardiography.

Modified from Cigarroa, J. E., Isselbacher, E. M., DeSanctis, R. W., and Eagle, K. A.: Diagnostic imaging in the evaluation of suspected aortic dissection: Old standards and new directions. N. Engl. J. Med. *328*:35, 1993. Copyright by the Massachusetts Medical Society.

The Role of Coronary Angiography

The importance of assessing the status of coronary artery patency prior to surgical repair of acute aortic dissection continues to be controversial. Some surgeons believe that obtaining this information prior to surgery is essential, whereas others are content to assess the coronaries intraoperatively. Two types of coronary artery involvement must be considered in the setting of aortic dissection. The first is acute proximal coronary narrowing or occlusion as a result of the dissection itself, often due to occlusion of the coronary ostia by the intimal flap. The second is the possible presence of chronic atherosclerotic coronary artery disease which, although generally independent of the dissection process, may complicate its surgical management.

In some cases, coronary involvement by the intimal flap is self-evident if the electrocardiogram shows evidence of acute myocardial ischemia or infarction. However, should this acute process not be clinically evident, TEE can effectively define the patency of the proximal coronaries in a majority of cases.[166] Aortography may also reveal such coronary artery involvement. A more comprehensive evaluation requires the performance of coronary angiography; however, this may be risky in patients with aortic dissection and often prolongs the time to aortic repair by several hours. Moreover, catheterization of the coronary arteries is sometimes unsuccessful in patients with proximal dissections and a dilated root, in which case the added procedural delay gains no potential benefit. In addition, such proximal coronary obstructions can usually be readily identified at the time of surgery.

Chronic coronary artery disease is seen in about one-quarter of patients presenting with aortic dissection. Identifying the presence of this underlying coronary disease is beyond the capability of any of the four imaging modalities discussed above. Furthermore, accurately defining such atherosclerotic disease intraoperatively is challenging, although Rizzo et al. have suggested the use of probing the proximal coronaries, epicardial palpation, and angioscopy as possible means to identify coronary stenoses.[173]

The impact of unrecognized coronary artery disease on outcome is not certain. In a 10-year review examining 54 patients undergoing urgent aortic repair, Kern et al. found that only 1 of 27 patients with a proximal dissection had a perioperative myocardial infarction; this patient had a prior history of coronary artery disease.[165] In addition, Rizzo et al. observed that of those patients in whom unrecognized coronary artery disease was discovered at autopsy, none died of coronary ischemia but several died of aortic rupture.[173] Accordingly, we and others[165] recommend avoiding preoperative coronary angiography unless a specific indication exists, such as a known history of coronary artery disease or the presence of ischemic electrocardiographic changes. Conversely, Creswell et al. report good outcomes when performing combined aortic repair and coronary artery bypass grafting in patients with underlying coronary artery disease, and therefore argue that all stable patients with acute proximal dissection should undergo preoperative coronary angiography.[175] While the debate continues unresolved, the trend in the literature has been a retreat from the routine performance of coronary angiography in acute aortic dissection.

Management

Therapy for aortic dissection is directed at halting the progression of the dissecting hematoma because lethal complications arise not from the intimal tear itself, but rather from the subsequent course taken by the dissecting aorta, e.g., vascular compromise or aortic rupture.[147a] Without treatment, aortic dissection has a high mortality. In a collective review of long-term survival in untreated aortic dissection, more than one-fourth of all patients died within the first 24 hours following onset of dissection, more than one-half died within the first week, more than three-fourths died within 1 month, and more than 90 per cent died within 1 year.[176]

The first surgical approach to aortic dissection was a fenestration procedure in which the dissected aorta was incised and a distal communication created between the true and false channels, thereby decompressing the false lumen.[177] This procedure is, in fact, still used by some surgeons in selected cases of dissection involving the descending aorta to relieve limb, renal, or mesenteric ischemia.[178] Definitive surgical therapy was pioneered by DeBakey et al. in the early 1950's.[179] Its purpose is to excise the intimal tear, obliterate the false channel by oversewing the aortic edges, reconstitute the aorta directly or with the interposition of a synthetic graft, and, in the case of proximal dissection, restore aortic valve competence either by resuspension of the displaced aortic leaflets or by prosthetic aortic valve replacement.

Aggressive medical treatment of aortic dissection was first advocated by Wheat et al.[180] They established the two primary goals for pharmacological therapy as reduction of systolic blood pressure and diminution of the force of left ventricular ejection (dP/dt). This force is thought to be a major stress acting upon the aortic wall, contributing to both the genesis and subsequent propagation of aortic dissection. Originally introduced for patients too ill to withstand surgery, medical therapy is now the initial treatment for virtually all patients with aortic dissection prior to definitive diagnosis and furthermore serves as the primary long-term therapy in a subset of patients, particularly those with distal dissections.

Immediate Medical Management

All patients in whom there is a strong suspicion of acute aortic dissection should immediately be placed in an acute care setting for hemodynamic stabilization and monitoring of blood pressure, cardiac rhythm, and urine output. Two large bore intravenous catheters should be inserted, to be used for intravenous medications and fluid resuscitation if necessary. An arterial line should be placed, preferably in the right arm so that it remains functional during surgery when the aorta is cross-clamped. However, in cases in which the blood pressure is significantly greater on the left than on the right, the arterial line should be placed on the left. In those with a lower likelihood of dissection who are hemodynamically stable, a automatic blood pressure cuff should suffice.

A central venous line or pulmonary arterial line should be considered in patients with hypotension or congestive heart failure, in order to monitor central venous pressure or pulmonary artery wedge pressure and cardiac output. Femoral lines and blood gases should be avoided if possible, in order to conserve these sites for bypass cannulation during a potential aortic repair. If a femoral line must be placed emergently, the opposite groin site should be protected from needle punctures.

BLOOD PRESSURE REDUCTION. Initial therapeutic goals include the elimination of pain and the reduction of systolic blood pressure to 100 to 120 mm Hg (mean 60 to 75 mm Hg), or to the lowest level commensurate with adequate vital organ (cardiac, cerebral, renal) perfusion. Simultaneously, arterial dP/dt, reflecting the force of left ventricular ejection, should be reduced through the use of beta blockade, regardless of whether pain or systolic hypertension is present. The use of long-acting medications should be avoided in patients who are surgical candidates, as this may complicate intraoperative arterial pressure management. Pain, which may itself exacerbate hypertension and tachycardia, should be promptly treated with intravenous morphine sulfate.

For the acute reduction of arterial pressure, the potent vasodilator sodium nitroprusside is very effective. It is initially infused at 20 μg/min with dosage titrated upward, as high as 800 μg/min, according to blood pressure response. When used alone, however, sodium nitroprusside can actually cause an increase in dP/dt, which in turn may potentially contribute to the propagation of the dissection. Therefore, when this drug is used the concomitant administration of adequate beta blockade is essential.

To reduce dP/dt acutely, an intravenous beta blocker should be administered in incremental doses until there is evidence of satisfactory beta blockade, usually indicated by a heart rate of 60 to 80 beats/min in the acute setting. Because propranolol was the first generally available beta blocker, it has been used most widely in treating aortic dissection. However, it is believed that other beta blockers are equally effective. Propranolol should be administered in intravenous doses of 1 mg every 3 to 5 minutes until the desired effect is achieved, although the maximum initial dose should not exceed 0.15 mg/kg (or approximately 10 mg). In order to maintain adequate beta blockade, as evidenced by heart rate, additional propranolol should be given intravenously every 4 to 6 hours, usually in doses somewhat lower than the total initial dose, i.e., 2 to 6 mg.

Labetalol, which acts as both an alpha- and beta-adrenergic receptor blocker, may be especially useful in the setting of aortic dissection[181] because it effectively lowers both dP/dt and arterial pressure. The initial dose of labetalol is 10 mg, administered intravenously over 2 minutes, followed by additional doses of 20 to 80 mg every 10 to 15 minutes (up to a maximum total dose of 300 mg) until heart rate and blood pressure have been controlled. Maintenance dosing may then be achieved with a continuous intravenous infusion, starting at 2 mg/min and titrating up to 5 to 20 mg/min.

The ultra–short-acting beta blocker esmolol may be particularly useful in patients with labile arterial pressure, especially if surgery is planned, as it can be abruptly discontinued if necessary.[182] It is administered as a 30-mg intravenous bolus followed by continuous infusion at 3 mg/min and titrated up to 12 mg/min. Esmolol may also be useful as a means to test beta blocker safety and tolerance in patients with a history of obstructive pulmonary disease who may be at uncertain risk for bronchospasm from beta blockade. In such patients, a cardioselective beta blocker, such as atenolol or metoprolol, may be considered.

When contraindications exist to the use of beta blockers —including sinus bradycardia, second- or third-degree atrioventricular block, congestive heart failure, or bronchospasm—other agents to reduce arterial pressure and dP/dt should be considered. Calcium channel antagonists, proven effective in managing hypertensive crisis,[183] are now used with increasing frequency in the treatment of aortic dissection. Sublingual nifedipine, successfully used in treating refractory hypertension associated with aortic dissection,[184] can be given immediately while other medications are being prepared. A key limitation of nifedipine, however, is that it has little negative chronotropic or inotropic effect. In contrast, the combined vasodilator and negative inotropic effects of both diltiazem and verapamil make these agents well suited for the treatment of aortic dissection. Moreover, both of these agents may be administered intravenously.

Refractory hypertension may result when a dissection flap compromises one or both of the renal arteries, thereby causing the release of large amounts of renin. In this situation the most efficacious antihypertensive may be the intravenous angiotensin-converting enzyme (ACE) inhibitor enalaprilat, which is administered initially in doses of 0.625 mg every 4 to 6 hours and then titrated upward.

If patients are normotensive rather than hypertensive on presentation, beta blockers may be used alone to reduce dP/dt or, if contraindicated, diltiazem or verapamil are alternatives.

In the event that the patient with suspected aortic dissection presents with significant hypotension, rapid volume expansion should be considered, given the possible presence of cardiac tamponade or aortic rupture. Before initiating aggressive treatment of such hypotension, however, the possibility of pseudohypotension, which occurs when the arterial pressure is being measured in an extremity whose circulation is selectively compromised by the dissection, should be carefully excluded. If vasopressors are absolutely required for refractory hypotension, norepinephrine (Levophed) or phenylephrine (Neo-Synephrine) are preferred. Dopamine should be reserved for improving renal perfusion and used only at very low doses, given that it may raise dP/dt.

Once appropriate medical therapy has been initiated and the patient sufficiently stabilized, a definitive diagnostic study should be promptly undertaken. If a patient remains unstable, a TEE is preferred because it can be performed at the bedside in the emergency department or intensive care unit, allowing both monitoring and therapeutic intervention to continue uninterrupted. When a patient with a strongly suspected dissection becomes extremely unstable, there is likely to be aortic rupture or cardiac tamponade and the patient should go directly to the operating room rather than delaying surgery for diagnostic imaging. In such situations an intraoperative TEE can be used both to confirm the diagnosis and to guide surgical repair.

MANAGEMENT OF CARDIAC TAMPONADE. Cardiac tamponade frequently complicates acute proximal aortic dissection and is one of the most common mechanisms of death in these patients. It is often the cause of hypotension when patients present with aortic dissection, and pericardiocentesis is commonly performed in this setting in an effort to stabilize patients while they await definitive surgical repair. However, in a retrospective series we found that pericardiocentesis may be harmful rather than beneficial in this setting, as it may precipitate hemodynamic collapse and death rather than stabilize the patient as intended.[185] Seven patients in this series were relatively stable at presentation (six hypotensive, one normotensive). Three of four who underwent successful pericardiocentesis died suddenly, secondary to acute electromechanical dissociation, between 5 and 40 minutes following the procedure. In contrast, none of the three patients without pericardiocentesis died prior to surgery. It may be that, in such patients, the increase in intraaortic pressure which follows pericardiocentesis causes a closed communication between the false lumen and pericardial space to reopen, leading to recurrent hemorrhage and lethal cardiac tamponade.

Therefore, when a patient with acute aortic dissection complicated by cardiac tamponade is relatively stable, the risks of pericardiocentesis likely outweigh the benefits and *every effort should be made to proceed as urgently as possible to the operating room for direct surgical repair of the aorta with intraoperative drainage of the hemopericardium.* However, when patients present with electromechanical dissociation or marked hypotension, an attempt to resuscitate the patient with pericardiocentesis is warranted. A prudent strategy in such cases might be to aspirate only enough pericardial fluid to raise blood pressure to the lowest acceptable level.[185]

Definitive Therapy

Despite minor variations from center to center, a reasonable consensus as to the definitive therapy of aortic dissection has evolved over the past several decades. It is universally agreed that surgical therapy is superior to medical therapy for acute proximal dissection.[186,187] With even limited progression of a proximal dissection, patients may suffer the potentially devastating consequences of aortic rupture or cardiac tamponade, acute aortic regurgitation, or neurological compromise. Thus, by controlling this risk, immediate surgical repair promises a better outcome. Occasional patients with proximal dissection who refuse surgery or for whom surgery is contraindicated (e.g., by age or prior debilitating illness) may potentially be treated successfully with medical therapy.[131,187]

Patients suffering acute distal aortic dissection, on the other hand, are generally at lower risk for early death from complications of the dissection than are those with proximal dissection.[131] Furthermore, as patients with distal dissection tend to be older and have a relatively increased prevalence of advanced atherosclerosis or cardiopulmonary disease, their surgical risk is often considerably higher. Early reports showed medical therapy to be as effective as surgery in this group,[115,131] and accordingly many centers advocated treating distal dissections medically. Nevertheless, agreement on this principle was not unanimous. Some investigators, reporting progressive improvement in surgical mortality, advocated surgical treatment of all dissections—both proximal and distal.[188] The debate was perpetuated by the notable absence of controlled prospective data on therapy and outcome. More recently, however, a large retrospective series involving patients from both Duke and Stanford Universities has, using multivariate analysis, suggested that medical therapy does provide an outcome equivalent to surgical therapy in patients with uncomplicated distal dissection.[189] As a consequence, medical therapy for such patients is currently favored by most groups. An important exception is that when a distal dissection is complicated by rupture, expansion, saccular aneurysm formation, vital organ or limb ischemia, or continued pain, the results of medical therapy are poor and surgery is therefore recommended.[178,187] Surgical therapy is also rec-

TABLE 45–4 INDICATIONS FOR DEFINITIVE SURGICAL AND MEDICAL THERAPY IN AORTIC DISSECTION

Surgical
1. Treatment of choice for acute proximal dissection
2. Treatment for acute distal dissection complicated by the following:
   a. Progression with vital organ compromise
   b. Rupture or impending rupture (e.g., saccular aneurysm formation)
   c. Aortic regurgitation (rare)
   d. Retrograde extension into the ascending aorta
   e. Dissection in the Marfan syndrome

Medical
1. Treatment of choice for uncomplicated distal dissection
2. Treatment for stable, isolated arch dissection
3. Treatment of choice for stable chronic dissection (uncomplicated dissection presenting 2 weeks or later after onset)

ommended for patients with the Marfan syndrome with either proximal or distal dissections.

Patients who present with chronic aortic dissection have, through self-selection, survived the early period of highest mortality and, whether treated medically or surgically, their subsequent hospital survival is approximately 90 per cent.[190,191] Accordingly, medical therapy is recommended for the management of all stable patients with chronic proximal and distal dissection, again unless complicated by rupture, aneurysm formation, aortic regurgitation, arterial occlusion, or extension or recurrence of dissection.

SURGICAL MANAGEMENT. The generally advocated indications for definitive surgical therapy are summarized in Table 45–4. Surgical candidacy should be determined whenever possible at the start of the patient's evaluation because this guides the selection of diagnostic studies. Surgical risk for all patients is increased by: age; comorbid disease (especially pulmonary emphysema); aneurysm leakage; cardiac tamponade; shock; or vital organ compromise as a result of such conditions as myocardial infarction, cerebrovascular accident, and particularly preexisting renal failure.[188]

Preoperative mortality in acute dissection ranges from 3 per cent when surgery is expedited to as high as 20 per cent when the preoperative evaluation is more prolonged.[173] These data reinforce the fact that prompt diagnosis and repair are essential to prevent even minimal progression of the dissection that might lead to further complications.[96]

The usual objectives of definitive surgical therapy include the resection of the most severely damaged segment of the aorta, excision of the intimal tear, and obliteration of entry into the false lumen by suturing the edges of the dissected aorta both proximally and distally. After resecting the diseased segment containing the intimal tear, typically a segment of the ascending aorta in proximal dissections or the proximal descending aorta in distal dissections, aortic continuity is reestablished by interposing a prosthetic sleeve graft between the two ends of the aorta (Fig. 45–18). Less commonly, following resection of the intimal tear, the edges of the aorta may be rejoined as a direct repair without the use of a graft.

Importantly, Miller et al. have found that the immediate and long-term survival of patients treated surgically was not significantly affected by failure to excise the intimal tear.[186,192] Some patients with proximal dissection have an intimal tear located in the aortic arch. Because surgical repair of the arch may increase the morbidity and mortality of the procedure and because resection of the tear may not necessarily improve mortality, many authors have elected not to repair the arch if the sole purpose of surgery is resecting the intimal tear.[192] However, with improvements in surgical technique during the last decade, several groups now suggest that even these challenging lesions can be resected with favorable results.[193,194]

When aortic regurgitation complicates aortic dissection, simple decompression of the false lumen is sometimes all that is required to allow resuspension of the aortic leaflets and restoration of valvular competence. More often, however, preservation of the aortic valve requires approximation of the two layers of dissected aortic wall and resuspension of the commissures with pledgeted sutures. This resuspension technique has had favorable results with a fairly low incidence of recurrent aortic regurgitation in long-term follow-up.[123,195] Preserving the aortic valve in this fashion may avoid the complications associated with pros-

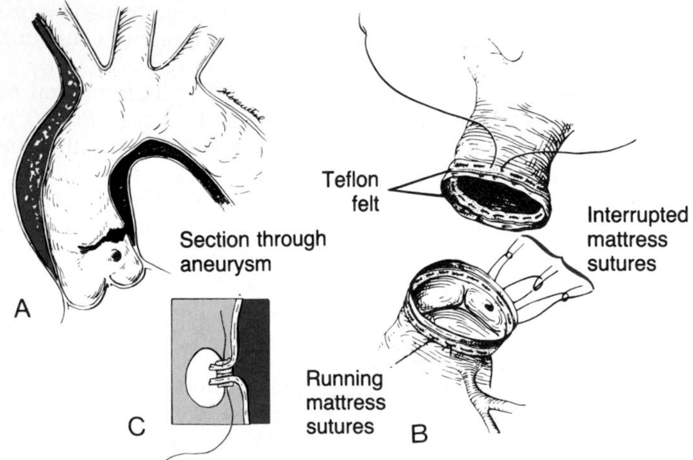

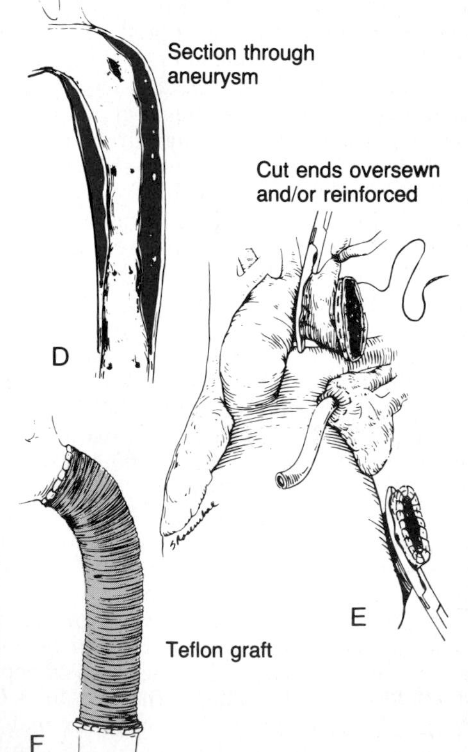

FIGURE 45–18. Several steps in the surgical repair of a proximal (*A*, *B*, and *C*) and a distal (*D*, *E*, and *F*) aortic dissection. *A* and *D* show the dissections and intimal tears. *B*, The aorta has been transected, and the ends of the aorta have been oversewn to obliterate the false lumen and have been buttressed with Teflon felt to prevent the sutures from tearing through the fragile tissue. *C*, The aortic ends are brought together in such a way that the Teflon is again used to reinforce the suture line between the two ends of the aorta and between the aorta and a sleeve graft, if such a graft is necessary for the reconstitution of the aorta. *E* shows resection of a distal dissection, with a Teflon graft interposed in *F*. (D, *E*, and *F* from Austen, W. G., and DeSanctis, R. W.: Surgical treatment of dissecting aneurysm of the thoracic aorta. N. Engl. J. Med. *272*:1314, 1965.)

thetic valve replacement, especially the requirement for oral anticoagulation that may pose an added risk in patients prone to future aortic rupture.

Prosthetic aortic valve replacement is frequently necessary, however, either because attempts at a valve repair are unsuccessful or in the setting of preexisting valvular disease or the Marfan syndrome.[195] Many surgeons are aggressive about replacing the aortic valve if it appears that even moderate aortic regurgitation will remain after the leaflets are resuspended, choosing to avoid the risk of having to replace the aortic valve at some later date in a second operation through a diseased aorta. When the proximal aorta is fragile or badly torn, most use the Bentall procedure, in which a composite prosthetic graft—a prosthetic aortic valve sewn onto the end of a Dacron tube graft—facilitates the replacement of both the ascending aorta and aortic valve together (Fig. 45–5). The coronary arteries are then reimplanted as buttons of aortic tissue into the graft wall.[196]

For repair of a proximal dissection, total cardiopulmonary bypass is necessary. On occasion, because of extensive dissection of the aorta, it may be difficult to find a safe site for placement of a perfusion cannula and, rarely, we have had to abandon plans for surgical repair of a proximal dissection for this reason. In the repair of dissections of the descending thoracic aorta, support of the distal circulation may be necessary and can be achieved either by partial left heart bypass or by use of a bypass conduit that carries blood from the proximal aorta to distal aorta, thereby circumventing the site of the dissection.

The operative procedure in aortic dissection is technically demanding. The wall of the diseased aorta is often friable, and the repair must be performed with meticulous care. The use of Teflon felt to buttress the wall and prevent sutures from tearing through the fragile aorta is essential (Fig. 45–18). An alternative surgical approach involves wrapping an unstable aortic arch dissection with Dacron.[197]

Determining the sources of vital organ perfusion distal to the surgical site by diagnostic imaging studies may be of critical importance. For example, if one or both renal arteries are supplied by the false lumen and are not going to be directly corrected surgically, the surgeon may leave communication between the true and false channel distal to the site of aortic repair so as not to jeopardize renal perfusion.

COMPLICATIONS. Bleeding, infection, pulmonary failure, and renal insufficiency constitute the most common early complications of surgical therapy. Spinal cord ischemia with paraplegia due to inadvertent interruption of blood supply from the anterior spinal or intercostal arteries is an uncommon but dreaded consequence of descending thoracic aortic repair. Late complications include progressive aortic regurgitation if the aortic valve has not been replaced, localized aneurysm formation, and recurrent dissection at the original site or at a secondary site.[192] With modern operative techniques, surgical survival is 80 to 90 per cent for proximal and distal dissections.

NEWER SURGICAL TECHNIQUES. Several innovative techniques for the surgical treatment of aortic dissection have been reported. The thromboexclusion procedure, applied typically in dissections of the descending aorta, consists of bypassing the dissected aorta with a long Dacron sleeve, ligating the aorta at the site of proximal extension of the dissection, and creating reversal of flow in the distal aorta to perfuse the major arterial branches arising from the dissected segment.[178] In most cases gradual thrombosis of the occluded aortic segment occurs, thereby reducing the risk of extension or rupture.[178]

As a modification of more standard operative techniques, several investigators have unified the layers of the dissected aortic wall using either a fibrin sealant[198] or gelatin-resorcine-formaldehyde glue.[199,200] After resection of the diseased aortic segment, this glue is used in place of pledgeted sutures to seal the false lumen of the aortic stumps, prior to implantation of the Dacron prosthesis. The glue not only hardens and reinforces the fragile dissected aortic tissue but also may simplify the operation, facilitate resuspension of the aortic valve, and potentially reduce the incidence of late aortic root aneurysm formation.[198] Another group has used such glue in carrying out direct surgical repair of the aorta without an interposing graft by first suturing the intimal tear, then applying the glue in the false lumen to unify the layers of the dissected aorta, and finally reattaching the free aortic ends. Although early reports show favorable morbidity and mortality with the use of these new techniques,[200,201] direct comparison with standard operative techniques is needed.

ENDOVASCULAR TECHNIQUES. One of the more promising avenues of investigation is the use of endovascular techniques for treating high-risk patients with aortic dissection. For example, because patients with renal or visceral artery compromise from dissection have operative mortality rates exceeding 50 per cent,[202,203] alternative management strategies are desirable. Walker et al. have successfully performed combined renal artery angioplasty and stent placement in five patients with aortic dissection, achieving immediate and sustained improvement of blood pressure control in four.[203] In another case, in order to improve peripheral perfusion, they successfully performed balloon dilation of a preexisting fenestration in the intimal flap, with favorable results.[203]

More definitive endovascular techniques have also been introduced. Sutureless intraluminal prostheses, placed during cardiopulmonary bypass, are intended to improve outcome by decreasing intraoperative and postoperative bleeding complications.[204] These devices have been used successfully with good outcomes in two small series of patients with proximal aortic dissections.[205,206] More recently, intraluminal stent-grafts, placed percutaneously by the transfemoral catheter technique, have been introduced as a potential alternative to aortic repair.[207,208] Kato et al. have recently demonstrated the efficacy of their self-expanding stent in an experimental canine model of distal aortic dissection, with angiographically confirmed closure of the entry site and thrombosis of the false lumen within 2 hours of device placement.[208] Again, such nonsurgical procedures may be particularly well suited for high-risk patients, but data on human trials of intraluminal stent-grafts for aortic dissection are not yet available.

DEFINITIVE MEDICAL MANAGEMENT. The indications for definitive medical therapy are summarized in Table 45–4. As discussed above, we prefer medical therapy for stable patients with uncomplicated acute distal dissection. However, surgery must clearly be performed in cases of medical management failure, such as rupture or impending rupture, progression of the dissection with vital organ compromise, aortic regurgitation (which is extremely rare), or an inability to control pain or blood pressure with medicines. Because of the extreme difficulty of surgery to repair the aortic arch when it is involved by the dissection, medical therapy is also usually advocated for distal dissections that either originate in the arch or extend retrograde into the arch. Operative therapy is again reserved for those with serious complications.

Medical therapy is also generally recommended for patients presenting with chronic aortic dissection, whether proximal or distal, unless late complications of the dissection, such as aortic regurgitation or localized aneurysm formation, necessitate surgery. Complications of medical therapy include orthostasis or more severe hypotension secondary to the medications. If unchecked, persistent hypotension may in turn precipitate acute tubular necrosis, cerebrovascular accident, or myocardial infarction.[131]

Long-Term Therapy and Late Follow-Up

Late follow-up of patients leaving the hospital with treated aortic dissection shows an actuarial survival rate not much worse than that of individuals of comparable age without dissection. There are no significant differences among discharged patients when comparing proximal versus distal dissection, acute versus chronic dissection, or medical versus surgical treatment.[131] Five-year survival rates for all of these groups are typically 75 to 82 per cent.[131,186,192] Thus, the initial success of surgical or medical therapy is usually sustained on long-term follow-up. Late complications include aortic regurgitation, recurrent dissection, and aneurysm formation or rupture.

Long-term medical therapy to control hypertension and reduce dP/dt is indicated for all patients who have sustained an aortic dissection, regardless of whether their in-hospital definitive treatment was surgical or medical. Indeed, one study found that late aneurysm rupture following aortic dissection was 10 times more common among patients with poorly controlled hypertension than among those with controlled blood pressure,[209] dramatically demonstrating the importance of aggressive life-long antihypertensive therapy. Systolic blood pressure should be maintained at or below 130 to 140 mm Hg. Preferred agents are beta blockers or other agents with a negative inotropic as well as a hypotensive effect, such as calcium channel antagonists, together with a diuretic if necessary to control blood pressure. Pure vasodilators, such as hydralazine and minoxidil, may cause an increase in dP/dt and should therefore be used only in conjunction with adequate beta blockade. ACE inhibitors are attractive antihypertensive agents for treating aortic dissection and may be of particular benefit in those with some degree of renal ischemia as a consequence of the dissection.

Up to 29 per cent of late deaths following surgery result from rupture of either the dissecting aneurysm or another aneurysm at a remote site. Moreover, the incidence of subsequent aneurysm formation at a site remote from the surgical repair is 17 to 25 per cent,[114,210] with these remote aneurysms accounting for many of the rupture-related deaths. The mean time interval from primary aortic dissection to the appearance of subsequent aneurysms is 18 months, with the majority appearing within 2 years.[210] Many such aneurysms occur from dilatation of the residual false lumen in the more distal aortic segments not resected at the time of surgery. Because the dissected aneurysm wall is relatively thin, consisting of only the outer half of the original aortic wall, these aneurysms rupture more frequently than do typical atherosclerotic thoracic aneurysms.[87,210] Thus, an aggressive approach to treating such late-appearing aneurysms may be indicated.

The high incidence of late aneurysm formation and rupture emphasizes both the diffuse nature of the aortic disease process in this population and the tremendous importance of careful follow-up. The primary goal of long-term surveillance is the early detection of aortic lesions that might require subsequent surgical intervention, such as the appearance of new aneurysms or rapid aneurysm expansion, progression or recurrence of dissection, aortic regurgitation, or peripheral vascular compromise.

Follow-up evaluation of patients after aortic dissection should include careful and repeated physical examinations, periodic chest roentgenograms, and serial aortic imaging with either TEE,[211] CT scanning,[187] or MRI.[178] We generally prefer MRI for serially following these patients because it is completely noninvasive and provides excellent anatomical detail that may be exceedingly helpful in evaluating interval changes.[212] Patients are at highest risk immediately following hospitalization and during the first 2 years, with the risk progressively declining thereafter. It is therefore important to have more frequent follow-up early on; for example, patients may be seen at 3 and 6 months initially, then return every 6 months for 2 years, after which time they may be reevaluated at 6- to 12-month intervals, depending on the given patient's risk.

Atypical Aortic Dissection

In recent years it has become increasingly clear that in addition to aortic dissection as classically described, there are two other closely related diseases of the aorta, *intramural hematoma* of the aorta and *penetrating atherosclerotic ulcer* of the aorta. These two conditions share with aortic dissection many of the predisposing risk factors and presenting symptoms, and indeed both may lead either to classic aortic dissection or to aortic rupture.

INTRAMURAL HEMATOMA. This is essentially a contained hemorrhage within the medial layer of the aortic wall. Although the pathogenesis of intramural hematoma is still uncertain, rupture of the vasa vasorum is believed to be the initiating event, resulting in hemorrhage into the outer media and extending into the adventitia.[213,213a] This may produce a localized or discrete hematoma, but more often the hemorrhage extends for a variable distance by dissecting along the outer media beneath the adventitia.[214] Intramural hematoma is distinguished from typical aortic dissection by the lack of an associated tear in the intima or direct communication between the media and aortic lumen; hence, some have termed it *aortic dissection without intimal rupture.*[213] Previous pathological studies of what were considered clinically to be aortic dissections have found that 3 to 13 per cent[112,113,215] did not have an identifiable intimal tear, and it is possible that such cases were in fact actually intramural hematomas. Moreover, it remains uncertain whether intramural hematoma is a distinct pathological entity or instead represents a reversible precursor of classic aortic dissection.

Clinically, intramural hematoma may be indistinguishable from true aortic dissection. The majority of patients are elderly with a history of hypertension and typically have extensive aortic atherosclerosis.[216,217] Almost all patients have the chest and back pain symptoms typical of classic aortic dissection. Aortic regurgitation and pulse deficits may be present. One-half of patients may have associated left pleural effusion[213,216] that may not appear until several days after the hematoma develops.[213] A pericardial effusion may appear when the ascending aorta is involved.[216]

Intramural hematoma is best diagnosed by CT scanning. On a non-contrast-enhanced CT scan (Fig. 45–19) it appears as a continuous, crescentic, high-attenuation area along the aortic wall without evidence of an intimal tear, false lumen, or associated intimal atherosclerotic ulcer.[214] This study is followed by a contrast-enhanced CT scan, which demonstrates failure of the intramural hematoma to enhance, thereby excluding communication with the aortic lumen. In some cases it may be difficult to distinguish intramural hematoma from aortic dissection with thrombosis of the false lumen or from mural thrombus within an aortic aneurysm.[213] However, with an intramural hematoma the aortic lumen retains its overall size and shape, unlike in aortic dissection.

On MRI, an intramural hematoma appears as a crescentic high-intensity area along the aortic wall.[213] On TEE it is manifested as a continuous crescentic or nearly concentric circular thickening of the aortic wall which, in some cases, may be difficult to distinguish from severe atherosclerotic thickening of the aortic wall.[218] Aortography may fail to detect an intramural hematoma because it does not usually compress the aortic lumen to produce recognizable aortographic signs such as are seen with aortic dissection.[213]

The natural history of intramural hematoma is not well defined. Involvement of the ascending aorta appears to carry a high risk of death or complications requiring surgical repair, whereas hematomas of the descending aorta have a more favorable prognosis. In a recent retrospective series, Nienaber et al. determined that 13 per cent of 195 patients presenting with aortic dissection–like syndromes in fact suffered intramural hematoma.[218] The actuarial survival rates were similar for the groups with intramural hematoma and overt aortic dissection.[218] Of those with proximal intramural hematoma, 30-day mortality was 80 per cent for those treated medically, compared with 0 per cent for those undergoing early repair. On the other hand, early mortality for distal intramural hematoma was 9 per cent and did not differ significantly between medical and surgical treatment.

Intramural hematomas may regress with time or even

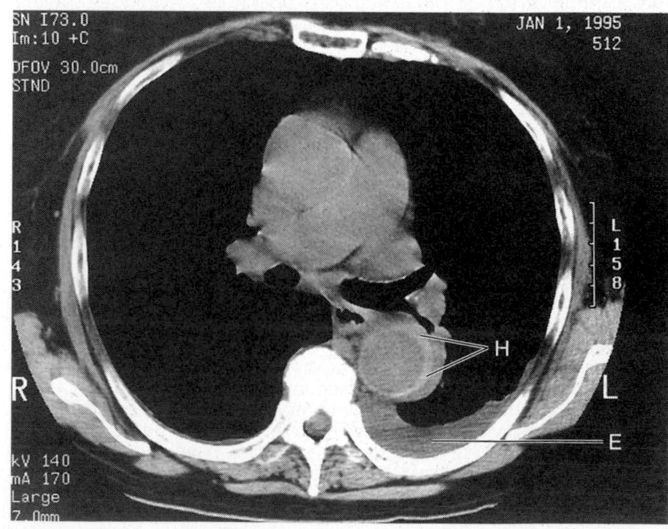

FIGURE 45–19. Intramural hematoma of the aorta. A CT scan without contrast enhancement demonstrates crescentic thickening of the aortic wall which is of increased density (H), consistent with an intramural hematoma of the aorta. A left pleural effusion (E) is also present.

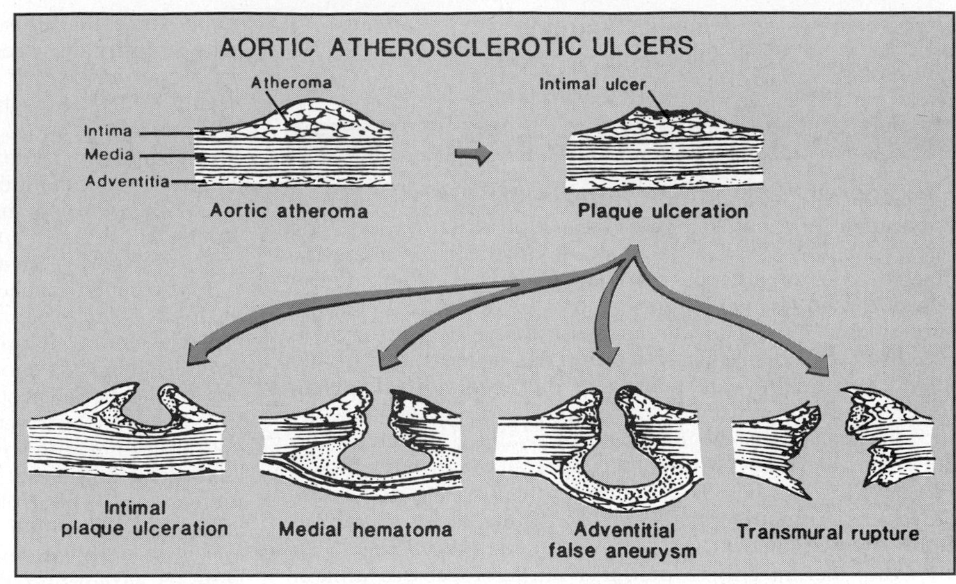

FIGURE 45–20. The evolution of a penetrating atherosclerotic ulcer of the aorta. Once an intimal ulcer has formed, it may then progress to a variable depth. Penetration through the intima causes a medial hematoma, whereas penetration through the media leads to the formation of a pseudoaneurysm and perforation through the adventitial layer results in aortic rupture. (From Stanson, A. W., Kazmier, F. J., Hollier, L. H., et al.: Penetrating atherosclerotic ulcers of the thoracic aorta: Natural history and clinicopathological correlations. Ann. Vasc. Surg. *1*:15, 1986.)

completely resolve on follow-up imaging[213] or, alternatively, may progress to overt aortic dissection within days[218,219] to months of initial presentation.[214] Nienaber et al. found progression to overt dissection, aortic rupture, or cardiac tamponade in one-third of patients.[218]

The limited data on the natural history of intramural hematoma suggest that it behaves very much like classic aortic dissection and should therefore be treated in a similar fashion. Thus surgical therapy is best for proximal hematomas, whereas medical therapy is reasonable for distal hematomas. There should be a low threshold, however, for proceeding to surgery in distal disease if symptoms persist or if there is evidence of progression. Medical management should therefore include serial imaging studies to follow the progression or regression of the intramural hematoma.

PENETRATING ATHEROSCLEROTIC ULCER. Penetrating atherosclerotic ulcer, first defined in the literature in 1986 by Stanson et al.,[220] is an ulceration of an atherosclerotic lesion of the aorta that penetrates the internal elastic lamina and allows hematoma formation within the media of the aortic wall (Fig. 45–20). Although such ulcerations occur almost exclusively in the descending thoracic aorta, with the majority located in its mid to distal portion,[221] they may rarely occur in the ascending aorta or arch.[222,223] The hematoma that results from a penetrating atherosclerotic ulcer usually remains localized or extends several centimeters in length but does not develop a false lumen.[224] These ulcers penetrate through the media in one-quarter of cases to cause aortic pseudoaneurysms, or through the adventitia in 8 per cent to cause transmural aortic rupture[222] (Fig. 45–20). Rarely, a penetrating atherosclerotic ulcer may progress to an extensive classic aortic dissection.[223] Over time, penetrating atherosclerotic ulcers frequently lead to the formation of saccular or fusiform aortic aneurysms.[225]

The patients who develop penetrating atherosclerotic ulcers tend to be elderly, with a history of hypertension and evidence of other atherosclerotic cardiovascular disease.[221] Presenting symptoms include chest and back pain similar to that of aortic dissection, but without associated pulse deficits, neurological deficits, or aortic regurgitation.[220] The majority are hypertensive at presentation.[221,226]

Chest roentgenogram often demonstrates a dilated descending thoracic aorta as well as left-sided or bilateral pleural effusions.[221] Aortography is the diagnostic standard for detecting a penetrating atherosclerotic ulcer, with the lesion appearing as contrast-filled outpouching in the descending aorta in the absence of an intimal flap or false lumen[222] (Fig. 45–21). On CT scanning[221] or MRI[227] the lesion appears as a focal ulceration, with thickening of the aortic wall and inward displacement of intimal calcification consistent with intramural hematoma. TEE may identify the presence of a culprit atherosclerotic ulcer in the setting of a visible intramural hematoma,[228] but diagnosis is difficult.[164]

The natural history of penetrating atherosclerotic ulcer remains largely unclear, and at present there is no definitive treatment strategy. Certainly, patients who are hemodynamically unstable or who have evidence of pseudoaneurysm formation or transmural rupture should undergo urgent surgical repair. Continued or recurrent pain, distal embolization, or progressive aneurysmal dilatation are also indications for surgery.[224] Those without such complications should be treated with antihypertensive medications and monitored closely with follow-up imaging studies, similar to the management of a patient with a distal aortic dissection.

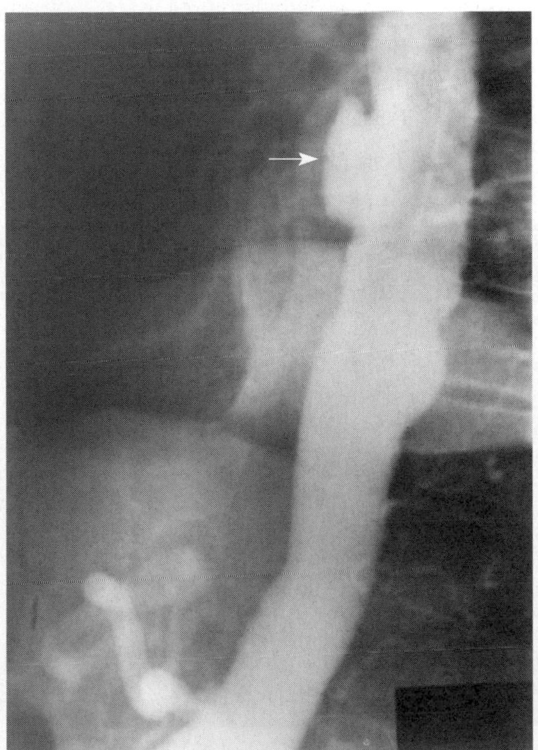

FIGURE 45–21. A thoracic aortogram demonstrating a penetrating atherosclerotic ulcer of the distal descending aorta (arrow). The hematoma of the aortic wall is evident as a localized contrast-filled outpouching of the aorta. The remainder of the aorta is diffusely atherosclerotic.

Aortic Trauma

See discussion on p. 1543.

AORTIC ATHEROMATOUS EMBOLI

AORTOGENIC ATHEROTHROMBOTIC EMBOLI. The clinical importance of atherosclerotic disease of the aorta has long been recognized, as atheromatous or fibrinous material, thrombi, or cholesterol particles dislodged from atherosclerotic plaques may cause cerebral or peripheral embolic phenomena.[229,229a] However, assessing the degree of such atherosclerotic disease ante mortem has been limited by the inability of the several imaging modalities to directly visualize the aortic intima.[230] Aortography demonstrates the aortic lumen rather than the aortic walls themselves and thus can only detect gross atherosclerotic changes, whereas CT scanning or MRI rarely detect protruding atheromas because the normal pulsatile motion of the aorta may limit definition of the aortic wall on the tomographic images. On the other hand, TEE is uniquely suited to assess atherosclerotic disease of the aorta in real time and has been demonstrated to have greater sensitivity for aortic arch atherosclerosis than chest roentgenography, aortography, or CT scanning.[230] On echocardiography, mild atherosclerosis appears as intimal thickening, irregularity, and calcification, whereas more severe disease appears as thick plaques with protruding atheromas (Fig. 45–22). In some cases protruding lesions have highly mobile components that may represent atheroma with superimposed thrombus.[231,232]

Risk factors for aortic atherosclerosis include age, hypertension, diabetes,[233] hyperlipidemia,[234] and other vascular disease.[235] Through the use of TEE, the prevalence and extent of macroscopic atherosclerotic disease have now been documented in a variety of patient populations.[235a] Atheromatous disease is least common in the ascending aorta, more common in the arch, and most common in the descending thoracic aorta.[236] Whereas aortic atheromas are detected in as few as 2 per cent of those without a history of stroke or known aortic disease, they are found in 38 per cent of those with significant carotid artery disease,[237] 60 per cent of those with ischemic stroke,[236] and up to 90 per cent of those with obstructive coronary artery disease.[238]

In an autopsy series Amarenco et al. found that the presence of ulcerated plaques in the aortic arch was a significant independent risk factor for stroke, particularly cryptogenic stroke,[235] and multiple clinical studies using TEE have found an association between aortic atherosclerosis and stroke as well as other peripheral embolic events.[229,234,239] In both retrospective and prospective studies, protruding aortic atheromas are detected in 7 to 8 per cent of patients undergoing routine TEE,[229,240] with about a 33 per cent incidence of embolic vascular events over a 2-year follow-up period.[240] The embolic risk is even higher among those with pedunculated or mobile lesions and those undergoing invasive aortic procedures.[229]

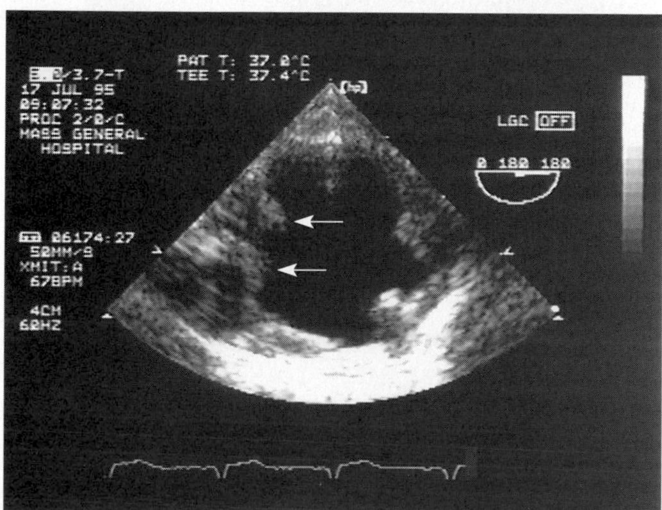

FIGURE 45–22. A cross-sectional transesophageal echocardiogram of the descending thoracic aorta demonstrating extensive atherosclerotic disease. This patient had recently suffered an embolic stoke of uncertain etiology. Multiple atheromatous plaques, up to 7 mm in thickness, protrude into the aortic lumen. When viewed in real-time, two plaques (arrows) had small mobile intraluminal components.

In a recent prospective case-control study, Amarenco et al. found atherosclerotic plaques of 4 mm or more in the ascending aorta or proximal arch in 14 per cent of patients with ischemic stroke, compared with only 2 per cent of controls. After adjustment for atherosclerotic risk factors, the odds ratio for stroke was 9.1 for ischemic stroke and 4.7 for cryptogenic stroke, with an even higher risk ratio for complex atheromas than for simple ones.[236] However, the increased risk of stroke was associated only with the large atheromas involving the ascending aorta and proximal arch, not with atheromas in the distal arch or descending aorta,[236] supporting the hypothesis that atheromas in the ascending aorta and proximal aortic arch embolize directly into the cerebral circulation to cause ischemic strokes in such patients.[241]

Little is known about the natural history of atheromatous lesions[242] of the aorta, and at present therapeutic strategies are limited. Potential approaches for chronic management include the use of antithrombotic[243,244] or antiplatelet[242] therapy to prevent thrombus formation. Some have reported the surgical removal, under hypothermic circulatory arrest, of protruding atheromas detected in patients following embolic events.[239] However, this surgery carries the risk of an early adverse outcome, and at present no controlled data suggest that it actually reduces the incidence of future embolization in this population.[245]

CARDIAC SURGERY AND ATHEROEMBOLISM. Perioperative dislodgment and embolization of atherosclerotic material from the aorta is a well-recognized hazard of cardiac surgery and has been increasingly implicated as an important cause of postoperative strokes and other embolic events in these patients. The incidence of cerebral ischemic events following cardiac surgery typically ranges from 1 to 3 per cent, with an increased risk among the elderly.[233,246] In an autopsy series of patients having undergone cardiac surgery, Blauth et al. identified atheroemboli in 22 per cent of cases.[247] Atheroembolic events occurred in 37 per cent of those with severe atherosclerosis of the ascending aorta, compared with only 2 per cent of those without significant ascending aortic atherosclerosis. Moreover, 96 per cent of patients suffering perioperative atheroemboli had severe atherosclerosis of their ascending aorta.[247] Mobile pedunculated lesions appear more prone to embolize.[229]

Mechanisms by which aortic atherosclerotic debris may be dislodged during cardiac surgery include external manipulation of the aorta during palpation,[246] cross-clamping, cannula placement, anastomosis of the bypass grafts to the aorta,[233] and the "sandblasting" effect of the high-velocity jet of blood that exits the aortic cannula and strikes the atherosclerotic intima of the opposite aortic wall.[246,247] Although surgeons have long relied on direct digital palpation to detect the presence of atherosclerosis in the ascending aorta, this method underestimates the incidence, severity, and extent of atherosclerotic disease.[248,249] In contrast, both TEE and intraoperative epiaortic ultrasonography appear to be superior techniques for delineating the presence and severity of atherosclerotic disease of the ascending aorta.[229]

Several studies have examined the potential role of aortic ultrasonography in identifying patients at highest risk for perioperative atheroemboli. In 8 to 17 per cent of cases, the ultrasonographic findings led to modifications in surgical technique such as changing the sites of aortic cannulation (with cannulation of the distal aorta or femoral artery instead), of cross-clamping, or of anastomosis of vein grafts.[233,246,248,250] The results of such procedural modifications have been promising, with several reports showing a trend toward reduction of stroke rates.

CHOLESTEROL EMBOLIZATION SYNDROME. Cholesterol embolization syndrome is caused by distal showering of cholesterol crystals from ulcerated atheromatous plaques in the aorta or iliac and proximal femoral arteries in patients with diffuse atherosclerosis. These cholesterol crystals then obstruct small peripheral arteries (100 to 300 μm in size), causing local tissue ischemia or necrosis, and frequently induce a local inflammatory reaction that may contribute to the arteriolar occlusive process.[251]

The precise mechanisms that precipitate cholesterol embolization are unclear. The syndrome is most commonly seen following instrumentation of the aorta, such as with cardiac catheterization, PTCA, angiography, or intraaortic balloon pump insertion.[252] The overall incidence following cardiac catheterization was 0.1 per cent in the Coronary Artery Surgery Study.[253] Cholesterol embolization may also complicate aortic surgery or cardiopulmonary bypass. At times, cholesterol embolization syndrome may occur spontaneously. Studies have suggested a causal relationship between warfarin therapy and such spontaneous cholesterol embolization.[254]

The clinical manifestations depend on the organs affected. Cutaneous manifestations, typically of the lower extremities, are most common and include livedo reticularis, gangrene, cyanosis, and ulceration.[255] Acute onset of pain with digital ischemia and small areas of cutaneous gangrene is often referred to as the "blue toe" or "purple toe syndrome."[254,256] The presence of preserved pedal pulses in the setting of peripheral ischemia distinguishes this syndrome from embolic occlusion of larger arteries.

Acute nonoliguric renal failure with or without hypertension is a common consequence of renal emboli, often presenting as a rise in creatinine over several weeks, followed by a slow but progressive worsening of renal function that may become severe and irreversible. Cholesterol embolization to the central nervous system is quite uncommon, but may present as focal neurological deficits, amaurosis fugax from retinal emboli, paralysis from spinal cord emboli, or a diffuse encephalopathy. Mesenteric embolization may present with abdominal pain, gastrointestinal bleeding, or pancreatitis. Finally, multiple organ systems may be simultaneously involved, mimicking vasculitis or bacterial endocarditis.[251]

When the cholesterol embolization syndrome occurs as a consequence of an invasive procedure, the temporal relation of events often suggests the diagnosis. In the case of spontaneous embolization, however, recognizing the syndrome remains extremely challenging, and diagnosis in the absence of cutaneous manifestations is especially difficult. An elevated erythrocyte sedimentation rate, eosinophilia, and a reduced complement level are helpful in suggesting the diagnosis, but making a definitive diagnosis requires a tissue biopsy. Paraffin-fixed sections reveal needle-shaped clefts in the arteriolar lumens, representing the spaces occupied by cholesterol particles prior to fixation.

No specific therapy effectively treats cholesterol embolization syndrome.[251,252] Because cholesterol embolization resembles other atheroembolic phenomena, some have advocated the use of anticoagulant therapy. However, such therapy is typically unsuccessful and may even exacerbate the condition,[257] whereas discontinuing anticoagulation may improve the condition in some cases.[258] Glucocorticoid therapy has also been tried without success. Surgical therapy is generally limited to the amputation of an ischemic or gangrenous extremity. Overall, the prognosis for those suffering cholesterol embolization syndrome is quite poor, with a mortality rate of 38 to 80 per cent.[259,260]

ACUTE AORTIC OCCLUSION

Acute aortic occlusion is an infrequent but potentially catastrophic condition with an early mortality of 31 to 52 per cent.[261–263] It is caused by either embolic occlusion of the infrarenal aorta at the bifurcation, known as a "saddle embolus," or acute thrombosis of the abdominal aorta. At least 95 per cent of aortic emboli originate from the left side of the heart,[262] typically as thrombus from the left atrium secondary to atrial fibrillation, particularly in the setting of rheumatic mitral stenosis, or from the left ventricle secondary to myocardial infarction, aneurysm, or dilated cardiomyopathy. Less common cardiac sources of emboli include atrial myxoma, prosthetic valve thrombus, and acute bacterial or fungal endocarditis.[264] Primary thrombosis accounts for the remaining 35 to 92 per cent[261,262] of acute aortic occlusions. Seventy-five to 80 per cent of thrombotic aortic occlusions occur in the setting of underlying severe aortoiliac occlusive disease, and they are frequently precipitated by a low-flow state secondary to heart failure or dehydration. In those without aortoiliac occlusive disease, a hypercoagulable state may precipitate thrombosis of an abdominal aortic aneurysm, leading to aortic occlusion.[261,262]

Acute aortic occlusion is in most cases heralded by the sudden onset of excruciating bilateral lower extremity pain —usually radiating from the mid-thigh distally—associated with weakness, numbness, and paresthesias. Nonclassic presentations include sudden onset of bilateral lower extremity weakness, severe hypertension from renal artery involvement, and abdominal pain from mesenteric ischemia. Persistent ischemia may lead to myonecrosis with secondary hypotension, hyperkalemia, myoglobinuria, and acute tubular necrosis. If perfusion is not reestablished within hours, death is almost inevitable.

DIAGNOSIS. Physical examination reveals cold pale extremities that are cyanotic and often exhibit a mottled, reticulated, and reddish blue appearance that may progress to the blue-black color of gangrene. Pulses are notably absent below the abdominal aorta, and capillary refill is absent. Signs of ischemic neuropathy are present and include symmetrical weakness, loss of all modalities of sensation (usually with demarcation at the level of the mid-thigh), and diminished or absent deep tendon reflexes. When neurological symptoms predominate, patients are often mistakenly thought to have spinal cord infarction or compression and their ischemic symptoms may initially be overlooked. In fact, as many as 11 to 17 per cent of such patients may initially undergo a neurological or neurosurgical evaluation before the vascular cause is recognized.[261,262]

The diagnosis of acute aortic occlusion is confirmed by aortography. Although some suggest that all stable patients should undergo the procedure,[261] others advise prompt surgical intervention without aortography if the diagnosis is strongly suspected,[262,263] because added delays increase the likelihood of irreversible ischemic damage to the limbs. Aortography is desirable if there is concomitant abdominal pain, hypertension, or anuria, to evaluate the possibility of renal and mesenteric arterial involvement.[262]

MANAGEMENT. Once a clinical diagnosis of acute aortic occlusion is made, intravenous heparin therapy should be initiated while awaiting immediate surgery. A saddle embolus can be removed using Fogarty balloon-tipped catheters inserted through a transfemoral arterial approach under local anesthesia. If the embolus cannot be retrieved with Fogarty catheters, removal by direct transabdominal aortotomy is undertaken. Patients with thrombotic occlusion generally undergo either direct aortic reconstruction or revascularization with aortofemoral or axillofemoral bypass. Operative mortality for acute aortic occlusion is 31 to 40 per cent[262,263] and as high as 85 per cent among those with severe left ventricular dysfunction or a hypercoagulable state.[261] Limb salvage rates are as high as 98 per cent.[262,263] Lifelong anticoagulant therapy is necessary following surgery in almost all cases to prevent recurrent emboli.[265]

AORTOARTERITIS SYNDROMES

Takayasu's Arteritis

Takayasu's arteritis is a chronic inflammatory disease of unknown etiology involving the aorta and its major branches, which was first noted in 1908 by the Japanese ophthalmologist Takayasu. This disease entity has been variously termed "aortic arch syndrome," "pulseless disease," "aortoarteritis," "occlusive thromboaortopathy," "young female arteritis," and "reversed coarctation," in addition to the familiar *Takayasu's arteritis*.

ETIOLOGY AND PATHOPHYSIOLOGY. Takayasu's arteritis occurs worldwide, although the large majority of cases are seen in Asia and Africa. The incidence in North American and European populations is 1.2 to 2.6 per million per year. A specific cause has not been found,[266] although the bulk of evidence favors an autoimmune etiology. It has been linked to rheumatic fever, streptococcal infections, rheumatoid arthritis, and other collagen vascular diseases. An association between the disease and certain HLA subtypes has been reported,[267,268] although it is of unclear significance.[266]

In the early stage of the disease there is active inflammation involving a granulomatous arteritis of the aorta and its branches, with secondary alterations in the media and adventitia. The disease progresses at variable rates to a later sclerotic stage in which there is intimal hyperplasia, medial degeneration, and adventitial fibrosis. The proliferative process leads to obliterative luminal changes in the aorta and other involved arteries.

Takayasu's arteritis most often involves the aortic arch and its major branches, with changes that are usually most marked at branch points in the aorta. It may present as multisegmental aortic disease with areas of normal wall between affected sites, as diffuse involvement of the aorta, or as disease of individual arteries arising from the aorta. The pulmonary artery may also be involved. Lesions are purely stenotic in 85 per cent of patients, purely dilatative in 2 per cent, and mixed in 13 per cent. The coronary arteries are affected in less than 10 per cent of patients. Aortic regurgitation as a consequence of disease of the proximal ascending aorta is seen in about one-quarter of cases. Ueno et al. have subdivided the disease into three types, depending on the predominant site of involvement[269] (Fig. 45–23). Type I involves primarily the aortic arch and its branches; type II spares the aortic arch, involving the thoracoabdominal aorta and its branches; type III combines the features of both. Lupi-Herrera et al. have suggested a fourth category, type IV, in which there is pulmonary arterial involvement.[270]

CLINICAL MANIFESTATIONS. The disease affects women much more frequently than men, in a ratio of 8:1.[271] The mean age at the time of diagnosis is 29 years. In as many as three-fourths of cases, onset is in the teenage years, although cases beginning from infancy to late middle-age have been reported.[271] Because the symptoms of Takayasu's arteritis are generally nonspecific, there may be a delay of months to years between the first appearance of symptoms and the time of diagnosis. In fact, only 6 per cent of the patients in the Mayo Clinic series were suspected of having Takayasu's arteritis at presentation.[272] More than half the patients with Takayasu's arteritis develop initial symptoms suggestive of a systemic inflammatory process, characterized by fever, anorexia, malaise, weight loss, night sweats, arthralgias, pleuritic pain, and fatigue. Localized pain and tenderness may be noted over affected arteries. The disease may occasionally present as fever of unknown origin.[273]

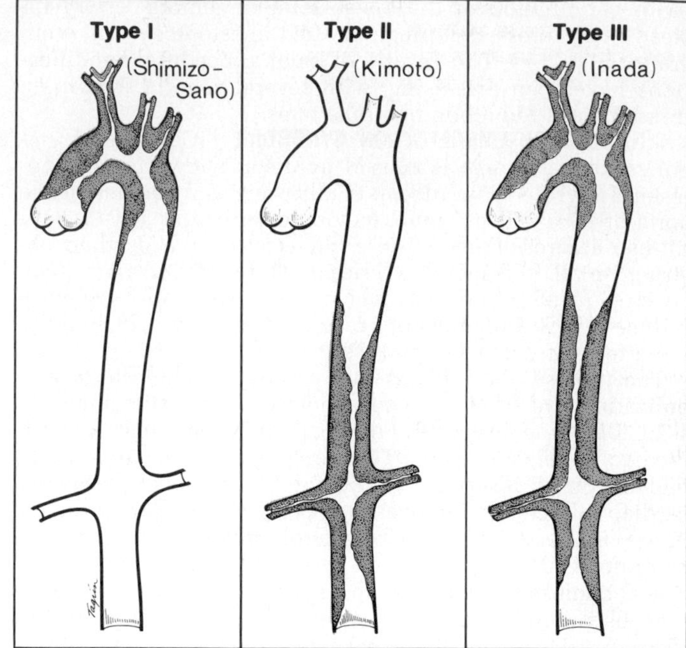

FIGURE 45–23. Types of Takayasu's arteritis. Type I involves primarily the aortic arch and brachiocephalic vessels. Type II affects the thoracoabdominal aorta and particularly the renal arteries. Type III combines features of both types I and II. Types I and III may be complicated by aortic regurgitation. The eponyms for each type are noted.

At the time of diagnosis, 85 to 96 per cent of patients have entered the sclerotic phase of the disease and have symptoms of vascular insufficiency of either the upper extremities or, less commonly, the lower extremities.[270] Patients with types I and III exhibit those findings most typical of the disease, namely "reversed" coarctation of the aorta with absent or diminished upper body pulses and barely detectable blood pressure in the arms, higher blood pressure in the lower extremities, bruits overlying diseased arteries, and manifestations of ischemia at various affected sites. Most have a pulse pressure difference of 30 mm Hg or more between their two arms, and many have postural dizziness or even syncope. The retinopathy originally described by Takayasu is seen in only about one-quarter of patients[271] and is usually associated with carotid artery involvement. Patients with type II arteritis may have abdominal angina and claudication of the limbs but also tend to develop hypertension because of renal artery involvement.

Hypertension complicates this disease in 50 to 60 per cent of cases[271] but may be difficult to recognize because of diminished pulses in the arms. Hypertension typically arises from renal artery stenosis and hemodynamically significant acquired coarctation of the aorta, although decreased aortic distensibility and reduced baroreceptor reactivity may also contribute.[274] Another major complication of Takayasu's arteritis is congestive heart failure, occurring in 28 per cent of cases[270] as a consequence of the systemic hypertension or, more rarely, aortic regurgitation.[275] Coronary artery involvement may cause angina or myocardial infarction.[276]

NATURAL HISTORY. The natural history of this uncommon disease has been best defined in a recent series by Ishikawa and Maetani, who followed 120 patients with Takayasu's arteritis for up to 15 years.[277] The overall 15-year survival was 83 per cent. Death usually resulted from cerebrovascular accidents, congestive heart failure, or myocardial infarction. The authors showed that the survival rate was only 66 per cent among those with major complications—severe hypertension, moderate or severe aortic regurgitation, aortic or arterial aneurysms, and

Takayasu's retinopathy—compared with a 96 per cent survival rate for those without such complications.[277]

DIAGNOSIS. Laboratory abnormalities during the acute systemic phase include an elevated sedimentation rate, a low-grade leukocytosis, and mild anemia of chronic disease. These return toward normal when the systemic phase resolves. IgG and IgM levels are elevated in more than half the patients.[266] Chest roentgenograms are usually unrevealing, although a rim of calcification is sometimes visible in the walls of involved arteries. Arteriography typically reveals findings of an irregular intimal surface, with stenoses of the aorta or its branch vessels, poststenotic dilatation, aortic or arterial aneurysms, and even complete occlusion of vessels (Fig. 45–24). The affected thoracic aorta has been described as having a narrowed, "rat-tail" angiographic appearance (Fig. 45–25).[278]

Proposed criteria for the clinical diagnosis of Takayasu's arteritis are shown in Table 45–5 (p. 1575).[279] An obligatory criterion is age 40 years or less at diagnosis. The two major criteria reflect involvement of either subclavian artery. A high probability of the disease exists if, in addition to age of 40 years or less, a patient meets two major criteria, one major criterion and two minor criteria, or four minor criteria.[279]

MANAGEMENT. Glucocorticoids in high doses (prednisone, 1 mg/kg body weight per day) are well established as the primary therapy of Takayasu's arteritis[266] and often dramatically improve the constitutional symptoms, halt disease progression in patients in the systemic inflammatory stage, and lower the sedimentation rate toward normal.[266,272] In fact, the sedimentation rate, usually an accurate indicator of systemic disease activity, is quite useful in directing therapy. When patients fail to respond to steroid therapy, cyclophosphamide (2 mg/kg/day) has been used with some success.[266] Alternatively, low-dose methotrexate (about 0.3 mg/kg/week) may enhance the efficacy of steroid therapy and facilitate steroid tapering.[280] Although medical therapy has been successful in improving symptoms in a majority of patients, it is not known whether it prevents the long-term complications of this disease or prolongs life.[266]

The indications for surgery in the treatment of Takayasu's arteritis are not well established. Given the diffuse nature of the arteritis, surgery often requires the bypass or reconstruction of multiple aortic or arterial segments. Surgery is generally performed to correct renovascular hypertension, relieve cerebral ischemia, repair aortic or arterial aneurysms, treat aortic regurgitation, or bypass coronary arteries. Renal artery stenosis is currently the most common indication. Surgery during the active phase of disease carries a significant risk of reocclusion and therefore, whenever possible, should be postponed until the inflammation has subsided. If surgery during the active phase is essential, postoperative steroid therapy is necessary.

One promising advance in the treatment of the obstructive lesions of Takayasu's arteritis is the use of percutaneous transluminal angioplasty. Tyagi et al. performed angioplasty for stenotic lesions of the aorta in a series of patients, with success in 94 per cent as indicated by an increase in aortic diameter, a decline in the pressure gradient across the stenosis, and a decline in blood pressure.[281] All patients with successful angioplasty had marked improvements in their symptoms. Tyagi et al. had similar success with renal artery angioplasty for management of hypertension in Takayasu's arteritis.[282]

Giant Cell Arteritis

Giant cell arteritis is one of the most common forms of vasculitis, occurring predominantly among older people and characteristically involving medium-sized arteries. The aorta and its branches, however, are affected in about 15 per cent of cases.[283] The disease is also referred to as "granulomatous arteritis," "temporal arteritis," and "cranial arteritis."

ETIOLOGY AND PATHOPHYSIOLOGY. Unlike Takayasu's arteritis, the highest incidence of giant cell arteritis is in the

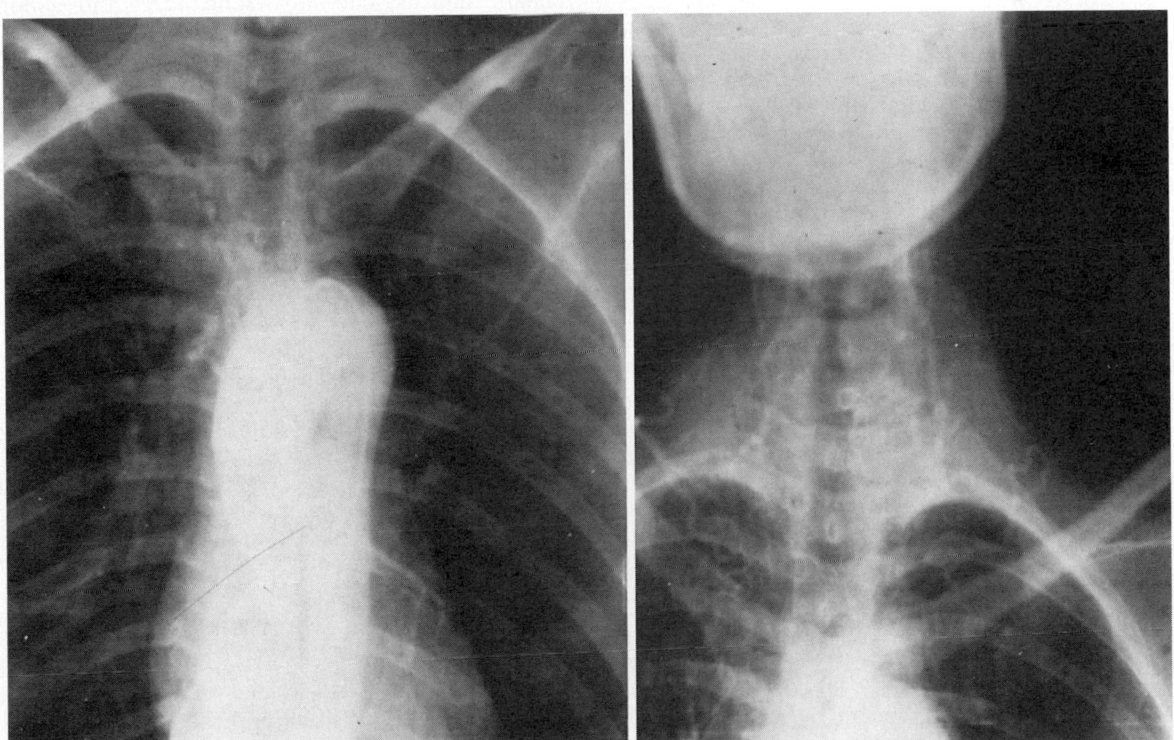

FIGURE 45–24. Thoracic aortogram *(left)* and late films of the head, neck, and upper thorax *(right)* in a 34-year-old Chinese woman with Takayasu's arteritis and no palpable pulses in the upper half of her body. The aortogram shows no direct filling of any of the major arteries arising from the aorta except the coronary arteries. In the delayed film *(right)* collateral channels faintly fill the carotid and vertebral systems.

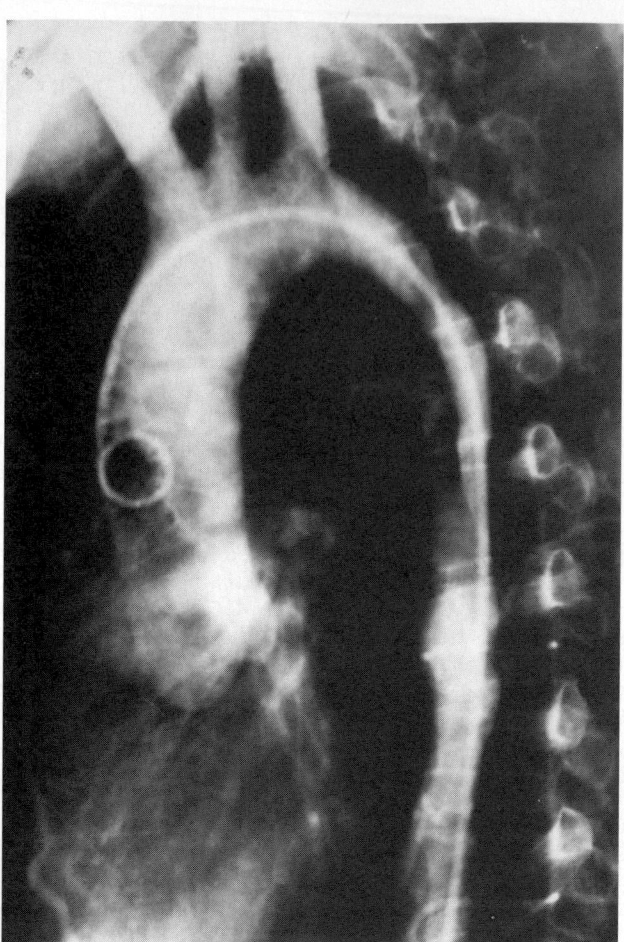

FIGURE 45–25. Thoracic aortogram in a 28-year-old Korean man with the clinical features of coarctation of the aorta that proved to be the result of Takayasu's arteritis. Note the typical "rat-tail" angiographic appearance of the descending aorta.

northern United States and Europe.[284] Its cause is unknown, although the generalized systemic manifestations of the disease and its occasional apparent temporal relationship to prior immunization or viral illness suggest a possible infectious or autoimmune origin.[285] Genetic factors may also play a role.[286]

The characteristic pathological lesion that distinguishes it from other arteritides is the granulomatous inflammation of the media of large and medium-caliber arteries,[287] about the size of the temporal artery. The disease has a special predilection for the branches of the proximal aorta, especially those supplying the head and neck, extracranial structures, and upper extremities.[284] Endarteritis is not an important feature, but the mural involvement can lead to obstruction of involved arteries. Involvement of the aorta[288] and its major branches usually coexists with the more classic and prevalent syndromes of temporal arteritis and polymyalgia rheumatica, although the aorta may rarely serve as the primary target of this disease. Narrowing or occlusions of the aorta are rare in giant cell arteritis.[287] Infrequently, the inflammatory process may weaken the aortic wall, leading to localized aneurysm formation, aortic annular dilatation, and aortic regurgitation.[289]

CLINICAL MANIFESTATIONS. Giant cell arteritis usually affects patients over the age of 50, with a mean age of 67, and occurs predominantly in women. The classic presentation is one of severe headaches, scalp or temporal artery tenderness, and constitutional symptoms. Headaches are often intense and almost unbearable, typically occurring over involved arteries (usually the temporal arteries). The area surrounding these arteries is exquisitely sensitive to pressure, and complaints such as being unable to rest the head comfortably against a pillow or to comb one's hair are common. Jaw claudication while chewing occurs in up to half of the patients.[271]

On *physical examination,* fever is quite common and patients frequently appear ill. Involved vessels are thickened and very tender. Pulses may be absent or diminished, and bruits may occur over sites of arterial occlusion. Signs of aortic regurgitation are occasionally present. Laboratory tests may be helpful in making the diagnosis. A markedly elevated sedimentation rate is virtually a sine qua non for this disease and is a valuable guide to disease activity. A moderate normochromic, normocytic anemia is the rule. Acute phase reactant levels are often elevated.[290]

The diagnosis is confirmed by biopsy of an involved artery, most often the temporal artery. However, false-negative biopsies occur in about 14 per cent[271] and therefore, if clinical suspicion persists, a second biopsy of another vessel should be performed. The rate of positive biopsies progressively declines after just a few days of glucocorticoid therapy, with as few as 10 per cent being positive after 1 week. Accordingly, biopsies should be performed without delay once the diagnosis is suspected and therapy initiated. In cases of larger vessel and aortic involvement, angiography may serve to differentiate arteritis from atherosclerosis.[283]

A serious complication is the onset of blindness from involvement of the ophthalmic artery. When visual loss occurs, progression to complete blindness is usually rapid and often irreversible. Overall, visual symptoms ranging from blurring to diplopia to vision loss occur in 36 to 58 per cent of patients.[271] In the milder form of giant cell arteritis, patients may complain only of generalized muscle aches and pains and unusual fatigue, the symptoms of polymyalgia rheumatica.

Narrowing or occlusion of the branch vessels of the thoracic aorta—often referred to as *aortic arch syndrome*—may be found in 9 to 14 per cent of cases,[283] producing symptoms similar to those of Takayasu's arteritis, such as decreased upper extremity pulses and blood pressure, arm or leg claudication, Raynaud's phenomenon, transient ischemic attacks, coronary ischemia,[291] and abdominal angina. Interestingly, in contrast with Takayasu's arteritis, renal artery involvement is almost never seen.[283] Aortic aneurysms, aortic regurgitation, and aortic dissection occur less commonly. In a recent series by Evans et al., aortic aneurysms occurred in 15 per cent of patients and at a median of 6 years after the giant cell arteritis was diagnosed.[287] Two-thirds were thoracic aortic aneurysms, with the majority located in the ascending aorta.[292] Almost one-half of those with thoracic aortic aneurysms died suddenly from aortic dissection, and one-third developed symptomatic aortic regurgitation.[287]

MANAGEMENT. High-dose glucocorticoid therapy (prednisone, 40 to 60 mg/day) is recommended in all patients with giant cell arteritis.[284] The goals of therapy are to reverse the disease and to prevent further progression, especially in the ophthalmic arteries in order to prevent blindness. Using constitutional symptoms, vascular symptoms, and the sedimentation rate as guides, the clinician can usually gradually reduce steroids to a maintenance dose for 1 to 2 years. The overall course of the disease is one of progressive improvement and eventual complete resolution, although in some patients it may be protracted for months to years. Methotrexate may be beneficial in patients with steroid-resistant symptoms, and both methotrexate and Dapsone may be useful as glucocorticoid-sparing agents in patients requiring protracted treatment.[286,293] Surgery, ideally performed while the disease is inactive and in the absence of steroid therapy, may be necessary in up to 41 per cent of those with thoracic aortic aneurysms.[292]

OTHER ARTERITIS SYNDROMES. In addition to the acute inflammation of Takayasu's and giant cell arteritis, isolated aortic regurgitation due to dilatation of the aortic annulus may occur during the

TABLE 45–5 PROPOSED CRITERIA FOR THE CLINICAL DIAGNOSIS OF TAKAYASU'S DISEASE*

CRITERION	DEFINITION
Obligatory Criterion	
Age ≤ 40 yr	Age ≤ 40 yr at diagnosis or at onset of "characteristic signs and symptoms"† of 1 month duration in patient history.
Two Major Criteria	
1. Left mid subclavian artery lesion	The most severe stenosis or occlusion present in the mid portion from the point 1 cm proximal to the left vertebral artery orifice to that 3 cm distal to the orifice determined by angiography.
2. Right mid subclavian artery lesion	The most severe stenosis or occlusion present in the mid portion from the right vertebral artery orifice to the point 3 cm distal to the orifice determined by angiography.
Nine Minor Criteria	
1. High ESR	Unexplained persistent high ESR ≥ 20 mm/h (Westergren) at diagnosis or presence of the evidence in patient history.
2. Carotid artery tenderness	Unilateral or bilateral tenderness of common carotid arteries by physician palpation: neck muscle tenderness is unacceptable.
3. Hypertension	Persistent blood pressure ≥ 140/90 mm Hg brachial or ≥ 160/90 mm Hg popliteal at age ≤ 40 yr or presence of the history at age ≤ 40 yr.
4. Aortic regurgitation	By auscultation or Doppler echocardiography or angiography.
or Annuloaortic ectasia	By angiography or two-dimensional echocardiography.
5. Pulmonary artery lesion	Lobar or segmental arterial occlusion or equivalent determined by angiography or perfusion scintigraphy; or presence of stenosis, aneurysm, luminal irregularity, or any combination in pulmonary trunk or in unilateral or bilateral pulmonary arteries determined by angiography.
6. Left mid common carotid lesion	Presence of the most severe stenosis or occlusion in the mid portion of 5 cm in length from the point 2 cm distal to its orifice determined by angiography.
7. Distal brachiocephalic trunk lesion	Presence of the most severe stenosis or occlusion in the distal third determined by angiography.
8. Descending thoracic aorta lesion	Narrowing, dilation or aneurysm, luminal irregularity, or any combination determined by angiography: tortuosity alone is unacceptable.
9. Abdominal aorta lesion	Narrowing, dilation or aneurysm, luminal irregularity, or any combination and absence of lesion in aortoiliac region consisting of 2 cm of terminal aorta and bilateral common iliac arteries determined by angiography; tortuosity alone is unacceptable.

* The proposed criteria consist of one obligatory criterion, two major criteria, and nine minor criteria. In addition to the obligatory criterion, the presence of two major criteria, or one major and two or more minor criteria, or four or more minor criteria suggests a high probability of the presence of Takayasu's disease.

† "Characteristic signs and symptoms" are explained in the reference text. ESR = erythrocyte sedimentation rate.

From Ishikawa, K.: Diagnostic approach and proposed criteria for the clinical diagnosis of Takayasu's arteriopath. J. Am. Coll. Cardiol. *12*:964, 1988.

course of ankylosing spondylitis,[294] psoriatic arthritis,[295] arthritis associated with ulcerative colitis, relapsing polychondritis, polyarteritis nodosa,[296] and Reiter's syndrome.[297] In addition, aneurysms of the aorta, pulmonary artery, and other major vessels can complicate Behçet's disease.[290]

Reported instances of aortitis complicating each of these diseases are rare. For example, aortic regurgitation has been documented in only 1 to 4 per cent of patients with ankylosing spondylitis, 2 per cent of patients with Behçet's disease,[299] and a small number of cases of Reiter's syndrome. Nevertheless, in these uncommon cases the symptoms of aortic regurgitation and ensuing congestive heart failure may eventually dominate the clinical picture.

The pathological features appear to be similar in each of the aforementioned diseases. In the early stage of inflammation there is marked dilatation of the aortic annulus with patchy elastic tissue disruption, an active inflammatory cell infiltrate, and subendothelial fibrosis.[300] These changes are most marked in the aortic root, which typically dilates but without frank aneurysm formation. The aortic valve cusps remain essentially normal in early stages but later become thickened and retracted.

The associated aortic regurgitation shares the clinical features of annuloaortic ectasia. The course of this condition is variable, with some patients exhibiting a rapidly progressive course of cardiac decompensation, whereas others have a more indolent and stable natural history. Thus, the development of aortic regurgitation does not necessarily signify an irreversible downhill course. Treatment is generally directed toward the underlying disease state. Aortic valve replacement should be performed when indicated, although, in contrast to annuloaortic ectasia, replacement of the ascending aorta itself is almost never necessary.

BACTERIAL INFECTIONS OF THE AORTA

Infected aortic aneurysms are rare, with as few as one case per year recently reported from a large medical center.[301] In an effort to avoid confusion with infections truly of fungal origin, the term "infected aneurysm" has gradually replaced the original designation "mycotic aneurysm" used by Osler to define the localized dilatation caused by sepsis in the wall of the aorta. Although saccular aneurysms are seen most commonly, infections can also cause fusiform and false aneurysms. In a minority of cases, infection may arise in a preexistent aortic aneurysm, typically atherosclerotic ones. Rarely, one may encounter nonaneurysmal bacterial aortitis.[301,302]

PATHOGENESIS. Aortic infection may arise by several mechanisms. Septic emboli from bacterial endocarditis were once the most common cause but have become rare in the era of efficacious antibiotic treatment of septicemia. Contiguous spread of infection from adjacent sites is also infrequently seen. The most common cause of infected aneurysm is the direct deposition of circulating bacteria in a diseased, atherosclerotic, or traumatized aortic intima,[301] after which organisms penetrate the aortic wall through breeches in intimal integrity to cause microbial arteritis. Recent reports suggest that the majority of aortic infections occur in patients with impaired immunity as a consequence of chronic disease, immunosuppressive therapy, or immune deficiency.[301,303]

MICROBIOLOGY. Although virtually any organism may infect the aorta, certain bacteria seem to have a proclivity for this site. *Staphylococcus aureus* and *Salmonella* species are consistently the most frequently identified organisms.[304] *Salmonella* commonly infects atherosclerotic arteries[302] but may also adhere to a normal aortic wall and directly penetrate an intact intima.[305] In fact, as many as one-quarter of patients over the age of 50 who experience *Salmonella* bacteremia may also develop secondary aortic infection.[305] Other gram-positive organisms, particularly pneumococcus, and gram-negative organisms may also cause infected aortic aneurysms. *Pseudomonas, Bacteroides fragilis, Campylobacter fetus, Neisseria gonorrhoeae*, and fungal infections are seen less often.[301,306] Aortic infections with unusual organisms are now seen with increasing frequency in the overtly immunocompromised population.[301]

CLINICAL MANIFESTATIONS. Most patients with infected aortic aneurysm are febrile, with extremely high fevers with rigors being common. Symptoms may arise from localized expansion of an infected aneurysm, which is palpable in as many as 50 per cent of patients and almost always tender.[307] A tender and pulsatile abdominal mass in a febrile patient should therefore be considered an infected aneurysm until proven otherwise.

Leukocytosis and an elevated erythrocyte sedimentation rate are present in most cases. When positive, blood cultures are helpful in suggesting the diagnosis and identifying the pathogen. In any patient with fever of unknown origin and documented *Salmonella* bacteremia, an arterial source of infection should be considered.[302] The absence of positive blood cultures, however, does not exclude the diagnosis of infected aortic aneurysm, as cultures have been found to be negative in one-quarter of cases.

Although abdominal ultrasonography may identify the presence of an aortic aneurysm, CT scanning is superior in demonstrating associated pathological findings suggestive of an infectious cause.[308,309] However, sometimes the aorta is normal in size when bacterial aortitis first presents, so lack of aneurysmal dilatation does not exclude the diagnosis.[304] In such cases, if a patient's fever, leukocytosis, and pain persist, follow-up imaging should be performed, as the aorta may rapidly dilate during the course of the infection. Aortography may also be used to make the diagnosis and is generally performed preoperatively to assist in surgical planning.

The natural history of infected aortic aneurysms is that of expansion and eventual rupture, with extremely rapid progression.[301,304] *Salmonella* and gram-negative infections have a greater tendency toward early rupture and death.[307] Overall mortality from infected aortic aneurysms is over 50 per cent, despite advances in therapy.[302,310]

MANAGEMENT. Infected aortic aneurysms are treated with intravenous antibiotics and surgical excision. The standard surgical approach involves resection of the infected aneurysm and infected retroperitoneal tissue, oversewing of the native aorta as stumps, and restoration of distal perfusion by placement of an extraanatomical bypass graft tunneled through unaffected tissue planes to avoid placing a graft in a contaminated region. Antibiotic therapy must be continued postoperatively for at least 6 weeks. Several reports suggest that in selected patients with localized infection and no gross pus, an effective and simpler surgical approach is the in situ reconstruction of the aorta with a prosthetic graft.[303,310]

PRIMARY TUMORS OF THE AORTA

Primary tumors of the aorta are quite rare, with only 45 cases reported in the literature from 1873 to the present. The frequency of such reports has increased significantly over the past decade, probably consequent to improvements in noninvasive imaging techniques. Most are diagnosed in the seventh to eighth decade of life. The thoracic and abdominal aorta are involved with equal frequency. In several cases aortic tumors have appeared in association with previously inserted Dacron aortic grafts.[311] Histologically, the majority of primary aortic tumors are classified as sarcomas, with the malignant fibrous histiocytoma subtype especially common.

The majority of primary aortic tumors arise in the intima[312] and grow along the intimal surface and into the aortic lumen to form polypoid masses (often with superimposed thrombus) but tend not to invade the aortic wall. Intimal tumors may present with symptoms of vascular obstruction from narrowing of the aortic lumen or, more typically, with signs and symptoms of peripheral embolization identical to those of atherothrombotic emboli. Emboli are commonly a mixture of tumor and thrombus, and the correct diagnosis may remain obscure until histological analysis of an embolectomy specimen is completed. Less commonly, aortic tumors arise in the medial or adventitial layers of the aortic wall. Such tumors tend not to invade the aortic lumen, but instead behave as aggressive mass lesions and present with constitutional symptoms or back pain.

Because primary aortic tumors are so uncommon and their presentation nonspecific, the diagnosis is rarely considered prior to surgical exploration or necropsy. However, several imaging modalities may be helpful in suggesting the diagnosis. Aortography demonstrates narrowing of the lumen or an intraluminal filling defect in the presence of an intimal tumor but may be negative if the tumor is adventitial.[313] An intraaortic biopsy of an intraluminal aortic mass using intravascular biopsy forceps guided by aortography has been reported.[314] CT scanning can detect intimal tumors but may not easily differentiate these from protruding atheromas.[313] MRI may better define both the tumor anatomy and the extent of invasion.[315] Lastly, the ability of TEE to image the aortic intima may make it especially useful in the detection of intimal tumors of the thoracic aorta (Fig. 45–26).[316]

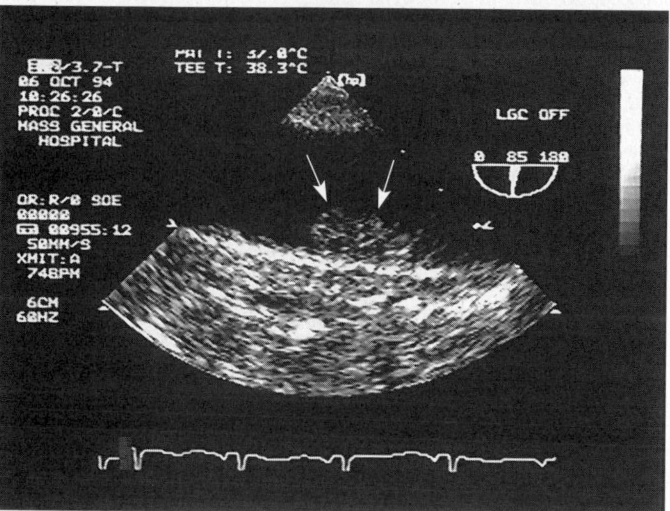

FIGURE 45–26. A transesophageal echocardiogram in long axis of the descending thoracic aorta demonstrating a primary tumor of the aorta (arrows) protruding into the lumen. The tumor, which is 3.5 cm in length, involves the intimal layer but does not appear to invade any further into the aortic wall.

Treatment of primary aortic tumors has met with little success. As the majority of patients present with metastatic disease, surgical approaches are often only palliative, i.e., to prevent further embolization. Many die secondary to the consequences of multiple emboli to vital organs. Of those undergoing surgical therapy, the large majority die within days to months postoperatively.

REFERENCES

THE NORMAL AORTA

1. Sonesson, B., Länne, T., Vernersson, E., and Hansen, F.: Sex differences in the mechanical properties of the abdominal aorta in human beings. J. Vasc. Surg. *20:*959, 1994.
2. Shimojo, M., Tsuda, N., Iwasaka, T., and Inada, M.: Age-related changes in aortic elasticity determined by gated radionuclide angiography in patients with systemic hypertension or healed myocardial infarcts and in normal subjects. Am. J. Cardiol. *68:*950, 1991.
3. Dart, A. M., Lacombe, F., Yeoh, J. K., et al.: Aortic distensibility in patients with isolated hypercholesterolemia, coronary artery disease, or cardiac transplant. Lancet *338:*270, 1991.
4. Mohiaddin, R. H., Underwood, S. R., Bogren, H. G., et al.: Regional aortic compliance studied by magnetic resonance imaging: The effects of age, training, and coronary artery disease. Br. Heart J. *62:*90, 1989.
5. Schlatmann, T. J. M., and Becker, A. E.: Histologic changes in the normal aging aorta: Implications for dissecting aortic aneurysm. Am. J. Cardiol. *39:*13, 1977.
6. Stefanadis, C., Vlachopoulos, C., Karayannacos, P., et al.: Effect of vasa vasorum flow on structure and function of the aorta in experimental animals. Circulation *91:*2669, 1995.
7. Urschel, C. W., Covell, J. W., Sonnenblick, E. H., et al.: Effects of decreased aortic compliance on performance of the left ventricle. Am. J. Physiol. *214:*298, 1968.
8. Kelly, R. P., Tunin, R., and Kass, D. A.: Effect of reduced aortic compliance on cardiac efficiency and contractile function of in situ canine left ventricle. Circ. Res. *71:*490, 1992.

AORTIC ANEURYSMS

9. Johnston, K. W., Rutherford, R. B., Tilson, M.D., et al.: Suggested standards for reporting on arterial aneurysms. J. Vasc. Surg. *13:*444, 1991.
10. Crawford, E. S., and Cohen, E. S.: Aortic aneurysm: A multifocal disease. Arch. Surg. *117:*1393, 1982.
11. Pressler, V., and McNamara, J. J.: Aneurysm of the thoracic aorta: Review of 260 cases. J. Thorac. Cardiovasc. Surg. *89:*50, 1985.
12. Bickerstaff, L. K., Pairolero, P. C., Hollier, L. H., et al.: Thoracic aortic aneurysms: A population based study. Surgery *92:*1103, 1982.
13. Bengtsson, H., Bergquist, D., and Sternby, N. H.: Increasing prevalence of abdominal aortic aneurysms: A necropsy study. Eur. J. Surg. *158:*19, 1992.
14. Bickerstaff, L. K., Hollier, L. H., Van Peenan, H. J., et al.: Abdominal aortic aneurysms: The changing natural history. J. Vasc. Surg. *1:*6, 1984.
15. Anidjar, S., and Kieffer, E.: Pathogenesis of acquired aneurysms of the abdominal aorta. Ann. Vasc. Surg. *6:*298, 1992.
16. Holmes, D. R., Liao, S., Parks, W. C., and Thompson, R. W.: Medial neovascularization in abdominal aortic aneurysms: A histopathologic marker of aneurysm degeneration with pathophysiologic implications. J. Vasc. Surg. *21:*761, 1995.
17. Webster, M. W., Ferrell, R. F., St. Jean, P. L., et al.: Ultrasound screening of first-degree relatives of patients with abdominal aortic aneurysm. J. Vasc. Surg. *13:*9, 1991.
18. Verloes, A., Sakalihassan, L., Koulischer, L., and Limet, R.: Aneurysms of the abdominal aorta: Familial and genetic aspects in three hundred thirteen pedigrees. J. Vasc. Surg. *21:*646, 1995.
19. Reilly, J. M., Brophy, C. M., and Tilson, M.D.: Characterization of an elastase from aneurysmal aorta which degrades intact aortic elastin. Ann. Vasc. Surg. *6:*499, 1992.
20. Anidjar, S., Dobrin, P. B., Eichorst, M., et al.: Correlation of inflammatory infiltrate with the enlargement of experimental aortic aneurysms. J. Vasc. Surg. *16:*139, 1992.
21. Newman, K. M., Jean-Claude, J., Li, H., et al.: Cytokines that activate proteolysis are increased in abdominal aortic aneurysms. Circulation *90*(Part 2):II-224, 1994.
22. Darling, R. C.: Ruptured arteriosclerotic abdominal aortic aneurysms. Am. J. Surg. *119:*397, 1970.
23. Rantakokko, V., Havia, T., Inberg, M. V., and Vänttinen, E.: Abdominal aortic aneurysms: A clinical and autopsy study of 408 patients. Acta Chir. Scand. *149:*151, 1983.
24. Astarita, D., Filippone, D. R., and Cohn, J. D.: Spontaneous major intra-abdominal arteriovenous fistulas: A report of several cases. Angiology *36:*656, 1985.
25. Muluk, S. C., Gertler, J. P., Brewster, D. C., et al.: Presentation and patterns of aortic aneurysms in young patients. J. Vasc. Surg. *20:*880, 1994.
26. Kiell, C. S., and Ernst, C. B.: Advances in the management of abdominal aortic aneurysm. Adv. Surg. *26:*73, 1993.
27. Marston, W. A., Ahlquist, R., Johnson, G., Jr., and Meyer, A. A.: Mis-

diagnosis of ruptured abdominal aortic aneurysms. J. Vasc. Surg. *16*:17, 1992.
28. Martinussen, H. J., Lolk, A., Rohr, N., et al.: Ruptured abdominal aortic aneurysm with fistula into the inferior vena cava. J. Cardiovasc. Surg. *27*:298, 1986.
29. Crew, J. R., Bashour, T. T., Ellertson, D., et al.: Ruptured abdominal aortic aneurysms: Experience with 70 cases. Clin. Cardiol. *8*:433, 1985.
30. Jenkins, A. M., Ruckley, C. V., and Nolan, B.: Ruptured abdominal aortic aneurysm. Br. J. Surg. *73*:395, 1986.
31. LaRoy, L. L., Cormier, P. J., Matalon, T. A. S., et al.: Imaging of abdominal aortic aneurysms. A. J. R. *152*:785, 1989.
32. Hollier, L. H., Taylor, L. M., and Ochsner, J.: Recommended indications for operative treatment of abdominal aortic aneurysms: Report of a subcommittee of the Joint Council of the Society for Vascular Surgery and of the North American Chapter of the International Society for Cardiovascular Surgery. J. Vasc. Surg. *15*:1046, 1992.
33. Ernst, C. B.: Abdominal aortic aneurysm. N. Engl. J. Med. *328*:1167, 1993.
34. Todd, G. J., Nowygrod, R., Benvenisty, A., et al.: The accuracy of CT scanning in the diagnosis of abdominal and thoracoabdominal aortic aneurysms. J. Vasc. Surg. *13*:302, 1991.
35. Pillari, G., Chang, J. B., Zito, J., et al.: Computed tomography of abdominal aortic aneurysm: An in vivo pathological report with a note on dynamic predictors. Arch. Surg. *123*:727, 1988.
36. Gomes, M. N., and Choyke, P. L.: Improved identification of the renal arteries in patients with aortic aneurysms by means of high-resolution computed tomography. J. Vasc. Surg. *6*:262, 1987.
37. Lederle, F. A., Wilson, S. E., Johnson, G. R., et al.: Variability in measurement of abdominal aortic aneurysms. J. Vasc. Surg. *21*:945, 1995.
38. Gomes, M. N., Davros, W. J., and Zemen, R. K.: Preoperative assessment of abdominal aortic aneurysm: The value of helical and three-dimensional computed tomography. J. Vasc. Surg. *20*:367, 1994.
39. Petersen, M. J., Cambria, R. P., Kaufman, J. A., et al.: Magnetic resonance angiography in the preoperative evaluation of abdominal aortic aneurysms. J. Vasc. Surg. *21*:891, 1995.
40. Campbell, J. J., Bell, D. D., and Gaspar, M. R.: Selective use of arteriography in the assessment of aortic aneurysm repair. Ann. Vasc. Surg. *4*:419, 1990.
41. Edelman, R. R.: MR angiography: Present and future. A. J. R. *161*:1, 1993.
42. Kandarpa, K., Piwnica-Worms, D., Chopra, P. S., et al.: Prospective double-blinded comparison of MR imaging and aortography in the preoperative evaluation of abdominal aortic aneurysms. J. Vasc. Intervent. Radiol. *3*:83, 1992.
43. Frame, P. S., Fryback, D. G., and Patteson, C.: Screening for abdominal aortic aneurysm in men ages 60 to 80 years: A cost-effectiveness analysis. Ann. Intern. Med. *119*:411, 1993.
44. Ingoldby, C. J. H., Wujanto, R., and Mitchell, J. E.: Impact of vascular surgery on community mortality from ruptured aortic aneurysm. Br. J. Surg. *73*:551, 1986.
45. Estes, J. E., Jr.: Abdominal aortic aneurysm: A study of one hundred and two cases. Circulation *2*:258, 1950.
46. Darling, R. C., Messina, C. R., Brewster, D. C., and Ottinger, L. W.: Autopsy study of unoperated abdominal aortic aneurysms: The case for early resection. Circulation *56*(Suppl. II):II-161, 1977.
47. Ouriel, K., Green, R. M., Donayre, C., et al.: An evaluation of new methods of expressing aortic aneurysm size: Relationships to rupture. J. Vasc. Surg. *15*:12, 1992.
48. Limet, R., Sakalihassan, N., and Adelin, A.: Determination of the expansion rate and incidence of rupture of abdominal aortic aneurysms. J. Vasc. Surg. *14*:540, 1991.
49. Gadowski, G. R., Pilcher, D. B., and Ricci, M. A.: Abdominal aortic aneurysm expansion rate: Effect of size and beta-adrenergic blockade. J. Vasc. Surg. *19*:727, 1994.
50. Katz, D. J., Stanley, J. C., and Zelenock, G. B.: Operative mortality rates for intact and ruptured abdominal aortic aneurysms in Michigan: An eleven-year statewide experience. J. Vasc. Surg. *19*:804, 1994.
51. Lederle, F. A., Wilson, S. E., Johnson, G. R., et al.: Design of the abdominal aortic aneurysm detection and management study. J. Vasc. Surg. *20*:296, 1994.
52. Johnston, K. W., and the Canadian Society for Vascular Surgery Aneurysm Study Group: Non-ruptured abdominal aortic aneurysm: Six-year follow-up results from the multicenter prospective Canadian aneurysm study. J. Vasc. Surg. *20*:163, 1994.
53. Parodi, J. C., Palmaz, J. C., and Barone, H. D.: Transfemoral intraluminal graft implantation for abdominal aortic aneurysms. Ann. Vasc. Surg. *5*:491, 1991.
54. Ruiz, C. E., Zhang, H. P., Douglas, J. T., et al.: A novel method for treatment of abdominal aortic aneurysms using percutaneous implantation of a newly designed endovascular device. Circulation *91*:2470, 1995.
55. Parodi, J. C.: Endovascular repair of abdominal aortic aneurysms and other arterial lesions. J. Vasc. Surg. *21*:549, 1995.
56. Hertzer, N. R.: Fatal myocardial infarction following abdominal aortic aneurysm resection: Three hundred forty-three patients followed 6–11 years postoperatively. Ann. Surg. *192*:671, 1980.
57. Hertzer, N. R., Beven, E. G., Young, Y. R., et al.: Coronary artery disease in peripheral vascular patients: A classification of 1000 coronary angiograms and results of surgical management. Ann. Surg. *199*:223, 1984.
58. Boucher, C. A., Brewster, D. C., Darling, R. C., et al.: Determination of cardiac risk by dipyridamole-thallium imaging before peripheral vascular surgery. N. Engl. J. Med. *312*:389, 1985.
59. Eagle, K. A., Singer, D. E., Brewster, D. C., et al.: Dipyridamole-thallium scanning in patients undergoing vascular surgery: Optimizing preoperative evaluation of cardiac risk. JAMA *257*:2185, 1987.
60. Levinson, J. R., Boucher, C. A., Coley, C. M., et al.: Usefulness of semiquantitative analysis of dipyridamole-thallium 201 redistribution for improving risk stratification before vascular surgery. Am. J. Cardiol. *66*:406, 1990.
61. Leppo, J., Plaja, J., Gionet, M., et al.: Noninvasive evaluation of cardiac risk before elective vascular surgery. J. Am. Coll. Cardiol. *9*:269, 1987.
62. Lalka, S. G., Sawada, S. G., Dalsing, M. C., et al.: Dobutamine stress echocardiography as a predictor of cardiac events associated with aortic surgery. J. Vasc. Surg. *15*:831, 1992.
63. Cambria, R. P., Brewster, D. C., Abbott, W. M., et al.: The impact of selective use of dipyridamole-thallium scans and surgical factors on the current morbidity of aortic surgery. J. Vasc. Surg. *15*:43, 1992.
64. Gersh, B. J., Rihal, C. S., Rooke, T. W., and Ballard, D. J.: Evaluation and management of patients with both peripheral vascular and coronary artery disease. J. Am. Coll. Cardiol. *18*:203, 1991.
65. Steinberg, J. B., Kresowik, T. F., and Behrendt, D. M.: Prophylactic myocardial revascularization based on dipyridamole-thallium scanning before peripheral vascular surgery. Cardiovasc. Surg. *1*:552, 1993.
66. Hertzer, N. R., Young, J. R., Beven, E. G., et al.: Late results of coronary bypass in patients with peripheral vascular disease. II. Five-year survival according to sex, hypertension, and diabetes. Cleve. Clin. J. Med. *54*:15, 1987.
67. Rihal, C. S., Eagle, K. A., Mickel, M. C., et al.: Surgical therapy for coronary artery disease among patients with combined coronary artery and peripheral vascular disease. Circulation *91*:46, 1995.
68. Pasternack, P. F., Grossi, E. A., Bauman, F. G., et al.: Silent myocardial ischemia monitoring predicts late as well as perioperative cardiac events in patients undergoing vascular surgery. J. Vasc. Surg. *16*:171, 1992.
69. Landesberg, G., Luria, M. H., Cotev, S., et al.: Importance of long-duration postoperative ST-segment depression in cardiac morbidity after vascular surgery. Lancet *341*:715, 1993.
70. Pasternack, P. F., Grossi, E. A., Bauman, F. G., et al.: Beta blockade to decrease silent myocardial ischemia during peripheral vascular surgery. Am. J. Surg. *158*:113, 1989.
71. Reigel, M. M., Hollier, L. H., Kazmier, F. J., et al.: Late survival in abdominal aortic aneurysm patients: The role of selective myocardial revascularization on the basis of clinical symptoms. J. Vasc. Surg. *5*:222, 1987.
72. Brophy, C., Tilson, J. E., and Tilson, M. D.: Propranolol delays the formation of aneurysms in the male blotchy mouse. J. Surg. Res. *44*:687, 1988.
73. Treiman, R. L., Hartunian, S. L., Cossman, D. V., et al.: Late results of small untreated abdominal aortic aneurysms. Ann. Vasc. Surg. *5*:359, 1991.
74. Pyeritz, R. E., and McKusick, V. A.: The Marfan syndrome: Diagnosis and management. N. Engl. J. Med. *300*:772, 1979.
75. Milewicz, D. M.: Ultrasonic characterization of the aortic architecture in Marfan patients. Circulation *91*(Edit.):1272, 1995.
76. Hollister, D. W., Goodfrey, M., Sakai, L. Y., and Pyeritz, R. E.: Immunohistologic abnormalities of the microfibrillar-fiber system in the Marfan syndrome. N. Engl. J. Med. *323*:152, 1990.
77. Jeremy, R. W., Huang, H., Hwa, J., et al.: Relation between age, arterial distensibility, and aortic dilatation in the Marfan syndrome. Am. J. Cardiol. *74*:369, 1994.
78. Marsalese, D. L., Moodie, D. S., Lytle, B. W., et al.: Cystic medial necrosis of the aorta in patients without Marfan's syndrome: Surgical outcome and long-term follow up. J. Am. Coll. Cardiol. *16*:68, 1990.
79. Emanuel, R., Ng, R. A., Marcomichelakis, J., et al.: Formes frustes of Marfan's syndrome presenting with severe aortic regurgitation: Clinicogenetic study of 18 families. Br. Heart J. *39*:190, 1977.
80. Johansson, G., Markström, U., and Swedenborg, J.: Ruptured thoracic aortic aneurysms: A study of incidence and mortality rates. J. Vasc. Surg. *21*:985, 1995.
81. Joyce, J. W., Fairbairn, J. F., II, Kincaid, O. W., and Juergens, J. L.: Aneurysms of the thoracic aorta: A clinical study with special reference to prognosis. Circulation *29*:176, 1964.
82. McNamara, J. J., and Pressler, V. M.: Natural history of arteriosclerotic thoracic aortic aneurysms. Ann. Thorac. Surg. *26*:468, 1978.
83. Bogey, W. M., Jr., Thomas, J. H., and Hermreck, A. S.: Aortoesophageal fistula: Report of a successfully managed case and review of the literature. J. Vasc. Surg. *16*:90, 1992.
84. Masuda, Y., Takanashi, K., Takasu, J., et al.: Expansion rate of thoracic aortic aneurysms and influencing factors. Chest *102*:461, 1992.
85. Dinsmore, R. E., Liberthson, R. R., Wismer, G. L., et al.: Magnetic resonance imaging of thoracic aortic aneurysms: Comparison with other diagnostic methods. A. J. R. *146*:309, 1986.
86. Pressler, V., and McNamara, J. J.: Thoracic aortic aneurysm: Natural history and treatment. J. Thorac. Cardiovasc. Surg. *79*:489, 1980.
87. Crawford, E. S., and DeNatale, R. W.: Thoracoabdominal aortic aneurysm: Observations regarding the natural course of disease. J. Vasc. Surg. *3*:578, 1986.
88. Hirose, Y., Hamada, S., Takamiya, M., et al.: Aortic aneurysms: Growth rate measured with CT. Radiology *185*:249, 1992.
89. Dapunt, O. E., Galla, J. D., Sadeghi, A. M., et al.: The natural history of thoracic aortic aneurysms. J. Thorac. Cardiovasc. Surg. *107*:1323, 1994.

90. Treasure, T.: Elective replacement of the aortic root in Marfan's syndrome. Br. Heart J. *69*(Edit.):101, 1993.
91. Verdant, A., Cossette, R., Page, A., et al.: Aneurysms of the descending thoracic aorta: Three hundred sixty-six consecutive cases resected without paraplegia. J. Vasc. Surg. *21*:385, 1995.
92. Livesay, J. J., Cooley, D. A., Ventemiglia, R. A., et al.: Surgical experience in descending thoracic aneurysmectomy with and without adjuncts to avoid ischemia. Ann. Thorac. Surg. *39*:37, 1985.
93. Gott, V. L., Gillinov, A. M., Pyeritz, R. E., et al.: Aortic root replacement: Risk factor analysis of a seventeen-year experience with 270 patients. J. Thorac. Cardiovasc. Surg. *109*:536, 1995.
94. David, T. E., Feindel, C. M., and Bos, J.: Repair of the aortic valve in patients with aortic insufficiency and aortic root aneurysm. J. Thorac. Cardiovasc. Surg. *109*:345, 1995.
95. Coselli, J. S., Büket, S., and Djukanovic, B.: Aortic arch operation: Current treatment and results. Ann. Thorac. Surg. *59*:19, 1995.
96. Svensson, L. G., Crawford, S., Hess, K. R., et al.: Dissection of the aorta and dissecting aortic aneurysms: Improving early and long-term survival results. Circulation *82*(Suppl. IV):IV-24, 1990.
97. Griepp, R. B., Stinson, E. B., Hollingsworth, J. F., and Buehler, D.: Prosthetic replacement of the aortic arch. J. Thorac. Cardiovasc. Surg. *70*:1051, 1975.
98. Crawford, E. S., Coselli, J. S., Svensson, L. G., et al.: Diffuse aneurysmal disease (chronic aortic dissection, Marfan, and mega aorta syndromes) and multiple aneurysm. Ann. Surg. *211*:521, 1990.
99. Kitamura, M., Hashimoto, A., Akimoto, T., et al.: Operation for type A aortic dissection: Introduction of retrograde cerebral perfusion. Ann. Thorac. Surg. *59*:1195, 1995.
100. Usui, A., Hotta, T., Hiroura, M., et al.: Retrograde perfusion through a superior vena caval cannula protects the brain. Ann. Thorac. Surg. *53*:47, 1992.
101. Heinemann, M. K., Buehner, B., Jurmann, M. J., and Borst, H.-G.: Use of the "elephant trunk technique" in aortic surgery. Ann. Thorac. Surg. *60*:2, 1995.
102. Crawford, E. S., Svensson, L. G., Coselli, J. S., et al.: Surgical treatment of aneurysm and/or dissection of the ascending aorta, transverse aortic arch, and ascending aorta and transverse arch: Factors influencing survival in 717 patients. J. Thorac. Cardiovasc. Surg. *98*:659, 1989.
103. Coselli, J. S., and Crawford, E. S.: Composite valve-graft replacement of aortic root using separate Dacron tube for coronary artery reattachment. Ann. Thorac. Surg. *47*:558, 1989.
104. Hollier, L. H., Symmonds, J. B., Pairolero, P. C., et al.: Thoracoabdominal aortic aneurysm repair: Analysis of postoperative morbidity. Arch. Surg. *123*:871, 1988.
105. Dake, M. D., Miller, D. C., Semba, C. P., et al.: Transluminal placement of endovascular stent-grafts for the treatment of descending thoracic aneurysms. N. Engl. J. Med. *331*:1729, 1994.
106. Moreno-Cabral, C. E., Miller, D. C., Mitchell, R. S., et al.: Degenerative and atherosclerotic aneurysms of the thoracic aorta. J. Thorac. Cardiovasc. Surg. *88*:1020, 1984.
107. Shores, J., Berger, K. R., Murphy, E. A., and Pyeritz, R. E.: Progression of aortic dilatation and the benefit of long-term β-adrenergic blockade in Marfan's syndrome. N. Engl. J. Med. *330*:1335, 1994.
108. Ellis, R. P., Cooley, D. A., and DeBakey, M. E.: Clinical considerations and surgical treatment of annulo-aortic ectasia. J. Thorac. Cardiovasc. Surg. *42*:363, 1961.
109. Lemon, D. K., and White, C. W.: Annuloaortic ectasia: Angiographic, hemodynamic, and clinical comparison with aortic valve insufficiency. Am. J. Cardiol. *41*:482, 1978.

AORTIC DISSECTION

110. Wheat, M. W., Jr.: Acute dissecting aneurysms of the aorta: Diagnosis and treatment—1979. Am. Heart J. *99*:373, 1980.
111. Roberts, W. C.: Aortic dissection: Anatomy, consequences, and causes. Am. Heart J. *101*:195, 1981.
112. Hirst, A. E., Jr., Johns, V. J., Jr., and Kime, S. W., Jr.: Dissecting aneurysm of the aorta: A review of 505 cases. Medicine *37*:217, 1958.
113. Wilson, S. K., and Hutchins, G. M.: Aortic dissecting aneurysms: Causative factors in 204 subjects. Arch. Pathol. Lab. Med. *106*:175, 1982.
114. DeBakey, M. E., McCollum, C. H., Crawford, E. S., et al.: Dissection and dissecting aneurysms of the aorta: Twenty-year follow-up of five hundred twenty-seven patients treated surgically. Surgery *92*:1118, 1982.
115. Daily, P. O., Trueblood, H. W., Stinson, E. B., et al.: Management of acute aortic dissections. Ann. Thorac. Surg. *10*:237, 1970.
116. VanMaele, R. G., De Bock, L., Van Schil, P. E., et al.: Limited acute dissections of the abdominal aorta: Report of five cases. J. Cardiovasc. Surg. *33*:298, 1992.
117. Spittell, P. C., Spittell, J. A., Jr., Joyce, J. W., et al.: Clinical features and differential diagnosis of aortic dissection: Experience with 236 cases (1980 through 1990). Mayo Clin. Proc. *68*:642, 1993.
118. Larson, E. W., and Edwards, W. D.: Risk factors for aortic dissection: A necropsy study of 161 patients. Am. J. Cardiol. *53*:849, 1984.
119. Shachter, N., Perloff, J. K., and Mulder, D. G.: Aortic dissection in Noonan's syndrome. Am. J. Cardiol. *54*:464, 1984.
120. Price, W. H., and Wilson, J.: Dissection of the aorta in Turner's syndrome. J. Med. Genet. *20*:61, 1983.
121. Om, A., Porter, T., and Mohanty, P. K.: Transesophageal echocardiographic diagnosis of acute aortic dissection complicating cocaine abuse. Am. Heart J. *123*:532, 1992.
122. Williams, G. M., Gott, V. L., Brawley, R. K., et al.: Aortic disease associated with pregnancy. J. Vasc. Surg. *8*:470, 1988.
123. Mazzucotelli, J.-P., Deleuze, P. H., Baureton, C., et al.: Preservation of the aortic valve in acute aortic dissection: Long-term echocardiographic assessment and clinical outcome. Ann. Thorac. Surg. *55*:1513, 1993.
124. Pumphrey, C. W., Fay, T., and Weir, I.: Aortic dissection during pregnancy. Br. Heart J. *55*:106, 1986.
125. Elkayam, U., Ostzega, E., Shotan, A., and Mehra, A.: Cardiovascular problems in pregnant women with the Marfan syndrome. Ann. Intern. Med. *123*:117, 1995.
126. Jacobs, L. E., Fraifeld, M., Kotler, M. N., and Ioli, A. W.: Aortic dissection following intraaortic balloon insertion: Recognition by transesophageal echocardiography. Am. Heart J. *124*:536, 1992.
127. Murphy, D. A., Craver, J. M., Jones, E. L., et al.: Recognition and management of ascending aortic dissection complicating cardiac surgical operations. J. Thorac. Cardiovasc. Surg. *85*:247, 1983.
128. Still, R. J., Hilgenberg, A. D., Akins, C. W., et al.: Intraoperative aortic dissection. Ann. Thorac. Surg. *53*:374, 1992.
129. Albat, B., and Thevenet, A.: Dissecting aneurysms of the ascending aorta occurring late after aortic valve replacement. J. Cardiovasc. Surg. *33*:272, 1992.
130. Slater, E. E., and DeSanctis, R. W.: The clinical recognition of dissecting aortic aneurysm. Am. J. Med. *60*:625, 1976.
131. Doroghazi, R. M., Slater, E. E., DeSanctis, R. W., et al.: Long-term survival of patients with treated aortic dissection. J. Am. Coll. Cardiol. *3*:1026, 1984.
132. Vilacosta, I., Castillo, J. A., San Román, J. A., et al.: New echo-anatomical correlations in aortic dissection. Eur. Heart J. *16*:126, 1995.
133. Hurak, A. M., and Konstadt, S. N.: Aortic intussusception: A rare complication of aortic dissection. Anesthesiology *82*:1292, 1994.
134. Fann, J. I., Sarris, G. E., Mitchell, R. S., et al.: Treatment of patients with aortic dissection presenting with peripheral vascular complications. Ann. Surg. *212*:705, 1990.
135. Zull, D. N., and Cydula, R.: Acute paraplegia: A presenting manifestation of aortic dissection. Am. J. Med. *84*:765, 1988.
136. Glower, D. D., Speier, R. H., White, W. D., et al.: Management and long-term outcome of aortic dissection. Ann. Surg. *214*:31, 1991.
137. Kamp, T. J., Goldschmidt-Clermont, P. J., Brinker, J. A., and Resar, J. R.: Myocardial infarction, aortic dissection, and thrombolytic therapy. Am. Heart J. *128*:1234, 1994.
138. Hartnell, G. G., Wakeley, C. J., Tottle, A., et al.: Limitations of chest radiography in discriminating between aortic dissection and myocardial infarction: Implications for thrombolysis. J. Thorac. Imaging *8*:152, 1993.
139. Cambria, R. P., Brewster, D. C., Moncure, A. C., et al.: Spontaneous aortic dissection in the presence of coexistent or previously repaired atherosclerotic aortic aneurysm. Ann. Surg. *208*:619, 1988.
140. Giannoccaro, P. J., Marquis, J.-F., Chan, K.-L., et al.: Aortic dissection presenting as upper airway obstruction. Chest *99*:256, 1991.
141. Roth, J. A., and Parekh, M. A.: Dissecting aneurysms perforating the esophagus. N. Engl. J. Med. *299*:776, 1978.
142. Logue, R. B., and Sikes, C.: A new sign in dissecting aneurysm of the aorta: Pulsation of a sternoclavicular joint. JAMA *148*:1209, 1952.
143. Murray, H. W., Mann, J. J., Genecin, A., and McKusick, V. A.: Fever with dissecting aneurysm of the aorta. Am. J. Med. *61*:10, 1976.
144. Hurley, D. V., Nishimura, R. A., Schaff, H. V., and Edwards, W. D.: Aortic dissection with fistula to right atrium: Noninvasive diagnosis by two-dimensional and Doppler echocardiography with successful repair: Case report and review of the literature. J. Thorac. Cardiovasc. Surg. *92*:953, 1986.
145. Perryman, R. A., and Gay, W. A.: Rupture of dissecting thoracic aortic aneurysm into the right ventricle. Am. J. Cardiol. *30*:277, 1972.
146. Oliveira, J. S. M., Bestetti, R. B., Marin-Neto, J. A., et al.: Ruptured aortic dissection into the left atrium: A rare cause of congestive heart failure. Am. Heart J. *121*:936, 1991.
147. Eagle, K. A., Quertermous, T., Kritzer, G. A., et al.: Spectrum of conditions initially suggesting acute aortic dissection but with negative aortograms. Am. J. Cardiol. *57*:322, 1986.
147a. O'Gara, P. T., and DeSanctis, R. W.: Acute aortic dissection and its variants: Toward a common diagnostic and therapeutic approach. Circulation *92*:1376, 1995.
148. Cigarroa, J. E., Isselbacher, E. M., DeSanctis, R. W., and Eagle, K. A.: Diagnostic imaging in the evaluation of suspected aortic dissection: Old standards and new directions. N. Engl. J. Med. *328*:35, 1993.
149. Wilbers, C. R., Carrol, C. L., and Hnilica, M. A.: Optimal diagnostic imaging of aortic dissection. Texas Heart Instit. J. *17*:271, 1990.
150. Petasnick, J. P: Radiologic evaluation of aortic dissection. Radiology *180*:297, 1991.
151. Earnest, F., IV, Muhm, J. R., and Sheedy, P. F., II: Roentgenographic findings in thoracic aortic dissection. Mayo Clin. Proc. *54*:43, 1979.
152. Erbel, R., Daniel, W., Visser, C., et al.: Echocardiography in diagnosis of aortic dissection. Lancet *1*:457, 1989.
153. Bansal, R. C., Chandrasekaran, K., Ayala, K., and Smith, D.: Frequency and explanation of false negative diagnosis of aortic dissection by aortography and transesophageal echocardiography. J. Am. Coll. Cardiol. *25*:1393, 1995.
154. Mugge, A., Daniel, W. G., Laas, J., et al.: False-negative diagnosis of proximal aortic dissection by computed tomography or angiography and possible explanations based on transesophageal echocardiographic findings. Am. J. Cardiol. *65*:527, 1990.

155. Nienaber, C. A., von Kodolitsch, Y., Nicolas, V., et al.: Definitive diagnosis of thoracic aortic dissection: The emerging role of noninvasive imaging modalities. N. Engl. J. Med. *328*:1, 1993.
156. Hamada, S., Takamiya, M., Kimura, K., et al.: Type A aortic dissection: Evaluation with ultrafast CT. Radiology *183*:155, 1992.
157. Zemen, R. K., Berman, P. M., Silverman, P. M., et al.: Diagnosis of aortic dissection: Value of helical CT with multiplanar reformation and three-dimensional rendering. A. J. R. *164*:1375, 1995.
158. White, R. D., Lipton, M. J., Higgins, C. B., et al.: Noninvasive evaluation of suspected thoracic aortic disease by contrast-enhanced computed tomography. Am. J. Cardiol. *57*:282, 1986.
159. Nienaber, C. A., Spielmann, R. P., von Kodolitsch, Y., et al.: Diagnosis of thoracic aortic dissection: Magnetic resonance imaging versus transesophageal echocardiography. Circulation *85*:434, 1992.
160. Kersting-Sommerhoff, B. A., Higgins, C. B., White, R. D., et al.: Aortic dissection: Sensitivity and specificity of MR imaging. Radiology *166*:651, 1988.
161. Shellock, F. G., and Curtis, J. S.: MR imaging and biomedical implants, materials, and devices: An updated review. Radiology *180*:541, 1991.
162. Adachi, H., Omoto, R., Kyo, S., et al.: Emergency surgical intervention of acute aortic dissection with the rapid diagnosis by transesophageal echocardiography. Circulation *84*(Suppl. III):III-14, 1991.
163. Evangelista, A., Garcia-del-Castillo, H., Gonzales-Alujas, T., et al.: Diagnosis of ascending aortic dissection by transesophageal echocardiography: Utility of M-mode in recognizing artifacts. J. Am. Coll. Cardiol. *27*:102, 1996.
164. Blanchard, D. G., Kimura, B. J., Dittrich, H. C., and DeMaria, A. N.: Transesophageal echocardiography of the aorta. JAMA *272*:546, 1994.
165. Kern, M. J., Serota, H., Callicoat, P., et al.: Use of coronary arteriography in the preoperative management of patients undergoing urgent repair of the thoracic aorta. Am. Heart J. *119*:143, 1990.
166. Ballal, R. S., Nanda, N. C., Gatewood, R., et al.: Usefulness of transesophageal echocardiography in assessment of aortic dissection. Circulation *84*:1903, 1991.
167. Erbel, R., Oelert, H., Meyer, J., et al.: Effect of medical and surgical therapy on aortic dissection evaluated by transesophageal echocardiography: Implications for prognosis and therapy. Circulation *87*:1604, 1993.
168. Granato, J. E., Dee, P., and Gibson, R. S.: Utility of two-dimensional echocardiography in suspected ascending aortic dissection. Am. J. Cardiol. *56*:123, 1985.
169. Chan, K.: Usefulness of transesophageal echocardiography in the diagnosis of conditions mimicking aortic dissection. Am. Heart J. *122*:495, 1991.
170. Yamada, E., Matsumura, M., Kyo, S., and Omoto, R.: Usefulness of a prototype intravascular ultrasound imaging in evaluation of aortic dissection and comparison with aortographic study, transesophageal echocardiography, computed tomography, and magnetic resonance imaging. Am. J. Cardiol. *75*:161, 1995.
171. Moon, M. R., Dake, M. D., Pelc, L. R., et al.: Intravascular stenting of acute experimental type B dissections. J. Surg. Res. *54*:381, 1993.
172. Banning, A. P., Ruttley, M. S. T., Musumeci, F., and Fraser, A. G.: Acute dissection of the thoracic aorta: Transesophageal echocardiography is the investigation of choice. Br. Med. J. *310*:72, 1995.
173. Rizzo, R. J., Aranki, S. F., Aklog, L., et al.: Rapid noninvasive diagnosis and surgical repair of acute ascending aortic dissection. J. Thorac. Cardiovasc. Surg. *108*:567, 1994.
174. Simon, P., Owen, A. N., Havel, M., et al.: Transesophageal echocardiography in the emergency surgical management of patients with aortic dissection. J. Thorac. Cardiovasc. Surg. *103*:1113, 1992.
175. Creswell, L. L., Kouchoukos, N. T., Cox, J. L., and Rosenbloom, M.: Coronary artery disease in patients with type A aortic dissection. Ann. Thorac. Surg. *59*:585, 1995.
176. Anagnostopoulos, C. E., Prabhakar, M. J. S., and Kittle, C. F.: Aortic dissections and dissecting aneurysms. Am. J. Cardiol. *30*:263, 1972.
177. Shaw, R. W.: Acute dissecting aortic aneurysms: Treatment by fenestration of the internal wall of the aneurysm. N. Engl. J. Med. *253*:331, 1955.
178. Elefteriades, J. A., Hartleroad, J., Gusberg, R. J., et al.: Long-term experience with descending aortic dissection: The complication-specific approach. Ann. Thorac. Surg. *53*:11, 1992.
179. DeBakey, M. E., Cooley, D. A., and Creech, O., Jr.: Surgical considerations of dissecting aneurysms of the aorta. Ann. Surg. *142*:586, 1955.
180. Wheat, M. W., Jr., Palmer, R. F., Barley, T. D., and Seelman, R. C.: Treatment of dissecting aneurysms of the aorta without surgery. J. Thorac. Cardiovasc. Surg. *50*:364, 1965.
181. Grubb, B. P., Sirio, C., and Zelis, R.: Intravenous labetalol in acute aortic dissection. JAMA *258*:78, 1987.
182. Fenner, S. G., Mahoney, A., and Cashman, J. N.: Repair of traumatic transection of the thoracic aorta: Esmolol for intraoperative control of arterial pressure. Br. J. Anaesth. *67*:483, 1991.
183. Frishman, W. H., Weinberg, P., Peled, H. B., et al.: Calcium entry blockers for the treatment of severe hypertension and hypertensive crisis. Am. J. Med. *77*(Suppl. 2B):35, 1984.
184. White, S. R., and Hall, J. B.: Control of hypertension with nifedipine in the setting of aortic dissection. Chest *88*:781, 1985.
185. Isselbacher, E. M., Cigarroa, J. E., and Eagle, K. A.: Cardiac tamponade complicating proximal aortic dissection: Is pericardiocentesis harmful? Circulation *90*:2375, 1994.
186. Miller, D. C., Stinson, E. B., Oyer, P. E., et al.: Operative treatment of aortic dissections: Experience with 125 patients over a sixteen-year period. J. Thorac. Cardiovasc. Surg. *78*:365, 1979.
187. Masuda, Y., Yamada, Z., Morooka, N., et al.: Prognosis of patients with medically treated aortic dissections. Circulation *84*(Suppl. III):III-7, 1991.
188. Miller, D. C., Mitchell, R. C., Oyer, P. E., et al.: Independent determinants of operative mortality for patients with aortic dissections. Circulation *70*(Suppl. I):153, 1984.
189. Glower, D. D., Fann, J. I., Speier, R. H., et al.: Comparison of medical and surgical therapy for uncomplicated descending aortic dissection. Circulation *82*(Suppl IV):IV-39, 1990.
190. Crawford, E. S., Svensson, L. G., Coselli, J. S., et al.: Aortic dissection and dissecting aortic aneurysms. Ann. Surg. *208*:254, 1988.
191. Cachera, J. P., Vouhe, P. R., Loisance, D. Y., et al.: Surgical management of acute dissections involving the ascending aorta. J. Thorac. Cardiovasc. Surg. *82*:576, 1981.
192. Haverich, A., Miller, D. C., Scott, W. C., et al.: Acute and chronic aortic dissections: Determinants of long-term outcome for operative survivors. Circulation *72*(Suppl. II):II-22, 1985.
193. Crawford, E. S., Kirklin, J. W., Naftel, D. C., et al.: Surgery for acute dissection of the ascending aorta: Should the arch be included? J. Thorac. Cardiovasc. Surg. *104*:46, 1992.
194. Yun, K. L., Glower, D. D., Miller, D. C., et al.: Aortic dissection resulting from tear of transverse arch: Is concomitant arch repair warranted? J. Thorac. Cardiovasc. Surg. *102*:355, 1991.
195. Fann, J. I., Glower, D. D., Miller, D. C., et al.: Preservation of aortic valve in type A aortic dissection complicated by aortic regurgitation. J. Thorac. Cardiovasc. Surg. *102*:62, 1991.
196. Culliford, A. T., Ayvaliotis, B., Shemin, R., et al.: Aneurysms of the descending aorta: Surgical experience in 48 patients. J. Thorac. Cardiovasc. Surg. *85*:98, 1983.
197. Kolff, J., Bates, R. J., Balderman, S. C., et al.: Acute aortic arch dissection: Reevaluation of the indications for medical and surgical therapy. Am. J. Cardiol. *39*:727, 1977.
198. Séguin, J. R., Picard, E., Frapier, J.-M., and Chaptal, P.-A.: Aortic valve repair with fibrin glue for type A acute aortic dissection. Ann. Thorac. Surg. *58*:304, 1994.
199. Weinschelbaum, E. E., Schamun, C., Caramutti, V., et al.: Surgical treatment of acute type A dissecting aneurysm, with preservation of the native valve and the use of biologic glue: Follow-up to 6 years. J. Thorac. Cardiovasc. Surg. *103*:369, 1992.
200. Bachet, J., Goudot, B., Teodori, G., et al.: Surgery of type A acute aortic dissection with gelatine-resorcine-formol biological glue: A twelve-year experience. J. Cardiovasc. Surg. *31*:263, 1990.
201. Séguin, J. R., Frapier, J.-M., Colson, P., and Chaptal, P.-A.: Fibrin sealant improves surgical results of type A acute aortic dissection. Ann. Thorac. Surg. *52*:745, 1991.
202. Cambria, R. P., Brewster, D. C., Gertler, J., et al.: Vascular complications associated with spontaneous aortic dissection. J. Vasc. Surg. *7*:199, 1988.
203. Walker, P. J., Dake, M. D., Mitchell, R. S., and Miller, D. C.: The use of endovascular techniques for the treatment of complications of aortic dissection. J. Vasc. Surg. *18*:1042, 1993.
204. Dureau, G., Villard, J., George, M., et al.: New surgical technique for the operative management of acute dissections of the ascending aorta. J. Thorac. Cardiovasc. Surg. *76*:385, 1978.
205. Liu, D. W., Lin, P. J., and Chang, C. H.: Treatment of acute type A aortic dissection with intraluminal sutureless prosthesis. Ann. Thorac. Surg. *57*:987, 1994.
206. Lemole, G. M., Strong, M. D., Spagna, P. M., and Karmilowicz, M. P.: Improved results for dissecting aneurysms: Intraluminal sutureless prosthesis. J. Thorac. Cardiovasc. Surg. *83*:249, 1982.
207. Yoshida, H., Yasuda, K., and Tanabe, T.: New approach to aortic dissection: Development of an insertable aortic prosthesis. Ann. Thorac. Surg. *58*:806, 1994.
208. Kato, M., Matsuda, T., Kaneko, M., et al.: Experimental assessment of newly devised transcatheter stent-graft for aortic dissection. Ann. Thorac. Surg. *59*:908, 1995.
209. Neya, K., Omoto, R., Kyo, S., et al.: Outcome of Stanford type B acute aortic dissection. Circulation *86*(Suppl. II):II-1, 1992.
210. Heinemann, M., Laas, J., Karck, M., and Borst, H. G.: Thoracic aortic aneurysms after type A aortic dissection: Necessity for follow-up. Ann. Thorac. Surg. *49*:580, 1990.
211. Khandheria, B. K.: Aortic dissection: The last frontier. Circulation *87*(Edit.):1765, 1993.
212. Laissy, J.-P., Blanc, F., Soyer, P., et al.: Thoracic aortic dissection: Diagnosis with transesophageal echocardiography versus MR imaging. Radiology *194*:331, 1995.
213. Yamada, T., Tada, S., and Harada, J.: Aortic dissection without intimal rupture: Diagnosis with MR imaging and CT. Radiology *168*:347, 1988.
213a. Nienaber, C. A., von Kodolitsch, Y., Petersen, B., et al.: Intramural hemorrhage of the thoracic aorta: Diagnostic and therapeutic implications. Circulation *92*:1465, 1995.
214. Lui, R. C., Menkis, A. H., and McKenzie, F. N.: Aortic dissection without intimal rupture: Diagnosis and management. Ann. Thorac. Surg. *53*:886, 1992.
215. Gore, I.: Pathogenesis of dissecting aneurysm of the aorta. Arch. Pathol. *53*:142, 1952.
216. Mohr-Kahaly, S., Erbel, R., Kearney, P., et al.: Aortic intramural hematoma visualized by transesophageal echocardiography: Findings and prognostic implications. J. Am. Coll. Cardiol. *23*:658, 1994.

217. Robbins, R. C., McManus, R. P., Mitchell, R. S., et al.: Management of patients with intramural hematoma of the thoracic aorta. Circulation *88*:1, 1993.
218. Nienaber, C. A., von Kodolitsch, Y., Petersen, B., et al.: Intramural hemorrhage of the thoracic aorta. Circulation *92*:1465, 1995.
219. Zotz, R. J., Erbel, R., and Meyer, J.: Noncommunicating intramural hematoma: An indication of developing aortic dissection? J. Am. Soc. Echocardiogr. *4*:636, 1991.
220. Stanson, A. W., Kazmier, F. J., Hollier, L. H., et al.: Penetrating atherosclerotic ulcers of the thoracic aorta: Natural history and clinicopathological correlations. Ann. Vasc. Surg. *1*:15, 1986.
221. Kazerooni, E. A., Bree, R. L., and Williams, D. M.: Penetrating atherosclerotic ulcers of the descending thoracic aorta: Evaluation with CT and distinction from aortic dissection. Radiology *183*:759, 1992.
222. Movsowitz, H. D., Lampert, C., Jacobs, L. E., and Kotler, M. N.: Penetrating atherosclerotic aortic ulcers. Am. Heart J. *128*:1210, 1994.
223. Benitez, R. M., Gurbel, P. A., Chong, H., and Rajasingh, C.: Penetrating atherosclerotic ulcer of the aortic arch resulting in extensive and fatal dissection. Am. Heart J. *129*:821, 1995.
224. Braverman, A. C.: Penetrating atherosclerotic ulcers of the aorta. Curr. Opin. Cardiol. *9*:591, 1994.
225. Harris, J. A., Bis, K. G., Glover, J. L., et al.: Penetrating atherosclerotic ulcers of the aorta. J. Vasc. Surg. *19*:90, 1994.
226. Hussain, S., Glover, J. L., Bree, R., and Bendick, P. J.: Penetrating atherosclerotic ulcers of the thoracic aorta. J. Vasc. Surg. *9*:710, 1989.
227. Yucel, E. K., Steinberg, F. L., Egglin, T. K., et al.: Penetrating atherosclerotic ulcers: Diagnosis with MR imaging. Radiology *177*:779, 1990.
228. Movsowitz, H. D., David, M., Movsowitz, C., et al.: Penetrating atherosclerotic ulcers: The role of transesophageal echocardiography in the diagnosis and clinical management. Am. Heart J. *126*:745, 1993.

AORTIC ATHEROMATOUS EMBOLI

229. Karalis, D. G., Chandrasekaran, K., Victor, M. F., et al.: Recognition and embolic potential of intraaortic atherosclerotic debris. J. Am. Coll. Cardiol. *17*:73, 1991.
229a. Halperin, J. L.: Atherosclerotic diseases of the aorta. *In* Fuster, V., Ross, R., and Topol, E. J. (eds.): Atherosclerosis and Coronary Artery Disease. Philadelphia, Lippincott-Raven, 1996, pp. 1625–1642.
230. Toyoda, K., Yasaka, M., Nagata, S., and Yamaguchi, T.: Aortogenic embolic stroke: A transesophageal echocardiography approach. Stroke *23*:1056, 1992.
231. Culliford, A. T., Colvin, S. B., Rohrer, K., et al.: The atherosclerotic ascending aorta and transverse arch: A new technique to prevent cerebral injury during bypass: Experience with 13 patients. Ann. Thorac. Surg. *41*:27, 1986.
232. Tunick, P. A., Perez, J. L., and Kronzon, I.: Protruding atheromas in the thoracic aorta and systemic embolization. Ann. Intern. Med. *115*:423, 1991.
233. Davila-Roman, V. G., Barzilai, B., Wareing, T. H., et al.: Intraoperative ultrasonographic evaluation of the ascending aorta in 100 consecutive patients undergoing cardiac surgery. Circulation *84*(Suppl. III):III-47, 1991.
234. Mitusch, R., Stierle, U., Tepe, C., et al.: Systemic embolism in aortic arch atheromatosis. Eur. Heart J. *15*:1373, 1994.
235. Amarenco, P., Duyckaerts, C., Tzourio, C., et al.: The prevalence of ulcerated plaques in the aortic arch in patients with stroke. N. Engl. J. Med. *326*:221, 1992.
235a. Montgomery, D. H., Ververis, J., McGorisk, G., et al.: Natural history of severe atheromatous disease of the thoracic aorta. A transesophageal echocardiographic study. J. Am. Coll. Cardiol. *27*:95, 1996.
236. Amarenco, P., Cohen, A., Tzourio, C., et al.: Atherosclerotic disease of the aortic arch and the risk of ischemic stroke. N. Engl. J. Med. *331*:1474, 1994.
237. Demopoulos, L. A., Tunick, P. A., Bernstein, N. E., et al.: Protruding atheromas of the aortic arch in symptomatic patients with carotid artery disease. Am. Heart J. *129*:40, 1995.
238. Fazio, G. P., Redberg, R. F., Winslow, T., and Schiller, N. B.: Transesophageal echocardiographically detected atherosclerotic aortic plaque is a marker for coronary artery disease. J. Am. Coll. Cardiol. *21*:144, 1993.
239. Tunick, P. A., Culliford, A. T., Lamparello, P. J., and Kronzon, I.: Atheromatosis of the aortic arch as an occult source of multiple systemic emboli. Ann. Intern. Med. *114*:391, 1991.
240. Tunick, P. A., Rosensweig, B. P., Katz, E. S., et al.: High risk for vascular events in patients with protruding aortic atheromas: A prospective study. J. Am. Coll. Cardiol. *23*:1085, 1994.
241. Jones, E. F., Kalman, J. M., Calafiore, P., et al.: Proximal aortic atheroma: An independent risk factor for cerebral ischemia. Stroke *26*:218, 1995.
242. Kistler, J. P.: The risk of embolic stroke: Another piece of the puzzle. N. Engl. J. Med. *331*(Edit.):1517, 1994.
243. Freedberg, R. S., Tunick, P. A., Culliford, A. T., et al.: Disappearance of a large intraaortic mass in a patient with prior systemic embolization. Am. Heart J. *125*:1445, 1993.
244. Bansal, R. C., Pauls, G. L., and Shankel, S. W.: Blue digit syndrome: Transesophageal echocardiographic identification of thoracic aortic plaque–related thrombi and successful outcome with warfarin. J. Am. Soc. Echocardiogr. *6*:319, 1993.
245. Culliford, A. T., Tunick, P. A., Katz, E. S., et al.: Initial experience with removal of protruding atheroma from the aortic arch: Diagnosis by transesophageal echo, operative technique, and follow-up. J. Am. Coll. Cardiol. *21*(Suppl. 2)(Abs.):342A, 1993.
246. Katz, E. S., Tunick, P. A., Rusinek, H., et al.: Protruding atheromas predict stroke in elderly patients undergoing cardiopulmonary bypass: Experience with intraoperative transesophageal echocardiography. J. Am. Coll. Cardiol. *20*:70, 1992.
247. Blauth, C. I., Cosgrove, D. M., Webb, B. W., et al.: Thromboembolism from the ascending aorta: An emerging problem in cardiac surgery. J. Thorac. Cardiovasc. Surg. *103*:1104, 1992.
248. Wareing, T. H., Davila-Roman, V. G., Barzilai, B., et al.: Management of the severely atherosclerotic aorta during cardiac operation: A strategy for detection and treatment. J. Thorac. Cardiovasc. Surg. *103*:453, 1992.
249. Barzilai, B., Marshall, W. G., Safitz, J. E., and Kouchoukos, N. T.: Avoidance of embolic complications by ultrasonic characterization of the ascending aorta. Circulation *80*(Suppl. I):I-275, 1989.
250. Duda, A. M., Letwin, L. B., Sutter, F. P., and Goldman, S. M.: Does routine use of aortic ultrasonography decrease the stroke rate in coronary artery bypass surgery? J. Vasc. Surg. *21*:98, 1995.
251. Om, A., Ellahham, S., and DiSciascio, G.: Cholesterol embolism: An underdiagnosed clinical entity. Am. Heart J. *124*:1321, 1992.
252. Colt, H. G., Begg, R. J., Saporito, J. J., et al.: Cholesterol emboli after cardiac catheterization: Eight cases and a review of the literature. Medicine *67*:389, 1988.
253. Davis, K., Kennedy, J. W., Kemp, H. G., Jr., et al.: Complications of coronary arteriography from the collaborative study of coronary artery surgery (CASS). Circulation *59*:1105, 1979.
254. Hyman, B. T., Landas, S. K., Ashman, R. F., et al.: Warfarin-related purple toes syndrome and cholesterol microembolization. Am. J. Med. *82*:1233, 1987.
255. Falanga, V., Fine, M. J., and Kapoor, W. N.: The cutaneous manifestations of cholesterol crystal embolization. Arch. Dermatol. *122*:1194, 1986.
256. Karmody, A. M., Powers, S. R., Monaco, V. J., and Leather, R. P.: "Blue toe" syndrome: An indication for limb salvage surgery. Arch. Surg. *111*:1263, 1976.
257. Arora, R. R., Magun, A. M., Grossman, M., and Katz, J.: Cholesterol embolization syndrome after intravenous tissue plasminogen activator for acute myocardial infarction. Am. Heart J. *126*:225, 1993.
258. Bruns, F. J., Segel, D. P., and Apler, S.: Control of cholesterol embolization by discontinuation of anticoagulant therapy. Am. J. Med. Sci. *275*:105, 1978.
259. Blankenship, J. C., Butler, M., and Garbes, A.: Prospective assessment of cholesterol embolization in patients with acute myocardial infarction treated with thrombolytic vs. conservative therapy. Chest *107*:662, 1995.
260. Fine, M. J., Kapoor, W., and Falanga, V.: Cholesterol crystal embolization: A review of 221 cases in the English literature. Angiology *38*:769, 1987.

ACUTE AORTIC OCCLUSION

261. Babu, S. C., Shah, P. M., and Nitahara, J.: Acute aortic occlusion: Factors that influence outcome. J. Vasc. Surg. *21*:567, 1995.
262. Dossa, C. D., Shepard, A. D., Reddy, D. J., et al.: Acute aortic occlusion: A 40-year experience. Arch. Surg. *129*:603, 1994.
263. Tapper, S. S., Jenkins, J. M., Edwards, W. H., et al.: Juxtarenal aortic occlusion. Ann. Surg. *215*:443, 1992.
264. Light, J. T., Hendrickson, M., Sholes, W. M., et al.: Acute aortic occlusion secondary to *Aspergillus* endocarditis in an intravenous drug abuser. Ann. Vasc. Surg. *5*:271, 1991.
265. Busuttil, R. W., Keehn, G., Milliken, J., et al.: Aortic saddle embolus: A twenty-two year experience. Ann. Surg. *197*:698, 1983.

AORTOARTERITIS SYNDROMES

266. Shelhamer, J. H., Volkman, D. J., Parrillo, J. E., et al.: Takayasu's arteritis and its therapy. Ann. Intern. Med. *103*:121, 1985.
267. Volkman, D. J., Mann, D. L., and Fauci, A. S.: Association between Takayasu's arteritis and a B-cell alloantigen in North Americans. N. Engl. J. Med. *306*:464, 1982.
268. Numano, F., Isohisa, I., Egami, M., et al.: HLA-DR MT and MB antigens in Takayasu disease. Tissue Antigens *21*:208, 1983.
269. Ueno, A., Awane, G., and Wakahayachi, A.: Successfully operated obliterative brachiocephalic arteritis (Takayasu) associated with the elongated coarctation. Jpn. Heart J. *8*:538, 1967.
270. Lupi-Herrera, E., Sanchez-Torres, G., Marcushamer, J., et al.: Takayasu's arteritis: Clinical study of 107 cases. Am. Heart J. *93*:94, 1977.
271. Procter, C. D., and Hollier, L. H.: Takayasu's arteritis and temporal arteritis. Ann. Vasc. Surg. *6*:195, 1992.
272. Hall, S., Barr, W., Lie, J. T., et al.: Takayasu arteritis: A study of 32 North American patients. Medicine *64*:89, 1985.
273. Wu, Y. J., Martin, B., Ong, K., et al.: Takayasu's arteritis as a cause of fever of unknown origin. Am. J. Med. *87*:476, 1989.
274. Takeshita, A., Tanaka, S., Orita, Y., et al.: Baroreflex sensitivity in patients with Takayasu's aortitis. Circulation *55*:803, 1977.
275. Akikusa, B., Kondo, Y., and Muraki, N.: Aortic insufficiency caused by Takayasu's arteritis without usual clinical features. Arch. Pathol. Lab. Med. *105*:650, 1981.
276. Hashimoto, Y., Numano, F., Maruyama, Y., et al.: Thallium-201 stress scintigraphy in Takayasu arteritis. Am. J. Cardiol. *67*:879, 1991.

277. Ishikawa, K., and Maetani, S.: Long term outcome for 120 Japanese patients with Takayasu's disease. Circulation *90:*1855, 1994.
278. Lande, A., and Rossi, P.: The value of total aortography in the diagnosis of Takayasu's arteritis. Radiology *114:*287, 1975.
279. Ishikawa, K.: Diagnostic approach and proposed criteria for the clinical diagnosis of Takayasu's arteriopathy. J. Am. Coll. Cardiol. *12:*964, 1988.
280. Hoffman, G. S., Leavitt, R. Y., Kerr, G. S., et al.: Treatment of glucocorticoid resistant or relapsing Takayasu arteritis with methotrexate. Arthritis Rheum. *4:*578, 1994.
281. Tyagi, S., Kaul, U. A., Nair, M., et al.: Balloon angioplasty of the aorta in Takayasu's arteritis: Initial and long term results. Am. Heart J. *124:*876, 1992.
282. Tyagi, S., Singh, B., Kaul, U. A., et al.: Balloon angioplasty for renovascular hypertension in Takayasu's arteritis. Am. Heart J. *125:*1386, 1993.
283. Klein, R. G., Hunder, G. G., Stanson, A. W., and Sheps, S. G.: Larger artery involvement in giant cell (temporal) arteritis. Ann. Intern. Med. *83:*806, 1975.
284. Hunder, G. G.: Giant cell (temporal) arteritis. Rheum. Dis. Clin. North Am. *16:*399, 1990.
285. Ghose, M. K., Shensa, S., and Lerner, P. I.: Arteritis of the aged (giant cell arteritis) and fever of unexplained origin. Am. J. Med. *60:*429, 1976.
286. Hunder, G. G., Lie, J. T., Goronzy, J. J., and Weyand, C. M.: Pathogenesis of giant cell arteritis. Arthritis Rheum. *36:*757, 1993.
287. Evans, J. M., O'Fallon, W. M., and Hunder, G. G.: Increased incidence of aortic aneurysm and dissection in giant cell (temporal) arteritis: A population based study. Ann. Intern. Med. *122:*502, 1995.
288. Perruquet, J. L., Davis, D. E., and Harrington, T. M.: Aortic arch arteritis in the elderly: An important manifestation of giant cell arteritis. Arch. Intern. Med. *146:*289, 1986.
289. Austen, W. G., and Blennerhassett, M. B.: Giant cell aortitis causing an aneurysm of the ascending aorta and aortic regurgitation. N. Engl. J. Med. *272:*80, 1965.
290. Malmvall, B. E., and Bengtsson, B. A.: Serum levels of immunoglobulin and complement in giant cell arteritis. JAMA *236:*1876, 1976.
291. Mitnick, H. J., Tunick, P. A., Rotterdam, H., and Esposito, R.: Antemortem diagnosis of giant cell arteritis. J. Rheumatol. *17:*708, 1990.
292. Evans, J. M., Bowles, C. A., Bjornsson, J., et al.: Thoracic aortic aneurysm and rupture in giant cell arteritis. Arthritis Rheum. *37:*1539, 1994.
293. Krall, P. L., Mazanec, D. J., and Wilke, W. S.: Methotrexate for corticosteroid-resistant polymyalgia rheumatica and giant cell arteritis. Cleve. Clin. J. Med. *56:*253, 1989.
294. Townend, J. N., Emery, P., Davies, M. K., and Littler, W. A.: Acute aortitis and aortic incompetence due to systemic rheumatological disorders. Int. J. Cardiol. *33:*253, 1991.
295. Muna, W. F., Roller, D. H., Craft, J., et al.: Psoriatic arthritis and aortic regurgitation. JAMA *244:*363, 1980.
296. Iino, T., Eguchi, K., Sakai, M., et al.: Polyarteritis nodosa with aortic dissection: Necrotizing vasculitis of the vasa vasorum. J. Rheumatol. *19:*1632, 1992.
297. Hoogland, Y. T., Alexander, E. P., Patterson, R. H., and Nashel, D. J.: Coronary artery stenosis in Reiter's syndrome: A complication of aortitis. J. Rheumatol. *21:*757, 1994.
298. González, T., Hernández-Beriain, J. A., Rodríguez-Lozano, B., and Martín-Herrera, A.: Severe aortic regurgitation in Behçet's disease. J. Rheumatol. *20:*10, 1993.
299. Koç, Y., Güllü, I., Akpek, G., et al.: Vascular involvement in Behçet's disease. J. Rheumatol. *19:*402, 1992.
300. Paulus, H. E., Pearson, C. M., and Pitts, W.: Aortic insufficiency in five patients with Reiter's syndrome: A detailed clinical and pathologic study. Am. J. Med. *53:*464, 1972.
301. Gomes, M. N., Choyke, P. L., and Wallace, R. B.: Infected aortic aneurysms: A changing entity. Ann. Surg. *215:*435, 1992.
302. Katz, S. G., Andros, G., and Kohl, R. D.: Salmonella infections of the abdominal aorta. Surg. Gynecol. Obstet. *175:*102, 1992.
303. Pasic, M., Carrel, T., von Segesser, L., and Turina, M.: In situ repair of mycotic aneurysm of the ascending aorta. J. Thorac. Cardiovasc. Surg. *105:*321, 1993.
304. Oz, M. C., Brener, B. J., Buda, J. A., et al.: A ten-year experience with bacterial aortitis. J. Vasc. Surg. *10:*439, 1989.
305. Cohen, O. S., O'Brien, T. F., Schoenbaum, S. C., and Mederos, A. A.: The risk of endothelial infection in adults with Salmonella bacteremia. Ann. Intern. Med. *89:*931, 1978.
306. Byard, R. W., Jimenez, C. L., Carpenter, B. F., and Hsu, E.: Aspergillus-related aortic thrombosis. Can. Med. Assoc. J. *136:*155, 1987.
307. Jarrett, F., Darling, R. C., Mundth, E. D., and Austen, W. G.: The management of infected arterial aneurysms. J. Cardiovasc. Surg. *17:*361, 1977.
308. Vogelzang, R. L., and Sohaey, R.: Infected aortic aneurysms: CT appearance. J. Comput. Assist. Tomogr. *12:*109, 1988.
309. Gomes, M. N., and Choyke, P. L.: Infected aortic aneurysms: CT diagnosis. J. Cardiovasc. Surg. *32:*4, 1991.
310. Robinson, J. A., and Johansen, K.: Aortic sepsis: Is there a role for in situ graft reconstruction? J. Vasc. Surg. *13:*677, 1991.
311. Fyfe, B. S., Quintana, C. S., Kaneka, M., and Griepp, R. B.: Aortic sarcoma four years after Dacron graft insertion. Ann. Thorac. Surg. *58:*1752, 1994.
312. Wright, E. P., Glick, A. D., Virmani, R., and Page, D. L.: Aortic intimal sarcoma with embolic metastases. Am. J. Surg. Pathol. *9:*950, 1985.
313. Navarra, G., Occhionorelli, S., Mascoli, F., et al.: Primary leiomyosarcoma of the aorta: Report of a case and review of the literature. J. Cardiovasc. Surg. *35:*33, 1994.
314. Ronaghi, A. H., Roberts, A. C., and Rosenkrantz, H.: Intraaortic biopsy of a primary aortic tumor. J. Vasc. Intervent. Radiol. *5:*777, 1994.
315. Higgins, R., Posner, M. C., Moosa, H. H., et al.: Mesenteric infarction secondary to tumor emboli from primary aortic sarcoma. Cancer *68:*1622, 1991.
316. Cziner, D. G., Freedberg, R. S., Tunick, P. A., et al.: Transesophageal echocardiographic diagnosis of a primary intraaortic tumor. Am. Heart J. *125:*1189, 1993.

In the Nurses Health Study,[25] *current oral contraceptive* users had a relative risk of 3.1, but past users had no increased risk of PE, after adjustment for coronary heart disease risk factors. Third-generation oral contraceptives (which use either desogestrel or gestodene as the progesterone component) are associated with about a doubled risk of venous thrombosis compared with other oral contraceptives.[25a] Postmenopausal estrogen use was not associated with increased risk of venous thrombosis. A case-control study also found no association between estrogen replacement therapy and the risk of venous thrombosis.[26]

PE is the most common medical cause of *maternal mortality* associated with live births.[27] Pregnancy and the puerperium alter the physiological balance between coagulation and fibrinolysis, thus predisposing women to a hypercoagulable state, especially during the first postpartum month.

Cancer is an acquired risk factor for venous thrombosis. The tumor may synthesize and secrete procoagulants. Furthermore, cancer patients often have concomitant predisposing factors for venous thrombosis such as surgery or immobility. Among 145 patients with venographically proven idiopathic venous thrombosis, cancer was diagnosed in 8 per cent during 2 years of follow-up. However, among those with idiopathic venous thrombosis who suffered a recurrence, the cancer incidence during this period was 17 per cent.[28] In a large Swedish case-control study, patients with venographically diagnosed DVT were 2.5 times more likely to develop cancer within the ensuing 6 months compared with controls who had normal venograms.[29] A similar relationship between PE and subsequent cancer risk has also been observed in a cohort study.[30]

Patients receiving *chemotherapy* for metastatic breast cancer are at risk of developing venous thromboembolic disease. In a randomized controlled trial of very low dose warfarin versus placebo, 4 per cent of the placebo group developed venous thrombosis during the average 6-month follow-up period.[31] Hemocysteinemia, which can be hereditary or acquired, appears to be a common risk factor for recurrent venous thrombosis.[31a]

Leg DVT is a common complication of *acute ischemic stroke*, particularly in the paralyzed limb. Even when patients receive 5000 units twice daily of unfractionated heparin for prophylaxis, the venous thrombosis rate is as high as 31 per cent.[32] With spinal cord injury there is also a high rate of venous thrombosis,[33] but devastating complications such as PE tend to occur more often.

Thrombotic complications due to indwelling central venous catheters are common and are often associated with catheter sepsis.[34] Thrombosis can be due to a fibrin sleeve or vascular occlusion. Soon after insertion, most indwelling vascular catheters become engulfed in a thrombin or fibrin sheath that can serve as a nidus for subsequent infection.

RELATIONSHIP BETWEEN DEEP VENOUS THROMBOSIS AND PULMONARY EMBOLISM. Most pulmonary emboli result from thrombi that originate in the pelvic or deep veins of the leg; occasionally, thrombi in the axillary or subclavian veins embolize to the pulmonary arteries. In an autopsy study of patients who died of PE, 83 per cent had leg DVT, but only 19 per cent had symptoms of DVT before death.[35] In a treatment trial of proximal leg DVT, Moser et al. found that nearly 40 per cent of patients had asymptomatic PE, based on concomitantly obtained ventilation–perfusion scans.[36] There is also a small but appreciable risk of asymptomatic PE due to isolated calf vein thrombosis[37] or upper extremity thrombosis.[38]

When venous thrombi become dislodged from their site of formation, they flow through the venous system to the pulmonary arterial circulation. If an embolus is extremely large, it may lodge at the bifurcation of the pulmonary artery, forming a saddle embolus (Fig. 46–2, *top*). More commonly, a major pulmonary vessel is occluded (Fig. 46–2, *bottom*).

RIGHT VENTRICULAR DYSFUNCTION. The extent of pulmonary vascular obstruction is probably the most important factor determining whether right ventricular dysfunction ensues. As obstruction increases, pulmonary artery pressures rise. Moreover, the release of vasoconstricting compounds (e.g., serotonin), reflex pulmonary artery vasoconstriction, and hypoxemia may further increase pulmonary vascular resistance and result in pulmonary hypertension.[39]

VENTRICULAR INTERDEPENDENCY. The sudden rise in pulmonary artery pressure reflects an abrupt increase in right ventricular afterload, with consequent elevation of right ventricular wall tension followed by right ventricular dilatation and dysfunction (Fig. 46–3). As the right ventricle dilates, the interventricular septum shifts toward the left ventricle, which may lead to underfilling of this chamber due to pericardial constraint.[40,41] In addition, right ventricular contractile dysfunction may decrease right ventricular cardiac output and further reduce left ventricular preload. As the right ventricle distends, coronary venous pressure increases and left ventricular diastolic distensibility decreases.[42]

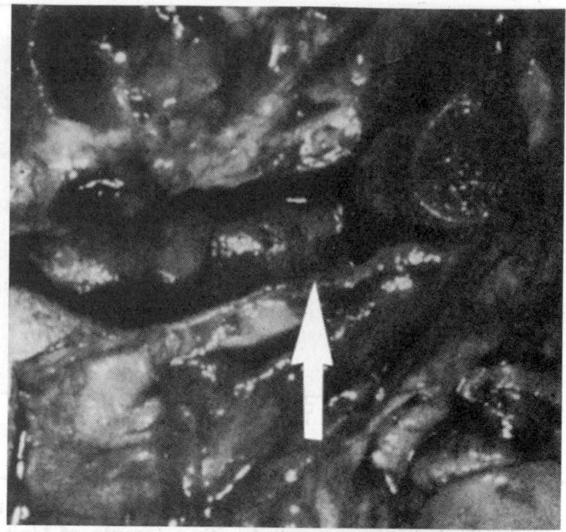

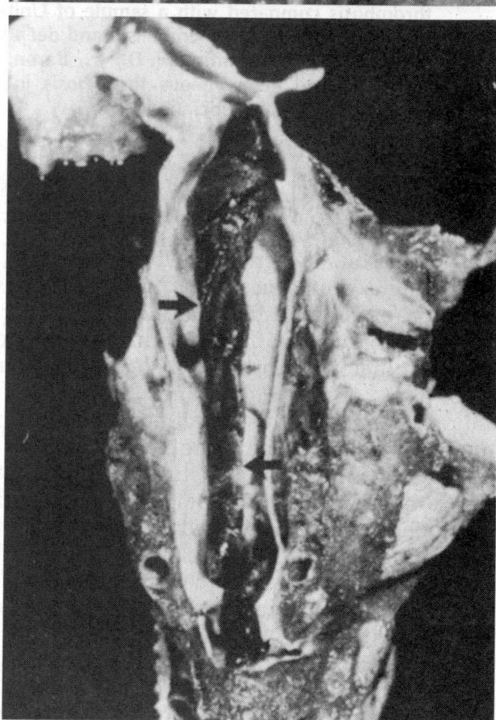

FIGURE 46–2. *Top,* saddle embolus (arrow) at the bifurcation of the pulmonary artery. *Bottom,* Pulmonary embolus in left lower lobe pulmonary artery, with minimal attachment to the wall of the vessel. The embolus was dark red, typical of venous thrombi, and had indentations believed to represent impressions of the venous valves (arrows). (From Godleski, J. J.: Pathology of deep venous thrombosis and pulmonary embolism. *In* Goldhaber, S. Z. [ed.]: Pulmonary Embolism and Deep Venous Thrombosis. Philadelphia, W. B. Saunders Company, 1985, p. 17.)

The reduction in left ventricular preload may also lead to interventricular septal shift toward the left ventricle. With underfilling of the left ventricle, systemic cardiac output and pressure both decrease, potentially compromising coronary perfusion and producing myocardial ischemia. Elevated right ventricular wall tension following massive PE reduces right coronary flow and increases right ventricular myocardial oxygen demand, which may result in ischemia and possibly cardiogenic shock. Perpetuation of this cycle can lead to right ventricular infarction, circulatory collapse, and death.

SUMMARY OF PATHOPHYSIOLOGY. Pulmonary embolism can have the following pathophysiological effects: (1) in-

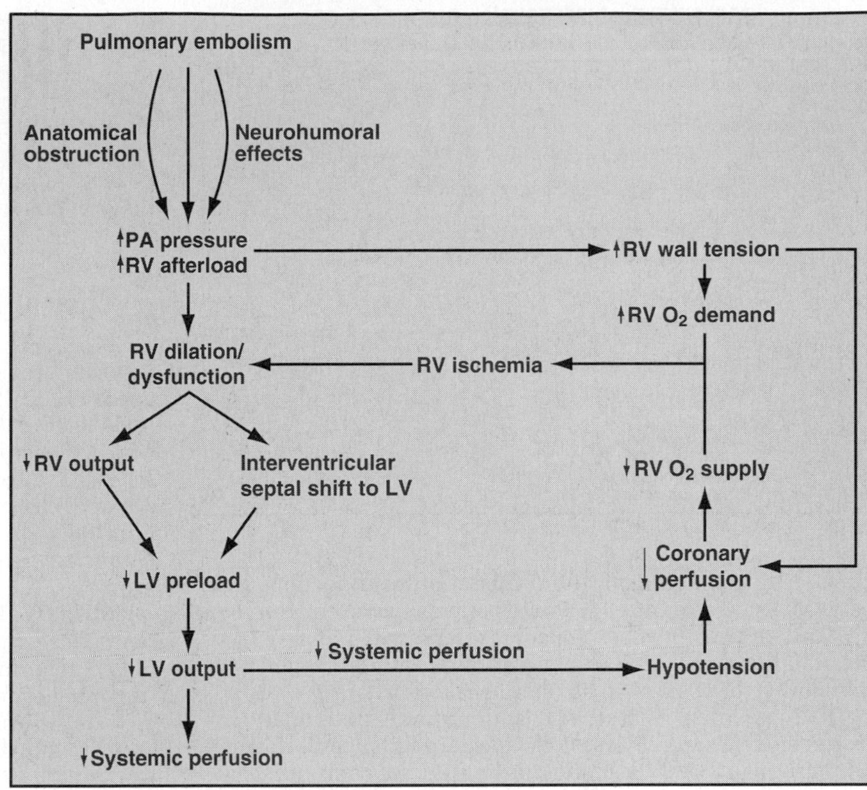

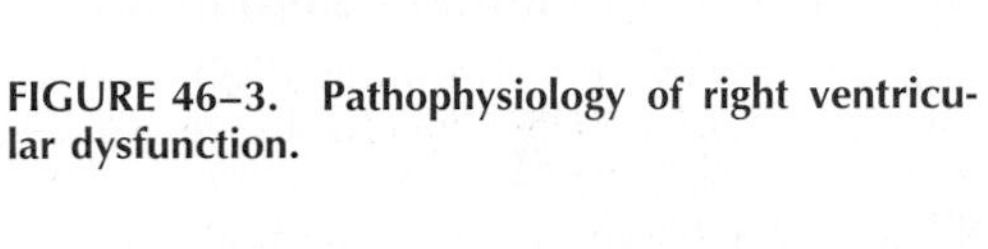
FIGURE 46–3. Pathophysiology of right ventricular dysfunction.

creased pulmonary vascular resistance due to vascular obstruction, neurohumoral agents, or pulmonary artery baroreceptors; (2) impaired gas exchange due to increased alveolar dead space from vascular obstruction and hypoxemia from alveolar hypoventilation, low V/Q units, and right-to-left shunting, as well as impaired carbon monoxide transfer due to loss of gas-exchange surface; (3) alveolar hyperventilation due to reflex stimulation of irritant receptors; (4) increased airway resistance due to bronchoconstriction; and (5) decreased pulmonary compliance due to lung edema, lung hemorrhage, and loss of surfactant.[39]

DIAGNOSIS

Diagnosis of PE is more difficult than treatment or prevention. For patients with PE, the most dangerous period is that preceding the establishment of the correct diagnosis. Fortunately, reliable noninvasive diagnostic approaches have become increasingly available—particularly venous ultrasound, plasma D-dimer ELISA, and echocardiography—and complement the more-established techniques of lung scanning and pulmonary angiography. Furthermore, procedures for pulmonary angiography have been developed that increase patient comfort and safety. The contemporary diagnosis of PE emphasizes a strategy that integrates the clinical findings with a variety of diagnostic methods.[43]

Clinical Presentation

Clinical suspicion of PE is of paramount importance in guiding diagnostic testing. Among patients without prior cardiopulmonary disease, dyspnea appears to be the most frequent symptom and tachypnea the most frequent sign of PE (Table 46–4). In general, dyspnea, syncope, or cyanosis portends a major life-threatening PE. However, pleuritic pain often signifies that the embolism is small and located in the distal pulmonary arterial system, near the pleural lining.

PE should be suspected in hypotensive patients when: (1) there is evidence of, or there are predisposing factors for, venous thrombosis and (2) there is clinical evidence of acute cor pulmonale (acute right ventricular failure) such as distended neck veins, an S_3 gallop, a right ventricular heave, tachycardia, or tachypnea, especially if (3) there is electrocardiographic evidence of acute cor pulmonale manifested by a new S_1-Q_3-T_3 pattern, new incomplete right bundle branch block, or right ventricular ischemia.[44]

DIFFERENTIAL DIAGNOSIS. The differential diagnosis of PE is broad and covers a spectrum from life-threatening dis-

TABLE 46–4 SYMPTOMS AND SIGNS OF PE IN 117 PATIENTS WITH NO PRIOR CARDIOPULMONARY DISEASE

SYMPTOMS	FREQUENCY (%)
Dyspnea	73
Pleuritic pain	66
Cough	37
Leg swelling	28
Leg pain	26
Hemoptysis	13
Palpitations	10
Wheezing	9
Angina-like pain	4
SIGNS	
Tachypnea (≥20/min)	70
Rales (crackles)	51
Tachycardia (>100/min)	30
Fourth heart sound	24
Increased pulmonary component of second sound	23
Clinically apparent deep venous thrombosis	11
Diaphoresis	11
Temperature > 38.5°C	7
Wheezes	5
Homans' sign	4
Right ventricular lift	4
Pleural friction rub	3
Third heart sound	3
Cyanosis	1

Reprinted with permission from Stein, P. D., Terrin, M. L., Hales, C. A., et al.: Clinical, laboratory, roentgenographic, and electrocardiographic findings in patients with acute pulmonary embolism and no pre-existing cardiac or pulmonary disease. Chest *100*:598, 1991.

TABLE 46–5 DIFFERENTIAL DIAGNOSIS OF PULMONARY EMBOLISM

Myocardial infarction
Pneumonia
Congestive heart failure ("left-sided")
Cardiomyopathy (global)
Primary pulmonary hypertension
Asthma
Pericarditis
Intrathoracic cancer
Rib fracture
Pneumothorax
Costochondritis
"Musculoskeletal pain"
Anxiety

ease such as acute myocardial infarction to innocuous anxiety states (Table 46–5). Some patients have concomitant PE and other illnesses. So, for example, if pneumonia or heart failure does not respond to appropriate therapy, the possibility of coexisting PE should be considered.

Distinguishing between PE and primary pulmonary hypertension (Chap. 25) deserves special vigilance (Table 46–6). Although both conditions ordinarily warrant anticoagulation, other advances in management (such as high doses of calcium channel blockers[45] and long-term prostacyclin infusions to treat primary pulmonary hypertension[46]) require differentiation between these two illnesses. Surprisingly, some patients will have a hybrid condition that is similar to primary pulmonary hypertension but that includes thrombi. Among these patients, large central pulmonary artery thrombi can develop.[47] Often it is impossible to determine whether these thrombi formed in situ or whether they embolized to the pulmonary arteries from a separate site.

TABLE 46–6 PRIMARY PULMONARY HYPERTENSION VS. RECURRENT PULMONARY EMBOLISM

SIMILARITIES		
Symptoms	Fatigue, dyspnea on exertion—most common; chest pain, syncope, hemoptysis, cyanosis—also common	
Clinical course	Progressive dyspnea, right-heart failure	
Hemodynamics	Elevated right-heart pressures, normal pulmonary capillary wedge pressure	
Histology	Thrombotic lesions usually present	
Treatment	Includes anticoagulation	
DIFFERENCES		
VARIABLE	**PPH**	**RECURRENT PE**
Age (years)	20–40	>50
Female/male ratio	4:1	1:1
Clinical course	Continued deterioration	Deterioration, with intermittent stabilization
Perfusion lung scan	No segmental perfusion defects	Segmental or larger perfusion defects
Pulmonary artery systolic pressure	> 60 mm Hg	< 60 mm Hg
Pulmonary angiogram	"Pruning"	Intraluminal filling defects
Confounding problems with angiogram	Thrombi may occur on or distal to PPH lesions	"Pruning" can also suggest PE
Diagnostic alternatives	Lung biopsy	Pulmonary angioscopy
Therapy	Anticoagulation; high-dose nifedipine or diltiazem; long-term continuous IV prostacyclin	Anticoagulation; IVC interruption; Thromboendarterectomy

Adapted from Goldhaber, S. Z.: Strategies for diagnosis. *In* Goldhaber, S. Z. (ed.): Pulmonary Embolism and Deep Vein Thrombosis. Philadelphia, W. B. Saunders Company, 1985, p. 89.

Clinical Syndromes of Pulmonary Embolism

Classification of PE into various syndromes (Table 46–7) is useful for prognostication and for deciding on subsequent clinical management.[48]

MASSIVE PULMONARY EMBOLISM. These patients are at risk of developing cardiogenic shock. They have thrombosis often affecting at least half of the pulmonary arterial system. Clot is almost always present bilaterally. Dyspnea is usually the cardinal symptom, and systemic arterial hypotension requiring pressor support is the predominant sign.

MODERATE TO LARGE PULMONARY EMBOLISM. These patients have right ventricular hypokinesis on echocardiography but normal systemic arterial pressure. Usually, perfusion lung scanning indicates that more than 30 per cent of the lung is not perfused. The condition of such patients was previously termed hemodynamically stable. However, this description is misleading because these patients have right ventricular hemodynamic instability that is masked

TABLE 46–7 SIX SYNDROMES OF ACUTE PULMONARY EMBOLISM

SYNDROME	PRESENTATION	RV DYSFUNCTION	THERAPY
Massive	Breathlessness, syncope, and cyanosis with persistent systemic arterial hypotension; typically greater than 50% obstruction of pulmonary vasculature	Present	Heparin plus thrombolytic therapy or mechanical intervention
Moderate to Large	Normal systemic arterial blood pressure; typically greater than 30% perfusion defect on lung scan	Present	Heparin plus thrombolytic therapy or mechanical intervention
Small to Moderate	Normal arterial blood pressure	Absent	Heparin
Pulmonary Infarction	Pleuritic chest pain, hemoptysis, pleural rub, or evidence of lung consolidation; typically small peripheral emboli	Rare	Heparin and NSAIDs
Paradoxical Embolism	Sudden systemic embolic event such as stroke	Rare	Variable*
Non-Thrombotic Embolism	Most commonly air, fat, tumor fragments, or amniotic fluid	Rare	Supportive

Adapted from Goldhaber, S. Z.: Treatment of acute pulmonary embolism. *In* Goldhaber, S. Z. (ed.): Cardiopulmonary diseases and cardiac tumors. Braunwald, E., Series ed. Atlas of Heart Diseases. Philadelphia, Current Medicine, 1995, vol. III, pp 7.1–7.12.

RV = right ventricular

NSAIDs = nonsteroidal antiinflammatory drugs

* Therapy depends on right ventricular function and presence or absence of contraindications to thrombolysis or heparin.

by normal systemic arterial pressure. Right ventricular dilatation and hypokinesis can be detected echocardiographically. It appears that these patients are at risk for recurrent (and possibly fatal) PE, even with adequate anticoagulation.[49] Therefore, these patients are receiving increasing consideration for primary therapy of PE with thrombolytics or embolectomy.

SMALL TO MODERATE PULMONARY EMBOLISM. This syndrome is characterized by both normal systemic arterial pressure and normal right ventricular function. Patients usually have a good prognosis if anticoagulation or an inferior vena caval filter is used to prevent recurrent PE.

PULMONARY INFARCTION. This syndrome is characterized by unremitting chest pain, occasionally accompanied by hemoptysis. The embolus usually lodges in the peripheral pulmonary arterial tree, near the pleura and close to the diaphragm.[50] Tissue infarction usually occurs 3 to 7 days after embolism. The syndrome at that time often includes fever, leukocytosis, and chest radiologic evidence of infarction.

PARADOXICAL EMBOLISM. This syndrome often presents with a sudden, devastating stroke and concomitant PE. Patients often have abnormally elevated pulmonary arterial pressure with a patent foramen ovale evident on echocardiography.[51] Among patients suspected of paradoxical embolism, occult leg vein thrombosis is frequently present and often is confined to the calves.[52]

NONTHROMBOTIC PULMONARY EMBOLISM. Sources of embolism other than thrombus are less commonly detected than thrombotic PE. Fat embolism syndrome is most often observed after blunt trauma complicated by long-bone fractures.[53] Among cancer patients, tumor embolism is more difficult to diagnose clinically than thrombotic PE because presenting symptoms and signs are similar in both conditions.[54] Air embolus can occur during placement or removal of a central venous catheter.[55] It has also been described from presumed inadvertent pressure placed on a partially empty plastic intravenous infusion bag.[56]

Intravenous drug abusers tend to inject inadvertently a variety of substances that contaminate their drug supply. Commonly found materials at autopsy include hair, talc, and cotton. These patients are also susceptible to septic PE, which may be accompanied by endocarditis of the tricuspid or pulmonic valves.

Nonimaging Diagnostic Methods

PLASMA D-DIMER ELISA. This is the most promising blood test for pulmonary embolism screening. An abnormally elevated level of *ELISA-determined plasma D-dimer* has more than 90 per cent sensitivity for identifying patients with PE proven by lung scan[57] or by angiogram (Fig. 46–4).[58] This test relies on the principle that most patients with PE have ongoing endogenous fibrinolysis that is not effective enough to prevent PE but that does break down some of the fibrin clot to D-dimers. These D-dimers can be assayed by monoclonal antibodies in commercially available kits.

Although elevated plasma concentrations of D-dimers are sensitive for the presence of PE, they are not specific. Levels are elevated in patients for at least 1 week postoperatively and are also increased in patients with myocardial infarction, sepsis, or almost any other systemic illness. Therefore the plasma D-dimer ELISA is best used in patients with suspected PE who have no coexisting acute systemic illness.

The usual D-dimer measurement obtained in hospital laboratories utilizes a latex agglutination assay to detect disseminated intravascular coagulation. Unlike the ELISA, the latex agglutination assay is simply not sensitive enough for reliable PE screening. Alternatively, a two-step approach can be used in which a latex D-dimer is obtained as an initial screening test. If it is elevated, the ELISA will also be elevated. However, if the latex D-dimer is normal, an ELISA D-dimer is required to help exclude PE.[59]

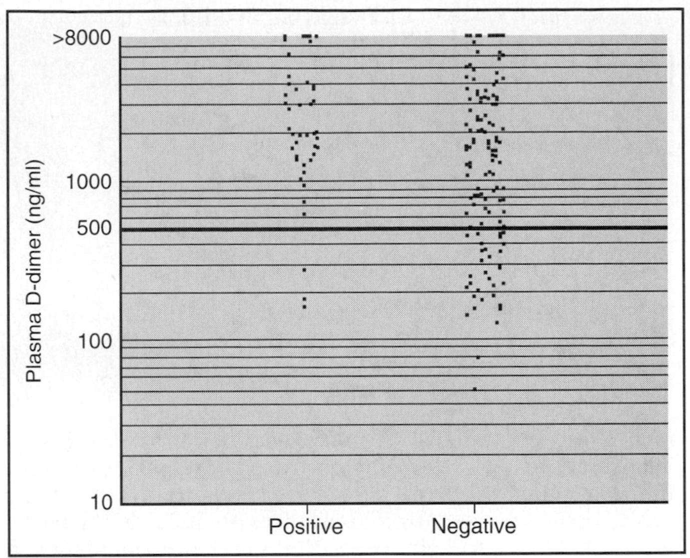

FIGURE 46–4. Distribution of plasma D-dimer levels, sorted according to pulmonary angiographic findings, among 173 patients with suspected acute pulmonary embolism. Plasma D-dimer levels < 500 ng/ml are rarely observed in patients with pulmonary angiographic evidence of PE. (Reprinted with permission from Goldhaber, S. Z., Simons, G. R., Elliott, C. G., et al.: Quantitative plasma D-dimer levels among patients undergoing pulmonary angiography for suspected pulmonary embolism. JAMA *270*:2819, 1993. Copyright 1993 the American Medical Association.)

ARTERIAL BLOOD GASES. Among patients suspected of PE who underwent angiography in the Prospective Investigation of Pulmonary Embolism Diagnosis (PIOPED) (see p. 1589), determination of the partial pressure of oxygen in arterial blood did not discriminate between those with and without PE. There was no difference between the average pO_2 (70 mm Hg) among patients with PE compared with those without PE (72 mm Hg) at angiography. Importantly, among patients with angiographically proven PE who had no prior cardiopulmonary disease, the pO_2 was ≥ 80 mm Hg in 26 per cent.[60] Furthermore, normal values of the alveolar–arterial oxygen gradient did not exclude the diagnosis of acute PE.[61] Therefore, obtaining arterial blood gases should not be part of the diagnostic strategy when investigating suspected PE.

ELECTROCARDIOGRAM (see p. 118). The electrocardiogram is useful not only to help exclude acute myocardial infarction but also for rapidly identifying some patients with large PE, who may have electrocardiographic manifestations of right-heart strain. In a series of 49 consecutive patients with subsequently proven PE, at least three of seven electrocardiographic features suggestive of right ventricular overload (Table 46–8) were identified on 76 per cent of electrocardiograms obtained at hospital admission.[62]

IMPEDANCE PLETHYSMOGRAPHY (IPG). This is a very indi-

TABLE 46–8 ELECTROCARDIOGRAPHIC FINDINGS IN PULMONARY EMBOLISM

Incomplete or complete right bundle branch block
S in Lead I and aVL > 1.5 mm
Transition zone shift to V5
Qs in leads III and aVF, but not in Lead II
QRS axis > 90° or indeterminate axis
Low limb lead voltage
T-wave inversion in leads III and aVF or in leads V1–V4

Modified from Sreeram, N., Cheriex, E. C., Smeets, J. L. R. M., et al.: Value of the 12-lead electrocardiogram at hospital admission in the diagnosis of pulmonary embolism. Am. J. Cardiol. *73*:298, 1994.

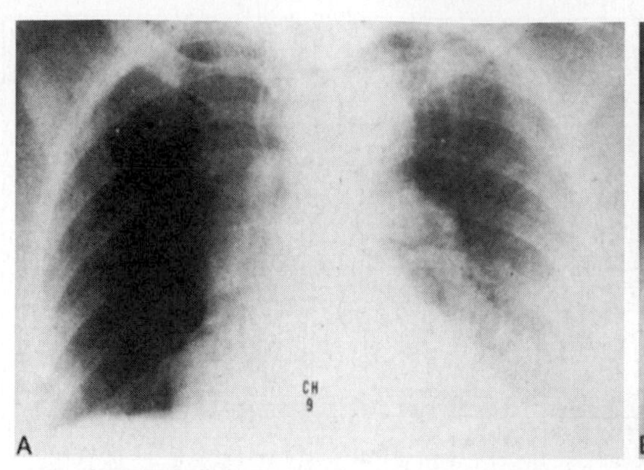

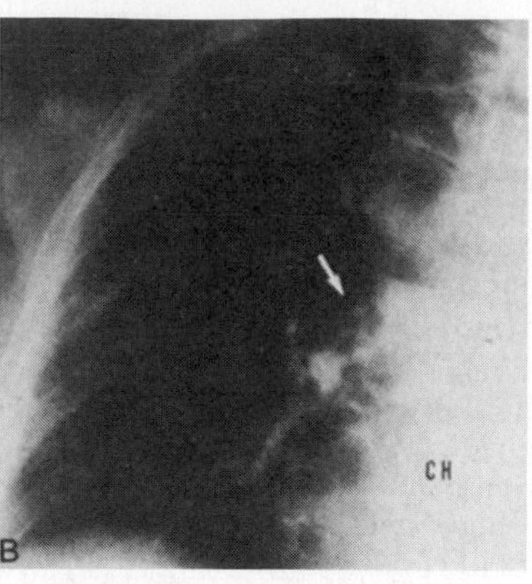

FIGURE 46–5. *A*, Chest film of patient with clinical signs of pulmonary embolism showing marked oligemia (Westermark's sign) in the entire right lobe. *B*, Arteriogram from same patient showing massive saddle embolus in the right main pulmonary artery (arrow). (Courtesy of Jack L. Westcott, M.D., The New York Hospital and Cornell University Medical College.)

rect approach to DVT diagnosis; it measures changes in electric resistance caused by obstruction to venous outflow. IPG was often used to detect DVT but now has only a limited role in special circumstances to help detect recurrence of DVT or to help assess the severity of venous insufficiency. In a study of consecutive patients with suspected DVT who underwent both IPG and contrast venography, IPG failed to detect 35 per cent of patients with proximal leg DVT.[63]

Imaging Methods

Chest Roentgenography

The chest radiograph is usually the first imaging study obtained in patients with suspected PE. Although more than half of patients with PE have an abnormal chest film examination, a near-normal radiograph in the setting of severe respiratory compromise is highly suggestive of massive PE. Classic chest film abnormalities are uncommon but include focal oligemia (Westermark's sign) (Fig. 46–5), indicating massive central embolic occlusion.[64] A peripheral wedge-shaped density above the diaphragm (Hampton's hump) (Fig. 46–6) usually indicates pulmonary infarction.[65] In PIOPED, PE patients with either a prominent central pulmonary artery or cardiomegaly had higher pulmonary arterial mean pressures than did patients with atelectasis, a pulmonary parenchymal abnormality, or pleural effusion.[66]

One should always search for subtle abnormalities such as distention of the descending right pulmonary artery. Often the vessel tapers rapidly after the enlarged portion. The chest radiograph can also help to identify patients with diseases that can mimic PE, such as lobar pneumonia or pneumothorax. Patients with these latter illnesses can also have concomitant PE.[67]

Venous Ultrasonography

The primary diagnostic criterion to establish the presence of DVT by ultrasonography is the loss of vein compressibility (Fig. 46–7). Normally the vein will collapse completely when gentle pressure is applied to the skin overlying it. Generally the applied pressure is kept below what is necessary to collapse the artery. The artery is not as affected because intraarterial pressure is much greater than venous pressure, and the structure of the arterial wall is more resistant to the pressure deformation than the venous wall. Upper extremity DVT may be more difficult to diagnose because the clavicle can hinder attempts to compress the subclavian vein. With acute DVT of either the upper extremity or leg, there is associated passive dilation of the vein.[68]

As many as half of PE patients have no imaging evidence of DVT. Therefore, if clinical suspicion of PE is high, patients without evidence of DVT should still be investigated for PE. For detection of DVT, ultrasound is more accurate than impedance plethysmography.[69] Suspected DVT may be most efficiently evaluated by developing a "critical pathway."[69a]

Ultrasonography is usually reliable in diagnosing proximal leg DVT in *symptomatic outpatients*.[70] The presence of newly detected DVT may sometimes be a useful surrogate for PE. At selected centers with special expertise, ultrasonography may also be dependable for evaluating suspected symptomatic infrapopliteal DVT.[71] Serial ultrasound measurement of thrombus mass after an episode of acute DVT may allow the subsequent correct identification of recurrent DVT.[72] Unfortunately, ultrasonography is unreliable because of its low sensitivity for screening of *asymptomatic patients* with possible DVT after orthopedic surgery[73] or after craniotomy.[74]

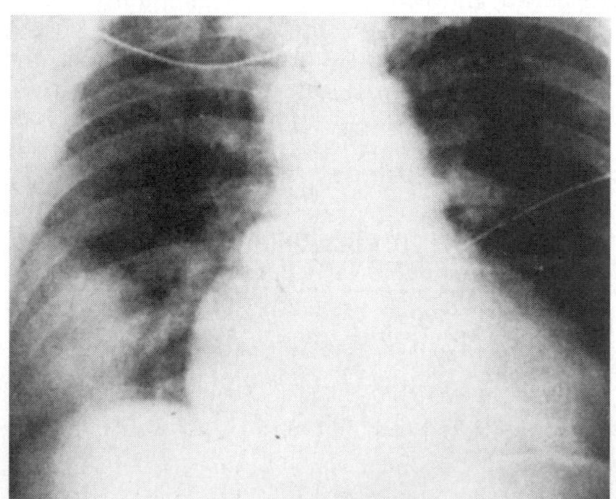

FIGURE 46–6. Posteroanterior chest film of patient with pulmonary embolism showing "Hampton's hump" in right lower lung field, a homogeneous, wedge-shaped density in the peripheral field, convex to the hilum. (Courtesy of Jack L. Westcott, M.D., The New York Hospital and Cornell University Medical College.)

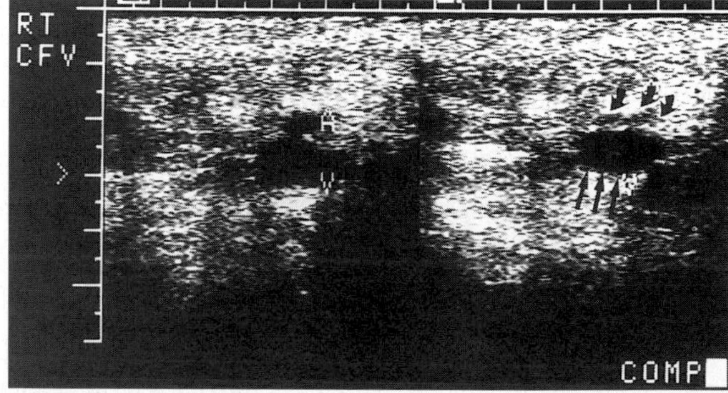

FIGURE 46–7. Right common femoral vein (RT CFV) thrombosis (transverse view) diagnosed by compression ultrasonography. The left half of the image is the baseline ultrasound examination demonstrating the artery (A) superior to the vein (V). During the examination, the artery can be seen to pulsate and appears to "wink" at the examiner. The vein is typically larger than the artery but normally is not severalfold larger. With compression (COMP) in the right half of the image, the artery is deformed (curved upper arrows), but the vein fails to compress (straight lower arrows).

TABLE 46–9 PIOPED: COMPARISON OF SCAN CATEGORY TO ANGIOGRAM FINDINGS

	PULMONARY EMBOLISM			NO	TOTAL
	Present	Absent	Uncertain	ANGIOGRAM	N
Scan category					
High	102	14	1	7	124
Intermediate	105	217	9	33	364
Low	39	199	12	62	312
Near-normal/ normal	5	50	2	74	131
Total	251	480	24	176	931

From the PIOPED Investigators: Value of the ventilation/perfusion scan in acute pulmonary embolism. JAMA *263*:2756, 1990.
PIOPED = Prospective Investigation of Pulmonary Embolism Diagnosis

CONTRAST PHLEBOGRAPHY. Although contrast phlebography has traditionally been considered the gold standard for DVT diagnosis,[75] venograms are now being obtained with less frequency because of the utility of ultrasonography. Venography is costly, invasive, and occasionally results in contrast allergy or contrast-induced phlebitis. Furthermore, there is considerable disagreement in the interpretation of contrast venograms among experienced readers.[76] Patients with massive leg DVT often have nondiagnostic venograms because the contrast agent simply cannot reach the totally obstructed deep leg veins. Consequently we reserve contrast phlebography for situations in which the ultrasound examination is equivocal or, alternatively, when the ultrasound examination is normal despite a high clinical suspicion for DVT.

LUNG SCANNING. Despite its limitations, lung scanning remains the principal test for diagnosing PE. Perfusion lung scintigraphy is sensitive but not specific for detecting pulmonary perfusion abnormalities. Small particulate aggregates of albumin or microspheres labeled with a gamma-emitting radionuclide are injected intravenously. The particles are trapped in the pulmonary capillary bed, reflecting pulmonary blood flow at the time of injection. Planar views of the chest are then obtained. Ventilation scans improve the specificity of the perfusion scan by indicating abnormal nonventilated lung, which could provide explanations for absence of perfusion other than acute PE.[67] If ventilation scanning cannot be performed, useful information can often be obtained from the perfusion scans alone if the scans either have multiple segmental perfusion defects or are normal or near normal.[77]

The diagnosis of PE is very unlikely in patients with normal and near-normal scans. High-probability scans usually indicate acute PE, but fewer than half of PE patients have a high-probability scan. Scans that fall between these extremes of the spectrum should be called intermediate probability. Many patients with low-probability scans but high clinical suspicion for PE do, in fact, have PE at angiography.[78] Therefore the term *low-probability scan* is a potentially lethal misnomer.[79]

Under the auspices of the National Heart, Lung, and Blood Institute, a multicenter study was undertaken to determine the diagnostic utility of the ventilation-perfusion lung scan in acute PE.[80] The PIOPED recruited 931 patients, of whom 81 per cent completed mandatory angiography within a day of having an abnormal lung scan. Among the 755 patients who completed angiography, 33 per cent had PE. The most important finding in PIOPED is that of the 251 patients with positive angiograms, only 102 (41 per cent) had high-probability lung scans. Therefore, because of the lung scan's low sensitivity, more than half (59 per cent) of patients with PE would not be recognized if high-probability lung scans were relied upon exclusively to establish the diagnosis of PE.

In PIOPED, the positive predictive value of lung scanning for PE at angiography was as follows: 87 per cent for high, 32 per cent for intermediate, 16 per cent for low, and 9 per cent for near-normal scans (Table 46–9). When the "clinical probability" was factored into the interpretation of the lung scan, it was evident that some patients suspected of PE would not require further work-up prior to making a disposition. For example, among patients who had both high probability lung scans and a clinical suspicion for PE of more than 80 per cent, the likelihood of PE at angiography was 96 per cent. Conversely, among patients who had both a low probability lung scan and a clinical suspicion for PE of less than 20 per cent, the likelihood of PE at angiography was only 4 per cent. Unfortunately, the majority of patients will not fit neatly into either of these categories. For example, patients with a high clinical suspicion of PE and a low probability scan had a 40 per cent likelihood of having PE at angiography (Table 46–10).

Retrospective analysis of the PIOPED data base has led to a slight revision of the initial PIOPED lung scan probability criteria (Table 46–11). For example, scans with a single moderate segmental mismatch are now classified as intermediate rather than low probability.[81]

ECHOCARDIOGRAPHY (see p. 95). Echocardiography is a rapid, practical, and sensitive technique for the identification of right ventricular overload following PE (Fig. 46–8).[82] The frequency of echocardiographic signs of PE (Table 46–12) depends on the population being studied. For example, Kasper et al. reported that the frequency of right ventricular dilatation exceeded 90 per cent when PE was accompanied by pulmonary hypertension; right ventricular free wall asynergy was present in 81 per cent with pulmonary hypertension, but in none with normal pulmonary artery pressures.[83] For those patients in whom transthoracic imaging is unsatisfactory, transesophageal echocardiography can be carried out.[84]

Patients with right ventricular dysfunction after PE have a worse prognosis and may be at increased risk for recurrent PE and death compared with those who have normal right ventricular function. Therefore, detection of right ventricular dysfunction at the time of presentation with PE is useful for risk stratification and prognostication. Echocar-

TABLE 46–10 PIOPED: PULMONARY EMBOLISM STATUS

	CLINICAL PROBABILITY (%)			
	80–100 No. PE/PTS (%)	20–79 No. PE/PTS (%)	0–19 No. PE/PTS (%)	ALL PROBABILITIES No. PE/PTS (%)
Scan category				
High	28/29 (96)	70/ 80 (88)	5/ 9 (56)	103/118 (87)
Intermediate	27/41 (66)	66/236 (28)	11/ 68 (16)	104/345 (30)
Low	6/15 (40)	30/191 (16)	4/ 90 (4)	40/296 (14)
Near-normal/normal	0/ 5 (0)	4/ 62 (6)	1/ 61 (2)	5/128 (4)
Total	61/90 (68)	170/569 (30)	21/228 (9)	252/887 (28)

From the PIOPED Investigators: Value of the ventilation/perfusion scan in acute pulmonary embolism. JAMA *263*:2757, 1990.
PIOPED = Prospective Investigation of Pulmonary Embolism Diagnosis.
80–100, 20–79, 0–19 represent the clinical probabilities of PE.
No. PE/PTS (%) represents the number and percentage of patients in each subgroup with PE.

TABLE 46–11 REVISED PIOPED V/Q SCAN CRITERIA

High Probability (≥ 80%)
- ≥ 2 Large mismatched segmental perfusion defects or the arithmetic equivalent in moderate or large + moderate defects*

Intermediate Probability (20%–79%)
- One moderate to two large mismatched segmental perfusion defects or the arithmetic equivalent in moderate or large + moderate defects*
- Single matched ventilation/perfusion defect with clear chest radiograph†
- Difficult to categorize as low or high, or not described as low or high

Low Probability (≤ 19%)
- Nonsegmental perfusion defects (e.g., cardiomegaly, enlarged aorta, enlarged hilum, elevated diaphragm)
- Any perfusion defect with a substantially larger chest radiographic abnormality
- Perfusion defects matched by ventilation abnormality† provided that there are: (1) clear chest radiograph and (2) some areas of normal perfusion in the lungs
- Any number of small perfusion defects with a normal chest radiograph

Normal
- No perfusion defects or perfusion outlines exactly the shape of the lungs seen on the chest radiograph (note that hilar and aortic impressions may be seen and the chest radiograph and/or ventilation study may be abnormal)

Reprinted with permission from Gottschalk, A., Sostman, D., Coleman, E., et al.: Ventilation-perfusion scintigraphy in the PIOPED study. Part II. Evaluation of the scintigraphic criteria and interpretations. J. Nucl. Med. *34*:1119, 1993.

PIOPED = Prospective Investigation of Pulmonary Embolism Diagnosis

* Two large mismatched perfusion defects are borderline for "high probability." Individual readers may correctly interpret individual scans with this pattern as "high probability." In general, it is recommended that more than this degree of mismatch be present for the "high probability" category.

† Very extensive matched defects can be categorized as "low probability." Single V/Q matches are borderline for "low probability" and thus should be categorized as "intermediate" in most circumstances by most readers, although individual readers may correctly interpret individual scans with this pattern as "low probability."

diograms done on normotensive patients with lung perfusion defects of greater than 30 per cent identify more than 90 per cent of patients with right ventricular dysfunction.[49]

Right ventricular dilatation and hypokinesis may occur in chronic pulmonary hypertension of any cause. Long-term elevation of right ventricular afterload is usually accompanied by right ventricular hypertrophy. In patients with chronic pulmonary hypertension, the velocity of the tricuspid regurgitant jet may be elevated to a greater level than in patients with acute PE and no underlying cardiopulmonary disease. Right ventricular infarction, cardiomyopathy, and right ventricular dysplasia may also result in right ventricular hypokinesis and dilatation on the echocardiogram. In these conditions, however, the velocity of tricuspid regurgitation is usually less than in acute PE.

It appears that right ventricular contractile dysfunction following PE has a distinct regional pattern in which wall excursion is hypokinetic from the base through the free wall but remains almost normal at the right ventricular apex (Fig. 46–8*B*). This pattern of right ventricular contractile dysfunction differs from the global dysfunction observed in primary pulmonary hypertension.[85] A possible explanation is that in PE the left ventricle may tether the right ventricular apex, thereby preserving near-normal wall motion in this region.

TABLE 46–12 ECHOCARDIOGRAPHIC SIGNS OF PULMONARY EMBOLISM

- Direct visualization of thrombus (rare)
- Right ventricular dilatation
- Right ventricular hypokinesis (with sparing of the apex)
- Abnormal interventricular septal motion
- Tricuspid valve regurgitation
- Pulmonary artery dilatation
- Lack of decreased inspiratory collapse of inferior vena cava

PULMONARY ANGIOGRAPHY. Selective pulmonary angiography is the most specific examination available for establishing the clinical diagnosis of PE.[86] Angiography should be undertaken as part of an integrated diagnostic approach that combines the clinical assessment with noninvasive diagnostic methods. Angiography tends to be most useful among patients in whom the clinical likelihood of PE differs substantially from the probability of PE based upon noninvasive testing. It is most often undertaken when the lung scan shows intermediate probability for PE.

Pulmonary angiography also has a role in primary therapy of PE. It is a first and necessary step prior to mechanical intervention in the catheterization laboratory with techniques such as suction catheter embolectomy or mechanical clot fragmentation.

PERFORMANCE OF PULMONARY ANGIOGRAPHY

As with any procedure, there is a learning curve for proper and safe performance of pulmonary angiography. Hospitals that perform fewer than several of these studies per month should probably refer their patients to centers that undertake this procedure more frequently. In PIOPED, complications from angiography resulted in death in five patients (0.5 per cent), two of whom were on ventilators and two of whom had severe heart failure prior to the procedure. Nine patients (1 per cent) had major nonfatal complications; respiratory distress occurred in four, renal failure in three, and hematoma requiring transfusion in two.[87] When a team of physicians and nurses is experienced in managing PE patients, even those with moderate or severe pulmonary hypertension can undergo pulmonary angiography safely. In a consecutive series of 67 such patients, 14 of whom had right ventricular end-diastolic pressure that equaled or exceeded 20 mm Hg, no major rhythm disturbances or systemic hypotension requiring therapy occurred, and there were no deaths.[88]

Contrast agents of lower osmolality are less toxic than conventional angiographic dye in patients with pulmonary hypertension. Furthermore, low osmolar contrast agents virtually abolish the heat sensation and urge to cough.[89] We employ low osmolar contrast agents rather than conventional angiographic dye to maximize patient comfort and to minimize repetition of the procedure because of patient coughing and consequent blurring of the films.

PREPARATION OF THE PATIENT. The rationale for performing pulmonary angiography should be explained carefully to the patient and the patient's family. The patient should be told that the procedure may cause discomfort.

A history of allergy to contrast medium should be sought. If present, high-dose oral corticosteroids should be administered both 12 hours and 2 hours before challenge with contrast agent.[90] Heparin can be discontinued immediately before the procedure, unless the clinical suspicion for PE is very high. Patients should avoid heavy meals for at least 4 hours before angiography.

THE ANGIOGRAPHIC PROCEDURE. The perfusion lung scan serves as a road map to the angiographer, who performs selective angiography rather than injecting into the main pulmonary artery. Obtaining accurate and high-quality recordings of right-heart pressures and waveforms is of paramount importance. If the pressure tracing "dampens" or "wedges" in the proximal pulmonary artery, anatomically massive PE should be suspected prior to injection of contrast agent. If the pulmonary artery systolic pressure exceeds approximately 50 mm Hg, the differential diagnosis should include chronic PE or acute superimposed upon chronic PE. Information gleaned from catheterization may occasionally make angiography unnecessary. For example, unexplained dyspnea might be due to cardiac tamponade or left ventricular failure rather than PE. Patients with dyspnea and pulmonary hypertension might have intracardiac shunting that can be defined most precisely with an oxygen saturation run.

Our preferred approach is via the right femoral vein. Percutaneous cannulation of the femoral vein (located 1 to 2 cm medial to the palpable femoral artery) permits rapid access to a large vessel and avoids the problems of using small brachial veins, which are prone to venospasm. To avoid inadvertent perforation of the right ventricle, a catheter with a pigtail configuration can be used rather than one with a straight end.[91] A pigtail catheter can usually be easily manipulated into the pulmonary artery (Fig. 46–9*A*).

Once the catheter has been positioned and the patient has been placed in the desired projection, a test dose of 5 to 10 ml of contrast agent is administered. A plain "scout" film is then obtained to ensure satisfactory exposure and field of view. Prior to the major contrast injection, the patient should be instructed carefully about proper breathing technique and should be reminded to try to suppress the urge to cough. Filming is carried out during maximal inspiration. Twenty to 25 ml of contrast medium per second is injected for 2

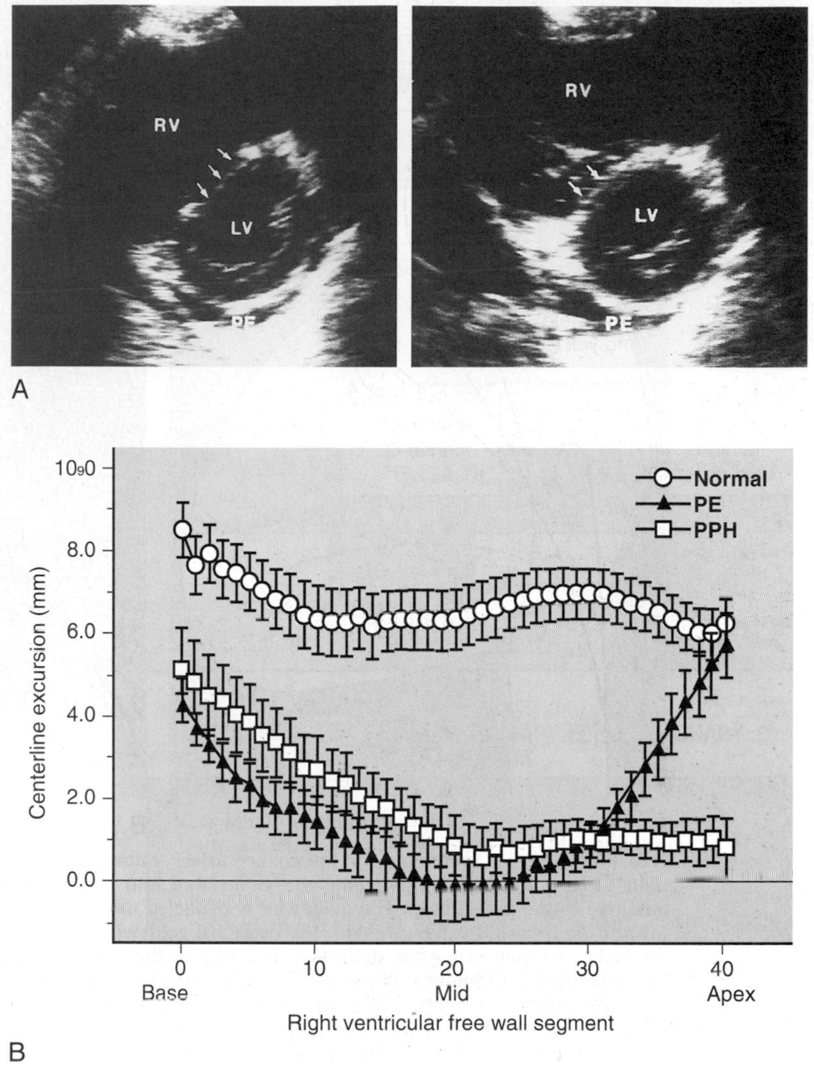

FIGURE 46–8. *A,* Parasternal short-axis views of the right ventricle (RV) and left ventricle (LV) in diastole *(left)* and systole *(right).* There is diastolic and systolic bowing of the interventricular septum (arrows) into the left ventricle compatible with right-ventricular volume and pressure overload, respectively. The right ventricle is appreciably dilated and markedly hypokinetic, with little change in apparent right-ventricular area from diastole to systole. PE = small pericardial effusion. (Reprinted with permission from Come, P. C.: Echocardiographic evaluation of pulmonary embolism and its response to therapeutic interventions. Chest *101*:151S, 1992.)

B, Segmental right ventricular free wall excursion (mean ± SEM) by centerline analysis in patients with acute pulmonary embolism (PE) or primary pulmonary hypertension (PPH) and in normal persons. The acute increase in afterload in PE results in regional right ventricular dysfunction predominantly affecting the mid free wall as it assumes a more spherical shape to equalize wall stress. The right ventricular apex is spared. In contrast, the chronic pressure overload of PPH results in more diffuse right ventricular dysfunction, with limited shape change of the hypertrophied right ventricle. (From McConnell, M. V., Rayan, M. E., Solomon, S. D., et al.: Echocardiographic diagnosis of acute pulmonary embolism: A distinct pattern of abnormal right ventricular wall motion. Am. J. Cardiol. *in press*).

seconds. The exposure rates for this phase are three per second for 3 seconds and then one per second for the pulmonary venous phase, which occurs 5 to 7 seconds after injection. After the selective pulmonary artery injection, pulmonary artery pressures are rechecked to monitor a possible pulmonary hypertensive response, and systemic arterial pressure should be rechecked (with a sphygmomanometer rather than an indwelling arterial cannula) to detect potential hypotension. This "large film" method offers high resolution, clarity of vascular detail, and versatility in field size. An alternative approach utilizes cineangiography.

Interpreting the Angiogram. Standard contrast pulmonary angiography can detect emboli as small as 1 to 2 mm. PE cannot be excluded unless the vasculature appears normal on two different views. Conversely, a definitive diagnosis of PE depends upon visualization of an intraluminal filling defect (Fig. 46–9*B*) in more than one projection. Secondary signs of PE reflect decreased perfusion and consist of abrupt occlusion ("cut off") of vessels, oligemia or avascularity of a segment, a prolonged arterial phase with slow filling and emptying of veins, and tortuous, tapering peripheral vessels.[92]

Not all pulmonary artery filling defects or occlusions are due to acute PE. In chronic PE, arteries may appear "pouched," and thrombus appears organized with a concave edge. Bandlike defects called webs may be present, in addition to intimal irregularities and abrupt narrowing or occlusion of lobar vessels.[93] Other causes of intraluminal filling defects include pulmonary Takayasu's arteritis (see p. 1572), angiosarcoma, and sarcoidosis.[67]

Angiographic methods for quantitating the severity of PE have been problematic. The Walsh scoring system,[94] which is most commonly used in the United States, does not take into account the impairment of peripheral perfusion. The Miller index,[95] which is commonly used in Europe, can overestimate the extent of pulmonary vascular obstruction among patients with massive PE. Both methods fail to differentiate adequately between clot size and the degree of vascular occlusion.

EVOLVING IMAGING METHODS

INTRAVASCULAR ULTRASOUND. Intravascular ultrasound is emerging as a useful technique for identifying patients with acute[96] and chronic[97] PE. Although the main pulmonary artery and large branches can be quickly accessed and examined, cannulation and visualization of peripheral branches are difficult to accomplish rapidly.

PULMONARY ANGIOSCOPY. Percutaneous pulmonary angioscopy using a guiding balloon catheter helps to differentiate among acute PE, chronic PE, and primary pulmonary hypertension.[98] Because aggressive interventional procedures for these three conditions are being undertaken with increasing frequency, the application of pulmonary angioscopy during the diagnostic work-up will probably increase.

SPIRAL COMPUTED TOMOGRAPHY. Spiral computed tomography (CT) allows continuous scanning of organ volumes during a single breath hold by advancing the patient through the roentgenography beam during continuous scanning. In a landmark study, 42 consecutive patients with suspected PE were prospectively evaluated with both spiral CT and selective pulmonary angiography. Patients received between 90 and 120 ml of contrast agent during the CT. All 23 patients with normal spiral CT also had normal pulmonary angiograms. Thromboemboli visualized with spiral CT were almost always seen on standard pulmonary angiography.[99] Spiral CT appears most effective in detecting emboli in the second to fourth division pulmonary vessels but may be ineffective in diagnosing smaller, peripheral PE.[100]

MAGNETIC RESONANCE IMAGING. Magnetic resonance pulmonary angiography provides images similar to catheter angiography, without the necessity of injecting iodinated contrast media.[101] For detecting DVT, magnetic resonance imaging (MRI) already compares favorably with venography and ultrasound. MRI is noninvasive and may be performed in patients with poor venous access, poor renal function, and contraindications to iodinated contrast. MRI is much less operator dependent than ultrasound, and MRI (unlike ultrasound) can provide good images of the inferior vena cava and iliac veins.[102]

Overall Strategy: An Integrated Diagnostic Approach

The diagnosis of PE requires an interdisciplinary effort, commonly involving cardiologist and radiologist. Unfortu-

ated heparin. LMWHs have not received Food and Drug Administration approval for PE or DVT treatment.

Heparin acts primarily by binding to antithrombin III (AT III), an enzyme that inhibits the coagulation factors thrombin (factor IIa), Xa, IXa, XIa, and XIIa. Heparin subsequently promotes a conformational change in AT III that accelerates its activity approximately 100- to 1000-fold.[111] This prevents additional thrombus formation and permits endogenous fibrinolytic mechanisms to lyse clot that has already formed. However, heparin does *not* directly dissolve thrombus that already exists.

One placebo-controlled randomized trial of heparin has been carried out in PE patients.[112] The mortality rate was significantly lower among the treated patients, and the trial was discontinued for ethical reasons. Nevertheless, the efficacy of heparin is limited because clot-bound thrombin is protected from heparin–antithrombin III inhibition.[113] Furthermore, heparin resistance can occur because unfractionated heparin binds to plasma proteins.[114]

MONITORING HEPARIN. An activated partial thromboplastin time (PTT) that is at least 1½ times greater than the control value should provide a minimum therapeutic level of heparin. However, there are many different PTT reagent kits and virtually no standardization of PTT levels.[115] Therefore, an individual hospital's target PTT range for heparin anticoagulation should correspond to a plasma heparin level of approximately 0.2 to 0.5 units/ml. At Brigham and Women's Hospital, we quantitatively measure the heparin level by having our chemistry laboratory use a HEPRN pack (Du Pont) in the automated clinical analyzer used for other chemistry tests. The plasma heparin level is a chromogenic assay based on the inhibition of factor X_a by heparin-activated antithrombin III. The HEPRN pack contains excess factor X_a and essentially analyzes the heparin level by means of an anti-factor X_a assay. Blood for this assay should be drawn into a citrated tube, placed on ice, centrifuged within 30 minutes, and analyzed within 4 hours.

The plasma heparin level is particularly useful in two situations: (1) monitoring heparin anticoagulation among patients with baseline elevated PTTs due to a lupus anticoagulant or anticardiolipin antibodies and (2) monitoring heparin among DVT and PE patients who require large daily doses of heparin.[116]

For patients in whom warfarin therapy has failed or who cannot take warfarin (e.g., pregnant women), we treat initially with continuous intravenous heparin and then teach self-administration of full-dose subcutaneous heparin. With subcutaneous injections, peak heparin levels are usually obtained at approximately 3 hours, and the effect may last for 8 to 12 hours if the heparin dose is adequate. To monitor heparin, the target is a midinterval PTT of approximately 50 to 90 seconds.[117] I rarely permit more than 15,000 units of unfractionated heparin per injection because of concern about possible poor absorption. This means that many patients require injections three times daily. If they object to this schedule, or if their heparin dosing regimen is difficult to adjust, I encourage ambulatory management with a continuous intravenous unfractionated heparin infusion.[118]

INITIATING HEPARIN THERAPY. Heparin is the cornerstone of treatment for acute PE. Before heparin therapy is begun, risk factors for bleeding should be considered, such as a prior history of bleeding with anticoagulation, thrombocytopenia, vitamin K deficiency, increasing age, underlying diseases, and concomitant drug therapy. The most frequently overlooked portion of the physical examination is a rectal examination for occult blood.

The Raschke regimen for achieving rapid, effective, and safe heparinization is presented in Table 46–13. In general, heparin infusion rates as high as 1500 to 2000 units per hour are quite commonly required to achieve adequate anticoagulation during the first few days of heparin administration.

Unless a severe bleeding problem such as active gastrointestinal bleeding is detected, heparin can be started prior to lung scanning or pulmonary angiography. In cases of severe bleeding, heparin therapy should be withheld, and nonpharmacological treatment (secondary prevention) with insertion of an inferior vena cava (IVC) filter should be considered if the diagnosis of PE is confirmed.

COMPLICATIONS. The most important adverse effect of heparin is hemorrhage. Major bleeding during anticoagulation may unmask a previously silent lesion, such as bladder or colon cancer. For most cases of moderate bleeding, cessation of heparin therapy will suffice, and the PTT will usually return to normal within 6 hours because the half-life of heparin is only 60 to 90 minutes. Resumption of heparin at a lower dose or implementing alternative therapy will depend on the severity of the bleeding, the risk of recurrent thromboembolism, and the extent to which bleeding may have resulted from excessive anticoagulation (i.e., a PTT greater than three times the baseline value). Risk factors for major in-hospital bleeding among anticoagulated patients include the presence of comorbid conditions, age greater than 60 years, or liver dysfunction that worsens during treatment.[119]

In the event of life-threatening or intracranial hemorrhage, protamine sulfate can be administered at the time heparin is discontinued. Protamine, a strongly basic protein, will immediately reverse anticoagulant activity by forming a stable complex with the acidic heparin. For life-threatening hemorrhage, the usual dose is approximately 1 mg/100 units of heparin, administered slowly (e.g., 50 mg over 10 to 30 minutes). Protamine sulfate may cause allergic reactions, particularly in diabetics who have had prior exposure to protamine after using neutral protamine Hagedorn (NPH) insulin.[111]

Heparin-associated thrombocytopenia can occur via two mechanisms. Platelet agglutination and aggregation that is rarely of clinical importance is more common but less ominous than immunologically mediated thrombocytopenia, which promotes platelet aggregation and subsequent destruction. Typically, platelet counts will decline below 100,000 per mm^3. This latter form of thrombocytopenia may be associated with either thrombocytopenic bleeding or with life-threatening arterial ("white clot syndrome") and venous thrombosis. Testing for heparin antibodies is specific but not sensitive.[111]

Patients receiving prolonged heparin therapy may develop osteopenia, osteoporosis, or pathological bone fractures. In most cases, asymptomatic osteopenia is the most severe adverse effect on bone metabolism. This finding is most readily assessed with bone densitometry.[120] Among women who have discontinued heparin after pregnancy, the osteopenia usually resolves within a year.[121]

Heparin-associated elevations in transaminase levels occur commonly, have no relation to whether the heparin is of bovine or porcine origin, and are rarely associated with clinical toxicity.[122,123] Heparin causes aldosterone depression by an unknown mechanism within 4 to 8 days after initiation of therapy. In patients with a normally functioning renin-angiotensin-aldosterone axis, this is probably of no clinical significance, although serum sodium levels may drop slightly. However, it may cause clinically important hyperkalemia in certain patients, such as those with diabetes or renal failure.[124]

Dextran

Dextran is a polysaccharide that inhibits erythrocyte aggregation, platelet adhesiveness, and leukocyte plugging. For patients in whom the hemorrhagic or thrombocytopenic risk of heparin is prohibitively high, the use of continuous infusion dextran can in some cases provide safe and immediate anticoagulation.[125] In practice, a test dose of 20 ml of dextran 1 is administered, followed by a continuous infusion of dextran 40 at approximately 20 ml/hr for as long as 5 days. During this period, patients can receive concomitant oral anticoagulation with warfarin.

Warfarin Sodium (see also p. 1818)

Warfarin is a vitamin K antagonist that prevents gamma carboxylation activation of coagulation factors II, VII, IX, and X. The full anticoagulant effect of warfarin may not be apparent for 5 days, even if the prothrombin time, used to monitor warfarin's effect, becomes elevated more rapidly. Elevation in the prothrombin time may initially reflect depletion of coagulation factor VII, which has a half-life of about 6 hours, whereas factor II has a half-life of about 5 days.

OVERLAP WITH HEPARIN. When warfarin therapy is initiated during an active thrombotic state, the levels of protein C and S decline, thus creating a thrombogenic potential. By overlapping heparin and warfarin for 5 days, the procoagulant effect of unopposed warfarin can be counteracted. In a Dutch study, patients with DVT were randomized to oral anticoagulation alone versus heparin plus oral anticoagulation. The recurrent DVT rate was three times higher in the group that received oral anticoagulation alone.[126] This study demonstrates that warfarin should be given with heparin coverage and overlap to patients with an active thrombotic state.

MONITORING WARFARIN. The prothrombin time, utilized to adjust the dose of warfarin, should be reported according to the International Normalized Ratio (INR), not the prothrombin time ratio or the prothrombin time expressed in seconds. Fewer bleeding complications occur when the INR is used to monitor warfarin dosing rather than the prothrombin time ratio.[131]

INTENSITY AND DURATION OF THERAPY. It is our practice to treat with 5 to 7 days of heparin and to initiate warfarin administration on the first hospital day after documenting a PTT within the therapeutic range.[127] It is clear that the recurrence rate after completion of anticoagulation is halved by utilizing 6 months of oral anticoagulation rather than 6 weeks.[127a] In otherwise healthy patients, I usually initiate warfarin therapy with 7.5 to 10 mg and then adjust the warfarin dose to achieve a target INR. Among systemically ill patients, however, vitamin K deficiency[128] may lead to marked overanticoagulation just after a single dose of warfarin. I tend to treat first-time DVT of the calf for 3 months,[130] proximal DVT for 6 months, and PE for 1 year. The target INR for first-time DVT is 2.0 to 3.0, but I tend to treat PE more intensively, with a target INR of at least 3.0. Whenever possible, patients with DVT or PE who also have the antiphospholipid-antibody syndrome should be maintained with a target INR of at least 3.0.[130a]

The optimal duration of therapy is unknown. In a prospective 12-year follow-up study of 58 low risk DVT patients in Zurich, 14 per cent and 24 per cent suffered recurrent venous thrombosis.[130b] In Padua, Italy, 355 consecutive DVT patients were treated with warfarin for 3 months and then followed long-term. The cumulative incidence of recurrent thrombosis at 2, 5, and 8 years was 18, 25, and 30 per cent, respectively.[129] For patients with recurrent thrombosis or underlying long-term risk factors for thrombosis (e.g., metastatic cancer or massive obesity), I often advise indefinite anticoagulation. Three ongoing trials are randomizing DVT patients to short-term (3 months) versus long-term anticoagulation with 1 to 3 years of warfarin.

COMPLICATIONS. The major toxic effect of warfarin is bleeding. The risk of bleeding increases as the INR increases. Risk factors for hemorrhage include severe hepatic or renal disease, alcoholism, drug interactions, trauma, malignant disease, and known previous bleeding sites in the gastrointestinal tract. Of 130 cases of bleeding in one study, 38 per cent were due to remediable lesions, half of which were occult prior to warfarin administration.[132] Among outpatients who develop intracranial hemorrhage with warfarin treatment, age is the most important risk factor other than the prothrombin time.[133]

Major life-threatening bleeding requires immediate treatment with enough cryoprecipitate or fresh frozen plasma (FFP) (usually 2 units) to normalize the INR and achieve immediate hemostasis. To treat less serious bleeding, vitamin K may be administered parenterally; a dose of 10 mg subcutaneously or intramuscularly will usually reverse the effects of warfarin in 6 to 12 hours. However, this approach will make the patient relatively refractory to warfarin for up to 2 weeks, so that reinstitution of warfarin becomes more difficult. Minor bleeding with a prolonged INR may merely require interruption of warfarin therapy, without administration of FFP, until the INR has returned to the therapeutic range. If bleeding occurs when the INR is within the therapeutic range, occult malignant disease should be suspected and ruled out. Evaluation of cases of minor bleeding and an INR above the therapeutic range is less productive.

Warfarin-induced skin necrosis[134] is a rare but important complication that may be related to warfarin-induced reduction of protein C. The "purple toes syndrome" is another rare complication of warfarin that appears to be caused by cholesterol microembolization.[135] In this syndrome, crystals are released from ulcerated atherosclerotic plaques. It appears that warfarin may worsen cholesterol microembolic disease by interfering with the healing of ulcerated atherosclerotic plaques.

During pregnancy, heparin should generally be used instead of warfarin because warfarin is associated with a 10-fold higher rate of congenital anomalies.[136] The fetus is particularly susceptible to warfarin embryopathy during the sixth through twelfth week of gestation.[137] The main features are saddle nose, nasal hypoplasia, frontal bossing, short stature, stippled epiphyses, optic atrophy, cataracts, mental retardation, and flexure contractures. Intracranial bleeding may also lead to secondary central nervous system deformities. Women can take warfarin post partum and breast feed safely. The level of warfarin in breast milk is so low (25 ng/ml)[138] that it cannot be detected in the baby's plasma.[138,139]

In the office setting, I routinely assess warfarin dosing with a machine that provides the INR result in 2 minutes by use of a drop of whole blood obtained from a fingertip puncture. Substantial saving of time has resulted, and patients leave the office with greater peace of mind and with a more accurate understanding of their warfarin dosing regimen. This device has the potential for home use,[140] but current Federal Clinical Laboratory Improvement Amendment of 1988 (CLIA) regulations make this approach impractical in the United States. Testing with fingertip puncture is also available for the PTT[141] and is particularly useful in patients (e.g., during pregnancy) who require long-term adjusted-dose heparin.

Aspirin

(see also p. 1818)

Aspirin exerts its antithrombotic effect by eliminating platelet prostaglandin synthesis, thereby blocking thromboxane A_2 formation and causing a moderate decrease in platelet function and a mild hemostatic defect.[142] Consequently, aspirin has at least a modest role in prevention of venous thrombosis.[143] I prescribe low-dose aspirin, usually 80 mg daily, for some patients who have finished their full course of warfarin. This strategy averts an abrupt transition from full anticoagulation to no anticoagulation.

Secondary Prevention: Inferior Vena Caval Interruption

The major indications for placement of an inferior vena caval (IVC) filter are listed in Table 46–15. Of note is that most "free-floating" DVTs rarely embolize and can be managed with heparin anticoagulation alone.[144] An IVC filter prevents PE, not DVT. Therefore, when a filter is inserted, anticoagulation should also be utilized, whenever possible, to prevent further thrombosis.[145] Recently a removable IVC filter has been tested with an infusion port that can be used to deliver thrombolytic therapy; the efficacy appeared promising, and the complication rate was low.[146]

Most IVC filters are placed below the renal veins. For suprarenal vein placement, the largest experience is with

TABLE 46–15 INDICATIONS FOR INFERIOR VENA CAVAL FILTERS

1. Anticoagulation contraindicated and PE is documented
   a. Active bleeding that might cause exsanguination (e.g., gastrointestinal)
   b. Feared bleeding that might be catastrophic (e.g., postoperative craniotomy)
   c. Ongoing complications of anticoagulation (e.g., heparin-associated thrombocytopenia)
   d. Planned intensive cancer chemotherapy (with anticipated pancytopenia or thrombocytopenia)
2. Anticoagulation failure despite documentation of adequate therapy (e.g., recurrent pulmonary embolism)
3. Prophylaxis in high-risk patients
   a. Extensive or progressive venous thrombosis
   b. In conjunction with catheter-based or surgical pulmonary embolectomy
   c. Severe pulmonary hypertension or cor pulmonale

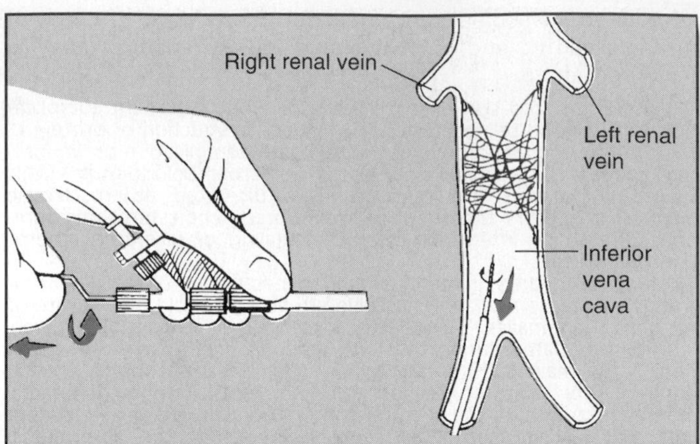

FIGURE 46–11. Inferior vena caval filters. Most filters are placed percutaneously via the right femoral vein. Our current preference is percutaneous placement of a Bird's Nest Filter (Cook Incorporated, Bloomington, IN), which has a low rate of failure, thrombogenicity, and occlusion. The smallness of its sheath may help minimize the risk of bleeding during and after the procedure. To insert the Bird's Nest Filter, the right-angled handle of the wire guide pusher is rotated counterclockwise for 10 to 15 turns to disengage it from the filter. Then the wire guide pusher is removed first, followed by the empty filter catheter. The introducing sheath is left in place so that a post-procedure venacavogram can be obtained. (Reprinted with permission from Goldhaber, S. Z.: Treatment of venous thrombosis. *In* Goldhaber, S. Z. (ed.): Cardiopulmonary Diseases and Cardiac Tumors. Braunwald, E., Series ed. Atlas of Heart Diseases. Philadelphia, Current Medicine, 1995, vol. III, pp. 12.1–12.14.)

the titanium Greenfield filter. Recently, however, unsatisfactory deployment of the titanium Greenfield filter legs has been reported, with wide gaps between the filter legs.[147] This problem has been associated with fatal PE.[48] At Brigham and Women's Hospital, we primarily use the Bird's Nest Filter (Fig. 46–11).

Primary Treatment

Thrombolysis

Thrombolytic therapy (Table 46–16) may be a useful adjunct to heparin in patients who have either systemic arterial hypotension or normal systemic arterial pressure with echocardiographic evidence of right ventricular dysfunction. Rapid improvement of right ventricular function and pulmonary perfusion, accomplished with thrombolytic therapy followed by heparin, may lead to a lower rate of death and recurrent PE.[49] Thrombolysis may (1) prevent the downhill spiral of right heart failure by physical dissolution of anatomically obstructing pulmonary arterial thrombus (Fig. 46–12); (2) prevent the continued release of serotonin and other neurohumoral factors that might otherwise lead to worsening pulmonary hypertension; and (3) dissolve much of the source of the thrombus in the pelvic or deep leg veins, thereby decreasing the likelihood of recurrent large PE.

TABLE 46–16 FDA-APPROVED THROMBOLYTIC REGIMENS FOR PULMONARY EMBOLISM

STREPTOKINASE: 250,000 IU as a loading dose over 30 min, followed by 100,000 U/hr for 24 hr—approved in 1977.
UROKINASE: 4400 IU/kg as a loading dose over 10 min, followed by 4400 IU/kg/hr for 12–24 hr—approved in 1978
rt-PA: 100 mg as a continuous peripheral IV infusion administered over 2 hr—approved in 1990

The potential benefits of immediately reversing right heart failure and preventing recurrent PE must be balanced by the risk of hemorrhage. Contraindications to thrombolysis, such as intracranial disease, recent surgery, or trauma, preclude its use in some patients who can safely receive heparin alone. There is about a 1 per cent risk of intracranial hemorrhage. Careful patient screening for contraindications to thrombolysis is the best way to minimize bleeding risk (see p. 1218).

The largest thrombolysis-versus-heparin-alone trial was carried out about 30 years ago when urokinase (UK) was compared with heparin alone in the Urokinase Pulmonary Embolism Trial (UPET).[148] Urokinase dissolved pulmonary arterial clot more rapidly than heparin alone and, in certain instances, reversed clinical shock. In UPET, it appeared that thrombolytic therapy followed by heparin might reduce the mortality and recurrent PE rate when compared with heparin alone. However, statistical significance was not demonstrated, possibly because of a relatively small sample size. Furthermore, among PE patients who survived for 1 week, there was no significant difference in lung scan improvement between the two treatments.

At Brigham and Women's Hospital, we have coordinated five trials of PE thrombolysis, including the second largest trial of thrombolysis versus heparin alone: 101 hemodynamically stable patients were randomized to rt-PA 100 mg/2 hours followed by intravenous heparin versus heparin alone.[149] The initial systolic arterial pressure was at least 90 mm Hg in every patient. Qualitative assessment of right ventricular wall motion demonstrated that 39 per cent of the rt-PA patients improved (Figs. 46–13*A* and 46–13*B*) and 2.4 per cent worsened, compared with 17 per cent improvement and 17 per cent worsening among those who received heparin alone ($p < 0.005$). Quantitative assessment showed that rt-PA patients had a significant decrease in right ventricular end-diastolic area during the 24 hours after randomization compared with none among those allocated to heparin alone ($p < 0.01$). rt-PA patients also had an absolute improvement in pulmonary perfusion of 14.6 per cent at 24 hours (Fig. 46–13*C* and 13*D*), compared with 1.5 per cent improvement among heparin-alone patients ($p < 0.0001$).

Most importantly, no clinical episodes of recurrent PE occurred among rt-PA patients, but there were five (two fatal and three non-

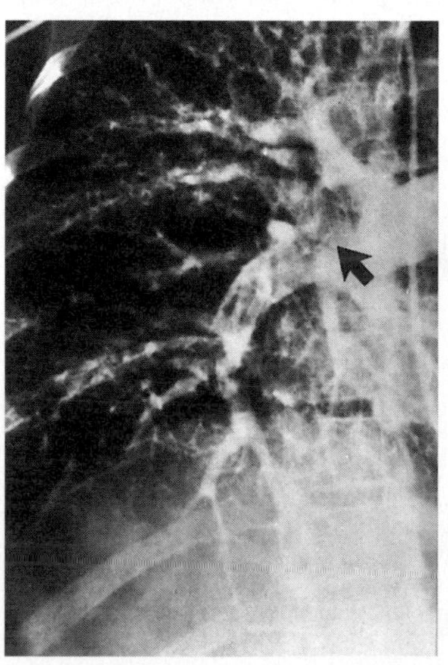

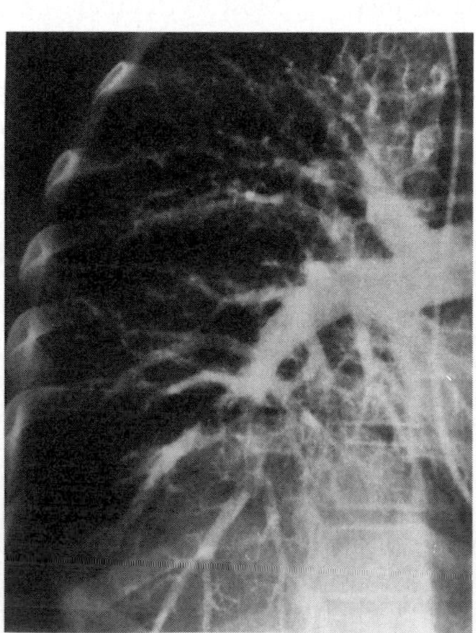

FIGURE 46–12. *Left,* A large embolus in the right pulmonary artery (arrow). *Right,* After a 2-hour infusion of rt-PA through a peripheral vein, there is pronounced resolution, with only a small amount of residual thrombus in segmental branches. (Reprinted with permission from Goldhaber, S. Z., Vaughan, D. E., Markis, J. E., et al.: Acute pulmonary embolism treated with tissue plasminogen activator. Lancet *2*:886, 1986.)

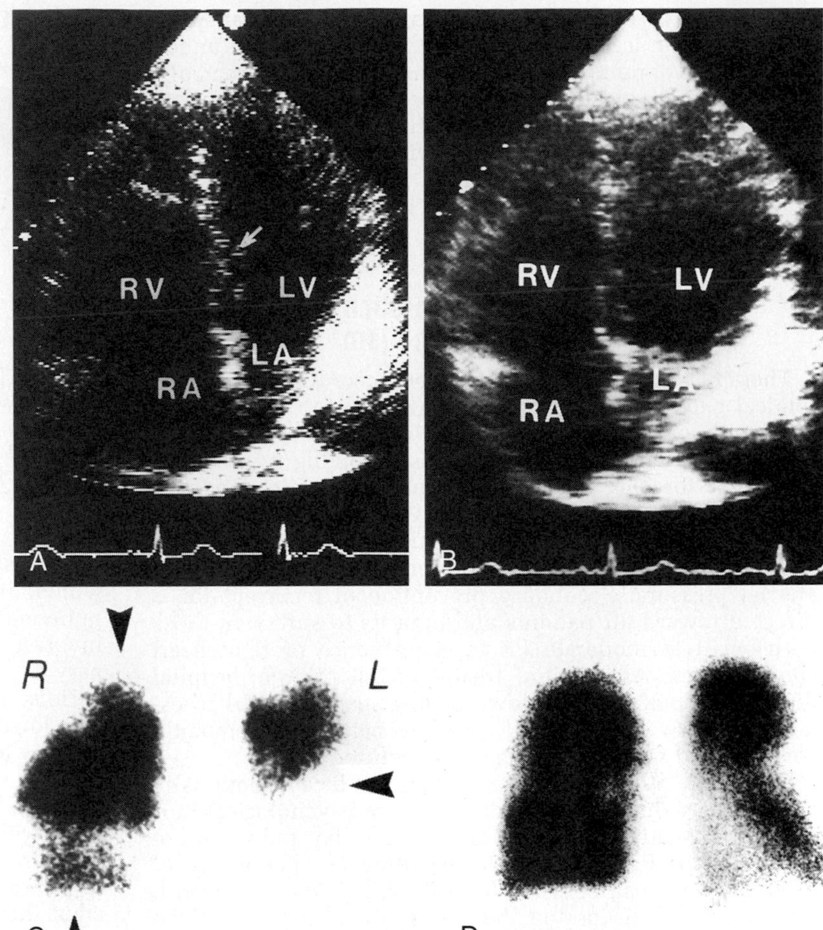

FIGURE 46–13. Echocardiograms (four-chamber view) and perfusion lung scans (anterior view) in a 53-year-old previously healthy man treated with rt-PA for PE. *A,* Right ventricular enlargement before treatment. The right ventricular end-diastolic area was 42.9 cm^2, and the interventricular septum (arrow) was displaced toward the left ventricle. There was moderately severe right ventricular hypokinesis. *B,* Three hours after initiation of rt-PA therapy, the size of the right ventricle normalized (with a planimetered area of 25.7 cm^2), and the interventricular septum resumed its normal configuration. Right ventricular wall motion normalized. *C,* The pretherapy lung scan *(left)* shows absence of perfusion in the right middle lobe (lower arrowhead) and in most of the right upper lobe, particularly the apical segment of the right upper lobe (upper arrowhead). The left lung shows absence of perfusion in the lingula and anterior segment of the left upper lobe (horizontal arrowhead), and irregular perfusion in the apical-posterior segment of the left upper lobe. *D,* The posttherapy scan *(right)* shows marked improvement in perfusion. (Reprinted with permission from Goldhaber, S. Z.: Treatment of acute pulmonary embolism. *In* Goldhaber, S. Z. (ed.): Cardiopulmonary Diseases and Cardiac Tumors. Braunwald, E., Series ed. Atlas of Heart Diseases. Philadelphia, Current Medicine, 1995, vol. III, pp. 3.1–3.25.

fatal) clinically suspected recurrent PEs within 14 days in patients randomized to heparin alone ($p < 0.06$). All five initially showed right ventricular hypokinesis on echocardiogram. This latter observation suggests that echocardiography may help identify a subgroup of PE patients at high risk of adverse clinical outcomes if treated with heparin alone. Such patients in particular would appear to be excellent candidates for thrombolytic therapy in the absence of contraindications.

There are currently three FDA-approved thrombolytic regimens from which to choose (Table 46–16).[150] We often can make the diagnosis of PE by lung scan without resorting to angiography. This makes PE thrombolysis safer because the risk is avoided of a major groin hematoma at the site of the femoral vein puncture.[108] Unlike myocardial infarction–thrombolysis patients, PE patients have a wide "window" for effective use of thrombolysis. Specifically, patients who receive thrombolysis 6 to 14 days after new symptoms or signs have as effective a response as those patients who receive thrombolytic therapy within 5 days after the onset of PE. Therefore, patients suspected of PE should be considered as potentially eligible for thrombolysis if they have had any new symptoms or signs within the 2 weeks before presentation.

DVT THROMBOLYSIS

Most patients with DVT have contraindications to thrombolysis.[151] Totally occlusive venous thrombosis usually does not lyse if the agent is administered through a peripheral vein.[152] Furthermore, the only FDA-approved regimen for DVT thrombolysis, 250,000 units of streptokinase followed by 100,000 units/hour for 24 to 72 hours, is not satisfactory because of frequent allergic reactions to prolonged streptokinase infusions and because the concentration of streptokinase usually has to be doubled or quadrupled to maintain a systemic lytic state. Newer thrombolytic regimens appear promising, including repeated administration of boluses of UK[153] and pro-UK.[154] For patients with iliofemoral venous thrombosis, catheter-directed thrombolysis[155] or thrombolysis plus venous angioplasty[156] may be successful.

Embolectomy

The results of embolectomy can be optimized if patients are referred for this procedure before the onset of cardiogenic shock. The Greenfield embolectomy device is probably the most frequently used catheter-based method of extracting pulmonary arterial thrombus (Fig. 46–14).[157] It consists of a 10F steerable catheter with a suction cup attached at the tip. Because of the cup's large size, a surgical venotomy is utilized, usually the right internal jugular vein. A steerable handle controls progression of the catheter through the right cardiac chambers and the pulmonary arterial branches.

Alternative catheterization methods include mechanical fragmentation of thrombus with a standard pulmonary artery catheter[158] or clot pulverization with an investigational rotating basket catheter. This 5F Teflon catheter has a distal tip that is divided into four 15-mm bends. The high-speed mechanical rotation of the catheter (about 100,000 revolutions per minute) causes centrifugal force to open the distal bends and form a soft flexible helical spiral that can disintegrate thrombus into microscopic particles within seconds.[159] Another approach is simultaneous mechanical clot fragmentation and pharmacological thrombolysis.[160] Finally, balloon angioplasty has also been utilized to improve pulmonary arterial flow among patients with PE.[161]

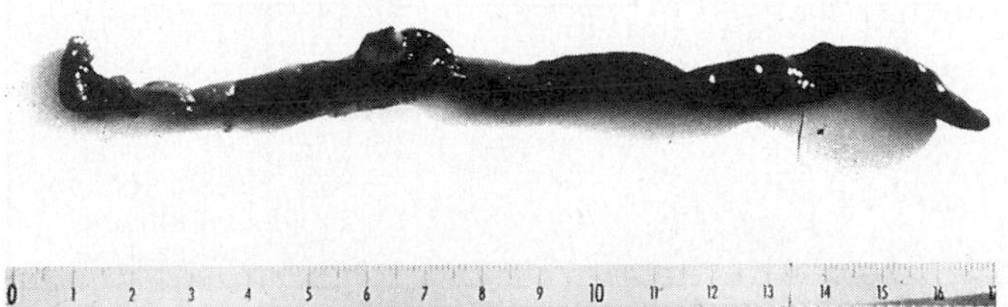

FIGURE 46–14. Philippe Reynaud, M.D., at the Laennec Hospital in Paris, used a Greenfield embolectomy catheter to remove this 17-cm thrombus from a severely compromised PE patient. Rapid hemodynamic improvement ensued. (Reprinted with permission from Meyer, G., Tamiser, D., Reynaud, P., and Sors, H.: Acute pulmonary embolectomy. *In* Goldhaber, S. Z. (ed.): Cardiopulmonary Diseases and Cardiac Tumors. Braunwald, E., Series ed. Atlas of Heart Diseases. Philadelphia, Current Medicine, 1995, vol. III, pp. 7.1–7.12.)

If catheter-based strategies fail, emergency surgical embolectomy with cardiopulmonary bypass can be undertaken.[162] A nonrandomized comparison of rt-PA thrombolysis versus surgical embolectomy indicated that both approaches can be lifesaving in the majority of patients with massive PE.[163] For patients with PE causing systemic arterial hypotension or right heart failure, pulmonary embolectomy in the catheterization laboratory or operating room should be considered when there are contraindications to thrombolysis or when thrombolysis has failed.[164]

Overall Management Approach for Acute Pulmonary Embolism

Therapy for PE should be tailored according to the anatomical extent of the embolus, the presence of underlying cardiopulmonary disease, and the detection of right-heart dysfunction. The echocardiogram is becoming increasingly important for risk stratification and prognostication (Fig. 46–15). Primary therapy frequently is being used for patients with right ventricular dilatation and hypokinesis on echocardiogram, even in the presence of normal systemic arterial pressure. Secondary prevention of recurrent PE is directed toward all patients and appears to suffice in those with small to moderate PE in the absence of right heart abnormalities. After initial treatment but prior to hospital discharge, obtaining a follow-up lung scan is useful to establish a new baseline, in case the patient subsequently complains of symptoms suggesting recurrent PE.

EMOTIONAL SUPPORT. Although PE can be as emotionally devastating as myocardial infarction, the psychological burden for PE patients may be greater. The lay public is not familiar with PE, particularly regarding the possibility of genetic predisposition, long-term disability, and recurrence of disease. By discussing the implications of PE with the patient and family, the emotional burden may be assuaged. We initiated a Pulmonary Embolism Support Group, co-led by a nurse-physician team, and have been gratified by the experience. Although these sessions have an educational component, the major emphasis is discussing the anxieties and living difficulties that occur in the aftermath of PE.

Chronic Pulmonary Embolism

Patients with chronic pulmonary hypertension due to previous PE may be virtually bedridden with breathlessness due to high pulmonary arterial pressures. They should be considered for pulmonary thromboendarterectomy, which, if successful, can reduce and at times even cure pulmonary hypertension (Table 46–17).[165] The operation involves a median sternotomy, institution of cardiopulmonary bypass, and deep hypothermia with circulatory arrest periods. Incisions are made in both pulmonary arteries into the lower-lobe branches. Pulmonary thromboendarterectomy is always bilateral, with removal of organized thrombus and endarterectomy plane from all involved vessels.

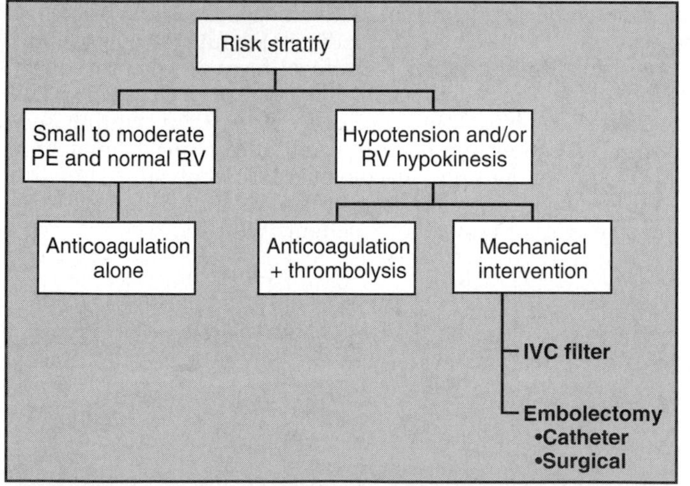

FIGURE 46–15. Proposed strategy for treatment of PE in which risk stratification, usually with echocardiography, is undertaken to assess right ventricular (RV) function. This evaluation helps to determine prognosis as well as appropriateness of aggressive intervention with thrombolysis or mechanical measures to remove thrombus. (From Goldhaber, SZ: Treatment of acute pulmonary embolism. *In* Goldhaber, SZ (ed.): Cardiopulmonary Diseases and Cardiac Tumors. *In* Braunwald, E.: Atlas of Heart Diseases, Vol. III. Current Medicine, 1995, pp. 3.1–3.25.)

TABLE 46–17 AVERAGE HEMODYNAMIC VALUES IN 34 PATIENTS BEFORE AND IMMEDIATELY AFTER THROMBOENDARTERECTOMY AND AT FOLLOW-UP

	PREOP	IMMEDIATE POSTOP	FOLLOW-UP*
Mean pulmonary artery pressure (mm Hg)	49	27	24
Mean pulmonary artery systolic pressure (mm Hg)	80	43	38
Cardiac output (liters/min)	3.8	5.9	4.9
Pulmonary vascular resistance (dynes-sec-cm^{-5})	997	230	272

* Follow-up 3 months to 16 years after thromboarterectomy.

Modified from Moser, K. M., Auger, W. R., and Fedullo, P. F.: Chronic major-vessel thromboembolic pulmonary hypertension. Circulation *81*:1735, 1990. Copyright 1990 the American Heart Association.

At the University of California at San Diego, 275 patients underwent pulmonary thromboendarterectomy between 1990 and 1993, with a mortality rate of 6 per cent. The two major causes of mortality are: (1) inability to remove sufficient thrombotic material at surgery, resulting in persistent postoperative pulmonary hypertension and right ventricular dysfunction; and (2) severe reperfusion lung injury.[166] Thus, at selected centers, pulmonary thromboendarterectomy can be performed with good results and at an acceptable risk among patients debilitated from chronic pulmonary hypertension due to PE (Fig. 46–16).

Prevention

PE is difficult to diagnose, expensive to treat, and occasionally lethal despite therapy. Therefore, preventive measures are of paramount importance.[167] A variety of mechanical measures and pharmacological agents can be utilized. The most recent innovation has been FDA approval of two different low molecular weight heparins, one (enoxaparin) for use in patients undergoing total hip or knee replacement and another (dalteparin) for patients undergoing high-risk abdominal or pelvic surgery.

In 1986, an NIH Consensus Development Conference strongly recommended prophylaxis against DVT and PE for most surgical patients.[168] Initially, physicians followed the specific guidelines only in a minority of instances. In one survey, two-thirds of high-risk patients did not receive prophylaxis.[169] More recently, however, the concept of prophylaxis has gained much wider acceptance. This is due, at least in part, to the medicolegal liability of physicians who omit prophylaxis among their hospitalized patients with risk factors for venous thrombosis.[170] Furthermore, a policy of prophylaxis is cost-effective. It is estimated that for every 1,000,000 patients undergoing operation who receive prophylaxis against DVT and PE, approximately $60,000,000 can be saved in direct health care costs.[171]

Mechanical Measures

GRADUATED COMPRESSION STOCKINGS. These provide continuous stimulation of blood flow and prevent dilation of the venous system in the legs. Graduated compression stockings (GCS) exert more compression at the ankles (usually 18 mm Hg) than at the popliteal fossa or upper thigh (usually 8 mm Hg). In an overview of 12 trials in moderate-risk surgery, GCS reduced the DVT rate by two-thirds.[172] Thus, GCS should be considered first-line prophylaxis for most hospitalized patients and should suffice for prophylaxis among low-risk patients.

INTERMITTENT PNEUMATIC COMPRESSION. Intermittent pneumatic compression (IPC) devices expel blood from the leg veins and thus prevent venous stasis. The mechanical force of compression appears to enhance systemic fibrinolytic activity.[173] IPC is particularly worthwhile among patients who have an absolute contraindication to anti-

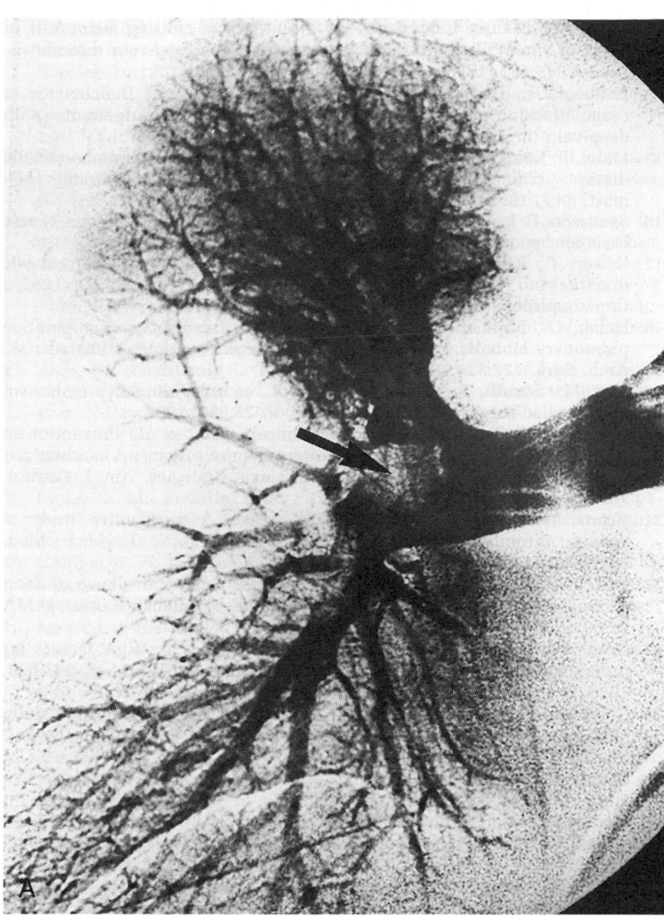

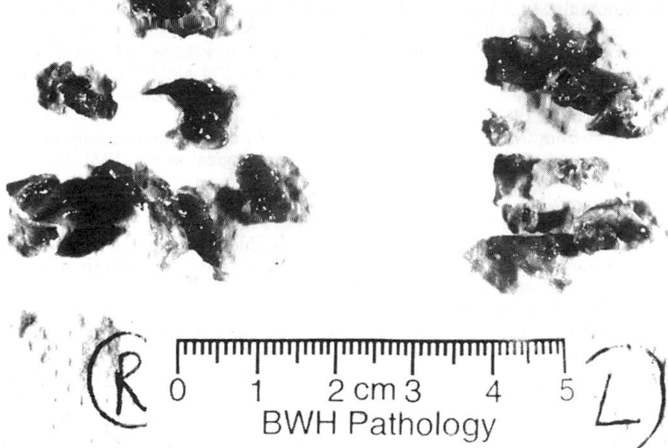

B

FIGURE 46–16. A 69-year-old woman who underwent pulmonary thromboendarterectomy at Brigham and Women's Hospital had a 1-month history of progressive dyspnea on exertion and recurrent syncope. *A*, Right-heart catheterization demonstrated pulmonary artery systolic pressure of 60 mm Hg. Right pulmonary arteriogram showed multiple filling defects clustered mainly around the hilum (arrow). *B*, At operation, large amounts of thrombus with focal organization were removed from the right and left pulmonary arteries. There were no postoperative complications. The subsequent course has been characterized by marked functional improvement.

coagulation, such as patients undergoing neurosurgery. In addition, for patients receiving postoperative warfarin prophylaxis, IPC devices have special utility because they are immediately useful, whereas warfarin requires 4 to 5 days of administration before it is entirely effective as an anticoagulant. IPC devices are, in general, used properly in intensive care units. However, in one survey, they were either not applied or applied improperly in the majority of patients after transfer from an intensive care to a regular general surgery unit.[174]

INFERIOR VENA CAVAL INTERRUPTION (see p. 1595). The most invasive mechanical prophylaxis measure that can be implemented is IVC filter placement. Use of an IVC filter might be appropriate for patients with recently diagnosed PE or DVT who must undergo major surgery that places them at high risk for suffering perioperative PE.

Pharmacological Agents

UNFRACTIONATED HEPARIN. The International Multicentre Trial studied pharmacological prophylaxis among 4121 patients undergoing elective major surgery. The intervention group received fixed-dose unfractionated heparin in a dose of 5000 units subcutaneously every 8 hours. The first injection was given 2 hours before the skin incision. Of autopsied subjects, 16 controls died of PE, compared with only 2 patients in the heparin group. Although more patients who received heparin prophylaxis had wound hematomas, the number of deaths due to hemorrhage was not increased among those who received heparin.[175] Collins et al. subsequently pooled data from 78 randomized controlled unfractionated heparin trials with 15,598 patients and confirmed the results of the International Multicentre Trial. Among patients who received heparin prophylaxis, there was a 40 per cent reduction in nonfatal PE and a 64 per cent reduction in fatal PE.[176] In more recent pharmacological prophylaxis trials, at times, prophylaxis has been deferred until the early postoperative period. Any loss of efficacy resulting from deferring prophylaxis until shortly after surgery is unlikely to be marked.[177]

LOW MOLECULAR WEIGHT HEPARIN. Low molecular weight heparin (LMWH) has a more predictable dose-response, more dose-independent mechanisms of clearance, and a longer plasma half-life than unfractionated heparin. LMWHs can achieve higher plasma heparin

TABLE 46–18 STRATEGIES FOR PREVENTION OF PULMONARY EMBOLISM AND DEEP VEIN THROMBOSIS

CONDITION	STRATEGY
Orthopedic surgery*	Coumadin (target INR 2.0–2.5 × 4–6 weeks IPC ± Coumadin Low molecular weight heparin × 5–14 days (e.g., enoxaparin 30 mg SC twice daily)
Nonorthopedic surgery	
Gynecologic cancer surgery	Coumadin (target INR 2.0–2.5) q IPC Unfractionated heparin 5000 U q8h ± IPC Dalteparin 2500 U SC once daily
Urological surgery	Coumadin (target INR 2.0–2.5) ± IPC
Thoracic surgery	IPC plus unfractionated heparin 5000 U q8h
High-risk general surgery (e.g., prior VTE, current cancer, or obesity)	IPC or graded-compression stockings plus unfractionated heparin 5000 U q8h Dalteparin 2500 U SC once daily
General, gynecological, or urological surgery (without prior VTE) for benign conditions	Graded-compression stockings plus unfractionated heparin 5000 q12h IPC alone
Neurosurgery, eye surgery, or other surgery when pharmacological prophylaxis is contraindicated	Graded-compression stockings ± IPC
Pregnancy	
Antepartum (with prior VTE)	Graded compression stockings plus daily exercise program plus serial leg examinations Subcutaneous unfractionated heparin
Peripartum (with prior VTE)	IPC ± subcutaneous unfractionated heparin
Postpartum (with prior VTE)	Coumadin (target INR 2.0–3.0) with subcutaneous unfractionated heparin continued until target INR attained
Medical conditions	Graded-compression stockings ± heparin 5000 q 8–12h IPC alone

* Especially total hip or knee replacement.
IPC = intermittent pneumatic compression
VTE = venous thromboembolism
INR = International Normalized Ratio

based intravascular ultrasound imaging of chronic thromboembolic pulmonary disease. Am. J. Cardiol. *67*:749, 1991.

98. Uchida, Y., Oshima, T., Hirose, T., et al.: Angioscopic detection of residual pulmonary thrombin in the differential diagnosis of pulmonary embolism. Am. Heart J. *130*:854, 1995.
99. Remy-Jardin, M., Remy, J., Wattinne, L., and Giraud, F.: Central pulmonary thromboembolism: Diagnosis with spiral volumetric CT with the single-breath-hold technique—comparison with pulmonary angiography. Radiology *185*:381, 1992.
100. Blum, A. G., Delfau, F., Grignon, B., et al.: Spiral-computed tomography versus pulmonary angiography in the diagnosis of acute massive pulmonary embolism. Am. J. Cardiol. *74*:96, 1994.
101. Wielopolski, P. A.: Pulmonary arteriography. M.R.I. Clin. North Am. *1*:295, 1993.
102. Spritzer, C. E., Norconk, J. J., Jr., Sostman, H. D., and Coleman, R. E.: Detection of deep venous thrombosis by magnetic resonance imaging. Chest *104*:54, 1993.
103. Ouderk, M., van Beek, E. J. R., van Putten, W. L. J., and Büller, H. R.: Cost-effectiveness analysis of various strategies in the diagnostic management of pulmonary embolism. Arch. Intern. Med. *153*:947, 1993.
104. Perrier, A., Bounameaux, H., Morabia, A., et al.: Contribution of D-dimer plasma measurement and lower-limb venous ultrasound to the diagnosis of pulmonary embolism: A decision analysis model. Am. Heart J. *127*:624, 1994.
105. Perrier, A., Bounameaux, H., Morabia, A., et al.: Diagnosis of pulmonary embolism by a decision analysis based strategy including clinical probability, D-dimer and ultrasonography: A management study. Personal communication, 1995.

MANAGEMENT

106. Cruickshank, M. K., Levine, M. N., Hirsh, J., et al.: A standard heparin nomogram for the management of heparin therapy. Arch. Intern. Med. *151*:333, 1991.
107. Raschke, R. A., Reilly, B. M., Guidry, J. R., et al.: The weight-based heparin dosing nomogram compared with a "standard care" nomogram: A randomized controlled trial. Ann. Intern. Med. *119*:874, 1993.
108. Stein, P. D., Hull, R. D., and Raskob, G.: Risks for major bleeding from thrombolytic therapy in patients with acute pulmonary embolism: Consideration of noninvasive management. Ann. Intern. Med. *121*:313, 1994.
109. Meyer, G., Tamiser, D., Reynaud, P., and Sors, H.: Acute pulmonary embolectomy. *In* Braunwald, E., and Goldhaber, S. Z. (eds.): Atlas of Heart Diseases. Vol. II, Cardiopulmonary Diseases and Cardiac Tumors. Philadelphia, Current Medicine, 1995, p. 6.1.
110. Estagnasié, P., Le Bourdellès, G., Mier, L., et al.: Use of inhaled nitric oxide to reverse flow through a patent foramen ovale during pulmonary embolism. Ann. Intern. Med. *120*:757, 1994.
111. Kondo, N. I., Maddi, R., Ewenstein, B. M., and Goldhaber, S. Z.: Anticoagulation and hemostasis in cardiac surgical patients. J. Cardiovasc. Surg. *9*:443, 1994.
112. Barritt, D. W., and Jordan, S. C.: Anticoagulant drugs in the treatment of pulmonary embolism: A controlled trial. Lancet *1*:1309, 1960.
113. Weitz, J. I., Hudoba, M., Massel, D., et al.: Clot-bound thrombin is protected from inhibition by heparin–antithrombin III but is susceptible to inactivation by antithrombin III–independent inhibitors. J. Clin. Invest. *86*:385, 1990.
114. Young, E., Prins, M., Levine, M. N., and Hirsh, J.: Heparin binding to plasma proteins, an important mechanism for heparin resistance. Thromb. Haemost. *67*:639, 1992.
115. Brill-Edwards, P., Ginsberg, J. S., Johnston, M., and Hirsh, J.: Establishing a therapeutic range for heparin therapy. Ann. Intern. Med. *119*:104, 1993.
116. Levine, M. N., Hirsh, J., Gent, M., et al.: A randomized trial comparing activated thromboplastin time with heparin assay in patients with acute venous thromboembolism requiring large daily doses of heparin. Arch. Intern. Med. *154*:49, 1994.
117. Hirsch, D. R., Lee, T. H., Morrison, R. B., et al.: Shortened hospitalization by means of adjusted-dose subcutaneous heparin for deep venous thrombosis. Am. Heart J. *131*:276, 1996.
118. Brabeck, M. C.: Ambulatory management of thromboembolic disease during pregnancy with continuous infusion of heparin. J. A. M. A. *257*:1790, 1987.
119. Landefeld, C. S., Cook, E. F., Flatley, M., et al.: Identification and preliminary validation of predictors of major bleeding in hospitalized patients starting anticoagulant therapy. Am. J. Med. *82*:703, 1987.
120. Ginsberg, J. S., Kowalchuk, G., Hirsh, J., et al.: Heparin effect on bone density. Thromb. Haemost. *64*:286, 1990.
121. Dahlman, T., Lindvall, N., and Hellgren, M.: Osteopenia in pregnancy during long-term heparin treatment: A radiological study post partum. Br. J. Obstet. Gynaecol. *97*:221, 1990.
122. Dukes, G. E., Sanders, S. W., Russo, J., et al.: Transaminase elevations in patients receiving bovine or porcine heparin. Ann. Intern. Med. *100*:646, 1984.
123. Goldhaber, S. Z., Meyerovitz, M. F., Green, D., et al.: Randomized controlled trial of tissue plasminogen activator in proximal deep venous thrombosis. Am. J. Med. *88*:235, 1990.
124. Oster, J. R., Singer, I., and Fishman, L. M.: Heparin-induced aldosterone suppression and hyperkalemia. Am. J. Med. *98*:575, 1995.
125. Bergqvist, D.: Dextran. *In* Goldhaber, S. Z. (ed.): Prevention of Venous Thromboembolism. New York, Marcel Dekker, 1993, p. 167.
126. Brandjes, D. P. M., Heijboer, H., Büller, H. R., et al.: Acenocoumarol and heparin compared with acenocoumarol alone in the initial treatment of proximal-vein thrombosis. N. Engl. J. Med. *327*:1485, 1992.
127. Pearson, S. D., Lee, T. H., McCabe-Hassan, S., et al.: A critical pathway to treat proximal lower extremity deep vein thrombosis. Am. J. Med. *100*:283, 1996.
127a. Schulman, S., Rhedin, A-S., Lindmarker, P., et al.: A comparison of 6 weeks with 6 months of oral anticoagulant therapy after a first episode of venous thromboembolism. N. Engl. J. Med. *332*:1661, 1995.
128. Shearer, M. J.: Vitamin K. Lancet *345*:229, 1995.
129. Prandoni, P., Lensing, A. W. A., Cogo, A., et al.: The clinical course of deep-vein thrombosis in symptomatic patients. Personal communication, 1995.
130. Lagerstedt, C. I., Olsson, C.-G., Fagher, B. O., et al.: Need for long-term anticoagulant treatment in symptomatic calf-vein thrombosis. Lancet *2*:515, 1985.
130a. Khamashta, M. A., Cuadrado, M. J., Mujic, F., et al.: The management of thrombosis in the antiphospholipid antibody syndrome. N. Engl. J. Med. *332*:993, 1995.
130b. Franzeck, U. K., Schalch, I., and Jager, K. A.: Prospective 12-year follow-up study of clinical and hemodynamic sequelae after deep vein thrombosis in low-risk patients. (Zurich Study). Circulation *93*:74, 1996.
131. Andrews, T. C., Peterson, D. W., Doeppenschmidt, D., et al.: Complications of warfarin therapy monitored by the international normalized ratio versus the prothrombin time ratio. Clin. Cardiol. *18*:80, 1995.
132. Landefeld, C. S., Rosenblatt, M. W., and Goldman, L.: Bleeding in outpatients treated with warfarin: Relation to the prothrombin time and important remediable lesions. Am. J. Med. *87*:153, 1989.
133. Hylek, E. M., and Singer, D. E.: Risk factors for intracranial hemorrhage in outpatients taking warfarin. Ann. Intern. Med. *120*:897, 1994.
134. Broekmans, A. W., Bertina, R. M., Leoliger, E. A., et al.: Protein C and the development of skin necrosis during anticoagulant therapy. Thromb. Haemost. *49*:251, 1983.
135. Hyman, B. T., Landas, S. K., Ashman, R. F., et al.: Warfarin-related purple toes syndrome and cholesterol microembolization. Am. J. Med. *82*:1233, 1987.
136. Hall, J. G., Pauli, R. M., and Wilson, K. M.: Maternal and fetal sequelae of anticoagulation during pregnancy. Am. J. Med. *68*:122, 1980.
137. Iturbe-Alessio, I., Fonseca, M. D. C., Mutchinick, O., et al.: Risks of anticoagulant therapy in pregnant women with artificial heart valves. N. Engl. J. Med. *315*:1390, 1986.
138. Orme, M. L. E., Lewis, P. J., de Swiet, M., et al.: May mothers given warfarin breast-feed their infants? B. M. J. *1*:1564, 1977.
139. McKenna, R., Cole, E. R., and Vasan, U.: Is warfarin sodium contraindicated in the lactating mother? J. Pediatr. *103*:325, 1983.
140. Anderson, D. R., Harrison, L., and Hirsh, J.: Evaluation of a portable prothrombin time monitor for home use by patients who require long-term oral anticoagulant therapy. Arch. Intern. Med. *153*:1441, 1993.
141. Vacek, J. L., Hibiya, K., Rosamond, T. L., et al.: Validation of a bedside method of activated partial thromboplastin time measurement with clinical range guidelines. Am. J. Cardiol. *68*:557, 1991.
142. Roth, G. J., and Calverley, D. C.: Aspirin, platelets, and thrombosis: Theory and practice. Blood *83*:885, 1994.
143. Antiplatelet Trialists' Collaboration: Collaborative overview of randomised trials of antiplatelet therapy—III: Reduction in venous thrombosis and pulmonary embolism by antiplatelet prophylaxis among surgical and medical patients. B. M. J. *308*:235, 1994.
144. Baldridge, E. D., Martin, M. A., and Welling, R. E.: Clinical significance of free-floating venous thrombi. J. Vasc. Surg. *11*:62, 1990.
145. Becker, D. M., Philbrick, J. T., and Selby, J. B.: Inferior vena cava filters: Indications, safety, effectiveness. Arch. Intern. Med. *152*:1985, 1992.
146. Dievart, F., Lefebvre, J. M., Fourrier, J. L., et al.: New infusion removable inferior vena caval filter catheter (Filcard RF 02) for protected thrombolytic treatment in deep venous thrombosis (DVT) and pulmonary embolism (PE): Results of an international multicentric study. J. Am. Coll. Cardiol. *95A*(Abs.):95a, 1994.
147. Sweeney, T. J., and Van Aman, M. E.: Deployment problems with the titanium Greenfield filter. JVIR *4*:691, 1993.
148. Urokinase Pulmonary Embolism Trial: A National Cooperative Study. Circulation *47* and *48* (Suppl. II):1, 1973.
149. Goldhaber, S. Z., Haire, W. D., Feldstein, M. L., et al.: Alteplase versus heparin in acute pulmonary embolism: Randomised trial assessing right-ventricular function and pulmonary perfusion. Lancet *341*:507, 1993.
150. Goldhaber, S. Z.: Contemporary pulmonary embolism thrombolysis. Chest *107*:45S, 1995.
151. Markel, A., Manzo, R. A., and Strandness, D. E., Jr.: The potential role of thrombolytic therapy in venous thrombosis. Arch. Intern. Med. *152*:1265, 1992.
152. Meyerovitz, M. F., Polak, J. F., and Goldhaber, S. Z.: Short-term response to thrombolytic therapy in deep venous thrombosis: Predictive value of venographic appearance. Radiology *184*:345, 1992.
153. Goldhaber, S. Z., Polak, J. F., Feldstein, M. L., et al.: Efficacy and safety of repeated boluses of urokinase in the treatment of deep venous thrombosis. Am. J. Cardiol. *73*:75, 1994.
154. Moia, M., Mannucci, P. M., Pini, M., et al.: A pilot study of pro-urokinase in treatment of deep vein thrombosis. Thromb. Haemost. *72*:430, 1994.
155. Comerota, A. J., Aldridge, S. C., Cohen, G., et al.: A strategy of aggressive regional therapy for acute iliofemoral venous thrombosis with con-

temporary venous thrombectomy or catheter-directed thrombolysis. J. Vasc. Surg. *20:*244, 1994.
156. Marache, P., Asseman, P., Jabinet, J. L., et al.: Percutaneous transluminal venous angioplasty in occlusive iliac vein thrombosis resistant to thrombolysis. Am. Heart J. *125:*362, 1993.
157. Greenfield, L. J., Proctor, M. C., Williams, D. M., and Wakefield, T. W.: Long-term experience with transvenous catheter pulmonary embolectomy. J. Vasc. Surg. *18:*450, 1993.
158. Brady, A. J. B., Crake, T., and Oakley, C. M.: Percutaneous catheter fragmentation and distal dispersion of proximal pulmonary embolus. Lancet *338:*1186, 1991.
159. Dievart, F., Fourrier, J. L., Lefebvre, J. M., et al.: Treatment of severe pulmonary embolism by means of a high speed rotational catheter (Angiocor Thrombolizer): First experience of mechanical thrombolysis in human beings. J. Am. Coll. Cardiol. *474*(Abs.):474a, 1994.
160. Essop, M. R., Middlemost, S., Skoularigis, J., and Sareli, P.: Simultaneous mechanical clot fragmentation and pharmacologic thrombolysis in acute massive pulmonary embolism. Am. J. Cardiol. *69:*427, 1992.
161. Voorburg, J. A. I., Cats, V. M., Buis, B., and Bruschke, A. V. G.: Balloon angioplasty in the treatment of pulmonary hypertension caused by pulmonary embolism. Chest *94:*1249, 1988.
162. Meyer, G., Tamisier, D., Sors, H., et al.: Pulmonary embolectomy: A 20-year experience at one center. Ann. Thorac. Surg. *51:*232, 1991.
163. Gulba, D. C., Schmid, C., and Borst, H.-G.: Medical compared with surgical treatment for massive pulmonary embolism. Lancet *343:*565, 1994.
164. Meyer, G., Tamisier, D., Reynaud, P., and Sors, H.: Acute pulmonary embolectomy. *In* Goldhaber, S. Z. (ed.): Cardiopulmonary diseases and cardiac tumors. Braunwald, E., Series ed. Atlas of Heart Diseases. Philadelphia, Current Medicine, Vol. 3, 1995, p. 6.1.
165. Moser, K. M., Auger, W. R., and Fedullo, P. F.: Chronic major-vessel thromboembolic pulmonary hypertension. Circulation *81:*1735, 1990.
166. Fedullo, P. F., Auger, W. R., Channick, R. N., et al.: A multidisciplinary approach to chronic thromboembolic pulmonary hypertension. *In* Braunwald, E., and Goldhaber, S. Z. (eds.): Atlas of Heart Diseases. Vol. III, Cardiopulmonary Diseases and Cardiac Tumors. Philadelphia, Current Medicine, 1995, p. 7.1.

PREVENTION

167. Goldhaber, S. Z. (ed.): Prevention of Venous Thromboembolism. New York, Marcel Dekker, Inc., 1993, 607 pp.
168. NIH Consensus Development Conference: Prevention of venous thrombosis and pulmonary embolism. J. A. M. A. *256:*744, 1986.
169. Anderson, F. A., Jr., Wheeler, H. B., Goldberg, R. J., et al.: Physician practices in the prevention of venous thromboembolism. Ann. Intern. Med. *115:*591, 1991.
170. Goldhaber, S. Z.: Malpractice claims relation to PE and DVT. Forum. Cambridge, MA, Risk Management Foundation of the Harvard Medical Institutions, Inc., 1994.
171. Landefeld, C. S., and Hanus, P.: Economic burden of venous thromboembolism. *In* Goldhaber, S. Z. (ed.): Prevention of Venous Thromboembolism. New York, Marcel Dekker, Inc., 1993, p. 69.
172. Wells, P. S., Lensing, A. W. A., and Hirsh, J.: Graduated compression stockings in the prevention of postoperative venous thromboembolism. Arch. Intern. Med. *154:*67, 1994.
173. Knight, M. T. N., and Dawson, R.: Effect of intermittent compression of the arms on deep venous thrombosis in the legs. Lancet *2:*1265, 1976.
174. Comerota, A. J., Katz, M. L., and White, J. V.: Why does prophylaxis with external pneumatic compression for deep vein thrombosis fail? Am. J. Surg. *164:*265, 1992.
175. Prevention of fatal postoperative pulmonary embolism by low doses of heparin: An international multicentre trial. Lancet *2:*45, 1975.
176. Collins, R., Scrimgeour, A., Yusuf, S., and Peto, R.: Reduction in fatal pulmonary embolism and venous thrombosis by perioperative administration of subcutaneous heparin: Overview of results of randomized trials in general, orthopedic, and urologic surgery. N. Engl. J. Med. *318:*1162, 1988.
177. Kearon, C., and Hirsh, J.: Starting prophylaxis for venous thromboembolism postoperatively. Arch. Intern. Med. *155:*366, 1995.
178. Leizorovicz, A., Haugh, M. C., Chapuis, F. R., et al.: Low molecular weight heparin in prevention of perioperative thrombosis. BMJ *305:*913, 1992.
179. Reis, S. E., Hirsch, D. R., Wilson, M. G., et al.: Program for the prevention of venous thromboembolism in high-risk orthopaedic patients. J. Arthroplasty *6:*S11, 1991.
180. Paiement, G. D., Wessinger, S. J., Hughes, R., and Harris, W. H.: Routine use of adjusted low-dose warfarin to prevent venous thromboembolism after total hip replacement. J. Bone Joint Surg. *75A:*893, 1993.
181. Paiement, G. D., Wessinger, S. J., and Harris, W. H.: Cost-effectiveness of prophylaxis in total hip replacement. Am. J. Surg. *161:*519, 1991.
182. Fordyce, M. J. F., Baker, A. S., and Staddon, G. E.: Efficacy of fixed minidose warfarin prophylaxis in total hip replacement. BMJ *303:*219, 1991.
183. RD Heparin Arthroplasty Group: RD heparin compared with warfarin for prevention of venous thromboembolic disease following total hip or knee arthroplasty. J. Bone Joint Surg. *76A:*1174, 1994.
184. Hull, R., Raskob, G., Pineo, G., et al.: A comparison of subcutaneous low-molecular-weight heparin with warfarin sodium for prophylaxis against deep-vein thrombosis after hip or knee implantation. N. Engl. J. Med. *329:*1370, 1993.
185. Ginsberg, J. S., Nurmohamed, M. T., Gent, M., et al.: Use of hirulog in the prevention of venous thrombosis after major hip or knee surgery. Circulation *90:*2385, 1994.
186. Barbour, L. A., and Pickard, J.: Controversies in thromboembolic disease during pregnancy: A critical review. Obstet. Gynecol. *86:*621, 1995.
187. Keane, M. G., Ingenito, E. P., and Goldhaber, S. Z.: Utilization of venous thromboembolism prophylaxis in the medical intensive care unit. Chest *106:*13, 1994.

Chapter 47
Cor Pulmonale*

HERBERT P. WIEDEMANN, RICHARD A. MATTHAY

ETIOLOGIES 1604

ANATOMICAL AND PATHOPHYSIOLOGICAL CORRELATES 1605
Right Ventricular Anatomy 1605
Right Ventricular Function 1605
Pulmonary Vascular Anatomy 1606

PHYSIOLOGY OF THE PULMONARY CIRCULATION 1607
Pressure–Volume Relations 1607
Pressure–Flow Relations 1607
Effects of Alveolar Gas Tension on the Pulmonary Circulation 1608

ASSESSMENT OF PATIENTS WITH COR PULMONALE 1608

ACUTE COR PULMONALE 1610
Pathophysiology 1610
Treatment 1612
Right Ventricular Preload Augmentation 1612
Right Ventricular Afterload Reduction 1613
Maintenance of Aortic Pressure 1613

CHRONIC COR PULMONALE 1613
Causes and Pathophysiology 1613
Pulmonary Vascular Disorders 1613
Disorders of the Neuromuscular Apparatus and Chest Wall 1613
Disorders of Ventilatory Control 1614
Upper Airway Obstruction 1615
Restrictive Lung Diseases 1615
Chronic Obstructive Pulmonary Disease 1615
Therapy 1617
Oxygen 1617
Digitalis 1619
Theophylline 1619
Beta-Adrenergic Agonists 1619
Vasodilators 1619
Phlebotomy 1620

REFERENCES 1620

Acute cor pulmonale is defined as right heart strain or overload secondary to acute pulmonary hypertension, often due to massive pulmonary embolism.[1–3] *Chronic cor pulmonale* is characterized by hypertrophy and dilatation of the right ventricle (RV) secondary to the pulmonary hypertension caused by disease of the pulmonary parenchyma and/or pulmonary vascular system between the origins of the main pulmonary artery and the entry of the pulmonary veins into the left atrium.[1–4] In this chapter, the anatomical and pathophysiological correlates of acute and chronic cor pulmonale are reviewed and the relevant principles of clinical management are discussed. Particular emphasis is given throughout the chapter to COPD. Primary pulmonary hypertension and pulmonary thromboembolism, two important causes of cor pulmonale, are discussed in Chapters 27 and 48, respectively.

ETIOLOGIES

The most frequent cause of *chronic* cor pulmonale in North America is chronic obstructive pulmonary disease (COPD) resulting from chronic obstructive bronchitis or emphysema, whereas the most important cause of *acute* cor pulmonale is pulmonary thromboembolism.[1–5] In addition to COPD and thromboembolic disease, a number of other disorders may cause cor pulmonale (Table 47–1).[5] Although many disorders may lead to cor pulmonale, the major mechanisms resulting in pulmonary hypertension are relatively few.[5] Alveolar hypoxia secondary to hypoventilation is the primary cause of pulmonary hypertension in neuromuscular diseases, thoracic cage deformities, and disorders of ventilatory control. Alveolar hypoxia is a potent stimulus for acute pulmonary vasoconstriction.[5] In addition, sustained vasoconstriction resulting from chronic hypoxia leads to structural alterations in the pulmonary vasculature that contribute to pulmonary hypertension.[6] Lung diseases, such as emphysema and interstitial fibrotic disorders, cause pulmonary hypertension not only through hypoxia but also by frank anatomical destruction of vessels.[5] Pulmonary hypertension frequently is observed in patients with the adult respiratory distress syndrome (ARDS), even after correction of arterial hypoxemia.[7,8] The mechanisms for this may include endothelial cell edema, diffuse microembolism or thrombosis, and fibrotic microvascular obliteration.[5] Primary disorders of the pulmonary circulation produce pulmonary hypertension through narrowing or obstruction of vessels.[5]

Because the normal pulmonary circulation is a low-resistance, high-compliance system with substantial reserve, considerable abnormality must occur before significant and sustained pulmonary hypertension develops.[5] This explains why the clinical appearance of cor pulmonale heralds a poor prognosis in chronic lung diseases,[9–12] primary pulmonary hypertension,[13] and neuromuscular disorders.[3]

The physiological significance of the muscular left ventricle (LV) and its role in human disease have long been appreciated. The thin-walled right ventricle (RV), however, has sometimes been considered a redundant, almost unnecessary, chamber (Fig. 47–1). This view originated from ani-

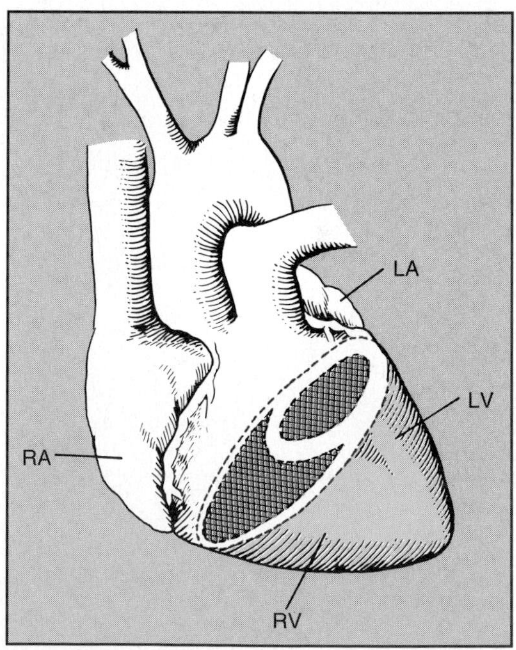

FIGURE 47–1. The anatomical relationship of the right ventricle (RV) to the left ventricle (LV), showing the globular shape of the LV and the half-moon shape of the RV. (Modified from Guyton, A. C.: The pulmonary circulation. *In* Guyton, A. C.: *Human Physiology and Mechanisms of Disease.* 4th ed. Philadelphia, W. B. Saunders Company, 1987, 124.)

* Portions of this chapter have been reproduced from the chapter on Cor Pulmonale in the 4th edition of *Heart Disease* with the gracious permission of its authors, McFadden and Braunwald.

TABLE 47–1 ETIOLOGY OF PULMONARY HEART DISEASE

I. DISEASES AFFECTING THE PULMONARY VASCULATURE
- A. Primary diseases of the arterial wall
  - (1) Primary pulmonary hypertension
  - (2) Granulomatous pulmonary arteritis
  - (3) Toxin-induced pulmonary hypertension
    - a. Aminorex fumarate
    - b. Intravenous drug abuse
  - (4) Chronic liver disease
  - (5) Peripheral pulmonic stenosis
- B. Thrombotic disorders
  - (1) Sickle cell diseases
  - (2) Pulmonary microthrombi
- C. Embolic disorders
  - (1) Thromboembolism
  - (2) Tumor embolism
  - (3) Other embolism (amniotic fluid, air)
  - (4) Schistosomiasis and other parasitic diseases

II. PRESSURES ON PULMONARY ARTERIES BY MEDIASTINAL TUMORS, ANEURYSMS, GRANULOMATA, OR FIBROSIS

III. DISEASES OF THE NEUROMUSCULAR APPARATUS AND CHEST WALL
- A. Neuromuscular weakness
- B. Kyphoscoliosis
- C. Thoracoplasty
- D. Pleural fibrosis
- E. Sleep apnea syndromes
- F. Idiopathic hypoventilation

IV. DISEASES AFFECTING AIR PASSAGES OF THE LUNG AND ALVEOLI
- A. Chronic obstructive pulmonary diseases
- B. Cystic fibrosis
- C. Congenital developmental defects
- D. Infiltrative or granulomatous diseases
  - (1) Idiopathic pulmonary fibrosis
  - (2) Sarcoidosis
  - (3) Pneumoconiosis
  - (4) Scleroderma
  - (5) Mixed connective tissue disease
  - (6) Systemic lupus erythematosus
  - (7) Rheumatoid arthritis
  - (8) Polymyositis
  - (9) Eosinophilic granuloma
  - (10) Malignant infiltration
  - (11) Radiation
- E. Upper airways obstruction
- F. Pulmonary resection
- G. High-altitude disease

Adapted from Rubin, L. J.: Introduction. Pulmonary Heart Disease. Boston, Martinus Nijhoff, 1984, p. 1.

mal studies conducted in the 1940's and 1950's, the results of which showed that the contractile function of the free wall of the RV is not required to maintain circulation over the short term, either at rest or under stress. Interest in the structure and function of the RV, however, has revived, primarily because RV dysfunction has been found to be critical in such important cardiopulmonary disorders as pulmonary embolism, COPD, ARDS, and coronary artery disease (RV ischemia or infarction).

ANATOMICAL AND PATHOPHYSIOLOGICAL CORRELATES

RIGHT VENTRICULAR ANATOMY

In humans born at or near sea level, the RV is the dominant chamber for the first 3 months of life. During this time, the RV is larger and heavier and has a greater end-diastolic volume than the LV.[3,14–18] The LV, however, gradually becomes dominant, and in adults, the RV is relatively thin walled and crescent shaped (Fig. 47–1).[3] At high altitude, the degree of RV predominance is greater at birth and after 3 months than that at lower altitude, and the relative RV enlargement may persist through the first decade of life.[17] Among adult natives living above 12,000 feet, 93 per cent showed some degree of RV enlargement in a necropsy series.[19] These morphological findings reflect the hemodynamic characteristics of persons living at high altitude and can be related to the degree of pulmonary artery hypertension.[20]

RIGHT VENTRICULAR HYPERTROPHY. The presence of RV hypertrophy and its severity have traditionally been determined by measuring ventricular weight and wall thickness.[3] However, many investigators believe that measuring the thickness of the ventricular wall is not sufficiently precise. Fulton et al.[21] have proposed widely used weight criteria, according to which the RV is dissected free and weighed, and the LV and the septum are weighed together. Right ventricular weight is then determined absolutely or relative to the weight of the LV plus the septum (S): (LV + S)/RV. By these criteria, a heart is considered normal only if the total ventricular weight is less than 250 gm, the free wall of the RV weighs less than 65 gm in men and 50 gm in women, and the value of (LV + S)/RV is between 2.3 and 3.3. If LV hypertrophy also is present, the ratio may be within normal limits or even raised. Using this method, Mitchell and colleagues[22] found that the upper limits of normal (defined by the mean plus two standard deviations) in men 40 years of age or older at death were 69 gm for the RV and 203 gm for the LV plus the septum. In this study, RV thickness was a relatively poor index of hypertrophy.

Other investigators have determined muscle fiber size morphometrically and found the distribution of myocardial fiber diameters to be uniform, with a distinct bell-shaped distribution for the RV, LV, and septum.[23] In pure RV hypertrophy, the distribution shifts so that the mean diameter of the muscle fibers from the RV exceeds that of the septum or normal LV.[3] An enlarged RV in cor pulmonale is shown in Figure 47–2.

Right Ventricular Function

Because RV hypertrophy is usually associated with long-standing pulmonary hypertension, an analogy often has been made between the LV in systemic hypertension and the RV in pulmonary hypertension.[3] The structure and the pumping action of the two ventricles are essentially the same before birth, and therefore the differences in the adult have been attributed to the flow resistance in the respective circulation.[24] As noted, the normal adult RV is thin walled and crescent shaped (see Fig. 47–1); its pumping action is similar to that of a bellows working in series with a low-pressure circuit in contrast to the concentric contraction of the LV.[25–27] The thin-walled RV is more compliant than the LV[27] and, compared with the LV, is better able to handle an increase in volume than in pressure. This latter finding was derived primarily from animal studies that measured the effects of increasing preload and afterload on RV and LV function.[28–31]

In the left panel of Figure 47–3, stroke volume is plotted as a function of various afterloads produced experimentally by constricting the main pulmonary artery and aorta in the dog.[28,29] Small increases in pulmonary artery pressure are associated with sharp decreases in right ventricular stroke volume. In contrast, the LV, which normally works against high initial pressure, maintains stroke volume despite substantial increases in systemic arterial pressure. The right panel of the figure shows the effects of increasing preload. These ventricular function curves were obtained by volume infusions in the atria of dogs.[31] The respective ventricular stroke work differs markedly as right and left atrial pressures are increased. For a fourfold increase in filling pres-

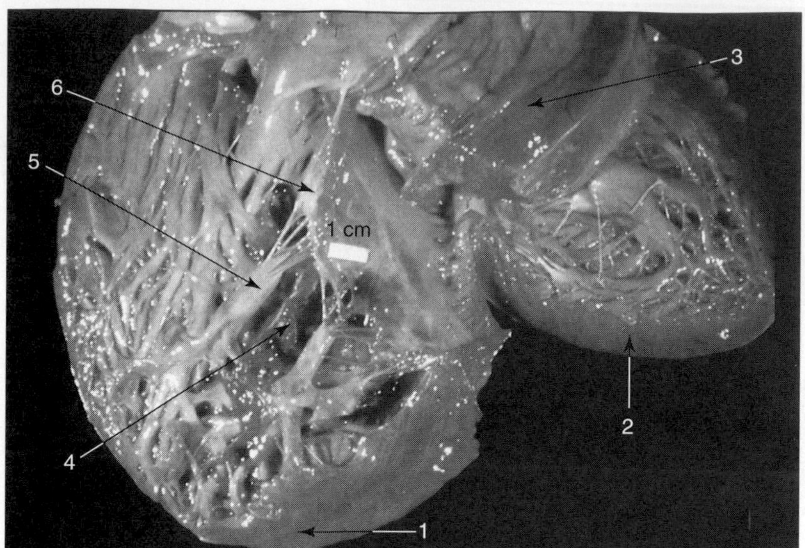

FIGURE 47–2. Heart specimen illustrating right ventricular enlargement and hypertrophy in a patient with cor pulmonale. (Number Key: 1, right ventricular free wall; 2, left ventricular free wall; 3, interventricular septum; 4, right ventricular chamber; 5, right ventricular papillary muscle; and 6, tricuspid valve.) The right ventricular free wall is markedly thickened, approximately 2.5 cm at widest diameter (normal ≤ 5 mm). Also, the right ventricular chamber and papillary muscles are significantly larger than the left ventricular chamber and papillary muscles. (From Matthay, R. A., and Berger, H. J.: Right and left ventricular performance in chronic obstructive pulmonary disease. Med. Clin. North Am. *65*:489, 1981.)

sure (e.g., from 5 to 20 cm H_2O), the increase in left ventricular work was about five times that of the right.

In response to chronic pressure loads, the structure, mass, and functional characteristics of the RV change significantly. The rate of such changes in humans, and the pressure needed to produce them, are unknown. Animal studies show that structure and function can change rapidly after experimental outflow tract obstruction. Spann et al.[32] observed a 71 per cent increase in RV weight in cats 2 days after the pulmonary artery was banded, and, within a month, RV weight had risen by 150 per cent of control. The response may not be as rapid in humans, but it is qualitatively similar.

The lumen of the main pulmonary artery can be reduced acutely by 60 to 80 per cent before aortic pressure declines as a consequence of a fall in cardiac output.[33–35] Because these experiments did not consider the effects of neurohumoral compensation that supports the systemic circulation, the impression has arisen that the acute RV response is abrupt and absolute. However, as suggested in Figure 47–3, RV decompensation is continuous.[28,31] At RV systolic pressures of 60 to 80 mm Hg, RV dilatation and failure occur with systemic hypotension and hypoperfusion.[36] The rate and absolute extent of outflow tract obstruction at which these changes develop can be greatly amplified or attenuated by respectively decreasing or increasing right coronary artery blood flow.[36] The effect of coronary artery blood flow in acute right heart failure in humans has not been determined.[3]

Pulmonary Vascular Anatomy

WALL STRUCTURE. From the pulmonary artery distally toward the capillaries, four structural regions can be identified: elastic, muscular, partially muscular, and nonmuscular[37] (see Fig. 25–16, p. 798). The main pulmonary artery and the first five generations are elastic, although less so than the aorta and major systemic arteries. These vessels have more than five elastic laminae in their media and in adults are more than 2000 μm in diameter. In the axial pathway, the next three generations are transitional.

Muscular arteries have two to five elastic laminae and a continuous muscle coat. These arteries constitute the majority of vessels in the lung and in adults range from 150 to 2000 μm in diameter. The medial muscle coat is much thinner than the arterioles in the systemic circulation. These vessels give way to partially muscular arteries in which the muscle is arranged in a spiral, so that in cross section it looks like a crescent, with the rest of the wall being like a capillary. Nonmuscular arteries are larger than capillaries, ranging from 30 to 75 μm in diameter in adults. Partially muscular and nonmuscular arteries lie within the alveolar units in adults. The smallest muscular and partially muscular arteries are probably the resistance arteries.[37]

Although the sizes of arteries that accompany conducting airways such as lobar bronchi vary greatly, arteries that follow the respiratory bronchi and alveolar ducts are muscular or partially muscular.[37] The implications for function of these observations are several-fold. Gas exchange occurs in respiratory bronchi and alveolar ducts through the arteries that accompany these structures.[38] In addition, hypoxia

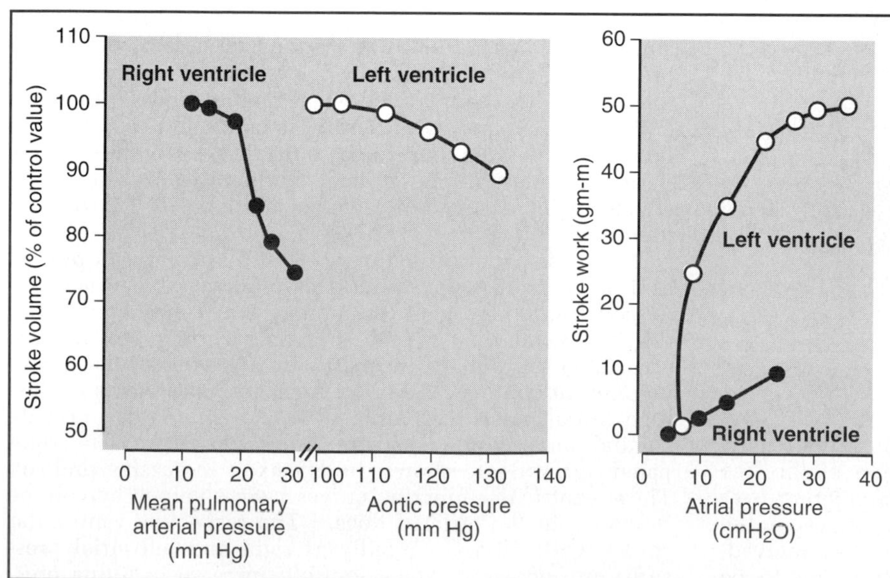

FIGURE 47–3. Effects of increasing preload and afterload on right and left ventricular function. The data in the left panel were obtained by constricting the main pulmonary artery and aorta in dogs. The right panel demonstrates the effect in increasing preloads.

induces constriction of the muscular arteries; therefore, this area of the lung evidently actively controls pulmonary blood flow. Furthermore, because the spiral of muscle in the partially muscular arteries is continuous with the muscle encircling the larger vessels, retrograde propagation of the hypoxic stimulus can occur in the intracellular pathways of the muscle syncytium,[37] thereby producing a wider and more severe response.

INNERVATION. Although the pulmonary circulation has both adrenergic and cholinergic fibers, they are sparse compared with those innervating systemic vessels of similar size, and they tend to be concentrated in the larger vessels at the hilum.[38,39] Evidence suggests that these nerves contain other neurotransmitters such as vasoactive intestinal peptide in parasympathetic fibers; substance P, the neurokinins, and calcitonin gene-related peptide in sensory fibers; and neuropeptide tyrosine in sympathetic fevers.[40] Some studies in children indicate that the predominant neuropeptide transmitter is tyrosine and that, during growth and development, the relative density of nerve fibers increases only in the arteries of the respiratory unit.[40] In this work, pulmonary hypertension in infants was associated with premature innervation of these arteries.

In summary, the structure of the pulmonary circulation conforms to its hemodynamics.[3] The thin-walled, sparsely innervated vessels that contain relatively small amounts of smooth muscle (see Fig. 25–15, p. 797) do not favor the development of marked vasomotor responses, and vasoconstriction alone is not sufficient to overload the RV to the point of producing acute cor pulmonale.[41] Therefore, in acute cor pulmonale, mechanical obstruction of the pulmonary circulation can be inferred, and in chronic cor pulmonale, structural alterations in the pulmonary vascular bed must be present.

PHYSIOLOGY OF THE PULMONARY CIRCULATION

(See also Chap. 25)

Most of the pulmonary vascular bed is contained within the parenchyma of the lung, and therefore the vessels are subject to external distending and compressive forces that are independent of any intrinsic properties of the vessels themselves.[3] In addition, the pulmonary circulation is in series with a pump that can develop only low pressures, yet it must accommodate the entire cardiac output under all states of physical activity.[3] Consequently, it must adjust to wide variations in blood flow without much change in pressure so as not to overload the RV.

PRESSURE–VOLUME RELATIONS. The pulmonary circulation was once thought to be highly elastic in order to accommodate increases in cardiac output, thus preventing an increase in pulmonary artery pressure in high-flow states.[42,43] Measurement of the compliance of the pulmonary vascular bed, however, has shown that it is significantly stiffer than its systemic counterpart[44,45] and that the large pulmonary vessels can accept only small increases in blood volume.[46–49] The increased blood flow and blood volume are primarily accommodated by the recruitment of previously unperfused vessels.[44,50] Morphological evidence suggests that, with an increase in pulmonary blood flow, both recruitment and distention occur and the transmural pressures to which the vessel is subjected determine which one predominates.[51] Recruitment appears to predominate in superior portions of the lung where the vessels are collapsed or where alveolar pressure is greater than pulmonary venous pressure, whereas distention is more important in dependent portions of the lung where pulmonary venous pressure is greater than alveolar pressure.

PRESSURE–FLOW RELATIONS. The pressure–flow relationship of the pulmonary circulation in normal humans is hyperbolic, with large changes in pulmonary blood flow being associated with small elevations in pulmonary artery pressure (Fig. 47–4*A*). The net result is that as flow increases, pulmonary vascular resistance decreases (Fig. 47–4*B*).[41] Consequently, whether distention or recruitment occurs, a low-pressure circuit is maintained during increased blood flow.

A U-shaped curve describes pulmonary vascular resistance as a function of lung volume (Fig. 47–4*C*).[48] At the extremes of lung volume at full inflation and deflation, vascular resistance is high, and it reaches its nadir at about the resting end-expiratory position (i.e., at functional residual capacity).

These findings can be explained by morphological changes in the alveolar and intrapulmonic but extra-alveolar vessels in response to the transmural pressures to which they are exposed.[3] The dimensions of the pulmonary vessels reflect the forces exerted on them by the pulmonary parenchyma. At low lung volumes, the extra-alveolar vessels tend to collapse because radial traction no longer supports them. Simultaneously, the alveolar vessels are pulled open by the increased recoil forces generated by the tendency of the alveoli to become smaller. As the lung is inflated above functional residual capacity, the larger vessels tend to be pulled open, but the resistance of the small vessels progressively increases as they are squeezed and lengthened by enlarging alveoli. In addition, changes in alveolar pressure also can dynamically affect the lumina of small vessels. When alveolar pressure is positive, as it is during expiration or with the Valsalva maneuver, vessels are compressed, whereas when pressure is negative, as it is during inspiration or with the Mueller maneuver, small

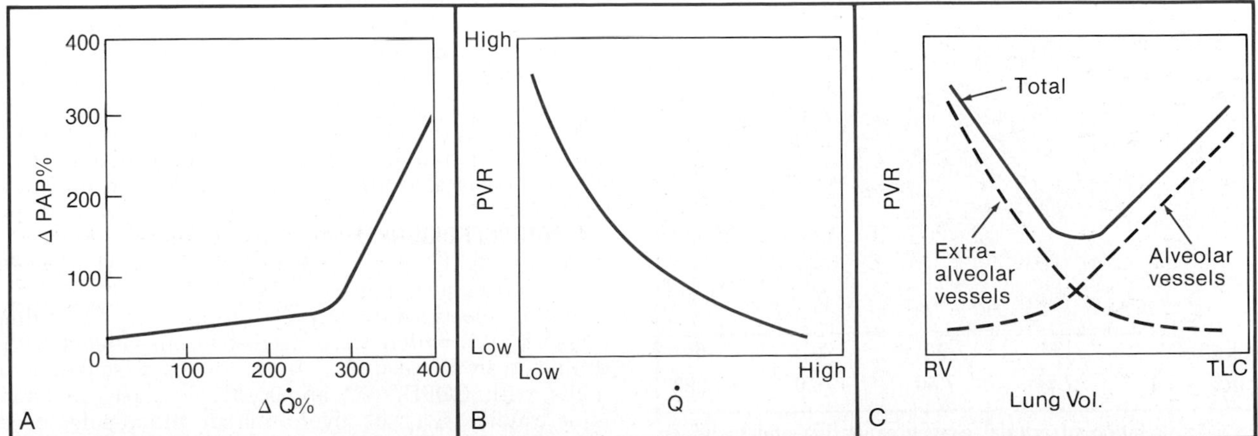

FIGURE 47–4. Some aspects of pulmonary vascular physiology. *A,* Pressure-flow relation. *B,* Resistance-flow relation. *C,* Pulmonary vascular resistance (PVR) as a function of lung volume for the total system and for extraalveolar and alveolar vessels. ΔPAP = percentage of change in mean pulmonary artery pressure from control; ΔQ̇ = percentage of change in cardiac output; 100 = normal cardiac output; RV = residual volume; TLC = total lung capacity.

vessels are distended. It is therefore apparent that alveolar pressure can play a crucial role in determining the distribution of pulmonary blood flow and, accordingly, gas exchange.[3]

Effects of Alveolar Gas Tension on the Pulmonary Circulation

HYPOXIA. The most potent stimulus for pulmonary vasoconstriction is alveolar hypoxia[38,52–54] (see Fig. 25–2, p. 782). Although acute vasoconstriction appears when the alveolar pO_2 is 60 mm Hg or lower, this response is found only in about two-thirds of normal subjects.[55] The subjects who respond to hypoxemia with pulmonary vasoconstriction may be prone to chronic cor pulmonale if they develop a disease that interferes with effective alveolar ventilation.[56] The pulmonary constrictor response to hypoxia appears to be locally mediated because it can be elicited in denervated lungs and isolated perfused lungs.

ACIDOSIS. Acidosis significantly increases pulmonary vascular resistance as well as acting synergistically with hypoxia.[57] In contrast, an increase in arterial pCO_2 seems to exert no direct effect but rather to operate by way of the induced increase in hydrogen-ion concentration. Hypoxia and acidemia frequently coexist, and their interaction, which is clinically important, follows a predictable pattern (Fig. 47–5). At minor degrees of oxygen unsaturation, pulmonary artery pressure is relatively insensitive to hydrogen-ion concentration but extremely sensitive to high levels of unsaturation. However, when the pH is high, the pressor effect of hypoxia is blunted.

Most studies indicate that the pulmonary vascular pressor response occurs in partially muscular arteries less than 200 μm in diameter.[37,52,58,59] The mechanism by which hypoxia causes pulmonary artery smooth muscle to constrict is unclear, but the likely alternatives are an indirect effect by which hypoxia causes endothelial cells to release eicosanoids or other cells in the pulmonary parenchyma to release vasoactive substances (e.g., histamine from mast cells) or a direct effect of hypoxia on pulmonary artery smooth muscle. Other influences may enhance hypoxic pulmonary vasoconstriction; for example, extrapulmonic reflexes or the adrenergic neurotransmitter norepinephrine may augment the pressor response.

CONSEQUENCES OF PULMONARY VASOCONSTRICTION. The mechanism that controls the resting tone of the pulmonary circulation is unknown. The smooth muscle and connective tissue elements in the walls of the vessels certainly contribute. The roles of other potential controlling factors have yet to be explored; these include the neuropeptides of the nonadrenergic noncholinergic nervous system or locally formed or circulating mediators such as the eicosanoids (prostacyclin, thromboxane, leukotrienes), catecholamines (epinephrine, norepinephrine), autocoids (histamine, bradykinin), and endothelial-derived relaxing and contrasting factors.[60]

Pulmonary vasoconstriction produces an acute elevation in pulmonary vascular pressure, and continuing constriction with pulmonary hypertension for even a few days is associated with structural changes in the vessels.[37] The lumen is narrowed by an increase in the thickness of the medial coat, endothelial swelling, muscular hypertrophy, and the appearance of muscle at more peripheral levels than normal. With continued insult, the cross-sectional area of the vascular bed is reduced in association with an increase in RV weight. These structural and functional changes occur with all forms of pulmonary hypertension, but the time sequences of development and ultrastructural patterns vary with different disease processes.

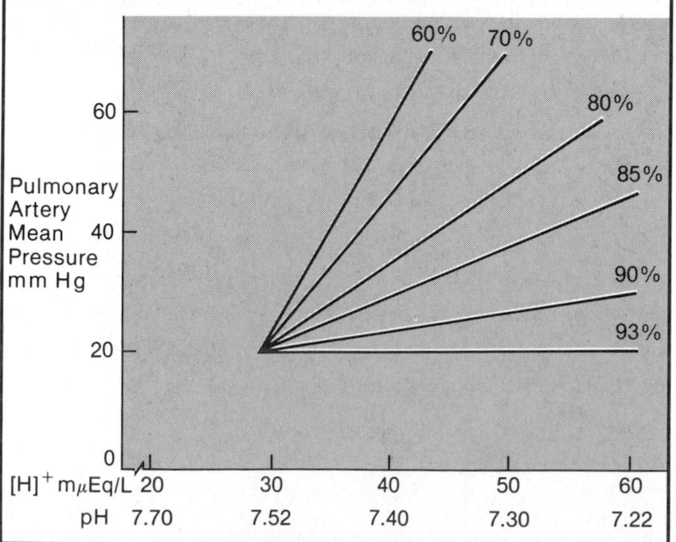

FIGURE 47–5. Relation of arterial oxygen saturation and hydrogen ion concentration to pulmonary artery pressure. (Reproduced from Enson, Y., et al.: The influence of hydrogen ion concentration and hypoxia on the pulmonary circulation. J. Clin. Invest. *43*:1146, 1964, by copyright permission of the American Society for Clinical Investigation.)

ASSESSMENT OF PATIENTS WITH COR PULMONALE

In patients with cor pulmonale, pulmonary hemodynamics and RV function are assessed by measuring pressure and flow, which requires the use of cardiac catheterization.[1] Because of the variable and irregular shape of the RV, even in normal subjects, measuring RV function and the chamber volumes is difficult.[1,61] Until recently, RV volume could be assessed only by contrast angiography,[1,62] an invasive technique that was not used widely in patients with cor pulmonale.[1] However, experience is now available with various noninvasive techniques including radionuclide ventriculography, echocardiography, and magnetic resonance imaging (MRI).

CLINICAL ASSESSMENT. The physical examination is insensitive for diagnosing cor pulmonale, especially in patients with COPD in whom hyperinflation of the chest usually obscures the typical signs of pulmonary hypertension or RV dysfunction.[1,3,63,64] For example, the intrathoracic pressure varies widely in such patients, making the jugular venous pressure difficult to assess. In addition, peripheral edema may be absent in patients with pulmonary artery hypertension or may be due to other causes such as hypoalbuminemia.[1] Other physical findings characteristic of cor pulmonale but not always present or frequently modified by hyperinflation include a systolic parasternal heave (indicating RV hypertrophy) and extra heart sounds or the murmur of tricuspid regurgitation (both suggesting RV dysfunction). Accentuation of the pulmonary component of the second heart sound, which usually suggests pulmonary hypertension, is also an insensitive finding in patients with COPD.[1]

ELECTROCARDIOGRAPHY (see also Chap. 4). Electrocardiography is highly specific but rather insensitive for detecting right ventricular hypertrophy.[1,65]

Classic electrocardiographic criteria for cor pulmonale (Table 47–2), which were derived from patients with congenital heart disease,[3,66,67] have not been sensitive in patients with COPD,[3,68,69] apparently because moderate RV hypertrophy is a late event in cor pulmonale, occurring only after prolonged dilatation of the RV.[70]

Assessing the effects of dynamic events on the electrocardiogram in 200 patients with COPD, Kilcoyn et al.[00] found that at least one of the following electrocardiographic changes occurred when arterial oxygen saturation fell

TABLE 47–2 ELECTROCARDIOGRAPHIC CHANGES IN COR PULMONALE

ECG CRITERIA FOR COR PULMONALE WITHOUT OBSTRUCTIVE DISEASE OF THE AIRWAYS*

1. Right-axis deviation with a mean QRS axis to the right of +110°
2. R/S amplitude ratio in $V_1 > 1$
3. R/S amplitude ratio in $V_6 < 1$
4. Clockwise rotation of the electrical axis
5. P-pulmonale pattern
6. S_1Q_3 or $S_1S_2S_3$ pattern
7. Normal voltage QRS

ECG CHANGES IN CHRONIC COR PULMONALE WITH OBSTRUCTIVE DISEASE OF THE AIRWAYS†

1. Isoelectric P waves in lead I or right-axis deviation of the P vector
2. P-pulmonale pattern (an increase in P-wave amplitude in II, III, AV_f)
3. Tendency for right-axis deviation of the QRS
4. R/S amplitude ratio in $V_6 < 1$
5. Low-voltage QRS
6. S_1Q_3 or $S_1S_2S_3$ pattern
7. Incomplete (and rarely complete) right bundle branch block
8. R/S amplitude ratio in $V_1 > 1$
9. Marked clockwise rotation of the electrical axis
10. Occasional large Q wave or QS in the inferior or mid-precordial leads, suggesting healed myocardial infarction

* Any one of the first three criteria suffices to raise suspicion of right ventricular hypertrophy. The diagnosis becomes more certain if two or more of these findings are present (2 and 7). The last four criteria commonly occur in cor pulmonale secondary to primary alveolar hypoventilation, interstitial diseases of the lung, or pulmonary vascular disease.

† The first seven criteria are suggestive but nonspecific; the last three are more characteristic of cor pulmonale in obstructive disease of the airways.

Reproduced with permission from Holford, F. D.: The electrocardiogram in lung disease. *In* Fishman, A. P. (ed.): Pulmonary Diseases and Disorders. New York, McGraw-Hill Book Co., 1980, p. 140.

below 85 per cent and mean pulmonary artery pressure rose to 25 mm Hg or greater: a rightward shift of the mean QRS axis of 30 degrees or more from its previous position; inverted, biphasic or flattened T waves in the precordial leads; depressed ST segments in leads II, III, and aV_f; and incomplete or complete right bundle branch block. These changes disappeared when arterial oxygen saturation increased. Transient T-wave changes in the right precordial leads and axis shifts to the right, which developed with only modest elevations in pulmonary artery pressure, persisted if pressure elevations were more severe and recurred frequently. If pulmonary function failed to improve, R-wave voltage increased in the right precordial leads and true right-axis deviation (a frontal plane axis greater than +90 degrees) developed. Increased R-wave voltage in the right precordial leads rarely returned to normal after improvement in arterial blood gases (Fig. 47–6).

In other studies of patients with chronic cor pulmonale, RV hypertrophy has been suggested by clockwise rotation, right-axis deviation, a qR pattern in aV_r, and electrocardiographic evidence of right atrial enlargement (P pulmonale) in that order.[3] In patients with COPD, the mean QRS axis is sometimes directed posteriorly, superiorly, and to the right with an apparent left-axis deviation in the standard limb leads.[3] This pattern, along with low voltage, has been associated most often with emphysema.[3] Electrocardiography is less accurate for detecting RV hypertrophy in patients with COPD than in patients with primary pulmonary artery hypertension. This is because COPD causes flattening of the diaphragm and hyperinflation of the lungs.[3,70]

CHEST RADIOGRAPHY (see also Chap. 7). The heart size may be normal on the plain chest radiograph in patients with cor pulmonale,[71] but in advanced disease, the heart may rotate counterclockwise and the aortic knob become less prominent.[71] Moreover, because the RV extends anteriorly and to the left, it infringes on the retrosternal space.[71,72] In the posteroanterior (PA) projection, the enlarged RV constitutes most of the left-heart border, forcing the LV to the rear and giving the left heart a lobular appearance.[71,72]

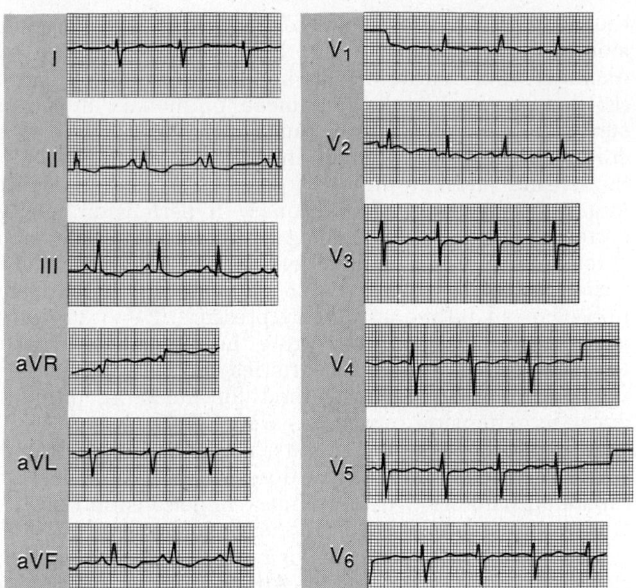

FIGURE 47–6. Electrocardiogram in a patient with emphysema and diffuse lung disease; there is right axis deviation, "P pulmonale," a qR pattern in V_1 and an rS pattern in V_6 (From McGowan, F. X., and Wagner, G. S.: The electrocardiogram in chronic lung disease. *In* Rubin, L. J. [ed.]: Pulmonary Heart Disease. Boston, Martinus Nijhoff, 1984, p. 117.)

On the plain chest radiograph, pulmonary hypertension is indicated by dilatation of the main pulmonary artery and its branches with concurrent underperfusion of the peripheral branches (Fig. 47–7).[71,73] In one study of patients with COPD, measurement of the widest diameter of the right and left descending pulmonary arteries on the plain chest ra-

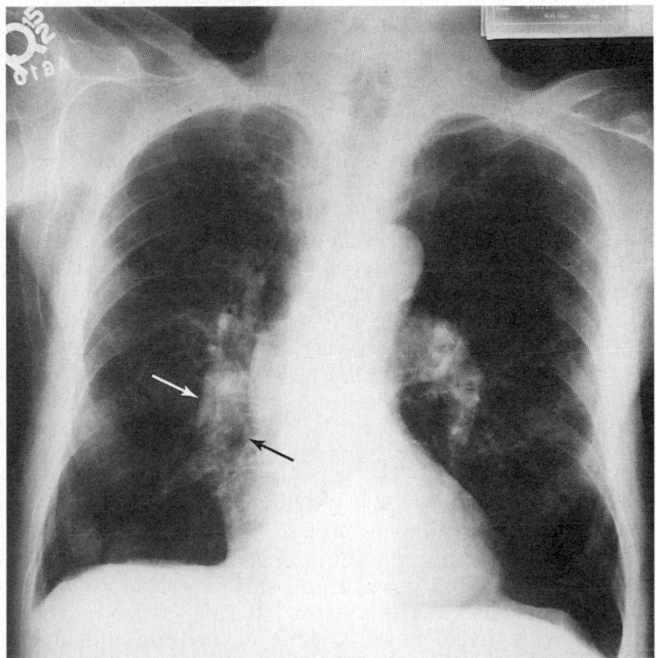

FIGURE 47–7. Upright chest radiograph in the posteroanterior (PA) projection in a man with severe COPD and pulmonary artery hypertension (mean pulmonary artery pressure = 47 mm Hg). The arrows indicate the widest dimensions of the enlarged right-descending pulmonary artery. Note also the enlarged main pulmonary artery in the central left hemithorax. An enlarged right-descending pulmonary artery (>15 mm) and an enlarged main pulmonary artery on the PA projection are indicative of pulmonary artery hypertension in patients with COPD.

diograph provided evidence of pulmonary artery hypertension (mean pulmonary artery pressure >20 mm Hg).[73] The diameter of both arteries was increased in 43 of 46 patients (93 per cent) with elevated mean pulmonary artery pressure. The right descending pulmonary artery was considered enlarged if it was more than 16 mm (Fig. 47–7),[74] and the left descending pulmonary artery if it was more than 18 mm.[73] Of 46 cases of pulmonary hypertension, 45 were correctly diagnosed by combining increased diameter measurements of the right and left descending pulmonary arteries. By these criteria, all 25 patients with a mild elevation of mean pulmonary artery pressure (21 to 30 mm Hg) were identified. Thus, measuring the diameter of right and left descending pulmonary arteries on the plain chest radiograph is a sensitive method for detecting pulmonary artery hypertension in patients with COPD.

In another study of patients with COPD,[75] a ≥20-mm widest diameter of the right-descending pulmonary artery separated patients with pulmonary hypertension from those without it. The hilar cardiothoracic ratio was an even more sensitive index: 95 per cent for pulmonary artery hypertension in patients with COPD.[68] Although these measures can indicate the presence of pulmonary artery hypertension, they cannot predict the precise pressures or the severity.

RADIONUCLIDE VENTRICULOGRAPHY (see also p. 299). Radionuclide ventriculography can measure the volume of the RV despite its variable and irregular shape.[76,77] An intravenous injection of technetium-99m-labeled erythrocytes or human serum albumin is detected in the central circuit by a gamma camera to produce a time-activity curve, either during the first pass of the radiolabeled tracer through the central circulation or by gating counts from several points throughout the cardiac cycle once the radiotracer has equilibrated in the blood pool.[1,76,78] Variation in the shape of the RV does not affect the measurement because radioactive counts are proportional to volume.[1]

Radionuclide ventriculography overcomes the problem of the variation in ventricular shape so problematic with contrast angiography and appears to be ideal for assessing RV function.[1,79–82] In patients with pulmonary hypertension, especially those with COPD, increases in pulmonary vascular resistance and pulmonary artery pressure are fairly accurately reflected in RV performance on radionuclide ventriculography.[76,82,83] In patients with COPD, the pulmonary artery pressure correlates inversely with the RV ejection fraction (RVEF).[82,84] Moreover, in one study, RVEF was abnormal in all patients with cor pulmonale due to COPD.[76] RVEF of less than or equal to 40 per cent on first-pass study indicates pulmonary arterial hypertension in patients with COPD.[76,83] Therefore, abnormal RVEF can help to identify patients with COPD who have pulmonary hypertension. RV performance on radionuclide angiocardiography can also be used to assess the efficacy of therapy (oxygen, vasodilators) in augmenting RVEF.[82]

THALLIUM IMAGING. Thallium-201 myocardial scintigraphy has been used to diagnose RV hypertrophy in patients with pulmonary artery hypertension.[1,85–90] Regional myocardial blood flow as well as myocardial mass determine the distribution of the radiotracer.[80] The large LV can be clearly visualized at rest, but the RV is usually not evident.[80] In one study, thallium imaging was 73 per cent sensitive for diagnosing RV pressure overload in 46 patients with COPD.[89] The clearest image usually occurs in patients with the highest RV systolic pressure and highest pulmonary vascular resistance, suggesting a correlation between RV hypertrophy and the degree of visualization.[80,90] However, thallium-201 scintigraphy is qualitative rather than quantitative, and because it offers no advantage over echocardiography, it has not been widely used clinically.[1]

ECHOCARDIOGRAPHY (see also Chap. 3). Doppler echocardiography has improved the assessment of pulmonary artery pressure.[1,91–99] The mean right atrial pressure and the peak systolic pressure gradient between the RV and the right atrium must be measured and the results added to estimate peak systolic pulmonary artery pressure.[1] The height of the jugular venous pulse is used to estimate the right atrial pressure.[1]

The tricuspid valve regurgitant jet can be assessed by Doppler echocardiography to measure the right ventricular-atrial gradient.[1,100,101] Tricuspid regurgitation occurs in normal subjects[1,102] and in patients with COPD.[1,101,103] By augmenting the signal with an intravenous infusion of saline, the quality of the signal to detect tricuspid regurgitation using continuous-wave Doppler echocardiography can be improved.[1,104,105] With the modified Bernoulli equation ($P = 4V^2$), using the peak velocity of the tricuspid regurgitant jet (V), peak pressure difference between the RV and atrium (P) can be calculated.[1,106] The systolic pulmonary artery pressure can be calculated, as stated above, by adding this pressure gradient to the mean right atrial pressure.[1,106]

Although continuous-wave Doppler echocardiography fails to produce an adequate assessment in 35 per cent of patients, even with intravenous saline contrast,[1,106] pulsed-wave Doppler echocardiography is even more sensitive for detecting tricuspid insufficiency.[1,92] In one study,[92] systolic pulmonary artery pressure could be measured in 91 per cent of patients with COPD. Moreover, the pulsed-wave Doppler echocardiographic technique can be used to assess changes in pulmonary artery pressure during exercise.[1,92] Cardiac catheterization results have been compared with those using echocardiographic measurements of pulmonary artery pressure and showed good correlations,[1,91–99] including in patients with COPD.[1,91]

The difficulty in differentiating the RV wall from its surrounding structures limits the use of echocardiography for detecting RV hypertrophy.[1] Echocardiographically measured RV wall thickness has correlated poorly with RV weight determined at autopsy.[1,107,108]

Unlike radionuclide ventriculography, echocardiography cannot readily show changes in RV function in patients with COPD and pulmonary arterial hypertension.[1] For a qualitative assessment, however, the position and the curvature of the interventricular septum give an indication of RV afterload.[1] Although the interventricular septum moves to the left during systolic ejection and to the right during diastolic filling in the normal heart, in patients with RV volume overload, this pattern reverses during cardiac ejection and filling.[1,109] Moreover, RV pressure overload displaces the septum further toward the LV.[1]

MAGNETIC RESONANCE IMAGING (see also Ch. 10). MRI produces the best images of the RV and is therefore considered by some authorities to be the gold standard for measuring ventricular dimensions.[1,110,111] Although MRI does not impose a radiation burden on the patient and is not invasive, it is expensive and is available only in specialized centers.[1] The RV free-wall volume determined by MRI correlates with both the pulmonary artery pressure ($r = 0.72$, $P < 0.01$) and the pulmonary vascular resistance ($r = 0.65$, $P < 0.01$) in patients with COPD.[111] In addition to being the best method for measuring RV dimensions,[111,112] MRI can be used to define RV hypertrophy in patients with COPD and to study the effects of therapy.[1,113,114]

ACUTE COR PULMONALE

Pathophysiology

RIGHT VENTRICULAR RESPONSE TO ACUTE PULMONARY HYPERTENSION. The foundation for the study of RV response to acute pulmonary hypertension was primarily established in animal experiments.[115] Figure 47–8 shows changes in mean systemic arterial pressure, mean pulmonary artery pressure, mean RV pressure, and mean right atrial pressure as the pulmonary artery of the dog is progressively constricted during a 4- to 5-minute period.[116] In response, the RV increased pressure and sustained cardiac output until the circulation suddenly and rapidly collapsed. When systemic pressure dropped below a critical value of about 60 mm Hg, progressive circulatory collapse ensued, even if the degree of pulmonary artery constriction remained constant. This finding, which has been reproduced by other investigators, suggests that acute increases in pressure load on the RV progress until a point at which a physiological "vicious circle" produces circulatory collapse.[115]

THE ROLE OF MYOCARDIAL ISCHEMIA. RV ischemia is likely a limiting factor in response to acute pressure

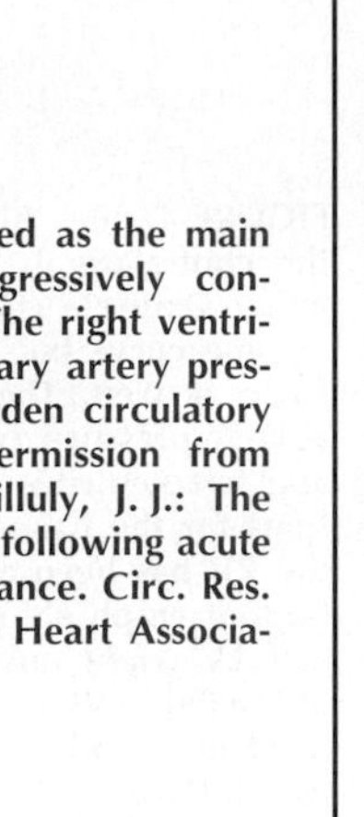

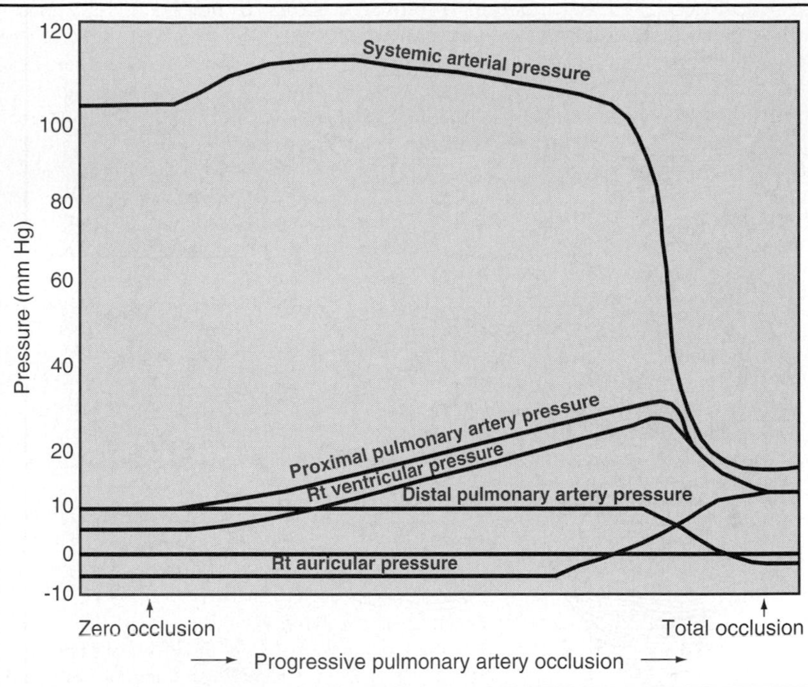

FIGURE 47–8. Mean pressures observed as the main pulmonary artery of the dog is progressively constricted over a 4- to 5-minute period. The right ventricle is unable to generate mean pulmonary artery pressures greater than 40 mm Hg, and sudden circulatory collapse occurs. (Reproduced with permission from Guyton, A. C., Lindsey, A. W., and Gilluly, J. J.: The limits of right ventricular compensation following acute increase in pulmonary circulatory resistance. Circ. Res. *2*:326, 1954. Copyright 1954 American Heart Association.)

load.[115,117] The right coronary artery, which supplies the RV free wall and a portion of the interventricular septum, originates in the aorta, and this fact may partially explain the frequent observation that LV function and systemic arterial pressure help determine whether the RV can continue to function despite pulmonary hypertension.[115,117]

Brooks et al.[118] showed that dogs with an acutely occluded right coronary artery had a diminished RV response to increased pressure load. As pulmonary artery pressure was increased above normal, cardiac output and aortic pressure fell and RV pressure rose more rapidly than in normal dogs. Such decompensation was reversible by perfusing the right coronary artery with higher than normal pressures. Spotnitz and colleagues[119] found that occluding the descending aorta with a balloon catheter reversed otherwise inexorable and fatal circulatory collapse in dogs with experimentally induced pulmonary embolism. The circulatory collapse was probably prevented by increased proximal aortic pressure and enhanced right coronary artery perfusion, although coronary blood flow was not measured.

RIGHT CORONARY ARTERY PERFUSION. Other studies in experimental animals directly assessed right coronary perfusion during progressive pulmonary hypertension and subsequent right ventricular failure.[120–123] Fixler et al.[120] and Cooper et al.[122] found that dogs with a degree of RV hypertension that leads to sudden circulatory collapse had inadequate right coronary blood flow relative to myocardial oxygen requirement (estimated from the RV tension-time index). Manohar et al.[121] caused RV pressure overload in pigs by inflating a cuff around the pulmonary artery trunk. By adjusting the degree of pulmonary artery constriction, they maintained a condition of RV dysfunction (a 30 per cent fall in cardiac output and a 15-mm Hg decrease in mean aortic pressure) without inducing sudden progressive circulatory collapse. Total blood flow to the RV free wall was markedly increased (91 per cent) over control conditions, despite a reduction in right coronary driving pressure (mean aortic pressure minus mean right ventricular pressure), indicating compensatory coronary vasodilation. Furthermore, infusion of adenosine (a vasodilator) increased right coronary flow. This occurred despite a further decrease in mean aortic pressure and therefore a decrease in right coronary driving pressure, indicating that there was coronary vasodilator reserve.

In similar experiments, Vlahakes et al.[123] constricted the pulmonary artery beyond the maximum pressure that could be generated by the RV (systolic pressure about 65 mm Hg), and irreversible circulatory collapse occurred. The point of collapse correlated with the sudden development of RV ischemia, manifested by loss of the normal endocardial-epicardial-blood-flow ratio, abnormal myocardial levels of metabolic markers (adenosine triphosphate, creatine kinase, lactate, and pyruvate), and loss of coronary vasodilator reserve. Infusion of phenylephrine after the onset of RV failure improved systolic function and alleviated the manifestations of ischemia. This effect was likely due to an increase in central aortic pressure and therefore a higher right coronary driving pressure.

Other investigators[124,125] showed in the dog that systemic infusion of norepinephrine, which increased aortic pressure, reversed RV failure and shock in acute pulmonary embolism. In these experiments, vasoconstrictor therapy was more effective than either volume expansion or isoproterenol. The mechanism of the beneficial effect of norepinephrine was presumed to be improved right coronary perfusion and alleviation of myocardial ischemia.

In contrast to these studies, Scharf et al.[126] suggest that ischemia may not be necessary for RV failure secondary to afterload stress. In their study, dogs were subjected to graded occlusion of the pulmonary artery until the circulation failed. Measurement of intramyocardial pH did not indicate myocardial ischemia at either the highest tolerated degree of occlusion or the point of frank circulatory failure. However, occluding the descending aorta, with an increase in central aortic pressure, increased RV load tolerance without any detectable change in right coronary arterial inflow, RV contractility, or intramyocardial pH. The mechanism for this effect on RV function is unexplained, but increased diastolic and systolic tension of the fibers of the LV, which occurs after aortic occlusion, may assist the RV, which shares some fibers with the larger LV.

VENTRICULAR INTERACTION. The RV distension that sometimes occurs abruptly in acute pulmonary hypertension may affect the LV pressure–volume relationship, thus causing the ventricles to compete for space within the pericardium.[115,127–132] The result is a form of LV diastolic "tamponade"[115,133] (Fig. 47–9).

Stool et al.[130] measured the dimensional changes of the LV during acute pulmonary hypertension in the dog and found that LV volume decreased progressively beginning at mean pulmonary artery pressures above 30 mm Hg. The LV became distorted and the septal–lateral wall axis became disproportionately shortened at both end diastole and end systole. Heart rate increased to maintain cardiac output as LV stroke volume decreased with increased pulmonary pressure. At a mean pulmonary artery pressure of 60 mm Hg, end-diastolic volume of the LV was reduced by 30 per cent from control conditions. If mean pulmonary artery pressure was maintained at this level or increased, circulatory collapse occurred, presumably partially because of reduced LV output.

ACUTE RIGHT VENTRICULAR FAILURE. As shown in Figure 47–10, the pathophysiology of acute RV failure can be viewed as a vicious circle. In response to mild or moderate pressure loading, right coronary flow increases despite a decrease in right coronary artery driving pressure because compensatory dilation of the coronary artery reduces resistance to flow.[115,117] Systolic function of the RV may be maintained, in part, by an augmentation of preload or end-diastolic volume; however, marked RV distention has adverse effects including increased wall tension (oxygen demand), decreased LV compliance, and tricuspid regurgitation.[115,117] The latter two effects may decrease cardiac

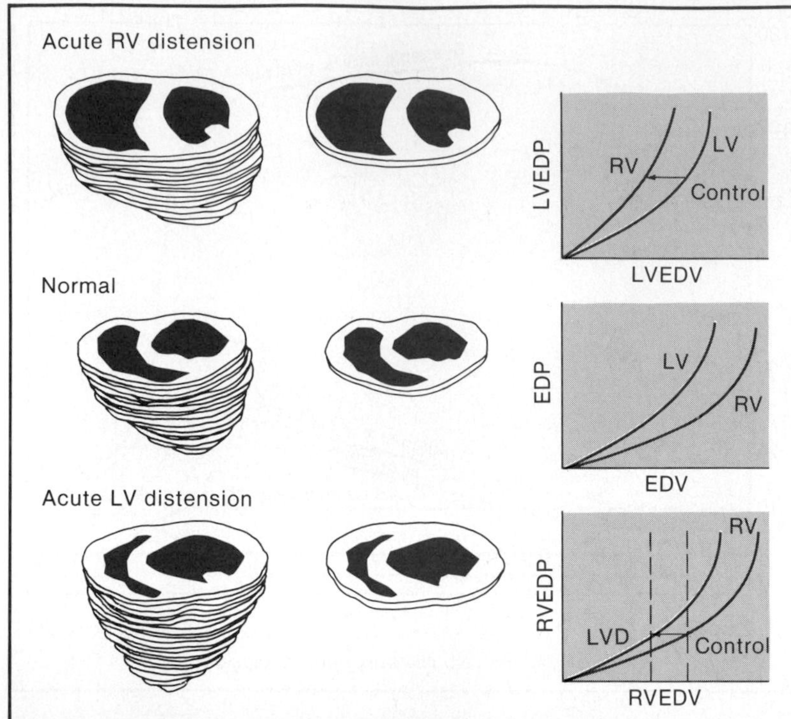

FIGURE 47–9. Alterations in compliance by distention of the contralateral ventricle. Note that acute distention of either ventricle changes not only that ventricle's pressure-volume curve but alters the compliance of the other ventricle as well. The middle graph shows the end-diastolic volume-pressure relationship for the right ventricle (RV) and left ventricle (LV). The top graph shows these relations for the LV with a normal RV *(right curve)* and after the RV has been acutely distended (RVD, *left curve*). The bottom graph shows the relations for the RV with a normal LV *(right curve)* and after the LV has been acutely distended (LVD). (From Weber, K. T., et al.: Contractile mechanics and interaction of the right and left ventricles. Am. J. Cardiol. *47*:686, 1981.)

output and aortic pressure, thereby further reducing right coronary driving pressure when the RV myocardium requires more oxygen. When vasodilatory reserve of the right coronary artery is exhausted, myocardial ischemia may ensue, with a resultant loss of RV function. At the critical point of RV decompensation, the circle irreversibly closes, and circulatory collapse rapidly follows.[115,117]

Treatment

Right Ventricular Preload Augmentation

Intravascular volume expansion helps maintain cardiac output in acute pulmonary hypertension.[115,134–137] For example, augmentation of RV preload enhances the circulation in acute pulmonary artery constriction[116] and in ARDS.[134] As venous volume increases, the systemic mean pressure rises, and peripheral edema is likely to develop.[115] If diuretic therapy is used to alleviate the edema, cardiac output may decline. Therefore, patients with reduced RV function may have to tolerate peripheral edema to maintain acceptable cardiac output.[115]

The use of RV preload augmentation to maintain cardiac output is theoretically limited. Increased RV volume potentially leads to reduced LV diastolic filling and tricuspid insufficiency. Although the RV is very compliant, increasing the volume also increases the wall tension and oxygen demand. In addition, the high systolic pressure necessary to overcome outflow resistance reduces right coronary artery driving pressure.

A number of studies[138–141] have shown that continued volume expansion against increasing pulmonary vascular resistance in anesthetized and ventilated dogs leads to circulatory deterioration. Molloy et al.[124] showed that volume expansion alone did not resuscitate dogs in shock caused by experimental pulmonary embolism. Sibbald et al.[134] showed that in ARDS patients with high pulmonary vascular resistance and very elevated RV volume, contractility was reduced compared with similar patients with lower pressure load and less chamber enlargement.

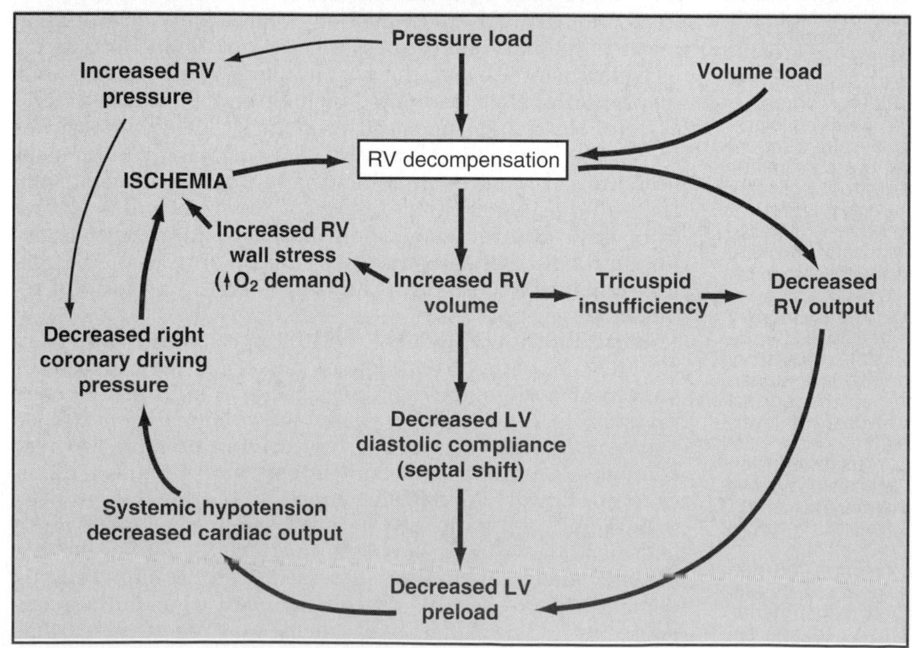

FIGURE 47–10. Pathophysiology of acute right ventricular failure: the vicious circle. (From Wiedemann, H. P., and Matthay, R. A.: Acute right heart failure. Crit. Care Clin. *1*:631, 1985.)

In patients with ARDS who have increased pulmonary capillary permeability, volume loading may aggravate pulmonary edema.[115] If RV volume is increased to the degree that LV diastolic compliance is altered, maintenance of LV preload, or volume, requires a higher filling pressure (wedge pressure); thus pulmonary edema worsens.[115] Therefore, in patients with RV dysfunction, volume expansion usually improves cardiac output initially, but volume expansion beyond a certain amount causes progressive deterioration of the circulation.[115] This condition should be suspected when volume infusion abruptly increases left- or right-sided filling pressure without improving cardiac output.[141]

Right Ventricular Afterload Reduction

OXYGEN THERAPY. Hypoxic pulmonary vasoconstriction may aggravate pulmonary hypertension in acute cor pulmonale, and therefore oxygen therapy may be beneficial by reducing right ventricular afterload. In patients with increased pulmonary vascular resistance due to obliterative anatomical lesions, supplemental oxygen therapy may be the only means of rapidly lowering afterload stress in acute RV failure.[115]

VASODILATOR THERAPY. Defining a beneficial hemodynamic response to pharmacological vasodilation in patients with pulmonary hypertension is complex.[115] Mean pulmonary artery pressure may remain unchanged as calculated pulmonary artery resistance decreases and cardiac output increases. In addition, vasodilator therapy may cause such adverse effects as systemic hypotension and decreased arterial oxygen saturation in patients with pulmonary hypertension.[142,143] Hypotension may result because most vasodilators affect the systemic circulation more than the pulmonary circulation.[115] In many patients with significant pulmonary hypertension and reduced right-sided cardiac output, systemic vasoconstriction helps maintain systemic arterial pressure. In such patients, selective dilation of the systemic vasculature may cause hypotension and precipitate RV failure (caused by decreased right coronary blood flow) and circulatory collapse.[117] Decreased arterial oxygen tension may result because of worsening ventilation-perfusion matching within the lung and increasing physiological shunting.[115,142,144]

Systemic vasodilator therapy for acute RV hypertension has been evaluated primarily in experimental studies of acute lung injury.[145–148] Vasodilators have been evaluated in this setting because patients with ARDS have elevated pulmonary vascular resistance, pulmonary hypertension, increased RV end-diastolic volume, and decreased RVEF.[134,149–152] In addition, in patients who survive ARDS, unlike nonsurvivors, the pulmonary vascular resistance usually progressively normalizes.[149] Nitric oxide (NO), a potent vasodilator, is becoming more widely used clinically. Inhaled NO has a rapid onset of action, and it is quickly inactivated after binding to hemoglobin. As a result, inhaled NO is a selective pulmonary vasodilator, and its vasodilator effect is greatest in well ventilated areas of the lung, thereby improving ventilation-perfusion matching. In patients with ARDS,[153] inhaled NO reduces pulmonary artery pressure and improves gas exchange. Controlled trials are in progress to test whether these physiological benefits improve outcome.

Maintenance of Aortic Pressure

The effective therapies for RV failure, including occlusion of the descending aorta,[115,126,154] intra-aortic balloon counterpulsation,[119] phenylephrine infusion,[155,156] and norepinephrine infusion,[124,140,141] all augment aortic pressure, which may be beneficial by increasing aortic pressure and thereby improving right coronary artery perfusion and alleviating myocardial ischemia.[126]

Therapies that may decrease systemic blood pressure should be used cautiously in patients with acute cor pulmonale.[115] For instance, vasodilators, by lowering aortic pressure, may adversely affect right coronary perfusion, an effect that might explain the instances of death after administration of hydralazine or diazoxide in patients with severe pulmonary hypertension.[142,143] Conversely, therapies directed at raising aortic pressure, such as norepinephrine infusion, should be considered if they are not contraindicated.

CHRONIC COR PULMONALE

Causes and Pathophysiology

The most common cause of chronic cor pulmonale in North America is COPD (emphysema, chronic obstructive bronchitis). The pathophysiology, natural history, and treatment of cor pulmonale secondary to COPD are discussed in detail in the later sections. Various other disorders associated with chronic cor pulmonale are shown in Table 47–1, and the pathogenetic mechanisms by which these disorders lead to pulmonary hypertension and cor pulmonale are summarized in Table 47–3.

Pulmonary Vascular Disorders

(See also Chap. 25)

Diseases such as primary pulmonary hypertension, which primarily affect the pulmonary vasculature and have little or no parenchymal involvement, clearly represent the pathogenetic progression from increased pulmonary vascular resistance resulting from gradual obliteration of the pulmonary vascular bed to pulmonary hypertension and RV overload. Patients with pulmonary vascular disorders invariably have dyspnea and very high pulmonary artery pressure, even though vital capacity and pulmonary gas exchange may be only minimally impaired.[157]

Disorders of the Neuromuscular Apparatus and Chest Wall

These disorders, which have in common the mechanical failure of the bellows apparatus, through weakness or paralysis of the respiratory muscles or distortion of the geometry of the thorax, can lead to cor pulmonale by failure of

TABLE 47–3 POTENTIAL PATHOGENETIC MECHANISMS LEADING TO PULMONARY ARTERIAL HYPERTENSION AND COR PULMONALE

MECHANISMS	EXAMPLE
Primary	
Anatomical decrease in cross-sectional area (vessel destruction; encroachment on lumen by hypertrophy) of the pulmonary resistance vessels	Interstitial fibrosis and granuloma
Vasoconstriction of pulmonary resistance vessels	Hypoxia and acidosis
Contributory	
Large increments in pulmonary blood flow	Exercise
Increased pressures on the left side of the heart and pulmonary veins	Left ventricular failure or pulmonary venoocclusive disease
Increased viscosity of the blood	Secondary polycythemia or chronic hypoxia
Unproved	
Compression of pulmonary resistance vessels by raised alveolar pressures in their vicinity	Asthmatic bronchitis
Bronchial arterial–pulmonary arterial anastomoses	Expanded bronchial circulation

From Fishman, A. P.: Pulmonary hypertension and cor pulmonale. *In* Fishman, A. P.: Pulmonary Diseases and Disorders, 2nd ed. New York, McGraw-Hill Book Co., 1988, p. 1001.

the neuromuscular apparatus, diaphragmatic paralysis, and distortion of the chest wall.[3]

FAILURE OF THE NEUROMUSCULAR APPARATUS. Weakness of the respiratory muscles can be caused by either generalized muscle diseases, such as myopathic infiltrating diseases or muscular dystrophy, or more commonly by such neurological disorders as a cord lesion at or below the third cervical vertebra, amyotrophic lateral sclerosis, myasthenia gravis, poliomyelitis, or Guillain-Barré syndrome.[3,157,158] These diseases result in *generalized alveolar hypoventilation.* The lungs and airways, although usually not affected primarily, may be injured by retained secretions and multiple aspirations. Cor pulmonale usually develops in response to the hypoxic and hypercapnic stimuli in patients with chronic forms of these disorders; consequently, cor pulmonale tends to be more common in patients with cord lesions than with the other disorders noted. Mechanical ventilatory support is the only therapy for the hypoventilation; a cuirass type of respirator is effective. In addition, vigorous bronchial toilet may alleviate the impaired handling of secretions.[3]

DIAPHRAGMATIC PARALYSIS. Bilateral diaphragmatic paralysis is an uncommon but often unrecognized cause of cor pulmonale.[3,159] When an affected patient is upright, ventilation may be normal or almost so, but when the patient is supine, gas exchange deteriorates. The diagnosis may be suspected in a patient with supine breathlessness, a disturbed sleep pattern, paradoxical (i.e., inward) motion of the abdomen on inspiration, and a low vital capacity in the upright position.[3] Therapy for this disorder consists of assisting ventilation when the patient is supine or during sleep, which is usually done by using a rocking bed; however, electrical pacing of the diaphragm may be necessary.[160] Diaphragmatic fatigue sometimes contributes to the respiratory failure of COPD.[161] Bilateral diaphragmatic paralysis may occur after cardiac surgery.[162] Ice cardioplegia can damage the phrenic nerves and lead to transitory respiratory failure that becomes manifest when the patient is removed from the ventilator. Diaphragmatic function usually returns in such patients.[3]

CHEST WALL DISORDERS. Common congenital or acquired abnormalities that distort the thoracic cage are kyphoscoliosis, pectus excavatum, pectus carinatum, and ankylosing spondylitis: Dyspnea is the major symptom of these disorders, but only kyphoscoliosis is associated with cor pulmonale.[3,163] Kyphosis consists of posterior angulation of the spine and scoliosis anterior angulation. Cor pulmonale may develop in a patient with a kyphotic angle exceeding 100 degrees or a scoliotic angle exceeding 120 degrees.[3,164] These structural abnormalities of the thorax cause repositioning and dysfunction of the respiratory muscles, compression of the lung and pulmonary vasculature, and abnormal gas exchange[163,165] (Fig. 47–11). In addition, scoliosis may interfere with the growth and development of alveoli and pulmonary arteries.[166]

Therapy for chest wall disorders is directed toward preventing infection; acute respiratory failure in such patients is treated with mechanical ventilation.[3] Surgical repair of the thoracic deformity often does not improve cardiorespiratory function.[167]

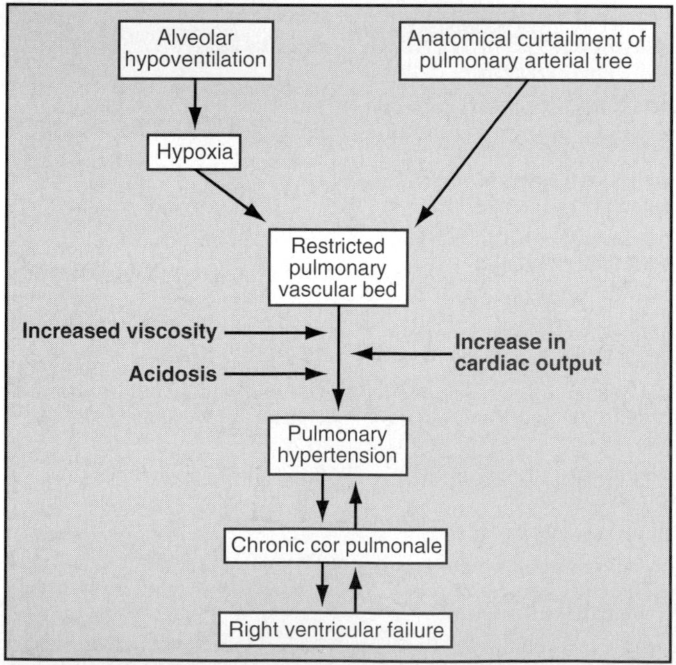

FIGURE 47–11. Pathogenesis of pulmonary hypertension and cor pulmonale in kyphoscoliosis and disorders of ventilatory control. (From Fishman, A. P.: Pulmonary hypertension and cor pulmonale. *In* Fishman, A. P. [ed.]: Pulmonary Diseases and Disorders. 2nd ed. New York, McGraw-Hill Book Co., 1988, p. 1033.)

Disorders of Ventilatory Control

These disorders produce pulmonary hypertension as the result of chronic hypoxemia and hypercapnia due to alveolar hypoventilation (Fig. 47–11). Patients with primary central hypoventilation ("Ondine's curse") have abnormally blunted ventilatory responses to hypercapnic and hypoxic stimulation; the pathogenesis of the congenital form of this disorder is unknown. The acquired disease may follow encephalitis, meningitis, or brain-stem injury or surgery.[168] A form of alveolar hypoventilation also occurs in some obese patients. The so-called pickwickian syndrome consists of the constellation of obesity, hypoventilation, somnolence, and peripheral edema.[169–171]

Treatment consists of weight reduction; respiratory stimulants, such as progesterone, may increase alveolar ventilation and thereby alleviate hypoxemia, hypercapnia, and cor pulmonale.[172,173] Patients with sleep-disordered breathing may have intermittent and repetitive nocturnal hypoxemia that can lead to pulmonary hypertension and cor pulmonale.[172,173] This is true even though most such patients have adequate ventilation and gas exchange while they are awake.

SLEEP APNEA SYNDROMES. These are classified into three general types: (1) central apnea, in which airflow stops in conjunction with cessation of all respiratory muscle effort; (2) obstructive apnea, in which upper airway obstruction causes cessation of airflow despite continuing efforts of the respiratory muscles; and (3) mixed apnea, in which airflow obstruction and respiratory effort both stop initially in the episode, followed first by a resumption of unsuccessful respiratory effort.[3,172,174,175] The upper airway obstruction in patients with sleep-disordered breathing may be due to a combination of such factors as discoordination and relaxation of the buccal and pharyngeal muscles, collapse of the walls of the pharynx and backward movement of the tongue due to inactivity of the genioglossus muscle, and anatomical factors such as enlarged tonsils and adenoids or narrowing due to marked obesity.[3,174]

Patients with sleep apnea may have 40 to 60 apneic episodes per hour,[174] which are associated with phasic hypoxemia and hypercapnia.[3] During the episodes, the pO_2 may fall to as low as 20 to 25 mm Hg, with saturation below 50 per cent.[3] Pulmonary and systemic arterial pressures rise with each episode, and stroke volume, heart rate, and cardiac output fall.[171] The pulmonary artery pressure progressively increases during the night,[171] and pulmonary hypertension is most severe in the morning. The pressure falls during the day but rises with sleep the next night.[3] Hypoxemia, hypercapnia, and pulmonary hypertension eventually become permanent and gradually worsen while the patient is awake.[3]

Patients with sleep apnea also often have severe bradyarrhythmias, which occur during apneic episodes, and tachyarrhythmias, which occur when breathing resumes.[176,177] The arrhythmias consist of sinus bradycardia, sinus arrest, long asystolic periods (ranging from 2 to 13 seconds), sinoatrial block, premature atrial contractions, atrial fibrillation, ventricular premature beats with bigeminy and trigeminy, multifocal premature beats, and ventricular tachycardia.[176–179] Pulmonary artery wedge pressure also may increase during episodes of apnea.[180] Clinical effects of apnea differ with the type, frequency, and intensity of the abnormal respiratory pattern.

Patients with sleep apnea rarely reach deep sleep and therefore are chronically sleep deprived.[3,181] Other common clinical manifestations are loud snoring, somnambulism, tremors, myoclonus, altered states of consciousness, nocturnal enuresis, morning headache, daytime hypersomnolence, hypnagogic hallucinations, and systemic hypertension.[3,181,182] Affected patients are usually not obese and breathe normally when awake. Patients with obstructive apnea tend to have milder hypoventilation and fewer hemodynamic abnormalities than patients with central apnea or mixed apnea. The diagnosis of sleep apnea is established by polysomnography.

About 20 per cent of patients with sleep apnea have COPD, and most of these eventually develop pulmonary hypertension.[183–186] Diagnosis of coexisting sleep apnea and COPD can be difficult, and both disorders must be treated to control symptoms.[3]

Etiology. The cause of sleep apnea is not always clear.[3] Obstructive apneas likely occur because of occlusion of the upper airway in the region of the pharynx.[173,187] Central apnea may have multiple mechanisms, including sleep-induced alteration in respiratory muscle drive, depressed central ventilatory output, or a change in the thresholds for sleep or arousal.[173,188]

Management. In patients with sleep apnea, sedatives and antihistamines should be assiduously avoided or withdrawn, and oxygen therapy should be used cautiously.[3] Narcoleptics and uncontrolled oxygen therapy have resulted in death in some patients.[174] Central apnea is treated with respiratory stimulants or nocturnal ventilatory support with respirators.[174,188] Phrenic nerve or diaphragmatic pacing also has been recommended.[159] Obstructive apnea is most often treated with nasal continuous positive airway pressure (CPAP) and far less commonly tracheostomy.[174,182] Tracheostomy bypasses the area of obstruction, whereas CPAP likely acts as a pneumatic splint that prevents upper airway collapse. Obese patients with obstructive apnea who lose weight may not need a permanent tracheal cannula.[3] Surgical removal of enlarged tonsils or adenoids or surgical enlargement of the entrance to the airway may also be efficacious.[3,182] In some patients, nocturnal oxygen therapy may reduce the duration of apneic episodes and decrease the arrhythmias, but, as noted, oxygen must be used cautiously in these patients.[189]

Upper Airway Obstruction

Obstruction of the upper airways may result in inadequate ventilatory drive, global alveolar hypoventilation, and cor pulmonale.[3] This disorder occurs primarily in children,[190] especially African-American children who have enlarged tonsils and adenoids, but cor pulmonale has been reported as a sequela of acute tonsillitis in adults.[191] Other causes of airway obstruction include vascular ring, macroglossia, micrognathia, laryngotracheomalacia, laryngeal web, Crouzon's disease, Hurler's syndrome, and severe Pierre Robin syndrome,[192,193] but the upper airways can become obstructed during sleep in both children and adults.[194] The mechanism for the hypoventilation is not clear, but an abnormally reactive pulmonary vascular bed, a defect in the central control of respiration, and an interference with normal sleep physiology (as in the sleep apnea syndrome), may alone or in combination have some effect. Ventilatory responsiveness to carbon dioxide is blunted in these patients and it is not normalized by therapy.[195]

The clinical features may mimic asthma, but affected patients usually have somnolence, stridor, and recurrent respiratory tract infection.[3] Treatment consists of surgical removal of the obstruction.[3]

Restrictive Lung Diseases

Pulmonary parenchymal disease, especially when associated with tissue fibrosis and secondary vascular changes, can eventually lead to severe pulmonary hypertension, although significant cor pulmonale usually occurs very late (Table 47–3). In some patients with scleroderma (especially patients with the so-called CREST variant), however, significant pulmonary vascular disease predominates[196,197] (p. 1781). These patients may develop severe pulmonary hypertension and cor pulmonale, even without significant lung fibrosis or restriction of lung mechanics.

Chronic Obstructive Pulmonary Disease

ETIOLOGY AND NATURAL HISTORY OF PULMONARY HYPERTENSION IN COPD. In patients with COPD, pulmonary vasoconstriction may be caused by hypoxia or acidosis, and the pulmonary vascular bed may contract owing to chronic hypoxia-induced structural narrowing and loss of capillaries from emphysema.[1,5] Pulmonary hypertension results as may increased cardiac output, increased pulmonary blood volume, increased blood viscosity, and increased intrathoracic pressure due to expiratory airflow limitation[3,5,198] (see Figs. 47–11, 47–12, and 47–13). Although LV failure cannot be a

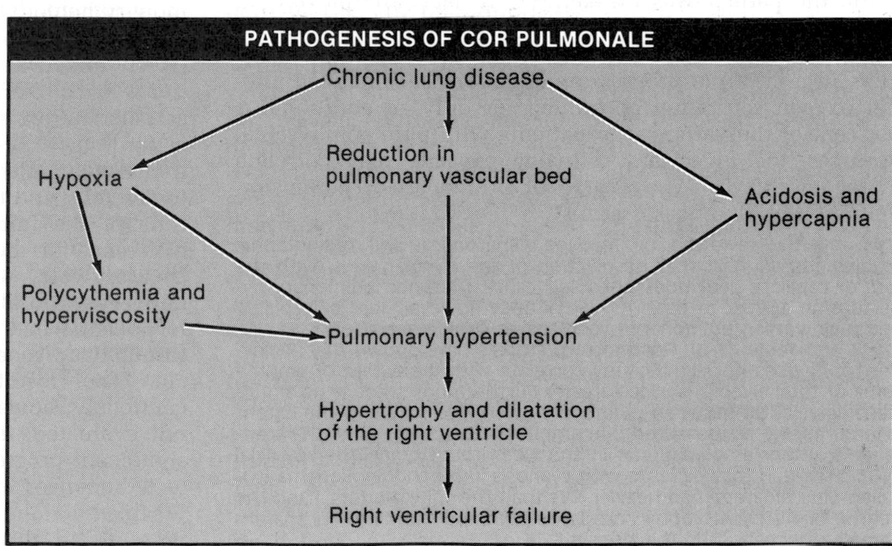

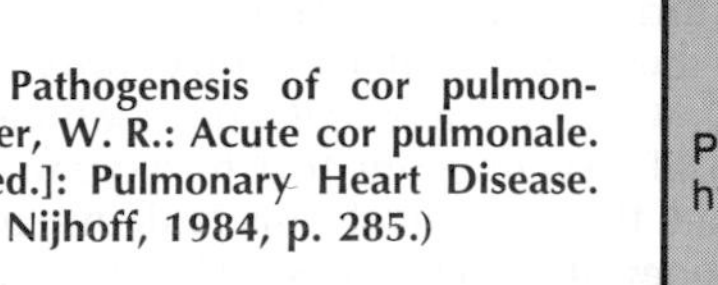
FIGURE 47–12. Pathogenesis of cor pulmonale. (From Summer, W. R.: Acute cor pulmonale. *In* Rubin, L. J. [ed.]: Pulmonary Heart Disease. Boston, Martinus Nijhoff, 1984, p. 285.)

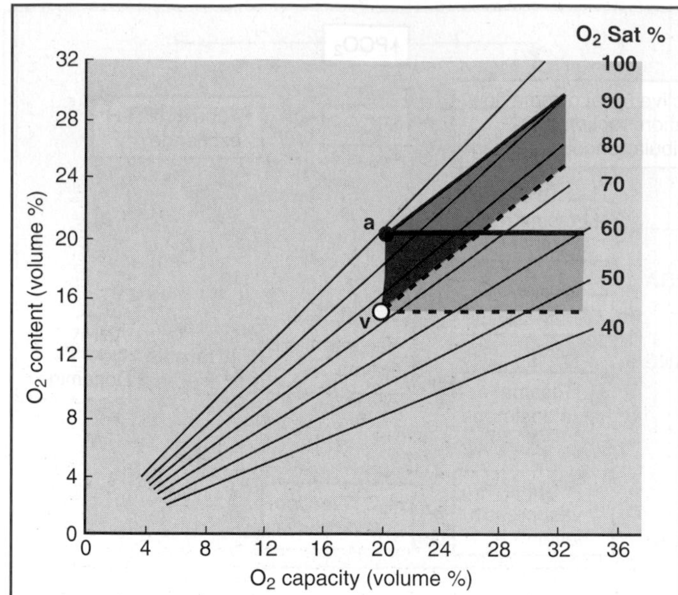

FIGURE 47–15. The relationships among oxygen content (ordinate), oxygen capacity or hemoglobin (Hb) concentration times 1.34 (abscissa), arterial and venous oxygen saturations, and arteriovenous oxygen content difference (CaO_2-CvO_2). A family of iso-oxygen saturation lines radiates from the origin. The normal arterial and venous points are labeled "a" and "v" (Hb, 15 g/dl blood; normal O_2 capacity, 20 ml/dl blood; full saturation is assumed to occur at pO_2 = 100 torr; normal CaO_2-CvO_2 = 5 ml/dl blood). The vertical separation between a pair of arterial and venous points is inversely related to cardiac output. The horizontal shaded band represents the situation in which the arterial oxygen content and the arteriovenous oxygen content difference are maintained constant in the face of progressive hypoxemia and "compensatory" polycythemia (keeping oxygen content stable) as may occur in COPD; i.e., this band represents constant oxygen delivery in the face of decreasing arterial saturation but increasing oxygen capacity. Notice that venous oxygen saturation is markedly decreased despite maintenance of oxygen delivery. The oblique lines extending up and to the right from points "a" and "v" show the degree of polycythemia necessary to maintain normal venous saturation (75 per cent) in the face of hypoxemia. It is clear that a severe degree of polycythemia would be necessary in response to even relatively mild hypoxemia, e.g., at the right end of this band, an arterial oxygen saturation of 90 per cent (PaO_2 = 60 mm Hg) would require an arterial oxygen capacity of about 32 volumes per cent (Hb, 24) to maintain normal mixed venous saturation. This is far in excess of what is observed clinically; furthermore, this assumes that cardiac output can be maintained at this high hemoglobin concentration. (From Tenney, S. M., and Mithoefer, J. D.: The relationship of mixed venous oxygenation to oxygen transport: With special reference to adaptations to high altitude and pulmonary disease. Am. Rev. Respir. Dis. *125*:474–479, 1982; with permission. Courtesy of the American Lung Association.)

chological benefits appear to be achieved only after at least 1 month of oxygen therapy.[240]

HEMODYNAMIC EFFECTS OF OXYGEN. How oxygen therapy improves survival is unknown. Two major hypotheses have been proposed: (1) oxygen relieves pulmonary vasoconstriction, decreasing pulmonary vascular resistance and thus enabling the right ventricle to increase stroke volume and (2) oxygen therapy improves arterial oxygen content, providing enhanced oxygen delivery to the heart, brain, and other vital organs.[115,242] These two hypotheses are not mutually exclusive, and each one has supporting evidence. Oxygen therapy clearly alleviates the progressive pulmonary hypertension of untreated COPD. Also, patients who exhibit a significant decrease in pulmonary artery pressure (>5 mm Hg) after acute oxygen therapy (28 per cent oxygen for 1 day) have a much greater rate of survival than patients who do not respond acutely when both groups of patients are subsequently treated with long-term continuous oxygen therapy.[243] In contrast, a study by Morrison and coworkers[242] suggested that enhanced RV performance during short-term oxygen therapy may be the direct result of improved tissue (e.g., myocardial) oxygenation rather than decreased pulmonary vascular resistance.

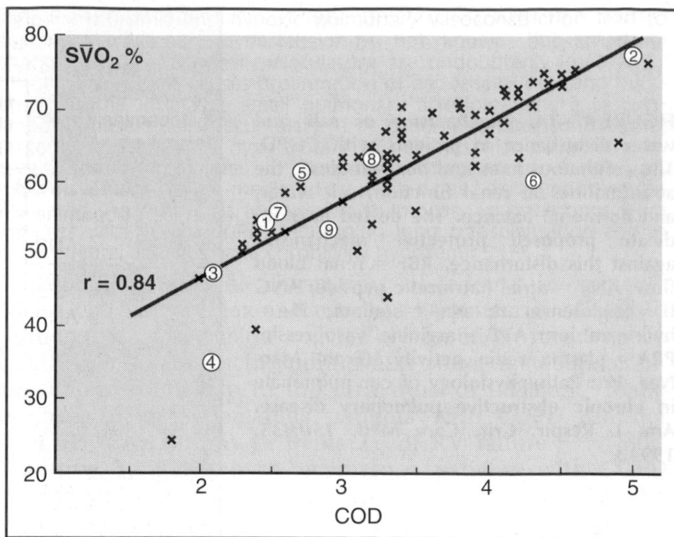

FIGURE 47–16. The relationship between mixed venous oxygen saturation ($S\bar{V}O_2$%) and the coefficient of oxygen delivery (COD) (the product of cardiac output and arterial oxygen content) in 68 patients with COPD at rest, breathing air. (From Tenney, S. M., and Mithoefer, J. C.: The relationship of mixed venous oxygenation to oxygen transport: with special reference to adaptations to high altitude and pulmonary disease. Am. Rev. Respir. Dis. *125*:474–479, 1982; with permission. Courtesy of the American Lung Association.)

RECOMMENDATIONS. Long-term oxygen therapy is warranted if the resting PaO_2 remains less than 55 mm Hg after a 3-week stabilization period on maximal medical therapy (e.g., bronchodilators, antimicrobial agents, diuretics).[115,220,244] Patients with a PaO_2 above 55 mm Hg should be considered for oxygen therapy if they are polycythemic[115,221] or have clinical evidence (e.g., electrocardiographic, physical examination) of pulmonary hypertension and cor pulmonale.[115] Hypoxemia should be documented after a stabilization period to avoid the cost of long-term oxygen therapy in patients who do not require it. In the NOTT study,[237] 45 per cent of hypoxemic patients initially selected for study improved enough during 3 to 4 weeks of observation and treatment to suspend plans for long-term oxygen therapy. An even longer observation period of 2 or 3 months may be necessary to exclude patients who eventually achieve acceptable PaO_2 values on medical therapy

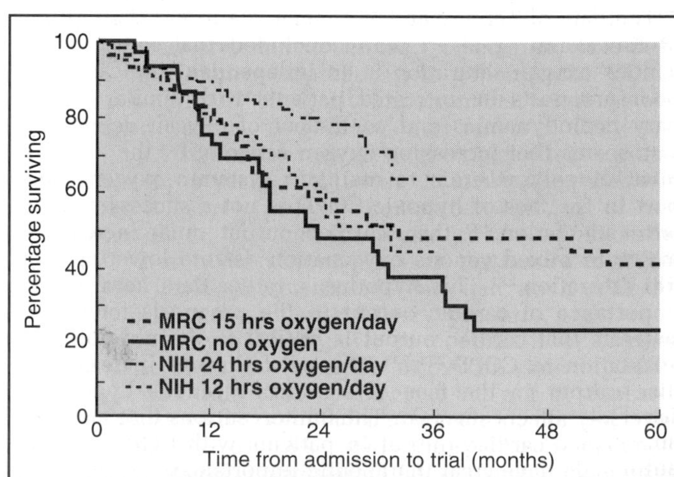

FIGURE 47–17. Survival curves in the MRC (British) and NIH (U.S.) long-term oxygen therapy trials in patients with severe hypoxemia and cor pulmonale. (From Flenley, D. C., and Muir, A. L.: Cardiovascular effects of oxygen therapy for pulmonary arterial hypertension. Clin. Chest Med. *4*:297, 1983.)

alone.[245] Nocturnal oxygen therapy may be important in patients with sleep desaturation.[238,246] Patients with desaturation only during exertion should receive supplemental oxygen during exercise, although the long-term benefits of such therapy remain unproven.[238]

Digitalis

(See also p. 484)

The effect of digitalis on RV function is complex.[5] The cardiac glycosides increase the contractility of the RV myocardium, but they also produce pulmonary vasoconstriction.[247] Furthermore, Sylvester et al.[248] showed that in dogs, digitalis increased the "unstressed reservoir volume" of the circulation through an effect on the peripheral vasculature. This effect reduces venous return and may adversely affect cardiac output.

Digitalis therapy should be used only in patients with cor pulmonale and coexistent LV failure.[200,249–254] For example, Mathur et al.[253] evaluated the effect of 8 weeks of digoxin therapy on resting RV function in patients with severe COPD. All patients were found to have a reduced RVEF at the start of the study. Digoxin therapy did not improve RVEF if the initial LV ejection fraction (LVEF) was normal; only patients with a reduced initial LVEF showed an improvement in RVEF with digoxin. A subsequent study of the effects of 2 weeks of therapy with oral digoxin (0.25 mg per day) in patients with COPD found no improvement in RVEF at rest or during exercise and no increase in maximal exercise performance.[250] Similarly, Mathur et al.[254] also found no improvement in exercise performance in patients with COPD who had had long-term digoxin therapy. Digitalis therapy also causes an increased incidence of adverse side effects (e.g. cardiac arrhythmias) in patients with obstructive lung disease, presumably in part owing to the effect of hypoxia.[255]

Although digoxin is not indicated in the routine hemodynamic management of cor pulmonale, one study indicated that intravenous digoxin improved diaphragm strength and blood flow in patients with COPD who had acute respiratory failure.[256] Therefore, there is a role for digoxin in the management of the acutely decompensated patient.

Theophylline

Theophylline is widely used for its bronchodilator activity.[5] However, sustained-release theophylline reduces dyspnea even in some patients with nonreversible obstructive airways disease.[257] This evidence supports the clinical impression that in some patients with COPD, theophylline may have salutary effects not directly related to bronchodilation.

Theophylline appears to have beneficial cardiovascular effects in patients with COPD with and without cor pulmonale.[221,258,259] Intravenous aminophylline acutely decreases pulmonary artery pressure and increases both RVEF and LVEF. The long-term consequences of oral theophylline therapy on RV function in patients with COPD are also favorable.[260] Eleven patients treated for an average of 4 months had a sustained improvement in RVEF (Fig. 47–18).[260] LVEF also increased slightly.

A combination of reduced afterload (lowered pulmonary and systemic vascular resistance) and enhanced myocardial contractility probably accounts for the improved biventricular pump function with theophylline therapy.[5,258] In isolated papillary muscle preparations, theophylline causes a shift upward and to the right in the force–velocity relationship.[261] In vivo studies in dogs also document an increase in cardiac contractility from aminophylline.[262,263] Other evidence indicates theophylline also probably acts directly to lower vascular resistance.[258,264] In dogs, however, aminophylline does not inhibit acute hypoxic pulmonary vasoconstriction.[265]

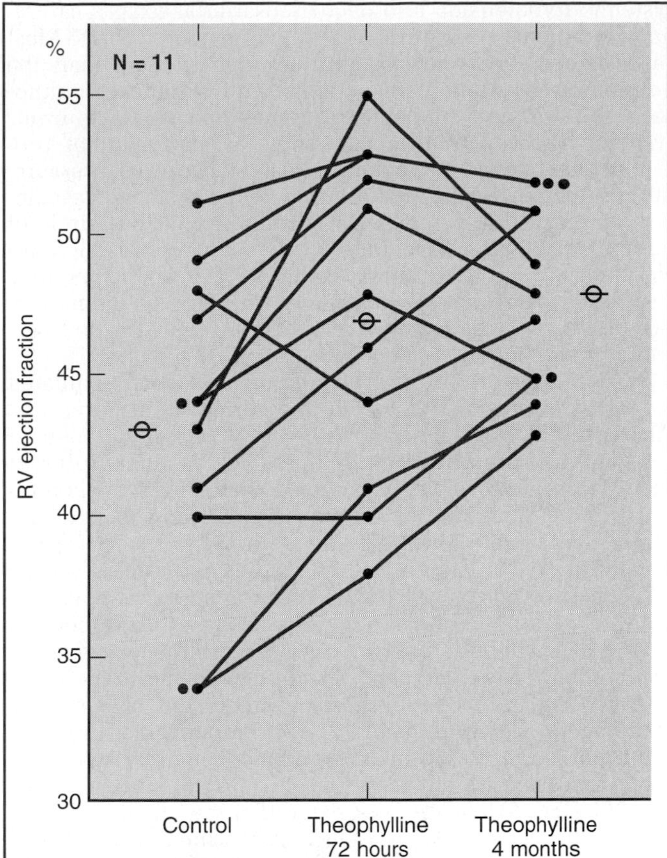

FIGURE 47–18. Oral long-acting theophylline (Theo Dur) significantly ($p < 0.05$) increased right ventricular ejection fraction (RVEF) after 72 hours and after an average of 4 months of therapy in 11 patients with COPD. (From Matthay, R. A. and Berger, H. J.: Cardiovascular function in cor pulmonale. Clin. Chest Med. *4*:269, 1983.)

Beta-Adrenergic Agonists

Although traditionally used as bronchodilators, the selective β_2-adrenergic receptor agonists may have salutary effects in cor pulmonale by causing pulmonary vasodilatation (the human pulmonary circulation contains β-adrenergic receptors) or direct inotropic action on myocardium.[5,221,266–268] In short-term studies, both terbutaline[269–272] and pirbuterol[5,266,273] have been shown to lower pulmonary vascular resistance, increase cardiac output, and increase RVEF and LVEF in most patients with COPD and cor pulmonale. However, these benefits are not sustained during chronic administration (longer than 6 months), especially in patients who are also receiving appropriate supplemental oxygen therapy.[273]

Vasodilators

Assessing the efficacy of vasodilators in COPD is difficult because the hemodynamic changes with therapy are complex, and it has not been established which changes are desirable.[115,221,274,275] Reducing pulmonary hypertension is often the goal of vasodilator therapy, but a fall in vascular resistance may be offset by a rise in cardiac output, leaving the pulmonary artery pressure unchanged.[115] Perhaps this is a beneficial effect (e.g., increased oxygen transport) despite the unrelieved pulmonary hypertension. Conversely, a medication that reduces venous return (nitroglycerin) or depresses RV function (nifedipine) may decrease pulmonary hypertension by lowering cardiac output.[115] This might not be beneficial despite the reduction in pulmonary artery pressure. Long-term studies are needed to evaluate the hemodynamic responses to vasodilators and to assess the overall survival effect of different agents.[115]

Vasodilator therapy may cause such adverse effects as

systemic hypotension and decreased arterial oxygen saturation in patients with pulmonary hypertension.[142,143,276] Most vasodilators affect the systemic circulation more than the pulmonary circulation. In patients with significant pulmonary hypertension and reduced right-sided cardiac output, systemic vasoconstriction may serve as an important protective mechanism to maintain systemic arterial pressure. In these patients, selective dilation of the systemic vasculature may cause hypotension and initiate a vicious circle of right ventricular failure (due to decreased right coronary blood flow) and circulatory collapse.[117] Vasodilators may also lead to arterial hypoxemia by disrupting pulmonary vascular tone, which helps maintain local ventilation-perfusion matching.[5]

The efficacy of various vasodilators has been evaluated in patients with COPD, including nitrates (nitroprusside, nitroglycerin),[266,277] hydralazine,[266,277–287] calcium channel antagonists (verapamil,[288] nifedipine,[289–291] nitrendipine,[292] and felodipine[293]), α-adrenergic antagonists (phentolamine,[294,295] urapidil,[296–298] prazosin[299]), angiotensin-converting enzyme inhibitors (captopril),[300–302] and prostaglandins.[303–305] The results of studies with these agents have been equivocal, and none of these agents is currently used in routine clinical practice. The nitrates appear to have essentially no role because both arterial oxygenation and cardiac index decrease. Therapy with currently available prostaglandins is limited by significant side effects. Some agents (including nifedipine, nitrendipine, urapidil, felodipine, and flosequinan) produce generally favorable short-term benefits, but these benefits are not sustained.

RECOMMENDATIONS. Vasodilator therapy should be considered in patients with COPD only when conventional therapy and oxygen have failed to alleviate signs of RV failure or pulmonary hypertension.[5] Because these agents have potentially adverse consequences,[286] their effects on hemodynamics and oxygenation must be carefully assessed; this usually requires invasive RV catheterization.

Rubin[274,275,306] provides the following guidelines to what constitutes a beneficial hemodynamic response to a vasodilator:

1. Pumonary vascular resistance is reduced by at least 20 per cent, *and*
2. Cardiac output is increased or unchanged, *and*
3. Pulmonary artery pressure is decreased or unchanged, *and*
4. Systemic blood pressure is not significantly reduced (e.g., no side effects.)

If vasodilator therapy produces these benefits, an affected patient should be reassessed after 4 or 5 months of therapy to determine whether the hemodynamic benefits are sustained.

Phlebotomy

Whether phlebotomy is efficacious in polycythemic patients with cor pulmonale is controversial.[5,115] Early studies by Segal and Bishop,[307] using exchange transfusions established that pulmonary artery pressure is more affected by blood volume than blood viscosity. After phlebotomy, in the resting patient, mean pulmonary pressure and pulmonary vascular resistance usually decrease, cardiac output does not significantly change, and systemic oxygen transport falls.[307–310] Despite the decrease in systemic oxygen transport, resting oxygen consumption remained unchanged in most investigations.[308,310] However, Segal and Bishop[307] reported that resting oxygen consumption was lower after phlebotomy, whereas Rakita and coworkers[311] found an increase in oxygen consumption 1 hour after phlebotomy.

The effect of phlebotomy on hemodynamic events during exercise may be more important than the changes observed at rest.[5] Many researchers have found that exercise performance significantly improves in polycythemic patients subjected to phlebotomy.[307,308,310] Weisse and coworkers[310] studied 12 patients with stable cor pulmonale and hematocrit values above 55 per cent. They were evaluated at baseline (mean hematocrit 61 per cent), after initial phlebotomy (mean hematocrit 50 per cent), and after a second phlebotomy (mean hematocrit 44 per cent). After the first reduction of hematocrit, exercise performance improved; however, no significant changes occurred with the further reduction in hematocrit to normal levels. Similarly, Chetty and colleagues[308] studied 15 patients with moderate to severe COPD (mean FEV_1 970 ml) and marked polycythemia (hematocrit above 55 per cent). Phlebotomy was performed until the hematocrit fell below 52 per cent and was at least five percentage points below the initial value. The mean workload, duration of exercise, and maximal oxygen consumption all increased significantly subsequent to phlebotomy.

In summary, reducing markedly elevated hematocrit to a value of about 50 per cent produces short-term salutary effects on circulatory hemodynamics, especially during exercise.[5] However, whether there are long-term benefits of repeated phlebotomy is unclear. Furthermore, the use of continuous oxygen therapy in appropriately selected patients should reduce the number of patients with COPD who become severely polycythemic. Phlebotomy should be reserved for adjunctive therapy in acute management of the markedly polycythemic patient who has an acute decompensation of cor pulmonale or in the rare patient who remains significantly polycythemic despite appropriate long-term oxygen therapy.[5]

REFERENCHES

ETIOLOGIES

1. MacNee, W.: Pathophysiology of cor pulmonale in chronic obstructive pulmonary disease (Part One). Am. J. Respir. Crit. Care Med. *150:*833, 1994.
2. Chronic cor pulmonale: Report of an expert committee. W. H. O. Tech. Rep. Ser. *213:*1, 1961.
3. McFadden, E. R., and Braunwald, E.: Cor pulmonale. *In* Braunwald, E. (ed.): Heart Disease, 4th ed. Philadelphia, W.B. Saunders Company, 1992, pp. 1581–1601.
4. Fowler, N. O.: Chronic cor pulmonale. *In* Fowler, N. O.: Diagnosis of Heart Disease, New York, Springer-Verlag, 1991, pp. 268–282.
5. Wiedemann, H. P., and Matthay, R. A.: Cor pulmonale in chronic obstructive pulmonary disease. Circulatory pathophysiology and management. Clin. Chest Med. *11:*523, 1990.
6. Reid, L. M.: Structure and function in pulmonary hypertension: New perceptions. Chest *89:*279, 1986.
7. Zapol, W., and Snider, M. T.: Pulmonary hypertension in severe acute respiratory failure. N. Engl. J. Med. *296:*476, 1977.
8. Sibbald, W. J., Driedger, A. A., Myers, M. L., et al.: Biventricular function in the adult respiratory distress syndrome: Hemodynamic and radionuclide assessment, with special emphasis on right ventricular function. Chest *84:*126, 1983.
9. Renzetti, Jr., A. D., McClement, J. H., and Litt, B. D.: The Veterans Administration Cooperative Study of Pulmonary Function III. Mortality in relation to respiratory function in chronic obstructive lung disease. Am. J. Med. *41:*115, 1966.
10. Fishman, A. P.: Chronic cor pulmonale. Am. Rev. Respir. Dis. *114:*775, 1976.
11. Stern, R. C., Borkat, G., Hirschfeld, S. S., et al.: Heart failure in cystic fibrosis: Treatment and prognosis of cor pulmonale with failure of the right side of the heart. Am. J. Dis. Child. *134:*267, 1980.
12. Moss, A. J.: The cardiovascular system in cystic fibrosis. Pediatrics *70:*728, 1982.
13. Hughes, J. D., and Rubin, L. J.: Primary pulmonary hypertension: An analysis of 28 cases and a review of the literature. Medicine *65:*56, 1986.

ANATOMICAL AND PATHOPHYSIOLOGICAL CORRELATES

14. Lewis, T.: Observations upon ventricular hypertrophy with special reference to preponderance of one or other chamber. Heart *5:*367, 1914.
15. Emery, J. L., and Mithal, A.: Weight of cardiac ventricles at and after birth. Br. Heart J. *23:*313, 1961.
16. Keen, E. N.: The post-natal development of the human cardiac ventricles. J. Anat. *89:*484, 1955.
17. Arias-Stella, J., and Recavarren, S.: Right ventricular hypertrophy in native children living at high altitude. Am. J. Pathol. *11:*55, 1962.
18. Mathew, R., Thilenius, O. G., and Arcilla, R. A.: Comparative response of right and left ventricles to volume overload. Am. J. Cardiol. *38:*239, 1976.

19. Recavarren, S., and Arias-Stella, J.: Right ventricular hypertrophy in people born and living at high altitudes. Br. Heart J. *26*:806, 1964.
20. Penaloza, D., Sime, F., Bancero, N., et al.: Pulmonary hypertension in healthy men born and living at high altitudes. Am. J. Cardiol. *11*:150, 1963.
21. Fulton, R. M., Hutchinson, E. C., and Jones, A. M.: Ventricular weight in cardiac hypertrophy. Br. Heart J. *14*:413, 1952.
22. Mitchell, R. S., Stanford, R. E., Silvers, G. W., and Dart, G.: The right ventricle in chronic airway obstruction: A clinicopathologic study. Am. Rev. Respir. Dis. *114*:147, 1976.
23. Ishikawa, S., Fattal, G. A., Popiewicz, J., and Wyatt, J. P.: Functional morphometry of myocardial fibers in cor pulmonale. Am. Rev. Respir. Dis. *105*:358, 1972.
24. Brecher, G. A., and Galletti, P. M.: Functional anatomy of cardiac pumping. *In* Hamilton, A. F., and Dow, P. (eds.): Handbook of Physiology: Circulation. Vol. II. Washington, D.C., American Physiological Society, 1963, p. 759.
25. Visner, M. S., Arenizen, C. E., O'Connor, M. J., et al.: Alterations in left ventricular three-dimensional dynamic geometry and systolic function during acute right ventricular hypertension in the conscious dog. Circulation *67*:353, 1983.
26. Barnard, D., and Alpert, J. S.: Right ventricular function in health and disease. Curr. Prob. Cardiol. *12*:417, 1987.
27. Laks, M. M., Garner, D., and Swan, H. J. C.: Volumes and compliances measured simultaneously in the right and left ventricles of the dog. Circ. Res. *20*:565, 1967.
28. Abel, F. L., and Waldhausen, J. A.: Effects of alterations in pulmonary vascular resistance on right ventricular function. J. Thorac. Cardiovasc. Surg. *54*:886, 1967.
29. Abel, F. L.: Effects of alterations in peripheral resistance on left ventricular function. Proc. Soc. Exp. Biol. Med. *120*:52, 1965.
30. Morrison, D., Goldman, S., Wright, A. L., et al.: The effect of pulmonary hypertension on systolic function of the right ventricle. Chest *84*:250, 1983.
31. Sarnoff, S. J., and Berglund, E.: Ventricular function. I. Starling's law of the heart studied by means of simultaneous right and left ventricular function curves in the dog. Circulation *8*:706, 1954.
32. Spann, J. R., Buccino, R. A., Sonnenblick, E. H., and Braunwald, E. B.: Contractile state of cardiac muscle obtained from cats with experimentally produced ventricular hypertrophy and heart failure. Circ. Res. *21*:341, 1967.
33. Haggard, G. E., and Walker, A. M.: The physiology of pulmonary embolism as disclosed by quantitative occlusion of the pulmonary artery. Arch. Surg. *5*:763, 1923.
34. Gibbons, J. H., Hopkinson, M., and Churchill, E. D.: Changes in the circulation produced by gradual occlusion of the pulmonary artery. J. Clin. Invest. *11*:543, 1932.
35. Fineberg, M. H., and Wiggens, C. J.: Compensation and failure of the right ventricle. Am. Heart J. *11*:255, 1936.
36. Brooks, H., Kirk, E. S., Bokonas, P. S., et al.: Performance of the right ventricle under stress: Relation to right coronary flow. J. Clin. Invest. *50*:2176, 1971.
37. Meyrick, B., and Reid, L. M.: Pulmonary hypertension: Anatomic and physiologic correlations. Clin. Chest Med. *4*:199, 1983.
38. Fishman, A. P.: The normal pulmonary circulation. *In* Fishman, A. P. (ed.): Pulmonary Diseases and Disorders. 2nd ed. New York, McGraw-Hill, 1991, p. 975–998.
39. Hebb, C.: Motor innervation of the pulmonary blood vessels of mammals. *In* Fishman, A. P., and Hecht, H. H. (eds.): The Pulmonary Circulation and the Interstitial Space. Chicago, University of Chicago Press, 1969, p. 195.
40. Allen, K. M., Wharton, J., Polak, I. M., and Chaworth, S. G.: A study of nerves containing peptides in the pulmonary vasculature of healthy infants and children and those with pulmonary hypertension. Br. Heart J. *62*:353, 1989.
41. Fishman, A. P.: Dynamics of the pulmonary circulation. *In* Hamilton, W. F., and Dow, P. (eds.): Handbook of Physiology: Circulation. Vol. II. Washington, D.C., American Physiological Society, 1963, p. 1667.
42. Bard, P.: The pulmonary circulation and respiratory variations in the systemic circulation. *In* Bard, P. (ed.): Medical Physiology. St. Louis, C. V. Mosby, 1961, p. 231.
43. Brofman, B. L., Charms, B. L., Kohn, P. M., et al.: Unilateral pulmonary artery occlusion in man: Control studies. J. Thorac. Surg. *34*:206, 1957.
44. Guyton, A. C.: Circulatory Physiology: Cardiac Output and its Regulation, Philadelphia, W.B. Saunders Company, 1963.
45. Maseri, A., Caldini, P., Howard, P., et al.: Determinants of pulmonary vascular volume-recruitment versus distensibility. Circ. Res. *31*:218, 1972.
46. Lanari, A., and Agrest, A.: Pressure-volume relationship in the pulmonary vascular bed. Acta Physiol. Lat. Am. *4*:116, 1954.
47. Caro, C. G.: Extensibility of blood vessels in isolated rabbit lung. J. Physiol. (Lond.) *178*:193, 1965.
48. Howell, J. B., Permutt, S., Proctor, D. F., and Riley, R. L.: Effect of inflation of the lung on different parts of the pulmonary vascular bed. J. Appl. Physiol. *16*:71, 1961.
49. Englebert, J., and DuBois, A. B.: Mechanics of pulmonary circulation in isolated rabbit lungs. Am. J. Physiol. *186*:401, 1959.
50. Maseri, A., Calcini, P., Permutt, S., and Zierler, K. L.: Pressure volume relationship in the pulmonary circulation. *In* Widimsky, J., Daum, S., and Herzog, H. (eds.): Progress in Respiration Research. Vol. 5, Basel, S. Karger, 1970, p. 53.
51. Glazier, J. B., Highes, J. M. B., Maloney, J. E., and West, J. B.: Measurements of capillary dimensions and blood volume in rapidly frozen lungs. J. Appl. Physiol. *26*:65, 1969.
52. Grover, R. F.: Chronic hypoxic pulmonary hypertension. *In* Fishman, A. P. (ed.): The Pulmonary Circulation: Normal and Abnormal. Philadelphia, University of Pennsylvania Press, 1990, pp. 283–299.
53. Fishman, A. P.: Hypoxia and its effects on the pulmonary circulation. Circ. Res. *38*:221, 1976.
54. Habb, P. E., and Duranad-Arczynska, W. Y.: Carbon monoxide effects on oxygen transport. *In* Crystal, R. G., and West, J. B. (eds.): The Lung: Scientific Foundations. New York, Raven Press, 1991, pp. 1267–1276.
55. Fowler, K. T., and Read, J.: Effect of alveolar hypoxia on zonal distribution of pulmonary blood flow. J. Appl. Physiol. *18*:244, 1963.
56. Lindsay, D. A., and Reed, J.: Pulmonary vascular responsiveness in the prognosis of chronic obstructive lung disease. Am. Rev. Repair. Dis. *105*:242, 1972.
57. Enson, Y., Guintini, C., Lewis, M. L., et al.: The influence of hydrogen ion concentration and hypoxia on the pulmonary circulation. J. Clin. Invest. *43*:1146, 1964.
58. Bergofsky, E. H.: Mechanisms underlying vasomotor regulation of regional pulmonary blood flow in normal and disease states. Am. J. Med. *57*:378, 1974.
59. Bergofsky, E. H., Haas, F., and Procelli, R. I.: Determination of the sensitive vascular sites from which hypoxia and hypercapnia elicit rises in pulmonary arterial pressure. Fed. Proc. *27*:1420, 1968.
60. Bergofsky, E. H.: Humoral control of the pulmonary circulation. Annu. Rev. Physiol. *42*:221, 1980.

ASSESSMENT OF PATIENTS WITH COR PULMONALE

61. Arcilla, R. A., Tsai, P., Thilenus, O., and Ranniger, K.: Angiographic method for volume estimation of the right and left ventricles. Chest *60*:446–454, 1971.
62. Gentzler, R., Briselli, M., and Gault, J.: Angiographic estimation of right ventricular volume in man. Circulation *4*:1, 1974.
63. Fishman, A. P.: State of the art: Chronic cor polmonale. Am. Rev. Respir. Dis. *114*:775–794, 1976.
64. Rubin, L. J.: Pulmonary Heart Disease. Boston, Martinus Nijhoff, 1984.
65. Lehtonen, J., Sutinen, S., Ikaheimo, P., and Paako, P.: Electrocardiographic criteria for the diagnosis of right ventricular hypertrophy verified at autopsy. Chest *93*:839, 1988.
66. McGowan, F. X., and Wagner, G. S.: The electrocardiogram in chronic lung disease. *In* Rubin, L. J. (ed.): Pulmonary Heart Disease. Boston, Martinus Nijhoff, 1984, p. 117.
67. Goodwin, J. F., and Abdin, Z. N.: The cardiogram of congenital and acquired right ventricular hypertrophy. Br. Heart. J. *21*:523, 1959.
68. Phillips, R. W.: The electrocardiogram in cor pulmonale secondary to pulmonary emphysema: A study of 18 cases proved by autopsy. Am. Heart J. *56*:352, 1958.
69. Kilcoyne, M. M., Davis, A. L., and Ferrer, M. I.: A dynamic electrocardiographic concept useful in the diagnosis of cor pulmonale. Circulation *42*:903, 1970.
70. Holford, F. D.: The electrocardiogram in pulmonary disease. *In* Fishman, A. P. (ed.): Pulmonary Diseases and Disorders. 2nd ed. New York, McGraw-Hill, 1991, pp. 471–478.
71. Matthay, R. A., and Shub, C.: Imaging techniques for assessing pulmonary artery hypertension and right ventricular performance with special reference to COPD. J. Thorac. Imaging *5*:47, 1990.
72. Matthay, R. A., and Berger, H. J.: Noninvasive assessment of right and left ventricular function in acute and chronic respiratory failure. Crit. Care Med. *11*:329, 1983.
73. Matthay, R. A., Schwarz, M. I., Ellis, H., Jr., et al.: Pulmonary artery hypertension in chronic obstructive pulmonary disease: Chest radiographic assessment. Invest. Radiol. *16*:95, 1981.
74. Chang, C. H.: The normal roentgenographic measurement of the right descending pulmonary artery in 1,085 cases. Am. J. Roentgenol. *87*:929, 1962.
75. Chetty, K. G., Brown, S. E., and Light, R. W.: Identification of pulmonary hypertension in chronic obstructive pulmonary disease from routine chest radiographs. Am. Rev. Respir. Dis. *126*:338, 1982.
76. Berger, H. J., Matthay, R. A., Loke, J., et al.: Assessment of cardiac performance with quantitative radionuclide angiography: Right ventricular ejection fraction with reference to findings in chronic obstructive pulmonary disease. Am. J. Cardiol. *41*:897, 1978.
77. Oliver, R. M., Fleming, J. S., and Waller, D. G.: Right ventricular function at rest and exercise in chronic obstructive pulmonary disease: Comparison of two radionuclide techniques. Chest *103*:74, 1993.
78. Maddahi, J., Bermon, D. S., Matsuoka, D. T., et al.: A new technique for assessing right ventricular ejection fraction using rapid multiple gated equilibrium cardiac blood pool scintigraphy. Circulation *60*:581, 1979.
79. Xue, Q. F., MacNee, W., Flenley, D. C., et al.: Can right ventricular performance be assessed by gated equilibrium ventriculography? Thorax *38*:486, 1983.
80. Matthay, R. A., and Berger, J. J.: Cardiovascular function in cor pulmonale. Clin. Chest. Med. *4*:269, 1983.
81. MacNee, W., Xue, Q. F., Hannan, W. J., et al.: Assessment by radionuclide angiography of right and left ventricular function in chronic bronchitis and emphysema. Thorax *38*:494–500, 1983.
82. Jain, D., and Zaret, B. J.: Assessment of right ventricular function: Role of nuclear imaging techniques. Cardiol. Clin. *10*:23, 1992.
83. Brent, B. N., Berger, H. J., Matthay, R. A., et al.: Physiologic correlates

of right ventricular ejection fraction in chronic obstructive pulmonary disease: A combined radionuclide and hemodynamic study. Am. J. Cardiol. *50*:255, 1982.
84. Brent, B. N., Mahler, D. A., Matthay, R. A., et al.: Noninvasive diagnosis of pulmonary arterial hypertension in chronic obstructive pulmonary disease: Right ventricular ejection fraction at rest. Am. J. Cardiol. *53*:1349, 1984.
85. Cohen, H. A., Baird, M. G., Rouleau, J. R., et al.: Thallium 201 myocardial imaging in patients with pulmonary hypertension. Circulation *54*:790, 1976.
86. Khaja, F., Alam, M., Goldstein, S., Anbe, D. T., and Marks, D. S.: Diagnostic value of visualization of the right ventricle using Thallium 201 myocardial imaging. Circulation *59*:182, 1979.
87. Ohsuzu, F., Handa, S., Kondo, M., et al.: Thallium 201 myocardial imaging to evaluate right ventricular overloading. Circulation *61*:620, 1980.
88. Berger, H., Wackers, F., Mahler, D., et al.: Right ventricular visualization of Thallium 201 myocardial images in chronic obstructive pulmonary disease: Relationship to right ventricular function and hypertrophy (abstract). Circulation *62*:111, 1980.
89. Weitzenblum, E., Moyses, B., Dickele, M., and Methlin, G.: Detection of right ventricular pressure overloading by Thallium 201 myocardial scintigraphy: Results in 57 patients with chronic respiratory diseases. Chest *85*:164, 1984.
90. Kondo, M., Unbo, A., Yamafaki, H., et al.: Thallium-201 myocardial imaging for evaluation of right ventricular overloading. J. Nucl. Med. *19*:1197, 1978.
91. Shiller, N. B., and Sahn, D. J.: Pulmonary pressure measurement by Doppler and two-dimensional echocardiography in adult and paediatric populations. *In* Weir, E. K., Archer, S. L., and Reeves, J. T. (eds.): The Diagnosis and Treatment of Pulmonary Hypertension. New York, Futura, 1992, pp. 41–59.
92. Migueres, M., Escamilla, R., Coca, F., et al.: Pulsed Doppler echocardiography in the diagnosis of pulmonary hypertension in COPD. Chest *98*:280, 1990.
93. Morpurgo, M., Saviotti, M., Dickele, M. C., et al.: Echocardiographic aspect of pulmonary arterial hypertension in chronic lung disease. Bull. Eur. Physiopathol. Respir. *20*:251, 1984.
94. Macharaoui, A., von Dryander, S., Hinrichsen, M., et al.: Two dimensional echocardiographic assessment of right cardiac pressure overload in patients with chronic obstructive airway disease. Respiration *60*:65, 1993.
95. Trivedi, H. S., Joshi, M. N., and Gamade, A. R.: Echocardiography and pulmonary artery pressure: Correlation in chronic obstructive pulmonary disease. J. Postgrad. Med. *38*:24, 1992.
96. Burghuber, O. C., Brummer, C. H., Schenk, P., and Weissel, M.: Pulsed Doppler echocardiography to assess pulmonary artery hypertension in chronic obstructive pulmonary disease. Monaldi Arch. Chest Dis. *48*:121, 1993.
97. Marangoni, S., Sealvini, S., Schena, M., et al.: Right ventricular diastolic function in chronic obstructive lung disease. Eur. Respir. J. *5*:438, 1992.
98. Yock, P. J., and Popp, R. L.: Non-invasive estimation of right ventricular systolic pressure by Doppler ultrasound in patients with tricuspid regurgitation. Circulation *70*:657, 1984.
99. Masuyama, T., Kodama, K., Kitabatakem, A., et al.: Continuous wave Doppler echocardiographic detection of pulmonary regurgitation and its application to noninvasive estimation of pulmonary arterial pressure. Circulation *74*:484, 1986.
100. Stevenson, G., Kawabori, I., and Guntheroth, W.: The validation of Doppler diagnosis of tricuspid regurgitation. Circulation *64*:255, 1981.
101. Tramarin, R., Torbicki, A., Marchandise, B., et al.: Doppler echocardiographic evaluation of pulmonary artery pressure in chronic obstructive pulmonary disease. A European multicentre study. Eur. Heart J. *12*:103, 1991.
102. Berger, M., Hecht, S., Van Tosh, A., and Lingam, U.: Pulse and continuous wave Doppler echocardiographic assessment of valvular regurgitation in normal subjects. J. Am. Coll. Cardiol. *113*:1540, 1989.
103. Morrison, D. A., Ovitt, T., and Hammermeister, K. E.: Functional tricuspid regurgitation and right ventricular dysfunction in pulmonary hypertension. Am. J. Cardiol. *62*:108, 1988.
104. Himelman, R. B., Stulbarg, K., Kircher, B., et al.: Noninvasive evaluation of pulmonary arterial pressure during exercise by saline enhanced Doppler echocardiography in chronic pulmonary disease. Circulation *79*:683, 1989.
105. Beard, J. T., and Byrd, B. F.: Saline contrast enhancement of trivial tricuspid regurgitation signals for estimating pulmonary artery pressure. Am. J. Cardiol. *62*:486, 1988.
106. Laaban, J. P., Diebold, B., Raffoul, H., et al.: Noninvasive estimation of systolic pulmonary arterial pressure (Pps) using continuous wave Doppler ultrasound in COPD. Am. Rev. Respir. Dis. *137*:150, 1988.
107. Mitchell, R. S., Stanford, R. E., Silvers, G. W., and Dart, G.: The right ventricle in chronic airway obstruction: A clinico-pathologic study. Am. Rev. Respir. Dis. *11*:147, 1976.
108. Murphy, M. L.: The pathology of the right heart in chronic hypertrophy and failure. *In* Fisk, R. L. (ed.): The Right Heart. Philadelphia, F. A. Davis, 1987, pp. 159–167.
109. Konstam, M. A., and Levine, H. A.: Effects of afterload and preload on right ventricular systolic performance. *In* Konstam, M. A., Isner, J. (eds.): The Right Ventricle. Boston, Kluwer Academic, 1988, pp. 17–35.
110. Langmore, D. B., Kerpstein, R. H., Underwood, S. R., et al.: Dimensional accuracy of magnetic resonance studies of the heart. Lancet *1*:1360, 1985.
111. Turnbull, L. W., Ridgeway, J. P., Biernacki, W., et al.: Assessment of the right ventricle by magnetic resonance imaging in chronic obstructive lung disease. Thorax *45*:597, 1990.
112. Wacker, C. M., Schad, L. R., Behling, U., et al.: The pulmonary artery acceleration time determined with the MR-RACE-technique: comparison to pulmonary artery mean pressure in 12 patients. Magn. Reson. Imaging *12*:25, 1994.
113. Saito, H., Dambura, T., Aiba, M., Suzuki, T., and Kira, S.: Evaluation of cor pulmonale on a modified short-axis section of the heart by magnetic resonance imaging. Am. Rev. Respir. Dis. *146*:1576, 1992.
114. Pattynama, P. M., Willems, L. N., Smith, A. H., et al.: Early diagnosis of cor pulmonale with MR imaging of the right ventricle. Radiology *182*:375, 1992.

ACUTE COR PULMONALE

115. Wiedemann, H. P., and Matthay, R. A.: The management of acute and chronic cor pulmonale. *In* Scharf, S. M., and Cassidy, S. S. (eds.): Heart-Lung Interactions in Health and Disease. New York, Marcel Dekker, Inc., 1989, pp. 915–981.
116. Guyton, A. C., Lindsey, A. W., and Gilluly, J. J.: The limits of right ventricular compensation following acute increases in pulmonary circulatory resistance. Circ. Res. *2*:326, 1954.
117. Wiedemann, H. P., and Matthay, R. A.: Acute right heart failure. Crit. Care Clin. *1*:631, 1985.
118. Brooks, H., Holland, R., and Al-Sadir, J.: Right ventricular performance during ischemia: An anatomic and hemodynamic analysis. Am. J. Physiol. *233*:500, 1977.
119. Spotnitz, H. M., Berman, M. A., and Epstein, S. E.: Pathophysiology and experimental treatment of acute pulmonary embolism. Am. Heart J. *82*:511, 1971.
120. Fixler, D. E., Archie, J. P., Ullyot, D. J., et al.: Effects of acute right ventricular systolic hypertension on regional myocardial blood flow in anesthetized dogs. Am. Heart J. *85*:491, 1973.
121. Manohar, M., Tranquilli, W. J., Parks, C. M., et al.: Regional myocardial blood flow and coronary vasodilator reserve during acute right ventricular failure due to pressure overload in swine. J. Surg. Res. *31*:382, 1981.
122. Cooper, N., Brazier, J., and Buckberg, G.: Effects of systemic-pulmonary shunts on regional myocardial blood flow in experimental pulmonary stenosis. J. Thorac. Cardiovasc. Surg. *70*:166, 1975.
123. Vlahakes, G. J., Turley, K., and Hoffman, J. I. E.: The pathophysiology of failure in acute right ventricular hypertension: Hemodynamic and biochemical correlations. Circulation *63*:87, 1981.
124. Molloy, W. D., Lee, K. Y., Girling, L., et al.: Treatment of shock in a canine model of pulmonary embolus. Am. Rev. Respir. Dis. *130*:870, 1984.
125. Ghignone, M., Girling, L., and Prewitt, R. M.: Volume expansion versus norepinephrine in treatment of a low cardiac output complicating an acute increase in right ventricular afterload in dogs. Anesthesiology *60*:132, 1984.
126. Scharf, S. M., Warner, K. G., Josa, M., et al.: Load tolerance of the right ventricle: Effect of increased aortic pressure. J. Crit. Care. *1*:163, 1986.
127. Laks, M. M., Garner, D., and Swan, H. J. C.: Volumes and compliances measured simultaneously in the right and left ventricles of the dog. Circ. Res. *20*:565, 1967.
128. Taylor, R. R., Covell, J. W., Sonnenblick, E. H., and Ross, J., Jr.: Dependence of ventricular distensibility on filling of the opposite ventricle. Am. J. Physiol. *213*:711, 1982.
129. Kelly, D. T., Spotnitz, H. M., Beiser, G. D., et al.: Effects of chronic right ventricular volume and pressure loading on left ventricular performance. Circulation *44*:403, 1971.
130. Stool, E. W., Mullins, C. B., Leshin, S. J., and Mitchell, J. H.: Dimensional changes of the left ventricle during acute pulmonary arterial hypertension in dogs. Am. J. Cardiol. *33*:868, 1974.
131. Weyman, A. E., Warn, S., Feigenbaum, H., and Dillon, J. C.: Mechanism of abnormal septal motion in patients with right ventricular volume overload: A cross-sectional echocardiographic study. Circulation *27*:594, 1963.
132. Goldstein, J. A., Vlahakes, G. J., Verrier, E. D., et al.: The role of right ventricular systolic dysfunction and elevated intrapericardial pressures in the genesis of low output in experimental right ventricular infarction. Circulation *65*:513, 1982.
133. Laver, M. B., Strauss, H. W., and Phost, G. M.: Right and left ventricular geometry: Adjustments during acute respiratory failure. Crit. Care Med. *7*:509, 1979.
134. Sibbald, W. J., Driedger, A. A., Myers, M. L., et al.: Biventricular function in the adult respiratory distress syndrome: Hemodynamic and radionuclide assessment, with special emphasis on right ventricular function. Chest *84*:126, 1983.
135. Guyton, A. C.: Determination of cardiac output by equating venous return curves with cardiac response curves. Physiol. Rev. *35*:123, 1955.
136. Goldberg, H. S., and Rabson, J.: Control of cardiac output by systemic vessels: Circultory adjustments to acute and chronic respiratory failure and the effect of therapeutic intervention. Am. J. Cardiol. *47*:696, 1981.
137. Rothe, C. F.: Physiology of venous return: An unappreciated boost to the heart. Arch. Intern. Med. *146*:977, 1986.
138. Ghignone, M., Girling, L., Prewitt, R. M.: Effect of increased pulmonary vascular resistance (PVR) and treatment on right ventricular perform-

ance in acute respiratory failure (ARF). Am. Rev. Respir. Dis. *125*:99, 1982.

139. Paetkau, D., Kettner, J., Girling, L., et al.: What is the appropriate therapy to maintain cardiac output as pulmonary vascular resistance increases? Anesthesiology *57*:A56, 1982.
140. Prewitt, R. M., and Ghignone, M.: Treatment of right ventricular dysfunction in acute respiratory failure. Crit. Care. Med. *11*:346, 1983.
141. Prewitt, R. M., Matthay, M. A., and Ghignone, M.: Hemodynamic management in the adult respiratory distress syndrome. Clin. Chest. Med. *4*:251, 1983.
142. Rubin, L. J.: Cardiovascular effects of vasodilator therapy for pulmonary arterial hypertension. Clin. Chest Med. *4*:309, 1983.
143. Packer, M.: Vasodilator therapy for primary pulmonary hypertension. Ann. Intern. Med. *103*:258, 1985.
144. Melot, C., Hallemans, R., Naeije, R., et al.: Deleterious effect of nifedipine on pulmonary gas exchange in chronic obstructive pulmonary disease. Am. Rev. Respir. Dis. *130*:612, 1984.
145. Harrison, W. D., Raizen, N., Ghignone, M., et al.: Treatment of canine low pressure pulmonary edema. Nitroprusside versus hydralazine. Am. Rev. Respir. Dis. *128*:857, 1983.
146. Benoit, A., Ducas, J., Girling, L., et al.: Acute cardiopulmonary effects of nitroglycerin in canine oleic acid pulmonary edema. Anesthesiology *62*:754, 1985.
147. Ghignone, M., Girling, L., and Prewitt, R. M.: Effects of vasodilators on canine cardiopulmonary function when a decrease in cardiac output complicates an increase in right ventricular afterload. Am. Rev. Respir. Dis. *131*:527, 1985.
148. Bishop, M. J., and Cheney, F. W.: Vasodilators worsen gas exchange in dog oleic-acid lung injury. Anesthesiology *64*:435, 1986.
149. Zapol, W. M., and Snider, M. T.: Pulmonary hypertension in severe acute respiratory failure. N. Engl. J. Med. *296*:476, 1977.
150. Martyn, J. A. J., Snider, M. T., Szyfelbein, S. K., et al.: Right ventricular dysfunction in acute thermal injury. Ann. Surg. *191*:330, 1980.
151. Her, C.: Right ventricular stroke-work: An index of distribution of pulmonary perfusion in acute respiratory failure. Chest *84*:719, 1983.
152. Sibbald, W. J., and Driedger, A. A.: Right ventricular function in acute disease states: Pathophysiologic considerations. Crit. Care Med. *11*:339, 1983.
153. Rossaint, R., Falke, K. J., and Lopez, F.: Inhaled nitric oxide for the adult respiratory distress syndrome. N. Engl. J. Med. *328*:399, 1993.
154. Parr, G. V. S., Pierce, W. S., Rosenberg, G., and Waldhausen, J. A.: Right ventricular failure after repair of left ventricular aneurysm. J. Thorac. Cardiovasc. Surg. *80*:79, 1980.
155. Prewitt, R. M., Girling, L., and Ghignone, M.: Effects of increased pulmonary vascular resistance (PVR) on right ventricular (RV) function in canine acute respiratory failure. Am. Rev. Respir. Dis. *125*:99, 1982.
156. Vlahakes, G. J., Turley, K., and Hoffman, J. I. E.: The pathophysiology of failure in acute right ventricular hypertension: Hemodynamic and biochemical correlations. Circulation *63*:87, 1981.

CHRONIC COR PULMONALE

157. Williams, M. H., Jr., Adler, J. J., and Colp, C.: Pulmonary function studies as an aid in the differential diagnosis of pulmonary hypertension. Am. J. Med. *47*:378, 1969.
158. White, J., Bullock, R. E., Hudgson, P., and Gibson, G. J.: Neuromuscular disease, respiratory failure and cor pulmonale. Postgrad. Med. J. *68*:820, 1992.
159. Davis, J. N., Goldman, M., Loh, L., et al.: Diaphragm function and alveolar hypoventilation. Q. J. Med. *45*:87, 1976.
160. Glenn, W. W. L., Holcomb, W. C., Hogan, J., et al.: Diaphragm pacing by radiofrequency transmission in the treatment of chronic ventilatory insufficiency: Present status. J. Thorac. Cardiovasc. Surg. *66*:606, 1973.
161. Aubier, M., DeTroyer, A., Sampson, M., et al.: Aminophylline improves diaphragmatic contractility. N. Engl. J. Med. *305*:249, 1981.
162. Chandler, K. W., Roxas, C. J., Kory, R. C., and Goldman, A. L.: Bilateral diaphragmatic paralysis complicating local cardiac hypothermia during open heart surgery. Am. J. Med. *77*:243, 1984.
163. Bergofsky, E. H.: Respiratory failure in disorders of the thoracic cage. Am. Rev. Respir. Dis. *119*:643, 1979.
164. Bergofsky, E. H., Turino, G. M., and Fishman, A. P.: Respiratory impairment and airway closure in patients with untreated idiopathic scoliosis. Medicine *38*:263, 1959.
165. Bijure, J., Grimby, G., Kasalicky, J., et al.: Respiratory impairment and airway closure in patients with untreated idiopathic scoliosis. Thorax *25*:451, 1970.
166. Davies, G., and Reid, L.: Effect of scoliosis on growth of alveoli and pulmonary arteries and on the right ventricle. Arch. Dis. Child. *46*:623, 1971.
167. Westgate, H. D., and Moe, J. H.: Pulmonary function in kyphoscoliosis before and after correction by the Harrington instrumentation method. J. Bone Joint Surg. *51*:935, 1969.
168. Mellins, R. B., Balfour, H. H., Jr., Turino, G. M., and Winters, R. W.: Failure of automatic control of ventilation (Ondine's curse). Medicine *49*:487, 1970.
169. Burwell, C. S., Robin, E. D., Whaley, R. D., and Bickelman, A. G.: Extreme obesity associated with alveolar hypoventilation: A pickwickian syndrome. Am. J. Med. *21*:811, 1956.
170. Rochester, D. F., and Enson, Y.: Current concepts in the pathogenesis of the obesity-hypoventilation syndrome. Am. J. Med. *57*:402, 1974.
171. Weil, J. V.: Pulmonary Hypertension and Cor Pulmonale in Hypoventilation. Mount Kisco, N.Y., Futura Publishing Co., 1984, p. 321.
172. Cherniack, N. S.: Respiratory dysrhythmias during sleep. N. Engl. J. Med. *305*:325, 1981.
173. Millman, R. P., and Fishman, A. P.: Sleep apnea syndromes. *In* Fishman, A. P. (ed.): Pulmonary Diseases and Disorders. 2nd ed. New York, McGraw-Hill Book Co., 1991, pp. 1347–1362.
174. Strohl, K. P., Cherniack, N. S., and Gather, B.: Physiologic basis of therapy in sleep apnea. Am. Rev. Respir. Dis. *134*:791, 1986.
175. Khoo, M. C. K.: Periodic breathing. *In* Crystal, R. G., and West, J. B. (eds.): The Lung: Scientific Foundations. New York, Raven Press, 1991, pp. 1419–1432.
176. Burrek, B.: The hypersomina-sleep apnea syndrome: Its recognition in clinical cardiology. Am. Heart J. *107*:543, 1984.
177. Shephard, J. W., Jr.: Hypotension, cardiac arrhythmias, myocardial infarction, and stroke in relation to obstructive sleep apnea. Clin. Chest Med. *13*:437, 1992.
178. Guilleminault, C., Cannally, S. J., and Winkler, R. A.: Cardiac arrhythmia and conduction disturbances during sleep in 400 patients with sleep apnea syndrome. Am. J. Cardiol. *52*:490, 1983.
179. Peiser, J., Ovnat, A., Uwyyed, K., et al.: Cardiac arrhythmias during sleep in morbidly obese sleep-apneic patients before and after gastric bypass surgery. Clin. Cardiol. *8*:519, 1985.
180. Buda, A. J., Schroeder, J. S., and Gulleminault, C.: Abnormalities of pulmonary wedge pressures in sleep-induced apnea. Int. J. Cardiol. *1*:67, 1981.
181. Moldofsky, H.: Evaluation of daytime sleepiness. Clin. Chest Med. *13*:417, 1992.
182. Kryger, M. H.: Management of obstructive sleep apnea. Clin. Chest Med. *13*:481, 1992.
183. Bradley, T. D.: Right and left ventricular functional impairment and sleep apnea. Clin. Chest Med. *13*:459, 1992.
184. Fletcher, E. C., Schaaf, J. W., Miller, J., and Fletcher, J. G.: Long term cardiopulmonary sequelae in patients with sleep apnea and chronic lung disease. Am. Rev. Respir. Dis. *135*:525, 1987.
185. Weitzenblum, E., Krieger, J., Apprill, M., et al.: Daytime pulmonary hypertension in patients with obstructive sleep apnea syndrome. Am. Rev. Respir. Dis. *138*:345, 1988.
186. Weitzenblum, E., Krieger, J., Oswald, M., et al.: Chronic obstructive pulmonary disease and sleep apnea syndrome. Sleep *15*(Suppl. 6):S33, 1992.
187. Hudgel, D. W.: The role of upper airway anatomy and physiology in obstructive sleep apnea. Clin. Chest Med. *13*:383, 1992.
188. Bradley, T. D., and Phillipson, E. A.: Central sleep apnea. Clin. Chest Med. *13*:493, 1992.
189. Martin, R. J., Sanders, M. H., Gray, B. A., and Pennock, B. E.: Acute and long-term ventilatory effects of hyperoxia in adult sleep apnea syndrome. Am. Rev. Respir. Dis. *125*:175, 1982.
190. Bland, J. W., Edwards, F. K., and Brainsfield, D.: Pulmonary hypertension and congestive heart failure in children with chronic upper airway obstruction: New concepts and etiologic factors. Am. J. Cardiol. *23*:830, 1969.
191. Randall, C. S., Braman, S. S., and Millman, R. P.: Rapid development of cor pulmonale following acute tonsillitis in adults. Chest *95*:462, 1989.
192. Noonan, J. A.: Pulmonary heart disease. Pediatr. Clin. North Am. *18*:1255, 1971.
193. Johnson, G. M., and Todd, D. W.: Cor pulmonale in severe Pierre Robin syndrome. Pediatrics *65*:152, 1980.
194. Glenn, W. W. L., Gee, J. B. L., Cole, D. R., et al.: Combined central alveolar hypoventilation and upper airway obstruction. Treatment by tracheostomy and diaphragm pacing. Am. J. Med. *64*:50, 1978.
195. Ingram, R. H., Jr., and Bishop, J. B.: Ventilatory response to carbon dioxide after removal of chronic upper airway obstruction. Am. Rev. Respir. Dis. *102*:645, 1970.
196. Ungerer, R. G., Tashkin, D. P., Furst, D., et al.: Prevalence and clinical correlates of pulmonary arterial hypotension in progressive systemic sclerosis. Am. J. Med. *75*:65, 1983.
197. Young, R. H., and Mark, G. S.: Pulmonary vascular changes in scleroderma. Am. J. Med. *64*:998, 1978.
198. Wright, J. L., Lawson, L., Pare, P. D., et al.: The structure and function of the pulmonary vasculature in mild chronic obstructive pulmonary disease: The effect of oxygen and exercise. Am. Rev. Respir. Dis. *128*:702, 1983.
199. Calverley, P. M., Howatson, R., Flenley, D. C., and Lamb, D.: Clinicopathological correlations in cor pulmonale. Thorax *47*:494, 1992.
200. Arroliga, A. C., Matthay, M. A., and Matthay, R. A.: Pulmonary thromboembolism and other pulmonary vascular diseases. *In* George, R. B., Light, R. W., Matthay, M. A., and Matthay, R. A. (eds.): Chest Medicine: Essentials of Pulmonary and Critical Care Medicine. 3rd ed. Baltimore, Williams and Wilkins, 1995, pp. 271–302.
201. Boushy, J. F., and North, L. B.: Hemodynamic changes in chronic obstructive pulmonary disease. Chest *72*:565, 1977.
202. Weitzenblum, E., Loisceau, A., Hirth, C., et al.: Course of pulmonary hemodynamics in patients with chronic obstructive pulmonary disease. Chest *75*:565, 1979.
203. Weitzenblum, E., Sautegeau, A., Ehrhart, M., et al.: Long-term course of pulmonary arterial pressure in chronic obstructive pulmonary disease. Am. Rev. Respir. Dis. *130*:993–998, 1984.
204. Bishop, J. M., and Cross, K. W.: Use of other physiological variables to predict pulmonary arterial pressure in patients with chronic respiratory disease: Multicenter study. Eur. Heart J. *2*:509, 1981.

205. Bishop, J. M., and Cross, K. W.: Physiological variables and mortality in patients with various categories of chronic respiratory disease: WHO multicenter study. Eur. Heart J. *2*:509, 1981.
206. Oswald-Mammosser, M., Apprill, M., Bachez, P., et al.: Pulmonary hemodynamics in chronic obstructive pulmonary disease of the emphysematous type. Respiration *58*:304, 1991.
207. Mahler, D. A., Brent, B. N., Loke, J., et al.: Right ventricular performance and central circulatory hemodynamics during upright exercise in patients with chronic obstructive pulmonary disease. Am. Rev. Respir. Dis. *130*:722, 1984.
208. Hicken, P., Brewer, D., and Heath, D.: The relation between the weight of the right ventricle of the heart and the internal surface area and the number of alveoli in the human lung in emphysema. J. Pathol. Bacteriol. *92*:529, 1966.
209. Biernacki, W., Gould, G. A., Whyte, K. F., and Flenley, D. C.: Pulmonary hemodynamics, gas exchange and the severity of emphysema as assessed by quantitative CT scan in chronic bronchitis and emphysema. Am. Rev. Respir. Dis. *139*:1509, 1989.
210. Jamal, K., Fleetham, J. A., and Thurlbeck, W. M.: Cor pulmonale: Correlation with central airways lesions, peripheral airways lesions, emphysema, and control of breathing. Am. Rev. Respir. Dis. *141*:1172, 1990.
211. Hasleton, P. S., Heath, D., and Brewer, D. B.: Hypertensive pulmonary vascular disease in states of chronic hypoxia. J. Pathol. Bacteriol. *95*:431, 1968.
212. Lamb, D.; Pathology of COPD. *In* Brewis, R. A. L., Gibson, G. J., and Geddes, D. M. (eds.): Respiratory Medicine. London, Baillière Tindall, 1990, pp. 497–507.
213. Wilkinson, M., Langhorn, C. A., Heath, D., et al.: A pathophysiological study of 10 cases of hypoxic cor pulmonale. Q. J. Med. *66*:65, 1988.
214. Wright, J. L., Lawson, L., Pare, P. D., et al.: The structure and function of pulmonary vasculature in mild chronic obstructive pulmonary disease: the effect of oxygen on exercise. Am. Rev. Respir. Dis. *128*:702, 1983.
215. Magee, F., Wright, J. L., Wiggs, B. R., et al.: Pulmonary vascular structure and function in chronic obstructive pulmonary disease. Thorax *43*:183, 1988.
216. Crawley, D. E., Liu, S. F., Evans, T. W., and Barnes, P. J.: Inhibitory role of endothelium-derived relaxing factor in rat and human pulmonary arteries. Br. J. Pharmacol. *101*:166, 1990.
217. Liu, S. F., Crawley, D. E., Barnes, P. J., and Evans, T. W.: Endothelium-derived relaxing factor inhibits hypoxic pulmonary vasoconstriction in rats. Am. Rev. Respir. Dis. *143*:32, 1991.
218. Dinh-Xuan, A. T.: Endothelial modulation of pulmonary vascular tone. Eur. Respir. J. *5*:757, 1992.
219. Din-Xuan, A. T., Higenbottam, T. W., Clelland, C. A., et al.: Impairment of endothelium-dependent pulmonary artery relaxation in chronic obstructive lung disease. N. Engl. J. Med. *324*:1539, 1991.
220. Adnot, S., Raffestin, B., Addahibi, S., et al.: Loss of endothelium-dependent relaxant activity in the pulmonary circulation of rats exposed to chronic hypoxia. J. Clin. Invest. *87*:155, 1991.
221. MacNee, W.: Pathophysiology of cor pulmonale in chronic obstructive pulmonary disease (Part 2). Am. J. Respir. Crit. Care Med. *150*:1158, 1994.
222. Weitzenblum, E., Apprill, M., Oswald, M., et al.: Pulmonary hemodynamics in patients with chronic obstructive pulmonary disease before and during an episode of peripheral edema. Chest *105*:1377, 1994.
223. Fulton, F. M., Hutchison, E. C., and Jones, A. M.: Ventricular weight in cardiac hypertrophy. Br. Heart J. *14*:413, 1952.
224. Heath, D., and Williams, D. R.: Man at High Altitude. Edinburgh, Churchill Livingstone, 1981.
225. Farber, M. O., Bright, T. P., Strawbridge, R. A., et al.: Impaired water handling in chronic obstructive lung disease. J. Lab. Clin. Med. *85*:41, 1975.
226. Farber, M. O., Kiblawi, S. S. O., Strawbridge, R. A., et al.: Studies on plasma vasopressin and the renin-angiotensin-aldosterone system in chronic obstructive lung disease. J. Lab. Clin. Med. *90*:373, 1977.
227. Campbell, E. J. M., and Short, D. S.: The cause of oedema in 'cor pulmonale.' Lancet *1*:1184, 1960.
228. Kawakami, Y., Kishi, F., Yamamoto, H., et al.: Relation of oxygen delivery, mixed venous oxygenation, and pulmonary hemodynamics to prognosis in chronic obstructive pulmonary disease. N. Engl. J. Med. *308*:1045, 1983.
229. Albert, R. K., Schrijen, F., and Poincelot, F.: Oxygen consumption and transport in stable patients with chronic obstructive pulmonary disease. Am. Rev. Respir. Dis. *134*:678, 1986.
230. Chappell, T. R., Rubin, L. J., Markham, R. V., Jr., et al.: Independence of oxygen consumption and systemic oxygen transport in patients with either stable pulmonary hypertension or refractory left ventricular failure. Am. Rev. Respir. Dis. *128*:30, 1983.
231. Tenney, S. M., and Mithoefer, J. D.: The relationship of mixed oxygenation to oxygen transport, with special reference to adaptations to high altitude and pulmonary disease. Am. Rev. Respir. Dis. *125*:474, 1982.
232. Mithoefer, J. C.: Assessment of tissue oxygenation. *In* Simmons, D. H. (ed.): Current Pulmonology. Vol. 4. New York, John Wiley and Sons, 1982, p. 215.
233. Bergorsky, E. H.: Tissue oxygen delivery and cor pulmonale in chronic obstructive pulmonary disease. N. Engl. J. Med. *308*:1092, 1983.
234. Burrows, B., Kettel, K. J., Niden, A. H., et al.: Patterns of cardiovascular dysfunction in chronic obstructive lung disease. N. Engl. J. Med. *286*:912, 1972.
235. Howard, P.: Drugs or oxygen for hypoxic cor pulmonale? Br. Med. J. *287*:1159, 1983.
236. Medical Research Council Working Party: Long term domiciliary oxygen therapy in chronic hypoxic cor pulmonale complicating chronic bronchitis and emphysema: A clinical trial. Lancet *1*:681, 1981.
237. Nocturnal Oxygen Therapy Trial Group: Continuous or nocturnal oxygen therapy in hypoxemic chronic obstructive lung disease. Ann. Intern. Med. *93*:931, 1980.
238. Anthonisen, N. R.: Long-term oxygen therapy. Ann. Intern. Med. *99*:519, 1983.
239. Flenley, D. C., and Muir, A. L.: Cardiovascular effects of oxygen therapy for pulmonary arterial hypertension. Clin. Chest. Med. *4*:297, 1983.
240. Heaton, R. K., Grant, I., McSweeny, A. J., et al.: Psychologic effects of continuous and nocturnal oxygen therapy in hypoxemic chronic obstructive pulmonary disease. Arch. Intern. Med. *143*:1941, 1983.
241. Wilson, D. K., Kaplan, R. M., Timms, R. M., and Dawson, A.: Acute effects of oxygen treatment upon information processing in hypoxemic COPD patients. Chest *88*:239, 1985.
242. Morrison, D. A., Henry, R., and Goldman, S.: Preliminary study of the effects of low flow oxygen on oxygen delivery and right ventricular function in chronic lung disease. Am. Rev. Respir. Dis. *133*:390, 1986.
243. Ashutosh, K., Mead, G., and Dunsky, M.: Early effects of oxygen administration and prognosis in chronic obstructive pulmonary disease and cor pulmonale. Am. Rev. Respir. Dis. *127*:399–404, 1983.
244. Petty, R. L.: Who needs home oxygen? Am. Rev. Respir. Dis. *131*:930, 1985.
245. Levi-Valensi, P., Weitzenblum, E., Pedinielli, J.-L., et al.: Three-month follow-up of arterial blood gas determination in candidates for long-term oxygen therapy. Am. Rev. Respir. Dis. *133*:547, 1986.
246. Flenley, D. C.: Long-term home oxygen therapy. Chest *87*:99, 1985.
247. Kim, Y. S., and Aviado, D. M.: Digitalis and the pulmonary circulation. Am. Heart J. *62*:680, 1961.
248. Sylvester, J. T., Goldberg, H. S., and Permutt, S.: The role of the vasculature in the regulation of cardiac output. Clin. Chest Med. *4*:222–236, 1983.
249. Berglund, E., Eidimsky, J., and Malmberg, R.: Lack of effect of digitalis in patients with pulmonary disease with and without heart disease. Am. J. Cardiol. *41*:897, 1978.
250. Brown, S. E., Pakron, F. J., Milne, N., et al.: Effects of digoxin on exercise capacity and right ventricular function during exercise in chronic airflow obstruction. Chest *85*:187, 1984.
251. Coates, A. L., Desmond, K., Asher, M. I., et al.: The effect of digoxin on exercise capacity and exercising cardiac function in cystic fibrosis. Chest *82*:543, 1982.
252. Jezek, V., and Schrijen, F.: Hemodynamic effect of deslanoside at rest and during exercise in patients with chronic bronchitis. Br. Heart J. *35*:2, 1973.
253. Mathur, P. N., Powles, A. C. P., Pugsley, S. O., et al.: Effect of long-term administration of digoxin on exercise performance in chronic airflow obstruction. Eur. J. Respir. Dis. *66*:273, 1985.
254. Mathur, P. N., Powles, A. C. P., Pugsley, S. O., et al.: Effect of digoxin on right ventricular function in severe chronic airflow obstruction. Ann. Intern. Med. *95*:283, 1981.
255. Green, L. H., and Smith, T. W.: The use of digitalis in patients with pulmonary disease. Ann. Intern. Med. *87*:459, 1977.
256. Aubier, M., Murciano, D., Viires, N., et al.: Effects of digoxin on diaphragmatic strength generation in patients with chronic obstructive pulmonary disease during acute respiratory failure. Am. Rev. Respir. Dis. *135*:544, 1987.
257. Mahler, D. A., Matthay, R. A., Snyder, P. E., et al.: Sustained-release theophylline reduces dyspnea in nonreversible obstructive airway disease. Am. Rev. Respir. Dis. *131*:22, 1985.
258. Matthay, R. A.: Effects of theophylline on cardiovascular performance in chronic obstructive pulmonary disease. Chest *88*(Suppl.):11S, 1985.
259. Matthay, R. A., and Berger, H. J.: Cardiovascular function in cor pulmonale. Clin. Chest Med. *4*:269, 1983.
260. Matthay, R. A., Berger, H. J., Davies, R., et al.: Improvement in cardiac performance by oral long-acting theophylline in chronic obstructive pulmonary disease. Am. Heart J. *104*:1022, 1982.
261. Marcus, M. L., Skelton, C. L., Grauer, L. E., et al.: Effects of theophylline on myocardial mechanics. Am. J. Physiol. *222*:1361, 1972.
262. DiMarco, A. F., Nochomovitz, M., DiMarco, M. S., et al.: Comparative effects of aminophylline on diaphragm and cardiac contractility. Am. Rev. Respir. Dis. *132*:800, 1985.
263. Rutherford, J. D., Vatner, S. E., and Braunwald, E.: Effects and mechanisms of action of aminophylline on cardiac function and regional blood flow distribution in conscious dogs. Circulation *63*:378, 1981.
264. Murphy, G. W., Schreiner, B. R., and Yu, P. M.: Effects of aminophylline on the pulmonary circulation and left ventricular performance in patients with valvular heart disease. Circulation *37*:361, 1968.
265. Benumof, J. L., and Trousdale, F. R.: Aminophylline does not inhibit canine hypoxic pulmonary vasoconstriction. Am. Rev. Respir. Dis. *126*:1017, 1982.
266. Brent, B. N., Berger, H. J., Matthay, R. A., et al.: Contrasting acute effects of vasodilators (nitroglycerin, nitroprusside, and hyralazine) on right ventricular performance in patients with chronic obstructive pulmonary disease and pulmonary hypertension: A combined radionuclide-hemodynamic study. Am. J. Cardiol. *51*:1682, 1983.
267. MacNee, W., Walthen, C. G., Hannan, W. J., et al.: Effects of pirbuterol and sodium nitroprusside on pulmonary haemodynamics in hypoxic cor pulmonale. Br. Med. J. *287*:1169–1172, 1983.

268. Whyte, K. F., and Flenley, D. C.: Can pulmonary vasodilators improve survival in cor pulmonale due to hypoxic chronic bronchitis and emphysema? Thorax *43:*1, 1988.
269. Brent, B. N., Mahler, D., Berger, H. J., et al.: Augmentation of right ventricular performance in chronic obstructive pulmonary disease by terbutaline. A combined radionuclide and hemodynamic study. Am. J. Cardiol. *50:*313, 1982.
270. Stockley, R. A., Finnegan, P., and Bishop, J. M.: Effect of intravenous terbutaline on arterial blood gas tensions, ventilation and pulmonary circulation in patients with chronic bronchitis and cor pulmonale. Thorax *32:*601, 1977.
271. Jones, R. M., Stockley, R. A., and Bishop, J. M.: Early effects of intravenous terbutaline on cardiopulmonary function in chronic obstructive bronchitis and pulmonary hypertension. Thorax *37:*746, 1982.
272. Teule, G. J. J., and Majid, P. A.: Hemodynamic effects of terbutaline in chronic obstructive airways disease. Thorax *35:*536, 1980.
273. Biernacki, W., Pruice, K., Whyte, K., et al.: The effect of six months of daily treatment with the beta-2 agonist oral pirbuterol on pulmonary hemodynamics in patients with chronic hypoxic cor pulmonale receiving long-term oxygen therapy. Am. Rev. Respir. Dis. *139:*492, 1989.
274. Rubin, L. J.: Vasodilators and pulmonary hypertension: Where do we go from here? Am. Rev. Respir. Dis. *135:*288, 1987.
275. Salvaterra, C. G., and Rubin, L. J.: Investigation and management of pulmonary hypertension in chronic obstructive pulmonary disease. Am. Rev. Respir. Dis. *148:*1414, 1993.
276. Packer, M.: Vasodilator therapy for primary pulmonary hypertension. Ann. Intern. Med. *103:*258, 1985.
277. Brent, B. N., Matthay, R. A., Mahler, D. A., et al.: Relationship between oxygen uptake and oxygen transport in stable patients with chronic obstructive pulmonary disease: Physiologic effects of nitroprusside and hydralazine. Am. Rev. Respir. Dis. *129:*682, 1984.
278. Corriveau, M. L., Minh, V.-D., and Dolan, G. F.: Long-term effects of hydralazine on ventilation and blood gas values in patients with chronic obstructive pulmonary disease hypertension. Am. J. Med. *83:*886, 1987.
279. Corriveau, M. L., Rosen, B. J., Keller, C. A., et al.: Effect of posture, hydralazine, and nifedipine on hemodynamics, ventilation, and gas exchange in patients with chronic obstructive pulmonary disease. Am. Rev. Respir. Dis. *138:*1494, 1988.
280. Dal Nogare, A. R., and Rubin, L. J.: The effects of hydralazine on exercise capacity in pulmonary hypertension secondary to chronic obstructive pulmonary disease. Am. Rev. Respir. Dis. *133:*385, 1986.
281. Keller, C. A., Shepard, J. W., Chun, D. S., et al.: Effects of hydralazine on hemodynamics, ventilation and gas exchange in patients with chronic obstructive pulmonary disease and pulmonary hypertension. Am. Rev. Repair. Dis. *130:*606, 1984.
282. Miller, M. J., Chappell, T. R., Cook, W., et al.: Effects of oral hydralazine on gas exchange in patients with cor pulmonale. Am. J. Med. *75:*937, 1983.
283. Rubin, L. J., and Peter, R. H.: Hemodynamics at rest and during exercise after oral hydralazine in patients with cor pulmonale. Am. J. Cardiol. *47:*116, 1981.
284. Lupi-Herrera, E., Seoane, M., and Verdejo, J.: Hemodynamic effect of hydralazine in advanced, stable chronic obstructive pulmonary disease with cor pulmonale: Immediate and short-term evaluation at rest and during exercise. Chest *85:*156, 1984.
285. McGoon, M. D., Seward, J. B., Vliestra, R. E., et al.: Haemodynamic response to intravenous hydralazine in patients with pulmonary hypertension. Br. Heart J. *50:*579, 1983.
286. Packer, M.: Greenberg, B., Massie, B., et al.: Deleterious effects of hydralazine in patients with pulmonary hypertension. N. Engl. J. Med. *306:*1326, 1982.
287. Tuxen, D. V., Powles, A. C. P., Mathur, P. N., et al.: Detrimental effects of hydralazine in patients with chronic air-flow obstruction and pulmonary hypertension: A combined hemodynamic and radionuclide study. Am. Rev. Respir. Dis. *129:*388, 1984.
288. Brown, S. E., Linden, G. S., Kling, R. R., et al.: Effects of verapamil on pulmonary haemodynamics during hypoxaemia, at rest, and during exercise in patients with chronic obstructive pulmonary disease. Thorax *38:*840, 1983.
289. Kalra, L., and Bone, M. F.: Effect of nifedipine on physiologic shunting and oxygenation in chronic obstructive pulmonary disease. Am. J. Med. *94:*419, 1993.
290. Domenighetti, G. M., and Saglini, V. G.: Short- and long-term hemodynamic effects of oral nifedipine in patients with pulmonary hypertension secondary to COPD and lung fibrosis: Deleterious effects in patients with restrictive disease. Chest *102:*708, 1992.
291. Kennedy, T. P., Michael, J. R., Huang, C.-K., et al.: Nifedipine inhibits hypoxic pulmonary vasoconstriction during rest and exercise in patients with chronic obstructive pulmonary disease. Am. Rev. Respir. Dis. *129:*544, 1984.
292. Rubin, L. J., and Moser, K.: Long-term effects of nitrendipine on hemodynamics and oxygen transport in patients with cor pulmonale. Chest *89:*141–145, 1986.
293. Sajkov, D., McEvoy, R. D., Cowie, R. J., et al.: Felodipine improves pulmonary hemodynamics in chronic obstructive pulmonary disease. Chest *103:*1354, 1993.
294. Geggel, R. L., Dozor, A. J., Fyler, D. C., et al.: Effects of vasodilators at rest and during exercise in young adults with cystic fibrosis and chronic cor pulmonale. Am. Rev. Respir. Dis. *131:*531, 1985.
295. Gould, L., Zahir, M., DeMartino, A., et al.: Haemodynamic effects of phentolamine in chronic obstructive pulmonary disease. Br. Heart J. *33:*445, 1971.
296. Spahn, F., Rottman, B., and Schmidt, U.: Effects of single intravenous administration of urapidil and diltiazem in patients with nonfixed pulmonary hypertension secondary to chronic obstructive lung disease. J. Cardiovasc. Pharmacol. *23:*517, 1994.
297. Adnot, S., DeFouilloy, C., Brun-Buisson, C., et al.: Hemodynamic effects of urapidil in patients with pulmonary hypertension: A comparative study with hydralazine. Am. Rev. Respir. Dis. *135:*288, 1987.
298. Adnot, S., Anrivet, P., Piquet, J., et al.: The effects of urapidil therapy on hemodynamics and gas exchange in exercising patients with chronic obstructive pulmonary disease and hypertension. Am. Rev. Respir. Dis. *137:*1068, 1988.
299. Vik-Mo, H., Walde, N., Jentoft, H., and Halvorsen, F. I.: Improved haemodynamics but reduced arterial oxygen tension at rest and during exercise after long-term oral prazosin therapy in chronic cor pulmonale. Eur. Heart J. *6:*1047, 1985.
300. Zielinski, J., Hawrylkiewicz, I., Gorecka, D., et al.: Captopril effects on pulmonary and systemic hemodynamics in chronic cor pulmonale. Chest *90:*562, 1986.
301. Burke, C. M., Harte, M., Duncan, J., et al.: Captopril and domiciliary oxygen in chronic airflow obstruction. Br. Med. J. *290:*1251, 1985.
302. Kastanos, N., Miro, R. E., and Agusti-Vidal, A.: Captopril in pulmonary hypertension. Br. Heart J. *49:*513, 1983.
303. Ishizaki, T., Miyabo, S., Mifune, J., et al.: OP-1206, A prostaglandin E^1 derivative: Effects of oral administration to patients with chronic lung disease. Chest *85:*382, 1984.
304. Jones, K., Higgenbottom, T., and Wallwork, J.: Pulmonary vasodilation and prostacyclin in primary and secondary pulmonary hypertension. Chest *96:*784, 1989.
305. Dujic, Z., Eterovic, D., Tocilj, J., et al.: About mechanisms of prostaglandin E^1 induced deterioration of pulmonary gas exchange in COPD patients. Clin. Physiol. *13:*497, 1993.
306. Rubin, J. J.: Cardiovascular effects of vasodilator therapy for pulmonary arterial hypertension. Clin. Chest Med. *4:*309, 1983.
307. Segal, N., and Bishop, J. M.: The circulation in patients with chronic bronchitis and emphysema at rest and during exercise, with special reference to the influence of changes in blood viscosity and blood volume on the pulmonary circulation. J. Clin. Invest. *45:*1555–1568, 1966.
308. Chetty, K. G., Brown, S. E., and Light, R. W.: Improved exercise tolerance of the polycythemic lung patient following phlebotomy. Am. J. Med. *74:*415, 1983.
309. Dayton, L. M., McCullough, R. E., Scheinhorn, D. J., et al.: Symptomatic and pulmonary response to acute phlebotomy in secondary polycythemia. Chest *68:*785, 1975.
310. Weisse, A. B., Moschos, C. B., Frank, M. S., et al.: Hemodynamic effects of staged hematocrit reduction in patients with stable cor pulmonale and severely elevated hematocrit levels. Am. J. Med. *58:*92, 1975.
311. Rakita, L., Gillespie, D. G., and Sancetta, S.: The acute and chronic effects of phlebotomy on general hemodynamics and pulmonary functions of patients with secondary polycythemia associated with pulmonary emphysema. Am. Heart. J. *70:*466, 1965.

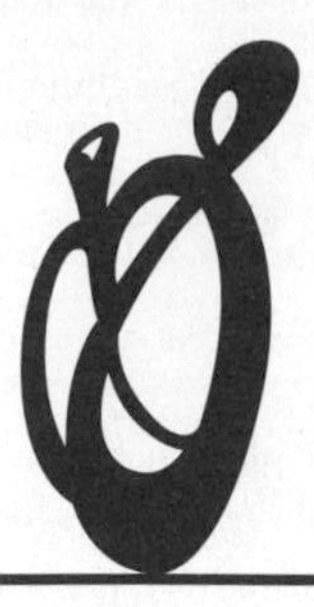

Part IV
Broader Perspectives on Heart Disease and Cardiologic Practice

Chapter 48
Principles of Cardiovascular Molecular and Cellular Biology

KENNETH R. CHIEN, ANDREW A. GRACE

RECOMBINANT PROTEIN THERAPY 1626
Tissue Plasminogen Activators 1627
Further Applications of Recombinant Protein Engineering 1628
RATIONAL DESIGN AND DEVELOPMENT OF PHARMACOLOGICAL ANTAGONISTS 1629
$\alpha_{IIb}\beta_3$ Platelet-Specific Integrin 1629
$\alpha_{IIb}\beta_3$ (II_b/IIIa) Inhibition 1630
LOCALIZATION OF CARDIOVASCULAR DISEASE GENES 1630
Molecular Genetics of Long Q-T Syndromes 1631
Molecular Genetics of Factor V Mutation 1633
GENETIC MODELS OF HUMAN CARDIOVASCULAR DISEASE 1634
Transgenic Technology 1635
Mouse Models of Atherosclerosis 1636
GENE THERAPY 1637
Technical Aspects 1637
Vector Development 1638
MOLECULAR ADVANCES IN CARDIAC HYPERTROPHY 1639
Activation of Cardiac Muscle Genes During Hypertrophy 1639
Identification of Cardiac Growth Factors and Cytokines 1641
Intracellular Signaling Pathways 1643
Familial Hypertrophic Cardiomyopathy . . .1644
Toward New Therapeutic Strategies for Heart Failure 1644
FUTURE PERSPECTIVES 1645
REFERENCES 1645

The past two decades of cardiovascular biology and medicine have been based largely upon the consideration of the heart and vasculature as an integrated physiological system, a view that has resulted in major therapeutic advances. With the advent of developments in gene transfer, mouse and human genetics, genetic engineering of intact animals, and molecular and cellular technology, cardiovascular medicine is now on the threshold of a molecular therapeutic era.[1] Major steps have been taken toward unraveling the molecular determinants of complex, integrative, and polygenic cardiovascular disease states, including atherosclerosis, hypertension, cardiac hypertrophy and failure, congenital heart disease, and coronary restenosis following balloon angioplasty. Our improved understanding of the fundamental basis of these important cardiovascular disease processes has established a scientific foundation for diagnostic, prognostic, and therapeutic advances in the mainstream of cardiovascular medicine.

This chapter provides a few selected examples that highlight the breadth and growing impact of the molecular sciences on the practice of cardiovascular medicine. A primer of basic molecular biology can also be found in a number of specialized texts and reviews devoted to molecular and cellular biology.[2–4] Although the scope of this chapter does not allow for a comprehensive analysis of this rapidly expanding area, a companion text[5] provides further background to the themes underlying the impact of molecular advances in cardiovascular medicine.

RECOMBINANT PROTEIN THERAPY

The production of clinically valuable recombinant proteins and their subsequent manipulation using protein engineering are among the major medical applications of recombinant DNA technology and have given rise to the biotechnology industry, which has been based upon the need for large-scale protein isolation and purification.[6] In medical applications, the recombinant protein can be the therapeutic agent, designed for replacement therapy where disease is based upon an acquired or genetic deficiency of a specific protein, as in diabetes mellitus or hemophilia. Alternatively, the therapeutic application may be based upon the promotion or inhibition of a specific biological pathway, e.g., stimulating erythrocytosis in chronic renal failure.[7] At present, a number of recombinant proteins have documented clinical utility, including insulin, factor VIII, erythropoietin, and hemopoietic growth factors.[7,8] Tissue plasminogen activator was the first product of protein engineering designed for clinical use in the cardiovascular field,[9,10] and a number of other potentially valuable proteins will be tested in the next few years.[11,12]

The techniques for large-scale production of proteins have necessitated industrial-scale approaches, but they fundamentally rely on conventional molecular technology utilizing gene cloning, expression, and mutagenesis to manipulate and match protein structure to particular tasks. Producing a recombinant protein first requires the cloning of the gene encoding the protein of interest, construction of an expression vector, and transfer of the gene construct into a surrogate cell system that is programmed for large-scale synthesis.[3]

Tissue Plasminogen Activators (t-PA)

CLONING OF THE t-PA GENE. Identification of a tissue source of t-PA[13] was followed only many years later by protein isolation from a human Bowes melanoma cell line[14] and subsequent purification and characterization of the enzyme.[15] The initial samples of t-PA for intracoronary thrombolysis came from this source, although conventional protein purification from the melanoma cell line was inadequate for purposes beyond small-scale clinical use.[10]

The therapeutic potential of thrombolytic agents and the availability of recombinant technology led to considerable efforts to genetically engineer t-PA[3,9] and has provided a paradigm for the industrial application of molecular technology. The project was initially pursued by two independent groups, using similar strategies to isolate and clone the t-pA gene.[16,17] The protein was isolated from the human melanoma cell line and the molecular weight identified at approximately 63,000 kDa. The amino acid sequence of a small stretch of the t-PA protein was determined, allowing the synthesis of oligonucleotides complementary to the DNA nucleotide sequence which encode defined portions of the molecule. The oligonucleotides were utilized as probes to isolate the t-PA cDNA from a library of sequences derived from Bowes melanoma cells.[3] The isolation of a full-length t-PA cDNA that followed served as the source for the recombinant t-PA that is currently used for thrombolytic therapy[10,18] (see pp. 1220 and 1907).

PRODUCTION OF RECOMBINANT t-PA IN CELL SYSTEMS. The techniques for the production of recombinant proteins harness the endogenous capacity of a surrogate cell system to be programmed to express the desired gene product and require the stable integration of an amplified expression vector.[3] A variety of bacterial, yeast, and mammalian cell systems have been used for this purpose. *Escherichia coli* is commonly used and displays several advantages of simplicity, short generation time, large yields, and relatively low cost.[3] Although this prokaryotic system is still standard for the production of recombinant products in the laboratory, the large-scale production of biologically active material usually requires more sophisticated methods, as the bacterial system can introduce folding defects and is unable to incorporate appropriate post-translational modifications (acetylation, glycosylation, phosphorylation), which can lead to functionally impaired products.[3]

The size, complexity, and maintenance of the proper folding of the t-PA protein provide a point of contrast with less complex proteins, such as insulin and growth hormone. The necessity for maintaining proper processing of t-PA led to the development of the Chinese hamster ovary (CHO) expression system, which has become standard in the field.[3] Transfection of a t-PA cDNA into these cells leads to the efficient generation of t-PA protein, which can be adapted to culture in large-scale fermenters (Fig. 48–1). Although the first mammalian expression systems displayed relatively low capacity, a novel modification increased expression of t-PA by gene amplification.[19] Resistance of cancer cells to methotrexate is associated with the rapid amplification of the dihydrofolate reductase *(dhfr)* gene. By fusing the t-PA gene to that of *dhfr* and exposing the CHO cells to serial increases in methotrexate, one can select for a CHO cell line displaying an increase in *dhfr* gene copy number with coamplification of the t-PA gene. These cells are programmed to release t-PA into the culture medium, thereby facilitating the large-scale isolation and purification of the t-PA protein.

PRINCIPLES UNDERLYING THE DEVELOPMENT OF t-PA VARIANTS. A number of limitations of native t-PA were observed in early evaluations and clinical trials—resistance to reperfusion (25 per cent), reocclusion (5 to 25 per cent), delayed reperfusion, occasional significant bleeding, and short plasma half-life—which spurred interests in modifying the molecule to optimize clinical efficacy.[18,20,21] Of course, the pressures of evolution had served to optimize t-PA only for a role in *endogenous* fibrinolysis and not for *clinical* thrombolysis. The generation of large quantities of t-PA allowed a detailed structure-function analysis of the native protein with regard to fibrin binding, catalytic action, and clearance.[10,22,23] This knowledge eventually resulted in the identification of the specific domains of the protein which account for these functional properties of the intact molecule (Fig. 48–2). Native t-PA was shown to provide a good example of a protein open to the rational application of recombinant molecular technology.[6,10,24] Par-

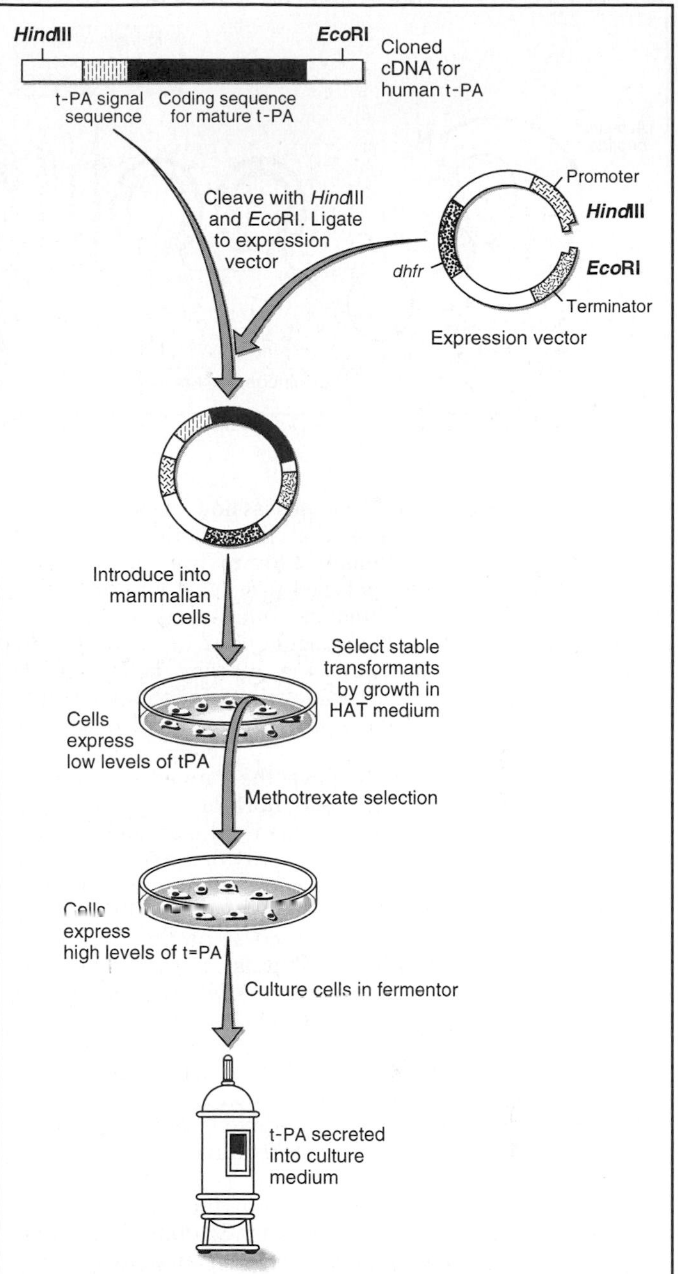

FIGURE 48–1. The production of t-PA in a mammalian cell (Chinese hamster ovary) system. The cloned cDNA for human t-PA was ligated into an expression vector under the control of a strong promoter and the vector stably transfected into the mammalian cell line (*HindIII* and *EcoRI* are endonuclease restriction sites). Initial transformants secreted low levels of t-PA into the culture medium, increased by the use of serial methotrexate selection for cells having the amplified dihydrofolate reductase *(dhfr)* gene linked to the t-PA expression cassette. High-expressing lines are grown in large-scale fermentors, with recombinant t-PA being purified from the culture medium. (Modified from Watson, J. D., Gilman, M., Witkowski, J., and Zoller, M.: Recombinant DNA. 2nd ed. © 1983, and 1992 by James D. Watson, Michael Gilman, Jan Witkowski, and Mark Zoller. New York, W. H. Freeman, 1992. Used with permission of W. H. Freeman and Co.)

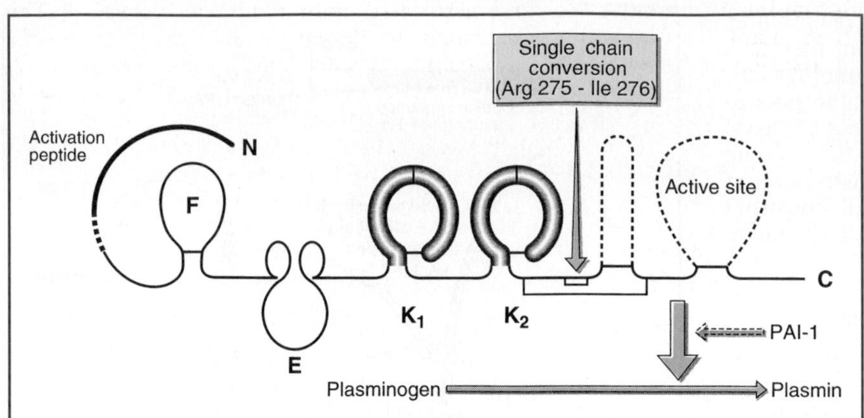

FIGURE 48–2. Structural domains of t-PA. The five distinct structural domains of the t-PA protein —finger (F) domain (residues 4 to 50 from the N-terminal region); growth factor (E) domain (residues 51 to 87); two kringle (K1/K2) domains (respectively, amino acids 87 to 176 and 176 to 262) with high-degree homology to five kringles of plasminogen; and serine protease catalytic domain (amino acids 276 to 527). These domains have structural homologies to other components of the plasminogen-plasmin system and other plasminogen activators. The finger and kringle domains confer the specificity for fibrin. Single-chain t-PA is synthesized and released from vascular endothelium; activity is further increased by conversion to the two-chain form after cleavage at Arg 275–Ile 276. The proteolytically active light chain region acts at Arg 560–Val 561 of plasminogen, resulting in the conversion to plasmin.

ticular advantages include the possession of several independent functional domains that have both independent and interdependent functions.[10,25] Improving the efficacy of the wild-type molecule was based upon the modification of the t-PA protein by site-directed mutagenesis of the structure of these domains.[25] The specific aims in re-engineering t-PA were directed at increasing efficacy by producing more rapid and persistent recanalization without rethrombosis, reducing hemorrhagic complications, and decreasing plasma clearance.[10]

Plasminogen activators all have the immediate function of cleaving plasminogen to yield fibrinolytic plasmin; the enzyme attacks fibrin to unravel a central component of the thrombotic latticework[10,22] (see p. 1815). t-PA is a serine protease catalyzing the cleavage of the common site single peptide bond (Arg560–Val561) of plasminogen.[10] The catalytic efficiency of t-PA is increased approximately 1000-fold in the presence of fibrin.[10] This is, in part, due to the high affinity of t-PA for fibrin (~10 nM), with selectivity being due to high-affinity fibrin-binding domains of the molecule.[10,22]

Structural analysis of human t-PA reveals a single polypeptide chain of 527 amino acids, and a complex binary and ternary structure has been predicted containing 16 disulphide bonds.[25] Five distinct structural domains are recognized: finger (F) domain (residues 4 to 50 from the N-terminal region) having homology to the fibrin affinity domain for fibronectin; growth factor (E) domain (residues 51 to 87) homologous to human epidermal growth factor; two kringle (K1/K2) domains (respectively, amino acids 87 to 176 and 176 to 262) with high-degree homology to five kringles of plasminogen; and a serine protease catalytic domain (amino acids 276 to 527). The full analysis of the three-dimensional structure of t-PA has not been achieved, although the crystal structure of the kringle-2 domain has been reported.[26] The integrated molecular structure, when solved, will facilitate understanding of how the function of the molecule is achieved in a dynamic fashion.[25]

Domain-deletion studies of t-PA have implicated the finger, growth factor, and second kringle domains in fibrin binding.[25] This fact produced attractive targets for modification using specific directed changes aimed at modifying both the structure and functional properties of t-PA and was encouraged by being ultimately therapeutically cleaner in view of preferential activation of plasminogen at the fibrin surface.[27] This contrasts with the systemic activation seen with streptokinase, anisolysated plasminogen streptokinase activated complex (APSAC), and urokinase, which could theoretically lead to a *lytic state.*[27]

t-PA MUTANTS WITH ALTERED FUNCTIONAL PROPERTIES. Despite considerable effort, the development of deletion/substitution functional domain mutants with altered properties of increased clot-specificity (targeting fibrin, uncovering either platelet epitopes or the covalent link between α_2-antiplasmin and fibrin) and decreased clearance (glycosylation, plasminogen activator inhibitor (PAI-1) resistance and so forth) has generally been disappointing.[10,24,28] Those mutants with improved pharmacokinetics achieved by the deletion of the F, E, and K_1 domains have tended toward decreased fibrinolytic activity.[22] Recently, the successful production of mutant t-PA with theoretically improved properties has, however, been described following sequential modification of the native t-PA molecule. The addition of a glycosylation site on kringle-1, termed T-t-PA, had the most promising pharmacokinetic profile; tetra-alanine substitution at amino acids 296 to 299 improved clearance and fibrin specificity (TK-t-PA); fibrin affinity was maintained with the additional mutation N117Q yielding TNK-t-PA.[29] These variants are now undergoing clinical trials. Clues to improvement of design have also come from other sources, such as the use of the plasminogen activator from the vampire bat *(Desmodus rotundus)* which is highly fibrin-specific, homologous to human t-PA, and lacks K-2 and the plasmin cleavage site for conversion to the two-chain form.[30]

The concept behind the development of *chimeric molecules* is that they would potentially enhance targeting with fewer systemic effects.[10] These conjugate hybrid proteins have been produced by chemical cross-linking or via recombinant technology by creating fusion proteins consisting of t-PA in conjunction with elements of other peptides (e.g., single-chain urokinase) to enhance fibrin affinity or to increase catalytic activity. In addition, monoclonal antibodies directed to the Bβ chain of fibrin and $\alpha_{IIb}\beta_3$ and thrombospondin have also been used to construct chimeras to allow targets of other components that contribute to thrombus formation.[22] In general, the approach has not yet produced agents of enhanced clinical value, instead having thrombolytic properties and fibrin selectivity generally similar but not superior to those of the component parts.[10]

Further Applications of Recombinant Protein Engineering

The production of sufficient quantities of clinical-grade t-PA for widespread use in thrombolysis represented a dramatic entrance for recombinant technology into the practice of cardiology. Second-generation plasminogen activators have followed, but truly rational protein design depends on three-dimensional structural analysis,[6,10] and it is not currently possible to precisely deduce tertiary protein structure from the primary amino acid sequences.[6] However, there have been technical advances in both the practical methods of protein structure determination, using both x-ray crystallography and nuclear magnetic resonance spectroscopy (which has the advantage of allowing structure determination in solution) and parallel advances in computer modeling that now allow improved prediction of ternary structure which should enhance rational approaches to protein engineering and should prove particularly valuable in regard to multidomain proteins such as t-PA.[6] Such approaches are likely to result in improvements in mutant design of existing molecules in addition to allowing the production of other recombinant molecules.

In this regard, several other recombinant proteins have been designed for cardiovascular use and are currently being tested in the appropriate clinical settings. Hirudin was initially isolated from the medical leech, *Hirudo medicinalis,* but recognition of therapeutic potential coincided with the leech becoming endangered.[11,12,33] Hirudin is the prototypic, direct thrombin inhibitor, binding both the active catalytic site and the substrate recognition site (anion exosite) of thrombin[12,32,33] (see p. 1820). It has several putative advantages over heparin, including an ability to inactivate clot-bound thrombin, and theoretical advantages of lack of inactivation by either heparinase or platelet factor 4, and no dependence on antithrombin-III.[12] The recombinant molecule has similar in vitro and in vivo anticoagulant, antiplatelet, and antithrombotic actions to those identified in the naturally occurring molecule.[11]

In addition to agents directed to the vessel wall, the development of recombinant peptide-derived growth factors that promote angiogenesis such as the fibroblast and vascular endothelial cell growth factors (FGF, VEGF)[34] or stimulate specific hematopoietic lineages such as thrombopoietin,[8] have potential clinical utility and will be examined in clinical studies in the next several years.

One other approach to rational antagonism uses genetically engineered monoclonal antibodies produced from cell lines secreting single antibody species of desired specificity.[35,36] This technology has been advanced by the development of mutant antibodies, antibodies of dual specificity, and rodent antibodies humanized by linking rodent immunoglobulin variable regions to human constant regions (chimeric humanized antibodies), thereby reducing immunogenicity.[37] The two major categories of monoclonal antibodies applied in cardiovascular medicine—antifibrin and antiplatelet antibodies ($\alpha_{IIb}\beta_3$ and thrombospondin), have, however, not yet found widespread application (see below).

RATIONAL DESIGN AND DEVELOPMENT OF PHARMACOLOGICAL ANTAGONISTS

Pharmaceutical development has traditionally relied on large-scale screening of natural sources for the identification of candidate compounds,[38] but molecular technology now indicates a likely change of fundamental approach. Recombinant protein and therapeutic antibody technology have had a clear impact on the development of new synthetic agonists and antagonists aimed at specific molecular targets causally related to disease phenotypes.[39] The molecular cloning of target molecules has led to rapid throughput screening approaches to identify appropriate antagonists. Molecular modeling of the compound and protein targets can now be employed to maximize the efficiency of identifying structure-function relationships and designing families of related compounds.[6,38]

In this regard, although the possibility of inhibition of intracellular signal transduction molecules has been raised,[38] inhibition of the ligand-surface receptor interaction (e.g., inhibition of the $\alpha_{IIb}\beta_3$ platelet receptor) remains the common principle for the development of many drugs with cardiovascular applications and serves as a prime example of the power of this approach.[40]

$\alpha_{IIb}\beta_3$ Platelet-Specific Integrin

The search for effective inhibitors of thrombosis has been a significant challenge of modern cardiovascular therapeutics, and the platelet has become a primary therapeutic target because it is a central component of thrombotic lesions.[41] Presently available antiplatelet agents all have problems, as they target individual pathways involved in platelet aggregation, leaving other pathways open which may then compensate via biologically redundant mechanisms[42] (see p. 1818). For example, aspirin, although of proven clinical utility in certain settings, has theoretical limitations, as it inhibits only thromboxane A_2–dependent mechanisms. The ideal target would be a molecule mediating final common pathways, where inhibition totally abrogates platelet adhesion, activation, and aggregation. The molecular identification of modulatory integrin receptors on the platelet surface has therefore presented a significant therapeutic opportunity.[43]

The platelet-specific integrin, most appropriately referred to as $\alpha_{IIb}\beta_3$[40,44–47] (also termed as GPIIb/IIIa), was the first integrin to be identified, purified, expressed in recombinant form, and associated with a human disease.[40] The functional importance of this molecule was first clearly shown in Glanzmann's thrombasthenia, where $\alpha_{IIb}\beta_3$ is either absent or dysfunctional and the clinical condition is characterized by mucocutaneous bleeding.[40]

The $\alpha_{IIb}\beta_3$ complex, a member of the widely distributed integrin supergene family of heterodimeric membrane proteins,[48] is an early specific marker of the megakarocyte lineage and the most abundant platelet integrin (density ~ 50,000 per platelet).[40] Integrins play key roles in cell adhesion events and are important in the migration, proliferation, and differentiation of several cell types.[44,45] Integrins are divided into three families, each possessing a common β subunit, but with different α subunits; $\alpha_{IIb}\beta_3$ is a β_3-cytoadherin family member along with the vitronectin receptor.[40] The receptor complex of $\alpha_{IIb}\beta_3$ has two components: the α subunit (GPIIb) is a 136-kDa glycoprotein with light and heavy chains and a disulfide bridge (Fig. 48–3). The light chain of 22 kDa allows anchorage, and the extracellular heavy chain has homologous sequences to calmodulin and troponin C.[40] The β subunit (GPIIIa) has a molecular weight of 90 to 105 kDa and is 90 per cent extracellular, with 41 residues in the cytoplasmic domain. The structure, as established by rotary shadowing electron microscopy, has a globular head and two tails. The recognition sites and ligand binding sites have been identified, which has facilitated the development of pharmacological antagonists.[40,47]

In view of their role in cell interaction and in thrombus formation, molecular characterization of $\alpha_{IIb}\beta_3$ and the structural basis of the $\alpha_{IIb}\beta_3$-ligand interaction, have become of great interest.[40] It has been established that in unstimulated platelets, $\alpha_{IIb}\beta_3$ has a random distribution and recognizes only immobilized fibrinogen. The binding of adhesive proteins stimulates platelets and activates $\alpha_{IIb}\beta_3$ with patches of $\alpha_{IIb}\beta_3$ becoming visible on the platelet surface, with a concomitant increase in platelet binding of fibrinogen von Willebrand factor (vWF), fibronectin, and thrombo-

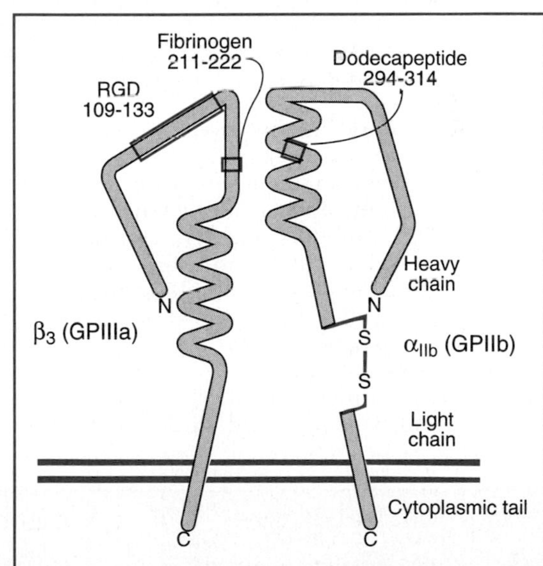

FIGURE 48–3. Schematic of structure and function of platelet membrane integrin $\alpha_{IIb}\beta_3$. Notable features of β_3 are the extracellular —NH_2 terminus, disulfide loop which binds —NH_2 to the midregion, typical transmembrane domain, and short cytoplasmic tail. α_{IIb} consists of disulfide linked heavy and light chains. The heavy chain has four Ca^{2+} binding repeats, and the light chain has a transmembrane segment and a short cytoplasmic tail. Three fibrinogen-binding sites are indicated: (1) β_3 109 to 130 has primary recognition for RGD sequences and secondary recognition for the fibrinogen gamma-chain sequence; (2) α_{IIb} 294 to 314 has the primary recognition for the gamma-chain sequence and secondary recognition for RGD; (3) β_3 211 to 222 recognition specificity has yet to be defined. The fibrinogen-binding sites provide potential targets for planned pharmacological intervention.

spondin. The dimeric structure of the molecule facilitates binding to platelets, leading to lattice formation and thrombus propagation.[40]

Two principal peptide recognition sequences on ligands interact with the platelet $\alpha_{IIb}\beta_3$ receptor complex. The arg-gly-asp (RGD) sequence was originally defined as the fibronectin sequence responsible for cell adhesion interactions[49] and has been shown to interact with a sequence localized to the amino-terminal part of the β subunit at residues 109 to 171.[47] Binding of RGD peptide recognition sequences in two molecules, vWF and fibrinogen, activates signals for the initiation of cell spreading, granular secretion, procoagulant activity, and conformational changes in the $\alpha_{IIb}\beta_3$ complex.[50] Conformational change results in exposure of the fibrinogen-binding site on the receptor complex. The second binding sequence is the lys-gln-ala-gly-asp-val sequence localized to the carboxy terminus of the γ chain of fibrinogen[47] and probably mediates the main binding mechanism for fibrinogen[40] (Fig. 48–3).

$\alpha_{IIb}\beta_3$ (II_b/IIIa) Inhibition

The approach to developing inhibitors of the $\alpha_{IIb}\beta_3$ system has employed a broad range of technologies, including the generation of monoclonal antibodies that can neutralize receptor function, the identification of naturally occurring antagonists,[51] and the development of synthetic antagonists based upon knowledge of the binding characteristics of the $\alpha_{IIb}\beta_3$ receptor RGD peptides, which may also function as partial agonists to generate high-affinity ligand-binding states.

Naturally occurring peptide inhibitors (disintegrins: echistatin, trigramin, apploggin, kistrin, bitan, barbourin[51–53]) isolated from puff adder and viper venoms, contain proteins, usually with the common RGD sequence that reversibly inhibits in vitro platelet aggregation. Binding is often rapid (kistrin) and has moderate affinity ($K_d \simeq 10^{-7}$ M). Barbourin displayed higher selectivity for $\alpha_{IIb}\beta_3$, which is conferred by a small change in the recognition sequence compared with other disintegrins.[54] The switch of the Lys to the Arg (KGD sequence) is responsible for this high selectivity, and the interaction of KGD with $\alpha_{IIb}\beta_3$ may be unique.[54]

Recognition of natural inhibitors and delineation of their binding characteristics and, in some cases, structural features[55] led to the development of synthetic peptides or peptidomimetics having higher affinity for the $\alpha_{IIb}\beta_3$ complex and enhanced inhibitory activity. The special properties of barbourin led to an investigation of KGD derivatives.[54] The synthetic heptapeptide, integrelin, has a modified KGD sequence and a high affinity and specificity for $\alpha_{IIb}\beta_3$.[54] The drug is potent, with a rapid onset of action and short biological half-life ($t_{1/2} \sim 10$ min), and, both in vitro and in vivo, inhibits platelet aggregation. The clinical utility of this agent is being tested clinically.[40,56] The possibility of the future development of peptide-specific inhibitors based on these approaches is likely to include synthetic peptidomimetic agents (e.g., Ro43-5054),[57] which may be more potent as $\alpha_{IIb}\beta_3$ inhibitors than RGD-containing peptides. Two peptidomimetics have been tested in clinical trials (MK-383; Ro4483) but appear to be less specific.[57]

Vascular-targeted monoclonal antibodies to the $\alpha_{IIb}\beta_3$ receptor are more potent than aspirin both ex and in vivo.[40] The technology may, however, be limited by potential immunogenicity problems with repeated exposure, therefore confining use to single administrations.[40] However, clinical trials have demonstrated the value of monoclonal antibodies in the context of acute coronary angioplasty[58,59] (Table 39–2, p. 1370).

LOCALIZATION OF CARDIOVASCULAR DISEASE GENES

The ability to characterize the genetic modifiers that maintain complex cardiovascular function, as well as to identify specific cardiovascular disease genes in monogenic disorders, is a central goal in molecular cardiology. The accelerated application of molecular genetics to human cardiovascular disease is covered in Chapter 49. Here, we review general principles, indicating how genetic information is extracted and then integrated with other data sources to allow mechanistic insights into cardiovascular physiology and pathology.

Principles of Gene Localization and Gene Product Analysis

The starting point for the identification of the gene responsible for a particular phenotype is the precise definition of that phenotype. The genetic study of human disease poses several problems but has the advantage of large numbers of well-characterized wild-type and mutant phenotypes.[60,61] The identification of human disease genes can follow one of two basic strategies (Fig. 48–4). *Functional cloning* allows the identification of the disease gene on the basis of functional knowledge, and the isolation of the gene is based upon the definition of a precise, usually biochemical, defect.[60] This method is not applicable to most mutations of the cardiovascular system, which have no biochemical or cytogenetic correlate that can be readily assayed from a clinical phenotype.[62] The major cardiovascular disease phenotypes each represent a complex interaction between genetic and environmental influences.[60]

Positional cloning assumes no functional information and instead depends on defining the position of the gene on a map of the entire human genome, the identification of the primary structure of the gene, and a determination of the

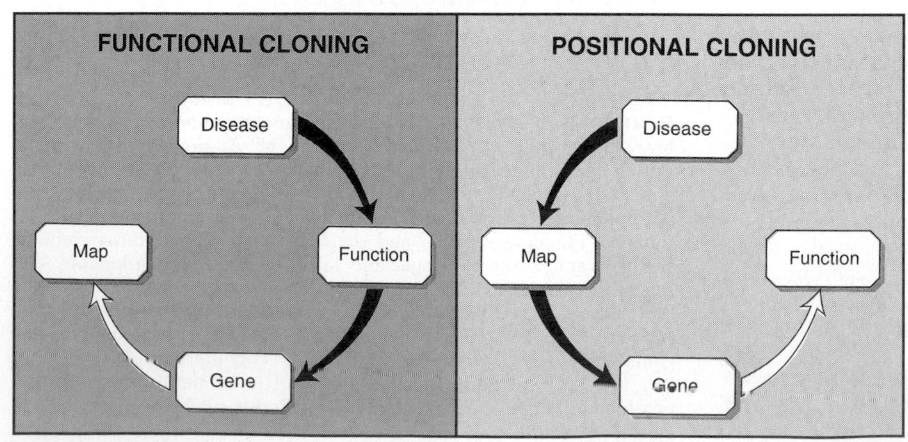

FIGURE 48–4. Paradigms for functional and positional cloning. Comparison of the functional and positional cloning of disease genes. In functional cloning, the study of the gene function precedes gene identification. In positional cloning, gene mapping precedes gene identification. The last step in each case (gene mapping and defining gene function, respectively) is not critical for the isolation of the disease gene itself. (Modified from Collins, F. S.: Positional cloning: Let's not call it reverse any more. Nature Genet. *1*:3, 1992.)

structure, tissue distribution, and expression of the gene product.[60,62] This approach had recently become dominant, but as information derived from the human genome project becomes available, the identification of candidate genes within a given region should greatly facilitate disease gene isolation (positional candidate approach).[60,62] It has been predicted that this modified approach, combining elements of both functional and positional cloning, will become the principal mode of disease gene identification.[62] This, in conjunction with appropriate biological assays for candidate gene expression, should allow further rapid advances in identifying single gene diseases that affect the cardiovascular system (Table 48–1).

THE HUMAN GENOME. The first step in the characterization of a human gene usually involves the identification of the position of that gene in the genome, the overall structure of which is best described by a map.[60] The premise upon which positional cloning is based suggests that the gene is located at a specific location on one of the chromosomes.[61] The requirement for the map is imposed by the size of the human genome.[63] The map may be physical or genetic and is constructed by observing the inheritance of markers that can be used as points of reference in offspring after well-characterized matings.[60] The quality and density of markers are the major determinants of its potential utility, but until recently markers were not ideal and the map of the human genome was characterized as being like a desert with only the occasional polymorphic oasis.[64] The first routinely used markers identified points of cleavage by restriction enzymes, known to vary within the population and termed restriction fragment length polymorphisms (RFLP).[60,65,66] These are resolved following the separation of endonuclease-generated fragments by gel electrophoresis and hybridization with appropriate probes using Southern blotting.[60]

The situation has been dramatically changed by the recognition that clusters of repeated sequences are present throughout the genome, allowing the construction of higher-resolution microsatellite-based maps.[64] These new maps, constructed around such short repeats, most notably containing cytosine and adenine (CA repeats) that occur approximately every 25 to 100 kb along the genome, are highly polymorphic.[64] In addition, they are reproducible, easily scored, and readily analyzed using amplification with the polymerase chain reaction and simple gel electrophoresis.[60,64]

POSITIONAL ASSIGNMENT. Mapping the position of a gene depends on defining the inheritance of genetic markers, along with the genes underlying the phenotype of interest. These show co-inheritance (genetic linkage) with markers in the immediate vicinity.[60,61] Conversely, genes that are far apart segregate independently, with an approximately linear relationship between the distance between genes and the probability of recombination.[60] In an individual family, the inheritance of a marker repeatedly with the disease phenotype implies a high probability that the marker is in the vicinity of the culprit gene. The concepts underlying localization are therefore simple, although in humans achieving linkage depends on prosaic considerations, particularly the size of a family pedigree and the quality of the available map.[60,61] The ideal is to develop a high-resolution map that covers the entire human genome, a goal of the Human Genome Project.[67] The delineation of such a map allows the definition of the position of any gene and thereby facilitates the analysis of the expression of that gene and, subsequently, of the gene product.[62,67] Present strategies require tracking a gene down to a chromosomal location of less than 1 to 3 million base pairs of DNA, containing only a few genes likely to be expressed in the relevant tissues. Once linkage is established, and now based on some knowledge of the disease, it is usually possible to search directly for the disease gene of interest with some likelihood of success.[60,61]

GENE CHARACTERIZATION. The identification of a specific gene location allows the nature of the genetic defect to be determined.[60] This is achieved either by identification of appropriate candidates, if known genes exist in that location, or by delivering the sequence of the gene in individuals having the disease phenotype and comparing these genotypes with normals. Sequencing can be manual but more recently has been automated with fluorescent markers and laser detection.[68] The mutation in the gene can cause the loss or change of function of a given gene via several mechanisms (deletions and duplications, base substitutions, expanding trinucleotide repeats), and these mutations provide important information, not only for the aberrant gene, but also regarding normal function and regulation.[60] Insights are then obtained into structure-function relationships of gene products and provide means to detect and analyze gene distribution in given families or in the general population.

The following sections provide two examples of the identification of important human cardiovascular disease genes and discusses recent insights gained into the relationship between the structure of the mutant protein and acquisition of the disease phenotype.

Molecular Genetics of Long Q-T Syndromes

(See also p. 1667)

The long Q-T syndromes often present clinically in the young with syncope, sudden cardiac death, abnormalities of ventricular repolarization, and torsades de pointes[69,70] (see p. 685). The condition is familial, with an autosomal dominant pattern of inheritance and high penetrance.[71] However, the incidence remains unknown, as minimal symptoms may go unrecognized, particularly in conjunction with a normal Q-T interval.[72] The gene frequency may therefore be much higher than suspected. Until recently, the electrophysiological mechanism responsible for this syndrome was unclear, and, as a result, management was empirical rather than rational.[70] This lack of a rational approach has nevertheless resulted in clinically effective approaches that have served to reduce the risks of the disease in those individuals that have been identified as being at risk.[70]

Within a single family, considerable heterogeneity in clinical presentation and electrocardiographic manifestations can be evident, thereby producing a problem in identifying affected individuals, which is the prelude to genetic dissection.[70,72] The application of a particularly stringent set of clinical criteria is usually required before successful linkage studies can be undertaken.[60] Published studies have used conservative approaches to a phenotypic assignment, characterizing patients in affected families as normal (if Q-T_c interval < 410 msec); abnormal (if Q-T_c interval > 450 msec with symptoms; or if asymptomatic, a Q-T_c interval > 470 msec); all other patients were classified as being of uncertain phenotype.[73]

POSITIONAL ASSIGNMENT. The first gene locus for the long Q-T syndrome was located by the availability of a large, well-characterized family with the condition.[73,74] The family had been based in a small town in Utah since the arrival of two brothers from the Netherlands in the mid-nineteenth century.[73] The lineage tree was constructed and DNA from the relatives examined using restriction digestion to establish RFLP linkage. Linkage of the long Q-T locus 1 (LQ-T_1) to the H-*ras* marker on the short arm of the chromosome 11 (11p15.5) with a Lod score of +16.43 was determined (the logarithm of the odds ratio for linkage (Lod) score is a logarithmic index of the likelihood that a disease gene is not linked to a particular genetic marker; here $1/10^{16.43}$). This finding pointed strongly to the H-*ras* gene as a potential candidate and also provided a putative mechanistic explanation in that both the p21 *ras* 1 protein and GAP (GTPase-activating protein) regulate cardiac muscarinic potassium channels.[73] However, H-*ras* was subsequently excluded for LQ-T_1, both by exclusion of this candidate gene from the region containing the disease gene[75] and with the sequencing of the entire segment containing H-*ras* showing no mutations. Moreover, this 1 million base region contains channel (KCNA4 and KCNC1) and dopamine receptor (DRD4) genes that have also been

TABLE 48–2 SOME MURINE TRANSGENIC MODELS OF ATHEROSCLEROSIS*

INTERVENTION	PHENOTYPIC FEATURES
	ATHEROSCLEROSIS-PRONE
Human apoAII overexpression	ApoAII 20% HDL protein content. Phenotype has no elevation in HDL-C. Despite normal HDL-C risk of atherosclerosis increases with fatty streak development even on low-fat diet. Indicates that qualitative features of HDL-C are also important.
Human CIII overexpression	First animal model of primary hypertryglyceridemia. Triglyceride level proportional to CIII expression. Primary abnormality decreased VLDL fractional catabolic rate.
Human AI, CIII, CETP overexpression	High triglyceride, low HDL-C phenotype. Comparable to most common lipoprotein disorder conferring susceptibility to CAD in humans.
Human apo(a) overexpression	Apo(a) mice developed 20 times greater area of lipid-rich lesions that control mice (outbred genetic background 3 months on atherogenic diet). $<5\%$ apo(a) associated with lipoprotein; suggested apo(a) produces pathology independently of LDL.
ApoE deficient	See text
LDL-receptor knockout	Homozygous mice have T_{chol} > twice normal litter mates with 7-9 times increase in LDL and IDL. Normal triglycerides. Correction with adenovirus-mediated gene transfer of LDL-R protein. Increased atherosclerosis.
	ATHEROSCLEROSIS-RESISTANT
ApoE overexpression	See text
Human LPL overexpression	LPL directed by the chick β-actin promoter produced accelerated VLDL clearance and resistance to diet-induced hypercholesterolemia.
Human LDL receptor overexpression	Radiolabeled LDL clearance increased 8-10 times compared with control mice. Resistant to high-fat high-cholesterol diet.
Human ApoAI overexpression	Major ($>70\%$) HDL protein. Selective doubling HDL-C. Useful model for examining effects of diet and drugs on HDL-C/apoA-I. Resistant to fatty streak development induced by atherogenic diet.

* Approximately 20 genes involved in human lipid transport have been overexpressed or knocked out in transgenic mice. Data from Breslow, J. L.: Transgenic mouse models of lipoprotein metabolism and atherosclerosis. Proc. Natl. Acad. Sci. *90*:8314, 1993; Ishibashi, S., et al.: Hypercholesterolemia in low density lipoprotein receptor knockout mice and its reversal by adenovirus-mediated gene delivery. J. Clin. Invest. *92*:883, 1993; Lawn, R. M., et al.: Atherogenesis in transgenic mice expressing human apolipoprotein (a). Nature *360*:670, 1992.

species are amenable to transgenic techniques, such as swine,[133] rabbit,[134] and rat,[122] most have been created in mice because of several intrinsic advantages, including the availability of ES cell technology, inbred strains, and the wealth of information on the mouse genome.[135] The development of apoE-deficient mice provides an example of the potential value of utilizing transgenic technology to engineer animal models of known cardiovascular disease.

Mouse Models of Atherosclerosis

The wild-type mouse, with some exceptions (e.g., strain C57BL/6), is generally resistant to atherosclerosis.[105,121,136] Nevertheless, by the creation of models with powerful analogies to human atherogenesis (Table 48–2), the mouse has become an important system for increasing our understanding of the human disease.[105,121] The generation of mouse models has been facilitated by the fact that human genes involved in lipoprotein metabolism are usually single-copy and have often been sequenced and mapped.[137,138] In addition to increasing understanding of the underlying processes,[105] these mice can also be used in the development of drugs directed against the atherosclerotic process which can be used to predict efficacy in clinical trials[119] and also for testing the applicability of other interventions directed at these processes.

The most atherogenic mouse strain is the apolipoprotein E (apoE)-deficient mouse, in which the apoE gene has been disrupted by homologous recombination.[139,140] apoE is the ligand that is responsible for LDL and chylomicron remnant uptake, playing an important role in the clearance of lipoprotein particles from the circulation.[105] The knockout of the gene for apoE results in a phenotype that is a true null mutation, with no expression of apoE, but has the considerable advantage that the homozygotes are both viable and fertile.[139,140] The pattern of disease is diet-responsive and the homozygotes fed a standard laboratory *chow diet* (0.01 per cent cholesterol, 4.5 per cent fat) have a serum cholesterol concentration of 400 to 500 mg/dl with the development of foam cell lesions at 10 weeks, whereas on a diet similar to that consumed in the United States (0.15 per cent cholesterol and 20 per cent fat) serum cholesterol rises to approximately 1800 mg/dl, mostly in the VLDL and IDL fractions, with triglycerides being minimally raised and with foam cells as early as 8 wks.[139,140]

Animals consuming both diets develop advanced lesions of atherosclerosis, with their distribution and histology being almost indistinguishable from those of human disease[141,142] (Figs. 48–8, 48–9). These mice also provide a

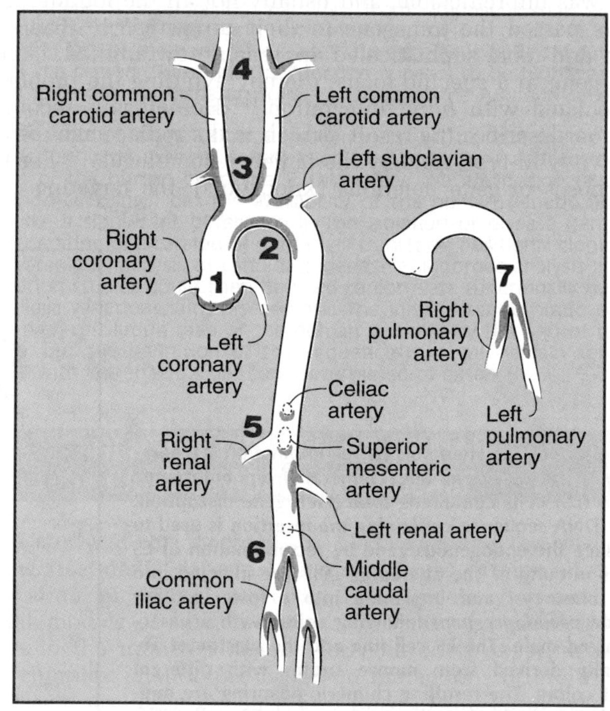

FIGURE 48–8. Extent of atheroma in the apoE-deficient mouse. Diagram of the arterial tree from apoE-deficient mice. The sites of lesion predilection are shown by shading: (1) Aortic root at the base of the valves; (2) lesser curvature of the aortic arch; (3) principal branches of the thoracic aorta; (4) carotid bifurcations; (5) principal branches of abdominal aorta; (6) aortic bifurcations and iliac arteries; (7) pulmonary arteries. The parallels to the distribution of human atheroma are clear. (From Nakashima, Y., Plump, A. S., Raines, E. W., et al.: ApoE-deficient mice develop lesions of all phases of atherosclerosis throughout the arterial tree. Arterioscler. Thromb. 14:133, 1994. Graphics prepared by Kris Carroll.)

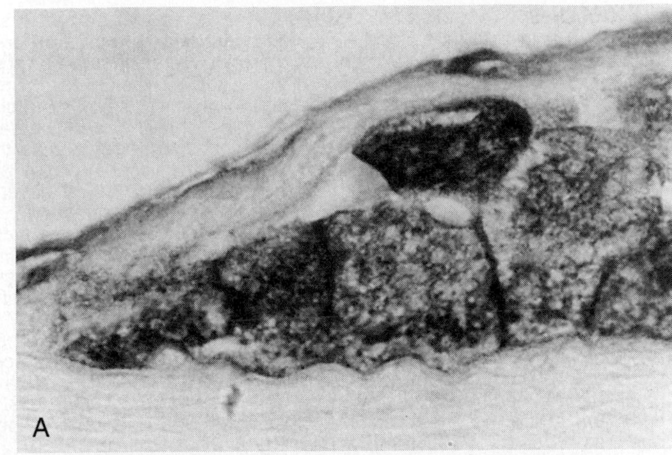

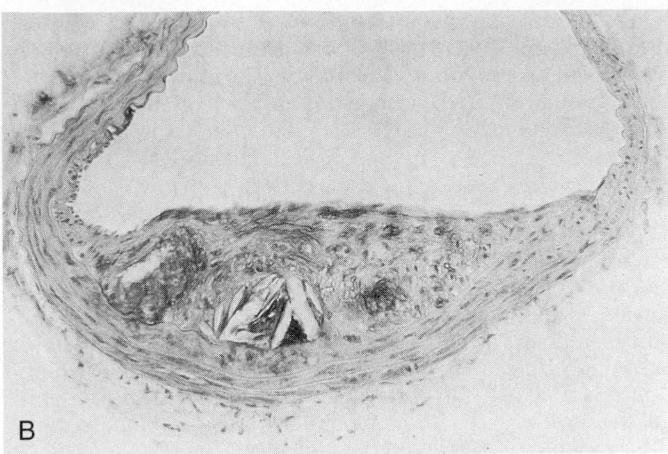

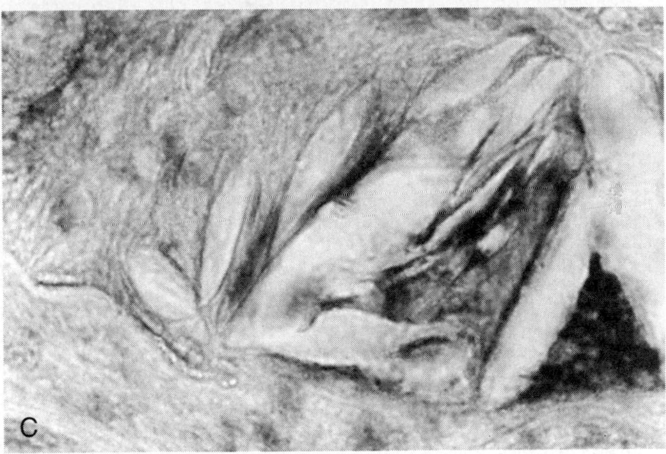

FIGURE 48–9. Photomicrographs showing histology of atherosclerosis in the apoE-deficient mouse. *A,* Transitional lesion in the aortic arch. In contrast to early lesions, consisting primarily of lipid accumulations and macrophages/macrophage-derived foam cells rich in oxidized lipoproteins, in later stages of atherosclerosis macrophages are found predominantly in the shoulder region of lesions, as shown here. *B,* Advanced lesion in the abdominal aorta immunostained for immunoglobulins G and M, showing an extensive necrotic core with cholesterol crystals. In murine models with extensive aortic lesions such as apoE- and LDL receptor-deficient mice, atherosclerotic lesions frequently involve the media, occasionally leading to aneurysms. ApoE-deficient mice have particularly high titers of circulating autoantibodies to epitopes of oxidized lipoproteins, which form immune complexes with oxidized proteins and lipoproteins with atherosclerotic lesions. *C,* Higher magnification of the necrotic core shown in *B,* showing cholesterol crystals and immunoglobulins in the vicinity of the internal elastic lamina. (Images courtesy of Wulf Palinski, M.D., adapted from Palinski, W., Ord, V. A., Plump, A. S., et al.: ApoE-deficient mice are a model of lipoprotein oxidation in atherogenesis. Arterioscler. Thromb. *14:*605, 1994. Copyright American Heart Association.)

model for the study of lipoprotein oxidation, with lesion oxidation–specific epitopes and antibodies to malondialdehyde-lysine in serum.[143,144] Heterozygotes have diminished apoE with normal fasting lipids and slightly delayed postprandial lipid clearance consistent with half-normal levels of E2 being sufficient to maintain normal serum lipids.[139] Interestingly, crossing these animals with mice that display overexpression of human transgene AI leads to an elevation of apo-AI, and HDL and apparently alleviates atherogenicity, as it does also with apo(a) overexpressing mice.[145]

The physiological role of apoE is exemplified in two other models. The human apoE3 Leiden variant (tandem duplication amino acids 120 to 126) leads to type III hyperlipoproteinemia[146,147]; overexpression of this gene in so-called E3 Leiden mice leads to a phenocopy of the human disease.[146] The apoE lipoprotein has also been overexpressed in transgenic mice, leading to fourfold increase in apoE levels. These animals have a severalfold increase in radiolabeled VLDL/LDL clearance and are resistant to diet-induced hypercholesterolemia.[148]

GENE THERAPY

The concept of gene therapy encompasses a broad range of diverse technologies having as a common aim the transfer and expression of specific genes to alleviate the fundamental consequences of a disease.[149,150] These aims are inextricably linked to the development of other molecular technologies which are required for the efficient, localized, and long-term expression of the transferred gene. In addition, molecular approaches are often required to identify candidate genes that have potential therapeutic value in experimental model systems.[149] Although the potential impact of gene therapy for cardiovascular medicine is clear, to date there has been no direct demonstration of the practical use for disease targets, cardiovascular or otherwise, within the clinical context.[151,152]

Indeed, significant challenges remain if gene therapy is to become a standard form of treatment for a subset of cardiovascular diseases.[151,152] The major contemporary problem is devising technically feasible methods for gene delivery, a task that requires the coordinate development of several individual technologies with proven value in appropriate animal models that have fidelity to human disease.[151,152] Once established, the specific questions that balance efficacy and safety, in comparison to existing treatments, also need to be addressed. The denominators of the risk-benefit equation are clearly going to be different in nonterminal diseases with high morbidity, such as cardiovascular disease, versus terminal diseases, such as the acquired immunodeficiency syndrome and cancer.[151,152] In addition, the minimal requirement for gene therapy must bear comparison to those of existing treatments having appropriate risk-benefit profiles.[149,153] Herein, we consider the technical issues involved in the application of cardiovascular gene therapy and early steps toward its implementation.

Technical Aspects

Before gene therapy will be achieved in the clinical setting, it is necessary to document the feasibility of the controlled, sustained expression at the appropriate level of therapeutic gene/product for the required duration in the chosen location.[149,153] Two general approaches to somatic gene therapy have been defined: (1) gene transfer ex vivo with removal of cells, followed by gene transduction and the in vivo reimplantation of the modified cells; (2) in vivo gene transfer employing a variety of gene delivery approaches and vectors that have been applied in animal models.[149,152,153] In the context of the cardiovascular system, such an approach implies transvascular delivery for which specialized catheters have been designed.[154] This could be applied for a local effect with delivery to the vessel wall or into myocardial vasculature to facilitate improved coronary flow or might provide a source for the release of cell-derived products for systemic gene replacement therapy, e.g., Factor VIII delivery.[152]

Vector Development

The vector is the agent carrying the gene to the desired site of action, and vector choice and optimization are therefore fundamental to achieve effective gene transfer.[149,153] The ideal vector would be relatively safe, highly efficient, display tissue- or cell-type tropism, and afford high but controllable levels of expression for a long duration. Vectors fall into two general categories—viral and nonviral—with other approaches using a combination of these delivery modes.

The main viruses considered are retroviruses and adenoviruses, with most others having confounding problems with limited host range, antigenicity, pathogenicity, problems with integration, and size constraints.[149,152,153] Replication-defective retroviruses have the advantages of a high (~100 per cent) transduction rate of transported DNA into the host genome. However, they are relatively labile and inactivated in vivo in humans by complement activation. In addition, the host cell range is limited by the requirement for cell division to allow viral integration, and not all mammalian cell types are persuasive for retroviral infection.[149,152,153] There is also an additional concern about long-term expression, with the risk of oncogene activation and neoplasia.[149,152] To date, the single most important advance in improving retroviral vectors has been the development of packaging cell lines able to produce high viral titers.

Adenoviruses have become important in view of the possibility of their use in vivo.[149,152,155] The two serotypes most commonly used (Ad2, Ad5) are minimally pathogenic and have been made replication-defective by the deletion of E1A/E1B gene components.[149,152] The viruses attach to the adenoviral glycoprotein receptor and undergo receptor-mediated endocytosis, escaping lysosomal degradation, to reach the nucleus where the delivered DNA persists unintegrated.[149,152] The adenoviral vectors display several advantages, including an ability to infect nondividing cells and the capability to transfer genes in situ. In addition, recombinant adenoviruses can accommodate large amounts of DNA (36 kb-pair genome), can be produced in high titers (10^{11}/ml), and do not integrate into the genome, thereby reducing the risk of malignant transformation. The main disadvantages are transient expression due to the humoral response following in vivo use facilitated by the presence of neutralizing antibodies in greater than 20 per cent of normal individuals. Humoral immunity reduces efficacy and increases pathogenicity, with tissue inflammation being a significant problem.[149,152]

Two other viruses have been considered in cardiovascular applications. Adeno-associated viruses (AAV) are relatively small, stable, nonpathogenic, and defective viruses that cannot go into the lytic stage and have broad host-range with site-specific integration (chromosome 19) *cf.* retrovirus.[156] It is proposed they have applications for both in vitro packaging and ex vivo use, although producing sufficiently high titers remains a problem.[156] Haemagglutin virus of Japan (HVJ) is an inactivated paramyxovirus that has been used with a liposome-complex (viral conjugate vector) entrapping DNA and has been suggested as an efficient way of introducing DNA into vascular tissues.[157]

Physical methods exploit natural endocytosis mechanisms to deliver the DNA-ligand complexes targeted to cell-type specific receptors.[149,158] Cationic liposomes are able to form large complexes with DNA, have low toxicity, and are nonimmunogenic, allowing the possibility of repeated high-level dosing, but have problems with low efficacy and transient expression.[158] In an effort to circumvent some of these, conjugates have used the whole virus or fusogenic viral peptides to disrupt endosomes or modifications of liposomal composition.[158] Direct injection of DNA has also been shown to be capable of allowing recombinant gene expression, although this has been seen in less than 1 per cent of cells around myocardial injection sites.[152,159] The advantages suggested are that this is not ex vivo; there are no infectious vectors; plasmid DNA does not integrate; and there is, in general, muscle-specific gene expression.[159] Polymer gels applied to the adventitial aspect of blood vessels have been used for the application of antisense oligonucleotides.[160,161]

Approaches to Specific Problems

Several potential clinical targets have been identified for cardiovascular gene therapy. However, the only clinical studies with direct cardiovascular relevance have been those related to the ex vivo therapy of monogenic familial hypercholesterolemia.[162,163] Below, two additional targets are considered, on which some experimental data are available:

ANGIOGENESIS. Angiogenesis, with new vessel formation and restoration of physiological blood flow, has been identified as a potential therapeutic option in both chronic coronary artery[164] and peripheral vascular disease.[165,166] The agenda here is clearly different from that for neoplastic disease and metastasis, in which the aim is inhibition of angiogenesis.[167] Two approaches to achieving new vessel growth have been identified. First, recombinant angiogenic growth factor formulations are administered directly to the vessels related to the underperfused region, to expedite or augment collateral development.[164,168] The second approach is based on gene transfer,[165,166] which has the theoretical advantage that the secreted gene product could have significant biological effects, with only relatively few cells transfected, following site-specific arterial gene transfer.[152] The genes encoding angiogenic factors, such as FGF and VEGF, have been cloned and mechanisms of action have been established in vitro.[134] However, in vivo efficacy has yet to be definitively established. The expression of PDGF-B, FGF-1, and TGF-β_1 genes following direct transfer into porcine arteries has been shown to induce intimal hyperplasia and neointimal angiogenesis.[165] Exploring the in vivo feasibility and efficacy of this angiogenic approach will undoubtedly be one area of research in coming years.

INHIBITION OF VASCULAR SMOOTH MUSCLE CELL PROLIFERATION. Vascular smooth muscle cell proliferation following PTCA is generally perceived as a target for gene delivery, an agenda that found particular urgency in the significant absence of proven pharmacological therapy.[40,151,152,169] Inhibition of vascular smooth muscle cell proliferation has been the principal aim, with other studies being designed to define the signaling pathways that mediate in vivo proliferation of vascular smooth muscle cells.[152,170]

The feasibility of gene transfection in vivo has been suggested following studies with retroviruses[171] and liposomes, although both methods have a low (<1 per cent) efficiency of transfer.[152] Adenoviruses have been reported to display an increased efficiency of reporter-gene expression (10- to 100-fold), but transient (7 to 14 days) expression is likely to limit utility.[152,172] One of the major determinants of gene transfer with both vector systems is the state of the vessel wall, with transfection in normal vessels being restricted to vascular endothelial cells,[172] whereas in balloon-injured vessels expression in medial cells is also seen. The two approaches currently in use include direct gene transfer with balloon delivery in vivo or the implantation of grafts after ex vivo gene transfer.[152]

Two novel methods for the selective inhibition of proliferation of actively dividing cells have been reported.[173,174] The first approach employed a herpes virus–associated thymidine kinase suicide gene in an adenoviral vector which was delivered into the injured pig femoral artery. The expression of thymidine kinase gene selectively in dividing cells converts gancyclovir to an active toxic form, resulting in cell death.[174] The second approach targeted another component of the nuclear cell cycle regulatory pathway.[173] The expression of the nonphosphorylable, constitutively active form of the retinoblastoma (Rb) gene product limited vascular smooth muscle cell proliferation in both rat carotid and pig femoral arteries at greater than 3 weeks following vascular injury.[173]

ANTISENSE OLIGONUCLEOTIDES. One further potential approach to vascular proliferation is the use of antisense oligonucleotides.[175,176] These are short chain nucleic acids (10 to 39 residues) which bind to a targeted complementary region of mRNA (sense strand) and prevent translation, thereby blocking the expression of specific gene.[175,177] This approach has the theoretical advantage of the inhibition of abnormal genes, while leaving normal genes intact, but their use has been associated with several technical difficulties.[177] The oligonucleotides cross the cell membrane with low efficiency, they are degraded rapidly in the circulation, and no efficient method of drug delivery has been devised.[175] In addition, the antisense oligonucleotides often display nonspecific activity at high concentrations, which complicates interpretation of experimental results.[177]

The published studies have thus far reported biological effects but no direct relevant effects on the production of either the protein or the mRNA.[175] The use of antisense oligonucleotides to the proto-oncogenes c-*myb*,[160] c-*myc*,[161] cdc2 kinase, and proliferating cell nuclear antigen[157] have been reported. The improvement of stability facilitating administration (e.g., chemical modification, liposomal conjugates), increases in in vivo biological half-life, and improved specificity will all be required before more widespread application.[175]

Prospects for Gene Therapy

Although currently immense difficulties need to be addressed to allow routine use of in vivo gene therapy in the cardiovascular system, this approach nevertheless represents one of the areas in which the molecular sciences could impact cardiology in the next millennium. Most likely, the first application of gene therapy will be in gene replacement for patients harboring specific genetic deficiencies of circulating proteins, such as Factor VIII deficiency (hemophilia). Vascular targets may continue to be attractive with regard to the inhibition of restenosis but

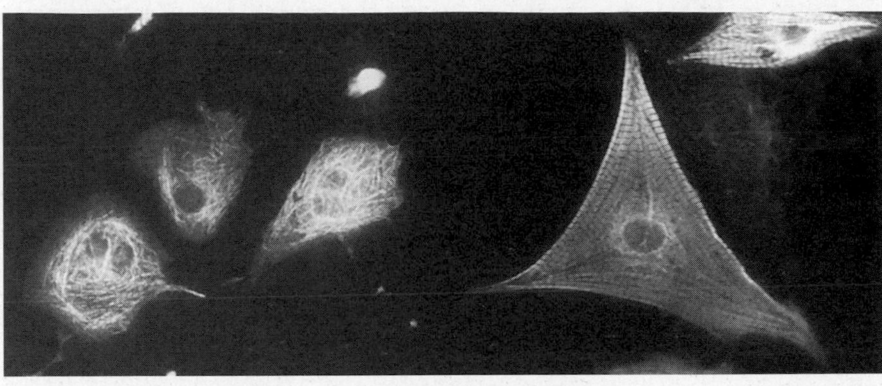

FIGURE 48–10. Hypertrophic cardiac myocyte. Alpha-adrenergic–mediated hypertrophy of cultured neonatal rat myocardial cells leads to the accumulation and assembly of individual contractile proteins into organized sarcomeric units. Myocardial cells were cultured using now standard techniques, with agonists being added to the media as required; here myocardial cells were harvested from indirect immunofluorescence analysis after 48 hours. The left panel shows control cells and the right following exposure to phenylephrine. (From Chien, K. R., Knowlton, K. U., Zhu, H., and Chien, S.: Regulation of cardiac gene expression during myocardial growth and hypertrophy: Molecular studies of an adaptive physiologic response. FASEB J. *5*:3037, 1991.)

will require critical comparison with other therapeutic approaches.[152] Cardiac muscle diseases clearly will be more difficult to approach, given the requirement for the transfer and long-term expression of a given gene in sufficient numbers of muscle cells to effect a global change in chamber function, and the potentially arrhythmogenic effects of heterogeneous expression.[159]

MOLECULAR ADVANCES IN CARDIAC HYPERTROPHY

During the past decade a large body of evidence has been accumulated from both basic and clinical research which is beginning to reshape our view of the failing heart[178,179] (see also Chap. 13). The result is that the heart failure syndrome can no longer be viewed as strictly a problem of altered peripheral hemodynamics and depressed cardiac contractility.[178] Two basic elements underlie this change in perspective. The first is the realization that heart failure is heterogeneous at both the molecular and cellular levels and this heterogeneity has significant physiological and clinical correlations. The second is that the course of both experimental and clinical heart failure is characterized by a series of physiological transitions.[178]

The activation of the cardiac hypertrophic response is characterized, and essentially defined, by increases in the size and contractile protein content of individual cardiac muscle cells[178] (see p. 399). The development of hypertrophy allows the heart to maintain cardiac work and follows as a response to several mechanical or hormonal cues.[180] It is an early milestone during the clinical course of heart failure and a significant risk factor for subsequent morbidity and mortality.[181] Agents that blunt the structural and clinical manifestations of hypertrophy may have beneficial effects on these outcomes.[181]

The pattern of hypertrophy depends on the context within which it develops. In pressure-overload hypertrophy (e.g., hypertensive heart disease, aortic stenosis), for example, additional sarcomeric proteins are assembled in parallel and the heart acquires a concentric pattern of hypertrophy with increased wall thickness, relative preservation of chamber volume, and maintained systolic function.[182] Conversely, in hypertrophy developing after chronic volume overload (e.g., aortic or mitral insufficiency), sarcomeric units become assembled in series, with increased individual myocyte length, global ventricular dilatation, and early-onset systolic dysfunction[182] (Fig. 48–10). Given such distinct morphological and physiological features, it is entirely possible that divergent signaling pathways mediate the development of these individual phenotypes[178] (Fig. 48–11).

The central importance of hypertrophy to the clinical phenotype of chronic heart failure indicates that unraveling the molecular signals that first trigger and then maintain the hypertrophic response may eventually hold the key to understanding the pathogenesis and mechanisms of progression of heart failure. Such understanding could lead to the identification of new therapeutic targets, the interruption of which may halt clinical deterioration.

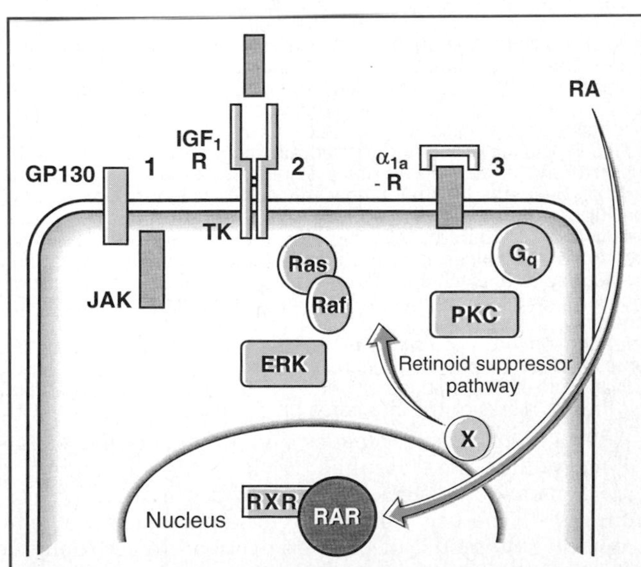

FIGURE 48–11. Signaling mechanisms of cardiac hypertrophy as identified in in vitro model. Three principal putative mechanisms (GP 130; Ras; G_q) leading to the hypertrophic phenotype are shown along with the retinoid suppressor pathway defined in vitro. Details are indicated in text. GP130 = glycoprotein cytokine signaling molecule; JAK = janus kinase; IGF_1R = insulin-like growth factor-1 receptor; TK = tyrosine kinase; α_{1a}-R = alpha-1 adrenoceptor; G_q = G protein (G_α) subunit; PKC = protein kinase C; Ras = signaling protein responsible for translocation Raf to cell membrane; Raf = principal effector of the ras pathway; ERK = mitogen activated protein kinase; RXR = retinoid X receptor; RAR = retinoid A receptor; RA = retinoids: all trans- and 9-cis retinoic acid.

Activation of Cardiac Muscle Genes During Hypertrophy

The activation of specific subsets of cardiac muscle genes is one of the first detectable phenotypic changes in the development of the hypertrophic response (Table 48–3), with the pattern of gene activation being related to the hypertrophic stimulus (pressure overload, volume overload, exercise-induced hypertrophy, hypertrophic cardiomyopathy).[178] These findings are consistent with the existence of distinct molecular phenotypes underlying clinical expressions of hypertrophy.[178] Under certain conditions, downregulation of a subset of cardiac muscle genes has also been observed, including the gene encoding the sarcoplasmic reticulum Ca^{++}-ATPase, which plays a central role in diastolic relaxation.[183]

TABLE 48–3 IN VITRO STIMULI, SIGNALING MOLECULES, AND GENE EXPRESSION THAT CHARACTERIZE THE HYPERTROPHIC RESPONSE

AGONISTS	TRANSDUCTION PATHWAYS	KINASES	NUCLEAR FACTORS	INDUCTION OF IMMEDIATE EARLY GENES	INDUCTION OF EMBRYONIC GENES	INDUCTION OF CONSTITUTIVE CONTRACTILE PROTEIN GENES
α adrenergic	ras	Protein kinase C	HF-1a/HF-1b	c-*fos*	ANF	MLC-2v
Angiotensin II	Gq	Raf-1 kinase	TEF-1	c-*jun*	Skeletal α-actin	Cardiac α-actin
Endothelin I	gp130	S6 kinase	SRF	*Egr*–1	β-MHC	
FGF		MAP kinases		*Jun*-B		
TGF-β		JAK kinases		Nur-77		
Cardiotrophin-1						
LIF						
Stretch						

Cardiac hypertrophy results in the induction of constitutively expressed sarcomeric protein genes, accounting for the increase in contractile protein content that is a necessary component of the phenotype.[178,180,182] In addition, the hypertrophic response is accompanied by ventricular reexpression of genes, which are ordinarily expressed in this location only in the fetus. In the embryonic heart, for example, atrial natriuretic factor (ANF) gene expression is observed in the atrium and ventricle.[184] Following birth there is selective downregulation of the ventricular gene, leading to restricted atrial expression.[184] However, hypertrophy invariably results in a rapid reinduction of ventricular ANF gene expression, and natriuretic peptide expression is increased in both hypertrophic[185] and dilated cardiomyopathy.[186] The constitutive activation of ANF in the hypertrophied heart is also thought to reflect the switching on of other embryonic genes.[187–189] In view of these findings, the ANF gene has become established as a well-characterized marker of the hypertrophic response in both in vitro and in vivo model systems and has been extensively used to map signaling pathways responsible for this adaptive physiological response.[124,184,190–193] These systems have also been used to identify the role of new and known growth factors in the activation of the hypertrophic response.[184,192,193]

IN VITRO ASSAY SYSTEM FOR MYOCARDIAL CELL HYPERTROPHY

Several laboratories have employed in vitro myocardial cell assays to determine which of the many phenotypic features of hypertrophy are under the control of particular signaling pathways (Table 48–4). The availability of a well-characterized cultured myocardial cell system that displays morphological and genetic features of the in vivo hypertrophic response[187,188,191,194–199] has led to the identification of a number of defined hormonal stimuli that can activate the hypertrophic phenotype in vitro, including alpha-adrenergic agonists,[195,196] angiotensin II,[197,200] and endothelin-1.[191,198,199] These systems have also been adapted to characterize specific elements of the hypertrophic response. For example, reproducible methods to stretch such cells both actively and passively have been successfully used to characterize signaling pathways activated following mechanical stimuli.[201,202] In addition, the in vitro myocardial cell assay system has been used to identify new paracrine sources of hypertrophic factors derived from cardiac fibroblasts[205]; and following transfer of the assay system to a rapid throughput, 96-well format has also allowed the isolation and cloning of a novel cytokine.[204]

TABLE 48–4 EXPERIMENTAL STRATEGY TO MAP SIGNALING PATHWAYS

1. Identify candidate signaling molecules and pathways in in vitro cultured myocardial cell model systems.
2. Develop and characterize a mouse-based model of hypertrophy.
3. Utilize miniaturized technology to monitor in vitro cardiac physiology in the living mouse.
4. Develop strategies for ventricular chamber–specific expression of transgenes.
5. Utilize combination of transgenic and gene-targeting approaches to assess role of individual candidate signaling molecules in in vivo hypertrophy in the mouse.

Adapted from Chien, K. R.: Cannon Award Lecture. Cardiac muscle diseases in genetically engineered mice: The evolution of molecular physiology. Am. J. Physiol. *269*:H755, 1995.

Combinations of cotransfection and microinjection techniques have been used to induce or block specific component molecules[205] and led to a skeleton plan of the downstream signaling pathways capable of activating phenotypic features of hypertrophy[205,206] (Fig. 48–11). Although clearly valuable in identifying known and novel candidate genes for the hypertrophic process, such in vitro studies do not address the question of whether activation of any of these signaling pathways is sufficient to promote a hypertrophic response in vivo. For example, whether the complex in vivo physiological stimulus of pressure overload can be adequately modeled by simple mechanical stretching of myocytes in vitro must remain an open question until correlative in vivo data are available.[202] Ultimately, the detailed modeling and evaluation of the role of specific signaling molecules in clinical hypertrophy and the cardiomyopathies and in the transition from hypertrophy to dilatation and systolic failure require study in vivo.[113]

In vivo Cardiac Hypertrophy Assay System in Genetically Manipulated Mice

One difficulty faced in defining signaling pathways in in vivo models of hypertrophy has been the limited ability to manipulate or control individual elements of the in vivo physiology of myocardial hypertrophy.[190] Inhibitors of various surface receptors and enzyme systems have been used to study the development of hypertrophy, but in many cases use of inhibitors, being nonspecific, has led to secondary physiological effects that confound clear interpretation of results.[178] Thus, the ability to genetically manipulate an in vivo animal hypertrophy model represents a significant advantage.[123] The final aim has been to document how mechanical triggers orchestrate a specific set of genetic events in the adult cardiac muscle cell within a multicellular content.[190] This endpoint could be achieved by the expression of a dominantly acting gene product or the neutralization of the activity of a specific signaling molecule without, ideally, interference with other components of a highly integrated network.[113] Subsequently, assessment can be made of the effects of such genetic alteration on the acquisition of specific molecular and cellular features of hypertrophy (e.g., increase in contractile protein content, activation of embryonic genes, increase in myocyte size) in addition to other hallmarks of the integrated physiological phenotype.[124,190,207]

Advances in mouse genetics and transgenic/gene-targeting technology have resulted in the mouse becoming an important model system to study cardiac hypertrophy and failure.[124,190] The use of microsurgical approaches has led to a reproducible model of pressure-overload hypertrophy despite the diminutive size of the murine heart and great vessels (Fig. 48–12).[124,190] Creating a constriction in the ascending thoracic aorta produces a stable 35-mm Hg gradient and a 35 per cent increase in heart weight with a greater than 20-fold increase in steady-state myocardial ANF mRNA expression.[124] The pattern of immediate early gene expression during pressure-overload hypertrophy in murine myocardium is identical with that elicited in other in vivo and in vitro model systems of hypertrophy.[124] In addition, the mouse hypertrophy model recapitulates other characteristic features of ventricular hypertrophy seen both in in vitro systems and clinically.[124,190,208] The onset of hy-

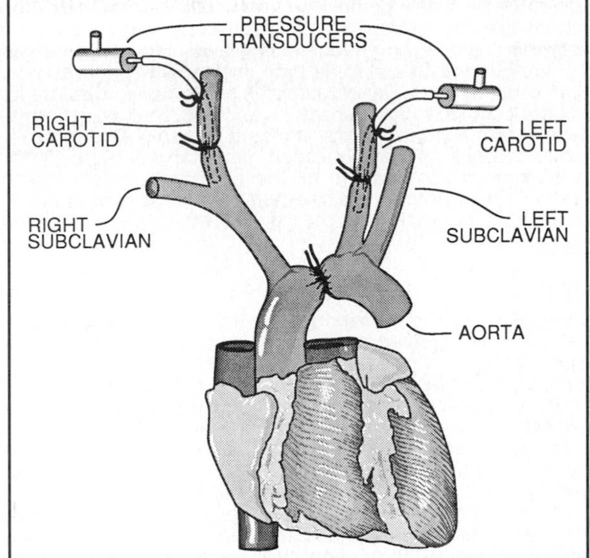

FIGURE 48–12. Microsurgical induction of transverse aortic constriction and associated cardiac hypertrophy in the mouse. Method for the production of stable transverse aortic constriction in mouse (see text for details). (From Rockman, H. A., Ross, R. S., Harris, A., et al.: Segregation of atrial specific and inducible expression of an ANF transgene in an in vitro murine model of cardiac hypertrophy. Proc. Natl. Acad. Sci. *88*:8277, 1991.)

pertrophy in the human setting, for example, is accompanied by a well-defined set of in vivo physiological phenotypes. In the initial stages of human hypertension, increased ventricular wall thickness is associated with decreased diastolic compliance and relative preservation of systolic function.[209] Subsequently, left ventricular ejection fraction decreases with ventricular dilatation and symptomatic heart failure associated with blunted beta-adrenergic responsiveness, as assessed by agonist-mediated increases in left ventricular dp/dt.[210,211] The ultimate utility of the mouse as a model system to study hypertrophic heart disease and heart failure rests upon documenting that these physiological phenotypes of impaired diastolic compliance, decreased systolic function, and basal and agonist-mediated increases in cardiac contractility and relaxation can be quantitatively assayed in the in vivo mouse context.[127,178] Miniaturized catheterization[207] with microangiography technology[125] to provide such quantitative assays is now available and has been routinely applied to characterize such physiological phenotypes in both transgenic and gene-targeted mice (Fig. 48–13).[123,212]

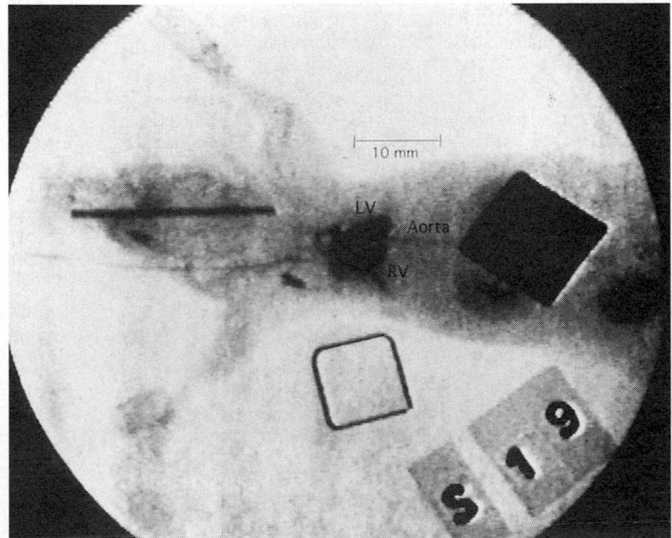

FIGURE 48–13. Digitized ventricular angiography for the in vivo assessment of hemodynamic function in the mouse. Cardiac catheter inserted from right jugular vein imaged in left anterior oblique. In addition to intracardiac opacification, renal shadow and bladder are visualized by contrast; tracheal cannula in situ. (From Chien, K. R.: Molecular advances in cardiovascular biology. Science *260*:916, 1993. Reprinted with permission, American Association for the Advancement of Science.)

Using observations from the in vitro model systems of hypertrophy, experimental strategies have been devised which should ultimately allow a definitive assessment of the roles of particular signaling molecules in the pathophysiology of cardiac hypertrophy and failure (Table 48–3). Candidate genes are identified in the in vitro model system, and their subsequent role in the in vivo context is evaluated in genetically manipulated mice produced with cardiac-specific promoters.[114,213] With the advent of tissue-specific knockout, conditional transgene expression,[131,132] and a variety of rescue strategies, future refinements in mouse genetic technology should eventually allow discrimination between primary and secondary events during the course of cardiac growth and development.[178]

Identification of Cardiac Growth Factors and Cytokines

The precise means by which hemodynamic stress is sensed by cardiac myocytes and the mechanisms of the subsequent activation of those growth-related signaling pathways that regulate the cardiac muscle gene program during myocardial hypertrophy are unknown.[178] The relative absence of hypertrophy in the right heart following aortic constriction[124] and the selective growth of the right ventricle after pulmonary artery banding[125] point against systemic circulating factors as principal mediators. The current general hypothesis is that growth factors are produced by cardiac nonmuscle cells or by myocytes themselves, in response to hemodynamic stress and, through specific signaling cascades, selectively regulate the transcription of genes leading to cardiomyocyte growth.[178,214]

The recent isolation and molecular cloning of numerous growth factors, the description of their expression in the heart, and the demonstration that cardiac myocytes are targets for peptide-derived growth factors have all supported a role for such locally produced diffusible factors initially in cardiac growth and later in myocardial failure[196,214,215] (Table 48–5). According to this perspective, the transition between compensated hypertrophy and overt cardiac dysfunction may reflect the action of different subsets of growth factors and/or cytokines. At any one time, the net structure and function of the heart might be the result of the integration of diverse paracrine stimuli that mediate distinct physiological phenotypes via control of various subsets of the cardiac gene program.[178] Under such circumstances, the pathogenesis of cardiac muscle failure could be viewed as a classical problem in growth and development, analogous to the process of cardiogenesis, in which specific molecular cues guide chamber morphogenesis with tight spatial and temporal regulation.[216,217] If such is the case, then new therapeutic approaches to heart failure could rest on the identification and manipulation of factors that promote physiological hypertrophy and inhibition of stimuli that activate phenotypic features of the failing heart.[178]

The absolute number of distinct growth factors expressed in the myocardium is not yet known, and therefore the identification of cardiac growth factors and their receptors remains an expanding area in cardiovascular research. Among those that have been identified in the heart include transforming growth factor-beta (TGF-β), insulin-like growth factor-1 (IGF-1), endothelin I, angiotensin II, and a burgeoning number of new growth factors and cytokines.[196,204,214,215] Some of the candidate growth factors that have been implicated in activating a hypertrophic response in cardiac model systems are discussed in Table 48–5.

TABLE 48–5 GROWTH FACTORS IMPLICATED IN ACTIVATING A HYPERTROPHIC RESPONSE

GROWTH FACTOR	ACTIVITY
Angiotensin II	⇑ release in in vitro stretch-induced hypertrophy ⇑ ANF, immediate early genes and skeletal α-actin expression in in vitro model ACE inhibition or AT_1 receptor antagonists block hypertrophy
Endothelin	Presence of binding sites on cardiac myocytes ⇑ mRNA pre-pro-endothelin-1 during cardiac hypertrophy ⇑ immediate early genes, ANF, and MLC_{2v} in in vitro model ET_A receptor antagonists block hypertrophy
TGF-β	⇑ mRNA during cardiac hypertrophy ⇑ β-MHC, α-skeletal actin, α-smooth muscle actin, ANF ⇓ α-MHC
IGF-1	⇑ IGF-1 mRNA and protein during hypertrophy ⇑ β-MHC, MLC_{2v}, troponin I ⇑ number of nascent myofibrils IGF-1 knockout mice show phenotype with impaired cardiac and skeletal muscle growth ⇑ Cardiac mass after in vivo administration

ANF = atrial natriuretic factor; AT = angiotensin; MLC = myosin light chain; MHC = myosin heavy chain. Adapted from Lembo, G., Hunter, J. J., and Chien, K. R.: Signaling pathways for cardiac growth and hypertrophy. Recent advances and prospects for growth factor therapy. Ann. N. Y. Acad. Sci. *752*:115, 1995.

ANGIOTENSIN II

The renin-angiotensin system is one of the principal regulators of intravascular volume, natriuresis, and systemic blood pressure[218–221] (see p. 413). The activity of the circulating system is significantly determined by the proteolytic enzyme renin, which is synthesized by the kidney and secreted into the circulation, where it hydrolyzes the decapeptide, angiotensin I, from the amino-terminal end of angiotensinogen. Angiotensin I is converted to the octapeptide, angiotensin II, by the dipeptidyl carboxypeptidase, angiotensin-converting enzyme. However, renin may not be the only rate-limiting step for angiotensin II production. Enzymes that can directly cleave angiotensinogen to release angiotensin II have been described, including cathepsin G, kallikrein, and tonin, and recently a chymotrypsin-like protease has been cloned from human heart (heart chymase[222]), which has been suggested to represent an alternative pathway for the conversion of angiotensin I to angiotensin II. In the heart, angiotensin-II binding sites have been described, and the recent development of nonpeptide angiotensin II antagonists has led to the characterization of two types of angiotensin-II receptors, designated AT_1 and AT_2.[223,224] The AT_1 receptor subtype is a seven transmembrane-domain protein that transmits angiotensin II effects through G protein–coupled pathways, but the AT_2 receptor does not appear to be G protein–linked, and its biological function remains unknown.[224]

ACTIONS ON THE MYOCARDIUM. Angiotensin II has both direct and indirect actions on the myocardium, modulating both cardiac contractility and hypertrophy.[218–221,225] Clinical and experimental studies have clearly indicated that ACE inhibitors or angiotensin receptor antagonists can cause regression of cardiac hypertrophy, an effect that in some experimental models seems independent from their effect on blood pressure.[225–227] Moreover, in the past decade, mounting experimental evidence suggests that the renin-angiotensin system is not solely an endocrine system but is present within several peripheral tissues, including the heart.[219,225] Renin and angiotensinogen mRNAs have been demonstrated in the four cardiac chambers,[220,225] and AT_1 mRNA is induced more than threefold in left ventricular myocardium from hypertrophied hearts.[228] Angiotensin II can diffuse from the myocardial microvasculature through the cardiac interstitium to activate receptors on cardiac myocytes, leading to increased contractility and/or growth.

Angiotensin II increases protein synthesis in chick cardiac myocytes[226] and is able to cause hypertrophy of rat cardiac myocytes and hyperplasia of cardiac nonmyocytes, both actions mediated by the AT_1 receptor.[197,224] Furthermore, in an in vitro model of stretch-induced cardiac hypertrophy, mechanical stretch causes release of angiotensin II from cardiac myocytes and may act as an initiator of the stretch-induced hypertrophic response.[229] Electron microscopy shows that immunoreactive angiotensin II is preferentially localized in what appear to be secretory granules in ventricular myocytes.[229] These observations are consistent with the hypothesis that locally produced angiotensin II acts as an endogenous growth factor regulating myocardial growth and, at the same time, may affect the level of expression of other growth factor genes.[218–221] However, because cardiac fibroblasts contain a high density of AT_1 receptors, whether the mechanical sensor for the stretch stimulus is within cardiac or noncardiac cells remains an open question. Gene-targeted mice with deletions of various components of the renin-angiotensin system are currently being characterized by a number of laboratories and should allow a direct evaluation of the role of this system in the hypertrophic response.[116,230]

ENDOTHELIN 1

As predicted by the primary structure of the full-length cDNA, endothelin 1 is synthesized as a pre-pro-peptide of approximately 200 residues, which is subsequently cleaved to a 38 to 39 residue *big endothelin* molecule.[231,232] Further proteolytic processing results in the mature, biologically active 21-amino acid peptide, which is highly conserved among species.[232] Although endothelin was initially thought to be localized exclusively in vascular endothelial cells, endothelin 1, endothelin 2, and endothelin 3 have now been found to be widely distributed in extravascular tissues.[233] Although the presence of high-affinity endothelin receptors on the surface of ventricular myocardial cells has been documented,[231] the role of endothelin 1 in the in vivo regulation of ventricular function has been the subject of some speculation, although it is clear that endothelin-1 is a potent stimulus for in vitro cardiac cell growth and hypertrophy.[191,198,199,234]

Because endothelin is released from endothelial cells that lie immediately adjacent to the myocytes within the intact myocardium, the activation of myocardial cell hypertrophy may represent another important paracrine mechanism for the regulation of cardiac growth.[178] Evidence to support such a phenomenon has been demonstrated in an animal model of coarctation of the aorta.[235] During the development of left ventricular hypertrophy, pre-pro-endothelin 1 mRNA was increased in banded compared with sham-operated control animals, peaking at 24 hours and returning to basal levels after 4 days.[235] It seems, therefore, that pressure-overload can upregulate endothelin-1 gene expression within the heart. When the animals were given a specific endothelin-1A receptor subtype antagonist (BQ123), despite the hemodynamic overload, genetic markers of cardiac hypertrophy (skeletal alpha-actin and ANF) were not induced, suggesting a specific role for endothelin-1 in the development of certain features of left ventricular hypertrophy.[235] The availability of well-characterized endothelin receptor antagonists should allow a further evaluation of the role of endothelin signaling pathways in the onset of cardiac muscle failure.[232,236]

INSULIN-LIKE GROWTH FACTOR-1 (IGF-1)

IGF-1 is a nonglycosylated, single-chain peptide of 70 amino acid residues with structural homology and biological function similar to those of proinsulin.[237] Although the pituitary secretion of growth hormone stimulates the production of IGF-1, primarily in the liver, most tissues synthesize IGF-1 locally. Recently, IGF-1 has also been shown to be a growth factor for cardiac myocytes.[238,239] In cultured cardiac myocytes, specific IGF-1 receptors are present and IGF-1 stimulation increases the mRNA for beta-MHC, MLC_2, and troponin I; protein synthesis is also enhanced by IGF-1 in adult cardiomyocytes.[240,241] More recently, it has been reported that IGF-1–treated adult cardiac myocytes showed a dramatic increase over controls in the number of nascent myofibrils.[238] An increase in both left ventricular IGF-1 mRNA and protein has been described in pressure-overload cardiac hypertrophy and in models of both high- and low-renin hypertension, suggesting that IGF-1 may be an important common mediator of an adaptive hypertrophic response.[242]

The association of IGF-1 administration in vivo with a physiological hypertrophic response in normal animals has suggested its potential value as a therapeutic agent to alter remodeling and improve global cardiac function in the setting of heart failure.[243] This supposition has been supported by the observation that IGF-1 can enhance cardiac size and improve cardiac performance during the development of experimental cardiac failure after myocardial infarction in the rat.[244] Whether these beneficial effects can be translated to improved therapy of heart failure is under investigation.[244a]

CYTOKINES INCLUDING CARDIOTROPHIN-1

The development of an in vitro assay system for myocardial cell hypertrophy has offered the possibility of isolating and characterizing both known and novel activities that might activate features of myocardial cell hypertrophy.[193,204,245] Totipotent mouse embryonic stem (ES) cells differentiate into multicellular, cystic embryoid bodies when cultured in the absence of a fibroblast feeder layer or with the removal of leukemia inhibitory factor (LIF).[246] Because these embryoid bodies spontaneously beat, display cardiac-specific markers, and are a source of ventricular myocytes, it has been suggested that they might serve as a valuable source of novel factors that can induce a hypertrophic response in vitro.[178] Embryoid bodies have now been shown to elaborate a factor that induces a hypertrophic response.[204] An expression cloning approach was used to characterize the protein responsible for this activity leading to the isolation of a cDNA clone encoding a 21.5-kDa protein, designated cardiotrophin-1 (CT-1), which can activate several features of in vitro cardiac hypertrophy.[204]

Amino acid similarity data indicate that CT-1 is a member of the leukemia inhibitory factor/ciliary neurotrophic factor/oncostatin-M/interleukin-6/interleukin-11 family of cytokines.[247] Several members of this family are known to signal through the transmembrane protein GP130 and can stimulate features of cardiac myocyte hypertrophy, in a manner similar to CT-1, suggesting the possibility that GP130-dependent signaling pathways may play a role in cardiac hypertrophy.[193] A 1.4-kb cardiotrophin-1 mRNA is expressed in the heart and several other mouse tissues.[248] Currently, a variety of experimental approaches are being taken to further evaluate the role of GP130-dependent pathways in the control of cardiac muscle cell hypertrophy in the in vivo context and define its relationship to the onset of cardiac muscle failure.[193,245,248]

Intracellular Signaling Pathways

(See also Chap. 12)

The finding that diverse growth factors and cytokines can activate distinct molecular and physiological phenotypes in cardiac myocytes has led to numerous studies examining the downstream signaling pathways, from the membrane to the nucleus, which activate specific subsets of the cardiac muscle gene program.[198,199,206,208,249,250] For the most part, these studies have focused on in vitro model systems employing cultured neonatal rat myocardial cells and well-defined downstream molecular markers, as noted previously. The cardiac muscle cell is endowed with many of the receptor-mediated signaling pathways, found in other cell types,[198,199,206,249,250] including G protein–coupled receptor pathways[251] (Fig. 12–17, p. 372), receptor tyrosine kinase pathways,[252] and GP130-dependent pathways.[193] Much of the downstream cell signaling machinery is also conserved between cardiac and other cell types, and, as such, much of this molecular machinery does not appear to be expressed in a cardiac cell–specific manner.[178] The question arises as to which of these conserved signaling pathways leads to defined phenotypic features of various forms of cardiac hypertrophy.

In this regard, recent studies in both cultured cells[206,249] and transgenic animals[123] have documented that *ras*-dependent pathways are sufficient to activate a hypertrophic response. p21 H-*ras* is a small, GTP-binding protein that functions as a critical molecular *switch* in mitogenic and differentiation signaling from a number of cell surface receptors, particularly members of the family of receptor tyrosine kinases.[253–255] Microinjection of oncogenic *ras* in cultured ventricular muscle cells leads to an increase in myocardial cell size, the organization of an individual contractile protein (MLC_2) into organized sarcomeric units, the induction of ANF gene expression, but no proliferation, all independent criteria of hypertrophy.[206,249] The questions remained as to whether *ras* was sufficient to activate a hypertrophic response in vivo and whether it would induce concomitant cardiac dysfunction analogous to that seen clinically.

By generating transgenic mice that harbor a MLC-*ras* fusion gene, direct evidence that *ras* is sufficient to activate in vivo cardiac hypertrophy has been obtained with appropriate structural, morphological, and genetic markers.[123] These include an increase in left ventricular mass/body weight ratio, an increase in myocardial cell size, and an increased expression of ANF and are qualitatively similar to murine pressure-overload hypertrophy[123,190] (Figs. 48–14 and 48–15). The response is massive, displaying an increase in wet heart weight (>50 per cent) comparable to that observed with a 100 mm Hg trans-stenotic gradient following thoracic aortic constriction.[190] Further, analysis of in vivo cardiac physiology in the mouse has demonstrated an effect of *ras* expression on diastolic dysfunction with reduced left ventricular compliance accompanied by a selective increase in left atrial size.[123] In contrast, basal and beta-adrenergic–stimulated contractile function remained intact. Moreover, as a genetically based model of cardiac

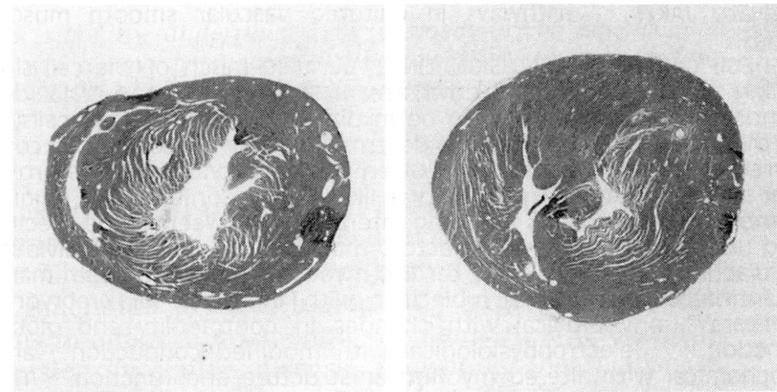

FIGURE 48–14. Hypertrophic heart in *ras* transgenic mouse. Representative histological sections from a wild-type mouse *(left)* and one harboring a MLC-2v-*ras* fusion gene *(right)*, showing increased wall thickness and ventricular chamber obliteration. (Courtesy of Dr. John Hunter, Department of Medicine, University of California, San Diego. Modified from Hunter, J. J., Tanaka, N., Rockman, H. A., et al.: Ventricular expression of an MLC-2v-*ras* fusion gene induces cardiac hypertrophy and selective diastolic dysfunction in transgenic mice. J. Biol. Chem. *270*:23173, 1995, with permission of publisher.)

muscle disease, these mice now permit dissection of the interaction of *ras* with other signaling pathways, through genetic crosses with other transgenic strains, and physiological and pharmacological manipulations that induce or impair the development of hypertrophy.[178]

The signaling pathways that lie downstream from *ras* are conserved in different eukaryotic cell types (e.g., yeast, muscle, cardiac, skeletal) and between widely divergent species (*Drosophila*, mouse, man). Since initial reports that *ras* is capable of activating a hypertrophic response,[206,249] a number of subsequent studies have suggested roles for both Raf and MAP kinase-dependent pathways using co-transfection–based approaches with well-defined reporter genes that are upregulated during the hypertrophic response.[199,256] Similarly, a role for a specific subset of the heterotrimeric G protein signaling pathways[251] via G_q has been documented, which appears to be parallel and co-dominant with the *ras*-dependent pathway.[249]

The activation of protein kinase C (PKC) has long been associated with hypertrophic response in cultured cell systems and represents one potential pathway by which these signals elicited from G protein–coupled receptors could be linked with downstream signaling pathways.[178,257–259] In addition, studies have recently demonstrated that GP130-dependent pathways can activate features of hypertrophy, including the upregulation of ANF, in cultured cardiac muscle cells.[193] In other cell types, this signaling pathway works through activation of JAK/STAT signaling pathways and eventually results in the regulation of specific subsets of cellular gene responses.[247,260,261] Interestingly, angiotensin II has also been shown to

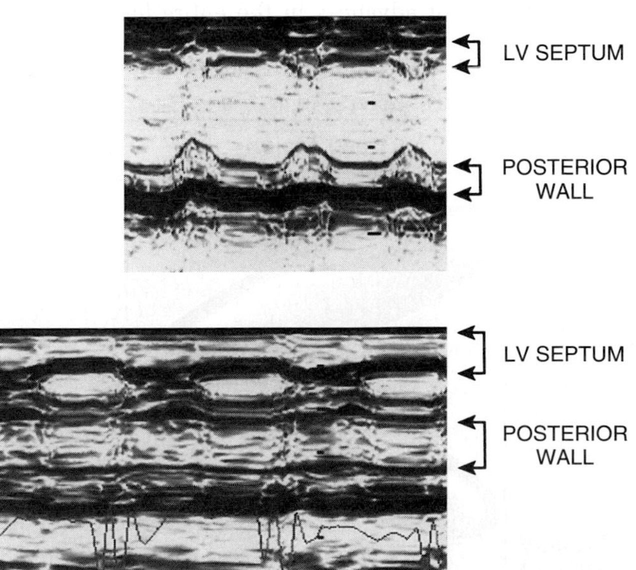

FIGURE 48–15. M-mode of ventricular hypertrophy in the *ras* overexpressing transgenic mouse. Representative M-mode echocardiograms from a wild-type mouse and one harboring a MLC-2v-*ras* fusion gene, showing increased wall thickness. (Courtesy of Dr. John Ross, Department of Medicine, University of California, San Diego.)

Chapter 49
Genetics and Cardiovascular Disease

REED E. PYERITZ

GENETIC FACTORS IN DISEASE 1650
Disorders Due to Microscopic Alterations in Chromosomes 1650
Disorders Due to Changes in Single Nuclear Genes 1651
Principles of Clinical Genetics 1654
Nonpathological Variation in the Cardiovascular System 1655
CARDIOVASCULAR DISORDERS ASSOCIATED WITH CHROMOSOME ABERRATIONS 1655
CONGENITAL HEART DISEASE 1657
Mendelian Disorders 1659
Teratogenic Effects 1663
CARDIOMYOPATHIES 1664
Hypertrophic Cardiomyopathy 1664
Dilated Cardiomyopathy 1665
Restrictive Cardiomyopathy 1665
Cardiomyopathies Secondary to Other Causes 1666
PRIMARY DISORDERS OF RHYTHM AND CONDUCTION 1667
DISORDERS OF CONNECTIVE TISSUE 1667
Marfan Syndrome 1669
Ehlers-Danlos Syndrome 1672
Pseudoxanthoma Elasticum 1673
INBORN ERRORS OF METABOLISM THAT AFFECT THE CARDIOVASCULAR SYSTEM . . 1673
Aminoacidopathies 1673
Disorders of Fatty Acid Metabolism 1673
Glycogenoses 1674
Hematological Disorders 1674
Mucopolysaccharidoses and Disorders of Targeting Lysosomal Enzymes 1675
Sphingolipidoses 1675
Familial Amyloidoses 1676
INHERITED DISORDERS OF THE CIRCULATION 1676
Hereditary Hemorrhagic Telangiectasia . . . 1676
Von Hippel–Lindau Syndrome 1676
Disorders Primarily Affecting Arteries 1676
Disorders Primarily Affecting Veins 1677
GENETIC FACTORS PREDISPOSING TO ATHEROSCLEROSIS 1677
ESSENTIAL HYPERTENSION 1677
REFERENCES 1679

GENETIC FACTORS IN DISEASE

Genes contribute to both the cause and the pathogenesis of virtually any abnormality of human physiology and behavior including, of course, disorders of the heart and vascular system. This statement carries two messages in addition to the obvious one. First, the pathology associated with even the most "environmental" of causes, such as trauma, malnutrition, and drug abuse, can be defined only in terms of the human body's response to the insult. How the stress of the initial insult is expressed (the *phenotype*) and how the patient suffers and perhaps recovers depend, to varying and as yet often poorly defined degrees, on the patient's *genotype.* This idea seems self-evident and verges on the trite, but it is frequently neglected. Some environmental insults, such as massive trauma or poisoning, are lethal to all, regardless of genotype. Nonetheless, as developments in fields such as *pharmacogenetics* and *ecogenetics* are defining genetic susceptibilities to human disease better and more simply, the physician must become increasingly attuned to the importance of the genotype.[1]

Second, the introductory statement stresses that genetic factors play roles in *both* cause and process; etiology and pathogenesis, although related, are conceptually distinct.[2] For example, the cause of sickle cell anemia is clearly a single mutant gene, whereas whether a patient homozygous for this mutation expresses all, some, or none of the manifestations of the disease depends on many other genetic and nongenetic factors. Conversely, the cause of pneumococcal pneumonia is equally evident, but the severity and resolution of the disease depend on the patient's immune competency (which in turn depends on genetic and nongenetic factors) as much as on treatment with an antibiotic.

The genotype, therefore, can be detrimental in at least two distinct ways. First, mutant genes can so upset embryology or physiology that a clinical abnormality occurs. Whereas the phenotype of any particular mutation depends on a host of factors, including which homeostatic systems are available to modulate the action of the defect, the genotype has the principal role in causing the disease. It is this class of mutations that are usually referred to as genetic diseases. Second, a mutation can facilitate the action of an extrinsic cause in producing disease. Inherited susceptibilities are part of the pathogenesis of disease and are one reason for taking the patient's family history. Until recently, the clinician could do little to pursue tantalizing facts, such as multiple relatives under age 50 suffering myocardial infarction. The long-touted prospect of detecting a patient's inherited susceptibilities and intervening before irreversible clinical sequelae occur is becoming reality.

Disorders Due to Microscopic Alterations in Chromosomes

Estimates of the total number of human genes range between 50,000 and 100,000. Two copies (termed *alleles*) of each gene are arrayed along 23 pairs of *chromosomes.* Twenty-two of the chromosomes are called *autosomes* (numbered 1 through 22), while the 23rd pair are the *sex chromosomes,* X and Y. Females have two X chromosomes and males have an X and a Y chromosome. Both autosomal alleles are potentially active in specifying RNA copies of their DNA sequences; whether a gene is active depends on the cell type, the developmental stage of the organism, and the regulatory molecules that interact with promoter and enhancer nucleotide sequences that control transcription of the gene. In cells with two X chromosomes (i.e., in all females, in the Klinefelter syndrome in which two X's and one Y occur, and in other rare conditions), only one X is active after early embryogenesis.

Human chromosomes can be examined by culturing cells capable of mitosis; T lymphocytes obtained from venous blood are the usual source, but fibroblasts, cells from chorionic villi, amniocytes, and leukocyte precursors present in bone marrow are also used clinically. Chromosomes are distinguished from one another by their size, shape (determined by the position of a constriction called the *centromere,* which functions as the attachment of the mitotic apparatus), and characteristic banding pattern as revealed by any of several staining techniques. The chromosomes are photographed, cut out, and arranged in pairs, from 1 through 22 and the sex chromosomes, in a display called the *karyotype.* This display and its interpretation are the end results of a clinical study of a patient's chromosomes. The chromosome constitution of a cell is designated by first specifying the number of chromosomes present (46 being normal in diploid cells), then specifying the sex chromosomes, and finally describing any abnormalities. For

TABLE 49–1 CONTIGUOUS GENE SYNDROMES

	REGION	LOCUS	CARDIOVASCULAR ABNORMALITIES
Syndromes with cardiovascular involvement			
Arteriohepatic dysplasia	AHD	del 20p11.23p12.2	Peripheral pulmonic stenosis/hypoplasia
Cat-eye syndrome	CES	dup22q11	Total anomalous pulmonary venous return
DiGeorge sequence	DGS	del 22q11	Truncus arteriosus, right aortic arch, TOF, PDA
Miller-Dieker syndrome	MDS	del 17p13	Patent ductus arteriosus ± complex anomalies
Prader-Willi syndrome	PWS/AS	del 15q12	Cor pulmonale (secondary to obesity and central apnea)
WAGR syndrome		del 11p13	Hypertension (secondary to Wilms tumor)
Syndromes without frequent cardiovascular involvement			
Angelman syndrome		del 15q12*	
Smith-Magenis syndrome		del 17p11.2	

TOF = tetralogy of Fallot; PDA = patent ductus arteriosus.
WAGR = Wilms' tumor, aniridia, genitourinary, and retardation.
* The deletion is indistinguishable at the cytogenetic level from that of the Prader-Willi syndrome; genetic imprinting is thought to account in part for the phenotypic differences. In Prader-Willi, the deleted chromosome is always the chromosome 15 inherited from father, whereas in Angelman syndrome, the deletion affects the maternal chromosome 15.

example, a normal male is designated 46,XY, and a female with an extra chromosome 21 is designated 46,XX,+21.

ANEUPLOIDY. Chromosome aberrations, especially too many or too few chromosomes *(aneuploidy),* are extremely common in human embryos; more than one-half of all conceptuses are spontaneously aborted in early pregnancy, and at least one-half of them are aneuploid. Among live-born infants, about 0.5 per cent have a chromosome aberration.

Gain or loss of chromosomes generally happens by nondisjunction, or the failure of a homologous pair of chromosomes to separate. Absence of one chromosome is termed *monosomy;* all autosomal monosomies are embryonic lethals, as is presence of only a Y sex chromosome. Presence of three chromosomes is *trisomy,* and presence of an entire extra set of chromosomes (for a total of 69) is *triploidy.* The most common autosomal aneuploidy, trisomy 21 associated with the Down syndrome, and aneuploidy for sex chromosomes are all compatible with survival into adulthood.

CHROMOSOME REARRANGEMENTS. A chromosome can break and rejoin within itself, potentially giving rise to an *inversion* of genetic material. Often no apparent phenotypic effect is seen in people with an inversion, but because inversions may disrupt chromosome pairing during meiosis, their offspring may have more profound aberrations.

DELETIONS AND DUPLICATIONS. Just as their names imply, these aberrations are losses or gains of chromosomal material. Many clinical syndromes have been associated with aberrations of specific chromosome regions.[3,4] The smallest deletion detectable by light microscopy is associated with loss of considerable DNA, on the order of one million base pairs, so more than one gene is potentially disrupted or lost.

A number of conditions, each initially thought to be due to a mutation in a single locus, are associated with small interstitial chromosome aberrations affecting a cluster of genes (Table 49–1). So rather than pleiotropic manifestations of one mutation, these conditions are likely to be due to the effects of several, and perhaps many, mutations and are therefore called *contiguous gene syndromes.*[5] Such defects are potentially heritable, and the occurrence of the disorder in a family behaves as a mendelian dominant.

Disorders Due to Changes in Single Nuclear Genes

(See also Chap. 48)

Mutations of genes located on the 22 pairs of autosomes and the two sex chromosomes produce phenotypes inherited according to the two principal tenets of Mendel: alleles segregate and nonalleles assort. The first statement refers to gametes receiving as a result of meiosis only one of the two alleles at a given locus. The second statement describes the results of recombination, the meiotic process of rearranging DNA between the two chromosomes of the pair *(homologous chromosomes);* if two loci are widely spaced along a chromosome, their chances of being separated by recombination are 50–50, and they are said to be *unlinked.*

More than 6500 individual loci have been identified on the basis of the phenotype that mutations in single genes produce. The presumption of single-gene defects is based in most instances on the pattern of inheritance in families; segregation of the phenotype according to mendelian principles is the central piece of evidence. For an increasing number of loci, however, molecular genetic techniques have mapped the phenotype to a single gene or even revealed the actual alteration in nucleotide sequence.[6,7] The range of known mendelian variation in humans and information about gene mapping and molecular defects are routinely catalogued[8] and available on-line.[9] Based on current estimates of the size of the human genome, about 5 to 10 per cent of loci have been identified through the effects their mutations have on phenotype.

More than 2000 loci have been mapped to a restricted region of the genome. Many of these loci cause specific mendelian disorders, and the genetic map of these loci represents the "morbid anatomy of the human genome." Many of the cardiovascular and hemostatic disorders that were mapped by early 1995 are shown in Figure 49–1.

DOMINANCE AND RECESSIVENESS. These related concepts are characteristics of the phenotype, *not of the gene.* A phenotype is dominant when the patient is *heterozygous* for a mutation, i.e., when one copy of the mutant allele, and one copy of the normal allele, are present; this holds for genes on both autosomes and the X chromosome. A phenotype is recessive when the patient has two mutant alleles at the locus causing the condition. If the mutant alleles are identical, the patient is *homozygous* at that locus, a situation usually present either when the allele is identical by descent through both parents (i.e., the parents had a common ancestor and are *consanguineous*) or when the mutant allele is common in the population (e.g., the most prevalent mutation for cystic fibrosis and the mutation for sickle cell anemia). Biochemical and molecular genetic assessment of mutant alleles has shown that the majority of recessive phenotypes are due to two distinct mutant alleles, a situation termed a *genetic compound,* indicative of the widespread heterogeneity in mutations at each locus. Males have but one X chromosome, and each locus is therefore *hemizygous;* a mutant locus is always expressed in the phenotype of a male. Dominance and recessiveness for X-linked traits refer to expression in heterozygous and homozygous women, respectively.

Whether a disorder is called dominant or recessive depends on how carefully the phenotype is assessed and how it is defined. For example, familial hypercholesterolemia is a relatively common hereditary disorder due to defects in the receptor for low-density lipoprotein (LDL, p. 1134). The vast majority of patients are heterozygous for a mutant allele at the *LDLR* locus on chromosome 19,[10] and the disease is inherited as a mendelian dominant trait. However, if a man and a woman, each heterozygous for an *LDLR* mutation, mate, they have a 25 per cent risk of having a child who inherits both of the mutant alleles and thereby is either homozygous or a genetic compound for *LDLR.* Such a child has a much more severe form of familial hypercholesterolemia (see p. 1142) that is inherited as a mendelian recessive trait. Similarly, homozygosity for the sickle hemoglobin mutation at the β-globin locus on chromosome 11 produces the familiar autosomal recessive disease, sickle cell anemia. However, heterozygosity for the same mutation rarely produces disease but produces sickling of erythrocytes if they are examined under conditions of low oxygen tension; this phenotype is transmitted as a dominant trait.

AUTOSOMAL RECESSIVE INHERITANCE. Nearly all deficiencies of enzymatic activity—the classic inborn errors of metabolism first defined by Archibald Garrod in 1903—cause recessive phenotypes. Most homeostatic systems, which include all metabolic pathways, have sufficient flexibility to function well if one of the enzymatic steps

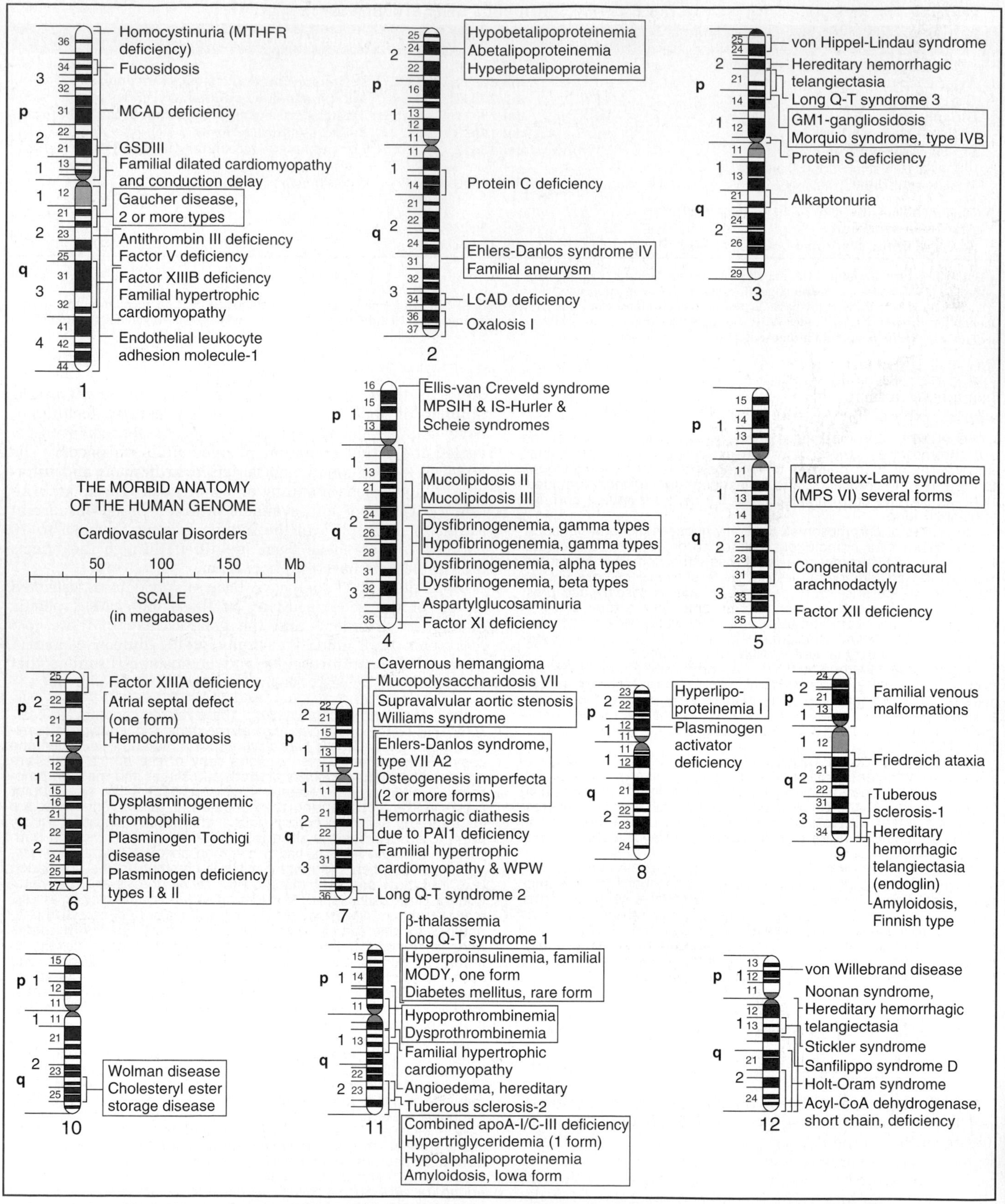

THE MORBID ANATOMY OF THE HUMAN GENOME

Cardiovascular Disorders

50 100 150 Mb

SCALE (in megabases)

Chromosome 1
Homocystinuria (MTHFR deficiency)
Fucosidosis
MCAD deficiency
GSDIII
Familial dilated cardiomyopathy and conduction delay
Gaucher disease, 2 or more types
Antithrombin III deficiency
Factor V deficiency
Factor XIIIB deficiency
Familial hypertrophic cardiomyopathy
Endothelial leukocyte adhesion molecule-1

Chromosome 2
Hypobetalipoproteinemia
Abetalipoproteinemia
Hyperbetalipoproteinemia
Protein C deficiency
Ehlers-Danlos syndrome IV
Familial aneurysm
LCAD deficiency
Oxalosis I

Chromosome 3
von Hippel-Lindau syndrome
Hereditary hemorrhagic telangiectasia
Long Q-T syndrome 3
GM1-gangliosidosis
Morquio syndrome, type IVB
Protein S deficiency
Alkaptonuria

Chromosome 4
Ellis-van Creveld syndrome
MPSIH & IS-Hurler & Scheie syndromes
Mucolipidosis II
Mucolipidosis III
Dysfibrinogenemia, gamma types
Hypofibrinogenemia, gamma types
Dysfibrinogenemia, alpha types
Dysfibrinogenemia, beta types
Aspartylglucosaminuria
Factor XI deficiency

Chromosome 5
Maroteaux-Lamy syndrome (MPS VI) several forms
Congenital contracural arachnodactyly
Factor XII deficiency

Chromosome 6
Factor XIIIA deficiency
Atrial septal defect (one form)
Hemochromatosis
Dysplasminogenemic thrombophilia
Plasminogen Tochigi disease
Plasminogen deficiency types I & II

Chromosome 7
Cavernous hemangioma
Mucopolysaccharidosis VII
Supravalvular aortic stenosis
Williams syndrome
Ehlers-Danlos syndrome, type VII A2
Osteogenesis imperfecta (2 or more forms)
Hemorrhagic diathesis due to PAI1 deficiency
Familial hypertrophic cardiomyopathy & WPW
Long Q-T syndrome 2

Chromosome 8
Hyperlipo-proteinemia I
Plasminogen activator deficiency

Chromosome 9
Familial venous malformations
Friedreich ataxia
Tuberous sclerosis-1
Hereditary hemorrhagic telangiectasia (endoglin)
Amyloidosis, Finnish type

Chromosome 10
Wolman disease
Cholesteryl ester storage disease

Chromosome 11
β-thalassemia
long Q-T syndrome 1
Hyperproinsulinemia, familial
MODY, one form
Diabetes mellitus, rare form
Hypoprothrombinemia
Dysprothrombinemia
Familial hypertrophic cardiomyopathy
Angioedema, hereditary
Tuberous sclerosis-2
Combined apoA-I/C-III deficiency
Hypertriglyceridemia (1 form)
Hypoalphalipoproteinemia
Amyloidosis, Iowa form

Chromosome 12
von Willebrand disease
Noonan syndrome,
Hereditary hemorrhagic telangiectasia
Stickler syndrome
Sanfilippo syndrome D
Holt-Oram syndrome
Acyl-CoA dehydrogenase, short chain, deficiency

FIGURE 49–1. Chromosomal location of human genes associated with disorders of the cardiovascular system. These genes affect the structure, function, and metabolism of the heart and blood vessels and hemostasis and have been identified by the deleterious effects of mutations. Numerous additional genes that encode structural proteins important to the cardiovascular system have been identified but not yet associated with disease. In the figure, brackets next to the chromosome show the regional localization of the gene causing a particular disorder. Brackets next to two or more disorders indicate that all of the genes causing the disorders map to the same region. Disorders surrounded by boxes are caused by different mutations at the same gene.

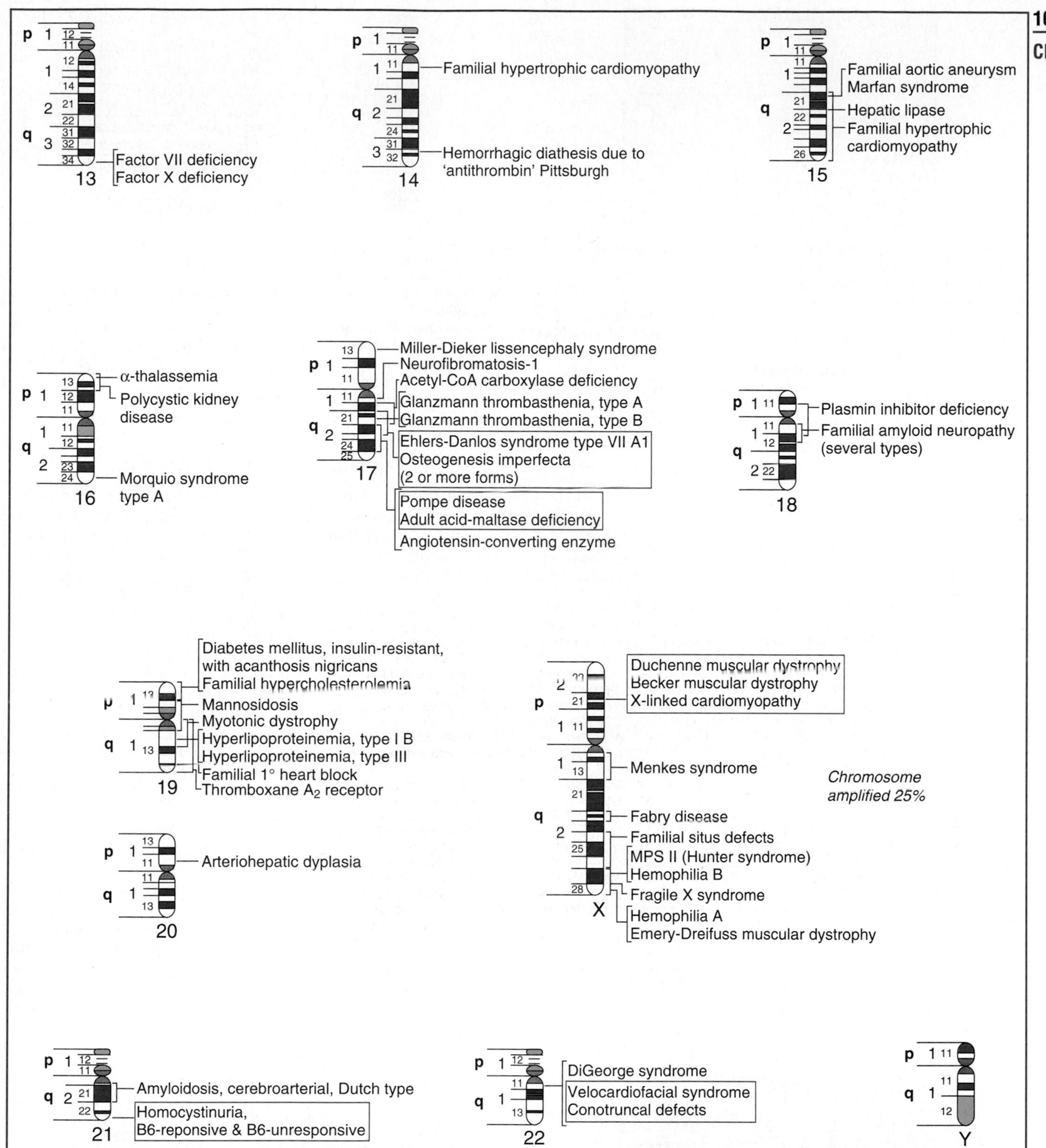

FIGURE 49–1 *See legend on opposite page*

function at half-normal efficiency, as would occur in heterozygosity for a mutant allele at a structural gene for an enzyme. However, homeostasis cannot cope if two mutant alleles cause a reduction in enzymatic activity to a few per cent or less of normal activity. The characteristics of autosomal recessive inheritance, features common to such phenotypes, and a typical pedigree are shown in Figure 49–2.

AUTOSOMAL DOMINANT INHERITANCE. Only a few enzyme deficiencies, but many disorders of development and structure, are inherited as dominant traits. The reasons for this are several. One possibility is that developmental homeostasis has a limited repertoire of responses to stress, and when a structural or regulatory macromolecule is reduced to only one-half normal amount, the system cannot cope. Another possibility, illustrated by mutations in procollagen molecules, pertains to gene products that must interact before becoming functional; an aberrant protein combined with a normal one would be a defective multimer, and the effect of being heterozygous for a mutation would be magnified—a *dominant-negative* effect.[7,11] The characteristics of autosomal dominant inheritance, features common to many such phenotypes, and a typical pedigree are shown in Figure 49–3.

Most human dominant traits are *incomplete*, in that the heterozygote is less severely affected than the homozygote. Defects of *LDLR* are illustrative, in which the heterozygote has classic type IIa hyperlipidemia, while the homozygote has a quantitatively worse form of the same disease.[10] It may well be that homozygosity for most alleles that cause dominant disorders is incompatible with life.

X-LINKED INHERITANCE. The characteristics of X-linked inheritance, features common to such phenotypes, and a typical pedigree are

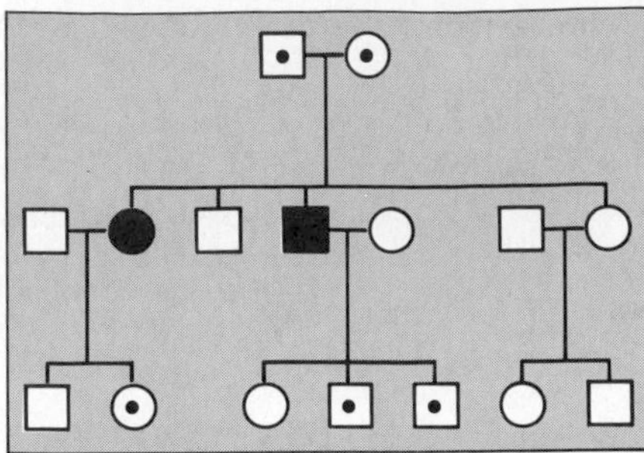

FIGURE 49–2. *Characteristics of autosomal recessive inheritance*
A single generation affected
Sexes affected equally frequently
Each parent heterozygous (a carrier)
Each offspring of two carriers has a 25% chance of being affected, a 50% chance of being a carrier, and a 25% chance of inheriting neither mutant allele
Two-thirds of clinically normal offspring are carriers
The rarer the phenotype, the greater the likelihood of consanguinity
Characteristics of autosomal recessive phenotypes
Often due to enzyme deficiencies
Often more severe than dominant disorders
Often early age of onset

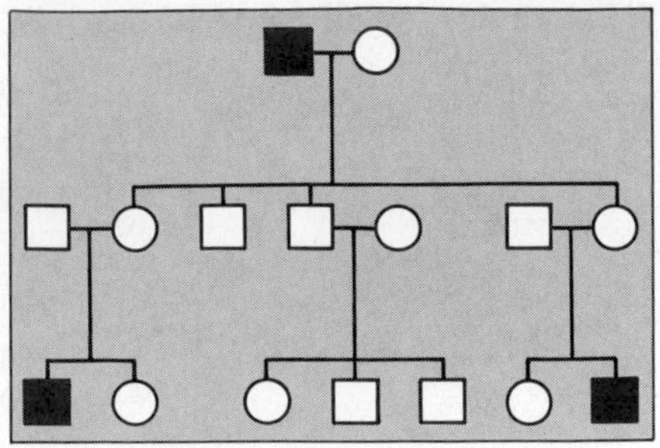

FIGURE 49–4. *Characteristics of X-linked inheritance*
No male-to-male transmission
All daughters of affected males are carriers
Sons of a carrier mother have a 50% chance of being affected; daughters have a 50% chance of being carriers
Some mothers of an affected male are not carriers, but they may have more affected sons if germinal mosaicism is present
Characteristics of X-linked phenotypes
More severe in males
Heterozygous females may be unaffected
Variable, especially in females

shown in Figure 49–4. Whereas virtually all diseases due to mutations on the X chromosome are more severe in hemizygous males, women heterozygous for the same mutations often show some manifestations, albeit less severe and of later age of onset. For example, most women carriers of α-galactosidase A deficiency (Fabry disease) eventually develop cerebrovascular disease or renal failure due to accumulation of sphingolipid.[12]

MITOCHONDRIAL INHERITANCE. Energy generation through oxidative phosphorylation occurs in mitochondria in the cytoplasm of most cell types. Numerous mitochondria, each containing a single chromosome, exist in each cell. Some of the enzymes of oxidative phosphorylation are encoded by genes on the nuclear chromosomes and the proteins transported into the mitochondrion; the rest of the proteins are encoded by genes on the mitochondrial chromosome. Thus, genetic defects of oxidative phosphorylation can be due to mutations of genes on the autosomes or the X chromosome, and the resulting diseases behave as mendelian recessive traits, or mutations of genes on the mitochondrial chromosome, in which case the resulting diseases do not behave as mendelian traits.[13,14] The differences are explicable by the events of conception. The spermatocyte contributes virtually no mitochondria to the zygote, and the entire complement of mitochondria that will ever be present in the fetus is derived from the mitochondria already present in the cytoplasm of the oocyte. Thus, phenotypes due to mutations of the mitochondrial chromosome show *maternal inheritance*, the characteristics of which are shown in Figure 49–5.

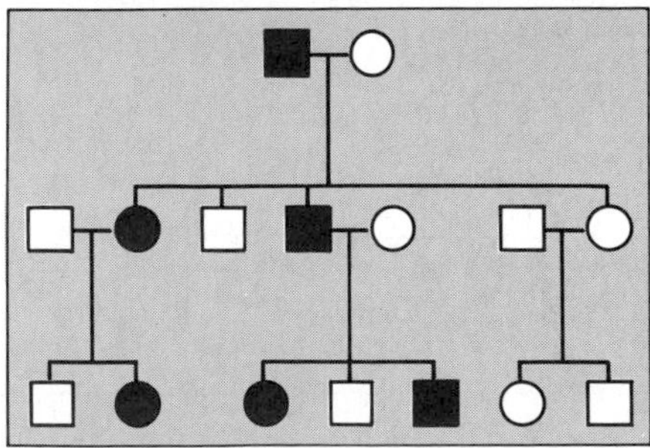

FIGURE 49–3. *Characteristics of autosomal dominant inheritance*
Multiple generations affected
Sexes affected equally frequently
In familial cases, only one parent need be affected
Male-to-male transmission occurs
Offspring of an affected parent has a 50% chance of being affected
Frequency of sporadic cases higher the more severe the condition
Paternal age effect of sporadic cases
Characteristics of autosomal dominant phenotypes
Often associated with malformations
Often pleiotropic
Usually variable
Often less severe than recessive phenotypes
Often age-dependent

Principles of Clinical Genetics

PLEIOTROPY. Most mutant alleles have effects on more than one organ system, and a mendelian phenotype frequently displays multiple, often diverse, manifestations.[15] For example, the Marfan syndrome (see p. 1669) is defined by abnormalities in the eye, skeleton, skin, heart, and aorta, and until the recent recognition of a defect in extracellular microfibrils,[7] the findings could not be linked either etiologically or pathogenetically.[16]

VARIABILITY. The effects of the same mutant allele on phenotype can be different among people heterozygous (for dominant traits), homozygous (for autosomal recessive traits), or hemizygous (for X-linked traits) for the allele. Variability can be described in terms of the frequency of a particular pleiotropic manifestation among patients with the mutation; the severity of the phenotype; and the age of onset of manifestations. If a person has the mutant allele(s) but shows no phenotypic effect, the trait is called *nonpenetrant.* To an important degree, whether or not a clinical phenotype is called nonpenetrant depends on the sensitivity of the techniques employed for detection. For example, two decades ago, based on bedside examination, cardiovascular abnormalities were thought to affect about half of people with the Marfan syndrome; echocardiography now reveals aortic dilatation in more than 90 per cent. The term *incomplete penetrance* should not be used with reference to individuals but to mean a prevalence of the phenotype is less than 100 per cent of people known to carry the muta-

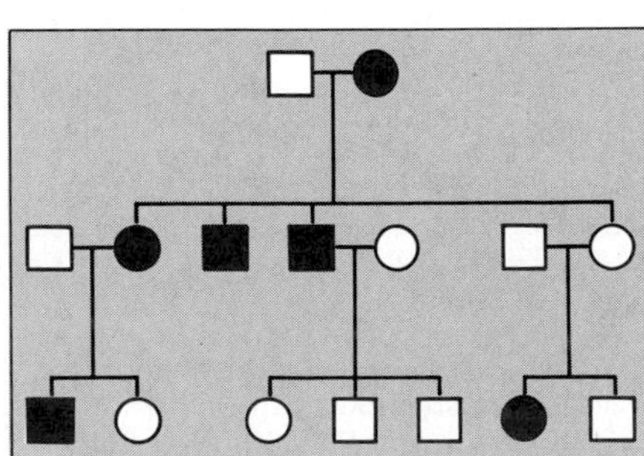

FIGURE 49–5. *Characteristics of disorders due to a mutation of the mitochondrial chromosome*
Sexes equally frequently and severely affected
Transmission only through women; offspring of affected men are unaffected
All offspring of an affected woman may be affected
Variability of expression can be extreme in a family, including apparent nonpenetrance
Phenotypes may be age-dependent

TABLE 49–2 CAUSES OF VARIABILITY OF GENE EXPRESSION

Genetic background
Age dependency
Sex influence
Sex limitation
Modifying loci: hypostasis and epistasis
Gene alteration
Somatic mutation
Somatic amplification
Transpositions and rearrangements
Mutations
Physiological rearrangements
Variation in X-inactivation*
Endogenous complementation*
Maternal factors
Effects of mitochondrial genome
Intrauterine environment
Imprinting
Exogenous and ecological factors
Ecology—temperature, diet
Teratogens
Medical intervention
Chance

* Pertains to female heterozygotes for X-linked disorders.

tion(s). The Holt-Oram syndrome (see p. 1661) is an instructive example. In this autosomal dominant syndrome of reduction anomalies of the upper limb and congenital heart defect, patients in the same family can have only arm anomalies, only a heart defect, or both. Moreover, the severity of the reduction defect varies widely, from a proximally placed thumb to near total absence of the arm. The cardiac feature is incompletely penetrant because only about 50 per cent of patients have it, but in any individual with the Holt-Oram allele, the heart is either structurally normal or not.

Numerous genetic and environmental factors can affect expression of a gene (Table 49–2), and it is often impossible to determine which of these factors are most important in a specific patient or particular disease. However, the pervasiveness of variable expression emphasizes that phenotypes determined by single genes are to some extent really "multifactorial."

GENETIC HETEROGENEITY. Similar or even identical phenotypes can be due to fundamentally distinct mutations, a phenomenon termed genetic heterogeneity. For example, Marfan syndrome and homocystinuria were long thought to be the same disorder, despite what now appear in retrospect to be obvious differences in inheritance pattern and intelligence.[17] As in the case of these two disorders, the causes may lie in two different genes whose products are functionally distinct. Osteogenesis imperfecta exemplifies a disorder in which mutations in two genes, $\alpha1$(I) and $\alpha2$(I) procollagen, can each produce the same phenotype because the two proteins interact to form type I collagen.[18] Genetic heterogeneity is pervasive at the intragenic level of analysis; except for sickle cell anemia and achondroplasia, virtually all single-gene disorders are due to a variety of mutations at a given locus.[8,11]

Nonpathological Variation in the Cardiovascular System

CARDIAC STRUCTURE AND PHYSIOLOGY. All aspects of the ontogeny of the cardiovascular system are dictated by the genome. If, as seems most credible, few genes have a large effect and many have small contributions, any specific aspect of "normal" cardiovascular phenotype—size, shape, function—exhibits multifactorial inheritance. In other words, to the extent that any given phenotype can be quantified, it shows a normal distribution within the population, and near-relatives are more similar to each other than they are to distant relatives and the rest of the population. The twin method should demonstrate a higher concordance of the trait in monozygotic than dizygotic twins. However, surprisingly few phenotypes have been examined.

Preliminary data on left ventricular dimensions measured echocardiographically showed higher correlations between parent and child than between matched controls, suggesting a genetic contribution[19]; however, as in many such studies, the effect of shared environment was not estimated. In an attempt to minimize environmental contributions, left ventricular sizes of twins who were not exercise trained were compared; the mean intrapair differences in echocardiographic dimensions were less in the monozygotic than in the dizygotic twins and nontwin sibs.[20] The caliber and branch geometry of coronary arteries show familial resemblance, and both parameters are much more similar in monozygotic twins than in other relatives.[21] Further support for the importance of genetic factors in normal development derives from studies that demonstrate ethnic differences in structure. For example, the thickness of the intima and the media of coronary arteries of children who died of noncardiovascular causes varied significantly with the ethnicity of the child.[22]

Measures of cardiac electrophysiology show familial resemblance. Studies of both nuclear families[23] and twins[24,25] suggest a genetic contribution to resting heart rate, conduction times, and repolarization time. Genetic control of normal cardiovascular function has been especially difficult to study because of the multitude of environmental (training, diet), stochastic (age), and clinical (subtle, unrecognized pathology) issues that confound comparisons of relatives and controls. Thus far, no strong genetic contribution to an individual's response to physical conditioning has emerged.[20]

VASCULAR SYSTEM. All members of certain inbred animal strains show little variation in arterial anatomy, especially branch angles, and considerable variation with other strains of the same species. Except for the studies of coronary arterial anatomy already noted[21] similar studies of humans have not been reported.

One intriguing question of clinical importance is whether certain people are predisposed to arterial spasm and whether this susceptibility has a genetic basis. An examination of hereditary pathological and polymorphic variation in factors elaborated by endothelial cells, platelets, and leukocytes to maintain patency of blood vessels, such as prostacyclin, endothelium-derived relaxing factor, and endothelin-1, may prove enlightening.[26,27] Similarly, is there genetic contribution to arterial stiffness or its variation with age and conditioning?

CARDIOVASCULAR DISORDERS ASSOCIATED WITH CHROMOSOME ABERRATIONS

Chromosome aberrations occur in 0.5 per cent of the population at birth and are common findings in tumors.[4,28] Visible alterations of the amount of chromosomal material cause primarily structural defects of the cardiovascular system that are evident in the newborn. The frequency of chromosome aberrations among live-born children with congenital heart defects has been found to range from 5 to 13 per cent.[29,30] Upward of 40 per cent of all fetuses with heart defects detected by ultrasonography at 18 to 20 weeks' gestation have chromosome aberrations; most are spontaneously aborted. Most forms of aneuploidy and most duplications and deletions of more than a chromosome band are associated with defects of the cardiovascular system[4,31] (Tables 49–1 and 49–3). Exceptions are 47,XXX, 47,XYY, and 47,XXY (Klinefelter syndrome), in which the incidence of congenital heart disease is probably not elevated over the population baseline.

ANEUPLOIDY. How the abnormal phenotypes caused by autosomal aneuploidy develop remains controversial. One view holds that disturbance of the dosage of the genes present on the specific aneuploid chromosome segments is the central issue. The other view is that any aneuploid state disturbs developmental homeostasis in a nonspecific manner. The former theory predicts some distinctiveness of phenotype among the trisomy syndromes that occur in live-born children, whereas the latter predicts shared manifestations. At a coarse level, the clinical pictures are similar, with grave problems of the craniofacies, central nervous system, genitalia, distal limbs, and heart usually present. But when a more refined examination of the phenotypes is obtained, considerable distinctiveness emerges.

The three most common autosomal trisomies—13, 18, and 21—can be distinguished readily at the bedside. In all three, membranous ventricular and atrial septal defects are common. However, the detailed accounting of cardiovascular lesions among large numbers of patients with these trisomies reveals important differences that suggest aneuploidy exerts more than a global effect on development. In

TABLE 49–3 CARDIOVASCULAR MANIFESTATIONS ASSOCIATED WITH CHROMOSOME ABERRATIONS

CHROMOSOME ABERRATION	EPONYM	CARDIOVASCULAR MANIFESTATIONS
Triploidy		
69,XXX (or XXY or XYY)		>50% have CHD: ASD and VSD
Aneuploidy		
+13	Patau	~80% have CHD; 75% of CHD is complex: PDA, VSD, ASD, PS, AS, dextrocardia, CoA
+18	Edwards	~90% have CHD: most CHD is complex: VSD, PDA, ASD, bicuspid PV and AV, CoA
+21	Down	~40% have CHD: ECD, TOF: MVP in ~20%; AR
+8 mosaicism		~25% have CHD, most of little clinical consequence: VSD, PDA, CoA, PS
+9 mosaicism		~70% have CHD, usually complex: VSD, PDA, PLSVC
45,X	Turner	~10% have clinically important CHD: 50% of these have CoA; mild CoA is likely much more common; also AS, ARD, VSD, ASD, dextrocardia
47,XXX		CHD not increased
47,XXY	Klinefelter	CHD possibly slightly increased; ? mild conduction changes; venous thromboembolic disease
47,XYY		CHD not increased; ? mild conduction changes
Deletions		
4p-	Wolf-Hirschhorn	~50% have CHD, usually complex: VSD, ASD, PDA, PS
5p-	Cri du chat	~20% have CHD, usually single: VSD, PDA, ASD, PS
7q-		~20% have CHD, various, often complex
13q-		CHD common, often severe, but depend on region deleted
18p-		CHD uncommon
18q-		~25% have CHD, usually single, of little consequence: VSD, PDA, ASD, PS
ring 18		~20% have CHD: CoA, PA hypoplasia, HLH, PLSVC
Duplications		
4p trisomy		~10% have CHD, usually single: no defect predominates
9 p trisomy		<10% have CHD: VSD, ASD, AS, PS
10p trisomy		~30% have CHD, usually single: no defect predominates
10q24–qter trisomy		~50% have CHD, usually complex: ECD, VSD, TOF
22pter–q11 trisomy or tetrasomy	Cat eye	~50% have CHD, usually complex: TAPVR, VSD, TOF
Other Aberrations		
Marker Xq27.3	Fragile X syndrome	~55% have aortic root dilatation, MVP, or both

CHD = congenital heart defect(s); ASD = atrial septal defect; VSD = ventricular septal defect; PDA = patent ductus arteriosus; PS = valvular pulmonic stenosis; AS = aortic stenosis; CoA = coarctation of aorta; PV = pulmonic valve; AV = aortic valve; ECD = endocardial cushion defect; TOF = tetralogy of Fallot; MVP = mitral valve prolapse; AR = aortic regurgitation; PLSVC = persistence of left superior vena cava; ARD = aortic root dilatation; PA = pulmonary artery; HLH = hypoplastic left heart; TAPVR = total anomalous pulmonary venous return.

this and most other analyses of congenital heart defects, the system of classification based on the presumed pathogenetic mechanisms proves most instructive and is a useful approach to comparing different causative factors (Table 49–4).

About one-quarter of the defects in trisomies 13 and 18 are due to cell migration abnormalities, and two-thirds are flow lesions; when combined, these two mechanisms account for considerably more of these classes of defects than in the general population with congenital heart disease. By contrast, in trisomy 21 left-sided flow lesions are much less common, whereas abnormal closure of endocardial cushions is strikingly frequent; indeed, in contrast to endocardial cushion defects without a chromosome 21 anomaly, left-sided flow lesions are rarely seen in Down syndrome patients with endocardial cushion defects.[29,32,38] Furthermore, the high incidence of endocardial cushion defects and low incidence of conotruncal and distal aortic anomalies have suggested a distinct pathogenetic mechanism in trisomy 21, potentially involving cell adhesiveness and the extracellular matrix.

TABLE 49–4 CLASSIFICATION OF CONGENITAL HEART DEFECTS BASED ON PATHOGENETIC MECHANISMS[35]

PATHOGENETIC MECHANISM	EXAMPLES OF DEFECTS
Embryonic blood flow defects	
Left-sided lesions	HLH; bicuspid aortic valve; IAA type A; CoA; PDA
Right-sided lesions	Secundum ASD; PS
Mesenchymal tissue migration defects	TOF; D-TGA
Extracellular matrix defects	ECD
Abnormal cellular death	Ebstein anomaly; muscular VSD
Defects of looping and situs	L-TGA
Abnormalities of targeted growth	TAPVR

HLH = hypoplastic left heart; IAA = interrupted aortic arch; CoA = coarctation of aorta; PDA = patent ductus arteriosus; ASD = atrial septal defect; PS = valvular pulmonic stenosis; TOF = tetralogy of Fallot; TGA = transposition of great arteries; ECD = endocardial cushion defect; VSD = ventricular septal defect; TAPVR = total anomalous pulmonary venous return.

TRISOMY 21—DOWN SYNDROME. This most common phenotype due to a human chromosome aberration occurs about once in every 600 births.[33] Most patients have trisomy 21, and the risk of this aberration is exponentially related to maternal age; the risk is lowest for young women and rises steeply after age 35, reaching 4 per cent for women over age 45. A small minority (3 per cent) of Down syndrome results from an extra copy of all or part of the long arm of chromosome 21 translocated to another chromosome. This situation is relatively more common in mothers under age 30. The phenotypes of the two forms of Down syndrome do not differ. The phenotype tends to be less severe if the trisomy is mosaic (3 per cent of Down syndrome) as a result of a mitotic nondisjunctional error in the embryo.

The most common causes of morbidity and mortality in Down syndrome patients are congenital heart defects present in 40 to 50 per cent of cases, hematological malignant disease, and duodenal atresia. If the patient either escapes or survives these problems, survival into the fifth decade and beyond is likely but is complicated by progressive dementia of the Alzheimer type. Premature aging may also affect the vasculature, although definitive studies are lacking.

The most characteristic cardiac anomaly in the Down syndrome is a defect of closure of the endocardial cushions (p. 898). Complicating the clinical problems in such patients and those with simple septal defects is a seeming predisposition to pulmonary hypertension in the face of elevated pulmonary blood flow.[36] About one-third of congenital heart defects are complex, and these patients tend not surprisingly to be the most ill patients. Mitral valve prolapse is found with a frequency exceeding that in age- and gender-matched controls.[37] The aortic and pulmonary valve cusps seem predisposed to fenestrations in adulthood.

Through the study of individuals trisomic for only a portion of the long arm of chromosome 21, the region crucial to the development of heart defects has been narrowed to 1.5 to 2.0 megabases (mb) of DNA in band 21q22.2 out of about 35 mb DNA on the entire long arm of chromosome 21 (J. R. Korenberg, personal communication).

The medical management of patients with Down syndrome has undergone evolution to more aggressive measures in recent years. Objections and hesitations on medical, societal, and ethical grounds to operative repair of heart defects in Down syndrome have been mollified substantially.[33,38] More follow-up data are becoming available, and early and late postoperative survival in Down syndrome patients appears to be no more different from that in other patients with similar defects.[36,38,39]

TRISOMY 18. *Edwards syndrome* is the second most common autosomal trisomy. Most cases are due to meiotic disjunction, and there is a strong relationship to maternal age. Routine prenatal diagnostic testing of women over age 34 would detect all aneuploid fetuses in them, but this would represent only one-third of all autosomal trisomies; less than one-half of all women of this advanced age undergo testing. Currently prenatal detection of trisomies followed by termination of pregnancy is having a small but measurable impact on decreasing the incidence of *Down, Edwards,* and *Patau* syndromes.

Although the severity of the phenotype rarely enables survival beyond a few months, 10 per cent of patients live to 1 year, and a few survive to adulthood, perhaps because of undetected mosaicism for a chromosomally normal cell line. However, central nervous system function is far less than that in the Down syndrome and leads to complex medical management and supportive care for long-term survivors.[40]

Cardiovascular defects occur in at least 90 per cent of cases and contribute to death. Complex lesions, usually involving septal defects, dysplastic valves that are rarely hemodynamically important, patent ductus arteriosus, and persistence of the left superior vena cava are common.[41,42] Right ventricular enlargement is common and may indicate not only shunting from left to right, but pulmonary hypertension due to anomalies of the pulmonary vasculature.[41] As in the Down syndrome, transposition of the great arteries is virtually unknown in trisomy 18.[42] Rarely should invasive diagnostic procedures or aggressive supportive measures be undertaken in Edwards syndrome.

TRISOMY 13. *Patau syndrome* occurs in about 0.01 per cent of live births and in progressively higher frequencies in stillbirths and spontaneous abortions. The external phenotype is usually severe, but occasionally not as characteristic as other trisomies; survival beyond a few weeks is rare, and the causes of death involve multiple organ systems, especially the heart. Cardiovascular anomalies are a bit less frequent than in trisomy 18 and have a slightly different spectrum.[31,41] Septal defects are the most common isolated lesions; dextrocardia and bicuspid semilunar valves occur in association with other anomalies.

Patients who survive beyond 1 month often are mosaic for a chromosomally normal cell line; thus, prognosis is fraught with uncertainty until detailed analysis is completed. Whether invasive cardiological studies are performed or aggressive management is undertaken can be determined by the severity of involvement of other organ systems, especially the brain, pending cytogenetic investigation.

TURNER SYNDROME. About one in every 2500 females lacks an X chromosome and has a 45,X karyotype. The frequency of a nonmosaic 45,X karyotype is much higher in spontaneous abortuses than in liveborns, and probably less than 2 per cent of such conceptuses come to term. The clinical phenotype is variable and often mild; the diagnosis is often not suspected until a child's short stature is evaluated or a woman complains of amenorrhea. Many cases are mosaic for cell lines with 46,XX or 46,XY constitutions. A variety of structural aberrations involving the X chromosome can cause partial or complete Turner syndrome.

Among patients with the 45,X karyotype, reported frequencies of congenital cardiovascular defects vary from 20 to 50 per cent, depending on how patients were ascertained. Fifty to 70 per cent of those with cardiovascular defects have clinically important aortic coarctation, usually of the postductal form.[43] As noninvasive imaging studies of asymptomatic patients became routine, the frequency of coarctation may increase. A variety of other cardiac malformations may occur, either singly or combined with coarctation. However, there is strong support for left-sided flow abnormalities as a major pathogenetic mechanism. Bicuspid aortic valve and dilatation of the ascending aorta (with a risk of dissection and histopathology showing elastic fiber disruption) occur even in the absence of coarctation,[44,45] and hypoplastic left heart has been reported.[46] Partial anomalous pulmonary venous drainage without an atrial septal defect is fairly common and should be suspected when right ventricular overload is detected on echocardiography.[47]

Postmortem examination of mid-trimester abortuses with 45,X showed a higher incidence of left-sided flow lesions than found at birth, suggesting an association between the pathogenesis of the cardiovascular anomalies and the uniform presence of lymphatic obstruction at the base of the heart.[43]

Blood pressure elevation is common, even without coarctation or after its repair; a high frequency of renal anomalies is one likely cause, but not the sole explanation, for the prevalence of hypertension.

In about two-thirds of cases, the retained X chromosome derives from the oocyte (maternal X). Because entire chromosomes or regions of a chromosome may be differentially regulated (imprinted)[48] by passage through oogenesis versus spermatogenesis, could some of the variability in phenotype among patients with Turner syndrome be due to the origin of the retained X or the origin of the lost X? In a study of 63 patients, 10 had severe cardiovascular features, and 9 of them had retained the maternal X.[49] This is an idea worthy of further pursuit. Women with mosaic karyotypes are less likely to have cardiovascular defects.

CONGENITAL HEART DISEASE

(See Chaps. 29 and 30)

In the past few decades, the reported incidence of structural heart defects in newborns has increased from 5 to 7 per 1000 live births, probably as the result of increased diagnostic sensitivity (especially cross-sectional and Doppler echocardiography and magnetic resonance imaging).[50–54] Supporting this explanation is the lack of change over the same period in the incidence of critical defects diagnosed neonatally at 3.1 to 3.5 per 1000.[50,51] This enhanced resolving power of noninvasive methods should prove particularly useful in the study of familial structural defects, because apparently unaffected relatives can be evaluated for subclinical evidence of anomalies. Few investigations to date have capitalized on this approach.[55,56]

As is evident from the previous section, gross aberrations of chromosomes produce an extensive and varied array of structural heart disease, an observation as true for spontaneous abortuses as for liveborn children.[57] Unfortunately, the complexity and inscrutability of the human genome severely limit the insight that cytogenetic aberrations provide into etiology and pathogenesis of congenital malformations. Better understanding comes from investigating the other two mechanisms by which genes cause congenital heart defects—multifactorial processes and mutations of single genes. The latter group should prove instructive soon, as the protein products of the mutant loci are identified and their normal function and regulation are defined. In addition to the mendelian syndromes discussed below, evidence for the involvement of genes of large effect derives from studies of incidence of congenital heart disease in populations with a high rate of inbreeding. The increased occurrence of defects in offspring of consanguineous matings suggests that mutations in one or more genes, when homozygous, strongly predispose to abnormal cardiovascular development.[58]

MULTIFACTORIAL PROCESSES. The empirical risks of recurrence of congenital heart defects have increased in recent years,[59,60] in keeping with the overall higher incidence noted above. However, this conclusion has been criticized because the studies focused on the offspring of women probands, in whom the recurrence risk appears higher than in men with congenital heart defects.[61] In addition to this unexplained maternal influence, other factors may be at work. For example, improved detection of subtle lesions, more faithful reporting of patients, and the assiduousness of epidemiologists may have shown a systematic variation. It is true that some patients with cardiovascular problems now survive[60–63] to bear children because of improved medical and surgical care; their offspring might be at increased risk because of the severity of the parents' problems, but some evidence against this idea exists.[64]

The familial aggregation of congenital heart defects supports many of the predictions of the threshold liability model of multifactorial inheritance.[56,65] In most studies, whether focused on populations or families, defects were classified by their pathology; for example, all ventricular septal defects were considered as one group. There has been bias in reporting families in which one type of defect aggregates, which has led to many reports of "familial atrial septal defect," "familial cardiomyopathy," and so on, without regard to the fact that not all septal defects or cardiopathies have the same structure on careful scrutiny, let alone the same cause.

A major advance has been the movement to examine familial aggregation of defects based on presumed pathogenesis.[66–68] The scheme developed by Clark[35] and since modified and expanded[69] (Table 49–4), has become widely used. Under this approach, some anatomically distinct lesions are related by common pathogenesis; if the pathogenetic mechanism has substantial genetic control, then the occurrence of distinct defects in the same family would still be consistent with a genetic model. Alternatively, defects unrelated by pathogenesis would require a different interpretation. This model also focuses on the examination of apparently unaffected relatives and hence increases the chances of detecting subtle manifestations of defective development of cardiovascular structures.

ERRORS IN MESENCHYMAL TISSUE MIGRATION. Included in this category are a wide range of anomalies of the outflow tract, some due to failure of fusion and others due to failure of septation. Relatives of probands with interruption of the aortic arch type B or truncus arteriosus, both uncommon conotruncal malformations, had 2.5 per cent and 6.6 per cent incidences, respectively, of congenital heart defects.[70] Both recurrence rates were higher than expected. The frequency of congenital malformations was much lower in relatives of patients with other forms of interrupted aortic arch. Moreover, relatives of probands with truncus arteriosus and other defects had a recurrence rate of 13 per cent, the majority in the spectrum of conotruncal lesions. Here is an instance in which refined empirical risk data should improve the accuracy of genetic counseling.

Categorizing anatomical defects by presumed pathogenesis emphasizes that all ventricular septal defects are not alike. If there is a strong genetic component to the etiology of tetralogy of Fallot, for example, one might find in close relatives an increased risk not only of tetralogy but of truncus arteriosus and supracristal ventricular septal defects, but not of other forms of septal defects.

Conotruncal Development. Considerable progress has been made over the past few years in identifying a region of chromosome 22 which plays a major role in development of the conotruncus, the branchial arches, and the face. Interest was first stimulated by detection of small deletions involving 22q11 in patients with *DiGeorge sequence*.[71–73] This condition includes developmental anomalies of the fourth branchial arch and derivatives of the third and fourth pharyngeal pouches. Hypoplasia of the thymus and parathyroids causes immune deficiency and hypocalcemia. The cardiac defects range from tetralogy of Fallot to ventricular septal defect, truncus arteriosus, interrupted aorta type B, and right aortic arch and are often lethal.

Subsequently, patients with *velocardiofacial syndrome* (VCF, also called Shprintzen syndrome) and what has been called in Japan the *conotruncal anomaly face syndrome* were found to have deletions in the same region, albeit generally smaller ones than in DiGeorge syndrome.[74] Because the deletion is often too small to be detected by routine cytogenetics, fluorescent in situ hybridization (FISH) with a DNA probe for the region is the assay of choice. The VCF syndrome is unlike the DiGeorge syndrome and includes an abnormal but characteristic facies, cleft palate, pharyngeal insufficiency, and conotruncal cardiac defects. The acronym CATCH22 (*c*ardiac anomaly, *a*bnormal facies, *t*hymic hypoplasia, *c*left palate, and *h*ypocalcemia) subsumes these related phenotypes.

This same region of chromosome 22 has been examined in patients with familial occurrence of various congenital cardiac defects and in patients with nonfamilial occurrence, nonsyndromic conotruncal defects. Although the prevalence figures are still soft, an important fraction of patients in both categories have submicroscopic deletions of 22q11.[75] Thus, a gene or genes in this region likely account for much of the recurrence risk of defects due to mesenchymal tissue migration abnormalities. Further, accurate counseling regarding recurrence risks for this broad range of defects necessitates FISH or molecular analysis for the presence of a deletion in the proband, and if present, in both parents.

Investigation of a strain of Keeshond dogs prone to conotruncal defects has shown that a single gene can be responsible for pathogenetically related defects of widely varying severity.[76]

FLOW DEFECTS. Left-sided flow lesions comprise a spectrum that includes hypoplastic left heart, congenital aortic stenosis, bicuspid aortic valve, interrupted aortic arch type A, and aortic coarctation. Various components of this spectrum can be present in the same patient.[71] Data from the Baltimore-Washington Infant Study,[51] a population-based case-control study of congenital cardiovascular malformations, were used to show that in first-degree relatives of probands with isolated hypoplastic left heart, incidence of bicuspid aortic valve was 12 per cent; most of the cases were asymptomatic and unrecognized before they were detected by echocardiography as part of this investigation.[55] In an exceptional family, four instances of aortic coarctation occurred in four generations.[77]

The association of coarctation of the aorta, bicuspid aortic valve, and dilatation of the ascending aorta, which may occur as part of the *Turner syndrome*,[44,45] is well known in the general population.[78] Several intriguing questions need to be addressed regarding the genetics and pathogenesis of this association. To what extent is the ascending aorta intrinsically abnormal, and hence predisposed to dilate, and to what extent is the dilatation simply a result of abnormal turbulence created by a bicuspid aortic valve? The fact that some patients with this association also have subtle evidence of a systemic connective tissue abnormality, reminiscent of Marfan syndrome, supports the former hypothesis. It will be of interest to extend the study of left-sided flow lesions to include probands with coarctation or congenital aortic stenosis and to evaluate close relatives with techniques capable of detecting the entire range of flow defects.

EXTRACELLULAR MATRIX ABNORMALITIES. Enough is known about the biochemistry and cell biology of cardiac embryology to state with some confidence that the extracellular matrix ("connective tissue") plays an important role. The endocardial cushions have received the most attention as an area where defects in the extracellular matrix might produce malformations.[35] The high frequency of endocardial cushion defects and atrioventricular septal defects in Down syndrome has been noted (see p. 1656). Of interest is the finding of increased adhesiveness of fibroblasts from trisomy 21 patients, a phenomenon that could reflect interaction with the extracellular matrix.[79] The distinctiveness of endocardial cushion defects in patients with normal chromosomes and in those with trisomy 21 has been suggested because of differences in associated cardiovascular malformations. However, of six families in which the proband had an endocardial cushion defect, three had recurrence of the same type of defect in a relative, including two with trisomy 21.[68]

SITUS AND LOOPING DEFECTS. This is an area fraught with difficulties of nomenclature, diagnosis, and heterogeneity of both etiology and pathogenesis. In analysis of clinical data, the most informative approach, but clearly arduous because of the large amount of data required, would be to categorize probands and their relatives by the type of situs (solitus, inversus, dextroversion, and levoversion, p. 946), and each of those by presence or absence of other cardiac and visceral defects. This has not been done on epidemiological cohorts, and in family studies relatives have rarely been subjected to evaluations sufficient to characterize their phenotypes in detail.[80] These variable phenotypes are grouped in a category, *heterotaxy*.

Several mendelian phenotypes point to single genes that have a major effect on determining laterality. In the autosomal recessive *Kartegener syndrome*, a randomization of lateralization of the heart (situs solitus and situs inversus are equally likely in homozygotes)[81] coexists with a defect in ciliary motility, which leads to sinusitis, bronchiectasis, and sperm immotility.[82]

Heterotaxy with splenic and other cardiac defects, particularly of the position of the great vessels, can be inherited as an autosomal recessive, as an autosomal dominant,[83] and as an X-linked recessive.[84] Some of the families with these apparently single-gene disorders have concordance of phenotype, but many do not, suggesting that in some cases various types of situs defects, polysplenia, and asplenia are different manifestations of the same mutation.[85,86]

In one family, complex heterotaxy involving abnormal abdominal situs, asplenia, polysplenia, simple dextrocardia, transposition, single ventricle and other cardiac anomalies, and a variety of other congenital malformations was inherited as an X-linked recessive trait.[84] The phenotype was mapped to Xq24-q27.1; still to be identified is the gene(s) responsible.

Two mouse mutants are instructive. Mice homozygous for the *iv* mutation, which maps to chromosome 12, are normal except that 50 per cent have situs inversus[87]; this is similar to the cardiac phenotype in Kartegener syndrome. Mice homozygous for a mutation at a different locus, *inv*, on chromosome 4, all have heterotaxy, with three-quarters showing situs inversus totalis.[88] Identification of the human homologues for these murine genes should further understanding of the control of human laterality.

There is a paucity of data on the recurrence risks of defects in the *cell death* (e.g., Ebstein anomaly) and *abnormal targeted growth* (e.g., anomalous pulmonary venous return) categories. Data from the Baltimore-Washington Infant Study do not show an increased risk of any cardiovascular defect in the relatives of a proband with a defect in either of these categories.[51] In one pedigree, nonsyndromic total anomalous pulmonary venous return was inherited as an autosomal

TABLE 49-5 DISORDERS OF UNCERTAIN CAUSE AND INHERITANCE THAT ARE ASSOCIATED WITH A HIGH INCIDENCE OF CARDIOVASCULAR ABNORMALITIES

DISORDER AND PHENOTYPE	MIM NO.*	CARDIOVASCULAR ABNORMALITIES†
Aase syndrome (Congenital anemia, triphalangeal thumbs)	205600	VSD
Bilateral left-sidedness sequence (Polysplenia syndrome)	208530	ASD
Bilateral right-sidedness sequence (Asplenia syndrome; Ivemark syndrome)	208530	Situs inversus, ECD, VSD
CHARGE association (*C*oloboma, *h*eart anomaly, choanal *a*tresia, *r*etardation, *g*enital, and *e*ar anomalies)	214800	TOF, PDA, ECD, VSD
Cornelia de Lange syndrome (Short stature, retardation, synophrys, hypertrichosis, micromelia, genital anomalies)	122470	~20% have CHD: VSD, PDA, ASD, PLSVC, TOF
DiGeorge sequence‡ (Abnormalities of derivatives of 3rd and 4th pharyngeal pouches and 4th branchial arch: hypoplastic thymus with cellular immune deficiency, hyoplastic parathyroids with hypocalcemia)	188400	CHD in ~100%: aortic arch anomalies (especially IAA type B and right-sided aortic arch); PDA, TOF
Goldenhar syndrome (Abnormalities of derivatives of 1st and 2nd branchial arch: hemifacial microsomia, microtia, vertebral anomalies)	141400, 164210, 257700	~50% have CHD: VSD, TOF, PDA, CoA, right-sided aortic arch, PLSVC
Klippel-Feil sequence (Short neck, limited rotation of the head, cervical anomalies)	118100, 148900, 214300	Variable estimates (5–70%) of CHD: VSD, dextrocardia
"Kabuki make-up" syndrome (Dwarfism, peculiar facies, scoliosis, mental retardation)	147920	30% have CHD: ASD, VSD, TOF, CoA, PDA
Pallister-Hall syndrome (Hypothalamic hamartoblastoma, hypopituitarism, imperforate anus, postaxial polydactyly)	146510	ECD
Poland sequence (Unilateral absence of sternocostal pectoralis major, ipsilateral synbrachydactyly)	173800	10% have dextrocardia or dextroversion
Rubinstein-Taybi syndrome (Short stature, retardation, microcephaly, characteristic facies, broad thumbs)	268600	~20% have CHD: ECD, ASD, TOF, PDA, VSD
VATER association (*V*ertebral defects, *a*nal atresia, *t*racheo-*e*sophageal fistula, *r*adial dysplasia, *r*enal anomaly)	192350	VSD

VSD = ventricular septal defect; ASD = atrial septal defect; TOF = tetralogy of Fallot; PDA = patent ductus arteriosus; ECD = endocardial cushion defect; CHD = congenital heart defect(s); PLSVC = persistence of left superior vena cava; IAA = interrupted aortic arch; CoA = coarctation of aorta; VSD = ventricular septal defect.

* None of these disorders is evidently due to a mutation in a single gene; however, most are listed in Mendelian Inheritance in Man (MIM),[8] and the MIM no. is provided as a ready source to the literature.

† Cardiovascular defects listed in approximate order of decreasing frequency.

‡ Most cases associated with del(22q11); likely a contiguous gene deletion defect.

dominant trait unassociated with other features in 14 relatives.[89] Linkage analysis localized the responsible gene to the centromere of chromosome 4 (4p13-q12).

DISORDERS OF UNCLEAR ETIOLOGY. A number of disorders include an important likelihood of malformation of the cardiovascular system but are of unclear cause (Table 49–5). Familial recurrence is so low to be *incompatible* with multifactorial inheritance. Several of these disorders deserve comment.

Certain congenital cardiac defects and other malformations occur together more frequently than expected by chance; this *association* of defects suggests a common cause, pathogenesis, or both, but the following disorders and those in Table 49–6 remain enigmatic on most of these counts. Designation as a *sequence* implies that some evidence exists for a common developmental problem to account for the features.

CHARGE Association (Table 49–5). Patients with this condition by definition have congenital heart defects.[90,91] The spectrum of cardiovascular malformations suggests not so much a common pathogenetic scheme as a common time of abnormal development. During gestational days 32 to 45, cardiac septation, fusion of the endocardial cushions and membranous ventricular septum, and formation of the outflow tracts and valves occur. An environmental insult or a breakdown in developmental homeostasis during this period could result in the malformation spectrum of this disorder. The defects in other systems could also arise during this embryological window and would be consistent with either environmental or intrinsic factors.

VATER Association (Table 49–5). This condition has expanded over the years to include *v*ertebral, *v*entricular septal, *a*nal, *t*racheo-*e*sophageal, *r*adial, and *r*enal defects. Omitted from the mnemonic is the single umbilical artery often present.[92] Cardiac defects are present in about one-half of patients with more than two components of this association but usually are not life threatening. Although infants with this condition often fail to thrive initially, the long-term prognosis for health and mental function is good, so aggressive management of the multiple malformations is warranted. It is important to separate as soon as possible those patients who have the features of trisomy 18 or 13q- chromosome aberrations, as prognosis in these cases is distinctly unfavorable.

Mendelian Disorders

Some congenital cardiovascular defects segregate in occasional families as predicted of a mendelian phenotype. There is strong bias favoring reporting such occurrences and an equally strong temptation to conclude that, at least in some cases, the defect is caused by mutation in a single gene. However, rarely and by chance alone, a multifactorial trait recurs in a family in a pattern mimicking mendelian segregation. This potential confusion and the resultant uncertainty in counseling patients and families pertains equally well to disturbances of conduction and rhythm, to various cardiomyopathies, to vascular anomalies, and to

TABLE 49–6 CONGENITAL HEART DEFECTS OCCASIONALLY SHOWING FAMILIAL AGGREGATION CONSISTENT WITH MENDELIAN INHERITANCE

DEFECT	MIM NO.*	DEFECT	MIM NO.
Aneurysm, intracranial berry	105800	Hypoplastic left heart	140500, 241550
Aneurysm, abdominal aortic	100070	Hypoplastic right heart	277200
Angioma	106050, 106070, 206570	Lymphedema, congenital	153000, 153100, 153400, 214900, 247440
ASD, ostium primum	209400		
ASD, ostium secundum	108800, 108900, 178650	Mitral valve prolapse	157700
Bicuspid aortic valve	109730	Patent ductus arteriosus	169100
Cardiomyopathy, dilated	108770, 115200, 115250, 212110	Pulmonary venous return, anomalous	106700
Cardiomyopathy, hypertrophic	192600		
Conotruncal defect	231060	Pulmonic stenosis	126190, 178650, 193520, 265500, 265600, 270460
Dextrocardia	244400, 304750		
Ebstein anomaly	224700	Subaortic stenosis	271950, 271960
Endocardial fibroelastosis	226000, 227280, 305300	Supravalvular aortic stenosis	185500, 194050
Hemangioma	106070, 140800, 140900, 234800	Tetralogy of Fallot	187500
Hemangioma, cavernous	116860, 140850	Ventricle, single	234750

* Data from McKusick, V. A.: Mendelian Inheritance in Man. 11th ed. Baltimore, John Hopkins University Press, 1994.

hypertension, all discussed subsequently. The true cause of the cardiovascular diseases in such families may not become clarified until each is investigated in detail, in concert with efforts to map and sequence the entire human genome.

The subject of this section can therefore be parsed into three broad classes of conditions: congenital cardiac defects that occasionally seem to be inherited as mendelian traits (Table 49–6), pleiotropic mendelian syndromes that always or frequently affect the structure of the cardiovascular system (Table 49–7), and mendelian syndromes that occasionally affect the cardiovascular system (Table 49–8).

PATENT DUCTUS ARTERIOSUS (PDA). Most instances of PDA are sporadic occurrences, and there is strong association with prematurity and all of its antecedents. However, a number of families have been reported in which PDA occurs as an autosomal dominant trait.[93] In some pedigrees, mild facial dysmorphism segregates with PDA; because the facial features differ among families, the number of syndromes remains unclear.[94,95]

FAMILIAL ATRIAL SEPTAL DEFECT. Two mendelian forms of atrial septal defect exist as autosomal dominant traits. One has no associated problems and has been described in few pedigrees.[96]

The second, and more common, condition has atrioventricular conduction delay as the only pleiotropic feature.[97,98] The defect is of the secundum type, and relatives do not seem to be at increased risk of other cardiac malformations. The severity of heart block rarely progresses to third degree. The electrocardiographic abnormality in a pa-

TABLE 49–7 MENDELIAN DISORDERS WITH CONGENITAL DEFECTS OF CARDIOVASCULAR STRUCTURE AS FREQUENT MANIFESTATIONS

DESCRIPTIVE NAME	EPONYM	MIM NO.*	CARDIOVASCULAR ABNORMALITIES
Adult polycystic kidney disease		173900	MVP, dilated aortic root, intracranial berry aneurysm
Arteriohepatic dysplasia	Alagille syndrome	118450	PPS
Cataract and cardiomyopathy		212350	HCM
Chondroectodermal dysplasia	Ellis–van Creveld syndrome	225500	ASD (ostium primum), common atrium
Deafness, mitral regurgitation, and short stature	Forney syndrome	157800	MR
Familial collagenoma syndrome		115250	DCM
Heart-hand syndrome	Holt-Oram syndrome	142900	ASD (ostium secundum), VSD, MVP, HLH
Keratosis palmoplantaris	Mal de Meleda	248300	DCM, dysrhythmia
Malignant hyperthermia and skeletal defects	King syndrome	145600	malignant hyperthermia → cardiac arrest
	Noonan syndrome	163950	PS, HCM
Pulmonic stenosis and deafness		178651	PS
	Smith-Lemli-Opitz syndrome	270400	PDA, ASD, VSD, TOF, ECD, CoA
Velocardiofacial syndrome	Shprintzen syndrome	192430	TOF, tortuous retinal vasculature

MVP = mitral valve prolapse; PPS = peripheral pulmonic stenosis; HCM = hypertrophic cardiomyopathy; ASD = atrial septal defect; MR = mitral regurgitation: DCM = dilated cardiomyopathy; VSD = ventricular septal defect; HLH = hypoplastic left heart, PS = valvular pulmonic stenosis; PDA = patent ductus arteriosus; TOF = tetralogy of Fallot; ECD = endocardial cushion defect; CoA = coarctation of aorta.

* Data from McKusick, V. A.: Mendelian Inheritance in Man. 11th ed. Baltimore, John Hopkins University Press, 1994.

TABLE 49–8 MENDELIAN DISORDERS WITH CARDIOVASCULAR ABNORMALITIES AS OCCASIONAL MANIFESTATIONS

SYNDROME	EPONYM	MIM NO.*	CARDIOVASCULAR ABNORMALITIES
Acrocephalosyndactyly type I	Apert syndrome	101200	PS, PPS, VSD, EFE
Acrocephalopolysyndactyly type II	Carpenter syndrome	201000	PDA, VSD, PS, TGA
Hereditary angioedema		106100	Coronary arteritis
Imperforate anus with hand, foot, and ear anomalies	Townes-Brocks syndrome	107480	Sporadic cases have CHD: VSD, ASD
Mandibulofacial dysostosis	Treacher Collins syndrome	154500, 248390	10% have CHD: variable
Neuronal ceroid lipofuscinosis	Batten disease	204200	HCM
Orofacial digital syndrome type II	Mohr syndrome	252100	Variable
Short rib–polydactyly syndrome	Saldino-Noonan syndrome	263530	TGA, ECD, hypoplastic right heart
Thrombocytopenia–absent radius syndrome		274000	TOF

PS = valvular pulmonic stenosis; PPS = peripheral pulmonic stenosis; VSD = ventricular septal defect; EFE = endocardial fibroelastosis; PDA = patent ductus arteriosus; TGA = transposition of great arteries; CHD = congenital heart defect(s); ASD = atrial septal defect; HCM = hypertrophic cardiomyopathy; ECD = endocardial cushion defect; TOF = tetralogy of Fallot.

* Data from McKusick, V. A.: Mendelian Inheritance in Man. 11th ed. Baltimore, John Hopkins University Press, 1994.

tient with apparently sporadic atrial septal defect should prompt a detailed family history and evaluation of close relatives. Attention should be directed to the upper limbs, particularly the thumbs, to rule out the Holt-Oram syndrome; radiographic examination of the entire limbs of the proband is helpful on this account.

When patients with atrial septal defect due to aneuploidy (a syndrome with extracardiac features), and one of the autosomal dominant forms is excluded, the recurrence risk of atrial septal defect is about 3 per cent, a value that conforms closely to the multifactorial threshold model. Several pleiotropic mendelian conditions have defects of the atrial septum as frequent manifestations.

HOLT-ORAM SYNDROME. This autosomal dominant condition, first elaborated in 1960, shows marked variability within a pedigree.[99] The cardinal manifestations are dysplasia of the upper limbs and atrial septal defect. In heterozygotes for the mutation, arm deformity ranges from undetectable through distally placed thumbs and hypoplastic thenar eminences, triphalangeal thumbs, anomalies of the carpus, and radial aplasia, to phocomelia and hypoplasia of the clavicles and shoulders. Upper extremity deformity is usually bilateral but may be asymmetrical in severity, with the left side the worse. Similarly, the atrial involvement ranges from none to a large secundum defect with early, severe hemodynamic compromise. Other cardiac malformations have been reported, with ventricular septal defects the most frequent. The skeletal and cardiac manifestations are not correlated in individuals, and how a parent is affected is not a reliable predictor of effects on offspring.[100] Prenatal diagnosis by ultrasonography was reported in a fetus with severe limb abnormalities; presumably a large septal defect could be detected as well. Other manifestations include dermatoglyphic abnormalities, pectus excavatum, hypoplastic peripheral arteries, and cardiac conduction disturbance, the last usually involving the AV node and present in patients with septal defects. Although the Holt-Oram syndrome bears some resemblance to the VATER association, the clear mendelian nature and lack of more extensive organ system involvement of the former indicate that the two conditions do not represent a pathogenetic spectrum.

The diagnosis of Holt-Oram syndrome is most likely to be missed in a patient with an unknown or unremarkable family history, a secundum septal defect, and minimal or no thumb anomaly. In any "sporadic" case of an atrial septal defect, the patient and the parents should be carefully examined for limb malformations and the family history studied in detail. Detection of a subtle limb defect alters the recurrence risk in offspring of the proband from the empirical risk of an isolated septal defect of 3 per cent to the 50 per cent of an autosomal dominant trait.

One gene for Holt-Oram syndrome has been mapped to 12q2, but the gene has not yet been identified.[100–102] In families with Holt-Oram syndrome linked to this locus, prenatal diagnosis is possible. Genetic heterogeneity exists, with some families not linked to this locus, and families with isolated atrial septal defect and conduction abnormalities without limb defects also unlinked.

ELLIS–VAN CREVELD SYNDROME (Fig. 49–6). This rare, autosomal recessive chondrodysplasia is found among the old order Amish because of a founder effect and consanguinity. Short stature, metaphyseal dysplasia, dysplastic nails and teeth, and postaxial polydactyly are the pleiotropic manifestations in addition to congenital heart disease.[103] The last is present in more than one-half of homozygotes, and most of the defects affect the atrial septum. The majority are defects of endocardial cushion closure, including ostium primum defects of widely varying size up to a single atrium. This disorder has long been thought to be due to an as yet unknown defect in the extracellular matrix, which would fit with the high frequency of endocardial cushion lesions. However, defects thought due to abnormal embryonic flow (coarctation, hypoplastic left heart, and patent ductus arteriosus) occur in about 20 per cent of cases. Ellis–van Creveld syndrome can be diagnosed prenatally by detection of polydactyly by ultrasonography.

FAMILIAL ATRIOVENTRICULAR CANAL DEFECTS. This spectrum of defects occasionally occurs in an autosomal dominant pattern in families and is unassociated with features in other systems. Because the cardiac defect is suggestive of that in the Down syndrome, linkage to chromosome 21 markers has been pursued, to no avail.[104,105]

VENTRICULAR SEPTAL DEFECT. This malformation does not seem to be inherited as an isolated mendelian malformation except when associated with CATCH22, and no syndromes include it as a common, isolated manifestation. One intriguing pedigree showed maternal transmission of a risk for atrial or ventricular septal defects to at least 11 of 13 offspring; the suggestion was made that phenotype was determined by the mitochondrial chromosome.[106] Subsequent study of the mitochondrial chromosome has not uncovered a candidate gene,[13] and the family has not been restudied.

Many other isolated defects have been described in families in patterns suggestive of mendelian inheritance, but only for supravalvular aortic stenosis and mitral valve prolapse is there convincing evidence for the action of a single mutant gene.

SUPRAVALVULAR AORTIC STENOSIS (see also p. 1662). This congenital lesion, which may be asymptomatic and detected long after birth because of an ejection murmur, occurs in at least three settings. It can be a sporadic anom-

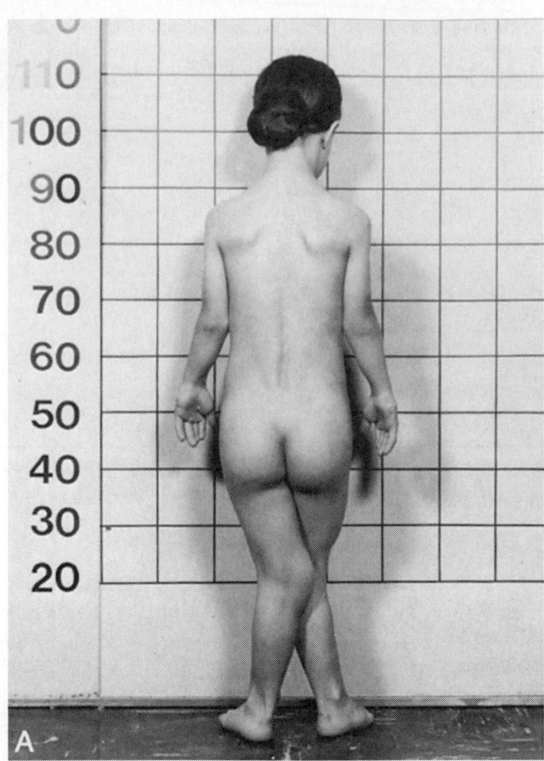

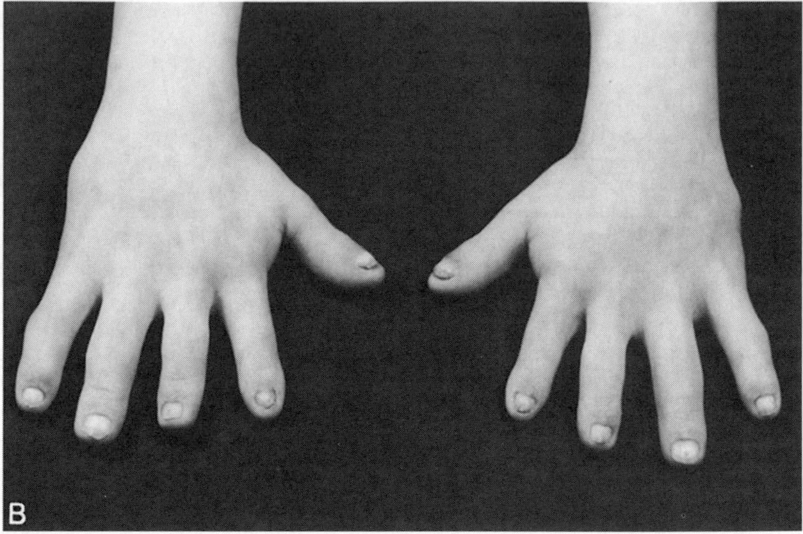

FIGURE 49–6. Ellis–van Creveld syndrome in a young woman. *A,* Note short stature, joint contractures at the elbows, and marked genu valgum. *B,* The fingers are short and the nails dysplastic. Note the protuberances along the ulnar edges of the hands where sixth digits were amputated.

aly, a component of Williams syndrome, or an autosomal dominant trait associated with peripheral pulmonic stenoses and a diffuse arteriopathy.

Williams syndrome is usually sporadic but, in more instances than previously recognized, is a highly variable autosomal dominant condition. The full spectrum includes infantile hypercalcemia, abnormal ("elfin") facies (Fig. 29–36, p. 920), mental deficiency, short stature, multiple peripheral pulmonic stenoses, and supravalvular aortic stenosis.[107] Occasional cardiovascular manifestations are mitral valve prolapse, bicuspid aortic valve, and hypertension.[108,109] Although patients usually survive the problems of infancy and show catch-up growth, progressive problems of joint contractures, genitourinary and gastrointestinal dysfunction, and psychosocial adjustment define the long-term prognosis.[110]

Supravalvular aortic stenosis (SVAS) is due to heterozygosity for a mutation in tropoelastin (see below). Because elastic fibers are intrinsic to the media of elastic and muscular arteries, a diffuse, progressive arteriopathy develops, with thickening of the wall and reduction of the lumen. The natural history of the arterial disease is just emerging as patients with Williams syndrome live longer and are followed prospectively.[111] A predisposition to cerebrovascular disease seems certain.[112,113]

Virtually all patients with Williams syndrome who have been tested have a deletion of the long arm of chromosome 7.[114] Those with SVAS have a deletion that involves the tropoelastin locus. The crucial gene(s) involved in the rest of the Williams phenotype lie telomeric to the tropoelastin locus; considerable effort is currently being directed at identifying these gene(s) that play a role in development of the face, in calcium metabolism, and in development of personality and cognitive capability.

Autosomal dominant SVAS is an entity distinct from Williams syndrome,[115–117] although some patients have subtle defects in personality and intelligence. Peripheral pulmonary artery stenoses may be present but rarely cause hemodynamic problems. The aortic lesion requires surgery in less than half of patients.

A patient with isolated SVAS was discovered to have a translocation involving chromosomes 6 and 7; although no macroscopic quantity of chromatin was apparently missing, any translocation carries the risk that the breakpoint disrupts a gene. This proved to be the case in this patient, who also had affected relatives; each person in this pedigree with SVAS also had the translocation.[118,119] Cloning of the breakpoint region showed that the tropoelastin locus at 7 was disrupted. Study of other patients, both sporadic and familial cases, none of whom had a visible chromosomal alteration, revealed that all with SVAS had one mutation or another in the tropoelastin gene. Most of the mutations involve a deletion that results in loss of function of the allele.[120] Thus, having only one copy of a functional tropoelastin allele during embryogenesis (developmental haploinsufficiency) is sufficient to produce SVAS and peripheral pulmonic stenosis and to set the stage for a diffuse arteriopathy later in life.[120] Is this a simple dosage effect, or is the pathogenesis much more complex?

MITRAL VALVE PROLAPSE (see also p. 1029). This trait is of heterogeneous cause and pathogenesis; although it has been called the most common abnormality of human heart valves,[121] mitral valve prolapse (MVP) is equally clearly not always an "abnormality." Here only the heritable forms of MVP are discussed. These can be classified into three groups. The first is an autosomal dominant form with minimal extracardiac involvement. The second is an autosomal dominant condition that is clinically variable, and at one end of its spectrum merges with the Marfan syndrome; it could just as well be discussed as a heritable disorder of connective tissue. The third category is composed of the various mendelian syndromes that include mitral valve prolapse as a pleiotropic manifestation.

The first category, which some have called mitral valve prolapse syndrome[122] or familial mitral valve prolapse,[123] includes a condition that is centered on the mitral valve. The development of actual prolapse shows the age- and gender-dependent behavior characteristic of the "idiopathic" form so common in the general population.[123,124] Formal genetic studies confirm *autosomal dominance with variable expression*. This category has been partitioned into those patients with billowing of the mitral leaflets and those with excessive systolic mitral annular expansion; because this phenotype breeds relatively true, two distinct autosomal dominant forms may exist.[125] The cause(s) of these entities is unknown.[126] Moreover, when and how the phenotype of this condition can be distinguished from the sporadic cases of MVP and the cases with obvious evidence of a systemic disorder of connective tissue are unclear. The only consistent extracardial manifestations are excessive arm span in women and relatively low body weight and systolic pressure.[127,128]

Many clinical geneticists and cardiologists have referred

patients with a suspicion of Marfan syndrome (see p. 1669) or Ehlers-Danlos syndrome (see p. 1672). Some of these patients do not meet minimal diagnostic criteria for a recognized connective tissue disorder[129] but clearly have extracardiac features consistent with a defect of the extracellular matrix described below. MVP is commonly but not always present; when it is, and evidence of a systemic abnormality of connective tissue is lacking, the patient should be considered to have the condition described in the preceding paragraph, what some call primary mitral valve prolapse.[130] The clinical spectrum of the patients with syndromic MVP includes abnormal striae atrophicae, excessive arm span and leg length, joint hypermobility, pectus excavatum, scoliosis, reduction in thoracic kyphosis ("straight back"), myopia, and mild aortic root dilatation.[131] Aortic dilatation beyond 3 SD above the mean for body surface area, aortic dissection, ectopia lentis, or a family history of any of these three features *removes* a patient from this category. For the remainder of patients, the acronym MASS phenotype, for *m*itral valve, *a*orta, *s*kin, and *s*keletal, describes what certainly is a heterogeneous grouping of patients and families. Aorta is mentioned specifically because of the appropriate concern that progressive dilatation and dissection will occur; in fact, neither has been the case, although prospective evaluation has been brief. Many of the associations between MVP and deformity of the thoracic cage and spontaneous pneumothorax are explained by the MASS phenotype.[132]

Finally, as described below, MVP frequently accompanies the Marfan syndrome, several of the Ehlers-Danlos syndromes, and cutis laxa and occurs more often than expected in osteogenesis imperfecta, Larsen syndrome, pseudoxanthoma elasticum, and other mendelian syndromes (see Table 49–11). In addition, occasional families with otherwise unclassified heritable disorders of connective tissue have prominent involvement of the mitral apparatus, with myxomatous deterioration or calcification, or both.[133]

NOONAN SYNDROME. Among the pleiotropic mendelian syndromes that have frequent cardiovascular involvement, the Noonan syndrome is important because of its relatively high prevalence and clinical variability. This autosomal dominant condition has been called the male Turner syndrome in the past because of the short stature, cubitus valgus, neck webbing, congenital lymphedema, and congenital heart defects that coexist in the 45,X Turner syndrome. However, the Noonan syndrome is distinct, not simply because both men and women are affected. Patients with Noonan syndrome often have an unusual deformity of the sternum, mental dullness, hypertelorism, ptosis, and cryptorchidism.[134] The cardiovascular defects, although widely varied, do not include an increased incidence of coarctation of the aorta. Because of the dysmorphism of the facies and the cardiac involvement, Noonan syndrome is often classified, along with the Williams, LEOPARD, King, and Watson syndromes, as a cardiofacial syndrome.

The entire phenotype of the Noonan syndrome is highly variable, and affected people can escape clinical problems (or accurate diagnosis), even if they have obvious manifestations.[135] Similarly, a wide range of cardiovascular involvement can occur. *Valvular pulmonic stenosis* was the first defect identified, and Noonan syndrome should always be considered in a patient with this lesion.[136] The valve cusps are thickened and dysplastic, even in the absence of hemodynamic compromise. Obstruction to right-sided flow can also occur in Noonan patients because of pulmonary artery hypoplasia or infundibular subvalvular changes. The latter finding reflects a generalized predisposition to hypertrophic cardiomyopathy, often asymmetrical, that can affect either ventricle.[137,138] *Atrial septal defect* occurs in about one-third of patients, usually in association with pulmonic stenosis. *Ventricular septal defects* and patent ductus arteriosus each occur in about 10 per cent. Congenital anomalies of coronary arteries are occasionally and unexpectedly found during evaluation of more obvious defects. The electrocardiogram often shows left anterior hemiblock and a deep precordial S wave, a pattern not common in pulmonic stenosis of other causes.

Lymphatic dysplasia, especially of the lower limbs, is common but causes clinical difficulties in less than 20 per cent.[134] While evidence of lymphedema often disappears during childhood, chylothorax and a protein-losing enteropathy represent the severe end of the spectrum.[139]

Noonan syndrome shares features with other cardiofacial syndromes, and in sporadic cases (which account for 50 per cent of Noonan syndrome) diagnosis can be difficult. All are *autosomal dominant,* so genetic counseling is somewhat easier. Affected males have reduced reproductive capabilities because of testicular abnormalities. Susceptibility to malignant hyperthermia can be detected by family history, elevated skeletal muscle creatine kinase levels, or muscle biopsy. Despite the relatively high frequency of the Noonan syndrome, estimated up to 1 per 1000, neither its cause nor its pathogenesis is clear. One gene has been mapped to the long arm of chromosome 12, but interlocus genetic heterogeneity is likely. Intriguing issues that may shed light on these uncertainties are the overlap in phenotype with type I neurofibromatosis[140,141] (the gene for which is on chromosome 17 and has been cloned) and the frequent coexistence of Noonan syndrome and deficiency of coagulation factor XI.[142]

Teratogenic Effects

A teratogen is any agent that adversely affects embryonic or fetal development, such as infectious vectors, radiation, drugs, and other chemicals (Table 49–9). Teratogenic effects on the cardiovascular system are considered in this chapter for several reasons: (1) The phenotypes are often reminiscent of those due to chromosomal aberrations and single-gene mutations. (2) Clinical geneticists and dysmorphologists are involved in diagnosing, managing, and investigating both teratogenic and genetic syndromes. (3) How the organism responds to an encounter with a potential teratogen is largely determined by its genome. The entire field of ecogenetics and part of pharmacogenetics are concerned with these issues.

The abilities to resist disruption of normal human embryogenesis and development involve systems quite distinct from physiological homeostasis and related only in part with developmental homeostasis. Genetic susceptibilities to teratogens can be illustrated by diverse mechanisms: reduced or inaccurate repair of radiation-induced DNA damage; enhanced receptiveness to viral entry or replication; immune deficiencies that prevent inactivation of infectious vectors or maintenance of immunity; slow inactivation of a compound that exerts a direct deleterious effect; or rapid conversion of an inoffensive drug to a teratogenic metabolite. These types of hereditary variation may be determined by single genes, with susceptibility inherited as a mendelian trait, or by many genes, each of small effect. Either situation can account for the well-known fact that

TABLE 49–9 CARDIOVASCULAR DEFECTS ASSOCIATED WITH PRENATAL EXPOSURE TO TERATOGENS

TERATOGEN	CARDIOVASCULAR ABNORMALITIES*
Ethanol	~50% have CHD: VSD (~50% close spontaneously), TOF, ASD, ECD, absence of a pulmonary artery
Hydantoin	~10% have CHD: VSD, ASD, PS
Lithium	<3% have Ebstein anomaly
Phenylalanine	~20% have CHD: TOF
Retinoic acid	>50% have CHD: TGA, TOF, VSD, IAA
Rubella	>50% have CHD: PDA with or without ASD, VSD, PPS, IAA
Trimethadione	~50% have CHD: complex combinations most frequent (involving VSD, ASD, PDA, AS, PS), VSD, TOF
Valproic acid	>50% have CHD: left- and right-sided flow lesions: CoA, HLH, ASD, VSD, pulmonary atresia
Vitamin D	Supravalvular aortic stenosis is the cardinal manifestation; PPS
Warfarin	~10% have CHD: PDA, PS; rarely, intracranial hemorrhage

CHD = congenital heart defect(s); VSD = ventricular septal defect; TOF = tetralogy of Fallot; ASD = atrial septal defect; ECD = endocardial cushion defect; PS = valvular pulmonic stenosis; TGA = transposition of great arteries; IAA = interrupted aortic arch; PPS = peripheral pulmonic stenosis; PDA = patent ductus arteriosus; AS = aortic stenosis; CoA = coarctation of aorta; HLH = hypoplastic left heart.

* Among patients with the full clinical spectrum associated with each teratogen; cardiovascular defects listed in decreasing order of prevalence.

only a fraction of pregnancies exposed to a given agent are affected adversely. Variation in dose and timing of exposure also confound interpretation of epidemiological and family data. It is not surprising, then, that the actual appearance of the abnormal phenotype is not amenable to traditional pedigree analysis. Rather, examination of the biochemical susceptibilities have proved, and will continue to prove, more enlightening.

Some teratogens, such as *warfarin,* have a clear action that explains how the pleiotropic manifestations emerge. The action of other teratogens, such as alcohol, is obscure. Finally, in some teratogenic syndromes, such as that in offspring of women with diabetes mellitus, the actual offensive agent is unclear, and multiple pathogenetic mechanisms seem to pertain.[143,144] Regardless of cause and pathogenetic mechanism, the phenotypes of many teratogens often share manifestations, especially prenatal growth retardation, abnormalities of the craniofacies, and mental retardation. The following syndromes have prominent consequences on the cardiovascular system.

FETAL ALCOHOL SYNDROME. Ethanol is the most common teratogen to which the human embryo and fetus are exposed. The period of greatest vulnerability is the first trimester, and the risks are clearly related to the amount of alcohol consumed; the risk of the fetal alcohol syndrome occurring in an offspring of a chronic alcoholic woman is 30 to 50 per cent. The features are highly variable and include growth retardation, mild to moderate mental retardation, hyperactivity, short palpebral fissures, a smooth philtrum with a thin upper lip, and small distal phalanges.[145] Congenital heart defects occur in more than one-half of children with the full spectrum of the phenotype; ventricular septal defects are most common and often insignificant, but atrial septal defects, tetralogy of Fallot, and aortic coarctation can occur.

FETAL HYDANTOIN SYNDROME. Virtually all antiseizure medications can affect the fetus. Hydantoin was the first to be identified as a teratogen. The risk to the fetus depends in part on the genotype of the fetus; defects in arene oxidase predispose to the full syndrome.[146,147] The features include prenatal and postnatal growth retardation, mild mental retardation, a broad face with a short nose, short distal phalanges with small nails, and hip dislocation. Cardiovascular defects, which are an inconstant part of the syndrome, include septal defects, right- and left-sided flow defects, and a single umbilical artery.

RETINOIC ACID EMBRYOPATHY. Isotretinoin was not recognized as a teratogen until after it was licensed for the treatment of acne. The vulnerable period extends from the first week through the fourth month of gestation. The risks of miscarriage and stillbirth are elevated. The phenotype includes anomalies of the craniofacies and gross neuroanatomical disruption. Cardiovascular defects are common and emphasize a variety of conotruncal malformations.[148] Liveborn infants often succumb to the cardiac and brain anomalies. Although the mechanism of action is not certain, vitamin A derivatives such as retinoic acid function as *morphogens* during embryogenesis, serving as signals for cell migration. The fact that the cardiovascular defects are primarily those of rotation and folding suggests disruption of a normal developmental homeostatic system.

WARFARIN EMBRYOPATHY. Coumarin-related vitamin K antagonists are usually prescribed for a variety of cardiovascular problems to women of childbearing age (see p. 1859) and can cause a variety of cardiovascular and other organ damage to the fetus. Coumarin interferes with embryogenesis directly when administered during gestational weeks 6 through 9. The most pronounced effects are on cartilage because of inhibition of enzymes of extracellular matrix metabolism. Congenital cardiac defects are perhaps increased in frequency but fit no specific pathogenetic mechanism.[149] The second pattern of coumarin effects involves exposure during the second and third trimester and includes spontaneous abortion, stillbirth, and various central nervous system defects. The last are not due simply to intracranial hemorrhage as was once assumed.[149]

What predisposes to the adverse fetal effects of coumarin remains to be discovered. First, more than 75 per cent of women who take coumarin derivatives throughout pregnancy have normal offspring; reassuring most women while identifying those at risk for adverse effects has obvious advantages. Second, placing all pregnant women on a regimen of heparin is not an acceptable solution, because heparin can cause stillbirth or premature fetal loss in about 20 per cent of exposures, is not as effective as coumarin in some indications for anticoagulation, and is more trouble to administer and regulate.

MATERNAL PKU. The inborn error of metabolism phenylketonuria produces severe mental retardation unless the phenylalanine content of the diet is markedly reduced soon after birth.[150] Deficiency of phenylalanine hydroxylase in the fetus produces no harm because fetal blood levels of phenylalanine are regulated by the heterozygous mother's enzyme. Because neonatal screening for this disease is now routine in all states, virtually all patients receive treatment and grow to adulthood with average intelligence. Many patients discontinue the rigorous dietary therapy during adolescence when the elevated phenylalanine levels have far less deleterious effects. The embryopathy occurs when a woman with homozygous deficiency for phenylalanine hydroxylase becomes pregnant and her fetus is exposed to high levels of the amino acid which overwhelm its ability to metabolize. The result is highly predictable if the mother does not restart dietary restriction of phenylalanine for the entire gestation: moderate to severe mental retardation, prenatal and postnatal growth retardation, microcephaly, and a variety of cardiovascular defects in 15 to 20 per cent.[151] This condition can largely be prevented by effective counseling of female patients with phenylketonuria.

FETAL RUBELLA EFFECTS (see p. 878). About 50 per cent of fetuses become infected with the rubella virus when the mother is infected during the first trimester. Not only does the infected fetus suffer varied and severe interference with development and organogenesis, but it acquires a chronic viral illness that can persist for years. The most common features of the embryopathy are mental deficiency, deafness, cataract, and cardiovascular defects. Patent ductus arteriosus is common, as are septal defects. Peripheral pulmonary stenosis and fibromuscular proliferation of medium and small arteries often improve postnatally.

CARDIOMYOPATHIES

(See also Chap. 41)

Each of the three clinical categories of primary cardiomyopathy—hypertrophic, dilated, and restrictive—can be caused by mutations in single genes as judged by mendelian inheritance of a consistent phenotype in multiple families. Many other mendelian and mitochondrial disorders also cause cardiomyopathies as a secondary consequence of their basic metabolic disturbance.

Hypertrophic Cardiomyopathy

(See also p. 1414)

In the more than 35 years since the recognition of hypertrophic cardiomyopathy as a clinical entity, many aspects of its natural history, pathology, and management have been substantially clarified. The phenotype is most clearly defined anatomically and histologically and consists of myocardial hypertrophy without secondary cause; cellular and myofiber disarray; myocardial fibrosis; and mediointimal proliferation of small coronary arteries. None of these features is pathognomonic; for example, myofiber disorganization is present in the normal human heart during embryogenesis and in congenital heart defects that place strain on the right-sided circulation.[152]

About half of probands with idiopathic hypertrophic cardiomyopathy of any segment of the left ventricle have affected first-degree relatives, and in those families the phenotype is inherited as an autosomal dominant, familial hypertrophic cardiomyopathy (FHC). There is wide variability of expression within a family, in part due to age-dependency of the trait.[152] Later generations of relatives in adolescence and childhood may not have developed echocardiographic evidence of hypertrophy. Hence, pedigree screening by phenotype for clinical, counseling, or investigative purposes should not be considered complete until the following criteria are satisfied: two-dimensional echocardiography is used to ensure that segmental hypertrophy is detected; a person at risk has a normal echocardiographic study and no evidence of electrocardiographic abnormality or important dysrhythmia after about age 20; and a person of any age has left ventricular hypertrophy without any other explanation, such as hypertension or aortic stenosis.

FHC is a disease of the sarcomere, with primary defects of thick and thin filaments now defined. Mutations of at least six and perhaps more loci cause FHC (Table 49–10, Fig. 41–15, p. 1417). The first locus identified was 14q1, and the cardiac β-myosin heavy chain gene was found to harbor mutations.[153] Depending on the population studied, about 50 per cent of all FHC mutations occur in this gene, *MYH7,* and more than 40 mutations have been described.[154] Patients with neither parent affected have also been shown

TABLE 49–10 FAMILIAL HYPERTROPHIC CARDIOMYOPATHY

VARIANT	MIM NO.*	GENE MAP	LOCUS	DEFECT
CMH1	192600	14q11	*MYH7*	β-Myosin HC
CMH2	115195	1 q3	*TNNT1*	Troponin T
CMH3	115196	15q2	*TPM1*	α-Tropomyosin
CMH4	115197	11p11.2	*MyBP-C*	Cardiac myosin binding protein-C
CMH5	115198	?		
CMH6		7q3	?	

* Data from McKusick, V. A.: Mendelian Inheritance in Man. 11th ed. Baltimore, Johns Hopkins University Press, 1994.

to have *MYH7* mutations, suggesting that the genetic alteration occurred in the egg or sperm of a parent.[155] Mutations that alter charge of the β-myosin heavy chain generally carry a worse prognosis in terms of age of detection, electrocardiographic abnormalities, and sudden death[156,157] (Fig. 41–16, p. 1418). Thus, defining the specific gene involved, followed by the specific mutation, has likely clinical importance. How the mutant protein interacts with other components of the sarcomere of both cardiac and skeletal muscle to produce the phenotype is another area of active research.[158]

While intergenic and intragenic heterogeneity account for much of the interfamilial variability in the FHC phenotype, there remains considerable variation among relatives who share the same mutation. Both environmental and genetic factors have impacts. A possible example of the latter is the angiotensin I-converting enzyme (ACE) genotype, with different polymorphic variants of ACE associated with more or less hypertrophy.[159]

Mutations in two genes specifying components of the thin filament, α-tropomyosin and cardiac troponin T, and in the gene encoding cardiac myosin binding protein-C, also cause FHC.[100–161b] A locus on chromosome 15q2 is associated with FHC indistinguishable from that caused by the loci with known mutations.[162] A family with Wolff-Parkinson-White syndrome and FHC shows linkage to markers at 7q3.[163] Finally, families with FHC are unlinked to any of these loci.

Dilated Cardiomyopathy

(See also p. 1407)

The prevalence of idiopathic dilated cardiomyopathy is about double that of the hypertrophic form, or about 2 to 8 per 100,000.[164–167] Although numerous occurrences of familial dilated cardiomyopathy are reported, few investigations have been conducted of an unselected series of probands for clinical and subclinical evidence of cardiac disease.[168] Thus, it is unclear what fraction of patients with idiopathic dilated cardiomyopathy have a mendelian disease, how many have a new mutation for a mendelian disease, and how many have phenocopies of nongenetic causes. Estimates of a positive family history, which could suggest a mendelian condition or a shared environmental cause, range from 7 to 30 per cent.[168–170]

Because of the risk of severe dysrhythmia in dilated cardiomyopathy, early detection of people with the disorder can be life saving.[171] Two-dimensional echocardiography is a sensitive method for detecting affected relatives with subclinical disease. Individuals who have equivocal left ventricular enlargement or dysfunction can have ambulatory electrocardiographic monitoring and, if the diagnosis is still uncertain, can have serial examinations. Certainly every patient with idiopathic dilated cardiomyopathy should have a detailed family history; about 20 per cent reveal an affected relative.[168] If any close relative has a history consistent with cardiomyopathy, dysrhythmia, or sudden death at a relatively young age, counseling about the risk of a familial disease and the potential benefits of pedigree screening should be offered.

The majority of instances of familial occurrence fit autosomal dominant inheritance.[168,171–174] Considerable clinical variability characterizes virtually all pedigrees; variation in severity, clinical phenotype, and age of onset is typical. Recurrence of congestive cardiomyopathy of early onset in an inbred pedigree is suggestive of an autosomal recessive condition.[175]

The causes of the autosomal dominant forms of dilated cardiomyopathy are unknown. In some families with autosomal dominant disease, a mild proximal skeletal myopathy of type I fibers coexists with cardiac involvement.[172,176] Skeletal muscle changes might serve not only as an early clinical marker of heterozygosity for the mutant gene in some individuals at risk but also indicate that the search for cause should address structural components or metabolites common to both cardiac and skeletal myofibers.

In one family, cardiomyopathy developed only in association with pregnancy.[179] Although peripartum cardiomyopathy is a well-recognized, usually sporadic, disorder, its occurrence in five women in two generations suggests a hereditary predisposition. One component of muscle that is not a common cause of idiopathic dilated cardiomyopathy is dystrophin.[177]

Histological examination of myocardium generally shows nonspecific hypertrophy and fibrosis. By electron microscopy, however, mitochondria are distinctly abnormal, a finding not seen in congestive heart failure of other causes.[178] Because the inheritance pattern in these cases does not suggest a mutation of the mitochondrial genome, focus could be directed on nuclear genes that encode structural components of the mitochondrion, components of the respiratory chain found in the mitochondrion, or enzymes that regulate and facilitate free fatty acid metabolism in the mitochondrion.

A number of laboratories are conducting linkage analysis across the human genome in pedigrees showing autosomal dominant inheritance of dilated cardiomyopathy. The first success occurred in a large pedigree that is somewhat unique in that conduction disease, rather than heart failure, is usually the first manifestation of cardiovascular disease.[179] The phenotype maps to the pericentromeric region of chromosome 1 (1p1-1q1), and all of the candidate genes already mapped to this region do not appear to be at fault.[180]

Some pedigrees show convincing evidence of X-linkage of dilated cardiomyopathy. At least three loci have been identified. In *Barth syndrome,* cardiac involvement is associated with skeletal myopathy, proportionate short stature, and neutropenia; the phenotype is linked to markers at Xq28.[181,182]

Many males with *Duchenne* and some with *Becker muscular dystrophy* develop myocardial dysfunction (see p. 1867).[183] In the Becker form, right ventricular involvement may be unassociated with left ventricular dysfunction.[184] Deletion of exon 49 of the dystrophin gene predisposes to cardiomyopathy. This pleiotropic feature in a disease that presents as a skeletal myopathy prompted evaluation of the dystrophin locus in pedigrees with apparently isolated cardiomyopathy. Mutations in the 5′ end of the dystrophin gene have been found to account for some instances of X-linked dilated cardiomyopathy.[185,186] Why some dystrophin mutations are selectively expressed in cardiac muscle (and other in brain) is unclear.

Emery-Dreifuss muscular dystrophy (see p. 1872) is distinguishable clinically from the Duchenne and Becker forms by absence of pseudohypertrophy of skeletal muscle, early involvement of the arms with elbow contractures, and early onset of cardiac conduction abnormalities and atrial dysrhythmia.[181,187] Female heterozygotes are also commonly affected, albeit more mildly than males. The disease was mapped to the distal region of Xq28, and a previously unknown gene, called emerin, was found to be mutated.[188] Hearts show replacement of myocardium, especially in the atria, with fat and fibrosis. Even though the conduction system is not primarily affected histologically, sudden death is common in both hemizygous men and heterozygous women; thus, carrier detection can be life saving.[189]

Restrictive Cardiomyopathy

(See also p. 1426)

The pathogenesis of the majority of cases of restrictive cardiomyopathy involves infiltration or replacement of the myocardium or both. The causes are varied and can be nongenetic or genetic; the latter are mostly metabolic diseases with secondary effects on the heart and are summarized in Table 49–11; some are reviewed subsequently. One form of restrictive cardiomyopathy that has primary genetic forms among many other causes is endocardial fibroelastosis. Other mutations produce restriction through pericardial constriction. Isolated pedigrees of primary myocardial fibrosis without secondary cause and leading to restrictive hemodynamics are not classifiable.[190,191]

ENDOCARDIAL FIBROELASTOSIS (see also p. 991). This abnormality is characterized by thickening of the endocardium, which leads to decreased compliance and impaired diastolic function. Primary forms, discussed here, are unassociated with other cardiac anomalies (Table 49–11). When congenital, endocardial fibroelastosis accounts for somewhat under 10 per cent of childhood deaths from heart disease. In infants there is often an indolent course of failure to thrive, tachypnea, and tachycardia, until a precipitant such as an upper respiratory infection leads to rapid cardiac decompensation. Treatment of children with primary endocardial fibroelastosis is ineffective; cardiac transplantation now offers some hope. Autopsy shows enlargement of the left ventricle and perhaps other chambers, no abnormality of lung vessels, and collapse of the left lower lobe. Histopathological study reveals extensive deposition of extracellular matrix, primarily collagen and elastic fibers, in the endocardium.

X-linked recessive inheritance is the most firmly established of the single-gene causes, and even here there may be heterogeneity. Some pedigrees show mainly small, contracted cardiac chambers, whereas others have chamber dilatation; both are compatible with the functional pathophysiology described by the term "restrictive." Males are affected earlier and more severely by both forms, with death in infancy not unusual.[192] In other families, the ventricles are dilated, and the condition is distinguished from X-linked dilated cardiomyopathy by the presence of endocardial fibroelastosis and an immune deficiency due to defective granulocyte function, a condition termed Barth syndrome (see also p. 1665).[181,182] Morphological abnormalities of mitochondria were present on ultrastructural studies of heart and leukocytes. Insufficient longitudinal experience is recorded to know whether females heterozygous for this mutation develop a dilated restrictive cardiomyopathy later in life.

Several pedigrees suggestive of autosomal recessive inheritance of primary endocardial fibroelastosis were reported before the routine availability of laboratory methods to diagnose metabolic derangements, especially defects in fatty acid catabolism.[193] The occurrence of hydrocephalus, endocardial fibroelastosis, and neonatal cataracts may be due to a single gene mutation but could represent sequelae of a viral infection.[194] Endocardial fibroelastosis can be a prominent finding at autopsy in patients with autosomal dominant dilated cardiomyopathy[195]; whether the endocardial changes are primary, representing yet another mendelian form of this disorder, or secondary is unclear.

Restrictive cardiomyopathy often occurs with both hemodynamic evidence of impaired diastolic filling and wall thickening; any of the conditions causing pseudohypertrophy of the myocardium can eventually exhibit restrictive pathophysiology. Hemochromatosis and the amyloidoses, both hereditary and acquired forms, are especially likely to present in this manner. Connective tissue replaces myocytes or infiltrates the interstitium in a number of conditions. Fibrosis of the myocardium may cause pseudohypertrophy, but the clinical consequences are more those of restriction. Disorders in this category are those that cause coronary artery disease (*diabetes mellitus*, the *hemoglobinopathies* associated with sickling, *Fabry disease* and the *mucopolysaccharidoses*) and some of the *muscular dystrophies*, in which myocardial fibers are replaced by extracellular matrix. Finally, a number of hereditary conditions are associated with endocardial fibroelastosis (Table 49–11).

CONSTRICTIVE PERICARDITIS (see also Chap. 43). Two rare autosomal recessive disorders include fibrous thickening of the pericardium as a manifestation. In both, signs and symptoms of constrictive pericarditis develop insidiously, and treatment by pericardiotomy is life saving. One condition was first described in Finland and given the name *MULIBREY nanism*, a combination of a mnemonic for *mu*scle, *li*ver, *bre*in, and *ey*e and an archaic word for dwarfism (nanism). Growth failure from an early age is common, and growth does not improve once pericardial constriction is abated. Subsequently, more than a dozen patients, generally with consanguineous parents, have been reported from around the world.[196]

The *arthropathy-camptodactyly syndrome* previously had been reported because of the skeletal and rheumatological manifestations before pericardial effusion and fibrous thickening of the pericardium were recognized as manifestations.[197] Its cause is unknown.

TABLE 49–11 DISORDERS ASSOCIATED WITH RESTRICTIVE CARDIOMYOPATHY

	MIM NO.*
Primary Endocardial Fibroelastosis	
Familial endocardial fibroelastosis	226000, 305300
Faciocardiorenal syndrome	227280
Secondary Endocardial Fibroelastosis	
as a relatively common manifestation	
Maternal lupus erythematosus	
Pseudoxanthoma elasticum	177850, 264800
Systemic carnitine deficiency	212140
Trisomy 18	
as a relatively infrequent manifestation	
Cornelia de Lange syndrome	122470
Rubinstein-Taybi syndrome	268600
Secondary Infiltrative Cardiomyopathy	
Familial amyloidoses I and III	176300
Fabry disease	301500
Gaucher's disease type I	230800
Glycogen storage disorder II	232300
Glycogen storage disorder III	232400
Hemochromatosis	235200
Mucopolysaccharidosis IH	252800
Mucopolysaccharidosis II	300000

* Data from McKusick, V. A.: Mendelian Inheritance in Man. 11th ed. Baltimore, John Hopkins University Press, 1994.

Cardiomyopathies Secondary to Other Causes

INBORN ERRORS OF METABOLISM. These can affect the left ventricle by various mechanisms (Table 49–12) and produce diverse anatomical, histological, and functional disturbances. The most common anatomical result is an apparent hypertrophic cardiomyopathy, which is actually *pseudohypertrophic*, because the thickened walls are not due to myocardial cell hypertrophy, but to cellular or interstitial infiltration by metabolites. Abnormalities of both systolic and diastolic function result, outflow obstruction may occur, and in some cases the hemodynamic characteristics resemble a restrictive cardiomyopathy. The offending metabolite may be an incompletely degraded macromolecule such as glycogen (*glycogen storage disorder II* [Pompe's disease] and *glycogen storage disorder III*), proteoglycan and glycosaminoglycan (*mucopolysaccharidoses I, III, IV, VI,* and *VII*), sphingolipid (*Fabry disease, Tay-Sachs disease, Farber's disease, Refsum's disease*, and *Gaucher's disease*), glycoprotein (*fucosidosis* and *mannosidosis*), and amyloid (*familial amyloidoses I* and *III*) or a small molecule such as iron in *hemochromatosis*. Some of these disorders are discussed later. True myocardial hypertrophy occurs as a part of mendelian syndromes, such as *Noonan syndrome, von Recklinghausen neurofibromatosis*,[200] and *LEOPARD syndrome*,[201,202] and monogenic errors of metabolism, notably those producing *hyperthyroidism* and *pheochromocytoma*. Any of the mendelian disorders that cause hypertension may, over time, produce true myocardial hypertrophy.

Dilated cardiomyopathy often results from inborn errors of energy production, especially fatty acid metabolism. Various disorders associated with *carnitine deficiency, mitochondrial* and *peroxisomal dysfunction*, and *muscle dysfunction* can present with symptoms of congestive heart failure or dysrhythmia.

PRIMARY DISORDERS OF RHYTHM AND CONDUCTION

Virtually every dysrhythmia and conduction abnormality has been reported to occur in relatives.[203] For example, *familial disturbance of conduction* occurs, without evident cause, at the sinus node,[204,205] atrioventricular node,[206,207] and bundle branches.[208,209] However, understanding the genetics of cardiac electrophysiology has been hampered by several characteristics of this extensive literature: Most families have been small, so that mode of inheritance, or even whether the inheritance is mendelian, is uncertain; many of the families show a mixture of different defects, partly because the disease is progressive[210,211]; and some specific conduction defects are associated with hereditary myocardial diseases, such as familial cardiomyopathy,[171,212] atrial cardiomyopathy,[213] and familial amyloidosis.[214] As noted earlier, there seems to be genetic control of normal electrical conduction, so it would not be surprising to find mutations in single genes that produced clinically important disturbance.

An important cause of complete heart block, although not mendelian, nonetheless involves genetic factors. The association between rheumatic diseases and heart block was clearly established when the offspring of mothers with acquired disorders of connective tissue, especially lupus erythematosus, were found to have complete heart block.[215–217] Many examples of "autosomal recessive" congenital heart block represent this familial, but nonmendelian, etiology. The risk is not related to severity of the maternal disease but is highest in children of women with antibodies to ribonucleoprotein (anti-Ro[SS-A])[218] and at least one allele for HLA-DR3.[219] Thus, it may be the maternal genotype that determines susceptibility to inflammation of the fetal heart at vulnerable periods, such as gestational weeks 3 to 4 when the atrioventricular node is forming. Genetic susceptibility to inflammation of the atrioventricular node of patients themselves is suggested by the relatively high association of HLA-B27 in adults requiring permanent pacemakers[220,221]; not all of these patients have overt evidence of HLA-B27–associated rheumatic diseases.

Familial dysrhythmia is also not uncommon. Nodal rhythm,[222] ventricular irritability,[223] and tachydysrhythmia associated with accessory atrioventricular pathways[163,224,225] have been reported in families. In one family, three generations were affected by a syndrome of ventricular extrasystoles and tachydysrhythmias with recurrent syncope, hypoplasia of the distal toes, and hypoplasia of the mandible (Robin sequence).[226] Hereditary cardiomyopathies are another cause of familial dysrhythmia, and a notable example is arrhythmogenic right ventricular dysplasia (ARVD), an autosomal dominant condition with variable expression[227,228] (see also p. 681). Although ARVD is uncommon, the familial form shows clusters of high incidence (0.4 per cent) in some regions of Italy and is an underappreciated cause of life-threatening dysrhythmia.[229] The right ventricle is involved primarily in most cases, with thinning and replacement of myocardium by fat and fibrosis (Fig. 41–2, p. 1405).[230] Dysrhythmia, usually ventricular but occasionally supraventricular, may precede signs of right ventricular dysfunction. About one-third of cases are familial, generally in an autosomal dominant pattern. Whether the primary process is homogeneous or not and whether true dysplasia, degeneration (due to a metabolic defect or muscular dystrophy), or inflammation plays the leading role are unclear. In addition to these disorders, several syndromes involving prolongation of the Q-T interval deserve comment.

WARD-ROMANO SYNDROME (see also p. 750). Familial syncope and sudden death have long been associated with ventricular dysrhythmia, but a distinct syndrome was not recognized until Ward[231] and Romano,[232] working independently three decades ago, reported the characteristic prolonged Q-T interval. Subsequent investigations of numerous families have clearly established that the defect in repolarization is inherited as an *autosomal dominant*. Although a long Q-T_c is consistently present, other abnormalities of conduction also occur, although they may not be evident on the resting electrocardiogram.[233] Ward-Romano syndrome, now generally called long Q-T syndrome, is distinguished from the Jervell and Lange-Nielsen syndrome by inheritance pattern and the absence of hearing deficiency. Long Q-T syndrome is generally unassociated with systemic abnormalities, but three patients with a negative family history for long Q-T had syndactyly of multiple fingers and toes.[234]

Long Q-T syndrome is genetically heterogeneous, and mutations of at least three loci can produce similar disorders. The first locus was mapped to 11p15.5,[235] and subsequently loci at 7q35-q36 and 3p21-p24[236] were identified. Because some families show recombination of long Q-T syndrome with all of these loci, a fourth gene, at a minimum, must be involved. Use of genotype to determine unequivocally who is heterozygous for the mutation has permitted assessment of the reliability of electrocardiographic criteria for diagnosis.[237] Not unexpectedly, the criterion of a corrected Q-T interval greater than 0.44 sec is good, but less than 90 per cent sensitive and specific. Treatment with beta-adrenergic blockade or an automatic implanted defibrillator is effective. Individuals heterozygous for the mutant gene should be identified through a detailed family history, clinical assessment and, if necessary, DNA testing, and counseled appropriately.

JERVELL AND LANGE-NIELSEN SYNDROME (see also p. 750). The association of familial syncope, sudden death, and congenital deafness was codified in 1957,[238] although as with most eponymous syndromes, reports of affected individuals occurred previously. As would be expected for a rare, autosomal recessive condition, the parents of affected children are more likely than average to be consanguineous. Although heterozygotes have normal hearing and no overt primary rhythm disturbance, the Q-T_c intervals may be slightly prolonged.[239] The frequency of a long Q-T_c among deaf children is about 1 per 100, so routine electrocardiographic screening of anyone with congenital deafness is warranted.

Neither the cause nor the pathogenesis is known. Fright and rage clearly precipitate syncope and sudden death, leading to the proposal of autonomic dysfunction as the basic defect. However, allotransplantation of the heart, thereby causing complete denervation, failed to correct the underlying problem in one patient.[240]

DISORDERS OF CONNECTIVE TISSUE

The two broad classes of disorders of connective tissue are those due to mutations in single genes that determine or somehow affect components of the extracellular matrix and those due to extrinsic factors affecting the extracellular matrix, such as rheumatoid arthritis and systemic lupus erythematosus. The former category includes many disorders that affect the cardiovascular system. Susceptibility to so-called acquired disorders of connective tissue is, in part, determined by genes, and this specific aspect is reviewed. Disorders due to intrinsic factors acting on the extracellular matrix are discussed in Chapter 56.

TABLE 49–12 MENDELIAN ERRORS OF METABOLISM WITH MANIFESTATIONS IN THE CARDIOVASCULAR SYSTEM

DISORDER	EPONYM OR COMMON NAME	MIM NO.*	PATHOGENESIS	CARDIOVASCULAR INVOLVEMENT	BIOCHEMICAL DEFECT	GENE LOCUS†	ANIMAL MODEL‡
Aminoacidopathies							
Alkaptonuria	Ochronosis	203500	Deposition of homogentisic acid in connective tissue	AS; atherosclerosis			
Cystinosis, nephropathic type		219800	Lysosomal storage	Hypertension from renal failure, vascular wall thickening	?	?	
Homocystinuria		236200	Unknown	Early CAD; venous thrombosis; pulmonary embolism	Cystathionine-β-synthase	CBS; 21q21-q22.1	
Oxalosis I	Hyperoxaluria	259900	Vascular and tissue accumulation of oxalate	Conduction defect; vascular occlusions; Raynaud phenomenon	Peroxisomal alanine: Glyoxylate aminotransferase	AGT	
Defects in Fatty Acid Metabolism							
Carnitine transport defect	Primary carnitine deficiency	212140	Lipid myopathy; defective energy generation	DCM: ECF	?	?	Syrian hamster
MCAD deficiency		201450	Lipid myopathy; defective energy generation	DCM	Medium-chain acyl-CoA dehydrogenase	ACADM,1p	
LCAD deficiency		201460	Lipid myopathy; defective energy generation	DCM	Long-chain acyl-CoA dehydrogenase	ACADL,7	
Glycogen Storage Disorders							
GSD I	Pompe	252300	Lysosomal storage	Pseudohypertrophic CM; short P-R interval; ECF	α-1,4-glucosidase	GAA: 17q21-q25	Canine and bovine
GSD II	Adult acid maltase deficiency	232300	Lysosomal storage	Primarily skeletal muscle; respiratory insufficiency; corpulmonale	α-1,4-glucosidase		
GSD III	Forbes; debrancher deficiency	232400	Intracellular glycogen accumulation fibrosis	Pseudohypertrophic CM	Amylo-1,6-glucosidase		
Phosphorylase kinase deficiency	GSD of the heart			DCM	Phosphorylase kinase		
Glycoproteinoses							
Fucosidosis, severe		230000	Lysosomal storage	Myocardial thickening	α-fucosidase	FUCA1; 1p34	
Fucosidosis, mild		230000	Lysosomal storage	Angiokeratoma	α-fucosidase	FUCA1; 1p34	
Mannosidosis		248500	Lysosomal storage	Myocardial thickening; valvular thickening; conduction disturbance	α-Mannosidase	MANB, 19p13.2-12	
Aspartylglycosaminuria		208400	Lysosomal storage	Valvular thickening	Aspartylglycosylamine amino hydrolase	AGA, 4q21-qter	
Mucolipidoses							
ML II	I-cell	252500	Lysosomal storage	Same as MPS IH	Acetylglucosamine-1-phosphotransferase	GNPTA; 4q21-q23	
ML III	Pseudo-Hurler polydystrophy	252500	Lysosomal storage	Valvular thickening and dysfunction, esp. AS, AR	Acetylglucosamine-1-phosphotransferase	GNPTA; 4q21-q23	
Mucopolysaccharidoses							
MPS IH	Hurler	252800	Lysosomal storage	Early CAD; PH and OAD → CP; valvular dysfunction, esp. MR, AR; pseudohypertrophic CM	α-L-Iduronidase	IDUA, 22q11-pter	Canine and feline
MPS IS	Scheie	252800	Lysosomal storage	Valvular dysfunction, esp. AS	α-L-Iduronidase	IDUA, 22q11-pter	
MPS IH/S	Hurler-Scheie	252800	Lysosomal storage	Same as MPS IH	α-L-Iduronidase	IDUA, 22q11-pter	
MPS II	Hunter	209900	Lysosomal storage	Same as MPS IH; less severe in mild MPS II variant	Sulfoiduronate sulfatase	IDS, Xq28	

TABLE 49–12 MENDELIAN ERRORS OF METABOLISM WITH MANIFESTATIONS IN THE CARDIOVASCULAR SYSTEM—*Continued*

DISORDER	EPONYM OR COMMON NAME	MIM NO.*	PATHOGENESIS	CARDIOVASCULAR INVOLVEMENT	BIOCHEMICAL DEFECT	GENE LOCUS†	ANIMAL MODEL‡
MPS III A	Sanfilippo A	252900	Lysosomal storage	Valvular thickening and occasional dysfunction	Heparin sulfate sulfatase	?	
MPS III B	Sanfilippo B	252920	Lysosomal storage	Valvular thickening and occasional dysfunction	N-Acetyl-α-D-glucosaminidase	?	
MPS III C	Sanfilippo C	252930	Lysosomal storage	Valvular thickening and occasional dysfunction	acetyl-CoA: α-glucosaminidase N-acetyl-transferase	?	
MPS III D	Sanfilippo D		Lysosomal storage	Valvular thickening and occasional dysfunction	N-Acetylglucosamine-6-sulfatase	G6S, 12q14	
MPS IV A	Morquio A	253000	Lysosomal storage	Valvular dysfunction, esp. AR	Galactosamine-6-sulfatase		
MPS IV B	Morquio B	253010	Lysosomal storage	Milder than MPS IV A	β-Galactosidase		
MPS VI	Maroteaux-Lamy	253200	Lysosomal storage	Same as MPS IH	Arylsulfatase B	5p11-qter	Feline
MPS VII	Sly	253220	Lysosomal storage	Valvular thickening	β-Glucuronidase	GUSB;7q	Mouse and canine
Sphingolipidoses							
α-Galactosidase A deficiency	Fabry	301500	Cellular accumulation of trihexosyl ceramide, esp. endothelium	Early CAD, valvular thickening and dysfunction; pseudohypertrophic CM; short P-R interval; arteriolar occlusion; angiokeratoma	α-Galactosidase A	GLA; Xq22	
Ceramidase deficiency	Farber	228000	Histiocytic infiltration	Nodular thickening of valves	Ceramidase	?	
Glucocerebrosidase deficiency	Gaucher, adult form	230800	Cellular accumulation of glucocerebroside	PH → CP; interstitial infiltration of myocytes by Gaucher cells; constrictive pericarditis	β-Glucocerebroside	GBA; 1q21	
Miscellaneous disorders							
Acid lipase deficiency	Wolman	278000	↑ Cholesterol; foam cell infiltration	Atherosclerosis	Lysosomal acid lipase	LIPA, 10q	
Acid lipase deficiency	Cholesterol ester storage disease	278000	↑ Cholesterol, foam cell infiltration	Atherosclerosis; PH	Lysosomal acid lipase	LIPA, 10q	
Geleophysic dysplasia		231050	Lysosomal storage	Valvular dysfunction	?		
Hereditary angioedema		106100	Complement and kinin activation	Angioedema	C1 esterase inhibitor ?	CINH, 11p11.2-q13	
Multiple sulfatase deficiency	Juvenile sulfatidosis	272200	Lysosomal storage				

CAD = coronary artery disease; DCM = dilated cardiomyopathy; ECF = endocardial fibroelastosis: CM = cardiomyopathy; AS = aortic stenosis; AR = aortic regurgitation; PH = pulmonary hypertension; OAD = obstructive airway disease; CP = cor pulmonale; MR = mitral regurgitation; GSD = glycogen storage disease.

* Data from McKusick, V. A.: Mendelian Inheritance in Man. 11th ed. Baltimore, John Hopkins University Press, 1994.

† Gene symbol followed by chromosomal locus.

‡ Naturally occurring mutants; does not include transgenic and knockout rodent models.

Mendelian Disorders of the Extracellular Matrix

Close to 200 distinct phenotypes now comprise this category, which was first defined less than four decades ago with fewer than 10 disorders.[241] Several reviews and textbooks describe the phenotypes, genetics, and causes of many of the conditions (Table 49–13).[18,242–245]

Marfan Syndrome

This *autosomal dominant* disorder is relatively frequent (~1 per 10,000), occurs in all races and ethnic groups, and is often not diagnosed during life.[245,246] In light of the classic phenotype, failure to diagnose the Marfan syndrome may seem surprising; however, marked clinical variability, age dependency of all of the manifestations, and a high (~30 per cent) rate of new mutation all conspire to make detection of mildly affected, young, sporadic patients challenging. Even with the discovery of the genetic and biochemical bases of the condition, the diagnosis of Marfan syndrome outside of families with the classic phenotype remains entirely clinical, for reasons described subsequently.[247] Current criteria (Table 49–14) depend on the manifestations in the cardinal organ systems—the eye, the skeleton, the heart, and the aorta—and other systems, and the family history[129] (Fig. 49–7). The presence of manifestations more specific for the Marfan syndrome, such as aortic dilatation, aortic dissection in a nonhypertensive young person, ectopia lentis, and dural ectasia, clearly is

TABLE 49–13 CARDIOVASCULAR MANIFESTATIONS OF HERITABLE DISORDERS OF CONNECTIVE TISSUE

DISORDER		MIM NO.*	CARDIOVASCULAR MANIFESTATIONS
Cutis laxa		219100	PS, PPS, CP
		123700	MVP
Ehlers-Danlos	I	130000	MVP
	II	130010	MVP
	III	130020	MVP
	IV	130050	Arterial rupture, MVP
	VI	225400	MVP
	VIII	130080	MVP
	X	225310	MVP, aortic root dilatation
Osteogenesis imperfecta	I	166200	MVP, mild aortic root dilatation
	II	166210	CP, arterial calcification
	III	259420	MVP
	IV	166220	Aortic root dilatation
Marfan syndrome		154700	MVP, aortic root dilatation, aortic dissection
MASS phenotype		157700	MVP, mild aortic root dilatation
Pseudoxanthoma elasticum		177850	Arteriolar sclerosis, claudication, myocordial infarction

PS = valvular pulmonic stenosis; PPS = peripheral pulmonic stenosis; CP = cor pulmonale; MVP = mitral valve prolapse

* Data from Mendelian Inheritance in Man.[8]

more important diagnostically than features common in other connective tissue disorders and in the general population, such as scoliosis, joint hypermobility, myopia, and MVP.

The most common cardiovascular features are MVP and dilatation of the sinuses of Valsalva.[246,248,249] Associated clinical problems of mitral regurgitation, aortic regurgitation, and aortic dissection account, if untreated, for most of the early mortality that results in an average age of death in the fourth and fifth decades.[250] Children tend to be more severely affected by mitral valve disease,[251–253] whereas aortic problems are progressive and more likely in adolescence and beyond.

TABLE 49–14 DIAGNOSTIC CRITERIA FOR THE MARFAN SYNDROME:[129] PHENOTYPIC MANIFESTATIONS*

Skeleton

Joint hypermobility, tall stature, pectus excavatum, reduced thoracic kyphosis, scoliosis, arachnodactyly, dolichostenomelia, pectus carinatum, erosion of the lumbosacral vertebrae from dural ectasia†

Eye

Myopia, retinal detachment, elongated globe, ectopia lentis†

Cardiovascular

Mitral valve prolapse, endocarditis, dysrhythmia, dilated mitral annulus, mitral regurgitation, tricuspid valve prolapse, aortic regurgitation, aortic dissection†, dilatation of the aortic root†

Pulmonary

Apical blebs, spontaneous pneumothorax

Skin and Integument

Inguinal hernias, incisional hernias, striae atrophicae

Central Nervous System

Attention deficit disorder, hyperactivity, verbal-performance discrepancy, dural ectasia†, anterior pelvic meningocele†

If the family history is positive for a close relative clearly affected by the Marfan syndrome, to make the diagnosis in the patient, manifestations should be present in the skeleton and one of the other organ systems, and the diagnosis confirmed by linkage analysis or mutation detection.

If the family history is negative or unknown, to make the diagnosis, the patient should have manifestations in the skeleton, the cardiovascular system, and one other system, and at least one of the manifestations indicated by †.

* Manifestations are listed within each organ system in increasing specificity for Marfan syndrome, although none is completely specific; those indicated by † are the most specific.

MITRAL VALVE INVOLVEMENT. MVP is age dependent and more common in women with the Marfan syndrome. The incidence reaches 60 to 80 per cent when patients are studied by two-dimensional echocardiography,[130] and generally the valve leaflets have an elongated and redundant appearance. Progression of severity, as judged by appearance or

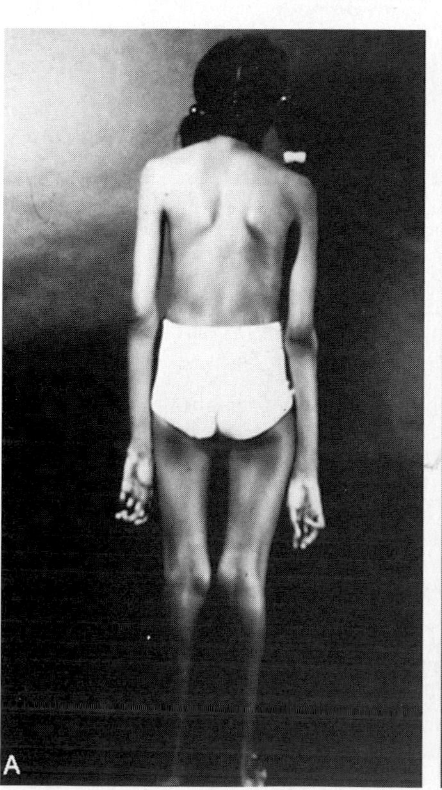

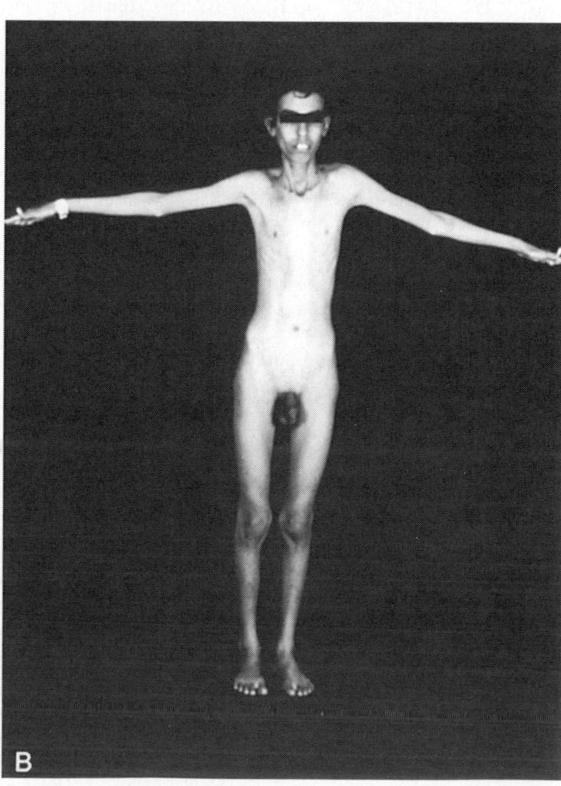

FIGURE 49–7. External phenotype of a boy with Marfan syndrome, showing long extremities and digits, tall stature, and pectus carinatum.

worsening of mitral regurgitation by clinical and echocardiographic criteria, occurs in at least one-quarter of patients,[254] a much higher rate than in MVP found in the general population.[249] The mitral annulus dilates and contributes to the regurgitation, as do stretching and occasional rupture of chordae. About 10 per cent of patients with marked prolapse have calcification of the mitral annulus. Standard treatment for chronic mitral regurgitation is indicated, but coexistent aortic root dilatation usually requires that increasing inotropy be avoided. When mitral regurgitation becomes severe enough to warrant surgical intervention, two considerations must be added to the balance: (1) Repair of the mitral apparatus is often successful and durable in the Marfan syndrome.[255,256] Repair is less easily accomplished when the cusps are extremely redundant, there is marked chordal damage, or the annulus is heavily calcified. (2) The aorta may be enlarged enough to permit concomitant replacement. We have often delayed mitral valve surgery for a time, carefully following ventricular function, until the sinuses of Valsalva dilated enough to make composite graft repair feasible. On the other hand, when operation is primarily because of aortic dilatation, a mitral annuloplasty can be performed if there is more than trivial mitral regurgitation.[257,258] In Marfan syndrome, as in virtually all of the heritable disorders of connective tissue, there is an increased susceptibility to dehiscence of prosthetic mitral valves, regardless of the care taken in placing them.

AORTIC ROOT INVOLVEMENT (see also p. 965). The sinuses of Valsalva are often dilated at birth, and the rate of progression varies widely among patients in general and also among relatives (Fig. 49–8). Thus, predicting long-term risks of developing aortic regurgitation (which is clearly positively associated with aortic root diameter[259]), suffering aortic dissection (which is less clearly associated with diameter), or requiring aortic surgery is fraught with uncertainty. Transthoracic echocardiography is sufficient for detecting and monitoring changes in diameter, because in the absence of dissection, dilatation is limited to the proximal ascending aorta, and the rate of change is slow, measured in millimeters per year. Rare exceptions of principal dilatation of the thoracic aorta can be followed with transesophageal echocardiography or magnetic resonance imaging. Patients with dilatation less than 1.5 times the mean diameter predicted for their body size[131,260] can be observed annually; as the diameter increases, more frequent evaluation is necessary. Aortic regurgitation often appears in adults at a diameter of 50 mm but may be absent at diameters of more than 60 mm.[259,261] The risk of dissection increases with the size of the aorta and fortunately occurs infrequently below a diameter of 55 mm in the adult. Many surgeons have adopted the criterion of a 50 to 55 mm maximal aortic root dimension for performing elective composite graft repair in Marfan syndrome patients, regardless of the severity of the aortic regurgitation,[258] although patients with a family history of aortic dissection should have surgery at the lower end of this range. The perioperative results of both elective and emergency repair of the aortic root have been excellent and a marked improvement from the pre–composite graft era that ended in the mid 1970's. Long-term results of operation are limited by the problems of endocarditis and anticoagulation, common to all prosthetic valves, but in the absence of chronic aortic dissection appear favorable for patients with Marfan syndrome.[262–264]

THORACIC ABNORMALITIES. Severe *pectus excavatum* may complicate cardiovascular surgery by making exposure of the heart by median sternotomy difficult. For elective cardiovascular surgery, repair of the sternal deformity some months in advance permits sufficient healing of the costochondral junctions that a stable and functionally and cosmetically improved thoracic cage will facilitate further surgery and postoperative recovery.[265] Simultaneous repair of cardiac and sternal defects, although possible, is a long procedure, and intraoperative bleeding from bone can be considerable because of the anticoagulation associated with cardiopulmonary bypass.

AORTIC DISSECTION (see also p. 1671). This complication usually begins just above the coronary ostia (type A in the Stanford scheme) and extends the entire length of the aorta (type I in the DeBakey scheme). About 10 per cent of dissections begin distal to the left subclavian (type B or III), but rarely is dissection limited to the abdominal aorta. Angiography (Fig. 45–12, p. 1561), magnetic resonance imaging (Fig. 10–22, p. 328), and transesophageal echocardiography all have a role in the diagnosis of acute dissection in the Marfan syndrome, with the capabilities and experience of the medical center and the stability of the patient important determinants of the approach. As many acute dissections of the ascending aorta in Marfan syndrome have a stuttering course that culminates in death from rupture or hemopericardium, rapid transfer to a facility prepared to perform immediate repair is essential.

Not all acute dissections in Marfan syndrome involve severe, tearing chest pain that radiates to the back; indeed, some extensive dissections have been occult.[258] This experience reinforces the need for a high index of suspicion by physicians whenever a tall, nearsighted young person with thoracic cage deformity arrives at an emergency department with vague complaints of lightheadedness, chest or abdom-

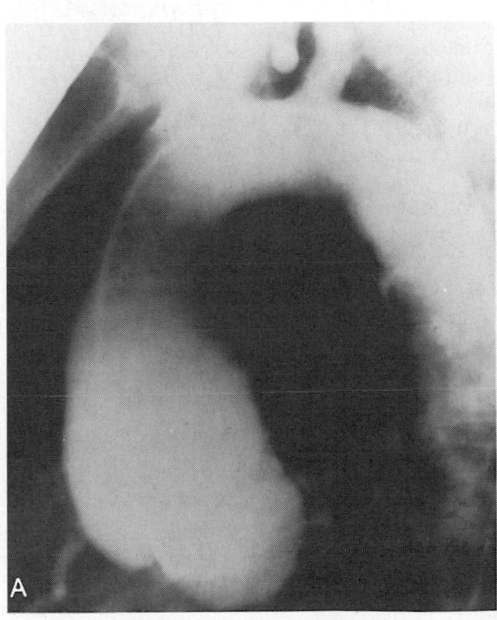

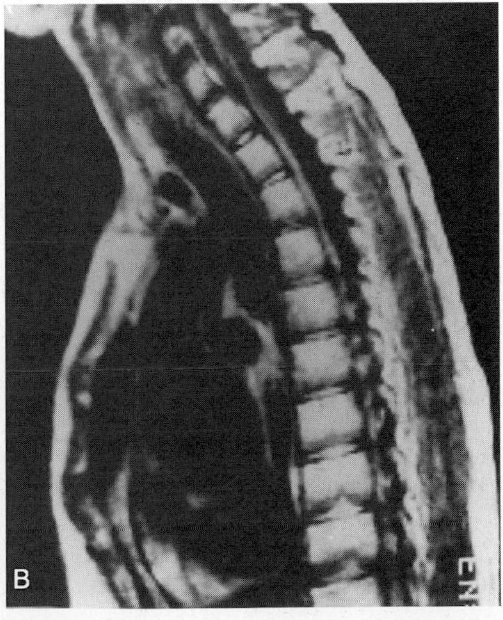

FIGURE 49–8. Dilatation of the aortic root in Marfan syndrome. *A*, Lateral angiogram of the ascending aorta showing dilatation of the sinuses of Valsalva and proximal ascending aorta and relatively normal caliber of the ascending aorta. *B*, Lateral magnetic resonance imaging of the same patient.

inal discomfort, or a murmur of aortic regurgitation. Similarly, patients known to have Marfan syndrome and their close relatives need to be educated about the signs and symptoms of aortic dissection. In general, the management of acute and chronic dissection in the Marfan syndrome follows standard practice,[266] with several departures. First, all dissections of the ascending aorta should be repaired promptly, preferably with a composite graft. Second, regular evaluation with magnetic resonance imaging is important, as the diameter of any region of dissected aorta is likely to expand over time.[267,268] Third, reduction of systolic blood pressure and administration of negative-inotropic doses of beta-adrenergic blockers should be even more strictly adhered to than in dissections without a connective tissue abnormality. In most instances, any region of the aorta should be repaired when complications of further dissection, branch vessel occlusion, or dilatation beyond about 50 mm occur. A staged approach to total replacement of the Marfan aorta is now both feasible and successful.[269]

DYSRHYTHMIAS. Some patients develop serious ventricular or supraventricular dysrhythmia. The latter often accompanies chronic mitral regurgitation, but the former may be of high grade and difficult to suppress when only MVP is present. Some patients have the syndrome of autonomic dysfunction, atypical chest pain, and palpitations seen in some patients with MVP unassociated with a flagrant connective tissue abnormality.

MANAGEMENT. The routine cardiological management of the Marfan syndrome is multifaceted: regular clinical and echocardiographic examinations; routine endocarditis prophylaxis for dental and other procedures; restriction of activity from heavy weightlifting, contact sports, and any exertion at maximal capacity; and chronic beta-adrenergic blockade form the basic approach, with individual variation often appropriate. Support for the role of beta-blockade comes from several prospective studies that show a reduction in the rate of aortic dilatation and the risk of aortic dissection in patients treated with negatively inotropic doses of propranolol or atenolol.[270,271] However, short-term administration of propranolol to patients with large sinus of Valsalva aneurysms, while reducing heart rate and peak systolic pressure, did not improve the impedance characteristics recorded in the ascending aorta.[272]

A woman with Marfan syndrome has two concerns regarding pregnancy (see also p. 1850). The first is the 50:50 risk that any child will inherit the condition; currently prenatal diagnosis can be attempted in selected situations. The second is the risk of dissection that the hemodynamic stresses of pregnancy place on the aorta. Several dozen case reports attest to the heightened incidence of dissection during the third trimester, parturition, and the first month post partum.[273,274] However, in the majority of instances, serious aortic dilatation was present. Prospective evaluation of 21 women through 45 pregnancies confirmed our earlier recommendation that the cardiovascular risks are relatively low if the aortic diameter does not exceed 40 mm and cardiac function is not compromised.[274]

ETIOLOGY. Marfan syndrome is caused by mutations in the gene that encodes fibrillin-1, the major constituent of microfibrils, components of the extracellular matrix that are widely dispersed and perform multiple function.[245,275,276]

Microfibrils form the scaffolding upon which elastin is deposited to form elastic fibers. Fragmentation and disorganization of elastic fibers in the aortic media have long been a histological marker (inappropriately called cystic medial necrosis) of Marfan syndrome,[246] although similar microscopic pathology occurs in familial aortic aneurysms and aging aortas of the normal population. A defect in microfibrils explains all of the pleiotropic manifestations of Marfan syndrome.[16,245]

After Marfan syndrome and fibrillin were mapped to the same region of chromosome 15,[277,278] it only remained to detect mutations in the *FBN1* gene to prove the cause.[279] Subsequently, over 100 distinct mutations in this gene have been found in different families, and only a couple have occurred, by chance, in unrelated patients.[7,245,280,281] Because *FBN1* is such a large gene (~10,000 nucleotides in the mRNA), finding a mutation is still not a simple matter. Once the mutation is identified, diagnosis in that family is straightforward. In families with multiple alive and cooperative affected people, linkage analysis can be used for presymptomatic and prenatal diagnosis.[247] The use of molecular testing is confounded, however, by the discovery that autosomal dominant ectopia lentis, familial tall stature, MASS phenotype, and familial aortic aneurysm are all phenotypes found to be due to mutations in *FBN1* and are exactly the conditions clinicians are interested in excluding in their patients of questionable diagnosis.[245,282,283]

Mutations in *FBN1* have distinct effects on microfibril formation: Some affect synthesis, others secretion, and others incorporation of fibrillin-1 monomers into the extracellular matrix.[281,284,285]

MITRAL VALVE PROLAPSE AND THE MASS PHENOTYPE. This heterogeneous group of conditions, described above (p. 1662) likely contains large numbers of patients and families who have a defect of the extracellular matrix underlying the phenotypes. Some, but not all, have mutations in *FBN1*.[245]

Ehlers-Danlos Syndrome

This group of heterogeneous conditions is linked by variable involvement of the skin and the joints, with hyperelasticity and fragility of the former occurring with hypermobility of the latter[8,18,129] (Fig. 49–9). Mitral valve prolapse is clearly increased in frequency in most of the clinical types,[243,286] but aortic root dilatation is an uncommon finding. The most serious cardiovascular problems occur in *Ehlers-Danlos type IV* in the form of spontaneous rupture of large- and medium-caliber arteries.

Various defects of type III collagen are the cause of the phenotype in virtually all patients studied.[18] In the classic syndrome, true aneurysms rarely form; rather, a rupture without dissection usually occurs

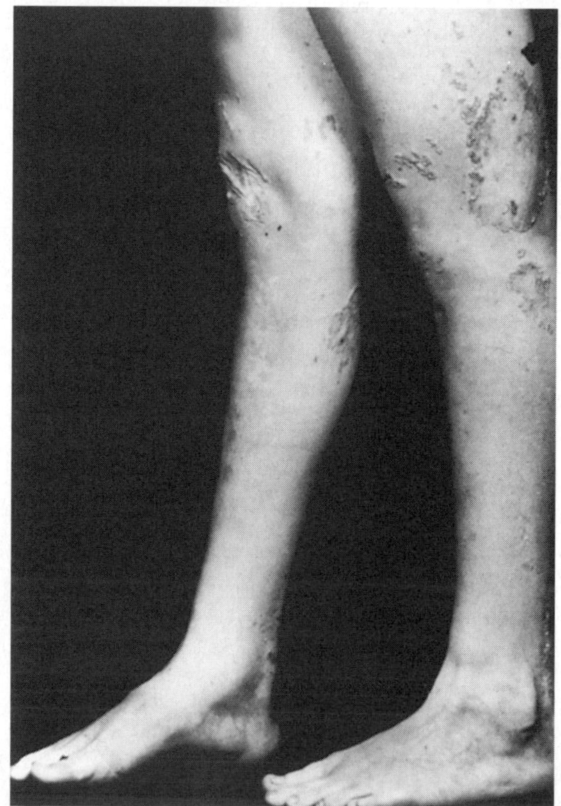

FIGURE 49–9. Legs of a patient with Ehlers-Danlos type IV who died of rupture of the subclavian artery. Note the mild joint hypermobility and the striking dermal abnormalities—elastosis perforans serpiginosa and thin, atrophic scars over areas of recurrent trauma.

as a catastrophic event. Most prone are the abdominal aorta and its branches, the great vessels of the aortic arch, and the large arteries of the limbs. False aneurysms and fistulas[18,243,287] may be one result in those patients who do not die of the initial rupture. Vascular surgery is difficult, as the normal-appearing vessels around the rent fail to hold sutures. As a consequence, elective surgery to repair vascular anomalies, such as false aneurysms, that are causing no immediate problem is contraindicated in most cases. Ehlers-Danlos type IV is often sporadic but, when familial, is usually autosomal dominant.

Prenatal diagnosis is possible by examining collagen production in amniocytes. However, pregnancy is particularly hazardous to women with Ehlers-Danlos type IV because of vascular rupture and should be avoided on medical grounds.[288]

Pseudoxanthoma Elasticum

This is a clinically variable and genetically heterogeneous disorder of unknown cause. Histopathological examination of affected tissues shows fragmentation and calcification of elastic fibers. The skin, the eye, the gastrointestinal system, and the cardiovascular system are the organs most severely affected.[129,244,289] The skin shows highly characteristic raised, yellowish papules (pseudoxanthoma) overlying areas of flexural stress, such as the neck, cubital and popliteal fossae, and groin (Fig. 49–10). Breaks in the elastic lamella, Bruch's membrane of the choroid, produce the funduscopic finding of angioid streaks. Gastrointestinal hemorrhage is common and potentially fatal; mucosal arterioles bleed, and because the calcified elastic fibers prevent effective vessel retraction, hemostasis is difficult. Selective arterial embolization was life saving in one instance.[290] The heart is affected in a number of ways. Endocardial fibroelastosis is common, but because primarily the atria are involved, a restrictive cardiomyopathy is uncommon. Mitral valve prolapse may be increased in frequency[291,292] but is rarely a clinical problem. Coronary artery disease with myocardial ischemia and infarction is the major problem and a common cause of early death.[293,294]

Elastic and muscular arteries, including the coronaries, develop a type of arteriosclerosis similar to Mönckeberg's; progressive luminal narrowing occurs and can produce complete occlusion. Initially this is most evident at the radial and ulnar arteries, where absence of pulses and a positive Allen test are noted early in the course.[293] Because narrowing progresses slowly, collaterals form, and peripheral ischemia is a late complication. Because the arterial stenoses tend to be diffuse, bypassing them often involves extensive surgery. One patient with marked endocardial fibroelastosis was helped by resection of calcified elastic bands within the left ventricle.[295] Because the basic defect is unknown (but does not involve the gene for elastin),[296] no specific treatment is available. Because of a positive association between phenotypic severity and dietary calcium intake, patients can be advised to restrict consumption of dairy products and to avoid calcium supplements.[297] Hypertension and all risk factors for atherosclerosis should be aggressively controlled.

Genetic Susceptibility to Acquired Disorders of Connective Tissue

Genetic factors are clearly implicated in the susceptibility to many of the rheumatic disorders and to specific complications of specific conditions. The cardiovascular manifestations of these disorders are particularly interesting in this regard (p. 1776). For example, study of HLA-DR antigen frequencies suggests that immune-response factors are involved in the pathogenesis of chronic rheumatic heart disease in blacks.[298]

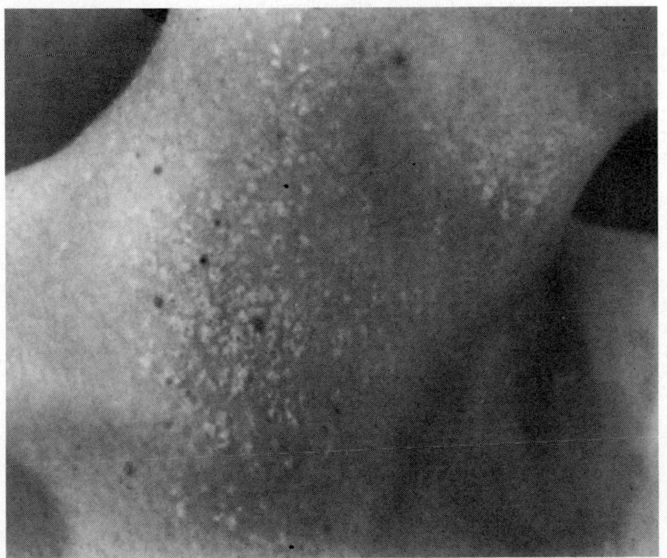

FIGURE 49–10. Skin of a young man with pseudoxanthoma elasticum. The neck is a typical location to notice the raised, yellowish papules from which the name of the condition derives.

INBORN ERRORS OF METABOLISM THAT AFFECT THE CARDIOVASCULAR SYSTEM

The hundreds of biochemical defects that affect human metabolism have direct or secondary impact on the cardiovascular system (Table 49–12). Several examples are reviewed, selected for their relevance to clinical practice or their instructive lessons about pathophysiology.

Aminoacidopathies

Inborn errors of amino acid metabolism result in the accumulation of precursors and a deficit of end products, either or both of which can be detrimental.

Alkaptonuria

An intermediate of tyrosine catabolism polymerizes to homogentisic acid, which readily accumulates in the extracellular matrix.[299] Over many years, connective tissue of cartilage, heart valves, and arteries becomes increasingly abnormal. Aortic stenosis and arteriosclerosis are the cardiological sequelae.

Homocystinuria

This condition is caused by a deficiency of cystathionine β-synthase; the pathogenesis of the pleiotropic manifestations is largely unknown.[17,300] Perhaps the amino acid sulfhydryl groups bind to collagen, fibrillin, and other macromolecules and interfere with cross-linking. The clinical features, once confused with the Marfan syndrome, include tall stature, skeletal deformity, ectopia lentis, mental retardation, psychiatric disturbances, and a predilection for venous and arterial thromboses. Those patients with mutations that render the enzyme activity able to be increased by pharmacological doses of pyridoxine are less severely affected; early treatment can prevent most aspects of the phenotype.[301] Patients unresponsive to pyridoxine can be helped by a low-protein diet to reduce intake of methionine.

Myocardial infarction, pulmonary embolism, and stroke are the most common causes of death. The pathogenesis of the vascular complications was once thought to involve abnormal platelet function, but platelet survival in untreated patients is normal.[302] Growing evidence supports a susceptibility of heterozygotes, who have none of the external phenotype of the disease, to atherosclerosis.[303–305] A variety of actions of homocysteine on endothelial receptors, stimulation of smooth muscle growth, and production of extracellular matrix components are being explored for clinical relevance.[306,307] Current therapeutic approaches are focused on maintaining physiological levels of the cofactors involved in metabolism of sulfurated amino acids—folate and vitamins B_6 and B_{12}.[308]

Disorders of Fatty Acid Metabolism

Although most organs can metabolize fatty acids when faced with hypoglycemia, only the heart depends on fatty acids as the primary source of energy generation. Thus, it is not surprising that virtually all genetic defects in fatty acid metabolism, including generalized defects in mitochondria and peroxisomes, are associated with myocardial dysfunction. Other substrates—glucose, lactate, and oxaloacetate—also generate energy in myocardial cells by entry into mitochondria and the tricarboxylic acid (Krebs) cycle. Thus, defects in conversion of pyruvate to acetyl coenzyme A and in any point along the tricarboxylic acid cycle and the respiratory chain have a major impact on myocardial energy generation. Quite likely, some sporadic and familial instances of idiopathic cardiomyopathy may represent undiagnosed or undefined metabolic disorders.

CARNITINE DEFICIENCIES. Carnitine is a required cofactor for entry of long-chain fatty acids into mitochondria and is both synthesized endogenously and available from dietary sources.[309] Deficiency of carnitine effectively blocks metabolism of long-chain fatty acids throughout the body and hepatic metabolism of ketones. Because of their relative dependency on fatty acids, muscle cells, including myocytes, suffer out of proportion to other tissue when carnitine levels are low for any reason. Cytoplasmic inclusions of lipid are characteristic findings in myocytes and hepatocytes.

Several mendelian defects produce primary or secondary carnitine deficiency. An autosomal recessive defect in carnitine palmitoyltransferase I leads to increased plasma carnitine and a skeletal muscle myopathy with little effect on the heart.[309] So-called systemic carnitine deficiency can be due to a variety of causes: primary deficiency of intake, synthesis, or function, and secondary deficiency, the majority now known to be a result of defects in fatty acid metabolism.[309–311] The latter group of conditions usually does not respond to pharmacological doses of carnitine.[311,312]

Primary carnitine deficiency usually presents in infancy with hypoglycemia, coma, and congestive heart failure due to dilated cardiomyopathy. In the few cases reported, problems largely resolve with carnitine treatment; they can be prevented from recurring by oral supplementation with L-carnitine[312,313] (p. 1447). Primary systemic carnitine deficiency is due to a defect in carnitine transport, which leads to excessive urinary loss and which affects muscle but not liver.[311] Thus, muscle cells still may be relatively deficient in carnitine, despite supplementation, and long-term prognosis is uncertain.

DEFECTS OF BETA-OXIDATION. At least 20 steps are involved when a molecule of free fatty acid leaves the plasma, enters the beta-oxidation spiral in the mitochondrion, and generates electrons and acetyl-CoA.[309] At each turn of the oxidation spiral, two carbons are removed from the fatty acid, and the enzymes involved in this step are specific for substrates of only certain chain length: long-chain, medium-chain, and short-chain acetyl-CoA dehydrogenases, or LCAD, MCAD, and SCAD. Thus far, patients with defects in nine of the steps have been characterized.

Patients homozygous for these generally autosomal recessive disorders develop episodic hypoketotic hypoglycemia, usually associated with fasting or intercurrent illness. Deficiency of MCAD is the most common cause and occurs in about 1 of every 7000 newborns in the United States. Hypoglycemic crises can rapidly progress to coma and death, and 50 to 60 per cent of affected infants die in the first 2 years of life.[165] Because infants between episodes or before a fatal crisis appear normal, MCAD deficiency accounts for a proportion of so-called sudden infant deaths.[314] Histopathological examination shows microvesicular accumulation of fat in cardiac and skeletal muscle. One mutation in MCAD (A985G) accounts for 90 per cent of all alleles that predispose to this lethal disorder, and various approaches to newborn screening are being investigated.

MITOCHONDRIAL MYOPATHIES. All of the enzymes of fatty acid oxidation are encoded by genes located on nuclear chromosomes, but the components of the electron transport chain are encoded by both nuclear and mitochondrial genes. Several syndromes involving various types of myopathies have been shown to be due to mutations in the mitochondrial chromosome.[13] The *Kearns-Sayre* syndrome includes pigmentary degeneration of the retina, ophthalmoplegia (Fig. 60–16, p. 1876), and cardiomyopathy as its most prominent manifestation; all of the affected tissue have nearly exclusive reliance on oxidative phosphorylation for energy generation.

The *MELAS syndrome* (*m*yopathy, *e*ncephalopathy, *l*actic *a*cidosis, and *s*troke-like episodes) is due to mutations in mitochondrial transfer RNA genes.[315–317] In addition to the features that define the acronym, hypertrophic cardiomyopathy and diffuse coronary angiopathy are common. A variety of other mtDNA mutations are associated with hypertrophic or dilated cardiomyopathy.[318,319]

Variations in both the actual mutations and the fraction of abnormal mitochondria in the cells of the different organs (heteroplasmy) account for many of the clinical differences in phenotype, severity, and age of onset among patients with this disorder. Inheritance is maternal for patients with mitochondrial mutations; apparent autosomal recessive and dominant inheritance may indicate that mutations of nuclear genes can impair electron transport similarly to mitochondrial mutations. Some patients have been treated with moderate success over the short term with coenzyme Q[320] and with cardiac transplantation in one case.[321]

Glycogenoses

Three of the glycogen storage disorders affect cardiac muscle.

GLYCOGEN STORAGE DISEASE II (see also p. 992). This autosomal recessive condition is due to deficiency of the lysosomal enzyme α-1,4-glucosidase and results in the lysosomal accumulation of glycogen in most tissues. Several allelic variants occur.[322] The condition with infantile onset is called *Pompe disease,* and cardiac involvement is profound.[323] The infant with Pompe disease appears well initially but soon fails to thrive and develops hypotonia, tachypnea, and tachycardia; the disease progresses during the first year to irreversible congestive heart failure and death from pneumonia or cardiopulmonary failure. Typically, auscultation reveals no murmurs until late in the course when obstruction develops, and hypoglycemia does not appear because the nonlysosomal pathway of glycogen catabolism is intact. The diagnosis is suggested by massive cardiomegaly on examination and chest radiography and by characteristic echocardiographic abnormalities of a short P-R interval and markedly increased QRS voltage.[324] Echocardiography shows tremendously thickened (pseudohypertrophic) ventricles, and Doppler interrogation or catheterization may reveal subaortic and subpulmonic pressure gradients characteristic of obstructive cardiomyopathy.

Reduced diastolic function of a restrictive cardiomyopathy develops eventually, and endocardial fibroelastosis is common.[324,325] With these findings, the diagnosis of Pompe disease is virtually certain, but it can be confirmed by analysis of α-1,4-glucosidase activity in cultured fibroblasts. Prenatal diagnosis is possible by enzymatic assay of amniocytes. Treatment is supportive, but cardiac transplantation could correct the cardiac problem; unfortunately, involvement of other organs, including the lungs, liver, and skeletal muscle, might eventually prove just as serious as the cardiomyopathy. Bone marrow transplantation might be a solution if performed early in the course. An animal model of α-1,4-glucosidase deficiency exists in cattle and develops cardiac pathology typical of human Pompe disease.[326]

Cardiomyopathy may develop in the juvenile-onset form of α-1,4-glucosidase deficiency,[327] but it is not invariable because of allelic heterogeneity. In one sibship without cardiac involvement, three brothers had extensive hepatic, skeletal muscle, and arterial smooth muscle accumulation of glycogen, and each died of rupture of a basilar artery aneurysm.[328] The adult-onset form usually presents with insidious onset of respiratory insufficiency, and clinically important cardiac disease is rare.[329]

GLYCOGEN STORAGE DISEASE III (see p. 1668). The striking clinical variability in phenotype associated with deficiency of α-1,4-glucosidase is due in large part to the extensive array of mutations that occur at the GAA locus,[330] which maps to 17q23. This autosomal recessive deficiency of amylo-1,6-glucosidase results in infantile- and juvenile-onset syndromes of muscular weakness, wasting, and hepatomegaly. Clinical cardiac disease is not common, although both cytoplasmic (nonlysosomal) and intermyofibril glycogen is routinely present in the heart and causes pseudohypertrophy and increased voltage on electrocardiography. The diagnosis has been established by enzymatic assay of an endomyocardial biopsy specimen.[331–333]

GLYCOGEN STORAGE DISEASE IV. This is caused by deficiency of α-1,4-glucan: α-1,4-glucan 6-glycosyl transferase. It usually causes a fatal disorder of early childhood characterized by hepatic failure; although extensive deposition of polysaccharide occurs in the heart, death intervenes before cardiac symptoms appear. As with all of the glycogen storage diseases, extensive allelic heterogeneity results in milder forms of the classic disorders. Patients with diagnosis later in adolescence tend to have more severe cardiomyopathy.[334,335] Liver transplant has been life saving in some cases and has, somewhat surprisingly, resulted in a reduction of glycogen deposits in the heart and skeletal muscles.[336,337]

CARDIAC PHOSPHORYLASE KINASE DEFICIENCY. Few cases of this enzyme deficiency have been reported: deposition of glycogen is confined to the heart, which may be massively thickened and enlarged, and leads to early death.[338,339]

GLYCOPROTEINOSES. As shown in Table 49–12, this group of disorders results in the lysosomal accumulation of a variety of compounds that cannot be catabolized further because of the specific enzyme deficiency. Some have prominent cardiac pathology, generally of pseudohypertrophy and valvular thickening, which present with congestive failure, valvular dysfunction, conduction defects, or dysrhythmia.

Hematological Disorders

(See Chap. 57)

HEMOCHROMATOSIS (see pp. 1430 and 1790). This is an autosomal recessive disorder of unknown cause that results in iron deposition in many tissues, including the myocardium. The manifestations include diabetes mellitus, skin hyperpigmentation, hypogonadism, hepatic failure with cirrhosis, hepatoma, and congestive heart failure; severity is considerably worse, and age of onset earlier, in women because of the autophlebotomy provided by menstruation.[340] The gene is located close to the HLA complex on chromosome 6, and presymptomatic diagnosis can be made in a family, even prenatally, by determining HLA antigen haplotypes and performing linkage analysis. Diagnosis in sporadic cases depends on finding increased serum iron, ferritin, and, especially, transferrin saturation in the absence of any obvious cause of excessive iron intake.[341] Fully 10 per cent of the population is heterozygous for the hemochromatosis mutation, suggesting that at an incidence of 2 to 3 per 1000, this disease is underdiagnosed.

Cardiac involvement often appears first as dysrhythmia or congestive heart failure. Dysrhythmia, conduction abnormalities, and low QRS voltage are typical electrocardiographic findings; cardiomegaly is seen on chest radiography, and a dilated cardiomyopathy with reduced systolic function can be documented on echocardiography.[342,343] Occasional patients have a restrictive pattern on cardiac catheterization.[344]

Treatment by repeated phlebotomy is most effective if begun before organ damage is irreversible. If a patient with congestive heart failure has not yet developed serious compromise in other organs, cardiac transplantation may be contemplated, as may combined heart-liver replacement.

HEMOGLOBINOPATHIES (see p. 1787). *Sickle cell disease* and other hemoglobinopathies associated with sickling can produce ischemia and infarction in multiple organs by occlusion of small vessels; however, the heart is relatively resistant.[345] Nonetheless, the combination of chronic hypoxemia and anemia produces a chronic high-output state that leads to congestive heart failure in many adults. The cardiovascular system can also be compromized by systemic hypertension from renal infarction, pulmonary embolism and infarction (the chest pain of which often causes concern about myocardial ischemia), pulmonary hypertension,[346] stroke, and hemosiderosis from chronic transfusions. In addition to a hyperdynamic congestive failure, iron overload is the principal risk to the myocardium in other causes of decreased erythrocyte production *(thalassemias)* and increased erythrocyte consumption *(hemolytic anemias)* requiring repeated transfusions.

Treatment with daily injections of deferoxamine can, if begun early, prevent the development of severe cardiac and hepatic disease.[347] Development of an oral iron chelator would greatly improve compliance and efficacy. Combined heart-liver transplantation has been used in a case of end-stage organ failure with homozygous β-thalassemia.[348]

Mucopolysaccharidoses and Disorders of Targeting Lysosomal Enzymes

Many of the specific disorders in these two groups share phenotypic manifestations and are caused by various defects in the ability of lysosomes to catabolize proteoglycan and glycosaminoglycan. Short stature, progressive coarsening of facial features, a skeletal dysplasia termed dysostosis multiplex, corneal clouding, and protean effects on the cardiovascular system are common[349–353] (Fig. 49–11). Only MPS IS (Scheie syndrome), the mild form of MPS IH (mild Hunter syndrome), MPS IV (Morquio syndrome), and MPS VI (Maroteaux-Lamy syndrome) have minimal or no mental impairment.

CARDIOVASCULAR MANIFESTATIONS. The cardiovascular complications (Table 49–12), which are all progressive and usually insidious, arise from engorgement of cells and tissues with macromolecular storage material.[354] First, the ventricular walls become pseudohypertrophic, and systolic function gradually deteriorates. The electrocardiogram shows reduced QRS voltages; rarely is any conduction disturbance present. Second, coronary arteries narrow because of intimal and medial thickening.[355] Myocardial infarction is common in MPS IH and the severe form of MPS II, although the patients are usually too retarded to complain of classic symptoms, and the diagnosis is made post mortem.[356] Third, valve leaflets thicken and cause progressive dysfunction that is oddly specific for individual disorders. For example, aortic stenosis is common in MPS IS, and mitral regurgitation is found frequently in MPS IH and MPS IV. Finally, narrowing of the upper and middle airways causes obstructive apnea, chronic hy-

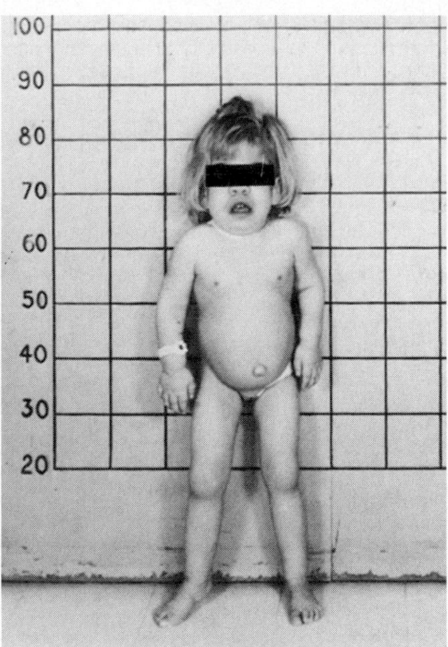

FIGURE 49–11. **The Hurler syndrome in a 4-year-old girl. Note short stature and coarse facial features.**

poxemia and hypercarbia, pulmonary hypertension, and eventually cor pulmonale.[357,358]

MANAGEMENT. Until recently, treatment of children with those conditions that caused mental retardation has been supportive. Increasing experience with bone marrow transplantation in many of the conditions shows that, in the relatively few survivors of the transplant, somatic accumulation of mucopolysaccharide can be reduced, with clinical improvement in cardiopulmonary function.[349,359,360] However, improvement of central nervous system function has been marginal or absent. Nonetheless, bone marrow transplantation may have a role, especially in MPS IV and MPS VI, in which cardiopulmonary compromise can greatly shorten otherwise productive lives. Attempts at cardiovascular surgery, indeed of any procedure requiring general anesthesia, are fraught with risks of difficult intubation, hyperextension of the neck with cervical cord damage (the odontoid process is often hypoplastic), and prolonged efforts to wean from mechanical ventilation.[357]

Sphingolipidoses

FABRY DISEASE (see also p. 1678). This X-linked condition deserves comment because the diagnosis is often not made until adulthood when serious end-organ damage has occurred.[12,361] As a result of deficiency of α-galactosidase A, ceramide trihexoside and other glycosphingolipids accumulate in lysosomes of many cells and organs, especially endothelial cells, glomerular and tubular cells of the kidney, and the heart. Microangiopathy causes the characteristic skin lesion, angiokeratoma, and may contribute, along with primary nerve involvement, to acroparesthesias and painful crises. Proteinuria and hypertension precede renal failure, which often has led to death in males and often leads by the fourth decade to the necessity for long-term dialysis or renal transplantation. A successful kidney allograft does not correct the systemic metabolic defect,[362] and the disease usually progresses in other organs.[349]

CARDIAC MANIFESTATIONS. Structural and functional cardiac involvement is similar qualitatively to that in the mucopolysaccharidoses. Thickening of the myocardium is pseudohypertrophy from deposition of glycosphingolipid in lysosomes; the diagnosis has been made by endocardial biopsy during the evaluation of unexplained ventricular hypertrophy or frank obstructive cardiomyopathy.[364,365] Chronic hypertension can exaggerate left ventricular dysfunction, as can ischemia and infarction from diffuse luminal narrowing of the coronary arteries. Two-dimensional echocardiography is useful for serial documentation of myocardial function.[366] Although valvular thickening and MVP are common, hemodynamically important mitral regurgitation is not.[366,367] The pulmonary vasculature becomes narrowed and right-sided pressures rise, but cor pulmonale is rarely a problem. The electrocardiogram often shows a shortened P-R interval, increased left ventricular voltages, and dysrhythmia. Medium-sized arteries throughout the body develop luminal narrowing, with cerebrovascular disease the most common cause of death after renal failure.

Heterozygous females generally show some clinical manifestations, especially in the eye, and at much later ages than hemizygous males develop renal, cerebrovascular, and cardiac disease.[12,366–368] Prenatal diagnosis is possible, and a detailed family history and genetic counseling are essential whenever the disease is found. A variety of mutations occur in the gene for α-galactosidase A and account for the clinical variability.[365,369]

Familial Amyloidoses

(See also p. 1427)

A variety of disorders, defined initially by clinical phenotype and due to progressive accumulation of amyloid in organs and tissues, are beginning to be categorized by the underlying biochemical and genetic defects.[370] The several conditions termed familial amyloidosis with polyneuropathy, and originally classified as separate autosomal dominant disorders, are now known to be due to different mutations in the same gene encoding transthyretin, a thyroxine- and retinol-binding protein also called prealbumin. Although polyneuropathy dominates the early course during young adulthood, renal failure and restrictive cardiomyopathy supervene later and cause death in most cases. The age of onset, severity, and predilection for kidney and cardiac involvement are determined by the type of mutation, with males affected earlier and more severely.[371–374]

Liver transplatation can prevent progression of the disease and potentially reverse some tissue accumulation[375]; when the myocardium is severely infiltrated, combined liver-heart transplant offers the only hope.

NEUROMUSCULAR DISORDERS

(See Chap. 60)

CARDIAC TUMORS

(See Chap. 42)

The three most common tumors that originate in the heart are myxomas, fibromas, and rhabdomyomas. All occur as part of hereditary syndromes and as sporadic events. The new occurrence of any of these tumors, especially in a child, may represent the first manifestation of a systemic condition, so a detailed general examination and family history are always indicated.[376,377] For example, 51 to 86 per cent of cardiac rhabdomyomas occur because of tuberous sclerosis.[378] Tumors due to hereditary disorders tend to be multiple and to recur after resection. An example is the NAME syndrome (see p. 1468) (for *n*evi, *a*trial myxoma, *m*yxoid neurofibromata, and *e*phelides, although the acronym ignores the multiple endocrine tumors), in which multiple myxoma can occur throughout the myocardium.[379–381]

INHERITED DISORDERS OF THE CIRCULATION

Hereditary Hemorrhagic Telangiectasia

This autosomal dominant condition, often called Osler-Rendu-Weber disease, is more common than appreciated. Because of marked intrafamilial and interfamilial variability, the condition may go undiagnosed in affected patients for years despite mild manifestations.[382,383] Mucocutaneous telangiectases, 0.5 to 3 mm in diameter, occur on the tongue, lips, and fingertips most commonly (Fig. 2–4, p. 17). Small and moderate-sized arteriovenous fistulas occur in the nose, leading to recurrent epistaxis, in the gastrointestinal system, where they cause recurrent bleeding and occult anemia, and in the lung, resulting in hypoxemia, hemoptysis, polycythemia, clubbing, paradoxical embolization through the right-to-left shunt, and a hyperdynamic circulation. Less common sites of vascular malformations are the brain,[384] liver,[385] and the kidney.[386] Diffuse ectasia of the coronary arteries was noted in one patient.[387] Bleeding is facilitated, even in the presence of normal platelet function and clotting function, because of the lack of resistance channels in the telangiectatic lesions.[388]

Patients with HHT, and their close relatives should be screened for pulmonary arteriovenous malformations through auscultation, arterial blood gas analysis, and chest radiography. A low arterial pO_2 should prompt consideration of angiography and therapeutic balloon occlusion of the feeding arteries of any sizable malformation to prevent systemic embolization, especially to the brain.[389] In a few patients, epistaxis and gastrointestinal blood loss have been reduced by antifibrinolytic therapy with danazol or aminocaproic acid.[390,392] Controlled trials of various approaches to chronic management, taking into account clinical and genetic variables, are sorely needed.

At least three genes are capable of causing HHT and two have been mapped, to 9q33-q34 and to 3p22.[393,394] The former locus encodes a transforming growth factor-β binding protein called endoglin, and a variety of mutations segregate with HHT in different families.[395] Thus, by mutation detection or linkage analysis, presymptomatic and prenatal diagnosis is available to a large number of patients with a potentially life-threatening disorder.

Von Hippel–Lindau Syndrome

The features of this autosomal dominant condition involve malformations and abnormal growth of small blood vessels. Retinal angioma, hemangioblastoma of the cerebellum, and hemangioma of the spinal cord occur in association with renal cell carcinoma, pancreatic and epididymal cystadenomas, and pheochromocytoma.[396,397] Secondary hypertension due to renal disease and pheochromocytoma, which is often bilateral, occurs and predisposes to subarachnoid hemorrhage. The cause is a tumor suppressor gene located on the short arm of chromosome 3. Patients inherit a germline mutation (and there is great diversity among families in the actual mutations) that is present in all cells. When a somatic mutation in the normal allele occurs in a susceptible cell, such as in the renal parenchyma or adrenal medulla, the cell becomes functionally homozygous for a lack of the gene product, and the cascade toward neoplasia is initiated.[398] How this gene product stimulates or permits angiomatous malformations is unclear.

Disorders Primarily Affecting Arteries

Mendelian disorders are associated with a diverse array of arterial pathology, and some have been described or catalogued earlier in this chapter. This section deals with two categories of disorders caused by a single mutant gene: pleiotropic syndromes better known for affecting organ systems other than the vasculature, and primary abnormalities of arteries.

ADULT POLYCYSTIC KIDNEY DISEASE (APKD). In the United States, this relatively common autosomal dominant disease affects 0.5 million people and accounts for 8 to 10 per cent of all long-term hemodialysis in the United States. Development of renal cysts is age dependent, and presymptomatic detection of heterozygotes, even by ultrasonography, can be uncertain into adulthood.[399,400] About one-half of patients are hypertensive, one-half have hepatic cysts, one-half eventually develop severe renal failure, and an unknown (but probably high) fraction have colonic diverticula. Elevated plasma renin levels contribute to hypertension long before renal failure occurs.[401] The cardiovascular manifestations include MVP in one-quarter, mild dilatation of the aortic root, occasional thoracic and abdominal aneurysms, and a predisposition to regurgitation of the aortic, mitral, and tricuspid valves.[402–404] The association of diverticula, organ cysts, and cardiovascular lesions reminiscent of, but milder than, the Marfan syndrome suggests some involvement of the extracellular matrix.

The most serious vascular problem is typical "berry" aneurysms of the cerebral circulation, which occur in about 10 per cent of heterozygotes but may remain asymptomatic throughout life. Hypertension predisposes to subarachnoid hemorrhage. How to screen for and treat intracranial aneurysms in patients without neurological symptoms remains controversial. Cerebral angiography carries higher risks in patients with APKD because of dissection and heightened vascular reactivity.[405] Magnetic resonance imaging detects most saccular aneurysms down to 2 to 3 mm in diameter. Whether to attempt prophylactic repair when a small aneurysm is detected has not been investigated systematically. Without question, aggressive blood pressure control is indicated in any patient with APKD.

At least three genes cause APKD. Most cases are due to mutations in a gene called *PBP* at the *PKD1* locus (16p13.3); the function of this gene is unclear.[406] In most of the rest of families, the disease maps to the *PKD2* locus in the region 4q13-q23.[407] Families affected by mutations in *PKD2* tend to develop renal failure later and have a milder course.[399] A French-Canadian family with disease typical of *PKD1* is unlinked to either locus, indicating that a *PKD3* gene exists.[408]

ARTERIOHEPATIC DYSPLASIA. An autosomal dominant disorder of marked variability, *Alagille syndrome* causes neonatal jaundice due to aplasia of intrahepatic bile ducts and congestive heart failure in the most severely affected infants but may be asymptomatic in heterozygous relatives.[409,410] The cardiovascular findings include peripheral pulmonic and systemic arterial stenoses in the majority, occasionally associated with septal defects or patent ductus arteriosus. Renal disease may produce hypertension. In some cases, a small deletion of the short arm of chromosome 20 involving the region p12.3-p11.23 occurs, suggesting that this complex phenotype is a contiguous gene deletion syndrome.[5]

ARTERIAL ANEURYSM, ECTASIA, OR DISSECTION. Pedigrees abound in which dilatation of the aortic root, aneurysm of the abdominal aorta, aortic dissection without dilatation, or a combination of these problems occurs in an autosomal dominant pattern without evidence of a recognized heritable disorder of connective tissue.[411–413] Because of the variable presentation and natural history of the aortic disease, presymptomatic detection of presumed heterozygotes is uncertain, as is reassurance of relatives at risk who are of childbearing age and would prefer not to pass this condition to offspring.

The association of dissection of the ascending aorta with bicuspid aortic valve is well known, although the cause and pathogenesis remain unclear. In such cases, the aortic wall shows abnormalities of elastic fibers.[414] A person with a congenitally bicuspid aortic valve should be screened for dilatation of the aortic root, and first-degree relatives should be screened for both lesions. This recommendation is based, in part, on bicuspid aortic valve being a congenital heart defect of the left-sided flow category, with a relatively high recurrence risk (see p. 964).

Until recently, no basic defects had been identified. In two families with autosomal dominant transmission of arterial aneurysms and mild increased skin fragility and bruisability, different mutations in the gene encoding type III procollagen occurred.[415,416] Thus, depending on the mutation, deficiency of type III collagen can cause the classic syndrome of Ehlers-Danlos type IV (see p. 1672) or a form of the much subtler but just as deadly syndrome, familial arterial rupture. For these families in which the mutations have been defined, reliable presymptomatic and prenatal diagnoses are at hand. However, suggestions that mutations in type III collagen would account for the majority of aortic aneurysms, including abdominal aneurysms in the elderly, have proven unfounded.[417]

A predisposition to cervical arterial dissection in young people was found to be associated with diffuse lentiginosis in several families, with a suggestion of autosomal recessive inheritance.[418] There also is an association between cervical dissection and intracranial hemorrhage.[419]

Formal genetic analysis of 91 families ascertained through a proband with abdominal aortic aneurysm suggests that an autosomal recessive predisposition exists for late-onset aneurysms.[420] This study provides a rationale for offering ultrasound screening to sibs of patients with abdominal aortic dilatation.

FAMILIAL ARTERIAL TORTUOSITY. This is a rare, possibly autosomal recessive, condition of unknown cause. Diffuse ectasia of all systemic arteries occurs with, paradoxically, peripheral pulmonic stenoses.[421]

FAMILIAL INTRACRANIAL HEMORRHAGE. In addition to adult polycystic kidney disease, three syndromes predispose to subarachnoid or cerebral hemorrhage. *Berry aneurysms* without pleiotropic manifestations in other organs are a rare, but well documented, autosomal dominant trait.[422] A defect in type III collagen was suggested by linkage analysis, but sequence analysis of the gene in 55 unrelated patients found no mutations.[423]

The *cerebral arterial type of familial amyloidosis* (type VI) is an autosomal dominant condition due to a defect in the proteinase inhibitor cystatin C.[424] This disease is rare outside of Iceland and Holland. The walls of cerebral arteries are thickened by a material resembling amyloid, and the vessels become tortuous and fragile. Recurrent cerebral hemorrhage is common in the fifth and sixth decades.[425]

Familial hemangiomas have been reported infrequently to occur as an autosomal dominant condition.[426] The brain and retina are the principal sites of vascular malformation, although in some pedigrees, cutaneous lesions occur. The intracranial hemangioma can be large and present with varied neurological symptoms, including hemorrhage.

FAMILIAL ARTERIAL OCCLUSIVE DISEASES. *Fibromuscular dysplasia* of the renal and other arteries occurs in *von Recklinghausen neurofibromatosis,* and along with pheochromocytoma can be a cause of hypertension.[427,428] Severe deficiency of α_1-antiprotease is another cause of fibromuscular dysplasia.[429] The arterial lesion can occur by itself in families and produce stroke, myocardial infarction, intermittent claudication, and hypertension at young ages ranging down to childhood.[430] Inheritance is most consistent with autosomal dominance.[431]

Familial hypoplasia of the carotid arteries,[432] *familial arteriopathy* caused by concentric thickening of systemic and pulmonic arteries,[433] and generalized *arterial calcification of infancy*[434] are all rare, possibly mendelian, syndromes of unknown cause.

FAMILIAL HEMIPLEGIC MIGRAINE. The migraine syndrome is commonly familial and occurs in multiple generations. A severe form, associated with recurrent hemiplegia, is inherited as an autosomal dominant trait and maps to the short arm of chromosome 9.[435] However, some families with hemiplegic migraine, and others with simple migraine, are unlinked to this locus.[436,437] In the same region of 19p is a locus causing autosomal dominant cerebral arteriopathy with subcortical infarcts.[438] Whether the two conditions are related through allelism is unclear.

FAMILIAL PULMONARY HYPERTENSION (see also p. 783). Primary pulmonary hypertension is occasionally familial.[439–441] Inheritance is most consistent with an autosomal dominant predisposition with sex influence favoring expression in females. The cause is unknown, but molecular defects favoring recurrent microemboli to the pulmonary circulation afford one area to explore.

Pulmonary hypertension can occur in *neurofibromatosis* due to pulmonary fibrosis.[442]

Disorders Primarily Affecting Veins

VARICOSE VEINS. Although a familial susceptibility to varicosities of the lower extremity clearly exists, and favors women in a ratio of 2:1, mendelian inheritance has not been confirmed. *Marfan syndrome,* various *Ehlers-Danlos syndromes,* and an autosomal recessive condition featuring distichiasis (a double row of eyelashes)[443] predispose to varicose veins.

ATRETIC VEINS. Some patients with the *Klippel-Trenaunay-Weber syndrome* of cutaneous hemangioma and hemihypertrophy have atresia of the deep venous system.[444] The concomitant superficial varicosities should not be stripped, lest the remaining venous drainage of the lower extremity be removed. This is a confusing syndrome that overlaps with several others; mendelian inheritance is uncertain. Renal arterial aneurysm and hemangioma occurred in one patient.[445]

CAVERNOUS ANGIOMAS. Cavernous angiomas represent at least 15 per cent of vascular malformations of the central nervous system, and familial occurrence is increasingly recognized.[446–450] These are not arteriovenous malformations, but primarily a tortuous collection of veins. Seizure is the most common presenting feature, followed by headache, stroke, and progressive neurologic deficit. Magnetic resonance (T_2-weighted) imaging is the procedure of choice because it is sensitive, and arteriography is not likely to detect the venous malformation. In some families, hepatic angiomas are an important feature.[451] At least one locus has been mapped.[452–453]

Disorders Primarily Affecting Lymphatics

Several forms of *hereditary lymphedema* exist, with the best studied inherited as autosomal dominants.[8] An early-onset form bears the eponym *Nonne-Milroy lymphedema* and can cause a protein-losing enteropathy and pleural effusion. *Meige lymphedema* does not appear until about the time of puberty and is most severe in the legs, although one family with late-onset edema had involvement of the arms and face.[454] The occurrence of lymphangiosarcoma in congenital[455] and late-onset lymphedema[456] suggests a predisposition to malignancy.

GENETIC FACTORS PREDISPOSING TO ATHEROSCLEROSIS

(See also Chap. 35)

A variety of genetic factors, in addition to the well-studied errors of lipid metabolism, clearly predispose to atherosclerosis. Few genes outside of those involved in lipid metabolism have such an overwhelming impact as to be identifiable from the family history. However, genes that predispose to hypertension and diabetes mellitus, control arterial diameter, reactivity, and branching angles, affect platelet adhesiveness, thrombosis, and fibrinolysis, and regulate endothelial and smooth muscle function can all be considered candidate genes for study in families predisposed to atherosclerosis.[457–459]

ESSENTIAL HYPERTENSION

(See also Chap. 26)

Blood pressure is a quantifiable trait that shows continuous variation within the population. Although many genes and environmental factors undoubtedly affect a person's

pathic dilated and hypertrophic cardiomyopathy: A population-based study in Olmsted County, Minnesota, 1975–1984. Circulation *80*:564, 1989.

165. Kelly, D. P., and Strauss, A. W.: Inherited cardiomyopathies. N. Engl. J. Med. *330*:913, 1994.
166. Dec, G. W., and Fuster, V.: Idiopathic dilated cardiomyopathy. N. Engl. J. Med. *331*:1564, 1994.
167. Manolio, T. A., Baughman, K. L., Rodeheffer, R., et al.: Prevalence and etiology of idiopathic dilated cardiomyopathy. Am. J. Cardiol. *69*:1458, 1992.
168. Michels, V. V., Moll, P. P., Miller, F. A., et al.: The frequency of familial dilated cardiomyopathy in a series of patients with idiopathic dilated cardiomyopathy. N. Engl. J. Med. *326*:77, 1992.
169. Fragola, P. V., Autore, C., Picelli, A., et al.: Familial idiopathic dilated cardiomyopathy. Am. Heart J. *115*:912, 1988.
170. Valantine, H. A., Hunt, S. A., Fowler, M. B., et al.: Frequency of familial nature of dilated cardiomyopathy and usefulness of cardiac transplantation in this subset. Am. J. Cardiol. *63*:959, 1989.
171. Graber, H. L., Unverferth, D. V., Baker, P. B., et al.: Evolution of a hereditary cardiac conduction and muscle disorder: A study involving a family with six generations affected. Circulation *74*:21, 1986.
172. Gardner, R. J. M., Hanson, J. W., Ionasescu, V. V., et al.: Dominantly inherited dilated cardiomyopathy. Am. J. Med. Genet. *27*:61, 1987.
173. Maclennan, B. A., Tsoi, E. Y., Maguire, C., et al.: Familial idiopathic congestive cardiomyopathy in three generations: A family study with eight affected members. Q. J. Med. *63*:335, 1987.
174. Schmidt, M. A., Michels, V. V., Edwards, W. D., et al.: Familial dilated cardiomyopathy. Am. J. Med. Genet. *31*:135, 1988.
175. Goldblatt, J., Melmed, J., and Rose, A. G.: Autosomal recessive inheritance of idiopathic dilated cardiomyopathy in a Madeira Portuguese kindred. Clin. Genet. *31*:249, 1987.
176. Caforio, A. L. P., Rossi, B., and Risaliti, R.: Type 1 fiber abnormalities in skeletal muscle of patients with hypertrophic and dilated cardiomyopathy: Evidence of subclinical myogenic myopathy. J. Am. Coll. Cardiol. *14*:1464, 1989.
177. Michels, V. M., Pastores, G. M., Moll, P. P., et al.: Dystrophin analysis in idiopathic dilated cardiomyopathy. J. Med. Genet. *30*:955, 1993.
178. Urie, P. M., and Billingham, M. E.: Ultrastructural features of familial cardiomyopathy. Am. J. Cardiol. *62*:325, 1988.
179. Voss, E. G., Reddy, C. V. R., Detrano, R., et al.: Familial dilated cardiomyopathy. Am. J. Cardiol. *54*:456, 1984.
180. Kass, S., McRae, C., Graber, H. L., et al.: A gene defect that causes conduction system disease and dilated cardiomyopathy maps to chromosome 1p1-q1. Nature Genet. *7*:546, 1994.
181. Barth, P. G., Scholte, J. A., Berden, J. A., et al.: An X-linked mitochondrial disease affecting cardiac muscle, skeletal muscle and neutrophil leukocytes. J. Neurol. Sci. *62*:327, 1983.
182. Christodoulou, J., McInnes, R. R., Jay, V., et al.: Barth syndrome: Clinical observations and genetic linkage studies. Am. J. Med. Genet. *50*:255, 1994.
183. Worton, R. G., and Brooke, M. H.: The X-linked muscular dystrophies. *In* Scriver, C. R., Beaudet, A. L., Sly, W. A., and Valle, D. (eds.): The Metabolic and Molecular Bases of Inherited Disease. New York, McGraw-Hill, 1995, p. 4195.
184. Melacini, P., Fanin, M., Danieli, G. A., et al.: Cardiac involvement in Becker muscular dystrophy. J. Am. Coll. Cardiol. *22*:1927, 1993.
185. Muntoni, F., Cau, M., Ganau, A., et al.: Deletion of the dystrophin muscle-promoter region associated with X-linked dilated cardiomyopathy. N. Engl. J. Med. *329*:921, 1993.
186. Towbin, J. A., Hejtmancik, J. F., Brink, P., et al.: X-linked dilated cardiomyopathy: Molecular genetic evidence of linkage to the Duchenne muscular dystrophy (dystrophin) gene at the Xp21 locus. Circulation *87*:1854, 1993.
187. Fishbein, M. C., Siegel, R. J., Thompson, C. E., et al.: Sudden death of a carrier of X-linked Emery-Dreifuss muscular dystrophy. Ann. Intern. Med. *119*:900, 1993.
188. Bione, S., Maestrini, E., Rivella, S., et al.: Identification of a novel X-linked gene responsible for Emery-Dreifuss muscular dystrophy. Nature Genet. *8*:323, 1994.
189. Östavik, K. H., Skjörten, F., Hellebostad, M., et al.: Possible X-linked congenital mitochondrial cardiomyopathy in three families. J. Med. Genet. *30*:269, 1993.
190. Aroney, C., Bett, N., and Radford, D.: Familial restrictive cardiomyopathy. Aust. N. Z. J. Med. *18*:877, 1988.
191. Fitzpatrick, A. P., Shapiro, L. M., Richards, A. F., et al.: Familial restrictive cardiomyopathy with atrioventricular block and skeletal myopathy. Br. Heart J. *63*:114, 1990.
192. Hodgson, S., Child, A., and Dyson, M.: Endocardial fibroelastosis: Possible X-linked inheritance. J. Med. Genet. *24*:210, 1987.
193. Opitz, J. M.: Genetic aspects of endocardial fibroelastosis. Am. J. Med. Genet. *11*:92, 1982.
194. Devi, A. S., Eisenfeld, L., Uphoff, D., et al.: New syndrome of hydrocephalus, endocardial fibroelastosis, and cataracts (HEC) syndrome. Am. J. Med. Genet. *56*:62, 1995.
195. Ross, R. S., Bulkley, B. H., Hutchins, G. M., et al.: Idiopathic familial myocardiopathy in three generations: A clinical and pathologic study. Am. Heart J. *96*:170, 1978.
196. Voorhees, M. L., Hussan, G. S., and Blackman, M. S.: Growth failure with pericardial constriction: The syndrome of mulibrey nanism. Am. J. Dis. Child. *130*:1146, 1976.
197. Martinez-Lavin, M., Buendia, A., Delgado, E., et al.: A familial syndrome of pericarditis, arthritis and camptodactyly. N. Engl. J. Med. *309*:224, 1983.
198. Laxer, R. M., Cameron, B. J., Chaisson, D., et al.: The camptodactyly-arthropathy-pericarditis syndrome: Case report and literature review. Arthritis Rheum. *29*:439, 1986.
199. Bulutlar, G., Yazici, H., Ozdogan, H., et al.: A familial syndrome of pericarditis, arthritis, camptodactyly, and coxa vara. Arthritis Rheum. *29*:436, 1986.
200. Fitzpatrick, A. P., and Emanuel, R. W.: Familial neurofibromatosis and hypertrophic cardiomyopathy. Br. Heart J. *60*:247, 1988.
201. Sommer, A., Contras, S. B., Craenen, J. M., et al.: A family study of the LEOPARD syndrome. Am. J. Dis. Child. *121*:520, 1971.
202. St. John Sutton, M. G., Tajik, A. J., Giuliani, E. R., et al.: Hypertrophic obstructive cardiomyopathy and lentiginosis: A little known neural ectodermal syndrome. Am. J. Cardiol. *47*:214, 1981.
203. Marks, M. L., and Keating, M. T.: Familial dysrhythmias. *In* Rimoin, D. L., Connor, J. M., and Pyeritz, R. E. (eds.): Principles and Practice of Medical Genetics. 3rd ed. New York, Churchill Livingstone, 1995.

DISORDERS OF RHYTHM AND CONDUCTION

204. Gambetta, M., Weese, J., Ginsburg, M., et al.: Sick sinus syndrome in a patient with familial PR prolongation. Chest *64*:520, 1973.
205. Surawicz, B., and Hariman, R. J.: Follow-up of the family with congenital absence of sinus rhythm. Am. J. Cardiol. *61*:467, 1988.
206. Balderston, S. M., Shaffer, E. M., Sondheimer, H. M., et al.: Hereditary atrioventricular conduction defect in a child. Pediatr. Cardiol. *10*:37, 1989.
207. Wolkowicz, J., and Burgess, J. H.: Complete heart block in an Inuit family. Can. J. Cardiol. *4*:352, 1988.
208. Stephan, E.: Hereditary bundle branch system defect: Survey of a family with four affected generations. Am. Heart J. *95*:89, 1978.
209. Lorber, A., Maisuls, E., and Naschitz, J.: Hereditary right axis deviation: Electrocardiographic pattern of pseudo left posterior hemiblock and incomplete right bundle branch block. Int. J. Cardiol. *20*:399, 1988.
210. Van Der Merwe, P.-L., Weymar, H. W., Torrington, M., et al.: Progressive familial heart block (type I): A follow up study after 10 years. S. Afr. Med. J. *73*:275, 1988.
211. Torrington, M., Weymar, H. W., van der Merwe, P.-L., et al.: Progressive familial heart block: Pt I. Extent of the disease. S. Afr. Med. J. *70*:354, 1986.
212. Kothari, S. S., Agrawal, S. M., and Kirshnaswami, S.: Familial complete heart block in hypertrophic cardiomyopathy. Int. J. Cardiol. *20*:294, 1988.
213. Stables, R. H., Bailey, C., and Ormerod, O. J. M.: Idiopathic familial atrial cardiomyopathy with diffuse conduction block. Q. J. Med. *264*:325, 1989.
214. Olofsson, B.-V., Eriksson, P., and Eriksson, A.: The sick sinus syndrome in familial amyloidosis with polyneuropathy. Int. J. Cardiol. *4*:71, 1983.
215. Winkler, R. B., Nora, A. H., and Nora, J. J.: Familial congenital complete heart block and maternal systemic lupus erythematosus. Circulation *56*:1103, 1977.
216. McCue, C. M., Mantakas, M. E., Tingelstad, J. B., et al.: Congenital heart block in newborns of mothers with connective tissue disease. Circulation *56*:82, 1977.
217. Chameides, L., Truex, R. C., Vetter, V., et al.: Association of maternal systemic lupus erythematosus with congenital complete heart block. N. Engl. J. Med. *297*:1204, 1977.
218. Scott, J. S., Maddison, P. J., Taylor, P. V., et al.: Connective-tissue disease, antibodies to ribonucleoprotein, and congenital heart block. N. Engl. J. Med. *309*:209, 1983.
219. Lockshin, M. D., Gibofsky, A., Peebles, C. L., et al.: Neonatal lupus erythematosus with heart block: Familial study of a patient with anti-SS-A and SS-B antibodies. Arthritis Rheum. *26*:210, 1983.
220. Bergfeldt, L., and Möller, E.: Complete heart block—another HLA B27 associated disease manifestation. Tissue Antigens *21*:385, 1983.
221. Bergfeldt, L., Vallin, H., and Edhag, O.: Complete heart block in HLA B27 associated disease. Electrophysiological and clinical characteristics. Br. Heart J. *51*:184, 1984.
222. Bacos, J. M., Eagan, J. T., and Orgain, E. S.: Congenital familial nodal rhythm. Circulation *22*:887, 1960.
223. Gault, J. H., Cantwell, J., Lev, M., et al.: Fetal familial cardiac arrhythmias. Am. J. Cardiol. *29*:548, 1972.
224. Chia, B. L., Yew, F. C., Chay, S. O., et al.: Familial Wolff-Parkinson-White syndrome. J. Electrocardiol. *15*:195, 1982.
225. Vidaillet, H. J., Pressley, J. C., Henke, E., et al.: Familial occurrence of accessory atrioventricular pathways: Preexcitation syndrome. N. Engl. J. Med. *317*:65, 1987.
226. Stoll, C., Kieny, J.-R., Dott, B., et al.: Ventricular extrasystoles with syncopal episodes, perodactyly, and Robin sequence in three generations: A new inherited MCA syndrome? Am. J. Med. Genet. *42*:480, 1992.
227. Laurent, M., Descases, C., Biron, Y., et al.: Familial form of arrhythmogenic right ventricular dysplasia. Am. Heart J. *113*:827, 1987.
228. Ruder, M. A.., Winston, S. A., Davis, J. C., et al.: Arrhythmogenic right ventricular dysplasia in a family. Am. J. Cardiol. *56*:799, 1985.
229. Wiesfeld, A. C. P., Crijns, J. G. M., Van Dijk, R. B., et al.: Potential role for endomyocardial biopsy in the clinical characterization of patients with idiopathic ventricular fibrillation. Am. Heart J. *127*:1421, 1993.
230. McKenna, W. J., Thiene, G., Nava, A., et al.: Diagnosis of arrhythmo-

genic right ventricular dysplasia/cardiomyopathy. Br. Heart J. *72*:215, 1994.
231. Ward, O. C.: A new familial cardiac syndrome in children. J. Ir. Med. Assoc. *54*:103, 1964.
232. Romano, C.: Congenital cardiac arrhythmia. Lancet *1*:658, 1965.
233. Greenspon, A. J., Kidwell, G. A., Barrasse, L. D., et al.: Hereditary long QT syndrome associated with cardiac conduction system disease. PACE *12*:479, 1989.
234. Marks, M. L., Whisler, S. L., Clericuzio, C., et al.: A new form of long QT syndrome associated with syndactyly. J. Am. Coll. Cardiol. *25*:59, 1995.
235. Keating, M., Atkinson, D., Dunn, C., et al.: Linkage of a cardiac arrhythmia, the long QT syndrome and Harvey *ras*-1 gene. Science *252*:704, 1991.
236. Jiang, C., Atkinson, D., Towbin, J. A., et al.: Two long QT syndrome loci map to chromosome 3 and 7 with evidence for future heterogeneity. Nature Genet. *8*:141, 1994.
237. Vincent, G. M., Timothy, K. W., Leppert, M., et al.: The spectrum of symptoms and QT intervals in carriers of the gene for the long-QT syndrome. N. Engl. J. Med. *327*:846, 1992.
238. Jervell, A., and Lange-Nielsen, F.: Congenital deaf-mutism, functional heart disease with prolongation of Q-T interval and sudden death. Am. Heart J. *54*:59, 1957.
239. Fraser, G. R., Froggatt, P., and Murphy, T.: Genetical aspects of the cardioauditory syndrome of Jervell and Lange-Nielsen (congenital deafness and electrocardiographic abnormalities). Ann. Hum. Genet. *28*:133, 1964.
240. Till, J. A., Shinebourne, E. A., Pepper, J., et al.: Complete denervation of the heart in a child with congenital long QT and deafness. Am. J. Cardiol. *62*:1319, 1988.

DISORDERS OF CONNECTIVE TISSUE

241. McKusick, V. A.: Heritable Disorders of Connective Tissue. St. Louis, C. V. Mosby Co., 1956.
242. Royce, P. M., and Steinmann, B. (eds.): Connective Tissue and Its Heritable Disorders: Molecular, Genetic and Medical Aspects. New York, Wiley-Liss, 1993.
243. Pyeritz, R. E.: Heritable disorders of connective tissue. *In* Pierpont, M. E., and Moller, J. H. (eds.): The Genetics of Cardiovascular Disease. Boston, Martinus Nijhoff Publishing, 1987, p. 265.
244. Beighton, P. (ed.): McKusick's Heritable Disorders of Connective Tissue. 5th ed. St. Louis, C. V. Mosby Co., 1993.
245. Pyeritz, R. E.: Disorders of fibrillins and microfibrilogenesis: Marfan syndrome, MASS phenotype, contractural arachnodactyly and related conditions. *In* Rimoin, D. L., Connor, J. M., and Pyeritz, R. E. (eds.): Principles and Practice of Medical Genetics. 3rd ed. New York, Churchill Livingstone, 1996.
246. McKusick, V. A.: The cardiovascular aspects of Marfan's syndrome: A heritable disorder of connective tissue. Circulation *11*:321, 1955.
247. Pereira, L., Levran, O., Ramirez, F., et al.: A molecular approach to the stratification of cardiovascular risk in families with Marfan's syndrome. N. Engl. J. Med. *331*:148, 1994.
248. Marsalese, D. L., Moodie, D. S., Vacante, M., et al.: Marfan's syndrome: Natural history and long-term follow-up of cardiovascular involvement. J. Am. Coll. Cardiol. *14*:422, 1989.
249. Child, J. S., Perloff, J. K., and Kaplan, S.: The heart of the matter: Cardiovascular involvement in Marfan's syndrome. J. Am. Coll. Cardiol. *14*:429, 1989.
250. Murdoch, J. L., Walker, B. A., Halpern, B. L., et al.: Life expectancy and causes of death in the Marfan syndrome. N. Engl. J. Med. *286*:804, 1972.
251. Sisk, H. E., Zahka, K. G., and Pyeritz, R. E.: The Marfan syndrome in early childhood: Analysis of 15 patients diagnosed less than 4 years of age. Am. J. Cardiol. *52*:353, 1983.
252. Gross, D. M., Robinson, L. K., Smith, L. T., et al.: Severe perinatal Marfan syndrome. Pediatrics *84*:83, 1989.
253. Morse, R. P., Rockenmacher, S., Pyeritz, R. E., et al.: Diagnosis and management of Marfan syndrome in infants. Pediatrics *86*:888, 1990.
254. Pyeritz, R. E., and Wappel, M. A.: Mitral valve dysfunction in the Marfan syndrome. Am. J. Med. *74*:797, 1983.
255. Crawford, E. S., and Coselli, J. S.: Marfan's syndrome: Combined composite valve graft replacement of the aortic root and transaortic mitral valve replacement. Ann. Thorac. Surg. *45*:296, 1988.
256. Cohn, L. H., DiSesa, V. J., Couper, G. S., et al.: Mitral valve repair for myxomatous degeneration and prolapse of the mitral valve. J. Thorac. Cardiovasc. Surg. *98*:987, 1989.
257. Gillinov, A. M., Hulyalkar, A., Cameron, D. E., et al.: Mitral valve operation in patients with the Marfan syndrome. J. Thorac. Cardiovasc. Surg. *107*:724, 1994.
258. Gott, V. L., Cameron, D. E., Pyeritz, R. E., et al.: Composite graft repair of Marfan aneurysm of the ascending aorta: Results in 150 patients. J. Cardiovasc. Surg. *9*:482, 1994.
259. Lima, S. D., Lima, J. A. C., Pyeritz, R. E., et al.: Relationship of mitral valve prolapse to left ventricular size in Marfan's syndrome. Am. J. Cardiol. *55*:739, 1985.
260. Henry, W. L., Gardin, J. M., and Ware, J. H.: Echocardiographic measurements in normal subjects from infancy to old age. Circulation *62*:1054, 1980.
261. Roman, M. J., Rosen, S. E., Kramer-Fox, R., et al.: Prognostic significance of the pattern of aortic root dilation in the Marfan syndrome. J. Am. Coll. Cardiol. *22*:1470, 1993.
262. Crawford, E. S.: Marfan's syndrome: Broad spectral surgical treatment: cardiovascular manifestations. Ann. Surg. *198*:487, 1983.
263. Svensson, L. G., Crawford, E. S., Coselli, J. S., et al.: Impact of cardiovascular operation on survival in the Marfan patient. Circulation *80*:233, 1988.
264. Silverman, D. I., Burton, K. J., Gray, J., et al.: Life expectancy in the Marfan syndrome. Am. J. Cardiol. *75*:157, 1995.
265. Arn, P. H., Scherer, L. R., Haller, J. A., Jr., et al.: Outcome of pectus excavatum in patients with Marfan syndrome and in the general population. J. Pediatr. *115*:954, 1989.
266. deSanctis, R., Doroghazi, R. M., Austen, W. G., et al.: Aortic dissection. N. Engl. J. Med. *317*:1060, 1987.
267. Schaefer, S., Peshock, R. M., Malloy, C. R., et al.: Nuclear magnetic resonance imaging in Marfan's syndrome. J. Am. Coll. Cardiol. *9*:70, 1987.
268. Soulen, R. L., Fishman, E., Pyeritz, R. E., et al.: Evaluation of the Marfan syndrome: MR imaging versus CT. Radiology *165*:697, 1987.
269. Crawford, E. S., Crawford, J. L., Stowe, C. L., et al.: Total aortic replacement for chronic aortic dissection occurring in patients with and without Marfan's syndrome. Ann. Surg. *199*:358, 1984.
270. Shores, J., Berger, K. R., Murphy, E. A., et al.: Chronic β-adrenergic blockade protects the aorta in the Marfan syndrome: A prospective, randomized trial of propranolol. N. Engl. J. Med. *330*:1335, 1994.
271. Salim, M. A., Alpert, B. S., Ward, J. C., et al.: Effect of beta-adrenergic blockade on aortic root rate of dilation in the Marfan syndrome. Am. J. Cardiol. *74*:629, 1994.
272. Yin, F. C. P., Brin, K. P., Ting, C.-T., et al.: Arterial hemodynamics in the Marfan syndrome. Circulation *79*:854, 1989.
273. Pyeritz, R. E.: Maternal and fetal complications of pregnancy in the Marfan syndrome. Am. J. Med. *71*:784, 1981.
274. Rossiter, J. P., Morales, A. J., Repke, J. T., et al.: A prospective longitudinal evaluation of pregnancy in the Marfan syndrome. Am. J. Obstet. Gynecol. *173*:1599, 1995.
275. Hollister, D. W., Godfrey, M., Sakai, L. Y., et al.: Marfan syndrome: Immunohistologic abnormalities of the elastin-associated microfibrillar fiber system. N. Engl. J. Med. *323*:152, 1990.
276. Sakai, L. Y., Keene, D. R., and Engvall, E.: Fibrillin, a new 350-kD glycoprotein, is a component of extracellular microfibrils. J. Cell. Biol. *103*:2499, 1986.
277. Kainulainen, K., Pulkkinen, L., Savolainen, A., et al.: The gene defect causing Marfan syndrome is located on chromosome 15. N. Engl. J. Med. *323*:935, 1990.
278. Dietz, H. C., Pyeritz, R. E., Hall, B. D., et al.: The Marfan syndrome locus: Confirmations of assignment to chromosome 15 and identification of tightly linked markers at 15q15-q21.3. Genomics *9*:355, 1991.
279. Dietz, H. C., Cutting, G. R., Pyeritz, R. E., et al.: Marfan syndrome caused by a recurrent *de novo* missense mutation in the fibrillin gene. Nature *352*:337, 1991.
280. Dietz, H. C., McIntosh, I., Sakai, L. Y., et al.: Four novel FBN1 mutations: Significance for mutant transcript level and EGF-like domain calcium binding in the pathogenesis of Marfan syndrome. Genomics *17*:468, 1993.
281. Kielty, C. M., Rantamaki, T., Child, A. H., et al.: Cystein-to-arginine mutation in a 'hybrid' eight-cysteine domain of FBN1: Consequences for fibrillin aggregation and microfibril assembly. J. Med. Genet. *(in press)*.
282. Milewicz, D. M., Grossfield, J., Cao, S.-N., et al.: A mutation in *FBN1* disrupts profibrillin processing and results in isolated skeletal features of the Marfan syndrome. J. Clin. Invest. *95*:2373, 1995.
283. Francke, U., Berg, M. A., Tynan, K., et al.: A Gly1127Ser mutation in an EGF-like domain of the fibrillin-1 gene is a risk factor for ascending aortic aneurysm and dissection in the absence of the Marfan syndrome. Am. J. Hum. Genet. *56*:1287, 1995.
284. Milewicz, D. Mc. G., Pyeritz, R. E., Crawford, E. S., et al.: Marfan syndrome: Defective synthesis, secretion and extracellular matrix formation of fibrillin by cultured dermal fibroblasts. J. Clin. Invest. *89*:79, 1992.
285. Aoyama, T., Francke, U., Dietz, H., et al.: Quantitative differences in biosynthesis and extracellular deposition of fibrillin in cultured fibroblasts distinguish five groups of Marfan syndrome patients and suggest distinct pathogenetic mechanisms. J. Clin. Invest. *94*:130, 1994.
286. Leier, C. V., Call, T. D., Fulkerson, P. K., et al.: The spectrum of cardiac defects in the Ehlers-Danlos syndrome, types I and III. Ann. Intern. Med. *92*:171, 1980.
287. Fox, R., Pope, F. M., Narcisi, P., et al.: Spontaneous carotid cavernous fistula in Ehlers-Danlos syndrome. J. Neurol. Neurosurg. Psychiatry *51*:984, 1988.
288. Rudd, N. L., Nimrod, C., Holbrook, K. A., et al.: Pregnancy complications in type IV Ehlers-Danlos syndrome. Lancet *1*:50, 1983.
289. Viljoen, D. L., Pope, F. M., and Beighton, P.: Heterogeneity of pseudoxanthoma elasticum: Delineation of a new form? Clin. Genet. *32*:100, 1987.
290. Cunningham, J. R., Lippman, S. M., Renie, W. A., et al.: Pseudoxanthoma elasticum: Treatment of gastrointestinal hemorrhage by arterial embolization and observations of autosomal dominant inheritance. Johns Hopkins Med. J. *147*:168, 1980.
291. Lebwohl, M. G., Distefano, D., Prioleau, P. G., et al.: Pseudoxanthoma elasticum and mitral-valve prolapse. N. Engl. J. Med. *307*:228, 1982.

292. Pyeritz, R. E., Weiss, J. L., Renie, W. A., et al.: Pseudoxanthoma elasticum and mitral-valve prolapse. N. Engl. J. Med. *307:*1451, 1982.
293. Goodman, R. M., Smith, E. W., Paton, D., et al.: Pseudoxanthoma elasticum: A clinical and histopathological study. Medicine *42:*297, 1963.
294. Lebwohl, M., Halperin, J., and Phelps, R. G.: Occult pseudoxanthoma elasticum in patients with premature cardiovascular disease. N. Engl. J. Med. *329:*1237, 1993.
295. Challenor, V. F., Conway, N., and Monro, J. L.: The surgical treatment of restrictive cardiomyopathy in pseudoxanthoma elasticum. Br. Heart J. *59:*266, 1988.
296. Raybould, M. C., Birley, A. J., Moss, C., et al.: Exclusion of an elastin gene (ELN) mutation as the cause of pseudoxanthoma elasticum (PXE) in one family. Clin. Genet. *45:*48, 1994.
297. Renie, W. A., Pyeritz, R. E., Combs, J., et al.: Pseudoxanthoma elasticum: High calcium intake in early life correlates with severity. Am. J. Med. Genet. *19:*235, 1984.
298. Maharaj, B., Hammond, M. G., Appadoo, B., et al.: HLA-A, B, DR, and DQ antigens in black patients with severe chronic rheumatic heart disease. Circulation *76:*259, 1987.

INBORN ERRORS OF METABOLISM THAT AFFECT THE CARDIOVASCULAR SYSTEM

299. La Du, B. N.: Alkaptonuria: *In* Scriver, C. R., Beaudet, A. L., Sly, W. A., and Valle, D. (eds.): The Metabolic and Molecular Bases of Inherited Disease. New York, McGraw-Hill, 1995, p. 1371.
300. Mudd, S. H., Levy, H. L., and Skovby, F.: Disorders of transsulfuration. *In* Scriver, C. R., Beaudet, A. L., Sly, W. A., and Valle, D. (eds.): The Metabolic and Molecular Bases of Inherited Disease. New York, McGraw-Hill, 1995, p. 1279.
301. Mudd, S. H., Skovby, F., Levy, H. L., et al.: The natural history of homocystinuria due to cystathionine beta-synthase deficiency. Am. J. Hum. Genet. *37:*1, 1985.
302. Hill-Zobel, R. L., Pyeritz, R. E., Scheffel, U., et al.: Kinetics and biodistribution of ^{111}In-labeled platelets in homocystinuria. N. Engl. J. Med. *307:*781, 1982.
303. Selhub, J., Jacques, P. F., Bostom, A. G., et al.: Association between plasma homocysteine concentrations and extracranial carotid-artery stenosis. N. Engl. J. Med. *332:*286, 1995.
304. Kang, S.-S., Passen, E. L., Ruggie, N., et al.: Thermolabile defect of methylenetetrahydrofolate reductase in coronary artery disease. Circulation *88:*1463, 1993.
305. Rolland, P. H., Friggi, A., Barlatier, A., et al.: Hyperhomocysteinemia-induced vascular damage in the minipig captopril-hydrochlorothiazide combination prevents elastic alterations. Circulation *91:*1161, 1995.
306. Hajjar, K. A.: Homocysteine-induced modulation of tissue plasminogen activator binding to its endothelial cell membrane receptor. J. Clin. Invest. *91:*2873, 1993.
307. Majors, A., Ehrhart, L. A., Pezacka, E. H.: Homocysteine as a risk factor for vascular disease: Enhanced collagen production and accumulation by smooth muscle cells. Proc. Natl. Acad. Sci. USA *(in press)*.
308. Stampfer, M. J., and Manilow, M. R.: Can lowering homocysteine levels reduce cardiovascular risk? N. Engl. J. Med. *332:*328, 1995.
309. Roe, C. R., and Coates, P. M.: Mitochondrial fatty acid oxidation disorders. *In* Scriver, C. R., Beaudet, A. L., Sly, W. A., and Valle, D. (eds.): The Metabolic and Molecular Bases of Inherited Disease. New York, McGraw-Hill, 1995, p. 1501.
310. Rebouche, C. J., and Engel, A. G.: Carnitine metabolism and deficiency syndrome. Mayo Clin. Proc. *58:*533, 1983.
311. Treem, W. R., Stanley, C. A., Finegold, D. N., et al.: Primary carnitine deficiency due to a failure of carnitine transport in kidney, muscle, and fibroblasts. N. Engl. J. Med. *319:*1331, 1988.
312. Waber, L. J., Valle, D., Neill, C., et al.: Carnitine deficiency presenting as familial cardiomyopathy: A treatable defect in carnitine transport. J. Pediatr. *101:*700, 1982.
313. Tripp, M. E., Katcher, M. L., Peters, H. A., et al.: Systemic carnitine deficiency presenting as familial endocardial fibroelastosis. N. Engl. J. Med. *305:*385, 1981.
314. Sato, W., Tanaka, M., Sugiyama, S., et al.: Cardiomyopathy and angiopathy in patients with mitochondrial myopathy, encephalopathy, lactic acidosis, and strokelike episodes. Am. Heart J. *128:*733, 1994.
315. Brackett, J. C., Sims, H. F., Steiner, R. D., et al.: A novel mutation in medium chain Acyl-CoA dehydrogenase causes sudden neonatal death. J. Clin. Invest. *94:*1477, 1994.
316. Anan, R., Nakagawa, M., Miyata, M., et al.: Cardiac involvement in mitochondrial diseases. A study of 17 patients with documented mitochondrial DNA defects. Circulation *91:*955, 1995.
317. Merante, F., Tein, I., Benson, L., et al.: Maternally inherited hypertrophic cardiomyopathy due to a novel T-to-C transition at nucleotide 9997 in the mitochondrial $tRNA^{glycine}$ gene. Am. J. Hum. Genet. *55:*437, 1994.
318. Van Hove, J. L. K., Shanske, S., Ciacci, F., et al.: Mitochondrial myopathy with anemia, cardiomyopathy and lactic acidosis: A distinct late onset mitochondrial disorder. Am. J. Med. Genet. *51:*115, 1994.
319. Wallace, D. C.: Mitochondrial genetics: A paradigm for aging and degenerative diseases? Science *256:*628, 1992.
320. Ogashara, S., Engel, A. G., Frens, D., et al.: Muscle coenzyme Q deficiency in familial mitochondrial encephalomyopathy. Proc. Natl. Acad. Sci. U.S.A. *86:*2379, 1989.
321. Channer, K. S., Channer, J. L., Campbell, M. J., et al.: Cardiomyopathy in the Kearns-Sayre syndrome. Br. Heart J. *59:*486, 1988.
322. Chen, Y.-T., and Burchell, A.: Glycogen storage diseases. *In* Scriver, C. R., Beaudet, A. L., Sly, W. A., and Valle, D. (eds.): The Metabolic and Molecular Bases of Inherited Disease. New York, McGraw-Hill, 1995, p. 935.
323. Ehlers, K. H., Hagstrom, J. W. C., Lukas, D. S., et al.: Glycogen-storage disease of the myocardium with obstruction to left ventricular outflow. Circulation *25:*96, 1962.
324. Bharati, S., Serratto, M., Du Brow, I., et al.: The conduction system in Pompe's disease. Pediatr. Cardiol. *2:*25, 1982.
325. Bonnici, F., Shapiro, R., Joffe, H. S., et al.: Angiocardiographic and enzyme studies in a patient with type II glycogenosis. S. Afr. Med. J. *58:*860, 1980.
326. Robinson, W. F., Howell, J. M., and Dorling, P. R.: Cardiomyopathy is generalised glycogenosis type II in cattle. Cardiovasc. Res. *17:*238, 1982.
327. Suzuki, Y., Tsuji, A., Omura, K., et al.: Km mutant of acid alpha-glucosidase in a case of cardiomyopathy without signs of skeletal muscle involvement. Clin. Genet. *33:*376, 1988.
328. Makos, M. M., McComb, R. D., Hart, M. N., et al.: Alpha-glucosidase deficiency and basilar artery aneurysm: Report of a sibship. Ann. Neurol. *22:*629, 1987.
329. Kretzschmar, H. A., Wagner, H., Hubner, G., et al.: Aneurysm and vacuolar degeneration of cerebral arteries in late-onset acid maltase deficiency. J. Neurol. Sci. *98:*169, 1990.
330. Martiniuk, F., Mehler, M., Tzall, S., et al.: Extensive genetic heterogeneity in patients with acid alpha glucosidase deficiency as detected by abnormalities of DNA and mRNA. Am. J. Hum. Genet. *47:*73, 1990.
331. Olson, L. J., Reeder, G. S., Noller, K. L., et al.: Cardiac involvement in glycogen storage disease III. Morphologic and biochemical characterization with endomyocardial biopsy. Am. J. Cardiol. *53:*980, 1984.
332. Coleman, R. A., Winter, H. S., Wolf, B., et al.: Glycogen debranching enzyme deficiency: Long-term study of serum enzyme activities and clinical features. J. Inherit. Metab. Dis. *15:*869, 1992.
333. Talente, G. M., Coleman, R. A., Alter, C., et al.: Glycogen storage diseases in adults. Ann. Intern. Med. *120:*218, 1994.
334. Servidei, S., Metlay, L. A., Chodosh, J., et al.: Fatal infantile cardiopathy caused by phosphorylase b kinase deficiency. J. Pediatr. *113:*82, 1988.
335. Schroder, J. M., May, R., Shin, Y. S., et al.: Juvenile hereditary polyglucosan body disease with complete branching enzyme deficiency (type IV glycogenosis). Acta Neuropathol. *85:*419, 1993.
336. Howell, R. R.: Continuing lessons from glycogen storage diseases. N. Engl. J. Med. *324*(Edit.):55, 1991.
337. Selby, R., Starzl, T. E., Yunis, E., et al.: Liver transplantation for type IV glycogen storage disease. N. Engl. J. Med. *324:*39, 1991.
338. Eishi, Y., Takemura, T., Sone, R., et al.: Glycogen storage disease confined to the heart with deficient activity of cardiac phosphorylase kinase: A new type of glycogen storage disease. Hum. Pathol. *16:*193, 1987.
339. Elleder, M., Shin, Y. S., Zuntova, A., et al.: Fatal infantile hypertrophic cardiomyopathy secondary to deficiency of heart specific phosphorylase b kinase. Virchows Arch. A *423:*303, 1993.
340. Bothwell, T. H., Charlton, R. W., and Motulsky, A. G.: Hemochromatosis. *In* Scriver, C. R., Beaudet, A. L., Sly, W. A., and Valle, D. (eds.): The Metabolic and Molecular Bases of Inherited Disease. New York, McGraw-Hill, 1995, p. 2237.
341. Edwards, C. Q.: Early detection of hereditary hemochromatosis. Ann. Intern. Med. *101:*707, 1984.
342. Olson, L. J., Baldus, W. P., and Tajik, A. J.: Echocardiographic features of idiopathic hemochromatosis. Am. J. Cardiol. *60:*885, 1987.
343. Porter, J., Cary, N., and Schofield, P.: Haemochromatosis presenting as congestive cardiac failure. Br. Heart J. *73:*73, 1995.
344. Cutler, D. J., Isner, J. M., Bracey, A. W., et al.: Hemochromatosis heart disease: An unemphasized cause of potentially reversible restrictive cardiomyopathy. Am. J. Med. *69:*923, 1980.
345. Weatherall, D. J., Clegg, J. B., Higgs, D. R., et al.: The hemoglobinopathies. *In* Scriver, C. R., Beaudet, A. L., Sly, W. A., and Valle, D. (eds.): The Metabolic and Molecular Bases of Inherited Disease. New York, McGraw-Hill, 1995, p. 3417.
346. Sutton, L. L., Castro, O., Cross, D. J., et al.: Pulmonary hypertension in sickle cell disease. Am. J. Cardiol. *74:*626, 1994.
347. Brittenham, G. M., Griffith, P. M., Nienhuis, A. W., et al.: Efficacy of deferoxamine in preventing complications of iron overload in patients with thalassemia major. N. Engl. J. Med. *331:*567, 1994.
348. Olivieri, N. F., Liu, P. P., Sher, G. D., et al.: Combination liver and heart transplantation for end-stage iron-induced organ failure in an adult with homozygous beta-thalassemia. N. Engl. J. Med. *330:*1125, 1994.
349. Neufeld, E. F., and Muenzer, J.: The mucopolysaccharidoses. *In* Scriver, C. R., Beaudet, A. L., Sly, W. A., and Valle, D. (eds.): The Metabolic and Molecular Bases of Inherited Disease. New York, McGraw-Hill, 1995, p. 2465.
350. Johnson, G. L., Vine, D. L., Cottrill, C. M., et al.: Echocardiographic mitral valve deformity in the mucopolysaccharidoses. Pediatrics *67:*401, 1981.
351. Gross, D. M., Williams, J. C., Caprioli, C., et al.: Echocardiographic abnormalities in the mucopolysaccharide storage diseases. Am. J. Cardiol. *61:*170, 1988.
352. John, R. M., Hunter, D., and Swanton, R. H.: Echocardiographic abnormalities in type IV mucopolysaccharidosis. Arch. Dis. Child. *65:*746, 1990.
353. Pyeritz, R. E.: Storage disorders. *In* Pierpont, M. E., and Moller, J. H.

(eds.): The Genetics of Cardiovascular Disease. Boston, Martinus Nijhoff Publishing, 1987, p. 215.

354. Nelson, J., Shields, M. D., and Mulholland, H. C.: Cardiovascular studies in the mucopolysaccharidoses. J. Med. Genet. *27:*94, 1990.
355. Brosius, F. C., III, and Roberts, W. C.: Coronary artery disease in the Hurler syndrome: Qualitative and quantitative analysis of the extent of coronary narrowing at necropsy in six children. Am. J. Cardiol. *47:*649, 1981.
356. Renteria, V. G., Ferrans, V. J., and Roberts, W. C.: The heart in the Hurler syndrome: Gross, histologic and ultrastructural observations in five necropsy cases. Am. J. Cardiol. *38:*487, 1976.
357. Semenza, G. L., and Pyeritz, R. E.: Respiratory complications of the mucopolysaccharide storage disorders. Medicine *67:*209, 1988.
358. Young, I. D., and Harper, P. S.: Long-term complications in Hunter's syndrome. Clin. Genet. *16:*125, 1979.
359. Armitage, J. O.: Bone marrow transplantation. N. Engl. J. Med. *330:*827, 1994.
360. Whitley, C. B., Belani, K. G., Chang, P.-N., et al.: Long-term outcome of Hurler syndrome following bone marrow transplantation. Am. J. Med. Genet. *46:*209, 1993.
361. Morgan, S. H., and Crawfurd, M. d'A.: Anderson-Fabry disease. A commonly missed diagnosis. BMJ *297:*872, 1988.
362. Spence, M. W., MacKinnon, K. E., Burgess, J. K., et al.: Failure to correct the metabolic defect by renal allotransplantation in Fabry's disease. Ann. Intern. Med. *84:*13, 1976.
363. Kramer, W., Thormann, J., Mueller, K., et al.: Progressive cardiac involvement by Fabry's disease despite successful renal allotransplantation. Int. J. Cardiol. *7:*72, 1985.
364. Colucci, W. S., Lorell, B. H., Schoen, F. J., et al.: Hypertrophic obstructive cardiomyopathy due to Fabry's disease. N. Engl. J. Med. *307:*926, 1982.
365. von Scheidt, W., Eng, C. M., Fitzmaurice, T. F., et al.: An atypical variant of Fabry's disease with manifestations confined to the myocardium. N. Engl. J. Med. *324:*395, 1991.
366. Goldman, M. E., Cantor, R., Schwartz, M. F., et al.: Echocardiographic abnormalities and disease severity in Fabry's disease. J. Am. Coll. Cardiol. *7:*1157, 1986.
367. Sakuraba, H., Yanagawa, Y., Igarashi, T., et al.: Cardiovascular manifestations in Fabry's disease: A high incidence of mitral valve prolapse in hemizygotes and heterozygotes. Clin. Genet. *29:*276, 1986.
368. Mutoh, T., Senda, Y., Sugimura, K., et al.: Severe orthostatic hypotension in a female carrier of Fabry's disease. Arch. Neurol. *34:*468, 1988.
369. Bernstein, H. S., Bishop, D. F., Astrin, K. H., et al.: Fabry disease: Six gene rearrangements and an exonic point mutation in the alpha-galactosidase gene. J. Clin. Invest. *83:*1390, 1989.
370. Benson, M. D., and Wallace, M. R.: Amyloidosis. *In* Scriver, C. R., Beaudet, A. L., Sly, W. S., and Valle, D. (eds.): The Metabolic Basis of Inherited Disease. 6th ed. New York, McGraw-Hill Book Co., 1989, p. 2439.
371. Benson, M. D.: Amyloidosis. *In* Scriver, C. R., Beaudet, A. L., Sly, W. A., and Valle, D. (eds.): The Metabolic and Molecular Bases of Inherited Disease. New York, McGraw-Hill, 1995, p. 4157.
372. Backman, C., and Olofsson, B. O.: Echocardiographic features in familial amyloidosis with polyneuropathy. Acta Med. Scand. *214:*273, 1983.
373. Eriksson, A., Eriksson, P., Olofsson, B.-O., et al.: The cardiac atrioventricular conduction system in familial amyloidosis with polyneuropathy: A clinico-pathologic study of six cases from Northern Sweden. Acta Pathol. Microbiol. Immunol. Scand. *91:*343, 1983.
374. Booth, D. R., Tan, S. Y., Hawkins, P. N., et al.: A novel variant of transthyretin, $59^{Thr \rightarrow Lys}$, associated with autosomal dominant cardiac amyloidosis in an Italian family. Circulation *91:*962, 1995.
375. Skinner, M., Lewis, W. D., Jones, L. A., et al.: Liver transplantation as a treatment for familial amyloidotic polyneuropathy. Ann. Intern. Med. *120:*133, 1994.
376. Vidaillet, H. J., Jr.: Cardiac tumors associated with hereditary syndromes. Am. J. Cardiol. *61:*1355, 1988.
377. Burke, A. P., Rosado-de-Christenson, M., Templeton, P. A., et al.: Cardiac fibroma: Clinicopathologic correlates and surgical treatment. J. Thorac. Cardiovasc. Surg. *108:*862, 1994.
378. Harding, C. O., and Pagon, R. A.: Incidence of tuberous sclerosis in patients with cardiac rhabdomyoma. Am. J. Med. Genet. *37:*443, 1990.
379. Liebler, G. A., Magovern, G. J., Park, S. B., et al.: Familial myxomas in four siblings. J. Thorac. Cardiovasc. Surg. *71:*605, 1976.
380. Carney, J. A., Gordon, H., Carpenter, P. C., et al.: The complex of myxomas, spotty pigmentation, and endocrine overactivity. Medicine *64:*270, 1985.
381. Handley, J., Carson, D., Sloan, J., et al.: Multiple lentigines, myxoid tumours and endocrine overactivity: Four cases of Carney's complex. Br. J. Dermatol. *126:*367, 1992.

INHERITED DISORDERS OF THE CIRCULATION

382. Peery, W. H.: Clinical specturm of hereditary hemorrhagic telangiectasia (Osler-Weber-Rendu disease). Am. J. Med. *82:*989, 1987.
383. Guttmacher, A. E., McKinnon, W. C., and Upton, M. D.: Hereditary hemorrhagic telangiectasia: A disorder in search of the genetics community. Am. J. Med. Genet. *52:*252, 1994.
384. Guillén, B., Guizar, J., de la Cruz, J., et al.: Hereditary hemorrhagic telangiectasia: Report of 15 affected cases in a Mexican family. Clin. Genet. *39:*214, 1991.
385. Nikolopoulos, N., Xynos, E., and Vassilakis, J. S.: Familial occurrence of hyperdynamic circulation status due to intrahepatic fistulae in hereditary hemorrhagic telangiectasia. Hepatogastroenterology *35:*167, 1988.
386. Cooke, D. A. P.: Renal arteriovenous malformation demonstrated angiographically in hereditary haemorrhagic telangiectasia (Rendu-Osler-Weber disease). J. R. Soc. Med. *79:*744, 1986.
387. Kurnik, P. B., and Heymann, W. R.: Coronary artery ectasia associated with hereditary hemorrhagic telangiectasia. Arch. Intern. Med. *149:*2357, 1989.
388. Braverman, I. M., Keh, A., and Jacobson, B. S.: Ultrastructure and three-dimensional organization of the telangiectases of hereditary hemorrhagic telangiectasia. J. Invest. Dermatol. *95:*422, 1990.
389. Terry, P. B., White, J. I., Jr., Barth, K. H., et al.: Pulmonary arteriovenous malformations: Physiologic observations and results of therapeutic balloon embolization. N. Engl. J. Med. *308:*1197, 1983.
390. Haq, A. U., Glass, J., Netchvolodoff, C. V., et al.: Hereditary hemorrhagic telangiectasia and danazol. Ann. Intern. Med. *109:*171, 1988.
391. Saba, H. I., Morelli, G. A., and Logrono, L. A.: Treatment of bleeding in hereditary hemorrhagic telangiectasia with aminocaproic acid. N. Engl. J. Med. *330:*1789, 1994.
392. Phillips, M. D.: Stopping bleeding in hereditary telangiectasia. N. Engl. J. Med. *330:*1822, 1994.
393. McDonald, M. T., Papenberg, K. A., Ghosh, S., et al.: A disease locus for hereditary haemorrhagic telangiectasia maps to chromosome 9q33-34. Nature Genet *6:*197, 1994.
394. Shovlin, C. L., Hughes, J. M. B., Tuddenham, E. G. D., et al.: A gene for hereditary haemorrhagic telangiectasia maps to chromosome 9q3. Nature Genet. *6:*205, 1994.
395. McAllister, K. A., Grogg, K. M. M., Johnson, D. W., et al.: Endoglin, a TGF-β binding protein of endothelial cells, is the gene for hereditary haemorrhagic telangiectasia type 1. Nature Genet. *8:*345, 1994.
396. Jennings, A. M., Smith, C., Cole, D. R., et al.: Von Hippel-Lindau disease in a large British family: Clinicopathological features and recommendations for screening and follow-up. Q. J. Med. *66:*233, 1988.
397. Lamiell, J. M., Salazar, F. G., and Hsia, Y. E.: Von Hippel-Lindau disease affecting 43 members of a single kindred. Medicine *68:*1, 1989.
398. Latif, F., Troy, K., Gnarra, J., et al.: Identification of the von Hippel-Landau disease tumor suppressor gene. Science *260:*1317, 1993.
399. Parfrey, P. S., Bear, J. C., Morgan, J., et al.: The diagnosis and prognosis of autosomal dominant polycystic kidney disease. N. Engl. J. Med. *323:*1085, 1990.
400. Gabow, P. A.: Autosomal dominant polycystic kidney disease. N. Engl. J. Med. *329:*332, 1993.
401. Chapman, A. B., Johnson, A., Gabow, P. A., et al.: The renin-angiotensin aldosterone system and autosomal dominant polycystic kidney disease. N. Engl. J. Med. *323:*1091, 1990.
402. Leier, C. V., Baker, P. B., Kilman, J. W., et al.: Cardiovascular abnormalities associated with adult polycystic kidney disease. Ann. Intern. Med. *100:*683, 1984.
403. Hossack, K. F., Leddy, C. L., Johnson, A. M., et al.: Echocardiographic findings in autosomal dominant polycystic kidney disease. N. Engl. J. Med. *319:*907, 1988.
404. Chapman, J. R., and Hilson, A. J. W.: Polycystic kidneys and abdominal aortic aneurysms. Lancet *1:*646, 1980.
405. Chapman, A. B., Rubinstein, D., Hughes, R., et al.: Intracranial aneurysms in autosomal dominant polycystic kidney disease. N. Engl. J. Med. *327:*916, 1992.
406. European Polycystic Kidney Disease Consortium: The polycystic kidney disease 1 gene encodes a 14 kb transcript and lies within a duplicated region on chromosome 16. Cell *77:*881, 1994.
407. Peters, D. J. M., Spruit, L., Saris, J. J., et al.: Chromosome 4 localization of a second gene for autosomal dominant polycystic kidney disease. Nature Genet. *5:*359, 1993.
408. Daoust, M. C., Reynold, D. M., Bichet, D. G., et al.: Evidence for a third genetic locus for autosomal dominant polycystic kidney disease. Genomics *25:*733, 1995.
409. Shulman, S. A., Hyams, J. S., Gunta, R., et al.: Arteriohepatic dysplasia (Alagille syndrome): Extreme variability among affected family members. Am. J. Med. Genet. *19:*325, 1984.
410. Dhorne-Pollet, S., Deleuze, J.-F., Hadchouel, M., et al.: Segregation analysis of Alagille syndrome. J. Med. Genet. *31:*453, 1994.
411. Nicod, P., Bloor, C., Godfrey, M., et al.: Familial aortic dissecting aneurysms. J. Am. Coll. Cardiol. *13:*811, 1989.
412. Toyama, M., Amano, A., and Kameda, T.: Familial aortic dissection: A report of rare family cluster. Br. Heart J. *61:*204, 1989.
413. Bixler, D., and Antley, R. M.: Familial aortic dissection with iris anomalies—a new connective tissue disease syndrome? Birth Defects *12*(5):229, 1976.
414. Roberts, C. S., and Roberts, W. C.: Dissection of the aorta associated with congenital malformation of the aortic valve. J. Am. Coll. Cardiol. *17:*712, 1994.
415. Kontusaari, S., Tromp, G., Kuivaniemi, H., et al.: Inheritance of RNA splicing mutation ($G^{+1\ IVS_{20}}$) in the type III procollagen gene (COL3AI) in a family having aortic aneurysms and easy bruisability: Phenotypic overlap between familial arterial aneurysms and Ehlers-Danlos syndrome type IV. Am. J. Hum. Genet. *47:*112, 1990.
416. Kontusaari, S., Tromp, G., Kuivaniemi, H., et al.: A mutation in the gene for type III procollagen (COL3AI) in a family with aortic aneurysms. J. Clin. Invest *86:*1465, 1990.
417. Tromp, G., Wu, Y., Prockop, D. J., et al.: Sequencing of cDNA from 50 unrelated patients reveals that mutations in the triple-helical domain of

type III procollagen are an infrequent cause of aortic aneurysms. J. Clin. Invest. *91*:2539, 1993.

418. Schievink, W. I., Michaels, V. V., Mokri, B., et al.: A familial syndrome of arterial dissections with lentiginosis. N. Engl. J. Med. *332*:576, 1995.
419. Majamaa, K., Portimojarvi, H., Sotaniemi, K. A., et al.: Familial aggregation of cervical artery dissection and cerebral aneurysm. Stroke *25*:1704, 1994.
420. Majumder, P. P., St. Jean, P. L., Ferrell, R. E., et al.: On the inheritance of abdominal aortic aneurysm. Am. J. Hum. Genet. *48*:164, 1991.
421. Pletcher, B. A., Fox, J. E., Boxer, R. A., et al.: Three siblings with arterial tortuosity syndrome: Description and review of the literature. Am. J. Med. Genet. *(in press)*.
422. Halal, F., Mohr, G., Toussi, T., et al.: Intracranial aneurysms: A report of a large pedigree. Am. J. Med. Genet. *15*:89, 1983.
423. Kuivaniemi, H., Prockop, D. J., Wu, Y., et al.: Exclusion of mutations in the gene for type III collagen (COL3A1) as a common cause of intracranial aneurysms or cervical artery dissections: Results from sequence analysis of the coding sequences of type III collagen from 55 unrelated patients. Neurology *43*:2652, 1993.
424. Abrahamson, M.: Human cysteine proteinase inhibitors: Isolation, physiological importance, inhibitory mechanism, gene structure and relation to hereditary cerebral hemorrhage. Scand. J. Clin. Lab. Invest. *48*:21, 1988.
425. Wattendorf, A. R., Bots, G. T. A. M., Went, L. N., et al.: Familial cerebral amyloid angiopathy presenting as recurrent cerebral haemorrhage. J. Neurol. Sci. *55*:121, 1982.
426. Pasyk, K. A., Argenta, L. C., and Erickson, R. P.: Familial vascular malformations: Report of 25 members of one family. Clin. Genet. *26*:221, 1984.
427. Stanley, J. C.: Arterial fibrodysplasia. Arch. Surg. *110*:561, 1975.
428. Kousseff, B. G., and Gilbert-Barness, E. F.: Vascular neurofibromatosis and infantile gangrene. Am. J. Med. Genet. *34*:221, 1989.
429. Schievink, W. I., Björnsson, J., Parisi, J. E., et al.: Arterial fibromuscular dysplasia associated with severe α_1-antitrypsin deficiency. Mayo Clin. Proc. *69*:1040, 1994.
430. Petit, H., Bouchez, B., Destee, A., et al.: Familial form of fibromuscular dysplasia of the internal carotid artery. J. Neuroradiol. *10*:15, 1983.
431. Rushton, A. R.: The genetics of fibromuscular dysplasia. Arch. Intern. Med. *140*:233, 1980.
432. Austin, J. G., and Stears, J. C.: Familial hypoplasia of both internal carotid arteries. Arch. Neurol. *24*:1, 1971.
433. McDonald, A. H., Gerlis, L. M., and Somerville, J.: Familial arteriopathy with associated pulmonary and systemic arterial stenoses. Br. Heart J. *31*:375, 1969.
434. Van Dyck, M., Proesmans, W., VanHollebeke, E., et al.: Idiopathic infantile arterial calcification with cardiac, renal and central nervous system involvement. Eur. J. Pediatr. *148*:374, 1989.
435. Joutel, A., Bousser, M-G., Biuosse, V., et al.: A gene for familial hemiplegic migraine maps to chromosome 19. Nature Genet. *5*:40, 1993.
436. Joutel, A., Ducros, A., Vahedi, K., et al.: Genetic heterogeneity of familial hemiplegic migraine. Am. J. Hum. Genet. *55*:1166, 1994.
437. Hovatta, I., Kallela, M., Färkkilä, M., et al.: Familial migraine: Exclusion of the susceptibility gene from the reported locus of familial hemiplegic migraine on 19p. Genomics *23*:707, 1994.
438. Tournier-Lasserve, E., Joutel, A., Melki, J., et al.: Cerebral autosomal dominant arteriopathy with subcortical infarcts and leukoencephalopathy maps to chromosone 19q12. Nature Genet. *3*:256, 1993.
439. Melmon, K. L., and Braunwald, E.: Familial pulmonary hypertension. N. Engl. J. Med. *269*:770, 1963.
440. Kingdon, H. S., Cohen, L. S., Roberts, W. C., et al.: Familial occurrence of primary pulmonary hypertension. Arch. Intern. Med. *118*:422, 1966.
441. Loyd, J. E., Primm, R. K., and Newman, J. H.: Familial primary pulmonary hypertension: Clinical patterns. Am. Rev. Respir. Dis. *129*:194, 1984.
442. Porterfield, J. K., Pyeritz, R. E., and Traill, T. A.: Pulmonary hypertension and interstitial fibrosis in von Recklinghausen neurofibromatosis. Am. J. Med. Genet. *25*:531, 1986.
443. Goldstein, S., Qazi, Q. H., Fitzgerald, J., et al.: Distichiasis, congenital heart defects and mixed peripheral vascular anomalies. Am. J. Med. Genet. *20*:283, 1985.
444. Lindenauer, S. M.: The Klippel-Trenaunay-Weber syndrome: Varicosity, hypertrophy and hemangioma with no arteriovenous fistula. Ann. Surg. *162*:303, 1965.
445. Campistol, J. M., Agusti, C., Torras, A., et al.: Renal hemangioma and renal artery aneurysm in the Klippel-Trenaunay syndrome. J. Urol. *140*:134, 1988.
446. Bicknell, J. M.: Familial cavernous angioma of the brain stem dominantly inherited in Hispanics. Neurosurgery *24*:102, 1989.
447. Dellemijn, P. L. I., and Vanneste, J. A. L.: Cavernous angiomatosis of the central nervous system: Usefulness of screening the family. Acta Neurol. Scand. *88*:259, 1993.
448. Dobyns, W. B., Michels, V. V., Groover, R. V., et al.: Familial cavernous malformations of the central nervous system and retina. Ann. Neurol. *21*:578, 1987.
449. Rigamonti, D., Hadley, M. N., Drayer, B. P., et al.: Cerebral cavernous malformations: Incidence and familial occurrence. N. Engl. J. Med. *319*:343, 1988.
450. Steichen-Gersdorf, E., Felber, S., Fuchs, W., et al.: Familial cavernous angiomas of the brain: Observations in a four generation family. Eur. J. Pediatr. *151*:861, 1992.
451. Drigo, P., Mammi, I., Battistella, P. A., et al.: Familial cerebral, hepatic, and retinal cavernous angiomas: A new syndrome. Child's Nerv. Sys. *10*:205, 1994.
452. Dubovsky, J., Zabramski, J. M., Kurth, J., et al.: A gene responsible for cavernous malformations of the brain maps to chromosome 7q. Hum. Molec. Genet. *4*:453, 1995.
452a. Gunel, M., Awad, I. A., Anson, J., et al.: Mapping a gene causing cerebral cavernous malformation to 7q11.2-q21. Proc. Nat. Acad. Sci. U.S.A. *92*:6620, 1995.
453. Marchuk, D. A., Gallione, C. J., Morrison, L. A., et al.: A locus for cerebral cavernous malformations maps to chromosome 7q in two families. Genomics *28*:311, 1995.
454. Herbert, F. A., and Bowen, P. A.: Hereditary late-onset lymphedema with pleural effusion and laryngeal edema. Arch. Intern. Med. *143*:913, 1983.
455. Offori, T. W., Platt, C. C., Stephens, M., et al.: Angiosarcoma in congenital hereditary lymphoedema (Milroy's disease). Clin. Exp. Dermatol. *18*:174, 1993.
456. Anderson, H. C., Parry, D. M., and Mulvihill, J. J.: Lymphangiosarcoma in late-onset hereditary lymphedema: Case report and nosological implications. Am. J. Med. Genet. *56*:72, 1995.
457. Cambien, F., Poirier, O., Lecerf, L., et al.: Deletion polymorphism in the gene for angiotensin-converting enzyme is a potent risk factor for myocardial infarction. Nature *359*:641, 1992.
458. Fowkes, F. G. R., Connor, J. M., Smith, F. B., et al.: Fibrinogen genotype and risk for peripheral atherosclerosis. Lancet *339*:693, 1992.
459. Ishigami, T., Umemura, S., Iwamoto, T., et al.: Molecular variant of angiotensinogen gene is associated with coronary atherosclerosis. Circulation *91*:951, 1995.
460. Burke, W., and Motulsky, A. G.: Hypertension. *In* King, R. A., Rotter, J. I., and Motulsky, A. G. (eds.): The Genetic Basis of Common Diseases. New York, Oxford University Press, 1992, p. 170.
461. Murphy, E. A., and Pyeritz, R. D.: Homeostasis: VII. A conspectus. Am. J. Med. Genet. *24*:735, 1986.
462. Parmer, R. J., Cervenka, J. H., and Stone, R. A.: Baroflex sensitivity and heredity in essential hypertension. Circulation *85*:497, 1992.
463. Lifton, R. P.: Genetic factors in hypertension. Curr. Opin. Nephrol. Hyperten. *2*:258, 1993.
464. Jeunemaitre, X., and Corvol, P.: Hypertension. *In* Rimoin, D. L., Connor, J. M., and Pyeritz, R. E. (eds.): Principles and Practice of Medical Genetics. 3rd ed. New York, Churchill Livingstone, 1996.
465. Lindpainter, K.: Genes, hypertension and cardiac hypertrophy. N. Engl. J. Med. *330*:1678, 1994.
466. McKusick, V. A.: Genetics and the nature of essential hypertension. Circulation *22*:857, 1960.
467. Shimkets, R. A., Warnock, D. G., Bositis, C. M., et al.: Liddle's syndrome: Heritable human hypertension caused by mutations in the β subunit of the epithelial sodium channel. Cell *79*:407, 1994.
468. Gordon, R. G., Klemm, S. A., Tunny, T. J., et al.: Primary aldosteronism: Hypertension with a genetic basis. Lancet *340*:159, 1992.
469. Gordon, R. D.: Heterogeneous hypertension. Nature Genet. *11*:6, 1995.
470. Lifton, R. P., Dluhy, R. G., Powers, M., et al.: A chimeric 11β-hydroxylase/aldosterone synthase gene causes glucocorticoid-remediable aldosteronism and human hypertension. Nature *355*:262, 1992.
471. Hata, A., Namikawa, C., Sasaki, M., et al.: Angiotensinogen as a risk factor for essential hypertension in Japan. J. Clin. Invest. *93*:1285, 1994.
472. Jeunemaitre, X., Soubrier, F., Kotelevtsev, Y. V., et al.: Molecular basis of human hypertension: Role of angiotensinogen. Cell *71*:169, 1992.
473. Caulfield, M., Lavendar, P., Farral, M., et al.: Linkage of the angiotensinogen gene to essential hypertension. N. Engl. J. Med. *33*:1629, 1994.
474. Barley, J., Carter, N., Crews, D., et al.: Angiotensin 1 converting enzyme (ACE) polymorphism in different groups and its association with hypertension, plasma renin activity and aldosterone. J. Med. Genet. *31*:172, 1994.
475. Morris, B. J., Zee, R. Y. L., and Schrader, A. P.: Different frequencies of angiotensin-converting enzyme genotypes in older hypertensive individuals. J. Clin. Invest. *94*:1085, 1994.
476. Jacob, H. J., Lindpainter, K., Lincoln, S. E., et al.: Genetic mapping of a gene causing hypertension in the stroke-prone spontaneously hypertensive rat. Cell *67*:213, 1991.
477. John, S. W. M., Krege, J. H., Oliver, P. M., et al.: Genetic decreases in atrial natriuretic peptide and salt-sensitive hypertension. Science *267*:679, 1995.
478. Cohen, L. S., Friedman, J. M., Jefferson, J. W., et al.: A reevaluation of risk of in utero exposure to lithium. JAMA 271:146, 1994.

Chapter 50

The Aging Heart: Structure, Function, and Disease

EDWARD G. LAKATTA, GARY GERSTENBLITH, MYRON L. WEISFELDT

STRUCTURE AND FUNCTION OF THE AGING HEART .1687
Aging in Animal Models 1687
Normal Aging Humans 1689
HEART DISEASE IN THE ELDERLY 1695
Chronic Ischemic Heart Disease 1696
Acute Myocardial Infarction 1697
Arrhythmias 1697
Valvular Disease 1698
Hypertension. .1699
Congestive Heart Failure 1699
Drug Use in the Elderly 1700
REFERENCES .1700

STRUCTURE AND FUNCTION OF THE AGING HEART

AGING IN ANIMAL MODELS

Cellular and molecular mechanisms that account for age-associated changes in myocardial performance have been studied largely in rodents (see reference 34 for review). In the normotensive rat, cardiac fibrosis increases with aging,[1,2] the number of myocytes decreases (Fig. 50–1*D*),[2,3] and myocyte size increases.[4] Variable degrees of left ventricular hypertrophy occur,[5,6] depending on the rodent strain, and this is due to ventricular dilatation with apparent preservation of normal ventricular wall thickness.[1] Functional, biophysical/biochemical, pharmacological, and molecular changes occur in the aging rat heart (Table 50–1).

There are coordinated changes in several key steps of excitation-contraction coupling that result in a prolonged Ca_i transient and a prolonged contraction. The transmembrane action potential (Fig. 50–1*A*) is prolonged approximately twofold in cardiac muscle isolated from senescent 24-month rats, compared with younger adult 6- to 8-month rats.[8–10] The L type sarcolemmal Ca^{++} current is not substantially increased in magnitude but inactivates more slowly[10] and could possibly account, in part, for the prolonged transmembrane action potential. However, it is likely that changes in outwardly directed K^+ currents[10] substantially contribute to the transmembrane AP prolongation. The cytosolic Ca^{++} transient following excitation (Fig. 50–1*C*) is prolonged in senescent rats.[16] The rate of Ca^{++} sequestration by the sarcoplasmic reticulum decreases in the senescent myocardium (Fig. 50–2*A*), and this may in part explain the prolonged Ca_i transient (Fig. 12–12, p. 368).[17,18] A reduction in the mRNA coding for the sarcoplasmic reticular Ca^{++}-ATPase[29,30] suggests that the diminished Ca^{++} accumulation rate could, in part, be secondary to a decrease in the sarcoplasmic reticular pump site density.[18] The myofilament force response to Ca^{++} is not altered by age.[34] However, marked shifts occur in the myosin heavy chain in rodents, i.e., the β or V_3 isozyme becomes predominant in senescent rat (85 per cent β versus 15 per cent α). Steady-state messenger RNA levels for α- and β-MHC parallel the age-associated changes in the myosin heavy chain proteins V_1 and V_3, and thus the isoenzyme shift appears to be transcriptionally regulated. The myosin Ca^{++}-ATPase activity declines (Fig. 50–3*A*) with the decline in V_i content. The altered cellular profile, which results in a contraction that exhibits a reduced velocity (Fig. 50–3*B*) and a prolonged time course (Fig. 50–1*B*), can be considered to be adaptive rather than degenerative in nature because the reduced velocity is energy efficient and prolonged contraction permits continued ejection for a longer period.[8,9,11,33]

Aggregate age-associated alterations in cytosolic Ca^{++} concentration, the Na-Ca exchanger, Na-K pump, and the sarcoplasmic reticular Ca^{++} pump, possibly in conjunction with nonspecific changes in sarcolemmal membrane ionic permeabilities, may predispose senescent myocardium to altered cell Ca^{++} homeostasis. Intriguingly, aged myocardium (and that chronically exposed to pressure overload) is more susceptible to Ca^{++} overload and spontaneous sarcoplasmic reticular Ca^{++} release than is young adult myocardium.[17,33,35] Aged myocardium demonstrates a reduced Ca^{++} threshold for diastolic afterdepolarizations and for ventricular fibrillation.[35] The former is caused by and the latter is preceded by an increase in spontaneous sarcoplasmic reticular oscillatory Ca^{++} release.[35]

Studies in isolated left ventricular muscle (Fig. 50–4*A*) and in individual rat ventricular cardiocytes, similar to recent studies in humans,[36,37] (Fig. 50–4*B*) indicate that a reduced contractile response to β_1-AR stimulation occurs with aging. This is due to failure of the intracellular Ca^{++} transient to increase in cells of senescent hearts to the same extent to which it increases in cells from younger adult hearts.[26] The blunted increase in the Ca^{++} transient in cells from the aged heart is attributed to a decrease in the ability of β_1-AR stimulation to increase L type sarcolemmal Ca^{++} channel availability in cells from senescent versus younger adult hearts[26] (Fig. 50–4*B*). The richly documented age-associated reduction in the postsynaptic response of myocardial cells to β_1-AR stimulation appears to be due to multiple changes in molecular and biochemical receptor coupling and postreceptor mechanisms rather than to a major modification of a single rate-limiting step, as might occur, for example, in a genetic defect (see reference 33 for review).

The multiple changes in cardiac excitation, myofilament activation, contraction mechanisms, and gene expression that occur with aging (Figs. 50–1 through 50–4 and Table 50–1) are interrelated. Many of these can be interpreted as adaptive in nature because they also occur in the hypertrophied myocardium of younger animals adapted to experimentally induced chronic hypertension[11,25,38–44] (Table 50–2). There is some evidence to suggest that the adaptive response to chronic passive loading declines with aging,[45–51] possibly in part because some of the adaptive capacity of the heart is used as a response to the aging process per se. Chronic exercise in older animals reverses some of the alterations in the cardiac function (prolonged contraction, reduced sarcoplasmic reticular function) that occur with aging.[12,18,23,43,52–55] Other aspects of cardiac func-

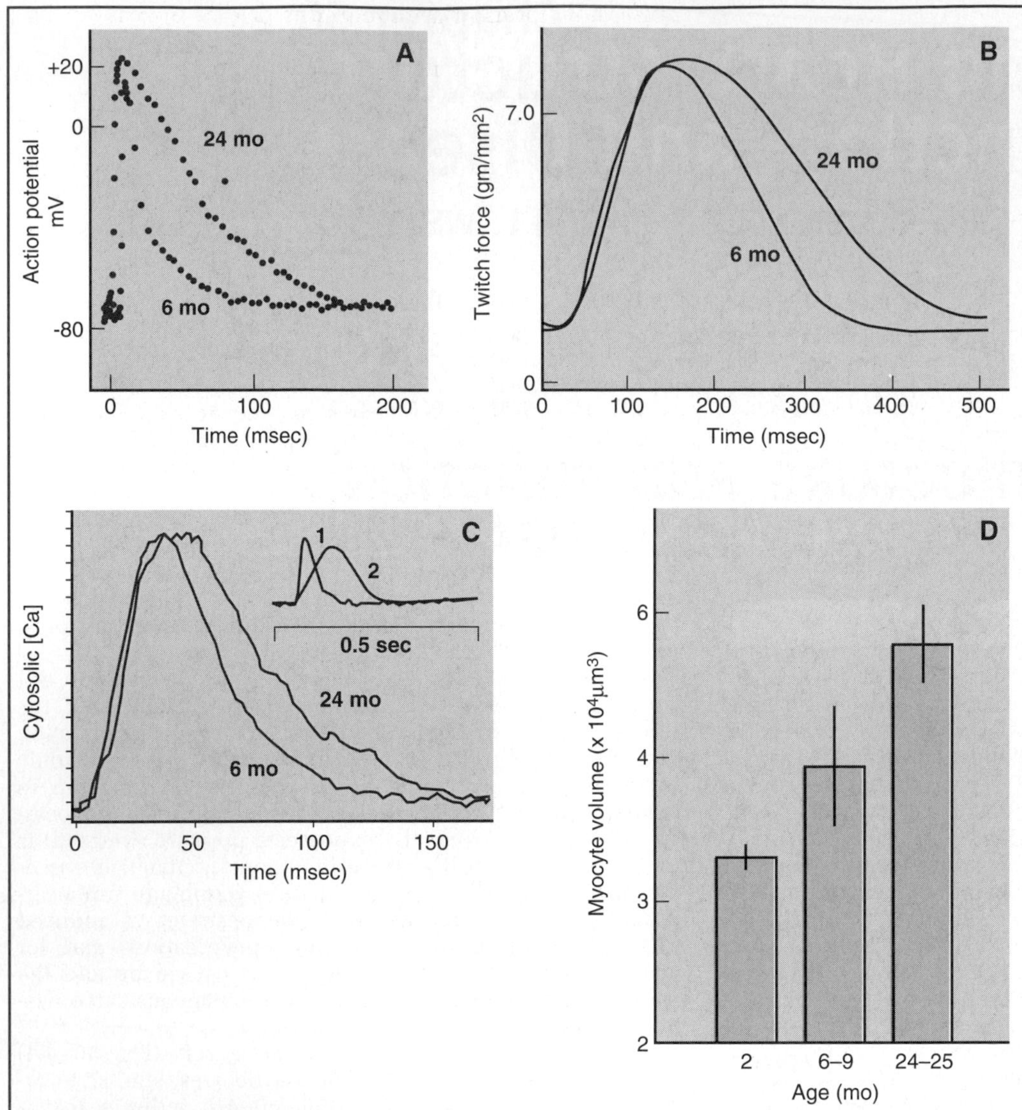

FIGURE 50–1. Action potential (Panel A), isometric twitch (Panel B), and Ca_i transient (Panel C), measured via aequorin luminescence, in isometric right ventricular papillary muscles isolated from the hearts of young adult and senescent Wistar rats. Inset in Panel C indicates the time course of the Ca_i transient[1] relative to that of the contraction.[2] (Panels A and B from Wei, J. Y., Spurgeon, H. A., and Lakatta, E. G.: Excitation-contraction in rat myocardium: Alterations with adult aging. Am. J. Physiol. *246*:H784, 1984. Panel C from Orchard, C. H., and Lakatta, E. G.: Intracellular calcium transients and developed tensions in rat heart muscle. A mechanism for the negative interval-strength relationship. J. Gen. Physiol. *86*:637, 1985.) Panel D, Left ventricular cell volume (single cells, isolated via collagenase dissection of hearts) measured via Coulter Counter technique increases with age. (Panel D from Fraticelli, A., Josephson, R., Danziger, R., et al.: Morphological and contractile characteristics of rat cardiac myocytes from maturation to senescence. Am. J. Physiol. *257*:H259, 1989.)

TABLE 50–1 MYOCARDIAL CHANGES WITH ADULT AGING

STRUCTURAL Δ	FUNCTIONAL Δ	IONIC, BIOPHYSICAL/BIOCHEMICAL MECHANISM(S)	MOLECULAR MECHANISMS
↑ Myocyte size[4]	Prolonged contraction[7–9]	Prolonged cystosolic Ca^{++} transient[16]	
↓ Myocyte number[2,3]		↓ SR Ca^{++} pumping rate[17,18] ↓ Pump site density[18]	↓ SR Ca^{++} pump mRNA[29,30] No Δ calsequestrin mRNA[29]
	Prolonged action[8–10] potential	↓ I_{Ca} inactivation[10] ↓ I_{To} density[10]	
	Diminished contraction[11] velocity	↓ α MHC protein[19,20] ↑ β MHC protein[19,20] ↓ Myosin ATPase activity[8,18,20,21]	↓ α MHC mRNA[17,19,31,32] ↑ β MHC mRNA[19,31,32] No Δ actin mRNA[33]
	Diminished β-adrenergic contractile response	↓ Coupling BAR-acyclase[22,23] ↓ TNI phosphorylation[24] ↓ Phospholamban phosphorylation[25] ↓ I_{Ca} augmentation[26] ↓ Ca_i transient augmentation[26]	
		↑ Enkephalin peptides[27]	↑ Proenkephalin mRNA[27]
↑ Matrix connective tissue[1,2]	↑ Myocardial stiffness[12–15]	↑ Atrial natriuretic peptide[28]	↑ Atrial natriuretic peptide mRNA[28]

Δ = change; ↑ = increased; ↓ = decreased.

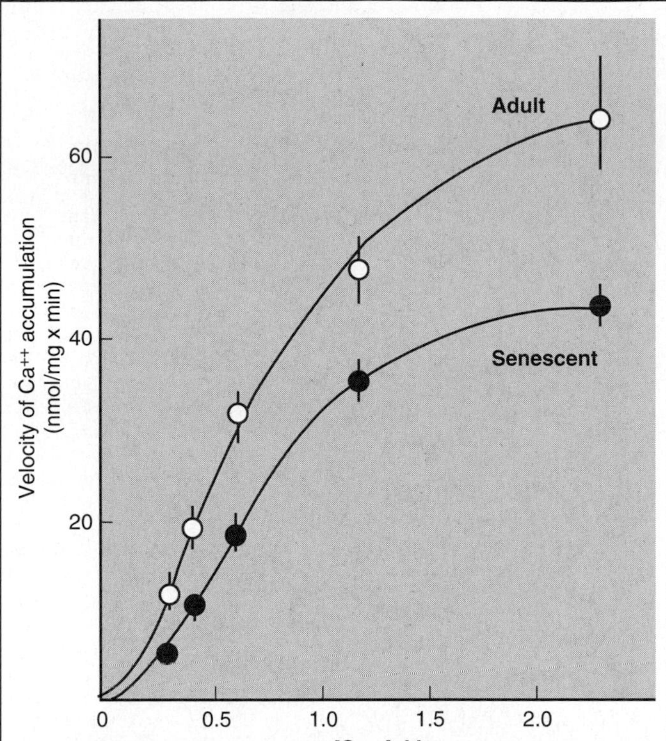

FIGURE 50–2. The effect of age on Ca^{++} accumulation velocity by sarcoplasmic reticulum isolated from senescent and adult Wistar rat hearts. (From Froehlich, J. P., Lakatta, E. G., Beard, E., et al.: Studies of sarcoplasmic reticulum function and contraction duration in young adult and aged rat myocardium. J. Mol. Cell. Cardiol. *10*:427, 1978.)

tion that change with aging (e.g., prolonged action potential, altered myosin isoform expression[18]) are not affected by chronic exercise.

NORMAL AGING HUMANS

Age changes in cardiac function in humans can be understood only by strictly segregating normal aging from the interplay of aging and disease. This is of importance because most forms of acquired heart disease increase in frequency and severity with age.

TABLE 50–2 ALTERED MYOCARDIAL GENE EXPRESSION IN ADVANCED AGE, HYPERTENSION, HEART FAILURE, OR AFTER GROWTH FACTORS*

	RODENT		GROWTH FACTORS†		
				FGF	
	Aging	Hypertension	*TGFβ*	*Acidic*	*Basic*
SR Ca^{++}-ATPase	↓	↓	↓	↓	↓
Calsequestrin	↔	↔			
Phospholamban		↑ (rabbit)			
α-Major histocompatibility complex	↓	↓	↓	↓	↓
β-Major histocompatibility complex	↑	↑	↑	↑	↑
β Tropomyosin	↓	↑‡			
α Skeletal actin	↓	↑§	↑	↓	↑
Atrial natriuretic factor	↑	↑	↑	↑	↑
Proenkephalin	↑				

* See references 33 and 34 for review.
† In neonatal cultured cardiocytes.
‡ In atrial tissue.
§ Only transient changes occur in situ following cardiac pressure loading.
SR = Sarcoplasmic reticulum.

Observed age changes in cardiovascular function in human subjects selected for the absence of demonstrable cardiovascular disease are direct extensions of the principal physiological changes that are documented in the experimental laboratory.[33] The major features of cardiac physiology in experimental animals that are well maintained with age are intrinsic cardiac muscle function under conditions of moderate stress and coronary perfusion. In males, studies using echocardiography and gated blood pool scans consistently show, in well-selected populations, only a small age-associated increase in left ventricular end-diastolic volume and end-systolic volume at rest, and therefore little change in ejection fraction.[56] Women show no increase in end-diastolic or end-systolic volume with age. During beta-adrenergic blockade there are no major age differences at rest.[57] Recent studies in several catheterization laboratories[58] measuring coronary sinus blood flow in subjects without coronary artery disease or other forms of heart disease show that maximal coronary vasodilating capacity or flow is unchanged with age. At rest, probably due to mild hypertrophy, coronary blood flow may increase slightly with age under physiological noncoronary vasodilated states.[58] Endothelial-dependent vasodilation is reduced with age, but the response to direct smooth muscle vasodilators is unchanged.[59]

In humans, as in experimental animals, there is evidence of modest left ventricular hypertrophy with age[60] (Fig. 50–5). In animal models, pressure load or impedance-induced hypertrophy results in prolonged cardiac muscle relaxation and the expected decrease in early left ventricular diastolic filling and maximal diastolic filling rates. The age-associated increase in impedance to left ventricular ejection is associated with left ventricular hypertrophy and prolonged relaxation. This age change in relaxation has important implications when the issue of aging and disease is addressed. With regard to normal cardiac physiology and response to exercise, there is no evidence that this prolonged relaxation has any detrimental effects on overall left ventricular function and capacity to augment cardiac performance during exercise. This is in part related to the slower heart rate during exercise, which allows a longer diastolic filling time and some sympathetic-induced increased relaxation rate during exercise. As a result, there is less potential for incomplete left ventricular relaxation between contractions.

As discussed in detail below, there are major and obvious age-associated changes in the hemodynamic response to exercise in humans without cardiovascular disease. These are entirely consistent with the two underlying mechanisms described in animals with age. The first is an age-associated increase in left ventricular load or impedance that results from stiffening of the central arterial system and the second is a decrease in general beta-sympathetic response leading to reduced augmentation of heart rate and contractility, or inotropic state, of ventricular myocardium and to diminished arterial vasodilation.

Increased Impedance to Left Ventricular Ejection

One of the most universally documented age changes in humans is the increase in pulse wave velocity within the arterial system (Fig. 50–6). The pulse wave is the rise in arterial pressure in the central aorta during left ventricular ejection of blood. This pressure wave travels in the central arterial system toward the brain, arms, and feet much faster in older than in younger individuals. This increase is quite linear with age, beginning essentially at birth and extending beyond 80 years of age.[61,62] Such changes in pulse wave velocity have been measured in many civilizations and cultures, both in populations in which hypertension and

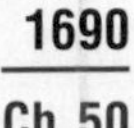

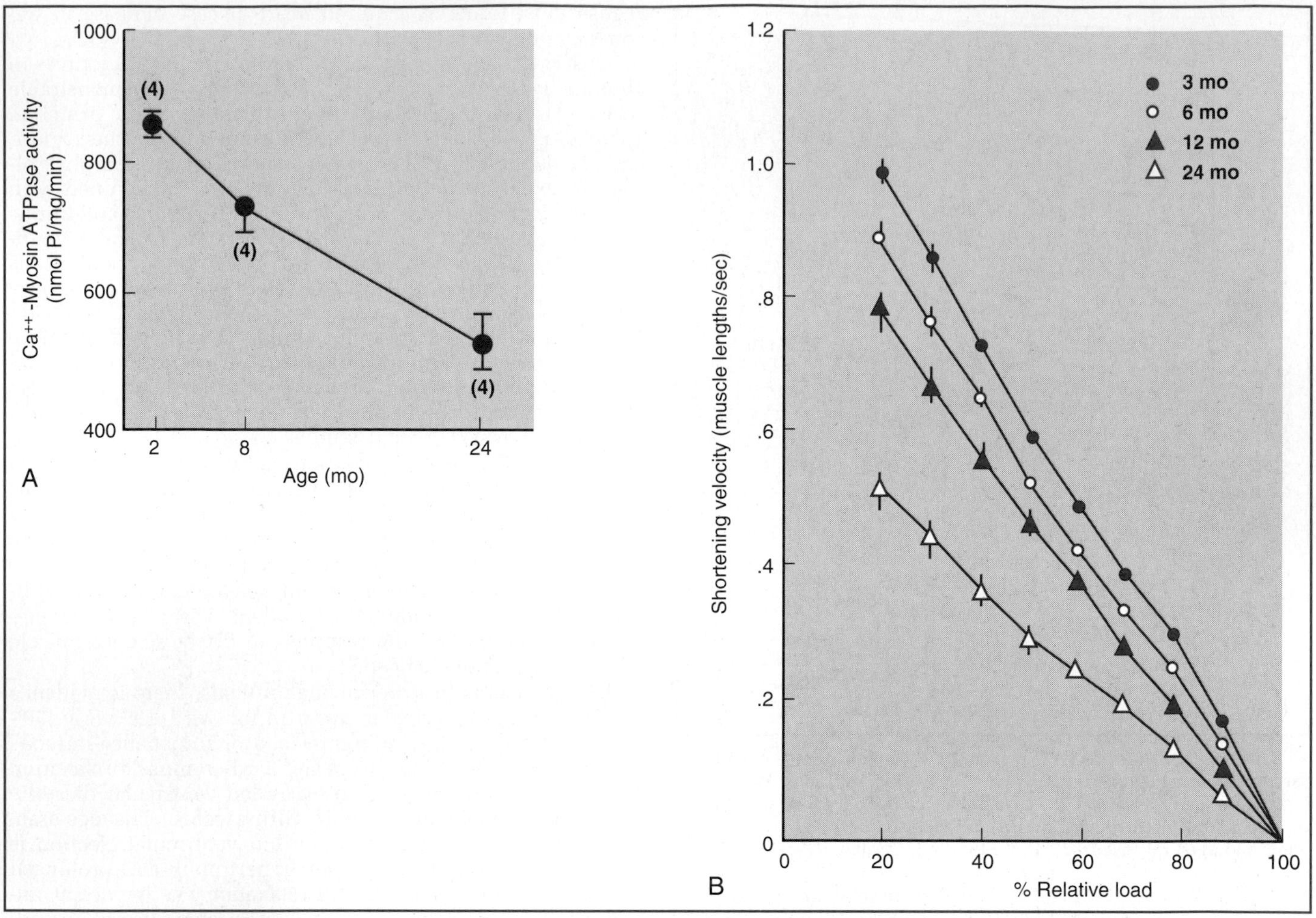

FIGURE 50–3. Panel A, Ca^{++}-activated myosin ATPase activity of Wistar rat hearts decreases with age. (From Effron, M. B., Bhatnagar, G. M., Spurgeon, H. A., et al.: Changes in myosin isoenzymes, ATPase activity, and contraction duration in rat cardiac muscle with aging can be modulated by thyroxine. Circ. Res. *60*:238, 1987.) Panel B, The velocity of shortening during lightly loaded isotonic contractions in isolated cardiac muscle from younger and older rats decreases with aging. (From Capasso, J. M., Malhotra, A., Remily, R. M., et al.: Effects of age on mechanical and electrical performance of rat myocardium. Am. J. Physiol. *245*:H72, 1983.)

atherosclerotic disease are prevalent and populations in which these disorders of the arterial vasculature are unusual.

This increase in pulse wave velocity is a reflection of changes in the compliance properties of the central arteries[63] due to age-associated alterations in the precise structure and composition of the collagen and ground substance in and around the blood vessels themselves. Some age-associated dilation of these arteries also occurs.[60] Thus, the artery functions on a stiffer portion of its pressure-volume relationship. Although one might speculate that these changes in aortic stiffness are due to alterations in the smooth muscle structure or function or to properties of the central arterial system, this evidence against this idea exists in experimental animals. Aortic and arterial rings have equal vasodilating properties when the arteries are stimulated with nitrates or other stimulants of the effects of endothelial-derived relaxing factor on vascular tone. There is some evidence of decreased endothelial-mediated vasodilation,[59] thus implying decreased endothelial vasodilator production, not response, with age.

Because the left ventricle is ejecting blood into a stiffer central aorta, the systolic blood pressure tends to be higher in older individuals, even the absence of disease. The higher systolic pressure in older individuals is even greater in the central aorta than it is in the periphery. This is because of the central superimposition of the direct pressure wave from ejection of blood from the left ventricle and the reflected wave returning to the central aorta from the periphery. O'Rourke demonstrated quite clearly in humans that the forward pulse wave in the arterial system reflects off the iliac bifurcation much like an ocean wave reflects off a dock.[64] In the case of the iliac bifurcation, the reflected wave moves backwards toward the central aorta. The actual movement of the direct pulse wave, as well as the reflected wave, is so much faster than in the central aorta there is superimposition of the direct and reflected waves *during* left ventricular ejection. In younger individuals, the reflected wave does not return to the central aorta until after aortic valve closure.

EFFECTS OF EXERCISE. The increase in left ventricular load is greater with age during exercise because of diminished arterial vasodilation mediated by beta-adrenergic receptor. Studies in chronically instrumented animals demonstrate that in the younger animal arterial vasodilation prevents an increase in impedance to left ventricular ejection during exercise, whereas in the older animal there is a further increase in impedance to ejection as exercise progresses (Fig. 50–7). This reflects a failure of beta-sympathetic–induced arterial vasodilatation.[65] After pharmacological beta blockade, young animals as well show an increase in impedance to left ventricular ejection of blood during exercise (Fig. 50–7). In a number of important respects exercise response is quite similar in adult and aged animals following beta-adrenergic blockade. This also appears to be the case in humans.

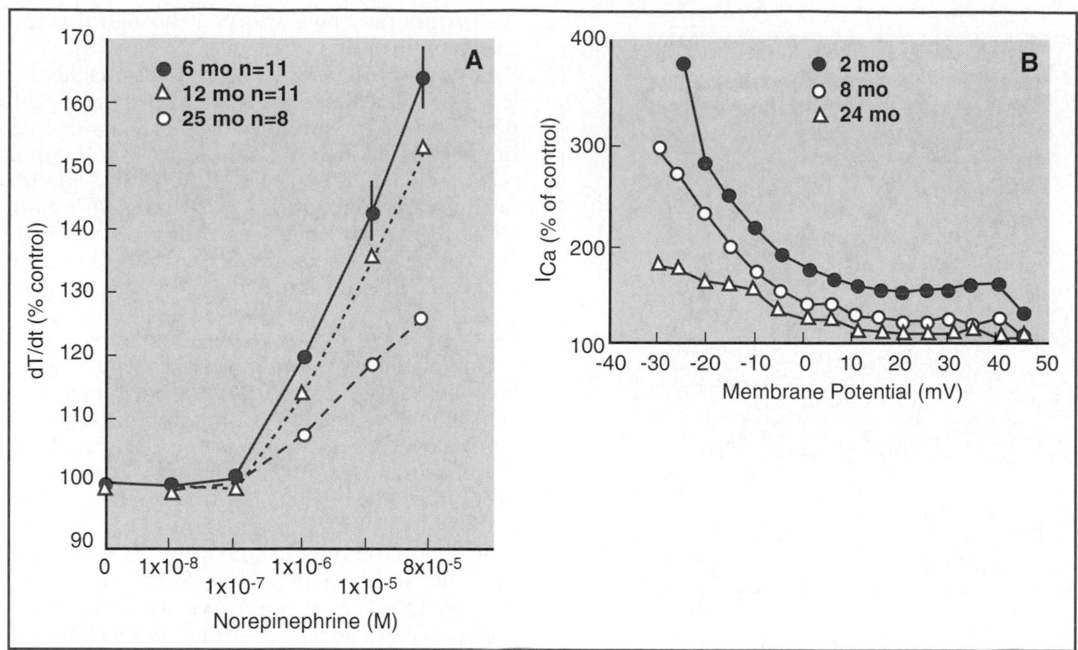

FIGURE 50–4. *A,* The effect of norepinephrine on the maximum rate of isometric tension development in isolated trabeculae from hearts of varying age. (Reproduced with permission from Lakatta, E. G., Gerstenblith, G., Angell, C. S., et al.: Diminished inotropic response of aged myocardium to catecholamines. Circ. Res. *36:*262, 1975. Copyright 1975 American Heart Association.) *B,* The effect of norepinephrine to increase the L type sarcolemmal channel current (I_{Ca}) across a range of activating steps to different membrane potentials in single vascular cells potential decline with aging, the norepinephrine concentration was 1×10^{-7} M. (From Xiao, R.-P., Spurgeon, H. A., O'Connor, F., and Lakatta, E. G.: Age-associated changes in β-adrenergic modulation on rat cardiac excitation-contraction coupling. J. Clin. Invest. *94:*2051, 1994, by permission of the American Society for Clinical Investigation.)

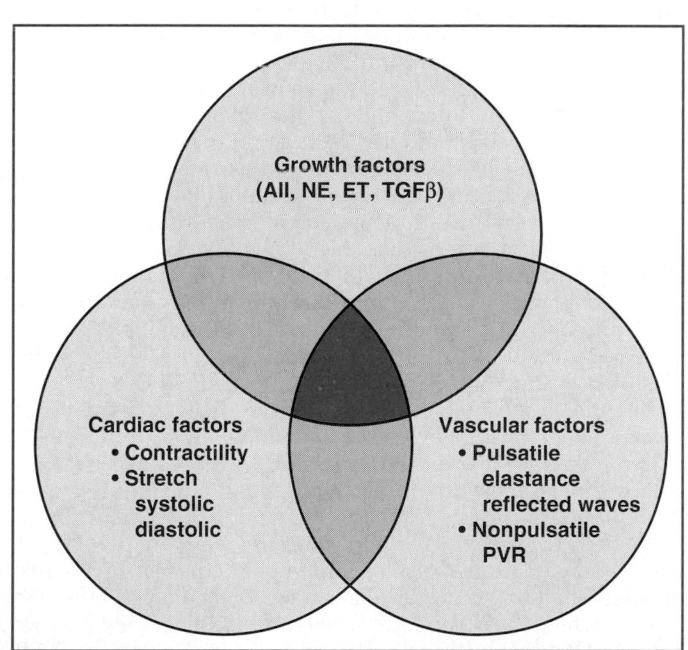

FIGURE 50–5. Acute and chronic regulation of myocardial function and structure. Cardiac factors (Ca^{++} activation of myofilaments, in part, regulated by fiber stretch prior to excitation) and vascular factors (peripheral vascular resistance [PVR], arterial elastance, and reflexed pulse waves) interact to determine the acute workload placed upon the heart and thus acutely modulate cardiac performance. Chronic increases in cardiac workload, due to any of the specific entities depicted within the cardiac and vascular factors, and growth factors interact to determine cardiac mass and long-term changes in cardiac function that accompany changes in cardiac structure. (AII = angiotensin II, NE = norepinephrine; ET = endothelin; TGFβ = transforming growth factor beta.)

STUDY OF AGE CHANGES IN CARDIAC FUNCTION IN THE ABSENCE OF DISEASE

Studies of "normal aging" are handicapped by an understandable reluctance to use invasive methodology in people who are thought to be free of cardiovascular disease. This resulted in two major limitations in some earlier work. First, it was difficult to exclude patients with occult coronary disease. This is an important consideration because the prevalence of autopsy-documented disease is much higher than the presence of clinically obvious disease.[66] Many individuals thought to be free of coronary disease on screening using routine history, physical examination, and resting electrocardiogram undoubtedly were not, and many older study participants with asymptomatic coronary disease were probably included as normal in the

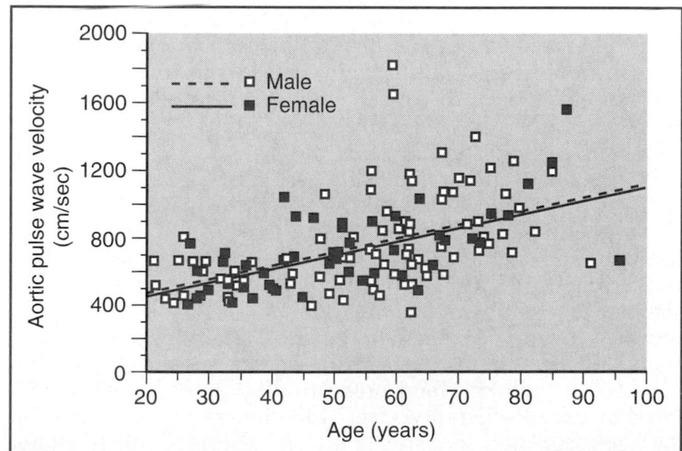

FIGURE 50–6. Aortic pulse wave velocity, an index of aortic stiffness, increases with age in healthy participants. (Reproduced with permission from Vaitkevicius, P. V., Fleg, J. L., Engel, J. H., et al.: Effects of age and aerobic capacity on arterial stiffness in healthy adults. Circulation *88:*1456, 1993. Copyright 1993 American Heart Association.)

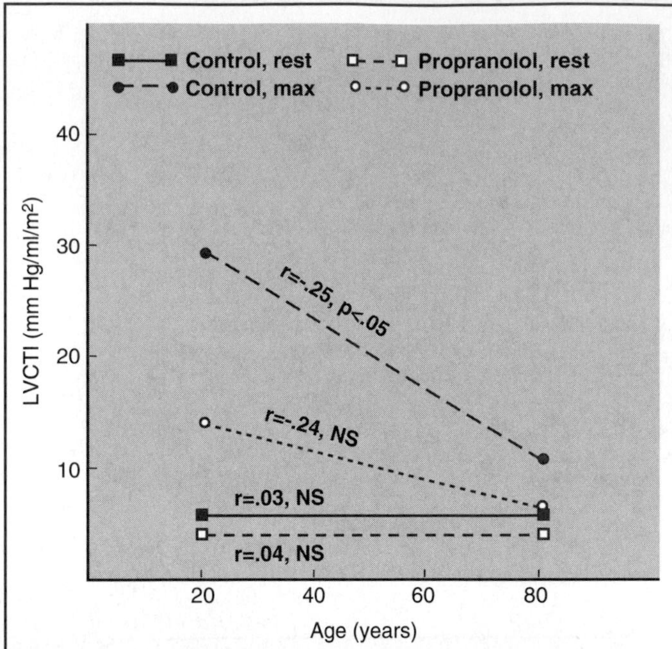

FIGURE 50–7. **Left ventricular contractility index (LVCTI) measured as the ratio of end-systolic arterial pressure and end-systolic volume index. Lines are the best fit, linear regressions at rest and during exercise in the presence and absence of β-adrenergic blockade with propranolol. (From Fleg, J. L., O'Connor, F., Gerstenblith, G., et al.: Impact of age on the cardiovascular response to dynamic upright exercise in healthy men and women. J. Appl. Physiol. *78*:890, 1995.)**

study protocols. This problem was overcome in a series of studies on well-selected and tested members of the Baltimore Longitudinal Study of Aging at the National Institute of Aging.[67,68]

The second limitation resulting from the hesitancy to use invasive methodology was an inability to measure central circulatory function (stroke volume or its determinants, left ventricular end-diastolic and end-systolic volumes) in relatively large numbers and volunteers. Previous studies used mainly Fick principle determination of cardiac output and derived only stroke volume. The introduction of nuclear cardiology and echocardiographic techniques, and the use of thallium scintigraphy to diagnose the presence of coronary disease, led to remarkable progress. Echocardiography and gated blood pool scans are able to estimate cardiac volume throughout the cardiac cycle at rest and during exercise, and thus have provided significant information concerning the effect of normal aging on cardiac function at rest and during stress.[56,69–72]

Hemodynamics at Rest

Although studies performed 30 years ago indicated that aging is associated with a decline in cardiac output at rest in men,[73] these results may have been due to selection of subjects not free of disease. Several of the studies involved hospitalized or disabled subjects not known to have alterations in resting cardiac function that are not age-related but rather condition-related. Studies using both echocardiography and gated blood pool scans at rest with and without beta-adrenergic blockade show that seated men at rest show a modest increase in the end-diastolic, end-systolic, and stroke volumes with age, but these volumes are not changed by aging in females (Fig. 50–8*A*). Once more, it should be emphasized that the most significant age-associated change in resting cardiovascular parameters is the increase in systolic blood pressure (Fig. 50–8*F*) with aortic dilation. As discussed above, this change is secondary to the age-associated increase in arterial stiffness and is likely responsible, at least in part, for the mild left ventricular hypertrophy associated with aging. Thus, the near-normal left ventricular volumes and preserved ejection fraction in seated persons at rest reflect the balance between the mild hypertrophy and the increase in vascular load and left ventricular size. At least in theory, normalized left ventricular wall stress may be preserved through this mild left ventricular hypertrophy.

Prolonged relaxation of cardiac muscle at rest with aging is reflected in these same studies using gated cardiac blood pool scanning techniques.[74] There is a decrease in the maximum rate of early diastolic filling, and, similarly, Doppler-recorded velocity of blood flow through the mitral valve during early diastole is also reduced.[75] Slowed early diastolic filling with age leads to greater contribution of atrial contraction to diastolic filling and the appearance of the "normal" S_4 sound and atrial enlargement.

Exercise Performance in the Elderly

One of the most universally accepted changes with aging is a decline in maximum work performance, which has as a consequence a decline in maximum oxygen consumption.[76] Many have interpreted this age-associated decrease in maximum work capacity and oxygen consumption to be a reflection of diminished cardiovascular performance and the ability of the heart to augment cardiac output during exercise. The reduction in maximum heart rate during exercise in older individuals, even following endurance training, support this.[77] However, noncardiac factors also contribute to the age-associated decline in maximum work capacity. These include a decline in maximum skeletal muscle performance parameters, a greater sense of muscle fatigue and discomfort, and/or a marked increase in the sensation of the work of breathing or dyspnea. Cardiovascular function is thought to limit oxygen consumption when oxygen consumption does not consistently increase at the highest levels of exercise. With aging, oxygen consumption often increases progressively with increasing workload performance. Data of this type raise the possibility that maximum work capacity in the elderly is limited by either skeletal muscle fatigue (or sense of fatigue) or the increased work of breathing. It is possible that differences in muscle mass, less diversion of blood flow to the exercising muscle, and/or reduced oxygen extraction may also be limiting factors. Age differences in maximum oxygen consumption are minimized when the values are adjusted for lean body mass.[78]

The mechanism for achieving the augmentation of cardiac output differs markedly with age. First, younger individuals augment heart rate considerably more than do older individuals, reflecting the age-associated decrease in the chronotropic response to beta-sympathetic stimulation (Fig. 50–8*D*). With gated cardiac blood pool scans, it is clear that the stroke volume in both male and female older individuals is maintained by end-diastolic dilatation. In contrast, end-diastolic volume in younger individuals does not increase measurably during vigorous exercise. Also, end-diastolic volume becomes exceedingly small in the younger individual, almost at the limits of the measurement techniques, whereas end-systolic volume in older individuals fails to decrease markedly (Fig. 50–8*B*). In younger individuals the marked sympathetic response at maximum workload maintains a small heart size and a high heart rate. Even though systemic blood pressure rises, end-systolic volume is small because of increased contractility. This response in the young is also aided by beta-sympathetic–central arterial vasodilatation, decreasing the impedance to left ventricular ejection of blood during exercise. The marked augmentation of heart rate (Fig. 50–8*D*) and relaxation velocity by beta-sympathetic stimulation allows the heart rate of the younger individual to increase from approximately one beat per second to three beats per second without compromising filling, and with each beat essentially ejecting the entire contents of the left ventricle into the aorta.

Age-Related Changes in Sympathetic Modulation

The impact of beta-adrenergic modulation of heart rate and cardiac volume during exercise can be determined

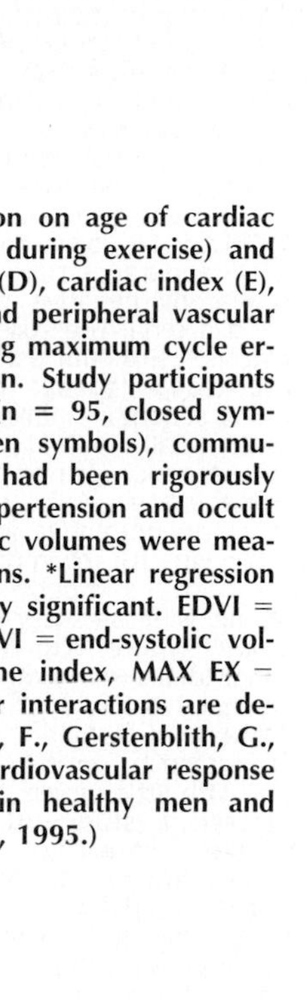

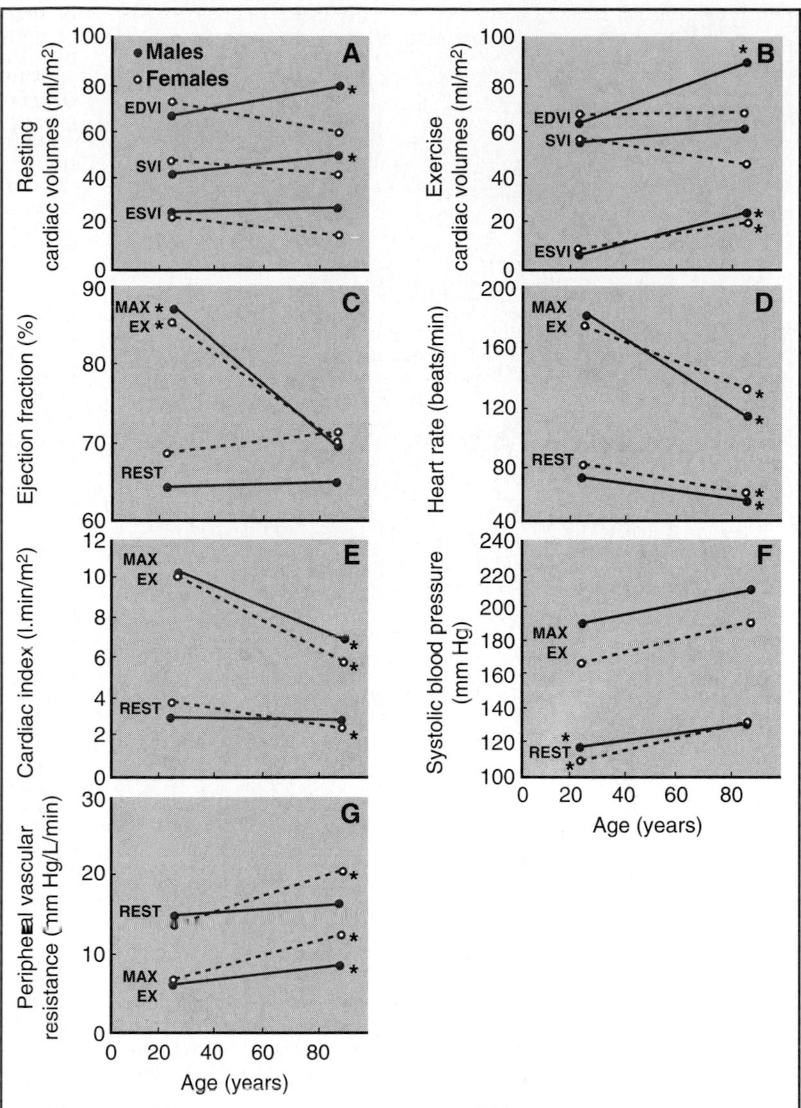

FIGURE 50–8. Linear regression on age of cardiac volume indices (A, at rest; B, during exercise) and ejection fraction (C), heart rate (D), cardiac index (E), systolic arterial pressure (F), and peripheral vascular resistance (G) at rest and during maximum cycle ergometry in the upright position. Study participants were healthy, sedentary male (n = 95, closed symbols) and female (n = 50, open symbols), community-dwelling volunteers who had been rigorously screened to exclude clinical hypertension and occult coronary artery disease. Cardiac volumes were measured via gated blood-pool scans. *Linear regression on age within sex is statistically significant. EDVI = end-diastolic volume index, ESVI = end-systolic volume index, SVI = stroke volume index, MAX EX = maximum exercise. (Age-gender interactions are described in Fleg, J. L., O'Connor, F., Gerstenblith, G., et al.: Impact of age on the cardiovascular response to dynamic upright exercise in healthy men and women. J. Appl. Physiol. *78*:890, 1995.)

when exercise is performed in the presence of beta adrenergic blockade. In young individuals, the same cardiac output is achieved during upright cycle exercise in the presence and absence of acute beta blockade with propranolol, but the hemodynamic profile differs: The increment in heart rate and the reduction in end-systolic volume are markedly less in the presence of beta blockade. However, the end-diastolic volume increases substantially during beta blockade, permitting a larger stroke volume.[57] The rate of early left ventricular filling and myocardial contractility are reduced. This altered hemodynamic pattern during acute beta blockade indicates the interaction among parameters that maintain cardiac output when a deficit in adrenergic modulation is present. Cardiac dilatation at end diastole augments stroke volume, which compensates for a reduction in heart rate.

An age-associated diminution in the effectiveness of sympathetic modulation of the cardiovascular response to exercise could contribute to many of the changes identified in the cardiovascular response to exercise in healthy older humans (Figs. 50–7, 50–8, and 50–9), including the decline in maximum heart rate, the increases in left ventricular end-diastolic and end-systolic volume indices, and decreased ejection fraction and left ventricular contractility. A recent study, in fact, demonstrated that the age-associated changes in left ventricular end-diastolic volume and stroke volume indices during upright cycle exercise do not occur in the presence of blockade and that the age-associated reduction in heart rate is markedly attenuated because of a greater effect of beta-adrenergic blockade to decrease heart rate and increase heart size in younger, rather than in older, subjects.[57] Age differences in the early diastolic filling rate and left ventricular contractility (Fig. 50–7) during exercise are also reduced or abolished when exercise is performed during beta-adrenergic blockade.[74] Thus, during stress the older heart is confronted with an increased impedance to ejection and greater venous return. The response is increased work performance, despite decreased contractility and heart rate, by left ventricular dilation during diastole. The Frank-Starling mechanism operates to augment stroke work and volume and meet the peripheral demands for increased blood flow (Fig. 50–9).

INTEGRATED RESPONSE TO EXERCISE

Thus, the overall picture of the cardiovascular response to exercise is entirely consistent with animal and human studies approaching aging as a selective process. Coronary perfusion and left ventricular function are well maintained with age, predicting that older individuals should be able to employ the Frank-Starling mechanism to augment cardiac function when other mechanisms fail. Cellular hypertrophy with age is clearly a helpful factor in maintaining left ventricular function. Although prolonged relaxation and delayed filling are present, in association with pressure overload hypertrophy, there is no evidence that left ventricular filling during exercise is compromised. Because end-diastolic volume is greater, end-diastolic pressure may be higher, and contribute to dyspnea and the increased work of breathing in older individuals. Finally, stiffening of central arteries with age and greater pulse wave velocity and earlier reflected waves increase the left ventricular workload during exercise more in the elderly than in the younger individual. This increase in load also reflects the diminished beta-sympathetic arterial vasodilat-

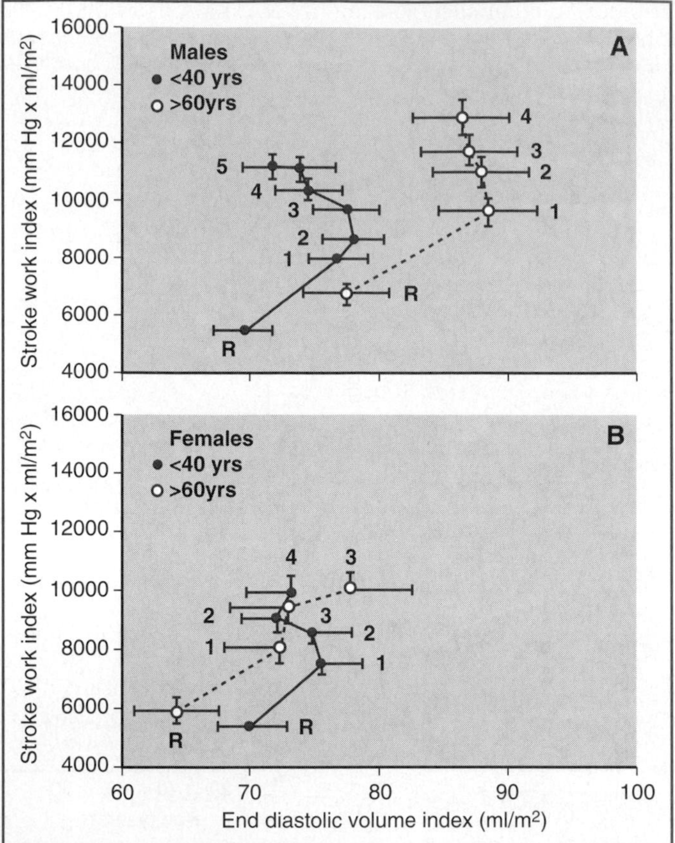

FIGURE 50–9. Left ventricular stroke work index (SWI) measured as the product of stroke volume index (SVI) and brachial systolic pressure at rest and during graded exercise in younger (< 40 yr) and older (> 60 yr) men *(top),* and women *(bottom)* of the study population depicted in Figure 17.7. R = seated rest. 1–5 = progressive increases in submaximal workload affected by increasing resistance to peddling on a cycle ergometer. (From Fleg, J. L., O'Connor, F., Gerstenblith, G., et al.: Impact of age on the cardiovascular response to dynamic upright exercise in healthy men and women. J. Appl. Physiol. *78*:890, 1995.)

ing response. In summary, the lower heart rate response and inotropic response and the increase in left ventricular workload due to arterial stiffness is compensated for by the intrinsic Frank-Starling mechanism in a remarkable and predictable manner in the elderly. During the transition from normal aging to aging and disease, it can easily be conceptualized that the older heart, using the Frank-Starling mechanism during exercise, has no further reserve. All of the compensatory mechanisms available to augment cardiac output are used during normal exercise. Thus, it would not be surprising if older individuals with a given severity of cardiovascular disease did worse during exercise than younger individuals who can utilize the Starling reserve mechanism after sympathetic reserve is exhausted.

EJECTION FRACTION AT REST AND DURING EXERCISE. It is of clinical interest that left ventricular ejection fraction increases during exercise in both young and old individuals who are free of disease. The exercise ejection fraction is greater in younger individuals, 80 to 90 per cent, than in older individuals, 60 to 80 per cent, respectively. This difference is due to a greater decrease in end-systolic volume in younger individuals than in older individuals during exercise. Recent studies in men and women during exercise at various ages indicate that the changes described above are more pronounced in older men than in older women.[51] It is not clear whether hormonal factors have an influence in the specific populations under study. In both young and old, a decline in ejection fraction during exercise is an abnormal response and is suggestive of the presence of disease.

Finally, the age-associated alterations in exercise response are not attributable to decreased catecholamine elaboration during exercise, because plasma levels of catecholamines are higher, not lower, in older humans during exercise.[79]

EFFECTS OF CHRONIC PHYSICAL CONDITIONING ON AEROBIC RESERVE

There is mounting evidence that some of the cardiovascular structural and functional changes that occur with aging in healthy humans can be modified by chronic exercise. The age-associated increases in pulse wave velocity and carotid pulse pressure augmentation are blunted in exercise-trained older individuals.[61,80] Additionally, it has recently been shown that arterial stiffness varies inversely with aerobic capacity in a healthy sedentary study population across a broad age range. This inverse relationship occurred over and above the effects of age to increase arterial stiffness and to decrease aerobic capacity.[61]

ENDURANCE TRAINING. In younger men, endurance training blunts the baroreceptor response, measured as the change in heart rate relative to arterial pressure during phenylephrine infusion or during lower body negative pressure.[81] In contrast, in healthy, rigorously screened sedentary middle-aged and older men, strenuous prolonged endurance training, sufficient to elicit large increases in maximal exercise capacity and small reductions in resting heart rate, appears to increase cardiac vagal tone at rest and not to alter arterial baroreflex control of heart rate, but it does result in a diminished forearm vasoconstrictor response to reductions in baroreflex sympatho-inhibition.[82] In endurance-trained older (60 to 80 years) individuals during lower body negative pressure, end-diastolic volume, stroke volume, and arterial pressure are better preserved than in age-matched controls.[83] This contrasts with a reduction in stroke volume during lower body negative pressure in young endurance-trained versus young sedentary individuals.[84]

In most[74,85–88] but not all studies, early diastolic left ventricular filling in chronically endurance-trained older men is slowed and similar to their sedentary age peers. Thus, slowed early diastolic filling appears to be intrinsic to normative aging and not secondary to the reduction in aerobic capacity accompanying the aging process.

Changes in both central and peripheral reflex mechanisms utilized during acute dynamic exercise occur with chronic endurance training in older individuals.[70,89,90] After high-intensity training of older (60 to 69 years of age) individuals for 10 months to 1 year, $\dot{V}O_{2max}$ increased by about 20 per cent (25.4 to 32.9 ml/kg/min). This was achieved primarily by an increase in peripheral oxygen utilization during treadmill exercise, manifested by an increase in estimated arteriovenous oxygen difference, with little increase in estimated maximum cardiac output.[77] In contrast, a study using the acetylene rebreathing method reported that stroke volume at peak *treadmill* exercise increased by 15 per cent in older (64 years) men following 12 months of endurance training.[53] This was accompanied by a 7 per cent increase in arteriovenous O_2 difference. In women, in contrast to men, increased $\dot{V}O_{2max}$ accompanying the training effect was achieved exclusively by an increase in exercise arteriovenous O_2 difference, as neither peak stroke volume nor maximum heart rate increased.[89]

In another study, similarly aged individuals (60 to 70 years), whose $\dot{V}O_{2max}$ increased by about 25 per cent (29.6 to 37.2 ml/kg/min) following training, had an 18 per cent increase in maximum cardiac output during *supine* cycle exercise. This increase in cardiac output following chronic endurance training was achieved by an increase in stroke volume, due to an increase in end-diastolic volume and to a greater reduction in end-systolic volume, resulting in augmentation of the ejection fraction achieved during exercise. As arterial pressure during the supine exercise testing was not affected by conditioning, the enhanced ejection fraction and reduced end-systolic volume after conditioning have been interpreted to reflect an increase in myocardial contractility induced by conditioning. A peculiarity of this study is that the estimated arteriovenous oxygen did not increase following exercise, in contrast to observations in similar training paradigms.[77] This may relate to the supine body position during this more recent study.[89] In contrast to the above study, less intense exercise paradigms in older individuals may not enhance cardiac performance (increased ejection fraction or reduced end-systolic volume) during cycle ergometry.[90]

In summary, it is quite clear that the aerobic capacity of both middle-aged and older individuals can increase following endurance training and that this is mediated by adaptations in both peripheral and cardiac mechanisms.

Conclusions

The mechanisms involved in the cardiovascular response to exercise are directly related to the age-associated alterations in central arterial stiffness and diminished sympathetic response. This is also true for the response to disease states such as congestive heart failure in which there is an increased emphasis on the importance of vasodilation in the elderly. Impedance to left ventricular ejection is markedly increased with age and dominates the clinical picture and potentially the therapeutic options available. The aging heart with its modest hypertrophy and consequent prolonged relaxation is, as most pressure-hypertrophied hearts, perhaps more sensitive to ischemic injury with more profound consequences.

The fact that cardiac function of younger individuals in the presence of beta blockade appears similar to that of older individuals supports the conclusion that the major factor contributing to age change in the cardiovascular system is a decreased beta-sympathetic response. During beta-adrenergic blockade, the cardiovascular response to exercise in young and old is very similar, with the Frank-Starling mechanism available to augment stroke volume.

Finally, the aged heart may be slower, or may have decreased capacity to hypertrophy and modify structure in response to long-term changes in load. This decreased hypertrophy response to hemodynamic stress may result in the decreased ability of the older heart to tolerate obstructive aortic valvular disease and/or alterations in left ventricular function such as acute myocardial infarction. Many other factors may change with age to a modest degree that does not interfere with physiological function. The fundamental mechanisms for the age-associated decrease in beta-sympathetic response and the decrease in hypertrophy response to stress remain to be entirely elucidated, although with regard to the sympathetic response, there appear to be mechanisms operating on a number of different levels, both at the receptor and within the myocardial or smooth muscle cell.

HEART DISEASE IN THE ELDERLY

Cardiovascular diseases, e.g., atherosclerosis, hypertension, heart failure, and stroke, reach epidemic proportions among older persons and, in this regard, are indicative of a failure of modern cardiology and medicine. One way to conceptualize why the clinical manifestations and the prognosis of these diseases worsen with age is that in older individuals the specific pathophysiological mechanisms that cause clinical disorders are superimposed on heart and vascular substrates that are modified by aging per se (Fig. 50–10). Imagine that age increases as one moves from the lower to the upper part of the figure, and that the line bisecting the top and bottom parts represents the clinical practice "threshold" for disease recognition. Thus, entities above the line are presently classified as "diseases" and lead to heart and brain failure. The vascular and cardiac changes presently thought to occur as a result of the "normal aging process" (i.e., those addressed in the previous sections) are depicted below the line. These age-associated changes in cardiac and vascular properties alter the substrate upon which cardiovascular disease is superimposed in several ways. First, they lower the extent of disease severity required to cross the threshold that results in clinically significant signs and symptoms. For example, a mild degree of ischemia-induced relaxation abnormalities that may be asymptomatic in a younger individual may cause dyspnea in an older individual, who, by virtue of age alone, has preexisting slowed and delayed early diastolic relaxation.

Age-associated changes may also alter the manifestations and presentation of common cardiac diseases. This usually occurs in patients with acute infarction in whom the diagnosis is delayed because of atypical symptoms resulting in increased time to onset of therapy. Age-associated changes, including those in beta-adrenergic responsiveness and in vascular stiffness, also influence the response to and therefore the selection of different therapeutic inventions in older individuals with cardiovascular disease. In one sense those processes below the line in Figure 50–10 ought not

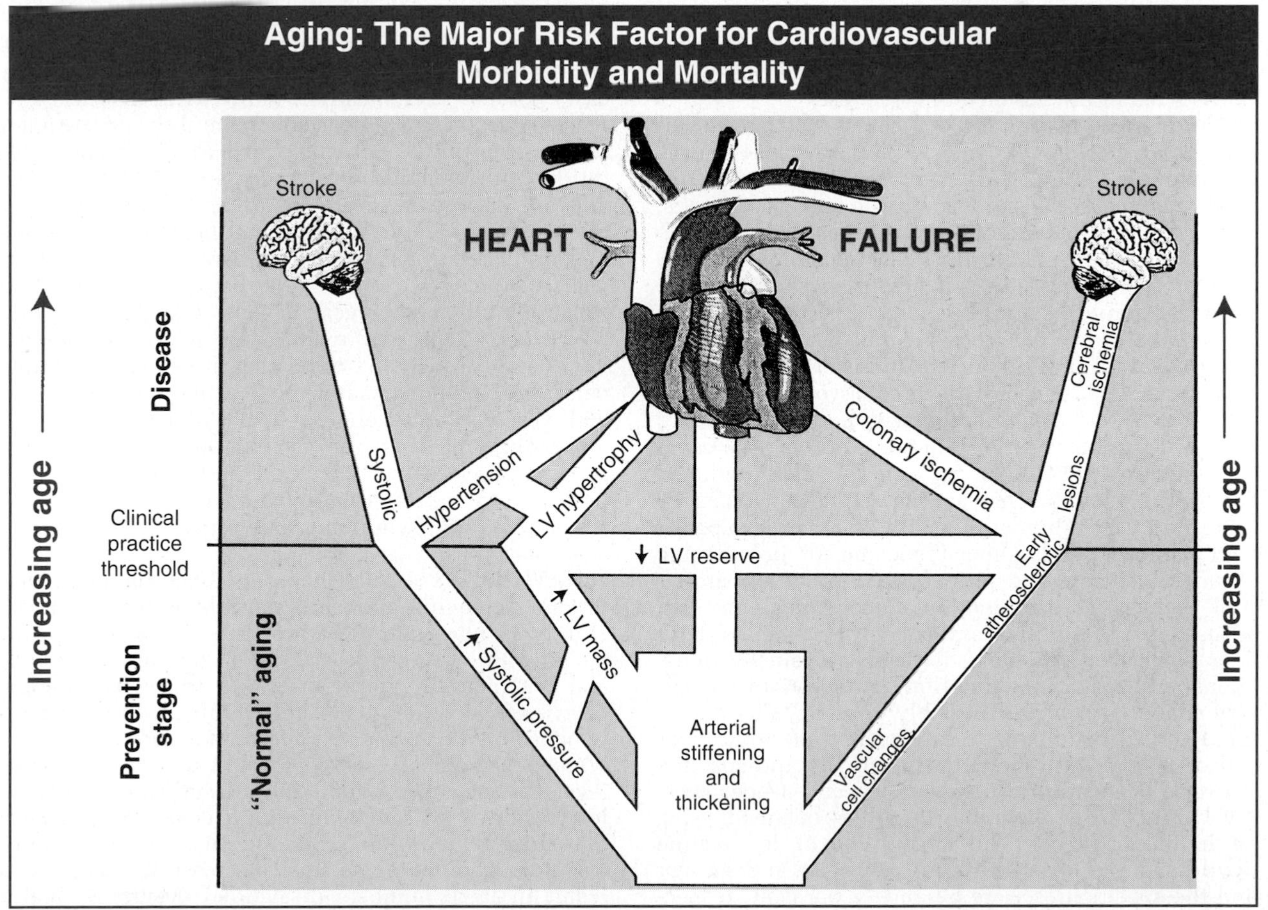

FIGURE 50–10. Changes in the vasculature and heart with aging in health may also be construed as risk factors for cardiovascular disease, leading to heart and brain disorders in older age (see text for details). (From Lakatta, E. G.: Aging effects on the vasculature in health. Risk factors for cardiovascular disease. Am. J. Geriatr. Cardiol. *3*:11–17, 1994.)

to be considered to reflect "normal" aging. Rather, they might be construed as specific risk factors for the diseases that they relate to, and thus might be targets of interventions designed to decrease the occurrence and/or manifestations of cardiovascular disease at later ages. Such a strategy would thus advocate treating "normal" aging. Additional studies of the specific risks of each "normal" age-associated change are required. In the following section the question of how aging influences the presentation and approach to the treatment of common cardiovascular diseases is reviewed, focusing on the influence and impact of the age-associated changes described above.

Chronic Ischemic Heart Disease

(See also Chap. 38)

DIAGNOSIS. Clinical Findings. The prevalence and severity of coronary atherosclerosis increase so dramatically with age that more than one-half of all deaths in persons aged 65 years or older are due to coronary disease and about three-fourths of all deaths from ischemic heart disease occur in older individuals.[91] The diagnosis of ischemic heart disease may be more difficult in the older individual since the prevalence of diagnosed disease is only one-third to one-half the prevalence of autopsy-documented significant atherosclerosis. The lack of classic symptomatology may be related to an age-associated decline in physical activity to the point at which ischemic symptoms are not present. In addition, dyspnea, rather than pain, may be the most prominent feature of the clinical picture in angina, as well as infarction, possibly because of the age-related changes in myocardial compliance and diastolic relaxation discussed above. The physical examination is of limited usefulness in the diagnosis of ischemic heart disease (see p. 1292). It should be remembered, however, that the transient features associated with acute ischemia (i.e., an S_4 gallop, reversed splitting of the second sound, and a systolic murmur secondary to mitral regurgitation) are often present in older individuals in the absence of ischemia.

Stress Testing (see also p. 1296). Stress tests are useful in the diagnosis of older patients with suspected coronary disease, although with certain caveats. The presence of resting ST-segment abnormalities or the use of digitalis, both of which are more common in the elderly, may invalidate the interpretation of the stress electrocardiogram and, in this setting, stress testing using thallium scintigraphy[92] or echocardiography is helpful. These techniques are also useful when the stress electrocardiogram is unexpectedly negative in an older individual whose history suggests the presence of ischemia, because the predictive accuracy of a negative test is low in a population with a high prevalence of disease. Finally, many elderly patients may not be capable of exercising to 85 to 90 per cent of their predicted maximum heart rate. In this setting a thallium scan or echocardiogram in conjunction with a pharmacological stress test using dipyridamole, adenosine, or dobutamine may provide diagnostic and prognostic information similar to that of an exercise examination. Echocardiography can also be used in the initial assessment of patients with known or suspected coronary disease to evaluate global and regional left ventricular function, left ventricular mass, and valve abnormalities, and possibly to distinguish nonviable from stunned or hibernating regions of left ventricular dysfunction. In a recent report, the sensitivity and specificity of exercise echocardiography were 88 and 82 per cent, respectively, and are comparable to values obtained using exercise thallium imaging. The sensitivities of dobutamine and dipyridamole echocardiography were 82 and 74 per cent, and the specificities were 82 and 77 per cent, respectively.[93]

MANAGEMENT. The treatment of angina in older and younger patients is similar (see p. 1299). After diagnosis, reversible factors should be identified and treated. Of these, anemia, hyperthyroidism, hypertension, congestive heart failure, and noncompliance with medication may all be more common and more difficult to diagnose in the elderly. It should also be remembered that atherosclerosis is a progressive disease, and although it has sometimes been stated that risk factor reduction is less important in the older patient, more recent evidence suggests that both successful treatment of hypertension[94–96] and cessation of smoking[97] decrease cardiovascular mortality in the elderly.

The goals of antiischemic medical therapy and the use of specific antiischemic agents are generally similar to those in the younger population. Older individuals may be more susceptible to symptoms related to any hypotensive effects of some antiischemics because of decreased sympathetic responsiveness. The degree to which ischemia may be mediated via a heart rate or contractility response to beta-adrenergic stimulation, and therefore the extent to which benefit may be achieved with beta blockers, may be decreased by the same age-associated change in sympathetic responsiveness. Although there are no controlled secondary prevention trials of aspirin in older populations, its effectiveness in the middle-aged group[98] and the low side effect profile support the use of low-dose therapy in the elderly with known coronary disease.

If medical therapy fails to control symptoms adequately, percutaneous transluminal coronary angioplasty (PTCA) should be considered in patients with appropriate anatomy (see Chap. 39). In the more elderly individuals, whose life span is limited regardless of therapy, and whose activity is restricted by other disease, treatment goals should be directed toward symptom alleviation and continuation of an independent life style. Although immediate success and complication rates in those 65 to 80 years of age are often similar to those in the younger age groups when angioplasty is performed by experienced individuals,[99,99a,99b] it is associated with a lower clinical success rate and higher vascular and cardiac complication rates in those over 80 years of age. This probably relates to more difficult access because of increased likelihood of peripheral vascular disease, coronary calcification, multivessel disease, renal impairment, and cerebrovascular complications. Angioplasty in one group of 26 patients over 90 years from seven institutions indicated a clinical success rate of only 65 per cent and six in-hospital deaths, four of which were related to the procedure.[100] A higher complication rate is also reported for rotational coronary atherectomy in those over 80 years of age.[101] There is also a distinction between success of coronary bypass surgery in those younger and older than 80 years.[102] This may relate again to the increased likelihood and severity of coexisting illnesses, including diabetes and pulmonary and renal disease as well as peripheral vascular and cerebrovascular disease. As is true of randomized trials in the general population, retrospective studies in those over 70 years undergoing PTCA and bypass surgery indicate that bypass surgery is associated with fewer recurrent symptoms and repeat procedures than is angioplasty.[103]

PREVENTION (see also Chap. 35). The importance of cholesterol screening and cholesterol-lowering therapy in the elderly is uncertain. The biphasic increase in cholesterol levels with advanced age, the high rate of coronary disease and outcomes in the elderly, and the most recent guidelines from the National Cholesterol Education Program,[104] which include age as a risk factor for coronary disease and which recommend screening and treatment of elevated levels in the older population all suggest that cholesterol-lowering therapy may be useful. It is also important to note that since the absolute risk of coronary events is so high in the older populations, a small decrease in *relative* risk may result in large numbers of avoided events. Several recent analyses, however, found no statistically significant relationship between elevated cholesterol levels and coronary outcomes in older individuals without known coronary disease. The analyses by Manolio,[105] Framingham data,[106] and Krumholz[107] suggest that the relationship declines over age 65 and that there may be no relationship between coronary outcomes and cholesterol levels in those over 80 years of age. In older individuals with known disease, however, the recent Scandinavian Simvastatin Survival Study results indicate that treatment of elevated cholesterol significantly reduces cardiovascular mortality and morbidity.[108] It seems reasonable, therefore, to screen and treat those older individuals with known coronary disease but not those without coronary artery disease, except for possibly men in their 70's with other known risk factors.[109]

Other prevalent risk factors in the older population are obesity and in women estrogen deficiency. A recent analysis of over 40,000 older women reported that the relationship between the waist to hip ratio and cardiovascular outcomes, as well as other causes of death, is strong and monotonic[110] (see p. 1706). The waist to hip ratio, but not the body mass index, was also the best marker for the metabolic hazards of obesity, including lipid levels and insulin resistance. There are several studies indicating that estrogen replacement therapy is associated with a decrease in the development of cardiovascular disease and cardiovascular mortality in postmenopausal women[111] (see p. 1708). Although the benefits of estrogen are often attributed to a favorable influence on the lipid profile, the Nurses' Health Study demonstrated a significant decrease in the development of cardiovascular disease, even after risk factor adjustment.[112] Other benefits of estrogen may include inhibition of endothelial hyperplasia[113] and, as demonstrated by Reis et al.,[114] attenuation of inappropriate coronary vasoconstriction in the setting of endothelial dysfunction. The latter may be particularly important because aging itself, i.e., in the absence of coronary disease and risk factors, is associated with decreased endothelium-dependent coronary vasodilation.[115]

Acute Myocardial Infarction

(See also Chap. 37)

MANAGEMENT. The treatment of acute infarction should be undertaken with the realization that in-hospital and subsequent mortality, reinfarction, and complications are all increased in the elderly. Although the large randomized thrombolytic trials show a survival benefit with thrombolysis in this age group, fewer older individuals are eligible for and actually receive thrombolytic therapy. Furthermore, in those who do not receive thrombolytic therapy, the age-related increase in mortality (of about 1.6 per cent per year), congestive heart failure, and recurrent infarctions is still present.[116–119] This may be related in part to atypical and delayed presentation, a higher incidence of non–Q wave infarcts, and increased perceived and real rates of bleeding.[116–118,120] A recent analysis of GISSI-2 data, in which all participants received thrombolytic therapy, indicates that although the size of the first infarction is not increased with age, the degree of left ventricular dysfunction is.[119] Electromechanical dissociation was a more common mechanism for death in the older-age group and ventricular fibrillation was less common. Autopsy data indicated no relation between age and the extent of fixed coronary atherosclerotic disease in this population of patients with a first infarction, but there was a marked increase in cardiac rupture, which was found in 86 per cent of those over age 70 at autopsy.

Analysis of the Thrombolysis in Myocardial Infarction-II (TIMI-II) data indicates an age-related increase in complications, mortality, and recurrent infarction in this population as well.[121] This may be explained, in part, by delay of administration of thrombolytics in the older-age groups and by the fact that fewer are eligible to receive beta blockers, probably because of coexisting illnesses. This analysis also indicated no difference in outcomes between the older individuals who were randomized to an early "invasive" strategy with routine catheterization and prophylactic revascularization following thrombolytic therapy, and those randomized to a "conservative" strategy, in which patients underwent these procedures only if there was subjective or objective evidence of recurrent ischemia during the early postinfarction period.

There are many limitations of thrombolytic therapy in the older population. More older individuals have relative or absolute contraindications to these agents, particularly hypertension, history of stroke, and gastrointestinal bleeding. In a subset analysis from the Global Utilization of Streptokinase and Tissue Plasminogen Activator for Occluded Coronary Arteries I (GUSTO I) trial, outcomes in 3600 patients 75 years of age or older showed that there was significantly increased risk of intracranial bleeding in the tissue plasminogen activatory (t-PA) group.[122] Thrombolysis is unsuccessful in about 20 per cent of patients, and less than 60 per cent achieve brisk flow in the infarct-related artery. These considerations prompted randomized trials of primary angioplasty versus thrombolysis for acute infarction.[123] A meta-analysis of some of these studies, performed by O'Neill, indicated a survival advantage in those over age 70 with primary angioplasty.[124] Of particular interest to those caring for older individuals is that a cerebrovascular accident occurred in 3.5 per cent of those in the thrombolytic groups and in none of those in the primary angioplasty groups.

Aging may also be associated with architectural or remodeling changes occurring subsequent to an infarction, including regional thinning at the site of the infarction and hypertrophy in regions remote from the infarction. These may result from preexisting changes in left ventricular wall thickness, increased peripheral impedance, increased collagen content of the infarct and remote areas, decreased capability of the remote region to undergo hypertrophy, and changes in the inflammatory and healing response of the infarct itself. It should also be noted that the elderly benefit as much as younger patients from the secondary prevention effects of beta blockade[125] and that reduction in fatal and nonfatal events following infarction in patients with ejection fractions of 40 per cent or less treated with angiotensin-converting enzyme inhibitors was the same in those over and under 65 years of age.[126]

Arrhythmias

(See also Chap. 22)

Because of the increasing prevalence of hypertension and coronary disease, arrhythmias occur more frequently and are more often associated with hemodynamic compromise in the older age groups. However, in one study, the incidences of supraventricular and ventricular ectopic activity (>100 beats/24 hr of ambulatory monitoring) were 26 and 17 per cent, respectively, in 98 healthy subjects 60 to 85 years of age.[127] Ventricular couplets occurred in 11 per cent but ventricular tachycardia in only 4 per cent of the population. In a larger population from the Cardiovascular Health Study, 15 per cent of women and 25 per cent of men over age 65 had ventricular arrhythmias, while 57 per cent of women and 58 per cent of men had supraventricular arrhythmias during 24 hours of ambulatory monitoring.[128] Although these are often asymptomatic in healthy individuals, they may be more ominous in the presence of disease. Any compromise of cardiac output and blood pressure may, in turn, be associated with more critical decreases in cerebral flow in older patients because of impaired beta-adrenergic cardiovascular responsiveness, an increased likelihood of preexisting cerebrovascular disease, and increased vascular stiffness. Older patients may also experience significant symptoms at a slower rate of ventricular tachycardia than do younger individuals because of prolonged relaxation time and because they are more dependent on atrial contribution to diastolic filling, which is lost in ventricular tachycardia.

ATRIAL FIBRILLATION (see p. 654). This is the most common supraventricular tachyarrhythmia in persons over 65 years of age, occurring in one study in 4.8 per cent of women and 6.2 per cent of men.[129] It is associated with chronic cardiovascular disease including hypertension, ischemia, and failure, and also acute illnesses such as pneumonia and other infections, surgery, and acute infarction. Atrial fibrillation may precipitate or worsen failure or ischemic symptoms in older patients and is associated with an increased risk of adverse long-term cardiovascular outcomes, particularly stroke.[130] The goals of therapy include decreasing the likelihood of systemic embolization (see p. 1582) and correction of hemodynamic compromise, which may require slowing the ventricular rate and restoring sinus rhythm. Echocardiographic predictors of stroke in atrial fibrillation include mitral annular calcification, left atrial size, and left ventricular dysfunction.[131,132]

A pooled analysis of five randomized controlled trials of antithrombotic therapy in atrial fibrillation indicates that age, a history of hypertension, diabetes, and a prior transient ischemic attack or stroke are associated with increased risk of stroke in the control groups[133] (see p. 1830). Warfarin decreased the annual stroke rate from 4.5 per cent in the control groups to 1.4 per cent.[133] The annual rate for major hemorrhage was 1.0 per cent in the control groups and 1.3 per cent in the warfarin groups. Hemorrhage was associated with age, excessive anticoagulation, and poorly controlled hypertension.[134] Although the risk of hemorrhage is age related, the benefit of warfarin outweighs the risk and it should be generally used in the older population. However, the target INR (International Normalized Ratio) should be kept below 3.0, and those with contraindications to anticoagulation and those who cannot reliably take medication should be treated with aspirin.

Although several agents may help in maintaining sinus rhythm, for reasons that are unclear a meta-analysis indicated increased mortality associated with quinidine.[135] *Flecainide* is useful for patients with supraventricular arrhythmias, but side effects preclude its use in patients with other forms of organic heart disease, which are usually present in the older age groups. *Sotalol* may also be considered but may be associated with undesirable side effects in patients with systolic dysfunction.[136] Low-dose *amiodarone* therapy, however, has been shown to preserve sinus rhythm with relatively few side effects over both short- and long-term follow-up periods.[137] It also has the advantage of slowing the ventricular response if atrial fibrillation does recur. If medical therapy is unsuccessful and/or not tolerated, atrioventricular functional ablation with radiofrequency energy or direct current (see p. 619) was reported to be 100 per cent successful in 37 patients 70 years of age or older with a complication rate of only 3 per cent.[138]

The diagnosis of an arrhythmia in an older patient differs only in that the index of suspicion should perhaps be higher for any complaints relating to transient cerebral ischemia, angina, heart failure, or mental status changes. Long-term ambulatory monitoring, particularly with loop recorders, is often useful. The urgency of therapy depends on the associated hemodynamic changes, and emergency treatment is the same in all age groups.

The routine work-up should include a search for associated and/or precipitating factors. Some of these, including electrolyte imbalance, digitalis excess, clinical or subclinical hyperthyroidism,[139] anemia, pulmonary embolism, and congestive heart failure, are more common in the older population. Specific therapy for the arrhythmia is guided by the severity of associated symptoms, the presence and type of underlying heart disease, and recognition of the age-associated changes in the pharmacokinetics of the antiarrhythmic drugs, as discussed below.

BRADYARRHYTHMIAS (see also p. 645). Sinus bradycardia is often present in older individuals in the presence or absence of cardiac disease. It may be related to age-associated histological changes in the sinus node, a hypersensitive carotid sinus reflex, or medications. Evaluation should be undertaken if the patient is symptomatic and, since other causes for neurological symptoms are often present in the elderly, to determine whether, in fact, the transient symptoms are related to the bradycardia. Long-term ambulatory monitoring, often with loop recorders, is most useful in this regard. There is also a group of older individuals with postprandial hypotension significant enough to result in syncope,[140] possibly from impaired postprandial autonomic modulation of systemic vascular resistance and heart rate.[141]

If the patient is symptomatic from the bradycardia, immediate therapy is dependent on the degree of hemodynamic compromise. Temporary emergency measures, including administration of atropine and isoproterenol and insertion of a temporary pacemaker, can be used. If no reversible factors are present, the only effective long-term therapy is permanent pacing. Pacemakers that allow for proper sequencing of atrial and ventricular events are particularly useful in the elderly because of increased reliance on late diastolic filling and hence atrial systole. This pacing mode is also associated with a decreased likelihood of stroke and development of atrial fibrillation in some patient subsets.[142] Idiopathic heart block without evidence of structural heart disease is also more common in older persons, probably because of age-associated fibrosis within the conducting system.

Valvular Disease

(See also Chap. 32)

The diagnosis of valvular disease in the elderly is often obscured by age-related but benign systolic murmurs, changes in S_2, and increased stiffness of the central arteries. The latter may prevent the appearance of the slow anacrotic shoulder and small pulse pressure that would otherwise be seen in significant aortic stenosis. The other findings, however, particularly the presence of a late peaking systolic murmur, electrocardiographic evidence of left ventricular hypertrophy, and echocardiographic demonstration of valve narrowing and calcification all retain their significance. Doppler examination may be particularly useful in assessing the severity of obstruction. The usual causes are calcification of a congenital bicuspid valve, and in those over 75 years of age, degenerative calcification.

Aortic valve replacement should be recommended for the usual indications, i.e., syncope, angina, and heart failure, and is often associated with low mortality and excellent quality of life. Older individuals with calcific aortic stenosis should be observed closely because hemodynamic compromise may develop rapidly with little hypertrophy. In patients over 70 years of age, operative mortality for aortic valve replacement is about 4 per cent[143] and 5-year actuarial survival in a group of patients over 80 years undergoing aortic valve replacement was 76 per cent.[54] Risk factors for operative mortality include left ventricular dysfunction, lack of sinus rhythm, associated cardiac procedures, and emergency status.[143–145] Aortic valvuloplasty provides only palliative relief in patients with aortic stenosis,[146] but should be considered in those with definite contraindications to surgery. The diagnosis of aortic regurgitation is not more difficult in the older age groups but the timing of aortic valve replacement may be, because of the often benign course of the disease. Surgery is usually recommended for those patients who continue to be symptomatic with medical therapy.

Mitral stenosis in the elderly is usually due to rheumatic disease, while regurgitation can be due to rheumatic disease as well as calcification of the mitral annulus, mitral valve prolapse, and ischemic papillary muscle dysfunction. Survival time is considerably shortened in the presence of atrial fibrillation and heart failure, and the results of mitral valve surgery are satisfactory in the elderly. Mitral valve repair is also associated with low operative mortality (3.8 per cent), successful elimination of mitral regurgitation (>90 per cent), and good long-term survival at 5 years without embolism, hemorrhage, or need for reoperation.[147] Balloon mitral valvuloplasty is associated with higher morbidity and mortality in elderly patients with heavily calcified valves than it is in younger patients with pliable valves and no subvalvular stenosis.[148]

Hypertension

(See also Chap. 26)

The importance of the diagnosis and effective treatment of hypertension in the elderly cannot be overemphasized.[149] The incidence of hypertension in the Third National Health and Nutrition Examination Survey was 54 per cent in those 65 to 74 years of age.[94] A recent meta-analysis of nine major trials that included more than 15,000 individuals 60 years of age or older demonstrated that antihypertensive therapy significantly improves survival and decreases stroke and cardiac mortality and morbidity in this population.[95] Isolated systolic hypertension, i.e., systolic elevations in the presence of normal pressure, accounts for 65 per cent of hypertension in the elderly.[94] The Systolic Hypertension in the Elderly Program (SHEP) trial demonstrated that treating those over age 60 with a systolic pressure of over 160 mm Hg but a normal diastolic pressure reduced nonfatal infarctions by 33 per cent, left ventricular failure by 54 per cent, and stroke by 36 per cent over a 4.5-year follow-up period.[96]

In considering the diagnosis of hypertension, it is important to note that pseudohypertension, due to increased stiffening of the brachial artery, and pseudohypotension, due to atherosclerotic disease in the subclavian artery, may be more common in the elderly. In older patients who suddenly develop severe pressure elevations despite their disease having been previously well controlled with a modest regimen, the possibility of a renovascular cause on the basis of atherosclerotic renal artery disease should be investigated.[150] It is also important to measure the pressure in the upright position before deciding to intensify any antihypertensive regimen since older individuals are more likely to experience orthostatic falls in pressure and because of age-related changes in cerebrovascular autoregulation that render them less able to compensate for any abrupt decline in perfusion pressure.

The target pressures for older patients are not clearly defined. Borderline isolated systolic hypertension, defined as systolic pressure between 140 and 159 mm Hg with diastolic pressure below 90 mm Hg is also common in those over 60 years of age and is associated with an increased risk of cardiovascular disease. The fifth report of the Joint National Committee on Detection, Evaluation, and Treatment of High Blood Pressure[94] (see p. 809) recommends considering treatment for those with systolic pressure greater than 150 mm Hg, although prospective trials have not yet demonstrated that antihypertensive therapy decreases risk for systolic levels between 150 and 160 mm Hg. The SHEP trial, which, as noted above, did demonstrate significant decreases in cardiovascular outcomes, targeted a pressure of less than 160 mm Hg for those with systolic pressure greater than 180 mm Hg and a reduction of 20 mm Hg for those with a pressure of 160 to 180 mm Hg. Although it is generally agreed that the target diastolic pressure should be less than 90 mm Hg, there are reports of a "J-shaped" relationship between treated diastolic pressure and clinical outcomes,[151] although this was not true of the SHEP results. Any J-shaped relationship may be due, in part, to the fact that most of coronary flow occurs in diastole and that such flow may be compromised by a lower diastolic pressure in individuals with obstructive coronary disease.

Antihypertensive therapy should consider not only the appropriate blood pressure goals but also the fact that hypertension is associated with other risk factors that independently predict cardiovascular outcomes. These include left ventricular hypertrophy, hyperlipidemia, and insulin resistance. Regarding specific therapy, it should be noted that thiazides were used as the step one antihypertensive agent in all of the major trials that documented a decline in cardiovascular morbidity and mortality. An increased incidence of cardiovascular deaths in hypertensive patients taking thiazides was not present in those also using potassium-sparing agents.[152] This benefit could not be mimicked by the addition of potassium supplements. It is not clear whether this is related to noncompliance with potassium supplements, the inability of supplements to adequately replete and/or maintain intracellular stores, or to other effects of thiazides.

Although beta blockers are effective antihypertensive agents in some populations, elderly patients respond less often than young hypertensives when beta blockers are used as single agents. In addition, beta blockers should be used cautiously in patients with systolic dysfunction, obstructive pulmonary disease, and peripheral vascular disease. Calcium channel blockers may be used in older hypertensives with associated ischemic disease, hypertrophy, and diastolic dysfunction; angiotensin-converting enzyme inhibitors in those with systolic dysfunction and diabetes; and alpha blockers in those with prostatic hypertrophy.

Congestive Heart Failure

(See also Chap. 17)

The evaluation and treatment of left ventricular dysfunction is an important consideration in the older population for several reasons. The incidence of congestive heart failure (9 per cent for those 80 to 89 years of age)[153] is the final common pathway of ischemic, hypertensive, and valvular disease and accounts for a large number of hospital admissions and office visits in this population. Congestive heart failure has a significant impact on survival as well as work status and quality of life. The mortality associated with congestive heart failure is approximately 50 per cent within 5 years of the diagnosis.[154] Although age-adjusted mortality due to coronary disease and that due to stroke have decreased in the older age groups over the past 20 years, the mortality due to congestive heart failure has increased significantly—by 29 per cent in those 65 to 74 years of age and by 45 per cent in those 75 to 84 years.[155]

The evaluation of symptoms suggestive of heart failure in older persons should include a determination of whether there is a predominant systolic or diastolic component (p. 447). This is particularly important in the older-age groups because up to 40 per cent of those over 60 years with these symptoms have normal systolic function. The distinction cannot be made easily by the history, the examination, or the chest film since both pathophysiological states often present with dyspnea, rales, and congestion on roentgenography. The distinction is best made with the echocardiogram or the gated blood pool examination. In the patient with predominant systolic dysfunction the cavity is dilated, the walls often thin, and the ejection fraction low. In the patient with predominant diastolic dysfunction, cavity size is normal, the walls often thick, and the ejection fraction normal or above normal, but indices of diastolic filling are reduced.

The evaluation should also consider whether there is an easily reversible precipitating factor, which is likely to be a superimposed illness in older persons. Pneumonia, anemia, renal failure, and supraventricular arrhythmia, for example, may all be present in the elderly with cardiac decompensation. Treating any superimposed illness may reverse the decompensation. An evaluation of underlying cardiac disorders should also be considered, and in the older individual, this is most likely to be hypertension and/or ischemic disease.

DIASTOLIC DYSFUNCTION. Predominant diastolic dysfunction often occurs in the presence of hypertension and is marked primarily by decreased early diastolic filling rates, elevated diastolic pressures, and increased dependence on atrial contribution. It is important to avoid antihypertensives that increase heart rate and thus compromise diastolic filling time. Although these patients often show evidence of a steep pressure/volume chamber and vascular relationship, and dramatic improvement with short-term diuretic and vasodilator administration, it is also necessary, as part of any long-term strategy, to maintain the preload that is needed to fill the stiff diastolic ventricle (see p. 378). Regression of left ventricular mass and improved diastolic function are often best achieved using long-term therapy with a calcium channel blocker or angiotensin-converting enzyme inhibitor. A report by Schulman et al. indicated that in hypertensive patients over 60 years of age a calcium channel blocker was better able to induce regression of left ventricular mass than was the beta blocker atenolol.[156] In this study, regression was associated with improved diastolic filling and did not impair either cardiac output or ejection fraction at rest or during mild upright bicycle exercise.

SYSTOLIC DYSFUNCTION. This occurs often in the setting of ischemic disease. In these patients, it is useful to keep in mind the entity of the "hibernating" myocardium (see p. 388) and that antiischemic interventions in this setting, including revascularization, may improve not only angina, but left ventricular function and failure symptoms as well. There are several goals of medical therapy. One is to decrease neurohormonal activation. Studies with angiotensin-converting enzyme inhibitors indicate improved survival and decreased morbidity in older, as well as younger, patients with systolic dysfunction.[156] Another goal is to favorably influence hemodynamics, primarily by decreasing preload and afterload. Diuretics are very useful, although it is usually necessary to use a higher dose to achieve a given efficacy in older patients because of age-associated decreases in glomerular filtration and tubular secretion.

Digitalis improves clinical outcomes in patients with systolic dysfunction, including those with sinus rhythm. Studies in experimental models indicate that the therapeutic/toxic window for digitalis is narrower in the older-age groups because of a decreased inotropic effect without a change in arrhythmogenic potential. Because of age-associated changes in renal function and pharmacokinetics, the maintenance dose of digitalis should be decreased in those over 70 years of age.

One particular problem in patients with congestive heart failure is frequent and early readmission. Close follow-up of weights and compliance with the medical and dietary regimens, as well as insuring that appropriate doses of the indicated agents are used, may be particularly useful.

Drug Use in the Elderly

As a consequence of the increased prevalence of cardiovascular and other diseases in the elderly, cardiovascular agents make up a higher fraction of total drug expenditure for older persons than they do in the general population. In considering the effects of age on the pharmacokinetics and pharmacodynamics of cardiovascular agents[157] it is important to note the heterogeneity of response in the older population. There are no strict age-related rules that apply to the entire geriatric population, and it is clear that the commitment of the physician to carefully assess the therapeutic results and side effects of medical therapy must be greater in older- than in younger-age groups.

Although age-related changes in gastric pH and absorptive surface are described, these have relatively unimportant effects for most cardiovascular drugs. The distribution of cardiovascular agents, however, is affected by age-associated decreases in serum albumin[158] and lean body mass[159] and increases in alpha-1-acid glycoproteins[160] and body fat.[159] A decrease in albumin results in increased free drug for those agents that are highly protein bound, which will, in turn, increase plasma concentrations for those agents whose metabolism is independent of the available free drug (e.g., lidocaine and propranolol). An increase in alpha-1-acid glycoprotein results in a decrease in the free fractions of acidic drugs. A change in body mass results in an increased distribution volume for fat-soluble drugs and a decreased distribution volume for water-soluble agents.

The effect of age on metabolism and excretion relates to age effects on renal and hepatic function. The influence of age on renal function has been extensively studied and a diminished glomerular filtration rate over a broad age range has been shown.[161] Decreased renal tubular secretion and concentration ability have also been demonstrated. Because lean body mass decreases with age, renal function cannot be indexed using serum creatinine alone in older persons. These age-related changes in renal function result in decreased clearance of quinidine, procainamide, digoxin, and the water-soluble beta blocker atenolol. Diminished tubular secretion of furosemide results in a diminished diuretic response to this drug and presumably other agents that act on the luminal side of the kidney tubule. The effect of age on hepatic metabolism has been evaluated less extensively, but it is undoubtedly affected by the decrease in hepatic mass, blood flow, and activity of the microsomal oxidizing system. These changes result in increased half-lives of lidocaine and the lipid-soluble beta blockers, including propranolol.

In addition to its effects on pharmacokinetics, aging may also influence the cardiac response to any given level of drug. Thus, a diminished response to beta agonists, beta blockers, and digitalis preparations is observed in human and/or animal models. The increased prevalence of other diseases associated with aging may render the older individual more sensitive to the side effect profile of cardiovascular agents as well. Preexisting decreased plasma volume and decreased baroreflex activity may render older patients more susceptible to the hypotensive effects of nitrates and diuretics. Preexisting conduction system disease or left ventricular dysfunction may also increase the likelihood of side effects of beta blockers and of some calcium antagonists.

In summary, the characterization of those cardiovascular changes in humans that are due to aging alone is difficult because of the age-related increasing prevalence of overt and latent cardiovascular disease and sedentary life style. It appears, however, that age does not significantly alter left ventricular performance except in the presence of superimposed stress, which can take the form of severe exercise or disease, particularly ischemia, a tachycardic arrhythmia, and hypertension. In these instances, impaired diastolic relaxation and systolic emptying, probably related to diminished responsiveness to beta-adrenoceptor stimulation, may occur. The diagnostic and therapeutic principles used in the management of cardiac disease do not differ in older and younger patients. The presence of other associated diseases, changed life style habits, and altered pharmacokinetics and pharmacodynamics, however, require more careful, skilled, conscientious, and often time-consuming application of these principles in the treatment of older patients.

REFERENCES

AGING IN ANIMAL MODELS

1. Weisfeldt, M. L., Loeven, W. A., and Shock, N. W.: Resting and active mechanical properties of trabeculae carneae from aged male rats. Am. J. Physiol. *220*:1921, 1971.

2. Anversa, P., Palackal, T., Sonnenblick, E. H., et al.: Myocyte cell loss and myocyte cellular hyperplasia in the hypertrophied aging rat heart. Circ. Res. *67*:871, 1990.
3. Anversa, P., Hiler, B., Ricci, R., et al.: Myocyte cell loss and myocyte hypertrophy in the aging rat heart. J. Am. Coll. Cardiol. *8*:1441, 1986.
4. Fraticelli, A., Josephson, R., Danziger, R., et al.: Morphological and contractile characteristics of rat cardiac myocytes from maturation to senescence. Am. J. Physiol. *257*:H259, 1989.
5. Yin, F. C. P., Spurgeon, H. A., Rakusan, K., et al.: Use of tibial length to quantify cardiac hypertrophy: Application in the aging rat. Am. J. Physiol. *243*:H941, 1982.
6. Yin, F. C. P., Spurgeon, H. A., Weisfeldt, M. L., and Lakatta, E. G.: Mechanical properties of myocardium from hypertrophied rat hearts. A comparison between hypertrophy induced by senescence and by aortic banding. Circ. Res. *46*:292, 1980.
7. Lakatta, E. G., Gerstenblith, G., Angell, C. S., et al.: Prolonged contraction duration in aged myocardium. J. Clin. Invest. *55*:61, 1975.
8. Capasso, J. M., Malhotra, A., Scheuer, J., and Sonnenblick, E. H.: Myocardial biochemical, contractile and electrical performance after imposition of hypertension in young and old rats. Circ. Res. *58*:445, 1986.
9. Wei, J. Y., Spurgeon, H. A., and Lakatta, E. G.: Excitation-contraction in rat myocardium: Alterations with adult aging. Am. J. Physiol. *246*:H784, 1984.
10. Walker, K. E., Lakatta, E. G., and Houser, S. R.: Age associated changes in membrane currents in rat ventricular myocytes. Cardiovasc. Res. *27*:1968, 1993.
11. Capasso, J. M., Malhotra, A., Remily, R. M., et al.: Effects of age on mechanical and electrical performance of rat myocardium. Am. J. Physiol. *245*:H72, 1983.
12. Spurgeon, H. A., Steinbach, M. F., and Lakatta, E. G.: Chronic exercise prevents characteristic age-related changes in rat cardiac contraction. Am. J. Physiol. *244*:H513, 1983.
13. Spurgeon, H. A., Thorne, P. R., Yin, F. C. P., et al.: Increased dynamic stiffness of trabeculae carneae from senescent rats. Am. J. Physiol. *232*:H373, 1977.
14. Starnes, J. W., and Rumsey, W. L.: Cardiac energetics and performance of exercised and food-restricted rats during aging. Am. J. Physiol. *254*:H599, 1988.
15. Templeton, G. H., Platt, G. H., Willerson, J. T., and Weisfeldt, M. L.: Influence of aging on left ventricular hemodynamics and stiffness in beagles. Circ. Res. *44*:189, 1979.
16. Orchard, C. H., and Lakatta, E. G.: Intracellular calcium transients and developed tensions in rat heart muscle. A mechanism for the negative interval-strength relationship. J. Gen. Physiol. *86*:637, 1985.
17. Froehlich, J. P., Lakatta, E. G., Beard, E., et al.: Studies of sarcoplasmic reticulum function and contraction duration in young adult and aged rat myocardium. J. Mol. Cell. Cardiol. *10*:427, 1978.
18. Tate, C. A., Taffet, G. E., Hudson, E. K., et al.: Enhanced calcium uptake of cardiac sarcoplasmic reticulum in exercise-trained old rats. Am. J. Physiol. *258*:H431, 1990.
19. Buttrick, P. A., Malhotra, A., Factor, S., et al.: Effect of aging and hypertension on myosin biochemistry and gene expression in the rat heart. Circ. Res. *68*:645, 1991.
20. Effron, M. B., Bhatnagar, G. M., Spurgeon, H. A., et al.: Changes in myosin isoenzymes, ATPase activity, and contraction duration in rat cardiac muscle with aging can be modulated by thyroxine. Circ. Res. *60*:238, 1987.
21. Bhatnagar, G. M., Effron, M. B., Ruano-Arroyo, G., et al.: Dissociation of myosin Ca^{2+}-ATPase activity from myosin isoenzymes and contractile function in rat myocardium. Fed. Proc. *44*(Abs.):826, 1985.
22. Scarpace, P. J., and Abrass, I. B.: Decreased beta-adrenergic agonist affinity and adenylate cyclase activity in senescent rat lung. J. Gerontol. *38*:143, 1983.
23. Scarpace, P. J.: Forskolin activation of adenylate cyclase in rat myocardium with age: Effects of guanine nucleotide analogs. Mech. Ageing Dev. *52*:169, 1990.
24. Sakai, M., Danziger, R. S., Staddon, J. M., et al.: Decrease with senescence in the norepinephrine-induced phosphorylation of myofilament proteins in isolated rat cardiac myocytes. J. Mol. Cell. Cardiol. *21*:1327, 1989.
25. Jiang, M. T., Moffat, M. P., and Narayanan, N.: Age-related alterations in the phosphorylation of sarcoplasmic reticulum and myofibrillar proteins and diminished contractile response to isoproterenol in intact rat ventricle. Circ. Res. *72*:102, 1993.
26. Xiao, R.-P., Spurgeon, H. A., O'Connor, F., and Lakatta, E. G.: Age-associated changes in β-adrenergic modulation on rat cardiac excitation-contraction coupling. J. Clin. Invest. *94*:2051, 1994.
27. Boluyt, M. O., Younes, A., Caffrey, J. L., et al.: Age-associated increase in rat cardiac opioid production. Am. J. Physiol. *265*:H212, 1993.
28. Younes, A., Boluyt, M. O., O'Neill, L., et al.: Age-associated alterations in atrial natiuretic factor gene expression in rat. Am. J. Physiol. *269*:H1003, 1995.
29. Lompre, A. M., Lambert, F., Lakatta, E. G., and Schwartz, K.: Expression of sarcoplasmic reticulum Ca^{2+}-ATPase and calsequestrin genes in rat heart during ontogenic development and aging. Circ. Res. *69*:1380, 1991.
30. Maciel, L. M. Z., Polikar, R., Rohrer, D., et al.: Age-induced decreases in the messenger RNA coding for the sarcoplasmic reticulum Ca^{2+}-ATPase of the rat heart. Circ. Res. *67*:230, 1990.
31. O'Neill, L., Holbrook, N. J., Fargnoli, J., and Lakatta, E. G.: Progressive changes from young adult age to senescence in mRNA for rat cardiac myosin heavy chain genes. Cardioscience *2*:1, 1991.
32. Schuyler, G. T., and Yarbrough, L. R.: Comparison of myosin and creatine kinase isoforms in left ventricles of young and senescent Fischer 344 rats after treatment with triiodothyronine. Mech. Ageing Dev. *56*:39, 1990.
33. Lakatta, E. G.: Cardiovascular regulatory mechanisms in advanced age. Physiol. Rev. *73*:413, 1993.
34. Bhatnagar, G. M., Walford, G. D., Beard, E. S., et al.: ATPase activity and force production in myofibrils and twitch characteristics in intact muscle from neonatal, adult, and senescent rat myocardium. J. Mol. Cell. Cardiol. *16*:203, 1984.
35. Hano, O., Bogdanov, K. Y., Sakai, M., et al.: Reduced threshold for myocardial cell calcium intolerance in the rat heart with aging. Am. J. Physiol. *269*:H1607, 1995.
36. White, M., Roden, R., Minobe, W., et al.: Age-related changes in β-adrenergic neuroeffector systems in the human heart. Circulation *90*:1225, 1994.
37. Harding, S. E., Jones, S. M., O'Gara, P., et al.: Isolated ventricular myocytes from failing and non-failing human heart: The relation of age and clinical status of patients to isoproterenol response. J. Mol. Cell. Cardiol. *24*:549, 1992.
38. Jacob, R., Kissling, G., Ebrecht, G., et al.: Adaptive and pathological alterations in experimental cardiac hypertrophy. *In* Chazov, E., Saks, V., and Rona, G. (eds.): Advances in Myocardiology. New York, Plenum, 1983, p. 55.
39. Lakatta, E. G.: Regulation of cardiac muscle function in the hypertensive heart. *In* Cox, R. H. (ed.): Cellular and Molecular Mechanisms of Hypertension. New York, Plenum, 1991, p. 149.
40. Lecarpentier, Y., Bugaisky, L. B., Chemla, D., et al.: Coordinated changes in contractility, energetics, and isomyosins after aortic stenosis. Am. J. Physiol. *252*:H275, 1987.
41. Michel, J. B., Heudes, D., Michel, O., et al.: Effect of chronic ANG I-converting enzyme inhibition on aging processes: II. large arteries. Am. J. Physiol. *267*:R-124, 1994.
42. Nagai, R., Zarain-Herzberg, A., Brandl, C. J., et al.: Regulation of myocardial Ca^{2+}-ATPase and phospholamban mRNA expression in response to pressure overload and thyroid hormone. Proc. Natl. Acad. Sci. USA *86*:2966, 1989.
43. Swynghedauw, B.: Remodelling of the heart in response to chronic mechanical overload. Eur. Heart J. *10*:935, 1989.
44. Yazaki, Y., and Komuro, I.: Molecular analysis of cardiac hypertrophy due to overload. J. Mol. Cell. Cardiol. (Suppl. III) *21*(Abs.):O.25, 1989.
45. Ding, O. H. L., Brooks, W. W., Conrad, C. H., et al.: Intracellular calcium transient in myocardium from spontaneously hypertensive rats during the transition to heart failure. Circ. Res. *68*:1390, 1991.
46. Boluyt, M. O., Opiteck, J. A., Esser, K. A., and White, T. P.: Cardiac adaptations to aortic-constriction in adult and aged rats. Am. J. Physiol. *257*:H643, 1989.
47. Isoyama, S., Grossman, W., and Wei, J. Y.: Effect of age on myocardial adaptation to volume overload in the rat. J. Clin. Invest. *81*:1850, 1988.
48. Kuroha, M., Isoyama, S., Ito, N., and Takishima T.: Effects of age on right ventricular hypertrophic response to pressure-overload in rats. J. Mol. Cell. Cardiol. *23*:1177, 1991.
49. Takahashi, T., Schunkert, H., Isoyama, S., et al.: Age-related differences in the expression of proto-oncogene and contractile protein genes in response to pressure overload in the rat myocardium. J. Clin. Invest. *89*:939, 1992.
50. Walford, G. D., Spurgeon, H. A., and Lakatta, E. G.: Diminished cardiac hypertrophy and muscle performance in older compared to younger adult rats with chronic atrioventricular block. Circ. Res. *63*:502, 1988.
51. Pfeffer, J. M., Pfeffer, M. A., Fishbein, M. C., and Frohlich, E. D.: Cardiac function and morphology with aging in the spontaneously hypertensive rat. Am. J. Physiol. *237*:H461, 1979.
52. Gwathmey, J. K., Slawsky, M. T., Perreault, C. L., et al.: The effect of exercise conditioning on excitation-contraction coupling in aged rats. J. Appl. Physiol. *69*:1366, 1990.
53. Farrar, R. P., Starnes, J. W., Cartee, G. D., et al.: Effects of exercise on cardiac myosin isozyme composition during the aging process. J. Appl. Physiol. *64*:880, 1988.
54. Oscai, L. B., Mole, P. A., and Holloszy, J. O.: Effects of exercise on cardiac weight and mitochondria in male and female rats. Am. J. Physiol. *220*:1944, 1971.
55. Starnes, J. W., Beyer, R. E., and Edington, D. W.: Myocardial adaptations to endurance exercise in aged rats. Am. J. Physiol. *245*:H560, 1983.

NORMAL AGING HUMANS

56. Fleg, J. L., O'Connor, F., Gerstenblith, G., et al.: Impact of age on the cardiovascular response to dynamic upright exercise in healthy men and women. J. Appl. Physiol. *78*:890, 1995.
57. Fleg, J. L., Schulman, S., O'Connor, F., et al.: Effects of acute β-adrenergic receptor blockage on age-associated changes in cardiovascular performance during dynamic exercise. Circulation *90*:2333, 1994.
58. Czernin, J., Muller, P., Chan, S., et al.: Influence of age and hemodynamics on myocardial blood flow and flow reserve. Circulation *88*:62, 1993.
59. Celermajer, D. S., Sorensen, K. E., Spiegelhalter, D. J., et al.: Aging is

associated with endothelial dysfunction in healthy men years before the age-related decline in women. J. Am. Coll. Cardiol. *24*:471, 1994.

60. Gerstenblith, G., Frederiksen, J., Yin, F. C. P., et al.: Echocardiographic assessment of a normal adult aging population. Circulation *56*:273, 1977.
61. Vaitkevicius, P. V., Fleg, J. L., Engel, J. H., et al.: Effects of age and aerobic capacity on arterial stiffness in healthy adults. Circulation *88*:1456, 1993.
62. Avolio, A. P., Chen, S. G., Wang, R. P., et al.: Effects of aging on changing arterial compliance and left ventricular load in a northern Chinese urban community. Circulation *68*:50, 1983.
63. Nichols, W. W., O'Rourke, M. F., Avolio, A. P., et al.: Effects of age-ventricular-vascular coupling. Am. J. Cardiol. *55*:1179, 1985.
64. O'Rourke, M. F.: Arterial Function in Health and Disease. New York, Churchill Livingstone, 1982, p. 275.
65. Yin, F. C. P., Weisfeldt, M. L., and Milnor, W. R.: Role of aortic input impedance in the decreased cardiovascular response to exercise with aging in dogs. J. Clin. Invest. *68*:28, 1981.
66. Elveback, L., and Lie, J. T.: Continued high incidence of coronary artery disease at autopsy in Olmsted County, Minnesota, 1950 to 1979. Circulation *70*:345, 1984.
67. Fleg, J. L., Gerstenblith, G., Zonderman, A. B., et al.: Prevalence and prognostic significance of exercise-induced silent myocardial ischemia detected by thallium scintigraphy and electrocardiography in asymptomatic volunteers. Circulation *81*:423, 1990c.
68. Fleg, J., Schulman, S. P., Gerstenblith, G., et al.: Additive effects of age and silent myocardial ischemia on the left ventricular response to upright cycle exercise. J. Appl. Physiol. *75*:499, 1993.
69. Ehsani, A. A., Ogawa, T., Miller, T. R., et al.: Exercise training improves left ventricular systolic function in older men. Circulation *83*:96, 1991.
70. Ogawa, T., Spina, R. J., Martin, W. H., III, et al.: Effects of aging, sex and physical training on cardiovascular responses to exercise. Circulation *86*:494, 1992.
71. Stratton, J. R., Cerqueira, M. D., Schwartz, R. S., et al.: Differences in cardiovascular responses to isoproterenol in relation to age and exercise training in healthy men. Circulation *86*:504, 1992.
72. Spina, R. J., Ogawa, R., Kohrt, W. M., et al.: Differences in cardiovascular adaptations to endurance exercise training between older men and women. J. Appl. Physiol. *75*:849, 1993.
73. Brandfonbrener, M., Landowne, M., and Shock, N. W.: Changes in cardiac output with age. Circulation *12*:557, 1955.
74. Schulman, S., Lakatta, E. G., Fleg, J. L., et al.: Age-related decline in left ventricular filling at rest and exercise. Am. J. Physiol. *263* (Heart Circ. Physiol. *34*):H1932, 1992.
75. Swinne, C. J., Shapiro, E. P., Lima, S. D., and Fleg, J. L.: Age-associated changes in left ventricular diastolic performance during isometric exercise in normal subjects. Am. J. Cardiol. *69*:823, 1992.
76. Bruce, R. A., and Hornsten, T. R.: Exercise stress testing in evaluation of patients with ischemic heart disease. Prog. Cardiovasc. Dis. *11*:371, 1969.
77. Seals, D. R., Hagberg, J. M., Hurley, B. F., et al.: Endurance training in older men and women. I. Cardiovascular responses to exercise. J. Appl. Physiol. *57*:1024, 1984.
78. Fleg, J. L., and Lakatta, E. G.: Role of muscle loss in the age-associated reduction in VO_{2max}. J. Appl. Physiol. *65*:1147, 1988.
79. Fleg, J. L., Tzankoff, S. P., and Lakatta, E. G.: Age-related augmentation of plasma catecholamines during dynamic exercise in healthy males. J. Appl. Physiol. *59*:1033, 1985.
80. Haber, P., Honiger, B., Klicpera, M., and Niederberger, M.: Effects in elderly people 67–76 years of age of three-month endurance training on a bicycle ergometer. Eur. Heart J. *5*(Suppl. E):37, 1984.
81. Smith, M. L., Graitzer, H. M., Hudson, D. L., and Raven, P. B.: Baroreflex function in endurance- and static exercise-trained men. J. Appl. Physiol. *64*:585, 1988.
82. Seals, D. R., and Chase, P. B.: Influence of physical training on heart rate variability and baroreflex circulatory control. J. Appl. Physiol. *66*:1886, 1989.
83. Fortney, S., Tankersley, C., Lightfoot, J. T., et al.: Cardiovascular response to lower body negative pressure in trained and untrained older men. J. Appl. Physiol. *73*:2693, 1992.
84. Smith, M. L., and Raven, P. B.: Cardiovascular responses to lower body negative pressure in endurance and static exercise-trained men. Med. Sci. Sports Exer. *18*:545, 1986.
85. Fleg, J. L., Shapiro, E. P., O'Connor, F., et al.: Failure of intensive long-term aerobic conditioning to prevent the age-associated decline in left-ventricular diastolic filling performance (*in press*).
86. Forman, D. E., Manning, W. J., Hauser, R., et al.: Enhanced left ventricular diastolic filling associated with long-term endurance training. J. Gerontol. Med. Sci. *47*:M56, 1992.
87. Levy, W. C., Cerqueira, M. D., Abrass, I. B., et al.: Endurance training augments diastolic filling at rest and during exercise in healthy young and older men. Circulation *88*:116, 1993.
88. Takemoto, K. A., Bernstein, L., Lopez, J. F., et al.: Abnormalities of diastolic filling of the left ventricle associated with aging are less pronounced in exercise trained individuals. Am. Heart J. *124*:143, 1992.
89. Ehsani, A. A., Ogawa, T., Miller, T. R., et al.: Exercise training improves left ventricular systolic function in older men. Circulation *83*:96, 1991.
90. Schocken, D. D., Blumenthal, J. A., Port, S., et al.: Physical conditioning and left ventricular performance in the elderly: Assessment by radionuclide angiocardiography. Am. J. Cardiol. *52*:359, 1983.
91. National Center for Health Statistics. Vital statistics of the United States, 1988, vol 2, mortality, part A. Washington, DC, Public Health Service, 1991.
92. Lam, J. Y. T., Chaitman, B. R., Glaenzer, M., et al.: Safety and diagnostic accuracy of dipyridamole-thallium imaging in the elderly. J. Am. Coll. Cardiol. *11*:585, 1988.
93. Beleslin, B. D., Ostojic, M., Stepanovic, J., et al.: Stress echocardiography in the detection of myocardial ischemia. Head-to-head comparison of exercise, dobutamine, and dipyridamole tests. Circulation *90*:1168, 1994.
94. Joint National Committee on Detection, Evaluation, and Treatment of High Blood Pressure: The fifth report of the Joint National Committee on Detection, Evaluation and Treatment of High Blood Pressure (JNC V). Arch. Intern. Med. *153*:154, 1993.
95. Insua, J. T., Sacks, H. S., Lau, T. S., et al.: Drug treatment of hypertension in the elderly: A meta-analysis. Ann. Intern. Med. *121*:355, 1994.
96. SHEP Cooperative Research Group: Prevention of stroke by antihypertensive drug treatment in older persons with isolated systolic hypertension. Final results of the Systolic Hypertension in the Elderly Program (SHEP). JAMA *265*:3255, 1991.
97. LaCroix, A. Z., Lang, J., Scherr, P., et al.: Smoking and mortality among older men and women in three communities. N. Engl. J. Med. *324*:1619, 1991.
98. Antiplatelet Trialists' Collaboration: Secondary prevention of vascular disease by prolonged antiplatelet treatment. Br. Med. J. *296*:320, 1988.
99. Thompson, R. C., Holmes, D. R., Gersh, B. J., and Bailey, K. R.: Predicting early and intermediate-term outcome of coronary angioplasty in the elderly. Circulation *88*:1579, 1993.

99a. Laster, S. B., Rutherford, B. D., Giorgi, L. V., et al.: Results of direct percutaneous transluminal coronary angioplasty in octogenarians. Am. J. Cardiol. 77:10, 1996.

99b. Thompson, R. C., Holmes, D. R. Jr., Grill, D. E., et al.: Changing outcomes of angioplasty in the elderly. J. Am. Coll. Cardiol. *27*:8, 1996.

100. Weyrens, F. J., Goldenberg, I., Mooney, J. F., et al.: Percutaneous transluminal coronary angioplasty in patients aged ≥ 90 years. Am. J. Cardiol. *74*:397, 1994.
101. Henson, K. D., Popma, J. J., Leon, M. B., et al.: Efficacy and safety of rotational coronary atherectomy in elderly patients. J. Am. Coll. Cardiol. *21*:214A, 1993.
102. Edmunds, L. H., Jr., Stephenson, L. W., Edie, R. N., et al.: Open-heart surgery in octogenarians. N. Engl. J. Med. *319*:131, 1988.
103. O'Keefe, J. H., Sutton, M. B., McCallister, B. D., et al.: Coronary angioplasty versus bypass surgery in patients >70 years old matched for ventricular function. J. Am. Coll. Cardiol. *24*:425, 1994.
104. Expert Panel on the Detection, Evaluation, and Treatment of High Blood Cholesterol in Adults: Summary of the second report of the National Cholesterol Education Program (NCEP) Expert Panel on Detection, Evaluation, and Treatment of High Blood Cholesterol in Adults (Adult Treatment Panel II). JAMA *269*:3015, 1993.
105. Manolio, T. A., Pearson, T. A., Wenger, N. K., et al.: Cholesterol and heart disease in older persons and women: Review of an NHLBI workshop. Ann. Epidemiol. *2*:161, 1992.
106. Krommal, R. A., Cain, K. C., Ye, Z., et al.: Total serum cholesterol levels and mortality risk as a function of age. A report based on the Framingham data. Arch. Intern. Med. *153*:1065, 1993.
107. Krumholz, H. M., Seeman, T. E., Merrill, S. S., et al.: Lack of association between cholesterol and coronary heart disease mortality and morbidity and all-cause mortality in persons older than 70 years. JAMA *272*:1335, 1994.
108. Scandinavian Simvastatin Survival Study Group: Randomised trial of cholesterol lowering in 4444 patients with coronary heart disease: The Scandinavian Simvastatin Survival Study (4S). Lancet *344*:1383, 1994.
109. Hulley, S. B., and Newman, T. B.: Cholesterol in the elderly. Is it important? JAMA *272*:1372, 1994.
110. Folsom, A. R., Kaye, S. A., Sellers, T. A., et al.: Body fat distribution and 5-year risk of death in older women. JAMA *269*:483, 1993.
111. Stampfer, M. J., and Colditz, G. A.: Estrogen replacement therapy and coronary heart disease: A quantitative assessment of the epidemiologic evidence. Prev. Med. *20*:47, 1991.
112. Stampfer, M. J., Colditz, G. A., Willett, W. C., et al.: Postmenopausal estrogen therapy and cardiovascular disease. Ten year follow-up from the Nurses' Health Study. N. Engl. J. Med. *325*:756, 1991.
113. Fischer, G. M., Cherian, K., and Swain, M. L.: Increased synthesis of aortic collagen and elastin in experimental atherosclerosis: Inhibition by contraceptive steroids. Atherosclerosis *39*:463, 1981.
114. Reis, S. E., Gloth, S. T., Blumenthal, R. S., et al.: Ethinyl estradiol acutely attenuates abnormal coronary vasomotor responses to acetylcholine in postmenopausal women. Circulation *89*:52, 1994.
115. Egashira, K., Inou, T., Hirooka, Y., et al.: Effect of age on endothelium-dependent vasodilation of resistance coronary artery by acetylcholine in humans. Circulation *88*:77, 1993.
116. Weaver, W. D., Litwin, P. E., Martin, J. S., et al.: Effect of age on use of thrombolytic therapy and mortality in acute myocardial infarction. J. Am. Coll. Cardiol. *18*:657, 1991.
117. Goldberg, R. J., Gurwitz, J., Yarzebski, J., et al.: Patient delay and re-

ceipt of thrombolytic therapy among patients with acute myocardial infarction from a community-wide perspective. Am. J. Cardiol. *70:*421, 1992.
118. Gore, J., Becker, R., Tiefenbrunn, A., et al.: The National Registry of Myocardial Infarction (NRMI) Investigators: Current trends in the treatment of elderly patients with acute myocardial infarction. J. Am. Coll. Cardiol. *21:*481A, 1993.
119. Maggioni, A. P., Maseri, A., Fresco, C., et al.: Age-related increase in mortality among patients with first myocardial infarction treated with thrombolysis. N. Engl. J. Med. *329:*1442, 1993.
120. Simoons, M. L., Maggioni, A. P., Knatterud, G., et al.: Individual risk assessment for intracranial haemorrhage during thrombolytic therapy. Lancet *342:*1523, 1993.
121. Aguirre, F. V., McMahon, R. P., Mueller, H., et al.: Impact of age on clinical outcome and postlytic management strategies in patients treated with intravenous thrombolytic therapy. Results from the TIMI II Study. Circulation *90:*78, 1994.
122. The GUSTO Investigators: An international randomized trial comparing four thrombolytic strategies for acute myocardial infarction. N. Engl. J. Med. *329:*673, 1993.
123. Grines, C. L., Browne, K. F., Marco, J., et al.: A comparison of immediate angioplasty with thrombolytic therapy for acute myocardial infarction. N. Engl. J. Med. *328:*673, 1993.
124. Grines, C. L., Griffin, J. J., Brodie, B. R., et al.: The second primary angioplasty for myocardial infarction study (PAMI-II): Preliminary Report. Circulation *90*(Suppl. I):433, 1994.
125. Gundersen, T., Abrahamsen, A. M., Kjekshus, J., et al.: Timolol-related reduction in mortality and reinfarction in patients ages 65–75 years surviving acute myocardial infarction. Circulation *66:*1179, 1982.
126. Pfeffer, M. A., Braunwald, E., Moye, L. A., et al.: Effect of captopril on mortality and morbidity in patients with left ventricular dysfunction after myocardial infarction. N. Engl. J. Med. *327:*669, 1992.
127. Fleg, J. L., and Kennedy, H. L.: Cardiac arrhythmias in a healthy elderly population: Detection by 24 hour ambulatory electrocardiography. Chest *81:*302, 1982.
128. Manolio, T. A., Furberg, C. D., Rautaharju, P. M., et al.: Cardiac arrhythmias on 24-hr ambulatory electrocardiography in older women and men: The Cardiovascular Health Study. J. Am. Coll. Cardiol. *23:*916, 1994.
129. Furberg, C. D., Psaty, B. M., Manolio, T. A., et al.: Prevalence of atrial fibrillation in elderly subjects (the Cardiovascular Health Study). Am. J. Cardiol. *74:*236, 1994.
130. Onundarson, P. T., Thorgeirsson, G., Jonmundsson, E., et al.: Chronic atrial fibrillation: Epidemiologic features and 14 year follow-up: A case-control study. Eur. Heart J. *8:*521, 1987.
131. Benjamin, E. F., Plehn, J. F., D'Agostino, R. B., et al.: Mitral annular calcification and the risk of stroke in an elderly cohort. N. Engl. J. Med. *327:*374, 1992.
132. The Stroke Prevention in Atrial Fibrillation Investigators: Predictors of thromboembolism in atrial fibrillation: II. Echocardiographic features of patients at risk. Ann. Intern. Med. *116:*6, 1992.
133. Atrial Fibrillation Investigators: Risk factors for stroke and efficacy of antithrombotic therapy in atrial fibrillation. Analysis of pooled data from five randomized controlled trials. Arch. Intern. Med. *154:*1449, 1994.
134. Albers, G. W.: Atrial fibrillation and stroke. Arch. Intern. Med. *154:*1443, 1994.
135. Coplen, S. E., Antman, E. M., Berlin, J. A., et al.: Efficacy and safety of quinidine therapy for maintenance of sinus rhythm after cardioversion. A meta-analysis of randomized control trials. Circulation *82:*1106, 1990.
136. Hohnloser, S. H., and Woosley, R. L.: Sotalol. N. Engl. J. Med. *331:*31, 1994.
137. Gosselink, A. T. M., Crijns, H. J. G. M., Van Gelder, I. C., et al.: Low-dose amiodarone for maintenance of sinus rhythm after cardioversion of atrial fibrillation or flutter. JAMA *267:*3289, 1992.
138. Epstein, L. M., Chiesa, N., Wong, M. N., et al.: Radiofrequency catheter ablation in the treatment of supraventricular tachycardia in the elderly. J. Am. Coll. Cardiol. *23:*1356, 1994.
139. Sawin, C. T., Geller, A., Wolf, P. A., et al.: Low serum thyrotropin concentrations as a risk factor for atrial fibrillation in older persons. N. Engl. J. Med. *331:*1249, 1994.
140. Vaitkevicius, P. V., Esserwein, D. M., Maynard, A. K., et al.: Frequency and importance of postprandial blood pressure reduction in elderly nursing-home patients. Ann. Intern. Med. *115:*865, 1991.
141. Lipsitz, L. A., Ryan, S. M., Parker, J. A., et al.: Hemodynamic and autonomic nervous system responses to mixed meal ingestion in healthy young and old subjects and dysautonomic patients with postprandial hypotension. Circulation *87:*391, 1993.
142. Sgarbossa, E. B., Pinski, S. L., Maloney, J. D., et al.: Chronic atrial fibrillation and stroke in paced patients with sick sinus syndrome. Relevance of clinical characteristics and pacing modalities. Circulation *88:*1045, 1993.
143. Aranki, S. F., Rizzo, R. J., Couper, G. S., et al.: Aortic valve replacement in the elderly. Effect of gender and coronary artery disease on operative mortality. Circulation *88*(Suppl. II):II-17, 1993.
144. Elayda, M. A., Hall, R. J., Reul, R. M., et al.: Aortic valve replacement in patients 80 years and older. Operative risks and long-term results. Circulation *88*(Suppl. II):II-11, 1993.
145. Logeais, Y., Langanay, T., Roussin, R., et al.: Surgery for aortic stenosis in elderly patients. A study of surgical risk and predictive factors. Circulation *90:*2891, 1994.
146. Litvack, F., Jakubowski, A. T., Buchbinder, N. A., and Eigler, N.: Lack of sustained clinical improvement in an elderly population after percutaneous aortic valvuloplasty. Am. J. Cardiol. *62:*270, 1088.
147. Jebara, V. A., Dervanian, P., Acar, C., et al.: Mitral valve repair using Carpentier techniques in patients more than 70 years old: Early and late results. Circulation *86*(Suppl. II):II-53, 1992.
148. Le Feuvre, C., Bonan, R., Lachurie, M. L., et al.: Balloon mitral commissurotomy in patients aged $\geq$ 70 years. Am. J. Cardiol. *71:*233, 1993.
149. Bennet, N. E.: Hypertension in the elderly. Lancet *344:*447, 1994.
150. Derkx, F. H. M.: Renal artery stenosis and hypertension. Lancet *344:*237, 1994.
151. Farnett, L., Mulrow, C. D., Linn, W. D., et al.: The J-curve phenomenon and the treatment of hypertension: Is there a point beyond which pressure reduction is dangerous? JAMA *265:*489, 1992.
152. Siscovick, D. S., Raghunathan, T. E., Psaty, B. M., et al.: Diuretic therapy for hypertension and the risk of primary cardiac arrest. N. Engl. J. Med. *330:*1852, 1994.
153. Kannel, W. B., and Belanger, A. J.: Epidemiology of heart failure. Am. Heart J. *121:*951, 1991.
154. Massie, B. M., and Conway, M.: Survival of patients with congestive heart failure: Past, present, and future prospects. Circulation *75*(Suppl. IV):IV-11, 1987.
155. Yusuf, S., Thom, T., and Abbott, R. D.: Changes in hypertension treatment and in congestive heart failure mortality in the United States. Hypertension *13*(Suppl. I):I-74, 1989.
156. Schulman, S. P., Weiss, J. L., Becker, L. C., et al.: The effects of antihypertensive therapy on left ventricular mass in elderly hypertensive patients. N. Engl. J. Med. *322:*1350, 1990.
157. Montamat, S. C., Cusack, B. J., and Vestal, R. E.: Management of drug therapy in the elderly. N. Engl. J. Med. *321:*303, 1989.
158. Dybkaer, R., Lauritzen, M., Krakauer, R., et al.: Relative reference values for clinical chemical and haematological quantities in "healthy" elderly people. Acta Med. Scand. *209:*1, 1981.
159. Bruce, A., Andersson, M., Arvidsson, B., and Isaksson, B.: Body composition. Prediction of normal body potassium, body water and body fat in adults on the basis of body height, body weight and age. Scand. J. Clin. Lab. Invest. *40:*461, 1980.
160. Abernathy, E. R., and Kerzner, L.: Age effects on alpha-1-acid glycoprotein concentration and imipramine plasma protein binding. J. Am. Geriatr. Soc. *32:*705, 1984.
161. Rowe, J. W., Andres, R., Tobin, J. D., et al.: Age-adjusted standards for creatinine clearance. Ann. Intern. Med. *84:*567, 1976.

Chapter 51
Coronary Artery Disease in Women

PAMELA S. DOUGLAS

EVALUATION OF CHEST PAIN 1704
Noninvasive and Invasive Diagnostic Testing 1705
Coronary Angiography 1706
CARDIAC RISK FACTORS AND THEIR MODIFICATION .1706
HORMONES AND HORMONAL THERAPY . . .1707
Oral Contraceptives 1707
Estrogen and Cardiac Risk Factor Modification 1707
MANAGEMENT OF CORONARY ARTERY DISEASE. 1709
Chronic Coronary Artery Disease 1709
Acute Myocardial Infarction 1710
CONCLUSIONS. .1711
REFERENCES .1711

For most of this century, cardiovascular disease has been the most common cause of death and disability in women of all ethnic and racial groups in the United States (Fig. 51–1).[1–3] The prevalence of cardiovascular disease in women increases dramatically with age (Fig. 51–2); as the population ages and women's life expectancy increases, the importance of these diseases will also increase.

While similar in many respects, men and women with coronary artery disease (CAD) demonstrate striking and clinically important differences in epidemiology, diagnosis, prognosis, treatment, and prevention. Clinical care is rapidly changing as evidence accumulates to suggest that estrogen has the potential to be among the most powerful cardiovascular drugs available. Proving this, understanding the underlying mechanisms of hormones' interaction with the cardiovascular system, and learning to use them optimally will take many years. An equally important challenge, however, involves recognition by both patients and their physicians of the enormous health risk that cardiovascular diseases pose for women.

EVALUATION OF CHEST PAIN

CLINICAL SYNDROMES. It has long been assumed that the clinical expression of CAD is similar in men and women, yet available information suggests that gender differences in presentation and disease manifestations exist and should be considered in the evaluation of the patient with chest pain. Several studies document that women are more likely than men to present with angina and less likely to present with a myocardial infarction as either the first or subsequent manifestations of CAD.[4,5] Further, women are on average 10 years older at the time of presentation. These results are closely linked to the finding that chest pain is a poor predictor of epicardial coronary disease in women. Perhaps even more than in men, the prevalence of angiographic coronary disease varies dramatically according to the nature of the chest pain, the patient's age, and the presence of coronary risk factors[6–8] (Fig. 51–2). This underlines the importance of good history taking and careful cardiovascular risk factor assessment in the evaluation of women with chest pain.

A variety of factors influence the evaluation of chest pain in women.[9] Although women seek medical care more often than men do, they also drastically underestimate their own risk of CAD. In addition, a woman's presentation style alters physicians' estimates of the likelihood of CAD, so that a woman whose demeanor was more business-like was judged to have a much higher probability of disease than one who behaved histrionically.[11] Compared with men, women with chronic stable angina are older and more likely to have hypertension, diabetes, and congestive heart failure but less likely to have had a myocardial infarction or revascularization.[10] While equally likely to have effort angina, such women are more likely to experience pain at rest, during sleep, or with mental stress. This patient pro-

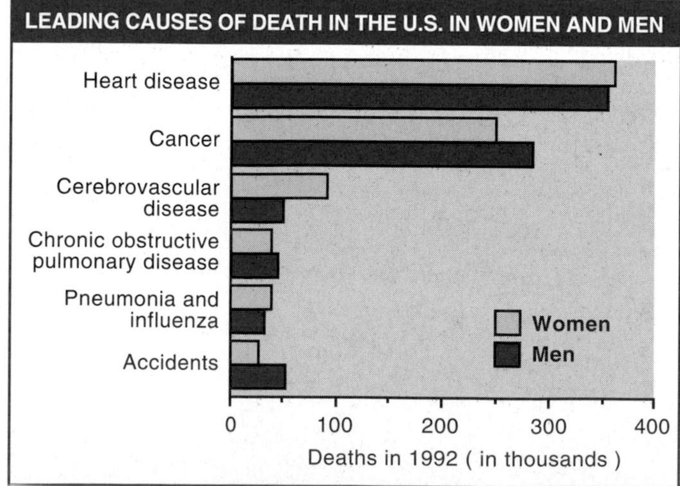

FIGURE 51–1. Number of deaths due to the six leading causes of death in women and men in the U.S. in 1992, ranked in order for women. (Data from Advance Report of Final Mortality Statistics for 1992, National Center for Health Statistics, 1995.)

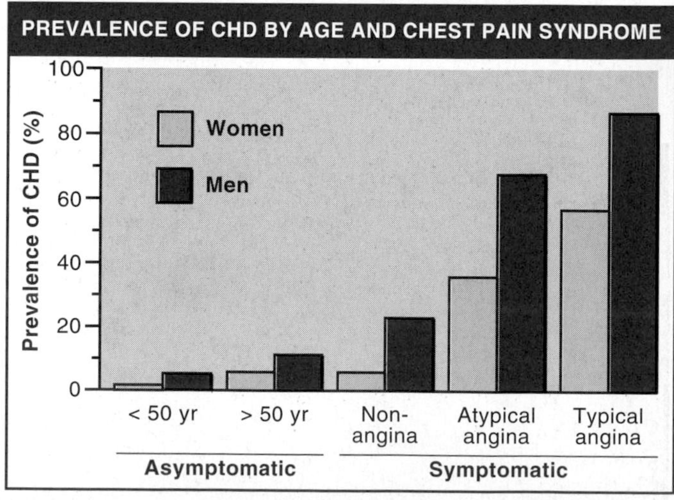

FIGURE 51–2. Prevalence of angiographically documented coronary heart disease in men and women according to age and chest pain syndrome. (Modified from DeSanctis, R.W.: Clinical manifestations of coronary artery disease: Chest pain in women. *In* Wenger, N.K., Speroff, L. and Packard, B. [eds.]: Cardiovascular Health and Disease in Women. Greenwich, CT, Le Jacq Communications, 1993, p. 68.)

file makes the evaluation of a new symptom or disability more complex.

The mechanisms by which ischemia is produced may help explain differences in anginal patterns. Women have higher prevalences than men do of vasospastic angina and of microvascular angina,[7,8,12] both of which are associated with atypical chest pain patterns, are often treated differently, and have a more favorable prognosis than epicardial coronary disease (Chap. 38). Even in the presence of angiographically documented disease, gender differences in plaque components, (more cellular and fibrous tissue in women) endothelial function (estrogen-induced coronary vasodilation) and hemostasis (higher fibrinogen and Factor VII levels in women) may influence the pathophysiology and therefore the clinical manifestations of coronary disease.[13,14] Finally, women more commonly have noncoronary chest pain syndromes, further complicating their clinical assessment.

NATURAL HISTORY AND PROGNOSIS. Women with angina are less likely to experience a subsequent myocardial infarction or coronary death than men.[5,15,16] Although overall age-adjusted rates of death or myocardial infarction in women with angina are less than those in men,[15] of subjects over age 65, women and men with exertional chest pain have the same relative risks of CAD death (2.7 vs 2.4).[17] Other data suggesting that the prognosis of coronary disease is not more benign in women include the similar (if not worse) early mortality after myocardial infarction in women.[18]

Thus, determination of the etiology of chest pain in women can be difficult, hampered by the onset of CAD later in life, the more common appearance of symptoms such as rest angina in patients with otherwise stable patterns, the poor predictive value of angina for angiographic coronary disease, and the higher likelihood of alternative mechanisms of chest pain and ischemia.

Noninvasive and Invasive Diagnostic Testing

While noninvasive diagnostic testing for CAD does not fully resolve the difficulties inherent in evaluating chest pain in women, careful test selection and interpretation can provide valuable information regarding the presence and severity of CAD in women. The general principles underlying noninvasive diagnostic testing do not differ in men and women (see Chap. 5). The simplest diagnostic test, the resting electrocardiogram, reveals a higher prevalence of repolarization (ST-T wave) abnormalities in women with suspected coronary disease than in men (32 vs 23 per cent).[6,19]

Treadmill exercise testing carries a higher false-positive rate in women, ranging from 38 to 67 per cent, than in men, 7 to 44 per cent in the same studies,[19] in part because of a lower pretest likelihood of disease.[7] However, women have a low false-negative rate (12 to 22 per cent) that compares favorably to that in men (12 to 40 per cent), and suggests that routine testing reliably *excludes* the presence of CAD in women with negative tests. The exercise electrocardiogram also provides useful prognostic information in women.[20] Variables contributing to test accuracy are resting ST-T wave abnormalities, peak exercise heart rate, number of diseased vessels, typical angina, age, gender, drug use (digitalis, diazepam, methyldopa), hyperventilation, conduction abnormalities, left ventricular hypertrophy, mitral valve prolapse, vasospasm, and hormonal influences. Although less common in women, false-negative studies may be contributed to by gender-specific characteristics including reduced exercise tolerance and the higher prevalence of single vessel disease in women.

The failure of many normal women to increase their ejection fraction during exercise directly affects the interpretation of the exercise radionuclide angiogram,[21] since disease detection is based on ejection fraction augmentation during exercise (see p. 434).

The addition of imaging to electrocardiographic stress testing markedly improves its accuracy in women. Planar thallium scans during treadmill exercise testing suggest moderate increases in sensitivity and specificity in women[22–31] (Table 51–1). The use of single-photon emission computed tomography (SPECT) may not improve accuracy in women as it does in men.[26] Much of the inaccuracy of thallium scanning in women has been attributed to breast attenuation, but the benefit of higher energy isotopes such as technetium-^{99m}-sestamibi has not yet been proved. Coupling exercise testing with echocardiographic visualization of wall motion (i.e., exercise echocardiography) also improves diagnostic accuracy in women[28,29,29a] (Table 51–1). This is particularly true when the resting electrocardiogram is abnormal or uninterpretable. The use of pharmacological stress agents (adenosine, dipyridamole dobutamine) in women coupled with either echocardiographic or nuclear imaging shows substantial improvements in test performance over electrocardiographic results alone.

Since few direct comparisons between exercise echocardiography and exercise-thallium or sestamibi testing have been reported, and none with adequate numbers of women, there is little objective basis for selecting one modality over another, and both appear more accurate than routine exercise electrocardiography testing. One approach,[23] which reduced both the number of thallium scans and angiographic procedures necessary without a loss of diagnostic accuracy, was the performance of treadmill exercise testing first in all women referred for noninvasive testing, with subsequent

TABLE 51–1 INCREMENTAL VALUE OF IMAGING TO EXERCISE STRESS TESTING FOR THE DIAGNOSIS OF CORONARY HEART DISEASE IN WOMEN

		STRESS ECG ALONE			WITH IMAGING	
STUDY, YEAR, REFERENCE	STRESS MODALITY	Sensitivity (%)	Specificity (%)	IMAGING MODALITY	Sensitivity (%)	Specificity (%)
Hung 1984[22]	Treadmill	73	59	Planar thallium	75	91
Melin 1985[23]	Bicycle	61	78	Planar thallium	70	93
Friedman 1982[24]	Treadmill	32	41	Planar thallium	75	88
Goodgold 1987[25]	Treadmill	N/A	N/A	Planar thallium	93	85
Fintel 1989[26]	N/A	N/A	N/A	Planar thallium SPECT thallium	84 86	90* 90*
Chae 1993[27]	Treadmill	66	60	SPECT thallium	71	65
Sawada 1989[28]	Treadmill/bicycle	29	83	Echo	86	86
Williams 1994[29]	Bicycle	67	51	Echo	88	84
Masini 1988[30]	Bicycle	72	52	Dipyridamole echo	79	93
Kong 1992[31]	N/A	N/A	N/A	Dipyridamole thallium	87	58

* Preset from receiver operator curves.

exercise thallium examination only in the 30 per cent with post test probabilities between 10 and 90 per cent (i.e., those in whom a reasonably certain diagnosis of CAD could not be reached or excluded on the basis of history, risk factors, and exercise electrocardiography. A recent theoretical analysis of accuracy and cost-effectiveness[32] considered seven different diagnostic testing strategies and suggested that one employing exercise *echocardiography* as the first test might be superior.

Coronary Angiography

Few studies have examined gender differences in invasive diagnostic testing. While it is reasonable to assume that the assessment of the extent and severity of angiographic coronary narrowing is similar in men and women, it has been suggested that coronary vasoconstriction is a more important mechanism of ischemia in women.[7,8,12] Women are more likely than men to experience vascular and renal complications from diagnostic angiography, possibly due to more advanced age and smaller body size[33]; the incidence of myocardial infarction, stroke, and death are similar.

GENDER BIAS. A 1987 study reporting that men with positive nuclear exercise tests were 6.3 times more likely to be referred to cardiac catheterization than women[34] gave rise to concerns that female patients were receiving inadequate or inappropriate care, a conclusion that has been supported by several subsequent studies. Coronary angiography is performed 28 to 45 per cent more often and revascularization 15 to 27 per cent more often in men than in women with a diagnosis of CAD.[35] In the Systolic Hypertension in the Elderly Program (SHEP), men with incident coronary disease were more likely to undergo revascularization by angioplasty or surgery than were women (26 vs 9 per cent in patients between 60 and 75; 6 vs. 2 per cent in those age 75 or older).[36] Other studies have suggested that gender differences in care may be due to overtreatment of low-risk men.[37,38]

It has been proposed that different treatment strategies in women might represent optimal care,[39] given the known differences in disease prevalence and the difficulties in noninvasively diagnosing coronary disease in women. This question has been addressed recently by examining the outcomes of patients undergoing diagnostic stress testing.[40] Although women were equally likely to have a positive stress electrocardiogram (29 per cent in women vs 30 per cent in men) or stress thallium examination (23 vs 27 per cent), they were less commonly referred for additional noninvasive testing (4 vs 20 per cent) or catheterization (34 vs 45 per cent). However, subsequent event rates were higher in women, whether they had a normal initial test (1.6 per cent/year death or myocardial infarction vs 0.8 per cent in men) or an abnormal one (14.3 per cent/year vs 6.0 per cent/year). Both male and female patients who did undergo revascularization had no events, while women who were not revascularized had a worse prognosis than similarly untreated men. These data demonstrate not only a gender-based difference in clinical practice but a worse patient outcome in women treated less aggressively.

CARDIAC RISK FACTORS AND THEIR MODIFICATION

(See also Chap. 35)

In the broadest sense, those factors associated with higher cardiac risk in men are also associated with increased cardiac risk in women, including age, family history, smoking, hypertension, lipoproteins, and diabetes mellitus.[41,42] However, they may have a different relative importance, and additional factors, such as hormonal status, are equally powerful predictors of CAD.

LIPIDS. In contrast to men, elevated total cholesterol and low-density lipoprotein (LDL) levels are only weakly associated with CAD in women, and only in women 65 years old or younger.[42–44] Instead, high-density lipoprotein (HDL) cholesterol is closely and inversely associated with CAD risk.[45] Triglycerides are an independent predictor of CAD in older women[46–48] but not in men. Lp(a), a composite of LDL, apo B-100, and apo(a), is also associated with higher cardiac risk in women.

Modification of lipoproteins is generally accomplished by the same life style changes and medications in men and women, although such interventions may be less effective in women.[50] While clinical trials have generally not included women in sufficient numbers for independent analysis, several recent studies employing aggressive, multifactorial treatment for lipid lowering have documented an equal or greater effect in women,[51–53] including angiographic regression of coronary atherosclerosis and reduction in coronary events, but not death.

In general, recommended dietary and pharmacological lipid-lowering strategies are similar in men and women. However, hormone replacement therapy may be a preferred primary therapy for postmenopausal women with low HDL and high LDL.[54] Effects of estrogen may be additive to or event supplant those of conventional lipid-lowering medications.[52] However, estrogen increases triglycerides in 20 to 25 per cent of women, particularly those with elevated baseline levels,[55] who may therefore be less likely to benefit from hormone replacement therapy. An elevated baseline level therefore mandates careful monitoring of lipid levels following institution of hormonal therapy.

Current recommendations for initiation of treatment and therapeutic goals (NCEP-II) are similar in men and women and are based on LDL levels[54] (see Table 35–6, p. 1138). Despite the fact that HDL is a more powerful determinant of CAD risk in women, the NCEP-II guidelines do not include HDL or triglyceride levels except as modifying factors. It is not clear how well these recommendations address the needs of women or the very elderly, who are predominantly female.[56]

DIABETES AND OBESITY (see also Chap. 60). Diabetes is a risk factor for the presence and severity of coronary heart disease in both men and women but carries a greater incremental risk in women, completely eliminating the "female advantage."[47,57] Even more than in men, diabetes dramatically increases the mortality of myocardial infarction in women.[58a]

Non–insulin-dependent diabetes is associated with obesity, abdominal and upper body fat distribution, hypertension, and insulin resistance, all of which have been associated with higher coronary heart disease risk.[57] It has been hypothesized that this complex of abnormalities may be causally related to high circulating insulin levels, but this remains unproved. More so than in men, obesity and body fat distribution appear to be independent coronary heart disease risk factors in women.[58a] Diabetes is also linked with the presence of hyperlipidemia (elevated triglycerides, reduced HDL), especially in women,[57] and the lipoprotein response to adequate diabetic treatment is variable.[59] Overall, it is unclear what effect diabetic treatment or weight loss have (if any) in modifying cardiovascular risk in women.

HYPERTENSION (see also Chap. 26). The prevalence of hypertension in women greatly increases with age so that nearly 80 per cent of women over age 75 are hypertensive.[60] Hypertension carries an independent coronary heart disease risk for both men and women and substantially enhances the risks associated with hyperlipidemia, smoking, obesity, and diabetes. While the benefits of antihypertensive treatment have not been well studied in women, it appears that therapy may reduce both overall mortality and cardiac morbidity as well as the incidence of stroke; these effects are most striking in the elderly.[61]

SMOKING. Smoking is a strong independent risk factor for coronary heart disease in both men and women; although smoking rates in the United States are falling overall, they are currently increasing among women.[62] This risk is present even with minimal exposure (1 to 4 cigarettes/day) and is not improved by use of low-yield cigarettes.[63] Smoking risk is strikingly synergistic with that of oral contraceptive use, especially in women over age 35, and often leads to an earlier menopause, another coronary heart disease risk unique to women.[64] Cessation of smoking appears to gradually eliminate the excess risk in women,[65] although women more often smoke to lose or maintain body weight and find it harder to quit than do men.

HEMOSTASIS. Elevated fibrinogen levels appear to be an independent cardiac risk factor in men and women, although women have not been as well studied.[66] The mechanism(s) by which fibrinogen enhances risk are poorly understood, although high fibrinogen levels have been associated with other CAD risk factors, including hypertension, diabetes, smoking, obesity, hyperlipidemia, and menopause, and lower levels have been associated with exercise, hormone replacement therapy, and high HDL.[67] Gender differences in platelet function and hemostasis are virtually unexplored.[68]

EXERCISE. A sedentary life style is associated with CAD in both men and women, although the data for women are sparse.[69] The reported beneficial effects of exercise on coronary heart disease risk profile are less marked in women compared with men,[69,70] with lesser increases in HDL and less weight loss resulting from similar exercise training. In prospective observational studies, a lower fitness level has been associated with a 4.7 fold-increased risk for all-cause mortality in women,[71] and higher activity levels have been associated with decreased relative risks for CAD (0.44) and stroke (0.51) compared with lower activity levels.[72] These results were independent of other vascular risk factors.[72]

PSYCHOSOCIAL. The interaction of psychosocial and biobehavorial factors and heart disease are complex, but perhaps have been more extensively studied in women than in men.[73–75] Several of the cardiovascular risk factors discussed above are related to behavior (obesity, smoking, exercise) and are treated with its modification. Perceived stress and its balance with situational control has been found to affect CAD risk in women as well as in men. Social networks and support influence CAD outcome both independently and through the likelihood of compliance with therapeutic strategies (e.g., cardiac rehabilitation). The lack of social support has been associated with a worse outcome in both men and women, but its impact may be greater in women.

HORMONES AND HORMONAL THERAPY

The ovary produces both estrogenic and androgenic hormones until the menopause, when production decreases gradually over several years but does not fully cease. The risk of CAD in women rises thereafter, equaling that in men by age 75. Women who have an early menopause and/or bilateral oophorectomy experience an accelerated risk of CAD. Menopause, or estrogen deprivation, is associated with detrimental changes in cardiovascular risk factors that help explain the increased risk. Chief among these is an increase in LDL cholesterol, a small decrease in HDL, and an increased total ratio of cholesterol to HDL.[76,77] Natural menopause seems to have little immediate effect on blood pressure, glucose tolerance, insulin levels, body weight, or physical activity other than that of advancing age.[77]

Oral Contraceptives

Oral contraceptives are perhaps the most commonly prescribed hormones today and generally contain a synthetic estrogen, such as ethinyl estradiol, and a synthetic progestin. Currently used low-dose oral contraceptives pose only a very neglible cardiovascular risk for most patients.[76] The risk of arterial and venous thrombosis is low in current low-dose formulations but is magnified by advancing age and especially by smoking. The risk of myocardial infarction is not increased by oral contraceptives unless the patient is over age 35 and/or smokes cigarettes,[78,79] and appears to be entirely caused by thromboembolism rather than by coronary atherosclerosis, since the angiographic coronary plaque burden is actually lower in oral contraceptive users.[80]

Because most regimens employ a combination of hormones, the effect of any given oral contraceptive on circulating lipoproteins represents the sum of estrogenic effects (higher HDL and triglycerides, lower LDL) and progestogenic effects (higher LDL, lower HDL). Newer agents such as norethindrone gestodine, desogestrel, and norgestinate have beneficial effects on lipoprotein levels as well as enhancing plasminogen levels, fibrinolytic activity, and platelet aggregation reduction.[81]

Estrogen and Cardiac Risk Factor Modification

Postmenopausal estrogen replacement has been proposed for the primary and secondary prevention of CAD in both men and women. Clinical trials of estrogen therapy in men in the 1950's and 1960's used high-dose conjugated estrogens (up to 10 mg/day) and generally uncovered poor drug tolerance, little in the way of favorable risk factor modification, and an excess of thrombophlebitis, cholecystitis, and embolic events without evidence of cardioprotection. Randomized trials in women are only now being undertaken; results will not be available for several years. Currently, the use of hormonal replacement therapy in women is based on its prospectively demonstrated beneficial effects on cardiac risk factors and observational evidence of primary protection.

In postmenopausal women, exogenous estrogen results in higher HDL (especially HDL_2, and apo AI, and lower LDL and apo B-100 and perhaps Lp (a)[76,82–85] (Table 51–2). Importantly, the PEPI trial showed that the addition of a progestin to estrogen did not interfere with the LDL cholesterol-lowering effect of the latter. The use of micronized progestin was associated with an increase in HDL cholesterol.[82] Triglycerides and LDL are often increased in a dose-dependent manner, and although the magnitude of these increases are highly variable, they may limit the use of estrogen in some patients. Transdermal estrogens appear to have lesser effects on all lipoproteins, suggesting that first-pass liver metabolism is important in mediating these effects, and that this mode of drug delivery may be preferred in women with marked triglyceride elevations in response to the oral route.[86]

Other effects of estrogen replacement include a relative decrease in thrombotic potential.[82,87] Reports of an idiosyncratic elevation of blood pressure and improved insulin sensitivity have not been confirmed by more recent studies.[82,85,88] Unopposed estrogen markedly increases the risk of endometrial hyperplasia, although the concomitant use of a progestin largely prevents this.[82]

Recently, important physiological effects of estrogen have been demonstrated in vascular smooth muscle and endothelium. Estrogen receptors are present in vascular smooth muscle cells in both men and women and are capable of altering gene transcription, suggesting a possible role of estrogen in the regulation of vascular smooth muscle cell proliferation.[89] Estrogen also acutely decreases the paradox-

TABLE 51–2 ALTERATIONS IN LIPOPROTEIN LEVELS WITH HORMONE REPLACEMENT THERAPY (%)

	PLACEBO	E ALONE	E + PA (CYCLIC)	E + PA (CONTINUOUS)	E + PA (CYCLIC)
TC	−11	−20	−36	−36	−20
LDL	−11	−37	−46	−43	−38
HDL	−3	+14	+4	+3	+11
Triglycerides	−4	+15	+14	+13	+15

E = conjugated equine estrogen 0.625 mg daily; E + PA (cyclic) = conjugated equine estrogen 0.625 mg daily plus medroxy progesterone acetate 10 mg/day for 12 days each month; E + PA (continuous) = E + PA 2.5 mg/day; E + P (cyclic) = E + micronized progesterone, 200 mg/d for 12 days each month.

Adapted from The Postmenopausal Estrogen/Progestin Interventions (PEPI) Trial: Effects of estrogen or estrogen/progestin regimens on heart disease risk factors in postmenopausal women. JAMA *273*:199, 1995. Copyright 1995 American Medical Association.

ical coronary vasoconstriction response to acetylcholine[90,91] and potentiates the endothelium-dependent vasodilation of conductance and resistance coronary beds and forearm vessels in women.[92,93] Estrogen decreases the atherogenic oxidation of LDL both in vivo and in vitro and decreases the incorporation of lipids into the vessel wall, suggesting additional protective mechanisms for estrogen replacement.[94,95] At present, which of the many beneficial effects of estrogen are most important for the prevention of coronary heart disease has not been determined.

PREVENTION OF CAD WITH ESTROGEN. To date, over 30 epidemiological studies have examined the utility of estrogen in the primary prevention of CAD, and the vast majority report a significant benefit.[76,96–98] The largest of these studies, the Nurses' Health Study, reported a relative risk of 0.56 for myocardial infarction or death in women currently using estrogen and 0.83 in ever-users, after adjustment for age and risk factors.[99] Recent meta-analyses[96,98] have determined composite relative risks of 0.50 to 0.65 for both the development of and death from CAD in estrogen users.

Other documented benefits of estrogen therapy include the alleviation of menopausal symptoms and prevention of osteoporosis and fatal hip fracture (relative risk for death from this common disease is 0.75 for users of estrogen).[76,96,97] A possible protective effect against stroke has been noted in several studies[100] but is not significant in others, including the large Nurses' Health Study (relative risk 0.97 for current users) and another recent meta-analysis.[96] It is possible that the relatively young cohorts examined may have influenced these findings (median age for stroke in women is 83 years).

The beneficial effect of reproductive hormones also extends to tamoxifen, an estrogen agonist/antagonist, which has been shown to have salutory effects on circulating lipoproteins[101] and to reduce the number of hospital admissions resulting from CAD, and death due to myocardial infarction and vascular causes.[102,103]

Only a very small number of studies have evaluated the utility of estrogen in the secondary prevention of coronary heart disease. Women who were current or ever-users of estrogen had less severe angiographic coronary artery disease than never-users, even after correction for age, cholesterol, smoking, diabetes, and hypertension.[104,105] Long-term survival in women with a similar extent of angiographically documented coronary disease or after coronary artery bypass grafting is greater in women taking estrogen (Table 51–3).[106,107]

While the benefits may seem large, there are methodological limitations in all available studies as well as significant risks associated with estrogen use and logistic problems with its prescription. Chief among the risks of estrogen use is *endometrial cancer,* for which unopposed estrogen therapy carries a five- to eightfold increased risk, associated with an estimated threefold increased risk of death.[96,97,97a] While the risk of this complication is obviously zero in women without a uterus, it has been proposed that the addition of a progestin also nullifies it. A potential detrimental effect on the cardioprotective action of estrogen of adding progestins is anticipated because of their androgenic effect on circulating lipids; however, recent studies suggest that this factor may have negligible effects or may even be beneficial.[82,97,98]

BREAST CANCER. Estrogen may increase breast cancer risk, with meta-analyses showing little increased risk for short-term therapy, whereas a higher relative risk, up to 1.5, has been associated with long-term use (over 10 years) in the Nurses' Health Study.[96,109,109a] If confirmed, this

TABLE 51–3 NET CHANGE IN LIFE EXPECTANCY FOR A 50-YEAR-OLD WHITE WOMAN TREATED WITH LONG-TERM HORMONE REPLACEMENT

CLINICAL CHARACTERISTICS	UNTREATED LIFE EXPECTANCY (YEARS)	NET CHANGE IN LIFE EXPECTANCY WITH RX: Estrogen**	E + P††	E + P‡‡
No cardiac risk factors, intact	82.8	+0.9	+1.0	+0.1
No risk factors and hysterectomy	82.8	+1.1	N/A	N/A
With history of CAD*	76.0	+2.1	+2.2	+0.9
With 1 or more CAD risk factors†	79.6	+1.5	+1.6	+0.6
At risk for breast cancer‡	82.3	+0.7	+0.8	−0.5
At risk for hip fracture§	82.4	+1.0	+1.1	+0.2

* Relative risk of dying of recurrent CAD estimated at 5.0.
† Relative risk of CAD death estimated as 2.5, as with smoking, hypertension, diabetes, or a sedentary life style.
‡ Breast cancer risk estimated as 2.0, as for a woman with a family history of breast cancer.
§ Hip fracture risk estimated as 3.0, as for a woman with low bone mineral density.
** Net change in life expectancy assumes that estrogen therapy carries the following relative risks; endometrial cancer death 3.0, breast cancer death 1.25, coronary heart disease death 0.65, hip fracture death 0.75, and death due to stroke 0.96.
†† E + P = Estrogen plus progesterone. These figures assume that the addition of progesterone to estrogen does not alter any relative risks, except to fully prevent the increased risk for endometrial cancer death (relative risk = 1.0).
‡‡ These figures assume that the addition of progesterone to estrogen reduces by one-third the benefit for CAD risk reduction (relative risk for CAD becomes 0.8) and that the relative risk for breast cancer increases to 2.0.

From Grady, D., Rubin, S. M., Pettiti, D. B., et al.: Hormone therapy to prevent disease and prolong life in postmenopausal women. Ann. Intern. Med. *117*:1016, 1992.

would represent a deterrent to estrogen replacement, especially in women with a personal or family history of breast cancer and a low likelihood of (i.e., no risk factors for) CAD. On the other hand, women with established CAD or with risk factors and no family history of breast cancer are the best candidates for estrogen replacement. The effects of the addition of progestins to estrogen in the incidence of breast cancer are unknown, but they appear to be minimal.[109a]

A recent meta-analysis of estrogen replacement reviewed all available data on its effects on endometrial and breast cancers, hip fracture, stroke, and coronary heart disease.[96] Combining these data with other information regarding the incidence and mortality of these diseases, detailed estimates of the gain/loss in life expectancy with hormone therapy for a hypothetical 50-year-old white woman with a variety of health risks were derived (Table 51–3). In most cases, estrogen replacement enhanced longevity.

BALANCING RISKS AND BENEFITS. Other considerations in the decision to use estrogen replacement include the drug's side effects, such as vaginal bleeding, the need for careful monitoring for breast and uterine cancers and endometrial hyperplasia, and the costs of therapy and of monitoring.[96,97,110,111] Thrombophlebitis is not a problem at the doses currently employed.[112] Compliance with estrogen replacement therapy taken to relieve menopause symptoms is poor; there is no reason to think that this will improve in asymptomatic women taking estrogen for the prevention of future disease.[113]

A full evaluation of the risks and benefits of estrogen replacement cannot be made without considering the methodological flaws inherent in all available data, and those crucial areas in which information is lacking. The lack of available results from any large observational studies raises issues of selection bias, especially because women using estrogen are more likely to see their physicians frequently, to adopt healthy behaviors such as exercise, prudent diet, and smoking cessation, and to be of higher socioeconomic status.[114]

The most commonly used estrogen is conjugated equine estrogens at a daily dose of 0.625 mg. There is no evidence that cardioprotection is enhanced or even preserved at a higher dose and side effects are often worse. In contrast, the optimal formulation, dosage, and regimen for progestins are unclear. The optimal timing of estrogen replacement is also unknown. Some workers suggest starting drug at menopause and continuing indefinitely for women at high risk. The usefulness of beginning therapy at a more advanced age (for example, with the first manifestation of CAD) is unknown, but this practice is likely to be of some benefit to those who have not been treated earlier.[115]

GUIDELINES FOR ESTROGEN REPLACEMENT THERAPY. The American College of Physicians recently published guidelines for counseling postmenopausal women about preventive hormone therapy that are well grounded in available knowledge.[116] These guidelines suggest that, based on available data, it is reasonable to state that estrogen replacement is likely of value in women with a high risk of developing osteoporosis or CAD and for secondary prevention in any woman currently with cardiovascular disease who is not at high risk for breast cancer. Because this includes all women with documented ischemia or infarction or those undergoing revascularization, this proposal represents an enormous potential change in cardiovascular therapeutics and practice. It is important to recognize that while salutary effects of estrogen replacement on lipids have been demonstrated in prospective randomized trials, clinical benefits thus far are limited to observational studies. Ongoing randomized trials of primary and secondary prevention will prove whether the wide use of estrogen replacement in postmenopausal women is a viable strategy.

MANAGEMENT OF CORONARY ARTERY DISEASE

Chronic Coronary Artery Disease

(See also Chap. 38)

Medical Therapy

Because few studies have examined the medical treatment of chronic CAD in women, there is little evidence as to whether women and men respond similarly to conventional therapy. Cross-sectional studies reveal that women with CAD are more likely than men to be receiving nitrates, calcium channel blockers, sedatives, diuretics, and other antihypertensive agents but are equally or less likely to have been prescribed aspirin and beta blockers.[10,40] The impact, if any, of these differences on the prognosis of coronary disease is unknown, although the Coronary Artery Surgery Study (CASS), shows that women treated medically had better 12-year survival with angiographically documented zero-, one-, or two-vessel disease than did men with similar anatomy.[117]

The use of aspirin is not as well proved in women as it is in men, and results cannot simply be extrapolated to women because gender may affect the antithrombotic and endothelial effects of aspirin.[14,18] The few observational studies in women have reported conflicting results regarding the effectiveness of aspirin for primary prevention. The most favorable, the Nurse's Health Study, showed a reduction in myocardial infarction risk of borderline statistical significance for women over 50 years taking one to six aspirin per week[119] but not in younger women or those taking higher doses. Other large studies have shown an increase in CAD risk in women with aspirin use.[120,121,121a] No study has yet demonstrated effective secondary prevention with aspirin in women.

Revascularization

In contrast to the paucity of data regarding medical therapy for CAD in women, many studies have addressed the relative effectiveness of revascularization procedures (angioplasty and coronary artery bypass grafting [CABG]) in men and women. Unfortunately, comparisons of the results of medical and invasive and operative management are few. Instead, these studies have focused on gender differences in the population under study, making difficult the application of these data to the optimal care of individual patients. Virtually all data for both angioplasty and CABG have been derived from post hoc subgroup analysis of studies designed to address other issues.

ANGIOPLASTY (see also p. 1371). Virtually all angioplasty studies note a greater prevalence of comorbidities in women, including advanced age, hypertension, congestive heart failure, diabetes, severe concomitant noncardiac disease, and hypercholesterolemia.[118,122–127] The severity of angina is also greater in women, the condition being more likely to be unstable or to be of Canadian Class III or IV severity.[122,124–126]

The likelihood of *angiographic success* of the application of balloon angioplasty or of new devices is similar in men and women in current series,[124–126] with lower success rates in women reported only in the older studies. In contrast, women experience higher complication and mortality rates, including groin complications, acute closure and death, but not myocardial infarction or emergency coronary artery bypass grafting[123] (Table 51–4). The difference in outcome has been variously attributed to women's older age, smaller body size, greater severity of angina, more fragile vessels, and perhaps greater comorbidity.[126]

The late outcome of angioplasty appears to be similar in men and women, with women more likely to experience angina and men more likely to experience cardiac events (myocardial infarction, revascularization, or death).[123–125,]

TABLE 51-4 GENDER DIFFERENCES IN EARLY OUTCOME OF ANGIOPLASTY

STUDY, YEAR, REFERENCE	SERIES	ANGIOGRAPHIC SUCCESS (%) W	ANGIOGRAPHIC SUCCESS (%) M	COMPLICATIONS (%) W	COMPLICATIONS (%) M	MORTALITY (%) W	MORTALITY (%) M
Cowley 1985[122]	NHLBI 1978–82	56.6	56.6	27.2	19.4	1.7	0.3
Kelsey 1993[123]	NHLBI 1985–86	89	89	29	20	2.6	0.3
Arnold 1994[124]	Cleveland Clinic 1980–88	93.6	93.3	9	7	1.1	0.3
Weintraub 1994[125]	Emory 1980–91	90.8	89.7	—	—	0.7	0.1
Bell 1993[126]	Mayo 1979–87	83	82	—	—	1.0	1.2
	Mayo Clinic 1988–90	87	90	—	—	2.9	1.4
Welty 1994[127]	Deaconess 1981–89	89.6	91.2	—	—	0.6	0.9

[127,128] Gender differences in angiographic restenosis rates have not been carefully examined.

CORONARY ARTERY BYPASS GRAFTING. Gender differences in outcome following CABG are well established.[118,129–135] As with angioplasty, virtually every study has shown women to have more comorbidities and less favorable patient characteristics preoperatively. Women are also more likely than men to undergo urgent or emergent surgery.[129,131,133] Women and men undergoing CABG are equally symptomatic but women are more likely to have preserved ventricular function and less likely to have multivessel or three-vessel disease.[129,130,132]

The mortality of women is higher than of men, with a risk ratio of 1.4 to 4.4.[118,129–135] In addition, women are less likely to receive internal mammary grafts or undergo complete revascularization and are more likely to experience the complications of heart failure, perioperative infarction, and hemorrhage.[129,131]

The causes of this higher mortality appear to be multiple, including technical factors such as smaller body size and coronary diameter, advanced age, comorbidities such as diabetes and hypertension, and clinical factors such as the urgency of the procedure.[129,130,132–134] Disease-related factors such as the extent and severity of angiographic stenoses and left ventricular dysfunction are also important in determining outcome, yet these factors tend to be more favorable in women. As with angioplasty, patient-related factors and comorbidities seem increasingly important to outcome, with more recent studies reporting widening gender differences in outcome.[130,134]

Women have a lower likelihood of being free of angina than do men[130] and experience greater physical disability and less return to work. Rates of long-term survival, infarction, and reoperation are similar.[130,132,135]

Acute Myocardial Infarction

(See also Chap. 37)

Although little is known of the pathophysiology underlying gender differences in acute myocardial infarction, it is clear that women have a different clinical presentation and respond differently to both medical and procedural therapies.

CLINICAL SYNDROMES. Women suffering from an acute myocardial infarction are likely to be older and more likely to have a history of hypertension, diabetes, unstable angina, hyperlipidemia, and congestive heart failure and are less likely to be smokers than their male counterparts.[136,139,141–150] Women are also more likely to experience neck and shoulder pain, abdominal pain, nausea, vomiting, fatigue, and dyspnea in addition to chest pain,[151] and are more likely to have silent infarctions.[5] Perhaps due in part to these more atypical symptoms, women seek medical attention more slowly[152] and even after hospital arrival may experience greater delays in receiving care.[145,147,153] Women are more likely to have experienced a nontransmural infarction.[141,150] Women with infarction have more serious presentations, with greater prevalences of tachycardia, rales, heart block, and a higher Killip class on initial presentation.[145,147,149,150,152] Nevertheless, women are less likely to receive thrombolysis (even after controlling for eligibility)[136,152,154,155,155a] and receive it later than do men.[147] Women are also less likely to be admitted to a coronary care unit[152,156] or to be hospitalized in an institution in which catheterization is available.[150] Most[150,151,153,154,156] but not all[137,157] women with acute infarction are less likely to undergo diagnostic catheterization during their hospital stay, even after controlling for age and a variety of clinical characteristics. Most studies have reported equal or near equal rates of angioplasty and bypass surgery among catheterized patients,[137,147,148,151,153] so that differences in treatment disappear once disease is documented angiographically.[158]

Women have higher rates of in-hospital complications from infarction, including bleeding, stroke, shock, myocardial rupture, and recurrent chest pain, than do men, although most of these differences disappear on correction for controlling for age and comorbidities.[138,141,147,148] Women with acute infarction are more likely to be treated with nitrates, digoxin, and diuretics than are men and are less likely to receive thrombolytics, antiarrhythmics, antiplatelet agents, and beta blockers.[141,146,152] Even after discharge,

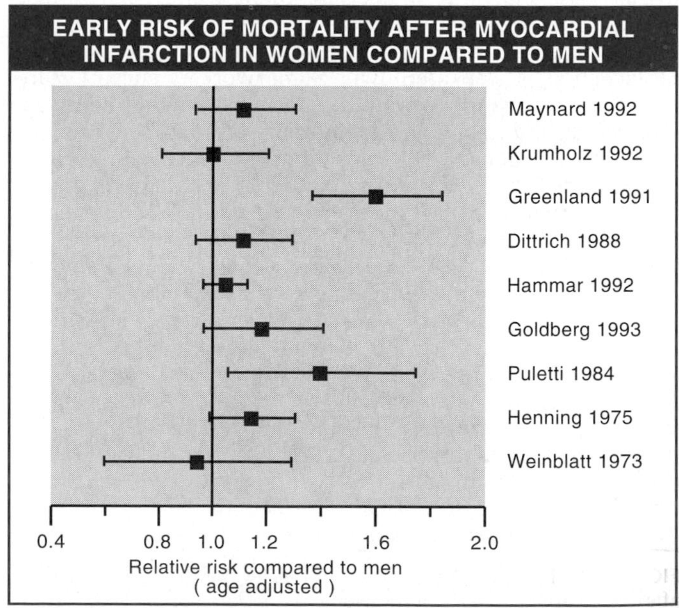

FIGURE 51-3. Relative risk of early mortality (in-hospital or first month) after myocardial infarction in women as compared to men. Data are shown as relative risk with 95% confidence interval. Three additional studies did not report 95% confidence intervals but were not significant. (Modified from Vaccarino, V., Krumholz, H.M., Berkman, L.F., Horvitz, R.I.: Sex differences in mortality after myocardial infarction. Circulation *91*:1861, 1995. Copyright 1995 American Heart Association.)

women are less likely to be scheduled for exercise tests or referred for cardiac rehabilitation, and recovery from infarction appears delayed with slower return to work and full resumption of all activities, with more sleep disturbance and psychiatric and psychosomatic complaints experienced.[159]

MORTALITY. Although early or in-hospital mortality in women appears to be greater than in men, most studies have shown that adjustment for age and/or clinical characteristics serves to reduce this difference but not to eliminate it fully (Fig. 51–3).[18,136–144,160] Mortality 1 to 3 years after hospital discharge is similar in men and women, and when adjustments are made for age and other baseline characteristics, women may actually do better.[18,139]

TREATMENT. Comparison of benefits from thrombolysis in men and women with acute myocardial infarction are difficult, but it appears that the reductions in mortality are similar (Fig. 51–4).[161–165] The efficacy of thrombolysis also appears similar in men and women with similar rates of infarct-related artery patency[145,148] and left ventricular function.[145,148,166] However, complication rates, particularly hemorrhagic stroke and recurrent myocardial infarction, appear to be higher in women.[147,148,167,168] Information on primary angioplasty is limited, but in the PAMI trial the improvement in women was impressive (Fig. 51–4).[170]

Medical treatment after hospital discharge appears to carry somewhat different benefits for men and women. Aspirin (see above) has not yet been proved to prevent reinfarction in women and calcium channel blockers have not been evaluated. Two studies suggest that men may experience more benefit than women when treated with angiotensin-converting enzyme inhibitors postinfarction.[171,172] In contrast, beta blockade clearly provides a substantial improvement in postinfarction survival in women that is equal to, if not greater than, that seen in men.[173–175] Unfortunately, women are less likely to be discharged on beta-blockers.[146,149,152]

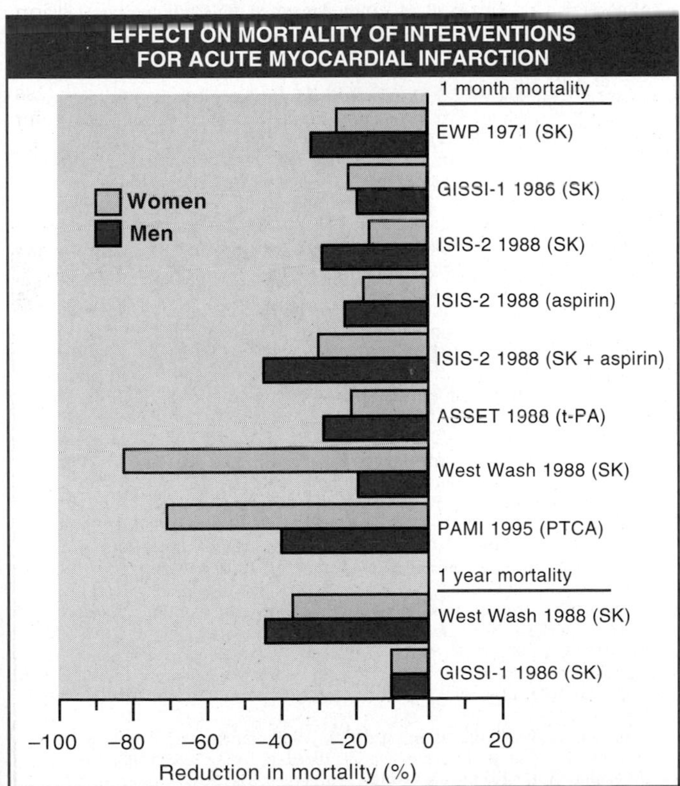

FIGURE 51–4. Comparison of reductions in early and late mortality after myocardial infarction in women and men with thrombolysis, aspirin and primary angioplasty. (EWP = European Working Party: GISSI-1 = Gruppo Italiano per lo Studio della Streptochinasi Nell' infarto Miocardico; ISIS-2 = Second International Study of Infarct Survival; ASSET = Anglo-Scandanavian Study of Early Thrombolysis; West Wash = Western Washington Intravenous Streptokinase in Acute Myocardial Infarction Trial; PAMI = Primary Angioplasty in Myocardial Infarction; SK = Streptokinase; t-PA = Tissue Plasminogen Activator.)

CONCLUSIONS

The time-honored observation of demographic differences in heart disease in men and women is now well supported by newer findings of gender-based differences in the clinical presentation, evaluation, and treatment of heart disease. While principles of diagnostic and therapeutic management of women are similar to those in men, the differences in diagnostic test characteristics and outcomes of interventions mandate careful consideration of risks and benefits for each individual.

Hormones and hormone replacement status are unique and important considerations of heart disease in women. The available epidemiological evidence suggests that such treatment should be a consideration in women at risk for cardiac disease or its recurrence. These clinical observations and elucidation of the underlying pathophysiology suggest new ways to improve upon all aspects of cardiovascular care for women.

REFERENCES

1. Eaker, E. D., Chesebro, J. H., Sacks, F. M., et al.: Cardiovascular disease in women. Circulation *88*:1999, 1993.
2. Higgins, M., and Thom, T.: Cardiovascular disease in women as a public health problem. *In* Wenger, N. K., Speroff, L., Packard, B. (eds.): Cardiovascular Health and Disease in Women. Greenwich, CT, Le Jacq Communications, Inc., 1993, p. 15.
3. Advance Report of Final Mortality Statistics for 1992 National Center for Health Statistics, 1995.
4. Reunanen, A., Suhonen, O., Aromaa, A., et al.: Incidence of different manifestations of coronary heart disease in middle-aged Finnish men and women. Acta Med. Scand. *218*:19, 1985.
5. Lerner, D. J., and Kannel, W. B.: Patterns of coronary heart disease morbidity and mortality in the sexes: 26-year follow-up of the Framingham population. Am. Heart J. *111*:383, 1986.
6. Weiner, D. A., Ryan, T. J., McCabe, C. H., et al.: Correlations among history of angina, ST-segment response and prevalence of coronary artery disease in the coronary artery surgery study (CASS). N. Engl. J. Med. *301*:230, 1979.
7. DeSanctis, R. W.: Clinical manifestations of coronary artery disease: Chest pain in women. *In* Wenger, N. K., Speroff, L., Packard B. (eds.): Cardiovascular Health and Disease in Women. Greenwich, CT, Le Jacq Communications, Inc., 1993, p. 67.
8. Sullivan, A. K., Holdright, D. R., Wright, C. A., et al.: Chest pain in women: Clinical, investigative, and prognostic features. Br. Med. J. *308*:883, 1994.
9. Fields, S. K., Savard, M. A., and Epstein, K. R.: The female patient. *In* Douglas, P. S. (ed.): Cardiovascular Health and Disease in Women. Philadelphia, W. B. Saunders Company, 1993, p. 3.
10. Pepine, C. J., Abrams, J., Marks, R. G., et al.: Characteristics of a contemporary population with angina pectoris. Am. J. Cardiol. *74*:226, 1994.
11. Birdwell, B. G., Herbers, J. E., and Kroenke, K.: Evaluating chest pain. Arch. Intern. Med. *153*:1991, 1993.
12. Cannon, R. O., Camici, P. G., and Epstein, S. E.: Pathophysiological dilemma of syndrome X. Circulation *85*:883, 1992.
13. Mautner, S. L., Lin, F., Mautner, G. C., and Roberts, W. C.: Comparison in women versus men of composition of atherosclerotic plaques in native coronary arteries and in saphenous veins used as aortocoronary conduits. J. Am. Coll. Cardiol. *21*:1312, 1992.
14. Weksler, B. B.: Hemostasis and thrombosis. *In* Douglas, P. S. (ed.): Cardiovascular Health and Disease in Women. Philadelphia, W. B. Saunders Company, 1993, p. 231.
15. Murabito, J. M., Evans, J. C., Larson, M. G., and Levy, D.: Prognosis after the onset of coronary heart disease. An investigation of differences in outcome between the sexes according to initial coronary disease presentation. Circulation *88*:2548, 1993.
16. Orencia, A., Bailey, K., Yawn, B. P., and Kottke, T. E.: Effect of gender on long-term outcome of angina pectoris and myocardial infarction/sudden unexpected death. JAMA *269*:2392, 1993.
17. LaCroix, A. Z., Guralnik, J. M., Curb, J. D., et al.: Chest pain and coronary heart disease mortality among older men and women in three communities. Circulation *81*:437, 1990.
18. Vaccarino, V., Krumholz, H. M., Berkman, L. F., and Horwitz, R. I.: Sex differences in mortality after myocardial infarction. Circulation *91*:1861, 1995.
19. Gibbons, R. F.: Exercise ECG testing with and without radionuclide

studies. *In* Wenger, N. K., Speroff, L., Packard, B. (eds.): Cardiovascular Health and Disease in Women. Greenwich, CT, Le Jacq Communications, Inc., 1993, p. 73.
20. Weiner, D. A., Ryan, T. J., Parsons, L., et al.: Long-term prognostic value of exercise testing in men and women from the coronary artery surgery study (CASS) registry. Am. J. Cardiol. *75:*865, 1995.
21. Higgenbotham, M. B., Morris, K. G., Coleman, E., et al.: Sex-related differences in normal cardiac response to supine exercise assessed by radionuclide angiography. J. Am. Coll. Cardiol. *13:*624, 1989.
22. Hung, J., Chaitman, B. R., Lam, J., et al.: Noninvasive diagnostic test choices for the evaluation of coronary artery disease in women: A multivariate comparison of cardiac fluoroscopy, exercise electrocardiography and exercise thallium myocardial perfusion scintigraphy. J. Am. Coll. Cardiol. *4:*8, 1984.
23. Melin, J. A., Wijns, W., Vanbutsele, R. J., et al.: Alternative diagnostic strategies for coronary artery disease in women: Demonstration of the usefulness and efficiency of probability analysis. Circulation *71:*535, 1985.
24. Friedman, T. D., Greene, A. C., Iskandrian, A. S., et al.: Exercise thallium-201 myocardial scintigraphy in women: Correlation with coronary arteriography. Am. J. Cardiol. *49:*1632, 1982.
25. Goodgold, H. M., Rehder, J. G., Samuels, L. D., and Chaitman, B. R.: Improved interpretation of exercise T1-201 myocardial perfusion scintigraphy in women: Characterization of breast attenuation artifacts. Radiology *165:*361, 1987.
26. Fintel, D. J., Links, J. M., Brinker, J. A., et al.: Improved diagnostic performance of exercise thallium-201 single photon emission computed tomography over planar imaging in the diagnosis of coronary artery disease: A receiver operating characteristic analysis. J. Am. Coll. Cardiol. *13:*600, 1989.
27. Chae, S. C., Heo, J., Iskandrian, A. S., et al.: Identification of extensive coronary artery disease in women by exercise single-photon emission computer tomographic (SPECT) thallium imaging. J. Am. Coll. Cardiol. *21:*1305, 1993.
28. Sawada, S. G., Ryan, T., Fineberg, N. S., et al.: Exercise echocardiographic detection of coronary artery disease in women. J. Am. Coll. Cardiol. *14:*1440, 1989.
29. Williams, M. J., Marwick, T. H., O'Gorman, D., and Foale, R. A.: Comparison of exercise echocardiography with an exercise score to diagnose coronary artery disease in women. Am. J. Cardiol. *74:*435, 1994.
29a. Marwick, T. H., Anderson, T., Williams, M. J., et al.: Exercise echocardiography is an accurate and cost-efficient technique for detection of coronary artery disease in women. J. Am. Coll. Cardiol. *26:*335, 1995.
30. Masini, M., Picano, E., Lattanzi, F., et al.: High-dose dipyridamole-echocardiography test in women: Correlation with exercise-electrocardiography test and coronary arteriography. J. Am. Coll. Cardiol. *12:*682, 1988.
31. Kong, B. A., Shaw, L., Miller, D. D., and Chaitman, B. R.: Comparison of accuracy for detecting coronary artery disease and side effect profile of dipyridamole thallium-201 myocardial perfusion imaging in women versus men. Am. J. Cardiol. *70:*168, 1992.
32. Anderson, T., Marwick, T., Williams, M. J., et al.: Exercise echocardiography is more cost efficient than exercise ECG as an initial test for evaluation of cardiac symptoms in women. J. Am. Coll. Cardiol. *25:*17A, 1995.
33. Steen, M. K., Jacobs, A. K., Freney, D., et al.: Gender related differences in complications during coronary angiography. Circulation 86 (Suppl I):254, 1992.
34. Tobin, J. N., Wassertheil-Smoller, S., Wexler, J. P., et al.: Sex bias in considering coronary bypass surgery. Ann. Intern. Med. *107:*19, 1987.
35. Ayanian, J. Z., and Epstein, A. M.: Differences in the use of procedures between women and men hospitalized for coronary heart disease. N. Engl. J. Med. *325:*221, 1991.
36. Bearden, D., Allman, R., McDonald, R., et al.: Age, race, and gender variation in the utilization of coronary artery bypass surgery and angioplasty in SHEP. SHEP cooperative research group. Systemic hypertension in the elderly program. J. Am. Geriatr. Soc. *42:*1143, 1994.
37. Bickell, N. A., Pieper, K. S., Lee, K. L., et al.: Referral patterns for coronary artery disease treatment: Gender bias or good clinical judgment? Ann. Intern. Med. *116:*791, 1992.
38. Green, L. A., and Ruffin, M. T.: A closer examination of sex bias in the treatment of ischemic cardiac disease. J. Fam. Pract. *39:*331, 1994.
39. Laskey, W. K.: Editorial. Gender differences in the management of coronary artery disease: Bias or good clinical judgment? Ann. Intern. Med. *116:*869, 1992.
40. Shaw, L. J., Miller, D. D., Romeis, J. C., et al.: Gender differences in the noninvasive evaluation and management of patients with suspected coronary artery disease. Ann. Intern. Med. *120:*559, 1994.
41. Kannel, W. B., and Vokonas, P. S.: Demographics of the prevalence, incidence, and management of coronary heart disease in the elderly and in women. Ann. Epidemiol. *2:*5, 1992.
42. Detection, Evaluation, and Treatment of High Blood Cholesterol in Adults (Adult Treatment Panel II). Circulation *89:*1329, 1994.
42a. Rich-Edwards, J. W., Manson, J. E., Hennekens, C. H., et al.: The primary prevention of coronary heart disease in women. N. Engl. J. Med. *332:*1758, 1995.
43. LaRosa, J. C.: Lipoproteins and lipid disorders. *In* Douglas, P. S. (ed.): Cardiovascular Health and Disease in Women. Philadelphia, W. B. Saunders Company, 1993, p. 175.
44. Eaker, E. D., and Castelli, W. P.: Coronary heart disease and its risk factors among women in the Framingham Study. *In* Eaker, E. D., Packer, B., Wenger, N., et al. (eds.): Coronary Heart Disease in Women. New York, Haymarket Doyma, 1987, p. 122.
45. Miller, V. T.: Lipids, lipoproteins, women and cardiovascular disease. Atherosclerosis *108:*S73, 1994.
46. Criqui, M. H., Heiss, G., Cohn, R., et al.: Plasma triglyceride level and mortality from coronary heart disease. N. Engl. J. Med. *328:*1220, 1993.
47. Wang, X. L., Tam, C., McCredie, R. M., and Wilcken, D. E. L.: Determinants of severity of coronary artery disease in Australian men and women. Circulation *89:*1974, 1994.
48. Bengtsson, C., Bjorkelund, C., Lapidus, L., and Lissner, L.: Associations of serum lipid concentrations and obesity with mortality in women: 20 year follow up of participants in prospective population study in Gothenburg, Sweden. Br. Med. J. *307:*1385, 1993.
49. Boston, A. G., Gagnon, D. R., Cupples, A., et al.: A prospective investigation of elevated lipoprotein (a) detected by electrophoresis and cardiovascular disease in women: The Framingham Heart Study. Circulation *90:*1688, 1994.
50. Bush, T. L., Fried, L. P., and Barrett-Connor, E.: Cholesterol, lipoproteins, and coronary heart disease in women. Clin. Chem. *34:*B60, 1988.
51. Kane, J. P., Malloy, M. J., Ports, T. A., et al.: Regression of coronary atherosclerosis during treatment of familial hypercholesterolemia with combined drug regimens. JAMA *264:*3007, 1990.
52. Blankenhorn, D. H., Azen, S. P., Kramsch, D. M., et al. and the MARS research group: The monitored atherosclerosis regression study (MARS): Coronary angiographic changes with lovastatin therapy. Ann. Intern. Med. *119:*969, 1993.
53. Scandinavian Simvastatin Survival Study Group (4S): Randomized trial of cholesterol lowering in 4444 patients with coronary heart disease: The Scandinavian Simvastatin survival study. Lancet *344:*1383, 1389, 1994.
54. Summary of the Second Report of the National Cholesterol Education Program (NCEP) Expert Panel on Detection, Evaluation, and Treatment of High Blood Cholesterol in Adults (Adult Treatment Panel II): Expert Panel on Detection, Evaluation and Treatment of High Blood Cholesterol in Adults. JAMA *269:*3015, 1993.
55. Walsh, B. W., Schiff, I., Rosner, B., et al.: Effects of postmenopausal estrogen replacement on the concentrations and metabolism of plasma lipoproteins. N. Engl. J. Med. *325:*1196, 1991.
56. Krumholz, H. M., Seeman, T. E., Merrill, S. S., et al.: Lack of association between cholesterol and coronary heart disease mortality and morbidity and all-cause mortality in persons older than 70 years. JAMA *272:*1335, 1994.
57. Spelsberg, A., Ridker, P. M., and Manson, J. E.: Carbohydrate metabolism, obesity, and diabetes. *In* Douglas, P. S. (ed.): Cardiovascular Health and Disease in Women. Philadelphia, W. B. Saunders Company, 1993, p. 191.
58. Zuanetti, G., Latini, R., Maggioni, A. P., et al.: Influence of diabetes on mortality in acute myocardial infarction: Data from the GISSI-2 study. J. Am. Coll. Cardiol. *22:*1788, 1993.
58a. Manson, J. E., Colditz, G. A., Stampfer, M. J., et al.: A prospective study of obesity and risk of coronary heart disease in women. N. Engl. J. Med. *322:*882, 1990.
59. Diabetes Control and Complications Trial Research Group: The effect of intensive treatment of diabetes on the development and progression of long-term complications in insulin-dependent diabetes mellitus. N. Engl. J. Med. *329:*977, 1993.
60. Bittner, V., and Oparil, S.: Hypertension. *In* Douglas, P. S. (ed.): Cardiovascular Health and Disease in Women. Philadelphia, W. B. Saunders Company, 1993, p. 63.
61. Dahloef, B., Lindholm, L., Hansson, L., et al.: Morbidity and mortality in the swedish trial in old patients with hypertension (STOP-hypertension). Lancet *338:*1281, 1991.
62. Fried, L. P., and Becker, D. M.: Smoking and cardiovascular disease. *In* Douglas, P. S. (ed.): Cardiovascular Health and Disease in Women. Philadelphia, W. B. Saunders Company, 1993, p. 217.
63. Colditz, G. A., Bonita, R., Stampfer, M. J., et al.: Cigarette smoking and risk of stroke in middle-aged women. N. Engl. J. Med. *318:*937, 1988.
64. Shapiro, S., Sloane, D., Rosenberg, L., et al.: Oral contraceptive use in relation to myocardial infarction. Lancet *1:*743, 1979.
65. Hermanson, B., Omenn, G. S., Kronmal, R. A., et al.: Beneficial six-year outcome of smoking cessation in older men and women with coronary artery disease. Results from the CASS registry. N. Engl. J. Med. *319:*1365, 1988.
66. Ernst, E., and Resch, K. L.: Fibrinogen as a cardiovascular risk factor: A meta-analysis and review of the literature. Ann. Intern. Med. *118:*956, 1993.
67. Kannel, W. B., Wolf, P. A., Castelli, W. P., and D'Agostino, R. B.: Fibrinogen and risk of cardiovascular disease. JAMA *258:*1183, 1987.
68. Weksler, B. B.: Hemostasis and Thrombosis. *In* Douglas, P. S. (ed.): Cardiovascular Health and Disease in Women. Philadelphia, W. B. Saunders Company, 1993, p. 231.
69. O'Toole, M. L.: Exercise and physical activity. *In* Douglas, P. S. (ed.): Cardiovascular Health and Disease in Women. Philadelphia, W. B. Saunders Company, 1993, p. 253.
70. Krummel, D., Etherton, T. D., Peterson, S., and Kris-Etherton, P. M.: Effects of exercise on plasma lipids and lipoproteins of women. Soc. Exp. Biology Med. *204:*123, 1993.
71. Blair, S. N., Kohl, H. W., Paffenbarger, R. S., et al.: Physical fitness and all-cause mortality. A prospective study of healthy men and women. JAMA *262:*2395, 1989.
72. Manson, J. E., Stampfer, M. J., Willet, W. C., et al.: Physical activity and

incidence of coronary heart disease and stroke in women. Circulation *91:*927, 1995.
73. Haynes, S. G., and Czajkowski, S. M.: Psychosocial and environmental correlates of heart disease. *In* Douglas, P. S. (ed.): Cardiovascular Health and Disease in Women. Philadelphia, W. B. Saunders Company, 1993, p. 269.
74. Frank, E., and Taylor, C. B.: Psychosocial influences on diagnosis and treatment plans of women with coronary heart disease. *In* Wenger, N. K., Speroff, L., Packard, B. (eds.): Cardiovascular Health and Disease in Women. Greenwich, CT, Le Jacq Communications, Inc., 1993, p. 231.
75. Berkman, L. F., Vaccarino, V., and Seeman, T.: Gender differences in cardiovascular morbidity and mortality: The contribution of social networks and support. *In* Wenger, N. K., Speroff, L., Packard, B. (eds.): Cardiovascular Health and Disease in Women. Greenwich, CT, Le Jacq Communications, Inc., 1993, p. 217.
76. Lobo, R. A.: Hormones, hormone replacement therapy, and heart disease. *In* Douglas, P. S. (ed.): Cardiovascular Health and Disease in Women. Philadelphia, W. B. Saunders Company, 1993, p. 153.
77. Matthews, K. A., Meilahn, E., Kuller, L. H., et al.: Menopause and risk factors for coronary heart disease. N. Engl. J. Med. *321:*641, 1989.
78. Croft, P., and Hannaford, P. C.: Risk factors for acute myocardial infarction in women: Evidence from the Royal College of General Practitioners' oral contraception study. Br. Med. J. *298:*165, 1989.
79. Stampfer, M. J., Willett, W. C., Colditz, G. A., et al.: A prospective study of past use of oral contraceptive agents and risk of cardiovascular diseases. N. Engl. J. Med. *319:*1313, 1988.
80. Engel, H. J., Engel, E., and Lichtlen, P. R.: Coronary atherosclerosis and myocardial infarction in young women—role of oral contraceptives. Eur. Heart J. *4:*1, 1983.
81. Daly, L., and Bonnar, J.: Comparative studies of 30 μg ethinyl estradiol combined with gestodene and desogestrel on blood coagulation, fibrinolysis, and platelets. Am. J. Obstet. Gynecol. *163:*430, 1990.
82. The Writing Group for the PEPI Trial: Effects of estrogen or estrogen/progestin regimens on heart disease risk factors in postmenopausal women. The Postmenopausal Estrogen/Progestin Interventions (PEPI) Trial. JAMA *273:*199, 1995.
83. Manolio, T. A., Furberg, C. D., Shemanski, L., et al.: Associations of postmenopausal estrogen use with cardiovascular disease and its risk factors in older women. The CHS Collaborative Research Group. Circulation *88:*2163, 1993.
84. Hong, M. K., Romm, P. A., Reagan, K., et al.: Effects of estrogen replacement therapy on serum lipid values and angiographically defined coronary artery disease in postmenopausal women. Am. J. Cardiol. *69:*176, 1992.
85. Nabulsi, A. A., Folsom, A. R., White, A., et al.: Association of hormone-replacement therapy with various cardiovascular risk factors in postmenopausal women. The Atherosclerosis Risk in Communities Study Investigators. N. Engl. J. Med. *328:*1069, 1993.
86. Crook, D., Cust, M. P., Gangar, K. F., et al.: Comparison of transdermal and oral estrogen-progestin replacement therapy: Effects on serum lipids and lipoproteins. Am. J. Obstet. Gynecol. *166:*950, 1992.
87. Gebara, O. C., Mittleman, M. A., Sutherland, P., et al.: Association between increased estrogen status and increased fibrinolytic potential in the Framingham Offspring Study. Circulation *91:*1952, 1995.
88. Barrett-Connor, E., and Laakso, M.: Ischemic heart disease risk in postmenopausal women. Effects of estrogen use on glucose and insulin levels. Arteriosclerosis *10:*531, 1990.
88a. Gerhard, M., and Ganz, M.: How do we explain the clinical benefits of estrogen? Circulation *92:*5, 1995.
89. Karas, R. H., Patterson, B. L., and Mendelsohn, M. E.: Human vascular smooth muscle cells contain functional estrogen receptor. Circulation *89:*1943, 1994.
90. Herrington, D. M., Braden, G. A., Williams, J. K., and Morgan, T. M.: Endothelial-dependent coronary vasomotor responsiveness in postmenopausal women with and without estrogen replacement therapy. Am. J. Cardiol. *73:*951, 1994.
91. Reis, S. E., Gloth, S. T., Blumenthal, R. S., et al.: Ethinyl estradiol acutely attenuates abnormal coronary vasomotor responses to acetylcholine in postmenopausal women. Circulation *89:*52, 1994.
92. Gilligan, D. M., Quyyumi, A. A., and Cannon, R. O. III: Effects of physiological levels of estrogen on coronary vasomotor function in postmenopausal women. Circulation *89:*2545, 1994.
93. Lieberman, E. H., Gerhard, M. D., Uehata, A., et al.: Estrogen improves endothelium-dependent, flow-mediated vasodilation in postmenopausal women. Ann. Intern. Med. *121:*936, 1994.
94. Sack, M. N., Rader, D. J., and Cannon, R. O. III: Oestrogen and inhibition of oxidation of low-density lipoproteins in postmenopausal women. Lancet *343:*269, 1994.
95. Keaney, J. F., Jr., Shwaery, G. T., Xu, A., et al.: 17-beta-estradiol preserves endothelial vasodilator function and limits low-density lipoprotein oxidation in hypercholesterolemic swine. Circulation *89:*2251, 1994.
96. Grady, D., Rubin, S. M., Petitti, D. B., et al.: Hormone therapy to prevent disease and prolong life in postmenopausal women. Ann. Intern. Med. *117:*1016, 1992.
97. Ravnikar, V. A.: Hormone replacement therapy in the primary prevention of cardiovascular disease: Benefits, risks, and compliance issues. *In* Wenger, N. K., Speroff, P., and Packard, B. (eds.): Cardiovascular Health and Disease in Women. Greenwich, CT, Le Jacq Communications, Inc., 1993, p. 181.
97a. Grady, D., Gebretsadik, T., Kerlikowske, K., et al.: Hormone replacement therapy and endometrial cancer risk: A meta-analysis. Obstet. Gynecol. *85:*304, 1995.
98. Stampfer, M. J., and Colditz, G. A.: Estrogen replacement therapy and coronary heart disease: A quantitative assessment of the epidemiologic evidence. Prev. Med. *20:*47, 1991.
99. Stampfer, M. J., Colditz, G. A., Willett, W. C., et al.: Postmenopausal estrogen therapy and cardiovascular disease. Ten-year follow-up from the Nurses' Health Study. N. Engl. J. Med. *325:*756, 1991.
100. Finucane, F. F., Madans, J. H., Bush, T. L., et al.: Decreased risk of stroke among postmenopausal hormone users. Results from a national cohort. Arch. Intern. Med. *153:*73, 1993.
101. Love, R. R., Newcomb, P. A., Wiebe, D. A., et al.: Effects of tamoxifen therapy on lipid and lipoprotein levels in postmenopausal patients with node-negative breast cancer. J. Natl. Cancer Inst. *82:*1327, 1990.
102. Rutqvist, L. E., and Mattsson, A.: Cardiac and thromboembolic morbidity among postmenopausal women with early-stage breast cancer in a randomized trial of adjuvant tamoxifen. The Stockholm Breast Cancer Study Group. J. Natl. Cancer Inst. *85:*1398, 1993.
103. Early Breast Cancer Trialists' Collaborative Group: Systemic treatment of early breast cancer by hormonal, cytotoxic, or immune therapy. 133 randomized trials involving 31,000 recurrences and 24,000 deaths among 75,000 women. Lancet *339:*1, 71, 1992.
104. Sullivan, J. M., Vander Zwaag, R., Lemp, G. F., et al.: Postmenopausal estrogen use and coronary atherosclerosis. Ann. Intern. Med. *108:*358, 1988.
105. Gruchow, H. W., Anderson, A. J., Barboriak, J. J., and Sobocinski, K. A.: Postmenopausal use of estrogen and occlusion of coronary arteries. Am. Heart J. *115:*954, 1988.
106. Sullivan, J. M., Vander Zwaag, R., Hughes, J. P., et al.: Estrogen replacement and coronary artery disease. Effect on survival in postmenopausal women. Arch. Intern. Med. *150:*2557, 1990.
107. Sullivan, J. M., El-Zeky, F., Vander Zwaag, R., and Ramanathan, K. K.: Estrogen replacement therapy after coronary artery bypass surgery: Effect on survival. Circulation *345:*669, 1995.
108. Bilezikian, J. P.: Major issues regarding estrogen replacement therapy in postmenopausal women. J. Women's Health *3:*273, 1994.
109. Henrich, J. B.: The postmenopausal estrogen/breast cancer controversy. JAMA *268:*1900, 1992.
109a. Colditz, G. A., Hankinson, S. E., Hunter, D. J., et al.: The use of estrogens and progestins and the risk of breast cancer in postmenopausal women. N. Engl. J. Med. *332:*1589, 1995.
110. Belchetz, P. E.: Hormonal treatment of postmenopausal women. N. Engl. J. Med. *330:*1062, 1994.
111. Martin, K. A., and Freeman, M. W.: Postmenopausal hormone-replacement therapy. N. Engl. J. Med. *328:*1115, 1993.
112. Devor, M., Barrett-Connor, E., Renvall, M., et al.: Estrogen replacement therapy and the risk of venous thrombosis. Am. J. Med. *92:*275, 1992.
113. Barrett-Connor, E.: Prevalence, initiation, and continuation of hormone replacement therapy. J. Women's Health *4:*143, 1995.
114. Posthuma, W. F. M., Westendorp, R. G. J., and Vandenbroucke, J. P.: Cardioprotective effect of hormone replacement therapy in postmenopausal women: Is the evidence biased? Br. Med. J. *308:*1268, 1994.
115. Henderson, B. E., Paganini-Hill, A., and Ross, R. K.: Estrogen replacement therapy and protection from acute myocardial infarction. Am. J. Obstet. Gynecol. *159:*312, 1988.
116. American College of Physicians: Guidelines for counseling postmenopausal women about preventive hormone therapy. Ann. Intern. Med. *117:*1038, 1992.
117. Edmond, M., Mock, M. B., Davis, K. B., et al.: Long-term survival of medically treated patients in the coronary artery surgery study (CASS) registry. Circulation *90:*2645, 1994.
118. Eysmann, S. B., and Douglas, P. S.: Coronary heart disease: Therapeutic principles. *In* Douglas, P. S. (ed.): Cardiovascular Health and Disease in Women. Philadelphia, W. B. Saunders Company, 1993, p. 43.
119. Manson, J. E., Stampfer, M. J., Colditz, G. A., et al.: A prospective study of aspirin use and primary prevention of cardiovascular disease in women. J. Am. Med. Assoc. *266:*521, 1991.
120. Paganini-Hill, A., Chao, A., Ross, R. K., and Henderson, B. E.: Aspirin use and chronic diseases: A cohort study of the elderly. Br. Med. J. *299:*1247, 1989.
121. Hammond, E. C., and Garfinkel, L.: Aspirin and coronary heart disease: Findings of a prospective study. Br. Med. J. *2:*269, 1975.
122. Cowley, M. J., Mullin, S. M., Kelsey, S. F., et al.: Sex differences in early and long-term results of coronary angioplasty in the NHLBI PTCA registry. Circulation *71:*90, 1985.
123. Kelsey, S. F., James, M., Holubkov, A. L., et al.: Results of percutaneous transluminal coronary angioplasty in women: 1985-1986 NHLBI coronary angioplasty registry. Circulation *87:*720, 1993.
124. Arnold, A. M., Mick, M. J., Piedmonte, M. R., and Simpfendorfer, C.: Gender differences for coronary angioplasty. Am. J. Cardiol. *74:*18, 1994.
125. Weintraub, W. S., Wenger, N. K., Kosinski, A. S., et al.: Percutaneous transluminal coronary angioplasty in women compared with men. J. Am. Coll. Cardiol. *24:*81, 1994.
126. Bell, M. R., Holmes, D. R., Berger, P. B., et al.: The changing in-hospital mortality of women undergoing percutaneous transluminal coronary angioplasty. JAMA *269:*2091, 1993.
127. Welty, F. K., Mittleman, M. A., Healy, R. W., et al.: Similar results of percutaneous transluminal coronary angioplasty for women and men with postmyocardial infarction ischemia. J. Am. Coll. Cardiol. *23:*35, 1994.

128. Greenberg, M. A., and Mueller, H. S.: Why the excess mortality in women after PTCA? Circulation *87:*1030, 1993.
129. King, K. B., Clark, P. C., and Hicks, G. L.: Patterns of referral and recovery in women and men undergoing coronary artery bypass grafting. Am. J. Cardiol. *69:*179, 1992.
130. Rahimtoola, S. H., Bennett, A. J., Grunkemeier, G. L., et al.: Survival at 15 to 18 years after coronary bypass surgery for angina in women. Circulation *88:*II-71, II-78, 1993.
131. O'Connor, G. T., Morton, J. R., Diehl, M. J., et al. for the Northern New England Cardiovascular Disease Study Group: Differences between men and women in hospital mortality associated with coronary artery bypass graft surgery. Circulation *88:*2104, 1993.
132. Eaker, E. D., Kronmal, R., Kennedy, J. W., and Davis, K.: Comparison of the long-term, postsurgical survival of women and men in the Coronary Artery Surgery Study (CASS). Am. Heart J. *117:*71, 1989.
133. Hannan, E. L., Bernard, H. R., Kilburn, H. C., and O'Donnell, J. F.: Gender differences in mortality rates for coronary artery bypass surgery. Am. Heart J. *123:*866, 1992.
134. Weintraub, W. S., Wenger, N. K., Jones, E. L., et al.: Changing clinical characteristics of coronary surgery patients: Differences between men and women. Circulation *88:*II-79, II-86, 1993.
135. Caracciolo, E. A., Davis, K. B., Sopko, G., et al.: Comparison of surgical and medical group survival in patients with left main coronary artery disease: Long-term CASS experience. Circulation *91:*2325, 1995.
136. Maynard, C., Litwin, P. E., Martin, J. S., and Weaver, W. D.: Gender differences in the treatment and outcome of acute myocardial infarction: Results from the myocardial infarction triage and intervention registry. Arch. Intern. Med. *152:*972, 1992.
137. Krumholz, H. M., Douglas, P. S., Lauer, M. S., and Pasternak, R. C.: Selection of patients for coronary angiography and coronary revascularization early after myocardial infarction: Is there evidence for a gender bias? Ann. Intern. Med. *116:*785, 1992.
138. Greenland, P., Reicher-Reiss, H., Goldbourt, U., and Behar, S.: In-hospital and 1-year mortality in 1,524 women after myocardial infarction: Comparison with 4,315 men. Circulation *83:*484, 1991.
139. Dittrrich, D., Gilpin, E., Nicod, P., et al.: Acute myocardial infarction in women: Influence of gender on mortality and prognostic variables. Am. J. Cardiol. *62:*1, 1988.
140. Hammar, N., Larsen, F. F., Sandberg, E., et al.: Time trends in survival from myocardial infarction in Stockholm County 1976-1984. Int. J. Epidemiol. *21:*1090, 1992.
141. Goldberg, R. J., Gorak, E. J., Yarzebski, J., et al.: A communitywide perspective of sex differences and temporal trends in the incidence and survival rates after acute myocardial infarction and out-of-hospital deaths caused by coronary heart disease. Circulation *87:*1947, 1993.
142. Puletti, M., Sunseri, L., Curione, M., et al.: Acute myocardial infarction: Sex-related differences in prognosis. Am. Heart J. *108:*63, 1984.
143. Henning, R., and Lundman, T.: The Swedish Cooperative Study, Part I: A description of the early stage. Acta Med. Scand. *586:*27, 1975.
144. Weinblatt, E., Shapiro, S., and Frank, C. W.: Prognosis of women with newly diagnosed coronary heart disease: A comparison with causes of disease among men. Am. J. Public Health *63:*577, 1973.
145. Jenkins, J. S., Flaker, G. C., Nolte, B., et al.: Causes of higher in-hospital mortality in women than in men after acute myocardial infarction. Am. J. Cardiol. *73:*319, 1994.
146. Wilkinson, P., Laji, K., Ranjadayalan, K., et al.: Acute myocardial infarction in women: Survival analysis in first six months. Br. Med. J. *309:*566, 1994.
147. White, H. D., Barbash, G. I., Modan, M., et al.: After correcting for worse baseline characteristics, women treated with thrombolytic therapy for acute myocardial infarction have the same mortality and morbidity as men except for a higher incidence of hemorrhagic stroke. The Investigators of the International Tissue Plasminogen Activator/Streptokinase Mortality Study. Circulation *88:*2097, 1993.
148. Lincoff, A. M., Califf, R. M., Ellis, S. G., et al.: Thrombolytic therapy for women with myocardial infarction: Is there a gender gap? Thrombolysis and angioplasty in myocardial infarction study group. J. Am. Coll. Cardiol. *22:*1780, 1993.
149. Fiebach, N. H., Viscoli, C. M., and Horwitz, R. I.: Differences between women and men in survival after myocardial infarction: Biology or methodology? JAMA *263:*1092, 1990.
150. Kostis, J. B., Wilson, A. C., O'Dowd, K. O., et al.: Sex differences in the management and long-term outcome of acute myocardial infarction: A statewide study. Circulation *90:*1715, 1994.
151. Maynard, C., and Weaver, W. D.: Treatment of women with acute MI: New findings from the MITI registry. J. Myocardial Ischemia *4:*27, 1992.
152. Clarke, K. W., Gray, D., Keating, N. A., and Hampton, J. R.: Do women with acute myocardial infarction receive the same treatment as men? Br. Med. J. *309:*563, 1994.
153. Behar, S., Gottlieb, S., Hod, H., et al.: Influence of gender in the therapeutic management of patients with acute myocardial infarction in Israel. Am. J. Cardiol. *73:*438, 1994.
154. Dellborg, M., and Swedberg, K.: Acute myocardial infarction: Difference in the treatment between men and women. Qual. Assur. Health Care *5:*261, 1993.
155. Pashos, C. L., Normand, S-L. T., Garfinkle, J. B., et al.: Trends in the use of drug therapies in patients with acute myocardial infarction: 1988 to 1992. J. Am. Coll. Cardiol. *23:*1023, 1994.
155a. Yarzebski, J., Col, N., Pagley, P., et al.: Gender differences and factors associated with the receipt of thrombolytic therapy in patients with acute myocardial infarction. A community-wide perspective. Am. Heart J. *131:*43, 1996.
156. Adams, J. N., Jamieson, M., Rawles, J. M., et al.: Women and myocardial infarction: Agism rather than sexism? Br. Heart J. *73:*87, 1995.
157. Funk, M., and Griffey, K. A.: Relation of gender to the use of cardiac procedures in acute myocardial infarction. Am. J. Cardiol. *74:*1170, 1994.
158. Healy, B.: The Yentl syndrome. N. Engl. J. Med. *325:*274, 1991.
159. Hamilton, G. A.: Recovery from acute myocardial infarction in women. Cardiology *77*(Suppl 2):58, 1990.
160. Lee, K. L., Woodlief, L. H., Topol, E. J., et al.: Predictors of 30-day mortality in the era of reperfusion for acute myocardial infarction: Results from an international trial of 41,021 patients. Circulation *91:*1659, 1995.
161. European Working Party: Streptokinase in recent myocardial infarction: A controlled multicentre trial. Br. Med. J. *3:*325, 1971.
162. Gruppo Italiano per lo studio della Streptochinasi nell'infarto miocardico (GISSI): Effectiveness of intravenous thrombolytic treatment in acute myocardial infarction. Lancet *1:*397, 1986.
163. ISIS-2 (Second International Study of Infarct Survival) Collaborative Group: Randomised trial of intravenous Streptokinase, oral aspirin, both, or neither among 17,187 cases of suspected acute myocardial infarction: ISIS-2. Lancet *1:*349, 1988.
164. Wilcox, R. G., Olsson, C. G., Skene, A. M., et al.: Trial of tissue plasminogen activator for mortality reduction in acute myocardial infarction: Anglo-Scandinavian Study of Early Thrombolysis (ASSET). Lancet *2:*525, 1988.
165. Kennedy, J. W., Martin, G. V., Davis, K. B., et al.: The Western Washington intravenous streptokinase in acute myocardial infarction randomized trial. Circulation *77:*345, 1988.
166a. The GUSTO Angiographic Investigators: The effects of tissue plasminogen activator, streptokinase, or both on coronary-artery patency, ventricular function, and survival after acute myocardial infarction. N. Engl. J. Med. *329:*1615, 1993.
167. Maggioni, A. P., Franzosi, M. G., Santoro, E., et al., and the Gruppo Italiano per lo studio della sopravvivenza nell'infarto miocardico II (GISSI-2), and the International Study Group: The risk of stroke in patients with acute myocardial infarction after thrombolytic and antithrombotic treatment. N. Engl. J. Med. *327:*1, 1992.
168. Becker, R. C., Terrin, M., Ross, R., et al., and the Thrombolysis in Myocardial Infarction Investigators: Comparison of clinical outcomes for women and men after acute myocardial infarction. Ann. Intern. Med. *120:*638, 1994.
169. Grines, C. L., Browne, K. F., Marco, J., et al., for the Primary Angioplasty in Myocardial Infarction Study Group: A comparison of immediate angioplasty with thrombolytic therapy for acute myocardial infarction. N. Engl. J. Med. *328:*673, 1993.
170. Stone, G. W., Grines, C. L., Browne, K. F., et al.: A comparison of in-hospital outcome in men versus women treated by either thrombolytic therapy or primary coronary angioplasty for acute myocardial infarction. Am. J. Cardiol. *75:*987, 1995.
171. Pfeffer, M. A., Braunwald, E., Moyé, L. A., et al., on behalf of the SAVE investigators: Effect of Captopril on mortality and morbidity in patients with left ventricular dysfunction after myocardial infarction: Results of the survival and ventricular enlargement trial. N. Engl. J. Med. *327:*669, 1992.
172. ISIS-4 (Fourth International Study of Infarct Survival) Collaborative Group: ISIS-4: A randomised factorial trial assessing early oral captopril, oral mononitrate, and intravenous magnesium sulphate in 58,050 patients with suspected acute myocardial infarction. Lancet *345:*669, 1995.
173. Rodda, B. E.: The Timolol myocardial infarction study: An evaluation of selected variables. Circulation *67:*I-101, I-106, 1983.
174. ISIS-1 Collaborative Group: Randomised trial of intravenous atenolol among 16,027 cases of suspected acute myocardial infarction. Lancet *ii:*57, 1986.
175. Yusuf, S., Peto, R., Lewis, J., et al.: Beta-blockade during and after myocardial infarction: An overview of the randomized trials. Progr. Cardiovasc. Dis. *27:*335, 1985.

Chapter 52

Medical Management of the Patient Undergoing Cardiac Surgery

ELLIOTT M. ANTMAN

PREOPERATIVE EVALUATION 1715
INTRAOPERATIVE MANAGEMENT 1720
POSTOPERATIVE MANAGEMENT 1721
Fluid, Electrolyte, and Acid-Base Balance .1721
Respiratory Management 1722
Hypertension .1723
Perioperative Myocardial Infarction 1723
Low-Output Syndrome and Shock States . .1725
Arrhythmias 1727
Hemostatic Disturbances 1731
Infection 1732
Peripheral Vascular Complications 1734
Other Complications 1734
REHABILITATION AND PREPARATION FOR DISCHARGE 1735
REFERENCES .1736

Several advances have occurred in cardiac surgery that make the operative repair of a variety of cardiac lesions a viable therapeutic alternative for an increasing number of patients with cardiovascular diseases. These include improvements in surgical and anesthesia techniques for myocardial revascularization, valve repair and replacement, and repair of complex congenital cardiac defects, as well as new approaches to management of patients with left ventricular dysfunction and cardiac arrhythmias.[1–8] In addition, perioperative medical and surgical supportive measures have progressed, including the proliferation of transesophageal echocardiography, ventricular assist devices, new inotropic agents, and new hemostatic drugs. Evidence suggests that translation of these improvements into routine surgical practice and institution of regular quality control surveillance measures have led to a reduction of risk-adjusted operative mortality for coronary artery bypass grafting (CABG) to less than 3 per cent for the general population and 5 to 6 per cent for the Medicare population.[9–13] However, the profile of patients referred for surgery has also changed, characterized by greater proportions of patients with advanced age, depressed left ventricular function, multiple comorbidities, prior revascularization operations, and failed acute interventional procedures leading to higher mortality rates in tertiary care referral centers that are called upon to operate on such cases with greater frequency.[14–22]

This chapter summarizes the information required by the cardiologist, whose important responsibilities include collaboration with the surgical team for both preoperative and postoperative care, especially of the medical complications that may develop. The indications for the operation, surgical options (e.g., valve repair versus replacement), and the relative advantages, costs, and limitations of surgery versus an interventional catheterization option (see Chap. 39) all must be considered.[23–28] The details of the decision process for referral for surgery are discussed in the chapters on the individual forms of heart disease.

PREOPERATIVE EVALUATION

The preoperative interview should be used to provide a sensitive and thoughtful review of the indications for the operation and an explanation of the postoperative procedures as well as to assess the patient's potential ability to comply with postoperative medical issues such as anticoagulation and follow-up procedures for permanent pacemakers and implanted defibrillators (see Chap. 23). Serious language barriers and lack of a family support system, especially in the elderly patient, can turn a surgical success into a postoperative failure.[29,30]

GENERAL MEDICAL CONDITION. Except for life-threatening conditions (e.g., proximal aortic dissection,[31] cardiogenic shock caused by ruptured papillary muscle in acute myocardial infarction, penetrating wound of the heart), it behooves the consulting cardiologist to assess the overall medical condition of the patient and advise the surgical team if postponement of the operation seems warranted (Tables 52–1 and 52–2).[32–43] Particular attention should be paid to the patient's potential for developing one or more of the following complications; (1) bleeding on cardiopulmonary bypass while heparinized or while anticoagulated after insertion of a mechanical heart valve prosthesis[44,45]; (2) deterioration of renal function; (3) development of arrhythmias because of electrolyte imbalance; (4) sepsis because of incompletely treated pulmonary, urinary tract, or dental infections, or dermatologic infections over the sternum or saphenous vein harvest site; (5) the need for prolonged ventilatory support postoperatively because of underlying pulmonary disease and preoperative malnutrition; and (6) development of exacerbation of a neurological deficit because of carotid artery disease or prior stroke.[35] Where perioperative intra-aortic balloon pump support may be needed, the status of the iliofemoral circulation should be assessed bilaterally. Of note, the risk of limb ischemia may be reduced by the use of sheathless, small-caliber balloon pump catheters.[46] Despite the increased risk of perioperative morbidity and mortality, recent data indicate that patients with combined coronary artery disease and peripheral vascular disease have greater likelihood of long-term survival and freedom from myocardial infarction with CABG surgery versus medical therapy, particularly in the presence of two- and three-vessel coronary artery disease.[47]

The *protein-calorie malnutrition* associated with cardiac cachexia has been shown to compromise cardiac function and is associated with a greater risk of respiratory failure, sepsis, and prolonged hospitalization.[30] If the clinical situation allows, patients diagnosed as having cardiac cachexia should receive 1 to 2 weeks of preoperative nutritional support before undergoing elective cardiac surgery. The general principles of nutritional support in cardiac surgical patients are outlined in Table 52–3.

The risk factors for morbidity and mortality after coronary revascularization surgery have been analyzed extensively.[48–53] A commonly employed, simple clinical severity scoring system is shown in Table 52–4.[48] Although patients with low risk scores (<3) may be considered candidates for "fast-track" cost saving measures such as admission on the day of surgery or early extubation postoperatively, those with higher risk scores (>6) are likely to require a longer intensive care unit stay and more consultations by specialists and consume a greater proportion of

TABLE 52–1 IMPORTANT ASPECTS OF PHYSICAL EXAMINATION IN PATIENTS SCHEDULED FOR CARDIAC SURGERY

PORTION OF PHYSICAL EXAMINATION	ABNORMAL FINDING	COMMENT
Head, eyes, ears, nose, throat	Dental caries, ENT infection	Risk of endocarditis in valvular surgery
Chest	Prior radical mastectomy	Previous mastectomy (especially left) may compromise thoracic blood supply[32] and therefore contraindicates use of internal mammary artery as conduit because of lack of patency or possible inadequate sternal wound healing.
Cardiovascular	Murmur of aortic regurgitation	Aortic regurgitation may worsen during cardiopulmonary bypass because of a jet from aortic cannulation; left ventricular distention may ensue. Intra-aortic balloon pump contraindicated.
Abdomen	Abdominal aortic aneurysm	Presence of abdominal aortic aneurysm or significant atherosclerosis may contraindicate use of intra-aortic balloon pump.
Extremities	1. Peripheral arterial insufficiency	1. May complicate use of intra-aortic balloon pump
	2. Extensive venous varicosities in lower extremities	2. Insufficient venous conduits may be available in lower extremities, necessitating use of arm veins. If this is the case, intravenous lines should not be inserted in the arm veins that will be harvested. For reoperation cases, cardiac catheterization should include imaging of the left internal mammary artery; noninvasive venous mapping of the lower extremities is advisable.
	3. Tinea pedis	3. Increased risk of lower-extremity cellulitis
Neurological	1. Carotid bruits	1. Cerebrovascular accident may occur perioperatively. Perform noninvasive studies of carotids preoperatively and consider combined carotid endarterectomy/CABG in symptomatic patients and those with history of prior stroke, severe bilateral carotid stenoses, or contralateral carotid occlusion.[33,34] Role of a combined or staged procedure in asymptomatic patients is unclear, but many surgeons opt for a combined procedure if high-grade carotid stenoses are present (>75%).[35,36]
	2. Preoperative neurological deficit(s)	2. Neurological status may deteriorate postoperatively because of compromised cerebral perfusion.

medical resources. By assembling and reviewing the data necessary for an accurate assessment of a patient's operative risk, cardiologists can help with the appropriate triage of patients to contain hospital costs and to facilitate consultations with other medical specialists (e.g., dialysis team) as needed. Patients at increased risk of mediastinal infection include the elderly and those suffering from diabetes mellitus, malnutrition, severe pulmonary disease that is likely to lead to prolonged postoperative ventilatory support, and macromastia in women.[54–56]

HEMODYNAMIC COMPENSATION. An especially important aspect of the preoperative evaluation of the cardiac surgical patient involves estimating the extent of underlying ventricular dysfunction. Evidence exists that unrevascularized viable myocardium after myocardial infarction serves as a substrate for recurrent ischemic events.[57–63] Also, patients with severe multivessel disease and akinetic myocardial zones who suffer from chronic congestive heart failure due to hibernating myocardium (see p. 1215) experience improved ventricular function after CABG.[57,60,61] Contemporary techniques that should be used for assessing myocardial viability in dysfunctional regions include imaging procedures that correlate perfusion with cell membrane integrity, metabolic activity, or contractile reserve.[57–58a] Because no large-scale randomized studies comparing PET scanning with stress-echocardiography are available for the preoperative evaluation of patients, clinicians should rely on those imaging modalities with which they are most familiar and which are available at their institution (see p. 1946).

Careful consideration should be given to the possibility of *right ventricular dysfunction* (Table 52–2), which should be suspected in patients with preoperative elevation of pulmonary artery systolic pressure (>60 mm Hg), a history of inferoposterior left ventricular infarction (which may be associated with right ventricular infarction), and longstanding tricuspid regurgitation. Patients with right ventricular dysfunction should be placed on maintenance digitalis and receive supplemental oxygen perioperatively in an attempt to lower pulmonary vascular resistance and improve right ventricular systolic performance. Intravenous nitrate infusions in the perioperative period also have been shown to reduce pulmonary hypertension and ameliorate right ventricular failure.

Patients with mitral regurgitation and severe heart failure should undergo preoperative afterload reduction with such agents as oral angiotensin-converting enzyme (ACE) inhibitors and intravenous sodium nitroprusside to a systolic pressure of about 90 to 100 mm Hg. Potential contraindications to such preoperative afterload reduction include concomitant severe aortic stenosis and hemodynamically significant cerebral or renal vascular disease.

RISK OF MYOCARDIAL ISCHEMIA. Acute thrombolytic and interventional catheterization treatment regimens for acute myocardial infarction may not successfully restore coronary perfusion because of inadequate thrombolysis, reocclusion of the infarct-related artery following initially successful thrombolysis, or dissection/acute thrombosis of the target vessel during angioplasty.[64–66] Identification of patients for referral for emergency bypass surgery and decisions regarding the timing of such surgery remain a challenging clinical problem, particularly in view of the high perioperative mortality rate for patients who require surgery within 24 to 48 hours of thrombolysis.[66–66a]

Potential indications for emergency bypass surgery following failed attempts at reperfusion in acute myocardial infarction include significant left main stenosis and inability to maintain patency of the infarct-related artery, severe multivessel coronary artery disease with anatomy unsuitable for angioplasty and ischemic dysfunction of noninfarct zones, and inability to maintain patency of an infarct-related artery that places a large amount of myocardium in jeopardy (proximal left anterior descending) in patients presenting with an infarct of less than 6 hours duration.[64–66] Although some clinical reports suggest that patients with cardiogenic shock who undergo urgent revascularization have an improved survival compared with those who are not revascularized, these series suffer from potential selection bias, and definitive recommendations regarding the management of cardiogenic shock and acute myo-

TABLE 52–2 PREOPERATIVE LABORATORY EVALUATIONS FOR PATIENTS UNDERGOING CARDIAC SURGERY

PREOPERATIVE LABORATORY TEST	ABNORMAL FINDING	COMMENT
Complete blood count	1. Anemia, especially Hct < 35%	1. Anticipate that hemodilution will occur on cardiopulmonary bypass and blood loss will occur intraoperatively. Preoperative RBC transfusions may be needed. In addition, patients with unstable angina, congestive heart failure, aortic stenosis, and left main coronary artery disease should be advised against autologous donation of blood in the preoperative period.
	2. WBC > 10,000	2. Search for possible infection.
Coagulation screen	1. Prolonged bleeding time 2. Elevated PT and/or PTT 3. Thrombocytopenia	All of these laboratory abnormalities suggest that the patient is at risk for bleeding postoperatively and may have excessive chest tube drainage. Corrective measures (e.g., vitamin K, fresh frozen plasma, platelet transfusions) should be considered preoperatively, and surgery may need to be postponed. Hematological consultation may be required if an inherited defect in coagulation (e.g., von Willebrand's factor deficiency) is suspected.
Chemistry profile	1. Elevated BUN/creatinine	1. Abnormal renal function that may worsen in perioperative period (caused by nonpulsatile flow on cardiopulmonary bypass and potential low flow postoperatively); this may necessitate temoporary or even permanent hemodialysis.
	2. Potassium < 4.0 mEq/liter and/or magnesium < 2.0 mEq/liter	2. Electrolyte deficits may place the patient at risk of arrhythmias perioperatively and should be corrected before induction of anesthesia.
	3. Abnormal liver function tests	3. Patient may clear anesthetic agents as well as other cardioactive drugs more slowly. Low albumin level may indicate a state of relative malnutrition that may need to be corrected with nutritional support perioperatively.
Stool hematest	Positive for occult blood	Because heparinization will take place while on cardiopulmonary bypass apparatus, the patient may be at risk for gastrointestinal (GI) bleeding perioperatively. The source of GI heme loss should be investigated preoperatively, if clinical circumstances permit. The potential for bleeding in the future may influence the choice of prosthetic valve inserted.
Pulmonary function	Reduced VC or prolonged FEV_1	Anticipate longer than usual process of weaning from ventilator postoperatively if FEV_1 < 65% VC or FEV_1 < 1.5–2.0 liters. Obtain baseline arterial blood gas analysis on room air to help guide respiratory management postoperatively.
Thyroid function	These tests are not ordered routinely but should be drawn in cases of suspected hypothyroidism or hyperthyroidism, known thyroid dysfunction on replacement therapy, and in patients with atrial fibrillation who have not undergone evaluation of thyroid function.	1. Hypothyroid patients require prolonged period of ventilatory support postoperatively because of slower clearance of anesthetic agents. 2. Hyperthyroid patients have a hypermetabolic state that places them at increased risk of myocardial ischemia, vasomotor instability, and poorly controlled ventricular rate in atrial fibrillation.
Cardiac catheterization	1. Elevated left ventricular end-diastolic pressure and pulmonary capillary wedge pressure	1. These may remain elevated in the early postoperative period and indicate a need for careful attention to maintenance of adequate preload postoperatively.
	2. Elevated right atrial pressure	2. This may reflect tricuspid regurgitation or right ventricular dysfunction from prior infarction. Such patients require vigorous volume expansion postoperatively to maintain an adequate cardiac output.
	3. Elevated pulmonary artery pressure (and pulmonary vascular resistance)	3. Fixed pulmonary vascular resistance should be suspected when the pulmonary artery diastolic pressure exceeds the mean pulmonary capillary wedge pressure. Vigorous oxygenation and pharmacological support with a pulmonary vasodilator (isoproterenol, prostaglandin E_1) are important in such cases. Patients with a pulmonary artery diastolic pressure equal to the pulmonary capillary wedge pressure usually have a more rapid resolution of pulmonary hypertension postoperatively.
	4. Left ventricular mural thrombus	4. Increased risk of stroke perioperatively.
	5. Status of internal mammary arteries	5. Highly desirable arterial conduits for planned revascularization surgery.[38–42] Particular care required during reoperation if patent internal mammary artery bypass is in place from previous surgery.
	6. Status of saphenous vein grafts	6. "Pseudoextravasation" of dye outside lumen in patent graft with slow flow probably represents thrombus-filled atherosclerotic aneurysm of graft.[43]

Hct, hematocrit; RBC, red blood cell; PT, prothrombin time; PTT, partial thromboplastin time; BUN, blood urea nitrogen; VC, vital capacity; FEV_1, volume of air expired at 1 second.

cardial infarction patients must await the results of ongoing randomized trials.[64,65]

Patients who are referred for emergency revascularization surgery should be supported by an intra-aortic balloon pump and, if technically feasible, an intracoronary perfusion catheter. Other methods for mechanical assistance of the failing circulation are described in Chapter 19. Because patients who undergo emergency bypass surgery within 6 to 12 hours of administration of a thrombolytic agent are at greater risk for intraoperative and postoperative hemorrhage, they should receive a hemostatic agent such as aprotinin (2 million KIU over 20 minutes followed by a continuous infusion of 500,000 KIU per hour).[67]

Patients with other presentations of an acute coronary

TABLE 52–3 PRINCIPLES OF NUTRITIONAL SUPPORT IN CARDIAC SURGICAL PATIENTS

I. **RECOGNIZE NUTRITIONALLY DEFICIENT PATIENT**
Current weight <10% of ideal body weight or unintentional, significant weight loss (≥10%) over past 6 months; inadequate daily caloric intake (<1000 calories) for ≥1 week, serum albumin <3.0 related to malnutrtion.

II. **CALCULATE DAILY CALORIE REQUIREMENTS**
A. Determine basal energy expenditure (BEE) in kcal/24 hr from the following Harris-Benedict formulae* (where W is body weight in kg, H is height in cm, and A is age in years):
$BEE_{men} = 66.5 + (13.8 \times W) + (5 \times H) - (6.8 \times A)$
$BEE_{women} = 655.1 + (9.6 \times W) + (1.8 \times H) - (4.7 \times A)$
B. Adjust for level of activity
1. Add (1.2 × BEE) for normal postoperative state.
2. Do not apply activity "factor" for patients who are at a reduced level of physical activity such as those who are on ventilators or comatose.
C. Adjust for stress (e.g., fever)
1. Add (0.13 × BEE) for each 1°C rise in temperature above normal (use [0.07 × BEE]/1°F).
2. Septic patients may need as much as (1.2–1.8 × BEE) added to their daily caloric intake.
D. Add additional calories if weight gain is desired (e.g., to treat cardiac cachexia); 500 kcal/day will result in a weight gain of 1 lb/wk.

III. **CALCULATE PROTEIN REQUIREMENTS**
A. For general cardiac surgical patient: 1.0 gm protein/kg body weight.
B. For nutritionally deficient or malnourished patient: 1.2–1.5 gm protein/kg body weight.
C. With renal or hepatic failure patient: may need to adjust protein.

IV. **DETERMINE ROUTE FOR NUTRITIONAL SUPPORT**
A. Functioning gastrointestinal tract
1. Adequate oral intake: Provide calculated calories in a diet that is 15–20% protein, 50–60% carbohydrate, and the remainder as fat.
2. Inadequate oral intake: Use enteral feeding to deliver daily caloric requirement (e.g., Osmolite = 1 cal/ml; Ensure Plus = 1.5 cal/ml). If renal or hepatic failure is present, use modified enteral feeding.
B. Nonfunctioning gastrointestinal tract or intolerance of enteral feedings
1. Insert sterile central line for parenteral nutrition and prescribe central parenteral nutrition in consultation with nutritional support service. Prescription may need to be modified daily.
2. For short-term feeding, peripheral parenteral nutrition (PPN) may be indicated. Should have normal renal function and be able to tolerate 2500 ml/day.

* The Harris-Benedict equation has recently been shown to overestimate BEE by 10–15%.

Adapted from data in Jeejeebhoy, K. N.: Nutrition in critical illness. *In* Shoemaker, W. C., Ayres, S., Grenovik, A., et al. (eds.): Textbook of Critical Care. Philadelphia, W. B. Saunders Co., 1989, pp. 1093–1118; Mifflin, M. D., St. Jeor, S. T., et al.: A new predictive equation for resting energy expenditure in healthy individuals. Am. J. Clin. Nutr. *51*:241, 1990.

syndrome such as active unstable angina may also be in a tenuous hemodynamic balance as they proceed to the operating room, particularly if significant left main coronary artery stenosis or severe three-vessel coronary artery disease associated with left ventricular dysfunction and/or mitral regurgitation is present. Delays while awaiting surgery and the time between the induction of anesthesia and the institution of cardiopulmonary bypass are high-risk periods during which a vicious spiral of myocardial ischemia and low-output syndrome can rapidly develop. Such patients should also be protected by an intra-aortic balloon pump inserted preoperatively and infusion of nitroglycerin intraoperatively.

ANESTHESIA FOR CARDIAC SURGERY. The details of the practice of cardiac anesthesia are beyond the scope of this

TABLE 52–4 PREOPERATIVE RISK FACTORS FOR ADVERSE OUTCOMES IN PATIENTS UNDERGOING CARDIAC SURGERY: A CLINICAL SEVERITY SCORING SYSTEM

PREOPERATIVE FACTORS	SCORE
Emergency case	6
Serum creatinine	
≥1.6 and ≤1.8 mg/dl	1
≥1.9 mg/dl	4
Severe left ventricular dysfunction	3
Reoperation	3
Operative mitral valve insufficiency	3
Age ≥65 and ≤74 years	1
Age ≥75 years	2
Prior vascular surgery	2
Chronic obstructive pulmonary disease	2
Anemia (hematocrit ≤0.34)	2
Operative aortic valve stenosis	1
Weight ≤65 kg	1
Diabetes, on oral or insulin therapy	1
Cerebrovascular disease	1

From Higgins, T., Estafanous, F., Lloyd, F., et al.: Stratification of morbidity and mortality outcome by preoperative risk factors in coronary artery bypass patients. A clinical severity score. JAMA *267*:2344, 1992. Copyright 1992, the American Medical Association.

chapter and are available in other sources.[70,71] High-dose synthetic narcotics, such as fentanyl and sufentanil, that do not cause vasodilatation have replaced morphine in many centers. Recently, early extubation has been proposed for patients with preserved ventricular function. Advocates of early extubation argue that the advantages include a decrease in respiratory complications, a decrease in ventilatory support, and a decrease in the length of stay in the Intensive Care Unit. In order to achieve early extubation within 6 hours of surgery, anesthetic techniques have included combinations of inhalational anesthetics—enflurane and isoflurane—together with low to moderate amounts of intravenous opioids—fentanyl and sufentanil—along with the intravenous anesthetic propofol. The newer, inhaled anesthetics that have replaced nitrous oxide still have the potential to cause vasodilatation. Patients with critical aortic stenosis, critical mitral stenosis, and large right-to-left shunts may experience a dramatic reduction in cardiac output as ventricular stroke volume falls with a reduction in preload. Preoperative volume expansion and even administration of vasopressor agents may be necessary to avoid this problem.

Cardiac Rhythm[72–89]

Although supraventricular arrhythmias after cardiac surgery are seldom life-threatening, they frequently provoke disturbing symptoms, may jeopardize hemodynamic stability, and are associated with an increased incidence of postoperative stroke, increased length of stay in the intensive care unit, and increased hospital costs.[72–74]

In the past it was a common preoperative practice in many institutions to administer digitalis prophylactically to all patients undergoing cardiac surgery, not only for inotropic support but also for "control" of the ventricular rate if atrial fibrillation occurred postoperatively.[74] There is little reason to believe that digoxin prevents the development of atrial fibrillation; indeed, clinical trials do not clearly substantiate either a lower incidence of atrial fibrillation or a slower ventricular rate in atrial fibrillation in patients

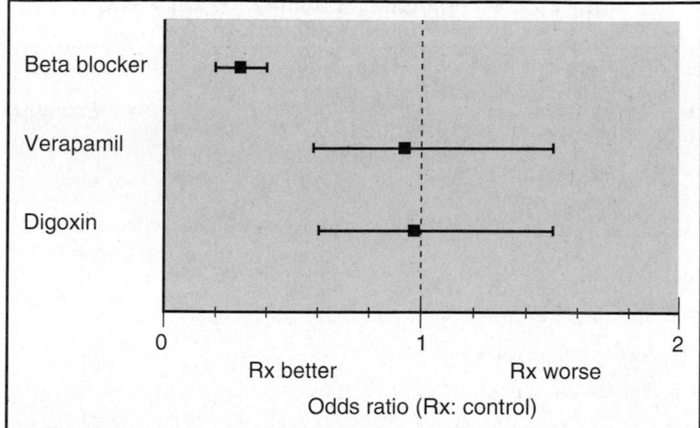

FIGURE 52–1. Meta-analysis of randomized control trials of therapies for prophylaxis against supraventricular arrhythmias in patients undergoing coronary artery bypass surgery. The pooled odds ratio for the development of supraventricular arrhythmias for treatment (Rx) with digoxin, verapamil, or beta blockers is shown. The width of the horizontal lines indicates the 95 per cent confidence intervals for the estimates of the odds ratios. (Reproduced with permission from Andrews, T. C., Reimold, S. C., Berlin, J. A., and Antman, E. M.: Prevention of supraventricular arrhythmias after coronary artery bypass surgery. A meta-analysis of randomized control trials. Circulation *84*:[Suppl. III]:236, 1991. Copyright 1991 American Heart Association.)

treated prophylactically with digoxin[75] (Fig. 52–1). Furthermore, hypoxia, hypokalemia, elevated catecholamine levels, and reduced clearance of digoxin are common postoperatively, and these may predispose the patient to digoxin toxicity.

ATRIAL FIBRILLATION

Because of the hazards of postoperative atrial fibrillation, considerable effort has been devoted to identifying preoperative factors associated with an increased risk of postoperative arrhythmia.[74] The preoperative factors most consistently found to be associated with an increased risk of this arrhythmia include advanced age and male gender. Recently it has been proposed that a prolonged P-wave duration recorded on a signal-averaged electrocardiogram and a greater than 70 per cent narrowing of the lumen of the right coronary artery are associated with an increased risk of postoperative atrial fibrillation.[76,77] However, for a substantial number of patients with postoperative atrial fibrillation, no apparent preoperative risk factor can be identified. Cox has presented clinical data suggesting that about one-third of patients undergoing cardiac operations are vulnerable to postoperative atrial fibrillation because of a mild nonuniformity in the distribution of their atrial refractory periods.[78] Intraoperative atrial ischemia associated with rapid rewarming of the atria during prolonged periods of cold cardioplegic arrest may increase the dispersion of refractoriness in the atria of such patients, increasing the risk of postoperative atrial fibrillation.

Because of difficulties in reliably identifying patients at risk of atrial fibrillation preoperatively, it is common clinical practice to provide prophylactic therapy to the majority of patients undergoing coronary artery bypass graft surgery. Beta-adrenoceptor blocking agents are most suitable for prophylaxis against atrial fibrillation.[74,75] This stems from a number of considerations: (1) A rebound phenomenon after withdrawal of such agents at the time of surgery may contribute to the appearance of arrhythmias in the postoperative period; (2) there is a heightened level of sympathetic nervous system tone in the postoperative period that may provoke supraventricular arrhythmias; and (3) the therapeutic index for digitalis glycosides is narrow.

Clinical trials with several beta blockers have shown statistically significant reductions not only in the frequency of supraventricular arrhythmias but also in the severity (duration, speed of ventricular response) of the arrhythmia when it does occur. In the *absence* of an ejection fraction less than 30 per cent, severe bronchospastic lung disease, or bradyarrhythmias, we advocate the use of prophylactic beta blockers in patients undergoing coronary artery bypass grafting.[75]

BRADYARRHYTHMIAS AND ATRIOVENTRICULAR AND INTRAVENTRICULAR BLOCK. Patients with high-grade (third-degree or type II second-degree) atrioventricular block and hemodynamic compromise (systolic pressure < 90 mm Hg) are at high risk for general anesthesia unless a temporary transvenous pacemaker wire is inserted preoperatively.

In patients in whom a permanent pacemaker has been implanted, its specifications (model, mode, and settings) and, if possible, a statement as to the pacemaker dependency of the patient should be noted in the medical record. The possibility of postoperative malfunction in the permanent pacing system should be anticipated because of the effects of anesthesia, electrocautery, and surgical manipulation of the leads (e.g., during caval cannulation).[88,89] Clinicians should have the appropriate pacemaker programming equipment available postoperatively because many problems (e.g., reversion to the VOO mode [see p. 728] because of electromagnetic interference from the electrocautery apparatus) can be quickly resolved by interrogation of the generator and reprogramming in the recovery area. It is currently recommended that all patients with a Telectronics AccuFIX atrial J lead have the lead removed at the time of atriotomy, regardless of fracture, because of the risk of retention wire fracture and protrusion.

The risk of permanent, complete heart block postoperatively is increased with multiple valve replacements, particularly in patients who have had previous valve surgery. However, there is rarely a need for implantation of a permanent epicardial pacing lead at the time of surgery because of the ease of implantation of a transvenous endocardial system postoperatively. An exception to this would be patients who are undergoing tricuspid valve replacement with a mechanical prosthesis, especially if they are simultaneously undergoing an aortic or mitral valve operation. Because of the contraindication to passing a transvenous lead through the mechanical tricuspid prosthesis, the surgical team should be alerted to the need for placement of permanent epicardial leads intraoperatively.

Patients with previously implanted cardioverter-defibrillator devices should have their unit disabled prior to surgery to minimize the risk of inappropriate shocks from sensing of electrocautery signals intraoperatively. Until the device is reactivated in the postoperative period, equipment for rapid external defibrillation should be available.

Perioperative Drug Therapy

With the exception of oral anticoagulation with warfarin, most medications can and should be continued up to the time of surgery. Clinical trials of patients receiving saphenous vein bypass grafts have demonstrated the importance of initiating antiplatelet therapy in the perioperative period.[90] Because of the increased risk of postoperative bleeding, some surgical groups discontinue aspirin for several days preoperatively in elective cases.[29,30] Many cardiologists are concerned about the risk of "breakthrough" episodes of ischemia if aspirin is discontinued preoperatively and prefer to continue it up to the time of operation, relying on preoperative donations of autologous red cells, cell-saver techniques, autotransfusion of shed blood intraoperatively and postoperatively, and drugs such as aprotinin to minimize the need for and potential hazards of homologous blood transfusion.[91] If asprin is witheld preoperatively, it should be restarted within 48 hours of surgery to reduce the risk of vein graft occlusion.[90] Warfarin therapy should be stopped 2 days preoperatively and, if necessary, treatment with heparin or low molecular weight dextran initiated.

Calcium antagonists previously prescribed for control of ischemic heart disease should be continued up to the time of operation to reduce the chance of myocardial ischemia from withdrawal of the drug. In the case of diltiazem and verapamil, the dose may need to be reduced because these agents may provoke bradycardia and a low-output syndrome postoperatively, especially if a beta blocker or amiodarone is given concurrently or the patient is elderly. Profound atropine- and isoproterenol-resistant bradyarrhythmias may occur postoperatively in patients on these calcium antagonists, particularly when the patient has not yet recovered from the hypothermia that is imposed intraoperatively; temporary dual-chamber pacing support should be available to manage such patients.

PROPHYLAXIS. Insufficient data are available to provide definitive recommendations for prophylaxis against atrial fibrillation in patients undergoing valve surgery. We individualize our recommendations for prophylaxis in such cases and usually do not start beta blockers in patients who have not received them chronically preoperatively. Patients under the age of 40 years undergoing isolated repair of an atrial septal defect or patent ductus arteriosus also need not receive prophylactic beta blockers preoperatively because they are likely to tolerate a postoperative supraventricular arrhythmia during the time it takes to initiate measures to slow the ventricular rate or terminate the arrhythmia.

Suggested doses of beta-adrenoceptor blockers for prophylaxis against atrial fibrillation are as follows: propranolol, 10 to 40 mg every 6 hours; metoprolol, 50 mg every 6 to 12 hours. For patients with depressed left ventricular function who cannot tolerate the negative inotropic effects of beta blockers, digoxin (0.25 to 0.375 mg/day) is frequently prescribed, although convincing data on its prophylactic benefit are limited.

Although oral verapamil (40 to 120 mg every 8 hours) or diltiazem (30 to 90 mg every 8 hours) also may be considered for prophylaxis against supraventricular arrhythmias, their use for that purpose is less well studied.[74,75] More commonly, intravenous verapamil or diltiazem is used for the acute postoperative management of supraventricular arrhythmias that may occur despite prophylaxis with other drugs.

HYPOMAGNESEMIA AND POSTOPERATIVE ARRHYTHMIAS. It has been shown that cardiopulmonary bypass produces hypomagnesemia postoperatively and that this is associated with an increased incidence of atrial dysrhythmias.[79] This observation has led to several small studies, the results of which suggest that maintenance of normomagnesemia (≥2.0 mEq/liter) by supplemental administration of magnesium perioperatively reduces the risk of postoperative atrial and ventricular arrhythmias.[80–83] These intriguing findings require confirmation in large-scale randomized trials to ascertain whether inclusion of magnesium in the cardiopulmonary bypass pump-priming solution or the routine administration of supplemental magnesium postoperatively is indicated for all patients undergoing coronary artery bypass surgery to prevent atrial fibrillation or only for specific subgroups of patients. At present, it seems prudent to correct any magnesium (and potassium) deficits preoperatively, monitor the patient's electrolytes carefully postoperatively, and promptly replete any electrolyte deficits that are detected.

CONTINUATION OF ANTIARRHYTHMICS. With the exception of amiodarone, antiarrhythmic drugs that have been prescribed for hemodynamically compromising or life-threatening ventricular tachyarrhythmias should be continued up to the time of operation because of the risk of "breakthrough" of a potentially lethal ventricular arrhythmia in the preoperative period.

Patients with a documented history of resuscitation from sudden cardiac death receiving amiodarone (see p. 613) should continue to receive this drug up to the time of operation. However, in cases where amiodarone was prescribed for a less overtly life-threatening arrhythmia (e.g., atrial fibrillation), the maintenance dosage has been >200 mg/day, and the patient has a history of lung disease, we recommend at least a 3-month period off the drug before subjecting the patient to elective cardiopulmonary bypass.

INTRAOPERATIVE MANAGEMENT

Important intraoperative surgical advances that have improved patient outcome, especially in cases of repeat CABG, include aortic root surface scanning with echo probes, transesophageal echocardiography, femoral cannulation for bypass, minimal dissection before bypass, antegrade and retrograde blood cardioplegia, and performance of all vascular anastomoses with a single aortic cross-clamp under cardioplegic arrest.[1,16,92–97a]

To achieve hemostasis more effectively, surgeons frequently use antifibrinolytic agents (tranexamic acid and aminocaproic acid), serine protease inhibitors (aprotinin), and bioactive surface-coated devices to which heparin is covalently bonded (Carmeda).[91,98–102] Table 52–5 provides a summary of the general sequence of cardiac surgical procedures, and Figures 52–2 and 52–3 provide examples of pump oxygenators and the usual monitoring devices in place when the patient returns from the operating room.

TABLE 52–5 GENERAL SEQUENCE OF ELECTIVE CARDIAC OPERATIONS

1. Preoperative medications (anxiolytic and narcotic) administered on call to operating room
2. Insertion/positioning of the following devices:
   a. Arterial line (usually radial artery)
   b. Central venous pressure or pulmonary artery catheter
   c. Urinary catheter
   d. ECG electrodes for oscilloscopic monitoring
   e. Grounding plate for electrocautery apparatus (over buttock)
3. Induction of anesthesia and endotracheal intubation
4. Skin preparation and draping of patient
5. Transesophageal echocardiogram may be performed for assessment of LV function and mitral valve insufficiency
6. Median sternotomy (with simultaneous harvesting of greater saphenous vein if coronary revascularization is to be performed)
7. Mobilization of internal mammary artery (usually left) if coronary revascularization is to be performed
8. Heparinization
9. Cannulation for cardiopulmonary bypass usually by one of the following routes:
   Venous: Right atrium, superior/inferior vena cava, femoral
   Arterial: ascending aorta; femoral artery
10. Initiation of cardiopulmonary bypass
11. Systemic cooling of patient to desired temperature
12. Cross-clamping of aorta
13. Myocardial protection: topical cooling, cold potassium cardioplegia solution injected by cannulae in root of aorta (antegrade cardioplegia) and coronary sinus (retrograde cardioplegia)
14. Operative procedure*
15. Initiate ventilation and begin weaning from extracorporeal circulation: rewarming by means of cardiopulmonary bypass apparatus, evacuation of air from left ventricle and aorta if heart has been entered. Discontinuation of bypass occurs by means of a gradual reduction of venous return and incremental volume loading of the heart. Reversal of anticoagulation by protamine with guidance by activated clotting time results intraoperatively. Removal of bypass cannulae
16. Placement of the following devices:
   a. Atrial, ventricular, and ground (subcutaneous) pacing electrodes
   b. Additional monitoring lines: right atrial, left atrial catheters (variable)
   c. Anterior and posterior mediastinal chest tubes; pleural tube if needed
17. Wire closure of sternum and skin closure
18. Transportation of recovery facility by team consisting of surgeon, anesthesiologist, and nurse. Temporary pacing box and defibrillator available during transportation

* The precise sequence of operative procedures such as valve replacement, aneurysm resection, and coronary revascularization is variable. Coronary revascularization usually is accomplished according to the following scheme: Distal venous anastomoses are performed (frequently followed by supplemental injection of cardioplegia solution down graft). Distal end of internal mammary artery is directly anastomosed to target coronary vessel. Aortic cross-clamp is removed. Proximal venous anastomoses to ascending aorta are performed. (The precise sequence is variable, with some surgeons preferring to perform the proximal and distal venous anastomoses first followed by internal mammary anastomosis.)

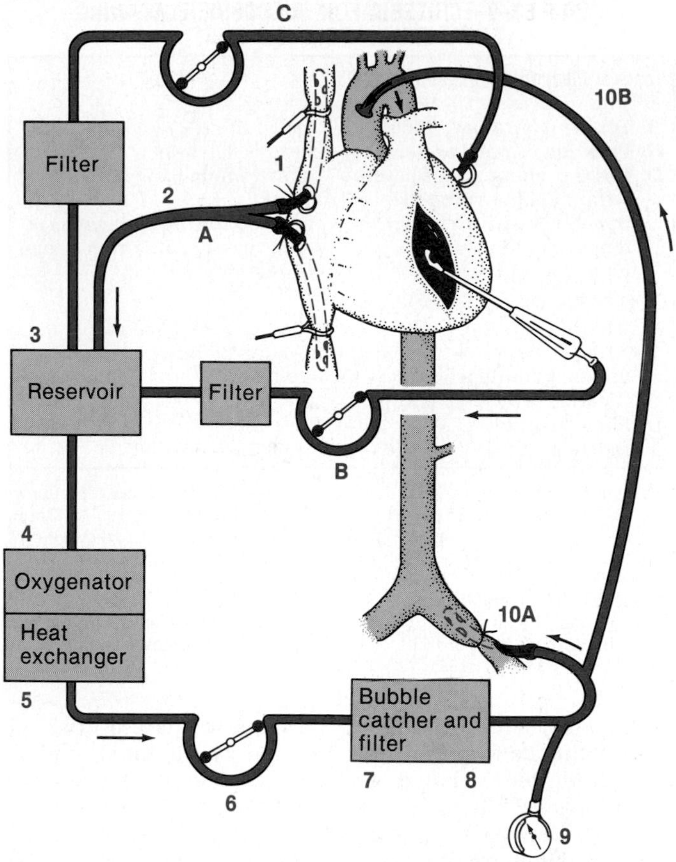

FIGURE 52–2. Schematic diagram of a typical cardiopulmonary bypass circuit. Blood is drained by gravity from the venae cavae (1) through venous cannula (2) into a venous reservoir (3). Blood from surgical field suction and from a ventricular vent (if used during operation) is pumped (*B, C*) into a cardiotomy reservoir (3). Venous blood is oxygenated (4), temperature adjusted (5), raised to arterial pressure (6), filtered (7–8), and returned to the patient by way of a cannula either in the aorta (10*B*) or femoral artery (10*A*). Arterial line pressure is monitored (9). (Modified from Nose, Y.: The Oxygenator. Vol. II. St. Louis, C. V. Mosby, 1973.)

POSTOPERATIVE MANAGEMENT

Fluid, Electrolyte, and Acid-Base Balance

After extracorporeal circulation there is an increase in extracellular fluid and total exchangeable sodium, along with a decrease in exchangeable potassium.[30] The cumulative experience in many centers has led to the following basic principles of management:

1. For the first 48 hours after operation, free water is limited to about 1000 ml/day and intravenous fluids are in the form of 5 per cent glucose in water. Sodium replacement varies with volume needs.

2. Serum potassium levels can fluctuate dramatically, and therefore frequent measurement of serum potassium is indicated, especially in diabetics. We attempt to maintain the serum potassium in the range of 4.5 ± 0.5 mEq/liter and magnesium at 2.0 mEq/liter or greater to minimize the chance of cardiac arrhythmias.

3. Serum glucose levels are frequently elevated (250–400 mg/dl), resulting from glucose-containing intravenous solutions and surgically induced increases in cortisol and catecholamine levels. In nondiabetic patients insulin therapy usually is not required, whereas it is routinely used in insulin-requiring diabetic patients to avoid uncontrolled hyperglycemia.

4. Mild metabolic acidosis or metabolic alkalosis may be present for the first 24 hours postoperatively, particularly during rewarming. These acid-base abnormalities usually do not require correction in the absence of preoperative renal dysfunction or acute renal failure developing postoperatively.[103]

5. Serum total calcium, phosphorus, and magnesium levels are frequently depressed for about 24 to 48 hours in the normally convalescing patient, owing in part to the effects of hemodilution. These electrolyte abnormalities usually are self-correcting, and replacement therapy usually is not required. A possible exception is hypomagnesemia, which may predispose to the development of cardiac arrhythmias.[74]

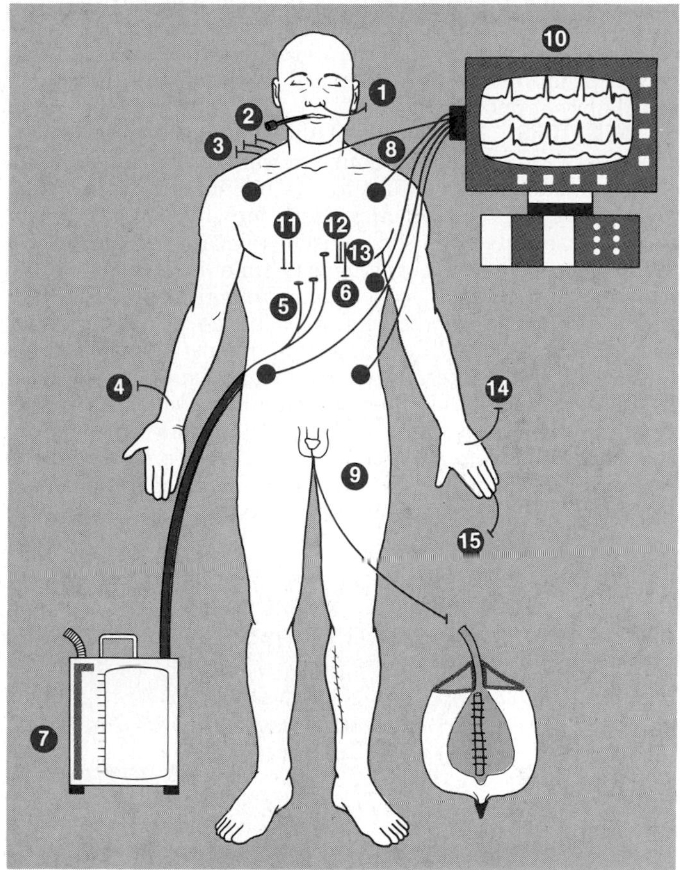

FIGURE 52–3. Schematic diagram of the various devices commonly used after cardiac surgery. (1) Nasogastric tube. (2) Endotracheal tube. (3) Central venous access catheter. This may have multiple ports for the simultaneous measurement of central venous pressure, pulmonary arterial pressure, and pulmonary capillary wedge pressure. Through a sheath introducer a triple-lumen catheter for drug administration and hyperalimentation also may be inserted. (4) Radial arterial pressure monitoring line. (5) Mediastinal chest tubes. One tube is positioned in the anterior mediastinum and the other in the posterior mediastinum. (6) Left pleural chest tube (the left pleural space having been entered during mobilization of the left internal mammary artery for bypass surgery). (7) Chest tube drainage apparatus. (8) Multiple-lead electrocardiograph cable. (9) Urinary drainage catheter. (10) Oscilloscopic monitor capable of the simultaneous recording of multiple electrocardiographic leads and pressures (systemic arterial, pulmonary arterial, central venous). Many contemporary monitoring systems provide modules for calculation of cardiac output by the thermodilution method, automated temperature, end-tidal CO_2 pressure measurements, and on-line help screens for calculations of the infusion rate of various medications and important hemodynamic variables, such as systemic and pulmonary vascular resistance. (11) Right atrial pacing wires. (12) Right ventricular pacing wires. (13) Subcutaneous "ground" (indifferent) pacing wire. The median sternotomy has been secured with stainless steel wires (not shown). The skin wounds from the median sternotomy and saphenous vein harvest site (left leg in this diagram) are typically covered with dry sterile dressings for the first several days postoperatively. (14) Peripheral intravenous line. (15) Pulse oximeter monitoring line. (Diagram courtesy of Cheryl Warrick-Brooks, R. N., Brigham and Women's Hospital, Boston.)

EFFECTS OF ANESTHESIA, STERNOTOMY, AND CARDIOPULMONARY BYPASS ON PULMONARY FUNCTION. Four broad areas should be considered, as outlined in Table 52–6.[104,105] Almost all patients experience alveolar dysfunction after open-heart surgery because of right-to-left intrapulmonary shunting of blood from various intrinsic alveolar abnormalities (e.g., atelectasis, edema, infection) and pulmonary vascular events (e.g., extravasation of fluid, inhibition of hypoxia-induced vasoconstriction). Central respiratory drive and respiratory muscle function are depressed postoperatively because of a combination of pharmacological effects and mechanical derangements of thoracic function. Patients with preexisting pulmonary disease may experience a more profound depression of respiratory function, necessitating vigorous pulmonary toilette and an extended period of ventilatory support.

VENTILATORS. Principles. Although most patients receive between 6 and 18 hours of ventilatory support, as already stated, early extubation (<6 hours) is possible if low-dose synthetic narcotics (e.g., fentanyl) and inhaled anesthetic agents are used, muscle relaxants are reversed, the total cardiopulmonary bypass time is less than 100 minutes, and the patient is hemodynamically stable and mentally alert and has a vital capacity equal to or greater than 10 cc/kg.[106] While intubated, the patient should be ventilated in the intermittent mandatory ventilation (IMV) mode, and arterial blood gases should be checked every hour for the first 8 hours to ensure adequate oxygenation and less frequently thereafter.[30] Positive end-expiratory pressure (PEEP), which is used to minimize the number of collapsed alveolar segments, should be applied cautiously in patients with obstructive pulmonary disease (risk of pneumothorax from air trapping and barotrauma), and is contraindicated in patients who have undergone operative procedures in which elevation of the right atrial pressure would be undesirable (e.g., total transposition of venous return, Fontan procedure, superior vena caval–right atrial anastomosis). PEEP may not be tolerated in patients with relative hypovolemia and inadequate preload (see p. 428).[107]

TABLE 52–6 ABNORMALITIES OF RESPIRATORY FUNCTION AFTER CARDIAC SURGERY

EFFECTS OF ANESTHESIA, THORACIC SURGERY, AND CARDIOPULMONARY BYPASS ON PULMONARY FUNCTION	POTENTIAL CAUSES
Alveolar dysfunction (e.g., widened alveolar-arterial oxygen gradient because of right-to-left intrapulmonary shunting)	a. Scattered regions of atelectasis with preserved perfusion b. Pulmonary edema (e.g., cardiogenic, noncardiogenic "post pump" alveolar capillary leak) c. Infection d. Inhibition of hypoxic pulmonary vasoconstriction by anesthetic agents e. Exacerbation of ventilation/perfusion mismatch by vasodilating agents used postoperatively (e.g., nitroprusside)
Decreased central respiratory drive	a. General anesthetics b. Narcotic analgesics c. Cerebral insult in perioperative period
Decreased respiratory muscle function	a. Thoracic pain (incision, chest tubes) b. Persistent effects of muscle relaxants c. Age d. Obesity e. Depressed cardiac function f. Primary diaphragmatic dysfunction (e.g., phrenic nerve injury)
Exacerbation of underlying chronic pulmonary disease	a. Increase in airway resistance b. Increased secretions and worsening bronchitis c. Pneumonia

TABLE 52–7 CRITERIA FOR SUCCESSFUL WEANING FROM VENTILATORY SUPPORT*

Tests of Mechanical Capability

A. Vital capcity >10–15 cc/kg body weight
B. Forced expiratory volume in 1 sec > 10 cc/kg body weight
C. Peak inspiratory pressure > −20 to −30 cm H_2O
D. Resting minute ventilation < 10 liters/min (can be doubled with maximal voluntary ventilation)
E. Spontaneous respiratory rate under 25 on intermittent mandatory ventilation (IMV) of 6 while resting comfortably, and no apparent increase in work of breathing

Tests of Oxygenation Capability

A. Alveolar-arterial gradient on 100% O_2 < 300–500 torr
B. Arterial Po_2 > 80 torr in the absence of intracardiac right-to-left shunting when the Fio_2 is ≤0.5
C. Arterial Pco_2 < 45 and pH > 7.37
D. Shunt fraction (Q_s/Q_t) < 10–20%
E. Dead space/tidal volume (V_d/V_t) < 0.55–0.60

* Modified from Snow, J. C.: Respiration and respiratory care. *In* Snow, J. C. (ed.): Manual of Anesthesia. Boston, Little, Brown and Co., 1977, pp. 317–331; Kirklin, J. K., Daggett, W. M., and Lappas, D. G.: Postoperative care following cardiac surgery. *In* Johnson, R. A., Haber, E., and Austen, W. G.: The Practice of Cardiology. The Medical and Surgical Cardiac Units at the Massachusetts General Hospital. Boston, Little, Brown and Co., 1980, pp. 110–113; and Yang, K., and Tobin, M.: A prospective study of indexes predicting the outcome of trials of weaning from mechanical ventilation. N. Engl. J. Med. *324*:1445, 1991.

Guidelines for Weaning. Suggested guidelines for identifying the patient who is ready to be weaned from the ventilator are shown in Table 52–7. Additional factors that may influence the decision to not extubate a patient, even if the pulmonary criteria are satisfied, include hemodynamic instability, recurrent malignant ventricular arrhythmias, postoperative bleeding that may require reoperation, ineffective cough, inadequate oxygen-carrying capacity of the blood (hemoglobin ≤10 gm/dl) and significant atelectasis, lobar consolidation, or pleural effusion on chest radiograph.[104–106]

During weaning, the IMV setting is progressively reduced to about two to four breaths per minute, and then the patient may be given a brief trial of T-tube ventilation (with or without continuous positive airway pressure or pressure support) before extubation occurs.

SPECIAL PROBLEMS

An increased alveolar-arterial (A-a) gradient postoperatively is a serious problem that demands a thorough evaluation. The ventilator settings should be checked and a chest radiograph obtained to ascertain the position of the tip of the endotracheal tube (to exclude, for example, intubation of the right mainstem bronchus) and to rule out pneumothorax, lobar atelectasis or pneumonia, or a large pleural effusion. Hemodynamic monitoring by means of a pulmonary artery catheter can cause pulmonary hemorrhage because of overinflation of the balloon, and bronchoscopy may need to be performed to diagnose and manage the problem (e.g., occlusion of the bronchus draining the bleeding segment of the lung).

PULMONARY EDEMA (see also Chap. 15). The most common cause of pulmonary edema postoperatively is elevated pulmonary venous pressure arising from left ventricular dysfunction and/or a valvular lesion (e.g., mitral regurgitation). Such patients require aggressive diuresis and vasodilator and inotropic support. Mechanical ventilation with PEEP is used until the patient's ventricular function improves. Repeat operation may be needed if pulmonary edema persists despite attempts to control severe mitral regurgitation medically.

In a minority of patients postcardiac surgery pulmonary edema is due to the adult respiratory distress syndrome (ARDS). In its most extreme form, this disorder is associated with a generalized whole-body *postpump syndrome,* characterized by increased capillary permeability, interstitial edema, fever, leukocytosis, renal dysfunction, and hemodynamic collapse. Although the inciting cause of ARDS in some patients may be sepsis, transfusion reactions, or anaphylaxis, in most cases it is the adverse consequences of exposure of the blood to foreign surfaces during prolonged cardiopulmonary bypass. Included among these are platelet clumping and capillary blockage by embolization, protein denaturation, liberation of free fat by lipoproteins, and activation of the coagulation cascade, fibrinolytic system, complement system (by way of C3a and C5a), and the kallikrein-bradykinin system. Generation of the anaphylatoxins C3a and C5a mediates leukocyte chemotaxis, aggregation, and enzyme release.[108–110] Pulmonary sequestration of activated leukocytes and platelets occurs with attendant damage to the pulmonary endothelium.[60]

There is a direct relation between the duration of cardiopulmonary bypass and administration of blood products and the development of the derangements of pulmonary and vascular integrity noted above.[104,105] Important early clues to the presence of ARDS are a diminished pulmonary compliance as determined by ventilator, elevated alveolar-arterial gradient with a clear chest radiograph, and increasing difficulty maintaining oxygenation utilizing conventional mechanical ventilatory modes.[104] Management of ARDS includes mechanical ventilation with PEEP (often for extended periods), minimization of the pulmonary capillary wedge pressure without compromising cardiac output, and nutritional support as needed (Table 52–3). Extreme cases may require extracorporeal membrane oxygenator support (ECMO).[111]

UNDERLYING CHRONIC LUNG DISEASE. General surgical preparation of patients with obstructive lung disease, including antibiotics, bronchodilators, and cessation of cigarette smoking, may help minimize the risk of respiratory failure from postoperative atalectasis and pneumonia.[104,105] Inhaled bronchodilators should be continued postoperatively. Refractory patients may require a short course of corticosteroids (e.g., methylprednisolone, 0.5 mg/kg every 6 hours for 3 days) to be weaned from the ventilator.[104] Previous enthusiasm for intravenous methylxanthines has waned because of evidence of limited efficacy and the risk of agitation, arrhythmias, and grand mal seizures.[112] Intravenous theophylline should therefore be reserved for extremely refractory cases and should be administered in a dose of 0.4 mg/kg/hr with careful monitoring of plasma levels to maintain them in the range of 10 to 15 μg/ml.

Patients with chronic obstructive pulmonary disease should be weaned from the ventilator slowly. It is helpful to maintain the arterial carbon dioxide tension close to the patient's baseline level to ensure an adequate respiratory drive.

DIAPHRAGMATIC FAILURE. Diaphragmatic dysfunction after cardiac surgical procedures usually occurs as a result of injury to the phrenic nerve(s). An elevated hemidiaphragm may be seen on postoperative roentgenograms in 25 per cent of patients who undergo myocardial preservation, including a topical ice slush and harvesting of an internal mammary artery.[113] A simple bedside test of diaphragmatic function is to ask the patient to protrude his or her umbilicus, a movement that requires diaphragmatic functional integrity. Of note, an elevated hemidiaphragm usually is not associated with increased postoperative morbidity or mortality; recovery of the hemidiaphragm to normal position occurs in 80 per cent of patients at 1 year and nearly all patients by 2 years postoperatively. Less than 1 per cent of patients develop clinically important diaphragmatic dysfunction after cardiac surgery because of unilateral or bilateral phrenic nerve injury.

Evidence of diaphragmatic failure includes the inability to wean the patient from the ventilator, a vital capacity less than 500 cc, and paradoxical movement of the diaphragm on fluoroscopy (abnormal "sniff" test[104]) or ultrasonography. Because it may take up to 6 weeks for an injured phrenic nerve to recover function, management includes a more prolonged period of mechanical ventilation and, for some patients, transition to a rocking bed.[114] In cases of permanent unilateral phrenic nerve damage, plication of the diaphragm may help to improve respiratory function.[115]

PROLONGED VENTILATORY INSUFFICIENCY. Patients who fail to wean from the ventilator within 48 hours require special attention. Such patients should be sedated and consideration given to neuromuscular blockade if the patient is not breathing synchronously with the respirator. Because of the risk of stress-induced gastritis, an H_2-receptor blocker (e.g., ranitidine, 50 mg intravenously every 8 to 12 hours) is administered. To maintain hemodynamic stability, such patients frequently receive large volumes of intravenous fluids; packed red blood cells should be used to maintain an adequate oxygen-carrying capacity. Nutritional support in the form of tube feedings (preferably as a continuous infusion with the patient positioned in the right lateral decubitous position) or parenteral feedings is critical to provide adequate metabolic needs and prevent catabolism of skeletal muscles (e.g., respiratory muscles) (Table 52–3).

If the patient remains intubated beyond 10 to 14 days, the risks of tracheal stenosis, vocal cord damage, retropharyngeal abscess formation, and tracheoesophageal fistula increase. High-compliance, low-pressure cuffs on endotracheal tubes have reduced the risk of such complications and permit patients to remain intubated continuously for up to 20 or even 30 days, provided that the cuff pressures are maintained below 20 mm Hg and meticulous respiratory care technique is used. Placement of a tracheostomy tube is not a trivial decision because it can be associated with a number of complications that may offset the advantages of improved endotracheal suctioning and reduced risk of upper airway damage, but tracheostomy usually is desirable if it is clear that the patient will remain intubated beyond 3 weeks.

Hypertension

(See also p. 830)

Postoperative hypertension has been defined variably in the literature,[116] but we consider it to be present if the systolic pressure exceeds 140 mm Hg.[117] The incidence of postoperative hypertension ranges from 40 to 60 per cent of patients.[118] It occurs more commonly in patients with a preoperative history of hypertension, prior maintenance therapy with a beta blocker, and well-preserved left ventricular function.[119] Postoperative hypertension is especially frequent after coronary artery bypass grafting and surgical relief of left ventricular outflow tract obstruction (e.g., aortic valve replacement, correction of coarctation of the aorta).[120]

The mechanism of postoperative hypertension probably varies from patient to patient, but usually includes: (1) a "rebound" effect from withdrawal of beta blockade administered preoperatively; (2) excessive sympathetic nervous system activity with elevations of circulating catecholamine levels (especially norepinephrine)[121]; (3) pressor reflexes originating in the heart, great vessels, or coronary arteries[122]; and (4) following correction of aortic coarctation, a drop in the aortic pressure proximal to the site of the prior coarctation with resultant stimulation of aortic and carotid baroreceptors by apparent "hypotension." The renin-angiotensin system is stimulated and peripheral resistance is increased. The sudden exposure of vascular beds downstream to the coarctation to "undamped" aortic pressure also has been reported to cause mesenteric arteritis.

The adverse consequences of elevated systemic pressure include an increased risk of postoperative bleeding, suture line disruption, and aortic dissection[103]; elevated left ventricular afterload and consequent reduction of left ventricular output; injury to aortocoronary bypass grafts and postoperative stroke.

MANAGEMENT. Although a variety of agents may be used for treating acute postoperative hypertension, we prefer those that are rapidly acting and titratable and have a short half-life. Such drugs include sodium nitroprusside (0.5 to 2.0 μg/kg/min), esmolol (50 to 250 μg/kg/min), labetalol (1 to 2 mg/min), and nitroglycerin (25 to 300 μg/min).[103,123] Initial reports suggest that an infusion of the dihyrdopyridine calcium antagonist isradipine (8–50 μg/min) is also a safe and effective means of treating postoperative hypertension.[124] Many centers are starting to use closed-loop systems designed to titrate the intravenous infusion rate of a drug to a preset pressure level that is constantly being monitored invasively.[125] The need for transition to oral antihypertensive therapy is assessed on an individual basis; chronic treatment usually is required only in the patient with a preoperative history of hypertension.

Perioperative Myocardial Infarction

Despite modern intraoperative myocardial protection and improvements in surgical techniques, some degree of ischemia occurs nearly uniformly during coronary artery bypass surgery. Only a minority of patients (5 to 15 per cent of patients undergoing coronary artery bypass graft surgery),

TABLE 52–8 DIAGNOSIS OF MYOCARDIAL INFARCTION AFTER CARDIAC SURGERY

DIAGNOSTIC FINDING	COMMENT
Symptoms	
Early (<48 hr postop)	Not reliable because of residual effects of anesthesia and postoperative analgesics
Late (>48 hr postop)	Potentially reliable but may be confused with incisional pain and pleuritic pain from chest tubes, pericarditis
Electrocardiogram	
New, persistent Q waves	This is the most reliable diagnostic finding but only if the Q waves persist on serial ECGs over several days.
Evolutionary ST-T changes	Supportive data favoring the diagnosis of MI only if a typical evolutionary pattern is observed. Because of the effects of cardiopulmonary bypass, hypothermia, postoperative pericarditis, mediastinal chest tubes, and medications (e.g., digitalis), a variety of nonspecific ST-T wave abnormalities may be seen and should not be relied on for diagnosing a perioperative MI.
Myocardial Specific Enzymes	
Total CK	Elevated total CK levels postoperatively may arise from multiple sources, including skeletal muscle in the thorax and calf as well as myocardium.
CK-MB	Myocardial-specific CK may be released from ischemia occurring during cardiopulmonary bypass as well as myocardial and aortic incisions made intraoperatively (e.g., right atrium for cannulation of cavae). Because of the nearly universal release of CK-MB, a diagnosis of MI should not be made unless the CK-MB is significantly elevated (e.g., >30 units/liter).
Echocardiogram	A regional wall motion abnormality is a helpful finding, particularly if it can be shown to be a new finding by comparison with a peroperative study. Paradoxical motion of the high anterior portion of the interventricular septum is a common finding postoperatively in the absence of MI and should not be taken as the sole evidence of new perioperative myocardial necrosis.

MI, myocardial infarction; CK, creatine kinase.

however, actually experience a *perioperative myocardial infarction,* even in tertiary care centers currently operating on higher risk patients, including those with failed interventional procedures.[126–129] The potential causes of myocardial ischemia and infarction in the perioperative period include incomplete revascularization; diffuse atherosclerotic disease of the distal coronary arteries; spasm, embolism, or thrombosis of the native coronary vessels or bypass grafts[130,131]; technical problems with graft anastomoses; inadequate myocardial preservation intraoperatively; increased myocardial oxygen needs, as in left ventricular hypertrophy; and hemodynamic derangements in the postoperative period (e.g., hypotension, hypertension, tachycardia). Although initially one might suspect that perioperative myocardial infarction results from occlusion of bypass grafts placed to diseased coronary arteries, autopsy studies have shown that bypass grafts usually are patent in patients dying of a perioperative myocardial infarction.[132] This observation lends support to the concept that a mismatch between myocardial oxygen supply and demand in the operating room accounts for much of the infarction noted postoperatively.

DIAGNOSIS. The diagnosis of a myocardial infarction after cardiac surgery is more difficult than at other times because of the nonspecific ST-T wave abnormalities on the electrocardiogram and nearly universal elevation of creatine-kinase (CK) levels postoperatively.[126] A number of diagnostic findings (Table 52–8) must be carefully interpreted and then integrated along the lines of the algorithm shown in Table 52–9.

A 12-lead electrocardiogram should be obtained immediately on the patient's arrival in the intensive care unit after operation and no less frequently than once every 24 hours for the first 3 postoperative days. Measurements of total CK and CK-MB should be made every 8 hours for the first 24 hours and every 24 hours thereafter for the first 3 postoperative days. If there is clinical suspicion of a perioperative myocardial infarction, the CK measurements are made more frequently (every 8 hours) during the second and third postoperative days.

TROPONIN (see also p. 1203). Experience with newer, more sensitive serum markers of cardiac injury, such as troponin I and troponin T, is limited.[133–134] However, initial reports suggest that cardiac-specific troponin I and troponin T are elevated postoperatively in virtually all patients who undergo coronary artery bypass graft surgery. Those patients who experience a perioperative myocardial infarction release greater quanitities of troponin such that serum measurements may remain 10- to 20-fold higher than the upper limit of the reference interval for at least 4 to 5 days postoperatively. Even in patients not experiencing perioperative myocardial infarctions by conventional diagnostic criteria, the relative increase in proteins such as cardiac troponin I over preoperative baseline values is greater than that of CK-MB, suggesting that troponin measurements can detect small amounts of myocardial tissue damage that are not detected by CK-MB. The clinical significance of detection of such episodes of minor myocardial damage postoperatively requires further investigation,

TABLE 52–9 ALGORITHM FOR DIAGNOSIS OF PERIOPERATIVE MI AFTER CARDIAC SURGERY

NEW Qs ON ECG	CK-MB > 30 IU/LITER	NEW RWMA ON ECHO*	DIAGNOSIS	COMMENT
Yes	Yes	Yes	Definite MI	
Yes	Yes	No	Probable MI	New zone of necrosis not evident on echo. The persistence of new Q waves and abnormally elevated CK-MB suggests that Q waves are not a "benign" postoperative finding.
Yes	No	Yes	Definite MI	CK-MB peak probably missed because of infrequent sampling.
Yes	No	No	Possible MI	New Q waves may be false-positive finding.
No	Yes	Yes	Probable MI	Non–Q wave MI.
No	Yes	No	MI unlikely	Small non–Q wave MI cannot be entirely excluded.
No	No	Yes	MI unlikely	Removal of "restraining" effect of pericardium may result in new RWMAs, especially in high anterior septal area.
No	No	No	No MI	Although small patchy areas of necrosis may be seen histologically, these are probably not of clinical significance.

* Perioperative echocardiography is not *required* for the diagnosis of a perioperative MI but can provide useful supportive data or aid in the diagnosis in unclear cases, especially if obtained acutely. RWMA, regional wall motion abnormality; MI, myocardial infarction.

and formal criteria for the diagnosis of a perioperative myocardial infarction using troponin I and troponin T have not been firmly established.

ECHOCARDIOGRAPHY. Beside echocardiograms (transthoracic and if necessary transesophageal) play an important role in establishing the diagnosis of a perioperative myocardial infarction by detecting new regional wall motion abnormalities in cases in which the electrocardiogram or serum marker measurements are unclear. It is especially helpful to compare new echocardiograms with the preoperative studies that are almost always available.

ELECTROCARDIOGRAPHY. The electrocardiogram is the most reliable tool for diagnosing a perioperative myocardial infarction. New and persistent Q waves accompanied by new, persistent, and evolutionary ST-T wave abnormalities are the most helpful criteria. Pathological Q waves owing to perioperative myocardial infarction may appear with an earlier time course (i.e., immediately on arrival from the operating room) than in the nonrevascularized patient; they should be considered diagnostic, however, only if they are seen on serial electrocardiograms once the early postoperative hypothermia, axis shifts, and any potentially reversible myocardial ischemia have resolved.[126]

RISKS AND CONSEQUENCES OF PERIOPERATIVE INFARCTION. Variables that have been found to correlate with the development of a perioperative myocardial infarction in patients undergoing coronary artery bypass grafting include emergency surgery, aortic cross-clamp time greater than 100 minutes, a recent myocardial infarction (within the prior week), and a history of previous revascularization (either PTCA or CABG surgery).[129] Earlier reports suggesting that an increased number of grafts are also correlated with myocardial infarction have not been substantiated in more recent series.

Although the unique circumstances of perioperative myocardial infarction (early reperfusion, revascularization of adjacent ischemic zones, potential for early intervention if complications should arise) may lessen the potential adverse impact of myocardial infarction on ventricular function, most patients with a perioperative myocardial infarction have an increased hospital mortality (about 10 to 15 per cent) compared with patients undergoing coronary bypass grafting who have not sustained a perioperative myocardial infarction (about 1 per cent).[129,135]

Characteristics of patients who are especially at risk of increased short-term mortality after a perioperative myocardial infarction include age over 65 years, unstable angina preoperatively, a myocardial infarction within 1 week before operation, left ventricular aneurysm, intraventricular conduction disturbance (e.g., left bundle branch block), and the need for reoperation for bleeding. About two-thirds of the postoperative mortality is due to pump failure and one-third is due to malignant ventricular tachyarrhythmias.[135] Perioperative myocardial infarction also adversely affects long-term prognosis, particularly if associated with inadequate revascularization and depressed left ventricular function.[136]

Low-Output Syndrome and Shock States

RECOGNITION. Sometimes diagnosis of the low-output syndrome and a shock state after cardiac surgery is difficult. Because cold extremities and mottled skin may result from hypothermia postoperatively, these observations lack sufficient specificity. Although reduced systolic pressure is the most striking manifestation of this disorder, a low-output syndrome may be present even if the arterial systolic pressure exceeds 100 mm Hg because an increased systemic vascular resistance (>1500 dynes-sec-cm^{-5}) may be supporting the peripheral perfusion pressure. It is important to recognize this syndrome because of the strong relation between the cardiac index in the early postoperative period and the probability of cardiac death after surgery. Common clinical features of the low-output syndrome and shock states after cardiac surgery include cold extremities, mottled skin, reduced systolic pressure (<90 mm Hg), decreased urine output (<30 ml/hr), low cardiac index (<2.0 liter/min/m^2), low mixed venous oxygen saturation (<50 per cent), and acidosis.

One should make careful hemodynamic measurements and integrate them with bedside echocardiographic recordings to confirm the diagnosis of a low-output syndrome and attempt to segregate the findings into one of the patterns (*reduced preload, cardiogenic,* or *septic*) in Table 52–10. Although there is overlap of the hemodynamic findings among these patterns, and coexistence of multiple disorders (e.g., bradycardia and hypovolemia) may blur the distinctions between patterns, they offer a clinically useful approach to the evaluation of the patient with a low-output syndrome. In addition to the specific treatment measures discussed below, a number of general measures are applicable to all patients who are in a shocklike condition after cardiac surgery, including prompt correction of any electrolyte and acid-base disturbances, transfusion to a hematocrit over 30 per cent for improved oxygen-carrying capacity of the blood, and a "low threshold" for mechanical ventilatory support to minimize the work of breathing and thereby reduce total body oxygen needs.

REDUCED PRELOAD. Hypovolemia. Low ventricular filling pressures, a normal systemic vascular resistance, and a reduced cardiac index, coupled with echocardiographic demonstration of small ventricular volumes with preserved systolic function, are indicative of *hypovolemia.* Possible causes include bleeding, excessive diuresis, the "leaky capillary state" associated with the postpump syndrome, and, less frequently, inadequate vascular volume because of insufficient return of fluids at the conclusion of cardiopulmonary bypass. Rarely, adrenal cortical insufficiency owing to perioperative hemorrhage into the adrenals has been reported as a cause of hypovolemic hypotension after cardiac surgery.

Therapeutic maneuvers include administration of intravenous fluids (normal saline solution, lactated Ringer's solution) transfusion with packed red blood cells if the hemoglobin is less than 10 gm/dl, and administration of colloid-type volume expanders. It also is important to discontinue any vasodilators or antihypertensives that may have been prescribed during a period when the patient was hypertensive. While waiting for the above measures to take effect, the patient may require a transient infusion of an inotropic pressor agent, usually dopamine (see p. 502).

Vasodilatation. Inhibition of sympathetic tone by the effects of anesthetic agents may cause peripheral vasodilatation. In combination with increased venous capacitance that may occur during rewarming, a low-output syndrome may develop owing to a markedly reduced systemic vascular resistance (<1000 dynes-sec-cm^{-5}). This situation is best treated by an infusion of a vasoconstrictor such as norepinephrine in a dose of 1 to 10 μg/min until the systemic vascular resistance returns to a normal level.

CARDIOGENIC SHOCK. When the right ventricular and left ventricular filling pressures are in the normal range and systemic vascular resistance is not reduced, a frequent cause of a cardiac index less than 2 liters/min/m^2 is *bradycardia.* Because cardiac index is the product of stroke volume and heart rate, this abnormality is easily corrected by atrial or atrioventricular pacing at 85 to 100 beats/min.

Left Ventricular Failure. The pattern of predominant *left ventricular failure* in the early postoperative state is characterized by a disproportionately elevated pulmonary capillary wedge pressure compared with right atrial pressure, low cardiac index, and normal or elevated systemic vascular resistance. Echocardiography usually reveals a dilated, poorly contractile left ventricle, often exhibiting multiple regional wall motion abnormalities. The differential diagnosis of left ventricular failure after cardiac surgery includes the following conditions (which may coexist in the same patient): preoperative left ventricular dysfunction, inadequate surgical correction of the cardiac lesion (e.g., persistent aortic valve gradient owing to mismatch between the patient's aortic ring and prosthesis, residual left ventricular outflow tract obstruction after repair of idiopathic

TABLE 52–10 LOW-OUTPUT SYNDROME AND SHOCK STATES AFTER CARDIAC SURGERY

	REDUCED PRELOAD		CARDIOGENIC SHOCK				SEPTIC
Causes	Hypovolemia	Vasodilatation	Bradycardia (Inappropriately slow HR postoperatively)	LV failure	RV failure	Cardiac tamponade	Sepsis
Hemodynamics							
RA	<8	<8	≤10	≥10	>10	>15	<10
PCW	<15	<15	>15	>20	≤15*	>15	<15
CI	<2.0	<2.0	<2.0	<2.0	<2.0	<2.0	≥2.0
SVR	>1200	<1000	>1200	>1000	>1000	>1000	<1000
Other			HR < 60		PCW > 15 if LV failure is present	RA = PCW = PAd (within 5 mm Hg) unless "asymmetric" tamponade occurs due to pericardial clots	Narrow AVO_2 difference
Echocardiogram	Small ventricular chambers with vigorous systolic contraction unless LV dysfunction was present preoperatively	Small ventricular chambers with normal systolic contraction unless LV dysfunction was present preoperatively	Normal-sized ventricular chambers with vigorous systolic contraction, albeit at a slow rate	Dilated LV with reduced systolic performance; regional wall motion abnormalities may reflect old or new myocardial ischemia and/or infarction.	Dilated RA and RV with reduced RV systolic contraction. TR often present on Doppler study. The contractile performance of LV is variable.	Small cardiac chambers with diastolic collapse of RA and RV. Systolic contraction of RV and LV usually normal unless dysfunction was present preoperatively or coexistent LV or RV failure has occurred postoperatively.	Small ventricular chambers with normal or slightly depressed contractile function (myocardial depressant factor)
Management	IV fluids Transfusion if Hgb < 10 inotropes	Vasopressors	Cardiac pacing	Search for correctible lesion, offending agent, or laboratory abnormality inotropes Vasopressors and vasodilators Mechanical assistance	Supplemental O_2 Pulmonary vasodilators inotropes Mechanical assistance	Reexploration Supportive measures: IV fluids, inotropes	IV fluids Antibiotics Vasopressors inotropes

LV, left ventricular; RV, right ventricular; RA, right atrial; PCW, pulmonary capillary wedge; CI, cardiac index; SVR, systemic vascular resistance; TR, tricuspid regurgitation.

hypertrophic subaortic stenosis, residual atrial or ventricular septal defect), complication of surgical procedure (e.g., prosthetic valve leak or thrombosis, depression of stroke volume after correction of mitral regurgitation caused by the elevation of afterload), dysrhythmia, depressant effect of pharmacological agent (e.g., antiarrhythmic drug), acid-base or electrolyte disturbance, or myocardial ischemia and/or infarction. Bedside echocardiography usually can help to identify mechanical disorders such as prosthetic valve dysfunction and dysrhythmias, and metabolic abnormalities and toxic drug levels can be readily recognized by electrocardiogram and laboratory measurements.[96a]

MANAGEMENT. The objectives of hemodynamic management of patients with *left ventricular failure* postoperatively are to correct hypotension if present, increase forward left ventricular output, and return left and right ventricular filling pressures to the normal range. These parameters are intimately related, and treatment may require careful titration of several intravenous agents for pharmacological support of the failing circulation. Boluses of calcium chloride (0.5 to 1.0 gm) increase myocardial contractility, but the effect is modest and short-lived. A continuous infusion of dopamine (5 to 10 μg/kg/min) is preferable if the primary goal is to increase systemic arterial pressure and cardiac output. Dobutamine (2 to 5 μg/kg/min), amrinone (bolus of 0.75 mg/kg and infusion of 5 to 10 μg/kg/min), or milrinone (bolus of 50 μg/kg/min and infusion of 0.375 to 0.75 μg/kg/min) also both augment cardiac output and should be selected if reduction of ventricular filling pressure is desired; systemic arterial pressure is usually unchanged or may even drop slightly because of the peripheral vasodilatory effects of these drugs.[103,123,137] A commonly used combination is dopamine (2 μg/kg/min) to achieve greater renal perfusion in conjunction with dobutamine (2 to 5 μg/kg/min) for augmentation of cardiac output. If the arterial pressure is equal to or greater than 90 mm Hg, vasodilator therapy with sodium nitroprusside or nitroglycerin increases forward cardiac output and lowers the pulmonary capillary wedge pressure further. When hypotension is profound (e.g., systolic pressure < 70 mm Hg), norepinephrine, 1 to 10 μg/min, may be necessary to prevent coronary hypoperfusion.[103,123]

We prefer to use an intra-aortic balloon pump (Chap. 19) for mechanical support of the circulation along with pharmacotherapy early in the course of management of postoperative left ventricular failure that does not respond to the initial pharmacological maneuvers already discussed. This has the advantages of avoiding a continuous upward titration of the dose of sympathomimetic inotropic agents and vasoconstrictors associated with downregulation of beta adrenoceptors and diminished perfusion of the renal, mesenteric, and coronary vascular beds. Also, intra-aortic balloon counterpulsation does not increase myocardial oxygen demand. The intra-aortic balloon pump is particularly helpful if significant mitral regurgitation is present but is contraindicated in the presence of aortic regurgitation and if an abdominal aortic aneurysm is present. If the patient fails to improve despite a combination of intra-aortic balloon pumping and pharmacotherapy, a left ventricular assist device may be inserted for temporary support or as a "bridge" to cardiac transplantation until a donor is located.[138,139] Serial evaluations of left ventricular function over time and under different loading conditions and supportive measures are best obtained with transesophageal echocardiograms.[140]

RIGHT VENTRICULAR FAILURE. The pattern of predominant *right ventricular failure* is characterized by a disproportionate elevation of the right atrial pressure in comparison with the pulmonary capillary wedge pressure. In severe cases of postoperative right ventricular failure, the right atrial pressure may exceed 20 mm Hg while the pulmonary capillary wedge pressure remains equal to or less than 15 mm Hg. When left ventricular failure is present simultaneously, the difference between the right atrial and pulmonary capillary wedge pressures lessens and differentiation from cardiac tamponade becomes difficult. Bedside echocardiography is useful for making a proper diagnosis (Table 52–10).

Postoperatively, predominant right ventricular failure may be seen as a result of one or more of the following conditions: elevated pulmonary vascular resistance (persistently elevated from preoperative elevations of pulmonary artery pressure; postoperative hypoxia, pulmonary embolus, or pneumothorax), primary right ventricular ischemia/infarction[141] or a mechanical lesion (tricuspid regurgitation, residual shunt flow, right ventriculotomy).

Massive pulmonary embolism is a rare occurrence after cardiac surgery (Chap. 46). The diagnosis should be suspected when sudden deterioration in oxygenation occurs in association with systemic hypotension, tachycardia, electrocardiographic abnormalities (unexplained right axis deviation, right bundle branch block, and right ventricular strain pattern), and elevation of right atrial pressure. Angiographic confirmation of the diagnosis is usually not necessary. Expeditious noninvasive confirmation by echocardiography is advisable in those patients in whom the diagnosis remains uncertain. Management consists of immediate intravenous heparin and emergency pulmonary embolectomy. Pulmonary emboli that cause limited hemodynamic compromise (right atrial pressure < 15 mm Hg, arterial pressure > 90 mm Hg, cardiac index ≥ 2 liters/min/m^2) can be treated with anticoagulation alone. An inferior vena caval filter should be inserted if venography reveals lower-extremity venous thrombosis and recurrences are detected, or if, after the index event, it is felt that the patient could not survive a recurrent embolus. Because a caval filter does not prevent embolization from right atrial or right ventricular thrombi, an echocardiogram should be performed with consideration of surgical removal of any large mobile, nonsessile right heart thrombi.

Management. Hemodynamic management of predominant right ventricular failure should focus on improvement of right ventricular output to allow adequate filling of the left ventricle. Supplemental oxygen is provided to lower the pulmonary artery pressure. Bradycardia (<60 beats/min) is corrected by atrial or atrioventricular pacing. Isoproterenol (1 to 2 μg/min in the average adult) increases right ventricular contractility and also causes pulmonary vasodilatation. Pulmonary hypertension also may be reduced by prostaglandin E_1[142] and intravenous nitroglycerin.[68] Further reduction in right ventricular afterload can be achieved by an infusion of dobutamine to decrease the pulmonary capillary wedge pressure and lower the driving force across the pulmonary vascular circuit.

Profound hypotension caused by right ventricular failure that does not respond to the above measures can be treated with an infusion of a pulmonary vasodilator (isoproterenol, phentolamine) directly into the pulmonary artery by way of a Swan-Ganz catheter or inhalation of nitric oxide.[143] Insertion of a counterpulsation balloon catheter directly into the pulmonary artery has been reported, but the survival rate in such cases has been poor. Mechanical support of the failing right ventricle is now being used more frequently. Rarely, pulmonary embolectomy may be considered in the presence of refractory failure or shock (see p. 1597).

Cardiac Tamponade (see p. 1486). Postoperative echocardiography has shown that virtually all patients have a pericardial effusion after cardiac surgery and that many such effusions are asymmetrical and loculated.[144,145] Even with mediastinal drains in place, it is possible for a patient to develop cardiac tamponade postoperatively; recognition of this condition requires a high index of suspicion and assessment of hemodynamics at the bedside.[146]

RECOGNITION. Important clinical features of tamponade, such as diminished heart sounds and pulsus paradoxus, may be obscured by mechanical ventilation. Asymmetrical, loculated accumulation of blood and clots in the mediastinum and pericardial space may cause isolated tamponade of one or two cardiac chambers, producing unusual elevations of diastolic pressures (e.g., right atrial tamponade with elevation of central venous pressure without an increase in right ventricular end-diastolic pressure or pulmonary capillary wedge pressure).[147] Bedside two-dimensional transthoracic and transesophageal echocardiography is extremely helpful for diagnosing pericardial effusions and assessing the hemodynamic significance of fluid collections.[148] Diastolic collapse of the right atrium and right ventricle is an indication of a hemodynamically significant external compressive force and should prompt urgent treatment.

TREATMENT. Although pericardiocentesis may be helpful in nonsurgical tamponade, it is unlikely to be successful in evacuating the organized pericardial and mediastinal material that develops after cardiac surgery; subxiphoid drainage and/or emergency sternotomy is preferred. Supportive measures that can be attempted in the interim include volume expansion with intravenous fluids (Plasmanate, whole blood), and inotropic agents (dobutamine).

SEPTIC SHOCK. Low ventricular filling pressures, a markedly reduced systemic vascular resistance, and a normal or unexpectedly high cardiac index in the setting of hypotension and a shocklike state should raise the suspicion of the early stages of *sepsis*. With progression of septic shock, a capillary leak syndrome develops (hypovolemia) and myocardial depression may occur, resulting in a somewhat reduced contractile pattern of the ventricles on echocardiography. Combined therapy with intravenous fluids, antibiotics, and inotropic agents is required to interrupt the vicious cycle of hypotension, acidosis, and diminished coronary perfusion. Most patients who are septic during the first 48 hours after cardiac surgery are infected with a skin organism (incision, monitoring lines) or from seeding the bloodstream from a pulmonary or urinary source. Broad antibiotic coverage with one of the following combinations should be instituted: vancomycin plus an aminoglycoside, or ampicillin plus oxacillin and an aminoglycoside. Because the offending organism is likely to be resistant to the prophylactic antibiotic given preoperatively, it is wise not to include it as one of the empiric antibiotics selected to treat sepsis.

Arrhythmias

EVALUATION AND TREATMENT. There appear to be two peaks in the incidence of arrhythmias perioperatively: the first occurs in the operating room (most commonly during induction of anesthesia, weaning from cardiopulmonary bypass, rewarming) and the second occurs in the intensive care unit between the second and fifth postoperative days. The electrophysiological mechanisms underlying perioperative arrhythmias are incompletely understood, but they can probably be ascribed to a combination of the effects of circulating catecholamines, alterations in autonomic nervous system tone, transient electrolyte imbalances, myocardial ischemia or infarction, and mechanical irritation of the heart.

The physician caring for the postoperative cardiac surgical patient is frustrated by the lack of clinical data on which to base treatment decisions. Most of the emphasis in the literature is placed on prophylaxis against supraventricular tachyarrhythmias with digoxin and extrapolation of the early (and now outdated) coronary care unit guidelines for treating "warning" ventricular arrhythmias to the postoperative cardiac surgical patient. The availability of newer antiarrhythmic agents (verapamil, diltiazem, esmolol, adenosine) with efficacy against supraventricular arrhythmias coupled with published reports of the successful use of atrial pacing techniques provide a more rational approach to *supraventricular arrhythmias*. The management of *ventricular arrhythmias* remains controversial, especially in light of data from the nonsurgical ischemic heart disease population that prophylactic and suppressive antiarrhythmic therapy for the asymptomatic or minimally symptomatic patient may be associated with an increased mortality (see Chap. 37). Studies of the prognostic significance of ventricular arrhythmias after cardiac surgery and the impact of antiarrhythmic therapy on postoperative mortality are limited.[74,149,150]

APPROACH TO THE PATIENT. In the absence of more definitive data, clinicians can only cautiously apply the information gleaned from arrhythmia-intervention trials in nonsurgical patients and individualize treatment decisions based on the specifics of the patient's medical history and the circumstances present in the intensive care unit. For example, a patient with depressed left ventricular function and a preoperative history of resuscitation from sudden cardiac death who has just undergone coronary revascularization requires an aggressive approach to prevent recurrent ventricular tachycardia or ventricular fibrillation. Alternatively, a young patient with normal left ventricular function who has undergone closure of an atrial septal defect or mitral valve repair for ruptured chordae tendineae probably does not require suppression of ventricular arrhythmias in the absence of sustained ventricular tachycardia causing hemodynamic compromise.

Several factors may predispose to the development of arrhythmias, including ventilatory dysfunction, fever, electrolyte imbalance (hypokalemia, hypomagnesemia, hypocalcemia), anemia, myocardial ischemia or infarction, low cardiac output and reflex increase in sympathetic tone, hypertension, pericardial inflammation, and toxic effects of cardioactive medications (e.g., digitalis toxicity, bradycardia induced by diltiazem).[74,149] *Every effort should be made to look for and eliminate any of the factors that may be provoking the arrhythmia.*

Although antiarrhythmic drug therapy and direct-current cardioversion are traditional methods for treating postoperative arrhythmias, cardiac pacing techniques have a number of advantages. These include a more rapid onset and offset of action, avoidance of potential drug toxicity—especially proarrhythmia, elimination of the need for anesthesia (required for cardioversion), reduced anxiety for the patient, greater safety in patients receiving digitalis, and, perhaps most important, the ability to repeat the pacing protocol if the arrhythmia should recur, a not infrequent event. In addition to terminating arrhythmias, cardiac pacing can be used to suppress arrhythmias in many patients by atrial, atrioventricular sequential, or ventricular stimulation at a critical rate (e.g., 85 to 100 beats/min).

Surface Electrocardiogram. The value of a 12-lead electrocardiogram and simultaneously recorded multiple standard electrocardiograph lead rhythm strips cannot be overemphasized if one is attempting to analyze a wide-complex tachycardia. Unfortunately, a number of the criteria for differentiating supraventricular tachycardia with aberrant conduction from ventricular tachycardia (see p. 678) may not be applicable to postoperative patients because of previous or newly acquired infarction patterns, transient conduction defects (seen in 5 to 15 per cent of patients in the early recovery period), and nonspecific repolarization patterns. Although carotid sinus massage and specialized electrocardiograph lead recordings to detect atrial activation may be helpful, it is important to take advantage of the additional recording capabilities provided by the atrial and ventricular epicardial electrodes placed at the conclusion of cardiopulmonary bypass (Fig. 52–4).

Epicardial Electrodes. It is desirable to place two wires high on the free wall of the right atrium to allow for bipolar atrial recording and pacing. The advantages of bipolar pacing include a smaller stimulus artifact, the ability to record a bipolar atrial electrogram during ventricular pacing, and a reduced likelihood of precipitating undesired atrial arrhythmias if an atrial wire is used as the indifferent electrode during unipolar ventricular pacing.[151] Schematic diagrams showing the suggested intrathoracic positioning of the right atrial wires and recordings of unipolar and bipolar atrial electrocardiograms are shown in Figures 52–5 and 52–6.

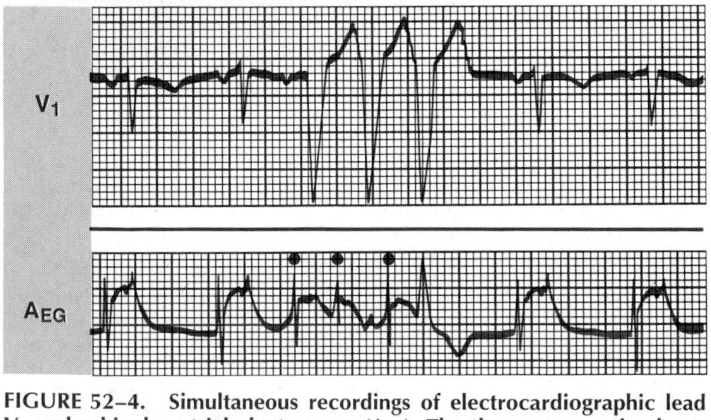

FIGURE 52–4. Simultaneous recordings of electrocardiographic lead V_1 and a bipolar atrial electrogram (A_{EG}). The three consecutive beats with wide QRS complexes recorded in the electrocardiogram do not represent ventricular tachycardia, but are due to aberrant ventricular conduction of three premature atrial beats (dots), as documented in the bipolar atrial electrogram. The appearance of a small ventricular complex after each atrial complex in the bipolar atrial electrogram recording helps to confirm the diagnosis. (From Waldo, A. L., and MacLean, W. A. H.: Diagnosis and Treatment of Cardiac Arrhythmias Following Cardiac Surgery. Mt. Kisco, N.Y., Futura Publishing Co., 1980.)

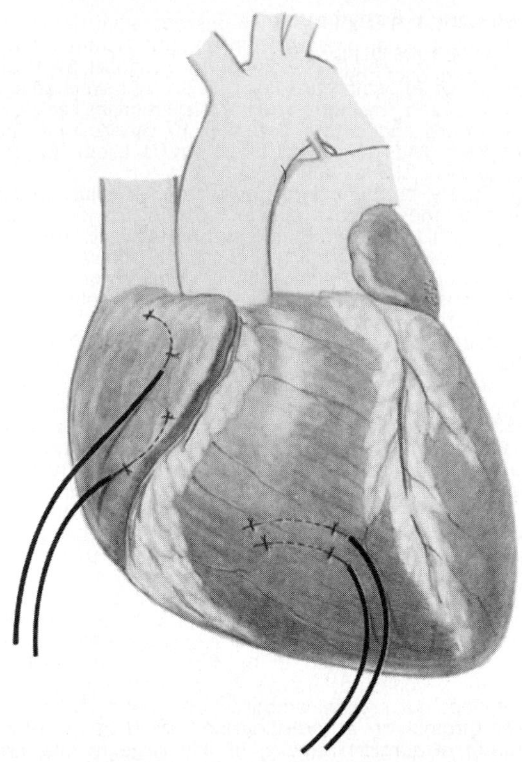

FIGURE 52–5. Placement of atrial and ventricular pacing wires during cardiac surgery. Although two atrial and ventricular electrodes are shown in this diagram (allowing bipolar recording and pacing), some surgeons place only one electrode in each of the sites (restricting recording and pacing to a unipolar configuration). Not shown in this diagram is an indifferent (ground) electrode that is placed in a subcutaneous position. The distal ends of the pacing wires are brought out to the skin through small stab wounds and positioned as shown in Figure 52–3. (From Behrendt, D. M., and Austen, W. G.: Patient Care in Cardiac Surgery. 4th ed. Boston, Little, Brown and Co., 1985.)

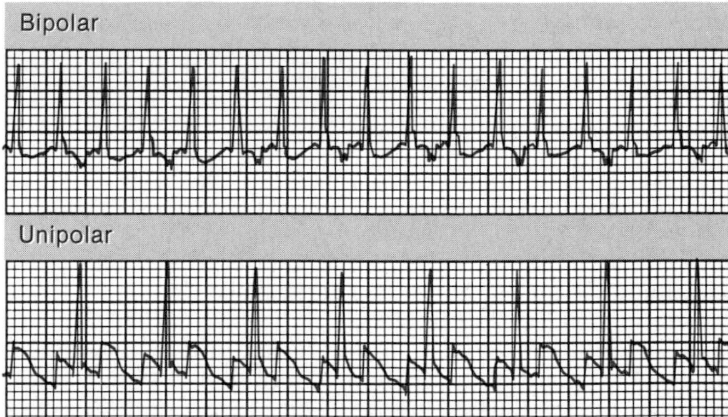

FIGURE 52–6. Simultaneous recording of bipolar and unipolar atrial electrograms utilizing a two-channel electrocardiograph machine with the standard right and left arm leads of the electrocardiograph patient cable attached to the two atrial wires and the recording selector set to the standard lead I (bipolar atrial electrogram) and standard lead II (unipolar atrial electrogram) positions. The rhythm disorder is type I (classical) atrial flutter with an atrial rate of 280 beats/min and 2:1 AV conduction. This type of atrial flutter is easily treated with rapid atrial pacing techniques. More rapid forms of atrial flutter (atrial rate 340 to 430 beats/min) are less responsive to atrial pacing and have been designated type II flutter. (From Waldo, A. L., and MacLean, W. A. H.: Diagnosis and Treatment of Cardiac Arrhythmias Following Cardiac Surgery. Mt. Kisco, N.Y., Futura Publishing Co., 1980.)

Supraventricular Arrhythmias

ATRIAL PREMATURE DEPOLARIZATIONS (see also p. 658). The hemodynamic consequences of atrial premature depolarizations are almost always minor, and one should resist the urge to suppress them with antiarrhythmic drugs. Instead, they should be considered a signal that the patient is possibly hypoxic or that an electrolyte imbalance is present, and a warning that the patient is at risk of developing a more serious arrhythmia, such as atrial fibrillation or atrial flutter. In the absence of such correctable abnormalities, one may want to administer a beta blocker to inhibit the effects of circulating catecholamines and also to slow the ventricular rate if atrial fibrillation should develop.

ATRIAL FLUTTER (see also p. 652). Control of the ventricular rate in atrial flutter is more difficult than atrial fibrillation because of the limited number of ventricular responses to atrial activation (usually 2:1, 4:1, but rarely an odd-numbered multiple). Atrial flutter may be difficult to terminate with antiarrhythmic agents. Cardioversion with an energy of 25 to 50 watt-seconds delivered as a single discharge can be expected to terminate atrial flutter in more than 90 per cent of patients.

Atrial flutter can also be terminated by rapid atrial pacing using the temporary epicardial atrial wires placed at the time of operation. The likelihood of success is increased if one uses sufficiently rapid rates of pacing (up to 140 per cent of the spontaneous atrial rate), a sufficient duration of pacing (10 to 30 seconds) with adequate strength (5 to 20 mA), and pretreats the patient with procainamide.[151,152] To achieve the high drive rates required, a special stimulator is utilized.[151] A bipolar pacing mode is preferred, although unipolar pacing can be attempted but with a lower chance of success. Difficulty also may be encountered if the spontaneous atrial rate is particularly rapid (i.e., >350 beats/min) and when pacing stimuli are delivered at a distance from the focus initiating the arrhythmia. In the latter instance the pacing protocol may be unable to penetrate and depolarize a portion of the reentrant circuit, allowing the flutter mechanism to persist. Examples of the diagnostic usefulness of atrial electrograms and the successful use of rapid atrial pacing for the termination of atrial flutter are shown in Figures 52–6 and 52–7.

ATRIAL FIBRILLATION (see also p. 654). Despite the fact that atrial fibrillation is an extremely common arrhythmia following cardiac surgery, the optimal management strategy has not been established. Despite prophylactic therapy with beta-adrenoceptor blockers, transient symptomatic atrial fibrillation occurs in at least 25 to 30 per cent of patients following coronary artery bypass grafting and 50 per cent of patients following valvular surgery, appearing with greatest incidence on the second or third postoperative day.[74]

Management. Unless hemodynamic collapse is present, in which case direct current cardioversion should be performed, the initial treatment of choice in the postoperative patient is to slow the ventricular rate. Although some textbooks and manuals of patient care continue to list digitalis glycosides as the drugs of choice, the therapeutic index is especially narrow in the postoperative patient and the likelihood of achieving a desired level of control of the ventricular rate is reduced in the presence of high circulating catecholamine levels. Provided that the patient's ventricular function is adequate, acute intravenous administration of beta blockers (e.g., metoprolol, 5 mg every 5 minutes for up to three doses), verapamil (e.g., 5-mg bolus every 5 to 10 minutes for three or four doses), or diltiazem (e.g., 0.25 to 0.35 mg/kg bolus over 2 minutes) are more desirable options. Esmolol, an ultrashort-acting cardioselective beta blocker, when administered intravenously in a dose of 50 to 250 μg/kg/min, provides the option of rapid onset; in the event of hemodynamic deterioration the effects of the drug are usually dissipated within 15 to 30 minutes after discontinuation of the infusion. In addition, the probability of conversion to sinus rhythm with esmolol appears to be better than with other agents such as verapamil.[153]

ANTICOAGULANTS. Epidemiological observations suggest that the development of postoperative atrial fibrillation is associated with a marked increase in the risk of stroke (odds ratio 3.0) and a prolonged hospitalization.[72–74,154] There is no consensus regarding the anticoagulation recommendations in patients with postoperative atrial fibrillation. The risks of hemorrhage in the early postoperative period must be weighed against the risk of systemic thromboembolism.[155] The level of risk for systemic embolization varies with the underlying cardiovascular pathology (valvular heart disease, dilated or hypertrophic cardiomyopathy, and CHF > nonvalvular heart disease > lone atrial fibrillation).[156] When atrial fibrillation develops beyond the second postoperative day, we generally advocate adherence to the guidelines established for nonsurgical patients and initiate anticoagulation (intravenous heparin followed by oral warfarin) in patients who have been in the arrhythmia for more than 48 hours, especially if the patient has a history of systemic embolism, or mitral valve disease or cardiomyopathy is present.[156]

Beyond the control of the ventricular rate acutely, the two treatment strategies for management of postoperative atrial fibrillation are similar to those for the nonsurgical patient: chronic anticoagulation while administering rate-controlling agents versus restoration of sinus rhythm and attempts at suppression of recurrences of atrial fibrillation. Because large-scale clinical trial data are not available to guide decision making in this area, therapeutic approaches must be individualized.[155] Although procainamide is frequently used for the treatment of atrial fibrillation after open heart surgery, evidence exists that it has limited effectiveness at suppressing recurrences of atrial fibrillation.[155a] Furthermore, any treatment decision formulated during hospitalization should be readdressed at the first postoperative visit (typically 4 to 6 weeks) to determine if it is still a desirable course of action once the inflammation and metabolic alterations of the postoperative state have dissipated.

Patients with depressed left ventricular function or striking ventricular hypertrophy who experience troublesome dyspnea and/or hypotension when in atrial fibrillation postoperatively are suitable candidates for a trial of restoration of sinus rhythm. It has been our experience that patients undergoing isolated coronary artery bypass surgery who have normal left ventricular function and no preoperative history of atrial fibrillation are likely to undergo spontaneous reversion to sinus rhythm by the time of the first postoperative visit and may therefore be adequately treated with a regimen of an oral beta-adrenoceptor blocker and a short term (1 to 2 months) of oral anticoagulation with warfarin (INR 1.5 to 2.0).

For those patients for whom a decision is made to attempt to restore sinus rhythm, we prefer to postpone the cardioversion procedure until 5 to 7 days postoperatively, when the risk of recurrent atrial fibrillation is decreased because pericardial and mediastinal inflammation have resolved somewhat and the level of sympathetic tone has decreased. Approximately 48 hours prior to cardioversion, antiarrhythmic treatment to possibly restore sinus rhythm pharmacologically (albeit successfully in only 5 to 15 per cent of patients) and suppress recurrences of atrial fibrillation is started. Because patients are most likely to relapse back into atrial fibrillation during the

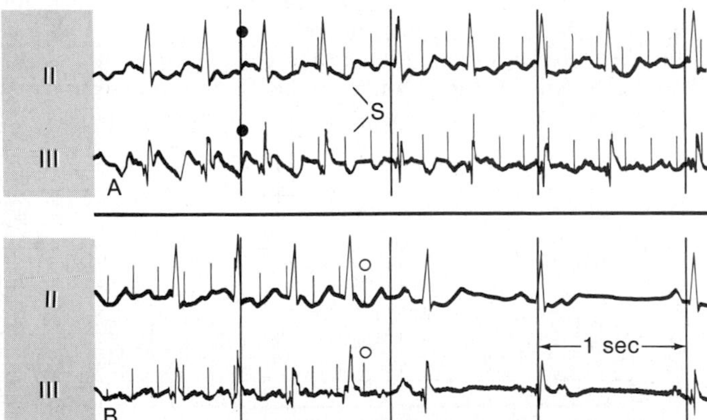

FIGURE 52–7. Recording of electrocardiographic leads II and III in a patient with atrial flutter. Panels A and B are not continuous tracings. The dots in Panel A mark the onset of rapid atrial pacing at 350 beats/min using a pacing stimulator capable of high drive rates. The morphology of the atrial complexes changes dramatically, such that by the end of the trace in Panel A, the atrial complexes are positive in leads II and III. Panel B shows the termination of 30 seconds of atrial pacing at 350 beats/min. The circles represent the last paced atrial beat. With abrupt termination of the rapid atrial pacing, sinus rhythm appears. S = stimulus artifact. Time lines are at 1-second intervals. (From Waldo, A. L., and MacLean, W. A. H.: Diagnosis and Treatment of Cardiac Arrhythmias Following Cardiac Surgery. Mt. Kisco, N.Y., Futura Publishing Co., 1980.)

first 1 to 2 months following cardioversion, it is important to administer suppressive antiarrhythmic therapy and oral anticoagulation during that period and then consider addressing the long-term need for further treatment.[156,157]

PERMANENT SUPPRESSIVE ANTIARRHYTHMIC THERAPY. This is often still necessary in patients with rheumatic heart disease and a preoperative history of atrial fibrillation despite successful aortic or mitral valve surgery even if sinus rhythm is present during the early postoperative period. Such patients typically have scarring of enlarged atria which places them at continued risk for intra-atrial reentry and atrial fibrillation. Patients with nonrheumatic mitral regurgitation (e.g., ruptured chordae tendineae) who have undergone mitral valve repair or replacement may not have a long-term need for suppressive antiarrhythmic therapy despite a preoperative history of atrial fibrillation because relief of the hemodynamic burden may decrease their propensity to atrial premature depolarizations and atrial fibrillation.

PAROXYSMAL SUPRAVENTRICULAR TACHYCARDIA (see p. 1763). The reentrant forms of paroxysmal supraventricular tachycardia (PSVT)—atrioventricular nodal reentry tachycardia and atrioventricular reentry tachycardia—occur less frequently in the postoperative patient than atrial fibrillation or atrial flutter, but fortunately retain their responsiveness to vagal maneuvers and pharmacotherapy to inhibit atrioventricular nodal conduction. The antiarrhythmic agent adenosine (see p. 619), an endogenous nucleoside, has a number of features that make it the drug of choice for treating PSVT in the postoperative patient.[158] A rapid (2 seconds) intravenous bolus of 6 mg terminates about 60 per cent of episodes of PSVT within 20 seconds; a subsequent bolus of 12 mg administered 1 to 2 minutes later terminates PSVT in virtually all those cases that failed to respond to the lower dose. Because adenosine is rapidly transported into the cell or degraded enzymatically to inosine, the physiological effects of adenosine are dissipated in less than 5 minutes. Untoward reactions such as flushing, chest pain, or dyspnea, although common, are mild and short-lived.

PSVT also may be diagnosed by atrial recordings, and terminated by burst atrial pacing or randomly delivered atrial or ventricular premature depolarizations that invade the reentrant circuit and interrupt the arrhythmia. The automatic form of PSVT (i.e., ectopic automatic atrial tachycardia) is sufficiently unusual postoperatively that its presence should strongly raise the suspicion of digitalis toxicity.

Ventricular Arrhythmias

VENTRICULAR PREMATURE DEPOLARIZATIONS (see p. 675). Isolated ventricular premature depolarizations (VPDs) commonly occur after cardiac surgery. There may be an increase in the density of VPDs in patients with a preoperative history of VPDs, or they may appear de novo in patients with no history of ventricular arrhythmias. Although there may be a fall in arterial pressure associated with isolated VPDs, this usually is extremely brief and of no significant hemodynamic consequence to the patient unless prolonged periods of bigeminy occur.

The emergence of frequent VPDs should trigger a search for any potentially correctable factors. Such a search would include measurement of serum electrolyte levels (potassium, calcium, magnesium), hematocrit, and blood pressure; assessment of the level of oxygenation; estimation of volume status (central venous pressure, pulmonary capillary wedge pressure, urine output); and screening for possible toxic levels of cardioactive agents (digitalis, theophylline).

As is the case with VPDs in acute myocardial infarction, there is no conclusive evidence that complex VPDs are harbingers of ventricular tachycardia (VT)/ventricular fibrillation (VF) or a poor outcome in the postoperative patient.[159,160] Nor is there evidence that prophylactic suppression of VPDs improves postoperative outcome.[161]

Sustained VT and VF in the early postoperative period are infrequent events and probably most often the result of transitory electrolyte disturbances or myocardial ischemia/infarction. Therefore, aggressive correction of electrolyte deficits and anti-ischemic therapy with intravenous nitroglycerin and beta blockers alone may be effective for preventing VF without exposing the patient to the potential hazards of antiarrhythmic therapy (myocardial depression, torsades de pointes).[74]

Management. We advocate a conservative approach focusing on prompt detection and correction of provocative factors, liberal use of beta blockers in patients with an ejection fraction greater than 30 per cent, overdrive atrial or atrioventricular sequential pacing between 85 and 100 beats/min, and restriction of suppressive antiarrhythmic therapy to patients with a preoperative history of serious ventricular tachyarrhythmias.[74] If the decision is made to suppress VPDs in a patient without a history of symptomatic ventricular arrhythmias, the treatment period should be brief (6 to 24 hours) and the patient should not be automatically converted to an oral antiarrhythmic drug regimen without careful reconsideration of the indications for treatment.

VENTRICULAR TACHYCARDIA (see p. 677). Many of the same arguments cited above for isolated VPDs can be applied for paroxysms of nonsustained VT. No definitive guidelines are available, but we believe that episodes of VT lasting for 15 to 30 seconds or more in the absence of correctable factors and attempts at overdrive atrial or atrioventricular sequential pacing are indications for antiarrhythmic therapy, especially if the episodes are associated with hemodynamic compromise. *Sustained VT* is a serious emergency that should be handled with an orderly approach. If the clinical situation permits, a 12-lead electrocardiogram should be obtained for future reference and confirmation of the diagnosis; simultaneous recording of surface electrocardiographic leads with electrograms from the epicardial wires may be helpful in establishing the mechanism of a wide complex tachycardia (Fig. 52–8).

Acute attempts at conversion of the tachycardia include the following maneuvers in the sequence listed: thumpversion, burst ventricular pacing (see p. 680), and boluses of antiarrhythmic agents (lidocaine, 100 mg; procainamide, up to 500 to 1000 mg over 20 minutes; bretylium, 500 to 1000 mg over 5 to 10 minutes; or amiodarone, 75 to 150 mg; infused over 10 minutes). In urgent circumstances synchronized direct-current cardioversion with a low-energy shock (25 to 50 watt-seconds) may be used. Unsynchronized shocks of 100 to 200 watt-seconds should be used if the tachycardia rate is greater than 160 beats/min and/or has a sinusoidal waveform on the electrocardiogram. After conversion a search for correctable disorders should be undertaken, and if none is found a continuous infusion of lidocaine (2 mg/min), procainamide (2 mg/min), bretylium (1 to 2 mg/min), or amiodarone (1.0 mg/min for 6 hours followed by maintenance infusion of 0.5 mg/min) is started.

VENTRICULAR FIBRILLATION (see p. 686). As in the nonsurgical patient, VF must be promptly treated with an unsynchronized direct-current shock. Extrapolating from experience in the electrophysiology laboratory, where VF frequently is provoked iatrogenically, it often can be reverted with shocks of 200 watt-seconds, provided the intervention is performed promptly. It should be possible to defibrillate postoperative patients in the intensive care unit expeditiously; therefore, the higher energies (360 to 400 watt-seconds) used in the "field" probably are unnecessary—at least initially. Emergency cardiopulmonary bypass in

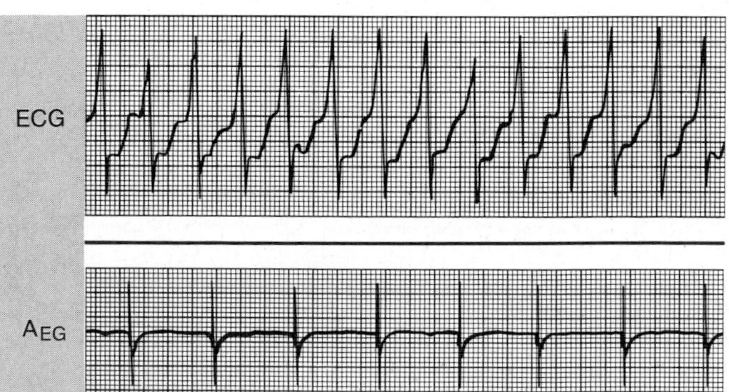

FIGURE 52–8. Monitor electrocardiographic lead recorded simultaneously with bipolar atrial electrogram (A_{EG}) during a wide QRS complex tachycardia at 155 beats/min. The A_{EG} demonstrates the presence of sinus rhythm at 90 beats/min. This observation in conjunction with AV dissociation and fusion beats (second and ninth QRS complexes) establishes that the wide QRS complex tachycardia is ventricular in origin. (From Waldo, A. L., and MacLean, W. A. H.: Diagnosis and Treatment of Cardiac Arrhythmias Following Cardiac Surgery. Mt. Kisco, N.Y., Futura Publishing Co., 1980.)

the cardiac surgical intensive care unit should be considered a potential life-saving measure in patients suffering postoperative cardiac arrest due to intractable VF.[162] Owing to the small number of patients experiencing unexpected sustained hemodynamically compromising VT or VF, epidemiological data on provocative factors and the prognosis of these arrhythmias are difficult to evaluate.[74,150,163] Evidence suggests that unexplained VT or VF occurring within 24 hours of coronary artery bypass graft surgery is associated with a very high in-hospital mortality, probably resulting from perioperative ischemia, infarction, and/or pump failure.[150] Episodes of VT or VF occurring more than 24 hours following bypass surgery have a slightly less ominous prognosis and may be due to reperfusion of previously ischemic zones or transmembrane shifts of electrolytes during the process of recovery.[164]

Risk stratification of patients experiencing VT or VF postoperatively should include assessment of left ventricular function, coronary arteriography if ischemia/infarction is suspected, and consideration of an electrophysiologic study to establish the most appropriate course of therapy.[164a] Because of the numerous metabolic fluxes taking place in the early postoperative period, electrophysiologic study should, if possible, be postponed until at least 5 to 7 days following surgery.[74]

ATRIOVENTRICULAR JUNCTIONAL RHYTHMS. Nonparoxysmal atrioventricular junctional rhythms (rate >45 beats/min) can be seen after mitral or aortic valve surgery. Trauma and tissue swelling from surgical debridement and suture placement are believed to be the provocative mechanisms. Such rhythms typically are transient (≤48 hours) and easily treated with atrial or atrioventricular sequential pacing at a rate above that of the intrinsic junctional mechanism.[165]

Bradyarrhythmias (See p. 1349)

Sinus bradycardia or sinus arrest with emergence of a slow atrioventricular junction escape rhythm may be seen postoperatively when one or more of the following factors are present: advanced age, hypothermia, drug effects (diltiazem, beta blocker, digitalis, procainamide), preoperative sinus node dysfunction, intraoperative trauma to the sinus node, and postoperative elevation of vagal tone.[166] In addition to modifying the dose or discontinuing offending drugs (such as those noted above), atrial pacing at 85 to 100 beats/min should be initiated to maintain an adequate cardiac output and urine flow. Checks of the intrinsic heart rate every 6 hours during the first 24 to 48 hours indicate when pacing may be discontinued.

Although up to 45 per cent of patients may develop a new conduction defect following cardiac surgery, the majority are usually transient and are related to the extensive use of cold cardioplegia, hypothermia, perioperative electrolyte shifts, or surgical trauma during valve repair/replacement or closure of septal defects.[167–169] Complete heart block occurs infrequently following CABG surgery.[169]

In the absence of a low cardiac output syndrome related to bradycardia, the development of a new fascicular block or bundle branch alone is not necessarily an indication for initiation of temporary pacing (although it is a common practice in many centers to attach the epicardial wires to an external generator that is either turned off or programmed in the VVI mode with a low escape rate, in the unlikely event that complete heart block occurs). As with nonsurgically related conduction defects, the prognosis of patients with postoperative conduction defects is closely related to the underlying ventricular function.

MANAGEMENT. The decision to insert a permanent pacemaker after cardiac surgery should be based on the hemodynamic consequences of bradycardia in the individual patient rather than on a specific heart rate. Most new conduction defects resolve in the early postoperative period, but some persist for as long as 2 weeks. Few data are available to guide the decision about timing of implantation of a permanent pacemaker. Although we are willing to observe a younger patient (<65 years) following CABG surgery with a temporary pacing system postoperatively to see if a conduction defect resolves, we have a low threshold for implanting a permanent pacemaker following aortic or mitral valve surgery or if antiarrhythmic therapy or beta blocker treatment is contemplated because these pharmacological measures might "stress" a diseased conduction system. We advocate early insertion of a permanent pacemaker in elderly patients with symptomatic bradycardia because the recuperative process is facilitated, the period of relative immobilization and electrocardiographic monitoring is minimized, and hospital stay is shortened.[170] Finally, we are more aggressive about implantation of permanent pacemakers in patients with persistent advanced atrioventricular block as compared to patients with isolated sinus bradycardia.

Cardioversion (See p. 619)

Direct-current cardioversion should be used in the postsurgical patient with the following additional considerations. The recent cardiotomy with resultant pericardial and mediastinal inflammation, presence of chest tubes and/or pleural effusions, and elevated catecholamine levels after surgery may all contribute to higher energy requirements for reversion of arrhythmias such as atrial fibrillation than are commonly required in patients who have not recently undergone cardiac surgery. To achieve the maximum trans-cardiac spread of current after a median sternotomy, the anterior paddle should be placed to the *right* of the sternum between the third and sixth intercostal spaces, and the other paddle should be positioned in the fourth to sixth intercostal space as far in the left axilla as possible or in a posterior location under the tip of the left scapula. Firm pressure is applied to the paddles to maintain contact with the chest wall as the discharge buttons are depressed.

Hemostatic Disturbances

(See Chap. 58)

All patients who undergo cardiopulmonary bypass develop a multifactorial derangement of the hemostatic system. These abnormalities are caused by exposure of the blood to artificial surfaces, hemodilution, and the effects of heparin (Table 52–11).[110,171–178] Platelet dysfunction is the most significant hemostatic abnormality that occurs after cardiopulmonary bypass, although diminution of coagulation factor levels may assume greater significance in patients with preoperative deficiencies of hemostasis. Administration of the following drugs before surgery may predispose the patient to excessive bleeding: aspirin, nonsteroidal anti-inflammatory agents, thrombolytic agents,[174] certain antibiotics (carbenicillin, ticarcillin, moxalactam, cefamandole, third-generation cephalosporins), dextran, amrinone, quinidine, cytotoxic agents, gold, phenylbutazone, and fish oils.[174] In some institutions, for patients who are undergoing a reoperation or are polycythemic (p. 1792), when the risk of early postoperative bleeding is increased, two units of fresh frozen plasma are administered prophylactically after cardiopulmonary bypass.

The most obvious evidence of bleeding in the postoperative cardiac surgical patient is by means of chest tube drainage. "Acceptable" rates of bleeding are usually less than 100 ml/hr. In our institution, guidelines for returning to the operating room because of excessive bleeding include more than 500 ml/hr for 1 hour, more than 300 ml/hr for 3 hours, and 200 to 300 ml/hr for 5 hours. These guidelines may be tempered by correctable extenuating circumstances, such as uncontrolled hypertension postoperatively, failure to achieve normothermia, or an abnormal coagulation status that is being corrected. Emergency medi-

TABLE 52–11 HEMOSTATIC DISTURBANCES FOLLOWING CARDIOPULMONARY BYPASS

ABNORMALITY	CAUSE
Exposure of blood to artificial surfaces	
1. Platelet dysfunction A. Prolonged bleeding time B. Decreased adhesiveness	1. Depletion of platelet alpha granules, reduced response to wound, and increased plasma levels of platelet factor 4 and beta-thromboglobulin.[171]
2. Inflammatory response	2. Activation of the complement, coagulation, fibrinolytic, and kallikrein cascades; activation of neutrophils with degranulation and protease enzyme release; oxygen free radical production; and synthesis of cytokines (tumor necrosis factor, interleukin-1, interleukin-6, interleukin-8).[110,172]
Hemodilution	
1. Thrombocytopenia	1. Priming of extracorporeal bypass circuit with crystalloid solutions. Heparin-mediated immune thrombocytopenia may occur in about 5% of patients.[173]
2. Coagulation factor depletion	2. Most coagulation factor levels are reduced by hemodilution by about 50%; Factor V is reduced to 20–30% of normal and Factor VIII is relatively unaffected. Factor levels usually return to normal within 12 hours after completion of cardiopulmonary bypass. Although plasminogen and fibrinogen levels are decreased by about 50%, fibrin degradation products usually do not appear in the plasma during bypass.[174]
Heparinization	Thrombus formation is inhibited and excessive bleeding is avoided intraoperatively by maintaining the activated clotting time (ACT) between 400–480 seconds.

* Note: reversal of heparin effects is accomplished with protamine sulfate. Vascular collapse has been reported in some patients during protamine treatment.[175] To avoid the problem of heparin induced thrombocytopenia and because heparin may not effectively inhibit all the thrombin generated during cardiopulmonary bypass ("heparin rebound"), novel antithrombins are being evaluated as alternatives to heparin during surgery.[176–178]

cal maneuvers that can be attempted after sending coagulation studies to the laboratory include the use of PEEP up to 10 cm H_2O for mediastinal tamponade; empirical "correction" of putative platelet dysfunction with desmopressin acetate (DDAVP, a synthetic analog of arginine vasopressin that increases plasma levels of von Willebrand factor), 0.3 μg/kg, infused over 15 to 30 minutes; and empirical administration of a small dose of protamine sulfate, 25 to 50 mg, because heparin may be liberated from the patient's fat stores as rewarming occurs.[179]

Once the coagulation profile returns, additional therapy in the form of platelet transfusions for a platelet count less than 100,000/mm^3 and fresh frozen plasma to correct an elevated prothrombin time can be prescribed. Recent reports suggest that aprotinin (2×10^6 KIU loading bolus followed by infusion of 0.5×10^6 KIU/hr for 4 hours) is helpful in cases of excessive postoperative bleeding by virtue of its ability to inhibit fibrinolysis and replenish platelet GPIb receptors and von Willebrand factor activity.[180,180a] When monitoring bleeding from a chest tube, it is important to be alert to a sudden cessation of hemorrhage. This may indicate that the chest tubes have clotted and the fluid is now draining into the mediastinum or the pleural spaces. Serial chest radiographs may be helpful while observing a patient during a bleeding episode. With correct medical management, only about 5 per cent of patients need to return to the operating room for control of bleeding; this should be accomplished within 3 to 4 hours of the original surgery, before hemodynamic destabilization occurs and large volumes of blood products are administered.

ANTITHROMBOTIC THERAPY IN PATIENTS WITH PROSTHETIC HEART VALVES (see pp. 1061 and 1834). Patients who have undergone implantation of a prosthetic heart valve are exposed to a lifelong risk of thromboembolism. The degree of risk varies with the type of valve implanted (mechanical > bioprosthetic), valve location (mitral > aortic), the presence of atrial fibrillation, the size of the left atrium, a history of thromboembolism or the presence of left atrial thrombi at the time of operation, and the adequacy of anticoagulation. For mechanical prosthetic heart valves it is strongly recommended that all patients undergoing implantation of a second-generation bileaflet or disc valve receive lifelong warfarin therapy to a target INR of 2.5 to 3.5.[181] (Patients with first-generation mechanical valves such as Starr-Edwards, standard Bjork-Shiley, and Omniscience should be anticoagulated to a target INR of 3.5 to 4.5.)[181]

Patients with bioprosthetic valves appear to be at greatest risk of thromboembolism in the first 3 months after valve implantation. For patients in sinus rhythm who have a bioprosthetic valve placed in the mitral position, we prescribe warfarin for 3 months, designed to prolong the prothrombin time to 1.3 to 1.5 times control; if atrial fibrillation persists, warfarin is continued permanently. We usually do not anticoagulate patients with bioprosthetic valves inserted in the aortic position, provided that the patient is in sinus rhythm.

Infection

FEVER. Despite its nonspecific nature, fever is the most common initial clinical sign of a postoperative infection.[182] It should be emphasized, however, that patients who experience a normal course of convalescence continue to show an elevated temperature for up to 6 days postoperatively.[183] In the absence of infection such early fevers are believed to be caused by alterations in blood components after cardiopulmonary bypass. In addition to infectious causes, fevers that occur beyond 6 days may be due to drug reactions, phlebitis at the site of intravenous lines, atelectasis, pulmonary emboli, or the postpericardiotomy syndrome.

WOUND AND INCISION. **Leg.** Infections of the leg wound typically present with fever, induration, pain, erythema, local warmth, and drainage from the suture line. The usual infectious agents include *Staphylococcus, Streptococcus,* and aerobic gram-negative bacilli. Wound aspiration and Gram's stain should be used to guide antibiotic treatment. More advanced cases require wound debridement and open drainage. Recurrent bacterial cellulitis in the leg used for saphenous vein harvest may be a recalcitrant problem that appears months to years after operation.[184] Antibiotic courses directed against staphylococcus and streptococcus species for each individual occurrence may be insufficient, and a long-term course of antibiotic therapy may be needed. It is important to search for evidence of superficial fungal infections in the affected leg because persistent tinea pedis infection has been reported to cause recurrent lower-extremity cellulitis.[185] If a fungal infection is identified, treatment with topical miconazole or clotrimazole should be given in addition to antibacterial therapy. Persistent fungal infections (owing to breaks in integrity of the dermal barrier) should be treated with either oral ketoconazole or griseofulvin.

Mediastinitis. Mediastinitis and sternal osteomyelitis are among the most serious complications of a median sternotomy.[54,186,187] If one excludes operations that occur after thoracic trauma, it is estimated that mediastinitis occurs in about 2 per cent of patients who undergo median sternotomy.

Most cases present within 2 weeks after sternotomy. Important diagnostic features of patients who develop mediastinitis early after cardiac surgery include persistent fever in excess of 101°F beyond the fourth postoperative day, a systemic toxic condition, leukocytosis, bacteremia, and a purulent discharge from the sternal wound. Wound erythema, abnormal sternal tenderness or instability, and mediastinal widening may all be absent or clinically unapparent early in the development of mediastinitis. Recognition of mediastinitis requires a high index of suspicion and a vigorous, repetitive search for evidence of sternal wound drainage in patients who are persistently febrile late into the first week after surgery and in whom there is no other obvious focus of infection, such as pneumonia or urinary tract infection.[188] The diagnosis can be confirmed by needle aspiration from the subxiphoid approach followed by Gram's stain and culture.

RISK FACTORS AND DIAGNOSIS. There are a number of intraoperative and postoperative risk factors for the development of mediastinitis. These include prolonged cardiopulmonary bypass time, excessive postoperative bleeding with reexploration for control of hemorrhage, and diminished cardiac output in the postoperative period. There is an increase in the development of mediastinitis when both internal mammary arteries are mobilized bilaterally for use as bypass conduits.[189] For that reason many surgeons prefer to use only the left internal mammary artery, particularly in elderly diabetic patients who may already be predisposed to delayed sternal wound healing.

The spectrum of microorganisms that cause mediastinitis includes *Staphylococcus* (*aureus* and *epidermidis*) in about 50 per cent of patients and a variety of gram-negative bacilli in about 40 per cent of cases.[188–191] Mixed infections and fungal infections are rare. The organism isolated frequently is resistant to the prophylactic antibiotic used preoperatively, especially if the isolate includes a gram-negative bacillus or a β-lactamase–producing *S. aureus*.

Definitive diagnosis of a sternal wound infection requires exploration of the wound and culture of suspicious areas. Specialized radiological techniques such as CT and MRI scanning also have been reported to be helpful in localizing the sites of infection. Although both closed and open methods of treatment of mediastinitis have been reported, most authorities comment on the need for experienced surgical judgment if the closed approach (debridement, reclosure, and antibiotic irrigation) is utilized. The open approach is more frequently used for chronic or extensive infections and often entails removal of involved bony or cartilaginous structures. Although previously the wound was allowed to heal by secondary intention, current strategy involves formation of a myocutaneous flap over the sternal area.[192] The patient is treated with nutritional (Table 52–3) and respiratory support as needed. With both the closed and open method, intravenous antibiotics and sternal antibiotic irrigation are continued for at least 10 to 14 days; 4 to 6 weeks of treatment may be needed in cases of documented sternal osteomyelitis.

The reported mortality associated with mediastinitis varies greatly and appears to be related to the delay in initiation of treatment; patients diagnosed and treated aggressively within 1 month of surgery have a mortality of about 10 per cent, whereas those treated later have a mortality of about 25 per cent.[188,190] Surprisingly, the presence of a mediastinal infection does not appear to reduce the likelihood of patency of coronary artery bypass grafts.[193]

INFECTIVE ENDOCARDITIS

(See Chap. 33)

It has been convincingly shown that perioperative antibiotic prophylaxis is of benefit in patients undergoing cardiac surgery.[194] Although the antibiotic regimen varies, in part related to local differences in microbiological flora and personal preference, it is directed against gram-positive cocci (the most frequent causative pathogen in infections after cardiac surgery) and usually contains a cephalosporin. The regimen utilized in our institution consists of 1 gm of cefazolin intravenously 30 minutes before the skin incision and then repeated at 8-hour intervals for 48 hours after operation.

Cardiac surgery does not appear to increase the risk of endocarditis in patients with abnormal native valves that are not repaired or replaced during the operative procedure, in patients with intracardiac shunts, or in patients with intravascular devices (e.g., permanent pacemaker wires or renal dialysis shunts).[195] Assuming no infection is present preoperatively, such patients need only receive the standard antibiotic prophylaxis regimen in force at the institution in which the surgery is being performed.

PROSTHETIC VALVE ENDOCARDITIS (see p. 1079). Prosthetic valve endocarditis is a rare but extremely serious complication of cardiac surgery, frequently arising from nosocomial bacteremias.[196–198] It is estimated to occur in only 2 to 4 per cent of patients; about half of the cases are classified as "early" (<60 days from the date of operation) and half as "late" (>60 days from the date of operation).[196–199] The pooled data from several series indicate that the organism responsible for early prosthetic valve endocarditis includes a *Staphylococcus* species in about 50 per cent of cases.[199] The remainder of early cases of prosthetic valve endocarditis are caused by gram-negative bacilli, diphtheroids, and fungi.

The microbiological spectrum of late prosthetic valve endocarditis is more characteristic of that seen with native valve endocarditis. Only 30 per cent of cases are due to either *S. epidermidis* or *S. aureus*, and slightly more than one-third are caused by *Streptococcus* species (*group D streptococci* and *Streptococcus pneumoniae*).

The nature of the pathology in prosthetic valve endocarditis varies, depending on the type of prosthesis.[199] Mechanical valves typically show a ring abscess or myocardial abscess, whereas porcine heterografts more commonly develop valvar stenosis or regurgitation as a result of the endocarditis.

Management. Features of prosthetic valve endocarditis that have been associated with increased mortality include invasive infection (i.e., extension into the myocardium), congestive heart failure resulting from dysfunction of the prosthesis, and the presence of antibiotic-resistant, virulent microorganisms or a fungal organism.[199] Appropriate antibiotic therapy for prosthetic valve endocarditis is discussed in Chapter 33.

Advances in the treatment of congestive heart failure and the current generation of antibiotics may allow postponement of surgery to achieve a healed status in the absence of any compelling indication for urgent operation.[200] Transthoracic and if needed transesophageal echocardiography should be employed to clarify the severity of the hemodynamic lesion and search for any endocarditis-associated complications such as vegetations and paravalvular abscesses that may influence the timing of operation and the choice of prosthesis at surgery (e.g., unstented aortic homograft if extensive aortic root reconstruction is required).[5] The following clinical characteristics indicate the need for early operative intervention: (1) moderate to severe congestive heart failure caused by prosthetic valve dysfunction (incompetence or stenosis); (2) signs of extension of the infection into the perivalvular tissue or formation of a myocardial abscess (new electrocardiographic conduction abnormalities, pericarditis, valve dehiscence, persistent unexplained fever beyond 10 days of antibiotic treatment); (3) infection caused by aggressive, invasive organisms or those that are difficult to eradicate (fungi, *S. aureus*, some cases of *S. epidermidis*); (4) persistently positive blood cultures despite appropriate antibiotic therapy; (5) relapse of the clinical syndrome of endocarditis after appropriate antibiotic therapy; and (6) recurrent systemic emboli.

VIRAL. Viral infections that occur after cardiac surgery are almost exclusively the result of infectious complications of transfusion therapy, and with the exception of human immunodeficiency virus, primarily result in hepatitis. The incidence of viral infections after cardiac operations is decreasing as a result of a reduction in the number of transfusions of blood bank products (e.g., cell-saver techniques and preoperative autologous blood donations) and improved screening techniques in contemporary blood bank practice. CMV infection is a febrile syndrome that typically presents 1 month postoperatively. It is characterized by high-spiking fevers, abnormalities of liver function tests, and arthralgias. A self-limited illness, it is best treated with antipyretics and supportive fluid therapy.

Hepatitis C is caused by an RNA virus and is characterized by a protracted course with fluctuating transaminase levels.[201] About 50 per cent of patients respond to a course of interferon therapy with a reduction in transaminase levels; half of the responders relapse over the long term.[202,203]

FUNGAL. Fungal infections that involve the heart are rare. They typically are seen in cases of fungemia and usually are fatal. Although the problem of fungemia is well described in the immunocompromised host (e.g., heart transplant recipient), in an autopsy study of 60 patients with fungal infections of the heart 25 per cent of cases occurred in association with conventional valvular surgery.[204] About half of fungal infections of the heart are confined to the endocardium, and half involve both the endocardium and the myocardium. Extracardiac involvement is common, with spread of the infection to the lungs, cerebrospinal fluid, urine, and skin. The most commonly encountered organisms, in descending order of frequency, are *Candida, Aspergillus,* and *Cryptococcus* species. Patients who appear at particular risk of fungal involvement of the heart are those who have received corticosteroids and long courses of antibiotic treatment postoperatively.

Peripheral Vascular Complications

Most adults who undergo cardiac surgery—especially coronary revascularization—have atherosclerosis of the peripheral vasculature (e.g., ileofemoral system) and may experience lower-extremity ischemia after surgery because of low flow in the perioperative period with in situ thrombosis, embolism from the heart or aorta, or vascular compromise from an intra-aortic balloon pump catheter. Management consists of anticoagulation and removal of indwelling catheters, if clinically feasible. Thrombectomy and even revascularization surgery of the lower extremities (e.g., femorofemoral, femoropopliteal, or axillofemoral bypass) may be required to salvage threatened limbs.

Asymptomatic deep venous thrombosis of the calf can develop before hospital discharge in about one-third to one-half of patients who receive saphenous vein bypass grafts. Occasionally, these thrombi propagate to the proximal leg veins; only rarely do they cause massive pulmonary embolism.[45,205] The best strategy is rigorous perioperative prophylaxis against venous thromboembolism in all such patients. "Minidose unfractionated heparin" (5000 units subcutaneously initiated 2 hours preoperatively and continued every 8 to 12 hours postoperatively) appears to be efficacious.

Other Complications

PERICARDITIS (see Chap. 43). Postoperative tamponade is discussed on p. 152. Pericardial friction rubs frequently are audible in the early postoperative period and probably are the result of mechanical irritation from the mediastinal chest tubes. They usually disappear by the second or third postoperative day and are asymptomatic because of the narcotic analgesics prescribed at that stage of recovery. Although some patients develop pericardial rubs toward the end of the first postoperative week, these usually are benign, do not indicate a need for prolongation of hospitalization, and do not require treatment. A separate clinical syndrome that appears late in the first postoperative month is the *postpericardiotomy syndrome* (p. 230).[206] The relation between the postpericardotomy syndrome and chronic constrictive pericarditis is not firmly established, but a number of patients with *postoperative constrictive pericarditis*[144] have a history of postpericardiotomy syndrome.

RENAL FAILURE (see Chap. 62). All patients who undergo cardiac surgery experience a reduction in renal blood flow and glomerular filtration rate (GFR) as a consequence of both anesthesia and cardiopulmonary bypass. Risk factors for the development of persistent renal failure after cardiac surgery include a preoperative history of renal dysfunction or left ventricular dysfunction, prolonged bypass time (>180 minutes), prolonged aortic cross-clamping (>40 minutes), perioperative hypotension, advanced age (>70 years), and the development postoperatively of medical complications.[207]

Most cases of acute renal failure after cardiac surgery result from renal ischemia that lowers the GFR directly (prerenal disease) or, if severe or prolonged, can induce acute tubular necrosis. Possible additional contributory factors include sepsis, nephrotoxic drugs, radiocontrast material injections, cholesterol plaque embolization to the renal circulation, increased urine free hemoglobin levels from hemolysis while on cardiopulmonary bypass, and the effects of ACE inhibitors on glomerular capillary pressure.[208] The detrimental effects of ACE inhibitors are most likely to occur when renal perfusion pressure is low because of renal artery stenosis or systemic hypotension caused by cardiac failure.

Urine output is variable in patients with postoperative acute renal failure. Anuria is uncommon and, if present, should raise the suspicion of urinary tract obstruction (e.g., occluded Foley catheter). More commonly patients are either oliguric (<400 mg/day) or nonoliguric. Oliguric acute renal failure occurs less frequently than nonoliguric renal failure, usually reflects more severe renal injury, and is associated with a greater probability of requiring dialysis during the acute phase.[208]

Differentiation Between Prerenal Azotemia and Acute Tubular Necrosis. Important diagnostic studies in all patients with acute renal failure include a urinalysis and estimation of pulmonary capillary wedge pressure and cardiac output by means of pulmonary artery catheterization. Prerenal azotemia should be suspected if the urine sodium level is less than 20 mEq/liter, the fractional excretion of sodium is less than 1 per cent, and the urine osmolality level is greater than 500 mOsm/liter. Acute tubular necrosis should be suspected if the urine sodium level is greater than 40 mEq/liter, the fractional excretion of sodium is greater than 2 per cent, and the urine osmolality level is less than 350 mOsm/liter.[208]

Treatment. Essential elements of treatment for both prerenal azotemia and acute tubular necrosis include optimization of intravascular fluid volume and cardiac output. The latter is best accomplished with vasodilators and inotropic agents (see p. 1935) rather than with vasopressors, to avoid further reductions in renal blood flow. Experimental studies suggest that several modalities may protect against the development of progressive renal failure in models of acute renal ischemic injury (e.g., renal artery clamping that simulates the effects of suprarenal aortic cross-clamping while on cardiopulmonary bypass). Mannitol (which washes out obstructing casts), a loop diuretic (which decreases energy requirements in the thick ascending limb of the loop of Henle, thereby decreasing ischemic injury), and the combination of dopamine and atrial natriuretic peptide (but neither alone) have all been effective.[209] There are, however, no good clinical trials to confirm the efficacy of these interventions. Several uncontrolled observations suggest that those patients who appear to be protected by a loop diuretic, mannitol, or dopamine were all treated within 12 to 24 hours of the onset of renal dysfunction.[208]

It is prudent to undertake a trial of furosemide and mannitol (only if the patient can tolerate the volume load of the latter) within the first 12 to 24 hours after the development of oliguria. The aim of such therapy is to increase urine output. Because of the renal vasodilating effects of dopamine (3 μg/kg/min), patients with both oliguric and nonoliguric renal failure may experience an increase in urine output.[210] There is, however, no evidence that dopamine alone given in this setting is helpful for recruiting salvageable but nonfunctioning nephrons.

If oliguria persists beyond 12 hours, a number of supportive measures must be activated, including careful attention to electrolyte balance, specifically avoiding hyperkalemia; excessive free water administration that might lead to hyponatremia; correction of acidosis (adding bicarbonate to daily fluids); and adjustment of medication dosages for delayed excretion if the drug is cleared by renal mechanisms. There seems little benefit to instituting dialysis prophylactically for a given level of blood urea nitrogen or creatinine. Rather, dialysis should be carried out for pericarditis, refractory hyperkalemia, uremic encephalopathy, or colitis. Continuous arteriovenous hemofiltration is a simpler modality that can be used to remove excess fluid.

Cardiac Surgery in the Patient with Chronic Renal Failure. Finally, the patient with chronic renal failure who undergoes surgery is at increased risk of exacerbation of renal dysfunction perioperatively. This may require temporary or even permanent hemodialysis, and these eventualities should be addressed with the patient and the cardiac surgical team preoperatively. Surgery can be safely performed in patients who are already on hemodialysis, but careful coordination of the surgical and dialysis schedules is essential to minimize postoperative problems with fluid and electrolyte management. Ultrafiltration can be performed while on cardiopulmonary bypass, to help minimize the intraoperative fluid load received by the patient.

GASTROINTESTINAL COMPLICATIONS (Table 52–12).[211–213] Serious gastrointestinal complications after cardiac surgery are rare (occurring in about 1 per cent of patients) and usually can be handled by a conservative approach. Only about 0.5 per cent of patients who undergo cardiac surgery require a general surgical operation for a gastrointestinal complication.[212–214] Patients with circulatory compromise and those who require intra-aortic balloon pump support are more likely to develop gastrointestinal complications. Despite their relative rarity, gastrointestinal complications are associated with a significant mortality (approaching 40 per cent in some series), highlighting the need for careful monitoring and repeated physical examination in high-risk patients.[212–213] Most complications occur within 7 days of surgery.

NEUROLOGICAL. Neurological complications after cardiac surgery are quite common, particularly in the elderly, if one is attentive to the subtle cognitive (short-term memory loss, lack of concentration) and psychological (depression, increased sense of dependency) changes seen early after operation.[35,215] A positive and supportive attitude on the part of the staff and enlistment of the aid of family members help to minimize these problems. Although many patients return to their postoperative state by 4 to 6 weeks after surgery, about 10 per cent continue to show deterioration of their neuropsy-

TABLE 52–12 GASTROINTESTINAL COMPLICATIONS AFTER CARDIAC SURGERY

COMPLICATIONS	COMMON CAUSES	EVALUATION	TREATMENT	COMMENT
Hyperbilirubinemia				
Early (1–10 days)	"Shock liver" syndrome	Check full chemistry profile	Maximize cardiac output, BP, and oxygenation	Markedly elevated enzyme levels are seen early after onset of shock state
	Hemolysis on cardiopulmonary bypass	↑ Plasma free hemoglobin	Observe	Isolated elevation of direct and indirect bilirubin without enzyme elevation
	Right heart failure	Chest x-ray, hemodynamic monitoring	Digitalis, diuretics, oxygen, consider isoproterenol infusion	Elevated direct bilirubin and alkaline phosphatase but without enzyme elevation
Late (10–90 days)	Infection (cytomegalovirus, hepatitis C)	Viral serology	Observe	Consider interferon for hepatitis C
	Cholecystitis	Ultrasound, biliary isotopic scan (e.g., HIDA, PIPIDA)	General surgical consultation	May require ERCP, cholecystectomy, cholesystotomy
Gastroduodenal disease				
Hemorrhage	Stress gastritis	Nasogastric aspirate (pH and Hematest), CBC	Nasogastric tube, antacids, H_2-receptor antagonists, transfusions	Because of the increased risk of developing this complication, it is important to provide prophylactic treatment (antacids, H_2-receptor antagonists) to patients with COPD and postoperative hypotension, bleeding, or reoperation. Early endoscopy and consideration of surgical intervention are strongly advised if supportive medical care is unsuccessful.
	Peptic ulcer disease	Nasogastric aspirate (pH and Hematest), CBC	Nasogastric tube, antacids, H_2-receptor antagonists, transfusions	Early endoscopy and consideration of surgical intervention are strongly advised if supportive medical care is unsuccessful.
Mesenteric ischemia	Combination of low cardiac output, embolization of atherosclerotic debris or thrombi, and vascular dissection by intra-aortic balloon pump	High index of suspicion and early surgical consultation	Early laparotomy with resection of affected bowel and embolectomy when possible	Mortality rate remains high.
Pancreatitis	Hypotension, thromboembolism of vascular supply, splanchnic vasoconstriction	Serum amylase measurements serially, abdominal ultrasonogram	Nasogastric suction and fluid support	Hyperamylasemia is common after cardiac surgery, but clinical pancreatitis is rare. Severe fulminating acute pancreatitis in postcardiac surgical patients has a poor prognosis despite aggressive surgical treatment.
Miscellaneous				
Intra-abdominal bleeding	Trauma (intraop, chest tubes) Preexisting lesion (e.g., hamartoma)	Abdominal lavage	General surgical consultation	
Lower gastrointestinal tract bleed	Colonic pathology (e.g., polyp)	Plain film of abdomen, colonoscopy		
Ileus	Narcotics Adhesions	Plain film of abdomen	Nasogastric suction	

CBC, complete blood count; COPD, chronic obstructive pulmonary disease; ERCP, endoscopic retrograde cholangiopancreatography.

chrological function over the next 6 months, especially if they are over age 65.[35,215] More serious neurological complications, such as stroke (Table 52–13), occur in 1 to 5 per cent of patients, but may be seen in as many as 10 per cent of patients over age 65.[35]

Symptomatic visual defects may be seen after cardiac surgery and result from retinal emboli, occipital lobe infarction, or anterior ischemic optic neuropathy. Risk factors for cerebrovascular accident (CVA) or transient ischemic attack (TIA) after cardiac surgery include preoperative carotid bruit, previous CVA or TIA, postoperative atrial fibrillation, prolonged cardiopulmonary bypass (>2 hours), and preoperative left ventricular mural thrombus.[35,216,217]

Neuropathies in the upper extremities have been reported after cardiac operations. The pattern of injury involving predominantly the ulnar nerve and medial antebrachial cutaneous nerve suggests that the lesion involves a brachial plexus compression or traction injury.[218] The average duration of symptoms after such an injury is 2 months, but some patients show a slower time course of improvement extending over 6 to 12 months.

CHYLOTHORAX, CHYLOPERICARDIUM. These are rare postcardiac surgical complications in adults, occurring in less than 0.5 per cent of cases. Treatment of chylothorax consists of prolonged chest tube drainage and dietary support with medium-chain triglycerides. Refractory cases of chylothorax have been successfully treated by the creation of a pleuroperitoneal shunt.[219] Chylopericardium may cause cardiac tamponade (see p. 1522) and is treated by creation of a pericardial window into the pleural space and management as above for chylothorax.[220] Persistent chyle leaks may necessitate thoracic duct ligation.

REHABILITATION AND PREPARATION FOR DISCHARGE

(See Chap. 40)

A coordinated, multidisciplinary cardiac exercise program is essential to overcome the physical deconditioning

TABLE 52–13 POSSIBLE CAUSES OF STROKE AFTER CARDIAC SURGERY[35,212,216]

Embolism
- Debridement or replacement of calcified aortic valve
- Dislodgment of atherosclerotic plaque during cannulation of aorta
- Introduction of air into the arterial circulation intraoperatively
- Dislodgment of atherosclerotic plaque from carotid artery stenosis by means of "jet effect" from aortic inflow cannula
- Arrhythmia (e.g., atrial fibrillation)
- Thrombosis of mechanical prosthetic valve
- Dissection of aorta during cannulation
- Left ventricular thrombus
- Dislodgment of fragment of left atrial myxoma
- Endocarditis
- Microaggregate formation on cardiopulmonary bypass

Hemorrhage
- Anticoagulation perioperatively
- Hypertension

Hypotension
- Hypoperfusion of cerebral circulation while on cardiopulmonary bypass
- Hypoperfusion of cerebral circulation during period of postoperative shock

and psychosocial upheaval associated with cardiac surgery.[220a] Emphasis should be placed on early mobilization and progressively more patient self-care, including in the intensive care unit during the first 48 hours postoperatively. After transfer out of the intensive care unit, the patient should be encouraged to engage in low-density (2 to 3 METS) isotonic activities such as walking and range-of-motion exercises.[221] The nursing staff should monitor the patient's progress, being alert to any undue acceleration of the heart rate (>120 beats/min) or hemodynamically compromising arrhythmias.

Patients should also participate in an education program focusing on instructions regarding postoperative medications and initiation of secondary measures targeted at preventing graft occlusion and progression of atherosclerosis (Table 52–14).[90,222,223] Because of the overwhelming evidence indicating that platelet inhibition is critical to prevention of graft occlusion, all patients undergoing bypass surgery should receive long-term therapy with aspirin unless contraindicated. Ticlopidine may be useful in aspirin-intolerant patients, but there is no evidence of significant benefit from the routine use of either dipyridamole or sulfinpyrazone. Finally, innovative strategies are needed to encourage patients to return to work and society to accept postcardiac surgical patients back into the work force.

TABLE 52–14 ASSESSMENT OF RISK FACTORS AND THERAPEUTIC GOALS IN THE PATIENT WHO HAS UNDERGONE CORONARY REVASCULARIZATION

RISK FACTOR	ASSESSMENT	THERAPEUTIC GOAL
Elevated LDL cholesterol	Fasting lipid profile	<100 mg/dl (<2.6 mmol/L)
Decreased HDL cholesterol	Fasting lipid profile	>35 mg/dl (>0.9 mmol/L)
Hypertension	Blood pressures confirmed on two visits	<140/90 mm Hg
Physical inactivity	Interview	>20 min of physical activity or level walking, 1.5–2 miles/day, three times per week as a minimum
Smoking	Interview	Complete cessation
Obesity	Body weight for height	<130% of ideal body weight
Diabetes	Fasting blood glucose	<140 mg/dl
Stress	Interview	Improved coping skills

LDL, low density lipoprotein; HDL, high density lipoprotein.

Adapted from Pearson, T., Rapaport, E., Criqui, M., et al.: Optimal risk factor management in the patient after coronary revascularization. A statement for healthcare professionals from an American Heart Association Writing Group. Circulation *90*:3125, 1994. Copyright 1994 American Heart Association.

REFERENCES

1. Savage, E. B., and Cohn, L. H.: 'No Touch' dissection, antegrade-retrograde blood cardioplegia, and single aortic cross-clamp significantly reduce operative mortality of reoperative CABG. Circulation *90*:II-140, 1994.

1a. Cameron, A., Davis, K. B., Green, G., et al.: Coronary bypass surgery with internal thoracic artery grafts—effects on survival over a 15 year period. N. Engl. J. Med. *334*:216, 1996.

2. Manapat, A., McCarthy, P., Lytle, B., et al.: Gastroepiploic and inferior epigastric arteries for coronary artery bypass: Early results and evolving applications. Circulation *90*:II-144, 1994.

3. Horvath, K., Mannting, F., and Cohn, L.: Improved myocardial perfusion and relief of angina after transmyocardial laser revascularization. Circulation *90*:I-640, 1994.

3a. Frazier, O. H., Cooley, D. A., Kadipasaoglu, K. A., et al.: Myocardial revascularization with laser: Preliminary findings. Circulation *92*:58, 1995.

3b. Robinson, C. L., Gross, D. R., Zeman, W., et al.: Minimally invasive coronary artery bypass grafting: A new method using an anterior mediastinotomy. J. Card. Surg. *10*:529, 1995.

4. Jamieson, W. R.: Modern cardiac valve devices—bioprostheses and mechanical prostheses: State of the art. J. Cardiac Surg. *8*:89, 1993.

5. Petrou, M., Wong, K., Albertucci, M., et al.: Evaluation of unstented aortic homografts for the treatment of prosthetic aortic valve endocarditis. Circulation *90*:II-198, 1994.

5a. Cohn, L. C., Kowalker, W., Bhatia, S., et al.: Comparative morbidity of mitral valve repair versus replacement for mitral regurgitation with and without coronary artery disease. Ann. Thorac. Surg. *60*:1452, 1995.

5b. Cohn, L. H., Rizzo, R. J., Adams, D. H., et al.: The effect of pathophysiology on the surgical treatment of ischemic mitral regurgitation: operative and late risks of repair versus replacement. Eur. J. Cardiothorac. Surg. *9*:568, 1995.

6. Carpentier, A., and Chachques, J.: Clinical dynamic cardiomyoplasty: Method and outcome. Semin. Thorac. Cardiovasc. Surg. *3*:136, 1991.

7. Bellotti, G., Moraes, A., Bocchi, E., et al.: Late effects of cardiomyoplasty on left ventricular mechanics and diastolic filling. Circulation *88*:II-304, 1993.

8. Glick, D. B., and Ferguson, T. B.: Surgery for cardiac arrhythmias. Curr. Opin. Cardiol. *9*:222, 1994.

9. Hannan, E., Kilburn, H., Racz, M., et al.: Improving the outcomes of coronary artery bypass surgery in New York state. JAMA *271*:761, 1994.

10. Rahimtoola, S., Bennett, A., Grunkemeier, G., et al.: Survival at 15-18 years after coronary bypass surgery for angina in women. Circulation *88*:II-71, 1993.

11. Peterson, E., Jollis, J., Bebchuk, J., et al.: Changes in the mortality after myocardial revascularization in the elderly: The national Medicare experience. Ann. Intern. Med. *121*:919, 1994.

12. Nugent, W., Schults, W., Plume, S., et al.: Designing an instrument panel to monitor and improve coronary artery bypass grafting. J. Clin. Outcomes Management *1*:57, 1994.

13. Hannan, E., Siu, A., Kumar, D., et al.: The decline in coronary artery bypass graft surgery mortality in New York state: The role of surgeon volume. JAMA *273*:209, 1995.

14. Aranki, S. F., and Cohn, L. H.: Coronary artery bypass grafting in the elderly. J. Myocard. Ischemia *6*:1, 1994.

15. Aranki, S., Rizzo, R., Couper, G., et al.: Aortic valve replacement in the elderly: Effect of gender and coronary artery disease on operative mortality. Circulation *88*:II-17, 1993.

16. Frank, R. A., and Mills, N. L.: Reoperative coronary artery bypass grafting. Curr. Opin. Cardiol. *9*:680, 1994.

17. Lieberman, E., Wilson, J., Harrison, J., et al.: Aortic valve replacement in adults after balloon aortic valvuloplasty. Circulation *90*:II-205, 1994.

18. Jones, E., Weintraub, W., Craver, J., et al.: Coronary bypass surgery: Is the operation different today? J. Thorac. Cardiovasc. Surg. *101*:108, 1991.

19. Zehr, K., Lee, P., Poston, R., et al.: Two decades of coronary artery bypass graft surgery in young adults. Circulation *90*:II-133, 1994.

20. Beyersdorf, F., Mitrev, Z., Sarai, K., et al.: Changing patterns of patients undergoing emergency surgical revascularization for acute coronary occlusion: Importance of myocardial protection techniques. J. Thorac. Cardiovasc. Surg. *106*:137, 1993.

21. Disch, D., O'Connor, G., Birkmeyer, J., et al.: Changes in patients undergoing coronary artery bypass grafting. Ann. Thorac. Surg. *57*:416, 1994.

22. Edwards, F., Clark, R., and Schwartz, M.: Coronary artery bypass grafting: The Society of Thoracic Surgeons National Database experience. Ann. Thorac. Surg. *57*:12, 1994.

23. Komeda, M., David, T., Rao, V., et al.: Late hemodynamic effects of the preserved papillary muscles during mitral valve replacement. Circulation *90*:II-190, 1994.
24. Mauldin, P., Weintraub, W., and Becker, E.: Predicting hospital costs for first-time coronary artery bypass grafting from preoperative and postoperative variables. Am. J. Cardiol. *74*:772, 1994.
25. Marwick, C.: Coronary bypass grafting economics, including rehabilitation. Curr. Opin. Cardiol. *9*:635, 1994.
26. Taylor, G., Mikell, F., Moses, H., et al.: Determinants of hospital charges for coronary artery bypass surgery: The economic consequences of postoperative complications. Am. J. Cardiol. *65*:309, 1990.
27. Smith, L., Milano, C., Molter, B., et al.: Preoperative determinants of postoperative costs associated with coronary artery bypass graft surgery. Circulation *90*:II-124, 1994.
28. Sculpher, M., Seed, P., Henderson, R., et al.: Health service costs of coronary artery angioplasty and coronary artery bypass surgery: The Randomised Intervention Treatment of Angina (RITA) trial. Lancet *334*:927, 1994.

PREOPERATIVE EVALUATION

29. Wagner, E., and Trexler, S.: Preoperative evaluation. *In* Baumgartner, W., Owens, S., Cameron, D., and Reitz, B. (eds.): The Johns Hopkins Manual of Cardiac Surgical Care. St. Louis, C. V. Mosby, 1994, p. 27.
30. Vlahakes, G. J., Lemmer, J. H., Behrendt, D. M., and Austen, W. G.: Handbook of Patient Care in Cardiac Surgery. Boston, Little, Brown and Co., 1994.
31. Rizzo, R., Aranki, S., Aklog, L., et al.: Rapid noninvasive diagnosis and surgical repair of acute ascending aortic dissection. J. Thorac. Cardiovasc. Surg. *108*:567, 1994.
32. Hanet, C., Marchand, E., and Keyeux, A.: Left internal mammary artery occlusion after mastectomy and radiotherapy. Am. J. Cardiol. *65*:1044, 1990.
33. Rizzo, R., Whittemore, A., Couper, G., et al.: Combined carotid and coronary revascularization: The preferred approach to the severe vasculopath. Ann. Thorac. Surg. *54*:1099, 1992.
34. Vassilidze, T., Cernaianu, A., Gaprindashvili, T., et al.: Simultaneous coronary artery bypass and carotid endarterectomy. Texas Heart Inst. J. *21*:119, 1994.
35. Hornick, P., Smith, P., and Taylor, K.: Cerebral complications after coronary bypass grafting. Curr. Opin. Cardiol. *9*:670, 1994.
36. Barnett, H. J. M., Eliasziw, M., and Meldrum, H. E.: Drugs and surgery in the prevention of ischemic stroke. N. Engl. J. Med. *332*:238 1995.
37. Moore, W., Barnett, H., Beebe, H., et al.: Guidelines for carotid endarterectomy: A multidisciplinary consensus statement from the ad hoc committee, American Heart Association. Circulation *91*:566, 1995.
38. Acinapura, A., Jacobowitz, I., Kramer, M., et al.: Internal mammary artery bypass: Thirteen years of experience: Influence of angina and survival in 5125 patients. J. Cardiovasc. Surg. *33*:554, 1992.
39. Velebit, V., Christenson, J., Maurice, J., et al.: A patent internal mammary artery graft decreases the risk of reoperative coronary artery bypass surgery. Texas Heart Inst. J. *21*:125, 1994.
40. Lytle, B. W., McElroy, D., McCarthy, P., et al.: Influence of arterial coronary bypass grafts on the mortality in coronary reoperations. J. Thorac. Cardiovasc. Surg. *107*:675, 1994.
41. Cameron, A., Green, G., Brogno, D., and Thornton, J.: Internal thoracic artery grafts: 20-year clinical follow-up. J. Am. Coll. Cardiol. *25*:188, 1995.
42. Edwards, F., Clark, R., and Schwartz, M.: Impact of internal mammary artery conduits on operative mortality in coronary revascularization. Ann. Thorac. Surg. *57*:27, 1994.
43. Liang, B., Antman, E., Taus, R., et al.: Atherosclerotic aneurysms of aortocoronary vein grafts. Am. J. Cardiol. *61*:185, 1988.
44. Cannegieter, S., Rosendaal, F., and Briet, E.: Thromboembolic and bleeding complications in patients with mechanical heart valve prostheses. Circulation *90*:635, 1994.
45. Kondo, N. I., Maddi, R., Ewenstein, B. M., and Goldhaber, S. Z.: Anticoagulation and hemostasis in cardiac surgical patients. J. Cardiac Surg. *9*:443, 1994.
46. Tatar, H., Cicek, S., Demirkilic, U., et al.: Vascular complications of intraaortic balloon pumping: Unsheathed versus sheathed insertion. Ann. Thorac. Surg. *55*:1518, 1993.
47. Rihal, C., Eagle, K., Mickel, M., et al.: Surgical therapy for coronary artery disease among patients with combined coronary artery and peripheral vascular disease. Circulation *91*:46, 1995.
48. Higgins, T., Estafanous, F., Lloyd, F., et al.: Stratification of morbidity and mortality outcome by preoperative risk factors in coronary artery bypass patients: A clinical severity score. JAMA *267*:2344, 1992.
49. Craddock, D., Iyer, V. S., and Russell, W. J.: Factors influencing mortality and myocardial infarction after coronary artery bypass grafting. Curr. Opin. Cardiol. *9*:664, 1994.
50. Findlay, I. N.: Coronary bypass surgery in women. Curr. Opin. Cardiol. *9*:650, 1994.
51. Latimer, R., and Mahmood, N.: Predicting the outcome from cardiac surgery: Trial or tribulation. Curr. Opin. Anaesthesiol. *7*:39, 1994.
52. Iyer, V., Russell, W., Leppard, P., and Craddock, D.: Mortality and myocardial infarction after coronary artery surgery: A review of 12003 patients. Med. J. Aust. *159*:166, 1993.
53. Tu, J. V., Jaglal, S. B., Naylor, C. D., and the Steering Committee of the Provincial Adult Cardiac Care Network of Ontario: Multicenter validation of a risk index for mortality, intensive care unit stay, and overall hospital length of stay after cardiac surgery. Circulation *91*:677, 1995.
54. Loop, F. D., Lytle, B. W., Cosgrove, D. M., et al.: Sternal wound complications after isolated coronary artery bypass grafting: Early and late mortality, morbidity, and cost of care. Ann. Thorac. Surg. *49*:179, 1990.
55. Copeland, M., Senkowski, C., Ulcickas, M., et al.: Breast size as a factor for sternal wound complications following cardiac surgery. Arch. Surg. *129*:757, 1994.
56. He, G. W., Ryan, W. H., Acuff, T. E., et al.: Risk factors for operative mortality and sternal wound infection in bilateral internal mammary artery grafting. J. Thorac. Cardiovasc. Surg. *107*:196, 1994.
57. Palazzo, R., and Barner, H. B.: Surgery for ischemic heart disease. Curr. Opin. Cardiol. *9*:216, 1994.
58. Ritchie, J. L., Bateman, T. M., Bonow, R. O., et al.: Guidelines for clinical use of cardiac radionuclide imaging. J. Am. Coll. Cardiol. *25*:521, 1995.
58a. Vanoverschelde, J.-L. J., Gerber, B. L., D'Hondt, A.-M., et al.: Preoperative selection of patients with severely impaired left ventricular function for coronary revascularization: Role of low-dose dobutamine echocardiography and exercise-redistribution-reinjection thallium SPECT. Circulation *92*:37, 1995.
59. Lee, K., Marwick, T., Cook, S., et al.: Prognosis of patients with left ventricular dysfunction, with and without viable myocardium after myocardial infarction: Relative efficacy of medical therapy and revascularization. Circulation *90*:2687, 1994.
60. vom Dahl, J., Eitzman, D., Al-Aouar, Z., et al.: Relation of regional function, perfusion, and metabolism in patients with advanced coronary artery disease undergoing surgical revascularization. Circulation *90*:2356, 1994.
61. Edmond, M., Mock, M., Davis, K., et al.: Long-term survival of medically treated patients in the coronary artery surgery study (CASS) registry. Circulation *90*:2645, 1994.
62. Lomboy, C., Schulman, D., Grill, H., et al.: Rest-redistribution thallium-201 scintigraphy to determine myocardial viability early after myocardial infarction. J. Am. Coll. Cardiol. *25*:210, 1995.
63. Foster, E., O'Kelly, B., LaPidus, A., et al.: Segmental analysis of resting echocardiographic function and stress scintigraphic perfusion: Implications for myocardial viability. Am. Heart J. *129*:7, 1995.
64. Kereiakes, D., Topol, E., George, B., et al.: Emergency coronary artery bypass surgery preserves global and regional left ventricular function after intravenous tissue plasminogen activator therapy for acute myocardial infarction. J. Am. Coll. Cardiol. *11*:899, 1988.
65. Moosvi, A. R., Khaja, F., Villanueva, L., et al.: Early revascularization improves survival in cardiogenic shock complicating acute myocardial infarction. J. Am. Coll. Cardiol. *19*:7, 1992.
66. Tardiff, B., Califf, R., Morris, D., et al.: Coronary revascularization surgery following myocardial infarction: Effect of bypass surgery on survival following thrombolysis *(in press)*.
66a. Braxton, J. H., Hammond, G. L., Letsou, G. V., et al.: Optimal timing of coronary artery bypass graft surgery after acute myocardial infarction. Circulation *92*:66, 1995.
67. Mannucci, P.: Nontransfusional modalities. *In* Loscalzo, J., and Schafer, A. (eds.): Thrombosis and Hemorrhage. Boston, Blackwell Scientific Publications, 1994, p. 1117.
68. Parsons, R. S., Mohandas, K., and Riaz, N.: The effects of an intravenous infusion of isosorbide dinitrate during open heart surgery. Eur. Heart J. *9*(Suppl. A):195, 1988.
69. Gersh, B. J., Chesebro, J. H., Braunwald, E., et al.: Coronary artery bypass graft surgery after thrombolytic therapy in the Thrombolysis in Myocardial Infarction Trial, Phase II (TIMI II). J. Am. Coll. Cardiol. *23*:395, 1995.
70. Lappas, D.: Anesthesia in cardiac and noncardiac surgery: Overview. Coronary Artery Dis. *4*:399, 1993.
71. Kirklin, J., and Barratt-Boyes, B.: Anesthesia for cardiovascular surgery. *In* Kirklin, J., and Barratt-Boyes, B. (eds.): Cardiac Surgery. New York, Churchill Livingstone, 1993, p. 167.
72. Creswell, L., Schuessler, R., Rosenbloom, M., and Cox, J.: Hazards of postoperative atrial arrhythmias. Ann. Thorac. Surg. *56*:539, 1993.
73. Aranki, S., Shaw, D., Adams, D., et al.: Predictors of atrial fibrillation following coronary artery surgery: Current trends and impact on hospital resources. Circulation *(in press)*.
74. Lauer, M., and Eagle, K.: Arrhythmias following cardiac surgery. *In* Podrid, P., and Kowey, P. (eds.): Cardiac Arrhythmia. Mechanisms, Diagnosis, and Management. Baltimore, Williams and Wilkins, 1995, p. 1206.
75. Andrews, T. C., Reimold, S. C., Berlin, J. A., and Antman, E. M.: Prevention of supraventricular arrhythmias after coronary artery bypass surgery: A meta-analysis of randomized control trials. Circulation *84*(Suppl. III):236, 1991.
76. Steinberg, J., Zelenkofske, S., Wong, S., et al.: Value of the P wave signal-averaged ECG for predicting atrial fibrillation after cardiac surgery. Circulation *88*:2618, 1993.
77. Mendes, L., Connelly, G., McKenney, P., et al.: Right coronary artery stenosis: An independent predictor of atrial fibrillation after coronary artery bypass surgery. J. Am. Coll. Cardiol. *25*:198, 1995.
78. Cox, J.: A perspective on postoperative atrial fibrillation in cardiac operations. Ann. Thorac. Surg. *56*:405, 1993.
79. Aglio, L. S., Stanford, G. G., Maddi, R., et al.: Hypomagnesemia is common following cardiac surgery. J. Cardiothorac. Vasc. Anesth. *5*:201, 1991.
80. Katholi, R., Woods, W., Womack, K., et al.: $MgCl_2$ replacement after

bypass surgery to prevent atrial fibrillation: A double blind, randomized trial. Circulation *82*:III-58, 1990.

81. England, M. R., Gordon, G., Salem, M., and Chernow, B.: Magnesium administration and dysrhythmias after cardiac surgery: A placebo-controlled double-blind, randomized trial. JAMA *268*:2395, 1992.
82. Fanning, W. J., Thomas, C., Jr., Roach, A., et al.: Prophylaxis of atrial fibrillation with magnesium sulfate after coronary artery bypass grafting. Ann. Thorac. Surg. *52*:529, 1991.
83. Casthely, P. A., Yoganathan, T., Komer, C., and Kelly, M.: Magnesium and arrhythmias after coronary artery bypass surgery. J. Cardiothorac. Vasc. Anesth. *8*:188, 1994.
84. Chassard, D., George, M., Giuraud, M., et al.: Relationship between preoperative amiodarone treatment and complications observed during anaesthesia for valvular cardiac surgery. Can. J. Anaesth. *37*:251, 1990.
85. Nalos, P. C., Kass, R. M., Gang, E. S., et al.: Life-threatening postoperative pulmonary complications in patients with previous amiodarone pulmonary toxicity undergoing cardiothoracic operations. J. Thorac. Cardiovasc. Surg. *93*:904, 1987.
86. Kupferschmid, J. P., Rosengart, T. K., McIntosh, C. L., et al.: Amiodarone-induced complications after cardiac operation for obstructive hypertrophic cardiomyopathy. Ann. Thorac. Surg. *48*:359, 1989.
87. Barbieri, E., Conti, F., Zampieri, P., et al.: Amiodarone and desethylamiodarone distribution in the atrium and adipose tissue of patients undergoing short- and long-term treatment with amiodarone. J. Am. Coll. Cardiol. *8*:210, 1986.
88. Lamas, G., Rebecca, G., Braunwald, N., and Antman, E.: Pacemaker malfunction after nitrous oxide anesthesia. Am. J. Cardiol. *56*:995, 1985.
89. Lamas, G., Antman, E., Gold, J., et al.: Pacemaker back-up mode reversion and injury during cardiac surgery. Ann. Throac. Surg. *41*:155, 1986.
90. Pearson, T., Rapaport, E., Criqui, M., et al.: Optimal risk factor management in the patient after coronary revascularization: A statement for healthcare professionals from an American Heart Association writing group. Circulation *90*:3125, 1994.
91. Murkin, J. M., Lux, J., Shannon, N. A., et al.: Aprotinin significantly decreases bleeding and transfusion requirements in patients receiving aspirin and undergoing cardiac operations. J. Thorac. Cardiovasc. Surg. *107*:554, 1994.

INTRAOPERATIVE MANAGEMENT

92. Kirklin, J. W., and Barratt-Boyes, B. G.: Cardiac Surgery. Morphology, Diagnostic Criteria, Natural History, Techniques, Results, and Indications. 2nd ed. New York, Churchill Livingstone, 1993.
93. D'Ambra, M.: Is intraoperative echocardiography a useful monitor in the operating room? Ann. Thorac. Surg. *56*:S83, 1993.
94. Aranki, S., Rizzo, R., Adams, D., et al.: Single-clamp technique: An important adjunct to myocardial and cerebral protection in coronary operations. Ann. Thorac. Surg. *58*:296, 1994.
95. Krukenkamp, I., Burns, P., Calderone, C., and Levitsky, S.: Perfusion and cardioplegia. Curr. Opin. Cardiol. *9*:247, 1994.
96. Hines, R. L.: Transesophageal echocardiography: Is it for everyone? J. Cardiac Surg. *5*:240, 1990.
96a. Joffe, I. I., Jacobs, L. E., Lampert, C., et al.: Role of echocardiography in perioperative management of patients undergoing open heart surgery. Am. Heart J. *131*:162, 1995.
97. Horvath, K., Smith, W., Laurence, R., et al.: Recovery and viability of an acute myocardial infarct after transmyocardial laser revascularization. J. Am. Coll. Cardiol. *25*:258, 1995.
97a. Flameng, W.: New strategies for intraoperative myocardial protection. Curr. Opin. Cardiol. *10*:577, 1995.
98. Aranki, S.: Cardiovascular surgery in the elderly. *In* Homburger, F. (ed.): The Rational Use of Advanced Medical Technology with the Elderly. New York, Springer-Verlag, 1994, p. 132.
99. Aprotonin to decrease bleeding in cardiac surgery. Med. Lett. *36*:50, 1994.
100. Videm, V., Svennevig, J., Fosse, E., et al.: Reduced complement activation with heparin-coated oxygenator and tubings in coronary bypass operations. J. Thorac. Cardiovasc. Surg. *103*:806, 1992.
101. Jones, D., Hill, R., Hollingsed, M., et al.: Use of heparin-coated cardiopulmonary bypass. Ann. Thorac. Surg. *56*:556, 1993.
102. Leung, J. M., Stanley, T. R., Mathew, J., et al.: An initial multicenter, randomized controlled trial on the safety and efficacy of acadesine in patients undergoing coronary artery bypass graft surgery: SPI Research Group. Anesth. Analg. *78*:420, 1994.

POSTOPERATIVE MANAGEMENT

103. Kirklin, J., and Barratt-Boyes, B.: Postoperative care. *In* Kirklin, J., and Barratt-Boyes, B. (eds.): Cardiac Surgery. New York, Churchill Livingstone, 1993, p. 195.
104. Lippmann, M., Goldberg, S., and Walkenstein, M.: Pulmonary complications of open heart surgery. *In* Kotler, M., and Alfieri, A. (eds.): Cardiac and Noncardiac Complications of Open Heart Surgery: Prevention, Diagnosis, and Treatment. Mt. Kisco, N.Y., Futura, 1992, p. 239.
105. Walden, S., and Meyer, P.: Pulmonary management. *In* Baumgartner, W., Owens, S., Cameron, D., and Reitz, B. (eds.): The Johns Hopkins Manual of Cardiac Surgical Care. St. Louis, C. V. Mosby, 1994, p. 161.
106. Quasha, A. C., Loeber, N., Feeley, T. W., et al.: Postoperative respiratory care: A controlled trial of early and late extubation following coronary artery bypass grafting. Anesthesiology *52*:135, 1980.
107. Cambier, B., Missault, L., Kockx, M., et al.: Influence of the breathing mode on the time course and amplitude of the cyclic inter-atrial pressure reversal in postoperative coronary bypass surgery patients. Eur. Heart J. *14*:920, 1993.
108. Svennevig, J., Geiran, O., Karlsen, J., et al.: Complement activation during extracorporeal circulation: In vitro comparison of duraflo-II heparin-coated and uncoated oxygenator circuits. J. Thorac. Cardiovasc. Surg. *106*:466, 1993.
109. Shafique, T., Johnson, R., Dai, H., et al.: Altered pulmonary microvascular reactivity after total cardiopulmonary bypass. J. Thorac. Cardiovasc. Surg. *106*:479, 1993.
110. Butler, J., Rocker, G. M., and Westaby, S.: Inflammatory response to cardiopulmonary bypass. Ann. Thorac. Surg. *55*:552, 1993.
111. Aranki, S., Adams, D., Rizzo, R., et al.: Femoral veno-arterial extracorporeal life support with minimal or no heparin. Ann. Thorac. Surg. *56*:149, 1993.
112. Lam, A., and Newhouse, M.: Management of asthma and chronic airflow limitation. Chest *98*:44, 1990.
113. Curtis, J. J., Weerachai, N., Walls, J. T., et al.: Elevated hemidiaphragm after cardiac operations: Incidence, prognosis, and relationship to the use of topical ice slush. Ann. Thorac. Surg. *48*:764, 1989.
114. Abd, G., Braun, N., Baskin, M., et al.: Diaphragmatic dysfunction after open heart surgery: Treatment with a rocking bed. Ann. Intern. Med. *111*:881, 1989.
115. Graham, D. R., Kaplan, D., Evans, C. C., et al.: Diaphragmatic plication for unilateral diaphragmatic paralysis: A 10-year experience. Ann. Thorac. Surg. *49*:248, 1990.
116. Weiss, S. J., and Longnecker, D. E.: Perioperative hypertension: An overview. Coronary Artery Dis. *4*:401, 1993.
117. Gray, R. J., Bateman, T. M., Czer, L. S., et al.: Use of esmolol in hypertension after cardiac surgery. Am. J. Cardiol. *56*:56, 1985.
118. Estafanous, F., and Tarazi, R.: Systemic arterial hypertension associated with cardiac surgery. Am. J. Cardiol. *46*:685, 1980.
119. Cooper, T. J., Clutton, B. T. H., Jones, S. N., et al.: Factors relating to the development of hypertension after cardiopulmonary bypass. Br. Heart J. *54*:91, 1985.
120. Rocchini, A., Rosenthal, A., Barger, A., et al.: Pathogenesis of paradoxical hypertension after coarctation resection. Circulation *54*:382, 1976.
121. O'Dwyer, J. P., Yorukoglu, D., and Harris, M. N.: The use of esmolol to attenuate the haemodynamic response when extubating patients following cardiac surgery—a double-blind controlled study. Eur. Heart J. *14*:701, 1993.
122. James, T., Hageman, G., and Urthaler, F.: Anatomic and physiologic considerations of a cardiogenic hypertensive reflex. Am. J. Cardiol. *44*:852, 1979.
123. Baumgartner, W., Owens, S., Cameron, D., and Reitz, B.: The Johns Hopkins Manual of Cardiac Surgical Care. St. Louis, C. V. Mosby, 1994, p. 546.
124. Leslie, J., Brister, N., Levy, J., et al.: Treatment of postoperative hypertension after coronary artery bypass surgery: Double-blind comparison of intravenous isradipine and sodium nitroprusside. Circulation *90*:II-256, 1994.
125. Ruiz, R., Borches, D., Gonzalez, A., and Corral, J.: A new sodium-nitroprusside-infusion controller for the regulation of arterial blood pressure. Biomed. Instrum. Technol. *27*:244, 1993.
126. Bruss, J., Meyerowitz, C., Greenspan, A., and Spielman, S.: The significance of the electrocardiogram after open heart surgery. *In* Kotler, M., and Alfieri, A. (eds.): Cardiac and Noncardiac Complications of Open Heart Surgery: Prevention, Diagnosis, and Treatment. Mt. Kisco, N.Y., Futura, 1992, p. 39.
127. Hamm, C. W., Reimers, J., Ischinger, T., et al.: A randomized study of coronary angioplasty compared with bypass surgery in patients with symptomatic multivessel coronary disease: German Angioplasty Bypass Surgery Investigation (GABI). N. Engl. J. Med. *331*:1037, 1994.
128. King, S. E., Lembo, N. J., Weintraub, W. S., et al.: A randomized trial comparing coronary angioplasty with coronary bypass surgery: Emory Angioplasty versus Surgery Trial (EAST). N. Engl. J. Med. *331*:1044, 1994.
129. Greaves, S., Rutherford, J., Aranki, S., et al.: Current incidence and determinants of perioperative myocardial infarction in coronary artery surgery. Am. Heart J. *(in press)*.
130. Lemmer, J. H., Jr., and Kirsh, M. M.: Coronary artery spasm following coronary artery surgery. Ann. Thorac. Surg. *46*:108, 1988.
131. Obarski, T. P., Loop, F. D., Cosgrove, D. M., et al.: Frequency of acute myocardial infarction in valve repairs versus valve replacement for pure mitral regurgitation. Am. J. Cardiol. *65*:887, 1990.
132. Bulkley, B. H., and Hutchins, G. M.: Myocardial consequences of coronary artery bypass graft surgery: The paradox of necrosis in areas of revascularization. Circulation *56*:906, 1977.
133. Katus, H., Schoeppenthau, M., Tanzeem, A., et al.: Non-invasive assessment of perioperative myocardial cell damage by circulating cardiac troponin T. Br. Heart J. *65*:259, 1991.
134. Mair, J., Larue, C., Mair, P., et al.: Use of cardiac troponin I to diagnose perioperative myocardial infarction in coronary artery bypass grafting. Clin. Chem. *40*:2066, 1994.
135. Bateman, T., Matloff, J., and Gray, R.: Myocardial infarction during coronary artery bypass surgery-benign event or prognostic omen? Int. J. Cardiol. *6*:259, 1984.
136. Force, T., Hibberd, P., Weeks, G., et al.: Perioperative myocardial infarction after coronary artery bypass surgery. Circulation *82*:903, 1990.
137. Feneck, R. O.: Intravenous milrinone following cardiac surgery: I. Ef-

fects of bolus infusion followed by variable dose maintenance infusion: The European Milrinone Multicentre Trial Group. J. Cardiothorac. Vasc. Anesth. *6*:554, 1992.

138. Lee, W. A., Gillinov, A. M., Cameron, D. E., et al.: Centrifugal ventricular assist device for support of the failing heart after cardiac surgery. Crit. Care Med. *21*:1186, 1993.
139. Oz, M., Rose, E., and Levin, H.: Selection criteria for placement of left ventricular assist devices. Am. Heart J. *129*:173, 1995.
140. Reichert, C. L., Koolen, J. J., and Visser, C. A.: Transesophageal echocardiographic evaluation of left ventricular function during intraaortic balloon pump counterpulsation. J. Am. Soc. Echocardiogr. *6*:490, 1993.
141. Reichert, C. L., Visser, C. A., Van den Brink, R. B., et al.: Prognostic value of biventricular function in hypotensive patients after cardiac surgery as assessed by transesophageal echocardiography. J. Cardiothorac. Vasc. Anesth. *6*:429, 1992.
142. Mikawa, K., Maekawa, N., Goto, R., et al.: Use of prostaglandin E1 to treat perianaesthetic pulmonary hypertension associated with mitral valve disease. J. Int. Med. Res. *21*:161, 1993.
143. Rich, G. F., Murphy, G. D., Jr., Roos, C. M., and Johns, R. A.: Inhaled nitric oxide: Selective pulmonary vasodilation in cardiac surgical patients. Anesthesiology *78*:1028, 1993.
144. D'Cruz, I. A., Overton, D. H., and Pai, G. M.: Pericardial complications of cardiac surgery: Emphasis on the diagnostic role of echocardiography. J. Cardiac Surg. *7*:257, 1992.
145. Pepi, M., Muratori, M., Barbier, P., et al.: Pericardial effusion after cardiac surgery: Incidence, site, size, and haemodynamic consequences. Br. Heart J. *72*:327, 1994.
146. Chuttani, K., Tischler, M. D., Pandian, N. G., et al.: Diagnosis of cardiac tamponade after cardiac surgery: Relative value of clinical, echocardiographic, and hemodynamic signs. Am. Heart J. *127*:913, 1994.
147. Russo, A. M., O'Connor, W. H., and Waxman, H. L.: Atypical presentations and echocardiographic findings in patients with cardiac tamponade occurring early and late after cardiac surgery. Chest *104*:71, 1993.
148. Schoebrechts, B., Herregods, M. C., Van, D. W. F., and De, G. H.: Usefulness of transesophageal echocardiography in patients with hemodynamic deterioration late after cardiac surgery. Chest *104*:1631, 1993.
149. Moore, S. L., and Wilkoff, B. L.: Rhythm disturbances after cardiac surgery. Semin. Thorac. Cardiovasc. Surg. *3*:24, 1991.
150. Gottipaty, V., Kocovic, D., Kinchla, N., et al.: Timing and impact on survival of in-hospital cardiac arrest after coronary artery bypass graft surgery. Circulation *88*:I-166, 1993.
151. Waldo, A. L., and MacLean, W. A.: Treatment of cardiac arrhythmias with emphasis on cardiac pacing. *In* Diagnosis and Treatment of Cardiac Arrhythmias Following Open Heart Surgery: Emphasis on the Use of Atrial and Ventricular Epicardial Wire Electrodes. Mt. Kisco, N.Y., Futura, 1980, p. 115.
152. Olshansky, B., Okumura, K., Hess, P. G., et al.: Use of procainamide with rapid atrial pacing for successful conversion of atrial flutter to sinus rhythm. J. Am. Coll. Cardiol. *11*:359, 1988.
153. Platia, E. V., Fitzpatrick, P., Wallis, D., et al.: Esmolol vs verapamil for the treatment of recent-onset atrial fibrillation/flutter. J. Am. Coll. Cardiol. *11*:170, 1988.
154. Reed, G. L., Singer, D. E., and Pilard, E. H.: Stroke following coronary artery bypass surgery: A case control estimate of the risk of carotid bruits. N. Engl. J. Med. *319*:1246, 1988.
155. Eckman, M. H., Levine, H. J., and Pauker, S. G.: Making decisions about antithrombotic therapy in heart disease: Decision analytic and cost-effectiveness issues. Chest *108*:457S, 1995.
155a. Raitt, M. H., Dolack, G. L., Kino, K., et al.: Procainamide has limited effectiveness for the treatment of atrial fibrillation after open heart surgery. Circulation *90*(Supp. 1):376, 1994.
156. Laupacis, A., Albers, G. W., Dalen, J. E., et al.: Antithrombotic therapy in atrial fibrillation. Chest *108*:352S, 1995.
157. Raitt, M., Dolack, G., Kino, K., et al.: Procainamide has limited effectiveness for the treatment of atrial fibrillation after open heart surgery. Circulation *90*:I-376, 1994.
158. Ganz, L., and Friedman, P.: Medical progress: Supraventricular tachycardia. N. Engl. J. Med. *332*:162, 1995.
159. Rubin, D., Nieminski, K., Monteferrante, J., et al.: Ventricular arrhythmias after coronary artery bypass graft surgery: Incidence, risk factors and long-term prognosis. J. Am. Coll. Cardiol. *6*:307, 1985.
160. Smith, R., Leung, J., Keith, F., et al.: Ventricular dysrhythmias in patients undergoing coronary artery bypass graft surgery: Incidence, characteristics, and prognostic significance. Am. Heart J. *123*:73, 1992.
161. Johnson, R., Goldberger, A., Thurer, R., et al.: Lidocaine prophylaxis in coronary revascularization patients: A randomized prospective trial. Ann. Thorac. Surg. *55*:1180, 1993.
162. Rousou, J., Engelman, R., Flack, J., III, et al.: Emergency cardiopulmonary bypass in the cardiac surgical unit can be a lifesaving measure in postoperative cardiac arrest. Circulation *90*(Suppl. II):280, 1994.
163. Carlson, M., Biblo, L., and Waldo, A.: Post open heart surgery ventricular arrhythmias. Cardiovasc. Clin. *22*:241, 1992.
164. Holman, W., Spruell, R., Vicente, W., and Pacifico, A.: Electrophysiological mechanisms for postcardioplegia reperfusion ventricular fibrillation. Circulation *90*:II-293, 1994.
164a. Costeas, X. F., and Schoenfeld, M. H.: Usefulness of electrophysiologic studies for new-onset sustained ventricular tachyarrhythmias shortly after coronary artery bypass grafting. Am. J. Cardiol. *72*:1291, 1993.
165. Scott, W. A.: Temporary DDD pacing after surgically induced heart block. Am. J. Cardiol. *71*:1123, 1993.
166. Hippeläinen, M., Mustonen, P., Manninen, H., and Rehnberg, S.: Predictors of conduction disturbances after coronary bypass grafting. Ann. Thorac. Surg. *57*:1284, 1994.
167. Baerman, J., Kirsh, M., de Buitleir, M., et al.: Natural history and determinants of conduction defects following coronary artery bypass surgery. Ann. Thorac. Surg. *44*:150, 1987.
168. Tuzcu, E. M., Emre, A., Goormastic, M., et al.: Incidence and prognostic significance of intraventricular conduction abnormalities after coronary bypass surgery. J. Am. Coll. Cardiol. *16*:607, 1990.
169. Emlein, G., Huang, S., Pires, L., et al.: Prolonged bradyarrhythmias after isolated coronary artery bypass graft surgery. Am. Heart J. *126*:1084, 1993.
170. Tsai, T., and Matloff, J.: Cardiac surgery in the elderly. *In* Matloff, R. G. A. J. (ed.): Medical Management of the Cardiac Surgical Patient. Baltimore, Williams and Wilkins, 1990, p. 27.
171. Kestin, A. S., Valeri, C. R., Khuri, S. F., et al.: The platelet function defect of cardiopulmonary bypass. Blood *82*:107, 1993.
172. Kalfin, R., Engelman, R., Rousou, J., et al.: Induction of interleukin-8 expression during cardiopulmonary bypass. Circulation *88*:II-401, 1993.
173. Cines, D. B., Tomaski, A., and Tannenbaum, S.: Immune endothelial-cell injury in heparin-associated thrombocytopenia. N. Engl. J. Med. *316*:581, 1987.
174. Kajani, M., and Waxman, H.: Hematologic problems after open heart surgery. *In* Kotler, M., and Alfieri, A. (eds.): Cardiac and Noncardiac Complications of Open Heart Surgery: Prevention, Diagnosis, and Treatment. Mt. Kisco, N.Y., Futura, 1992, p. 219.
175. Cormack, J. G., and Levy, J. H.: Adverse reactions to protamine. Coronary Artery Dis. *4*:420, 1993.
176. Brister, S. J., Ofosu, F. A., and Buchanan, M. R.: Thrombin generation during cardiac surgery: Is heparin the ideal anticoagulant? Thromb. Haemost. *70*:259, 1993.
177. Walenga, J., Bakhos, M., Messmore, H., et al.: Potential use of recombinant hirudin as an anticoagulant in a cardiopulmonary bypass model. Ann. Thorac. Surg. *51*:271, 1991.
178. Mossad, E., and Estafanous, F.: Blood use in cardiac surgery and the limitations of hemodilution. Curr. Opin. Cardiol. *10*:584, 1995.
179. Baumgartner, W., and Owens, S.: Hemorrhage and tamponade. *In* Baumgartner, W., Owens, S., Cameron, D., and Reitz, B. (eds.).: The Johns Hopkins Manual of Cardiac Surgical Care. St. Louis, C. V. Mosby, 1994, p. 183.
180. Kallis, P., Tooze, J. A., Talbot, S., et al.: Aprotinin inhibits fibrinolysis, improves platelet adhesion and reduces blood loss: Results of a double-blind randomized clinical trial. Eur. J. Cardiothorac. Surg. *8*:315, 1994.
180a. Royston, D.: Aprotinin in patients having coronary artery bypass graft surgery. Curr. Opin. Cardiol. *10*:591, 1995.
181. Stein, P. D., Alpert, J. S., Copeland III, J. G., et al.: Antithrombotic therapy in patients with mechanical and biological prosthetic heart valves. Chest *108*:371S, 1995.
182. Verkkala, V., Valtonen, V., Jarvinen, A., and Tolppanen, E.: Fever, leukocytosis and C-reactive protein after open-heart surgery and their value in the diagnosis of postoperative infections. Thorac. Cardiovasc. Surg. *35*:78, 1987.
183. Livelli, F., Johnson, R., McEnany, M., et al.: Unexplained in-hospital fever following cardiac surgery: Natural history, relationship to post-pericardiotomy syndrome, and a prospective study of therapy with indomethacin versus placebo. Circulation *57*:968, 1978.
184. Baddour, L., and Bisno, A.: Recurrent cellulitis after saphenous venectomy for coronary bypass surgery. Ann. Intern. Med. *97*:493, 1982.
185. Greenberg, J., DeSanctis, R. W., and Mills, R. M. J.: Vein-donor-leg cellulitis after coronary artery bypass surgery. Ann. Intern. Med. *97*:565, 1982.
186. Spencer, F. C., and Grossi, E. A.: Mediastinitis after cardiac operations. Ann. Thorac. Surg. *49*:506, 1990.
187. Demmy, T. L., Park, S. B., Liebler, G. A., et al.: Recent experience with major sternal wound complications. Ann. Thorac. Surg. *49*:458, 1990.
188. Greenblatt, J., and Fischer, R.: Complications of cardiac surgery: Infections. *In* Kotler, M., and Alfieri, A. (eds.): Cardiac and Noncardiac Complications of Open Heart Surgery: Prevention, Diagnosis, and Treatment. Mt. Kisco, N.Y., Futura, 1992, p. 145.
189. Kouchoukos, N. T., Wareing, T. H., Murphy, S. F., et al.: Risks of bilateral internal mammary artery bypass grafting. Ann. Thorac. Surg. *49*:210, 1990.
190. Bor, D. H., Rose, R. M., Modlin, J. F., et al.: Mediastinitis after cardiovascular surgery. Rev. Infect. Dis. *5*:885, 1983.
191. Kernodle, D. S., Classen, D. C., Burke, J. P., and Kaiser, A. B.: Failure of cephalosporins to prevent *Staphylococcus aureus* surgical wound infections. JAMA *263*:961, 1990.
192. Omura, K., Misaki, T., Takahashi, H., et al.: Omental transfer for the treatment of sternal infarction after cardiac surgery: Report of three cases. Surg. Today *24*:67, 1994.
193. Macmanus, Q., and Okies, J. E.: Mediastinal wound infection and aortocoronary graft patency. Am. J. Surg. *132*:558, 1976.
194. Hall, J., Christiansen, K., Carter, M., et al.: Antibiotic prophylaxis in cardiac operations. Ann. Thorac. Surg. *56*:916, 1993.
195. Keys, T. F.: Antimicrobial prophylaxis for patients with congenital or valvular heart disease. Mayo Clin. Proc. *57*:171, 1982.
196. Threlkeld, M., and Cobbs, C.: Infectious disorders of prosthetic valves and intravascular devices. *In* Mandell, G., Douglas, R., and Bennett, J. (eds.): Principles and Practice of Infectious Diseases. New York, Churchill-Livingstone, 1990, p. 706.
197. Hall, T., and Reitz, B.: Valve replacement and repair. *In* Baumgartner,

W., Owens, S., Cameron, D., and Reitz, B. (eds.): The Johns Hopkins Manual of Cardiac Surgical Care. St. Louis, C. V. Mosby, 1994, p. 365.

198. Fang, G., Keys, T., Gentry, L., et al.: Prosthetic valve endocarditis resulting from nosocomial bacteremia: A prospective multicenter study. Ann. Intern. Med. *119:*560, 1993.

199. Cowgill, L. D., Addonizio, V. P., Hopeman, A. G., and Harken, A. H.: A practical approach to prosthetic valve endocarditis. Ann. Thorac. Surg. *43:*450, 1987.

200. Aranki, S., Santini, F., Adams, D., et al.: Aortic valve endocarditis: Determinants of early survival and late morbidity. Circulation *90:*II-175, 1994.

201. Tremolada, F., Casarin, C., Alberti, A., et al.: Long-term follow-up of non-A, non-B (type C) post-transfusion hepatitis. J. Hepatol. *16:*273, 1992.

202. Davis, G., Balart, L., Schiff, E., et al.: Treatment of chronic hepatitis C with recombinant interferon alfa: A multicenter randomized, controlled trial. N. Engl. J. Med. *321:*1501, 1989.

203. DiBisceglie, A. M., Martin, P., Kassiandes, C., et al.: Recombinant interferon ALFA therapy for chronic hepatitis C. N. Engl. J. Med. *321:*1506, 1989.

204. Atkinson, J. B., Connor, D. H., Robinowitz, M., et al.: Cardiac fungal infections: Review of autopsy findings in 60 patients. Hum. Pathol. *15:*935, 1984.

205. Gillinov, A. M., Davis, E. A., Alberg, A. J., et al.: Pulmonary embolism in the cardiac surgical patient. Ann. Thorac. Surg. *53:*988, 1992.

206. Khan, A. H.: The postcardiac injury syndromes. Clin. Cardiol. *15:*67, 1992.

207. Kellerman, P. S.: Perioperative care of the renal patient. Arch. Intern. Med. *154:*1674, 1994.

208. Kobrin, S., and Tobias, S.: Renal complications of open heart surgery. *In* Kotler, M., and Alfieri, A. (eds.): Cardiac and Noncardiac Complications of Open Heart Surgery: Prevention, Diagnosis, and Treatment. Mt. Kisco, N.Y., Futura, 1992, p. 311.

209. Rose, B.: Acute renal failure-prerenal disease versus acute tubular necrosis. *In* Rose, B. (ed.): Pathophysiology of Renal Disease. New York, McGraw-Hill Book Co., 1987, p. 63.

210. Casale, A., and Ulrich, S.: Complications in other organ systems. *In* Baumgartner, W., Owens, S., Cameron, D., and Reitz, B. (eds.): The Johns Hopkins Manual of Cardiac Surgical Care. St. Louis, C. V. Mosby, 1994, p. 271.

211. Kelberman, I., and Levine, G.: Gastroenterologic complications of open heart surgery. *In* Motler, M., and Alfieri, A. (eds.): Cardiac and Noncardiac Complications of Open Heart Surgery: Prevention, Diagnosis, and Treatment. Mt. Kisco, N.Y., Futura, 1992, p. 177.

212. Egleston, C. V., Wood, A. E., Gorey, T. F., and McGovern, E. M.: Gastrointestinal complications after cardiac surgery. Ann. R. Coll. Surg. Engl. *75:*52, 1993.

213. Tsiotos, G. G., Mullany, C. J., Zietlow, S., and Van, H. J. A.: Abdominal complications following cardiac surgery. Am. J. Surg. *167:*553, 1994.

214. Zeithofer, J., Asenbaum, S., Spiss, C., et al.: Central nervous system function after cardiopulmonary bypass. Eur. Heart J. *14:*885, 1993.

215. Kallis, P., Unsworth-White, J., Munsch, C., et al.: Disability and distress following cardiac surgery in patients over 70 years of age. Eur. J. Cardiothorac. Surg. *7:*306, 1993.

216. Taylor, G. J., Malik, S. A., Colliver, J. A., et al.: Usefulness of atrial fibrillation as a predictor of stroke after isolated coronary artery bypass grafting. Am. J. Cardiol. *60:*905, 1987.

217. Kuroda, Y., Uchimoto, R., Kaieda, R., et al.: Central nervous system complications after cardiac surgery: A comparison between coronary artery bypass grafting and valve surgery. Anesth. Analg. *76:*222, 1993.

218. Seyfer, A. E., Grammer, N. Y., Bogumill, G. P., et al.: Upper extremity neuropathies after cardiac surgery. J. Hand. Surg. [Am.] *10:*16, 1985.

219. Murphy, M. C., Newman, B. M., and Rodgers, B. M.: Pleuroperitoneal shunts in the management of persistent chylothorax. Ann. Thorac. Surg. *48:*195, 1989.

220. Chan, B. B., Murphy, M. C., and Rodgers, B. M.: Management of chylopericardium. J. Pediatr. Surg. *25:*1185, 1990.

220a. Pearson, S. D., Goulart-Fisher, D., and Lee, T. H.: Critical pathways as a strategy for improving care: Problems and potential. Ann. Intern. Med. *123:*941, 1995.

REHABILITATION AND PREPARATION FOR DISCHARGE

221. Fletcher, G., Balady, G., Froelicher, V., et al.: Exercise standards: A statement for healthcare professionals from the American Heart Association. Circulation *91:*580, 1995.

222. van der Meer, J., Hillege, H., Koostra, G., et al.: Prevention of one-year vein-graft occlusion after aortocoronary-bypass surgery: A comparison of low-dose aspirin, low-dose aspirin plus dipyridamole, and oral anticoagulants. Lancet *342:*257, 1993.

223. Daida, H., Yokoi, H., Miyano, H., et al.: Relation of saphenous vein graft obstruction to serum cholesterol levels. J. Am. Coll. Cardiol. *25:*193, 1995.

Chapter 53
Cost-Effective Strategies in Cardiology

LEE GOLDMAN

QUANTITATIVE ANALYSES OF COSTS AND EFFECTIVENESS 1741
Calculation of Costs 1742
DIAGNOSTIC TESTING 1743
PREVENTION AND TREATMENT 1745
Detection and Treatment of Hyperlipidemia 1745
Detection and Treatment of Hypertension 1747
Cigarette Smoking 1747
Obesity 1748
Physical Activity 1748
Prevention of Infective Endocarditis in Valvular Heart Disease 1748
Prehospital Emergency Services 1748
Acute Myocardial Infarction 1749
Coronary Artery Revascularization 1750
SUMMARY 1751
REFERENCES 1751

The availability of an increasing number of diagnostic and therapeutic technologies, coupled with concerns over the rising costs of health care, has generated growing interest in determining the cost and effectiveness of cardiological care. Cost-effectiveness analysis, which initially had been used principally by economists and policymakers, is a potentially useful technique for evaluating how best to diagnose, prevent, and treat medical illnesses. Such analyses highlight the important issues that should guide the physician-decision maker. They can help in identifying gaps in knowledge and establishing priorities for research to be carried out by clinical investigators. To appreciate the implications of the emerging literature on cost-effectiveness in cardiology, it is important to understand the basic concepts that underlie formal cost-effectiveness analysis.

QUANTITATIVE ANALYSES OF COSTS AND EFFECTIVENESS

Analysts commonly distinguish between *cost-benefit analysis,* in which both costs and benefits are expressed in the same units (such as dollars), and *cost-effectiveness analysis,* in which the costs are commonly expressed in monetary terms while the effectiveness is expressed in terms of the health benefit.[1] The health benefit commonly is measured in units such as the number of lives that are saved, the years of life gained, the quality-adjusted years of life saved,[1–7] the days of disability avoided, or other suitable measurements.

SENSITIVITY ANALYSIS. Cost-effectiveness analyses are critically dependent on the accuracy of the assumptions on which they are based. Therefore, the analysis should include a "sensitivity analysis," in which the calculations are repeated with varying assumptions to determine whether the conclusions are altered.[1–4] It is vital to determine whether the final conclusions are critically dependent on a tenuous estimate by determining whether reasonable variations in important assumptions make major differences in the results of the analysis.

For example, in an analysis of the cost-effectiveness of admitting patients with chest pain and possible uncomplicated acute myocardial infarction in the absence of ST-segment elevation to a full-fledged coronary care unit as opposed to a nonintensive care unit bed with telemetry monitoring, it would be critical to estimate the relative difference, if any, in the rate of successful resuscitation from primary ventricular fibrillation in the two settings. The larger the estimated difference, the more cost-effective the coronary care unit would appear. If the two settings were assumed to be equally effective, the additional cost of the coronary care unit would not yield additional effectiveness for this purpose. Because no randomized controlled data address this issue, any analysis of the relative cost-effectiveness of care of patients with possible myocardial infarction in these two settings depends on the estimates that are made. When a sensitivity analysis was performed, the nonintensive care bed with telemetry monitoring remained the more cost-effective option for patients whose probability of acute myocardial infarction was about 20 per cent or less. Only patients with ST-segment elevation or with ischemic ST-T changes had probabilities sufficiently high to warrant a coronary care unit to rule out a myocardial infarction, unless other complications requiring intensive care were already evident.[8]

THE CLINICAL DECISION TREE. Some cost-effectiveness analyses address difficult clinical problems for which no clear agreement exists, often because available data are not adequate even for the experienced clinician. In such situations, cost-effectiveness analysis may not yield clear answers, usually because the relative differences between competing strategies are small. For example, it may be difficult to decide whether or not to implant a permanent pacemaker in an elderly patient who has symptoms that are suggestive of a pacemaker-responsive arrhythmia but in whom the relation between arrhythmia and symptoms has not been proved. The therapeutic options can be displayed using a decision tree (Fig. 53–1) that explicitly outlines the various possibilities.[9] In this decision analysis, estimates about the relative cost-effectiveness of various therapeutic strategies would depend on the patient's subjective assessment of the quality of life under different scenarios, including persistent symptoms and no pacemaker, persistent symptoms despite a pacemaker, and the pacemaker without symptoms. Because small changes in the assessment of quality of life[10] under these different circumstances would alter the preferred strategy, this particular analysis could not provide a definitive solution for all cases involving this therapeutic dilemma. Nevertheless, this analysis demonstrated that empirical pacing was an attractive option in an elderly patient with unexplained syncope even when there was only about a 25 per cent chance that the syncope was caused by a pacemaker-responsive arrhythmia.

The goal of cost-effectiveness analysis is not to find the greatest possible benefit for the lowest possible cost, because it is not possible to achieve both simultaneously.[2,11] Instead, it is necessary either to determine the resources that are available and then find the greatest possible effectiveness that can be purchased for those resources or to determine the desired effectiveness and then find the lowest cost to achieve it. In either case, it is important to have a preconceived idea of the desirable or acceptable relative ratio of cost to effectiveness. Although cost-effectiveness analyses determine the ratio of cost to effectiveness, two strategies with the same ratio may have quite different absolute costs and absolute effectiveness. For example, a pro-

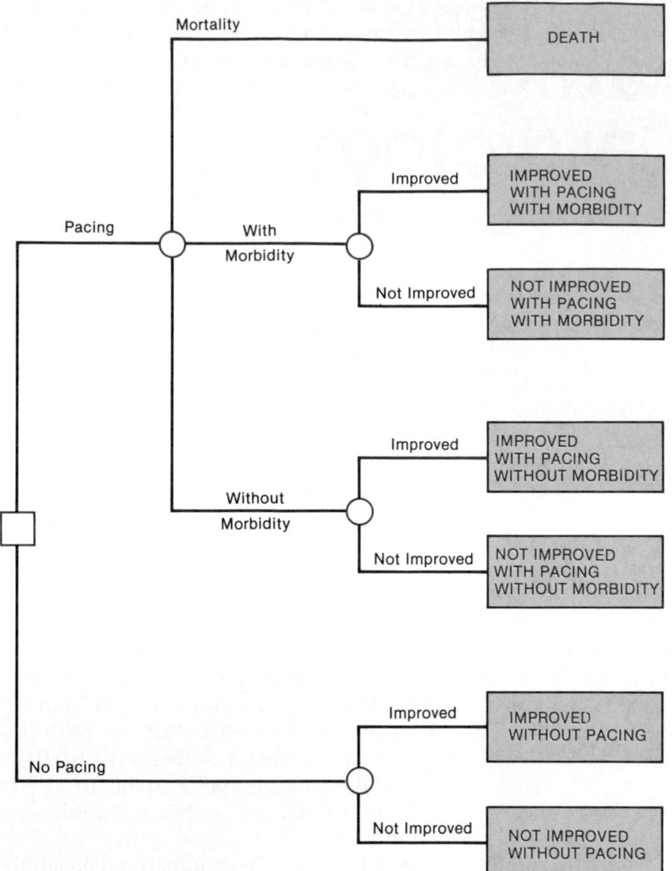

FIGURE 53–1. Decision tree for whether or not to perform empirical pacing in the elderly patient with syncope that may or may not be caused by a pacemaker-responsive arrhythmia. Branches of this decision tree explicitly detail the potential outcomes from the various options. The square denotes the outcome of decisions that the physician must make, whereas the circles denote events over which the physician has no control, i.e., occur "by chance." In constructing the decision tree, physicians would use either their own judgment or probabilities derived from the literature to estimate the likelihood of each of the events that can occur at a "chance" node. The sum of the probabilities of these chance events is always 100 per cent. In a cost-effectiveness analysis, each of the potential outcomes, as displayed in the rectangles in the right column, would be assigned a cost and a "utility." The utility would denote how highly the outcome is valued compared with perfect health, which traditionally has a value of 1.0, versus death, which traditionally has a value of 0. Cost-effectiveness calculations would compute the average expected costs and utilities for each of the various options that might be chosen by the physician, in this case the "pacing" and "no pacing" options that emanate from the initial square node. (From Kwoh, C. K., Beck, J. R., and Pauker, S. G.: Repeated syncope with negative diagnostic evaluation. Med. Decis. Making *4*:351, 1984.)

gram that saves 100 lives for $10,000 has the same cost-effectiveness ratio as one that saves 10,000 lives for $1,000,000, but the two programs' absolute costs and absolute effectiveness vary 100-fold. In cost-effectiveness analyses, any potentially new strategy usually is compared with the current, or baseline, strategy by calculating the *incremental cost/incremental effectiveness* ratio.[1–3]

Calculation of Costs

In determining costs, several types must be considered.[1–3] *Operating costs* may include both direct costs such as salaries and indirect costs such as overhead, including utilities and maintenance. Costs also can be categorized as *fixed* versus *variable* costs. For example, the first 100 cardiac scans carried out in an imaging center may cost $100,000 for an average cost of $1000 per scan because of the high capital costs of the equipment. If the laboratory were to "increase its output," the incremental cost for the next 100 scans would be much less than the cost for the first 100 scans because the capital costs of the equipment would be nearly the same regardless of whether 100 scans or 200 scans were performed. Thus one could distinguish between the *incremental* cost of performing the second 100 scans versus the *average* cost of all 200 scans. In many medical analyses, true costs are not available, and charges are used in the calculation of "cost" effectiveness. Because charges often are the same regardless of volume, they usually do not consider fully the important differences between average and incremental costs.

In calculating net health care costs, a useful approach is shown in Table 53–1. Unfortunately many cost-effectiveness analyses have concentrated only on direct medical costs, without fully taking into account the other terms in the equation.

DISCOUNTING. In virtually all cost analyses, it is important to consider the time frame during which costs and effects will be achieved. Because current dollars or benefits are more highly valued than a promise of future dollars or health benefits, a cost or benefit achieved immediately is more highly valued than one that is achieved later.[1] For example, one would be more willing to spend $10,000 today to prevent a death that otherwise would occur tomorrow than to spend $10,000 today to prevent a death that otherwise would occur in 10 years, even if there were no inflation and if there were no interest to be earned on the dollars. There is a preference to achieve an immediate benefit for several reasons. First, other events may intercede so that the projected future death may not occur or might be avoided as a consequence of newly available options that cost less than $10,000. Second, another illness could terminate life during the intervening period. Also, the $10,000 might be spent during the intervening 10 years in ways that are deemed more valuable. Furthermore, there is always a lingering doubt that the money spent now will not actually achieve the desired effect 10 years hence. This principle, by which the promise of future events is less valued than known immediate events, is termed "discounting," and is independent of monetary inflation. It is common practice to "discount" both future costs and future benefits by about 5 per cent per year.

In discussions of costs and effectiveness, several common misconceptions occur.[11] Cost-effective should not be equated with cost-saving because one often must spend to achieve a real benefit. Although a strategy that saves money *and* achieves an equal or better outcome is obviously cost-effective, a program is also cost-effective if it yields an additional benefit that is worth the additional cost. The definition of "worth the cost" may be somewhat arbitrary because it is difficult to place a monetary value on years of life and productivity. In many analyses, the approximately $35,000 to $40,000 per year cost in 1995 dollars of renal dialysis,[12] a program that the United States has decided to support with tax dollars, has been used as the benchmark for the amount of cost that the public appears willing to bear to prolong useful life by 1 year.

Although physicians must be aware of the relative cost-

TABLE 53–1 CALCULATION OF NET HEALTH CARE COSTS FOR A PROGRAM

Net costs = direct medical costs*
+ health care costs associated with the adverse effects of treatment
− savings of health care, rehabilitation, and custodial costs owing to prevention or alleviation of disease
+ costs of treating disease that would not have occurred if the patient had not lived longer as a result of the original treatment

* Costs of hospitalization, physician time, medications, laboratory services, and other ancillary services.

effectiveness of various diagnostic and therapeutic options if they are to make optimal choices for their patients, decisions about the number of dollars that *should* be spent to achieve specific health care benefits will ultimately be determined by society. Physicians have a critical role to play in developing appropriate data on cost-effectiveness issues, but the individual physician's primary responsibility is to the patient, within the confines of the economic limitations that may be imposed on both the physician and the patient by society.

One example of societal constraints on medical care expenditures is the diagnosis-related groups (DRG) system of prospective reimbursement. By defining in advance the number of dollars that a hospital will be reimbursed for the care of certain types of patients, the physician, the hospital, and the patient may all become more concerned with issues of cost-effectiveness. In an analogous manner, capitation systems, in which physicians are prepaid a fixed sum to assume the care of a patient, place an increased emphasis on the determination of cost-effective strategies.

DIAGNOSTIC TESTING

Modern cardiology includes an impressive armamentarium of diagnostic tests. Good clinical judgment requires that the physician choose tests in a cost-effective manner, in which the tests individually or sequentially may lead to improved diagnosis and management. The cost-effective use of diagnostic tests requires the physician to proceed logically through evaluation of the patient, selection of diagnostic tests, integration of the test with clinical data, and formulation of management strategies.[13,14] Each of these steps must be carefully considered for the proper utilization of diagnostic testing.

THE ESTIMATION OF CLINICAL PROBABILITIES. Regardless of the condition in question, the physician must utilize data from the medical history and physical examination to estimate the likelihood of its presence. For example, in evaluating the patient with chest pain, the physician may consider the patient's age and gender, as well as the typicality of the discomfort for angina pectoris.[13,14] The symptom may be categorized as typical angina pectoris, atypical angina pectoris, or nonanginal chest discomfort on the basis of its character, location, provocation, and response to rest or nitroglycerine (see p. 1290). Similarly, in estimating the probability of the presence of hemodynamically significant aortic stenosis in an adult with a systolic murmur, one would consider factors such as the intensity, location, and radiation of the murmur, the volume and rate of upstroke of the carotid arterial pulse, and the second heart sound (see p. 1039). Although these estimates of clinical probabilities can be based on the judgment of an experienced physician, in some circumstances, the physician can be aided by accumulated data from large series of patients in whom the clinical probability of conditions such as significant coronary artery disease[15] or acute myocardial infarction[16,17] has been determined.

ORDERING A DIAGNOSTIC TEST. When considering ordering a test, the physician must determine whether the test is effective and sufficiently accurate for indications for which it is being considered, that no other test with acceptable efficacy is less hazardous or less expensive, and that this is the most appropriate time for ordering the test.[13,18] In one such study carried out in 1977, soon after cardiac nuclear medicine scans became clinically available, 35 per cent were found *not* to have been ordered appropriately.[18] By comparison, the utility of two-dimensional echocardiograms was substantially better when studied in the 1990's, well after the test had been widely used and appreciated by clinicians.[19]

Tests may be ordered for such indications as to plan or monitor therapy, to establish a diagnosis, to define the extent of a known disease, to estimate prognosis, or to reassure the physician or the patient.[18,20] Although each of these indications can be a legitimate reason for ordering a diagnostic test, test results that may influence therapeutic action usually are the most valued and are certainly the most cost-effective.

When assessing the accuracy of a test, one must understand terms such as sensitivity, specificity, and positive predictive value (see Table 5–2, p. 161).[13] For some tests, such as a thallium scintiscan, the result is often dichotomized into "normal" versus "abnormal," even though it is understood that the precise distinction between normal and abnormal may be difficult and somewhat arbitrary. Other tests, such as the ejection fraction, commonly are reported on a continuous scale. In some circumstances, such as with the exercise electrocardiogram, a continuous result (e.g., the extent of ST-segment depression) often is dichotomized into normal or abnormal to facilitate the test's interpretation. When a continuous result is dichotomized, an increase in its sensitivity, or the likelihood of a positive test result among patients with the condition, can be obtained only at the expense of decreasing specificity, or the likelihood of a normal test result in patients without the condition.[13] For example, the sensitivity of the exercise electrocardiogram for detecting patients with coronary artery disease can be increased by reducing the depth of ST-segment depression required for a "positive" test result. However, as the definition of a "positive" test result is changed from 2 mm of ST-segment depression to 1 mm of ST-segment depression, the resulting increase in apparent sensitivity will be at the expense of a decreased specificity because patients who have between 1 and 2 mm of ST-segment depression and who do not have coronary artery disease now will be misclassified.

In an era of cost consciousness, the physician often must be asked to decide between two tests that may offer similar types of information. For example, a radionuclide ventriculogram may provide a more accurate assessment of the left ventricular ejection fraction than a two-dimensional echocardiogram, but the latter frequently provides a sufficiently accurate estimate of left ventricular function to obviate the need for the more expensive radionuclide study.

INTEGRATING THE TEST RESULT WITH CLINICAL DATA. To use diagnostic tests efficiently, the physician should decide the threshold probability above or below which the future diagnostic or management strategy would be altered.[14,21] For example, consider that a patient has recurrent chest pain, and on the basis of history and physical examination, the physician estimates that there is a 50 per cent probability that it is caused by coronary artery disease. The physician also knows that coronary arteriography would be required to decide whether coronary artery bypass grafting or percutaneous transluminal coronary angioplasty should be carried out if coronary artery disease were present. For cost-effective test ordering, the physician then must estimate how unlikely coronary artery disease would have to be for this strategy to be altered. If the physician would proceed with catheterization provided that the probability of coronary artery disease were as low as 10 per cent (or higher), then a test such as an exercise radionuclide ventriculogram, whose negative result might reduce the probability of coronary artery disease to 30 per cent, would not be helpful in decision-making.

Threshold Approach. This concept has been called the "threshold approach" to test utilization and decision-making.[13,21] In essence, it emphasizes that a test is potentially helpful only if its result would change the pretest probability of disease to a degree that could be sufficient to alter the approach to the patient. If it is highly unlikely that the available diagnostic test could move the probability of disease across such a threshold, the test would not be cost-effective and ordinarily would not be ordered. In some situations, the diagnostic threshold may be redefined because of

TABLE 53–2 HOW THE POSITIVE AND NEGATIVE PREDICTIVE VALUES OF THE SAME TEST VARY DEPENDING ON THE PRIOR PROBABILITY OF DISEASE

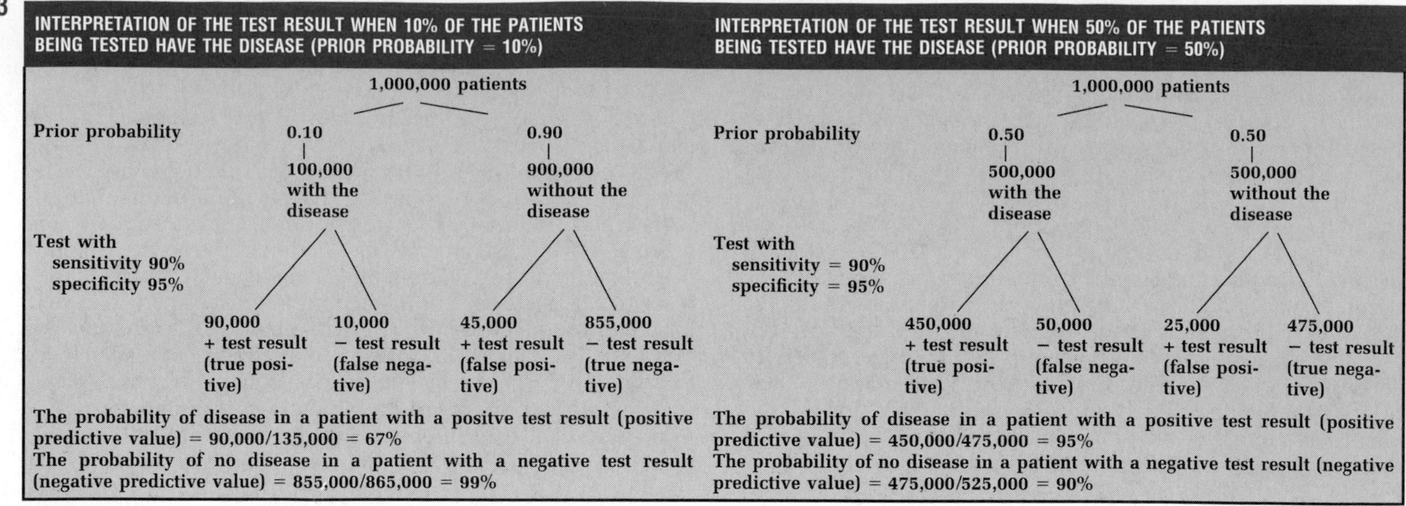

INTERPRETATION OF THE TEST RESULT WHEN 10% OF THE PATIENTS BEING TESTED HAVE THE DISEASE (PRIOR PROBABILITY = 10%)

1,000,000 patients

Prior probability: 0.10 — 100,000 with the disease; 0.90 — 900,000 without the disease

Test with sensitivity 90% specificity 95%

90,000 + test result (true positive); 10,000 − test result (false negative); 45,000 + test result (false positive); 855,000 − test result (true negative)

The probability of disease in a patient with a positve test result (positive predictive value) = 90,000/135,000 = 67%

The probability of no disease in a patient with a negative test result (negative predictive value) = 855,000/865,000 = 99%

INTERPRETATION OF THE TEST RESULT WHEN 50% OF THE PATIENTS BEING TESTED HAVE THE DISEASE (PRIOR PROBABILITY = 50%)

1,000,000 patients

Prior probability: 0.50 — 500,000 with the disease; 0.50 — 500,000 without the disease

Test with sensitivity = 90% specificity = 95%

450,000 + test result (true positive); 50,000 − test result (false negative); 25,000 + test result (false positive); 475,000 − test result (true negative)

The probability of disease in a patient with a positive test result (positive predictive value) = 450,000/475,000 = 95%

The probability of no disease in a patient with a negative test result (negative predictive value) = 475,000/525,000 = 90%

From Goldman, L.: Quantitative aspects of clinical reasoning. *In* Wilson, J. D., et al. (eds.): Harrison's Principles of Internal Medicine. 13th ed. New York, McGraw-Hill Book Co., 1994. © 1994 The McGraw-Hill Companies, Inc.

the special characteristics of the patient at hand. For example, it would be considered important to rule out significant coronary artery disease in an otherwise healthy airline pilot who has atypical chest pain. In this situation, the combination of a normal exercise electrocardiogram and a normal exercise thallium scintiscan would make the presence of coronary disease unlikely. If it were argued that the airline pilot's occupational responsibilities would require even a greater degree of certainty, it would be preferable to proceed directly to the test that usually is considered the benchmark, in this case, coronary arteriography, if it were necessary to be as certain as possible that coronary disease was not present.

BAYES' THEOREM (see p. 162). One way to understand the concepts of prior probability, thresholds, and the impact of diagnostic tests is through Bayes' theorem.[1,13] When the prior probability (prevalence) of the disease is known in patients who are similar to the patient under consideration, and when the sensitivity and specificity of the test to be ordered are known, the post-test probability that the disease is present can be calculated. Table 53–2 emphasizes how the physician must consider both the prior (pretest) probability that the patient has a disease and the test result in estimating the post-test probability. For example, if a test has a sensitivity of 90 per cent and a specificity of 95 per cent, a patient whose prior probability of disease was 10 per cent and who has a positive test result would have a 67 per cent probability of disease after the test. By comparison, the same test result in a patient whose prior probability was 50 per cent would yield a post-test probability of 95 per cent.

A test is potentially useful if it changes the probability of disease sufficiently to cross the threshold for decision-making. Unfortunately, available data do not always provide precise guidelines for establishing such appropriate thresholds for diagnostic decision-making. Nevertheless, common clinical judgment is often a sufficient guide. For example, using pooled data from the literature, the effects of exercise electrocardiography and exercise thallium testing can be estimated for a patient with typical angina pectoris (Fig. 53–2), a patient with atypical angina (Fig. 53–3), and a patient with presumably nonanginal chest pain (Fig. 53–4). These estimated probabilities correspond well to the actual probability of disease in patients who have been evaluated.[22]

NONINVASIVE TESTING IN PATIENTS WITH POSSIBLE ANGINA PECTORIS (see p. 1295). The patient with symptoms typical for angina pectoris already has a high probability of coronary artery disease on the basis of the history alone (80 to 85 per cent); the probability becomes even higher (95 per cent) if the exercise electrocardiogram is positive and becomes overwhelming (99 per cent) after a confirmatory exercise thallium scan. For diagnosing the presence or absence of coronary disease, however, the exercise thallium scan adds little to the results of the exercise test. Although the exercise thallium test appears to have additional prog-

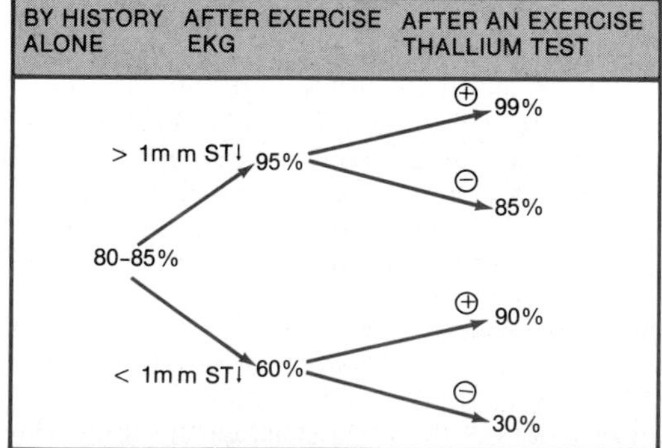

FIGURE 53–2. Approximate probabilities of coronary artery disease in a patient with typical angina pectoris before and after the sequential use of an exercise electrocardiogram and an exercise thallium test. (From Lee, T. H., and Goldman, L.: Non-invasive tests In cardiology. *In* Branch, W., Jr. [ed.]: Office Practice of Medicine. 3rd ed. Philadelphia, W. B. Saunders Company, 1994.)

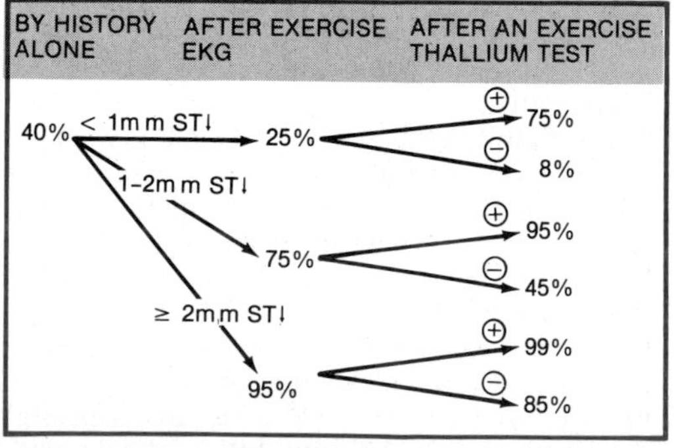

FIGURE 53–3. Approximate probabilities of coronary artery disease in a patient with atypical anginal symptoms before and after the sequential use of an exercise electrocardiogram and an exercise thallium test. (From Lee, T. H., and Goldman, L.: Non-invasive tests in cardiology. *In* Branch, W., Jr. [ed.]: Office Practice of Medicine. 3rd ed. Philadelphia, W. B. Saunders Company, 1994.)

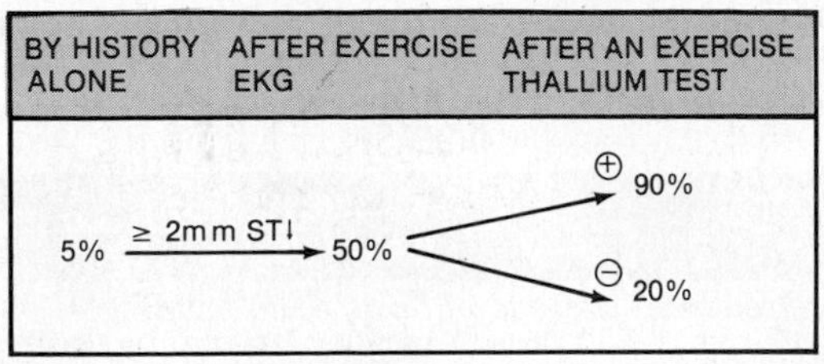

FIGURE 53–4. Approximate probabilities of coronary artery disease in an asymptomatic subject in the coronary artery disease age range before and after the sequential use of an exercise electrocardiogram and an exercise thallium test. (From Lee, T. H., and Goldman, L.: Non-invasive tests in cardiology. *In* Branch, W., Jr. [ed.]: Office Practice of Medicine. 3rd ed. Philadelphia, W. B. Saunders Company, 1994.)

nostic value,[23,24] in most situations, the results of the exercise thallium test would be unlikely to add substantial independent information regarding the diagnosis of the presence of coronary artery disease. If the exercise electrocardiogram and exercise thallium test give conflicting information, the probability of coronary artery disease in the patient with typical angina pectoris remains similar to what it was before either test was obtained (80 to 90 per cent). If both tests are negative, the patient with typical angina pectoris still has a reasonable probability of having significant coronary artery disease (30 per cent). Thus even two negative tests have not "ruled out" coronary artery disease in a patient with typical angina to an extent to which one could simply reassure the patient, even though they imply a favorable prognosis if coronary artery disease should be present.[23–25] Thus, if one were trying to rule out coronary artery disease in a patient with typical angina pectoris, coronary arteriography still would be required.[14,26]

In the patient with atypical angina (Fig. 53–3), positive results on both exercise electrocardiography and exercise thallium testing would raise the probability of coronary artery disease from 40 to 95 to 99 per cent. Conversely, negative results on both tests would lower the probability of coronary artery disease substantially (to 8 per cent), perhaps to a low enough level that one would not feel compelled to obtain coronary arteriography except in unusual circumstances. If the two tests give conflicting results, the probability of the disease has not been altered appreciably by the two tests.

In asymptomatic healthy people, a resting electrocardiogram appears to have little value as a screening test.[27] Similarly, screening exercise tests have too small a yield to justify their use in healthy people.[28] If, however, an asymptomatic subject who is in the age range in which coronary disease usually occurs has a strongly positive exercise electrocardiogram, the probability of coronary disease is increased substantially (from about 5 to about 50 per cent), and a subsequent negative exercise thallium test is not sufficiently reassuring to eliminate the possibility of coronary disease. Thus one cannot simply use the negative exercise thallium scan to "prove" that the exercise electrocardiogram was a false-positive result. Coronary arteriography is required to determine whether the exercise electrocardiogram was a true- or false-positive result, and this frequent need to proceed to invasive testing greatly increases the cost of any program that uses screening exercise electrocardiography.

It is beyond scope of this chapter to discuss the precise guidelines for the most cost-effective use of each of the various types of cardiac diagnostic tests for each possible indication. Nevertheless, test ordering becomes more cost-effective if the physician estimates the pretest probability of disease, orders the appropriate test, and properly integrates the test results with the available clinical information. A test is helpful only to the extent that it provides nonredundant information (i.e., information above and beyond what was previously available).[13] It must be emphasized, however, that a test can add incremental information regardless of whether its result is "positive" or "negative."[13,29]

Cost-effective medicine requires that tests be ordered only if their incremental information will have a positive impact on patient care. The finding that major variations in resource utilization often do not correlate with discernible differences in health outcome suggests that many tests and treatments do not meet such criteria.[30,31] Substantial financial savings can be realized by reducing the utilization of low- or moderate-cost tests as well as by reducing the utilization of expensive procedures.[32]

PREVENTION AND TREATMENT

The current and projected future costs of heart disease are substantial. The rate of death from coronary heart disease has been declining in the United States since the late 1960's,[33–35] but the increase in the total population and especially its age portends a rise in the total absolute number of cases of coronary heart disease unless there are major declines in risk factors.[36] Furthermore, the high cost of medical care for prevalent cases of coronary heart disease indicates that coronary disease will remain a major cost for the American public.[36,37]

Among the various preventive and therapeutic modalities in cardiology, some have been studied by means of formal cost-effectiveness analysis, whereas others have been studied in a more qualitative manner. In evaluating the cost-effectiveness of any program, it must be compared with a baseline or standard current approach. In the following sections, selected data on the costs and effectiveness of several modalities for the diagnosis, prevention, and treatment of heart disease are considered.

Detection and Treatment of Hyperlipidemia

(See also Chap. 35)

Substantial data indicate that the serum cholesterol level is significantly correlated with the risk of coronary artery disease (see p. 1127), and after controlling for the cholesterol level, the triglyceride level probably is not an important independent predictor.[38–40] The ratio of the high-density lipoprotein cholesterol fraction to the low-density lipoprotein fraction is more important than either level alone[41] for prediction. For primary care settings, a prudent screening technique is to obtain a total serum cholesterol level. If it is elevated, fasting levels of total cholesterol, low-density and high-density lipoprotein cholesterol, and triglycerides can be obtained to define risk more precisely and to determine the hyperlipidemia pattern to guide future dietary and perhaps drug therapy.[38,39]

The increased risk of hypercholesterolemia begins by early adulthood,[42] leading some to suggest screening by this age.[39] Others, however, argue against early screening because the risk of coronary events remains low until men reach their 40's and women reach their 50's and because intervention to lower cholesterol is efficacious within about 2 years.[38,43] Most agree that children and adolescents should not be screened except when the family history is compelling.[43–45]

Cholesterol is clearly a risk factor for coronary disease in women under age 65.[46] However, because coronary disease is not a dominant cause of death in younger women, cholesterol is not as strong a correlate of total mortality in middle-aged women as in middle-aged men.[47]

Despite some data and opinions to the contrary,[48,49] cholesterol appears to be a risk factor in the elderly. Even though the relative risk associated with hypercholesterolemia appears to be somewhat lower in the elderly,[46] their higher absolute risk of coronary disease implies that the incremental risk attributable to cholesterol is at least as high in the elderly.

The potential noncoronary hazards of low cholesterol and of reducing an individual's cholesterol level are unclear[47,50–52] but are proportionately of more potential relevance in persons with lower risks for coronary disease such as women and younger men, individuals without other coronary risk factors, and those with moderate hypercholesterolemia.[53–55] Furthermore, even small decrements in quality of life from being labeled as having hypercholesterolemia, from dietary changes, or from side effects of medications could outweigh the benefits of cholesterol screening and treatment in people with only mildly elevated risk.[56]

Despite these caveats, much is to be gained by addressing cholesterol abnormalities because each 1 per cent reduction in serum cholesterol is associated with at least a 2 per cent reduction in coronary risk,[57–60] and each 1 per cent increase in HDL cholesterol is associated with a 2 to 3 per cent decrease in risk.[61] Coronary risk reductions of similar magnitude have been observed in randomized intervention trials for both primary and secondary prevention.[62–71] Because up to 52 million Americans may be candidates for dietary interventions to reduce cholesterol and 13 million might be candidates for drug therapy,[39,72] cost-effectiveness assessments are of substantial relevance.[40]

A number of analyses have assessed the cost-effectiveness of interventions to lower serum cholesterol.[40,73–78] The most cost-effective use of medications for cholesterol-lowering is for secondary prevention in patients with existing coronary disease. In this setting, cholesterol reduction clearly reduces the risks of coronary disease and lowers all-cause mortality.[63–68] Because patients with existing coronary disease are at high risk for recurrent events and death, aggressive cholesterol-lowering therapy can sometimes save costs as well as lives and tends to be well worth the cost across a wide range of secondary prevention settings (Table 53–3). Of note is that the predicted benefits and favorable cost-effectiveness ratios for secondary prevention are relatively unaffected by varying assumptions regarding possible noncoronary hazards of lowering cholesterol, because about 80 per cent of deaths in patients with existing coronary disease are caused by coronary events.[63]

By comparison, aggressive cholesterol-lowering therapy has relatively less favorable cost-effectiveness ratios when used for primary prevention in individuals without coronary disease. The risks of coronary disease and hence the expected benefits from cholesterol reduction depend not only on the cholesterol level but also on the presence of other risk factors, such as age, gender, cigarette smoking, hypertension, and glucose intolerance. When cholesterol reduction for primary prevention is specifically targeted at individuals with multiple coronary risk factors or with marked elevation of serum cholesterol,[71,74,76–79] the effectiveness of treatment increases and cost-effectiveness ratios are more reasonable (Table 53–4). Cost-effectiveness ratios tend to be more favorable with more efficacious medications, such as HMG-CoA reductase inhibitors, than with less efficacious and equally expensive drugs, such as cholestyramine. Cost-effectiveness ratios are more favorable when medications become less expensive, such as substituting bulk cholestyramine for the drug in packets,[77] or if the costs of medications fall because of competition or when generic formulations become available.[79] In general, nicotinic acid and HMG-CoA reductase inhibitors have been estimated to be more cost-effective than other medications.

TABLE 53–3 ESTIMATED COST (IN DOLLARS) PER YEAR OF LIFE SAVED FOR LOVASTATIN AS SECONDARY PREVENTION

	AGE (YEARS)				
	35–44	45–54	55–64	65–74	75–84
Pretreatment cholesterol level ≥ 250 mg/dl					
Men					
Lovastatin 20 mg/d	*	*	1,600	10,000	19,000
Lovastatin 40 mg/d	14,000	86,000	17,000	27,000	38,000
Women					
Lovastatin 20 mg/d	4,500	3,500	8,100	12,000	15,000
Lovastatin 40 mg/d	49,000	30,000	29,000	30,000	29,000
Pretreatment cholesterol level < 250 mg/dl					
Men					
Lovastatin 20 mg/d	38,000	16,000	17,000	25,000	30,000
Lovastatin 40 mg/d	120,000	57,000	48,000	53,000	58,000
Women					
Lovastatin 20 mg/d	210,000	73,000	36,000	30,000	23,000
Lovastatin 40 mg/d	310,000	150,000	81,000	62,000	45,000

* Therapy estimated to save both lives and money.

From Goldman, L., et al.: The cost-effectiveness of programs to lower serum cholesterol. *In* Rifkind, B. M. (ed.): Lowering Cholesterol in High-Risk Individuals and Populations. New York, Marcel Dekker, 1995, p. 311.

TABLE 53–4 COST-EFFECTIVENESS RATIO (DOLLARS PER YEAR OF LIFE SAVED) OF 20 mg/d OF LOVASTATIN FOR PRIMARY PREVENTION OF CORONARY HEART DISEASE

	AGE (YEARS)				
	35–44	45–54	55–64	65–74	75–84
Men, pretreatment cholesterol level > 300 mg/dl					
High risk*	24,000	13,000	15,000	23,000	66,000
Moderate risk*	130,000	49,000	29,000	32,000	92,000
Low risk*	330,000	110,000	58,000	58,000	150,000
Women, pretreatment cholesterol level > 300 mg/dl					
High risk*	195,000	62,000	34,000	39,000	67,000
Moderate risk*	480,000	140,000	62,000	46,000	87,000
Low risk*	1,500,000	320,000	130,000	68,000	110,000

* High risk = diastolic blood pressure > 105 mm Hg, smoker, weight > 130% of ideal; moderate risk = diastolic blood pressure 95–104 mm Hg, nonsmoker, weight 110–129% of ideal; low risk = diastolic blood pressure < 95 mm Hg, nonsmoker, weight < 110% of ideal.

From Goldman, L., et al.: The cost-effectiveness of programs to lower serum cholesterol. *In* Rifkind, B. M. (ed.): Lowering Cholesterol in High-Risk Individuals and Populations. New York, Marcel Dekker, 1995, p. 311.

Because aggressive medications are not cost-effective in the primary prevention setting except in very high risk individuals, an alternative approach is population-based interventions. Such programs are especially attractive because half or more of the cases of new coronary disease occur in individuals with serum cholesterol levels below 250 mg/dl.[80] Population-wide education programs in northern California and in Finland were able to reduce serum cholesterol levels by up to 4 per cent, combined with other favorable changes in other risk factors, and at an estimated annual cost of less than $10 per person.[81,82] Unless it is assumed that there are major negative effects on noncardiac mortality in reducing cholesterol levels, population-wide cholesterol reduction programs emphasizing dietary interventions appear to have very favorable cost-effectiveness ratios.[40,78]

Although existing analyses are limited by the fact that they have not considered how medications or the avoidance of coronary events affects quality of life, they nevertheless provide reasonable economic guidelines to hypercholesterolemia: aggressive medications for secondary prevention and targeted medications for primary prevention in very high risk individuals superimposed on population-wide programs for everyone. These recommendations based on cost-effectiveness results suggest strategies that are somewhere between those recommended by Canadian and American consensus groups[38,39] and support the screening strategies discussed previously.[38,39,83]

Detection and Treatment of Hypertension

(See also Chaps. 26 and 27)

Most epidemiological data emphasize that the systolic blood pressure is an independent significant predictor of coronary heart disease but that the diastolic blood pressure is not (after controlling for the systolic blood pressure). Nevertheless, it has been common practice to define the threshold for treating hypertension on the basis of the diastolic blood pressure, and, until recently, virtually all treatment trials used definitions that were based on the diastolic blood pressure level.

An estimated 50 million Americans have hypertension, defined as a systolic blood pressure of 140 mm Hg or above, or a diastolic blood pressure of 90 mm Hg or above, or the use of antihypertensive medication.[84] Current recommendations of the US Joint National Committee are that all people with moderate hypertension (systolic blood pressure 160 to 169 mm Hg or diastolic blood pressure of 100 to 109 mm Hg) and mild hypertension (systolic blood pressure 140 to 159 mm Hg or diastolic blood pressure 90 to 99 mm Hg) be treated.[84]

Recent research has emphasized the importance of even mild systolic hypertension. Individuals with systolic blood pressures of 140 to 159 mm Hg and diastolic blood pressures below 90 mm Hg have elevated relative risks of about 1.5 for cardiovascular disease, 1.4 for coronary heart disease, 1.4 for stroke or transient ischemic attacks, 1.6 for congestive heart failure, and 1.6 for cardiovascular death (all $P < 0.05$) compared with age-matched normotensive controls.[85] The striking results of the Systolic Hypertension in the Elderly Program (SHEP) Trial emphasized the benefits of treating isolated systolic hypertension.[86]

Although physicians have historically been hesitant to treat hypertension aggressively in the elderly, three randomized trials[86–88] of about 10,000 patients have shown that treatment with diuretics or beta-adrenoceptor blockers, with added medications when needed, can reduce all-cause mortality by 12 per cent, stroke mortality by 36 per cent, and coronary mortality by 25 per cent.[89] Of note is that only about 20 elderly patients had to be treated for 5 years to avoid one cardiac or cerebrovascular event.[90]

Early studies that first demonstrated the benefit of antihypertensive medications for reducing cerebrovascular events tended not to show any benefit in terms of coronary events. However, cumulative meta-analysis of these large trials for the treatment of mild to moderate hypertension demonstrates that treated patients have a relative risk of 0.84 for coronary heart disease events, 0.84 for coronary heart disease death, 0.62 for cerebrovascular attacks, and 0.79 for all-vascular mortality (all $P < 0.01$).[91] The inability of the individual studies to find such differences in coronary mortality was probably based on their small sample size and relatively short duration of follow-up.

Although nonpharmacological therapy for hypertension is inherently attractive, medications are truly preferable to placebo.[92] Monotherapy is often successful in patients with mild to moderate hypertension.[92] Diltiazem may be somewhat more efficacious in African-Americans, captopril in young whites, and beta-blockers in elderly whites, but these differences are modest and cannot predict responses in individuals. Of note is that angiotensin-converting enzyme inhibitors at low doses are generally no more effective, and sometimes less effective, than low doses of diuretics.[93]

Screening to detect and treat hypertension appears to be relatively cost-effective for men and women of all ages.[94] The marginal cost per quality-adjusted year of life gained ranged from about $8000 for men aged 60 to about $29,000 for men aged 20. For women, the cost ranged from about $12,000 at age 60 to about $44,000 at age 20. The results of the analysis were affected relatively little when the authors varied many of the assumptions inherent in their analysis, except that the results were dependent on the cost of medication.

Weinstein and Stason used data from the Framingham Heart Study to calculate the cost-effectiveness of the treatment of mild hypertension.[95] They concluded that the reduction in direct medical care costs for stroke and coronary heart disease would offset about 22 per cent of the cost of treating moderate to severe diastolic hypertension (105 mm Hg and above) and about 15 per cent of the cost for treating mild hypertension (95 to 104 mm Hg), an estimate similar to those made by Stokes and Carmichael.[96] These cost-effectiveness estimates also are similar to those of Littenberg et al.,[94] who found that a program that would screen for hypertension and treat if the diastolic blood pressure was 95 mm Hg or greater would cost about $41,000 per quality-adjusted year of life gained. Treatment programs aimed at people with diastolic blood pressures of 105 mm Hg or greater would be more cost-effective: The cost would be only about $20,000 per year of life gained.

Edelson et al. reported that the cost of primary prevention to treat people 35 to 60 years of age with diastolic blood pressures of 95 mm Hg or greater and no known coronary heart disease was about $11,000 per year of life saved for propranolol and about $16,000 for hydrochlorothiazide.[97] Once again, however, cost-effectiveness was highly dependent on the cost of the medication, and the costs per year of life saved were not estimated to be nearly as favorable for the newer, more expensive medications.

Thus several analyses indicate that screening and treating people with hypertension is reasonably cost-effective and is in the range of the annual cost of hemodialysis for chronic renal failure.[12] Although hypertension detection and treatment are most cost-effective when performed by the patients' own physicians as part of routine medical care,[94,98] worksite programs for the detection and treatment of hypertension can more than pay for themselves by reducing direct medical costs and absenteeism.[99]

Cigarette Smoking

(See also Chap. 35)

Cigarette smoking is an independently significant correlate of the risk of developing coronary heart disease (p. 1147) and also is a major risk factor for several types of cancer. Many of these risks appear to be reversed after smokers stop smoking. Tsevat used data from a variety of sources to estimate that smoking cessation could increase life expectancy by 2 to 5 years.[100]

Although it is not possible to design a trial in which patients are randomized to continue smoking or to guarantee smoking cessation, substantial data confirm that discontinuing smoking improves prognosis.[101–105]

There are a variety of interventions to reduce smoking. On average, about 5 per cent of smokers discontinue the habit for 1 year after receiving a physician's advice, although the rate of quitting is higher in more highly motivated cohorts.[106,107] Nicotine gum or transdermal patches may increase the 1-year likelihood of smoking cessation by 30 to 100 per cent,[108,109] suggesting that the cost of a physician's advice plus the availability of nicotine gum per year of life saved will range from about $5700 to $9200 in men aged 35 to 69 and from about $9800 to $13,000 in women aged 35 to 69 in 1990 dollars.[110–113]

Group counseling can increase rates of quitting.[113,114] Public programs also are effective, with television advertisements against smoking among the most cost-effective.[115,116] Physicians should not be discouraged by the relatively low rate of quitting that occurs immediately after their advice because this advice is among the most cost-effective of all the interventions and may be a necessary psychological prelude to the patient's response to subsequent interventions. Nurse-managed smoking cessation programs may be especially effective and may cost as little as $220 per year of life saved when utilized in survivors of a myocardial infarction.[117]

Obesity

In long-term follow-up of the Framingham cohort,[118] obesity emerged as an independently significant risk factor for the development of coronary artery disease (see p. 0000). Unfortunately, it is extremely difficult for most adults to lose weight and to maintain the weight loss over the long term. Programs in schools or at the worksite commonly can help to achieve weight losses of 2 to 5 kg at costs that are about $10 to $30 per kilogram lost, which would be highly cost-effective.[119,120] Lay organizations such as Weight Watchers also can aid in producing similar losses at similar costs and are clearly cost-effective despite the high attrition rate. More intensive weight-loss programs for motivated people may still be very cost-effective for those people for whom simpler measures are ineffective.[121] Although physicians may become discouraged over the inability of their patients to lose weight, the usual effects of these other programs are not substantially greater than what may be achieved simply by a physician's advice. Furthermore, it often is a physician's advice that influences patients to try other interventions that might not be considered if the physician had not identified overweight as a medical problem.

Physical Activity

(See Chap. 40)

Substantial data indicate that physical activity reduces coronary heart disease and all-cause mortality, partly because of its beneficial effects on other risk factors but apparently partly independently.[122–128] Unfortunately, physicians often do not recommend exercise for their patients. Many patients, however, both want and expect their physicians to make recommendations regarding physical activity, and a substantial proportion of active people ascribed their activity in large part to the advice of a physician.

Worksite exercise programs also are potentially cost-effective independent of their possible effect on the development of clinical coronary artery disease. In one study, employees in the experimental exercise program group missed fewer days of work, were more likely to remain employed, and had fewer hospital days and fewer medical claims, thus resulting in substantial health care savings.[129,130] In fact, some employers have decided to pay their employees directly for participating in exercise programs, such as jogging, and some managed health care plans include membership in health clubs as one of their covered services. Unlike antismoking campaigns, media campaigns advocating exercise seem to encourage people to seek out other programs in the community but not to lead to direct changes in behavior by themselves.[131] Thus it appears that a physician's encouragement of increased physical activity, especially if combined with direct guidance on how to implement the suggestion, can lead to major changes in health behavior. Although it is difficult to determine the exact degree of effectiveness to be gained for the cost, there are substantial data linking physical activity to other cardiovascular risk factors and apparently independently to cardiovascular and all-cause mortality.[122–128] These data suggest that efforts to increase physical activity have the potential for being highly cost-effective.[132]

Cardiac rehabilitation in patients who have suffered a myocardial infarction (see Chap. 40) appears to lower by about 25 per cent the subsequent rates of reinfarction, cardiovascular mortality, and total mortality.[133] These programs improve the functional and symptomatic status of patients, and the exercise programs themselves are associated with a very small risk of major adverse events.[133] Such programs also can help patients return to work earlier after uncomplicated myocardial infarction,[134] and, as a result, can both reduce costs of medical care and increase productivity.[135] Thus the combination of cardiac rehabilitation services and occupational work evaluations appears to be very cost-effective for the post-myocardial infarction patient.

Prevention of Infective Endocarditis in Valvular Heart Disease

(See also Chaps. 32 and 33)

By extrapolation from cost-effectiveness analyses, penicillin prophylaxis to prevent bacterial endocarditis in patients with rheumatic valvular heart disease appears to have a cost-effectiveness of about $13,000 per year of life gained.[136,137] In patients with prosthetic heart valves, in whom the risk of endocarditis is higher, the cost-effectiveness is likely to be even more favorable. By comparison, two detailed cost-effectiveness analyses indicate that penicillin prophylaxis before dental work to prevent bacterial endocarditis is *not* cost-effective for patients with mitral valve prolapse[136,137] (see p. 1035). Using the most likely assumptions, people are as likely to die of penicillin reactions as they are to die of endocarditis, and even given the most optimistic assumptions, it is estimated that routine penicillin prophylaxis for dental procedures in patients with mitral valve prolapse would cost more than $1 million to save a year of life. In most studies of mitral valve prolapse, the risk of endocarditis is substantially higher in patients with murmurs of mitral regurgitation. Although the cost-effectiveness in this subpopulation of patients with mitral valve prolapse is unclear, the use of prophylactic antibiotics in the presence of a murmur of mitral valve prolapse is often recommended.[138]

Prehospital Emergency Services

(See also Chaps. 24 and 37)

Prehospital emergency services range from basic life support to advanced life support services. Advanced life support programs, which include interventions such as defibrillation, endotracheal intubation, and intravenous or intramuscular medications, have been instituted throughout much of the United States. Because about 60 per cent of patients whose death certificates list the cause of death as myocardial infarction die outside of the hospital, advances in prehospital emergency services, such as better training in the community or dispatcher-assisted instruction, could have a substantial impact on survival.[139]

Prehospital emergency care appears to be extremely successful in patients who have ventricular fibrillation and who are seen very soon after cardiac arrest (see p. 761). For example, in pooled data, about two-thirds of patients who are seen within 5 minutes of a ventricular fibrillation arrest survive to leave the hospital.[140–142] Unfortunately, many arrests are not caused by ventricular fibrillation, and even the most successful prehospital emergency services often cannot deliver care within 5 minutes. Thus, results in many urban and rural areas have been disappointing.[143–146] Only about 15 to 20 per cent of prehospital cardiac arrest patients commonly survive to leave the hospital in even the best programs,[141,142] and the rates are 1 to 5 per cent in many parts of the country.[143–146] Higher success rates are achieved principally through advanced life support programs utilizing paramedics, which appear to increase the likelihood of reaching the hospital alive from about 19 to 34 per cent and the likelihood of being discharged alive from the hospital from 7 to 17 per cent,[147] and through very rapid response times. However, the prognosis after hospital discharge of patients who were resuscitated from prehospital arrest is only about 75 per cent as high as age-

and sex-matched comparison groups who have survived myocardial infarction without prehospital arrest, and it is only about 60 per cent as high as for age- and gender-adjusted members of the general population.[141]

The cost-effectiveness of prehospital emergency programs is difficult to estimate. One analysis estimated that a mobile coronary care unit has an incremental cost of about $25,000 (in 1991 dollars) per life saved above and beyond the cost of the ambulance system itself.[142] Another analysis estimated that the incremental cost-effectiveness of a mobile coronary care unit was about $100,000 (in 1991 dollars) per life saved and $50,000 (in 1991 dollars) per year of life saved, but this analysis included only the incremental costs of the mobile coronary care unit program and not the costs of the existing emergency medical technician and community training program to which it was added.[148]

Analyses of the cost-effectiveness of prehospital emergency services depend on assumptions about the mean response time and the patients' prognoses, both in terms of life expectancy and in terms of quality of life and neurological impairment.[149] For example, the longer the response time, the more likely it is that survivors of prehospital cardiac arrest will have neurological impairment. If the years of life expectancy that are gained are compromised by such neurological impairment, then the *quality* of those years of life will not be the same as the quality of the years of life that might be gained from preventive measures that delay the onset of disease. Thus, when the calculation of cost-effectiveness is adjusted for the years of life that are gained without major neurological impairment, the apparent benefit of prehospital resuscitation is reduced. Furthermore, patients whose lives are saved by prehospital emergency services are likely to require careful medical follow-up, sometimes including expensive interventions such as coronary bypass grafting. Most studies[150–152] have not clearly considered the fact that the survivors of out-of-hospital cardiac arrest will have costs other than those included in the first term of the equation in Table 53–1, such as the costs for rehabilitative and custodial care and the costs for additional diagnosis and therapy of the substantial coronary disease that may have precipitated the arrest. When these costs are taken into account, the relative cost-effectiveness of prehospital emergency services programs becomes less appealing, although upgrading to paramedic services, either as the first responder or as the second part of a two-tier system, appears to be worthwhile from a cost-effectiveness standpoint.[153]

Acute Myocardial Infarction

(See also Chap. 37)

CORONARY CARE UNITS (see also p. 1226). These were originally designed to provide the ready availability of resuscitative services to patients with obvious acute myocardial infarction, for which there were no other therapies known to be effective at the time. The mission of coronary care units subsequently broadened in several ways. First, large numbers of patients were admitted with a suspicion of myocardial infarction so that they might have access to resuscitative facilities should they develop definitive evidence of infarction. Second, coronary care units became cardiac intensive care units, where patients could receive acute interventions to treat ischemia, pump failure, or other complications. The advent of thrombolysis and the availability of emergency percutaneous transluminal coronary angioplasty (PTCA) have further redefined the modern coronary care unit. At the same time, financial considerations have led to the development of alternative management strategies for low-risk patients who need diagnostic or monitoring facilities rather than intensive interventions.

REPERFUSION THERAPY (see also p. 1213). Reperfusion therapy with thrombolytic agents is most successful when it is given as soon as possible after the onset of symptoms in patients with acute myocardial infarction. Prehospital thrombolysis, which provides treatment about 55 minutes earlier, on average, than treatment that begins in the hospital, can significantly reduce both the cardiac death rate and overall mortality from the acute myocardial infarction by about 17 per cent compared with treatment begun in the hospital.[154] Although precise cost data are not currently available, intravenous thrombolysis provided either at home in systems such as are available in Great Britain[155] or in an ambulance[154,156,157] appears to afford benefits that are likely to be well worth the cost.

Meta-analysis[158] indicates a benefit from thrombolysis when it is administered as late as 7 to 12 hours after the onset of symptoms. Among patients treated more than 12 hours after the onset of symptoms, results remain inconclusive.[158–160] Although the costs of thrombolysis are higher and the relative benefits somewhat lower in the elderly, the higher absolute mortality rates from acute myocardial infarction in the elderly translate into overall benefits that are easily equivalent to those found in younger patients.[161]

Accelerated tissue plasminogen activator (t-PA) appears to be somewhat more efficacious than streptokinase for opening the infarct-related artery[162] at 90 minutes and hence has been associated with a lower mortality rate than streptokinase.[163] Despite substantial ongoing debate,[164,165] these incremental benefits would translate into a cost of about $25,000 to $30,000 per year of life saved.[166]

Although the methods have varied among different cost-effectiveness analyses for acute thrombolytic therapy, all have shown intravenous thrombolysis with streptokinase to be well worth the cost under a variety of assumptions in patients of all age ranges[161] and even in high-risk patients in whom an acute myocardial infarction could not be definitively diagnosed at the time the treatment was begun.[161,167–171] The incremental cost-effectiveness of t-PA compared with streptokinase is also more appealing in higher risk patients, in whom its relative advantages would translate into larger absolute benefits.[166]

PRIMARY PERCUTANEOUS TRANSLUMINAL CORONARY ANGIOPLASTY (see also p. 1221). Emergent primary PTCA appears to result in an even higher rate of effective reperfusion than intravenous thrombolysis.[172] As a result, it is not surprising that primary PTCA has been associated with a significant reduction in mortality in several randomized trials.[173–175] Most notably, primary PTCA was not more costly because patients tended to be discharged from the hospital more quickly.[174] Although feasibility of extending primary PTCA to an increased proportion of the population remains uncertain at the present time, this treatment appears to be the most effective and cost-effective option when it can be provided immediately by a highly skilled physician.[172]

An analysis of these various recent studies indicates that the benefits of prehospital versus in-hospital thrombolysis result in about a 17 per cent reduction in mortality, each hour earlier that the thrombolysis is administered results in about a 10 to 15 per cent relative mortality reduction, and accelerated t-PA versus streptokinase results in about a 12 per cent relative mortality reduction. Emergent PTCA on demand by highly skilled operators, on average at about 1 hour after hospital arrival and thus no more than 1 hour later than thrombolysis would have been given, results in about a 63 per cent relative reduction in mortality. Each of these mortality reductions appears to be worth the cost, based on currently available data. The choices among them and decisions regarding the development of the most appropriate system depend on local factors and the results of future research.

SUBSEQUENT TREATMENT AND RISK STRATIFICATION AFTER ACUTE MYOCARDIAL INFARCTION (see also p. 1258). After thrombolysis, conservative treatment, in which invasive procedures are used only for patients with symptoms such as recurrent ischemia, is just as good as routine cardiac catheterization followed by revascularization of significant stenoses.[176] Although post-myocardial infarction risk stratification is widely recommended,[177] formal testing with rest and exercise electrocardiograms, stress thallium scintigraphy, radionuclide ventriculograms, and 24-hour electrocardiographic recordings is limited by the abilities of any of these tests to predict which patients will subsequently have a clinical event.[178,179] Substantially less aggressive strategies, such as practiced in Canada, result in rates of survival and reinfarction equivalent to those with more aggressive United States practices, although patients treated in Canada tend to have a higher frequency of angina that limits their activities.[180] The relative cost-effectiveness of various strategies to stratify risk and base therapies upon these risks in the post-myocardial infarction patient is not well defined.

LONG-TERM TREATMENT. In addition to the known beneficial effects of cholesterol reduction therapy for secondary prevention in patients after myocardial infarction,[63,68] other therapies appear to be effective and cost-effective. Oral anticoagulation with warfarin or coumarin derivatives reduces recurrent cardiac deaths,[181] but there is no evidence that such therapy is more effective than aspirin, which is less expensive and probably safer.[182,183] Treatment with angiotensin-converting enzyme inhibitors, beginning acutely soon after a myocardial infarction or up to 6 weeks later, results in a 19 to 27 per cent benefit in reducing mortality at 30 to 48 months after the infarction,[184–186] and this treatment saves a year of life for less than $25,000 in most patients.[187] Long-term therapy with beta-adrenoceptor inhibitors confers a 25 per cent or so reduction in the relative risk of reinfarction and cardiac death and is associated with a cost-effectiveness ratio of well less than $10,000 per year of life saved for high- and medium-risk patients and no more than $30,000 per year of life saved in even the lowest risk patients.[188]

POTENTIAL COST-EFFECTIVE ALTERNATIVES TO CORONARY CARE UNIT ADMISSION. Patients who are evaluated for symptoms that may potentially represent acute myocardial infarction present a difficult diagnostic and therapeutic dilemma: Should they be admitted to intensive facilities for diagnosis and monitoring even though the risks of complications are low, or can they be managed in lower cost ways that do not appreciably increase their risk? In general, admission to a coronary intensive care unit is not a cost-effective alternative unless the probability of myocardial infarction is close to 20 per cent. This suggests that such an option be limited to patients who have electrocardiographic evidence of acute myocardial infarction or acute cardiac ischemia, unless the patient has an otherwise uninterpretable electrocardiogram (for example, left bundle branch block or a paced rhythm) and has very high risk clinical characteristics.[8] Clinical algorithms that are based on routine information from the history, physical examination, and electrocardiogram can stratify patients into various risk groups.[16,17,189,190] Decisions based on these predictive probabilities can improve coronary care unit admission practices[17,189–191] and help guide which patients should be admitted to less intensive units, where they will receive more cost-effective care.[192,193] Although echocardiography[194,195] and technetium-99m sestamibi myocardial imaging can also be used to identify higher versus lower risk patients,[196,197] the logistics and cost-effectiveness of these approaches remain uncertain at this time.

Newer enzymatic assays show great promise in improving the rapid diagnosis of acute myocardial infarction.[198,199] Measurements of CK isoforms,[200] troponin I,[201] or troponin T[202] can result in more sensitive and specific diagnoses of acute myocardial infarction or complicated unstable angina more quickly than conventional CK-MB isoenzyme assays. Although the true costs of these new enzyme assays are not yet clearly known, the potential to use these assays to shorten the diagnostic evaluation period for patients with suspected myocardial ischemia suggests that they are likely to have favorable cost-effectiveness ratios and ultimately to replace currently used enzyme assays.

In patients who are at low risk for acute myocardial infarction but are admitted to the hospital, the absence of major complications or a definitive diagnosis of acute myocardial infarction within 12 to 24 hours implies a low-risk status and the safety of discharge from the coronary care unit. In patients whose initial risk for an acute myocardial infarction is below about 10 per cent, a 12-hour or perhaps even a 6-hour period of sequential electrocardiograms and cardiac enzymes to rule out acute myocardial infarction is adequate.[16,17,203–204] After thrombolysis, low-risk patients can be discharged from the hospital as early as 4 days after admission.[205] Use of practice guidelines and reminders is an effective way to increase the early transfer of patients from more intensive to less intensive settings and to facilitate early hospital discharge.[206–208]

Coronary Artery Revascularization

(See also Chap. 39)

Directional atherectomy can result in a greater increase in coronary lumen than traditional PTCA (see p. 1376) but with early complication rates that are about twofold higher.[209,210] Rates of clinical restenosis may be slightly lower for directional atherectomy, but death rates and costs do not appear to be significantly different between the two procedures.[209,210]

Coronary stenting with balloon-expandable stents also can increase the postprocedure coronary diameter and reduce the rate of clinical restenosis.[211,212] However, the initial larger coronary diameter is achieved at the cost of a higher rate of acute complications and of longer hospital admissions.[211,212] The cost-effectiveness of stenting may be worthwhile[213] when compared with routine PTCA, but longer-term clinical and economic follow-up is required to derive precise cost-effectiveness ratios.

Although coronary artery bypass grafting (CABG) has probably accounted for only about 3 per cent of the decline in coronary heart disease mortality,[214] the benefits of CABG compared with medical treatment in many subgroups of patients is clear.[215] However, many CABG procedures are performed for indications in which the benefits are uncertain, even though few are used in truly inappropriate situations.[216,217] Centers that perform a large volume of procedures generally have better outcomes,[217,218] and feedback of information regarding coronary artery bypass mortality can result in marked improvements in outcome.[219]

For single-vessel disease, PTCA results in better symptomatic status than medical treatment (see p. 1373).[220] When PTCA is compared with coronary bypass grafting for patients with single-vessel or multivessel disease, the PTCA

TABLE 53–5 ESTIMATED APPROXIMATE COST PER GAIN IN ONE QUALITY-ADJUSTED YEAR OF LIFE FOR CORONARY ARTERY BYPASS GRAFTING

	ONE-VESSEL	TWO-VESSEL	THREE-VESSEL	LEFT MAIN DISEASE
Very mild angina	*	$86,000	$14,000	$6,300
Mild angina	$850,000	$55,000	$13,500	$6,600
Severe angina	$55,000	$32,000	$13,000	$7,000

* Quality-adjusted life expectancy is reduced.

From Weinstein, M. C., and Stason, W. B.: Cost-effectiveness of coronary artery bypass surgery. Circulation *66*(Suppl. III):56, 1982.

patients generally have higher rates of repeat revascularization and angina but similar rates of death, myocardial infarction, employment, and overall costs.[221–224] Nonrandomized data from a large data bank suggest that CABG may be better than PTCA for improving the survival of patients with three-vessel disease or severe two-vessel disease, whereas the choice is between PTCA and medical treatment in patients with less severe disease.[225] The estimated cost-effectiveness of CABG depends on the patient's symptomatic status and extent of disease (Table 53–5).[226]

SUMMARY

The gratifying reduction in mortality from ischemic heart disease usually is regarded as testimony to the effectiveness of a variety of primary and secondary preventive and therapeutic measures. It will be necessary, however, for current and future interventions to be carefully analyzed, so that the benefit of medical care to reduce cardiovascular morbidity and mortality can be maximized within the constraints of the resources that will be available.

Physicians should not view the current emphasis on cost-effective care as contradictory to excellent care. Patients should not be treated as numbers, and optimal medical care cannot be routinely derived from equations. The physician's principal responsibility is to render the best possible medical care to the patient as an individual. An understanding of the principles of cost-effectiveness should allow the physician to improve the choice of diagnostic and therapeutic strategies, and it should assist the physician's ability to determine strategies that are optimal in the aggregate and to adopt or adapt them for the person at hand. In such a context, more cost-effective care implies better care for the individual patient as well as the conservation of resources to improve care for the population as a whole.

REFERENCES

QUANTITATIVE ANALYSES OF COSTS AND EFFECTIVENESS

1. Weinstein, M. C., and Fineberg, H. V.: Clinical Decision Analysis. Philadelphia, W. B. Saunders Co., 1980.
2. Weinstein, M. C., and Stason, W. B.: Foundations of cost-effectiveness analysis for health and medical practices. N. Engl. J. Med. *296:*716, 1977.
3. Detsky, A. S., and Naglie, J. G.: A clinician's guide to cost-effectiveness analysis. Ann. Intern. Med. *113:*147, 1990.
4. Kupersmith, J., Holmes-Rovner, M., Hogan, A., et al.: Cost-effectiveness analysis in heart disease, Part I: General principles. Prog. Cardiovasc. Dis. *37:*161, 1994.
5. Udvarhelyi, I. S., Colditz, G. A., Rai, A., and Epstein, A. M.: Cost-effectiveness and cost-benefit analyses in the medical literature. Ann. Intern. Med. *116:*238, 1992.
6. Russell, L. B.: Some of the tough decisions required by a national health plan. Science *246:*892, 1989.
7. Goldman, L. G.: Cost awareness in medicine. *In* Isselbacher, K. J., et al. (eds.): Harrison's Principles of Internal Medicine. 13th ed. New York, McGraw-Hill Book Co., 1994, p. 38.
8. Tosteson, A. N. A., Goldman, L., Udvarhelyli, I. S., and Lee, T. H.: Cost-effectiveness of a coronary care unit versus a stepdown unit for emergency department patients with acute chest pain. Circulation (*In press*).
9. Kwoh, C. K., Beck, J. R., and Pauker, S. G.: Repeated syncope with negative diagnostic evaluation. To pace or not to pace? Med. Decis. Making *4:*351, 1984.
10. Fryback, D. G., Dasbach, E. J., Klein, R., et al.: The Beaver Dam Health Outcomes Study: Initial catalog of health-state quality factors. Med. Decis. Making *13:*89, 1993.
11. Doubilet, P., Weinstein, M. D., and McNeil, B. J.: Use and misuse of the term "cost-effective" in medicine. N. Engl. J. Med. *314*(Edit):253, 1986.
12. Iglehart, J. K.: The American health care system. The end-stage renal disease program. N. Engl. J. Med. *328:*366, 1993.

DIAGNOSTIC TESTING

13. Goldman, L.: Quantitative aspects of clinical reasoning. *In* Isselbacher, K. J., et al. (eds.): Harrison's Principles of Internal Medicine. 13th ed. New York, McGraw-Hill Book Co., 1994, p. 43.
14. Goldman, L.: Noninvasive tests in cardiology. *In* Branch, W. T., Jr. (ed.): Office Practice of Medicine. 3rd ed., Philadelphia, W. B. Saunders Company, 1994, p. 40.
15. Diamond, G. A., Staniloff, H. M., Forrester, J. S., et al.: Computer-assisted diagnosis in the noninvasive evaluation of patients with suspected coronary artery disease. J. Am. Coll. Cardiol. *1:*444, 1983.
16. Lee, T. H., Juarez, G., Cook, E. F., et al.: Ruling out acute myocardial infarction: Prospective multicenter validation of a 12 hour strategy for low risk patients. N. Engl. J. Med. *324:*1239, 1991.
17. Goldman, L., Cook, E. F., Brand, D.A., et al.: A computer protocol to predict myocardial infarction in emergency department patients with chest pain. N. Engl. J. Med. *318:*797, 1988.
18. Goldman, L., Feinstein, A. R., Batsford, W. P., et al.: Ordering patterns and clinical impact of cardiovascular nuclear medicine procedures. Circulation *62:*680, 1980.
19. Krumholz, H., Douglas, P. S., Goldman, L., and Waksmonski, C.: Clinical utility of transthoracic two-dimensional and Doppler echocardiography. J. Am. Coll. Cardiol. *24:*125, 1994.
20. Sox, H. C., Margulies, I., and Sox, C. H.: Psychologically mediated effects of diagnostic tests. Ann. Intern. Med. *95:*680, 1981.
21. Pauker, S. G., and Kassirer, J. P.: The threshold approach to clinical decision-making. N. Engl. J. Med. *302:*1109, 1980.
22. Weintraub, W. S., Madeira, S. W., Bodenheimer, M. M., et al.: Critical analysis of the application of Bayes' theorem to sequential testing in the noninvasive diagnosis of coronary artery disease. Am. J. Cardiol. *54:*43, 1984.
23. Pamelia, F. X., Gibson, R. S., Watson, D. D., et al.: Prognosis with chest pain and normal thallium-201 exercise scintigrams. Am. J. Cardiol. *55:*920, 1985.
24. Zaret, B. L., and Wachers, F. J.: Nuclear cardiology. N. Engl. J. Med. *329:*775, 1993.
25. Gordon, D. J., Ekelund, L., Karon, J. M., et al.: Predictive value of the exercise tolerance test for mortality in North American men: The Lipid Research Clinics Mortality Follow-up Study. Circulation *74:*252, 1986.
26. Patterson, R. E., Eng, C., Horowitz, S. F., et al.: Bayesian comparison of cost-effectiveness of different clinical approaches to diagnose coronary artery disease. J. Am Coll. Cardiol. *4:*278, 1984.
27. Sox, H. C., Garber, A. M., and Littenberg, B.: The resting electrocardiogram as a screening test: A clinical analysis. Ann. Intern. Med. *111:* 489, 1989.
28. Sox, H. C., Littenberg, B., and Garber, A. M.: The role of exercise testing in screening for coronary artery disease. Ann. Intern. Med. *110:*456, 1989.
29. Gorry, G. A., Pauker, S. G., and Schwartz, W. B.: The diagnostic importance of the normal finding. N. Engl. J. Med. *298:*486, 1978.
30. Wennberg, J. E., Freeman, J. L., and Culp, W. J.: Are hospital services rationed in New Haven or over-utilised in Boston? Lancet *1:*1185, 1987.
31. Fineberg, H. V., and Hiatt H. H.: Evaluation of medical practices. The case for technology assessment. N. Engl. J. Med. *301:*1086, 1979.
32. Eagle, K. S., Mulley, A. G., Field, T. S., et al.: Variation in intensive care unit practices in two community hospitals. Med. Care *29:*1237, 1991.
33. Gillum, R. F.: Trends in acute myocardial infarction and coronary heart disease death in the United States. J. Am. Coll. Cardiol. *23:*1273, 1993.
34. DeStefano, F., Merritt, R. K., Anda, R. F., et al.: Trends in nonfatal coronary heart disease in the United States, 1980 through 1989. Arch. Intern. Med. *153:*2489, 1993.

PREVENTION AND TREATMENT

35. Sytkowski, P. A., Kannel, W. B., and D'Agostino, R. B.: Changes in risk factors and the decline in mortality from cardiovascular disease. The Framingham Heart Study. N. Engl. J. Med. *322:*1635, 1990.
36. Weinstein, M. C., Coxson, P. G., Williams, L. W., et al.: Forecasting coronary heart disease incidence, mortality, and cost: The coronary heart disease policy model. Am. J. Public Health *77:*1417, 1987.
37. Wittels, E. H., Hay, J. W., and Gotto, A. M.: Medical costs of coronary artery disease in the United States. Am. J. Cardiol. *65:*432, 1990.
38. Canadian Task Force on the Periodic Health Examination: Periodic health examination, 1993 update: 2. Lowering the blood total cholesterol level to prevent coronary heart disease. Can. Med. Assoc. J. *148:*521, 1993.
39. Expert Panel on Detection, Evaluation, and Treatment of High Blood Cholesterol in Adults: Summary of the Second Report of the National Cholesterol Education Program (NCEP) Expert Panel on Detection, Evaluation, and Treatment of High Blood Cholesterol in Adults (Adult Treatment Panel II). JAMA *269:*3015, 1993.
40. Goldman, L., Gordon, D.J., Rifkind, B. M., et al.: Cost and health implications of cholesterol lowering. Circulation *85:*1960, 1992.
41. Stampfer, M. J., Sacks, F. M., Salvini, S., et al.: A prospective study of cholesterol, apolipoproteins, and the risk of myocardial infarction. N. Engl. J. Med. *325:*373, 1991.
42. Klag, M. J., Ford, D. E., Mead, L. A., et al.: Serum cholesterol in young men and subsequent cardiovascular disease. N. Engl. J. Med. *328:*313, 1993.
43. Hulley, S. B., Newman, T. B., Grady, D., et al.: Should we be measuring blood cholesterol levels in young adults? JAMA *269:*1416, 1993.
44. Newman, T. B., Browner, W. S., and Hulley, S. B.: Childhood cholesterol screening: Contraindications. JAMA *267:*100, 1992.

45. Newman, T., Browner, W., and Hulley, S.: The case against childhood cholesterol screening. JAMA *264:*3039, 1990.
46. Manolio, T. A., Pearson, T. A., Wenger, N. K., et al.: Cholesterol and heart disease in older persons and women. Review of an NHLBI Workshop. Ann. Epidemiol. *2:*161, 1992.
47. Jacobs, D., Blackburn, H., Higgins, M., et al.: Report of the Conference on Low Blood Cholesterol: Mortality Associations. Circulation *86:*1046, 1992.
48. Krumholz, H. M., Seeman, T. E., Merrill, S. S., et al.: Lack of association between cholesterol and coronary heart disease mortality and morbidity and all-cause mortality in persons older than 70 years. JAMA *272:*1335, 1994.
49. Hulley, S. B., and Newman, T. B.: Cholesterol in the elderly. Is it important? JAMA *272:*1372, 1994.
50. Stamler, J., Stamler, R., Brown, W. V., et al.: Serum cholesterol. Doing the right thing. Circulation *88:*1954, 1993.
51. Jacobs, D. R., and Blackburn, H.: Models of effects of low blood cholesterol on the public health. Implications for practice and policy. Circulation *87:*1033, 1993.
52. LaRosa, J. C.: Cholesterol lowering, low cholesterol, and mortality. Am. J. Cardiol. *72:*776, 1993.
53. Smith, G. D., Song, F., and Sheldon, T. A.: Cholesterol lowering and mortality: The importance of considering initial level of risk. Br. Med. J. *306:*1367, 1993.
54. Frank, J. W., Reed, D. M., Grove, J. S., and Benfante, R.: Will lowering population levels of serum cholesterol affect total mortality? Expectations from the Honolulu heart program. J. Clin Epidemiol. *45:*333, 1992.
55. McIsaac, W. J., Naylor, C. D., and Basinski, A.: Mismatch of coronary risk and treatment intensity under the National Cholesterol Education Program Guidelines. J. Gen. Intern. Med. *6:*518, 1991.
56. Krahn, M., Naylor, C. D., Basinski, A. S., and Detsky, A. S.: Comparison of an aggressive (U.S.) and a less aggressive (Canadian) policy for cholesterol screening and treatment. J. Gen. Intern. Med. *115:*248, 1991.
57. Stamler, J., Wentworth, D., and Neaton, J. D.: Is relationship between serum cholesterol and risk of premature death from coronary heart disease continuous and graded? Findings in 356,222 primary screenees of the Multiple-Risk Factor Intervention Trial (MRFIT). JAMA *256:*2823, 1986.
58. MacMahon, S., Peto, R., Cutler, J., et al.: Blood pressure, stroke, and coronary heart disease: Part I. Prolonged differences in blood pressure: Prospective observational studies corrected for the regression dilution bias. Lancet *335:*765, 1990.
59. Lipid Research Clinics Program: The Lipid Research Clinics Coronary Primary Prevention Trial results. II. The relationship of reduction in incidence of CHD to cholesterol lowering. JAMA *251:*365, 1984.
60. Davis, C. E., Rifkind, B. M., Brenner, H., and Gordon, D. J.: A single cholesterol measurement underestimates the risk of coronary heart disease. JAMA *264:*3044, 1990.
61. Gordon, D. J., Probstfield, J. L., Garrisons, R. J., et al.: High-density lipoprotein cholesterol and cardiovascular disease. Four prospective American studies. Circulation *79:*8, 1989.
62. Lipid Research Clinics Program: The Lipid Research Clinics Coronary Primary Prevention Trial results: I. Reduction in incidence of coronary heart disease. JAMA *251:*351, 1984.
63. Roussouw, F. E., Lewis, B., and Rifkind, B. M.: The value of lowering cholesterol after myocardial infarction. N. Engl. J. Med. *323:*1112, 1990.
64. Brown, G., Albers, J. J., Fisher, L. D., et al.: Regression of coronary artery disease as a result of intensive lipid-lowering therapy in men with high levels of apoliprotein B. N. Engl. J. Med. *323:*1289, 1990.
65. Buchwald, H., Varco, R. L., Matts, J. P., et al.: Effect of partial ileal bypass surgery on mortality and morbidity from coronary heart disease in patients with hypercholesterolemia. N. Engl. J. Med. *323:*946, 1990.
66. Cashin-Hemphill, L., Mack, W. J., Pagoda, J. M., et al.: Beneficial effects of colestipol-niacin on coronary atherosclerosis. JAMA *264:*3013, 1990.
67. Kane, J. P., Malloy M. J., Ports, T., et al.: Regression of coronary atherosclerosis during treatment of familial hypercholesterolemia with combined drug regimens. JAMA *264:*3007, 1990.
68. Scandinavian Simvastatin Survival Study Group: Randomised trial of cholesterol lowering in 4444 patients with coronary heart disease: The Scandinavian Simvastatin Survival Study (4S). Lancet *344:*1383, 1994.
69. Canner, P. L., Berge, K. G., Wenger, N. K., et al.: Fifteen year mortality in coronary drug project patients; long-term benefits with niacin. J. Am. Coll. Cardiol. *8:*1245, 1986.
70. Frick, M. H., Elo, O., Haapa, K., et al.: Helsinki Heart Study: Primary-prevention trial with gemfibrozil in middle-aged men with dyslipidemia. N. Engl. J. Med. *317:*1237, 1987.
71. Shepherd, J., Cobbe, S. M., Ford, I., et al.: Prevention of coronary heart disease with pravastatin in men with hypercholesterolemia. N. Engl. J. Med. *333:*1301, 1995.
72. Sempos, C. T., Cleeman, J. I., Carroll, M. D., et al.: Prevalence of high blood cholesterol among US adults. An update based on guidelines from the Second Report of the National Cholesterol Education Program Adult Treatment Panel. JAMA *269:*3009, 1993.
73. Schulman, K. A., Kinosian, B., Jacobson, T. A., et al.: Reducing high blood cholesterol level with drugs: Cost-effectiveness of pharmacologic management. JAMA *264:*3025, 1990.
74. Oster, G., and Epstein, A. M.: Cost-effectiveness of antihyperlipemic therapy in the prevention of coronary heart disease: The case of cholestyramine. JAMA *258:*2381, 1987.
75. Goldman, L., Weinstein, M. C., Goldman, P. A., and Williams, L. W.: Cost-effectiveness of HMG-CoA reductase inhibition for primary and secondary prevention of coronary heart disease. JAMA *265:*1145, 1991.
76. Hay, J. W., Wittels, E. H., and Gotto, A. M.: An economic evaluation of lovastatin for cholesterol lowering and coronary artery disease reduction. Am. J. Cardiol. *67:*780, 1991.
77. Kinosian, B. P., and Eisenberg, J. M.: Cutting into cholesterol: Cost-effective alternatives for treating hypercholesterolemia. JAMA *259:*2249, 1988.
78. Kristiansen, I. S., Eggen, A. E., and Thelle, D. S.: Cost-effectiveness of incremental programmes for lowering serum cholesterol concentration: Is individual intervention worthwhile? Br. Med. J. *302:*1119, 1991.
79. Goldman, L., Goldman, P., Williams, L., and Weinstein, M. C.: Cost-effectiveness considerations in the treatment of heterozygous familial hypercholesterolemia with medications. *In* Proceedings of the National Heart, Lung, and Blood Institute Workshop on Identification and Management of Heterozygous Familial Hypercholesterolemia. Am. J. Cardiol. *72:*75D, 1993.
80. Goldman, L., Weinstein, M. C., and Williams, L. W.: Relative impact of targeted versus populationwide cholesterol interventions on the incidence of coronary heart disease. Circulation *80:*254, 1989.
81. Farquhar, J. W., Fortmann, S. P., Flora, J. A., et al.: Effects of community-wide education on cardiovascular disease risk factors. The Stanford Five-City Project. JAMA *264:*359, 1990.
82. Puska, P., Salonen, J. T., Nissinen, A., et al.: Change in risk factors for coronary heart disease during 10 years of a community intervention programme (North Karelia project). Br. Med. J. *287:*1840, 1983.
83. Garber, A. M., Sox, H. C., and Littenberg, B.: Screening asymptomatic adults for cardiac risk factors: The serum cholesterol level. Ann. Intern. Med. *110:*622, 1989.

HYPERTENSION

84. The Fifth Report of the Joint National Committee on Detection, Evaluation, and Treatment of High Blood Pressure (JNC V). Arch. Intern. Med. *153:*154, 1993.
85. Sagie, A., Larson, M. G., and Levy, D.: The natural history of borderline isolated systolic hypertension. N. Engl. J. Med. *329:*1912, 1993.
86. SHEP Cooperative Research Group: Prevention of stroke by antihypertensive drug treatment in older persons with isolated systolic hypertension: Final results of the Systolic Hypertension in the Elderly Program (SHEP). JAMA *265:*3255, 1991.
87. Dahlof, B., Lindholm, L. H., Hansson, L., et al.: Morbidity and mortality in the Swedish Trial in Old Patients with Hypertension (STOP-Hypertension). Lancet *338:*1281, 1991.
88. Medical Research Council Working Party: MRC trial of treatment of mild hypertension: Principal results. Br. Med. J. *291:*97, 1985.
89. Insua, J. T., Sacks, H. S., Lau, T., et al.: Drug treatment of hypertension in the elderly: A meta-analysis. Ann. Intern. Med. *121:*355, 1994.
90. Mulrow, C. D., Cornell, J. A., Herrera, C. R., et al.: Hypertension in the elderly. Implications and generalizability of randomized trials. JAMA *272:*1932, 1994.
91. Hebert, P. R., Joser, M., Mayer, J., et al.: Recent evidence on drug therapy of mild to moderate hypertension and decreased risk of coronary heart disease. Arch. Intern. Med. *153:*578, 1993.
92. Materson, B. J., Reda, D. J., Cushman, W. C., et al.: Single-drug therapy for hypertension in men: A comparison of six antihypertensive agents with placebo. N. Engl. J. Med. *328:*914, 1993.
93. Neaton, J. D., Grimm, R. H., Prineas, R. J., et al.: Treatment of mild hypertension study: Final results. JAMA *270:*713, 1993.
94. Littenberg, B., Garber, A. M., and Sox, H. C.: Screening for hypertension. Ann. Intern. Med. *112:*192, 1990.
95. Weinstein, M. C., and Stason, W. B.: Hypertension: A Policy Perspective. Cambridge, Mass., Harvard University Press, 1976.
96. Stokes, J., III, and Carmichael, D. C.: A Cost-Benefit Analysis of Model Hypertension Control. Bethesda, National Heart, Lung and Blood Institute, 1975.
97. Edelson, J. T., Weinstein, M. C., Tosteson, A. N. A., et al.: Long-term cost-effectiveness of various initial monotherapies for mild to moderate hypertension. JAMA *263:*408, 1990.
98. Three-Community Hypertension Control Program. V. Cost-effectiveness of intervention. Mayo Clin. Proc. *56:*11, 1981.
99. Hannan, E. L., and Graham, J. K.: A cost-benefit study of hypertension screening and treatment program at the work setting. Inquiry *15:*345, 1978.
100. Tsevat, J.: Impact and cost-effectiveness of smoking interventions. Am. J. Med. *93*(Suppl. 1A):43, 1992.
101. Hermanson, B., Omenn, G. S., Kronmal, R. A., and Gersh, B. J.: Beneficial six-year outcome of smoking cessation in older men and women with coronary artery disease. N. Engl. J. Med. *319:*1365, 1988.
102. Rosenberg, L., Palmer, J. R., and Shapiro, S.: Decline in the risk of myocardial infarctions among women who stop smoking. N. Engl. J. Med. *322:*213, 1990.
103. Bartecchi, C. E., MacKenzie, T. D., and Schrier, R. W.: The human costs of tobacco use (first of 2 parts). N. Engl. J. Med. *330:*907, 1994.
104. MacKenzie, T. D., Bartecchi, C. E., and Schrier, R. W.: The human costs of tobacco use (second of 2 parts). N. Engl. J. Med. *330:*975, 1994.
105. Grover, S. A., Gray-Donald, K., Joseph, L., et al.: Life expectancy fol-

lowing dietary modification or smoking cessation. Estimating the benefits of a prudent lifestyle. Arch. Intern. Med. *154:*1697, 1994.
106. Cohen, S. J., Stookey, G. K., Katz, B. P., et al.: Encouraging primary care physicians to help smokers quit. Ann. Intern. Med. *110:*648, 1989.
107. Cummings, S. T., Coates, T. J., Richard, R. J., et al.: Training physicians in counseling and smoking cessation: A randomized trial of the "Quit for Life" program. Ann. Intern. Med. *110:*640, 1989.
108. Silagy, C., Mant, D., Fowler, G., and Lodge, M.: Meta-analysis on efficacy of nicotine replacement therapies in smoking cessation. Lancet *343:*139, 1994.
109. Kenford, S. L., Fiore, M. C., Jorenby, D. E., et al.: Predicting smoking cessation. Who will quit with and without the nicotine patch? JAMA *271:*589, 1994.
110. Oster, G., Huse, D. M., Delea, T. E., and Colditz, G. A.: Cost effectiveness of nicotine gum as an adjunct to physician's advice against cigarette smoking. JAMA *256:*1315, 1986.
111. Hughes, J. R., Gust, S. W., Keenan, R. M., et al.: Nicotine vs placebo gum in general medical practice. JAMA *261:*1300. 1989.
112. Abelin, T., Muller, P., Buehler, A., et al.: Controlled trial of transdermal nicotine patch in tobacco withdrawal. Lancet *1:*7, 1989.
113. Tonnesen, P., Fryd, V., Hansen, M., et al.: Effect of nicotine chewing gum in combination with group counseling on the cessation of smoking. N. Engl. J. Med. *318:*15, 1988.
114. Lando, H. A., McGovern, P. G., Barrios, F. X., and Etringer, B. D.: Comparative evaluation of American Cancer Society and American Lung Association smoking cessation clinics. Am. J. Public Health *80:*554, 1990.
115. Danaher, B. G., Berkanovic, E., and Gerger, B.: Mass media-based health behavior change: Televised smoking cessation program. Addict. Behav. *9:*245, 1984.
116. Pierce, J. P., Macaskill, P., and Hill, D.: Long-term effectiveness of mass media led antismoking campaigns in Australia. Am. J. Public Health *80:*565, 1990.
117. Krumholz, H. M., Cohen, B. J., Tsevat, J., et al.: Cost-effectiveness of a smoking cessation program after myocardial infarction. J. Am. Coll. Cardiol. *22:*1697, 1993.
118. Hubert, H. B., Feinleib, M., McNamara, P. M., and Castelli, W. P.: Obesity as an independent risk factor for cardiovascular disease: A 26-year follow-up of participants in the Framingham Heart Study. Circulation *67:*968, 1983.
119. Brownell, K. D., and Kaye, F. S.: A school-based behavior modification, nutrition, education, and physical activity program for obese children. Am. J. Clin. Nutr. *35:*277, 1982.
120. Brownell, K. D., Stunkard, A. J., and McKeon, P. E.: Weight reduction at the worksite: A promise partially fulfilled. Am. J. Psychiatry *142:*47, 1985.
121. Stunkard, A. J.: The current status of treatment for obesity in adults. *In* Stunkard, A. J., and Stellar, E. (eds.): Eating and Its Disorders. New York, Raven Press, 1984.
122. Blair, S. N., Kohl, H. W., Paffenbarger, R. S., et al.: Physical fitness and all-cause mortality: A prospective study of healthy men and women. JAMA *262:*2395, 1989.
123. Slattery, M. L., Jacobs, D. R., and Nichaman, M. Z.: Leisure time physical activity and coronary heart disease death. The US Railroad Study. Circulation *79:*304, 1989.
124. Ekelund, L. G., Haskell, W. L., Johnson, J. L., et al.: Physical fitness as a predictor of cardiovascular mortality in asymptomatic North American men. N. Engl. J. Med. *310:*1379, 1988.
125. Paffenbarger, R. S., Jr., Hyde, R. T., Wing, A. L., et al.: The association of changes in physical-activity level and other lifestyle characteristics with mortality among men. N. Engl. J. Med. *328:*538, 1993.
126. Sandvik, L., Erikssen, J., Thaulow, E., et al.: Physical fitness as a predictor of mortality among healthy, middle-aged Norwegian men. N. Engl. J. Med. *328:*533, 1993.
127. Lakka, T. A., Venalainen, J. M., Rauramaa, R., et al.: Relation of leisure-time physical activity and cardiorespiratory fitness to the risk of acute myocardial infarction in men. N. Engl. J. Med. *330:*1549, 1994.
128. Rodriguez, L., Curb, J. D., Burchfiel, C. M., et al.: Physical activity and 23-year incidence of coronary heart disease morbidity and mortality among middle-aged men. The Honolulu Heart Program. Circulation *89:*2540, 1994.
129. Cox, M., Shepard, R. J., and Corey, P.: Influence of an employee fitness programme upon fitness, productivity, and absenteeism. Ergonomics *24:*795, 1981.
130. Shepard, R. J., Corey, P., Renzland, P., and Cox, M.: The influence of an employee fitness and lifestyle modification upon medical care costs. Can. J. Public Health *73:*259, 1982.
131. Oldridge, N. B.: Adherence to adult exercise fitness programs. *In* Matarazzo, J. D., Miller, N. E., Herd, J. A., and Weiss, S. M. (eds.): Behavioral Health: A Handbook of Health Enhancement and Disease Prevention. New York, John Wiley and Sons, 1984, pp. 467–487.
132. Hatziandreu, E. I., Koplan, J. P., Weinstein, M. C., et al.: A cost-effectiveness analysis of exercise as a health promotion activity. Am. J. Public Health *78:*1417, 1988.
133. Oldridge, N. B., Guyatt, G. H., Fischer, M. E., and Rimm, A. A.: Cardiac rehabilitation after myocardial infarction. Combined experience of randomized clinical trials. JAMA *260:*945, 1988.
134. Dennis, C. A., Houston-Miller, N., Schwartz, R. G., et al.: Early return to work after uncomplicated myocardial infarction: Results of a randomized trial. JAMA *260:*214, 1988.
135. Picard, M. H., Dennis, C., Schwartz, R. G., et al.: Cost-benefit analysis of early return to work after uncomplicated acute myocardial infarction. Am. J. Cardiol. *63:*1308, 1989.
136. Bor, D. H., and Himmelstein, D. U.: Endocarditis prophylaxis for patients with mitral valve prolapse. A quantitative analysis. Am. J. Med. *76:*711, 1984.
137. Clemens, J. D., and Ransohoff, D. F.: A quantitative assessment of predental antibiotic prophylaxis for patients with mitral valve prolapse. J. Chron. Dis. *37:*531, 1984.
138. Durack, D. T.: Prevention of infective endocarditis. N. Engl. J. Med. *332:*38, 1995.
139. Kellerman, A. L., Hackman, H. B., and Somes, G.: Dispatcher-assisted cardiopulmonary resuscitation—validation of efficacy. Circulation *80:*1231, 1989.
140. Crampton, R. S., Aldrich, R. F., Gascho, J. A., et al.: Reduction of prehospital, ambulance, and community coronary death rates by the community-wide emergency cardiac care system. Am. J. Med. *58:*151, 1975.
141. Eisenberg, M. S., Hallstrom, A., and Bergner, L.: Long-term survival after out-of-hospital arrest. N. Engl. J. Med. *306:*1340, 1982.
142. Cummins, R. O., and Eisenberg, M. S.: Prehospital cardiopulmonary resuscitation: Is it effective? JAMA *253:*2408, 1985.
143. Bachman, J. W., McDonald, G. S., and O'Brien, P. C.: A study of out-of-hospital cardiac arrests in Northeastern Minnesota. JAMA *256:*477, 1986.
144. Lombardi, G., Gallagher, J., and Gennis, P.: Outcome of out-of-hospital cardiac arrest in New York City. The Pre-Hospital Arrest Survival Evaluation (PHASE) study. JAMA *271:*678, 1994.
145. Becker, L. B., Ostrander, M. P., Barrett, J., and Kondos, G. T.: Outcome of CPR in a large metropolitan area. Where are the survivors? Ann. Emerg. Med. *20:*48, 1991.
146. Solomon, N. A.: What are representative survival rates for out-of-hospital cardiac arrest? Insights from the New Haven (Conn) Experience. Arch. Intern. Med. *153:*1218, 1993.
147. Eisenberg, M. S., Bergner, L., and Hallstrom, A.: Out-of-hospital cardiac arrest: Improved survival with paramedic services. Lancet *1:*812, 1980.
148. Urban, N., Bergner, L., and Eisenberg, M. S.: The costs of a suburban paramedic program in reducing deaths due to cardiac arrest. Med. Care *19:*379, 1981.
149. Roine, R. O., Kajaste, S., and Kaste, M.: Neuropsychological sequelae of cardiac arrest. JAMA *269:*237, 1993.
150. Ornato, J. P., Craren, E. J., Gonzalez, E. R., et al.: Cost-effectiveness of defibrillation by emergency medical technicians. Am. J. Emerg. Med *6:*108, 1988.
151. Valenzuela, T. D., Criss, E. A., Spaite, D., et al.: Cost-effectiveness analysis of paramedic emergency medical services in the treatment of prehospital cardiopulmonary arrest. Ann. Emerg. Med. *19:*1407, 1990.
152. Jakobsson, J., Nyquist, O., Rehnqvist, N., and Norberg, K. A.: Cost of a saved life following out-of-hospital cardiac arrest resuscitated by specially trained ambulance personnel. Acta Anaesthesiol. Scand. *31:*426, 1987.
153. Weisfeldt, M. L., Kerber, R. E., McGoldrick, P., et al.: American Heart Association report on the Public Access Defibrillation Conference, December 8–10, 1994. Circulation *92:*2740, 1995.

ACUTE MYOCARDIAL INFARCTION

154. The European Myocardial Infarction Project Group: Prehospital thrombolytic therapy in patients with suspected acute myocardial infarction. N. Engl. J. Med. *329:*383, 1993.
155. GREAT Group: Feasibility, safety, and efficacy of domiciliary thrombolysis by general practitioners: Gramian region early anistreplase trial. Br. Med. J. *305:*548, 1992.
156. Arntz, H.-R., Stern, R., Linderer, T., and Schroder, R.: Efficiency of a physician-operated mobile intensive care unit for prehospital thrombolysis in acute myocardial infarction. Am. J. Cardiol. *70:*4170, 1992.
157. Weaver W. D., Cerqueira, M., Halstrom, A. P., et al.: Prehospital-initiated vs hospital-initiated thrombolytic therapy. The Myocardial Infarction Triage and Intervention Trial. JAMA *270:*1211, 1993.
158. Fibrinolytic Therapy Trialists' Collaborative Group: Indications for fibrinolytic therapy in suspected acute myocardial infarction: Collaborative overview of early mortality and major morbidity results from all randomised trials of more than 1000 patients. Lancet *343:*311, 1994.
159. EMERAS (Estudio Multicentrico Estreptoquinasa Republicas de America del Sur) Collaborative Group: Randomised trial of late thrombolysis in patients with suspected acute myocardial infarction. Lancet *342:*767, 1993.
160. LATE Study Group: Late Assessment of Thrombolytic Efficacy (LATE) study with Alteplase 6-24 hours after onset of acute myocardial infarction. Lancet *342:*759, 1993.
161. Krumholz, H. M., Pasternak, R. C., Weinstein, M. C., et al.: Cost-effectiveness of thrombolytic therapy with streptokinase in elderly patients with suspected acute myocardial infarction. N. Engl. J. Med. *327:*7, 1992.
162. The GUSTO Angiographic Investigators: The effects of tissue plasminogen activator, streptokinase, or both on coronary-artery patency, ventricular function and survival after acute myocardial infarction. N. Engl. J. Med. *329:*1615, 1993.
163. The GUSTO Investigators: An international randomized trial comparing four thrombolytic strategies for acute myocardial infarction. N. Engl. J. Med. *329:*673, 1993.

164. Lee, K. L., Califf, R. M., Simes, J., et al. for the GUSTO Investigators: Holding GUSTO up to the light. Ann. Intern. Med. *120*:876, 1994.
165. Ridker, P. M., O'Donnell, C. J., Marder, V. J., and Hennekens, C. H.: A response to "Holding GUSTO up to the light." Ann. Intern. Med. *120*:882, 1994.
166. Mark, D. B., Hlatky, M. A., Califf, R. M., et al.: Cost-effectiveness of thrombolytic therapy with tissue plasminogen activator as compared with streptokinase for acute myocardial infarction. N. Engl. J. Med. *332*:1418, 1995.
167. Goel, V., and Naylor, C. D.: Potential cost-effectiveness of intravenous tissue plasminogen activator versus streptokinase for acute myocardial infarction. Can. J. Cardiol. *8*:31, 1992.
168. Simoons, M. L., Vos, J., and Martens, L. L.: Cost-utility analysis of thrombolytic therapy. Eur. Heart J. *12*:694, 1991.
169. Brody, B., Wray, N., Bame, S., et al.: The impact of economic considerations on clinical decisionmaking: The case of thrombolytic therapy. Med. Care *29*:899, 1991.
170. Midgett, A. S., Wong, J. B., Beshansky, J. R., et al.: Cost-effectiveness of streptokinase for acute myocardial infarction: A combined meta-analysis and decision analysis of the effects of infarct location and of likelihood of infarction. Med. Decis. Making *14*:108, 1994.
171. Laffel, G. L., Fineberg, H. V., and Braunwald, E.: A cost-effectiveness model for coronary thrombolysis/reperfusion therapy. J. Am. Coll. Cardiol. *10*:79, 1987.
172. Goldman, L.: Cost and quality of life: Thrombolysis and primary angioplasty. J. Am. Coll. Cardiol. *25*:38s–41s, 1995.
173. Grines, C. L., Browne, K. F., Marco, J., et al.: A comparison of immediate angioplasty with thrombolytic therapy for acute myocardial infarction. N. Engl. J. Med. *328*:673, 1993.
174. Ziljstra, F., de Boer, M. J., Hoorntje, J. C. A., et al.: A comparison of immediate coronary angioplasty with intravenous streptokinase in acute myocardial infarction. N. Engl. J. Med. *328*:680, 1993.
175. Gibbons, R. J., Holmes, D. R., Reeder, G. S., et al. for the Mayo Coronary Care Unit and Catheterization Laboratory Groups: Immediate angioplasty compared with the administration of a thrombolytic agent followed by conservative treatment for myocardial infarction. N. Engl. J. Med. *328*:685, 1993.
176. Williams, D. O., Braunwald, E., Knatterud, G., et al.: One-year results of the Thrombolysis in Myocardial Infarction Investigation (TIMI) Phase II Trial. Circulation *85*:533, 1992.
177. Pitt, B.: Evaluation of the postinfarct patient. Circulation *91*:1855, 1995.
178. Myers, M. G., Baigrie, R. S., Charlat, M. L., and Morgan, C. D.: Are routine noninvasive tests useful in prediction of outcome after myocardial infarction in elderly people? Lancet *342*:1069, 1993.
179. Moss, A. J., Goldstein, R. E., Hall, W. J., et al.: Detection and significance of myocardial ischemia in stable patients after recovery from an acute coronary event. JAMA *69*:2379, 1993.
180. Rouleau, J. L., Moye, L. A., Pfeffer, M. A., et al.: A comparison of management patterns after acute myocardial infarction in Canada and the United States. N. Engl. J. Med. *328*:779, 1993.
181. Anticoagulants in the Secondary Prevention of Events in Coronary Thrombosis (ASPET) Research Group: Effect of long-term oral anticoagulant treatment on mortality and cardiovascular morbidity after myocardial infarction. Lancet *343*:499, 1994.
182. van Bergen, P. F. M. M., Jonker, J. J. C., van Hout, B. A., et al.: Costs and effects of long-term oral anticoagulant treatment after myocardial infarction. JAMA *273*:925, 1995.
183. Cairns, J. A., and Markham, B. A.: Economics and efficacy in choosing oral anticoagulants or aspirin after myocardial infarction. JAMA *273*(Edit.):965, 1995.
184. Pfeffer, M. A., Braunwald, E., Moye, L. A., et al.: Effect of captopril on mortality and morbidity in patients with left ventricular dysfunction after myocardial infarction: Results of the Survival and Ventricular Enlargement Trial. N. Engl. J. Med. *327*:669, 1992.
185. The Acute Infarction Ramipril Efficacy (AIRE) Study Investigators: Effect of ramipril on mortality and morbidity of survivors of acute myocardial infarction with clinical evidence of heart failure. Lancet *342*:821, 1993.
186. Gruppo Italiano per lo Studio della Sopravvivenza nell'Infarto Miocardico (GISSI):GISSI-3: Effects of lisinopril and transdermal glyceryl trinitrate singly and together on 6-week mortality and ventricular function after acute myocardial infarction. Lancet *343*:1115, 1994.
187. Tsevat, J., Duke, D., Goldman, L., et al.: Cost-effectiveness of captopril therapy after myocardial infarction. J. Am. Coll. Cardiol. *26*:914, 1995.
188. Goldman, L., Sia, S. T. B., Cook, E. F., et al.: Cost-effectiveness of routine long-term beta-adrenergic antagonist therapy following acute myocardial infarction. N. Engl. J. Med. *319*:152, 1988.
189. Pozen, M. W., D'Agostino, R. B., Mitchell, J. B., et al.: The usefulness of a predictive instrument to reduce inappropriate admissions to the coronary care unit. Ann. Intern. Med. *92*:238, 1980.
190. Pozen, M. W., D'Agostino, R. B., Selker, H. P., et al.: A predictive instrument to improve coronary-care-unit admission practices in acute ischemic heart disease: A prospective multicenter clinical trial. N. Engl. J. Med. *310*:1273, 1984.
191. Sarasin, F. P., Reymond, J.-M., Griffith, J. L., et al.: Impact of the Acute Cardiac Ischemia Time-Insensitive Predictive Instrument (ACI-TIPI) on the speed of triage decision making for emergency department patients presenting with chest pain. A controlled clinical trial. J. Gen. Intern. Med. *9*:187, 1994.
192. Gaspoz, J. M., Lee, T. H., Cook, E. F., et al.: Outcomes of rule-out myocardial infarction patients admitted to a new short-stay unit. Am. J. Cardiol. *68*:1459, 1991.
193. Gaspoz, J. M., Lee, T. H., Weinstein, M. C., et al.: Cost-effectiveness of a new short-stay unit to "rule-out" acute myocardial infarction in low risk patients. J. Am. Coll. Cardiol. *24*:1249, 1994.
194. Berning, J., Launbjerg, J., and Appleyard, M.: Echocardiographic algorithms for admission and predischarge prediction of mortality in acute myocardial infarction. Am. J. Cardiol. *69*:1538, 1992.
195. Fleischmann, K. E., Goldman, L., Robiolio, P., et al.: Echocardiographic correlates of survival in chest pain patients. J. Am. Coll. Cardiol. *23*:1390, 1994.
196. Hilton, T. C., Thompson, R. C., Williams, H. J., et al.: Technetium-99m sestamibi myocardial perfusion imaging in the emergency room evaluation of chest pain. J. Am. Coll. Cardiol. *23*:1016, 1994.
197. Varetto, T., Cantalupi, D., Altieri, A., and Orlandi, C.: Emergency room technetium-99m sestamibi imaging to rule out acute myocardial ischemic events in patients with nondiagnostic electrocardiograms. J. Am. Coll. Cardiol. *22*:1804, 1993.
198. Adams, J. E., III, Abendschein, D. R., and Jaffe, A. S.: Biochemical markers of myocardial injury. Is MB creatine kinase the choice for the 1990s? Circulation *88*:750, 1993.
199. Roberts, R., and Kleiman, N. S.: Earlier diagnosis and treatment of acute myocardial infarction necessitates the need for a "new diagnostic mind-set." Circulation *89*:872, 1994.
200. Puleo, P. R., Meyer, D., Wathen, C., et al.: Use of a rapid assay of subforms of creatine kinase MB to diagnose or rule out acute myocardial infarction. N. Engl. J. Med. *331*:561, 1994.
201. Adams, J. E., III, Bodor, G. S., Davila-Roman, V. G., et al.: Cardiac troponin I. A marker with high specificity for cardic injury. Circulation *88*:101, 1993.
202. Hamm, C. W., Ravkilde, J., Gerhardt, W., et al.: The prognostic value of serum troponin T in unstable angina. N. Engl. J. Med. *327*:146, 1992.
203. Lee, T. H., Rouan, G. W., Weisberg, M. C., et al.: Sensitivity of routine clinical criteria for diagnosing myocardial infarction within 24 hours of hospitalization. Ann. Intern. Med. *106*:181, 1987.
204. Mulley, A. G., Thibault, G. E., Hughes, R. A., et al.: The course of patients with suspected myocardial infarction: The identification of low-risk patients for early transfer from intensive care. N. Engl. J. Med. *302*:943, 1980.
205. Mark, D. B., Sigmon, K., Topol, E. J., et al.: Identification of acute myocardial infarction patients suitable for early hospital discharge after aggressive interventional therapy. Results from the Thrombolysis and Angioplasty in Acute Myocardial Infarction Registry. Circulation *83*:1186, 1991.
206. Weingarten, S., Ermann, B., Bolus, R., et al.: Early "step-down" transfer of low-risk patients with chest pain. Ann. Intern. Med. *113*:283, 1990.
207. Weingarten, S. R., Riedinger, M. S., Conner, L., et al.: Practice guidelines and reminders to reduce duration of hospital stay for patients with chest pain. Ann. Intern. Med. *120*:257, 1994.
208. Ellrodt, A. G., Conner, L., Riedinger, M., and Weingarten, S.: Measuring and improving physician compliance with clinical practice guidelines. Ann. Intern. Med. *122*:277, 1995.
209. Topol, E. J., Leya, F., Pinkerton, C. A., et al.: A comparison of directional atherectomy with coronary angioplasty in patients with coronary artery disease. N. Engl. J. Med. *329*:221, 1993.
210. Adelman, A. G., Cohen, E. A., Kimball, B. P., et al.: A comparison of directional atherectomy with balloon angioplasty for lesions of the left anterior descending coronary artery. N. Engl. J. Med. *329*:228, 1993.
211. Serruys, P. W., de Jaegere, P., Kiemeneij, F., et al.: A comparison of balloon-expandable-stent implantation with balloon angioplasty in patients with coronary artery disease. N. Engl. J. Med. *331*:489, 1994.
212. Fischman, D. L., Leon, M. B., Baim, D. S., et al. for the Stent Restenosis Study Investigators: A randomized comparison of coronary-stent placement and balloon angioplasty in the treatment of coronary artery disease. N. Engl. J. Med. *331*:496, 1994.
213. Cohen, D. J., Breall, J. A., Ho, K. K., et al.: Evaluating the potential cost-effectiveness of stenting as a treatment for symptomatic single-vessel coronary disease: Use of a decision-analytic model. Circulation *89*:1859, 1994.
214. Doliszny, K. M., Luepker, R. V., Burke, G. L., et al.: Estimated contribution of coronary artery bypass graft surgery to the decline in coronary heart disease mortality: The Minnesota Heart Survey. J. Am. Coll. Cardiol. *24*:95, 1994.
215. Yusuf, S., Zucker, D., Peduzzi, P., et al.: Effect of coronary artery bypass graft surgery on survival: Overview of 10-year results from randomised trials by the Coronary Artery Bypass Graft Surgery Trialists Collaboration. Lancet *344*:565, 1994.
216. Bernstein, S. J., Hilborne, L. H., Leape, L. L., et al.: The appropriateness of use of coronary angiography in New York State. JAMA *269*:766, 1993.
217. Leape, L. L., Hilborne, L. H., Park, R. E., et al.: The appropriateness of use of coronary artery bypass graft surgery in New York State. JAMA *269*:753, 1993.
218. Cromwell, J., Mitchell, J. B., and Stason, W. B.: Learning by doing in CABG surgery. Med. Care *28*:6, 1990.
219. Hannan, E. L., Kilburn, H., Racz, M., et al.: Improving the outcomes of coronary artery bypass surgery in New York State. JAMA *271*:761, 1994.
220. Parisi, A. F., Folland, E. D., and Hartigan, P. on behalf of the Veterans

Affairs ACME Investigators: A comparison of angioplasty with medical therapy in the treatment of single-vessel coronary artery disease. N. Engl. J. Med. *326*:10, 1992.

221. RITA Trial Participants: Coronary angioplasty versus coronary artery bypass surgery: The Randomised Intervention Treatment of Angina (RITA) trial. Lancet *341*:573, 1993.
222. Goy, J. J., Eeckhout, E., Burnand, B., et al.: Coronary angioplasty versus left internal mammary artery grafting for isolated proximal left anterior descending artery stenosis. Lancet *343*:1449, 1994.
223. Hamm, C. W., Reimers, J., Ischinger, T., et al. for the German Angioplasty Bypass Surgery Investigation: A randomized study of coronary angioplasty compared with bypass surgery in patients with symptomatic multivessel coronary disease. N. Engl. J. Med. *331*:1037, 1994.
224. King, S. B., III, Lembo, N. J., Weintraub, W. S., et al.: A randomized trial comparing coronary angioplasty with coronary bypass surgery. N. Engl. J. Med. *331*:1044, 1994.
225. Mark, D. B., Nelson, C. L., Califf, R. M., et al.: Continuing evolution of therapy for coronary artery disease. Initial results from the era of coronary angioplasty. Circulation *89*:2015, 1994.
226. Weinstein, M. C., and Stason, W. B.: Cost-effectiveness of coronary artery bypass surgery. Circulation *66*(Suppl. III):56, 1982.

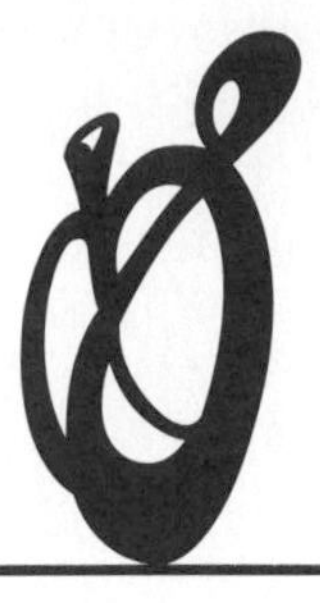

Part V
Heart Disease and Disorders of Other Organ Systems

Chapter 54
General Anesthesia and Noncardiac Surgery in Patients with Heart Disease

LEE GOLDMAN

ANESTHESIA 1756
General Anesthesia 1757
Spinal and Epidural Anesthesia 1757
Intraoperative Hemodynamics and Arrhythmias 1757
The Operation 1758
INFLUENCE OF UNDERLYING CARDIOVASCULAR DISEASE. 1758
Ischemic Heart Disease 1758
Hypertension .1761
Valvular Heart Disease and Cardiomyopathy 1761
Congenital Heart Disease 1762
Congestive Heart Failure. 1762
Arrhythmias 1763
General Medical Problems 1763
POSTOPERATIVE COMPLICATIONS 1763
THE ROLE OF THE MEDICAL CONSULTANT .1764
REFERENCES .1766

The cardiovascular system of patients undergoing general anesthesia and noncardiac surgical procedures is subject to multiple stresses owing to depression of myocardial contractility and respiration as well as fluctuations in temperature, arterial pressure, ventricular filling pressures, blood volume, and activity of the autonomic nervous system. Complications of anesthesia and operation, such as hemorrhage, infection, fever, pulmonary embolism, and myocardial infarction, impose additional burdens on the cardiovascular system. The patient with cardiac disease who is compensated preoperatively may be unable to meet these increased demands during the perioperative period, in which case arrhythmias, myocardial ischemia, and/or heart failure may develop.[1–3] As a consequence, a substantial proportion of all deaths in most series of noncardiac operations results from cardiovascular complications.

Because both the frequency and the seriousness of cardiovascular complications of general anesthesia and operation are considerably increased in the patient with known cardiovascular disease, the magnitude of these risks must be appreciated to decide on the advisability of noncardiac surgery in the cardiac patient. In addition, both the life expectancy and the quality of life of the patient must be taken into account. For instance, a noncardiac surgical procedure with a high risk, directed to correct a disorder that is not life threatening, may be difficult to justify if the patient's cardiac condition precludes a survival period sufficient to allow the patient to reap the benefits of the operation. Obviously the dangers and disability of the disease for which an operation is being proposed must also be balanced against the risk of the operation itself.

ANESTHESIA

Changes in cardiovascular function during general anesthesia are due to many factors, including direct effects of the anesthetic agent(s) and indirect effects mediated primarily through the autonomic nervous system. In addition, if respiration is inadequately maintained, the resulting hypoxemia, hypercarbia, and acidosis may further depress myocardial contractility and increase cardiac irritability. The interplay of these several variables may produce changes in arterial and central venous pressures, cardiac output, and rate and rhythm. To minimize the risk of operation in the patient with a compromised cardiovascular system, it is essential to minimize these changes.[3]

The choice of the anesthetic approach and the specific anesthetic agents to be used should be made by a qualified anesthesiologist, commonly after careful evaluation of the patient's medical and cardiac condition and often after consultation with the surgeon and the internist or cardiologist. Different anesthesiologists may prefer different anesthetic techniques, and the anesthesiological literature clearly indicates that there is little, if any, correlation between the anesthetic route or agents and the likelihood of major clinical complications. Thus, the skill and experience of the anesthesiologist, including the ability to monitor hemodynamics and respond quickly, are far more important than the specific agent that is used. Although the cardiological consultant should not expect to dictate the anesthetic approach, the quality of the consultation will be improved if the consultant appreciates the clinical pharmacology of the anesthetic agent and the effects of intubation and extubation.

General Anesthesia

The induction of anesthesia is usually accomplished with intravenous anesthetics. With the exception of ketamine, the agents used for the induction of anesthesia commonly lower systemic arterial pressure by about 20 to 30 per cent in healthy patients, but sometimes by a greater amount in hypertensive patients.[4] During laryngoscopy and tracheal intubation, blood pressure can increase by 20 to 30 mm Hg,[4] but such increases can be avoided by adequate topical anesthesia or by nasal intubation because the hypertension appears to be caused by the laryngoscopy rather than by the passage of a tube into the trachea.

INHALATION AGENTS. These agents enter the bloodstream by way of the alveoli and are excreted across the alveoli essentially unchanged. In most major operations a combination of inhalation agents and/or intravenous anesthetics is used.[5]

Nitrous oxide usually is used to supplement other intravenous or inhalation agents. It causes a modest decrease of about 15 per cent in cardiac output but usually does not cause substantial hypotension because of reflex vasoconstriction.

Halothane and related agents also cause a reduction in myocardial contractility,[6] but unlike nitrous oxide, they are not associated with substantial reflex vasoconstriction. Thus, when halothane is added to nitrous oxide, there are often further reductions in arterial pressure because of reductions in cardiac output without concomitant vasoconstriction. Halothane also appears to sensitize the myocardium to catecholamines, sometimes resulting in arrhythmias. *Enflurane* has properties similar to halothane; it appears to result in less sensitization to catecholamines but potentially more risks of hypotension than with halothane. *Isoflurane* appears to have less of a negative inotropic effect than halothane or enflurane, but it can be associated with marked decreases in systemic vascular resistance, and hence a fall in systemic blood pressure.

INTRAVENOUS ANESTHETICS. Among the narcotic analgesics, *morphine* is generally well tolerated, although it does cause venodilation, thereby decreasing preload and cardiac output. *Fentanyl* is less likely to cause as much hypotension or vasodilation as morphine, and it has a shorter duration of action.[7] Like morphine, it tends not to have major effects on myocardial contractility, but it is more likely than morphine to cause bradycardia. *Sufentanil* and *alfentanil* have cardiovascular effects that are generally similar to those of fentanyl.

Short-acting barbiturates, especially *thiopental,* often cause a fall in blood pressure because of depressive actions on myocardial contractility and sympathetic tone.[8] In patients who have severe hypovolemia or severe cardiac dysfunction, serious reductions in cardiac output can occasionally occur after a small dose of thiopental.

Benzodiazepines, including midazolam, can achieve adequate sedation with only mild cardiovascular depression. However, occasionally patients may become apneic or hypotensive after small doses. *Droperidol* causes vasodilation because of its alpha-adrenergic blocking action and its effect on the central nervous system.

Ketamine is unlike other commonly used intravenous anesthetics in that it does not cause cardiovascular depression. Although it does cause some direct myocardial depression, this is commonly counterbalanced by direct stimulation of the central nervous system and by an increase in circulating catecholamines.

MUSCLE RELAXANTS. Drugs used for muscle relaxation also may have cardiovascular effects. *Succinylcholine* can cause bradycardia, which can be reversed or prevented by the administration of atropine. In patients anesthetized with halothane, *pancuronium* and *gallamine* cause an increase in heart rate, arterial pressure, and cardiac output, while *tubocurarine* and *metocurine* result in a fall in mean arterial pressure with mild elevations in heart rate and little, if any, change in cardiac output. *Vecuronium* has essentially no cardiovascular side effects.

Spinal and Epidural Anesthesia

Spinal and epidural anesthesia cause sympathetic denervation, which produces peripheral arteriodilation and venodilation. Systemic vascular resistance may be reduced by 10 to 15 per cent. Venodilation may cause a marked reduction in right ventricular preload as a consequence of sympathetic denervation. Under these circumstances, right ventricular preload depends critically on the effects of gravity on the patient's position, and on the total blood volume.

REGIONAL AND LOCAL ANESTHESIA. Regional and local anesthesia cause cardiovascular effects only to the extent that the agents are absorbed into the bloodstream or where there is sympathetic blockade accompanying the local sensory block. A major concern with local or regional anesthesia is whether the technique is adequate for the planned procedure; the cardiological consultant should not underestimate the cardiovascular consequences of inadequate anesthesia.

Complications of General Anesthetics

In a prospective randomized trial comparing enflurane, fentanyl, halothane, and isoflurane carried out in over 17,000 patients, severe ventricular arrhythmias were more common with halothane, severe hypertension was more common with fentanyl, and severe tachycardia was more common with isoflurane. However, these four agents were not associated with significantly different overall rates of death, myocardial infarction, or stroke, perhaps because the rates of these events were so low.

As of this writing, the potential benefit of regional anesthesia compared with general anesthesia is uncertain,[10–12] in part because the decline in systemic blood pressure from regional anesthesia can cause transient myocardial ischemia.[13] Combined epidural and general anesthesia and analagesia can attenuate sympathetic nervous system hyperactivity, reduce the need for parenteral analgesia, reduce coagulation abnormalities, improve postoperative ventilatory function, and reduce the duration of intensive care unit stay in patients undergoing major vascular surgery.[14,15] In a randomized trial of 173 patients, however, there were no differences in cardiac complications among patients who underwent abdominal aortic surgery with combined epidural and light general anesthesia compared with general anesthesia alone.[16]

Intraoperative Hemodynamics and Arrhythmias

During the operative procedure, it is not uncommon for systolic blood pressure to fall into the range of 95 to 105 mm Hg. Such blood pressure reductions are often brief and may respond to a lightening of the anesthesia or, in 20 to 30 per cent of patients, either to a brisk fluid challenge or the use of intravenous sympathomimetic agents. Any severe reduction in arterial pressure in patients with ischemic heart disease can reduce coronary flow and precipitate myocardial ischemia. In general, such reductions in blood pressure are not associated with major cardiac complications, such as myocardial infarction, unless they are marked and sustained. For example, increased complication rates have been reported for reductions in systolic arterial pressures that exceed approximately 33 per cent of the preoperative blood pressure and that persist for 10 or more minutes, or are more than 50 per cent below the preoperative blood pressure, or for mean arterial pressure reductions of 20 mm Hg or greater for 60 or more minutes, or for 20-mm Hg increases in mean arterial pressure sustained for 15 or more minutes.[17-19] Fluids that are administered to maintain intraoperative blood pressure can potentially cause postoperative fluid overload.

The risk of unplanned intraoperative hypotension is at least as great with spinal or epidural anesthesia as with general anesthesia.[20] However, because spinal and epidural anesthesia are not direct myocardial depressants, they may be advantageous in patients with very severe myocardial dysfunction; but even in those circumstances, well-balanced general anesthesia, sometimes including ketamine, has been used successfully.

Transient bradycardias, such as sinus bradycardia and junctional rhythm, may occur during periods of vagal stimulation. These bradyarrhythmias commonly respond to a lightening of the anesthesia or to the administration of atropine or $beta_1$-adrenoceptor agonists such as isoproterenol or epinephrine. Tachyarrhythmias may result from hypovolemia or vasodilation as well as from sensitization of the myocardium to catecholamines that are circulating and/or released by sympathetic nerve endings in the heart. Tachycardia is poorly tolerated by patients with mitral stenosis (see p. 1007) and may cause myocardial ischemia in patients with coronary artery disease. Therapy with specific antiarrhythmic medications is usually indicated only when the arrhythmia causes circulatory compromise and does not respond to changes in the depth of anesthesia or to attention to problems such as hypoxemia, hypovolemia, hypotension, or the potentially precipitating surgical manipulation.

Positive-pressure ventilation during general anesthesia reduces the return of blood to the right side of the heart and tends to reduce ventricular preload. Fluid that is administered during positive-pressure ventilation does not increase preload to the extent that it would in the patient who is ventilating spontaneously. When the positive-pressure ventilation of general anesthesia ceases, ventricular preload increases, often abruptly, and hypertension or pulmonary congestion may result. Analogous physiological changes can occur with the cessation of spinal or epidural anesthesia because the venodilation caused by these agents also reduces right ventricular preload.

MONITORING. In patients with severe underlying heart disease undergoing noncardiac surgery, it is mandatory to monitor cardiac function during anesthesia,[21] including cardiac rate and rhythm and directly recorded arterial blood pressure. A radial artery line permits not only monitoring of intra-arterial pressure but also frequent sampling for determination of blood gases. In the presence of peripheral vasoconstriction, indirect (cuff) blood pressure measurements may greatly underestimate true arterial pressure. Monitoring of the pulmonary artery (or, preferably, pulmonary artery wedge) pressure and cardiac output is often desirable in patients who are critically ill, who have marginal cardiovascular reserve, who are to undergo prolonged operative procedures in which major blood losses might occur, and in whom hypotensive anesthesia is to be used. Both pulmonary artery wedge pressure and cardiac output can be measured with the aid of a multiple-lumen balloon flotation catheter (Swan-Ganz) and the thermodilution method (see Chap. 6). For detection of intraoperative myocardial ischemia, multiple-lead electrocardiography is preferable and data suggest that transesophageal echocardiography can be reserved for patients with a recent myocardial infarction, unstable angina, advanced heart failure, tight aortic stenosis, or a thoracic aortic aneurysm. Pulmonary capillary wedge pressure is a poor marker of ischemia, but the pulmonary capillary wedge pressure remains the best index of fluid balance.[22] In one randomized, unblinded study, aggressive preoperative optimization of cardiac hemodynamics was associated with a reduced risk of postoperative cardiac morbidity and graft occlusion after peripheral vascular surgery, but the regimen provoked a preoperative myocardial infarction in 2 of 68 patients.[23] In seriously ill patients, urine output should be monitored with a Foley catheter.

The Operation

Just as consultant cardiologists must understand the pharmacological effects of anesthesia, they must also recognize the physiological effects of surgery, including the direct consequences of the operation and the expected responses to postoperative recuperation.

NATURE OF THE OPERATION. Although ophthalmological surgery[24] and transurethral prostatic resection[25] long have been known almost always to be safe, even in patients with a history of serious cardiac disease, general surgical mortality is often 25 to 50 per cent higher in patients with underlying cardiovascular conditions than in patients with normal cardiac function.[17,20,26-29] Among noncardiac surgical procedures, the highest cardiovascular complication rates are commonly associated with abdominal aortic aneurysm surgery,[26,30] which causes substantial myocardial stress because of aortic cross-clamping and major shifts in fluid and electrolytes. The risk of cardiac complications is also higher in other major abdominal and thoracic procedures than in procedures on the extremities, in large part because of the more difficult postoperative course. Patients who undergo operation for aortic aneurysm, carotid arterial disease, or peripheral vascular disease often have substantial coronary artery disease as well, and the extent of the latter may be underestimated because of the limitations caused by the peripheral arterial disease.

DURATION. The risk of cardiovascular mortality and morbidity is generally correlated with the duration of anesthesia, but this is principally because the longest operations are more often on the aorta or in the abdomen or chest than on the extremities. The risk of major cardiovascular complications does not appear to correlate with the duration of surgery after controlling for the type of surgery, unless the operation is prolonged because of intraoperative complications.

EMERGENCY OPERATION. When an operation is carried out under emergency conditions, it is associated with greatly increased mortality in patients with cardiovascular disease. The risk of postoperative cardiac complications, including postoperative myocardial infarction or cardiac death, is increased anywhere from 2.5- to 4-fold in emergency compared with elective surgery.[20,26,28,31] Part of this increased risk is because patients undergoing emergency operations may often have poorly controlled or unappreciated general medical problems, such as fluid and electrolyte imbalance or hepatic dysfunction.[26,28] However, emergency surgery appears to be an important correlate of postoperative complications, even after controlling for the underlying medical disease.[26,28,31]

The application of careful selection criteria and aggressive hemodynamic monitoring to noncardiac surgical procedures in patients with severe underlying heart disease may reduce the risk of intraoperative and postoperative cardiovascular complications. Thus the risk of a new infarction was reduced by about 40 per cent or more when patients with a history of infarction were aggressively monitored compared with when minimal invasive monitoring was used in the period from 1973 to 1976.[32,33] Although these nonrandomized studies did not control for other secular changes in medical care, it should not be surprising that the application of cardiovascular anesthesiological techniques to noncardiac surgery would have a beneficial effect. Thus, in patients who have suffered a myocardial infarction within the past 3 months, who have angina that is more severe than Canadian Class II (see pp. 12, 13), who have severe heart failure, or who are at very high risk based on indices such as the multifactorial index of cardiac risk in noncardiac surgery[26,28,34-36] (see p. 1765), available data support the use of intra-arterial and pulmonary artery catheters for careful hemodynamic monitoring. In other patients, even those undergoing abdominal aortic surgery, the value of pulmonary artery catheters is unproven.[37-39]

INFLUENCE OF UNDERLYING CARDIOVASCULAR DISEASE

Ischemic Heart Disease

Assessment of Risk

CLINICAL. Ischemic heart disease is a major determinant of perioperative morbidity and mortality. The incidence of perioperative myocardial infarction is increased 10- to 50-fold in patients who have previously suffered infarcts compared with patients who do not have a clinical history of coronary disease.

During the 1970's, several studies reported about a 30 per cent risk of reinfarction or cardiac death when patients were operated on within 3 months of the previous myocardial infarction, about a 15 per cent risk when the operation was performed 3 to 6 months after a prior infarction, and about a 5 per cent risk when the operation was performed more than 6 months after the infarction.[17,20] However, more recent data indicate that the application of invasive hemodynamic monitoring and careful regulation of oxygenation, electrolytes, volume status, and the hematocrit have markedly reduced the complication rate. For example, Rao et al.[32] reported only a 6 per cent reinfarction rate within 3 months after preoperative myocardial infarction and only a 2 per cent reinfarction rate between 3 and 6 months after a myocardial infarction, and then confirmed these low risks in a subsequent report.[33]

Obviously, truly life-saving procedures must be performed almost regardless of the cardiac risk, and purely elective surgery should commonly be delayed for 6 months after infarction, when the cardiovascular risks will have returned to a stable, long-term baseline risk. The more difficult issue is in patients in whom the operation is not truly emergent but is also not purely elective, for example, a patient with severe symptomatic peripheral vascular disease or a patient with a potentially resectable malignant tumor. In such situations one would like to delay operation sufficiently long for cardiac risk to be reduced but not wait a full 6 months. Because full healing of a myocardial infarction usually takes about 4 to 6 weeks, one rational approach is to evaluate the patient with post-myocardial infarction prognostic studies, such as a submaximal exercise tolerance test (Chap. 5)[37] and to use the patient's clinical and cardiological conditions as the guide for surgery sometime between 4 weeks and 3 months after the infarction.

A recent preoperative myocardial infarction increases a patient's relative risk of reinfarction with operation, but the absolute risk depends on a variety of factors in addition to the timing of the infarction. In general, one should be influenced less by whether or not a preoperative myocardial infarction was associated with the development of new Q waves than by the state of left ventricular function and the severity of preoperative angina. Thus, patients who have good exercise tolerance and left ventricular function after infarction and who can resume normal activity levels within 4 to 6 weeks after infarction should be able to undergo operation with relatively small absolute risks, even if their relative risk might be slightly lower if one could wait the full 6 months. By comparison, risks are likely to be substantially higher in patients who have postinfarction angina, large reversible defects on thallium scintigraphy, reduced left ventricular function, marked ST-segment depression with exercise, or other evidence of easily induced ischemia (see p. 1260).

When the patient with angina pectoris is evaluated, the patient's current (preoperative) exercise tolerance should be ascertained and an assessment made as to whether the anginal pattern is stable or unstable (see p. 1290). In patients who can carry objects such as two grocery bags or a young child up a flight of stairs without stopping and without appreciable symptoms, most surgical procedures are generally well tolerated.[40] Physicians should avoid relying on the *frequency* of angina because patients who voluntarily reduce their activity level may also greatly reduce their symptoms. This phenomenon is especially true in patients whose surgical conditions, such as orthopedic disorders or peripheral vascular disease, limit ambulation.

LABORATORY. *Exercise treadmill testing* is an objective means for assessing exercise tolerance and is especially beneficial if the history is unreliable. Unfortunately, the limited sensitivity and specificity of standard electrocardiographic exercise tolerance testing limit the use of this test for diagnosing coronary artery disease (see Chap. 5). In two studies of vascular surgery patients,[41,42] postoperative cardiac complications were significantly less in patients who exercised to higher heart rates and cardiac workloads. The prognostic value of limited exercise tolerance has also been reported in persons over age 65[43,44] in whom the inability to perform 2 minutes of bicycle exercise in a supine position and to raise the heart rate above 99 beats per minute was an independent important predictor of cardiac complications in noncardiac surgery. Of note was that poor exercise capacity was an independent predictor of cardiac complications, but electrocardiographic changes with exercise were not. Although some investigators have used radionuclide ventriculography to predict risk,[45] in other studies data from resting and/or exercise radionuclide ventriculography did not add important independent information for predicting overall perioperative cardiac risk.[43,46–48]

In patients who are unable to exercise because of noncardiac disability (e.g., intermittent claudication or orthopedic abnormalities), dipyridamole thallium imaging, ambulatory ischemia monitoring, or stress echocardiography can be used to assess perioperative risk. Dipyridamole thallium imaging (see Chap. 10) has been successful in identifying high-risk patients among selected subgroups of patients who are referred for the test prior to undergoing vascular surgery, and it is especially appealing for patients who have abnormal resting electrocardiograms or are taking medications such as digoxin that make electrocardiographic monitoring unreliable for the detection of ischemia.

Among 1410 patients in the five largest series of such patients,[49–53] a reversible defect on thallium scintigraphy had a sensitivity of 85 per cent for predicting postoperative cardiac complications and a specificity of 60 per cent; the relative risk of cardiac complications in a patient with a reversible defect was 9.0. However, when dipyridamole thallium scintigraphy was used in *unselected*, consecutive patients having abdominal aneurysm or major vascular surgery, it was *not* proven useful for predicting perioperative myocardial infarction, myocardial ischemia, or cardiac death.[48,54] In the largest single series of 451 *consecutive*, unselected patients, the presence of a reversible thallium defect had a sensitivity of just 36 per cent, a specificity of 65 per cent, and a relative risk of 1.0 (i.e., it was of no value whatsoever) for predicting major perioperative cardiac events.

Ambulatory electrocardiographic (Holter) monitoring can identify up to 90 per cent of patients who will develop major postoperative ischemic complications.[55] Patients with asymptomatic preoperative ischemia or asymptomatic postoperative ischemia have as high as a 30 per cent risk of developing a clinical event, including myocardial infarction, unstable angina, ischemic pulmonary edema, or cardiac death.[55–57] In contrast, asymptomatic intraoperative ischemia is less predictive.[57,58] Asymptomatic postoperative ischemia, which is found in a substantial minority of patients with or at risk for atherosclerotic disease,[59,60] commonly precedes a clinical event by an hour or more[58,61]; longer episodes of postoperative ischemia are associated with a higher risk of a major clinical event.[61] Patients with perioperative ischemia also have more late cardiac events well after surgery.[58,62]

Although routine transthoracic echocardiography adds little for the prediction of postoperative complications,[63] stress echocardiography after exercise or agents such as dipyridamole or dobutamine can be used to identify patients at markedly increased risk based on the provocation of left ventricular wall motion abnormalities with stress.[64–68] Stress echocardiography appears to be at least as good as dipyridamole thallium scintigraphy or ambulatory ischemia monitoring for predicting complications.

The utility of dipyridamole thallium imaging, ambulatory ischemia monitoring, and stress echocardiography can be improved when these techniques are used in appropriate patient subsets, such as patients with known coronary disease or patients who are undergoing major vascular surgery *and* are over age 70, have ventricular ectopic activity requiring treatment, or have diabetes mellitus requiring treatment.[49] In other types of patients, the lower risk of complications and the lower predictive values of the tests lead to unattractive cost-effectiveness ratios, especially because good results have been reported in series in which preoperative testing has been limited to patients with unstable angina pectoris, uncontrolled arrhythmias, or severe congestive heart failure.[69]

PRIOR CORONARY REVASCULARIZATION. Patients who have undergone successful coronary revascularization can undergo major noncardiac surgical procedures with a low mortality rate,[70] except perhaps in the first 30 days postoperatively. An alternative is percutaneous transluminal coronary angioplasty (PTCA),[71] which can more easily be performed during the course of the same admission.[72] It must be remembered, however, that the operative mortality rate for major noncardiac surgery in patients with stable angina and good exercise tolerance is relatively low, usually in the range of 2 per cent. No randomized controlled trials are available to assess the value of coronary artery bypass grafting or PTCA preoperatively in patients with stable angina pectoris who are about to undergo noncardiac surgery. An analysis of patients in the Coronary Artery Surgery Study registry[70] showed that total operative mortality was 2.4 per cent in 458 patients who had significant coronary artery disease and underwent noncardiac operations without prior coronary artery bypass grafting. By comparison, operative mortality was 0.9 per cent among 399 patients who had had a coronary artery bypass grafting procedure performed before noncardiac surgery. The mortality was higher in patients who had more severe left ventricular dysfunction or dyspnea on exertion and in patients who used nitrates, were older, and had diabetes. The risk of myocardial infarction, however, was not significantly different between the patients with and without preoperative coronary artery bypass grafting, and the cardiac death rates were only 1.3 per cent and 0.4 per cent, respectively, in the two groups. Furthermore, if one considers the mortality associated with coronary artery bypass grafting, which was 1.4 per cent in the Coronary Artery Surgery Study, the overall mortality from combined coronary artery bypass grafting and noncardiac surgery (2.3 per cent) would be as high as for the noncardiac surgery done in the non-bypassed group (2.4 per cent). Thus the data do not argue in favor of prophylactic coronary artery bypass grafting for patients whose symptoms would not otherwise warrant revascularization, who have stable angina with good exercise tolerance, and who do not have other factors that define a high-risk status (Table 54–1).

TABLE 54–1 RECOMMENDATIONS FOR SPECIAL PERIOPERATIVE CARDIAC EVALUATION AND MANAGEMENT*

	PREOPERATIVE DIAGNOSTIC RECOMMENDATIONS	SPECIAL PERIOPERATIVE CARDIAC TREATMENT RECOMMENDATIONS
1. No known CAD Good cardiac functional status† Class I-II on the cardiac risk index[28] or its equivalent (regardless of CAD risk factors or type of surgery)	None	None
2. Known stable CAD with good (Class I or early Class II) functional status†	None	Conservative treatment Continue cardiac medications Postoperative electrocardiogram day 1 and again prior to hospital discharge and to rule out myocardial infarction after any suspicious perioperative events
3. Known CAD, functional status unclear	Noninvasive testing Exercise thallium testing if patient can exercise Other tests (dipyridamole thallium, stress echocardiography, or ambulatory ischemia monitor) if patient cannot exercise	If test is negative: Conservative treatment (see above) If test is positive: Aggressive medical treatment or angiography 1. Intensify preoperative CAD medications, identify and address non-CAD risk factors, and consider repeating noninvasive test if major changes have been made (if now negative, use conservative treatment; if still positive, proceed to 2 or 3). 2. More intensive perioperative monitoring and perioperative medications to control blood pressure and pulse or 3. Coronary angiography and revascularization as indicated
4. Known CAD, poor cardiac functional status	None	Aggressive medical treatment or angiography (see above)
5. Poor noncardiac functional status, no CAD or CAD status unclear		
No or few risk factors‡	None	None
Multiple risk factors	Noninvasive testing (see above)	If test is negative: Conservative treatment (see above) If test is positive: Aggressive medical treatment or angiography (see above)
6. CAD and Class III or IV on the cardiac risk index or its equivalent	None	Aggressive medical treatment or angiography (see above)

* Does not include procedure-specific decisions regarding routine use of intraoperative electrocardiographic monitoring, arterial catheters, and so on.

† Cardiac functional Class I or early Class II—can walk up a flight of stairs carrying objects weighing 10 to 20 pounds without cardiac symptoms.

‡ Risk factors include age over 70, diabetes mellitus, congestive heart failure, important atrial or ventricular arrhythmias, known vascular disease, or aortic, abdominal, or thoracic surgery.

CAD = coronary artery disease defined as a clinical diagnosis of angina, a prior myocardial infarction, or a positive coronary angiogram.

From Mangano, D. T., and Goldman, L.: Preoperative assessment of the patient with known or suspected coronary disease. N. Engl. J. Med. *333*:1750, 1995.

APPROACH TO RISK ASSESSMENT. A practical approach to the patient with known ischemic heart disease or with specified high-risk characteristics[49] should utilize information from the history as well as diagnostic tests.[73–77] If the patient's history indicates reliably that Class I or Class II activities can be performed (see p. 1741), the patient will commonly be raising the double product (the heart rate multiplied by the systolic blood pressure) above the range to be expected with general anesthesia and surgery, and hence should be able to withstand the stress of the procedure.[40,70] If the history is unreliable, exercise testing to assess physical function[41–44] will aid in risk assessment. If the patient is unable to exercise because of noncardiac conditions, ambulatory ischemia monitoring (in a patient with a normal resting electrocardiogram who is not receiving medication such as digoxin), dipyridamole thallium imaging, or stress echocardiography should be used.

Patients who can exercise to Class I or II levels, or who have normal ambulatory ischemia monitoring, dipyridamole thallium imaging, or stress echocardiography can undergo most operations with acceptable risk. Patients who cannot perform Class I or II activities or who have positive ambulatory ischemia monitoring or dipyridamole thallium images should have their medical regimens intensified, if possible, and then have repeat testing. If tests remain positive or physical functioning remains limited after optimization of medical management, coronary arteriography will usually be indicated prior to elective surgery to determine whether coronary revascularization, with either PTCA or coronary bypass surgery, would be feasible.[74] The decision to proceed with revascularization depends more on the functional limitations that result from the coronary lesions than on their anatomical severity. Although the latter is important for long-term prognosis, the former is probably the more relevant correlate of perioperative risk.

USE OF BETA BLOCKERS, CALCIUM ANTAGONISTS, AND NITRATES. Although some concern has been expressed about the use of general anesthesia in patients receiving beta-adrenocepter blocking agents and calcium antagonists, no clinical data indicate that such medications should routinely be discontinued preoperatively. Intravenous esmolol is clearly effective for reducing perioperative tachycardia and hypertension,[78,79] although it is less effective in preventing perioperative ischemia.[78] Aggressive perioperative medication regimens, with special emphasis on beta-adrenoceptor blockers and nitrates, may reduce clinical ischemic events in patients with asymptomatic perioperative ischemia.[80] Intravenous beta-adrenoceptor blockers should be used in patients with a prior history of severe angina that required beta-adrenoceptor blocking agents for its control or in patients who have evidence of postoperative myocardial ischemia or otherwise unexplained hypertension or tachycardia.

Nifedipine can be given sublingually, and nitrates can be given sublingually, topically, or intravenously, to aid in the management of the early postoperative patient with angina. However, these agents cannot substitute for beta-adrenoceptor blockers in patients who have relied on the latter for the control of their ischemic heart disease.

Hypertension

Several studies have documented that patients with hypertension have higher risks of suffering major cardiac complications during or shortly after noncardiac operation than do patients who have always been normotensive. However, most, if not all, of this increased risk is because of the ischemic heart disease, left ventricular dysfunction, renal failure, or other abnormalities that often occur in patients with hypertension. Thus, in patients with mild to moderate hypertension, diastolic pressures below 100 mm Hg, and no evidence of serious end-organ damage, general anesthesia and major noncardiac surgery are generally well tolerated.[18] Halothane anesthesia may be more likely than other anesthetic agents to induce intraoperative hypotension in patients with a history of hypertension,[18] and hypertensive patients are at higher risk for labile blood pressures and for hypertensive episodes during surgery and especially just after extubation.

Although uncontrolled early studies suggested that the continuation of any hypertensive agents might increase the risk of perioperative hypotension, substantial subsequent data from more careful studies indicate that patients whose hypertension is well controlled do at least as well, if not better, if their medications are, in fact, continued up to the time of operation.[18,81] Thus, although it is neither mandatory nor desirable to delay noncardiac operation for the weeks or months that may be required to achieve ideal blood pressure control in the stable patient with mild to moderate hypertension who has no complications of the hypertension, there is also no apparent benefit, and some potential harm, from discontinuing successful antihypertensive therapy before surgery.

Thiazide and other diuretics cause some degree of chronic volume depletion, and patients receiving these drugs may require more fluid administration early during the operative procedure. If severe perioperative hypertension develops in a patient who has previously been receiving clonidine, and if the clonidine cannot be given orally, it can be administered intramuscularly in doses about one-half as large as the patient's usually daily dose or it can be administered topically,[82] or the patient can be treated with sublingual captopril, with methyldopa, or with a beta blocker. Although it may be desirable to use propranolol, metoprolol, or esmolol intravenously in patients who rely on beta-adrenoceptor blockers for the control of ischemic heart disease, these agents usually need not be given intravenously for prophylaxis in patients who take them for their antihypertensive effects. Intravenous esmolol,[83] labetalol,[84] or nitroprusside can be used for acute episodes of hypertension and methyldopa for nonacute situations.

Valvular Heart Disease and Cardiomyopathy

Patients with valvular heart disease undergoing anesthesia and noncardiac operation are subject to many potential hazards: heart failure, infection, tachycardia, and embolization. As might be expected, patients with no or only mild limitation of activity (i.e., those in Class I or II) tolerate operation well[85] and probably require little more than careful perioperative care and prophylaxis for infective endocarditis (see p. 1099). Those with more serious impairment of cardiac reserve (i.e., those in Class III or IV) tolerate major noncardiac operations poorly, and their prognosis for surviving major surgery is distinctly worse,[20,29] although as is the case for patients with rheumatic heart disease who face the stress of pregnancy (see p. 1848), the risk of operation depends on the functional state of the heart. Patients with symptomatic critical aortic[28] or mitral stenosis are especially prone to sudden death or acute pulmonary edema during the perioperative period; this may occur if demands on cardiac output are suddenly increased or if atrial fibrillation and a rapid ventricular rate are precipitated by anesthesia or operation. Every effort should be made to treat heart failure preoperatively. Patients with severe stenotic or regurgitant valve disease should undergo corrective valvular surgery before an elective operation, whereas those who require an emergency noncardiac operation may benefit from intraoperative hemodynamic monitoring, afterload reduction, and preload augmentation.[86] In some patients with mitral or aortic stenosis, balloon valvuloplasty (see p. 1385) may offer relief of severe obstruction at a low risk when it might not be desirable to carry out valve replacement.[87,88]

HYPERTROPHIC CARDIOMYOPATHY. Patients with hypertrophic cardiomyopathy are intolerant of hypovolemia, which may lead to both a reduction in the elevated preload necessary to maintain cardiac output and an increase in the obstruction to left ventricular outflow (see p. 1414). With careful perioperative, intraoperative, and postoperative care, however, the risk of major cardiac complications in such patients is small. In one series of 56 operations in patients with hypertrophic cardiomyopathy, there were no deaths and the only major complication was a myocardial infarction with congestive heart failure in a patient who also had underlying coronary artery disease. Intraoperative or postoperative hypotension requiring vasoconstrictors occurred in less than 10 per cent of patients.[81,89] It has been suggested that spinal anesthesia may be relatively contraindicated in patients with hypertrophic obstructive cardiomyopathy because of its tendency to reduce systemic vascular resistance and increase venous pooling and thereby increase the severity of obstruction to outflow.[89] Hemodynamic monitoring is not routinely required but may be helpful when these patients undergo major aortic, abdominal, or thoracic procedures.

PROSTHETIC HEART VALVES. Most patients with mechanical prosthetic heart valves receive anticoagulants on a long-term basis to prevent thromboembolic complications (see p. 1066). If these medications are continued through the period of noncardiac operation, hemostasis, hematoma formation, and persistent postoperative bleeding may ensue. Anticoagulants can be temporarily discontinued during the perioperative period with minimal risk of thrombosis. In one study,[90] no thromboembolic complications occurred in 159 patients with prosthetic valves undergoing 180 noncardiac operations when warfarin was discontinued an average of 2.9 days preoperatively and resumed 2.7 days postoperatively.[90] Using a similar approach, Katholi et al. did not observe thromboembolic complications in 25 noncardiac operations on patients with prosthetic aortic valves[91]; however, two such complications occurred in the 10 patients with mitral valve prostheses when anticoagulants were discontinued for noncardiac operations, although these patients had Kay-Shiley caged-disc valves, which are associated with a somewhat higher risk of thromboembolic complications. Because there is a distinct risk of hemorrhagic complications in patients whose anticoagulants have been discontinued for only 2 or 3 days,[90] prothrombin time should be restored to within 20 per cent of normal before one proceeds with the noncardiac surgery.[92] Low molecular weight dextran can be used in the postoperative period to minimize thrombotic complications during the 2 to 3 days when the risk of hemorrhagic complications from resuming anticoagulation is relatively higher. In patients with prostheses that are at high risk for thrombosis, such as caged-disc valves, we recommend discontinuing warfarin, allowing the prothrombin time to come to within about 2 to 3 seconds of normal, using intravenous heparin until about 6 hours before the operation, restarting the heparin about 36 to 48 hours after surgery, and switching to warfarin about 2 to 5 days later. Recent analyses indicate that these various anticoagulation regimens are cost-effective provided that they do not result in lengthening the hospitalization.[93] Even one day of additional hospitalization is relatively costly, and the daily risk of thromboembolic complications is low. Thus, perioperative anticoagulation management should focus on regimens that provide reasonable protection from thromboembolic disease but that permit the patient to be discharged when the surgical condition itself permits.[93]

ENDOCARDITIS PROPHYLAXIS. Patients with valvular heart disease and those with prosthetic heart valves should receive prophylactic antibiotics for surgical procedures likely to be complicated by bacteremias.[94] These include incision and drainage of an infected site; oral, lower gastrointestinal, and gallbladder surgery; and genitourinary procedures. Penicillin can be used before operation involving the upper respiratory tract, with erythromycin or vancomycin an acceptable alternative for patients with a penicillin allergy. For gastrointestinal and genitourinary surgery, which can be complicated by either enterococci or gram-negative bacteremia, gentamicin or streptomycin is required in addition to penicillin. (Suggested doses are given on p. 1099.)

The value of antibiotic prophylaxis before noncardiac operation in patients with *mitral valve prolapse* is controversial (see p. 1035). Most studies indicate that patients with this condition who have murmurs of mitral regurgitation are at substantially higher risk than patients who do not have murmurs,[95] and cost-effectiveness analyses argue *against* routine antibiotic prophylaxis in patients without a murmur.[96,97] At the present time a reasonable compromise is to use antibiotic prophylaxis before surgery in patients with mitral valve prolapse who have clinical evidence of mitral regurgitation.

Congenital Heart Disease

Depending on the nature of the malformation, the patient with congenital heart disease may be subject to one or more potentially serious complications, such as infection, bleeding, hypoxemia, and paradoxical embolization during general anesthesia and operation. As is the case for patients with valvular heart disease, patients with congenital heart disease who are to undergo a surgical procedure require prophylaxis to prevent infective endocarditis (see p. 1098). Patients with cyanotic congenital heart disease and secondary polycythemia are at increased risk of intraoperative and postoperative hemorrhage as a consequence of coagulation defects and thrombocytopenia (see p. 884); this risk can be reduced with careful preoperative phlebotomy, usually to a hematocrit of 50 to 55 per cent.[93]

Patients with cyanotic congenital heart disease tolerate systemic hypotension poorly because this increases the right-to-left shunt and the severity of hypoxemia. In one large series, induction was commonly accomplished using ketamine or fentanyl to avoid hypotension, and anesthesia was maintained with morphine and nitrous oxide or with large doses of fentanyl with or without nitrous oxide. Halothane in very low concentrations can be used in patients with less severe degrees of cyanosis.[99] With use of careful anesthetic techniques, the risk of major anesthetic complications is extremely low even in very ill and cyanotic patients. However, spinal anesthesia, which causes peripheral arterial vasodilation and reduces venous return, can have deleterious hemodynamic effects in patients with cyanotic congenital heart disease. Occasionally, infusion of a vasoconstrictor such as phenylephrine may be required to raise systemic vascular resistance and thereby decrease the magnitude of the right-to-left shunt. Because patients with right-to-left shunts are subject to the risk of paradoxical emboli, including air emboli, meticulous techniques with regard to intravenous solutions and injections are mandatory to prevent such complications.

Congestive Heart Failure

Congestive heart failure is a major determinant of perioperative risk, irrespective of the nature of the underlying cardiac disorder. Mortality with noncardiac surgery increases with worsening cardiac class[20,40] and with the presence of pulmonary congestion,[20,26] especially when a third heart sound is noted.[28] Because the perioperative mortality rate appears to depend more on the patient's condition at the time of operation than on the most severe depression of cardiovascular status the patient has ever experienced, it is clearly advisable to treat the congestive heart failure before the contemplated major elective noncardiac surgery. However, because such a therapeutic regimen almost always includes a diuretic, both hypovolemia and hypokalemia are potential problems for patients treated just before operation. It is therefore desirable, if possible, to stabilize the patient's condition by treating heart failure for approximately 1 week rather than for only 1 or 2 days before the contemplated operation. Also, great care should be taken to avoid dehydration because hypovolemic patients may be especially likely to experience marked hypotension during the early phases of anesthesia. Perioperative cardiogenic pulmonary edema develops in about 2 per cent of patients over age 40 undergoing major noncardiac surgery without prior congestive heart failure, in about 6 per cent of patients whose heart failure is well controlled, and in about 16 per cent of patients whose heart failure persists on physical examination or chest radiograph before surgery.[20]

Although digitalis can counteract the myocardial depressant actions of many general anesthetic agents,[93] the value of digitalis in patients with congestive heart failure appears to be limited to certain subsets of patients, especially those who have a third heart sound.[94] Digitalis is one of the most common causes of iatrogenic complications in hospitalized patients, and it may be associated with a higher risk of intraoperative bradyarrhythmias.[20] Therefore, preoperative digitalization is *not* recommended except in patients whose congestive heart failure is sufficiently severe that they would normally meet the criteria for long-term digitalization (see p. 499).

Arrhythmias

Arrhythmias may be a manifestation of the severity of underlying left ventricular dysfunction and of coronary artery disease and hence are frequently markers for the likelihood of perioperative cardiac complications. Because patients who have ventricular premature contractions but no evidence of underlying heart disease on detailed examination have an apparently normal cardiac prognosis,[102] ventricular premature contractions in the *absence* of underlying heart disease should not be considered a risk factor for cardiac complications with noncardiac surgery. Atrial arrhythmias are often a manifestation of atrial enlargement, and a supraventricular rhythm other than sinus appears to be a risk factor for the development of perioperative complications.[28]

Although it would be ideal for arrhythmias to be well controlled preoperatively, the risks associated with arrhythmias appear to be related more to the underlying cardiac disease than to the arrhythmias per se. Therefore, there currently is no evidence that asymptomatic ventricular premature contractions require aggressive preoperative control or prophylactic intraoperative suppression. Similarly, in the patient with well-controlled atrial fibrillation, cardioversion need not be carried out specifically because of planned noncardiac surgery if such a management option would not otherwise be appropriate.

Patients who are most at risk for the development of postoperative supraventricular tachyarrhythmias include elderly patients undergoing pulmonary surgery, patients with subcritical valvular stenoses, and patients with prior histories of supraventricular tachyarrhythmias. Although data are less than decisive, digitalis may reduce the risk of the development of postoperative supraventricular tachycardia in such patients,[103] and the rate of the supraventricular tachycardia may be slower in the digitalized patient.[20] Thus, prophylactic preoperative digitalization is reasonable in elderly patients undergoing major pulmonary surgery, patients with subcritical valvular stenoses, and patients with a prior history of symptomatic supraventricular tachycardias, except if the latter are already taking other medications for the control of such arrhythmias. Another alternative is to use verapamil or adenosine to treat arrhythmias acutely when they occur.

CONDUCTION DEFECTS. The patient with *complete heart block* (see p. 687) must respond to the demands for an increased cardiac output by augmenting stroke volume, but this compensatory response is prevented in many patients by a concurrent impairment of cardiac contractility. In addition, most anesthetic agents depress myocardial contractility and/or produce peripheral vasodilatation. Furthermore, anesthesia may cause further depression of the automaticity, and therefore the ventricular rate, of the patient with heart block. Thus patients with untreated complete heart block may be unable to meet the increased demands placed on the cardiovascular system by anesthesia and operation, and a permanent or temporary pacemaker should be inserted before general anesthesia, even in asymptomatic patients (Chap. 24).

Another problem is presented by the patient with *chronic bifascicular block* (see p. 121).[20,104] A significant fraction of patients developing this abnormality in the course of an acute myocardial infarction progress to complete heart block, often accompanied by sudden severe hemodynamic compromise (see p. 1233). In several series, progression from bifascicular to complete heart block has not been documented during the perioperative period in patients without a previous history of third-degree heart block. Therefore, we do *not* recommend prophylactic pacemaker placement for such patients or for patients with first-degree atrioventricular (AV) block or type I second-degree AV block (Wenckebach), although a pacemaker should always be available in the operating room for emergency placement. However, in patients who have bifascicular block, and either type II second-degree AV block or a history of unexplained syncope or transient third-degree AV block, the risk of development of complete heart block is much higher, and a temporary pacemaker should be inserted preoperatively.

THE PATIENT WITH A PERMANENT PACEMAKER. When a patient with a permanent pacemaker in situ is about to undergo operation, the device should be carefully evaluated to ensure that it is functioning properly preoperatively (Chap. 24). Demand pacemakers are sensitive to electromagnetic interference, such as that produced by the electrocautery, which may result in failure to pace. The danger of this potentially hazardous interaction can be reduced by placing the indifferent plate of the cautery unit as far as possible from the lead and pulse generator, and the electrocautery should be used in brief bursts rather than continuously. Also, a magnet should be available in the operating room to convert the pacemaker from the demand to the fixed-rate mode. Because the cautery may also interfere with the electrocardiographic monitor and render it temporarily uninterpretable, arterial pressure should be monitored directly when the cautery is being used on patients with permanent pacemakers.

In general, a prophylactic *temporary pacemaker* should be inserted before noncardiac operations only if the patient meets the indications for permanent pacemaker insertion (see p. 707) and the operation should not be delayed for the time required for a permanent pacemaker insertion, or if the operative course is likely to be complicated by transient bacteremia. In such situations a temporary pacemaker should be placed initially, and the permanent pacemaker can be inserted after the operation. The occasional exception is the patient who has a severe bradycardic response to vagal stimuli and who might be difficult to manage during a major operation without a pacemaker.

General Medical Problems

Patients with heart disease whose general medical status is complicated by diabetes, renal insufficiency, hepatic abnormalities, hypoxemia, or electrolyte abnormalities have a higher risk of cardiac complications, presumably because these nonmedical conditions exacerbate the stress placed on the heart by the operation.[20,26,28] Morbidity is also higher in markedly obese patients[105] because obesity is often associated with abnormal cardiorespiratory function, metabolic function, and hemostasis. Every effort should be made to correct any of these noncardiac problems before operation, and the potential long-term benefits of surgery must also be interpreted in light of the patient's general prognosis.

POSTOPERATIVE COMPLICATIONS

MYOCARDIAL INFARCTION. Transient intraoperative ischemia does not appear to be a major correlate of postoperative ischemic events in patients undergoing noncardiac surgery,[57,58] but most clinical postoperative ischemic events are preceded by asymptomatic episodes of postoperative ischemia that can be detected by ambulatory ischemic monitoring.[56–59,61] Although series from before 1980 showed a peak in the risk of myocardial infarction on about the third postoperative day,[106] more recent series show that a combination of frequent electrocardiograms and cardiac enzymes detects many non–Q-wave infarctions in the first 24 hours postoperatively.[55,107–110] Although care must be taken in interpreting cardiac enzymes in the perioperative period,[109] it may be that supply-demand imbalances cause an early peak in non–Q-wave postoperative infarctions, whereas the hypercoagulable postoperative state leads to a later (3 to 5 days postoperatively) peak in Q-wave infarctions. For both types of infarction, postoperative stresses include general surgical complications, hypoxia and other pulmonary complications, fluid and electrolyte abnormalities, and the stresses of modern postoperative ambulation protocols. Substantial data indicate that prophylactic anticoagulation with low-dose heparin reduces the risk of postoperative thromboembolic complications,[111] and such therapy is routinely indicated in most cardiac patients who undergo noncardiac operations. In fact, such anticoagulation regimens may permit a more gradual postoperative ambulation protocol in cardiac patients, and hence possibly lower the incidence of postoperative myocardial infarction.

Myocardial infarction occurring in the perioperative period is often painless. Obviously, then, the incidence of perioperative infarction is underestimated if electrocardiograms and serial estimations of serum creatine kinase isoenzyme (MB fraction) are not obtained routinely during the postoperative period in high-risk patients.[106]

HYPERTENSION. Postoperative hypertension is most likely to occur soon after the cessation of positive-pressure ventilation or in the recovery room, and it is more common after carotid endarterectomy and major abdominal vascular procedures.[18]

Common precipitants include fluid overload after cessation of positive-pressure ventilation, hypoxemia, anxiety, and pain. The principal therapeutic approaches should therefore concentrate on assuring adequate oxygenation, pain control, and fluid control. In general, supplemental oxygen, morphine, and diuretics are the mainstays of the treatment of postoperative hypertension. Nitroprusside (see p. 858) and labetalol[84] (see p. 854) are the preferred medications for more severe hypertension. Intravenous hydralazine in small doses is effective for treating postoperative hypertension, but it has the potential of precipitating supraventricular tachyarrhythmias.

CONGESTIVE HEART FAILURE. Although postoperative heart failure may be precipitated by myocardial infarction or ischemia, a substantial proportion of the cases are directly caused by excess fluid administration. Heart failure tends to occur soon after cessation of positive-pressure ventilation and again at about 24 to 48 hours after operation, when the fluid that was given in the perioperative period is mobilized from the extravascular sites. Diuretics, often given intravenously, and rarely supplemented by digitalis glycosides, are usually sufficient therapy for postoperative congestive heart failure.

POSTOPERATIVE ARRHYTHMIAS. Arrhythmias are common after operation and are often a manifestation of a noncardiac complication, such as bleeding, infection, or an acid-base or electrolyte imbalance occurring in a patient with heart disease. Management of such arrhythmias often requires recognition and correction of extracardiac factors.

In one study of 916 patients with sinus rhythm throughout the course of major noncardiac surgery, 35 patients (4 per cent) developed new supraventricular tachyarrhythmias postoperatively.[112] Of these 35 patients, 46 per cent had acute cardiac conditions, 31 per cent had major infections, 29 had preexisting hypotension, 26 per cent had anemia, 23 per cent had metabolic derangements, 23 per cent had received new parenteral drugs that could be implicated, and 20 per cent were hypoxic. Forty per cent of the patients required no new therapy with cardiac medications, and only two patients required electrical cardioversion; the arrhythmias of all treated patients reverted to sinus rhythm. No deaths were related to the supraventricular tachyarrhythmias per se, but a substantial proportion of the patients in whom these arrhythmias occurred died as a result of the concurrent medical problems. Thus, a new postoperative supraventricular tachyarrhythmia should prompt a search for remediable medical problems. Direct antiarrhythmic therapy is often unnecessary and is usually secondary in importance to correction of the underlying cause of the arrhythmia.

Sinus tachycardia is the most common rhythm disturbance in the postoperative patient. Multiple noncardiac etiological factors have been identified, including pain, hypovolemia, hypervolemia, fever, anemia, hypoxemia, pulmonary emboli, anxiety, infection, hypotension, and electrolyte abnormalities (especially hypokalemia). These noncardiac factors are much more common causes of sinus tachycardia in the postoperative cardiac patient than is either myocardial infarction or heart failure. Sinus tachycardia not caused by congestive heart failure does not slow with cardiac glycosides. The therapeutic/toxic ratio of these drugs is actually reduced by most of the above-mentioned noncardiac causes of sinus tachycardia, and therefore digitalis glycosides are not considered appropriate for postoperative patients unless the sinus tachycardia is caused by impaired cardiac function.

Atrial fibrillation is also a common postoperative arrhythmia. Atrial dilatation, which lowers the threshold for development of this arrhythmia, may result from heart failure, mitral valve disease, and/or hypervolemia. Noncardiac precipitants include pneumonia, atelectasis, and pulmonary emboli. Initially, the postoperative patient with atrial fibrillation should be treated with a digitalis glycoside or verapamil; in addition, a beta-adrenoceptor blocker can be used to help gain rapid control of the ventricular rate. Cardioversion is usually delayed until the precipitating factors have been eliminated, because in the patient who has cardioversion before clearing of the atelectasis or pneumonia there is frequently reversion to atrial fibrillation, whereas in the patient whose pulmonary problem or congestive heart failure is adequately treated there is often spontaneous reversion to sinus rhythm.

Atrial flutter is often poorly tolerated because of the rapid ventricular rate and the difficult pharmacological management. Cardioversion is the treatment of choice.

IMPLICATIONS OF POSTOPERATIVE COMPLICATIONS FOR LONG-TERM MANAGEMENT. When a patient develops a perioperative myocardial infarction, the evaluation and the recuperative process generally should be analogous to when a myocardial infarction occurs in other patients (see Chap. 37). Because postoperative congestive heart failure is commonly precipitated by iatrogenic fluid overload, the patient commonly does not need long-term therapy for congestive heart failure. Similarly, perioperative arrhythmias are often precipitated by specific stimuli, and the patient with a postoperative arrhythmia should not automatically be consigned to long-term antiarrhythmic therapy. In patients who develop either postoperative congestive heart failure or arrhythmias, it is often appropriate to discontinue new cardiac therapies several days before discharge and observe the patient to see whether long-term therapy is indicated.

THE ROLE OF THE MEDICAL CONSULTANT

The physician called on to evaluate the status of a patient with suspected or overt cardiac disease before elective or emergency noncardiac surgery must first determine whether cardiovascular disease is present and, if it is, must identify those factors that may increase the risk of operation. It may be necessary to invest considerable time and effort to prepare the patient for operation. In addition, the patient must be followed carefully after operation to detect and manage the cardiac problems that frequently complicate the postoperative period.

ESTIMATION OF RISK. A few patients have such compelling reasons for operation (e.g., rupturing aortic aneurysm, perforated or necrotic bowel, life-threatening hemorrhage, or some forms of intestinal obstruction) that estimation of operative risk is an academic exercise, because failure to operate almost certainly will result in the patient's death. Often, however, the timing or even the performance of an operation is elective, and under these circumstances estimation of risk is an important aspect of the medical consultant's role. Certain cardiovascular problems, such as recent myocardial infarction (less than 1 month), inadequately treated congestive heart failure, and severe mitral or aortic stenosis, are *absolute contraindications* to *elective* surgery. *Relative contraindications,* which commonly require further clinical or laboratory evaluation or treatment before elective surgery, include more remote myocardial infarction (1 month to 6 months previously), angina pectoris, mild heart failure, cyanotic congenital heart disease with severe polycythemia, and a coagulation abnormality. Several other problems should be recognized and treated before operation: anemia, hypovolemia, polycythemia, pulmonary disease causing hypoxemia, adrenal hyporesponsiveness secondary to long-term administration of adrenal steroids, hypertension, electrolyte abnormalities, as well as the entire gamut of cardiac arrhythmias. Considerable judgment must be exercised when one or more of the above-mentioned problems are present and when a patient requires prompt surgical treatment but the situation is not a true emergency, as for neoplastic disease.

To identify those preoperative factors associated with the development of cardiac complications after major noncardiac operation in patients over 40 years of age, one analysis[20] identified nine independently significant correlates of life-threatening and fatal cardiac complications. When these factors were weighted based on their relative significance as predictors of cardiac outcome, a multifactorial index was developed for predicting perioperative risk. Other investigations of relatively unselected patients have noted similar risk factors[26,35] (Table 54–2).

The value of the information in this index has been confirmed in large prospective series of general surgical patients,[26,34,35] in a large series of patients who had prior coronary or valvular heart surgery,[113] and in several other studies.[43,107,114,115] In one series,[35] risk stratification was equally good when several minor modifications were made in point assignment and when a prior history of Class III or IV angina, unstable angina, and pulmonary edema was included in the index.

However, because the index was derived from unselected general surgical patients above age 40, it appears to underestimate risk by about 40 per cent in patients who undergo

TABLE 54–2 THREE COMMONLY USED CARDIAC RISK INDICES

	ORIGINAL INDEX (Goldman et al.)[28]		DETSKY et al†[35]		LARSEN et al‡[26]	
FACTOR	Definition	Points	Definition	Points	Definition	Points
1. Ischemic heart disease	MI within 6 months	10	MI within 6 months MI more than 6 months ago Canadian Cardiovascular Society angina Class III Class IV Unstable angina within 6 months	10 5 10 20 10	MI within 3 months No, but older infarction and/or angina pectoris	11 3
2. Congestive heart failure	S_3 gallop or jugular venous distention	11	Pulmonary edema Within 1 week Ever	 10 5	Persistent pulmonary congestion No, but previous pulmonary edema Neither, but previous heart failure	12 8 4
3. Cardiac rhythm	Rhythm other than sinus or PACs on last preoperative ECG >5 PVCs/min documented at any time before operation	7 7	Rhythm other than sinus or sinus plus PACs on last preoperative ECG >5 PVCs/min at any time prior to surgery	5 5		
4. Valvular heart disease	Important aortic stenosis	3	Suspected critical aortic stenosis	20		
5. General medical status	pO_2 < 60 or pCO_2 > 50 mm Hg, K < 3.0 or HCO_3 < 20 mEq/L, BUN > 50 or Cr > 3.0 mg/dl, abnormal AST, signs of chronic liver disease or bedridden from noncardiac causes	3	Same as for original	5	Serum creatinine above 0.13 mmol/L^{-1} Diabetes mellitus	2 3
6. Age	Age > 70 yr	5	Age over 70	5		
7. Type of surgery	Intraperitoneal, intrathoracic, or aortic operation Emergency operation	3 4	Emergency operation	10	Emergency operation Aortic operation Other intraperitoneal/pleural operation	3 5 3

MI = myocardial infarction; PAC = premature atrial contraction; PVC = premature ventricular contraction.

* Derived from 1001 consecutive unselected patients over age 40 undergoing major noncardiac surgery using multivariable analysis.

† Modification of original index based on the clinical judgments of the authors.

‡ Derived from 2609 patients over age 40 undergoing non-minor noncardiac surgery using multivariable analysis.

Complications were defined as myocardial infarction, cardiogenic pulmonary edema, sustained ventricular tachycardia or ventricular fibrillation, or cardiac death.

Grouping and outcomes for the various indices—original index: Class I = 0 to 35 points, Class II = 6 to 12 points, Class III = 13 to 25 points, Class IV = >25 points (see Fig. 54–1); Detsky et al.: points integrated with prior probability to compute a continuous score; Larsen et al.: 0 to 5 points = 11 (0.5%) complications in 2022 patients; 6 to 7 points = 12 (3.8%) complications in 317 patients; 8 to 14 points = 27 (11%) complications in 239 patients; > 15 points = 18 (58%) complications in 31 patients. For the original index, the area under the receiver operating characteristic curve (ROC) (a summary measure of both sensitivity and specificity where 1.0 indicates perfect discrimination of complicated versus uncomplicated patients, while a value of 0.5 indicates discrimination that is not better than chance) was 0.81 in the original derivation set of patients, 0.80 (34) and 0.77 (26) (estimated) in other studies of unselected consecutive patients, 0.81 in patients with prior coronary or valvular surgery (113), 0.69 in patients having medical consultations (35,116), and 0.63 in patients undergoing abdominal aortic aneurysm surgery (30). All of these ROC values were significantly better than chance. From Mangano, D. T., and Goldman, L.: Preoperative assessment of the patient with known or suspected coronary disease. N. Engl. J. Med. *333*:1750, 1995.

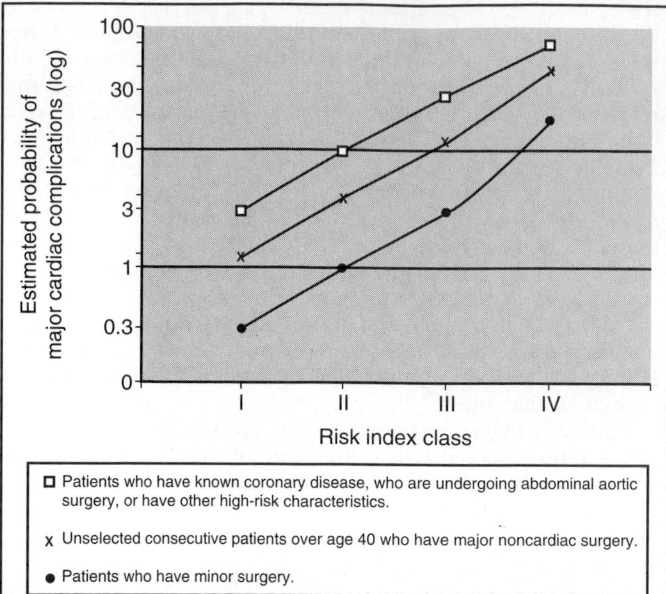

FIGURE 54–1. Approximate risk of major cardiac complications in different types of patients as adjusted using the original multifactorial index.[28] The risks of major complications, which are defined as pulmonary edema and arrhythmic cardiac arrest, as well as myocardial infarction and cardiac death, were calculated by multiplying the prior odds of complications times the likelihood ratio for each class. Classes are defined as follows: Class I = 0 to 5 points; Class II = 6 to 12 points; Class III = 13 to 25 points; and Class IV = 26 or more points. Points are calculated as follows: myocardial infarction within 6 months = 10; age over 70 = 5; S_3 gallop or jugular venous distention = 11; important aortic stenosis = 3; rhythm other than sinus or sinus plus APBs on last preoperative ECG = 7; more than 5 premature ventricular beats per minute at any time preoperatively = 7; poor general medical status [$pO_2 < 60$ mm Hg; $pCO_2 > 50$ mm Hg; $K^+ < 3.0$ mEq/L; $HCO_3 < 20$ mEq/L; BUN > 50 mg/dl (18 mmol/L); creatinine > 3 mg/dl (260 mmol/L); abnormal SGOT or signs of liver disease; bedridden from noncardiac causes] = 3; intraperitoneal, intrathoracic, or aortic surgery = 3; emergency operation = 4. (From Mangano, D. T., and Goldman, L.: Preoperative assessment of the patient with known or suspected coronary disease. N. Engl. J. Med. *333*:1750, 1995. Copyright Massachusetts Medical Society.)

resection of an abdominal aortic aneurysm,[30] and it also underestimates risk in patients who are selected on the basis of any high-risk status such as patients with stable coronary artery disease, in whom the risk of a major event is 2 to 4 per cent, even in the absence of other risk factors. One way to take into account the fact that some patients have higher baseline risks is to know the baseline probability of cardiac complications for specific types of patients or types of surgery and then to modify these "pre-test" probabilities on the basis of the patient's cardiac condition.[35,73,74,116,117] As shown in Figure 54–1, this can be a useful approach to estimating the risk of major cardiac complications. Even at its best, however, any index for predicting cardiac complications should be viewed as an aid and not as a crutch; it should supplement, not substitute for, clinical judgment.

PREPARATION OF THE PATIENT FOR ANESTHESIA AND OPERATION. Careful preparation of the cardiac patient for operation may diminish the frequency and seriousness of intraoperative and postoperative complications. The medical consultant should, after appropriate discussion with the surgeon, be prepared to urge postponement or cancellation of an elective operation or to insist on sufficient time to institute any measures that are necessary to minimize risk. The consultant should attempt to be brief and to the point, and to provide a limited number of explicit, relevant suggestions.[118] The cardiological consultant should work closely with the anesthesiologist and the surgeon so that their talents may be combined to maximize the likelihood of a favorable outcome.

REFERENCES

ANESTHESIA

1. Breslow, M. J., Miller, C. F., and Rogers, M. (eds.): Perioperative Management. St. Louis, C. V. Mosby Co., 1990.
2. Mangano, D. T. (ed.): Perioperative Cardiac Assessment. Philadelphia, J. B. Lippincott Co., 1990.
3. Rogers, M. C., Tinker, J. H., Covino, B. G., and Longnecker, D. E. (eds.): Principles and Practice of of Anesthesiology. St. Louis, Mosby-Year Book, 1993.
4. Derbyshire, D. R., Chmielewski, A., Fell, D., et al.: Plasma catecholamine responses to endotracheal intubation. Br. J. Anaesth. *55*:855, 1983.
5. Longnecker, D. E., and Miller, F. L.: Pharmacology of inhalational anesthetics. *In* Rogers, M. C., Tinker, J. H., Covino, B. G., and Longnecker, D. E. (eds.): Prinicples and Practice of Anesthesiology. St. Louis, Mosby-Year Book, 1993, p. 1053.
6. Rusy, B. F., and Komai, H.: Anesthetic depression of myocardial contractility: A review of possible mechanisms. Anesthesiology *67*:745, 1987.
7. Philbin, D. M., Rosow, C. E., Schneider, R. C., et al.: Fentanyl and sufentanil anesthesia revisited: How much is enough? Anesthesiology *73*:5, 1990.
8. White, P. F.: Clinical uses of intravenous anesthetic and analgesic infusions. Anesth. Analg. *68*:161, 1989.
9. Forrest, J. B., Cahalan, M. K., Redher, K., et al.: Multicenter study of general anesthesia. II. Results. Anesthesiology *72*:262, 1990.
10. Scott, N. B., and Kehlet, H.: Regional anaesthesia and surgical morbidity. Br. J. Surg. *75*:299, 1988.
11. Yeager, M. P.: Regional anesthesia for the patient with heart disease. Pro: Regional anesthesia is preferable to general anesthesia for the patient with heart disease. J. Cardiothorac. Anesth. *3*:793, 1989.
12. Beattie, C.: Regional anesthesia for the patient with heart disease. Con: Regional anesthesia is not preferable to general anesthesia for the patient with heart disease. J. Cardiothorac. Anesth. *3*:797, 1989.
13. Saada, M., Duval, A. M., Bonnet, F., et al.: Abnormalities in myocardial segmental wall motion during lumbar epidural anesthesia. Anesthesiology *71*:26, 1989.
14. Her, C., Kizelshteyn, G., Walker, V., et al.: Combined epidural and general anesthesia for abdominal aortic surgery. J. Cardiovasc. Anesth. *4*:552, 1990.
15. Tuman, K. J., McCarthy, R. J., March, R. J., et al.: Effects of epidural anesthesia and analgesia on coagulation and outcome after major vascular surgery. Anesth. Analg. *73*:696, 1991.
16. Baron, J. F., Bertrand, M., Barre, E., et al.: Combined epidural and general anesthesia versus general anesthesia for abdominal aortic surgery. Anesthesiology *75*:611, 1991.
17. Steen, P. A., Tinker, J. H., and Tarhan, S.: Myocardial reinfarction after anesthesia and surgery. JAMA *239*:2566, 1978.
18. Goldman, L., and Caldera, D. L.: Risks of general anesthesia and elective surgery in the hypertensive patient. Anesthesiology *50*:285, 1979.
19. Charlson, M. E., MacKenzie, C. R., Gold, J. P., et al.: The preoperative and intraoperative hemodynamic predictors of postoperative myocardial infarction or ischemia in patients undergoing noncardiac surgery. Ann. Surg. *210*:637, 1989.
20. Goldman, L., Caldera, D. L., Southwick, F. S., et al.: Cardiac risk factors and complications in non-cardiac surgery. Medicine *57*:357, 1978.
21. Eisenberg, M. J., London, M. J., Leung, J. M., et al.: Monitoring for myocardial ischemia during noncardiac surgery. A technology assessment of transesophageal echocardiography and 12-lead electrocardiography. JAMA *268*:210, 1992.
22. Van Daele, M. E. R. M., Sutherland, G. R., Mitchell, M. M., et al.: Do changes in pulmonary capillary wedge pressure adequately reflect myocardial ischemia during anesthesia? Circulation *81*:865, 1990.
23. Berlauk, J. F., Abrams, J. H., Gilmour, I. J., et al.: Preoperative optimization of cardiovascular hemodynamics improves outcome in peripheral vascular surgery. A prospective, randomized clinical trial. Ann. Surg. *214*:289, 1991.
24. Backer, C. L., Tinker, J. H., Robertson, D. M., and Vliestra, R. E.: Myocardial reinfarction following local anesthesia for ophthalmic surgery. Anest. Analg. *59*:257, 1980.
25. Erlik, D., Valero, A., Birkhan, J., and Gersh, I.: Prostatic surgery and the cardiovascular patient. Br. J. Urol. *40*:53, 1968.
26. Larsen, S. F., Olesen, K. H., Jacobsen, E., et al.: Prediction of cardiac risk in non-cardiac surgery. Eur. Heart J. *8*:179, 1987.
27. Ashton, C. M., Petersen, N. J., Wray, N. P., et al.: The incidence of perioperative myocardial infarction in men undergoing noncardiac surgery. Ann. Intern. Med. *118*:504, 1993.
28. Goldman, L., Caldera, D. L., Nussbaum, R. R., et al.: Multifactorial index of cardiac risk in noncardiac surgical procedures. N. Engl. J. Med. *297*:845, 1977.
29. Forrest, J. B., Rehder, K., Cahalan, M. K., and Goldsmith, C. H.: Multi-

center study of general anesthesia. III. Predictors of severe perioperative adverse outcomes. Anesthesiology *76*:3, 1992.
30. Jeffrey, C. C., Kunsman, J., Cullen, D. J., and Brewster, D. C.: A prospective evaluation of cardiac risk index. Anesthesiology *58*:462, 1983.
31. Shah, K. B., Kleinman, B. S., Rao, T. L. K., et al.: Angina and other risk factors in patients with cardiac diseases undergoing noncardiac operations. Anesth. Analg. *70*:240, 1990.
32. Rao, T. L. K., Jacobs, K. H., and El-Etr, A. A.: Reinfarction following anesthesia in patients with myocardial infarction. Anesthesiology *59*:499, 1983.
33. Shah, K. B., Kleinman, B. S., Sami, H., et al.: Reevaluation of perioperative myocardial infarction in patients undergoing noncardiac operations. Anesth. Analg. *71*:231, 1990.

INFLUENCE OF UNDERLYING CARDIOVASCULAR DISEASE

34. Zeldin, R. A.: Assessing cardiac risk in patients who undergo noncardiac surgical procedures. Can. J. Surg. *27*:402, 1984.
35. Detsky, A. S., Abrams, H. B., McLaughlin, J. R., et al.: Predicting cardiac complications in patients undergoing non-cardiac surgery. J. Gen. Intern. Med. *1*:211, 1986.
36. Shah, K., Kleinman, B., Rao, T., et al.: Reduction in mortality from cardiac causes in Goldman class IV patients. J. Cardiothorac. Anesth. *2*:789, 1988.
37. Isaacson, I. J., Lowdon, J. D., Berry, A. J., et al.: The value of pulmonary artery and central venous monitoring in patients undergoing abdominal aortic reconstructive surgery: A comparative study of two selected, randomized groups. J. Vasc. Surg. *12*:754, 1990.
38. Garnett, R. L.: Pro: A pulmonary artery catheter should be used in all patients undergoing abdominal aortic surgery. J. Cardiothorac. Vasc. Anesth. *7*:750, 1993.
39. Ellis, J. E.: Con: Pulmonary artery catheters are not routinely indicated in patients undergoing elective abdominal aortic reconstruction. J. Cardiothorac. Vasc. Anesth. *7*:753, 1993.
40. McPhail, N., Menkis, A., Shariatmadar, A., et al.: Statistical prediction of cardiac risk in patients who undergo vascular surgery. Can. J. Surg. *28*:404, 1985.
41. McPhail, N., Calvin, J. E., Shariatmadar, A., et al.: The use of preoperative exercise testing to predict cardiac complications after arterial reconstruction. J. Vasc. Surg. *7*:60, 1988.
42. Cutler, B. S., Wheeler, H. B., Paraskos, J. A., and Cardullo, P. A.: Applicability and interpretation of electrocardiographic stress testing in patients with peripheral vascular disease. Am. J. Surg. *141*:501, 1981.
43. Gerson, M. C., Hurst, J. M., Hertzberg, V. S., et al.: Cardiac prognosis in noncardiac geriatric surgery. Ann. Intern. Med. *103*:832, 1985.
44. Gerson, M. C., Hurst, J. M., Hertzberg, V. S., et al.: Prediction of cardiac and pulmonary complications related to elective abdominal and noncardiac thoracic surgery in geriatric patients. Am. J. Med. *88*:101, 1990.
45. Pasternack, P. F., Imparato, A. M., Riles, T. S., et al.: The value of the radionuclide angiogram in the prediction of perioperative myocardial infarction in patients undergoing lower extremity revascularization procedures. Circulation *72*(Suppl. 2):13, 1985.
46. Franco, C. D., Goldsmith, J., Veith, F. J., et al.: Resting gated pool ejection fraction: A poor predictor of perioperative myocardial infarction in patients undergoing vascular surgery for infrainguinal bypass grafting. J. Vasc. Surg. *10*:656, 1989.
47. McCann, R. L., and Wolfe, W. G.: Resection of abdominal aortic aneurysm in patients with low ejection fractions. J. Vasc. Surg. *10*:240, 1989.
48. Baron, J. F., Mundler, O., Bertrand, M., et al.: Dipyridamole-thallium scintigraphy and gated radionuclide angiography to assess cardiac risk before abdominal aortic surgery. N. Engl. J. Med. *330*:663, 1994.
49. Eagle, K. A., Coley, C. M., Newell, J. B., et al.: Combining clinical and thallium data optimizes preoperative assessment of cardiac risk before major vascular surgery. Ann. Intern. Med. *110*:859, 1989.
50. Brown, K. A., and Rowen, M.: Extent of jeopardized viable myocardium determined by myocardial perfusion imaging best predicts perioperative cardiac events in patients undergoing noncardiac surgery. J. Am. Coll. Cardiol. *21*:325, 1993.
51. Hendel, R. C., Whitfield, S. S., Villegas, B. J., et al.: Prediction of late cardiac events by dipyridamole thallium imaging in patients undergoing elective vascular surgery. Am. J. Cardiol. *70*:1243, 1992.
52. Lette, J., Waters, D., Cerino, M., et al.: Preoperative coronary artery disease risk stratification based on dipyridamole imaging and a simple three-step, three-segment model for patients undergoing noncardiac vascular surgery or major general surgery. Am. J. Cardio. *69*:1553, 1992.
53. Bry, J. D. L., Belkin, M., O'Donnell, T. F., Jr., et al.: An assessment of the positive predictive value and cost-effectiveness of dipyridamole myocardial scintigraphy in patients undergoing vascular surgery. J. Vasc. Surg. *19*:112, 1994.
54. Mangano, D. T., London, M. J., Tubau, J. F., et al.: Dipyridamole thallium-201 scintigraphy as a preoperative screening test. A re-examination of its predictive potential. Circulation *84*:493, 1991.
55. Raby, K. E., Goldman, L., Creager, M. A., et al.: Correlation between preoperative ischemia and major cardiac events after peripheral vascular surgery. N. Engl. J. Med. *321*:1296, 1989.
56. Pasternack, P. F., Grossi, E. A., Baumann, F. G., et al.: Silent myocardial ischemia monitoring predicts late as well as perioperative cardiac events in patients undergoing vascular surgery. J. Vasc. Surg. *16*:171, 1992.
57. Mangano, D. T., Browner, W. S., Hollenberg, M., et al.: Association of perioperative myocardial ischemia with cardiac morbidity and mortality in men undergoing noncardiac surgery. N. Engl. J. Med. *323*:1781, 1990.
58. Raby, K. E., Barry, J., Creager, M. A., et al.: Detection and significance of intraoperative and postoperative myocardial ischemia in peripheral vascular surgery. JAMA *268*:222, 1992.
59. Mangano, D. T., Hollenberg, M., Fegert, G., et al.: Perioperative myocardial ischemia in patients undergoing noncardiac surgery—I. Incidence and severity during the 4 day perioperative period. J. Am. Coll. Cardiol. *17*:843, 1991.
60. Mangano, D. T., Wong, M. G., London, M. J., et al.: Perioperative myocardial ischemia in patients undergoing noncadiac surgery—II. Incidence and severity during the first week after surgery. J. Am. Coll. Cardiol. *17*:851, 1991.
61. Landesberg, G., Luria, M. H., Cotev, S., et al.: Importance of long-duration postoperative ST-segment depression in cardiac morbidity after vascular surgery. Lancet *341*:715, 1993.
62. Mangano, D. T., Browner, W. S., Hollenberg, M., et al., for the *McSPI* Research Group: Long-term cardiac prognosis following noncardiac surgery. JAMA *268*:233, 1992.
63. Halm, E. A., Browner, W. S., Tubau, J. F., et al., for the *McSPI* Research Group: Echocardiography for preoperative assessment of cardiac risk in noncardiac surgery. J. Gen. Intern. Med. *9*:31, 1994.
64. Tischler, M. D., Lee, T. H., Hirsch, A. T., et al.: Prediction of major cardiac events after peripheral vascular surgery using dipyridamole echocardiography. Am. J. Cardiol. *68*:593, 1991.
65. Langan, A. M., Youkey, J. R., Franklin, D. P., et al.: Dobutamine stress echocardiography for cardiac risk assessment before aortic surgery. J. Vasc. Surg. *18*:905, 1993.
66. Poldermans, D., Fioretti, P. M., Forster, T., et al.: Dobutamine stress echocardiography for assessment of perioperative cardiac risk in patients undergoing major vascular surgery. Circulation *87*:1506, 1993.
67. Poldermans, D., Arnese, M., Fioretti, P. M., et al.: Improved cardiac risk stratification in major vascular surgery with dobutamine-atropine stress echocardiography. J. Am. Coll. Cardiol. *26*:648, 1995.
68. Davila-Roman, V. G., Waggoner, A. D., Sicard, G. A., et al.: Dobutamine stress echocardiography predicts surgical outcome in patients with an aortic aneurysm and peripheral vascular disease. J. Am. Coll. Cardiol. *21*:957, 1993.
69. Taylor, L. M., Yeager, R. A., Moneta, G. L., et al.: The incidence of perioperative myocardial infarction in general vascular surgery. J. Vasc. Surg. *15*:52, 1991.
70. Foster, E. D., Davis, K. B., Carpenter, J. A., et al.: Risk of noncardiac operation in patients with defined coronary disease. The Coronary Artery Surgery Study (CASS) registry experience. Ann. Thorac Surg. *41*:42,1986.
71. Elmore, J. R., Hallett, J. W., Jr., Gibbons, R. J., et al.: Myocardial revascularization before abdominal aortic aneurysmorrhaphy: Effect of coronary angioplasty. Mayo Clin. Proc. *68*:637, 1993.
72. Huber, K. C., Ebans, M. A., Bresnahan, J. F., et al.: Outcome of noncardiac operations in patients with severe coronary artery disease successfully treated preoperatively with coronary angioplasty. Mayo Clin. Proc. *67*:15, 1992.
73. Goldman, L.: Cardiac risk in noncardiac surgery: An update. Anesth. Anal. *80*:810, 1995.
74. Mangano, D. T., and Goldman, L.: Preoperative assessment of the patient with known or suspected coronary disease. N. Engl. J. Med. *333*:1750, 1995.
75. Fleisher, L. A., and Barash, P. G.: Preoperative cardiac evaluation for noncardiac surgery: A functional approach. Anesth. Analg. *74*:586, 1992.
76. Granieri, R., and Macpherson, D. S.: Perioperative care of the vascular surgery patient. The perspective of the internist. J. Gen. Intern. Med. *7*:102, 1992.
77. Wong, T., and Detsky, A. S.: Preoperative cardiac risk assessment for patients having peripheral vascular surgery. Ann. Intern. Med. *116*:743, 1992.
78. Neustein, S. M., Bronheim, D. S., Lasker, S., et al.: Esmolol and intraoperative myocardial ischemia: A double-blind study. J. Cardiothorac. Vasc. Anesth. *8*:273, 1994.
79. Kataja, J. H. K., Kukinen, S., Vinamaki, O. V. K., et al.: Esmolol for treatment of hypertension and tachycardia in patients during and after abdominal aortic surgery. J. Cardiothorac. Anesth. *4*:37, 1990.
80. Andrews, T. C., Goldman, L., Creager, M. A., et al.: Identification and treatment for myocardial ischemia in patients undergoing peripheral vascular surgery. J. Vasc. Med. Biol. *5*:8, 1994.
81. Prys-Roberts, C.: Hypertension and anesthesia—fifty years on. Anesthesiology *50*:281, 1979.
82. Bruce, D. L., Croley, T. F., and Lee, J. S.: Preoperative clonidine withdrawal syndrome. Anesthesiology *51*:90, 1979.
83. Kataria, B., Dubois, M., Lea, D., et al.: Evaluation of intravenous esmolol for treatment of postoperative hypertension. J. Cardiothorac. Anesth. *4*:13, 1990.
84. Orlowski, J. P., Vidt, D. G., Walker, S., and Haluska, J. F.: The hemodynamic effects of intravenous labetalol for postoperative hypertension. Cleve. Clin. J. Med. *56*:29, 1989.
85. O'Keefe, J. H., Shub, C., and Rettke, S. R.: Risk of noncardiac surgical procedures in patients with aortic stenosis. Mayo Clin. Proc. *64*:400, 1989.

86. Stone, J. G., Hoar, P. F., Calabro, J. R., et al.: Afterload reduction and preload augmentation improve the anesthetic management of patients with cardiac failure and valvular regurgitation. Anesth. Analg. *59:*737, 1980.
87. Hayes, S. N., Holmes, D. R., Jr., Nishimura, R. A., and Reeder, G.S.: Palliative percutaneous aortic balloon valvuloplasty before noncardiac operations and invasive diagnostic procedures. Mayo Clin. Proc. *64:*753, 1989.
88. Roth, R. B., Palacios, I. F., and Block, P. C.: Percutaneous aortic balloon valvuloplasty: Its role in the management of patients with aortic stenosis requiring major noncardiac surgery. J. Am Coll. Cardiol. *13:*1039, 1989.
89. Thompson, R. C., Liberthson, R. R., and Lowenstein, E.: Perioperative anesthetic risk of noncardiac surgery in hypertrophic obstructive cardiomyopathy. J.A.M.A. *254:*2419, 1985.
90. Tinker, J. H., and Tarhan, S.: Discontinuing anticoagulant therapy in surgical patients with cardiac valve prostheses. J.A.M.A. *239:*738, 1978.
91. Katholi, R. E., Nolan, S. P., and McGuire, L. B.: Living with prosthetic heart valve. Subsequent noncardiac operations and the risk of thromboembolism or hemorrhage. Am. Heart J. *92:*162, 1976.
92. Tinker, J. H., Noback, C. R., Vliestra, R. E., and Frye, R. L.: Management of patients with heart disease for noncardiac surgery. J.A.M.A. *246:*1348, 1981.
93. Eckman, M. H., Beshansky, J. R., Durand-Zaleski, I., et al.: Anticoagulation for noncardiac procedures in patients with prosthetic heart valves. J.A.M.A. *263:*1513, 1990.
94. Durack, D. T.: Prevention of infective endocarditis. N. Engl. J. Med. *332:*38, 1995.
95. Clemens, J. D., Horwitz, R. I., Jaffe, C. C., et al.: A controlled evaluation of the risk of bacterial endocarditis in persons with mitral-valve prolapse. N. Engl. J. Med *307:*776, 1982.
96. Bor, D. H., and Himmelstein, D. U.: Endocarditis prophylaxis for patients with mitral valve prolapse. Am. J. Med. *76:*711, 1984.
97. Clemens, J. D., and Ransohoff, D. F.: A quantitative assessment of predental antibiotic prophylaxis for patients with mitral valve prolapse. J. Chronic Dis. *37:*531, 1984.
98. Sommerville, J., McDonald, L., and Edgill, M.: Postoperative haemorrhage and related abnormalities of blood coagulation in cyanotic congenital heart disease. Br. Heart J. *27:*440, 1965.
99. Hickey, P. R., Hansen, D. D., Norwood, W. I., and Castaneda, A. R.: Anesthetic complications in surgery for congenital heart disease. Anesth. Analg. *63:*657, 1984.
100. Goldberg, A. H., Maling, H. M., and Gaffney, T. E.: The value of prophylactic digitalization in halothane anesthesia. Anesthesiology *23:*207, 1962.
101. Lee, D. C., Johnson, R. A., Bingham, J. B., et al.: Heart failure in outpatients. A randomized trial of digoxin versus placebo. N. Engl. J. Med. *306:*699, 1982.
102. Kennedy, H. L., Whitlock, J. A., Sprague, M. K., et al.: Long-term follow-up of asymptomatic healthy subjects with frequent and complex ventricular ectopy. N. Engl. J. Med. *312:*193, 1985.
103. Bergh, N. P., Dottori, O., and Malmberg, R.: Prophylactic digitalis in thoracic surgery. Scand. J. Resp. Dis. *48:*197, 1967.
104. Pastore, J. O., Yurchak, P. M., Janis, K. M., et al.: The risk of advanced heart block in surgical patients with right bundle branch block and left axis deviation. Circulation *57:*677, 1978.
105. Pasulka, P. S., Bistrian, B. R., Benotti, P. N., and Blackburn, G. L.: The risks of surgery in obese patients. Ann. Intern. Med. *104:*540, 1986.

POSTOPERATIVE COMPLICATIONS

106. Salem, D. N., Homans, D. C., and Isner, J. M.: Management of cardiac disease in the general surgical patient. *In* Harvey, W. P. (ed.): Current Problems in Cardiology. Vol. 5. Chicago, Year Book Medical Publishers, 1980.
107. Charlson, M. E., MacKenzie, C. R., Ales, K. L., et al.: Surveillance for postoperative myocardial infarction after noncardiac operations. Surg. Gynecol. Obstet. *167:*407, 1988.
108. Charlson, M. E., MacKenzie, C. R., Ales, K. L., et al.: The post-operative electrocardiogram and creatine kinase: Implications for diagnosis of myocardial infarction after non-cardiac surgery. J. Clin. Epidemiol. *42:*25, 1989.
109. Rettke, S. R., Shub, C., Naessens, J. M., et al.: Significance of mildly elevated creatine kinase (myocardial band) activity after elective abdominal aortic aneurysmectomy. J. Cardiothorac. Vasc. Anesth. *5:*425, 1991.
110. Adams, J. E., III, Scicard, G. A., Allen, B. T., et al.: Diagnosis of perioperative myocardial infarction with measurement of cardiac troponin I. N. Engl. J. Med. *330:*670, 1994.
111. Oster, G., Tuden, R. L., and Colditz, G. A.: Prevention of venous thromboembolism after general surgery. Cost-effectiveness analysis of alternative approaches to prophylaxis. Am. J. Med. *82:*889, 1987.
112. Goldman, L.: Supraventricular tachyarrhythmias in hospitalized adults after surgery. Chest *73:*450, 1978.

THE ROLE OF THE MEDICAL CONSULTANT

113. Michel, L. A., Jamart, J., Bradpiece, H. A., and Malt, R. A.: Prediction of risk in noncardiac operations after cardiac operations. J. Thorac. Cardiovasc. Surg. *100:*595, 1990.
114. Perry, M. O., and Calcagno, D.: Abdominal aortic aneurysm surgery: The basic evaluation of cardiac risk. Ann. Surg. *208:*738, 1988.
115. Rivers, S. P., Scher, L. A., Gupta, S. K., and Veith, F. J: Safety of peripheral vascular surgery after recent acute myocardial infarction. J. Vasc. Surg. *11:*70, 1990.
116. Detsky, A. S., Abrams, H. B., Forbath, N., et al.: Cardiac assessment for patients undergoing noncardiac surgery. A multifactorial clinical risk index. Arch. Intern. Med. *146:*2131, 1986.
117. Goldman, L.: Multifactorial index of cardiac risk in noncardiac surgery: Ten-year status report. J. Cardiothorac. Anesth. *1:*237, 1987.
118. Lee, T. H., and Goldman, L.: Role of consultant. *In* Breslow, M. J., Mullen, C. F., and Rogers, M. (eds.): Perioperative Management. St. Louis, C. V. Mosby Co., 1990.

Chapter 55
Rheumatic Fever

ADNAN S. DAJANI

Epidemiology 1769
Pathogenesis 1769
Pathology 1770
DIAGNOSIS 1770
Major Clinical Manifestations 1770
Antecedent Group A Streptococcal Infection 1772
TREATMENT 1772
PREVENTION 1772
REFERENCES 1774

Rheumatic fever (RF) is generally classified as a connective tissue or collagen-vascular disease. Its anatomical hallmark is damage to collagen fibrils and to the ground substance of connective tissue. The rheumatic process is expressed as an inflammatory reaction that involves multiple organs: primarily the heart, the joints, and the central nervous system. The clinical manifestations of acute RF follow a group A streptococcal (GAS) infection of the tonsillopharynx after a latent period of approximately 3 weeks. The major importance of acute RF is its ability to cause fibrosis of heart valves, leading to crippling hemodynamics of chronic heart disease.

RF is the most common cause of acquired heart disease in children and young adults worldwide. Although the incidence of RF declined sharply in many developed countries, the disease remains a major problem in many developing countries. The precise reasons for the fluctuations in the incidence of the disease remain only partly understood. Although RF has been studied extensively, the pathogenesis of the disease is not well defined.

Epidemiology

The incidence of RF and prevalence of rheumatic heart disease are markedly variable in different countries.[1,2] At the turn of the century, the incidence of RF in the United States was over 100 per 100,000 population, ranged between 40 and 65 per 100,000 between 1935 and 1960, and is currently estimated at less than 2 per 100,000. Beginning in 1984, several outbreaks of acute RF were reported from a number of geographically distinct areas in the United States.[3–14] These focal outbreaks were not associated with a national increase in the incidence of RF.[15] The decline in the incidence of RF in the industrialized countries is in sharp contrast to the persistent high incidence of the disease in nonindustrialized countries.

In many developing countries, the incidence of acute RF approaches or exceeds 100 per 100,000.[1] In keeping with the falling incidence of RF in industrialized countries, the prevalence of rheumatic heart disease has declined. Table 55–1 compares the prevalence of rheumatic heart in school-age children in different regions of the world.

The decline in incidence of RF and prevalence of rheumatic heart disease has been attributed to several factors. Although the decline preceded the introduction of antimicrobial agents for the treatment of streptococcal pharyngitis, some reports suggest that the use of these agents may have enhanced the rate of this decline.[16] Improved economic standards, better housing conditions, decreased crowding in homes and schools, and access to medical care are often credited, at least in part, for the marked decline in RF.[1] Epidemiological observations in the United States[17] and the United Kingdom[18] show periodic shifts in the appearance and disappearance of specific M types in a particular geographical location. Such shifts may be another explanation for the decline and resurgence of RF in some parts of the world.

Because of the causal relationship between RF and GAS pharyngitis, the epidemiologies of the two illnesses are very similar. Initial attacks of RF occur most commonly between the ages of 6 and 15 years, and RF is rarely seen before the age of 5 years.[19] The risk of RF is increased in populations at high risk for streptococcal pharyngitis such as military recruits, persons living in crowded conditions, and those in close contact with school-age children.[20] The incidence of RF is equal in male and female patients. The seasonal incidence of RF also parallels that of streptococcal pharyngitis. The peak incidence of RF in Europe and the United States is in spring. Although RF used to be considered a disease of temperate climates, it is now more common in warm tropical climates, particularly in developing countries.

TABLE 55–1 RHEUMATIC HEART DISEASE IN SCHOOL-AGE CHILDREN

LOCATION	PREVALENCE PER 1000
United States	0.6
Japan	0.7
Asia (other)	0.4–21.0
Africa	0.3–15.0
South America	1.0–17.0

Pathogenesis

The evidence that GAS is the agent causing initial and recurrent attacks of RF is strong but indirect. It is based on clinical, epidemiological, and immunological observations. Factors that contribute to the pathogenesis of RF are related to both the putative causative agent and the host (Table 55–2).

THE ETIOLOGICAL AGENT. An untreated GAS tonsillopharyngitis is the antecedent event that precipitates RF.[21,22] RF does not follow streptococcal skin infection (impetigo). Proper antimicrobial treatment of the streptococcal pharyngitis with eradication of the organism virtually eliminates the risk of RF.[21] In situations conducive to epidemic streptococcal pharyngitis (such as the military population, crowding), as many as 3 per cent of untreated acute streptococcal sore throats may be followed by rheumatic fever.[23] Endemic infections result in much lower attack rates. It has been well documented that about one-third of all cases of acute RF follow mild, almost asymptomatic, pharyngitis. The lack of symptomatic pharyngitis was particularly striking in most of the recent outbreaks of acute RF in which

TABLE 55–2 PATHOGENESIS OF RHEUMATIC FEVER

GROUP A STREPTOCOCCUS
Tonsillopharyngeal infection, not other sites
Intensity of the infection
Brisk antibody response
Persistence of the organism
Rheumatogenic strains
M types 1, 3, 5, 6, 14, 18, 19, 27, and 29
Distinct structural characteristics of M proteins
Long terminal antigenic domain
Epitopes that are shared with human heart tissue
Heavily encapsulated, forming mucoid colonies
Resist phagocytosis
Do not produce opacity factor
SUSCEPTIBLE HOST
Genetic predisposition
Presence of specific B cell alloantigen
High incidence of class II HLA antigens

the majority of patients (58 per cent) had no history of pharyngitis.[2] This is an alarming observation, because the primary prevention of acute RF relies on the identification and proper treatment of streptococcal pharyngitis.

The major factors that are related to the risk of RF are the magnitude of the immune response to the antecedent streptococcal pharyngitis and persistence of the organism during convalescence.[23] Variations in the rheumatogenicity of GAS strains are a factor influencing the attack rate of RF.[24] The concept that RF is associated with infections due to virulent encapsulated (mucoid) strains capable of inducing strong type-specific immune responses to M protein and other streptococcal antigens[25] has been strengthened by observations made during the outbreaks of acute RF in the mid 1980's. The streptococci isolated from patients with RF and their sibling contacts during these outbreaks were primarily strains belonging to M types 1, 3, 5, 6, and 18.[26] M proteins of rheumatogenic streptococci show distinct structural characteristics: they share a long terminal antigenic domain[27] and contain epitopes that are shared with human heart tissue, particularly sarcolemmal membrane proteins and cardiac myosin.[28,29]

THE HOST. Although only a small proportion of individuals with untreated streptococcal pharyngitis may develop RF (3 per cent), the incidence of the disease following streptococcal pharyngitis in patients who have had a previous episode of RF is substantially more (about 50 per cent). Numerous epidemiological studies also indicate familial predisposition to the disease. These observations and more recent studies strongly suggest a genetic basis for susceptibility to RF. A specific B-cell alloantigen, identified by monoclonal antibodies, has been described in almost all patients (99 per cent) with RF but only in a small number (14 per cent) of controls.[30] Furthermore, susceptibility to RF has been linked with HLA-DR 1, 2, 3, and 4 haplotypes in various ethnic groups.[31]

Pathology

The acute phase of RF is characterized by exudative and proliferative inflammatory reactions involving connective or collagen tissue. Although the disease process is diffuse, it affects primarily the heart, joints, brain, and cutaneous and subcutaneous tissues. A generalized vasculitis affecting small blood vessels is commonly noted, but unlike the vasculitis of some other connective tissue disorders, thrombotic lesions are not seen in RF.

The basic structural change in collagen is fibrinoid degeneration. The interstitial connective tissue becomes edematous and eosinophilic, with fraying, fragmentation, and disintegration of collagen fibers. This is associated with infiltration of mononuclear cells including large modified fibrohistiocytic cells (Aschoff cells). Some of the histiocytes are multinucleated and form Aschoff giant cells.

The Aschoff nodule in the proliferative stage is considered pathognomonic of rheumatic carditis. These nodules have been described almost invariably in the autopsies of patients who died of rheumatic carditis; however, more recent observations indicate that the Aschoff nodules are observed in only 30 per cent to 40 per cent of biopsies from patients with primary or recurrent episodes of RF.[32] Aschoff bodies may be seen in any area of the myocardium but not in other affected organs such as joints or brain. They are most often noted in the interventricular septum, the wall of the left ventricle, or the left atrial appendage. Aschoff nodules persist for many years after a rheumatic attack, even in patients with no evidence of recent or active inflammation.

Inflammation of valvular tissue accounts for the more commonly recognized clinical manifestations of rheumatic carditis. Initial inflammation leads to valvular insufficiency. The histological findings in endocarditis consist of edema and cellular infiltration of the valvular tissue and the chordae tendineae. Hyaline degeneration of the affected valve leads to the formation of verrucae at its edge, preventing total approximation of the leaflets. Fibrosis and calcification of the valve occur if inflammation persists. Eventually, this process may lead to valvular stenosis.

DIAGNOSIS

There is no specific clinical, laboratory, or other test that establishes the diagnosis of RF. In 1944, T. Duckett Jones formulated his criteria for the diagnosis of RF[33]; these criteria are still valuable. The criteria have been modified, revised, edited, and updated by the Committee on Rheumatic Fever, Endocarditis, and Kawasaki Disease of the Council on Cardiovascular Disease in the Young (American Heart Association).[34] The most recent guidelines (Table 55–3) emphasize the diagnosis of *initial attacks* of RF. Dividing clinical and laboratory findings into major and minor manifestations is based on the diagnostic importance of a particular finding. If supported by evidence of preceding GAS infection, the presence of two major manifestations or of one major and two minor manifestations indicates a high probability of acute RF.

Major Clinical Manifestations

CARDITIS. Rheumatic carditis is a pancarditis affecting the endocardium, myocardium, and pericardium to varying degrees. Clinically, rheumatic carditis is almost always associated with a murmur of valvulitis. The severity of carditis is variable. In its most severe form, death from cardiac failure may occur. More commonly, carditis is less intense, and the predominant effect is subsequent scarring of the heart valves. Evidence of carditis may be very subtle; signs of valvular involvement may be mild and transient and may be easily missed on auscultation. Baseline studies, including electrocardiographs and echocardiographs, should be obtained in patients in whom RF is suspected. Patients who show no clear evidence of carditis on initial examination should be monitored closely over a few weeks to assess cardiac involvement.

Carditis is often regarded as the most specific manifestation of RF. It is noted in at least 50 per cent of patients with acute RF (Fig. 55–1). Recent outbreaks in the United States suggested that the frequency of carditis was somewhat higher than traditionally reported and may be in part due to more sophisticated diagnostic methods.[2] In one report,[3] carditis was diagnosed in 72 per cent of cases by auscultation and in 91 per cent of cases by Doppler ultrasonography. The risk of overdiagnosing valvular incompetence by echocardiography should be emphasized, and over-reliance on this tool in diagnosing rheumatic carditis should be avoided.

Valvulitis (endocarditis) involving mitral and aortic valves and the chordae of the mitral valve is the most characteristic component of rheumatic carditis. Mitral in-

TABLE 55–3 GUIDELINES FOR THE DIAGNOSIS OF INITIAL ATTACKS OF RHEUMATIC FEVER (JONES CRITERIA, UPDATED 1992)

MAJOR MANIFESTATIONS	MINOR MANIFESTATIONS
Carditis	Clinical findings
Polyarthritis	Arthralgia
Chorea	Fever
Erythema marginatum	Laboratory findings
Subcutaneous nodules	Elevated acute phase reactants
	Erythrocyte sedimentation rate
	C-reactive protein
	Prolonged P–R interval
SUPPORTING EVIDENCE OF ANTECEDENT GROUP A STREPTOCOCCAL INFECTION	
Positive throat culture or rapid streptococcal antigen test	
Elevated or rising streptococcal antibody titer	

From Dajani, A. S., Ayoub, E. M., Bierman, F. Z., et al.: Guidelines for the diagnosis of rheumatic fever: Jones Criteria, updated 1992. JAMA *268*:2069, 1992. Copyright 1992 American Medical Association.

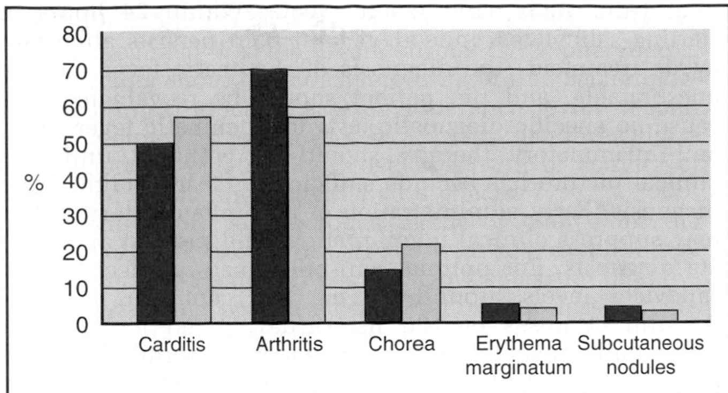

FIGURE 55–1. Relative frequency of major manifestations of rheumatic fever in earlier *(dark bars)* and more recent reports in the 1980s *(light bars)*.

sufficiency is the hallmark of rheumatic carditis. Aortic insufficiency is less common and usually associated with mitral insufficiency. The pulmonic and tricuspid valves are rarely involved. Residual valvular damage is a major concern in patients with RF and may lead to intractable cardiac failure requiring surgical intervention.

Myocarditis or pericarditis in the *absence* of valvulitis is *not* likely to be due to RF. Tachycardia is an early sign of myocarditis but may also be due to fever or cardiac failure. Transient arrhythmias may occur in patients with myocarditis. Severe myocarditis or valvular insufficiency may lead to cardiac failure. Cardiac enlargement occurs when severe hemodynamic changes result from valvular, myocardial, or pericardial disease. Inflammation of the visceral and parietal surfaces of the pericardium occurs, resulting in pericarditis and the accumulation of pericardial fluid.

ARTHRITIS. Polyarthritis is the most common major manifestation of RF (Fig. 55–1), but the least specific. It is almost always asymmetric, migratory, and involves larger joints (knees, ankles, elbows, and wrists). Characteristically there is swelling, redness, heat, severe pain, limitation of motion, and tenderness to touch. The arthritis of RF is benign and does not result in permanent joint deformity. Joint fluid shows findings characteristic of inflammation (not infection). In untreated cases, arthritis usually lasts 2 to 3 weeks. A striking feature of rheumatic arthritis is its dramatic response to salicylates. Indeed, if a patient does not improve substantially after 48 hours of adequate salicylate treatment, the diagnosis of RF should be in doubt.

Some patients may develop arthritis and other multisystem manifestations following acute streptococcal pharyngitis that do not fulfill the Jones criteria for the diagnosis of acute RF. This "syndrome" has been referred to as poststreptococcal reactive arthritis (PSRA). The arthritis of PSRA does not respond dramatically to anti-inflammatory agents. Some patients with PSRA may have silent or delayed-onset carditis[35]; therefore, these patients should be observed carefully for several months for the subsequent development of carditis.

CHOREA. Sydenham's chorea, St. Vitus' dance, or chorea minor occurs in about 20 per cent of patients with RF (see Fig. 55–1). The rheumatic inflammatory process in the central nervous system specifically involves the basal ganglia and caudate nuclei. Chorea is a *delayed* manifestation of RF, usually appearing in 3 months or longer after the onset of the precipitating streptococcal infection. This is in sharp contrast to the latent period of carditis or arthritis, which is usually 3 weeks. As such, chorea is frequently the only manifestation of RF. Furthermore, evidence of a recent GAS infection may be difficult to document and other supporting historical, clinical, or laboratory findings to fulfill the Jones criteria may be lacking. The diagnosis of RF can be made in a patient with chorea without strictly adhering to the Jones criteria.

Sydenham's chorea is characterized clinically by purposeless and involuntary movements, muscular incoordination and weakness, and emotional lability. The manifestations are more evident when the patient is awake and under stress and may disappear during sleep. All muscles may be involved, but primarily muscles of the face and extremities. Speech may be affected, being explosive and halting. Handwriting deteriorates, and the patient becomes uncoordinated and easily frustrated. The symptoms of Sydenham's chorea must be distinguished from tics, athetosis, conversion reactions, hyperkinesis, and behavior problems. Symptoms usually resolve in 1 to 2 weeks, even without treatment.

ERYTHEMA MARGINATUM. This distinctive rash is a rare manifestation of RF occurring in less than 5 per cent of patients. It is an evanescent, erythematous, macular, nonpruritic rash with pale centers and rounded or serpiginous margins. Lesions vary greatly in size and occur mainly on the trunk and proximal extremities, not on the face. The rash may be induced by application of heat.

SUBCUTANEOUS NODULES. These are firm, painless, freely movable nodules that measure 0.5 to 2 cm. They are rarely seen in patients with RF (about 3 per cent); when present, they are most seen in patients with carditis. They are usually located over extensor surfaces of the joints (particularly elbows, knees, and wrists), in the occipital scalp, or over spinous processes. The overlying skin is freely movable, shows no discoloration, and is not inflamed.

Minor Manifestations

CLINICAL FINDINGS. Fever and arthralgia are nonspecific, common findings in patients with acute RF. Their diagnostic value is limited because they are encountered commonly in a variety of other diseases. They are used to support the diagnosis of RF when only a single major manifestation is present. Fever is noted during the acute stages of the disease and has no characteristic pattern. Arthralgia is pain in one or more large joints without objective findings on examination and must not be considered a minor manifestation if arthritis is present. Epistaxis and abdominal pain may also occur but are not included as minor diagnostic criteria for RF.

LABORATORY FINDINGS. Elevated acute phase reactants offer objective but nonspecific indications of tissue inflammation. The erythrocyte sedimentation rate (ESR) and C-reactive protein (CRP) level are almost always elevated during the acute stages of the disease in patients with carditis or polyarthritis, but are usually normal in patients with chorea. The ESR is very useful in following the course of the disease; it usually returns to normal as the rheumatic activity subsides. The ESR may be elevated in patients with anemia and may be suppressed to normal levels in patients with congestive cardiac failure. Unlike the ESR, the CRP is unaffected by anemia or cardiac failure.

A common finding in patients with acute RF is a prolonged P-R interval for age and rate on electrocardiography. This finding alone is not diagnostic of carditis and does not correlate with the ultimate development of chronic rheumatic cardiac disease. Other findings on electrocardiography include tachycardia, atrioventricular block, and QRS–T changes suggestive of myocarditis; these changes are not considered minor manifestations.

Leukocytosis may be observed in the acute stages of RF, but the leukocyte count is variable and not dependable. Anemia is usually mild or moderate and normocytic normochromatic in morphology (anemia of chronic inflammation). Chest roentgenograms are useful in assessing cardiac size; however, a normal chest roentgenogram does not exclude the presence of carditis. Pericarditis, pulmonary edema, and increased pulmonary vascularity are also detected by this examination. Echocardiography may be help-

UNUSUAL CARDIAC MANIFESTATIONS. *Pulmonary hypertension* due to pulmonary vasculitis is an uncommon complication of rheumatoid arthritis. Chloroquine or hydroxychloroquine therapy, disease-modifying drugs used in rheumatoid arthritis, may occasionally result in the development of *cardiomyopathy*. Endomyocardial biopsy is diagnostic with characteristic curvilinear bodies, myelin bodies, and large secondary lysosomes demonstrated upon electron microscopy.[12]

STILL'S DISEASE. Still's disease (systemic onset juvenile arthritis) is an uncommon inflammatory disorder occurring in children and rarely in adults. As in adult rheumatoid arthritis, the most common cardiac manifestation is pericarditis, which may lead to tamponade. Other rare manifestations include myocarditis, dilated cardiomyopathy, and symptomatic aortic and mitral valve disease. Aggressive treatment of the underlying illness with corticosteroids and disease-modifying drugs, with appropriate surgical intervention for tamponade or valve replacement, may be necessary.[13]

SYSTEMIC LUPUS ERYTHEMATOSUS

The cardiac manifestations of systemic lupus erythematosus (SLE) are varied (Table 56–2) and are found more commonly at autopsy than clinically. William Osler first noted cardiac involvement as part of the group of diseases called *exudative erythema,* which clinically describes patients with SLE.[14] The incidence of cardiac involvement varies with the mode of detection. With two-dimensional and Doppler echocardiography, 57 per cent of patients had echocardiographic abnormalities including valvular abnormalities, pericardial disease, and myocardial abnormalities.[15] The incidence of coronary artery involvement differs between the pre- or post-steroid era, with a marked acceleration of coronary atherosclerosis in the post-steroid era.[16] Although the cardiac lesions in SLE are presumably due to immune deposits in the walls of blood vessels, the myocardium, or the pericardium,[17] newer studies have sought to define an association between SLE and antiphospholipid antibodies.[18]

PERICARDITIS. The most common cardiac manifestation of SLE is pericarditis, presenting in up to 30 per cent of patients with active disease.[16,19] Pericarditis may be asymptomatic or may present with typical chest pain, pericardial rub, fever, and tachycardia. Electrocardiograms may demonstrate diffuse ST-segment elevation, but sinus tachycardia and atrial arrhythmias are often seen. Symptomatic patients usually have pericardial effusions. Pericardial tamponade may occur in SLE, but the incidence of this complication is less than 1 per cent. Serum hypocomplementemia and/or high-titer antinuclear antibody/anti-DNA antibodies uniformly accompany this complication.[20] Pericardial fluid is often exudative and may be hypocomplementemic. The pathology of the pericardium may show fibrosis and acute inflammation, but frank vasculitis also may be seen.[16,19]

Drug-induced SLE causes pericarditis, presumably due to pathogenic mechanisms similar to those in native SLE. Constrictive pericarditis is very rare in SLE and has been reported in both native SLE and drug-induced SLE.[20]

Management. The treatment of pericarditis in SLE depends on the degree of hemodynamic compromise. NSAIDs are quite effective. For symptomatic serositis 10 to 20 mg per day of prednisone is usually sufficient. In the setting of tamponade, aggressive treatment, including daily systemic corticosteroids at doses of 1 to 2 mg per kg of prednisone and pericardiocentesis to normalize hemodynamics, is recommended. Most patients will require pericardiotomy or a pericardial window for long-term relief.

TABLE 56–2 CARDIAC MANIFESTATIONS OF SYSTEMIC LUPUS ERYTHEMATOSUS

PERICARDITIS
Cardiac tamponade
Constrictive pericarditis
Drug-induced pericarditis
MYOCARDITIS
Rare manifestation
? Association with myositis, anti-RNP
ENDOCARDIAL/VALVULAR LESIONS
Libman-Sacks endocarditis
Regurgitant and stenotic lesions (aortic and mitral)
Secondary bacterial endocarditis, embolization
Inflammatory valvulitis (vasculitis)
CORONARY ARTERY DISEASE
Coronary arteritis uncommon
Increased artherogenesis
Coronary artery spasm
CONDUCTION SYSTEM ABNORMALITIES
Varying degrees of atrioventricular block
Complete heart block
Anti-Ro/La-associated fetal heart block
PULMONARY HYPERTENSION
ANTIPHOSPHOLIPID ANTIBODY SYNDROME
Valvular (regurgitant) lesions
Cerebrovascular events
Coronary artery disease
Pulmonary hypertension
Dilated cardiomyopathy
Endocardial thrombi

MYOCARDITIS. Myocarditis is clinically diagnosed in up to 10 per cent of patients with SLE.[21] The incidence of myocarditis in autopsy studies, however, approaches 40 per cent.[20,22] Immunofluorescent findings in cardiac tissue are more diffuse and more frequent than histological findings. Immune deposits are found in myocardial vessels, suggesting a role for immune complex deposition as a factor in myocardial injury.[17] Echocardiographic studies in SLE confirm the relative lack of clinically active myocarditis.

In a retrospective review of 140 consecutive patients with SLE, five had myocarditis, and each also had skeletal myositis. The most striking finding was the presence of antibodies to nuclear ribonucleoprotein (RNP) in all five patients.[21] Endomyocardial biopsies in patients with SLE myocarditis show moderate-to-marked lymphocytic infiltrate in the interstitium and fibrous tissue around blood vessels.[23] The treatment of myocarditis is similar to treatment of other cardiomyopathies. However, aggressive therapies with prednisone, and possibly immunosuppressive drugs, should also be administered.

ENDOCARDITIS. In 1924, Libman and Sacks first described endocardial involvement in SLE.[24] Libman-Sacks endocarditis is present in up to 50 per cent of hearts at autopsy, but clinical manifestations are rare.[22] Verrucous vegetations 3 to 4 mm in size may appear on the valvular or mural endocardial surface; any valve may be involved, but the posterior leaflet of the mitral valve is the most common site (Fig. 56–4). Mitral and aortic regurgitation are the most common clinically important lesions, although mitral stenosis, aortic stenosis and tricuspid stenosis, and regurgitation have all been described. Despite the appearance of fragility, these vegetations rarely embolize to the brain or the coronary arteries.[22]

The pattern and outcome of patients with endocardial damage secondary to SLE appears to be changing with the advent of steroid therapy, valve replacement, and the increased longevity of these patients. In a classic autopsy series, Bulkley and Roberts report that in the post-steroid era, the Libman-Sacks type of endocardial lesions were smaller, fewer in number, mainly left sided, and pathologically were either partly or completely healed.[16] Other causes of valve dysfunction in SLE include valvulitis, vasculitis in valve tissue, thrombus formation upon the valve, and nodular calcification within the valve.[25]

The frequency of valvular involvement in SLE ranges from 18 per cent using standard echocardiography (Fig. 56–5) to as high as 74 per cent using transesophageal echocardiography.[26,27] Patients with valve thickening and dysfunction, rather than classic verrucous lesions, may have more hemodynamic compromise and a higher incidence of associated antiphospholipid antibodies.[26,27] The presence of endocardial lesions in patients with SLE may increase the likelihood of bacterial endocarditis and possible embolic disease.[27] Steroids have no role in the treatment of valve disease per se and may, in fact, exacerbate outcomes.[25]

Management of the valve disease is dependent on the

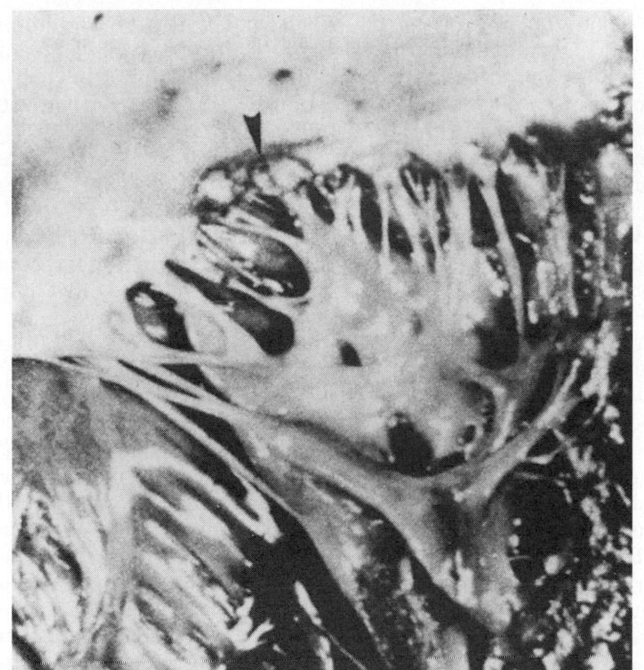

FIGURE 56–4. Verrucous endocarditis of Libman and Sacks involving the chordal attachments of an atrioventricular valve in a patient with systemic lupus erythematosus. The vegetations are usually 1 to 4 mm in diameter, may occur in clusters, and involve mural endocardium as well as valvular tissue. (From McAllister, H.A.: Collagen vascular diseases and the cardiovascular system. *In* Silver, M.D. [ed.]: Cardiovascular Pathology. New York, Churchill Livingstone, 1983.)

extent of hemodynamic compromise. Some series report that the mortality and morbidity from valve replacement in patients with SLE is quite high, but others report an improving outcome.[25,28]

CORONARY ARTERY DISEASE. In the pre-steroid era, myocardial infarction and coronary artery disease (CAD) were quite rare. In a major pathological comparison of SLE patients pre- and post-steroid use, there were no atherosclerotic plaques in patients treated less than 1 year with steroids, but plaques were found in over 40 per cent of those patients treated more than 1 year with steroids.[16] Whether corticosteroids have an independent role in atherogenesis is unclear. Increased atherogenesis may be due to hypertension, hyperlipidemia, and prolonged survival, all possibly related to the use of corticosteroids.[29,30]

Coronary artery involvement in SLE may also be due to active arteritis, which, in one small series, occurred in 50 per cent of patients.[31] Other causes of CAD in patients with SLE include coronary artery spasm and the hypercoagulable state secondary to antiphospholipid antibodies.[32] Management of patients with CAD and SLE requires attempts to decrease the dosage of prednisone and control hypercholesterolemia, hypertension, obesity, and other coronary risk factors.[30]

CONDUCTION SYSTEM ABNORMALITIES/CONGENITAL HEART BLOCK. Heart block of all degrees is a relatively rare manifestation of SLE. Atrial arrhythmias and, occasionally, ventricular arrhythmias, may be associated with accompanying myocarditis, coronary artery disease, or pericarditis.

Neonatal lupus may present as complete heart block; women who carry anti-Ro and anti-La antibodies have increased risk of giving birth to children with complete heart block.[33] Myocardial inflammation and fibrosis of the conduction system occur in infants with this syndrome.[34] The treatment of a fetus with congenital heart block secondary to maternal anti-Ro/La antibodies may include treatment of the mother with steroids and/or intravenous gamma globulin or a temporary or permanent pacemaker in the neonate.[35] Although the risk for developing complete heart block in the offspring of an anti-Ro–positive mother is quite low, mothers at risk for such an occurrence should be closely monitored with the use of fetal ultrasounds to detect complete heart block or myocarditis before delivery.

MISCELLANEOUS. Cardiac manifestations of SLE also include pulmonary hypertension, which has been estimated to occur in up to 5 per cent of patients. This may be related to vasospasm and/or vasculitis, and cor pulmonale may result.

ANTIPHOSPHOLIPID ANTIBODY SYNDROME. Clinical manifestations of this syndrome (which may occur independent of SLE) include thrombotic disorders including venous and arterial thrombosis, fetal loss in the late first trimester and second trimester, thrombocytopenia, premature stroke, and other neurological and cardiac manifestations. Patients with SLE who possess antiphospholipid antibodies or the lupus anticoagulant have an apparent increased risk of cardiac abnormalities. Valvular involvement is more common in patients with the antiphospholipid antibody and SLE. SLE valvular lesions tend to be both regurgitant and stenotic. Valve lesions in antiphospholipid antibody syndrome (APS) are more often regurgitant.[27,36–38] In patients with APS, there is an increased risk of embolic cerebrovascular complications.[36,39]

Approximately 5 per cent of patients with APS may develop myocardial infarction, especially patients under age 45.[39] Other cardiac manifestations of APS with SLE include pulmonary hypertension and cardiomyopathy, with bland thrombotic occlusions of the microcirculation without vasculitis. Anticoagulation in the setting of regurgitant disease, myocardial infarction, and pulmonary hypertension is indicated, and it is suggested that the international normalized ratio should be greater than 3.0.[40]

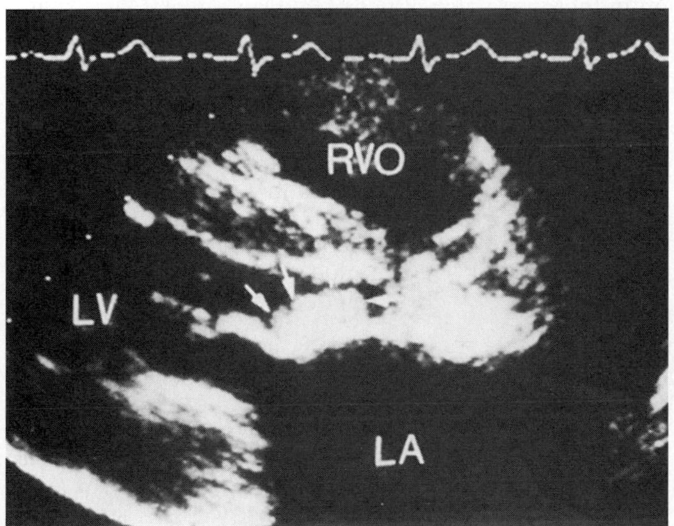

FIGURE 56–5. Parasternal long-axis view of the heart from a patient with systemic lupus erythematosus and high levels of anticardiolipin antibodies. A massive vegetation on ventricular surface of the anterior mitral leaflet *(arrows)* not interfering with the valve mobility, is clearly visualized. LA = left atrium, LV = left ventricle, RVO = right ventricular outflow. (Reproduced with permission from Nihoyannopoulos, N., et al.: Cardiac abnormalities in systemic lupus erythematosus: Association with raised anticardiolipin antibodies. Circulation *82*:369, 1990. Copyright 1990 American Heart Association.)

Polymyositis/Dermatomyositis

The cardiac manifestations of polymyositis and dermatomyositis include electrocardiographic changes with varying degrees of atrioventricular and interventricular block, atrial and ventricular tachyarrhythmias, sick sinus syndrome, congestive heart failure secondary to acute myocarditis, and/or end-stage myocardial fibrosis. Rare manifestations of polymyositis include coronary vasculitis, acute pericarditis and tamponade, and constrictive pericarditis.[41,42]

Numerous studies in the past two decades have revealed that cardiac involvement is common in polymyositis and may be associated with a poor prognosis.[41] In a series of 20 autopsy cases, myocarditis was detected in six patients; four had congestive heart failure.[43] In another autopsy series of 16 patients with polymyositis/dermatomyositis syndromes, 43 per cent had congestive heart failure, 25 per cent with histological evidence of myocarditis and 25 per cent with focal myocardial fibrosis.[44]

CONDUCTION SYSTEM INVOLVEMENT. In an electrocardiographic study of 77 patients with polymyositis, 32 per cent had an abnormal electrocardiogram; 13 per cent had left anterior hemiblock, and 9 per cent had right-bundle branch block.[45] Other electrocardiographic abnormalities, including atrioventricular conduction disturbances, atrial and ventricular arrhythmias, sick sinus syndrome, progressive fascicular block requiring pacemaker therapy, atrial fibrillation, and ventricular tachycardia, have been observed, but these are only rarely the cause of death.[46]

MYOCARDITIS. Myocardial involvement similar to that in skeletal muscle can result in congestive heart failure but is only rarely a cause of serious morbidity. Heart failure may be due to atherosclerotic disease and/or corticosteroid- and hypertension-related disorders or myocarditis. Pathology of heart failure includes myocardial fibrosis, inflammatory myocarditis, or, rarely, vasculitis with small vessel involvement.[43,44] The onset of heart failure secondary to myocarditis usually occurs in patients with active peripheral muscle involvement. However, it may rarely be the presenting symptom of polymyositis or may develop in the setting of improving peripheral myositis.[47]

If myocarditis is confirmed, treatment with prednisone or its equivalent at 1 to 1.5 mg/kg/day for at least 6 to 8 weeks is recommended. If there is no response, methotrexate should be added, although other drugs such as azathioprine, cyclophosphamide, and cyclosporin have been used.[46] Endomyocardial biopsy should be performed if myocarditis is the initial presenting manifestation or to clarify the degree of myocardial inflammation or fibrosis. If fibrosis predominates, steroids and immunosuppressive agents may be withheld.

OTHER CARDIAC MANIFESTATIONS. Pericarditis and/or pericardial effusions diagnosed by echocardiography may be found in up to 25 per cent of patients.[41] However, the incidence of pericarditis is greater in patients who have overlap syndromes and significantly higher in children with dermatomyositis.[48] Rarely, dermatomyositis has been associated with constrictive pericarditis and pericardial tamponade.[42,48] Clinical pericardial involvement is rare; treatment with nonsteroidal agents and/or corticosteroids (less than 0.5 mg/kg/day) may be beneficial.

Other manifestations of polymyositis heart disease include mitral valve prolapse, unexplained high-output cardiac failure, pulmonary hypertension, and systemic vasculitis. Complete heart block secondary to polymyositis induced by D-penicillamine has been described.[49] Cardiac involvement is one of the most significant clinical factors associated with impaired prognosis in polymyositis.

SPONDYLOARTHROPATHIES

The inflammatory aspect of cardiac disease in this group of diseases differs from rheumatoid arthritis by the higher frequency of aortic valve involvement, the relative lack of pericardial involvement, and relatively characteristic echocardiographic findings in a small subset of patients with aortic insufficiency.

Ankylosing Spondylitis

It was not until 1958 that ankylosing spondylitis and rheumatoid arthritis were recognized as distinct clinical entities. Therefore, pathological data regarding cardiac involvement before this time was based upon mixed data from patients with various inflammatory polyarthropathies.

AORTIC FINDINGS (see also p. 1575). The seminal pathological description of the cardiac manifestations of ankylosing spondylitis was published in 1973.[50] In this study, the pathological findings were described in eight patients with combined ankylosing spondylitis and aortic regurgitation. The aorta in ankylosing spondylitis is histologically similar to that in syphilitic aortitis. There is adventitial scarring, intimal proliferation with scarring of the media, and the vasa vasora are narrowed and surrounded by lymphocytes and plasma cells. The adventitial scarring extends below the base of the aortic valve. This thickening is particularly prominent behind the commissures of the aortic valve cusp and form a fibrous commissural bump.[50] Aortic regurgitation therefore results from shortening and thickening of the aortic valve cusps, displacement of the cusps by the "fibrous tissue bump," and dilatation of the aortic root. Similarly, one can rarely observe mitral regurgitation secondary to dilatation of the left ventricle from aortic regurgitation and from thickening of the basal portion of the anterior mitral valve leaflet.[50] In an echocardiographic study of patients who had ankylosing spondylitis greater than 10 years, 29 per cent had cardiac abnormalities.[51] This included aortic insufficiency (8 per cent), conduction system abnormalities (12 per cent), and pericardial effusions (4 per cent).

VALVULAR INVOLVEMENT. Aortic valve disease has been reported in up to 10 per cent in patients with ankylosing spondylitis[52] (Fig. 56–6). Rarely, aortic insufficiency may be the presenting manifestation. Subacute infective endocarditis is an uncommon complication. Aortic regurgitation may be progressive and require aortic valve replacement. Mitral regurgitation is relatively uncommon in ankylosing spondylitis; it may be secondary to mitral valve prolapse[53] as well as the extension of the "subaortic ridge or bump" affecting the basal portion of the anterior leaflet of the mitral valve.[54] Mitral valve replacement may be required if there is no improvement with standard medical therapy.

CONDUCTION SYSTEM DISORDER. Cardiac conduction disturbances are quite frequent in ankylosing spondylitis, occurring in up to 33 per cent of patients, and are more frequently observed in patients with aortic valve disease.[52] Conduction system abnormalities may be associated with the HLA-B27 antigen; the frequency of HLA-B27–positive men without spondylitis with permanent pacemakers is higher than in controls, suggesting an increased prevalence of heart block associated with this antigen alone.[55] Pathological changes in the aorta of patients with HLA-B27 heart disease without spondylitis are identical to the changes seen in patients with ankylosing spondylitis. The atrioventricular node and the bundle are distorted by fibrous tissue, consistent with extension of the same fibrotic process.[50,56] There is a wide spectrum of cardiac conduction disturbances, including Wolff-Parkinson-White syndrome, to all degrees of atrioventricular block.[57,58] These conduction system abnormalities may be intermittent, asymptomatic, and may spontaneously resolve.

It is speculated that although fibrosis contributes to the conduction system lesions, inflammatory infiltrates also contribute.[58] A trial of aggressive antiinflammatory medication may therefore be advisable to see if the inflammatory component resolves before permanent pacemaker implantation in those patients with complete heart block.

OTHER CARDIAC MANIFESTATIONS. Myocardial disease has been recognized as part of the spectrum of ankylosing

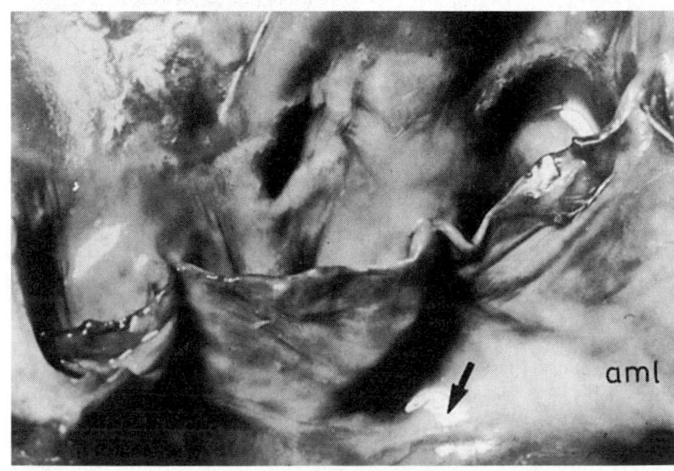

FIGURE 56–6. The aortic valve and sinus of Valsalva cut open in a patient with ankylosing spondylitis who was HLA-B27–positive. The base of the cusps is thickened. The orifice of the right coronary artery is distorted. Aortic regurgitation had been present during life. aml = anterior mitral leaflet. (From Bergfeldt, L.: HLA-B-27–associated heart disease. Am. J. Med. *77*:961, 1984.)

spondylitis. In one echocardiographic study, 53 per cent of patients, although asymptomatic, had left ventricular abnormalities. The left ventricular dysfunction is presumably related to excess connective tissue in the myocardium.[59] Significant left ventricular dysfunction has been reported in less than 1 per cent of patients. Pericarditis, cor pulmonale, and aortic arch syndromes may occur rarely.

REITER'S SYNDROME. The cardiac manifestations of Reiter's syndrome are similar to those of ankylosing spondylitis. Although unusual, aortitis and aortic regurgitation have been described in Reiter's syndrome. Fulminant aortic regurgitation requiring aortic valve replacement has been observed.[60] The pathology of the aorta is similar to that in ankylosing spondylitis, with aortic dilatation leading to aortic regurgitation. Reiter's syndrome rarely will present with angina, with aortitis leading to narrowing of the coronary ostia.[61]

Varying degrees of heart block, including complete heart block, are common in Reiter's syndrome and may be an early manifestation. Indeed, 25 per cent of patients with Reiter's syndrome develop conduction system abnormalities.[62] Pericarditis may occur at a somewhat higher frequency than in ankylosing spondylitis. As with ankylosing spondylitis, treatment depends upon the severity of the manifestations. Corticosteroids and/or NSAIDs may forestall the need for permanent pacemaker therapy in the setting of acute Reiter's syndrome and complete heart block.

PSORIATIC ARTHRITIS. Isolated aortitis causing aortic regurgitation potentially requiring aortic valve replacement has been described in psoriatic arthritis, although this complication is exceedingly rare.[63] Mitral valve prolapse has also been reported to occur at an increased frequency in psoriatic arthritis.[64]

PROGRESSIVE SYSTEMIC SCLEROSIS AND ITS VARIANTS

In 1943 it was recognized that cardiac dysfunction occurred in scleroderma and characteristic myocardial lesions were seen in a classic autopsy study.[65] Scleroderma may also cause pulmonary hypertension and/or systemic hypertension; cardiac manifestations may be difficult to interpret because one may not be able to differentiate primary myocardial disease from changes secondary to systemic and/or pulmonary hypertension. Pathological observations in scleroderma do show significant primary myocardial lesions, with a clear increase in myocardial fibrosis compared to controls, especially in patients who died in their fourth decade.[66]

PATHOGENESIS. The pathogenesis of the cardiac lesion in scleroderma is controversial. An intriguing concept is one of repetitive vascular insults secondary to cold induced perfusion changes. Classic pathological changes of contraction band necrosis seen in scleroderma are similar to the findings in hearts subjected to prolonged ischemia and subsequent reperfusion.[67] There appears to be a reversible component to myocardial perfusion deficits, and calcium channel blockers can, to some extent, blunt these responses.[68]

PERICARDIAL INVOLVEMENT. Autopsy series report pericardial involvement in up to 50 per cent of patients with systemic sclerosis. Pericardial involvement includes fibrinous pericarditis, pericardial adhesions, and pericardial effusions. Symptomatic pericarditis, however, was present in only 16 per cent of patients with diffuse scleroderma but was present in over 30 per cent of patients with CREST syndrome (*c*alcinosis, *R*aynaud's, *e*sophageal dysfunction, *s*clerodactylia, *t*elangiectasia) or limited scleroderma. Clinical presentation varies from chest pain, fever, and dyspnea to, rarely, tamponade and/or constrictive pericarditis.[69,70] Pericardial fluid may be exudative, but there is no evidence for autoantibodies or complement depletion in the fluid implying a different pathogenesis than that in rheumatoid arthritis or SLE.[71]

The treatment of acute pericarditis is therapy with NSAIDs with careful observation of renal function. Corticosteroids may be used, but their use is of concern in patients with scleroderma. Patients rarely need pericardiocentesis or surgical intervention.

MYOCARDIAL INVOLVEMENT. Myocardial lesions and fibrosis, which are found in up to 80 per cent of patients upon autopsy, may be patchy, may present in both ventricles, and may bear no relationship to myocardial perfusion.[66,69] In an autopsy study of nine patients with progressive systemic sclerosis and sudden cardiac death, extensive myocardial necrosis was found in seven and scarring in nine although the coronary arteries were otherwise normal; seven patients had contraction-band necrosis.[72]

Myocardial dysfunction occurs often, although clinical congestive heart failure occurs in less than 5 per cent of patients with progressive systemic sclerosis. Using extensive noninvasive techniques, left ventricular dysfunction and myocardial perfusion defects can be detected in up to 75 per cent of patients[73] (Fig. 56–7). Restrictive and dilated cardiomyopathies rarely occur in adults and children with diffuse scleroderma. Inflammatory myocarditis may occur but is rare.[74]

MANAGEMENT. The treatment of patients with scleroderma heart disease is not unlike the treatment of cardiomyopathy or congestive heart failure of other causes. Steroids are usually withheld in severe scleroderma for the fear of potentiating renal crisis, but in the setting of proven myocarditis, they may be life saving. Additionally, the use of D-penicillamine and immunosuppressive agents, such as methotrexate or azathioprine, has been suggested, but there is no convincing evidence that these agents will prevent further myocardial damage. The main therapeutic advance in the treatment of scleroderma myocardial dysfunction has been the aggressive control of hypertension, particularly with an angiotensin-converting enzyme (ACE) inhibitor. Calcium antagonists have been shown to improve perfusion defects (Fig. 56–8).

CONDUCTION SYSTEM DISEASE. The electrocardiogram may be abnormal in 50 per cent of patients with scleroderma.[75] A wide variety of electrocardiographic abnormalities have been described and include all degrees of heart block, septal infarction pattern, ventricular tachycardia, and supraventricular tachycardias.[72] The extent of the electrocardiographic abnormality correlates with the degree of presumed myocardial fibrosis.

OTHER CARDIAC MANIFESTATIONS. Valvular abnormalities in progressive systemic sclerosis include nonspecific thickening of the mitral and aortic valves.[66,67] Pulmonary hypertension is a leading cause of morbidity and mortality in patients with scleroderma (diffuse and localized).

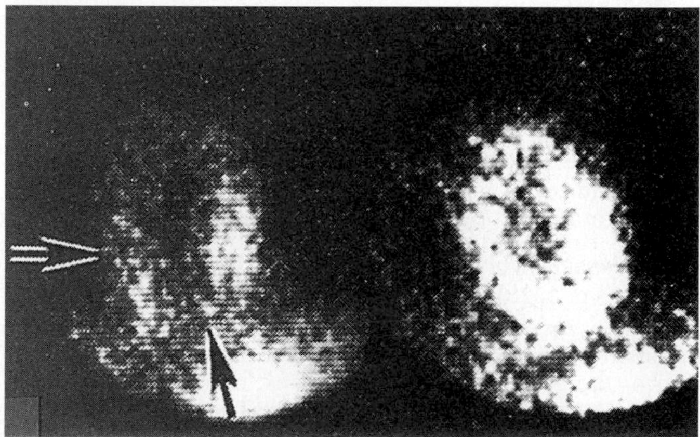

FIGURE 56–7. Thallium scintigrams obtained from a patient with scleroderma obtained immediately after immersion of the patient's hand in ice water for 2 minutes (*left*) and after 3 hours of redistribution (*right*). Images were obtained in the 40° left anterior oblique view and demonstrate a septal and inferoapical perfusion defect (*arrows*) that completely resolved with redistribution. (Modified from Alexander, E.L., et al.: Reversible cold-induced abnormalities in myocardial perfusion and function in systemic sclerosis. Ann. Intern. Med. *105*:661–668, 1986.)

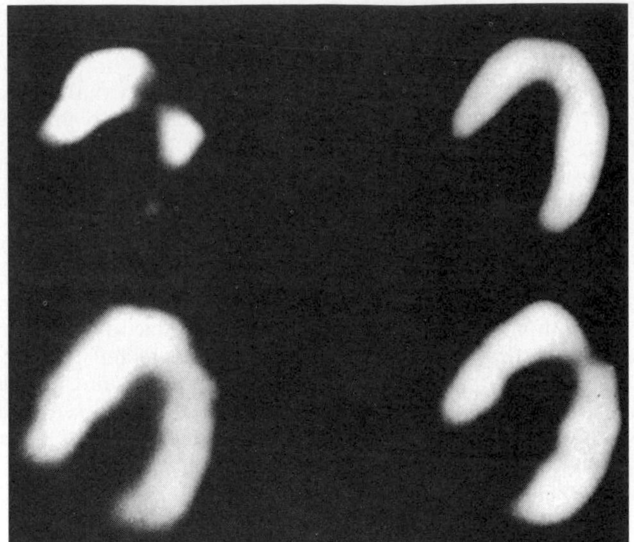

FIGURE 56–8. Positron emission tomographic images of a mid-left ventricular slice in a representative patient with systemic sclerosis showing ^{38}K myocardial uptake at baseline *(upper left)*. ^{38}K myocardial uptake after treatment with nifedipine *(lower left)*. These reflect increased perfusion and erduced ischemia, respectively. ^{18}F-Fluorodeoxyglucose (^{18}FDG) myocardial uptake at baseline *(upper right)* and ^{18}FDG myocardial uptake after treatment with nifedipine *(lower right)*. An increase in ^{38}K myocardial uptake and a decrease in ^{18}FDG myocardial uptake are seen after treatment with nifedipine. (From Duboc, D., et al.: The effect of nifedipine on myocardial perfusion and metabolism in systemic sclerosis. Arthritis Rheum. *34:*198, 1991; with permission.)

MIXED CONNECTIVE TISSUE DISEASE

The cardiac pathology of mixed connective tissue disease (MCTD) is similar to scleroderma. These patients often develop significant pulmonary hypertension as a result of an underlying pulmonary vasculopathy with marked intimal proliferation and luminal narrowing of the small pulmonary arterioles.[76] Pericarditis, pleuritis, massive pericardial effusions, myocarditis, and arrhythmias, have also been described.[77]

SJÖGREN'S SYNDROME

The incidence of primary myocardial and pericardial involvement in Sjögren's syndrome is low. Primary Sjögren's syndrome can result in verrucous endocarditis, similar to that seen in SLE. Conduction defects may also develop and fetal heart block may occur in the offspring of mothers' with primary Sjögren's syndrome who are anti-Ro positive.[78]

SYSTEMIC VASCULITIS

The clinical manifestations of vasculitis depend primarily on the size of the blood vessel involved and its location. A high index of suspicion for cardiac disease in any patient with pathologically defined vasculitis must be considered.

Large Vessel Involvement/Giant Cell Arteritis

(See also p. 1573)

Cardiac involvement in giant cell arteritis includes inflammation of the aorta with dilatation and/or inflammation of the aortic valve and its cusps, coronary arteritis, as well as pericarditis and myocarditis. The incidence of involvement of the aorta or its major branches approaches 13 per cent in some studies.[79] Inflammation of the vessel wall may become extensive enough to weaken the wall and produce a thoracic aortic aneurysm, and subsequent dilation may lead to aortic insufficiency. Prolonged inflammation of the vessel wall may lead to aortic rupture and death.[79,80] Occlusion of the aorta or its branches can occur along the course of the ascending, thoracic, or descending aorta, producing an aortic arch syndrome. Initial symptoms of thoracic aortic aneurysms secondary to giant cell arteritis (GCA) include exertional dyspnea and other symptoms of congestive heart failure, chest pain secondary to aortic dissection, angina, limb claudication and arterial bruits. In one study of patients with thoracic aortic aneurysms, 34 per cent were asymptomatic when the aneurysm was discovered.[81] The vast majority had GCA for an average of 2 years. Mortality from aortic dissection was 50 per cent. Patients with GCA or polymyalgia rheumatica should be examined carefully to ascertain that there are no pulse deficits, thoracic symptoms, or any symptoms or signs of limb ischemia.

Aortic regurgitation can rarely occur in giant cell arteritis, as an initial or a late complication.[82] The aortic regurgitation is usually due to aortitis resulting in destruction of elastic fibers within the arterial wall with marked inflammation and/or giant cells (Fig. 56–9). This inflammation leads to dilatation and distortion of the valve ring and the aortic root causing aortic regurgitation. When the aortic regurgitation is severe, aortic valve replacement is necessary and may be life saving.

Treatment of giant cell arteritis consists of high-dose corticosteroids (1 to 1.5 mg/kg/day of prednisone) and if there is no sign of improvement within 6 to 8 weeks, and if large vessel symptoms are suspected, cytotoxic therapies should be used.

Coronary vasculitis may rarely occur in giant cell arteritis. The pathology reveals granulomatous arteritis of epicardial coronary arteries and of intramural branches of the coronary arteries and arterioles.[83] Pericarditis and myocarditis are rare manifestations of giant cell arteritis. The treatment of these cardiac manifestations are similar to the treatment of GCA alone.

Behçet's Disease

Cardiac manifestations of Behçet's disease have classically included occlusion of the subclavian artery, aneu-

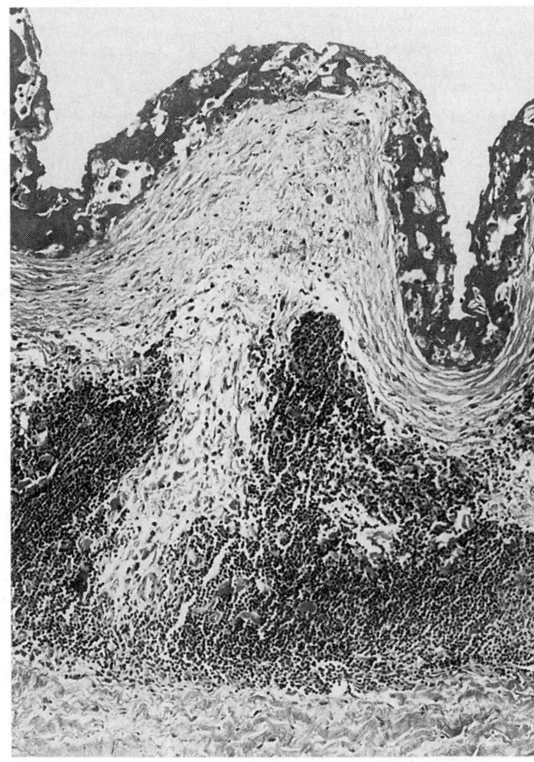

FIGURE 56–9. Active aortitis with perivascular lymphoplasmacytic infiltrate in the adventitia, unorganized periadventitial fibrin and secondary infarcts and patchy scarring involving approximately 50 per cent of the media in giant cell arteritis. (Courtesy of Frederick J. Schoen, M.D., Ph.D.)

rysms of the common carotid artery, aortic arch syndromes, and abdominal aortic aneurysms.[84] Diffuse aortitis with resultant proximal aortic dilatation may lead to severe aortic regurgitation requiring valve replacement.[85] The aortic wall pathology reveals endarteritis obliterans, with a normal aortic valve cusp. Other manifestations of Behçet's include pericarditis, myocarditis, conduction-system abnormality, and, rarely, formation of spontaneous arterial aneurysm, resulting in myocardial infarction or rupture.[86,87] The incidence of cardiac abnormalities in Behçet's disease is unclear. Recent studies using echocardiography in 65 patients revealed no significant difference in the prevalence of cardiac findings between a group of patients with Behçet's disease and controls, putting the true incidence of cardiac involvement in Behçet's disease in doubt.[88]

Medium Size Vessel Involvement

Polyarteritis Nodosa

The incidence of cardiac involvement in polyarteritis nodosa (PAN) has been misunderstood because it is confused with other medium-size vasculitides. In a clinicopathologic study of PAN, 50 per cent of patients had either active or healed coronary arteritis.[89] Of this group, only 19 per cent had evidence of active coronary arteritis of multiple vessels. The vessels involved usually included small subepicardial vessels rather than deep intramyocardial arteries. Formation of aneurysm was also seen; arteritis observed in the heart was milder than observed in other organs. Interstitial myocarditis was occasionally observed. Gross infarcts were identified in only 11 per cent. Pericarditis appeared in 19 per cent of these patients, but all had renal involvement.

In the past, cardiac involvement was commonly cited as a leading cause of death in patients with PAN, more recent studies discount this involvement.[89] It is possible that the combined use of corticosteroids and immunosuppressive drug therapies, as well as improved treatment of resultant hypertension, congestive heart failure, and renal insufficiency, have contributed to increased longevity.

CHURG-STRAUSS SYNDROME. Cardiac manifestations of the Churg-Strauss syndrome include acute pericarditis, chronic constrictive pericarditis, tamponade, cardiac failure, arrhythmias, and myocardial infarction.[90] The frequency of cardiac involvement in the steroid era is probably greater than 50 per cent, with cardiac disease accounting for one-half of deaths caused by Churg-Strauss syndrome.

Myocardial involvement includes either an obliterative or restrictive type of cardiomyopathy that later may develop into endomyocardial fibrosis. The myocardium may also show eosinophilic myocarditis, vasculitis, or fibrosis. Endomyocardial biopsy may help guide treatment by determining the degree of inflammation or fibrosis present. Appropriate steroids and immunosuppressive therapy (cyclophosphamide) has resulted in reversal of myocardial impairment.[91] Coronary artery involvement may occur in Churg-Strauss syndrome in the setting of systemic vasculitis or as an isolated eosinophilic coronary arteritis.

WEGENER'S GRANULOMATOSIS. Cardiac involvement is rare in Wegener's granulomatosis. Pericarditis may occur in 6 per cent of patients.[92] This only rarely requires pericardiocentesis and pericardiectomy.[92] Retrospective reviews, prior to the advent of C-antineutrophil cytoplasmic antibody (C-ANCA) reveal more frequent cardiac involvement including coronary arteritis, myocarditis, valvulitis of the mitral or aortic valve, varying degrees of heart block, and myocardial infarction.[93] With the advent of earlier diagnosis and aggressive treatment with cyclophosphamide, cardiac manifestations are quite rare.

SMALL VESSEL VASCULITIDES. Cardiac involvement in the small vessel vasculitides is rare and includes pericarditis, tamponade, and aortic and mitral regurgitation.[94,95]

MISCELLANEOUS VASCULITIDES

COGAN'S SYNDROME. This is a rare disease manifested by interstitial keratitis and hearing loss, tinnitus, and vertigo. Aortic regurgitation is the most severe cardiac lesion. Valvulitis or aortitis may occur in up to 10 per cent of cases.[96] Rare cases of aortitis have been associated with myocardial infarction due to either vasculitis or embolization.

RELAPSING POLYCHONDRITIS. This condition may involve noncartilage-containing tissues, such as the aorta and sclera, which have a high content of mucopolysaccharide. Loss of the supporting structures and elastic tissue from the aortic root lead to aneurysmal dilatation at the aorta, with dilatation of the valve ring and secondary aortic regurgitation. However, relapsing polychondritis may also be associated with significant arterial inflammation with inflammatory aortic aneurysms and systemic vasculitis.

The most significant cardiac manifestations of relapsing polychondritis include aortic aneurysms and aortic regurgitation, which may include significant necrotizing inflammation of the cardiac valves and coronary arterial vasculitis.[97] Aortic regurgitation may occur in up to 6 per cent of patients with relapsing polychondritis and may be progressive, requiring aortic valve replacement. This may occur when the disease itself seems to be inactive.[98] Myxomatous degeneration of the mitral valve, pericarditis, myocarditis, myocardial ischemia, and complete heart block may occur rarely.[97,98]

The treatment of relapsing polychondritis must be aggressive if cardiac disease and vasculitis is suspected. There is a significant morbidity rate with aortic valve replacement due to involvement of supporting structures. Treatment with corticosteroids and/or immunosuppressive therapies should be considered for patients with life-threatening organ involvement.

REFERENCES

1. Lange, L. G., and Schreiner, G. F.: Immune mechanisms of cardiac disease. N. Engl. J. Med. *330:*1129, 1994.

RHEUMATOID ARTHRITIS

2. Hora, K. S., Ballard, D. J., Ilstrup, D. M., et al.: Rheumatoid pericarditis: Clinical features and survival. Medicine *69:*81, 1990.
3. Maione, S., Valentin, G., Giunta, A., et al.: Cardiac involvement in rheumatoid arthritis. Cardiology *83:*234, 1993.
4. Escalonte, A., Kaufman, R. L., Quismorio, F. P., and Beardmore, T. D.: Cardiac compression in rheumatoid pericarditis. Semin. Arthritis Rheum. *20:*148, 1990.
5. Thould, A. K.: Constrictive pericarditis in rheumatoid arthritis. Ann. Rheum. Dis. *45:*89, 1986.
6. Leibowitz, W. B.: The heart in rheumatoid arthritis. Ann. Intern. Med. *58:*102, 1963.
7. Roberts, W. C., Kehoe, J. A., Carpenter, D. F., and Golden, A.: Cardiac valvular lesions in rheumatoid arthritis. Arch. Intern. Med. *122:*141, 1968.
8. Mody, G., Stevens, J. E., and Meyers, O. L.: The heart in rheumatoid arthritis: A clinical and echocardiographic study. Q. J. Med. *247:*921, 1987.
9. Slack, J. D., and Waller, B.: Acute congestive heart failure due to the arteritis of rheumatoid arthritis. Early diagnosis by endocardial biopsy: A case report. Angiology *37*(6):477, 1986.
10. Ahern, M., Lever, J. V., and Cosh, J.: Complete heart block in rheumatoid arthritis. Ann. Rheum. Dis. *42:*389, 1983.
11. Gravallese, E., Corson, J., Coblyn, J. S., et al.: Rheumatoid aortitis: A rarely recognized but clinically significant entity. Medicine *68:*95, 1989.
12. Ratliff, N. B., Estes, M. L., Myles, J. L., et al.: Diagnosis of chloroquine cardiomyopathy by endomyocardial biopsy. N. Engl. J. Med. *316:*191, 1987.
13. Goldenberg, J., Ferraz, M. B., Fonseca, A. S., et al.: Symptomatic cardiac involvement in juvenile rheumatoid arthritis. Int. J. Cardiol. *34:*57, 1992.

SYSTEMIC LUPUS ERYTHEMATOSUS

14. Osler, W.: On the visceral manifestations of the erythema group of skin diseases. Am. J. Med. Sci. *127:*629, 1895.
15. Cervera, R., Font, J., Paré, C., et al.: Cardiac disease in systemic lupus erythematosus: Prospective study of 70 patients. Ann. Rheum. Dis. *51:*156, 1992.
16. Roberts, W. C., and Bulkley, B. H.: The heart in systemic lupus erythematosus and the changes induced in it by corticosteroid therapy: A study of 36 necropsy patients. Am. J. Med. *58:*243, 1975.
17. Bidani, A. K., Roberts, J. L., Schwartz, M. M., and Lewis, E. J.: Immunopathology of cardiac lesions in fatal systemic lupus erythematosus. Am. J. Med. *69:*849, 1980.
18. Nihoyannopoulos, P., Gomez, P. M., Joshi, J., et al.: Cardiac abnormalities in systemic lupus erythemotosus: Association with raised anticardiolipin antibodies. Circulation *82:*369, 1990.
19. Kahl, L.: The spectrum of pericardial tamponade in systemic lupus erythematosus. Arthritis Rheum. *35:*1343, 1992.
20. Doherty, N. E., and Siegel, R. J.: Cardiovascular manifestations of systemic lupus erythematosus. Am. Heart J. *110:*1257, 1985.
21. Bornstein, D. G., Fye, W. B., Arnett, F. C., and Stevens, M. B.: The myocarditis of systemic lupus erythematosus: Association with myositis. Ann. Intern. Med. *89*(Part I):619, 1978.
22. Ansari, A., Larson, P. H., and Bates, B. D.: Cardiovascular manifestations of systemic lupus erythematosus. Prog. Cardiovasc. Dis. *27:*421, 1985.
23. Fairfax, M. J., Osborn, J. G., Williams, G. A., et al.: Endomyocardial biopsy in patients with systemic lupus erythematosus. J. Rheumatol. *15:*593, 1988.

24. Libman, E., and Sacks, B.: A hitherto undescribed form of valvular and mural endocarditis. Arch. Intern. Med. *33*:701, 1924.
25. Straaton, K. V., Chatham, W. W., Reveille, J. D., et al.: Clinically significant valvular heart disease in systemic lupus erythematosus. Am. J. Med. *85*:645, 1988.
26. Galve, E., Condill-Riera, J., Pigrau, C., et al.: Prevalence, morphologic types, and evolution of cardiac valvular disease in systemic lupus erythematosus. N. Engl. J. Med. *319*:817, 1988.
27. Roldan, C., Shirley, B., Lau, C. C., et al.: Systemic lupus erythematosus valve disease by transesophageal echocardiography and the role of antiphospholipid antibodies. J. Am. Coll. Cardiol. *20*:1127, 1992.
28. Alameddine, A. K., Schoen, F. J., Yaragi, H., et al.: Aortic or mitral valve replacement in systemic lupus erythematosus. Am. J. Cardiol. *70*:955, 1992.
29. Haidir, Y. S., and Roberts, W. C.: Coronary arterial disease in systemic lupus erythematosus: Quantification of degrees of narrowing in 22 necropsy patients (21 women) aged 16 to 37 years. Am. J. Med. *70*:775, 1981.
30. Petri, M., Spence, D., Bone, L., and Hochberg, M. C.: Coronary artery disease risk factors in the Johns Hopkins Lupus Cohort: Prevalence, recognition by patients and preventive practices. Medicine *71*:291, 1992.
31. Homcy, C. J., Liberthson, R. P., Fallon, J. J., et al.: Ischemic heart disease in systemic lupus erythematosus in the young patient: Report of six cases. Am. J. Med. *49*:478, 1982.
32. Wilson, V. E., Eck, S. L., and Bates, E. R.: Evaluation and treatment of acute myocardial infarction complicating systemic lupus erythematosus. Chest *101*:420, 1992.
33. Scott, J. S., Maddison, P. J., Taylor, P. V., et al.: Connective tissue-disease, antibodies to ribonucleoprotein, and congenital heart block. N. Engl. J. Med. *309*:209, 1983.
34. Silverman, E., Mamula, M., Hardin, J. A., and Laxer, R.: Importance of the immune response to the Ro/La particle in the development of congenital heart block and neonatal lupus erythematosus. J. Rheumatol. *18*:120, 1991.
35. Kaaja, R., Julkuren, H., Ammala, P., et al.: Congenital heart block: Successful prophylactic treatment with intravenous gamma globulin and corticosteroid therapy. Am. J. Obstet. Gynecol. *165*:1333, 1991.
36. Kaplan, S. D., Chartash, E. K., Pizzarello, R. A., and Furie, R. A.: Cardiac manifestations of the antiphospholipid syndrome. Am. Heart. J. *124*:1331, 1992.
37. Galve, E., Ord, J., Barquinero, J., et al.: Valvular heart disease in primary antiphospholipid syndrome. Ann. Intern. Med. *116*:293, 1992.
38. Vianna, J. L., Khamashta, M. A., Ordi-Ros, J., et al.: Comparison of the primary and secondary antiphospholipid syndrome: A European multicenter study of 114 patients. Am. J. Med. *96*:3, 1994.
39. Asherson, R. A., and Cervera, R.: Antiphospholipid antibodies and the heart: Lessons and pitfalls for the cardiologist. Circulation *84*:920, 1991.
40. Khamashta, M. A., Cuadrado, M. J., Mujic, F., et al.: The management of thrombosis in the anti-phospholipid-antibody syndrome. N. Engl. J. Med. *332*:993, 1995.

POLYMYOSITIS/DERMATOMYOSITIS

41. Askari, A. D.: Inflammatory disorders of muscle: Cardiac abnormalities. Clin. Rheum. Dis. *10*:131, 1984.
42. Yale, S. H., Adlakha, A., and Stanton, M. S.: Dermatomyositis with pericardial tamponade and polymyositis with pericardial effusion. Am. Heart J. *126*:997, 1993.
43. Denbow, C. E., Lie, J. J., Tancredi, R. G., and Burch, J. W.: Cardiac involvement in polymyositis: A clinicopathologic study of 20 autopsied patients. Arthritis Rheum. *27*:1088, 1979.
44. Haupt, H. M., and Hutchins, G. M.: The heart and cardiac conduction system in polymyositis-dermatomyositis: A clinicopathologic study of 16 autopsied patients. Am. J. Cardiol. *50*:998, 1982.
45. Stern, R., Godbold, J. H., Chess, Q., and Kagen, L.: ECG abnormalities in polymyositis. Arch. Intern. Med. *144*:2185, 1984.
46. Plotz, P. H., Dalakas, M., Leff, R. L., et al.: Current concepts in the idiopathic inflammatory myopathies: Polymyositis, dermatomyositis and related disorders. Ann. Intern. Med. *111*:143, 1989.
47. Rechavia, E., Rotenberg, Z., Fuch, J., and Strasberg, B.: Polymyositis heart disease. Chest *88*:309, 1985.
48. Tami, L. F., and Bhasin, S.: Polymorphism of the cardiac manifestations in dermatomyositis. Clin. Cardiol. *16*:260, 1992.
49. Wright, C. D., Wilson, C., and Bell, A.: D-Penicillamine-induced polymyositis causing complete heart block. Clin. Rheum. Dis. *13*:80, 1994.

SPONDYLOARTHROPATHIES

50. Bulkley, B. H., and Roberts, W. C.: Ankylosing spondylitis and aortic regurgitation: Description of the characteristic cardiovascular lesion from study of eight necropsy patients. Circulation *48*:1014, 1973.
51. O'Neill, T. W., King, G., Graham, J. M., et al.: Echocardiographic abnormalities in ankylosing spondylitis. Ann. Rheum. Dis. *5*:652, 1992.
52. O'Neill, T. W.: The heart in ankylosing spondylitis. Ann. Rheum. Dis. *51*(6):705, 1992.
53. Alves, M. G., Espirito-Santo, J., Queiroz, M. V., et al.: Cardiac alterations in ankylosing spondylitis. Angiology *39*:567, 1988.
54. Shah, A.: Echocardiographic features of mitral regurgitation due to ankylosing spondylitis. Am. J. Med. *82*:353, 1987.
55. Bergfeldt, L., and Moller, E.: Complete heart block: Another HLA-B27 associated disease manifestation. Tissue Antigens *21*:385, 1983.
56. Bergfeldt, L., Edhay, O., and Rajs, J.: HLA-B27 associated heart disease: Clinicopathologic study of three cases. Am. J. Med. *77*:961, 1984.
57. Bergfeldt, L., Vallin, H., Edhay, O.: Complete heart block in HLA-B27 associated disease: Electrophysiological and clinical characteristics. Br. Heart. J. *51*:184, 1984.
58. Bergfeldt, L., Edhay, O., and Vallin, H.: Cardiac conduction disturbances: An underestimated manifestation in ankylosing spondylitis. Acta Med. Scand. *212*:217, 1982.
59. Brewerton, D. A., Goddard, D. H., Moore, R. B., et al.: The myocardium in ankylosing spondylitis: A clinical echocardiographic and histopathologic study. Lancet *1*(8540):995, 1987.
60. Misukiewicz, P., Carlson, R. W., Rowan, L., et al.: Acute aortic insufficiency in a patient with presumed Reiter's syndrome. Ann. Rheum. Dis. *51*(5):686, 1992.
61. Hoagland, Y. T., Alexander, E. P., Patterson, R. H., et al.: Coronary artery stenosis in Reiter's syndrome: A complication of aortitis. J. Rheumatol. *21*(4):757, 1994.
62. Havermain, J. F., Albada-Kuipers, G. A. V., Dohmen, H. J. M., and Dijkmons, B. A. C.: Atrioventricular conduction disturbance as an early feature of Reiter's syndrome. Ann. Rheum. Dis. *47*:1017, 1988.
63. Muna, W. F., Roller, D. H., Craft, J., et al.: Psoriatic arthritis and aortic regurgitation. JAMA *244*:363, 1980.
64. Pines, A., Ehrenfeld, M., Fishman, E. Z., et al.: Mitral valve prolapse in psoriatic arthritis. Arch. Intern. Med. *146*:1371, 1986.

PROGRESSIVE SYSTEMIC SCLEROSIS AND ITS VARIANTS

65. Weiss, S., Stead, E. A., Warren, J. V., and Bailey, O. T.: Scleroderma heart disease, with a consideration of certain other visceral manifestations of scleroderma. Arch. Intern. Med. *71*:749, 1943.
66. D'Angelo, W. A., Fries, J. F., Masi, A. T., and Shulman, L. E.: Pathologic observations in systemic sclerosis: A study of 58 autopsy cases and 58 matched controls. Am. J. Med. *46*:428, 1969.
67. Bulkley, B. H., Rudolfi, R. L., Salyer, W. R., and Hutchins, G. M.: Myocardial lesions of progressive systemic sclerosis: A cause of cardiac dysfunction. Circulation *53*:483, 1976.
68. Ellis, W. W., Baer, A. N., Robertson, R. M., et al.: Left ventricular dysfunction induced by cold exposure in patients with systemic sclerosis. Am. J. Med. *80*:385, 1986.
69. Botstein, G. R., and LeRoy, E. C.: Primary heart disease in systemic sclerosis (scleroderma): Advances in clinical and pathologic features, pathogenesis, and new therapeutic approaches. Am. Heart J. *102*:913, 1981.
70. Satter, M. A., Guindi, R. T., and Vajcik, J.: Pericardial tamponade and limited cutaneous systemic sclerosis (CREST syndrome). Br. J. Rheumatol. *29*:306, 1990.
71. Gladman, P. D., Gordon, D. A., Urowitz, M. B., and Levy, H. L.: Pericardial fluid analysis in scleroderma (systemic sclerosis). Am. J. Med. *60*:1064, 1976.
72. Bulkley, B. H., Klacsmann, P. G., and Hutchins, G. M.: Angina pectoris, myocardial infarction and sudden cardiac death with normal coronary arteries: A clinicopathologic study of nine patients with progressive systemic sclerosis. Am. Heart J. *95*:563, 1978.
73. Anuari, A., Graninger, W., Schneider, B., et al.: Cardiac involvement in systemic sclerosis. Arthritis Rheum. *35*:1356, 1992.
74. Kerr, L. D., and Spiera, H.: Myocarditis as a complication in scleroderma patients with myositis. Clin. Cardiol. *16*:895, 1993.
75. Follansbee, W. P., Curtiss, E. I., Rahko, P. S., et al.: The electrocardiogram in systemic sclerosis: Study of 102 consecutive cases with functional correlations and review of the literature. Am. J. Med. *79*:183, 1985.
76. Suzuki, M., Homada, M., Semkiya, M., et al.: Fatal pulmonary hypertension in a patient with mixed connective tissue disease: Report of an autopsy case. Intern. Med. *31*:74, 1992.
77. Beier, J. M., Neilsen, H. L., and Nieilsen, D.: Pleuritis-pericarditis-an unusual manifestation of mixed connective tissue disease. Eur. Heart J. *13*:859, 1992.
78. Veille, J. C., Sunderland, C., and Bennett, R. M.: Complete heart block in fetus associated in the maternal Sjogren's Syndrome. Am. J. Obstet. Gynecol. *151*:660, 1985.

SYSTEMIC VASCULITIS

79. Klem, R. G., Hunder, G. G., Stenson, A. W., and Sheps, S. G.: Large artery involvement in giant cell (temporal) arteritis. Ann. Intern. Med. *83*:806, 1975.
80. Hunder, G. G.: Giant cell (temporal) arteritis. Clin. Rheumatol. *16*:399, 1990.
81. Evans, J. M., Bowles, C. A., Bjornsson, J., et al.: Thoracic aortic aneurysms and rupture in giant cell arteritis. Arthritis Rheum. *37*:1539, 1994.
82. Costello, J. M., and Nicholson, W. J.: Severe aortic regurgitation as a late complication of temporal arteritis. Chest *98*:875, 1990.
83. Lie, J. T., Failoni, D. D., and Davis, D. C.: Temporal arteritis with giant cell aortitis, coronary arteritis, and myocardial infarction. Arch. Pathol. Lab. Med. *110*:857, 1986.

84. Shimizu, T., Ehrlich, G. E., Inaba, G., and Hayash, K.: Behçet's disease (Behçet's syndrome). Semin. Arthritis Rheum. *8:*223, 1979.
85. Tai, Y.-T., Fong, P. C., Ng, W. F., et al.: Diffuse aortitis complicating Behçet's disease leading to severe aortic regurgitation. Cardiology *79:*156, 1991.
86. Jones, D. G., and Thomson, A.: Recognition of the diverse cardiovascular manifestations in Behçet's disease. Am. Heart J. *82:*457, 1982.
87. Bowles, C. A., Nelson, A. M., Hammill, S. C., and O'Duffy, J. D.: Cardiac involvement in Behçet's disease. Arthritis Rheum. *28:*345, 1985.
88. Ozkon, M. D., Emil, O., Ozdemir, M., et al.: M-mode, 2-D and Doppler echocardiographic study in 65 patients with Behçet's syndrome. Eur. Heart J. *13:*638, 1992.
89. Schrader, M. L., Hochman, J. S., and Bulkley, B. H.: The heart in polyarteritis nodosa: A clinicopathologic study. Am. Heart J. *109:*1313, 1985.
90. Hasley, P. G., Follansbee, W. P., and Coulehan, J. L.: Cardiac manifestation of Churg-Strauss syndrome: Report of a case and review of the literature. Am. Heart J. *120:*996, 1990.
91. Renaldini, E., Spandrio, S., Cerudilli, B., et al.: Cardiac involvement in Churg-Strauss syndrome: A follow-up of three cases. Eur. Heart J. *14:*1717, 1993.
92. Hoffman, G. S., Kerr, G. S., Leavitt, R. Y., et al.: Wegener's granulomatosis: An analysis of 158 patients. Ann. Intern. Med. *116:*488, 1992.
93. Grant, S. C. D., Levy, R. D., Venning, M. C., et al.: Wegener's granulomatosis and the heart. Br. Heart J. *71:*82, 1994.
94. Babajanianis, A., Chung-Park, M., and Visnieski, J.: Recurrent pericarditis and cardiac tamponade in a patient with hypocomplementemic urticarial vasculitis syndrome. J. Rheumatol. *18:*752, 1991.
95. Palazzo, E., Bourgeois, P., Meyer, O., et al.: Hypocomplementemic urticarial vasculitis syndrome, Jaccoud's syndrome, valvulopathy: A new syndrome combination. J. Rheumatol. *20:*7:1236, 1993.
96. Vollerstein, R. S.: Vasculitis and Cogen's syndrome. Rheum. Dis. Clin. North Am. *16:*433, 1990.
97. Bowness, P., Hawley, I. C., Morris, T., et al.: Complete heart block and severe aortic incompetence in relapsing polychondritis: Clinicopathologic findings. Arthritis Rheum. *34:*97, 1991.
98. Buckley, L. M., and Ades, P.: Progressive aortic inflammation occurring despite apparent remission of relapsing polychondritis. Arthritis Rheum. *35:*812, 1992.

Chapter 57
Hematological-Oncological Disorders and Heart Disease

LAWRENCE N. SHULMAN, EUGENE BRAUNWALD,
DAVID S. ROSENTHAL

ANEMIA AND CARDIOVASCULAR DISORDERS 1786
Cardiac Disorders Associated With Hemolytic Anemia 1787
HEMOCHROMATOSIS AND HEMOSIDEROSIS 1790
DISORDERS ASSOCIATED WITH INCREASED BLOOD VISCOSITY 1792
Polycythemia .1792
CARDIAC MANIFESTATIONS OF NEOPLASTIC DISEASE. 1794
CARDIAC EFFECTS OF RADIATION THERAPY AND CHEMOTHERAPY. 1799
HEMATOLOGICAL ABNORMALITIES RELATED TO CARDIAC DRUGS. 1804
REFERENCES .1805

The higher frequency of cardiovascular abnormalities in patients with hematological and neoplastic disorders and, conversely, of blood disorders in patients being treated for a variety of cardiovascular diseases has led to increasing interaction between cardiologists and hematologist-oncologists. Blood dyscrasias often complicate the use of cardiac medications and prosthetic heart valves and cardiovascular surgery. Hematologist-oncologists must often consult cardiologists regarding clinical problems that range from interpreting abnormal physical findings and electrocardiographic and echocardiographic changes in their patients to obtaining advice about how to treat heart failure, pericardial effusion, or other cardiac complications common among patients with anemia and hematological malignant diseases.

ANEMIA AND CARDIOVASCULAR DISORDERS

(See also p. 460)

Anemia is one of the most common causes of increased cardiac output and when extremely severe sometimes results in heart failure due to a high-output state in the absence of heart disease. As discussed in Chapter 15, tissue hypoxia combined with reduced blood viscosity leads to a reduction in systemic vascular resistance, which is associated with an increase in cardiac output.[1] Acutely induced anemia lowers coronary vascular resistance, whereas chronic anemia enhances formation of intercoronary collaterals and causes increases in preload and reduction of afterload.[2] When the normal hemoglobin concentration is restored, all signs and symptoms of cardiovascular disease usually disappear. The gradual development of severe anemia may lead to cardiac hypertrophy, by causing vasodilation, which increases venous return (and thereby preload) and causes volume overload. It reduces peripheral resistance (and thereby afterload). Left ventricular end-diastolic volume is increased in patients with chronic anemia, and afterload reduction, as reflected in left ventricular end-systolic stress, has been demonstrated. Such changes may favor maintaining a sufficiently high stroke volume (Chap. 14). Another mechanism of enhanced left ventricular function in chronic anemia has been attributed to increased levels of catecholamine and noncatecholamine inotropic factors in plasma.[3]

CARDIAC SYMPTOMS OF ANEMIA. The severity of reduction of cardiac reserve, of fatigue, exertional dyspnea, and edema depend on the severity of the anemia and the presence of an underlying cardiovascular disorder such as myocardial, coronary arterial, or valvular heart disease. Severely anemic patients without heart disease have few if any cardiac symptoms. When hemoglobin values decline below 9 gm/dl, resting cardiac output increases.[4,5] Symptoms also depend on the rapidity with which the anemia develops, as well as the physical activity of the patient. For example, if the anemia develops gradually in a normal person, patients with hemoglobin levels as low as 7 gm/dl may be able to carry out all but the most strenuous activities, whereas in the presence of coronary artery disease, anemia lowers the threshold for development of angina pectoris, so that patients with mild anemia may develop intensified angina.

Although uncommon, congestive heart failure with pulmonary edema can occur *solely* on the basis of very severe anemia (Hb $<$ 4 gm/dl) even in the absence of underlying heart disease. It may be difficult to distinguish congestive heart failure secondary to chronic anemia from that related to myocardial iron infiltration secondary to transfusion-related hemosiderosis (see p. 1790). However, the symptoms of reduced cardiac reserve secondary to anemia alone are usually relieved when the anemia is corrected and a normal red cell mass has been restored.

Electrocardiographic findings are not uncommon as the anemia progresses. With hemoglobin levels below 7 gm/dl, T-wave depression and inversion may be found, simulating myocardial disease. With transfusions, these findings usually return to normal.

Studies in anesthetized dogs have shown that maximal myocardial oxygen delivery far exceeds the supply at all levels of hematocrit. When one is plotting maximum oxygen transport against hematocrit, an "inverted U-shaped" relationship results (Fig. 57–1).[6] In otherwise normal subjects, the gradual occurrence of severe anemia rarely if ever results in myocardial hypoxia, because of several compensatory mechanisms, including the development of coronary collaterals and increased concentration of 2,3-diphosphoglycerate (2,3-DPG) in red cells, and its effect on the hemoglobin-oxygen dissociation curve,[7] as described below.

OXYGEN DISSOCIATION AND LEVELS OF 2,3-DIPHOSPHOGLYCERATE IN RED CELLS

Normally, 1 gm of hemoglobin binds 1.34 ml of O_2. With a hemoglobin concentration of 15 gm/dl, 100 ml of arterial blood contains 20 ml of O_2. As can be calculated from the Hb-O_2 dissociation curve (Fig. 57–2), 100 ml of mixed venous blood having a PO_2 of 40 mm Hg will contain 15.5 ml of O_2. The difference (i.e., 4.5 ml of O_2 per 100 ml of arterial blood) would be available for delivery to tissues.

SHIFTS OF THE HEMOGLOBIN-OXYGEN DISSOCIATION CURVE. In most patients with anemia, the Hb-O_2 dissociation curve shifts to the right, and more oxygen is released from hemoglobin as the PO_2 declines. The red cell concentrations of 2,3-diphosphoglycerate (2,3-DPG), profoundly affect the binding and release of O_2 by hemoglobin.[7] Deoxygenated hemoglobin, which is more alkaline than oxyhemoglobin, stimulates the production of 2,3-DPG, a byproduct of glycolysis. As a consequence, the intraerythrocytic ratio of deoxyhemoglobin to oxyhemoglobin serves as a critical regulator of 2,3-DPG concentration. For example, the decreased oxygen affinity present in chronic anemia can be accounted for by this increase in red cell 2,3-DPG. At a normal

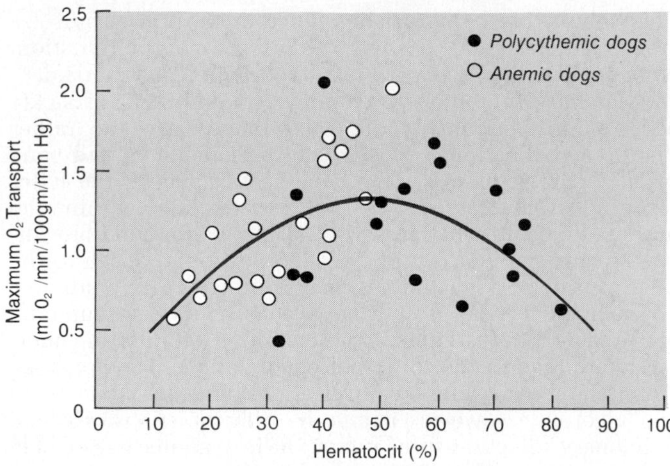

FIGURE 57–1. Maximum oxygen transport adjusted per unit perfusion pressure is shown as a function of hematocrit in anemic and polycythemic dogs. (From Baer, R. W., et al.: Maximum myocardial oxygen transport during anemia and polycythemia in dogs. Am. J. Physiol. *252*:H1086, 1987.)

arterial PO_2, arterial oxygen saturation remains high despite the reduction in oxygen affinity. However, at the lower PO_2 in the venous blood, elevated 2,3-DPG displaces the Hb-O_2 dissociation curve to the right, enabling greater release of oxygen from the cells at any level of PO_2. Oski et al. have calculated that decreased oxygen affinity mediated by increased red cell 2,3-DPG may compensate for up to half the oxygen deficit in anemia.[8] High levels of 2,3-DPG have also been found in subjects exposed to altitude[9] and in patients with pulmonary disease.[10]

The position of the Hb-O_2 dissociation curve can be expressed by the value of P_{50}, i.e., the partial pressure of O_2 at which hemoglobin is 50 per cent saturated. A reduction of the oxygen affinity of hemoglobin, i.e., a shift of the dissociation curve to the right, is reflected in an elevation of P_{50}. With a P_{50} of 34 mm Hg (instead of the normal P_{50} of 26.5 mm Hg), 3.3 ml of O_2 is unloaded per 100 ml of blood. As a consequence, an anemic individual with a 50 per cent reduction in red cell mass would suffer only a 27 per cent reduction in oxygen unloading.

RESPONSE TO HYPOXIA. Figure 57–2 summarizes the factors responsible for oxygenation in response to hypoxia. O_2 delivery to the metabolizing tissues depends directly on three principal factors: (1) blood flow; (2) hemoglobin concentration (i.e., the O_2-carrying capacity of the blood), and (3) the O_2 unloaded per unit of blood, as represented by the difference between arterial and venous blood oxygen saturations. Each of these three factors varies independently. Blood flow to any tissue is a function of total cardiac output and its fractional distribution. The red cell mass is regulated by erythropoietin in response to tissue oxygenation. The position of the Hb-O_2 dissociation curve is determined primarily by red cell 2,3-DPG levels and blood pH. Chronic anemia is usually well tolerated when these compensatory mechanisms operate effectively, i.e., with an increased cardiac output, redistribution of blood flow, and decreased O_2 affinity.

CARDIAC EXAMINATION. The cardiac enlargement that develops with severe, chronic anemia usually results from dilatation and eccentric hypertrophy with a normal ratio of wall thickness to cavity diameter, as occurs in other forms of volume overload (see Fig. 13–10, p. 401). The precordium is usually hyperactive, not unlike that in mitral regurgitation. Third and fourth heart sounds are frequently present, and a midsystolic murmur, maximal at the left sternal border, is usually audible.[11] The murmur is probably secondary to the combined effects of increased velocity of blood flow across the pulmonic and aortic valve orifices and reduced blood viscosity. Less frequently, an early, midsystolic rumbling murmur may be heard at the apex or along the left sternal border. This diastolic murmur is probably related to the increase in blood flow across the mitral or tricuspid valves and may be difficult to distinguish from the murmurs of mitral or tricuspid stenosis, although the murmur follows a third heart sound rather than an opening snap. Accurate diagnosis may require echocardiography as well as reexamination after correction of the anemia.

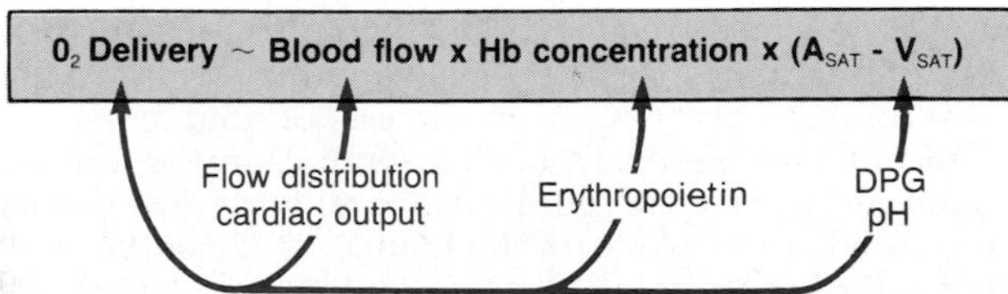

FIGURE 57–2. Oxygen delivered to an organ or tissue is directly proportional to blood flow, hemoglobin concentration, and the difference in oxygen saturation between arterial and venous blood. Patients with various types of hypoxia may compensate in the following ways: (1) Blood flow distribution may be altered to maintain oxygenation of vital organs, with an increase in total cardiac output when hypoxia is severe. (2) Increased erythropoietin production may stimulate erythropoiesis. (3) Oxygen unloading may be enhanced by a shift to the right in the oxygen dissociation curve, mediated by an increase in red cell 2,3-DPG. (From Bunn, H. F.: Pathophysiology of the anemias. *In* Isselbacher, K. J., et al. [eds.]: Harrison's Principles of Internal Medicine. 13th ed. New York, McGraw-Hill, 1994, p. 1720. © 1994 The McGraw-Hill Companies, Inc.)

In patients with chronic anemia whose hearts are compensated at a reduced concentration of hemoglobin, blood volume expansion achieved by the transfusion of whole blood may be poorly tolerated. Expanding the blood volume and augmenting left ventricular filling pressure will risk precipitating or aggravating heart failure. Therefore, the slow infusion of packed red blood cells accompanied by the administration of a diuretic is desirable.

Cardiac Disorders Associated With Hemolytic Anemia

Cardiomegaly, congestive heart failure, and sudden death have been reported frequently in patients with chronic hemolytic anemias such as sickle cell disease and thalassemia. In addition, hemolysis secondary to cardiac disease (see below) may cause cardiac failure.

Hemoglobinopathies

SICKLE CELL DISEASE. Sickle hemoglobin results from a mutation in the codon for the sixth amino acid of the beta globin chain from glutamic acid to valine. This single mutation causes sickle hemoglobin to polymerize when it becomes deoxygenated, leading to all the manifestations of the disease as described.[12,13] It is likely that the sickle gene was selected during evolution in central Africa because persons with sickle trait (one affected beta globin gene) appear to be more resistant to the effects of falciparum malaria. In central Africa the sickle gene frequency may be as high as 20 per cent. Eight to 10 per cent of black Americans are heterozygous for this trait.

PATHOPHYSIOLOGY OF SICKLE CELL DISEASE. When sickle hemoglobin becomes deoxygenated it polymerizes, giving sickle cells their characteristic shape. The degree of sickling is related to both the intracellular concentration of sickle hemoglobin and the intracellular oxygen tension. Polymerization is initially reversible, and if the cell is quickly and sufficiently reoxygenated, hemoglobin will return to its normal configuration and sickling will resolve. With prolonged deoxygenation polymerization and sickling become irreversible.

The propensity of a cell to sickle is affected by the concentration of sickle hemoglobin. When one beta gene is mutated to produce sickle hemoglobin (sickle trait) there is insufficient sickle hemoglobin to polymerize, except in the most hypoxic of conditions. Therefore, patients with sickle trait (AS) are generally not anemic and do not suffer the complications of sickle cell anemia. On the other hand, if both genes are affected, as in sickle cell disease (SS), red cells will sickle in minimally hypoxic circumstances, often in the venous capillary bed leading to microvascular occlusion.

Classical sickle cell anemia (SS disease) is a severe disease manifested by significant anemia and sickle crises from an early age. Generally patients have hematocrits of 20 to 22 per cent, with reticulocyte counts of 5 to 20 per cent. Variations of sickle cell disease occur when one beta chain has the sickle mutation and the other beta chain has another abnormal gene such as hemoglobin C or a thalassemic variant. SC disease is not as severe as SS disease, and the sickle-thalassemia syndromes vary depending on the amount of beta globin produced by the thalassemic gene. Particularly in the case of the sickle–beta thalassemia syndromes, because of the reduction in beta chain production from the thalassemic gene, intracellular hemoglobin concentrations are reduced. In turn, the propensity for these cells to sickle under hypoxic conditions is decreased.

In addition, many blacks are heterozygous for alpha-thalassemia and the concurrence of alpha-thalassemia trait and sickle cell disease makes the sickle cell disease less severe because of more balanced globin chain production, and because the red cell hemoglobin concentration is lower, resulting in less sickling.

The clinical manifestations of sickle cell disease relate to the effects of sickled cells and their propensity to become sequestered in the microvasculature, and to their short life span resulting in a chronic hemolytic anemia.

When sickling occurs in the capillary bed, the sickled cells become trapped in the microvasculature, leading to vascular occlusion. This is the result of both the rigid nature of sickle cells making transport through the microcirculation difficult, and the fact that sickled cells have a membrane that is particularly sticky, leading the cells to adhere to vessel walls. When additional cells become trapped they become progressively deoxygenated. If not quickly released from the microcirculation to become re-oxygenated in the pulmonary bed, they become irreversibly sickled. When they become permanently entrapped in the microcirculation a sickle cell crisis may result due to vascular insufficiency in the area of vascular occlusion. This is associated with severe pain and can be associated with local tissue damage such as bone infarcts, strokes, and pulmonary infarcts.

Red cells from patients with homozygous sickle disease (SS) that are not entrapped in the microcirculation nevertheless become damaged because of polymerized hemoglobin and membrane alterations. These cells have a very short half-life and are rapidly destroyed in the spleen or other reticuloendothelial organs. Therefore, patients with homozygous sickle cell disease are chronically anemic, in spite of vigorous red cell production as demonstrated by high reticulocyte counts. Otherwise well patients with sickle cell anemia (SS disease) maintain hematocrits between 19 and 22 per cent with a high compensatory reticulocyte count, but in cases of bone marrow suppression due to bacterial or viral infections, a suppression of the reticulocyte count can lead to an acute worsening of the anemia.

Cardiopulmonary Manifestations. The cardiopulmonary system is frequently involved in sickle cell anemia.[14–17] As in other chronic anemias, both cardiac output and oxygen extraction by tissues are increased, and the reduced oxygen content of these red cells leads to further sickling. A normal left ventricle is able to tolerate the volume overload of chronic, moderately severe anemia for indefinite periods with no deterioration in functional capacity.[16] The increased preload and decreased afterload characteristic of chronic anemia (Fig. 57–3) compensate for any left ventricular dysfunction and maintain a normal ejection fraction and high cardiac output in sickle cell anemia.[17] When cardiac decompensation occurs in patients with sickle cell anemia, it is usually the result of other coexisting complications of the SS disease or the presence of underlying cardiovascular abnormalities. Deaths secondary to congestive heart failure occurring in children and young adults with sickle cell anemia are usually precipitated by chronic renal failure, pulmonary thrombosis, or infections.[18]

Acute myocardial infarction is a rare complication of sickle cell disease and has been confirmed at postmortem examination in a few patients without significant coronary atherosclerosis.[14,19] More O_2 is extracted by the myocardium than by any other tissue, and transmural infarction due to in situ thrombosis by sickled cells is rare. However, infarction of the papillary muscles of the heart does occur.

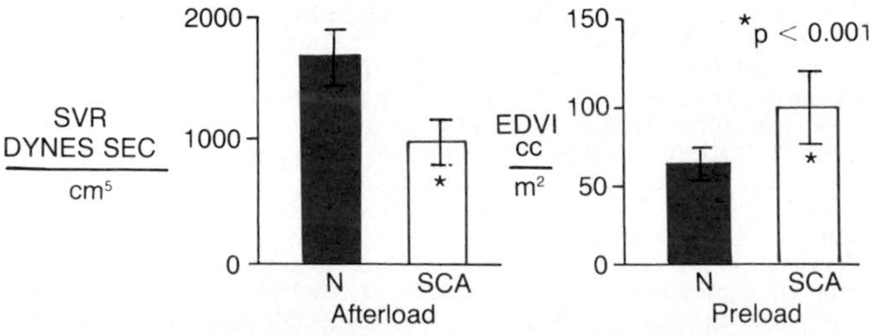

FIGURE 57–3. Loading conditions in 11 patients with sickle cell anemia (SCA) and 11 normal subjects (N). *Left,* Afterload, as indicated by systemic vascular resistance (SVR), was significantly decreased in patients with SCA. *Right,* Preload, as indicated by end-diastolic volume index (EDVI), was significantly increased in patients with SCA. (From Dennenberg, B. S., et al.: Cardiac function in sickle cell anemia. Am. J. Cardiol. *51*:1675, 1983.)

This should not be surprising, since the papillary muscles are at the terminal portion of the coronary circulation, where collateral vessels are scant and hypoxia is marked.

Pulmonary infarction, a common complication of sickle cell anemia, is probably due to thrombosis in situ rather than to embolization.[20,21] Although infrequent, fat and bone marrow emboli to the lungs have been reported, the latter resulting from necrosis caused by sickling within the marrow sinusoids. Patients with sickle cell anemia are unusually susceptible to infection. In addition, damage to the lung caused by repeated vascular insults creates a suitable milieu for bacterial growth; as a consequence, pneumonia is a frequent and serious complication. Mortality and morbidity are high in the setting of pneumonia and hypoxia, so that treatment of these complications must be immediate and vigorous. However, it may be difficult to differentiate pulmonary infection from infarction in patients with sickle cell anemia. Although impaired pulmonary function in sickle cell anemia is common, pulmonary hypertension and cor pulmonale are rarely encountered.

In almost all patients with sickle cell anemia the heart ultimately becomes enlarged, and at autopsy strikingly high heart weights are noted in a majority of patients despite the absence of other causes of cardiomegaly such as hypertension, atherosclerosis, or coronary artery disease.[1] In patients who have received multiple blood transfusions, myocardial iron deposition (hemosiderosis) may contribute both to the cardiac enlargement and to the associated impairment of cardiac function. However, this complication occurs much less frequently in sickle cell anemia than in homozygous thalassemia (see below). Histological studies have suggested that the increase in heart weight is secondary to fibrosis, presumably caused by the combination of anemia and papillary muscle infarction. With time, children with sickle cell disease exhibit progressive cardiac chamber enlargement with a progressive increase in left ventricular mass.[21]

There are no specific electrocardiographic changes in sickle cell anemia. However, almost 80 per cent of patients with sickle cell anemia have an abnormal electrocardiogram. These abnormalities include left ventricular hypertrophy and first-degree atrioventricular (AV) block as well as nonspecific ST-segment and T-wave changes and abnormal septal Q waves; this last finding is believed to be secondary to excessive septal thickness.[22] Arrhythmias rarely occur with sickle cell anemia, although continuous electrocardiographic monitoring during painful crises has revealed both atrial and ventricular arrhythmias in the majority of patients.[23] Echocardiographic measurements in patients with cardiac symptoms are useful in documenting both cardiac hyperactivity and depressed left ventricular performance.[24] Radiological studies may be entirely normal. With exercise, cardiac dysfunction may be manifested by an abnormal ejection fraction response, abnormalities of wall motion, and slowed left ventricular filling.[24–26] M-mode echocardiographic studies demonstrated an incidence of mitral valve prolapse in 25 per cent of SS patients,[15,27] far in excess of that expected. More recent two-dimensional echo and Doppler ultrasonography performed in adult patients with SS disease demonstrated a 22 per cent incidence of diastolic murmurs but no instances of myxomatous valvular degeneration or mitral valve prolapse.[15]

THALASSEMIC SYNDROMES. The thalassemic syndromes are a group of inherited disorders caused by mutations of either the alpha or beta globin genes resulting in a decrease in the production of the respective globin chain.[28] Hemoglobin is composed of two alpha and two beta chains. This tetramer binds iron and carries oxygen. There are four alpha genes and a mutation of one or more of them will cause a decrease in alpha chain production, resulting in alpha-thalassemia. There are two beta genes, and abnormalities in one or both will result in a beta thalassemia syndrome. Alpha thalassemia is primarily a disease of the Far East, though alpha-thalassemia trait can occur in Africans. Beta-thalassemia is a disease concentrated in those ethnic groups from the Mediterranean area.

In each case, when production of one of the globin chains is reduced, there are reduced levels of hemoglobin and an imbalance in beta and alpha chain production. The red cells are hypochromic reflecting the reduced concentration of hemoglobin, and are often misshapen due to precipitated globin chains, which are removed with excess red cell membrane by the reticuloendothelial system.

The severity of the thalassemic syndromes depends on the degree of reduction of either alpha or beta chain production. In the case of alpha-thalassemia, the deletion of one or two of the four genes results in microcytosis, but not in substantial anemia. Mutations in three of the four alpha genes leads to severe anemia. Total absence of the four alpha globin genes usually results in fetal or neonatal death.

The mutations that occur in the beta genes are variable, some leading to no beta chain production (β^o) or a reduced beta chain production (β^+). Beta-thalassemia can range from mild, when only one beta chain is affected, resulting in microcytosis but no significant anemia, to very severe, when both beta genes are affected and produce little beta globin (thalassemia major, or Cooley's anemia).

The clinical manifestations of the severe thalassemias relate to the significant degree of anemia. Thalassemic red cells can have a very short life span due to their low hemoglobin concentration, excess membrane, and globin chain precipitates caused by imbalanced alpha and beta chain production. Extreme erythroid hyperplasia is present in the bone marrow, causing bone marrow expansion, often pronounced in the facial bones. Transfusions are often required to correct the anemia, resulting in iron overload, and because of the severe anemia, iron is also hyperabsorbed by the small intestine. Iron overload is one of the important complications of the disease, particularly in relation to the heart, as described below. The combination of hemosiderosis of the heart, and severe anemia requiring increased cardiac output, leads to cardiac morbidity and mortality as a prime cause of illness and death in these patients.

CARDIAC ABNORMALITIES IN THALASSEMIA. Cardiac complications are the major cause of death in patients with thalassemia.[29–31] As with sickle cell disease, these events may be due in part to chronic anemia. In addition, cardiac siderosis is a frequent problem in thalassemia, unlike the situation in sickle cell anemia or many other chronic anemias.[32,33] Iron overload results from a combination of extravascular hemolysis, frequent transfusions, and an inappropriate increase in intestinal iron absorption. Consequently, heart failure and arrhythmias are the common causes of death in children with this condition.[28] Although anemia per se undoubtedly contributes to cardiomegaly, iron overload of the heart, with its attendant impairment of systolic and diastolic function, is the most likely cause of myocardial damage.[33–35]

Prior to the era of hypertransfusion and chelation therapy,[1] patients with transfusion-dependent, chronic, severe refractory thalassemia regularly manifested serious cardiac involvement, usually by the second decade of life. Although most died within months of the development of congestive heart failure, occasionally patients died suddenly, presumably secondary to an arrhythmia. Intensive treatment of heart failure and antiarrhythmic therapy do not appear to change the natural history. At postmortem examination, widespread iron deposition characteristic of hemochromatosis is found in all viscera, including the heart, which is hypertrophied and sometimes twice its normal weight; it is often a deep brown, with large quantities of iron in myocardial cells, demonstrated by staining with Prussian blue dye. The sinoatrial node is usually spared, but the AV node is frequently involved. Apparently cardiac dysfunction depends on the quantity of iron deposited in the ventricles, and it has been suggested that myocardial damage results from iron-induced release of acid hydrolases from lysosomes.[10]

Pericarditis occurs in about half of all patients with thalassemia and is often recurrent and associated with fever, precordial pain, and electrocardiographic changes characteristic of acute pericarditis (see p. 1481). Pericardial effusion is common; in rare cases, creation of a pericardial window is necessary to relieve tamponade or a recurrent effusion.

The *electrocardiogram* often shows left ventricular hypertrophy, nonspecific ST-segment and T-wave abnormalities, supraventricular or ventricular premature contractions, and first- or second-degree AV block. The His bundle electrogram may show prolongation of the P-R interval, signifying abnormal conduction through the AV node. The chest roentgenogram may show slight to moderate cardiac enlargement, and *echocardiographic* assessment may disclose increased left ventricular end-diastolic, left atrial, and aortic root dimensions as well as a thickened left ventricular wall[44] and diastolic abnormalities. At cardiac catheterization, the usual findings comprise a normal or elevated cardiac index with moderate elevations in left ventricular end-diastolic pressure and volume and end-systolic volume with a reduced ejection fraction.

There has been considerable interest in defining abnormalities of cardiac performance noninvasively in asymptomatic patients. Valdes-Cruz et al. have reported that in asymptomatic children with thalassemia major[36] the left ventricular posterior wall thinned more slowly than normal during diastole. Utilizing the relationship between ventricular fractional shortening and end-systolic pressure (see p. 430), Borow et al. identified preclinical left ventricular dysfunction (Fig. 57–4),[37,38] an approach that may be useful in the serial assessment of left ventricular contractility in response to chelation therapy.

Management. Supportive therapy consisting primarily of an adequate transfusion program (and even hypertrans-

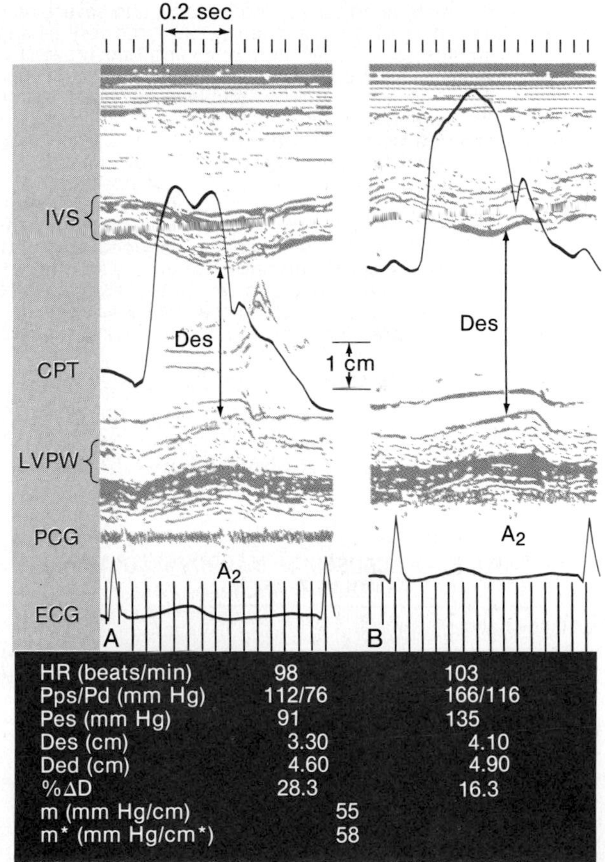

	A	B
HR (beats/min)	98	103
Pps/Pd (mm Hg)	112/76	166/116
Pes (mm Hg)	91	135
Des (cm)	3.30	4.10
Ded (cm)	4.60	4.90
%ΔD	28.3	16.3
m (mm Hg/cm)	55	
m* (mm Hg/cm*)	58	

FIGURE 57–4. Recordings from a 16-year-old patient with thalassemia major during baseline conditions *(A)* and at peak methoxamine effect *(B)*. Both the actual and corrected slope values (m and m*) were abnormal despite normal resting fractional shortening (%ΔD). The 44-mm Hg increase in end-systolic pressure (Pes) resulted in a 0.80-cm increase in end-systolic dimension (Des). For the control population, a comparable change in Pes resulted in a 0.40 ± 0.05-cm increase in Des. IVS = interventricular septum; LVPW = left ventricular posterior wall; A_2 = aortic component of the second heart sound; HR = heart rate; Pps = peak systolic pressure; Pd = aortic diastolic pressure; %ΔD = per cent fractional shortening; m = slope; m* = corrected slope. (Reproduced with permission from Borow, K. M., et al.: The left ventricular end-systolic pressure-dimensions relation in patients with thalassemia major. A new noninvasive method for assessing contractile state. Circulation *66:*980, 1982. Copyright 1982 American Heart Association.)

fusions), splenectomy, and early treatment of infections has prolonged the life of many patients with thalassemia.[1,28] Roentgenographic evidence of cardiomegaly in children often regresses when hemoglobin is maintained above 10 gm/dl. Indeed, in one study, in four of seven patients with significant cardiomegaly, heart size returned to normal 1 week after multiple transfusions restored hemoglobin to near-normal levels. The use of chelating agents for both treatment and prevention of iron overload and left ventricular systolic function is necessary and is discussed on page 1792).

HEMOLYTIC ANEMIA IN PATIENTS WITH VALVULAR HEART DISEASE. In 1964, Dameshek described an interesting patient with aortic, mitral, and tricuspid stenosis and mitral regurgitation who had hemolytic anemia with distorted and fragmented red cells, including helmet cells, burr cells, and schistocytes.[39] At autopsy, numerous calcified excrescences were present on the mitral valve and the free margins of the aortic valve. The presence of excess iron deposits in the kidney suggested intravascular hemolysis, but it could not be established whether the cardiac abnormalities were the cause. Subsequently, shortened red cell survival was demonstrated in other patients with aortic valve disease, some of whom had anemia.[40] In patients with rheumatic aortic valve disease with mild hemolytic anemia, red cell survival may be significantly reduced during periods of exercise.[44] Although this form of hemolytic anemia is probably uncommon, it should be considered in patients with valvular heart disease and unexplained anemia.

HEMOLYTIC ANEMIA AFTER CARDIAC SURGERY. The potentially serious nature of the hemolytic anemia associated with an intracardiac prosthesis was not really appreciated until chronic and severe hemolytic anemia characterized by microangiopathic red cell changes (consisting of fragmented red cells, burr cells, and schistocytes) was noted after a Teflon patch repair of an ostium primum atrial septal defect.[41] Chromium-51 red cell survival studies confirmed that the half-life of not only autologous red cells but also of donor cells was shortened, indicating a defect extrinsic to the red cell. In keeping with intravascular hemolysis, high concentrations of hemoglobin in the plasma and urine were noted along with hemosiderinuria. At reoperation a jet of blood was found regurgitating through a cleft in the mitral valve that had been impinging on the prosthetic interatrial Teflon patch. Part of the septum had become denuded of endothelium and had formed a small cul-de-sac in contact with the jet of blood. With repair of the cul-de-sac and reendothelialization of the area, hemolysis ceased. Torn cusps of porcine mitral valve or dehiscence of an implanted mitral ring can also cause the sudden onset of a hemolytic anemia.[42,43]

MICROANGIOPATHIC HEMOLYTIC ANEMIA. This condition has now been reported in association with many cardiac defects (Table 57–1). Its incidence after valve surgery depends on many variables, including the specific operation, the surgical technique, and the tests used to determine hemolysis, and varies widely. In many instances, diurnal variations occur, with greater intravascular hemolysis during physical activity.[44]

Clinical Presentation. With newer surgical techniques and prosthetic valves, the incidence of microangiopathic hemolytic anemia appears to be declining.[45] Symptoms and signs may develop suddenly or gradually, usually with no associated splenomegaly. Rarely, a vicious circle develops in a patient with a perivalvular leak: the resultant shear stress produces hemolytic anemia, increasing stroke volume and shear stress, and in turn intensifying the anemia. While it is agreed that direct mechanical trauma to the red cells is the cause of hemolysis, the relative contributions of valve closure, denuded endothelium, turbulence, and the development of antierythrocyte autoantibodies are still not clear and probably vary among patients. In some instances, the hemolytic anemia observed in the early postoperative period is probably due simply to multiple intraoperative transfusions or to the lymphocyte-splenomegaly syndrome (post–pump-oxygenator syndrome) associated with cytomegaloviral infection.

Excessive blood turbulence is the most common feature of all hemolytic anemias associated with valvular disease and cardiac surgery. For example, after insertion of a prosthetic valve, perivalvular regurgitation will increase the stroke volume and therefore the turbulence of flow through the narrowed orifice.

Definitive treatment of the hemolytic syndrome secondary to turbulence consists of surgical repair of the cardiac abnormality, i.e., either replacement or correction of the prosthesis or correction of the perivalvular leak. If a patient is not readily operable, rest should alleviate the condition, and iron and folate replacement may be helpful.

TABLE 57–1 CAUSES OF MACROVASCULAR HEMOLYTIC ANEMIA

A. Without Surgery
  1. Aortic stenosis
  2. Ruptured sinus of Valsalva
  3. Ruptured chordae tendineae
  4. Coarctation of aorta
  5. Aortic aneurysm

B. Following Surgery
  1. "Patching" operations
    a. Ostium primum repair, especially if mitral regurgitation present
    b. Aortic aneurysm repair (aortofemoral bypass)
    c. Hemodialysis shunt
  2. Valvular replacement
    a. Uncomplicated
      (1) Outflow too small
      (2) Large area of exposed plastic
      (3) Cloth-covered struts
      (4) Two or more valves replaced
      (5) Xenograft
    b. Complicated
      (1) Ball variance
      (2) Regurgitation around seating of valve
      (3) Rupture of cloth-covered strut

From Erslev, A. J.: Traumatic cardiac hemolytic anemia. *In* Williams, W. J., et al. (eds.): Hematology. 4th ed. New York, McGraw-Hill Book Co., 1990, p. 656.

HEMOCHROMATOSIS AND HEMOSIDEROSIS

(See also p. 1430)

Normal iron homeostasis is carefully protected by the body, in both its absorption and its storage. Iron deficiency can cause anemia, and a number of important enzymes utilize iron as a cofactor. Excess iron is stored in tissues in ferritin. The liver, heart, pancreas, brain, skin, and other tissues become iron overloaded when body iron stores are very high, and excess iron in these tissues is a highly toxic state that can lead to local cellular damage.

Iron overload occurs either as a result of an inappropriate excess iron absorption, as in the case of primary hemochromatosis, or due to multiple transfusions. In some cases of chronic anemia, such as thalassemia, there is intestinal hyperabsorption of iron related to the chronic anemia. Some of the more common conditions leading to hemochromatosis are shown in Table 57–2.

NONCARDIAC MANIFESTATIONS OF IRON OVERLOAD. In the iron overload state iron is stored as ferritin in many body organs including the skin, liver, pancreas, brain, and heart (Fig. 57–5). Cellular damage results from release of lysoso-

TABLE 57–2 CAUSES OF IRON OVERLOAD

PRIMARY
  A. Primary hemochromatosis–genetically transmitted
    1. Men affected more severely than women
    2. Alcohol increases iron absorption and worsens disease

SECONDARY
  A. Transfusion-related with intestinal hyperabsorption
    1. Thalassemias, alpha and beta
  B. Transfusion related without intestinal hyperabsorption
    1. Aplastic anemia
    2. Pure red cell aplasia
    3. Refractory anemia (myelodysplastic syndrome)

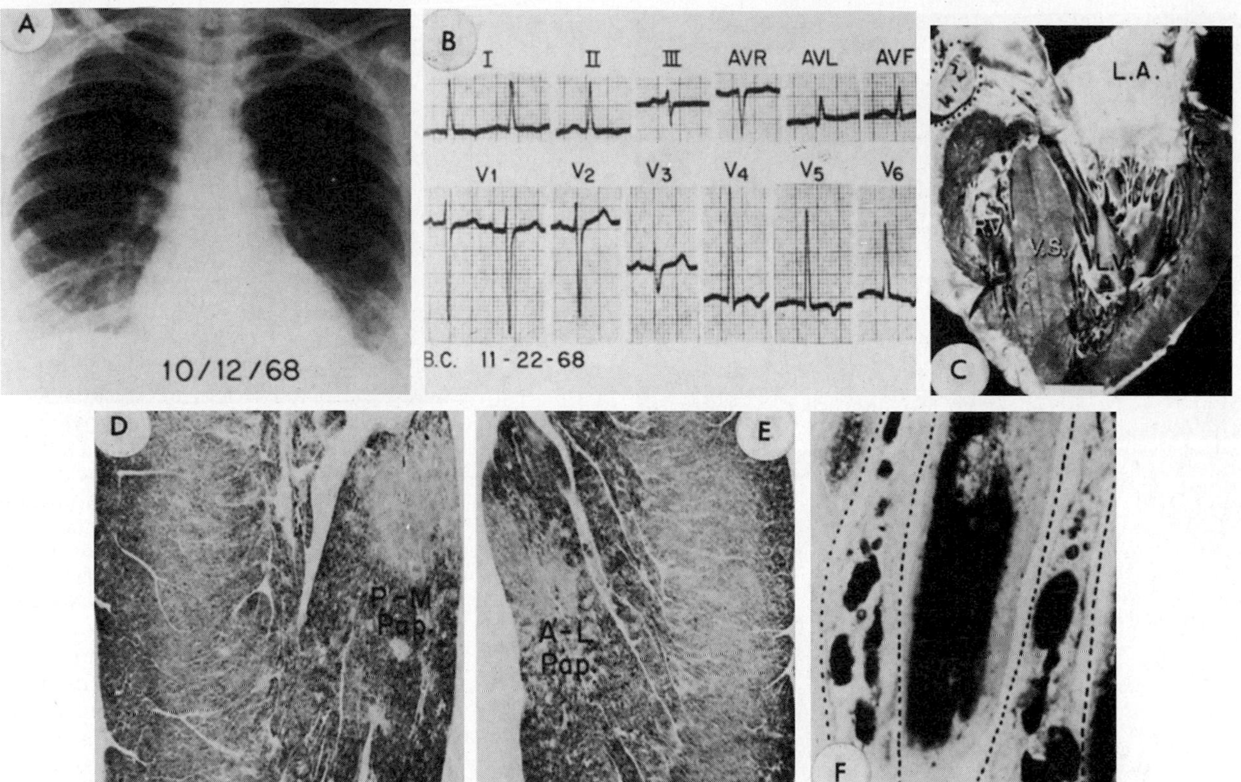

FIGURE 57–5. Observations in a 42-year-old woman with sickle cell anemia who developed congestive heart failure after cumulative transfusions of 260 units of blood. By the time of death, she had received a total of 359 units of blood (90 gm iron). *A,* Chest roentgenogram 2 weeks prior to death, showing cardiomegaly. *B,* Ischemic ST-segment and T-wave changes can be seen on the electrocardiogram. *C,* At autopsy the walls of the right (R.V.) and left (L.V.) ventricles and left atrium (L.A.) and the atrial and ventricular (V.S.) septa were rusty brown, owing to extensive iron deposits. The right atrial wall (partially enclosed by dotted line), in contrast, was tan; only minute particles of iron were present on microscopic examination. *D* and *E,* Large areas of replacement fibrosis (pale areas) were present in both left ventricular papillary muscles. *F,* Severely degenerated myocardial fibers (enclosed by dotted lines) that also contained iron deposits were often found adjacent to viable myocardial fibers. (Prussian blue stains.) (From Buja, L. M., and Roberts, W. C.: Iron in the heart. Am. J. Med. *51*:209, 1971.)

mal acid hydrolases.[46] Patients develop a "bronzed" appearance from the accumulation of iron in the skin. Liver failure due to cirrhosis ensues, and patients with hemochromatosis involving the liver are at risk for the development of malignant hepatomas. Pancreatic involvement may lead to diabetes, and pituitary involvement can lead to loss of libido and other endocrine abnormalities.

CARDIAC MANIFESTATIONS. Cardiac abnormalities develop when there is sufficiently high myocardial iron concentrations over prolonged periods of time. Cardiac manifestations are significant in about one-third of patients with hemochromatosis,[31] and about that percentage of patients with hemochromatosis die of cardiac complications. Both atrial and ventricular arrhythmias and heart block are common in these patients, presumably due to both myocardial dysfunction and iron deposition in the AV node and conduction system.[47,48] Biventricular enlargement and heart failure eventually ensue with characteristics of a restrictive cardiomyopathy.[49,50]

Cardiac manifestations of early stages of hemochromatosis can be reversed by reduction in myocardial iron content. Because body stores of iron are in equilibrium with serum iron, this is accomplished by the removal of serum iron either by phlebotomy, as in the case of primary hemochromatosis or chelation therapy, as in the case of transfusional related hemochromatosis, as discussed below. In either case, reduction in total body iron stores may result in improvement in the cardiac manifestations of hemochromatosis, making early recognition and treatment of this entity essential.[30,50–57]

DIAGNOSIS. The diagnosis of hemochromatosis is suggested by an elevated serum ferritin and increased ratio of iron to total iron binding capacity (TIBC). There are no definitive values for either of these tests that confirm the diagnosis, and the most definitive test is measurement of iron concentration in the liver by liver biopsy. Magnetic resonance imaging (MRI) scans can also be suggestive because of the "blackness" of iron laden organs as seen on these scans, but the specificity of this test is still uncertain. Some studies have shown good correlations between MRI scans of the liver, serum ferritin values, and liver biopsy iron concentrations.[58,59] MRI is also used as a diagnostic tool for cardiac involvement[60] (Fig. 57–6).

Cardiac iron deposition can be assessed by endomyocardial biopsy.[61] Although cardiac dysfunction can be evaluated on echocardiography, findings are nonspecific and similar to those of other cardiomyopathies.[62]

PRIMARY HEMOCHROMATOSIS. This is a genetic disorder of increased intestinal absorption of iron (see also p. 1674). The gene has been localized to chromosome 6, close to the HLA locus, and exhibits variable expression.[63] The disease is almost never evident before the age of 20, because children are chronically iron deficient as they grow and expand their red cell mass. Environmental factors, such as alcohol intake and dietary iron intake, affect iron absorption and therefore the severity of disease. Alcohol, which increases iron absorption, is a particularly significant risk factor for the development of hemochromatosis in persons bearing an affected gene. Women are relatively protected until menopause because of blood (and iron) loss from menses, and therefore men tend to be more severely affected and affected at younger ages.

Treatment. The iron overload state of primary hemochromatosis as well as its complications can be easily

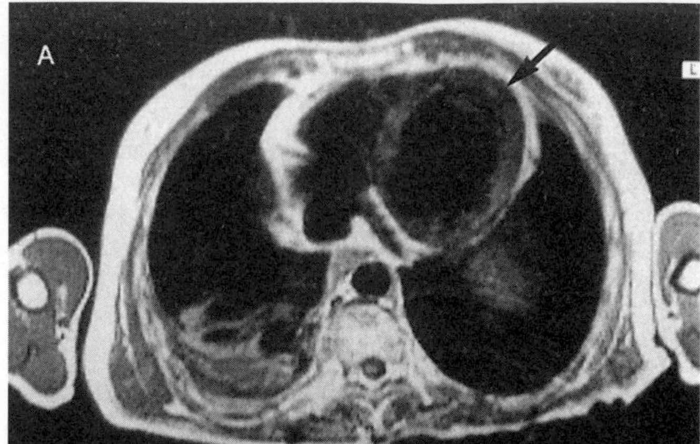

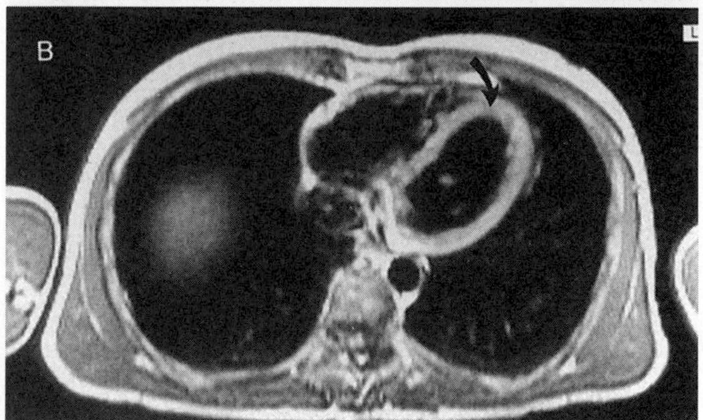

FIGURE 57–6. *A,* MRI shows signal hypointensity of left ventricular myocardium resulting from susceptibility effect (arrow) in hemochromatosis. Signal value = 280; myocardial/skeletal ratio = 0.59. Incidental right pleural effusion is visualized. *B,* MRI of healthy control shows normal signal intensity of left ventricular myocardium (arrow). (From Waxman, S., et al.: Myocardial involvement in primary hemochromatosis demonstrated by magnetic resonance imaging. Am. Heart J. *128:*1047, 1994.)

prevented by repeated phlebotomy. This is particularly true if the disease is identified early, before there is accumulation of high levels of iron in tissues. Even if early organ damage is present, iron unloading by phlebotomy can result in improved organ function. Because red blood cell production is intact, the patient replaces those red cells removed by phlebotomy. Each unit removed results in the loss of approximately 200 to 250 mg of iron. Phlebotomy is performed as frequently as required to maintain the body stores of iron in a normal range, which can be assessed by serum ferritin levels.

SECONDARY OR TRANSFUSION-RELATED HEMOCHROMATOSIS. Patients with severe anemia that is caused by poor red cell production and increased destruction, such as in the thalassemias or in bone marrow failure states such as aplastic anemia or refractory anemia, require frequent red cell transfusions to maintain the hematocrit in a reasonable range. Even with transfusion they tend to remain significantly anemic, and this, in combination with iron overload and its resultant cardiomyopathy, can cause life-threatening cardiac failure.

Each unit of transfused red blood cells contains 200 to 250 mg of iron, and between 50 and 100 units of red cells lead to a severe iron overload state and progressive impairment of left ventricular function (Fig. 57–7). Because these patients have defective red cell production and require red cell transfusions to remain compensated from the hemodynamic point of view, phlebotomy is not an option for treatment. Chronic iron chelation with the parenteral drug desferrioxamine can remove modest amounts of iron; this treatment must be initiated early in the disease to prevent organ damage.[30,31,54,56–58] Because this method of iron re-

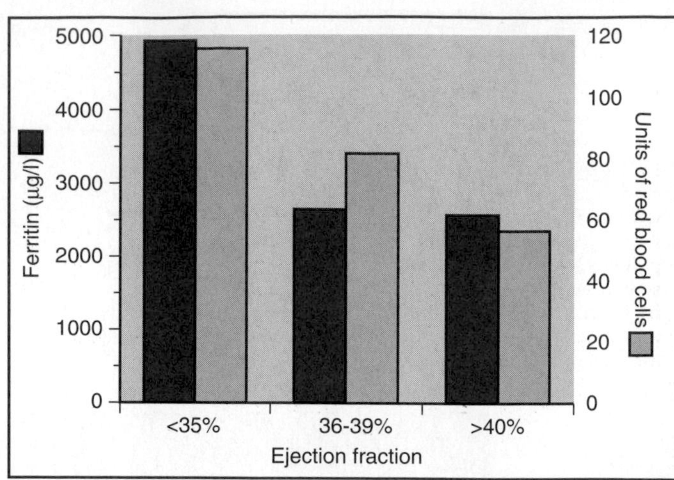

FIGURE 57–7. Correlation of cardiac ejection fraction with serum ferritin and number of transfusions in patients with iron overload. (From Bridges, K. R., and Seligman, P. A.: Disorders of iron metabolism. *In* Handin, R. I., et al. [eds.]: Blood: Principles and Practice of Hematology. Philadelphia, Lippincott-Raven, 1995, pp. 1433–1472.)

moval is inefficient, it is difficult to remove sufficient amounts of iron if it is begun when iron overload is extreme. Ascorbic acid may enhance the removal of iron by desferrioxamine; the latter must be administered parenterally and over extended periods of time (8- to 15-hour infusions) on a regular basis (3 to 7 times/week) to chelate sufficient iron, which makes this therapy a burden for the patient. On the other hand, it provides life-saving relief from the effects of iron overload, as shown in Figure 57–8. Oral chelators are currently under trial in Europe but are not available in the United States.[59]

DISORDERS ASSOCIATED WITH INCREASED BLOOD VISCOSITY

As discussed on p. 1786, delivery of oxygen to an organ or tissue is directly proportional to blood flow, hemoglobin concentration, and the difference in oxygen saturation between arterial and venous blood (Fig. 57–2). In anemic patients, an increase in blood flow, due in part to reduced blood viscosity, and enhanced oxygen delivery through elevated levels of red cell 2,3-DPG compensate for the reduced hemoglobin levels. In contrast, conditions associated with increased viscosity cause an increase in resistance to flow and a reduction in blood flow. Disorders with increased viscosity and abnormal blood rheology include the erythrocytoses, such as polycythemia vera, and disease states associated with hypergammaglobulinemia, such as multiple myeloma and cryoglobulinemia.

Polycythemia

Polycythemia is characterized by an increase in red cells, as determined by hematocrit, hemoglobin, and/or red blood cell count.[64] However, the terms *polycythemia* and its synonym *erythrocytosis* do not refer to a specific disease entity but to a variety of conditions. *Absolute* polycythemias refer to conditions in which there is an absolute increase in red cell mass (as measured by ^{51}Cr labeling or other dilution techniques). The absolute erythrocytoses are subclassified as primary or secondary, depending whether the elevation in red cell mass is autonomous (primary) or under hormonal (erythropoietin) control. *Primary* polycythemia, i.e., polycythemia vera, is part of the spectrum of myeloproliferative disorders. *Secondary* polycythemia is further classified into those disorders which cause an appropriate increase in erythropoietin secretion (e.g., disorders associated with hypoxemia, such as cyanotic forms of congenital heart

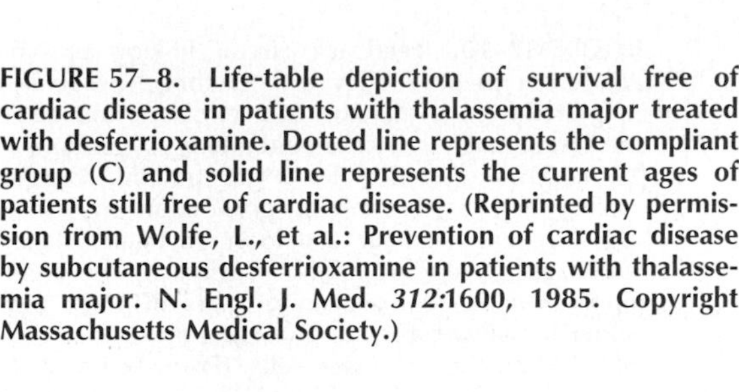

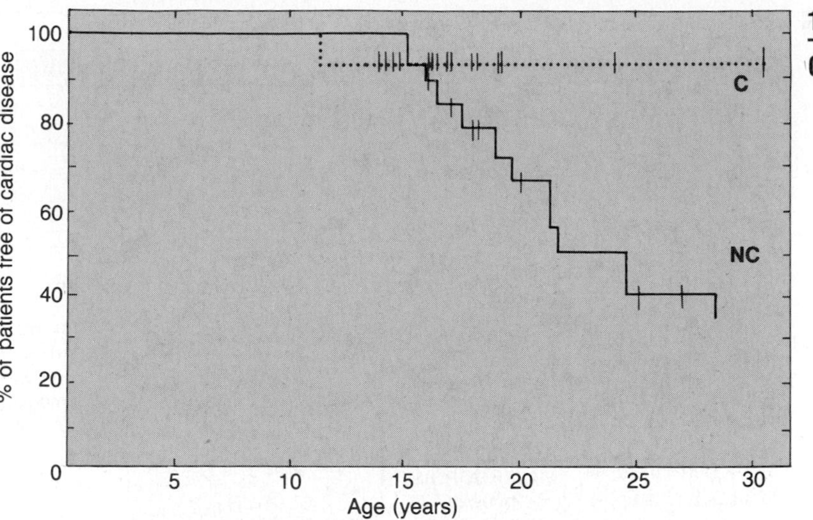

FIGURE 57–8. Life-table depiction of survival free of cardiac disease in patients with thalassemia major treated with desferrioxamine. Dotted line represents the compliant group (C) and solid line represents the current ages of patients still free of cardiac disease. (Reprinted by permission from Wolfe, L., et al.: Prevention of cardiac disease by subcutaneous desferrioxamine in patients with thalassemia major. N. Engl. J. Med. *312:*1600, 1985. Copyright Massachusetts Medical Society.)

disease and pulmonary disease) and those which cause an inappropriate increase in erythropoietin production, as occurs with tumors and a variety of renal diseases. In the *relative* polycythemias, red cell mass is normal but plasma volume is decreased, causing hematocrit, hemoglobin, and red cell values to be elevated.

Although the symptoms of polycythemia depend on the underlying disease state, they are also usually a consequence of increased blood volume and viscosity; the latter increases exponentially with increased hematocrit.[1] When flow rate through a capillary tube is determined at various levels of hematocrit, flow decreases as an essentially linear function of hematocrit (Fig. 57–9). The product of flow rate and arterial oxygen content provides a relative measure of the rate of oxygen transport through a single blood vessel; optimal hematocrit is just below 40 per cent. Delivery of oxygen to the body depends on the product of total blood flow and the oxygen content of arterial blood, which tends to be high in polycythemia vera, in which blood volume, cardiac output, and arterial blood oxygen content are all increased, despite the increase in viscosity. Although the increases in oxygen content, blood volume, and cardiac output in polycythemia vera are not required for adequate tissue oxygenation, in the polycythemias secondary to hypoxemia the increases in blood oxygen content and cardiac output represent an attempt to improve oxygen delivery.

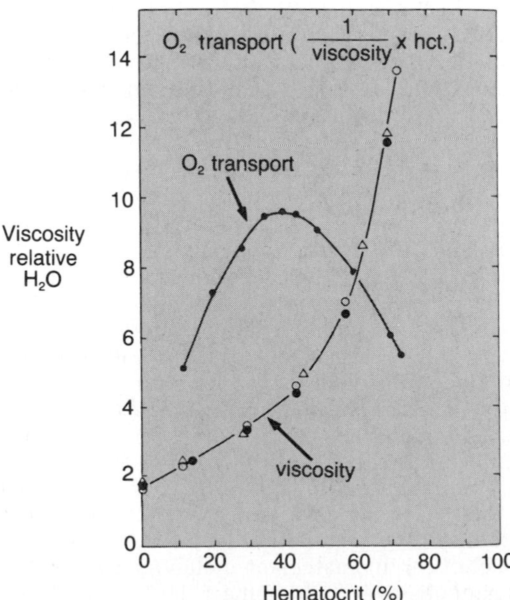

FIGURE 57–9. Viscosity of heparinized normal blood related to hematocrit. Viscosity was measured with an Ostwald viscosimeter at 37°C and expressed in relation to viscosity of water. Oxygen transport was calculated from the product of hematocrit and 1/viscosity and is recorded in arbitrary units. (From Williams, W. J. [ed.]: Hematology. 4th ed. New York, McGraw-Hill, 1990, p. 351.)

POLYCYTHEMIA VERA

Polycythemia vera is a clonal, malignant proliferation of an early hemopoietic stem cell, and is classified as a myeloproliferative disorder because increased numbers of mature cells are produced.[65] In polycythemia vera there is disregulated clonal growth not only of red cells but also of neutrophils and platelets. Splenomegaly is usually present owing to the presence of extramedullary hematopoiesis. In addition to an elevated red cell mass, leukocytosis, thrombocytosis, and elevations of the leukocyte alkaline phosphatase, LDH, and serum B_{12} are common findings in this disease.

CLINICAL MANIFESTATIONS. Patients often complain of sweats, fevers, and weight loss, hypermetabolic symptoms due to an increased bone marrow mass. In addition, pruritus—often exacerbated by hot showers—can be severe. The major symptoms and morbidity and mortality of the disease result from polycythemia and abnormal platelet function. With increased hematocrit, there is increased blood viscosity and decreased oxygen transport. Blood viscosity rises quickly as hematocrits rise above 50 per cent, and it has been shown that reduction of the hematocrit below 45 per cent results in improved blood flow, particularly in the brain.[66] Severe polycythemia can cause headache and/or confusion, plethora and dyspnea, as well as stroke.

Thrombotic and hemorrhagic events can occur as well.[66a] Thrombosis occurs due to increased viscosity and blood stasis, and hemorrhage can occur from local ischemia due to reduced or absent blood flow and vascular break down. Thrombosis and hemorrhage can still occur when the hematocrit has been reduced to normal levels because platelets in polycythemia vera are derived from the malignant clone and aggregate abnormally. They can behave unpredictably, particularly when the platelet count is high, and in some circumstances thrombosis and hemorrhage will occur simultaneously.

TREATMENT. Patients with significant polycythemia should undergo urgent phlebotomy to hematocrits of 45 per cent or less, particularly if symptoms or signs of polycythemia are present. In addition, treatment with antiproliferative agents such as hydroxyurea reduces the platelet count and red blood cell production, decreasing the need for phlebotomy. More importantly, it has been shown that treatment with agents such as hydroxyurea also significantly reduce the risk of thrombosis and hemorrhage.[67] However, some of these agents, such as chlorambucil and radioactive phosphorus, can also cause polycythemia vera to undergo a leukemic transformation. It is not certain whether hydroxyurea increases the likelihood of conversion to acute leukemia. Nonetheless, in cases of advanced polycythemia vera patients should rapidly undergo phlebotomy to an hematocrit level of under 45 per cent, and many physicians would recommend simultaneous treatment with hydroxyurea.

SECONDARY POLYCYTHEMIAS

The secondary polycythemias may be divided into two subgroups: (1) those in which the increased red cell mass compensates for a reduction in oxygen transport with appropriate stimulation by erythropoietin and (2) those in which erythrocytosis is associated with an inappropriate increase in erythropoietin production. It has been suggested that any hypoxic stimulus will cause production of the enzyme erythrogenin in the kidney, which generates erythropoietin by acting enzymatically on a proposed plasma protein substrate, possibly of hepatic origin (Fig. 57–10). If an individual living at sea level is transported to a high altitude, hemoglobin concentrations will rise[68]

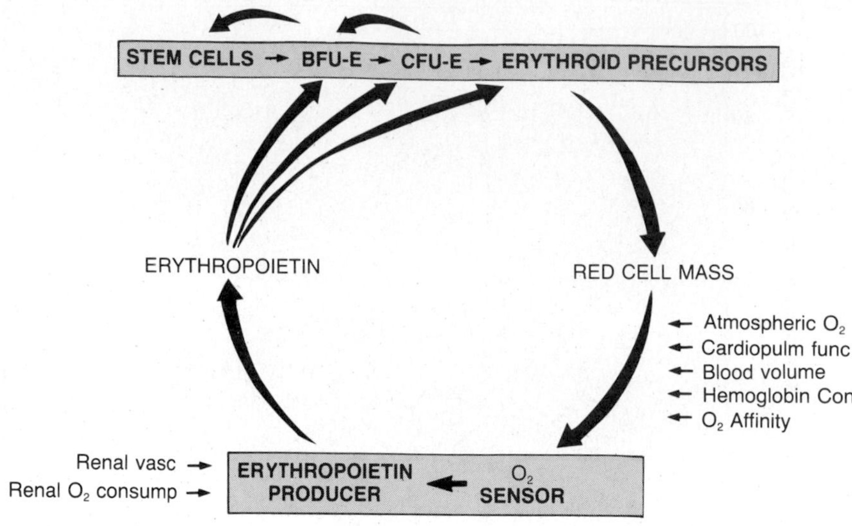

FIGURE 57–10. Feedback circuit linking an oxygen sensor in the kidney with erythroid progenitor cells in the bone marrow. The circuit is moved in one direction by red cells containing oxygen and in the opposite direction by erythropoietin. Oxygen sensing and erythropoietin production may also take place in the liver and in some macrophages. The target for erythropoietin is primarily the erythropoietin-dependent progenitor cells (CFU-E), with milder actions on the burst-forming progenitor cells (BFU-E) and the precursor cells. (From Erslev, A. J.: Production of erythrocytes. *In* Williams, W. J., et al. [eds.]: Hematology. 4th ed. New York, McGraw-Hill, 1990, p. 395. © 1990 The McGraw-Hill Companies, Inc.)

accompanied by an increase in erythropoietin. Similarly, with severe degrees of chronic hypoxemia in chronic obstructive pulmonary disease, an arterial PO_2 less than 60 mm Hg usually leads to an increase in red cell mass. In cyanotic congenital heart disease, red cell mass increases as resting arterial oxygen saturation falls (see p. 891). Hematocrits as high as 86 per cent may be seen with red blood cell masses almost three times normal.[69] Although plasma volume may be diminished, total blood volume remains significantly elevated because of the striking increase in red cell mass.

CLINICAL MANIFESTATIONS. Signs and symptoms of hyperviscosity generally occur as hematocrit exceeds 60 per cent; cardiac function may be compromised because of the combination of hypervolemia and the constant volume load and augmented vascular resistance secondary to the increased viscosity of the blood. Ruddy cyanosis, headache, dizziness, roaring in the ears, thrombotic episodes, and bleeding are the major clinical findings and may be treated with phlebotomy.[65] Careful monitoring of arterial pressure, heart rate, and general condition is necessary during phlebotomy, and the acute reduction in blood volume may have to be avoided by the simultaneous administration of plasma expanders.[70] After isovolemic phlebotomy to reduce the hematocrit from the 70's to the 60's, cardiac output rises, and despite the fall in arterial oxygen content, systemic oxygen transport usually increases. These favorable changes are attributed to the reduced blood viscosity and vascular resistance. Although the erythrocytosis is a homeostatic mechanism compensating for the chronic arterial hypoxemia, greatly increased hematocrits are generally undesirable. Studies by Erslev and Caro suggest that secondary polycythemia is not necessarily a boon but could be a burden, and that secondary erythrocytosis cannot always be considered optimal for overall oxygen transport.[71] Secondary polycythemia due to cyanotic congenital heart disease has been reported to cause myocardial infarction without manifestations of coronary atherosclerosis.[72]

MANAGEMENT (see also p. 972). Phlebotomy, or preferably erythropheresis, in secondary polycythemia reduces blood viscosity, increases systemic oxygen transport without lowering peripheral oxygen consumption, and simultaneously increases effective renal plasma flow.[73] The optimal hematocrit for patients with cyanotic congenital heart disease and other chronically hypoxemic states is poorly defined and presents an interesting and perplexing dilemma. The clinical presentation of the patient must be carefully considered. Cerebral blood flow is reduced in secondary erythrocytosis as well as in polycythemia vera and improves with phlebotomy.[74] As might be expected from the decreased oxygen transport associated with right-to-left shunts, P_{50} and red cell 2,3-DPG are increased, but the relationship between decreased arterial PO_2 and the rise in P_{50} and red cell 2,3,-DPG varies greatly.[75] Successful surgical correction of the cardiac defect will result in normal saturation and obviate the adaptive mechanism, and hematocrit and blood volume will return to normal.

HEMOGLOBIN VARIANTS WITH INCREASED AFFINITY FOR OXYGEN. In 1966, it was first recognized that a hemoglobin variant with *increased* oxygen affinity could be associated with erythrocytosis.[76] These variants, which generally have amino acid substitutions at structural sites crucial to hemoglobin function and individually are quite rare, now number over 40. They are transmitted in an autosomal dominant fashion and cause a shift in the oxygen dissociation curve to the left with reduced levels of P_{50}.

RELATIVE POLYCYTHEMIA. This is a distinct and commonly encountered entity that is also referred to as *spurious polycythemia, Gaisböck syndrome,* and *stress erythrocytosis.* It is not a primary disease process and may be merely a physiological state in which the plasma volume is slightly reduced and the red cell mass is slightly increased. Hematocrit rarely exceeds 60 per cent, and other blood constituents are normal. Patients are often hypertensive, prone to thromboembolic complications,[77,78] and obese; however, these complications appear to be unrelated to the hematological changes, so that reducing the red cell mass by phlebotomy, radiation therapy, or chemotherapy is not appropriate. When present, hypertension and thromboembolic complications should be treated in the usual manner.

THROMBOCYTOSIS

Occasionally thrombocytosis value may be seen alone as a manifestation of a myeloproliferative disorder without an increased hematocrit. Essential thrombocytosis has been associated in several instances of sudden catastrophic events such as massive arterial thrombosis in the cerebral and coronary arteries, occurring even in young adults without underlying atherosclerosis.[79–82] Such complications rarely occur in the thrombocytosis secondary to nonmyeloproliferative states such as iron deficiency or postsplenectomy states unless coexistent with severe anemia.

CARDIAC MANIFESTATIONS OF NEOPLASTIC DISEASE

INCIDENCE. Primary tumors of the heart, which are discussed in Chap. 42, are rare, occurring in less than 0.1 per cent of autopsies. Here we deal with tumors metastatic to the pericardium or heart, which are far more common, ranging from 1.5 to 20.6 per cent (average 6 per cent) of autopsies on patients with malignant diseases.[83–87] The frequency with which various tumors metastasize to the heart is shown in Figure 57–11 and the frequency at which various tumors are represented among cardiac metastases are shown in Figure 57–12. Prolonged survival of cancer patients may be the reason for this higher incidence. Usually the metastases involve the pericardium and myocardium, with the valves or endocardium rarely affected, and the right side of the heart appears to be affected more frequently than the left.[88,89] Solitary metastases to the heart are rare. Although metastatic nodules in the heart are generally multiple (Fig. 57–13), they may become diffuse and lead to the manifestations of restrictive cardiomyopathy (see p. 1426). The mode of spread to the heart may be by direct extension, as occurs in lung cancer; via the hematogenous route,[90] as in malignant melanoma; or through lymphatic channels, as in lymphoma.

The most common primary tumor producing cardiac metastases is carcinoma of the lung (Fig. 57–13), with carcinoma of the breast, malignant melanoma, lymphomas, and leukemias next in order of frequency (Table 57–3). At autopsy, 15 to 35 per cent of patients dying with primary

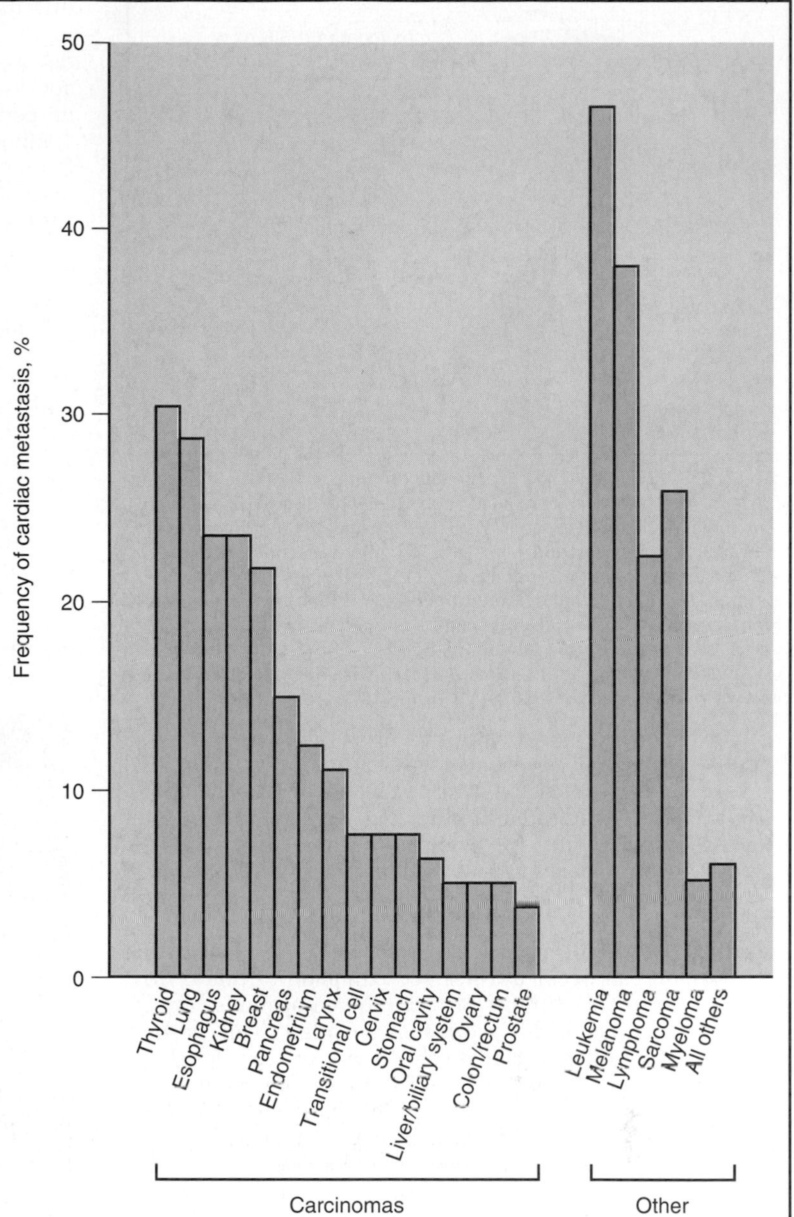

FIGURE 57–11. Frequency of metastatic tumors of the heart and pericardium found in one large autopsy series between 1950 and 1970 in one metropolitan area of the United States. (From English, J. C., et al.: Metastatic tumors of the heart. *In* Goldhaber, S. Z. [ed.]: Cardiopulmonary Diseases and Cardiac Tumors. *In* Braunwald, E. (series ed.): Atlas of Heart Diseases. Vol. 3. Philadelphia, Current Medicine, 1995, pp. 116.1–116.16. Adapted from McAllister, H. A., and Fenoglio, J. J.: Tumors of the cardiovascular system. *In* Atlas of Tumor Pathology. 2nd ed. Washington, D.C., Armed Forces Institute of Pathology, 1978, pp. 111–119.)

lung cancer show cardiac involvement, while over 60 per cent of patients with melanoma have cardiac metastases.[90] Hematological malignant tumors, especially lymphomas, have been reported to account for 15 per cent of all cardiac and pericardial metastases,[91] and about 15 per cent of patients dying of malignant lymphomas show metastases to the heart. Metastatic cardiac lesions secondary to mesothelioma and sarcoma, as well as melanoma and breast cancer, are all increasing in number.

TABLE 57–3 TUMORS ASSOCIATED WITH PERICARDIAL INVOLVEMENT

TUMORS OF THE THORAX, OFTEN WITH DIRECT EXTENSION TO PERICARDIUM
1. Lung cancer, non-small-cell and small-cell carcinoma
2. Large-cell lymphoma of the mediastinum
3. Hodgkin's disease with mediastinal involvement
4. Malignant mesothelioma
EXTRATHORACIC TUMORS MANIFESTING PERICARDIAL INVOLVEMENT—HEMATOGENOUS SPREAD OF TUMOR TO PERICARDIUM
1. Breast cancer
2. Metastatic malignant melanoma
3. Pancreatic cancer
4. Gastric cancer

Clinical Manifestations

Many metastatic cardiac lesions are clinically silent and are found only at necropsy. For example, despite massive heart involvement with melanoma ("charcoal heart"), sometimes there is surprisingly little evidence of cardiac dysfunction.[92] Specific clinical manifestations of cardiac involvement by cancer may be divided into those due to pericardial, myocardial, or endocardial involvement; cardiac compression by extracardiac tumors; indirect consequences of tumor complications of circulating mediators; embolization in patients in a hypercoagulable state; or the effects of specific tumor therapy, such as chemotherapy and radiation therapy (Table 57–4).[89] The most common clinical manifestations result from pericardial effusion with tamponade, tachyarrhythmias, AV block,[93] or congestive heart failure.[94] Metastatic cardiac disease is rarely the presenting symptom of a tumor. The mode of spread may be by direct extension, the hematogenous route, or through

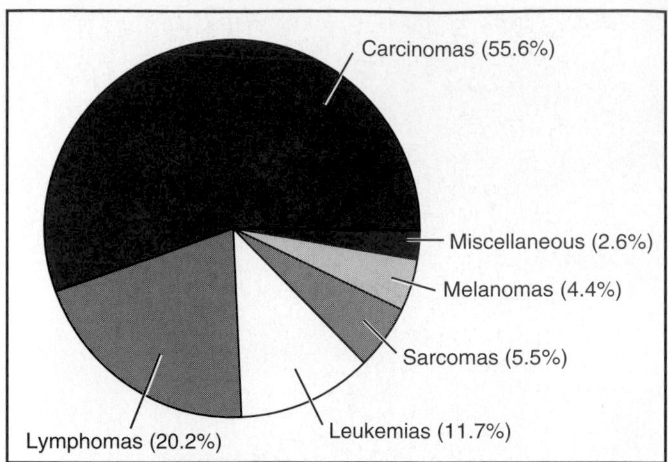

FIGURE 57–12. When the frequency of tumors that have metastasized to the heart is evaluated according to the type of tumor, carcinomas—themselves common—were clearly the most common metastases to the heart (56 per cent). Lymphomas (about 20 per cent) and leukemias (about 12 per cent) were the second and third most common types of neoplasia found during evaluation for metastasis. (From English, J. C., et al.: Metastatic tumors of the heart. *In* Goldhaber, S. Z. [ed.]: Cardiopulmonary Diseases and Cardiac Tumors. *In* Braunwald, E. (series ed.): Atlas of Heart Diseases. Vol. 3. Philadelphia, Current Medicine, 1995, pp. 116.1–116.16.)

lymphatic channels. Routine chest radiographs, computed chest tomography, magnetic resonance imaging, echocardiography, and/or radionuclide imaging with gallium or thallium are often helpful in diagnosis (Chap. 10). Osteogenic sarcoma, which may metastasize to the heart, is unique because the metastases contain bone and may be radiographically visible.[94]

PERICARDIAL INVOLVEMENT (see also p. 1514). Pericardial involvement can occur from direct extension of tumor from the lung or mediastinum, or from hematogenous spread. Involvement from direct extension is often seen in lung cancer and lymphoma (Hodgkin's disease or non-Hodgkin's lymphoma) involving the mediastinum. Hematogenous spread is frequently a complication of malignant metastatic melanoma and metastatic breast cancer. Recently, subclinical pericardial involvement may be more frequently recognized early in the course of malignancy since CT scans have become an integral part of staging evaluations for patients with systemic cancer such as lung cancer and lymphoma.

Malignant pericardial involvement can take several forms. The pericardium can be minimally involved with tumor, retaining its relative elasticity, but a large primarily reactive effusion can be present. The pericardium can be extensively involved with tumor and thickened but not adherent to the myocardium, causing both an effusion and a restrictive picture even without a large volume of pericardial fluid. The pericardium can be thickened and adherent to the myocardium, sometimes with direct infiltration of the myocardium leading to constrictive pericardial tamponade as well as myocardial dysfunction, often with little or no pericardial fluid present.

Etiology. Lung cancer and breast cancer are the most frequent causes of malignant pericardial disease.[95] Lymphomas of the mediastinum also frequently involve the pericardium, with 50 per cent of patients with large cell lymphoma of the mediastinum demonstrating pericardial involvement in one series.[96] Tumors which most frequently involve the pericardium are shown in Table 57–3.

Symptoms and Signs. Dyspnea is by far the most common symptom of patients with malignant pericardial involvement. Dyspneic symptoms may worsen dramatically with exertion because the heart cannot increase its cardiac output to meet the increased oxygen demand of exercise. Unexplained tachycardia is also a frequent sign of tamponade, and minimal exertion can substantially increase the heart rate. In the patient with dyspnea and tachycardia who has a relatively normal resting oxygen saturation, pericardial tamponade should be suspected. Cough and chest pain can also be signs of pericardial involvement with tumor. Pulsus paradoxus and paradoxical movement of the jugular venous pulse are important clinical signs of

TABLE 57–4 CLINICAL MANIFESTATIONS OF CARDIAC INVOLVEMENT IN MALIGNANT DISEASE

Manifestation
Pericardial involvement
Pericarditis
Cardiac tamponade
Superior vena caval syndrome
Arrhythmias
Supraventricular tachycardia
Carotid sinus syncope
Atrioventricular block
Cardiomegaly and congestive heart failure
Unexplained heart murmur
Unexplained hypotension
Noninfective (marantic) endocarditis

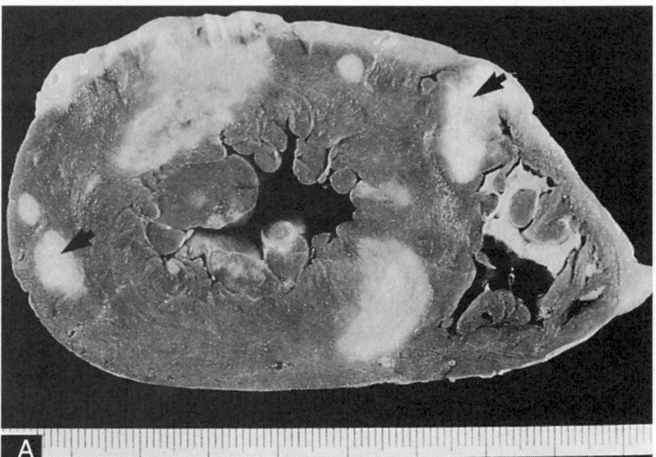

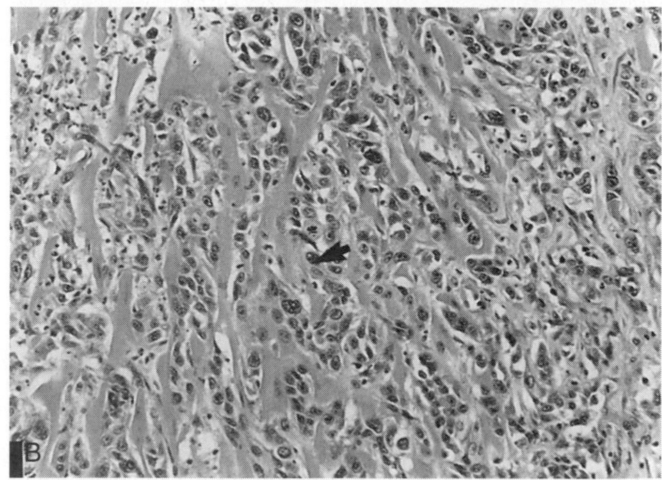

FIGURE 57–13. ***A,* Transverse section of the left and right ventricular myocardium shows extensive involvement of the myocardium by several well-circumscribed tumor nodules in a patient with carcinoma of the thyroid (arrows). *B,* Photomicrograph of a representative tumor nodule in the myocardium showing a poorly differentiated carcinoma with marked cellular pleomorphism and evident mitotic activity (arrow; hematoxylin and eosin × 100). (From English, J. C., et al.: Metastatic tumors of the heart. *In* Goldhaber, S. Z. [ed.]: Cardiopulmonary Diseases and Cardiac Tumors. *In* Braunwald, E. (series ed.): Atlas of Heart Diseases. Vol. 3. Philadelphia, Current Medicine, 1995, pp. 116.1–116.16.)**

tamponade but are not invariably present, even when tamponade is significant. The cardiac impulse is usually imperceptible. Frequently only some symptoms or signs of tamponade are present, and the clinician must have a high suspicion of tamponade in the patient with a known malignancy.[97] It is possible for the patient to be asymptomatic, without any clinical signs of tamponade until cardiac decompensation occurs.

Diagnosis. The diagnosis is almost always confirmed by echocardiography, which can demonstrate an effusion or pericardial thickening. Physiological signs of tamponade can be evaluated on echocardiography. As intrapericardial pressure rises, right atrial collapse will occur. With further increase in pressure, right ventricular collapse occurs, and this correlates well with clinically significant tamponade.[97]

Rarely, CT scans will demonstrate pericardial involvement not seen by echocardiography, although echocardiography can better delineate the functional compromise of pericardial involvement whereas CT scan cannot.[98] CT scans are particularly helpful in cases of pericardial thickening and constriction without effusion. Because CT scans are frequently used as staging procedures for many malignancies, they are often the first test to suggest pericardial involvement (Fig. 10–41, p. 341).

In the patient with a pericardial effusion who has previously received chest radiation therapy, malignant pericardial involvement must be distinguished from radiation induced pericardial effusion. Malignant effusions tend to be larger and are more likely to cause tamponade physiology than radiation induced effusions.[99,100] Radiation induced effusions can occur any time after radiation therapy but most frequently occur within the first year, as discussed later.

Treatment. Management of malignant pericardial disease depends on the severity of the effusion, the type of tumor, and previous treatment.[101–102a] In a patient with untreated mediastinal large cell lymphoma and minimal signs of tamponade, chemotherapy usually results in rapid resolution of the effusion and signs of tamponade. Malignant pericardial disease caused by lung cancer, on the other hand, almost always requires surgical drainage. Percutaneous catheter drainage can be a temporizing procedure but rarely results in lasting relief of tamponade in patients with malignant effusions.[103,104] Thoracotomy, subxiphoid pericardiectomy, and video-assisted thoracoscopic surgical (VATS) approaches have all been successfully utilized. Subxiphoid pericardiectomy appears to be more effective and safer than anterior thoracotomy. In one nonrandomized series comparing the subxiphoid approach with anterior thoracotomy, no patients undergoing the subxiphoid approach had recurrent effusions or major complications.[105] Fifty per cent of patients undergoing anterior thoracotomy had major complications including pulmonary embolism, disseminated intravascular coagulation, acute renal failure, pneumonia, and recurrent pericardial and pleural effusions. Although this was not a randomized study, the patient groups undergoing these two procedures appeared comparable.

VATS, a more recent procedure, has been highly effective as reported in one series in which all 22 patients treated had relief of their effusions without morbidity or mortality.[106] The ability to open both the anterior and posterior pericardium may be an advantage to this procedure as well.

MYOCARDIAL METASTASES. Direct myocardial or endocardial involvement by tumor such as lung cancer, lymphoma, or melanoma may result in arrhythmias, congestive heart failure, ventricular outflow tract obstruction, and peripheral emboli.[91,107] Cardiac metastases can be detected on two-dimensional echocardiography (Figs. 57–14 and 57–15),[136] computed tomography, and magnetic resonance imaging (Fig. 10–17, p. 326).[108]

VENA CAVAL OBSTRUCTION. Tumors of the mediastinum, including lung cancer, and Hodgkin's and non-Hodgkin's lymphoma, can compress the superior vena cava resulting in obstruction, frequently leading to thrombosis of the vena cava.[109,110] Facial plethora and headache are frequent signs. Facial and arm edema occur, and collateral vessels become more prominent and numerous, as can be ascertained on examination of the anterior chest wall. Rarely is superior vena caval obstruction life-threatening, although it can result in impeded filling of the right atrium and ventricle when severe, and particularly if accompanied by inferior vena caval obstruction, which can occur from retroperitoneal, hepatic, and renal tumors. Treatment of the obstruction by radiation therapy and/or chemotherapy may or may not relieve the symptoms and signs of vena caval obstruction, depending on whether thrombosis is also present.

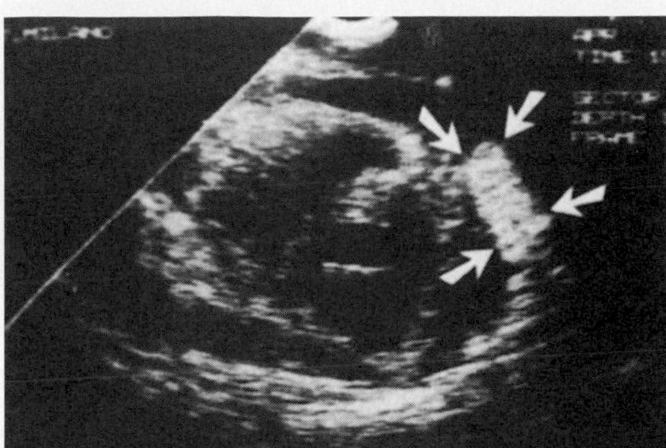

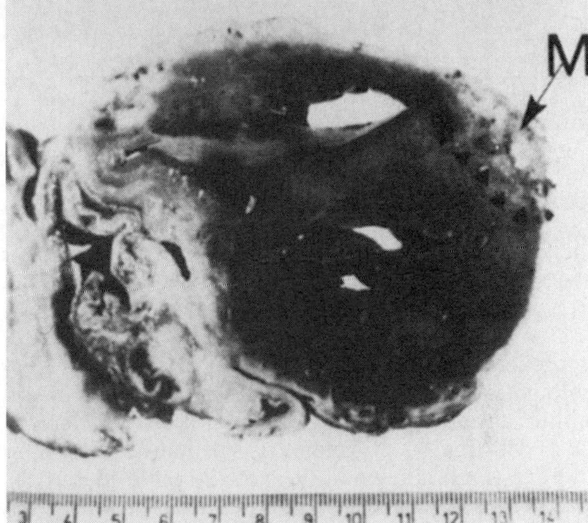

FIGURE 57–14. *Top,* Echocardiogram in parasternal short-axis view. A large echogenic mass *(arrows)* infiltrates the left lateral ventricular wall and the septum. *Bottom,* Postmortem specimen (cross section). The neoplastic mass (M) infiltrates the epicardium and the subepicardial myocardium. (From Lestuzzi, C., et al.: Secondary neoplastic infiltration of the myocardium diagnosed by two-dimensional echocardiography in seven cases with anatomic confirmation. J. Am. Coll. Cardiol. *9:*439, 1987.)

CARDIAC AMYLOIDOSIS (see also p. 1427). The heart is involved in the majority of cases of primary amyloidosis and also in many instances of amyloidosis secondary to multiple myeloma. Symptoms often include congestive heart failure, hypotension, arrhythmias, and conduction disturbances.[111,112] Echocardiographic examination, contrast tomography, and endomyocardial biopsy have made it easier to confirm this diagnosis. A low myocardial density on contrast-aided tomography, diffuse myocardial thickening, and diffuse hypokinetic wall motion may be the result of cardiac amyloidosis and may simulate hypertrophic cardiomyopathy. Endomyocardial biopsy may be necessary to confirm the diagnosis.[113]

ELECTROCARDIOGRAPHIC AND ROENTGENOGRAPHIC FINDINGS. Arrhythmias and a wide variety of electrocardiographic changes are common in patients with metastatic disease. Although they may certainly be caused by tumor involvement of the heart, they are more often due to concomitant factors, such as altered electrolyte concentrations, anemia,

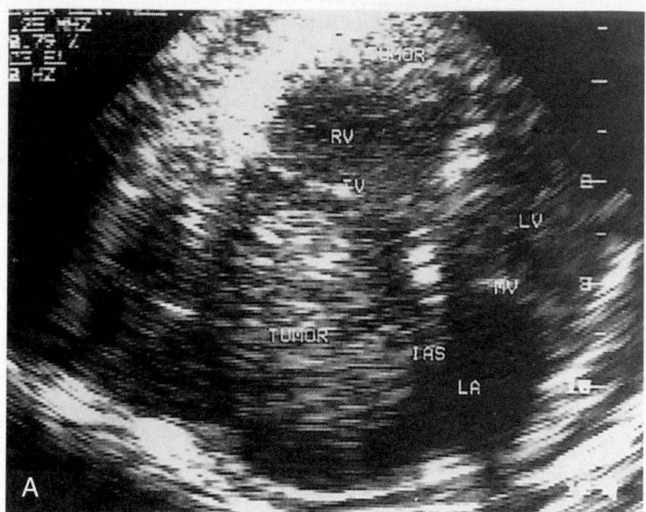

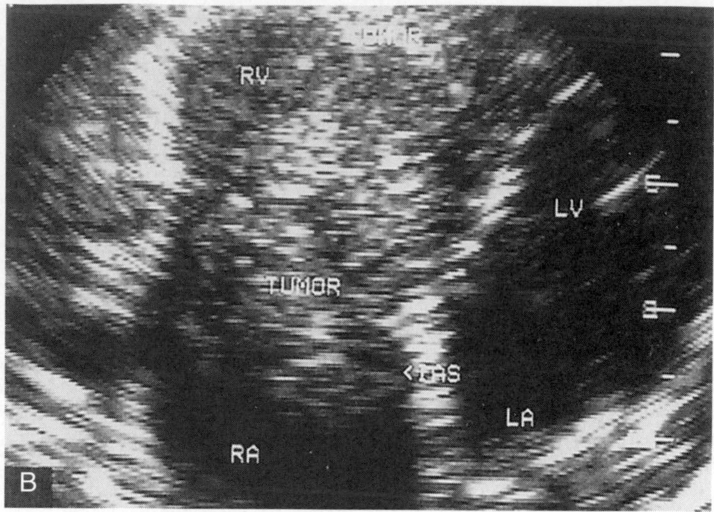

FIGURE 57–15. Echocardiograms of carcinoma that has metastasized from the cervix. *A,* The four-chamber view demonstrates that the tumor virtually fills the right atrium (RA); an attachment point on the interatrial septum (IAS) can be seen. Additional tumor mass can also be visualized in the right ventricular (RV) apex. *B,* In diastole, the atrial tumor mass prolapses through the tricuspid valve (TV) to contact the RV apical tumor mass. (From English, J. C., et al.: Metastatic tumors of the heart. *In* Goldhaber, S. Z. [ed.]: Cardiopulmonary Diseases and Cardiac Tumors. *In* Braunwald, E. (series ed.): Atlas of Heart Diseases. Vol. 3. Philadelphia, Current Medicine, 1995, pp. 116.1–116.16.)

and hypoxia. Nonspecific ST-segment and T-wave changes, low voltage, and sinus tachycardia are frequent electrocardiographic abnormalities and cannot be considered diagnostic.[114] Clinically it may be difficult to determine whether any such abnormality is attributable to cardiac metastases or is due to an associated cardiac problem, irradiation, or the cardiotoxic effects of drugs. Atrial arrhythmias, such as fibrillation and flutter, may occur secondary to either neoplastic involvement of autonomic fibers supplying the atria or tumor invasion of the coronary arteries perfusing the atria, with resulting atrial infarction, or to neoplastic infiltration of the atrial myocardium or sinus node. Similarly, electrocardiographic changes of acute myocardial infarction can be produced by tumor infiltration or hemorrhage into the ventricle or occlusion of one of the coronary arteries. Occasionally, the exact area of tumor involvement may be pinpointed based on the acute electrocardiographic changes.[115] Involvement of the AV node is a rare cause of complete heart block but may be the presenting symptom of the tumor.[116] In addition, tumor involvement of cervical lymph nodes without mediastinal involvement has been associated with carotid sinus syncope.[117]

Roentgenographic evidence of cardiac enlargement and the development of congestive heart failure may be the only clinical signs of malignant involvement of the heart. New systolic murmurs may occur with intraluminal invasion or external compression of the carotid or pulmonary arteries by the tumor. In addition to coincidental atherosclerosis, coronary artery disease in cancer patients can be caused by tumor emboli, extrinsic compression of the coronary arteries or ostia, or thromboemboli brought about by tumor-associated coagulation disorders.

If myocardial metastases are suspected from clinical or electrocardiographic data, a two-dimensional echocardiogram is often helpful diagnostically.

MYOCARDIAL INFARCTION. In a necropsy study of 816 patients with solid tumors, 33 (4 per cent) died of myocardial infarction.[118] Patients with carcinoma of the lung, malignant lymphoma, and leukemia are most commonly afflicted; less frequently affected were patients with cancer of the breast and gastrointestinal tract and malignant melanoma.[119] The etiology of coronary artery disease in patients with cancer is most frequently coincidental spontaneous atherosclerosis.[120] The most common cause of tumor-related myocardial infarction is extrinsic compression of a coronary artery, occurring in 60 per cent of cases, whereas tumor emboli are responsible for about 35 per cent.[119,121] Widespread thromboses, including coronary artery thromboses due to disseminated intravascular coagulation, occasionally occur in patients with metastatic tumors, most commonly mucin-secreting adenocarcinomas. Rarely, cardiac metastases present as acute myocardial infarction.[122] Approximately half of all patients with acute myocardial infarction secondary to malignant disease had a history of typical chest pain prior to death. An acute myocardial infarction in a patient with advanced malignant disease is a particularly poor prognostic sign, since more than two-thirds of such patients die within 3 weeks of the event.

VALVULAR EFFECTS: NONBACTERIAL THROMBOTIC ENDOCARDITIS (NBTE). Metastatic tumors may affect cardiac valves in a variety of ways, including direct invasion of valves, interference with valvular function by compression, valvular dysfunction secondary to malignant carcinoid (see p. 1434), but most commonly by NBTE.[123–125] Although the pathogenesis is unclear, this condition is associated with adenocarcinomas—especially of the pancreas and lung—as well as hematological malignant disease and lymphomas.[125] It has been suggested that immune complexes elicited by the underlying malignant process play a role in the formation of thrombi.[126] Other causes of NBTE include disseminated intravascular coagulation and non-neoplastic causes of debilitation and cachexia.[126] The fibrin matrix is attached to, but does not destroy, valve leaflets that may be normal or show degenerative changes.[123] NBTE involves principally the aortic and mitral valves equally. (The pulmonic valve may be involved in patients with catheters in place for long periods in the right heart and pulmonary artery.[127])

Patients may have clinical evidence of arterial embolization and microembolic events resembling those of infective endocarditis (see p. 1083), and changing murmurs, often without fever or leukocytosis (unless an unrelated infection is present). The most serious complications are cerebral emboli with neurological sequelae. Rarely coronary embolization may occur, causing myocardial infarction.

The diagnosis is aided immensely by two-dimensional echocardiography. Antiplatelet therapy with aspirin or anticoagulants has been employed to prevent recurrent embolization, but its effectiveness has yet to be demonstrated.

THE HYPEREOSINOPHILIC SYNDROMES WITH ENDOCARDIAL INVOLVEMENT (see also p. 1432). The hypereosinophilic syndromes are a group of diseases characterized by hypereosinophila in the peripheral blood, as well as tissue infiltration with eosinophils. The etiology of these diseases is not understood, and the course and prognosis is very variable. When severe, the bone marrow as well as other organs including the heart are infiltrated. In a series of 50 patients from the National Institutes of Health, 54 per cent had cardiac involvement, 64 per cent neurologic involvement, 56 per cent skin involvement, 40 per cent pulmonary involvement and 32 per cent hepatic involvement.[128] The NIH also prospectively followed 26 patients with hypereosinophilic syndrome and related cardiac disease and found that 42 per cent of patients complained of dyspnea and 27 per cent of chest pain.[129] Thirty-five per cent of patients developed cardiomegaly and 38 per cent developed signs of congestive heart failure. Echocardiography demonstrated cardiomegaly with increased left ventricular wall thickness and signs of restrictive cardiomyopathy. Pathologically there was endomyocardial infiltration with eosinophils and myocardial fibrosis. Left ventricular mural thrombi were also common.

CARDIAC EFFECTS OF RADIATION THERAPY AND CHEMOTHERAPY

With the advent of intensive radiation therapy and aggressive chemotherapy, cardiac toxicity of antitumor treatment has increased greatly. Formerly, the heart was considered one of the most radioresistant organs and seemed to be spared most of the side effects of chemotherapy. However, radiation can cause myocardial damage. The incidence of cardiovascular complications has risen sharply with the use of curative forms of radiation therapy for Hodgkin's disease and non-Hodgkin's lymphoma involving the mediastinum and the addition of one of the most potent classes of chemotherapeutic agents, the anthracyclines. The addition of growth factors and cytokines such as interferon and interleukin-2 to the armamentarium of the therapist has also brought on unexpected cardiac complications.

Radiation Therapy

Therapeutic radiation can cause acute and chronic cardiac damage. The pericardium, myocardium, endocardium, valves and coronary arteries can be affected by radiation (Table 57–5).[130–134] The successful treatment of Hodgkin's disease frequently using chest (mantle) radiation, and other childhood cancers successfully treated with radiation has left a large number of adults who are long-term survivors and are at risk for the development of cardiac abnormalities from radiation. It has been estimated that 15 per cent of all patients with cardiomyopathy had received treatment for cancer during childhood, and that as many of 40% of those patients treated with mediastinal radiation have some demonstrable cardiac abnormality.[135]

TABLE 57–5 CLASSIFICATION OF RADIATION-RELATED CARDIAC DISEASE

1. Acute pericarditis (caused by necrosis of tumor adjacent to the heart)
2. Delayed pericarditis
   a. Acute radiation-induced pericarditis, without effusion
   b. Acute radiation-induced pericarditis, without effusion, with/without cardiac tamponade
   c. Chronic effusive pericarditis
   d. Effusive constrictive pericarditis
   e. Chronic pericardial constriction
   f. Occult constrictive pericarditis
3. Myocardial fibrosis
4. Occlusive coronary artery disease
5. Conduction abnormalities
6. Valvular regurgitation or stenosis

Radiation can cause cardiac damage by two mechanisms: (1) It can produce direct cellular damage, resulting in a loss of myocardial tissue; (2) it can also cause endothelial damage, which can lead to microvascular changes resulting in ischemia, secondary cellular loss and progressive fibrosis.

PERICARDIAL EFFECTS (see also p. 1516). Acute and delayed pericarditis can occur in association with radiation therapy. Of 635 patients below the age of 21 years treated at Stanford University, 19 per cent had cardiac events, including 12 patients with fatal events and 106 with non-fatal cardiac events.[136] Eight patients developed acute pericarditis during radiation therapy and 30 patients developed pericardial disease 3 months to 18 years (mean 6 years) after treatment for an incidence of pericardial disease of 6 per cent. Twelve patients required pericardiectomy for symptomatic tamponade. The finding that pericardial effusion can occur very late after radiation therapy has been confirmed by others.

In a group of 49 patients treated for Hodgkin's disease studied with pulsed Doppler echocardiography, 39 per cent had pericardial thickening, although none had demonstrable effusions.[137] This suggests that pericardial damage is common after mediastinal radiation, but in only a minority of patients does it become clinically significant.

MYOCARDIAL, VASCULAR AND VALVULAR EFFECTS OF RADIATION. Radiation therapy can have profound effects on the heart leading to microvascular cardiomyopathy, coronary artery disease and valvular disease. Accelerated coronary artery narrowing unassociated with atherosclerotic plaque and composed of intima fibrous thickening and adventitial scarring suggests that radiation damage causes vascular lesions sufficient to result in myocardial infarction and sudden death.[130, 131, 138–142] In young patients examined at autopsy, proximal portions of the coronary arteries are more severely narrowed than distal portions.[139] It is possible that this is due to the design of mediastinal radiation ports that often extend over the base of the heart and the origins of the coronary arteries, but not lower.

Children appear to be particularly sensitive to the effects of irradiation. Stanford reported follow-up of 635 children below the age of 21 years treated for Hodgkin's disease and found the relative risk of death from acute myocardial infarction to be 41.5 (95 per cent) CI 18.1–82.1).[136] For males it was 35.6 (95 per cent CI 13.0–79.1) and for females 70.4 (95 per cent CI 11.7–23.3). The absolute risk was 10.4 excess cases per 10,000 patient-years.

Cardiac effects can also be seen in children irradiated for diseases other than Hodgkin's disease. In a group of children between the ages of 2 and 12 years receiving spinal radiation that included the heart, 75 per cent had maximal cardiac indices below the fifth percentile.[143]

Adults appear less sensitive to the effects of cardiac irradiation, but those who receive mediastinal irradiation do have a significantly increased risk of both acute myocardial infarction and sudden death. In a series of 4665 patients from several centers the relative risk of acute myocardial infarction was 4.09 (95 per cent CI 1.54–10.89).[144] Age at time of radiation, sex, interval between radiation and cardiac event, and standard cardiac risk factors such as smoking and hypertension did not significantly alter the relative risk in these patients.

Using pulsed Doppler echocardiography on patients treated for Hodgkin's disease, reduced ejection fraction can be demonstrated in 14 per cent of patients in one series, as well as valvular thickening in 42 per cent.[137]

Chemotherapy

Since the late 1960's there have been major advances in the management of a variety of neoplastic disorders using combination chemotherapy. Therapies have become more intensive and new agents have been introduced, resulting in significant responses and longer survival. Unfortunately, concomitant with this increased response rate has been an increase in toxicity. Although most complications due to drugs are limited to rapidly proliferating tissues such as the bone marrow and gastrointestinal tract, cardiotoxicity, both early and late, has been recognized with increasing frequency (Table 57–6).[145–149,149a]

For many years, the only notable cardiopulmonary complications of chemotherapy for neoplastic disease were orthostatic hypotension and the rare myocardial infarctions that occurred in the course of therapy with vincristine, a periwinkle alkaloid, and the interstitial lung disease and mild pulmonary hypertension secondary to pulmonary fibrosis created by bleomycin or busulfan. However, with the use of higher doses of conventional therapy for curative intent and the addition of the anthracycline group of drugs (doxorubicin, daunorubicin), the incidence of cardiac toxicity as a consequence of chemotherapy for neoplastic disease has increased greatly.

Anthracycline Cardiotoxicity

The anthracyclines (doxorubicin, daunorubicin, and idarubicin) and the anthracenedione mitoxantrone have become important and widely used agents in the treatment of cancer. These drugs are crucial in the treatment of the acute leukemias, Hodgkin's and non-Hodgkin's lymphoma, and breast cancer, all of which can occur in young people and can be cured. The importance of these agents in cancer therapy cannot be overstated, and not only are they being used with increasing frequency but they are being given in higher dosages in an attempt to improve treatment results.

These agents intercalate into DNA, therefore interfering with both DNA and RNA polymerase activity. They must be administered intravenously and are metabolized in the liver.

MECHANISM OF TOXICITY. The exact mechanism of anthracycline-induced myocardial cell injury is not known, but it may relate to the production of free radicals, reactive oxygen species leading to speculation that free-radical scavengers such as vitamin E and the bispiperazine ICRF-187 might be protective of this toxicity, although this remains controversial.[150] Anthracyclines may also interfere with the sarcolemmal sodium-potassium pump and may hinder the mitochondrial electron-transport chain. This may explain the propensity for myocardial toxicity from the anthracyclines because the heart is a mitochondrial-rich organ and also may be poorly suited to combat oxidative damage by free radicals because its peroxide-reducing potential resides solely in the glutathione-glutathione peroxidase cycle.[150,151]

TABLE 57–6 MAJOR CARDIOVASCULAR COMPLICATIONS OF CHEMOTHERAPEUTIC AGENTS

AGENT	CARDIAC TOXICITY
Amsacrine	Arrhythmia, cardiomyopathy
Busulfan	Pulmonary fibrosis
	Pulmonary hypertension
	Endocardial fibrosis
Cisplatin	ECG changes, vaso-occlusion
Cyclophosphamide	Cardiac necrosis, cardiomyopathy
Cytosine arabinoside	Congestive heart failure
	Pericarditis
Diethylstilbestrol	Cardiovascular deaths
Doxorubicin	ECG changes, cardiomyopathy
Etoposide	Myocardial infarction
5-Fluorouracil	Vaso-occlusion, myocarditis
Methotrexate	ECG changes
Mitomycin	Myocardial damage
Mitoxantrone	Cardiomyopathy
Vincristine	Hypotension

On pathological analysis of the myocardium after exposure to anthracyclines myocytes are partially or totally devoid of myofibrillar content.[152] Swelling of the sarcoplasmic reticulum can lead to their coalescence into vacuoles. These findings are shown in Figure 57–16. With more severe injury there is mitochondrial and nuclear degeneration. Several grading systems have been devised to classify the severity of injury, and one is shown in Table 57–7.

Acute injury can be demonstrated on endomyocardial biopsy after a single injection of doxorubicin.[153] Increased nuclear chromatin clumping and abnormal nucleoli with fewer fibrillar centers and less evident nucleolonema were most evident four hours after drug administration, and many of these abnormalities resolved by 24 hours suggesting cellular repair. With additional exposure to doxorubicin these changes may become irreversible.

CLINICAL ASPECTS OF TOXICITY. With very high single

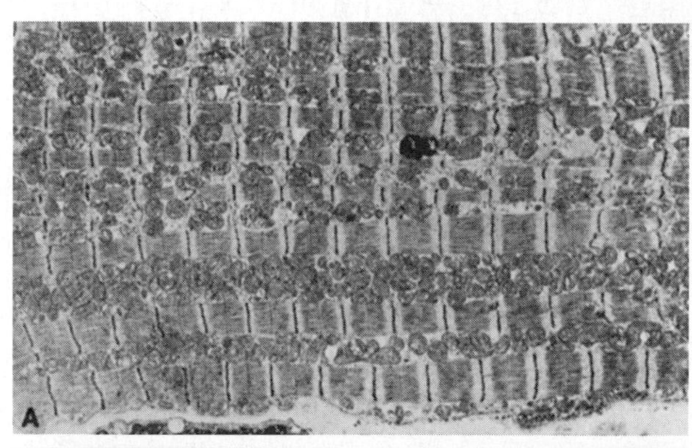

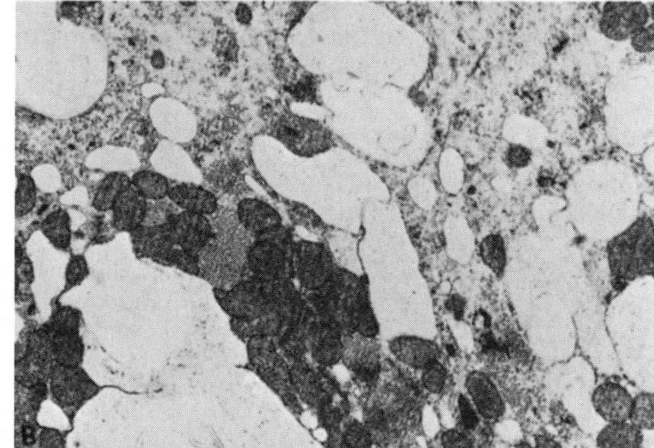

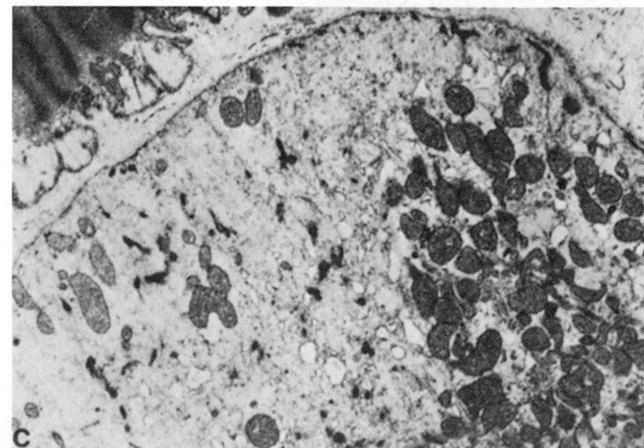

FIGURE 57–16. Electron microscopic images of cardiac biopsy specimens. *A,* Normal cardiac muscle fiber (grade O). *B,* Vacuolation. *C,* Myofibrillar dropout (× 3,575). *B* and *C* follow doxorubicin treatment. (From Ali, M. D., and Ewer, M. S.: Cancer and the Cardiopulmonary System. New York, Raven Press, 1984, pp. 62 and 63.)

TABLE 57–7 SEMIQUANTITATIVE SCALE OF BIOPSY-DETERMINED ANTHRACYCLINE MYOCARDIAL DAMAGE

BIOPSY GRADE	HISTOPATHOLOGICAL FEATURES
0	No detectable change from normal
1	Scant number of cells (≤5%) showing distended sarcoplasmic reticulum and/or early myofibrillar loss
1.5	Small numbers of cells (5 to 15%), some showing definite cytoplasmic vacuolization and/or myofibrillar loss
2	Groups of cells (16 to 25%), some showing definite cytoplasmic vacuolization and/or myofibrillar loss
	Biopsy grades up to 2 carry <10% risk of heart failure with 100 mg/m² incremental dose of doxorubicin
2.5	Groups of cells (26 to 35%), some showing definite cytoplasmic vacuolization and/or marked myofibrillar loss
	Biopsy grade of 2.5 carries a 10 to 25% risk of heart failure with 100 mg/m² incremental dose of doxorubicin
3	Diffuse cell injury (>35%) showing advanced loss of organelles, total loss of myofibrils, and mitochondrial and nuclear degeneration
	Biopsy grade 3 is associated with >25% risk of heart failure if more doxorubicin is given

From Fowles, R. E.: Cardiac catheterization and endomyocardial biopsy. *In* Kapoor, A. S. (ed.): Cancer and the Heart. New York, Springer-Verlag, 1986, p. 48.

doses, there can be acute cardiac toxicity usually manifested by atrial and ventricular arrhythmias. More commonly, a cardiomyopathy results from myocyte damage as described above, leading to congestive heart failure.

Anthracycline cardiomyopathy is clearly related to total cumulative exposure to these agents, as well as acute peak levels, age at exposure, and the concurrent administration of other cardiotoxic antineoplastic agents. Factors known to be associated with the development of cardiac toxicity from these agents are shown in Table 57–8.

The most powerful predictor of anthracycline cardiotoxicity is the total cumulative dosage administered (Fig. 57–17). Clinically apparent cardiotoxicity due to doxorubicin is rare below cumulative doses of 400 mg/m², then becomes increasingly frequent with higher dosages. However, subclinical cardiac toxicity can be demonstrated by more sensitive testing, with high frequency, at much lower cumulative doses. Bristow et al. studied 33 patients receiving doxorubicin using echocardiography, cardiac catheterization, and endomyocardial biopsy.[152] Twenty-seven of 29 patients receiving greater than 272 mg/m² had endomyocardial biopsies showing myocyte damage, although one patient had biopsy-proved evidence of doxorubicin-induced damage after only 45 mg/m². Another patient had no evidence of myocyte damage on biopsy after receiving 400 mg/m². On the other hand, preejection period to left ventricular ejection time ratio (PEP/LVET) was increased only in patients who had received greater than 400 mg/m² of doxorubicin.

TABLE 57–8 RISK FACTORS FOR THE DEVELOPMENT OF ANTHRACYCLINE CARDIOTOXICITY

1. High total cumulative dose of drug administered
2. High peak serum levels of drug
3. Previous or concurrent mediastinal or heart irradiation
4. Concurrent administration of other cardiotoxic antineoplastic drugs such as high-dose cyclophosphamide
5. Age at time of exposure—very young and very old are most susceptible
6. History of cardiac disease, particularly coronary artery disease

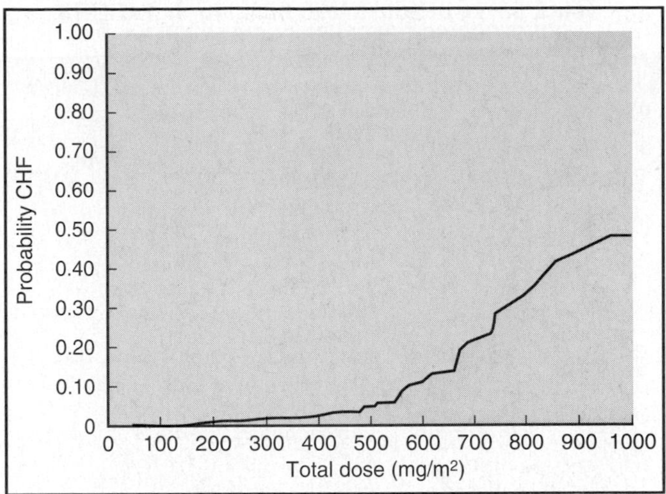

FIGURE 57–17. Cumulative probability of developing doxorubicin-induced congestive heart failure versus total cumulative dose of doxorubicin in 3941 patients of whom 88 developed congestive heart failure. (From Von Hoff, D. D., et al.: Risk factors for doxorubicin-induced congestive heart failure. Ann. Intern. Med. *91*:710, 1979.)

Gottdiener et al. studied 32 patients with radionuclide cineangiography who had been treated with between 480 and 550 mg/m² of doxorubicin for sarcomas.[154] All patients were asymptomatic, without signs of cardiomyopathy. The mean ejection fraction at rest for all patients was 49 per cent as compared with 57 per cent for normal controls. With maximal exercise, patients treated with doxorubicin had a mean ejection fraction of 52 per cent compared with 71 per cent for normal subjects, suggesting that these patients had a moderate decrease in ejection fraction after treatment with doxorubicin. The relative reduction in ejection fraction during maximal exercise suggests that the doxorubicin-treated heart is less able to keep up with increased demand than is the normal heart. In another study 18 patients were examined by radionucleotide angiography before and after treatment with 500 mg/m² of doxorubicin.[155] Pretreatment ejection fractions averaged 60.4 per cent and post-treatment ejection fractions averaged 49.8 per cent, a difference that was highly significant. Myocardial damage was assessed using monoclonal antibodies to myosin labeled with indium 111. Abnormal uptake was present in all patients, but only those with high uptake were likely to have a decreased ejection fraction and/or clinically apparent congestive heart failure. This supports the hypothesis that all patients receiving doxorubicin have some evidence of myocardial damage, but in only a subset is this clinically significant.

MONITORING OF PATIENTS RECEIVING ANTHRACYCLINES. Because anthracyclines have become such an integral part of cancer chemotherapy and are often best used in high cumulative doses, considerable effort has been expended in determining criteria to evaluate those patients suitable for anthracycline therapy, particularly among patients with known heart disease and to evaluate patients during therapy to reduce the risk of developing congestive heart failure. This is important because the total cumulative dose of an anthracycline that can lead to heart failure in an individual patient is highly variable. Grading systems for severity of heart failure have been proposed, though most studies do not report their results using these recommendations. One such system is shown in Table 57–9.

Investigators at Yale reviewed records of 1487 patients undergoing chemotherapy who had serial radionuclide angiocardiograms and identified 282 patients who were thought to be at high risk for developing anthracycline-in-

TABLE 57–9 HEMODYNAMIC GRADING OF PATIENTS UNDERGOING DOXORUBICIN CHEMOTHERAPY

GRADE	HEMODYNAMIC FINDINGS
0 Normal	Mean RA < 7 mm Hg RVEDP < 8 mm Hg LVEDP/Mean PAW < 12 mm Hg Cardiac index > 2.5 L/min/m² Exercise factor > 5.0
1 Mildly abnormal	Any of the following: Mean RA = 7 to 10 mm Hg RVEDP = 8 to 12 mm Hg at rest with increase on exercise = 5 to 9 mm Hg LVEDP/Mean PAW = 12 to 15 mm Hg at rest with increase on exercise = 5 to 11 mm Hg Cardiac index = 2.2 to 2.5 L/min/m² Exercise factor = 4.0 to 5.0
2 Moderately abnormal	Any of the following: Two or more grade 1 features Mean RA = 10 to 15 mm Hg RVEDP = 12 to 17 mm Hg at rest with increase on exercise ≥ 9 mm Hg Cardiac index = 1.8 to 2.2 L/min/m² Exercise factor < 4.0
3 Severely abnormal	Any of the following: Two or more grade 2 features Mean RA ≥ 16 mm Hg RVEDP ≥19 mm Hg LVEDP/Mean PAW ≥ 20 mm Hg Cardiac index < 1.8 L/min/m²

RA = right atrium; RVEDP and LVEDP = right and left end-diastolic pressure, respectively; PAW = pulmonary artery wedge pressure. Abnormal cardiac index is accompanied by elevated AV oxygen content difference (>5 vol%). Exercise factor = increase in cardiac output (ml/min)/increase in total body oxygen consumption.

From Bristow, M. R., et al.: Efficacy and the cost of cardiac monitoring in patients receiving doxorubicin. Cancer *50*:32, 1982.

TABLE 57–10 GUIDELINES FOR ADMINISTRATION AND MONITORING OF PATIENTS RECEIVING DOXORUBICIN

1. Patients with pre-treatment LVEF ≥ 50%
   A. Repeat LVEF after 350–300 mg/m².
   B. Repeat LVEF after 400 mg/m² in patients with known heart disease, heart irradiation or cyclophosphamide therapy, or after 450 mg/m² in patients without these risk factors.
   C. Repeat LVEF measurements after each subsequent dose of doxorubicin.
   D. Discontinue doxorubicin therapy if LVEF declines by ≥10% to a value of less than 50%.
2. Patients with pre-treatment LVEF < 50%
   A. Do not administer doxorubicin at all to patients with baseline LVEF of ≤30%.
   B. In patients with LVEF of between 30 and 50%, repeat LVEF prior to each dose.
   C. Discontinue doxorubicin therapy if LVEF declines by ≥10% and/or to a value of less than 30%.

LVEF = Left ventricular ejection fraction, measured by radionuclide cardioangiography

Adapted from Schwartz, R. G., et al.: Congestive heart failure and left ventricular dysfunction complicating doxorubicin therapy: Seven-year experience using serial radionucleotide angiocardiography. Am. J. Med. *82*:1112, 1987.

duced cardiomyopathy.[156] High-risk patients were defined as those with either a decline of ≥10 per cent in absolute left ventricular ejection fraction (LVEF) from a normal baseline to an LVEF of 50 per cent or less, a total cumulative dose of doxorubicin of 450 mg/m² or more, or a pretreatment LVEF of <50 per cent. Clinically apparent heart failure occurred in 49 patients (17 per cent). The 49 patients who developed heart failure received total cumulative doses of doxorubicin of between 75 to 1,095 mg/m² as compared with those who did not develop heart failure who received doses between 30 and 880 mg/m², demonstrating that total doxorubicin dose alone is insufficient to predict the development of this complication. Pretreatment LVEF was similar in patients who developed CHF as compared with those who did not—57 and 58 per cent, respectively. Decline in LVEF during therapy was greater in those patients developing CHF than in those who did not; 23 and 12 per cent.

Guidelines for administration and monitoring of doxorubicin therapy are shown in Table 57–10. When these guidelines were applied to the cohort of 282 patients at high risk for the development of doxorubicin cardiomyopathy there was fourfold reduced risk of developing heart failure in the group treated according to these guidelines as compared with those whose management was discordant with the guidelines as shown in Figure 57–18.

OUTCOME OF PATIENTS WITH ANTHRACYCLINE CARDIOMYOPATHY. It was once thought that anthracycline cardiomyopathy was uniformly rapidly progressive and fatal for most patients.[157] Others have suggested some patients will do well with conventional heart failure management. Of 16 patients studied by Schwartz et al., 87 per cent improved with standard therapy for heart failure, whereas 11 per cent remained stable and only one patient worsened.[156] In another series, 19 patients with anthracycline-induced heart failure were evaluated and followed.[158] The mean onset from the last dose of anthracycline to the development of heart failure was 4 weeks with a range of 1 to 17 weeks. For the 7 patients who died of heart failure, the median time to death was 6 weeks with a range of 1 to 15 weeks. Sixty-three per cent of patients survived with improved symptomatology with a median follow-up of 3 years. The authors could not identify any predisposing factors which would predict fatal outcome from anthracycline-induced heart failure, although none of the patients who died had cumulative anthracycline doses of <300 mg/m², whereas 5 of 12 of the survivors were given doses below this value.

A number of case reports exist suggesting that viral illnesses or other stresses can have severe and sometimes fatal outcomes in patients with seemingly well-compensated anthracycline-induced heart failure indicate that these patients have little cardiac reserve to compensate for these stresses or that minimal additional cardiac toxicity can cause a patient with well-compensated heart failure to decompensate and die.

ANTHRACYCLINE CARDIOTOXICITY IN CHILDREN. It is now known that children are at particular risk for the late de-

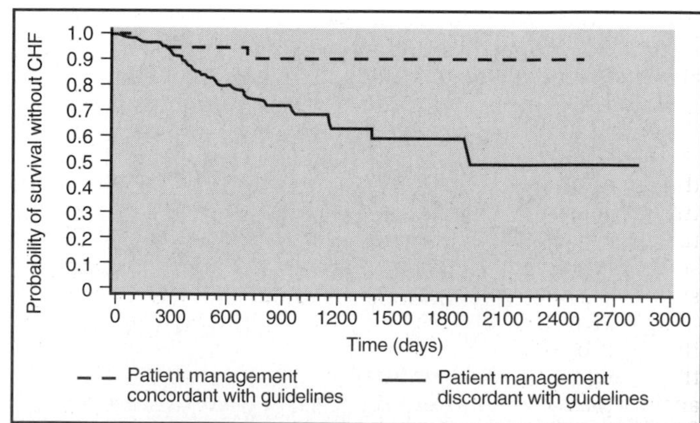

FIGURE 57–18. Kaplan-Meier plot demonstrating the probability of survival without congestive heart failure in patients whose management was either concordant or discordant with guideline criteria shown in Table 57–10. (From Schwartz, R. G., et al.: Congestive heart failure and left ventricular dysfunction complicating doxorubicin therapy: Seven-year experience using serial radionuclide angiocardiography. Am. J. Med. *82*:1109, 1987.)

velopment of cardiotoxicity from anthracyclines, and those who receive anthracyclines before the age of 4 years may be at specially high risk.[159] Eleven (10 per cent) of 115 children between the ages of 7 months and 19 years treated with doxorubicin for acute lymphoblastic leukemia developed heart failure. All patients improved with standard heart failure therapy and eventually all were able to discontinue cardiac medications. Five of the 11 patients had recurrent heart failure 3 to 10 years after the initial episode and two patients required cardiac transplantation. Similar results have been observed in another series of 30 children between the ages of 4 and 16 years treated with a mean of 317 mg/m^2 of doxorubicin.[160] Fractional shortening declined from pretreatment levels of 34.9 to 32.0 ($p < .0001$) at the conclusion of chemotherapy, although all of these children were clinically well at this time. However, seven of these patients developed late cardiac decompensation, five during an acute viral illness, raising concern about the role of viral illnesses in causing cardiac decompensation in these patients.

Among children treated with anthracyclines, females are much more sensitive to the cardiotoxic effects of this agent than males, although the reason for this is unknown. In a study of 120 patients who had received doxorubicin during childhood for either acute lymphoblastic leukemia or osteogenic sarcoma, for any given cumulative dose of doxorubicin females had a higher probability of depressed left ventricular contractility.[160a] This difference was most marked at higher cumulative doses of doxorubicin.

REDUCED ANTHRACYCLINE-INDUCED CARDIAC TOXICITY FROM LOW-DOSE OR INFUSIONAL REGIMENS. It has been suggested that either more frequent lower-dose doxorubicin schedules or continuous infusion schedules would produce less cardiotoxicity for any given cumulative dose without compromising antitumor activity.[161–166] The mechanism of reduction of cardiotoxicity for these regimens is not known, although it has been hypothesized that toxicity is related in part to peak serum levels.

Doxorubicin toxicity was compared by endomyocardial biopsy in 98 patients receiving standard doses every 3 weeks, and 27 patients receiving lower doses weekly.[164] In both groups total cumulative dose was predictive of myocardial damage on biopsy specimens, but for any given total cumulative dose, patients receiving low dose weekly doxorubicin had less damage. Another study compared doxorubicin given by standard bolus injection every 3 weeks to patients receiving infusional doxorubicin over 48 or 96 hours.[165] Patients receiving continuous infusion received higher total cumulative doses of doxorubicin than those receiving bolus administration, and for any given total cumulative dose of doxorubicin, less severe myocardial changes were seen on biopsy in the patients receiving infusional therapy. Shorter infusions, over 6 hours for instance, have not shown cardiac sparing effects.[166]

5-Fluorouracil

Vaso-occlusive complications, including acute myocardial infarction, often occur in patients with malignant tumors. There is increasing suspicion that chemotherapeutic agents such as 5-fluorouracil (5-FU)[149,167,168] may be the sole precipitating factor of this complication in a small but significant percentage of cases.

The incidence and severity of these complications, and the link to 5-FU itself has been difficult to discern because this agent is often administered in conjunction with other antineoplastic agents, and often to patients who are very ill from manifestations of their malignancy. In a recent review of 135 cases of suspected 5-FU cardiotoxicity angina and electrocardiographic changes occurred in the majority of patients and congestive heart failure occurred transiently in 33 patients.[168] The patients who developed heart failure responded well to therapy. The overall incidence of these events, and their effect on quality and duration of survival of cancer patients remains unclear since the denominator from which these 135 cases were drawn is not known.

Cyclophosphamide

As noted in Table 57–7, cardiomyopathies have been reported secondary to high doses of intravenous cyclophosphamide.[146,168–170] In contrast to doxorubicin, the cardiotoxicity of cyclophosphamide is acute and not due to cumulative doses. It causes reductions in ECG voltage and systolic function and an increase in myocardial mass, presumably secondary to edema. Cyclophosphamide may also cause acute pericarditis. A prior history of heart failure and a pretreatment ejection fraction less than 50 per cent correlate with clinical cardiotoxicity. Although mortality is appreciable, survivors exhibit no residual cardiac abnormalities.[171]

Ifosfamide, an active compound related to cyclophosphamide, may also cause cardiac side effects in the form of supraventricular arrhythmias and ST-T wave changes.[172] When administered in high doses, between 10 and 18 mg/m^2, arrhythmias and congestive heart failure are common. Of 52 consecutive patients treated at the NIH with this agent at these doses, 9 developed heart failure between 6 and 23 days after drug administration.[173] Eight required admission to an intensive care unit. One patient died of cardiogenic shock, and one had pulseless ventricular tachycardia requiring emergent cardioversion and survived. Of the eight patients who survived their heart failure, all recovered cardiac function in 1 to 2 weeks, and three patients who are long-term survivors had return of normal cardiac function.

Other Antineoplastic Agents

Ischemic coronary complications have also been reported after treatment with cisplatinum,[146,173] bleomycin,[174] and vinca alkaloids,[175] such as vincristine, vinblastine, and VP-16-213 (etoposide). Acute endothelial injury, vasospasm and/or autonomic dysfunction, hypomagnesemia, autoimmune response, increases in platelet aggregability, and a synergistic effect of irradiation to the heart are all possible mechanisms. *Amsacrine* (AMSA) has been associated with acute cardiac arrhythmias and cardiomyopathy. Although AMSA-related cardiac events are frequent, they are less common than those due to doxorubicin. Manifestations of toxicity include ECG abnormalities, sudden death, and congestive heart failure. Hypokalemia appears to be a risk factor for the development of severe arrhythmias with this agent.[176–178]

Bone marrow transplantation, either allogeneic or autologous, involves the combination of large doses of whole-body irradiation therapy with high-dose chemotherapy. Cardiac complications are frequent during these transplant procedures and may be an important factor in limiting the success rate.[179] Fatal cardiomyopathies, pericarditis, and significant arrhythmias are not infrequent. High-dose cyclophosphamide and cytosine arabinoside are commonly associated with cardiotoxicity. In addition, the effect of whole-heart irradiation in conjunction with anthracycline drugs and cyclophosphamide appears to be additive.

The glycoproteins of the interferon and interleukin family are used with increasing frequency in treating many refractory cancers. Interferon alpha is effective against hairy cell leukemia, chronic myelogenous leukemia, and condyloma acuminatum and also is approved for use in treating Kaposi's sarcoma. In high doses, interferon can cause a severe congestive cardiomyopathy with severe myocardial dysfunction, usually reversible with discontinuation of the agents.[179–182]

BIOLOGIC RESPONSE MODIFIERS. Biologic response modifiers such as interleukin-2, now FDA approved for the treatment of renal cancer, and the investigational agent interleukin-1 have become part of the oncologist's armamentarium. These agents have potent effects on the immune system, but also have significant toxicity. Both cause fever and myalgias. More importantly, both cause capillary leak syndromes that can result in tissue edema, vascular hypovolemia and hypotension, noncardiogenic pulmonary edema, myocardial infarction, and renal failure.[183–185] These effects are largely dose dependent but can, even at low doses, result in death. Aggressive fluid and pressor support is often required during periods of administration of these agents.

HEMATOLOGICAL ABNORMALITIES RELATED TO CARDIAC DRUGS

Blood dyscrasias are frequent complications of drugs used to treat cardiac disorders. The development of unexplained anemia, leukopenia, or thrombocytopenia in a patient receiving a diuretic, antihypertensive, or antiarrhythmic agent should immediately raise the suspicion that a drug used in the treatment of cardiac disease might be responsible.

Many different types of blood dyscrasias occur secondary to drug ingestion. The anemias may be of the aplastic, hemolytic, megaloblastic, or sideroblastic type; other disorders may include granulocytopenia and agranulocytosis, thrombocytopenia, thrombocytosis, defects of platelet function, and a variety of miscellaneous disorders (Table 57–11). Underlying mechanisms include suppression of one or more of the three cellular elements in the bone marrow as well as a variety of immune phenomena with increased peripheral destruction of the formal elements. The drug effect may be dose related or idiosyncratic.

APLASTIC ANEMIA. Many chemical agents are capable of suppressing marrow function and producing hypoplasia or aplasia. Chloramphenicol, benzene, cytostatic agents used in the treatment of malignant disease, and phenylbutazone are the drugs most commonly implicated. Less frequently involved, and perhaps less well documented, are antibiotics such as sulfonamides, hypoglycemic agents, and insecticides. Among drugs used to treat cardiovascular disease, the antiarrhythmic agent phenytoin (see p. 608), the diuretic agent acetazolamide, and the angiotensin-converting enzyme inhibitor captopril[186] (see p. 855) have been reported, on rare occasion, to lead to such reactions. The onset of aplastic anemia is usually insidious, and the symptoms are directly related to the degree of pancytopenia. If the causative agent is immediately discontinued upon detection of the blood dyscrasia, the latter can often be reversed.

MEGALOBLASTIC ANEMIA. A pancytopenia characterized by macrocytic red cells due to impairment of DNA synthesis may be caused by vitamin B_{12} or folate deficiency or by purine and pyrimidine inhibitors. Most commonly, drugs cause megaloblastic anemia by impairing the absorption of folic acid or acting as folate antagonists. Phenytoin, oral contraceptives, and a variety of other drugs can impair folate absorption by interfering with the liver conjugases needed to break down the polyglutamate structure of naturally occurring folates to the monoglutamate form appropriate for absorption by the gastrointestinal tract. Triamterene, a potassium-sparing diuretic (see p. 477), is a pteridine analog that exhibits antifolate activity, similar to aminopterin, in vitro. Its propensity to produce a megaloblastic anemia appears to be dose related.

IMMUNOHEMOLYTIC ANEMIAS. There are four different causes for the development of a positive direct Coombs' or antiglobulin test, two of which involve cardiac medications: the first mechanism, which is uncommon, involves some drugs that bind to plasma protein and thereby become antigenic, including quinidine and the sulfonamides. The resultant antigen-antibody complex may deposit on the red cell surface and cause agglutinability by anticomplement sera. Hemolysis may be severe, but rapid improvement follows withdrawal of the drug.

The second type of reaction that results in a positive Coombs' test involves the antihypertensive drug alpha-methyldopa[187] (see p. 852). The mechanism of antibody formation is unknown, but presumably antibody induced by alpha-methyldopa has an affinity for the Rh locus of the red cell, similar to that of IgG antibodies in idiopathic

TABLE 57–11 BLOOD DYSCRASIAS ASSOCIATED WITH CARDIAC MEDICATIONS

	ANEMIA					
	Aplastic	Megaloblastic	Hemolytic	NEUTROPENIA	THROMBOCYTOPENIA	OTHER
Antiarrhythmics						
Digitoxin	–	–	–	–	+	L
Phenytoin	+	+	–	+	+	L, P
Procainamide	–	–	–	+(A)	–	–
Propranolol	–	–	–	+	–	–
Quinidine	–	–	+	+	+	–
Tocainide	+	–	–	+(A)	–	–
Moricizine	–	–	–	–	+	–
Propafenone	–	–	–	+(A)	–	–
Anticoagulants						
Heparin	+*	–	–	–	+	–
Phenindione	–	–	–	+	–	–
Antihypertensives						
Captopril	+	–	–	+	+	–
Glutethimide	+*	–	–	–	–	P
Hydralazine	–	–	–	–	+	L
Methyldopa	–	–	+	+	+	P
Reserpine	–	–	–	–	+	–
Diuretics						
Acetazolamide	+	–	–	+	+	–
Chlorothiazide	–	–	–	–	+	–
Chlorthalidone	–	–	–	+	+	–
Diazoxide	–	–	–	–	+	–
Ethacrynic acid	–	–	–	+	–	–
Hydrochlorothiazide	–	–	–	+	–	–
Mercurials	–	–	–	+	+	–
Spironolactone	–	–	–	–	+	–
Triamterene	–	+	–	–	–	–
Coronary Dilators						
Amyl nitrite	–	–	–	–	–	M
Nitroglycerin	–	–	–	–	–	M
Other						
Amrinone	–	–	–	–	+	–

* Pure red cell aplasia.
L = lupus-like syndrome; P = porphyria; A = agranulocytosis; M = methemoglobinemia.

immunohemolytic anemia. The frequency of positive results on Coombs' test varies from 11 per cent for patients who are receiving 0.75 gm per day for over 3 months to 40 per cent for those receiving 2 gm per day for the same time. Fortunately, the affinity of the alpha-methyldopa antibody for red cells is low, and fewer than 1 per cent of patients whose antiglobulin test is positive will manifest significant hemolytic anemia. Nonetheless, alpha-methyldopa surpasses all other drugs in causing immunohemolytic anemia. On withdrawal of the drug, hemolysis improves within 1 or 2 weeks, with full recovery in 1 month, although the positive Coombs' test may persist for 6 to 24 months. A positive Coombs' test without hemolysis is not an indication to discontinue alpha-methyldopa if its administration is otherwise indicated in the treatment of hypertension.

The other two mechanisms of drug-related positive antiglobulin reactions do not involve cardiovascular drugs. The third is represented by penicillin, in which the drug binds to the red cell membranes, creating a cell-drug complex and antigenic stimulation of an IgG antibody. The fourth mechanism involves cephalothin, which is bound to the red cell membrane; normal serum proteins adhere nonspecifically to red cell membranes.

GRANULOCYTOPENIA AND AGRANULOCYTOSIS. A reduction in circulating neutrophils is the most toxic hematological effect of drugs. It may be secondary to depression of the marrow, or it may be an immune mechanism causing peripheral destruction. When there is immune suppression, examination of the marrow reveals active myeloid precursors, whereas the absence of myeloid elements suggests suppression of synthesis. The marrow-depressive effect is dose related. Anticoagulants such as phenindione, antiarrhythmics such as procainamide and tocainide,[188,189] antihypertensives such as captopril, and diuretics such as the thiazides have all been reported to produce granulocytopenia. Procainamide and its relative tocainide are the most dangerous and most frequently implicated cardiac drugs in granulocytopenia.[190] Presenting symptoms may include a sore throat, ulcerations of mucous membranes, fever, malaise, fatigue, and weakness. Discontinuation of the drug may be followed by a rebound in the white blood cell count and occasionally a leukemoid picture. Because laboratory tests are not conclusive for white cell antibodies, an accurate definition of the immune mechanism responsible for white cell destruction remains unclear.

DRUG-INDUCED THROMBOCYTOPENIA. Many of the drugs used to treat cardiovascular disorders may cause thrombocytopenia, either by a direct effect on the bone marrow or by inducing formation of drug-specific antibody.[191] For example, the thiazide diuretics (p. 849) directly suppress megakaryocyte production. Thiazide-induced thrombocytopenia is usually mild, with the platelet count rarely falling below 50,000/μl. This condition is unique, since it persists for 6 to 8 weeks after drug withdrawal. Thrombocytopenia caused by amrinone, a positive inotropic agent with vasodilator properties (see p. 484), is less well studied but is clearly related to the total dose of drug administered and to peripheral destruction of platelets.[192] Other common agents like alcohol and some estrogen preparations may cause thrombocytopenia by a direct depressant effect on the bone marrow.

Shortened platelet survival secondary to antibody or complement binding to platelets can cause severe thrombocytopenia and life-threatening hemorrhage. The onset is abrupt and is not related to the dose of medication or the duration of its use. In most cases of immunological thrombocytopenia, the offending agent induces a specific antibody. The resulting drug-antibody complex then binds to the platelet, thereby shortening its survival. Quinidine, one of the first cardiac drugs to produce this response, has been well studied as a cause of thrombocytopenia. The defect can be transferred to a normal individual by administering serum from a patient with quinidine-induced thrombocytopenia, followed by a quinidine challenge to the normal subject. A similar defect can be caused by antibodies to quinine, including the small quantities present in tonic drinks. Acetaminophen (a common analgesic given to cardiac patients), acetazolamide, digitoxin, phenytoin, ethacrynic acid, alpha-methyldopa, and spironolactone have all been implicated in various cases of suspected drug-induced thrombocytopenia, although the mechanism has not always been well defined.

Although in vitro laboratory tests for drug-dependent platelet antibody are available, the results do not always correlate with clinical events. The best proof of drug-induced thrombocytopenia is prompt recovery of the platelet count after drug withdrawal followed by a second episode of thrombocytopenia upon readministration of the suspected drug. (Because of this potential hazard, the drug challenge is not advised.) If serious hemorrhage persists after the drug is withdrawn, treatment with 1 mg/kg prednisone or its equivalent may be necessary. Corticosteroids may hasten the return of a normal platelet count and may also protect capillaries and small vessels even without altering the platelet count. Platelet transfusions are not usually helpful but can be tried in desperate situations in which hemorrhage is life threatening. They are most useful if thrombocytopenia persists well after the drug-antibody complex has been cleared. In this situation, a gratifying elevation in platelet count sometimes occurs.

HEPARIN-INDUCED THROMBOCYTOPENIA (see also p. 1594). Treatment with this drug is one of the most important causes of thrombocytopenia in cardiac patients. The incidence of thrombocytopenia in patients receiving heparin has been reported from 0 to 30 per cent.[193] A review of pooled data from the literature estimates the incidence of heparin-induced thrombocytopenia at 1.1 per cent for porcine heparin and 2.9 per cent for beef heparin.[194]

The heparin-induced thrombocytopenia (HIT) syndromes have been divided into two types, Type I HIT, and Type II HIT on the basis of both severity of disease, and pathophysiology.[195–197] Type I HIT is a mild disease, with platelet counts often between 100,000 and 150,000/mm^3. This syndrome is likely due to direct heparin-induced platelet aggregation. Thromboembolic phenomena are usually not seen.[198] No treatment is required and the thrombocytopenia will usually resolve even if heparin is continued. Heparin is usually stopped, however, because of the inability to distinguish, early on, this from type II HIT.

Type II HIT is more severe than type I HIT, with greater degrees of thrombocytopenia, and frequent thromboembolic complications from platelet thrombi. This has clearly been shown to be an autoimmune disease, with production of IgG that binds to platelets and causes both clearance of platelets by the reticuloendothelial system, and platelet activation leading to platelet aggregation and microthrombotic complications.[199] In cases of type II HIT, heparin must be stopped, and oral anticoagulants or thrombolytic agents must be substituted depending on the clinical needs.

OTHER HEMATOLOGICAL ABNORMALITIES CAUSED BY CARDIAC DRUGS. Amyl nitrite, sodium nitrite, and nitroglycerin can oxidize hemoglobin to methemoglobin, which cannot effectively carry oxygen. The patient with methemoglobinemia appears cyanotic but has a normal arterial PO_2, and oxygen therapy will not improve the pallor. Although symptomatic methemoglobinemia may occur in adults, most cases are seen in children who accidentally ingest medications prescribed for adults. Occasionally, adults with mild congenital methemoglobinemia will become markedly symptomatic when exposed to small doses of these same medications. With the increasing use of intravenous nitroglycerin, this complication may become more frequent.[194] If venous blood is chocolate brown and this color persists after the blood is shaken in air, the diagnosis of methemoglobinemia is almost certain. The diagnosis is confirmed by the addition of a few drops of 10 per cent potassium cyanide, which results in the rapid production of the bright red cyanmethemoglobin. Symptoms are nonspecific and consist of dyspnea, headache, fatigue, and dizziness. They are usually self-limited if the responsible drugs are discontinued, since normal red cells can enzymatically reduce the methemoglobin. In severe cases or in patients with enzyme defects, methylene blue may be administered to stimulate reduction of the methemoglobin.

Other medications may interfere with oxygen delivery to tissues. For example, sodium nitroprusside used to treat hypertensive emergencies and to reduce afterload in the management of heart failure may cause fatigue, nausea, abnormal behavior, and muscle spasm as the agent reacts with oxyhemoglobin, producing cyanmethemoglobin and free cyanide ions.[195]

Hydralazine (p. 1052), procainamide (p. 594), and rarely phenytoin (p. 1051) can cause a lupus erythematosus-like syndrome, with urticaria, erythema multiforme, photosensitivity, delirium, and immune-mediated blood cell destruction.[196] Although patients with drug-induced lupus have positive antinuclear antibody tests and many of the clinical manifestations of the systemic form, renal function is not usually impaired, and all these manifestations usually remit within several months if the drugs are discontinued. The syndrome is of particular importance in cardiac patients, since the onset of chest pain, pleurisy, or pericardial effusion in the patient with heart disease could lead to an erroneous diagnosis unless drug-induced lupus is suspected.

REFERENCES

ANEMIA AND CARDIOVASCULAR DISORDERS

1. Handin, R. I., Lux, S. E., and Stossel, T. P.: Blood: Principles and Practice of Hematology. Philadelphia, J. B. Lippincott, 1995.
2. Eckstein, R. W.: Development of interarterial coronary anastomoses by chronic anemia. Disappearance following correction of anemia. Circ. Res. *3*:306, 1955.
3. Florenzano, F., Diaz, G., Regonesi, C., and Escobar, E.: Left ventricular function in chronic anemia: Evidence of noncatecholamine positive inotropic factor in the serum. Am. J. Cardiol. *54*:638, 1984.
4. Varat, M. A., Adolph, R. J., and Fowler, N. O.: Cardiovascular effects of anemia. Am. Heart J. *83*:415, 1972.
5. Asimacopoulos, P. J., Groves, M. D., Fischer, D. K., et al.: Pernicious anemia manifesting as angina pectoris. South. Med. J. *87*:671, 1994.
6. Baer, R. W., Vlahakes, G. J., Uhlig, P. N., and Hoffman, I. E.: Maximum myocardial oxygen transport during anemia and polycythemia in dogs. Am. J. Physiol. *252*:H1086, 1987.
7. Torrance, J. D., Jacobs, P., Restrepo, A., et al.: Intraerythrocyte adaptation to anemia. N. Engl. J. Med. *283*:165, 1970.
8. Oski, F. A., Marshall, B. D., Cohen, P. J., et al.: Exercise with anemia. The role of the left or right shifted oxygen-hemoglobin equilibrium curve. Ann. Intern. Med. *74*:44, 1971.
9. Lenfant, C., Torrance, J., English, E., et al.: Effect of altitude on the oxygen binding by hemoglobin and on organic phosphate levels. J. Clin. Invest. *47*:2652, 1968.

10. Oski, F. A., Gottlieb, A. J., Delivoria-Papadopoulos, M., and Miller, W. W.: Red-cell 2,3-diphosphoglycerate levels in subjects with chronic hypoxemia. N. Engl. J. Med. *280:*1165, 1969.
11. Harris, T. N., Friedman, S., Tuncali, M. T., and Hallidie-Smith, K. A.: Comparison of innocent murmur of childhood with cardiac murmurs in high output states. Pediatrics *33:*341, 1964.
12. Bunn, H. F.: Disorders of hemoglobin. *In* Wilson, J., and Braunwald, E., et al. (eds.): Harrison's Principles of Internal Medicine, 12th ed. New York, McGraw-Hill, 1991, pp. 1543–1552.
13. Buchanan, G. R.: Sickle cell disease: Recent advances. Curr. Probl. Pediatr. *23:*219, 1993.
14. Powars, D. R.: Sickle cell anemia and major organ failure. Hemoglobin *14:*573, 1990.
15. Simmons, B. E., Santhanam, V., Castaner, A., et al.: Sickle cell heart disease. Two dimensional echo and doppler ultrasonographic findings in the hearts of adult patients with sickle cell anemia. Arch. Intern. Med. *148:*1526, 1988.
16. Gaffney, J. W., Bierman, F. Z., Donnelly, C. M., et al.: Cardiovascular adaptation to transfusion/chelation therapy of homozygote sickle cell anemia. Am. J. Cardiol. *62:*121, 1988.
17. Estrade, G., Pointrineau, D., Bernasconi, F., et al.: Left ventricular function and sickle-cell anemia. Echocardiographic Study. Arch. Mal. Coeur *82:*1975, 1989.
18. Gerry, J. L., Bulkley, B. H., and Hutchins, G. M.: Clinicopathologic analysis of cardiac dysfunction in 52 patients with sickle cell anemia. Am. J. Cardiol. *42:*211, 1978.
19. McCormick, W. F.: Massive nonatherosclerotic myocardial infarction in sickle cell anemia. Am. J. Forensic Med. Pathol. *9:*151, 1988.
20. Francis, R. B., Jr.: Platelets, coagulation and fibrinolysis in sickle cell disease: Their possible role in vascular occlusion. Blood Coagul. Fibrinolysis *2:*341, 1991.
21. Balfour, I. C., Covitz, W., Davis, H., et al.: Cardiac size and function in children with sickle cell anemia. Am. Heart J. *108:*345, 1984.
22. Lippman, S. M., Niemann, J. T., Thigpen, T., et al.: Abnormal septal Q waves in sickle cell disease. Prevalence and causative factors. Chest *88:*543, 1985.
23. Maisel, A., Friedman, H., Flint, J., et al.: Continuous electrocardiographic monitoring in patients with sickle cell anemia during pain crisis. Clin. Cardiol. *6:*339, 1983.
24. Covitz, W., Eubig, C., Balfour, I. C., et al.: Exercise-induced cardiac dysfunction in sickle cell anemia. Radionuclide study. Am. J. Cardiol. *51:*570, 1983.
25. Manno, B. V., Burka, E. R., Hakki, A., et al.: Biventricular function in sickle cell anemia: Radionuclide angiographic and thallium-201 scintigraphic evaluation. Am. J. Cardiol. *52:*584, 1983.
26. Willens, H. J., Lawrence, C., Frishman, W. H., and Strom, J. A.: A noninvasive comparison of left ventricular performance in sickle cell anemia and chronic aortic regurgitation. Clin. Cardiol. *6:*542, 1983.
27. Lippman, S. M., Ginzton, L. E., Thigpen, T., et al.: Mitral valve prolapse in sickle cell disease: Presumptive evidence for a linked connective tissue disorder. Arch. Intern. Med. *145:*435, 1985.
28. Forget, B. G., and Pearson, H. A.: Hemoglobin synthesis and the thalassemias. *In* Handin, R. I., Lux, S. E., and Stossel, T. P. (eds.): Blood: Principles and Practice of Hematology. Philadelphia, J. B. Lippincott, 1995.
29. Sanakul, D., Thakerngpol, K., and Pacharee, P.: Cardiac pathology in 76 thalessemic patients. Birth Defects *23:*177, 1988.
30. Wacker, P., Halperin, D. S., Balmer-Ruedin, D., et al.: Regression of cardiac insufficiency after ambulatory intravenous deferoxamine in thalassemia major. Chest *103:*1276, 1993.
31. Aldouri, M. A., Wonke, B., Hoffbrand, A. V., et al.: High incidence of cardiomyopathy in betathalassaemia patients receiving regular transfusion and iron chelation: Reversal by intensified chelation. Acta Haematol. *84:*113, 1990.
32. Ehlers, L. H., Levin, A. R. Klein, A. A., et al.: The cardiac manifestations of thalassemia major: Natural history, noninvasive cardiac diagnostic studies, and results of cardiac catheterization. *In* Engle, M. A. (ed.): Pediatric Cardiovascular Disease. Cardiovascular Clinics II. Philadelphia, F. A. Davis Co., 1981, pp. 171–186.
33. Spirito, P., Lupi, G., Melevendi, C., and Vecchio, C.: Restrictive diastolic abnormalities identified by Doppler echocardiography in patients with thalassemia major. Circulation *82:*88, 1990.
34. Sapoznikov, D., Lewis, N., Rachmilewitz, E. A., et al.: Left ventricular filling and emptying patterns in anemia due to beta-thalassemia. A computer-assisted echocardiographic study. Cardiology *69:*276, 1982.
35. Lau, K. C., Li, A.M.C., Hui, P. W., and Yeung, C. Y.: Left ventricular function in β thalassemia major. Arch. Dis. Child *64:*1046, 1989.
36. Valdes-Cruz, L. M., Reinecke, C., Rutkowski, M., et al.: Preclinical abnormal segmental cardiac manifestations of thalassemia major in children on transfusion-chelation therapy: Echographic alterations of left ventricular posterior wall contractions and relaxation patterns. Am. Heart J. *103:*505, 1982.
37. Borow, K. M., Propper, R., Bierman, F. Z., et al.: The left ventricular end-systolic pressure-dimensions relation in patients with thalassemia major. A new noninvasive method for assessing contractile state. Circulation *66:*980, 1982.
38. Canale, C., Terrachini, V., Vallebena, A., et al.: Thalassemic cardiomyopathy: Echocardiographic difference between major and intermediate thalassemia at rest and during isometric effort: Yearly follow-up. Clin. Cardiol. *11:*563, 1988.
39. Dameshek, W., and Roth, S. I.: Case Records of the Massachusetts General Hospital—Weekly Clinicopathological exercises. Case 52. N. Engl. J. Med. *271:*898, 1964.
40. Westring, D. W.: Aortic valve disease and hemolytic anemia. Ann. Intern. Med. *65:*203, 1966.
41. Sonaer, D. H., Cheng, T. O., and Aaron, B. L.: Hemolytic anemia and acute mitral regurgitation caused by a torn cusp of a porcine mitral prosthetic valve 7 years after its implantation. Am. Heart J. *113:*404, 1987.
42. Enzenauer, R. J., Berenberg, J. L., and Cassell, P. F., Jr.: Microangiopathic hemolytic anemia as the initial manifestation of porcine valve failure. South. Med. J. *83:*912, 1990.
43. Mok, P., Lieberman, E. H., Lilly, L. S., et al.: Severe hemolytic anemia following mitral valve repair. Am. Heart J. *117:*1171, 1989.
44. Sears, A. D., and Crosby, W. H.: Intravascular hemolysis due to intracardiac prosthetic devices. Diurnal variations related to activity. Am. J. Med. *39:*341, 1965.
45. DiSosa, V. J., Collins, J. J., Jr., and Cohn, C. H.: Hematological complications with the St. Jude valve and reduced-dose coumadin. Ann. Thorac. Surg. *48:*280, 1989.

HEMOCHROMATOSIS AND HEMOSIDEROSIS

46. Schafer, A. I.: Iron overload. *In* Fairbanks, V. F. (ed.): Current Hematology. New York, John Wiley and Sons, 1981, pp. 191–218.
47. Rosenqvist, M., and Hultcrantz, R.: Prevalence of haemochromatosis among men with clinically significant bradyarrhythmias. Eur. Heart J. *10:*473, 1989.
48. James, T. N.: Pathology of the cardiac conduction system in hemochromatosis. N. Engl. J. Med. *271:*92, 1964.
49. Wasserman, A. J., Richardson, D. W., Baird, C. L., and Wyso, E. M.: Cardiac hemochromatosis simulating constrictive pericarditis. Am. J. Med. *32:*316, 1962.
50. Westra, W. H., Hruban, R. H., Baughman, K. L., et al.: Progressive hemochromatotic cardiomyopathy despite reversal of iron deposition after liver transplantation. Am. J. Clin. Pathol. *99:*39, 1993.
51. Rivers, J., Garrahy, P., Robinson, W., and Murphy, A.: Reversible cardiac dysfunction in hemochromatosis. Am. Heart J. *113:*216, 1987.
52. Wolfe, L., Olivieri, N., Sallan, D., et al.: Prevention of cardiac disease by subcutaneous deferoxamine in patients with thalassemia major. N. Engl. J. Med *312:*1600, 1985.
53. Maurer, H. S., Lloyd-Still, J. D., Ingrisano, C., et al.: A prospective evaluation of iron chelation therapy in children with severe beta-thalassemia. A six year study. Am. J. Dis. Child. *142:*287, 1988.
54. Freeman, A. P., Giles, R. W., Berdoukas, V. A., et al.: Sustained normalization of cardiac function by chelation therapy in thalassemia major. Clin. Lab. Haematol. *11:*299, 1989.
55. Strack, M. F., and Hannah, E. E.: Venesection responsive cardiomyopathy in a patient with idiopathic haemochromatosis. N. Z. Med. J. *105:*360, 1992.
56. Lerner, N., Blei, F., Bierman, F., et al.: Chelation therapy and cardiac status in older patients with thalassemia major. Am. J. Pediatr. Hematol. Oncol. *12:*56, 1990.
57. Russo, G.: Iron chelating therapy in thalassemia: Current problems. Haematologica *75*(Suppl. 5):84, 1990.
58. Jensen, P. D., Jensen, F. T., Christensen, T., and Ellegaard, J.: Non-invasive assessment of tissue iron overload in the liver by magnetic resonance imaging. Br. J. Haematol. *87:*171, 1994.
59. Kaltwasser, J. P., Gottschalk, R., Schalk, K. P., and Hartl, W.: Non-invasive quantitation of liver iron-overload by magnetic resonance imaging. Br. J. Haematol. *74:*360, 1990.
60. Wasman, S., Eustace, S., and Hartnell, G. G.: Myocardial involvement in primary hemochromatosis demonstrated by magnetic resonance imaging. Am. Heart J. *128:*1047, 1994.
61. Olson, L. J., Edwards, W. D., Holmes, D. R., et al.: Endomyocardial biopsy in hemochromatosis: Clinicopathologic correlates in six cases. J. Am. Coll. Cardiol. *13:*116, 1989.
62. Candell-Riera, J., Permanger-Miralda, G., and Soler-Soler, J.: Cardiac hemochromatosis. Primary Cardiol. *12*(October):123, 1986.
63. Edwards, C. Q., Griffen, L. M., Goldgar, D., et al.: Prevalence of hemochromatosis among 11,065 presumably healthy blood donors. N. Engl. J. Med. *318:*1355, 1988.
64. Venegoni, P., and Cyprus, G.: Polycythemia and the heart. Tex. Heart Inst. J. *21:*198, 1994.
65. Fruchtman, S. M., and Berk, P. D.: Polycythemia vera and agnogenic myeloid metaplasia. *In* Handin, R. I., Lux, S. E., and Stossel, T. P.: Blood: Principles and Practice of Hematology. Philadelphia, J. B. Lippincott, 1995.

DISORDERS ASSOCIATED WITH ABNORMAL BLOOD FLOW DISTRIBUTION OR INCREASED VISCOSITY

66. Thomas, D. J., Marshall, J., Russell, R. W., et al.: Effect of hematocrit on cerebral blood flow in man. Lancet *2:*941, 1977.
66a. Al-Saif, S., Bhat, R. P., Hijazi, A.: Left ventricular and aortic valve thrombosis caused by polycythemia rubra vera successfully treated with streptokinase. Am. Heart J. *131:*397, 1996.
67. Kaplan, M. E., Mack, K., Goldberg, J. D., et al.: Long-term management of polycythemia vera with hydroxyurea: A progress report. Semin. Hematol. *23:*167, 1986.
68. Messinezy, M., Aubry, S., O'Connell, G., et al.: Oxygen desaturation in apparent and relative polycythaemia. BMJ *302:*216, 1991.

69. Rosenthal, A., Button, L. N., and Nathan, D. G.: Blood volume changes in cyanotic congenital heart disease. Am. J. Cardiol. *29*:162, 1971.
70. Rosenthal, A., Nathan, D. G., Marty, A. T., et al.: Acute hemodynamic effects of red cell production in polycythemia of cyanotic congenital heart disease. Circulation *42*:197, 1970.
71. Erslev, A. J., and Caro, J.: Secondary polycythemia: A boon or a burden? Blood Cells *10*:177, 1984.
72. Grant, P., Patel, P., and Singh, S.: Acute myocardial infarction secondary to polycythemia in a case of cyanotic congenital heart disease. Int. J. Cardiol. *9*:108, 1985.
73. Wallis, P. J., Skehan, J. D., Newland, A. C., et al.: Effects of erythropheresis on pulmomary hemodynamics and oxygen transport in patients with secondary polycythemia and cor pulmonale. Clin. Sci. *70*:91, 1986.
74. York, E. L., Junes, R. L., Menon, D., and Sproule, B. J.: Effects of secondary polycythemia on cerebral flood flow in chronic obstructive pulmonary disease. Am. Rev. Respir. Dis. *121*:813, 1980.
75. Rosenthal, A., Mentzer, W. C., and Eisenstein, E. B.: The role of red blood cell organic phosphates in adaptation to congenital heart disease. Pediatrics *47*:537, 1971.
76. Charache, S., Weatherall, D. J., and Clegg, J. B.: Polycythemia associated with hemoglobinopathy. J. Clin. Invest. *45*:813, 1966.
77. Weinreb, N. J., and Shih, C. F.: Spurious polycythemia. Semin. Hematol. *12*:397, 1975.
78. Schwarcz, T. H., Hogan, L. A., Endean, E. D., et al.: Thromboembolic complications of polycythemia: polycythemia vera versus smokers' polycythemia. J. Vasc. Surg. *17*:518, 1993.
79. Saffitz, J. E., Phillips, E. R., Temesy-Armos, P. N., and Roberts, W. C.: Thrombocytosis and fatal coronary heart disease. Am. J. Cardiol. *52*:651, 1983.
80. Koh, K. K., Cho, S. K., Kim, S. S., et al.: Coronary vasospasm, multiple coronary thrombosis, unstable angina, and essential thrombocytosis. Int. J. Cardiol. *41*:168, 1993.
81. Mitus, A. J., Barbui, R., Shulman, L. N., et al.: Hemostatic complications in young patients with essential thrombocythemia. Am. J. Med. *88*:371, 1990.
82. Rosenthal, D. S., and Murphy, S.: Thrombocytosis. *In* Handin, R. I., Lux, S. E., Stossel, T. P. (eds.): Blood: Principles and Practice of Hematology. Philadelphia, J. B. Lippincott, 1995.
83. McAllister, H. A., and Fenoglio, J. J.: Tumors of the cardiovascular system. *In* Atlas of Tumor Pathology. 2nd ed. Washington, D.C.: Armed Forces Institute of Pathology; 1978.
84. MacGee, W.: Metastatic and invasive tumors involving the heart in a geriatric population: A necropsy study. Virchows Arch. A. Pathol. Anat. Histopathol. *419*:183, 1991.
85. Abraham, J. M.: Neoplasms metastatic to the heart: Review of 3314 consecutive autopsies. Am. J. Cardiovasc. Pathol. *3*:195, 1990.
86. Lam, K. Y., Dickens, P., and Chan, A.C.L.: Tumors of the heart: A 20-year experience with a review of 12,485 consecutive autopsies. Arch. Pathol. Lab. Med. *117*:1027, 1993.
87. English, J. C., Allard, M. F., Babul, S., and McManus, B. M.: Metastatic tumors of the heart, *In* Goldhaber, S. Z.: Cardiopulmonary Diseases and Cardiac Tumors, Atlas of Heart Diseases. Vol. 3. Philadelphia, Current Medicine, 1995.

CARDIAC MANIFESTATIONS OF NEOPLASTIC DISEASE

88. Israeli, A., Rein, A.J.J.T., Kriski, M., et al.: Right ventricular outflow tract obstruction due to extracardiac tumors: A report of three cases diagnosed and followed up by echocardiographic studies. *149*:2105, 1989.
89. Kapoor, A. S.: Clinical manifestations of neoplasia of the heart. *In* Kapoor, A. S. (ed.): Cancer and the Heart. New York, Springer-Verlag, 1986, pp. 21–25.
90. Roberts, W. C., Glancy, D. L., and DeVita, V. T.: Heart in malignant lymphoma. A study of 196 autopsy cases. Am. J. Cardiol. *22*:85, 1968.
91. Petersen, C. D., Robinson, Q. A., and Kurnich, J. E.: Involvement of the heart and pericardium in the malignant lymphomas. Am. J. Med. Sci. *272*:161, 1976.
92. Waller, B. F., Gottdiener, J. S., Virmni, R., and Roberts, W. C.: Structure-function correlations in cardiovascular and pulmonary diseases. The charcoal heart. Chest *77*:671, 1980.
93. Almange, C., Lebrestec, T., Louvet, M., et al.: Bloc auriculo-ventriculaire complet par metastase cardiaque: A propos dune observation. Sem. Hop. Paris *54*:1419, 1978.
94. Seibert, K. A., Rettenmier, C. W., Waller, B. F., et al.: Osteogenic sarcoma metastatic to the heart. Am. J. Med. *73*:136, 1982.
95. Kralstein, J., and Frishman, W.: Malignant pericardial disease: Diagnosis and treatment. Am. Heart J. *113*:785, 1987.
96. Kirn, D., Mauch, P., and Shaffer, K., et al.: Large-cell and immunoblastic lymphoma of the mediastinum: Prognostic features and treatment outcome in 57 patients. J. Clin. Oncol. *11*:1336, 1993.
97. Singh, S., Wann, S., Schuchard, G. H., et al.: Right ventricular and right atrial collapse in patients with cardiac tamponade: A combined echocardiographic and hemodynamic study. Circulation *70*:966, 1984.
98. Isner, J. M., Carter, B. L., Bankoff, M. S., et al.: Computed tomography in the diagnosis of pericardial heart disease. Ann. Intern. Med. *97*:473, 1982.
99. Buck, M., Ingle, J. N., Giuliani, E. R., et al.: Pericardial effusion in women with breast cancer. Cancer *60*:263, 1987.
100. Posner, M. R., Cohen, G. I., and Skarin, A. T.: Pericardial disease in patients with cancer. The differentiation of malignant from idiopathic and radiation-induced pericarditis. Am. J. Med. *71*:407, 1981.
101. Hancock, E. W.: Neoplastic pericardial disease. Cardiol. Clin. *8*:673, 1990.
102. Press, O. W., and Livingston, R.: Management of malignant pericardial effusion and tamponade. JAMA *256*:2301, 1987.
102a. Laham, R. J., Cohen, D. J., Kuntz, R. E., et al.: Pericardial effusion in patients with cancer: Outcome with contemporary management strategies. Heart *75*:67, 1996.
103. Snow, N., and Lucas, A.: Subxiphoid pericardiotomy: A safe, accurate, diagnostic and therapeutic approach to pericardial and intrapericardial disease. Am. Surg. *49*:249, 1983.
104. Osuch, J. R., Khandekar, J. D., and Fry, W. A.: Emergency subxiphoid pericardial decompression for malignant pericardial effusion. Am. Surg. *51*:298, 1985.
105. Park, J. S., Tentschler, R., and Wilbur, D.: Surgical management of pericardial effusion in patients with malignancies. Cancer *67*:76, 1991.
106. Mack, M. J., Landreneau, R. J., Hazelrigg, S. R., and Acuff, T. E.: Video thoracoscopic management of benign and malignant pericardial effusions. Chest *103*:390s, 1993.
107. Gouldesbrough, D. R., and Carder, P. J.: Rapidly progressive cardiac failure due to lymphomatous infiltration of the myocardium. Postgrad. Med. J. *65*:668, 1989.
108. Lestuzzi, C., Biasi, S., Nicolosi, G. L., et al.: Secondary neoplastic infiltration of the myocardium diagnosed by two-dimensional echocardiography in seven cases with anatomic confirmation. J. Am. Coll. Cardiol. *9*:439, 1987.
109. Perez, C. A., Presant, C. A., and Amburg, A. L.: Management of superior vena caval syndrome. Semin. Oncol. *5*:123, 1978.
110. Lopez, M. I., and Vincent, R. J.: Malignant superior vena cava syndrome. *In* Kapoor, A. S. (ed.): Cancer and the Heart. New York, Springer-Verlag, 1986, p. 206.
111. Wahlin, A., Olofsson, B., Eriksson, A., and Backman, C.: Myeloma-associated cardiac amyloidosis. Acta Med. Scand. *215*:189, 1984.
112. Alpert, M. A.: Cardiac amyloidosis. *In* Kapoor, A. S. (ed.): Cancer and the Heart. New York, Springer-Verlag, 1986, p. 162.
113. Ursell, P. C., and Fenogolio, J. J.: Spectrum of cardiac disease diagnosed by endomyocardial biopsy. Pathol. Annu. *19*:197, 1984.
114. Koiwaya, Y., Nakamura, M., and Yamamoto, K.: Progressive ECG alterations in metastatic cardiac mural tumor. Am. Heart J. *105*:339, 1983.
115. Hartman, R. B., Clark, P. I., and Schulman, P.: Pronounced and prolonged ST segment elevation. A pathognomonic sign of tumor invasion of the heart. Arch. Intern. Med. *142*:1917, 1982.
116. Cole, T. O., Attah, E. D., and Onyemelukwe, G. C.: Burkitt's lymphoma presenting with heart block. Br. Heart J. *37*:94, 1975.
117. Ballentyne, F., VanderArk, C. R., and Holick, M.: Carotid sinus syncope and cervical lymphoma. Wis. Med. J. *74*:91, 1975.
118. Inagaki, R., Rodriguez, V., and Brody, G. P.: Causes of death in cancer patients. Cancer *33*:568, 1974.
119. Kopelson, G., and Herwig, K. J.: The etiologies of coronary artery disease in cancer patients. Int. J. Radiat. Oncol. Biol. Phys. *4*:895, 1978.
120. Stewart, J. R., and Fajardo, L. F.: Cancer and coronary artery disease. Int. J. Radiat. Oncol. Biol. Phys. *4*:915, 1978.
121. Ackerman, D. M., Hyma, B. A., and Edwards, W. D.: Malignant neoplastic emboli to the coronary arteries. Report of two cases and review of the literature. Hum. Pathol. *18*:955, 1987.
122. Kountz, D. S.: Isolated cardiac metastasis from cervical carcinoma: Presentation as acute anteroseptal myocardial infarction. South. Med. J. *86*:228, 1993.
123. Parker, B. M.: Valvular involvement in cancer. *In* Kapoor, A. S. (ed.): Cancer and the Heart. New York, Springer-Verlag, 1986, p. 64.
124. Blanchard, D. G., Ross, R. S., and Dittrich, H. C.: Nonbacterial thrombotic endocarditis. Assessment by transesophageal echocardiography. Chest *102*:954, 1992.
125. Chino, F., Kodama, A., Otake, M., and Dock, D. S.: Nonbacterial thrombotic endocarditis in a Japanese autopsy sample. A review of eighty cases. Am. Heart J. *90*:190, 1975.
126. Gonzalez Quintela, A., Candela, M. J., Vidal, C., et al.: Nonbacterial thrombotic endocarditis in cancer patients. Acta Cardiologica *XLVI*:1, 1991.
127. Lehto, V. P., Stenman, S., and Somer, T.: Immunohistological studies on valvular vegetations in nonbacterial thrombotic endocarditis. Arch. Pathol. Microbiol. Scand. *90*:207, 1982.
128. Fauci, A. S., Harley, J. B., Roberts, W. C., et al.: The idiopathic hypereosinophilic syndrome: Clinical, pathophysiologic, and therapeutic considerations. Ann. Intern. Med. *97*:78, 1982.
129. Parrillo, J. E., Borer, J. S., Henry, W. L., et al.: The cardiovascular manifestations of the hypereosinophilic syndrome: Prospective study of 26 patients, with review of the literature. Am. J. Med. *67*:572, 1979.

CARDIAC EFFECTS OF RADIATION THERAPY AND CHEMOTHERAPY

130. Geist, B. J., Lauk, S., Bornhausen, M., and Trott, K.-R.: Physiologic consequences of local heart irradiation in rats. Int. J. Radiat. Oncol. Biol. Phys. *18*:1107, 1990.
131. Om, A., Ellahham, S., and Vetrovec, G. W.: Radiation-induced coronary artery disease. Am. Heart J. *124*:1598, 1992.
132. Carlson, R. G., Mayfield, W. R., Normann, S., and Alexander, J. A.: Radiation-associated valvular disease. Chest *99*:538, 1991.
133. Arsenian, M. A.: Cardiovascular sequelae of therapeutic thoracic radiation. Prog. Cardiovasc. Dis. *33*:299, 1991.
134. Schultz-Hector, S.: Radiation-induced heart disease: Review of experi-

mental data on dose response and pathogenesis. Int. J. Radiat. Biol. *61*:149, 1992.

135. Lipshultz, S. E., and Sallan, S. E.: Cardiovascular abnormalities in long-term survivors of childhood malignancy. J. Clin. Oncol. *11*:1199, 1993.
136. Hancock, S. L., Donaldson, S. S., and Hoppe, R. T.: Cardiac disease following treatment of Hodgkin's disease in children and adolescents. J. Clin. Oncol. *11*:1208, 1993.
137. Kreuser, E.-D., Voller, H., Behles, C., et al.: Evaluation of late cardiotoxicity with pulsed Doppler echocardiography in patients treated for Hodgkin's disease. Br. J. Haematol. *84*:614, 1993.
138. McReynolds, R. A., Gold, G. L., and Roberts, W. C.: Coronary heart disease after mediastinal irradiation for Hodgkin's disease. Am. J. Med. *60*:39, 1976.
139. Brosius, F. C., Waller, B. F., and Roberts, W. C.: Radiation heart disease: Analysis of 16 young (aged 15 to 33 years) necropsy patients who received over 3500 rads to the heart. Am. J. Med. *7*:519, 1981.
140. Joesuu, H.: Acute myocardial infarction after heart irradiation in young patients with Hodgkin's disease. Chest *95*:388, 1989.
141. Green, D., Gingell, R. L., Pearce, J., et al.: The effect of mediastinal irradiation on cardiac function of patients treated during childhood and adolescence for heart disease. J. Clin. Oncol. *5*:239, 1987.
142. O'Donnell, L. O., O'Neill, T., Toner, M., et al.: Myocardial hypertrophy, fibrosis and infarction following exposure of the heart to radiation for Hodgkin's disease. Postgrad. Med. J. *62*:1055, 1986.
143. Boivin, J.-F., Hutchison, G. B., Lubin, J. H., and Mauch, P.: Coronary artery disease mortality in patients treated for Hodgkin's disease. Cancer *69*:1241, 1992.
144. Jakacki, R. I., Goldwein, J. W., Larsen, R. L., et al.: Cardiac dysfunction following spinal irradiation during childhood. J. Clin. Oncol. *11*:1033, 1993.
145. Perry, M. C.: Effects of chemotherapy on the heart. *In* Kapoor, A. S. (ed.): Cancer and the Heart. New York, Springer-Verlag, 1986, p. 223.
146. Icli, F., Karaoguz, H., Dincol, D., et al.: Severe vascular toxicity associated with cisplatin-based chemotherapy. Cancer *72*:587, 1993.
147. Ayash, L. J., Wright, J. E., Tretyakov, O., et al.: Cyclophosphamide pharmacokinetics: Correlation with cardiac toxicity and tumor response. J. Clin. Oncol. *10*:995, 1992.
148. Watts, R. G.: Severe and fatal anthracycline cardiotoxicity at cumulative doses below 400 mg/m^2: Evidence for enhanced toxicity with multiagent chemotherapy. Am. J. Hematol. *36*:217, 1991.
149. de Forni, M., and Armand, J. P.: Cardiotoxicity of chemotherapy. Curr. Opin. Oncol. *6*:340, 1994.
149a. Frishman, W. H., Sung, H. M., Yee, H. C. M., et al.: Cardiovascular toxicity with cancer chemotherapy. Curr. Prob. Cardiol. *21*:225, 1996.
150. Doroshow, J. H.: Doxorubicin-induced cardiac toxicity. N. Engl. J. Med. *324*:843, 1991.
151. Doroshow, J. H., Locker, G. Y., and Myers, C. E.: Enzymatic defenses of the mouse heart against reactive oxygen metabolites: Alterations produced by doxorubicin. J. Clin. Invest. *65*:128, 1980.
152. Bristow, M. R., Mason, J. W., Billingham, M. E., and Daniels, J. R.: Doxorubicin cardiomyopathy. Evaluation by phonocardiography, endomyocardial biopsy, and cardiac catheterization. Ann. Intern. Med. *88*:168, 1978.
153. Unverferth, B. J., Magorien, R. D., Balcerzak, S. P., et al.: Early changes in human myocardial nuclei after doxorubicin. Cancer *52*:215, 1983.
154. Gottdiener, J. S., Mathisen, D. J., Barer, J. S., et al.: Doxorubicin cardiotoxicity: Assessment of late left ventricular dysfunction by radionuclide cineangiography. Ann. Intern. Med. *94*:430, 1981.
155. Estorch, M., Carrio, I., Martinez-Duncker, D., et al.: Myocyte cell damage after administration of doxorubicin or mitoxantrone in breast cancer patients assessed by indium 111 antimyosin monoclonal antibody studies. J. Clin. Oncol. *7*:1264, 1993.
156. Schwartz, R. G., McKenzie, W. B., Alexander, J., et al.: Congestive heart failure and left ventricular dysfunction complicating doxorubicin therapy. Seven-year experience using serial radionuclide angiocardiography. Am. J. Med. *82*:1109, 1987.
157. Von Hoff, D. D., Layard, M. W., Basa, P., et al.: Risk factors for doxorubicin-induced congestive heart failure. Ann. Intern. Med. *91*:710, 1979.
158. Moreb, J. S., and Oblon, D. J.: Outcome of clinical congestive heart failure induced by anthracycline chemotherapy. Cancer *70*:22637, 1992.
159. Lipshultz, S. E., Colan, S. D., Gelber, R. D., et al.: Late cardiac effects of doxorubicin therapy for acute lymphoblastic leukemia in childhood. N. Engl. J. Med. *324*:808, 1991.
160. Ali, M. K., Ewer, M. S., Gibbs, H. R., et al.: Late doxorubicin-associated cardiotoxicity in children: The possible role of intercurrent viral infection. Cancer *74*:182, 1994.
160a. Lipshultz, S. E, Lipsitz, S. R., Mone, S. M., et al.: Female sex and higher drug dose as risk factors for late cardiotoxic effects of doxorubicin therapy for childhood cancer. N. Engl. J. Med. *332*:1738, 1995.
161. Anders, R. J., Shanes, J. G., and Zeller, F. P.: Lower incidence of doxorubicin cardiomyopathy by one-a-week low-dose administration. Am. Heart J. *111*:755, 1986.
162. Shapira, J., Gotfried, M., Lishner, M., et al.: Reduced cardiotoxicity of doxorubicin by a 6-hour infusion regimen. A prospective randomized evaluation. Cancer *65*:870, 1990.
163. Valdirieso, M., Burgess, M. A., Awer, M. S., et al.: Increased therapeutic index of weekly doxorubicin in the therapy of non small cell lung cancer; A prospective randomized study. J. Clin. Oncol. *2*:207, 1984.
164. Torti, F. M., Bristow, M. R., Howes, A. E., et al.: Reduced cardiotoxicity of doxorubicin delivered on a weekly schedule: Assessment by endomyocardial biopsy. Ann. Intern. Med. *99*:745, 1983.
165. Legla, S. S., Benjamin, R. S., MacKay, B., et al.: Reduction of doxorubicin cardiotoxicity by prolonged continuous intravenous infusion. Ann. Intern. Med. *96*:133, 1982.
166. Speyer, J. L., Green, M. D., Dubin, N., et al.: Prospective evaluation of cardiotoxicity during a six-hour doxorubicin infusion regimen in women with adenocarcinoma of the breast. Am. J. Med. *78*:555, 1985.
167. Ensley, J. F., Patel, B., Kloner, R., et al.: The clinical syndrome of 5-fluorouracil cardiotoxicity. Invest. New Drugs *7*:101, 1989.
168. Robben, N. C., Pippas, A. W., and Moore, J. O.: The syndrome of 5-fluorouracil cardiotoxicity: An elusive cardiopathy. Cancer *71*:493, 1993.
169. Goldberg, M. A., Antin, J. H., Guinan, E. C., and Rappeport, J. M.: Cyclophosphamide cardiotoxicity. An analysis of dosing as a risk factor. Blood *68*:1114, 1986.
170. Braverman, A. C., Antin, J. H., Plappert, M. T., et al.: Cyclophosphamide cardiotoxicity: A prospective evaluation of new dosing regimens. (Submitted for publication.)
171. Gottdiener, J. S., Applebaum, F. R., Ferrans, V. J., et al.: Cardiotoxicity associated with high dose cyclophosphamide therapy. Arch. Intern. Med. *141*:758, 1981.
172. Kandylis, K., Vassilomanolakis, M., Tsoussis, S., and Efremidis, A. P.: *Ifosfamide* cardiotoxicity in humans. Cancer Chemother. Pharmacol. *24*:395, 1989.
173. Quezado, Z. M. N., Wilson, W. H., Cunnion, R. E., et al.: High-dose ifosfamide is associated with severe, reversible cardiac dysfunction. Ann. Intern. Med. *118*:31, 1993.
174. Burkhardt, A., Haltje, W. J., and Gebbens, J. O.: Vascular lesions following perfusion with bleumycin: Electron-microscopic observations. Virchows Arch. Pathol. Anat. *372*:227, 1976.
175. Aisner, J., VanEcho, D. A., Whitacre, M., and Wiernik, P. H.: A phase-I trial of continuous infusion VP-16-213 *(etoposide)*. Cancer Chemother. Pharmacol. *7*:157, 1982.
176. Steinherz, L. J., Steinherz, P. G., Mangiacasale, D., et al.: Cardiac abnormalities after AMSA administration. Cancer Treat. Rep. *66*:483, 1982.
177. Lindpainter, K., Lindpainter, L. S., Wentworth, M., and Burns, C. P.: Acute myocardial necrosis during administration of amsacrine. Cancer *57*:1284, 1986.
178. Weiss, R. B., Grillo-Lopez, A. J., Marsoni, S., et al.: Amsacrine-associated cardiotoxicity: An analysis of 82 cases. J. Clin. Oncol. *4*:919, 928, 1986.
179. Cazin, V., Gorin, C., Laport, J. P., et al.: Cardiac complications after bone marrow transplantation. A report on a series of 63 consecutive transplantations. Cancer *57*:2061, 1986.
180. Cohen, M. C., Huberman, M. S., and Nesto, R. W.: Recombinant alpha-2 interferon-related cardiomyopathy. Am. J. Med. *85*:549, 1988.
181. Deyton, L. R., Walker, R. E., Kovacs, J. A., et al.: Reversible cardiac dysfunction associated with interferon alpha therapy in AIDS patients with Kaposi's sarcoma. N. Engl. J. Med. *321*:1246, 1989.
182. Schechter, D., and Nagler, A.: Recombinant interleukin-2 and recombinant interferon-alpha immunotherapy cardiovascular toxocity (editorial). Am. Heart J. *123*:1736, 1992.
183. Rosenberg, S. A., Lotze, M. T., Muul, L. M., et al.: A progress report on the treatment of 157 patients with advanced cancer using lymphokineactivated hilar cells and interleukin-2 or high dose interleukin-2 alone. N. Engl. J. Med. *316*:889, 1987.
184. Osanto, S., Cluitman, F. H. M., Franks, C. R., et al.: Myocardial injury after interleukin-2 therapy. Lancet *2*:48, 1988.
185. Nora, R., Abrams, J. S., Tait, N. S., et al.: Myocardial toxic effects during recombinant interleukin-2 therapy. J. Natl. Cancer Inst. *81*:59, 1989.

HEMATOLOGICAL ABNORMALITIES RELATED TO CARDIAC DRUGS

186. Gavras, F., Graff, L. G., Rose, B. D., et al.: Fatal pancytopenia associated with the use of captopril. Ann. Intern. Med. *94*:58, 1981.
187. Lundh, B., and Hasselgren, K. H.: Hematological side effects from antihypertensive drugs. Acta Med. Scand. (Suppl.)*628*:73, 1979.
188. Soff, G. A., and Kadin, M. E.: Tocainide-induced reversible agranulocytosis and anemia. Arch. Intern. Med. *147*:598, 1987.
189. Morrill, G. B., and Gibson, S. M.: Tocainide-induced aplastic anemia (letter). Drug Intell. Clin. Pharm. *23*:90, 1989.
190. Volosin, K., Greenberg, R. M., and Grenspon, A. J.: Tocainide-associated agranulocytosis. Am. Heart J. *109*:1392, 1985.
191. Hackett, T., Kelton, J. G., and Powers, P.: Drug-induced platelet destruction. Semin. Thromb. Hemostas. *8*:116, 1982.
192. Ansell, J., McCue, J., Tiarks, C., et al.: Amrinone-induced thrombocytopenia. Blood *58*(Suppl. 1):187a, 1981.
193. Bell, W. R., and Royall, R. M.: Heparin-associated thrombocytopenia: A comparison of three heparin preparations. N. Engl. J. Med. *303*:902, 1980.
194. Schmitt, P. B., and Adelman, B.: Heparin-associated thrombocytopenia: A critical review and a pooled analysis. Am. J. Med. Sci. *305*:208, 1993.
195. Green, D.: Heparin-induced thrombocytopenia. Med. J. Aust. *144*:37, 1986.
196. Chong, B. H.: Heparin-induced thrombocytopenia. Aust. N. Zeal. J. Med. *22*:145, 1992.
197. Chong, B. H.: Heparin-induced thrombocytopenia. Br. J. Haematol. *89*:431, 1995.
198. Salzman, E. W., Rosenberg, R. D., Smith, M. H., et al.: Effect of heparin and heparin fractions on platelet aggregation. J. Clin. Invest. *65*:64, 1980.
199. Warkentin, T. E., and Kelton, J. G.: Heparin-induced thrombocytopenia. Ann. Rev. Med. *40*:31, 1989.

Chapter 58
Hemostasis, Thrombosis, Fibrinolysis, and Cardiovascular Disease

VALENTIN FUSTER, MARC VERSTRAETE

HEMOSTASIS, FIBRINOLYSIS, ANTITHROMBOTICS, AND THROMBOLYTICS 1809
Hemostasis. 1809
The Fibrinolytic System and Its Control . . .1814
Antithrombotic Drugs 1816
Thrombolytic Drugs 1821
ANTITHROMBOTIC AND THROMBOLYTIC THERAPY IN CARDIAC DISEASE 1822
Antithrombotic Therapy in Coronary Artery Disease 1823
Antithrombotic Therapy for Cardiac Chamber Thromboembolism 1829
Antithrombotic Therapy in Prosthetic Heart Valve Replacement 1834
REFERENCES .1836

Over the last 2 decades, much evidence has indicated that thrombosis plays a crucial role in many cardiovascular events. It also is becoming apparent that variations in plasma levels of coagulation and fibrinolytic components may determine the individual's response to vascular changes, including fissuring of atherosclerotic plaques. Such cardiovascular patients could benefit from antithrombotic drugs, while thrombolytic agents are indicated in others with acute vascular occlusions. In the first section of this chapter, relevant aspects of the normal coagulation and fibrinolytic systems and their main defects associated with cardiovascular disorders are discussed; this section includes a discussion of registered antithrombotic and thrombolytic drugs. In the second section, the recent antithrombotic and thrombolytic clinical trials are reviewed and the specific approaches to antithrombotic and thrombolytic therapy are discussed.

HEMOSTASIS, FIBRINOLYSIS, ANTITHROMBOTICS, AND THROMBOLYTICS

HEMOSTASIS

The Vessel Wall With Focus on the Endothelium

The vast majority of blood vessels are capillaries that have no smooth muscle cells, and hemostasis depends on direct sealing. The first event in hemostasis (Fig. 58–1) in response to vascular injury of arterioles and venules is contraction of smooth muscle cells, soon followed by local perivascular and intravascular activation of platelets and coagulation components.

One of the unsolved mysteries of hemostasis and thrombosis is why platelets do not, or hardly ever, adhere to normal (unstimulated) endothelial cells in vivo. One possible answer is that both platelets and endothelium have a negative charge and thus would be mutually repulsive. The negative electric charge of endothelial cells is due to a pronounced glycocalyx, consisting of proteoglycans, of which heparan sulfate (a heparin-like substance that binds

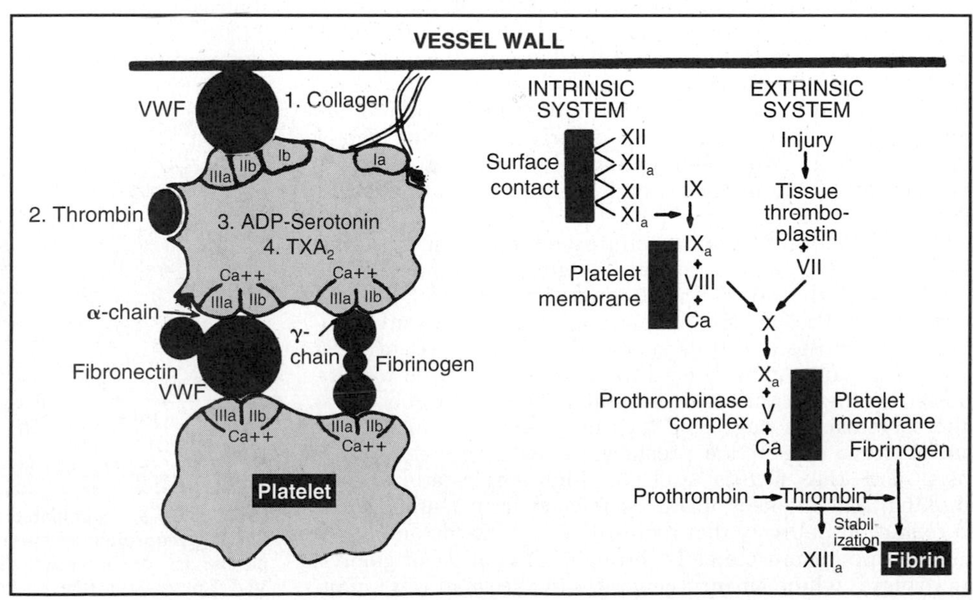

FIGURE 58–1. Interactions among platelet membrane receptors (glycoproteins Ia, Ib, and IIb/IIIa), adhesive macromolecules, and the disrupted vessel wall *(left)* and a flow chart of the intrinsic and extrinsic systems of the coagulation cascade *(right)*. On the left, Arabic numerals indicate the pathways of platelet activation that are dependent on collagen (1), thrombin (2), ADP and serotonin (3), and thromboxane A_2 (TXA_2) (4); there are also some reports that suggest the binding of von Willebrand factor (VWF) (polymeric protein) to collagen or heparin. Note the interaction at the right between clotting factors (XII, XIIa, XI, XIa, IX, IXa, VII, VIII, X, Xa, V, and XIIIa) and the platelet membrane. (From Fuster, V., et al.: N. Engl. J. Med. *326:*315, 1992. Copyright Massachusetts Medical Society.)

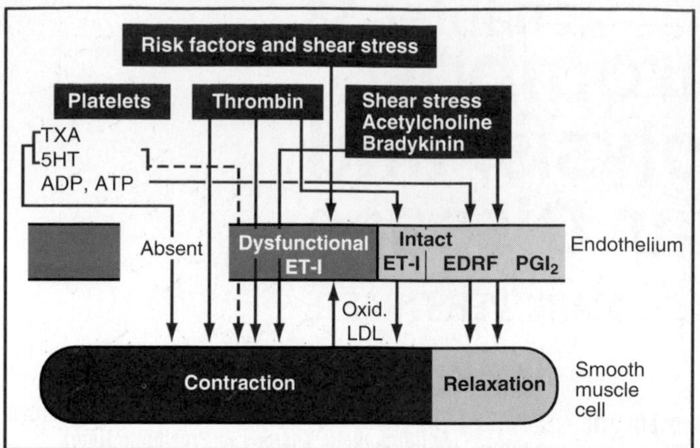

FIGURE 58–2. The effects of shear stress, acetylcholine, and bradykinin lead intact endothelium to generate and release endothelium-derived relaxing factor (EDRF) and prostacyclin (PGI_2), which in turn causes relaxation of the smooth muscle. The effect of thrombin leads the intact endothelium to generate endothelin-1 (ET-1), which causes vasoconstriction of the smooth muscle. After minor endothelial injury or damage (i.e., induced by risk factors), dysfunctional endothelium may not generate relaxing substances; in these circumstances, all of the above-mentioned stimulants exert a vasoconstrictive effect, either through the enhancement of endothelium-derived contracting factors or directly. As a result of severe endothelial injury or damage in areas of deendothelialization (Absent), thrombin and the platelet products thromboxane A_2 and serotonin (5-HT) induce direct vasoconstriction of the smooth muscle. (Modified from Fuster, V., et al.: The pathogenesis of coronary artery disease and the acute coronary syndrome. N. Engl. J. Med. *326*:313, 1992. Copyright Massachusetts Medical Society.)

antithrombin III) is the most important. Stimulated or injured endothelial cells lose their negative surface charge or anionic property.

Normal endothelial cells are much more than a semipermeable barrier between the blood and the vascular smooth muscle. They can be regarded as a highly active metabolic and endocrine organ that plays a major role in maintaining a proper balance between the formation of hemostatic plugs and the avoidance of intraluminal thrombi (see p. 1121). Endothelial cells inactivate vasoactive substances and have an important function on vasomotor tone.[1,2] For instance, carrier mechanisms in their cell membrane specifically transport serotonin, adenosine, and adenine nucleotides into the cell where they are metabolized. Angiotensin-converting enzyme on the outer surface of the cell inactivates bradykinin, a potent vasodilator. Perhaps a more crucial function is the synthesis of active substances that intervene in important physiological and pathological processes (Fig. 58–2).[3] Larger substances than those depicted in Figure 58–2 include fibronectin, heparan sulfate, tissue plasminogen activator, interleukin-1, and various growth factors. Smaller molecules synthesized by endothelial cells include prostacyclin (PGI_2), endothelium-derived relaxing factor (EDRF or nitric oxide, NO), endothelium-derived constricting factor(s) (endothelin-1), and platelet activating factor (PAF).

The production of prostacyclin by endothelium is stimulated by contact with activated platelets or leukocytes, by stretching of the arterial wall (pulsatile pressure), and by some drugs. Prostacyclin has strong antiplatelet and vasodilator properties and thus acts as the biological antagonist of thromboxane A_2. A direct link between impaired biosynthesis of prostacyclin in the vessel wall and thrombosis or atherosclerosis is suggested by the decreased capacity of endothelium to generate prostacyclin with age, atherosclerosis, and risk factors such as high cholesterol, heavy smoking, and diabetes. EDRF is formed from L-arginine by an oxidation pathway that requires several co factors. EDRF relaxes smooth muscle cells through stimulation of guanylate cyclase, which in turn generates cyclic guanosine monophosphate (cyclic GMP).[3] By the same mechanism it is also a potent inhibitor of adhesion and aggregation of platelets. There is a clear synergism between prostacyclin and EDRF in preventing platelet activation. EDRF is effective only in the immediate vicinity of its site of release because hemoglobin almost immediately inactivates any EDRF that enters the bloodstream. It has been suggested that a deficiency in EDRF production contributes to the pathogenesis of atherosclerosis and to the development of complications of diabetes. Endothelin-1 is a 21-residue peptide that is slowly released from endothelial cells by various stimuli and acts as a local hormone to induce vasodilation at low concentrations and vasoconstriction at high concentrations. Cleavage of a larger propeptide (big endothelin) by a putative endopeptidase (endothelin-converting enzyme) produces the active peptide. Its possible role in the pathophysiology of cardiovascular diseases is currently under intense scrutiny. Synthesis of platelet-activating factor (PAF), a strong stimulator of platelet aggregation, may be activated by thrombin that is locally generated if a break occurs in the endothelial lining. Thrombomodulin is a transmembranous protein that serves as an endothelial receptor for free thrombin.[4] In the complex that is formed and that does not require calcium, thrombin loses its procoagulant activity and expresses its anticoagulant role by activating protein C.

Thus, apart from a metabolic function with respect to the synthesis of vasoactive substances, the primary role of endothelium is in maintaining the patency of the blood vessels and the fluidity of blood. However, endothelium also has the potential to enhance and amplify the formation of a hemostatic plug initiated by a local endothelial lesion.

Platelets

In normal conditions, platelets are quiescent and circulate freely in the blood, because they do not attach to normally functioning endothelium. Vessel injury, however, exposes subendothelial connective tissue with various elements to which platelets can adhere.[5,6] Collagen and fibronectin interact readily with platelets, particularly with their membrane glycoproteins Ia/IIa and Ic/IIa (Fig. 58–3). von Willebrand factor, which has two collagen-binding sites, is an absolute requirement for platelets in flowing blood to adhere to the vascular wall. Adhered platelets lose their discoid shape, form pseudopods, and spread out over the injured surface. Through the action of activators such as collagen and eventually thrombin and norepinephrine, the adhered platelets soon become activated, which in turn expresses other platelet receptors and releases several mediators.[7] Phospholipase C hydrolyzes platelet membrane

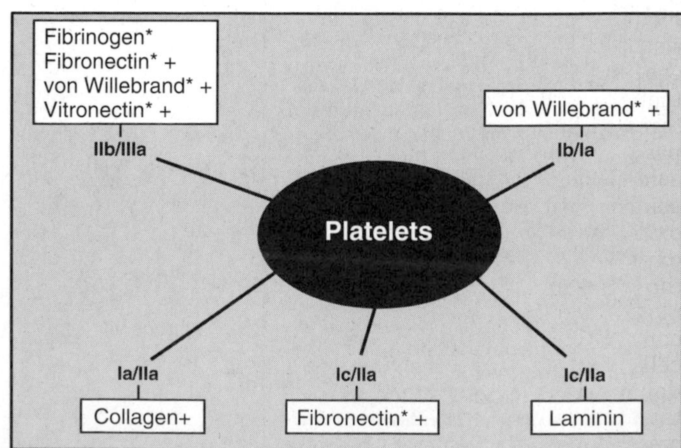

FIGURE 58–3. Stimulated platelets express on their membrane different glycoprotein receptors (integrins) that bind to ligands present in plasma (*) or in endothelial basement membranes (+). GPIa-IIa = VLA-2 or $\alpha_2\beta ii$; Ic/IIa = VLA-5 or $\alpha_5\beta ii$; IIB/IIIA = $\alpha_{11}\beta\beta_3$.

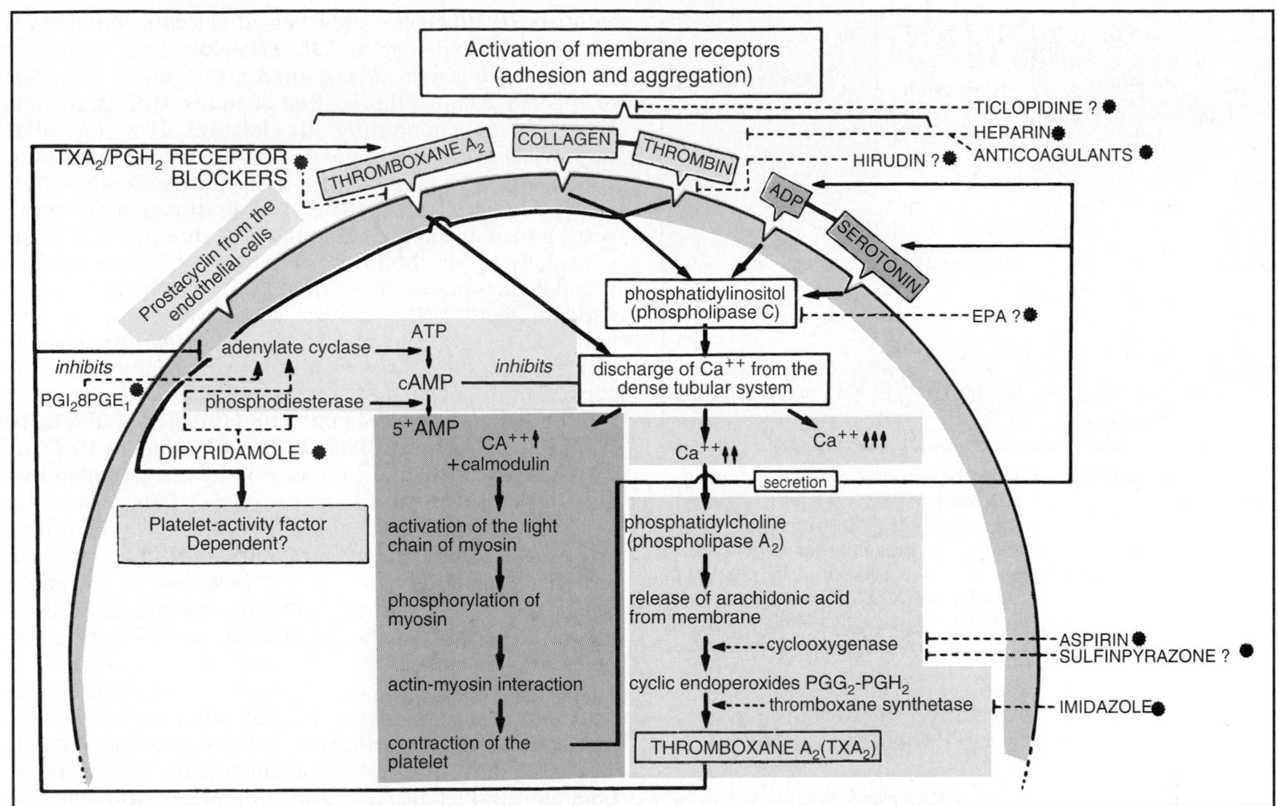

FIGURE 58–4. Mechanisms of platelet activation and presumed sites of action of various platelet inhibitor agents. Platelet agonists lead to the mobilization of calcium (Ca^{++}), which functions as a mediator of platelet activation through metabolic pathways dependent on adenosine diphosphate (ADP), thromboxane A_2 (TXA_2), thrombin, and collagen. Cyclic adenosine monophosphate (cAMP) inhibits calcium mobilization from the dense tubular system. Note that thrombin and collagen may independently activate platelets by means of platelet activating factor. • = a platelet inhibitor. Dashed line = a presumed site of drug action. ATP = adenosine triphosphate; EPA = eicosapentaenoic acid; PGE_1 = prostaglandin E_1; PGH_2 = prostaglandin H_2; PGI_2 = prostaglandin I_2 or prostacyclin. (From M. Verstraete and J. Vermylen: Thrombosis. Pergamon Press, 1984, p. 11. Modified by Stein, B., et al.: Platelet inhibitor agents in cardiovascular disease: An update. Reprinted by permission from the American College of Cardiology. J. Am. Coll. Cardiol. *14*:813, 1989.)

phosphatidylinositol, which leads to release of calcium from the dense tubular system (Fig. 58–4). Calcium in turn activates a protein kinase that phosphorylates intra-platelet regulatory proteins; activation of the actin-myosin system results in platelet contraction with release of adenosine diphosphate (ADP) and serotonin from the platelet dense granules and of thromboxane A_2.[8,9]

These potent inducers of platelet aggregation are capable of recruiting circulating platelets, which in turn adhere and transform the initial monolayer of platelets into an aggregate. The platelet glycoproteins IIb-IIIa on the platelet membrane undergo a conformational change in the activation process, so that they can interact with plasma fibrinogen and other adhesive proteins as fibronectin and endothelial thrombospondin, which serve to link platelets together into a tighter aggregate.[10,11] In addition, phospholipase A_2 acts on phosphatidylcholine to release arachidonic acid from the platelet membrane (Fig. 58–4). Arachidonic acid is converted to proaggregating prostaglandin endoperoxide intermediates (prostaglandins G_2 and H_2) by cyclooxygenase. Thromboxane A_2 is formed by the action of thromboxane synthase on prostaglandin H_2; it further promotes platelet activation, thrombus growth and local vasoconstriction. On the other hand, the vascular endothelial cells synthesize prostacyclin (PGI_2) starting from arachidonic acid or from platelet derived prostaglandin G_2. Prostacyclin stimulates adenylate cyclase and leads to an increased level of cyclic adenosine monophosphate (cyclic AMP) in the platelet. Cyclic AMP, in turn, inhibits the discharge of calcium from the dense tubular system and thus prevents platelet aggregation and secretion. Phosphodiesterase enhances the breakdown of cyclic AMP.

Coagulation

Activated platelets rearrange their surface lipoproteins so that phospholipids, on which coagulation factors can concentrate, are now exposed to the bloodstream. Thus, activated platelets, which lose their electronegativity in the process, markedly accelerate the formation of thrombin. Thrombin occupies a central position in the coagulation process. It is formed as the end result of a chain of reactions that transform, in sequence, a number of coagulation factors present as precursors (zymogens) in plasma into activated factors. The reactions occur mainly on the membrane of activated platelets and other stimulated cells and on tissue factor (a membrane protein that is exposed to the blood, e.g., after trauma) on which coagulation factors bind. Because of the low concentration of these factors in plasma and because of the abundant presence of circulating inhibitors, the interaction of procoagulants and their subsequent activation would proceed only slowly in the fluid phase of blood.

The traditional coagulation scheme distinguishes an "intrinsic" from an "extrinsic" activation pathway.

THE "INTRINSIC" PATHWAY OF THE COAGULATION SYSTEM. All factors participating in the intrinsic pathway are present in the circulating blood, and the reaction sequence is initiated by contact of platelets and/or coagulation components with a subendothelial tissue. Antigen-antibody complexes and activated platelets may serve this purpose, as can fissured atherosclerotic plaques and foreign surfaces such as those in an extracorporeal circulation or renal dialysis. This initial contact phase involves the interaction of factor XII (Hageman factor), prekallikrein, and high molec-

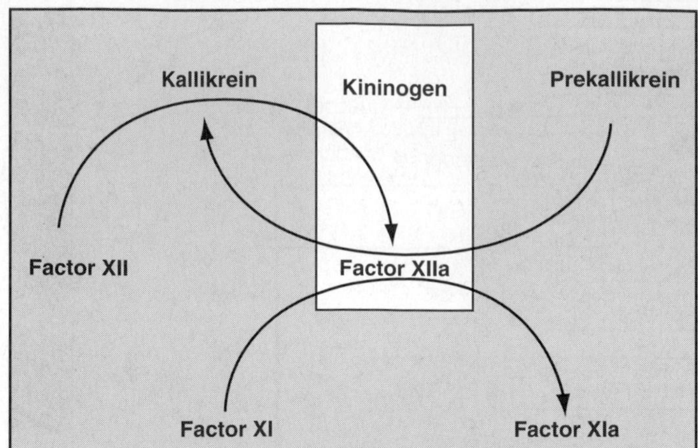

FIGURE 58–5. The contact phase of the intrinsic activation pathway. The initial event in vitro is the adsorption of factor XII to a negatively charged surface where it undergoes a conformational change to expose its active site. Factor XIIa converts prekallikrein to kallikrein. Additional factor XIIa and kallikrein are then generated by reciprocal activation. Factor XIIa also activates factor IX. Both prekallikrein and factor XI bind to a co-factor, high molecular weight kininogen, which serves to anchor them to the charged surface.

ular weight kininogen. However, the precise mechanism of the initial firing spark triggering the contact activation remains elusive.

Factor XII circulates in plasma; its heavy chain has great affinity for negatively charged surfaces such as glass and kaolin. Upon adsorption, bound factor XII now exerts traces of biological activity (Figs. 58–5 and 58–6). The actual activation of factor XII is facilitated by kallikrein. Factor XIIa converts the next factor of the coagulation cascade, factor XI, from its zymogen form to its enzymatic constellation (factor XIa).

Factor XIa bound to the surfaces by high molecular weight kininogen interacts upon activation with factor IX in a calcium-dependent two-step reaction. Activated factor IX, thrombin-modified factor VIII, negatively charged phospholipid (i.e., phospholipids of activated platelets), and calcium ions form a complex called tenase because it activates factor X (Fig. 58–6).

THE "EXTRINSIC" PATHWAY OF THE COAGULATION SYSTEM. In the "extrinsic" system, membrane-bound tissue factor starts off the chain of events by forming a complex with factor VII in the presence of calcium ions (Fig. 58–6). The tissue factor–factor VIIa complex then combines with the substrate (factor X), producing a further conformational change in factor VIIa, so that it binds still more tightly to tissue factor, precluding dissociation of factor VIIa from tissue factor.[12] The tissue factor–factor VIIa complex activates primarily factor X but also factors IX and XI, which interconnects the intrinsic and extrinsic activation pathways and plays a "prima ballerina" role in the activation of coagulation.[13] It should be noted that phospholipids of the platelet membrane, in conjunction with factor Xa, can also activate factor VII—another bridge between the intrinsic and extrinsic pathways. Thus, the earlier concepts of clearly separate intrinsic and extrinsic activation systems are becoming obsolete.

THE PATHWAY IN COMMON: THE FORMATION OF PROTHROMBINASE, THE ENZYME CONVERTING PROTHROMBIN TO THROMBIN. Factor X stands at the intersection of the so-called extrinsic and intrinsic activation pathways.[14,15] This means that factor X can be activated either by the tenase complex or by the tissue factor–factor VIIa complex. The presence of proteolytically modified factor VIII (whether by thrombin, factor Xa, or factor IXa) enhances 10,000-fold the rate of activation of factor X by factor IXa. Factor VIII is thus a helper protein (a co-factor).[16]

To be fully active, factor Xa has to form a stoichiometric 1:1 complex with factor Va; the latter molecule enhances the activation of prothrombin by factor Xa 300,000-fold. The association of factor Va with factor Xa on an anionic phospholipid is termed prothrombinase and has been reported to position the active site at a proper distance above the membrane for optimal enzymatic activity.

THE ACTION OF PROTHROMBINASE ON PROTHROMBIN. Prothrombinase initially cleaves the Arg-Ile bond in the prothrombin molecule, producing thrombin. This intermediate molecule remains membrane bound through the retained glutamic acid (Gla)-domain linkage and activates protein C but lacks procoagulant properties either on platelets or on fibrinogen. To obtain the latter property, another arginine bond (Arg-Thr) has to be cleaved, yielding alpha-thrombin.

THE PIVOTAL ROLE OF THROMBIN. Thrombin represents the culmination of the coagulation cascade; its action on fibrinogen is most dramatic because thrombus formation is a visible process. Thrombin itself is responsible for its own nonlinear generation caused by positive feedback activation, whereby thrombin enhances new formation of throm-

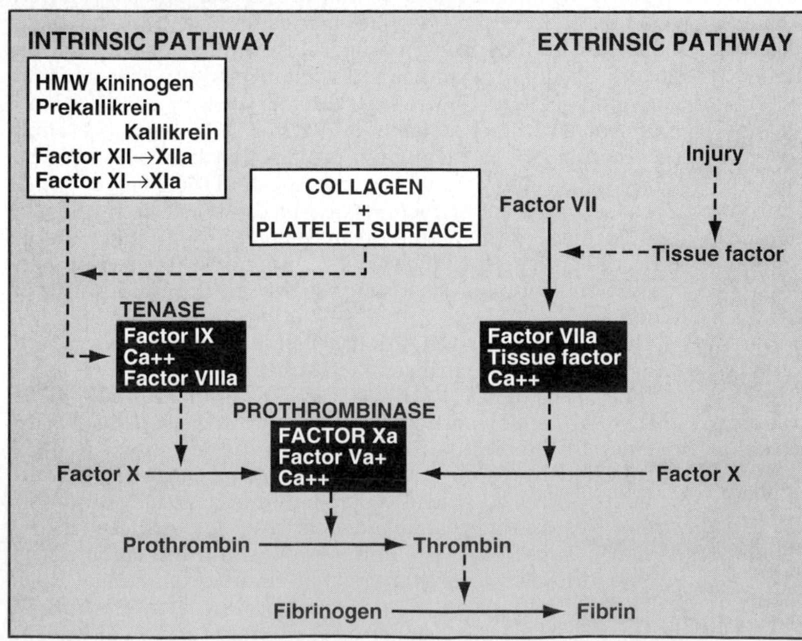

FIGURE 58–6. Clotting factor interactions. Coagulation is initiated by either an intrinsic or extrinsic pathway. In the intrinsic pathway, negatively charged surfaces initiate the contract activation and the phospholipid is furnished by platelets. In the extrinsic system, the phospholipid portion of tissue thromboplastin functions in conjunction with factor VIIa on the activation of factor X. From factor Xa on, both pathways converge upon a common path. Omitted from the diagram are inhibitors of the various steps, the augmentation of action of each pathway by activated factors, and the interaction between the intrinsic and extrinsic systems.

bin. In addition, thrombin is a pivotal molecule for numerous other functions (Fig. 58–7). The action of thrombin on platelets results in the release of platelet factor V exteriorization and in the transbilayer movement of its inner membrane surface (flip-flop reaction). Thrombin activates three of the four co-factor or helper proteins (factors V and VIII, thrombomodulin, but not tissue factor). Thrombin furthermore activates factor XIII, which increases the strength and renders the fibrin more resistant to thrombolysis; thrombin also releases prostacyclin, nitric oxide (NO, endothelial-derived relaxing factor), von Willebrand factor, and ADP from the normal endothelium, protecting the microcirculation against thrombosis. Thrombin inhibits its own production by a negative feedback mechanism via the thrombomodulin proteins C and S system.

THE CONVERSION OF FIBRINOGEN TO FIBRIN. Fibrinogen is a large paired molecule held together by disulfide bridges. Each symmetrical half-molecule consists of one set of three different polypeptide chains termed Aα, Bβ, and Gγ. Thrombin splits an arginine-glycine bond, first at the amino end of the two Aα chains and later at the amino end of each of the two Bβ chains so that each molecule releases two small aminopeptides A (FPA) and two small fibrinopeptides B (FPB) from fibrinogen and thus converts this molecule to fibrin monomers that are still soluble. The fibrinopeptide A release exposes a polymerization site in the central region of the fibrinogen molecule (E domain) that subsequently aligns with a complementary site in the outer region (D domain) of another fibrin monomer to form staggered overlapping two-stranded fibrils. Coupled monomers of fibrin, called polymers, are still soluble unless they become too large and precipitate; the resulting gel of fibrin forms the skeleton of a thrombus and traps red and white cells.

The structural stability of the fibrin network is achieved through covalent crosslinking.[17] Thrombin activates factor XIII, a transglutaminase that in the presence of calcium forms peptide bonds between side chains of suitable lysine (donors) and glutamic acid (acceptors) residues. The result of such a lysine crosslink is that the thrombus becomes firmer and more resistant to thrombolysis. It should be noted that fibrin-bound thrombin (approximately 40 per cent of the thrombin generated) retains its coagulant and platelet activating properties and is protected from inactivation by heparin-antithrombin III).[18] During thrombolysis, fibrin-bound thrombin is released and can cause rethrombosis. Hirudin, hirulog, and similar synthetic compounds that are smaller than heparin can inhibit fibrin-bound thrombin.

CONNECTIONS BETWEEN THE INTRINSIC AND EXTRINSIC PATHWAYS. The strict separation of the coagulation system into the intrinsic and extrinsic pathways of activation that merge in a common pathway from the activation of factor X is a didactic schematization that is rendered obsolete by more recent findings.[13] It is obvious that both systems are interconnected. For example, the factor VIIa–tissue factor complex can activate factors IX and XI directly; factor IXa and Xa can activate factor VII.

COAGULATION—SURFACE-CATALYZED EVENTS. The coagulation factors are present in the fluid phase of blood at very low concentrations, with the exception of fibrinogen, prothrombin, and plasminogen. Their encounter in solution is possible and their interaction slow, though this can be accelerated up to 100,000-fold after adsorption and concentration on surfaces. Modified endothelium, stimulated platelets, denuded subendothelial structures (e.g., collagen), and fissured atherosclerotic plaques and foreign surfaces (extracorporeal circulation conduits) allow attachment of passing platelets (adhesion) and adsorption of coagulation proteins. Assembly on surfaces increases the local concentration of clotting factors considerably and creates an optimal steric relationship (better alignment) for their interaction. Inhibitors of activated coagulation factors are much less effective in binding to phospholipid surfaces, and thus binding of activated coagulation factors to such a surface protects them from being inhibited.[19]

REGULATION OF THE COAGULATION PROCESS. A number of proteins circulate in the blood to inhibit the coagulation process at various stages of the cascade. Two of them appear particularly important in preventing thrombosis: antithrombin III and protein C.

Antithrombin III is an inhibitor of thrombin and of factor Xa.[20] Thrombin forms a tightly bound complex with antithrombin III; this occurs at a relatively slow rate that is enormously enhanced by heparin (see below) and also appreciably by heparan sulfate, a substance very similar to heparin that is found on the intraluminal surface of vascular endothelial cells. The inhibition of factor Xa is the result of the formation of a binary complex between antithrombin III and factor Xa.

Protein C is a proenzyme formed in the liver; vitamin K is required in its synthesis. Protein C is activated by thrombin to become a serine protease that inhibits factor Va and VIIIa (Fig. 58–8). Complex formation between thrombin and thrombomodulin, a potent co-factor present on the endothelial surface, catalyzes the activation of protein C. Protein S is another vitamin K-dependent protein that functions as a co-factor for activated protein C by facilitating its binding to membrane phospholipids.[21] In addition to being a powerful anticoagulant, activated protein C initiates fibrinolysis by releasing tissue plasminogen activator (t-PA) from the endothelium and neutralizing plasminogen activator inhibitor.

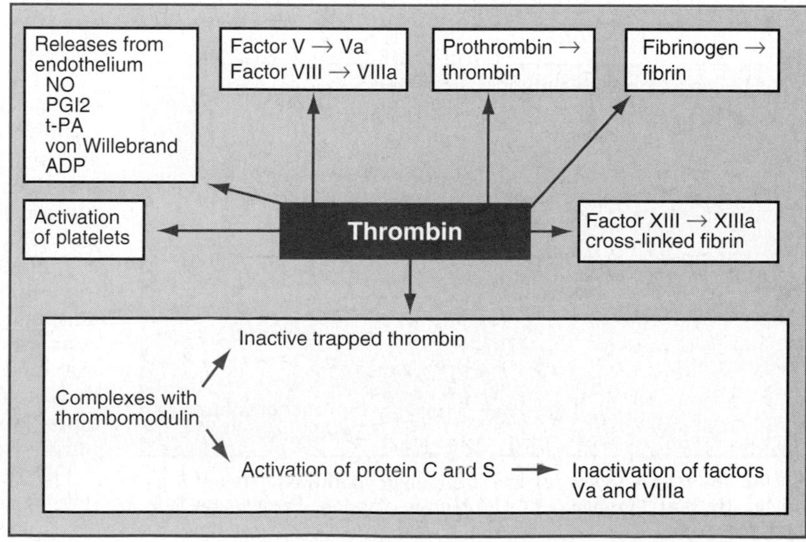

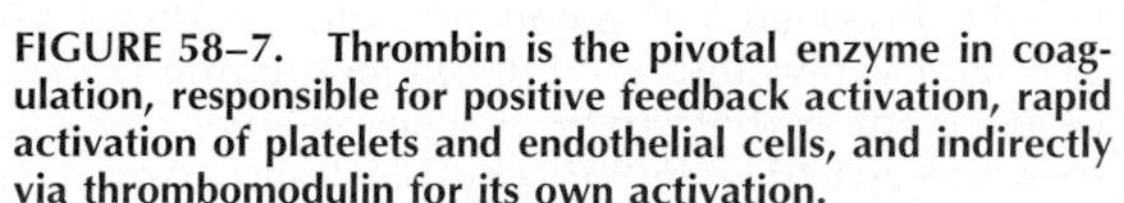
FIGURE 58–7. Thrombin is the pivotal enzyme in coagulation, responsible for positive feedback activation, rapid activation of platelets and endothelial cells, and indirectly via thrombomodulin for its own activation.

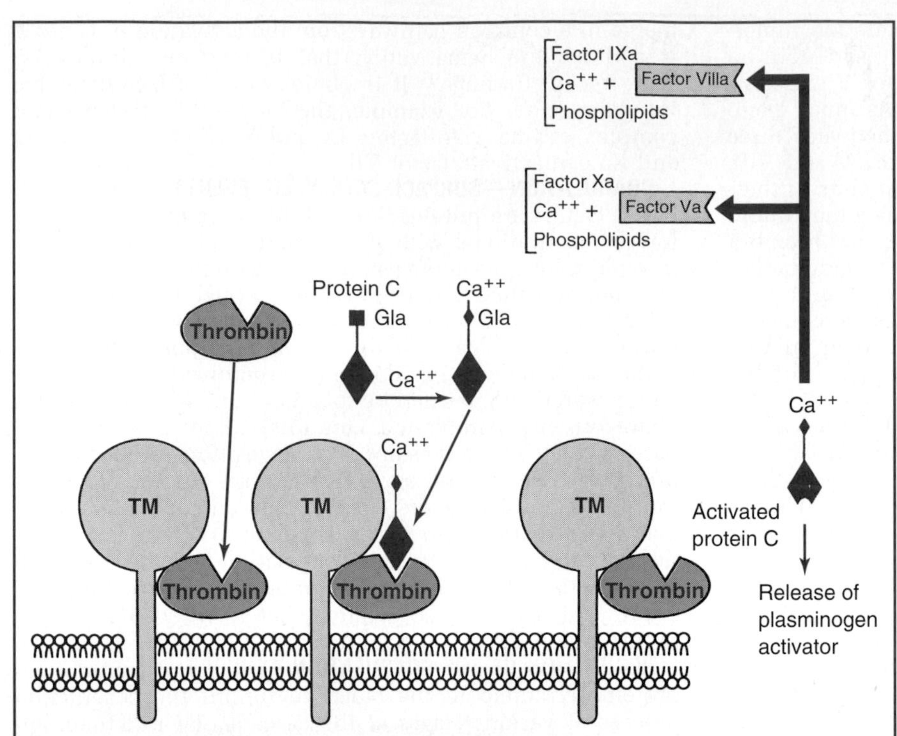

FIGURE 58–8. Thrombin forms a complex with the endothelium-bound protein thrombomodulin (TM). This complex activates circulating protein C, which inhibits factor Va and VIIIa and releases tissue-plasminogen activator from the endothelial cells. Binding of activated protein C to phospholipids is facilitated by protein S. Gla = γ-carboxyglutamic acid.

Tissue factor–factor VII complex is inactivated by the tissue factor pathway inhibitor (TFPI).[13,14,19,22] Factor VIIa cannot be neutralized effectively unless it is bound to tissue factor.[13] This is in contrast to other coagulation components, which are neutralized more effectively as free reactants than after they interact in complexes.[22]

THE FIBRINOLYTIC SYSTEM AND ITS CONTROL

Components of the Fibrinolytic System

(Fig. 58–9)

PLASMINOGEN. Plasminogen is present in human plasma at a concentration of about 2 μM, which is about twice the concentration of α_2-antiplasmin. The native molecule is a single-chain glycoprotein, organized in seven structural domains (Fig. 58–10).[23] From the NH2-terminal end, there is a "preactivation peptide" (animo acid residues 1–77), five sequential homologous kringle domains (about 90 residues each), and the proteinase domain (residues 562–791) with the catalytic site composed of His603, Asp646, and Ser741.[24–26] Plasminogen is converted to the two-chain serine proteinase plasmin by cleavage of a single Arg561-Val562 peptide bond between kringle 5 and the proteinase domain.

Tissue-type plasminogen activator
Urokinase-type plasminogen activator
Plasminogen activator inhibitor-1
Plasminogen activator inhibitor-2
Plasminogen → Plasmin
α2-Antiplasmin
Fibrin → Fibrin degradation products

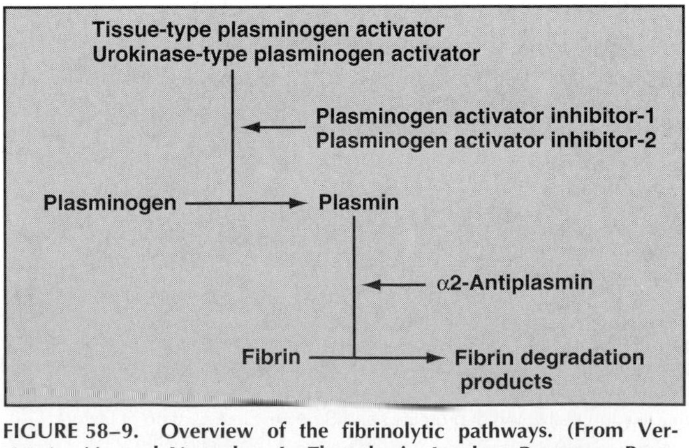

FIGURE 58–9. Overview of the fibrinolytic pathways. (From Verstraete, M., and Vermylen, J.: Thrombosis. London, Pergamon Press, 1984, p. 41.)

PLASMINOGEN ACTIVATORS. Tissue-type plasminogen activator (t-PA) is a 70 kDa serine proteinase, which consists of a single polypeptide chain in its native form. t-PA is converted by plasmin to a two-chain form by hydrolysis of the Arg275-Ile276 peptide bond. In contrast to most single-chain forms of serine proteinases, single-chain t-PA possesses significant catalytic activity. The aminoterminal region is composed of several domains with homologies to other proteins: a finger domain (residues 4-50), a growth factor domain (residues 50-87), and two kringles (residues 87–176 and 176–262) (Fig. 58–11).[27,28] The region constituted by residues 276-527 represents the serine proteinase part with the catalytic site.

Single-chain urokinase-type plasminogen activator (scu-PA) is a 54 kDa glycoprotein containing 411 amino acids. The plasma concentration of scu-PA is about 2 ng/ml. Upon proteolytic cleavage of the Lys158-Ile519 peptide bond, the molecule is converted to a two-chain derivative (tcu-PA, urokinase). The u-PA receptor is essential for localization of u-PA–mediated plasmin formation to the pericellular environment.[29,30] A low molecular weight scu-PA (32 kDa) can be generated by proteolytic cleavage of the Glu143–Leu144 peptide bond.[28]

INHIBITORS. Alpha$_2$-antiplasmin (α-plasmin inhibitor) and plasminogen activator inhibitors belong to the serine proteinase inhibitor superfamily (serpins).[31] Alpha$_2$-antiplasmin is present in plasma at a concentration of about 1 μM. It is a 67 kDa glycoprotein containing 464 amino acids and about 13 per cent carbohydrate.[32] The reactive site of the inhibitor is the Arg364-Met365 peptide bond. Alpha$_2$-antiplasmin (plasminogen-binding form) becomes partly converted in the circulating blood to a non-plasminogen-binding, less reactive form (about 30 per cent of the total), that lacks the 26 carboxyterminal residues. Two forms of alpha$_2$-antiplasmin are present in about equal amounts in purified preparations of the inhibitor.

The two most important plasminogen activator inhibitors (PAI's) are PAI-1 and PAI-2. PAI-1 is a 52 kDa single chain glycoprotein consisting of 379 amino acids.[33,34] The reactive

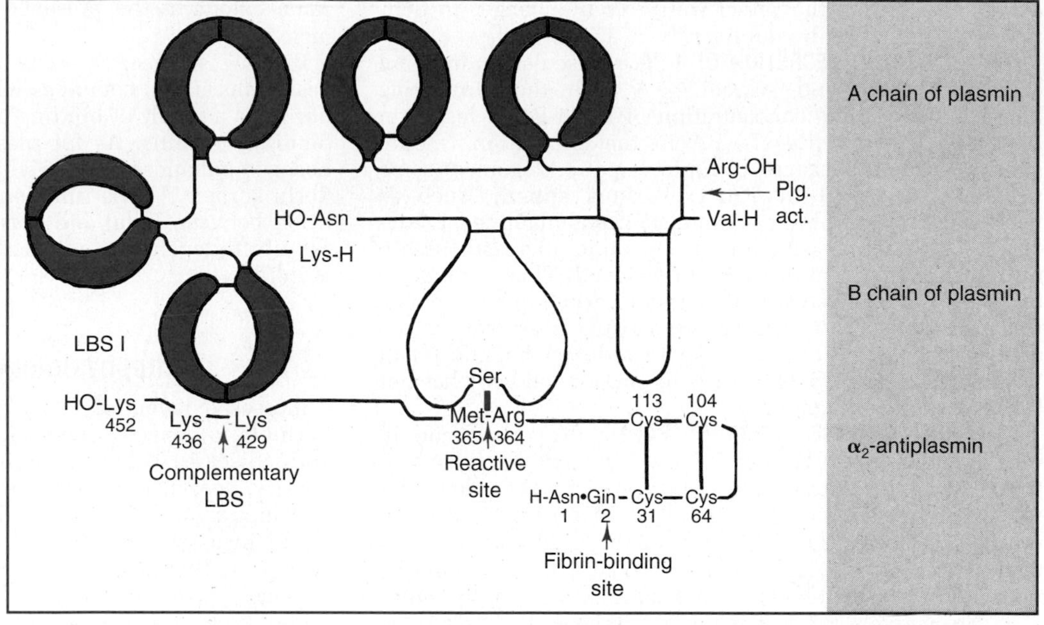

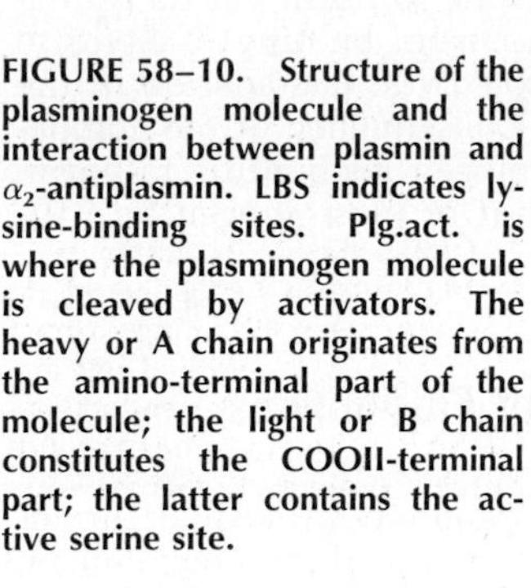

FIGURE 58–10. Structure of the plasminogen molecule and the interaction between plasmin and α_2-antiplasmin. LBS indicates lysine-binding sites. Plg.act. is where the plasminogen molecule is cleaved by activators. The heavy or A chain originates from the amino-terminal part of the molecule; the light or B chain constitutes the COOH-terminal part; the latter contains the active serine site.

site of the inhibitor is the Arg346-Met347 peptide bond. PAI-1 is stabilized by a tight binding to the cell adhesive protein vitronectin. PAI-2 exists in two different forms with comparable kinetic properties and is detected only in pregnant women.[35]

UROKINASE RECEPTOR. The specific cell surface receptor for urokinase plasminogen activator (u-PAR) is a heterogeneously glycosylated protein of 50–60 kDa synthesized as a 313 amino acid polypeptide.[36–38]

Regulation of the Fibrinolytic System

The physiologic fibrinolytic system is regulated by controlled activation and inhibition (Fig. 58–9). Activation of plasminogen by t-PA is enhanced in the presence of fibrin or at the endothelial cell surface. Inhibition of fibrinolysis may occur at the level of plasminogen activation or at the level of plasmin. Fibrinolysis is also regulated as a result of increased or decreased synthesis and/or secretion of t-PA

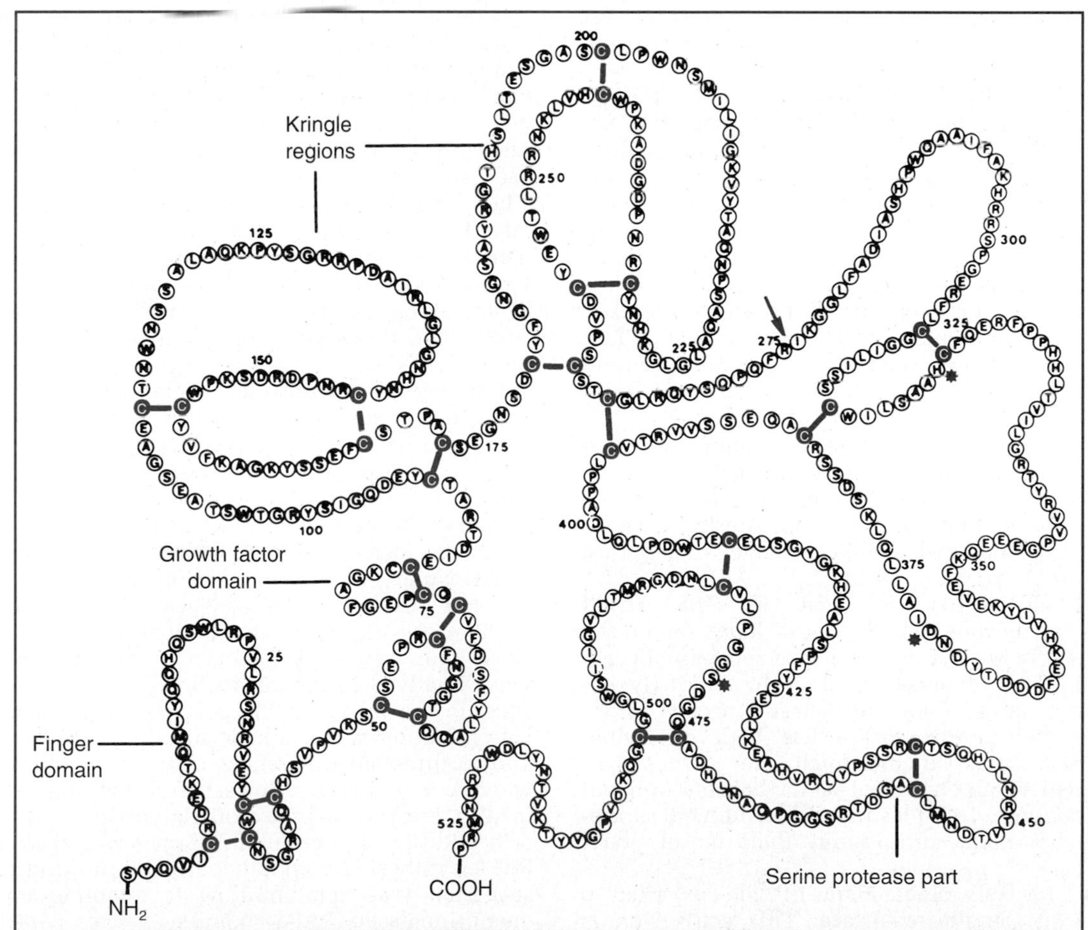

FIGURE 58–11. Primary structure of t-PA. The amino acids are represented by their single-letter symbols, and the black bars indicate disulfide bonds. * = active site residues His[322], Asp[371], and Ser[478]; arrow = plasmin cleavage site for conversion of single-chain t-PA to two-chain t-PA.

and of PAI-1 from the vessel wall,[39] or by changes in their rates of elimination by the liver.[40]

SYNTHESIS AND SECRETION OF t-PA. Vascular endothelial cells synthesize and secrete t-PA into the circulating blood.[39] The plasma concentration of free t-PA is less than 1 ng/ml. The half-life of t-PA in the circulation is only about 5 minutes because of rapid hepatic clearance; some t-PA is inactivated by PAI-1. Various stimuli, such as venous occlusion, physical exercise, catecholamines, bradykinin, or desmopressin, produce a rapid increase (within minutes) in the level of t-PA in the blood. This response is too rapid to represent increased synthesis, but may reflect release of t-PA from cellular storage pools as well as decrease in hepatic clearance due to reduced hepatic blood flow.[41–43] A storage pool of t-PA in endothelial cells has not been conclusively identified.[42]

SYNTHESIS AND SECRETION OF PAI-1. PAI-1 is found in plasma, platelets, placenta, and in the extracellular matrix.[44] The concentration in plasma is in the picomolar range, but may increase to about 2 nM during pregnancy, most likely as a result of release of the inhibitor from placenta. Both active and latent PAI-1 are cleared rapidly, with half-lives in rabbits of approximately 15 and 5 minutes, respectively.[45,46] For unknown reasons, PAI-1 exhibits a circadian variation; the plasma concentration peaks in the morning and reaches a trough in the late afternoon and evening[47]; t-PA exhibits a diurnal variation, which is opposite to that observed for PAI-1.

INHIBITION OF PLASMIN BY ALPHA$_2$-ANTIPLASMIN. Alpha$_2$-antiplasmin forms an inactive 1:1 stoichiometric complex with plasmin. The half-life of plasmin molecules on the fibrin surface, which have both their lysine-binding sites and active site occupied, is estimated to be 2 to 3 orders of magnitude longer than that of free plasmin.

INHIBITION OF PLASMINOGEN ACTIVATORS BY PAI-1. PAI-1 reacts very rapidly with single-chain and two-chain t-PA and with two-chain u-PA (tcu-PA).[48,49] PAI-2 primarily inhibits tcu-PA.[48]

Like other serpins, PAI-1 inhibits its target proteinases by formation of a 1:1 stoichiometric reversible complex, followed by covalent binding between the hydroxyl group of the active site serine residue of the proteinase and the carboxyl group of the P1 residue at the reactive center ("bait region") of the serpin. The rapid inhibition of both t-PA and u-PA by PAI-1 involves a reversible high-affinity second-site interaction that does not depend on a functional active site. In the presence of fibrin, single-chain t-PA is protected from rapid inhibition by PAI-1. It has, however, also been reported that PAI-1 binds to fibrin and that fibrin-bound PAI-1 may inhibit t-PA–mediated fibrin clot lysis.[50]

The active form of PAI-1 converts to a latent form that can be partially reactivated by denaturing agents. In addition, inhibitory PAI-1 may not only convert to latent PAI-1, which can be reactivated, but also to substrate PAI-1, which may be irreversibly degraded by target proteinases, including t-PA, u-PA, and thrombin.[51]

PLASMINOGEN ACTIVATION BY t-PA AT THE FIBRIN SURFACE. The main role of t-PA most likely is in the dissolution of fibrin.[52] t-PA is a poor enzyme in the absence of fibrin, but the presence of fibrin strikingly enhances the activation rate of plasminogen.[53] Plasmin formed on the fibrin surface has both its lysine-binding sites and active site occupied and is thus only slowly inactivated by alpha$_2$-antiplasmin (half-life of about 10–100 s); in contrast, free plasmin, when formed, is rapidly inhibited by alpha$_2$-antiplasmin (half-life of about 0.1 s).

During fibrin clot lysis, single-chain t-PA is converted to two-chain t-PA at the fibrin surface. This conversion is probably of little physiological relevance, since the activity of single-chain t-PA and two-chain t-PA is enhanced to the same extent in the presence of fibrin or fragment X-polymer.[54]

Binding studies,[55,56] as well as kinetic studies, have revealed that Lp(a) competes with plasminogen for binding to fibrin, as a result of binding of Lp(a) to fibrin via its lysine-binding domains. As for plasminogen, binding of Lp(a) to fibrin is enhanced by partial proteolytic degradation of the fibrin surface.[55] As a functional consequence of the competition between Lp(a) and plasminogen for binding to fibrin, the fibrin-dependent enhancement of plasminogen by t-PA is inhibited.[56,57]

Pathophysiology of Fibrinolysis

Increased levels of PAI-1 activity resulting in decreased fibrinolytic capacity have been reported in several thrombotic disease states, including venous thromboembolism, obesity, sepsis, coronary artery disease, and acute myocardial infarction.[47,56] Increased levels of PAI-1 have also been found in association with the insulin resistance syndrome (see p. 1340), in which significant correlation was found between plasma PAI-1 levels and body mass index, triglyceride levels, insulin levels, and systolic blood pressure.[57] Obese people—particularly those with android obesity—also have high PAI-1 levels.[57]

Increased plasma levels of PAI-1 are one of the major disturbances of the hemostatic system in patients with coronary heart disease, and multiple interrelations with established metabolic risk factors have been observed. Increased PAI-1 levels have also been demonstrated in atherosclerotic lesions within the vessel wall. Therefore, both systemically and locally increased PAI-1 concentrations could have a pathogenic role in the development of atherosclerotic disease.[41,58–60]

Many case-control or cross-sectional studies have demonstrated high plasma PAI-1 levels in patients who have had a myocardial infarction or have had unstable angina. A relationship between deficient fibrinolysis due to high PAI activity levels and recurrent (within 3 years) myocardial infarction was demonstrated in young men who had survived a first myocardial infarction.[61] On the other hand, PAI activity was not predictive of recurrent infarction (nor was t-PA antigen) in a group of older patients followed over 5 years. In a cohort of patients with angina pectoris, high basal t-PA antigen levels were found to be associated with an increased risk of myocardial infarction, while no correlation was observed with PAI activity.[62]

Attempts to demonstrate a relationship between plasma PAI-1 levels and the severity of vessel wall damage have led to conflicting results in cross-sectional studies.[59] Recent analysis of the data of the ECAT angina pectoris study[63] demonstrated that there was a weak distinction between patients with and patients without significant coronary stenosis; the former had significantly higher plasma levels of PAI-1. No association could be observed with the extent of coronary atherosclerosis.

There are multiple interrelations between plasma PAI-1 levels and other risk factors of atherothrombosis such as those involved in the metabolic syndrome of insulin resistance. In the ECAT angina pectoris study, in which insulin determination was available for almost 1500 patients, twofold to threefold differences in PAI-1 levels were observed when comparing the lowest and the highest quintile of insulin, body mass index, or triglyceride.[64]

In addition, lipoprotein(a) (Lp[a]) was shown to enhance PAI-1 synthesis by endothelial cells in culture, and it was suggested that Lp(a) binding to endothelium and subsequent increased PAI-1 expression may contribute to the generation of a specific prothrombotic endothelial phenotype.[65]

ANTITHROMBOTIC DRUGS

Unfractionated Heparin, Low Molecular Weight Heparins, and Heparinoids

UNFRACTIONATED HEPARIN (Table 58–1). The term *heparin* refers not to a single structure but rather to a family of mucopolysaccharide chains of varying length and composition.[65a] Heparin by itself has no anticoagulant property. It accelerates the action of two naturally occurring plasma inhibitors, forming a 1:1 stoichiometric complex with antithrombin III (an inhibitor of thrombin and activated factors X, IX, and XI) and, at very high doses, with heparin co-factor II, which acts only on thrombin decay. Heparin contains a unique pentasaccharide that has a high-affinity binding sequence for antithrombin III. This sequence is present in only one-third of heparin molecules and is not required for binding to heparin co-factor II.

Factor Xa bound to platelets and thrombin bound to the endothelium or to fibrin (thrombus) are protected from inactivation by heparin-antithrombin III complex.[66,67] In plasma, approximately 20 times more heparin is needed to inactivate fibrin-bound thrombin than to inactivate free thrombin.[66] This explains why more heparin is needed to prevent the extension of venous thrombosis than to prevent formation of the initial thrombus.

Heparin is not absorbed by the gastrointestinal mucosa. When in the bloodstream after parenteral administration, heparin binds to endothelial cells, mononuclear macrophages, and numerous plasma proteins. Some of these neutralize anticoagulant activity (e.g., platelet factor 4, vitronectin), while others such as von Willebrand factor lose their function. Elevated levels of these heparin-binding proteins explain the different individual heparin dose requirements to obtain the same antithrombotic effect and the so-called heparin resistance in patients with inflammatory and malignant diseases.[67] Binding of heparin to the endothelium and various plasma proteins reduces bioavailability at low concentrations and causes variability of response to fixed doses of anticoagulant.[67]

The pharmacokinetics of heparin are complicated; suffice it to say that the anticoagulant response increases disproportionately in intensity and duration as the dose increases. This explains why the anticoagulant effect of heparin has to be closely monitored. At present, no completely satisfactory test measuring the generation of thrombin and the levels of antithrombin is available. The most commonly used test is the activated partial thromboplastin time (APTT), which is sensitive to the inhibitory effect of heparin on thrombin, factor X, and factor IX. Unfortunately, the different commercial APTT reagents vary in their response to heparin, and there are technical variables. The therapeutic level of the APTT should therefore be established in each clinical laboratory to correspond to 0.2 to 0.4 units of heparin per milliliter plasma by protamine titration[67] or to 0.2 to 0.7 units of factor Xa per milliliter plasma by the chromogenic substrate assay for the determination of antifactor Xa activity.[68] A nomogram may help, but should be adapted to the responsiveness of the reagent and APTT test system in use in the local laboratory.[68]

The most common and major side effect of heparin is bleeding. The risk is higher when unfractionated heparin is given by intermittent (14.2 per cent) rather than continuous infusion (6.8 per cent) or subcutaneous route (4.1 per cent). Also, the dose of heparin, the patient's anticoagulant response, serious concurrent illness, and chronic consumption of alcohol may predispose to bleeding. Heparin-induced thrombocytopenia (HIT) occurs in 2.4 per cent of patients receiving therapeutic heparin and 0.3 per cent receiving prophylactic heparin. In addition, vascular occlusion occurs in 0.4 per cent.[67] Rare complications are osteoporosis, alopecia, skin necrosis, urticaria, and transient increase of hepatic transaminases.

TABLE 58–1 COMPARISON OF SOME PROPERTIES OF UNFRACTIONATED HEPARIN, LMW HEPARIN AND HIRUDIN

UNFRACTIONATED HEPARIN	LMW HEPARIN	HIRUDIN
Inhibits to the same extent thrombin and factor VII, much less IXa and XIa	Inhibits mainly factor Xa, thrombin to some extent	Specific and potent inhibitor of thrombin
Antithrombin III-dependent	Antithrombin III-dependent	Antithrombin III-independent
Neutralized by heparinase, several plasma proteins, platelet factor 4, and endothelium	Neutralized by heparinase, weak endothelium, binding	Not neutralized by heparinase, endothelium, macrophages, fibrin monomer, and plasma proteins
Does not inactivate clot-bound thrombin and factor VII	Does not inactivate clot-bound thrombin and factor VII	Inactivates clot-bound thrombin
Inhibits platelet function	Inhibits platelet function	Prevents thrombin-induced aggregation but not other platelet agonists
Induced thrombocytopenia not rare	Can induce thrombocytopenia	Does not induce thrombocytopenia
Bioavailability after sc injection 30%	Bioavailability after sc injection > 90%	Good bioavailability after sc injection, about 85%
Poor dose-effect response	Fair dose-effect response	Fair dose-effect response
Not immunogenic	Not immunogenic	Not or barely immunogenic
Transient increase of liver enzymes common	Transient increase of liver enzymes possible	No liver toxicity
Increases vascular permeability	No increase of vascular permeability	No increase of vascular permeability

LMW = low molecular weight; SC = subcutaneous.

LOW MOLECULAR WEIGHT HEPARINS. Some of the limitations of unfractionated heparin can be overcome with low molecular weight (LMW) heparins (mean MW 4000 to 5000; range 1000 to 10,000) (Table 58–1). These LMW heparins produce their major anticoagulant effect by binding to antithrombin III through the same high-affinity pentasaccharide sequence of unfractionated heparin, which, however, is present in only one-third of the LMW molecules. A minimum additional chain length of 15 saccharides (MW > 5400) is required for the inactivation of thrombin, but the inactivation of factor X requires only the pentasaccharide. Unfractionated heparin has by definition an antifactor Xa to antithrombin-III ratio of 1:1, which is between 4:1 and 2:1 for the various LMW heparins. Drugs with high antifactor Xa activity were indeed designed based on the hypothesis that inhibition of earlier steps in the blood coagulation system would be associated with a more potent antithrombotic effect than inhibiting subsequent steps. This is because of the amplification process inherent in the coagulation cascade; that is, a single factor Xa molecule can lead to the generation of multiple thrombin molecules.

The advantages of LMW heparins over unfractionated heparin are numerous (Table 58–1). Factor Xa bound to the platelet membrane in the prothrombinase complex is resistant to inactivation by unfractionated heparin, but is not resistant to inactivation by LMW heparins. Also, LMW heparins have lesser binding characteristics to platelet factor 4, other plasma proteins, and endothelial cells, resulting in higher bioavailability (after subcutaneous injection > 90 versus 30 per cent for unfractionated heparin); reduced plasma clearance, which is independent of dose and plasma concentration; a longer half-life (anti-Xa activity between 3 and 4 hours for LMW heparins versus 30 to 150 minutes for unfractionated heparin); and less interindividual variability of the anticoagulant response.[70] LMW heparins have lower affinity for von Willebrand factor,[71] increase vascular permeability less than unfractionated heparin, and have a weak effect on platelet function. These differences could explain why LMW heparins produce less bleeding than unfractionated heparin with equivalent or higher antithrombotic effect in experimental animals[70] and in some clinical studies.[72–75]

The long half-life of LMW heparins and their predictable anticoagulant response to weight-adjusted doses allow once-daily subcutaneous administration without laboratory monitoring.[70]

It has been observed that thrombocytopenia is more common with unfractionated heparin than with low molecular weight heparin.[76,77]

HEPARINOIDS: MIXTURE OF LOW MOLECULAR WEIGHT SULFATE GLYCOSAMINOGLYCANS. Danaparoid sodium (Org 10172) is a low molecular weight heparinoid (6 kDa) and consists of a polydisperse mixture comprising sulfated glycosaminoglycuronans derived from animal mucosa, heparan sulfate (83 per cent w/w), of which 4 to 5 per cent has high affinity for antithrombin III dermatan sulfate (12 per cent w/w) and a minor amount of chondroitin sulfate (5 per cent w/w).[78–81] Its anticoagulant profile is characterized by a high ratio of anti-factor Xa/antithrombin activity (14 over < 0.5), resulting in effective inhibition of thrombin generation. The anti-Xa activity is mediated by antithrombin III and is not inactivated by endogenous heparin-neutralizing factors. The low antithrombin activity is mediated by heparin co-factor II and antithrombin III. In contrast to heparin, danaparoid sodium shows hardly any or no effect on blood platelet function in vitro or in vivo. Danaparoid sodium is essentially free of contaminating heparin, has minimal cross reactivity in in vitro assays for HIT, and has been used successfully in patients with this complication.

After intravenous and subcutaneous administration of danaparoid sodium the antithrombin activity half-life of danaparoid sodium is shorter (1.8 hours) than its anti-factor Xa half-life (17.6 hours). Danaparoid sodium has absolute bioavailability of 100 per cent after subcutaneous administration.

Danaparoid sodium is effective in the prevention of deep vein thrombosis in patients with thrombotic stroke and after elective hip surgery or hip fracture.[82] The long half-life of danaparoid sodium, which is not effectively neutralized by protamine, has been rather difficult to manage clinically.

Coumarin-Type Oral Anticoagulants

Warfarin sodium and related coumarin congeners are effective antithrombotic compounds that differ in speed in their inhibition of vitamin K-2,3 epoxide within hepatic chromosomes.[65a] These compounds depress the synthesis of four vitamin K–dependent procoagulants (factors II, VII, IX, and X) and of two natural inhibitor proteins, C and S. The plasma concentration of these proteins will decrease in accord with their half-life. The coagulation components with the shortest half-life are the procoagulant factor VII and the endogenous anticoagulant protein C. This may cause frank imbalance at the start of treatment and lead to thrombosis of skin capillaries and venules with cutaneous necrosis.[83]

MONITORING OF COUMARIN THERAPY. The intensity of the effect of warfarin on the synthesis of coagulation factors differs among patients; moreover, in the same individual it may, over time, vary considerably. This explains the need for close monitoring by having daily blood tests in the first week of treatment with warfarin. The test used is the *prothrombin time,* a term that leads to confusion because the assay depends in fact on the global activity of five coagulation factors (prothrombin, factors V, VII, IX and X). Among the six factors whose synthesis is inhibited by coumarin derivatives, three (prothrombin and factors VII and X) are effectively measured by this test, but not factor IX and the anticoagulant proteins C and S. On the other hand, the prothrombin time is also sensitive to factor V, a coagulation protein independent of vitamin K.

To determine the prothrombin time a tissue extract (thromboplastin) and calcium are added to citrated plasma, and the time to fibrin formation is measured. Commercial thromboplastin reagents extracted by different methods from various organs and species vary extensively in their sensitivity to reductions in levels of vitamin K–dependent factors. To standardize prothrombin time determinations, and thus allow direct comparison of results obtained with different thromboplastins, the International Normalized Ratio (INR) is recommended but not yet universally applied.[84]

At the start of warfarin treatment the prothrombin time is first prolonged by factor VII depletion because factor VII has a half-life much shorter than the other vitamin K–dependent coagulation factors (II, IX, and X). Thus, in the beginning of warfarin treatment, the prothrombin time is prolonged while the intrinsic and common coagulation pathways are still uninfluenced. This explains why in switching from heparin to warfarin, heparin should be continued unabated for at least 1 day after the prothrombin time (INR) has reached therapeutic values. Also, during long-term warfarin therapy, prothrombin times should be checked regularly, as many drugs and foods can enhance or decrease the warfarin effect. Certain intercurrent diseases (hepatic failure, heart failure, hyperthyroidism) may also modify warfarin dose requirements. Bleeding is the most important side effect, and the risk may vary from patient to patient, depending upon the presence of co-morbid conditions (hypertension, malignant disease, older age, recent surgery) and the intensity of anticoagulation. Patients with intensive anticoagulation (INR 2.5 to 4) have during the first 3 months a risk of clinically important bleeding over 2 times greater (14 versus 6 per cent) than those with less intensive anticoagulation (INR 2.0 to 2.5).[85] On average, the overall annual risk of bleeding is 6 per cent, with major and fatal bleeding incidence estimated to be 2 and 0.8 per cent, respectively.

A rare, nonhemorrhagic side effect of warfarin is coumarin-induced skin necrosis, an unexplained complication that occurs between the third and eighth day of therapy. The rapid decline in protein C level is postulated to play a role in the obscure pathogenesis of thrombosis of skin venules and capillaries within the subcutaneous fat, usually in the lower part of the body.[83] Coumarin drugs readily cross the placenta and may be teratogenic, particularly during the first trimester of pregnancy.[86]

In conclusion, vitamin K antagonists are effective antithrombotic drugs with a narrow risk/benefit ratio that require regular monitoring and a disciplined patient. Their main virtues are oral administration and low cost.

Inhibitors of Platelet Function

Several strategies are currently being used to reduce platelet function[65a] (Fig. 58–4). These include inhibition of platelet enzyme prostaglandin synthase (aspirin, sulfinpyrazone, flurbiprofen, indobufen), inhibition of thromboxane synthase, blockade of endoperoxide-thromboxane receptors or inhibition of the activation pathway of GPIIb/IIIa (ticlopidine, clopidogrel). Inhibition of platelet function was also obtained by modulation of platelet adenylate or guanylate cyclase (stable prostacyclin analogs), interference with the function of the platelet glycoprotein Ib-IX receptor (monoclonal antibodies to GP1b-IX, synthetic peptides to the A1 von Willebrand factor domain, recombinant von Willebrand fragments covering the A1 domain, aurin tricarboxylic acid), specific blockers of the IIb/IIIa receptor (monoclonal antibodies, natural antagonists, synthetic peptides containing the Arg-Gly-Asp [RGD] sequence or nonpeptide inhibitors), and peptides that bind to but do not activate the platelet-receptor domain that interacts with thrombin. In this chapter, only platelet inhibitors that have been investigated in therapeutic trials are discussed. Several reviews on inhibitors of platelet function have recently been published.[87–91]

ASPIRIN. Several pathways lead to platelet aggregation (Fig. 58–12). Aspirin very selectively inhibits thromboxane (TXA2) formation but only partially impedes platelet aggregation induced by ADP, collagen, and low concentrations of thrombin. Aspirin does not inhibit adherence of the initial layer of platelets to the subendothelium or atherosclerotic plaques, and the release of granule contents is not opposed. Thus the effects of platelet-derived growth factors and other mitogens on smooth muscle cells are not inhibited (Table 58–2).[92]

The ideal dose of aspirin for primary or secondary prevention of cardiovascular disease is not determined. Doses between 324 and 1300 mg daily seem to induce a similar reduction of cardiovascular complications, while doses between 1 and 2 mg/kg daily produce virtually complete inhibition of cyclo-oxygenase–dependent platelet aggregation.[93] Slow-release aspirins are associated with few gastrointestinal side effects, particularly when an enteric coated preparation is used. There is increasing evidence that the antithrombotic effect of aspirin is due not only to its inhibition of platelet oxygenase. Aspirin also impairs thrombinogenesis by a mechanism that seems to be unrelated to platelet cyclo-oxygenase; for instance, the acetylation of GTP-binding proteins, thrombin receptors, and prothrombin.[94,95] The salicylate moiety of aspirin also antagonizes the lipoxygenase pathway of arachidonate metabolism in platelets, and the demonstration of two cyclo-oxygenase enzymes (COX-1, COX-2)[96] may further elucidate the antithrombotic mechanism of aspirin.[97]

TICLOPIDIN, CLOPIDOGREL. These two thienopyridine derivatives can be considered bioprecursors, since they are inactive in vitro but potent antiaggregating agents in vivo, indicating the importance of at least one active transient metabolite. Ticlopidine and its chemical analog clopidogrel are noncompetitive but selective antagonists of ADP-induced platelet aggregation and act by specifically blocking glycoprotein IIb/IIIa (GPIIb/IIIa) activation specific for the ADP pathway (Fig. 58–4). Since the two compounds are chemically related, their mechanism of action is considered similar.[98,99] The binding of fibrinogen to GPIIb/IIIa complex, triggered by ADP, is dramatically inhibited; this inhibition is not due to direct modification of the glycoprotein complex.[100]

TABLE 58–2 ASPIRIN AS PLATELET INHIBITOR

Inhibits only TXA_2 pathway; much less inhibition of platelet activation by thrombin, ADP, and collagen and not by PAF
Provides no inhibition of platelet adhesion
Has no effect on smooth muscle cell proliferation
Prolongs bleeding time
Can induce gastrointestinal problems
Can induce allergy (rare)

ADP = adenosine diphosphate; PAF = platelet activating factor.

Clopidogrel is approximately 40 to 100 times as active as ticlopidine in inhibiting ADP-induced platelet aggregation in animal models, but about 6 times as potent as ticlopidine in inhibition of ADP-induced aggregation of human platelets.

The effectiveness of ticlopidine has been convincingly demonstrated in patients at high risk of arterial thromboembolic events, i.e., those with transient ischemic cerebral attacks and stroke, peripheral arterial or ischemic heart disease.[101–103] A trial in more than 3000 patients has shown that ticlopidine has a more pronounced effect on death from all causes or nonfatal stroke than aspirin.[104,105]

The most potentially serious problem of ticlopidine is bone marrow depression (leukopenia, thrombocytopenia, pancytopenia); close monitoring is therefore essential for at least the first 12 weeks of ticlopidine therapy.[101] Ticlopidine has also been associated with an increase in total cholesterol levels by 9 per cent.[104] Clopidogrel was developed because this compound was not toxic to bone marrow pluripotent stem cells in the mouse (Till and McCullogh test).

THROMBOXANE SYNTHASE INHIBITORS. Thromboxane synthase inhibitors have been developed with the expectation of not only suppressing TXA_2 biosynthesis but also sparing or even enhancing the formation of prostacyclin (PGI_2) by the vascular endothelium (Fig. 58–4). Most thromboxane synthase inhibitors have moderate potency and short duration of action and do not result in sufficiently sustained inhibition of TXA_2 production to be clinically effective.[106] Although thromboxane synthase inhibitors have shown some benefit in experimental models, their effects in clinical trials in patients with coronary artery disease have been disappointing.

THROMBOXANE RECEPTOR BLOCKERS. The more recently developed thromboxane receptor blockers specifically impede the action of both TXA_2 and endoperoxides on their presumed common receptors on platelets and prevent vasoconstriction induced by TXA_2 (Fig. 58–4). These agents leave the normal pattern of thromboxane and PGI_2 for-

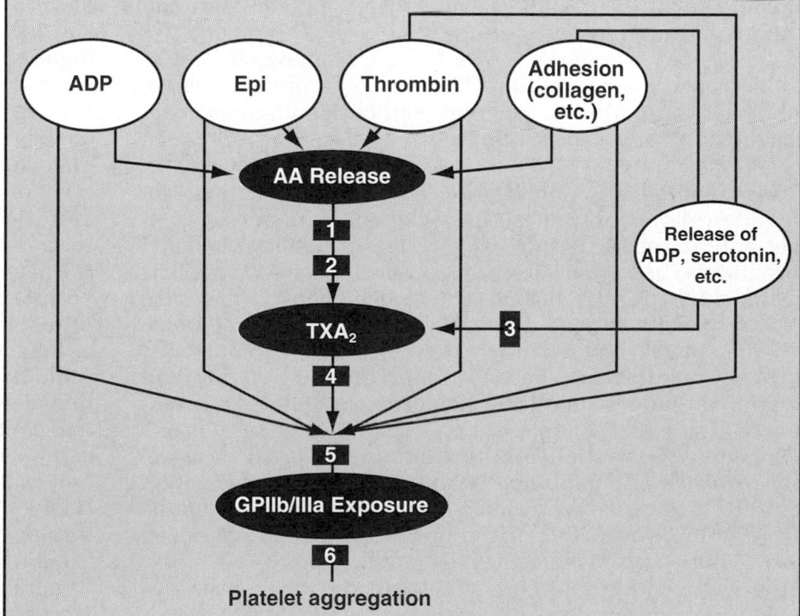

FIGURE 58–12. Pathways of platelet activation. Exposure of GPIIb/IIIa receptors at the platelet surface is the final common endpoint of all pathways. AA = arachidonic acid; ADP = adenosine diphosphate; Epi = epinephrine; TXA_2 = thromboxane A_2.

mation unaltered. Thromboxane receptor antagonists prolong bleeding time more than thromboxane synthase inhibitors. As expected, TXA_2 synthesis is not inhibited, and PGI_2 generation is not augmented by specific thromboxane/endoperoxide receptor antagonists.

Several of the thromboxane/endoperoxide receptor blockers are relatively short acting, and the magnitude of their blockade is modest.[106]

COMBINED THROMBOXANE SYNTHASE INHIBITORS AND RECEPTOR BLOCKERS. Some compounds have a dual activity. Ridogrel is a potent TXA_2 synthase inhibitor with modest additional TXA_2/prostaglandin endoperoxide receptor antagonist properties (at least 100-fold less).[107] Although the animal pharmacology was very promising, the preclinical evaluation has been disappointing.[106] Picotamide is a rather weak thromboxane synthase inhibitor and receptor blocker.[108]

BLOCKERS OF THE PLATELET GLYCOPROTEIN IIb/IIIa RECEPTOR (Figs. 58–1 and 58–12). Exposure of GPIIb/IIa receptors at the platelet surface is the final common endpoint of all pathways leading to platelet aggregation (Fig. 58–1).

Monoclonal Antibodies (7E3). The first platelet GPIIb/IIIa antagonists to be developed were murine monoclonal antibodies.[109] In vitro, these antibodies completely inhibit platelet aggregation and, in animal models of angioplasty injury and thrombolysis, prevent thrombosis and augment the activity of thrombolytic agents. Because of concerns about their immunogenicity, the derivative product chimeric monoclonal 7E3Fab (c7E3Fab, abciximab) was created via genetic recombination. This new molecule consists of the mouse-derived variable regions from the original molecule linked to the constant region derived from human immunoglobulin IgG. Data from a dose-escalation study[110] and a pilot therapeutic trial[111] suggested an abciximab dosing regimen that was evaluated in patients with high-risk percutaneous transluminal coronary angioplasty (PTCA)[112,113] (Table 39–2, p. 1370). As compared with placebo, an abciximab bolus of 0.25 mg/kg followed by an infusion of 10 μg/kg/hour for 12 hours in 2099 patients resulted in a 35 per cent reduction in the rate of the primary endpoints (death, nonfatal myocardial infarction, unplanned surgical revascularization, unplanned repeat PTCA, stent or balloon pump for refractory ischemia.) However, bleeding episodes and transfusions were more frequent in patients treated with abciximab. At 6 months, the absolute difference in patients with a major ischemic event or elective revascularization was 8.1 per cent between the placebo group and abciximab bolus-plus-infusion group.

To be effective, more than 90 per cent of the GPIIb/IIIa receptors have to be blocked. This is associated with a very prolonged bleeding time and risk of bleeding without an antidote being available. Moreover, even chimeric monoclonal antibodies contain some murine proteins and can still be immunogenic.

The same drawbacks prevail for cysteine-rich single-chain snake venom peptides binding to GPIIb/IIIa, which, moreover, have a lower potency than chimeric monoclonal abciximab. Their shorter half-life may be an advantage in case of bleeding.

Synthetic IIb/IIIa Inhibitors. The synthetic antiplatelet peptides, particularly those in cyclic configuration, are potent antithrombotic agents when tested in platelet-mediated thrombosis in various experimental animals. While short cyclic synthetic peptides have a higher potency, they also lack specificity for the GPIIb/IIIa receptors and recognize receptors on several integrins. The most potent compounds, at doses required for effective inhibition of in vivo thrombus formation, also induce a hemorrhagic tendency as witnessed by marked prolongation of the bleeding time.[114] Structure-activity studies have resulted in partial dissociation between the inhibition of ex vivo platelet aggregation and bleeding time prolongation and suggest that it might be possible to obtain GPIIb/IIIa antagonists with an optimized antithrombotic versus hemorrhagic ratio.[114]

The nonpeptide inhibitors are reversible antagonists and have obvious advantages compared to monoclonal antibodies as their effects are much shorter (3 hours for tirofiban [MK-383] versus 3 days for abciximab), they have no immunogenicity and have the potential to be active orally. Lamifiban (RO43-5054) is a nonpeptide, low molecular weight GPIIb/IIIa antagonist almost 1000 times more active than RGDS (Arg-Gly-Asp-Ser) in inhibiting platelet aggregation in human platelet-rich plasma.[115]

SC-5468A is a prodrug of a nonpeptide mimetic of the tetrapeptide RGDS. The active metabolite SC-54701A, is a potent inhibitor of GPIIb/IIIa receptors and exhibits specificity for this receptor with respect to other integrins.[116] Fradafibran (BIBU 104XX) is the orally available prodrug of the GPIIb/IIIa receptor antagonist BIBU 52 and has a mean residence time of approximately 12 hours.[117] At these oral doses GPIIb/IIIa receptors were blocked by more than 80 per cent in a reversible and dose-proportional manner.

Specific Thrombin Inhibitors

HIRUDIN (Table 58–1). Natural hirudin is a single-chain, carbohydrate-free polypeptide containing three intramolecular disulfide bridges and a sulfated tyrosine residue. The polypeptide chain contains 65 amino acids with a molecular weight of approximately 7000 daltons. Recombinant hirudin has been obtained using *Escherichia coli* and yeast. With both methods, hirudin is expressed as desulfatohirudin lacking the sulfate residue on tyrosine 63. The nonsulfated molecules result in about a 10-fold reduction in thrombin affinity.[118] Unlike heparin, which requires endogenous co-factors for activity (mainly antithrombin III, heparin co-factor II), hirudin does not need a co-factor for its anticoagulant activity and therefore is still active in states of deficiency of these proteins.

Hirudin is a specific potent inhibitor of thrombin to which it binds with extraordinary tightness (KD 2 × 10 − 14 M) near the active center at the substrate recognition site. In addition, there are multiple other contacts between hirudin and thrombin over an extended area of the molecule forming a highly stable noncovalent complex. All known functions of thrombin are inhibited.

The terminal half-life of r-hirudin in healthy young volunteers is 50 to 65 minutes, with a half-life of its effect on the APTT of about 2 hours.[119–122] Recombinant hirudin appears to be a weak allergen. Hirudin-specific IgE antibodies were rarely seen in 163 immunocompetent healthy volunteers receiving recombinant hirudin twice at an interval of 1 month.[123]

In contrast to unfractionated and LMW heparins, hirudin penetrates the thrombus and neutralizes thrombin bound to fibrin. Hirudin, but not heparin, reduces platelet deposition and thrombus growth on deep wall injury at both low- and high-shear rate conditions. As hirudin is not inhibited by plasma proteins and endothelium, while unfractionated heparin is, the anticoagulant effect of hirudin is more predictable. Hirudin, a specific inhibitor of thrombin, prevents platelet aggregation induced by thrombin but does not oppose platelet aggregation by other agonists. Unfractionated and LMW heparins can induce thrombocytopenia; this untoward effect has not been observed with hirudin.

On the negative side, there is no antidote for hirudin. Furthermore, hirudin inhibits also the interaction between thrombin and thrombomodulin, a prerequisite for activation of the endogenous coagulation inhibitory proteins C and S.

HIRULOG. Hirulog is a bifunctional 20-amino acid peptide designed on the structure of hirudin. It combines a fragment of the C-terminus of hirudin (interacting with the anion-binding exosite of thrombin) with an N-terminus fragment [D-Phe-Pro-Arg-Pro(Gly)], which interacts with the catalytic site of thrombin.[124,125] There is no antidote for hirulog.

ARGATROBAN. This arginine derivative that binds to thrombin with intermediate affinity (KD 3.9 × 10 − 8 M) is a competitive antagonist inhibiting fibrinogen cleavage and platelet activation by thrombin. Compared to heparin, argatroban is significantly more effective in the prevention of platelet-rich thrombi after vascular injury and was effective at APTTs of only 2 to 3 × baseline control.[126,127]

THROMBOLYTIC DRUGS

STREPTOKINASE. This is a nonenzyme protein produced by several strains of hemolytic streptococci; it consists of a single polypeptide chain of 414 amino acids with a molecular weight of 47,000 to 50,000. Streptokinase cannot directly cleave peptide bonds, but it activates plasminogen to plasmin indirectly, following a three-step mechanism.[128] In the first step, streptokinase forms an equimolar complex with plasminogen. This complex undergoes a conformational change resulting in the exposure of an active site in the plasminogen moiety. In the second step, this active site catalyzes the activation of plasminogen to plasmin. In a third step, plasminogen-streptokinase molecules are converted to plasmin-streptokinase complexes.[129] The active site residues in the plasmin-streptokinase complex are the same as those in the plasmin molecule. However, plasmin is unable to activate plasminogen, whereas the plasmin(ogen)-streptokinase complex is not inhibited by alpha$_2$-antiplasmin.

Most individuals have measurable circulating streptokinase-neutralizing antibodies, which may result from previous infections with beta-hemolytic streptococci. Therefore, during thrombolytic therapy, sufficient streptokinase must be infused to neutralize these antibodies. A few days after streptokinase administration, the antistreptokinase titer rises rapidly to 50 to 100 times the preinfusion value and remains high for 4 to 6 months, during which period renewed treatment with streptokinase is impracticable.[130]

ANISOYLATED PLASMINOGEN-STREPTOKINASE COMPLEX. Anisoylated plasminogen-streptokinase activator complex (APSAC, anistreplase) was constructed with the aim of controlling the enzymatic activity of the plasmin(ogen)-streptokinase complex by a specific reversible chemical protection of its catalytic center (i.e., by titration with a p-anisoyl group).[131] Deacylation of anistreplase uncovers the catalytic center, which converts plasminogen to plasmin. A plasma half-life of 70 minutes was found for anistreplase compared with 25 minutes for the plasminogen-streptokinase complex formed in vivo after administration of streptokinase.[132] Patients with a high titer of streptokinase antibodies do not respond to anistreplase, and anistreplase causes a marked increase in the streptokinase antibody titer within 2 to 3 weeks, which persists for months.

UROKINASE. Two-chain urokinase-type plasminogen activator (tcu-PA), a trypsin-like serine proteinase composed of two polypeptide chains (Mr 20,000 and 34,000) has been isolated from human urine[133] and from cultured human embryonic kidney cells.[134] Extensive plasminogen activation and depletion of α_2-antiplasmin may occur following treatment of thromboembolic diseases with tcu-PA, leading to degradation of several plasma proteins, including fibrinogen, factor V, and factor VIII.

PROUROKINASE. Single-chain urokinase-type plasminogen activator (scu-PA, pro-urokinase) is a naturally occurring human protein first isolated from natural sources and then produced through recombinant DNA technology.[135,136] scu-PA is the native zymogenic precursor of urokinase. Limited hydrolysis by plasmin or kallikrein of the Lys158-Ile159 peptide bond converts the molecule to two-chain urokinase-type plasminogen activator (tcu-PA, urokinase), which is held together by one disulfide bond that is essential for the thrombolytic activity. A fully active tcu-PA derivative is obtained after additional proteolysis at position Lys135-Lys136.

TISSUE-TYPE PLASMINOGEN ACTIVATOR (see also p. 1816). Native tissue-type plasminogen activator (t-PA) is a serine proteinase with a molecular weight of about 70,000, composed of one polypeptide chain containing 527 amino acids with serine as aminoterminal amino acid[137] (Fig. 58–11). t-PA is converted by plasmin to a two-chain form by hydrolysis of the Arg275-Ile276 peptide bond. The two-chain form is held together by one interchain disulfide bond. t-PA for clinical use is presently produced by recombinant DNA technology (Activase, Genentech Inc., or Actilyse, Boehringer Ingelheim GmbH, Germany) and consists mainly of the single-chain form.

The activation of plasminogen by t-PA, both in the presence and in the absence of fibrin, follows Michaelis-Menten kinetics.[53] Although different kinetic constants were obtained by several investigators, there is a consensus that the presence of fibrin enhances the efficiency of plasminogen activation by t-PA by 2 to 3 orders of magnitude.[53] The kinetic data support a mechanism in which fibrin provides a surface to which t-PA and plasminogen adsorb in a sequential and ordered way, yielding a cyclic ternary complex. Fibrin essentially increases the local plasminogen concentration by creating an additional interaction between t-PA and its substrate. The high affinity of t-PA for plasminogen in the presence of fibrin thus allows efficient activation on the fibrin clot, while no efficient plasminogen activation by t-PA occurs in plasma.

Plasmin formed on the fibrin surface has both its lysine-binding sites and active sites occupied and is thus only slowly inactivated by α_2-antiplasmin (half-life about 10 to 100 s); free plasmin, when formed, is rapidly inhibited by α_2-antiplasmin (half-life about 0.1 s). The fibrinolytic process thus seems to be triggered by and confined to fibrin.

MUTANTS AND VARIANTS OF t-PA

Several mutants of recombinant tissue-type plasminogen activator (rt-PA) have been constructed with interesting properties, including slower clearance from the circulation, more selective binding to fibrin, stronger stimulation by fibrin, and resistance to plasma protease inhibitors.[138,139]

RETEPLASE. This is a single-chain nonglycosylated deletion variant of r-PA consisting only of the kringle 2 and the protease domain of human t-PA. Production of reteplase in *Escherichia coli* leads to formation of inactive protein aggregates (inclusion bodies). The isolation of the inclusion bodies, the refolding, and the chromatographic purification of reteplase have been described.[140,141] The active site of the protease domain of reteplase and of t-PA, and their plasminogenolytic activity in the absence of a stimulator, do not differ, but the plasminogenolytic activity of reteplase in the presence of CNBr fragments of fibrinogen as a stimulator was fourfold lower compared to t-PA, whereas the binding of reteplase to fibrin was five times lower. These differences in plasminogenolytic activity and fibrin binding between the two molecules might possibly be due to the missing finger domain in reteplase. It is known that fibrin binding is mediated through both the finger domain and the lysine-binding site in the kringle 2 domain of t-PA.

Reteplase and t-PA are inhibited by PAI-1 to a similar degree, but the affinity of reteplase for binding to endothelial cells and monocytes is reduced, probably as a consequence of deletion of the finger and epidermal growth factor domains in reteplase, which seem to be involved in the interaction with endothelial cell receptors. The thrombolytic properties of reteplase and alteplase (recombinant t-PA) were compared in the rabbit jugular vein thrombosis model. The effective dose for 50 per cent thrombolysis (ED50) was 163 kU/kg (0.28 mg/kg) for reteplase, and 871 kU/kg (1.09 mg/kg) for alteplase, indicating 5.3 (3.9)-fold higher potency of reteplase. At equipotent doses (50 per cent thrombolysis), the residual concentration of fibrinogen was 74.2 per cent with reteplase and 76.5 per cent with alteplase. Pharmacokinetic analysis of plasma activity at a dose of 400 kU/kg in the rabbit revealed a half-life of 18.9 ± 1.5 minutes for reteplase and 2.1 ± 0.1 minutes for alteplase. Plasma clearance for reteplase was 4.3-fold slower than for alteplase (4.7 versus 1.2 ml/min/kg). One may therefore conclude that the higher potency of reteplase is due to its slower clearance.[141] An initial half-life of 14 to 18 minutes was also observed with reteplase in healthy human volunteers[142,143] and in patients with acute myocardial infarction.[144]

Dose-ranging studies of bolus reteplase were performed in a multicenter trial.[145] With a dose of 10 million units (MU) of reteplase, a patent infarct-related coronary artery (TIMI-3) was obtained at 30 minutes in 46 per cent, at 60 minutes in 48 per cent, at 90 minutes in 52 per cent, and at 24 to 48 hours in 88 per cent of patients with acute myocardial infarction. With 15 MU a higher angiographic patency rate at the same time intervals was obtained (38, 58, 69, and 85 per cent). Because there was a 20 per cent (10 MU) and 12.5 per cent (15 MU) reocclusion rate between the 30-minute and 90-minute angiogram, the administration of a second smaller bolus of reteplase (5 MU) 30 minutes after the initial bolus (10 MU) was investigated in an open uncontrolled study.[146] Patency rates (TIMI-3) reached 50 per cent at 60 minutes, 58 per cent at 90 minutes, and 84 per cent at 24 to 48 hours. Only 1 of the 50 patients studied had reocclusion in the first 24 to 48 hours. In a controlled study in 605 patients with acute myocardial infarction, different bolus doses of reteplase (single dose of 15 MU, 10 MU and 5 MU 30 minutes later, 10 MU and 10 MU 30 minutes later) were compared with the conventional-dose regimen of alteplase (100 mg over 3 hours). TIMI-3 patency rates at 90 minutes were obtained with the given reteplase regimen in 42.7, 45.4, 62.9 per cent, respectively, and in 47.6 per cent of patients treated with alteplase.[147] The difference between the 10 MU + 10 MU reteplase and alteplase arms is significant (p = 0.01). Recently, a direct comparison of reteplase versus frontloading t-PA (100 mg over 90 minutes) was completed. A large-scale, double-blind trial in 6010 patients with acute myocardial infarction demonstrates that there is a nonsignificant difference between 35-day mortality in patients treated with streptokinase (1.5 MU over 60 minutes) and reteplase (two boluses of 10 MU given 30 minutes apart [9.53 and 9.02 per cent, respectively]).[148]

rt-PA-TNK. An rt-PA mutant in which Thr103 is substituted by Asn (code rt-PA-T) and the sequence Lys296-His-Arg-Arg is mutagenized to Ala-Ala-Ala-Ala (code rt-PA-K) was found to have both a prolonged half-life and resistance to PAI-1.[149] This mutant has increased potency on platelet-rich arterial thrombi (rich in PAI-1) in a canine model of coronary thrombosis. Additional substitution in this mutant of Asn117 by Gln (code rt-PA-N) resulted in a t-PA variant with 8-fold slower clearance and 200-fold enhanced resistance to PAI-1. These three combinations in a single molecule are referred to as rt-PA-TNK. In in vivo models of thrombolysis in rabbits, rt-PA-TNK was shown to have increased thrombolytic potency on platelet-rich clots, to conserve fibrinogen, and to be effective upon bolus administration at half the dose of rt-PA.[149] Similar results were obtained in a combined arterial and venous thrombosis model in the dog.[150] A pilot dose-finding clinical trial was recently completed (TIMI 10) and large scale clinical trials in patients with acute myocardial infarction are planned.

RECOMBINANT CHIMERIC PLASMINOGEN ACTIVATORS. Recombinant chimeric plasminogen activators have been constructed primarily using different regions of t-PA and scu-PA, although several alternative combinations have been evaluated to some extent.[138,139] Only a small feasibility study of coronary thrombolysis with K1K2Pu has been performed in patients with acute myocardial infarction.[151]

DESMODUS SALIVARY PLASMINOGEN ACTIVATOR. The subsistence of vampire bats on a diet of fresh blood is apparently contingent on their ability to interfere with the hemostatic system of the blood donor. The saliva of vampire bats contains a variety of factors that presumably satisfy two essential requirements: to maintain prolonged bleeding from the wound and to preserve blood fluidity following ingestion of a meal.[152] Different molecular forms of the *Desmodus* salivary plasminogen activator (DSPA) have been purified, characterized, cloned, and expressed.[153]

STAPHYLOKINASE. Mature staphylokinase consists of 136 amino acids in a single polypeptide chain without disulfide bridges. Staphylokinase, like streptokinase, is not an enzyme, but it forms a 1:1 stoichiometric complex with plasmin(ogen) that activates other plasminogen molecules.[154] Streptokinase and plasminogen produce a complex that exposes the active site in the plasminogen molecule without proteolytic cleavage, whereas generation of plasmin is required for exposure of the active site in the complex with staphylokinase.[154] Pilot trials with recombinant staphylokinase are presently being conducted in patients with acute myocardial infarction and recent occlusion of leg arteries.[154a,b]

ANTITHROMBOTIC AND THROMBOLYTIC THERAPY IN CARDIAC DISEASE

Risk Stratification—The Concept of Relative Versus Absolute Reduction of Events

Preexisting cardiovascular disease is considered a most powerful risk factor for coronary events.[155] For example, as shown in the Lipid Research Clinics Program Prevalence Study, high LDL or low HDL in preexisting cardiovascular disease predicts subsequent mortality in men 40 to 69 years of age to a much greater extent than high LDL or low HDL in an otherwise healthy population.[156] Accordingly, the impact of lipid-modifying strategies is much more evident in secondary prevention or in patients with known cardiovascular disease than in primary prevention or in the general apparently healthy population.[156–158] Similar rationale should apply to antithrombotic therapy for the prevention of coronary events.[159]

Conceptually, and assuming no use of antithrombotic agents (aspirin or anticoagulants), in 1989 we defined patients with coronary artery disease at high risk for coronary events as those with an acute coronary syndrome, in whom the incidence of a recurrent event of coronary occlusion is higher than 6 per cent per year (Table 58–3). We defined patients at medium risk as those with stable angina, when the incidence of a coronary event is about 2 to 6 per cent per year. And finally, we defined patients at low risk as those without previous evidence of cardiovascular disease, in whom the incidence of a coronary event is less than 2 per cent per year.[160] If these three groups of patients are treated with aspirin, we assume that there will be about a 25 to 30 per cent relative reduction of coronary events (i.e., 10 per cent becomes about 7 per cent in high-risk patients, 4 per cent becomes about 3 per cent in medium-risk patients, and 1 per cent becomes about 0.7 per cent in the

TABLE 58–3 RISK STRATIFICATION IN CARDIOVASCULAR DISEASE: ROLE OF ASPIRIN AND ANTICOAGULANTS

	THROMBOEMBOLIC RISK		
PATHOGENESIS	High (> 6%/yr)	Medium (2–6%/yr)	Low (< 2%/yr)
Arterial Platelets and fibrin (PI and/or A/C)	ACS, PTCA ASA + A/C	Stable CAD ASA or A/C	Primary prevention PI?
Chambers Fibrin (A/C)	A-fib-emboli A-fib-M. stenosis INR 2.5–3.5	A-fib-valv, nonvalv Anterior MI-early Dilated cardiomyopathy INR 2.0–3.0	A-fib—lone Chronic LV aneurysm No therapy
Prostheses Fibrin more than platelets (A/C > PI)	Old mechanical Previous emboli Extensive atherosclerosis INR 3.0–4.5 or INR 2.5–3.5 + ASA	Recent mechanical Bioprosthesis.-A-fib Mech-INR 2.5–3.5 Bio-INR 2.0–3.0	Biopr.-NSR No therapy

Modified from Stein, B., Fuster, V., Halperin, J. L., Chesebro, J. H.: Antithrombotic therapy in cardiac disease: An emerging approach based on pathogenesis and risk. Circulation *80*:1501, 1989.

PI = platelet inhibitor (i.e., aspirin); A/C = anticoagulants; ACS = acute coronary syndrome; PTCA = percutaneous transluminal coronary angioplasty; ASA = aspirin; CAD = coronary artery disease; A-fib = atrial fibrillation; MI = myocardial infarction; LV = left ventricle; INR = international normalized ratio.

low-risk subset). In other words, with aspirin use, the *relative* decrease of coronary events is about the same regardless of risk.[93,160] However, the *absolute* reduction or clinical impact is very different; thus, a decrease in events from 10 to 7 per cent—or for each 1000 patients treated, 30 are benefited—in the high-risk population with an acute coronary syndrome is much more striking than a decrease from 1 to 0.7 per cent—or for each 1000 treated patients only 3 benefited—in the lowest-risk patients without previous evidence of cardiovascular disease. Thus, what matters most is *not* the proportional reduction in risk, but the absolute reduction in risk. Furthermore, conceptually, because of the high incidence of events, the clinical impact in the high-risk population could even be improved by combining aspirin and anticoagulants, while in the low-risk population even the use of aspirin alone might be debatable in terms of risk/benefits.

We further defined the pathogenesis of thrombosis and thromboembolic risk in various cardiovascular entities (Table 58–3).[160] Thrombosis within the coronary arteries involves activation of both platelets and the coagulation system. With fibrin deposition, thromboembolism in patients with diseases of the cardiac chambers (i.e., atrial fibrillation or ventricular dysfunction) or valves (i.e., prosthetic devices) is related primarily to hemodynamic abnormalities, in which activation of the coagulation system with fibrin deposition predominates over that of platelets. Finally, thrombosis within the venous system is mostly related to blood stasis and endothelial damage, leading to activation of the clotting system. A systemic approach to the patient at risk for a thromboembolic event has been proposed,[160] allowing the selection of the most appropriate antithrombotic therapy based on pathogenetic principles and the risk of thromboembolism. In general, the higher the risk, the more intensive the recommended antithrombotic approach.

ANTITHROMBOTIC THERAPY IN CORONARY ARTERY DISEASE

Unstable Angina

(See also p. 1331)

EFFICACY OF ANTIPLATELET AGENTS ALONE (Table 58–4). Antiplatelet agents have been found to reduce acute myocardial infarction and short- and long-term death in four large trials of unstable angina. In the Veterans Administration Cooperative Study, men with unstable angina were randomized to receive aspirin or placebo for 12 weeks. During the treatment period the aspirin group demonstrated a risk reduction of 51 per cent, and the overall benefits of aspirin were maintained during the 1-year follow-up period.[161] In the Canadian Multicenter Trial, patients with unstable angina were randomized to receive aspirin, sulfinpyrazone, the combination of both, or placebo. The incidence of death and myocardial infarction was reduced in the aspirin groups from 17 to 8.6 per cent or a 51 per cent reduction; sulfinpyrazone demonstrated no benefit.[162]

TABLE 58–4 MAJOR ASPIRIN TRIALS IN UNSTABLE ANGINA

STUDY	NO. PATIENTS	DOSE (mg/day)	DURATION OF FOLLOW-UP	RELATIVE RISK REDUCTION (%)
Lewis et al.[161]	1338	324	3 months	51
Cairns et al.[162]	555	1300	24 months	51
Theroux et al.[163]	479	650	6 days	72
RISC[164]	796	75	5 days 3 months	57 68

In the Montreal Heart Institute Study, aspirin reduced the rate of myocardial infarction by 72 per cent compared to placebo.[163] In the European RISC study group,[164] patients with unstable angina or non-Q-wave infarction were randomized to receive 75 mg/day of aspirin for 3 months, intravenous heparin for 5 days, both, or neither. At the end of 3 months, the incidence of death or myocardial infarction was significantly reduced by aspirin and, to a greater extent, by the combination of aspirin and heparin.

EFFICACY OF ANTICOAGULANTS (HEPARIN) ALONE AND WITH ASPIRIN (Table 58–5). The use of heparin for the treatment of unstable angina was suggested by Teleford and Wilson.[165] They demonstrated an 80 per cent reduction in myocardial infarction in patients with unstable angina treated with heparin for 7 days. The most convincing evidence comes from the Montreal Heart Institute Study[163] in which heparin reduced the total cardiac event rate by 57 per cent ($P = 0.001$) and fatal and nonfatal myocardial infarction by 85 per cent. (Aspirin also reduced the incidence of fatal and nonfatal myocardial infarction by 72 per cent, as mentioned previously.) The combination of aspirin and heparin was superior to aspirin alone, but had no increased benefit compared to heparin alone (Fig. 38–24, p. 1337). There was a trend toward less frequent myocardial infarction in the heparin group compared to the aspirin group. An extension of this study was subsequently performed that randomized patients to either aspirin or heparin. The combined results of these studies demonstrated the greater reduction in the rate of myocardial infarction with heparin over aspirin.[166]

It is important to be aware of a rebound phenomenon that may occur when heparin is discontinued. This effect may be blunted when aspirin is given as concomitant therapy.[164] The RISC[167] study examined patients with unstable angina or non-Q-wave myocardial infarction. Patients were randomized to receive aspirin and/or intermittent intravenous heparin. Aspirin therapy compared to no aspirin therapy significantly reduced the risk ratios of fatal or nonfatal myocardial infarction. Heparin did not show such benefit. However, the group treated with combination heparin and aspirin showed the lowest event rate at 5 days. The more recent ATACS trial[168] randomized patients, with either unstable angina or non-Q-wave myocardial infarction, to receive aspirin alone or aspirin plus anticoagulation (Fig. 58–13). There was significant reduction in total ischemic events in the combination group versus aspirin (3.8 versus 8.3 per cent, $P = 0.004$) at the end of 14 days. At the end of 12 weeks, there was a trend toward reduction in total ischemic events (13 versus 25 per cent, $P = 0.06$). In a more recent British trial, the combination of aspirin and heparin did not reveal further benefit than aspirin alone.[169]

Ticlopidine was examined in patients with unstable angina.[170] The administration of ticlopidine in a dose of 250 mg twice a day for 6 months was found to reduce the incidence of death and myocardial infarction by 46 per cent.

In *summary,* there is ample evidence to suggest that the use of aspirin or heparin in the early phase of unstable angina reduces the incidence of death and myocardial infarction. The combination of aspirin and heparin in unstable angina and non-Q-wave myocardial infarction may be more effective than either drug alone in reducing total ischemic events in the early phase of such unstable syndromes.[171]

DIRECT THROMBIN INHIBITORS AND IIb/IIIa PLATELET RECEPTOR BLOCKERS. Given the central role of thrombin in the coagulation process, there is much enthusiasm for the development of direct thrombin inhibitors for use in acute coronary syndromes. Several small studies have examined the efficacy of these agents in unstable angina.[172–174] Results of these studies were encouraging. However, the larger studies of hirudin, GUSTO II[175] in unstable angina and other acute coronary syndromes, and TIMI-9[176] in acute

TABLE 58–5 MAJOR ANTICOAGULANT (HEPARIN) TRIALS IN UNSTABLE ANGINA

TRIAL	NO. PATIENTS	FOLLOW-UP	DRUG	REDUCTION IN DEATH OR MI (%)	P
Teleford and Wilson[165]	214	7 days	Heparin	80	< .05
Theroux et al.[163–167]	479	6 days	Heparin	85	< .001
			Heparin + aspirin	88	.001
RISC[164]	796	3 months	Heparin	5	NS
			Heparin + aspirin	68	< .0005
ATACS[168]	214	5 days	Aspirin	—	—
			Heparin + aspirin	46	.06
Holdright et al.[169]	285	6 days	Aspirin	—	—
			Heparin + aspirin	—	NS

MI = myocardial infarction.

myocardial infarction required reduction of the planned dose because of an observed increase in hemorrhagic stroke. In addition, HIT III[177] in acute myocardial infarction was terminated because of excessive bleeding with hirudin. With a change in dosage, the large trials GUSTO IIb and TIMI 9B have been completed and the results are being tabulated.

Most importantly, following the promising pilot studies in variable angina,[177a–c] platelet receptor blockade (c7E3) has just been preliminarily reported to be of most benefit in patients with refractory unstable angina (the CAPTURE study).

THROMBOLYTICS. At the present time there is little experimental evidence to support the use of thrombolytic therapy in unstable angina. There are many small and inconclusive studies conducted during the 1980–1990 period evaluating the use of thrombolytic therapy in unstable angina.[178] Many of these studies are difficult to evaluate because of different patient populations, timing of angiography, dose, and route of administration of the thrombolytic agent.

Two large recent trials evaluating thrombolytics give important insight into the issue of thrombolytic agents in unstable angina. The Unstable Angina Study using Eminase (UNASEM) trial was a large, randomized, placebo-controlled trial designed to evaluate both the angiographic and clinical outcome of the use of APSAC in unstable angina.[179] The improvement with APSAC of the occluded arteries (26 per cent of the APSAC group and 18 per cent of the placebo group had total occlusion of the artery) accounted for a favorable statistical difference in degree of stenosis before and after therapy. Despite a possible difference in angiographic appearance between the two groups, there was no significant difference in clinical outcome in the two groups. The TIMI-IIIB[180] study was designed to evaluate the use of t-PA and early angiography and revascularization for patients with unstable angina. At 42 days and 1 year, there were no differences in death and infarction between the two groups.

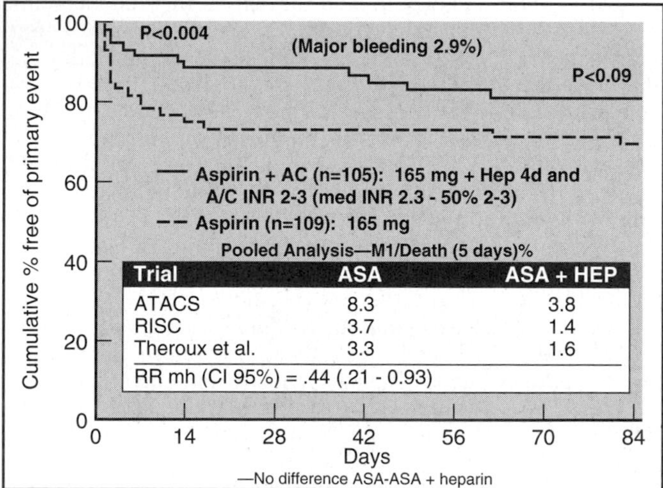

FIGURE 58–13. Data from the ATACS trial examining the use of aspirin versus aspirin plus anticoagulation in unstable angina and non-Q-wave myocardial infarction demonstrates improvement in event-free survival in the combination therapy group. Pooled analysis from ATACS, RISC, and the Theroux study groups demonstrates relative risk reduction (RR) of 0.44 in the combination group. ASA = aspirin; Hep = heparin. (From Holdright, D., Patel, D., Cunningham, D., et al.: Comparison of the effect of heparin and aspirin versus aspirin alone on transient myocardial ischemia and in-hospital prognosis in patients with unstable angina. J. Am. Coll. Cardiol. *24*:39, 1994. Reprinted by permission from the American College of Cardiology.)

Possible reasons for the failure of thrombolytic therapy to improve outcome in unstable angina as opposed to acute infarction relate to pathophysiological observations in unstable angina. In unstable angina, the incidence of total occlusion of the culprit vessel is significantly lower than in acute myocardial infarction. In addition, Falk[181] found partial organization and layering of the thrombus in patients with unstable angina. Thus much of the thrombus formation in unstable angina may be beneath the fibrous cap, rather than within the lumen of the artery. This may allow only small amounts of thrombus to be accessible to the thrombolytic agent.

RECOMMENDATIONS. All patients with unstable angina should immediately receive at least 75 mg of chewable aspirin and intravenous heparin (bolus followed by continuous infusion in doses sufficient to raise the PTT to approximately 85 seconds). The combination of aspirin and heparin is probably more efficacious than either agent alone.[182] This is particularly true when one takes into account aspirin's ability to blunt the rebound phenomenon at the time of discontinuation of heparin. Ticlopidine can be used as an alternative treatment in patients intolerant or allergic to aspirin. At the present time there is little clinical evidence to recommend the administration of thrombolytic therapy to patients with unstable angina.

Acute Myocardial Infarction

Thrombolytic Therapy

(See also p. 1215)

INTRAVENOUS THROMBOLYTIC VERSUS CONVENTIONAL THERAPY[183] (Fig. 58–14). A definitive overview[184] of 24 trials of intravenous thrombolytic therapy conducted between 1959 and 1979 found that the pooled odds reduction of mortality was 22 ± 5 per cent ($P < 0.001$). However, generalizations to clinical practice were of uncertain relevance, and subsequent trials were designed to be of sufficient size individually to allow the evaluation of mortality.

Three published, well-designed prospective trials have demonstrated mortality reduction by intravenous streptoki-

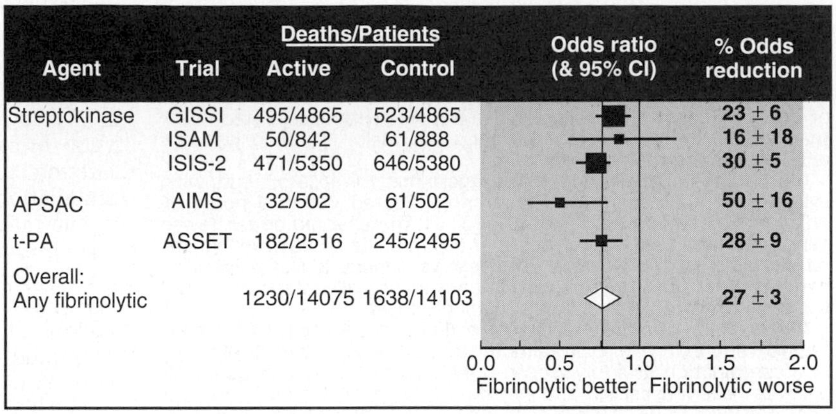

FIGURE 58–14. Reduction in mortality (3–5 weeks) among patients with myocardial infarction treated within 6 hours of symptom onset in the five major placebo-controlled trials of thrombolytic therapy. ci = confidence interval. (From Granger, et al.: Thrombolytic therapy for acute myocardial infarction: A review. Drugs *44(3)*:293, 1992. With permission.)

Agent	Trial	Deaths/Patients Active	Deaths/Patients Control	% Odds reduction
Streptokinase	GISSI	495/4865	523/4865	23 ± 6
	ISAM	50/842	61/888	16 ± 18
	ISIS-2	471/5350	646/5380	30 ± 5
APSAC	AIMS	32/502	61/502	50 ± 16
t-PA	ASSET	182/2516	245/2495	28 ± 9
Overall: Any fibrinolytic		1230/14075	1638/14103	27 ± 3

Odds ratio (& 95% CI): 0.0 0.5 1.0 1.5 2.0 — Fibrinolytic better / Fibrinolytic worse

nase (SK).[185–187] The GISSI-I study[185] randomized patients to SK or conventional therapy (i.e., no placebo control). Hospital mortality was significantly reduced from 13.0 to 10.7 per cent, an 18 per cent risk reduction. The ISIS-II study,[186] using placebo controls, randomized patients to SK, aspirin (160 mg enteric coated daily for 1 month, the first tablet chewed at the time of study entry), both, or neither, according to factorial design. The 5-week vascular mortality was significantly reduced from 12.0 to 9.2 per cent, a 23 per cent risk reduction by SK when compared with no SK, and from 13.2 to 8 per cent, a 39 per cent risk reduction by the combination of SK and ASA when compared to no SK or aspirin. The ISAM Study with SK showed 16 per cent risk reduction.[187]

The AIMS[188,189] randomized patients to APSAC or placebo, and 30-day mortality was significantly reduced from 12.1 to 6.4 per cent, a 50.5 per cent odds reduction of mortality. However, the trial was stopped early by the Data Monitoring Committee, so the magnitude of the true benefit may have been overestimated.

The ASSET trial[190,191] randomized patients to intravenous rt-PA or placebo. All patients received intravenous heparin for 24 hours. The 1-month all-cause mortality was significantly reduced by rt-PA from 9.8 to 7.2 per cent, a 28 per cent odds reduction. The European Cooperative Trial[192] randomized patients to rt-PA (100 mg single chain) or placebo infusion over 3 hours, all patients receiving heparin and low-dose aspirin. At 21 days, there was a nonsignificant difference in mortality (3.7 per cent with rt-PA versus 6.8 per cent with placebo).

The Fibrinolytic Therapy Trialists' (FTT) Collaborative Group reported on an overview of the results of all trials of fibrinolytic therapy versus control that randomized more than 1000 patients with suspected acute mycoardial infarction.[193] Among the 58,600 patients included in these trials, mortality at 35 days was reduced from 11.5 to 9.6 per cent, and 18 per cent odd reduction (Fig. 37–26, p. 1217).

STUDIES COMPARING INTRAVENOUS THROMBOLYTIC AGENTS[182] (Table 58–6). The clot specificity of rt-PA compared to SK offered the promise of greater efficacy and fewer complications from bleeding, hypotension, and allergic reaction. APSAC also offered promise because of its relative clot specificity compared to SK. However, no distinct advantages of any available thrombolytic agent emerged from the individual placebo-controlled trials, and it became clear that direct comparisons in large trials were necessary to determine relative efficacies and side effect profiles.

GISSI-2 TRIAL. This was a multi-center, randomized open-label trial designed to compare SK to alteplase (single-chain rt-PA).[194] In this 2 × 2 factorial design, patients were also randomly allocated to heparin (12,500 units subcutaneously, beginning at 12 hours, and repeated every 12 hours to hospital discharge) or usual therapy. Oral acetylsalicylic acid (ASA) (300 to 325 mg/day) was recommended for all patients. Hospital mortality was not significantly different at 8.6 per cent with SK and 9 per cent with rt-PA. Use of heparin did not alter the results. The International TPA/SK Mortality Trial[195] was a collaboration of the Italian GISSI-2 centers and those in several additional countries following the GISSI-2 protocol. Again there was no difference in hospital mortality between patients treated with SK and rt-PA.

ISIS-3. This was a multi-center, randomized trial, designed to address the following questions[196]: (1) Which of the three commonly used thrombolytic agents (SK, APSAC, and rt-PA), if any, is the most effective? (2) What are the effects of adding heparin to thrombolytic/aspirin regimens? Patients were further randomized in a factorial design to calcium heparin (12,500 units subcutaneously, the first dose about 4 hours postrandomization, and then every 12 hours for 7 days), or no heparin. All patients were expected to receive ASA (162 mg/day). Among the patients randomized, the vascular mortality rates at 35 days postrandomization were not as significant among the three groups: rt-PA, 10.3 per cent; SK, 10.6 per cent; APSAC, 10.5 per cent. Mortality was similar among the heparin-treated patients at 10.3 per cent, and the non-heparin-treated patients at 10.6 per cent. An overview[196] of the GISSI-2 and ISIS-3 data, based upon an analysis of 48,293 patients, found that 35 day mortality was 10.5 per cent with both rt-PA and SK.

GUSTO-I. The Global Utilization of Streptokinase and Tissue plasminogen activator for Occluded coronary arteries (GUSTO) trial[197] sought to determine whether a regimen designed to produce rapid and sustained infarct vessel recanalization was associated with improved survival. All patients received chewable aspirin, two 80 mg tablets, as soon as possible. They were randomized to one of four regimens: (1) rt-PA (alteplase) intravenous 15-mg bolus, then 0.75 mg/kg over 30 minutes, not to exceed 50 mg, then 0.5 mg/kg over 60 minutes, not to exceed 35 mg, the total dose not to exceed 100 mg. Simultaneously, heparin was begun with a 5000-unit intravenous bolus, followed by a continuous infusion of 1000 to 1200 units/hour for at least 48 hours, maintaining APTT at 60 to 85 seconds; (2) streptokinase 1.5 million units (MU) intravenously over 1 hour *plus* heparin intravenously in an identical regimen to that for the rt-PA group; (3) SK 1.5 MU intravenously over 1 hour *plus* heparin 12,500 units subcutaneously beginning 4 hours after initiation of SK and repeated every 12 hours for 7 days (or until prior discharge); (4) rt-PA 1.0 mg/kg intravenously over 60 minutes, maximum total dose 90 mg, including an initial bolus of 10 per cent of the total amount, *plus* simultaneously SK 1.0 intravenously over 60 minutes, *plus* heparin in an identical regimen to that for the rt-PA group. Mortality at 24 hours and 30 days was, respectively, for rt-PA 2.3 and 6.3 per cent; for rt-PA/SK 2.8 and 7.0 per cent; for SK (subcutaneous heparin) 2.8 and 7.2 per cent; and for SK (intravenous heparin) 2.9 and 7.4 per cent. The relative mortality reduction with accelerated rt-PA versus the SK alone group

TABLE 58–6 DEATH, TOTAL STROKE, AND CEREBRAL HEMORRHAGE IN THREE LARGE-SCALE MORTALITY TRIALS

	DEATH (%)	TOTAL STROKE (%)	HEMORRHAGE CEREBRAL (%)
GISSI-2 (n = 20,891)			
SK	9.2	0.94	0.29
t-PA	9.6	1.33	0.42
ISIS-3 (n = 41,299)			
SK	10.6	1.04	0.24
t-PA	10.3	1.39	0.66
APSAC	10.5	1.26	0.55
GUSTO-1 (n = 41,021)			
SK + SC heparin	7.2	1.22	0.49
t-PA + IV heparin	6.3	1.55	0.72
SK + IV heparin	7.4	1.40	0.54
t-PA + SK + IV heparin	7.0	1.64	0.94

From Hennekens, C. H., et al.: Current issues concerning thrombolytic therapy for acute myocardial infarction. J. Am. Coll. Cardiol. *25*(Suppl. 1):18S, 1995. With permission.

was 14 per cent, and the absolute mortality reduction was 1 per cent, which was significant. As shown in Table 8–6, hemorrhagic and total stroke were significantly more common with the accelerated rt-PA than the SK alone groups (0.72 per cent versus 0.52 per cent, P = 0.03), and 1.55 per cent versus 1.31 per cent). The composite outcome of death or nonfatal disabling stroke was less with accelerated rt-PA than SK (6.9 per cent versus 7.8 per cent). Major bleeding was not different among the four regimens.

The findings of the GUSTO trial suggest that for 1000 patients with evidence of acute myocardial infarction, treated within 6 hours of onset using accelerated rt-PA rather an SK, there would be ten fewer deaths, or nine fewer occurrences of a composite of death or nonfatal disabling stroke. However, the relative benefit is less evident in patients older than 75 years with inferior myocardial infarction, when therapy is initiated after 6 hours of infarct onset.[197]

TIMI-4. This trial[198] randomized patients to front-loaded rt-PA (GUSTO regimen), APSAC 30 units intravenously over 2 to 5 minutes, or a combination of a lower-dose rt-PA plus APSAC 20-unit bolus. All patients received aspirin and heparin. In-hospital mortality was 2.2 per cent with rt-PA, 8.8 per cent with APSAC, and 7.2 per cent with the combination (rt-PA versus APSAC, significant; rt-PA versus combination, nonsignificant).

RECOMMENDATIONS. As of this writing, according to the above information and taking into account the higher cost of rt-PA, accelerated rt-PA would appear to offer reasonably cost-effective therapy and be preferable to SK for patients under age 75 years with large infarctions, when therapy can be initiated within 6 hours of onset of acute myocardial infarction.[183,199]

TIME DELAY TO THROMBOLYTIC THERAPY.[183] There is considerable clinical evidence to indicate that thrombolytic therapy begun within the first few hours after the onset of acute myocardial infarction results in greater benefit than when it is begun many hours after the onset (Fig. 37–28, p. 1219). Indeed, the highest priority in the thrombolytic treatment of myocardial infarction is to minimize the delays in the initiation of therapy, regardless of the agent used. In regard to late initiation of thrombolytic treatment, patients seen between 6 and 12 hours may still be good candidates for therapy, particularly those with anterior or large infarctions.[199]

Adjuvant Antithrombotic Therapy

ASPIRIN. The rationale for the use of aspirin along with thrombolytic therapy lies in the relatively high risk of reocclusion of 5 to 30 per cent, and a rate of reinfarction of about 4 per cent when aspirin is not used.[199] The ISIS-2 trial,[186] reviewed above, demonstrated a 5-week significant reduction in the odds of death of 23 per cent with aspirin, 25 per cent with SK, and 42 per cent with the combination. Among patients receiving SK, the reinfarction rate was reduced from 4 to 2 per cent. The addition of aspirin to SK caused less than a 1 per cent absolute increase of minor bleeding and no increase in major bleeding, while stroke incidence fell significantly. Although there has been no evaluation of the contribution of aspirin to the treatment with APSAC or rt-PA, the combined use has become standard. The Antiplatelet Trialists' overview[93] indicated that aspirin may be expected to reduce the odds of vascular mortality by about 15 per cent, and of fatal and nonfatal vascular events by about 25 per cent over an approximate 2-year period following the in-hospital phase of acute myocardial infarction. These observations indicate that additional benefits of aspirin may be anticipated if it is continued beyond the 1 month protocol of the ISIS-2 study.

HEPARIN (Table 58–7). Low-dose, subcutaneous heparin (i.e., 7500 units), given until full ambulation, reduces calf vein thrombosis among patients with acute myocardial infarction, particularly those at risk (i.e., cardiac failure, late ambulation).[182]

The International Study Group,[195] and ISIS-3,[196] reviewed above, revealed minimal evidence for a benefit of subcutaneous heparin over placebo in patients treated with SK, rt-PA, or APSAC. Concerns that the heparin regimens employed in GISSI-2 and ISIS-3 may have been suboptimal prompted the use of aggressive intravenous regimens along with three of the four thrombolytic regimens evaluated in the GUSTO trial.[197] Heparin as a bolus of 5000 units intravenously was given immediately and followed by an infusion of 1000 to 1200 units/hour to maintain APTT at 60 to 85 seconds, in the accelerated rt-PA, the rt-PA/SK combination, and in one SK group. The other SK group received heparin subcutaneously according to the ISIS-3 protocol. Among the SK-treated patients, there was no difference in mortality, reinfarction, major hemorrhage, cerebral hemorrhage, patency, or reocclusion in relation to the heparin regimen. Hence, there was no evidence to indicate that intravenous heparin is superior to subcutaneous heparin among patients receiving SK.

RECOMMENDATIONS. According to the above information, there is no reason to routinely administer heparin along with SK, and it appears rational to reserve its use for those patients at high risk of systemic embolization because of congestive heart failure, large infarction, or atrial fibrillation. There has been no study among patients receiving rt-PA that has assessed the value of adjunctive heparin in relation to important patient outcomes. However, the results from the angiographic trials,[200–202] together with the short half-life and lesser systemic fibrinolytic effect of rt-PA, provide a rationale for adjunctive heparin for about 48 hours following administration of rt-PA.

Coronary Revascularization Procedures[203]

(See also Chaps. 38 and 39)

Atherothrombosis is not only the basis of coronary disease leading to the need for coronary artery bypass grafting and percutaneous coronary angioplasty, but it is also an important factor in the early complication rate of such interventions.

SAPHENEOUS VEIN BYPASS GRAFT DISEASE (see p. 1317) Vein graft disease can be divided into three phases: an early postoperative phase, within 1 month of thrombotic occlusion; an intermediate phase, within the first postoperative year, characterized by intimal hyperplasia resulting in a form of accelerated atherosclerosis that may have a superimposed thrombotic tendency; and a late phase, after the first postoperative year, composed of graft atherosclerosis similar to that affecting the native coronary arteries.[204] Accordingly, in the original Mayo Clinic trial on saphenous

TABLE 58–7 DATA FROM DIRECT COMPARISON OF ANTITHROMBOTIC REGIMENS: GISSI-2, ISIS-3, AND GUSTO-1

	GISSI-2 AND ISIS-3 (ASA PLUS ANY THROMBOLYTIC AGENT)		GUSTO-1 (ASA PLUS SK)	
Outcome	No Heparin (n = 31,050)	SC Heparin (n = 31,017)	SC Heparin (n = 9971)	IV Heparin (n = 10,377)
Death	10.2	10.0	7.2	7.4
Reinfarction	3.3	3.0	3.4	4.0
Total stroke	1.2	1.2	1.3	1.4
Hemorrhagic stroke	0.4	0.5	0.5	0.5
Major bleeding	0.7	1.0	0.3	0.5

From O'Donnell, C. J., et al.: Antithrombotic therapy for acute myocardial infarction. J. Am. Coll. Cardiol. 25(Suppl. I):23S, 1995.
ASA = aspirin; SK = streptokinase; SC = subcutaneous; IV = intravenous.

vein bypass grafting, patients received dipyridamole (100 mg four times daily) for 2 days before surgery, followed by aspirin (325 mg) and dipyridamole (75 mg) three times daily, starting 7 hours after surgery and continuing for 1 year. There was no increased incidence of bleeding complications in the treatment group. At vein graft angiography 1 month after surgery, there was significant reduction in graft occlusion in the treated group, from 10 per cent to 2 per cent distal graft anastomosis, and from 22 to 6 per cent per patient.[205,206] Reviews of all reported studies to date have convincingly demonstrated the importance of initiating platelet inhibitor therapy in the perioperative period, preferably before but not later than 48 hours after surgery. Indeed, when therapy was not started 48 hours after surgery, no reduction in the vein graft occlusion rate was observed.[207]

In the Veterans Administration Cooperative Study, patients receiving saphenous vein grafts were randomly assigned into five groups, taking 325 mg aspirin per day, 325 mg aspirin three times daily, 325 mg aspirin plus 75 mg dipyridamole three times daily, 267 mg sulfinpyrazone three times daily, or placebo. Early graft patency at a median of 9 days was significantly higher in the aspirin-treated group (92 per cent) than in those given placebo (85 per cent).[208] At 1 year, benefit was seen only in patients at high risk of graft occlusion (those with vein grafts placed to vessels ≤1.5 mm in diameter) taking aspirin.[209] It is important to note that one daily dose of aspirin was as effective as three daily doses. Dipyridamole conferred no additional benefit over aspirin alone.

In another Veterans Affairs Cooperative Study, preoperative aspirin use was associated with increased bleeding complications and no additional benefit in early vein graft patency compared with aspirin started 6 hours after surgery.[210] Other trials of antithrombotic therapy within the first year of saphenous vein bypass grafting have provided information of some interest: (1) Aspirin also, at the low dose of 100 mg/day, was found by Lorenz and colleagues[211] to be effective in reducing vein graft closure. (2) In one study, ticlopidine (250 mg twice daily), started on the second postoperative day, significantly reduced the incidence of vein graft occlusion by approximately 40 per cent, as assessed angiographically at 10, 180, and 360 days after surgery.[212] (3) Indobufen, a reversible inhibitor of platelet cyclooxygenase, in two recent 1-year studies appeared to be as effective as the combination of aspirin and dipyridamole in maintaining graft patency and was associated with a lower incidence of gastrointestinal side effects.[213,214] (4) Heparin and oral anticoagulants have been shown to be of some benefit for the prevention of graft occlusion in various trials[215,216]; however, the perioperative use of anticoagulants may be undesirable because of the risk of surgical bleeding.[216]

RECOMMENDATIONS. Platelet inhibitor therapy appears mandatory for prevention of early thrombotic occlusion of saphenous vein bypass grafts.[216] Aspirin should be started immediately after surgery and continued for at least 1 year and probably indefinitely. Ticlopidine can be used as an alternative treatment in patients intolerant or allergic to aspirin. No currently available agent prevents graft atherosclerosis, although control of risk factors such as hyperlipidemia and cigarette smoking may be beneficial.[217,218] In a new trial sponsored by the National Institutes of Health for prevention of vein graft atherosclerosis, the use of aspirin and lipid-lowering therapy, either alone or in combination, is being tested.

OCCLUSION FOLLOWING CORONARY ANGIOPLASTY. As discussed in more detail in Chapter 39, thrombosis plays a major role among the several multifactorial pathophysiological processes responsible for early occlusion after percutaneous transluminal coronary angioplasty (which without technical and pharmacological precautions occurs in about 7 to 20 per cent of patients).[219]

RECOMMENDATIONS. Based on six reported studies, pretreatment with aspirin, combined with adequate heparinization throughout the procedure, is strongly recommended.[220] Ticlopidine can be used as alternative treatment in patients intolerant or allergic to aspirin. The results of clinical trials of use of different antiplatelet drugs and anticoagulant agents aimed at reducing the re-stenosis rate have been disappointing. However, interest in using the class of agents that act by inhibiting fibrinogen binding to the platelet GP IIb/IIIa receptor has been stimulated by a recent report (the EPIC study) that showed a reduced incidence of acute complications and delayed complications, including restenosis, following PTCA in the group of patients receiving the 7E3 antibody directed against the GPIIb/IIIa receptor complex.[112,113] This approach should be considered in patients at "high risk" for ischemic complications following angioplasty.[220] However, preliminary data on an interventional study (the EPILOG study) also suggest significant benefit in "lower-risk" patients.

In patients undergoing stent implantation, the use of aspirin and heparin, followed by short-term coumadin, is presently recommended. Less aggressive anticoagulation regimens, including only antiplatelet therapy (i.e., aspirin alone or in combination with ticlopidine), are not recommended in patients at high risk for subacute thrombosis after stent replacement.[220]

Postmyocardial Infarction and Stable Coronary Disease

Survivors of acute myocardial infarction are at moderate risk of recurrent infarction or cardiac death. Because morbidity and mortality following a mycoardial infarction may be related to arrhythmias, left ventricular dysfunction, and recurrent myocardial infarction, proving that antithrombotic therapy is beneficial in these patients has been difficult.

ASPIRIN AND OTHER PLATELET INHIBITORS (Table 58–8). Multiple trials examining the use of aspirin for the secondary prevention of myocardial infarction have been

TABLE 58–8 ASPIRIN IN CARDIOVASCULAR DISEASE

CATEGORY OF TRIAL	NO. TRIALS	MI, STROKE, OR VASCULAR DEATH		Odds Ratio and Confidence Interval	% Odds Reduction (SD)
		Antiplatelet (%)	Controls (%)		
Prior MI	11	13.5	17.1		25 (4)
Acute MI	9	10.6	14.4		29 (4)
Prior stroke/TIA	18	18.4	22.2		22 (4)
Other high risk	104	6.9	9.2		32 (4)
All high risk (4 main categories)	142	11.4	14.7		27 (2)
All low risk (primary prevention)	3	4.46	4.85		10 (6)
All trials (high or low risk)	145	9.5	11.9		25 (2)
				0 0.5 1.0 1.5 2.0 better | worse Treatment effect 2P < 0.00001	

Data from Antiplatelet Trialists' Collaboration: Collaborative overview of randomised trials of antiplatelet therapy: I. Prevention of death, myocardial infarction, and stroke by prolonged antiplatelet therapy in various categories of patients. Br. Med. J. *306*:81, 1994. With permission.
SD = standard deviation; MI = myocardial infarction; TIA = transient ischemic attack.

conducted. However, no single study has provided definitive results. The results of a meta-analysis that included more than 18,000 patients revealed that platelet inhibitor therapy reduced cardiovascular mortality by 13 per cent, nonfatal reinfarction by 31 per cent, and nonfatal stroke by 42 per cent,[93] with overall risk reduction of 25 per cent. Aspirin alone was at least as effective as the combination of aspirin and dypyridamole and more effective than sulfinpyrazone. Available data do not justify the additional cost and frequency of administration of drugs other than aspirin in this group of patients. Medium-dose aspirin (75 to 325 mg) was as efficacious as higher-dose aspirin. No studies on the use of ticlopidine for secondary prevention are available.

Evidence from a 5-year trial of aspirin (975 mg/day) plus dipyridamole (225 mg/day) for prevention of progression of coronary disease in patients with stable angina revealed that these platelet inhibitors reduced new lesion formation as detected angiographically (with no effect on the progression of existing lesions) and reduced the incidence of myocardial infarction from 12 to 4 per cent (a 67 per cent reduction).[221] In a study of 333 men with chronic stable angina, aspirin alone (125 mg every other day) reduced the incidence of myocardial infarction by 87 per cent compared with placebo; there was only a slight trend toward decreased mortality, but the risk of stroke, presumed to be hemorrhagic, increased.[222] Similar favorable effects of aspirin in patients with stable coronary disease were reported in another study.[223]

ANTICOAGULANTS. Numerous studies have assessed the usefulness of anticoagulants in the secondary prevention of cardiovascular disease after myocardial infarction. The Warfarin and Reinfarction Study (WARIS) is the second largest study to date of anticoagulants in the secondary prevention of myocardial infarction (Fig. 58–15).[224] In this placebo-controlled, double-blind trial, patients were randomized after initial acute myocardial infarction to warfarin (target INR 2.8–4.8) or placebo. Patients were advised not to take aspirin during the trial. At mean follow-up of 37 months, warfarin resulted in significant reductions of mortality, total reinfarctions, nonfatal infarctions, and total strokes. Although four fatal intracranial hemorrhages occurred in the warfarin group compared to none in the placebo group, ten nonhemorrhagic fatal strokes occurred in the placebo group compared to none in the warfarin group.

The ASPECT trial,[225] the largest study of anticoagulants in secondary prevention following myocardial infarction, was conducted concurrently with the WARIS trial, but was completed at a later date. Patients were randomized to phenprocoumon or acenocoumarol or placebo. The anticoagulant therapy was titrated to achieve an INR of 2.8 to 4.8, and the mean follow-up was 37 months. There was a significant reduction in recurrent myocardial infarction in the anticoagulant-treated group compared to the placebo-treated group (114 versus 242 patients; risk reduction, 53 per cent). There was, however, no significant difference in mortality between the placebo and anticoagulant groups. The anticoagulant-treated group experienced a larger number of hemorrhagic events than the placebo-treated group, and gastrointestinal-related bleeding accounted for half of the major bleeding episodes.

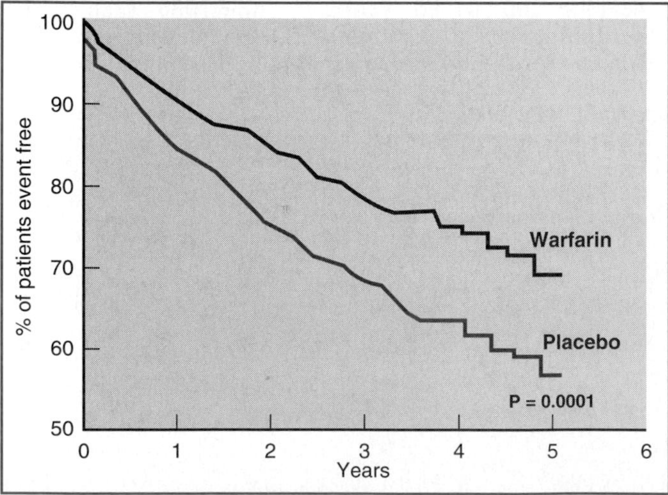

FIGURE 58–15. The WARIS Trial Study of anticoagulants in the secondary prevention of myocardial infarction. Cumulative rates (Kaplan-Meier) of total mortality, recurrent myocardial infarction, and stroke. (From Smith, P., Arnesen, H., and Holme, I.: The effect of warfarin on mortality and reinfarction after myocardial infarction. N. Engl. J. Med. *323:*147, 1990. Copyright Massachusetts Medical Society.)

To study anticoagulation for patients with stable coronary disease, the Sixty Plus Reinfarction Study involved patients over 60 years of age who had been taking anticoagulants for a median time of 6 years after infarction. Patients were randomly assigned to continue anticoagulant therapy or placebo substitute for 2 more years. By intention-to-treat analysis, patients receiving anticoagulant therapy had a 26 per cent lower death rate (11.6 per cent compared with 15.7 per cent) and an impressive 51 per cent lower rate of reinfarction (4.1 per cent compared with 8.4 per cent) than patients taking placebo. A trend toward reduced frequency of cerebrovascular events was observed in the group receiving anticoagulant therapy.[226]

Two clinical trials compared warfarin with aspirin in secondary prevention of myocardial infarction. In the German-Austrian Myocardial Infarction Study (GAMIS), patients were randomized after acute myocardial infarction to open label phenprocoumon (target INR 2.5 to 5.0), aspirin 1.5 mg/day, or placebo.[227] No difference in mortality or reinfarction was observed between groups. The French Enquete de Prevention Secondaire de l'Infarctus de Myocarde (EPSIM)[228] revealed no difference in death or reinfarction in patients receiving either oral anticoagulants or aspirin. However, there was 54 per cent more patients with gastrointestinal events with aspirin and four times more severe hemorrhagic events with warfarin.

In the Aspirin Versus Coumadin in the Prevention of Reocclusion and Recurrent Ischemia After Successful Thrombolysis (APRICOT) trial, patients were randomized to either 325 mg/day of aspirin or to heparin followed by warfarin (target INR 2.8 to 4.0) after an initial angiogram < 48 hours after acute myocardial infarction revealed a patent infarct-related artery.[229] At 3 months there was no significant difference in reocclusion rates among the aspirin, warfarin, and placebo arms (25, 30, and 32 per cent, respectively). Aspirin significantly reduced reinfarction in comparison to placebo, but not to warfarin (3, 11, and 8 per cent respectively). Mortality did not differ between the groups.

Currently there are two randomized studies examining the unsolved issue of the combination of anticoagulants and antiplatelet regimens after acute myocardial infarction.[230] The CARS trial is studying patients randomized to three treatment regimens: (1) 160 mg/day of aspirin; (2) 80 mg/day of aspirin plus 3 mg of warfarin; (3) a combination pill of 80 mg of aspirin plus 1 mg of warfarin per day. The CHAMP study is randomizing patients to receive either 160 mg/day of aspirin or 80 mg of aspirin plus Coumadin to achieve an INR of 1.5 to 2.5.

RECOMMENDATIONS. When the results of trials of aspirin and anticoagulant therapy for secondary prevention in survivors of myocardial infarction and in patients with stable coronary disease are analyzed together, both treatments appear to confer protection against death and reinfarction. Thus, for most patients the advantage of aspirin over anticoagulant agents is not higher effectiveness but lower costs, ease of administration, and less need for monitoring. For patients intolerant of aspirin, at risk of embolism from the left ventricle (i.e., those with mural thrombi or severe myo-

TABLE 58–9 ASPIRIN IN PRIMARY PREVENTION (U.S. PHYSICIANS' HEALTH STUDY AND BRITISH DOCTORS' TRIAL RESULTS)

ENDPOINT	REDUCTION (% ± SD) U.S. Physicians' Health Study	British Doctors' Trials	Overview of Both Trials	P VALUE
Nonfatal myocardial infarction	39 ± 9	3 ± 19	32 ± 8	<0.0001
Nonfatal stroke	↑19 ± 15	↑13 ± 24	↑18 ± 13	NS
Total cardiovascular deaths	2 ± 15	7 ± 14	5 ± 10	NS
Any vascular event	18 ± 7	4 ± 12	13 ± 6	$P < .05$

Hennekens, C. H., Buring, J. E., Sandercock, P., et al.: Aspirin and other antiplatelet agents in the secondary and primary prevention of cardiovascular disease. Circulation *80*:749, 1989.

cardial dysfunction) or left atrium (i.e., those with atrial fibrillation), or with prior embolism, oral anticoagulant treatment is preferred.

Primary Prevention

ASPIRIN. Because aspirin has a significant protective effect in secondary prevention of vascular disease, the possible benefit of aspirin in primary prevention has also been tested. Two randomized trials, the United States Physicians' Health Study[231,232] and the British Doctors' Trial,[233] have been conducted (Table 58–9).

Results from the United States trial of more than 22,000 male physicians, aged 40 to 84 years, assigned to receive aspirin (325 mg every other day) or placebo for 5 years, revealed a 44 per cent reduction in the incidence of myocardial infarction, from approximately 0.4 per cent to 0.2 per cent per year. This effect was limited to those older than 50 years. Over the 5-year period, the incidence of cardiovascular death was similar in the aspirin and placebo groups; in the aspirin-treated group there was a slight increase in hemorrhagic stroke that was not statistically significant (0.2 per cent in the aspirin group compared with 0.1 per cent in the placebo group), but there was a significant increase in gastrointestinal hemorrhage requiring transfusion (0.5 per cent in the aspirin group compared with 0.3 per cent in the placebo group).

In the British primary prevention trial of more than 5000 male physicians, ages 50 to 78 years, two-thirds were randomly assigned to take aspirin (500 mg/day) and one-third were instructed to avoid it (no placebo used). After 6 years, no difference in the rate of myocardial infarction or cardiovascular death was detected; however, as in the American study, there was a slight increase in disabling strokes among those assigned to aspirin.

Overall, the prevalence of cardiovascular events was quite low among the relatively healthy physicians who participated in these primary prevention trials. Even analyzing the most striking data, such as the rate of nonfatal myocardial infarction in the American study being reduced by 44 per cent, the absolute risk reduction was less than two events per 1000 per year. Thus, as previously discussed, there are clear problems in reporting risk reduction as a percentage when the absolute prevalence of events is low. Furthermore, in the more favorable American study, for the combined endpoints of all important cardiovascular events (myocardial infarction, stroke, and death), the risk reduction favoring aspirin was only 18 per cent. Therefore, based on these studies the use of aspirin in an overall healthy population for primary prevention of coronary events is not justified.

Although in these relatively low-risk apparently healthy populations the per cent reduction in the rate of myocardial infarction was similar whether or not risk factors for coronary disease were present, it seems important to consider the absolute prevalence of events. The rate of myocardial infarction was consistently higher among patients with these risk factors than among those without—ranging from 1.4-fold in those with a parental history of coronary disease to 5-fold in those with diabetes, with intermediate increments associated with smoking, hypercholesterolemia, and hypertension. Thus, in primary prevention the absolute impact is greater in groups with a high-risk factor profile.[234]

RECOMMENDATIONS. Given the available data, it now seems reasonable to advocate the use of aspirin in a dose of 75 to 325 mg/day (body weight may be a guide) or every other day in patients with clinical manifestations of coronary disease, if no specific contraindications are present.[182] For primary prevention, aspirin should be considered only in men over the age of 50 with uncontrolled risk factors for the development of coronary events.[182] However, aspirin should be used cautiously, if at all, in patients with poorly controlled hypertension. Furthermore, aspirin should be viewed as a possible adjunct, rather than as an alternative to the management of coronary risk factors. Most important, although the short-term benefit of aspirin in these populations appears to outweigh its risk, the long-term advantages and toxicity of the drug remain uncertain.

Observational epidemiological studies in primary prevention have suggested a possible benefit of aspirin in women[235]; however, definitive recommendations for women, particularly in those with uncontrolled risk factors, will have to await the results of the Women's Health Study, a large randomized trial of low-dose aspirin use among more than 40,000 female nurses 45 years old and older. In an ongoing thrombosis prevention trial among men at high risk of coronary heart disease,[236,237] the effects of low-dose aspirin (75 mg/day), low-dose warfarin, and the combination of both agents in being evaluated. The results of this trial will define further the role of antithrombotic agents in primary prevention.

ANTITHROMBOTIC THERAPY FOR CARDIAC CHAMBER THROMBOEMBOLISM

(Table 58–3)

Atrial Thrombosis

Atrial thrombosis occurs in patients with valvular heart disease and with nonvalvular atrial fibrillation. The pathogenesis is probably dominated by stasis and the generation of fibrin, but endocardial abnormalities and activation of platelets may contribute under some circumstances. Standard techniques are much less reliable for detecting thrombi in the atrium than in the ventricle. Two-dimensional echocardiography detected 30 to 60 per cent of thrombi in the body of the left atrium[238,239] but did not detect thrombosis in the left atrial appendage and most small thrombi in the body of the atrium. Transesophageal echocardiography has permitted excellent imaging of both atria and atrial appendages and appears to be sensitive for the detection of thrombi.[240] However, this technique has not been used to determine the frequency of atrial thrombi in large-scale clinical studies. Consequently the prevalence of left atrial thrombosis in various cardiovascular disease is uncertain. On the basis of autopsy studies in patients with rheumatic heart disease, about half of patients with atrial fibrillation have atrial thrombi (range 24.5 to 55.2 per cent) compared with 15 per cent of patients with sinus rhythm (range 6.5 to 22 per cent).[241] With the use of transesophageal echocardiography, new insights may be gained into the prevalence of atrial thrombosis and risk of thromboembolism in valvular heart disease and nonvalvular atrial fibrillation.

Valvular Heart Disease

MITRAL STENOSIS (see p. 1009). The incidence of thromboembolism complicating mitral stenosis is reported to be 1.5 to 4.7 per cent per year.[242] Up to 75 per cent of clinically significant embolic episodes involve the cerebral circulation, and this may be the initial manifestation of disease in more than 10 per cent of cases. The risk of emboli increases with age and correlates inversely with cardiac output, but it is unrelated to left atrial size, valve area, or functional class.[242,243] The most significant risk factors are atrial fibrillation and previous embolism. The risk of embolism in mitral stenosis increases by 7-fold to 18-fold with the onset of atrial fibrillation, and nearly 75 per cent of the patients who have emboli have chronic atrial fibrillation.[242,243] Up to 30 per cent of emboli occur in the first month of onset of atrial fibrillation, and 66 per cent occur within the first year.[242,243] Thus, it is important to anticipate atrial fibrillation, or detect it early, so that prophylactic anticoagulant therapy can be administered. There is recurrence of emboli in up to 65 per cent of cases, mostly in the first 6 to 12 months, resulting in a substantial mortality.[242,243]

No prospective randomized studies have evaluated the effectiveness of anticoagulants in preventing systemic thromboemboli in mitral stenosis. However, several descriptive studies report that warfarin appears to be effective in preventing recurrent emboli.[242]

MITRAL REGURGITATION (see p. 1020). This valvular lesion is associated with a somewhat lower risk of systemic emboli than is mitral stenosis.[242,243] Systemic embolism occurred at the rate of one to 2 events per 100 patient years when the lesion is relatively mild and isolated, but it occurred at the rate of up to 4 events per 100 patient years when regurgitation was severe, or when mixed stenosis and regurgitation were present.[242,243] Up to 14 to 18 per cent of such patients may ultimately suffer thromboembolic complications. In the Mayo Clinic study of patients with severe isolated mitral regurgitation, a moderately high incidence of 2.9 thromboembolic events per 100 patient years was found.[244] The risk of embolism with mitral regurgitation is much higher in the presence of atrial fibrillation. In the series of Coulshed and associates of over 800 patients with rheumatic mitral disease, 7.7 per cent of those with predominant regurgitation with sinus rhythm had emboli, compared with 22 per cent of patients with atrial fibrillation. In contrast, when mitral stenosis was the dominant lesion, 8 per cent of patients with sinus rhythm had emboli, compared with 32 per cent with atrial fibrillation.[243]

MITRAL VALVE PROLAPSE (see p. 1031). This condition is very prevalent in the general population; it is usually well tolerated and asymptomatic. In a small percentage of patients, however, serious symptoms may occur, including transient or permanent cerebral ischemic events, which may be recurrent.[242,245] The pathogenesis of these adverse events has been linked to abnormalities of the valvular endocardium detected at autopsy, including thickening, endocardial denudation, and inflammatory changes.[242] Deposits of fibrin and platelet aggregates have been detected on the surface of valves in patients dying of embolic complications.[242] Echocardiographically these changes are manifested as valvular leaflet redundancy, which in one study was suggested to predict embolic risk.[246] Nevertheless, in this study, of 10 patients with embolism, only 2 experienced embolic complications in the absence of other risk factors, including atrial fibrillation, left ventricular thrombus, or infective endocarditis. This latter observation supports the common view that there is a low risk of thromboembolism with mitral valve prolapse in the absence of other predisposing conditions. Accordingly, routine prophylaxis is unwarranted in patients with mitral valve prolapse in the absence of other conditions that predispose to thromboembolism, such as atrial fibrillation or left ventricular dysfunction.

AORTIC VALVE DISEASE (see p. 1037). Very few long-term studies are available to define what appears to be a very low incidence of thromboembolism in aortic valve disease. In one study, 68 patients with moderate to severe aortic regurgitation were observed for 10 years; embolic complications occurred in 4.4 per cent for a low overall event rate of 0.083 per cent per 100 patient years.[247] In aortic stenosis, accurate diagnosis of embolic events may be confounded by the frequent occurrence of neurological symptoms due to abnormal hemodynamics or arrhythmias. Additionally, many of the emboli that are detected are probably calcific. Calcareous emboli have been found in up to 19 per cent of cases at autopsy[248]; although clinically significant embolic events have been reported involving the retinal circulation,[249] most calcific emboli are probably small and subclinical.

RECOMMENDATIONS.[242,250] 1. Patients with mitral regurgitation or mixed lesions (stenosis and regurgitation) with atrial fibrillation are at moderate risk for systemic embolism and should receive long-term oral anticoagulation to maintain the INR at 2.0 to 3.0. Patients with mitral stenosis and atrial fibrillation, and those with valvular heart disease and a prior thromboembolic event, are at higher risk and should receive anticoagulants with an INR of about 2.5 to 3.5.

2. In patients with mitral valve prolapse, if a transient ischemic attack (TIA) occurs, aspirin may be advised at a dose of 325 mg daily. However, in such cases, other causes of the cerebral symptoms should first be excluded. Few data are available upon which to base antithrombotic recommendations in the setting of clinically convincing recurrent TIAs or a definitive cerebral embolus in the patient with mitral valve prolapse; long-term anticoagulation with warfarin is justified in such cases at the lower intensity of an INR 2.0 to 3.0.

3. Routine anticoagulant therapy is not warranted in patients with aortic valve disease in the absence of other risk factors, such as atrial fibrillation.

4. Anticoagulant therapy is not warranted in infective endocarditis of a native valve. On the other other hand, anticoagulant therapy is recommended in nonbacterial thrombotic endocarditis.

Nonvalvular Atrial Fibrillation

Atrial fibrillation is a common cardiac arrhythmia of the elderly (p. 654), and stroke is its most devastating complication. The high risks of thromboembolism in atrial fibrillation associated with mitral stenosis and prosthetic mitral valves have long been appreciated (Table 58–3). However, atrial fibrillation carries a substantially increased risk of ischemic stroke even in the absence of these valvular disorders.[251] The rate of ischemic stroke among elderly people with atrial fibrillation averages 5 per cent a year, about six times that of people without atrial fibrillation.[252,253] Considering transient ischemic attacks (often causing radiographic evidence of brain infarction) and clinically occult stroke detected radiographically, the rate of brain ischemia accompanying nonvalvular atrial fibrillation exceeds 7 per cent a year—an impressive threat to the brain.[254,255] However, the absolute rate of stroke varies importantly with patient age and coexistent cardiovascular disease.[256–258] Stratification of atrial fibrillation patients into those at high and low risk of thromboembolism is a crucial determinant of optimal antithrombotic prophylaxis, as discussed in detail below.

Most ischemic strokes associated with atrial fibrillation

are probably due to embolism of stasis-induced thrombi forming in the left atrium, and particularly its appendage. Transesophageal echocardiography shows left atrial thrombi to be more frequent in atrial fibrillation patients who have suffered an ischemic stroke compared with atrial fibrillation patients without a stroke. However, perhaps 25 per cent of atrial fibrillation–associated stroke is due to associated intrinsic cerebrovascular diseases, other cardiac sources of embolism, or aortic arch atheroma.[259,260] Thus, about half of elderly atrial fibrillation patients have chronic hypertension, a major risk factor for primary cerebrovascular disease.[253] About 12 per cent of elderly atrial fibrillation patients harbor cervical carotid artery stenosis, but the frequency of carotid artery stenosis is not substantially greater in atrial fibrillation patients with stroke, suggesting that carotid artery stenosis is a minor contributor to atrial fibrillation–associated stroke.[251]

ATRIAL FIBRILLATION PATIENTS WITH HIGH AND LOW RATES OF THROMBOEMBOLISM (Table 58–10). The absolute rate of ischemic stroke in atrial fibrillation patients is crucially influenced by coexistent cardiovascular disease.[252] Identification of subpopulations of atrial fibrillation patients who have relatively high or low absolute rates of stroke determine which patients gain the greatest benefit from anticoagulant therapy. Two prospective studies included sufficient numbers of patients and stroke, analyzed by multivariable techniques, and provide the most reliable stratification schemes available.[253,254] The differences in the two schemes (presence of age versus heart failure) are not contradictory or even substantially conflicting, as clinical variables overlap (age is related to heart failure, hypertension, and diabetes). Interestingly, intermittent (i.e., paroxysmal) atrial fibrillation was *not* an independent predictor of thromboembolic risk in either study. In summary, the five clinical variables listed in Table 58–10 are independently predictive of thromboembolic risk and are clinically useful in characterizing atrial fibrillation patients with high and low risks for stroke.

Echocardiographic predictors of increased thromboembolic risk in atrial fibrillation are enlarged left atrial size (mitigated by mitral regurgitation) and impaired left ventricular function.[258,259] Impaired left ventricular function may contribute further to stasis within the left atrium in patients with atrial fibrillation.[260] Indeed, transthoracic echocardiographic findings can be combined with clinical risk stratifiers to identify atrial fibrillation patients with very low inherent rates of thromboembolism.[258] Transesophageal echocardiography offers better visualization of the left atrium and its appendage than conventional transthoracic echocardiography. With use of transesophageal echocardiography, left atrial appendage thrombi and spontaneous echogenic densities ("smoke"), possibly indicative of stasis, are more often found in atrial fibrillation patients with thromboembolism.[240] However, the predictive value of transesophageal echocardiographic findings for subsequent stroke has yet to be validated by adequate clinical studies.

ANTITHROMBOTIC THERAPEUTIC METHODS TO PREVENT STROKE. Anticoagulation with oral vitamin K antagonists such as warfarin is highly effective for reducing ischemic stroke in atrial fibrillation patients.[252,252a] Five recent randomized clinical trials using INR ranges of approximately 1.8 to 4.2 showed a mean reduction in ischemic stroke of nearly 70 per cent of patients assigned anticoagulation (Fig. 58–16); on-therapy analysis indicated an even greater benefit.[253] Furthermore, warfarin is particularly effective in subgroups of atrial fibrillation patients with a high inherent risk of thromboembolism (see Table 58–10).[253,261] The incremental risk of serious bleeding was < 1 per cent/year among anticoagulated patients selected for participation in these clinical trials and who were followed carefully on protocols. Low-intensity anticoagulation (INR 2.0 to 3.0) clearly confers benefit.[253,262]

The safety and tolerability of long-term anticoagulation titrated to conventional levels has not been well defined in the very elderly (age > 75 years), the age group encompassing perhaps half of atrial fibrillation–associated stroke. All but one of the placebo-controlled trials testing anticoagulation enrolled atrial fibrillation patients with a mean age in the late 60s.[253] The single placebo-controlled trial involving atrial fibrillation patients with a mean age of 75 years reported a 38 per cent withdrawal rate from anticoagulation after 1 year.[253,263] A relatively recent clinical trial comparing anticoagulation in atrial fibrillation patients under and over age 75 years found that the risk of major hemorrhage during anticoagulation (INR range 2.0 to 4.5, mean INR = 2.7) was substantially increased in patients over 75 years compared with younger ones anticoagulated to similar intensities.[253] While the very elderly have a

TABLE 58–10 RISK STRATIFICATION IN ATRIAL FIBRILLATION*: INDEPENDENT PREDICTORS OF THROMBOEMBOLIC RISK

	SPAF-I PLACEBO PATIENTS[118]	AFI POOLED ANALYSIS[114]
Number of patients	568	1236
Number of events	46	81
High-risk variables	History of hypertension Prior stroke/TIA Diabetes Recent heart failure	History of hypertension Prior stroke/TIA Diabetes Age > 65 years
Thromboembolic rate (95% CI)		
Low risk	1.4%/yr (0.05–3.7)	1.0%/yr (0.3–3.1)
High risk	> 7%/yr	> 5%/yr
Percentage of cohort "low risk"	38%	15%

* Large, prospectively acquired data sets analyzed by multivariable techniques. The SPAF-I placebo data set[118] was included in the pooled analysis of clinical trials by the Atrial Fibrillation Investigators.[114]

SPAF = Stroke Prevention in Atrial Fibrillation study, AFI = Atrial Fibrillation Investigators, CI = confidence interval.

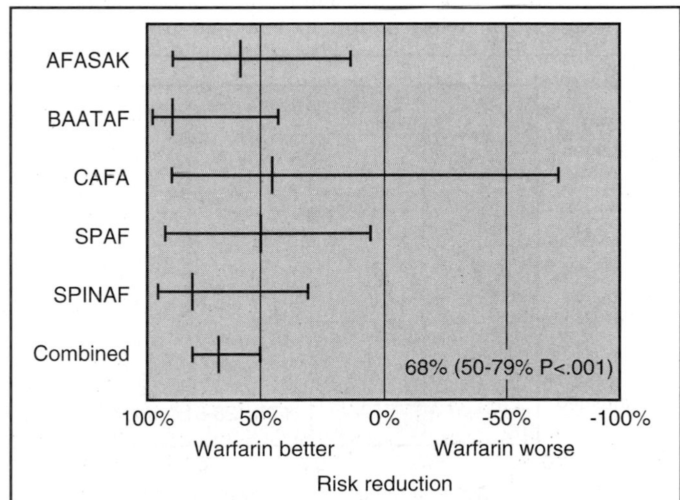

FIGURE 58–16. Risk-reduction plot of the results of five randomized clinical trials comparing warfarin with control for prevention of ischemic stroke in atrial fibrillation patients. Horizontal lines indicate the 95% confidence intervals around the point estimates (vertical lines) for each trial. The combined risk reduction was 68% (95% confidence interval, 50% to 79%; P < 0.991). See Atrial Fibrillation Investigators' pooled analysis for specific data. AFASAK = Atrial Fibrillation, Aspirin and Anticoagulant Therapy study; BAATAF = Boston Area Anticoagulation Trial for Atrial Fibrillation; CAFA = Canadian Atrial Fibrillation Anticoagulation study; SPAF = Stroke Prevention in Atrial Fibrillation study; and SPINAF = Stroke Prevention in Nonrheumatic Atrial Fibrillation study.

thromboembolic rate at 3.5 events per 100 patient years—occurring in 14 per cent of patients with sinus rhythm and 33 per cent of patients with atrial fibrillation. Overall, in retrospective uncontrolled studies, great variation has been reported in the annual incidence of clinically apparent embolization, which ranged from less than 1 per cent to 12 per cent.[290–294] The risk is greatest in patients with severe left ventricular dysfunction (ejection faction ≤ 35 per cent), established or paroxysmal atrial fibrillation, a history of thromboembolism, or echocardiographic evidence of thrombus.[291,294]

Pulmonary embolism is reported to occur with a frequency of 5 to 11 per cent[295,296] and is associated with significant mortality.[296,297] No prospective randomized trials of anticoagulation in dilated cardiomyopathy have been conducted. However, in the Mayo Clinic study, patients receiving anticoagulants had no thromboembolic events in 101 patient years of follow-up[290]; other observational studies suggest similar protective effects of anticoagulants (Table 58–11).

In ischemic cardiomyopathy, the incidence of systemic emboli appears to be significantly lower than in nonischemic cardiomyopathy,[298] perhaps because in ischemic cardiomyopathy akinetic regions predispose to thrombosis and not to emboli, while in nonischemic cardiomyopathy myocardial dysfunction and stasis predispose to thrombosis,[298] and also to emboli because of some degree of global contractility.[291,293,299] This different pathophysiology may explain in part the controversy in left ventricular failure whether anticoagulants are of benefit (nonischemic cardiomyopathy?)[290,291,294] or whether they are not (ischemic cardiomyopathy?).[300–302]

Recommendations. (1) In nonischemic dilated cardiomyopathy, in view of the moderate risk of embolism in these patients and the apparent efficacy of anticoagulants in its prevention, medium-intensity anticoagulant therapy (INR 2.0 to 3.0) is recommended pending further studies; this indication is stronger in the presence of atrial fibrillation, significant left ventricular dysfunction and/or failure, or history of thromboembolism and/or left ventricular thrombus at echocardiography. (2) In patients with ischemic dilated cardiomyopathy, cardiac failure alone may not be an indication for anticoagulation, unless there is atrial fibrillation or history of thromboembolism and/or left thrombus at echocardiography.[242,280]

TABLE 58–11 THROMBOEMBOLISM IN NONISCHEMIC CARDIOMYOPATHY

AUTHOR	SYSTEMIC EMBOLI INCIDENCE % NO A/C	% A/C
Fuster, V., et al.[290] (n = 104)	18	0
Gottdiener, J. S., et al.[289] (n = 123)	11	
Kyrle, P. A., et al.[290a] (1985) (n = 38)	44	0
Roberts, W. C. et al.[290b] (1987) (n = 152 autopsy)	39 (clinical)	
Ciaccheri, M., et al.[290c] (1989) (n = 126)	8	0
Yokota, Y., et al.[290d] (1989) (n = 40) (n = 17 autopsy)	20	0

A/C = anticoagulants.

Modified from Falk, R. H., Foster, E., and Coats, M. H.: Ventricular thrombi and thromboembolism in dilated cardiomyopathy: A prospective follow-up study. Am. Heart J. *123*:136, 1992.

ANTITHROMBOTIC THERAPY IN PROSTHETIC HEART VALVE REPLACEMENT

Incidence of Thromboembolism With and Without Appropriate Anticoagulation

(See also pp. 1835 to 1836)

The overall incidence of ischemic thromboembolism in patients taking anticoagulants, as expressed per 100 patients times years of exposure, is about 2.5 per cent for the Starr-Edwards and Omniscience prostheses, 2 per cent for the Medtronic Hall prosthesis, 1.5 per cent for the St. Jude Medical prosthesis, and 1 per cent for the pericardial and porcine bioprostheses.[303,304] Without anticoagulation, the incidence tends to double. The incidence of thromboembolism is cumulative, and the risk is persistent throughout the years of follow-up. However, recent observations have revealed that the highest incidence of thromboembolism is within the first 30 postoperative days (being particularly high within the first 10 days) for both bioprosthetic and mechanical prosthetic valves.[305,306] Patients with a prior embolus are also at great risk for recurrence. In the Mayo Clinic series, 20 per cent of patients with mitral prostheses and 27 per cent with aortic prostheses had recurrent embolism.[304] A history of an embolus preceding surgery was also predictive of an increased risk of postoperative embolus.[304] This has also been found in patients with nonvalvular trial fibrillation and suggests that some persons may be predisposed in some way to thromboembolic complications. Overall there has been a decreasing risk of thromboembolism after valve replacement in recent years, probably as a result of factors involving both patients and valves.[304] Patients now are usually operated on when their disease is less advanced than in the past. This means that the incidence of atrial fibrillation is generally lower, left atrial size is smaller, and left ventricular function is better at operation. Also, the mechanical prosthetic valves themselves have been improved, with design modifications that result in less turbulent flow and better hemodynamics.

Maintenance of adequate anticoagulation is also critical in the prevention of valvular thrombosis. In patients who were not treated or were inadequately treated with anticoagulants, valvular thrombosis has been reported in approximately 5 to 6 per cent of Bjork-Shiley valves in the mitral position and 2 to 3 per cent of such valves in the aortic position.[304] Even the St. Jude Medical valve, which is widely held to be less thrombogenic than other mechanical prostheses, was associated with a 5 per cent rate of valve thrombosis in patients who did not receive anticoagulants.[304] In contrast, adequately treated patients have a risk of valve thrombosis of 0.2 to 1.8 per cent per year, regardless of valve model or position.[304,307]

OPTIMIZATION OF ORAL ANTICOAGULANTS. The optimal anticoagulant regimen may be defined as that intensity of anticoagulation that leads to the lowest incidence of valve thrombosis, or systemic embolism, with the minimum number of bleeding episodes. It appears from retrospective studies of late postoperative thromboembolic and bleeding complications that the generally recommended INR of 3.0 to 4.5 may not be necessary after aortic and/or mitral valve replacement with mechanical prostheses.[308,309] Thus, for mechanical prostheses, an INR of 2.5 to 3.5 may be adequate (Table 58–3) (Fig. 58–19); a lower level of anticoagulation with an INR of 2.0 to 3.0 may suffice in bioprosthetic valves in atrial fibrillation or no anticoagulation at all (sinus rhythm) in bioprosthetic valves in sinus rhythm. A large-scale, prospective, randomized trial (GELIA) has been started, therefore, to provide conclusive evidence regarding the optimum level of anticoagulation after valve replacement with the St. Jude Medical prosthesis.

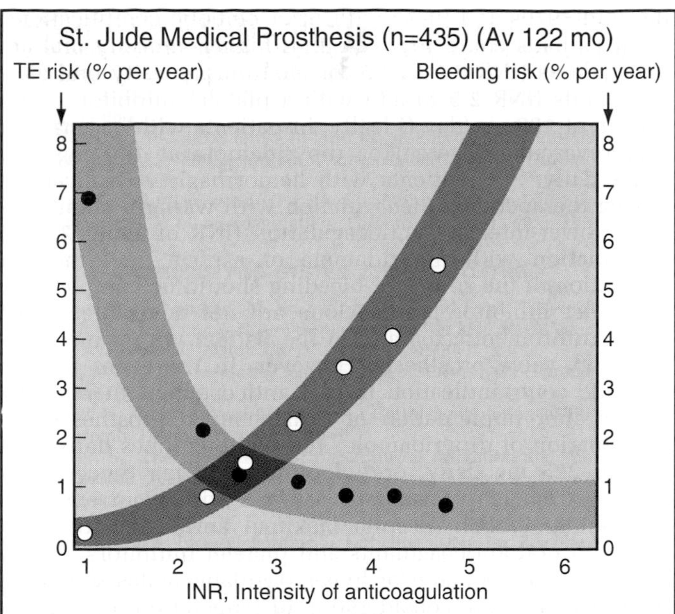

FIGURE 58–19. Thromboembolic and bleeding risks with different anticoagulation regimens in 435 consecutive patients with St. Jude valve replacement. (Modified from Piper, C., Schulte, H. D., and Horstkotte, D.: Optimization of oral anticoagulation for patients with mechanical heart valve prostheses. J. Heart Valve Dis. *4*:127, 1995. With permission.)

PLATELET INHIBITOR THERAPY ALONE AND COMBINED WITH ANTICOAGULANTS. No randomized placebo-controlled clinical trials have tested the use of platelet inhibitors alone as an antithrombotic regimen in mechanical heart valve replacement. However, the use of combination antiplatelet therapy with dipyridamole and aspirin, or pentoxifylline and aspirin, was associated with a significantly higher incidence of thromboembolism when compared with warfarin in an open prospective randomized trial of patients with mitral or aortic Starr-Edwards valves.[310] In addition, in other nonrandomized series, aspirin alone, dipyridamole alone, or the combination of both did not show a significant protective effect.[242] Results in several small nonrandomized trial suggest that platelet inhibitors may provide adequate protection for children with normal sinus rhythm and mechanical prostheses in the aortic position, but such findings must be considered preliminary pending further investigation.[304] Once again, data are very limited concerning the use of platelet inhibitors in patients with bioprosthetic heart valve replacements, and no randomized or placebo-controlled study has been conducted.

Although consistent and optimal anticoagulant therapy is critical for patients with mechanical heart valve prostheses, there is still a relatively high residual risk of systemic thromboembolism. As a result, five randomized controlled trials have been conducted comparing the antithrombotic efficacy of warfarin plus dipyridamole versus warfarin alone in recipients of mechanical ball or tilting disc valves. In three trials, combination therapy was significantly better than warfarin alone, resulting in a 70 to 92 per cent reduction in embolic events. In two other trials the addition of dipyridamole to the warfarin regimen resulted in a 40 to 50 per cent decrease in embolic episodes compared with warfin therapy alone. However, with relatively low event rates in both groups, as is characteristic of more recently operated-on patients, these differences did not achieve statistical significance.[304] Aspirin did lead to a decrease in systemic embolism in three trials when combined with warfarin in doses of 500 to 1000 mg/day.[304]

In each of these trials, this combination led to a significant increase in serious hemorrhage requiring blood transfusion, and the combination of warfarin with high-dose aspirin (500 to 1000 mg) is, therefore, not recommended. However, a very interesting recent study by Turpie et al.[311] tested the combination of anticoagulation with warfarin (INR 3.0 to 4.5) with aspirin in doses of 100 mg/daily. This trial studied 370 patients with prosthetic heart valves implanted between 1987 and 1991, 75 per cent of whom had mechanical heart valve prostheses. A comparison of the combination of warfarin and aspirin with warfarin alone showed a statistically significant reduction in annualized event rates for the endpoints of major systemic embolism and vascular death (1.9 versus 8.5 per cent, $P < 0.01$) and death alone (2.8 versus 7.4 per cent, $P = 0.01$). Although the risk of hemorrhagic events was higher in the combination therapy group compared to warfarin alone (35 per cent per year versus 22 per cent per year, $P = 0.02$), this difference was largely the result of minor bleeding, and the rates of major hemorrhagic events were not significantly different.

Several interesting points emerged from this study: The addition of aspirin to warfarin led to a highly significant reduction in embolism and vascular death, even in patients operated on with late-model prosthetic heart valves, usually a lower-risk cohort. Critical review of the data suggests that a main effect of aspirin might have been a decrease in myocardial infarction in a population at risk for coronary events. In fact, the annual rate of major systemic embolism or death in the warfarin group appears relatively high. Although the intended INR was 3.0 to 4.5, the actual mean INR was only 3.1 in the warfarin group and 3.0 in the combination group, perhaps an attempt to lower hemorrhagic complications; whether this contributed to a higher thrombotic risk in patients without adjunctive platelet inhibition is unclear. Similar conclusions can be drawn from a recent Japanese study in which warfarin was combined with dipyridamole, aspirin, or ticlopidine.[312]

Special Situations Concerning the Use of Antithrombotic Therapy

(Prosthetic valve endocarditis and anticoagulation during pregnancy are described in Chapters 33 and 59, respectively.)

REQUIREMENTS FOR NONCARDIAC SURGERY. In patients with prosthetic heart valves, temporary discontinuation of oral anticoagulants for 7 to 10 days appears to be associated with low overall risk when a patient requires noncardiac therapy.[313] However, as noted previously, in many series most thromboembolic events have occurred when anticoagulants were temporarily discontinued or the level of anticoagulation had fallen to a suboptimal range. Thus, in the high-risk patient, it is advisable either to lower anticoagulation to an INR of about 2.0[314] or to stop oral anticoagulants 3 to 4 days before surgery and start intravenous heparin to maintain the activated partial thromboplastin time at twice the control level; the heparin may be infused up to 4 to 5 hours before surgery and resumed as soon as possible after surgery until oral anticoagulant therapy can be reestablished at optimal levels.

ANTICOAGULATION AFTER AN EMBOLIC EVENT. A difficult clinical decision is the appropriate time to begin anticoagulation when a patient with a prosthetic heart valve experiences an aseptic cardiogenic cerebral embolus. Aggregate data suggest that up to 12 per cent of patients will have a recurrent embolus within the first 2 weeks, the risk being equally distributed over this period at approximately 1 per cent per day.[304,315] Aggregate data from nonrandomized and retrospective series suggest that immediate anticoagulation may decrease this risk, but immediate anticoagulation is associated with an increased risk of hemorrhagic transformation of cerebral infarction.[304,315] However, patients with large cerebral infarcts seem to be at greatest risk of hemorrhagic transformation, which occurs most commonly in the first 48 hours, although it may occur later.[315]

Clinical picture related to long-term prognosis. Acta. Med. Scand. *199:*399, 1976.
296. Hamby, R. J.: Primary myocardial disease. Medicine *49:*55, 1970.
297. The European Working Group on Echocardiography: The European Co-operative Study on clinical significance of right heart thrombi. Eur. Heart J. *10:*1046, 1989.
298. Yamamoto, K., Ikeda, U., Furuhashi, K., et al.: The coagulation system is activated in idiopathic cardiomyopathy. J. Am. Coll. Cardiol. *25:*1634, 1995.
299. Sawada, S. G., Ryan, T., Segar, D., et al.: Distinguishing ischemic cardiomyopathy from nonischemic dilated cardiomyopathy with coronary echocardiography. J. Am. Coll. Cardiol. *19:*1223, 1992.
300. Tsevat, J., Eckman, M. H., McNutt, R. A., and Pauker, S. G.: Warfarin for dilated cardiomyopathy: A bloody tough pill to swallow? Med. Decis. Making *9:*162, 1989.
301. Baker, D. W., and Wright, R. F.: Management of heart failure: IV. Anticoagulation for patients with heart failure due to left ventricular systolic dysfunction. JAMA *272:*1614, 1994.
302. Richardson, W. S., and Detsky, A. S., for the Evidence-Based Medicine Working Group: Users' guides to the medical literature. VII. How to use a clinical decision analysis. A. Are the results of the study valid? JAMA *273:*1292, 1995.

ANTITHROMBOTIC THERAPY IN PROSTHETIC HEART VALVE REPLACEMENT

303. Fuster, V., Badimon, L., Badimon, J. J., and Chesebro, J. H.: Prevention of thromboembolism induced by prosthetic heart valves. Semin. Thromb. Hemost. *14:*50, 1988.
304. Israel, D. H., Sharma, S. K., and Fuster, V.: Antithrombotic therapy in prosthetic heart valve replacement. Am. Heart J. *127:*400, 1994.
305. Heras, M., Chesebro, J. H., Fuster, V., et al.: High risk of thromboembolic early after bioprosthetic cardiac valve replacement. J. Am. Coll. Cardiol. *25:*1111, 1995.
306. Butchart, E. G.: Thrombogenicity, thrombosis and embolism. *In* Butchart, E. G., Bodnar, E. (eds.): Current Issues in Heart Valve Disease: Thrombosis, Embolism and Bleeding. London, ICR Publishers, 1992, p. 293.
307. Horstkotte, D., and Burckhardt, D.: Prosthetic valve thrombosis. J. Heart Valve Dis. *4:*141, 1995.
308. Piper, C., Schulte, H. D., and Horstkotte, D.: Optimization of oral anticoagulation for patients with mechanical heart valve prostheses. J. Heart Valve Dis. *4:*127, 1995.
309. Butchart, E. G.: Rationalizing antithrombotic management for patients with prosthetic heart valves. J. Heart Valve Dis. *4:*106, 1995.
310. Mok, D. C., Boey, J., Wang, R., et al.: Warfarin versus dipyridamole-aspirin and pentoxifylline-aspirin for the prevention of prosthetic heart valve thromboembolism: A prospective randomized clinical trial. Circulation *72:*1059, 1985.
311. Turpie, A. G. G., Gent, M., Laupacis, A., et al.: A comparison of aspirin with placebo in patients treated with warfarin after heart valve replacement. N. Engl. J. Med. *329:*524, 1993.
312. Hayashi, J. I., Nakazawa, S., Oguma, F., et al. Combined warfarin and antiplatelet therapy after St. Jude Medical valve replacement for mitral valve disease. J. Am. Coll. Cardiol. *23:*672, 1994.
313. Tinker, J. H., and Tarhan, S.: Discontinuing anticoagulation therapy in surgical patients with cardiac valve prostheses: Observation in 180 operations. JAMA *239:*738, 1978.
314. Butchart, E. G.: Anticoagulation management during non-cardiac surgery—time for common sense. J. Heart Valve Dis. *3:*313, 1994.
315. Sherman, D. G., Dyken, M. L., Gent, M., et al.: Antithrombotic therapy in cerebrovascular disorders. Chest *108*(Suppl. Oct):371S, 1995.
316. Hoylaerts, M., Kijken, D. C., Lijnen, H. R., and Collen, D.: Kinetics of the activation of plasminogen by human tissue plasminogen activator. Role of fibrin. J. Biol. Chem. *257:*2912, 1982.
317. Canneigieter, S. C., and Rosendaal, F. R.: Thromboembolic and bleeding complications in patients with mechanical heart valve prostheses. Circulation *89:*635, 1994.
318. Lengyel, M., Fuster, V., Keltai, M., et al.: Guidelines for the management of left-sided prosthetic valve thrombosis. Am. J. Cardiol. *(submitted for publication.)*
319. Roudaut, R., Labbe, T., Lorient-Roudaut, M. F., et al.: Mechanical cardiac valve thrombosis. Is fibrinolysis justified? Circulation *86:*8, 1992.
320. Vilanyi, J., Wladika, Z. S., Bartek, I., and Lengyel, M.: Diagnosis and treatment of tricuspid mechanical prosthetic valve dysfunction. Eur. Heart J. *13:*2190, 1992.
321. Birdi, I., Angelini, G. D., and Bryan, A. J.: Thrombolytic therapy for left-sided prosthetic heart valve thrombosis. J. Heart Valve Dis. *4:*154, 1995.
322. Stein, P. D., Albert, J. S., Copeland, J., et al.: Antithrombotic therapy in patients with mechanical and biological prosthetic heart valves. Chest *108*(Suppl. Oct):371S, 1995.

Chapter 59
Pregnancy and Cardiovascular Disease

URI ELKAYAM

CARDIOVASCULAR PHYSIOLOGY DURING PREGNANCY AND THE PUERPERIUM 1843
CARDIAC EVALUATION DURING PREGNANCY 1844
CONGENITAL HEART DISEASE 1846
RHEUMATIC HEART DISEASE 1848
OTHER CONDITIONS AFFECTING THE VALVES, AORTA, AND MYOCARDIUM 1850
Hypertension in Pregnancy 1852
CORONARY ARTERY DISEASE. 1853
ARRHYTHMIAS 1854
OTHER CARDIOVASCULAR DISORDERS . . . 1855
Cardiac Surgery during Pregnancy 1856
CARDIOVASCULAR DRUGS IN PREGNANCY . 1857
REFERENCES 1860

CARDIOVASCULAR PHYSIOLOGY DURING PREGNANCY AND THE PUERPERIUM

Pregnancy and the peripartum period are associated with substantial cardiocirculatory changes. In the woman with heart disease, these changes can lead to rapid clinical deterioration. The approach to the cardiac patient during pregnancy therefore requires an understanding of the alteration in cardiovascular physiology during gestation, labor, delivery, and the puerperium. Hemodynamic changes occurring during pregnancy are summarized in Table 59–1.

BLOOD VOLUME. Blood volume increases substantially during pregnancy, starting as early as the sixth week, rising rapidly until midpregnancy, when the rise continues, but at a much slower rate.[1] The degree of volume expansion varies considerably in the individual patient (20 to 100 per cent) and averages 50 per cent. This increase is reported to correlate with fetal weight, placental mass, weight of the products of conception, neonatal weight, and maternal weight. A higher increment in blood volume is reported in multigravidas and in women with multiple pregnancies.[1]

Because increase in blood volume is more rapid than increase in red blood cell mass (Fig. 59–1), hemoglobin concentration falls during pregnancy, causing the "physiological anemia of pregnancy."[2] Hematocrit and hemoglobin levels are frequently as low as 33 to 38 per cent and 11 to 12 gm/100 ml, respectively, and can be partially corrected with iron therapy.[1] Changes in blood volume during pregnancy are attributable to estrogen-mediated stimulation of the renin-aldosterone system,[3] which results in sodium and water retention.[2] Chorionic somatomammotropin, a hormone-like substance in the placenta, may also be a factor.

TABLE 59–1 HEMODYNAMIC CHANGES DURING NORMAL PREGNANCY

PARAMETER	1st TRIMESTER	2nd TRIMESTER	3rd TRIMESTER
Blood volume	↑	↑↑	↑↑↑
Cardiac output	↑	↑↑ to ↑↑↑	↑↑↑ to ↑↑
Stroke volume	↑	↑↑↑	↑, ↔, or ↓
Heart rate	↑	↑↑	↑↑ or ↑↑↑
Systolic blood pressure	↔	↓	↔
Diastolic blood pressure	↓	↓↓	↓
Pulse pressure	↑	↑↑	↔
Systemic vascular resistance	↓	↓↓↓	↓↓

Modified from Elkayam, U., and Gleicher, N.: Hemodynamics and cardiac function during normal pregnancy and the puerperium. *In* Elkayam, U., and Gleicher, N. (eds.): Cardiac Problems in Pregnancy: Diagnosis and Management of Maternal and Fetal Disease. 2nd ed. New York, Alan R. Liss, Inc., 1990, p. 5.

↔ = no change compared with nonpregnant level; ↑ = small increase; ↑↑ = moderate increase; ↑↑↑ = large increase; ↓ = small decrease; ↓↓ = moderate decrease; ↓↓↓ = large decrease.

CARDIAC OUTPUT, STROKE VOLUME, AND HEART RATE. Augmentation of blood volume alters stroke volume and cardiac output (Table 59–1). Cardiac output during pregnancy is estimated to exceed the output during the nonpregnant state by 30 to 50 per cent.[1,2,4] It begins to rise around the fifth week and peaks between the middle of the second and the third trimesters, when it plateaus. Body position can substantially influence cardiac output, with levels rising in the lateral position and declining in the supine position, owing to caval compression by the gravid uterus and decrease in venous return to the heart. The increase in cardiac output early in pregnancy is predominantly due to augmentation in stroke volume, whereas in the third trimester it is largely due to an accelerated heart rate, while stroke volume declines toward prepregnancy values as a result of caval compression.

Rise in heart rate peaks during the third trimester with an average increase of 10 to 20 beats/min,[4,5] although on occasion it may be markedly faster. Pregnancy of multiple fetuses is associated with an even higher heart rate. The heart rate may decrease slightly in the lateral position in comparison with the supine position.[1]

BLOOD PRESSURE AND SYSTEMIC VASCULAR RESISTANCE. Systemic arterial pressure begins to fall during the first trimester, reaches a nadir in midpregnancy, and returns

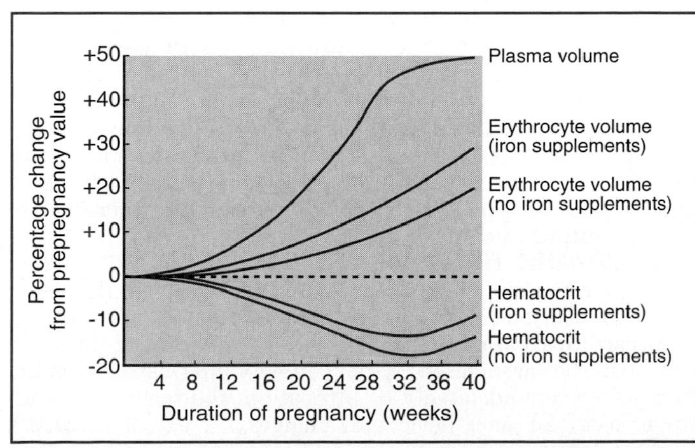

FIGURE 59–1. Changes in plasma volume, erythrocyte volume, and hematocrit during pregnancy. Increase in plasma volume is more rapid than increase in erythrocyte volume, causing the "physiological anemia of pregnancy," which can be partially corrected with iron supplements. (From Pitkin, R. M.: Nutritional support in obstetrics and gynecology. Clin. Obstet. Gynecol. *19*:489, 1976, with permission.)

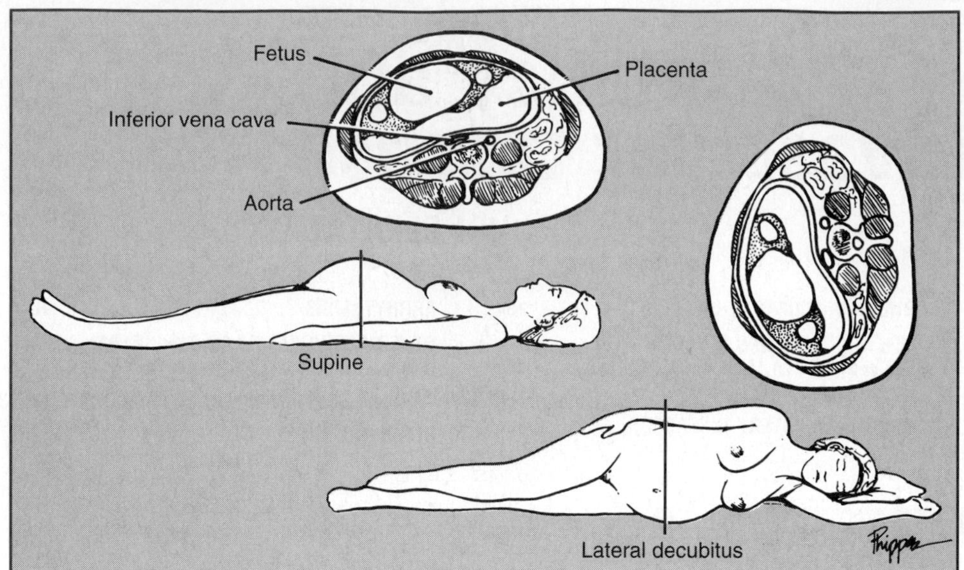

FIGURE 59–2. Venocaval compression of the inferior vena cava and abdominal aorta by the gravid uterus can lead to decreased cardiac output due to reduced venous return and to supine hypotensive syndrome. (From Lee, W., Shah, P. K., Amin, D. K., et al.: Hemodynamic monitoring of cardiac patients during pregnancy. *In* Elkayam, U., Gleicher, N. [eds.]: Cardiac Problems in Pregnancy, 2nd ed., New York, Alan R. Liss, Inc., 1990, p. 61.)

toward pregestational levels before term.[1] Because diastolic blood pressure decreases substantially more than systolic pressure, the pulse pressure widens.[1,6] Reduction in blood pressure is caused by a decline in systemic vascular resistance due to vasodilation,[1] probably mediated by (1) gestational hormonal activity, increased levels of circulating prostaglandins,[7] and atrial natriuretic factor[8]; (2) increased heart production by the developing fetus; and (3) the creation of low-resistance circulation in the pregnant uterus. A phenomenon unique to pregnancy and described as the supine hypotensive or the uterocaval syndrome of pregnancy occurs with significant decreases in heart rate and blood pressure in up to 11 per cent of pregnant women.[1] These hemodynamic changes are associated with weakness, lightheadedness, nausea, dizziness, and even syncope and are explained by acute occlusion of the inferior vena cava by the enlarged uterus (Fig. 59–2). When the supine position is abandoned, these hemodynamic effects and symptoms usually are promptly relieved.

HEMODYNAMIC CHANGES DURING LABOR AND DELIVERY. Anxiety, pain, and uterine contractions all alter hemodynamics substantially during labor and delivery. Oxygen consumption increases threefold. Cardiac output rises by up to 50 per cent during contractions, mainly owing to changes in stroke volume,[9] and it is higher in the lateral position than in the supine position. The effect of uterine contractions on the heart rate varies[13] and may be influenced by body position during labor and the form of sedation used. Both systolic and diastolic blood pressures increase markedly during contractions, with greater augmentation during the second stage.[1,9] Hemodynamic changes during labor and delivery are greatly influenced by the form of anesthesia and analgesia.[10] Reduction of pain and apprehension by local and caudal anesthesia may limit the rise in oxygen consumption, hemodynamic changes, and cardiac output, but does not prevent the increase in cardiac output related to uterine contractions.

HEMODYNAMIC EFFECTS OF CESAREAN SECTION. To avoid the hemodynamic changes associated with vaginal delivery, cesarean section is frequently recommended for women with cardiovascular disease. However, this form of delivery can also be associated with considerable hemodynamic fluctuation related largely to intubation, the technique, and drugs used for anesthesia and analgesia[10]; extent of blood loss; abdominal surgery; the relief of caval compression; extubation; and postoperative awakening.[1,10]

HEMODYNAMIC CHANGES POST PARTUM. Clinical status often deteriorates in the immediate postpartum period when venous return increases after the fetus is removed and caval compression is relieved.[1] In addition, blood shifting from the contracting, emptied uterus into the systemic circulation (autotransfusion) increases the preload. This change in effective blood volume occurs despite blood loss during delivery and leads to a substantial rise in ventricular filling pressure, stroke volume, and cardiac output immediately after delivery. Within the first hour, however, the reduction in heart rate decreases cardiac output, which falls to prepregnancy levels 24 hours post partum as stroke volume normalizes.[9]

HEMODYNAMIC RESPONSE TO EXERCISE. Exercise-mediated increase in cardiac output is limited during gestation and in the third trimester may be more than 20 per cent lower than it is in nonpregnant women.[11] This attenuated rise in cardiac output is due to the lower responses of heart rate and stroke volume; the latter is probably the result of reduction in venous return during pregnancy. Uterine blood flow is also reduced (25 per cent) in the third trimester during mild exercise. Such reductions may be associated with fetal hypoxia, manifested by brief episodes of fetal bradycardia.[12] Strenuous physical activity may therefore be associated with fetal compromise and is not recommended during pregnancy.

CARDIAC EVALUATION DURING PREGNANCY

The evaluation of cardiac disease in pregnancy may be complicated by the normal anatomical and functional changes of the cardiovascular system. Such changes may result in signs and symptoms that can either simulate or obscure heart disease.[13] It is therefore imperative in many cases to use additional diagnostic tools to obtain objective and reliable information about cardiac status. The selection of such diagnostic tools should be influenced by the potential risk to the fetus posed by certain methods.

History and Physical Examination

(Table 59–2).

Normal pregnancy is often accompanied by symptoms of fatigue, decreased exercise capacity, hyperventilation, dyspnea, lightheadedness, and even syncope.[14,15] In addition, distention of the jugular veins due to increased blood volume and leg edema, often observed in late pregnancy, could lead to an erroneous diagnosis of heart failure or overestimation of its severity. Systemic arterial pulses are full and collapsing and are similar to those palpated in patients with aortic regurgitation or hyperthyroidism. A left ventricular impulse is easily detected in most women in late pregnancy; usually it is hyperactive and brisk. The

TABLE 59–2 CARDIAC SYMPTOMS AND PHYSICAL FINDINGS DURING NORMAL PREGNANCY

SYMPTOMS
Decreased exercise capacity
Tiredness
Dyspnea
Orthopnea
Lightheadedness
Syncope
PHYSICAL FINDINGS
Inspection
Hyperventilation
Peripheral edema
Distended neck veins with prominent A and V waves and brisk x and y descents
Capillary pulsation
Precordial palpation
Brisk, diffuse, and displaced left ventricular impulse
Palpable right ventricular impulse
Palpable pulmonary trunk impulse
Auscultation
Increased S_1 with exaggerated splitting
Persistent splitting of S_2
Midsystolic ejection-type murmurs at lower left sternal edge and/or over pulmonary area radiating to left side of neck
Continuous murmurs (cervical venous hum, mammary souffle)
Diastolic murmurs (rare)

Modified from Elkayam, U., and Gleicher, N.: Changes in cardiac findings during normal pregnancy. *In* Elkayam, U., and Gleicher, N. (eds.): Cardiac Problems in Pregnancy: Diagnosis and Management of Maternal and Fetal Disease. 2nd ed. New York, Alan R. Liss, Inc., 1990, p. 31.

quality of the impulse may simulate a volume overload state such as that seen in aortic or mitral valve regurgitation. The pulmonary trunk, right ventricle, and pulmonic valve closure are often palpable, and this group of findings may result in difficulty in assessing the presence and/or severity of pulmonary hypertension.

CARDIAC AUSCULTATION. Especially after the first trimester, auscultation often reveals an increased first heart sound (S_1) with exaggerated splitting that may be misinterpreted as S_4 or as a systolic click.[13] The physiological increase in the amplitude of the second component of S_1 with inspiration should help differentiate it from an abnormal auscultatory event. S_2 is often increased in late pregnancy and may exhibit persistent splitting when the patient is examined in the lateral position. These changes in S_2 may be interpreted as signs of pulmonary hypertension (loud S_2) or atrial septal defect (fixed splitting of S_2). Auscultation of S_3 and S_4 sounds is uncommon in normal pregnancy, and their presence warrants further investigation to detect possible underlying disease.[13]

Innocent Systolic Murmurs. These can be heard in most pregnant women and are the result of the hyperkinetic circulation of pregnancy.[13] Murmurs are usually midsystolic and soft, heard best at the lower left sternal edge and over the pulmonic area, radiating to the suprasternal notch and to the left and, at times, also to the right side of the neck.[13,16] Not uncommonly the benign murmur of pregnancy may be louder or longer and may sound like those associated with atrial septal defect or stenosis of one of the semilunar valves.[16] In such cases an echocardiographic and Doppler evaluation is warranted to rule out an abnormal cardiac condition. Two benign continuous murmurs that may be heard during gestation are the cervical venous hum and the mammary souffle. The venous hum is usually heard maximally over the right supraclavicular fossa but can radiate to the contralateral area and sometimes to the area below the clavicle. The mammary souffle may be either systolic or continuous, is heard over the breast late in gestation or in the lactating woman, and is caused by increased flow in the mammary vessels. Characteristically the murmur decreases or vanishes when pressure is applied to the stethoscope or when the patient moves into the upright position.[13] Diastolic murmurs may be heard in normal pregnant women due to increased blood flow through the atrioventricular valve.[13] Such a finding, however, is infrequent in the healthy pregnant woman and therefore requires careful diagnostic work-up to rule out organic disease.

Increases in blood volume and flow across the various cardiac valves may augment systolic murmurs of aortic or pulmonic stenosis and the diastolic murmur of mitral stenosis. In contrast, the murmurs associated with mitral or aortic regurgitation may decrease in intensity because of a reduction in systemic vascular resistance during pregnancy. In addition, the change in volume may abolish the systolic click and murmur commonly heard in patients with mitral valve prolapse[17] and may decrease the systolic murmur typical of obstructive hypertrophic cardiomyopathy.[18]

Laboratory Examinations

ELECTROCARDIOGRAPHY (Table 59–3). In normal pregnancy, QRS axis may shift to either the left or the right, but it usually stays within normal limits.[13] Slight ST-segment depressions and T-wave changes may be seen. A small Q wave and an inverted P wave in lead III that vary with respiration as well as a greater R-wave amplitude in lead V_2 are often present. A high incidence of ST-segment depression mimicking myocardial ischemia but not associated with wall motion abnormalities has been described relatively recently in patients undergoing cesarean section.[19] Increased susceptibility to arrhythmias during pregnancy can be manifested by the frequent finding of sinus tachycardia and atrial and/or ventricular premature beats.[20]

CHEST RADIOGRAPHY (Table 59–3). Although the radiation dose associated with a routine chest X-ray examination is minimal (the average dose to the skin in the primary beam is 70 to 150 mrad, while the estimated dose to the uterus is 0.2 to 43.0 mrad),[21] this diagnostic test is best avoided during pregnancy because of the potential for adverse biological effects from any amount of radiation. When chest radiography is performed, the pelvic area should be shielded by protective lead material.

Changes seen on chest films in normal pregnancy may simulate cardiac disease and should be interpreted with caution.[13,14] Straightening of the left upper cardiac border because of prominence of the pulmonary conus is often seen. The heart may seem enlarged because of its horizontal positioning secondary to the elevated diaphragm. In addition, an increase in lung markings may simulate a pattern of flow redistribution seen with increased pulmonary venous pressure due to left ventricular failure or mitral valve disease. Pleural effusion is often found early post partum[22]; it is usually small and resorbs 1 to 2 weeks after delivery.

DOPPLER ECHOCARDIOGRAPHY (Table 59–3). Gestational use of both

TABLE 59–3 FINDINGS ON ELECTROCARDIOGRAM, CHEST X-RAY, AND ECHO-DOPPLER DURING NORMAL PREGNANCY

ELECTROCARDIOGRAM
QRS-axis deviation
ST-segment and T-wave changes
Small Q wave and inverted P wave in lead III (abolished by inspiration)
Increased R-wave amplitude in lead V_2
Frequent sinus tachycardia
Increased incidence of arrhythmias
CHEST X-RAY
Straightening of left upper cardiac border
Horizontal position of heart
Increased lung marking
Small pleural effusion early post partum
ECHO-DOPPLER
Increased left and right ventricular dimensions
Unchanged or slightly increased size and systolic function of left ventricle
Mild increase in left and right atrial size
Small pericardial effusion
Increased diameter of tricuspid annulus
Functional tricuspid, pulmonary, and mitral insufficiency

Modified from Elkayam, U., and Gleicher, N.: Changes in cardiac findings during normal pregnancy. *In* Elkayam, U., and Gleicher, N. (eds.): Cardiac Problems in Pregnancy: Diagnosis and Management of Maternal and Fetal Disease. 2nd ed. New York, Alan R. Liss, Inc., 1990, p. 31.

maternal and fetal cardiac ultrasound is considered safe.[23] Transesophageal echocardiography has been increasingly used in pregnancy and seems to be well tolerated by both mother and fetus.[24] Normal gestational changes in the cardiovascular system are reflected echocardiographically and should be taken into consideration. Examination in the left lateral position often shows enlarged dimensions of cardiac chambers, especially the right atrium and ventricle.[5,25,26] These changes progress with the pregnancy but return to baseline dimensions post partum. Left ventricular systolic dimensions and function are either unchanged or slightly increased during pregnancy.

Pericardial effusion, usually small or minimal, has been noted in 40 per cent of normal pregnant women late in pregnancy.[27] Studies have demonstrated mild regurgitation of the tricuspid and pulmonary valves in the majority of normal pregnant women at term and of the mitral valve in approximately one-third.[25,26] These findings seem to be related to chamber enlargement and dilatation of the valve annulus. Repeat examination 3 to 6 weeks post partum still demonstrated tricuspid and pulmonary regurgitation in 70 to 80 per cent of women.[26] These findings, although not clinically important, need to be considered in the interpretation of Doppler echocardiograms obtained during pregnancy.

STRESS TESTING. An exercise test using bicycle ergometry or a treadmill may be carried out during pregnancy to help establish the diagnosis of ischemic heart disease and to assess functional capacity and cardiac reserve. The safety of such testing in pregnancy has not been fully established. Because fetal bradycardia has been reported with maximal but not with submaximal exercise,[12] a low-level exercise protocol allowing heart rate increase to 75 per cent of maximal predicted heart rate with fetal monitoring is recommended when stress testing is indicated.[13]

RADIONUCLIDE IMAGING. A potential limitation of these techniques during pregnancy is radiation exposure to the fetus. The dose estimated to reach the fetus with the radiopharmaceuticals generally used for cardiac imaging is equal to or less than 800 mrad.[28] However, calculations of the dose to the fetus are only approximations and can vary from person to person owing to differences in the uptake of radionuclides by maternal organs and in placental uptake and transfer. Because of these uncertainties and the potential risk, use of radionuclide imaging during gestation and in particular during the first trimester should be limited to cases in which the information desired cannot be obtained by other noninvasive techniques.

MAGNETIC RESONANCE IMAGING. Magnetic resonance imaging has been used in pregnancy for the assessment of congenital heart disease and aortic dissection.[29,30] Experience with this technique is limited, however, and its safety has not been fully established. This technique should therefore be used only when evaluation cannot be delayed until after pregnancy, and if possible after the first trimester.[31]

PULMONARY ARTERY CATHETERIZATION. Hemodynamic monitoring with the aid of a pulmonary artery catheter can be of great help in managing patients at high risk during pregnancy, labor, delivery, and the postpartum period. The ability to insert and position the flotation catheter under pressure monitoring without the need for fluoroscopy makes it particularly attractive for use during pregnancy.[32] Hemodynamic monitoring can provide useful diagnostic and prognostic information and therapeutic guidance and should be used without hesitation at any time during pregnancy if a noninvasive cardiac work-up does not provide conclusive information.

Hemodynamic monitoring is recommended throughout labor and delivery for any patient with symptomatic cardiac disease during pregnancy or with the potential for deterioration due to valvular, vascular, myocardial, or ischemic heart disease. Since significant circulatory changes that may lead to hemodynamic deterioration occur in the early postpartum period,[1] hemodynamic monitoring should be continued for at least several hours after delivery to assure stability.

CARDIAC CATHETERIZATION. When cardiac decompensation occurs during pregnancy, particularly if cardiac surgery, coronary angioplasty, or balloon valvuloplasty is being considered, cardiac catheterization may be required. Although this technique provides high-quality images, it is associated with a relatively high dose of radiation. The median dose to the skin is 47 rads per examination with 10 to 15 per cent exposure to an unshielded abdomen and approximately 500 mrad estimated dose to the conceptus, even with an appropriate pelvic shield.[21]

The potentially deleterious effect of ionizing radiation is linearly proportional to the absorbed dose and is present at all times after fertilization. The type and likelihood of this effect vary with the stage of fetal development and the dose of radiation. Increased incidence of fetal malformation appears to be highly unlikely with doses below 5 rads, even when these are delivered at a time when the induction of any specific type of maldevelopment is critical.[33] In general, radiation exposure during the first week of pregnancy may result in absorption or resorption of the preimplanted blastocyst, whereas the risk of teratogenic effects predominates during the second to sixth weeks of gestation. Developing brain cells can be affected by radiation during the seventh to fifteenth weeks, which may lead to alterations in neurological function or behavior. In addition, irradiation at any time during the entire pregnancy may increase the risk for childhood cancer[34]; this risk seems to be higher with exposure during the first trimester.

Cardiac catheterization during gestation should be performed only if information cannot be obtained by alternative noninvasive methods. To minimize radiation to the pelvic and abdominal areas, the brachial rather than the femoral approach is preferred. Appropriate shielding should be used, and roentgen exposure should be kept to a minimum. To minimize the use of ionizing radiation, as much information as possible should be obtained by noninvasive techniques such as contrast[35] and Doppler echocardiography.

CONGENITAL HEART DISEASE (CHD)

(See also Chaps. 29 and 30)

PRECONCEPTION COUNSELING. This should include an accurate diagnostic and functional evaluation and counseling of both the patient and her family regarding contraceptive alternatives, potential maternal and fetal risks of pregnancy, and, when appropriate, expected long-term maternal morbidity and survival as well as the risk of transmitting CHD to the offspring. In addition, guidance concerning anticoagulation and prophylactic antibiotics, if needed, should be provided.[36,37]

MATERNAL AND FETAL OUTCOME. In general, a good maternal outcome can be expected in most cases with noncyanotic congenital heart disease. Maternal outcome is determined by the nature of the disease, surgical repair, presence and severity of cyanosis, level of hemoglobin, increased pulmonary vascular resistance, and functional capacity.[36–38] Unfavorable outcome, including development of congestive heart failure, arrhythmias, and hypertension, is commonly seen in patients with impaired functional status and with cyanosis.[38] Other reported complications include angina, infective endocarditis, and thromboembolic phenomena. Factors that may increase likelihood of cardiovascular deterioration include exercise, heat, humidity, anemia, infections, and cardiac arrhythmias.[39]

Maternal functional capacity and cyanosis also determine fetal outcome. Fetal wastage was reported in 45 per cent of cyanotic mothers compared with 20 per cent in acyanotic mothers with CHD.[38] Low birth weight for gestational age and prematurity are common in cyanotic mothers and correlate with maternal hemoglobin and hematocrit values.[40] Risk of CHD is increased for the offspring of mothers with CHD with a reported incidence of about 10 per cent (3.4 to 16.1 per cent).[38–42] In addition, there are a greater number of noncardiac abnormalities as well as mental and physical impairments in children born to mothers with CHD.[38]

LABOR AND DELIVERY. Elective induction of labor when fetal maturity is confirmed may be used in high-risk patients for better planning of hemodynamic monitoring and availability of expert personnel.[39] Cesarean section is not indicated in most patients with CHD[36,38,39] and should be performed primarily for obstetrical reasons or in response to deteriorating maternal status. Oxygen should be given to hypoxemic mothers, and hemodynamic as well as blood gas monitoring is recommended in patients with impaired functional capacity, cardiac dysfunction, pulmonary hypertension, and cyanotic malformations.[32]

ANTIBIOTIC PROPHYLAXIS. Official recommendations by the American Heart Association do *not* include patients with CHD undergoing uncomplicated vaginal delivery unless they have a prosthetic heart valve or a surgically constructed systemic-to-pulmonary shunt.[43] Because of the difficulties in predicting complicated deliveries and the potential devastating consequences of endocarditis, we recommend antibiotic prophylaxis for vaginal delivery for patients with CHD, with the exception of those with an isolated secundum type of atrial septal defect and those ≥ 6 months after ligation and division of a patent ductus arteriosus. There is no need for antibiotic prophylaxis for cesarean section delivery.

Specific Malformations

(See also p. 976)

ATRIAL SEPTAL DEFECT (ASD) (see also pp. 966 and 970). This condition is usually well tolerated in pregnancy, even among patients with large left-to-right shunts. The development of pulmonary hypertension and atrial arrhythmias rarely occurs in the childbearing age. Because endocarditis is rare, antibiotic prophylaxis is not indicated in patients with secundum-type ASD. Recommendations concerning pregnancy in patients with ASD should be made on an individual basis, considering accompanying lesions, functional status, and the level of pulmonary vascular resistance.[42]

VENTRICULAR SEPTAL DEFECT (VSD) (see also p. 967). Women with isolated VSD usually tolerate pregnancy well, although congestive heart failure and arrhythmias have been reported.[42] The risk posed by pregnancy after closure of an uncomplicated VSD should not differ from that in patients without heart disease. The incidence of CHD in offspring of women with VSD was found to be as high as 22 per cent among live-born offspring in one report; 50 per cent of them had VSD.[38] Marked reduction in blood pressure during or after delivery as a result of blood loss or anesthesia may lead to shunt reversal in patients with pulmonary hypertension. The use of vasopressors and volume replacement to stabilize blood pressure promptly should prevent further complications.

PATENT DUCTUS ARTERIOSUS (PDA) (see p. 966). Maternal outcome in patients with PDA with left-to-right shunt is usually favorable[36,42]; however, clinical deterioration and congestive heart failure may occur in some patients.[42] There were no maternal deaths among a large number of patients with PDA.[36,42,44] The occasional patient with heart failure should be treated with bed rest, diuretics, digitalis, and vasodilators. The need for surgical intervention during pregnancy is rare. A fall in systemic vascular resistance during gestation and hypotension early post partum may lead to shunt reversal in women with pulmonary hypertension. Peripartum decrease in systemic blood pressure should be corrected by means of vasopressor agents.

CONGENITAL AORTIC VALVE DISEASE (see p. 969). These abnormalities may lead to significant aortic stenosis and regurgitation in women of childbearing age. Obstruction of left ventricular outflow can also result from unicuspid or tricuspid valve stenosis or supravalvular and subvalvular obstruction. Aortic stenosis, especially if mild, can easily be missed on physical examination, because murmur may be attributed to the flow-related systolic murmur commonly heard in the normal pregnant woman. The presence of a sustained left ventricular impulse, aortic ejection sound, maximum murmur intensity heard in the second right intercostal space, S_4, and radiation of the murmur to both sides of the neck should raise the level of suspicion.

Most patients with aortic stenosis should have favorable outcome of pregnancy provided that they receive early diagnosis and appropriate care, including hemodynamic monitoring during labor and delivery, and appropriate anesthesia.[42] At the same time, however, worsening of symptoms during pregnancy, especially in women with severe aortic stenosis, is not uncommon.[45–48] Symptoms usually develop in the second or third trimester and may include exertional dyspnea, chest pain, lightheadedness, syncope, and pulmonary edema. A high incidence (20 per cent) of cardiac defects has been reported in live-born infants of mothers with left ventricular outflow obstruction.[38] Because of the risk involved, patients with severe aortic stenosis (aortic valve area < 1.0 cm^2) should undergo valve replacement prior to pregnancy. Optional management of a pregnant patient with severe aortic stenosis includes (1) early abortion followed by valve replacement and repeat pregnancy and (2) continuation of pregnancy and plan for percutaneous balloon valvuloplasty or surgical intervention in patients who show clinical deterioration not controlled by medical therapy.

Both replacement of aortic valve and percutaneous balloon valvuloplasty have been performed successfully in pregnant women with aortic stenosis.[46–49] These procedures, however, are not free of complications. While valvuloplasty obviates the general anesthesia and cardiopulmonary bypass required for surgery, it can be associated with prolonged radiation exposure and hemodynamic fluctuations that may lead to immediate and late fetal complications. Surgical replacement of the aortic valve during pregnancy may be associated with increased incidence of fetal loss.[49] For these reasons, these procedures should be considered only in patients with severe disease and symptoms not manageable with medical therapy, and they should be avoided when possible during the first trimester.

COARCTATION OF THE AORTA (see p. 971). Available information[38] as well as our experience indicates a favorable outcome of pregnancy in most women with uncomplicated coarctation. At the same time, however, complications such as hypertension, congestive heart failure, and angina have been reported. In addition, aortic dissection and rupture, as well as rupture of an aneurysm of the circle of Willis,[36] have also been associated with coarctation of the aorta during pregnancy. Also, a higher incidence of infective endocarditis in the mother and of CHD in the fetus has been shown in cases with surgically uncorrected compared with corrected coarctation.[36,38] For all of these reasons, it seems advisable to correct aortic coarctation prior to pregnancy.

Treatment to reduce the incidence of aortic rupture and cerebral aneurysms during pregnancy consists of limiting physical activity and controlling blood pressure. Excessive blood pressure reduction, however, may compromise uteroplacental blood flow and should be avoided. Surgical correction of coarctation has been performed successfully during pregnancy[50] and may be indicated in patients with severe uncontrollable systolic hypertension or heart failure.

PULMONIC STENOSIS (see also p. 965). Although complications such as congestive heart failure and syncope have been described, women with pulmonic valve stenosis, even if severe, usually tolerate pregnancy well.[36,51,52] When possible, however, severe stenosis should be corrected prior to conception. In the rare instance of progressive right ventricular failure or symptoms clearly related to the stenotic valve despite appropriate drug therapy, surgical or percutaneous balloon valvotomy should be considered.

TETRALOGY OF FALLOT (see p. 968). Hemodynamic changes associated with pregnancy may become severe and cause clinical deterioration in women with surgically uncorrected or only partially corrected tetralogy of Fallot. Increases in blood volume and venous return to the right atrium raise right ventricular pressure, which combined with a fall in systemic vascular resistance can produce or exacerbate a right-to-left shunt and cyanosis.

Maternal hematocrit above 60 per cent, arterial oxygen saturation below 80 per cent, right ventricular hypertension, and syncopal episodes are poor prognostic signs. Close monitoring of systemic blood pressure and blood gases during labor and delivery is recommended for cyanotic or symptomatic patients. Although reports of pregnancies in 37 women with corrected tetralogy of Fallot described no maternal deaths,[38] worsening of the clinical condition necessitating interruption of the pregnancy is not uncommon. Incidence of cardiac defects reported in born infants ranges between 3 and 17 per cent.

Because maternal and fetal outcomes seem to be markedly improved after surgical repair, this procedure should be performed prior to conception.[36] Patients who have undergone only palliative procedures or who have significant residual defects after repair are still at higher risk during pregnancy. Although mortality associated with complete repair is slightly increased in older patients who have previously undergone a palliative procedure,[38] surgical repair is recommended prior to pregnancy. Since revision of an incompletely repaired defect is recommended in patients with residual VSD when the pulmonary/systemic flow ratio is greater than 1.5:1, in those with right ventricular outflow obstruction (right ventricular systolic pressure >60 mm Hg), and in those with right ventricular failure due to pulmonic regurgitation, such revision should be performed prior to conception in a woman who plans to conceive.[42]

Inhalation analgesia and paracervical or pudendal block have been recommended for labor and vaginal delivery.[53] Epidural block could result in systemic hypotension and shunt reversal and should therefore be used with great care. To minimize potential hemodynamic problems, a segmental epidural block for the first stage of labor with pudendal or caudal block for the second stage has been recommended along with opiates to decrease the concentration of anesthetics injected epidurally.

EISENMENGER'S SYNDROME (see p. 799). This condition continues to be associated with high risk for maternal morbidity and mortality. A relatively recent review of 24 women with this syndrome revealed a mortality rate of 38 per cent.[42] Several cases published since 1990 confirm the risk associated with pregnancy in patients with this syndrome.[41,54–58] Maternal mortality often occurs in the first few days after delivery and is preceded by desaturation and hemodynamic deterioration. Eisenmenger's syndrome is also associated with a poor fetal outcome and a high incidence of fetal loss, prematurity, intrauterine growth retardation, and perinatal death.[42,54,57,59]

Because of the high risk of maternal mortality, patients with Eisenmenger's syndrome should be advised against pregnancy. Abortion should be recommended for patients who are already pregnant. Management of a patient who decides to proceed to term must include close follow-up for early detection of clinical deterioration and restriction of physical activity to minimize the hemodynamic burden. Because of the increased incidence of peripartum thromboembolic events—which are often fatal in such patients[42,59] —anticoagulent therapy seems indicated for at least the third trimester of gestation and for 4 weeks post partum. Since premature delivery is common, women with Eisenmenger's syndrome should be hospitalized for any sign of premature uterine activity. For this reason and to assure restriction of activity and close follow-up, early elective hospitalization is recommended. Spontaneous labor is preferred to induction and should lower the chance of prematurity or the need for cesarean section. Blood pressure, electrocardiographic, and blood gas monitoring are essential during labor and delivery to ensure early detection and correction of problems; high concentrations of oxygen may be helpful. Most patients in stable condition will tolerate vaginal delivery; however, an attempt should be made to shorten the second stage of labor by the use of forceps or vacuum extraction.

Because epidural anesthesia may lead to peripheral vasodilation and increased shunting from right to left, epidural block should be titrated carefully with local anesthetics.[53] Delivery has been successful with lumbar epidural block for the first stage of labor and caudal block for delivery; other authors have preferred the use of systemic medications, inhalation analgesia, and paracervical or pudendal block. For cesarean section, general anesthesia with drugs having a minimal negative inotropic effect is recommended. In addition, segmental epidural anesthesia has been used successfully for cesarean section in patients with Eisenmenger's syndrome.[53]

EBSTEIN'S ANOMALY. Most patients with Ebstein's anomaly survive to childbearing age. Long-term prognosis depends on the severity of tricuspid regurgitation, the presence of right ventricular failure, and the presence and degree of cyanosis due to shunting from right to left. Successful pregnancies have been reported in the majority of patients with Ebstein's anomaly.[60] However, complications such as right ventricular failure, infective endocarditis, and paradoxical embolism can occur.[42] The incidence of maternal and fetal complications is increased among cyanotic patients.[38] The approach to labor and delivery in symptomatic or cyanotic patients with Ebstein's anomaly includes antibiotic prophylaxis, oxygen administration, hemodynamic and blood gas monitoring, and efforts to prevent a drop in systemic blood pressure in response to peripheral vasodilation or blood loss.

COMPLEX CYANOTIC CHD. The more widespread use of palliative and corrective surgical procedures for complex cyanotic congenital cardiac anomalies has allowed more women who are so affected to reach childbearing age.[42] Although successful pregnancies have been reported in patients with partially corrected and uncorrected cyanotic heart disease including pulmonary and tricuspid atresia,[41,54] transposition of the great vessels,[41,61] truncus arteriosus,[54,62] single ventricle,[41,63] double-outlet right ventricle,[64] and double-inlet left ventricle,[65] pregnancy is associated with increased risk in these patients. A recent report[41] of 96 pregnancies in 44 patients with cyanotic heart disease but without Eisenmenger's reaction demonstrated cardiovascular complications in 32 per cent of the patients. These complications included heart failure, thromboembolic events, supraventricular tachycardia, and peripartum bacterial endocarditis resulting in postpartum maternal death in one patient. In addition, a high incidence of fetal wastage (57 per cent), premature deliveries, small-for-gestational-age newborns, and both cardiac and noncardiac congenital malformations has been reported.[38,41]

Hemoglobin and arterial oxygen saturation prior to pregnancy were found to be best predictors for fetal outcome.[41] When serious risk to the mother is predicted, pregnancy should be discouraged prior to conception or should be interrupted early if it has already begun. If the patient wishes to continue the pregnancy, restriction of physical activity and early detection and management of heart failure and/or arrhythmias are essential. Because of potential for severe thromboembolic events,[41,55] anticoagulation is recommended at least during the third trimester and 1 month post partum. Diuretics, if indicated, should be used carefully because of rise of hemoconcentration in the cyanotic patients. Antibiotic prophylaxis and oxygen therapy are strongly recommended for delivery,[41] as well as hemodynamic and blood gas monitoring. Although vaginal delivery appears to be tolerated by most women,[41,42,65] attempts should be made to shorten the second stage by the use of forceps or vacuum extraction.

During labor and delivery, systemic hypotension due to vasodilation or blood loss should be expeditiously corrected to avoid increasing right-to-left shunt.[42,63] Regional anesthetic techniques should be used cautiously. Systemic medications, inhalation analgesia, nerve blocks, and intrathecal morphine have been recommended.[53,56]

RHEUMATIC HEART DISEASE

Although the incidence of rheumatic heart disease is declining in the United States, the disease continues to be prevalent in many parts of the world and may be associated with significant morbidity and even mortality during pregnancy.[66–68]

ACUTE RHEUMATIC FEVER (see Chap. 55). This disease occurs most commonly in children, before puberty, and may recur during pregnancy. Acute rheumatic fever associated with carditis and congestive heart failure may be fatal in the pregnant woman.[66] The incidence of Sydenham's chorea, like acute rheumatic fever itself, has been reported to be increased in pregnancy (chorea gravidarum) and can cause preterm labor and fetal and maternal death. Because of the problems faced by women with recurrent rheumatic fever during pregnancy, it is prudent to continue antibiotic prophylaxis against streptococcal infection in the pregnant patient with a history of this condition. The recommended antibiotic regimen is discussed in detail on page 1773.

Chronic Rheumatic Valvular Disease

(See also Chap. 32)

Patients with chronic rheumatic valvular disease should be managed individually according to the site and severity of the lesion. However, certain general guidelines apply to the care of all patients. These include restriction of physical activity in symptomatic patients, to reduce cardiovascular load and prevent hemodynamic and symptomatic worsening, and prophylactic antibiotic treatment to prevent streptococcal infection and recurrence. Although antibiotic prophylaxis during labor and delivery has not been uniformly recommended,[43] it is commonly used for vaginal and abdominal deliveries.[66] Hemodynamic monitoring is strongly recommended from the onset of labor to approxi-

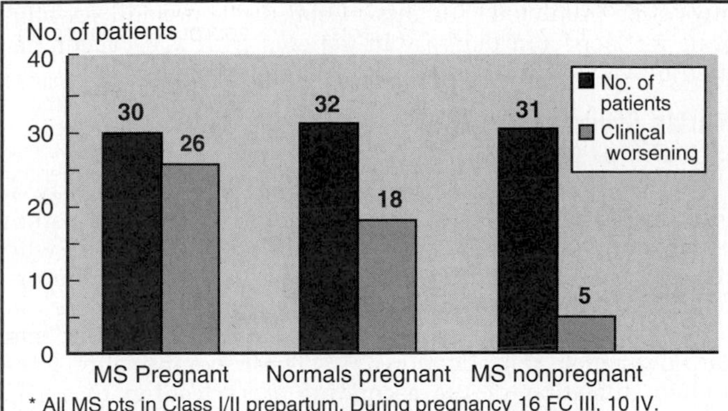

FIGURE 59–3. Worsening in functional classification in patients with mitral stenosis (MS). Twenty-six of 30 patients with MS reported worsening of symptoms during pregnancy. However, more than 50 per cent of women without heart disease also described similar symptoms and impairment of functional capacity during normal pregnancy. Only 5 of 31 nonpregnant patients with MS reported clinical worsening over a similar period. (Modified from Avila, W. S., Grinberg, M., Cardoso, L. F., et al.: Course of pregnancy and puerperium in women with mitral valve stenosis. Rev. Assoc. Med. Bras. *38*:195, 1992.)

mately 24 hours post partum in any patient who experiences symptoms of heart failure during pregnancy and for those with severe valvular disease, left ventricular dysfunction, or pulmonary hypertension.[32]

MITRAL STENOSIS. This condition is the most common rheumatic valvular lesion in pregnancy.[44,68] The majority of patients with moderate to severe mitral stenosis demonstrate worsening of clinical status during gestation (Fig. 59–3).[69] Although mitral stenosis is often accompanied by some degree of mitral regurgitation, hemodynamic problems are related predominantly to flow obstruction. The pressure gradient across the narrowed mitral valve may increase greatly secondary to the physiological increase in heart rate and blood volume of pregnancy.[1] Increased left atrial pressure may result in atrial flutter or fibrillation, substantially accelerating ventricular rate and further elevating left atrial pressure. In addition, decreased serum colloid osmotic pressure during pregnancy and excessive peripartum intravenous fluid administration can both predispose to pulmonary edema.

The therapeutic approach to patients with significant mitral stenosis should aim to reduce the heart rate and decrease blood volume. Both heart rate and symptoms can be controlled effectively by restricting physical activity and administering beta-adrenergic receptor blockers.[69,70] In patients with atrial fibrillation, digoxin may also be useful for control of ventricular rate. Blood volume can be decreased through restriction of salt intake and the use of oral diuretics; aggressive use of diuretic agents should, however, be avoided to prevent hypovolemia and reduction of uteroplacental perfusion.

Vaginal delivery can be permitted in most patients with mitral stenosis. In symptomatic patients or those with moderate or severe stenosis (mitral valve area <1.5 cm^2), hemodynamic monitoring is recommended during labor and delivery. Initiation of monitoring at onset of labor allows hemodynamic optimization by means of intravenous diuretics, digoxin (in case of atrial fibrillation), beta blockers, or nitroglycerin and prevention of a rise in left atrial pressure during labor and delivery.[71] With delivery and thus relief of venocaval obstruction due to the gravid uterus, there is an immediate increase in venous return, which may lead to a substantial increase in pulmonary artery wedge pressure.[32] For this reason, hemodynamic monitoring should be continued for at least several hours post partum.

Epidural anesthesia is the most appropriate form of analgesia in patients with mitral stenosis[53,71,72] for both vaginal and abdominal delivery. This form of anesthesia is often associated with a significant fall in pulmonary arterial and left atrial pressures due to systemic vasodilation. With this approach, the great majority of patients with mitral stenosis, even if it is severe, can be delivered with few complications.

Mitral Valve Repair or Replacement. My experience with a large number of patients with moderate and severe mitral stenosis as well as experience of other investigators indicates that careful medical therapy, with particular emphasis on lowering the heart rate,[70] allows successful completion of pregnancy in the great majority of women without the need for valve correction or replacement during pregnancy (Fig. 59–4). Repair or replacement of the valve during pregnancy, however, may be indicated in some patients with severe symptomatic mitral stenosis in spite of adequate medical therapy.[67,70,72] In both mitral valve commissurotomy (open or closed) and replacement, the risk in pregnant patients is comparable to that in nonpregnant patients. In contrast, however, open commissurotomy and valve replacement are likely to result in increased fetal loss.[68] Closed mitral commissurotomy is associated with only minimal risk to the fetus; it is therefore preferable to the open technique.[73] However, it should be recommended only in centers where it is performed routinely.

Percutaneous Mitral Balloon Valvuloplasty (see also p. 1386). The use of this procedure during pregnancy has recently been reported in an increasing number of pregnant patients with mitral stenosis.[74–79] In the majority of cases, hemodynamic and symptomatic improvement has been achieved without apparent untoward maternal and fetal effects. At the same time, however, serious complications have occasionally been reported, including initiation of uterine contraction,[76] maternal arrhythmia leading to fetal distress,[78] cardiac tamponade requiring surgical intervention, and systemic embolization.[79] In addition, this procedure is associated with some risk to the fetus secondary to unavoidable ionizing radiation. This information suggests that percutaneous mitral balloon valvuloplasty is an attractive alternative to surgery during pregnancy, but is limited by the exposure to radiation and possible complications that may result in fetal distress or require surgical intervention during pregnancy.

For all of the aforementioned reasons, mitral valve repair or replacement during pregnancy should be considered only in cases with severe mitral stenosis (mitral valve area <1.0 cm^2) refractory to optimal medical therapy and should be avoided if possible during the first trimester.[80]

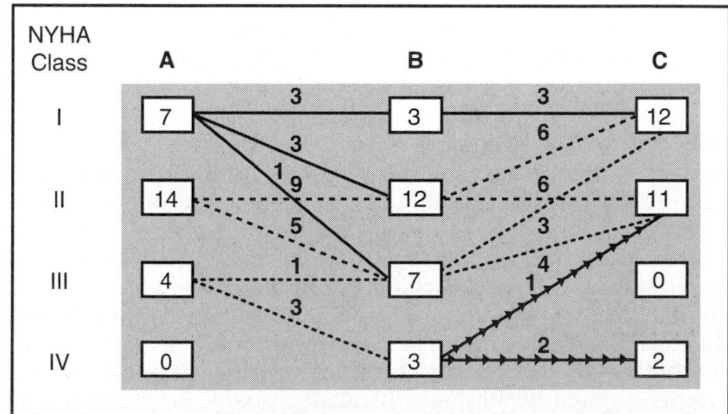

FIGURE 59–4. Effect of beta-blockade therapy on New York Heart Association functional class in 25 pregnant patients with symptomatic mitral stenosis (mean valve area 1.1 ± 0.25 cm^2). *A*, before pregnancy; *B*, during pregnancy before initiation or increase of beta-blockade therapy; *C*, during pregnancy with adequate beta blockade. (From Al Kasab, S. M., Sabag, T., Al Zaibag, et al.: B-adrenergic receptor blockade in the management of pregnant women with mitral stenosis. Am. J. Obstet. Gynecol. *169*:37, 1990.)

Balloon valvuloplasty should be done under echocardiographic guidance if possible and with abdominal and pelvic shielding if fluoroscopy is used. When valve replacement is indicated, selection of the type of prosthesis should be based on its hemodynamic profile and durability and the need for anticoagulation.

MITRAL REGURGITATION. This condition is usually well tolerated in pregnancy, presumably because of left ventricular unloading secondary to the physiological fall in systemic vascular resistance. In symptomatic patients, drug therapy with diuretics is indicated, and digoxin may be useful in those with impaired left ventricular systolic function. Because hydralazine has been shown to be safe for use during pregnancy,[81] it may be used for further reduction of left ventricular afterload and prevention of hemodynamic worsening associated with isometric exercise during labor.[82]

Bicuspid aortic valve is the most common cause for aortic valve disease during gestation.[68] Rheumatic aortic valve involvement occurs in conjunction with mitral valve disease in approximately 5 per cent of pregnant patients with rheumatic valvular disease.[68]

AORTIC STENOSIS. Although most patients with aortic stenosis and valve area greater than 1.0 cm^2 tolerate pregnancy well, patients with more severe stenosis may demonstrate clinical deterioration with exertional dyspnea, near-syncope, or syncope and pulmonary edema.[83–85] Development of serious symptoms during pregnancy, especially if resistant to medical therapy, may require termination of pregnancy or repair of valve either surgically (valve replacement) or by percutaneous balloon valvuloplasty.[83–86]

AORTIC REGURGITATION. Similar to mitral regurgitation, aortic regurgitation is also well tolerated during pregnancy, probably because of reduced systemic vascular resistance and increased heart rate, which results in shortening of diastole. In symptomatic patients, diuretics, digoxin, and hydralazine for afterload reduction can be safely used. Since hydralazine has been shown to prevent an increase in pulmonary artery wedge pressure during isometric exercise in patients with aortic regurgitation,[87] it may be used for this purpose during labor and delivery.

OTHER CONDITIONS AFFECTING THE VALVES, AORTA, AND MYOCARDIUM

Mitral Valve Prolapse (MVP)

(See also p. 1029)

Diagnosed by M-mode echocardiography, MVP was reported in approximately 15 per cent of women of childbearing age. However, when the diagnosis was based on two-dimensional (2-D) echocardiographic criteria, the incidence was reported to be only about 2 per cent.[17] In a review of heart disease in pregnancy, MVP was found in only two of 145 pregnant women and suspected in 1.2 per cent of women examined in prenatal clinics.[17] A combined experience involving 158 pregnant women showed that MVP has no effect on maternal or fetal outcome.[17,88,89]

Pregnancy may reduce the incidence of prolapse-related auscultatory and echocardiographic changes as a result of an increase in left ventricular end-diastolic volume.[17] For the few patients with MVP with chest pain or cardiac arrhythmias, the emphasis should be on reassurance and attempts to avoid the use of medications. Beta-adrenergic blocking agents are recommended when therapy is indicated,[89] with periodic reassessment of the need to continue drug therapy. Patients with MVP, especially those with a thickened mitral valve and mitral regurgitation, are at increased risk for infective endocarditis. Although antibiotic prophylaxis for uncomplicated vaginal delivery has not been uniformly recommended, the development of bacteremia during vaginal delivery and cesarean section cannot always be predicted. For this reason, I recommend prophylaxis for labor and delivery in patients with MVP accompanied by valve thickening and/or regurgitation.

Marfan Syndrome

(See also p. 1672)

Pregnancy in women with Marfan syndrome poses a twofold problem: a potential catastrophic and often lethal acute aortic dissection and a risk of having a child who will inherit the condition.[90] Review of available literature published since 1980 reveals the description of 15 cases of pregnancy in Marfan patients, the majority of whom had cardiovascular complications.[90,91] These complications included dilatation of the ascending aorta leading to aortic regurgitation and heart failure and proximal and distal aortic dissections (Fig. 59–5). The majority of patients developed their complications in the later phase of pregnancy. Aortic dissection resulted in maternal death in three cases; in three other cases live babies were delivered by cesarean section before successful surgery; and in two cases surgery was performed during pregnancy. In contrast to these selected reports of complications, a retrospective analysis of 105 unselected pregnancies among 26 women with this syndrome revealed only one death from endocarditis in a patient with severe mitral regurgitation.[92]

The management of pregnancy in women with Marfan syndrome should include preconception counseling to discuss potential maternal and fetal risks.[90] Women with significant cardiac involvement—in particular, dilatation of the aorta—are at high risk for complications during gestation and should be advised against conception or, if they are already pregnant, to have an early abortion. In contrast, the risk is significantly lower in patients without cardiac complications and a normal aortic diameter. Still, a favorable outcome is not guaranteed, and aortic dissection can

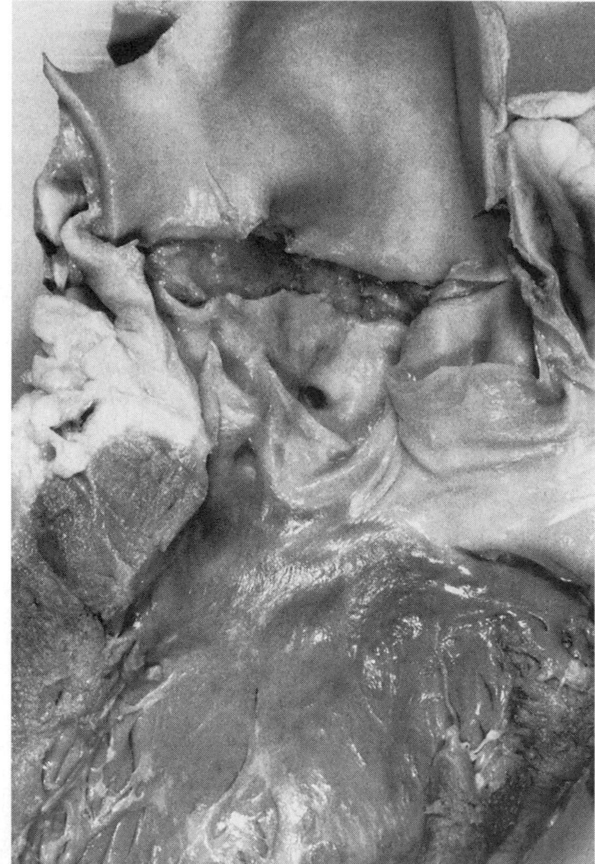

FIGURE 59–5. Just above the cusps of the aortic valve is a transverse tear across nearly the entire diameter of the ascending aorta in a 34-year-old woman with the Marfan syndrome who died suddenly 2 days post partum.

occur, albeit infrequently, in patients with a normal sized aorta.[90] Preconceptual echocardiographic assessment of the aorta and periodic follow-up during pregnancy are highly recommended. Since aneurysm and dissection of the aorta can occasionally involve the descending aorta, the use of transesophageal seems preferred to transthoracic echocardiography.[93] During pregnancy, physical activity should be limited. Beta blockers, which have been shown to reduce the rate of aortic dilatation and the risk of complications in patients with the Marfan syndrome, should be administered.[94] In case of substantial dilatation of the aorta during pregnancy, therapeutic abortion or surgical intervention should be considered.[90,95] In women with aortic dilatation, aortic dissection, or other cardiac complications, abdominal delivery by cesarean section should be the preferred mode of delivery to minimize hemodynamic changes associated with vaginal delivery.

Cardiomyopathies

HYPERTROPHIC CARDIOMYOPATHY (HC) (see also p. 1414). Reported experience in 89 pregnancies among 42 patients with hypertrophic cardiomyopathy (HC) reveals a favorable outcome in most cases but at the same time a potential for increased morbidity and even mortality.[96–100] New onset or worsening of congestive heart failure has been reported in 25 per cent of cases, and a few patients experienced chest pain, palpitations, dizzy spells, and syncope. Three patients had ventricular arrhythmias, which proved fatal in one,[96] and in one patient sudden death occurred at 28 weeks while she was running upstairs.[99] Fetal outcome in most cases does not seem to be affected by maternal HC; however, premature labor and delivery have been reported.[97,100] In addition, the risk of inheriting the disease may be as high as 50 per cent in familial cases and less in sporadic cases.[99]

The therapeutic approach to the pregnant patient with HC depends on the presence of symptoms and left ventricular outflow obstruction. In the symptomatic patient with obstructive HC, blood loss during delivery, vasodilation, and sympathetic stimulation during anesthesia must be avoided. Indications for drug therapy include symptoms and the presence of arrhythmias. Symptoms associated with elevated left ventricular filling pressure should be treated with beta-adrenergic blocking agents, with diuretics and calcium antagonists added if beta blockers alone are not sufficient.[99] Dual-chamber pacemaker may be considered in the patients who develop symptoms in the early phase of pregnancy.[100] Because of the arrhythmogenic effect of pregnancy, implantation of an automatic defibrillator should be considered in patients with HC with a history of sudden death, syncope, or life-threatening arrhythmias.

Vaginal delivery has been shown to be safe in women with HC.[96] In those with symptoms or outflow obstruction, the second stage of labor may be shortened by the use of forceps. The use of prostaglandins to induce uterine contractions may be unfavorable in a patient with obstructive HC owing to their vasodilatory effect, whereas oxytocin should be well tolerated. Since tocolytic agents with beta-adrenergic receptor activity may aggravate left ventricular outflow tract obstruction, magnesium sulfate is preferred. Similarly, spinal and epidural anesthetics should be used with great caution in obstructive HC because of their vasodilatory effect, and excessive blood loss should be avoided or replaced promptly with intravenous fluid or blood.[96]

Because the risk for infective endocarditis is increased in HC, especially the obstructive form, and in patients with mitral valve abnormality, antibiotic prophylaxis should be considered for labor and delivery.

PERIPARTUM CARDIOMYOPATHY. Peripartum cardiomyopathy (PPCM) is a form of dilated cardiomyopathy (see p. 1407) with left ventricular systolic dysfunction that results in signs and symptoms of heart failure. Symptoms usually occur during the last trimester of gestation, and diagnosis is usually made in the peripartum period (Fig. 59–6).[101] Since there is no specific test available for the diagnosis of PPCM, it is established by exclusion of other causes of left ventricular dilatation and systolic dysfunction. The reported incidence of the disease in the United States is approximately 1 in 10,000, with a higher incidence—up to 1 in 100—in certain parts of Africa.[102]

Common symptoms and signs are shortness of breath, fatigue, chest pain, palpitations, weight gain, peripheral edema, and occasionally peripheral or pulmonary embolization.[101–108] Physical examination often reveals an enlarged heart, S_3, and murmurs of mitral and tricuspid regurgitation.[102] The electrocardiogram may show left ventricular hypertrophy, ST-T changes, conduction abnormalities, and arrhythmias. Chest x-ray examination may reveal cardiomegaly, pulmonary venous congestion with interstitial or alveolar edema, and occasionally pleural effusion. Doppler echocardiography shows that all four chambers are enlarged, with marked reduction in left ventricular systolic function. Small-to-moderate pericardial effusion and mitral, tricuspid, and pulmonic regurgitation may be evident. The clinical presentation and hemodynamic changes are indistinguishable from those found in other forms of dilated cardiomyopathy.[101,107] A few patients with high-output heart failure have been reported.[109]

The incidence of PPCM is greater in women with twin pregnancies, in multiparas, in women over 30 years of age, and in African-American women.[102] Although the etiology of PPCM is still unknown, the unique nature of this syndrome is suggested by its occurrence at a relatively young age when compared with other forms of dilated cardiomyopathy, the recovery of cardiac size and function in a large number of patients, and its relation to pregnancy.[107] It has been postulated that PPCM may be due to nutritional deficiency, small-vessel coronary artery abnormalities, hormonal effects, toxemia, maternal immunological response to fetal antigen, or myocarditis. The association between myocarditis and PPCM was suggested by some investigators who reported a high incidence of myocarditis documented by endomyocardial biopsy.[110] Later reports, however, have indicated a low incidence of myocarditis in patients with PPCM that was comparable to that found in an age- and sex-matched nonpregnant, control population with idiopathic dilated cardiomyopathy.[104,107,108,111]

The clinical course of PPCM varies with approximately 50 to 60 per cent of patients showing complete or near-complete recovery of clinical status and cardiac function,

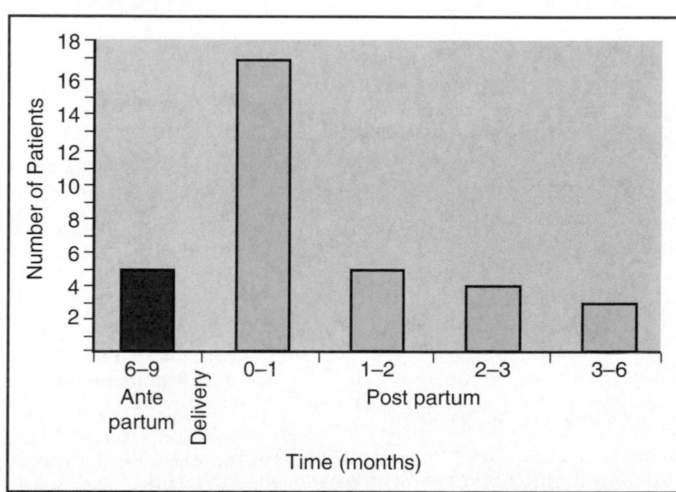

FIGURE 59–6. Time of onset of symptoms in relation to time of delivery in 34 patients with peripartum cardiomyopathy. (From Rizeq, M. N., Rickenbacher, P. R., Fowler, M. B., et al.: Incidence of myocarditis in peripartum cardiomyopathy. Am. J. Cardiol. *74*:474, 1994.)

usually within the first 6 months post partum[106]; the rest of the patients demonstrate either continuous clinical deterioration, leading to cardiac transplantation or early death, or persistent left ventricular dysfunction and chronic heart failure.[102,104–106]

Management. Acute heart failure should be treated vigorously with oxygen, diuretics, digitalis, and vasodilator agents. The use of hydralazine as an afterload-reducing agent is safe during pregnancy.[81] The use of organic nitrates, dopamine, dobutamine, or milrinone has been reported in pregnancy in a limited number of cases. Nitroprusside has been used successfully during pregnancy, but experiments in animals have shown the potential for fetal toxicity.[112] Angiotensin-converting enzyme inhibitors have a teratogenic effect on the fetus, may cause fetal renal dysfunction, and should therefore not be used during pregnancy (see p. 1859).[113] Because of the increased incidence of thromboembolic events in PPCM, anticoagulant therapy is recommended. Since the disease may be reversible, the temporary use of an intraaortic balloon pump or left ventricular assist device may help stabilize the patient's condition pending improvement.[114]

Although a beneficial effect of immunosuppressive therapy has been suggested in patients with PPCM, reported failure of such treatment even in patients with histological evidence of myocarditis[107] and clinical as well as cardiac improvement in patients given supportive therapy alone raise doubt regarding the efficacy of immunosuppression in patients with this disease. Predictors for clinical deterioration post partum are older age, higher parity, severe left ventricular dilatation, later onset of symptoms after delivery, high pulmonary arterial and pulmonary artery wedge pressures, and conduction defects on the surface ECG.[106] Because of the high risk of mortality and morbidity among patients who do not recover early, such patients should be considered for cardiac transplantation.[114,115]

Subsequent pregnancies in women with PPCM are often associated with relapses and a high risk for maternal morbidity and mortality. Although the likelihood of such relapse is greater in patients with persistently abnormal heart size and/or function,[101,116] it has also been reported in women in whom left ventricular function is restored after the first episode.[105,117] For these reasons, subsequent pregnancies should be discouraged in patients with PPCM who have persistent cardiac dysfunction; women with recovered cardiac function after an episode of PPCM should be informed that subsequent pregnancy may not be risk free.

Hypertension in Pregnancy

(See also p. 830)

Hypertension in pregnancy is defined as increments in systolic and diastolic blood pressure of ≥30 and ≥15 mm Hg respectively or a diastolic pressure of ≥90 mm Hg as measured on more than one occasion.[118,119] Hypertension complicates 8 to 10 per cent of all pregnancies and is an important cause of maternal mortality and morbidity, including abruptio placentae, disseminated intravascular coagulation, cerebral hemorrhage, hepatic failure, and acute renal failure. The recommended classification by the working group on high blood pressure in pregnancy[119] identified the following categories: (1) chronic hypertension; (2) preeclampsia-eclampsia; (3) preeclampsia-eclampsia superimposed on chronic hypertension; and (4) transient hypertension.

CHRONIC HYPERTENSION. Defined as blood pressure ≥140/90 mm Hg diagnosed (1) prior to pregnancy; (2) before the 20th gestational week; and (3) during pregnancy and persisting beyond the 42nd postpartum day. Chronic hypertension is associated with increased complications (15 per cent) such as fetal growth retardation, premature delivery, abruption, acute renal failure, and hypertensive crisis; most of these complications occur in patients older than 30 years with a longer duration of hypertension or those who develop superimposed preeclampsia. Drug therapy is recommended for diastolic pressure ≥100 mm Hg or ≥90 mm Hg in patients with renal disease or evidence of end-organ involvement. Guidelines for antihypertension drug therapy for chronic hypertension in pregnancy are shown in Table 59–4.

PREECLAMPSIA-ECLAMPSIA. Preeclampsia usually occurs after 20 weeks' gestation in the first pregnancy and near term in multiparous women. It is characterized by hypertension accompanied by proteinuria (≥0.3 gm/24 hours), edema, or both. Hypertension in this condition is defined as (1) increased systolic blood pressure ≥30 mm Hg; or (2) increased diastolic blood pressure ≥15 mm Hg from values before 20 weeks' gestation. If prior blood pressure is not known, values ≥140/90 mm Hg after 20 weeks' gestation are diagnostic. Preeclampsia is always associated with increased risk to both mother and fetus; certain signs and symptoms are predictors for complications and are listed in Table 59–5.[118,120] Preeclampsia may progress to eclampsia, a life-threatening convulsive phase. Preeclampsia usually regresses within 24 to 48 hours post partum. In the minor-

TABLE 59–4 ANTIHYPERTENSIVE DRUGS USED TO TREAT CHRONIC HYPERTENSION IN PREGNANCY

DRUG	COMMENT
α_2-Adrenergic receptor agonists	Methyldopa is the most extensively used drug in this group, its safety and efficacy supported in randomized trials, and there is a 7.5-yr follow-up study of children born to treated mothers. Methyldopa is the drug of choice recommended by the Working Group.
β-Adrenergic receptor antagonists	These drugs, especially atenolol and metoprolol, appear safe and efficacious in late pregnancy, but fetal growth retardation has been noted when treatment was started in early or midgestation. Fetal bradycardia can occur, and animal studies suggest the fetus' ability to tolerate hypoxic stress may be compromised.
α- and β-Adrenergic receptor antagonists	Labetalol appears as effective as methyldopa, but there is little or no follow-up information on children born to mothers treated with labetalol, and there is concern for maternal hepatotoxicity.
Arteriolar vasodilators	Hydralazine is used frequently as adjunctive therapy with methyldopa and β-adrenergic receptor antagonists. Rarely, neonatal thrombocytopenia has been reported. Trials with calcium channel blockers look promising. Experience with minoxidil is limited; this drug is not recommended.
Converting enzyme inhibitors	Captopril causes fetal death in diverse animal species, and several converting enzyme inhibitors have been associated with renal failure in the newborn when administered to humans. Do not use in pregnancy.
Diuretics	Many authorities discourage their use, but others continue these medications if they were prescribed before gestation or if a chronic hypertensive patient appears quite salt sensitive. The latter views have been endorsed by the Working Group.

From Lindheimer, M. D.: Hypertension in pregnancy. Hypertension *22*:127, 1993.

TABLE 59–5 PREDICTORS FOR HIGH RISK IN WOMEN WITH PREECLAMPSIA

1. Systolic blood pressure ≥160 mm Hg or diastolic blood pressure ≥110 mm Hg
2. New proteinuria ≥2.0 gm/24 hr (2+ or 3+ on qualitative examination)
3. New increased serum creatinine levels (>2.0 mg/dl)
4. Platelet count <100,000/liter or evidence of microangiographic hemolytic anemia (e.g., schistocytes and/or increased lactic acid dehydrogenase and direct bilirubin levels)
5. Elevated hepatic enzymes (alanine aminotransferase or aspirate aminotransferase)
6. Upper abdominal pain (especially epigastric and right upper quadrant)
7. Headache and other cerebral or visual disturbances
8. Cardiac decompensation (e.g., pulmonary edema)
9. Retinal hemorrhage, exudates, or papilledema*
10. Intrauterine growth retardation and decreased urine volumes

Modified from Lindheimer, M. D.: Hypertension in pregnancy. Hypertension *22*:127, 1993.
* Unlikely to occur without other major signs of severity.

ity of cases, postpartum eclampsia with hypertension, proteinuria, and convulsions occurs within 10 days post partum.

Hospitalization is recommended in preeclamptic patients. If the patient is near term (34 to 36 weeks), labor should be induced after control of hypertension and preventive antieclamptic treatment; if the fetus is immature, delay of delivery should be considered. Patients with severe hypertension in spite of 24 to 48 hours of therapy and any high-risk manifestations (Table 59–5) should be delivered regardless of gestational age. Drug therapy is recommended if diastolic blood pressure is 105 to 110 mm Hg,[118] which should be reduced to 90 to 104 mm Hg. Guidelines for drug treatment of severe hypertension near term or during labor are shown in Table 59–6.

TRANSIENT HYPERTENSION. Defined as the development of elevated blood pressure during pregnancy or in the first 24 hours post partum without preexisting hypertension and without other signs of preeclampsia. This condition is predictive for future development of hypertension.

PREGNANCY AFTER CARDIAC TRANSPLANTATION

A recent study conducted to determine the outcome of pregnancy in cardiac allograft recipients identifed 30 such cases.[121] Maternal hemodynamic changes during gestation were well tolerated by all patients, and rejection episodes were rare. At the same time, however, a high incidence of maternal complications was reported, including chronic hypertension, preeclampsia, and infections.[121–123] Although fetal death did not occur, fetal growth retardation was found in 20 per cent, and 40 per cent of births were preterm. None of the newborns was found to have congenital malformations, supporting a lack of teratogenic effect of immunosuppressive agents.[123] There were no maternal deaths during pregnancy, but three patients died within 30 months after delivery. This limited information suggests, therefore, that pregnancy in women after cardiac transplantation is not associated with increased maternal mortality; however, it results in increased maternal morbidity, preterm deliveries, and fetal growth retardation. In addition, the patients and their families should be informed regarding potential limited life span after delivery in patients after heart transplantation.

CORONARY ARTERY DISEASE

PATHOGENESIS. Coronary artery disease (CAD) is rare among women of childbearing age, and the occurrence of peripartum acute myocardial infarction (AMI) is anecdotal.[124]

Risk factors for CAD in women under the age of 50 years include high levels of total plasma cholesterol, low levels of high-density lipoproteins, cigarette smoking, diabetes mellitus, hypertension, a family history of CAD, toxemia of pregnancy, and the use of oral contraceptives.[125] The combination of heavy smoking and concurrent use of oral contraceptives has been shown to be a powerful predictor of AMI.[126] In addition, increased risk has been related to the patient's age at the time of her first delivery (below the age of 20 years)[127] and to a lifelong irregular pattern of menstruation.[128]

Several mechanisms have been proposed to explain the relationship between oral contraceptives and AMI. These drugs may trigger clot formation and embolization, as suggested by the increased incidence of venous thrombosis, pulmonary embolism, and cerebral thromboembolism.[124] In addition, oral contraceptives may raise serum levels of triglycerides, total cholesterol, and low-density lipoprotein; lower the level of high-density lipoprotein; increase the incidence of hypertension; and precipitate the ulceration of atherosclerotic plaques.[124] To reduce the risk for AMI, oral contraceptives should be avoided or formulations with lower effective doses of estrogen should be used in women over the age of 35, cigarette smokers, and those who develop hypertension while using this form of birth control.

Peripartum AMI is often associated with normal coronary angiographic findings[129–133] and may be due to a decrease in coronary perfusion caused by spasm or in situ thrombosis. Although the cause of spasm is not clear, it has often been associated with pregnancy-induced hypertension and in some instances with the use of ergot derivatives—oxytocin,[132] and prostaglandin[134]—to suppress lactation or uterine bleeding.[134,135] Coronary arterial dissection during pregnancy or immediately post partum is another relatively common cause of peripartum AMI[136–139] (Fig. 59–7). The dissection involves the left anterior descending artery in approximately 80 per cent of cases and the right coronary artery in most other cases.[138] Multiple coronary artery dissections have been recently reported in two cases (Fig. 59–8).[137,139] Other potential causes of AMI during pregnancy have been collagen vascular disease,[140,141] Kawasaki's disease,[142] sickle cell anemia,[143] and pheochromocytoma.[144]

DIAGNOSIS. The diagnostic approach to ischemic myocardial disease in pregnancy is influenced to some extent

TABLE 59–6 GUIDELINES FOR TREATING SEVERE HYPERTENSION NEAR TERM OR DURING LABOR

REGULATION OF BLOOD PRESSURE

The degree to which blood pressure should be decreased is disputed. The Working Group's Consensus Report recommends maintaining diastolic levels between 90 and 105 mm Hg.[119]

DRUG THERAPY

1. Hydralazine administered intravenously is the drug of choice. Start with low doses (5 mg IV bolus), then administer 5 to 10 mg every 20 to 30 min to avoid precipitous decreases. Side effects include tachycardia and headache. Neonatal thrombocytopenia has been reported.
2. Diazoxide is recommended for the occasional patient whose hypertension is refractory to hydralazine. Use 30 mg miniboluses because precipitous hypotension may result with higher doses. Side effects include arrest of labor and neonatal hypoglycemia.
3. Experience with labetalol is growing, and some use this agent instead of diazoxide as a second-line drug.
4. Favorable results have been reported with calcium channel blockers. However, if magnesium sulfate is being infused, the magnesium ion may potentiate the effect of the calcium channel blockers, resulting in precipitous and severe hypotension.
5. Refrain from using nitroprusside, because fetal cyanide poisoning has been reported in animal models. However, in the final analysis, maternal well-being will dictate therapy choice.

The Working Group retained parenteral magnesium sulfate as the drug of choice for preventing impending eclamptic convulsions. Therapy should continue for 12 to 24 hr into the puerperium, because one-third of patients with eclampsia have their convulsion after childbirth.

From Lindheimer, M. D.: Hypertension in pregnancy. Hypertension *22*:127, 1993.

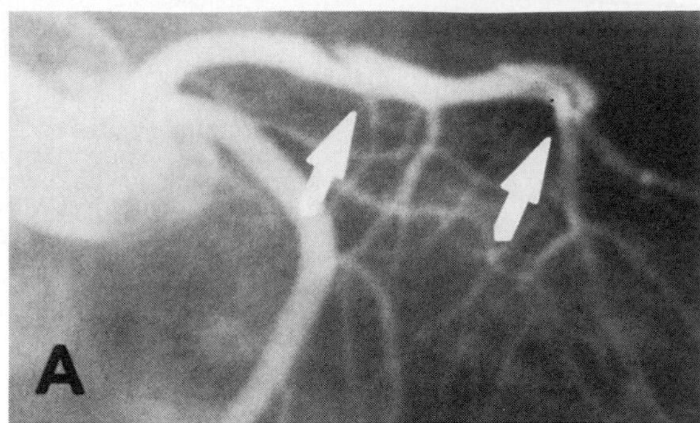

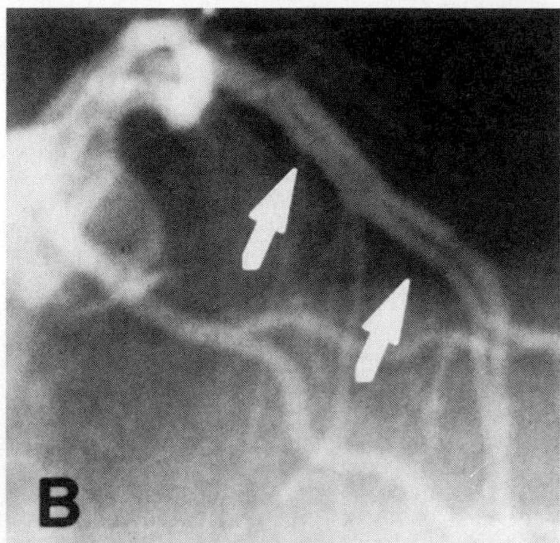

FIGURE 59–7. ***A* and *B*, A long dissection in the left anterior descending artery (arrows) in a 44-year-old woman with acute anterior myocardial infarction in the early postpartum period. (Courtesy of Y. Almagor, M. D., and S. Goldberg, M. D.)**

by whether a diagnostic procedure could harm the fetus and by normal changes seen during pregnancy that may mimic pathological changes. T-wave inversion, Q wave in lead III, and increased R/S ratio in lead V_2 are commonly seen in normal pregnancy.[13] ST-segment depression not associated with chest pain or echocardiographic wall motion abnormalities has been described during elective cesarean section and can mimic myocardial ischemia (Fig. 59–8).[19] Since fetal bradycardia has been reported during maximal exercise in normal women, a submaximal exercise protocol with fetal monitoring is recommended for the evaluation of ischemic myocardial disease during pregnancy.[13] Radionuclide myocardial perfusion scans and radionuclide ventriculography expose the fetus to radiation and should be used only when the potential benefits seem to outweigh fetal risk.[13] For similar reasons, cardiac catheterization involving fluoroscopy and cineangiography should be used only when relevant information cannot be obtained by other, noninvasive methods. It should be noted that the diagnosis of myocardial ischemia and infarction has been reported to be delayed during pregnancy because of the low level of suspicion.[132]

MANAGEMENT. Both maternal and fetal considerations should influence the therapeutic approach to ischemic heart disease during pregnancy. Because of their safety in pregnancy, beta blockers appear to be the most appropriate drugs of choice. The use of organic nitrates and calcium antagonists in patients with acute myocardial ischemia or infarction has been described in a limited number of patients.[131,135,137,145–147] These drugs should be given cautiously to prevent maternal hypotension and potential fetal distress.[145,148,149] Use of high-dose aspirin during pregnancy is debatable, since it has been reported to cause bleeding in the neonate and in the mother,[150] as well as growth retardation in the fetus.[151] Use of low-dose aspirin, however, is safe during pregnancy.[148,150] Although only limited experience is available regarding thrombolytic therapy during pregnancy, it has been safely used in several cases[151,152] and should be considered in high-risk patients with AMI. Coronary reperfusion by means of percutaneous transluminal coronary angioplasty or coronary artery bypass graft surgery has been reported to be successful during pregnancy,[154] although experience is still limited. Such procedures should be avoided during the first trimester, if possible, owing to the potential deleterious fetal effects due to ionizing radiation as well as cardiopulmonary bypass.

Risk stratification after AMI during pregnancy should be determined by noninvasive methods. Coronary angiography should be done only in cases in which coronary angioplasty or bypass surgery seems indicated during pregnancy.[149,155] Management should focus on reducing cardiovascular stress during pregnancy and the peripartum period. Termination of pregnancy may be required in patients with intractable ischemia or heart failure in the early phase of gestation.[147] Pulmonary artery catheterization with hemodynamic monitoring can help in the early detection and correction of hemodynamic abnormalities during labor and delivery.[146,147,155] During labor, adequate analgesia and supplemental oxygen should be given, and if desired, cardiac output can be increased by placing the patient in the left lateral decubitus position (Fig. 59–2). Labor in the supine position, however, may decrease venous return and thus reduce right atrial and left ventricular filling pressures. Low forceps can be used to shorten the second stage of labor.

Although elective cesarean section is not indicated in every case, it should be used in patients with active ischemia or hemodynamic instability despite adequate medical therapy.[146] Epidural anesthesia can reduce hemodynamic fluctuations during labor and is associated with left ventricular unloading due to vasodilation. If general anesthesia is indicated, halothane should be avoided in patients with depressed left ventricular systolic function. In addition, atropine and ketamine should be used with caution to prevent tachycardia. Continued hemodynamic monitoring is advisable for several hours post partum to detect hemodynamic worsening associated with the postpartum hemodynamic changes described earlier.

ARRHYTHMIAS

Pregnancy is associated with an increased incidence of arrhythmias in women both with and without organic heart disease.[155–157] In healthy women, multiple and even frequent atrial and ventricular premature beats may occur, usually without effect on either the mother or the fetus. Although palpitations, dizziness, and even syncope are relatively common in pregnancy, a relation to arrhythmias can be found in only the minority of cases.[156] At the same time, however, symptomatic and hemodynamically significant ventricular and supraventricular tachycardia have been reported in patients with a normal heart during gestation.[157] Reduction in blood pressure occasionally associated with such arrhythmias may result in fetal bradycardia[160] and necessitate immediate treatment with antiarrhythmic drugs, electric cardioversion, or immediate cesarean section. New onset or exacerbation of an arrhythmia has been demonstrated during pregnancy in patients with an antepartum history of arrhythmias,[158] preexcitation,[159] and other forms of acquired congenital heart disease.[161]

ATRIAL FLUTTER AND FIBRILLATION. These arrhythmias are rare during normal pregnancy and are usually associated with rheumatic mitral valve disease. Recent reports have described atrial fibrillation during gestation accompanied by treatment with magnesium sulfate[162] and in a patient with preexcitation.[163] Ventricular tachycardia or fibrillation is also rare in pregnancy and is usually associated with structural heart disease, drugs,[164,165] electrolyte abnormalities,[166] or

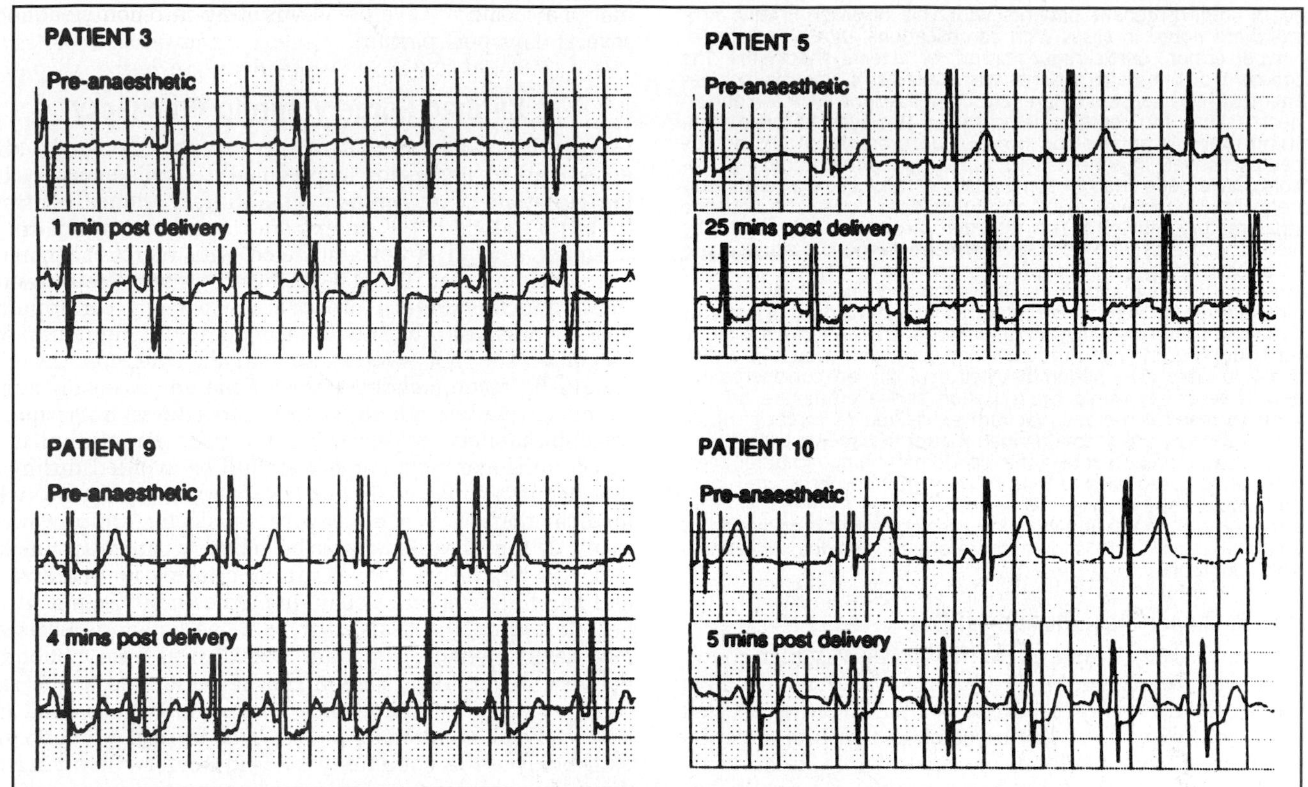

FIGURE 59–8. ST-segment depression recorded in healthy women during cesarean section. These changes were not associated with ventricular wall motion abnormalities. (From McLintic, A. J., Pringle, S. D., Lilley, S., et al.: Electrocardiographic changes during cesarean section under regional anesthesia. Anesth. Analg. *74*:51, 1992.)

eclampsia.[167] Uneventful pregnancy has been reported in women with long QT syndrome.[168,169]

COMPLETE HEART BLOCK. This condition has been described during pregnancy; although usually congenital,[170–172] it can be acquired as a result of myocarditis, congenital heart disease, acute myocardial infarction, or infective endocarditis.[173,174] Patients with complete heart block may remain asymptomatic during pregnancy and have an uncomplicated labor and delivery without treatment.[170] Improvement of atrioventricular nodal conduction during two successive uncomplicated pregnancies in a patient with congenital heart block has been reported.[175] Symptomatic patients with conduction abnormalities, including bifascicular block,[176] second-degree atrioventricular block,[177] and complete heart block,[170,173] have been treated during pregnancy with either temporary or permanent pacemakers, and numerous pregnancies have been reported in patients after pacemaker implantation.[174,178] A rate-adaptive pacemaker seems to be indicated in women of childbearing age.[166] In an attempt to reduce exposure to ionizing radiation, placement of a pacemaker during pregnancy has been done with electrocardiographic and echocardiographic guidance.[171,177] Reports of skin irritation and ulceration at the implant site due to enlargement of the breast and abdomen during pregnancy have led to placement of the battery under the breast in such women.

A complete evaluation is indicated in a case of arrhythmias during pregnancy to rule out either a cardiac or a noncardiac cause such as electrolyte imbalance, thyroid disease, and arrhythmogenic effects of drugs, alcohol, caffeine, and cigarette smoking. An identified cause should be treated and antiarrhythmic drug therapy initiated only if arrhythmia is symptomatic, hemodynamically important, or life threatening. When drug therapy seems necessary, the smallest therapeutic dose of drugs known to be safe for the fetus should be used. Therapeutic blood levels and the indication for continuous drug therapy should be reevaluated periodically. In cases of persistent arrhythmias resulting in symptoms and/or hemodynamic effect that do not respond to short-term drug intervention, electric cardioversion can be performed.[161,165,179–181] Electrophysiological evaluation is usually postponed till the postpartum period but can be performed under echocardiographic guidance if indicated during pregnancy.[102] Because of the unpredictable exposure to ionizing radiation, catheter ablation procedures should be performed after delivery.[161]

OTHER CARDIOVASCULAR DISORDERS

Aortic Dissection

(See also p. 1556)

A predisposition to aortic dissection during gestation has been suggested.[30] Over the last 50 years, approximately 200 cases of aortic dissection in association with pregnancy have been reported. The incidence is increased among multiparous women older than 30 years with coarctation of the aorta and the Marfan syndrome. Pregnancy-related aortic dissection seems to occur most often during the third trimester and peripartum period.

Transesophageal echocardiography provides a powerful and safe tool for establishing the diagnosis of aortic dissection during pregnancy. This method is preferable to computed tomography, which involves radiation exposure, and to magnetic resonance imaging, the safety of which during gestation has not been fully established.

The combination of nitroprusside and propranolol is currently recommended for the control of hypertension in nonpregnant patients with aortic dissection. Since nitroprusside may result in fetal toxicity it should be used only post partum or in patients refractory to other drugs during pregnancy. Hydralazine should be substituted for nitroprusside for blood pressure reduction in pregnant women with aortic dissection. To avoid blood pressure elevation associated with labor and vaginal delivery in women with aortic dissection, cesarean section using epidural anesthesia is recommended.[30]

TAKAYASU'S ARTERITIS (see p. 1572). Our review of the literature revealed 118 pregnancies in 91 women with Takayasu's disease.[183–185] Cerebral hemorrhage, heart failure, and even death have been reported in some pregnant patients with this disorder.[183] Low birth weights were noted in cases with complications, including retinopathy, hypertension, aortic regurgitation, or arterial aneurysms. The management of pregnant patients with Takayasu's arteritis includes treatment of hypertension to prevent complications such as congestive heart failure and cerebral hemorrhage. However, to avoid compromising uteroplacental blood flow, blood pressure should not be reduced excessively in patients with aortic narrowing. Adrenal glucocorticoids have been used in some cases of Takayasu's arteritis during pregnancy[184]; however, since pregnancy does not seem to change the inflammatory activity of this disorder, glucocorticoids should be reserved for patients who become pregnant during the acute phase of the disease. Prophylactic antibiotics may be given for labor and delivery in patients with aortic regurgitation and vascular stenoses.

Vaginal delivery is likely to be tolerated in the majority of patients with Takayasu's arteritis. However, a marked increase in systolic blood pressure during uterine contractions may occur and should be anticipated and treated.[183,184] Abdominal delivery may be considered for those with severe systemic hypertension and heart failure not responding to medical therapy. Vacuum extraction or forceps should be used to shorten the second stage of labor in patients with hypertension. In patients with substantial aortic narrowing, epidural anesthesia should be used with caution to prevent blood pressure reduction and compromise of placental perfusion.

The use of oral contraceptives may accelerate the progression of Takayasu's arteritis[183] and should therefore be avoided in patients with this condition.

Primary Pulmonary Hypertension (PPH)

PPH (see p. 783) is one of the few cardiovascular conditions in which pregnancy may be associated with a high maternal mortality rate. A review of the literature as well as of our own experience has revealed peripartum maternal mortality of approximately 40 per cent.[186–189] Clinical deterioration or death during pregnancy cannot always be predicted on the basis of the patient's preconceptual clinical status. Symptomatic deterioration usually occurs in the second trimester and is manifested by fatigue, dyspnea, syncope, chest pain, and right ventricular failure. Death occurs most often during late gestation or in the early postpartum period. Because hemodynamic or electrocardiographic information has not been available, the exact cause of death in patients with PPH is not clear. However, right ventricular ischemia and failure, cardiac arrhythmias, and pulmonary embolism are likely mechanisms. In addition to high maternal risk, PPH is associated with poor fetal outcome with high incidence of fetal loss, prematurity, and fetal growth retardation.

Because of the potentially deleterious effect of pregnancy both on mothers with PPH and their fetuses, pregnancy should be avoided in these patients. Since an etiological link between pulmonary hypertension and estrogen-containing oral contraceptives has been suggested, this form of birth control is not recommended for women with PPH.[190] Tubal ligation should provide maximum protection against the undesired risks of pregnancy. Early abortion is indicated in PPH patients who become pregnant. If the patient elects to continue the pregnancy, physical exertion should be restricted to reduce the circulatory load. The incidence of premature deliveries is increased in patients with PPH and should be anticipated.

Because of the beneficial effect of anticoagulation in patients with PPH[191] and the increased incidence of thromboembolism during pregnancy, such therapy is recommended throughout gestation or at least during the third trimester and early postpartum phase. Hemodynamic monitoring and blood gas measurements should be performed continuously during labor and delivery. Oxygen should be provided to prevent hypoxemia, and every effort should be made to prevent or immediately replace blood lost during delivery.[186]

Segmental epidural anesthesia and intrathecal morphine have been successful in relieving pain in these patients.[186,192] Because right ventricular dysfunction is likely, anesthetics having a negative inotropic effect should be avoided in patients with PPH. Most patients can tolerate vaginal delivery, and spontaneous labor is preferable to induction. Because of the high rate of early postpartum maternal death,[186,187] close monitoring is recommended for several days post partum.

Cardiac Surgery during Pregnancy

Since heart disease that requires surgery is usually diagnosed and treated prior to pregnancy, cardiac surgery during gestation is uncommon, and the experience continues to be anecdotal.[193–197] In general, cardiac surgery in the pregnant woman is not associated with increased maternal risk, but may lead to fetal wastage.[193] The effects of anesthesia and the surgical procedure, especially cardiopulmonary bypass, on the uteroplacental circulation and fetal outcome are not well understood. Therefore, surgery should be recommended only for patients who do not respond to medical therapy, and procedures not requiring cardiopulmonary bypass are preferred. To minimize the risk of teratogenicity, surgery should be avoided during the first trimester. Because heart surgery is indicated when medical therapy has not led to satisfactory improvement, many of these patients will be hemodynamically unstable and will require hemodynamic monitoring for stabilization and careful anesthetic technique. Anesthetic agents should be selected on the basis of their hemodynamic effects and fetal safety. When the patient is at or near term, abdominal delivery by cesarean section can be performed at the same time as cardiac surgery, once fetal maturity has been confirmed. Fetal monitoring is essential for early detection of fetal bradycardia commonly seen in surgery involving cardiopulmonary bypass. This finding most likely indicates fetal distress due to a decrease in placental blood flow and can frequently be managed by increasing the flow rate.[198]

Pregnancy in Patients with Valve Prostheses

The risk of pregnancy in women with a valve prosthesis is multifactorial and should be assessed and discussed with the patient and her family prior to conception. Potential problems may be related to an increased hemodynamic load, the hypercoagulable state of pregnancy with increased likelihood of thromboembolic events, accelerated deterioration of bioprostheses, and risk to the fetus due to anticoagulants and other cardiovascular drugs. Most patients with NYHA functional classes I and II with an adequately functioning valve prosthesis, including those with two and three prosthetic valves, can tolerate the hemodynamic load of pregnancy.[152,199,200] Pregnancy with a higher functional class or severe cardiac dysfunction is risky and should be avoided. In questionable cases, evaluation of exercise capacity before conception may be used to predict whether a patient with a prosthetic heart valve can tolerate the increased hemodynamic load of pregnancy.

VALVE SELECTION (see also p. 1065). The selection of a prosthetic valve for pregnant patients or women of childbearing age involves a number of difficult issues. Because it is desirable to avoid anticoagulation during pregnancy, the use of tissue valves is often recommended.[199] However, the long-term durability of these valves is limited, resulting in the need for reoperation within several years. In addition, there is strong and increasing evidence for pregnancy-related accelerated deterioration of tissue valves, leading to the need for valve replacement either during pregnancy or shortly after.[152,201] A mechanical valve is recommended for patients who are willing to follow a strict regimen of anticoagulation and for those who require anticoagulation therapy for other conditions such as thrombophlebitis, atrial fibrillation, rheumatic mitral valve disease with enlargement of the left atrial diameter, intracardiac thrombus, or a history of pulmonary embolism. It should be noted, however, that significant changes in the levels of coagulation factors increase the risk for thrombosis during gestation.[202] Thrombosis of prosthetic valves during pregnancy has been reported in several cases despite anticoagulation.[152,199,203] Salazar et al.[199] and Iturbe-Alessio et al.[200] reported thromboembolic events in 6 of 165 pregnant patients with mechanical mitral prostheses (3.6 per cent) and in none of 37 patients with aortic prostheses.[203] A recent retrospective survey reported thromboembolic events in 19 of 141 pregnancies (13.5 per cent) in women with a mechanical prosthesis in spite of anticoagulation; 12 women had mitral valve thrombosis, 4 cases were fatal, 5 required emergency surgery, and 4 were managed medically with thrombolytic therapy.[152] Ten of the patients were treated with heparin; the level of anticoagulation was not reported. The majority of these patients had first-generation mechanical valves (Starr-Edwards, Björk-Shiley).

Based on the available information, it seems therefore that there is no safe method of anticoagulation during pregnancy in women with a mechanical heart valve. The use of oral anticoagulation may be associated with an increased incidence of spontaneous abortion, prematurity, and still birth and a 4 to 10 per cent risk of fetal deformity (coumadin embryopathy),[199,200,204,205] while the subcutaneous use of adjusted-dose heparin may result in a higher incidence of valve thrombosis.[152] The potential limitations of the various approaches to anticoagulation in pregnancy should be discussed with the patient prior to conception. Because of the disturbing increased risk of valve thrombosis and death with use of heparin, the use of oral anticoagulation throughout pregnancy, aiming at an INR between 2.0 and 3.0, with in-hospital intravenous administration of heparin for the last 3 to 4 weeks of gestation may be considered in high-risk patients, including women with first-generation mechanical valves in the mitral position and patients with a history of thromboembolism.[206] Patients with an aortic mechanical prosthesis and newer generation mechanical valves in the mitral position may be treated with adjusted subcutaneous doses of heparin to maintain a partial thromboplastin time (PTT) at 2.0 to 2.5 times the control from conception to week 13 and during the last 3 to 4 weeks of gestation. The patient should be admitted to the hospital for initiation and adjustment of heparin therapy, and the dose of heparin should be adjusted to achieve prolongation of activated PTT to twice the control value at midinterval 6 hours after the morning dose. PTT should be carefully and frequently checked, and the dose of heparin adjusted accordingly.

Because of the potential limitations and risk involved in the selection of anticoagulation regimen, the choice of treatment should involve the patient and her family.

Heparin should be withdrawn at the onset of labor. If onset of labor occurs when the patient is treated with oral anticoagulation, performance of a cesarean section to avoid fetal bleeding associated with vaginal delivery is recommended. If there are no hemorrhages, heparin administration can be resumed a few hours post delivery. Breast feeding is permitted in the mother treated with anticoagulation, since coumadin does not affect the newborn.

CARDIOVASCULAR DRUGS IN PREGNANCY

Because of their potentially unfavorable effects on the developing fetus, all drugs should be avoided, if possible, during pregnancy. When drugs are needed, however, risk/benefit ratio must be evaluated carefully, and the smallest effective dose should be used (Table 59–7). Another source of concern is the transfer of drugs into breast milk and subsequently to the neonate during lactation. Generally, 1 to 2 per cent of the maternal dose appears in breast milk.[207] Most data regarding drug excretion in human milk are anecdotal, and except for some drugs that are clearly contraindicated, there is not enough information to permit or prohibit breast feeding in mothers receiving medications. Because the mechanisms involved in drug excretion into breast milk are complex, the various models and formulas used to estimate plasma:milk ratios are of limited clinical value. Close monitoring of the infant's ingested dose and plasma levels, as well as close observation for adverse effects or toxicity, is necessary to ensure safety.

CARDIAC GLYCOSIDES

Digoxin alone or combined with other drugs has been employed to treat maternal as well as fetal supraventricular arrhythmias and con-

TABLE 59–7 SAFETY AND ADVERSE EFFECTS OF CARDIOVASCULAR DRUGS DURING PREGNANCY

DRUG	POTENTIAL FETAL ADVERSE EFFECTS	SAFETY
Digoxin	Low birth weight	Safe
Quinidine	Toxic dose may induce premature labor and damage to fetal eighth cranial nerve	Safe
Procainamide	None reported	*
Disopyramide	May initiate uterine contractions	*
Lidocaine	In high blood levels and fetal acidosis may cause central nervous system depression	Safe
Mexiletine	Fetal bradycardia, IUGR, low Apgar score, neonatal hypoglycemia, neonatal bradycardia, and neonatal hypothyroidism	*
Flecainide	One reported fetal death	*
Propafenone	None reported	*
Adenosine	None reported. Use during first trimester limited to a few patients.	Safe
Amiodarone	IUGR, prematurity, hypothyroidism	Unsafe
Calcium antagonists	Fetal distress due to maternal hypotension	*
Beta-adrenergic blocking agents	IUGR, apnea at birth, bradycardia, hypoglycemia, hyperbilirubinemia; $beta_2$ blockade may initiate uterine contractions	Safe
Sodium nitroprusside	Potential thiocyanate toxicity with high dose, fetal mortality in animal studies	Potentially unsafe
Organic nitrates	Fetal heart rate deceleration and bradycardia	*
ACE inhibitors	Skull ossification defect, IUGR, premature deliveries, low birth weight, oligohydramnios, neonatal renal failure, anemia and death, limb contractures, patent ductus arteriosus	Unsafe
Diuretic agents	Impairment of uterine blood flow, thrombocytopenia, jaundice, hyponatremia, bradycardia	Potentially unsafe

* To date, only limited information is available, and safety during pregnancy cannot be established.
IUGR = intrauterine growth retardation.

gestive heart failure.[208,209] The fetomaternal serum digoxin concentration ratio has been shown to range from 0.5 to 1.0.[208] Pregnancy, especially when complicated by hypertension, is associated with increased levels of digoxin-like substances,[208,209] which can cause errors of up to 2 μg/ml in measurements of digoxin serum concentration.

Gestational use of digoxin is considered safe and without teratogenic effect. Caution is advised in digitalis administration, however, since overdose can be detrimental to the mother and may be lethal to the fetus. Potential side effects of cardiac glycosides in pregnancy include low birth weight, which has been postulated to be secondary to digoxin effect on amino acid transport through the placenta, with consequent growth retardation.[209] However, since the duration of pregnancy has been noted to be shorter in mothers with long-term digoxin therapy, it is possible that low birth weight has been due to prematurity rather than intrauterine growth retardation.

Digoxin is excreted in breast milk with a reported milk/plasma ratio ranging from 0.59 to 0.90.[206] The total amount of digoxin ingested daily by the infant has been estimated to be approximately 1/100 of the pediatric recommended dose. No apparent clinical effects have been demonstrated in newborns, so digoxin therapy of the mother should not affect breast feeding decisions.

ANTI-ARRHYTHMICS

QUINIDINE. Substantial clinical experience with quinidine for the treatment of maternal as well as fetal supraventricular arrhythmias[210,211] has established both its efficacy and safety. Potential side effects include fetal thrombocytopenia and minimal oxytocic activity reported mostly during development of spontaneous uterine contractions. Toxic doses of quinidine, however, may cause premature labor, abortion, or damage to the fetal eighth cranial nerve. Quinidine is secreted in breast milk, with a milk/plasma ratio of 0.71.[207] The calculated total dose of quinidine likely to be ingested by the infant is far below the recommended therapeutic daily pediatric dose.

PROCAINAMIDE. The drug has been successfully used to treat maternal and fetal supraventricular tachycardia.[210–212] Fetomaternal drug level ratios have been found to be 0.28 and 1.32 in two different patients. No teratogenic effects have been reported; however, because of limited experience with procainamide, quinidine should be used as the IA antiarrhythmic drug of choice during pregnancy.

A milk/plasma ratio of 4.3 ± 2.4 was reported for procainamide and 3.8 ± 1.8 for *N*-acetylprocainamide (NAPA). Although the high ratio may indicate accumulation in the milk, the amount of both procainamide and NAPA ingested daily by the infant is considered to be clinically insignificant.[210]

DISOPYRAMIDE. Reports regarding disopyramide treatment in pregnancy are limited to only several patients treated for ventricular and supraventricular arrhythmias.[210,213] The drug crosses the placenta, and the fetal/maternal ratio is 0.39.[214] No teratogenic effects have been described; however, disopyramide was reported to trigger uterine contractions[215] in one patient.

Disopyramide is secreted in breast milk in concentrations similar to those in plasma.[213] The estimated dose likely to be ingested by the infant is less than 2 mg/kg/day.[209] The drug is probably safe for use during pregnancy[210]; however, because of limited available information, disopyramide should be used in patients not tolerating or not responding to treatment with quinidine.

LIDOCAINE. This drug has been used during pregnancy mainly for epidural or local anesthesia; occasional reports have described its use as an antiarrhythmic agent.[210,211,215] or in acute myocardial infarction.[216] The fetomaternal plasma concentration ratio of lidocaine is 0.5 to 0.7. The available data indicate that lidocaine is safe for use during pregnancy as long as blood levels are closely monitored. Elevated lidocaine levels may cause infant central nervous system depression and apnea, hypotonia, dilation of pupils, seizures and bradycardia. As a weak base, lidocaine may be trapped by an acidic environment. Caution should be exercised, therefore, in cases with fetal distress when fetal acidosis is likely and may be associated with increased blood levels of the drug and likelihood of toxicity. Lidocaine use during pregnancy has not been associated with teratogenic effects.

MEXILETINE. A limited number of pregnant women have been treated with mexiletine in doses between 600 and 800 mg/day.[217,218] The reported fetomaternal ratio ranged from 0.7 to 1.0. Fetal bradycardia, infants small for gestational age, low Apgar score, and neonatal hypoglycemia have all been reported in cases of maternal treatment wth mexiletine. Despite these concerns, no teratogenic or long-term adverse effects have been reported. Mexiletine was found in breast milk in concentrations equal to or higher than that in maternal plasma (milk/plasma ratio varied between 0.8 and 1.9)[207]; however, the calculated daily quantity ingested by the infant appears to be below the therapeutic range, and drug levels were undetectable in infants' blood. Owing to very limited information and its reported untoward effects, mexiletine cannot be recommended for use during gestation; its safety must be investigated further.

FLECAINIDE. This drug has been used during pregnancy for both maternal and fetal tachyarrhythmias.[210,221] The drug seems to be effective for conversion of fetal supraventricular tachycardia and devoid of teratogenic effects. One reported fetal death[221]; however, raises some questions regarding its safety, although the death could not be attributed with certainty to flecainide. More information is needed before the safety of flecainide can be established.

PROPAFENONE. Teratogenicity studies in animals have been negative.[210] In humans this drug has been used in a few cases during the second and third trimester of pregnancy for the treatment of maternal arrhythmias.[210,211,222] There is a clear evidence that propafenone and its metabolite, 5-hydroxypropafenone, cross the placenta, reaching approximately 30 to 40 per cent of maternal blood levels. Because of the limited available data, the safety of propafenone during pregnancy is unknown.

AMIODARONE. The use of amiodarone during pregnancy for the treatment of maternal and fetal arrhythmias has been reported by several investigators.[207,223–225] Transplacental transfer of amiodarone and its metabolite desethylamiodarone has been reported to be 10 to 25 per cent.

In a review of 34 pregnancies associated with amiodarone therapy,[223] 53 per cent of the neonates had an uncomplicated course and 15 per cent had minor side effects, including bradycardia and prolonged Q-T interval. However, a substantial number of neonates showed more serious complications such as hypothyroidism (9 per cent), prematurity (12 per cent), and small for gestational age (21 per cent), casting doubts on amiodarone's safety during pregnancy. Pending further studies, amiodarone should be used only in refractory cases of maternal or fetal tachyarrhythmias. Close monitoring of maternal and neonatal thyroid size and function is important for early detection of abnormalities.

Amiodarone is secreted in breast milk in quantities significant enough to be detected in the infant's blood.[207] The effect of long-term amiodarone exposure in infants is unknown; however, because of the well-known potential side effects of this drug, breast feeding is not recommended in women being treated with amiodarone.

CALCIUM ANTAGONISTS

VERAPAMIL. This drug has been used in pregnancy for maternal and fetal supraventricular arrhythmias, premature labor, preeclampsia, and severe gestational proteinuric hypertension.[226–228]

Rapid intravenous injection of verapamil may cause maternal hypotension and fetal distress and should be avoided.[210] More data are required to establish the safety of long-term therapy during pregnancy. Verapamil is excreted in breast milk[210]; its concentration ranges from 23 to 94 per cent of maternal blood level. The estimated total amount of verapamil secreted in milk is less than 0.01 to 0.04 per cent of the administered dose, and no pharmacological effects have been observed in neonates.

NIFEDIPINE. There is increasing experience with the use of nifedipine during pregnancy, mainly in long-term treatment of hypertension but also in preeclampsia, hypertensive emergencies, myocardial ischemia, and tocolysis.[155,229–231] Multiple studies have suggested the efficacy and safety of this drug. Sublingual administration of nifedipine in one case, however, resulted in maternal hypotension and fetal distress.[150]

DILTIAZEM. Use of this drug during pregnancy has been reported in a limited number of patients, primarily for relief of myocardial ischemia and treatment of supraventricular arrhythmias and hypertension.[211,232,233] No adverse effects on the fetus have been described. Diltiazem is secreted in breast milk. In a single reported case, maternal blood and milk concentrations closely correlated, and peak milk concentration exceeded 200 μg/liter.[235]

BETA-ADRENOCEPTOR BLOCKING AGENTS

PROPRANOLOL. This drug has been extensively used in pregnancy for treatment of cardiac arrhythmias, hypertrophic cardiomyopathy, mitral stenosis, and hyperthyroidism.[69,210,235] Propranolol readily crosses the placenta; at delivery, fetal serum concentrations are equal to or lower than maternal concentrations. Because of decreased hepatic metabolism and altered protein binding, serum concentration and half-life may be increased in the neonate during the first 10 days of life. Several adverse effects on the fetus and neonate have been reported, including intrauterine growth retardation, delayed onset of respiration in the newborn, bradycardia, hypoglycemia, and hyperbilirubinemia. Although increasing experience with the use of propranolol in pregnancy has demonstrated the rarity of these side effects, they should be anticipated by the clinician. Since blockade of myometrial beta$_2$-adrenergic receptors with propranolol may stimulate uterine contractions, selective beta$_1$-receptor blockers may be preferable for use during gestation.

Propranolol is excreted in breast milk, with a milk/plasma ratio of approximately 0.5 to 1.0.[209] No adverse effects were observed in infants breast-fed by mothers treated with propranolol. However, careful observation of such infants is recommended, since propranolol may accumulate as a result of the immature hepatic microsomal enzyme system of the neonate.

METOPROLOL. The use of metoprolol in pregnancy is primarily to control hypertension or tachyarrhythmias without causing teratogenic or major side effects.[235] Since metoprolol's metabolism is increased during pregnancy, its half-life serum concentration and bioavailability are decreased. The drug crosses the placenta, and the fetomaternal serum concentration ratio is approximately 1.0. Use of metoprolol in the treatment of hypertension was not associated with fetal growth retardation. Metoprolol is secreted in breast milk[209]; however, the daily quantity ingested by the neonate is very small. Unless hepatic function in the newborn is markedly impaired, breast feeding is probably safe.

ATENOLOL. Several studies have reported the use of atenolol in the treatment of hypertension during gestation.[235] Transplacental transfer of atenolol has been well documented with a fetomaternal ratio of 1.0.[209] Although available data indicate that the safety of atenolol during pregnancy is similar to that of other beta blockers, some of the published studies have reported low birth weight in association with its use during pregnancy.[112] Atenolol is secreted in breast milk. No adverse effects have been noted, however, in babies exposed to breast milk of women treated with atenolol, so that breast feeding need not be discontinued.

SOTALOL. This drug has been used during pregnancy in several cases for treatment of maternal hypertension and maternal and fetal arrhythmias.[236] The drug has been shown to cross the placenta, and levels in the fetal circulation have been found to be approximately 85 per cent of the maternal circulation.[237] Sotalol is secreted in breast milk, and the milk–serum concentration has been found to be 1.57 to 5.64. Breast feeding was not associated with fetal bradycardia.[237]

VASODILATORS

SODIUM NITROPRUSSIDE. During pregnancy, nitroprusside (NP) has been used to control blood pressure and heart failure in patients with intracranial aneurysm or severe gestational hypertension or in those undergoing surgery.[112] Data concerning the effect of NP on uterine blood flow are conflicting. The drug has been demonstrated to cross the placenta, both in animals and in humans. In pregnant ewes, maternal and fetal levels achieved equilibrium within 20 minutes. In the limited number of patients treated with NP during pregnancy, no unfavorable drug-related effect on the fetus was noticed. A large dose of NP in animals, however, resulted in significant accumulation of maternal and fetal cyanide and in fetal death. NP has been employed in pregnancy mostly in severely ill patients, and the data available are minimal. Until further studies clarify its safety during pregnancy, caution is recommended.

ORGANIC NITRATES. Intravenous as well as oral nitrates have been used in pregnancy for the treatment of hypertension, myocardial ischemia, and heart failure and for uterine relaxation in the postpartum patient with retained placenta.[133,155,215,216,233,238,239] In two patients in whom blood pressure was suddenly lowered with nitroglycerin, fetal heart rate deceleration, bradycardia, and attenuation of spontaneous beat-to-beat variability were reported. It appears, therefore, that as with the use of other vasodilators, careful monitoring of systemic blood pressure is required when nitrates are used during pregnancy.

ANGIOTENSIN-CONVERTING ENZYME (ACE) INHIBITORS

Numerous reports both in animals and in humans have been published in the last decade describing use of ACE inhibitors in pregnancy.[113,240] There is evidence in humans that captopril, enalapril, and lisinopril cross the placenta. Available experience indicates a high degree of morbidity and even mortality in fetuses or newborns exposed to ACE inhibitors during pregnancy. Reported complications include oligohydramnios, intrauterine growth retardation, premature labor, fetal and neonatal renal failure, bony malformations, limb contractures, persistent patent ductus arteriosus, pulmonary hypoplasia, respiratory distress syndrome, prolonged hypotension, and neonatal death. The FDA recently has warned against the use of ACE inhibitors during the second and third trimester of pregnancy.[241] Even more recently, Shotan et al. extended this warning to all trimesters of pregnancy and recommended discontinuation of the drugs prior to anticipated conception.[113]

DIURETIC AGENTS

Diuretics have been used in pregnancy for the management of hypertension, heart failure, and fluid retention and to prevent preeclampsia.[81,112] Because of the benign nature of dependent edema in pregnancy and the potential impairment of uterine blood flow and placental perfusion due to decreased blood volume, diuretics are not recommended for dependent edema. The prophylactic use of diuretics has not been proved effective in patients with preeclampsia; moreover, further volume restriction with these drugs may be deleterious. Because of the potential for a decrease in placental perfusion, initiation of treatment with diuretics during pregnancy is not recommended. However, continuation of diuretic therapy initiated prior to conception does not seem unfavorable. Although no teratogenic effects have been described, case reports of neonatal thrombocytopenia, jaundice, hyponatremia, and bradycardia have been reported with the use of thiazides. Recent data have shown, however, that thiazide diuretics are safe and effective when used in combination with methyldopa. Placental transfer of both hydrochlorothiazide and furosemide has been documented, with similar maternal and fetal serum levels.

ANTITHROMBOTIC AGENTS

Antithrombotic therapy may be necessary to prevent or control the following cardiovascular conditions during pregnancy; venous thrombophlebitis, hypertension, pulmonary embolism, rheumatic mitral valve disease, prosthetic heart valves, peripartum cardiomyopathy, primary pulmonary hypertension, ischemic heart disease, complex congenital heart disease, and Eisenmenger's syndrome.[242] However, the use of both antithrombotic agents, i.e., coumadin and heparin, may not be without complications, both for the mother and the fetus.[152,242]

COUMADIN. Because of its large molecular size, heparin does not cross the placenta, is relatively safe for the fetus[243] and is therefore the drug of choice during pregnancy. The use of Coumadin during pregnancy is associated with substantial risk, including fetal wastage due to spontaneous abortion and stillbirths; central nervous system disease such as optic nerve atrophy and blindness, mental retardation, microcephaly, and spasticity; and even death secondary to intracranial hemorrhage.[242] Use of this drug during the first trimester has been associated with "coumarin embryopathy" in 4 to 10 per cent of newborns.[180,200,201,204] This syndrome includes nasal bone hypoplasia and epiphyseal stippling (chondrodysplasia punctata).[242] Labor and delivery while the patient is taking Coumadin places both the mother and fetus at risk of hemorrhage and is an indication for cesarean section. Because the half-life is longer in the fetus, the effect of Coumadin may persist for 7 to 10 days after its discontinuation.

HEPARIN. Patients of childbearing age who are taking anticoagulants on a long-term basis should be advised prior to conception regarding the maternal and fetal risks of these agents. If pregnancy is planned, close monitoring and early diagnosis of pregnancy are essential. As soon as pregnancy is diagnosed, oral anticoagulants should be discontinued and subcutaneous heparin started. A brief period of hospitalization is advisable to establish the required heparin dose and ensure continuity of effective anticoagulation. Self-injection of an adjusted dose of heparin subcutaneously for the duration of pregnancy is the preferred approach in all cases, except in patients with mechanical heart valve. Heparin is administered into the lower abdominal subcutaneous tissue at 12-hour intervals, with dose adjustment to prolong the activated partial thromboplastin time to 1.5 to 2.0 times normal. To reduce pain, concentrated heparin (20,000 units/ml) should be used.

Complications related to long-term heparin therapy may occur and include sterile abscesses and hematomas in the abdominal wall, thrombocytopenia, and osteoporosis.[242,243] To reduce the risk of bleeding at delivery, subcutaneous heparin should be replaced in the hospital with intravenous heparin at 36 weeks' gestation. If needed, heparin can be substituted with oral Coumadin, adjusted to increase INR 2.0 to 3.0 times normal value, at the end of the first trimester. Heparin and Coumadin should be given concomitantly until a therapeutic level of Coumadin is achieved.

Heparin should be discontinued at the onset of labor to prevent bleeding during and after delivery and to allow safe prudential and epidural anesthesia. Hemostatic stitches should be used to avoid bleeding in patients undergoing episiotomy, and uterine contraction

TABLE 59–8 ANTIBIOTIC PROPHYLAXIS FOR LABOR AND DELIVERY

DRUG	DOSAGE REGIMEN
	STANDARD REGIMEN
Ampicillin, gentamicin, and amoxicillin	Intravenous or intramuscular administration of ampicillin, 2.0 gm, plus gentamicin, 1.5 mg/kg (not to exceed 80 mg), 30 min before procedure; followed by amoxicillin, 1.5 gm orally 6 hr after initial dose; alternatively, parenteral regimen may be repeated once 8 hr after initial dose
	AMPICILLIN/AMOXICILLIN/PENICILLIN–ALLERGIC PATIENT REGIMEN
Vancomycin and gentamicin	Intravenous administration of vancomycin, 1.0 gm, over 1 hr plus intravenous or intramuscular administration of gentamicin, 1.5 mg/kg (not to exceed 80 mg), 1 hr before procedure; may be repeated once 8 hr after initial dose
	ALTERNATE LOW-RISK PATIENT REGIMEN
Amoxicillin	3.0 gm orally 1 hr before procedure; then 1.5 gm 6 hr after initial dose

From Dajani, A. S., Bisno, A. L., Chung, K. J.: Prevention of endocarditis recommendations by the American Heart Association. JAMA *264*:2919, 1990.

should be stimulated after delivery by massage and Pitocin or ergot derivatives. It should be noted that heparin therapy may cause persistent anticoagulation for up to 28 hours after administration.[244] For this reason, discontinuation of heparin therapy 24 hours before elective induction of labor or judicious use of protamine sulfate to reduce the risk of bleeding and allow the use of epidural analgesia has been recommended.[150] Intravenous administration of heparin can be resumed after delivery once hemostasis is deemed adequate, and oral anticoagulation therapy can be started 24 hours post partum after bleeding and hemorrhage have been ruled out.[242] Low molecular weight heparin has been used during pregnancy mostly for the treatment of deep vein thrombosis.[245–247] The safety and efficacy of this drug need to be further established before it can be recommended for use in pregnancy and the lactating period. Both regular heparin and oral anticoagulation can be safely used after delivery, even in lactating women.[150] For recommendations of anticoagulation in the patient with prosthetic valves during pregnancy, see page 1066.

PROPHYLACTIC ANTIBIOTICS

Antibiotics are indicated to prevent recurrent acute rheumatic fever in patients with a history of this disease and to prevent bacterial endocarditis in patients with certain types of underlying heart disease.

The recommended regimen for the prevention of rheumatic fever is the same as in the nongravid state and includes 1.2 million units of benzathine penicillin G intramuscularly every 4 weeks, 250,000 units of oral penicillin V twice a day, or 1 gm/day of sulfadiazide.[248] Because of predisposition to kernicterus with the use of sulfadiazine, these drugs are not recommended during the third trimester of pregnancy and in women with a previous history of children with neonatal jaundice or blood-group incompatibility.

As in the nongravid state, antibiotic prophylaxis for infective endocarditis is indicated during gestation in patients with prosthetic heart valves, previous bacterial endocarditis, most congenital cardiac malformations, rheumatic valvular disease, obstructive hypertrophic cardiomyopathy, and mitral valve prolapse with thickened mitral valve and mitral insufficiency who are undergoing procedures likely to result in bacteremia.[43] Since the incidence of bacteremia associated with uncomplicated vaginal delivery has been reported to be low (0 to 5 per cent), the Committee on Bacterial Endocarditis, formed by the American Heart Association, has recommended routine prophylaxis for vaginal delivery in the presence of infection but not for uncomplicated vaginal delivery and for cesarean section. Despite these recommendations, and since complications and bacteremia are not always predictable, we routinely administer prophylactic antibiotics for vaginal delivery to all patients susceptible to bacterial endocarditis. The antibiotic regimens recommended for labor and delivery are shown in Table 59–8.

REFERENCES

CARDIOVASCULAR PHYSIOLOGY DURING PREGNANCY AND THE PUERPERIUM

1. Elkayam, U., and Gleicher, N.: Hemodynamics and cardiac function during normal pregnancy and the puerperium. *In* Elkayam, U., and Gleicher, N. (eds.): Cardiac Problems in Pregnancy: Diagnosis and Management of Maternal and Fetal Disease. 2nd ed. New York, Alan R. Liss, Inc., 1990, p. 5.
2. Longo, L. D.: Maternal blood volume and cardiac output during pregnancy: A hypothesis of endocrinologic control. Am. J. Physiol. *245:*R720, 1983.
3. Plouin, P. F., Cudek, P., Arnal, J. F., et al.: Immunoradiometric assay of active renin versus determination of plasma renin activity in the clinical investigation of hypertension, congestive heart failure, and liver cirrhosis. Horm. Res. *34:*138, 1990.

3a. Cheek, D. B., Petrucco, O. M., Gillespie, A., et al.: Muscle cell growth and the distribution of water and electrolyte in human pregnancy. Early Hum. Dev. *11:*293, 1985.

4. Robson, S. C., Hunter, S., Boys, R. J., et al.: Serial study of factors influencing changes in cardiac output during human pregnancy. Am. J. Physiol. *256:*H1060, 1989.
5. Metcalfe, J., and Ueland, K.: Maternal cardiovascular adjustments to pregnancy. Prog. Cardiovasc. Dis. *16:*363, 1974.
6. Creasy, P. K., and Resnik, R.: Maternal-fetal medicine: Principles and Practice. 2nd ed. Philadelphia, W. B. Saunders Co., 1989.
7. Gerber, J. G., Payne, N. A., Murphy, R. R., et al.: Prostacyclin produced by the pregnant uterus in the dog may act as a circulating vasodepressor substance. J. Clin. Invest. *67:*632, 1981.
8. Itoh, H., Sagawa, N., Mori, T., et al.: Plasma brain natriuretic peptide level in pregnant women with pregnancy-induced hypertension. Obstet. Gynecol. *82:*71, 1993.
9. Robson, S. C., Dunlop, W., Boys, R. J., et al.: Cardiac output during labour. Br. Med. J. *295:*1169, 1987.
10. Morgan, M.: Anesthetic choice for the cardiac obstetric patient. N. Engl. J. Anesth. *10:*621, 1990.
11. Artal, R.: Cardiopulmonary responses to exercise in pregnancy. *In* Elkayam, U., and Gleicher, N. (eds.): Cardiac Problems in Pregnancy: Diagnosis and Management of Maternal and Fetal Disease. 2nd ed. New York, Alan R. Liss, Inc., 1990, p. 25.
12. Carpenter, M. W., Sady, S. P., Hoegsberg, B., et al.: Fetal heart rate response to maternal exertion. JAMA *259:*3006, 1988.

CARDIAC EVALUATION DURING PREGNANCY

13. Elkayam, U., and Gleicher, N.: The evaluation of the cardiac patient. *In* Gleicher, N. (ed.): Principles and Practice of Medical Therapy in Pregnancy. 2nd ed. Norwalk, Conn., Appleton and Lange, 1992, p. 759.
14. Avila, W. S., Grinberg, M., Cardoso, L. F., et al.: Course of pregnancy and puerperium in women with mitral valve stenosis. Rev. Assoc. Med. Bras. *38:*195, 1992.
15. Zeldis, S. M.: Dyspnea during pregnancy: Distinguishing cardiac from pulmonary causes. Clin. Chest Med. *13:*567, 1992.
16. Mishra, M., Chambers, J. B., and Jackson, G.: Murmurs in pregnancy: An audit of echocardiography. Br. Med. J. *304:*1413, 1992.
17. Rayburn, W. F.: Mitral valve prolapse and pregnancy. *In* Elkayam, U., and Gleicher, N. (eds.): Cardiac Problems in Pregnancy: Diagnosis and Management of Maternal and Fetal Disease. 2nd ed. New York, Alan R. Liss, Inc., 1990, p. 181.
18. Kumar, A., and Elkayam, U.: Hypertrophic cardiomyopathy in pregnancy: *In* Elkayam, U., and Gleicher, N. (eds.): Cardiac Problems in Pregnancy: Diagnosis and Management of Maternal and Fetal Disease. 2nd ed. New York, Alan R. Liss, Inc., 1990, p. 129.
19. McLintic, A. J., Pringle, S. D., Lilley, S., et al.: Electrocardiographic changes during cesarean section under regional anesthesia. Anesth. Analg. *74:*51, 1992.
20. Widerhorn, J., Rahimtoola, S. H., and Elkayam, U.: Cardiac rhythm disorders. *In* Gleicher, N. (ed.): Principles and Practice of Medical Therapy in Pregnancy. 2nd ed. Norwalk, Conn., Appleton and Lange, 1992, p. 135.
21. Wagner, C. K., Leser, R. G., and Saldana, L. R.: Exposure of the pregnant patient to diagnostic radiation. A Guide to Medical Management. Philadelphia, J. B. Lippincott Co., 1985, p. 52.
22. Austin, J. H. M.: Postpartum pleura effusions. Ann. Intern. Med. *98:*555, 1983.
23. Bioeffects Committee of the American Institute of Ultrasound in Medicine. J. Ultrasound Med. Biol. *2:*R14, 1983.
24. Stoddard, M. F., Longaker, R. A., Vuocolo, L. M., and Dawkins, P. R.: Transesophageal echocardiography in the pregnant patient. Am. Heart. J. *124:*785, 1992.
25. Limacher, M. C., Ware, J. A., O'Meara, M. E., et al.: Tricuspid regurgitation during pregnancy. Am. J. Cardiol. *55:*1059, 1985.
26. Campos, O., Andrade, J. L., Bocanegra, J., et al.: Physiological multivalvular regurgitation during pregnancy: A longitudinal Doppler echocardiographic study. Intern. J. Cardiol. *40:*265, 1993.
27. Enein, M., Aziz, A., Zima, A., et al.: Echocardiography of the pericardium in pregnancy. Obstet. Gynecol. *69:*851, 1987.
28. Kereiakes, J. J., and Rosenstein, M.: Handbook of radiation doses in nuclear medicine and diagnostic x-ray. Boca Raton, Fla., CRC Press, 1980, p. 70.
29. Kupferminc, M. J., Lessing, J. B., Vidne, B. A., and Peyser, M. R.: Feto-maternal blood flow measurements and management of combined coarctation and aneurysm of the thoracic aorta in pregnancy. Acta Obstet. Gynecol. Scand. *72:*398, 1993.
30. Elkayam, U., and Shotan, A.: Aortic dissection. *In* Gleicher, N., Elkayam, U., Galbraith, R. M., et al. (eds.): Principles of Medical Therapy in Pregnancy. 2nd ed. Norwalk, Conn., Appleton and Lange, 1992, p. 823.
31. Colletti, P. M., and Platt, L. D.: Obstetric MRI acceptable under specific criteria. Diagn. Radiol. *11:*84, 1989.
32. Lee, W., Shah, P. K., Amin, D. K., and Elkayam, U.: Hemodynamic monitoring of cardiac patients during pregnancy. *In* Elkayam, U., and Gleicher, N. (eds.): Cardiac Problems in Pregnancy: Diagnosis and Management of Maternal and Fetal Disease. 2nd ed. New York, Alan R. Liss, Inc., 1990, p. 47.
33. Medical Radiation Exposure of Pregnant and Potentially Pregnant Women: Recommendations of the National Council on Radiation Protection and Measurements. Washington, National Council on Radiation Protection and Measurements, 1977, p. 13.
34. Bithell, J. F., and Steward, A. M.: Prenatal irradiation and childhood malignancy: A review of British data from the Oxford survey. Br. J. Cancer *31:*271, 1975.
35. Elkayam, U., Kawanishi, D., Reid, C. L., et al.: Contrast echocardiography to reduce ionizing radiation associated with cardiac catheterization during pregnancy. Am. J. Cardiol. *52:*213, 1983.

CONGENITAL HEART DISEASE

36. Perloff, J. K.: Congenital heart disease. *In* Gleicher, N. (ed.): Principles and Practice of Medical Therapy in Pregnancy, 2nd ed., Norwalk, Conn., Appleton and Lange, 1992, p. 788.
37. Uzark, K.: Counseling adolescents with congenital heart disease. J. Cardiovasc. Nurs. *6:*65, 1992.
38. Whittemore, R., Hobbins, J. C., and Engle, M. A.: Pregnancy and its outcome in women with and without surgical treatment of congenital heart disease. Am. J. Cardiol. *50:*641, 1982.
39. Pitkin, R. M., Perloff, J. K., Koos, B. J., and Beall, M. H.: Pregnancy and congenital heart disease. Ann. Intern. Med. *112:*445, 1990.
40. Presbitero, P., Somerville, J., Stone, S., et al.: Pregnancy in cyanotic congenital heart disease: Outcome of mother and fetus. Circulation *89:*2673, 1994.

41. Weiss, B. M., and Atanassoff, P. G.: Cyanotic congenital heart disease and pregnancy: Natural selection, pulmonary hypertension and anesthesia. J. Can. Anesth. *5*:332, 1993.
42. Elkayam, U., Cobb, T., and Gleicher, N.: Congenital heart disease and pregnancy. *In* Elkayam, U., and Gleicher, N. (eds.): Cardiac Problems in Pregnancy: Diagnosis and Management of Maternal and Fetal Disease. 2nd ed. New York, Alan R. Liss, Inc., 1990, p. 73.
43. Dajani, A. S., Bisno, A. L., Chung, K. J., et al.: Prevention of bacterial endocarditis. Recommendations by the American Heart Association. JAMA *264*:2191, 1990.
44. McFaul, P. B., Dorman, J. C., Lamki, H., et al.: Pregnancy complicated by maternal heart disease. A review of 519 women. Br. J. Obstet. Gynecol. *95*:861, 1988.
45. Easterling, T., Chadwick, H. S., Otto, C., and Benedetti, T.: Aortic stenosis in pregnancy. Obstet. Gynecol. *72*:1131, 1988.
46. Banning, A. P., Pearson, J. F., and Hall, R. J. C.: Role of balloon dilatation of the aortic valve in pregnant patients with severe aortic stenosis. Br. Heart. J. *70*:544, 1993.
47. Lao, T. T., Sermer, M., MaGee, L., et al.: Congenital aortic stenosis and pregnancy—a reappraisal. Am. J. Obstet. Gynecol. *169*:540, 1993.
48. Lao, T. T., Adelman, A. G., Sermer, M., and Colman, J. M.: Balloon valvuloplasty for congenital aortic stenosis in pregnancy. Br. J. Obstet. Gynaecol. *100*:1141, 1993.
49. Ben-Ami, M., Battino, S., Rosenfeld, T., et al.: Aortic valve replacement during pregnancy: A case report and review of the literature. Acta Obstet. Gynecol. Scand. *69*:651, 1990.
50. Kupferminc, M. J., Lessing, J. B., Jaffa, A., et al.: Fetomaternal blood flow measurements and management of combined coarctation and aneurysm of the thoracic aorta in pregnancy. Acta Obstet. Gynecol. Scand. *72*:398, 1993.
51. Togo, T., Sugishita, Y., Tamura, T., et al.: Uneventful pregnancy and delivery in a case of multiple peripheral pulmonary stenosis. Acta Cardiol. *18*:143, 1983.
52. Larsen-Disney, P., Price, D., Meredith, I.: Undiagnosed maternal Fallot tetralogy presenting in pregnancy. Aust. N. Z. J. Obstet. Gynaecol. *32*:169, 1992.
53. Geller, E., Rudick, V., and Niv, D.: Analgesia and anesthesia during pregnancy. *In* Elkayam, U., and Gleicher, N. (eds.): Cardiac Problems in Pregnancy: Diagnosis and Management of Maternal and Fetal Disease. 2nd ed. New York, Alan R. Liss, Inc., 1990, p. 283.
54. Patton, D. E., Lee, W., Cotton, D. B., et al.: Cyanotic maternal heart disease in pregnancy. Obstet. Gynecol. Surv. *45*:594, 1990.
55. Fong, J., Druzin, M., Gimbel, A. A., and Fisher, J.: Epidural anaesthesia for labour and caesarean section in a parturient with a single ventricle and a transposition of the great arteries. Can. J. Anaesth. *37*:680, 1990.
56. Gilman, D. H.: Caesarean section in undiagnosed Eisenmenger's syndrome. Anaesthesia *46*:371, 1991.
57. Jackson, G. M., Dildy, G. A., Varner, M. W., and Clark, S. L.: Severe pulmonary hypertension in pregnancy following successful repair of ventricular septal defect in childhood. Obstet. Gynecol. *82*:680, 1993.
58. Jeyamalar, R., Sivanesaratnam, V., and Kuppuvelumani, P.: Eisenmenger syndrome in pregnancy. Aust. N. Z. J. Obstet. Gynaecol. *32*:275, 1992.
59. Pollack, K. L., Chestnut, D. H., and Wenstrom, K. D.: Anesthetic management of a parturient with Eisenmenger's syndrome. Anesth. Analg. *70*:212, 1990.
60. Connolly, H. M., and Warnes, C. A.: Ebstein's anomaly: Outcome of pregnancy. J. Am. Coll. Cardiol. *23*:1194, 1994.
61. Megerian, G., Bell, J. G., Huhta, J. C., et al.: Pregnancy outcome following mustard procedure for transposition of the great arteries: A report of five cases and review of the literature. Obstet. Gynecol. *83*:512, 1994.
62. Perry, C. P.: Childbirth after surgical repair of truncus arteriosus. J. Reprod. Med. *5*:65, 1990.
63. Sumner, D., Melville, C., Smith, C. D. R., et al.: Successful pregnancy in a patient with a single ventricle. Eur. J. Obstet. Gynecol. Reprod. Biol. *44*:239, 1992.
64. Rowbottom, S. J., Gin, T., and Cheung, L. P.: General anesthesia for caesarean section in a patient with uncorrected complex cyanotic heart disease. Anaesth. Intensive Care *22*:74, 1994.
65. Walsh, T., Savage, R., and Hess, D. B.: Successful pregnancy in a patient with a double inlet left ventricle treated with a septation procedure. South. Med. J. *83*:358, 1990.

RHEUMATIC HEART DISEASE

66. Ueland, K.: Rheumatic heart disease and pregnancy. *In* Elkayam, U., and Gleicher, N. (eds.): Cardiac Problems in Pregnancy: Diagnosis and Management of Maternal and Fetal Disease. 2nd ed. New York, Alan R. Liss, Inc., 1990, p. 99.
67. Stephen, S. J.: Changing patterns of mitral stenosis in childhood and pregnancy in Sri Lanka. J. Am. Coll. Cardiol. *19*:1276, 1992.
68. Guleria, R., Vasisht, K., Dhall, G. I., et al.: Pregnancy with heart disease: Experience at Postgraduate Institute of Medical Education and Research, Chandigarh. J. Assoc. Physicians India, *38*:902, 1990.
69. Avila, W. S., Grinberg, M., D'ecourt, L. V., et al.: Clinical course of women with mitral valve stenosis during pregnancy and puerperium. Arq. Bras. Cardiol. *58*:359, 1992.
70. Al Kasab, S. M., Sabag, T., Al Zaibag, M., et al.: B adrenergic receptor blockade in the management of pregnant women with mitral stenosis. Am. J. Obstet. Gynecol. *163*:37, 1990.
71. Jacobi, P., Adler, Z., Zimmer, E. Z., et al.: Effect of uterine contractions on left atrial pressure in pregnant women with mitral stenosis. Br. J. Med. *298*:27, 1989.
72. Ziskind, Z., Etchin, A., Frenkel, Y., et al.: Epidural anesthesia with the Trendelenburg position for cesarean section with or without a cardiac surgical procedure in patients with severe mitral stenosis: A hemodynamic study. J. Cardiothorac. Anesth. *4*:354, 1990.
73. De Swiet, M., and Deverall, P.: Editorial note: Pregnancy—Still an indication for closed mitral valvotomy. Int. J. Cardiol. *26*:323, 1990.
74. Esteves, C. A., Ramos, A. I. O., Braga, S. L. N., et al.: Effectiveness of percutaneous balloon mitral valvotomy during pregnancy. Am. J. Cardiol. *68*:930, 1991.
75. Farhat, M. B., Maatouk, F., Betbout, F., et al.: Percutaneous balloon mitral valvuloplasty in eight pregnant women with severe mitral stenosis. Eur. Heart. J. *13*:1658, 1992.
76. Lung, B., Cormier, B., Elias, J., et al.: Usefulness of percutaneous balloon commissurotomy for mitral stenosis during pregnancy. Am. J. Cardiol. *73*:398, 1994.
77. Ribeiro, P. A., Fawzy, M. E., Awad, M., et al.: Balloon valvotomy for pregnant patients with severe pliable mitral stenosis using the Inoue technique with total abdominal and pelvic shielding. Am. Heart. J. *124*:1558, 1992.
78. Glantz, J. C., Pomerantz, R. M., Cunningham, M. J., and Woods, J. R.: Percutaneous balloon valvuloplasty for severe mitral stenosis during pregnancy: A review of therapeutic options. Obstet. Gynecol. Surv. *48*:503, 1993.
79. Sharma, S., Loya, Y. S., Desai, D. M., and Pinto, R. J.: Percutaneous mitral valvotomy in 200 patients using Inoue balloon—immediate and early haemodynamic results. Indian Heart J. *45*:169, 1993.
80. Ribeiro, P. A., and Al Zaibag, M.: Mitral balloon valvotomy in pregnancy (editorial). J. Heart Valve Dis. *1*:206, 1992.
81. Myers, S. A.: Antihypertensive drug use during pregnancy. *In* Elkayam, U., and Gleicher, N. (eds.): Cardiac Problems in Pregnancy: Diagnosis and Management of Maternal and Fetal Disease. 2nd ed. New York, Alan R. Liss, Inc., 1990, p. 381.
82. Roth, A., Shotan, A., and Elkayam, U.: A randomized comparison between the hemodynamic effects of hydralazine and nitroglycerin alone and in combination at rest and during isometric exercise in patients with chronic mitral regurgitation. Am. Heart J. *125*:155, 1993.
83. Banning, A. P., Pearson, J. F., and Hall, R. J. C.: Role of balloon dilatation of the aortic valve in pregnant patients with severe aortic stenosis. Br. Heart J. *70*:544, 1993.
84. McIvor, R. A.: Percutaneous balloon aortic valvuloplasty during pregnancy. Int. J. Cardiol. *32*:1, 1991.
85. Peterson, J. J., Owen, J., and Aldrich, M.: The antepartum patient in the CCU: Educational preparation for nursing staff. Crit. Care Nurse *11*:82, 1991.
86. Lao, T. T., Sermer, M., MaGee, L., et al.: Congenital aortic stenosis and pregnancy—A reappraisal. Am. J. Obstet. Gynecol. *169*:540, 1993.
87. Elkayam, U., McKay, C. R., Weber, L., et al.: Favorable effects of hydralazine on the hemodynamic response to isometric exercise in chronic severe aortic regurgitation. Am. J. Cardiol. *53*:1603, 1984.

OTHER CONDITIONS AFFECTING THE VALVES, AORTA, AND MYOCARDIUM

88. Tank, L. C. H., Chan, S. Y. W., Wong, V. C. W., et al.: Pregnancy in patients with mitral valve prolapse. Int. J. Gynaecol. Obstet. *23*:217, 1985.
89. Kral, J., Spacil, J., Hradec, J., and Cech, E.: Pregnancy and labor in women with mitral valve prolapse. Cas. Lek. Cesk. *129*:1029, 1990.
90. Elkayam, U., Ostrzega, E., Shotan, A., and Mehra, A.: Cardiovascular problems in pregnant women with the Marfan syndrome. Ann. Int. Med. *(in press).*
91. Kotter-Thomsem, I., Weisner, D., Lehmann-Willenbrock, E., et al.: Marfan-syndrom und Schwangerschaft, kompliziert durch das aneurysma dissecans. Geburtshilfe Frauenheilkd. *51*:653, 1991.
92. Pyeritz, R. E.: The Marfan syndrome. Am. Fam. Physician *34*:83, 1986.
93. Simpson, I. A., deBelder, M. A., Treasure, T., et al.: Cardiovascular manifestations of Marfan's syndrome: Improved evaluation by transesophageal echocardiography. Br. Heart J. *69*:104, 1993.
94. Shores, J., Berger, K. R., Murphy, E. A., and Pyeritz, R. E.: Progression of aortic dilatation and the benefit of long-term beta adrenergic blockade in Marfan's syndrome. N. Engl. J. Med. *330*:1335, 1994.
95. Treasure, T.: Elective replacement of the aortic root in Marfan's syndrome. Br. Heart J. *69*:101, 1993.
96. Kumar, A., and Elkayam, U.: Hypertrophic cardiomyopathy in pregnancy. *In* Elkayam, U., and Gleicher, N. (eds.): Cardiac Problems in Pregnancy: Diagnosis and Management of Maternal and Fetal Disease. 2nd ed. New York, Alan R. Liss, Inc., 1990, p. 129.
97. van Kasteren, Y. M., Kleinhout, J., Smit, M. A., et al.: Hypertrophic cardiomyopathy and pregnancy: A report of three cases. Eur. J. Obstet. Gynecol. Reprod. Biol. *38*:63, 1990.
98. Tessler, M. J., Hudson, R., Naugler-Colville, M. A., and Biehl, D. R.: Pulmonary edema in two parturients with hypertrophic obstructive cardiomyopathy (HOCM). Can. J. Anaesth. *37*:469, 1990.
99. Pelliccia, F., Cianfrocca, C., Gaudig, C., and Reale, A.: Sudden death during pregnancy in hypertrophic cardiomyopathy. Eur. Heart. J. *13*:421, 1992.

100. Rowe, T.: Hypertrophic cardiomyopathy in pregnancy: A case study. J. Cardiovasc. Nurs. *8*:69, 1994.
101. Elkayam, U., Ostrzega, E., and Shotan, A.: Peripartum cardiomyopathy. *In* Gleicher, N. (ed.): Principles and Practice of Medical Therapy in Pregnancy. 2nd ed. Norwalk, CT, Appleton and Lange, 1992, p. 131.
102. Ribner, H. S., and Silverman, R. I.: Peripartal cardiomyopathy. *In* Elkayam, U., and Gleicher, N. (eds.): Cardiac Problems in Pregnancy: Diagnosis and Management of Maternal and Fetal Disease. 2nd ed. New York, Alan R. Liss, Inc., 1990, p. 115.
103. Rolfe, M., Tang, C. M., Walker, R. W., et al.: Peripartum cardiac failure in the Gambia. J. Trop. Med. Hyg. *95*:192, 1992.
104. Leonard, R. B., Schwartz, E., Allen, D. A., and Alson, R. L.: Peripartum cardiomyopathy: A case report. J. Emerg. Med. *10*:157, 1992.
105. Nwosu, E. C., and Burke, M. F.: Cardiomyopathy of pregnancy. Br. J. Obstet. Gynecol. *100*:1145, 1992.
106. Ravikishore, A. G., Kaul, U. A., Sethi, K. K., and Khalilullah, M.: Peripartum cardiomyopathy: Prognostic variables at initial evaluation. Int. J. Cardiol. *32*:377, 1991.
107. van Hoevan, K. H., Kitsis, R. N., Katz, S. D., and Factor, S. M.: Peripartum versus idiopathic dilated cardiomyopathy in young women—A comparison of clinical, pathological and prognostic features. Int. J. Cardiol. *40*:57, 1993.
108. Oakley, C. M., and Nihoyannopoulos, P.: Peripartum cardiomyopathy with recovery in a patient with coincidental Eisenmenger ventricular septal defect. Br. Heart J. *67*:190, 1992.
109. Marin-Neto, J. A., Maciel, B. C., Teran Urbanetz, L. L., et al.: High output failure in patients with peripartum cardiomyopathy: A comparative study with dilated cardiomyopathy. Am. Heart J. *121*:134, 1990.
110. Midei, M. C., DeMent, S. H., Feldman, A. M., et al.: Peripartum myocarditis and cardiomyopathy. Circulation *81*:922, 1990.
111. Rizeg, M. N., Rickenbacher, P. R., Fowler, M. B., and Billingham, M. E.: Incidence of myocarditis in peripartum cardiomyopathy. Am. J. Cardiol. *74*:474, 1994.
112. Widerhorn, J., Widerhorn, A. L. M., and Elkayam, U.: Cardiovascular pharmacotherapy in pregnancy and lactation. *In* Gleicher, N. (ed.): Principles and Practice of Medical Therapy in Pregnancy. 2nd ed. Norwalk, CT, Appleton and Lange, 1992, p. 767.
113. Shotan, A., Widerhorn, J., Hurst, A., and Elkayam, U.: Risks of angiotensin-converting enzyme inhibition during pregnancy: Experimental and clinical evidence, potential mechanisms, and recommendations for use. Am. J. Med. *96*:451, 1994.
114. Hovsepian, P. G., Ganzel, B., Sohi, G. S., et al.: Peripartum cardiomyopathy treated with a left ventricular assist device as a bridge to cardiac transplantation. South Med. J. *82*:527, 1989.
115. Liljestrand, J., Lindstrom, B.: Chidlbirth after post partum cardiac insufficiency treated with cardiac transplant. Acta Obstet. Gynecol. Scand. *72*:406, 1993.
116. St. John Sutton, M. S. J., Cole, P., Plappert, M., et al.: Effects of subsequent pregnancy on left ventricular function in peripartum cardiomyopathy. Am. Heart J. *121*:1776, 1991.
117. Garla, P. G. N.: Epidural fentanyl for cesarean section in postpartal cardiomyopathy. W. Va. Med. J. *86*:11, 1990.
118. Lindheimer, M. D.: Hypertension in pregnancy. Hypertension *22*:127, 1993.
119. National High Blood Pressure Education Program Working Group Report on High Blood Pressure in Pregnancy. Am. J. Obstet. Gynecol. *163*:1689, 1990.
120. Svenson, A.: Hypertension in pregnancy. Clin. Exp. Hypertens. *15*:1353, 1993.
121. Scott, J. R., Wagoner, L. E., Olsen, S. E., et al.: Pregnancy in heart transplant recipients: Management and outcome. Obstet. Gynecol. *82*:324, 1993.
122. Liljestrand, J., and Lindstrom, B.: Childbirth after post partum cardiac insufficiency treated with cardiac transplant. Acta Obstet. Gynecol. Scand. *72*:406, 1993.
123. Laifer, S. A.: Pregnancy after transplantation. *In* Lee, R. V., Barron, W. M., Cotton, D. B., et al. (eds.): Current Obstetric Medicine, Vol. 2. St. Louis, C. V. Mosby, 1993, p. 1.

CORONARY ARTERY DISEASE

124. Goldman, M. E., and Meller, J.: Coronary artery disease in pregnancy. *In* Elkayam, U., and Gleicher, N. (eds.): Cardiac Problems in Pregnancy: Diagnosis and Management of Maternal and Fetal Disease. 2nd ed. New York, Alan R. Liss, Inc., 1990, p. 153.
125. La Vecchia, C., Franceschi, S., Decarli, A., et al.: Risk factors for myocardial infarction in young women. Am. J. Epidemiol. *125*:832, 1987.
126. Croft, P., and Hannaford, P. C.: Risk factors for acute myocardial infarction in women: Evidence from the Royal College of General Practitioners' Oral Contraception Study. Br. Med. J. *298*:165, 1989.
127. La Vecchia, C., Decarli, A., Franceschi, S., et al.: Menstrual and reproductive factors and the risk of myocardial infarction in women under fifty-five years of age. Am. J. Obstet. Gynecol. *157*:1108, 1987.
128. Raymond, R., Lynch, J., Underwood, E., et al.: Myocardial infarction and normal coronary arteriography: A 10-year clinical and risk analysis of 74 infants. J. Am. Coll. Cardiol. *11*:471, 1988.
129. Donnelly, S., McKenna, P., McGing, P., and Sugrue, D.: Myocardial infarction during pregnancy. Br. J. Obstet. Gynaecol. *100*:781, 1993
130. Etienne, Y., Jobic, Y., Houel, J. F., et al.: Papillary fibroelastoma of the aortic valve with myocardial infarction: Echocardiographic diagnosis and surgical excision. Am. Heart J. *127*:443, 1994.
131. Maekawa, K., Ohnishi, H., Hirase, T., et al.: Acute myocardial infarction during pregnancy caused by coronary artery spasm. J. Intern. Med. *235*:489, 1994.
132. Menegakis, N. E., and Amstey, M. S.: Case report of myocardial infarction in labor. Am. J. Obstet. Gynecol. *165*:1383, 1991.
133. Skeikh, A. U., and Harper, M. A.: Myocardial infarction during pregnancy: Management and outcome of two pregnancies. Am. J. Obstet. Gynecol. *169*:279, 1993.
134. Delay, M., Genestal, M., Carrie, D., et al.: Arrêt cardiocirculatoire après administration de l'association mifepristone (Mifegyne) sulprostone (Nalador) pour interruption de grossesse. Arch. Mal. Coeur. *85*:105, 1992.
135. Liao, J. K., Cockrill, B. A., and Yurchak, P. M.: Acute myocardial infarction after ergonovine administration for uterine bleeding. Am. J. Cardiol. *68*:823, 1991.
136. Efstratiou, A., and Singh, B.: Combined spontaneous postpartum coronary artery dissection and pulmonary embolism with survival. Cathet. Cardiovasc. Diagn. *31*:29, 1994.
137. Emori, T., Goto, Y., Maeda, T., et al.: Multiple coronary artery dissections diagnosed in vivo in a pregnant woman. Chest *104*:289, 1993.
138. Kearney, P., Singh, H., Hutter, J., et al.: Spontaneous coronary artery dissection: A report of three cases and review of the literature. Postgrad Med. J. *69*:940, 1993.
139. Verkaaik, A. P. K., Visser, W., Deckers, J. W., Lotgering, F. K.: Multiple coronary artery dissections in a woman at term. Br. J. Anaesth. *71*:301, 1993.
140. Rallings, P., Exner, I., and Abraham, R.: Coronary artery vasculitis and myocardial infarction associated with antiphospholipid antibodies in a pregnant woman. Aust. N. Z. J. Med. *19*:347, 1989.
141. Parry, G., Goudevenos, J., and Williams, D. O.: Coronary thrombosis postpartum in a young woman with Still's disease. Clin. Cardiol. *15*:305, 1992.
142. Nolan, T. E., and Savage, R. W.: Peripartum myocardial infarction from presumed Kawasaki's disease. South. Med. J. *83*:1360, 1990.
143. Van Enk, A., Visschers, G., Jansen, W., and Van Eps, L. W. S.: Maternal death due to sickle cell chronic lung disease. Br. J. Obstet. Gynaecol. *99*:162, 1992.
144. Jessurun, C. R., Adam, K., Moise, K. J., and Wilansky, S.: Pheochromocytoma-induced myocardial infarction in pregnancy. A case report and literature review. Tex. Heart Inst. J. *20*:120, 1993.
145. Hands, M. E., Johnson, M. D., Saltzman, D. H., and Rutherford, J. D.: The cardiac, obstetric and anesthetic management of pregnancy complicated by acute myocardial infarction. J. Clin. Anesth. *2*:258, 1990.
146. Kannan, P., Raman, S., Ramani, V. S., and Jeyamalar, R.: Myocardial infarction in a young Indian grandmultipara. Aust. N. Z. J. Obstet. Gynaecol. *33*:424, 1993.
147. Sheikh, A. U., and Harper, M. A.: Myocardial infarction during pregnancy: Management and outcome of two pregnancies. Am. J. Obstet. Gynecol. *169*:279, 1993.
148. Viinikka, L., Hartikainen-Sorri, A. L., Lumme, R., et al.: Low dose aspirin in hypertensive pregnant women: Effect on pregnancy outcome and prostacyclin-thromboxane balance in mother and newborn. Br. J. Obstet. Gynaecol. *100*:809, 1993.
149. Impey, L.: Severe hypotension and fetal distress following sublingual administration of nifedipine to a patient with severe pregnancy induced hypertension at 33 weeks. Br. J. Obstet. Gynaecol. *100*:959, 1993.
150. Ginsberg, J. S., and Hirsch, J.: Use of antithrombotic agents during pregnancy. Chest *108*:305S, 1995.
151. Corby, D. G.: Aspirin in pregnancy and fetal effects. Pediatrics 62:930, 1978.
151a. Shores, J., Berger, K. R., Murphy, E. A., and Pyeritz, R. E.: Progression of aortic dilatation and the benefit of long-term beta adrenergic blockade in Marfan's syndrome. N. Engl. J. Med. *330*:1335, 1994.
152. Sbarouni, E., and Oakley, C. M.: Outcome of pregnancy in women with valve prostheses. Br. Heart. J. *71*:196, 1994.
153. Tissot, H., Vergnes, C., Rougier, P., et al.: Fibrinolytic treatment with urokinase and streptokinase for recurrent thrombosis in two valve prostheses for the aortic and mitral valves during pregnancy. J. Gynecol. Obstet. Biol. Reprod. *20*:1093, 1991.
154. Cowan, N. C., de Belder, M. A., and Rothman, M. T.: Coronary angioplasty in pregnancy. Br. Heart J. *59*:588, 1988.
155. Shalev, Y., Ben-Hur, H., Hagay, Z., et al.: Successful delivery following myocardial ischemia during the second trimester of pregnancy. Clin. Cardiol. *16*:754, 1993.

ARRHYTHMIAS

156. Mehra, A., Ostrzega, E., Widerhorn, J., et al.: Arrhythmias in pregnancy: Prevalence and effect on fetal and maternal outcome in a large group of asymptomatic women. Clin. Res. (Abs)*39*:79a, 1991.
157. Brodsky, M., Doria, R., Allen, B., et al.: New-onset ventricular tachycardia during pregnancy. Am. Heart J. *123*:933, 1992.
158. Tawam, M., Levine, J., Mendelson, M., et al.: Effect of pregnancy on paroxysmal supraventricular tachycardia. Am. J. Cardiol. *72*:838, 1993.
159. Widerhorn, J., Widerhorn, A. L. M., Rahimtoola, S. H., and Elkayam, U.: WPW syndrome during pregnancy: Increased incidence of supraventricular arrhythmias. Am. Heart J. *124*:796, 1992.
160. Field, L. M., Barton, F. L.: The management of anaesthesia for caesarean section in a patient with paroxysmal ventricular tachycardia. Anaesthesia *48*:593, 1993.
161. Gras, D., Mabo, P., Kermarrec, A., et al.: Radiofrequency ablation of

atrioventricular conduction during the 5th month of pregnancy. Arch. Mal. Coeur. V. *85:*1873, 1992.
162. Oettinger, M., and Pelitz, Y.: Asymptomatic paroxysmal atrial fibrillation during intravenous magnesium sulfate treatment in preeclampsia. Gynecol. Obstet. Invest. *36:*244, 1993.
163. Penkala, M., and Hancock, E. W.: Wide-complex tachycardia in pregnancy. Hos. Pract. Jul. 63, 1993.
164. Feldman, J. M.: Cardiac arrest after succinylcholine administration in a pregnant patient recovered from Guillain-Barré syndrome. Anesthesiology *72:*942, 1990.
165. Swartjes, J. M., Schutte, M. F., and Bleker, O. P.: Management of eclampsia: Cardiopulmonary arrest resulting from magnesium sulfate overdose. Eur. J. Obstet. Gynaecol. Reprod. Biol. *47:*73, 1992.
166. Varon, M. E., Sherer, D. M., Abramowicz, J. S., and Akiyama, T.: Maternal ventricular tachycardia associated with hypomagnesemia. Am. J. Obstet. Gynecol. *167:*1352, 1992.
167. Naidoo, D. P., Bhorat, I., Moodley, J., et al.: Continuous electrocardiographic monitoring in hypertensive crises in pregnancy. Am. J. Obstet. Gynecol. *164:*530, 1991.
168. Plotz, J., Heidegger, H., von Hugo, R., et al.: Hereditary prolonged QT interval (Romano-Ward syndrome) in a female patient with nonelective cesarean section. Anaesthetist *41:*88, 1992.
169. Wilkinson, C., Gyaneschwar, R., and McCusker, C.: Twin pregnancy in a patient with idiopathic long QT syndrome. Case report. Br. J. Obstet. Gynecol. *98:*1300, 1991.
170. Dalvi, B. V., Chaudhuri, A., Kulkarni, H. L., and Kale, P. A.: Therapeutic guidelines for congenital complete heart block presenting in pregnancy. Obstet. Gynecol. *79:*802, 1992.
171. Lau, C. P., Lee, C. P., Wong, C. K., et al.: Rate responsive pacing with a minute ventilation sensing pacemaker during pregnancy and delivery. PACE *13:*158, 1990.
172. Ramsewak, S., Persad, P., Perkins, S., and Narayansingh, G.: Twin pregnancy in a patient with complete heart block. Clin. Exp. Obstet. Gynecol. *19:*166, 1992.
173. Rosen, A., Klein, M., Ambros, O., and Pfemeter, G.: Implantation eines herzschrittmachers in der 25.SSW bei erworbenem AV block III. Grades. Gerburtshilfe Frauenheilkd. *51:*239, 1991.
174. Walsh, T., Savage, R., and Hess, D. B.: Successful pregnancy in a patient with a double inlet left ventricle treated with a septation procedure. South. Med. J. *83:*358, 1990.
175. Holdright, D. R., and Sutton, G. C.: Restoration of sinus rhythm during two consecutive pregnancies in a woman with congenital complete heart block. Br. Heart J. *64:*338, 1990.
176. Emori, T., Goto, Y., Maeda, T., et al.: Multiple coronary artery dissections diagnosed in vivo in a pregnant woman. Chest *104:*289, 1993.
177. Jordaens, L. J., Vandenbogaerde, J. F., Van De Bruaene, P., and De Buyzere, M.: Transesophageal echocardiography for insertion of a physiological pacemaker in early pregnancy. PACE *13:*955, 1990.
178. Terhaar, M., and Schakenbach, L.: Care of the pregnant patient with a pacemaker. J. Perinat. Neonat. Nurs. *5:*1, 1991.
179. Elkayam, U., Goodwin, T. M.: Adenosine therapy for supraventricular tachycardia during pregnancy. Am. J. Cardiol. *75:*521, 1995.
179a. Gilson, G. J., Knieriem, K. J., Smith, J. F., et al.: Short acting beta-adrenergic blockade and the fetus. A case report. J. Reprod. Med. *37:*277, 1992.
180. Doig, J. C., McComb, J. M., and Reid, D. C.: Incessant atrial tachycardia accelerated by pregnancy. Br. Heart J. *67:*266, 1992.
181. Treakle, K., Kostic, B., and Hulkower, S.: Supraventricular tachycardia resistant to treatment in a pregnant woman. J. Fam. Pract. *35:*581, 1992.
182. Lee, M. S., Evans, S. J. L., Blumberg, S., et al.: Echocardiographically guided electrophysiologic testing in pregnancy. J. Am. Soc. Echocardiogr. *7:*182, 1994.

OTHER CARDIOVASCULAR DISORDERS

183. Elkayam, U., Rose, J., Jamison, M.: Vascular aneurysms and dissections during pregnancy. *In* Elkayam, U., and Gleicher, N. (eds.): Cardiac Problems in Pregnancy: Diagnosis and Management of Maternal and Fetal Disease. 2nd ed. New York, Alan R. Liss, Inc., 1990, p. 215.
184. Del Corso, L., De Marco, S., Vannini, A., and Pentimone, F.: Takayasu's arteritis: Low corticosteroid dosage and pregnancy—A case report. Angiology *44:*827, 1993.
185. Hampl, K. F., Schneider, M. C., Skarvan, K., et al.: Spinal anesthesia in a patient with Takayasu's disease. Br. J. Anaesth. *72:*129, 1994.
186. Elkayam, U., and Gleicher, N.: Primary pulmonary hypertension and pregnancy. *In* Elkayam, U., and Gleicher, N. (eds.): Cardiac Problems in Pregnancy: Diagnosis and Management of Maternal and Fetal Disease. 2nd ed. New York, Alan R. Liss, Inc., 1990, p. 189.
187. Pfisterer, J., Runge, H. M., Kommoss, F., et al.: Primare pulmonale hypertronie und Schwangerschaft. Gerburtshilfe Frauenheilkd. *51:*236, 1991.
188. Torres, P. J., Gratacos, E., Magrina, J., et al.: Primary pulmonary hypertension and pre-eclampsia: A successful pregnancy. Br. J. Obstet. Gynaecol. *101:*163, 1994.
189. Kiss, H., Egarter, C., Asseryanis, E., et al.: Primary pulmonary hypertension in pregnancy: A case report. Am. J. Obstet. Gynecol. *172:*1052, 1995.
190. Wilson, N. J., and Neutze, J. M.: Adult congenital heart disease: Principles and management guidelines. Part I. Aust. N. Z. J. Med. *23:*498, 1993.
191. Fuster, V., Steele, P. M., Edwards, W. D., et al.: Primary pulmonary hypertension: Natural history and the importance of thrombosis. Circulation *70:*580, 1984.
192. Abboud, T. K., Raya, J., Noueihed, R., et al.: Intrathecal morphine for relief of labor pain in a parturient with severe pulmonary hypertension. Anesthesiology *59:*477, 1983.
193. Gazzaniga, A.: Cardiac surgery during pregnancy. *In* Elkayam, U., and Gleicher, N. (eds.): Cardiac Problems in Pregnancy: Diagnosis and Management of Maternal and Fetal Disease. 2nd ed. New York, Alan R. Liss, Inc., 1990, p. 259.
194. Kupferminc, M. J., Lessing, J. B., Vidne, B. A., and Peyser, M. R.: Fetomaternal blood flow measurements and management of combined coarctation and aneurysm of the thoracic aorta in pregnancy. Acta Obstet. Gynecol. Scand. *72:*398, 1993.
195. Pamulapati, M., Treague, S., Stelzer, P., and Thadani, U.: Successful surgical repair of a ruptured aneurysm of the sinus of Valsalva in early pregnancy. Ann. Intern. Med. *115:*880, 1991.
196. Said, S. A. M., Veerbeek, A., van der Wieken, L. R.: Dextrocardia, situs inversus and severe mitral stenosis in a pregnant woman: Successful closed commissurotomy. Eur. Heart J. *12:*825, 1991.
197. Westaby, S., Parry, A. J., Forfar, J. C.: Reoperation for prosthetic valve endocarditis in the third trimester of pregnancy. Ann. Thorac. Surg. *53:*263, 1992.
198. Levy, D. L., Warriner, R. A., and Burgess, G. E.: Fetal response to cardiopulmonary bypass. Obstet. Gynecol. *56:*112, 1980.
199. Salazar, E., Zajarias, A., Guiterrez, N., et al.: The problem of cardiac valve prosthesis, anticoagulants and pregnancy. Circulation *70*(Suppl. 1):169, 1984.
200. Iturbe-Alessio, I., Del Carmen Fonseca, M., Mutchinik, O., et al.: Risks of anticoagulant therapy in pregnant women with artificial heart valve. N. Engl. J. Med. *315:*1390, 1986.
201. Lee, C. N., Wu, C. C., Lin, P. Y., et al.: Pregnancy following cardiac prosthesis valve replacement. Obstet. Gynecol. *83:*353, 1994.
202. Bick, R. L., and Pegram, M.: Syndrome of hypercoagulability and thrombosis: A review. Semin. Thromb. Hemost. *20:*109, 1994.
203. Elkayam, U., and Gleicher, N.: Anticoagulation in pregnant women with artificial heart valves. N. Engl. J. Med. *316:*1663, 1987.
204. Sareli, P., England, M. J., Berk, M. R., et al.: Maternal and fetal sequelae of anticoagulation during pregnancy in patients with mechanical heart valve prostheses. Am. J. Cardiol. *63:*1462, 1989.
205. Born, D., Martinez, E. E., Almeida, P. A. M., et al.: Pregnancy in patients with prosthetic heart valves: The effects of anticoagulation on mother, fetus, and neonate. Am. Heart J. *124:*413, 1992.
206. Ad Hoc Committee of the Working Group on Valvular Heart Disease, European Society of Cardiology: Guidelines for prevention of thromboembolic events in valvular heart disease. J. Heart Valve Dis. *2:*298, 1993.

CARDIOVASCULAR DRUGS IN PREGNANCY

207. Mitani, G. M., Steinberg, I., Lien, E., et al.: The pharmacokinetics of antiarrhythmic agents in pregnancy and lactation. Clin. Pharmacokinet. *12:*253, 1987.
208. Gleicher, N., and Elkayam, U.: Intrauterine therapy of rhythm and rate disorders and heart failure. *In* Elkayam, U., and Gleicher, N. (eds.): Cardiac Problems in Pregnancy: Diagnosis and Management of Maternal and Fetal Disease. 2nd ed. New York, Alan R. Liss, Inc., 1990, p. 749.
209. Mitani, G. M., Harrison, E. C., Steinberg, I., et al.: Digitalis glycosides in pregnancy. *In* Elkayam, U., and Gleicher, N. (eds.): Cardiac Problems in Pregnancy: Diagnosis and Management of Maternal and Fetal Disease. 2nd ed. New York, Alan R. Liss, Inc., 1990, p. 417.
210. Cox, J. L., and Gardner, M. J.: Treatment of cardiac arrhythmias during pregnancy. Prog. Cardiovasc. Dis. *36:*137, 1993.
211. Widerhorn, J., Shotan, A., Widerhorn, A. L. M., et al.: Antiarrhythmias. *In* Lee, R. V., Garner, P. R., Barron, W. M., et al. (eds.): Curr. Obstet. Med. *3:*95, 1995.
212. Treakle, K., Kostic, B., and Hulkower, S.: Supraventricular tachycardia resistant to treatment in a pregnant woman. J. Fam. Pract. *35:*581, 1992.
213. Ellsworth, A. J., Horn, J. R., Raisys, V. A., et al.: Disopyramide and *N*-monodesalkyl disopyramide in serum and breast milk. Drug Intell. Clin. Pharm. *23:*56, 1989.
214. Tadmor, O. P., Keren, A., Rosenak, D., et al.: The effect of disopyramide on uterine contractions during pregnancy. Am. J. Obstet. Gynecol. *162:*482, 1990.
215. Juneja, M. M., Ackerman, W. E., Kaczorowski, D. M., et al.: Continuous epidural lidocaine infusion in the parturient with paroxysmal ventricular tachycardia. Anesthesiology *71:*305, 1989.
216. Hands, M. E., Johnson, M. D., Saltzmann, D. H., and Rutherford, J. D.: The cardiac, obstetric and anesthetic management of pregnancy complicated by acute myocardial infarction. J. Clin. Anesth. *2:*258, 1990.
217. Lownes, H. E., and Ives, T. J.: Mexiletine use in pregnancy and lactation. Am. J. Obstet. Gynecol. *157:*446, 1987.
218. Gregg, A. R., and Tomich, P. G.: Mexiletine use in pregnancy. J. Perinat. *8:*33, 1988.
219. Wagner, X., Jouglard, J., Moulin, M., et al.: Coadministration of flecainide acetate and sotalol during pregnancy: Lack of teratogenic effects, passage across the placenta, and excretion in human breast milk. Am. Heart J. *119:*700, 1990.
220. Perry, J. C., Ayres, N. A., Carpenter, R. J.: Fetal supraventricular tachycardia treated with flecainide acetate. J. Pediatr. *118:*303, 1991.

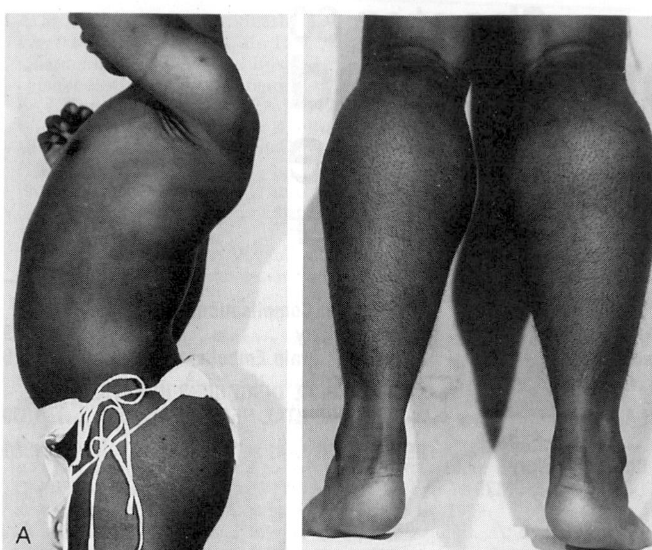

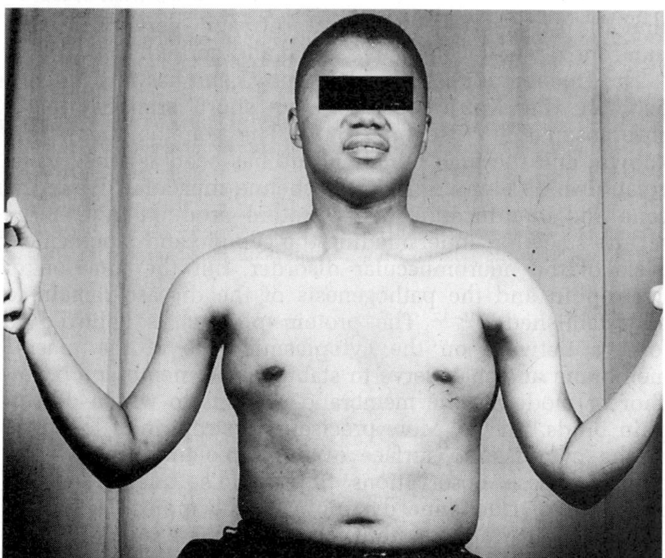

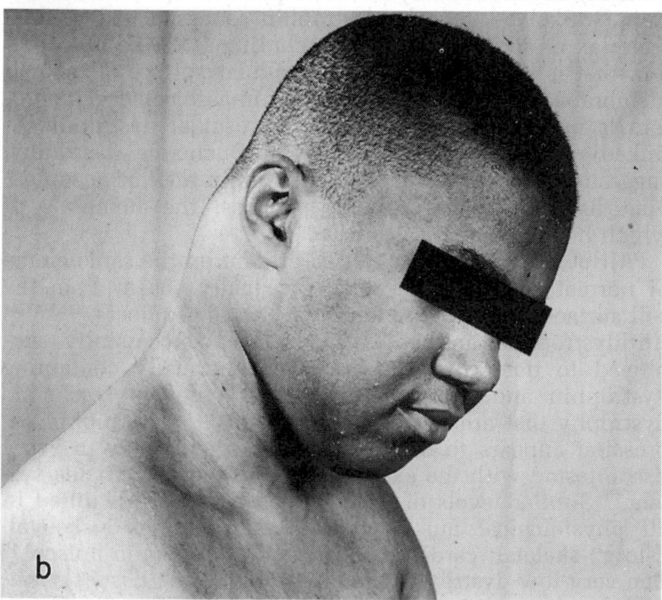

FIGURE 60–1. *A,* Classic X-linked muscular dystrophy. *Left,* exaggerated lumbar lardosis. *Right,* calf pseudohypertrophy and shortening of the Achilles tendons. *B,* Seventeen-year-old male with Duchenne muscular dystrophy. *Upper,* there is striking enlargement (hypertrophy/pseudohypertrophy) of the deltoid and pectoralis major muscles and *(lower)* of the trapezius. There was also striking enlargement of both calves, not shown.

tain similar amounts of dystrophin, should be equally vulnerable to necrosis based upon dystrophin content per se, but that clearly is not the case.[10]

Polyclonal antibodies used to assess the quantity and quality of dystrophin not only provide a laboratory method for the diagnosis of Duchenne dystrophy, but represent a major step forward in identification of female carriers.[9,22] Highly accurate prenatal diagnosis is now possible with Southern analysis using Duchenne muscular dystrophy cDNA and genomic clones.[9]

Rare cases of clinical Duchenne muscular dystrophy in female patients have been attributed to X translocation of a single mutant gene.[25,26] The normal X is inactivated, so the mutant X-linked recessive gene expresses itself.

CLINICAL MANIFESTATIONS. Overt clinical manifestations of Duchenne muscular dystrophy typically begin in the second year of life, although there is histological and enzymatic evidence that the disease is present at birth.[6] Skeletal muscle enzymes are copiously released into the plasma. Creatinine kinase (CK) elevations are present at birth, peak in 1 to 2 years, and precede the onset of overt clinical disease. Because the disorder exists at birth, it is present in utero.[27] Distinctive profiles of an isozyme such as MB-CK cannot be used to identify myocardial dystrophy because the isozyme originates in dystrophic skeletal muscle, compromising the specificity of the determination.[28,29]

In a child just learning to walk, the clumsy, waddling gait and frequent falls may go unnoticed, and the boy's difficulty in rising from the floor using the device of "climbing up" himself (Gowers' sign) tends to be ignored initially by parents and physicians. Because of what is interpreted as good muscle development (early enlargement of the calves) (Fig. 60–1*A*), reduced strength is not ascribed to an abnormality of skeletal muscle. Rarely, regional muscle enlargement (hypertrophy/pseudohypertrophy) in Duchenne dystrophy is striking in muscle groups other than the calves (Fig. 60–1*B*). Lumbar lordosis, hyperextension of the knees, and shortening of the Achilles tendons contribute to a precarious balance on the toes (Fig. 60–1*A*). Kyphoscoliosis becomes progressively more marked, and in the terminal stages of the disease, the patient sits in a wheelchair, twisted like a pretzel, with the head lolling unsupported because of inadequate neck-muscle strength.

Dystrophy of thoracic muscles and diaphragm together with kyphoscoliosis compromise coughing and breathing. Diaphragmatic dysfunction together with respiratory muscle weakness may result in hypercapnia that profoundly worsens with the use of supplemental oxygen therapy.[30] Patients are likely to succumb to pulmonary infection in the second decade, although cardiac involvement is an important and sometimes dramatic cause of death. Rapidly progressive preterminal heart failure may follow years of circulatory stability during which the chief, if not only, suspicion of cardiac involvement is the typical electrocardiogram (Fig. 60–2). Pulmonary emboli have been reported in patients with end-stage Duchenne dystrophy, and systemic emboli sometimes originate in a dilated, hypokinetic left ventricle.[31,32]

Physical examination. There are thoracic deformities and a high diaphragm of diaphragmatic dystrophy, features confirmed in the chest roentgenogram. A reduction in anteroposterior chest dimension is often striking and is commonly responsible for a systolic impulse at the left sternal border, a grade 1-3/6 short impure midsystolic murmur in the second left interspace, and a relatively loud pulmonary component of the second heart sound. These signs should not be mistaken for evidence of pulmonary hypertension, which if present at all, occurs in the terminal stage of the disease in conjunction with respiratory failure.[33] An increase in transverse heart size in the chest roentgenogram is more often than not caused by the high diaphragm and decreased anteroposterior chest dimen-

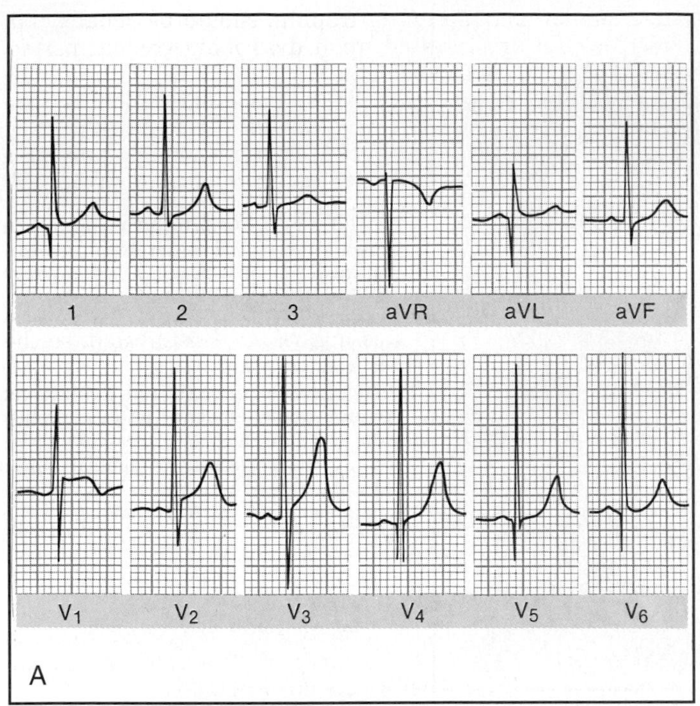

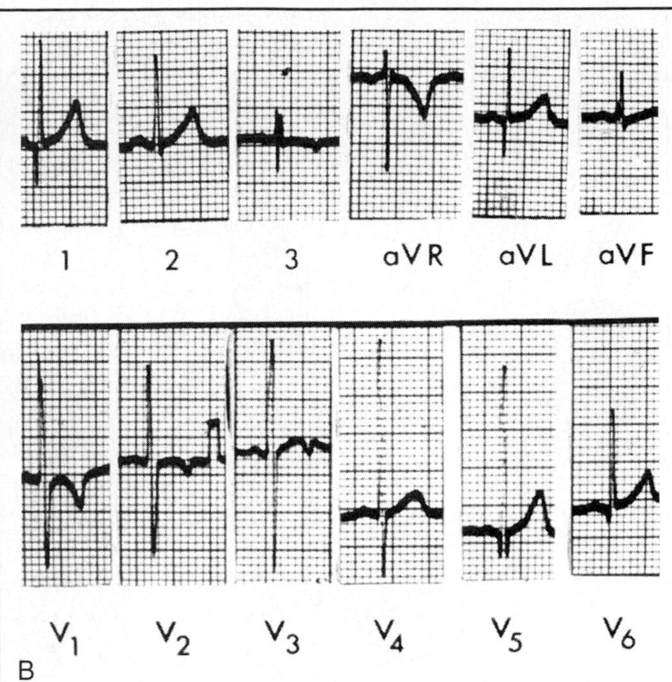

FIGURE 60–2. Electrocardiogram from a 10-year-old boy with classic Duchenne muscular dystrophy. The P–R interval is short (100 msec in lead 2). The QRS complex is typical of Duchenne dystrophy, showing an anterior shift in the right precordial leads and deep but narrow Q waves in leads I, aVL, and V_{4-6}. (From Perloff, J. K.: Cardiac rhythm and conduction in Duchenne's muscular dystrophy. Reprinted by permission of the American College of Cardiology. J. Am. Coll. Cardiol. 3:1263, 1984.) *B,* Twelve-lead scalar electrocardiogram in an obligate female carrier of the Duchenne muscular dystrophy gene. The tracing is similar, if not identical, to the typical scalar electrocardiogram in boys who overtly express Duchenne muscular dystrophy. The tall right precordial R waves and deep but narrow Q waves in leads I, aVL, and V_5 reflect posterolateral left ventricular extension of myocardial dystrophy in the female carrier. (From Perloff, J. K.: Cardiac manifestations of neuromuscular disease. *In* Abelmann, W. H. [ed.]: Cardiomyopathies, Myocarditis, and Pericardial Disease. *In* Braunwald, E. (series ed.): Atlas of Heart Diseases. Vol. 2. Philadelphia, Current Medicine, 1995, pp. 6.1–6.19.)

sion rather than by ventricular dilatation.[1] The murmur of mitral regurgitation has a relatively firm anatomical basis related to dystrophic involvement of the posterior papillary muscle and contiguous posterobasal left ventricular wall.[34,35]

CK quantification is a useful but limited means of identifying female carriers and families with Duchenne dystrophy.[36,37] Female carriers sometimes manifest occult or overt muscle weakness and mild calf pseudohypertrophy[37] in addition to electrocardiographic evidence of cardiac involvement.[36–40] Electrocardiograms in female carriers differ significantly from those of normal adult women, with larger R/S ratios in leads V_{1-2} in the carrier group.[37,41] Cardiac involvement in female carriers is occasionally expressed overtly as dilated cardiomyopathy.[38,40,41]

The standard scalar *electrocardiogram* is the simplest and most reliable tool for detecting cardiac involvement in Duchenne dystrophy.[1,34,42,43] Abnormal electrocardiograms are present in early childhood.[43,44] Tall right precordial R waves and increased R/S amplitude ratios together with deep Q waves in leads 1, aVL, and $V_{5,6}$ are characteristic of the classic, rapidly progressive pseudohypertrophic X-linked dystrophy of Duchenne (Fig. 60–2).[34,45–47] A reduction or loss of electromotive force caused by myocardial dystrophy in the posterobasal left ventricular wall (anterior shift of the QRS) and contiguous lateral wall (deep Q waves in leads 1, aVL and $V_{5,6}$) is believed to be responsible for the characteristic electrocardiogram.[1,34,45] At necropsy, these regions are the initial and most extensive sites of myocardial dystrophy (Fig. 60–3),[34,45,46] which is preceded by ultrastructural (subcellular) abnormalities.[40]

Electron microscopic examination of right ventricular endomyocardial biopsy specimens has identified abnormalities of mitochondria, C bands, sarcoplasmic reticulum, and nuclei.[48] The initial posterobasal involvement spreads to the epicardial third of the contiguous lateral left ventricular free wall, with transmural progression and fibrous replacement.[45,49] There is relative sparing of the ventricular septum and comparatively little involvement of right ventricular and atrial myocardium.[34,45,49] Duchenne dystrophy is an unusual form of heart disease characterized by a predilection for specific regions of the myocardium: the posterobasal and posterolateral left ventricular walls.[1,34,45,47,50] Relevant to this discussion are the scalar electrocardiographic abnormalities in the dystrophic hamster[51] and particularly in the canine model of Duchenne dystrophy.[52] Dystrophic dogs have deep Q waves and tall right precordial R waves that develop in animals older than 6 months, corresponding to hyperechoic regions in the posterobasal left ventricular wall in two-dimensional echocardiograms.[52]

ANATOMICAL CHANGES. The following hypothesis has been proposed to explain the posterobasal localization of myocardial involvement in Duchenne muscular dystrophy.[50] Cardiac myocytes are mononuclear and branched, whereas skeletal myocytes are multinuclear and linear. Skeletal muscle generates force exclusively along its major axis because of its linear configuration. Cardiac muscle generates force radially because of its branched configuration, although the vector of force is principally along its major axis. The force generated by cardiac myocytes is also distributed around the cell, owing to its rich sarcolemmal connections to fibroblasts and collagen. Because the forces acting upon skeletal myocytes are directed almost entirely axially, whereas the forces acting upon cardiac myocytes are more broadly distributed, strain upon the sarcolemma is more uniformly directed in skeletal muscle than in cardiac muscle.

In the anterior wall of the left ventricle, the muscle bundles are "mesh-like," whereas in the posterior wall, the bundles run in a parallel manner, especially in the epicardial half of the posterior wall, which is the site of orgin of myocardial involvement in Duchenne muscular dystrophy. Longitudinal shortening in the posterior wall is far greater during ventricular systole than in the anterior wall. If the role of dystrophin is to reinforce the sarcolemma against axial force, then absence of dystrophin (as in Duchenne muscular dystrophy), would cause a loss in structural integrity of those myocytes with the highest degree of axial forces. It is therefore postulated that the

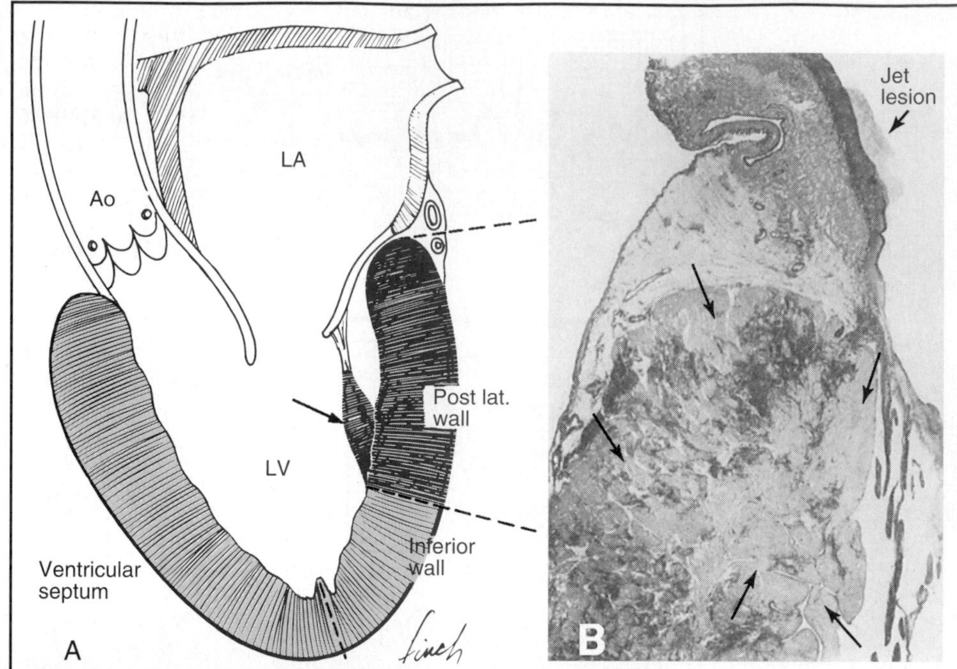

FIGURE 60–3. *A,* Schematic illustration showing the typical posterobasal myocardial involvement with lateral extension in classic Duchenne muscular dystrophy. The posterolateral papillary muscle is involved (arrow). LA = left atrium; LV = left ventricle; Ao = aorta. *B,* Necropsy section showing posterobasal involvement (arrows) of the left ventricle (LV) in a boy with classic Duchenne muscular dystrophy. The posterolateral papillary muscle was involved resulting in mitral regurgitation and the jet lesion shown in the upper right.

posterior left ventricular wall is the initial site of cardiac involvement in Duchenne muscular dystrophy.[50]

POSITRON EMISSION TOMOGRAPHY. Accelerated use of exogenous glucose (^{18}Fluorodeoxyglucose) in the posterobasal and contiguous lateral left ventricular walls (Fig. 60–4) provide evidence of a regional myocardial metabolic abnormality in Duchenne dystrophy.[2,53] $^{13}NH_3$ activity is reduced in wall segments in which uptake of exogenous glucose is accelerated (Fig. 60–4). These wall segments correspond to the sites of primary initial dystrophic involvement found at necropsy as described above.[34,45,46]

THALLIUM SCINTIGRAPHY. Regional perfusion defects demonstrated by thallium scintigraphy and thallium-201 myocardial SPECT are sometimes detected in older patients with Duchenne dystrophy.[2,54,55] Necropsy studies (light microscopy) have not identified luminal narrowing of extramural or intramural coronary arteries in these involved segments, despite the existence of a small vessel coronary arteriopathy.[34] Although reduction or loss of posterobasal/posterolateral left ventricular electrical forces is believed to be the cause of the distinctive electrocardiogram in Duchenne dystrophy,[1,34,45] this loss of forces does not require transmural replacement of myocardium by connective tissue. Increased ^{18}Fluorodeoxyglucose concentrations in these regions together with normal regional wall motion imply the presence of abnormal but viable (metabolically active) contracting myofibers or the preservation of a sufficient population of normal myofibers.[2]

Investigations of cardiac involvement in classic progressive X-linked Duchenne muscular dystrophy have focused chiefly upon gross morphological, histological, ultrastructural, and regional metabolic abnormalities of ventricular myocardium. Disorders of impulse formation and conduction arising or potentially arising from specialized cardiac tissue have received less attention, and there is only scant morphological information on the cardiac impulse and conduction system.[45,56–58] The following remarks focus upon the electrophysiological expressions related to impulse formation and conduction in Duchenne dystrophy.

ELECTROPHYSIOLOGICAL FINDINGS. At least two fundamental variables are relevant to cardiac electrophysiological involvement in Duchenne dystrophy, namely, the small vessel coronary arteriopathy, and abnormalities believed to originate in specialized cardiac tissues. There is a small vessel coronary arteriopathy characterized principally by striking hypertrophy of media with luminal narrowing (Fig. 60–5), less commonly by coexisting cystic degeneration and mucopolysaccharide material in the vessel wall, including small arteries that supply the sinus node and atrioventricular nodes.[34] Dystrophin content of vascular smooth muscle cells has been found to be similar to that of striated myofibers.[10]

An unanswered question is why the dystrophin deficiency in vascular smooth muscle expresses itself chiefly as hypertrophy rather than necrosis. It may be relevant that the earliest clinical expression (phenotype) of human Duchenne muscular dystrophy in skeletal muscle is enlargement of the calves, generally termed "pseudohypertrophy," because the enlargement results from extensive infiltration if not replacement with connective tissues and fat. However, before 2 years of age, connective tissue and fat are often minimal in enlarged calves that almost certainly exhibit true hypertrophy rather than pseudohypertrophy.[11] Rarely, regional muscle enlargement (hypertrophy/pseudohypertrophy) in Duchenne dystrophy can be striking in muscle groups other than the calves. Interestingly, in the cat model of Duchenne dystrophy, hypertrophy is especially striking in skeletal muscle in animals that exhibit dramatic elevations of serum CK but little evidence of overt muscle necrosis.[59] Whether vascular smooth muscle shares in the hypertrophy of the cat model is not clear. Relevant to our concerns is whether a relationship exists between the coronary arteriopathy (medial smooth muscle hypertrophy) and certain electrophysiologic disorders.

A second concern fundamental to an understanding of cardiac electrophysiological involvement in Duchenne muscular dystrophy centers upon the *specialized cardiac tissues.*[56] Specialized cardiac tissues and cardiac muscle have close embryologic origins, although the specialized tissues are believed to be so designated ab origine in the embryonic heart.[60] If there is an embryologic kinship between cardiac muscle and specialized cardiac tissue, does the plasma membrane of the latter normally contain dystrophin as does the cell membrane of cardiac muscle? Immunocytochemical staining has identified dystrophin localized to the membrane surface of normal human cardiac Purkinje fibers.[61,62] Little or no light has been shed upon this question, but if cell membranes of normal cardiac specialized tissues contain dystrophin, it is reasonable to hypothesize that in Duchenne dystrophy, cell membranes of specialized tissues may be dystrophin deficient.[56,61] Should that be the case, how might dystrophin deficiency affect specialized tissue viability, and how might that interplay manifest itself as overt electrophysiological disturbances? The presence of well-defined plasma cell membranes in neurogenic and myogenic specialized cardiac tissues provide a morphologic basis that lends credence to a dystrophin-deficiency hypothesis for certain electrophysiological disorders in Duchenne dystrophy.

CARDIAC ARRHYTHMIAS

The electrophysiological abnormalities that have been documented in human Duchenne dystrophy are expressed as disturbances in rhythm and conduction.[56–58,63] The most common rhythm disturbance is inappropriate sinus tachycardia (rate acceleration without discernible cause).[64] Two types of sinus tachycardia occur: (1) persistent sinus acceleration (minimal heart rate during a 24-hour period of not less than 100 beats/min in patients older than 12 years of age or not less than 110 beats/min in younger patients) and (2) labile sinus tachycardia during waking hours or sleep, so designated because a labile rate acceleration without change in P-wave morphology is unprovoked by a definable circumstantial cause. Episodes of labile sinus tachycardia are either gradual in onset (brief warm-up) or abrupt (within one beat). The mechanism(s) of sinus tachycardia, persistent or labile, gradual or abrupt, have not been established, but may reflect an increase in sympathetic activity and/or a decrease in parasympathetic activity.[56] Studies of the autonomic nervous system, although less than ideal, thus far have not provided convincing evidence of autonomic dysfunction, and observations of sleep hypoxemia have shed little or no light on the sinus tachycardia.[56]

Heart rate variability in the time and frequency domain[64] may yield further information. Mild-to-marked sinus arrhythmia (not necessarily sleep related) is common in Duchenne dystrophy.[63] Morphological observations also leave the above disturbances in sinus rhythm unresolved. The nutrient artery to the sinus node has been described in a limited number of patients as thick-walled (medial hypertrophy with small lumen), less commonly as having cystic medial degeneration and endothelial proliferation.[34] Histological observations on the sinus

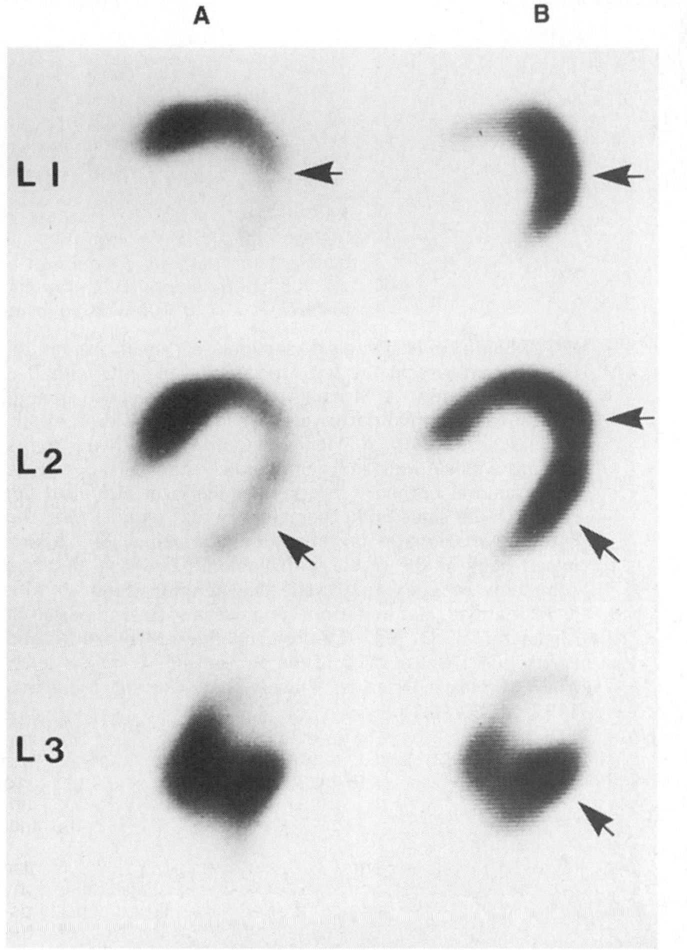

FIGURE 60–4. Regional myocardial uptake of $^{13}NH_3$ (A) and ^{18}F fluorodeoxyglucose (B) visualized in three contiguous positron CT images (L1, L2, L3) of left ventricular myocardium in a 24-year-old man with classic Duchenne dystrophy. There is a segmental decrease in $^{13}NH_3$ activity in the posterolateral wall (arrows) with a discordant increase in ^{18}F fluorodeoxyglucose concentration in the same region (arrows). This patient had a moderate posterolateral thallium-201 defect, posterolateral akinesis on technetium-99m radionuclide imaging, and a left ventricular ejection fraction of 46 per cent. (Reproduced by permission from Perloff, J. K., et al.: Alterations in regional myocardial metabolism, perfusion, and wall motion in Duchenne muscular dystrophy studied by radionuclide imaging. Circulation *69*:33, 1984. Copyright 1984 The American Heart Association.)

node have disclosed occasional mild fibrosis.[58] In a limited study, sinus node myofibers varied in size and showed vacuolization, fatty encroachment, and nuclear pyknosis, with focal areas of fibrosis in the presence of a normal sinus node artery.[57] It is unclear whether the morphological changes in the sinus node cause an increase in intercellular resistance, reduce electrotonic effects, and accelerate pacemaker activity, producing sinus tachycardia.

The most important disturbance in atrial rhythm is flutter, a rare tachyarrhythmia in children, but a relatively common preterminal tachyarrhythmia in Duchenne muscular dystrophy.[34,63,65] In addition, atrial premature beats, intermittent atrial ectopic rhythms, intermittent junctional rhythm, and sustained supraventricular tachycardia have been observed.[51,56] Recall the focal areas of fibrosis at the cellular level and a loss of thick and thin myofilaments at the subcellular level together with P terminal force evidence of prolonged intra-atrial conduction.[57,63] Focal areas of fibrosis are associated with increased intracellular resistance and slowed conduction, which facilitate reentrant arrhythmias.[66–68] Slowed intra-atrial conduction is the electrophysiologic substrate associated with atrial fibrillation and atrial flutter.[68,69]

The incidence of ventricular electrical instability appears to be increased in Duchenne dystrophy, especially in older patients with depressed left ventricular function.[63,70–72] Ventricular ectopic rhythms include premature ventricular complexes (uniform or multiform), couplets, and nonsustained ventricular tachycardia. The clinical substrate for an increased incidence of ventricular ectopic rhythms appears to be duration of disease and depressed left ventricular function.[70–72] But what are the morphological and electrophysiological substrates of ventricular ectopic rhythms? There is little evidence that the metabolically abnormal but viable posterobasal left ventricular myocardium in young patients (Fig. 60–3) is electrically unstable even though the zone generates decreased electromotive force. In the late stages of the disease, these regional zones of abnormal but viable myocardium are replaced with connective tissue containing islands of muscle cells. The left ventricle and ventricular septum then have focal areas with variability of myofibrillar size, some atrophic fibers surrounded by fibrosis and islands of fat, some adjacent fibers that are normal and others hypertrophic. In addition, degenerative changes have been reported in the peripheral conduction tissue fibers (Purkinje).[58] Do areas of regional or focal myocardial scarring result in slow conduction that provides the electrophysiological substrate for reentrant ventricular tachycardia as has been shown to be the case with ventricular tachycardia originating from myocardial infarction scars? Late potentials recorded on signal-averaged electrocardiograms in older patients with Duchenne muscular dystrophy have been found to be associated with left ventricular wall-motion abnormalities and left ventricular dysfunction. The significance of these late potentials in Duchenne dystrophy is not clear; a correlation with ventricular tachcyardia or sudden death has not been established.[71]

Procainamide and phenytoin may reinforce muscle weakness, and intravenous verapamil has resulted in fatal respiratory arrest.[65,73] Malignant hyperthermia and cardiac arrest have occurred during anesthesia in a number of children with Duchenne muscular dystrophy after the use of halothane, suxamethonium, isoflurane, and succinylcholine.[74,75]

Now let us turn to *abnormalities of conduction*. The terminal force of the P wave, especially in lead V_1, may be abnormal or less commonly, the P wave in lead 2 may be broad and notched, implying prolongation of interatrial or left-atrial conduction. Focal areas of fibrosis at the cellular level, and minimal loss of thick and thin myofilaments at the subcellular level occur in the left atrium and have been proposed as explanations for prolonged left-atrial conduction and abnormal P waves.[57,63]

Early reports of atrioventricular conduction in Duchenne dystrophy commented upon an increase in the P-R interval,[1] an observation that has been confirmed in the relatively late stage of the disease.[2] More systematic observations have disclosed a prevalence of short P-R intervals indicating accelerated AV conduction.[2,45,57] As in the case of the sinus node, the short P-R interval in Duchenne dystrophy may reflect accelerated conduction from intrinsic properties within the AV node.

Intranodal conduction defects take the form of minor right ventricular conduction delay, left posterior fascicular block, left anterior fascicular block, right bundle branch block, and exceptionally bifascicular block.[2,57] Histopathological studies of the atrioventricular bundle have disclosed abnormalities that varied from mild fibrosis and fatty infiltration to focal areas of fibrosis and vascular degeneration involving the penetrating portion and branching portion of AV node.[57,58]

Becker Muscular Dystrophy

Becker muscular dystrophy is considered a milder allelic variant of Duchenne muscular dystrophy, but the clinical expression—both the phenotype and the presence and degree of cardiac involvement—are much more variable.[76–79] Becker dystrophy and Duchenne muscular dystrophy are

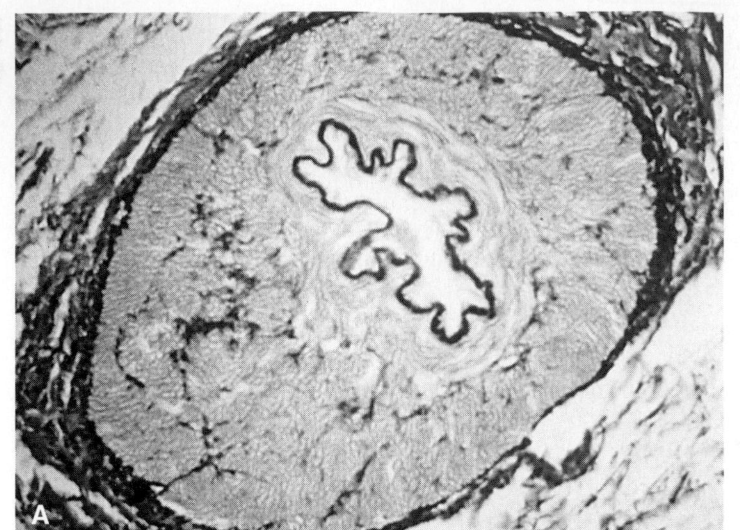

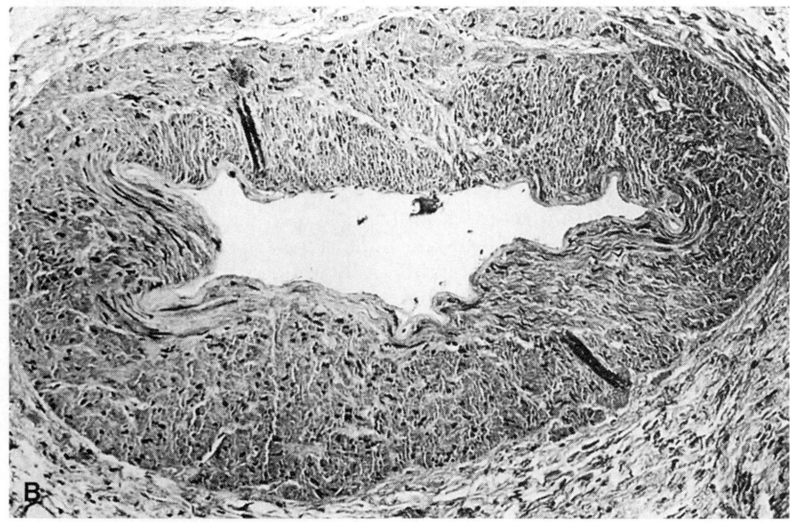

FIGURE 60–5. Histological sections of small intramural coronary arteries in the left atria of two patients with Duchenne dystrophy. *A,* Striking hypertrophy of medial smooth muscle with luminal narrowing (Verhoeff-von-Gieson elastic tissue stains, ×260). *B,* Medial smooth muscle hypertrophy causing a thick wall and a moderately narrowed lumen in an intramural coronary artery from the right atrium in the region of the sinus node (hematoxylin and eosin, ×25). The coronary arteriopathy is characterized principally by striking hypertrophy of the media with luminal narrowing, and less commonly by coexisting cystic degeneration (From Perloff, J. K.: Cardiac manifestations of neuromuscular disease. *In* Abelmann, W. H. [ed.]: Cardiomyopathies, Myocarditis, and Pericardial Disease. Vol. 2. *In* Braunwald, E. (series ed.): Atlas of Heart Diseases. Philadelphia, Current Medicine, 1995, pp. 6.1–6.19.)

both believed to be caused by mutations of the Duchenne muscular dystrophy gene.[24,80] Mutations have different effects on dystrophin expression and clinical severity, reflecting a number of functional roles for the dystrophin domains.[79] The Becker dystrophy gene is expressed in both skeletal muscle and cardiac muscle.[24,76,78,81] Becker dystrophy can be distinguished from Duchenne dystrophy by immunohistochemical dystrophin assays of skeletal muscle biopsies.[79,80] In Becker dystrophy, dystrophin is present in skeletal muscle but is abnormal in molecular weight, whereas in Duchenne dystrophy, the protein product is absent or scanty but is of normal molecular weight.[10,22] The dystrophin abnormality has been identified with immunostaining of endomyocardial biopsies in patients with Becker muscular dystrophy.[82]

Becker dystrophy is later in onset and slower in progression than Duchenne dystrophy. Most patients remain ambulant into adulthood[6,83] (Fig. 60–6), but Becker dystrophy exhibits a considerable variation in clinical expression, both in skeletal and cardiac muscle.[76–78] Cardiac involvement may occur at an early age and is unrelated to the extent of the musculoskeletal disorder.[78,84,85] Appreciable cardiac involvement can occur in patients without significant muscular disability,[79,86–88] while other patients with progressive muscular atrophy and weakness have comparatively little cardiac involvement, at least overtly.[77,79] X-linked dilated cardiomyopathy without clinical signs of skeletal myopathy is believed to be due, at least in part, to the Becker gene on the short arm of the X chromosome.[89,90] Severe familial dilated cardiomyopathy occurs in the context of Becker progressive muscular dystrophy.[91]

Because the diagnosis of Becker dystrophy was not secure before the advent of current molecular diagnostic techniques, reports on the incidence and type of associated heart disease have been open to question. The severity of cardiac involvement is not related to age,[84] but patients who reach adulthood generally have cardiomyopathy and may succumb to it.[86,88,91] Involvement of both ventricles culminates in dilatation and failure (Fig. 60–7*A*,*B*).[86–88] Abnormalities of the His bundle and of infranodal conduction express themselves as fascicular block, right bundle branch block, left bundle branch block, and complete heart block[86–88] (Fig. 60–5*C*). Defective dystrophin expression in specialized cardiac tissues may be responsible for these conduction defects in Becker dystrophy, as hypothesized for Duchenne dystrophy.[56,61] Serious ventricular arrhythmias have been documented in patients with Becker dystrophy and are believed to play a role in sudden death.

LIMB–GIRDLE DYSTROPHY OF ERB

Neuromuscular disorders designated "limb-girdle dystrophy" represent a poorly defined group within the major muscular dystrophies. The term *limb-girdle syndromes* has sometimes been applied.[6,92] There is variation in mode of inheritance, age of onset, progression of illness, and distribution of muscle weakness. Two forms of autosomal dominant limb-girdle muscular dystrophy have been proposed. One variety, Bethlem myopathy,[93] is well documented but rare and thus far has been devoid of cardiac involvement.[78] The other variety is relatively heterogeneous with late onset and slow progression.[94] The pelvic girdle is chiefly affected, the upper limbs and shoulder girdle less so, and the face is spared. Because of disproportionate pelvic involvement, patients are often confined to a wheelchair.[6] Limb-girdle dystrophy with calf pseudohypertrophy can now be distinguished from Becker dystrophy by dystrophin and molecular genetic analysis.[95,96]

The type and prevalence of heart disease are uncertain because the diagnosis of limb-girdle dystrophy has been poorly defined. If cardiac

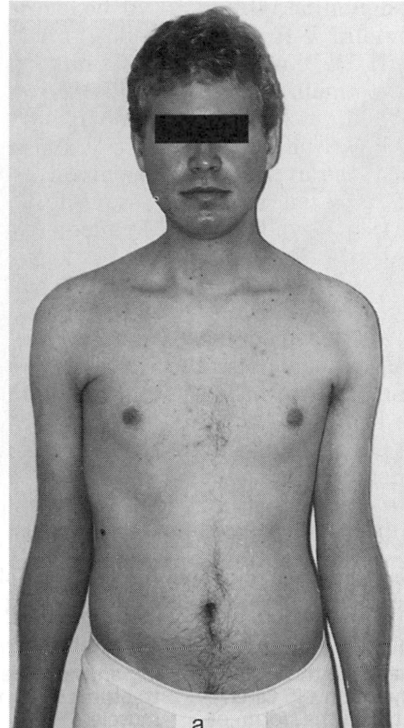

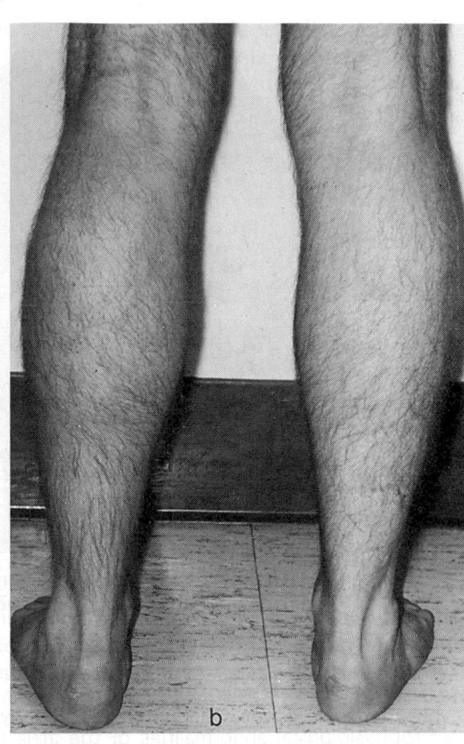

FIGURE 60–6. A 22-year-old man with late onset, slowly progressive Becker muscular dystrophy. *A,* There is dystrophy of the shoulder girdle, arms, and pelvic girdle (latter not shown). *B,* Asymmetric calf pseudohypertrophy, greater on the left than on the right. Dystrophy of proximal leg muscles is not shown.

involvement occurs, it is generally occult (asymptomatic).[96] Disorders of cardiac conduction have been reported, especially intraventricular conduction defects and fascicular block.[96,97] A unique case of limb-girdle dystrophy with dilated cardiomyopathy has been described.[98]

FACIOSCAPULOHUMERAL DYSTROPHY OF LANDOUZY-DEJERINE

Facioscapulohumeral dystrophy is inherited as an autosomal dominant with strong penetrance and an incidence estimated at one in 20,000.[99] The genetic locus has been mapped to the long arm of chromosome 4 in the region of 4q35.[100,101] The disease typically becomes overt at the end of the first decade or the beginning of the second decade. Facial weakness may be signaled by no more than an inability to whistle or drink through a straw. More distinctive and troublesome is the inability to close the eyes, even during sleep. The face ultimately becomes smooth and the forehead unlined; loss of the normal upward curvature of the lower lip creates a pouting appearance, and the only marks on an otherwise expressionless face are the dimples on either side of the angles of the mouth, creating an enigmatic smile (Fig. 60–8*A*). Concurrently, the muscles of the arms and shoulders (scapulohumeral) are involved, and winging of the scapulae become apparent (Fig. 60–8*B*). Infrequently, the disease expresses itself in infancy and runs a rapid course with death in adolescence.[102] Asymptomatic or minimally affected parents may have severely affected offspring with the infantile form of the disease.[102]

Cardiac Findings. The type of cardiac abnormality previously ascribed to the adult form of facioscapulohumeral dystrophy was a unique variety of heart disease: permanent atrial paralysis. However,

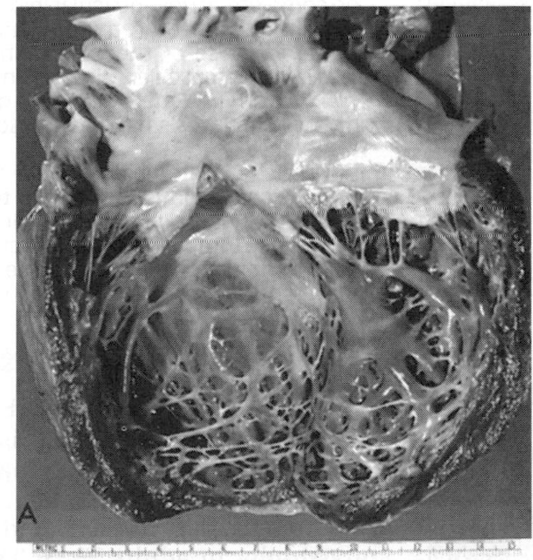

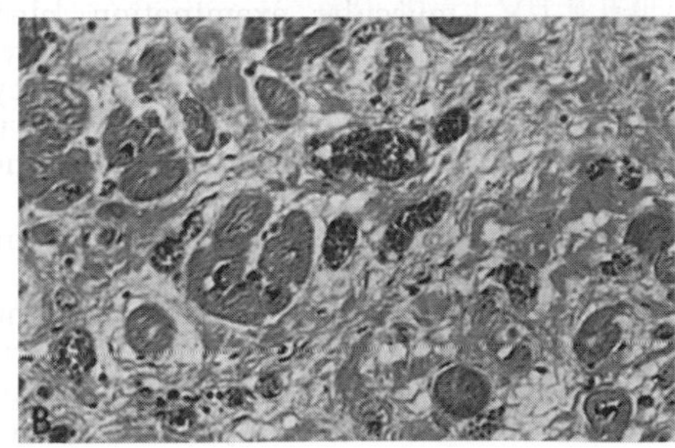

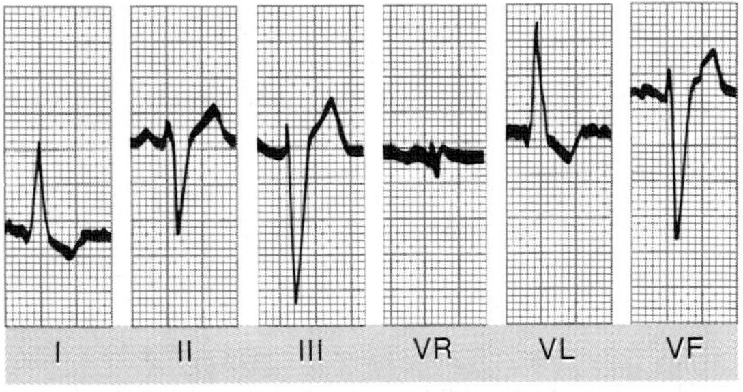

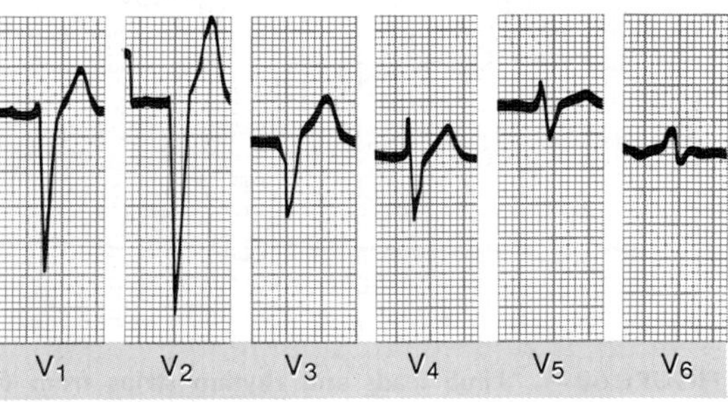

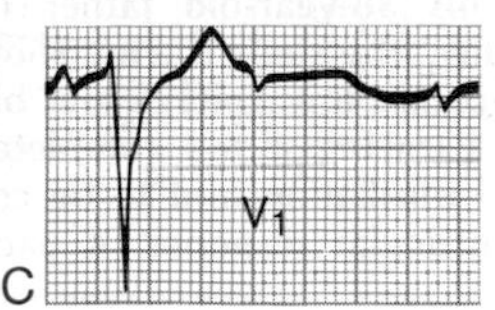

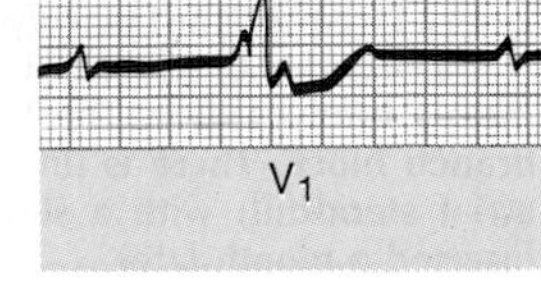

FIGURE 60–7. Gross and microscopic cardiac pathological specimens and the electrocardiogram from a 45-year-old man with late-onset, slowly progressive Becker muscular dystrophy. *A,* Dilated, flabby left ventricle with focal endocardial thickening. *B,* Microscopic section from the left ventricle shows marked confluent scarring with variations in fiber size; there was no significant coronary artery disease. *C,* Electrocardiogram recorded at age 40 years. The 12-lead tracing shows left-axis deviation, a QRS of 0.14 sec, small Q waves in leads I and aVL and loss of R waves in leads V_2 and V_3. The lower tracings, taken 4 years later (a year before death), show complete heart block with a variable QRS configuration. (Reproduced by permission from Perloff, J. K., et al.: The cardiomyopathy of progressive muscular dystrophy. Circulation *33*:625, 1966. Copyright 1966 The American Heart Association.)

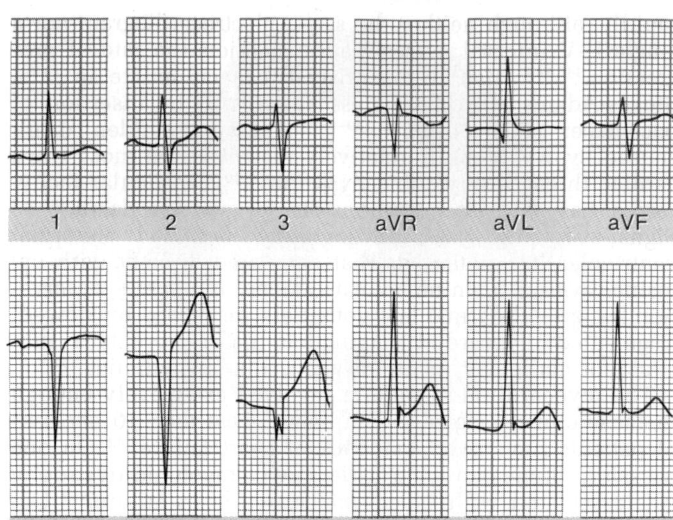

FIGURE 60–11. Electrocardiogram from a 38-year-old man with myotonic muscular dystrophy. Prominent QS deformities are present in leads V1-3. The P–R interval is 0.21 sec, and the frontal plane QRS axis is horizontal. (From Perloff, J. K., et al.: Cardiac involvement in myotonic muscular dystrophy [Steinert's disease]: A prospective study of 25 patients. Am. J. Cardiol. *54:*1074, 1984.)

fected children have characteristic facies with the upper lip forming a cupid's bow. Studies on cardiac involvement in these children are limited, but have reportedly disclosed atrioventricular and intraventricular conduction defects, less commonly reduced left ventricular systolic function.[159,160] Apart from genetic transmission from the mother (cytoplasmic inheritance), pregnancy is hazardous to the gravida with myotonic dystrophy.[130,153]

MYOTONIA CONGENITA (THOMSEN'S DISEASE) AND PARAMYOTONIA CONGENITA. This must be distinguished from myotonic muscular dystrophy.[130,132] Thomsen's disease is characterized by myotonia without dystrophy and by skeletal muscles that are well developed, even hypertrophied.[6,130] Because the natural history of Thomsen's disease is benign, longevity permits conclusions regarding cardiac involvement, which is conspicuously absent, although in a single case, cardiac conduction abnormalities similar to those found in myotonic dystrophy were reported.[161] Paramyotonia congenita is an uncommon to rare autosomal dominant disorder characterized by a prolonged myotonic reaction to cold.[6,132,162,163] Dystrophy of skeletal muscle is absent, and cardiac involvement is unknown.

Friedreich's Ataxia

The hereditary ataxias are divided into (1) the spinocerebellar ataxia of Friedreich, (2) ataxia with muscular atrophy (Roussy-Lévy syndrome), (3) spinocerebellar ataxia, and (4) olivopontocerebellar atrophy.[164] Despite a century of lively interest, Friedreich's ataxia has resisted precise clinical and biochemical definition, and there is still disagreement on where this spinocerebellar degenerative disease fits into the complex framework of the hereditary ataxias.[164–166] It is important to underscore that the disorder is essentially neurological rather than myopathic.[164–166] Friedreich's ataxia is inherited as an autosomal recessive trait and is characterized by ataxia of the limbs and trunk, absence of tendon reflexes, extensor plantar responses, and loss of proprioceptive sensations in the limbs.[166] There are no remissions; instead, ataxia of gait and weakness of muscle progress relentlessly, affecting first the lower limbs and then all four extremities. Pes cavus (Friedreich's foot) (Fig. 60–12) and kyphoscoliosis develop within a few years of onset.

CARDIAC MANIFESTATIONS. When strict neurological and genetic criteria were used to identify a clinically homogeneous group of patients with Friedreich's ataxia, the incidence of cardiac involvement exceeded 90 per cent.[4,167–173] Severe ataxia occurs long before overt heart disease, and there is no relationship between the degrees of neurological and cardiac involvement.[4] Nevertheless, cardiac disease is often the cause of death.[4,174] There is reason to believe that phenotypically identical Friedreich patients are not genetically homogeneous, so the cardiac expressions might be expected to vary. This proved to be the case in a prospective study of 75 patients.[4] Cardiac involvement, usually occult and asymptomatic, is the rule.[174,175] Scalar electrocardiography and echocardiography detected one or more abnormalities in 95 per cent of study patients.[4]

HYPERTROPHIC CARDIOMYOPATHY. The most common echocardiographic finding is concentric (symmetrical) left ventricular hypertrophy (Fig. 60–13). Asymmetric septal thickening occurs, but less frequently.[169,171,176–178] Left ventricular outflow gradients are present in some cases with disproportionate septal thickness[171] but not in others.[169] Importantly, septal cellular disarray—the histological hallmark of genetic hypertrophic cardiomyopathy (see p. 1664)—has been absent or only focal in necropsy studies of Friedreich's ataxia.[167,170,179,180] The potentially malignant ventricular arrhythmias common in genetic hypertrophic cardiomyopathy are essentially unknown in Friedreich's ataxia.[181] In the hypertrophic cardiomyopathy of Friedreich's ataxia, systolic ventricular function is normal, not supernormal, and diastolic function is not depressed as in genetic hypertrophic cardiomyopathy.[182,183]

DILATED CARDIOMYOPATHY. A second and much less common form of cardiac involvement in Friedreich's ataxia is dilated cardiomyopathy, which may initially express itself as global hypokinesis with normal left ventricular internal dimensions (Fig. 60–14)[4,178] There is one report of dilated cardiomyopathy, chiefly involving the right ventricle, with ventricular tachyarrhythmias.[184] In contrast to the favorable prognosis of Friedreich's ataxia with hypertrophic cardiomyopathy, the outlook is poor in dilated cardiomyopathy patients who experience relentless, progressive cardiac deterioration.[4,178] There is convincing evidence that the dilated form of cardiomyopathy in Friedreich's ataxia is distinct from the hypertrophic form: i.e., not a transition from one to the other, and that it represents a fundamentally different type of cardiac involvement designated dystrophic.[4] This view is supported by the flabby myocardium with normal wall thickness in necropsy cases that exhibited premortem progression on echocardiography from normal to dilated globally hypofunctional left ventricles with normal wall thickness (Fig. 60–14).[4] The initial force deformities on electrocardiograms and vectorcardiograms (Fig. 60–15)[4,172] are believed to represent areas of regional ventricular myocardial dystrophy which, if sufficiently widespread, might result in depressed systolic function.[4] Atrial arrhythmias (flutter, fibrillation) and ventricular arrhythmias are features of the dilated cardiomyopathy of Friedreich's ataxia.[4,184] Disease of the coronary arteries, especially small intramural coronary arteries, has been reported,[180] but a relationship between the coronary arteriopathy and regional wall abnormalities has not been established.

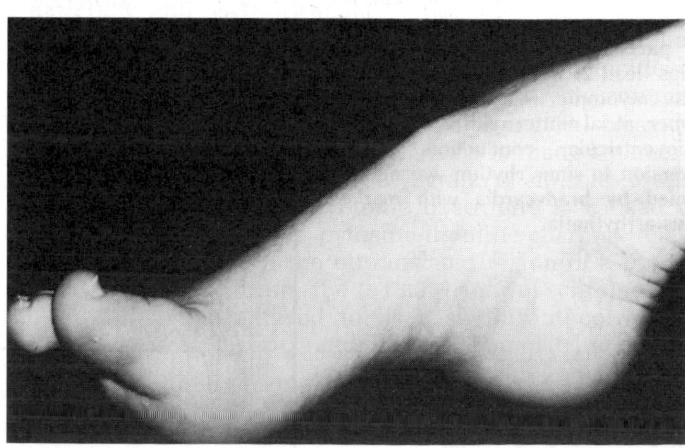

FIGURE 60–12. Pes cavus with hammer toe: Friedreich's foot.

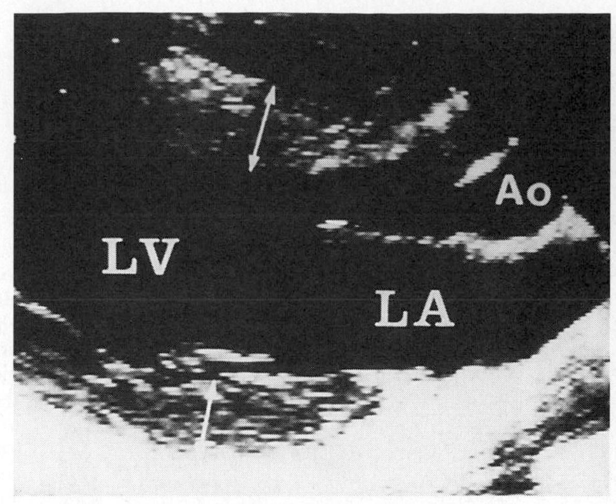

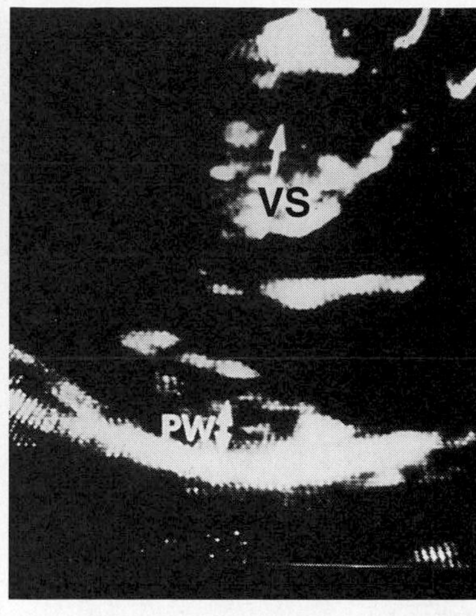

FIGURE 60–13. *A,* Two-dimensional echocardiogram (parasternal long axis diastolic frames) from a 14-year-old girl with Friedreich's ataxia and concentric hypertrophy (arrows) of the left ventricle (LV). *B,* Two-dimensional echocardiogram (parasternal long axis) from a 17-year-old boy with Friedreich's ataxia and hypertrophic cardiomyopathy characterized by disproportionate thickness (arrows) of the ventricular septum (VS) compared with the posterior wall (PW). Ao = aorta; LA = left atrium. (From Perloff, J. K.: Cardiac manifestations of neuromuscular disease. *In* Abelmann, W. H. [ed.]: Cardiomyopathies, Myocarditis, and Pericardial Disease. Vol. 2. *In* Braunwald, E. (series ed.): Atlas of Heart Diseases. Philadelphia, Current Medicine, 1995, pp. 6.1–6.19.)

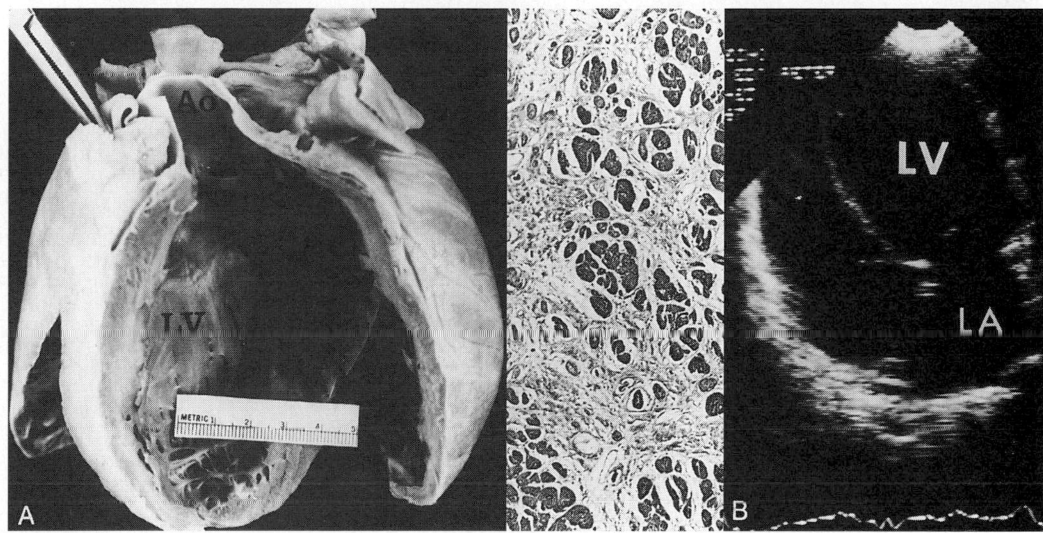

FIGURE 60–14. *A,* Gross and histological specimens from a 17-year-old boy with Friedreich's ataxia whose echocardiogram progressed from normal at age 13 years to a minimally dilated, hypocontractile left ventricle 3 to 4 years later. The gross specimen shows a mildly dilated left ventricle (LV) with normal wall thickness; the walls were flabby. The microscopic section from the left ventricular free wall shows marked connective tissue replacement. Although specifically sought, small-vessel coronary artery disease was not identified. *B,* Two-dimensional echocardiogram (apical window) showing the mildly dilated, thin-walled left ventricle (LV). LA = left atrium. (From Child, J. S., et al.: Cardiac involvement in Friedreich's ataxia. Reprinted by permission of the American College of Cardiology. J. Am. Coll. Cardiol. *7*:1370, 1986.)

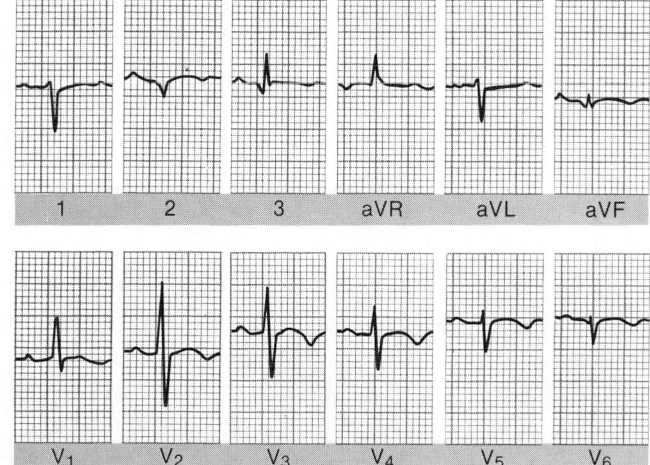

FIGURE 60–15. Electrocardiogram in a 28-year-old man with Friedreich's ataxia. The QRS shows marked right-axis deviation. There are 40-msec Q waves in leads 2, 3, and aVL. A prominent 60-msec R wave appears in lead V1. A vectorcardiogram and echocardiogram showed no evidence of right ventricular hypertrophy. The electrocardiograph pattern reflects loss of inferior and posterior electrical forces without a corresponding regional wall motion abnormality on echocardiography. (From Child, J. S., et al.: Cardiac involvement in Friedreich's ataxia. Reprinted by permission of the American College of Cardiology. J. Am. Coll. Cardiol. *7*:1370, 1986.)

Other Neuromyopathic Diseases Associated with Heart Disease

PERONEAL MUSCULAR ATROPHY (CHARCOT-MARIE-TOOTH SYNDROME). Peroneal muscular atrophy includes several genetic disorders (the hereditary motor and sensory neuromyopathies) characterized by distal weakness of the legs with predilection for muscles innervated by the peroneal nerves, particularly the everters of the foot and occasionally intrinsic muscles of the hands.[185] Peroneal muscular atrophy is autosomal dominant. One type begins during the first 20 years of life, whereas the other type begins later, sometimes not until middle age. Arrhythmias, conduction abnormalities and dilated heart failure have been sporadically reported in patients with peroneal muscular atrophy,[186–190] but are believed to be chance associations.[191]

MYOTUBULAR MYOPATHY (CENTRONUCLEAR MYOPATHY). Centronuclear myopathy typically exhibits internal nuclei that structurally resemble fetal myotubes (rows of nuclei separated by spaces).[192,193] The disorder is characterized clinically by slow but progressive wasting and weakness of skeletal muscle beginning at birth. Ptosis is the rule. Patients are hyporeflexic or areflexic. Few examples are available for study, but presumptive evidence indicates that myotubular myopathy can be associated with extensive myocardial fibrosis, cardiac dilatation, and early death.[192] In an illustration in one report on skeletal muscle in "idiopathic cardiomyopathy," numerous internal nuclei could be seen.[194] Centronuclear myopathy had apparently presented as cardiomyopathy before the neuromuscular disease was identified.

CARDIAC INVOLVEMENT IN MITOCHONDRIAL DISEASES. Mitochondrial diseases are important from a genetic point of view because mitochondria contain their own DNA and are capable of synthesizing a small but vital set of proteins.[195] The vast majority of mitochondrial proteins are encoded by nuclear DNA and have to be imported from the cytoplasm into mitochondria through a complex translocation

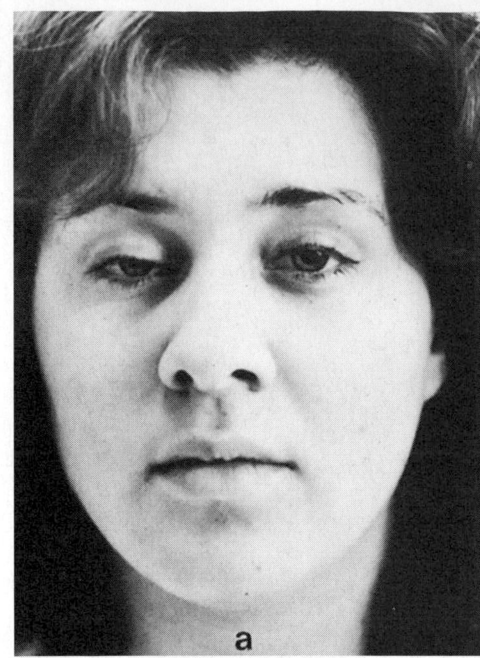

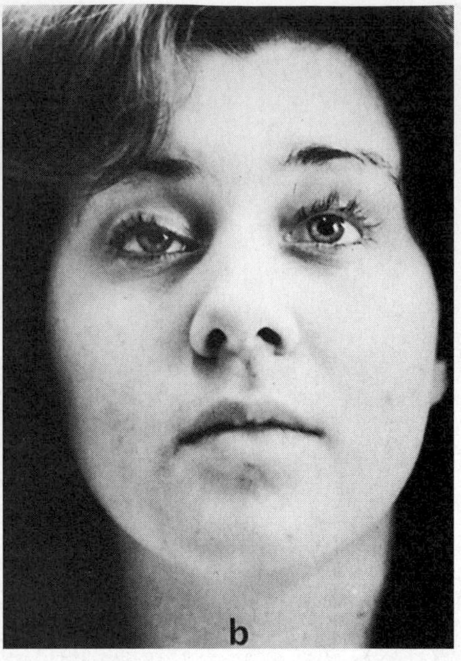

FIGURE 60–16. An 18-year-old girl with Kearns-Sayre syndrome and bilateral asymmetrical ptosis. Within 24 months, her electrocardiogram changed from normal to bifascicular block (complete right bundle branch block, and left anterior fascicular block). *A,* The asymmetrical ptosis when the patient looks straight ahead. *B,* Ptosis of the right lid persists when the patient looks up. She also had typical pigmentary retinopathy.

machinery which is under the control of the nuclear genome.[195] The human mitochondrial genome is a circular double-stranded DNA.[196] Mitochondrial myopathy, defined as a disease caused by mitochondrial DNA mutations, has been proposed, and is believed to represent a state of premature cardiac aging wherein the somatic mutations of mitochondrial DNA are abnormally accelerated because of a patient's germ-aligned mutations.[197] Mutations of mitochondrial DNA are responsible for human mitochondrial diseases that involve many but not all organ systems.[196] Examples include Kearns-Sayre syndrome, ocular myopathy, myoclonic epilepsy with ragged red fibers, and mitochondrial myopathy, encephalopathy, lactic acidosis, and stroke-like episodes.[196]

KEARNS-SAYRE SYNDROME. The most important of these mitochondrial diseases, certainly from the point of view of cardiac involvement, is Kearns-Sayre syndrome, characterized by progressive external ophthalmoplegia (Fig. 60–16), pigmentary retinopathy, and heart block.[198–200] Morphological alterations in skeletal muscle can be identified in the trichrome stain as ragged-red fibers.[198] Cardiac involvement primarily afflicts the specialized conduction pathways.[201,202] Clinically overt myocardial disease is the exception, despite well-documented myocardial ultrastructural abnormalities, especially of mitochondria.[203–205] Occasionally patients exhibit dilated cardiomyopathy with progressive heart failure,[203–205] but the chief risk resides in abnormalities of the specialized conduction pathways.

Two derangements in cardiac conduction coexist: (1) gradually progressive impairment of infranodal conduction (left anterior hemiblock, right bundle branch block, complete heart block) (Fig. 60–17), and (2) concomitant enhancement of AV nodal conduction.[201,206] The morphological basis for impaired infranodal conduction lies in extensive distal His bundle abnormalities that extend to the origins of the bundle branches.[206] Evidence of enhanced AV nodal conduction has been identified by His bundle electrocardiograms (Fig. 60–15).[201] A short or relatively short P-R interval cannot be used as evidence against risk inherent in the trifascicular disease of patients with Kearns-Sayre syndrome, right bundle branch block and left anterior hemiblock.[201] Pacemaker implantation is often necessary.

GUILLAIN-BARRÉ SYNDROME. This disorder is the most common of the acquired demyelinative neuropathies.[207] The incidence gradually increases with age, but the disease may occur at any age, and both sexes are equally affected. The syndrome often appears days to weeks after a viral respiratory or gastrointestinal infection, with neurological symptoms consisting of symmetrical weakness of the limbs often accompanied by paresthesias. The incidence af the acute polyneuropathy is higher in patients with Hodgkin's disease, and the disorder may be precipitated by pregnancy, general surgery, or vaccinations. Myocardial infarction was believed to be the precipitating cause in two cases.[208] Important and characteristic features of the syndrome are flaccid motor paralysis with a distinctive tendency to ascend (Landry's ascending paralysis), together with elevation of cerebrospinal fluid protein without an increase in the number of white blood cells. Involvement of thoracic muscles often requires assisted ventilation. Despite respiratory support, the Guillain-Barré syndrome is fatal in approximately 20 per cent of children when there is significant involvement of trunk muscles and associated pulmonary insufficiency.[209]

Cardiac Findings. Postmortem studies have shed little or no light on the cause of sudden death in Guillain-Barré syndrome. There is substantial evidence, however, that deaths are often not invariably related to cardiac arrhythmias.[209–211] Bradyarrhythmias (sinus arrest, complete heart block) and tachyarrhythmias (supraventricular and ventricular) as well as premature atrial and ventricular beats are common and are increased by the use of a respirator.[210] Autonomic dysfunction, especially sympathetic hyperactivity, is manifested by orthostatic hypotension, transient hypertension, wide fluctuations in blood pressure and heart rate, and variations in the R-R interval.[212–214] Pacemaker support may be required because of recurrent syncope.[210] Tracheal aspiration has produced an idioventricular rhythm of 40 beats/min that reverted to sinus rhythm when aspiration ceased.[209] Cardiac monitoring is advisable, especially when the Guillain-Barré syndrome is sufficiently severe to warrant assisted ven-

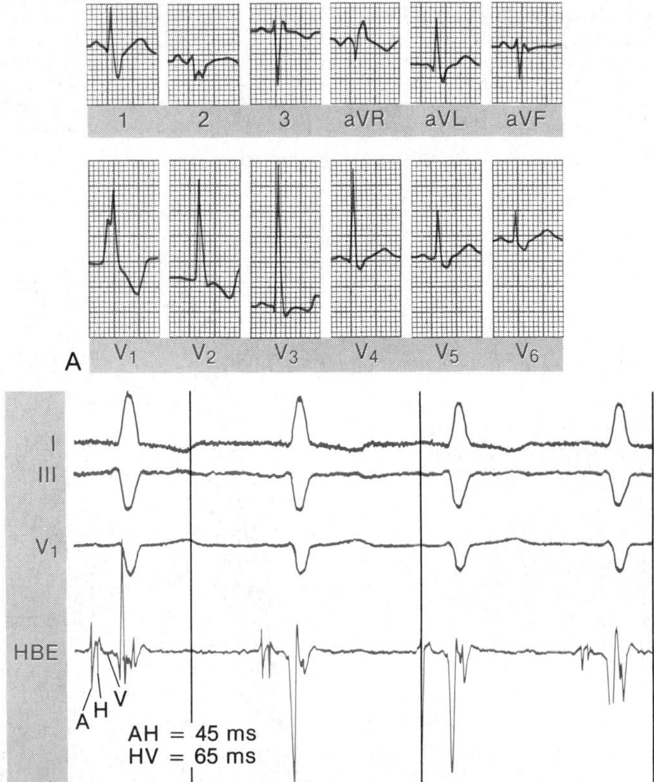

FIGURE 60–17. *A,* Electrocardiogram from a 13-year-old boy with Kearns-Sayre syndrome. There is a short P–R interval (110 msec), left anterior hemiblock, and complete right bundle branch block. *B,* Leads I, III, and V_1 with His bundle electrogram (HBE) in a 21-year-old woman with Kearns-Sayre syndrome. Time lines are at 1-sec intervals. The A-H interval is 45 msec (short) and the H–V interval is 65 msec (prolonged). (From Roberts, J. K., et al.: Cardiac conduction in Kearns-Sayre syndrome. Am. J. Cardiol. *44:*1396, 1979).

tilation.[209] The electrocardiogram occasionally shows widespread, deep T-wave inversions.[214]

NEMALINE MYOPATHY. This disorder is characterized by myriad small, rodlike particles in striated muscle.[215–217] Inheritance is either autosomal dominant or recessive, with occasional sporadic cases. The most common clinical manifestation is hypotonia with diffuse weakness of limbs and trunk beginning at an early age. Children are often dysmorphic with an elongated, narrow face, high arched palate, and slender musculature.[6] Alternatively, symptoms may begin in adolescence or adult life and are characterized by scapuloperoneal weakness and footdrop.[218] Nemaline myopathy is only rarely associated with cardiac involvement, but nemaline rods have been found in the myocardium and in cardiac conduction tissues, and held responsible for ventricular dilatation and conduction defects.[219,220]

MYASTHENIA GRAVIS. This is a "neuroimmunological" disease caused by an abnormality of neuromuscular transmission due to antibodies to acetylcholine receptors.[221,222] The abnormality may become manifest at any age, but is most common in the second to fourth decades. Overt pathological evidence of myasthenia gravis resides primarily in the thymus, which shows lymphoid hyperplasia and numerous lymphoid follicles with germinal centers in the medulla. Ocular muscles are affected first. Weakness characteristically fluctuates during the course of a single day, sometimes within minutes. The association of myocardial disease with thymoma, especially malignant thymoma, is generally accepted, whereas the association of myasthenia gravis with heart disease is less clear despite a considerable body of suggestive evidence.[223] Specific cardiac involvement is unproved even though clinical, electrocardiographic, and vectorcardiographic data implicate the myocardium.[223]

Early in this century, quinine was used as a provocative diagnostic test for myasthenia gravis. Quinidine and procainamide, like quinine, have anticholinergic properties that depress neuromuscular conduction.[224] These antiarrhythmic agents can unmask previously unsuspected myasthenia gravis and can exacerbate symptoms in well-controlled patients.[224,225] Accordingly, quinidine and procainamide should be avoided.

McARDLE SYNDROME. This is a disorder of myophosphorylase deficiency.[6,226] A defect in the enzyme prevents use of glycogen as an energy source during heavy or intensive short-term exercise when glycogen is normally the chief substrate.[6,226] McArdle's disease was the first enzyme defect suspected on clinical grounds. It is inherited as an autosomal recessive, or rarely as an autosomal dominant, and is more common in male children. Mild aching in the legs usually begins before age 10 years, ultimately becomes severe, and is provoked by the mildest exercise. Pain may last for hours, and is accompanied by Burgundy-colored urine because of myoglobinuria. The typical cardiac manifestation is rapid inappropriate acceleration of heart rate (sinus tachycardia) and hyperventilation immediately after the onset of exercise[5,189] (Fig. 60–18). Less commonly, the scalar electrocardiogram reveals sinus bradycardia, increased QRS voltage, and PR interval prolongation. The precise diagnosis depends upon biochemical and histochemical documentation that phosphorylase is absent in skeletal muscle.

KUGELBERG-WELANDER SYNDROME. The proximal spinal muscular atrophies are autosomal recessive.[227] The childhood form is subdivided into the acute Werdnig-Hoffmann, the intermediate Werdnig-Hoffmann, and the Kugelberg-Welander.[227] The latter variety is characterized by onset in childhood or adolescence, atrophy and weakness principally of proximal limb muscles, a slowly progressive course, development of fasciculations, and evidence of neurogenic changes in the electromyogram and on muscle biopsy. There are a few reports of cardiac involvement in the Kugelberg-Welander syndrome including atrial fibrillation, atrial standstill, conduction defects (H-V prolongation, complete AV block), and dilated heart failure.[228]

POLIOMYELITIS. Cardiac involvement is believed to occur only rarely in childhood poliomyelitis, but may be clinically occult.[229,230] In adults, the infrequency of symptomatic involvement of the heart contrasts with a relatively high incidence of electrocardiographic abnormalities, especially of rhythm and conduction.[229,230] Disturbances of rhythm take the form of premature beats (atrial and ventricular), atrial fibrillation or atrial flutter. Disturbances in conduction are manifested by impaired AV conduction (first-, second-, and third-degree heart block) and abnormalities of infranodal conduction (left-axis deviation and bundle branch block).[229,230] Respiratory failure can provoke hypoxemia-induced pulmonary hypertension[231] and multifocal atrial tachycardia.

At necropsy, the sinoatrial node, distal His bundle, and left and right bundle branches show infiltration, degeneration, and fibrous replacement that wholly or in part account for the conduction defects.[229,230] Pathological changes in the myocardium tend to be similar to those in skeletal muscle, including diffuse mononuclear cell infiltration and myofibril degeneration, regeneration, and fibrosis.

PERIODIC PARALYSIS. The disorder is characterized by recurrences of flaccid weakness and by either abnormally high or abnormally low levels of serum potassium.[232,233] *Hypokalemic attacks* typically begin in late childhood or adolescence, usually occur at night, tend to be severe, and last a day or longer.[233] *Hyperkalemic attacks* have their onset at a younger age. Episodes occur more frequently than with hypokalemia, but tend to be milder and shorter (minutes or hours). Many features are common to both varieties of periodic paralysis, including familial recurrence (autosomal dominant inheritance),

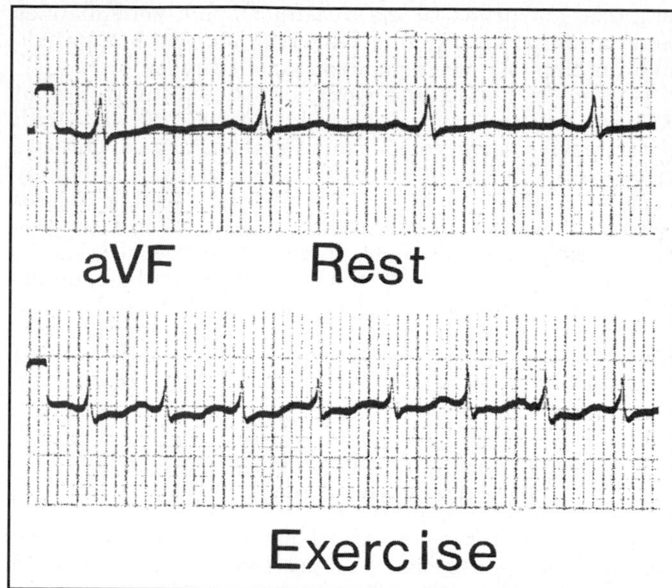

FIGURE 60–18. Rhythm strip (aVF) from a 37-year-old woman with McArdle disease. At the very onset of exercise, there was a sudden sustained acceleration of cardiac rate represented by sinus tachycardia *(lower strip)* accompanied by hyperventilation and aching in the leg muscles.

heightened susceptibility immediately after ceasing strenuous exercise, termination of incipient attacks by *mild* exercise, onset of weakness in the lower extremities with progression to arm muscles but not to respiratory muscles, intensification by cold, and persistent weakness between attacks even though potassium levels may be normal.[232,234] During hyperkalemia, the electrocardiogram exhibits peaked T waves. During hypokalemia, the T waves are low voltage, and there is digitalis sensitivity.

More important are the cardiac arrhythmias that accompany periodic paralysis including ventricular ectopic beats, ventricular bigeminy, and fusion beats producing multiform complexes.[233–235] Of particular interest is bidirectional tachycardia that is believed to originate in the left ventricle, is refractory to antiarrhythmic therapy, occurs independent of attacks of muscle weakness, exhibits no correlation with serum electrolytes, and is consistently converted to sinus rhythm with mild exercise.[236,237] Hypokalemic episodes are best treated with oral potassium and hyperkalemic episodes with glucose and insulin, but it should be underscored that administration of potassium does not necessarily suppress ventricular electrical instability during hypokalemic attacks.[235]

ALCOHOLIC CARDIOMYOPATHY (see also p. 1412). Dilated cardiomyopathy associated with chronic ingestion of large amounts of ethyl alcohol may be accompanied by clinically occult skeletal myopathy.[238,239] Alcohol withdrawal is occasionally accompanied by "rum fits."[240] The teratogenic potential of alcohol, exemplified by the fetal alcohol syndrome, afflicts the fetal central nervous system but not the myocardium, although congenital malformations of the heart are not uncommon in the offspring of alcoholic mothers.[241]

ACUTE CEREBRAL DISORDERS CAUSED BY CARDIOVASCULAR ABNORMALITIES

Acute cerebral injury can provoke cardiovascular abnormalities, and abnormalities of the heart can set the stage for acute cerebral injury. A connection between certain acute cerebral events—subarachnoid hemorrhage, intracranial hemorrhage—and overt cardiovascular abnormalities has been recognized for nearly a century, and a relationship between head trauma and cardiac abnormalities was proposed more than 60 years ago.[242] In 1938, Aschenbrenner and Bodechtel reported that neurological lesions could be associated with electrocardiographic abnormalities in young patients without heart disease,[243] and in 1947 Byer, Ashman, and Toth described large upright T waves and long Q-T intervals following subarachnoid hemorrhage.[244] A more systematic study was published in 1954 by Burch,[245] who concluded that the principal offending cerebral lesions were intracerebral or subarachnoid hemorrhage, and that the principal electrocardiographic abnormalities were prolongation of the Q-T interval, increased amplitude and duration of T waves and abnormal U waves.

Neurogenic pulmonary edema occurs with a variety of disorders of the central nervous system[246,247] and with brain-stem hemorrhage. A rise in systemic blood pressure in response to cerebral injury[248] was known to Harvey Cushing at the turn of the century (the Cushing pressor response),[249] and experimentally induced intense cerebral compression in rats evokes a marked increase in systemic vascular resistance, a profound decrease in cardiac output, and hemorrhagic pulmonary edema.[246] In human subjects, interest has also focussed upon myocardial injury, especially severe brain damage caused by craniocerebral trauma.[250–255]

Arrhythmias, Conduction Defects, and Repolarization Abnormalities

Approximately 90 per cent of patients with acute cerebral accidents—especially intracerebral or subarachnoid hemorrhage or acute cerebral trauma—exhibit electrocardiographic abnormalities that consist chiefly of disturbances of cardiac rhythm and repolarization.[253,254,256–267] Abnormalities in rhythm include sinus bradycardia (sometimes profound), sinus tachycardia, atrial arrhythmias (ectopic beats, fibrillation, flutter, or supraventricular tachycardia), junctional rhythms, and ventricular arrhythmias (ectopic beats, ventricular tachycardia, or fibrillation).[259,268,269] Repolarization abnormalities closely resemble those of ischemic heart disease and consist chiefly of abnormalities of ST segments and T waves in addition to prominent U waves, and prolonged Q-T interval.[256,257,262,269] ST segments may be dramatically elevated and T waves dramatically inverted (Fig. 60–19). Conduction disturbances include first-, second-, or third-degree AV block.[254]

There is little information in human subjects regarding a relationship between specific stroke location and disturbances in cardiac rhythm, conduction and repolarization,[257] but some experimental evidence is available.[270,271] The left insular cortex of the rat contains a site of cardiac chronotropic representation.[270] Prolonged phasic stimulation within the insular cortex of the rat results in atrioventricular block, prolongation of the Q-T interval, and ST-segment depression.[271]

Because the left insular cortex of the rat contains a site of cardiac representation, Oppenheimer postulated that there might be a difference in cardiac expression between right- and left-sided lesions.[257] There is evidence that asymmetries in brain function influence the heart through ipsilateral pathways, and there is a reported association between right-hemisphere strokes and tachyarrhythmias of supraventricular origin and left hemisphere strokes and arrhythmias of ventricular origin.[272] More recent reports call attention to the cardiovascular effects of human insular cortex stimulation,[273] and there is a reported association between a neurosurgical intervention in the region of the left insular cortex, premature ventricular complexes, and prolonged Q-T interval.[274] (The insular cortex in humans lies beneath the frontoparietal and superior temporal opercula.)

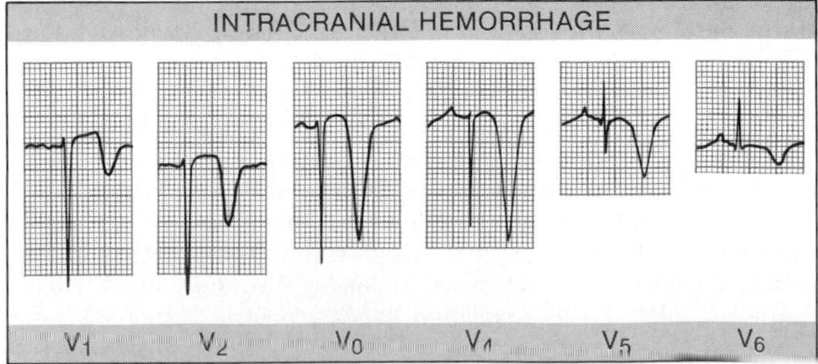

FIGURE 60–19. Deep, symmetrical T-wave inversions in precordial leads of a patient with a cerebral hemorrhage. (Courtesy of John H. Phillips, M. D., Tulane Medical Center, New Orleans, Louisiana.)

Migraine-related stroke—migrainous cerebral infarction—has been firmly established.[275] Less well known and perhaps less firmly established are atrial arrhythmias—atrial fibrillation, sinoatrial block—that are believed to be provoked by the autonomic discharge accompanying migraine headache.[276]

MYOCARDIAL INJURY. There is substantial evidence that the "catecholamine storm"—characterized by copious release of norepinephrine from cardiac beta-1 receptor sites—during acute cerebral accidents is responsible for myocardial damage, reflected in a rise of cardiac enzymes (CK-MB), left-ventricular wall motion abnormalities,[255] evidence of myofibrillar degeneration on light microscopy, and subendocardial injury.[248,252,265] Steroids combined with catecholamines have been implicated in the genesis of myocardial stress injury.[259] The myocardial damage associated with acute cerebral injury puts patients at additional risk. Subarachnoid hemorrhage can be associated with abnormal myocardial perfusion[277] and reversible left-ventricular wall motion abnormalities.[278] It is important to emphasize that the major sources of donor organs for heart and heart and lung transplantation are victims of motor vehicle accidents or gunshot wounds that cause acute cerebral damage. Those patients have necessarily suffered massive cerebral injury and, in all probability, have varying degrees of catecholamine- and stress-induced myocardial and lung injury.[253,275]

NEUROGENIC PULMONARY EDEMA AND CARDIOPULMONARY ARREST. Cerebrogenic hemorrhagic pulmonary edema has been experimentally induced by cranial compression in rats,[246] and neurogenic pulmonary edema sometimes accompanies acute cerebral injury in patients[246,247,256] (see p. 466). Myocardial damage may aggravate the pulmonary edema but is not necessary for its genesis. Respiratory arrest without circulatory collapse is more common than cardiac arrest in response to acute cerebral injury.[279] Cardiac arrest is likely to be triggered by disturbances in ventricular rhythm. Cerebrogenic arrhythmias and neurogenic pulmonary edema occasionally follow generalized tonic-clonic epileptic seizures without acute cerebral injury.[280,281] Acute injury to the cervical spinal cord without cerebral damage is frequently accompanied by disturbances in cardiac rhythm and conduction and occasionally by sudden death.[282] Bradyarrhythmias are most common, but supraventricular and ventricular tachyarrhythmias and AV block also occur in addition to marked hypotension. The cardiac abnormalities are believed to arise from acute autonomic imbalance imposed on the heart by the cervical cord injury.[282]

COEXISTING CEREBROVASCULAR AND CORONARY HEART DISEASE

The preceding section emphasized that acute cerebrovascular accidents in patients with normal hearts—i.e., without coronary artery disease—were often accompanied by electrocardiographic abnormalities resembling those of myocardial ischemia or infarction, by release of MB-creatinine phosphokinase (CPK) and by abnormal myocardial perfusion. In older patients experiencing an acute cerebrovascular accident, however, the same abnormalities may in fact represent an acute myocardial ischemic event caused by coexisting atherosclerotic coronary artery disease.[283] Because ST-segment elevations, deep T-wave inversions, and a rise in MB-CPK occur with cerebrovascular accidents in patients *without* ischemic heart disease, those criteria cannot be relied upon to diagnose ischemic injury due to coexisting coronary artery obstruction.

Although earlier estimates of the incidence of acute myocardial infarction in patients with acute cerebrovascular accidents were less than reliable,[285] it is now clear that cerebrovascular disease and coronary artery disease have similar risk factors and often coexist.[286] Differential diagnosis is important, because mortality is high in patients who simultaneously experience an acute cerebrovascular accident and acute myocardial infarction. After presentation with threatened stroke, patients may be at higher risk for a subsequent myocardial infarction than for stroke. However, the presence of coronary artery disease adversely affects survival in stroke patients.[286] Another important relationship is the prevalence of significant coronary artery disease and coronary events among patients with transient ischemic attacks, small strokes, asymptomatic carotid arterial murmurs, or carotid stenosis.[286]

One of the mechanisms believed to be responsible for transient ischemic attacks is embolization from carotid plaques.[287] Recent attention has focused upon ulcerated plaques in the ascending aorta and aortic arch as a source of cerebral embolic events.[288] Nearly one-half of patients with either symptomatic or asymptomatic cerebrovascular disease as just defined were found to have abnormal thallium-201 scans induced by exercise or pharmacological stress.[286] The primary cause of death following the onset of transient ischemic attacks is coronary artery disease.[287]

CAROTID ARTERIAL DISEASE AND CORONARY ARTERY DISEASE. Patients with symptomatic atherosclerotic coronary artery disease may have occult carotid artery disease, and patients with symptomatic carotid artery disease may have occult atherosclerotic coronary artery disease.[286] Cervical arterial murmurs have been found in 4.4 to 12.6 per cent of subjects 45 years of age and older with no history of stroke, transient cerebral ischemia, or overt ischemic heart disease.[289–291] The incidence of asymptomatic cervical murmurs (asymptomatic atherosclerotic carotid artery disease) increases with age. Thirty per cent of persons over age 50 years have some evidence of carotid artery disease.[292] The prevalence of carotid disease relates to the same risk factors as coronary artery disease, especially hypertension, cigarette smoking, hyperlipidemia, and diabetes mellitus.[293] Nevertheless, it is important to distinguish between mild carotid stenosis with an exceedingly low risk of stroke and severe carotid stenosis in which the risk of even nonfatal cerebral infarction is appreciable.[291,294,295] An early Framingham study called attention to the relative frequency of cerebral infarction in vascular territories different from those predicted by an asymptomatic carotid arterial murmur.[293] Embolization from ulcerated carotid or proximal aortic plaques may in part account for this observation.[287,288,293]

Symptoms ascribed to carotid artery lesions represented by stenosis or plaque ulceration include transient or persistent monocular visual loss, hemispheric transient ischemic attacks, and frank ischemic stroke.[293] Patients with transient ischemic attacks related to severe carotid stenosis confront stroke risk at a rate of 12 per cent within the first year after onset of symptoms, and a cumulative stroke risk of 30 to 35 per cent at 5 years.[293] After an initial stroke, the risk of subsequent cerebral events is approximately 7 per cent per year, with approximately 35 per cent of patients experiencing another stroke within 5 years after the original event.[293]

Auscultation should be routinely used for the detection of carotid arterial murmurs, but the presence of a murmur does not identify a critical carotid lesion, and a critical carotid lesion is not always associated with a murmur.[293] Ultrasound technology using color-coded Doppler and B-mode ultrasonography should be used as a screening test. However, carotid arteriography is required for precise definition because ultrasonographic measurements are currently less than precise.[292]

MANAGEMENT. Expert opinion regarding the indications for carotid endarterectomy to prevent stroke has varied widely[295] and has resulted in many retrospective reviews, natural history studies, position papers, and, more recently, in prospective randomized trials.[292,293] Relevant to this chapter is the problem of the coexistence of carotid artery stenosis and coronary artery disease. A number of relatively current and well conceived publications address this problem,[296–298] but optimal strategy for the management of patients with *combined* coronary artery stenosis and carotid disease awaits a well-designed prospective randomized trial.[293] In patients with combined carotid and coronary disease, surgical options include operating upon the carotid lesion first with an increased risk of morbidity and mortality from myocardial infarction; coronary artery bypass grafting first with an increased risk of perioperative stroke; or operating upon both lesions at the same time.[293] Meta-analysis findings indicate that perioperative stroke rate was similar if carotid and coronary surgery were combined or if carotid surgery preceded coronary bypass grafting.[293] The frequency of stroke was significantly greater if coronary bypass grafting preceded carotid surgery, and the frequency of myocardial infarction and death was greater when carotid surgery preceded coronary bypass grafting.[293] Simultaneous performance of coronary artery bypass grafting and carotid endarterectomy carries an increased risk that is warranted when patients present with recent symptoms of severe carotid artery stenosis and a compelling reason for coronary artery bypass grafting.[292,293,296,297,299] If a patient presents with symptomatic severe carotid artery stenosis, carotid endarterectomy should be done initially, and a month later, if necessary, the coronary artery disease can be addressed by bypass grafting or balloon dilatation.[292] If a patient with asymptomatic cerebrovascular disease that requires carotid endarterectomy needs urgent coronary revascularization, a staged procedure commencing with the latter can be carried out. Often, coronary angioplasty can be performed first, followed in 2 to 4 weeks by carotid endarterectomy. Patients who have simultaneous unstable coronary and carotid arterial disease can be considered for a combined procedure.

NEUROLOGICAL COMPLICATIONS OF CORONARY BYPASS SURGERY. An important corollary is the incidence of neurological complications unassociated with obstruction of the carotid artery in patients undergoing coronary artery bypass grafting.[297,299–302] These complications are in addition to and apart from those accompanying open-heart surgery.[303,304] Major central nervous system events are associated with coronary bypass operations in 1 to 2 per cent of cases.[299,301,302] The majority of these cerebral events are related to embolization of atheromatous material from the ascending aorta or to embolization from a postinfarction left ventricular mural thrombus.[299,302]

Cardiogenic Brain Embolism

Aggregate clinical data regarding cardiac sources of embolic stroke include "nonvalvular" atrial fibrillation, ischemic heart disease (acute myocardial infarction, healed myocardial infarction with ventricular aneurysm), mechanical prosthetic valves, and rheumatic heart disease (mitral stenosis)[305,306] (see p. 1009). Important but less common sources of cardiogenic embolism to the brain include nonischemic dilated cardiomyopathy, infective endocarditis, nonbacterial thrombotic vegetations, myxomatous mitral valve, paradoxical embolism, atrial septal aneurysm, left atrial myxoma, mitral annular calcification, and calcific aortic stenosis.[305,306] Nonvalvular atrial fibrillation encompasses a wide spectrum from "lone atrial fibrillation" that occurs without other clinical evidence of heart disease to atrial dilatation with congestive heart failure. Nonvalvular atrial fibrillation is the most common cardiac substrate for cardiogenic embolism, accounting for almost one-half of cardiogenic embolic strokes.[305–309] Both warfarin anticoagulation and aspirin are effective in reducing the risk of systemic embolism in patients with nonvalvular atrial fibrillation.[306,308,309] The approximate reduction achieved with warfarin anticoagulation is 70 per cent; the approximate reduction achieved with aspirin is 42 per cent.[306,309] Aspirin is safer, cheaper, and easier to administer than warfarin and has been recommended in patients 75 years or younger[308] (see Fig. 58-17, p. 1832).

Embolic stroke from left ventricular mural thrombi accompanies acute myocardial infarction generally within the first weeks (see p. 1256). In 90 per cent of cases, the infarct is anterior.[305] Persistent left ventricular dyskinesis or ventricular aneurysm in healed myocardial infarction are also important sources of ventricular mural thrombi and cardiogenic cerebral embolism.[305]

In patients with mechanical prosthetic heart valves, the risk of embolism is 2 to 4 per cent per year, with higher rates for mitral prostheses, especially in the presence of atrial fibrillation[305,306] (see p. 655). Focal neurological signs occasionally occur in patients with myxomatous mitral valves (mitral valve prolapse) (see p. 1032) and are believed to be embolic (platelet aggregates, sterile thrombi).[306,310,311] Aspirin is recommended as the initial antithrombotic therapy.[306]

Left atrial myxoma results in peripheral emboli in about 45 per cent of cases, and the brain is involved in one-half (see p. 867). Patients with left atrial myxoma are sometimes seen first by a neurologist because of presenting neurological manifestations.[312]

Nonischemic dilated cardiomyopathy with mural thrombi is more likely to cause cerebral emboli than are mural thrombi associated with myocardial infarction.[238] Infants with endocardial fibroelastosis of the dilated type suffer strokes caused by emboli from left ventricular endocardial thrombi.[313]

Atheromatous plaques or platelet-fibrin aggregates originating in the ascending aorta[288] or in the carotid arteries[287] are important and often unrecognized sources of cardiogenic brain embolism. Transient ischemic attacks associated with carotid disease often originate from plaques rather than impaired perfusion.[287]

INFECTIVE ENDOCARDITIS. This condition gives rise to a host of neurological complications including cerebral embolic events (transient ischemic attacks/stroke), intraparenchymal hemorrhage, subarachnoid hemorrhage, meningitis/meningoencephalitis, cerebral abscess, mycotic aneurysm, seizures and encephalopathy[314-318] (see p. 1085). *Prosthetic valve infective endocarditis* (see p. 1079) typically involves mechanical prostheses, especially in the mitral location, and is associated with high mortality.[315,317] The incidence of focal neurological events ranges from 11 to 44 per cent in patients with prosthetic valve infective endocarditis, much higher than the thromboembolic rate of 1 to 4 per cent per year for anticoagulated patients with prosthetic valves but without infective endocarditis.[315] Neurological complications are of special concern because of the risk of intracranial hemorrhage associated with anticoagulation. Septic cerebral emboli may result in intracranial hemorrhage or cerebral abscess after a misleading quiescent interval. A septic cerebral aneurysm is potentially catastrophic because of rupture.[318]

In patients with nonbacterial thrombotic vegetations, bland cerebral emboli are not uncommon.[319] The aortic valve is the usual site of the noninfectious thrombotic vegetations.

Drug abuse not only causes infective endocarditis but, depending on the drug and vehicle (embolization from foreign matter), may be associated with intracranial or subarachnoid hemorrhage, cerebral emboli, and ischemic stroke.[320]

PARADOXICAL EMBOLI. These reach the brain when peripheral venous blood enters the systemic arterial circulation via right-to-left shunts of cyanotic congenital heart disease.[313,321] An important variation on this theme are paradoxical emboli in acyanotic patients with interatrial communications: patent foramen ovale or ostium secundum atrial septal defect.[322-324,324a] Inferior vena caval streaming directs blood toward the midportion of the atrial septum and —in the presence of a defect—into the left atrium and systemic circulation. Especially vulnerable are pregnant women with an ostium secundum atrial septal defect and an increased incidence of emboli from peripheral and pelvic veins.[325] Recent interest has focused upon younger adults with embolic stroke caused by paradoxical emboli through a patent foramen ovale[322,326] (Fig. 60–20). The incidence of patent foramen ovale in a necropsy study of 965 autopsy specimens of human hearts was 27.3 per cent ranging from 34.3 per cent during the first three decades of life to 22.2 per cent during the ninth and tenth decades.[327] Another source of cerebral embolization is from an atrial septal aneurysm, a highly mobile malformation of the interatrial septum that briskly oscillates from right atrium to left atrium.[324,328]

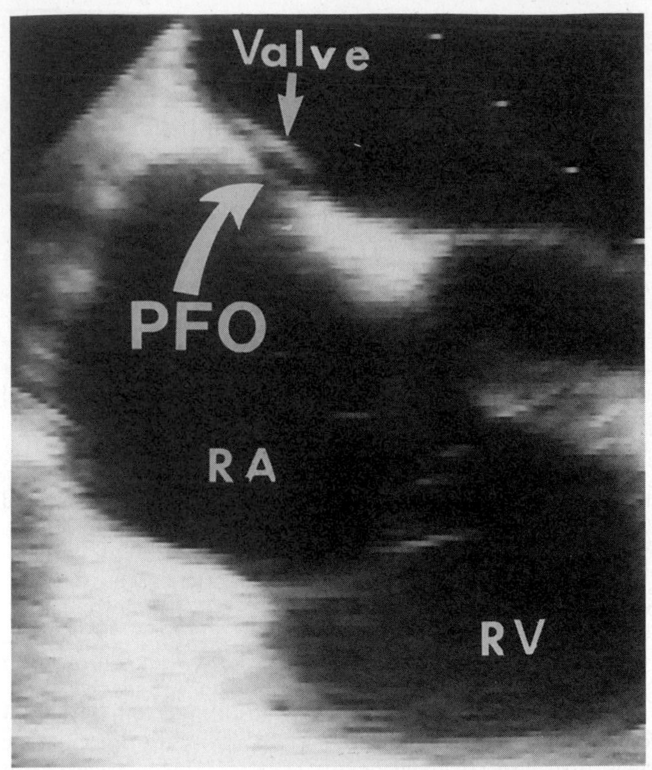

FIGURE 60–20. Transesophageal echocardiogram from a 22-year-old woman who came to attention because of a transient cerebral event. A patent foramen ovale (PFO) guarded by its valve were identified. Following a Valsalva maneuver, transient right-to-left shunting was identified with color flow imaging. RA = right atrium; RV = right ventricle.

Focal neurological deficits are well known sequelae of cerebral emboli. Less well known are diffuse cerebral symptoms believed to result from recurrent multiple small cortical emboli that cause agitated confusion, dulled sensorium, and seizures.[329]

NEUROLOGICAL DISORDERS IN PATIENTS WITH CONGENITAL HEART DISEASE

(See Chap. 29)

NEUROLOGICAL COMPLICATIONS AFTER CARDIAC ARREST

Neurological outcomes vary considerably, ranging from complete recovery to a vegetative state.[330-333] A reversible "metabolic encephalopathy" occurs in patients with brief episodes of circulatory arrest and mild degrees of cerebral hypoxia. Recovery is rapid and complete. In contrast, patients with severe cerebral hypoxia suffer structural damage to specific areas of the brain as if they had a stroke and, on awakening, manifest permanent focal or multifocal motor, sensory, and intellectual deficits.[330,331,333] Patients with more widespread brain injury remain hospitalized in a state of wakefulness without awareness (vegetative) or die a neurological (brain) death. Serious neurologic deficits occur in only about 10 per cent of patients who are discharged because severe postarrest neurological complications so often culminate in in-hospital or preadmission death.[332] Preexisting neurological deficits are ominous for survivors of cardiopulmonary resuscitation. Early return of consciousness and return of cranial nerve function and electroencephalographic function imply a better cerebral prognosis but do not guarantee a good outcome.[332] Delayed electroencephalographic return signifies a poor neurologic prognosis.

CARDIAC COMPLICATIONS OF DRUGS USED IN TREATING NEUROMUSCULAR DISEASE

Methysergide prescribed for migraine headache is occasionally accompanied by inflammatory retroperitoneal fibrosis and by a similar fibrotic disease of pleura, systemic arteries, cardiac valves, endocardium, and pericardium.[334-336] Methysergide-induced lesions cause little or no damage to underlying cardiac structures but result in a layer of fresh collagen upon the surfaces of otherwise unharmed cardiac tissue.[335] The aortic valve disorder induced by methysergide is stenosis or regurgitation, whereas the mitral lesion generally causes regurgitation. If the drug is continued, the valvular abnormalities generally progress. Regression or complete disappearance (at least of the cardiac murmurs) may follow discontinuation of methysergide.[335]

In *Parkinson's disease,* neurons are selectively destroyed and cannot release the neurotransmitter dopamine.[337] Accordingly, levodopa (L-dopa), the precursor of dopamine, is used in treatment. A relatively large dose is required for a therapeutic response because only a small percentage of oral L-dopa crosses the blood-brain barrier. Large doses are seldom tolerated without side effects. Cardiovascular effects are mediated by the action of L-dopa on the central and peripheral nervous systems. L-Dopa provokes hypotension (supine and postural) as well as ventricular ectopic beats.[337] The drug must therefore be used cautiously in patients with cerebral ischemia, angina pectoris, recent myocardial infarction, or cardiac arrhythmias, although after weeks (sometimes months) of use, tolerance improves and side effects diminish.

Bromocriptine, an ergot derivative, stimulates dopamine-sensitive receptors and is also useful in parkinsonism.[337] In high doses, the drug may cause a significant postural fall in blood pressure. The hypotensive effect may persist for as long as 6 weeks. Rarely, severe hypotension, both supine and erect, occurs after the initial dose of bromocriptine.

NEUROLOGICAL COMPLICATIONS OF THERAPY FOR CARDIOVASCULAR DISEASE

Certain therapies for cardiovascular disease can result in serious neurological impairment such as the sequelae of cardiac arrest and resuscitation. Systemic emboli related to cardioversion for chronic atrial fibrillation can occur either at the time of reversion to sinus rhythm or upon recurrence of atrial fibrillation. If an anticoagulant is used, it must precede cardioversion and be maintained until stable sinus rhythm seems assured.[338]

Cyclosporine neurotoxicity is only one of the neuropathological concerns in the management of cardiac transplantation.[339,340] Cyclosporine may produce a wide range of neurological disorders including coma, encephalopathy, cortical blindness, tremor, ataxia, peripheral neuropathy, and paraparesis.[339,340] There is no necessary correlation between blood levels and neurotoxic effects of the drug. However, withdrawal of cyclosporine or dose reduction generally results in resolution of the signs and symptoms, but cases of fatal convulsions and coma have been reported.[339] Perioperative neurological complications of cardiac transplantation (first 2 weeks) include cerebrovascular disorders, encephalopathy, acute psychosis, and mononeuropathy.[341,342] Late neurological complications are related primarily to the use of chronic immunosuppression, with cerebrovascular disorders becoming less frequent.[341,342]

Several commonly used cardiac drugs have important, although relatively rare, central or peripheral nervous system effects. The adverse responses to quinidine and procainamide in patients with myasthenia gravis were mentioned earlier. *Lidocaine neurotoxicity* (see p. 607) includes drowsiness, dizziness, dysarthria, blurred vision, muscular fasciculations, and occasionally convulsions.[343] Beta-adrenoceptor blockers (see p. 1306), in addition to causing drowsiness and lightheadedness, sometimes result in mental depression. Even digitalis glycosides are not exempt from neurotoxic effects[344] (see p. 484). William Withering reported that, "The Foxglove when given in very large and quickly repeated doses occasions giddiness, confused vision, objects appearing green or yellow . . . cold sweats, convulsions, syncope, death."[345]

CARDIAC DENERVATION

The most common cause of cardiac denervation is transplantation of the heart (see Chap. 18). Less well known is the remarkable denervation of the heart's intrinsic nervous system that occurs with Chagas' disease (see p. 1442).[346,347] Chagasic dysautonomia is associated with pathological changes in the cardiovascular, digestive, and autonomic nervous systems.[347] The cardioneuropathy is characterized by bradycardia, absent postural reflexes, hypotension, and an abnormal hyperventilatory response.[347] The increased capacity of the coronary arteries (judged at necropsy by the volume of barium sulfate-gelatin mass occupied by the coronary arterial bed relative to heart weight) has been attributed to relative sympathetic overdrive.[346]

REFERENCES

HEREDOFAMILIAL NEUROMYOPATHIC DISORDERS

1. Perloff, J. K., deLeon, A. C., and O'Doherty, D.: The cardiomyopathy of progressive muscular dystrophy. Circulation *33:*625, 1966.
2. Perloff, J. K., Henze, E., and Schelbert, H. R.: Alterations in regional myocardial metabolism, perfusion and wall motion in Duchenne muscular dystrophy studied by radionuclide imaging. Circulation *69:*33, 1984.
3. Perloff, J. K., Stevenson, W. G., Roberts, N. K., et al.: Cardiac involvement in myotonic muscular dystrophy (Steinert's disease): A prospective study of 25 patients. Am. J. Cardiol. *54:*1074, 1984.
4. Child, J. S., Perloff, J. K., Bach, P. M., et al.: Cardiac involvement in Friedreich's ataxia. J. Am. Coll. Cardiol. *7:*1370, 1986.
5. Melacini, T., Fanin, M., Danieli, G. A., et al.: Cardiac involvement in Becker muscular dystrophy. Am. J. Cardiol. *22:*1927, 1993.
6. Brooke, M. H.: A Clinician's View of Neuromuscular Disease. 2nd ed. Baltimore, Williams and Wilkins Co., 1986.
7. Kunkel, L. M.: Analysis of deletions in DNA from patients with Becker and Duchenne muscular dystrophy. Nature *322:*73, 1986.
8. Koenig, M., Hoffman, E. P., Bertelson, C. J., et al.: Complete cloning of the Duchenne muscular dystrophy (DMD) cDNA and preliminary genomic organization of the DMD gene in normal and affected individuals. Cell *50:*509, 1987.
9. Chamberlain, J. S., Gidbs, R. A., Rainier, J. E., et al.: Deletion screening of the Duchenne muscular dystrophy locus via multiplex DNA amplification. Nucleic Acids Res. *16:*11, 141, 1988.
10. Worton, R.: Muscular dystrophies: Diseases of the dystrophin-glycoprotein complex. Science *270:*755, 1995.
11. Hoffman, E. P., and Gorospe, M.: The animal models of Duchenne muscular dystrophy: Windows on the pathophysiological consequences of dystrophin deficiency. Curr. Top. Membr. *38:*113, 1991.
12. Lansman, J. B., and Franco, A.: What does dystrophin do in normal muscle. Muscle Res. Cell Motil. *12:*409, 1991.
13. Hoffman, E. P., and Kunkel, L. M.: Dystrophin abnormalities in Duchenne/Becker muscular dystrophy. Neuron *2:*1019, 1989.
14. Towbin, J. A., Hejtmanck, F., Brink, P., et al.: X-linked dilated cardiomyopathy: Molecular genetic evidence of linkage to the Duchenne muscular dystrophy (dystrophin gene at the Xp21 locus). Circulation *87:*1154, 1993.
15. Rojas, C. V., and Hoffman, E. P.: Recent advances in dystrophin research. Curr. Opin. Neurobiol. *1:*420, 1992.
16. Hoffman, E. P., Brown, R. H., and Kunkel, L. M.: Dystrophin: The protein product of the Duchenne muscular dystrophy locus. Cell *51:*919, 1987.
17. Koenig, M., Monaco, A. P., and Kunkel, L. M.: The complete sequence of dystrophin predicts a rod-shaped cytoskeletal protein. Cell *53:*219, 1988.
18. Love, D. R., Morris, G. E., Ellie, J. M., et al.: Tissue distribution of the dystrophin-related gene product and expression in the mdx and dy mouse. Proc. Natl. Acad. Sci. USA *88:*3243, 1991.
19. Bonilla, E., Samitt, C. F., Mirande, A. F., et al.: Duchenne muscular dystrophy: Deficiency of dystrophin at the muscle cell surface. Cell *54:*447, 1988.
20. Roland, L. P.: Biochemistry of muscle membranes in Duchenne muscular dystrophy. Muscle Nerve *3:*3, 1980.
21. Pons, F., Augier, N., Heilig, R., et al.: Isolated dystrophin molecules as seen by electron microscopy. Proc. Natl. Acad. Sci. USA *87:*7851, 1990.
22. Ervasti, J. M., Ohlendieck, K., Kahl, S. D., Gaver, M. G., and Campbell, K. P.: Deficiency of a glycoprotein component of the dystrophin complex in dystrophic muscle. Nature *345:*315, 1990.
23. Ervasti, J. M., and Campbell, K. P.: Membrane organization of the dystrophin-glycoprotein complex. Cell *66:*1121, 1991.
24. Hoffman, E. P., Fishbeck, K. H., Brown, R. H., et al.: Characterization of dystrophin in muscle-biopsy specimens from patients with Duchenne's or Becker's muscular dystrophy. N. Engl. J. Med. *318:*1363, 1988.
25. Boyd, Y., Buckle, V., Holt, S., Munro, E., Hunter, D., and Craig, I.: Muscular dystrophy in girls with X; autosome translocations. J. Med. Genet. *23:*484, 1986.
26. Boyd, Y. and Buckle, V. J.: Cytogenetic heterogeneity of translocations associated with Duchenne muscular dystrophy. Clin. Genet. *29:*108, 1986.
27. Valentine, B. A., Cooper, B. J., deLahunta, A., et al.: Canine X-linked muscular dystrophy. Neurol. Sci. *88:*69, 1988.
28. Pennington, R. J. T.: Serum enzymes. *In* Rowland, L. P. (ed.): Pathogenesis of Human Muscular Dystrophies. Amsterdam-Oxford, Excerpta Medica, 1977, p. 341.
29. Sutton, T. M., O'Brien, J. F., Kleinberg, F., et al.: Serum levels of creatine phosphokinase and its isoenzymes in normal and stressed neonates. Mayo Clin. Proc. *56:*150, 1981.
30. Gay, P. C., and Edmonds, L. C.: Severe hypercapnia after low-flow oxygen therapy in patients with neuromuscular disease and diaphragmatic dysfunction. Mayo Clin. Proc. *70:*327, 1995.
31. Riggs, T.: Cardiomyopathy and pulmonary emboli in terminal Duchenne's muscular dystrophy. Am. Heart J. *119:*690, 1990.
32. Gaffney, J. F., Kingston, W. J., Metlay, L. A., and Gramiak, R.: Left ventricular thrombus and systemic emboli complicating the cardiomyopathy of Duchenne's muscular dystrophy. Arch. Neurol. *46:*1249, 1989.
33. Yotsukura, M., Miyagawa, M., Tsuya, T., Ishihara, T., and Ishikawa, K.: Pulmonary hypertension in progressive muscular dystrophy of the Duchenne type. Jpn. Circ. J. *52:*321, 1988.
34. Perloff, J. K., Roberts, W. C., deLeon, A. C., and O'Doherty, D.: The distinctive electrocardiogram of Duchenne's progressive muscular dystrophy. Am. J. Med. *42:*179, 1967.
35. Sanyal, S. K., Johnson, W. W., Dische, M. R., et al.: Dystrophic degeneration of papillary muscle and ventricular myocardium: A basis for

mitral valve prolapse in Duchenne's muscular dystrophy. Circulation *62*:430, 1980.
36. Yoshioka, M.: Clinically manifesting carriers in Duchenne muscular dystrophy. Clin. Genet. *20*:6, 1981.
37. Lane, R. J. M., Gardner-Medwin, D., and Roses, A. D.: Electrocardiographic abnormalities in carriers of Duchenne muscular dystrophy. Neurology *30*:497, 1980.
38. Mann, O., deLeon, A. C., Perloff, J. K., et al.: Duchenne's muscular dystrophy: The electrocardiogram in female relatives. Am. J. Med. Sci. *255*:376, 1968.
39. Paillonry, M., Citron, B., Hersch, B., et al.: Electrocardiograms of women carriers of Duchenne-type muscular dystrophy. Ann. Cardiol. Angiol. *31*:47, 1982.
40. Wiegand, V., Rahlf, G., Meinck, M., and Kreuzer, H.: Cardiomyopathy in female carriers of the Duchenne gene. Z. Kardiol. *73*:188, 1984.
41. Mirabella, M., Serbidei, S., Manfredi, G., et al.: Cardiomyopathy may be the only clinical manifestation in female carriers of Duchenne muscular dystrophy. Neurology *43*:342, 1993.
42. Skyring, A., and McKusick, V. A.: Clinical, genetic and electrocardiographic studies in childhood muscular dystrophy. Am. J. Med. Sci. *242*:54, 1961.
43. Slucka, C.: The electrocardiogram in Duchenne's progressive muscular dystrophy. Circulation *38*:933, 1968.
44. Fitch, C. W., and Ainger, L. E.: The Frank vectorcardiogram and the electrocardiogram in Duchenne muscular dystrophy. Circulation *35*:1124, 1967.
45. Sanyal, S. K., Johnson, W. W., Thapar, M. K., and Pitner, S. E.: An ultrastructural basis for the electrocardiographic alterations associated with Duchenne's progressive muscular dystrophy. Circulation *57*:1122, 1978.
46. Rubler, S., Perloff, J. K., and Roberts, W. C.: Clinical Pathological Conference—Duchenne's muscular dystrophy. Am. Heart J. *94*:776, 1977.
47. Ronan, J. A., Perloff, J. K., Bowen, P. J., and Mann, O.: The vectorcardiogram in Duchenne's progressive muscular dystrophy. Am. Heart J. *84*:588, 1972.
48. Wakai, S., Minami, R., Kameda, K., et al.: Electron microscopic study of the biopsied cardiac muscle in Duchenne muscular dystrophy. J. Neurol. Sci. *84*:167, 1988.
49. Frankel, K. A., and Rosser, R. J.: The pathology of the heart in progressive muscular dystrophy. Hum. Pathol. *7*:375, 1976.
50. Cziner, D. G., and Levin, R. I.: The cardiomyopathy of Duchenne's muscular dystrophy and the function of dystrophin. Med. Hypotheses *40*:169, 1993.
51. Bhattacharya, S. K., Crawford, A. J., and Pate, J. W.: Electrocardiographic, biochemical, and morphologic abnormalities in dystrophic hamsters with cardiomyopathy. Muscle Nerve *10*:168, 1987.
52. Moise, N. S., Valentine, B. A., Brown, C. A., et al.: Duchenne's cardiomyopathy in a canine model: Electrocardiographic and echocardiographic studies. Am. Coll. Cardiol. *17*:812, 1991.
53. Schelbert, H. R., Benson, L., Schwaiger, M., and Perloff, J. K.: Positron emission tomography. Cardiol. Clin. *1*:501, 1983.
54. Nagamachi, S., Jinnouchi, S., Ono, S., et al.: Tl-201 myocardial SPECT in patients with Duchenne's muscular dystrophy: A long-term follow-up. Clin. Nucl. Med. *14*:827, 1989.
55. Tamura, T., Shivuya, N., Hashiba, K., et al.: Evaluation of myocardial damage in Duchenne's muscular dystrophy with thallium-201 myocardial SPECT. Jpn. Heart J. *34*:51, 1993.
56. Perloff, J. K., Moise, N. S., Stevenson, W. G., and Gilmour, R. F.: Cardiac electrophysiology in Duchenne muscular dystrophy: From basic science to clinical expression. J. Cardiovasc. Electrophysiol. *3*:394, 1992.
57. Sanyal, S. K., Johnson, W. W.: Cardiac conduction abnormalities in children with Duchenne progressive muscular dystrophy: Electrocardiographic features and morphologic correlates. Circulation *66*:853, 1982.
58. Nomura, H., Hizawa, K.: Histopathological study of the conduction system of the heart in Duchenne progressive muscular dystrophy. Acta Pathol. Jpn. *32*:1027, 1982.
59. Gaschen, F. P., Hoffman, E. P., Goroscope, M. Jr., et al.: Dystrophin deficiency causes lethal muscle hypertrophy in cats. J. Neurosci. *110*:149, 1992.
60. James, T. N.: Cardiac conduction system: Fetal and postnatal development. Am. J. Cardiol. *25*:213, 1970.
61. Bies, R. D., Friedman, D., Roberts, R., et al.: Expression and localization of dystrophin in human cardiac Purkinje fibers. Circulation *86*:147, 1992.
62. Pons, F., Robert, A., Fabbricio, E., et al.: Utrophin localization in normal and dystrophin-deficient heart. Circulation *90*:369, 1994.
63. Perloff, J. K.: Cardiac rhythm and conduction in Duchenne's muscular dystrophy. J. Am. Coll. Cardiol. *3*:1263, 1984.
64. Bigger, J. T. Jr., Fleiss, J. L., Steinman, R. C., et al.: Frequency domain measures of heart rate period variability and mortality after myocardial infarction. Circulation *85*:164, 1992.
65. Zalman, F., Perloff, J. K., Durant, N. N., and Campion, D. S.: Acute respiratory failure following intravenous verapamil in Duchenne's muscular dystrophy. Am. Heart J. *105*:510, 1983.
66. Spach, M. S., and Dolber, P. C.: Relating intracellular potentials and their derivatives to anisotropic propagation at a microscopic level in human cardiac muscle. Circ. Res. *58*:356, 1986.
67. Ursell, P. C., Gardner, P. I., Alvala, A., et al.: Structural and electrophysiological changes in the epicardial border zone of canine myocardial infarcts during infarct healing. Circ. Res. *56*:436, 1985.
68. Shimizu, A., Nobaki, A., Rudy, Y., et al.: Onset of induced atrial flutter in the canine pericarditis model. J. Am. Coll. Cardiol. *17*:1223, 1991.
69. Cosio, F. G., Aribas, F., Placios, J., et al.: Fragmented electrocardiograms and continuous electrical activity in atrial flutter. Am. J. Cardiol. *57*:1309, 1986.
70. D'Orsogna, L., O'Shea, L. P., and Miller, G.: Cardiomyopathy of Duchenne muscular dystrophy. Pediatr. Cardiol. *9*:205, 1988.
71. Yotsukura, M., Ishizuka, T., Shimada, T., et al.: Late potentials in progressive muscular dystrophy of the Duchenne type. Am. Heart J. *121*:1137, 1991.
72. Mori, H., Utsunomiya, T., Ishijima, M., et al.: The relationship between 24-hour total heart beats or ventricular arrhythmias and cardiopulmonary function in patients with Duchenne's muscular dystrophy. Can. Anaesth. Soc. J. *33*:492, 1986.
73. Ilan, Y., Hillman, M., Oren, R.: Intravenous verapamil for tachyarrhythmia in Duchenne's muscular dystrophy. Pediatr. Cardiol. *11*:177, 1990.
74. Chalkiadis, G. A., and Branch, K. G.: Cardiac arrest after isoflurane anaesthesia in a patient with Duchenne's muscular dystrophy. Anaesthesia *45*:22, 1990.
75. Sethna, N. F., and Rockoff, M. A.: Cardiac arrest following inhalation induction of anaesthesia in a child with Duchenne's muscular dystrophy. Can. Anaesth. Soc. J. *33*:799, 1986.
76. Beggs, A. H., Hoffman, E. P., Snyder, J. R., et al.: Exploring the molecular basis for variability among patients with Becker muscular dystrophy: Dystrophin gene and protein studies. Am. J. Hum. Genet. *49*:54, 1991.
77. Yoshiba, K., Ikeda, S., Nakamura, A., et al.: Molecular analysis of the Duchenne muscular dystrophy gene in patients with Becker muscular dystrophy presenting with dilated cardiomyopathy. Muscle Nerve *16*:1161, 1993.
78. de Visser, M., de Voogt, W. G., la Riviere, G. V.: The heart in Becker muscular dystrophy, facioscapulohumeral dystrophy, and Bethlem myopathy. Muscle Nerve *15*:591, 1992.
79. Comi, G. T., Prelle, A., Bresolin, N., et al.: Clinical variability in Becker muscular dystrophy: Genetic, biochemical and immunohistochemical correlates. Brain *117*:1, 1994.
80. Hoffman, E. P., and Kunkel, L. M.: Dystrophin abnormalities in Duchenne/Becker muscular dystrophy. Neuron *2*:1019, 1989.
81. Anan, R., Higuchi, I., Ichinari, K., et al.: Myocardial patchy staining of dystrophin in Becker's muscular dystrophy associated with cardiomyopathy. Am. Heart J. *123*:1088, 1992.
82. Maeda, M., Nakao, S., Miyacato, H., et al.: Cardiac dystrophin abnormalities in Becker muscular dystrophy assessed by endomyocardial biopsy. Am. Heart J. *129*:702, 1995.
83. Markand, O. N., North, R. R., D'Agostino, A. N., and Daly, D. D.: Benign sex-linked muscular dystrophy. Neurology *19*:617, 1969.
84. Steare, S. E., Dubowitz, V., and Banater, A.: Subclinical cardiomyopathy in Becker muscular dystrophy. Br. Heart J. *68*:304, 1992.
85. Nigro, G., Comi, L. I., Politano, L., et al.: Evaluation of the cardiomyopathy in Becker muscular dystrophy. Muscle Nerve *18*:283, 1995.
86. Yazawa, M., Ikeda, S., Owa, M., et al.: A family of Becker's progressive muscular dystrophy with severe cardiomyopathy. Eur. Neurol. *27*:13, 1987.
87. Levin, R. N., and Narahara, K. A.: Right axis deviation and anterior wall thallium-201 defect in Becker's muscular dystrophy. Am. J. Cardiol. *56*:203, 1985.
88. Melacini, P., Fanin, M., Danieli, D. A., et al.: Cardiac involvement in Becker muscular dystrophy. J Am. Coll. Cardiol. *22*:1927, 1993.
89. Towbin, J. A., Hejtmancik, F., Drink, P., et al.: X-linked dilated cardiomyopathy: Molecular genetic evidence of linkage to the Duchenne muscular dystrophy (dystrophin) gene at the Xp21 locus. Circulation *87*:1854, 1993.
90. Muntoni, F., Cau, M., Ganau, A., et al.: Deletion of the dystrophin muscle-promoter region associated with X-linked dilated cardiomyopathy. N. Engl. J. Med. *329*:921, 1993.
91. Nigro, G., Comi, L. I., Limonselli, F. M., et al.: Prospective study of X-linked progressive muscular dystrophy in Campania. Muscle Nerve *6*:253, 1983.
92. Panegyres, P. K., Mastaglia, F. L., and Kakulas, B. A.: Limb-girdle syndromes: Clinical, morphological and electrophysiological studies. J. Neurol. Sci. *95*:201, 1990.
93. Bethlem, J., and Wijngaarden, G. K.: Benign myopathy with autosomal dominant inheritance. Brain *99*:91, 1976.
94. Manconi, G., Pizzi, A., Arimondi, C. G., et al.: Limb-girdle muscular dystrophy with autosomal dominant inheritance. Acta Neurol. Scand. *83*:234, 1991.
95. Miller, G., Beggs, A. H., and Towfighi, J.: Early onset autosomal dominant progressive muscular dystrophy presenting in childhood as a Becker phenotype: The importance of dystrophin and molecular genetic analysis. Neuromuscul. Disord. *2*:121, 1992.
96. Stubegen, J.: Limb-girdle muscular dystrophy: A non-invasive cardiac evaluation. Cardiology *83*:324, 1993.
97. Hoshio, A., Kotake, H., Saitoh, M., et al.: Cardiac involvement in a patient with limb-girdle muscular dystrophy. Heart Lung *16*:439, 1987.
98. Kawashima, S., Ulno, M., Kondo, T., et al.: Marked cardiac involvement in limb girdle muscular dystrophy. Am. J. Med. Sci. *299*:411, 1990.
99. Lunt, P. W., and Harper, P. S.: Genetic counseling in facioscapulohumeral muscular dystrophy. J. Med. Genet. *28*:655, 1991.

100. Wijmenga, C., Sandkuijl, L. A., Moerer, P., et al.: Genetic linkage map of facioscapulohumeral muscular dystrophy and five polymorphic loci on chromosome 4q35-qter. Am. J. Hum. Genet. *51:*411, 1992.
101. Haraguchi, Y., Chung, A. B., Torroni, A., et al.: Genetic mapping of human heart-skeletal muscle adenine nucleotide translocator and its relationship to the facioscapulohumeral muscular dystrophy locus. Genomics *61:*479, 1993.
102. Bailey, R. O., Marzulo, D. C., and Hans, M. B.: Infantile facioscapulohumeral muscular dystrophy: New observations. Acta Neurol. Scand. *74:*51, 1986.
103. Bloomfield, D. A., and Sinclair-Smith, B. C.: Persistent atrial standstill. Am. J. Med. *39:*335, 1965.
104. Caponnetto, S., Patorini, C., and Tirelli, G.: Persistent atrial standstill in a patient affected with facioscapulohumeral dystrophy. Cardiologia *53:*341, 1968.
105. Baldwin, A. J., Talley, R. C., Johnson, C., and Nutter, O.: Permanent paralysis of the atrium in a patient with facioscapulohumeral muscular dystrophy. Am. J. Cardiol. *31:*649, 1973.
106. Stevenson, W. G., Perloff, J. K., Weiss, J. N., and Anderson, T. L.: Facioscapulohumeral muscular dystrophy: Evidence for selective, genetic electrophysiologic cardiac involvement. J. Am. Coll. Cardiol. *15:*292, 1990.
107. Emery, A. E. H., and Dreifuss, F. E.: Unusual type of benign X-linked muscular dystrophy. J. Neurol. Neurosurg. Psychiatr. *29:*338, 1966.
108. Emery, A. E. H.: X-linked muscular dystrophy with early contractures and cardiomyopathy (Emery-Dreifuss type). Clin. Genet. *32:*360, 1987.
109. Hopkins, L. C., Jackson, J. A., and Elsas, L. J.: Emery-Dreifuss humeroperoneal muscular dystrophy: An X-linked myopathy with unusual contractures and bradycardia. Ann. Neurol. *10:*230, 1981.
110. Bialer, M. G., and Kelly, T. E.: Localization of the gene for Emery-Dreifuss muscular dystrophy to X-q28. Am. J. Hum. Genet. *45:*(Suppl A)130, 1989.
111. Fenichel, G. M., Sul, Y. C., Kilroy, A. W., and Blouin, R.: An autosomal-dominant dystrophy with humeropelvic distribution and cardiomyopathy. Neurology *32:*1399, 1982.
112. Takamoto, K., Hirose, K., and Nonaka, I.: A genetic variant of Emery-Dreifuss disease. Arch. Neurol. *41:*1292, 1984.
113. Tanaka, K., Yoshimura, T., Muratani, H., et al.: Familial myopathy with scapulohumeral distribution, rigid spine, cardiomyopathy and mitochondrial abnormality. J. Neurol. *236:*52, 1989.
114. Bergia, B., Sybers, H. D., and Butler, I. J.: Familial lethal cardiomyopathy with mental retardation and scapuloperoneal muscular dystrophy. J. Neurol. *49:*1433, 1990.
115. Wooliscroft, J., and Tuna, N.: Permanent atrial standstill: The clinical spectrum. Am. J. Med. *49:*2037, 1982.
116. Ward, D. E., Ho, S. Y., and Shinebourne, E. A.: Familial atrial standstill and inexcitability in childhood. Am. J. Cardiol. *53:*965, 1984.
117. Disertori, M., Guarnerio, M., Vergara, G., et al.: Familial endemic persistent atrial standstill in a small mountain community. Eur. Heart J. *4:*354, 1983.
118. Levy, S., Pougot, B., Demurat, M., et al.: Partial atrial electrical standstill: Report of three cases and review of clinical and electrophysiological features. Eur. Heart J. *1:*107, 1980.
119. Effendy, F. N., Bolognesi, R., Bianchi, G., and Visioli, O.: Alternation of partial and total atrial standstill. J. Electriocardiol. *12:*121, 1979.
120. Shah, M. K., Subramanyan, R., Tharakan, J., et al.: Familial total atrial standstill. Am. Heart J. *123:*1379, 1992.
121. Miller, R. G., Layzer, R. B., Mellenthin, M. A., et al.: Emery-Dreifuss muscular dystrophy with autosomal dominant transmission. Neurology *35:*1230, 1985.
122. Rowland, L. P., Fetell, M., Alarte, M., et al.: Emery-Dreifuss muscular dystrophy. Ann. Neurol. *5:*111, 1979.
123. Dickey, P. P., Ziter, F. A., and Smith, R. A.: Emery-Dreifuss muscular dystrophy. J. Pediatr. *104:*555, 1984.
124. Oswald, A. H., Goldblatt, J., Horak, A. R., and Beighton, P.: Lethal cardiac conduction defects in Emery-Dreifuss muscular dystrophy. S. Afr. Med. J. *72:*567, 1987.
125. Wyse, D. G., Nath, F. C., and Brownell, A. K. W.: Benign X-linked (Emery-Dreifuss) muscular dystrophy is not benign. PACE *10:*533, 1987.
126. Yoshioka, M., Saida, K., Itagaki, Y., and Kamiya, T.: Follow up study of cardiac involvement in Emery-Dreifuss muscular dystrophy. Arch. Dis. Child. *64:*713, 1989.
127. Hopkins, L. C., Jackson, J. H., and Elsas, L. J.: Emery-Dreifuss humeroperoneal muscular dystrophy: An X-linked myopathy with unusual contractures and bradycardia. Ann. Neurol. *10:*230, 1981.
128. Bialer, M. G., McDaniel, N. L., and Kelly, T. E.: Progression of cardiac disease in Emery-Dreifuss muscular dystrophy. Clin. Cardiol. *14:*411, 1991.
129. Bartlett, R. J., Pericak-Vance, M. A., Yamaoka, L., et al.: A new probe for the diagnosis of myotonic muscular dystrophy. Science *235:*1648, 1987.
130. Harper, P. S.: Myotonic Dystrophy. 2nd ed. Philadelphia, W. B. Saunders Co., 1989.
131. Wieringa, B., Brunner, H., Hulsebos, T., et al.: Genetic and physical demarcation of the locus for dystrophia myotonica. Adv. Neurol. *48:*47, 1988.
132. Rudel, R., and Lehmann-Horn, F.: Membrane changes in cells from myotonic patients. Physiol. Rev. *65:*310, 1985.
133. Mahadevan, M., Tsilfidis, C., Sabourin, L., et al.: Myotonic muscular dystrophy mutation: An unstable CTG repeat in the 3′ untranslated region of the gene. Science *255:*1253, 1992.
134. Annane, D., Duboc, D., Mazoyer, B., et al.: Correlation between decreased myocardial glucose phosphorylation and the DNA mutation size in myotonic dystrophy. Circulation *90:*2629, 1994.
135. Tokgozoglu, L. S., Ashizaina, T., Pacifico, A., et al.: Cardiac involvement in a large kindred with myotonic dystrophy. Quantitative assessment and relation to size of CTG repeat expansion. JAMA *274:*813, 1995.
136. Ono, S., Inoue, K., Mannen, T., et al.: Neuropathological changes of the brain in myotonic dystrophy: Some new observations. Neurol. Sci. *81:*301, 1987.
137. Bharati, S., Bump, F. T., Bauernfeind, R., and Lev, M.: Dystrophica myotonia: Correlative electrocardiographic, electrophysiologic and conduction system study. Chest *86:*444, 1984.
138. Moorman, J. R., Coleman, R. E., Packer, D. L., et al.: Cardiac involvement in myotonic muscular dystrophy. Medicine *64:*371, 1985.
139. Fragola, P. V., Luzi, M., Calo, L., et al.: Cardiac involvement in myotonic dystrophy. Am. J. Cardiol. *74:*1070, 1994.
140. Fragola, P. V., Autore, C., Magni, G., et al.: The natural course of cardiac conduction disturbances in myotonic dystrophy. Cardiology *79:*93, 1991.
141. Hawley, R. J., Milner, M. R., Gottdiener, J. S., and Cohen, A.: Myotonic heart disease: A clinical follow-up. Neurology *41:*259, 1991.
142. Nguyen, H. H., Wolfe, J. T. III, Holmes, D. R. Jr., and Edwards, W. D.: Pathology of the cardiac conduction system in myotonic dystrophy: A study of 12 cases. J. Am. Coll. Cardiol. *11:*662, 1988.
143. Hiromasa, S., Ikeda, T., Kubota, K., et al.: Myotonic dystrophy: Ambulatory electrocardiogram, electrophysiologic study, and echocardiographic evaluation. Am. Heart J. *113:*1482, 1987.
144. Hiromasa, S., Ikeda, T., Kubota, K., et al.: A family with myotonic dystrophy associated with diffuse cardiac conduction disturbances as demonstrated by His bundle electrocardiography. Am. Heart J. *111:*85, 1986.
145. Olofsson, B., Forsberg, H., Andersson, S., et al.: Electrocardiographic findings in myotonic dystrophy. Br. Heart J. *59:*47, 1988.
146. Grigg, L. E., Chan, W., Mond, H. G., et al.: Ventricular tachycardia and sudden death in myotonic dystrophy: Clinical, electrophysiologic and pathologic features. Am. J. Cardiol. *6:*254, 1985.
147. Hiromasa, S., Ikeda, T., Kubota, K., et al.: Ventricular tachycardia and sudden death in myotonic dystrophy. Am. Heart J. *115:*914, 1988.
148. Prystowsky, E. N., Pritchett, E. L. C., Roses, A. D., and Gallagher, J. J.: The natural history of conduction system disease in myotonic muscular dystrophy as determined by serial electrophysiologic studies. Circulation *60:*1360, 1979.
149. Melacini, T., Buja, G., Fasoli, G., et al.: The natural history of cardiac involvement in myotonic dystrophy: An eight-year follow-up in 17 patients. Clin. Cardiol. *11:*231, 1988.
150. Uemura, N., Tanaka, H., Niimura, T., et al.: Electrophysiological and histological abnormalities of the heart in myotonic dystrophy. Am. Heart J. *86:*616, 1973.
151. Petkovitch, N. J., Dunn, M., and Reed, W.: Myotonia dystrophica with AV dissociation and Stokes-Adams attacks. Am. Heart J. *68:*391, 1964.
152. Melacini, P., Villanova, C., Menegazzo, E., et al.: Correlation between cardiac involvement and CTG trinucleotide repeat length in myotonic dystrophy. J. Am. Coll. Cardiol. *25:*239, 1995.
153. Fall, L. H., Young, W. W., Power, J. A., et al.: Severe congestive heart failure and cardiomyopathy as a complication of myotonic dystrophy in pregnancy. Obstet. Gynecol. *76:*481, 1990.
154. Hartwig, G. R., Ran, K. R., Radoff, F. M., et al.: Radionuclide angiocardiographic analysis of myocardial function in myotonic muscular dystrophy. Neurology *33:*657, 1983.
155. Motta, J., Guilleminault, C., Billingham, M., et al.: Cardiac abnormalities in myotonic dystrophy: Electrophysiologic and histopathologic studies. Am. J. Med. *67:*467, 1979.
156. Ludatscher, R. M., Kerner, H., Amikam, S., and Gellei, B.: Myotonia dystrophica with heart involvement: An electron microscopic study of skeletal, cardiac, and smooth muscle. J. Clin. Pathol. *31:*1057, 1978.
157. Tanaka, N., Tanaka, H., Takeda, M., et al.: Cardiomyopathy in myotonic dystrophy: A light and electron microscopic study of the myocardium. Jpn. Heart J. *14:*202, 1973.
158. Child, J. S., and Perloff, J. K.: Diastolic properties of the left ventricle in myotonic muscular dystrophy (Steinert's disease). Am. Heart J. *129:*982, 1995.
159. Forsberg, H., Olofsson, B., Eriksson, A., and Andersson, S.: Cardiac involvement in congenital myotonic dystrophy. Br. Heart J. *63:*119, 1990.
160. Forsberg, H., Olofsson, B., Eriksson, A., and Andersson, S.: Cardiac involvement in congenital myotonic dystrophy. Br. Heart J. *63:*119, 1990.
161. Anderson, M.: Probable Thomsen's disease with cardiac involvement. J. Neurol. *214:*301, 1977.
162. Subramony, S. H., Malhotra, C. P., and Mishra, S. K.: Distinguishing paramyotonia congenital and myotonia congenita by electromyography. Muscle Nerve *6:*374, 1983.
163. Streib, F. W., Sun, S. F., and Hanson, M.: Paramyotonia congenita: Clinical and electrophysiologic studies. Electromyogr. Clin. Neurophysiol. *23:*315, 1983.
164. Rosenberg, R. N.: Hereditary ataxias. *In* Rowland, L. P. (ed.): Merritt's Textbook of Neurology. Philadelphia, Lea and Febiger, 1984, p. 499.

165. Barbeau, A.: Friedreich's ataxia 1980. Our overview of the pathophysiology. J. Can. Sci. Neurol. *7*:455, 1980.
166. Harding, A. E.: Friedreich's ataxia: A clinical and genetic study of 90 families with an analysis of early diagnostic criteria and intrafamilial clustering of clinical features. Brain *104*:589, 1981.
167. Brumback, R. A., Panner, B. J., and Kingston, W. J.: The heart in Friedreich's ataxia. Arch. Neurol. *43*:189, 1986.
168. Grenadier, E., Goldberg, S. J., Stern, L. Z., and Feldman, J.: M-mode and two-dimensional echocardiographic examination of patients with Friedreich's ataxia. J. Cardiovasc. Ultrasonogr. *3*:5, 1984.
169. Gottdiener, J. S., Hawley, R. J., Maron, B. J., et al.: Characteristics of the cardiac hypertrophy in Friedreich's ataxia. Am. Heart J. *103*:525, 1982.
170. Barbeau, A.: Pathophysiology of Friedreich's ataxia. *In* Matthews, W. B., and Glaser, G. H. (eds.): Recent Advances in Clinical Neurology, No. 3. Edinburgh, Churchill Livingstone, 1982, p. 129.
171. Pastertac, A., Drol, R., Petitclerc, R., et al.: Hypertrophic cardiomyopathy in Friedreich's ataxia: Symmetric or asymmetric? J. Can. Sci. Neurol. *7*:379, 1980.
172. Harding, A. E., and Hewer, R. L.: The heart disease of Friedreich's ataxia: A clinical and electrocardiographic study of 115 patients, with an analysis of serial electrocardiographic changes in 30 cases. Q. J. Med. *28*:489, 1983.
173. Zimmermann, M., Gabathuler, J., Adamec, R., and Pinget, L.: Unusual manifestations of heart involvement in Friedreich's ataxia. Am. Heart J. *111*:184, 1986.
174. Barbeau, A.: Quebec cooperative study of Friedreich's ataxia. J. Can. Sci. Neurol. *3*:2779, 1976.
175. Unverferth, D. V., Schmidt, W. R., Baker, P. B., and Wooley, C. F.: Morphologic and functional characteristics of the heart in Friedreich's ataxia. Am. J. Med. *82*:5, 1987.
176. Smith, E. R., Sangalang, V. E., Heffernan, L. P., et al.: Hypertrophic cardiomyopathy: The heart disease of Friedreich's ataxia. Am. Heart J. *94*:428, 1977.
177. Hawley, R. J., and Gottdiener, J. S.: Five-year follow-up of Friedreich's ataxia cardiomyopathy. Arch. Intern. Med. *146*:483, 1986.
178. Alboliras, E. T., Shub, C., Gomez, M. R., et al.: Spectrum of cardiac involvement in Friedreich's ataxia: Clinical, electrocardiographic and echocardiographic observations. Am. J. Cardiol. *58*:518, 1986.
179. Pentland, B., and Fox, K. A. A.: The heart in Friedreich's ataxia. J. Neurol. Neurosurg. Psychiatr. *46*:1138, 1983.
180. James, T. N., Cobbs, B. W., Coghlan, H. C., et al.: Coronary disease, cardioneuropathy, and conduction system abnormalities in the cardiomyopathy of Friedreich's ataxia. Br. Heart J. *57*:446, 1987.
181. Spach, N. S., and Kootsey, J. M.: The nature of electrical propagation in cardiac muscle. Am. J. Physiol. *244*:H3, 1983.
182. Palagi, B., Picozzi, R., Casazza, F., et al.: Biventricular function in Friedreich's ataxia: A radionuclide angiographic study. Br. Heart J. *59*:692, 1988.
183. Giunta, A., Maione, S., Biagini, R., et al.: Noninvasive assessment of systolic and diastolic function in 50 patients with Friedreich's ataxia. Cardiology *75*:321, 1988.
184. Zimmermann, M., Gabathuler, J., Adamec, R., and Pinget, L.: Unusual manifestations of heart involvement in Friedreich's ataxia. Am. Heart J. *111*:184, 1986.
185. Pleasure, D. E., and Schotland, D. L.: Hereditary neuropathies. *In* Rowland, L. P. (ed.): Merritt's Textbook of Neurology. Philadelphia, Lea and Febiger, 1984.
186. Leak, D.: Paroxysmal atrial flutter in peroneal muscular atrophy. Br. Heart J. *23*:326, 1961.
187. Littler, W. A.: Heart block and peroneal muscular atrophy. Q. J. Med. *39*:431, 1970.
188. Kaj, J. M., Littler, W. A., and Meade, J. B.: Ultrastructure of the myocardium in familial heart block and peroneal muscular atrophy. Br. Heart J. *34*:1081, 1972.
189. Lowry, P. I., and Littler, W. A.: Peroneal muscular atrophy associated with cardiac conduction tissue disease. Postgrad. Med. J. *59*:530, 1983.
190. Martin-Du Pan, R. C., Juse, C., and Perrenoud, J. J.: Congestive cardiomyopathy and pyruvate elevation in a case of Charcot-Marie-Tooth disease. Schweiz. Med. Wochenschr. *5*:114, 1984.
191. Isner, J. M., Hawley, R. J., Weintraub, A. B., and Engel, W. K.: Cardiac findings in Charcot-Marie-Tooth disease. Arch. Intern. Med. *139*:1161, 1979.
192. Spiro, A. J., Shy, G. M., and Gonatas, N. K.: Myotubular myopathy. Arch Neurol. *14*:1, 1966.
193. Verhiest, W., Brucher, J. M., Goddeeris, P., et al.: Familial centronuclear myopathy associated with cardiomyopathy. Br. Heart J. *38*:504, 1976.
194. Shafiq, S. A., Sande, M. A., Carruthers, R. R., et al.: Skeletal muscle in idiopathic cardiomyopathy. J. Neurol. Sci. *15*:303, 1972.
195. di Mauro, S., and Moraes, C. T.: Mitochondrial encephalopathies. Arch. Neurol. *50*:1197, 1993.
196. Anan, R., Nakagawa, M., Miyata, M., et al.: Cardiac involvement in mitochondrial diseases: A study on 17 patients with documented mitochondrial DNA defects. Circulation *91*:955, 1995.
197. Ozawa, T., Katsumata, K., Hayakawa, M., et al.: Genotype and phenotype of severe mitochondrial cardiomyopathy: A recipient of heart transplantation and the genetic control. Biochem. Biophys. Res. Com mun. *207*:613, 1995.
198. Berenberg, R. A., Pellock, J. M., DiMauro, S., et al.: Lumping or splitting? "Ophthalmoplegia-plus" or Kearns-Sayre syndrome? Ann. Neurol. *1*:37, 1977.
199. Lowes, M.: Chronic progressive external ophthalmoplegia, pigmentary retinopathy and heart block (Kearns-Sayre syndrome). Acta Ophthalmol. *53*:610, 1975.
200. Charles, R., Holt, S., Kay, J. M., et al.: Myocardial ultrastructure and the development of atrioventricular block in Kearns-Sayre syndrome. Circulation *63*:214, 1981.
201. Roberts, N. K., Perloff, J. K., and Kark, P.: Cardiac conduction in Kearns-Sayre syndrome. Am. J. Cardiol. *44*:1396, 1979.
202. Schwartzkopff, B., Frenzel, H., Losse, B., et al.: Heart involvement in progressive external ophthalmoplegia (Kearns-Sayre syndrome): Electrophysiologic, hemodynamic and morphologic findings. Z. Kardiol. *75*:161, 1986.
203. Schwartzkopff, B., Frenzel, H., Breithardt, G., et al.: Ultrastructural findings in endomyocardial biopsy of patients with Kearns-Sayre syndrome. J. Am. Coll. Cardiol. *12*:1522, 1988.
204. Channer, K. S., Channer, J. L., Campbell, M. J., and Rees, J. R.: Cardiomyopathy in the Kearns-Sayre syndrome. Br. Heart J. *59*:486, 1988.
205. Kenny, D., and Wetherbee, J.: Kearns-Sayre syndrome in the elderly: Mitochondrial myopathy with advanced heart block. Am. Heart J. *120*:440, 1990.
206. Clark, D. S., Myerburg, R. J., Morales, R. R., et al.: Heart block and Kearns-Sayre: Electrophysiologic-pathologic correlation. Chest *68*:727, 1975.
207. Pleasure, D. E., and Schotland, D. L.: Acquired neuropathies. *In* Rowland, L. P. (ed.): Merritt's Textbook of Neurology. 7th ed. Philadelphia, Lea and Febiger, 1984.
208. McDonagh, A. J. G., and Dawson, J.: Guillain-Barré syndrome after myocardial infarction. Br. Med. J. *294*:613, 1987.
209. Emmons, P. R., Blume, W. T., and DuShane, J. W.: Cardiac monitoring and demand pacemaker in Guillain-Barré syndrome. Arch. Neurol. *32*:59, 1975.
210. Greenland, P., and Griggs, R. C.: Arrhythmic complications in the Guillain-Barré syndrome. Arch. Intern. Med. *140*:1053, 1980.
211. Narayam, D., Huang, M. T., and Matthew, P. K.: Bradycardia and asystole requiring pacemaker in Guillain-Barré syndrome. Am. Heart J. *108*:426, 1984.
212. Fagius, J., and Wallin, B. G.: Microneurographic evidence of excessive sympathetic outflow in the Guillain-Barré syndrome. Brain *106*:589, 1983.
213. Persson, A., and Solders, G.: R–R variations in Guillain-Barré syndrome: A test of autonomic dysfunction. Acta Neurol. Scand. *67*:294, 1983.
214. Palferman, T. G., Wright, I., Doyle, D. V., and Amiel, S.: Electrocardiographic abnormalities and autonomic dysfunction in Guillain-Barré syndrome. Br. Med. J. *284*:1231, 1982.
215. Shy, G. M., Engel, W. K., Somers, J. E., and Wanko, T.: Nemaline myopathy; A new congenital myopathy. Brain *86*:793, 1963.
216. Conen, P. E., Murphy, G. E., and Donohue, W. L.: Light and electron microscopic studies of "myogranules" in a child with hypotonia and muscle weakness. Can. Med. Assoc. J. *89*:983, 1963.
217. Ishibashi-Veda, H., Imakita, M., Yutani, C., et al.: Congenital nemaline myopathy with dilated cardiomyopathy: An autopsy study. Hum. Pathol. *21*:77, 1990.
218. Kinoshita, M., and Satoyoshi, E.: Type I fiber atrophy and nemaline bodies. Arch. Neurol. *31*:423, 1974.
219. Meier, C., Gertsch, M., Zimmerman, A., et al.: Nemaline myopathy presenting as cardiomyopathy. N. Engl. J. Med. *308*:1536, 1983.
220. Meier, C., Voellmy, W., Gertsch, M., et al.: Nemaline myopathy appearing in adults as cardiomyopathy: A clinicopathologic study. Arch. Neurol. *41*:443, 1984.
221. Penn, A. S., and Rowland, L. P.: Neuromuscular junction. *In* Rowland, L. P. (ed.): Merritt's Textbook of Neurology. 7th ed. Philadelphia, Lea and Febiger, 1984, p. 561.
222. Barnes, D. M.: Nervous and immune system disorders linked in a variety of diseases. Science *232*:160, 1985.
223. Gibson, T. C.: The heart in myasthenia gravis. Am. Heart J. *90*:389, 1975.
224. Kornfeld, P., Horowitz, S. H., Genkins, G., and Papatestas, A.: Myasthenia gravis unmasked by antiarrhythmic agents. Mt. Sinai J. Med. *43*:10, 1976.
225. Niakan, E., Bertorini, T. E., Acchiardo, S. R., and Werner, M. F.: Procainamide-induced myasthenia-like weakness in a patient with peripheral neuropathy. Arch. Neurol. *38*:378, 1981.
226. Ratinov, G., Baker, W. P., and Swaiman, K. F.: McArdle's syndrome with previously unreported electrocardiographic and serum enzyme abnormalities. Ann. Intern. Med. *62*:328, 1965.
227. Melki, J., Abdelhak, S., Sheth, P., et al.: Gene for chronic proximal spinal muscular atrophies maps to chromosome 5q. Nature *344*:767, 1990.
228. Kimura, S., Yokota, H., Tateda, K., et al.: A case of the Kugelberg-Welander syndrome complicated with cardiac lesions. Jpn. Heart J. *21*:417, 1980.
229. Gottdiener, J. S., Sherber, H. S., Hawley, R. J., and Engel, W. K.: Cardiac manifestations in polymyositis. Am. J. Cardiol. *41*:1141, 1978.
230. Singsen, B., Goldreyer, B., Stanton, R., and Hanson, V.: Childhood polymyositis with cardiac conduction defects. Am. J. Dis. Child. *131*:72, 1976.
231. Farber, H. W., and Make, B.: Physiologic closure of a symptomatic

patent foramen ovale with oxygen therapy. Am. Rev. Respir. Dis. *131*:181, 1985.
232. Lisak, R. P., Lebeau, J., Tucker, S. H., and Rowland, L. P.: Hyperkalemic periodic paralysis and cardiac arrhythmias. Neurology *22*:810, 1972.
233. Buruma, O. J., Schipperheyn, J. J., and Bots, G. T.: Heart muscle disease in familial hypokalemic periodic paralysis. Circulation *64*:12, 1981.
234. Klein, R., Ganelin, R., Marks, J. F., et al.: Periodic paralysis with cardiac arrhythmia. J. Pediatr. *62*:371, 1963.
235. Kastor, J. A., and Goldreyer, B. N.: Ventricular origin of bidirectional tachycardia. Circulation *48*:897, 1973.
236. Karpawich, P. P., Hart, Z. H., Perry, B. L., et al.: Childhood periodic paralysis with dysrhythmias: Electrophysiologic and histopathologic evaluation. Am. Heart J. *114*:186, 1987.
237. Fukuda, K., Ogawa, S., Yokozuka, H., et al.: Long-standing bidirectional tachycardia in a patient with hypokalemic periodic paralysis. J. Electrocardiol. *21*:71, 1988.
238. Perloff, J. K. (ed.): The Cardiomyopathies. Philadelphia, W. B. Saunders Co., 1988.
239. Rubin, E.: Alcoholic myopathy in heart and skeletal muscle. N. Engl. J. Med. *301*:28, 1979.
240. Meyer, J. G., and Urban, K.: Electrolyte changes and acid-base balance after alcohol withdrawal. With special reference to rum fits and magnesium depletion. J. Neurol. *215*:135, 1977.
241. Clarren, S. K., and Smith, D. W.: The fetal alcohol syndrome. N. Engl. J. Med. *298*:1063, 1978.

ACUTE CEREBRAL DISORDERS

242. Bramwell, C.: Can head injury cause auricular fibrillation? Lancet *1*:8, 1934.
243. Aschenbrenner, R., and Bodechtel, G.: Ueber EKG veranderungen veihirntumorkranken. Klin. Wochenschr. *17*:298, 1938.
244. Byer, E., Ashman, R., Toth, L. A.: Electrocardiogram with large upright T waves and long QT intervals. Am. Heart J. *33*:796, 1947.
245. Burch, G. E., Meyers, R., Abildskov, J. A.: A new electrocardiographic pattern observed in cerebrovascular accidents. Circulation *9*:719, 1954.
246. Chen, H. I., Liao, J. F., and Ho, S. T.: Centrogenic pulmonary hemorrhagic edema induced by cerebral compression in rats. Circ. Res. *47*:366, 1980.
247. Schell, A. R., Shenoy, M. M., Friedman, S. A., and Patel, A. R.: Pulmonary edema associated with subarachnoid hemorrhage. Arch. Intern. Med. *147*:591, 1987.
248. Robertson, C. S., Clifton, G. L., Taylor, A. A., and Grossman, R. G.: Treatment of hypertension associated with head injury. J. Neurosurg. *59*:455, 1983.
249. Cushing, H.: Concerning a definite regulatory mechanism of the vasomotor center which controls blood pressure during cerebral compression. Bull. Johns Hopkins Hosp. *12*:390, 1901.
250. Sciarra, D.: Head injury. *In* Rowland, L. P. (ed.): Merritt's Textbook of Neurology. 7th ed. Philadelphia, Lea and Febiger, 1984, p. 277.
251. Hackenberry, L. E., Miner, M. E., Rea, G. L., et al.: Biochemical evidence of myocardial injury after severe head trauma. Crit. Care Med. *10*:641, 1982.
252. Clifton, G. L., Robertson, C. S., Kyper, K., et al.: Cerebrovascular response to severe head injury. J. Neurosurg. *59*:447, 1983.
253. McLeod, A. A., Neil-Dwyer, G., Meyer, C. H. A., et al.: Cardiac sequelae of acute head injury. Br. Heart J. *47*:221, 1982.
254. Tobias, S. L., Bookatz, B. J., and Diamond, T. H.: Myocardial damage and electrocardiographic changes in acute cerebrovascular hemorrhage: A report of three cases and review. Heart Lung *16*:521, 1987.
255. Pollick, C., Cujec, B., Parker, S., and Tator, C.: Left ventricular wall motion abnormalities in subarachnoid hemorrhage: An echocardiographic study. J. Am. Coll. Cardiol. *12*:600, 1988.
256. Yamour, B. J., Sridharan, M. R., Rice, J. F., and Flowers, N. C.: Electrocardiographic changes in cerebrovascular hemorrhage. Am. Heart J. *99*:294, 1980.
257. Oppenheimer, S. M., and Hachinski, V. C.: The cardiac consequences of stroke. Neurol. Clin. *10*:167, 1992.
258. Baur, H. R., Gobel, F. L., and Pierach, C. A.: Electrocardiographic changes after cervical laminectomy. Int. J. Cardiol. *1*:37, 1981.
259. Samuels, M. A.: Electrocardiographic manifestations of neurologic disease. Semin. Neurol. *4*:453, 1984.
260. Carruth, J. E., and Silverman, M. E.: *Torsades de pointes* atypical ventricular tachycardia complicating subarachnoid hemorrhage. Chest *78*:886, 1980.
261. Mikolich, J. R., Jacobs, W. C., and Fletcher, G. F.: Cardiac arrhythmias in patients with acute cerebrovascular accidents. JAMA *246*:1314, 1981.
262. Goldberger, A. L.: Recognition of ECG pseudoinfarct patterns. Mod. Concepts Cardiovasc. Dis. *49*:13, 1980.
263. Taylor, A. L., and Fozzard, H. A.: Ventricular arrhythmias associated with CNS disease. Arch. Intern. Med. *142*:232, 1982.
264. Gould, L., Reddy, R. C., Kollali, M., et al.: Electrocardiographic normalization after cerebral vascular accident. J. Electrocardiol. *14*:191, 1981.
265. Myers, M. G., Norris, J. W., Hachinski, V. C., et al.: Cardiac sequelae of acute stroke. Stroke *13*:838, 1982.
266. Stober, T., Anstätt, T., Sen, S., et al.: Cardiac arrhythmias in subarachnoid haemorrhage. Acta Neurochir. *93*:37, 1988.
267. Rudehill, A., Olsson, G. L., Sundqvist, K., and Gordon, E.: ECG abnormalities in patients with subarachnoid haemorrhage and intracranial tumours. J. Neurol. Neurosurg. Psychiatr. *50*:1375, 1987.
268. Melin, J., and Fogelhohm, R.: Electrocardiographic findings in subarachnoid hemorrhage. Acta Med. Scand. *213*:5, 1983.
269. Gascon, P., Ley, T. J., Toltzis, R. J., and Bonow, R. O.: Spontaneous subarachnoid hemorrhage simulating acute transmural myocardial infarction. Am. Heart J. *105*:511, 1983.
270. Oppenheimer, S. M., and Cechetto, D. F.: Cardiac chronotropic organization of the rat insular cortex. Brain Res. *533*:66, 1990.
271. Oppenheimer, S. M., Wilson, J. X., Guiraudon, C., et al.: Insular cortex stimulation produces lethal cardiac arrhythmias: A mechanism of sudden death? Brain Res. *550*:115, 1991.
272. Lane, R. D., Wallace, J. D., Petrosky, P. P., et al.: Supraventricular tachycardia in patients with right hemisphere strokes. Stroke *23*:362, 1992.
273. Oppenheimer, S. M., Gelvagirvin, J. P., et al.: Cardiovascular effects of human insular cortex stimulation. Neurology *42*:1727, 1992.
274. Svigelj, V., Grad, A., and Tekavcic, I.: Cardiac arrhythmia associated with reversible damage to insula in a patient with subarachnoid hemorrhage. Stroke *25*:1053, 1994.
275. Welch, K. M. A., and Levine, S. R.: Migraine-related stroke in the context of the International Headache Society classification of head pain. Arch. Neurol. *47*:458, 1990.
276. Oppenheimer, S. M., Cechetto, D. F., and Hachinski, V. C.: Cerebrogenic cardiac arrhythmias: Cerebral electrocardiographic influences and their role in sudden death. Arch. Neurol. *47*:513, 1990.
277. Szabo, M. D., Crosby, G., Hurford, W. E., and Strauss, H. W.: Myocardial perfusion following acute subarachnoid hemorrhage in patients with an abnormal electrocardiogram. Anesth. Analg. *76*:253, 1993.
278. Handlin, L. R., Kindred, L. H., Beauchamp, G. D., et al.: Reversible left ventricular dysfunction after subarachnoid hemorrhage. Am. Heart J. *126*:235, 1993.
279. Tabbaa, M. A., Ramirez-Lassepas, M., and Snyder, B. D.: Aneurysmal subarachnoid hemorrhage presenting as cardiorespiratory arrest. Arch. Intern. Med. *147*:1661, 1987.
280. Fredberg, U., Bøtker, H. E., and Rømer, F. K.: Acute neurogenic pulmonary oedema following generalized tonic clonic seizure: A case report and a review of the literature. Eur. Heart J. *9*:933, 1988.
281. Oppenheimer, S. M., Cechetto, D. F., and Hachinski, V. C.: Cerebrogenic cardiac arrhythmias. Arch. Neurol. *47*:513, 1990.
282. Lehmann, K. G., Lane, J. G., Piepmeier, J. M., and Batsford, W. P.: Cardiovascular abnormalities accompanying acute spinal cord injury in humans: Incidence, time course and severity. J. Am. Coll. Cardiol. *10*:46, 1987.
283. Komrad, M. S., Coffey, C. E., Coffey, K. S., et al.: Myocardial infarction and stroke. Neurology *34*:1403, 1984.
284. Chin, P. L., Kaminski, J., and Rout, N.: Myocardial infarction coincident with cerebrovascular accidents in the elderly. Age Ageing *6*:29, 1977.
285. Gillum, R. F., Fortmann, S. P., Prineas, R. J., and Kottke, T. E.: International diagnostic criteria for acute myocardial infarction and acute stroke. Am. Heart J. *108*:150, 1984.
286. Love, B. S., Grover-McKay, M., Biller, J., et al.: Coronary artery disease and cardiac events with asymptomatic and symptomatic cerebrovascular disease. Stroke *23*:939, 1992.
287. Scheinberg, P.: Transient ischemic attacks: An update. J. Neurol. Sci. *101*:133, 1991.
288. Davila-Roman, V. G., Barzilai, B., Waring, T. H., et al.: Atherosclerosis of the ascending aorta: Prevalence and role as an independent predictor of cerebrovascular events in cardiac patients. Stroke *25*:2010, 1994.
289. Sandok, B. A., Whisnant, J. P., Furlan, A. J., and Mickell, J. L.: Carotid arterial bruits. Mayo Clin. Proc. *57*:224, 1982.
290. Heyman, A., Wilkinson, W. E., Heyden, S., et al.: Risk of stroke in asymptomatic persons with cervical arterial bruits. N. Engl. J. Med. *302*:838, 1980.
291. Sundt, T. M. Jr., Whisnant, J. P., Houser, O. W., and Fode, N. C.: Prospective study of the effectiveness and durability of carotid endarterectomy. Mayo Clin. Proc. *65*:625, 1990.
292. Barnett, H. J. M., Eliasziw, M., and Meldrum, H. E.: Drugs and surgery in the prevention of ischemic stroke. N. Engl. J. Med. *332*:238, 1995.
293. Moore, W. S., Barnett, H. J. M., Beebe, H. G., et al.: Guidelines for carotid endarterectomy: A multidisciplinary consensus statement from the ad hoc committee, American Heart Association. Circulation *91*:566, 1995.
294. Busuttil, R. W., Baker, J. D., Davidson, R. K., and Machleder, H. I.: Carotid arterial stenosis: Hemodynamic significance and clinical course. JAMA *245*:1438, 1981.
295. Matchar, D. B.: Decision making in the face of uncertainty: The case of carotid endarterectomy. Mayo Clin. Proc. *65*:756, 1990.
296. Chang, B. B., Darling, C., Shah, D. M., et al.: Carotid endarterectomy can be safely performed with an acceptable mortality and morbidity in patients requiring coronary artery bypass grafts. Am. J. Surg. *168*:94, 1994.
297. Kaul, T. K., Fields, B. L., Wyatt, D. A., et al.: Surgical management in patients with coexisting coronary and cerebrovascular disease. Chest *106*:1349, 1994.
298. Kouchoukos, N. T., Daily, B. B., Wareing, T. H., and Murphy, S. F.:

Hypothermic circulatory arrest for cerebral protection during combined carotid and cardiac surgery in patients with bilateral carotid artery disease. Ann. Surg. *219*:699, 1994.
299. Vermeulen, F. E. E., Hamerlijnck, R. P. H. M., Defau, H. A. M., and Ernest, S. M. G. P.: Synchronous operation for ischemic cardiac and cerebrovascular disease: Early results and long-term follow-up. Ann. Thorac. Surg. *53*:381, 1992.
300. Breuer, A. C., Hanson, M. R., Furlan, A. J., et al.: Central nervous system complications of myocardial revascularization: A prospective analysis of 400 patients. Stroke *11*:136, 1980.
301. Gonzalez-Scarano, F., and Hurtig, H. I.: Neurologic complications of coronary artery bypass grafting: Case-control study. Neurology *31*:1032, 1981.
302. Bojar, R. M., Najafi, H., De Laria, G. A., et al.: Neurological complications of coronary revascularization. Ann. Thorac. Surg. *36*:427, 1983.
303. Sotaniemi, K. A.: Brain damage and neurological outcome after open heart surgery. J. Neurol. Neurosurg. Psychiatr. *43*:127, 1980.
304. Ferry, P. C.: Neurologic sequelae of cardiac surgery in children. Am. J. Dis. Child. *141*:309, 1987.
305. Cardiogenic brain embolism: Cerebral embolism task force. Arch. Neurol. *43*:71, 1986.
306. Hart, R. G.: Cardiogenic embolism to the brain. Lancet *339*:589, 1992.
307. Kopecky, S. L., Gersh, B. J., McGoon, M. D., et al.: The natural history of lone atrial fibrillation. N. Engl. J. Med. *317*:669, 1987.
308. Stroke Prevention in Atrial Fibrillation Study Group Investigators: Preliminary report of the stroke prevention in atrial fibrillation study. N. Engl. J. Med. *322*:863, 1990.
309. Maladies attributed to myxomatous mitral valve. Circulation *83*:328, 1991.
310. Perloff, J. K., and Child, J. S.: Clinical and epidemiological issues in mitral valve prolapse. Am. Heart J. *113*:1324, 1987.
311. Wolf, P. A., and Sila, C. A.: Cerebral ischemia with mitral valve prolapse. Am. Heart J. *113*:1308, 1987.
312. Yufe, R., Karpati, G., and Carpenter, S.: Cardiac myxoma: A diagnostic challenge for the neurologist. Neurology *26*:1060, 1976.
313. Perloff, J. K.: The Clinical Recognition of Congenital Heart Disease. 4th ed. Philadelphia, W. B. Saunders Co., 1994, p. 302.
314. Selky, A. K., and Roos, K. L.: Neurologic complications of infective endocarditis. Semin. Neurol. *12*:225, 1992.
315. Tunkel, A. R., and Kaye, D.: Neurologic complications of infective endocarditis. Neurol. Clin. *11*:419, 1993.
316. Kanter, M. C., and Hart, R. G.: Neurologic complications of infective endocarditis. Neurology *41*:1015, 1991.
317. Kaeyser, D. L., Biller, J., Coffman, T. T., and Adams, H. P.: Neurologic complications of late prosthetic valve endocarditis. Stroke *21*:472, 1990.
318. Meyer, F. B., Morita, A., Puumala, M. R., and Nichols, D. A.: Medical and surgical management of intracranial aneurysms. Mayo Clin. Proc. *70*:153, 1995.
319. Fujishima, S., Okada, Y., Irie, K., et al.: Multiple brain infarction and hemorrhage by nonbacterial thrombotic endocarditis in occult lung cancer. Angiology *45*:161, 1994.
320. Caplan, L. R., Hier, D. B., and Banks, G.: Stroke and drug abuse. Curr. Concepts Cerebrovasc. Dis. *17*:9, 1982.

COEXISTING CEREBROVASCULAR AND CORONARY HEART DISEASE

321. Biller, J., Johnson, M. R., Adams, H. P. Jr., et al.: Further observations on cerebral or retinal ischemia in patients with right-left intracardiac shunts. Arch. Neurol. *44*:740, 1987.
322. Lechat, P., Mas, J. L., Lascault, G., et al.: Prevalence of patent foramen ovale in patients with stroke. N. Engl. J. Med. *318*:1148, 1988.
323. Harvey, J. R., Teague, S. M., Anderson, J. L., et al.: Clinically silent atrial septal defects with evidence for cerebral embolization. Ann. Intern. Med. *105*:695, 1986.
324. Cabanes, L., Mas, J. L., Cohen, A., et al.: Atrial septal aneurysm and patent foramen ovale as risk factors for cryptogenic stroke in patients less than 55 years of age. Stroke *24*:1865, 1993.
324a. Stone, D. A., Godard, J., Corretti, M. C., et al.: Patent foramen ovale: Association between the degree of shunt by contrast transesophageal echocardiography and the risk of future ischemic neurologic events. Am. Heart J. *131*:158, 1996.
325. Perloff, J. K.: Congenital heart disease and pregnancy. Clin. Cardiol. *17*:579, 1994.
326. Karnik, R., Stollberger, C., Valentin, A., et al.: Detection of patent foramen ovale by transcranial contrast Doppler ultrasound. Am. J. Cardiol. *69*:560, 1992.
327. Hagen, P. T., Scholz, D. G., and Edwards, W. D.: Incidence and size of patent foramen ovale during the first ten decades of life: An autopsy study of 965 normal hearts. Mayo Clin. Proc. *59*:17, 1984.
328. Schneider, B., Hanrath, P., Vogel, P., and Meinertz, T.: Improved morphologic characterization of atrial septal aneurysm by transesophageal echocardiography: Relation to cerebrovascular events. J. Am. Coll. Cardiol. *16*:1000, 1990.
329. Dodge, R. P., Richardson, E. P., and Victor, M.: Recurrent convulsive seizures as a sequel to cerebral infarction. Brain *77*:610, 1959.
330. Rosenberg, M., Wang, C., Hoffman-Wilde, S., and Hickman, D.: Results of cardiopulmonary resuscitation. Arch. Intern. Med. *153*:1370, 1993.
331. McIntyre, K. M.: Failure of "predictors" of cardiopulmonary resuscitation outcomes to predict cardiopulmonary resuscitation outcomes. Arch. Intern. Med. *153*:1293, 1993.
332. Bircher, N. G.: Neurologic management following cardiac arrest. Neurol. Crit. Care *5*:773, 1989.
333. Bircher, N. G.: Brain resuscitation. Resuscitation *18*:S1, 1989.
334. Orlando, R. C., Moyer, P., and Barnett, T. B.: Methysergide therapy and constrictive pericarditis. Ann. Intern. Med. *88*:213, 1978.
335. Bana, D. S., MacNeal, P. S., LeCompte P. M., et al.: Cardiac murmurs and endocardial fibrosis associated with methysergide therapy. Am. Heart J. *88*:640, 1974.
336. Dorne, H. L., and Satin, R.: Methysergide-induced lower extremity arterial insufficiency. J. Can. Assoc. Radiol. *37*:210, 1986.
337. Yahr, M. D.: Parkinsonism. *In* Rowland, L. P. (ed.): Merritt's Textbook of Neurology, 7th ed. Philadelphia, Lea and Febiger, 1984, p. 526.
338. Francis, D. A., Heron, J. R., and Clarke, M.: Ambulatory electrocardiographic monitoring in patients with transient focal cerebral ischaemia. J. Neurol. Neurosurg. Psychiatr. *47*:256, 1984.
339. de Prada, J. A. V., Nartin-Duran, R., Garcia-Monco, C., et al.: Cyclosporine neurotoxicity in heart transplantation. J. Heart Lung Transplant *9*:581, 1990.
340. McManus, R. P., O'Hair, D. P., Schweiger, S., et al.: Cyclosporine-associated central neurotoxicity after heart transplantation. Ann. Thorac. Surg. *53*:326, 1992.
341. Hotson, J. R., and Enzmann, D.R.: Neurologic complications of cardiac transplantation. Neurol. Clin. *6*:349, 1988.
342. Ang, L. C., Gillett, J. M., and Kaufmann, J. C. E.: Neuropathology of heart transplantation. Can. J. Neurol. Sci. *16*:291, 1989.
343. Benorvitz, N. L.: Clinical applications of the pharmacokinetics of lidocaine. Cardiovasc. Clin. *6*:77, 1974.
344. Weidler, D. J., Jallad, N. S., Keener, D. B., et al.: The effects of acute focal cerebral ischemia on digoxin toxicity and pharmacokinetics. Pharmacology *20*:188, 1980.
345. Withering, W.: An Account of the Foxglove. *In* Willius, F. A., and Keys, T. E.: Classics of Cardiology. Vol. 1. Malabar, Fla., Robert E. Krieger Publishing Co., 1983, p. 244.
346. Oliveira, J. S. M., dos Santos, J. C. M., Muccillo, G., and Ferreira, A. L.: Increased capacity of the coronary arteries in chronic Chagas' heart disease: Further support for the neurogenic pathogenetic concept. Am. Heart J. *109*:304, 1985.
347. Iosa, D., DeQuattro, V., Lee, D. D., et al.: Plasma norepinephrine in Chagas' cardioneuromyopathy: A marker of progressive dysautonomia. Am. Heart J. *117*:882, 1989.

Chapter 61
The Heart in Endocrine and Nutritional Disorders

GORDON H. WILLIAMS, LEONARD S. LILLY, ELLEN W. SEELY

ACROMEGALY 1887
Cardiovascular Manifestations 1888
Acromegalic Cardiomyopathy 1889
THYROID DISEASE 1890
Relation Between the Thyroid and the Sympathetic Nervous System 1890
Effect of Thyroid Hormone on the Heart 1891
Hyperthyroidism 1891
Hypothyroidism 1894
DISEASES OF THE ADRENAL CORTEX 1895
Cushing's Syndrome 1896
Hyperaldosteronism 1896
Adrenal Insufficiency 1897
PHEOCHROMOCYTOMA 1897
Effects of Catecholamines on the Cardiovascular System 1897
PARATHYROID DISEASE 1899
Cardiovascular Manifestations of Parathyroid Diseases 1899
DIABETES MELLITUS 1900
Cardiovascular Changes in Diabetes 1901
Treatment of Diabetes 1904
OBESITY 1905
Cardiovascular Consequences of Severe Obesity 1905
Treatment 1906
MALNUTRITION 1907
Cardiovascular Manifestations of Vitamin Deficiency 1907
HEART AND GONADAL HORMONES 1908
REFERENCES 1908

In 1835, Robert Graves described "three cases of violent and long-continued palpitation in females" with thyrotoxicosis.[1] Twenty years later, Thomas Addison reported that patients with disease of the "suprarenal capsules" had a "pulse, small and feeble . . . excessively soft and compressible." As the disease progressed, "the body wastes . . . the pulse becomes smaller and weaker, and . . . the patient at length gradually sinks and expires."[2] Thus, since the mid-19th century, it has been known that deranged hormonal secretion can significantly alter cardiovascular function. The purpose of this chapter is to summarize the more important cardiovascular manifestations of endocrine and nutritional diseases.

ACROMEGALY

The anterior pituitary gland secretes at least seven polypeptide hormones. Four (ACTH and related peptides, FSH, LH, and TSH) primarily produce their biological effect indirectly by altering hormonal secretion from a specific target gland (adrenal cortex, gonad, or thyroid). Thus, the pathophysiological manifestations of a derangement in their secretion are the same as those of their target organs and will be discussed later. There are no cardiovascular manifestations of altered prolactin secretion, but acromegaly (growth hormone excess) is associated with a number of clinical signs and symptoms related to the cardiovascular system.

ACTIONS OF GROWTH HORMONE. Growth hormone is only one of a family of peptides whose overall function is to regulate growth of the organism.[3,4] Two hormones secreted by the hypothalamus (somatotropin-releasing hormone and somatostatin) regulate the release of growth hormone from the anterior pituitary.[5,6] After growth hormone is released into the circulation, it stimulates the production of insulin-like growth factors (IGF-I and IGF-II).[7] Thus, growth hormone can exert its effect on tissues both directly and via the production of IGF-I and IGF-II.

In humans, the gene for IGF-I is located on chromosome 12 and that for IGF-II on chromosome 11 near the insulin gene. Expression of mRNAs from these genes occurs in many tissues, particularly in the fetus. They are homologues of the pro-insulin molecule and therefore have biological effects that are qualitatively similar to those of insulin.[8] Post-partum, mRNA levels are highest in the liver but also are found in a number of other tissues. IGF is synthesized in the liver in response to growth hormone and, for the most part, is bound to one of four specific binding proteins. Because the production of these binding proteins can be regulated by growth factors, they may play a functional role by producing a readily available circulating reservoir of growth factors. It is uncertain whether either or both IGFs can be produced in the absence of growth hormone, although currently available data suggest that at least IGF-II, the weaker growth-promoting hormone, may not require growth hormone for synthesis. Thus, it is likely that IGF-I (somatomedin C) may be the major final mediator of growth hormone's biological effects.[3] It feeds back on the pituitary, modifying mRNA levels in the pituitary and growth hormone secretion.[9] In this chapter, by convention the term *growth hormone effects* is used, although most of these effects are probably mediated by the insulin-like growth factors, particularly somatomedin C.

Growth hormone effects influence many metabolic processes, but the net effect is anabolic. Thus, when growth hormone is administered to a growth hormone–deficient individual, positive nitrogen balance, with retention of calcium, sodium, potassium, magnesium, and chloride, is manifest within days.[3,4]

Growth hormone also induces changes in both fat and carbohydrate metabolism.[3,4] When administered for a short time, it increases the uptake and utilization of glucose by fat cells, thus increasing lipogenesis. However, when administered over a long period, it promotes lipolysis, thus increasing plasma free fatty acid levels and their oxidation and promoting ketogenesis, particularly in diabetic patients or animals. Growth hormone reduces glucose uptake by fat and muscle cells, increases gluconeogenesis, and increases peripheral resistance to insulin; as a consequence, plasma glucose levels rise. Because of this reduced tissue uptake of glucose and the increased blood levels of free fatty acids and ketones, those tissues, like the myocardium, that are able to use these latter compounds as energy substrates do so. Interestingly, if IGF-I is administered to patients with non–insulin-dependent diabetes mellitus, glycemic control improves and insulin sensitivity increases, in contrast to the effects of growth hormone administration.[11] Thus, it is unclear what mediates the reduced insulin sensitivity associated with excess growth hormone production. Growth hormone also increases the synthesis and/or accumulation of sulfated mucopolysaccharides in connective tissue.

EFFECT OF GROWTH HORMONE AND SOMATOSTATIN ON THE HEART. Animal studies have clarified both the acute and chronic effects of growth hormone administration. Growth hormone or IGF-I induces the expression of genes for specific contractile proteins and also those responsible for myocyte hypertrophy. Growth hormone also increases the force of contraction and shifts the myosin form to the low ATPase activity V_3 isoform[10] (see p. 406). Short-term administration of growth hormone to normal subjects, which produces changes in growth hormone levels similar to those observed in patients with mild acromegaly, increases heart rate and myocardial contractility, the latter reflected in fractional shortening of the left ventricle and mean circumferential shortening of velocity, determined by echocardiography.[12] There is no effect on mean arterial blood pressure. In adults with growth hormone deficiency, replacement therapy also modifies cardiac function, but the changes differ from those observed in normal subjects given growth hormone. Left ventricular mass, stroke volume, and cardiac output increase significantly, whereas total peripheral resistance and arterial pressure decrease. However, systolic blood pressure does not change either at rest or during exercise.[13]

Somatostatin has an effect on the heart beyond that induced by its effect on growth hormone secretion. Infusion of somatostatin causes bradycardia and a fall in cardiac output. Furthermore, in some cases of supraventricular arrhythmias somatostatin administration restores sinus rhythm.[14] Finally, cardiac nerves have been shown to contain somatostatin, suggesting that this hormone may be an important physiological regulator of cardiac conduction.[15]

CLINICAL AND BIOCHEMICAL MANIFESTATIONS. Acromegaly is almost invariably the result of a growth hormone–producing chromophobic or eosinophilic pituitary adenoma, although rarely it may be secondary to ectopic production of growth hormone or somatotropin-releasing hormone.[16,17]

A derangement in carbohydrate metabolism is the most common metabolic consequence of chronic overproduction of growth hormone. Impaired glucose tolerance is found in half the patients, and hyperinsulinism is present in nearly all; thus a state of insulin resistance exists. However, clinical diabetes mellitus is present in only 20 to 30 per cent of patients, which suggests that only those who are predisposed and have limited insulin reserve actually develop overt disease.[16] The insulin-resistant state also may contribute to other features of the disease, e.g., the hypertension. Nearly three-quarters of the subjects are overweight. Thus, it might be anticipated that hyperlipidemia would be common in acromegaly. Yet, it is in fact infrequently observed except in patients with clinical diabetes mellitus.[3,4,17] Even in these patients, it is probably secondary to the decreased secretion of insulin rather than to the increased secretion of growth hormone.

Cardiovascular Manifestations

The cardiac manifestations of acromegaly include cardiac enlargement that is greater than would be anticipated for the generalized organomegaly. In addition, the frequency of a number of other cardiovascular disorders is increased in acromegaly: hypertension, premature coronary artery disease, congestive heart failure, and cardiac arrhythmias, particularly frequent ventricular premature beats and intraventricular conduction defects.[10,18] Indeed, because of the frequent occurrence of congestive heart failure and cardiac arrhythmias in patients who otherwise have no predisposing factors (e.g., no hypertension or arteriosclerosis), it has been suggested that a specific acromegalic cardiomyopathy exists[19] (see below).

CARDIOMEGALY. Nearly all patients with acromegaly have cardiomegaly (Fig. 61–1), particularly after the fifth decade.[10,18,20] Echocardiographic assessment suggests that frequently there is an increase in cardiac mass, particularly asymmetrical septal hypertrophy, and in a sizable minority left ventricular dilatation and a reduced ejection fraction.[18,20,21] Although the cardiomegaly may be related to the generalized effect of growth hormone on protein synthesis, some data suggest that other factors may also be important. For example, enlargement of the heart is often greater than that of other organs. Furthermore, there is no direct relationship between the degree of cardiomegaly and the level of circulating growth hormone.[18,20] Although there is a correlation between the duration of acromegaly and the severity of cardiac hypertrophy,[19] other factors that may be important in the genesis of cardiomegaly include hypertension and atherosclerosis, both of which occur with increased frequency in acromegaly. Focal cardiac interstitial fibrosis and a myocarditis with lymphocytic infiltrate also have been reported in the majority of cases.[10,19] The former is probably due to the effect of growth hormone on collagen synthesis. Additionally, small-vessel disease of the myocardium occasionally may be present.[19] The resultant dysfunction in cardiac contraction secondary to any of these pathological changes could also contribute to the cardiac enlargement. Finally, the cardiomyopathy characteristic of acromegaly may also contribute to the cardiomegaly.

HYPERTENSION. This is the most common cardiovascular manifestation of acromegaly, occurring in 25 to 50 per cent of patients if individuals with hypopituitarism are excluded. Hypertensive acromegalic patients tend to be older and to have had their acromegaly longer than nonhypertensive acromegalic patients. The underlying pathophysiology is uncertain. However, the hypertension usually is mild, uncomplicated, and readily responsive to drugs.[17] Most investigators either have searched for factors other than growth hormone that could cause hypertension or have attempted to determine how growth hormone itself may produce hypertension. In many respects, in patients with acromegaly there appears to be volume expansion; the presence of an increase in glomerular filtration rate, renal plasma flow, extracellular fluid volume and sodium space, and reduction in plasma renin activity all support this hypothesis.[4,22–24] Indeed, there is a striking increase in plasma volume in active acromegaly that is reduced following treatment.

A number of studies have suggested that growth hormone itself may be responsible for the hypertension. Thus, pituitary irradiation or hypophysectomy significantly reduces arterial pressure in hypertensive acromegalic patients, even when full glucocorticoid replacement is carried out, unless growth hormone levels are not normalized.[20] Indeed, the apparent volume expansion may be directly related to the elevated growth hormone levels because administration of growth hormone can produce retention of sodium, expansion of extracellular fluid volume, and abnormalities in white blood cell sodium transport.[25] It has been proposed that the pathophysiology of the hypertension in acromegaly may be similar to that in essential hypertension. In both conditions, there may be initial elevation of cardiac output secondary to expansion of extracellular fluid volume (see Chap. 26). This could elevate arterial pressure and lead ultimately to changes in the peripheral vasculature producing fixed hypertension.

ATHEROSCLEROSIS. In view of the alterations in carbohydrate and lipid metabolism caused by growth hormone (see above) as well as the high incidence of hypertension, it is not surprising that premature atherosclerosis occurs in pa-

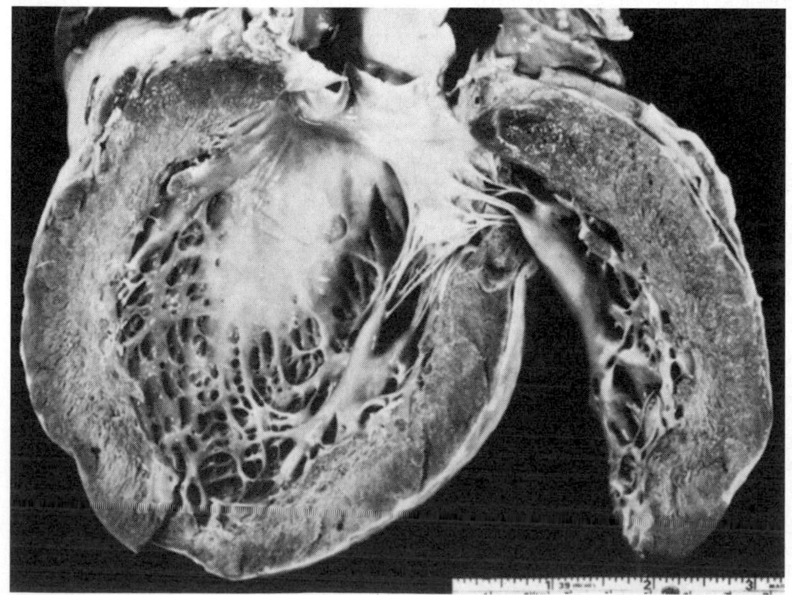

FIGURE 61–1. Opened left ventricle of the heart of an acromegalic patient showing the marked dilatation and hypertrophy, with fibrosis in the left septal endocardium. (From Rossi, L., et al.: Dysrhythmias and sudden death in acromegalic heart disease. A clinicopathologic study. Chest *72*:496, 1977.)

tients with acromegaly. What is uncertain is its frequency.[19] Coronary atherosclerosis could also contribute to the cardiomegaly observed in these patients.

Acromegalic Cardiomyopathy

Some patients with acromegaly without evidence of hypertension or atherosclerosis have significant cardiac dysfunction.[19] They primarily have cardiomegaly, congestive heart failure, and/or cardiac dysrhythmias[10,26]; the congestive heart failure is particularly resistant to conventional therapy. It has been suggested that these are manifestations of an acromegalic cardiomyopathy which is related to the higher collagen content per gram of heart than in normal myocardium.[19] Histological observations show cellular hypertrophy, patchy fibrosis, and myofibrillar degeneration (Fig. 61–2). Sudden death has been associated with inflammatory and degenerative damage to the sinoatrial perinodal nerve plexus and degeneration of the AV node.

It is not clear whether acromegalic cardiomyopathy is a specific entity. The evidence favoring this view, although indirect, comes from five types of observations: (1) Nearly 50 per cent of acromegalic patients have electrocardiographic abnormalities.[26,27] The most common findings are ST-segment depression with or without T-wave abnormalities, patterns consistent with left ventricular hypertrophy, intraventricular conduction disturbances—specifically, bundle branch block—and, supraventricular or ventricular ectopic rhythms. Indeed, in one controlled study, 48 per cent of acromegalic patients had Lown grade III or IV complex ventricular arrhythmias, compared with 12 per cent of normal subjects. Although no correlation has been found between the severity of ventricular arrhythmias and growth hormone levels, the frequency of premature ventricular contractions increases with the duration of acromegaly.[26] Although hypertension or signs of atherosclerosis are present in many, 10 to 20 per cent of patients with acromegaly and electrocardiographic changes have no evidence of these conditions. (2) Ten to 20 per cent of acromegalics have overt congestive heart failure. In perhaps a fourth of these there is no known predisposing cause. (3) The majority of patients with acromegaly but without hypertension or atherosclerosis have subclinical evidence for cardiac, particularly diastolic, dysfunction.[18] (4) Approximately half of all patients with acromegaly, including patients without hypertension, have echocardiographic evidence of left and right ventricular hypertrophy.[18,29,30] These patients have growth hormone levels that are significantly higher than those of patients without left ventricular hypertrophy. Half of the patients with left ventricular hypertrophy exhibit asymmetrical septal hypertrophy, and these patients have a significantly greater percentage of internal dimensional shortening during systole than either the patients with concentric hypertrophy or those without left ventricular hypertrophy.

(5) The most compelling evidence for a specific effect of growth hormone hypersecretion inducing cardiac abnormalities comes from the impact of administration of a somatostatin analog, octreotide, which inhibits secretion of growth hormone on cardiac function. In one study, seven patients with acromegaly, three of whom had refractory congestive heart failure, were given octreotide subcutaneously three times daily. Right heart catheterization performed before and after 3 months of therapy showed an 18 per cent increase in stroke volume and a return of the cardiac index to normal. Within 40 days of treatment, the three patients with congestive heart failure had a dramatic clinical improvement, which was sustained for up to 3 years.[31] In a second study, within 1 week of initiating octreotide therapy, left ventricular mass was reduced, as assessed by echocardiography.[32] In a third study in 11 normotensive patients with active acromegaly, 6 months of octreotide therapy produced a significant reduction in left ventricular mass index, mean wall thickness, and isovolumic relaxation time, as well as a significant increase in the ratio of early to late peak velocity of right ventricular filling. This improvement in diastolic function was not accompanied by significant differences in systolic function indices.[33] However, improvement in left ventricular function does not universally occur following correction of the excess growth hormone production. In some patients who have had longstanding active acromegaly, left ventricular

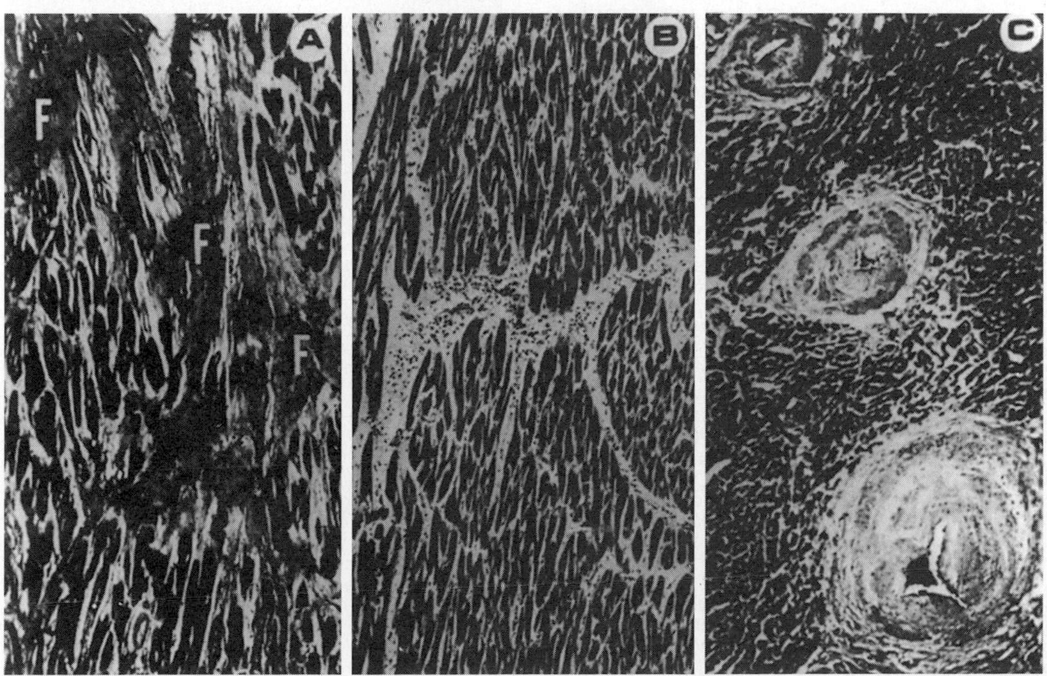

FIGURE 61–2. Histopathological features of acromegalic heart disease. *A*, Nonspecific myocardial hypertrophy and interstitial fibrosis (F). *B*, Myocarditis with predominantly lymphomononuclear cell infiltrate. *C*, Small-vessel disease (proliferative fibrous wall thickening) or intramural coronary artery branches. (Reproduced with permission from Lie, J. T.: Acromegaly and heart disease. Primary Cardiol. *7*:53, 1981. Copyright PW Communications, Inc.)

filling abnormalities may be only partly reversible. In these patients, presumably nonreversible interstitial fibrosis prevents the correction of the growth hormone–induced cardiomyopathy.[34]

DIAGNOSIS AND TREATMENT

The *diagnosis* of acromegaly is established by documenting the nonsuppressibility of serum growth hormone levels following glucose loading.[3,4] In most laboratories, growth hormone concentrations in normal subjects are less than 2 ng/ml 120 minutes after the oral administration of 100 gm of glucose. It is also important to evaluate the integrity of the other pituitary hormones, and, in hypertensive patients, to rule out an associated pheochromocytoma or aldosteronoma. The presence of sinus tachycardia or atrial fibrillation in a patient with acromegaly warrants a careful search for coexisting hyperthyroidism.

Surgery and irradiation remain the mainstays of treatment. The surgical approach is more often transsphenoidal rather than transfrontal; heavy particle (proton beam) instead of conventional irradiation is often used.[3] Because of the delayed reduction in growth hormone levels with the latter method, progression of cardiovascular disease in acromegalics continues even though growth hormone levels are falling if they are not normal.[20] The secretion of growth hormone can be suppressed in some acromegalics with the dopamine agonist bromocriptine and somatostatin, the latter with considerable success.[31–33] Whether these agents have any effect on tumor growth, however, is unclear.

Acromegalic patients with cardiovascular abnormalities usually respond to conventional therapeutic measures for hypertension, heart failure, and arrhythmias. Two caveats: (1) those with hypertension appear to be particularly responsive to volume-depleting maneuvers, i.e., diuretics and sodium restriction, perhaps even more so than patients with essential hypertension; (2) on the other hand, some patients with congestive heart failure, primarily those *without* underlying hypertensive heart disease (i.e., those who are considered to have acromegalic cardiomyopathy), appear to be particularly resistant to therapy.

THYROID DISEASE

Thyroid hormone has a profound effect on a number of metabolic processes in virtually all tissues, with the heart being particularly sensitive to its effects. Therefore, it is not surprising that thyroid dysfunction can produce dramatic cardiovascular effects, often mimicking primary cardiac disease.

ACTION OF THYROID HORMONE. Two biologically active hormones are secreted by the thyroid: thyroxine (T_4) and tri-iodothyronine (T_3). Most studies support the hypothesis that T_3 is the final mediator and that T_4 is a prohormone, primarily because of the universal presence of T_3 but not T_4 nuclear receptors in tissues responsive to thyroid hormone, specifically the heart.[35–38]

Nuclear-Mediated Effects of Thyroid Hormone. Investigations over the past decade have established that the majority of thyroid hormone's effects are mediated via a change in expression of responsive genes. This process begins with the diffusion of T_4 and T_3 across the plasma membrane because of their lipid solubility. In the cytosol, T_4 is converted into T_3 by the action of 5′ monodeiodinase, the concentration of which varies from tissue to tissue in direct relationship to the tissue's responsiveness to thyroid hormone. Then the circulating and newly synthesized T_3 passes through the nuclear membrane to bind to specific thyroid hormone receptors (THRs), which are attached to chromatin tissue. The THR is part of the nuclear receptor superfamily of proteins, which also include proteins that act as receptors for steroids, vitamin D, and retinoic acid.

There are at least two thyroid hormone receptor genes—one located on chromosome 17 and the other on chromosome 3. The predominant THR form in the heart is the alpha-1, whereas the predominant receptor form in the pituitary and liver is the beta isoform. Several other isoforms also have been reported, the functions of which are unclear.[39] The thyroid hormone receptor is located almost exclusively within the nucleus. After interacting with T_3 and other protein transcription factors, the entire complex binds to thyroid response elements (TREs) located on the promoter region on specific genes (for additional details, the reader is referred to the review by Tsai and O'Malley[40]).

Thyroid hormone's effect on the synthesis of specific proteins can be either direct or indirect. Indirect effects include a change in production of an intermediate factor necessary for the function or activity of a more distant targeted protein. Thyroid hormone can have a positive or negative effect on regulating gene transcription. Positive effects have been documented for the following genes: myosin heavy-chain alpha[41]; Ca^{2+} ATPase[42]; Na^+, K^+-ATPase[43]; beta$_1$-adrenergic receptor[44]; glucose transporter (Glut-4)[45]; cardiac troponin I[46,47]; and atrial natriuretic protein.[48] Thyroid hormone also can negatively regulate genes, e.g., myosin heavy-chain beta and the glucose transporter Glut-1, at least neonatally.[45]

Thyroid Extranuclear Actions. Whereas the predominant effects of thyroid hormone are via its effect in regulating gene expression as noted above, there has been clear documentation that thyroid hormone also has extranuclear effects. For example, T_3 increases both glucose and calcium uptake by the heart. Although some of these effects could be nuclear-mediated events, some studies suggest that thyroid hormone must also have a membrane effect. Evidence supporting this includes the rapid onset (for calcium uptake, maximum effect is achieved within 30 seconds); independence from new protein synthesis; and thyroid hormone specificity in that analogs of thyroid hormone which have no biological effect do not produce similar changes.[37,49,50]

In summary, thyroid hormone's nuclear and extranuclear effects on the heart lead to changes in the proportion of myosin heavy chain protein from beta to alpha, thereby increasing myosin V_1 and decreasing myosin V_3 isoenzyme levels (see p. 363), leading to an increased velocity of contraction and diastolic relaxation. It also increases transcription of the calcium ATPase gene. Extranuclear effects include thyroid hormone's direct effect on calcium current and cytosolic calcium changes induced by inotropic factors, including isoproterenol and external calcium concentration.[51,52]

As a secondary event, thyroid hormone also increases ATP consumption. However, less of the chemical energy is used in the contractile process and more is dissipated as heat, resulting in less efficient myocardial metabolism.[35,51,52]

RELATION BETWEEN THE THYROID AND THE SYMPATHETIC NERVOUS SYSTEM

While the effects of thyroid hormone on the heart are varied and complex, it has been proposed that some of them are indirect, being secondary to changes in the activity of the sympathetic nervous system (Table 61–1). For example, many of the cardiovascular effects of hyperthyroidism, i.e., tachycardia, systolic hypertension, increased cardiac output, and myocardial contractility, can be abolished or re-

TABLE 61–1 CLINICAL FEATURES OF HYPERTHYROIDISM

DIRECT THYROID HORMONE EFFECT†	BETA-ADRENERGIC-LIKE EFFECT†
Resting heart rate > 90/min (90%)	Resting heart rate > 90/min (90%)
Palpitations (85%)	Palpitations (85%)
Atrial fibrillation (10%)	Exertional dyspnea (80%)
Pedal edema (30%)	Increased pulse pressure (systolic hypertension)
Increased oxygen consumption (basal metabolism)	Active apical impulse
Weight loss	Loud first heart sound and pulmonic component of second heart sound
Skeletal muscle myopathy	Midsystolic murmur, usually basal
Increased bone turnover (occasional osteoporosis or hypercalcemia)	Third heart sound (occasional)
Fair skin	Means-Lerman scratch (rare)‡
Fine brittle hair	Tremor
Brittle nails	Brisk reflexes
Oligomenorrhea or amenorrhea	Increased perspiration
Increased bowel frequency	Heat intolerance
	Insomnia
	Anxiety
	Stare, lid lag§

The numbers in parentheses are approximate prevalences of the findings, compiled from several large series. Goiter is almost always present, although in elderly patients the thyroid enlargement may be minimal or absent.

† Both types of effects contribute to the tachycardia and palpitations.

‡ A systolic scratch or click in the second left intercostal space that is probably generated by the pleura and pericardium rubbing together.

§ These reflect upper-lid retraction. Infiltrative ophthalmyopathy with exophthalmos is found only when Graves' disease is the cause of the hyperthyroidism and is not related to the hyperthyroid state per se.

Reproduced with permission from Kaplan, M. M.: The thyroid and the heart: How do they interact? J. Cardiovasc. Med. *7*:893, 1982.

duced by blocking the activity of the sympathetic nervous system.[53] It has been proposed that thyroid hormone may alter the relationship between the sympathetic nervous and cardiovascular systems, either by increasing the activity of the sympathoadrenal system or by enhancing the response of cardiac tissue to normal sympathetic stimulation.[54] Also, it has been suggested that sympathetic stimuli merely exert a direct additive effect on cardiovascular function above that produced by thyroid hormone. On the other hand, there is also evidence that hyperthyroidism reduces the sensitivity of cardiac tissue to sympathetic stimuli.[55]

Thus the results of experiments on the relationship between the sympathoadrenal system and hyperthyroidism have evoked considerable controversy. Three areas have been explored in an attempt to unravel the conflicting data: thyroid hormone's effect on adrenergic output; thyroid hormone's effect on adrenergic receptors; and thyroid hormone's action on adrenergic transduction mechanisms. The plasma and urine levels of norepinephrine, epinephrine, dopamine, and beta-hydroxylase are either low or normal in hyperthyroidism and either normal or elevated in hypothyroidism.[56] These data suggest that the sympathomimetic features of hyperthyroidism cannot be due simply to an overall increase in adrenergic activity but rather are due to a change in the affinity of catecholamines for their receptors or to a modification of a postreceptor mechanism. Previously such changes were difficult to document, primarily because thyroid hormone appears to have different effects on adrenoceptors in different tissues. For example, the effect of thyroid hormone in the rat liver is different from that in the rat heart. Thyroid hormones reduce beta-adrenoceptor number in the rat liver, and hypothyroid animals show an increase in these receptors.[57] In contrast, in the rat heart, which has been the organ most extensively studied, administration of thyroid hormone causes both an increase in the number of receptors and their affinity for their ligand, while hypothyroidism induces the opposite effect.[54,58] Finally is the documentation that thyroid hormone increases the mRNA level for the beta$_1$-adrenergic receptor.[44]

These changes in receptor number and affinity lead to appropriate changes in sensitivity of the myocardium to beta-adrenoceptor agonists. For example, stimulation of adenylate cyclase activity by isoproterenol is increased in hyperthyroidism and reduced in hypothyroidism. Finally, there are also changes in the force of contraction with increased sensitivity of the ventricular muscle to isoproterenol-induced contraction in hyperthyroidism and reduction in hypothyroidism.[54] That this effect is specific is shown by an unaltered change in calcium-stimulated contractility in hypothyroid animals. These effects were also observed in vivo in dogs in which propranolol-induced reductions of heart rate and myocardial contractility were greater in hyperthyroid than in euthyroid animals.[59]

Further support comes from the study by Guarnieri et al., who showed that hyperthyroid rats have enhanced activation of protein kinase and contractile response following administration of a threshold dose of the beta-adrenoceptor agonist isoproterenol.[60] In the aforementioned study in conscious hyperthyroid dogs,[59] however, no alteration in the sensitivity of the inotropic response to isoproterenol and norepinephrine was found.

Circulating blood elements have also provided additional evidence in support of the concept that thyroid hormone "up-regulates" beta-adrenoceptors. When patients are used as their own control, both the number of beta-adrenoceptors and the sensitivity of adenylate cyclase to isoproterenol stimulation in mononuclear cells are increased by thyroid hormone.[61] Additionally, in circulating reticulocytes of hypothyroid animals, the number of receptors is decreased.[62]

The evidence supporting an additional effect of thyroid hormone in modifying the transduction mechanisms mediating adrenergic effects is less clear. In cultured developing rat myocardial cells, the addition of T_3 increased the level of $G_{s\alpha}$ protein while reducing $G_{i\alpha}$ and the β subunits of G proteins. These results suggest that thyroid hormone elevates G protein subunits that activate adenylate cyclase and suppresses those that inhibit it. However, Levine et al. could not document an effect of thyroid hormone on $G_s\alpha$ subunits using adult rat ventricles, although an apparent inhibitory effect of thyroid hormone on $G_{i\alpha}$ 2 and 3, and $G\beta$ 1 and 2 protein, polypeptide, and mRNA levels was confirmed.[64] Similar effects have been reported for adipose tissue,[65] probably explaining the reduced lipolytic response to catecholamines in hypothyroidism.[66] Thus, thyroid hormone has a complex interaction with the adrenergic nervous system. Hyperthyroidism increases the number, and potentially the affinity, of beta-adrenergic receptors and also modifies the intracellular G protein milieu so as to enhance the transduction potential of agonists binding to the adrenergic receptor.

Effect of Thyroid Hormone on the Heart

There is abundant evidence that thyroid hormone may alter cardiac function directly, as noted above. Additionally, the increased heart rate and myocardial contractility observed in experimental hyperthyroidism are not completely reversed by either sympathetic or parasympathetic blockade.[55,59] Finally, T_4 enhances the rate of contraction of cardiac muscle even in the presence of adrenergic blockade.[67] Right ventricular papillary muscles isolated from cats rendered hyperthyroid exhibited augmented myocardial contractility, as reflected in an upward shift of the myocardial force-velocity curve,[55] with a greatly increased velocity of myocardial fiber shortening, a reduced time to peak tension during isometric contraction, and an augmented peak tension development. Single ventricular myocytes isolated from hyperthyroid rats exhibited a marked augmentation of twitch velocity and abbreviated both the time required for contraction and relaxation.[68] Prior catecholamine depletion by pretreatment of the hyperthyroid cats with reserpine did not alter this inotropic effect of hyperthyroidism, providing further evidence for a direct cardiac effect.[55] This hypothesis has been assessed in intact conscious animals. The results suggest that the major actions of T_4 on the left ventricle are (1) a direct positive inotropic effect and (2) an increase in the size of the ventricular cavity without a change in the end-diastolic pressure or length of the sarcomere in diastole, although hypothyroidism does not necessarily impair pump function.[69]

The available data suggest that the direct effect of thyroid hormone on the heart is primarily mediated via a change in protein synthesis, as described above. Specifically, there is a change in synthesis of the myosin heavy chains from the β to the α form, thereby increasing the level of the more mobile myosin isoenzyme (V_1). With the reduction in mRNA level for the beta myosin heavy chain, the slower V_3 myosin isoform is substantially reduced. Goto et al. demonstrated in the hyperthyroid rabbit heart that the increase in myosin isoform V_1/V_3 ratio is associated with decreased contractile efficiency and increased energy cost of excitation-contraction coupling.[70] This change produces a less efficient system, thereby leading to more heat production per contractile response.

Thyroid hormone's effect on cardiac contractility also appears to be mediated in part by changes in intracellular calcium handling. Thyroid hormone increases the expression of the sodium-calcium ATPase, which augments transsarcolemmal calcium influx in cultured ventricular cells.[71]

In ferret ventricular muscle, hypothyroidism reduces peak tension and prolongs the duration of contraction in association with changes in cytosolic calcium that are decreased and prolonged in relation to ventricular muscle obtained from euthyroid animals (Fig. 61–3). Hyperthyroidism produces the opposite changes. Thus, alteration in intracellular calcium handling, specifically related to recycling of calcium by the sarcoplasmic reticulum, may account for the thyroid-induced changes in myocardial contractile function.[72,73] Finally, the effect of thyroxine on myosin isoenzyme appears to be localized primarily to the ventricles, with atrial isoenzymes relatively unaltered by changes in thyroid hormone.[74] Thus, while thyroid hormone itself has a major direct effect on modifying protein synthesis, the changes in cardiac workload may also contribute. Studies using heterotrophic cardiac isografts suggest that the changes in myosin enzyme levels may in part be secondary to changes in workload.[75]

The tachycardia observed in hyperthyroidism appears to be due to a combination of an increased rate of diastolic depolarization and a decreased duration of the action potential in the sinoatrial node cells.[76] The propensity for the development of atrial fibrillation may be due to the shortened refractory period of atrial cells.[77]

Hyperthyroidism

Hyperthyroidism is the clinical state resulting from the excess production of T_3, T_4, or both. The most common cause is a diffuse toxic goiter (Graves' disease). Although the etiology of this condition is still unknown, the hyperproduction of T_4 and T_3 is thought to result from circulating IgG autoantibodies that bind to the thyrotropin receptor on the thyroid gland. The second most common form of hyperthyroidism is nodular toxic goiter, a condition in which localized areas of the gland function excessively and autonomously.[78]

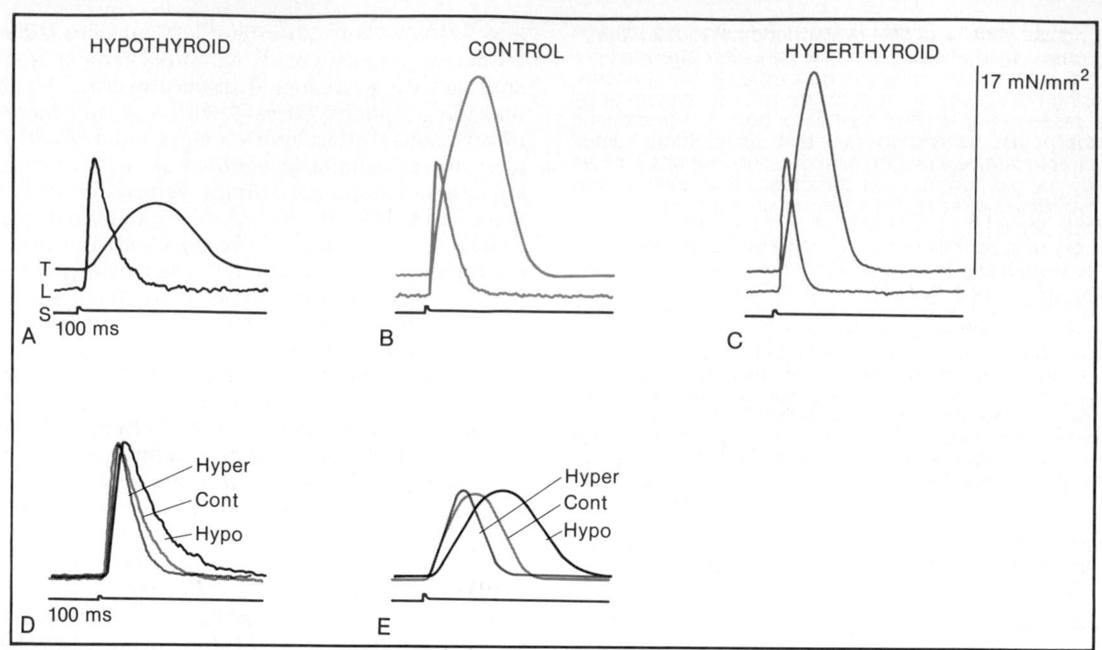

FIGURE 61–3. The thyroid state influences the time course of the isometric contraction and the Ca^{++} transient. The isometric tension (T) and the aequorin light signal, reflecting intracytoplasmic $[Ca]^{++}$ (L), were recorded from myocardium obtained from a hypothyroid *(A)*, euthyroid *(B)*, and hyperthyroid *(C)* ferret at 30°C; 0.33 Hz stimulation. I is expressed in milliNewtons/m² muscle cross-sectional area. The Ca^{++} transients (aqueorin signals) are scaled to equal amplitudes and superimposed in *D*. In *E*, the tensions have been scaled to equal amplitudes and superimposed. The time from the beginning of the stimulus sweep (S) to the stimulus represents 100 msec. (Reproduced with permission from MacKinnon, R., et al.: Modulation by the thyroid state of intracellular calcium and contractility in ferret ventricular muscle. Circ. Res. *63*:1084, 1988. Copyright 1988 American Heart Association.)

Hyperthyroidism is a relatively common disease, occurring four to eight times more commonly in women than in men, with a peak incidence in the third and fourth decades. The commonly associated signs and symptoms (Table 61–1) include fatigue, hyperactivity, insomnia, heat intolerance, palpitations, dyspnea, increased appetite with weight loss, nocturia, diarrhea, oligomenorrhea, muscle weakness, tremor, emotional lability, increased heart rate, systolic hypertension, hyperthermia, warm moist skin, lid lag, stare, and brisk reflexes. T_3 levels are invariably elevated, and serum T_4 levels are usually increased as well.

CARDIOVASCULAR MANIFESTATIONS. The heart is among the most responsive organs in thyroid disease, and cardiovascular signs and symptoms are therefore important clinical features of hyperthyroidism.[78,79] Palpitations, dyspnea, tachycardia, and systolic hypertension are common findings. Diastolic hypertension can also occur. Typically, there is a hyperactive precordium with a loud first heart sound, an accentuated pulmonic component of the second heart sound, and a third heart sound; occasionally, a systolic ejection click is heard. Midsystolic murmurs along the left sternal border are common, and a systolic scratch, the so-called Means-Lerman scratch, is occasionally heard in the second left intercostal space during expiration. It is presumed to be secondary to the rubbing together of normal pleural and pericardial surfaces by the hyperdynamic heart.

As would be anticipated, and as described on page 447, cardiac and stroke volume index, mean systolic ejection rate, velocity and extent of wall shortening (Fig. 61–4), and coronary blood flow[80] are all increased, the systolic ejection period and preejection period are abbreviated, the pulse pressure is widened, and systemic vascular resistance is reduced in hyperthyroidism.[81] The changes in left ventricular performance induced by thyroid hormone appear to be secondary to augmented contractility rather than to alterations in loading conditions or change in heart rate.[82] If the hyperthyroidism is relatively mild, many of the indices of left ventricular function are normal, with exercise needed to bring out abnormalities.[79,83] It has been suggested that many of the changes in cardiac function are secondary to the increased metabolic demands of peripheral tissue. However, the increase in cardiac output is greater than would be predicted on the basis of the increased total body oxygen consumption, supporting the view that thyroid hormone exerts a direct cardiac stimulant action independent of its effect on general tissue metabolism, as noted above. Furthermore, normalization of myocardial contractile response to exercise may not occur until several months after normalization of thyroid function.[84] However, it is likely that the overall pathological consequences associated with

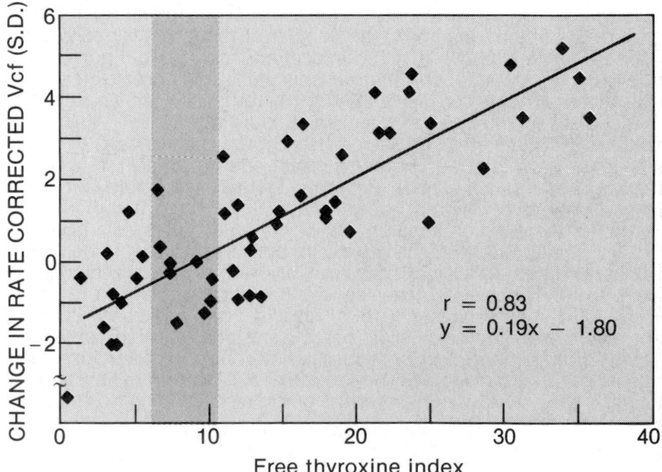

FIGURE 61–4. Rate-corrected velocity of shortening (V_{cf}) in SD units from the normal mean regression line obtained from 11 patients at varying levels of the free thyroxine index. There is a strong positive correlation between the level of thyroid hormone and the change in contractile state. The shaded area represents the normal range for serum free thyroxine index. (From Feldman, T., et al.: Myocardial mechanics in hyperthyroidism; Importance of left ventricular loading conditions, heart rate and contractile state. By permission of the American College of Cardiology. J. Am. Coll. Cardiol. *7*:972, 1986.)

thyrotoxicosis result from an interaction between the effect of thyroid hormone on the heart and its effect on the circulation (Fig. 61–5).

Roentgenographic and electrographic changes are common but are nonspecific in hyperthyroidism.[79] Thus the left ventricle, the aorta, and the pulmonary artery are prominent, and, in some cases, there is generalized cardiac enlargement, which may be accompanied by signs and symptoms of heart failure. In patients with sinus rhythm, the magnitude of the tachycardia, in general, parallels the severity of the disease. Sinus tachycardia, i.e., a rate exceeding 100 beats/min, is present in 40 per cent of patients with hyperthyroidism, occurring most frequently in the younger age groups, and often at night.[85] Fifteen to 25 per cent of patients with hyperthyroidism have persistent atrial fibrillation, which is often heralded by one or more transient episodes of this arrhythmia.[86] There is shortening of the A-V conduction time and functional refractory period, resulting in an increased frequency at which the A-V conduction system transmits rapid atrial impulses.[86] Intra-atrial conduction disturbances, manifested by prolongation or notching of the P wave and prolongation of the P-R interval in the absence of treatment with digitalis, occur in 15 per cent and 5 per cent of patients with hyperthyroidism, respectively. Occasionally, second- or third-degree heart block may result. The cause of the A-V conduction disturbance is not clear because animal experiments have shown that the functional refractory period of the A-V conduction system and the conduction time were shortened in dogs with hyperthyroidism and prolonged in dogs with hypothyroidism.[87] Intraventricular conduction disturbances, most commonly right bundle branch block, occur in about 15 per cent of patients with hyperthyroidism without associated heart disease of other etiology. Paroxysmal supraventricular tachycardia and flutter are rare in hyperthyroidism. Finally, occult thyrotoxicosis may underlie either chronic or paroxysmal isolated atrial fibrillation.[86,88]

Both angina pectoris and heart failure occur in patients with hyperthyroidism, and for many years it was assumed that these were seen only in the presence of underlying cardiovascular disease. Support for this position came primarily from the absence of these symptoms in young persons with significant hyperthyroidism. More recently, however, five lines of evidence have suggested otherwise: (1) Congestive heart failure has been produced in experimental animals by simply administering T_4. (2) Children with thyrotoxicosis without underlying cardiac disease may develop congestive heart failure.[89] (3) Angina has been reported in a hyperthyroid patient with normal coronary arteries, presumably secondary to thyroid-induced coronary artery spasm.[90] (4) Abnormal left ventricular function observed during exercise in hyperthyroid subjects is not reversed by beta blockade but is reversed by treating the hyperthyroidism.[91] (5) Finally, Ebisawa et al. reported that the cardiomyopathy in patients with thyrotoxicosis may be irreversible. Four patients with this condition had increased left ventricular end-diastolic volumes and reduced ejection fractions, even 13 to 15 years following treatment of their hyperthyroidism. Myocardial biopsies, performed in two patients, showed no specific light microscopic abnormalities.[92]

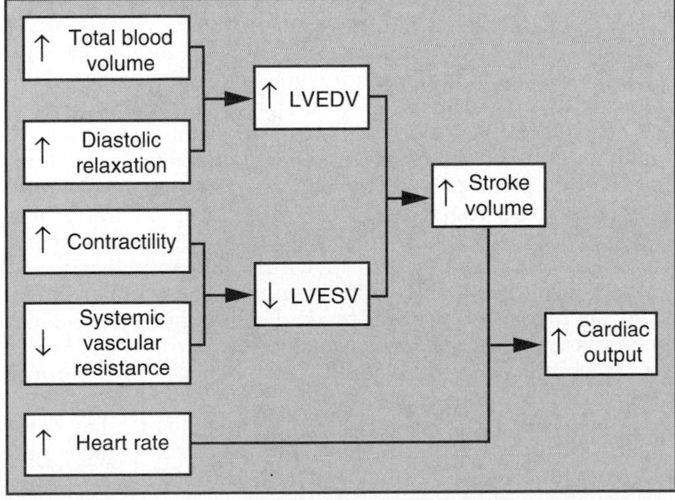

FIGURE 61–5. Cardiovascular effects of hyperthyroidism. Cardiac output is increased as a result of thyroid hormone augmentation of the hemodynamic parameters indicated in the figure. LVEDV = Left ventricular end-diastolic volume; LVESV = left ventricular end-systolic volume. (Modified from Woeber, K. A.: Thyrotoxicosis and the heart. N. Engl. J. Med. *327*:94, 1992. Copyright Massachusetts Medical Society.)

Thus, when it is severe and persistent, thyrotoxicosis can overtax even the normal heart, although, in most instances, the development of clinical manifestations of heart failure and myocardial ischemia in patients with hyperthyroidism signifies the presence of underlying cardiac or coronary vascular disease. There is also increased frequency of hyperthyroidism in patients with familial hypertrophic cardiomyopathy. In one kindred, 3 of 17 members with hypertrophic cardiomyopathy also had hyperthyroidism.[93] Finally, in one study hyperthyroidism was associated with mitral value prolapse in more than a third of cases.[94]

TREATMENT OF CARDIOVASCULAR DISEASE IN HYPERTHYROIDISM. Hyperthyroid patients with cardiovascular disease are particularly resistant to therapy. For example, it has been well documented that both heart failure and arrhythmias are resistant to conventional doses of the cardiac glycosides. Although the specific mechanisms underlying these altered responses remain obscure, they may be related to both systemic and local effects.[95] First, serum levels of cardiac glycosides are diminished in hyperthyroidism, not because there is an augmentation of its metabolism but because there is an increase in its volume of distribution. Second, experimental hyperthyroidism reduces the enhancement of the myocardial contractile force and the prolongation of the atrioventricular nodal refractory period produced by these agents.[95] Because of this decreased sensitivity to cardiac glycosides, toxicity may develop at a dose that has relatively little therapeutic effect.

DIAGNOSIS AND THERAPY OF HYPERTHYROIDISM

The diagnosis is made on the basis of a suppressed TSH level (reflecting elevated levels of thyroid hormone in the blood). Because only serum T_3 is increased in some individuals, it is important to obtain serum levels of *both* T_3 and T_4 and an index of the thyroid-binding capacity of the patient's serum (resin thyroxine uptake).

The definitive treatment of hyperthyroidism is surgical removal of the gland or irradiation using radioactive iodide. In severely ill patients, particularly those with thyroid storm or significant cardiovascular symptoms or both, neither of these therapies is appropriate. Thus, medical therapy is directed at reducing both the production and biological effect of thyroid hormone.[96] Because many of the cardiovascular symptoms of thyrotoxicosis are related to increased beta-adrenoceptor activity, treatment with beta-adrenoceptor blocking agents has been useful.[97] Tachycardia, palpitations, tremor, restlessness, muscle weakness, and heat intolerance are reversed by these agents, which offer the additional benefit of inhibiting the conversion of T_4 to the biologically active T_3 in peripheral tissues.

TREATMENT OF CARDIOVASCULAR MANIFESTATIONS OF HYPERTHYROIDISM. Prompt treatment of the hyperthyroid state can significantly reduce, if not eliminate, the associated cardiovascular symptoms. About half of patients with concurrent onset of hyperthyroidism and angina pectoris experience complete remission of this symptom after treatment of hyperthyroidism.[98,99] Furthermore, in 62 per cent of 163 thyrotoxic patients with atrial fibrillation sustained for 1 week or longer, spontaneous reversion to sinus rhythm was found when they became euthyroid.[100,101] In elderly patients with apathetic hyperthyroidism, cardiovascular manifestations, specifically atrial fibrillation and/or congestive heart failure, predominate, and therefore evaluation of thyroid function in such patients is particularly important. However, it should be noted that these individuals are particularly resistant to cardiac glycosides.

Beta blockers (see p. 502) can be administered orally or intravenously, but because these drugs interfere with the effects of sympathetic stimulation on the heart, they must be used with caution in patients with congestive heart failure. However, if the heart failure is in part related to the tachycardia, beta blockade may be beneficial.[97] Beta-blocking drugs and cardiac glycosides act synergistically to slow ventricular rate in atrial fibrillation. Correction of the basic metabolic defect requires specific therapy directed at reducing the production of thyroid hormone.[97,99] The most useful agents are the thionamides, such as propylthiouracil,[96] which inhibit thyroid hormone synthesis. Iodine inhibits the release of thyroid hormones from the thyrotoxic gland, and its beneficial effects occur more rapidly than the thionamides. It is therefore useful in the rapid amelioration of the hyperthyroid state in patients with thyroid heart disease. Ipodate may be particularly useful for this purpose.[102] Iodine may also be utilized along with antithyroid agents to control thyrotoxicosis following ^{131}I treatment until the radioactive iodide has had time to take effect. Most hyperthyroid patients, however, escape from the effects of iodide after 10 to 14 days.

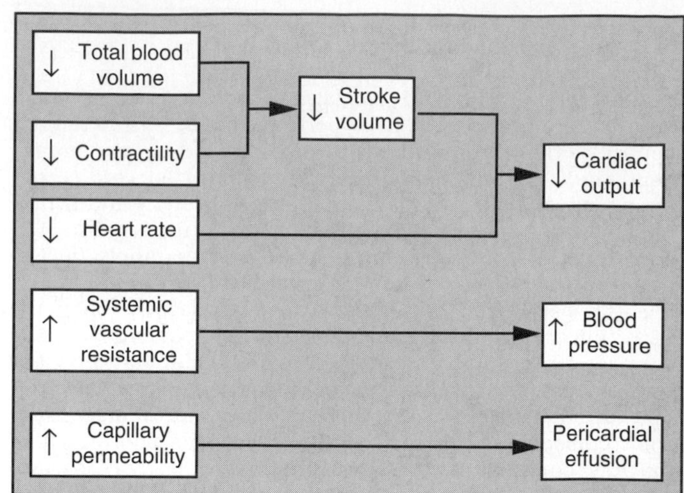

FIGURE 61–6. Cardiovascular effects of hypothyroidism. Cardiac output is decreased because of diminished total blood volume, impaired left ventricular contractility, and bradycardia. Hypertension results from increased systemic vascular resistance. Pericardial effusion results from increased capillary permeability and interstitial protein leak.

Hypothyroidism

Hypothyroidism results from reduced secretion of both T_4 and T_3, occurring in most cases as a consequence of destruction of the thyroid gland itself, usually by an inflammatory process. In some cases, it is secondary to decreased secretion of TSH, due to either pituitary or hypothalamic disease. In secondary hypothyroidism, the signs and symptoms associated with deficiency of other pituitary hormones are also usually present. The incidence of hypothyroidism peaks between the ages of 30 and 60 years, and it is twice as common in women as in men. The following signs and symptoms are common: cold intolerance, dryness of the skin, weakness, impairment of memory, personality changes, shortness of breath, constipation, hoarseness, menorrhagia and other forms of menstrual dysfunction, and, occasionally, heart failure.

EFFECTS OF AMIODARONE ON THYROID FUNCTION. The antiarrhythmic agent amiodarone (see p. 613) has three effects on thyroid function. Its first effect is to antagonize thyroid hormone action on pituitary cells by binding to the intranuclear thyroid hormone receptor, and it thereby inhibits T_3-induced changes in mRNA levels and TSH response to TRH.[103,104] Its second effect is to inhibit peripheral conversion of T_4 to T_3. Thus, in nearly all patients who receive long-term treatment with this drug, there is reduction in serum T_3 levels and a transient rise in TSH. Within a few days to weeks this causes an increase in serum T_4 levels and a return of serum TSH to normal. Clinically and metabolically, these patients are euthyroid even though their T_4 levels are elevated.[105] Amiodarone's third effect is due to its high iodide content (35 per cent by weight). Thus, when it is metabolized there is a massive increase in the available inorganic iodide, resulting in acute inhibition of thyroid organification. Depending upon the state of iodine intake before its administration, patients may develop either hypothyroidism (common in the United States) or thyrotoxicosis (more common in Europe).[105–107]

In susceptible individuals this agent can also induce a marked increase in Ia-positive T cells (an abnormality found in patients with spontaneous Graves' disease). These T-cell abnormalities disappear after discontinuation of the amiodarone. Thus, amiodarone may induce T-cell abnormalities leading to an autoimmune state.[108] Because of amiodarone's long half-life, the biochemical and clinical abnormalities can persist for months after it is stopped.

CARDIOVASCULAR MANIFESTATIONS (Fig. 61–6). The heart in overt myxedema is often pale, flabby, and grossly dilated. Histological examination discloses myofibrillar swelling, loss of striations, and interstitial fibrosis. With the early detection and treatment of hypothyroidism, the classic findings of cardiac enlargement, cardiac dilatation, significant bradycardia, weak arterial pulses, hypotension, distant heart sounds, low electrocardiographic voltages, nonpitting facial and peripheral edema, and evidence of congestive heart failure, such as ascites, orthopnea, and paroxysmal dyspnea, are now seen only infrequently. However, exertional dyspnea and easy fatigability continue to be common complaints.

Myxedema is associated with increased capillary permeability and subsequent leakage of protein into the interstitial space, resulting in pericardial effusion, a common clinical finding in overt myxedema, occurring in about one-third of all patients (see p. 1521). Rarely, it is complicated by cardiac tamponade.[109] Echocardiography is the most useful method of establishing the diagnosis (see p. 93). The effusions disappear with thyroid replacement therapy.[110] Myxedema-associated cardiogenic shock has also rarely been reported. It, too, responds to thyroid replacement therapy.[111]

The electrocardiographic changes include sinus bradycardia and prolongation of the Q-T interval. The P-wave amplitude is usually very low. It is possible that hypothermia may contribute to reentrant ventricular arrhythmias.[112] The incidence of atrioventricular and intraventricular conduction disturbances is about three times greater in patients with myxedema than in the general population. Incomplete or complete right bundle branch block has been observed, and a primary myocardial abnormality suggestive of a cardiomyopathy has been reported.[113] Other electrocardiographic changes are those associated with pericardial effusion[110] (see p. 1485).

There is increased frequency of hypertension in patients with hypothyroidism, although not in severe myxedema.[114] In one study of 477 patients, 15 per cent of hypothyroid subjects had a blood pressure greater than 160/95, compared with 5.5 per cent in age-matched euthyroid subjects. Replacement of thyroid hormone resulted in substantial reduction in blood pressure in the hypertensive patients.[115] In a study of 688 consecutive hypertensive patients, hypothyroidism was found in 25 (3.5 per cent). In nearly one-third of this subgroup, treatment of the hypothyroidism lowered the blood pressure to within the normal range.[114] Thus, individuals with mild to moderate hypothyroidism have an increased possibility of developing hypertension, particularly diastolic hypertension, whereas individuals with severe hypothyroidism are more likely to have normal or slightly low blood pressures.[114–116]

MYOCARDIAL EFFECTS. Hypothyroid patients have reduced cardiac output, stroke volume, and blood and plasma volumes.[117,118] Right and left heart filling pressures are usually within normal limits unless they are elevated by a pericardial effusion. There is a redistribution of blood flow with mild reductions in cerebral and renal flow and significant reductions in cutaneous flow. Ventricular isovolumetric relaxation time is prolonged and is normalized during T_4 replacement.[119,120] The impact of hypothyroidism on cardiac function can occur quickly in patients rendered hypothyroid for assessment of thyroid status in the treatment of thyroid cancer. Two weeks after discontinuing thyroid medication the left ventricular end-diastolic diameter and peak velocity of early diastolic filling, as well as heart rate, were reduced. There were no changes in systolic or diastolic blood pressure.[121]

Cardiac muscle isolated from cats with experimentally produced hypothyroidism exhibited reduced contractility, characterized by a depression of the myocardial force-velocity curve, a reduction of the rate of tension development, and a prolongation of the contractile response.

There is little evidence that congestive heart failure is common in myxedema or that it occurs in the absence of other cardiac disease.[122] Presumably the depressed myocardial contractility is sufficient to sustain the reduced workload placed on the heart in hypothyroidism. However, it may be difficult to distinguish between symptoms of myxedema and heart failure. Dyspnea, edema, effusions, cardiomegaly, and T-wave changes occur in both conditions. In left heart failure, pulmonary arterial pressure is usually elevated during exercise, cardiac output fails to rise normally, and the Valsalva response is normal, whereas the opposite occurs in myxedema.[122] Also, the hemodynamic changes in myxedema respond to thyroid hormone administration.

Cardiac catecholamine levels are not reduced in hypothyroidism. Neither the sensitivity of the mechanical performance of the heart to sympathetic nerve stimulation nor the response of the cardiac adenylate cyclase to norepinephrine is altered in hypothyroidism. However, there is a reduction in the total number of myocardial beta receptors.[62,63] Both isoproterenol-stimulated contractility and the accumulation of cyclic AMP are reduced in hearts obtained from hypothyroid rats.[123] In experimental hypothyroidism, calcium in isolated myocardial sarcoplasmic reticulum particles is reduced, which may explain the altered contractile state.[70]

ATHEROSCLEROSIS. It has been suggested that patients with hypothyroidism are at increased risk of developing atherosclerosis, because this disease is accompanied by significant changes in lipid metabolism. Thus, hypercholesterolemia and hypertriglyceridemia, which are associated with the development of premature coronary artery disease, are found in patients with hypothyroidism.[124] Furthermore, treatment of patients with hypothyroidism corrects the abnormal lipid pattern. For example, Arem and Patsch noted a 22 per cent reduction in mean LDL cholesterol concentration after 4 months of thyroid replacement therapy.[125] HDL cholesterol levels did not change appreciably. Support for a connection between hypothyroidism and atherosclerosis has come from several sources, including the documentation that the latter occurs with twice the frequency in patients with myxedema than in age- and sex-matched controls and that the development of atherosclerosis in cholesterol-fed animals is enhanced by the presence of hypothyroidism and reduced when thyroid hormone is administered.[126,127] Yet myocardial infarction and angina pectoris are relatively uncommon in hypothyroidism. The latter was present in only 7 per cent of a group of such patients.[128] This low frequency of cardiac complications from atherosclerosis may simply reflect the decreased metabolic demand on the myocardium in hypothyroidism. However, the known effects of hypothyroidism on serum enzyme concentrations do complicate the assessment of chest pain in patients with myxedema.[129]

DIAGNOSIS AND TREATMENT OF HYPOTHYROIDISM

Caution must be exercised in treating hypothyroid patients who are elderly and who may have underlying heart disease, to avoid precipitating myocardial infarction or severe congestive heart failure; a slow replacement program is indicated in these individuals.

The treatment of congestive heart failure is particularly difficult in patients with myxedema, both because of the effect of thyroid hormone on the heart and because the heart's response to cardiac glycosides is altered.[95] Patients with severe angina pectoris and untreated myxedema pose a difficult clinical dilemma because angina may be exacerbated by thyroid hormone replacement, and the usual medical management of angina with beta blockers may induce severe bradycardia. Coronary arteriography often shows severe coronary artery disease in these patients, and an excellent surgical team can perform successful coronary revascularization with minimal thyroid replacement. Full thyroid replacement can then be safely achieved during the postoperative period, without the recurrence of angina.[130–132]

DISEASES OF THE ADRENAL CORTEX

Since Addison's description in 1849 of adrenal insufficiency,[2] it has been appreciated that steroids secreted by the adrenal cortex exert a significant effect on the cardiovascular system, primarily by altering blood pressure. Adrenal insufficiency is characterized by significant hypotension, whereas excessive production of adrenal steroids is often accompanied by hypertension.

Three classes of steroids are secreted by the adrenal cortex: glucocorticoids, e.g., cortisol; mineralocorticoids, e.g., aldosterone; and androgens, e.g., dehydroepiandrosterone. In this section, the physiology and pathophysiology of glucocorticoid and mineralocorticoid secretion are addressed.

HORMONE ACTIONS

CORTISOL. The primary glucocorticoid, cortisol, is synthesized from cholesterol in the inner layers of the adrenal cortex. Its average plasma concentration is 15 μg/dl in the morning, falling to 5 μg/dl by early evening.[133] The fundamental mechanism of action of the glucocorticoids is similar to that of other steroid hormones. They enter a target tissue by diffusion and combine with a specific high-affinity cytoplasmic receptor protein. The receptor-cortisol complex is then transferred to specific acceptor sites on nuclear chromatin tissue (promoter region) where it produces an increase in RNA and later protein synthesis. The major action of glucocorticoids is to promote gluconeogenesis, and, in that respect, they are both catabolic and anti-insulin.

Glucocorticoids also have anti-inflammatory properties related to their effects on both the microvasculature and the lymphatic system. They maintain normal vascular responsiveness to circulating vasoconstrictors, such as norepinephrine, and have a major effect on both the distribution and excretion of body water.

ALDOSTERONE. The major mineralocorticoid produced by the human adrenal gland is aldosterone. It is also synthesized from cholesterol but almost exclusively in the outer layer (glomerulosa) of the adrenal cortex. Aldosterone has two important functions: (1) it is a major regulator of extracellular fluid volume by its effect on sodium retention, and (2) it is a major determinant of potassium metabolism. Aldosterone acts predominantly on the distal convoluted tubule and/or collecting duct of the kidney, where it promotes the reabsorption of sodium. Potassium then diffuses into the lumen of the tubules because of the change in electrochemical gradient produced by the active reabsorption of the positively charged sodium ion. Hydrogen ion may also be more freely excreted because of this change in the electrochemical gradient. Although aldosterone also acts on salivary and sweat glands and on the endothelial cells of the gastrointestinal tract, these have little impact on total body sodium and potassium homeostasis.

There are three well-defined control mechanisms for aldosterone release.[133,134]

1. The renin-angiotensin system is the major system for the control of extracellular fluid volume by regulating aldosterone secretion. Aldosterone is linked in a negative feedback loop with the renin-angiotensin system. Thus, during periods registered as volume deficiency there is increased release of the enzyme renin from the juxtaglomerular cells of the kidney. Renin then increases the production of angiotensin I from its substrate. Angiotensin I is rapidly converted into the biologically active angiotensin II, which increases aldosterone secretion. Angiotensin II also produces vasoconstriction, thereby raising blood pressure and reducing blood flow to a variety of tissues, especially the kidney.
2. Potassium ion also regulates aldosterone secretion independent of the renin-angiotensin system; elevation of potassium concentration increases aldosterone secretion and vice versa. The adrenal cortex is very sensitive to changes in potassium concentration with as little as 0.1 mEq/liter increment producing significant changes in the plasma aldosterone levels.
3. ACTH also has been documented to affect aldosterone secretion profoundly. However, because the control of aldosterone release is not appreciably altered in patients who have been on a long-term regimen of steroid therapy, ACTH probably has a smaller role than the other two factors in maintaining normal aldosterone secretion.

In addition to these major stimuli controlling aldosterone secretion, salt-losing hormones such as atrial natriuretic peptide (see p. 1917) and dopamine inhibit aldosterone secretion, particularly in response to angiotensin II.[134] Finally, the poor dietary intake of both sodium and potassium alters the magnitude of the aldosterone response to acute stimulation, sodium restriction, and potassium loading, both enhancing the response of the adrenal, perhaps by modifying the local (adrenal) renin-angiotensin system.[133,134]

Diseases of the adrenal cortex, therefore, primarily affect the cardiovascular system via changes in blood pressure or volume homeostasis. However, aldosterone, and perhaps angiotensin II itself, also can have a direct effect on collagen metabolism in cardiac fibroblasts. In both primary aldosteronism and renal vascular hypertension, there is a reactive perivascular and interstitial fibrosis that does not seem to be due to pressure overload alone. Documentation of this effect has been provided by in vitro studies using cardiac fibroblasts. Both angiotensin II and aldosterone increase the collagen synthesis and collagenase activity. These effects could be completely abolished by either type I or type II angiotensin II receptor antagonists or the competitive aldosterone antagonist, spironolactone.[135]

Cushing's Syndrome

(See also p. 829)

In 1932 Harvey Cushing reported a syndrome characterized by truncal obesity, hypertension, fatigue, weakness, amenorrhea, hirsutism, purple abdominal striae, glucosuria, edema, and osteoporosis.[136] The majority of cases are secondary to bilateral adrenal hyperplasia, with the predominant feature being excess production of glucocorticoids and androgens.[133] Some cases are due to ACTH-producing tumors of either the pituitary gland (Cushing's disease) or nonendocrine tissue (ectopic ACTH production). Fifteen to 20 per cent of the cases are due to primary adrenal neoplasia, either adenoma or carcinoma. Most patients have the typical body habitus: central obesity and slender extremities with proximal muscle weakness. Hypertension is present in 80 to 90 per cent of patients, and diabetes occurs in 20 per cent, probably in those individuals with a predisposition.[133] Evidence of androgen excess may also be present, including hirsutism, amenorrhea, and clitoromegaly.

Laboratory tests disclose evidence of excess production of both glucocorticoids and androgens in the majority of cases. Thus, urinary metabolites of these steroids, 17-ketosteroids and 17-hydroxysteroids, are characteristically increased. Most patients show some evidence of glycosuria or hyperglycemia.

CARDIOVASCULAR MANIFESTATIONS. Prior to the development of effective treatment for Cushing's syndrome, accelerated atherosclerosis was a common finding. Early death usually occurred from myocardial infarction, congestive heart failure, or stroke. Even with more effective treatment, the mortality of patients with Cushing's syndrome is still significantly higher than in the general population, primarily owing to an increased risk of cardiovascular disease.[137] Although the pathophysiology of the accelerated atherosclerosis is not clear, the hypertensive process probably contributes. Chronic excess production of cortisol leads to hyperlipidemia and hypercholesterolemia, both of which may promote the development of atherosclerosis.[133]

The pathophysiology of the hypertension in Cushing's syndrome has been much debated. Early studies suggested that it was secondary to volume expansion due to cortisol's mineralocorticoid properties. Support for this comes from the demonstration of increased levels of atrial natriuretic hormone in patients with Cushing's syndrome, suggesting a volume-expanded state.[138] However, recent studies have not supported this hypothesis. Alternative hypotheses include glucocorticoid potentiation of response of vascular smooth muscle to vasoconstrictive agents and ACTH- or cortisol-induced increases in renin substrate.[133] The latter thesis suggests that the increased blood pressure is secondary to increased generation of angiotensin II. Support for the potentiation hypothesis comes from a documented increased vascular response to both angiotensin II and catecholamines in patients with Cushing's syndrome compared with normal subjects.[139,140] Thus, the pathophysiology of the hypertension may be multifactorial, being related to volume expansion, increased production of vasoactive agents, e.g., angiotensin II, and increased sensitivity of vascular smooth muscle to vasoactive agents.

The hemodynamic, electrocardiographic, and roentgenographic studies of patients with Cushing's syndrome have revealed no specific abnormalities except those that are, in general, associated with either hypertension or hypokalemia. The P-R intervals tend to be shorter than normal. Echocardiograms have shown ventricular hypertrophy with asymmetrical septal thickening. The frequency of these abnormalities is greater than that of those seen in patients with essential hypertension with equivalent levels of blood pressure.[141]

Over the past several years, a new familial syndrome has been described: Cushing's syndrome and cardiac myxoma occurring in the same individual (see p. 1467). In addition to having these two conditions, 80 per cent of the patients have a cutaneous abnormality. In most it is a pigmented lesion; in some it is a subcutaneous myxoma. Histologically the adrenal glands show nodular hyperplasia.[142]

DIAGNOSIS AND TREATMENT. The diagnosis of Cushing's syndrome is established by the lack of appropriate suppression of cortisol secretion by dexamethasone. The best screening test is the administration of 1 mg of dexamethasone at bedtime with measurement of plasma cortisol between 7 and 10 the next morning.[133] In normal subjects cortisol levels are less than 5 μg/dl. Some patients, particularly the obese, may have false-positive responses, but false-negative responses occur only rarely. The definitive diagnosis of Cushing's syndrome is made by administration of 0.5 mg of dexamethasone every 6 hours for 2 days, with measurement either of plasma cortisol levels at the end of the second day (normal <5 μg/dl) or of the 24-hour cortisol excretory rate on the second day of dexamethasone suppression (normal <30 μg/24 hours).[133]

Therapy of Cushing's syndrome is usually directed at the specific cause. Thus, patients with adrenal carcinoma or adenoma or an ACTH-producing pituitary tumor are treated surgically. In some cases, patients with adrenal carcinoma have nonresectable lesions, and therefore surgery is combined with chemotherapy. The treatment of patients with bilateral hyperplasia without an evident ACTH-producing tumor is controversial, because the cause is often unknown. In some centers, bilateral adrenalectomy is the treatment of choice, while more commonly, therapy directed at the pituitary (either surgery or irradiation) is used.[133]

The treatment of the *cardiovascular abnormalities* associated with Cushing's syndrome is directed at lowering blood pressure and correcting the hypokalemia if present. Caution should be exercised in treating the hypertension with potassium-losing diuretics because of the tendency for these patients to develop hypokalemia. Thus, potassium-sparing diuretics or potassium supplements are often required. As in all clinical conditions in which hypokalemia may be present, cardiac glycosides should be used with caution in patients with Cushing's syndrome.

The hypertension is often resistant to conventional antihypertensive programs. Fallo et al. reported that only 15 per cent of their hypertensive patients with Cushing's syndrome had control of blood pressure using conventional medications: diuretics, calcium antagonists, angiotensin-converting enzyme inhibitors either as single agents or in combination. In 12 patients who failed conventional therapy, treatment with ketoconazole, an adrenal enzyme inhibitor, normalized blood pressure in all but one subject. In that one subject cortisol levels were not decreased. Thus, specific therapy directed at lowering cortisol production appears to be more effective than conventional antihypertensive therapy in controlling the hypertension in patients with Cushing's syndrome.[143]

Hyperaldosteronism

(See also p. 827)

CLINICAL AND BIOCHEMICAL MANIFESTATIONS. Aldosteronism is a syndrome associated with hypersecretion of aldosterone. Primary aldosteronism signifies that the stimulus for the excess aldosterone production resides within the adrenal. In secondary aldosteronism, the stimulus is of extra-adrenal origin.

In patients with primary aldosteronism, which most commonly is due to an aldosterone-producing adrenal adenoma, hypertension, hypokalemia, and metabolic alkalosis are common.[133,144] Polyuria may exist because of the hypokalemia, and glucose intolerance is increased in frequency. Muscle cramps due to the hypokalemia may be present, but little else distinguishes this from other forms of hypertension. Laboratory studies confirm the presence of hypokalemic alkalosis with a low specific gravity of urine and normal levels of adrenal glucocorticoids. The incidence of primary aldosteronism is between 0.5 and 2 per cent of the hypertensive population and it occurs twice as frequently in females as in males, with an initial presentation usually between the ages of 30 and 50 years.[133]

CARDIOVASCULAR MANIFESTATIONS. Many of the cardiovascular effects of aldosteronism are nonspecific, being related to aldosterone's effect on atrial pressure and potassium balance. Thus, T-wave flattening or U-wave prominence on the electrocardiogram and the presence of premature ventricular contractions and other arrhythmias due to hypokalemia are observed.[27] Evidence of left ventricular hypertrophy, either on the electrocardiogram or by echocardiography, may also be present in patients with longstanding hypertension and hyperaldosteronism. Malignant hypertension and changes in renal function secondary to severe hypertensive angiopathy are infrequent.

DIAGNOSIS AND TREATMENT. The diagnosis of primary aldosteronism is made by the presence of diastolic hypertension without edema, hypersecretion of aldosterone that fails to suppress appropriately during volume expansion, hyposecretion of renin, and hypokalemia with inappropriate urinary potassium loss during salt loading. The state of the renin-angiotensin system is often used to distinguish primary aldosteronism from other conditions that produce hypertension and hypokalemia. For example, hypertension and hypokalemia may be part of the clinical picture of secondary aldosteronism that accompanies malignant or accelerated hypertension or is associated with renal artery stenosis. Secondary aldosteronism can be readily distinguished from primary aldosteronism by the plasma renin activity, which is increased in the former and reduced in the latter. However, the combination of hypertension and a low plasma renin activity does not necessarily mean primary aldosteronism. Between 15 and 30 per cent of patients with essential hypertension have low renin levels, so-called low-renin essential hypertension.[144] The possibility of excess mineralocorticoid secretion has been extensively evaluated in these patients; however, no definitive evidence for such exists (Chap. 26).

Another entity that mimics primary aldosteronism is glucocorticoid-remediable aldosteronism (GRA) (see p. 827). This condition is an inherited hypertensive disorder with dysregulation of aldosterone secretion secondary to a gene mutation. The mutation is a fusion gene product between two genes coding for the enzymes responsible for the last step in biosynthesis of aldosterone and cortisol, i.e., 11β-hydroxylase/aldosterone synthase. This chimeric enzyme is expressed in the fasciculata cells, thereby leading to ACTH control of aldosterone synthase—a condition that normally does not occur. These patients can be distinguished by either genetic assessment or measurement of unique 18-hydroxycortisol steroids in the urine.[145]

The principal treatment for primary aldosteronism is surgical removal of the aldosterone-producing adenoma. In some cases, this is not possible because of the excessive risk imposed by the general physical status of the patient; then, spironolactone, which pharmacologically blocks the effects of aldosterone, is used long term. This form of therapy may be of limited benefit in men because compliance is reduced by the undesirable side effects of gynecomastia and impotence, particularly when doses greater than 200 mg per day are required.[133]

In some patients, primary aldosteronism is due not to a solitary adenoma but to bilateral hyperplasia.[144] Although the clinical characteristics of these two conditions are similar, their responses to surgery are different. In both cases hypokalemia is corrected, but patients with bilateral hyperplasia often do not exhibit reduction in arterial pressure. Patients with bilateral hyperplasia are best treated with spironolactone and other antihypertensive agents. Thus, preoperative distinction between bilateral hyperplasia and an adrenal adenoma, using adrenal venography or adrenal scanning, is important.

Adrenal Insufficiency

Clinically, patients with adrenal insufficiency can be divided into four types:[133] (1) the most common, primary insufficiency (Addison's disease); (2) secondary insufficiency due to a lack of ACTH; (3) selective hypoaldosteronism; and (4) enzyme deficiency (congenital adrenal hyperplasia).

Addison's disease may occur at any age and affects both genders equally. It is commonly due to a destructive process involving both adrenal glands; this process is sometimes infectious, but most often it is autoimmune.[146] Nearly all patients with primary adrenal insufficiency have weakness, increased skin pigmentation, significant weight loss, anorexia, nausea, vomiting, and hypotension, particularly postural. As the disease progresses, there is a gradual reduction in serum levels of sodium, chloride, and bicarbonate and an increase in potassium levels.

CARDIOVASCULAR MANIFESTATIONS. The most common cardiovascular finding in adrenal insufficiency is arterial hypotension. In severe cases the pressure may be in the range of 80/50 mm Hg, with postural accentuation. Indeed, syncope occurs in a significant percentage of patients. In severe cases, heart size and peripheral pulses decrease. The most common electrocardiographic abnormalities are low or inverted T waves, sinus bradycardia, prolonged Q-T_c interval, and low voltage. Conduction defects also occur, with first-degree block present in 20 per cent of patients. Changes secondary to the hyperkalemia are not common, and cardiac failure is unusual.[147,148]

DIAGNOSIS AND TREATMENT. Decreased response of the adrenal cortex to ACTH establishes the diagnosis of Addison's disease. The best screening test is the administration of synthetic ACTH (cosyntropin), 0.25 mg intramuscularly or intravenously, with measurement of plasma cortisol levels 30 to 60 minutes later. Cortisol levels double or increase by 10 μg/dl in normal subjects. Definitive evaluation is by prolonged (usually 24-hour) infusion of ACTH with assessment of either plasma cortisol or excretion of cortisol or both.[133]

It is possible to differentiate primary adrenal insufficiency from secondary adrenal insufficiency, isolated hypoaldosteronism, or congenital adrenal hyperplasia because one of the adrenal hormonal functions is normal in each of the latter three conditions.

An increasingly common form of hypoaldosteronism is that associated with *hyporeninism.* Most commonly this syndrome is observed in older diabetic patients with a mild degree of renal impairment and hypertension; acidosis is also common. Usually these patients present with unexplained hyperkalemia. The cause is unknown but may be secondary to damage to the juxtaglomerular apparatus and/or reduced conversion of a renin precursor into the active enzyme.[149] This clinical syndrome is particularly important in the presence of cardiovascular diseases. Furthermore, commonly used drugs (beta blockers and calcium antagonists) can exacerbate this condition by further compromising aldosterone release.[150]

The treatment of adrenal insufficiency is accomplished by replacement of the deficient steroid. In adults with primary or secondary insufficiency, hydrocortisone, 20 to 30 mg daily, is administered in divided doses, usually two-thirds in the morning and one-third in midafternoon. In those patients with associated aldosterone deficiency, 9α-fluorohydrocortisone, 0.05 to 0.10 mg daily, is given. During periods of significant stress (surgery, infection, or trauma), the dose of glucocorticoids should be increased.[151,152]

PHEOCHROMOCYTOMA

(See also p. 829)

Effects of Catecholamines on the Cardiovascular System

The adrenal medulla and sympathetic nervous system are linked morphologically, biochemically, and physiologically and are often referred to as the sympathoadrenal system.[153,154] In addition to their important effects on the cardiovascular system, catecholamines also have significant metabolic effects, stimulating glycogenolysis and gluconeogenesis, that is, increasing the production of glucose from glycogen and amino acid precursors and stimulating lipolysis.

CLINICAL AND BIOCHEMICAL MANIFESTATIONS. A pheochromocytoma is a catecholamine-producing tumor derived from chromaffin cells. Those arising from extra-adrenal chromaffin cells are called nonadrenal pheochromocytomas or paraganglionomas. Probably less than 0.1 per cent of patients with hypertension have a pheochromocytoma. Despite the fact that it is an uncommon disease, pheochromocytomas generate a great deal of interest, largely because the morbidity and mortality associated with these tumors are significant, with detection often resulting in cure. Pheochromocytomas are highly vascular tumors; less than 10 per cent are malignant as indicated by local invasion or metastasis, but, as with other endocrine tumors, malignancy cannot always be determined by microscopic appearance alone.

Although the vast majority of tumors occur sporadically, approximately 5 per cent are inherited as an autosomal trait, by which they are often part of a pluriglandular neoplastic syndrome,[153] which, in addition to pheochromocytoma, may consist of medullary carcinoma of the thyroid, parathyroidadenoma, and retinal or cerebellar hemangioblastomas. Most pheochromocytomas are solitary adrenal tumors, with 10 per cent being bilateral and 10 per cent nonadrenal. However, in the familial form of pheochromocytoma nearly half the patients have bilateral adrenal tumors.

CARDIOVASCULAR MANIFESTATIONS. Hypertension is the major cardiovascular manifestation of pheochromocytoma. The features that suggest pheochromocytoma in hypertensive patients are (1) paroxysmal attacks of any kind, (2) headaches, (3) excessive sweating, (4) signs of hypermetabolism, (5) orthostatic hypotension, and (6) unusual blood pressure elevations due to trauma or operation.[154] Many of the features are similar to those of hyperthyroidism. Although paroxysmal attacks are the hallmark of pheochromocytoma, more than half the patients have fixed hypertension and nearly 10 per cent are normotensive.

The lability of blood pressure in patients with pheochromocytoma has been suggested to be due not only to episodic discharge of catecholamines but also to a reduction in plasma volume, as well as to impaired sympathetic reflexes. A number of observations suggest that chronic volume depletion is present.[155] For example, alpha-adrenoceptor blockade or removal of the tumor produces severe hypotension, which is correctable by volume expansion.[153] Cardiac output has been reported to be normal, whereas heart rate is increased, and orthostatic hypotension is accompanied by decreased stroke volume and inadequate adjustments in peripheral resistance indicative of impaired peripheral vascular reflexes.[155] An occasional patient has markedly elevated central aortic pressure and severe systemic hypotension due to severe arterial vasoconstriction. Patients with pheochromocytoma may also have acute pulmonary edema.[156] In some patients with pheochromocytoma, hemodynamic features are indistinguishable from those with essential hypertension. These results suggest that long-term exposure to high circulating levels of catecholamines may produce a different clinical picture than that observed with acute administration. These differences may be due to desensitization induced by chronic exposure to catecholamines.[157]

The electrocardiogram is abnormal in as many as 75 per cent of patients with pheochromocytoma.[27] The changes consist of T-wave inversion, left ventricular hypertrophy, sinus tachycardia, and, in some cases, other alterations in rhythm, such as frequent supraventricular ectopic beats or paroxysmal supraventricular tachycardia.[158] An occasional patient has a short P-R interval and a narrow QRS complex, suggesting that catecholamines are modifying the A-V conduction system. When arterial pressure increases markedly, changes suggestive of myocardial damage, including transient ST-segment elevations, marked diffuse T-wave inversions, and depression of ST segments, are present. These changes are usually transient, and the electrocardiographic pattern reverts to normal after removal of the tumor or pharmacological blockade.[153,159] Some of the electrocardiographic abnormalities are presumably due to hypertensive heart disease or myocardial ischemia. However, a specific catecholamine-induced myocarditis and/or cardiomyopathy has also been suggested.[160,161] Interestingly, a patient with catecholamine-induced cardiomyopathy was treated with captopril, with resolution of the cardiomyopathy within 2 weeks.[162] In rats with pheochromocytomas, treatment with captopril also markedly attenuated the cardiomyopathy but did not modify contraction of isolated rings of the thoracic aorta in response to either epinephrine or angiotensin II.[163] The mechanism by which captopril produced these beneficial effects is unclear but could be related to inhibiting angiotensin II–induced cardiac fibrosis.[135]

The echocardiogram often shows left ventricular hypertrophy with normal left ventricular systolic function.[164] During a hypertensive crisis it may show systolic anterior involvement of the anterior mitral leaflet, paradoxical septal motion, and proximal excursion of the posterior wall.[165]

Myocarditis. Pathologically, the myocarditis consists of focal necrosis with infiltration of inflammatory cells, perivascular inflammation, and contraction band necrosis[166] (Fig. 61–7), finally resulting in fibrosis. In some studies, 50 per cent of patients who died of pheochromocytoma had myocarditis, usually accompanied by left ventricular failure and pulmonary edema. Although coronary atherosclerosis is usually present, medial thickening is the most characteristic lesion of the coronary arteries. When norepinephrine is infused into the rabbit, there is sustained coronary vasoconstriction that within 48 hours leads to histologically documented myocardial damage.[167] Occasionally, patients with pheochromocytoma have manifestations of cardiomyopathy which may be reversed when the tumor is removed[160,161] (Fig. 61–8). The myositis is not necessarily limited to the myocardium, as it also may occur in skeletal muscle.[168]

DIAGNOSIS AND TREATMENT. The diagnosis of pheochromocytoma is established by documenting increased urinary or plasma levels of catecholamines or one of their metabolites.[153] Three tests are commonly employed: (1) total catecholamines, (2) vanillylmandelic acid (VMA), and (3) metanephrine. The last two are metabolites of catecholamine and were first used to screen for pheochromocytoma because they are present in greater quantities. When reliably performed, these tests are probably equivalent in accuracy. The probability of pheochromocytoma being present in a hypertensive patient with a single normal urine level is less than 5 per cent. It is most desirable to measure both the catecholamines and one of the two metabolites, preferably metanephrine, in screening for pheochromocytoma. If the blood pressure fluctuates, it is particularly important to collect the urine at a time when the pressure is elevated. Specific pharmacological tests to screen for pheochromocytoma are of limited benefit, usually hazardous, and therefore warranted only in unusual circumstances. Clonidine has been proposed as a useful definitive test for pheochromocytoma, although it is necessary only in unusual cases. Catecholamine levels are suppressed in normal subjects via stimulation of central alpha-adrenoceptors; following clonidine administration in patients with pheochromocytoma they are not.[153] Unfortunately, profound and prolonged hypotension has been reported in some patients during the course of this test.

Once the diagnosis of pheochromocytoma is established, specific pharmacological blockade should be initiated.[153] Administration of phenoxybenzamine hydrochloride should be begun, with the initial dosage 10 mg every 12 hours; the dose is then gradually increased every 2 to 3 days until the arterial pressure is restored to normal. Alternatively, prazosin may be used. However, it should be noted that alpha-adrenoceptor blockade may induce a decline in arterial pressure accompanied by serious postural hypotension, presumably because of the vasodilatation occurring in the presence of hypovolemia. This hypotensive response can be prevented by adequate sodium intake; if the response is very striking, infusion of saline may be required. Adequate control of arterial pressure is essential prior to any arteriographic procedure before initiating beta-adrenoceptor blockade, and before operation. Calcium an-

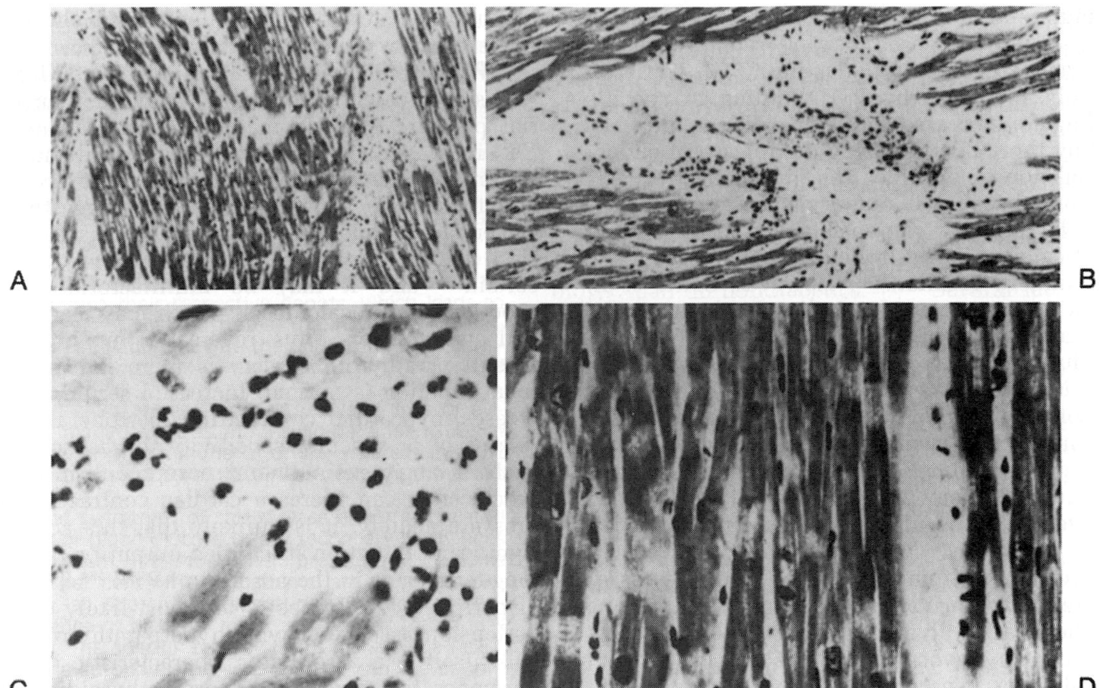

FIGURE 61–7. Left ventricular myocardium with acute myocarditis and contraction band necrosis in a patient with pheochromocytoma dying of catecholamine crisis. *A,* Diffuse infiltration by inflammatory cells through myocardium. *B,* Perivascular inflammation. *C,* Close-up of the inflammatory infiltrate. *D,* Contraction-band necrosis of myocytes. H&E; original magnification ×20 *(A),* ×45 *(B),* ×540 *(C),* ×330 *(D).* (From McManus, B. M., et al.: Fatal catecholamine crisis in pheochromocytoma: Curable cause of cardiac arrest. Am. Heart J. *102:*930, 1981.)

tagonists may be useful both in treating the hypertension associated with pheochromocytoma and in reducing catecholamine production.[169]

Beta-adrenoceptor blockade is useful in patients with pheochromocytoma who have significant tachycardia, palpitations, and catecholamine-induced arrhythmias. However, beta blockade with a drug affecting $beta_2$ receptors must not be initiated prior to inadequate alpha blockade, since severe *hypertension* may occur as a result of unopposed alpha-stimulating activity of the circulating catecholamines.

Definitive treatment is surgical removal of the tumor, usually after localization with computed tomography, arteriography, or scanning using a radioactive iodide derivative of guanethidine as the scanning agent.[153] Scanning may be particularly important in localizing extra-adrenal, e.g., thoracic, pheochromocytomas. Precise definition of the anatomical boundaries of this tumor is important preoperatively if surgery is to be successful.[170] In those patients with inoperable lesions, long-term use of the combination of alpha- and beta-adrenoceptor blockers has been helpful.

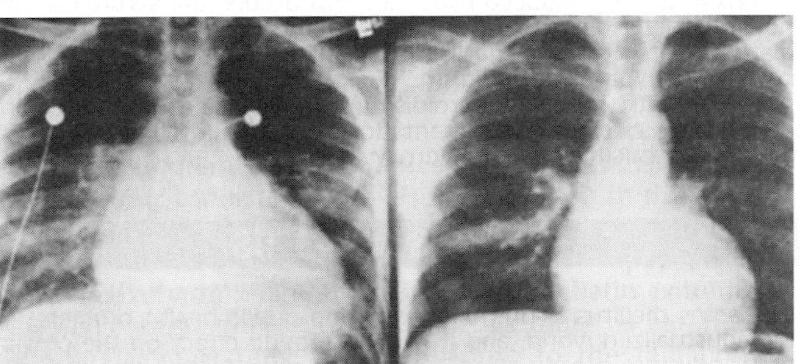

FIGURE 61–8. Pheochromocytoma-induced cardiomyopathy. *Left,* Chest x-ray on admission. Cardiomegaly, right pleural effusion, and signs of congestive heart failure. *Right,* One month after removal of the tumor. No signs of congestion and significant decrease of the heart size. (From Velasquez, G., et al.: Phaeochromocytoma and cardiomyopathy. Br. J. Radiol. *57:*89, 1984.)

Drugs that inhibit the biosynthesis of catecholamines, such as alpha-methyltyrosine, and generalized chemotherapeutic agents have also been used in patients with malignant pheochromocytoma.[153] Although rare, of particular importance to the cardiologist is the presence of a cardiac pheochromocytoma (see p. 1897).

PARATHYROID DISEASE

Disordered parathyroid secretion is associated with two cardiovascular disturbances, cardiac arrhythmias and hypertension. Changes in calcium metabolism as well as a direct effect of parathyroid hormone on the cardiovascular system appear to be responsible.

CLINICAL AND BIOCHEMICAL MANIFESTATIONS. Parathyroid hormone (PTH) is a single-chain polypeptide of 84 amino acids. Its major biological effect is to increase mobilization of calcium into the extracellular fluid from a variety of tissues; this action is linked in a negative feedback loop with serum unbound calcium concentration. Thus, an increase in serum calcium concentration reduces PTH release and vice versa.[171] PTH also increases urinary excretion of phosphate, augments bone resorption, and reduces the urinary excretion of calcium.

Primary hyperparathyroidism, the excess production of PTH, is usually secondary to a solitary parathyroid adenoma. Occasionally, generalized parathyroid hyperplasia exists, and infrequently, carcinoma of the parathyroid gland is found. The signs and symptoms of primary hyperparathyroidism are related to direct effects of PTH on kidney or bone or those associated with the hypercalcemia. Nearly half the patients have signs and symptoms of renal dysfunction, such as polyuria, nocturia, renal stones, and, in severe cases, nephrocalcinosis and renal failure.

Cardiac hypertrophy is found with increased frequency in patients with hyperparathyroidism, even in the absence of hypertension. In one study, 5 of 18 patients with hypertrophic cardiomyopathy had raised serum PTH levels but normal serum calcium levels. In contrast, left ventricular hypertrophy did not occur in six patients with hypercalcemia alone.[171]

Cardiovascular Manifestations of Parathyroid Diseases

(See also p. 830)

CARDIAC EFFECTS. Although most of the effects of PTH on the heart are probably secondary to a change in ex-

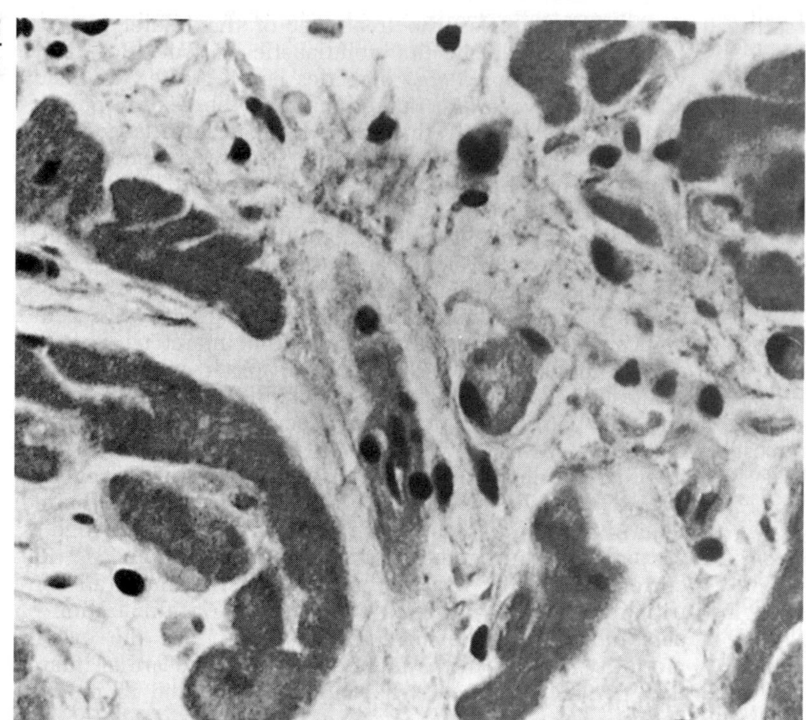

FIGURE 61–10. Myocardium of diabetic patient showing atrophied myocytes on right side (compare with more normal fibers on left), increased interstitial fibrous tissue, and thickening of small arteriolar walls. H & E × 300. (From Sutherland, C. G. G., et al.: Endomyocardial biopsy pathology in insulin-dependent diabetic patients with abnormal ventricular function. Histopathology *14*:596, 1989.)

sudden death in diabetics with abnormal autonomic function tests.[206]

CONGESTIVE HEART FAILURE. Diabetes mellitus appears to increase the likelihood of the development of congestive heart failure from all causes. The role of diabetes in congestive heart failure was analyzed in the Framingham Study,[196] and the risk of developing heart failure was found to be increased substantially. Even when patients with prior coronary or rheumatic heart disease were excluded, diabetic subjects had a four- to fivefold increased risk of congestive heart failure. Furthermore, this increased risk persisted after age, blood pressure, weight, and cholesterol values, as well as coronary heart disease, were taken into account. On the basis of these findings it appeared that the excessive risk of heart failure in diabetic patients is caused by factors other than accelerated atherogenesis and coronary heart disease. One suggested possibility is a diabetes-induced cardiomyopathy.

Diabetic Cardiomyopathy. There is a substantial increase in the coincidence of diabetes mellitus and cardiomyopathy. The cardiomyopathy may occur in patients who have no evidence of large-vessel disease or abnormalities in myocardial capillary basal lamina documented by endomyocardial biopsies.[206,207] The most common histological abnormalities are interstitial fibrosis (Fig. 61-10) and arteriolar hyalinization (Fig. 61–11). Evidence supporting the presence of cardiomyopathy even in children with diabetes mellitus has been reported. Both systolic and diastolic dysfunctions have been observed. The severity of dysfunction is related to the degree of metabolic control, even when there is no clinical evidence of cardiovascular or microvascular disease.[208] Taken together, these studies strongly sug-

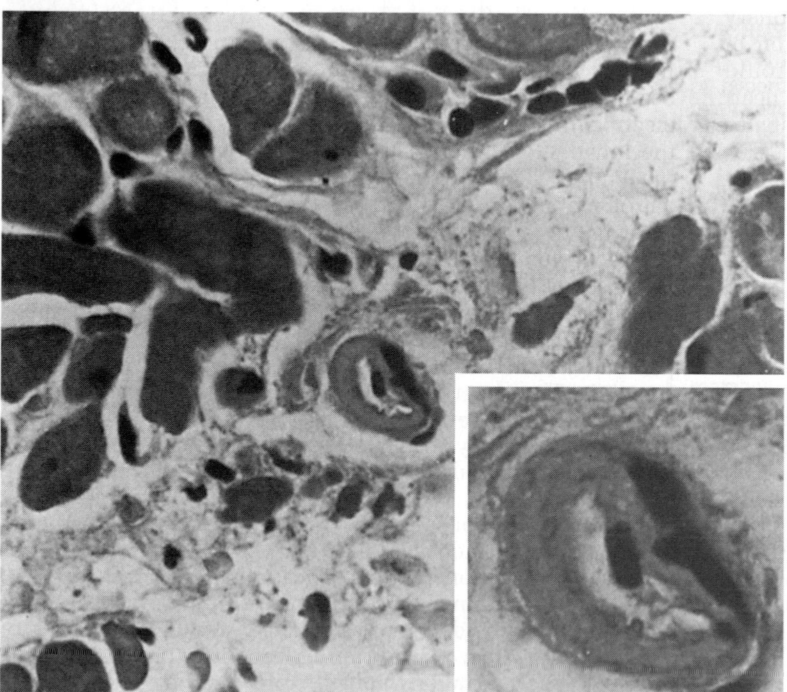

FIGURE 61–11. Hyalinization without luminal narrowing of small arteriole in myocardium of diabetic patient. H&E, ×300. Inset, Same arteriole. (H&E, ×750). (From Sutherland, C. G. G., et al.: Endomyocardial biopsy pathology in insulin-dependent diabetic patients with abnormal ventricular function. Histopathology *14*:597, 1989.)

gest that in some diabetic patients there is a nonischemic cardiomyopathic process.

ABNORMALITIES OF VENTRICULAR FUNCTION. Several abnormalities of ventricular function, using echocardiographic techniques, have been reported in diabetics.

In young asymptomatic patients, the ratio of early to peak filling velocity is significantly decreased while atrial filling velocity is significantly increased (Fig. 61-12). There is no relationship between the left ventricular diastolic filling abnormalities and evidence of severity of the diabetes, i.e., retinopathy, nephropathy, or peripheral neuropathy.[209] Other reported abnormalities in diabetic subjects include left ventricular asynergy on two-dimensional echocardiograms,[209,210] reduction in the peak diastolic filling rate[211]; an abnormal left ventricular ejection fraction in response to exercise[212,213]; and evidence of diastolic dysfunction, even in normotensive diabetic patients.[214,215]

Several factors have been reported to contribute to the abnormalities in left ventricular function in diabetics: (1) The role of hypertension with a concomitant increase in left ventricular mass.[216] (2) The potential role of growth hormone. Patients with difficult-to-control diabetes often have increased growth hormone levels. Several investigators have reported that this metabolic abnormality could account for the increased collagen levels present in the left ventricular wall of diabetic humans and animals[217] (Fig. 61-12). Regan et al., however, have reported that in experimental diabetes induced in dogs the collagen accumulation in the myocardium is not related to or dependent on an increase in plasma growth hormone levels.[218] (3) The increased cardiac sorbitol level.[219] (4) The impairment in Ca^{2+} handling with hypersensitivity of the myocardium to Ca^{2+} secondary to increased sarcolemmal Ca^{2+} ATPase activity[220,221] (Fig. 61-13). In a rat model of non–insulin-dependent diabetes mellitus, the abnormalities in myocardial Ca^{2+} ATPase activity have also been demonstrated.[222] Further support for this hypothesis comes from the beneficial effect of a calcium antagonist (verapamil), which prevented diabetes-induced myocardial changes in experimental diabetes.[223] (5) Finally, Okumura et al. have suggested that increased 1,2-diacylglycerol levels with resultant activation of protein kinase C may underlie the cardiomyopathy, at least in experimentally induced diabetes.[224] Despite these observations in experimental models, it should be noted that when insulin is administered, the cardiac abnormality is not necessarily corrected. Thus, the relationship between the hyperglycemic state and the abnormalities in myocardial function and metabolism present in experimental diabetes is still unclear.

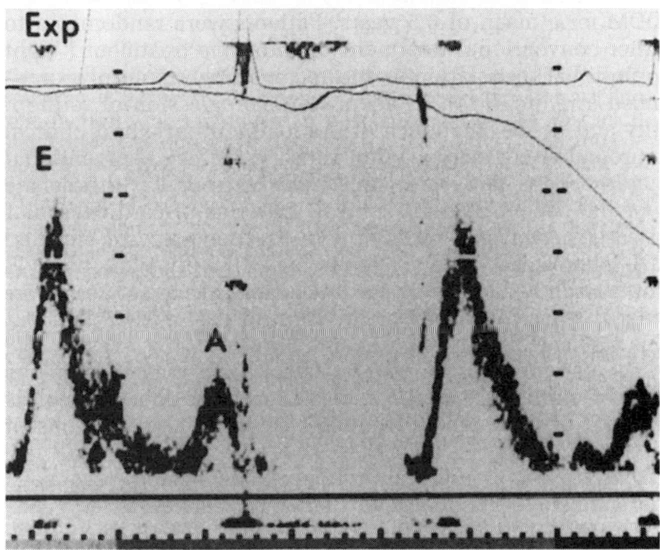

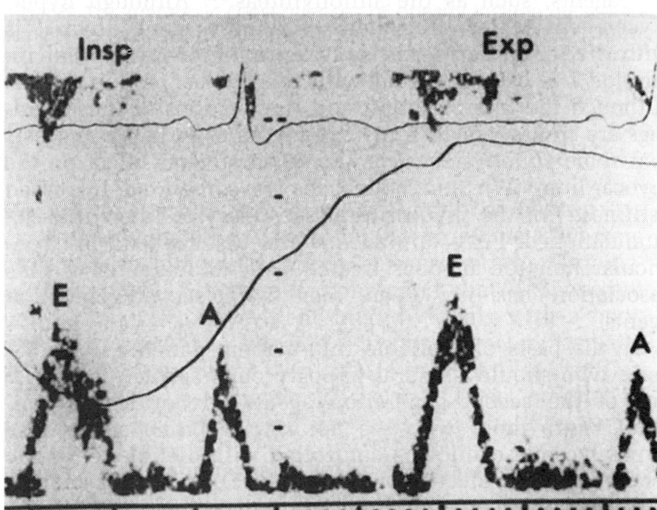

FIGURE 61–12. *A,* Transmitral Doppler echocardiogram obtained from a normal adolescent patient. The early phase of ventricular filling (E wave) is greater than the late diastolic A wave. *B,* In this diabetic adolescent, the early phase of atrial filling (E wave) is less prominent and the late diastolic A wave is taller, with a lower E/A ratio than in the normal patient. These findings are consistent with impaired diastolic filling in the diabetic patient. Exp = End-expiration; Insp = end-inspiration. (From Riggs, T. W., and Transue, D.: Doppler echocardiographic evaluation of left ventricular diastolic function in adolescents with diabetes mellitus. Am. J. Cardiol. *65*:899, 1990. Copyright 1990 by Excerpta Medica Inc.)

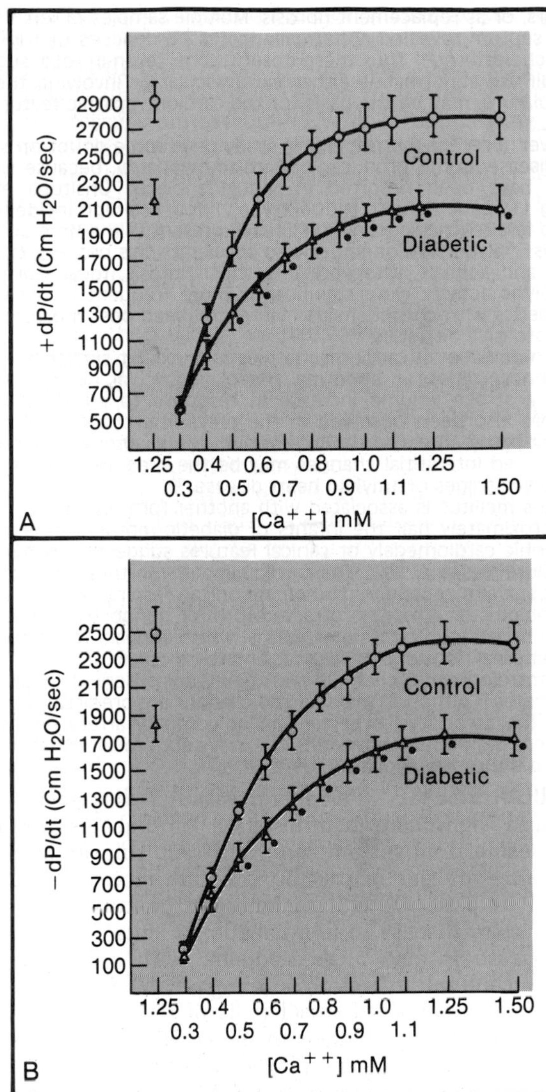

FIGURE 61–13. Effect of non–insulin-dependent diabetes mellitus on myocardial contractility (+ dp/dt). Hearts from 12-month-old diabetic rats (triangles) and the age-matched controls (circles) were perfused during the initial 20-minute stabilization period with Krebs-Henseleit buffer. Each data point represents mean ± SE of five to seven hearts. Similar reductions in − dp/dt (an index of relaxation) were noted in diabetic hearts. Significant difference from control ($P < .05$). (From Schaffer, S. W., et al.: Basis for myocardial mechanical defects associated with non–insulin-dependent diabetes. Am. J. Physiol. *256*:E27, 1989. Reproduced by permission of the American Physiological Society.)

PATHOLOGICAL CHANGES. In postmortem studies of 11 diabetic patients, 9 of whom were without significant obstructive disease of the proximal coronary arteries and had died of cardiac failure, all exhibited positive periodic acid-Schiff (PAS) staining material in the interstitium, but none had luminal narrowing of the intramural vessels. Collagen accumulation was present in perivascular loci, between the

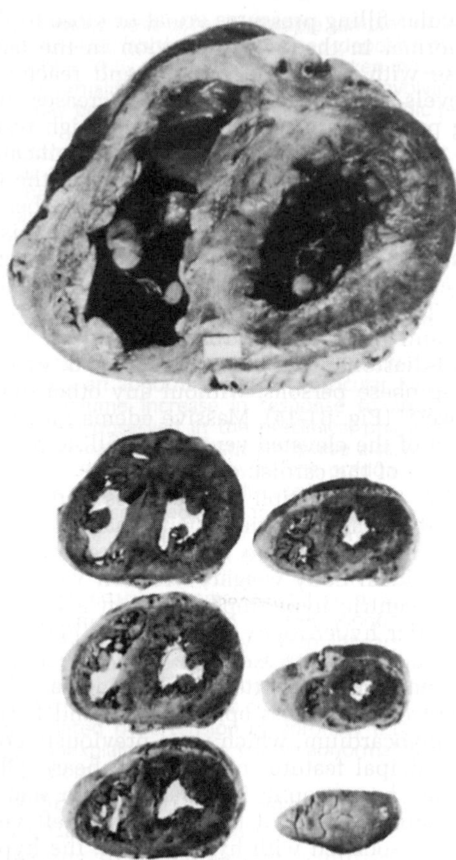

FIGURE 61–15. Cross section of the heart of a 34-year-old man who weighed more than 500 lbs. Both ventricular walls are hypertrophied and both cavities are dilated. The heart weight (825 gm) was greatly increased. (From Warnes, C. A., and Roberts, W. C.: The heart in massive [more than 300 pounds or 136 kilograms] obesity: Analysis of 12 patients studied at necropsy. Am. J. Cardiol. *54*:1090, 1984. Copyright 1984 by Excerpta Medica Inc.)

evidence of other heart disease and that, in the absence of the obesity hypoventilation syndrome, which may also complicate obesity (see p. 801), cor pulmonale is not a presenting feature.

HYPERTENSION. Hypertension is common in the obese,[247] although it must be recognized that indirect measurement of blood pressure frequently leads to overestimation of the arterial pressure by the standard cut-off method. Nonetheless, direct measurement of arterial pressure frequently shows moderate elevations. The Second National Health and Examination Survey (NHANES II) demonstrated an increased risk of hypertension of 2.9 times in overweight compared with normal weight individuals.[257] This increased risk may be secondary to the accompanying hyperinsulinemia, resulting in increased tubular reabsorption of sodium, increased catecholamine activity, and altered cellular ion transport.[258] *Syndrome X* has been defined as insulin resistance, hyperlipidemia, and obesity and is frequently associated with hypertension. This syndrome appears to play an important role in coronary artery disease.[259]

CORONARY ARTERY DISEASE. Obesity is associated with coronary artery disease by increasing several of its risk factors. These include hypertension, hyperinsulinemia, hyperlipidemia, and diabetes mellitus. Obesity may also have an independent effect that differs depending on the location of the body fat (see p. 1152). A study of more than 7600 individuals in the Honolulu Heart Program demonstrated that central obesity was a risk factor for coronary heart disease independent of body mass index.[260] In addition, analysis of data from the Nurses' Health Study demonstrated an increased risk of coronary heart disease (myocardial infarction and angina) in mildly to moderately overweight women.[261]

CONGESTIVE HEART FAILURE. Heart failure in the markedly obese is usually chronic. The pulmonary and systemic congestion with symptoms of dyspnea and edema are, at first, simply related to the reductions in ventricular compliance and elevations of filling pressures. Later, these symptoms are related also to increases in ventricular end-diastolic volume and the reduction of myocardial contractility. Thus, the marked chronic increase in cardiac work, i.e., in cardiac output and arterial pressure, ultimately leads to heart failure.

CARDIAC BENEFITS OF WEIGHT LOSS. Fortunately, weight reduction is beneficial in the majority of patients.[261a] It usually improves the exercise capacity of patients with chronic exogenous obesity and decreases total body oxygen uptake, the cardiothoracic ratio on chest roentgenogram, systemic arterial pressure, blood volume, cardiac output, arteriovenous oxygen difference, and left ventricular filling pressure at rest.[262] MacMahon et al. have documented that weight loss of as little as 8 kg is associated with a significant decrease in left ventricular mass, particularly the thickness of the posterior and central walls.[263] Alpert and colleagues, studying cardiac function in grossly obese individuals, noted a substantial reduction in left ventricular chamber enlargement and an improvement in systolic function with an average weight loss of 55 kg.[264] However, they were unable to show a change in septal or posterior wall thickness, suggesting that some of the beneficial effects of weight loss on cardiac function may occur only if the obesity is mild or of short duration. Supporting this conclusion is the persistence of elevated left ventricular filling pressure with exercise in obese patients following weight reduction.[265]

BLOOD PRESSURE BENEFITS OF WEIGHT LOSS. The Framingham Study has shown a decrease in systolic blood pressure by 10 per cent with a 15 per cent decrease in body weight in men. In the Evans County longitudinal study, an 8-kg weight loss was associated with a 13 mm Hg decrease in diastolic blood pressure. A fall in blood pressure can occur even if ideal body weight is not achieved.[266]

Treatment

Most cases of adult-onset obesity are the result of imbalance between intake and output. Thus, reduction of intake

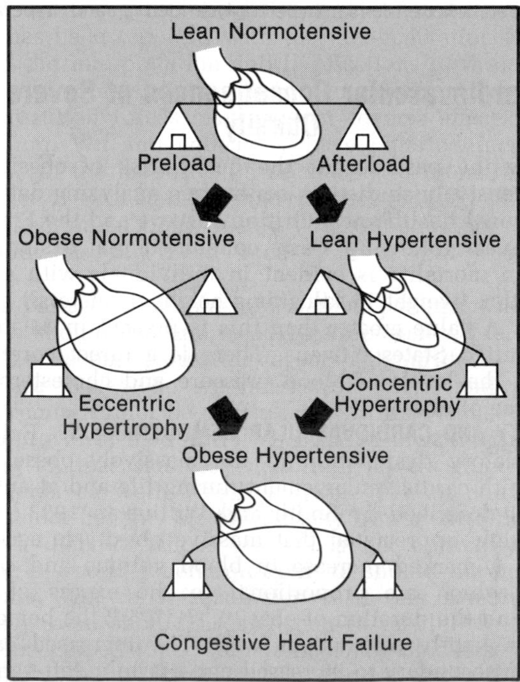

FIGURE 61–16. Adaptation of the heart to obesity and hypertension. (From Messerli, F. H.: Cardiovascular effects of obesity and hypertension. Lancet *1*:1165, 1982. © by The Lancet Ltd.)

is the most significant factor in treating this disease. Although abnormalities in endocrine function, particularly of the thyroid or adrenal, have often been implicated in the pathophysiology of obesity, this thesis is rarely substantiated by detailed evaluation. The quantity and rate of weight loss with a given level of caloric restrictions depend on the degree of energy expenditure. Energy expenditure depends on both the physical activity and mass of the individual. Thus, with a fixed level of intake and activity, the rate of weight loss decreases as the total weight decreases. There is no evidence that a specific type of diet has any intrinsic benefit except as it is related to its caloric regimen.

CARDIAC COMPLICATIONS OF WEIGHT LOSS. Rapid weight loss has been associated with cardiac arrhythmias and sudden death.[267] In some cases, this is probably secondary to inadequate electrolyte supplementation. In others, it may be related to a reduction in myocardial protein and cardiac atrophy, similar to what has been reported in severe malnutrition[268] (see below). Although initially associated with a liquid protein diet, sudden death may occur under any circumstance in which there is rapid weight loss.[269] In nearly all cases, prolongation in the Q-T interval as well as ventricular arrhytmias has been reported, providing strong support for the need for an electrocardiogram in any patient undergoing significant rapid weight loss.

MALNUTRITION

Malnutrition, particularly protein-calorie deficiency, is prevalent in many underdeveloped areas of the world. However, in recent years, it has also become a concern in developed countries in those individuals who have chronic diseases, in whom it exists as a result of both anorexia and hypermetabolism and in otherwise healthy individuals with anorexia nervosa. The clinical picture is similar to that of adult kwashiorkor reported from underdeveloped countries, described below.

Protein-calorie malnutrition of childhood refers to syndromes of nutritional deficiency, which range from marasmus to kwashiorkor and which result from a stress like a serious infection superimposed upon an inadequate diet.[270] *Marasmus* is a state of malnutrition in an infant who has been weaned early and fed a diet grossly deficient in calories, protein, and other essential nutrients. *Kwashiorkor* usually occurs in children 1 to 4 years of age and is due to deficiency of protein relative to calories.

CARDIAC CHANGES IN MALNUTRITION. The circulatory status of patients with severe nutritional depletion and electrolyte imbalance is precarious; the cardiac output, systolic pressure, and pulse pressure are abnormally low, and there may be massive, generalized edema; the P-R interval may be shortened (Table 61-2). There is loss of subcutaneous fat and general wasting and atrophy of most organs, including the heart, which is thin-walled, pale, and flabby on gross examination. Histological study reveals atrophy of the muscle fibers, sometimes with interstitial edema. In experimental chronic protein-calorie undernutrition, not only is the heart atrophic, but also left ventricular function may be normal. In the dog there are reductions in left ventricular compliance and contractility, the latter secondary to loss of cardiac tissue, not altered function,[271] whereas in the rat this apparently does not occur, although there is striking atrophy of the heart.[272] The treatment of the dehydrated or severely anemic patient with protein-calorie malnutrition involves correction of hematological, fluid, and electrolyte imbalance and the treatment of infection. Congestive failure can be avoided if care is taken to avoid overloading with sodium, water, or blood. Digitalis must be given cautiously when these patients are in heart failure because of their sensitivity to glycosides.

In parts of the world where pediatric kwashiorkor is common, there are also cases of adults with similar clinical features. These include loss of subcutaneous fat and muscle with edema, weakness, depression, anorexia, diarrhea, abdominal distention, hair loss, and thinning of the skin. Classically, plasma albumin and amino acid levels are low, as are serum concentrations of sodium, magnesium, and phosphorus. Urinary excretion of nitrogen is reduced, as is total body potassium. On the other hand, total body and extracellular water and plasma volume are usually increased. The primary pathophysiological event is protein malnutrition. All the clinical signs and symptoms are related to this basic defect.

Anorexia Nervosa. This condition is more frequently observed in developed countries but produces symptoms similar to those observed in kwashiorkor. Hypomagnesemia with hypocalcemia and hypokalemia frequently occurs in this condition, resulting in arrythmias, heart failure, and sometimes sudden death.[273] Compared with normal weight or constitutionally thin women, in women with anorexia nervosa, cardiac index is decreased secondary to low stroke index and heart rate. There also are reduced left ventricular mass, systolic dysfunction, and mitral valve motion abnormalities.[274] Sinus bradycardia is common and appears to be secondary to increased vagal tone.[275] Anorexia nervosa also has been associated with a prolonged Q-T interval compared with age- and gender-matched controls. The prolonged Q-T interval may predispose to arrhythmias.[276] Congestive heart failure may occur, particularly in the early refeeding phases, probably secondary to an exacerbation of the hypophosphatemia when hyperalimentation and/or oral intake is rich in glucose.

TABLE 61–2 SPECTRUM OF CARDIAC EFFECTS DUE TO STARVATION AND ANOREXIA NERVOSA

Cellular
Diminished protein synthesis
Activation of calcium-dependent proteinase
Mitochondrial swelling
Decreased glycogen content
Interstitial edema
Myofibrillar atrophy and destruction
Physiological
Decreased contractile force
Decreased cardiac output
Diminished diastolic compliance
Clinical
Bradycardia
Relative hypertension
Nonspecified electrocardiographic changes
Ectopic rhythms
Mitral valve prolapse
Diminished exercise capacity
Heart failure, worsened or precipitated by refeeding

Adapted from Schocken, D. D., Holloway, J. D., and Powers, P. S.: Weight loss and the heart. Effects of anorexia nervosa and starvation. Arch. Intern. Med. *149*:878, 1989.

MALNUTRITION IN CARDIAC DISEASE. The protein-calorie nutritional status in cardiac patients has not been extensively evaluated. However, there has been increasing awareness that some patients with cardiovascular disease have clinical features similar to those with primary malnutrition described above. In these cases, instead of involuntary protein deprivation, anorexia plays a significant role. For example, chronic heart failure leads to cellular hypoxia as well as hypermetabolism. Gastrointestinal hypoxia produces anorexia, which then initiates a vicious circle. Decreased protein intake produces cardiac atrophy, increased right atrial pressure, tricuspid regurgitation, and increasing heart failure, which produces more cellular hypoxia, greater anorexia, and finally death.[277]

A similar condition has been described in some patients undergoing open-heart surgery for correction of rheumatic valvular disease. In some malnourished patients the mortality reaches 20 per cent, significantly greater than the 1 to 2 per cent in normally nourished patients undergoing the same procedure. The underlying pathophysiology is uncertain but probably includes (1) decreased cardiac mass, (2) impairment of this biosynthetic activity of liver, (3) poor healing due to reduced levels of substrate, and (4) impairment of cell-mediated immunity.[278] As a result, wound healing is retarded, skin ulcers occur, and requirements for artificial ventilation are prolonged. Abel and colleagues have suggested that hyperalimentation in the immediate postoperative period does not significantly alter the increased morbidity.[279] This has led Blackburn et al. to suggest that both preoperative and concurrent nutritional support are necessary.[278]

Cardiovascular Manifestations of Vitamin Deficiency

THIAMINE DEFICIENCY

(See p. 461)

OTHER VITAMIN DEFICIENCIES. Deficiencies of other vitamins have not led to specifically definable cardiovascular abnormalities, except for the hypocalcemia-accompanied vitamin D deficiency. However, vitamin deficiencies, particularly of the B group and folic acid, have been diagnosed with increasing frequency in patients with cardiovascular disease. For example, nearly a third of infants and children with congenital heart disease have been reported to be deficient in a number of the B vitamins.[280] Folic acid deficiency has been documented in a significant number of patients with congestive heart failure. Although the deficient state may simply be related to decreased intake, abnormal intestinal absorption or increased rates of excretion may also contribute.

THE HEART AND GONADAL HORMONES

There are no specific cardiovascular abnormalities associated with altered gonadal function except for occasional cardiac structural abnormalities in Kallman's syndrome, a genetic form of hypogonadotropic hypogonadism, and a rare form of cardiomyopathy associated with primary hypogonadism. Men have an increased risk of coronary heart disease of approximately twice that of women, as demonstrated in the 26-year follow-up of the Framingham population. With increasing age, the coronary heart disease mortality rate in women approaches that of men, becoming almost equal by age 75[281] (see p. 1707). Of note, however, is the dramatic increase in coronary heart disease in women that occurs at age 45 to 55. Because these years encompass the average time of menopause in the United States, it is postulated that hormones of the premenopausal woman are protective against coronary heart disease. Several risk factors for coronary heart disease increase following menopause, including hypertension and a more atherogenic lipid profile, which may be secondary to the loss of estrogen. Estrogens increase HDL cholesterol, which represented much of its cardiovascular benefit in the Lipid Research Clinics Trial.[282] Natural estrogen may also lower blood pressure.[283] Much of the belief to the contrary is based on outdated oral contraceptive literature, which used higher doses of estrogens and various progestins. In addition, estrogen may have direct effects that impact on coronary heart disease. For example, estrogens may act as direct vasodilators in the coronary vessels and thereby improve ischemia in women with coronary heart disease.[284] Finally, estrogen appears to lower levels of plasminogen activator inhibitor (PAI-1), which could lead to greater fibrinolytic activity.[285]

In 1985, two major conflicting studies were published addressing the issue of hormone replacement therapy's effect on cardiovascular disease. Whereas analysis of the Framingham population demonstrated an increased risk of coronary heart disease without a concomitant increased mortality associated with estrogen use,[286] analysis of the Nurses' Health Study[287] showed a benefit for the use of estrogen. The majority of prospective studies, however, have found a *reduction* in risk of coronary heart disease with estrogen use (reviewed in ref. 288). The more recent analysis of 10 years of follow-up in the Nurses' Health Study supported the earlier finding of a benefit of estrogen on cardiovascular disease.[289] Of the 48,470 women followed prospectively, those who were current users of estrogen for hormone replacement therapy had an approximately 50 per cent lower risk of fatal cardiovascular disease with no increase in stroke, compared with those who had never used estrogen. The reason for the discrepancy between the Framingham Study and the majority of other studies is unclear. The Framingham population did report higher estrogen doses than those of other studies. This conflict illustrates the potential limitations of epidemiological *versus* clinical trial approaches to answer critical therapeutic questions.

In summary, most studies demonstrate a benefit for estrogen use against coronary heart disease. In practice, however, estrogen is given with a progestin to protect against endometrial hyperplasia in women who have not undergone hysterectomy. The effect of the use of both an estrogen and progestin on coronary heart disease has been less well studied. A recent cross-sectional study of 4958 postmenopausal women taking estrogen alone, and women taking estrogen and progestin, demonstrated persistent or even greater benefit in terms of lipid profiles with the addition of progestin.[290]

A prospective 3-year study of 875 postmenopausal women who received estrogen alone or in combination with a progestin confirmed the results of the cross-sectional study. Women who received estrogen alone and those who received both estrogen and a progestin showed an improvement in lipoprotein profiles and a lowering in fibrinogen levels, whereas the former group alone had a high rate of endometrial hyperplasia not seen in the latter.[291] Treatment with estrogen alone also led to a greater increase in HDL cholesterol. Future studies of the impact of the combined use of estrogen and progestin on actual coronary heart disease are necessary.

TAMOXIFEN. This drug, an estrogen receptor partial agonist with antiestrogenic activity on the breast, is frequently used for the treatment of breast cancer, particularly in postmenopausal women. Several studies have suggested a cardiovascular benefit to tamoxifen. A retrospective review of women in the Scottish adjuvant tamoxifen trial, compared 1070 women who were randomized to tamoxifen given as adjuvant prophylactically versus only on recurrence. The incidence of fatal myocardial infarction was significantly lower in the women given adjuvant tamoxifen for at least 5 years. The Stockholm Breast Cancer Study group found that in over 1000 women receiving tamoxifen, there was a significant decrease in hospital admissions for cardiac disease compared with 1000 who were not. There was greater benefit seen with 5 than with 2 years of use.[293] One mechanism whereby tamoxifen may provide cardiovascular benefit is through a fall in total cholesterol and LDL, as demonstrated in the Wisconsin Tamoxifen Study.[294]

ORAL CONTRACEPTIVES. The literature on the association between oral contraceptive use and coronary heart disease is controversial. The controversy is due in large part to the decreasing estrogen content in oral contraceptives over the past 40 years as well as the incorporation of varying progestins with different androgenic potencies. The changing spectrum of oral contraceptive composition also makes it difficult to extend data based on earlier agents to today's preparations. Several studies have shown an increased risk of myocardial infarction in oral contraceptive users.[295–297] However, prior oral contraceptive use does not confer an increased risk for cardiovascular disease.[298] Studies of the effect of newer contraceptive agents are not available.

BLOOD PRESSURE EFFECTS OF ORAL CONTRACEPTIVES AND HORMONAL REPLACEMENT THERAPY

Oral contraceptive use has been associated with a rise in blood pressure since their widespread use in the 1960's. When blood pressure rises, it usually remains within the normotensive range; rarely, it increases into the hypertensive (>140/90 mm Hg) range. Even with the earlier generation oral contraceptives, which used higher estrogen dose and varied progestins, there were conflicting data as to whether blood pressure rises or not.[299–301] Differences in responses to oral contraceptives may depend on quantity of estrogen, type of progestin, and race and genetic background of the user. Studies of the new generation of oral contraceptives, which contain no greater than 35 μg ethinyl estradiol and less androgenic progestins, are more limited. Available data on desogestrel-containing oral contraceptives include a multicenter trial of more than 1600 women followed over 23,000 cycles. No significant change in mean blood pressure over 2 years of use was observed and only a 0.3 per cent incidence of hypertension was noted.[302] Other studies of this agent have revealed similar results.[303,304] Although activation of the renin-angiotensin-aldosterone axis occurs in oral contraceptive users, the degree of activation may be greater in those who remain normotensive than those who became hypertensive.[305] Thus, the etiology of oral contraceptive–induced hypertension remains unclear.

The belief that estrogens used for hormone replacement therapy induce hypertension is largely based on the older oral contraceptive literature. In fact, the use of estrogen in many trials is associated with no change in blood pressure. It is likely that estrogens differ in their effect on blood pressure. Estrone, a natural estrogen, may actually lead to a fall in blood pressure.[306]

REFERENCES

1. Graves, R. J.: Clinical lectures. London Med. Surg. J. (Part II) *7*:516, 1835.
2. Addison, T.: On the constitutional and local effects of diseases of the suprarenal capsules. London, Highley, 1855.

3. Daughaday, W. H.: Growth hormone, insulin-like growth factors, and acromegaly. *In* DeGroot, L. J., et al. (eds.): Endocrinology, Vol. 1. 3rd ed. Philadelphia, W.B. Saunders Company, 1995, p. 303.
4. Strobl, J. S., and Thomas, M. J.: Human growth hormone. Pharmacol. Rev. *46*:1, 1994.
5. Hartman, M. L., Veldhuis, J. D., and Thorner, M. O.: Normal control of growth hormone secretion. Horm. Res. *40*:37, 1993.
6. Wass, J. A. H.: Somatostatin. *In* DeGroot, L. J., et al. (eds.): Endocrinology, Vol. 1. 3rd ed. Philadelphia, W.B. Saunders Company, 1995, p. 266.
7. Rotwein, P.: Structure, evolution, expression and regulation of insulin-like growth factors I and II. Growth Factors *5*:3, 1991.
8. Clemmons, D. R.: Insulin-like growth factor binding proteins. Trends Endocrin. Metab. *1*:412, 1990.
9. Yamashita, S., Weiss, M., and Melmed, S.: Insulin-like growth factor I regulates growth hormone secretion and messenger ribonucleic acid levels in human pituitary cells. J. Clin. Endocrinol. Metab. *62*:730, 1986.
10. Sacca, L., Cittadini, A., and Fazio, S.: Growth hormone and the heart. Endocr. Rev. *15*:55, 1994.
11. Froesch, E. R., Zenobi, P. D., and Hussain, M.: Metabolic and therapeutic effects of insulin-like growth factor I. Horm. Res. *42*:66, 1994.
12. Thuesen, L., Christiansen, J. S., Sorensen, J. O. L., et al.: Increased myocardial contractility following growth hormone administration in normal man. Danish Med. Bull. *35*:183, 1988.
13. Caidahl, K., Eden, S., and Bengtsson, B. A.: Cardiovascular and renal effects of growth hormone. Clin. Endocrinol. *40*:393, 1994.
14. Greco, A. V., Ghirlanda, G., Barone, C., et al.: Somatostatin in the paroxysmal supraventricular and junctional tachycardia. Br. Med. J. *288*:28, 1984.
15. Day, S. M., Gu, J., Polak, J. M., and Bloom, S. R.: Somatostatin in the human heart and comparison with guinea pig and rat heart. Br. Heart J. *53*:153, 1985.
16. Thorner, M. O., Perryman, R. L., Cronin, M. J., et al.: Somatotroph hyperplasia: Successful treatment of acromegaly by removal of a pancreatic islet tumor secreting a growth hormone–releasing factor. J. Clin. Invest. *70*:965, 1982.
17. Ezzat, S., Forster, M. J., Berchtold, P., et al.: Acromegaly. Clinical and biochemical features in 500 patients. Medicine *73*:233, 1994.
18. Fazio, S., Cittadini, A., Cuocolo, A., et al.: Impaired cardiac performance is a distinct feature of uncomplicated acromegaly. J. Clin. Endocrinol. Metab. *79*:441, 1994.
19. Lie, J. T., and Grossman, S. J.: Pathology of the heart in acromegaly: Anatomic findings in 27 autopsied patients. Am. Heart J. *100*:41, 1980.
20. Hradec, J., Marek, J., Kral, J., et al.: Long-term echocardiography follow-up of acromegalic heart disease. Am. J. Cardiol. *72*:204, 1993.
21. Cuocolo, A., Nicolai, E., Fazio, S., et al.: Impaired left ventricular diastolic filling in patients with acromegaly: Assessment with radionuclide angiography. J. Nucl. Med. *36*:196, 1995.
22. Deray, G., Chanson, P., Maistre, E., et al.: Atrial natriuretic factor in patients with acromegaly. Eur. J. Clin. Pharmacol. *38*:409, 1990.
23. Kraatz, C., Benker, G., Weber, F., et al.: Acromegaly and hypertension: Prevalence and relationship to the renin-angiotensin-aldosterone system. Klin. Wochenschr. *68*:583, 1990.
24. Moore, T. J., Thein-Wai, W., Dluhy, R. G., et al.: Abnormal adrenal and vascular responses to angiotensin II and an angiotensin antagonist in acromegaly. J. Clin. Endocrinol. Metab. *51*:215, 1980.
25. Ng, L. L., and Evans, D. L.: Leukocyte sodium transport in acromegaly. Clin. Endocrinol. *26*:471, 1987.
26. Kahaly, G. Olshausen, K. V., Mohr-Kahaly, S., et al.: Arrhythmia profile in acromegaly. Eur. Heart J. *13*:51, 1992.
27. Surawicz, B., and Mangiardi, M. L.: Electrocardiogram in endocrine and metabolic disorders. *In* Rios, J. G. (eds.): Clinical Electrocardiographic Correlations. Philadelphia, F. A. Davis Co., 1977, p. 243.
28. Hayward, R. P., Emanuel, R. W., and Navarro, J. D. N.: Acromegalic heart disease: Influence of treatment of the acromegaly on the heart. Q. J. Med. *62*:41, 1987.
29. Rodrigues, E. A., Caruana, M., Lahiri, A., et al.: Subclinical cardiac dysfunction in acromegaly: Evidence for a specific disease of heart muscle. Br. Heart J. *62*:185, 1989.
30. Fazio, S., Cittadini, A., Sabatini, D., et al.: Evidence for biventricular involvement in acromegaly: A Doppler echocardiographic study. Eur. Heart J. *14*:26, 1993.
31. Chanson, P., Timsit, J., Masquet, C., et al.: Cardiovascular effects of the somatostatin analog octreotide in acromegaly. Ann. Intern. Med. *113*:921, 1990.
32. Lim, M. J., Barkan, A. L., and Buda, A. J.: Rapid reduction of left ventricular hypertrophy in acromegaly after suppression of growth hormone hypersecretion. Ann. Intern. Med. *117*:719, 1992.
33. Merola, B., Cittadini, A., Colao, A., et al.: Chronic treatment with the somatostatin analog octreotide improves cardiac abnormalities in acromegaly. J. Clin. Endocrinol. Metab. *77*:790, 1993.
34. Rossi, E., Zuppi, P., Pennestri, F., et al.: Acromegalic cardiomyopathy. Left ventricular filling and hypertrophy in active and surgically treated disease. Chest *102*:1204, 1992.
35. Dillmann, W. H.: Biochemical basis of thyroid hormone action in the heart. Am. J. Med. *88*:626, 1990.
36. Polikar, R., Burger, A. G., Scherrer, U., and Nicod, P.: The thyroid and the heart. Circulation *87*:1435, 1993.
37. Davis, P. J., and Davis, F. B.: Acute cellular actions of thyroid hormone and myocardial function. Ann. Thorac. Surg. *56*:S16, 1993.
38. Dillmann, W. H.: Cardiac function in thyroid disease: Clinical features and management considerations. Ann. Thorac. Surg. *56*:S9, 1993.
39. Lazar, M. A.: Thyroid hormone receptors: Multiple forms, multiple possibilities. Endocrinol. Rev. *14*:184, 1993.
40. Tsai, M. J., and O'Malley, B. W.: Molecular mechanisms of action of steroid/thyroid receptor superfamily members. Ann Rev. Biochem. *63*:451, 1994.
41. Tsika, R. W., Bahl, J. J., Leinwand, L. A., and Morkin, E.: Thyroid hormone regulates expression of a transfected human α-myosin heavy chain fusion gene in fetal rat heart cells. Proc. Natl. Acad. Sci. U.S.A. *87*:379, 1990.
42. Zarain-Herzberg, A., Marques, J., Sukovich, D., and Periasamy, M.: Thyroid hormone receptor modulates the expression of the rabbit cardiac sarco (endo) plasmic reticulum Ca(2+)-ATPase gene. J. Biol. Chem. *269*:1460, 1994.
43. Orlowski, J., and Lingrell, J. B.: Thyroid and glucocorticoid hormones regulate the expression of multiple Na, K-ATPase genes in cultured neonatal rat cardiac myocyte. J. Biol. Chem. *265*:3462, 1990.
44. Bahouth, S. W.: Thyroid hormones transcriptionally regulate the β-1 adrenergic receptor gene in cultured ventricular myocyte. J. Biol. Chem. *266*:15863, 1991.
45. Castello, A., Rodriguez-Manazaneque, J. C., Camps, M., et al.: Perinatal hypothyroidism impairs the normal transition of GLUT4 and GLUT1 glucose transporters from fetal to neonatal levels in heart and brown adipose tissue. Evidence for tissue-specific regulation of GLUT4 expression by thyroid hormone. J. Biol. Chem. *269*:5905, 1994.
46. Averyhart-Fullard, V., Fraker, L. D., Murphy, A. M., and Solaro, R. J.: Differential regulation of slow-skeletal and cardiac troponin I mRNA during development and by thyroid hormone in rat heart. J. Mol. Cell Cardiol. *26*:609, 1994.
47. Dieckman, L. J., and Solaro, R. J.: Effect of thyroid status on thin-filament Ca^{2+} regulation and expression of troponin I in perinatal and adult rat hearts. Circ. Res. *67*:344, 1990.
48. Fullerton, M. J., Stuchbury, S., Krozowski, Z. S., and Funder, J. W.: Altered thyroidal status and the *in vivo* synthesis of atrial natriuretic peptide in the rat heart. Mol. Cell Endocrinol. *69*:227, 1990.
49. Segal, J.: Acute effect of thyroid hormone on the heart: An extranuclear increase in sugar uptake. J. Mol. Cell Cardiol. *21*:323, 1989.
50. Segal, J.: Calcium is the first messenger for the action of thyroid hormone at the level of the plasma membrane: First evidence for an acute effect of thyroid hormone on calcium uptake in the heart. Endocrinology *126*:2693, 1990.
51. Morgan, J. P.: Thyroid hormone effects on intracellular calcium and inotropic responses of rat ventricular myocardium. Am. J. Physiol. *267*:H1112, 1994.
52. Han, J., Leem, C., So, I., et al.: Effects of thyroid hormone on the calcium current and isoprenaline-induced background current in rabbit ventricular myocytes. J. Mol. Cell. Cardiol. *26*:925, 1994.
53. Levey, G. S., and Klein, I.: Catecholamine-thyroid interactions and the cardiovascular manifestation of hyperthyroidism. Am. J. Med. *88*:642, 1990.
54. Hammond, H. K., White, F. C., Buxton, I. L. O., et al.: Increased myocardial beta-receptors and adrenergic responses in hyperthyroid pigs. Am. J. Physiol. *252*:H283, 1987.
55. Buccino, R. A., Spann, J. F., Pool, P. E., and Braunwald, E.: Influence of the thyroid state on the intrinsic contractile properties and the energy stores of the myocardium. J. Clin. Invest. *46*:1669, 1967.
56. Nishizawa, Y., Hamada, N., Fujii, S., et al.: Serum dopamine beta-hydroxylase activity in thyroid disorders. J. Clin. Endocrinol. Metab. *39*:599, 1974.
57. Malbon, C. C., and Greenberg, M. L.: 3, 3′,5′-Triiodothyronine administration in vivo modulates the hormone sensitive adenylate cyclase system of rat hepatocytes. J. Clin. Invest. *69*:414, 1982.
58. Whitsett, J. A., Pollinger, J., and Matz, S.: β-Adrenergic receptors and catecholamine-sensitive adenylate cyclase in developing rat ventricular myocardium: Effect of thyroid status. Pediatr. Res. *16*:463, 1982.
59. Rutherford, J. P., Vatner, S. F., and Braunwald, E.: Adrenergic control of myocardial contractility in conscious hyperthyroid dogs. Am. J. Physiol. *237*:590, 1980.
60. Guarnieri, T., Filburn, C. R., Beard, E. S., and Lakatta, E. G.: Enhanced contractile response and protein kinase activation to threshold levels of β-adrenergic stimulation in hyperthyroid rat heart. J. Clin. Invest. *65*:861, 1980.
61. Andersson, R. G. G., Nilsson, O. R., and Kuo, J. F.: β-Adrenoreceptor adenosine 3′-5′-monophosphate system in human leukocytes before and after treatment for hyperthyroidism. J. Clin. Endocrinol. Metab. *56*:42, 1993.
62. Stiles, G. L., Stadel, J. M., DeLean, A., and Lefkowitz, R. J.: Hypothyroidism modulates beta-adrenergic receptor adenylate cyclase interactions in rat reticulocytes. J. Clin. Invest. *68*:1450, 1981.
63. Bahouth, S. W.: Regulation of steady-state levels of beta-adrenergic re-

ceptors and G-proteins by thyroid hormones in cultured rat myocardial cells. FASEB J. *4*:A1779, 1990.
64. Levine, M. A., Feldman, A. M., Robishaw, J. D., et al.: Influence of thyroid hormone status on expression of genes encoding G protein subunits in the rat heart. J. Biol. Chem. *265*:3553, 3560, 1990.
65. Rapiejko, P. J., Watkins, D. C., Ros, M., and Malbon, C. C.: Thyroid hormones regulate G-protein beta-subunit mRNA expression in vivo. J. Biol. Chem. *264*:16183, 1989.
66. Ling, E., O'Brien, P. J., Salerno, T., et al.: Effects of different thyroid treatments on the biochemical characteristics of rabbit myocardium. Can. J. Cardiol. *4*:301, 1988.
67. Murayama, M., and Goodkind, M. J.: Effect of thyroid hormone on the frequency-force relationship of atrial myocardium from the guinea pig. Circ. Res. *23*:743, 1968.
68. Josephson, R. A., Spurgeon, H. A., and Lakatta, E. G.: The hyperthyroid heart: An analysis of systolic and diastolic properties in single rat ventricular myocytes. Circ. Res. *66*:773, 1990.
69. Goldman, S., Olajos, M., Friedman, H., et al.: Left ventricular performance in conscious thyrotoxic calves. Am. J. Physiol. *242*:H113, 1982.
70. Goto, Y., Slinker, B. K., and LeWinter, M. M.: Decreased contractile efficiency and increased nonmechanical energy cost in hyperthyroid rabbit heart: Relation between O_2 consumption and systolic pressure-volume area or force-time interval. Circ. Res. *66*:999, 1990.
71. Kim, D., Smith, T. W., and Marsh, J. D.: Effect of thyroid hormone on slow calcium channel function in cultured chick ventricular cells. J. Clin. Invest. *80*:88, 1987.
72. MacKinnon, R., Gwathmey, J. K., Allen, P. D., et al.: Modulation by the state of intracellular calcium and contractility in ferret ventricular muscle. Circ. Res. *63*:1080, 1988.
73. Poggesi, C., Everets, M., Polla, B., et al.: Influence of thyroid state on mechanical restitution of rat myocardium. Circ. Res. *60*:142, 1987.
74. Samuel, J. L., Rappaport, L., Syrovy, L., et al.: Differential effect of thyroxine on atrial and ventricular isomyosins in rats. Am. J. Physiol. *250*:H333, 1986.
75. Korecky, B., Zak, R., Schwartz, K., et al.: Role of thyroid hormone in regulation of isomyosin composition, contractility, and size of heterotypically isotransplanted rat heart. Circ. Res. *60*:824, 1987.
76. Johnson, P. N., Freedberg, A. S., and Marshall, J. M.: Action of thyroid hormone on the transmembrane potentials from sinoatrial cells and atrial muscle cells in isolated atria of rabbits. Cardiology *58*:273, 1973.
77. Arnsdorf, M. D., and Childers, R. W.: Atrial electrophysiology in experimental hyperthyroidism in rabbits. Circ. Res. *26*:575, 1970.
78. McKenzie, J. M., and Zakarija, M.: Hyperthyroidism. *In* DeGroot, J. L., et al. (eds.): Endocrinology, Vol. 1. 3rd ed. Philadelphia, W.B. Saunders Company, 1995, p. 676.
79. Woeber, K. A.: Thyrotoxicosis and the heart. N. Engl. J. Med. *327*:94, 1992.
80. Talafih, K., Briden, K. L., and Weiss, H. R.: Thyroxine-induced hypertrophy of the rabbit heart. Effect on regional oxygen extraction, flow and oxygen consumption. Circ. Res. *52*:272, 1983.
81. Friedman, M. J., Okada, R. D., Ewy, G. A., and Hellman, D. J.: Left ventricular systolic and diastolic function in hyperthyroidism. Am. Heart J. *104*:1303, 1982.
82. Feldman, T., Borow, K. M., Sarne, D. H., et al.: Myocardial mechanics in hyperthyroidism: Importance of left ventricular loading conditions, heart rate and contractile state. J. Am. Coll. Cardiol. *7*:967, 1986.
83. Maciel, B. C., Gallo, L., Marin-Neto, J., et al.: Autonomic control of heart rate during dynamic exercise in human hyperthyroidism. Clin. Sci. *75*:209, 1988.
84. Forfar, J. C., Matthews, D. M., and Toft, D. A.: Delayed recovery of left ventricular function after antithyroid treatment: Further evidence for reversible abnormalities on contractility in hyperthyroidism. Br. Heart J. *52*:215, 1984.
85. Olshausen, K., Bischoll, S., Kahaly, G., et al.: Cardiac arrhythmias and heart rate in hyperthyroidism. Am. J. Cardiol. *63*:930, 1989.
86. Ciaccheri, M., Cecchi, F., Arcangeli, C., et al.: Occult thyrotoxicosis in patients with chronic and paroxysmal isolated atrial fibrillation. Clin. Cardiol. *7*:413, 1984.
87. Goel, B. G., Hanson, C. S., and Han, J.: A-V conduction in hyper- and hypothyroid dogs. Am. Heart J. *83*:504, 1972.
88. Seibers, M. J., Drinka, P. J., and Vergauwen, C.: Hyperthyroidism as a cause of atrial fibrillation in long-term care. Arch. Intern. Med. *152*:2063, 1992.
89. Cavallo, A., Joseph, C. J., and Casta, A.: Cardiac complications in juvenile hyperthyroidism. Am. J. Dis. Child. *138*:479, 1984.
90. Featherstone, H. J., and Stewart, D. K.: Angina in thyrotoxicosis: Thyroid-related coronary artery spasm. Arch. Intern. Med. *143*:554, 1983.
91. Forfar, J. C., Muir, A. L., Sawers, S. A., and Toft, A. D.: Abnormal left ventricular function in hyperthyroidism: Evidence for a possible reversible cardiomyopathy. N Engl. J. Med. *307*:1165, 1982.
92. Ebisawa, K., Ikeda, U., Maruta, M., et al.: Irreversible cardiomyopathy due to thyrotoxicosis. Cardiology *84*:274, 1994.
93. Wilson, R., Gibson, T. C., Terrien, C. M., and Levy, A. M.: Hyperthyroidism and familial hypertrophic cardiomyopathy. Arch. Intern. Med. *143*:378, 1983.
94. Noah, M. S., Sulimani, R. A., Famuyiwa, F. O., et al.: Prolapse of the mitral valve in hyperthyroid patients in Saudi Arabia. Int. J. Cardiol. *19*:217, 1988.
95. Morrow, D. H., Gaffney, T. E., and Braunwald, E.: Studies on digitalis: VIII. Effect of autonomic innervation and of myocardial catecholamine stores upon the cardiac action of ouabain. J. Pharmacol. Exp. Ther. *140*:236, 1963.
96. Klein, I., Becker, D. V., and Levey, G. S.: Treatment of hyperthyroid disease. Ann. Intern. Med. *121*:281, 1994.
97. Geffner, D. L., and Hershman, J. M.: β-Adrenergic blockade for the treatment of hyperthyroidism. Am. J. Med. *93*:61, 1992.
98. Sandler, G., and Wilson, G. M.: The nature and prognosis of heart disease in thyrotoxicosis. A review of 150 patients treated with ^{131}I. Q.J. Med. *28*:347, 1959.
99. Ladenson, P. W.: Recognition and management of cardiovascular disease related to thyroid dysfunction. Am. J. Med. *88*:638, 1990.
100. Nakazawa, H. K., Sakurai, K., Hamada, N., et al.: Management of atrial fibrillation in the post-thyrotoxic state. Am. J. Med. *72*:903, 1982.
101. Staffurth, J. S., Gibberd, M. C., and Fui, S. T.: Arterial embolism in thyrotoxicosis with atrial fibrillation. Br. Med. J. *2*:688, 1977.
102. Chopra, I. J., Huang, T.-S., Hurd, R. E., and Solomon, D. H.: A study of cardiac effects of thyroid hormones: Evidence for amelioration of the effects of thyroxine by sodium ipodate. Endocrinology *114*:2039, 1984.
103. Norman, M. F., and Lavin, T. N.: Antagonism of thyroid hormone action by amiodarone in rat pituitary tumor cells. J. Clin. Invest. *83*:306, 1989.
104. Lambert, M., Burger, A. G., DeNayer, P., et al.: Decreased TSH response to TRH induced by amiodarone. Acta Endocrinol. *118*:449, 1988.
105. Gammage, M. D., and Franklyn, J. A.: Amioradone and the thyroid. Q.J. Med. *62*:83, 1987.
106. Martino, E., Bartalena, L., Mariotti, S., et al.: Radioactive iodine thyroid uptake in patients with amioradone iodine-induced thyroid dysfunction. Acta Endocrinol. *119*:167, 1988.
107. Kasim, S. E., Bagchi, N., Brown, T. R., et al.: Effect of amiodarone on serum lipids, lipoprotein lipase, and hepatic triglyceride lipase. Endocrinology *120*:1991, 1987.
108. Rabinowe, S. L., Larsen, P. R., Antman, E. M., et al.: Amioradone therapy and autoimmune thyroid disease. Am. J. Med. *81*:53, 1986.
109. Zimmerman, J., Yahalom, J., Bar-On, H.: Clinical spectrum of pericardial effusion as the presenting feature of hypothyroidism. Am. Heart J. *106*:770, 1983.
110. Khaleeli, A. A., and Memon, N.: Factors affecting resolution of pericardial effusions in primary hypothyroidism: A clinical, biochemical and echocardiographic study. Postgrad. Med. J. *58*:1073, 1982.
111. Mackerrow, S. D., Osborn, L. A., Levey, H., et al.: Myxedema-associated cardiogenic shock treated with intravenous thyronine. Ann. Intern. Med. *117*:1014, 1992.
112. Kumar, A., Bhandari, A. K., and Rahimtoola, S. H.: Torsade de pointes and marked QT prolongation in association with hypothyroidism. Ann. Intern. Med. *106*:712, 1987.
113. Shenoy, M. M., and Goldman, J. M.: Hypothyroid cardiomyopathy: Echocardiographic documentation of reversibility. Am. J. Med. Sci. *294*:1, 1987.
114. Streeten, D. H. P., Andersen, G. H., Howland, T., et al.: Effects of thyroid function on blood pressure: Recognition of hypothyroid hypertension. Hypertension *11*:78, 1988.
115. Saito, I., Kunihiko, I., and Saruta, T.: Hypothyroidism as a cause of hypertension. Hypertension *5*:112, 1983.
116. Fouron, J. C., Bourgin, J. H., Letarte, J., et al.: Cardiac dimensions and myocardial function of infants with congenital hypothyroidism: An echocardiographic study. Br. Heart J. *47*:584, 1982.
117. Graettinger, J. S., Muenster, J. J., and Checchia, C.: A correlation of clinical and hemodynamic studies in patients with hypothyroidism. J. Clin. Invest. *37*:502, 1958.
118. Wieshammer, S., Keck, F. S., Waitzinger, J., et al.: Left ventricular function at rest and during exercise in acute hypothyroidism. Br. Heart J. *60*:204, 1988.
119. Vora, J., O'Malley, B. P., Petersen, S., et al.: Reversible abnormalities of myocardial relaxation in hypothyroidism. J. Clin. Endocrinol. Metab. *61*:269, 1985.
120. Hillis, W. S., Bremmer, W. F., Lawrie, T. D. V., and Thomson, J. A.: Systolic time intervals in thyroid disease. Clin. Endocrinol. *4*:617, 1975.
121. Grossman, N. G., Wieshammer, S., Keck, F. S., et al.: Doppler echocardiographic evaluation of left ventricular diastolic function in acute hypothyroidism. Clin. Endocrinol. *40*:227, 1994.
122. McBrion, D. J., and Hindle, W.: Myxedema and heart failure. Lancet *1*:1065, 1963.
123. Levey, G. S., Skelton, C. L., and Epstein, S. E.: Decreased myocardial adenyl cyclase activity in hypothyroidism. J. Clin. Invest. *48*:2244, 1969.
124. Elder, J., McLelland, A., O'Reilly, D. S., et al.: The relationship between serum cholesterol and serum thyrotropin, thyroxine and tri-iodothyronine concentrations in suspected hypothyroidism. Ann. Clin. Biochem. *36*:110, 1990.
125. Arem, N., and Patsch, W.: Lipoprotein and apolipoprotein levels in subclinical hypothyroidism. Arch. Intern. Med. *150*:2097, 1990.
126. Steinberg, A. D.: Myxedema and coronary artery disease—a comparative autopsy study. Ann. Intern. Med. *68*:338, 1968.
127. Karlsberg, R. P., Friscia, D. A., Aronow, W. S., and Sekhon, S. S. Deleterious influence of hypothyroidism on evolving myocardial infarction in conscious dogs. J. Clin. Invest. *67*:1024, 1981.
128. Keating, F. R., Parkin, T. W., Selby, J. B., and Dickinson, L. S.: Treatment of heart disease associated with myxedema. Prog. Cardiovasc. Dis. *3*:364, 1960.

129. Griffiths, P. D.: Serum enzymes in diseases of the thyroid gland. J. Clin. Pathol. *18*:660, 1965.
130. Drucker, D. J., and Burrow, G. N.: Cardiovascular surgery in the hypothyroid patient. Arch. Intern. Med. *145*:1585, 1985.
131. Hamblin, P. S., Dyer, S. A., Mohr, V. S., et al.: Relationship between thyrotropin and thyroxine changes during recovery from severe hypothyroxinemia of critical illness. J. Clin. Endocrinol. Metab. *62*:717, 1986.
132. Brent, G. A., and Hershman, J. M.: Thyroxine therapy in patients with severe nonthyroidal illnesses and low serum thyroxine concentration. J. Clin. Endocrinol. Metab. *63*:1, 1986.

DISEASES OF THE ADRENAL CORTEX

133. Williams, G. H., and Dluhy, R. G.: Diseases of the adrenal cortex. *In* Isselbacher, K., et al. (eds.): Harrison's Principles of Internal Medicine. 13th ed. New York, McGraw-Hill Book Co., 1994, p. 1953.
134. Mortensen, R. M., and Williams G. H.: Aldosterone action: Physiology. *In* DeGroot, L. J., et al. (eds.): Endocrinology, Vol. 1. 3rd ed. Philadelphia, W.B. Saunders Company, 1995, p. 1668.
135. Brilla, C. G., Zhou, G., Matsubara, L., and Weber, K. T.: Collagen metabolism in cultured rat cardiac fibroblasts: Response to angiotensin II and aldosterone. J. Mol. Cell Cardiol. *26*:809, 1994.
136. Cushing, H.: The basophil adenomas of the pituitary body and their clinical manifestations (pituitary basophilism). Bull. Johns Hopkins Hosp. *50*:137, 1932.
137. Etxabe, J., and Vazquez, J. A.: Morbidity and mortality in Cushing's disease: An epidemiological approach. Clin. Endocrinol. *40*:479, 1994.
138. Soszynski, P., Slowinska-Srzednicka, J., Kasperlik-Zaluska, A., and Zglicaynski, S.: Endogenous natriuretic factors: Atrial natriuretic hormone and digitalis-like substance in Cushing's syndrome. J. Endocrinol. *129*:453, 1991.
139. Mantero, F., and Boscaro, M.: Glucocorticoid-dependent hypertension. J. Steroid Biochem. Mol. Biol. *43*:409, 1992.
140. Yasuda, G., Shionoiri, H., Umeura, S., et al.: Exaggerated blood pressure response to angiotensin II in patients with Cushing's syndrome due to adrenocortical adenomas. Eur. J. Endocrinol. *131*:582, 1994.
141. Sugihara, N., Shimizu, M., Kita, Y., et al.: Cardiac characteristics and post-operative courses in Cushing's syndrome. Am. J. Cardiol. *69*:1475, 1992.
142. Carney, J. A., Gordon, H., Carpenter, P. C., et al.: The complex of myxomas, spotty pigmentation, and endocrine overactivity. Medicine *64*:270, 1985.
143. Fallo, F., Paoletta, A., Tona, F., et al.: Response of hypertension to conventional antihypertensive treatment and/or steroidogenesis inhibitors in Cushing's syndrome. J. Intern. Med. *234*:595, 1993.
144. Conlin, P. R., Dluhy, R. G., and Williams, G. H.: Disorders of the renin-angiotensin-aldosterone system. *In* Schrier, R. W. (ed.): Renal and Electrolyte Disorders. 4th ed. Boston, Little, Brown & Co., 1992, p. 405.
145. Lifton, R. P., Dluhy, R. G., Powers, M., et al.: A chimeric 11 β-hydroxylase/aldosterone synthase gene causes glucocorticoid-remediable aldosteronism in human hypertension. Nature *355*:262, 1992.
146. Rabinowe, S. L., Jackson, R. A., Dluhy, R. G., and Williams, G. H.: Ia-positive T lymphocytes in recently-diagnosed idiopathic Addison's disease. Am. J. Med. *77*:597, 1984.
147. Knowlton, A. L., and Baer, L.: Cardiac failure in Addison's disease. Am. J. Med. *74*:829, 1983.
148. Dorin, R. I., and Kearns, P. J.: High output circulatory failure in acute adrenal insufficiency. Crit. Care Med. *16*:296, 1988.
149. Schambelan, M., Sebastian, A., and Biglieri, E. G.: Prevalence, pathogenesis and functional significance of aldosterone deficiency in hyperkalemic patients with chronic renal insufficiency. Kidney Int. *17*:89, 1980.
150. Lee, T. H., Salomon, D. R., Rayment, C. M., and Antman, E.: Hypotension and sinus arrest with exercise-induced hyperkalemia and combined verapamil/propranolol therapy. Am. J. Med. *80*:1203, 1986.
151. Mannisi, J. A., Weisman, H. F., Bush, D. E., et al.: Steroid administration after myocardial infarction promotes early infarct expansion. J. Clin. Invest. *79*:1431, 1987.
152. Alford, W. C., Meador, C. K., Mihalevich, J., et al.: Acute adrenal insufficiency following cardiac surgical procedures. J. Thorac. Cardiovasc. Surg. *78*:489, 1979.

PHEOCHROMOCYTOMA

153. Gifford, R. W., Manger, W. M., and Bravo, E. L.: Pheochromocytoma. Endocrinol. Metab. Clin. North. Am. *23*:387, 1994.
154. Wurtman, R. J., and Axelrod, J.: Control of enzymatic synthesis of adrenaline in the adrenal medulla by adrenal cortical steroids. J. Biol. Chem. *241*:2301, 1966.
155. Levenson, J. A., Safar, M. E., London, G. M., and Simon, A. C.: Haemodynamics in patients with phaeochromocytoma. Clin. Sci. *58*:349, 1980.
156. Sardesai, S. H., Marinde, A. J., Sivathandon, Y., et al.: Phaeochromocytoma and catecholamine-induced cardiomyopathy presenting as heart failure. Br. Heart J. *63*:234, 1990.
157. Bravo, E., Fouad-Tarazi, F., Rossi, G., et al.: A reevaluation of the hemodynamics of pheochromocytoma. Hypertension *15*:I128, 1990.
158. Strenson, G., and Swedberg, K.: QRS amplitudes, QT intervals, and ECG abnormalities in pheochromocytoma patients before, during and after treatment. Acta Med. Scand. *224*:231, 1988.
159. Haas, G. J., Tzagournis, M., and Boudoulas, H.: Pheochromocytoma: Catecholamine-mediated electrocardiographic changes mimicking ischemia. Am. Heart J. *116*:1363, 1988.
160. Scott, I., Parkes, R., and Cameron, D. P.: Pheochromocytoma and cardiomyopathy. Med. J. Aust. *148*:94, 1988.
161. Behrana, A. J., Haselton, P., Leen, C. I. S., et al.: Multiple extra-adrenal paragangliomas associated with catecholamine cardiomyopathy. Eur. Heart J. *10*:182, 1989.
162. Slathe, M., Weiss, P., and Ritz, R.: Rapid reversal of heart failure in a patient with phaeochromocytoma and catecholamine-induced cardiomyopathy who was treated with captopril. Br. Heart J. *68*:527, 1992.
163. Hu, Z. W., Billingham, M., Tuck, M., and Hoffman, B. B.: Captopril improves hypertension and cardiomyopathy in rats with pheochromocytoma. Hypertension *15*:210, 1990.
164. Schub, C., Gueto-Carcia, L., Sheps, S. G., et al.: Echocardiographic findings in pheochromocytoma. Am. J. Cardiol. *57*:971, 1986.
165. Cueto, L., Arriaga, J., and Zinser, J.: Echocardiographic changes in pheochromocytoma. Chest *76*:600, 1979.
166. McManus, B. M., Fleury, T. A., Roberts, W. C.: Fatal catecholamine crisis in pheochromocytoma. Curable form of cardiac arrest. Am. Heart J. *102*:930, 1981.
167. Simons, M., and Downing, S. E.: Coronary vasoconstriction and catecholamine cardiomyopathy. Am. Heart J. *109*:297, 1985.
168. Bhatnagar, D., Carey, P., and Pollard, A.: Focal myositis and elevated creatinine kinase levels in a patient with phaeochromocytoma. Postgrad. Med. J. *62*:197, 1986.
169. Serfas, D., Shoback, D. M., and Lorrell, B. H.: Phaeochromocytoma and hypertrophic cardiomyopathy: Apparent suppression of symptoms and noradrenaline secretion by calcium-channel blockade. Lancet *2*:711, 1983.
170. Jebara, V. A., Uva, M. S., Farge, A., et al.: Cardiac pheochromocytomas. Ann. Thorac. Surg. *53*:356, 1992.
171. Brown, E. M.: Physiology of calcium metabolism. *In* Becker, K. L. (ed.): Principles and Practice of Endocrinology and Metabolism. Philadelphia, J. B. Lippincott, Co., 1990, p. 423.
172. Bogin, E., Massry, S. G., and Harary, I.: Effect of parathyroid hormone on rat heart cells. J. Clin. Invest. *67*:1215, 1981.
173. Katoh, Y., Klein, K. L., Kaplan, R. A., et al.: Parathyroid hormone has a positive inotropic action in the rat. Endocrinology *109*:2252, 1981.
174. Palmieri, G. M., Nutting, D. F., Bhattacharya, S. K., et al.: Parathyroid ablation in dystrophic hamsters: Effects of Ca content and histology of heart, diaphragm, and rectus femoris. J. Clin. Invest. *68*:646, 1981.
175. Gafter, U., Battler, A., Eldar, M., et al.: Effect of hyperparathyroidism on cardiac function in patients with end-stage renal disease. Nephron *41*:30, 1985.
176. Vered, I., Vered, Z., Perez, J. E., et al.: Normal left ventricular performance documented by Doppler echocardiography in patients with long-standing hypocalcemia. Am. J. Med. *86*:413, 1989.
177. Giles, T. D., Iteld, B. J., and Rires, K. L.: The cardiomyopathy of hypoparathyroidism. Chest *79*:225, 1981.
178. Ellison, D. H., and McCarron, D. A.: Structural prerequisites for the hypotensive action of parathyroid hormone. Am. J. Physiol. *246*:F551, 1984.
179. Roberts, W. C., and Waller, B. F.: Effect of chronic hypercalcemia on the heart: An analysis of 18 necropsy patients. Am. J. Med. *71*:371, 1981.
180. Roberts, W. C., and Waller, B. F.: Chronic hypercalcemia as a risk factor for coronary atherosclerosis. Cardiovasc. Rev. Rep. *4*:1275, 1983.
181. Slavich, G. A., Antonucci, F., and Sponza, E.: Primary hyperparathyroidism and angina pectoris. Int. J. Cardiol. *19*:266, 1988.
182. Csanady, M., Forster, T., and Julesz, J.: Reversible impairment of myocardial function in hypoparathyroidism causing hypocalcaemia. Br. Heart J. *63*:58, 1990.
183. Kleerekoper, M., Rao, D. S., and Frame, B.: Hypercalcemia, hyperparathyroidism and hypertension. Cardiovasc. Med. *3*:1283, 1978.
184. Daniels, J., and Goodman, A. D.: Hypertension and hyperparathyroidism: Inverse relation of sodium phosphate level and blood pressure. Am. J. Med. *75*:17, 1983.

PARATHYROID DISEASE

185. Hatton, D. C., Xue, H., DeMerritt, J. A., and McCarron, D. A.: $1,25(OH)_2$ vitamin D_3-induced alterations in vascular reactivity in the spontaneously hypertensive rat. Am. J. Med. Sci. *307*:S154, 1994.
186. Benishin, C. G., Lewanczuk, R. Z., and Pang, P. K.: Purification of parathyroid hypertensive factor from plasma of spontaneously hypertensive rats. Proc. Natl. Acad. Sci. U.S.A. *88*:6372, 1991.
187. Benishin, C. G., Labeda, T., Guo, D. D., et al.: Identification and purification of parathyroid hypertensive factor from organ culture of parathyroid glands from spontaneously hypertensive rats. Am. J. Hypertens. *6*:134, 1993.
188. Pang, P. K., Benishin, C. G., Shan, J., and Lewanczuk, R. Z.: PHF: The new parathyroid hypertensive factor. Blood Press. *3*:148, 1994.
189. Lewanczuk, R. Z., Benishin, C. G., Shan, J., and Pang, P. K.: Clinical aspects of parathyroid hypertensive factor. J. Cardiovasc. Pharmacol. *23*:S23, 1994.
190. Lewanczuk, R. Z., Resnick, L. M., Ho, M. S., et al.: Clinical aspects of parathyroid hypertensive factor. J. Hypertens. (Suppl). *12*:S11, 1994.

191. Halban, P. A., and Weir, G. C.: Islet cell hormones: Production and degradation. *In* Becker, K. L. (ed.): Principles and Practice of Endocrinology and Metabolism. Philadelphia. J. B. Lippincott Co., 1990, p. 1068.
192. Eisenbarth, G. S., and Kahn, C. R.: Etiology and pathogenesis of diabetes mellitus. *In* Becker, K. L. (ed.): Principles and Practice of Endocrinology and Metabolism. Philadelphia, J. B. Lippincott Co., 1990, p. 1074.
192a. Aronson, D., and Rayfield, E. J.: Diabetes and obesity. *In* Fuster, V., Ross, R., and Topol, E. J. (eds.): Atherosclerosis and Coronary Artery Disease. Philadelphia, Lippincott-Raven, 1996, pp. 327–362.
193. Woods, K. L., Samanta, A., and Burden, A. C.: Diabetes mellitus as a risk factor for acute myocardial infarction in Asians and Europeans. Br. Heart J. *62:*118, 1989.
194. Stone, P. H., Muller, J. E., Hartwell, T., et al.: The effect of diabetes mellitus on prognosis and serial left ventricular function after acute myocardial infarction: Contribution of both coronary disease and diastolic left ventricular dysfunction to the adverse prognosis. J. Am. Coll. Cardiol. *14:*49, 1989.
195. Herlitz, J., Malmberg, K., Karlson, B. W., et al.: Mortality and morbidity during a five-year follow-up of diabetics with myocardial infarction. Acta Med. Scand. *224:*31, 1988.
196. Bradley, R. F., and Schanfield, H.: Diminished pain in diabetic patients with acute myocardial infarction. Geriatrics *17:*322, 1962.
197. Kannel, W. B.: Silent myocardial ischemia and infarction: Insights from the Framingham study. Cardiol. Clin. *4:*583, 1986.
198. Savage, M. P., Krolewski, A. S., Kenien, G. G., et al.: Acute myocardial infarction in diabetes mellitus and significance of congestive heart failure as a prognostic factor. Am. J. Cardiol. *62:*665, 1988.
199. Gunderson, T., and Kjekshus, J.: Timolol treatment after myocardial infarction in diabetic patients. Diabetes Care *6:*285, 1983.
200. Ceremuzynski, L.: Hormonal and metabolic reactions evoked by acute myocardial infarction. Circ. Res. *48:*767, 1981.
201. Roy, T. M., Peterson, H. R., Snider, H. L., et al.: Autonomic influence on cardiovascular performance in diabetic subjects. Am. J. Med. *87:*382, 1989.
202. Ewing, D. J., and Clarke, B. F.: Diagnosis and management of diabetic autonomic neuropathy. Br. Med. J. *285:*916, 1982.
203. Ambepityia, G., Kopelman, P. G., Ingram, D.: Exertional myocardial ischemia in diabetes: A quantitative analysis of anginal perceptual threshold and the influence of autonomic function. J. Am. Coll. Cardiol. *15:*72, 1990.
204. Zola, B., Kahn, J. K., Juni, J. E., and Vinik, A. I.: Abnormal cardiac function in diabetic patients with autonomic neuropathy in the absence of ischemic heart disease. J. Clin. Endocrinol. Metab. *63:*208, 1986.
205. Weise, F., Heydenreich, F., Gehrig, W., and Runge, U.: Heart rate variability in diabetic patients during orthostatic load—a spectral analytic approach. Klin. Wochenschr. *68:*26, 1990.
206. Zoneraich, S.: Diabetes and the Heart. Springfield, Ill., Charles C Thomas, Publisher, 1978, p. 303.
207. Sutherland, C. G. G., Fisher, B. M., Frier, B. M., et al.: Endomyocardial biopsy pathology in insulin-dependent diabetic patients with abnormal ventricular function. Histopathology *14:*593, 1989.
208. Hausdorf, G., Rieger, U., and Koepp, P.: Cardiomyopathy in childhood diabetes mellitus: Incidence, time of onset, and relation to metabolic control. Int. J. Cardiol. *19:*225, 1988.
209. Zarich, S. W., Arbuckle, B. E., Cohen, L. R., et al.: Diastolic abnormalities in young asymptomatic diabetic patients assessed by pulsed Doppler echocardiography. J. Am. Coll. Cardiol. *12:*114, 1988.
210. Takenakam, K., Sakamoto, T., Amano, K., et al.: Left ventricular filling determined by Doppler echocardiography in diabetes mellitus. Am. J. Cardiol. *61:*1139, 1988.
211. Ruddy, T. D., Shumak, S. L., Liu, P. P., et al.: The relationship of cardiac diastolic dysfunction to concurrent hormonal and metabolic status in Type I diabetes mellitus. J. Clin. Endocrinol. Metab. *66:*113, 1988.
212. Mustonen, J. N., Usitupa, M. I. J., Tahvanainen, K., et al.: Impaired left ventricular systolic function during exercise in middle-aged insulin-dependent and noninsulin-dependent diabetic subjects without clinically evident cardiovascular disease. Am. J. Cardiol. *62:*1273, 1988.
213. Danielsen, R., Nordrehaug, J. E., and Vik-Mo, H.: Left ventricular function in young long-term Type I (insulin-dependent) diabetic men during exercise assessed by digitized echocardiography. Eur. Heart J. *9:*395, 1988.
214. Bouchard, A., Sanz, N., Botvinick, E. H., et al.: Noninvasive assessment of cardiomyopathy in normotensive diabetic patients between 20 and 50 years old. Am. J. Med. *87:*160, 1989.
215. Paillole, C., Dahan, M., Paycha, F., et al.: Prevalence and significance of left ventricular filling abnormalities determined by Doppler echocardiography in young Type I (insulin-dependent) diabetic patients. Am. J. Cardiol. *64:*1010, 1989.
216. Danielsen, R.: Factors contributing to left ventricular diastolic dysfunction in long-term Type I diabetic subjects. Acta Med. Scand. *224:*249, 1988.
217. Ramandaham, S., Rodrigues, B., and McNeill, J. H.: Growth hormone and diabetes-induced cardiomyopathy. J. Lab. Clin. Med. *110:*257, 1987.
218. Regan, T. J., Altszuler, N., Eaddy, C., et al.: Relation of growth hormone and myocardial collagen accumulation in experimental diabetes. J. Lab. Clin. Med. *110:*274, 1987.
219. Nakada, T., and Kwee, I. L.: Sorbitol accumulation in heart: Implication for diabetic cardiomyopathy. Life Sci. *45:*2491, 1989.
220. Schaffer, S. W., Mozaffari, M. S., Artman, M., et al.: Basis for myocardial mechanical defects associated with noninsulin-dependent diabetes. Am. J. Physiol. *256:*E25, 1989.
221. Borda, E., Pascual, J., Wald, M., et al.: Hypersensitivity to calcium associated with an increased sarcolemmal Ca^{++}-ATPase activity in diabetic rat heart. Can. J. Cardiol. *4:*97, 1988.
222. Pierce, G. N., Lockwood, K., and Eckhert, C. D.: Cardiac contractile protein ATPase activity in a diet induced model of noninsulin dependent diabetes mellitus. Can. J. Cardiol. *5:*117, 1989.
223. Afzal, N., Ganguly, P. K., Dhalla, K. S., et al.: Beneficial effects of verapamil in diabetic cardiomyopathy. Diabetes *37:*936, 1988.
224. Okumura, K., Akiyama, N., Hashimoto, H., et al.: Alteration of 1,2 diacyglycerol content in myocardium from diabetic rats. Diabetes *37:*1168, 1988.
225. Sunni, S., Bishop, S. P., Kent, S. P., and Geer, J. C.: Diabetic cardiomyopathy. Arch. Pathol. Lab. Med. *110:*375, 1986.
226. Unsitupa, M., Siitonen, O., Pyorala, K., and Lansimies, E.: Left ventricular function in newly diagnosed noninsulin-dependent (type 2) diabetes evaluated by systolic time intervals and echocardiography. Acta Med. Scand. *217:*379, 1985.
227. Fein, F. S., Capasso, J. M., Aronson, R. S., et al.: Combined renovascular hypertension and diabetes in rats: A new preparation of congestive cardiomyopathy. Circulation *70:*318, 1984.
228. Regan, T. J., Wu, C. F., Weisse, A. B., et al.: Acute myocardial infarction in toxic cardiomyopathy without coronary obstruction. Circulation *51:*453, 1975.
229. Deorari, A. K., Saxena, A., Singh, M., et al.: Echocardiographic assessment of infants born to diabetic mothers. Arch. Dis. Child. *64:*721, 1989.
230. Sheehan, J. P., Sisam, D. A., and Schumacher, O. P.: Insulin-induced cardiac failure. Am. J. Med. *79:*147, 1985.
231. Zatz, R., Dunn, B. R., Meyer, T. W., et al.: Prevention of diabetic glomerulopathy by pharmacological amelioration of glomerular capillary hypertension. J. Clin. Invest. *77:*1925, 1986.
232. Marre, M., Leblanc, H., Suarez, L., et al.: Converting enzyme inhibition and kidney function in normotensive diabetic patients with persistent microalbuminuria. Br. Med. J. *294:*1448, 1987.
233. Sowers, J. R., Sowers, P. S., and Peuler, J. D.: Role of insulin resistance and hyperinsulinemia in development of hypertension and atherosclerosis. J. Lab. Clin. Med. *123:*647, 1994.
234. The Working Group on Hypertension in Diabetes: Statement on hypertension in diabetes mellitus. Final report. Arch. Intern. Med. *147:*830, 1987.
235. Ferrannini, E., and DeFronzo, R. A.: The association of hypertension, diabetes, and obesity: A review. J. Nephrol. *1:*3, 1989.
236. Reaven, G. M., and Hoffman, B. B.: Hypertension as a disease of carbohydrate and lipoprotein metabolism. Am. J. Med. *87:*2S, 1989.
237. Williams, G. H.: Converting enzyme inhibitors in the treatment of hypertension. N. Engl. J. Med. *319:*1517, 1988.
238. Houston, M. C.: Treatment of hypertension in diabetes mellitus. Am. Heart. J. *118:*819, 1989.
239. The Diabetes Control and Complications Trial Research Group: The effect of intensive treatment of diabetes on the development and progression of long-term complications in insulin-dependent diabetes mellitus. N. Engl. J. Med. *329:*977, 1993.
240. University Group Diabetes Program: A study of the effects of hypoglycemic agents on vascular complications in patients with adult onset diabetes. V. Evaluation of phenoformin therapy. Diabetes *24*(Suppl. I):65, 1975.
241. Wu, C. F., Haider, B., Ahmed, S. S., et al.: The effects of tolbutamide on the myocardium in experimental diabetes. Circulation *55:*200, 1977.
242. Regan, T. J.: Cardiac disease in the older diabetic: Management considerations. Geriatrics *44:*91, 1989.
243. United Kingdom Prospective Diabetes Study Group: United Kingdom prospective diabetes study (UKPDS) 13: Relative efficacy of randomly allocated diet, sulphonylurea, insulin, or metformin in patients with newly diagnosed non-insulin dependent diabetes followed for three years. Br. Med. J. *310:*83, 1995.
244. Bielefeld, D. R., Pace, C. S., and Boshell, B. R.: Hyperosmolarity and cardiac function in chronic diabetic rat heart. Am J. Physiol. *245:*E568, 1983.

OBESITY

245. Salan, S.: The obesities. *In* Felig, P., et al. (eds.): Endocrinology and Metabolism. 2nd ed. New York, McGraw-Hill Book Co., 1987, p. 1203.
246. Hirsch, J.: The adipose cell hypothesis. N. Engl. J. Med. *294:*389, 1976.
247. Foster, W. R., and Burton, B. T. (eds.): Health implications of obesity: NIH consensus development conference. Ann. Intern. Med. *103:*979, 1985.
248. Smith, H. L., and Willius, R. A.: Adiposity of the heart. A clinical and pathological study of one hundred and thirty-six obese patients. Ann. Intern. Med. *52:*911, 1933.
249. De Divitis, O., Fazio, S., Petitto, M., et al.: Obesity and cardiac function. Circulation *64:*477, 1981.
250. Egan, B., Fitzpatrick, M. A., Juni, J., et al.: Importance of overweight in studies of left ventricular hypertrophy and diastolic function in mild systemic hypertension. Am. J. Cardiol. *64:*752, 1989.
251. Nakajima, T., Fujioka, S., Tokunaga, K., et al.: Correlation of intraab-

dominal fat accumulation and left ventricular performance in obesity. Am. J. Cardiol. *64*:369, 1989.
252. Zack, P. M., Wiens, R. D., and Kennedy, H. L.: Left-axis deviation and adiposity: The United States health and nutrition examination survey. Am. J. Cardiol. *53*:1129, 1984.
253. Ventura, H. O., Messerli, F.H., Dunn, F. G., and Frohlich, E. D.: Left ventricular hypertrophy in obesity: Discrepancy between echo and electrocardiogram. J. Am. Coll. Cardiol. *1*:682, 1983.
254. Warnes, C. A., and Roberts, W. C.: The heart in massive (more than 300 pounds or 136 kilograms) obesity: Analysis of 12 patients studied at necropsy. Am. J. Cardiol. *54*:1087, 1984.
255. Lavie, C. J., Amodeo, C., Ventura, H. O., et al: Left atrial abnormalities indicating diastolic ventricular dysfunction in cardiopathy of obesity. Chest *92*:1042, 1987.
256. Rossi, M., Marti, G., Ricordi, L., et al.: Cardiac autonomic dysfunction in obese subjects. Clin. Sci. *76*:567, 1989.
257. National High Blood Pressure Education Program: The Fifth Report of the Joint National Committee on detection, evaluation and treatment of high blood pressure. Bethesda, MD, NIH Publication No. 93-1088.
258. Reaven, G. M.: Role of insulin resistance in human disease. Diabetes *37*:1495, 1988.
259. Reaven, G. M.: Insulin resistance and compensatory hyperinsulinemia: Role in hypertension, dyslipidemia, and coronary heart disease. Am. Heart J. *121*:1283, 1991.
260. Donahue, R. P., Abbott, R. D., Bloom, E., et al.: Central obesity and coronary heart disease in men. Lancet *1*:821, 1987.
261. Manson, J. E., Colditz, G. A., Stampher, M. J., et al.: A prospective study of obesity and risk of coronary heart disease in women. N. Engl. J. Med. *322*:882, 1990.
261a. Himeno, E., Nishino, K., Nakashima, Y., et al.: Weight reduction regresses left ventricular mass regardless of blood pressure level in obese subjects. Am. Heart J. *131*:313, 1996.
262. Reisin, E., Frohlich, E. D., Messerli, F. H., et al.: Cardiovascular changes after weight reduction in obesity hypertension. Ann. Intern. Med. *98*:315, 1983.
263. MacMahon, S. W., Wilcken, D. E. L., and Macdonald, G. J.: The effect of weight reduction on left ventricular mass: A randomized controlled trial in young, overweight hypertensive patients. N. Engl. J. Med. *314*:334, 1986.
264. Alpert, M. A., Terry, B. E., and Kelley, D. L.: Effect of weight loss on cardiac chamber size, wall thickness and left ventricular function in morbid obesity. Am. J. Cardiol. *55*:783, 1985.
265. Backman, L., Freyschuss, U., Hallberg, D., and Melcher, A.: Reversibility of cardiovascular changes in extreme obesity: Effects of weight reduction through jejunoileostomy. Acta Med. Scand. *205*:367, 1979.
266. Pi-Sunyer, F. X.: Short-term medical benefits and adverse effects of weight loss. Ann. Intern. Med. *119*:722, 1993.
267. Frank, A., Graham, C., and Frank, S.: Fatalities on the liquid protein diet: An analysis of possible causes. Int. J. Obes. *5*:243, 1981.

MALNUTRITION

268. Webb, J. G., Kiess, M. C., and Chan-Yan, C. C.: Malnutrition and the heart. Can. Med. Assoc. J. *135*:753, 1986.
269. Pringle, T. H., Scobie, I. N., Murray, R. G., et al.: Prolongation of the QT interval during therapeutic starvation: A substrate for malignant arrhythmias. Int. J. Obes. *7*:253, 1983.
270. Bergman, J. W., Human, D. G., DeMoor, M. M. A., et al.: Effect of kwashiorkor on the cardiovascular system. Arch. Dis. Child. *63*:1359, 1988.
271. Alden, P. B., Madoff, R. D., Stahl, T. J., et al.: Left ventricular function in malnutrition. Am. J. Physiol. *253*:H380, 1987.
272. Nutter, D. O., Murray, T. G., Heymsfield, S. T., and Fuller, E. O.: The effect of chronic protein-calorie undernutrition in the rat on myocardial function and cardiac function. Circ. Res. *45*:144, 1979.
273. Isner, J. M., Roberts, W. C., Heymsfield, S. B., and Yager, J.: Anorexia nervosa and sudden death. Ann. Intern. Med. *102*:49, 1985.
274. de Simone, G., Scalfi, L., Galderisi, M., et al.: Cardiac abnormalities in young women with anorexia nervosa. Br. Heart J. *71*:287, 1994.
275. Kollai, M., Bonyhay, I., Jokkel, G., and Szanyi, L.: Cardiac vagal hyperactivity in adolescent anorexia nervosa. Eur. Hypertens. J. *15*:113, 1994.
276. Cooke, R. A., Chambers, T. B., Singh, R., et al.: Q T interval in anorexia nervosa. Br. Heart J. *72*:69, 1994.

THE HEART AND GONADAL HORMONES

277. Carr, J. G., Stevenson, L. W., Walden, J. A., et al.: Prevalence and hemodynamic correlates of malnutrition in severe congestive heart failure secondary to ischemic or idiopathic dilated cardiomyopathy. Am. J. Cardiol. *63*:709, 1989.
278. Blackburn, G. L., Gibbons, G. W., Bothe, A., et al.: Nutritional support in cardiac cachexia. J. Thorac. Cardiovasc. Surg. *73*:489, 1977.
279. Abel, R. M., Fischer, J. E., Buckley, M. J., et al.: Malnutrition in cardiac surgical patients. Arch. Surg. *111*:45, 1976.
280. Steier, M., Lopez, R., and Cooperman, J. M.: Riboflavin deficiency in infants and children with hearth disease. Am. Heart J. *92*:139, 1976.
281. Lerner, D. J., and Kannel, W. B.: Patterns of coronary heart disease, morbidity and mortality in the sexes: A 26 year follow-up of the Framingham population. Am. Heart J. *111*:383, 1986.
282. Bush, T. L., Barrett-Connor, E., Cowan, L. D., et al.: Cardiovascular mortality and non-contraceptive use of estrogen in women. Results from the Lipid Research Clinics Program follow-up. Circulation *75*:1102, 1987.
283. Wren, B. G.: The effect of estrogen on the female cardiovascular system. Med. J. Aust. *157*:204, 1992.
284. Rosano, G. M. C., Sarrel, P. M., Poole-Wilson, P. A., and Collins, P.: Beneficial effect of oestrogen on exercise-induced myocardial ischemia in women with coronary artery disease. Lancet *342*:133, 1993.
285. Gebara, O. C. E.: Association between increased estrogen status and increased fibrinolytic potential in the Framingham Offspring Study. Circulation *91*:1952, 1995.
286. Gordon, T., Kannel, W. B., Hjortland, M. C., and McNamara, P. M.: Menopause and coronary heart disease. The Framingham Study. Ann. Intern. Med. *89*:157, 1978.
287. Stampfer, M. J., Willett, W. C., Colditz, C. A., et al.: A prospective study of post-menopausal estrogen therapy and coronary heart disease. N. Engl. J. Med. *313*:1044, 1985.
288. Stampfer, M. J., and Colditz, C. A.: Estrogen replacement therapy and coronary heart disease: A quantitative assessment of the epidemiologic evidence. Prev. Med. *20*:47, 1991.
289. Stampfer, M. J., Colditz, G. A., Willett, W. C., et al.: Postmenopausal estrogen therapy and cardiovascular disease. Ten-year follow-up from the Nurses' Health Study. N. Engl. J. Med. *325*:756, 1991.
290. Nabulsi, A. A., Folsom, A. R., White, A., et al.: Association of hormone-replacement therapy with various cardiovascular risk factors in post-menopausal women. N. Engl. J. Med. *328*:1069, 1993.
291. The Writing Group for the PEPI Trial: Effects of estrogen or estrogen/progestin regimens on hearty disease risk factors in post-menopausal women. The post-menopausal estrogen/progestin interventions (PEPI) trial. JAMA *273*:199, 1995.
292. McDonald, C. C., and Stewart, H. J.: Fatal myocardial infarction in the Scottish adjuvant tamoxifen trial. The Scottish Breast Cancer Committee. BMJ *303*:435, 1991.
293. Rutqvist, L. E., and Mattsson, A.: Cardiac and thromboembolic morbidity among postmenopausal women with early-stage breast cancer in a randomized trial of adjuvant tamoxifen. The Stockholm Breast Cancer Study Group. J. Natl. Cancer Inst. *85*:1298, 1993.
294. Love, R. R., Wiebe, D. A., Newcomb, P. A., et al.: Effects of tamoxifen on cardiovascular risk factors in post-menopausal women. Ann. Intern. Med. *115*:860, 1991.
295. Webber, L. S., Hunter, S. M., Baugh, J. G., et al.: The interaction of cigarette smoking, oral contraceptive use, and cardiovascular risk factor variables in children: The Bogalusa Heart Study. Am. J. Publ. Health *72*:266, 1982.
296. Jaffe, M. D.: Effect of oestrogens on postexercise electrocardiogram. Br. Heart J. *38*:1299, 1976.
297. Merians, D. R., Haskell, W. L., Vranizan, K. M., et al.: Relationship of exercise, oral contraceptive use, and body fat to concentrations of plasma lipids and lipoprotein cholesterol in young women. Am. J. Med. *78*:913, 1985.
298. Stampfer, M. J., Willett, W. C., Colditz, G. A., et al.: A prospective study of past use of oral contraceptive agents and risk of cardiovascular diseases. N. Engl. J. Med. *319*:1313, 1988.
299. Ramcharan, S., Pellegrin, F. A., and Hoag, E. J.: The occurrence and course of hypertensive disease in users and nonusers of oral contraceptive drugs. *In* The Walnut Creek Contraceptive Drug Study: A prospective study of the side effects of oral contraceptives, Vol. 2. Edited by Ramcharan, S. U.S. Department of Health, Education, and Welfare Publications No. (NIH) 76-563. Washington, DC, Government Printing Office, 1976, p. 1.
300. Prentice, R. L.: On the ability of blood pressure effects to explain the relation between oral contraceptives and cardiovascular disease. Am. J. Epidemiol. *127*:213, 1988.
301. Blumenstein, B. A., Douglas, M. B., and Hall, W. D.: Blood pressure changes and oral contraceptive use: A study of 2676 black women in the southeastern United States. Am. J. Epidemiol. *112*:539, 1980.
302. Rekers, H.: Multicenter trial of a monophasic oral contraceptive containing ethinyl estradiol and desogestrel. Acta Obstet. Gynecol. Scand. *67*:171, 1988.
303. Walling, M.: A multicenter efficacy and safety study of an oral contraceptive containing 150 μg desogestrel and 30 μg ethinyl estradiol. Contraceptive *46*:313, 1992.
304. Shoupe, D.: Multicenter randomized comparison of two low-dose triphasic combined oral contraceptive containing desogestrel or norethindrone. Obstet. Gynecol. *83*:679, 1994.
305. Laragh, J. H., Sealey, J. E., Ledingham, J. G. G., and Newton, M. A.: Oral contraceptives: Renin, aldosterone, and high blood pressure. JAMA *201*:918, 1967.
306. Wren, B. G., and Routledge, D. A.: Blood pressure changes: Oestrogens in climacteric women. Med. J. Aust. *2*:528, 1981.

Chapter 62
Renal Disorders and Heart Disease

CARL V. LEIER, HARISIOS BOUDOULAS

CARDIOVASCULAR CONDITIONS THAT AFFECT RENAL FUNCTION 1914
Heart Failure 1914
Infective Endocarditis 1921
Thromboembolic Disease 1922
Other Cardiovascular Conditions 1922
EFFECTS OF RENAL FAILURE ON THE CARDIOVASCULAR SYSTEM..............1923
Cardiac Failure Caused by Renal Failure . .1923
Hypertrophic Cardiomyopathy 1924
Accelerated Coronary Atherosclerosis 1924
Cardiovascular Calcification 1927
Heart Murmurs and Valvular Heart Disease 1927
Pericardial Disease 1928
Systemic Hypertension 1928
Cardiac Arrhythmias................1928
Cardiovascular Drug Therapy in Patients with Renal Disease 1935
Cardiovascular Complications During Dialysis 1935
REFERENCES 1936

The kidney can be viewed as a component of the circulatory system. Within this integrated system, the function, regulation, and adjustments of the heart and vasculature are closely linked to those of the kidneys. Renal dysfunction and failure adversely affect cardiovascular function, frequently leading to a cardiovascular disorder or failure and, consequently, further impairment of renal performance. Cardiovascular disease, dysfunction, and failure, in turn, can disturb renal function, occasionally to the point of evoking acute or chronic renal failure, which then causes further deterioration of the cardiovascular condition. Clinicians have for years appreciated the fact that failure of one component of the cardiorenal system (e.g., renal failure) greatly amplifies the difficulty in clinical management of the failure of another component (e.g., heart failure).

This chapter presents the principal cardiovascular disorders that commonly affect renal performance and the primary renal conditions responsible for altering cardiovascular structure and function.

CARDIOVASCULAR CONDITIONS THAT AFFECT RENAL FUNCTION

HEART FAILURE

The development of cardiac dysfunction and failure evokes a series of pathophysiological events affecting renal function. The renal responses to these events in turn contribute heavily to the overall pathophysiology and clinical manifestations of congestive heart failure. The nature and degree of renal involvement is largely related to the acuity and severity of cardiac decompensation.

Chronic Low-Output Congestive Heart Failure

The principal pathophysiological forces that bring the kidney into the syndrome of chronic congestive heart failure (CHF) are a reduction in renal blood flow (Fig. 62–1) and progressive activation of a number of hormonal and other regulatory systems (e.g., sympathetic nervous system, renin-angiotensin-aldosterone axis, atrial natriuretic peptide [ANP], arginine vasopressin) (Table 62–1). The mechanisms controlling and activating these events, systems, and factors in CHF are presented in more detail in Chapter 15.

Cardiovascular and Systemic Events Influencing Renal Function in Chronic Heart Failure

DISTRIBUTION OF CARDIAC OUTPUT TO THE KIDNEYS (RENAL BLOOD FLOW). For most CHF patients, the fall in effective renal blood flow is proportional to the reduction in cardiac output. Renal blood flow in normal subjects (age range of 20 to 80 years) averages 600 to 660 ml/min/m^2, comprising 14 to 20 per cent of simultaneously measured cardiac output.[1,2] Within a wide spectrum of CHF severity (and without intrinsic renal disease), renal blood flow is depressed to an average range of 250 to 450 ml/min/m^2, but still representing 12 to 18 per cent of the cardiac output.[1,3–5] These data indicate that for human chronic CHF, renal vascular resistance increases to a similar extent as overall systemic vascular resistance, and that for most patients with this condition, the renal share of cardiac output is not substantially redistributed to other "more vital" organs or regions.

Although not precisely delineated in human heart failure, renal blood flow in this condition appears to be strongly influenced by systemic and intrarenal renin-angotensin and by autonomic nervous system tone. Major modulation of renal blood flow by angiotensin II is supported by the finding that angiotensin-converting enzyme inhibition substantially augments renal blood flow in chronic heart failure.[4,6] Renal flow, in striking contrast to hepatosplanchnic and limb blood flow, is influenced only modestly by alpha-adrenergic blockade.[7] This indicates that the mechanisms (or the relative contribution of each mechanism) adjusting renal vascular resistance and blood flow in human chronic heart failure are not the same as those influencing the vascular resistance and blood flow in other regions of the body. The findings that renal blood flow on an average does not fall below its usual share of cardiac output and that it may plateau as cardiac output drops below 2.0 liters/m^2/min[1] support the view that renal blood flow in chronic heart failure is also influenced by a number of local mechanisms and substances, including endothelial modulators of vascular tone (e.g., nitric oxide [EDRF], endothelin), prostaglandin (PGE_2, PGI_2) production and release, tubuloglomerular feedback, myogenic tone, and other "autoregulatory" responses.

Renal blood flow should not be equated with renal function. The functional reserve of the kidneys is such that renal blood flow can be chronically reduced by at least 30 to 40 per cent without substantially affecting overall renal performance. For most patients with chronic heart failure, the disparity between renal blood flow and renal function is related to the relative dissociation of renal blood flow and glomerular filtration rate[4,5,8] (Fig. 62–1). As heart failure evolves and renal blood flow falls, glomerular filtration rate is maintained by enhanced constriction of the efferent arteriole (postglomerulus) relative to the afferent arteriole (preglomerulus). Thus, filtration fraction (ratio of glomerular filtration rate to renal plasma flow) tends to rise as patients advance from mild to moderately severe stages of chronic CHF.

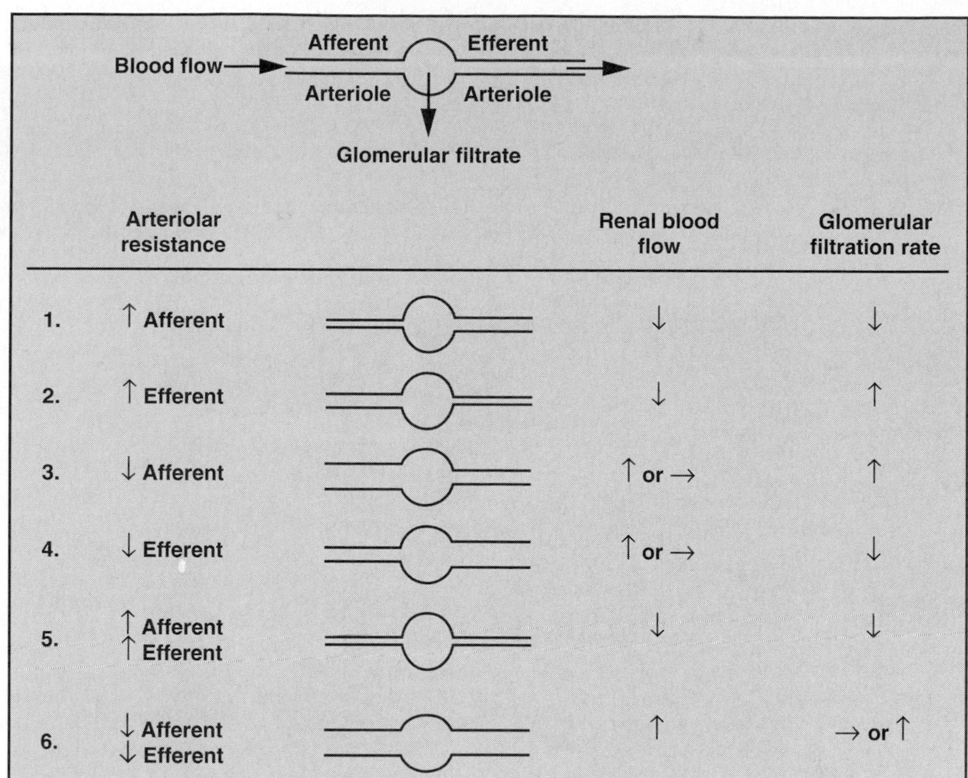

FIGURE 62–1. The renal vascular determinants of renal blood flow are not necessarily the same as those adjusting glomerular filtration rate. Situation 2 applies to most patients with heart failure, a condition accompanied by activation of systemic and intrarenal renin-angiotensin, elevated plasma atrial natriuretic peptide levels, and increased intrarenal prostaglandin activity. Situations 1 and 5 apply to patients with severe reduction in renal perfusion and marked increase of sympathetic nervous system activity and endothelin release, as seen in terminal, end-stage heart failure and/or circulatory shock. Converting enzyme inhibitors can evoke responses 4 and 6 in congestive heart failure. (Adapted from Leier, C. V., and Boudoulas, H.: Cardiorenal Disorders and Diseases. Armonk, N.Y., Futura Publishing Co., 1992.)

Preferential constriction of the efferent arteriole by angiotensin II and dilation of the afferent arteriole by ANP and prostaglandins appear to be the major mechanisms for maintaining glomerular filtration rate (GFR) as renal blood flow declines[4,9–11]; this also explains why GFR and overall renal function can decrease despite a rise in renal blood flow in some CHF patients receiving angiotensin-converting enzyme inhibitors (resultant ↓ angiotensin II).[12,13]

ADVANCED HEART FAILURE. The extremely advanced, terminal stage of chronic CHF is usually accompanied by marked reduction in cardiac output and renal blood flow. At this stage, substantial vasoconstriction of the afferent arteriole occurs to depress glomerular filtration rate (Fig. 62–1). Renal dysfunction in this setting is exacerbated by a concomitant fall in mean systemic blood pressure below 70 to 75 mm Hg and consequent drop in renal perfusion pressure.[14] Low urine output, fluid volume retention, and edema refractory to standard orally administered medication and azotemia now complicate the clinical setting.

Management. Higher doses of diuretics and combined use of loop and tubule diuretics (e.g., furosemide and thiazide) are frequently required (see Chap. 17). Strategies to enhance renal function by increasing renal blood flow and glomerular filtration rate are still generally limited to drugs requiring intravenous administration. Dopamine at doses $\leq 5.0\ \mu g/kg/min$ can augment renal blood flow and function via stimulation of renal dopaminergic receptors (renal arteriolar dilatation) and some increase in cardiac output.[15,16] In certain instances, vasopressor doses of dopamine ($\geq 6.0\ \mu g/kg/min$) may be required to bring renal perfusion pressure into an acceptable range (mean systemic arterial pressure ≥ 70 mm Hg). Dobutamine and nitroprusside can improve renal blood flow and function, principally by increasing cardiac output and perhaps, by evoking some renal vasodilation in severely vasoconstricted states.[15,17–19] It is reasonable to employ dobutamine-dopamine or nitroprusside-dopamine combinations in these desperate clinical situations in an attempt to optimally improve cardiac output, renal hemodynamics and function, and renal responsiveness to diuretic therapy. For the patient on a heart transplant waiting list, the failure to respond adequately to these interventions often necessitates the placement of a mechanical assist device. Unless complicated by considerable renal dysfunction and failure, hemodialysis and related methods have not yet earned a role in the long-term management of chronic CHF.

HORMONAL AND OTHER ENDOGENOUS SUBSTANCES MODULATING RENAL FUNCTION. Heart failure activates a number of hormonal and regulatory systems, which greatly influence renal function. The major hormones and systems so affected and their regulation and renal effects in heart failure are presented in Table 62–1. Basically, as patients move from mild heart failure to moderate to severe stages, the protective vasodilatory and natriuretic properties of increased ANP (and perhaps renal prostaglandins and bradykinin) are overwhelmed by the vasoconstricting and salt and water–retaining effects of the progressively activated sympathetic nervous system, renin-angiotensin-aldosterone axis, arginine vasopressin, and adrenocorticotropin-corticosteroid axis.[20–36] This imbalance is exacerbated in heart failure by gradual attenuation of the vascular and renal responses to atrial natriuretic peptide and by development of a disordered vascular endothelium (increased endothelin production and release with loss of endothelium-derived vasodilation).[37,38]

Renal Responses in Chronic Congestive Heart Failure

The renal responses to the aforementioned cardiovascular-systemic consequences of chronic low-output CHF are reduced excretion of salt, water, and metabolic products (e.g., BUN, creatinine) and enhanced urinary loss of potassium and magnesium. These renal responses account for many of the clinical manifestations and for the "congestive" component of CHF. In untreated chronic CHF, whole-body sodium increases 5 to 40 per cent and water 5 to 45 per cent above normal and whole-body potassium decreases by 5 to 20 per cent.[24,39]

SODIUM RETENTION. The avid retention of sodium by the kidney in CHF is multifactorial in mechanism and basically a result of the antinatriuretic forces in this clinical condition overwhelming the natriuretic properties of circulating ANP and renal prostaglandins (Table 62–1 and Fig. 62–2).

Intrarenal physical factors and fluid dynamics contribute to sodium retention in CHF. A fall in cardiac output, effective blood volume, and renal blood flow is accompanied by activation of specific substances (e.g., angiotensin II, ANP,

TABLE 62–1 MAJOR HORMONAL AND OTHER ENDOGENOUS SUBSTANCES AFFECTING RENAL FUNCTION IN HUMAN HEART FAILURE

SUBSTANCE	INCREASED PRODUCTION RELEASE	DECREASED PRODUCTION RELEASE	RENAL EFFECTS	OTHER PROPERTIES RELEVANT TO RENAL FUNCTION
RENIN-ANGIOTENSIN-ALDOSTERONE SYSTEM				
Renin	Reduced renal perfusion pressure Reduced "effective" blood volume Low sodium diet Beta-adrenergic stimulation Reduced NaCl delivery to macula densa Prostaglandins (PGE_2, PGI_2) ACTH Endothelin Diuretic therapy Certain vasodilators ACE inhibitors	Normal or increased renal perfusion pressure Alpha-adrenergic stimulation Increased NaCl delivery to macula densa Increased serum [K+] Angiotensin II ANP Vasopressin Dopamine Digitalis Beta-adrenergic blockade	Mediated via increases in intrarenal and vascular angiotensin II production and elevated circulating angiotensin II and aldosterone levels	Converts angiotensinogen to angiotensin I, which is converted to angiotensin II by circulating and local tissue (e.g., vascular, renal)-converting enzyme
Angiotensin II	Renin	ACE inhibitors	Maintains glomerular filtration rate as renal blood flow falls by preferentially vasoconstricting efferent arteriole (> afferent arteriole) Promotes sodium reabsorption by proximal tubule Counters many renal actions of atrial natriuretic peptide Promotes renal vascular remodeling Possibly increases renal interstitial fibrosis	Increases production and release of aldosterone from adrenal gland May evoke release of arginine vasopressin from CNS May stimulate thirst center Augments sympathetic nervous system effects Proximal tubule produces angiotensinogen, and brush border contains converting enzyme
Aldosterone	Angiotensin II ACTH Vasopressin Increased serum [K+] Endothelin Beta-endorphin	ANP Dopamine ACE inhibitors Angiotensin II inhibitors	Increases sodium reabsorption by distal tubule and collecting duct Evokes potassium and magnesium loss from distal tubule	Increases whole body NaCl-H_2O content, and lowers whole body potassium
SYMPATHETIC NERVOUS SYSTEM TONE				
Norepinephrine Release	Activation of high- and low-pressure baroreceptors by reduced blood pressure, volume, or flow "Ineffective" blood volume Angiotensin II Certain vasodilators	Central alpha-adrenergic agonists and other sympatholytic agents ACE inhibitors Digitalis	Increases renin production and release Increases sodium reabsorption by proximal tubule Evokes modest kaliuresis Intense SNS activation: a. Reduces renal blood flow and GFR by vasoconstricting afferent (> efferent) arteriole b. May shift cortical blood flow to medullary region	Evokes production and release of: Arginine vasopressin ANP ACTH Corticosteroids Intrarenal prostaglandins Endothelin
Arginine Vasopressin	Various nonosmotic stimuli in heart failure, including: a. Sympathetic nervous system activation and catecholamines b. Reduction in blood pressure, flow or volume or "ineffective" blood volume c. Angiotensin II	Hypo-osmolar state	Acts on V_2 receptor of distal tubule and collecting duct to allow water reabsorption from tubular filtrate	Antagonistic to tubular effects of renal prostaglandins

TABLE 62–1 MAJOR HORMONAL AND OTHER ENDOGENOUS SUBSTANCES AFFECTING RENAL FUNCTION IN HUMAN HEART FAILURE *(continued)*

SUBSTANCE	INCREASED PRODUCTION RELEASE	DECREASED PRODUCTION RELEASE	RENAL EFFECTS	OTHER PROPERTIES RELEVANT TO RENAL FUNCTION
	d. Parasympathetic withdrawal(?) Reduced hypo-osmolar negative feedback Reduced clearance Elevation of serum osmotic pressure Endothelin(?)			
Atrial Natriuretic Peptide	Elevation of intraatrial pressure and atrial dilatation Vasopressin, endothelin, and increased sympathetic nervous system activity(?)	Interventions that improve central hemodynamics and lower atrial pressures and volume	Renal vasodilation with afferent > efferent arteriolar dilatation: ↑ Renal blood flow ↑ GFR Relaxation of mesangium Suppression of: Renin release Angiotensin II production and renal effects Inhibition of tubular sodium channels and sodium transport to reduce NaCl reabsorption Inhibition of tubuloglomerular feedback	Some afterload-preload reduction via vasodilatory and renal effects Cardiovascular and renal effects of ANP become attenuated in moderate to severe chronic CHF
Renal prostaglandins (PGE_2, PGI_2)	Renal vasoconstriction Reduced renal blood flow and perfusion pressure Reduced or "ineffective" blood volume Renin-angiotensin Norepinephrine Vasopressin Bradykinin	Cyclo-oxygenase inhibitors (e.g., acetylsalicylic acid, nonsteroidal antiinflammatory drugs)	Renal vasodilation with afferent > efferent arteriolar dilatation: ↑ Renal blood flow ↑ GFR Inhibition of tubular NaCl reabsorption Inhibition of vasopressin-mediated water uptake by tubule and collecting duct	Possible augmentation of renin production and release
Endothelin	Increased experimentally by a rise in local concentrations of: Norepinephrine Angiotensin II Arginine vasopressin Bradykinin Various cytokines Thrombin Platelet-activating factor Changes in blood flow over endothelial cells Local ischemia		Increases renal vascular resistance with preferential afferent (> efferent) arteriolar constriction: ↓ Renal blood flow ↓ GFR ↓ Sodium excretion ↓ Urine volume Mesangial contraction	Acts on local endothelial cells to increase production of prostacyclin and nitric oxide(?) Contributes heavily to development of acute renal failure in cardiogenic-shock states(?) Elevates: Renin Aldosterone Arginine vasopressin Atrial natriuretic peptide

ACE = angiotensin-converting enzyme; ANP = atrial natriuretic peptides; (?) = possible but unproven; CHD = congestive heart disease; GFR = glomerular filtration rate; SNS = sympathetic nervous system.

and renal prostaglandins) that augment the vascular tone of the glomerular efferent arteriole relative to that of the afferent arteriole (Fig. 62–1). The perfusion pressure in the glomerular capillaries is thereby maintained, thus preserving glomerular-tubular filtrate (as measured by the glomerular filtration rate [GFR]); filtration fraction, defined as glomerular filtration rate/renal blood flow, increases.[20,23,26,40] The increase in filtration fraction leads to a substantial rise in the oncotic pressure and a fall in the hydrostatic pressure of blood leaving the glomerulus to enter the peritubular capillaries. These physical factors (elevated oncotic and reduced hydrostatic pressures) lead to enhanced NaCl-H_2O uptake into the postglomerular peritubular capillary network from the proximal renal tubules and adjacent interstitial space.

Several other local events contribute to sodium retention. If the balance of afferent to efferent arteriolar tone fails to maintain GFR at an adequate level, a fall in GFR delivers less NaCl-H_2O into the tubule, allowing greater proximal tubular reabsorption of sodium via aforementioned physical and hormonal (e.g., angiotensin II, catecholamines) mechanisms. At this point, tubuloglomerular feedback likely serves as a countermeasure[20,23,40,41]; reduced tubular filtrate and flow evoke feedback augmentation of efferent > afferent arteriolar tone to try to increase and maintain GFR. Second, as filtrate and sodium delivery to the distal tubule falls, it is believed that the macula densa cells of the distal tubule send a signal to adjacent juxtaglomerular cells to secrete more renin (with consequent increase of angiotensin II and aldosterone), further intensifying the vascular (glomerular), physical, and hormonal forces promoting sodium reabsorption.[41] Third, although not proven in human chronic CHF, it is possible that in severe stages some of the cortical blood flow is shifted to medullary nephrons, which have an even greater capacity to reabsorb NaCl-H_2O.[14,42]

ROLE OF HORMONES (Table 62–1). Elevated concentrations of certain hormones in CHF constitute powerful mechanisms for sodium retention.[11,20,21,43] Increased aldosterone concentrations cause NaCl reabsorption by the distal tubule and collecting duct, while angiotensin II and norepinephrine augment sodium reabsorption by the proxi-

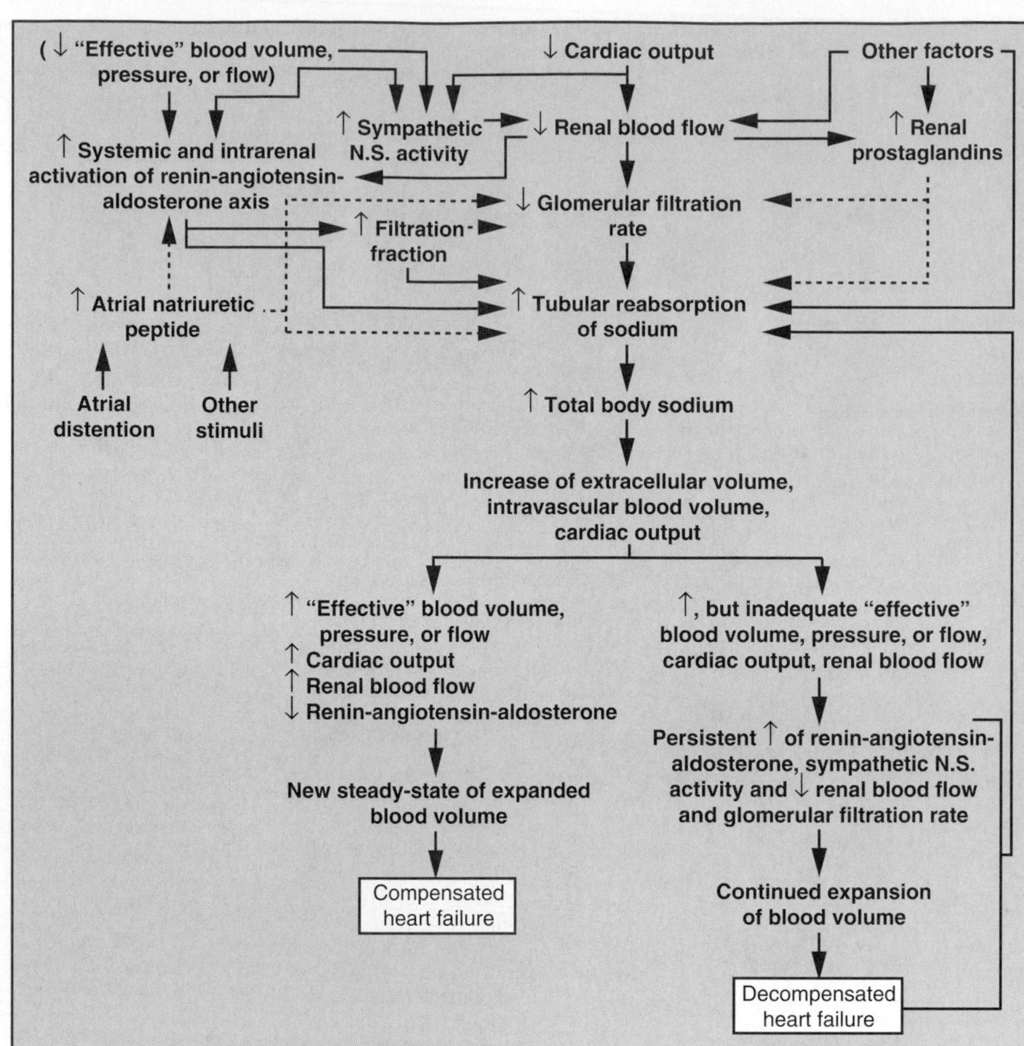

FIGURE 62–2. Schema of the known major mechanisms for enhanced sodium retention in congestive heart failure. Solid connecting lines indicate positive influence or stimulus, and dashed lines indicate negative input or feedback. N.S. = nervous system (Adapted from Leier, C. V., and Boudoulas, H.: Cardiorenal Disorders and Diseases. Armonk, N.Y., Futura Publishing Co., 1992.)

mal tubule. When elevated, circulating corticosteroids retain sodium at the distal tubule. In severe CHF, increased circulating concentrations and enhanced local release of endothelin probably contribute to the fall in glomerular filtration rate and sodium clearance.[34,35]

Elevated circulating ANP levels and intrarenal production of PGE_2 and PGI_2 represent the primary endogenous natriuretic forces in CHF.[28–30,32,36] Experimentally, ANP inhibits renin, aldosterone, arginine vasopressin, and norepinephrine release; inhibits the renal effects of angiotensin II, aldosterone, and arginine vasopressin, and tubular sodium reabsorption; and favorably affects glomerular arteriolar tone (preferential relaxation of afferent arteriole) and GFR (Table 62–1). PGE_2 and PGI_2 augment renal blood flow, preferentially dilate afferent glomerular arterioles to increase GFR, and inhibit tubular NaCl-H_2O reabsorption and the renal effects of arginine vasopressin. In mild CHF, ANP, PGE_2, and PGI_2 probably contribute substantially to proper NaCl balance and overall cardiovascular compensation. As CHF advances, the favorable effects of ANP wane and the antinatriuretic forces intensify, resulting in a progressive rise in whole-body NaCl-H_2O content and an expanded extracellular volume.

WATER RETENTION. The major mechanisms responsible for water retention in CHF[20,26,27,44–46] are presented in Figure 62–3. In health and disease, water is an obligatory component of NaCl reabsorption. In CHF, local renal factors enhance water uptake; these include a reduction in the delivery of filtrate to the distal tubule and, as filtration fraction increases, a fall in the hydrostatic pressure and rise in oncotic pressure of postglomerular blood as it enters peritubular capillaries. Water retention in moderate to severe heart failure is also mediated by an absolute or relative increase in circulating arginine vasopressin[20,45,46]; this represents the predominant mechanism for excessive water retention (often greater than sodium retention) by the kidneys, even in the presence of reduced serum sodium concentrations and serum osmolality. In other words, the various nonosmotic stimuli for vasopressin release (Table 62–1) become quite prominent and overwhelm osmotic-osmoreceptor mechanisms. Suppression of arginine vasopressin with a water load and the kidney's capacity to eliminate a water load are also significantly reduced in CHF patients.[46] Thirst, provoked in large part by elevated angiotensin II levels, exacerbates the water imbalance with continued water intake in the face of hypo-osmolality, dilutional hyponatremia, and whole body fluid volume overload.

These mechanisms and derangements intensify as CHF increases in severity and account for the rather common occurrence of hyponatremia in advanced stages of the condition.[44–47] Therefore, hyponatremia in CHF usually indicates more severe stages of CHF, marked activation of sympathetic nervous, renin-angiotensin-aldosterone, and arginine vasopressin systems, and if one includes the entire spectrum of CHF patients, probably a higher mortality rate as well.[44,45,47] The hyponatremic CHF patient depends heavily on the renin-angiotensin-aldosterone and vasopressin systems for support of central and peripheral hemodynamics, blood pressure, renal perfusion, and GFR and thus is quite susceptible to the hypotensive and potentially adverse renal effects (fall in GFR, azotemia) of angiotensin-converting enzyme inhibitors.[48]

LOSS OF POTASSIUM AND MAGNESIUM. Excessive urinary loss of potassium is a consistent feature of CHF[24,39] (Fig. 62–4). Aldosterone-induced sodium reabsorption by the distal tubule is accompanied by a 1:1 exchange for potassium or hydrogen ion and consequent urinary loss. Respiratory and metabolic alkalosis, not uncommon in CHF, further augments potassium loss by causing the distal tubule to preferentially retain hydrogen ions. Interventions that increase delivery of sodium to the distal tubule (e.g., diuretics) invariably enhance exchange for potassium and thereby promote kaliuresis.

Thus a number of factors predispose the CHF patient to potassium depletion and its threatening consequences (e.g., dysrhythmias). Potassium supplementation (KCl), potas-

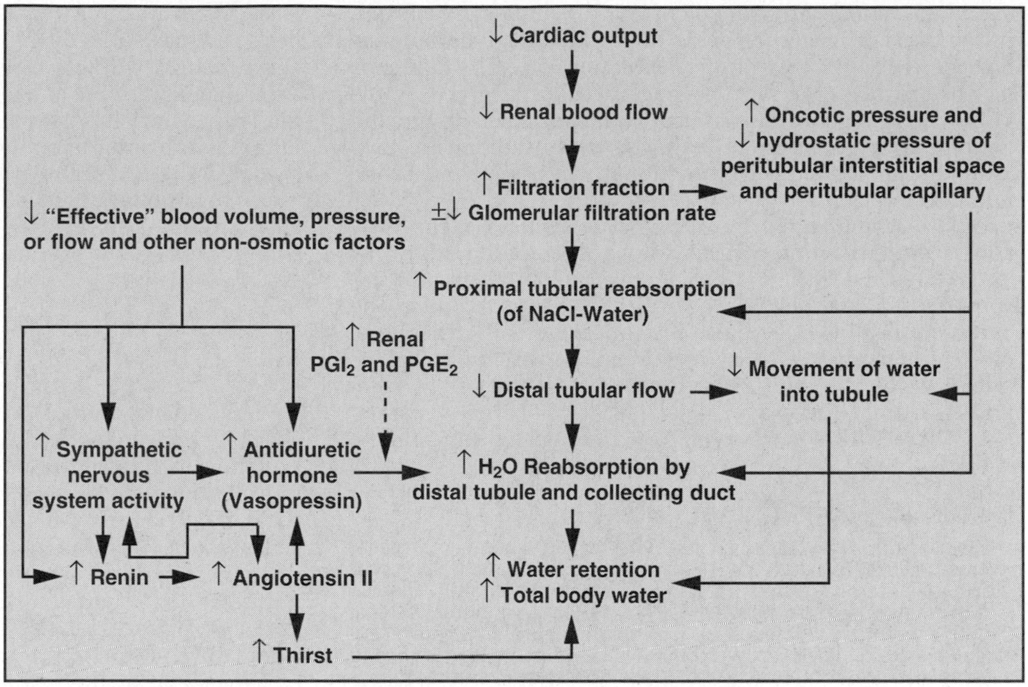

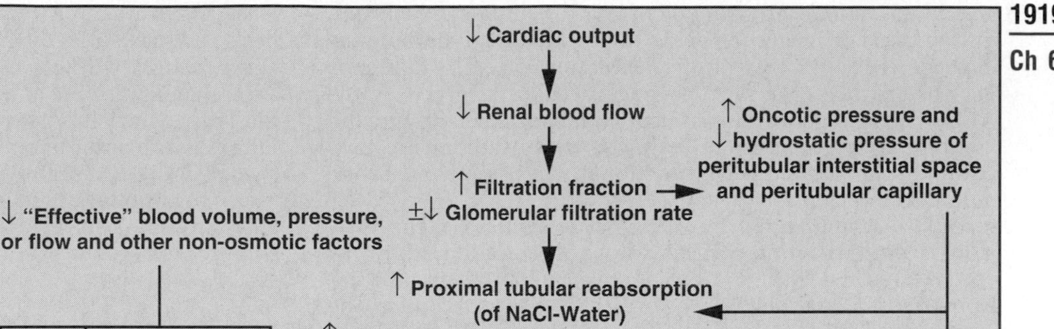

FIGURE 62–3. Major mechanisms for enhanced water retention in heart failure. In advanced stages of heart failure, the degree of water retention can exceed that of sodium retention to cause hyponatremia. Dashed connecting line indicates inhibition or negative feedback. (Adapted from Leier, C. V., and Boudoulas, H.: Cardiorenal Disorders and Diseases. Armonk, N.Y., Futura Publishing Co., 1992.)

sium-sparing diuretics, and angiotensin-converting enzyme inhibitors (by reducing aldosterone) are strategies used to treat this complication of CHF and CHF management.

Generally, the renal loss of magnesium is not quite as problematic for most CHF patients.[49] However, excessive loss and hypomagnesemia do occur in patients with advanced CHF, particularly when treated with high-dose diuretics for an extended period.

AZOTEMIA. Azotemia (increased blood urea nitrogen [BUN]) can occur in moderate to severe CHF or as a consequence of CHF therapy.[24,39,50] A common clinical situation in chronic CHF is in the patient in a state of decompensation who enters the hospital with an elevated BUN (generally > 30 mg/dl), which steadily falls toward normal values with supportive therapy and hemodynamic improvement, but progressively rises again as a phase of inadvertent overdiuresis (relative volume depletion) is entered or a state of decompensation returns.

Tubular urea movement generally follows that of water. Therefore, as renal uptake of NaCl-H_2O increases in CHF, more urea is retained by the kidneys. BUN levels will still generally remain in the normal range or increase only slightly as long as GFR, tubular flow, and urine output are maintained within a near-normal range. A fall in GFR and urine output, as may occur in severe CHF or as a consequence of certain therapeutic measures, will be accompanied by a rise in BUN. Excretion of creatinine occurs via filtrate plus active tubular secretion. Because renal elimination of creatinine is less dependent on tubular flow, serum creatinine will generally not increase until GFR falls below 30 ml/min. Therefore, unless a patient has intrinsic renal disease or marked depression of GFR, the azotemia of CHF is invariably "prerenal" in character, that is, greater retention of BUN than of creatinine with a serum BUN to creatinine ratio of >10:1.

Because of the physiological adjustments required of the kidneys to maintain adequate renal function in heart failure, this organ system in CHF is quite vulnerable to any type of pharmacological, hemodynamic, or structural disturbance. As noted, for patients with moderate to severe heart failure, maintenance of GFR in the face of reduced renal blood flow depends on the proper balance of afferent to efferent arteriolar tone.

ROLE OF THERAPEUTIC AGENTS IN EXACERBATING AZOTEMIA. Angiotensin II plays a major role in this compensatory mechanism by preferentially vasoconstricting the efferent arteriole. By lowering angiotensin II, converting enzyme inhibitors can lower GFR in spite of a concomitant increase in renal blood flow. For most CHF patients, this response will not significantly reduce overall renal performance, or it may increase BUN modestly. However, in the face of severe CHF or low-output hypotension (when GFR and renal function are greatly dependent on angiotensin II), hyponatremia (indicative of high renin-angiotensin and vasopressin activity), relative volume depletion (diuretics), or intrinsic renal disease (e.g., concomitant diabetes mellitus, longstanding systemic hypertension), a reduction of angiotensin II following angiotensin-converting enzyme inhibition, particularly if accompanied by a significant fall in systemic blood pressure and renal perfusion, will often evoke a substantial rise in BUN.[10,12,13,48,51,52] However, converting enzyme inhibitors are still indicated in these situations, but dosing must be initiated at a lower level with appropriate adjustment of diuretic therapy (usually lowered until the dosage of the converting enzyme inhibitor is optimized).

Renal function in CHF is vulnerable to diuretic therapy (see p. 480). Even closely monitored diuretic therapy is associated with additional activation of neurohormonal systems (probably via reduced "effective" blood volume, flow, or pressure), and if overdiuresis occurs, significant reduction in renal blood flow and GFR results and is manifested as a rising BUN.[50,53] In moderate to severe heart failure, renal performance also depends on activation of its prostaglandin system (to dilate the afferent arteriole and reduce tubular NaCl-H_2O reabsorption). It is not uncommon in a CHF patient for clinical decompensation to result from fluid retention, and for azotemia to develop and occasionally advance to renal failure after the administration of cyclo-oxygenase inhibitors (e.g., nonsteroidal antiinflammatory drugs).[54]

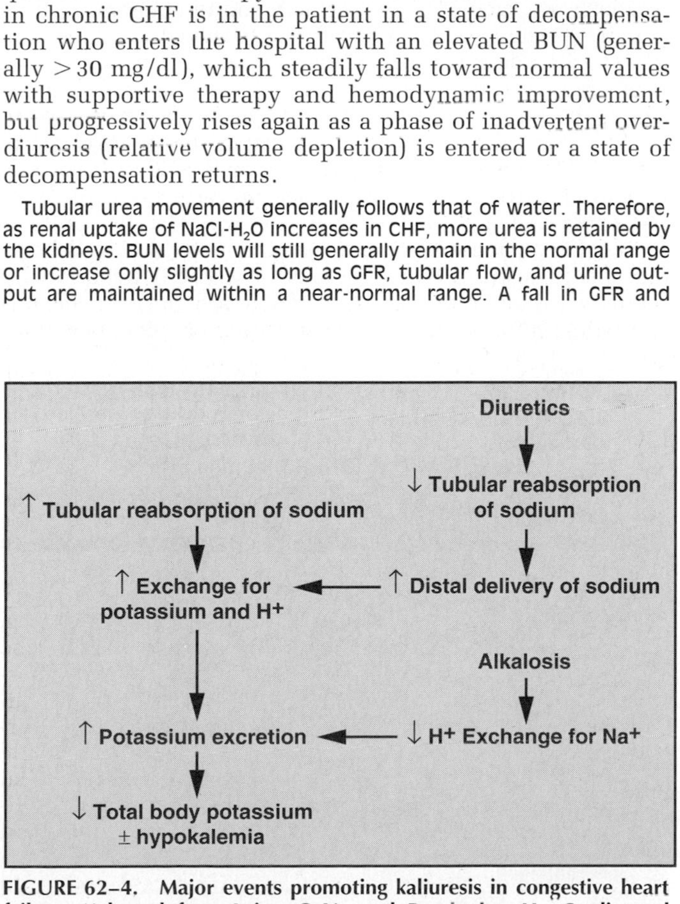

Diuretics
↓ Tubular reabsorption of sodium
↑ Tubular reabsorption of sodium
↑ Exchange for potassium and H^+
↑ Distal delivery of sodium
Alkalosis
↑ Potassium excretion
↓ H^+ Exchange for Na^+
↓ Total body potassium ± hypokalemia

FIGURE 62–4. Major events promoting kaliuresis in congestive heart failure. (Adapted from Leier, C. V., and Boudoulas, H.: Cardiorenal Disorders and Diseases. Armonk, N.Y., Futura Publishing Co., 1992.)

Management of Azotemia in Heart Failure. The general approach to azotemia in CHF is optimization of therapy to provide the best central and renal hemodynamic status possible and elimination of precipitating factors (e.g., overdiuresis, cyclo-oxygenase inhibitors). If the azotemia (and often accompanying refractory edema) is substantial, is secondary to hemodynamic decompensation, and does not respond to optimal adjustment of orally administered drugs, intravenous drug support (e.g., dopamine, dobutamine) may be required[15,16,18]; this clinical situation generally portends a poor prognosis. Dosage of drugs primarily cleared by the kidney (e.g., digoxin, potassium, certain antiarrhythmic and antibiotic agents) must be adjusted downward as the CHF kidney becomes more dysfunctional, GFR falls, and azotemia develops.

Unless accompanied by intrinsic renal disease, the BUN and serum creatinine concentrations in chronic CHF rarely exceed 100 mg/dl and 4 mg/dl, respectively. It is also uncommon for patients who have azotemia secondary to chronic CHF to experience uremic symptoms. Therefore, dialysis is rarely necessary in the patient with chronic CHF unless excessive fluid retention or threatening hyperkalemia refractory to therapy, renal failure, or perhaps marked elevation of BUN (≥100 mg/dl) complicates the clinical course.

CHRONIC HIGH-OUTPUT HEART FAILURE

This condition is discussed on pages 460 to 462. A number of mechanisms gradually convert the initial asymptomatic condition of persistent high cardiac output (e.g., vascular fistulas, chronic anemia) into high-output heart failure.[19,20,55,56] A major contributor is renal NaCl-H_2O retention. Detection by low- and high-pressure baroreceptors of a state of "ineffective" blood volume, pressure, and flow, and in some instances, the diversion of blood flow away from the kidneys provoke chronic activation of the sympathetic nervous system, the renin-angiotensin-aldosterone axis, and arginine vasopressin. Chronic volume overload secondary to renal NaCl-H_2O retention, continuous neurohormonal activation, and persistent increase of myocardial work and energy expenditure gradually cause ventricular enlargement, remodeling, and failure.

Many of the high-output conditions, if untreated, eventually evolve into chronic low-output heart failure with the accompanying renal pathophysiology described above for chronic CHF. Needless to say, the optimal therapeutic approach is to eradicate the underlying cause for the persistently increased cardiac output as soon as it is identified and before it leads to irreversible cardiac dysfunction and failure.

The kidney itself can serve as a primary cause of high-output heart failure.[19,55,56] The kidney is one of the more common sites for arteriovenous fistula formation; this lesion can occur as a complication of renal biopsy and surgery, arterial aneurysmal penetration, and renal neoplasia. Because of concomitant anemia, a sizable arteriovenous access shunt, and chronic tachycardia, the clinical course of chronic renal failure can be further complicated by the development of high-output heart failure.

Acute Heart Failure

The systemic and hormonal responses just described for chronic CHF are also activated in acute heart failure,[57–60] but at a far faster rate of recruitment. Although not well studied in acute human heart failure, the full pathophysiological expression of acute renin-angiotensin-aldosterone activation—particularly that of aldosterone—is not likely to develop within the first 1 to 2 hours of the acute precipitating event. Whole body fluid volume overload is thus not a major component of the very early course but does become important thereafter if the precipitating lesion and acute heart failure are not corrected and as the full impact of acute renin release takes hold. Therefore, the very early, often dramatic, clinical presentation is predominantly related to the extent of myocardial damage or disruption, the intensity of consequent sympathetic nervous system activation, and the circulating and tissue levels of angiotensin II, endothelin, and other vasoactive substances at that point. However, many of these patients do have markedly elevated ventricular filling pressures, acute "congestive" heart failure, and pulmonary edema within minutes of the cardiac event, suggesting that central blood volume (albeit not whole body fluid volume) is indeed excessive at this stage; the mechanisms include peripheral-to-central redistribution of blood volume and an acute rise in ventricular afterload, superimposed on significant cardiac disruption (e.g., large infarct, valvular regurgitation).

The kidney via renal artery stenosis (and consequent release of renin) can serve as the precipitating cause of acute heart failure. This diagnosis should be suspected in the aging patient with a recent history of poorly controlled severe hypertension and new onset or episodic acute pulmonary edema. In this setting, renal insufficiency or asymmetry, a dramatic reduction in blood pressure or the occurrence of renal failure following angiotensin-converting enzyme inhibitor therapy, evidence of atherosclerotic vascular disease elsewhere, or an upper abdominal bruit should also arouse clinical suspicion of renal artery stenosis.

Cardiogenic Shock

(See also p. 1725)

Prerenal azotemia is a common feature of cardiogenic shock and near-shock. The mechanisms causing prerenal azotemia in this setting are generally similar to those discussed above for severe chronic CHF. Unfortunately, acute renal failure is also an occasional complication of cardiogenic shock. For the oliguric or azotemic shock patient, distinguishing between prerenal causation and acute renal failure is important for the optimal management of these critically ill individuals. Prerenal azotemia is approached by treating the reversible conditions that elevate BUN and by agents and methods that improve renal perfusion. Acute renal failure in this setting is managed by avoiding fluid volume, potassium, and protein overload and with dialysis for problematic fluid volume overload, hyperkalemia, uremic symptoms, or plasma creatinine levels ≥7.0 mg/dl.

Table 62–2 presents the laboratory studies useful in distinguishing the azotemia and oliguria of prerenal causes from those of acute renal failure. The principal structural defect of acute renal failure in cardiogenic shock is tubular injury and necrosis. As such, the characteristics of the urine in acute renal failure generally approach those of glomerular filtrate, because the filtrate is modified little by the defective tubules. Thus, urinary sodium content will be high (>40 mEq/liter) and osmolality low (<350 mOsm) despite the oliguric state, and the urinary concentrations of BUN and creatinine will be low despite elevated serum values, because of the inability of the tubules to reabsorb, secrete, and/or concentrate (reduced water uptake) these metabolites. The plasma BUN:creatinine ratio will usually remain at ≤10:1, with an average daily increase of 15 to 20 mg/dl and 1.5 to 2.0 mg/dl respectively. In contrast, prerenal azotemia and oliguria are characterized by laboratory findings indicative of intense NaCl-H_2O retention by normally functioning tubules, which are under considerable stimulation from an activated renin-angiotensin-aldo-

TABLE 62–2 LABORATORY FINDINGS USED TO DISTINGUISH AZOTEMIA AND OLIGURIA OF PRERENAL CAUSES (E.G., HEART FAILURE) FROM AZOTEMIA AND OLIGURIA OF ACUTE RENAL FAILURE

LABORATORY PARAMETER	PRERENAL*	RENAL FAILURE
Urine		
Osmolality	>400 mOsm	<350 mOsm
Na^+ content	<15 mEq/liter	>40 mEq/liter
Sediment	Normal or a small number of nonpigmented granular or hyaline casts	Substantial number of renal tubular cell casts and/or pigmented casts
Urine/plasma ratios of		
BUN	>8	<3
Creatinine	>40	<20
Serum		
BUN:Creatinine	>10:1	10:1

* These laboratory results can be substantially altered by diuretic therapy and/or underlying renal disease.

sterone axis and increased vasopressin. The urine will therefore have a low sodium concentration (<15 to 20 mEq/liter), high osmolality, and high urea and creatinine concentrations. Plasma creatinine levels stay normal unless renal perfusion and GFR fall considerably or the patient has intrinsic renal disease. With the reduction in urine flow, BUN rises to increase the serum BUN : creatinine ratio to $>10:1$. A not unusual urinary sediment or a small number of granular, proteinaceous, or hyaline casts is typical for prerenal azotemia, whereas the sediment of acute renal failure often shows pigmented or tubular cell casts.

Two situations commonly distort the aforementioned laboratory findings. First, diuretics or concomitant renal disease can increase the urinary sodium and water content of patients with prerenal azotemia such that the urinary sodium and osmolality data can be difficult to interpret. Second, oliguria (urine flow <600 ml/24 hr) is not a mandatory feature of acute renal failure. Nonoliguric renal failure is a variant of acute renal failure; these patients have a urine output of 1000 to 6000 ml/24 hr, accompanied by a steady rise in serum BUN and creatinine indicative of ongoing renal failure. Although high urine output can occasionally occur in the early phase of acute renal failure, it usually follows a period of oliguric renal failure. Urinary sodium concentration is still elevated and urinary osmolality depressed in nonoliguric acute renal failure, rendering the pathophysiological impression that the nephrons have reestablished flow, but the tubular cells remain dysfunctional.

Following reversal of cardiogenic shock, the usual clinical course of shock-induced acute renal failure consists of a 1- to 8-week period of intermittent dialysis and eventual recovery. The status of an occasional patient, particularly one with previous renal disease or one who experienced a prolonged period of renal hypoperfusion-ischemia, may proceed into permanent renal failure requiring long-term dialysis or renal transplantation. Although acute renal failure still carries a mortality rate of 10 to 15 per cent, the long-term clinical course and prognosis in patients who experience acute renal failure secondary to cardiogenic shock are usually related to the nature, extent, and reversibility of the cardiac injury and the residual cardiovascular function.

MECHANISM OF RENAL FAILURE. The precise mechanisms leading to the development of acute renal failure during cardiogenic shock in humans have not yet been definitively established.[34,61–63] The potential pivotal role of endothelin in the pathogenesis of acute renal failure in shock conditions is suggested by the results of preliminary studies in animal models, which indicate that inhibition of this substance significantly reduces the prevalence and severity of ischemia-induced renal failure.[34,63] The drop in cardiac output and renal blood flow, intense activation of the sympathetic nervous system, increased circulating and intrarenal renin-angiotensin, and the endothelial release of endothelin can reduce renal blood flow in cardiogenic shock to ≤ 15 per cent of normal with possible diversion of flow from the renal cortex to medulla as well. Low tissue oxygen tension and depleted energy substrate depress tubular function and membrane transport. Renal tubular cells undergo ischemic injury and death and aggregate with tubular filtrate and proteinaceous exudation (across glomeruli or from the interstitium) to obstruct the tubules and collecting ducts. An increase in interstitial edema and pressure leads to compression of nephrons with additional impairment of tubular flow.

INFECTIVE ENDOCARDITIS

(See also Chap. 33)

In the preantibiotic era, 10 to 15 per cent of deaths from infective endocarditis were attributable to renal failure. Early recognition, precise identification of the infecting organism, and prompt, aggressive antibiotic therapy specifically directed at the offending organism have greatly reduced the renal complications of infective endocarditis, particularly renal failure. Nevertheless, more than 60 per cent of patients with documented infective endocarditis have clinical, laboratory, or biopsy evidence of renal involvement.[64–66] The manifestations of endocarditic renal disease range from none to hematuria, pyuria, proteinuria, and occasional renal failure; the prevalence and severity of these manifestations are generally related to the duration of endocarditis prior to cure.

The deposition of immune complex material in glomeruli represents the most common mechanistic link between infective endocarditis and its renal consequences. Circulating immune complexes and their subsequent deposition in kidneys (and elsewhere) account for the common laboratory finding of reduced serum levels of certain complements (e.g., C3, C4, C1q) in affected individuals. The resultant glomerular lesions are generally proliferative in histological type with demonstrable immune deposits of IgG, IgM, and C3 along the basement membrane and in the mesangium. The distribution of the glomerular lesions ranges from focal/segmental to diffuse and their clinical behavior from subclinical to rapidly progressive.

FOCAL/SEGMENTAL PROLIFERATIVE GLOMERULONEPHRITIS. This is the most commonly encountered glomerulopathy in bacterial endocarditis and represents a wide spectrum of involvement, including focal inflammation of single tufts of glomeruli, sporadic glomerular inflammation and fibrosis, and inflammation and fibrosis of most glomeruli within a renal segment(s) in the midst of normal appearing kidney.[64,65] In addition to neutrophil and round cell infiltration and varying degrees of fibrosis, glomerular pathology often includes focal necrosis, fibrin deposition, enlargement and proliferation of endothelial, epithelial, and mesangial cells, and occasional crescent formation. The demonstration of immune complex components in the involved glomeruli and the observation that similar glomerular lesions can occur in isolated right-heart endocarditis, nonendocarditic infections, and noninfectious inflammatory conditions implicate immunological mechanisms as the cause for the focal/segmental glomerulonephritis of infective endocarditis. The focal/segmental glomerulonephritis can be rather widespread, such that occasionally it is indistinguishable using clinical, laboratory, and biopsy criteria from diffuse proliferative glomerulonephritis. Although the urine of focal/segmental glomerulonephritis may not be unusual, it customarily shows microscopic hematuria, sterile pyuria, or mild proteinuria. Moderate to marked proteinuria (over 2 gm/24 hr), systemic hypertension, or renal failure can develop in extensive or recurrent focal/segmental glomerulonephritis, but these manifestations are more commonly associated with diffuse proliferative glomerulonephritis.

DIFFUSE PROLIFERATIVE GLOMERULONEPHRITIS. This lesion, viewed by many to simply represent a more severe and extensive form of focal/segmental glomerulonephritis, attacks most glomeruli with a very proliferative cellular process, usually involving the entire glomerulus. The clinical consequences of systemic hypertension, nephritic proteinuria, and chronic renal failure are considerably more prevalent with the diffuse forms of proliferative glomerulonephritis. Hematuria, sterile pyuria, proteinuria, and heme or red blood cell casts are common features on urinalysis.

Renal biopsy reveals considerable proliferation and swelling of endothelial, epithelial, and mesangial cells, giving the typically involved glomerulus a packed cellular, even avascular, appearance. Neutrophils and round cells can be scattered throughout the glomerulus and interstitium. Fibrous replacement of the glomerulus and tubular atrophy and loss are common histological findings in more advanced stages. Immunofluorescent staining shows deposition of IgG, IgM, and C3 in subendothelial, subepithelial, and mesangial regions. Rapidly progressive glomerulonephritis with widespread glomerular crescent formation can occasionally occur in infective endocarditis and is often the explanation for rapid loss of renal function.

MANAGEMENT. Prompt identification and aggressive antibiotic treatment of the infecting organism are the principal means of preventing endocarditic renal disease. Antibiotic therapy has lowered the incidence of diffuse proliferative glomerulonephritis during infective endocarditis from 55 to 80 per cent to less than 15 per cent.[64,65] Pharmacological control of systemic hypertension and dialysis for renal failure occasionally are necessary supportive measures.

RENAL EMBOLIZATION. While evidence of renal embolization is found at necropsy in 60 to 70 per cent of patients who die of infective endocarditis, less than 25 per cent have clinically recognizable renal emboli.[64,65] Hematuria is the most common sign of renal emboli. Back or flank pain and renal hemorrhage, rarely fatal, can occur with a large embolus and sizable renal infarction. Larger emboli most often originate from prosthetic valves or from valvular infections caused by *Staphylococcus aureus, Neisseria gonococcus, Streptococcus pneumoniae,* or fungi. On rare occasions, an infected embolus can evolve into a renal abscess.

Cortical necrosis may occur when infective endocarditis is complicated by a coagulopathy, and acute tubular necrosis can be precipitated by concomitant cardiogenic shock or the use of nephrotoxic agents. Interstitial nephritis can occur in infective endocarditis, but generally in combination with glomerulonephritis. If interstitial nephritis develops as the predominant renal lesion in this clinical setting, a reaction to drug therapy must be considered.

CAUSES. Table 62–3 presents the major cardiovascular conditions responsible for renal embolization. Because 14 to 20 per cent of cardiac output passes through the kidneys and because of their direct proximity to the commonly diseased aorta, the kidneys represent favorite targets for arterial embolization.[67–73] The atherosclerotic aorta is a common source of fibrin, plaque, and cholesterol emboli. Suprarenal aneurysms, aortic surgery, intraaortic balloon counterpulsation, cardiac or aortic catheterization, anticoagulation, and thrombolytic therapy increase the risk of renal embolization from the atherosclerotic aorta (see p. 1570). Massive embolization to skeletal muscle can exacerbate or cause renal dysfunction and failure via myoglobinemia-myoglobinuria. The more common cardiac conditions serving as embolic sources are atrial fibrillation, mural thrombi of the left ventricle, mitral stenosis, and prosthetic heart valves (Table 62–3).

Renal pathology ranges from isolated occlusion of an arteriole with minimal histological change, to segmental infarction ("white infarcts" and scarring), to complete occlusion of a renal artery with unilateral loss of renal function and mass. Cholesterol clefts and calcified debris are histological features of atherosclerotic emboli. Capsular rupture and retroperitoneal hemorrhage can complicate a large infarction.

Similar to embolization elsewhere, the majority are not likely to be detected clinically. Clinical manifestations include varying degrees of hematuria, proteinuria, back or flank pain, systemic hypertension (secondary to elevated plasma renin), and renal dysfunction. Extensive embolization to both kidneys or a large embolus of a sole functioning kidney can result in anuria. Eosinophilia, depressed serum levels of C3 and C4, and rarely, lipid droplets floating in a urine sample can occur with cholesterol emboli.

TABLE 62–3 MAJOR CARDIOVASCULAR SOURCES, CAUSES, AND PREDISPOSING FACTORS FOR EMBOLIZATION TO KIDNEYS

AORTA
Atherosclerotic disease
Extensive atherosclerotic plaque formation; rupture, thrombus and cholesterol embolization
Suprarenal aortic aneurysm
Cardiac and aortic catheterization
Intraaortic balloon counterpulsation therapy
Anticoagulation
Thrombolytic therapy
Aortic surgery
ATRIA
Atrial fibrillation
Atrial enlargement
Cardiomyopathy
Atrial septal aneurysms
Paradoxical embolization
Myxoma (less commonly located in ventricles and on valves)
States of hypercoagulation (e.g., neoplastic diseases; protein C, protein S, or antithrombin III deficiency)
VENTRICLES
Mural thrombus
Myocardial infarction
Cardiomyopathy
Cardiac tumors
States of hypercoagulation (see Atria above)
VALVES
Mitral stenosis (via atrial or valvular thrombus)
Prosthetic valves
Endocarditis
Infective
Marantic (noninfective thrombotic)
Mitral annular calcification

The renal manifestations of atherosclerotic or cholesterol emboli are commonly part of an embolic multisystem "polyarteritis" presentation. Clinical suspicion of renal emboli is raised in patients with an obvious predisposition (e.g., prosthetic heart valve, atherosclerotic aorta, aortic surgery, recent cardiovascular catheterization). Perfusion defects secondary to large emboli are detectable with renal radionuclide scanning. Renal arteriography generally shows a cutoff sign at the point of occlusion with few vascular markings distal to the occlusion. The "rim sign" (subcapsular contrast overlying regions of noncontrast) may be seen with extensive or large embolization.

MANAGEMENT. This is generally directed at correcting the source of embolization with supportive therapy for accompanying systemic hypertension or renal failure. For large renal emboli, local thrombolytic therapy, angioplasty, retrieval via catheter, or surgical embolectomy are the principal interventional options.[72,73] The approach to atherosclerotic-cholesterol emboli is somewhat limited; an obvious source (e.g., suprarenal atherosclerotic aortic disease or aneurysm) should be considered for resection with the understanding that the aorta is usually diffusely involved with atherosclerosis and that further embolization may occur during and after surgery. Whether long-term anticoagulation for atheroembolic renal disease offers effective therapy or exacerbation of the problem remains unresolved; prolonged aspirin therapy is a reasonable option and skirts this controversy.

OTHER CARDIOVASCULAR CONDITIONS

Aortic Aneurysm and Dissection

(See also Chap. 45)

The atherosclerotic aneurysm can threaten renal function in a number of ways including thromboembolism from a suprarenal location (see Thromboembolic disease, above), reduction of renal blood flow by local involvement or encroachment, rupture with hypovolemic shock, aortorenal vein fistula, ureteral obstruction, and the consequences of its surgical repair.[67,74–76] Ten to 20 per cent of atherosclerotic aortic aneurysms are complicated by renal artery stenosis. Clinical suspicion of renal involvement by an atherosclerotic aneurysm is prompted by recent onset or acceleration of systemic hypertension, location near the renal arteries, hematuria, proteinuria, occasional eosinophilia (in cases of atheroemboli), and renal dysfunction and failure. Aneurysmectomy with renal revascularization (when renal arteries are involved) is generally the treatment of choice.

Renal involvement by aortic dissection takes the form of renal artery occlusion or renal dysfunction secondary to compromised hemodynamics from hemorrhagic-hypovolemic shock, cardiac tamponade, or acute heart failure caused by acute aortic valvular insufficiency or acute myocardial infarction.[77] Partial or total renal artery occlusion can occur via an ostial flap or displacement of the intima-media into the lumen as the dissecting hematoma moves into the renal artery. Renal manifestations can include proteinuria, hematuria, systemic hypertension (high plasma renin), renal infarction, azotemia, and renal failure. Anuria should bring bilateral renal artery occlusion (unilateral for a sole functioning kidney) into consideration. Operative correction of the dissection with renal revascularization remains the intervention of choice in most instances.

Congenital Heart Disease

CYANOTIC CONGENITAL DISEASE. The clinical course of cyanotic congenital heart disease is often accompanied by the development of renal dysfunction.[78–80] Although the mechanism for the renal dysfunction is not known, its severity appears to be related to the level and duration of arterial desaturation, the degree of polycythemia, age, severity of right-heart failure, and elevation of systemic venous pressure. Histologically, the glomeruli enlarge ("glomerulomegaly") with mesangial hypercellularity, capillary congestion, focal glomerulosclerosis, and localized thickening of the basement membrane. Functionally, the disorder behaves as a glomerulopathy with proteinuria occurring in 30 per cent and microscopic hematuria in 15 to 20 per cent of patients.[79] Five to 10 per cent develop considerable proteinuria and occasionally the nephrotic syndrome, usually after the age of 21 years.[79,80] Tubular dysfunction can occur. Because of increased uric acid production during polycythemia and the tubular dysfunction, hyperuricemia is a common metabolic complication of cyanotic heart disease. A reduction in renal blood flow, GFR, and urea clearance also occurs over time. Most of the glomerular lesions, renal dysfunction, and urinary findings are reversible and usually return toward normal after successful surgical correction of the cardiac defect and subsequent improvement in hemodynamics, oxygen delivery, and hematocrit.

COARCTATION OF THE AORTA. This malformation has a significant impact on renal physiology and function.[81–83] The lower renal perfusion pressure (distal to the coarctation) evokes sustained release of renin, which contributes to the characteristic hypertension present in the vascular system located above the coarctation. Depending somewhat on the age of the patient and duration of the condition, surgical or angioplasty correction usually does not immediately lower systemic blood pressure (in fact, it may initially increase) and systemic hypertension can persist long-term after correction in up to one-third of the patients.[81,82] Congestive heart failure, infective endocarditis, and aortic dissection are other complications of coarctation, which in addition to post-repair systemic hypertension, can adversely affect renal function. Fibromuscular dysplasia and developmental hypoplasia of the renal arteries have been reported in association with coarctation or hypoplasia of the abdominal aorta.[83]

EFFECTS OF RENAL FAILURE ON THE CARDIOVASCULAR SYSTEM

CARDIAC FAILURE CAUSED BY RENAL FAILURE

Left ventricular dysfunction and CHF are common complications of chronic renal failure.[19,84–92] Factors that contribute to myocardial damage and dysfunction in patients with this condition are depicted in Figure 62–5. Because it is usually difficult to attribute a predominant causative role to any one of these factors or events, the term *uremic cardiomyopathy* is often used to identify the cardiac disorder resulting from the integration of the various disruptive factors of chronic renal failure.

Factors Contributing to the Development of Congestive Heart Failure

The conditions contributing to the development of CHF in patients with chronic renal failure are presented in Figure 62-6.

VOLUME OVERLOAD. Loss of renal function allows salt and fluid retention and the development of volume overload. Other factors that contribute to volume overload are chronic anemia and the arteriovenous (AV) access fistula. Normochromic, normocytic anemia is common in chronic renal failure, with nontreated hematocrits ranging from 20 to 30 per cent and hemoglobin from 7 to 9 gm/dl; the introduction of erythropoietin therapy in chronic renal failure has reduced the degree and consequences of anemia. In general, the overall hemodynamic effect of the typical upper extremity AV access fistula is small; however, the fistula may contribute to the development of CHF in patients with left ventricular (LV) dysfunction.

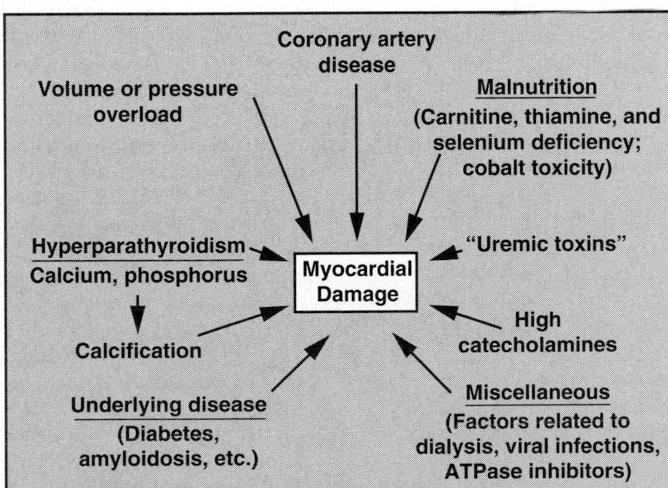

FIGURE 62–5. Factors contributing to myocardial damage in patients with chronic renal failure. (Modified from Leier, C. V., and Boudoulas, H.: Cardiorenal Disorders and Diseases. Armonk, N.Y., Futura Publishing Co., 1992.)

The contribution of volume overload to the development of CHF in chronic renal failure is related to the magnitude and time course of volume expansion and to the concomitant status of cardiac function. A sudden rise in plasma volume can increase LV end-diastolic pressure to levels that produce pulmonary edema, even in the presence of normal resting LV systolic function. In contrast, a gradual increase in plasma volume can allow compensatory ventricular dilatation and hypertrophy with less immediate elevations in LV diastolic pressure.

PRESSURE OVERLOAD. Systemic hypertension, a common finding in patients with chronic renal failure, contributes considerably to the generation of acute and chronic CHF by placing an excessive afterload burden on the dysfunctional heart. Increased afterload in chronic renal failure is also a result of reduced compliance of the aorta and large arteries.[93] Renal artery stenosis with secondary or concomitant chronic renal failure can cause episodic, marked systemic hypertension and consequently evoke intermittent acute heart failure and pulmonary edema.[94]

NEGATIVE INOTROPIC EFFECTS. Several factors in chronic renal failure may decrease myocardial contractility. These include hypoxemia (often present during hemodialysis), subendocardial ischemia, certain buffers (e.g., acetate) added to the hemodialysis fluid, elevated parathormone levels, various metabolic and electrolyte abnormalities, and "uremic toxins."

EFFECTS OF DIALYSIS AND RENAL TRANSPLANTATION ON THE HEART

DIALYSIS. During dialysis, changes in preload, afterload, arterial pO_2, adrenergic activity, concentrations of electrolytes, ionized calcium, "uremic toxins," and other metabolites and the composition of the dialysis solution affect cardiac-ventricular performance (Fig. 62–7).[19,84] The baseline status of LV function prior to the initiation of dialysis therapy is a major determinant of LV performance during dialysis. In general, patients with normal LV function experience little change or a modest decrease in LV performance during dialysis, whereas LV performance in those with baseline systolic dysfunction often improves during the procedure. These observations are due in part to the fact that the preload reduction of dialysis has less effect on LV systolic performance in the dysfunctional (systolic) LV com-

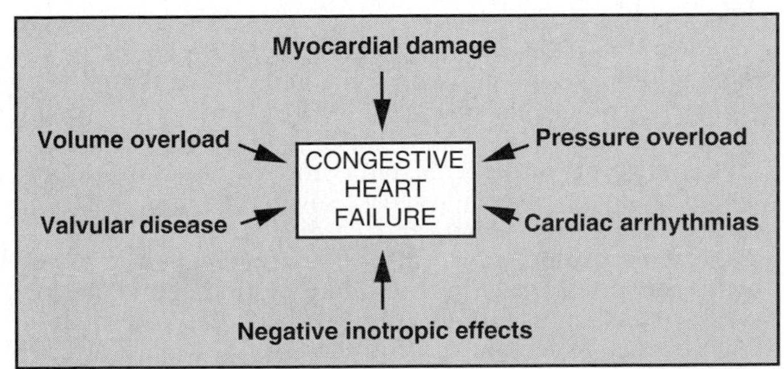

FIGURE 62–6. Factors contributing to the development of congestive heart failure in patients with chronic renal failure. (Modified from Leier, C. V., and Boudoulas, H.: Cardiorenal Disorders and Diseases. Armonk, N.Y., Futura Publishing Co., 1992.)

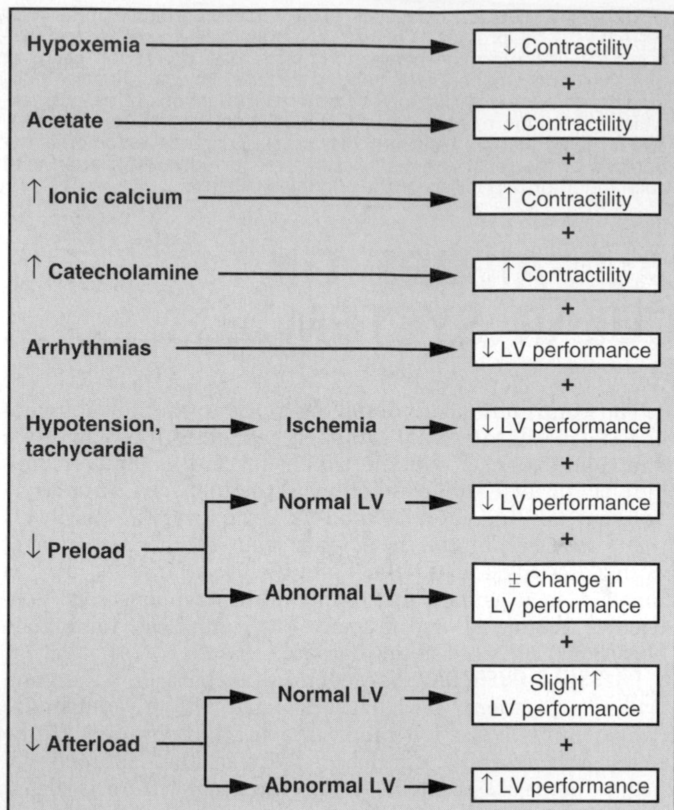

FIGURE 62–7. Effects of multiple factors and events during dialysis on left ventricular (LV) performance. (Modified from Leier, C. V., and Boudoulas, H.: Cardiorenal Disorders and Diseases. Armonk, N.Y., Futura Publishing Co., 1992.)

pared to the normal LV, while the opposite responses occur during shifts in afterload. Preload reduction during dialysis can adversely affect LV systolic performance and overall hemodynamics in patients with predominant LV diastolic dysfunction.

Changes in preload and afterload during peritoneal dialysis are more gradual and less in magnitude, and thus its effects on LV performance are not as marked as those of hemodialysis. However, large amounts of intraperitoneal fluid can impair LV systolic performance by reducing venous return and raising afterload.

RENAL TRANSPLANTATION. LV systolic and diastolic volumes and ventricular mass decrease and ejection fraction generally increases over 3 to 4 months after renal transplantation. These changes are likely related to favorable alterations of LV preload and afterload, an increase in hematocrit value, and correction of the various metabolic/endocrinological abnormalities already discussed.[19,88,89] Because commonly used immunosuppressive agents (e.g., cyclosporine) can evoke systemic hypertension, blood pressure should be checked regularly and treated appropriately in the post-transplant patient.

Management of Heart Failure in Patients with Renal Failure

The clinical presentation and evaluation of CHF in chronic renal failure patients are similar to those of patients without this condition (see Chap. 15). As in patients without chronic renal failure, the principles of CHF management in CRF include correcting remedially reversible lesions (e.g., operable occlusive coronary disease), improving contributory conditions (e.g., severe anemia), and optimizing preload, afterload, and cardiac rhythm. Restriction of dietary sodium to ≤ 2 gm/day is recommended. Angiotensin-converting enzyme inhibitors, digitalis, and vasodilators are often useful in this setting.[19] The duration of dialysis may be lengthened to increase fluid removal or to remove the usual amount of fluid volume more gradually and thus avoid hypotension. Peritoneal dialysis should be considered if problematic hypotension occurs during hemodialysis in the CRF patient with CHF. Erythropoietin is an effective and safe means of increasing the hematocrit of CRF anemia, and an oversized AV access shunt may have to be modified. Long-term administration of 1α-hydrocholecalciferol may improve LV performance by reducing circulating parathormone and improving cellular calcium, phosphorous, and magnesium metabolism. Renal transplantation usually improves LV performance, hemodynamics, and CHF symptoms. In select patients with end-stage myocardial and kidney disease, combined cardiac and renal transplantation, preferably from the same donor, should be considered.[88,95]

HYPERTROPHIC CARDIOMYOPATHY

For yet undetermined reasons, hypertrophic cardiomyopathy and asymmetrical septal hypertrophy are not uncommon complications of CRF.[19] Patients with CRF with hypertrophic cardiomyopathy also invariably have LV diastolic dysfunction, which, when combined with a LV outflow tract gradient, makes them particularly vulnerable to the occurrence of systemic hypotension during hemodialysis. Special care must be taken to avoid volume depletion during hemodialysis in these patients, with consideration for peritoneal dialysis in those who experience problematic hypotension. If symptoms or complications during dialysis appear to be exacerbated by high adrenergic tone, beta-adrenergic blockade is a reasonable option.

ACCELERATED CORONARY ATHEROSCLEROSIS

Atherogenic Factors in Chronic Renal Failure

CHRONIC RENAL FAILURE AND DIALYSIS. Cardiovascular mortality remains high in these patients. This is in large part related to aging of the affected population and to the increased number of diabetic patients undergoing long-term dialysis. Thirty to 35 per cent of patients on long-term dialysis management have overt diabetes mellitus. Women with chronic renal failure develop coronary artery disease (CAD) as frequently and severely as age-matched men with chronic renal failure, perhaps because of earlier menopause and alterations in the pituitary-gonadal axis in these women.[19,89–92] For yet unknown reasons, patients with chronic pyelonephritis or interstitial renal disease develop CAD more frequently than patients with other forms of chronic renal failure.

Carbohydrate and lipid abnormalities occur early in chronic renal insufficiency (serum creatine levels >3 mg/dl) and persist as the patient's condition advances into end-stage renal failure and necessitates long-term dialysis. Glucose intolerance and insulin resistance have been demonstrated in a large proportion of chronic renal failure patients who are not overtly diabetic, and patients undergoing long-term dialysis develop carbohydrate and lipid disturbances similar to those of diabetes mellitus (insulin resistance, glucose intolerance, increased triglycerides). While the total cholesterol concentration in serum of chronic renal failure patients on maintenance dialysis can be normal, the level of the high-density lipoproteins is usually depressed. Caucasian men with chronic renal failure have lower levels of high-density lipoproteins than African-American men so affected, which may account for the higher incidence of CAD in the former group.[19,96–102] Other abnormalities that likely augment the atherosclerotic process include carnitine deficiency (adversely affects lipoprotein metabolism), secondary hyperparathyroidism, vascular calcification, increased homocystine, various states of hypercoagulation, and enhanced fibrin and platelet deposition (Fig. 62–8). Depressed endothelium-derived vasodilation and elevated local and circulating levels of endothelin in

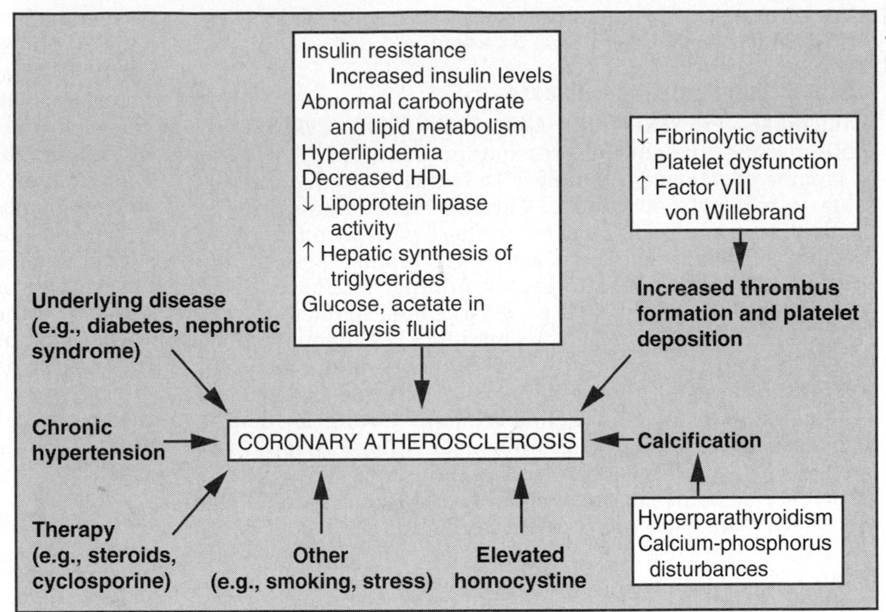

FIGURE 62–8. Factors contributing to the development and acceleration of coronary atherosclerosis in patients with chronic renal failure. HDL = high-density lipoproteins. (Modified from Leier, C. V., and Boudoulas, H.: Cardiorenal Disorders and Diseases. Armonk, N.Y., Futura Publishing Co., 1992.)

patients with chronic renal failure may also play a role.[103,104]

NEPHROTIC SYNDROME. Elevation of serum lipid values is a major feature of the nephrotic syndrome. Total cholesterol and low-density lipoprotein cholesterol concentrations are generally elevated, and high-density lipoprotein cholesterol is normal or low.[105] These lipid derangements can persist for some time after remission of the nephrotic syndrome, particularly in children. Chronic hypertension and corticosteroid therapy further accelerate atherosclerosis in this subgroup of patients.

RENAL TRANSPLANTATION. Cardiovascular disease contributes heavily to mortality following kidney transplantation. Many chronic renal failure patients have generalized arteriosclerosis-atherosclerosis at the time of transplantation and thus their pre-transplant and post-transplant cardiovascular disease represents a continuum, perpetuated by the persistence, worsening, and accumulation of risk factors (e.g., age, hypertension, diabetes, hyperlipidemia, immunosuppressive drugs)[19,106,107] (Fig. 62–8). The number of acute rejection episodes is also linked as an independent risk factor to the development of cardiovascular disease.[19] Significant proteinuria occurs in 10 to 15 per cent of transplantation patients and usually indicates varying degrees of graft rejection or failure; urinary protein excretion >0.5 gm daily in the post-transplant patient is associated with a significant rise in low-density and very low-density lipoprotein cholesterol and in total triglycerides. Immunosuppressive therapy with corticosteroids evokes insulin resistance and hyperlipoproteinemia. Cyclosporine increases total cholesterol by elevating the level of low-density lipoprotein cholesterol.[106,107] Therefore the cumulative atherogenic risk factors—long-term dialysis, renal transplantation, and periodic graft rejection—account for the high prevalence of morbid cardiovascular disease in renal transplant patients.

FACTORS AFFECTING MYOCARDIAL OXYGEN SUPPLY AND DEMAND IN CHRONIC RENAL FAILURE

Although the general determinants of myocardial oxygen supply and demand in these patients are similar to those of patients without renal failure (see p. 381), chronic renal failure adds several conditions that can evoke myocardial ischemia, even without occlusive CAD. Chronic renal failure adversely affects coronary perfusion pressure, diastolic perfusion time, and oxygen-carrying capacity of blood (Fig. 62–9). Volume and pressure overload increase ventricular diastolic pressure and thus can decrease coronary perfusion pressure (coronary perfusion pressure during diastole equals coronary artery pressure minus LV diastolic pressure). In the presence of occlusive coronary artery disease, coronary artery pressure distal to a high-grade obstruction is not only low but is also not affected significantly by the usual changes in aortic diastolic pressure. Therefore, distal to an obstruction, only changes in LV diastolic pressure can significantly alter coronary perfusion pressure in that region of the heart. An increase in heart rate (as occurs with dialysis, AV shunt, or anemia) reduces myocardial blood flow simply by decreasing diastolic perfusion time.

Since the majority of coronary blood flow occurs in diastole and the duration of diastole (diastolic perfusion time) has a nonlinear inverse relationship with heart rate, even small increases in heart rate can substantially reduce diastolic perfusion time.[108] Anemia, a common feature of chronic renal failure, reduces the oxygen-carrying capacity of blood. Hemodialysis with accompanying hypotension, tachycardia, and leftward shift in the arterial hemoglobin-oxygen dissociation curve can be especially threatening to myocardial oxygena-

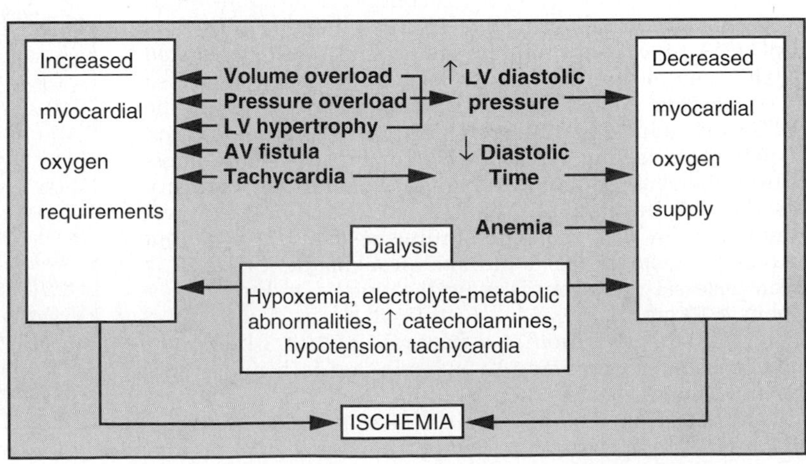

FIGURE 62–9. Factors affecting myocardial oxygen supply and oxygen requirements in patients with chronic renal failure. AV = arteriovenous, LV = left ventricle. (Modified from Leier, C. V., and Boudoulas, H.: Cardiorenal Disorders and Diseases. Armonk, N.Y., Futura Publishing Co., 1992.)

tion. Coronary blood flow has been shown to decrease in some patients during hemodialysis.[109]

Chronic Coronary Artery Disease

CLINICAL PRESENTATION AND DIAGNOSTIC EVALUATION. CRF modifies the clinical presentation of chronic CAD with a greater prevalence of painless ischemia, partially attributable to a large proportion of chronic renal failure patients with diabetes mellitus, and with chest pain secondary to a variety of nonischemic causes (e.g., uremic pericarditis, neuritis).[19,110] Electrocardiographic findings similar to those of myocardial ischemia (e.g., ST-segment depression, T-wave inversion) are present in many CRF patients without significant CAD (especially during and after dialysis), thereby limiting the specificity of this diagnostic method. The sensitivity of radionuclide exercise testing for detecting obstructive CAD in chronic renal failure is low, perhaps because of generally poor exercise capacity,[111] and there are insufficient data in this condition regarding the sensitivity and specificity of radionuclide-perfusion imaging after dipyridamole administration. Dobutamine-stress echocardiography has recently been shown to be a promising means of detecting significant CAD in chronic renal failure.[112] Coronary arteriography is often required in these patients with suspected or problematic CAD to define their coronary artery anatomy and pathology and to develop the most appropriate management plan.

USE OF CONTRAST RADIOGRAPHY. To minimize the renal complications of radiocontrast angiography in patients with serum creatinine concentrations greater than 2 mg/dl who are not yet undergoing long-term dialysis, preprocedural hydration and postprocedural volume replacement (saline solution for urine volume) are the most effective interventions.[113] The routine administration of 20 per cent mannitol solution is no longer advocated in this clinical setting. The smallest possible amount of radiocontrast agent should be used, because the degree of nephrotoxicity is closely related to the quantity injected. Patients with renal artery stenosis are especially susceptible to contrast-induced nephropathy. The osmotic and volume load of radiocontrast material can also provoke acute pulmonary edema in chronic renal failure patients with underlying volume overload or LV dysfunction. Nonionic contrast material evokes less intravascular volume expansion and should generally be employed in chronic renal failure. To further reduce the amount and risk of administered radiocontrast agent, information regarding ventricular size and function should be obtained via two-dimensional echocardiography or radionuclide angiography.

MANAGEMENT. The general management approach to CAD in chronic renal failure is similar to that of patients without this condition (Ch. 38); management aspects unique to chronic renal failure patients are presented below.[19,114–117] A diet weighted with polyunsaturated fats and a carbohydrate content of approximately 20 per cent of total caloric intake is generally recommended. Lipid-lowering agents are usually effective in this clinical setting, and HMG-CoA reductase inhibitors are generally better tolerated in CRF than most other agents. Because of an increased risk of developing skeletal myopathy and rhabdomyolysis, the HMG-CoA reductase inhibitors must be used with caution in patients receiving cyclosporine. Disturbed calcium-phosphorus metabolism and resultant peripheral and coronary vascular calcification are approached with long-time oral administration of phosphate-binding agents (e.g., calcium carbonate, calcium acetate). For problematic CAD, it is often necessary to administer erythropoietin to keep hemoglobin ≥10 gm/dl.

Oxygen administration at a flow rate of 2 to 3 liters/min may be useful in reducing hypoxemia and ischemic events during hemodialysis. When possible, sodium bicarbonate instead of sodium acetate should be employed as the dialysis buffer. This produces resultant improvement in arterial oxygenation, less provocation of hypotension, and reduction in the tendency of this procedure to precipitate myocardial ischemia. Certain patients with severe CAD and ventricular dysfunction cannot tolerate hemodialysis because of problematic dialysis-induced reduction in cardiac output or blood pressure; some of these patients require cardioactive drug support (e.g., dopamine, dobutamine) during hemodialysis, and others are best managed with peritoneal dialysis.

Percutaneous transluminal coronary angioplasty (PTCA) can be performed in these patients; however, the restenosis rate is rather high.[115] Chronic renal failure patients, whether or not they are undergoing long-term dialysis and prerenal or postrenal transplantation, can undergo coronary artery bypass surgery with acceptable risk and with an expectation for significant improvement of ischemic symptoms, exercise tolerance, and, perhaps for some, survival.[114,117]

PERIOPERATIVE MANAGEMENT

Table 62–4 lists the major recommendations for the perioperative management of the chronic renal failure patient undergoing cardiac surgery. Intravascular volume, serum potassium, hematocrit, and drug administration must be carefully monitored during the perioperative period.[19,114,117] Preoperatively, daily dialysis (usually of shorter duration) against a low potassium bath should be considered to control serum and whole body potassium content. Hemoglobin and hematocrit should be raised to ≥10 gm/dl and ≥30 per cent, respectively, with erythropoietin administration or via red cell transfusion during dialysis in more urgent situations. The patient should go to surgery at near "dry weight." Intravenously administered fluids are kept to a minimum with little or no potassium administration. To prevent excessive hemodilution during cardiopulmonary bypass, both blood and Ringer's lactated solution are used to prime the extracorporeal pump. Beta-adrenergic blockade should be continued throughout the perioperative period to avert the myocardial and dysrhythmic complications of the hyperadrenergic state of cardiac surgery. Intraoperative hemofiltration can be used to treat any excessive intravascular volume accumulated during cardiopulmonary bypass.

Postoperatively, dialysis is employed to reverse hyperkalemia, significant azotemia, or volume overload. Regional heparinization or citration should be considered during the first 5 to 10 postoperative days as a means of controlling bleeding complications during hemodialysis. The perioperative management used for CRF patients undergoing lengthy dialysis also applies to nondialyzed CRF patients undergoing cardiac surgery; renal function in the latter patients may have to be supported with dialysis over several postoperative days, but function usually returns to its preoperative status by 10 to 15 days after surgery. Patients with a functioning transplanted kidney can be managed in a near-routine (nonchronic renal failure) manner with special attention directed at providing adequate corticosteroid support, avoiding nephrotoxic drugs, and maintaining adequate urine output.

Pericarditis is a common complication; total pericardiectomy

TABLE 62–4 PERIOPERATIVE MANAGEMENT OF CHRONIC RENAL FAILURE IN PATIENTS UNDERGOING CARDIAC SURGERY

PREOPERATIVE
Dental evaluation and correction
Decrease intake of sodium, potassium, and fluid volume
Short dialysis daily (low potassium bath)
Beta-blockade therapy throughout perioperative period
Antibiotic prophylaxis (start immediately before surgery and continue for 2 days after surgery)
Raise hemoglobin/hematocrit above 10 gm per dl/30 per cent
INTRAOPERATIVE
Keep fluid administration to minimum
Do not administer potassium
Special effort to preserve arm vessels and AV access fistula
Hemodynamic monitoring (during and after surgery) as needed
POSTOPERATIVE
Determine serum potassium levels and arterial blood gases every 4 hr during first 24 hr
Perform dialysis as indicated
Use regional anticoagulation during dialysis over first 5 to 10 postoperative days

AV = arteriovenous.

should be considered as a reasonable elective addition to the cardiac surgical procedure in patients with chronic renal failure.

Acute Myocardial Ischemic Syndromes

The clinical presentation, diagnostic steps, and therapeutic measures for these patients with acute ischemic syndromes are generally similar to those directed at patients without chronic renal failure (Ch. 37). Unfortunately, chronic renal failure patients also frequently exhibit abnormal electrocardiographic ST-segment and T-wave abnormalities and elevated serum cardiac enzyme values in the absence of myocardial ischemia-necrosis. Because of impaired renal clearance, total creatine phosphokinase (CPK) and lactic dehydrogenase levels are often elevated. However, the total CPK is usually composed of brain band CPK (CPK-BB, increased in about 30 per cent of patients with CRF) or skeletal muscle band (CPK-MM). Therefore, when myocardial ischemia and infarction is suspected, careful monitoring of the myocardial band (CPK-MB) over the ensuing 24 to 48 hours becomes important; new or transient elevation of the CPK-MB fraction can usually be regarded as an indication of acute myocardial necrosis.[118]

In the chronic renal failure patient with acute myocardial infarction who has end-stage renal disease or is nonresponsive to intravenous administration of loop diuretics in moderate to high doses, fluid overload is approached with dialysis. Hemodynamic monitoring with a flow-directed indwelling pulmonary artery catheter is appropriate when a low perfusion state or heart failure develops. Electrolyte and metabolic abnormalities are controlled with dietary measures and dialysis as needed.

CARDIOVASCULAR CALCIFICATION

Dystrophic (metastatic) calcification commonly occurs in CRF patients receiving maintenance dialysis and can involve all tissues, including heart, vasculature, and kidneys. Hyperphosphatemia with elevation of the calcium X phosphorus product, shifts in plasma and tissue pH during and following dialysis, and secondary hyperparathyroidism are regarded as the most important factors responsible for tissue calcification in CRF (Table 62–5).[19,119] The calcification is exacerbated by excessive intake of milk, use of certain antacids, and calcium extraction from calcium polystyrene materials and surfaces (e.g., certain dialysis units).

The mitral annulus and valve and aortic valve are the preferential cardiac sites for dystrophic calcification in chronic renal failure (Table 62–5). Consequently, hemodynamically significant valvular stenosis and/or regurgitation, usually manifested clinically as murmurs and occasionally as symptoms and signs of heart failure, are common complications of cardiac calcification in chronic renal failure. Myocardial calcification can evoke conduction abnormalities (most commonly atrioventricular or bundle branch block), various arrhythmias, ventricular dysfunction, and CHF. Significant annular, valvular, and coronary artery calcification and regions of dense calcification elsewhere in the heart are usually detectable by image-amplified fluoroscopy, echocardiography, or magnetic resonance imaging. Technetium pyrophosphate scintigraphy may demonstrate uptake in areas of myocardial calcification. Diffuse myocardial calcification can occasionally be detected with special histological processing of myocardial biopsy specimens. Pericardial calcification, usually microscopic in degree, contributes to the pathological process of uremic pericarditis. Dense pericardial calcification is not a feature of chronic renal failure and implicates another disease process.

TABLE 62–5 METASTATIC CALCIFICATION OF CHRONIC RENAL FAILURE: CONTRIBUTING FACTORS AND COMMON CARDIOVASCULAR SITES OF INVOLVEMENT

POSSIBLE CONTRIBUTING FACTORS	CARDIOVASCULAR SITES
Hyperphosphatemia	Mitral annulus and valve
Increased ionized calcium	Aortic valve
Increased calcium-phosphorus product	Atrioventricular node/conduction system
Increased parathormone levels	Myocardium
Acute changes in blood pH	Interventricular septum
Increased calcium ingestion	Coronary arteries
Certain antacids	Pericardium
Extraction from calcium-containing polymers and materials	
Vitamin D preparations	

Modified from Leier, C. V., and Boudoulas, H.: Cardiorenal Disorders and Diseases. Armonk, N. Y., Futura Publishing Co., 1992.

Prevention of cardiovascular calcification is an important component of chronic renal failure management. Phosphate-binding agents and dietary measures (restriction of phosphate and avoidance of excessive calcium intake) are employed for this purpose. Regression of nonvisceral calcification has been achieved by lowering serum phosphorus with oral phosphate-binding agents, parathyroidectomy, and renal transplantation; visceral calcification (including cardiovascular) does not appear to be as readily reversible. Management of the congestive heart failure, atrioventricular block, and cardiac arrhythmias caused by cardiac calcification is directed at controlling symptoms.

HEART MURMURS AND VALVULAR HEART DISEASE

Heart murmurs and acquired valvular abnormalities are common in these patients. Dystrophic calcification, infectious and noninfectious endocarditis, and certain renal diseases (e.g., polycystic kidney disease) are associated with structural abnormalities of heart valves.[19,120-122] However, heart murmurs are frequently noted in chronic renal failure without obvious underlying valvular abnormalities and are probably evoked by anemia, the AV access fistula, hyperadrenergic tone, and volume and pressure overload. Early diastolic murmurs of functional aortic or pulmonic regurgitation, generally related to pressure and volume overload, can appear during advanced stages of renal failure and often disappear following hemodialysis. An occasional murmur audible over the anterior chest may be transmitted from an AV access fistula located in the upper limb. In patients with forearm shunt access, bruits can be heard in the ipsilateral axillary, clavicular, and cervical regions. Cervical venous hums are also common in these patients. Thus, murmurs in chronic renal failure can represent valvular disease, functional pulmonic or aortic valvular flow or regurgitation, transmission from an AV fistula, or a venous hum.

As in other conditions, each murmur requires clinical assessment to define the underlying cause, and if associated with valvular or congenital heart disease, evaluation of the severity of the lesion. A precordial systolic murmur secondary to high flow or transmission from the AV fistula can be easily distinguished from other murmurs by observing the response of the murmur to transient obstruction of the fistula. Functional murmurs secondary to pressure or volume overload decrease considerably with control of hypertension, reduction of fluid overload, correction of anemia, and so forth. Venous hums are usually audible throughout the cardiac cycle; are loudest at the base of the neck, in the upright position and during inspiration; and are abolished by compression of the neck veins or by the Valsalva maneuver.

Laboratory evaluation and overall management of valvular heart disease in affected patients is similar to that recommended for patients without chronic renal failure (see Ch. 32). Cardiac valve replacement can be done with acceptable operative mortality and reasonably good cardiac rehabilitation in patients undergoing prolonged hemodialysis. Long-term survival for most of these patients is still limited by the clinical course and complications of chronic renal failure, but quality of life is generally improved after valve replacement.

Preoperative dental evaluation is mandatory, and dental treatment should be completed several weeks before cardiac surgery. The patient should arrive at operation at near "dry weight," and with a hematocrit of ≥30 per cent and a serum potassium level of 3.5 to 4.5 mEq/liter (Table 62–4). Serum potassium and arterial blood gases should be measured every 4 to 6 hours during the first postoperative day. Hemodialysis may be required to manage fluid overload, azotemia, or hyperkalemia. Chronic renal failure patients undergoing open-heart surgery—especially placement of prosthetic heart valves—are at high risk for infective endocarditis. In the perioperative period, *Staphylococcus aureus*, coagulase-negative staphylococci, and diphtheroids are the most common infecting organisms. No single antibiotic agent is effective against all of these organisms, and prolonged use of broad-spectrum antibiotics predisposes patients to superinfection with unusual or resistant organisms. Thus, antibiotic prophylaxis at the time of valvular surgery is primarily directed against staphylococci and should be started immediately before the operative procedure and continued postoperatively for approximately 2 days. The choice of mechanical versus bioprosthetic valve for replacement in chronic renal failure remains controversial.[19,121,122] When technically feasible, reconstructive valvular repair should be considered for problematic mitral regurgitation.[120,121]

PERICARDIAL DISEASE

Pericardial disease remains a relatively common complication in these patients. The contributory factors are depicted in Figure 62–10, and the evaluation and management of pericardial disorders are presented in Chapter 43.

SYSTEMIC HYPERTENSION

HYPERTENSION ASSOCIATED WITH CHRONIC RENAL FAILURE (see also p. 824). Systemic hypertension occurs in more than 80 per cent of these patients prior to initiation of dialysis. Chronic renal failure patients who remain normotensive most often have tubular and interstitial disease or obstructive uropathy as the underlying pathological process. In contrast, arterionephrosclerosis and glomerulonephritis are usually associated with hypertension, often marked. The various factors that likely contribute to the development of systemic hypertension in chronic renal failure are presented in Figure 62–11.

HYPERTENSION ASSOCIATED WITH RENAL TRANSPLANTATION. The incidence of systemic hypertension after renal transplantation varies widely (25 to 80 per cent) and is highest during the early months after transplantation. The incidence 5 years after transplantation is about 40 to 50 per cent. Renal graft failure is increased considerably in the

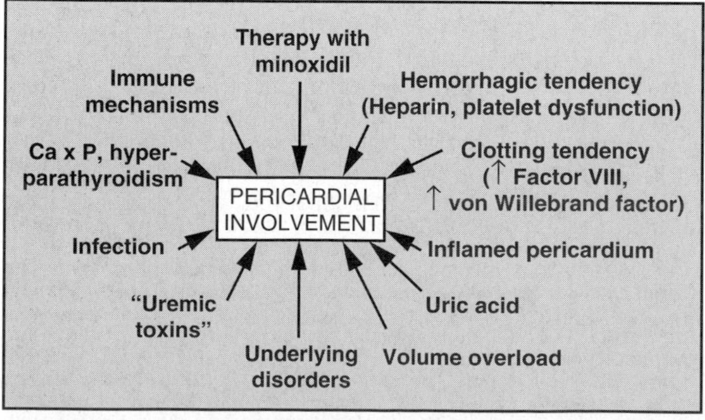

FIGURE 62–10. Factors contributing to the development of pericardial disease in patients with chronic renal failure. Ca = calcium, P = phosphorus. (Modified from Leier, C. V., and Boudoulas, H.: Cardiorenal Disorders and Diseases. Armonk, N.Y., Futura Publishing Co., 1992.)

setting of poorly controlled systemic hypertension.[123] Renal artery stenosis (of the transplanted kidney or native kidneys), chronic rejection, native kidney disease, therapy with corticosteroids or cyclosporine, and essential hypertension prior to transplantation are the leading causes for systemic hypertension in the post-transplant patient. Recipients of cadaveric kidneys from donors with a family history of essential hypertension are also more likely to experience post-transplant hypertension. On the other hand, essential hypertension can undergo remission for up to 8 to 10 years after successful transplantation of a kidney from a normotensive donor.

MANAGEMENT. Diagnostic studies should be undertaken in patients with renal failure and hypertension to exclude a reversible renovascular cause (see Chap. 26) and determine the nature of the underlying renal disease. Distinguishing hypertension secondary to renal parenchymal disease from essential hypertension with resultant hypertensive renal disease is often quite difficult at this stage. The medical history may identify patients who have had longstanding essential hypertension and a familial tendency for such, diabetes mellitus, or an episode of glomerulonephritis prior to developing renal failure.

The treatment of systemic hypertension in patients with active glomerulonephritis and/or chronic renal failure is similar to that of essential hypertension (Chap. 27). However, for chronic renal failure patients, the dosage schedule of drugs cleared by the kidney has to be modified to match renal function to avoid the deleterious effects of accumulated drug or metabolite. Dialysis should be considered in patients with a substantial reduction of renal function and hypertension refractory to medical management (Fig. 62–12). Early initiation of dialysis decreases the consequences of uremia, allows easier control of hypertension, and reduces the complications of chronic hypertension.

Bilateral nephrectomy is reserved for the severely hypertensive chronic renal failure patient whose hypertension is refractory to aggressive hemodialysis and optimal drug therapy. The results of nephrectomy are best in patients with markedly elevated plasma renin activity. The major, but correctable, disadvantages of nephrectomy are a further drop in the hemoglobin and hematocrit (reduced erythropoietin) and exacerbation of renal osteodystrophy (depressed generation of certain forms of vitamin D). The availability of potent oral antihypertensive agents, such as central sympatholytic drugs (e.g., clonidine), high-dose angiotensin-converting enzyme inhibitors, and minoxidil, has now made bilateral nephrectomy an uncommon procedure in chronic renal failure.

The management of systemic hypertension is often complicated by concomitant drug therapy; this is particularly relevant to the post-transplant patient.[19,124] Corticosteroids adversely affect hypertension control by increasing blood volume and insulin resistance and blunting responsiveness to antihypertensive drugs. Cyclosporine commonly provokes or exacerbates systemic hypertension, occasionally to extremely high levels of blood pressure; calcium channel blocking drugs are usually effective in controlling cyclosporine-induced hypertension. A marked and often refractory increase in systemic blood pressure and occasionally renal interstitial disease can follow the administration of nonsteroidal antiinflammatory agents.

Because spontaneous improvement of systemic hypertension in post-transplant patients with obstructing renal artery lesions (usually at the site of vascular anastomosis) is not uncommon, conservative management is generally recommended of the transplantation patient with stable, adequate renal function whose hypertension is amenable to medications. When stenosis-induced hypertension becomes difficult to control or renal function falls, percutaneous transluminal angioplasty of the arterial lesion becomes a therapeutic option. Surgical intervention may become necessary if angioplasty is not feasible or is unsuccessful. Effective treatment of post-transplant hypertension is very important for the long-term health and survival of both graft and patient.[123]

CARDIAC ARRHYTHMIAS

Cardiac arrhythmias constitute a major clinical problem in chronic renal failure because of their increased prevalence and potentially serious complications; their episodic nature also makes identification and characterization difficult. A multicenter study of longstanding hemodialyzed pa-

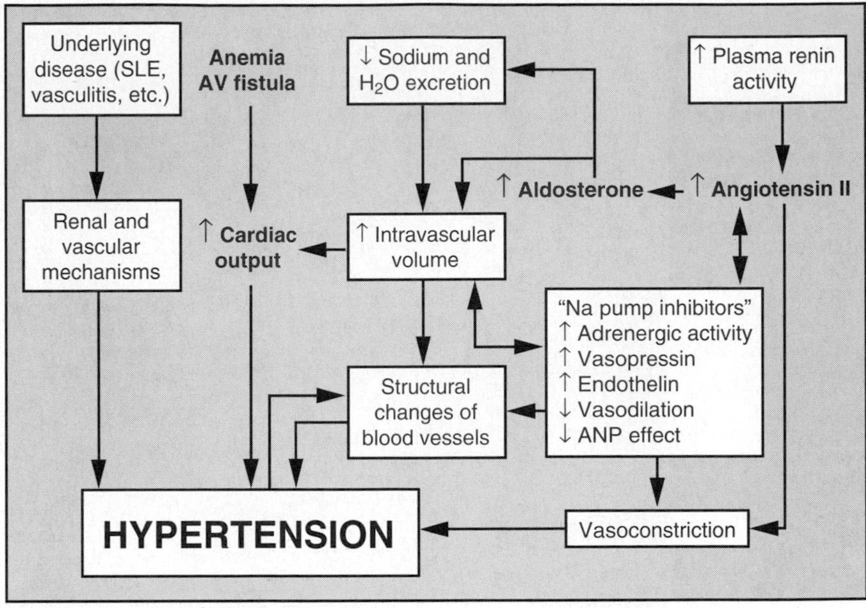

FIGURE 62–11. Pathophysiological mechanisms contributing to the development of systemic hypertension in patients with parenchymal renal disease and failure. ANF = atrial natriuretic peptide, SLE = systemic lupus erythematosus. (Modified from Leier, C. V., and Boudoulas, H.: Cardiorenal Disorders and Diseases. Armonk, N.Y., Futura Publishing Co., 1992.)

tients showed that ventricular arrhythmias, as assessed by 48-hour ambulatory monitoring, were present in 76 per cent of patients[125]; 39 per cent had two or more events of two or more sequential ventricular ectopic beats (i.e., couplets or nonsustained ventricular tachycardia) per hour. The frequency of ventricular arrhythmias rose significantly after the second hour of hemodialysis and lasted up to 5 hours following dialysis. The independent risk factors for the presence of ventricular arrhythmias were age over 55 years and LV dysfunction. The frequency of ventricular ectopic beats also appeared to vary directly with resting heart rate. 69 per cent of the CRF patients undergoing long-term dialysis had supraventricular arrhythmias, mostly nonsustained. Table 62–6 lists the major factors in chronic renal failure likely to contribute to the development of cardiac arrhythmias.

MANAGEMENT. While a detailed discussion of arrhythmia management is not within the scope of this chapter, a few general principles are important in managing these patients. As in other patients, the initial approach is directed at treating remedial cardiac disease and at reversing contributory factors (Table 62–6). Caffeine and other cardiac stimulants should be avoided by CRF patients with tachyarrhythmias. If arrhythmias are related to hemodialysis, attention should be directed to the potassium concentration of the dialysis bath. A low potassium concentration of the dialysate can lead to hypokalemia and serious rhythm disturbances, particularly in patients who are receiving digitalis or are afflicted with CAD, LV hypertrophy, or LV dysfunction. A dialysate potassium concentration of 3.5 mEq/liter usually abolishes dialysis-related ventricular arrhythmias. If the dialysate potassium concentration exceeds 3.5 mEq/liter, dietary potassium restriction is usually necessary between hemodialysis runs to prevent life-threatening hyperkalemia. Arrhythmias secondary to pericarditis tend to respond to treatment of the inflammatory component, when present.

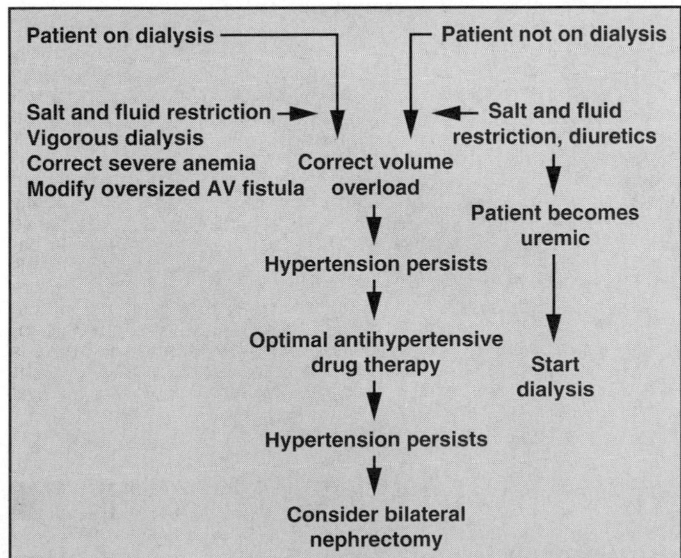

FIGURE 62–12. General management of arterial hypertension caused by renal parenchymal disease. AV = arteriovenous. (Modified from Leier, C. V., and Boudoulas, H.: Cardiorenal Disorders and Diseases. Armonk, N.Y., Futura Publishing Co., 1992.)

PREDISPOSITION FOR CARDIOVASCULAR INFECTIONS

Infections are common in patients with end-stage renal disease. Because these patients undergo dialysis 100 to 180 times a year, it is not surprising that infections often involve the AV access site or the abdominal catheter in patients receiving peritoneal dialysis. It is estimated that up to 6 per cent of hemodialysis patients will develop infective endocarditis sometime during the course of their disease; the most common culprit organism is *Staphylococcus aureus*, followed by *Streptococcus viridans* and enterococci; the aortic valve is the usual target followed by the mitral valve.[19]

Proper sterile technique during the entire dialysis procedure is mandatory to prevent infectious disease in this very susceptible patient population. Patients should maintain good oral health and personal hygiene to reduce other potential sources for bacteremia and infective endocarditis. Skin flora of the dialysis patient and the dialysis staff should be controlled with bactericidal soap. The staff (via nasal discharge, skin, and other sites) is not an uncommon source for culprit organisms.[126] Patients undergoing long-term hemodialysis who have prosthetic valves and those who have had renal transplantation should receive antibiotics prophylactically.

Recurrent or prolonged bacteremia and septicemia in chronic renal failure patients receiving dialysis implicates persistent infection of the access shunt or catheter or infective endocarditis. Appropriate antibiotic therapy, based on blood culture and antibiotic-sensitivity data, should be initiated as soon as possible in these patients. Surgi-

TABLE 62–6 FACTORS CONTRIBUTING TO DEVELOPMENT OF CARDIAC ARRHYTHMIAS IN PATIENTS WITH CHRONIC RENAL FAILURE

UNDERLYING CARDIAC DISEASE
Myocardial disease (left ventricular hypertrophy, left ventricular dysfunction)
Coronary artery disease—myocardial ischemia
Pericardial disease—myocardial inflammation
Cardiac calcification
HEMODIALYSIS
Rapid changes in serum electrolytes
Rapid changes in blood pH
Hypoxemia
HYPERADRENERGIC STATE
HIGH CALCIUM X PHOSPHORUS PRODUCT
HIGH PARATHORMONE LEVELS(?)

From Leier, C. V., and Boudoulas, H.: Cardiovascular Disorders and Diseases. Armonk, N. Y., Futura Publishing Co., 1992, with permission.

Text continues on page 1935

TABLE 62–7 CARDIOVASCULAR DRUG THERAPY IN RENAL FAILURE

DRUG	THERAPEUTIC RANGE/ml (PLASMA LEVELS)	ELIMINATION AND METABOLISM	HALF-LIFE—hr		PROTEIN BINDING %		ADJUSTMENT FOR RENAL FAILURE	REMOVAL BY DIALYSIS	COMMENTS
			Normal	Renal Failure	Normal	Renal Failure			
CARDIAC GLYCOSIDES									
Digoxin	0.8–2.0 ng	75% Renal	45	72–96	25	18	Yes	No	Radioimmunoassay may overestimate serum levels in renal failure
Digitoxin	20–35 ng	95% Hepatic	145	Unchanged	90–97	86–97	Decrease dose when creatinine clearance < 10 ml/min	No	8% converted to digoxin; protein binding decreases slightly by dialysis
ANTIARRHYTHMIC AGENTS									
Procainamide	4.0–10.0 μg	50% Renal 50% Hepatic	3–4	11–20	15–20	Unchanged	Yes	Yes, hemodialysis	Some patients require higher plasma concentrations (10–25 μg/ml)
N-Acetylprocainamide	10–20 μg	Renal	6–8	35–70	10	Unchanged	Yes	Yes, hemodialysis	Active metabolite of procainamide
Quinidine	2.0–5.0 μg	85% Hepatic 15% Renal	6	5–14	80–85	↑	No	Yes, hemodialysis	May increase serum digoxin levels
Disopyramide	0.5–2.0 μg	60% Renal 40% Hepatic	5–7	10–18	40–90	—	Yes	Yes, hemodialysis	Protein binding concentration dependent
Lidocaine	1.5–5.0 μg	90% Hepatic	1.2–2.2	1.3–3	60–66	Unchanged	No	No	Protein binding may be concentration dependent
Tocainide	4–10 μg	40% Renal	15	—	10	—	Yes	—	—
Mexiletine	2–7 μg	Hepatic Renal	7–11	↑	57–69	—	Yes	—	—
Phenytoin	10.0–18.0 μg	Hepatic	24	May be shorter	90–95	70–85	No	No	Protein binding in renal failure decreased
Encainide	250 μg	Hepatic (93% population)	2.3	—	60–80	—	No	—	—
		Hepatic-Renal (7% population)	11.3	—	70–80	—	Yes	—	—
a. O-desmethylencainide	30 μg	Hepatic (90%) Renal	3.5	—	—	—	Yes	—	—
b. 3-Methoxy-O-desmethylencainide	100 ng	Hepatic Renal	6.4	—	—	—	Yes	—	—
Flecainide	0.4–0.8 μg	Hepatic Renal (40%)	8–14	↑	50–70	—	Yes	—	—
Propafenone	—	Hepatic	2–10	—	85–87	—	—	—	—
Moricizine	—	Hepatic	—	—	85	—	Yes	—	—
Amiodarone	0.5–3.0 μg	Hepatic	53 days	—	> 95	—	—	—	—
Bretylium	—	80% Renal 20% Nonrenal	6.0	13.6	—	—	Yes	—	Avoid when creatinine clearance < 10 ml/min

TABLE 62–7 CARDIOVASCULAR DRUG THERAPY IN RENAL FAILURE *(continued)*

DRUG	THERAPEUTIC RANGE/ml (PLASMA LEVELS)	ELIMINATION AND METABOLISM	HALF-LIFE—hr		PROTEIN BINDING %		ADJUSTMENT FOR RENAL FAILURE	REMOVAL BY DIALYSIS	COMMENTS
			Normal	Renal Failure	Normal	Renal Failure			
BETA-ADRENERGIC BLOCKERS									
Acebutolol	—	Hepatic	8	22	15–20	—	No	Yes, hemodialysis	Accumulation of active metabolite diacetolol
Alprenolol	—	Hepatic	1–3	2–3	85	—	No	—	—
Atenolol	—	Renal	6–9	15–35	<5	—	Yes	Yes, hemodialysis	Significant accumulation in renal failure
Metoprolol	—	Hepatic	2.5	4.5	12	—	No	Yes, hemodialysis	
Nadolol	—	Renal	14–24	45	25–30	—	Yes	Yes, hemodialysis	Significant accumulation in renal failure
Oxprenolol	—	Hepatic	2–3	2–3	80	—	No	—	—
Pindolol	—	Hepatic Renal	3–4	3–4	40–55	—	No	—	—
Propranolol	—	Hepatic	2–4	2–4	90–95	—	No	Yes, hemodialysis	Active metabolites may accumulate
Sotalol	—	Renal (60%) Hepatic	8	15–50	50	—	Yes	Yes, hemodialysis	—
Timolol	—	Hepatic	4–6	4–6	10	—	No	Yes, hemodialysis	—
Esmolol	—	Hepatic	.06–2	—	55	—	No	—	For IV use only
Labetolol	—	Mostly hepatic	6–8	—	50	—	—	No	—
Carteolol	—	60–70% Renal	6	—	23–30	—	Yes	—	—
Penbutolol	—	Hepatic	5	5	80–98	—	—	—	—
Betaxolol	—	Primarily hepatic, renal	14–22	30–40	50	—	Yes	Small amount	—
CALCIUM CHANNEL BLOCKERS									
Verapamil	—	Hepatic	3	?7	90	≈ 90	No	Yes	—
Diltiazem	—	Hepatic	2	?8	83	—	No	—	—
Nifedipine	—	Hepatic	4	?5.5	95	—	No	—	—
Nicardipine	—	Hepatic	1–1.6	—	89–99	—	No	—	—
Nimodipine	—	Hepatic	8–9	—	95; binding concentration dependent	—	No	—	—
Bepridil hydrochloride	—	Liver 70%; urine excretion of metabolites	Early 2 Terminal 26–64	—	99	—	—	—	Type 1A antiarrhythmic properties
Isradipine	—	Hepatic	Early 1.5–2 Terminal 8	—	95	—	—	—	—
Felodipine	—	Hepatic	11–16	—	>99	—	No	—	—

TABLE 62–7 CARDIOVASCULAR DRUG THERAPY IN RENAL FAILURE *(continued)*

DRUG	THERAPEUTIC RANGE/ml (PLASMA LEVELS)	ELIMINATION AND METABOLISM	HALF-LIFE—hr		PROTEIN BINDING %		ADJUSTMENT FOR RENAL FAILURE	REMOVAL BY DIALYSIS	COMMENTS
			Normal	Renal Failure	Normal	Renal Failure			
ANTIHYPERTENSIVES									
Methyldopa	—	Mostly renal	5–8	7–16	<15	—	May be necessary when creatinine clearance <50 ml/min	Yes, peritoneal and hemodialysis	Retention of active metabolites in renal failure
Clonidine	—	Renal	6–23	39–42	20–40	—	Yes, when creatinine clearance <10 ml/min	No	Rebound hypertension can occur if drug stopped abruptly
Guanfacine	—	Hepatic Renal	12–24	—	—	—	—	—	Withdrawal syndrome may appear
Guanabenz	—	Hepatic	4–6	—	—	—	—	—	—
Trimethaphan	—	—	—	—	—	—	—	—	Ganglionic blocking drug for IV use with short duration of action
Mecamylamine	—	Renal	—	—	—	—	Contraindicated in uremic patients	—	—
Guanethidine	—	Mostly renal, less nonrenal	48–72	96–196	0	—	Yes	—	Orthostatic hypotension common side effect
Reserpine	—	Hepatic, nonrenal	50–170	87–320	40	—	Avoid when creatinine clearance <10 ml/min	No	Long biologic half-life
Minoxidil	—	Hepatic	2.8–4.2	—	0	—	No	Yes, hemodialysis	May induce pericardial effusion and pericarditis
Hydralazine	—	Hepatic, nonrenal	2.5–5	7–16	87	—	May be necessary when creatinine clearance <50 ml/min	No	—
Diazoxide	—	Mostly renal	17–31	>30	>90	Decreased	No	Yes, peritoneal dialysis, hemodialysis	May produce sodium and water retention and hyperglycemia; protein binding decreased in renal failure
Prazosin	—	Mostly hepatic, some renal	2–3	—	97	—	No	No	—
Doxazosin	—	Liver	22	—	98	—	—	Yes	—
Terazosin	—	10% Urine	12	—	90–94	—	—	—	—
Nitroglycerin (sublingual)	—	Hepatic	2–4 (min)	2–4 (min)	—	—	No	—	—
Isosorbide-2-mononitrate	—	Hepatic	1.5–2.4		—	—	Yes	—	—
Isosorbide-5-mononitrate	—	Hepatic	4.0–5.0		—	—	—	—	—
Nitroprusside	—	Nonrenal	<10 min.	<10 min.	—	—	No	Hemodialysis	Thiocyanate and cyanide may accumulate

TABLE 62–7 CARDIOVASCULAR DRUG THERAPY IN RENAL FAILURE *(continued)*

DRUG	THERAPEUTIC RANGE/ml (PLASMA LEVELS)	ELIMINATION AND METABOLISM	HALF-LIFE—hr		PROTEIN BINDING %		ADJUSTMENT FOR RENAL FAILURE	REMOVAL BY DIALYSIS	COMMENTS
			Normal	Renal Failure	Normal	Renal Failure			
CONVERTING ENZYME INHIBITORS									
Captopril	—	Mostly renal, some hepatic	1.9	Prolonged	25–30	—	May be necessary when creatinine clearance < 10 ml/min	Yes, hemodialysis	Deterioration of renal function in patients with bilateral renal artery stenosis
Enalapril	—	Mostly renal	11	—	—	—	When creatinine clearance < 30 ml/min	—	Deterioration of renal function in patients with bilateral renal artery stenosis
Lisinopril	—	Renal	12	—	—	—	When creatinine clearance < 30 ml/min	—	—
Enalaprilat	—	Renal	11	—	—	—	When creatinine clearance < 30 ml/min	Yes	For IV injection
Benazepril	—	—	10–11	96.7	—	—	When plasma creatinine > 3 mg/dl	—	—
Fosinopril sodium	—	50% Urine	12	≥95	—	—	No	—	—
Ramipril	—	60% Urine	13–17	—	—	—	When plasma creatinine > 2.5 mg/dl	—	—
DIURETICS									
Thiazides	—	Renal	1–2	4–6	70	—	Yes	—	May be ineffective when creatinine clearance < 30 ml/min
Metolazone	—	—	—	—	—	—	—	—	Can produce marked diuresis
Furosemide	—	Mostly renal	1	3	95	—	—	Yes, hemodialysis	Large doses necessary in renal failure
Ethacrynic acid	—	Renal, hepatic	3	—	90	—	Yes	Yes, hemodialysis	Large doses necessary in renal failure
Bumetanide	—	Renal, hepatic	1	—	90	—	No	—	Can be effective in patients with renal failure
Acetazolamide	—	Renal	8	Prolonged	80	—	Yes	—	Ineffective when GFR < 10 ml/min
Amiloride	—	Renal	7.5	Prolonged	Low	—	Yes	—	May cause hyperkalemia
Triamterene	—	Hepatic, renal	2–12	10	60	Decreased	Yes, avoid when creatinine clearance < 30 ml/min	—	Active metabolites have long half-life; may cause hyperkalemia
Spironolactone	—	Hepatic	10–35	10–35	98	—	Yes, avoid when creatinine clearance < 30 ml/min	—	May cause hyperkalemia
Indapamide	—	Mostly renal, some hepatic	14	—	71–79	—	—	—	Oral antihypertensive-diuretic; has little or no diuretic effect in renal failure
ANTICOAGULANTS									
Heparin	—	Nonrenal	0.3–2.0	0.5–3.0	> 90	—	No	Yes, hemodialysis and peritoneal dialysis	May potentiate uremic bleeding
Warfarin	—	Hepatic	40	40	99	Decreased	No	—	May decrease protein binding of other drugs; may potentiate uremic bleeding

TABLE 62–7 CARDIOVASCULAR DRUG THERAPY IN RENAL FAILURE *(continued)*

DRUG	THERAPEUTIC RANGE/ml (PLASMA LEVELS)	ELIMINATION AND METABOLISM	HALF-LIFE—hr		PROTEIN BINDING %		ADJUSTMENT FOR RENAL FAILURE	REMOVAL BY DIALYSIS	COMMENTS
			Normal	Renal Failure	Normal	Renal Failure			
THROMBOLYTICS									
Streptokinase	—	—	0.38	—	—	—	No	—	May potentiate uremic bleeding
Anistreplase	—	—	1–2	—	—	—	—	—	May potentiate uremic bleeding
Urokinase	—	Hepatic	0.33	—	—	—	—	—	May potentiate uremic bleeding
Tissue plasminogen activators (t-PA)	—	Hepatic	0.05	—	—	—	—	—	May potentiate uremic bleeding
LIPID-LOWERING AGENTS									
Cholestyramine	—	Not absorbed	—	—	—	—	No	—	May cause hyperchloremic acidosis
Colestipol	—	Not absorbed	—	—	—	—	No	—	May cause hyperchloremic acidosis
Clofibrate	—	Renal (40–60%), hepatic	17	46–110	96	—	Yes	Hemodialysis	Restricted use because of high profile of adverse effects
Gemfibrozil	—	Renal, fecal	1.5	—	Low	—	Yes	—	
Nicotinic acid	—	Hepatic, renal	0.5–1.0	—	—	—	Yes	—	Frequent adverse effects in patients with renal failure; aspirin may reduce flushing
Lovastatin	—	Hepatic Renal	—	—	95	—	—	—	—
Probucol	—	Hepatic	—	—	—	—	—	—	—

Modified from Leier, C. V., and Boudoulas, H.: Cardiovascular Disorders and Diseases. Armonk, N. Y., Futura Publishing Co., 1992, with permission.

cal consultation is indicated when access shunts show abscess or aneurysm formation, thrombosis, or bleeding. Clinical recognition of infective endocarditis in the setting of chronic renal failure is often difficult, because many features (e.g., recurrent bacteremia, anemia, and encephalopathy) can occur in patients with end-stage renal failure without infective endocarditis. It is prudent to suspect infective endocarditis in any such patient with fever, leukocytosis, or bacteremia, particularly if associated with an infected access site. The appearance of new murmurs or changes in murmurs increases the likelihood of infective endocarditis. Demonstration of valvular vegetations by echocardiography is most informative and can be diagnostic in the presence of other clinical manifestations of infective endocarditis.

AUTONOMIC DYSFUNCTION

Derangements of the autonomic nervous system in chronic renal failure, most commonly manifested as postural or dialysis-induced hypotension, abnormal hemodynamic responses to Valsalva and other maneuvers, impairment of perspiration, and alterations in gastric motility, can evoke major symptoms and disability. The cause of autonomic dysfunction in these patients is multifactorial and attributable in some cases to the underlying cause of chronic renal failure (e.g., diabetic mellitus, amyloidosis), antihypertensive drugs (e.g., sympatholytic agents), aluminum intoxication from certain antacids, and the uremic syndrome itself.[127-129] Determination of the specific type of autonomic dysfunction can be difficult and may require additional diagnostic testing (e.g., nerve conduction, bladder and sphincter function, tilt studies). Informative yet simple and inexpensive clinical maneuvers include blood pressure and heart rate responses to upright posture or the Valsalva maneuver and heart rate response to normal and deep inspiration.[127] In general, specific therapy for the autonomic dysfunction of renal disease is rather limited, and symptomatic therapy is employed in most instances.

CARDIOVASCULAR DRUG THERAPY IN PATIENTS WITH RENAL DISEASE

Patients with renal failure are often treated with drugs primarily cleared or metabolized by the kidneys. In comparison to patients with normal renal function, any dose or dosage schedule of such agents in patients with renal failure usually produces higher plasma concentrations for longer duration. In addition, patients with renal failure can react unpredictably and atypically to pharmacological agents; thus, the adverse effects of a drug in this clinical setting are often related to factors other than plasma drug concentration. For example, nausea and vomiting after ingestion of certain agents (e.g., analgesics, potassium elixirs) occur more frequently in chronic renal failure patients because of preexisting chronic inflammation of the gastrointestinal mucosa, and the adverse effects of digitalis and antiarrhythmic agents are exacerbated by abnormalities in serum potassium, magnesium, and calcium; hypoxemia; and the hyperadrenergic state of renal disease and dialysis. Side effects of a drug must always be considered when a chronic renal failure patient experiences unexpected or unusual symptoms.

Renal failure often modifies the pharmacokinetics and pharmacodynamics of a drug[19,130-133]; many of these variations, however, are not directly linked to the simple reduction in renal function and GFR. The pharmacokinetic-pharmacodynamic modifications of chronic renal failure are also related to greater variability in drug absorption, protein binding, metabolism, and receptor affinity, sensitivity, and responsiveness. Lower protein binding for many agents is related to hypoproteinemia or hypoalbuminemia, an alteration of the protein molecule, or competition for protein-binding sites by endogenous substances and other types of CRF therapy. Nonesterified fatty acids, increased in chronic renal failure and with heparin administration, can displace certain drugs from their binding sites. Anemia with reduced red cell binding increases the plasma concentration of certain drugs. Patients with renal failure are commonly treated with several agents; drug-drug interactions can affect gastrointestinal absorption, protein binding, tissue distribution, drug metabolism and clearance, and pharmacodynamic properties.

For drugs cleared by the kidney, dosing is adjusted for renal function. Three dosing modifications can be employed: the dosing interval can be lengthened without altering the dose amount, the dose amount can be lowered without changing the dosing schedule, or a combination of both. The second approach is preferable in most patients because it averts wide swings in plasma drug concentration. Precise adjustment of dosing is usually not necessary for drugs with few adverse effects and a large therapeutic index (safety margin). Pharmacokinetic and dose-adjustment information for the use of the more commonly employed cardiovascular drugs in renal disease is presented in Table 62–7. In most instances, the application and monitoring of drug therapy in chronic renal failure is based on pharmacodynamic and clinical responses, occasionally supplemented by determination of the drug's plasma concentration (e.g., digitalis) or another laboratory endpoint (e.g., prothrombin time for warfarin).

The therapeutic objectives are fairly well defined for most cardiovascular drugs. For example, for drugs used to control systemic hypertension or edema, the therapeutic endpoints are clear (decrease arterial pressure, reduce edema) and are best followed by clinical observations (blood pressure, physical examination, body weight) for proper drug and dose selection. Angiotensin-converting enzyme inhibitors, most vasodilators, and calcium channel blockers have reasonably well defined clinical endpoints (e.g., decrease arterial pressure, reduce pulmonary congestion, improve symptoms of heart failure, control angina pectoris). The therapeutic objectives of beta-adrenergic blocking drugs can be followed clinically in most patients (e.g., reduce arterial pressure, myocardial ischemia, and angina; control cardiac rhythms). For digitalis and antiarrhythmic drugs the clinical endpoints are more elusive and are threatened by potentially serious adverse effects; determination of plasma drug concentrations for such agents often becomes an important component of optimally effective, safe dosing.

CARDIOVASCULAR COMPLICATIONS DURING DIALYSIS

SYSTEMIC HYPOTENSION. Removal of fluid volume, redistribution of plasma volume, baroreceptor disturbances, dysfunction of the autonomic nervous system, depressed responsiveness to alpha-adrenergic receptor stimulation, concomitant drug therapy (e.g., antihypertensive agents), and LV diastolic dysfunction contribute to the propensity of the chronic renal failure patient to develop hypotension during hemodialysis. Interestingly, some renal disease patients with dialysis-induced hypotension have higher plasma concentrations of atrial natriuretic peptide and lower norepinephrine levels compared to chronic renal failure patients without hypotension.[134]

Symptomatic depletion of fluid volume during dialysis can be averted by allowing a modest amount of weight gain between dialysis treatments. When feasible, antihypertensive therapy and other potential hypotension-inducing drugs (e.g., nitrates) can be withheld 4 to 6 hours before dialysis to minimize their contribution to the problem. Of the antihypertensive agents, minoxidil is least likely to cause unpredictable changes in blood pressure during hemodialysis; however, drug-induced hirsutism and occasional pericarditis make this drug unacceptable to some patients, particularly females. Small doses of noncardioselective beta-adrenergic blocking drugs can be effective in maintaining acceptable arterial pressure; the $beta_1$- and $beta_2$-receptor blockade allows circulating norepinephrine to evoke unopposed alpha-adrenergic receptor stimulation and vasoconstriction. Either peritoneal dialysis or renal transplantation is the best option for chronic renal failure patients who poorly tolerate hemodialysis because of hypotension.

HYPOXEMIA. The mechanisms for hemodialysis-induced hypoxemia have not been definitively established; leading explanations include nonbicarbonate buffers (e.g., acetate) used in the dialysis bath, Cupraphane membranes, and pulmonic ventilation and perfusion mismatch elicited by systemic hypotension. Acetate buffer evokes a significant leftward shift in the hemoglobin-oxygen dissociation curve and can disturb ventilation/perfusion of the lungs through its vasodilatory properties. Activation of complement along Cupraphane exchange membranes can result in sequestration of leukocytes within pulmonary vessels, ventilation and perfusion abnormalities, and hy-

time with various pharmacologic agents. Implications for myocardial perfusion. Circulation *60:*164, 1979.
109. Kenny, A., Sutters, M., Evans, D. B., and Shapiro, L. M.: Effects of hemodialysis on coronary blood flow. Am. J. Cardiol. *74:*291, 1994.
110. Kremastinos, D., Paraskevaidis, I., Voudiklari, S., et al.: Painless myocardial ischemia in chronic hemodialysed patients: A real event? Nephron *60:*164, 1992.
111. Holley, J. L., Fenton, R. A., and Arthur, R. S.: Thallium stress testing does not predict cardiovascular risk in diabetic patients with end-stage renal disease undergoing cadaveric renal transplantation. Am. J. Med. *90:*563, 1991.
112. Reis, G., Marcovitz, P. A., Leichtman, A. B., et al.: Usefulness of dobutamine stress echocardiography in detecting coronary artery disease in end-stage renal disease. Am. J. Cardiol. *75:*707, 1995.
113. Soleman, R., Werner, C., Mann, D., et al.: Effects of saline, mannitol, and furosemide on acute decreases in renal function induced by radiocontrast agents. N. Engl. J. Med. *331:*1416, 1994.
114. Manske, C. L., Wang, Y., Rector, T., et al.: Coronary revascularization in insulin-dependent diabetic patients with chronic renal failure. Lancet *340:*998, 1992.
115. Reusser, L. M., Orebon, L. A., White, H. J., et al.: Increased morbidity after coronary angioplasty in patients on chronic hemodialysis. Am. J. Cardiol. *73:*965, 1994.
116. Thomas, M. E., Harris, K. P., Ramaswamy, C., Hattersley, J. M., Wheeler, D. C., Varghese, Z., Williams, J. D., Walls, J., and Moorhead, J. F.: Simvastatin therapy for hypercholesterolemic patients with nephrotic syndrome or significant proteinuria. Kidney Int. *44:*1124, 1993.
117. Ilson, B. E., Bland, P. S., Jorkasky, D. K., et al.: Intraoperative versus routine hemodialysis in end-stage renal disease patients undergoing open-heart surgery. Nephron *61:*170, 1992.
118. Adams, J. E., Abendschein, D. R., and Jaffe, A. S.: Biochemical markers of myocardial injury: Is MB creatinine kinase the choice for the 1990s? Circulation *88:*750, 1993.
119. Wade, M. R., Chen, Y. J., Soliman, M., et al.: Myocardial texture and cardiac calcification in uremia. Miner. Electrolyte Metab. *19:*21, 1993.
120. Sim, E. K., Mestres, C. A., Lee, C. N., and Adebo, O.: Mitral valve repair in patients on chronic hemodialysis. Ann. Thorac. Surg. *52:*341, 1992.
121. Straumann, E., Meyer, B., Misteli, M., et al.: Aortic and mitral valve disease in patients with end-stage renal failure on long-term haemodialysis. Br. Heart J. *67:*236, 1992.
122. Lucke, J. C., Samy, R. N., Atkins, Z., et al.: Results of valve replacement with mechanical versus biological prosthesis in patients on chronic renal dialysis. J. Am. Coll. Cardiol. *25*(Abs.):429, 1995.
123. Cosio, F. G., Dillon, J. J., Falkenhain, M. E., et al.: Racial differences in renal allograft survival: The role of systemic hypertension. Kidney Int. *47:*1136, 1995.
124. Carter, P. L.: Dosing of antihypertensive medications in patients with renal failure. J. Clin. Pharmacol. *35:*81, 1995.
125. Gruppo Hemodialisi E Pathologie Cardiovascolari: Multicenter, cross-sectional study of ventricular arrhythmias in chronically hemodialyzed patients. Lancet *2:*305, 1988.
126. Luzar, M. R., Coles, G. A., Faller, B., et al.: Staphylococcus aureus nasal carriage and infection in patients on continuous ambulatory peritoneal dialysis. N. Engl. J. Med. *322:*505, 1990.
127. Robertson, D., Hollister, A. S., Biaggioni, I., et al.: The diagnosis and treatment of baroreflex failure. N. Engl. J. Med. *329:*1449, 1993.
128. Converse, R. L., Jr., Jacobsen, T. N., Toto, R. D., et al.: Sympathetic overactivity in patients with chronic renal failure. N. Engl. J. Med. *327:*1912, 1992.
129. Crum, R., Fairchild, R., Bronsther, O., et al.: Neuroendocrinology of chronic renal failure and renal transplantation. Transplantation *52:*818, 1991.

CARDIOVASCULAR DRUG THERAPY IN RENAL FAILURE

130. Hoyer, J., Schulte, K. L., and Lentz, T.: Clinical pharmacokinetics of angiotensin converting enzyme (ACE) inhibitors in renal failure. Clin. Pharmacokinet. *24:*230, 1993.
131. Ujhelyi, M. R., Robert, S., Cummings, D. M., et al.: Influence of digoxin immune fab therapy and renal dysfunction on the disposition of total and free digoxin. Ann. Intern. Med. *119:*273, 1993.
132. Kovarik, J. M., Mueller, E. A., Gaber, M., et al.: Pharmacokinetics of cyclosporine and steady-state aspirin during coadministration. J. Clin. Pharmacol. *33:*513, 1993.
133. Talbert, R. L.: Drug dosing in renal insufficiency. J. Clin. Pharmacol. *34:*99, 1994.
134. Morrissey, E. C., Wilner, K. D., Barager, R. R., et al.: Atrial natriuretic factor in renal failure and posthemodialytic postural hypotension. Am. J. Kidney Dis. *12:*510, 1988.
135. Arnow, P., Bland, L. A., Garcia-Houchings, S., et al.: An outbreak of fatal fluoride intoxication in a long-term hemodialysis unit. Ann. Intern. Med. *121:*339, 1994.
136. Burhop, K. E., Johnson, R. J., Simpson, J., et al.: Biocompatibility of hemodialysis membranes: Evaluation in an ovine model. J. Lab. Clin. Med. *121:*276, 1993.
137. Verresen, L., Waer, M., Vanrenterghen, Y., and Michaelson, P.: Angiotensin converting enzyme inhibitors and anaphylactoid reaction to high-flux membrane dialysis. Lancet *2:*136, 1990.

Chapter 63
Practice Guidelines in Cardiovascular Medicine

THOMAS H. LEE

NONINVASIVE TESTS AND PROCEDURES . . 1940
Electrocardiography 1940
Exercise Testing 1940
Echocardiography 1942
Cardiac Radionuclide Imaging 1943
Ambulatory Electrocardiography 1946
In-hospital Cardiac Monitoring 1948
INVASIVE TESTS AND PROCEDURES 1949
Cardiac Catheterization and Coronary Angiography 1949
Percutaneous Transluminal Coronary Angioplasty 1954
Coronary Artery Bypass Graft Surgery 1957
Electrophysiological Procedures 1959
Pacemakers, Antiarrhythmia Devices and Implanted Automatic Defibrillators 1963
CLINICAL SYNDROMES 1967
Acute Chest Pain 1967
Acute Myocardial Infarction 1970
Unstable Angina 1979
Heart Failure 1985
Perioperative Cardiovascular Evaluation for Noncardiac Surgery 1989
PREVENTION OF CORONARY DISEASE 1990
Secondary Prevention of Coronary Artery Disease 1990
High Blood Cholesterol 1991
Hypertension 1991
REFERENCES 1993

In recent years, practice guidelines in cardiovascular medicine have become ubiquitous for a number of reasons, the most prominent of which is intense pressure for cost-containment. Health services research has demonstrated marked variability in the rate of performance of cardiovascular procedures among patient subsets, types of facilities, and regions.[1–10] Practice guidelines seek to standardize management around strategies likely to lead to high-quality, cost-effective care.[11]

Although this basic theme underlies most practice guidelines, there is considerable variability in their sources, specific goals, and methods of application. Agencies of the federal government such as the United States Agency for Health Care Policy and Research have convened multidisciplinary expert panels to develop practice guidelines for unstable angina[12] and congestive heart failure.[13] An extensive series of guidelines in cardiovascular medicine has been formulated by expert panels convened by the American College of Cardiology, the American Heart Association, and other professional societies. Insurance companies and for-profit companies have also developed guidelines aimed at assessing the appropriateness of hospital admissions and procedures as well as targeting lengths of stay. Additionally, as financial risk for health care is progressively transferred to the actual providers of health care, an increasing number of physicians and their organizations have developed their own guidelines and algorithms for the care of specific clinical syndromes.

These different types of guidelines often bear little resemblance to each other, in part because the organizations behind them have different goals. The guidelines that are the focus of this chapter seek to define *optimal care*—that is, management strategies that yield the best possible patient outcomes while reducing inappropriate and possibly harmful use of tests and therapies. These guidelines are evidence-based, that is, derived from analysis of published studies and emphasizing, when available, randomized trials. When data are not available, expert opinion is invoked.

Guidelines developed by task forces sponsored jointly by the American College of Cardiology and American Heart Association generally divide indications into three classes according to their appropriateness: Class I conditions are those for which there is general agreement that a test or procedure is useful. Class II conditions are those for which the test or procedure is often used, but for which there is disagreement as to its appropriateness. Class III indications are those for which there is general agreement that the test or procedure is inappropriate.

In many instances, the expert panels that developed and approved such guidelines have been exclusively or predominantly cardiovascular specialists. The guidelines are often highly detailed because of the perceived need to define most or all circumstances in which use of cardiovascular resources would be reasonable; as a result, such guidelines tend to err on the side of minimizing the percentage of cases for which care would be called "inappropriate."

In contrast, guidelines that have been developed or applied by payers do not seek to define the optimal management of patients with a syndrome. Instead, these guidelines are intended to serve as a *screening test* to detect patients for whom further evaluation should occur before planned procedures or other resources are used. When applied retrospectively to the medical records of patients who have already received cardiovascular services, these guidelines can be used to identify physicians whose practice patterns differ from those of their colleagues. For example, an appropriateness protocol for cardiac catheterization[14–16] could be used to identify physicians or hospitals with unusually low thresholds for performing this procedure.

Like any medical test, these "appropriateness protocols" have a sensitivity and a specificity and false-positive and -negative rates.[17] For example, when an appropriateness protocol for the use of a cardiac procedure is applied to a patient population, there will inevitably be some percentage of patients for whom a cardiac procedure is potentially beneficial but for whom the procedure will be categorized by the protocol as inappropriate. Similarly, there will be some patients for whom the procedure is actually inappropriate, yet it will be classified as appropriate by the protocol.

Just as physicians should weigh the sensitivity and specificity of a diagnostic test in interpreting its results, organizations that use appropriateness protocols as screening tests should consider their "performance characteristics" before adopting them. Extremely "tight" criteria for appropriateness—that is, guidelines that are highly sensitive for the detection of unnecessary resource use—reduce the chances that inappropriate procedures will be performed but have a high "false-positive" rate and therefore increase the percentage of cases that must be reviewed and discussed. On the other hand, "loose" criteria that identify only the most inappropriate use of resources are likely to allow approval of many referrals and procedures that are equivocal at best.

Yet another form of practice guideline is a *critical pathway,* also known by other names such as *clinical pathways* and *care maps.* These pathways attempt to define an optimal management strategy in detail, including time frames for specific outcomes and actions.[18] By achieving consensus around these plans, and collecting data on the frequency and causes of deviations from the pathways, critical pathways can help decrease length of stay and overall costs while improving quality of care by standardizing management.

Although practice guidelines are now extremely common in cardiovascular medicine, their impact has been highly variable.[19–22] In some cases, physicians disagree with the content of the guidelines,[23] suspect that they could be used against them in malpractice litigation,[24] or believe that these guidelines might compromise professional autonomy and satisfaction with medical practice.[25] Nevertheless, practice guidelines are likely to continue to proliferate, and a literature about the methods of their development is emerging.[26–28] They are used increasingly by payers and assessors of the quality of care.

This chapter summarizes the principal features of the guidelines for the use of important cardiovascular tests and procedures, as well as the management of major clinical syndromes. The series of practice guidelines jointly developed by the American College of Cardiology and American Heart Association are emphasized. For the complete guidelines, readers are referred to the original references, which are given in the text.*

* An up-to-date listing and copies of the American College of Cardiology/American Heart Association and other American College of Cardiology guidelines can be obtained by calling 800-247-4740 or by Internet (http://acc.org).

NONINVASIVE TESTS AND PROCEDURES

ELECTROCARDIOGRAPHY

(See Chap. 4)

Electrocardiograms are among the most commonly performed tests in medicine and are "the procedure of first choice" in the evaluation of chest pain, syncope, or dizziness.[29] Beyond diagnosis of cardiovascular conditions, electrocardiograms can be used to detect metabolic abnormalities, including side effects of some medications. Electrocardiograms also are frequently obtained to establish a "baseline" against which future tracings can be compared.

Guidelines published in 1992 by a task force of the American College of Cardiology and American Heart Association described conditions for which there is general agreement that electrocardiograms are useful (Class I), conditions for which opinion diverges with respect to their usefulness (Class II); and conditions for which general agreement exists that electrocardiograms are of little or no use (Class III). These guidelines addressed categories of patients defined by whether they had (1) known, (2) suspected, or (3) no evidence of cardiovascular disease. For each category of patients, the guidelines evaluated the use of the electrocardiogram as a baseline test, as a measure of response to therapy for follow-up, and before surgery.

PATIENTS WITH KNOWN CARDIOVASCULAR DISEASE OR DYSFUNCTION. The electrocardiogram is so crucial to the evaluation of all cardiovascular conditions that this test was considered appropriate (Class I) for all patients during the initial evaluation and to evaluate the short- and long-term responses to therapy known to produce electrocardiographic changes. The guidelines offer no specific recommendations about the frequency of follow-up electrocardiograms, but note that, for several acute cardiovascular problems, serial electrocardiograms are warranted until the patient has returned to a stable condition. Even in the absence of new symptoms or signs, ECGs are considered appropriate for follow-up of patients with several conditions, including syncope or near-syncope, chest pain, and unexplained fatigue. The electrocardiogram was not considered appropriate for patients with mild chronic cardiovascular conditions that were not considered likely to progress (e.g., mild mitral valve prolapse). Obtaining electrocardiograms at *each* visit was considered inappropriate for patients with stable heart disease who were seen frequently (e.g., within 4 months) and had no evidence of clinical change.

The ACC/AHA guidelines considered electrocardiograms appropriate before cardiac or noncardiac surgery, for all patients with known cardiovascular disease or dysfunction except those with significant or mild conditions such as mild systemic arterial hypertension.

PATIENTS WITH SUSPECTED OR AT HIGH RISK FOR DEVELOPING CARDIOVASCULAR DISEASE. The electrocardiogram was considered an appropriate baseline test for all patients with suspected cardiovascular conditions and those at high risk for developing such conditions. It was also considered an appropriate test after administration of any drug known to influence cardiac structure of function. Follow-up electrocardiograms more often than once per year were not recommended for patients who remained clinically stable, as long as they had not been previously demonstrated to have cardiac disease. However, for patients known to be at increased risk for the development of heart disease, electrocardiograms every 1 to 5 years were considered appropriate (Class I). Electrocardiograms were considered appropriate before cardiac or noncardiac surgery for all patients in this population.

PATIENTS WITHOUT KNOWN OR SUSPECTED HEART DISEASE. For patients without evidence suggesting cardiovascular disease, electrocardiograms were considered appropriate during the baseline evaluation in the ACC/AHA guidelines for those aged 40 or more years. The ACC/AHA guidelines also recommended electrocardiograms for patients for whom drugs with a high incidence of cardiovascular effects (e.g., chemotherapy) or exercise testing are planned, and for people of any age in occupations with high cardiovascular demands or whose cardiovascular status might affect the well-being of many other people (e.g., airline pilots).

These guidelines are similar to those of the U.S. Preventive Services Task Force,[30] which suggested electrocardiographic screening for persons at increased risk for coronary disease and for those with occupations in which their cardiovascular health might jeopardize the lives of others. The U.S. Preventive Services Task Force guidelines specifically state that electrocardiograms are not necessary for young adults who have no evidence of heart disease and are about to embark on an athletic program.

Different guidelines for the use of the baseline ECG have been offered by other organizations. A different expert panel commissioned by the American Heart Association recommended in 1987 that ECGs be obtained at ages 20, 40, and 60 years in persons with normal blood pressure,[31] while a task force assembled by the Canadian government has discouraged the use of *any* screening electrocardiograms.[32] The frequency of follow-up electrocardiograms in asymptomatic people without evidence of cardiovascular disease is not explicitly addressed in any guidelines.

The practice of obtaining electrocardiograms before any surgical procedure in patients of all ages does not draw support from any of the major guidelines. Before cardiac or noncardiac surgery, the ACC/AHA guidelines recommend electrocardiograms for all people aged 40 years or more,[29] and electrocardiograms are considered equivocal in appropriateness (Class II) for surgical patients aged 30 to 40 years. Guidelines issued from the American College of Physicians[33] recommend electrocardiograms preoperatively and upon hospital admission for men age 40 years or more and women age 50 years or more, as well as for all patients having elective intrathoracic, intraperitoneal, or aortic surgery; elective major neurosurgery; or emergency operations under general or regional anesthesia.

EXERCISE TESTING

(See Chap. 5)

Exercise testing is performed for several reasons, including to diagnose coronary artery disease, to assess prognosis, to determine functional capacity, and to evaluate the effects of therapy. Exercise electrocardiography is safe and inexpensive compared with invasive technology for diagnosis of coronary disease. However, the interpretation of exercise electrocardiography results and subsequent management is often variable, and "false-positive" exercise tests can lead to coronary angiography and even revascularization procedures in patients who have a low risk for complications of ischemic heart disease. Therefore, managed care organizations have sought to ensure the appropriateness of use of exercise tests. At least some health maintenance organizations have experimented with a strategy in which only cardiologists are allowed to order exercise tests and other noninvasive cardiology tests. A more common trend is the use of guidelines for the appropriateness of exercise tests.

One of the first sets of guidelines developed by ACC/AHA task forces focused on exercise testing and was published in 1986.[34] These guidelines rate the appropriateness of this test in various patient subsets according to three levels of appropriateness (Table 63–1), including condi-

TABLE 63–1 ACC/AHA GUIDELINES FOR EXERCISE TESTING

	CLASS I (APPROPRIATE)	CLASS II (POSSIBLY APPROPRIATE)	CLASS III (INAPPROPRIATE)
Patients with symptoms or signs suggestive of coronary artery disease or with known coronary artery disease	**1.** To assist in the diagnosis of coronary disease in male patients with symptoms that are atypical for myocardial ischemia. **2.** To assess functional capacity and to aid in assessing the prognosis of patients with known coronary disease. **3.** To evaluate patients with symptoms consistent with recurrent, exercise-induced cardiac arrhythmias.	**1.** To assist in the diagnosis of coronary disease in women with a history of typical or atypical angina pectoris. **2.** To assist in the diagnosis of coronary disease in patients taking digitalis. **3.** To assist in the diagnosis of coronary disease in patients with complete right bundle branch block. **4.** To evaluate the functional capacity and response to therapy with cardiovascular drugs in patients with coronary disease or heart failure. **5.** To evaluate patients with variant angina. **6.** To follow serially (at 1 year or longer intervals) patients with known coronary disease.	**1.** To evaluate patients with simpler premature ventricular depolarizations on the resting ECG but no other evidence of coronary disease. **2.** To evaluate functional capacity serially in the course of an exercise cardiac rehabilitation program. **3.** To assist in the diagnosis of coronary artery disease in patients who demonstrate preexcitation (Wolff-Parkinson-White) syndrome or complete left bundle branch block on the resting ECG.
Screening apparently healthy individuals	None	**1.** To evaluate asymptomatic male patients over age 40 in special occupations (pilots, firemen, police officers, bus or truck drivers, railroad engineers). **2.** To evaluate asymptomatic male patients over age 40 with two or more of the following increased risk factors for coronary artery disease: • serum cholesterol $>$ 240 mg/dl • blood pressure $\geq$ 160/ $\geq$ 90 • cigarette smoking • diabetes mellitus • family history of coronary disease with onset under the age of 55 years **3.** To evaluate male patients over age 40 who are sedentary and plan to enter a vigorous exercise program.	**1.** To evaluate asymptomatic, apparently healthy men or women with no risk factors for coronary artery disease. **2.** To evaluate men or women with a history of chest discomfort not thought to be of cardiac origin.
Patients with hypertension or cardiac pacemakers	None	To evaluate the blood pressure response of patients being treated for systemic arterial hypertension who wish to engage in vigorous dynamic or static exercise.	**1.** To evaluate patients with severe, uncontrolled systemic hypertension. **2.** To evaluate the blood pressure response to exercise in patients treated for hypertension who are not engaging in vigorous exercise. **3.** To evaluate pacemaker function in patients with cardiac pacemakers.

Class I: Conditions for which or patients for whom there is general agreement that exercise testing is useful.
Class II: Conditions for which or patients for whom exercise testing is frequently used but there is divergence of opinion with respect to its usefulness (possibly appropriate).
Class III: Conditions for which or patients for whom there is general agreement that exercise testing is of little or no usefulness.
From Schlant, R. C., Blomqvist, C. G., Brandenburg, R. O., et al.: Guidelines for exercise testing. A report of the American College of Cardiology/American Heart Association Task Force on Assessment of Cardiovascular Procedures (Subcommittee on Exercise Testing). Reprinted with permission from the American College of Cardiology. J. Am. Coll. Cardiol. *8*:725, 1986.

tions for which or patients for whom there is general agreement that exercise testing is useful (Class I), conditions for which or patients for whom exercise testing is frequently used but there is divergence of opinion with respect to its usefulness (Class II), and conditions for which or patients for whom there is general agreement that exercise testing is of little or no usefulness (Class III).

PATIENTS WITH KNOWN OR SUSPECTED CORONARY ARTERY DISEASE. The ACC/AHA guidelines for exercise testing reflect the lower positive predictive value for this test in women compared with men (see p. 169). According to the guidelines, exercise testing is appropriate (Class I) for assessment of male patients with symptoms atypical for myocardial ischemia, but of equivocal appropriateness (Class II) in women with a history of typical or atypical angina pectoris. Use of the exercise test is also of uncertain value (Class II) in other settings in which its diagnostic performance is less than ideal, such as in patients who take digitalis or who have right bundle branch block on their baseline electrocardiogram. It is considered an *inappropriate* test for the diagnosis of coronary disease in patients with preexcitation syndrome or complete left bundle branch block because of the difficulties of interpreting electrocardiographic changes.

The exercise test is considered valuable for assessment of prognosis for patients with coronary disease, and the guidelines indicate that repetition at approximately 1-year intervals is a reasonable if unproven (Class II) strategy. The use of exercise tests to evaluate the response to therapy with cardiovascular drugs is also considered a Class II indication. However, the ACC/AHA task force *discouraged* the use of serial exercise tests to assess functional capacity in the course of an exercise rehabilitation program.

APPARENTLY HEALTHY INDIVIDUALS. Because the specificity of the exercise test is about 90 per cent in apparently healthy individuals, the positive predictive value of an abnormal exercise test result is poor when it is applied to patients at low risk for coronary artery disease. Therefore, the ACC/AHA guidelines do not support the use of exercise testing in any setting to screen apparently healthy individuals or those with chest discomfort not thought to be of cardiac origin. However, the guidelines acknowledge that the test may have a role (Class II) in evaluation of asymptomatic patients with special occupations or of those over the age of 40 with two or more major risk factors for coronary artery disease. The exercise test is also considered to be of equivocal appropriateness for patients over age 40 who are sedentary and about to embark on a vigorous exercise program.

AFTER MYOCARDIAL INFARCTION (see p. 165). Exercise testing before hospital discharge for patients with acute myocardial infarction was still a relatively recent innovation when the ACC/AHA guidelines were published in 1986, and the guidelines refer to predischarge testing as occurring 10 to 14 days after uncomplicated infarction. Over a decade later, the average hospital length of stay for patients with uncomplicated myocardial infarctions is half that time at many hospitals, and predischarge exercise tests must therefore be performed on the fourth hospital day or even earlier. The ACC/AHA guidelines caution against performance of this test in patients who are unstable because of ischemia, left ventricular dysfunction, or arrhythmias. In these patients, whose clinical data indicate a high risk for complications, exercise testing frequently will not alter management. The task force indicated that the greatest contribution of postinfarction exercise testing was in patients with a low clinical risk for complications.

Performance of a limited exercise test before discharge from the hospital does not preclude the use of exercise testing several weeks later. The guidelines do not directly support the use of both predischarge and postdischarge exercise testing but note that predischarge exercise tests are often halted when a patient reaches a specified level of exertion (e.g., 5 METS). In contrast, a full, symptom-limited test performed a few weeks later presumably has greater sensitivity for detecting ischemic myocardium. The guidelines supported performance of symptom-limited tests 21 days or more after infarction. Patients whose exercise tests did not indicate ischemia at a workload of at least 7 METS after an uncomplicated acute myocardial infarction were considered generally capable of resuming their usual occupational tasks within the next 2 to 3 weeks. For patients whose occupations demand heavy physical effort, exercise testing 6 to 8 weeks after infarction was supported by the guidelines.

AFTER ANGIOPLASTY OR CARDIAC SURGERY. The ACC/AHA task force considered exercise testing appropriate for evaluation of coronary artery revascularization either by surgery or coronary angioplasty. These tests can be used to document that improvement has occurred and to serve as a baseline against which later tests can be compared. Full, symptom-limited exercise testing should usually be delayed for at least 3 months after surgery, so that chest and leg wounds do not cause pain during testing. Exercise testing can be performed with safety 2 to 5 days after angioplasty, according to these guidelines. Exercise testing at 3 and 6 months can be used to identify patients who have had restenosis.

PATIENTS WITH OTHER CONDITIONS. Exercise testing is not supported for routine use in patients with valvular heart disease, hypertension, or cardiac pacemakers. The ACC/AHA guidelines caution against use of exercise tests for patients with symptomatic critical aortic valve stenosis, hypertrophic obstructive cardiomyopathy, and uncontrolled hypertension, all of which are considered Class III indications because of the danger of complications during testing. An equivocal (Class II) indication for exercise testing is evaluation of functional capacity in patients with valvular heart disease, because serial exercise tests at 1- to 3-year intervals might demonstrate a decline in exertional capacity that is not detected through the patient history. Another Class II indication for exercise testing is assessment of blood pressure response with exertion in patients with hypertension who wish to engage in an exercise program.

ECHOCARDIOGRAPHY

(See also Chap. 3)

Echocardiography has evolved in many ways into an ideal testing technology: it is portable, provides information on cardiovascular structure and function, and, particularly when performed via the transthoracic approach, causes minimal discomfort and no risk to the patient. This test is regarded as so useful that guidelines published by an ACC/AHA task force in 1991[35] did not identify any disease states in which use of echocardiography was regarded as inappropriate except borderline hypertension without evidence of heart disease (Table 63–2). According to the guidelines, echocardiography is an appropriate test for patients with any valvular heart disease or other structural abnormalities, such as cardiac masses and possible primary myocardial diseases.

Echocardiography is not a test that should be performed for every patient, however, in part because of its personnel and equipment costs. Echocardiography and other noninvasive tests also prolong hospitalization when performed on patients with low risk for complications, therefore incurring additional costs beyond those of the test itself.[36] Furthermore, there are now various forms of echocardiography, including transesophageal and exercise echocardiography. These variations provide different types of information, although at higher costs and with additional risks and discomfort for the patient. There are few data on selection of cases in which these newer echocardiographic-based tests should be used instead of more traditional tests such as transthoracic echocardiography.

Another cause of difficulty in defining appropriate use of echocardiography is the lack of standardization in what strategies physicians pursue in response to echocardiographic data. There have been no randomized trials in which outcomes were compared in patients who did and did not undergo echocardiography. Nevertheless, guidelines for performance of this test are based on the assumption that echocardiography is likely to be used more appropriately under two conditions: (1) when physicians have a specific question to be answered by the test, and (2) if results from the test might alter management.

The ACC/AHA guidelines consider echocardiography to be the noninvasive technique of choice for several issues, including evaluation of valvular heart disease, detection of intracardiac thrombi, and detection of the cardiac effects of hypertension. For many questions, such as detection of ischemic heart disease, echocardiography must compete with other techniques, and the superiority of echocardiography has not been demonstrated.

EVALUATION OF SYMPTOMS. The appropriateness of echocardiography for diagnosis of the etiology of various symptom complexes is less clear than when echocardiography is used for evaluation of specific disease states. The ACC/AHA guidelines stress the importance of a careful history and physical examination and do not recommend echocardiography if, on the basis of that evaluation, the physician considers the probability of cardiac abnormalities to be low.

For example, echocardiographic abnormalities are often present in patients with *dyspnea* due to pulmonary disease, and the echocardiogram can provide important information in patients with dyspnea due to congestive heart failure, such as chamber sizes and myocardial and valvular function. However, dyspnea is a common symptom in patients without heart disease, and the ACC/AHA task force therefore concludes that this test is *not* recommended as an initial diagnostic study in patients with normal blood pressure and physical examinations.

For patients with *chest pain,* echocardiography can sometimes contribute to diagnosis and prediction of risk of future complications. The task force noted, however, that most patients with coronary artery disease have essentially normal findings on rest echocardiography; hence, echocardiography does little to exclude this diagnosis. At some medical centers, echocardiography is used for patients with acute chest pain as part of the emergency department or chest pain observation protocols.[37,38] However, because of the costs of this test, the logistic difficulties of providing echocardiography in the emergency department, and the high frequency of acute chest pain, this test is not part of routine care for patients with acute chest pain at most institutions.

Stress echocardiography is now in use at an increasing number of institutions; the stress used to induce ischemia can be exercise or pharmacological (see p. 86). The ACC/AHA guidelines note, however, that the addition of echocardiography substantially increases the cost of a routine stress test.

For patients with *heart murmurs,* routine clinical data are usually sufficient to determine its cause and significance. The ACC/AHA guidelines emphasize that patients with murmurs and a low probability of heart disease do not routinely require echocardiography. However, echocardiography can be an appropriate test when used in patients with probable organic heart disease and can provide information on coexisting abnormalities such as left ventricular dysfunction. In patients with a low probability of coronary artery disease, cardiac valve surgery can often be safely performed on the basis of data from the echocardiogram without prior cardiac catheterization (see section on cardiac catheterization).

Emboli originating in the heart are believed to account for 15 per cent of *cerebrovascular ischemic strokes*[39] (see p. 1878), and echocardiography is therefore an appropriate test for patients with cerebral embolism and clinical evidence of heart disease. Because of a lower likelihood of cerebrovascular atherosclerosis as a cause of ischemic stroke in younger patients, echocardiography is also considered an appropriate test in patients with a cerebrovascular event who are younger than age 45. In such patients, potential embolic sources include mitral valve prolapse or an intraatrial communication.

A major unresolved question is whether transesophageal echocardiography should be used instead of transthoracic echocardiography, because the transesophageal approach provides better images of the left atrium, left atrial appendage, and mitral valve. The optimal use of these testing techniques is uncertain and not addressed by the ACC/AHA guidelines. One algorithm has been proposed by DeRook et al., although it has not been formally tested.[40]

The ACC/AHA guidelines do not support routine use of echocardiography for all patients with *syncope* (Chap. 28). This test is considered appropriate (Class I) for patients with murmurs consistent with significant valvular heart disease or hypertrophic obstructive cardiomyopathy, but these are rare causes compared with vasodepressor reflexes or cardiac arrhythmias. Even rarer cardiac causes of syncope such as atrial myxoma may be detected with echocardiography (see p. 94), but these guidelines recommend that echocardiography should not be a "first-line" test for patients with syncope.

CARDIAC RADIONUCLIDE IMAGING

(See also Chap. 9)

Guidelines for the use of cardiac radionuclide imaging have been difficult to develop and apply for several reasons. As is true for most diagnostic tests, there have been no randomized trials comparing outcomes for patients who did and those who did not undergo nuclear cardiology tests, nor have there been large trials comparing these tests with competing techniques. Furthermore, there has been rapid evolution in radionuclide imaging techniques, which has increased both the number and the complexity of choices for clinicians.

These tests are considerably more expensive than treadmill exercise electrocardiography or echocardiography, however, and therefore interest in increasing the appropriateness of their use has intensified in recent years. An ACC/AHA task force initially published guidelines for cardiac radionuclide imaging in 1986[41]; because of developments, including pharmacological stress testing, new isotopes (technetium- and rubidium-based perfusion agents), and progress in single-photon emission computed tomography (SPECT) and positron emission tomography (PET), the ACC/AHA task force issued revised guidelines in 1995.[42] These guidelines are scheduled to be reviewed in 1997 and yearly thereafter—a reflection of the rate of change in this discipline.

As is true of most ACC/AHA guidelines, this task force designated some indications for cardiac radionuclide imaging as generally appropriate (Class I) and generally inappropriate (Class III). However, these guidelines subdivided the equivocal indications for nuclear cardiology tests into two groups: Class IIa (weight of evidence in favor of usefulness); and Class IIb (can be helpful but not well established by evidence).

TABLE 63–2 ACC/AHA GUIDELINES FOR ECHOCARDIOGRAPHY

SETTING	CLASS I (APPROPRIATE)	CLASS II (EQUIVOCAL)	CLASS III (INAPPROPRIATE)
Valvular heart disease	**1.** Native cardiac valve disease. **2.** Prosthetic cardiac valve disease. **3.** Suspected or proven infective endocarditis.	None	None
Ischemic heart disease	**1.** *Rest echocardiography:* Myocardial infarction when there is a specific question that can be resolved by echocardiography. **2.** *Stress echocardiography:* None	**1.** *Rest echocardiography:* Clinical evidence of coronary artery disease. **2.** *Stress echocardiography:* Whenever there is a high pretest probability that an indicated standard exercise stress test would be inadequate, nondiagnostic, or false-positive.	**1.** *Rest echocardiography:* Screening test for coronary disease in the general population. **2.** *Stress echocardiography:* Routine screening of the general population without significant coronary risk factors.
Disease of the heart muscle	**1.** Establishment of the morphological diagnosis and assessment of hemodynamic status of patients with cardiomyopathies. **2.** Systemic illness associated with cardiac involvement, with clinical symptoms. **3.** Exposure to cardiotoxic agents.	**1.** Systemic illness with high incidence of cardiac involvement but no clinical evidence of cardiac involvement. **2.** Clinical evidence suggesting cardiomyopathy. **3.** Family history of genetically transmitted cardiac disease.	Systemic illness with low incidence of cardiac involvement and no clinical evidence of cardiac involvement.
Pericardial disease	Patients with clinical manifestations of or suspected pericardial disease.	Follow-up studies	None
Cardiac masses	Evaluation of patients with suspected cardiac masses.	None	None
Diseases of the great vessels	**1.** Acute aortic root dilation or clinical suspicion of aortic dissection. **2.** First-degree relatives of patients with genetically transmitted connective tissue disorders.	**1.** Chronic aortic root dilation. **2.** Suspected connective tissue disorder in athletes. **3.** All other suspected disease of the great vessels.	None
Pulmonary disease	**1.** Unexplained pulmonary hypertension. **2.** Pulmonary emboli and suspected clots in the right atrium or ventricle.	**1.** Lung disease with clinical suspicion of cardiac involvement. **2.** Pulmonary emboli	None
Hypertension	Hypertension with clinical evidence of heart disease	Hypertension without signs or symptoms of heart disease.	Borderline hypertension without signs or symptoms of heart disease.

ACUTE MYOCARDIAL INFARCTION (see Chap. 37). The ACC/AHA guidelines indicate that nuclear cardiology tests have a limited role in the diagnosis of acute myocardial infarction, and should be used only when the history, electrocardiogram, and chemistry tests are less reliable. Technetium-99m pyrophosphate scanning is considered potentially useful (Class IIa) for patients who present more than 24 hours and less than 7 days after the onset of symptoms, and radionuclide angiography can be used to support the diagnosis of right ventricular infarction by demonstrating a reduced right ventricular ejection fraction and right ventricular asynergy. However, nuclear tests are considered inappropriate for routine use for diagnosis.

For evaluation of prognosis after acute myocardial infarction, stress myocardial perfusion imaging is considered appropriate (Class I) to assess whether more myocardium is in jeopardy (Table 63–3). The stress used to provoke ischemia can be physical exercise or pharmacological, although these guidelines noted that the safety of dipyridamole and adenosine testing that is performed 2 to 3 days after admission remains to be established. The guidelines do not address settings in which radionuclide imaging would be preferred over standard exercise electrocardiography.

Radionuclide angiography is considered useful for assessment of ventricular function after acute myocardial infarction and also can help detect aneurysms and mechanical complications such as an infarct-related ventricular septal defect. However, the ACC/AHA guidelines imply that, for assessment of mechanical complications, nuclear cardiology tests are second-choice techniques that should be used when echocardiography is not available or definitive.

UNSTABLE ANGINA (see Chap. 38). The ACC/AHA task force identified two principal issues for which radionuclide imaging techniques are potentially useful in patients with unstable angina: assessment of myocardial viability and prediction of future cardiac events in patients whose angina is successfully stabilized with medical therapy. Therefore, the two indications considered clearly appropriate (Class I) are use of stress myocardial perfusion imaging to detect ischemia and use of radionuclide angiography to assess baseline left ventricular function. Myocardial perfusion imaging is also considered potentially useful (Class IIa) for patients with ongoing ischemia who undergo imaging at rest. The use of rest myocardial perfusion imaging is considered less proven (Class IIb) in patients in whom the diagnosis of myocardial ischemia was uncertain after consideration of routinely available clinical data.

CHRONIC ISCHEMIC HEART DISEASE (see Chap. 38). The ACC/AHA guidelines considered exercise or pharmacological myocardial perfusion imaging to be appropriate (Class I) for identification of the extent and severity of ischemia and localization of ischemia in patients with chronic ischemic heart disease. The guidelines consider thallium-201 and technetium-99m to be sufficiently similar to be used interchangeably in this patient population.[43]

TABLE 63–2 ACC/AHA GUIDELINES FOR ECHOCARDIOGRAPHY—*Continued*

SETTING	CLASS I (APPROPRIATE)	CLASS II (EQUIVOCAL)	CLASS III (INAPPROPRIATE)
Dyspnea	None	**1.** Dyspnea with clinical evidence or suspicion of heart disease. **2.** Unexplained dyspnea.	**1.** Dyspnea without clinical evidence of heart disease, pulmonary hypertension or significant lung disease. **2.** Hyperventilation syndrome.
Chest pain	Chest pain with clinical evidence of valvular, pericardial or primary myocardial disease.	Known or suspected coronary artery disease.	Noncardiac chest pain
Murmurs	**1.** An organic murmur in a patient with cardiorespiratory symptoms. **2.** A murmur in an asymptomatic patient if the clinical features indicate at least a moderate probability that the murmur is organic.	A murmur in an asymptomatic patient in whom there is low probability of heart disease but in whom the diagnosis of heart disease cannot be reasonably excluded by standard cardiovascular clinical evaluation.	A typically innocent murmur in an asymptomatic patient without any other reason to suspect heart disease.
Neurological ischemic syndromes	**1.** Patients with cerebral embolism and clinical evidence of heart disease. **2.** Patients <45 with a cerebrovascular event.	Patients >45 with suspicion of cardiogenic brain embolism but without clinical evidence of heart disease.	Patients with known noncardiac causes of the neurological disorder.
Syncope	Patients with a murmur suggestive of significant valvular heart disease or obstructive cardiomyopathy.	Patients without clinical evidence of heart disease and normal findings on evaluation for noncardiac causes of syncope.	Patients with known noncardiac causes of syncope.
Evaluation of ventricular function	**1.** To evaluate global left ventricular function. **2.** To evaluate regional left ventricular function. **3.** Qualitative right ventricular function.	Diastolic left ventricular function	Quantitative right ventricular function (except in children).
Screening	Patients with a family history of cardiovascular disease that is clearly inheritable.	Competitive athletes	General population

Class I: Conditions for which or patients for whom there is general agreement that echocardiography is appropriate.
Class II: Conditions for which or patients for whom echocardiography is frequently used but there is a divergence of opinion with respect to its appropriateness.
Class III: Conditions for which or patients for whom there is general agreement that echocardiography is not appropriate.
From Ewy, G. A., Appleton, C. P., Demaria, A. N., et al.: ACC/AHA guidelines for the clinical application of echocardiography. A report of the American College of Cardiology/American Heart Association Task Force on Assessment of Diagnostic and Therapeutic Cardiovascular Procedures (Subcommittee to Develop Guidelines for the Clinical Application of Echocardiography). Reprinted with permission from the American College of Cardiology. J. Am. Coll. Cardiol. *16*:1505, 1990.

TABLE 63–3 INDICATIONS FOR USE OF EXERCISE OR PHARMACOLOGICAL MYOCARDIAL PERFUSION IMAGING

CLASS I (APPROPRIATE)

1. Prognostic stratification after acute myocardial infarction.
2. Identification of ischemia in patients with unstable angina.
3. Identification of extent and severity of ischemia in symptomatic patients and selected patients with asymptomatic myocardial ischemia.
4. Planning PTCA—identifying lesions causing myocardial ischemia if not otherwise known.
5. Risk stratification for selected patients before noncardiac surgery.
6. Assessment for restenosis after PTCA for symptomatic patients.
7. Assessment of ischemia in symptomatic patients after CABG.
8. Assessment of selected asymptomatic patients after PTCA or CABG, such as patients with an abnormal electrocardiographic response to exercise or those with rest electrocardiographic changes precluding identification of ischemia during exercise.

CLASS IIA

1. Identification of severity/extent of disease in patients whose angina is satisfactorily stabilized with medical therapy.
2. Diagnosis of anomalies of coronary circulation in adults with congenital heart disease.
3. Detection and assessment of functional significance of concomitant coronary artery disease in valvular heart disease patients.

CLASS IIB

1. Assessment of drug therapy upon myocardial perfusion.
2. Assessment of coronary arteriopathy after cardiac transplantation.

CLASS III (INAPPROPRIATE)

1. Screening of asymptomatic patients with low likelihood of ischemic heart disease.

From Guidelines for Clinical Use of Cardiac Radionuclide Imaging. A Report of the American College of Cardiology/American Heart Association Task Force on Assessment of Cardiovascular Procedures (Committee on Nuclear Imaging). Reprinted with permission from the American College of Cardiology. J. Am. Coll. Cardiol. *25*:521, 1995.

The difficult question of when radionuclide tests should be used instead of exercise electrocardiography was addressed in a separate set of guidelines issued in 1990 by a subcommittee of the American College of Physicians.[44] This group concluded that thallium scintigraphy is most clearly preferable to exercise electrocardiography alone when the resting electrocardiogram shows abnormalities impairing interpretation of changes or when information on the reversibility of ischemia in specific myocardial segments is needed to evaluate the potential impact of revascularization therapy.

Because of marked differences in complexity and costs, choices among scanning techniques are reviewed in the ACC/AHA guidelines. SPECT is considered preferable to planar imaging, although the task force noted that SPECT gamma cameras are not always available, and many patients cannot tolerate lying on the SPECT table. Positron emission tomography scanning using dipyridamole and either rubidium-92 or N-13 ammonia has been found in some studies to offer better diagnostic accuracy than thallium SPECT[45,46]; however, a review of available data by an American Heart Association committee in 1991 concluded that PET had *not* been demonstrated to be clearly superior to SPECT.[47] Noting the high costs of PET technology, the ACC/AHA task force concluded that PET should be considered for routine diagnostic purposes only if its costs are equivalent to or less than the costs of SPECT imaging in the same community.

Review of data on the three most commonly used agents in pharmacological perfusion imaging (dipyridamole, adenosine, and dobutamine) led the ACC/AHA task force to conclude that their diagnostic performances are in the same range as exercise testing.

ASYMPTOMATIC PATIENTS. The ACC/AHA guidelines do *not* consider cardiac radionuclide imaging an appropriate routine test for diagnosis of coronary artery disease in patients who are not symptomatic. However, a stress radionuclide test (either perfusion imaging or radionuclide angiography) can be useful for determining the need for coronary angiography in asymptomatic patients with positive exercise electrocardiography tests. The use of a stress radionuclide test can also be valuable in asymptomatic patients with known coronary artery disease to determine the presence and severity of inducible ischemia.

BEFORE NONCARDIAC SURGERY. Several studies have demonstrated that abnormal dipyridamole or adenosine thallium-201 scintigraphy identifies patients at increased risk for cardiovascular complications associated with noncardiac surgery (see Chap. 54). Most of these investigations have focused on vascular surgery procedures, but some data indicate that these tests can also be expected to help stratify patients according to the risk associated with other types of major operations.[48] However, because the overall risk of elective noncardiac surgery is low, the positive predictive value of abnormal tests is only between 15 and 30 per cent.[42] Therefore the ACC/AHA guidelines conclude that noninvasive testing is not needed in most patients undergoing nonvascular surgery if their cardiac risk is low.

BEFORE AND AFTER REVASCULARIZATION INTERVENTIONS. Myocardial perfusion imaging can be useful in planning percutaneous transluminal coronary angioplasty (PTCA) procedures by providing insight into the functional impact of single or multiple coronary artery stenoses. These tests can also be used after PTCA to assess whether restenosis has occurred and for patients who are symptomatic after coronary artery bypass graft (CABG) surgery to determine whether grafts may have occluded. However, the ACC/AHA guidelines do *not* endorse routine testing for patients who are asymptomatic after PTCA or CABG because of the lack of data that outcomes are improved with this approach.

MYOCARDITIS AND CARDIOMYOPATHIES (see Chap. 41). With the exception of assessment of ventricular function with radionuclide angiography, there are *no* indications for the use of nuclear cardiology tests in patients with myocarditis and cardiomyopathies that are considered clearly appropriate (Class I) by the ACC/AHA task force. Thallium-201 scintigraphy is believed to be potentially useful (Class IIa) for the purpose of differentiating ischemic and dilated cardiomyopathy and assessment of myocardial ischemia in patients with hypertrophic cardiomyopathy. Other indications for testing in patients with myocarditis or cardiomyopathies, such as gallium-67 imaging to demonstrate myocardial inflammation, are considered possibly useful but are unproven.

OTHER CONDITIONS. Echocardiography is the imaging technique of choice for patients with congenital heart disease; first-pass radionuclide angiography and lung perfusion scanning can be used to detect, localize, and quantify shunts. For patients who have undergone cardiac transplantation, the use of radionuclide tests to detect rejection or coronary arteriopathy is not well established (Class IIb). Similarly, cardiac nuclear tests are not considered to be directly useful for assessment of valvular heart disease, except for left ventricular function.

AMBULATORY ELECTROCARDIOGRAPHY

(See also p. 1345)

Ambulatory electrocardiography is often used for confirmation of arrhythmias as the cause of patients' symptoms; it is also used for the evaluation of the efficacy of therapy, assessment of prognosis, and detection of myocardial ischemia. For many of the "endpoints" for which ambulatory electrocardiography is ordered, there are no "gold standards." Hence, data on the sensitivity, specificity, and cost-effectiveness of this test in various settings are sparse. The lack of certainty about the impact of ambulatory electrocardiography and the heterogeneity of the outcomes of patients who undergo this test leads to considerable variability in its application. Therefore, an ACC/AHA task force published guidelines in 1989[49] that described conditions for which there was general agreement that ambulatory electrocardiography is useful and reliable (Class I); for which there was divergence of opinions about its usefulness (Class II); and for which there was agreement that the test is not useful (Class III) (Table 63–4). Similar recommendations were issued by a subcommittee of the American College of Physicians in 1990.[50]

Among patients who undergo ambulatory electrocardiography for assessment of symptoms that may be related to arrhythmias, the positive predictive value of abnormal findings depends on the nature of the symptoms. Therefore the ACC/AHA and the American College of Physicians guidelines consider ambulatory electrocardiography an appropriate test for symptoms such as palpitation, syncope, or dizziness, which have a high likelihood of being due to arrhythmia. However, the indications for this test are considered by the ACC/AHA task force to be less certain (Class II) for symptoms that are less frequently caused by arrhythmia, such as shortness of breath, chest pain, and fatigue.

Regardless of whether symptoms of arrhythmia are present, the ACC/AHA task force considers ambulatory electrocardiography useful for patients who have medical conditions associated with life-threatening arrhythmias. Therefore, this test is considered appropriate (Class I) for patients with idiopathic hypertrophy and patients with left ventricular dysfunction after acute myocardial infarction. The American College of Physicians guidelines, however, noted that antiarrhythmic therapy in asymptomatic patients is of unproven value; hence, these guidelines discourage use of ambulatory monitoring after acute myocardial infarction in asymptomatic patients.

TABLE 63–4 ACC/AHA GUIDELINES FOR AMBULATORY ELECTROCARDIOGRAPHY

SETTING	CLASS I (APPROPRIATE)	CLASS II (EQUIVOCAL)	CLASS III (INAPPROPRIATE)
Symptoms	**1.** Palpitation **2.** Syncope **3.** Dizziness	**1.** Shortness of breath **2.** Chest pain or fatigue not otherwise explained, episodic and strongly suggestive of arrhythmia as the cause because of a relation of the symptom with palpitation.	Symptoms not reasonably expected to be due to arrhythmia.
Assessment of R-R interval characteristics	**1.** Sleep apnea. **2.** Visceral diabetic neuropathy.	For prognostic assessment of R-R interval in coronary artery disease.	None
Prognostic stratification in patients with and without symptoms of arrhythmia	**1.** Patients with idiopathic hypertrophic cardiomyopathy, with or without symptoms. **2.** Postmyocardial infarction patients with left ventricular dysfunction.	**1.** Patients with known stable coronary artery disease or who have undergone coronary bypass surgery or angioplasty and have evidence for myocardial dysfunction or arrhythmia. **2.** Wolff-Parkinson-White syndrome **3.** Long Q-T intervals **4.** Documented significant aortic valve disease and symptoms suggestive of arrhythmia. **5.** Patients with dilated cardiomyopathy and symptoms suggestive of arrhythmia.	**1.** Patients with known coronary artery disease without evidence for myocardial dysfunction or arrhythmia. **2.** Asymptomatic mitral valve prolapse. **3.** Asymptomatic persons without known heart disease about to embark on an exercise program. **4.** Asymptomatic persons who require assessment of risk for potentially disabling arrhythmias because their occupation might place others in jeopardy if an arrhythmia were to occur.
Assessment of efficacy of antiarrhythmic therapy	Patients with baseline high-frequency, reproducible sustained symptomatic premature ventricular complexes, supraventricular arrhythmias, or ventricular tachycardia.	**1.** Patients with known episodic or reverted atrial fibrillation to determine efficacy of arrhythmia control. **2.** Patients with premature ventricular complexes of variable frequency and complexity or relatively infrequent brief salvos of ventricular or supraventricular arrhythmias. **3.** Patients with Wolff-Parkinson-White syndrome. **4.** Assessment of proarrhythmia effects. **5.** Assessment of tachycardias, bradycardias and conduction defects related to drug administration.	None
Detection of myocardial ischemia in patients with chest pain	Patients with chest pain suggestive of Prinzmetal's angina.	Symptomatic patients who are unable to be tested by treadmill or bicycle.	**1.** Patients whose description of chest pain is classic for angina pectoris and who have one or more risk factors for coronary artery disease. **2.** Patients with atypical chest pain and one or more risk factors. **3.** Patients with chest pain atypical for myocardial ischemia in the absence of coronary artery disease risk factors.
Detection of ischemia in the asymptomatic individual	None	None	**1.** Primary detection of ischemia in the asymptomatic individual with known risk factors for coronary artery disease. **2.** Detection of ischemia in the asymptomatic individual without identifiable coronary artery disease risk factors.
Primary detection of asymptomatic ischemia in the patient with known coronary artery disease	None	**1.** Postmyocardial infarction patients who have been known to have premature ventricular complexes. **2.** Patients with chronic stable angina to assess efficacy of antiischemic therapy.	**1.** For routine use after acute myocardial infarction. **2.** For routine use in the postrevascularization patient. **3.** For patients entering a cardiovascular rehabilitation program.

Class I: Conditions for which or patients for whom there is general agreement that an ambulatory electrocardiogram is a useful and reliable test.
Class II: Conditions for which or patients for whom ambulatory electrocardiography is frequently used but there is a divergence of opinion with respect to its usefulness.
Class III: Conditions for which or patients for whom there is general agreement that ambulatory electrocardiography is not a useful test.

From Knoebel, S. B., Crawford, M. H., Dunn, M. I., et al.: Guidelines for ambulatory electrocardiography. A report of the American College of Cardiology/American Heart Association Task Force on Assessment of Diagnostic and Therapeutic Cardiovascular Procedures (Subcommittee on Ambulatory Electrocardiography). Reprinted with permission from the American College of Cardiology. J. Am. Coll. Cardiol. *13*:249, 1989.

Both task forces discourage the test in persons with low risks for arrhythmic complications, e.g., those with known coronary disease without complicating left ventricular dysfunction or arrhythmia, or asymptomatic mitral valve prolapse. In the ACC/AHA guidelines, equivocal (Class II) indications include conditions that carry an intermediate risk for major arrhythmic complications, such as Wolff-Parkinson-White syndrome.

The ACC/AHA guidelines do *not* support the use of ambulatory electrocardiography for asymptomatic persons in occupations in which others might be endangered if an arrhythmia occurs. Major arrhythmic events are so uncommon in this population that the capability of ambulatory electrocardiography to identify high-risk patients is very limited.

Ambulatory electrocardiography is also used to assess prognosis in several ways. Several studies have shown that beat-to-beat changes in heart rate or cycle length (R-R intervals) provide information on prognosis for patients with myocardial infarction and other cardiovascular conditions.[51,52] R-R interval variability can also contribute to evaluation of sleep apnea and visceral diabetic neuropathy, in which abrupt marked changes in heart rate may occur.

This test is considered an appropriate strategy by both the ACC/AHA and the American College of Physicians task forces for assessing the impact of pharmacological therapy for ventricular arrhythmias that cause symptoms or appear life threatening. The underlying assumption for this recommendation is that a decrease in the frequency of arrhythmias detected with ambulatory electrocardiography is associated with either a decrease in symptomatic events or improved survival. However, subsequent data from the Electrophysiologic Study Versus Electrocardiographic Monitoring (ESVEM) Trial have raised questions about this assumption. In this trial,[53] suppression of spontaneous ventricular ectopy did *not* identify patients with a better outcome. Furthermore, there is no agreement as to which magnitude of reduction in arrhythmia constitutes a reasonable target. Therefore, evaluation of the efficacy of antiarrhythmic therapy remains a difficult challenge, with ambulatory electrocardiography the most easily performed of imperfect alternative tests.

Pacemaker function is also often assessed with ambulatory electrocardiography, which has the advantage over other technologies of providing data on pacemaker function as the patient performs activities of daily living. The appropriateness of ambulatory electrocardiography is considered uncertain (Class II) for routine evaluation of pacemaker function immediately after implantation and other routine follow-up of patients with pacemakers.

DETECTION OF ISCHEMIA. Modifications of ambulatory electrocardiography that allow accurate measurement of ST-segment deviation have introduced new functions for this technique—diagnosis and prognostic stratification of ischemic heart disease. The ACC/AHA guidelines consider ambulatory electrocardiography an appropriate test for patients with suspected Prinzmetal's angina, since exercise stress tests or even coronary angiography might miss this diagnosis. Ambulatory electrocardiography is also considered a potential test for the diagnosis of ischemia in patients who are unable to perform exercise tests (Class II).

The dominant theme of the ACC/AHA comments on the use of ambulatory electrocardiography for detection of ischemia is that there are too few data to recommend routine use of this test in many settings, especially for patients with atypical chest pain or for asymptomatic patients. The American College of Physicians guidelines also do not support routine use of this technique for either diagnosis or management of coronary disease. These assessments of the role of ambulatory electrocardiography for detection of ischemia may be subject to revision as a result of subsequent research demonstrating the usefulness of ambulatory electrocardiography in settings such as before major vascular surgery.[54] The use of this test would also likely increase markedly if research supports benefit from treatment of asymptomatic ischemia[55–57] (see p. 1345).

IN-HOSPITAL CARDIAC MONITORING

(See also p. 1226)

Few data are available on the value and limitations of in-hospital cardiac monitoring,[58–63] and most published studies have been rendered outdated by technological advances and the transition of coronary care to settings outside the coronary care unit, such as intermediate care units and chest pain emergency units. The availability of electrocardiographic monitoring in a variety of settings has been accompanied by a trend toward the use of monitors in many patients with a low risk for arrhythmic complications. Although the per-diem costs of monitors are low, the costs of personnel who are appropriately trained to observe monitors are high. Therefore, an ACC committee recommended guidelines for the use of this method that were published in 1991.[63] These guidelines assume that there is adequate surveillance of the monitors 24 hours a day by personnel trained and qualified in electrocardiographic recognition of cardiac rhythm disturbances.

Cardiac monitoring is considered to be appropriate (Class I indication) for most if not all patients because of a high risk of immediate, life-threatening arrhythmias. Although in general these guidelines do not specify the duration for which monitoring should be continued, the guidelines endorse monitoring for the first 3 days of hospitalization for patients with acute myocardial infarction or who undergo cardiac surgery. For patients who suffer clinically important complications after myocardial infarction, monitoring for 2 or more days is considered appropriate.

Monitoring is also considered to be appropriate for patients with a variety of other conditions associated with arrhythmias, including suspected myocardial infarction, until that diagnosis had been excluded; ingestion of agents with cardiac toxicity; myocarditis; and, for patients with potentially life-threatening arrhythmias, during initiation of therapy with Type I or Type III antiarrhythmic drugs. Electrocardiographic monitoring is recommended for patients with unstable angina and those with high-risk coronary artery lesions who are scheduled for urgent revascularization.

The use of monitoring was less clear-cut in populations with a lower risk of complications, such as patients with acute myocardial infarction who were without complications during their first 3 hospital days; patients with a non-life-threatening arrhythmia undergoing initiation of Type I or Type III antiarrhythmic agents; and patients with pericarditis without myocarditis. Syncope and other neurological events that might have a cardiac cause are also considered equivocal (Class II) indications for electrocardiographic monitoring, implying that some but not all such patients should receive this care.

The guidelines specify only a few situations in which monitoring is not indicated, as in patients who have undergone routine uncomplicated coronary angiography, patients with chronic stable atrial fibrillation, and patients with stable asymptomatic ventricular premature contractions. After uncomplicated surgery, young patients and obstetrical patients often do not need monitoring, according to these guidelines. The guidelines indicate that monitoring can be stopped for patients whose cardiac syndrome has been stabilized and who have been free of arrhythmia for 3 days.

INVASIVE TESTS AND PROCEDURES

CARDIAC CATHETERIZATION AND CORONARY ANGIOGRAPHY

(See also Chaps. 6 and 8)

Because of high costs and rising rates of utilization, cardiac catheterization and coronary angiography have been the focus of numerous guidelines. The developers of these guidelines include national organizations[64,65] as well as individual provider and payer organizations. One goal of these guidelines is to ensure appropriate use of these procedures, because investigations have demonstrated considerable variability in their use. Therefore, some guidelines seek to standardize which patients are considered appropriate for cardiac catheterization.[14–16]

In addition to *who* undergoes cardiac catheterization, guidelines also seek to decrease variability in *how* the procedure is performed. In many regions of the United States, cardiac catheterization laboratories have been almost totally unregulated, and these facilities are used for a widening range of diagnostic and interventional procedures. Ambulatory cardiac catheterizations are now frequently performed in many laboratories, including facilities that do not have surgical back-up on site. Mobile cardiac catheterization laboratories are also used for performance of cardiac catheterization in regions without hospital-based facilities. Finally, guidelines from professional organizations have addressed specific issues related to cardiac catheterization, including the volume of procedures that operators must perform to maintain clinical skills and use of non-ionic contrast agents.

Appropriateness of Coronary Angiography

Detailed guidelines for the use of coronary angiography were published in 1987 by a task force of the American College of Cardiology and American Heart Association.[64] (The process of revising these guidelines began in 1995.)

The two principles underlying these guidelines are:

1. Coronary angiography should be performed for patients in whom the presence or absence of coronary disease should be determined with reasonable probability in order to improve management.
2. Patients who are at high risk for complications of ischemic heart disease should be identified.

Although accurate diagnosis of coronary disease is believed to contribute to improved management, the guidelines note that performance of coronary angiography in all patients with suspected coronary disease would be very costly, and that noninvasive tests can be used to establish diagnoses and assess prognosis in many patients. The noninvasive criteria for "high risk" were adopted from a joint ACC/AHA Task Force report.[66] These high-risk criteria were chosen for their correlation with poor overall prognosis, left main or multivessel coronary artery disease, and with impaired left ventricular function (Table 63–5).

ASYMPTOMATIC PATIENTS. Asymptomatic patients are considered to have "known" coronary disease if they have had a previous myocardial infarction or have undergone coronary bypass surgery or angioplasty. Asymptomatic patients have "suspected" coronary disease if they have rest- or exercise-induced electrocardiographic abnormalities suggesting "silent" ischemia.

Among these, coronary angiography is considered an appropriate procedure in those with markedly abnormal noninvasive tests for ischemic heart disease (Table 63–6).

For patients in whom noninvasive tests indicate a high probability of coronary disease but in whom these "high-risk" criteria are not present, there were varying opinions about the appropriateness of coronary angiography among

TABLE 63–5 EXERCISE TEST PARAMETERS ASSOCIATED WITH POOR PROGNOSIS AND/OR INCREASED SEVERITY OF CORONARY ARTERY DISEASE

EXERCISE ELECTROCARDIOGRAM

Duration of symptom-limited exercise
- Failure to complete Stage II of Bruce protocol or equivalent work load ($\leq$6.5 METS) with other protocols

Exercise heart rate at onset of limiting symptoms
- Failure to attain heart rate $\geq$ 120/min (off beta blockers)

Time of onset, magnitude, morphology and postexercise duration of abnormal horizontal or downsloping ST-segment depression
- Onset at heart rate $<$ 120/min or $\leq$ 6.5 METS
- Magnitude $\geq$ 2.0 mm
- Postexercise duration $\geq$ 6 min
- Depression in multiple leads

Systolic blood pressure response during or following progressive exercise
- Sustained decrease of $>$ 10 mm Hg or flat blood pressure response ($\leq$130 mm Hg) during progressive exercise

Other potentially important determinants
- Exercise-induced ST-segment elevation in leads other than AVR
- Angina pectoris during exercise
- Exercise-induced U wave inversion
- Exercise-induced ventricular tachycardia

THALLIUM SCINTIGRAPH

Abnormal thallium distribution in more than one vascular region at rest or with exercise that redistributes at another time
- Abnormal distribution associated with increased lung uptake produced by exercise in the absence of severely depressed left ventricular function at rest.
- Enlargement of the cardiac pool of thallium with exercise.

RADIONUCLIDE VENTRICULOGRAM
- A fall in left ventricular ejection fraction of $\geq$ 0.10 during exercise
- A rest or exercise left ventricular ejection fraction of $<$ 0.50, when suspected to be due to coronary artery disease.

Data from Schlant, R. C., Blomqvist, C. G., Brandenburg, R. O., et al.: Guidelines for exercise testing. A report of the American College of Cardiology/American Heart Association Task Force on Assessment of Cardiovascular Procedures (Subcommittee on Exercise Testing). J. Am. Coll. Cardiol. *8*:725, 1986.

From Pepine, C. J., Allen, H. D., Bashore, T. M., et al.: ACC/AHA Guidelines for cardiac catheterization and cardiac catheterization laboratories. American College of Cardiology/American Heart Association Ad Hoc Task Force on Cardiac Catheterization. Reprinted with permission from the American College of Cardiology. J. Am. Coll. Cardiol. *18*:1149, 1991.

TABLE 63–6 ACC/AHA GUIDELINES FOR CORONARY ANGIOGRAPHY

SETTING	CLASS I (APPROPRIATE)	CLASS II (EQUIVOCAL)	CLASS III (INAPPROPRIATE)
Asymptomatic patients with known or suspected coronary disease	**1.** Evidence of high risk on noninvasive testing (see Table 63–5). **2.** Individuals whose occupation involves the safety of others. **3.** Individuals in certain occupations that frequently require sudden vigorous activity. **4.** After successful resuscitation from cardiac arrest that occurred without obvious precipitating cause when a reasonable suspicion of coronary artery disease exists.	**1.** Presence of ≥ 1 but < 2 mm of ischemic ST depression during exercise, confirmed as ischemia by an independent noninvasive stress test. **2.** Presence of two or more major risk factors and a positive exercise test in male patients without known coronary heart disease. **3.** Presence of prior myocardial infarction with normal left ventricular function at rest and evidence of ischemia by noninvasive testing, but without high-risk criteria. **4.** Before high-risk noncardiac surgery in patients with evidence of ischemia by noninvasive testing.	**1.** As a screening test for coronary artery disease in patients who have not had appropriate noninvasive testing. **2.** After coronary bypass surgery or percutaneous transluminal angioplasty when there is no evidence of ischemia, unless with informed consent for research purposes. **3.** Presence of an abnormal ECG exercise test alone, excluding categories listed in Classes I and II.
Symptomatic patients with known or suspected coronary artery disease	**1.** Angina pectoris that is *inadequately responsive* to medical treatment, percutaneous transluminal angioplasty, thrombolytic therapy, or coronary bypass surgery. **2.** Unstable angina pectoris **3.** Prinzmetal's or variant angina pectoris **4.** Angina pectoris in association with any of the following: • Evidence of high risk on noninvasive testing • Intolerance to medical therapy because of uncontrollable side effects • Occupation or lifestyle that involves unusual risk or "need to know" for insurance or job-related purposes **5.** Before major vascular surgery if angina pectoris or objective evidence of myocardial ischemia is present. **6.** After resuscitation from cardiac arrest or sustained ventricular tachycardia in absence of acute myocardial infarction.	**1.** Angina pectoris in the following groups: • Female patients < 40 years of age with objective evidence of myocardial ischemia by noninvasive testing. • Male patients < 40 • Patients < 40 with previous myocardial infarction. • Patients requiring major nonvascular surgery if there is objective evidence of myocardial ischemia. • Patients showing a progressively abnormal exercise ECG or other noninvasive stress test on serial testing. **2.** Patients who cannot be risk stratified by other means; e.g., those unable to exercise because of amputation, arthritis, limb deformity, or peripheral vascular disease.	**1.** The presence of mild, clinically stable (Canadian Class I or II) angina pectoris in patients who do not have impaired ventricular function, or exercise studies suggesting high-risk or other criteria listed under Classes I and II. **2.** The presence of well-controlled angina pectoris (Canadian Class I or II) in patients who are clearly not candidates for bypass surgery or angioplasty because of age or life expectancy limited by other illnesses.
Atypical chest pain of uncertain origin	**1.** Atypical chest pain when ECG or radionuclide stress tests indicate that high-risk coronary disease may be present. **2.** When the presence of atypical chest pain due to coronary artery spasm is suspected. **3.** When there are associated symptoms or signs of abnormal left ventricular function or failure.	**1.** Atypical chest pain when noninvasive studies are equivocal or cannot be adequately performed. **2.** When noninvasive tests are negative but symptoms are severe and management requires that significant coronary artery disease be excluded.	Atypical chest pain in patients without objective signs of ischemia who have had an earlier technically satisfactory normal coronary angiogram for the same chest pain.
Completed myocardial infarction (after the initial 6 hours up to but not including predischarge evaluation)	**1.** Recurrent episodes of ischemic chest pain, particularly if accompanied by ECG changes. **2.** Suspected mitral regurgitation or ruptured interventricular septum causing heart failure or shock. **3.** Suspected subacute cardiac rupture (pseudoaneurysm)	**1.** Thrombolytic therapy during the evolving phase, particularly with evidence of reperfusion.* **2.** Congestive heart failure or hypotension or both, during intensive medical therapy. **3.** Recurrent ventricular tachycardia or ventricular fibrillation, or both, during intensive antiarrhythmic therapy. **4.** Cardiogenic shock	Myocardial infarction in which no acute mechanical or surgical intervention is contemplated.

TABLE 63–6 ACC/AHA GUIDELINES FOR CORONARY ANGIOGRAPHY—*Continued*

SETTING	CLASS I (APPROPRIATE)	CLASS II (EQUIVOCAL)	CLASS III (INAPPROPRIATE)
Valvular heart disease	**1.** When valve surgery is being considered in the adult patient with chest discomfort or ECG changes, or both, suggesting coronary artery disease. **2.** When valve surgery is being considered in male patients ≥35 years of age. **3.** When valve surgery is being considered in postmenopausal female patients.	**1.** During left heart catheterization when aortic or mitral valve surgery is being considered in male patients <35 years of age. **2.** During left heart catheterization when aortic or mitral valve surgery is being considered in female patients ≥40. **3.** When one or more major risk factors for coronary artery disease are present in adult patients of any age being considered for valve surgery.	**1.** When cardiac surgical treatment is planned for infective endocarditis in patients who are <35 and have no evidence of coronary embolization. **2.** When aortic or mitral valve surgery is being considered in female patients <40 who have no evidence suggesting coronary artery disease.
Known or suspected congenital heart disease	**1.** Evaluation of patients with congenital heart disease who have signs or symptoms suggesting associated atherosclerotic coronary artery disease. **2.** Suspected congenital coronary anomalies such as congenital coronary artery stenosis, coronary arteriovenous fistula, supravalvular aortic stenosis, an anomalous origin of left coronary artery, provided that aortography is not diagnostic. **3.** When corrective open heart surgery for congenital heart disease is being planned in male patients >40 or postmenopausal female patients.	The presence of forms of congenital heart disease frequently associated with coronary artery anomalies that may complicate surgical management (e.g., tetralogy of Fallot, truncus arteriosus, transposition complexes, and corrected [levo] transposition), provided that aortography is not diagnostic.	Coronary angiography is not routinely indicated in the evaluation of congenital heart disease.

* Subsequent trials suggest revision of these recommendations may be appropriate. See text.
Class I: Conditions for which or patients for whom there is general agreement that coronary angiography is justified.
Class II: Conditions for which or patients for whom coronary angiography is frequently used but there is a divergence of opinion with respect to its justification in terms of value and appropriateness.
Class III: Conditions for which or patients for whom there is general agreement that coronary angiography is not ordinarily justified.
From Ross, J., Jr., Brandenburg, R. O., Dinsmore, R. E., et al.: Guidelines for coronary angiography. A report of the American College of Cardiology/American Heart Association Task Force on Assessment of Diagnostic and Therapeutic Cardiovascular Procedures (Subcommittee on Coronary Angiography). Reprinted with permission from the American College of Cardiology. J. Am. Coll. Cardiol. *10*:935, 1987.

the developers of these guidelines. Hence, test results such as ST depression more than 1 mm but less than 2 mm are considered Class II indications for coronary angiography. In these patients, occupation and life style are important determinants of the appropriateness of angiography. Coronary angiography is considered appropriate (Class I) among individuals whose occupation involves the safety of others (such as airline pilots, bus drivers, truck drivers, air traffic controllers) and individuals in occupations that frequently require sudden vigorous activity (such as firefighters, police officers, and athletes).

Coronary angiography is also considered appropriate for survivors of cardiac arrest, because such patients frequently have extensive coronary disease. Particularly if the cardiac arrest has occurred outside the setting of an acute myocardial infarction, these patients are at high risk for recurrent sudden death[67]; hence, an invasive evaluation is considered appropriate for planning therapy for such patients.

The use of coronary angiography varies markedly for patients undergoing major noncardiac surgery (e.g., abdominal or thoracic aneurysmectomy, ileofemoral bypass surgery). There continues to be progress in noninvasive techniques for the identification of high-risk patients, and patients with normal results with preoperative noninvasive tests such as dipyridamole thallium scintigraphy and ambulatory ischemia monitoring have a low risk for major cardiac complications (see Chap. 54). Strategies for preoperative use of these invasive and noninvasive tests remain uncertain; therefore the appropriateness of coronary angiography in this setting is considered Class II.

Coronary angiography is considered *inappropriate* (Class III) as a screening test in patients who had not undergone appropriate noninvasive testing, or did not have evidence of ischemia on such tests sufficiently severe to place them in Classes I or II.

SYMPTOMATIC PATIENTS. ACC/AHA guidelines for the use of coronary angiography among symptomatic patients reflect the high probability of relief of severe symptoms with coronary artery bypass graft surgery or percutaneous transluminal coronary angioplasty. Coronary angiography is therefore considered appropriate in patients for whom medical or invasive therapy has proved inadequate—that is, when "patient and physician agree that angina significantly interferes with a patient's occupation or ability to perform his or her usual activities."[64] *All* of the "high-risk" noninvasive criteria in Table 63–5 are considered Class I indications for coronary angiography in patients with symptoms of coronary disease, including failure to complete Stage II of the Bruce protocol or equivalent workload (≤6.5 METS). Coronary angiography is also considered appropriate for patients with unstable or variant angina, and for patients with even mild angina who have high-risk occupations or are to undergo major vascular surgery. Another Class I indication is evaluation after resuscitation from cardiac arrest or sustained ventricular tachycardia that occurred outside the setting of acute myocardial infarction.

The appropriateness of coronary angiography is considered more equivocal (Class II) in patients with angina pectoris if they are under age 40 or have responded well to medical therapy. The guidelines also acknowledge that coronary angiography is frequently performed before major nonvascular surgery in patients with evidence of myocardial ischemia, in patients with progressively more abnormal noninvasive tests for ischemia, and in patients who cannot undergo risk stratification using noninvasive tests. However, these patients are considered to be at lower risk for poor outcomes than those in Class I patient subsets; hence these settings are considered Class II indications for coronary angiography.

Coronary angiography is considered *inappropriate* in patients with mild angina who do not have adverse prognostic factors such as high-risk exercise test results. The guidelines also do *not* support use of coronary angiography in patients with well-controlled angina who are not candidates for revascularization because of diseases limiting life expectancy, such as malignant disease, or because of advanced "biological" age.

ATYPICAL CHEST PAIN. Coronary angiography is considered appropriate (Class I) for patients with atypical chest pain, i.e., "single or recurrent episodes of chest pain suggestive, but not typical, of the pain of myocardial ischemia," with high-risk noninvasive tests using the same criteria as for asymptomatic patients with known or suspected coronary disease. Coronary angiography is also considered appropriate for patients in whom coronary spasm is suspected or patients with left ventricular dysfunction associated with atypical chest pain. In such cases, coronary angiography might prove useful in defining the pathophysiology.

Coronary angiography is considered to be equivocally appropriate (Class II) in patients in whom the diagnosis of coronary disease could not be adequately excluded with noninvasive tests or in patients with intractable symptoms in whom definitive demonstration of normal coronary arteries might be useful.

ACUTE MYOCARDIAL INFARCTION. The 1987 ACC/AHA guidelines considered coronary angiography to be of uncertain appropriateness (Class II) during the initial hours of acute myocardial infarction, whether or not thrombolytic therapy had been carried out. However, since the publication of these guidelines, randomized trials have demonstrated excellent and possibly superior outcomes for patients treated with primary angioplasty for acute myocardial infarction.[68–70] Therefore, revisions of these guidelines can be expected to consider coronary angiography to be appropriate in the early hours after the onset of infarction, assuming that the goal of the procedure is to identify patients for whom angioplasty can be performed.

After the initial 6 hours, when the myocardial infarction can be considered "complete," coronary angiography has the goal not of reducing infarct size but of identifying patients at high risk for poor outcomes, and whose outcomes can be improved with revascularization. Therefore, coronary angiography is considered appropriate for patients with evidence of recurrent ischemia, hemodynamic dysfunction due to acute mitral regurgitation or rupture of the interventricular septum, or suspected subacute cardiac rupture.

The guidelines also acknowledge that coronary angiography is frequently used in other settings after acute myocardial infarction, including routinely after thrombolytic therapy or in patients with hemodynamic dysfunction or life-threatening arrhythmia. However, because the role of coronary angiography is not clearly established in such patients, these indications are considered equivocal (Class II). Since the publication of the ACC/AHA guidelines, studies[71–73] have shown that routine early PTCA does *not* improve outcome and actually increases the need for urgent coronary artery bypass surgery. Furthermore, the TIMI II study showed that the strategy of elective catheterization and PTCA did not improve outcomes compared with "watchful waiting"[74] (see Chap. 37). Therefore, future revisions of these guidelines are *unlikely* to recommend *routine* coronary angiography in patients without clinical indications of increased risk for poor outcomes during the hospitalization. However, some data indicate that "rescue" PTCA may improve outcome for patients with persistent occlusion of the infarct-related artery after thrombolytic therapy,[75,76] so that the use of coronary angiography in this patient population is likely to be considered possibly appropriate.

In the convalescent period after myocardial infarction (i.e., from hospital discharge up to 8 weeks), coronary angiography is again considered most appropriate for patients who demonstrate clinical evidence of increased risk, including those with angina pectoris at rest or with minimal activities, evidence indicative of myocardial ischemia on noninvasive tests, heart failure, or non-Q-wave infarction. The appropriateness of the procedure is considered equivocal (Class II) in patients with mild angina. Coronary angiography is considered inappropriate for patients for whom revascularization is unlikely to improve survival, such as patients with a poor prognosis due to noncardiac disease.

VALVULAR HEART DISEASE. The ACC/AHA guidelines for the use of coronary angiography for patients with valvular heart disease reflect two key facts: (1) Patients with significant coronary disease that is not treated with coronary artery bypass graft surgery at the time of cardiac valvular procedures have higher rates of adverse outcomes[77] and (2) many patients with valvular heart disease who have concomitant coronary artery disease do not have angina pectoris. Therefore, coronary angiography is considered appropriate (Class I) in any adult in whom valve surgery is being considered who has clinical evidence suggestive of ischemic heart disease, who is a male over the age of 35 years or a postmenopausal woman. Coronary angiography is often performed before major valvular surgery in younger patients without evidence of ischemic coronary disease, but the guidelines considered the appropriateness of such procedures equivocal (Class II). Coronary angiography is considered *inappropriate* (Class III) in women patients younger than age 40 without clinical evidence of coronary artery disease and in patients younger than age 35 who require operation for infective endocarditis without signs of coronary artery embolization.

KNOWN OR SUSPECTED CONGENITAL HEART DISEASE. Patients with congenital heart disease are at increased risk for congenital coronary anomalies that can cause symptoms and complications, including sudden death after exertion without warning (see Chaps. 29 and 30). Coronary angiography is therefore considered appropriate (Class I) in patients with congenital disease with symptoms suggestive of atherosclerotic coronary artery disease or any other evidence of coronary anomalies.

The use of coronary angiography in patients with congenital heart disease is also directed at ensuring the safe performance of corrective cardiac surgery; hence, coronary angiography is considered appropriate before surgery in male patients over age 40 years and in postmenopausal female patients. Anomalous coronary artery positions may also lead to injury of the vessels at the time of corrective surgery; therefore, preoperative coronary angiography is often performed when aortography does not allow definitive localization of the site of the coronary arteries.

OTHER CONDITIONS. The ACC/AHA guidelines consider coronary angiography an appropriate procedure when surgery is planned for other cardiac and major vascular conditions in which patients have a high risk of coronary artery disease, such as patients with aortic aneurysms. The guidelines do not consider coronary angiography necessary for all patients with aortic dissection, whereas they note that definition of coronary anatomy may be important for patients with dissections of the ascending aorta because of the risk of involvement of the origins of the coronary arteries.

Coronary angiography is also considered potentially appropriate for patients with other vascular diseases that may involve the coronary arteries (e.g., Takayasu's arteritis, Kawasaki disease). Whether coronary angiography should be performed in patients with Kawasaki disease who have coronary artery aneurysms detected by echocardiography is uncertain (Class II).

Coronary angiography is considered potentially appropriate for other patients in whom the etiology of anginal symptoms or congestive heart failure is uncertain. Thus, Class I indications for coronary angiography include normal left ventricular systolic function but clinical evidence of left ventricular failure. Coronary angiography is also considered appropriate for patients with hypertrophic cardiomyopathy if they are men over age 35 years or postmenopausal women in two settings: (1) if they have symptoms of angina pectoris uncontrolled by medical therapy and (2) if surgery is planned to relieve outflow obstruction. On the other hand, coronary angiography is *not* considered to be clearly appropriate for routine evaluation of dilated cardiomyopathy. Coronary angiography is frequently performed in this patient population to determine whether the left ventricular dysfunction results from coronary disease and therefore might improve with revascularization. However, the ACC/AHA guidelines note that the distinction between ischemic and idiopathic cardiomyopathy can usually be made on the basis of available clinical data. The most appropriate role for coronary angiography in this population is in patients with dilated cardiomyopathy who also have symptoms of angina pectoris or left ventricular aneurysm or evidence of reversible ischemia.

Site of Cardiac Catheterization

ACC/AHA guidelines for cardiac catheterization and cardiac catheterization laboratories that were published in 1991 cover a broad range of topics related to the provision of these procedures, with particular emphasis on the site of cardiac catheterization.[65] This focus was stimulated by the increasing performance of ambulatory cardiac catheterization and the use of mobile laboratories. These "nontraditional" strategies and settings for cardiac catheterization have the potential to reduce costs for procedures and make cardiac catheterization more accessible to patients who live or are hospitalized in rural areas. However, these advantages must be weighed against the possible increase in risk for complications and the potential for overuse of catheterization for patients who have low probability of benefiting from this procedure.

These guidelines therefore attempt to define which patients can safely undergo coronary angiography in which settings. "Ambulatory" patients are those who do not stay in the hospital overnight either before or after the procedure. In general, these patients should be those who are at low risk for complications from the procedure and also have low probability of instability due to the underlying disease process. These guidelines dictate that ambulatory catheterization can be considered for diagnostic coronary angiography or evaluation of valvular, congenital, or myocardial disease. However, the guidelines indicate that PTCA should not be performed on an outpatient basis and, as a general rule, endorse ambulatory catheterization only for patients with stable cardiovascular symptomatic status.

Previous studies of ambulatory cardiac catheterization have reported that postprocedure hospitalizations occur frequently even among "low-risk" patients.[78,79] Therefore, no guidelines can identify a patient population for whom outpatient catheterization can be expected to be completely free of complications. As a result, the ACC/AHA guidelines stress that formal protocols for urgent hospitalization and special care are essential to the performance of ambulatory catheterization.

Several clinical conditions were identified that render the patient *inappropriate* (Class III) or of *uncertain appropriateness* (Class II) for ambulatory cardiac catheterization (Table 63–7). These conditions reflect predictors of complications during cardiac catheterization. Some of these factors (e.g., morbid obesity and severe peripheral vascular disease) increase a patient's risk for vascular complications. Others reflect increased risk for systemic complications (e.g., severe insulin-dependent diabetes mellitus and renal insufficiency).

Ambulatory cardiac catheterization should also be used with caution in patients whose underlying cardiovascular disease places them at increased risk for hemodynamic and other cardiovascular complications after coronary angiography. Therefore, the guidelines consider patients with noninvasive tests suggestive of high risk (see Table 63–6), recent cerebrovascular events, or severe pulmonary hypertension to be *inappropriate* for ambulatory cardiac catheterization.

The guidelines for use of outpatient catheterizations that were published in 1991 by the ACC/AHA are similar in content to those reported in 1992 by the Society for Cardiac Angiography and Interventions.[80] These latter guidelines describe in detail standards for the preprocedural preparation and the performance of the procedure itself. In addition to the conditions that were cited by the ACC/AHA task force as rendering patients inappropriate for outpatient cardiac catheterization, the Society for Cardiac Angiogra-

TABLE 63–7 ACC/AHA CRITERIA FOR EXCLUSION FROM AMBULATORY CARDIAC CATHETERIZATION

CLASS II (EQUIVOCAL)
1. History of contrast material allergy
2. Older than age 75
3. Severe obesity
4. Generalized debility or dementia
5. Frequent ventricular arrhythmia
6. Renal insufficiency (serum creatinine more than 2 mg/dl)
CLASS III (INAPPROPRIATE)
1. Geographic remoteness (>1-hour drive) from laboratory with inadequate or unreliable follow-up likely over next 24 hours.
2. Interventional therapeutic procedure (e.g., PTCA, valvuloplasty)
3. Infancy
4. Noncandidacy for cardiac catheterization because of other circumstances (e.g., fever, active infection, severe anemia or electrolyte imbalance, bleeding diathesis, uncontrolled systemic hypertension, or digitalis toxicity).
5. Transient cerebral ischemic episodes or recent stroke (less than one month before).
6. Suspected severe pulmonary hypertension
7. Severe peripheral vascular disease
8. Severe insulin dependent diabetes
9. Noninvasive testing data suggesting that detected ischemia may be associated with a high risk for adverse outcome (see Table 63–5).

From Pepine, C. J., Allen, H. D., Bashore, T. M., et al.: ACC/AHA Guidelines for cardiac catheterization and cardiac catheterization laboratories. American College of Cardiology/American Heart Association Ad Hoc Task Force on Cardiac Catheterization. Reprinted with permission from the American College of Cardiology. J. Am. Coll. Cardiol. *18*:1149, 1991.

phy and Interventions added (1) ventricular ectopy requiring antiarrhythmic prophylaxis, (2) severe aortic stenosis, (3) known bleeding disorders, and (4) emotional lability.

CATHETERIZATION IN DIFFERENT TYPES OF FACILITIES. The ACC/AHA guidelines indicate that stricter criteria should be used to identify candidates for ambulatory catheterization in settings with less capability to treat complications. In this respect, hospital-based facilities without surgical support are intermediate in capability between full-service hospitals and mobile catheterization laboratories. Hospital-based facilities permit prolonged monitoring of patients after the procedure and ready access to at least noncardiac surgical management of vascular complications.

For *suspected coronary artery disease,* patients with severe symptoms of ischemia or congestive heart failure are considered *inappropriate* for ambulatory catheterization, as are those with acute myocardial infarction within the last 7 days or a history of pulmonary edema thought due to transient ischemia. These guidelines consider the indications for ambulatory catheterization to be equivocal (Class II) for patients with noninvasive test data suggestive of high-risk coronary disease, if the procedure is performed in a full-service institution. However, catheterization of such patients in a hospital-based facility without immediate cardiac surgical capability is considered *inappropriate* (Class III).

For patients with suspected *valvular heart disease,* the ACC/AHA guidelines consider ambulatory catheterization *inappropriate* in *any* facility for patients with conditions including poor functional class, severe right ventricular failure or pulmonary hypertension, suspected severe aortic valve disease, active endocarditis, and need for continuous anticoagulation. Left ventricular puncture should be performed only at full-service hospitals. Transseptal procedures (Class II), as well as catheterizations in patients with an ejection fraction less than or equal to 35 per cent, are considered inappropriate for facilities without immediate access to cardiac surgical services.

OTHER ISSUES RELATED TO CARDIAC CATHETERIZATION. The ACC/AHA and other organizations have also recommended that physicians who perform cardiac catheterization in adults maintain a caseload of approximately 150 cases per year.[65,81] The guidelines note that, in some cases, the laboratory director may decide that a physician's skills are such that this minimum number of cases is not mandatory. The guidelines also recommend that physicians who begin performing cardiac catheterization after a prolonged hiatus first undergo a period of preceptorship involving at least 25 cases with a variety of diagnoses.

PERCUTANEOUS TRANSLUMINAL CORONARY ANGIOPLASTY

(See also Chaps. 38 and 39)

The development of guidelines for percutaneous transluminal coronary angioplasty (PTCA) is complicated by several trends, including technological innovations (e.g., stents, rotational and directional atherectomy), broadening of the patient population to which this procedure is applied, and the lack of data identifying populations in which PTCA confers a survival advantage. As physicians have become more expert in performing this procedure, they have also become more aggressive, and PTCA is now frequently used for patients with acute myocardial infarction and patients with multivessel coronary artery disease. An additional reason for uncertainty over the optimal role for PTCA is that it is an alternative to more than one major strategy—medical therapy or coronary artery bypass graft surgery. Hence, trials in which PTCA is directly compared with one other strategy[82–86] do not address the full range of choices for the clinicians.

Available guidelines do not address the issue whether patients with coronary disease requiring revascularization should undergo PTCA or CABG (see Chap. 38). Therefore, available guidelines do not present the optimal management for various subsets of patients with coronary disease. Instead, guidelines provide expert opinion on the yes-no question whether PTCA is likely to be regarded as appropriate (Class I), equivocal (Class II), or inappropriate (Class III).

An ACC/AHA task force published guidelines for PTCA in 1993[87] (Table 63–8) that defined contraindications to *elective* angioplasty, which include the relative contraindications to coronary angiography. These guidelines stress that PTCA may be appropriate even in patients with these contraindications who are severely symptomatic and not candidates for coronary bypass surgery.

Absolute contraindications include:

1. Absence of a lesion that causes a 50 per cent or greater reduction in coronary diameter;
2. Presence of significant left main coronary disease unless this coronary distribution is protected by at least one nonobstructed bypass graft;
3. Absence of a formal cardiac surgical program in the institution.

Relative contraindications include:

1. Conditions associated with unacceptable risks of serious bleeding or thrombotic occlusion or a recently dilated vessel;
2. Diffusely diseased saphenous vein grafts without a focal dilatable lesion;
3. Diffusely diseased native coronary arteries with distal vessels suitable for bypass grafting;
4. The vessel under consideration is the sole remaining source of myocardial perfusion;
5. Chronic total occlusions with clinical features suggesting a very low anticipated success rate;
6. Borderline stenotic lesion (usually less than 50 per cent stenosis);
7. Procedure proposed for a non-infarct-related artery in patients with multivessel disease who are undergoing direct angioplasty for acute myocardial infarction.
8. ACC/AHA guidelines also consider anatomical features that increase the risk for abrupt closure (see Chap. 39) to be relative contraindications to PTCA.

Many of these absolute and relative contraindications to PTCA will require reevaluation before new guidelines for this procedure are issued because of changes in interventional techniques. Coronary stents can prevent abrupt closure after attempted dilations of complex lesions, and new devices such as rotational atherectomy catheters have the potential to address lesions that previously would have been considered unlikely to yield to a balloon catheter. The guidelines that are described in this section were developed for balloon angioplasty, and it seems unlikely that they can or should be extended without change to these new techniques.

Because of the risk for complications with angioplasty, the ACC/AHA guidelines consider mandatory for all *elective* PTCA procedures the presence of an experienced cardiovascular surgical team within the hospital to perform emergency coronary bypass surgery should the need arise. However, the task force considers PTCA reasonable under some circumstances even if surgical back-up is not available. For patients at high risk for acute myocardial infarction in whom thrombolytic therapy is contraindicated, emergency PTCA is deemed "acceptable treatment" even if the patient cannot be transferred expeditiously to a center with surgical back-up. However, the guidelines note that patients with unstable angina should usually be transferred to an institution with a cardiac surgical program before consideration of PTCA.

TABLE 63–8 ACC/AHA GUIDELINES FOR PERCUTANEOUS TRANSLUMINAL CORONARY ANGIOPLASTY

SETTING	CLASS I (APPROPRIATE)	CLASS II (EQUIVOCAL)	CLASS III (INAPPROPRIATE)
Single-vessel coronary artery disease — Asymptomatic or mildly symptomatic patients with or without medical therapy	Patients who have a significant (≥50%) lesion in a major epicardial artery that subtends a *large* area of viable myocardium, and who: **1.** Show evidence of severe myocardial ischemia during laboratory testing, i.e., ischemia induced by low-level exercise (Bruce Stage I or <4.0 METS, or heart rate <100 beats/min) **2.** Have been resuscitated from cardiac arrest or from sustained ventricular tachycardia in the absence of acute myocardial infarction, or **3.** Must undergo high-risk noncardiac surgery, if angina is present or there is objective evidence of ischemia as described above.	Patients with mild or no symptoms, single-vessel coronary disease in a major epicardial artery that subtends at least a *moderate-sized* area of viable myocardium, and show objective evidence of myocardial ischemia during laboratory testing† and • Have at least a moderate likelihood of successful dilation, and • Have a low risk of abrupt vessel closure, and • Are at low risk for morbidity and mortality.	Patients with mild or no symptoms and single-vessel coronary disease who do not meet Class I or Class II criteria; e.g., those who: **1.** Have only a small area of viable myocardium at risk, or **2.** Do not manifest evidence of myocardial ischemia during laboratory testing,† **3.** Have borderline lesions (50 to 60% diameter reduction) and have no inducible ischemia, or **4.** Are at moderate or high risk for morbidity and mortality.
Single-vessel coronary artery disease — Symptomatic patients with angina pectoris (functional Classes II to IV, unstable angina) with medical therapy	Patients who have a significant lesion in a major epicardial artery that subtends at least a moderate-sized area of viable myocardium and who: **1.** Show evidence of myocardial ischemia while on medical therapy (including ECG monitoring at rest), or **2.** Have angina pectoris inadequately responsive to medical treatment, or **3.** Are intolerant of medical therapy because of uncontrollable side effects.	Patients who have a significant lesion in a major epicardial artery that subtends at least a moderate-sized area of viable myocardium and who: **1.** Show evidence of myocardial ischemia during laboratory testing† and have one or more complex (type B or C morphology) lesions in the same vessel or its branches or **2.** Have disabling symptoms and a small area of viable myocardium at risk.	All other symptomatic patients with single-vessel disease who do not fulfill criteria for Class I or Class II. Examples include patients who: **1.** Have no or only a small area of viable myocardium at risk in the absence of disabling symptoms, or **2.** Have clinical symptoms not likely to be indicative of ischemia, or **3.** Have a very low likelihood of successful dilation, or **4.** Are at high risk for morbidity and mortality, or **5.** Have no symptoms or objective evidence of myocardial ischemia during high-level stress testing (≥12 METS)
Multivessel coronary artery disease — Asymptomatic or mildly symptomatic patients with or without medical therapy	Patients who have one significant lesion in a major epicardial artery that could result in nearly complete revascularization because the additional lesion subtends a small viable or nonviable area of myocardium. Also, patients in this category must: **1.** Have a *large* area of viable myocardium at risk, and **2.** Show evidence of severe myocardial ischemia while on medical therapy during laboratory testing, or **3.** Have been resuscitated from cardiac arrest or from sustained ventricular tachycardia in the absence of acute myocardial infarction.	**1.** Patients who are similar to those in Class I but who: • Have a *moderate-sized* area of viable myocardium at risk, or • Have objective evidence of myocardial ischemia during laboratory testing, or **2.** Who have significant lesions in two or more major epicardial arteries, each of which subtends at least a *moderate-sized* area of viable myocardium.	All other patients with multivessel disease and mild or no symptoms who do not fulfill the above criteria for Class I or Class II. Examples include patients who: **1.** Have only a small area of viable myocardium at risk, or **2.** Have chronic total occlusions in major epicardial vessels subtending moderate or large areas of viable myocardium, or **3.** Are at high risk for morbidity or mortality.
Multivessel coronary artery disease — Symptomatic patients with angina pectoris (functional Classes II to IV, unstable angina) with medical therapy	Patients who have significant lesions in two or more major epicardial arteries both subtending at least *moderate-sized* areas of viable myocardium and who: **1.** Show evidence of myocardial ischemia while on medical therapy during laboratory testing† **2.** Have unstable angina or angina pectoris that has proved inadequately responsive to medical therapy, or **3.** Are intolerant of medical therapy because of uncontrollable side effects.	Patients who have significant lesions in two or more major epicardial arteries that subtend at least *moderate-sized* areas of viable myocardium and who: **1.** Are similar to patients in Class I but who are at moderate risk for morbidity and mortality, or have angina pectoris but do not necessarily have objective evidence of myocardial ischemia during laboratory testing. **2.** Have disabling angina proved inadequately responsive to medical therapy, and are considered poor candidates for surgery because of advanced physiologic age or coexisting medical disorders	All other symptomatic patients with multivessel disease who do not fulfill the preceding criteria in Class I or Class II. Examples include patients who: **1.** Have only a small area of myocardium at risk in the absence of disabling symptoms, or **2.** Have lesion morphology with a low likelihood of successful dilation and subtending moderate or large areas of viable myocardium, or **3.** Are at high risk for morbidity or mortality, or both.

Table continues on the following page

TABLE 63–8 ACC/AHA GUIDELINES FOR PERCUTANEOUS TRANSLUMINAL CORONARY ANGIOPLASTY—*Continued*

SETTING	CLASS I (APPROPRIATE)	CLASS II (EQUIVOCAL)	CLASS III (INAPPROPRIATE)
Direct immediate coronary angioplasty for evolving acute myocardial infarction	Patients who can be managed in the *appropriate laboratory setting* and who: **1.** Are within 0 to 6 hours of onset of a myocardial infarction **2.** Are within 6–12 hours of onset of a myocardial infarction but who have continued symptoms of ongoing myocardial ischemia, or **3.** Are in cardiogenic shock with or without previous thrombolytic therapy and within 12 hours after onset of symptoms.	Patients who: **1.** Are within 6–12 hours of onset of an acute myocardial infarction and have no symptoms of myocardial ischemia but have a large area of myocardium at jeopardy and/or are in a higher-risk clinical category **2.** Are within 12–24 hours of onset of an acute myocardial infarction but who have continued symptoms of ongoing myocardial ischemia.	**1.** Angioplasty of a non-infarct-related artery at the time of acute myocardial infarction. **2.** Patients who are at more than 12 hours after onset of acute myocardial infarction at the time of admission and who have no symptoms of myocardial ischemia, or **3.** Patients who have had successful thrombolytic therapy within the past 24 hours and have no symptoms of myocardial ischemia.
After acute myocardial infarction (Angioplasty during initial hospitalization)	Patients who have one or more lesions that predict a high (>90) success rate and are at low risk for morbidity and mortality, and: **1.** Have recurrent episodes of ischemic chest pain, particularly if accompanied by ECG changes (postinfarction angina), or **2.** Show objective evidence of myocardial ischemia during laboratory testing performed before discharge from the hospital, or **3.** Have recurrent sustained ventricular tachycardia or ventricular fibrillation, or both, while receiving intensive medical therapy.	Patients who: **1.** Are similar to patients in Class I but: • Have more complex lesions with at least a moderate likelihood of successful dilation, or • undergo multivessel angioplasty. **2.** Have survived cardiogenic shock in the period before discharge or **3.** Are asymptomatic but have a significant residual lesion in the infarct-related artery supplying a large or moderate area of angiographically functioning myocardium, or **4.** Have had a non-Q-wave myocardial infarction, and have a large area at risk or objective evidence of myocardial ischemia.	All other patients in the immediate postinfarction period who do not fulfill the criteria for Class I and Class II. Examples include: **1.** Dilation of borderline residual lesions (50 to 60% diameter reduction) in the absence of spontaneous or stress-induced ischemia, or **2.** Dilation of chronic total occlusions subtending nonviable myocardium, or **3.** Angioplasty in patients at high risk for morbidity and mortality.

† Evidence for myocardial ischemia during laboratory testing includes the following, with or without exercise-induced angina pectoris:
a. Ischemic ST segment depression ≥1 mm, or
b. One or more stress-induced reversible nuclear perfusion defects and/or exercise-induced reduction in the ejection fraction and/or wall motion abnormalities on radionuclide ventriculographic or stress echocardiographic studies.

Class I: Conditions for which there is general agreement that coronary angioplasty is justified. A Class I indication does not mean that coronary angioplasty is the only acceptable therapy.
Class II: Conditions for which there is a divergence of opinion with respect to the justification for coronary angioplasty in terms of value and appropriateness.
Class III: Conditions for which there is general agreement that coronary angioplasty is not ordinarily indicated.

From Ryan, T. J., Bauman, W. B., Kennedy, J. W., et al.: Guidelines for percutaneous transluminal coronary angioplasty. A report of the American College of Cardiology/American Heart Association Task Force on Assessment of Diagnostic and Therapeutic Cardiovascular Procedures (Subcommittee on Percutaneous Transluminal Coronary Angioplasty). Reprinted with permission from the American College of Cardiology. J. Am. Coll. Cardiol. *22*:2033, 1993.

The experience of the operator is also a crucial factor in determining the outcome for PTCA. Therefore, several task forces have provided similar recommendations for the minimum number of cases during PTCA training and for the minimum annual volume required to maintain competency.[87–90] All recommend that a structured fellowship program in PTCA involve a minimum of 125 coronary angioplasty procedures, including at least 75 in which the trainee was the primary operator. Estimates of the number of PTCA cases per year required to maintain competency range from 50 to 75. The ACC/AHA task force recommends that PTCA operators who did not meet these requirements be required to discontinue performance of the procedure. The task force also recommends that institutions offering PTCA perform at least 200 such procedures annually and indicates that an initial success rate of 90 per cent or more for single-lesion dilations is a reasonable expectation.

Indications for PTCA

The ACC/AHA task force developed assessments of the appropriateness of PTCA in various clinical settings according to the same three classes used in other ACC/AHA guidelines.[87]

SINGLE-VESSEL CORONARY DISEASE. For patients who are *asymptomatic* or only mildly symptomatic, regardless whether they have received medical therapy, PTCA is considered appropriate (Class I) in those who have a lesion resulting in a 30 per cent or greater reduction in the diameter of a coronary artery that supplies a large area of viable myocardium *and* myocardial ischemia induced by low levels of exercise during noninvasive testing (Bruce Stage 1 or less or less than 4.0 METS, *or* heart rate less than 100 beats/min). Other Class I indications for PTCA include prior cardiac arrest or sustained ventricular tachycardia in the absence of acute myocardial infarction; and the need to undergo major vascular surgery (such as aortic aneurysm repair, iliofemoral bypass, or carotid artery surgery) in patients with clinical evidence of ischemic heart disease.

The appropriateness of single-vessel angioplasty is less clear-cut in asymptomatic patients with less myocardium in jeopardy. PTCA is considered inappropriate (Class III) for patients with only a small area of viable myocardium at risk, or no evidence of ischemia, or a moderate-to-high risk for complications.

For patients who are *symptomatic* from single-vessel coronary disease despite medical therapy, the ACC/AHA guidelines consider PTCA appropriate (Class I) even if only a moderate amount of myocardium is supplied by the stenosed vessel—if they exhibit ischemia despite medical therapy, have angina pectoris that is inadequately responsive to medical treatment, or are intolerant of medical therapy. "Inadequately responsive" indicates that angina significantly interferes with the patient's occupation or ability to perform usual activities. These patients should have at least a moderate likelihood of successful dilation and be at low or moderate risk for morbidity and mortality for PTCA to be considered clearly appropriate.

PTCA is considered to be of equivocal appropriateness (Class II) in patients with increased risk for complications or failure of the procedure. The ACC/AHA guidelines do not deem PTCA to be appropriate in patients with no or only a small area of myocardium at risk in the absence of disabling symptoms or in patients with a high risk of procedural failure or complications.

MULTIVESSEL CORONARY DISEASE. For *asymptomatic* patients with multivessel disease, the guidelines indicate that PTCA is appropriate (Class I) if dilation of a single major coronary artery could lead to nearly complete revascularization, and the patients have a moderate or high chance of success. PTCA is considered inappropriate (Class IV) if patients had only a small amount of viable myocardium at risk, had chronic total occlusions, or had a high risk for complications.

For *symptomatic* patients with multivessel coronary disease, appropriate (Class I) indications for PTCA are similar to those for symptomatic patients with single-vessel disease except that these indications include lesions in two or more major arteries affecting at least moderate-sized areas of viable myocardium.

DIRECT CORONARY ANGIOPLASTY FOR EVOLVING ACUTE MYOCARDIAL INFARCTION. This topic is also addressed in guidelines for management of acute myocardial infarction (see p. 1221), and current recommendations reflect findings from recent randomized trials comparing direct angioplasty with intravenous thrombolytic therapy in patients with acute myocardial infarction.[68–70]

The 1993 guidelines for PTCA by the ACC/AHA task force reflect the promise as well as the uncertainty of this procedure for patients with evolving myocardial infarction. Percutaneous transluminal coronary angioplasty is considered appropriate for patients with continuing symptoms of ischemia within the first 6 hours after the onset of myocardial infarction, and from 6 to 12 hours after onset. It is also regarded as an effective therapy for patients within 12 hours of the onset of infarction who are in cardiogenic shock, even if they have had thrombolytic therapy.

The appropriateness of PTCA according to the ACC/AHA guidelines diminishes as time elapses; hence the use of this procedure 6 to 12 hours after the onset of infarction is considered an equivocal (Class II) indication, and its use more than 12 hours after the onset of infarction is considered inappropriate unless the patients have symptoms of ongoing ischemia. To minimize PTCA-related complications, the ACC/AHA guidelines recommend against the dilatation of non-infarct related arteries at the time of PTCA for acute infarction.

AFTER ACUTE MYOCARDIAL INFARCTION. Data from several trials do not support a strategy of routine performance of coronary angiography and PTCA after successful thrombolytic therapy for acute myocardial infarction.[71–74] Other studies, however, have shown that PTCA can be performed successfully in most patients in whom thrombolytic therapy has failed[75,76] and that patients with evidence of recurrent ischemia or other complications after myocardial infarction have a poorer prognosis. Therefore, the ACC/AHA guidelines for use of PTCA consider it appropriate for patients with evidence of ischemia or life-threatening arrhythmias if they have lesions that suggest a high success rate for the procedure.

For patients with coronary lesions associated with a worse success rate or greater complication rate, the indications for PTCA after myocardial infarction are considered uncertain (Class II). The guidelines also consider the use of PTCA equivocal for patients who are asymptomatic but have a large or moderate area of myocardium threatened by a residual lesion in the infarct-related artery, and for patients with a non-Q-wave myocardial infarction and further myocardium at risk.

CORONARY ARTERY BYPASS GRAFT SURGERY

(See also Chap. 38)

Coronary artery bypass graft surgery (CABG) is indicated for relief of symptoms that are unresponsive to medical treatment (or to coronary angioplasty), and for some patient subsets, to increase life expectancy. Guidelines published by an ACC/AHA task force on performance of CABG in 1991[91] are based on the comparative benefits of surgery versus medical therapy. These benefits are assumed to be dependent on (1) the number and type of coronary arteries whose stenoses can be "neutralized" by bypass surgery and (2) the expected survival of the patient with medical therapy. An implication of this approach is that CABG may be most beneficial in patient subsets with high surgical mortality if outcomes with medical therapy are even worse. Conversely, patient subsets with low surgical mortality often have excellent outcomes with medical therapy—implying that the comparative benefit from CABG may be low. For example, patients with left ventricular dysfunction have higher surgical mortality but a greater potential benefit from CABG than patients without left ventricular dysfunction.

These guidelines preceded trials published in 1993–1994 comparing outcomes for patients with multivessel disease who were randomized to CABG or PTCA[82–85]; they do not provide direct guidance on which form of revascularization should be used for specific patient subsets. However, subsequent data have not demonstrated clear differences in outcomes, such as ability to return to work, for CABG or PTCA for most patient subsets that could reasonably be considered for either approach[92]; hence the choice between these two alternatives must continue to be determined on a case-by-case basis.

The ACC/AHA guidelines are summarized in Table 63–9. These tables were developed to apply to patients with an ejection fraction greater than 20 per cent, because the benefits of surgery versus medical therapy in patients with lower ejection fractions have not been well defined in prospective trials. Class I indications are those for which surgery has a demonstrated advantage over medical treatment either in terms of longevity or relief of symptoms or both. Class II indications are those for which surgery is acceptable treatment, but for which its advantages over medical therapy have not been defined. Class III indications are those for which the operation is usually considered not indicated. Exceptions to the overall appropriateness classification system are made for patients with severe proximal stenoses of the left anterior descending coronary artery, which have a more serious prognostic implication than lesions more distal in this artery or in the left circumflex or right coronary artery.[93–95] Therefore, in the ACC/AHA guidelines, surgery is generally considered more appropriate for patients with severe proximal left anterior descending coronary artery obstructions than for patients with stenoses in other locations.

INDICATIONS FOR PATIENT SUBSETS. Certain subsets of coronary anatomy have been found to have better prognoses with surgical than medical therapy and therefore are considered indications for CABG regardless of the patient's symptomatic status and severity of ischemia on noninvasive testing (Table 63–9). In the ACC/AHA guidelines, CABG surgery is considered appropriate (Class I) for all patients with any of these criteria: (1) significant stenosis (greater than 50 per cent) of the left main coronary artery, (2) three-vessel disease and moderate to severe left ventric-

TABLE 63–9 ACC/AHA GUIDELINES FOR CORONARY ARTERY BYPASS GRAFT SURGERY: INDICATION CLASSES

	LEFT VENTRICULAR DYSFUNCTION			
CORONARY DISEASE	None	Mild	Moderate	Severe (but Ejection Fraction > 0.20)
I. Asymptomatic Patients				
1. No or Mild Myocardial Ischemia With Noninvasive Stress Testing				
Left main	I	I	I	I
3 vessel	II[a]	II[a]	I	I
2 vessel	III[b]	III[b]	II	II
1 vessel	III[b]	III[b]	III[b]	III[b]
2. Moderate or Severe Myocardial Ischemia With Noninvasive Stress Testing				
Left main	I	I	I	I
3 vessel	II[c]	II[c]	I	I
2 vessel	II[c]	II[c]	II[c]	II[c]
1 vessel	III[b]	III[b]	II[c]	II[c]
II. Patients With Chronic Stable Class I or II Angina				
1. No or Mild Myocardial Ischemia With Noninvasive Stress Testing				
Left main	I	I	I	I
3 vessel	II[c]	II[c]	I	I
2 vessel	II[c]	II[c]	II[c]	II[c]
1 vessel	III[b]	III[b]	II[c]	II[c]
2. Moderate or Severe Myocardial Ischemia With Noninvasive Stress Testing				
Left main	I	I	I	I
3 vessel	I	I	I	I
2 vessel	II[c]	II[c]	II[c]	II[c]
1 vessel	III[b]	III[b]	II[c]	II[c]
III. Patients With Chronic Stable Class III or IV Angina (regardless of severity of ischemia on exercise testing)				
Left main	I	I	I	I
3 vessel	I	I	I	I
2 vessel	II[c]	II[c]	II[c]	II[c]
1 vessel	II[c]	II[c]	II[c]	II[c]

[a] Class I if there is severe proximal large left anterior descending and left circumflex coronary artery stenoses.
[b] Class II if there is severe proximal stenosis in a large left anterior descending coronary artery.
[c] Class I if there is severe proximal stenosis in a large left anterior descending coronary artery.
Class I: Conditions for which the operation is indicated on the basis of a demonstrated advantage over medical treatment in terms of longevity or relief of symptoms, or both.
Class II: Conditions for which the operation is acceptable treatment but for which its advantages over medical therapy have not yet been fully defined.
Class III: Conditions for which the operation is not generally considered to be indicated.
From Kirklin, J. W., Akins, C. W., Blackstone, E. H., et al.: Guidelines and indications for coronary artery bypass graft surgery. A report of the American College of Cardiology/American Heart Association Task Force on Assessment of Diagnostic and Therapeutic Cardiovascular Procedures (Subcommittee on Coronary Artery Bypass Graft Surgery). Reprinted with permission from the American College of Cardiology. J. Am. Coll. Cardiol. *17*:543, 1991.

ular dysfunction, and (3) three-vessel disease that includes a severe proximal left anterior descending stenosis, regardless of the severity of left ventricular dysfunction. For patients with asymptomatic coronary disease and no or only mild evidence of ischemia on exercise testing, this last criterion is modified so that three-vessel disease must include involvement of both the proximal left anterior *and* the left circumflex coronary arteries.

Asymptomatic Patients. The ACC/AHA task force considers CABG *inappropriate* for most asymptomatic patients with one- or two-vessel disease with no or only mild myocardial ischemia on noninvasive stress testing. Exceptions are patients with severe proximal left anterior descending coronary artery stenoses or a combination of two-vessel disease and moderate to severe left ventricular dysfunction. For these patients, CABG was considered acceptable but unproven (Class II).

A lower threshold for performing CABG is described for asymptomatic patients who have moderate or severe myocardial ischemia with exercise testing. In this population the ACC/AHA task force considers surgery appropriate (Class I) if there is two-vessel disease involving the proximal left anterior descending coronary artery. Surgery is considered *inappropriate* (Class III) for patients with one-vessel disease and good left ventricular function, as long as there is no involvement of the proximal left anterior descending coronary artery. Otherwise, CABG is considered acceptable if unproven (Class II) for such patients with one- or two-vessel disease.

Patients with Chronic Stable Class I or II Angina.

Relief of symptoms is not usually justification for operation in patients with stable mild angina. Therefore the ACC/AHA task force concludes that the indications for CABG in this population should be dictated by the same factors as in asymptomatic patients.

For patients with moderate or severe myocardial ischemia with noninvasive stress testing, however, surgery is considered appropriate (Class I) for patients in several major categories, including all patients with (1) left main disease, (2) three-vessel disease, (3) two-vessel disease with proximal left anterior descending coronary artery involvement, (4) isolated left anterior descending coronary artery involvement associated with moderate to severe left ventricular dysfunction.

Surgery is considered *inappropriate* only for patients with good left ventricular function and one-vessel disease that does not involve the proximal left anterior descending coronary artery.

Patients with Chronic Stable Class III or IV Angina. Patients with Class III or IV angina usually represent failures of medical therapy and often cannot undergo noninvasive stress testing because of concern of risk for complications. In this population, CABG can often improve symptomatic status, and therefore surgery is *not* considered inappropriate for any patient subset. The ACC/AHA guidelines deem surgery to be clearly appropriate (Class I) for all patients except those with one- or two-vessel disease that does not include involvement of the left anterior descending coronary artery.

Unstable Angina. The ACC/AHA guidelines recommend CABG on an emergency basis only when intensive medical management fails to relieve the unstable angina. (See p. 1336 for unstable angina guidelines.) Once medical therapy has led to control of anginal symptoms, recent unstable angina predisposes a patient to further cardiovascular complications.[96] Therefore the ACC/AHA task force concludes that a recent history of unstable angina should lower the threshold for performing CABG.

Acute Myocardial Infarction. The ACC/AHA guidelines discourage use of CABG for patients with uncomplicated Q wave acute myocardial infarction, and recommend that patients with non-Q-wave infarctions be considered for bypass surgery according to the same criteria as patients with unstable angina. For patients with hemodynamic deterioration after acute myocardial infarction, the ACC/AHA guidelines recognize that an aggressive approach including CABG surgery probably improves outcomes in comparison with noninterventional strategies.

CARE OF PATIENTS AFTER CABG. The ACC/AHA task force makes several explicit recommendations aimed at optimization of the patient's recovery after surgery, promotion of graft patency, and control of risk factors. These include (1) cessation of cigarette smoking, (2) a program of daily exercise, (3) antiplatelet therapy, and (4) counseling about risk factor reduction. Although formal cardiac rehabilitation is described as often useful, it is not endorsed for routine care. Electrocardiographic stress testing is considered *possibly useful* 6 weeks to 6 months after surgery, particularly for patients who had silent ischemia.

ORGANIZATIONAL CONSIDERATIONS. The ACC/AHA guidelines offer specific recommendations about the responsibilities and qualifications of key personnel. The cardiac surgeon usually should be certified by the American Board of Thoracic Surgery or an equivalent certifying body, and a CABG surgery program should include at least two qualified cardiac surgeons. A minimum case load of 200 to 300 cases per year was recommended by the Inter-Society Commission for Heart Disease Resources in 1972,[97] the American College of Surgeons in 1984,[98] and the ACC/AHA task force in 1991.[91] Individual surgeons should perform a minimum of 100 to 150 open-heart operations, the majority of which are CABG operations. The ACC/AHA guidelines recognize that surgeons in densely and in sparsely populated areas may require different guidelines.

ELECTROPHYSIOLOGICAL PROCEDURES

(See also Chap. 21)

ACC/AHA guidelines for the use of intracardiac electrophysiological procedures were first published in 1989.[99] Because of rapid evolution in this field, these guidelines were revised in 1995.[100] This version of these guidelines reflects the emerging importance of catheter ablation as a primary treatment option for most forms of paroxysmal supraventricular tachycardias and preexcitation syndromes, and in patients with monomorphic ventricular tachycardia and structurally normal hearts. The new guidelines also demonstrate progress in understanding the role of electrophysiological studies for risk stratification of patients with tachyarrhythmias, while emphasizing consideration of whether or not the test is likely to influence management decisions.

The ACC/AHA task force identifies a narrow list of indications for which electrophysiological testing is clearly appropriate for guiding drug therapy (Table 63–10): sustained ventricular tachycardia or cardiac arrest, especially among patients with prior myocardial infarction, and supraventricular tachyarrhythmias associated with reentry loops and/or accessory pathways. However, the ACC/AHA guidelines reflect the increasing importance of electrophysiological testing as a prelude to interventions such as the insertion of implantable electric devices and catheter ablation.

EVALUATION OF SINUS NODE FUNCTION. Clinical evaluation of sinus node function is often difficult because of the episodic nature of symptomatic abnormalities and the finding that asymptomatic patients frequently have wide variability in sinus node rates. Invasive tests of sinus node function can assess the ability of the sinus node to recover from overdrive suppression (sinus node recovery time) and assess sinoatrial conduction by introducing atrial extrastimuli or by atrial pacing. These tests can be used to complement data from noninvasive testing, including ambulatory electrocardiography, exercise testing, and tilt-table testing to assess chronotropic incompetence.

The ACC/AHA guidelines consider electrophysiological studies of sinus node function most appropriate for patients in whom dysfunction is suspected but not proven despite noninvasive evaluation; conversely, such studies would be inappropriate (Class III) when bradyarrhythmias had been proven the cause of symptoms, and electrophysiological studies would not alter treatment. When bradyarrhythmias are recognized as the cause of the patient's symptoms, electrophysiological studies are considered to have possible but uncertain appropriateness (Class II) when data might refine treatment choices. These procedures are deemed inappropriate for asymptomatic patients who have bradyarrhythmias observed only during sleep.

ACQUIRED ATRIOVENTRICULAR BLOCK. Electrophysiological studies permit evaluation of conduction above, within, and below the His bundle. This information can be useful to clinicians because patients with atrioventricular (AV) block that is lower in the conduction system tend to have a worse prognosis. Both prognosis and the level at which AV block is occurring often can be predicted from the surface electrocardiogram, however. Therefore the ACC/AHA guidelines emphasize that electrophysiological studies are inappropriate (Class III) when electrocardiographic findings correlate with symptoms, and the findings from electrophysiological studies are unlikely to alter therapy. For example, if a patient warrants implantation of a pacemaker because of documented symptomatic advanced AV block (see p. 687), documentation of His bundle conduction will rarely contribute to management. Similarly, electrophysio-

TABLE 63–10 ACC/AHA GUIDELINES FOR CLINICAL INTRACARDIAC ELECTROPHYSIOLOGICAL STUDIES

SETTING	CLASS I (APPROPRIATE)	CLASS II (EQUIVOCAL)	CLASS III (INAPPROPRIATE)
Evaluation of sinus node function	Symptomatic patients in whom sinus node dysfunction is suspected to be the cause of symptoms but a causal relation between an arrhythmia and the symptoms has not been established after appropriate evaluation.	**1.** Patients who have documented sinus node dysfunction in whom evaluation of AV or VA conduction or susceptibility to arrhythmias may aid in selection of the most appropriate pacing modality. **2.** Patients with electrocardiographically documented sinus bradyarrhythmias to determine if abnormalities are due to intrinsic disease, autonomic nervous system dysfunction, or the effects of drugs to help select therapeutic options.	**1.** Symptomatic patients in whom an association between symptoms and a documented bradyarrhythmia has been established and the choice of therapy would not be affected by EP study results. **2.** Asymptomatic patients with sinus bradyarrhythmias or sinus pauses observed only during sleep, including sleep apnea.
Patients with acquired atrioventricular block	**1.** Symptomatic patients in whom His-Purkinje block, suspected as a cause of symptoms, has not been established. **2.** Patients with 2nd- or 3rd-degree AV block treated with a pacemaker who remain symptomatic, and in whom another arrhythmia is suspected as a cause of symptoms.	**1.** Patients with 2nd or 3rd degree AV block, in whom knowledge of the site of block or its mechanism, or response to pharmacological or other temporary intervention, may help to direct therapy or assess prognosis. **2.** Patients with premature concealed junctional depolarizations suspected as a cause of 2nd or 3rd degree AV block pattern (i.e., pseudo AV block).	**1.** Symptomatic patients in whom the symptoms and the presence of AV block are correlated by ECG findings. **2.** Asymptomatic patients with transient AV block associated with sinus slowing (e.g., nocturnal type I 2nd degree AV block).
Patients with chronic intraventricular conduction delay	Symptomatic patients in whom the cause of the symptoms is not known.	Asymptomatic patients with bundle branch block in whom pharmacological therapy is contemplated with a drug that could increase the conduction delay or produce heart block.	**1.** Asymptomatic patients with intraventricular conduction delay. **2.** Symptomatic patients in whom the symptoms can be correlated with, or excluded by, ECG events.
Patients with a narrow QRS tachycardia (QRS complex < 0.12 sec)	**1.** Patients with frequent or poorly tolerated episodes of tachycardia not adequately responding to drug therapy in whom information about site of origin, mechanism, and electrophysiological properties of the tachycardia pathways is essential for choosing appropriate therapy (drugs, catheter ablation, pacing, or surgery). **2.** Patients who prefer ablative therapy to pharmacological management.	Patients with frequent episodes of tachycardia requiring drug treatment in whom there is concern about proarrhythmia or the effects of the antiarrhythmic drug on the sinus node or on AV conduction.	Patients whose tachycardias are easily controlled by vagal maneuvers and/or well-tolerated drug therapy and who are not candidates for nonpharmacological forms of therapy.
Patients with wide complex tachycardias	Patients with wide QRS tachycardias when the correct diagnosis is unclear after analysis of available ECG tracings and knowledge of the correct diagnosis is necessary for appropriate patient care.	None	Patients with ventricular tachycardia or SVT with aberrant conduction or preexcitation syndromes diagnosed with certainty by ECG criteria and in whom invasive electrophysiological data would not influence therapy. Data obtained at baseline electrophysiological study in these patients might be appropriate to guide subsequent therapy (see sections on therapy).
Patients with ventricular premature complexes, couplets, and nonsustained ventricular tachycardia	None	**1.** Patients with other risk factors for future arrhythmic events, e.g., a low ejection fraction, positive signal-averaged ECG, and nonsustained ventricular tachycardia on ambulatory ECG recordings. **2.** Patients with highly symptomatic, uniform morphology ventricular premature complexes, couplets, and nonsustained ventricular tachycardia.	Asymptomatic or mildly symptomatic patients with premature ventricular complexes, couplets, and nonsustained ventricular tachycardia without other risk factors for sustained arrhythmias.
Patients with unexplained syncope	Patients with syncope that remains unexplained after appropriate evaluation, and who have suspected structural heart disease.	Patients with recurrent unexplained syncope without structural heart disease and a negative head-up tilt test.	Patients with known cause of syncope in whom treatment will not be guided by electrophysiological testing.
Survivors of cardiac arrest	**1.** Patients surviving an episode of cardiac arrest without evidence of an acute Q-wave myocardial infarction. **2.** Patients surviving an episode of cardiac arrest occurring ≥ 48 hours after acute myocardial infarction.	**1.** Patients surviving cardiac arrest due to bradyarrhythmia. **2.** Patients surviving cardiac arrest thought to be associated with a congenital repolarization abnormality (long Q-T syndrome) in whom the results of noninvasive diagnostic testing are equivocal.	**1.** Patients surviving a cardiac arrest that occurred during the acute phase (< 48 hours) of myocardial infarction. **2.** Patients with cardiac arrest resulting from clearly definable specific causes such as reversible ischemia, severe valvular aortic stenosis, or noninvasively defined congenital or acquired long Q-T syndrome.

TABLE 63–10 ACC/AHA GUIDELINES FOR CLINICAL INTRACARDIAC ELECTROPHYSIOLOGICAL STUDIES—*Continued*

SETTING	CLASS I (APPROPRIATE)	CLASS II (EQUIVOCAL)	CLASS III (INAPPROPRIATE)
Guidance of drug therapy	**1.** Patients with sustained ventricular tachycardia or cardiac arrest, especially those with prior myocardial infarction. **2.** Patients with atrioventricular nodal reentrant tachycardia, AV reentrant tachycardia using an accessory pathway or atrial fibrillation associated with an accessory pathway in whom chronic drug therapy is involved.	**1.** Patients with sinus node reentrant tachycardia, atrial tachycardia, atrial fibrillation or atrial flutter without ventricular preexcitation syndrome in whom chronic drug therapy is planned. **2.** Patients with arrhythmias not inducible during control electrophysiologic study in whom drug therapy is planned.	**1.** Patients with isolated atrial or ventricular premature complexes. **2.** Patients with ventricular fibrillation with a clearly identified reversible cause.
Patients who are candidates for, or who have, implantable electrical devices	**1.** Patients with tachyarrhythmias, prior to and during implantation, and final (predischarge) programming of an electrical device, to confirm ability of the system to perform as anticipated. **2.** Patients in whom an electrical antitachyarrhythmia device has been implanted in whom changes in status or therapy may have influenced continued safety and efficacy of the device.	Patients with previously documented indications for pacemaker implantation to test for the most appropriate chronic pacing mode and sites to optimize symptomatic improvement and hemodynamics.	Patients who are not candidates for device therapy.
Indications for catheter ablation procedures	**1.** Patients with symptomatic atrial tachyarrhythmias who have inadequately controlled ventricular rates *unless* primary ablation of the atrial tachyarrhythmia is possible. **2.** Patients with symptomatic atrial tachyarrhythmias such as those in No. 1 above but when drugs are not tolerated, or the patient does not wish to take them, even though the ventricular rate can be controlled. **3.** Patients with symptomatic nonparoxysmal junctional tachycardia that is drug resistant, drugs are not tolerated, or the patient does not wish to take them. **4.** Patients resuscitated from sudden cardiac death due to atrial flutter or atrial fibrillation with a rapid ventricular response in the absence of an accessory pathway.	Patients with a dual chamber pacemaker and pacemaker-mediated tachycardia that cannot be treated effectively by drugs or by reprogramming the pacemaker.	Patients with atrial tachyarrythmias responsive to drug therapy that is acceptable to the patient.
Radiofrequency catheter ablation for AV nodal reentrant tachycardia, (AVNRT)	Patients with symptomatic sustained AVNRT that is drug resistant or when the patient is drug intolerant or does not desire long-term drug therapy.	**1.** Patients with sustained AVNRT identified during electrophysiological study or catheter ablation of another arrhythmia. **2.** The finding of dual AV nodal pathway physiology and atrial echos but without AV nodal reentrant tachycardia during electrophysiological study in a patient suspected to have AV nodal reentrant tachycardia clinically.	**1.** Patients with AVNRT that is responsive to drug therapy, that is well tolerated and preferred by the patient to ablation. **2.** The finding of dual AV nodal pathway physiology (with or without echo complexes) during electrophysiological study in a patient in whom AV nodal reentrant tachycardia is not suspected clinically.
Ablation of atrial tachycardia, flutter, and fibrillation: atrium/atrial sites	**1.** Patients with atrial tachycardia that is drug resistant or when the patient is drug intolerant or does not desire long-term drug therapy. **2.** Patients with atrial flutter that is drug resistant or when the patient is drug intolerant or does not desire long-term drug therapy.	**1.** Atrial flutter/atrial tachycardia associated with paroxysmal atrial fibrillation when the tachycardia is drug resistant or when the patient is drug intolerant or does not desire long-term drug therapy. **2.** Patients with atrial fibrillation in whom there is evidence of (a) localized site(s) of origin when the tachycardia is drug resistant or when the patient is drug intolerant or does not desire long-term drug therapy.	**1.** Patients with atrial arrhythmia that is responsive to well-tolerated drug therapy that the patient prefers to ablation. **2.** Patients with multiform atrial tachycardia.

Table continues on the following page

TABLE 63–10 ACC/AHA GUIDELINES FOR CLINICAL INTRACARDIAC ELECTROPHYSIOLOGICAL STUDIES—*Continued*

SETTING	CLASS I (APPROPRIATE)	CLASS II (EQUIVOCAL)	CLASS III (INAPPROPRIATE)
Ablation of atrial tachycardia, flutter, and fibrillation: accessory pathways	**1.** Patients with symptomatic AV reentrant tachycardia that is drug resistant or when the patient is drug intolerant or does not desire long-term drug therapy. **2.** Patients with atrial fibrillation (or other atrial tachyarrhythmia) and a rapid ventricular response via the accessory pathway when the tachycardia is drug resistant or when the patient is drug intolerant or does not desire long-term drug therapy.	**1.** Patients with AV reentrant tachycardia or atrial fibrillation with rapid ventricular rates identified during electrophysiological study of another arrhythmia. **2.** Asymptomatic patients with ventricular preexcitation whose livelihood, profession, important activities, insurability, mental well-being, or the public safety would be affected by spontaneous tachyarrhythmias or by ECG abnormality. **3.** Patients with atrial fibrillation and a controlled ventricular response via the accessory pathway. **4.** Patients with a family history of sudden cardiac death.	Patients who have accessory pathway-related arrhythmias responsive to drug therapy that is well tolerated and preferable to ablation by the patient.
Ablation of ventricular tachycardia	**1.** Patients with symptomatic sustained monomorphic ventricular tachycardia when the tachycardia is drug resistant or when the patient is drug intolerant or does not desire long-term drug therapy. **2.** Patient with bundle branch ventricular reentrant tachycardia. **3.** Patients with sustained monomorphic ventricular tachycardia and an implantable cardioverter-defibrillator who are receiving multiple shocks not manageable by reprogramming or concomitant drug therapy.	Nonsustained ventricular tachycardia that is symptomatic when the tachycardia is drug resistant or when the patient is drug intolerant or does not desire long-term drug therapy.	**1.** Patients with ventricular tachycardia that is responsive to drug, ICD, or surgical therapy and that therapy is well tolerated and preferable to ablation by the patient. **2.** Unstable, or rapid, or multiple, or polymorphic ventricular tachycardia that cannot be adequately localized by present mapping techniques. **3.** Asymptomatic and clinically benign nonsustained ventricular tachycardia.

Class I: Conditions for which there is general agreement that the electrophysiological study provides information that is useful and important for patient management. Experts agree that patients with these conditions are likely to benefit from electrophysiological studies.

Class II: Conditions for which electrophysiological studies are frequently performed but there is less certainty regarding the usefulness of the information that is obtained. Experts are divided in their opinion as to whether these conditions are likely to benefit from electrophysiological study.

Class III: Conditions for which there is general agreement that electrophysiological studies do not provide useful information. Experts agree that electrophysiological studies are not warranted in patients with these conditions.

From Zipes, D. P., DiMarco, J. P., Gillette, P. C., et al.: Guidelines for Clinical Intracardiac Electrophysiological Studies and Catheter Ablation Procedures. A report of the American College of Cardiology/American Heart Association Task Force on Practice Guidelines (Subcommittee to Assess Clinical Intracardiac Electrophysiological and Catheter Ablation Procedures). Reprinted with permission from the American College of Cardiology. J. Am. Coll. Cardiol. *26*:555, 1995.

logical studies are not appropriate for asymptomatic patients with mild degrees of AV block who are not likely to warrant pacemaker implantation. According to these guidelines, electrophysiological studies of AV conduction *should* be performed when the relationship between symptoms and AV block has not been proven; in such patients, another arrhythmia could be the cause of symptoms.

CHRONIC INTRAVENTRICULAR CONDUCTION DELAY. Patients with prolonged H-V intervals have an increased risk for developing complete trifascicular block, but the specificity of the H-V interval for predicting the development of complete block among patients with bifascicular block is only about 63 per cent.[101] The use of rapid atrial pacing can improve the specificity of this test, but the annual incidence of progression to complete trifascicular block is low. Therefore, the main role for electrophysiological testing in this population, according to the ACC/AHA guidelines, is not to predict future complications but to determine whether symptoms of arrhythmia are due to conduction delays or some other arrhythmia.

The only Class I (clearly appropriate) indication for electrophysiological testing in patients with intraventricular conduction delays according to the guidelines is in the determination of the cause of symptoms. The guidelines *discourage* the use of electrophysiological testing in asymptomatic patients with conduction system delays.

NARROW AND WIDE COMPLEX QRS TACHYCARDIAS. In narrow QRS tachycardia, the site of abnormal impulse formation or the reentry circuit can be located in the sinus node, the atria, or in the AV node–His bundle axis. The correct diagnosis can often be made using information from the 12-lead surface electrocardiogram, particularly when the electrocardiogram is combined with vagal maneuvers. In contrast, wide QRS tachycardias can be caused by ventricular or supraventricular arrhythmias, and identifying the site of origin of the tachycardia is frequently impossible using electrocardiographic tracings alone. As a result, electrophysiological testing plays different roles in these two types of tachycardias. In patients with *wide complex tachycardias,* electrophysiological testing permits accurate diagnosis in virtually all patients. Because knowledge of the mechanism of the arrhythmia is essential for the selection of the best therapeutic strategy, use of electrophysiological testing is considered appropriate (Class I) by the ACC/AHA task force for diagnosis of wide complex tachycardias. However, when the diagnosis is already clear from other data, electrophysiological testing is unlikely to influence therapy, and these procedures are not generally useful.

In patients with narrow QRS tachycardias, electrophysiological testing is considered more appropriate as a guide to therapy than as a tool for diagnosis. Therefore, the Class I indications for such testing include poorly controlled tachycardia in which data from electrophysiological testing may help clinicians choose among drug therapy, catheter ablation, pacing, and surgery. The ACC/AHA task force, however, does not believe that electrophysiological testing is useful for patients who have narrow complex tachycardias that are well controlled with medications and who are not candidates for nonpharmacological therapy.

OTHER CONDITIONS. Prolonged Q-T Intervals. The ACC/AHA task force concludes that electrophysiological testing has a limited role in the evaluation of congenital or acquired forms of prolonged Q-T syndrome. The results of such testing have only modest predictive value.[102] Whether catecholamine infusion during testing can unmask patients who are at high risk for complications[103] or whether electrophysiological testing can be used to evaluate proarrhythmic effects[104] in this population is unclear. Therefore, no indication for electrophysiological testing for this problem is clearly appropriate.

Wolff-Parkinson-White Syndrome. Electrophysiological studies can be used in patients with this syndrome to determine the mechanism of arrhythmia, to assess the electrophysiological properties of the accessory pathway, and to evaluate the location and response to drugs of accessory pathways. Therefore, electrophysiological studies are considered appropriate by the ACC/AHA task force for patients who were candidates for catheter or surgical ablation, who have had cardiac arrest or unexplained syncope, or whose management might be altered by knowledge of the electrophysiological properties of the accessory pathway and normal conduction system. For asymptomatic patients, however, electrophysiological testing was deemed inappropriate except in special situations, such as patients with high-risk occupations and those with a family history of sudden cardiac death.

Nonsustained Ventricular Tachycardia. The usefulness of electrophysiological testing is compromised by the lack of therapeutic strategies that have been shown to improve outcome in patients with ventricular premature beats, couplets, and nonsustained ventricular tachycardia. There are no indications in this patient population for which the ACC/AHA task force agreed that electrophysiological testing is clearly useful. Therefore, these tests are considered inappropriate for patients with no symptoms or only mild ones.

Unexplained Syncope. Arrhythmia is an important cause of syncope—and a worrisome prognostic sign in patients with structural heart disease. Therefore, electrophysiological testing is highly useful for evaluation of syncope in this patient population. In contrast, among patients without structural heart disease, an arrhythmic cause of syncope is uncommon, and the yield of electrophysiological testing is low.[105] Consequently the ACC/AHA guidelines recommend a higher threshold for use of electrophysiological testing in patients without known heart disease and suggest that head-up tilt-testing may provide more useful data in this population.

Survivors of Cardiac Arrest. In patients who have survived cardiac arrest, electrophysiological testing is frequently used to assess prognosis and identify drugs that suppress inducible arrhythmia. The assumption that these data can be used to improve patient outcome has been called into question by data from the ESVEM trial.[53] Nevertheless, electrophysiological testing is considered appropriate by the ACC/AHA task force for patients who have survived cardiac arrest without evidence that the event was directly provoked by ischemia or myocardial infarction. These tests are deemed *inappropriate* when the cardiac arrest was closely associated with acute ischemic syndromes or other specific causes.

Unexplained Palpitations. The procedure of choice to determine the cause of palpitations, according to the ACC/AHA guidelines, is ambulatory electrocardiography. Electrophysiological testing should be reserved for patients with associated syncope or those in whom ambulatory electrocardiography has failed to capture a cause of palpitations but who have been noted by medical personnel to have a rapid pulse rate. Electrophysiological testing is of equivocal value in patients whose symptoms are so sporadic that they cannot be documented while ambulatory electrocardiography is being performed.

Appropriateness of Catheter Ablation Procedures

Catheter ablation of the AV junction or accessory pathways is a rapidly advancing technique that has been reviewed in guidelines and position papers from several organizations, including the American Medical Association,[106] the American College of Cardiology,[107] the North American Society of Pacing and Electrophysiology,[108] and an ACC/AHA task force.[100] The ACC/AHA task force identified several conditions for which they consider catheter ablation an appropriate strategy (Table 63–10). The characteristics that are common among appropriate indications include supraventricular arrhythmias that are symptomatic; that cannot be controlled with medications either because of limited effectiveness, side effects, or inconvenience; or that have caused sudden cardiac death. Catheter ablation is also useful for some patients with ventricular tachycardia, although patients with extensive structural heart disease tend to have multiple sites of origin of their arrhythmia and therefore are poor candidates for this procedure.

PACEMAKERS, ANTIARRHYTHMIA DEVICES, AND IMPLANTED AUTOMATIC DEFIBRILLATORS

(See also Chaps. 21 and 23)

INDICATIONS FOR PERMANENT CARDIAC PACING. Cardiac pacemakers are implanted to relieve symptoms and prevent sudden death. These goals are reflected in ACC/AHA guidelines published in 1991,[109] which evaluate potential indications for pacemaker implantation (Table 63–11). For patients with acquired AV block, bifascicular or trifascicular block, or sinus node dysfunction, permanent pacing is considered appropriate when the abnormality causes complications and is not precipitated by a drug that could be discontinued. Examples of complications include symptomatic bradycardia, congestive heart failure, and confusional states. Permanent pacing is also deemed appropriate for asymptomatic patients at high risk for the subsequent development of complications, such as patients with complete heart block and periods of asystole of 3 seconds or more or a slow escape rate or patients with bifascicular or trifascicular block with intermittent second-degree AV block.

Indications for permanent pacing for patients who do not have symptoms or complications are less certain. In asymptomatic patients, complete heart block with a ventricular escape rate of 40 or more beats/min or type II second-degree AV block are considered equivocal (Class II) indications for permanent pacing. Bifascicular or trifascicular block in patients with syncope is also not a clear indication for permanent pacing but is regarded as acceptable if unproven if other possible causes for syncope cannot be identified. Pacemakers are explicitly discouraged for patients with mild asymptomatic conduction abnormalities, such as type I second-degree AV block at the supra-His level; fascicular block with no or only first-degree AV block, and sinus node dysfunction.

Symptoms do not play as important a role in determination of the appropriateness of permanent pacing after acute myocardial infarction because of poor prognosis and the high incidence of sudden death in postinfarction patients with conduction system disturbances. The ACC/AHA task force has emphasized that the requirement for temporary pacing after acute myocardial infarction (see p. 1252) is not in itself an indication for permanent pacing, but it considers pacemakers to be appropriate for patients with persistent advanced-degree AV block or complete heart block with block in the His-Purkinje system. Although the usefulness of permanent pacemakers for patients with advanced block at the AV node is less clear (Class II), permanent

TABLE 63–11 ACC/AHA GUIDELINES FOR IMPLANTATION OF CARDIAC PACEMAKERS AND ANTIARRHYTHMIA DEVICES

SETTING	CLASS I (APPROPRIATE)	CLASS II (EQUIVOCAL)	CLASS III (INAPPROPRIATE)
Permanent pacing in acquired AV block in adults	**A.** Complete heart block, permanent or intermittent, at any anatomical level, associated with any one of the following complications: **1.** Symptomatic bradycardia **2.** Congestive heart failure **3.** Ectopic rhythms and other medical conditions that require drugs that suppress the automaticity of escape pacemakers and result in symptomatic bradycardia. **4.** Documented periods of asystole ≥3.0 sec or any escape rate <40 beats/min in symptom-free patients. **5.** Confusional states that clear with temporary pacing. **6.** Post AV junction ablation, myotonic dystrophy. **B.** 2nd degree AV block, permanent or intermittent, regardless of the type or the site of block, with symptomatic bradycardia. **C.** Atrial fibrillation, atrial flutter or rare cases of supraventricular tachycardia with complete heart block or advanced AV block, bradycardia, and any of the conditions described under A. The bradycardia must be unrelated to digitalis or drugs known to impair AV conduction.	**A.** Asymptomatic complete heart block, permanent or intermittent, at any anatomical site, with ventricular rates of 40 beats/min or faster. **B.** Symptomatic type II second degree AV block, permanent or intermittent. **C.** Asymptomatic type I second degree AV block at intra-His or infra-His levels.	**A.** 1st degree AV block **B.** Asymptomatic type I 2nd degree AV block at the supra-His (AV node) level.
Permanent pacing after myocardial infarction	**A.** Persistent advanced 2nd degree AV block or complete heart block after acute myocardial infarction with block in the His-Purkinje system (bilateral bundle branch block). **B.** Patients with transient advanced AV block and associated bundle branch block.	Patients with persistent advanced AV block at the AV node.	**A.** Transient AV conduction disturbances in absence of intraventricular conduction defects. **B.** Transient AV block in the presence of isolated left anterior hemiblock. **C.** Acquired left anterior hemiblock in absence of AV block. **D.** Patients with persistent 1st degree AV block in the presence of bundle branch block not demonstrated previously.
Permanent pacing in bifascicular and trifascicular block	**A.** Bifascicular block with intermittent complete heart block associated with symptomatic bradycardia. **B.** Bifascicular or trifascicular block with intermittent type II second degree AV block without symptoms attributable to the heart block.	**A.** Bifascicular or trifascicular block with syncope not proved to be due to complete heart block, but other possible causes for syncope are not identifiable. **B.** Markedly prolonged HV (>100 msec). **C.** Pacing-induced infra-His block.	**A.** Fascicular block without AV block or symptoms. **B.** Fascicular block with 1st degree AV block without symptoms.
Permanent pacing in sinus node dysfunction	Sinus node dysfunction with documented symptomatic bradycardia.	Sinus node dysfunction, occurring spontaneously as a result of necessary drug therapy, with heart rates <40 beats/min when a clear association between significant symptoms consistent with bradycardia and the actual presence of bradycardia has not been documented.	**A.** Sinus node dysfunction in asymptomatic patients, including those in whom substantial sinus bradycardia (heart rate <40 beats/min) is a consequence of long-term drug treatment. **B.** Sinus node dysfunction in patients in whom symptoms suggestive of bradycardia are clearly documented not to be associated with a slow heart rate.

TABLE 63–11 ACC/AHA GUIDELINES FOR IMPLANTATION OF CARDIAC PACEMAKERS AND ANTIARRHYTHMIA DEVICES—*Continued*

SETTING	CLASS I (APPROPRIATE)	CLASS II (EQUIVOCAL)	CLASS III (INAPPROPRIATE)
Permanent pacing in hypersensitive carotid sinus and neurovascular syndromes	Recurrent syncope associated with clear, spontaneous events provoked by carotid sinus stimulation; minimal carotid sinus pressure induces asystole of >3 sec duration in the absence of any medication that depresses the sinus node or AV conduction.	**A.** Recurrent syncope without clear provocative events and with a hypersensitive cardioinhibitory response. **B.** Syncope with associated bradycardia reproduced by a head-up tilt with or without isoproterenol or other forms of provocative maneuvers and in which a temporary pacemaker and a second provocative test can establish the likely benefits of a permanent pacemaker.	**A.** A hyperactive cardioinhibitory response to carotid sinus stimulation in the absence of symptoms. **B.** Vague symptoms (e.g., dizziness or lightheadedness or both) with a hyperactive cardioinhibitory response to carotid sinus stimulation. **C.** Recurrent syncope, lightheadedness, or dizziness in the absence of a cardioinhibitory response.
Pacing for tachyarrhythmia Permanent pacemakers that automatically detect and pace to terminate tachycardias	**A.** Symptomatic recurrent supraventricular tachycardia when drugs fail to control arrhythmia or produce intolerable side effects. **B.** Symptomatic recurrent ventricular tachycardia after an automatic defibrillator has been implanted or incorporated in the device and recurrence of ventricular tachycardia is not prevented by drug therapy or when no other therapy is applicable.	Recurrent supraventricular tachycardia as an alternative to drug therapy.	**A.** Tachycardias accelerated or converted to fibrillation by pacing. **B.** The presence of accessory pathways having the capacity for rapid anterograde conduction whether or not the pathways participate in the mechanism of the tachycardia.
Pacing for tachyarrhythmia Externally manually activated antitachyarrhythmia devices that act to terminate tachycardia	Recurrent, symptomatic ventricular tachycardia uncontrolled by drugs when surgery, catheter ablation, or the implantation of an automatic pacemaker or cardioverter-defibrillator is not indicated.	None	Recurrent tachycardia that produces syncope.
Pacing for tachyarrhythmia Overdrive or atrial synchronous ventricular pacemakers intended to prevent tachycardia occurrence	Atrioventricular reentrant or AV node reentrant supraventricular tachycardia unresponsive to medical therapy.	**A.** Sustained ventricular tachycardia in other conditions when all other therapies are ineffective or inapplicable and efficacy of pacing is thoroughly documented. **B.** Long Q-T syndrome	**A.** Frequent or complex ventricular ectopic activity without sustained ventricular tachycardia associated with coronary artery disease, cardiomyopathy, mitral valve prolapse; or a normal heart and in the absence of long Q-T syndrome. **B.** Long Q-T syndrome due to remediable causes.
Implantation of automatic defibrillator devices	**A.** One or more documented episodes of hemodynamically significant ventricular tachycardia or ventricular fibrillation in a patient in whom electrophysiological testing and ambulatory monitoring cannot be used to accurately predict efficacy of therapy. **B.** One or more documented episodes of hemodynamically significant ventricular tachycardia or ventricular fibrillation in a patient in whom no drug was found to be effective or no drug currently available and appropriate was tolerated. **C.** Continued inducibility at electrophysiological study of hemodynamically significant ventricular tachycardia or ventricular fibrillation despite the best available drug therapy or despite surgery or catheter ablation if drug therapy has failed.	**A.** One or more documented episodes of hemodynamically significant ventricular tachycardia or ventricular fibrillation in a patient in whom drug efficacy testing is possible. **B.** Recurrent syncope of undetermined origin in a patient with hemodynamically significant ventricular tachycardia or ventricular fibrillation induced at electrophysiological study in whom no effective or no tolerated drug is available or appropriate.	**A.** Recurrent syncope of undetermined cause in a patient without inducible tachyarrhythmias. **B.** Arrhythmias not due to hemodynamically significant ventricular tachycardia or ventricular fibrillation. **C.** Incessant ventricular tachycardia or fibrillation.
Single-chamber pacemakers Atrial-AAI	Symptomatic sinus node dysfunction (sick sinus syndrome), provided AV conduction is shown to be adequate by appropriate studies.	Hemodynamic enhancement through rate adjustment in patients with bradycardia and symptoms of impaired cardiac output, provided AV conduction is shown to be adequate by appropriate tests.	**A.** Preexisting AV conduction delay or block or if decremental AV conduction is demonstrated by appropriate tests. **B.** Inadequate intracavitary atrial complexes.

Table continues on the following page

TABLE 63–11 ACC/AHA GUIDELINES FOR IMPLANTATION OF CARDIAC PACEMAKERS AND ANTIARRHYTHMIA DEVICES—*Continued*

SETTING	CLASS I (APPROPRIATE)	CLASS II (EQUIVOCAL)	CLASS III (INAPPROPRIATE)
Single-chamber pacemakers Ventricular-VVI	Any symptomatic bradyarrhythmia but particularly when there is: **1.** No significant atrial hemodynamic contribution (persistent or paroxysmal atrial flutter/fibrillation, giant atria). **2.** No evidence of pacemaker syndrome due to loss of atrial contribution or negative atrial kick.	Symptomatic bradycardia where pacing simplicity is a prime concern in cases of: **1.** Senility (for life-sustaining purposes only) **2.** Terminal disease **3.** Domicile remote from a follow-up center **4.** Absent retrograde ventriculoatrial (VA) conduction	**A.** Known pacemaker syndrome or symptoms produced by temporary ventricular pacing at the time of initial pacemaker implantation. **B.** The need for maximum atrial contribution because of **1.** Congestive heart failure **2.** Special need for rate response
Dual-chamber pacemakers VDD	Requirements for ventricular pacing when adequate atrial rates and adequate intracavitary atrial complexes are present. This includes the presence of complete AV block when: **A.** Atrial contribution is needed for hemodynamic benefit. **B.** Pacemaker syndrome had existed or is anticipated.	Normal sinus rhythm and normal AV conduction in patients needing ventricular pacing intermittently.	**A.** Frequent or persistent supraventricular tachyarrhythmias, including atrial fibrillation or flutter. **B.** Inadequate intracavitary atrial complexes. **C.** Intact VA conduction.
Dual-chamber pacemakers DVI	**A.** The need for synchronous atrial-ventricular contraction in symptomatic bradycardia and a slow atrial rate. **B.** Previously documented pacemaker syndromes.	**A.** Frequent supraventricular arrhythmias in which combined pacing and drugs have been shown to be therapeutically effective. **B.** Bradycardia-tachycardia syndrome, provided adjustment of atrial rate and AV interval terminates or prevents the emergence of supraventricular arrhythmias with or without concomitant drug administration.	Frequent or persistent supraventricular tachyarrhythmias, including atrial fibrillation or flutter.
Dual-chamber pacemakers DDD	Requirement for AV synchrony over a wide range of rates such as **A.** The active or young patient with atrial rates responsive to clinical need. **B.** Significant hemodynamic need. **C.** Pacemaker syndrome during previous pacemaker experience or a reduction in systolic blood pressure >20 mm Hg during ventricular pacing at the time of pacemaker implantation (with or without evidence of VA conduction).	**A.** Complete heart block or sick syndrome and stable atrial rates. **B.** When simultaneous control of atrial and ventricular rates can be shown to inhibit tachyarrhythmias or when the pacemaker can be adjusted to a mode designed to interrupt the arrhythmia.	**A.** Frequent or persistent supraventricular tachyarrhythmias, including atrial fibrillation or flutter. **B.** Inadequate intracavitary atrial complexes. **C.** Angina pectoris aggravated by rapid heart rates.

Class I: Conditions for which there is general agreement that permanent pacemakers or antitachycardia devices should be implanted, or that a mode of pacing is appropriate.
Class II: Conditions for which permanent pacemakers or antitachycardia devices are frequently used but there is divergence of opinion with respect to the necessity of their insertion, or for which a given mode of pacing may be used but there is divergence of opinion with respect to the necessity of that mode of pacing.
Class III: Conditions for which there is general agreement that pacemakers or antitachycardia devices are unnecessary or that such a mode of pacing is inappropriate.

From Dreifus, L. S., Fisch, C., Griffin, J. C., et al.: Guidelines for implantation of cardiac pacemakers and antiarrhythmia devices. A report of the American College of Cardiology/American Heart Association Task Force on Assessment of Diagnostic and Therapeutic Cardiovascular Procedures (Committee on Pacemaker Implantation). Reprinted with permission from the American College of Cardiology. J. Am. Coll. Cardiol. *18*:1, 1991.

Addenda
Atrial-AAI: Atrial pacing inhibited by sensed atrial activity
Ventricular-VVI: The classic prototypical pacing mode; ventricular pacing inhibited by sensed spontaneous ventricular activity.
VDD: Ventricular pacing in synchrony with sensed atrial activity inhibited by sensed ventricular activity.
DVI: Pacing of both chambers at a preselected rate with both outputs inhibited by ventricular but not atrial complexes.
DDD: Pacing of both chambers, sensing of both chambers, inhibition of atrial or ventricular output by sensed atrial or ventricular activity; triggering of ventricular output by sensed atrial activity.

pacing is discouraged if the sole indication is transient AV conduction disturbances or left anterior hemiblock.

The ACC/AHA guidelines also define explicit criteria for appropriateness of permanent pacing in patients with hypersensitive carotid sinus and neurovascular syndromes. The only Class I indication is recurrent syncope associated with clear, spontaneous events provoked by carotid sinus stimulation. In such patients, minimal carotid sinus pressure should induce asystole of 3 seconds or more in the absence of medications that depress the sinus node.

ANTITACHYCARDIA DEVICES. Antitachycardia devices include permanent pacemakers that can be programed to interrupt reentrant arrhythmias or prevent their occurrence, and automatic defibrillator devices. The ACC/AHA guidelines stress that these devices should be implanted only after careful evaluation by experienced electrophysiologists.

Permanent pacemakers are recommended for use for recurrent supraventricular tachycardias in symptomatic patients whose arrhythmias cannot be controlled with drug therapy. For patients with symptomatic ventricular tachycardia, permanent pacemakers are considered appropriate only after an automatic defibrillator has been implanted, and symptoms cannot be controlled by drug therapy. If such patients remain symptomatic even after a permanent pacemaker has been implanted, use of an externally manually activated antitachycardia device is considered appropriate. These devices are considered inappropriate in settings in which pacing might lead to complications such as conversion of a tachyarrhythmia to fibrillation.

The threshold for implanting automatic defibrillator devices has been decreasing because of three major developments: disappointing data on the lack of beneficial impact on survival of antiarrhythmic medications; inability of ambulatory electrocardiographic monitoring or electrophysiological testing data to predict subsequent efficacy of therapy[53]; and the availability of new defibrillator systems that do not require a thoracotomy for implantation. Because of rapid evolution and the promise of this technique, the ACC/AHA task force defined indications that it termed fairly liberal, implying an expectation that the range of appropriate indications for these devices will continue to expand. However, the task force stressed that patients should not be considered for an automatic defibrillator unless they have experienced an arrhythmia that has been demonstrated to be life threatening by producing sudden death, syncope, or severe hemodynamic compromise. Furthermore, remedial causes of the arrhythmia such as drugs, electrolyte imbalances, or ischemia must be excluded.

A special case directly addressed by the ACC/AHA task force is that of the patient who has been resuscitated from a documented sudden death episode who does not have an inducible arrhythmia during subsequent electrophysiological testing. The guidelines consider an automatic defibrillator appropriate (Class I) in such patients even if electrophysiological testing and ambulatory monitoring cannot be used to predict the efficacy of the therapy. Because the ability of such tests to predict drug efficacy is in question,[53] future guidelines might consider automatic defibrillators appropriate for most patients who have documented hemodynamically significant sustained ventricular tachycardia or ventricular fibrillation. However, these devices are not considered appropriate for patients who have these arrhythmias incessantly, because of the intolerable effects of repeated discharges of the defibrillators.

CHOICE OF PACING MODE AND DEVICE. Clinicians can choose among several types of pacemakers and modes of pacing to seek the best functional outcome for patients. However, the costs for different types of pacemakers vary markedly, and pacemakers that adapt their rate in response to physical, chemical, or other stimuli are particularly expensive. Therefore, ACC/AHA guidelines seek to identify patients most likely to benefit from the more advanced techniques. A key unresolved issue in this effort is whether dual-chamber pacing can increase life expectancy by decreasing the incidence of atrial fibrillation and stroke. Research to address this issue is currently under way, and, if dual-chamber pacing is found to improve survival, the indications for its use can be expected to broaden considerably.

The ACC/AHA guidelines recommend that the decision between pacemakers with and without adaptive rate functions be based on factors including the nature of the conduction abnormality, comorbid medical conditions, presence of coronary heart disease and angina, degree of left ventricular dysfunction, impact of drug therapy, level of anticipated activity, availability of support services, expertise of implant teams, and costs. The primary goal of adaptive-rate pacemakers is to permit the heart rate to increase in the absence of an appropriate spontaneous rise in heart rate; the definition of chronotropic incompetence used by this group is failure of the heart rate to reach 100 beats/min in response to an exercise test. In general, adaptive-rate pacemakers are recommended for patients with an anticipated moderate to high level of physical activity but are contraindicated in settings in which they might precipitate tachyarrhythmias via retrograde VA conduction or aggravate angina pectoris or congestive heart failure.

Single-chamber pacing is recommended by the ACC/AHA task force as a "default" for patients with symptomatic bradyarrhythmias that are not due to medications or other reversible causes. Ventricular single-chamber pacing is considered particularly appropriate when there is no significant atrial hemodynamic contribution, as is the case in patients with atrial flutter or fibrillation. Ventricular pacing is also recommended for patients without evidence of "pacemaker syndrome," which includes lightheadedness, syncope, episodic weakness, inadequate cardiac output, or patient awareness of beat-to-beat variation in cardiac contractile sequence related to absence of AV asynchrony.

When patients have a high likelihood of benefiting from AV synchrony and single-chamber atrial pacing cannot achieve that goal, dual-chamber pacing is appropriate. The choice among various dual-chamber pacing modes should be made by an experienced pacemaker specialist, but the ACC/AHA guidelines emphasize that patients with frequent or persistent supraventricular tachyarrhythmias, including atrial fibrillation, are generally inappropriate choices for these devices.

CLINICAL SYNDROMES

ACUTE CHEST PAIN

(See also Chap. 37)

In patients with acute myocardial infarction who are discharged from the emergency department the short-term mortality is about 25 per cent—about double what might be expected with inpatient care.[110] As a result, missed myocardial infarctions are the greatest source of dollar losses in emergency department malpractice cases,[111] and admission of patients with myocardial infarction to a coronary care unit or intermediate care unit where they undergo electrocardiographic monitoring is generally considered an accepted standard of care.[112] Researchers have studied a wide range of issues related to increasing the efficiency of management of this patient population, including the development of decision aids,[112–116] the use of intermediate care units and special chest pain evaluation units for patients who are at low risk of needing the facilities and personnel of a coronary care unit,[117–121] shorter "rule-out" protocols for low-risk patients,[122] and the early use of diagnostic techniques for risk stratification.[123–126]

The major emphasis from this recent research is rapid identification of which patients are *safe* for discharge; however, a risk that is inherent in any strategy that seeks to accomplish earlier discharges and shorter lengths of hospital stay is that patients with unstable ischemic syndromes might suffer preventable complications. Many standards for the initial evaluation and subsequent management aimed at reducing that risk for patients with chest pain are addressed in guidelines developed by a multidisciplinary panel sponsored by the Agency for Health Care Policy and Research (AHCPR).[12] The recommendations regarding the entry of the patient with chest pain into medical care include:

1. The initial evaluation of symptoms that suggest a possible acute ischemic syndrome should not be carried out over the telephone but in a facility equipped to perform electrocardiography.

2. Patients with duration of symptoms longer than 20 minutes, hemodynamic instability, or recent loss of consciousness should generally be referred to an emergency department (as opposed to an outpatient office).

Emergency Department Evaluation

Standards of care of the initial evaluation in the patient with acute chest pain are provided in a "policy statement" issued by the American College of Emergency Physicians (ACEP) in 1990 and revised in 1995[127] (Table 63–12). The statement stresses that the decision to admit the patient must be based primarily on clinical judgment. This policy statement does not make recommendations about levels of care (coronary care unit versus intermediate care or chest pain unit) for different patient subsets.

The ACEP statement provide "rules" and "guidelines" about the data that should be obtained and recorded as part of the evaluation and the actions that should follow from certain findings. *Rules* are considered actions that reflect principles of good practice in most situations. When circumstances dictate that these rules cannot be followed, the ACEP statement asserts, the deviation from the rule should be justified in writing. *Guidelines* in the ACEP document are actions that should be considered but are not always followed; there is no implication that failure to follow a guideline is improper care.

The ACEP policy indicates that routine evaluation of nontraumatic chest pain should include a history that obtains data on character of pain, age, associated symptoms, and past history. The physical examination should include vital signs, a cardiovascular examination, and a pulmonary examination. Recommendations and rules for what tests should be performed—and initial responses to some data—are summarized in Table 63–12. An electrocardiogram is recommended for men over 33 years of age, women over age 40, and patients with risk factors for coronary disease, but the electrocardiogram is considered standard care (i.e., a rule) for patients with a prior history of coronary disease.

The National Heart Attack Alert Program (NHAAP) report also includes guidelines for specific functions related to evaluation and treatment in patients with chest pain; they are aimed at improving the speed with which patients with acute myocardial infarction are identified and treated,[95] including recommendations for which patient subsets should be placed on the acute myocardial infarction protocol. For registration staff, the NHAAP guidelines recommend that patients over age 30 with the following chief complaints receive immediate assessment by the triage nurse and be referred for further evaluation:

- Chest pain, pressure, tightness, or heaviness. Radiating pain in neck, jaw, shoulders, back, or one or both arms
- Indigestion or "heartburn"/nausea and/or vomiting
- Persistent shortness of breath
- Weakness, dizziness, lightheadedness, loss of consciousness

The triage nurse should immediately assess patients for initiation of the myocardial infarction protocol and obtain an electrocardiogram if they have any of the following:

- Chest pain
- Associated dyspnea
- Associated nausea/vomiting
- Associated diaphoresis

For physicians, the NHAAP guidelines offer several clinical recommendations and explicitly note that use of a "GI cocktail" (usually including an antacid) as a diagnostic test to differentiate between gastrointestinal and cardiac causes of the patient's symptoms is "inappropriate," because it frequently leads to erroneous conclusions.

Initial Triage and Management

The actions in response to the data that are collected during this evaluation are intended to lead to timely care for patients with acute myocardial infarction, unstable an-

TABLE 63–12 EVALUATION OF ACUTE CHEST PAIN; EXCERPTS FROM THE CLINICAL POLICY OF THE AMERICAN COLLEGE OF EMERGENCY PHYSICIANS (ACEP)

VARIABLE	FINDING	RULE (STANDARD)	GUIDELINE (RECOMMENDED)
Pain	Ongoing and severe and crushing and substernal or same as previous pain diagnosed as myocardial infarction.	IV access Supplemental oxygen ECG Aspirin Nitrates Management of ongoing pain Admit	Serum cardiac markers Chest X-ray Anticoagulation
	Severe or pressure or substernal or exertional or radiating to jaw, neck, shoulder, or arm.	ECG	IV access Supplemental oxygen Cardiac monitor Serum cardiac markers Chest X-ray Nitrates Management of ongoing pain Admit
	Tearing, severe, radiating to back	Large-bore IV access Supplemental oxygen Cardiac monitor Chest X-ray ECG	Differential upper extremity blood pressures Aortic imaging Management of ongoing pain Admit
	Similar to that of previous pulmonary embolus	IV access Supplemental oxygen Cardiac monitor ABG and oximetry Anticoagulation Pulmonary vascular imaging ECG	Chest X-ray Admit

TABLE 63–12 EVALUATION OF ACUTE CHEST PAIN; EXCERPTS FROM THE CLINICAL POLICY OF THE AMERICAN COLLEGE OF EMERGENCY PHYSICIANS (ACEP)—*Continued*

VARIABLE	FINDING	RULE (STANDARD)	GUIDELINE (RECOMMENDED)
	Indigestion or burning epigastric	None	ECG
	Pleuritic	None	Chest X-ray ECG
Age	Male > 33 years Female > 40 years	None	ECG
Associated symptoms	Syncope or near-syncope	ECG	Cardiac monitor Hct.
	Shortness of breath, dyspnea on exertion, paroxysmal nocturnal dyspnea, or orthopnea	ECG	ABG/oximetry Chest X-ray
Past medical history	Previous myocardial infarction, coronary artery bypass surgery, angioplasty, cocaine use within last 96 hours, previous positive cardiac diagnostic studies	ECG	
	Major risk factors for coronary artery disease		ECG
Assessment	Unstable angina—new-onset, exertional	ECG, aspirin	IV access Supplemental oxygen Cardiac monitor Nitrates Consult/Admit
	Unstable angina—Ongoing or recurrent ischemia ECG showing new ST-segment depressions or T-wave inversions consistent with ischemia	IV access Supplemental oxygen Cardiac monitor Anticoagulation Aspirin Nitrates Management of ongoing pain Admit	Serial serum cardiac markers Chest X-ray Cardiac imaging Serial ECGs Beta blockers
	High clinical suspicion of myocardial infarction with nondiagnostic ECG	IV access Supplemental oxygen Cardiac monitor Anticoagulation Aspirin Nitrates Management of ongoing pain Admit	Serial serum cardiac markers Chest X-ray Cardiac imaging Serial ECGs Magnesium therapy Beta blockers
	High clinical suspicion of myocardial infarction with diagnostic ECG or bundle branch block	IV access Supplemental oxygen Cardiac monitor Anticoagulation Assessment for thrombolytic therapy or other reperfusion techniques Anticoagulation Aspirin Nitrates Management of ongoing pain Admit	Serial serum cardiac markers Chest X-ray Cardiac imaging Serial ECGs Magnesium therapy if not given thrombolytics Beta blockers
	Aortic dissection	Large-bore IV access Supplemental oxygen Cardiac monitor Blood type and crossmatch ECG Management of blood pressure/cardiac contractility Management of ongoing pain Immediate surgical consultation Admit	Aortic imaging
	Pericarditis/myocarditis	ECG	Serum cardiac markers Chest X-ray/echocardiography Consult/admit

From American College of Emergency Physicians. Clinical policy for the initial approach to adults presenting with a chief complaint of chest pain, with no history of trauma. Ann. Emerg. Med. *25*:274, 1995.

gina, aortic dissection, and pulmonary embolus. Patients with possible or probable acute myocardial infarction as suggested by the description of their pain or electrocardiographic findings are expected to be admitted and receive interventions, including aspirin, nitrates, and—in the presence of ST-segment elevation on the electrocardiogram—anticoagulation, thrombolysis, and/or other therapy aimed at achieving reperfusion.

Performance of electrocardiography and initiation of aspirin therapy are strongly recommended for patients with new-onset angina that is exertional, but admission is not considered mandatory in the ACEP policy statement. The AHCPR guidelines also indicate that not all patients with unstable angina require admission but recommend that patients with unstable angina be monitored electrocardiographically during their evaluation and that those with ongoing rest pain should be placed at bed rest during the initial phase of stabilization[12] (see p. 1336).

Admission should be considered but is also not a rule for pericarditis and myocarditis. The ACEP policy statement indicates that patients who are discharged should be provided a referral for follow-up care and instructions regarding treatment and circumstances that require a return to the emergency department.

The ACEP policy statement includes in its appendix forms that can be used to assess compliance with their rules and to remind clinicians of their content.

ACUTE MYOCARDIAL INFARCTION

(See also Chap. 37)

Advances in the treatment of acute myocardial infarction have accelerated in recent years, with a particularly intense focus on the beneficial impact of thrombolytic therapy and percutaneous transluminal angioplasty in the early hours after the onset of infarction. Recent research, however, has also provided important insights into the limitations of interventions such as routine performance of angioplasty after myocardial infarction. To define practice patterns likely to achieve the optimal patient outcomes without subjecting patients to unnecessary procedures, guidelines for the management of acute myocardial infarction have been developed by the National Heart Attack Alert Program (NHAAP)[128] and an ACC/AHA task force.[129] These guidelines have complementary focuses: The NHAAP guidelines define a goal for time-to-treatment with thrombolytic therapy and provide practical strategies for reaching that goal. These recommendations from the NHAAP are essentially a "critical path" for treatment of acute myocardial infarction that defines time frames for the performance of specific tasks. The ACC/AHA task force examines a range of interventions that might be considered for patients with acute myocardial infarction and classifies them according to their appropriateness.

DIAGNOSIS OF MYOCARDIAL INFARCTION. Several alternative markers for myocardial injury are now available, but the ACC/AHA guidelines recommend basing the diagnosis of myocardial infarction upon creatine kinase (CK) -MB determinations in combination with serial electrocardiograms and a chest X-ray study. According to these guidelines, electrocardiograms should be obtained daily until the nature of evolution of the infarction is clear, and longer if patients have complications. Sampling of total CK and CK-MB is recommended at 6-hour intervals for the first 24 hours, and then daily until the diagnosis is established. Routine use of other enzyme assays, such as lactate dehydrogenase, is not recommended. The AHCPR guidelines for unstable angina[12] (see Tables 63–15, 63–16 and 63–17) offer slightly different, but qualitatively similar, recommendations:

> Total CK and CK-MB measured every 6 to 8 hours for the first 24 hours
>
> Serial lactate dehydrogenase (LDH) isoenzymes should be considered for patients presenting 24 to 72 hours after symptom onset if CK and CK-MB levels are normal.

More conservative recommendations for the use of cardiac enzyme assays are endorsed by the American College of Physicians.[130] These guidelines recommend a sampling interval of 12 hours, and do not support measurement of cardiac enzymes each day or until abnormal levels return to baseline. However, patients with unstable angina or electrocardiographic changes suggestive of active ischemic syndromes have a higher probability of acute myocardial infarction than the general population of patients with acute chest pain, and a strategy with increased frequency of enzyme sampling that is more sensitive for detecting CK-MB elevations is reasonable for a higher-risk population.

Initial Triage and Use of Thrombolytic Therapy

The NHAAP was initiated by the National Heart, Lung, and Blood Institute to promote rapid identification and treatment of acute myocardial infarction. The multidisciplinary expert panel examined the factors responsible for delay in administration of thrombolytic therapy and focused its main recommendations on decreasing the time between the patient's presentation at the hospital and the administration of thrombolytic therapy to 30 minutes or less. This target is similar to the 30- to 60-minute goal recommended by the American Heart Association.[131] The long-range goal of the NHAAP is to decrease the time from onset of symptoms to treatment to 60 minutes, but that effort will require community interventions that lead to earlier presentation to the hospital of patients with myocardial infarction.

Although these time targets have been described as guidelines, they more appropriately might be called recommended goals. Administration of thrombolytic therapy *more* than 30 minutes after presentation of a patient with acute myocardial infarction would not represent a deviation from a guideline or a variation from the standard of care. These time goals are instead intended to be used by institutions to understand whether they need to improve their system of care. To achieve this goal, the NHAAP recommends measuring the time at which four specific events occur for patients with acute myocardial infarction:

1. Presentation to the emergency department
2. Recording of the electrocardiogram
3. Decision whether to administer thrombolytic therapy
4. Actual infusion of the thrombolytic agent

These four time points can be used to define three intervals. In one multicenter thrombolytic trial, the median time from emergency department arrival to recording the electrocardiogram was 6 minutes; from recording the electrocardiogram to decision to use thrombolytic therapy, 20 minutes; from decision to drug administration, 20 minutes.[132]

Another crucial issue is who gives the order to administer thrombolytic therapy. ACEP guidelines recommend that emergency department physicians be given the authority to administer thrombolytic therapy.[127]

ELIGIBILITY FOR THROMBOLYTIC THERAPY. Eligibility criteria for administration of thrombolytic therapy according to the NHAAP guidelines are presented in Table 63–13. Similar criteria are endorsed by the AHCPR guidelines for unstable angina.[12] The eligibility criteria supported by the ACC/AHA task force[129] (see Table 63–14) recommend a lower threshold for administration of thrombolytic therapy for patients less than age 70 years and for those presenting in less than 6 hours after the onset of pain. There was little support for the use of thrombolytic therapy more than 6 hours after the onset of symptoms in these 1990 guidelines. Since then, a meta-analysis of studies of thrombolytic therapy concluded that mortality rates were significantly re-

TABLE 63–13 ELIGIBILITY/EXCLUSION CRITERIA FOR THROMBOLYTIC THERAPY

1. ELIGIBILITY CRITERIA

Clinical:
Chest pain or chest-pain-equivalent syndrome consistent with acute myocardial infarction ≤ 12 hours from symptom onset with:

ECG
- ≥1 mm ST elevation in ≥2 contiguous limb leads
- ≥2 mm ST elevation in ≥2 contiguous precordial leads
- New bundle branch block

Cardiogenic shock: emergency catheterization and revascularization if possible; consider thrombolysis if catheterization not immediately available.

2. CONTRAINDICATIONS

Absolute contraindications
- Altered consciousness
- Active internal bleeding
- Known spinal cord or cerebral arteriovenous malformation or tumor
- Recent head trauma
- Known previous hemorrhagic cerebrovascular accident
- Intracranial or intraspinal surgery within 2 months
- Trauma or surgery within 2 weeks, which could result in bleeding in a closed space
- Persistent blood pressure >200/120 mm Hg
- Known bleeding disorder
- Pregnancy
- Suspected aortic dissection
- Previous allergy to streptokinase (but not a contraindication to use of other thrombolytic agents)

Relative contraindications
- Active peptic ulcer disease
- History of ischemic or embolic cerebrovascular accident
- Current use of oral anticoagulants
- Major trauma or surgery >2 weeks, <2 months
- History of chronic, uncontrolled hypertension (diastolic >100 mm Hg), treated or untreated
- Subclavian or internal jugular venous cannulation

From National Heart Attack Alert Program Coordinating Committee 60 Minutes to Treatment Working Group. Emergency Department: Rapid Identification and Treatment of Patients with Acute Myocardial Infarction. NIH Publication No. 93-3278. Washington, D.C., National Heart, Lung and Blood Institute, Public Health Service, U.S. Department of Health and Human Services, Sept. 1993.

duced by this therapy for patients treated 7 to 12 hours after the onset of symptoms (11.1 versus 12.7 per cent), while the difference was not significant for patients treated 13 to 24 hours after onset of symptoms.[133]

The NHAAP contraindications to thrombolytic therapy[128] (Table 63–13) are similar to those noted by the ACC/AHA task force,[129] which also include as absolute contraindications prolonged or traumatic cardiopulmonary resuscitation and diabetic hemorrhagic retinopathy or other hemorrhagic ophthalmic condition. Significant liver dysfunction is included as a relative contraindication to thrombolytic therapy by the ACC/AHA guidelines.

Both NHAAP and ACC/AHA guidelines were written before the publication of the Global Utilization of Streptokinase and Tissue Plasminogen Activator for Occluded Coronary Arteries (GUSTO) study, which demonstrated a 1 per cent reduction in mortality for patients treated with accelerated tissue plasminogen activator (t-PA) versus streptokinase.[134] Two 1995 cost-effectiveness analyses based on data from GUSTO concluded that the cost-effectiveness of t-PA compares favorably with that of other accepted medical interventions.[135,136] Therefore, future guidelines may directly comment on the choice between these two agents.

Other Specific Interventions

ACC/AHA guidelines addressing several specific interventions often used for treatment of acute myocardial infarction were first published in 1990 and were undergoing revision in 1996. Like most ACC/AHA guidelines, the 1990 recommendations identify class I (appropriate) and class III (inappropriate) indications, but divide the class II interventions, which are considered acceptable but of uncertain efficacy, into two subclasses. Class IIa interventions are those for which the weight of evidence is in favor of their usefulness; Class IIb interventions are those that are not well established by evidence, may be useful, and probably are not harmful. Recommendations for interventions are summarized in Table 63–14.

ELECTROCARDIOGRAPHIC MONITORING. The duration of electrocardiographic monitoring in patients with uncomplicated myocardial infarction is a major determinant of cost, since the need for monitoring often dictates the level of care (and intensity of nursing) for the patient. The ACC/AHA guidelines recommend 48 to 72 hours of electrocardiographic monitoring, with longer periods for patients who have hemodynamic, ischemic, or arrhythmic complications. These guidelines consider 12 to 36 hours of monitoring appropriate for patients who are admitted with suspected myocardial infarction. Recent research indicates that shorter periods are safe for selected low-risk patients[120,125]; hence this guideline should not be interpreted as indicating that monitoring periods of 12 hours or more to "rule out" myocardial infarction are mandatory for all patients who are admitted.

HEMODYNAMIC MONITORING. Although hemodynamic monitoring with a balloon flotation right-heart catheter and/or arterial pressure line can provide useful data for management of patients with hypotension and other hemodynamic complications, both of these interventions are associated with a risk of vascular complications. Therefore, the ACC/AHA guidelines do not support use of hemodynamic monitoring in patients who are hemodynamically stable. Balloon flotation right-heart catheters are considered possibly useful (Class IIb) for patients with evidence of mild pulmonary congestion and probably useful (Class IIa) for patients with hypotension not responding to fluid administration, even in the absence of evidence of pulmonary congestion. Use of an arterial line is considered appropriate (Class I) or usually indicated (Class IIa) in patients receiving vasopressor, vasodilator, or inotropic agents.

LIDOCAINE. Lidocaine is the drug of choice for management of ventricular arrhythmias after acute myocardial infarction, but trials have failed to demonstrate that this therapy reduces overall mortality.[137] Furthermore, lidocaine can cause side effects, including sinus arrest and central nervous system depression. Therefore, the ACC/AHA guide-

Text continues on page 1978

TABLE 63–14 ACC/AHA GUIDELINES FOR THE EARLY MANAGEMENT OF ACUTE MYOCARDIAL INFARCTION

ISSUE	CLASS I—USUALLY INDICATED	CLASS II—ACCEPTABLE, OF UNCERTAIN EFFICACY: A. Evidence Favors Efficacy	CLASS II—ACCEPTABLE, OF UNCERTAIN EFFICACY: B. Not Well Established By Evidence	CLASS III—NOT INDICATED
Atropine use in first 6 to 8 hours after onset of myocardial infarction	**1.** Sinus bradycardia with evidence of low cardiac output and peripheral hypoperfusion or frequent premature ventricular contractions at onset of symptoms of acute myocardial infarction. **2.** Acute inferior infarction with symptomatic type I 2nd degree AV block. **3.** Bradycardia and hypotension after nitroglycerin administration. **4.** For nausea and vomiting associated with morphine administration. **5.** Asystole	**1.** Administration concomitantly with (before or after) morphine in the presence of sinus bradycardia, even without evidence of low cardiac output or peripheral hypoperfusion. **2.** Asymptomatic patients with inferior infarction and type I 2nd degree heart block or 3rd degree heart block at the level of the AV node (see Class III-2.)	None	**1.** Sinus bradycardia >40 beats/min without signs or symptoms of hypoperfusion or frequent premature ventricular contractions. **2.** AV block at the His-Purkinje level (i.e., type II AV block and 3rd degree AV block with new wide QRS complex).
Electrocardiographic monitoring	**1.** Patients with acute myocardial infarction during the initial 48 to 72 hours. **2.** Patients >72 hours after acute myocardial infarction who have hemodynamic instability, persistent ischemia, or arrhythmia. **3.** Patients with suspected myocardial infarction ("rule out" myocardial infarction) during the initial 12 to 36 hours. **4.** Patients who have a temporary transvenous pacemaker.	**1.** Patients >72 hours after acute myocardial infarction with a high likelihood of intermittent ischemia or complex ventricular arrhythmias. **2.** Patients with chest pain in whom there is a low likelihood of myocardial infarction.	Monitoring >72 hours after myocardial infarction, particularly if the patient has undergone thrombolysis or angioplasty.	Patients with or without known heart disease in whom there is no evidence of myocardial ischemia, recent infarction, or arrhythmia.
Right heart catheterization	**1.** Severe or progressive congestive heart failure. **2.** Cardiogenic shock or progressive hypotension. **3.** Mechanical complications of acute infarction, such as a ventricular septal defect or papillary muscle rupture.	**1.** Hypotension not responding rapidly to fluid administration in a patient without evidence of pulmonary congestion. **2.** Before giving a fluid challenge in a patient with circulatory insufficiency and suspected pulmonary congestion. **3.** As a diagnostic tool when there is suspicion of an intracardiac shunt, acute mitral insufficiency, or pericardial tamponade.	Patients with acute myocardial infarction who are hemodynamically stable but have evidence of mild pulmonary congestion.	Patients with acute myocardial infarction who are hemodynamically stable and without evidence of cardiac or pulmonary congestion.
Intraarterial pressure monitoring	**1.** Patients with severe hypotension (systolic <80 mm Hg) or cardiogenic shock. **2.** Patients receiving vasopressor agents.	**1.** Patients receiving intravenous nitroprusside or other powerful arterial dilating agents. **2.** Hemodynamically stable patients receiving intravenous vasodilators for myocardial ischemia. **3.** Patients receiving intravenous inotropic agents. **4.** Patients with life-threatening arrhythmias.	None	Patients with acute myocardial infarction who are hemodynamically stable.
Lidocaine use	**1.** In patients with acute myocardial ischemia or infarction, or both, with ventricular premature beats that are: **a.** frequent (>6/min) **b.** closely coupled (R on T), **c.** multiform in configuration, or **d.** occurring in short bursts of three or more in succession.	In patients with suspected acute myocardial infarction or ischemia or both, with indications as in Class I.	Prophylactic administration in the presence of uncomplicated acute myocardial ischemia or infarction or both, without ventricular premature beats in patients <70 and within the first 6 hours of onset of symptoms.	Patients with proved allergic or hypersensitivity reactions to lidocaine.

TABLE 63–14 ACC/AHA GUIDELINES FOR THE EARLY MANAGEMENT OF ACUTE MYOCARDIAL INFARCTION—*Continued*

ISSUE	CLASS I—USUALLY INDICATED	CLASS II—ACCEPTABLE, OF UNCERTAIN EFFICACY A. Evidence Favors Efficacy	CLASS II—ACCEPTABLE, OF UNCERTAIN EFFICACY B. Not Well Established By Evidence	CLASS III—NOT INDICATED
Lidocaine use—*Continued*	**2.** In patients with ventricular tachycardia or ventricular fibrillation or both, in association with defibrillation and cardiopulmonary resuscitation as indicated.			
Temporary pacemaker implantation	**1.** Asystole **2.** Complete heart block **3.** Right bundle branch block with left anterior or left posterior hemiblock developing in acute myocardial infarction. **4.** Left bundle branch block developing in acute myocardial infarction. **5.** Type II 2nd degree AV block. **6.** Symptomatic bradycardia not responsive to atropine.	**1.** Type I 2nd degree AV block with hypotension not responsive to atropine. **2.** Sinus bradycardia with hypotension not responsive to atropine. **3.** Recurrent sinus pauses not responsive to atropine. **4.** Atrial or ventricular overdrive pacing for incessant ventricular tachycardia.	**1.** Left bundle branch block with 1st degree heart block of unknown duration. **2.** Bifascicular block of unknown duration.	**1.** First degree heart block. **2.** Type I 2nd degree AV block with normal hemodynamics. **3.** Accelerated idioventricular rhythm causing AV dissociation. **4.** Bundle branch block known to exist before the myocardial infarction.
Transfer to a tertiary care facility equipped for angioplasty and cardiovascular surgery	**1.** Patients with recurrent pain. **2.** Patients with hemodynamic instability as manifested by persistent congestive heart failure, arterial hypotension or cardiogenic shock. **3.** Patients with resistant, recurrent ventricular arrhythmias (ventricular tachycardia or fibrillation)	**1.** Patients with high-risk myocardial infarction and contraindications to thrombolytic therapy but in whom it is reasonable to expect that reperfusion can be accomplished by percutaneous transluminal coronary angioplasty or coronary artery bypass grafting within 6 hours. **2.** Patients who are stable late in initial hospitalization but who are to be evaluated for angioplasty or bypass grafting before discharge. **3.** Patients in the early hours of acute myocardial infarction who have had prior bypass grafting and who may be candidates for angioplasty or regrafting.	**1.** Patients in stable condition in the early hours of acute myocardial infarction after thrombolysis but are in a facility in which coronary angioplasty or surgery cannot be performed. **2.** Stable patients with early acute transmural infraction and extensive ST-T changes.	
Echocardiography in the early phase of acute myocardial infarction	**1.** Myocardial infarction associated with shock or profound pump failure consistent with extensive myocardial dysfunction or a potentially surgically remediable lesion. **2.** Myocardial infarction associated with extensive infarction (ECG localization and peak MB CK > 150 IU/liter [or total CK > 1.000 IU/liter]). **3.** Myocardial infarction accompanied by clinical complications suggestive of pump failure, refractory angina or pericardial tamponade, associated valvular or congenital heart disease, or suspected pericarditis or pericardial effusion, or in patients being or to be treated with calcium antagonists or beta blockers in whom left ventricular function may be compromised.	**1.** Myocardial infarction superimposed on previous infarction or associated with ECG phenomena such as left bundle branch block or posterior locus that may obscure diagnosis, in which case delineation of regional wall motion abnormalities may help confirm the diagnosis and provide prognostically important information. **2.** Myocardial infarction with suspected concomitant right ventricular infarction (such as true posterior infarction) to define the severity of right ventricular involvement as a guide to management and to exclude pericardial tamponade.	Myocardial infarction of modest extent without clinical complications for evaluation of prognosis.	None

Table continues on the following page

TABLE 63–14 ACC/AHA GUIDELINES FOR THE EARLY MANAGEMENT OF ACUTE MYOCARDIAL INFARCTION—*Continued*

ISSUE	CLASS I—USUALLY INDICATED	CLASS II—ACCEPTABLE, OF UNCERTAIN EFFICACY: A. Evidence Favors Efficacy	CLASS II—ACCEPTABLE, OF UNCERTAIN EFFICACY: B. Not Well Established By Evidence	CLASS III—NOT INDICATED
Early IV beta blockade	**1.** Patients, including those receiving thrombolytic therapy, with reflex tachycardia or systolic hypertension or both, without signs of congestive heart failure or contraindication to beta blockade. **2.** Patients with continuing or recurrent ischemic pain, tachyarrhythmias such as atrial fibrillation with a rapid ventricular response, or an enzyme elevation thought to represent recurrent injury with no contraindication to beta blockade. **3.** Postinfarction angina while awaiting study in patients without contraindications.	**1.** Other patients without contraindication to beta blockade who can be treated within the first 12 hours from the onset of chest pain. **2.** Non-Q-wave myocardial infarction	None	Patients with moderate to severe left ventricular failure and other contraindications to beta blockade.
Long-term beta blockade in secondary prevention	All but low-risk patients who do not have a clear contraindication to beta blockade. Treatment should ordinarily begin within the first few days of infarction and should be continued for at least 2 years.	Low-risk patients who do not have a clear contraindication to beta blockade.	None	Patients with contraindications to beta blockade.
Calcium channel blockers	Symptomatic treatment of postinfarction angina while awaiting cardiac catheterization and therapy based on angiographic findings.	**1.** Diltiazem in patients with non-Q-wave infarction in whom no contraindication exists. **2.** After angioplasty, a calcium channel blocker to prevent coronary vasospasm.	A calcium channel blocker may be used in transmural (Q-wave) infarction for treatment of postinfarction angina, especially if contraindications to proceeding with coronary arteriography and more definitive treatment exist.	Calcium channel blockers that suppress ventricular function in patients with myocardial infarction complicated by pulmonary congestion or left ventricular dysfunction.
Anticoagulation and platelet inhibitory agents Prevention of deep vein thrombosis and pulmonary embolism	**1.** Immediate subcutaneous heparin (5,000 U every 12 hours) for the first 24 to 48 hours unless full-dose anticoagulant therapy has been initiated in association with thrombolytic therapy or for the prevention of systemic emboli. **2.** Continued low-dose subcutaneous heparin in high-risk patients (age >70, large acute myocardial infarction, previous myocardial infarction, heart failure or shock, necessity for immobilization for >3 days, prior deep venous thrombosis or pulmonary emboli, obesity, or evidence of chronic venous insufficiency) until fully ambulatory.	None	None	None
Anticoagulation and platelet inhibitory agents Prevention of arterial embolism	**1.** Immediate high-dose SC or IV heparin in a dosage sufficient to prolong the activated partial thromboplastin time to 1.5 to 2.0 times control in patients with a large anterior transmural myocardial infarction. Heparin should be continued until discharge. **2.** Oral anticoagulants administered at a dose sufficient to prolong the prothrombin time to 1.3 to 1.5 times the control value (INR = 2.0 to 3.0) after heparin in patients who have a	Long-term (indefinite) oral anticoagulant therapy in patients with a diffusely dilated and poorly contracting left ventricle. (Prolong prothrombin time to 1.3 to 1.5 times the control value, or INR = 2.0 to 3.0.)	In patients with anterior myocardial infarction requiring anticoagulation up to 3 months for the prevention of systemic emboli, low-dose aspirin (80 to 160 mg/day) to prevent coronary events may be added to the anticoagulants and then continued alone indefinitely.	None

TABLE 63–14 ACC/AHA GUIDELINES FOR THE EARLY MANAGEMENT OF ACUTE MYOCARDIAL INFARCTION—*Continued*

ISSUE	CLASS I—USUALLY INDICATED	CLASS II—ACCEPTABLE, OF UNCERTAIN EFFICACY A. Evidence Favors Efficacy	CLASS II—ACCEPTABLE, OF UNCERTAIN EFFICACY B. Not Well Established By Evidence	CLASS III—NOT INDICATED
	ventricular mural thrombus or a large akinetic region of the apex of the left ventricle. Anticoagulant therapy should be continued for at least 3 months.			
Anticoagulation and platelet inhibitory agents The reduction of early recurrence or extension of myocardial infarction and mortality in patients not receiving thrombolytic therapy	Short-term aspirin begun immediately and continued for at least 1 month at a dose of 160 mg/day. After 1 month, aspirin should be continued at a dose of 160 to 325 mg/day.	Heparin followed by oral anticoagulant therapy for at least 1 month after infarction (prolong prothrombin time to 1.3 to 1.5 times control value).	None	None
Anticoagulation and platelet inhibitory agents Reduction in early reocclusion and in mortality after successful reperfusion with thrombolytic therapy	**1.** Aspirin (160 mg/day) started as soon as the patient is admitted and given daily until hospital discharge, at which time it can be continued at 160 to 325 mg daily. **2.** Heparin should be administered together with or immediately after thrombolysis to maintain the activated partial thromboplastin time approximately 1.5 to 2.0 times the control value for 24 to 72 hours.	None	None	None
Anticoagulation and platelet inhibitory agents Secondary prevention of late recurrence of myocardial infarction and death	Aspirin (160 to 325 mg daily) if not associated with significant side effects.	Oral anticoagulant therapy with warfarin (prothrombin time 1.3 to 1.5 times the control value, or INR = 2.0 to 3.0) rather than aspirin for long-term prevention of myocardial infarction recurrence.	None	None
Percutaneous transluminal coronary angioplasty Angioplasty after IV thrombolysis	Dilation of a significant lesion suitable for coronary angioplasty in the infarct-related artery in patients who are in the low-risk group for angiographic-related morbidity and mortality who have a type A lesion and: **1.** Have recurrent episodes of ischemic chest pain particularly if accompanied by ECG changes (postinfarction angina). **2.** Show evidence of myocardial ischemia while on optimal medical therapy during submaximal stress testing performed before hospital discharge or on maximal stress testing in the early posthospital period. **3.** Have recurrent ventricular tachycardia or ventricular fibrillation or both, convincingly related to ischemia while on antiarrhythmic therapy.	Dilation of significant lesions in patients who: **1.** Are similar to those in class I but who have type B lesions (anticipated success rate 60 to 85%). **2.** Are within 18 hours of onset of acute infarction and have cardiogenic shock or pump failure. **3.** Before hospital discharge in those who have survived cardiogenic shock or pump failure.	Dilation of a lesion in patients who: **1.** Have an occluded coronary artery after attempted thrombolytic therapy. **2.** Require multivessel angioplasty. **3.** Have >90% diameter proximal narrowing of an infarct-related artery with a large area of viable myocardium still at risk.	All patients in the immediate postinfarct period who do not fulfill Class I or II criteria such as: **1.** Patients within the early hours of an evolving myocardial infarction and have <50% residual stenosis of the infarct-related artery after receiving a thrombolytic agent. **2.** Lesions in vessels other than the infarct-related artery within early hours of infarction. **3.** Residual lesions that are borderline in severity (50 to 70% diameter narrowing) of the infarct-related artery without demonstration of ischemia on functional testing.

Table continued on the following page

ISSUE	CLASS I—USUALLY INDICATED	CLASS II—ACCEPTABLE, OF UNCERTAIN EFFICACY: A. Evidence Favors Efficacy	CLASS II—ACCEPTABLE, OF UNCERTAIN EFFICACY: B. Not Well Established By Evidence	CLASS III—NOT INDICATED
Intraaortic balloon counterpulsation or other circulatory assist devices	**1.** Cardiogenic shock or pump failure not responding promptly to pharmacological therapy. **2.** Right ventricular infarction with pump failure or shock not responding to volume infusion and appropriate pharmacological therapy. **3.** Refractory postinfarction angina for stabilization before and during angiography. **4.** Intractable recurrent tachycardia in patients with hemodynamic instability during the arrhythmia.	**1.** Ventricular septal rupture **2.** Acute mitral insufficiency **3.** Persistent ischemic pain **4.** Progressive congestive heart failure despite pharmacological therapy, particularly as a bridge to more definitive therapy.	None	**1.** A patient who is reasonably stable and in whom balloon insertion may delay more definitive therapy. **2.** Severe peripheral vascular disease and fewer indications than in Class I.
Emergency or urgent coronary bypass surgery in early management of myocardial infarction	**1.** Failed angioplasty with persistent pain or hemodynamic instability. **2.** Postinfarct angina with left main or 3-vessel disease or where coronary angioplasty is not indicated, with 2-vessel disease involving the proximal left anterior descending coronary artery or 2-vessel disease and poor left ventricular function.	**1.** At the time of surgical repair of ventricular septal defect or acute mitral insufficiency. **2.** Cardiogenic shock not suitable for angioplasty.	None	Where the available surgical mortality rate exceeds the mortality rate associated with appropriate medical therapy.
Emergency or urgent cardiac repair	**1.** Papillary muscle rupture (emergency). **2.** Ventricular septal defect or free wall rupture (urgent). **3.** Aneurysmal infarction with intractable ventricular arrhythmias or pump failure (urgent), or both. **4.** Acute mitral insufficiency with intractable failure (urgent). **5.** Intractable ventricular tachycardia (urgent).	**1.** Ventricular septal defect or free wall rupture (emergency). **2.** Severe mitral insufficiency with controlled failure (urgent).	None	**1.** Acute infarctectomy in hemodynamically stable patients. **2.** Surgery when the operative mortality rate exceeds the expected mortality rate associated with conservative therapy.
Implantable ventricular assist devices	None	None	As a bridge in a patient with intractable pump failure who would be a reasonable candidate for cardiac transplantation.	None
Noninvasive evaluation of patients at low risk by clinical indicators†	**1.** Stress ECG **a.** Before discharge for prognostic assessment (submaximal at 6 to 10 days or symptom-limited at 10 to 14 days). **b.** Early after discharge for prognostic assessment and functional capacity (3 weeks). **c.** Late after discharge (3 to 8 weeks) for functional capacity and prognosis if early stress was submaximal. **2.** Exercise thallium-201 scintigraphy (whenever baseline abnormalities of the ECG compromise its interpretation).	**1.** Exercise thallium-201 scintigraphy; before discharge for prognostic assessment with symptom-limited exercise at 10 to 14 days. **2.** Dipyridamole thallium-201 scintigraphy (before discharge for prognostic assessment in patients judged to be unable to perform exercise). **3.** Exercise radionuclide ventriculography predischarge at 10 to 14 days or early after discharge for prognostic assessment. **4.** Exercise two-dimensional echocardiography (before discharge or early after discharge for prognostic assessment).	**1.** Stress ECG **a.** In patients with baseline ECG abnormalities or coexisting medical problems that limit ability to achieve maximal exertion. **b.** Before discharge or early after discharge to evaluate patients who have sustained complicated myocardial infarction but who have subsequently "stabilized" and for whom a decision for invasive evaluation has not been made. **2.** Exercise thallium-201 myocardial scintigraphy (late after discharge at 6 to 8 weeks for prognostic assessment).	**1.** Stress ECG **a.** Within 72 hours of acute myocardial infarction. **b.** At any time to evaluate patients having unstable postinfarction angina pectoris. **c.** At any time to evaluate patients with acute myocardial infarction who have uncompensated congestive heart failure, cardiac arrhythmia, or noncardiac conditions that severely limit their ability to exercise. **d.** Before discharge to evaluate patients who have already been selected for cardiac catheterization.

TABLE 63–14 ACC/AHA GUIDELINES FOR THE EARLY MANAGEMENT OF ACUTE MYOCARDIAL INFARCTION—*Continued*

		CLASS II—ACCEPTABLE, OF UNCERTAIN EFFICACY		
ISSUE	CLASS I—USUALLY INDICATED	A. Evidence Favors Efficacy	B. Not Well Established By Evidence	CLASS III—NOT INDICATED
Noninvasive evaluation of patients at low risk by clinical indicators†— *Continued*			**3.** Dipyridamole thallium or dobutamine thallium before discharge in patients judged unable to exercise.	
Rest radionuclide ventriculography	Predischarge rest radionuclide ventriculography to determine the high-risk subset unless determination of ventricular function has been made by other means.	For shunt detection in patients with suspected ventricular septal defect (pulmonary artery injection).	None	**1.** Predischarge radionuclide ventriculography to detect left ventricular thrombus. **2.** Where similar information can be derived from other tests already performed or scheduled.
Two-dimensional echocardiography at rest	Detection or confirmation of suspected complications of infarction; tissue rupture, aneurysm or pseudoaneurysm formation, infarct extension or expansion, mural thrombus, and right ventricular infarction.	For evaluation of left ventricular function in predicting a low-risk subgroup for ambulation and early discharge from CCU.	Prediction of patients with multivessel coronary artery disease by the detection of remote asynergy.	Where similar information has been obtained from other tests already performed or scheduled.
Ambulatory electrocardiographic monitoring	None	After myocardial infarction, in patients with moderate to severe left ventricular dysfunction, or with significant ventricular ectopic activity in the CCU or stepdown telemetry unit for prognostic assessment.	**1.** After myocardial infarction, in patients to determine heart rate variability for prognostic assessment. **2.** In high-risk postmyocardial infarction as screened for silent ischemia.	Uncomplicated ambulatory patients after discharge as a routine screen.
Coronary angiography Late evolving MI (after the initial 6 hours)	**1.** Patients with recurrent episodes of ischemic chest pain, particularly if accompanied by ECG changes. **2.** Patients suspected of acute mitral regurgitation or a ruptured interventricular septum causing heart failure or shock. **3.** Patients suspected of developing subacute cardiac rupture (pseudoaneurysm). **4.** Patients with cardiogenic shock or severe pump failure.	**1.** Patients with congestive heart failure during intensive medical therapy. **2.** Patients with recurrent ventricular tachycardia or ventricular fibrillation or both during intensive antiarrhythmic therapy.	Asymptomatic patients who were given thrombolytic therapy during the evolving phase.	Patients with uncomplicated completed myocardial infarction in whom no acute mechanical or surgical intervention is contemplated.
Coronary angiography Convalescent myocardial infarction (immediate predischarge up to 8 weeks after discharge)	**1.** Postinfarction angina pectoris. **2.** Patients with evidence of myocardial ischemia on laboratory testing.	**1.** Patients with the need to return to unusually active and vigorous physical employment. **2.** Patients with a left ventricular ejection fraction < 40%.	**1.** As a routine in patients receiving thrombolytic therapy during the evolving phase of infarction. **2.** Otherwise uncomplicated and asymptomatic patients who are < 45. **3.** Patients with uncomplicated non-Q-wave infarction without evidence of myocardial ischemia on noninvasive laboratory testing.	**1.** Patients judged to have a debilitating disease or conditions that preclude invasive intervention. **2.** Patients with very advanced left ventricular dysfunction (ejection fraction <20%) in the absence of angina pectoris or evidence of ischemia. **3.** Patients with ventricular arrhythmias who have no evidence of ischemia symptomatically or during exercise testing, well-preserved exercise tolerance, and no suggestion of aneurysm formation.

* Likely to be affected by subsequent randomized trials. † Timing likely to be modified by trend toward shorter hospital stay.

Class I: Usually indicated, always acceptable, and considered useful/effective.

Class II: Acceptable, of uncertain efficacy and may be controversial. a: Weight of evidence usefulness/efficacy. b: Not well established by evidence; can be helpful, probably not harmful.

Class III: Not indicated and may be harmful.

From Gunnar, R. M., Bourdillon, P. D. V., Dixon, D. W., et al.: Guidelines for the early management of patients with acute myocardial infarction. A report of the ACC/AHA Task Force on Assessment of Diagnostic and Therapeutic Cardiovascular Procedures. Reprinted with permission from the American College of Cardiology. J. Am. Coll. Cardiol. *16*:249, 1990.

Addenda: Long-term beta blockers: Treatment to begin within the first few days of infarction and continued for at least 2 years. Decisions concerning beta blockade withdrawal (or dose reduction) because of drug side effects should take into account the risk status of the individual patient (that is, the decision to reduce or discontinue should be controlled by weighing side effects more heavily as one moves from high- to low-risk patients).

lines consider lidocaine therapy appropriate (Class I) for patients with acute myocardial ischemia or infarction who have ventricular premature beats with characteristics that suggest a high risk for cardiac arrest. Use of lidocaine is discouraged (Class IIb) in uncomplicated acute myocardial ischemia or infarction without ventricular premature beats in patients less than 70 years of age and within the first 6 hours of the onset of symptoms.

USE OF TEMPORARY PACEMAKERS. The ACC/AHA guidelines recommend temporary pacemakers for patients with asystole and complete heart block or with conduction disturbances with a high risk of progressing to these catastrophic arrhythmias. Pacemakers are also supported for bradycardia that causes symptoms or hypotension and is not responsive to atropine. The ACC/AHA task force also considers use of pacemakers to overdrive incessant ventricular tachycardia an acceptable if unproven strategy (Class IIa). However, these guidelines do not support the use of pacemakers for conduction abnormalities that do not cause symptoms or hemodynamic compromise. Guidelines for the use of permanent pacemakers are reviewed on page 1963.

TRANSPORTATION. The decision to transfer a patient to a facility that can perform interventions such as angioplasty and coronary artery bypass graft surgery requires weighing potential benefits against the risk of complications during the transfer. The ACC/AHA guidelines support transfer to a tertiary care facility of patients with major ischemic, hemodynamic, or arrhythmic complications, all of which are deemed Class I indications for transfer. This task force considers transfer acceptable and probably beneficial (Class IIa) for patients who might benefit from reperfusion therapy with either angioplasty or coronary artery bypass graft surgery either early or late in the hospitalization. However, routine transfer of stable patients to tertiary facility is not recommended.

BETA-ADRENERGIC BLOCKING DRUGS. Randomized trials have now demonstrated that beta-adrenergic blocking agents can both limit myocardial damage when administered during the first few hours of infarction and reduce the risk of reinfarction or death when administered after infarction. The ACC/AHA guidelines therefore are generally supportive of the early and late use of beta blockers after myocardial infarction in patients without contraindications. Specific *contraindications* to beta blockers include:

- Heart rate less than 60 beats/min
- Systolic blood pressure less than 100 mm Hg
- Moderate to severe left ventricular failure
- Signs of peripheral hypoperfusion
- P-R interval more than 0.22 second
- Type I and II AV block or complete heart block
- Severe chronic obstructive pulmonary disease

Relative contraindications include history of asthma, severe peripheral vascular disease, and difficult to control insulin-dependent diabetes.

The guidelines do not express a preference between cardioselective and nonselective beta blockers, but recommend avoiding agents with intrinsic sympathomimetic activity. Daily dosages of the beta blockers, such as 180 mg to 240 mg/day of propranolol, have been high in randomized trials,[138] but studies have not defined the lowest possible dose that is efficacious. A period of treatment of at least 2 years is supported by the guidelines.

CALCIUM CHANNEL BLOCKERS. Randomized trials have not demonstrated that calcium channel blocking agents are beneficial after acute myocardial infarction[139] except in the subset of patients with non-Q-wave infarction in which early reinfarction and recurrent angina were reduced in patients given diltiazem 90 mg every 6 hours.[140] Therefore, the ACC/AHA guidelines do not support use of this class of drugs after myocardial infarction except for patients with postinfarction angina. Acceptable other indications (Class IIa) include use of diltiazem after angioplasty to prevent coronary spasm and in patients with non-Q-wave infarction. In the latter setting, diltiazem should be started during the first 48 hours and continued through the hospital phase and the first postinfarction year.

ANTICOAGULATION AND PLATELET INHIBITORY AGENTS. The ACC/AHA guidelines support administration of intravenous heparin and aspirin for several indications in patients with acute myocardial infarction:

- To prevent reocclusion of the infarct artery: Intravenous heparin and aspirin are both considered appropriate (Class I) for patients who receive thrombolytic therapy.
- To prevent deep venous thrombosis: Immediate subcutaneous heparin is recommended for the first 24 to 48 hours, with continued treatment for patients at increased risk for venous thrombosis.
- To prevent arterial embolism: "Therapeutic" anticoagulation for periods up to 3 months is considered appropriate for patients with large anterior transmural myocardial infarctions, ventricular mural thrombus, or a large akinetic region of the apex of the left ventricle (Table 63–14). For patients at high risk for arterial embolism, continued anticoagulation is recommended for at least 3 months.
- Reduction of early and late recurrence or extension of myocardial infarction: For patients who do not receive thrombolytic therapy, immediate initiation of aspirin is considered appropriate. Continued use of aspirin is endorsed for patients who do not have side effects from this medication. Anticoagulation with heparin followed by warfarin therapy is considered acceptable and probably useful (Class IIa).

PERCUTANEOUS TRANSLUMINAL CORONARY ANGIOPLASTY. The ACC/AHA guidelines for acute myocardial infarction and for PTCA were both developed before publication of randomized trials indicating that primary PTCA was effective and potentially superior therapy for acute myocardial infarction compared with thrombolysis.[68–70] The 1990 ACC/AHA guidelines considered primary PTCA clearly appropriate only for patients in whom thrombolytic therapy is clearly contraindicated, and only when a large amount of myocardium is at risk. Revisions of the myocardial infarction guidelines can be expected to provide more support for primary PTCA. The choice between thrombolytic therapy and PTCA when both therapies are available should be influenced by the time frame in which PTCA can be performed. The 1990 ACC/AHA guidelines for acute myocardial infarction considered performance of PTCA within 1 hour "acceptable" (Class IIb), but subsequent and future research may provide better insight into what can be considered an appropriate time goal for invasive revascularization. See previous section of guidelines for PTCA for further discussion of more recent (1993) ACC/AHA guidelines for the role of PTCA after acute myocardial infarction (see p. 1954).

INTRAAORTIC BALLOON COUNTERPULSATION OR OTHER CIRCULATORY ASSIST DEVICES. Pump failure and cardiogenic shock indicate a poor prognosis for patients with acute myocardial infarction, and ACC/AHA guidelines for acute myocardial infarction recommend that all patients with pump failure be transferred to facilities equipped to perform angioplasty and cardiovascular surgery, particularly if the patient is seen during the first 12 to 24 hours after onset of infarction. These guidelines emphasize that these patients need early angiographic evaluations so that interventions can be undertaken before hemodynamic deterioration becomes irreversible.

Intraaortic balloon counterpulsation or other circulatory assist devices can be used to stabilize the condition of patients until such evaluations can be completed. The ACC/AHA guidelines consider use of these devices appropriate in patients with cardiogenic shock that does not respond promptly to pharmacological therapy, and for patients with refractory postinfarction angina or recurrent ventricular tachycardia leading to hemodynamic instability. The use of these devices is considered acceptable and probably useful (Class IIb) for mechanical complications such as ventricular septal rupture and acute mitral insufficiency and for patients with persistent ischemic pain or progressive congestive heart failure. The guidelines do not support use of these devices in patients whose condition was stable after myocardial infarction.

CORONARY ARTERY BYPASS SURGERY. The use of emergency coronary artery bypass graft surgery as primary therapy for acute myocardial infarction is discouraged by both the 1990 ACC/AHA guidelines for acute myocardial infarction and the 1991 ACC/AHA guidelines for coronary artery bypass graft surgery. Thrombolysis and angioplasty are instead regarded as first choice strategies, with CABG reserved for patients with failed PTCA or postinfarction angina that is found to be due to coronary anatomy configurations that do not lend themselves to angioplasty. CABG is also considered appropriate for patient subsets in which this procedure has been found to increase survival, compared with medical therapy.

Coronary bypass surgery is endorsed, however, as an emergent or urgent treatment for severe mechanical or arrhythmic complications. The use of ventricular assist devices as bridge therapy for patients who might be candidates for cardiac transplantation is considered acceptable but unproven (Class IIb).

Postinfarction Evaluation

The ACC/AHA guidelines for acute myocardial infarction describe three strategies for risk stratification of patients after infarction, all of which are based on identifying patients whose clinical characteristics place them at high risk for subsequent complications, directing them toward early invasive evaluations. For risk stratification of other patients, the next step in the evaluation is a submaximal exercise test performed before discharge or a full symptom-limited test after discharge from the hospital. These 1990 guidelines were based on the assumption that patients without major complications remain in the hospital for 7 to 14 days, whereas shorter stays have become more common in recent years. Therefore, revisions of these guidelines can be expected to modify the time frame in which exercise tests are performed.

Choices among the techniques used to detect ischemia (electrocardiography, radionuclide imaging, echocardiography) and the methods used to provoke ischemia (exercise, pharmacological agent) are not the subject of explicit recommendations in the ACC/AHA guidelines. These guidelines also do not address directly which patients *should* undergo which tests (if any) to assess left ventricular function or the presence of asymptomatic arrhythmia. Instead, the guidelines endorse as appropriate or acceptable the use of these techniques in various clinical settings in which the probability of detecting abnormalities is greater.

The appropriateness of coronary angiography in the early or late periods after acute myocardial infarction is directly related to the appropriateness of revascularization procedures such as PTCA. The ACC/AHA guidelines discourage coronary angiography for patients having uncomplicated courses or as routine after intravenous thrombolytic therapy. Coronary angiography is also not supported for patients with cardiac or noncardiac conditions that render them unlikely to benefit from invasive revascularization therapy.

UNSTABLE ANGINA

(See also Chap. 38)

Practice guidelines for the treatment of unstable angina were issued in 1994 by a multidisciplinary panel sponsored by the Agency for Health Care Policy and Research (AHCPR). These guidelines differ qualitatively from the series of guidelines developed by the ACC/AHA task forces, which tend to rate the appropriateness of use of an intervention in various settings. In contrast, the AHCPR guidelines seek to describe optimal overall management strategies and to rate the strength of the evidence supporting specific recommendations. Hence the AHCPR guidelines include flow sheets that schematically summarize management plans, and use the following grading scale to describe the data addressing a specific issue:

- A = at least one randomized controlled trial as part of a body of literature of overall good quality and consistency
- B = well-conducted clinical studies but no randomized clinical trials
- C = absence of directly applicable clinical studies of good quality

These guidelines include a broad spectrum of illness under the topic of unstable angina. Three basic presentations include symptoms of angina at rest, usually prolonged for more than 20 minutes, new-onset (less than 2 months) exertional angina that is Canadian Cardiovascular Society Class (CCSC) III or IV in severity, and recent (less than 2 months) acceleration of angina, with an increase in severity of at least one CCSC class to CCSC class III or IV. Variant angina, non-Q-wave myocardial infarction, and angina occurring more than 24 hours after acute myocardial infarction are also considered unstable angina.

The overall management strategy of the AHCPR guidelines is summarized in Figure 63–1. Principal conclusions of the guidelines include:

1. Many patients suspected of having unstable angina can be discharged home after adequate initial evaluation. Further outpatient evaluation should be concluded within 72 hours after initial evaluation.
2. Patients with unstable angina who are judged to be at intermediate or high risk of complications should be hospitalized and receive aspirin, heparin, nitroglycerin, and beta blocker therapy.
3. Intravenous thrombolytic therapy should not be administered to patients without evidence of acute myocardial infarction.
4. Noninvasive testing can often guide therapy selection.

Initial Evaluation and Treatment

The AHCPR guidelines rely on early assessment of the probability that a patient has coronary disease and the patient's risk of death or myocardial infarction. Combinations of features that place patients in groups with high, intermediate, and low probabilities of these outcomes are summarized in Tables 63–15 and 63–16. As noted in the section on Acute Chest Pain (see p. 1967), the guidelines emphasize that ECG data are crucial for this assessment; hence this evaluation cannot be made over the telephone. In patients with prolonged pain (more than 20 minutes), hemodynamic instability, or symptoms of arrhythmia, evaluation should take place in an emergency department. The guidelines recommend that evaluation in such patients, including the electrocardiogram, be completed within 20 minutes of arrival at the medical facility. In the absence of these adverse prognostic signs, the evaluation can sometimes be performed in an outpatient office.

During the initial evaluation, the guidelines recommend the use of continuous electrocardiographic monitoring, and

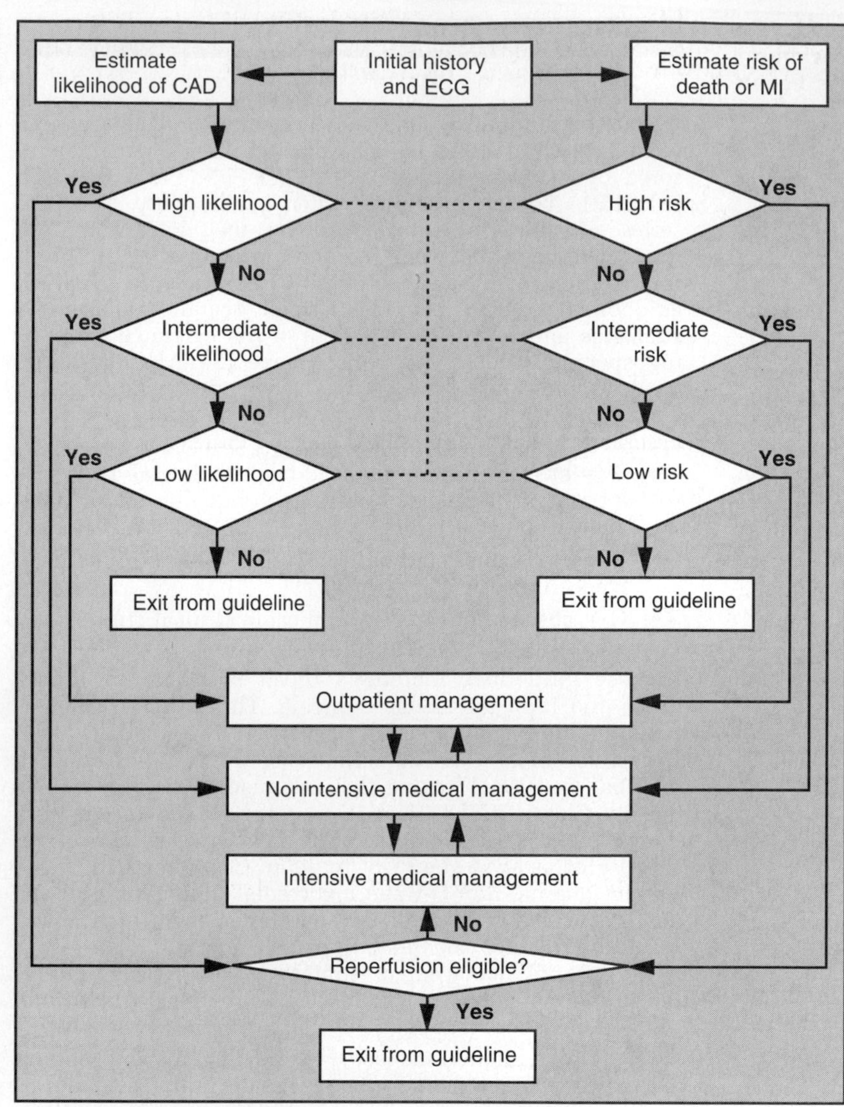

FIGURE 63–1. Overall strategy for diagnosis and risk stratification for patients with unstable angina according to AHCPR guidelines.

TABLE 63–15 LIKELIHOOD OF SIGNIFICANT CORONARY ARTERY DISEASE IN PATIENTS WITH SYMPTOMS SUGGESTING UNSTABLE ANGINA

HIGH LIKELIHOOD (e.g., 0.85–0.99)	INTERMEDIATE LIKELIHOOD (e.g., 0.15–0.84)	LOW LIKELIHOOD (e.g., 0.01–0.14)
Any of the following features:	**Absence of high likelihood features and any of the following:**	**Absence of high or intermediate likelihood features but may have:**
History of prior MI or sudden death or other known history of CAD	Definite angina: males <60 or females <70	Chest pain classified as probably not angina
Definite angina: males ≥60 or females ≥70	Probable angina: males ≥60 or females ≥70	One risk factor other than diabetes
Transient hemodynamic or ECG changes during pain	Chest pain probably not angina in patients with diabetes	T-wave flattening or inversion <1 mm in leads with dominant R waves
Variant angina (pain with reversible ST-segment elevation)	Chest pain probably not angina and two or three risk factors other than diabetes	Normal ECG
ST-segment elevation or depression ≥1 mm	Extracardiac vascular disease	
Marked symmetrical T-wave inversion in multiple precordial leads.	ST depression 0.05 to 1 mm or T-wave inversion ≥1 mm in leads with dominant R waves	

From Braunwald, E., Mark, D. B., Jones, R. H., et al.: Unstable Angina: Diagnosis and Management. Clinical Practice Guideline Number 10 (amended) AHCPR Publication No. 94-0602. Rockville, Md., Agency for Health Care Policy and Research and the National Heart, Lung, and Blood Institute, Public Health Service, US Department of Health and Human Services, May 1994.

TABLE 63–16 SHORT-TERM RISK OF DEATH OR NONFATAL MYOCARDIAL INFARCTION IN PATIENTS WITH UNSTABLE ANGINA

HIGH RISK	INTERMEDIATE RISK	LOW RISK
At least one of the following features must be present:	**No high-risk feature but must have any of the following:**	**Absence of high or intermediate likelihood features but may have any of the following features:**
Prolonged ongoing (≥20 min) rest pain	Prolonged (>20 min) rest angina, now resolved, with moderate or high likelihood of coronary artery disease	Increased angina frequency, severity, or duration
Pulmonary edema, most likely related to ischemia	Rest angina (>20 min or relieved with rest or sublingual nitroglycerin)	Angina provoked at a lower threshold
Angina at rest with dynamic ST changes ≥1 mm	Nocturnal angina	New-onset angina with onset 2 weeks to 2 months before presentation
Angina with new or worsening mitral regurgitation murmur	Angina with dynamic T-wave changes	Normal or unchanged ECG
Angina with S3 or new/worsening rales	New-onset Canadian Cardiovascular Society Class III or IV angina in the past 2 weeks with moderate or high likelihood of CAD	
Angina with hypotension	Pathological Q waves or resting ST depression ≤1 mm in multiple lead groups (anterior, inferior, lateral)	
	Age >65 years	

From Braunwald, E., Mark, D. B., Jones, R. H., et al.: Unstable Angina: Diagnosis and Management. Clinical Practice Guideline Number 10 (amended). AHCPR Publication No. 94-0602. Rockville, Md., Agency for Health Care Policy and Research and the National Heart, Lung, and Blood Institute, Public Health Service, US Department of Health and Human Services, May 1994.

for patients with ongoing rest pain, placement at bed rest. If it is concluded that a patient has unstable angina, aspirin should be given unless there is contraindication, such as evidence of ongoing major hemorrhage, a significant risk for bleeding complications, or a clear history of severe hypersensitivity to aspirin.

The guidelines recommend that antiischemia medications should be initiated in the emergency department for patients with unstable angina and titrated to dosages that are adequate to relieve symptomatic ischemia without causing excessive bradycardia or hypotension. For patients at high or intermediate risk of complications (Table 63–16), intravenous heparin is recommended. The guidelines suggest an initial dose of 80 units/kg by intravenous bolus followed by an infusion of 18 units/kg/hour, maintaining the activated partial thromboplastin time (aPTT) at 1.5 to 2.5 times control. The use of thrombolytic therapy is not supported in the absence of acute ST-segment elevation or left bundle branch block.

A major theme of the AHCPR guidelines is involvement of patients in their care, and the initial treatment recommendations urge that patients be encouraged to participate in monitoring the relief of symptoms. Throughout the course of treatment, the guidelines specifically recommend that the health care team should keep the patient and the patient's family informed of the probable diagnosis, most reasonable treatment strategies, and most likely outcomes.

After initial treatment and stabilization, the AHCPR guidelines recommend triage of patients with a high risk for complications (Table 63–16) if possible to an ICU bed, while intermediate-risk patients can be managed in an ICU or other monitored bed. The guidelines support management of patients who fall into low-risk subsets as outpatients, however. These low-risk patients should undergo follow-up outpatient evaluations within 72 hours.

Outpatient Care of Low-Risk Patients

Patients with unstable angina who are at low risk for complications tend to be those with new-onset angina or with worsening of symptoms due to ischemia, but without severe, prolonged, or rest pain. At the follow-up evaluation, the guidelines recommend that the physician determine whether a patient's symptoms have worsened, in which case the patient should be admitted. A search for noncardiac causes of pain should be undertaken, but if the leading diagnosis is still ischemic heart disease, the evaluation should be directed at further risk stratification.

Exercise or pharmacological stress testing usually should be part of this evaluation but need not be performed for patients with a very low probability of coronary disease or complications from ischemic disease. Conversely, stress testing would be excessively risky for patients who have a high clinical risk for complications, such as those with significant left ventricular dysfunction or worsening of symptoms despite medical therapy. In such cases, referral of the patient for coronary angiography may be the most appropriate course. The guidelines recognize that coronary angiography may be useful for some low-risk patients who believe their symptoms are due to ischemia despite reassurance and noninvasive test results to the contrary.

The treatment guidelines for low-risk patients recommend beginning with instruction in the proper use of sublingual nitroglycerin tablets, followed by oral beta blockers. The guidelines suggest starting with one major antianginal medication, preferably a long-acting preparation, and adding a second only if the symptoms are not adequately controlled. For most low-risk outpatients, therapy with aspirin and one antianginal medication is sufficient initial treatment. Patients with contraindications to aspirin can be treated with ticlopidine 250 mg twice a day as an alternative.

Intensive Medical Treatment

Patients with unstable angina and either intermediate or high risk for complications should receive intensive medical therapy aimed at relieving their symptoms. According to the AHCPR guidelines, this therapy should include beta blockers and nitrate preparations, including intravenous nitroglycerin for nonhypotensive patients with high-risk unstable angina (Table 63–17). A patient whose pain cannot be controlled should be referred for catheterization and revascularization.

Patients whose angina is controlled for 24 hours by intravenous nitroglycerin can be switched to other nitrate preparations. Whereas prolonged exposure to nitrates can cause tolerance to their effects, responsiveness to nitrates can be

TABLE 63–17 SELECTED RECOMMENDATIONS AND STRENGTH OF EVIDENCE FOR MANAGEMENT OF UNSTABLE ANGINA (AHCPR)

TOPIC	RECOMMENDATION	STRENGTH OF EVIDENCE
Initial treatment	• All patients with unstable angina should receive regular ASA 160 to 324 mg as soon as possible after presentation unless a definite contraindication is present. • IV heparin should be started as soon as a diagnosis of intermediate- or high-risk unstable angina is made.	A A
Triage	• High-risk unstable angina patients should be admitted initially to an ICU bed whenever possible. • Intermediate-risk unstable angina patients should be admitted to an ICU or monitored cardiac bed. • Low-risk unstable angina patients may be managed as outpatients with planned early follow-up evaluations.	B C C
Intensive medical treatment: Nitrates	• Patients whose symptoms are not fully relieved with three sublingual nitroglycerin (NTG) tablets and initiation of beta blocker therapy (when possible), as well as all nonhypotensive high-risk unstable angina patients, may benefit from IV NTG. IV NTG should be started at a dose of 5 to 10 μg/min by continuous infusion and titrated up by 10 μg/min every 5 to 10 min until relief of symptoms or limiting side effects occur. • Patients on IV NTG should be switched to oral or topical nitrate therapy once they have been symptom-free for 24 hours.	B C
Morphine sulfate	Morphine sulfate at a dose of 2 to 5 mg IV is recommended for any patient whose symptoms are not relieved after three serial sublingual NTG tablets or whose symptoms recur with adequate antiischemic therapy unless contraindicated by hypotension or intolerance. Morphine may be repeated every 5 to 10 min as needed to relieve symptoms and maintain patient comfort.	C
Beta blockers	IV (for high-risk patients) or oral (for intermediate- and low-risk patients) beta blockers should be started in the absence of contraindications.	B
Calcium channel blockers	• Calcium channel blockers may be used to control ongoing or recurring ischemic symptoms in patients already on adequate doses of nitrates and beta blockers or in patients unable to tolerate adequate doses of one or both of these agents or in patients with variant angina. Calcium channel blockers should be avoided in patients with pulmonary edema or evidence of LV dysfunction. • Nifedipine should not be used in the absence of concurrent beta blockage.	B A
Aspirin	ASA to be taken once/day at a dose of 80 to 324 mg, should be continued indefinitely following presentation with unstable angina.	A
Ticlopidine and other antiplatelet agents	• Patients unable to take ASA may be started on ticlopidine 250 mg twice per day as a substitute. • Heparin infusion should be continued for 2 to 5 days or until revascularization is performed.	B C
Laboratory testing	• Total CK and CK-MB should be measured every 6 to 8 hours for the first 24 hours after admission. • Lactate dehydrogenase isoenzymes may be useful in patients presenting 24 to 72 hours after symptom onset if serial CK and CK-MB levels are normal. • Serum lipid levels within 24 hours of admission unless patients have had a recent determination or are on chronic therapy for hyperlipidemia. • Follow-up ECG 24 hours after admission and whenever the patient has recurrent symptoms or a change in clinical status. • Chest film. • Assessment of left ventricular function within 72 hours.	C
Emergency/urgent cardiac catheterization	If chest discomfort with objective evidence of ischemia persists for $\geq$1 hour after aggressive medical therapy, triage to emergency cardiac catheterization should be strongly considered.	B
	Urgent cardiac catheterization should be considered in patients with unstable angina who have recurrent ischemic episodes despite appropriate medical therapy or who have high-risk unstable angina.	B
Acute revascularization	Acute revascularization is indicated for patients with refractory pain ($\geq$1 hour on aggressive medical therapy) who are found at catheterization to have an acutely occluded major coronary vessel, or severe subtotal occlusion of a culprit vessel, or severe multivessel disease with impaired LV function.	B
Use and timing of noninvasive tests	Exercise or pharmacological stress testing should generally be an integral part of the outpatient evaluation of low-risk patients with unstable angina.	B
	Unless cardiac catheterization is indicated, noninvasive exercise or pharmacological stress testing should be performed in low- or intermediate-risk patients (see Table 63–16) hospitalized with unstable angina who have been free of angina and congestive heart failure for a minimum of 48 hours.	B

TABLE 63–17 SELECTED RECOMMENDATIONS AND STRENGTH OF EVIDENCE FOR MANAGEMENT OF UNSTABLE ANGINA (AHCPR)—*Continued*

TOPIC	RECOMMENDATION	STRENGTH OF EVIDENCE
Selection of stress testing modality	The exercise treadmill test should be the standard mode of stress testing employed in patients with a normal ECG who are not taking digoxin. Patients with widespread resting ST depression ($\geq$1 mm), ST changes secondary to digoxin, left ventricular hypertrophy, LBBB/significant intraventricular conduction deficit (IVCD), or preexcitation usually should be tested using an imaging modality. Patients unable to exercise due to physical limitations should undergo pharmacological stress testing in combination with an imaging modality.	B
Use of noninvasive test results in patient management	• Patients with a low-risk exercise test result (predicted average annual cardiac mortality $<$1%/year) can be managed medically without need for referral to cardiac catheterization. • Patients with a high-risk exercise test result (predicted average annual cardiac mortality $\geq$4%/year) should be referred for prompt cardiac catheterization. • Patients with intermediate-risk exercise test result (predicted average annual cardiac mortality 2–3%/year) should be referred for additional testing, either cardiac catheterization or an (alternative) exercise imaging study • A stress test result of intermediate risk combined with evidence of left ventricular dysfunction should prompt referral to cardiac catheterization.	B B C C
Cardiac catheterization	• *Early invasive strategy:* cardiac catheterization is performed routinely in all hospitalized patients without contraindications, usually within 48 hours of presentation. • *Early conservative strategy:* cardiac catheterization is performed routinely in patients admitted to the hospital with unstable angina who are candidates for a revascularization procedure and have one or more of the following high-risk indicators: prior revascularization (PTCA or CABG); associated congestive heart failure or depressed left ventricular function (EF $<$ 0.50) by noninvasive study; malignant ventricular arrhythmia; persistent or recurrent pain/ischemia; and/or a functional study indicating high risk.	A A
Myocardial revascularization	• Patients found at catheterization to have significant left main disease ($\geq$50%) or significant ($\geq$70%) 3-vessel disease with depressed left ventricular function (EF $<$ 0.50) should be referred promptly for CABG surgery. • Patients with 2-vessel disease with proximal severe subtotal stenosis ($\geq$95%) of the left anterior descending artery and depressed left ventricular function should be referred promptly for CABG or PTCA. • Patients with significant coronary artery disease should be considered for prompt revascularization (PTCA or CABG) if they have any of the following: failure to stabilize with medical treatment; recurrent angina/ischemia at rest or with low-level activities; and/or ischemia accompanied by congestive heart failure symptoms, and S3 gallop, new or worsening mitral regurgitation, or definite ECG changes. • For patients with significant coronary artery disease not included in the above recommendations, two strategies are possible: early invasive and early conservative. In early invasive strategy, revascularization is performed only on those patients meeting criteria for failure of initial therapy necessitating cardiac catheterization. Medical therapy without revascularization is continued for patients without criteria for failure of therapy.	A B C B S
Discharge from hospital and postdischarge care	Patients should continue on ASA, 80 mg to 324 mg per day, indefinitely after discharge.	B

From Braunwald, E., Mark, D. B., Jones, R. H., et al.: Unstable Angina: Diagnosis and Management. Clinical Practice Guideline Number 10 (amended). AHCPR Publication No. 94-0602. Rockville, Md., Agency for Health Care Policy and Research and the National Heart, Lung, and Blood Institute, Public Health Service, US Department of Health and Human Services, May 1994. (For definition of A, B, C and S see p. 1979.)

restored by increasing the dose or giving the patient topical, oral, or buccal nitrates with a 6- to 8-hour nitrate-free interval. Morphine sulfate can be used to relieve symptoms in patients whose pain is not controlled with three sublingual nitroglycerin tablets or whose symptoms recur.

Beta blockers can be given orally for most patients with unstable angina, but intravenous administration should be considered for patients who are at high risk for complications. A patient at risk for adverse effects from beta blockers because of pulmonary disease, left ventricular dysfunction, or severe bradycardia should be treated initially with a short-acting beta blocker. The value of beta blockers is sufficiently impressive that the guidelines recommend a trial of a short-acting agent at a reduced dose (e.g., 2.5 mg metoprolol intravenously, 12.5 mg metoprolol orally, or 25 ug/kg/min esmolol as initial doses), rather than complete avoidance of beta blocker therapy, in patients with mild wheezing or a history of chronic obstructive pulmonary disease.

Calcium channel blockers are the next class of drugs used to control symptoms after nitrates and beta blockers. This class of drugs can relieve ischemic symptoms[141] but does not appear to change mortality or rates of nonfatal myocardial infarction.[142,143] Because of the negative inotropic effects of these agents, the AHCPR guidelines discourage their use in patients with pulmonary edema or left ventricular dysfunction. The guidelines also recommend that nifedipine not be used in patients who are not also receiving a beta blocker because of randomized trial data demonstrating an increased risk of myocardial infarction or recurrent angina in such settings.[144]

As noted above, the AHCPR guidelines also recommend that all patients with unstable angina receive aspirin or other antiplatelet agents unless they have contraindications to such drugs. Intravenous heparin therapy should be continued for at least 2 days.

Laboratory Testing

Guidelines from the AHCPR, ACC/AHA, and American College of Physicians for the use of cardiac enzyme assays are reviewed on page 1970. None of these guidelines provides recommendations regarding the use of newer markers such as cardiac troponin I and T,[123,124] which may be useful markers for myocardial injury. For example, troponin T appears to improve risk stratification of patients with unstable angina,[124] and troponin I has demonstrated high specificity for cardiac damage.[123] These new markers are just beginning to enter the market, however, and strategies for their use have not yet been addressed by guidelines.

The AHCPR guidelines recommend serial CK and CK-MB sampling for 24 hours, and an electrocardiogram 24 hours after admission. This 24-hour period exceeds the duration of hospitalizations currently used for many patients admitted for acute chest pain,[122] but these shorter observation periods were developed and evaluated for patients with a low risk for acute myocardial infarction and cardiovascular complications. Data support the use of a 24-hour observation period for patients with electrocardiographic changes or worsening of ischemic syndromes, and even longer enzyme sampling periods for patients who have recurrent ischemic pain in the hospital.[122]

The AHCPR guidelines support obtaining a chest film upon admission, particularly in patients with hemodynamic instability, and suggest assessment of left ventricular function with either echocardiography or radionuclide ventriculography within 72 hours of admission unless the patient undergoes early cardiac catheterization. These data can provide insight into the patient's left ventricular function, which is an important predictor of prognosis and therefore a factor in the consideration of who should undergo coronary angiography.

Initiation of secondary prevention strategies during the hospitalization is a major priority of the AHCPR guidelines, but these interventions can get overlooked when the focus of management is on questions such as whether or not the patient needs coronary revascularization. The AHCPR guidelines therefore recommend measurement of serum lipid levels within 24 hours of admission unless there has been a recent determination or the patient is receiving long-term therapy for hyperlipidemia. Levels obtained later in the hospitalization may not reflect the patient's usual lipid profile.

Early Assessment and Management

The goal of initial therapy for patients with unstable angina is to institute a regimen that includes aspirin, intravenous heparin adjusted to maintain an aPTT value of 1.5 to 2.5 times control, plus nitrates and a beta blocker. Calcium blockers should be considered for patients with refractory ischemia, significant hypertension, or variant angina, according to the AHCPR. Failure of these measures to control ischemia should prompt consideration of urgent cardiac catheterization.

For patients who have ischemia refractory to medical management, *intraaortic balloon pumping* may be useful if coronary angiography is not possible or for stabilization until the patient can reach the catheterization laboratory or operating room. *Urgent or emergency cardiac catheterization* is recommended if patients have evidence of ischemia persisting for more than 1 hour after institution of aggressive medical therapy, and in patients who have recurrent ischemic episodes despite appropriate treatment or who have high-risk unstable angina. Acute revascularization with either PTCA or CABG should be used for patients with refractory pain and acute vessel occlusions, severe subtotal occlusion of a culprit vessel, or severe multivessel disease with impaired left ventricular function.

For patients whose course is uncomplicated for at least 24 hours, the AHCPR guidelines recommend that intravenous medications can be switched to nonparenteral regimens. As the patient is mobilized, counseling should include assessment of the patient's life situation, anxiety level, and coping skills. The guidelines recommend that the health care team observe the patient as activity is increased to a level that allows performance of activities of daily living. During this period, the patient and family should receive education about and begin working toward risk-factor modification goals.

Use of Noninvasive Testing

The AHCPR guidelines support use of exercise or pharmacological stress testing to improve risk stratification of patients with unstable angina once they are sufficiently stable to undergo such testing. For low-risk patients who may not have been admitted to the hospital or who were discharged early, the guidelines recommend that these tests be performed within 72 hours. For hospitalized patients with a low or intermediate risk for complications, the guidelines recommend testing when the patient has been free of angina and congestive heart failure for 48 hours. The guidelines recommend exercise electrocardiography as the first-choice method for noninvasive assessment of ischemic heart disease. When electrocardiographic abnormalities such as left bundle branch block render the electrocardiogram an unreliable test for ischemia, an imaging method should be used; when patients are unable to exercise, a pharmacological stressor should be employed.

Data from the noninvasive tests help determine the subsequent management strategy for patients whose condition remains clinically stable. The AHCPR guidelines include a nomogram for prediction of annual mortality on the basis of exercise-induced ST-segment deviation, the degree of angina observed during exercise, and the duration of exercise[145] (Fig. 5–12, p. 166). Medical therapy without cardiac catheterization is recommended for patients with a predicted annual cardiac mortality of less than 1 per cent per year, while prompt catheterization is recommended for those with an estimated average annual mortality of 4 per cent or more. For patients with an intermediate risk after exercise testing, the AHCPR guidelines suggest cardiac catheterization if those patients have left ventricular dysfunction; in the absence of left ventricular dysfunction, the guidelines recommend further risk stratification either with cardiac catheterization or alternative noninvasive tests.

Early Invasive and Conservative Strategies

The AHCPR guidelines proposed two alternative treatment strategies, which were termed early invasive and early conservative strategies. Published research has not demonstrated an advantage of one approach over the other, so the guidelines recommend basing the decision of which strategy to use on factors including the patient's estimated risk of complications, available facilities, and patient preferences. In the early invasive strategy, patients admitted to the hospital for unstable angina routinely undergo coronary angiography, usually within 48 hours of presentation. In the conservative strategy, catheterization is performed in admitted patients who have at least one of several high-risk indicators (Table 63–17). Cardiac catheterization is *not* performed in patients who are not candidates for revascularization or who have extensive comorbidity that would render them unlikely to benefit from the procedure.

Figure 63–2 shows a schematic integration of early invasive and conservative strategies and the recommended management according to the results of the coronary angiograms. Coronary artery bypass graft surgery is recommended for patients with left main coronary disease or significant three-vessel disease with depressed left ventricular function. Revascularization with PTCA or CABG should be performed for patients with two-vessel disease

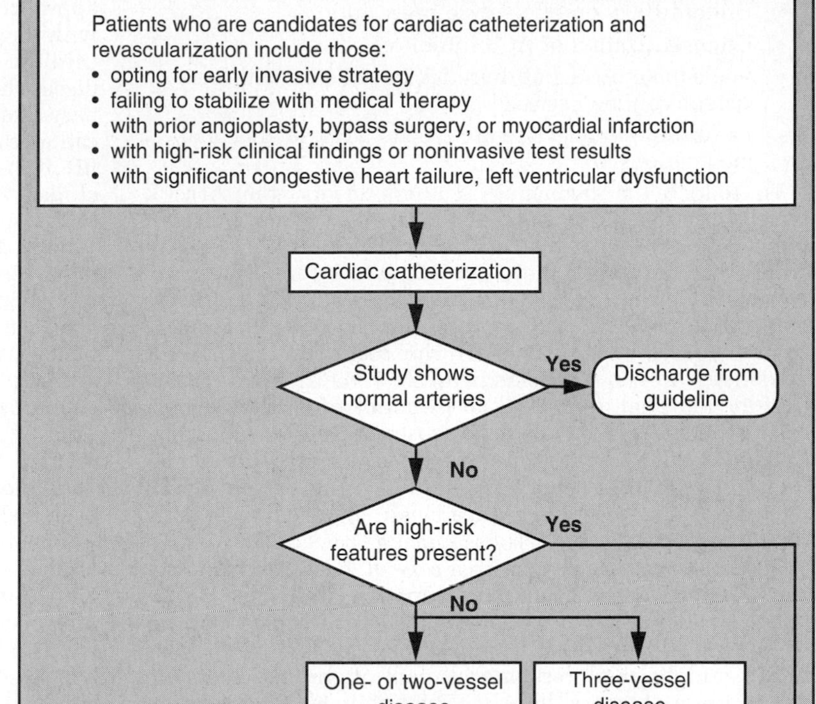

FIGURE 63–2. Cardiac catheterization and myocardial revascularization in unstable angina according to AHCPR guidelines. (From Braunwald, E., Mark, D. B., Jones, R. H., et al.: Unstable Angina: Diagnosis and Management. Clinical Practice Guideline Number 10 [amended]. AHCPR Publication No. 94-0602. Rockville, Md., Agency for Health Care Policy and Research and the National Heart, Lung, and Blood Institute, Public Health Service, US Department of Health and Human Services, May 1994.)

with proximal severe subtotal stenosis of the left anterior descending coronary artery and depressed left ventricular function. These procedures should also be performed for other patients with coronary disease if they have high-risk factors (Table 63–17). For patients without these high-risk factors, the patient and physician should choose between an early invasive strategy, in which revascularization is performed, and an early conservative strategy, in which revascularization is performed only if the patient's symptoms are not controlled with medical therapy.

Hospital Discharge and Postdischarge Care

Throughout the hospitalization—and after discharge—patients and their families should be kept fully informed of the patient's status, crucial issues, options, and probable outcomes. In the absence of contraindications, the AHCPR guidelines recommend use of aspirin indefinitely, as well as continuation of medications needed to achieve adequate symptom control. Those patients with signs or symptoms of ischemia should receive instruction in the use of sublingual nitroglycerin. Patients with successful revascularization without recurrent ischemia do not require postdischarge antianginal therapy.

The AHCPR guidelines recommend that low-risk patients and patients with successful CABG or PTCA be seen in an outpatient facility at 2 to 6 weeks, and higher-risk patients should return in 1 to 2 weeks. Follow-up care should emphasize secondary prevention, with appropriate continued management of risk factors including hypertension, hyperlipidemia, smoking, and physical inactivity. Patients should be given advice on specific physical activities, including resumption of work, driving, and sexual activity. The guidelines recommend consideration of an outpatient cardiac rehabilitation program but gave a low grade (C) to the strength of evidence supporting this intervention for patients with unstable angina.

HEART FAILURE

(See also Chap. 17)

Heart failure was one of the first three topics chosen by the AHCPR for the development of practice guidelines; these guidelines were released in 1994. Among the reasons for choosing heart failure were its high prevalence, poor prognosis, and high costs. More than two million Americans suffer from heart failure, and 5-year mortality rates are in the range of 50 per cent. The estimated cost to society exceeds $10 billion per year.[13] Research has demonstrated that improved management can decrease mortality and improve functional status for patients with heart failure, and there is considerable variation in the strategies used by physicians in the care of heart failure.[146] Among the common errors in management and testing cited by the AHCPR panel are:

- Overuse of testing techniques
- Inadequate treatment of coexistent hypertension
- Inadequate education for patient, family, and caregivers
- Inappropriate treatment of heart failure not due to systolic dysfunction
- Suboptimal patient involvement in care and compliance

- Delayed referral for transplantation
- Underutilization of exercise prescriptions
- Underutilization of ACE inhibitors
- Inadequate dosing of diuretics in patients with persistent volume overload
- Failure of clinicians to appreciate adverse effects of medications

To reduce the frequency of these errors, the AHCPR panel formulated recommendations for a wide range of topics[13] (excerpted in Table 63–18). The multidisciplinary group that developed these guidelines used an A-B-C system to grade the strength of evidence to support their recommendations similar to that used for the AHCPR unstable angina guidelines (p. 1979).[12] The focus of the AHCPR guidelines was on patients with left ventricular systolic dysfunction leading to volume overload or inadequate tissue perfusion, but one of their most specific recommendations was aimed at preventing this syndrome—the guidelines recommend use of ACE inhibitors in patients with moderately or severely reduced left ventricular systolic function even if they are asymptomatic.

Guidelines for care of patients with heart failure associated with left ventricular dysfunction were also developed by the American College of Cardiology/American Heart Association Task Force on Practice Guidelines.[147] These guidelines address management of chronic and acute heart failure, whereas the AHCPR guidelines focus more on the management and prevention of chronic heart failure.

Initial Evaluation

As summarized in the ACC/AHA guidelines, the initial evaluation in patients with heart failure should seek to distinguish diastolic from systolic function and to determine the cause. Of particular importance is excluding ischemic heart disease as the cause of heart failure, since patients with coronary disease might benefit from revascularization.

The AHCPR guidelines identify symptoms that should trigger consideration of an evaluation for heart failure, the most crucial of which are paroxysmal nocturnal dyspnea, orthopnea, or new-onset dyspnea on exertion. Unless the patient has clear evidence of a noncardiac cause for these symptoms, the AHCPR guidelines indicate that echocardiography or radionuclide ventriculography should be used to evaluate left ventricular function—even if physical signs of heart failure are not present. Other symptoms that suggest this diagnosis are lower extremity edema, decreased exercise tolerance, unexplained confusion or fatigue, and abdominal symptoms associated with ascites and/or hepatic engorgement.

Several tests are recommended by both AHCPR and ACC/AHA guidelines for the initial evaluation of patients with heart failure, and the goals of this testing include assessment of severity and identification of causes of the myocardial dysfunction (Table 63–18). If the patients would be candidates for revascularization, the ACC/AHA guidelines recommend performance of a noninvasive stress test to detect ischemia in two groups of patients: (1) patients without angina but with a high probability of coronary artery disease and (2) patients with a previous infarction but with no angina. Performance of noninvasive stress testing to detect ischemia in all patients with unexplained heart failure who are potentially candidates for revascularization was considered to be of uncertain appropriateness (Class II). These guidelines also consider exercise testing, usually with respiratory gas analysis, to determine whether patients are candidates for heart transplantation, to be an appropriate test for patients with severe heart failure.

The ACC/AHA guidelines were equivocal (Class II) about the appropriateness of coronary arteriography for *all* patients with unexplained heart failure who might be candidates for revascularization but considered catheterization appropriate (Class I) for patients with heart failure and with angina or large areas of ischemic or hibernating myocardium, as well as patients at risk for coronary artery disease who are to undergo surgical correction of noncoronary cardiac lesions. These guidelines deemed cardiac catheterization and stress testing to be inappropriate (Class III) if patients have previously had coronary disease excluded as a cause of left ventricular dysfunction and no objective evidence of ischemia has developed.

Both sets of guidelines emphasize that screening evaluations for arrhythmias such as ambulatory electrocardiography should not be performed routinely for all patients with heart failure; instead, this test should be reserved for patients with a history of syncope, near-syncope, or other symptoms suggestive of arrhythmia. This recommendation is supported by data from the Cardiac Arrhythmia Suppression Trial,[148,149] which found increased mortality in patients with ejection fractions of 40 per cent or less who were treated with moricizine, encainide, and flecainide. These findings have led to reservations about treating any but the most serious ventricular arrhythmias in this patient population.

One arrhythmia that may be *undertreated* in patients with heart failure is atrial fibrillation. The AHCPR guidelines recommend attempting cardioversion for patients with left atrial diameter less than 50 mm and less than a 1-year history of atrial fibrillation. No recommendations are offered on the drug of choice, although the guidelines comment that amiodarone may emerge as the preferred agent.

Routine use of myocardial biopsy was not supported by *both* guidelines because of lack of evidence that this information leads to improved management or outcomes. The ACC/AHA guidelines were uncertain (Class II) about the appropriateness of endomyocardial biopsy for patients (1) with recent onset of rapidly deteriorating cardiac function or other clinical indications of myocarditis; (2) receiving chemotherapy with Adriamycin or other myocardial toxic agents; and (3) with a systemic disease and possible cardiac involvement.

The ACC/AHA guidelines also considered measurement of circulating neurohormone levels to be of little value in routine management and evaluation.

Inpatient and Outpatient Management

The AHCPR guidelines provide specific criteria for admission to the hospital and also offer standards for outcomes to be achieved before patients with heart failure are discharged from the hospital (Table 63–18). These recommendations reflect the importance of discharge planning and an adequate system of outpatient care. Readmission rates as high as 57 per cent within 90 days have been reported in elderly patients with heart failure.[150] In that study, factors associated with readmission were failed social support systems, inadequate follow-up, failure to seek medical attention promptly when symptoms recurred, and noncompliance with diet and medications. Such findings led to a series of recommendations regarding patient and family education and counseling. Many of these interventions, such as support groups, have not been part of the traditional focus of physicians; hence, these guidelines imply close collaboration of a team of providers for patients with heart failure. Among the topics for patient education specifically cited were:

- Nature of heart failure
- Drug regimens
- Dietary restrictions
- What to do if symptoms occur
- Prognosis
- Completion of advanced directives
- Smoking and chewing of tobacco

TABLE 63–18 SELECTED RECOMMENDATIONS FROM GUIDELINES FOR HEART FAILURE (AHCPR)

TOPIC	RECOMMENDATION	STRENGTH OF EVIDENCE
Prevention in asymptomatic patients	Asymptomatic patients with moderately or severely reduced left-ventricular systolic function (ejection fraction <35–40%) should be treated with an angiotensin-converting enzyme (ACE) inhibitor to reduce the chance of developing clinical heart failure.	A
Initial evaluation	Patients with symptoms highly suggestive of heart failure should undergo echocardiography or radionuclide ventriculography to measure left ventricular function even if physical signs of heart failure are absent.	C
Diagnostic testing	Practitioners should perform a chest x-ray; ECG; complete blood count (CBC); serum electrolytes, serum creatinine, serum albumin, liver function tests; and urinalysis for all patients with suspected or clinically evident heart failure. A T_4 and thyroid-stimulating hormone (TSH) level should also be checked in all patients over age 65 with heart failure and no obvious etiology, and in patients who have atrial fibrillation or other signs or symptoms of thyroid disease. Routine use of myocardial biopsy is not recommended.	C
Screening for arrhythmias	Screening evaluation for arrhythmias such as ambulatory electrocardiography is not routinely warranted.	A
Hospital admission criteria	Presence or suspicion of heart failure and any of the following findings usually indicates a need for hospitalization: • Clinically or ECG evidence of acute myocardial ischemia. • Pulmonary edema or severe respiratory distress. • Oxygen saturation below 90% (not due to pulmonary disease). • Severe complicating medical illness (e.g., pneumonia). • Anasarca. • Symptomatic hypotension or syncope. • Heart failure refractory to outpatient therapy. • Inadequate social support for safe outpatient management.	C
Hospital discharge criteria	Patients with heart failure should be discharged from the hospital only when: • Symptoms of heart failure have been adequately controlled. • All reversible causes of morbidity have been treated or stabilized. • Patients and caregivers have been educated about medications, diet, activity and exercise recommendations, and symptoms of worsening heart failure. • Adequate outpatient support and follow-up care have been arranged	C
Activity recommendations	Regular exercise should be encouraged for all patients with stable NYHA Class I-III heart failure.	B
Cardiac rehabilitation	There is insufficient evidence at this time to recommend the routine use of supervised rehabilitation programs for patients with heart failure.	C
Diet	Dietary sodium should be restricted to as close to 2 grams per day as possible.	C
	People who drink alcohol should be advised to consume no more than one drink per day.	C
Discussion of prognosis	All patients should be encouraged to complete a durable power of attorney for health care or another form of advanced directive.	N/A
The initial pharmacological management	Patients with heart failure and signs of significant volume overload should be started immediately on a diuretic. Patients with mild volume overload can be managed adequately on thiazide diuretics, whereas those with more severe volume overload should be started on a loop diuretic.	C
ACE inhibitors	Patients with heart failure due to left ventricular systolic dysfunction should be given a trial of ACE inhibitors unless specific contraindications exist: (1) history of intolerance or adverse reactions to these agents, (2) serum potassium greater than 5.5 mEq/liter that cannot be reduced, or (3) symptomatic hypotension. Patients with systolic blood pressure less than 90 mm Hg have a higher risk of complications and should be managed by a physician experienced in utilizing ACE inhibitors in such patients. Caution and close monitoring are also required for patients who have a serum creatinine greater than 3.0 mg/dl or an estimated creatinine clearance of less than 30 ml/min; half the usual dose should be used in this setting.	B
Digoxin	Digoxin should be used routinely in patients with severe heart failure and should be added to the medical regimen of patients with mild or moderate heart failure who remain symptomatic after optimal management with ACE inhibitors and diuretics.	C
Hydralazine/isosorbide dinitrate	Isosorbide dinitrate and hydralazine is an appropriate alternative in patients with contraindications or intolerance to ACE inhibitors.	B
Anticoagulation	Routine anticoagulation is not recommended.	C
Beta blockers	This form of treatment should be considered experimental at this time.	B
Patient follow-up	Patients should be instructed to call if they experience an unexplained weight gain greater than 3–5 pounds since their last clinical evaluation.	C

From Konstam, M., Dracup, K., Baker, D., et al.: Heart Failure: Evaluation and care of patients with left-ventricular systolic dysfunction. Clinical Practice Guideline No. 11. AHCPR Publication No. 94-0612. Rockville, Md.; Agency for Health Care Policy and Research, Public Health Service, U.S. Department of Health and Human Services, June 1994. (For definition of A, B, & C see p. 1979.)

- Importance of influenza and pneumococcal vaccination
- Sexual activity
- Alcohol use

Regular physical activity programs are recommended for all patients except those with NYHA Class IV heart failure, but the guidelines do not explicitly endorse the use of cardiac rehabilitation programs for all patients with heart failure.

Management

Both the ACC/AHA and AHCPR guidelines provide a strong endorsement of the use of angiotensin-converting enzyme (ACE) inhibitors for patients with left ventricular systolic dysfunction in the absence of specific contraindications (Table 63–18), and make similar recommendations regarding several other medications. Diuretic use for patients with signs of volume overload should be immediate according to both sets of guidelines, and the AHCPR guidelines also suggest that patients with mild volume overload can be managed adequately with thiazide diuretics, which cause a less acute diuresis than does furosemide.[150,151] For patients without volume overload, ACE inhibitors may be considered as the sole initial therapy. The prominent roles of ACE inhibitors and diuretics in the AHCPR guidelines are reflected in its flow sheet summarizing pharmacological management (Fig. 63–3).

The guidelines also support use of digoxin, despite the uncertainty regarding its impact on mortality. The ACC/AHA guidelines considered routine use of digoxin for all patients with left ventricular systolic function to be of uncertain appropriateness (Class II). Because of data demonstrating that digoxin can improve physical function and decrease symptoms in at least some patients with heart failure,[152] both sets of guidelines recommend that it be used routinely for patients with heart failure who remain symptomatic despite diuretics and ACE inhibitors. The ACC/AHA guidelines also note that digoxin is appropriate (Class I) for patients with heart failure and atrial fibrillation.

The AHCPR task force concludes that anticoagulation is not justifiable as part of routine therapy for heart failure, but that it should be reserved for patients with thromboembolic disease, atrial fibrillation, or mobile left ventricular thrombi. The guidelines also do not support use of beta-

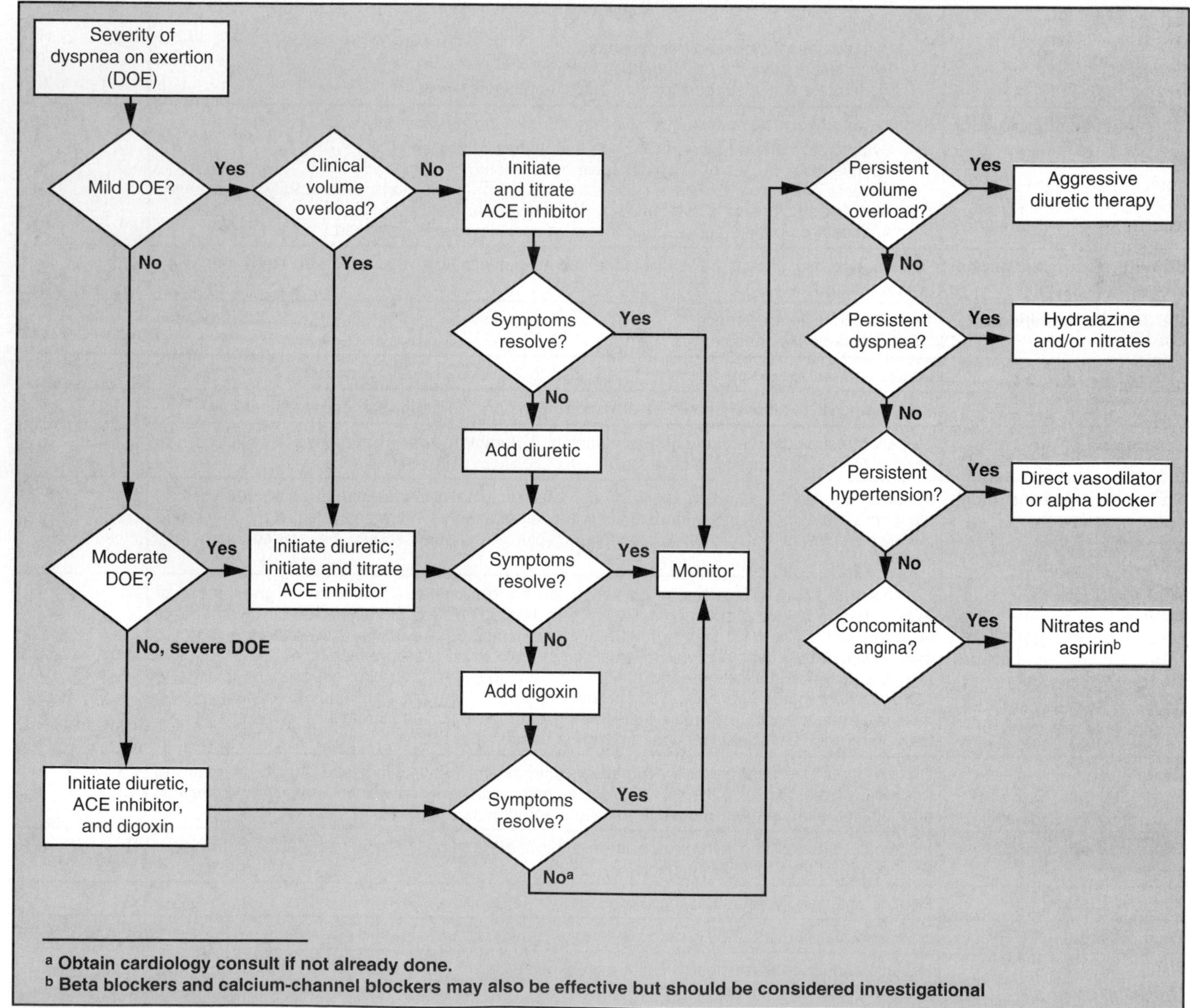

FIGURE 63–3. Flow sheet from AHCPR guidelines for heart failure describing strategy for using pharmacological measures. (From Konstam, M., Dracup, K., Baker, D., et al.: Heart Failure: Evaluation and Care of Patients with Left-Ventricular Systolic Dysfunction. Clinical Practice Guideline Number 11. AHCPR Publication No. 94-0612. Rockville, Md., Agency for Health Care Policy and Research and the National Heart, Lung, and Blood Institute, Public Health Service, US Department of Health and Human Services, June 1994.)

adrenergic blockers, despite the promising findings from some studies. Which patients are appropriate for trials of beta blockers remains uncertain; hence, the guidelines conclude that beta blockers are "an experimental, albeit promising, therapy." Similar conclusions were reached by the ACC/AHA expert panel, which also commented that use of calcium channel blockers in the absence of coexisting angina or hypertension was inappropriate.

Although revascularization of ischemic myocardium either by PTCA or CABG does not directly improve heart failure in most patients, this strategy can improve survival because patients with severe coronary disease and left ventricular dysfunction have a poor prognosis with medical therapy alone. Therefore, the guidelines support performance of coronary angiography in heart failure patients with exercise-limiting angina, rest angina, or recurrent episodes of acute pulmonary edema.

Should left ventricular function be irreversibly and severely damaged, patients may be considered for cardiac transplantation. The AHCPR guidelines do not provide recommendations for the evaluation of this patient population.

Even though the ACC/AHA guidelines also focus on systolic dysfunction, these guidelines make specific recommendations for the treatment of diastolic dysfunction. These guidelines considered appropriate (Class I) the use of diuretic drugs, nitrates, drugs suppressing AV conduction to control ventricular rate in patients with atrial fibrillation, and anticoagulation in patients with atrial fibrillation or prior embolization. Class II therapy included calcium channel blockers, beta blockers, ACE inhibitors, and anticoagulation in patients with intracardiac thrombus. Class III (inappropriate) interventions included drugs with positive inotropic effects in the absence of systolic dysfunction and treatment of asymptomatic arrhythmia.

Interventions for Acutely Ill Patients

The ACC/AHA guidelines offer recommendations regarding the management of patients with acute syndromes including pulmonary edema and cardiogenic shock. In addition to the tests already described, these guidelines comment that cardiac catheterization is appropriate for patients with acute pulmonary edema and suspected coronary artery disease (1) if acute intervention for myocardial injury or infarction is anticipated, or (2) to determine the cause for refractory pulmonary edema.

Pulmonary artery balloon catheters are recommended for consideration in patients with pulmonary edema: (1) if the patient's condition is deteriorating; (2) recovery from the acute presentation is not occurring as anticipated; (3) high-dose nitroglycerin or nitroprusside is required; (4) dobutamine or dopamine is needed to augment systemic blood pressure and peripheral perfusion; or (5) there is uncertainty regarding the diagnosis. Indwelling arterial cannula and transesophageal echocardiography are of uncertain (Class II) appropriateness.

For patients with cardiogenic shock, the ACC/AHA guidelines recommend a rapid infusion of intravenous fluids unless there is evidence of volume overload. If there is not a satisfactory response to this infusion, hemodynamic monitoring should include a pulmonary artery balloon flotation catheter and an indwelling arterial cannula. Intraaortic balloon counterpulsation is also considered appropriate (Class I) for patients with cardiogenic shock or pulmonary edema who do not respond to fluid volume or pharmacological therapy and in patients with acute heart failure accompanied by refractory ischemia.

Outcome Assessment and Follow-up

The most important judge of whether therapeutic interventions have led to improvement is the patient, not a noninvasive test. Therefore, the AHCPR guidelines emphasize the importance of follow-up of patient data such as physical functioning, mental health, sexual function, and the ability to perform usual work and social activities. Between visits to their physicians, patients should keep track of their own weight, and contact their provider if their weight goes up more than 3 to 5 pounds.

PERIOPERATIVE CARDIOVASCULAR EVALUATION FOR NONCARDIAC SURGERY

An ACC/AHA task force issued guidelines in 1996 for the evaluation and management of patients undergoing noncardiac surgery.[153] Few issues related to this topic have been subjected to randomized or controlled trials; thus, these guidelines do not classify many interventions as clearly appropriate or inappropriate. Instead, these guidelines synthesize the literature and offer recommendations for some common clinical issues. A theme that characterizes these recommendations is that interventions are rarely necessary simply to reduce the risk for complications during noncardiac surgery unless the intervention is indicated as part of the routine care of the patient.

These guidelines also emphasize that the goal of the evaluation is not to "clear" the patient but to perform an evaluation of the patient's medical status and to make recommendations regarding the risk of cardiac problems over the entire perioperative period. A specific recommendation is that coronary bypass surgery and coronary angioplasty are almost never appropriate unless they would otherwise be indicated to improve survival and quality of life.

Tests are discouraged unless they are likely to influence patient management. Preoperative noninvasive evaluation of left ventricular function, for example, is considered appropriate (Class I) in these guidelines for patients with current or poorly controlled congestive heart failure, but of equivocal (Class II) appropriateness in other patients with heart failure and patients with dyspnea of unknown etiology.

For most patients who are candidates for noninvasive tests for ischemia, the guidelines conclude that the "test of choice" is exercise electrocardiography, which can provide data on functional status as well as detection of ischemia. For patients who cannot undergo this test because of abnormal electrocardiograms, no specific recommendation is issued regarding the choice of stress echocardiography versus myocardial perfusion imaging. The guidelines do not support the use of ambulatory electrocardiography as the only diagnostic test to identify candidates for coronary angiography.

Indications for coronary angiography before noncardiac surgery are summarized in Table 63–19. These are adapted from 1987 ACC/AHA guidelines for the use of coronary angiography[64] and incorporate the nature of the procedure to be undertaken. "High-risk" procedures are those with a reported cardiac risk that is usually over 5 per cent, including emergency major operations, particularly in the elderly, aortic and other major vascular procedures, and operations with an anticipated large fluid shift and/or blood loss. "Intermediate-risk" procedures include carotid endarterectomy, head and neck surgery, intraperitoneal and intrathoracic procedures, orthopedic procedures, and prostate operations. The guidelines for coronary angiography also rely on stratification of patients according to their risk for complications, with major predictors of risk including unstable coronary syndromes, decompensated heart failure, significant arrhythmias, and severe valvular disease.

Recommendations for the use of revascularization procedures before noncardiac surgery are tempered by the lack of data demonstrating beneficial impact from revascularization. Therefore, the ACC/AHA guidelines conclude that the timing of revascularization procedures in patients for whom they are otherwise indicated must be determined by the urgency of the noncardiac procedure. Revascularization

TABLE 63–19 INDICATIONS FOR CORONARY ANGIOGRAPHY IN THE PERIOPERATIVE EVALUATION OF PATIENTS WITH SUSPECT OR PROVEN CORONARY ARTERY DISEASE*

I. APPROPRIATE

1. High-risk results on noninvasive testing.
2. Angina pectoris unresponsive to adequate medical therapy.
3. Most patients with unstable angina pectoris.
4. Nondiagnostic or equivocal noninvasive test in a high-risk patient undergoing a high-risk noncardiac surgical procedure.

II. EQUIVOCAL

1. Intermediate risk results on noninvasive testing.
2. Nondiagnostic or equivocal noninvasive test in a lower-risk patient undergoing a high-risk noncardiac surgical procedure.
3. Urgent noncardiac surgery in a patient convalescing from acute myocardial infarction.
4. Perioperative myocardial infarction.

III. INAPPROPRIATE

1. Low-risk noncardiac surgery in a patient with known coronary artery disease and low-risk results on noninvasive testing.
2. Screening for coronary artery disease without appropriate noninvasive testing.
3. Asymptomatic after coronary revascularization, with excellent exercise capacity (≥7 METS).
4. Mild stable angina in patients with good left ventricular function, low-risk noninvasive test results.
5. Patient not candidate for coronary revascularization because of concomitant medical illness.
6. Prior technically adequate normal coronary angiogram within 5 years.
7. Severe left ventricular dysfunction and patient not considered candidate for revascularization procedure.
8. Patient unwilling to consider coronary revascularization procedure.

* If results will affect management.
Modified from Eagle, K. A., Brundage, B. H., Chaitman, B. R., et al.: Guidelines for perioperative cardiovascular evaluation for noncardiac surgery. Report of the American College of Cardiology/American Heart Association Task Force on Practice Guidelines (Committee on Perioperative Cardiovascular Evaluation for Noncardiac Surgery). Reprinted with permission from the American College of Cardiology. J. Am. Coll. Cardiol. *27*:910, 1996.

before noncardiac elective surgical procedures of high or intermediate risk was supported for patients who are found to have high-risk coronary anatomy in whom long-term outcome would likely be improved by PTCA or CABG.

Specific recommendations were not made for the use of intraoperative pulmonary artery catheters, computerized ST-segment monitoring, or intraaortic balloon counterpulsation. Routine testing to detect evidence of myocardial injury after surgery was discouraged. In patients with known or suspected coronary disease who undergo surgical procedures with a high risk for complications, the ACC/AHA guidelines recommend electrocardiograms at baseline, immediately after the procedure, and daily on the first 2 postoperative days. Measurement of cardiac enzymes is recommended for high-risk patients or those who demonstrate clinical evidence of cardiovascular dysfunction.

PREVENTION OF CORONARY ARTERY DISEASE

SECONDARY PREVENTION OF CORONARY ARTERY DISEASE

(See also Chap. 35)

Although many guidelines described in this chapter have the goal of decreasing the use of tests and procedures by defining appropriate indications, some guidelines seek to decrease *underutilization* of interventions that may improve patient outcome through prevention. Clinical trial data are now available to support several measures aimed at preventing or slowing the progression of coronary artery disease, and these interventions are generally most cost-effective when used for secondary prevention, that is, for patients with known coronary disease.[154] Secondary prevention tends to be more cost-effective than primary prevention—that is, intervention for patients without known coronary disease—because patients with known disease are at higher risk of subsequent complications and therefore have a higher probability of benefiting from an effective preventive measure.

Specific recommendations for the use of preventive interventions were provided in a 1995 consensus panel statement from the American Heart Association,[155] which was also endorsed by the American College of Cardiology. These recommendations provide explicit goals for a wide range of topics including smoking cessation, lipid management, physical activity, weight management, blood pressure control, and the use of several key medications. Particularly noteworthy are recommendations that:

- Patients with coronary disease start the American Heart Association Step II Diet (≤30 per cent fat, <7 per cent saturated fat, <200 mg/dl cholesterol), as recommended by the National Cholesterol Education Program (NCEP) Adult Treatment Panel II[156]
- For cholesterol management, drug therapy should be added to diet for coronary disease patients with LDL cholesterol levels greater than 130 mg/dl and considered for those with LDL cholesterol levels between 100 and 130 mg/dl (Fig. 35–4, p. 1138). This recommendation is also consistent with the NCEP definitions of desirable levels of serum lipids in patients with known coronary disease as an LDL cholesterol level less than 100 mg/dl, HDL cholesterol level greater than 35 mg/dl, and triglycerides less than 200 mg/dl.[156]
- Patients perform a minimum of 30 to 60 minutes of moderate-intensity activity three or four times weekly, supplemented by an increase in daily life style activities
- Aspirin 80 mg to 325 mg per day should be started in the absence of contraindications.

- The goal of blood pressure management is to reduce systolic pressure below 140 mm Hg and diastolic pressure below 90 mm Hg.

A similar but separate set of preventive guidelines directed specifically at patients who had undergone coronary revascularization were issued by an AHA panel in 1994.[157]

HIGH BLOOD CHOLESTEROL

(See also Chap. 35)

The most influential guidelines for detection and treatment of serum lipid abnormalities were revised and published by the National Cholesterol Education Program (NCEP) in 1993.[156] As was true in previous guidelines from this NHLBI-sponsored group, LDL cholesterol is the most important determinant of cholesterol-lowering strategy. However, these revisions emphasize the emerging recognition of age and low HDL cholesterol as important risk factors for coronary heart disease and describe different strategies for groups at various risks of ischemic complications.

In the revised guidelines, screening evaluations of HDL cholesterol level are recommended, and HDL cholesterol levels below 35 mg/dl are considered a major risk factor for coronary heart disease. High HDL cholesterol levels (>60 mg/dl) are considered a "negative" risk factor that reduces the count of total risk factors.

Age also influences risk assessment in the new guidelines. Men below age 35 years and premenopausal women are considered to be at low risk for coronary heart complications, and delays in initiation of drug therapy for LDL cholesterol levels in the range of 160 to 220 mg/dl are recommended. (Pharmacotherapy is supported for patients in these age groups who have higher LDL cholesterol levels.) In contrast, age over 45 years for men and over 55 years for women is considered a major risk factor for coronary heart disease. Other major risk factors include family history of premature coronary heart disease, cigarette smoking, hypertension, and diabetes mellitus.

These risk factors and the patient's history are used to divide patients into one of three risk categories:

1. Patients with high blood cholesterol who are otherwise at low risk
2. Patients without evidence of coronary heart disease who are at increased risk because of high blood cholesterol together with multiple other risk factors
3. Patients with known coronary heart disease or other atherosclerotic disease

Different thresholds and goals for initiation of diet and drug therapy for these three groups are recommended in the NCEP guidelines.

The guidelines also encourage more stringent dietary measures for higher-risk patients. The NCEP's eating pattern recommendation for the general public is similar to an American Heart Association Step I diet. This diet includes an intake of saturated fat of 8 to 10 per cent of total calories, 30 per cent or less of calories from total fat, and cholesterol intake less than 300 mg/day.

For patients with known coronary heart disease or other atherosclerotic disease, the guidelines recommend a Step II diet. This diet calls for saturated fat intake of less than 7 per cent of total calories, and total cholesterol intake of less than 200 mg/day. The Step II Diet generally requires intervention by a trained nutritionist. Patients who are unable to meet lipid goals with the Step I Diet and other nonpharmacological goals should also attempt the Step II Diet.

With these diets, total cholesterol levels should be measured and adherence assessed after 4 to 6 weeks and at 3 months of therapy. The guidelines recommend a minimum of 6 months of intensive dietary therapy and counseling before initiation of drug therapy, unless patients have severe elevations of LDL cholesterol (≥220 mg/dl).

Although the NCEP guidelines do not make explicit recommendations about the sequence in which drugs are tried, they note that there are fewer long-term data available on the safety and efficacy of the statins compared with older agents such as the bile acid sequestrants and nicotinic acid. However, recent data demonstrating decreased mortality with this class of drugs may lead to more support for statins as an initial choice in future versions of these guidelines.

HYPERTENSION

(See also Chap. 26)

Guidelines for the treatment of high blood pressure in adults have been issued periodically for more than 20 years by the Joint National Committee on Detection, Evaluation, and Treatment of High Blood Pressure, which published its fifth report (also known as JNC-V) in 1994.[158] These guidelines include a new classification system (Table 63–20) for blood pressure that replaced the traditional terms of "mild" and "moderate" hypertension with stages. "Optimal" blood pressure is systolic blood pressure less than 120 mm Hg and diastolic blood pressure less than 80 mm Hg. Classifications should be based on two or more readings taken at each of two or more visits following initial screening.

The response to an initial elevated blood pressure reading—and the timing of that response—should be dictated by factors including the magnitude of the blood pressure elevation, presence of cardiovascular disease, and risk factors. The JNC-V guidelines for follow-up that are summarized in Table 63–21 provide recommendations for when patients should get immediate treatment (systolic pressure ≥210 mm Hg and/or diastolic pressure ≥120 mm Hg), and how quickly other patients should be asked to return for further evaluation. During these evaluations, recommended tests include urinalysis; complete blood count; blood glucose, potassium, calcium, creatinine, uric acid, total and high-density lipoprotein cholesterol and triglyceride levels; and electrocardiography.

TABLE 63–20 CLASSIFICATION OF BLOOD PRESSURE FOR ADULTS (JNC-5)

CATEGORY	SYSTOLIC (mm Hg)	DIASTOLIC (mm Hg)
Normal	<130	<85
High normal	130–139	85–89
Stage 1 (mild) hypertension	140–159	90–99
Stage 2 (moderate) hypertension	160–179	100–109
Stage 3 (severe) hypertension	180–209	110–119
Stage 4 (very severe) hypertension	≥210	≥120

When systolic and diastolic pressures fall into different categories, the higher category should be selected to classify the individual's blood pressure status.

From National High Blood Pressure Education Program: The Fifth Report of the Joint National Committee on Detection, Evaluation, and Treatment of High Blood Pressure. Bethesda, Md., National Heart, Lung, and Blood Institute, 1993. U.S. Department of Health, Education, and Welfare publication NIH 93-1088.

TABLE 63–21 RECOMMENDATIONS FOR FOLLOW-UP BASED ON INITIAL SET OF BLOOD PRESSURE MEASUREMENTS (JNC-5)

INITIAL SCREENING BLOOD PRESSURE (mm Hg*)		
Systolic	**Diastolic**	**Follow-up Recommended**
<130	<85	Recheck in 2 years
130–139	85–89	Recheck in 1 year
140–159	90–99	Confirm within 2 months
160–179	100–109	Evaluate or refer to source of care within 1 month
180–209	110–119	Evaluate or refer to source of care within 1 week
≥210	≥120	Evaluate or refer to source of care immediately

* If the systolic and diastolic categories are different, follow recommendation for the shorter time follow-up.
From National High Blood Pressure Education Program: The Fifth Report of the Joint National Committee on Detection, Evaluation, and Treatment of High Blood Pressure. Bethesda, Md., National Heart, Lung, and Blood Institute, 1993. U.S. Department of Health, Education, and Welfare publication NIH 93-1088.

A more explicit set of recommendations for the definition and management of mild hypertension (systolic pressure 140 to 180 mm Hg and/or diastolic pressure 90 to 105) was revised and published in 1993 by the World Health Organization/International Society of Hypertension Liaison Committee[159] (Fig. 63–4). These guidelines suggest repeat measurement to confirm the diagnosis on at least two occasions over a 4-week period, with regular follow-up for patients whose blood pressure was below 140/90 on remeasurement. Drug treatment is recommended for those whose repeat measurements show diastolic blood pressures greater than 100 mm Hg or systolic pressures greater than 160 to 180 mm Hg with diastolic pressures of 95 or more. For patients with blood pressure between these two levels, observation periods with non-drug antihypertensive measures were recommended. The threshold for initiation of drug therapy varies according to blood pressure levels and presence of other coronary risk factors.

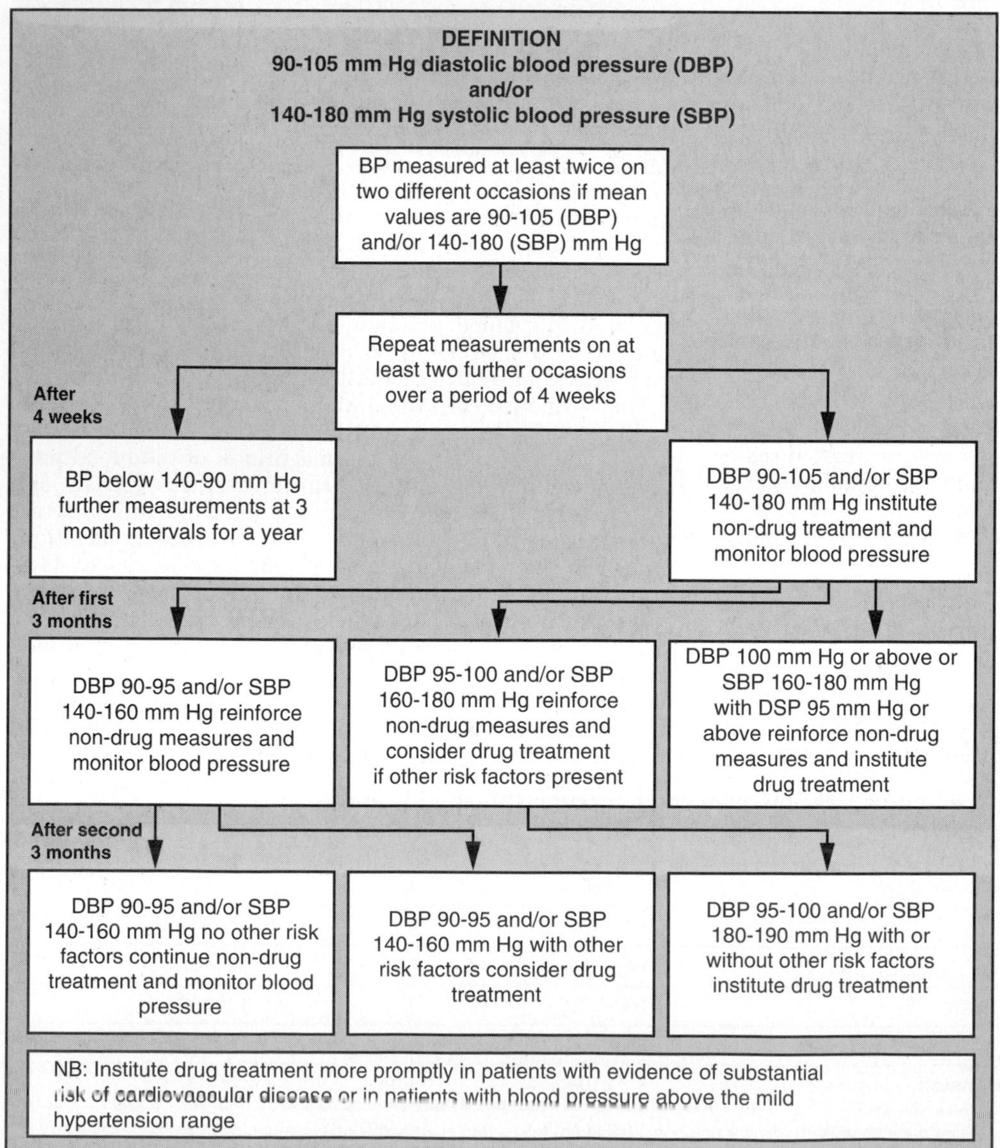

FIGURE 63–4. Recommendations or the definition and management of mild hypertension (systolic pressure 140 to 180 mm Hg and/or diastolic pressure 90 to 105). (Reproduced by permission from The Guidelines Subcommittee of the WHO/ISH Mild Hypertension Liaison Committee: 1993 guidelines for the management of mild hypertension. Memorandum from a World Health Organization/International Society of Hypertension meeting. Hypertension *22*:392, 1993. Copyright 1993 American Heart Association.)

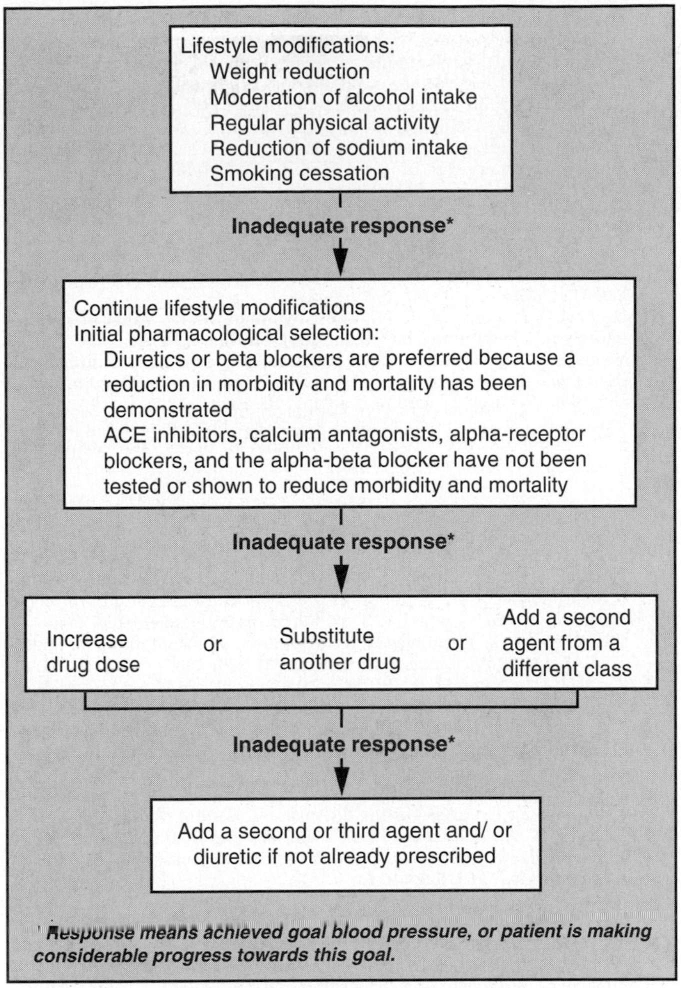

Lifestyle modifications:
Weight reduction
Moderation of alcohol intake
Regular physical activity
Reduction of sodium intake
Smoking cessation

Inadequate response*

Continue lifestyle modifications
Initial pharmacological selection:
Diuretics or beta blockers are preferred because a reduction in morbidity and mortality has been demonstrated
ACE inhibitors, calcium antagonists, alpha-receptor blockers, and the alpha-beta blocker have not been tested or shown to reduce morbidity and mortality

Inadequate response*

Increase drug dose | or | Substitute another drug | or | Add a second agent from a different class

Inadequate response*

Add a second or third agent and/ or diuretic if not already prescribed

*Response means achieved goal blood pressure, or patient is making considerable progress towards this goal.

FIGURE 63–5. JNC-5 guidelines for initiation of antihypertensive therapy. (From National High Blood Pressure Education Program: The Fifth Report of the Joint National Committee on Detection, Evaluation, and Treatment of High Blood Pressure. Bethesda, Md.: National Heart, Lung, and Blood Institute, 1993. US Department of Health, Education, and Welfare publication NIH 93-1088.)

The JNC-V guidelines for initiation of therapy (Fig. 63–5) also emphasize a trial of nonpharmacological measures and, if these measures do not lead to satisfactory reduction in blood pressure, initiation of drug therapy. These guidelines recommend diuretics or beta blockers as first-choice agents, because trials have demonstrated reduction in morbidity and mortality with these agents.[160] Alternative drugs include calcium antagonists, ACE inhibitors, $alpha_1$-receptor blockers, and an alpha-beta blocker. Should the chosen agents not reduce blood pressure to the target level during the next 1 to 3 months, the clinician has three options, including increasing the drug dose, substituting another drug, and adding a second agent from a different class.

REFERENCES

1. Chassin, M. R., Brook, R. H., Park, R. E., et al.: Variations in the use of medical and surgical services by the Medicare population. N. Engl. J. Med. *314*:285, 1986.
2. Wenneker, M. B., and Epstein, A. M.: Racial inequalities in the use of procedures for patients with ischemic heart disease in Massachusetts. JAMA *261*:253, 1989.
3. Ayanian, J. Z., Udvarhelyi, I. S., Gastonis, C. A., Pashos, C. L., and Epstein, A. M.: Racial differences in the use of revascularization procedures after coronary angiography. JAMA *269*:2642, 1993.
4. Whittle, J., Conigliaro, J., Good, C. B., and Lofgren, R. P.: Racial differences in the use of invasive cardiovascular procedures in the Department of Veterans Affairs medical system. N. Engl. J. Med. *329*:600, 1993.
5. Johnson, P. A., Lee, T. H., Cook, E. F., et al.: Effect of race on the presentation and management of patients with chest pain. Ann. Intern. Med. *118*:593, 1993.
6. Ayanian, J. Z., and Epstein, A. M.: Differences in the use of procedures between women and men hospitalized for coronary heart disease. N. Engl. J. Med. *325*:1221, 1991.
7. Tobin, J. N., Wassertheil-Smoller, S., Wexler, J. P., et al.: Sex bias in considering coronary bypass surgery. Ann. Intern. Med. *107*:19, 1987.
8. Wenneker, M. B., Weissman, J. S., and Epstein, A. M.: The association of payer with utilization of cardiac procedures in Massachusetts. JAMA *264*:1255, 1990.
9. Rouleau, J. L., Moye, L. A., Pfeffer, M. A., et al.: A comparison of management patterns after acute myocardial infarction in Canada and the United States. N. Engl. J. Med. *328*:779, 1993.
10. Every, N. R., Larson, E. B., Litwin, P. E., et al.: The association between on-site cardiac catheterization facilities and the use of coronary angiography after acute myocardial infarction. N. Engl. J. Med. *329*:546, 1993.
11. Institute of Medicine Committee to Advise the Public Health Service on Practice Guidelines: Clinical Practice Guidelines: Directions for a New Agency. Washington, D.C., National Academy Press, 1990.
12. Braunwald, E., Mark, D. B., Jones, R. H., et al.: Unstable Angina: Diagnosis and Management. Clinical Practice Guideline Number 10 (amended). AHCPR Publication No. 94-0602. Rockville, Md., Agency for Health Care Policy and Research and the National Heart, Lung, and Blood Institute, Public Health Service, US Department of Health and Human Services, May 1994.
13. Konstam, M., Dracup, K., Baker, D., et al.: Heart Failure: Evaluation and Care of Patients with Left-Ventricular Systolic Dysfunction. Clinical Practice Guidelines No. 11. AHCPR Publication No. 94-0612. Rockville, Md., Agency for Health Care Policy and Research and the National Heart, Lung, and Blood Institute, Public Health Service, US Department of Health and Human Services, June 1994.
14. Bernstein, S. J., Hilborne, L. H., Leape, L. L., et al.: The appropriateness of use of coronary angiography in New York State. JAMA *269*:766, 1993.
15. Brook, R. H., Park, R. E., Chassin, M. R., et al.: Predicting the appropriate use of carotid endarterectomy, upper gastrointestinal endoscopy, and coronary angiography. N. Engl. J. Med. *323*:1173, 1990.
16. Bernstein, S. J., Laouri, M., Hilborne, L. H., et al.: Coronary Angiography. A literature review and ratings of appropriateness and necessity. Santa Monica, Calif., RAND, 1992.
17. Phelps, C. E.: The methodological foundations of studies of the appropriateness of medical care. N. Engl. J. Med. *329*:1241, 1993.
18. Pearson, S. D., Goulart-Fisher, D., and Lee, T. H.: Critical pathways: potential and pitfalls. Ann. Intern. Med. *123*:941, 1995.
19. Lomas, J., Anderson, G. M., Domnick-Pierre, K., et al.: Do practice guidelines guide practice? The effect of a consensus statement on the practice of physicians. N. Engl. J. Med. *321*:1306, 1989.
20. Kosecoff, J., Kanouse, D. E., Rogers, W. H., et al.: Effects of the National Institutes of Health Consensus Development Program on physician practice. JAMA *258*:2708, 1987.
21. Hill, M. N., Levine, D. M., and Whelton, P. K.: Awareness, use and impact of the 1984 Joint National Committee Consensus Report on High Blood Pressure. Am. J. Public Health. *78*:1190, 1988.
22. Ellrodt, A. G., Conner, L., Riedinger, M., and Weingarten, S.: Measuring and improving physician compliance with clinical practice guidelines. A controlled interventional trial. Ann. Intern. Med. *122*:277, 1995.
23. Zyzanski, S. J., Stange, K. C., Kelly, R., et al.: Family physicians' disagreements with the US Preventive Services Task Force recommendations. J. Fam. Pract. *39*:140, 1994.
24. Hyams, A. L., Brandenburg, J. A., Lipsitz, S. R., et al.: Practice guidelines and malpractice litigation: a two-way street. Ann. Intern. Med. *122*:450, 1995.
25. Tunis, S. R., Hayward, R. S., Wilson, M. C., et al.: Internists' attitudes about clinical practice guidelines. Ann. Intern. Med. *120*:956, 1994.
26. Woolf, S. H.: Practice guidelines: A new reality in medicine: I. Recent developments. Arch. Intern. Med. *150*:1811, 1990.
27. Woolf, S. H.: Practice guidelines: A new reality in medicine: II. Methods of developing guidelines. Arch. Intern. Med. *152*:946, 1992.
28. Audet, A. M., Greenfield, S., and Field, M.: Medical practice guidelines: Current activities and future directions. Ann. Intern. Med. *113*:709, 1990.

NONINVASIVE TESTS AND PROCEDURES

29. Schlant, R. C., Adolph, R. J. DiMarco, J. P., et al.: Guidelines for electrocardiography. A report of the American College of Cardiology/American Heart Association Task Force on Assessment of Diagnostic and Therapeutic Cardiovascular Procedures (Committee on Electrocardiography. J. Am. Coll. Cardiol. *19*:473, 1992.
30. U.S. Preventive Task Force Guide to Clinical Preventive Services. Baltimore, Williams and Wilkins, 1989.
31. Grundy, S. M., Greenland, P., Herd, A., et al.: Cardiovascular and risk factor evaluation of healthy American adults: A statement for physicians by an ad hoc committee appointed by the Steering Committee, American Heart Association. Circulation *75*:1340A, 1987.
32. Hayward, R. S. A., Steinberg, E. P., Ford, D. E., et al.: Preventive care guidelines: 1991. Ann. Intern. Med. *114*:758, 1991.
33. Goldberger, A. L., and O'Konski, M. S.: Utility of the routine electrocardiogram before surgery and on general hospital admission. Critical re-

view and new guidelines. *In* Sox, H. C., Jr. (ed.): Common Diagnostic Tests. Use and Interpretation. 2nd ed. Philadelphia, American College of Physicians, 1990, pp. 67–78.
34. Schlant, R. C., Blomqvist, C. G., and Brandenburg, R. O., et al.: Guidelines for exercise testing. A report of the American College of Cardiology/American Heart Association Task Force on Assessment of Cardiovascular Procedures (Subcommittee on Exercise Testing). J. Am. Coll. Cardiol. *8:*725, 1986.
35. Ewy, G. A., Appleton, C. P., Demaria, A. N., et al.: ACC/AHA guidelines for the clinical application of echocardiography. A report of the American College of Cardiology/American Heart Association Task Force on Assessment of Diagnostic and Therapeutic Cardiovascular Procedures (Subcommittee to Develop Guidelines for the Clinical Application of Echocardiography). J. Am. Coll. Cardiol. *16:*1505, 1990.
36. Udvarhelyi, I. S., Goldman, L., Komaroff, A. L., and Lee, T. H.: Determinants of resource utilization for patients admitted for evaluation of acute chest pain. J. Gen. Intern. Med. *7:*1, 1992.
37. Gibler, W. B., Runyon, J. P., Levy, R. C., et al.: Evaluation of patients with chest pain in an emergency department rapid diagnosis and treatment unit. Ann. Emerg. Med. *25:*1, 1995.
38. Sabia, P., Abott, R. D., Afrookteh, A., et al.: Importance of two-dimensional echocardiographic assessment of left ventricular systolic function in patients presenting to the emergency room with cardiac-related symptoms. Circulation *84:*1615, 1991.
39. Cardiogenic brain embolism. Cerebral Embolism Task Force. Arch. Neurol. *43:*71, 1986.
40. DeRook, F. A., Komess, K. A., Albers, G. W., and Popp, R. L.: Transesophageal echocardiography in the evaluation of stroke. Ann. Intern. Med. *117:*922, 1992.
41. Guidelines for Clinical Use of Cardiac Radionuclide Imaging, December 1986.: A Report of the American College of Cardiology/American Heart Association Task Force on Assessment of Cardiovascular Procedures. J. Am. Coll. Cardiol. *8:*1471, 1986.
42. Ritchie, J. L., Bateman, T. M., Bonow, R. O., et al.: Guidelines for clinical use of cardiac radionuclide imaging. Report of the American College of Cardiology/American Heart Association Task Force on Assessment of Diagnostic and Therapeutic Cardiovascular Procedures (Committee on Radionuclide Imaging), developed in collaboration with the American Society of Nuclear Cardiology. J. Am. Coll. Cardiol. *25:*521, 1995.
43. Maddahi, J., Kiat, H., Friedman, J. D., et al.: Technetium-99m-sestamibi myocardial perfusion imaging for evaluation of coronary artery disease. *In* Zaret, B. L. and Beller, G. A., (eds.): Nuclear Cardiology: State of the Art and Future Directions. St. Louis, C. V. Mosby, 1993, pp. 191–200.
44. American College of Physicians.: Efficacy of exercise thallium-201 scintigraphy in the diagnosis and prognosis of coronary artery disease. Ann. Intern. Med. *113:*703, 1990.
45. Go, R. T., Marwick, T. H., MacIntyre, W. J., et al.: A prospective comparison of rubidium-82 PET and thallium-201 SPECT myocardial perfusion imaging utilizing a single dipyridamole stress in the diagnosis of coronary artery disease. J. Nucl. Med. *31:*1899, 1990.
46. Stewart, R. E., Schwaiger, M., Molina, E., et al.: Comparison of rubidium-82 positron emission tomography and thallium-201 SPECT imaging for detection of coronary artery disease. Am. J. Cardiol. *67:*1303, 1991.
47. Bonow, R. O., Berman, D. S., Gibbons, R. J., et al.: Cardiac positron emission tomography: A report for health professionals from the Committee on Advanced Cardiac Imaging and Technology of the Council on Clinical Cardiology, American Heart Association. Circulation *84:*447, 1991.
48. Shaw, L., Miller, D. D., Kong, B. A., et al.: Determination of perioperative cardiac risk by adenosine thallium-201 myocardial imaging. Am. Heart J. *124:*861, 1992.
49. Knoebel, S. B., Crawford, M. H., Dunn, M. I., et al.: Guidelines for ambulatory electrocardiography. A report of the American College of Cardiology/American Heart Association Task Force on Assessment of Diagnostic and Therapeutic Cardiovascular Procedures (Subcommittee on Ambulatory Electrocardiography). J. Am. Coll. Cardiol. *13:*249, 1989.
50. American College of Physicians.: Ambulatory electrocardiographic (Holter) monitoring. Ann. Intern. Med. *113:*77, 1990.
51. Kleiger, R. E., Miller, J. P., Bigger, J. T., Moss, A. J., and The Multicenter Post-Infarction Research Group.: Decreased heart rate variability and its association with increased mortality after acute myocardial infarction. Am. J. Cardiol. *59:*256, 1987.
52. Martin, G. J., Magid, N. M., Myers, G., et al.: Heart rate variability and sudden death. Am. J. Cardiol. *59:*256, 1987.
53. Reiter, M. J., Mann, D. E., Reiffel, J. E., et al.: Significance and incidence of concordance of drug efficacy predictions by Holter monitoring and electrophysiological study in the ESVEM Trial. Electrophysiologic Study versus Electrocardiographic Monitoring. Circulation *91:*1988, 1995.
54. Raby, K. E., Goldman, L., Creager, M. A., et al.: Correlation between preoperative ischemia and major cardiac events after peripheral vascular surgery. N. Engl. J. Med. *321:*1296, 1989.
55. Pepine, C. J., Cohn, P. F., Deedwania, P. C., et al.: Effects of treatment on outcome in mildly symptomatic patients with ischemia during daily life. The Atenolol Silent Ischemia Study. Circulation *90:*762, 1994.
56. Knatterud, G. L., Bourassa, M. G., Pepine, C. J., et al.: Effects of treatment strategies to suppress ischemia in patients with coronary artery disease; 12-week results of the Asymptomatic Cardiac Ischemia Pilot (ACIP) Study. J. Am. Coll. Cardiol. *24:*11, 1994.
57. Stone, P. H., Gibson, R. S., Glasser, S. P., et al.: Comparison of propranolol, diltiazem, and nifedipine in the treatment of ambulatory ischemia in patients with stable angina. Differential effects on ambulatory ischemia, exercise performance, and angina symptoms. The ASIS Study Group. Circulation *82:*1962, 1990.
58. Hubner, P. J. B., Goldberg, M. J., and Lawson, C. W.: Value of routine cardiac monitoring in the management of acute myocardial infarction outside a coronary care unit. Br. Med. J. *1:*815, 1969.
59. Macy, J., and James, T. N.: The value and limitations of computer monitoring in myocardial infarction. Prog. Cardiovasc. Dis. *13:*495, 1971.
60. Lindsay, J., and Bruckner, N. V.: Conventional coronary care unit monitoring—nondetection of transient rhythm disturbances. JAMA *232:*51, 1975.
61. Lipskis, D. J., Dannehl, K. N., and Silverman, M. E.: Value of radiotelemetry in a community hospital. Am. J. Cardiol. *53:*1284, 1984.
62. Vismara, L. A., DeMaria, A. N., Hughes, J. L., et al.: Evaluation of arrhythmias in the late hospital phase of acute myocardial infarction compared to coronary care unit ectopy. Br. Heart J. *37:*598, 1975.
63. Jaffe, A. S., Atkins, J. M., Field, J. M., et al.: Recommended guidelines for in-hospital cardiac monitoring of adults for detection of arrhythmia. J. Am. Coll. Cardiol. *18:*1431, 1991.

INVASIVE TESTS AND PROCEDURES

64. Ross, J., Jr., Brandenburg, R. O., Dinsmore, R. E., et al.: Guidelines for coronary angiography. A report of the American College of Cardiology/American Heart Association Task Force on Assessment of Diagnostic and Therapeutic Cardiovascular Procedures (Subcommittee on Coronary Angiography). J. Am. Coll. Cardiol. *10:*935, 1987.
65. Pepine, C. J., Allen, H. D., Bashore, T. M., et al.: ACC/AHA Guidelines for cardiac catheterization and cardiac catheterization laboratories. American College of Cardiology/American Heart Association Ad Hoc Task Force on Cardiac Catheterization. J. Am. Coll. Cardiol. *18:*1149, 1991.
66. ACC/AHA Task Force on Assessment of Cardiovascular Procedures.: Guidelines for Exercise Testing. J. Am. Coll. Cardiol. *8:*725, 1986.
67. Schaffer, W. A., and Cobb, L. A.: Recurrent ventricular fibrillation and modes of death in survivors of out-of-hospital ventricular fibrillation. N. Engl. J. Med. *293:*259, 1975.
68. Grines, C. L., Browne, K. F., Marco, J., et al. for the Primary Angioplasty in Myocardial Infarction Study Group.: A comparison of immediate angioplasty with thrombolytic therapy for acute myocardial infarction. N. Engl. J. Med. *328:*673, 1993.
69. Zijlstra, F., de Boear, M. J., Hoornthje, J. C. A., et al.: A comparison of immediate coronary angioplasty with intravenous streptokinase in acute myocardial infarction. N. Engl. J. Med. *328:*680, 1993.
70. Gibbons, R. J., Holmes, D. R., Reeder, G. S., et al., for the Mayo Coronary Care Unit and Catheterization Laboratory Groups.: Immediate angioplasty compared with the administration of a thrombolytic agent followed by conservative treatment for myocardial infarction. N. Engl. J. Med. *328:*685, 1993.
71. Topol, E. J., Califf, R. M., George, B. S., et al.: A randomized trial of immediate versus delayed elective angioplasty after intravenous tissue plasminogen activator in acute myocardial infarction. N. Engl. J. Med. *317:*581, 1987.
72. Simoons, M. L., Arnold, A. E. R., Betriu, A., et al.: Thrombolysis with tissue plasminogen activator in acute myocardial infarction: No additional benefit from immediate percutaneous coronary angioplasty. Lancet *1:*197, 1988.
73. Rogers, W. J., Baim, D. S., Gore, J. M., et al.: Comparison of immediate invasive, delayed invasive, and conservative strategies after tissue-type plasminogen activator. Results of the Thrombolysis in Myocardial Infarction (TIMI). Phase II—A trial. Circulation *81:*1457, 1990.
74. The TIMI Study Group.: Comparison of invasive and conservative strategies after treatment with intravenous tissue plasminogen activator in acute myocardial infarction. Results of the Thrombolysis in Myocardial Infarction (TIMI) Phase II Trial. N. Engl. J. Med. *320:*618, 1989.
75. Ellis, S. G., Ribeiro da Silva, E., Heyndrickx, G. R., et al.: Final results of the randomized RESCUE study evaluating PTCA after failed thrombolysis for patients with anterior infarction. Circulation *88:*I-106, 1993.
76. Belenkie, I., Traboulsi, M., Gall, C. A., et al.: Rescue angioplasty during myocardial infarction has a beneficial effect on mortality: A tenable hypothesis. Can. J. Cardiol. *8:*357, 1992.
77. Czer, L. S., Gray, R. J., DeRoberts, M. A., et al.: Mitral valve replacement: Impact of coronary artery disease and determinants of prognosis after revascularization. Circulation *70* (suppl. I):I-198, 1984.
78. Block, P. C., Ockene, I., Goldberg, R. J., et al.: A prospective randomized trial of outpatient versus inpatient cardiac catheterization. N. Engl. J. Med. *319:*1251, 1988.
79. Klinke, W. P., Kubac, G., Talibi, T., and Lee, S. J. K.: Safety of outpatient cardiac catheterizations. Am. J. Cardiol. *56:*639, 1985.
80. Clark, D. A., Moscovich, M. D., Vetrovec, G. W., and Wexler, L.: Guidelines for the performance of outpatient catheterization and angiographic procedures. Cathet. Cardiovasc. Diagn. *27:*5, 1992.
81. Society for Cardiac Angiography, Laboratory Performance Standards Committee.: Guidelines for approval of professional staff for privileges in the cardiac catheterization laboratory. Cathet. Cardiovasc. Diagn. *10:*199, 1984.

82. Rodriguez, A., Boullon, F., Perez-Balino, N., et al.: Argentine randomized trial of percutaneous transluminal coronary angioplasty versus coronary artery bypass surgery in multivessel disease (ERACI): In-hospital results and 1-year follow-up. J. Am. Coll. Cardiol. *22*:1060, 1993.
83. Hamm, C. W., Reimers, J., Ischinger, T., et al., for the German Angioplasty Bypass Surgery Investigation.: A randomized study of coronary angioplasty compared with bypass surgery in patients with symptomatic multivessel coronary disease. N. Engl. J. Med. *331*:1037, 1994.
84. Hamptom, J. R., Henderson, R. A., Julian, D. G., and the RITA trial participants.: Coronary angioplasty versus coronary artery bypass surgery: The Randomised Intervention Treatment of Angina (RITA) trial. Lancet *341*:573, 1993.
85. King, S. B., III, Lembo, N. J., Weintraub, W. S., et al.: A randomized trial comparing coronary angioplasty with coronary bypass surgery: The Emory Angioplasty versus Surgery Trail. N. Engl. J. Med. *331*:1044, 1994.
86. Parisi, A. F., Folland, E. D., and Hartigan, P., for the Veterans Affairs ACME Investigators.: A comparison of early invasive and conservative strategies in unstable angina and non-Q-wave myocardial infarction. Circulation *89*:1545, 1994.
87. Ryan, T. J., Bauman, W. B., Kennedy, J. W., et al.: Guidelines for percutaneous transluminal coronary angioplasty. A report of the American College of Cardiology/American Heart Association Task Force on Assessment of Diagnostic and Therapeutic Cardiovascular Procedures (Subcommittee on Percutaneous Transluminal Coronary Angioplasty). J. Am. Coll. Cardiol. *22*:2033, 1993.
88. Society for Cardiac Angiography.: Guidelines for credentialing and facilities for performance of coronary angioplasty. Cathet. Cardiovasc. Diagn. *15*:136, 1988.
89. Ryan, T. J., Klocke, F. J., and Reynolds, W. A.: Clinical competence in percutaneous transluminal coronary angioplasty: A statement for physicians from the ACP/ACC/AHA Task Force on Clinical Privileges in Cardiology. J. Am. Coll. Cardiol. *15*:1469, 1990.
90. 17th Bethesda Conference: Adult Cardiology Training. November 1–2, 1985. J. Am. Coll. Cardiol. *7*:1191, 1986.
91. Kirklin, J. W., Akins, C. W., Blackstone, E. H., et al.: Guidelines and indications for coronary artery bypass graft surgery. A report of the American College of Cardiology/American Heart Association Task Force on Assessment of Diagnostic and Therapeutic Cardiovascular Procedures (Subcommittee on Coronary Artery Bypass Graft Surgery) J. Am. Coll. Cardiol. *17*:543, 1991.
92. Mark, D. B., Lam, L. C., Lee, K. L., et al.: Effects of coronary angioplasty, coronary bypass surgery, and medical therapy on employment in patients with coronary artery disease. A prospective comparison study. Ann. Intern. Med. *120*:111, 1994.
93. Varnauskas, E., and the European Coronary Surgery Study Group: Twelve-year follow-up of survival in the randomized European Coronary Surgery Study. N. Engl. J. Med. *319*:332, 1988.
94. Chaitman, B. R., Davis, K. B., Kaiser, G. C., et al.: The role of coronary bypass surgery for 'left main equivalent' coronary disease: The Coronary Artery Surgery Study Registry. Circulation *74* (suppl. III):III-17, 1986.
95. Chaitman, B. R., Davis, K., Fisher, L. D., et al.: A life table and Cox regression analysis of patients with combined proximal left anterior descending and proximal left circumflex coronary artery disease: Non-left main equivalent lesions (CASS). Circulation *68*:1163, 1983.
96. Parisi, A. F., Khuri, S., Deupree, R. H., et al.: Medical compared with surgical management of unstable angina; five-year mortality and morbidity in the Veterans Administration study. Circulation *80*:1176, 1989.
97. Wright, I. S., and Fredrickson, D. T. (eds.): Cardiovascular Disease. Guidelines for Prevention and Care. Reports of the Inter-Society Commission for Heart Disease Resources. Washington, D. C., U. S. Government Printing Office, 1972.
98. Subcommittee on Cardiac Surgery Standards of the Cardiovascular Committee and the Advisory Council for Cardiothoracic Surgery of the American College of Surgeons.: Guidelines for minimal standards in cardiac surgery. ACS Bulletin, 1984, pp. 67–69.
99. Zipes, D. P., Akhtar, M., Denes, P., et al.: Guidelines for clinical intracardiac electrophysiologic studies. A report of the American College of Cardiology/American Heart Association Task Force on Assessment of Diagnostic and Therapeutic Cardiovascular Procedures (Subcommittee to Assess Clinical Intracardiac Electrophysiologic Studies). J. Am. Coll. Cardiol. *14*:1827, 1989.
100. Zipes, D. P., DiMarco, J. P., Gillette, P. C., et al.: Guidelines for clinical intracardiac electrophysiologic and catheter ablation procedures. A report of the American College of Cardiology/American Heart Association Task Force on Practice Guidelines (Subcommittee on Clinical Intracardiac Electrophysiologic and Catheter Ablation Procedures). J. Am. Coll. Cardiol. *26*:555, 1995.
101. Dhingra, R. C., Palileo, E., Strasberg, B., et al.: Significance of the HV interval in 517 patients with chronic bifascicular block. Circulation *64*:1265, 1981.
102. Bhandari, A. K., Shapiro, W. A., Morady, F., et al.: Electrophysiologic testing in patients with the long QT syndrome. Circulation *71*:63, 1985.
103. Jackman, W. M., Friday, K. J., Anderson, J. L., et al.: The long QT syndromes: A critical review, new clinical observations, and a unifying hypothesis. Prog. Cardiovasc. Dis. *31*:115, 1988.
104. Myerburg, R. J., Kessler, K. M., Kimura, S., and Castellanos, A.: Sudden cardiac death: Future approaches based upon identification and control of transient risk factors. J. Cardiovasc. Electrophysiol. *3*:626, 1992.
105. Gulamhusein, S., Naccarelli, G. V., and Ko, P. T.: Value and limitations of clinical electrophysiologic study in assessment of patients with unexplained syncope. Am. J. Med. *73*:700, 1982.
106. Diagnostic and therapeutic technology assessment (DATTA).: Radiofrequency catheter ablation of aberrant conducting pathways of the heart. JAMA *268*:2091, 1992.
107. Fisher, J. D.: American College of Cardiology Cardiovascular Technology Assessment Committee. Catheter ablation for cardiac arrhythmias: Clinical applications, personnel and facilities. J. Am. Coll. Cardiol. *24*:828, 1994.
108. Scheinman, M. M.: Catheter ablation for cardiac arrhythmias, personnel and facilities. North American Society of Pacing and Electrophysiology Ad Hoc Committee on Catheter Ablation. PACE Pacing Clin. Electrophysiol. *15*:715, 1992.
109. Dreifus, L. S., Fisch, C., Griffin, J. C., et al.: Guidelines for implantation of cardiac pacemakers and antiarrhythmia devices. A report of the American College of Cardiology/American Heart Association Task Force on Assessment of Diagnostic and Therapeutic Cardiovascular Procedures (Committee on Pacemaker Implantation) J. Am. Coll. Cardiol. *18*:1, 1991.

CLINICAL SYNDROMES

110. Lee, T. H., Rouan, G. W., Weisberg, M. C., et al.: Clinical characteristics and natural history of patients with acute myocardial infarction sent home from the emergency room. Am. J. Cardiol. *60*:219, 1987.
111. Rusnak, R. A., Stair, T. O., Hansen, K., and Fastow, J. S.: Litigation against the emergency physician: Common features in cases of missed myocardial infarction. Ann. Emerg. Med. *14*:1029, 1989.
112. Lee, T. H., and Goldman, L.: The coronary care unit turns 25: Historical trends and future directions. Ann. Intern. Med. *108*:887, 1988.
113. Goldman, L., Cook, E. F., Brand, D. A., et al.: A computer protocol to predict myocardial infarction in emergency department patients with chest pain. N. Engl. J. Med. *318*:797, 1988.
114. Pozen, M. W., D'Agostino, R. B., Selker, H. P., et al.: A predictive instrument to improve coronary-care-unit admission practices in acute ischemic heart disease. A prospective multicenter clinical trial. N. Engl. J. Med. *310*:1273, 1984.
115. Selker, H. P., Griffith, J. L., and D'Agostino, R. B.: A tool for judging coronary care unit admission appropriateness, valid for both real-time and retrospective use. A time-insensitive predictive instrument (TIPI) for acute cardiac ischemia: a multicenter study. Med. Care. *29*:610, 1991.
116. Baxt, W. G.: Use of an artificial neural network for the diagnosis of myocardial infarction. Ann. Intern. Med. *115*:843, 1991.
117. Fiebach, N. H., Cook, E. F., Lee, T. H., et al.: Outcomes of patients with myocardial infarction who are initially admitted to stepdown units: data from the Multicenter Chest Pain Study. Am. J. Med. *89*:15, 1990.
118. Gaspoz, J. M., Lee, T. H., Cook, E. F., et al.: Outcome of patients who were admitted to a new short-stay unit to "rule-out" myocardial infarction. J. Am. Coll. Cardiol. *68*:145, 1991.
119. Gaspoz, J. M., Lee, T. H., Weinstein, M. C., et al.: Cost-effectiveness of a new short-stay unit to rule out acute myocardial infarction in low risk patients. J. Am. Coll. Cardiol. *24*:1249, 1994.
120. Gibler, W. B., Runyon, J. P., Levy, R. C., et al.: A rapid diagnostic and treatment center for patients with chest pain in the emergency department. Ann. Emerg. Med. *25*:1, 1995.
121. Graff, L., Zun, L. S., Leikin, J., et al.: Emergency department observation beds improve patient care: Society for Academic Emergency Medicine debate. Ann. Emerg. Med. *21*:967, 1992.
122. Lee, T. H., Juarez, G., Cook, E. F., et al.: Ruling out acute myocardial infarction. A prospective multicenter validation of a 12-hour strategy for patients at low risk. N. Engl. J. Med. *324*:1239, 1991.
123. Adams, J. E., III, Bodor, G. S., Davila-Roman, V. G., et al.: Cardiac troponin I: A marker with high specificity for cardiac injury. Circulation *88*:101, 1993.
124. Hamm, C. W., Ravkilde, J., Gerhardt, W., et al.: The prognostic value of serum troponin T in unstable angina. N. Engl. J. Med. *327*:146, 1992.
125. Lewis, W. R., et al.: Utility and safety of immediate exercise testing of low risk patients admitted to the hospital for suspected acute myocardial infarction. Am. J. Cardiol. *74*:987, 1994.
126. Sabia, P., Afrookteh, A., Touchstone, D. A., et al.: Value of regional wall motion abnormality in the emergency room diagnosis of acute myocardial infarction. A prospective study using two-dimensional echocardiography. Circulation *84* (suppl. I):I-85, 1991.
127. American College of Emergency Physicians.: Clinical policy for the initial approach to adults presenting with a chief complaint of chest pain, with no history of trauma. Ann. Emerg. Med. *25*:274, 1995.
128. National Heart Attack Alert Program Coordinating Committee 60 Minutes to Treatment Working Group.: Emergency Department: Rapid Identification and Treatment of Patients with Acute Myocardial Infarction. NIH Publication No. 93-3278. National Heart, Lung and Blood Institute, Public Health Service, U.S. Department of Health and Human Services. September 1993.
129. Gunnar, R. M., Bourdillon, P. D. V., Dixon, D. W., et al.: Guidelines for the early management of patients with acute myocardial infarction. A report of the American College of Cardiology/American Heart Association Task Force on Assessment of Diagnostic and Therapeutic Cardiovascular Procedures (Subcommittee to Develop Guidelines for the Early Management of Patients with Acute Myocardial Infarction). J. Am. Coll. Cardiol. *16*:249, 1990.

130. Lee, T. H., and Goldman, L.: Serum enzyme assays in the diagnosis of acute myocardial infarction. Recommendations based on a quantitative analysis. *In* Sox, H. C., Jr., (ed.): Common Diagnostic Tests. Use and Interpretation. 2nd ed. Philadelphia, American College of Physicians, 1990, pp. 36–66.
131. American Heart Association/Emergency Cardiac Care Committee and Subcommittees: Guidelines for cardiopulmonary resuscitation and emergency cardiac care, III: Adult advanced cardiac life support. JAMA *268:*2199, 1992.
132. Gonzalez, E. R., Jones, L. A., Ornato, J. P., et al. (Virginia Thrombolytic Study Group): Hospital delays and problems with thrombolytic administration in patients receiving thrombolytic therapy: A multicenter prospective assessment. Ann. Emerg. Med. *21:*1215, 1992.
133. Fibrinolytic Therapy Trialists' Collaborative Group.: Indications for fibrinolytic therapy in suspected acute myocardial infarction: Collaborative overview of early mortality and major morbidity results from all randomized trials of more than 1000 patients.Lancet *343:*311, 1994.
134. The GUSTO Investigators: An international randomized trial comparing four thrombolytic strategies for acute myocardial infarction. N. Engl. J. Med. *329:*673, 1993.
135. Mark, D. B., Hlatky, M. A., Califf, R. M., et al.: Cost-effectiveness of thrombolytic therapy with tissue plasminogen activator as compared with streptokinase for acute myocardial infarction. N. Engl. J. Med. *332:*1418, 1995.
136. Kalish, S. C., Gurwitz, J. H., Krumholz, H. M., and Avorn, J.: A cost-effectiveness model of thrombolytic therapy for acute myocardial infarction. J. Gen. Intern. Med. *10:*321, 1995.
137. MacMahon, S., Collins, R., Peto, R., et al.: Effects of prophylactic lidocaine in suspected acute myocardial infarction: An overview of results from the randomized controlled trials. JAMA *260:*1910, 1988.
138. Beta-Blocker Heart Attack Trial Research Group.: A randomized trial of propranolol in patients with acute myocardial infarction: I. Mortality results. JAMA *247:*1707, 1982.
139. Moss, A. J.: Secondary prevention with calcium channel-blocking drugs in patients after myocardial infarction: A critical review. Circulation *75*(Suppl. V):V-148, 1987.
140. The Multicenter Diltiazem Postinfarction Trial Research Group.: The effect of diltiazem on mortality and reinfarction after myocardial infarction. N. Engl. J. Med. *319:*385, 1988.
141. Theroux, P., Taeymans, Y., Morissette, D., et al.: A randomized study comparing propranolol and diltiazem in the treatment of unstable angina. J. Am. Coll. Cardiol. *5:*717, 1985.
142. Held, P. H., Yusuf, S., and Furberg, C. D.: Calcium channel blockers in acute myocardial infarction and unstable angina: An overview. Br. Med. J. *299:*1187, 1989.
143. Yusuf, S., Wittes, J., and Friedman, L.: Overview of results of randomized clinical trials in heart disease: II. Unstable angina, heart failure, primary prevention with aspirin, and risk factor modification. JAMA *260:*2259, 1988.
144. Lubsen, J., and Tijssen, J. G.: Efficacy of nifedipine and metoprolol in the early treatment of unstable angina in the coronary care unit: Findings from the Holland Interuniversity Nifedipine/metoprolol Trial (HINT). Am. J. Cardiol. *60:*18A, 1987.
145. Mark, D. B., Shaw, L., Harrell, F. E., et al.: Prognostic value of a treadmill exercise score in outpatients with suspected coronary disease. N. Engl. J. Med. *325:*849, 1991.
146. Fleg, J. L., Hinton, P. C., Lakatta, E. G., et al.: Physician utilization of laboratory procedures to monitor outpatients with congestive heart failure. Arch. Intern. Med. *149:*393, 1989.
147. Williams, J. F., Bristow, M. R., Fowler, M. B., et al.: Guidelines for the evaluation and management of heart failure. Report of the American College of Cardiology/American Heart Association Task Force on Practice Guidelines (Committee on Evaluation and Management of Heart Failure). J. Am. Coll. Cardiol. *26:*1376, 1995.
148. The Cardiac Arrhythmia Suppression Trial II Investigators.: Effect of the antiarrhythmic agent moricizine on survival after myocardial infarction. N. Engl. J. Med. *327:*227, 1992.
149. The Cardiac Arrhythmia Suppression Trial (CAST) Investigators.: Preliminary report: Effect of encainide and flecainide on mortality in a randomized trial of arrhythmia suppression after myocardial infarction. N. Engl. J. Med. *321:*406, 1989.
150. Vinson, J. M., Rich, M. W., Sperry, J. C., et al.: Early readmission of elderly patients with congestive heart failure. J. Am. Geriatr. Soc. *38:*1290, 1990.
151. Kupper, A. J., Fintelman, H., Huige, M. C., et al.: Cross-over comparison of the fixed combination of hydrochlorothiazide and triamterene and the free combination of furosemide and triamterene in the maintenance treatment of congestive heart failure. Eur. J. Clin. Pharmacol. *30:*341, 1986.
152. Packer, M., Gheorghiade, M., Young, D., et al.: Withdrawal of digoxin from patients with chronic heart failure treated with angiotensin-converting-enzyme inhibitors. N. Engl. J. Med. *329:*1, 1993.
153. Eagle, K. A., Brundage, B. H., Chaitman, B. R., et al.: Guidelines for perioperative cardiovascular evaluation for noncardiac surgery. Report of the American College of Cardiology/American Heart Association Task Force on Practice Guidelines (Committee on Perioperative Cardiovascular Evaluation for Noncardiac Surgery). J. Am. Coll. Cardiol. *27:*910, 1996.

PREVENTION OF CORONARY ARTERY DISEASE

154. Tengs, T. O., Adams, M. E., Pliskin, J. S., et al.: Five-hundred life-saving interventions and their cost-effectiveness. Risk Analysis *15:*369, 1995.
155. Smith, S. C., Blair, S. N., Criqui, M. H., et al.: Preventing heart attack and death in patients with coronary disease. J. Am. Coll. Cardiol. *26:*292, 1995.
156. Summary of the Second Report of the National Cholesterol Education Program (NCEP) Expert Panel on Detection, Evaluation, and Treatment of High Blood Cholesterol in Adults (Adult Treatment Panel II). JAMA *269:*3015, 1993.
157. Pearson, T. D., Rapaport, E., Criqui, M., et al.: Optimal risk factor management in the patient after coronary revascularization: A statement for healthcare professionals from an American Heart Association writing group. Circulation *90:*3215, 1994.
158. National High Blood Pressure Education Program.: The Fifth Report of the Joint National Committee on Detection, Evaluation, and Treatment of High Blood Pressure. Bethesda, Md.: National Heart, Lung, and Blood Institute, 1993. U. S., Department of Health, Education, and Welfare publication NIH 93-1088.
159. The Guidelines Subcommittee of the WHO/ISH Mild Hypertension Liaison Committee. 1993 guidelines for the management of mild hypertension. Memorandum from a World Health Organization/International Society of Hypertension meeting. Hypertension *22:*392, 1993.
160. Alderman, M. H.: Which antihypertensive drugs first—and why! JAMA *267:*2786, 1992.

Index

Note: Page numbers in *italics* indicate illustrations; those followed by t indicate tables. **Boldface page numbers** indicate main discussion. **Plate numbers** indicate color plates.

Aase syndrome, 1659t
Abdomen, examination of, 17–18
in myocardial infarction, 1201
Abdominojugular reflux, 18, 19
Aberration, intraventricular, acceleration-dependent (tachycardia-dependent aberrancy, phase 3 aberrancy), electrocardiography in, 125–126, *125*
deceleration-dependent (bradycardia-dependent aberrancy, phase 4 aberrancy), electrocardiography in, 126, *126*
electrocardiography in, 124–126, *124–126*
ABO compatibility, in heart transplantation, 518
Abrupt vessel closure, with percutaneous transluminal coronary angioplasty, 1314, 1368–1370, *1369*, 1369t, 1370t
Abscess, brain, in congenital heart disease, 885, 973
Accelerated idioventricular rhythm, 641t–642t, 683–684, *684*
electrocardiography of, 683–684, *684*
in myocardial infarction, 1245t, 1246–1247
treatment of, 598t, 684
Accelerated junctional escape, 143
Accelerated junctional rhythm, in myocardial infarction, 1254
Acceleration-dependent aberrancy, electrocardiography in, 125–126, *125*
Accentuated antagonism, 645
Accuracy, of diagnostic tests, 1743
Acebutolol, in arrhythmias, 610–613, 611t
in renal failure, 1931t
pharmacodynamic properties of, 487t
pharmacology of, 1307t
Acetaminophen (Tylenol), in pediatric cardiology, 1000t
Acetate, carbon-11–labeled, for myocardial metabolism assessment, 306, **Plate 8**
Acetazolamide, hematological abnormalities with, 1804t
in heart failure, 477t
in renal failure, 1933t
Acetylcholine, *1165*
atrioventricular node stimulation by, 552
in contraction-relaxation cycle, 374–375, *374*, 375t
in coronary blood flow regulation, 1164, *1164*, 1165, *1165*, *1166*
in Prinzmetal's variant angina, 1342
pulmonary vascular effects of, 782–783
sinoatrial node stimulation by, 548, 563, *563*
Acetyl-CoA dehydrogenase, defects of, 1668t, 1674
N-Acetylprocainamide, in renal failure, 1930t
Acetylsalicylic acid. See *Aspirin (acetylsalicylic acid).*
Achromobacter xylosoxidans, in infective endocarditis, 1094
Acid lipase deficiency, 1669t
Acid-base balance, cardiac glycoside effects on, 500
diuretic effects on, 480
in congenital heart disease, 885–886
in contraction-relaxation cycle, 371, *371*
postoperative, 1721
Acidemia, in congenital heart disease, 886
Acidosis, in pulmonary vasoconstriction, 1608, *1608*
Acquired immunodeficiency syndrome (AIDS), myocarditis in, 989, 1438–1439, *1438*, 1438t
electrocardiography in, 135, *149*
pericarditis in, 1506–1508
pulmonary hypertension in, 786
tuberculous pericarditis in, 1507–1508
Acrocephalopolysyndactyly, genetic factors in, 1661t
Acrocephalosyndactyly, genetic factors in, 1661t
Acromegaly, 1887–1890
atherosclerosis in, 1888–1889
cardiomegaly in, 1888, *1888*
cardiomyopathy in, 1889–1890, *1889*
diabetes mellitus in, 1888
diagnosis of, 1890
growth hormone in, 1887, 1889
hypertension in, 1888
somatostatin in, 1887
systemic hypertension in, 830
treatment of, 1890
Actin filament, 361
structure of, 364–365, *364*
Actinobacillus actinomycetemcomitans, in infective endocarditis, 1092, 1093t
Actinomyces israelii, in pericarditis, 1511
Actinomycosis, myocarditis in, 1441
Action potential, 555–563, 555t, *558*
during ischemia, 1178
fast-response, 559–561, 561t, 562t
depressed, *562*, 564
in heart failure, 404–405, *405*
inward currents of, 559–561, 561t, 562t
outward currents of, 559–561, 561t, 562t
phase 0 (rapid depolarization) of, 555t, 557–561, *557–560*, 561t, *562*
calcium channels in, 557–559, *557*, *559*
rate of, 555t, 557
sodium channels in, 557–559, *557*, *559*
phase 1 (early rapid repolarization) of, 559–560
phase 2 (plateau) of, 563
phase 3 (final rapid repolarization) of, 563
phase 4 (resting) of, 555–556, 555t, *556*, *557*, 563, *563*
reduction of, 564–565, *565*
slow-response, 559–561, 561t, 562t
tetrodotoxin effect on, *562*
upstroke of, 559–561, 561t, 562t
verapamil effect on, *562*
Activated protein C, in familial thrombosis, 1633–1634, *1634*
Acute coronary syndromes, 1185–1189, *1187*, *1188*. See also *Angina pectoris; Myocardial infarction.*
Addison's disease, 1897
Adenoma, aldosterone-producing, 1896–1897
Adenosine, adverse effects of, 619
dosage of, 618
electrophysiological actions of, 601t, 602t–603t, 618
for angina reproduction, 1290
for stress myocardial perfusion imaging, 289, 289t
in arrhythmia, 594t–595t, 601t, 602t–603t, 618–619
in atrial flutter, 654
in atrioventricular nodal reentrant tachycardia, 664
Adenosine *(Continued)*
in contraction-relaxation cycle, 375–376
in coronary blood flow regulation, 1163, *1163*
in ischemia, 386, *387*
in pulmonary hypertension testing, 793, *793*
indications for, 618
pharmacokinetics of, 618
receptors for, in contraction-relaxation cycle, 375–376
Adenosine diphosphate, *1165*
in myocardial ischemia, 1178
Adenosine diphosphate–adenosine triphosphate carrier, in heart failure, 407
Adenosine monophosphate, cyclic (cAMP), *1165*
in contraction-relaxation cycle, 373–374, *373*, *374*
inhibition of, 374, *374*
Adenosine triphosphate (ATP), in heart failure, 407
in myocardial ischemia, 1178
Adenosine triphosphate (ATP)–binding pocket, of myosin filament, 363, *364*, *365*
Adenovirus vector, for gene therapy, 1638
Adenylate cyclase, in heart failure, 411–412
Adolescents. See also *Children.*
hypertension in, 810, 810t, 822, 822t
Adrenal cortex, disease of, 1895–1897
in myocardial infarction, 1197
Adrenal hyperplasia, congenital, 1678t
hypertension in, 829
Adrenal insufficiency, 1897
Adrenal medulla, catecholamine secretion by, in myocardial infarction, 1197
Adrenalin (epinephrine), in congenital heart disease–related heart failure, 891t
in hypertension, 819
in pediatric cardiology, 1000t
myocardial oxygen consumption and, 1162
Adrenergic inhibitors, 851–854, *851*, 851t
β-Adrenergic receptor kinase, in heart failure, 411, *411*
α-Adrenoceptor, in coronary blood flow regulation, 1170, 1171
β-Adrenoceptor, in contraction-relaxation cycle, 372–374, *372–374*
in coronary blood flow regulation, 1170
in heart failure, 376, *376*, 410–411, *411*, 411t
in idiopathic dilated cardiomyopathy, 1409
physiological actions of, 1304, 1305t
α-Adrenoceptor agonists, in coronary artery disease, 1149t
β-Adrenoceptor agonists, in cor pulmonale, 1619
in myocardial infarction, 1237
α-Adrenoceptor blockers, 848t
in coronary artery disease, 1149t
in systemic hypertension, 851t, 852–853
β-Adrenoceptor blockers, 610–613, *611*, 611t, 848t
after myocardial infarction, 1264, *1264*
α-adrenoceptor blocking activity of, 1306
antiarrhythmic actions of, 1305
cardioselectivity of, 853, *853*, 1305–1306, 1306t
classification of, 853, *853*
clinical effects of, 853
contraindications to, 1306, 1308, 1308t
digoxin interaction with, 483t
dosage of, 594t–595t, 612, 1306, 1307t
electrophysiological actions of, 611–612

β-Adrenoceptor blockers *(Continued)*
  exercise stress testing effects of, 170
  hemodynamic effects of, 612
  hydrophilicity of, 1305–1306
  in angina pectoris, 1301, 1304–1308, *1305*, 1305t, 1306t, 1307t, 1308t, 1311–1312, 1312t, 1337, 1982t, 1983
  in anxiety, 854
  in aortic dissection, 1564–1565
  in arrhythmias, 610–613, *611*, 611t
  in arteriography, 245
  in coronary artery disease, 1149t, 1301
  in elderly, 1699
  in heart failure, 412, 486–488, *487*, 487t, 502–503
  in hyperkinetic hypertension, 854
  in hypertrophic cardiomyopathy, 1425
  in idiopathic dilated cardiomyopathy, 1411
  in ischemic heart disease, 853
  in Marfan syndrome, 1554
  in myocardial infarction, 1211–1212, 1228–1229, *1228*, 1974t, 1978
  in pheochromocytoma, 1899
  in pregnancy, 854
  in Prinzmetal's variant angina, 1342
  in syncope, 874
  in syndrome X, 1344
  indications for, 612–613
  intrinsic sympathomimetic activity of, 853, 1305, 1306t
  lipid solubility of, 853, *854*
  mechanism of, 853
  membrane-stabilizing activity of, 1306
  myocardial oxygen consumption and, 1306t
  noncardiac surgery and, 1761
  oxidation phenotype of, 1306
  pharmacokinetics of, 594t–595t, 612
  pharmacology of, 486, 487t
  potency of, 1305
  selectivity of, 853, *853*, 1305–1306, 1306t
  serum lipid effects of, 1306
  side effects of, 613, 854, 1303t, 1306, 1308
  toxicity of, 11
  withdrawal from, 1308
Adrenocorticotropic hormone (ACTH), in aldosterone secretion, 1895
Adriamycin (doxorubicin), cardiotoxicity of, 11, 997, *997*, 1800–1803, *1800–1803*, 1801t, 1802t
    radionuclide angiocardiography in, 302–303, 303t
  pericarditis with, 1515, 1519
Adult polycystic kidney disease, 1676–1677
  genetic factors in, 1660t
Adult respiratory distress syndrome (ARDS), pulmonary edema in, 463t, 464, 465
  pulmonary hypertension in, 1604
Adventitia, 1106, *1106*, 1546
African sleeping sickness, 989, 1444
Afterdepolarization, delayed, in arrhythmogenesis, 567–568, *568*, 568t
  early, in arrhythmogenesis, 566–567, *566*, 567t
Afterload, 378, 421
  aortic impedance and, 380
  in heart failure, 399–400, 402
  in left ventricular function, 422, *422*, 428–429, *428*, *429*
  in myocardial infarction, 1195, 1236–1237
  in myocardial oxygen uptake, 381, *381*
  reduction of, in heart failure, 495
    in myocardial infarction, 1236–1237
  wall stress and, 380
Afterload mismatch, in heart failure, 399–400, 402
Aging heart, **1687–1700,** *1695*
  animal models of, 1687–1689, *1688–1691*, 1688t, 1689t
  arrhythmias of, 1697–1698
  atrial fibrillation of, 1698
  bradyarrhythmias of, 1698
  calcium sequestration in, 1687, *1689*
  chronic ischemic heart disease of, 1696–1697
  contractile response of, 1687, *1691*
  diastolic dysfunction of, 1700
  drug effects on, 1700
  failure of, 1699–1700. See also *Heart failure.*
  hypertension and, 1699
  myocardial infarction of, 1697
  myosin Ca⁺⁺-ATPase in, 1687, *1690*
  normal, 1689–1695
Aging heart *(Continued)*
    exercise effects on, 1690, *1692*
    exercise performance and, 1692–1694, *1693*, *1694*
    hemodynamics of, 1692, *1693*
    left ventricular ejection in, 1689–1690, *1691*, *1692*
    pulse wave velocity in, 1689–1690, *1691*, *1692*
    sympathetic modulation in, 1692–1693, *1694*
  systolic dysfunction of, 1700
  transmembrane action potential in, 1687, *1688*
  valvular disease of, 1698–1699
Agranulocytosis, drug-induced, 1805
A-H interval, in arrhythmias, 643, *644*
Air embolism, in renal failure, 1936
  in sudden death, 752
Airway, in cardiac arrest, 763
  obstruction of, in cor pulmonale, 1615
Alagille syndrome (arteriohepatic dysplasia), 880t, 1651t, 1660t, 1677, 1678t
Alanine aminotransferase (ALT), in heart failure, 456
Albright syndrome (fibrous dysplasia), heart failure in, 462
Albuterol, digoxin interaction with, 483t
Alcohol, fetal effects of, 881t
  in coronary artery disease, 1153–1154
  in hypertension, 821, 845–846
  toxicity of, 11
Alcoholic cardiomyopathy, 1412–1414, 1877
Aldactone. See *Spironolactone (Aldactone).*
Aldomet. See *Methyldopa (Aldomet).*
Aldosterone, 1895
  heparin-associated levels of, 1594
  in heart failure, 1916t
  in myocardial infarction, 1197
Aldosteronism, 1678, 1678t, 1896–1897
  diagnosis of, 828, *828*
  etiology of, 828, *828*
  hypertension in, 827–829, *828*
  treatment of, 828–829
Alfentanil, for anesthesia, 1757
Aliasing, 57
Alkalosis, hypochloremic, diuretics and, 480
Alkaptonuria, 1668t, 1673
Allen test, in cardiac catheterization, 186
Allergy, radiocontrast, 245
Alpha thalassemia, 1788–1790
Alpha$_2$-antiplasmin, plasmin inhibition by, 1816
Alpha-Tocopherol, Beta Carotene Cancer Prevention Study, 1154–1155
Alport syndrome, 1678t
Alprenolol, in myocardial infarction, 1228–1229, *1228*
  in renal failure, 1931t
Alteplase. See *Plasminogen activator(s), tissue-type.*
Alveolar proteinosis, in pulmonary hypertension, 801
Alveolar-capillary membrane, in pulmonary edema, 462, 463t, 464
Amebiasis, in pericarditis, 1511
Amiloride, in heart failure, 477t
  in renal failure, 1933t
Aminoacidopathy, 1668t, 1673
ε-Aminocaproic acid (Amicar), in pediatric cardiology, 1000t
6-Amino-9-D-psicofuranosylpurine, pericarditis with, 1519
Aminophylline, in pediatric cardiology, 1000t
Aminorex, pulmonary hypertension with, 786
Amiodarone, adverse effects of, 614–615
  after myocardial infarction, 1265–1266, *1266*
  digoxin interaction with, 483t
  dosage of, 614
  exercise stress testing effects of, 170
  hemodynamic effects of, 613
  in arrhythmia, 594t–595t, 601t, 602t–603t, 613–615
  in atrial fibrillation, 656
  in atrial flutter, 654
  in cardiac arrest, 766
  in elderly, 1698
  in heart failure, 505
  in hypertrophic cardiomyopathy, 1426
  in myocardial infarction, 1254, 1265–1266, *1266*
  in pediatric cardiology, 1000t
  in pregnancy, 1858
  in renal failure, 1930t
Amiodarone *(Continued)*
  in trypanosomiasis, 1444
  in ventricular tachycardia, 1248
  indications for, 614
  pharmacokinetics of, 613
  pulmonary toxicity of, 614
  thyroid effects of, 1894
Amlodipine, in angina pectoris, 1309t, 1311
  in heart failure, 472t
  pharmacokinetics of, 1309t
  side effects of, 1303t
Ammonium chloride, in pediatric cardiology, 1000t
Amniocentesis, 977
Amplatz catheters, for arteriography, 242, *243*
Amrinone, hematological abnormalities with, 1804t
  in heart failure, 472t, 484–485, 502, 891t
  in myocardial infarction, 1237–1238
Amsacrine, cardiac effects of, 1803
Amyl nitrate, with cardiac catheterization, 198–199
Amyl nitrite, auscultatory effects of, *48*, 49
  hematological abnormalities with, 1804t
Amylo-1,6-glucosidase deficiency, 1668t, 1674
Amyloidosis, 324, 1797
  familial, 1427–1428, 1676, 1678t
    cerebral hemorrhage in, 1677
    echocardiography in, 92–93, *92*, *1428*, 1429
  restrictive cardiomyopathy of, 1427–1429
  sudden cardiac death in, 749
Anaerobic threshold, in exercise, 154, *154*
Analgesic nephropathy, hypertension in, 825
Anaphylaxis, radiocontrast-induced, 245
Anectine chloride (succinylcholine chloride), for anesthesia, 1757
  in pediatric cardiology, 1002t
Anemia, **1786–1790**
  aplastic, 1804
  cardiac examination in, 1787
  cardiac symptoms of, 1786, *1787*
  drug-induced, 1804–1805
  hemoglobin-oxygen dissociation curve in, 1786–1787
  hemolytic, 1787–1790
    after cardiac surgery, 1790
    drug-induced, 1804–1805
    microangiopathic, 1790
  hypoxia response in, 1787, *1787*
  immunohemolytic, 1804–1805
  in high-output heart failure, 460–462
  in myocardial infarction, 1213
  in rheumatic fever, 1771
  megaloblastic, 1804
  treatment of, 460
Anesthesia, 1756–1758
  complications of, 1757
  epidural, 1757
  for cardiac surgery, 1718
  general, 1757
  in hypertensive patient, 857
  inhalation agents for, 1757
  intraoperative arrhythmias and, 1758
  intraoperative hemodynamics and, 1757–1758
  intravenous agents for, 1757
  local, 1757
  monitoring of, 1758
  muscle relaxants for, 1757
  pulmonary edema after, 466
  regional, 1757
  spinal, 1757
Aneuploidy, 1651, 1655–1656, 1656t
Aneurysm, aortic, 1547–1554. See also *Aortic aneurysms.*
  congenital, of circle of Willis, 965, *965*
    of sinus of Valsalva, 910–911, *911*, 967, 971
  coronary, in Kawasaki disease, 995–996, *996*
  false, magnetic resonance imaging of, 321, *321*
  intracranial, genetic factors in, 1660t
    in adult polycystic kidney disease, 1676
  mycotic, in adult congenital heart disease, 974, *974*
    in infective endocarditis, 1096
  septal, atrial, 83, 87–88
      echocardiography in, 58–59, *59*
      in secundum-type atrial septal defect, 898
  ventricular, left, 228
      computed tomography of, 336–337, *337*
      in coronary artery disease, 1347–1348, *1347*

Aneurysm *(Continued)*
in mitral regurgitation, 1017
in myocardial contusion, 1538, *1538*
in myocardial infarction, 136, *150*, *1242*, 1256
palpation in, 25
post-traumatic, 1542
T wave in, 136, *150*
treatment of, 1348, *1348*, 1833
Angelman syndrome, 1651t
Anger, in stable angina pectoris, 1293
Angina pectoris, 4
angiography in, 1295, 1296, 1321–1323, 1338
practice guidelines for, 1951–1952
cost-effective noninvasive testing in, 1744–1745, *1744*
drug-induced, 12t
effort, 4t
endothelin-1 in, 1168
endothelium-dependent coronary vasodilation in, *1167*, 1168
equivalents of, 3, 4
in aortic stenosis, 1039
in children, 11, 888
in elderly, 1696–1697
in hyperthyroidism, 1893
in women, 1704–1705, 1704t
microvascular, *1289*, 1343–1344. See also *Syndrome X.*
noncardiac surgery and, 1758–1761
postinfarction, 1254–1255, *1255*
practice guidelines for, 1951–1952, 1979–1985, *1980*, 1980t, *1985*
precipitation of, 7
rest, 4t
silent myocardial ischemia in, 1344–1346, *1345*, *1346*
stable, **1290–1316**
alpha receptor–mediated coronary vasoconstriction in, 1171
angiography in, 1295, 1296, 1951–1952
asymptomatic, 1297–1298
atypical, 1298, *1744*, 1745
biochemical tests in, 1298
blood pressure in, 1292
cardiac examination in, 1292
characteristics of, 1290–1292, 1291t
chest roentgenography in, 1298
clinical manifestations of, 1290–1292, 1291t
computed tomography in, 1298
corneal arcus in, 1292
coronary blood flow in, 1299
differential diagnosis of, 1291–1292, 1291t
earlobe crease in, 1292
echocardiography in, 1296–1297
electrocardiography in, 1295–1296
exercise electrocardiography in, 1295–1296
exercise radionuclide angiography in, 1296
fixed, 1293, *1294*
gender differences in, 1297
grading of, 1294–1295
left ventricular function in, 1298–1299
management of, 1304–1331
amlodipine in, 1309t, 1311
angiotensin-converting enzyme inhibitors in, 1301
antihypertensive therapy in, 1299
antioxidants in, 1300
aspirin in, 1301
bepridil in, 1309t, 1311
beta-adrenoceptor blocking agents in, 1301, 1304–1308, *1305*, 1305t, 1306t, 1307t, 1308t
contraindications to, 1306, 1308, 1308t
dosage of, 1306
selectivity of, 1305–1306
side effects of, 1303t, 1306, 1308, 1308t
vs. calcium antagonists, 1311–1313, 1312t
calcium channel blocking agents in, 1308–1313, 1309t, 1312t
antiatherogenic action of, 1308
vs. beta-adrenoceptor blocking agents, 1311–1313, 1312t
cholesterol-lowering therapy in, 1300, 1321
coronary artery bypass graft surgery in, 1316–1331, 1958–1959, 1958t
antiplatelet therapy after, 1321
carotid artery disease and, 1331
Angina pectoris *(Continued)*
cholesterol-lowering therapy after, 1321
complications of, 1318, 1319–1320
disease progression after, 1320–1321
graft patency after, 1320
in diabetic patients, 1329
in elderly, 1328
in women, 1328
in younger patients, 1328
internal mammary artery for, 1317–1319, *1317*, *1318*
left ventricular function depression and, 1326–1328, *1326*, *1327*, 1328t
myocardial hibernation and, *1326*, 1327–1328, *1327*, 1328t
myocardial infarction after, 1326
outcome of, 1319–1321, 1323–1329, *1324*, *1325*, 1325t, *1326*, *1327*, 1328t
patient selection for, 1321–1323, 1321t, *1322*, 1329
peripheral vascular disease and, 1331
reoperation after, 1328
technical considerations in, 1316–1319, *1317*, *1318*
venous conduits for, 1317, *1317*
vs. percutaneous transluminal coronary angioplasty, 1329–1331, *1329*, 1330t
counseling in, 1301
diltiazem in, 1309t, 1310–1311
estrogen replacement therapy in, 1300
exercise in, 1300–1301
felodipine in, 1309t, 1311
isradipine in, 1309t, 1311
nicardipine in, 1309t, 1311
nifedipine in, 1308, 1309t, 1310
nitrates in, 1302–1304, *1302*, 1303t
side effects of, 1303, 1303t
tolerance to, 1304
percutaneous transluminal coronary angioplasty in, 1313–1316
abrupt closure after, 1314
acute outcome of, 1313–1314
coronary bypass graft and, 1316
in elderly, 1316
left ventricular dysfunction and, 1314–1315
patient selection for, 1313, 1316, *1316*
restenosis after, 1315–1316
vs. coronary artery bypass graft surgery, 1329–1331, *1329*, 1330t
vs. medical therapy, 1314, *1314*, *1315*
smoking cessation in, 1299–1300
verapamil in, 1309t, 1310
mixed, 1294, *1294*
murmurs in, 1292
myocardial metabolism in, 1299
myocardial oxygen demand in, 1293
myocardial oxygen supply in, 1293, *1293*
noninvasive stress testing in, 1295–1298, 1297t, 1744–1745, *1744*
pathogenesis of, *1289*
pathophysiology of, *1289*, 1293–1295, *1293*, *1294*
patient history in, 1295
pharmacological stress echocardiography in, 1297
physical examination in, 1292
resting electrocardiography in, 1295
risk assessment in, 1297, 1297t
stress myocardial perfusion imaging in, 1296
typical, 1298
variable-threshold, 1293–1294, *1294*
vs. biliary colic, 1291
vs. cervical radiculitis, 1291
vs. costosternal syndrome, 1291
vs. esophageal disorders, 1291, 1291t
vs. esophageal motility disorders, 1291
vs. gastroesophageal reflux, 1291
vs. myocardial infarction, 1291–1292
vs. pericarditis, 1292
vs. pulmonary embolism, 1292
vs. pulmonary hypertension, 1292
xanthelasma in, 1292
supply, 1293
unstable, *1187*, 1188, *1188*, **1331–1339.** See also *Myocardial infarction.*
angioscopy in, 1335
arteriography in, 240–241, 265, *266*, 268, 1335
Angina pectoris *(Continued)*
autopsy studies of, 1335
chest pain in, 5
classification of, 1331–1332, 1332t
coronary constriction in, 1333–1334
definition of, 1331
diagnosis of, 1979–1981, *1980*, 1980t, 1981t
electrocardiographic monitoring in, 1334–1335
electrocardiography in, 134, 1334–1335, *1334*
exercise stress testing in, 165, 1336
hospital discharge after, 1985
hospitalization for, 1198
intracoronary thrombus in, 268
arteriography in, 265, *266*
laboratory testing in, 1984
management of, 1336–1339, 1981–1985, *1985*
angiography in, 1338
antithrombotic agents in, 1338, 1823–1824, 1823t
aspirin in, 1337, 1823, 1823t
beta-adrenoceptor blocking agents in, 1337, 1982t, 1983
calcium channel blocking agents in, 1337, 1982t, 1983
cardiac catheterization in, 1338, 1982t, 1983t, 1984, *1985*
coronary artery bypass graft surgery in, 1339, *1339*
glycoprotein IIb/IIIa receptor blockers in, 1823–1824
heparin in, 1337, *1337*, 1823, *1824*, 1824t
intraaortic balloon counterpulsation in, 535, 1338, 1984
medical, 1336–1338, 1981–1984, 1982t–1983t
nitrates in, 1336–1337
percutaneous transluminal coronary angioplasty in, 1338–1339
practice guidelines for, 1981–1984, 1982t–1983t, *1985*
thrombolytic therapy in, 1337–1338, 1824
ticlopidine in, 1337, 1823
myocardial perfusion imaging of, 288
natural history of, 1336
noninvasive testing in, 1744–1745, 1983t, 1984
pathogenesis of, *1289*
pathophysiology of, 1332–1334
physical examination in, 1334
plaque fissuring in, 1166
platelet aggregation in, 1333
practice guidelines for, 1979–1985, *1980*, 1980t, *1985*
radionuclide imaging in, 1944
risk stratification for, 1979–1981, *1980*, 1980t, 1981t
severity of, 268, 1332, 1332t
symptoms of, 1334
thrombosis in, 1333, *1333*
ventricular function in, 1335–1336
variant (Prinzmetal's), **1340–1343**
acetylcholine injection in, 1342
arteriography in, 1341–1342
clinical manifestations of, 1340–1341
coronary spasm in, 1171
electrocardiography in, 1340–1341, *1341*
ergonovine test in, 1342
hemodynamic features of, 1341–1342
hyperventilation in, 1342
management of, 1342–1343
mechanisms of, *1289*, 1340
myocardial perfusion imaging in, 1342
pathogenesis of, *1289*
precipitation of, 7
ST segment in, *137*
T wave in, *137*
warm-up, 1214, 1290
Angiocardiography, radionuclide, 297–303, *302*, 303t. See also *Angiography.*
equilibrium, 297–300, *297–299*
first-pass, 300–301
Angioedema, hereditary, 1661t, 1669t
with angiotensin-converting enzyme inhibitors, 474
Angiogenesis, gene therapy–induced, 1638
Angiography. See also *Arteriography.*
after cardiac arrest, 1951

Angiography *(Continued)*
after coronary bypass, 253–255, *254, 255*
before noncardiac surgery, 1951
CT, 339, *339*
exercise stress testing correlation with, 162
for coronary blood flow measurement, 199
in abdominal aortic aneurysm, 1549
in angina pectoris, 1321–1323, 1338, 1951–1952
in aortic dissection, 1563–1564, 1563t
in aortic regurgitation, 1050, 1051
in aortic stenosis, 1041, 1042
in asymptomatic patients, 1949, 1950t
in atrioventricular septal defect, 899, 900
in cardiac tumor, 1474–1475
in chest pain, 1950t, 1952
in chronic coronary artery disease, 1295
in chronic obstructive pulmonary disease, 303
in congenital heart disease, 1951t, 1952
in congenitally corrected transposition of great arteries, 941, *942*
in constrictive pericarditis, 1503–1504, *1504*
in coronary artery disease, 1295, 1296, 1321–1323, *1322*, 1706, 1949–1954, 1950t–1951t
in double-outlet right ventricle, 943, *943*
in doxorubicin monitoring, 302–303, 303t
in Ebstein's anomaly, 935
in endomyocardial fibrosis, 1433
in heart failure, 302–303
in hypertrophic cardiomyopathy, 1423
in idiopathic dilated cardiomyopathy, 1411
in Kawasaki disease, 995, *996*
in mitral regurgitation, 1024, *1024*, 1025, *1025*
in mitral stenosis, 1012, 1013–1014
in mitral valve prolapse, 1033–1034
in myocardial infarction, 302–303, *302*, 1241, 1950t, 1952, 1977t
in pulmonary embolism, 1590–1591, *1592*
in pulmonary hypertension, 790, *790*, 887
in renal failure, 1926
in Takayasu's arteritis, 1573, *1573, 1574*
in tetralogy of Fallot, 931
in transposition of great arteries, 937–938, 941, *942*
in tricuspid atresia, 933
in tricuspid regurgitation, 1058, *1058*
in trypanosomiasis, 1443–1444
in valvular heart disease, 303, 1950t, 1951t, 1952
MRI, 321, *322, 323*
of saphenous vein bypass graft, 253–254, *254*
practice guidelines for, 1949–1954, 1949t, 1950t–1951t, 1953t
Angioma, 1471
cavernous, 1677
genetic factors in, 1660t
Angioplasty. See *Percutaneous transluminal coronary angioplasty (PTCA).*
Angiosarcoma, 1471, *1472*
Angioscopy, 1384
in pulmonary embolism, 1591
in unstable angina, 1335
Angiotensin, cardiovascular actions of, 472–473
inotropic effects of, 472
receptors for, 471–472
in heart failure, 414
Angiotensin II, in azotemia, 1919
in heart failure, 1916t
in myocyte hypertrophy, 1640t, 1642, 1642t
in vasoconstriction, 472, 783
receptors for, antagonists of, 474
renal actions of, 473, *473*
Angiotensin-converting enzyme (ACE), *1165*
gene for, 1679
Angiotensin-converting enzyme (ACE) inhibitors, 848t
action of, 474, 856
clinical use of, 474, 856
cost-benefit ratio of, 497
cough with, 497
doses of, 497–499
first-dose effects of, 497
in angina pectoris, 1301
in coronary artery disease, 1149t
in heart failure, 494, 495–497, *496*
in hypertension, 827, 855–856, *855*
in myocardial infarction, 1213, 1229–1230, *1229, 1230*, 1264
in pregnancy, 1859
in valvular regurgitation, 497
quality of life and, 497
Angiotensin-converting enzyme (ACE) inhibitors *(Continued)*
renal function and, 473–474, *473*
side effects of, 856
synthesis of, 474
tissue actions of, 474
Angiotensinogen, in blood pressure regulation, 1678–1679
Anisotropic model of reentry, *571*, 572, *577*
Anisoylated plasminogen-streptokinase activator complex (APSAC, anistreplase), 1220, 1821. See also *Thrombolytic therapy.*
in myocardial infarction, 1824–1826, *1825*, 1825t
in renal failure, 1934t
Ankylosing spondylitis, 1575, 1780–1781, *1780*
Annuloaortic ectasia, aortic regurgitation in, *226*
aortography in, *1552*, 1554
Annulus, aortic, calcifications of, 221–223, *222*
mitral, calcification of, 221–223, *222*
echocardiography in, 78
in mitral regurgitation, 1017–1018, 1024
in mitral stenosis, 1007
dilatation of, in mitral regurgitation, 1017
Anomalous muscle bands, in right ventricular obstruction, 928–929
Anomalous pulmonary origin of coronary artery, 909–910
diagnosis of, 909–910, *910*
management of, 910
pathophysiology of, 909, *909*
Anomalous pulmonary venous connection, genetic factors in, 1660t
in secondary pulmonary hypertension, 801
partial, 946
in atrial septal defect, 897
total, 944–946
anatomy of, *944*, 944t
cardiac catheterization in, 945
chest roentgenography in, 945, *945*
clinical manifestations of, 945
echocardiography in, 83, 945
hemodynamics of, 944–945
laboratory findings in, 945, *945*
management of, 945–946
morphology of, 944, *944*, 944t
sites of, *944*, 944t
Anorexia, in heart failure, 455
in patient history, 10
Anorexia nervosa, 1907, 1907t
heart size in, 215, *217*
Anorexigens, pulmonary hypertension with, 786
Anoxia, definition of, 1161
Antacids, digoxin interaction with, 483t
Antagonism, accentuated, 645
Anthracyclines, cardiac effects of, 997, *997*, 1800–1803, *1800–1803*, 1801t, 1802t
in children, 1802–1803
infusional, 1803
low-dose, 1803
monitoring of, 1801–1802, 1802t
Antiarrhythmic agents, **593–619**
absorption of, 593–594
after myocardial infarction, 1265–1266, *1266*
bioavailability of, 594t–595t, 595
cardiac arrest with, 767
class IA, 594t–595t, 601–605, 601t, 602t–603t
class IB, 594t–595t, 601t, 602t–603t, 605–608
class IC, 594t–595t, 601t, 602t–603t, 608–610
class II, 610–613, *611*, 611t
class III, 601t, 602t–603t, 613–616
class IV, 594t–595t, 601t, 602t–603t, 616–618
classification of, 597–598, 598t, 599t
distribution of, 594–595, *596*
dosages of, 594t–595t
drug interactions of, 600, 600t
elimination of, 594t–595t, 596–597
half-life of, 593, 594t–595t, 596–597
Holter monitoring of, 579
in idiopathic dilated cardiomyopathy, 1411
in myocardial infarction, 1254, 1265–1266, *1266*
mechanism of, 599–600, 599t
metabolism of, 596–597, 600
one-compartment model of, 595
pharmacokinetics of, 593–597, 594t–595t, *595*
plasma concentration of, 594t–595t, 595–597, *595, 590*
proarrhythmic effects of, 600–601, 752
side effects of, 600
steady-state concentration of, 597
Antiarrhythmic agents *(Continued)*
stereoselectivity of, 600
systemic availability of, 594
therapeutic concentrations of, 593, 594t–595t
two-compartment model of, 595–597, *595, 596*
use-dependence of, 598–599
volume of distribution of, 596, *596*
Antibiotic, in acute pericarditis, 1484
in pregnancy, 1846, 1859t, 1860
Antibiotic prophylaxis, against endocarditis, 1097–1099, 1097t, 1098t, 1099t
in aortic stenosis, 918
in congenital heart disease, 887–888, 888t, 918
in mitral regurgitation, 1026
in mitral stenosis, 1012–1013
in mitral valve prolapse, 1035, 1762
in noncardiac surgery, 1762
in rheumatic fever, 1774
in rheumatic heart disease, 1012–1013
Antibiotic resistance, in infective endocarditis, 1081
Antibody (antibodies), anti–beta-adrenoceptor, in idiopathic dilated cardiomyopathy, 1409
antidigoxin, 484
antimyosin, after heart transplantation, 520
antinuclear, in pulmonary hypertension, 786
antiphospholipid, in systemic lupus erythematosus, 1779
in venous thrombosis, 1582t
dystrophin, in Duchenne muscular dystrophy, 1865–1866
Anticoagulant therapy. See also *Heparin; Warfarin sodium (Coumadin).*
coumarin-type, 1818
for cardioversion, 1832
in atrial fibrillation, 1831–1832, *1831, 1832*
in heart failure, 509
in idiopathic dilated cardiomyopathy, 1411–1412
in infective endocarditis, 1096
in mitral stenosis, 1830
in myocardial infarction, 1265, *1265*, 1828, *1828*, 1974t–1975t, 1978
in pericarditis, 1484
in prosthetic valve replacement, 1066, 1732, 1834–1836, *1835*, 1836t
in pulmonary hypertension, 795
in rheumatic heart disease, 1013
in trypanosomiasis, 1444
Antidepressants, toxicity of, 11
Antidigoxin immunotherapy, 484
Antidromic tachycardia, 670, *672*
Antihypertensive agents, 846–849. See also specific agents, e.g., *Captopril (Capoten).*
combinations of, 847, *847*
guidelines for, 846t
once daily dosing with, 847, *848*
selection of, 847–849, 848t
starting dosages for, 846–847, *847*
Antimony, myocardial effects of, 1447
Antimyosin antibody imaging, in idiopathic dilated cardiomyopathy, 1410
in myocardial infarction, 296–297, *296*
Antimyosin antibody test, after heart transplantation, 520
Antinuclear antibodies, in pulmonary hypertension, 786
Antioxidants, in atherosclerosis, 1116
in coronary artery disease, 1154–1155, 1300
in myocardial infarction, 1232
Antiphospholipid antibodies, in systemic lupus erythematosus, 1779
in venous thrombosis, 1582t
Antiplatelet therapy, 1818–1820, *1819*, 1819t
after coronary artery bypass surgery, 1321
in myocardial infarction, 1225, *1225*, 1264, 1827–1828, 1827t, 1974t–1975t, 1978
in prosthetic valve replacement, 1835
Antisense oligonucleotides, in vascular proliferation, 1638
Antitachycardia devices, 1966–1967. See also *Pacemaker(s).*
Antithrombin III, 1813
in venous thrombosis, 1582t
Antithrombotic therapy, **1817–1836,** 1817t, *1819*, 1819t. See also specific drugs, e.g., *Heparin.*
in aortic valve disease, 1830
in atrial fibrillation, 655–656, 1830–1832, *1831*, 1831t, *1832*
in atrial thrombosis, 1829–1830
in dilated cardiomyopathy, 1833–1834, 1834t

Antithrombotic therapy *(Continued)*
in left ventricular aneurysm, 1833
in mitral regurgitation, 1830
in mitral stenosis, 1830
in mitral valve prolapse, 1830
in myocardial infarction, 1826, 1826t, 1832–1833, *1833*
in prosthetic valve replacement, 1834–1836, *1835*, 1836t
in saphenous vein bypass graft disease, 1826–1827
in unstable angina, 1338, 1823–1824, 1823t, *1824*
in ventricular thrombosis, 1832–1834
risk stratification for, 1822–1823, 1822t
Anti-thymocyte globulin (ATGAM), in heart transplantation rejection, 522
Anxiety disorders, dyspnea in, 451
syncope and, 865, 872
Aorta, **1546–1576**
abdominal, aneurysm of, 1547–1550. See also *Aortic aneurysms, abdominal.*
atherosclerosis of, 18, 1106, 1114
acute occlusion of, 1571–1572
aging of, 1546
anatomy of, 1546
aneurysm of, 1547–1554. See also *Aortic aneurysms.*
arch of, 1546
aneurysm of, 1553
ascending, 1546
on plain chest radiography, *205*, 211
postoperative pseudoaneurysm of, 230, *231*
atherosclerotic disease of, 1547, 1570–1571, *1570*
echocardiography in, 97
bacterial infection of, 1575–1576
calcifications of, 224–225
in Takayasu's aortitis, *223*, 224
coarctation of. See *Coarctation of aorta.*
descending, 1546
dilatation of, echocardiography of, 96, *96*
dissection of. See *Aortic dissection.*
distension of, 1546
elasticity of, 1546
enlargement of, on plain chest radiography, *207*
examination of, 1546–1547
function of, 1546
imaging of, in abdominal aortic aneurysm, 1548–1549
in annuloaortic ectasia, *1552*, 1554
in aortic dissection, 1559, *1559–1561*
in hypoplastic left heart syndrome, 921
in thoracic aortic aneurysm, 1551–1552, *1552*
in cardiac malposition, 946–947
inflammation of, 1572–1576
giant cell, 1782
in Cogan's syndrome, 1783
in rheumatoid arthritis, 1777–1778, *1777*
in thoracic aortic aneurysm, 1551
syphilitic, 1349
in myocardial infarction, 1193
Takayasu's, 1572, *1572*, *1573*, 1575t. See also *Takayasu's arteritis.*
occlusion of, 1571–1572
on M-mode echocardiography, *64*
palpation of, 28
root of, 1546
rupture of, 1543–1544, *1543*, 1543t
systolic pressure of, 1546
thoracic, 1546
aneurysm of, 1550–1554. See also *Aortic aneurysms, thoracic.*
atherosclerosis of, 1550–1551
endothelium of, *1107*
trauma to, *1542*, 1543–1544, *1543*, 1543t
aortic dissection and, 1556
tumors of, 1576, *1576*
Aortic aneurysms, **1547–1554**
abdominal, 1547–1550
aortography in, 1548–1549
atherosclerosis and, 18
clinical manifestations of, 1548–1549, *1548*
computed tomography in, 1548, *1548*
diagnosis of, 1548–1549, *1548*
etiology of, 1547
follow-up for, 1550
genetic factors in, 1660t, 1677
management of, 1549–1550
Aortic aneurysms *(Continued)*
natural history of, 1549
pathogenesis of, 1547
physical examination in, 1548
rupture of, 1548, 1549
computed tomography of, 343, *343*, 1548, *1548*, 1552
echocardiography of, 96
false, 1547
fusiform, 1547
multiple, 1547
proteolytic enzymes and, 1547
renal function and, 1922
saccular, 1547
thoracic, 1550–1554
annuloaortic ectasia and, 1554
atherosclerosis and, 1550–1551
chest pain in, 5
clinical manifestations of, 1551–1552, *1551*
composite graft replacement for, 1552–1553, *1553*
cystic medial degeneration in, 1550
diagnosis of, 1551–1552, *1551*, *1552*
etiology of, 1550
expansion of, 1552
infectious aortitis and, 1551
management of, 1552–1554, *1553*
complications of, 1553, 1554
endovascular stent-graft in, 1553–1554
natural history of, 1552
pathogenesis of, 1550
rupture of, 1551
syphilis and, 1551
thoracoabdominal, 1550
Aortic annulus, calcifications of, 221–223, *222*
Aortic arch(es), computed tomography of, 342
congenital abnormalities of, 342, 911–914, *912–914*
double, 342
embryology of, 882–883, *882*
giant aneurysm of, *207*
hypoplasia of, 913–914
obstruction of, 911–914, *912–914*
on plain chest radiography, 204–205, *206*, *207*, 213
right, 205, *207*
Aortic arch interruption, 913–914
Aortic arch syndrome, in giant cell arteritis, 1574
Aortic dissection, **1554–1569**
acute pericarditis in, 1484
aortic regurgitation in, 1557, *1557*, 1566–1567
atypical, 1568–1569, *1568*, *1569*
calcification in, 1558, *1558*
cardiac tamponade in, 1521
chest pain in, 5, 1556
chest roentgenography in, *207*, 1557–1558, *1558*
classification of, 1554–1555, *1555*, 1555t
clinical manifestations of, 1556–1558, *1557*
complications of, 1567–1568
computed tomography in, 342–343, *343*, 1559–1560, *1561*, 1563, 1563t
coronary artery disease in, 1563–1564, 1563t
cystic medial degeneration in, 1555–1556, *1555*
diagnosis of, 1558–1564, 1563t
aortography in, 1559, *1559–1561*
computed tomography in, 342–343, *343*, 1559–1560, *1561*, 1563, 1563t
coronary angiography in, 1563–1564, 1563t
echocardiography in, 96, *96*, 1561–1563, *1562*, 1563t, **Plate 4, Plate 10, Plate 11**
intravascular ultrasonography in, 1562–1563
laboratory findings in, 1557–1558, *1558*
magnetic resonance imaging in, 328–329, *328*, *329*, 1560–1561, *1562*
physical findings in, 1556–1557, *1557*
transesophageal echocardiography in, 1561–1563, *1562*, 1563t
transthoracic echocardiography in, 1561
disease associations of, 1556
etiology of, 1555–1556
extension of, 1557
follow-up of, 1567–1568
genetic factors in, 1677
hemopericardium with, 1521
hypertension in, 1567
hypotension in, 1556
in Marfan syndrome, 1671–1672
in pregnancy, 1556, 1855–1856
incidence of, 1556
Aortic dissection *(Continued)*
intramural hematoma in, 1554, *1555*, 1568–1569, *1568*
magnetic resonance imaging in, 328–329, *328*, *329*, 1563, 1563t
management of, 1564–1568
blood pressure reduction in, 1564–1565
cardiac tamponade in, 1565
follow-up for, 230, 1567–1568
medical, 1564–1565, 1566t, 1567
mortality and, 1557
surgical, 230, 1566–1567, *1566*, 1566t
mortality from, 1557
murmur in, 1556
pain in, 1199
pathogenesis of, 1555–1556
penetrating atherosclerotic ulcer in, 1569, *1569*
pleural effusion in, 1558
pulse deficit in, 1556–1557
renal function and, 1922
symptoms of, 1556
syncope in, 867
transesophageal echocardiography in, 1561–1562, 1563, 1563t
transthoracic echocardiography in, 1561
vs. myocardial infarction, 1557
with intraaortic balloon counterpulsation, 536
without intimal rupture, 1568–1569, *1568*
Aortic impedance, afterload and, 380
Aortic isthmus, 1546
Aortic pressure, 188t, 189, *189*, 191t
Aortic regurgitation, **1045–1053**
acute, *1048*, 1048–1051, 1049t
aortic root disease in, *1045*, 1046
arterial pulse in, 22
auscultation in, 1049–1050
Austin Flint murmur of, 49
bicuspid, 1046
noncardiac surgery and, 981
chest radiography in, 225–226, *226*
chronic, 1048–1049, 1049t
clinical manifestations of, 1048–1050
congenital, 922
Corrigan (water-hammer) pulse of, 22, 1049
diastolic murmur in, 41, *41*, *48*, 49
during pregnancy, 1850
Duroziez's sign in, 22
echocardiography in, 75–76, *76*, 1050–1051, **Plate 2**
electrocardiography in, 1050, *1051*
etiology of, 1045–1046, *1045*
experimental, 1048
Hill's sign in, 22
imaging in, 1050, 1051
in aortic dissection, 1557, *1557*, 1566–1567
in Cogan's syndrome, 1783
in giant cell arteritis, 1782, *1782*
in psoriatic arthritis, 1781
in relapsing polychondritis, 1783
in subvalvular aortic stenosis, 919
in Takayasu's arteritis, 1572
infective endocarditis in, 1046
laboratory examination in, 1050–1051, *1051*
left ventricular dilatation in, *210*
left ventricular function in, 1047–1048
left ventricular tension in, 426, *426*
magnetic resonance imaging of, 330–331, *331*, *332*, 1051
mitral regurgitation and, 1061
mitral stenosis and, 1060
murmur in, 1050
noncardiac surgery and, 981
palpation in, 25
pathophysiology of, 1046–1048, *1046*, *1047*
patient history in, 1048–1049
physical examination in, 1049–1050
precordial motion in, 24t
pregnancy and, 975
Quincke's sign in, 22
Traube's sign in, 22
trauma in, 1046
treatment of, 1051–1053
angiotensin-converting enzyme inhibitors in, 497
medical, 1052
surgical, 1052–1053, *1053*
results of, 1053
ventricular septal defect and, 903–904, *904*
vs. mitral regurgitation, 1019
Aortic root, 1546
in Marfan syndrome, 1671, *1671*

Aortic root disease, in aortic regurgitation, *1045*, 1046
Aortic sclerosis, midsystolic murmur of, 36–37, *37*, 38
Aortic septal defect, 205, *208*, 906–907
Aortic shelf, in juxtaductal coarctation, 911–913, *912*
Aortic sinus, aneurysm of, 910–911, *911*, 967, 971
echocardiography in, 96–97
congenital aneurysm of, 910–911, 967
in adult, 971
coronary artery origin from, 260–261, *261*, *262*
sudden cardiac death and, 747
fistula of, 910–911, *911*
left circumflex artery origin from, 261–262, *262*
Aortic stenosis, **1035–1045**
acquired, 1036–1037
angina in, 1039
angiography in, 1041, 1042
arterial pulse in, 1040
atherosclerotic, 1036
auscultation in, 1040–1041, 1040t
bicuspid, 1036
pregnancy and, 975
calcific, 1036, *1037*
plain film radiography of, 221, *222*
cardiac impulse in, 1040
cardiac output in, 1038, 1040
cerebral emboli in, 1040
clinical manifestations of, 1039–1041, 1040t
congenital, **914–918**, 1035–1036, *1037*, 1040t
balloon valvuloplasty in, 918, 1386
cardiac catheterization in, 917–918, *917*
diagnosis of, 916–918, *916*, *917*
echocardiography in, 916–917, *917*
electrocardiography in, 916, *916*
exercise and, 978
heart sounds in, *30*
hemodynamics of, 914–915
in adult, 969, *969*
in children, 915–916
in infants, 915
management of, 918, 1386
morphology of, 914
natural history of, 918
plain film radiography in, 221, *222*, 225, 916, 1041
subvalvular, 918–919, *919*
supravalvular, 919–921, *920*, *921*
surgical treatment of, 918, 1386
vs. subvalvular stenosis, 918–919, *919*
degenerative, 1036, *1037*
diastolic pressure-volume curve in, 403
diastolic properties in, 1039
differential diagnosis of, 1023t
echocardiography in, 74–75, *74*, *75*, 79, 84, 916–917, *917*, 1041–1042
electrocardiography in, 916, *916*, 1041
etiology of, 1035–1037, *1037*
gastrointestinal bleeding in, 1040
gender differences in, 1038, *1038*
genetic factors in, 1660t
heart sounds in, *30*, 1040–1041, 1040t
in hemolytic anemia, 1790
infective endocarditis in, 1040
ischemia in, 1039
jugular venous pulse in, 1040
laboratory examination in, 1041–1042
left ventricular alternans in, 1040
left ventricular end-diastolic volume in, 1038
left ventricular hypertrophy in, *210*, 1036–1037
midsystolic murmur in, 36–37, *37*
mitral regurgitation and, 1061
mitral stenosis and, 1060–1061
murmur in, 36–37, *37*, 49, 1023t, 1041
myocardial function in, 1038–1039, *1039*
natural history of, 1042, *1042*
noncardiac surgery and, 1761
pathophysiology of, 1037–1039, *1038*
patient history in, 1039–1040
physical examination in, 1040–1041, 1040t
plain film radiography in, 221, *222*, 225, 916, 1041
precordial motion in, 24t
pregnancy and, 975, 976, 1850
pressure gradients in, 193, *194*
pulsus alternans in, *23*
Aortic stenosis *(Continued)*
right ventricular failure in, 1040
subvalvular, 918–919, *919*
sudden cardiac death in, 749–750
supravalvular, arterial pulse in, 22
echocardiography in, 84
genetic factors in, 1660t, 1661–1662
syncope in, 1039–1040
treatment of, 1042–1045
balloon aortic valvuloplasty in, 915, 1044–1045, *1044*, 1385–1386, *1385*
medical, 1042
surgical, 1043–1044, *1043*
indications for, 1043
results of, 1043–1044
tricuspid valves in, 1036
unicuspid valves in, 1036
vs. intracavitary gradient, 195
Aortic valve, area of, calculation of, 194–195
in aortic stenosis, 917
bicuspid, congenital, 964–965, *964*
calcification of, *222*
echocardiography of, 79, *79*
genetic factors in, 1660t
noncardiac surgery and, 981
stenosis of, 975, 1036
calcification of, 221–223, *222*
in aortic regurgitation, 1050
in congenital stenosis, 914
plain film radiography of, 221, *222*
closure of, palpation of, 28
in ankylosing spondylitis, 1780, *1780*
in rheumatoid arthritis, 1776, *1777*
on myocardial perfusion imaging, 277
replacement of, 1065t
in aortic dissection, 1567
in aortic regurgitation, 1053
in aortic stenosis, 918, 1043–1044, *1043*
in elderly, 1698
systemic hypertension after, 830
resistance of, calculation of, 195
stenosis of, **1035–1045.** See also *Aortic stenosis.*
trauma to, 1541–1542, *1541*
Aortic valvuloplasty, 1044–1045, *1044*, 1385, *1385*, 1386
Aorticopulmonary septal defect, 906–907
on plain chest radiography, 205, *208*
Aortic-ventricular coupling, in contraction-relaxation cycle, 385
Aortitis, 1572–1576
giant cell, 1573–1576, *1574*, 1782
in Cogan's syndrome, 1783
in rheumatoid arthritis, 1777–1778, *1777*
in thoracic aortic aneurysm, 1551
syphilitic, 1349
in myocardial infarction, 1193
Takayasu's, 1572, *1572*, *1573*, 1575t. See also *Takayasu's arteritis.*
Aortography, in abdominal aortic aneurysm, 1548–1549
in annuloaortic ectasia, *1552*, 1554
in aortic dissection, 1559, *1559–1561*
in hypoplastic left heart syndrome, 921
in thoracic aortic aneurysm, 1551–1552, *1552*
Apathetic hyperthyroidism, 461
Apert syndrome, 880t, 1661t
Apex, dyskinetic bulges of, in angina pectoris, 1292
infarction of, 1195
malpositions of, 946–947
palpation of, in mitral stenosis, 1010
Apex beat, 25, *26*
Apical impulse, in hypertrophic cardiomyopathy, 1420
Aplastic anemia, drug-induced, 1804
Apnea, in cyanosis, 892
APO A-1/APO C-III deficiency, low high-density lipoprotein in, 1144
APO $A\text{-}I_{Milano}$, low high-density lipoprotein in, 1144
Apolipoprotein B-100, familial defect of, 1143
Apolipoprotein E–deficient mouse, for atherosclerosis model, 1636–1637, *1636*, 1636t, *1637*
Appearance, in physical examination, 15–17, *17*, *18*
Apresoline. See *Hydralazine (Apresoline)*
APSAC (anisoylated streptokinase plasminogen activator complex), 1220, 1821
APSAC *(Continued)*
in myocardial infarction, 1824–1826, *1825*, 1825t
in renal failure, 1934t
AR wave, in pulmonary venous flow velocity, 438, *438*
Aramine (metaraminol), in atrioventricular nodal reentrant tachycardia, 664
in pediatric cardiology, 1001t
ARDS (adult respiratory distress syndrome), pulmonary edema in, 463t, 464, 465
pulmonary hypertension in, 1604
Area-length method, of left ventricular measurement, 424–425, *425*, 425t
Arfonad. See *Trimethaphan camsylate (Arfonad).*
Argatroban, 1820–1821
Arginine vasopressin, in heart failure, *408*, 414, 1916t
receptors for, 414
Arm crank ergometry, in exercise stress testing, 155
Arrestins, in heart failure, 376
Arrhythmia(s), **548–585, 640–695,** 641t–642t. See also specific arrhythmias, e.g., *Sinus tachycardia.*
autonomic nervous system and, 553
congenital, 949–951, *950*
diagnosis of, 577–583
baroreceptor reflex sensitivity testing in, 585
body surface mapping in, 583
cardiac mapping in, 583
carotid sinus massage in, 641–642
electrocardiography in, 583–584, *584*, 643
long-term, 578–579, *578*
practice guidelines for, 1946–1948, 1947t
electrophysiological studies in, 579–583, *580–583*, 643, *644*
esophageal electrocardiography in, 583
exercise stress testing in, 577–578. See also *Exercise stress testing.*
heart rate variability in, 579
patient history in, 640
physical examination in, 640–642
signal-averaging techniques in, 583–584, *584*
T-wave alternans in, 579
upright tilt test in, 584–585, 585t
digitalis-induced, 11, 12t, 142–143, 484, *645*, 661
electrocardiography of, 142–143, *151*
treatment of, 598t
drug-induced, 11, 12t, 142–143, 484, 600–601, *645*, 661
exercise-induced, 578
genesis of, 565–568, 565t
anatomical reentry in, 570–571, *570*
deceleration-dependent block in, 569
decremental conduction in, 569
delayed afterdepolarizations in, 567–568, *568*, 568t
early afterdepolarizations in, 566–567, *566*, *567*, 567t, *568*
functional reentry in, 571–572, *572*
impulse conduction disorders in, 569–577, *570*, *571*, *573–577*
impulse formation disorders in, 565–568, 565t, *566*, *567*, 567t, *568*, 568t
parasystole in, 568, *569*
reentry in, 569–577, *570*, *571*, *573–577*
tachycardia-dependent block in, 569
triggered activity in, 565t, 566–568, *566*, *567*, 567t
in Becker muscular dystrophy, 1870
in cardiac rehabilitation, 1396
in coronary artery disease, 1349
in Duchenne muscular dystrophy, 1868–1869
in elderly, 1697–1698
in Emery-Dreifuss muscular dystrophy, 1872, *1872*
in heart failure, 449, *458*, 459, 504–507, 504t
in mitral valve prolapse, 1033, 1034
in myocardial contusion, 1537
in myocardial infarction, 1245–1257, 1245t
in myotonic muscular dystrophy, 1873, *1873*
in periodic paralysis, 1877
in pregnancy, 1854–1855
in renal failure, 1928–1929, 1929t, 1935
in rheumatic heart disease, 1013
in sarcoidosis, 1431
in syncope, 869–870
intraoperative, 1758

Arrhythmia(s) *(Continued)*
lethal, *745, 754,* 755–756. See also *Cardiac arrest; Sudden cardiac death.*
management of, **593–631,** 643–645
chemical ablation in, 628
direct current cardioversion in, 619–620, *620*
drugs in, 593–597, 594t–595t, 598t, 599t
absorption of, 593, 595
bioavailability of, 595
class IA, 594t–595t, 601–605, 601t, 602t–603t
class IB, 594t–595t, 601t, 602t–603t, 605–608
class IC, 594t–595t, 601t, 602t–603t, 608–610
class II, 610–613, *611,* 611t
class III, 601t, 602t–603t, 613–616
class IV, 594t–595t, 601t, 602t–603t, 616–618
classification of, 597–598
interactions of, 600, 600t
kinetics of, 595
mechanisms of, 599–600
metabolites of, 600
one-compartment model of, 595
side effects of, 600
steady state of, 597
two-compartment model of, 595–597, *595, 596*
use-dependence of, 598–599
electrical, 619–628, *620–628*
implantable electrical devices in. See *Pacemaker(s).*
radiofrequency catheter ablation in, 621–628, *621–628*
indications for, 623
pathway location for, 621–622, *621*
results of, 623
site selection for, 622, *622*
surgical, 628–631, *629, 630*
noncardiac surgery and, 1763
postoperative, 1720, 1727–1731, *1728,* 1764
electrocardiography in, 1728, *1728*
evaluation of, 1727–1728, *1728*
in tetralogy of Fallot, 931–932
reperfusion, 755–756, 1214
tapping rhythm of, 640
trigger of, 640, *641*
Arrhythmogenic right ventricular dysplasia, 681–682, *681,* 1413–1414, *1413,* 1667
Arsenic, myocardial effects of, 1448
Arterial blood gases, in cyanosis, 892t, 893
Arterial calcification of infancy, 1677, 1678t
Arterial compliance, aging and, 1690
Arterial continuous murmur, *44,* 45
Arterial end-systolic elastance, 428–429, *429*
Arterial fibromuscular dysplasia, 1678t
Arterial input impedance, calculation of, 428, *428*
Arterial pulse, 20–23
abnormal, 22
anacrotic, *21,* 22
dicrotic, *21,* 22
in aortic stenosis, 22, 1040
in atrioventricular dissociation, 22
in coarctation of aorta, 18
in mitral regurgitation, 1022
in mitral stenosis, 1010, 1022
in stable angina pectoris, 1292
normal, 21–22, *21*
palpation of, 20–23, *21,* 23
percussion wave of, 21–22
tidal wave of, 21–22
Arterial switch operation, in transposition of great arteries, 939, *940*
Arterial tortuosity, familial, 1677
Arteriography, **240–269.** See also *Angiography.*
after cholesterol reduction, 268–269
after coronary bypass, 253–255, *254, 255*
after heart transplantation, 241
Amplatz catheters for, 242, *243*
angiographic projections for, 247, *248, 249*
anteroposterior view for, 247
atropine in, 245
beta-adrenoceptor blockers in, 245
brachial artery approach for, 244
catheters for, 241–242, *242, 243*
complications of, 241t, 259
contraindications to, 241, 241t
Arteriography *(Continued)*
contrast media for, 245–246
inadequate filling by, 255–256
equipment for, 241–243, *242, 243,* 245–246, *246*
femoral approach for, 243–244, *244,* 244t
femoral sheath for, 242–243, *243*
gastroepiploic artery catheterization for, 255, *255*
guidewires for, 243
heparin in, 245
in aortic stenosis, 1042
in chest pain, 240, 2343–2344
in idiopathic dilated cardiomyopathy, 1411
in mitral valve prolapse, 1035
in myocardial infarction, 241, 265–266, *266*
in Prinzmetal's variant angina, 1341–1342
in unstable angina, 240–241, 265, *266,* 268, 1335
indications for, 240–241
internal mammary artery catheterization for, 254–255, *255*
interpretation of, 255–259, *256–259*
interventional, 265–269, *266, 267*
intraaortic balloon counterpulsation in, 245
Judkins catheters for, 241–242, *242*
Judkins technique for, 184–185, *185*
left anterior descending artery anatomy on, *248,* 250–251
left anterior oblique view for, 247, *249*
left circumflex artery anatomy on, 251–252
left coronary artery anatomy on, *248,* 250–252
left coronary artery catheterization for, 249
left main coronary artery anatomy on, 250
manifold for, 242
mechanical ventilation before, 245
monitoring during, 245
multipurpose catheters for, 242, *243*
nitroglycerin in, 245
normal, 1343–1344
of branch superimposition, *256, 257,* 258, *258*
of branch-point obstruction, *257,* 258
of cholesterol reduction, 268–269
of coronary artery enlargement, 258, *258*
of coronary artery fistulas, 259–260, *260*
of coronary artery spasm, 264–265
of coronary artery stenosis, 255–257, *256, 257*
of coronary collateral circulation, 262–263, *263, 264*
of coronary dissection, 266–267, *267*
of coronary thrombus, 265–266, *266*
of eccentric stenoses, 256–257, *257*
of left circumflex artery origin from right aortic sinus, 261–262, *262*
of left coronary artery origin from aortic sinus, 260–261, *261, 262*
of left coronary artery origin from left aortic sinus, 260–261, *262*
of left coronary artery origin from pulmonary artery, 260–262, *260*
of left coronary artery origin from right aortic sinus, 260–261, *261*
of left main coronary artery stenosis, 255, *256*
of myocardial blood flow, 262
of myocardial bridging, 258–259, *258*
of pseudolesions, 267–268, *267*
of recanalization, 259, *259*
of total occlusions, 267, *267*
of unrecognized occlusions, *257,* 258
patient preparation for, 241
prednisone in, 245
quantitative, 246–247, *247*
radial artery approach for, 244
right anterior oblique view for, 247, *248*
right coronary artery anatomy on, *249,* 253
right coronary artery catheterization for, 252–253
saphenous vein bypass graft catheterization for, 254, *254*
sedation for, 244–245
timing of, 241
Arteriohepatic dysplasia (Alagille syndrome), 880t, 1651t, 1660t, 1677, 1678t
Arteriovenous continuous murmur, 45
Arteriovenous fistula, 908–909
acquired, in heart failure, 460–461
congenital, in heart failure, 461
diastolic pressure-volume curve in, 403
in renal failure, 1936
post-traumatic, 1542–1543
Arteriovenous fistula *(Continued)*
pulmonary, 967, *968*
systemic, in heart failure, 460–461
Arteriovenous oxygen difference, 439, *439*
Arteriovenous pressure difference, 780
Arteritis, giant cell, 1573–1576, *1574,* 1782, *1782*
clinical manifestations of, 1574
etiology of, 1573–1574
management of, 1574
pathophysiology of, 1574
in polyarteritis nodosa, 1783
in pulmonary hypertension, 787, 787t
Takayasu's, 1572–1573, *1572–1574,* 1575t. See also *Takayasu's arteritis.*
Artery (arteries), 1105–1106, *1106*
adventitia of, 1106, *1106*
bronchial, 780
endothelium of, 1106–1108, *1106–1108*
intima of, 1105–1106, *1106*
macrophages in, 1110, *1110*
media of, 1106, *1106*
platelets in, 1110–1111, *1111*
smooth muscle of, 1108–1110, *1109*
T-lymphocytes in, 1111
Arthritis, in rheumatic fever, 1771, *1771*
psoriatic, 1781
rheumatoid, 1776–1778, 1776t. See also *Rheumatoid arthritis.*
Arthropathy camptodactyly syndrome, 1666
Artificial heart, 534, 544–545, *544, 545*
Asbestos, pericarditis with, 1519
Aschoff nodule, in rheumatic fever, 1770
Ascites, 18
edema with, 10
in heart failure, 455
Ashman phenomenon, 124, *124,* 125
Aspartate aminotransferase (AST), in heart failure, 456
in myocardial infarction, 1204
Aspartylglycosaminuria, 1668t
Aspergillosis, myocarditis in, 1441, *1442*
Aspergillus, in infective endocarditis, 1000
Aspirin (acetylsalicylic acid), 1819, *1819,* 1819t
after coronary artery bypass surgery, 1321
as platelet inhibitor, 1818–1819, 1819t
in atrial fibrillation, 1832, *1832*
in coronary artery disease, 1301
in Kawasaki disease, 997, 997t
in myocardial infarction, 1210, 1225, *1225,* 1257, 1264, 1265, 1826, 1827–1828, 1974t–1975t
in pediatric cardiology, 1000t
in primary prevention, 1829, 1829t
in prosthetic valve replacement, 1835
in PTCA-related abrupt vessel closure, 1369
in pulmonary embolism, 1595
in rheumatic fever, 1772
in unstable angina, 1337, *1337,* 1338, 1823, 1823t, *1824,* 1982t
perioperative, 1719
postinfarction, 1264, 1265, 1827–1828, 1827t
protective effects of, 1829, 1829t
Asplenia, 1659t
cardiac anomalies with, 946
AST (aspartate aminotransferase), in heart failure, 456
in myocardial infarction, 1204
Asthenia, neurocirculatory, chest pain in, 5
Asthma, bronchial, vs. cardiogenic pulmonary edema, 465
cardiac, 451
Asystole, in myocardial infarction, 1253
Ataxia, Friedreich's, 880t, *1874, 1875,* 1894
Atenolol, in arrhythmias, 610–613, 611t
in myocardial infarction, 1228–1229, *1228*
in pregnancy, 1859
in renal failure, 1931t
pharmacodynamic properties of, 487t
pharmacology of, 1307t
ATGAM (anti-thymocyte globulin), in heart transplantation rejection, 522
Atheroembolism, diffuse, after coronary artery bypass surgery, 1331
Atherosclerosis, **1105–1122.** See also *Coronary artery disease.*
after heart transplantation, 525–526, *526*
apolipoprotein E–deficient mouse model of, 1636–1637, *1636,* 1636t, *1637*
cytokines in, 1116–1117
cytomegalovirus in, 525

Atherosclerosis *(Continued)*
  diffuse intimal thickening in, 1113
  endothelial cell dysfunction in, *1164*
  fatty streak of, 1112–1113, *1112*, 1118, *1119*
  genetic factors in, 1677
  growth factors in, 1116–1117
  hypertension and, 813–814, 814t
  imaging of, 354, 354t, 1122
  in acromegaly, 1888–1889
  in diabetes mellitus, 1904
  in hypothyroidism, 1895
  in thoracic aortic aneurysm, 1550–1551
  lesions of, 1111–1114, *1112*, *1113*
    cellular events of, 1117–1121, *1117–1120*
  lipids in, 1116
  lipoproteins in, 1116
  lovastatin in, *1167*
  of heart transplant, 525–526, *526*
  phases of, 1111–1114, *1112*, *1113*
  plaque of, 1113–1114, *1113*, 1185–1189, *1186*, *1187*
  platelet-derived growth factor-B protein in, 1115, **Plate 9**
  regression of, 1121
  response-to-injury hypothesis of, 1114–1116, *1115*
  risk factors for, 1105
  sudden death in, 1121
  thrombosis in, 1121–1122
  transgenic mouse model of, 1117, 1636–1637, *1636*, 1636t, *1637*
Atherosclerotic ulcer, penetrating, 1569, *1569*
Athletes, hypertrophic cardiomyopathy in, 1424–1425, 1424t
  sudden cardiac death in, 752
Athlete's heart, vs. hypertrophic cardiomyopathy, 1415, *1415*
ATP (adenosine triphosphate), in heart failure, 407
  in myocardial ischemia, 1178
Atrial beats, ectopic, *644*
Atrial fibrillation, 641t–642t, 654–656
  accessory pathway in, *671*
  after coronary artery bypass surgery, 1320
  anticoagulation in, 655–656
  clinical features of, 655
  electrocardiography in, 116, *146*, *151*, 654–655, *654*
  embolism with, 655–656
  exercise stress testing in, 168, *168*
  genesis of, 572
  in aortic stenosis, 1042
  in constrictive pericarditis, 1500
  in elderly, 1698
  in heart failure, 506–507, 1986
  in mitral stenosis, 1009, 1013
  in myocardial contusion, 1538
  in myocardial infarction, 1245t, 1253–1254
  in pregnancy, 1854–1855
  in Wolff-Parkinson-White syndrome, 672, *673*
  mid-diastolic murmur in, 41, *42*
  murmur in, 41, *42*, 1011
  postoperative, 1729–1730, 1764
    prophylaxis against, 1720
    risks for, 1719
  reentry in, 572
  syncope in, 867
  thromboembolic risk in, 1831, 1831t
  treatment of, 656
    antithrombotic therapy in, 1830–1832, *1831*, 1831t
    aspirin in, 1832, *1832*
    digitoxin in, *151*
    electrical cardioversion in, 619–620
    radiofrequency catheter ablation in, 625, 627
    warfarin in, 1831–1832, *1831*, *1832*
Atrial flutter, 641t–642t, 652–654
  carotid sinus massage in, 652, *653*
  clinical features of, 652–654, *653*
  congenital, 951
  electrocardiography in, 652, *653*, *654*
  flecainide effect on, 654, *654*
  genesis of, 572
  in aortic stenosis, 1042
  in Duchenne muscular dystrophy, 1869
  in hydrops fetalis, 951
  in myocardial infarction, 1245t, 1253–1254
  in pregnancy, 1854–1855
  postoperative, *1728*, 1729, *1729*, 1764
  prevention of, 654
  quinidine effect on, *653*

Atrial flutter *(Continued)*
  reentry in, 572
  sinus rhythm and, *653*
  syncope in, 867
  treatment of, 654
    drugs in, 598t
    electrical cardioversion in, 620
    radiofrequency catheter ablation in, 624–627, *625*
Atrial natriuretic peptide, gene for, 1640
  in heart failure, 405, *405*, *408*, 414, 478, *548*, 1917t
  in myocardial infarction, 1197
  in systemic hypertension, 818
Atrial parasystole, 693, 695, *695*
Atrial premature depolarization, postoperative, 1729
Atrial pressure, 188t, 189, *189*
  in constrictive pericarditis, 1502, *1502*
  left, 188t, 189, *189*, 190t
    in mitral stenosis, 1009
  right, 188t, 189, *189*, 190t
Atrial reentry, *650*
  clinical features of, 658
  electrocardiography of, *650*, 658
Atrial septal defect, 1847
  closure of, hypertension after, 830
  echocardiography in, 81–83, *82–83*, 897, *897*, **Plate 4**
  exercise and, 979
  familial, 1660–1661, 1660t
  in Noonan syndrome, 1663
  magnetic resonance imaging in, *334*
  mitral stenosis and, 967
  ostium primum, echocardiography in, 81, *83*
    pulmonary blood flow in, *218*
  ostium secundum, 896–898
    cardiac catheterization in, 897
    chest roentgenography in, 232–233, *232*, 897
    clinical findings in, 896–897
    echocardiography in, 81–83, *82*, *83*, **Plate 4**
    electrocardiography in, 897, *897*
    electrophysiological studies in, 898
    heart sounds in, *32*, 33, *33*
    hemodynamics of, 896
    in adult, 966, *966*, 970
    management of, 897–898, *898*
    midsystolic murmur of, *32*, 37
    morphology of, 896, *896*
    noncardiac surgery and, 981
    operative repair of, 897–898, *898*
    pregnancy and, 975, 976
  physical examination in, 896–897
  precordial motion in, 24t
  pulmonary hypertension with, 786
  sinus venosus type, echocardiography in, 82
Atrial septostomy, in congenital heart disease, 895
  in pulmonary hypertension, 795
  in transposition of great arteries, 939
  in tricuspid atresia, 933
Atrial (venous) switch operation, in transposition of great arteries, 939
Atrial tachycardia, 656–658
  automatic, *650*, 657–658, *657*
    clinical features of, 657–658
    electrocardiography in, *650*, 657
  chaotic, 658, *658*
  clinical features of, 657
  electrocardiography in, *650*, 656–657, *657*
  practice guidelines for, 1961t–1962t
  reentry, 658
  treatment of, 598t, 657
    radiofrequency catheter ablation in, 624–627
  with block, 641t–642t, 657
atrio-Hisian tracts, in Wolff-Parkinson-White syndrome, *668*, 669
Atrioventricular block, 688–691
  clinical features of, 692
  complete, 641t–642t, 687, 691–692
    clinical features of, 691–692, *691*, *692*
    electrocardiography in, 691, *691*
    in children, 691–692
  congenital, 949–950, 1667
    in adult, 966
    in systemic lupus erythematosus, 1779
    noncardiac surgery and, 981
    pacemaker in, 707, 708t
    pregnancy and, 976
  drug-induced, 12t

Atrioventricular block *(Continued)*
  electrocardiography in, 124, *124*, 127, 579, *580*, 691, *691*
  exercise stress testing in, 168
  first degree, 641t–642t, 687, 688, *688*
    in myocardial infarction, 1250
  in ankylosing spondylitis, 1780
  in myocardial infarction, 1245t, 1250–1251, 1251t
  in rheumatoid arthritis, 1777
  inducible, pacemaker in, 707, 708t
  management of, 692
  pacemaker in, 707–708, 708t
    practice guidelines for, 1964t
  paroxysmal, 691
  practice guidelines for, 1959, 1960t, 1962
  second degree, 641t–642t, *644*, 687, 688–691, *688*
    in myocardial infarction, 1250
    Mobitz type I (Wenckebach), 687, 688–691, *689*, *690*
      electrocardiography in, *124*
      in myocardial infarction, 1250
    Mobitz type II, 687, 688–691, *689*, *690*
      in myocardial infarction, 1250
      pacemaker in, 707–708, 708t
  sudden cardiac death in, 750
  temporary pacing in, 706
  third-degree, in myocardial infarction, 1250–1251, 1251t
  Wolff-Parkinson-White syndrome and, 127
Atrioventricular canal, unbalanced, 899
Atrioventricular canal defect. See *Atrioventricular septal defect.*
Atrioventricular conduction, in Duchenne muscular dystrophy, 1869
  in hyperthyroidism, 1893
  radiofrequency catheter ablation of, 627
Atrioventricular dissociation, 692–693, *692*
  arterial pulse in, 22
  classification of, 692–693, *692*
  clinical features of, 693
  electrocardiography in, 693
  in ventricular tachycardia, 678
  management of, 693
  mechanisms of, 693
  physical findings in, 640
Atrioventricular junctional area, 548–553, *549–551*
  cells of, 550–552, *551*
Atrioventricular junctional beat, *644*
Atrioventricular junctional complexes, premature, 658–659, *659*
Atrioventricular junctional escape beat, 658
Atrioventricular junctional rhythm, 641t–642t, 658–659, *659*
  in myocardial infarction, 1254
  postoperative, 1731
Atrioventricular junctional tachycardia, nonparoxysmal, 641t–642t, 659–661
    clinical features of, 660–661
    electrocardiography in, *650*, 659–660, *660*
    management of, 661
Atrioventricular nodal reentrant tachycardia, 661–665
  clinical features of, 663–664
  dual pathways in, *662*, 663
  electrocardiography in, *650*, *651*, 661
  electrophysiological features of, 661–663, *662*, *663*
  fast pathways in, 661, 663
  management of, 664–665, 664t
  postoperative, 1730
  prevention of, 664–665
  retrograde atrial activation in, 663
  slow pathways in, 661, 663
  treatment of, atrial pacing in, 664
    drugs in, 598t
    fast-pathway ablation in, 623, *623*
    radiofrequency catheter ablation in, 623–624, *623*, *624*
    slow-pathway ablation in, 623–624, *624*
Atrioventricular nodal reentry, 572–574, *573–575*, 641t–642t, *650*
  atrial dissociation in, 574, *575*
  atrial preexcitation in, 573, *573*
  pathways in, 573–574, *574*
  uncommon form of, 573
Atrioventricular node, anatomy of, 550–551, *550*, *551*
  cells of, 550

Atrioventricular node *(Continued)*
  cystic tumor of, 1471
  dead-end pathways of, 550
  in cardiac activation, 110, *110*
  innervation of, 552–553, *553*
Atrioventricular pacing, in syncope, 874
Atrioventricular reciprocating tachycardia, antidromic, 670, *671*
  concealed accessory pathway in, *663*, 665–667, *666–668*
    clinical features of, 665–666
    management of, 666–667
  genesis of, 574–575, *576*
  permanent form of, 670, 672, *672*, *673*
  septal accessory pathway in, 665
Atrioventricular septal defect, 898–901
  complete, 899–901
    diagnosis of, 899–900, *900*
    echocardiography in, 899, *899*, 900, *900*
    management of, 900–901, *901*
    morphology of, 899, *900*
    operative repair of, 900–901, *901*
  familial, 1661
  ostium primum (partial), 898–899
Atrioventricular synchrony, in cardiac pacing, 722
  restoration of, 723
Atrium (atria), calcifications of, 221, *221*
  embryology of, 879, *879*, *882*
  enlargement of, 115–116, *115*, *209*, *213*, *215*
  infarction of, 1192–1193, 1206. See also *Myocardial infarction.*
  left, echocardiography of, *64*, 68
    enlargement of, electrocardiography in, 115–116, *115*
      in mitral stenosis, *213*, *215*
      on plain chest radiography, *209*
    in contraction-relaxation cycle, 384–385
    on plain chest radiography, 207–208, *209*, 211
    palpation of, 28
  right, echocardiography of, *60*, 68
    enlargement of, electrocardiography in, 115, *115*
      on plain chest radiography, *209*
    in contraction-relaxation cycle, 384–385
  rupture of, 1538–1529, *1539*
  single, 947
  volume of, 427
Atropine, in arteriography, 245
  in myocardial infarction, 1972t
  in pediatric cardiology, 1000t
  in sinus bradycardia, 1249
Auscultation, 28–35, *29*. See also *Heart sound(s); Murmur(s).*
  drug effects on, 46t, *48*, 49
  dynamic, 46–49, 46t
  early diastolic sounds on, *29*, 33–34
  early systolic sounds on, *29*, 30–31, *30*, *31*
  first heart sound on, 29–30, *29*, *30*
  fourth heart sound on, *29*, 34–35, *34*
  in aortic regurgitation, 1049–1050
  in aortic stenosis, 1040–1041, 1040t
  in mitral regurgitation, 1022–1024, 1023t
  in mitral stenosis, 1010–1011
  in mitral valve prolapse, 1032–1033
  in myocardial infarction, 1200–1201
  in pulmonic valve disease, 1059
  in tricuspid regurgitation, 1057
  in tricuspid stenosis, 1055
  late diastolic sounds on, *29*, 34–35
  late systolic sounds on, *29*, 31–32, *31*, *32*
  mid-diastolic sounds on, *29*, 34–35
  midsystolic sounds on, *29*, 31–32, *31*, *32*
  of aorta, 1547
  of supraclavicular systolic arterial murmur, 40, *40*
  patient position for, 28, *29*, 47–49, *48*, *49*
  pharmacological effects on, 46t, *48*, 49
  principles of, 28–29
  second heart sound on, *29*, 32–33, *32*
    abnormal splitting of, 32–33, *32*, *33*
  technique of, 28–29, *29*
  third heart sound on, *29*, 34–35, *34*
Auscultatory gap, in arterial pressure measurement, 20
Austin Flint murmur, *42*
  in aortic regurgitation, 1050
Autoantibodies, anti beta-adrenoceptor, in idiopathic dilated cardiomyopathy, 1409
Autoimmune disease, pericarditis in, 1519
Automatic atrial tachycardia, *650*, 657–658, *657*
  clinical features of, 657–658
  electrocardiography in, *650*, 657
Automaticity, 563–564
  abnormal, 566
  in sinus nodal cells, 563–564
  in ventricular tachycardia, 577
Automobile accident, 1535. See also *Traumatic heart disease.*
Autonomic dysfunction, in diabetes mellitus, 1901–1902
Autoregulation, of coronary blood flow, 1168–1169, *1168*
Axial cineangiography, in tetralogy of Fallot, 931
Azathioprine, toxicity of, in heart transplantation, 525
Azide, myocardial effects of, 1448
Azithromycin, in rheumatic fever, 1773, 1773t
Azotemia, in heart failure, 1919–1920
  prerenal, in cardiogenic shock, 1920–1921, 1920t
Azygos vein, on plain chest radiography, 211, *211*

Babesia microti, in pericarditis, 1511
Bachmann's bundle, 548
Back pain, in abdominal aortic aneurysm, 1548
Bangungut, 752
Barbourin, 1630
Baroreceptor, in heart failure, *396*, 410
Baroreceptor reflex, cardiac glycoside effect on, 482
  in arrhythmia diagnosis, 585
Barth syndrome, 1665
Bartonella, in infective endocarditis, 1082
Bartter syndrome, 1678t
Basement membrane, 1107–1108
Basic fibroblast growth factor, in collateral vessel development, 1174–1175
Bat wing edema, plain film radiography of, 219, *219*, 221
Batten disease, genetic factors in, 1661t
Bayes theorem, in diagnostic testing, 1744, *1744*, 1744t, *1745*
  in exercise stress testing, 162–163, *162*
Beall mitral valve prosthesis, on plain radiography, *217*
Becker muscular dystrophy, 1632t, 1665, 1869–1870, *1871*
Bed rest, in unstable angina, 1336
Behavior, Type A, in cardiac rehabilitation, 1398
  in coronary artery disease, 1154
  in sudden cardiac death, 745
Behçet's disease, 1782–1783
  aortitis in, 1575
Benazepril, in renal failure, 1933t
Bendroflumethiazide, in heart failure, 477–478, 477t
Benzimidazole, in trypanosomiasis, 1444
Benzodiazepines, for anesthesia, 1757
Benzthiazide, in heart failure, 477–478, 477t
Bepridil, digoxin interaction with, 483t
  in angina pectoris, 1309t, 1311
  in renal failure, 1931t
  pharmacokinetics of, 1309t
  side effects of, 1303t
Beriberi, heart failure in, 461–462, 461t
  infantile, 993–994
  pulmonary hypertension with, 786
  vs. alcoholic cardiomyopathy, 1412
Bernheim effect, in contraction-relaxation cycle, 385
Bernoulli equation, in Doppler measurements, 69, *69*
Bernstein test, in gastroesophageal reflux, 1291
Beta thalassemia, 1788–1790
Beta-oxidation, defects of, 1668t, 1674
Betaxolol, in renal failure, 1931t
  pharmacodynamic properties of, 487t
  pharmacology of, 1307t
Bevantolol, in arrhythmias, 610–613, 611t
  pharmacodynamic properties of, 487t
Bezafibrate, in dyslipidemia, 1141–1142
Bezold-Jarisch reflex, in myocardial infarction, 1199
BIBU 104XX, 1820
Bicarbonate sodium, in pediatric cardiology, 1000t
Bicarbonate/chloride exchanger, in contraction-relaxation cycle, 371
Bicycle ergometry, in exercise stress testing, 155
Bifid T wave, 139
Bigeminy, definition of, 676
Bile-acid sequestrants, in dyslipidemia, 1139–1140, 1139t, 1140t
Biliary colic, vs. angina pectoris, 1291
Biliary disease, pain in, 4t
Biologic response modifiers, cardiac effects of, 1803–1804
Biological death, 742–743, *742*, 743t, 758–759
Biopsy, endomyocardial, 1404–1406. See also *Endomyocardial biopsy.*
  lung, in pulmonary hypertension, 887
  pericardial, 1496
    in acute pericarditis, 1484
    in pericardial effusion, 1496
    in tuberculous pericarditis, 1507
Bioptomes, for endomyocardial biopsy, 186, *187*
Bio-Pump centrifugal pump, 537t, 538, *538*
Bipolar limb leads, 110
Bisferious (bisferiens) pulse, *21*
  in aortic regurgitation, 1049
  in hypertrophic obstructive cardiomyopathy, *21*
Bishydroxycoumarin (Dicumarol), in pediatric cardiology, 1000t
Bisoprolol, in arrhythmias, 610–613, 611t
  pharmacodynamic properties of, 487t
  pharmacology of, 1307t
Blacks, hypertension in, 815, 821–822
  left ventricular hypertrophy in, 815
Blastomycosis myocarditis, 1441
Bleeding. See also *Hemorrhage.*
  after coronary artery bypass surgery, 1319
Blindness, in giant cell arteritis, 1574
Blood, culture of, in infective endocarditis, 1086, 1087, 1093, 1096
  viscosity of, in myocardial infarction, 1198
Blood count, preoperative, 1717t
Blood flow, cerebral, in hypertensive crises, 832–833, *833*
  coronary, **1161–1176.** See also *Myocardial ischemia.*
    angiographic assessment of, 262
    collateral, 1174–1176, *1175*
    Doppler echocardiography of, 68–71, *68–70*
    effective, 197
    endocardial:epicardial ratio of, 1170, *1170*
    in atherosclerosis, 1171–1174, *1171–1173*
    in coronary artery disease, 1299
    in stable angina pectoris, 1293–1294, *1294*
    magnetic resonance imaging of, 318–319, *319*, *320*, *323*, 331–332, *332–334*
    maximal, 1173–1174, *1173*
    measurement of, 197, 199–200, *199*
    myocardial oxygen consumption and, 1163, *1163*
    nitroglycerin effects on, 1302
    positron emission tomography of, 307
    regulation of, 1163–1176
      adenosine in, 1163, *1163*
      autoregulation in, 1168–1169, *1168*
      endothelial, 1164–1168, *1164–1167*
      endothelium-dependent vasodilation in, 1165–1166, *1165*, *1166*
      endothelium-derived constricting factors in, 1167–1168
      endothelium-derived relaxing factor in, 1164, *1164*, *1165*
      extravascular compressive forces in, 1169
      metabolic, 1163, *1163*
      neural, 1170–1171
    reserve of, 1173–1174, *1173*
    subendocardial:subepicardial ratio of, 1170
    transmural distribution of, 1169–1170, *1169*, *1170*
  pulmonary, asymmetrical, 220, *220*
    calculation of, 197
    cephalization of, 219, *220*
    decrease in, 220
    in pulmonary arterial hypertension, 218–219, *219*
    in transposition of great arteries, 936–937
    increase in, 217–218, *218*
    on plain chest radiography, 217–221, *218–220*
    primary pulmonary hypertension and, 786
  renal, 1914–1915
  systemic, 197
Blood gases, in pulmonary embolism, 1587

Blood pressure, basal, 20
borderline elevated, 810
exercise and, 163–164, 809
high, 808–810, *808*. See also *Hypertension*.
high normal, 809, 810t
in aortic dissection, 1564–1565
in children, 857, 997–998, *998*, *999*
in elderly, 823
in exercise stress testing, 163–164
in heart failure, 456
in myocardial infarction, 1200
in pheochromocytoma, 1898
in pregnancy, 830–832, 831t, 1843–1844, *1844*
in stable angina pectoris, 1292, 1293–1294
in stroke, 815
intraoperative, 1757–1758
measurement of, 20, 810t
in children, 997–998, *998*, *999*
in hypertension, 809–810, 810t
indirect, 20
nocturnal fall in, 809
normal, 810t
in children, *998*, 999, *999*
out-of-office measurement of, 808–809
peripheral, 189
smoking cessation and, 1148
variability in, 808, *808*
weight loss and, 1906
Blood transfusion, hemochromatosis after, 1792, *1792*
Blood urea nitrogen, preoperative, 1717t
Blue sclerae, 15
Body surface mapping, in arrhythmia diagnosis, 583
Bone, heparin effects on, 1594
Borg scale, in exercise training, 1396, 1396t
Borrelia burgdorferi, 989–990, 1511
Bosentan, in heart failure, 415
Boundary potential, on electrocardiography, 109–110, *109*
Bowditch effect, in contraction-relaxation cycle, 380, *380*
BQ123, in heart failure, 415
Brachial artery technique, for cardiac catheterization, 185–186
Bradyarrhythmia, after coronary artery bypass surgery, 1320
in elderly, 1698
postoperative, 1320, 1731
preoperative, 1719
Bradycardia, fetal, 950, *950*
in heart failure, 449
intraoperative, 1758
syncope in, 867
Bradykinin, *1165*
Brain abscess, in congenital heart disease, 885, 973
Brain death, in heart donor, 517–518
Brain natriuretic peptide, in heart failure, 414
in myocardial infarction, 1197
Bran, digoxin interaction with, 483t
Branham's sign, 460
Breast cancer, cardiac metastases from, 1794–1799, *1795*, 1795t, *1796*, 1796t
electrocardiography in, 135, *136*
chemotherapy for, venous thrombosis and, 1584
estrogen replacement therapy and, 1708–1709
pericarditis with, 1513–1516
Breast feeding, 977
Breast tissue, on myocardial perfusion imaging, 278, 279, *280*, 281
Bretylium tosylate, adverse effects of, 615
dosage of, 594t–595t, 615
electrophysiological actions of, 601t, 602t–603t, 615
hemodynamic effects of, 615
in arrhythmia, 592t, 594t–595t, 602t–603t, 615
in infarction-related ventricular fibrillation, 1249
in pediatric cardiology, 1000t
in renal failure, 1930t
indications for, 615
pharmacokinetics of, 594t–595t, 615
Brevibloc. See *Esmolol (Brevibloc)*.
Broadbent's sign, in constrictive pericarditis, 25
Brockenbrough maneuver (premature ventricular beat), with cardiac catheterization, 198
Bromocriptine, cardiac complications of, 1881
Bronchial circulation, 780
Bronchiolitis obliterans, after lung transplantation, 530, 796
Bronchitis, in pulmonary hypertension, 798–799
Bruce protocol, for exercise stress testing, 155–156, *156*
Brucella, in infective endocarditis, 1082, 1094
Brucellosis, myocarditis in, 1439
Bucindolol, in arrhythmias, 610–613, 611t
in heart failure, 472t, 487–488
pharmacodynamic properties of, 487t
Bulboventricular loop, in cardiac malposition, 946
Bullet injury, 1539–1541, *1540*
aortic, 1543
Bumetanide, in heart failure, 477t
in renal failure, 1933t
Bundle branch, 550, *551*
Bundle branch block. See also *Left bundle branch block (LBBB); Right bundle branch block (RBBB)*.
bilateral, 123, *124*
masquerading, 123, *123*
pacemaker in, 707–708, 708t
Bundle branch block alternans, 123
Bundle of His, 550, *551*
innervation of, 552–553
Bundles of Kent, 668
in sudden cardiac death, 750
Butterfly wing edema, plain film radiography of, 21, 219, *219*
BVS 5000 Bi-ventricular Support System, 537t, 538, *539*

Cable properties, of membrane, 564
Cachexia, in heart failure, 455
Cafe coronary, 752
Caffeine, in hypertension, 845
Calcification(s), annular, 1017–1018, 1024
plain film radiography of, 221–223, *222*
arterial, computed tomography of, 338–339, *339*
plain film radiography of, 223, *223*
atrial, in myocardial infarction, 221
plain chest radiography of, 221, *221*
dystrophic, in renal failure, 1927, 1927t
fluoroscopic evaluation of, 213–215, *217*
in aortic dissection, 1558, *1558*
in cardiac myxoma, 1468
in cardiac tumor, 1468, 1473
in pericarditis, 225
in pulmonary arterial hypertension, *219*
of aortic annulus, 221–223, *222*
of aortic valve, 221, *222*, 914, 1050
of mitral annulus, 221–223, *222*, 1017–1018, 1024
pericardial, computed tomography of, 340, *340*
plain film radiography of, *224*, 225
plain chest radiography of, 221–225, *221–224*
tumor, 1468, 1473
plain film radiography of, *224*, 225
valvular, 221–223, *222*, 1017–1018, 1024, 1050
Calcium, in contraction-relaxation cycle, 362–363, *362*, *365*
in crossbridge cycling, 363–364, *365*, *366*
in heart failure, 403, 403t, 404–406, *405*
in hyperparathyroidism, 1900, *1900*
in hypoxia-induced vasoconstriction, 781
in ischemia, 386, *386*
in myocardial ischemia, 1178–1179
in myocardial stunning, 388–389, 388t, *389*
in reperfusion, 388, 388t, *389*
in resting potential, *556*, 557
myocardial concentration of, 554t
myocardial oxygen consumption and, 1162
Calcium channel, currents of, 560–561, 561t, 562t
in action potential phase 0, 557–559, *557*, *559*
inactivation of, *559*
L-type, 369–370, *369*
selectivity of, 560
T-type, 370
voltage-dependent, in heart failure, 406
Calcium channel blockers, 594t–595t, 601t, 602t–603t, 616–618, 848t
antiatherogenic action of, 1308
exercise stress testing effects of, 170
in angina pectoris, 1308–1313, 1309t, 1312t
in aortic dissection, 1565
in coronary artery disease, 1149t
Calcium channel blockers *(Continued)*
in elderly, 1699
in heart failure, 472t, 475
in hypertension, 855, 855t
in hypertrophic cardiomyopathy, 1425
in idiopathic dilated cardiomyopathy, 1411
in myocardial infarction, 1198, 1231, 1265, 1974t, 1978
in Prinzmetal's variant angina, 1342–1343
in pulmonary hypertension, *793*
in pulmonary hypertension testing, 794–795, *794*
in syndrome X, 1344
in unstable angina, 1337, 1982t, 1983
myocardial oxygen consumption effects of, 1306t
noncardiac surgery and, 1761
preoperative, 1719–1720
Calcium chloride, in pediatric cardiology, 1000t
Calcium gluconate, in cardiac arrest, 766
in pediatric cardiology, 1000t
Calcium pump, of sarcoplasmic reticulum, 368–369, *368*
Calcium release channel (ryanodine receptor), 360, *363*
in heart failure, 405–406
of sarcoplasmic reticulum, 367–368, *367*, *368*
Calcium supplementation, in hypertension, 845
Calcium-sensitizing drugs, in heart failure, 485
Caliprolol, pharmacodynamic properties of, 487t
Calrectulin, 369
Calsequestrin, 361, 369
in heart failure, 406
Canadian Cardiovascular Society, cardiovascular disability assessment system of, 12t, 13
Canadian Coronary Atherosclerosis Intervention Trial, in hypercholesterolemia prevention, 1132
Cancer. See *Tumor(s)*.
Candida, in endocarditis, 1082, 1092–1093, 1094
in myocarditis, 1441
in pericarditis, 1510–1511
Candoxatrilat, in heart failure, 414
Canrenone, in heart failure, 477t
Capillary hemangiomatosis, in pulmonary hypertension, 787–788, 787t
Captopril (Capoten), digoxin interaction with, 483t
during pregnancy, 1852t
first-dose effects of, 497
hematological abnormalities with, 1804t
in congenital heart disease–related heart failure, 890, 891t
in heart failure, 472t, 495–497, *496*, 890, 891t
in hypertension, 855–856, *855*
in myocardial infarction, 1229–1230, *1229*, *1230*
in pediatric cardiology, 1000t
in renal failure, 1933t
Captopril challenge test, in renovascular hypertension, 827
Capture threshold, of pacemaker, 710–711, *710*, *711*
Carbohydrate intolerance, diuretics and, 480
Carbomedics valve, 1061, *1062*, 1065
Carbon dioxide, on exercise stress testing, 439–440, *440*
Carbon monoxide, myocardial effects of, 1447
Carbonic anhydrase inhibitors, in heart failure, 476, 477t
Carcinoid syndrome, 1434
patient history in, 11
tricuspid regurgitation in, 1056, *1057*
Cardene. See *Nicardipine (Cardene)*.
Cardiac activation, 110, *110*
Cardiac arrest, *742*, **742–756**, 743t. See also *Sudden cardiac death*.
antiarrhythmic agent precipitation of, 767
asystolic, 756, 758–759
management of, 766
out-of-hospital, 761
bradyarrhythmic, 756, 758–759
management of, 766
out-of-hospital, 761
central nervous system injury in, 759
circulation in, 763–765, *763*, 764t–765t
clinical features of, 758, 758t
coronary thrombosis in, 753, 755
drug precipitation of, 767
in myocardial infarction, 766–767
in-hospital, 767

Cardiac arrest *(Continued)*
management of, 760–772
advanced life support in, 764t–765t, 765–766
airway clearance in, 763
algorithm for, 771–772, *771, 772*
antiarrhythmic drugs in, 768–769
basic life support in, 762–765
cardiopulmonary resuscitation in, 763–765, *763*, 764t–765t
bystander, 762
mortality after, 758, 758t, 762
community-based, 760–762, *761, 762*
defibrillation-cardioversion in, 764t, 765–766
initial assessment in, 762
long-term, 768
mouth-to-mouth respiration in, 763
pharmacotherapy in, 766
practice guidelines for, 1960t, 1963
stabilization in, 766
thumpversion in, 762–763
neurological complications of, 1880
onset of, 757–758, 757t
out-of-hospital, 759–760, *759, 760*
early defibrillation for, 762, *762*
electrical mechanisms in, 761–762, *761, 762*
emergency medical services for, 760–762, *761, 762*
survivors of, 760–761, *761*, 767–768
practice guidelines for, 1960t, 1963
prodromal symptoms in, 757
progression of, 758–759
public safety and, 772
recurrent, 760, *760*
prevention of, 768–771, *769*
ambulatory electrocardiographic monitoring for, 770
antiarrhythmic drugs in, 768–769
implantable devices for, 770–771
programmed electrical stimulation in, 769–770
surgical intervention for, 770
secondary, 767
survivors of, 758, 759–760, *759, 760*, 766–768
hospital course of, 759–760, *759, 760*
Cardiac catheterization, **177–200,** 178t
aortic pressure with, 189, *189*, 191t
arteries for, *183*, 185–186
atrial pressure with, 188t, 189, *189*, 190t
cardiac output measurements with, 189, 191–193
Fick technique for, 192, *192*
indicator-dilution techniques for, 191
thermodilution techniques for, 191–192
cardiac perforation with, 1521
catheters for, 182, 188
complications of, 179–180, 179t
contrast media for, 180, 180t
coronary blood flow measurments with, 199–200, *199*, 1173–1174
death from, 179–180
direct left ventricular puncture for, 186
dynamic exercise with, 198
equipment for, 181, *181*
exercise with, 198
femoral vein technique for, 182–183, *183, 184*
flow reserve measurement during, 1173–1174, *1173*
great vessel pressures with, 188t, 189, *189*, 191t
hemodynamic component of, 187–200, 188t, *189*, 190t–191t, *192, 194, 197, 199*
history of, 177
hypotension after, 180
in adult congenital heart disease, 980–981
in aortic sinus aneurysm, 911, *911*
in atrial septal defect, 897
in cardiac tamponade, 1492–1493, *1493*, 1521
in congenital aortic stenosis, 917–918, *917*
in congenital heart disease, 178t, 179, 895, 971t
in congenital pulmonic stenosis, 926
in congenitally corrected transposition of great arteries, 941
in cor triatriatum, 791t
in Ebstein's anomaly, 935
in endomyocardial fibrosis, 1433
in hypertrophic cardiomyopathy, 1422–1423
in idiopathic dilated cardiomyopathy, 1411
in Löffler endocarditis, 1433

Cardiac catheterization *(Continued)*
in mitral regurgitation, 791t
in mitral stenosis, 791t, 1013–1014
in neoplastic pericarditis, 1515
in partial anomalous pulmonary venous connection, 946
in pericardial effusion, 1492–1493, *1493*
in pericarditis, 1502–1504, *1502, 1503*
in persistent truncus arteriosus, 908
in pregnancy, 1846
in pulmonary hypertension, 790–791, 791t
in shunt evaluation, 196–198, *197*
in tetralogy of Fallot, 930–931, *930, 931*
in total anomalous pulmonary venous connection, 945
in transposition of great arteries, 937–938, 941
in tricuspid atresia, 933
in unstable angina, 1338, 1982t, 1983t, 1984, *1985*
in women, 1706, 1846
indications for, 177–179, 178t
isometric exercise and, 198
laboratory facilities for, 180
practice guidelines for, 1954
left heart, 181, 184–185, *185*
myocardial infarction risk with, 180
pacemaker use during, 181–182
pacing tachycardia with, 198
patient preparation for, 181
percutaneous brachial artery technique of, 185–186
percutaneous radial artery technique of, 186
personnel for, 180–181
pharmacological maneuvers with, 198–199
physiologic monitors for, 181
physiologic stress with, 198
practice guidelines for, 1953–1954, 1953t
preoperative, 1717t
pressure measurements with, 188–192, 188t, *189*, 190t–191t
abnormal, 189, 190t–191t
in valvular regurgitation, 195–196
in valvular stenosis, 193–195, *194*
normal, 188–189, 188t, *189*
protocol for, 181–182, 182t
pulmonary artery pressure with, 190t
pulmonary capillary wedge pressure with, 188t, 189, *189*
radiation safety for, 181
radiographic equipment for, 181, *181*
right heart, 181, 182–184, 182t, *183, 184*
complications of, 184, *184*
transseptal, 186
vagal reactions to, 180
vascular resistance measurement with, 192–193
ventricular pressure with, 188t, 189, *189*, 191t
Cardiac compression, in rheumatoid arthritis, 1776
Cardiac cycle. See *Contraction-relaxation cycle.*
Cardiac examination, **24–45.** See also *Physical examination.*
aortic palpation in, 28
auscultation in, 28–35, *29*. See also *Auscultation.*
inspection in, 24
left atrium palpation in, 28
left ventricle palpation in, 25–27, *26, 27*
murmurs in, 35–45. See also *Murmur(s).*
continuous, 43–45, *44*
diastolic, 40–43, *40*
early diastolic, 40–41, *40, 41*
early systolic, *36*, 38–39, *39*
holosystolic, *36*, 38, *38, 39*
late diastolic, 43, *43, 44*
late systolic, 39–40, *39*
mid-diastolic, *40*, 41–43, *42*
midsystolic, 36–38, *36, 37*
systolic, 35, 36–40, *36*
systolic arterial, 40, *40*
palpable sounds in, 28
palpation in, 24–28, 24t, *26, 27*
vs. percussion, 28
pericardial rubs in, 45
right ventricle palpation in, *26*, 27–28
thrills in, 28
Cardiac herniation, 1522
Cardiac impulse, in aortic stenosis, 1040
in mitral regurgitation, 1022
Cardiac index, of aging heart, 1692, *1693*
Cardiac mapping, in arrhythmia diagnosis, 583

Cardiac output, 191–193
during exercise, 153
in aortic stenosis, 1038, 1040
in chronic obstructive pulmonary disease, 1616–1617
in heart failure, 394, 446, 447, 452
in hyperthyroidism, 1892
in mitral regurgitation, 1020–1021
in mitral stenosis, 1007–1008, 1009
in pregnancy, 1843, 1843t, *1844*
in ventricular septal defect, 904
measurement of, 189, 191–193, 439
Fick technique for, 195
indicator-dilution technique of, 191
thermodilution technique of, 191–192
of aging heart, 1692
to kidneys, 1914–1915
Cardiac rehabilitation, **1392–1401,** 1735–1736, 1736t
cost-effectiveness analysis of, 1748
counseling in, 1400
education in, 1400
exercise in, 1392–1397, *1393, 1394*, 1400–1401
effects of, 1394, *1394*
patient selection for, 1394–1397, 1395t, 1397t
prescription for, 1395–1396, 1396t
risks of, 1396–1397, 1397t
safety of, 1397
iatrogenic factors and, 1392
inpatient, 1399–1400
left ventricular dysfunction and, 1392–1393, *1393*
morbidity and, 1394, *1394*
myocardial ischemia and, 1393–1394
myocardial performance and, 1394
outcomes of, 1401
outpatient, 1400–1401
physical capacity in, 1392
physical conditioning in, 1392–1394, *1393*
physiological factors and, 1392
psychological factors in, 1398
reemployment after, 1399
secondary prevention in, 1397–1398
self-efficacy and, 1398
sexual activity in, 1400
skeletal muscle performance and, 1394
smoking cessation in, 1397–1398
vocational, 1398–1399
Cardiac resuscitation. See *Cardiopulmonary resuscitation; Cardioversion.*
Cardiac rupture, 1536t, 1538–1539, *1539*
Cardiac surgery, **1715–1736,** 1720t. See also specific procedures.
cardiopulmonary bypass circuit for, *1721*
complication(s) of, 1715
arrhythmias as, 1727–1731, *1728–1730*
gastrointestinal, 1734, 1735t
hemostatic, 1731–1732
hypertension as, 1723
infectious, 1732–1734
ischemic, 1723–1725, 1724t
neurological, 1734–1735, 1736t
pericardial, 1734
peripheral, 1734
renal, 1734
respiratory, 1722–1723, 1722t
risk factors for, 1718t
shock states as, 1725–1727, 1726t
discharge after, 1735–1737, 1736t
general sequence of, 1720t
hemolytic anemia after, 1790
in chronic renal failure, 1734
intraoperative management of, 1720, 1720t, *1721*
monitoring devices for, *1721*
nutritional support for, 1715, 1718t
postoperative management of, 1721–1735
acid-base balance in, 1721
antiarrhythmic agents in, 1730
anticoagulant agents in, 1729–1730
antithrombotic therapy in, 1732
arrhythmias in, 1727–1731, *1728*
atrial fibrillation in, 1729
atrial flutter in, 1729
atrioventricular junctional rhythms in, 1731
bradyarrhythmias in, 1731
cardiac tamponade in, 1727
cardioversion in, 1731
chronic lung disease in, 1723

- Cardiac surgery *(Continued)*
    - chylopericardium in, 1735
    - chylothorax in, 1735
    - diaphragmatic failure in, 1723
    - echocardiography in, 1725
    - electrocardiography in, 1725, 1728, *1728*
    - electrolytes in, 1721
    - fever in, 1732
    - fluids in, 1721
    - fungal infection in, 1733–1734
    - gastrointestinal complications in, 1734, 1735t
    - hemostatic disturbances in, 1731–1732, 1732t
    - hypertension in, 1723
    - hypovolemia in, 1725
    - incision infection in, 1732–1733
    - infection in, 1732–1734
    - infective endocarditis in, 1733–1734
    - left ventricular failure in, 1725–1726
    - leg infection in, 1732
    - low-output syndrome in, 1725–1727
    - mediastinitis in, 1732–1733
    - myocardial infarction in, 1723–1725, 1724t
    - neurological complications in, 1734–1735, 1736t
    - paroxysmal supraventricular tachycardia in, 1730
    - pericarditis in, 1734
    - peripheral vascular complications in, 1734
    - prosthetic valve endocarditis in, 1733
    - prosthetic valves in, 1732
    - pulmonary edema in, 1722–1723
    - pulmonary embolism in, 1727
    - renal failure in, 1734
    - respiratory function in, 1722–1723, 1722t
    - right ventricular failure in, 1726–1727
    - septic shock in, 1727
    - shock states in, 1725–1727
    - sternal osteomyelitis in, 1732–1733
    - supraventricular arrhythmias in, *1728*, 1729–1730, *1729*
    - troponin levels in, 1724–1725
    - vasodilatation in, 1725
    - ventilators in, 1722, 1722t
    - ventilatory insufficiency in, 1723
    - ventricular arrhythmias in, 1730–1731
    - ventricular fibrillation in, 1730–1731
    - ventricular premature depolarizations in, 1730
    - ventricular tachycardia in, 1730, *1730*
    - viral infection in, 1733
    - wound infection in, 1732–1733
  - preoperative evaluation for, 1715–1720
    - anesthesia and, 1718
    - antiarrhythmic agents in, 1720
    - atrial fibrillation in, 1719
    - atrioventricular block in, 1719
    - bradyarrhythmias in, 1719
    - cardiac rhythm in, 1718–1719, *1719*
    - drug therapy in, 1719–1720
    - hemodynamic, 1716
    - hypomagnesemia in, 1720
    - intraventricular block in, 1719
    - medical, 1715–1716, 1716t, 1717t, 1718t
    - myocardial ischemia risk and, 1716–1718
  - rehabilitation after, 1735–1737, 1736t
- Cardiac syncope, 866–867. See also *Syncope.*
  - outcomes of, 867–868
- Cardiac tamponade, **1486–1495,** 1498t, 1535. See also *Traumatic heart disease.*
  - cardiac catheterization in, 1492–1493, *1493*, 1521
  - chest roentgenography in, 1490
  - chylopericardium in, 1522
  - clinical manifestations of, 1489–1490, 1489t
  - consequences of, 1486–1488, *1487*
  - echocardiography in, 93–94, *93*, 1490–1492, *1491*, 1491t
  - electrocardiography in, 1490, *1490*
  - etiology of, 1489, 1489t
  - in aortic dissection, 1521, 1565
  - in postinfarction pericarditis, 1511
  - in postpericardiotomy syndrome, 1520
  - in rheumatoid arthritis, 1518
  - in systemic lupus erythematosus, 1518
  - laboratory studies in, 1490–1492, *1490*, 1491t
  - low-pressure, 1490
  - myocardial ischemia and, 1487
  - patient history in, 11
- Cardiac tamponade *(Continued)*
  - percutaneous balloon pericardiotomy in, 1495–1496, *1495*
  - pericardial biopsy in, 1496
  - pericardiectomy in, 1496
  - pericardiocentesis in, 1493–1495, *1494*
  - pericardioscopy in, 1496
  - physical examination in, 1489–1490
  - postoperative, 1521, 1727
  - pulsus paradoxus in, 1488–1490, *1488*
  - regional, 1487
  - right atrial collapse in, 1487–1488
  - superior vena cava obstruction and, 1515
  - tension pneumopericardium in, 1490
  - ventricular collapse in, 1487–1488
  - ventricular pressure-volume relationships in, 404
  - vs. constrictive pericarditis, 1498t, 1503
  - vs. shock, 1490, 1512
  - vs. superior vena cava syndrome, 1493
- *Cardiobacterium hominis*, in infective endocarditis, 1092, 1093t
- Cardiogenic shock, *1195*, 1725–1726, 1726t
  - appearance in, 1199
  - definition of, 535t
  - diagnosis of, 1239
  - hypotension in, 1200
  - in heart failure, 1988
  - in myocardial infarction, *1195*, 1238–1240, *1238*
  - intraaortic balloon counterpulsation in, 535, 1239
  - management of, 1239
  - piecemeal necrosis in, 1238
  - postcardiotomy, intraaortic balloon counterpulsation in, 535
    - ventricular assist device in, 541–542, 541t, 543, 543t
  - postoperative, 1725–1726, 1726t
  - prerenal azotemia in, 1920–1921, 1920t
  - reperfusion in, 1240
  - surgical treatment of, 1240
  - vs. cardiac tamponade, 1512
- Cardiomegaly, in acromegaly, 1888, *1888*
  - in heart failure, 455
- Cardiomyopathy, **1404–1449,** 1405t
  - acromegalic, 1889–1890, *1899*
  - alcoholic, 1412–1414, 1877
  - diabetic, 1902–1903, *1902*
  - dilated, 1404, 1406t, **1407–1414**
    - alcoholic, 1412–1414, 1877
      - clinical manifestations of, 1412–1413
      - laboratory examination in, 1412–1413
      - management of, 1413
      - physical examination in, 1412
    - cobalt, 1413
    - diastolic function in, 1415t
    - during pregnancy, 1665, 1851–1852, *1851*
    - echocardiography in, 92
    - embolism in, 1834, 1834t, 1880
    - G_1 protein in, 412
    - genetic factors in, 1660t, 1665–1666
    - idiopathic, **1407–1412,** *1407*, *1408*
      - angiography in, 1411
      - cardiac catheterization in, 1411
      - clinical manifestations of, 1409–1411, *1410*
      - diagnosis of, 991
      - echocardiography in, 1410
      - electrocardiography in, 1410
      - etiology of, 1407–1408, 1409, *1409*
      - familial, 1409
      - histology of, *1405*, 1408
      - in children, 990–991, *991*
      - incidence of, 1407
      - iodine-123–labeled metaiodobenzylguanidine imaging of, 303
      - management of, 991, 1411–1412, 1411t
      - metoprolol in, 487, *487*
      - pathology of, *1406*, *1407*, 1408
      - patient history in, 1409–1410
      - physical examination in, 1410
      - radionuclide ventriculography in, 1411
      - survival with, 1408, *1408*, 1408t
    - in Friedreich's ataxia, 1874, *1875*
    - in systemic lupus erythematosus, *227*
    - magnetic resonance imaging of, 323–324
    - precordial motion in, 24t
    - pulmonary embolism in, 1834, 1834t
    - right atrial enlargement in, *209*
- Cardiomyopathy *(Continued)*
    - right ventricular, 749, 1413–1414, *1413*
    - sudden cardiac death in, 748, 749
    - systolic function in, 1415t
    - thrombus in, 1833–1834, 1834t
    - ventricular pressure-volume relationships in, *433*
    - ventricular tachycardia in, 682
    - X-linked, 1665
  - diphtheritic, 989
  - drug-induced, 12t
  - hypertrophic, 880t, 1404, 1406t, **1414–1426,** *1414*, 1415t
    - angiography in, 1423
    - beta-adrenoceptor blockers in, 1425
    - bisferious pulse in, *21*, 22
    - calcium antagonists in, 1425
    - cardiac catheterization in, 1422–1423
    - chest roentgenography in, 1421
    - clinical manifestations of, 1418–1422, 1419t, *1420*
    - computed tomography in, *336*
    - coronary artery abnormalities in, 1416
    - diastolic function in, 1415, 1415t, 1418, *1419*, 1422
    - diastolic pressure-volume curve in, 403
    - during pregnancy, 1851
    - dyspnea in, 1419
    - echocardiography in, 79–80, 91–92, *91*, *92*, 1421–1422
    - electrocardiography in, 1421
    - electrophysiological testing in, 1421
    - etiology of, 1417, *1417*, *1418*, 1419t
    - exercise in, 1426
    - familial, 1416, *1416*, 1417, *1417*, *1418*, 1632t, 1664–1665, 1665t
    - genetic factors in, 1417, *1417*, *1418*, 1632t, 1660t, 1664–1665, 1665t
    - heart sounds in, 1420
    - hypertensive, 1416
    - imaging in, 228–229, 354
    - in athletes, 1424–1425, 1424t
    - in children, 1424, *1424*
    - in elderly, 1416, 1419
    - in Friedreich's ataxia, 1874, *1875*
    - in renal failure, 1924
    - left ventricular end-systolic pressure-volume relation in, *433*
    - left ventricular outflow gradient in, 1420, 1420t, 1422–1423
    - magnetic resonance imaging in, 323, *323*
    - management of, 1425–1426
    - mitral leaflet systolic anterior motion in, 1418, *1418*, 1422
    - murmurs in, 1041, 1420, 1420t
    - myofibrillar disarray in, 1416, *1416*
    - natural history of, 1423–1426, *1424*, 1424t
    - noncardiac surgery and, 1761–1762
    - pacemaker in, 709
    - palpation in, 25, *27*
    - pathology of, 1415–1416, *1415*, *1416*
    - pathophysiology of, 1418, *1418*, *1419*
    - patient history in, 11
    - physical examination in, 1420–1421, 1420t
    - plain chest radiography in, 228–229
    - precordial motion in, 24t
    - progression of, 1423–1426, *1424*, 1424t
    - pulsus bisferiens in, *21*
    - Q wave in, 135, *136*, *149*
    - radionuclide scanning in, 1422
    - sudden death in, 747–748, 1424–1425, 1424t
    - symptoms of, 1418–1420, *1420*, 1420t
    - syncope in, 866
    - systolic function in, 1415, 1415t, 1418, *1418*, 1422
    - systolic murmurs in, *28*, 1023t
    - ventricular tachycardia in, 682
    - vs. athlete's heart, 1415, *1415*
    - vs. fixed orifice obstruction, 1420–1421
    - vs. mitral valve prolapse, 1033
  - imaging in, 354t, 356
    - practice guidelines for, 1946
  - in coronary artery disease, 1346–1347
  - in rheumatoid arthritis, 1778
  - inborn errors of metabolism and, 1666–1667, 1668t–1669t
  - ischemic, 1346–1347, 1404, 1833–1834, 1834t
  - magnetic resonance imaging of, 323–324, *323*
  - pheochromocytoma-induced, 1898, *1899*

Cardiomyopathy *(Continued)*
  restrictive, 1404, 1406t, **1426–1434**
    amyloidosis in, 1427–1429, *1428*
    classification of, 1426–1427, 1427t
    clinical manifestations of, 1427, *1428*
    echocardiography in, 92–93, *92*, 1427, *1428*
    endomyocardial, 1431–1434, *1432*
    genetic factors in, 1666, 1666t
    hemodynamics of, 1427
    in carcinoid heart disease, 1434
    in endomyocardial fibrosis, 1433–1434
    in Fabry disease, 1430, *1430*
    in Gaucher disease, 1430
    in glycogen storage disease, 1431, *1431*
    in hemochromatosis, 1430
    in hypereosinophilic syndrome, 1432–1433, *1432*
    in Löffler endocarditis, 1432–1433, *1432*
    in sarcoidosis, 1431
    infiltrative disorders in, 1430–1431, *1430*
    magnetic resonance imaging of, 324
    radiography in, 229
    vs. constrictive pericarditis, 1503t
    vs. pericardial constriction, 235
  secondary, 1404
    in anthracycline toxicity, 997
    in glycogen storage disease, 992–993, *993*
    in infantile beriberi, 993–994
    in infants of diabetic mothers, 992
    in Kawasaki disease, 994–997
    in neonatal thyrotoxicosis, 993
    in protein-calorie malnutrition, 994
    in tropical endomyocardial fibrosis, 994
Cardiopulmonary bypass, *1721*
  in aortic dissection, 1567
  pulmonary edema after, 466
Cardiopulmonary exercise testing. See *Exercise stress testing.*
Cardiopulmonary resuscitation, 763–765, *763*, 764t–765t
  bystander, 762
  complications of, 1530
  defibrillation-cardioversion in, 764t–765t, 765–766
  in out-of-hospital cardiac arrest, 762
  pharmacotherapy in, 766
Cardiorespiratory murmur, 45
Cardiotrophin-1, in myocyte hypertrophy, 1640t, 1642–1643
Cardioversion, 762, *762*, 764t–765t, 765–766
  anticoagulation for, 1832
  for arrhythmia, 619–620, *620*
  for atrial flutter, 654
  for atrioventricular nodal reentrant tachycardia, 664
  for ventricular tachycardia, 680
  pacemaker effects of, 728
  postoperative, 1731
  pulmonary edema after, 466
Cardioverter-defibrillator, for cardiac arrest prevention, 505–506
  for out-of-hospital cardiac arrest, 762, *762*
  implantable, 732–736, *733*
    after cardiac arrest, 770–771
    antitachycardia pacing by, 733, *734*
    arrhythmia sensing of, 732–733
    complications of, 734
    drug effects on, 733
    effectiveness of, 735
    electrogram analysis of, 735, *735*, *736*
    follow-up for, 734–736, *735*, *736*
    indications for, 732, 732t
    low-energy synchronized cardioversion by, 733–734
    methods of, 733
    transvenous, 733
  in cardiac arrest, 762, *762*, 764t–765t, 765–766
  pacemaker effects of, 728
  preoperative disabling of, 1719
Carditis. See also *Myocarditis.*
  rheumatic, 1770–1771, *1771*
Care map. See *Practice guidelines.*
Carey-Coombs murmur, 1011
Carney syndrome, 1467–1468, *1468*, 1468t
Carnitine deficiency, 1447, 1668t, 1674
  in idiopathic dilated cardiomyopathy, 1409
Carnitine palmitoyltransferase I, defect in, 1668t, 1674
Carotid artery, disease of, cerebrovascular accident and, 1879
  coronary artery bypass surgery and, 1331
  familial hypoplasia of, 1677
Carotid pulse, abnormal, 22
  in myocardial infarction, 1200
  palpation of, 21, *21*
Carotid sinus, hypersensitivity of. See *Hypersensitive carotid sinus syndrome.*
  in coronary blood flow regulation, 1170–1171
Carotid sinus massage, 642
  in arrhythmia evaluation, 641–642, 642t
  in atrial flutter, 652, *653*
  in hypersensitive carotid sinus syndrome, 647–648, *648*
  in syncope evaluation, 869
Carotid sinus syncope, 865. See also *Syncope.*
Carpenter syndrome, genetic factors in, 1661t
Carpentier-Edwards valve, 1063, *1063*
Carteolol, in arrhythmias, 610–613, 611t
  in renal failure, 1931t
  pharmacodynamic properties of, 487t
  pharmacology of, 1307t
Carvallo's sign, in tricuspid regurgitation, *31*, 38
Carvedilol, in arrhythmias, 610–613, 611t
  in heart failure, 472t, 487–488
  pharmacodynamic properties of, 487t
Casoni skin test, in echinococcal cyst, 1444
Catapres (clonidine), in hypertension, 852
  in pediatric cardiology, 1000t
  in renal failure, 1932t
CATCH 22 (*c*ardiac anomaly, *a*bnormal facies, *t*hymic hypoplasia, *c*left palate, and *h*ypocalcemia) association, 1658
Catecholamine(s), cardiovascular effects of, 11, 1447, 1897–1899, *1899*
  in congenital heart disease–related heart failure, 890, 891t
  in contraction-relaxation cycle, *373*, 374, 375t
  in hypertension, 819
  in myocardial infarction, 1197
  in pheochromocytoma, 1898
Catecholamine storm, in cerebrovascular accident, 1878
Cat-eye syndrome, 1651t, 1656t
Catheter(s), Amplatz, 242, *243*
  for arteriography, 241–242, *242*, *243*
  for cardiac catheterization, 182, 188
  Judkins, 241–242, *242*
  micromanometer, 188
  multipurpose, 242, *243*
  postoperative assessment of, 229–230, *229*
Catheter ablation, 621–628, *621–628*. See also *Radiofrequency catheter ablation.*
Catheterization, cardiac, **177–200.** See also *Cardiac catheterization.*
Cavernous angioma, 1677
c7E3 Fab (abciximab), in PTCA-related abrupt vessel closure, 1369
Celiprolol, in arrhythmias, 610–613, 611t
Cell membrane (sarcolemma), action potential of, 555–563
    loss of, 564–565
    phase 0 (rapid depolarization) of, 557–561, *557–559*, 561t, *562*, 562t
    phase 1 (early rapid depolarization) of, 559–560
    phase 2 (plateau) of, 563
    phase 3 (final rapid repolarization) of, 563
    phase 4 (resting) of, 555–556, 555t, *556*, *557*, 563, *563*
  electrophysiology of, 553–555, *554*, 554t
  gap junctions of, 555, *555*
  intercalated discs of, 554–555
  passive electrical properties of, 564–565, *565*
Cell transport, in hypertension, 818, *818*
Center line method, of left ventricular regional wall motion analysis, 427, *427*
Central nervous system, in cyanotic congenital heart disease, 973–974
  in heart failure, 452
  in sudden cardiac death, 751
Central venous catheterization, venous thrombosis and, 1584
Centrifugal pumps, 537t, 538, *538*
Centronuclear myopathy, 1875
Cephalosporin, in rheumatic fever, 1773, 1773t
Ceramidase deficiency, 1669t
Cerebral blood flow, in hypertensive crises, 832–833, *833*
Cerebral embolism, cardiogenic, 1879–1880
  in aortic stenosis, 1040
  in infective endocarditis, 1095
  in mitral valve prolapse, 1034
  paradoxical, 1880, *1880*
    in adult congenital heart disease, 973–974
  practice guidelines for, 1943
Cerebral hemorrhage, familial, 1667
  in adult congenital heart disease, 974, *974*
Cerebral infarction, after myocardial infarction, 1832–1833
  in atrial fibrillation, 1830–1832, *1831*, 1831t
  venous thrombosis and, 1584
Cerebral thrombosis, in congenital heart disease, 885
Cerebrovascular accident, cardiac emboli in, 1879–1880
  cardiovascular abnormalities and, 1877–1878, *1878*
  carotid artery disease and, 1879
  coronary artery bypass grafting and, 1879
  coronary artery disease and, 1878–1881
  in aortic dissection, 1557
  infective endocarditis and, 1880
  paradoxical emboli and, 1880, *1880*
  pulmonary edema in, 1878
Cervical arterial dissection, genetic factors in, 1677
Cervical cancer, cardiac metastases from, 1794–1799, *1795*, 1795t, *1796*, 1796t, *1798*
Cervical disc, herniation of, pain in, 4t
  inflammation of, vs. angina pectoris, 1291
Cesarean section, hemodynamic effects of, 1844
  ST-segment depression during, 1854, *1855*
Chagas' disease, 989
  cardiac denervation in, 1881
  myocarditis in, 1442–1444, *1442*, *1443*
Charcot-Marie-Tooth syndrome, 1875
CHARGE (*c*oloboma, *h*eart anomaly, choanal *a*tresia, *r*etardation, *g*enital, and *e*ye anomalies) association, 881t, 1659, 1659t
Chemical contamination, in renal dialysis, 1936
Chemodectoma, 829
Chemoreceptors, in coronary blood flow regulation, 1170–1171
Chemotherapy, cardiac effects of, 1799–1804, *1800–1802*, 1800t, 1801t, 1802t
  pericarditis with, 1515, 1516
  venous thrombosis and, 1584
Chest, examination of, 17–18, 24
  in myocardial infarction, 1200
  shield, 24
Chest pain, 3–7. See also *Angina pectoris.*
  acute, emergency department evaluation of, 1968, 1968t
    evaluation of, 1968–1970, 1969t
    practice guidelines for, 1967–1970, 1968t–1969t
    triage for, 1968, 1970
  angiography in, 1950t, 1952
  cardiac catheterization in, 178t. See also *Cardiac catheterization.*
  coronary arteriography in, 240
  differential diagnosis of, 7, 1290, 1291–1292, 1291t
  drug-induced, 12t
  duration of, 6–7
  functional, 5
  hemoptysis with, 7
  in acute pericarditis, 1481–1482, 1482t, 1484
  in aortic dissection, 1556
  in children, 888
  in chronic coronary artery disease, 1290
  in congenital heart disease, 888
  in exercise stress testing, 164
  in mitral stenosis, 1010
  in myocardial contusion, 1538
  in patient history, 3–7
  in syndrome X, 1343–1344
  in women, 1704–1705, 1704t
  location of, 5–6, *5*
  mechanisms of, 1290–1291, 1291t
  noncardiac, 5t
  normal coronary arteriography and, 1343–1344
  pleuritic, 5
  practice guidelines for, 1943, 1950t, 1952, 1967–1970, 1968t–1969t
  precipitation of, 7
  psychogenic, 5
  quality of, 4–5, 4t

Chest pain *(Continued)*
relief of, 7
shortness of breath with, 7
sweating with, 7
Chest roentgenography, in alcoholic cardiomyopathy, 1412
in amyloidosis, 1429
in aortic dissection, *207,* 1557–1558, *1558*
in aortic stenosis, 916, 1041
in atrial septal defect, 232–233, *232,* 897
in atrioventricular septal defect, 899
in carcinoid heart disease, 1434
in cardiac metastases, 1797–1798
in cardiac tamponade, 1490
in cardiac tumor, 1473, 1797–1798
in congenital aortic stenosis, 916
in congenital heart disease, 893–894
in congenital pulmonic stenosis, 926
in congenitally corrected transposition of great arteries, 941
in constrictive pericarditis, 1499–1500, *1499*
in cor pulmonale, 1609–1610, *1609*
in coronary artery disease, 1298
in endomyocardial fibrosis, 1433
in glycogen storage disease, 993, *993*
in heart failure, 456–457
in hydatid cyst, 1444
in hypertrophic cardiomyopathy, 1421
in idiopathic dilated cardiomyopathy, 1410
in juxtaductal coarctation, 912
in Löffler endocarditis, 1432
in mitral regurgitation, 1024
in mitral stenosis, 1012
in myocardial infarction, 1206–1207
in neoplastic pericarditis, 1514
in penetrating atherosclerotic ulcer, 1569, *1569*
in pericardial effusion, 1485–1486, *1485*
in pericarditis, 1484, 1499–1500, *1499*
in postpericardiotomy syndrome, 1520
in pregnancy, 1845, 1845t
in pulmonary embolism, 1588, *1588*
in pulmonary hypertension, 789
in pulmonic valve disease, 926, 1060, *1060*
in rheumatic fever, 1771
in rheumatoid arthritis, 1776
in single ventricle, 947
in SLE-associated pericarditis, 1518
in stable angina pectoris, 1298
in tetralogy of Fallot, 930
in thoracic aortic aneurysm, 1551, *1551*
in total anomalous pulmonary venous connection, 945, *945*
in transposition of great arteries, 937, *937,* 941
in tricuspid regurgitation, 1057
in tricuspid stenosis, 1055
in trypanosomiasis, 1443
in unstable angina, 1335
in ventricular septal defect, 902
of aorta, 1547
Chest wall, disorders of, in cor pulmonale, 1614, *1614*
in secondary pulmonary hypertension, 801
Cheyne-Stokes respiration, in heart failure, 455, 509
Children. See also *Congenital heart disease; Infant.*
atrioventricular block in, 691–692
bacterial pericarditis in, 1509
blood pressure values in, 857, 997–998, *998,* *999*
cardiomyopathy in, 990–997
anthracycline toxicity and, 997
beriberi and, 993–994
dilated, 990–991, *991*
diphtheritic, 989
glycogen storage disease and, 992–993, *993*
hypertrophic, 1424, *1424*
Kawasaki disease and, 994–997, *995,* 995t, *996,* 996t, 997t
maternal diabetes and, 992
primary, 990–992, *991*
protein-calorie malnutrition and, 994
secondary, 992–997, 992t, *993, 995,* 995t, *996, 997,* 997t
thyrotoxicosis and, 993
tropical endomyocardial fibrosis and, 994
chest pain in, 888
constrictive pericarditis in, 1498
cyanosis in, 11
dysphagia in, 11
Children *(Continued)*
endocardial fibroelastosis in, 991–992, *992*
exertional angina in, 11
glycogen storage disease in, 992–993, *993*
heart transplantation in, 528
human immunodeficiency virus myocarditis in, 989
hypercholesterolemia in, 1002t, 1003–1004, *1003*
hyperlipidemias in, 1003–1004, *1003*
hypertension in, 810, 810t, 812, 822, 822t, 857, 997–1003, *998,* 998t, *999,* 1000t–1002t
idiopathic dilated cardiomyopathy in, 990–991, *991*
infective endocarditis in, 1078. See also *Infective endocarditis.*
infective myocarditis in, 988–990
infective pericarditis in, 990
juxtaductal coarctation of aorta in, 912–913, *912*
Lyme disease myocarditis in, 989–990
murmurs in, 11
nonrheumatic inflammatory disease in, 988–990
pericardiocentesis in, 1495
pneumonia in, 11
postpericardiotomy syndrome in, 990
sudden cardiac death in, 752
syncope in, 9
triglycerides in, 1002t
trypanosomal myocarditis in, 989
viral myocarditis in, 988–989
Chills, in patient history, 10
Chimeric molecules, 1628
Chlamydia pneumoniae, in pericarditis, 1511
Chlamydia psittaci, in pericarditis, 1511
Chloride, myocardial concentration of, 554t
Chloroquine, myocardial effects of, 1446–1447
Chlorothiazide (Diuril), hematological abnormalities with, 1804t
in heart failure, 477–478, 477t
in pediatric cardiology, 1000t
Chlorthalidone, hematological abnormalities with, 1804t
in heart failure, 477–478, 477t
in pediatric cardiology, 1000t
Cholesterol. See also *Hypercholesterolemia.*
levels of, in children, 1002t
in elderly, 1696–1697
in myocardial infarction, 1204
in women, 1706
mortality and, 1133–1134
Cholesterol embolization syndrome, 1571
Cholesterol ester storage disease, 1669t
Cholesterol Lowering Atherosclerosis Study, 1145
Cholesterol pericarditis, 1522
Cholestyramine (Questran), digoxin interaction with, 483t
in dyslipidemia, 1139–1140, 1139t, 1140t
in hypercholesterolemia prevention, 1129–1130, 1131
in pediatric cardiology, 1000t
in renal failure, 1934t
Cholinergic receptors, in contraction-relaxation cycle, 374–375, *374,* 375t
Chondroectodermal dysplasia, genetic factors in, 1660t, 1661, *1662*
Chordae tendineae, abnormalities of, in mitral regurgitation, 1018
rupture of, in mitral regurgitation, 1024
in mitral valve prolapse, 1034
Chorea, in rheumatic fever, 1771
Chromosome(s), aberrations of, 881t, 1655–1657, 1656t
deletions of, 1651, 1656t
duplications of, 1651, 1656t
homologous, 1651
microscopic alterations in, 1650–1651, 1651t
mitochondrial, mutations of, 1654, *1654*
rearrangements of, 1651
unlinked, 1651
Chromosome 22, in conotruncus development, 1658
Chronic obstructive lung disease (COLD), electrocardiography in, 118–119, *118, 119*
Chronic obstructive pulmonary disease (COPD), 1604. See also *Cor pulmonale.*
beta-adrenergic agonists in, 1619
cardiac output in, 1616–1617
Chronic obstructive pulmonary disease (COPD) *(Continued)*
cor pulmonale in, *1614–1616,* 1615–1619, *1618, 1619*
digitalis in, 1619
hypoxia in, 1616
oxygen therapy in, 1617–1619, *1618*
oxygen transport in, 1616–1617, *1618*
peripheral edema in, 1616, *1617*
phlebotomy in, 1619
radionuclide angiocardiography in, 303
theophylline in, 1619, *1619*
vasodilators in, 1619–1620
venous oxygenation in, 1616–1617, *1618*
Chronotropic incompetence, in coronary artery disease, 1392
Churg-Strauss syndrome, 1432, 1783
Chylomicron, 1127t, 1145
Chylomicron remnants, 1127t, 1145
Chylomicronemia, familial, 1146
Chylopericardium, 1522
postoperative, 1735
Chylothorax, postoperative, 1735
Cigarette smoking, abdominal aortic aneurysm and, 1550
cessation of, cost-effectiveness analysis of, 1747–1748
in cardiac rehabilitation, 1397–1398, 1401
in hypertension, 844, *845*
in coronary artery disease, 1147–1148, 1299–1300, 1707
in hypertension, 821, 844, *845*
in Prinzmetal's variant angina, 1340
in stable angina pectoris, 1299–1300
sudden cardiac death and, 745
Cinchonism, 602
Cineangiography, axial, in tetralogy of Fallot, 931
ventricular, in trypanosomiasis, 1443–1444
Ciprofibrate, in dyslipidemia, 1141–1142
Circadian periodicity, in myocardial infarction, 1187, 1198
Circle of Willis, congenital aneurysm of, 965, *965*
Circulatory failure, 394. See also *Cardiogenic shock; Heart failure; Shock.*
Circumferential wall stress, of left ventricle, 426–427, *426*
Circumflex artery, left, anatomy of, *248,* 251–252, *252*
from right aortic sinus, 261–262, *262*
obtuse marginal branches of, 252
Cirrhosis, pulmonary hypertension and, 786
Climate, in heart failure, 449
Clinical decision tree, in cost-effectiveness analysis, 1741–1742, *1742*
Clinical pathway. See *Practice guidelines.*
Clofibrate, in dyslipidemia, 1140t, 1141–1142
in hypercholesterolemia prevention, 1129
in renal failure, 1934t
Clonidine (Catapres), in hypertension, 852
in pediatric cardiology, 1000t
in renal failure, 1932t
Clopidogrel, 1819
Clostridia, in myocarditis, 1439–1440
Clubbing, 17, *17*
in congenital heart disease, 885, 972
in tetralogy of Fallot, 930
C-natriuretic peptide, in heart failure, 414
Coagulation, 1811–1814. See also *Anticoagulant therapy.*
coagulation factors in, 1812, *1812,* 1813
extrinsic pathway of, 1812, *1812*
fibrinogen in, 1813
in cyanotic congenital heart disease, 972
in myocardial infarction, 1197–1198
in pulmonary embolism, 1582–1585, 1582t, 1583t
intrinsic pathway of, 1811–1812, *1812*
postoperative, 1731–1732, 1732t
preoperative, 1717t
prothrombinase in, 1812
regulation of, 1813–1814, *1814*
thrombin in, 1812–1813, *1813*
Coagulation factor(s), 1153, 1732t, 1812, *1812,* 1813
Coagulation necrosis, *1189,* 1191
Coagulative myocytolysis, 1191, *1191*
Coarctation of aorta, 965, *965,* 1847
arterial pulse in, 18, 22
E sign in, 232, *232*
echocardiography in, 84

Coarctation of aorta *(Continued)*
exercise and, 978
hypertension in, 830
in adult, 971
juxtaductal, 911–913, *912*
clinical findings in, 911–912
complications of, 913
in children, 912–913, *912*
in infants, 912
management of, 913
morphology of, 911
pathogenesis of, 911, *912*
recurrence of, 913
magnetic resonance imaging of, 327–328, *328*, 332
pregnancy and, 975, 976
radiography in, 231–232, *232*
renal function and, 1923
rib notching in, 232
Coarctation of aortic isthmus, systolic arterial murmur in, 40
Cobalt cardiomyopathy, 1413
Cocaine, in myocardial infarction, 1193
in Prinzmetal's variant angina, 1340
myocardial effects of, 11, 1445, *1445*, *1446*
Coccidioidomycosis, myocarditis in, 1441
pericarditis in, 1510–1511
Cockayne syndrome, 880t
Codeine, in pediatric cardiology, 1000t
Cogan's syndrome, 1783
Cognition, postoperative, 1734–1735, 1736t
Colchicine, in acute pericarditis, 1485
in cyanotic congenital heart disease, 972
Cold pressor testing, with cardiac catheterization, 198
Colestipol, in dyslipidemia, 1139–1140, 1139t, 1140t
in hypercholesterolemia prevention, 1130
in renal failure, 1934t
Collagen, smooth muscle cell formation of, 1109, *1109*
Collateral vessels, 1174–1176
arteriography of, 262–263, *263*, *264*
density of, 1174
development of, 263
coronary obstruction in, 1174
enhancement of, 1175–1176, *1175*
exercise in, 1174
pharmacological effects on, 1174–1175
vascular endothelial growth factor and, *1175*
during percutaneous transluminal coronary angioplasty, 1175
function of, 263, 1175
in coronary artery disease, 1298
in myocardial infarction, 1193
maturation of, 1174
nitric oxide effects on, 1175
nitroglycerin effects on, 1302
percutaneous transluminal coronary angioplasty of, 263
prostacyclin effects on, 1175
Collimation, in radionuclide imaging, 273, 275
Complement-fixation test, in trypanosomiasis, 1444
Complete blood count, preoperative, 1717t
Compression stockings, graded, in pulmonary embolism prophylaxis, 1598, 1599t
Computed tomography, **335–344**
cine mode for, 335, *336*
contrast for, 335
in abdominal aortic aneurysm, 1548, *1548*
in aortic aneurysm, 343, *343*, 1548, *1548*, 1552
in aortic dissection, 342–343, *343*, 1559–1560, *1561*, 1563, 1563t
in cardiac tumor, 341–342, *341*, 1474
in congenital heart disease, 340, 342
in constrictive pericarditis, 340, *340*, 1501
in coronary arterial calcification, 223, 338–339, *339*
in coronary artery disease, 1298
in effusive-constrictive pericarditis, 340–341, *341*
in hypertrophic cardiomyopathy, *336*
in intramural aortic hematoma, 1568, *1568*
in ischemic heart disease, 336–339, *337*
in myocardial infarction, 336–337, *337*, 337–338, 1206–1207
in neoplastic pericarditis, 1515
in pericardial cysts, 340
in pericardial disease, 235, 339–341, *340*, *341*, 1501, *1501*, 1515

Computed tomography *(Continued)*
in pericardial masses, 341
in pericarditis, 340–341, *340*, 1501, *1501*
in pulmonary embolism, 344, *344*, 1591, 1591
in stable angina pectoris, 1298
in thoracic aortic aneurysm, 1552
of aortic arch, 342
of coronary arteries, 339, *339*
of coronary artery bypass grafts, 338, *338*
of coronary thrombus, 337, 342
of intracardiac masses, 341–342, *341*
of intracardiac thrombus, 342
of left ventricular aneurysm, 336–337, *337*
of myocardial perfusion, 337
of pericardial fluid, 340
of regional wall motion, 337, *337*
of right ventricle, 210, *210*, 342
of stroke volume, 336
principles of, 335, *335*, *336*
spiral, 335
in pulmonary embolism, 1591
triggered mode for, 335
ultrafast, 335, *335*, 336, *336*, 342
volume mode for, 335
Computer, in radionuclide imaging, 273
Concealed conduction, *124*, 126, 693, *695*
Conductance, definition of, 558
familial disturbance of, 1667
Conductance catheter, for left ventricular volume measurement, 423–424, *424*
Conduction, anisotropic, 554–555
atrioventricular, radiofrequency catheter ablation of, 627
concealed, *124*, 126, 693, *695*
decremental, in arrhythmogenesis, 569
in Duchenne muscular dystrophy, 1869
in hyperthyroidism, 1893
internodal, 548–549
intraatrial, 548–549
supernormal, 693, *694*
Conduction system, anatomy of, 548–553, *549–551*
intraventricular, 548–553, *550–551*
specialized, in sudden cardiac death, 753
Congenital heart disease, **877–951,** 1657–1664, 1846–1848. See also specific defects, e.g., *Atrial septal defect.*
acid-base imbalance in, 885–886
adult, **963–984**
cyanotic, 971–974, *973*, 973t, *974*
noncardiac surgery and, 981–982
pregnancy and, 976
employability and, 980
exercise and, 978–980, *978*
historical perspectives on, 963
infective endocarditis and, 974–975
noncardiac surgery and, 981–982
noncardiovascular residua of, 983
pregnancy and, 975–978, *975*, 975t
psychosocial considerations in, 980
radiography in, 231
treatment of, 971–984
cardiac catheterization in, 980–981
multidisciplinary, 963–964
surgical, *790*, 968–971, *969*, 980–981
residua of, 982–983, 982t, *983*
sequelae of, 983–984, 983t
unoperated survival in, 964–967, *964–968*
vascular residua of, 983
ventricular residua of, 983, *983*
arterial embryology in, 882–883, *882*
atrial embryology in, 879, *879*, *882*
balloon valvuloplasty in, 918, 1386
cardiac catheterization in, 178t, 179, 791t, 895. See also *Cardiac catheterization.*
cardiac reserve in, 889, *889*
chest pain in, 888
chromosome 22 in, 1658
computed tomography in, 342
conotruncal development in, 1658
cyanotic, 885–886, 891–894, *892*, 892t
complex, 1848
renal function and, 1922–1923
deductive echocardiography in, 78–79
definition of, 877–878
echocardiography in, 78–85, *79–85*, 894–895, *894*
electrophysiological studies in, 895
embryology of, 879, *879*, 882–883, *882*
etiology of, 878–883, *879*, 880t–881t, *882*
extracellular matrix abnormalities in, 1658

Congenital heart disease *(Continued)*
fetal circulation in, 883–884, *883*
fetal echocardiography in, 894, *894*
fibroelastosis in, 991
flow defects in, 1658
genetic factors in, 878, 880t–881t
growth impairment in, 886
heart failure in, 884–885, 884t, 889–891
treatment of, 889–891, 890t, 891t
imaging in, 354t, 355–356
in trisomy 21, 1656–1657
incidence of, 878, 878t, 1657
infective endocarditis in, 887–888, 888t, 1078
looping defects in, 1658–1659
magnetic resonance imaging of, 327–328, *327*, *328*
mesenchymal tissue migration errors in, 1658
multifactorial processes in, 1657–1659
noncardiac surgery and, 1762
patient history in, 11
practice guidelines for, 1951t, 1952
prevention of, 879
pulmonary embryology in, 882
pulmonary hypertension in, 886–887
situs defects in, 1658–1659
sudden death in, 750, 888
syncope in, 888
teratogenic effects in, 1663–1664, 1663t
transitional circulation in, 883–884
ventricular embryology in, 879
Congestive heart failure. See *Heart failure.*
Connective tissue disease, 880t, 1349, 1667–1673, 1668t–1669t
Connexins, 555, *555*
Conotruncal anomaly face syndrome, 1658
Conotruncus, development of, 1658, 1660t
Conradi-Hünermann syndrome, 880t
Consanguinity, 1651
Contiguous gene syndromes, 1651
Continuous positive airway pressure, in sleep apnea syndromes, 1615
Contraceptives, oral, cardiovascular effects of, 1908
coronary artery disease and, 1707
hypertension with, 823–824
clinical features of, 823
incidence of, 823
management of, 824
mechanisms of, 824
pulmonary embolism and, 1583, 1584
Contraction band necrosis, 1191, *1191*
Contraction-relaxation cycle, **376–386,** *377*, 377t
acid-base homeostasis in, 371, *371*
adenosine signaling in, 375–376
aortic-ventricular coupling, 385
atrial function in, 384–385
beta-adrenoceptors in, 372–374, *372–374*
calcium ion fluxes in, 366–369, *367*, *368*
chemical synapse theory of, 366–369, *367*, *368*
cholinergic receptors in, 374–375, *374*, 375t
contractile proteins of, 361–366, *364–366*
contractility (inotropic state) in, 381–383, *382*, *383*
cyclic adenosine monophosphate in, 373–374, *373*, *374*
cyclic guanosine monophosphate in, 374–375, *374*
cytosolic calcium in, 383–384, *384*
1,2-diacylglycerol in, 375, *375*
diastole of, 377–378, 378t, 384, *384*, 384t, 385
endocardium in, 385–386
force-frequency relationship in, 380–381, *380*
force-velocity relationship in, 382, *382*
Frank-Starling relationship in, 366, *366*, 378–379, *378*, *379*, 433, *434*
G proteins in, 375, *375*
G-protein signal transduction in, 372–373, *372*
heart rate and, 380, *380*, 381
homeometric autoregulation of, 379
in heart failure, 376, *376*
in hibernating heart, 388, 388t
in ischemia, 386–388, *386–388*, 388t
in myocardial stunning, 388–389, 388t, *389*
inositol triphosphate in, 375, *375*
ion channels in, 369–370, *369*
ion exchangers in, 370–371, *370*, *371*
isovolumic relaxation phase of, 384, *384*, 384t
left atrium in, 384–385
left ventricle contraction of, 376–377, *377*
left ventricular filling of, 377

Contraction-relaxation cycle *(Continued)*
left ventricular pressure-volume loop of, 421, *422*
left ventricular relaxation of, 377
length-dependent activation in, 366, *366*, 378–379, *378*, *379*
molecular basis of, 363, *364*
nitric oxide in, 375
oxygen uptake and, 381, *381*
pericardium in, 385
phospholipase C signal transduction in, 375, *375*
pressure-volume loop measurements of, 383, *383*
protein kinase C in, 375, *375*
quadruple-rhythm, 34
sarcoplasmic reticulum calcium-induced calcium release in, 366–369, *367*, *368*
signal transduction in, 372–376, *372–375*, 375t, *376*
sodium pump in, 371–372
sodium-calcium exchanger in, 370–371, *370*, *371*
sodium-proton exchange in, 371, *371*
stretch receptors in, 376
systole of, 377–378, 378t
treppe effect in, 382
triple-rhythm, 34
vascular compliance in, 385
ventricular interaction in, 385
vs. crossbridge cycling, 366
wall stress in, 379–380, *379*
Contrast media, allergy to, 245
in arteriography, 245–246, 255–256
in cardiac catheterization, 180, 180t
Contrast-induced nephropathy, in renal failure, 1926
Contusion, myocardial, 1536–1538, 1536t, *1537*, 1538t
arrhythmias in, 1537, *1537*
echocardiography in, 1537, *1537*
prognosis for, 1537–1538, *1538*
radionuclide imaging in, 1537
serum enzymes in, 1537
treatment of, 1537–1538, 1538t
ventricular aneurysm in, 1538, *1538*
Conus artery, 254
Convulsions, in congenital heart disease, 885
Cor bovinum, in aortic regurgitation, 1047
Cor pulmonale, **1604–1620**
acute, 1610–1613
aortic pressure maintenance in, 1613
electrocardiography in, 118, *118*
myocardial ischemia in, 1610–1611
oxygen therapy in, 1613
pathophysiology of, 1610–1612, *1611*
right coronary artery perfusion in, 1611
right ventricular afterload reduction in, 1613
right ventricular failure in, 1611–1612, *1613*
right ventricular response in, 1610, *1611*
treatment of, 1612–1613
vasodilator therapy in, 1613
ventricular interaction in, 1611, *1612*
anatomical correlates of, 1605–1607, *1606*
assessment of, 1608–1610, *1609*, 1609t
chest radiography in, 1609–1610, *1609*
chronic, 1613–1620, 1613t
chest wall disorders and, 1614, *1614*
chronic obstructive pulmonary disease and, *1614*, 1615–1617, *1615–1617*. See also *Chronic obstructive pulmonary disease (COPD).*
diaphragmatic paralysis and, 1614
neuromuscular apparatus disorders and, 1613–1614
pulmonary vascular disorders and, 1613
restrictive lung diseases and, 1615
sleep apnea syndromes and, 1614–1615
treatment of, 1617–1620
beta-adrenergic agonists in, 1619
digitalis in, 1619
oxygen in, 1617–1619, *1618*
phlebotomy in, 1620
theophylline in, 1619, *1619*
vasodilators in, 1619–1620
upper airway obstruction and, 1615
ventilatory control disorders and, 1614–1615
clinical assessment of, 1608
echocardiography in, 1610
electrocardiography in, 118–119, *118*, *119*, 1608–1609, 1609t
Cor pulmonale *(Continued)*
etiology of, 1604–1605, *1604*, 1605t
in chronic obstructive pulmonary disease, *1614*, 1615–1617, *1615–1617*
magnetic resonance imaging in, 1610
pathogenesis of, *1615*
pathophysiology of, 1605–1607, *1606*
patient history in, 11
pressure-flow relations in, 1607–1608, *1607*
pressure-volume relations in, 1607
pulmonary circulation in, 1607–1608, *1607*, *1608*
pulmonary vascular anatomy in, 1606–1607
pulmonary vasoconstriction in, 1608, *1608*
radionuclide ventriculography in, 1610
right ventricular function in, 1605–1606, *1606*
right ventricular hypertrophy and, 1605, *1606*
thallium imaging in, 1610
Cor triatriatum, 923, *923*
cardiac catheterization in, 791t
echocardiography in, 81, *81*, 923, *923*
in secondary pulmonary hypertension, 798
vs. primary pulmonary hypertension, 791
Corneal arcus, in stable angina pectoris, 1292
Cornelia de Lange syndrome, 881t, 1659t
Coronary artery (arteries). See also *Coronary artery disease.*
aberrant, exercise and, 978, *978*
abnormalities of, in sudden cardiac death, 747, 748t
anatomy of, imaging of, 351t, 352
nonpathological variation in, 1655
on myocardial perfusion imaging, *279*, *281*
anomalous pulmonary origin of, 909–910, *909*, *910*
anterior descending, anatomy of, *248*, 250–251
angiographic projections for, *248*, 251
atresia of, congenital, 260
blood flow of. See *Blood flow, coronary.*
calcification of, computed tomography of, 223, 338–339, *339*
plain film radiography of, 223, *223*
tram track pattern of, 223, *223*
catheterization of. See *Arteriography; Cardiac catheterization.*
collateral. See *Collateral vessels.*
computed tomographic angiography of, 339, *339*
congenital abnormalities of, 160, 260
in coronary artery disease, 1349
in sudden cardiac death, 747, 748t
diameter of, 246, *247*
dissection of, 1349
arteriography of, 266–267, *267*
sudden cardiac death in, 747
echocardiography of, in ischemic heart disease, 89–90, *89*, *90*
ectasia of, in coronary artery disease, 1298
embolism to, sudden cardiac death and, 747
fistula of, arteriography of, 259–260, *260*
congenital, in adult, 967
in cyanotic congenital heart disease, 973
in hypertrophic cardiomyopathy, 1416
left, anatomy of, *248*, 250–251
angiographic projections for, 247, *248*
anomalous origin of, sudden cardiac death and, 747
branches of, superimposition of, arteriography of, *256*, 258, *258*
catheterization of, 249
computed tomographic angiography of, 339, *339*
dominance of, 249, *252*
fistula of, arteriography of, 259–260, *260*
magnetic resonance imaging of, *322*, *323*
myocardial bridging of, arteriography of, 258–259, *258*
pulmonary artery origin of, 260, *260*, 909–910, *909*, *910*
septal branches of, enlargement of, arteriography of, 258, *258*
magnetic resonance angiography of, 321, *322*, *323*
main, left, anatomy of, 250
anomalous pulmonary artery origin of, 909–910, *909*, *910*
stenosis of, arteriography in, 255, *256*
trifurcation of, 251
normal, chest pain with, *1289*, 1343–1344. See also *Syndrome X.*
Coronary artery (arteries) *(Continued)*
obstruction of, branch-point, arteriography of, *257*, 258
electrocardiography in, 133–134
left ventricular end-systolic pressure-volume relation in, 431, *432*
sudden cardiac death in, 747
total, arteriography of, 267, *267*
origin of, from aortic sinus, 260–261, *261*, *262*
from pulmonary artery, 260, *260*, 909–910, *909*, *910*
via multiple aortic sinus ostia, 262
pacing via, 706
pseudolesions of, arteriography of, 267–268, *267*
recanalization of, arteriography of, 259, *259*
right, angiographic projections for, 247, *249*, 253
anomalous origin of, sudden cardiac death and, 747
catheterization of, 252–253
dominance of, 249, *250*, *251*, 253
high anterior origin of, 262
obstruction of, arteriography of, 267, *267*
perfusion of, in pulmonary hypertension, 1611
posterior descending, *249*, 253
pseudolesions of, arteriography of, 267–268, *267*
recanalization of, arteriography of, 259, *259*
shepherd's crook of, *267*
superdominant, 251
single, 262
spasm of, arteriography of, 264–265
genetic factors in, 1655
in cardiac arrest, 747, 753
in myocardial infarction, 1193
mechanisms of, 264
stenosis of, arteriography of, 255–257, *256*, *257*
congenital, 260
eccentric, arteriography of, 256–257, *257*
magnetic resonance imaging of, 321, *322*
myocardial blood flow in, positron emission tomography of, 307
radiation-induced, 1349
traumatic injury to, 1542–1543
Coronary artery bypass graft surgery, **1316–1331**, 1958–1959, 1958t
angiography after, 253–255, *254*, *255*
antiplatelet therapy after, 1321
antithrombotic therapy in, 1826–1827
arteriography after, 253–255, *254*, *255*
care after, 1959
carotid artery disease and, 1331
cholesterol-lowering therapy after, 1321
complications of, 1318, 1319–1320
computed tomography of, 338, *338*
cost-effectiveness analysis of, 1750
deep venous thrombosis after, 1583
disease progression after, 1320–1321
emergency, indications for, 1716–1718
exercise testing after, practice guidelines for, 1942
graft patency after, 231, 1318–1319, *1318*, 1320
hypertension after, 830
in asymptomatic patients, 1958, 1958t
in diabetic patients, 1329
in elderly, 1328
in Kawasaki disease, 997
in myocardial infarction, 1223, 1959, 1976t, 1978–1979
in Prinzmetal's variant angina, 1343
in PTCA-related abrupt vessel closure, 1370
in unstable angina, 1339, *1339*, 1958t, 1959
in women, 1328, 1710
in younger patients, 1328
internal mammary artery for, 1317–1319, *1317*, *1318*
left ventricular function depression and, 1326–1328, *1326*, *1327*, 1328t
magnetic resonance imaging of, 321–323, *322*, *323*
myocardial hibernation and, *1326*, 1327–1328, *1327*, 1328t
myocardial infarction after, 1326
myocardial perfusion imaging after, 294
neurologic complications of, 1879
outcome of, 1319–1321, 1323–1329, *1324–1327*, 1325t, 1328t
patient selection for, 1321–1323, 1321t, *1322*, 1329

Coronary artery bypass graft surgery *(Continued)*
  peripheral vascular disease and, 1331
  personnel for, 1959
  practice guidelines for, 1942, 1957–1959, 1958t
  reoperation after, 1328
  survival after, 1318, *1318*
  technical considerations in, 1316–1319, *1317*, *1318*
  venous conduits for, 1317, *1317*
  vs. percutaneous transluminal coronary angioplasty, 1316, 1329–1331, *1329*, 1330t
Coronary artery disease, **1289–1349.** See also *Sudden cardiac death.*
  age and, 1152–1153
  alcohol in, 1153–1154
  aneurysms in, 1298, 1347–1348, *1347*, *1348*
  angina pectoris and, 1289–1316. See also *Angina pectoris.*
  angiography in, 1295, 1321–1323, *1322*
    practice guidelines for, 1949–1954, 1950t–1951t
  antioxidant level in, 1154–1155
  arrhythmias in, 1349
  cerebrovascular accident and, 1878–1881
  chronotropic incompetence in, 1392
  cigarette smoking and, 1299
  coagulation factor VII in, 1153
  collateral vessels in, 1298
  coronary artery bypass graft surgery in, 1316–1331. See also *Coronary artery bypass graft surgery.*
  coronary artery ectasia in, 1298
  coronary blood flow in, 1299
  diabetes mellitus in, 1150–1151
  diagnosis of, arteriography in, 240–269. See also *Arteriography.*
      normal, 1343–1344
    biochemical tests in, 1298
    cardiac catheterization in, 177–179, 178t, 1298–1299. See also *Cardiac catheterization.*
    chest roentgenography in, 1298
    computed tomography in, 1298
    echocardiography in, 1296–1297
    exercise electrocardiography in, 1295–1296, 1323
    gated positron emission tomography in, 307
    gender differences in, 1297
    high-risk positivity in, 1297, 1297t
    in asymptomatic persons, 1297–1298
    in atypical angina, 1298
    noninvasive testing in, 1295–1298, 1297t, 1323
    normal arteriography in, 1343–1344
    positron emission tomography in, 307–308, 307t
    thallium-201 imaging in, 307
  dobutamine stress echocardiography in, 1297
  dyslipidemia in, 1126–1147, 1127t
  echocardiography in, 89–90, *89*, *90*, 1296–1297
  elevated lipoprotein(a) in, 1146–1147
  esophageal disease and, 1291
  exercise electrocardiography in, 1295–1296, 1323
  exercise stress testing in, 165, *166*
    practice guidelines for, 1942
  family history in, 1152–1153
  fibrinogen in, 1153
  fibrinolytic activity in, 1153
  gender in, 1153, 1297
  genetic factors in, 1152
  heart failure in, 1346–1349
  hemostatic factors in, 1153
  high-risk, stress myocardial perfusion imaging in, 291, *291*, **Plate 6, Plate 7**
  homocysteine in, 1153
  hypercholesterolemia in, 1127–1143
    Canadian Coronary Atherosclerosis Intervention Trial in, 1132
    Cholesterol Lowering Atherosclerosis Study in, 1130
    clinical evaluation of, 1136
    Coronary Drug Project study in, 1129
    detection of, 1135
    familial, 1142–1143
    Familial Atherosclerosis Treatment Study in, 1130, *1131*
    Helsinki Heart Study in, 1128
    interventional studies of, 1127–1133, 1129t
Coronary artery disease *(Continued)*
    Life Style Heart Trial in, 1131–1132
    Lipid Research Clinics Coronary Primary Prevention Trial in, 1127–1128
    low-density lipoprotein metabolism and, 1134
    Monitored Atherosclerosis Regression Study in, 1132
    mortality and, 1133–1134
    Multicentre Anti-Atheroma Study in, 1133
    National Heart, Lung, and Blood Institute Type II Coronary Intervention Study in, 1129–1130, 1129t
    observational studies of, 1127
    Oslo Study Diet and Antismoking Trial in, 1128
    polygenic, 1143
    Pravastatin Limitation of Atherosclerosis in the Coronary Arteries study in, 1132
    prevention of, 1135–1136, *1136–1138*
    Program on the Surgical Control of the Hyperlipidemias study in, 1131
    Regression Growth Evaluation Statin Study in, 1132–1133
    St. Thomas' Atherosclerosis Regression Study in, 1131
    Scandinavian Simvastatin Survival Study in, 1133
    treatment of, 1136–1142, 1300
      angiographic studies of, 268–269
      bile-acid sequestrants in, 1139–1140, 1140t
      dietary, 1136–1138, 1137t, 1138t
      estrogen in, 1142
      fibric-acid derivatives in, 1141–1142
      gene therapy in, 1143
      HMG-CoA reductase inhibitors in, 1141
      liver transplantation in, 1143
      low-density lipoprotein apheresis in, 1143
      nicotinic acid in, 1140–1141
      pharmacologic, 1138–1142, 1139t
      probucol in, 1142
    University of California, San Francisco, Arteriosclerosis Specialized Center of Research Intervention Trial in, 1130–1131
    West of Scotland Coronary Prevention Study in, 1128
    World Health Organization Cooperative Trial in, 1128
  hypertension in, 815, 1148–1150, 1149t, 1299
  hypertriglyceridemia in, 1144–1146
    detection of, 1145
    epidemiology of, 1145
    familial, 1146
    treatment of, 1145–1146
  in aortic dissection, 1563–1564, 1563t
  in APO A-1/APO C-III deficiency, 1144
  in diabetes mellitus, 1901
  in elderly, 1696–1697
  in pregnancy, 1853–1854, *1854*
  in renal failure, 1926
  in rheumatoid arthritis, 1776–1777
  in sudden cardiac death, 744, 746–747, *746*, 752–755, 752t, *754*, *755*
  in systemic lupus erythematosus, 1779
  in women, 1704–1711. See also *Women, coronary artery disease in.*
  ischemic cardiomyopathy in, 1346–1347
  left ventricular aneurysm in, 1347–1348, *1347*, *1348*
  left ventricular function in, 1298–1299
  low high-density lipoprotein cholesterol in, 1143–1144
  mitral regurgitation in, 1019, 1348–1349
  mitral valve prolapse in, 1299
  mortality in, 1126, 1133–1134
  murmurs in, 1292
  myocardial bridging in, 1298
  myocardial hibernation in, 1299
  myocardial metabolism in, 1299
  myocardial perfusion imaging in, 288–295, *288*, 1296, 1323
  myocardial viability in, positron emission tomography for, 306, 306t
  nonatheromatous, 1349
  noncardiac surgery and, 1758–1761, 1760t
  noninvasive testing in, 1295–1298, 1297t, 1323
  normal arteriography in, 1343–1344
  obesity in, 1152, 1906
  of left main coronary artery, 1322, *1323*, 1325
Coronary artery disease *(Continued)*
  percutaneous transluminal coronary angioplasty in, 1313–1316. See also *Percutaneous transluminal coronary angioplasty (PTCA).*
    practice guidelines for, 1954–1957, 1955t–1956t
  personality type in, 1154
  pharmacological nuclear stress testing in, 1296
  physical examination in, 1292
  physical inactivity in, 1151, *1152*
  plasminogen activator inhibitor 1 in, 1153
  precordial motion in, 24t
  prevention of, practice guidelines for, 1990–1993, 1991t, *1992*, 1992t, *1993*
  Prinzmetal's variant angina and, 1340–1343. See also *Prinzmetal's variant angina.*
  prognosis for, stress myocardial perfusion imaging and, 291–294, *292*, *293*
  progression of, after coronary artery bypass surgery, 1320–1321
    arteriographic assessment of, 268–269
  radionuclide angiography in, 1296
  regional wall motion in, 1299
  rehabilitation in, **1392–1401**
    counseling in, 1400
    education in, 1400
    exercise in, 1392–1397, *1393*, *1394*, 1400–1401
      effects of, 1394, *1394*
      patient selection for, 1394–1397, 1395t, 1397t
      prescription for, 1395–1396, 1396t
      risks of, 1396–1397, 1397t
      safety of, 1397
    iatrogenic factors and, 1392
    inpatient, 1399–1400
    left ventricular dysfunction and, 1392–1393, *1393*
    morbidity and, 1394, *1394*
    myocardial ischemia and, 1393–1394
    myocardial performance and, 1394
    outcomes of, 1401
    outpatient, 1400–1401
    physical capacity in, 1392
    physical conditioning in, 1392–1394, *1393*
    physiological factors and, 1392
    psychological factors in, 1398
    reemployment after, 1399
    secondary prevention in, 1397–1398
    self-efficacy and, 1398
    sexual activity in, 1400
    skeletal muscle performance and, 1394
    smoking cessation in, 1397–1398
    vocational, 1398–1399
  resting electrocardiography in, 1295
  risk for, diastolic blood pressure and, 812–813, *812*, *813*
    stratification of, 1822–1823, 1822t
  silent myocardial ischemia in, 1344–1346, *1345*, *1346*
  stress in, 1154
  stress myocardial perfusion imaging in, 288–295, *288*
    sensitivity of, 295
  ST-segment depression in, 1296
  sudden cardiac death and, 747
  survival with, 1321–1326, *1322*, *1324*, *1325*, 1325t
  tobacco use in, 1147–1148, 1147t
  treatment of. See also *Coronary artery disease, hypercholesterolemia in, treatment of.*
    angiotensin-converting enzyme inhibitors in, 1301
    antioxidants in, 1300
    aspirin in, 1301
    beta blockers in, 1149t, 1301
    counseling in, 1301
    estrogen replacement therapy in, 1300
    exercise in, 1300–1301
    life style changes in, 1301
  type A personality in, 1154
  unstable angina in, 1331–1339. See also *Angina pectoris, unstable.*
Coronary atherectomy, 1376–1378, 1376t
  directional, 1376–1378, *1376*, 1376t, *1377*
    cost-effectiveness analysis of, 1750
  extraction, 1376t, 1378
  rotational, *1376*, 1376t, 1378, *1378*
Coronary blood flow, **1163–1176**
  adenosine and, 1163, *1163*

Coronary blood flow *(Continued)*
autoregulation of, 1168–1169, *1168*
collateral, 1174–1176
endogenous vasodilators and, 1175
enhancement of, 1175–1176, *1175*
exercise in, 1174
functional capacity of, 1175
hereditary factors in, 1174
in humans, 1175
obstruction in, 1174
pharmacological effects and, 1174–1175
coronary vascular tone and, 1164–1168, *1164–1167*
diastolic compressive forces and, 1169
digital subtraction angiography of, 199
endothelial dysfunction and, 1166–1167, *1166, 1167*
endothelium-dependent vasodilation and, 1165–1166, *1165, 1166*
endothelium-derived constricting factors and, 1167–1168
endothelium-derived relaxing factor and, 1164, *1164, 1165*
extravascular compressive forces and, 1169
flow reserve of, 200, 1173–1174, *1173*
in coronary artery disease, 1299
in stable angina pectoris, 1294, *1294*
metabolic regulation of, 1163, *1163*
myocardial oxygen consumption and, 1163
neurotransmitter regulation of, 1170–1171
reflex regulation of, 1170–1171
stenosis and, 1171–1174, *1171–1173*
systolic compressive forces and, 1169
tonic coronary vasoconstriction and, 1171
transmural distribution of, 1169–1170, *1169, 1170*
Coronary care unit (CCU), cost-effectiveness analysis of, 1749
for myocardial infarction, 1226–1228, 1227t
intermediate, for myocardial infarction, 1227–1228
mobile, for myocardial infarction, 1208
Coronary Drug Project, in hypercholesterolemia prevention, 1129
Coronary flow reserve, 200, 1173–1174, *1173*
absolute, 1174
in coronary artery disease, 1299
in stable angina pectoris, 1294, *1294*
measurement of, 1173–1174
relative, 1174
Corrigan (water-hammer) pulse, in aortic regurgitation, 22, 1049
Corticosteroids, in heart transplantation, 524–525
in Löffler endocarditis, 1433
in myocarditis, 1437
Cortisol, 1895
in Cushing's syndrome, 1896
Corynebacterium, in infective endocarditis, 1082, 1092–1093
Cost(s), average, 1742
calculation of, 1742–1743, 1742t
fixed, 1742
incremental, 1742
operating, 1742
variable, 1742
Cost-benefit analysis, vs. cost-effectiveness analysis, 1741
Cost-effectiveness analysis, 1741–1743
Bayes theorem in, 1744, *1744*, 1744t, *1745*
calculation of costs in, 1742–1743, 1742t
clinical decision tree in, 1741–1742, *1742*
clinical probabilities in, 1743
discounting in, 1742–1743
of angina testing, 1744–1745, *1744*
of cigarette smoking prevention, 1747–1748
of coronary artery revascularization, 1750–1751, 1750t
of coronary care units, 1749
of diagnostic testing, 1743–1745, *1744*, 1744t, *1745*
of endocarditis prevention, 1748
of hyperlipidemia prevention, 1745–1746, 1746t
of hypertension prevention, 1747
of obesity prevention, 1748
of percutaneous transluminal coronary angioplasty, 1749–1750
of physical activity programs, 1748
of prehospital emergency services, 1748–1749
of reperfusion therapy, 1749
sensitivity analysis in, 1741
Costochondritis, chest pain in, 5
Costosternal syndrome, vs. angina pectoris, 1291
Cough, 10
in heart failure, 450
in myocardial infarction, 1200
with angiotensin-converting enzyme inhibitors, 474, 497
Cough syncope, 864. See also *Syncope.*
Cough-version, in cardiac arrest, 763
Coumadin. See *Warfarin sodium (Coumadin).*
Coumarin, 1818
Counseling, in cardiac rehabilitation, 1400
in stable angina pectoris, 1301
Coxiella burnetii, in infective endocarditis, 1082, 1093
in pericarditis, 1506
Coxsackievirus, in myocarditis, 988, 1437
in pericarditis, 1505–1507. See also *Pericarditis, viral.*
C-reactive protein, in rheumatic fever, 1771
Creatine kinase, in heart failure, 407
in myocardial contusion, 1537
in myocardial infarction, 1202–1203, *1202*, 1202t, 1207
Creatine phosphate, in myocardial ischemia, 1178
Creatine phosphokinase, in acute pericarditis, 1484
Creatinine, preoperative, 1717t
Creatinine kinase, in Duchenne muscular dystrophy, 1866
CREST (*c*alcinosis, *R*aynaud's phenomenon, *e*sophageal dysfunction, *s*clerodactyly, *t*elangiectasia) association, in secondary pulmonary hypertension, 799
pericarditis in, 1781
Cri du chat syndrome, 881t, 1656t
Critical pathway. See *Practice guidelines.*
Cromakalim, in heart failure, 475–476
Cromolyn sodium, pericarditis with, 1519
Crossbridge cycling, binding states in, 362–363, *365*
cytosolic calcium in, 363–364, *365, 366*
in contraction-relaxation cycle, 361, *365*
vs. contraction-relaxation cycle, 366
Crosstalk, pacemaker, 715, *715*
Crouzon's syndrome, 880t
Cryptococcosis, myocarditis in, 1441
Cuff sphygmomanometry, for intracardiac pressure measurement, 422–423
Culture, blood, in infective endocarditis, 1086, 1087, 1093, 1096
Cushing's syndrome, 1896
hypertension in, 829
Cutis laxa, 880t
Cyanosis, 7–8
apnea in, 892
blood gases in, 892t, 893
cardiac examination in, 893
central, 7–8
clubbing in, 17, *17*
in congenital heart disease, 891, *892*
differential, 17
in congenital heart disease, 891, *892*
reversed, 17
differential diagnosis of, 892–894, *892*, 892t
electrocardiography in, 893
in congenital heart disease, 8, 11, 885–886, 891–894, *892*, 892t
in myocardial infarction, 1201
in primary pulmonary hypertension, 789
in tetralogy of Fallot, 930
in transposition of great arteries, 937
peripheral, 7
in congenital heart disease, 891, *892*
pH in, 893
respiratory patterns in, 892–893
tachypnea in, 892–893
Cycle, cardiac. See *Contraction-relaxation cycle.*
Cyclophosphamide, cardiac effects of, 11, 13, 1448, 1803
in Takayasu's arteritis, 1573
Cyclosporine, digoxin interaction with, 483t
toxicity of, 1881
in heart transplantation, 524
Cyst(s), hydatid, myocarditis with, 1444
pericardial, 1522, *1523*
imaging of, 236, *236*, 240
Cystathionine β-synthase deficiency, 1668t, 1673
Cystic fibrosis, 880t
Cystic medial degeneration, in annuloaortic ectasia, 1554
in aortic dissection, 1555–1556, *1555*
in thoracic aortic aneurysm, 1550
Cystic tumor, of atrioventricular node, 1471
Cystinosis, 1668t
Cytochromes, in heart failure, 407
Cytokines, in heart failure, 415, *415*
Cytomegalovirus, after heart transplantation, 524, 525
in graft atherosclerosis, 525
in myocarditis, 1437
in pericarditis, 1506
postoperative, 524, 525, 1733
Cytoplasm, 361
Cytosol, 361

D wave, in pulmonary venous flow velocity, 438, *438*
Da Costa syndrome, chest pain in, 5
Damping, in pressure measurements, 188
Damus-Kaye-Stansel procedure, in single ventricle, 949
Danaparoid sodium, 1818
Dantrolene sodium, pericarditis with, 1519
Daunorubicin, cardiac effects of, 11, 997, *997*, 1515, 1519, 1800–1803, 1801t, 1802t
De Musset's sign, 15
in aortic regurgitation, 1049
Deafness, familial, 880t
Death, biological, 742–743, *742*, 743t, 758–759
brain, in heart donor, 517–518
during cardiac catheterization, 179–180
voodoo, 751
Deceleration-dependent block, in arrhythmogenesis, 569
Deceleration-dependent intraventricular aberration, electrocardiography in, 126, *126*
Decision tree, in cost-effectiveness analysis, 1741–1742, *1742*
Decremental conduction, in arrhythmogenesis, 569
Deep venous thrombosis, postoperative, 1734
Defecation syncope, 864. See also *Syncope.*
Dehydroemetine, myocardial effects of, 1446
Dengue myocarditis, 1437
Dental procedures, prophylactic antibiotics for, in congenital heart disease, 888t
Depolarization, on electrocardiography, 100, 109, *109*, 139
Depression, after myocardial infarction, 1263
syncope with, 865, 872
therapy for, in cardiac rehabilitation, 1398
Dermatomyositis, 1779–1780
Deslanoside, in atrial flutter, 654
O-Desmethylencainide, in renal failure, 1930t
Desmodus salivary plasminogen activator, 1822
Desmopressin acetate (DDAVP), postoperative, 1732
DeVega annuloplasty, in tricuspid regurgitation, 1058
Dexamethasone (Decadron), in pediatric cardiology, 1000t
Dexamethasone suppression test, in Cushing's syndrome, 829
Dexfenfluramine, pulmonary hypertension with, 786
Dextran, in pulmonary embolism, 1594
Dextrocardia, 946
genetic factors in, 1660t
Diabetes mellitus, 1900–1905
autonomic dysfunction in, 1901–1902
cardiomyopathy in, 1902–1903, *1902*
coronary artery bypass surgery and, 1329
coronary artery disease in, 1150–1151, 1706, 1901
echocardiography in, 1903, *1903*
heart failure in, 1902–1903, *1902*
hypertension in, 823, 825, *825*
in acromegaly, 1888
maternal, neonatal cardiomyopathy and, 992
myocardial infarction in, 1217, *1217*, 1901
peripheral vascular disease in, 1904
treatment of, 1904–1905
ventricular function in, 1903–1904, *1903*
Diabetic nephropathy, hypertension in, 825, *825*
1,2-Diacylglycerol, in contraction-relaxation cycle, 375, *375*

Dialysis. See *Kidney dialysis.*
Dialyzable current of injury, in hyperkalemia, 141
Diameter, cardiac, 215, *217*
Diaphragm, in cor pulmonale, 1614
  in Duchenne muscular dystrophy, 1866
  postoperative failure of, 1723
Diastole, 377–378, 378t, 383–384, *384*
  in coronary blood flow, 1169
  in elderly, 1700
  in hypertrophic cardiomyopathy, 385, 1415, 1415t, 1418, *1419*
  measurement of, 385
  pericardial effects on, 385
Diastolic asynchrony, in heart failure, 403
Diastolic asynergy, in heart failure, 403
Diastolic compressive forces, in coronary blood flow, 1169
Diastolic current of injury, in ischemia, 127, *128*
Diastolic overload, Q wave in, 117, *146*
Diastolic pericardial knock, in constrictive pericarditis, 1499
Diastolic reserve, in young heart, 889
Diastolic ventricular interference, in contraction-relaxation cycle, 385
Diatrizoic acid, for arteriography, 245
Diazepam (Valium), for arteriography, 244
Diazoxide (Hyperstat), hematological abnormalities with, 1804t
  in heart failure, 472t
  in hypertensive crisis, 858t, 1003
  in pediatric cardiology, 1000t
  in renal failure, 1932t
Dichlorphenamide, in heart failure, 477t
Dicumarol (bishydroxycoumarin), in pediatric cardiology, 1000t
Diet, fish oil, 1121, 1145–1146
  in atherosclerosis regression, 1121
  in dyslipidemia, 1136–1138, 1137t, 1138t
  in hypertension, 844–846
  in hypertriglyceridemia, 1145–1146
  in myocardial infarction, 1226, 1227t
  preoperative, 1715, 1718t
Diffuse intimal thickening, 1113
DiGeorge syndrome, 880t, 1651t, 1658
  aortic arch interruption in, 914
  truncus arteriosus in, 907
Digital subtraction angiography, for coronary blood flow measurement, 199
Digitalis. See *Digoxin.*
Digitalis toxicity, 500–501, 661
  age and, 501
  electrocardiography in, *151*
  nonrespiratory sinus arrhythmia in, *645*
  renal, 501
Digitoxin, *151*
  hematological abnormalities with, 1804t
  in renal failure, 1930t
Digits, clubbing of, 17, *17*
    in congenital heart disease, 885, 972
    in tetralogy of Fallot, 930
Digoxin, drug interaction with, 483t
  electrocardiographic effects of, 142–143
  exercise stress testing effects of, 170
  in amyloidosis, 1429
  in aortic stenosis, 1042
  in atrial fibrillation prophylaxis, 1720
  in atrial flutter, 654
  in atrioventricular nodal reentrant tachycardia, 664
  in congenital heart disease–related heart failure, 890, 890t
  in cor pulmonale, 1619
  in coronary artery disease, 501
  in elderly, 1700
  in heart failure, 410, **480–484,** *481*, *483*, 483t, 494, 499–501, *500*, 890, 890t, 1987t
  in hypertrophic cardiomyopathy, 1423, 1425
  in myocardial infarction, 501, 1237
  in pediatric cardiology, 1000t
  in pregnancy, 1857–1858
  in pulmonary hypertension, 792
  in renal failure, 1930t
  in respiratory disease, 501
  in thyroid disease, 501
  individual sensitivity to, 500–501
  pharmacokinetics of, 482–484
  prophylactic, 1720
    preoperative, 1718–1719, *1719*
  therapeutic monitoring of, 482–484, 482t, *483*, 483t
Digoxin *(Continued)*
  toxicity of, 11, 142–143, 484, 661
    electrocardiography of, 142–143, *151*
    nonrespiratory sinus arrhythmia and, *645*
    treatment of, 598t
Digoxin immune Fab fragments (Ovine), in pediatric cardiology, 1000t
Dihydropyridines, in hypertension, 855, 855t
Dilantin. See *Phenytoin (Dilantin).*
Dilevalol, in arrhythmias, 610–613, 611t
Diltiazem, digoxin interaction with, 483t
  dosage of, 594t–595t, 617, 1311
  drug interactions of, 483t, 1311
  electrophysiological actions of, 601t, 602t–603t, 616
  hemodynamic effects of, 617
  in angina pectoris, 1309t, 1310–1312, 1312t
  in arrhythmias, 594t–595t, 601t, 602t–603t, 616–618
  in atrial fibrillation prophylaxis, 1720
  in atrial flutter, 654
  in hypertension, 855, 855t
  in hypertrophic cardiomyopathy, 1425
  in idiopathic dilated cardiomyopathy, 1411
  in myocardial infarction, 1231
  in pregnancy, 1858
  in renal failure, 1931t
  indications for, 617
  myocardial oxygen consumption effects of, 1306t
  pharmacokinetics of, 594t–595t, 617, 1309t
  preoperative, 1719–1720
  side effects of, 11, 618, 1303t, 1311
2,3-Diphosphoglycerate, in anemia, 1786–1787
  in heart failure, 397
Diphtheria, 989
  cardiomyopathy in, 989
  myocarditis in, 1440
Diprenorphine, carbon-11–labeled, for positron emission tomography, 308
Dipyridamole, in coronary artery bypass surgery, 1321
  in stress myocardial perfusion imaging, 289, 289t
Disability, cardiovascular, assessment of, 12t, 13
Discounting, in cost-effectiveness analysis, 1742
Disopyramide, adverse effects of, 605
  digoxin interaction with, 483t
  dosage of, 594t–595t, 605
  electrophysiological actions of, 601t, 602t–603t, 604–605
  hemodynamic effects of, 605
  in arrhythmias, 594t–595t, 601t, 602t–603t, 604–605
  in hypertrophic cardiomyopathy, 1425–1426
  in pregnancy, 1858
  in renal failure, 1930t
  in syncope, 874
  indications for, 605
  pharmacokinetics of, 605
  stereochemical properties of, 604
  toxicity of, 11
Distention, cardiac, 1480
Diuretics, 848t, **849–851,** 849t, *850*
  clinical effects of, 849
  complications of, 479–480
  digoxin interaction with, 483t
  dosage for, 849, 849t
  exercise stress testing effects of, 170
  hypercalcemia with, 851
  hyperglycemia with, 850
  hyperlipidemia with, 850
  hyperuricemia with, 850
  hypokalemia with, 849–850
  hypomagnesemia with, 850
  impotence with, 851
  in azotemia, 1919
  in coronary artery disease, 1149t, 1151
  in elderly, 499
  in heart failure, 476–480, *476*, 477t, *478*, 479t, 494, 498–499
  in hypertrophic cardiomyopathy, 1425
  in myocardial infarction, 1236
  in pulmonary hypertension, 792
  loop, 849t, 851
    in heart failure, 476–477, 477t
  mechanism of action of, 849
  osmotic, in heart failure, 476, 477t
  potassium-sparing, 849t, 851
    in heart failure, 477t, 478
  resistance to, 478–479, *478*
Diuretics *(Continued)*
  side effects of, 849–851, *850*
  thiazide, 849t
    in coronary artery disease, 1151
    in heart failure, 477–478, 477t
    in renal failure, 1933t
Diuril (chlorothiazide), hematological abnormalities with, 1804t
  in heart failure, 477–478, 477t
  in pediatric cardiology, 1000t
Diverticulum of Kommerall, on plain chest radiography, *207*
Dobutamine (Dobutrex), in congenital heart disease–related heart failure, 891t
  in heart failure, 472t, 485–486, 502, 891t
  in myocardial infarction, 1237
  in pediatric cardiology, 1000t
  in pulmonary embolism, 1593
  in stress myocardial perfusion imaging, 289–290, 289t
Dopamine (Intropin), in congenital heart disease–related heart failure, 891t
  in heart failure, 472t, 486, 502, 891t
  in myocardial infarction, 1237
  in pediatric cardiology, 1000t
Dopamine β-hydroxylase deficiency, 1678t
Dopexamine, in heart failure, 486
Doppler echocardiography. See also *Echocardiography; Echocardiography, Doppler.*
Doppler flow meter, for coronary blood flow measurement, 199–200, *199*
Double-outlet left ventricle, 944
Double-outlet right ventricle, 941–944, *943*
  angiography in, 943, *943*
  clinical manifestations of, 943
  definitions of, 941–943
  diagnosis of, 943, *943*
  echocardiography in, 943
  morphology of, 941
  surgical treatment of, 943–944
  Taussig-Bing form of, 943
Down syndrome (trisomy 21), 881t, 1656–1657, 1656t
Doxazosin, in hypertension, 852–853
  in renal failure, 1932t
Doxorubicin (Adriamycin), cardiotoxicity of, 11, 997, *997*, 1800–1803, *1800–1803*, 1801t, 1802t
    radionuclide angiocardiography in, 302–303, 303t
  pericarditis with, 1515, 1519
Dressler syndrome, 1256, 1511–1512, 1519–1520
  plain film radiography in, 228
  vs. recurrent myocardial infarction, 1520
Droperidol, for anesthesia, 1757
Drug(s). See specific drug or drug group.
Drug abuse, intravenous, in secondary pulmonary hypertension, 801
    infective endocarditis and, 1078–1079, 1079t
Drug-induced heart disease, 11–13, 12t
Duchenne muscular dystrophy, 1665, 1865–1869
  anatomic changes of, 1867–1868
  arrhythmias in, 1868–1869
  atrial flutter in, 1869
  atrioventricular conduction in, 1869
  clinical manifestations of, 1866–1869, *1866*, *1867*
  conduction abnormalities in, 1869
  electrocardiography in, 1867, *1867*
  electrophysiological findings in, 1868, *1869*
  genetics of, 1632t, 1865, *1865*
  intranodal conduction defects in, 1869
  myocardial perfusion imaging in, 1868
  pathogenesis of, 1865–1866
  physical examination in, 1866–1867, *1867*, *1868*
  positron emission tomography in, 1868, *1869*
  small vessel coronary arteriopathy in, 1868, *1869*
  specialized cardiac tissues in, 1868
  subcellular abnormalities in, 1867, *1868*
Ductus arteriosus, at birth, 883–884
  echocardiography of, *904*, 906
  of premature infant, 905
  patent, 905–906, *906*
    transcatheter closure of, 906, *906*
Ductus diverticulum, on plain chest radiography, 205
Ductus venosus, patent, 884
Duroziez's sign, 460
  in aortic regurgitation, 22, 1049

Dyrenium. See *Triamterene (Dyrenium).*
Dysautonomia, in Chagas disease, 1881
Dysbetalipoproteinemia, 1146
Dyslipidemia, 1126–1147. See also *Hypercholesterolemia.*
clinical evaluation of, 1136
detection of, 1135
in angina pectoris, 1300
in diabetes, 1150–1151
primary prevention of, 1135, *1136, 1137*
secondary prevention of, 1135–1136, *1138*
treatment of, 1136–1142
cholestyramine in, 1139–1140, 1139t, 1140t
clofibrate in, 1140t, 1141–1142
colestipol in, 1139–1140, 1139t, 1140t
dietary, 1136–1138, 1137t, 1138t
estrogen-replacement therapy in, 1142
fibric-acid derivatives in, 1141–1142
fluvastatin in, 1140t, 1141
gemfibrozil in, 1140t, 1141–1142
lovastatin in, 1140t, 1141
nicotinic acid in, 1140–1141, 1140t
pharmacologic, 1138–1142, 1139t, 1140t
pravastatin in, 1140t, 1141
probucol in, 1140t, 1142
simvastatin in, 1140t, 1141
Dysphagia, in infant, 11
Dysplasia, chondroectodermal, genetic factors in, 1660t, 1661, *1662*
Dyspnea, 2–3, 3t
as anginal equivalent, 3, 4
cardiac, 450–451, 450t
vs. pulmonary dyspnea, 451
echocardiography in, 1943
edema with, 9–10
exertional, 2, 450
in coronary artery disease, 1290
expiratory, 2
functional origin of, 2
in anxiety neurosis, 451
in asthma, 2
in heart failure, 2–3, 450–451, 450t
in hypertrophic cardiomyopathy, 1419
in malignant pericardial disease, 1796–1797
in mitral stenosis, 1008, 1010
in neoplastic pericarditis, 1514
in panic attacks, 2
in patient history, 2–3, 3t
in pericarditis, 1482, 1514
inspiratory, 2
malingering and, 451
mechanisms of, 450–451, 450t
mediastinal emphysema and, 3
nocturnal, paroxysmal, 3
in heart failure, 450
pneumothorax and, 3
pulmonary embolism and, 3
pulmonary function testing in, 451
sudden development of, 2, 3
Dysrhythmias. See also *Arrhythmia(s).*
familial, 1667
in Marfan syndrome, 1672
Dystrophin, in Becker muscular dystrophy, 1870
in Duchenne muscular dystrophy, 1865–1866, 1868
in idiopathic dilated cardiomyopathy, 1409

E sign, in coarctation of aorta, 232, *232*
Earlobe crease, 15
in stable angina pectoris, 1292
Ebstein's anomaly, 934–935, *934*, 1658, 1848
accessory pathways in, 673
angiocardiography in, 935
cardiac catheterization in, 935
clinical manifestations of, 934–935
echocardiography in, 79, *80*, 935, *935*
genetic factors in, 1660t
in adult, 966–967, 969–970
laboratory findings in, 935
management of, 935
noncardiac surgery and, 981, 982
plain chest radiography of, 233–234, *234*
pregnancy and, 976
tricuspid regurgitation in, 1056
Echinococcosis, in myocarditis, 1444
in pericarditis, 1511
Echocardiographic score, in balloon mitral valvuloplasty, 1016, *1016*
Echocardiography, **53–97**
advantages of, 59
after heart transplantation, 520
contrast, 58–59, *59*, 90, *90*
deductive, 78–79
Doppler, 56–57, *56*, *57*, 1384, **Plate 1**
for intracardiac pressure measurement, 423
in aortic dissection, 96, *97*
in aortic regurgitation, 75–76, *76*, **Plate 2**
in aortic stenosis, 74, *75*
in atrial septal defect, **Plate 4**
in cardiac performance evaluation, 67, *67*
in congenital heart disease, 894–895, *894*
in constrictive pericarditis, 1500, *1500*, 1503–1504, *1504*
in cor pulmonale, 1610
in hemodynamic evaluation, 68–71, *68–70*
in infective endocarditis, 1088
in mitral regurgitation, 72–73, *72*, 1025, **Plate 2**
in mitral stenosis, 71, *72*, 1012
in myocardial infarction, 1206
in patent ductus arteriosus, 84, *84*, **Plate 4**
in pregnancy, 1845–1846, 1845t
in pressure gradient measurement, 68–70, *69*
in tricuspid regurgitation, 1058
intracardiac pressure, 68–70, *69*
intracoronary, 1384
of coronary blood flow, 68–71, *68–70*
of normal heart, 63–64, *64*, *65*
of prosthetic valves, 78, **Plate 3**
spectral, 57
vs. electrocardiography, *64*
fetal, 894, *894*
ground-glass appearance on, 1421
in abdominal aortic aneurysm, 1548
in acquired valvular heart disease, 71–78, *71–78*
in amyloidosis, 92–93, *92, 1428*, 1429
in anomalous pulmonary venous connection, 83, 945
in aortic aneurysm, 96, 1548, 1552
in aortic atheromatous emboli, 1570–1571, *1570*
in aortic atherosclerosis, 97
in aortic dilatation, 96, *96*
in aortic dissection, 96, *96*, 1561–1563, *1562*, **Plate 4, Plate 10, Plate 11**
in aortic regurgitation, 75–76, *76*, 1050–1051, **Plate 2**
in aortic sinus aneurysm, 96–97
in aortic stenosis, 74–75, *74*, *75*, 79, 84, 916–919, *917*, 1041–1042
in atrial septal aneurysm, 58–59, *59*
in atrial septal defect, 81–83, *82–83*, 897, *897*, **Plate 4**
in atrioventricular septal defect, 899, *899*, 900, *900*
in carcinoid heart disease, 1434
in cardiac metastasis, 95
in cardiac performance evaluation, 67, *67*
in cardiac shunt, 81–84, *81*, *82*, **Plate 3**
in cardiac tamponade, 93–94, *93*, 1490–1492, *1491*, 1491t, 1521
in cardiac tumor, 94, *94*, *95*, *1472*, 1473–1474
in cardiomyopathy, 79–80, 91–93, *91*, *92*, 990–991, *991*, 1410–1411, 1421–1422, *1427*, *1428*
in cerebral embolism, 1943
in coarctation of aorta, 84
in congenital absence of pericardium, 94, 1523, *1523*
in congenital aortic stenosis, 916–917, *917*
in congenital heart disease, 78–85, *79–85*, 894–895, *894*
in congenital pulmonic stenosis, 79, *79*, 926, *926*
in congenitally corrected transposition of great arteries, 941
in constrictive pericarditis, 94, 1500–1501, *1500*
in cor pulmonale, 1610
in cor triatriatum, 81, *81*, 923, *923*
in coronary artery disease, 89–90, *89*, *90*, 1296–1297
in coronary thrombus, 88, *88*, 94, *95*
in coxsackievirus myocarditis, 1437
in deep venous thrombosis, 1588, *1588*
in diabetes mellitus, 1903, *1903*
in double-outlet right ventricle, 943
in Dressler syndrome, 1520
in dyspnea, 1943
Echocardiography *(Continued)*
in Ebstein's anomaly, 79, *80*, 935, *935*
in endocardial fibroelastosis, 991
in endomyocardial fibrosis, 1433
in Fabry disease, 1430
in fetus, 59
in flail mitral leaflet, 74, *74*
in Friedreich's ataxia, *1875*
in hemodynamic evaluation, 68–71, *68–70*
in hereditary amyloidosis, 92–93, *92*
in hypertrophic cardiomyopathy, 91–92, *91*, *92*, 1421–1422
in idiopathic dilated cardiomyopathy, 990–991, *991*, 1410–1411
in infective endocarditis, 77–78, *77*, 1086–1089
in ischemic heart disease, 85–90, *86–90*
in Kawasaki disease, 995, *996*
in left atrial thrombi, 94, *95*
in left atrial tumors, 94, *94*, *95*
in Löffler endocarditis, 1432–1433
in Marfan syndrome, 96, *96*
in mitral annulus calcification, 78
in mitral regurgitation, 57, 72–74, *72–74*, 1024–1025, **Plate 1, Plate 2**
in mitral stenosis, 71–72, *71*, *72*, 79, 1012, *1012*
in mitral valve prolapse, 73–74, *73*, *74*, 1033, *1034*
in myocardial contusion, 1537, *1537*
in myocardial infarction, *86*, 87–90, *87–89*, 1206, *1206*, 1241, 1725, *1725*, 1973t, 1977t
in myocardial infarction–associated pseudoaneurysm, 87, *87*
in myocardial ischemia, 85–86, *86*, *87*
in myocarditis, 1436, 1437
in neoplastic pericarditis, 1515
in nonrheumatic mitral regurgitation, 73–74, *73*, *74*
in papillary muscle dysfunction, 74
in patent ductus arteriosus, 84, *84*, *904*, 906, **Plate 4**
in pediatric idiopathic dilated cardiomyopathy, 990–991, *991*
in pericardial cyst, 1522, *1523*
in pericardial effusion, 93–94, *93*, 1486
in pericarditis, 94, 94, 1484, *1484*, 1500–1501, *1500*, 1503–1504, *1504*, 1513, 1515
in postpericardiotomy syndrome, 1520
in pregnancy, 1845–1846, 1845t
in pressure gradient measurement, 68–70, *69*
in pulmonary artery clots, 95
in pulmonary embolism, 1589–1591, 1590t
in pulmonary hypertension, 789–790
in pulmonic stenosis, 79, *79*, 926, *926*
in pulmonic valve absence, 932, *932*
in pulmonic valve disease, 926, *926*, 1060
in restrictive cardiomyopathy, 92–93, *92*, 1427, *1428*
in rheumatic fever, 1771–1772
in rheumatoid arthritis, 1776
in rheumatoid arthritis–related pericarditis, 1518
in right atrial masses, 94
in sarcoidosis, 1431
in septal aneurysm, 58–59, *59*, 83, *83*, 87–88
in single ventricle, 947–948, *948*
in sinus of Valsalva aneurysm, 96–97, *97*
in SLE-associated pericarditis, 1518
in stable angina pectoris, 1296–1297
in subvalvular aortic stenosis, 918–919
in subvalvular obstruction, 79–81, *80*, *81*
in supravalvular aortic stenosis, 84, 921, *921*
in surgically corrected congenital heart disease, 85, *85*
in syncope, 1943
in systemic lupus erythematosus, 1518, 1778, *1779*
in tetralogy of Fallot, 84, *84*, 930, *930*, 932, *932*
in thoracic aortic aneurysm, 1552
in total anomalous pulmonary venous connection, 83, 945
in transposition of great arteries, 84–85, *85*, 937, *938*, *939*
in tricuspid atresia, 79, *80*, 933, *933*
in tricuspid regurgitation, 76, *77*, 1057–1058
in tricuspid stenosis, 76, 1055, *1056*
in trypanosomiasis, 1443
in uremic pericarditis, 1513
in valvular tumors, 95

Echocardiography *(Continued)*
in ventricular septal defect, 81, *82*, *83*, 901–902, **Plate 3**
in ventricular tumors, 94–95
in women, 1705, 1705t, 1845–1846, 1845t
intravascular, 58, *58*, *1377*, *1378*, *1381*, 1383–1384, *1383*
in pulmonary embolism, 1591
limitations of, 59
M-mode, 54, *54*, *55*
aorta on, *64*
cardiac dimensions on, 63, 64t
in cardiac performance evaluation, 64–65, *64*, 64t
in congenital heart disease, 894, *894*
in mitral stenosis, 71, *71*
of normal heart, 63, *63*, *64*, 64t
of valve motion, 70, *70*
of bicuspid aortic valve, 79, *79*
of cardiac performance, 64–71, 64t, *66–70*, 86–87
of coronary arteries, 89–90, *89*, *90*
of ductus arteriosus, *904*, 906
of hibernating myocardium, 89
of inferior vena cava, 70–71, *70*
of murmurs, 1943
of myocardial hibernation, 89
of myocardial perfusion, 90, *90*
of myocardial stunning, 89
of myocardial viability, 1328
of normal heart, 59–64, *59–61*, 61t, *62–64*, 64t, *65*
of prosthetic valves, 78, *78*, **Plate 3**
of pulmonic valve, 70, *70*
of stunned myocardium, 89
postoperative, 1725
practice guidelines for, 1942–1943, 1944t–1945t
preoperative, for noncardiac surgery, 1759
principles of, 53–59
stress, in cardiac performance evaluation, 67–68
transesophageal, 57–59, *57–59*, 78, *78*, **Plate 1**
in aortic atheromatous emboli, 1570, *1570*
in aortic atherosclerosis, 97
in aortic dissection, 96, 1561–1563, *1562*, 1563t, **Plate 4, Plate 10, Plate 11**
in atrial septal aneurysm, 58–59, *59*
in cardiac tumor, *1472*, 1474
in infective endocarditis, 1088
in mitral regurgitation, 1025
in postoperative cardiac tamponade, 1521
in thoracic aortic aneurysm, 1552
of coronary arteries, 90
of prosthetic valves, 78, *78*
transthoracic, in aortic dissection, 1561
in infective endocarditis, 1088
of coronary arteries, 90, *90*
two-dimensional, 54, *55*, *56*
apical, 61, *61*
four-chamber view in, 60, *60*, 61, *61*
in aortic stenosis, 74, *74*
in cardiac performance evaluation, 65–67, *66*
in flail mitral leaflet, 74, *74*
in hereditary amyloidosis, 92–93, *92*
in hypertrophic obstructive cardiomyopathy, 91–92, *91*, *92*
in ischemic heart disease, 85–86, *86*, *87*
in Marfan syndrome, 96, *96*
in mitral stenosis, 71, *72*
in tricuspid regurgitation, 76, *77*
long-axis, 60, *60*, *61*
of inferior vena cava, 70–71, *70*
of normal heart, 59–63, *59–61*, 61t, *62*, *63*
short-axis view in, 60, *60*, 61
subcostal, 61–62, *62*
suprasternal, 62–63, *63*
transducer locations for, 59–63, *60*, *61*, 61t, *62*, *63*
two-chamber, 61, *61*
venous, in deep venous thrombosis, 1588, *1588*
Echovirus, in pericarditis, 1505–1507. See also *Pericarditis, viral.*
Eclampsia, 832, 1852–1853, 1852t, 1853t
pulmonary edema in, 466
Ectopic beats, *644*
Edecrin. See *Ethacrynic acid (Edecrin).*
Edema, 9–10
ascites with, 10

Edema *(Continued)*
bat wing, plain film radiography of, 21, 219, *219*
drug-induced, 12t
dyspnea with, 9–10
extremity, 17
in heart failure, 453–455
in patient history, 9–10
localization of, 9
peripheral, in chronic obstructive pulmonary disease, 1616, *1617*
in myocardial infarction, 1201
pulmonary. See *Pulmonary edema.*
Edrophonium chloride (Tensilon), in atrioventricular nodal reentrant tachycardia, 664
in pediatric cardiology, 1000t
EDTA (ethylenediaminetetraacetic acid), in pediatric cardiology, 1000t
Education, in cardiac rehabilitation, 1400
Edwards syndrome (trisomy 18), 881t, 1656t, 1657
Efficiency of work, in myocardial oxygen uptake, 381
Effusive-constrictive pericarditis, 1493, 1505
Ehlers-Danlos syndrome, 880t, 1672–1673, *1672*
coronary artery disease in, 1349
cystic medial degeneration in, 1550
genes for, 1632t
varicose veins in, 1677
Eikenella corrodens, in infective endocarditis, 1092, 1093t
Eisenmenger complex, 800
Eisenmenger syndrome, 799–801, 1848
clinical features of, 800
pathology of, 799–800, *800*
pathophysiology of, 799
vs. primary pulmonary hypertension, 791
Ejection fraction. See *Left ventricular ejection fraction.*
Ejection fraction–end-systolic stress relationship, in myocardial contractility, 430–431, *430*
Ejection phase indices, of myocardial contractility, 430–431, *430*
Ejection sounds, 30–31, *30*, *31*
Elastin gene, in Williams syndrome, 920
Elderly patient. See *Aging heart.*
Electric pulsatile blood pumps, 537t, 540–541, *540*
Electric total artificial heart, 544–545, *545*
Electrical alternans, *138*, 140–141
in cardiac tamponade, 1490, *1490*
in heart failure, 455
Electrical potential, body surface mapping of, 114–115
on electrocardiography, 108–109, *109*. See also *Electrocardiography.*
Electrocardiogram, 12-lead, 111–114
P wave on, 111–112, 111t, *112*
P-R interval on, 112
Q wave on, 111t, 135–136, *136*, *150*
QRS axis on, 112–113, *113*
QRS complex on, 112–114, *112*, *113*, 140–141, *140*
Q-T interval on, 114, *136*, 136–139, *140*
R wave on, 111t
S wave on, 111t
ST segment on, 113, 136, *137*, *138*, 139, 139t
T wave on, 111t, 113–114, 136–139, *137*, *138*, 139t
U wave on, 114, 139, *150*
normal, 108–115
Ta segment on, 111–112, *112*
Electrocardiography, **108–143**, 1940–1941
activation sequence in, 110, *110*
after myocardial infarction, 1261–1263
after out-of-hospital cardiac arrest, 760
ambulatory, in myocardial infarction, 1977t
in silent myocardial ischemia, 1345, *1345*
in syncope, 869–870
practice guidelines for, 1946–1948, 1947t
boundary potential on, 109–110, *109*
depolarization on, 109, 139
digitalis-induced changes on, 142–143
during pacing, 712–714, *713*
exercise, 156–157, *157–160*
in angina pectoris, 1295–1296, 1323
in coronary artery disease, 1295–1296, 1323
frequency domain analysis in, 584
in accelerated idioventricular rhythm, 683–684, *684*

Electrocardiography *(Continued)*
in acceleration-dependent aberration, 125–126, *125*
in African trypanosomiasis, 1444
in alcoholic cardiomyopathy, 1412–1413
in amyloidosis, 1429
in anemia, 1786
in anomalous pulmonary origin of coronary artery, 909, *910*
in antimony-associated myocardial changes, 1447
in aortic dissection, 1558
in aortic regurgitation, 1050, *1051*
in aortic stenosis, 915, 916, *916*, 1041
in arrhythmias, 578–579, *578*, 583–584, *584*, 643, 1728, *1728*, 1946–1948, 1947t
in Ashman phenomenon, 125
in atrial fibrillation, 116, *146*, *151*, 654–655, *654*
in atrial flutter, 652, *653*, *654*
in atrial septal defect, 897, *897*
in atrial tachycardia, *650*, 656–657, *657*
in atrioventricular block, 124, *124*, 127, 579, *580*, 691, *691*
in atrioventricular dissociation, 693
in atrioventricular septal defect, 899
in automatic atrial tachycardia, *650*, 657
in bilateral bundle branch block, 123, *124*
in bundle branch block alternans, 123
in carcinoid heart disease, 1434
in cardiac metastases, 135, *136*, 1797–1798
in cardiac tamponade, 1490, *1490*
in cardiomyopathy, 1410, 1412–1413, 1421
in cerebral hemorrhage, 1878, *1878*
in chronic obstructive lung disease, 118–119, *118*
in concealed conduction, *125*, 126
in congenital aortic stenosis, 915, 916, *916*
in congenital heart disease, 893
in congenital pulmonic stenosis, 925–926
in congenitally corrected transposition of great arteries, 941
in constrictive pericarditis, 1500, *1500*
in cor pulmonale, 118–119, *118*, 1608–1609, 1609t
in coronary artery disease, 1295–1296, 1323
in coronary artery obstruction, 133–134
in coxsackievirus myocarditis, 1437
in cryptococcosis, 1441
in cyanosis, 893
in deceleration-dependent aberration, 126, *126*
in digitalis-induced arrhythmias, 142–143, *151*
in divisional (fascicular) blocks, 121–123, *123*
in Dressler syndrome, 1520
in Duchenne muscular dystrophy, 1867, *1867*
in Emery-Dreifuss muscular dystrophy, 1872, *1872*
in emetine-associated myocardial changes, 1446
in endomyocardial fibrosis, 1433
in exercise stress testing, 156–160, *157–160*
in Fabry disease, 1430
in fascicular block, 121–123, *121*, *122*, *147*
in Friedreich's ataxia, *1875*
in glycogen storage disease, 993, *993*
in hepatitis myocarditis, 1437
in hydatid cyst, 1444
in hypercalcemia, 142, *142*
in hyperkalemia, 141–142, *141*, *150*, *151*
in hypermagnesemia, 142
in hyperparathyroidism, 1900
in hypersensitive carotid sinus syndrome, 647, *648*
in hypertrophic cardiomyopathy, 1421
in hypocalcemia, 142, *142*
in hypokalemia, *141*, 142
in hypoplastic left heart syndrome, 921, *922*
in hypothyroidism, 1894
in idiopathic dilated cardiomyopathy, 1410
in intraventricular aberration, 124–126, *124–126*
in intraventricular conduction defect, 123, *147*
in ischemia, 128, *128*, *129*, *147*, *148*, 1295, 1947t, 1948
in juxtaductal coarctation, 912
in Kearns-Sayre syndrome, 1876, *1876*
in kidney disease, *138*
in left atrial enlargement, 115–116, *115*
in left bundle branch block, 119–121, *120*, 132–133, *133*, 136, *148*

Electrocardiography *(Continued)*
in left ventricular hypertrophy, 116–117, *116*, 136
in Löffler endocarditis, 1432
in long Q-T syndromes, *684*, 685
in masquerading bundle branch block, 123, *123*
in mitral regurgitation, *184*, 1024
in mitral stenosis, *150*, 1011–1012
in mitral valve prolapse, 1033
in myocardial contusion, 1536–1537
in myocardial depression, *125*, 126
in myocardial infarction, 116, 127–135, *128–135*, 129t, 713–714, 1189, 1202, 1205–1210, *1206*, *1209*, 1240–1241, 1725, 1971, 1972t
in myocarditis, 1435–1436, 1437, 1439, 1440, 1445
in myotonic dystrophy, 1873, *1873*, *1874*
in neoplastic pericarditis, 1514
in nonparoxysmal atrioventricular junctional tachycardia, *650*, 659–660, *660*
in pericardial effusion, 1486
in pericarditis, 1483–1484, *1483*, 1483t, 1500, *1500*, 1511–1512, 1514, 1518
in periinfarction block, 133, *133*
in pheochromocytoma, 1898
in poliomyelitis myocarditis, 1439
in polymyositis, 1780
in posterior left ventricular infarction, 134–135, *135*
in postextrasystolic aberration, 126
in postinfarction pericarditis, 1511–1512
in postoperative arrhythmias, 1728, *1728*
in postoperative myocardial infarction, 1725
in postoperative ventricular tachycardia, 1730, *1730*
in pregnancy, 1845, 1845t
in preinfarction block, 133, *133*
in premature atrial complexes, 650–652, *651*
in premature excitation, 125
in premature ventricular complexes, 675–676, *676*
in Prinzmetal's variant angina, 1340–1341, *1341*
in pulmonary embolism, 118, *118*, 1587, 1587t
in pulmonary hypertension, 789
in pulmonic stenosis, 925–926
in pulmonic valve disease, 1059
in rheumatoid arthritis, 1776
in rheumatoid arthritis–related pericarditis, 1518
in right atrial enlargement, 115, *115*
in right bundle branch block, 121, *121*, *122*, 123, *146*, *147*
in right ventricular hypertrophy, 117–118, *117*
in right ventricular infarction, 134, *134*
in salmonella myocarditis, 1440
in sarcoidosis, 1431
in scleroderma, 1781
in scorpion sting, 1448
in septal infarction, 134
in sickle cell disease, 1788
in single ventricle, 947
in sinus bradycardia, 645–646, *645*
in sinus tachycardia, 645, *645*
in SLE-associated pericarditis, 1518
in stable angina pectoris, 1295–1296, 1321, 1323
in streptococcus myocarditis, 1440
in supravalvular aortic stenosis, 921
in syncope, 869–870
in tetralogy of Fallot, 930
in thalassemia, 1789, *1789*
in torsades de pointes, 684–685, *684*
in total anomalous pulmonary venous connection, 945
in transposition of great arteries, 937
in trichinosis myocarditis, 1445
in tricuspid atresia, 933
in tricuspid regurgitation, 1057
in tricuspid stenosis, 1055
in truncus arteriosus, 907–908, *908*
in trypanosomiasis, 1443, 1444
in unstable angina, 131, 1334–1335, *1334*
in ventricular fibrillation, 686, *686*
in ventricular flutter, 686, *686*
in ventricular hypertrophy, 116–119, *116–119*, 136, 139, *150*
Electrocardiography *(Continued)*
in ventricular tachycardia, 677–678, *678*, 678t, 1730, *1730*
in Wolff-Parkinson-White syndrome, 126–127, *126*, *127*, 136, *146*, *147*, *150*, 667–669, *668*
in women, 1705
intraoperative, 1758
intrinsic deflection in, 109
intrinsicoid deflection in, 117
leads for, 110–114, *111*, 111t, *112*, *113*
myocardial perfusion imaging with, 285, **Plate 5, Plate 6, Plate 7**
Osborne wave on, *140*, 141
postoperative, 1725, 1728, *1728*
practice guidelines for, 1940–1941, 1946–1948, 1947t
preoperative, for noncardiac surgery, 1759
Q wave on, 135–136, *136*, *150*
QRS complex on, 140–141, *140*
Q-T interval on, 139–140, *140*
redepolarization on, 109
repolarization on, 139
resting, as screening test, 1744–1745, *1744*
in angina pectoris, 1321
in coronary artery disease, 1295
in myocardial ischemia, 1295
in stable angina pectoris, 1295
signal-averaged, in arrhythmia diagnosis, 583–584, *584*
in syncope, 869
ST-segment on, 136, *137*, *138*, 139, 139t
T wave on, 136–139, *137*, *138*, 139t
technical errors in, 141
theory of, 108–111, *109*
time domain analysis in, 584
U wave on, 139, *150*
vs. Doppler echocardiography, *64*
Electrocautery, pacemaker effects of, 728
Electrodes, electrocardiographic, 110–111, *111*
Electrolytes, cardiac glycoside effects on, 500
in heart failure, 456
in renal failure, 1936
postoperative, 1721
Electromagnetic flow meter, for coronary blood flow measurement, 199
Electrophysiological studies. See also *Electrocardiography; Electrophysiology.*
in arrhythmias, 579–583, *580–583*, 643, *644*
in atrioventricular nodal reentrant tachycardia, 661–663, *662*, *663*
in congenital heart disease, 895
in Duchenne muscular dystrophy, 1868, *1869*
in hypertrophic cardiomyopathy, 1421
in intraventricular conduction defect, 580, 1960t, 1962
in secundum-type atrial septal defect, 898
in supraventricular tachycardia, 581–582, *582*, 1960t, 1962
in syncope, 582, 870, 1960t, 1963
in tachyarrhythmias, 581–582, *582*, *583*
in ventricular tachycardia, 581–582, *582*, *583*, 678–679, *679*, *680*, 1960t, 1962t, 1963
in Wolff-Parkinson-White syndrome, *668*, 669–673, *669–674*, 1963
of palpitations, 582–583, 1963
practice guidelines for, 1959–1963, 1960t–1962t
Electrophysiology, of adenosine, 601t, 602t–603t, 618
of beta-adrenoceptor blockers, 611–612
of bretylium tosylate, 601t, 602t–603t, 615
of cell membrane (sarcolemma), 553–555, *554*, 554t
of diltiazem, 601t, 602t–603t, 616
of disopyramide, 601t, 602t–603t, 604–605
of flecainide acetate, 608–609
of mexiletine, 601t, 602t–603t, 607
of moricizine hydrochloride, 601t, 602t–603t, 610
of myocardial ischemia, 561, 755–756, 1178
of phenytoin, 601t, 602t–603t, 608
of procainamide, 601t, 602t–603t, 603
of propafenone, 601t, 602t–603t, 609
of propranolol, 611–612
of quinidine, 601, 601t, 602t–603t
of sotalol, 615–616
of sudden cardiac death, 750–751, *751*
of torsades de pointes, 685
Elfin facies, of Williams' syndrome, 920, *920*
ELISA-determined plasma D-dimer, in pulmonary embolism, 1587, *1587*
Ellis–van Creveld syndrome, 880t, 1660t, 1661, *1662*
Embolectomy, in pulmonary embolism, 1597–1598, *1597*
Embolism, atherothrombotic, aortogenic, 1570–1571, *1570*
cerebral, cardiogenic, 1879–1880
in aortic stenosis, 1040
in infective endocarditis, 1095
in mitral valve prolapse, 1034
paradoxical, 1880, *1880*
in adult congenital heart disease, 973–974
practice guidelines for, 1943
cholesterol, 1571
in atrial fibrillation, 655–656
in mitral stenosis, 1010
in myocardial infarction, 1193
paradoxical, in congenital heart disease, 885
pulmonary. See *Pulmonary embolism.*
renal, 1921–1923, 1922t
systemic, in infective endocarditis, 1085, 1095
tumor, 1465–1466, *1465*
with ventricular assist device, 542
Embolization, tumor, 1468–1469
Embryology, 879, *879*, 882–883, *882*
Emery-Dreifuss muscular dystrophy, 1665–1666, 1872, *1872*
Emetine, myocardial effects of, 1446
Eminase, in unstable angina, 1824
Emotional state, in myocardial infarction, 1201
Emphysema, chest pain in, 5
in secondary pulmonary hypertension, 798–799
plain chest radiography in, *213*
Employment, in cardiac rehabilitation, 1398–1399
Enalapril maleate (Vasotec), first-dose effects of, 497
in heart failure, 472t, 495–497, *496*
in hypertensive crisis, 858t
in pediatric cardiology, 1000t
in renal failure, 1933t
Encainide, after myocardial infarction, 1265
in heart failure, 505
in renal failure, 1930t
Encephalopathy, hypertensive, 832–833, *833*, 1003
Endless-loop tachycardia, with dual-chamber pacemaker, 717–720, *719*, *720*
Endocardial cushion defects. See *Atrioventricular septal defect.*
Endocardial fibroelastosis, 991–992, *992*
contracted form of, 991–992
genetic factors in, 1660t, 1666, 1666t
in hypoplastic left heart syndrome, 921
Endocarditis, bacterial pericarditis in, 1508–1509
in systemic lupus erythematosus, 1778–1779, *1779*
infective, **1077–1099.** See also *Infective endocarditis.*
rheumatic, 1770–1771, 1774
sudden cardiac death in, 750
thrombotic, nonbacterial, 1082–1083
tumor-related, 1798
Endocardium, in contraction-relaxation cycle, 385–386
Endocrine tumors, 1471
Endometrial cancer, estrogen replacement therapy and, 1708
Endomyocardial biopsy, 186–187, *187*, 1404–1406, *1405*, 1405t, 1406t, 1407t
after heart transplantation, 520–522, *521*, 521t, 522t
complications of, 187
Dallas criteria for, 1406
in amyloidosis, 1429
in constrictive pericarditis, 1504
in endocardial fibroelastosis, 991
in endomyocardial fibrosis, 1434
in Fabry disease, 1430
in glycogen storage disease, 1431, *1431*
in myocarditis, *1405*, 1436
in rheumatoid arthritis, 1778
in sarcoidosis, 1431
indications for, 187, 1406t, 1407t
Endomyocardial fibrosis, 1433–1434
biventricular, 1433
endomyocardial biopsy in, 1434
tropical, 994
Endoscopic sclerotherapy, hemopericardium with, 1521

Endothelial cells, in atherosclerosis, 1106–1108, *1106–1108*, 1114–1116, *1115*, 1118–1121, *1119*, *1120*
  in heart failure, 397, *397*
  in hypercholesterolemia, *1164*
  in hypertension, 820, *821*
  in myocardial ischemia, 1166–1167, *1166*, *1167*
  in pulmonary hypertension, 784, *784*
  lipoprotein modification by, 1108
  obligate monolayer growth of, 1108
  platelet-derived growth factor formation by, 1108
  receptors of, 1108
  transcytosis of, 1107
  transendothelial channels of, 1107
Endothelin(s), in coronary blood flow, 1167–1168
  in heart failure, 415, 1917t
  in pulmonary hypertension, 784
  in systemic hypertension, 820, *821*
Endothelin-1 (ET-1), *1165*
  in coronary blood flow, 1167–1168
  in heart failure, 415
  in myocyte hypertrophy, 1640t, 1642, 1642t
Endothelin-2 (ET-2), 1167
Endothelin-3 (ET-3), 1167
Endothelin converting enzymes, *1165*
Endothelium. See also *Endothelial cells.*
  in hemostasis, 1809–1810, *1809*, *1810*
  in hypoxia-induced vasoconstriction, 781, *782*
Endothelium-derived contracting factors, in systemic hypertension, *821*
Endothelium-derived hyperpolarizing factor, *1165*
Endothelium-derived relaxing factor. See also *Nitric oxide (endothelium-derived relaxing factor).*
  formation of, 1108
  in coronary blood flow regulation, 1164, *1164*, *1165*
  in hypoxia-induced vasoconstriction, 781, *782*
  in pulmonary hypertension, 781
  in systemic hypertension, *821*
  in vasodilation, *782*, *783*
Endotracheal tube, postoperative, 1723
Endovascular stents, in abdominal aortic aneurysm, 1549
  in aortic dissection, 1567
  in thoracic aortic aneurysm, 1553–1554
End-systolic diameter, in mitral regurgitation, 1020, *1020*
End-systolic elastance, 421, *422*
End-systolic pressure-volume relation, left ventricular, 421, *422*
    errors in, 432
    in myocardial contractility, 431–432, *431–433*
  right ventricular, 438–439
Endurance training, in elderly, 1694
Energy production, in heart failure, 407
Energy window, for thallium-201 imaging, 275
Enflurane, for anesthesia, 1757
Enterobacter, in infective endocarditis, 1093
Enterococci, in infective endocarditis, 1080, 1081, 1090–1091, 1090t, 1091t
Enterococcus faecalis, in infective endocarditis, 1080, 1081
Enterococcus faecium, in infective endocarditis, 1081
Eosinophils, in Löffler endocarditis, 1432
Ephedrine sulfate, in pediatric cardiology, 1000t
Epicardial pacing, 706
Epinephrine (Adrenalin), in congenital heart disease–related heart failure, 891t
  in pediatric cardiology, 1000t
  in systemic hypertension, 819
  myocardial oxygen consumption and, 1162
Epsilon wave, *681*
Epsilon-aminocaproic acid (aprotinin), in coronary artery bypass surgery, 1319
Equilibrium radionuclide angiocardiography, 297–300, *297–299*
  ambulatory, 300, *300*
Erb, limb-girdle dystrophy of, 1870–1871
Ergometry, arm, in exercise stress testing, 155
Ergonovine, with cardiac catheterization, 199
Ergonovine test, in Prinzmetal's variant angina, 1342
Erythema marginatum, in rheumatic fever, 1771
Erythrocyte sedimentation rate, in infective endocarditis, 1087–1088
Erythrocyte sedimentation rate *(Continued)*
  in myocardial infarction, 1205
  in rheumatic fever, 1771
Erythrocytosis, 1792–1794, *1793*
  compensated, 972
  decompensated, 972
  in congenital heart disease, 885, 972
  stress, 1794
Erythromycin, digoxin interaction with, 483t
  in rheumatic fever, 1773, 1773t
Escherichia coli, in infective endocarditis, 1082, 1093
Esmolol (Brevibloc), in aortic dissection, 1565
  in arrhythmias, 610–613, 611t
  in hypertensive crisis, 858t
  in myocardial infarction, 1228–1229, *1228*
  in renal failure, 1931t
  indications for, 612, 613
  perioperative, 854
  pharmacodynamic properties of, 487t
Esophageal motility, disorders of, 1291
Esophageal pain, 4t, 1291, 1291t
  vs. chest pain, 7
Esophageal reflux, 4t, 7
Esophageal spasm, 4t, 7
Esophageal varices, endoscopic sclerotherapy for, hemopericardium with, 1521
Esophageal ventricular pacing, 705
Esophagus, disorders of, 4t, 7, 1291, 1291t
  on plain chest radiography, 211, *213*
  rupture of, pericarditis with, 1522
Estrogen, coronary artery disease and, 1908
Estrogen replacement therapy, 1707–1709, 1908
  after myocardial infarction, 1266
  breast cancer and, 1708–1709
  endometrial cancer and, 1708–1709
  guidelines for, 1709
  hypertension with, 824
  in coronary artery disease, 1300
  in dyslipidemia, 1142
  in syndrome X, 1344
  lipid levels and, 1697, 1706, 1708t
Ethacrynic acid (Edecrin), hematological abnormalities with, 1804t
  in congenital heart disease–related heart failure, 890t
  in heart failure, 477t, 890t
  in pediatric cardiology, 1000t
  in renal failure, 1933t
Ethanol, teratogenicity of, 1663t, 1664
Ethmozine. See *Moricizine hydrochloride (Ethmozine).*
Ethylenediaminetetraacetic acid (EDTA), in pediatric cardiology, 1000t
Excimer laser, 1382–1383
Excitation, supernormal, 693, *694*
Excitation-contraction coupling, in crossbridge cycling, 362–363, *365*
  in heart failure, 404–406, *405*
Exercise. See also *Physical activity; Physical inactivity.*
  arteriovenous oxygen difference in, 439
  atrial septal defect and, 979
  blood pressure response to, 809
  coarctation of aorta and, 978
  congenital aortic stenosis and, 978
  coronary artery disease and, 1707
  coronary artery response to, 1166
  cost-effectiveness analysis of, 1748
  during pregnancy, 1844
  dynamic (isotonic), in exercise stress testing, 155–156, *156*
    left ventricular wall thickness with, 400
    with cardiac catheterization, 198
  Fallot's tetralogy and, *780*, 979
  Fontan procedure and, 979–780
  for stress myocardial perfusion imaging, 288–289
  in aberrant coronary artery, 978, *978*
  in adult congenital heart disease, 978–980, *978*, *980*
  in aging animal, 1690, *1692*
  in cardiac rehabilitation, 1392–1397, *1393*, *1394*, 1395t, 1396t, 1397t
  in collateral vessel development, 1174
  in congenital heart block, 978
  in coronary artery disease, 1151, *1152*, 1300–1301
  in elderly, 1692–1694, *1693*, *1694*
  in hypertension, 846
Exercise *(Continued)*
  in hypertrophic cardiomyopathy, 1424–1425, 1424t, 1426
  in myocardial infarction, 1198
  in pulmonary hypertension, 791
  in radionuclide angiocardiography, 302
  in restrictive cardiomyopathy, 1427
  in systemic hypertension, 821
  left ventricular wall thickness with, 400
  pacing rate during, 722
  patent ductus arteriosus and, 979
  physiology of, 153–155, *154*
  pulmonary stenosis and, 978–979
  static (isometric), auscultatory effects of, 48–49
    in exercise stress testing, 155
    left ventricular wall thickness with, 400
    with cardiac catheterization, 198
  submaximal, in exercise stress testing, 164
  transplant heart response to, 527–528, *527*
  transposition of great arteries and, 979–780
  ventricular septal defect and, 979
  with cardiac catheterization, 198
Exercise factor, 198
Exercise index, 198
Exercise prescription, in cardiac rehabilitation, 1395–1396, 1396t
Exercise stress testing, **153–174,** 439–441, *440*, 440t
  after cardiac pacemaker insertion, 172
  after cardiac transplantation, 171–172, *172*
  after coronary revascularization, 170–171
  after out-of-hospital cardiac arrest, 760
  anaerobic threshold in, 154, *154*
  arm ergometry for, 155
  Bayesian theory for, 162–163, *162*
  bicycle ergometry for, 155
  blood pressure during, 163–164
  carbon dioxide output on, 439–440, *440*
  chest discomfort during, 164
  complications of, 173–174
  contraindications to, 173–174, 173t
  coronary angiography correlation with, 162
  diagnostic use of, 161–163, 161t, *162*, 162t
  drug effects on, 170
  electrocardiography in, 156–160
    computer-assisted analysis of, 158–159
    lead systems in, 156–157, *157*
    R wave on, 163
    ST segment on, 157–160, *157–160*, 163
    ST segment/heart rate slope on, 163
    T wave on, 157–158
  evaluation of, 161–163, 161t, *162*, 162t
  heart rate during, 163, 164
  heart rate–systolic blood pressure product during, 164
  in angina pectoris, 1295–1296
  in arrhythmias, 167, *168*, 577–578
  in asymptomatic population, 164–165
  in atrial fibrillation, 168, *168*
  in atrioventricular block, 168
  in cardiac rehabilitation, 1395, 1395t, 1399
  in coronary artery disease, 1295–1296
  in elderly patients, 172, 1696
  in heart failure, 170, *171*, 451–452, *548*
  in hypertension, 170, 174
  in left bundle branch block, 168, *169*
  in myocardial infarction, 165–167, *167*, 1261
  in preexcitation syndrome, 169, *169*
  in pregnancy, 1846
  in Prinzmetal's variant angina, 1341
  in right bundle branch block, 168–169
  in sick sinus syndrome, 168
  in silent myocardial ischemia, 165
  in supraventricular arrhythmias, 167–168
  in symptomatic population, 165, *166*
  in syndrome X, 1344
  in unstable angina, 165, 1336, 1983t
  in valvular heart disease, 172
  in ventricular arrhythmias, 167, *168*
  in ventricular septal defect, 904–905
  in women, 165, 169, *170*, 1705, 1705t
  indications for, 160, 161t
  limitations of, 441
  maximal work capacity in, 164
  metabolic equivalent in, 154–155
  multivariate analysis of, 163
  oxygen uptake on, 439–441, *440*
  postdischarge, 1400
  practice guidelines for, 1941–1942, 1941t
  preoperative, for noncardiac surgery, 1759
  protocols for, 155–156, *156*

Exercise stress testing *(Continued)*
ramp protocol for, 156
report of, 173, 173t
risks of, 173–174, 173t
safety of, 173–174, 173t
six-minute walk test for, 156
submaximal, 164
technique of, 160–161
termination of, 172–173, 172t
treadmill protocol for, 155–156, *156*
Exercise training, contraindications to, 1395
cost-effectiveness analysis of, 1748
in cardiac rehabilitation, 1394, *1394*, 1400–1401
in elderly patient, 1694
monitoring for, 1397, 1397t
patient selection for, 1394–1397, 1395t
risks of, 1396–1397, 1397t
safety of, 1397
Exertional syncope, 866–867. See also *Syncope.*
Exit block, with pacemaker, 711
Exophthalmos, 15
Exploring electrode, 110
Extracorporeal shock wave lithotripsy, hypertension with, 824
Extracorporeal ultrafiltration, in heart failure, 480
Extremities, arterial pressure measurement in, 20
edema of, 17
examination of, 16–17
in myocardial infarction, 1201
Eyes, examination of, 15–16, *16*

Fabry disease, 1675, 1678t
restrictive cardiomyopathy of, 1430, *1430*
Face, physical examination of, 15
Facies, elfin, 920, *920*
mitral, 1010
Facioscapulohumeral dystrophy of Landouzy-Dejerine, 1871, *1872*
Factor V, gene for, mutation of, 1582t, 1583, 1633–1634, *1634*
Factor VIIa, 1814
Factor VIII, in coronary artery disease, 1153
Factor XIa, 1812, *1812*
Factor XII, 1812, *1812*
Fallot's tetralogy. See *Tetralogy of Fallot.*
False tendons, 552, *552*
Familial arteriopathy, 1677
Familial collagenoma syndrome, 1660t
Fascia adherens, of intercalated discs, 554
Fascicular block, 707
anterior, electrocardiography in, 121–122, *121*, *122*, *147*
in myocardial infarction, 1251–1252
in myocardial infarction, 1251–1252
noncardiac surgery and, 1763
pacemaker in, practice guidelines for, 1964t
posterior, electrocardiography in, 122–123, *122*
in myocardial infarction, 1252
right bundle branch block and, electrocardiography of, *121*, *122*, 123, *147*
ventricular hypertrophy in, 119
Fascicular tachycardia, 683, *683*
Fasciculoventricular fibers, in Wolff-Parkinson-White syndrome, *668*, 669
Fatigue, in acceleration-dependent aberrancy, 126
in heart failure, 449, 452
in patient history, 10
Fatty acid(s), metabolism of, disorders of, 1668t, 1673–1674
myocardial oxygen consumption and, 1162–1163
SPECT imaging of, 303
Fatty acid binding proteins, in myocardial infarction, 1202t
Fatty streak, 1111–1113, 1118, *1119*
cell composition of, *1112*, 1113
Felodipine, in angina pectoris, 1309t, 1311
in heart failure, 472t
in Prinzmetal's variant angina, 1343
in renal failure, 1931t
pharmacokinetics of, 1309t
Femoral sheath, for arteriography, 242–243, *243*
Femoral vein, for right heart catheterization, 182–183, *183*, *184*
Fenfluramine, pulmonary hypertension with, 786
Fenofibrate, in dyslipidemia treatment, 1141–1142
Fenoldopam, in heart failure, 486
Fentanyl, for anesthesia, 1757
Fetal alcohol syndrome, 878, 1664
Fetal circulation, 883–884, *883*
Fetal hydantoin syndrome, 1664
Fetal rubella syndrome, 878, 881t, 1663t, 1664
myocarditis in, 1439
pulmonary artery stenosis in, 924
Fetus, cardiac circulation of, 883–884, *883*
echocardiography in, 59
heart disease of. See *Congenital heart disease.*
heart of, 883
maternal congenital heart disease and, 977–978
pulmonary circulation in, 883
radionuclide exposure of, 1846
Fever, in heart failure, 455
in infective endocarditis, 1084, 1084t
in patient history, 10
postoperative, 1732
rheumatic, 1769–1783. See also *Rheumatic fever.*
Fibric-acid derivatives, in dyslipidemia, 1140t, 1141–1142
Fibrillin-1, in Marfan syndrome, 1672
Fibrin, formation of, 1813
Fibrinogen, in coagulation, 1813
in coronary artery disease, 1153, 1707
in myocardial infarction, 1197
Fibrinolysis, 1814–1816
in coronary artery disease, 1153
inhibitors of, 1814–1815
pathophysiology of, 1816
plasminogen activators in, 1814, *1815*
plasminogen in, 1814–1815, *1814*, *1815*
plasminogen inhibitors in, 1814–1815
regulation of, *1814*, 1815–1816
urokinase receptor in, 1815
Fibrinopeptide A, in myocardial infarction, 1197
Fibroblast growth factor, in myocyte hypertrophy, 1640t
Fibroelastosis, endocardial, 991–992, *992*
contracted form of, 991–992
genetic factors in, 1660t, 1666, 1666t
in hypoplastic left heart syndrome, 921
surgical, 984
Fibroma, 1470–1471
genetic factors in, 1676
Fibronectin, in infective endocarditis, 1083
Fibrosarcoma, 1471
Fibrosis, endomyocardial, 1433–1434
biventricular, 1433
endomyocardial biopsy in, 1434
tropical, 994
Fibrous dysplasia (Albright syndrome), heart failure in, 462
Fibrous histiocytoma, malignant, 1471
Fick technique, of cardiac output measurement, 192, *192*, 195
Figure-of-8 model of reentry, *571*, 572
Fingers, clubbing of, 17, *17*
in congenital heart disease, 885, 972
in tetralogy of Fallot, 930
First-pass radionuclide angiocardiography, 300–301
Fish oil, in atherosclerosis regression, 1121
in hypertriglyceridemia, 1145–1146
Fish-eye disease, low high-density lipoprotein in, 1144
Fistula, arteriocameral, post-traumatic, 1542
arteriovenous, coronary, 908–909
post-traumatic, 1542–1543
pulmonary, 967, *968*
coronary artery, congenital, 967
FK-506 (tacrolimus), in heart transplantation rejection, 523
Flail mitral leaflet, 74, *74*
Flamm formula, 197
Flecainide acetate (Tambocor), adverse effects of, 609
after myocardial infarction, 1265
atrial flutter effect of, 654, *654*
digoxin interaction with, 483t
dosage of, 609
electrophysiological actions of, 608–609
hemodynamic effects of, 609
in arrhythmias, 608–609
in elderly, 1698
Flecainide acetate (Tambocor) *(Continued)*
in heart failure, 505
in pediatric cardiology, 1000t
in pregnancy, 1858
in renal failure, 1930t
indications for, 609
pharmacokinetics of, 609
Flow meter, Doppler, for coronary blood flow measurement, 199–200, *199*
electromagnetic, for coronary blood flow measurement, 199
Fludrocortisone, in orthostatic hypotension, 874
Fluid, postoperative, 1721
Fluid retention. See also *Edema; Pulmonary edema.*
in heart failure, 446, 449
Fluorinated hydrocarbons, myocardial effects of, 1447
Fluoro-2-deoxyglucose, fluorine-18–labeled, 304–306, 304t
Fluorodopamine, fluorine-18–labeled, 308
6-Fluorometaraminol, fluorine-18–labeled, 308
Fluoromisonidazole, fluorine-18–labeled, 304
Fluoroscopy, 213–215, *217*
in pulmonary hypertension, 789
of aorta, 1547
5-Fluorouracil, cardiac effects of, 13, 1448, 1803
Fluvastatin, in dyslipidemia, 1140t, 1141
Foam cells, 1109, *1112*, 1113, 1118, *1119*
Fontan procedure, 971
exercise and, 979–780
in single ventricle, 949
in tricuspid atresia, 933–934, *934*
pregnancy and, 976
Food and Drug Administration, ventricular assist device regulation by, 537
Force-frequency relationship, in contraction-relaxation cycle, 380–381, *380*
negative, 398
positive, 398
Force-velocity relationship, beta-adrenergic effects on, 383, *383*
in contraction-relaxation cycle, 382, *382*
Forney syndrome, 1660t
Fosinopril sodium, in renal failure, 1933t
Fradafibran, 1820
Fragile X syndrome, 1656t
Frank-Starling relationship, in contraction-relaxation cycle, 366, *366*, 378–379, *378*, *379*, 433, *434*
in heart failure, 394–396, *395*
in pulmonary edema, 463t, 464
Free radicals, in myocardial infarction, 1214
Friedreich's ataxia, 880t, 1874, *1874*, *1875*
Frontal view, for plain chest radiography, 204–211, *205–211*
Fucosidosis, 1668t
Fundus (fundi), examination of, 15–16, *16*
in myocardial infarction, 1201
in systemic hypertension, 814
Fungus (fungi), in infective endocarditis, 1082, 1092–1093, 1094
in pericarditis, 1510–1511
postoperative infection with, 524, 1733–1734
Furifosmin, technetium-99m–labeled, 274, 275t
Furosemide (Lasix), in congenital heart disease–related heart failure, 890, 890t
in heart failure, 477t, 890, 890t
in myocardial infarction, 1236
in pediatric cardiology, 1000t
in renal failure, 1933t
postoperative, 1734

G proteins, in contraction-relaxation cycle, 372–373, *372*, 375, *375*
in heart failure, 411–412
in preconditioning, 387–388, *388*
Gaisböck syndrome, 1794
α-Galactosidase A deficiency, 1669t
Gallamine, for anesthesia, 1757
Gallavardin dissociation, in aortic valve stenosis, 36–37, *37*
Gallop sounds, in heart failure, 455
in idiopathic dilated cardiomyopathy, 1410
Gallstones, in cyanotic congenital heart disease, 972–973, *973*
Gamma camera, 273

Gamma-globulin, in Kawasaki disease, 997, 997t
  in myocarditis, 989
Gap junctions, connexins of, 555, *555*
  of intercalated discs, 554, 555, *555*
  of sinus node cells, 548
Gastritis, postoperative, 1735t
Gastroepiploic artery, catheterization of, 255, *255*
  in coronary artery bypass surgery, 254, *255*, 1318–1319
Gastroesophageal reflux, pain in, 1291, 1291t
Gastrointestinal tract, bleeding of, in aortic stenosis, 1040
  disorders of, in heart failure, 452
  postoperative complications of, 1734, 1735t
  surgery on, prophylactic antibiotics for, 888t
Gaucher disease, restrictive cardiomyopathy of, 1430
Geleophysic dysplasia, 1669t
Gemfibrozil, in dyslipidemia, 1140t, 1141–1142
  in renal failure, 1934t
Gender differences. See also *Women.*
  in coronary artery disease, 1153
  in exercise stress testing, 165, 169, *170*
Gene(s), *1652–1653*. See also *Phenotype.*
  cloning of, 1630–1631, *1630*
  for adult polycystic kidney disease, 1676–1677
  for alkaptonuria, 1668t, 1673
  for aminoacidopathies, 1668t, 1673
  for amyloidosis, 1676
  for aortic dissection, 1677
  for arrhythmogenic right ventricular dysplasia, 1632t
  for arterial aneurysm, 1677
  for arterial occlusive diseases, 1677
  for arterial tortuosity, 1677
  for arteriohepatic dysplasia, 1677
  for atherosclerosis, 1677
  for atretic veins, 1677
  for atrial natriuretic factor, 1640
  for atrial septal defect, 1660–1661
  for atrioventricular canal defects, 1661
  for Becker muscular dystrophy, 1632t
  for beta-oxidation defects, 1668t, 1674
  for cardiac tumors, 1676
  for carnitine deficiency, 1668t, 1674
  for cavernous angiomas, 1677
  for conduction disorders, 1667
  for congenital heart disease, 1660–1663, 1660t
  for connective tissue disorders, 1667–1673, 1668t–1669t
  for dilated cardiomyopathy, 1665–1666
  for Duchenne muscular dystrophy, 1632t, 1865
  for Ehlers-Danlos syndrome, 1632t, 1672–1673
  for Ellis–van Creveld syndrome, 1661
  for essential hypertension, 1677–1679, 1678t
  for Factor V, 1633–1634, *1634*
  for familial hypertrophic cardiomyopathy, 1632t, 1644, *1644*, 1664–1665, 1665t
  for fatty acid metabolic disorders, 1668t, 1673–1674
  for fibrillin-1, 1672
  for glycogen storage diseases, 1668t, 1674
  for hemiplegic migraine, 1677
  for hemochromatosis, 1674–1675
  for hemoglobinopathies, 1675
  for hereditary hemorrhagic telangiectasia, 1676
  for Holt-Oram syndrome, 1655, 1661
  for homocystinuria, 1668t, 1673
  for hypertrophic cardiomyopathy, 1632t, 1664–1665, 1665t
  for insulin-like growth factor, 1887
  for intracranial hemorrhage, 1677
  for long Q-T syndrome, 1631–1633, 1632t, *1633*
  for lymphatic disorders, 1677
  for Marfan syndrome, 1632t, 1667–1672, *1670*, 1670t, *1671*
  for mitochondrial myopathy, 1668t, 1674
  for mitral valve prolapse, 1662–1663
  for mucopolysaccharidoses, 1668t–1669t, 1675
  for myocyte hypertrophy, 1639–1640, 1640t, 1643, *1643*, 1645t
  for myotonic dystrophy, 1632t
  for Noonan syndrome, 1663
  for obesity-diabetes syndrome, 1634
  for Osler-Rendu-Weber disease, 1632t, 1676
  for osteogenesis imperfecta, 1655
  for patent ductus arteriosus, 1660
  for pseudoxanthoma elasticum, 1673
  for pulmonary hypertension, 1677
Gene(s) *(Continued)*
  for Rendu-Weber-Osler syndrome, 1632t, 1676
  for restrictive cardiomyopathy, 1666, 1666t
  for sphingolipidosis, 1675–1676
  for supravalvular aortic stenosis, 1632t, 1661–1662
  for tissue plasminogen activator, 1627–1628, *1627, 1628*
  for tropoelastin, 1662
  for varicose veins, 1677
  for ventricular septal defect, 1661
  for von Hippel–Lindau syndrome, 1676
  for William's syndrome, 1632t
  functional cloning of, 1630–1631, *1630*
  linkage of, 1631
  localization of, 1630–1634
    in familial thrombosis, 1633–1634, *1634*
    in long Q-T syndromes, 1631–1633, 1632t, *1633*
    positional assignment in, 1631
    principles of, 1630–1631, *1630*
  mutations of, 1651–1654, *1652–1654*
    incomplete penetrance of, 1654–1655
    nonpenetrant, 1654
  positional cloning of, 1630–1631, *1630*
  ras, in cardiac hypertrophy, 1643, *1643*
  reporter, 1635
  teratogenic effects on, 1663–1664, 1663t
Gene therapy, 1637–1639
  in angiogenesis, 1638
  in familial hypercholesterolemia, 1143
  in vascular smooth muscle inhibition, 1638
  prospects for, 1638–1639
  technical aspects of, 1637–1638
  vectors for, 1638
Genetic compound, 1651
Genetic markers, 1631. See also *Gene(s).*
Genitourinary tract procedures, prophylactic antibiotics for, 888t
Genome, human, 1631, *1652–1653*
Gestational hypertension, 830–832, 831t, 1852–1853, 1852t, 1853t
  clinical features of, 831, 831t
  prognosis for, 832
  treatment of, 831–832
Giant cell arteritis, 1573–1574, 1782, *1782*
  clinical manifestations of, 1574
  etiology of, 1573–1574
  management of, 1574
  pathophysiology of, 1574
Giant cell myocarditis, 1449
Gianturco-Roubin stent, 1379–1380, *1379, 1380*
Glenn operation, bidirectional, 971
  in hypoplastic left heart syndrome, 922
Glomerular filtration rate, in heart failure, 476
Glomerulonephritis, proliferative, 1921
  systemic hypertension in, 824
Glossopharyngeal neuralgia, 865
Glucagon, in pediatric cardiology, 1000t
α 1,4-Glucan 6-glycosyl transferase deficiency, 1668t, 1674
Glucocerebrosidase deficiency, 1669t
Glucocorticoid(s), in giant cell arteritis, 1574
  in Takayasu's arteritis, 1573
Glucocorticoid-remediable aldosteronism, 1897
Glucocorticosteroids, in myocardial infarction, 1197
Glucose, postoperative, 1721
Glucose 50%, in pediatric cardiology, 1000t
Glucose 50% + insulin, in pediatric cardiology, 1000t
Glucose tolerance, in myocardial infarction, 1197
Glucose utilization, fluorine-18–labeled fluoro-2-deoxyglucose imaging of, 304t, 305–306, **Plate 7**
Glucose-insulin-potassium infusion, in myocardial infarction, 1232, *1232*
α-1,4-Glucosidase deficiency, 1668t, 1674
amylo-1,6-Glucosidase deficiency, 1668t, 1674
Glutethimide, hematological abnormalities with, 1804t
Glycerol, in heart failure, 477t
Glycogen storage disease, 1668t, 1674
  cardiomyopathy in, 992–993, *993*, 1431, *1431*
Glycoprotein IIb/IIIa. See *Platelet-specific integrin $\alpha_{IIb}\beta_3$ (GPIIb/IIIa).*
Glycoproteinoses, 1668t, 1674
Glycosides, cardiac. See also *Digoxin.*
  electrophysiologic effects of, 482
Glycosides *(Continued)*
  in heart failure, 480–484, *481*, *483*, 483t, 499–501
  mechanisms of action of, 480–481
  pharmacokinetics of, 482–484
  positive inotropic effect of, 481–482, *481*
  sympathetic nervous system effects of, 482
  therapeutic endpoints for, 500
  therapeutic monitoring of, 482–484, 482t, *483*, 483t
  toxicity of, 482
Goldenhar syndrome, 1659t
Goldman constant-field equation, 556
Gorlin formula, for valve area, 194–195
  in mitral stenosis, 1008
Gorlin syndrome, 1470
Gowers' sign, in Duchenne muscular dystrophy, 1866
GPIIb/IIIa. See *Platelet-specific integrin $\alpha_{IIb}\beta_3$ (GPIIb/IIIa).*
Graded compression stockings, in pulmonary embolism prophylaxis, 1598, 1599t
Graham Steell murmur, *31*, 41
  in pulmonic valve disease, 1059
Granulocytopenia, drug-induced, 1805
Gravity, in pulmonary circulation, 463, *463*
Group A streptococcus, in rheumatic fever, 1769–1770, 1769t, 1772–1773, 1773t
  treatment of, 1772–1773, 1773t
Growth, cardiac, pericardium and, 1481
  congenital heart disease and, 886
Growth factors, in atherosclerosis, *1108–1110*, 1116–1117
  in heart failure, 399, *400*
  in hypertension, 818–819, *818*
  macrophage, 1110, *1110*
  platelet, 1110–1111, *1111*
Growth hormone, 1887
  in acromegaly, 1889
Guanabenz, in hypertension, 852
  in renal failure, 1932t
Guanadrel, in coronary artery disease, 1140t
Guanethidine, in coronary artery disease, 1149t
  in hypertension, 852
  in renal failure, 1932t
Guanfacine, in hypertension, 852
  in renal failure, 1932t
Guanosine monophosphate, cyclic (cGMP), *1165*
  in contraction-relaxation cycle, 374–375, *374*
Guidewires, for arteriography, 243
  for cardiac catheterization, 182
Guillain-Barré syndrome, 1876–1877
Gull-wing configuration, in tetralogy of Fallot, 931, *931*
Gunshot injury, 1539–1541, *1540*

HACEK organisms, in infective endocarditis, 1081–1082, *1082*, 1092, 1093t
Haemophilus aphrophilus, in infective endocarditis, 1081, 1092, 1093t
Haemophilus parainfluenzae, in infective endocarditis, 1081, 1092, 1093t
Haloperidol, in myocardial infarction, 1226
Halothane, for anesthesia, 1757
Hampton's hump, in pulmonary embolism, 1588, *1588*
Head, physical examination of, 15
Heart. See also at *Cardiac; Myocardial.*
Heart block, **687–693**
  advanced, 687
  atrioventricular, 688–691. See also *Atrioventricular block.*
  genetic factors in, 1667
  in pregnancy, 1855
  in Reiter's syndrome, 1781
  in systemic lupus erythematosus, 1779
  in ventricular septal defect, 904
  noncardiac surgery and, 1763
  postoperative, 1719
  presystolic murmurs in, 44
  sinoatrial, 647, *647*
  ventricular. See *Fascicular block; Left bundle branch block (LBBB); Right bundle branch block (RBBB).*
Heart failure, **394–415,** *395*, 395t, 446–447, 446t, 1920
  adaptive mechanisms in, 394–397, *395–397*

Heart failure *(Continued)*
  adenylate cyclase in, 411–412
  adrenergic activity in, 412, 453
  adrenergic blockade effects on, 412, *412*
  afterload in, 399–400, 402, 495
  alanine aminotransferase in, 456
  anemia and, 1786
  angiotensin II in, 1642
  angiotensin receptors in, 414
  arginine vasopressin in, *408*, 414
  arrhythmias in, 449, 449t, 504–507, 504t
    prevention of, 505–506
  ascites in, 455
  aspartate aminotransferase in, 456
  asymptomatic, treatment of, 493, 493t
  atrial fibrillation in, 506–507, 1986
  atrial natriuretic factor in, *408*
  atrial stretch receptors in, 410
  autonomic nervous system in, 408–410, *408*, *409*
  backward, 445–446
  baroreflex in, 410
  beta-adrenergic receptor–G protein–adenylate cyclase pathway in, 410–413, *411*, 411t
  beta-adrenergic receptors in, 410–411, *411*, 411t
  cachexia in, 455
  calcium channel in, 406
  calcium in, 404–406, *405*
  calcium release channel in, 405–406
  calsequestrin in, 406
  cardiac findings in, 455–456
  cardiac growth factors in, 1641–1643, 1642t
  cardiac infection in, 449
  cardiac inflammation in, 449
  cardiac muscle gene activation in, 1639–1640, 1640t, 1645t
    in vitro assay for, 1640, 1640t
    in vivo assay for, 1640–1641, *1641*
    intracellular signaling pathways and, 1643–1644, *1643*
    suppressor pathways and, 1644
  cardiac output in, 446
  cardiomegaly in, 455
  cardiotrophin-1 in, 1642–1643
  cerebral symptoms in, 452
  chest roentgenogram in, 456–457
  Cheyne-Stokes respiration in, 455
  classification of, 445–448, 446t, *447*, 448t, 452–453
  contractile apparatus in, 406–407, *406*
  contraction-relaxation cycle in, 376, *376*
  cytokines in, 415, *415*, 1642–1643
  definition of, 394, 445, 445t
  development of, 400–401, *401*, 401t
  diastolic, 447–448, *447*, 448t
    cardiomyopathy in, 404
    collagen in, 404
    ischemic heart disease in, *403*, 404, *404*
    pathophysiology of, 402–404, *402–404*
    pericardial disease in, 404
    treatment of, 503–504, 504t
    ventricular diastolic pressure-volume relationship in, 403–404
    ventricular filling in, 403, *403*
    ventricular relaxation in, 402–403, *402*
  2,3-diphosphoglycerate in, 397
  drug-induced, 12t, 449
  dyspnea in, 450–451, 450t
  edema in, 453–455
  emotional stress in, 449
  endothelial dysfunction in, 397, *397*
  endothelin in, 415
  endothelin 1 in, 1642
  end-stage, management of, 517. See also *Heart transplantation.*
  environmental factors in, 449
  etiology of, 448–449, 449t
  excitation-contraction coupling in, 404–406, *405*
  exercise capacity in, 451–452
  exercise stress testing in, 170, *171*, 451–452. See also *Exercise stress testing.*
  exertional dyspnea in, 450
  exhaustion phase of, 401, 401t
  fatigue in, 452
  fever in, 455
  fluid retention in, 446, 453–455
  forms of, 445–448, 446t, *447*, 448t
  forward, 446

Heart failure *(Continued)*
  Frank-Starling mechanism in, 394–396, *395–397*
  functional classification of, 452–453
  G proteins in, 411–412
  gallop sounds in, 455
  general appearance in, 453
  growth factors in, 399, *400*
  heart transplantation in, 517. See also *Heart transplantation.*
  hepatojugular reflux in, 453
  hepatomegaly in, 453
  high-output, 447
    anemia and, 460
    chronic, 1920
    clinical aspects of, 460–462
    hyperthyroidism and, 461
    in secondary pulmonary hypertension, 801
    Paget's disease and, 462
    patient history in, 11
    systemic arteriovenous fistula and, 460–461
    thiamine deficiency and, 461–462, 461t
  high-output states in, 449
  hydrothorax in, 455
  hyperbilirubinemia in, 456
  hypertension in, 858
  in alcoholic cardiomyopathy, 1413
  in amyloidosis, 1429
  in cardiac rehabilitation, 1396
  in congenital aortic stenosis, 915
  in congenital heart disease, 884–885, 884t, 889–891, 890t, 915
  in coronary artery disease, 1346–1349, *1347*, *1348*
  in diabetes mellitus, 1902, *1902*
  in elderly, 1699–1700
  in hyperthyroidism, 1893
  in idiopathic dilated cardiomyopathy, 1409–1410
  in infant, 884–885, 884t, 889–891, 890t
  in infective endocarditis, 1086
  in myocardial contusion, 1537
  in myocardial infarction, 1213
  in neonatal thyrotoxicosis, 993
  infection in, 449, 449t
  insulin-like growth factor-1 in, 1642
  laboratory findings in, 456, *567*
  lactic dehydrogenase in, 456
  left ventricular output redistribution in, 396–397, *396*
  left ventricular wall thickness in, 399–400, *401*
  left-sided, 446
  liver in, 456
  low-output, 447
  maximal exercise capacity in, 451
  molecular mechanisms of, 1639, *1639*
  murmurs in, 455
  myocardial contractility in, 397–399, *398*, *399*
    experimental study of, 397–398, *398*
  myocardial energetics in, 407
  myocardial hypertrophy in, 399–402, *399–401*, 401t, *402*
  myosin ATPase in, 406
  myosin isoform in, 406
  Na^+/Ca^{++} exchanger in, 406
  natriuretic peptides in, 414
  natural history of, 492, *492*
  neurohormonal alterations in, 407–415, *408*, *409*, *411*, 411t, *412*, *413*, *415*
  noncardiac surgery and, 1762–1763
  nonsustained ventricular tachycardia in, 506
  norepinephrine in, 396, 408–410, *408*, 412, *412*
  obesity and, 1906
  orthopnea in, 450
  P_2 in, 455
  pacemaker in, 709
  parasympathetic function in, 413
  paroxysmal nocturnal dyspnea in, 450–451, 450t
  patient appearance in, 453
  pericardium in, 1481
  physical findings in, 453–456
  postoperative, 1725–1726, 1764
    radiologic assessment of, 230
  practice guidelines for, 1985–1989, 1987t, *1988*
  precipitating causes of, 448–449, 449t
  premature ventricular complex in, 506
  prognosis for, 457–459

Heart failure *(Continued)*
    biochemical factors in, 458–459, *458*
    clinical factors in, 457, *457*, 457t, *458*, *459*
    electrophysiological factors in, 459
    hemodynamic factors in, 458, *459*
  pulmonary blood flow cephalization in, 219, *220*
  pulmonary congestion in, 456
  pulmonary edema in, 462–467
    alveolar-capillary membrane in, 462, 463t, 464
    classification of, 463–466, 463t
    diagnosis of, 464–465
      differential, 466–467, 466t
    gravity in, 463, *463*
    lymphatics in, 462
    mechanism of, 462–463
    pulmonary artery wedge pressure in, 465
    stages of, 463, 464–465
    Starling forces imbalance in, 463t, 464
    vs. bronchial asthma, 465
  pulmonary embolism in, 449
  pulmonary function testing in, 451
  pulmonary rales in, 453
  pulsus alternans in, *23*, 455
  quality of life in, 453, *454*
  radionuclide angiocardiography in, 302
  ras gene in, 1643, *1643*
  refractory, hemodynamic monitoring in, 508–509, 508t
    treatment of, 507–509, *508*
  regulatory protein alterations in, 406–407
  renal circulation in, 410
  renal function in, 413–414, *413*, 1914–1921, *1915*
    aldosterone and, 1916t
    angiotensin II and, 1916t
    arginine vasopressin and, 1916t
    atrial natriuretic peptide and, 1917t
    azotemia and, 1919–1920
    endothelin and, 1917t
    hormonal effects on, 1915, 1916t–1917t, 1917–1918
    management of, 1915
    norepinephrine and, 1916t
    potassium loss and, 1918–1919, *1919*
    prostaglandins and, 1917t
    renin and, 1916t
    sodium retention and, 1915, 1917–1918, *1918*
    water retention and, 1918, *1919*
  renin in, *408*, 1916t
  renin-angiotensin system in, 413–414, *413*
  respiratory distress in, 450–451
  retinoid-inducible suppressor genes in, 1644
  right-sided, 446, 452
  sarcoplasmic reticulum Ca^{++}-ATPase in, 405, *405*
  sarcoplasmic reticulum in, 369, 405, *405*
  serum electrolytes in, 456
  six-minute walk test in, 452, *452*
  splanchnic circulation in, 410
  submaximal exercise capacity in, 451–452
  sudden cardiac death in, 748, 748t
  sudden death in, 504–507, 504t, 748, 748t
  sympathetic activity in, *396*, 408–409, *408*
  symptoms of, 450–457, 450t, *452*, *454*
  syncope in, 506
  systemic infection in, 449, 449t
  systolic, 447–448, 448t
  systolic murmurs in, 455
  tension-independent heat in, 405
  treatment of, **471–511**
    acetazolamide in, 476, 477t
    adrenergic agonists in, 485–486
    afterload reduction in, 495, *495*
    amiloride in, 477t
    amlodipine in, 472t
    amrinone in, 472t, 484–485
    angiotensin-converting enzyme inhibitors in, 471–474, *471*, 472t, *473*, 473t, 493–497, *493*
      cough and, 497
      first-dose effects of, 497
      valvular regurgitation and, 497
    bendroflumethiazide in, 477–478, 477t
    beta-adrenoceptor blockers in, 486–488, *487*, 502–503
      pharmacology of, 486–487, 487t
    bucindolol in, 472t

Heart failure *(Continued)*
bumetanide in, 476–477, 477t
calcium channel blockers in, 472t, 475
calcium-sensitizing drugs in, 485
canrenone in, 477t
captopril in, 472t
carbonic anhydrase inhibitors in, 476, 477t
cardiac glycosides in, 480–484, 499–501
age and, 501
clinical efficacy of, 499–500
disease severity and, 500–501
electrophysiologic actions of, 482
mechanisms of, 480–482
pharmacokinetics of, 482–484
positive inotropic effects of, 481–482, *481*
potassium homeostasis and, 500
pulmonary disease and, 501
renal failure and, 501
sympathetic nervous system effects of, 482
therapeutic endpoints for, 500
therapeutic monitoring of, 482t, 483–484, *483*, 483t
thyroid disease and, 501
toxicity of, 482, 484
carvedilol in, 472t
chlorothiazide in, 477–478, 477t
chlorthalidone in, 477–478, 477t
cromakalim in, 475–476
diazoxide in, 472t
dichlorphenamide in, 476, 477t
diuretics in, 476–480, *476*, 477t, 498–499
acid-base disturbances with, 480
carbohydrate intolerance with, 480
complications of, 479–480
hyperlipidemia with, 480
hypomagnesemia with, 479
hyponatremia with, 479–480
in elderly, 499
loop, 476–477, 477t
osmotic, 476, 477t
potassium-sparing, 477t, 478
renal insufficiency and, 480
resistance to, 478–479, *478*
thiazide, 477–478, 477t
dobutamine in, 472t, 485–486, 502
dopamine in, 472t, 486, 502
dopaminergic agonists in, 485–486
dopexamine in, 486
enalapril in, 472t
ethacrynic acid in, 476–477, 477t
extracorporeal ultrafiltration in, 480
felodipine in, 472t
follow-up after, 1989
furosemide in, 476–477, 477t
general approach to, 492–494
glycerol in, 476, 477t
goals of, 492
hemodynamic monitoring in, 494, 494t
hydralazine in, 472t, 475, 498
hydrochlorothiazide in, 477–478, 477t
hydroflumethiazide in, 477–478, 477t
inappropriate reduction in, 448–449
indapamide in, 477–478, 477t
isosorbide dinitrate in, 472t, 498
labetalol in, 472t
lisinopril in, 472t
losartan in, 472t
mannitol in, 476, 477t
methazolamide in, 476, 477t
methyclothiazide in, 477–478, 477t
metolazone in, 477–478, 477t
milrinone in, 472t, 484–485
minoxidil, 472t
molecular, 1644–1645
molsidomine in, 475
natriuretic peptides in, 478
nicorandil in, 472t, 475–476
nifedipine in, 472t
nitroglycerin in, 472t
nitroprusside in, 472t, 474–475, 497–498
nitrovasodilators in, 472t, 474–476, 497–498
tolerance to, 475
organic nitrates in, 475
phentolamine in, 472t
phosphodiesterase inhibitors in, 472t, 484–485, 502
pinacidil in, 475–476
piretanide in, 476–477, 477t
polythiazide in, 477–478, 477t
potassium channel activators in, 475–476

Heart failure *(Continued)*
practice guidelines for, 1986, 1988, *1988*
prazosin in, 472t
preload reduction in, 494–495, *495*
pulmonary artery balloon catheter in, 1989
quinapril in, 472t
quinethazone in, 477–478, 477t
ramipril in, 472t
spironolactone in, 477t
sympatholytics in, 472t
sympathomimetics in, 502
targets of, 492, 493t
torsemide in, 476–477, 477t
transplantation in, 509–511, 510t, 511t. See also *Heart transplantation*.
triamterene in, 477t
trichlormethiazide in, 477–478, 477t
vasodilators in, 471–476, *471*, 472t, *473*, 473t, 494–498, *495*
vasopressin antagonists in, 478
vesnarinone in, 472t, 485, 502
treatment reduction in, 448–449, 449t
troponin-T in, *406*, 407
unrelated illness in, 449
urinary symptoms in, 452
Valsalva maneuver in, 456
vascular wall changes in, 397
venous hypertension in, 453
venous pressure in, 456
ventricular ectopy in, 506
voltage-dependent calcium channel in, 406
vs. circulatory failure, 394
vs. myocardial failure, 394
weakness in, 452
Heart rate, 421
after heart transplantation, 527
in arrhythmia diagnosis, 579
in contraction-relaxation cycle, 380, *380*, 381
in Duchenne muscular dystrophy, 1868–1869
in exercise stress testing, 163, 164
in heart failure, 410, 413
in infant, 889, *889*
in myocardial infarction, 1199–1200
in myocardial oxygen uptake, 381, *381*, 1162t
in pregnancy, 1843, 1843t
of aging heart, 1692, *1693*
Heart rate reserve, of infant, 889, *889*
Heart rate–systolic blood pressure product, in exercise stress testing, 164
Heart retransplantation, 528–529, *529*
Heart rhythm, 421
Heart sound(s), **29–35.** See also *Murmur(s)*.
early diastolic, *29*, 33–34, *33*
early systolic, *29*, 30–31, *30*, *31*
ejection, 30–31, *30*, *31*
respiration effects on, 47
first, 29–30, *29*, *30*
in mitral regurgitation, 1024
in mitral stenosis, 1010–1011, 1024
splitting of, 29–30, *29*
fourth, *29*, *30*, 34–35, *34*, *35*
abnormal, 35, *35*
in myocardial infarction, 1201
in unstable angina, 1334
loudness of, 35
respiration effects on, 47
gallop, in heart failure, 455
in idiopathic dilated cardiomyopathy, 1410
in anemia, 460, 1787
in aortic stenosis, 916, 1040–1041, 1040t
in cardiac tumor, 1472–1473
in congenital aortic stenosis, 916
in congenital pulmonic stenosis, 925
in cyanosis, 893
in Ebstein's anomaly, 935
in heart failure, 455
in hyperthyroidism, 1892
in hypertrophic cardiomyopathy, 1420
in idiopathic dilated cardiomyopathy, 1410
in mitral regurgitation, 1022–1024, 1023t
in mitral stenosis, 1010–1011
in mitral valve prolapse, 1032–1033
in myocardial infarction, 1200–1201
in pregnancy, 1845
in pulmonary hypertension, 788, 789
in stable angina pectoris, 1292
in total anomalous pulmonary venous connection, 945
in tricuspid regurgitation, 1057
in unstable angina, 1334

Heart sound(s) *(Continued)*
isometric exercise effects on, 48–49
late diastolic (presystolic), *29*, 34–35, *34*
late systolic, *29*, 31–32, *31*
mid-diastolic, *29*, 34–35, *34*
midsystolic, *29*, 31–32, *32*
pharmacological effects on, 46t, *48*, 49
physiological effects on, 46–49, 46t
postural effects on, 47–49, *48*, *49*
respiration effects on, 47
second, *29*, 32–33
fixed splitting of, 33
in arrhythmias, 641
in mitral stenosis, 1011
in stable angina pectoris, 1292
loudness of, 33, *33*
paradoxical splitting of, 33
persistent splitting of, 33
splitting of, 32–33
third, *29*, 34–35, *34*
in angina pectoris, 1321
in heart failure, 455
in mitral regurgitation, 1022, 1024
in myocardial infarction, 1201
in unstable angina, 1334
loudness of, 35
respiration effects on, 47
Heart transplantation, **515–530**
age limit on, 516t
arteriography after, 241
arteriopathy after, 1349
atherosclerosis of, 525–526, *526*
candidates for, 509–511, *510*, 515–517, *516*, 516t
age and, 516, 516t
clinical considerations in, 516–517
coexisting diseases and, 517
peak oxygen consumption and, 517
pulmonary vascular disease and, 516
centers for, 515
contraindications to, 516t
cost of, 528
denervation effects in, 527–528
donor evaluation for, 517–519, 518t
early postoperative recovery in, 519–520, 520t
exercise stress testing after, 171–172, *172*
exercise stress testing before, 171, *172*
heart preservation for, 518
heart size in, 518
heterotopic, 519
history of, 515
hypertension after, 830
immunosuppression for, 519–520, 520t
complications of, 523–525
in children, 528
in myocarditis, 989
indications for, 509–510, 515–516, *516*
infection after, 523–525
intraaortic balloon counterpulsation in, 517, 535. See also *Intraaortic balloon counterpulsation*.
late follow-up for, 526–527, 526t
neoplasms after, 525
physiology of, 527–528, *527*
postoperative imaging in, 231
pregnancy after, 1853
preoperative management in, 517
rejection of, 520–522
echocardiography of, 520
endomyocardial biopsy in, 520–522, *521*, 521t, 522t
hyperacute, 522
lymphocyte measurements in, 520
mild, *521*, 523
moderate, *521*
persistent, 523
radionuclide tests of, 520
severe, *521*, 522–523
treatment of, 522–523, *522*
algorithm for, *522*
repeat of, 528–529, *529*
status I recipients in, 517
status II recipients in, 517
survival after, 527, *527*
technique of, 518–519, *519*
ventricular assist device in, 517, 542, 542t, 543–544. See also *Ventricular assist device*.
waiting list for, 510–511
Heartburn, 1291, 1291t

Heart-hand syndrome, 17, 880t
genetic factors in, 1655, 1660t, 1661
Heart-lung transplantation, 529–530, *529*
in pulmonary hypertension, 795–796
postoperative assessment of, 231
HeartMate 1000 LVAS pump, 537t, 538–539, *539*
HeartMate 1000 VE LVAS blood pump, 537t, 540–541
Heat stroke, myocardial effects of, 1449
Helsinki Heart Study, 1145
in hypercholesterolemia prevention, 1128
Hemangioendothelioma, hepatic, heart failure in, 461
Hemangioma, familial, 1677
genetic factors in, 1660t
Hemangiomatosis, capillary, in pulmonary hypertension, 787–788, 787t
Hematocrit, in cyanotic congenital heart disease, 972
in pregnancy, 1843, *1843*
Hematoma, intramural, in aortic dissection, 1554, *1555*, 1568–1569, *1568*
pericardial, magnetic resonance imaging of, 324–325, *325*
postoperative, 230
Hemiplegic migraine syndrome, 1677
Hemizygosity, genetic, 1651
Hemochromatosis, 1674–1675, 1790–1792
cardiac manifestations of, 1791
diagnosis of, 11, 1791, *1792*
patient history in, 11
pigmentation of, 16
primary, 1791–1792
restrictive cardiomyopathy of, 1430
secondary, 1792, *1793*
transfusion-related, 1792, *1792*
Hemodialysis. See *Kidney dialysis.*
Hemoglobin, in myocardial infarction, 1197
in pregnancy, 1843, *1843*
variants of, 1794
Hemoglobinopathy, 1675, 1787–1788
Hemoglobin-oxygen dissociation curve, in anemia, 1786–1787, *1787*
Hemolysis, in renal failure, 1936
Hemolytic anemia, 1675, 1787–1790
after cardiac surgery, 1790
microangiopathic, 1790
Hemopericardium, postoperative, 1521
Hemoptysis, 10
chest pain with, 7
in congenital heart disease, 885
in differential diagnosis, 10
in mitral stenosis, 1010
Hemorrhage, cerebral, familial, 1677
in adult congenital heart disease, 974, *974*
exsanguinating, 1535. See also *Traumatic heart disease.*
gastrointestinal, 1735t
heparin-associated, 1594
in infective endocarditis, 1085, *1085*
in mitral stenosis, 1010
in myocardial infarction, 1198
intracranial, familial, 1677
in adult congenital heart disease, 974, *974*
thrombolytic therapy and, 1220
mediastinal, postoperative, 230
reperfusion-induced, 1179
retinal, 1085, *1085*
splinter, 17, 1085, *1085*
subungual, 1085, *1085*
warfarin-associated, 1595
with ventricular assist device, 542
Hemorrhagic shock, in abdominal aortic aneurysm, 1548
Hemosiderosis, 1790–1792, 1790t
Hemostasis, 1809–1814
coagulation in, 1811–1814, *1811–1814*. See also *Coagulation.*
endothelium in, 1809–1810, *1809*, *1810*
in cyanotic congenital heart disease, 972
platelets in, 1810–1811, *1811*
Heparin, after myocardial infarction, 1832–1833
collateral blood flow and, 1176
complications of, 1224, 1594
exercise stress testing effects of, 170
hematological abnormalities with, 1804t
in arteriography, 245
in myocardial infarction, 1223–1225, 1257, 1826, 1826t, 1974t–1975t
in pediatric cardiology, 1001t
in pregnancy, 977, 1859–1860
Heparin *(Continued)*
in PTCA-related abrupt vessel closure, 1369
in pulmonary embolism, 1592–1594, 1593t
in pulmonary embolism prophylaxis, 1598, 1599–1600, 1599t
in renal failure, 1933t
in unstable angina, *1337*, 1338, 1823, *1824*, 1824t
low molecular weight, 1817–1818, 1817t
pharmacokinetics of, 1817
side effects of, 1817
unfractionated, 1817, 1817t
Heparinization, postoperative, 1732t
Heparinoids, 1818
Hepatitis. See also *Liver.*
myocarditis in, 1437
postoperative, 1733
Hepatojugular reflux, in heart failure, 453
Hepatomegaly, in constrictive pericarditis, 1499
in heart failure, 452, 453
Hereditary angioedema, 1669t
Hereditary hemorrhagic telangiectasia (Osler-Weber-Rendu disease), 16, *17*, 1676
heart failure in, 461
Herniation, cardiac, 1522
Heroin overdose, pulmonary edema in, 465–466
Herpes zoster, infection with, chest pain in, 5
Heterotaxy, 1658
Heterozygosity, genetic, 1651
Hibernating myocardium, 388, 388t, 1176, 1215
after coronary artery bypass surgery, 1327–1328, *1327*, 1328t
contractile reserve in, 1327, *1327*
detection of, 1327–1328, *1327*, 1328t
echocardiography of, 89
in coronary artery disease, 1299
High altitude, pulmonary arterial pressure at, 783
pulmonary edema at, 465, *466*
syncope at, 865
High-density lipoprotein deficiency, xanthomas with, 1144
Hill's sign, in aortic regurgitation, 22, 1049
Hirudin, 1628–1629, 1817t, 1820
in myocardial infarction, 1224
Hirulog, 1820
His bundle, 550, *551*
innervation of, 552–553
His-Purkinje system, disease of, sudden cardiac death in, 750–751
Histamine, in hypoxia-induced vasoconstriction, 781, *782*, 783
Histiocytoma, fibrous, malignant, 1471
Histoplasmosis, myocarditis in, 1441
pericarditis in, 1510–1511
History, **1–13**
anorexia in, 10
chest pain in, 3–7, 4t, 5t, *6*
cough in, 10
cyanosis in, 7–8
dyspnea in, 2–3, 3t
edema in, 9–10
fatigue in, 10
hemoptysis in, 10
in cardiomyopathy, 11
in childhood, 11
in congenital malformations, 11
in cor pulmonale, 11
in disability assessment, 12t, 13
in drug-induced heart disease, 11–13, 12t
in endocarditis, 11
in high-output heart failure, 11
in myocarditis, 11
in pericarditis, 11
nocturia in, 10
palpitation in, 9, 9t
role of, 1
syncope in, 8–9, 8t
technique of, 1–2
HMG-CoA reductase inhibitors, in dyslipidemia, 1140t, 1141
Hodgkin's disease, pericardial effusion in, 1514
radiation pericarditis in, 1516–1517
Hoffman-Rigler sign, 211
Holiday heart syndrome, 752
Holmium laser, 1383
Holter monitor, in arrhythmia diagnosis, 570–579
Holt-Oram syndrome, 880t
extremities in, 17
genetic factors in, 1655, 1660t, 1661
Homocysteine, in coronary artery disease, 1153
Homocystinuria, 880t, 1668t, 1673
coronary artery disease in, 1349
Homozygosity, genetic, 1651
Hormone replacement therapy. See *Estrogen replacement therapy.*
Human genome, 1631, *1652–1653*. See also *Gene(s).*
Human immunodeficiency virus (HIV), infection with, myocarditis in, 135, *150*, 989, 1438–1439, *1438*, 1438t
pericarditis in, 1506–1508
pulmonary hypertension with, 786
tuberculous pericarditis in, 1507–1508
Hunter syndrome, 881t, 1668t, 1675
Hurler syndrome, 881t, 1349, 1668t, 1675, *1675*
Hurler-Scheie syndrome, 1668t
H-V interval, in arrhythmias, 643, *644*
Hydantoin, teratogenicity of, 1663t, 1664
Hydatid cyst, myocarditis with, 1444
Hydralazine (Apresoline), during pregnancy, 1852t
hematological abnormalities with, 1804t
in aortic regurgitation, 1052
in congenital heart disease–related heart failure, 890, 891t
in heart failure, 472t, 475, 498, 890, 891t, 1987t
in hypertension, 855, 858t
in pediatric cardiology, 1001t
in renal failure, 1932t
pericarditis with, 1519
Hydrocarbons, myocardial effects of, 1447
Hydrochlorothiazide, hematological abnormalities with, 1804t
in heart failure, 477–478, 477t
in pediatric cardiology, 1001t
Hydrocortisone sodium succinate (Solu-Cortef), in pediatric cardiology, 1001t
Hydroflumethiazide, in heart failure, 477–478, 477t
Hydrops fetalis, aortic valve stenosis and, 915
atrial flutter in, 951
17-Hydroxycorticosteroids, in myocardial infarction, 1197
Hydroxyephedrine, carbon-11–labeled, 308
11-Hydroxylase deficiency, 829
17-Hydroxylase deficiency, 829
11-β-Hydroxysteroid dehydrogenase deficiency, 828
5-Hydroxytryptamine (serotonin), 783, *1165*
Hyperaldosteronism, 1896–1897
Hyperbilirubinemia, in heart failure, 456
postoperative, 1735t
Hyperbradykininism, 1678t
Hypercalcemia, diuretic-induced, 851
electrocardiography in, 142, *142*
Hypercholesterolemia, **1127–1143**
abdominal aortic aneurysm and, 1550
endothelial cell dysfunction in, *1164*
familial, 1142–1143
genetic factors in, 1651
tendinous xanthomas in, 16, *17*
fatty streaks in, 1118, *1119*
hypertension and, 813
in atherosclerosis, 1114, 1116
observational studies of, 1127
PDGE-B protein in, **Plate 9**
pediatric, 1002t, 1003–1004, *1003*
polygenic, 1143
prevention of, 1127–1133
Canadian Coronary Atherosclerosis Intervention Trial, 1132
Cholesterol Lowering Atherosclerosis Study in, 1130
cholestyramine in, 1129–1130, 1131
clofibrate in, 1129
colestipol in, 1130
Coronary Drug Project in, 1128
Familial Atherosclerosis Treatment Study in, 1130, *1131*
Helsinki Heart Study in, 1128
ileal bypass surgery in, 1131
interventional studies in, 1127–1133, 1129t
Life Style Heart Trial in, 1131–1132
Lipid Research Clinics Coronary Primary Prevention Trial in, 1127–1128
lovastatin in, 1130, 1132
Monitored Atherosclerosis Regression Study in, 1132
Multicenter Anti-Atheroma Study in, 1133

Hypercholesterolemia *(Continued)*
National Heart, Lung, and Blood Institute Type II Coronary Intervention Study in, 1129–1130
nicotinic acid in, 1129, 1130
Oslo Study Diet and Antismoking Trial in, 1128
practice guidelines for, 1990–1991
pravastatin in, 1132–1133
Pravastatin Limitation of Atherosclerosis in the Coronary Arteries study in, 1132
Program on the Surgical Control of the Hyperlipidemias in, 1131
Regression Growth Evaluation Statin Study in, 1132–1133
St. Thomas' Atherosclerosis Regression Study in, 1131
Scandinavian Simvastatin Survival Study in, 1133
University of California, San Francisco, Arteriosclerosis Specialized Center of Research Intervention Trial in, 1130–1131
West of Scotland Coronary Prevention Study in, 1128
World Health Organization Cooperative Trial in, 1128
retinopathy in, 15, *16*
treatment of, 1121, 1136–1142
after myocardial infarction, 1263–1264
angiographic studies of, 268–269
bile-acid sequestrants in, 1139–1140, 1139t, 1140t
cholestyramine in, 1139–1140, 1139t, 1140t
clofibrate in, 1140t, 1141–1142
colestipol in, 1139–1140, 1139t, 1140t
cost-effectiveness analysis of, 1745–1746, 1746t
dietary, 1136–1138, 1137t, 1138t
endothelial dysfunction reversal in, *1167*, *1168*
estrogen replacement therapy in, 1142
fibric-acid derivatives in, 1141–1142
fluvastatin in, 1140t, 1141
gemfibrozil in, 1140t, 1141–1142
lovastatin in, 1140t, 1141
nicotinic acid in, 1140–1141, 1140t
pharmacologic, 1138–1142, 1139t, 1140t
positron emission tomography of, 308
practice guidelines for, 1990–1991
pravastatin in, 1140t, 1141, 1300
probucol in, 1140t, 1142
simvastatin in, 1140t, 1141
Hyperemia, reactive, in myocardial ischemia, 1173–1174, *1173*
Hypereosinophilic syndrome, 1432–1433, *1432*
tumor-related, 1798–1799
Hyperglycemia, diuretic-induced, 850, *850*
in myocardial infarction, 1197
Hyperinsulinemia, in hypertension, 820, *820*
in Prinzmetal's variant angina, 1340
Hyperkalemia, electrocardiography in, *137*, 141–142, *141*, *150*, *151*
in heart failure, 456
in periodic paralysis, 1877
with diuretics, 479
Hyperlipidemia, after coronary artery bypass surgery, 1321
combined, familial, 1143, 1146
diuretic-induced, 480, 850, *850*
familial, 1143, 1146
coronary artery bypass surgery and, 1328
Fredrickson classification of, 1127t
in atherosclerosis, 1114
pediatric, 1002t, 1003–1004, *1003*
treatment of, after coronary artery bypass surgery, 1321
cost-effectiveness analysis of, 1745–1746, 1746t
type III, 1146
Hypermagnesemia, electrocardiography in, 142
Hyperoxaluria, 1668t
Hyperparathyroidism, systemic hypertension in, 830
Hypersensitive carotid sinus syndrome, 647–648, 865
carotid sinus massage in, 647–648, *648*
clinical features of, 647–648
electrocardiography in, 647, *648*
pacemaker in, 708, 709t
practice guidelines for, 1965t
Hypersensitivity drug reactions, 1448–1449, 1448t
Hyperstat. See *Diazoxide (Hyperstat).*
Hypertension, **807–834,** 811t
abdominal aortic aneurysm and, 1550
accelerated-malignant, 832
after coronary artery bypass surgery, 1319
coronary artery disease and, 812–813, *812*, *813*, 1706–1707
coronary blood flow autoregulation in, 1168
critical degree of, 832–834, 832t, *833*, 833t, 834t
diastolic pressure-volume curve in, 403
drug-induced, 12t
emergency treatment of, 832–834, 832t, *833*, 833t, 834t
exercise stress testing in, 170, 174
gestational, 830–832, 831t, 1852–1853, 1852t, 1853t
clinical features of, 831, 831t
prognosis for, 832
treatment of, 831–832
in acromegaly, 1888
in aortic dissection, 1567
in congestive heart failure, 858
in coronary artery disease, 1148–1150, 1149t, 1299–1300
in Cushing's disease, 1896
in elderly, 857–858, 857t, 1699
in hyperparathyroidism, 1900
in hypothyroidism, 1894
in ischemic heart disease, 858
in myocardial infarction, 1200
in renal failure, 1923, 1928, *1929*
in stable angina pectoris, 1299
in Takayasu's arteritis, 1572
mineralocortical, 827–829, *828*
natural history of, 816–817
noncardiac surgery and, 1761
obesity and, 1906
pediatric, 810, 810t, 812, 812t, 822, 822t, 857, 997–1003, 998t
assessment of, 999–1000, 1002, 1002t
management of, 1000t–1002t, 1002–1003
portal, in pulmonary hypertension, 786
postoperative, 1723, 1764
pregnancy and, 830–832, 831t, 1852–1853, 1852t, 1853t
prevention of, 807, 813
practice guidelines for, 1991–1993, 1991t, *1992*, 1992t, *1993*
primary, **807–823**
alcohol intake in, 821
borderline, 810
cardiac involvement in, 814–815, *814*, *815*
cell membrane dysfunction in, 818, *818*
cerebral involvement in, 815
cigarette smoking in, 821
complications of, 813–814, 814t
definition of, 808–810, *808*, *809*
documentation of, 809–810, 810t
endothelial cell dysfunction in, 820, *821*
endothelin in, 820, *821*
fetal environment in, 817, *817*
fundus involvement in, 814
genetic factors in, 1677–1679, 1678t
genetic predisposition to, 817
hematologic findings in, 821
hemodynamic patterns in, 816–817
hyperinsulinemia in, 820, *820*
hyperuricemia in, 821
in adolescents, 810, 810t, 822, 822t
in blacks, 821–822
in children, 810, 810t, 812, 812t, 822, 822t
in diabetes mellitus, 823
in elderly, 822–823
in obesity, 820–821
in sleep apnea, 821
in women, 822
insulin resistance in, 820, *820*
mechanisms of, 816–820, *816*
natural history of, 812–813, 815
nitric oxide in, 820
physical inactivity in, 821
plasma renin in, 815
pressor mechanisms in, 818–819, *818*
prevalence of, *807*, 811–812, *811*
prognosis for, plasma renin in, 815
renal involvement in, 815, 817–818, 817t
renin-angiotensin system in, 819–820, *819*
risk for, 813, *813*, 816
Hypertension *(Continued)*
sodium retention in, 817–818, 817t
sympathetic nervous hyperactivity in, 819
vascular hypertrophy in, 818–819, *818*
pulmonary, **783–801.** See also *Pulmonary hypertension.*
pulmonary hypertension with, 786
renovascular, 825–827, 826t
classification of, 826t
diagnosis of, 826–827, 826t
mechanisms of, 826
resistant, treatment of, 856–857, 857t
retinopathy of, 15, *16*
screening for, cost-effectiveness analysis of, 1747
secondary, 811, 811t, **823–834,** 998t
adrenal disease in, 827–830, *828*
after heart surgery, 830
during pregnancy, 830–832, 831t, 1852–1853, 1852t, 1853t
in aldosteronism, 827–829, *828*
in analgesic nephropathy, 825
in coarctation of aorta, 830
in congenital adrenal hyperplasia, 829
in Cushing's syndrome, 829
in diabetic nephropathy, 825, *825*
in extracorporeal shock wave lithotripsy, 824
in glomerulonephritis, 824
in kidney dialysis, 825
in kidney transplantation, 825
in oliguric renal failure, 824
in pheochromocytoma, 829–830, 830t
in polycystic kidney disease, 824
in pyelonephritis, 824
in renal parenchymal disease, 824–825, *825*
in vasculitis, 824
oral contraceptives and, 823–824
postmenopausal estrogens and, 823–824
renovascular, 825–827, 826t
classification of, 826, 826t
diagnosis of, 826–827, 826t
management of, 827
mechanisms of, 826
stroke risk and, 812–813, *812*
sudden cardiac death and, 745
treatment of, 813, **840–859**
adequacy of, 807, *807*, 840, 856–857, 857t
adrenergic inhibitors in, 851–854, *851*, 851t, *853*, *854*
alcohol moderation in, 845–846
antihypertensive therapy guidelines in, 846–849, 846t, *847*, *848*, 848t
benefits of, 840–842, *841*, *842*
calcium supplementation in, 845
captopril in, 855–856, *855*
cost-effectiveness analysis of, 1747
dietary changes in, 845–846
dihydropyridines in, 855, 855t
diltiazem in, 855, 855t
diuretics in, 849–851, 849t, *850*
goal of, 844
guanabenz in, 852
guanethidine in, 852
guanfacine in, 852
hydralazine in, 855
in elderly, 843, *843*
J-curve in, 844
lifestyle modifications in, 844–846
magnesium supplementation in, 845
methyldopa in, 852
minoxidil in, 855
nifedipine in, 855
outcomes of, 840–842, *841–843*
physical exercise in, 846
potassium supplementation in, 845
prazosin in, 852
relaxation techniques in, 846
reserpine in, 852
risk assessment in, 816
sodium restriction in, 844–845
threshold for, 842–843, *843*
tobacco avoidance in, 844, *845*
vasodilators in, 854–856, 854t, *855*, 855t
verapamil in, 855, 855t
weight reduction in, 844
venous, in heart failure, 453, 456
white coat, 808–809
Hypertensive crises, 832–834
course of, 833–834
definition of, 832, 832t
differential diagnosis of, 834, 834t

Hypertensive crises *(Continued)*
incidence of, 832
manifestations of, 833–834, 833t
pathophysiology of, 832–833, *833*
treatment of, 858–859, 858t
Hyperthermia, malignant, genetic factors in, 1660t
Hyperthyroidism, 1890t, 1891–1894
apathetic, 461
cardiovascular manifestations of, 1892–1894, *1892*, *1893*
diagnosis of, 1893
digoxin in, 501
heart failure in, 461
pulmonary hypertension with, 786
sympathoadrenal system and, 1891
Hypertriglyceridemia, 1144–1146
detection of, 1145
epidemiology of, 1145
familial, 1146
treatment of, 1145–1146
Hypertrophic cardiomyopathy, 1414–1426. See also *Cardiomyopathy, hypertrophic.*
Hyperuricemia, diuretic-induced, 850, *850*
in cyanotic congenital heart disease, 972
in hypertension, 821
Hyperventilation, chest pain in, 4t
in myocardial infarction, 1197
in Prinzmetal's variant angina, 1342
Hyperviscosity, erythrocyte, 1792–1794, *1793*
Hypervitaminosis D, experimental, supravalvular aortic stenosis in, 920
Hypoalbuminemia, in pulmonary edema, 463t, 464
Hypocalcemia, electrocardiography in, 142, *142*
myocardial effects of, 1447
Hypochloremic alkalosis, diuretics and, 480
Hypokalemia, diuretic-induced, 479, 849–850, *850*
electrocardiography in, *141*, 142, *151*
in heart failure, *458*, 459
in myocardial infarction, 1248
in periodic paralysis, 1877
U wave in, 139
ventricular fibrillation and, 1248
Hypokinesis, in mitral stenosis, 1009
Hypomagnesemia, cardiac glycosides and, 500
diuretic-induced, 479, 850, *850*
in myocardial infarction, 1248–1249
myocardial effects of, 1447
postoperative, 1720
ventricular fibrillation and, 1248–1249
with diuretics, 479
Hyponatremia, diuretic-induced, 479–480
in heart failure, 456, *458*, 549
Hypoperfusion, with ventricular assist device, 542–543
Hypophosphatemia, myocardial effects of, 1447
Hypoplastic left heart syndrome, 921–922, *922*
Hyporeninism, 1897
Hypotension. See also *Syncope.*
drug-induced, 12t
in amyloidosis, 1429
in aortic dissection, 1556
in elderly, 822–823
in myocardial infarction, 1200, 1212–1213, 1234–1235, 1241
in pulmonary embolism, 1585
in renal failure, 1935
intraoperative, 1758
Hypothermia, myocardial effects of, 1449
Osborne wave in, *140*, 141
Hypothyroidism, 1894–1895, *1894*
atherosclerosis in, 1895
cardiovascular manifestations of, 1894, *1894*
diagnosis of, 1895
hypertension in, 830
myocardial effects of, 1894–1895
treatment of, 1895
Hypoventilation, alveolar, in cor pulmonale, 1614–1615
in secondary pulmonary hypertension, 801
Hypovolemia, in hypertrophic cardiomyopathy, 1423
in myocardial infarction, 1235
postoperative, 1725, 1726t
Hypoxemia, in myocardial infarction, *1195*, 1196–1197, 1212, 1236
in renal failure, 1935–1936
Hypoxia, definition of, 1161
in anemia, 1787, *1787*
Hypoxia *(Continued)*
in chronic obstructive pulmonary disease, 1616
in pulmonary vasoconstriction, 781, *782*, 1608
Hypoxic spells, in congenital heart disease, 885

Ibopamine, in heart failure, 486, 499–500
Ice pick injury, 1539–1541, *1540*
Idarubicin, cardiac effects of, 1800–1803, 1801t, 1802t
Idiopathic dilated cardiomyopathy, 1407–1414. See also *Cardiomyopathy, dilated, idiopathic.*
Idiopathic hypertrophic subaortic stenosis. See *Cardiomyopathy, hypertrophic.*
Idiopathic orthostatic hypotension, 865
Idiopathic ventricular fibrillation, 682–683
Idioventricular rhythm, accelerated, 641t–642t, 683–684, *684*
electrocardiography in, 683–684, *684*
management of, 684
Ifosfamide, cardiac effects of, 1803
Ileal bypass surgery, in hypercholesterolemia prevention, 1131
Ileus, postoperative, 1735t
Imaging, **349–357.** See also specific methods, e.g., *Magnetic resonance imaging (MRI).*
anatomic assessment by, 352
computer-assisted, 350–351
costs of, 356–357, 357t
energy form for, 350, 350t
goals of, 351–354, 351t
left ventricular function assessment by, 352
myocardial metabolism assessment by, 353–354
myocardial perfusion assessment by, 353, *353*
myocardial tissue assessment by, 354
of aortic disease, 354t, 356
of cardiomyopathy, 354t, 356
of congenital heart disease, 354t, 355–356
of infective endocarditis, 354t, 356
of intracardiac masses, 354t, 356
of ischemic heart disease, 354–355, 354t
of pericardial disease, 354t, 356
of traumatic heart disease, 354t, 356
of valvular heart disease, 354t, 355
planar, 349–350
projection, 349–350
relative diagnostic yields of, 351–354, 351t
right ventricular function assessment by, 352
scope of, 349–351, 349t, 350t
standard, 350
tomographic, 350
valvular function assessment by, 352–353
ventricular function assessment by, 352
Imdur (isosorbide-5-mononitrate), doses of, 1303–1304, 1303t
in renal failure, 1932t
Immune system, in atherosclerosis, 1110, 1111
in endocarditis, 1084
in idiopathic dilated cardiomyopathy, 1409, *1409*
in myocarditis, 988, 1435
in postpericardiotomy syndrome, 990, 1520
in trypanosomiasis, 1442
Immunization, before heart transplantation, 523
Immunoglobulin G (IgG), in atherosclerosis, 1120
Immunohemolytic anemia, drug-induced, 1804–1805
Immunosuppression, in heart transplantation, 519–520, 520t, 523–525
Immunotherapy, antidigoxin, 484
Impedance plethysmography, in pulmonary embolism, 1587–1588, 1587t
Imperforate anus, genetic factors in, 1661t
Impotence, diuretic-induced, 851
Incontinentia pigmenti, 880t
Incremental cost/incremental effectiveness ratio, 1742
Indapamide, in coronary artery disease, 1149t
in heart failure, 477–478, 477t
in renal failure, 1933t
Inderal. See *Propranolol (Inderal).*
Indicator-dilution technique, of cardiac output measurement, 191
Indomethacin, in pediatric cardiology, 1001t
Infant. See also *Children; Congenital heart disease.*
apnea in, 892
Infant *(Continued)*
cyanosis in, 8, 891–894, 891t, *892*
heart failure in, 884–885, 884t
juxtaductal coarctation in, 912
patent ductus arteriosus of, 905–906, *906*
respiratory patterns in, 892
systolic arterial murmurs in, 40
tachypnea in, 892–893
ventricular septal defect in, 902
Infection, after heart transplantation, 523–525
after lung transplantation, 530
bacterial, after heart transplantation, 523–524
of aorta, 1575–1576
fungal, after heart transplantation, 524
postoperative, 1733–1734
in renal failure, 1929, 1935
metastatic, in infective endocarditis, 1084
postoperative, 523–525, 530, 1732–1734, 1733
systemic, in heart failure, 449
viral, after heart transplantation, 524
postoperative, 1733
Infectious mononucleosis, myocarditis in, 1439
Infective endocarditis, **1077–1099**
antibiotic resistance in, 1081
Aspergillus in, 1082
bacteremia in, 1086–1087, 1087t
Bartonella in, 1082
blood culture in, 1087
Candida albicans in, 1082
chemoprophylaxis against, 1098t, 1099, 1099t
clinical classification of, 1078–1082, 1079t, *1080*, *1082*
clinical features of, 1084–1086, 1084t, *1085*
coagulase-negative staphylococci in, 1081
complications of, 1095–1096
Corynebacterium in, 1082
Coxiella burnetii in, 1082
culture-negative, 1093
definition of, 1077
diagnosis of, 1086–1089, 1087t
echocardiography in, 77–78, *77*, 1088–1089
emboli in, 1085
embolization in, 1084
enterococci in, 1081, 1090–1091, 1090t, 1091t
epidemiology of, 1077–1078, 1077t
erythrocyte sedimentation rate in, 1087–1088
fungi in, 1082
gram-negative bacteria in, 1081–1082, *1082*
heart failure in, 1086
hemorrhages in, 1085, *1085*
imaging in, 354t, 356
immune system in, 1084
in adult congenital heart disease, 974–975
in adults, 1078
in aortic stenosis, 1040
in children, 1078
in congenital heart disease, 887–888
in heart failure, 449
in intravenous drug abusers, 1058, 1078–1079, 1079t
in mitral regurgitation, 1017
in mitral stenosis, 1010
in mitral valve prolapse, 1034, 1078
laboratory examination in, 1087–1089
Listeria monocytogenes in, 1082
magnetic resonance imaging in, 1089
microbiology of, 1077–1082, 1077t, 1079t
mortality rates in, 1096–1097
musculoskeletal symptoms in, 1085
mycotic aneurysm in, 1096
Neisseria gonorrhoeae in, 1082
neurologic complications of, 1880
neurologic symptoms in, 1085–1086
nonbacterial thrombotic endocarditis in, 1082–1083
nosocomial, 1080
of prosthetic valve, 1733
Osler's nodes in, 1085
pathogenesis of, 1082–1083
pathophysiology of, 1083–1084, *1084*
patient history in, 11
penicillin-resistant streptococci in, 1090, 1090t
petechiae in, 1085, *1085*
postoperative, 1733–1734
preexisting cardiac disorders and, 1098, 1098t
prevention of, 1097–1099, 1097t, 1098t, 1099t
cost-effectiveness analysis of, 1748
prophylaxis against, in rheumatic fever, 1774
noncardiac surgery and, 1762
prosthetic valve, 1079–1080
microbiology of, 1079, 1079t

Infective endocarditis *(Continued)*
pathology of, 1079–1080, *1080*
treatment of, 1092–1093, 1092t, 1093t
Pseudomonas aeruginosa in, *1082*
recurrence of, 1097
renal failure and, 1921
renal insufficiency in, 1086
rheumatoid factor in, 1084
Roth spots in, 1085, *1085*
scintigraphy in, 1089
septic arteritis in, 1096
serological tests in, 1088
spleen in, 1085, 1095–1096
splenic abscess in, 1095–1096
staphylococci in, 1081, 1091–1092, 1092t
Staphylococcus aureus in, 1095
streptococci in, 1081, 1089–1090, 1090t
Streptococcus bovis in, 1081, 1089–1090, 1090t
Streptococcus pneumoniae in, 1081, 1090, 1090t
Streptococcus pyogenes in, 1090, 1090t
Torulopsis glabrata in, 1082
treatment of, 1089–1097
anticoagulant, 1096
antimicrobial, 1089–1093, 1090t, 1091t, 1092t, 1093t
monitoring of, 1093
outpatient, 1093–1094
timing of, 1093
response to, 1096–1097
surgical, 1094–1095, 1094t
antimicrobial treatment after, 1095
timing of, 1095
urine analysis in, 1088
viridans streptococci in, 1080–1081, 1089–1090, 1090t
Inferior vena cava, echocardiography of, 70–71, *70*
in constrictive pericarditis, 1500
in pulmonary embolism, 1595–1596, 1595t
Inflammation, myocardial. See *Myocarditis*.
pericardial. See *Pericarditis*.
Influenza, myocarditis in, 1439
Infundibular stenosis, subpulmonic, 928
Inhalation anesthesia, 1757
Injury, cardiac, 1535–1544. See also *Traumatic heart disease*.
Innovar (fentanyl citrate & droperidol), in pediatric cardiology, 1001t
Inositol triphosphate (IP_3), in contraction-relaxation cycle, 375, *375*
Inositol triphosphate (IP_3) receptor, of sarcoplasmic reticulum, 368, *368*
Insertional mutagenesis, in transgenic technology, 1635, *1635*
Inspection, in cardiac examination, 24
Inspiration, paradoxical jugular venous pressure rise with (Kussmaul's sign), 19
in cardiac catheterization, 198
in constrictive pericarditis, 1497
in heart failure, 453
Insulin, 1900–1901
in hypertension, 818–819, *818*
Insulin resistance, diuretic-induced, 850, *850*
in coronary artery disease, 1150
in hypertension, 820, *820*
in Prinzmetal's variant angina, 1340
Insulin-like growth factor, 1887
Insulin-like growth factor-1, in myocyte hypertrophy, 1642, 1642t
Intact valve, 1063
Integrelin, 1630
in myocardial infarction, 1225
Intensive care unit. See also *Coronary care unit (CCU)*.
deep venous thrombosis occurrence in, 1583
Intercalated discs, of cell membranes, 554–555
Intercellular adhesion molecule-1 (ICAM-1), in atherosclerosis, 1108
Intercostal vein, on plain chest radiography, *206*
Interferon-alpha (IFN-α), myocardial effects of, 1445–1446
Interferon-gamma (IFN-γ), in atherosclerotic plaque changes, 1187
Interleukin-1 (IL-1), in heart failure, 415
Interleukin-2 (IL-2), cardiac effects of, 1446, 1803–1804
Interleukin-6 (IL-6), in cardiac myxoma, 1464–1465
Internodal atrial myocardium, 548–549
Internodal pathways, 548–549
Interstitial pressure, in pulmonary edema, 463t, 464
Interstitial pulmonary fibrosis, progressive, in secondary pulmonary hypertension, 799
Interventional catheterization, 1366–1387. See also specific techniques, e.g., *Percutaneous transluminal coronary angioplasty (PTCA)*.
history of, 1366
Interventricular septum, rupture of, in myocardial infarction, 1241t, 1243, *1244*
traumatic, 1536t, 1538, 1541, *1541*
vs. mitral regurgitation, 1244
Intima, 1105–1106, *1106*, 1546
diffuse thickening of, 1113
Intraaortic balloon counterpulsation, 534, 535–536, *535*
balloon insertion for, 187, *535*, 536
balloon removal after, 536
complications of, 187, 536
contraindications to, 536
in end-stage heart failure, 517
in myocardial infarction, 1232, 1239, 1976t, 1978–1979
in unstable angina, 538, 1338, 1984
indications for, 535–536
Intracardiac pressures, Doppler echocardiography of, 68–70, *69*
measurement of, 422–423, *423*
Intracavitary gradient, 195
Intracoronary stents, 1378–1382, *1380*
implantation of, 1381–1382, *1381*
Palmaz-Schatz, *1379*, 1380–1381, 1380t, *1381*
Wallstent, 1379, *1379*
Intrapericardial pressure, 1479–1480
Intravenous anesthetics, 1757
Intraventricular aberration, electrocardiography in, 124–126, *124–126*
Intraventricular block, in myocardial infarction, 1245t, 1251–1252
Intraventricular conduction defect (IVCD), electrocardiography in, 123
electrophysiological studies in, 580
practice guidelines for, 1960t, 1962
nonspecific, 123
Intraventricular conduction delay, electrocardiography in, *147*
Intraventricular pressure gradient, measurement of, 195
Intraventricular right ventricular obstruction, 928–929, *928*
Intropin. See *Dopamine (Intropin)*.
Intubation, in cardiac arrest, 763
postoperative, 1723
Iohexol, for arteriography, 245
Ion channels, 553–555, *554*, 554t
cycle of, 553, *554*
in action potential phase 0, 557–559, *557*, *559*
proteins of, 553, *554*
Ion exchangers, in contraction-relaxation cycle, 370–371, *370*, *371*
Iopamidol, for arteriography, 245
Iron, in cyanotic congenital heart disease, 972
Iron deficiency, in cyanotic congenital heart disease, 972
Iron overload, 1790–1792, 1790t, *1792*
Ischemia. See *Myocardial ischemia*.
Ischemic preconditioning, in myocardial infarction, 1214
Isoflurane, for anesthesia, 1757
Isoproterenol hydrochloride (Isuprel hydrochloride), for upright tilt testing, 871
in congenital heart disease–related heart failure, 891t
in hypertrophic cardiomyopathy evaluation, 1423
in pediatric cardiology, 1001t
infusion of, with cardiac catheterization, 198
pulmonary vascular effects of, 782
Isopten. See *Verapamil (Isopten)*.
Isosorbide dinitrate, doses of, 1303, 1303t
in heart failure, 472t, 475, *476*, 498, 1987t
Isosorbide mononitrate, in heart failure, 475
Isosorbide-2-mononitrate, in renal failure, 1932t
Isosorbide-5-mononitrate (Imdur), doses of, 1303–1304, 1303t
in renal failure, 1932t
Isovolumetric phase indices, of myocardial contractility, 430, *430*
Isovolumetric relaxation, of left ventricle, 435–436, *435*
Isradipine, in angina pectoris, 1309t, 1311
in renal failure, 1931t
pharmacokinetics of, 1309t
Isuprel hydrochloride. See *Isoproterenol hydrochloride (Isuprel hydrochloride)*.
Ivemark syndrome, 1659t

Janeway lesions, 17
Jarvik-7-100 heart, 544
Jaundice, 16
in heart failure, 456
Jervell syndrome, 1667
Judkins catheters, for arteriography, 241–242, *242*
Judkins technique, for left heart catheterization, 184–185, *185*
Jugular vein, in cardiac tamponade, 1489
Jugular venous pulse, 18–20
a wave of, *18*, 19–20
elevation of, 19–20, *19*
examination of, 18–20, *18*, *19*
H wave of, *18*, 19
in aortic stenosis, 1040
in constrictive pericarditis, *19*, 20, 1498, *1499*
in mitral stenosis, *19*, 1010
in myocardial infarction, 1200
in tricuspid regurgitation, *18*, 20
normal, *18*
v wave of, *18*, 19
Junctional escape, accelerated, 143
Junctional rhythms, in myocardial infarction, 1245t, 1254
Juxtaductal coarctation of aorta, 911–913, *912*
clinical findings in, 911–912
complications of, 913
in children, 912–913, *912*
in infants, 912
management of, 913
morphology of, 911
pathogenesis of, 911, *912*
recurrence of, 913

Kabuki make-up syndrome, 1659t
Kaolin-pectin, digoxin interaction with, 483t
Kartagener syndrome, 880t, 1658
Kawasaki disease (mucocutaneous lymph node syndrome), 994–997
angiography in, 995, *996*
cardiac manifestations of, 995–996, *996*, 996t
clinical features of, 995t
coronary aneurysm in, 995–996, *996*
coronary artery disease in, 1349
echocardiography in, 995, *996*
management of, 996–997, 997t
natural history of, 994–995
sudden cardiac death in, 747
Kearns-Sayre syndrome, 1674, 1876, *1876*
Kent, bundles of, 668, 750
Keratosis palmoplantaris, genetic factors in, 1660t
Kerley A lines, 227
Kerley B lines, *226*
in mitral stenosis, 1012
in pulmonary edema, 220
Kerley C lines, 227
Ketamine, for anesthesia, 1757
Ketosteroids, in myocardial infarction, 1197
Kidney(s). See also *Renal* entries.
cardiac output to, 1914–1915
circulation of, in heart failure, 410
contrast media–induced dysfunction of, in cardiac catheterization, 180
digoxin effect on, 501
disease of, electrocardiography in, *138*
pain in, 4t
polycystic, 824
diuretic-induced dysfunction of, 480
embolization of, 1921–1923, 1922t
examination of, 18
failure of, 1923–1935. See also *Renal failure*.
in cardiogenic shock, 1920–1921, 1920t
in cyanotic congenital heart disease, 972
in heart failure, 476, 1914–1920, *1915*, 1916t–1917t, *1918*, *1919*
in hypertension, 815, 817–818, 817t
in infective endocarditis, 1086, 1921

Kidney(s) *(Continued)*
in thromboembolic disease, 1922–1923, 1922t
polycystic disease of, 824
sodium retention by, 817–818, 817t
transplantation of, 1924, 1925, *1925*
hypertension and, 825, 1928
Kidney dialysis, 1923–1925, *1924*, 1935–1936
air embolism and, 1936
cardiovascular complications during, 1935–1936
coronary atherosclerosis and, 1924–1925, *1925*
hemolysis and, 1936
hypertension and, 825
hypotension and, 1935
hypoxemia and, 1935–1936
metabolic abnormalities and, 1936
pericarditis in, 1512–1513
prosthetic valves and, 1066
systemic hypertension during, 825
Kinetic work, in myocardial oxygen uptake, 381
King syndrome, genetic factors in, 1660t
Kingella kingii, in infective endocarditis, 1092, 1093t
Kistrin, 1630
Klebsiella, in infective endocarditis, 1093
Klinefelter syndrome, 1656t
Klippel-Feil sequence, 1659t
Klippel-Trenaunay-Weber syndrome, atretic veins in, 1677
Knife injury, 1539–1541, *1541*, 1543
Korotkoff sounds, of arterial pressure measurement, 20
Kugelberg-Welander syndrome, 1877
Kussmaul's sign, 19
in constrictive pericarditis, 1497
in heart failure, 453
with cardiac catheterization, 198
Kwashiorkor, 994
Kyphoscoliosis, 17

Labetalol (Normodyne, Trandate), alpha-blocking potency of, 1306
during pregnancy, 1852t
in aortic dissection, 1564–1565
in arrhythmias, 610–613, 611t
in coronary artery disease, 1149t
in heart failure, 472t, 487
in hypertensive crisis, 858t
in renal failure, 1931t
indications for, 613
pharmacodynamic properties of, 487t
pharmacology of, 1307t
Labor, 977, 1846. See also *Pregnancy.*
Lactate dehydrogenase, in myocardial infarction, *1202*, 1202t, 1204
Lactic dehydrogenase, in heart failure, 456
Ladder diagram, in arrhythmia evaluation, 643, *644*
LAME (*l*entigines, *a*trial *m*yxoma, and *b*lue nevi) association, 1468
Lamifiban, 1820
Landouzy-Dejerine, facioscapulohumeral dystrophy of, 1871–1872, *1872*
Lange-Nielsen syndrome, 1667
Laplace law, in contraction-relaxation cycle, 379–380, *379*
Laryngeal nerve, recurrent, in mitral stenosis, 1010
Laser angioplasty, 1382–1383
Lasix. See *Furosemide (Lasix).*
Lassa fever, myocarditis in, 1439
Lateral view, for plain chest radiography, 211, *212*, *213*
Laurence-Moon-Biedl-Bardet syndrome, 880t
Lead, myocardial effects of, 1447
Lead(s), electrocardiographic, 110–111, *111*
for exercise stress testing, 156–157, *157*
reversal of, 141
Lead impedance, of pacemaker, 711
Leading circle model of reentry, 571–572, *571*
Lecithin:cholesterol acyltransferase deficiency, low high-density lipoprotein in, 1144
Lecompte procedure, in transposition of great arteries, 940
Left anterior oblique view, for plain chest radiography, 212–213, *216*
Left bundle branch, *551*
anatomy of, 550, *551*
Left bundle branch block (LBBB). See also *Fascicular block.*
electrocardiography in, 119–121, *120*, 136, *148*
exercise stress testing in, 168, *169*
incomplete, electrocardiography in, 121, *122*
myocardial infarction and, electrocardiography in, 132–133, *133*
T wave in, 138
temporary pacing in, 706
vectorcardiography in, 121
ventricular hypertrophy in, 119
Left ventricular ejection, of aging heart, 1689–1690, *1691*, *1692*
Left ventricular ejection fraction, 425, 425t, 434, *434*
in elderly, 1694
in heart failure, 458, *459*
in myocardial infarction, 166
in sudden cardiac death, 746
Left ventricular pressure-volume loop, 421, *422*
Leg, ischemia in, with intraaortic balloon counterpulsation, 536
postoperative infection of, 1732
Legionnaires' disease, myocarditis in, 1440
Leiden factor V mutation, 1582t, 1583
Lenegre's disease, sudden cardiac death in, 750
Length constant, of cable, 564
Lentigines, 16
multiple, 880t
LEOPARD syndrome, 880t
Leptospirosis, myocardial involvement in, 1440
Leukemia, cardiac metastases in, 1794–1799, *1795*, 1795t, *1796*, 1796t
Leukocytes, in adult respiratory distress syndrome, 465
in myocardial infarction, 1198, 1204–1205
indium-111–labeled, for infarct imaging, 296
Leukocytosis, in rheumatic fever, 1771
Levine sign, in myocardial infarction, 1199
Levodopa, cardiac complications of, 1881
in heart failure, 486
Levosimendan, in heart failure, 485
Lev's disease, sudden cardiac death in, 750
Liddle's syndrome, 1678, 1678t
Lidocaine (Xylocaine hydrochloride), adverse effects of, 607
dosage of, 594t–595t, 606, *606*
in AMI-related ventricular tachycardia, 1248
in arrhythmias, 594t–595t, 601t, 602t–603t, 605–607
in cardiac arrest, 766
in myocardial infarction, 1246, *1247*, 1248, 1971, 1972t–1973t, 1978
in pediatric cardiology, 1001t
in pregnancy, 1858
in renal failure, 1930t
indications for, 607
neurotoxicity of, 1881
Life Change Units, in myocardial infarction, 1198
Life Style Heart Trial, in hypercholesterolemia prevention, 1131–1132
Lifestyle, modifications in, after myocardial infarction, 1263
in hypertension, 844–846, *845*
Lillehei-Kaster valve, 1061
Limb-girdle dystrophy, 1870–1871
Lipid(s). See also *Dyslipidemia; Hypercholesterolemia.*
in atherosclerosis, 1116
in children, 1002t
Lipid Research Clinic Trials, 1116
Lipid Research Clinics Coronary Primary Prevention Trial, in hypercholesterolemia prevention, 1127–1128
Lipodystrophy, intestinal, myocardial involvement in, 1440
Lipoma, 1471
Lipoprotein, endothelial cell modification of, 1108
high-density, 1127t
deficiency of, xanthomas with, 1144
estrogen replacement therapy and, 1708t
in myocardial infarction, 1204
in women, 1706
low levels of, 1143–1144
tobacco effects on, 1147–1148
in atherosclerosis, 525, 1116
in children, 1002t
in graft atherosclerosis, 525
intermediate-density, 1127t
low-density, 1127t, 1134
Lipoprotein *(Continued)*
apheresis of, in familial hypercholesterolemia, 1143
estrogen replacement therapy and, 1708t
in atherosclerosis, 1108, 1110, 1111, 1116, 1134
in women, 1706
oxidized, in atherosclerosis, 1108, 1110, 1111, 1116, 1134
very-low-density, 1127t
Lipoprotein(a), in atherogenesis, 1111
in coronary artery disease, 1146–1147
plasminogen activator inhibitor-1 synthesis and, 1816
Lisinopril, in heart failure, 472t
in myocardial infarction, 1229–1230, *1230*
in renal failure, 1933t
Listeria monocytogenes, in infective endocarditis, 1082
Lithium, 11
in Ebstein's anomaly, 934
myocardial effects of, 1447
teratogenicity of, 881t, 934, 1663t
tricuspid valve effects of, 878
Liver. See also *Hepatitis*; *Hepato-* entries.
biopsy of, in heart failure, 456
enlargement of, in constrictive pericarditis, 1499
in heart failure, 452, 453
examination of, 17–18
hemangioendothelioma of, heart failure in, 461
in heart failure, 452, 453, 456
preoperative function of, 1717t
transplantation of, in familial hypercholesterolemia, 1143
Löffler endocarditis, 1432–1433, *1432*
Long Q-T syndromes, *684*, 685–686, 881t, 1667
acquired, 567, 686
clinical features of, 685–686
electrocardiography in, *684*, 685
genetic factors in, 685, 1632t
idiopathic (congenital), 567, 685–686, 951
locus 1 for, 1631, 1633
locus 2 for, 1633
locus 3 for, 1633, *1633*
management of, 686
molecular genetics of, 1631–1633, 1632t, *1633*
repolarization in, 567
Losartan, in heart failure, 472t, 474
Lovastatin, in atherosclerosis, *1167*
in dyslipidemia, 1140t, 1141
in hypercholesterolemia prevention, 1130
in renal failure, 1934t
Low birth weight, in hypertension, 817, *817*
Lown-Ganong-Levine syndrome, 669
Low-output syndrome, postoperative, 1725–1727, 1726t
Lung(s). See also *Pulmonary* entries.
amiodarone toxicity to, 614
biopsy of, in pulmonary hypertension, 887
cancer of, cardiac metastases from, 1794–1799, *1795*, 1795t, *1796*, 1796t
pericarditis with, 1513–1516
embryology of, 882
in heart failure, 456
in myocardial infarction, 1196–1197
on myocardial perfusion imaging, 282
transplantation of, 529–530, *529*
bronchiolitis obliterans after, 530
donor for, 529
in pulmonary hypertension, 795–796, *795*
indications for, 529, *529*
infection after, 530
rejection of, 530
Lung scan, in pulmonary embolism, 1589, 1589t, 1590t
in pulmonary hypertension, *789*, 790
Lupus anticoagulant, 799
Lutembacher's syndrome, 896, 967
Lyme carditis, 989–990, 1440–1441
Lymphatic system, in adult respiratory distress syndrome, 465
in pulmonary edema, 462, 463t
Lymphedema, hereditary, 1660t, 1677
Lymphocytes, after heart transplantation, 520
in adult respiratory distress syndrome, 465
T, 1111
Lymphoma, 1471–1472
cardiac metastases from, 1794–1799, *1795*, 1795t, *1796*, 1796t
mediastinal, pericardial effusion in, 1514

M cells, repolarization characteristics of, 562
Machado-Guerrerio test, in trypanosomiasis, 1444
Macrophages, 1110, *1110*
growth factor secretion by, 1110, *1110*
in atherosclerosis, 1114, 1115, 1118, *1119*, *1120*
Macula adherens (desmosome), of intercalated discs, 554
Magnesium, diuretic effects of, 479
in hypertension, 845
in myocardial infarction, 1214, 1231–1232, *1231*
Magnesium sulfate, in cardiac arrest, 766
in Prinzmetal's variant angina, 1340
Magnesium sulfate 3%, in pediatric cardiology, 1001t
Magnetic resonance angiography, of coronary arteries, 321, *322*, *323*
Magnetic resonance imaging (MRI), **317–335**
blood flow effects on, 318–319, *319*, *320*
cine, 319
breath-hold, 328, *329*
velocity-encoded, 331–332, *332–334*
contrast agents for, 332–333
ECG-gated, 319
echoplanar, 317, 320, *334*, 335
fast gradient-echo techniques of, 319–320
gating with, 319
gradient-echo sequence in, 317
hydrogen density in, 317
in abdominal aortic aneurysm, 1549
in aortic dissection, 328–329, *328*, *329*, 1560–1563, *1562*, 1563t
in aortic regurgitation, 1051
in atherosclerosis, 1122
in bacterial endocarditis, 329
in cardiac tumor, *1473*, 1474
in cardiomyopathies, 323–324, *323*
in coarctation of aorta, 327–328, *328*, 332
in congenital heart disease, 327–328, *327*, *328*
in constrictive pericarditis, 1501, *1501*
in cor pulmonale, 1610
in coronary artery bypass grafts, 321–323, *322*, *323*
in coronary artery stenosis, 321, *322*
in dilated cardiomyopathy, 323–324
in hemochromatosis, 1791, *1792*
in hypertrophic cardiomyopathy, 323, *323*
in infective endocarditis, 1089
in intramural aortic hematoma, 1568
in ischemic heart disease, 320–323, *320–323*
in Marfan syndrome, 329
in mitral regurgitation, 331, *333*, 1024
in myocardial infarction, 320–321, *320*, *321*, 1207
in neoplastic disease, 325–327, *326*, 1514, *1514*, 1515, *1515*
in pericardial disease, 235, *236*, 324–325, *325*, *1514*, *1515*
in pregnancy, 1846
in pulmonary embolism, 1591
in restrictive cardiomyopathy, 324
in right ventricular dysplasia, 324, *324*
in thoracic aortic aneurysm, 1551, *1551*
in transposition of great arteries, 327, *327*
in valvular regurgitation, 330–331, *331*
in ventricular sarcoma, 326, *326*
in ventricular thrombus, 326, *326*
magnetic susceptibility agents for, 333, 334–335
multislice, 319
myocardial tagging methods with, 330, *330*
of blood flow velocity, 331–332, *332*, *333*
of cardiovascular function, 329–330, *329*, *330*
of coronary blood flow, 318–319, *319*, *320*, *323*, 331–332, *332–334*
of left ventricular function, 329–330, *329*, *330*
of mammary artery, *323*
of right ventricular function, 329
of stroke volume, 331
pacemaker effects of, 729
paramagnetic agents for, 317, 333–334
principles of, 318–320, *319*, *320*
radiofrequency signal localization in, 318
relaxation times for, 318
relaxing agents for, 332–333
spin-echo sequence in, 318
terminology of, 317–318
velocity-flow mapping with, 331, *332*
Magnetic susceptibility agents, for magnetic resonance imaging, 333, 334–335
Mahaim fibers, in sudden cardiac death, 750
Major histocompatibility complex, in pulmonary hypertension, 787
Mal de Meleda, genetic factors in, 1660t
Malaria, myocardial changes in, 1444
Malignant hyperthermia, genetic factors in, 1660t
Malingering, dyspnea in, 451
Mallory-Weiss syndrome, chest pain in, 7
Malnutrition, 1907–1908, 1907t
preoperative, 1715
protein-calorie, 994, 1715, 1907–1908, 1907t
Malposition, cardiac, 946–947, 1660t
Mammary artery, catheterization of, 254–255, *255*
in coronary artery bypass surgery, 1317–1319, *1317*, *1318*
magnetic resonance imaging of, *323*
Mammary souffle, 40, 45
Mandibulofacial dysostosis, genetic factors in, 1661t
Manifold, for arteriography, 242
Mannitol, in heart failure, 476, 477t
in pediatric cardiology, 1001t
postoperative, 1734
Mannosidosis, 1668t
Marasmus, 994
Marfan syndrome, 880t, 1669–1672, *1670*, 1670t
aortic dissection in, 1671–1672
aortic root involvement in, 1671, *1671*
beta blockers in, 1554
coronary artery disease in, 1349
cystic medial degeneration in, 1550, 1556
diagnosis of, 1669–1670, 1670t
during pregnancy, 1850–1851, *1850*
dysrhythmias in, 1672
etiology of, 1672
extremities in, 17
genes for, 1632t
left ventricular dilatation in, *210*
magnetic resonance imaging in, 329
management of, 1672
mitral valve in, 1670–1671
thoracic abnormalities in, 1671
two-dimensional echocardiography in, 96, *96*
varicose veins in, 1677
Maroteaux-Lamy syndrome, 881t, 1669t, 1675
Masquerading bundle branch block, electrocardiography in, 123, *123*
Maximal work capacity, in exercise stress testing, 164
McArdle syndrome, 1877, *1877*
Means-Lerman scratch, in hyperthyroidism, 461
Mecamylamine, in renal failure, 1932t
Mechanical ventilation, in pulmonary embolism, 1593
postoperative, 1722, 1722t
Media, 1106, *1106*, 1546
Mediastinum, infection of, postoperative, 1732–1733
lymphoma of, pericardial effusion in, 1514
radiation to, in myocardial infarction, 1193
Medical consultation, for noncardiac surgery, 1764–1766, 1765t
Medtronic-Hall valve, 1062, *1062*, 1065
Megaloblastic anemia, drug-induced, 1804
Meige lymphedema, 1677
Melanoma, cardiac metastases from, 1794–1799, *1795*, 1795t, *1796*, 1796t
MELAS (*m*yopathy, *e*ncephalopathy, *l*actic *a*cidosis, and *s*troke-like episodes) syndrome, 1674
Meningococcus, in myocarditis, 1440
in pericarditis, 1509
Menopause. See *Women*.
Mental status, in myocardial infarction, 1201
in syncope, 872
postoperative, 1734–1735, 1736t
Meperidine hydrochloride (Demerol), in myocardial infarction, 1211
in pediatric cardiology, 1001t
Mercurials, hematological abnormalities with, 1804t
Meridional wall stress, of left ventricle, 426–427, *426*
Mesenteric ischemia, postoperative, 1735t
Mesocardia, 946
Mesothelioma, 1471
MET, 154–155, 1392
Metabolic acidosis, in renal failure, 1936
Metabolic equivalent, 154–155, 1392
Metabolic syndrome X, in coronary artery disease, 1150
Metabolism, inborn errors of, 880t–881t, 1666–1667, 1668t–1669t, 1673–1676
Metaiodobenzylguanidine, iodine-123–labeled, 303–304
Metalloproteinases, in atherosclerotic plaque changes, 1187
Metanephrine, in pheochromocytoma, 1898
Metaraminol (Aramine), in atrioventricular nodal reentrant tachycardia, 664
in pediatric cardiology, 1001t
Methacholine, in Prinzmetal's variant angina, 1342
Methazolamide, in heart failure, 477t
Methemoglobinemia, nitroglycerin-associated, 1230, 1303
Methotrexate, in Takayasu's arteritis, 1573
Methoxamine (Vasoxyl), auscultatory effects of, 49
in atrioventricular nodal reentrant tachycardia, 664
3-Methoxy-O-desmethylencainide, in renal failure, 1930t
Methyclothiazide, in heart failure, 477–478, 477t
Methyldopa (Aldomet), during pregnancy, 1852t
hematological abnormalities with, 1804t
in coronary artery disease, 1149t
in hypertension, 852
in pediatric cardiology, 1001t
in renal failure, 1932t
myocardial effects of, 1448
side effects of, 852
Methylglucamine, for arteriography, 245
Methylglucamine–sodium ioxaglate, for arteriography, 245
Methylprednisolone (Solu-Medrol), in pediatric cardiology, 1001t
Methysergide, cardiac complications of, 1881
myocardial effects of, 1446
Metocurine, for anesthesia, 1757
Metolazone, in heart failure, 477–478, 477t
in renal failure, 1933t
Metoprolol, in arrhythmias, 610–613, 611t
in cardiac arrest, 766
in dilated cardiomyopathy, 487, *487*
in myocardial infarction, 1211–1212, 1228–1229, *1228*, 1264, *1264*
in pregnancy, 1858–1859
in renal failure, 1931t
indications for, 612
oxidative metabolism of, 1306
pharmacodynamic properties of, 487t
pharmacology of, 1307t
Mexiletine, adverse effects of, 607
dosage of, 607
electrophysiological actions of, 601t, 602t–603t, 607
hemodynamic effects of, 607
in arrhythmias, 601t, 602t–603t, 607
in pediatric cardiology, 1001t
in pregnancy, 1858
in renal failure, 1930t
indications for, 607
pharmacokinetics of, 607
MICE (*m*esothelial/monocytic *i*ncidental *c*ardiac *e*xcrescens), 1469
Micromanometer catheters, 188
Micturition syncope, 864. See also *Syncope*.
Midnodal cells, of atrioventricular node, *551*
Midsystolic click, in stable angina pectoris, 1292
Migraine, familial, 1677
syncope in, 866
Miller-Dieker syndrome, 1651t
Milrinone, in heart failure, 472t, 484–485, 502
in myocardial infarction, 1237–1238
Mineralocorticoid hypertension, 827–829, *828*
Minipress. See *Prazosin (Minipress)*.
Minoxidil, in heart failure, 472t
in pediatric cardiology, 1001t
in renal failure, 1932t
in systemic hypertension, 855
pericarditis with, 1519
Mitochondria, 360
Mitochondrial diseases, 1875–1876
Mitral annulus, calcification of, 221–223, *222*, 1017–1018, 1024
reconstruction of, in idiopathic dilated cardiomyopathy, 1412
Mitral commissurotomy, in mitral stenosis, 1015

Mitral E point septal separation, 65
Mitral incompetence, systolic murmur in, *28*
Mitral leaflet systolic anterior motion, in hypertrophic cardiomyopathy, 1418, *1418*, 1422
Mitral regurgitation, **1017–1029**, 1025t
acute, *1021*, 1025–1026, 1025t
surgical treatment of, 1029
after myocardial infarction, 535, 1027
annulus calcification in, 1017–1018
annulus dilatation in, 1017
aortic regurgitation and, 1061
aortic stenosis and, 1061
arterial pulse in, 22, 1022
asymptomatic, 1029
auscultation in, 1022–1024, 1023t
cardiac catheterization in, 791t
chordae tendineae abnormalities in, 1018
clinical manifestations of, 1021–1024, *1022*, 1023t
congenital, 923–924
differential diagnosis of, 1023–1024, 1023t
during pregnancy, 1850
early systolic murmur of, 38, *39*
echocardiography in, 57, 73–74, *73*, *74*, 1024–1025, **Plate 1**, **Plate 2**
electrocardiography in, *184*, 1024
end-systolic diameter in, 1020, *1020*
end-systolic volume in, 1020
etiology of, 1017–1019, 1018t
prognosis and, 1029
hemodynamics in, 1020–1021, *1020*
holosystolic murmur in, 38, *38*, *42*
in coronary artery disease, 1019, 1348–1349
in hemolytic anemia, 1790
in mitral valve prolapse, 1034
in secondary pulmonary hypertension, 798
intraaortic balloon counterpulsation in, 535
ischemic, 1027
laboratory examination in, 1024–1026, *1024*
left atrial compliance in, 1021, *1021*
left ventricular angiocardiography in, 1024, *1024*
left ventricular compensation for, 1019
magnetic resonance imaging in, 331, *333*, 1024
midsystolic murmur of, 38
mitral valve reconstruction in, 1026–1028, *1027*, *1028*
mitral valve replacement in, 1026–1028, *1027*
murmur in, 38, *38*, *39*, *42*, 49, 1022–1024, 1023t
myocardial contractility in, 1020
myocardial oxygen consumption in, 1020
natural history of, 1022
papillary muscle dysfunction in, 1018–1019, *1019*
pathology of, 1017–1019, *1019*
pathophysiology of, 1019–1021, *1020*, *1021*
patient history in, 1021–1022
physical examination in, 1022–1024, *1022*, 1023t
plain chest radiography in, 227–228, *227*, *228*
precordial motion in, 24t
pulmonary edema in, 227, *228*
radiological findings in, 1024
radionuclide angiography in, 1025
systolic murmur of, 49
transesophageal echocardiography in, 57, **Plate 1**
treatment of, 1026–1029
angiotensin-converting enzyme inhibitors in, 497
antithrombotic, 1830
medical, 1026
surgical, 1026–1029, *1026–1028*
results of, 1028–1029, *1028*
valve leaflet abnormalities in, 1017
ventricular hypertrophy in, 1020, *1020*
vs. aortic regurgitation, 1019
vs. interventricular septum rupture, 1244
Mitral stenosis, **1007–1017**
angiography in, 1012, 1013–1014
aortic regurgitation and, 1060
aortic stenosis and, 1060–1061
arrhythmias in, 1013
arterial pulse in, 1022
atrial contraction in, 1008
atrial fibrillation in, 1009, 1013
atrial septal defect and, 967
auscultation in, 1010–1011
cardiac catheterization in, 791t, 1013–1014
cardiac output in, 1009
Mitral stenosis *(Continued)*
chest pain in, 1010
clinical manifestations of, 1010–1011
commissurotomy in, 1015
congenital, 79, 923
diagnosis of, 797–798
diastolic murmur of, 49
differential diagnosis of, 1011
Doppler echocardiography in, 1012
during pregnancy, 1849–1850, *1849*
echocardiography in, 71–72, *71*, *72*, 79, 1012, *1012*
electrocardiography in, *150*, 1011–1012
etiology of, 1007
fish mouth appearance of, 1007, *1008*
Gorlin formula in, 1008
heart sounds in, 33–34, *33*, 1024
hemoptysis in, 1010
in elderly, 1698–1699
in hemolytic anemia, 1790
in secondary pulmonary hypertension, 797–798, *798*
infective endocarditis in, 1010
intracardiac pressures in, 1008–1009
intravascular pressures in, 1008–1009
jugular venous pulse in, *19*
Kerley B lines in, 1012
laboratory examination in, 1011–1012, *1012*
laryngeal nerve compression in, 1010
left atrial enlargement in, *209*, *213*, *215*
left atrial pressure pulse in, 1009
left ventricular diastolic pressure in, 1008–1009, *1009*
mid-diastolic murmur of, *33*, 41
murmur of, *33*, 41, 43, *43*, 49, 1011, 1024
myocardial contractility in, 1009
natural history of, 1013, *1013*
noncardiac surgery and, 1761
opening snap in, 1011
palpation in, 25
pathology of, 1007, *1008*
pathophysiology of, 1007–1009, *1009*
patient history in, 1010
physical examination in, 1010–1011
plain chest radiography in, 226–227, *226*, *227*
precordial motion in, 24t
pressure gradients in, 194, *194*
presystolic murmur of, *33*, 43, *43*
pulmonary arterial pressure in, 1009
pulmonary edema in, 798
pulmonary hypertension in, 1009
radiological findings in, 1012
recurrence of, 1014, 1015
thromboembolism in, 1010
transvalvular pressure gradient in, 1008
treatment of, 1012–1017
antithrombotic, 1830
balloon mitral valvuloplasty in, *1015*, 1016–1017, *1016*, *1017*, 1385–1386, *1385*
medical, 1012–1013
surgical, 1013–1017
indications for, 1013–1014
techniques of, 1014–1015
valvotomy in, 1014–1015
vectorcardiography in, 1012
Mitral valve, area of, 194–195
calcifications of, 221–223, *222*, 1017–1018, 1024
closure of, palpation of, 28
cross-sectional area of, 1007
in rheumatoid arthritis, 1776
M-mode echocardiography of, 63, *63*
myxomatous, in mitral regurgitation, 1030–1031, *1031*
on myocardial perfusion imaging, 277
opening snap of, in mitral stenosis, 1011
parachute deformity of, 919, 923
reconstruction of, 1385–1386, *1385*
in idiopathic dilated cardiomyopathy, 1412
in mitral regurgitation, 1026–1028, *1027*, *1028*
in mitral valve prolapse, 1035
replacement of, 1065t
in hypertrophic cardiomyopathy, 1426
in mitral regurgitation, 1026–1028, *1027*
in mitral stenosis, 1015
on plain radiography, *217*
trauma to, 1542
Mitral valve prolapse, **1029–1032**
after myocardial infarction, 1031–1032
angiography in, 1033–1034
Mitral valve prolapse *(Continued)*
asymptomatic, 1035, 1035t
auscultation in, 1032–1033
chest pain in, 4t
clinical manifestations of, 1032–1033
definition of, 1029–1030, 1030t
diagnosis of, 1029–1030, 1030t
during pregnancy, 1850
echocardiography in, 73–74, *73*, *74*, 1033, *1034*
electrocardiography in, 1033
electron microscopy in, 1030–1031, *1031*
etiology of, 1030
genetic factors in, 1660t, 1662–1663
heart sounds in, *31*
hereditary factors in, 1031
in children, 888
in coronary artery disease, 1299
in Marfan syndrome, 1670–1671
infective endocarditis in, 1078, 1098, 1098t
laboratory examination in, 1033–1034, *1034*
late systolic murmur of, 39–40
murmurs in, 39–40, 1023t
myocardial perfusion imaging in, 1033
natural history of, *1030*, 1034
parasternal view in, 1030
pathology of, 1030–1032, *1031*
patient history in, 1032
pectus excavatum with, *213*
physical examination in, 1032
preoperative antibiotic prophylaxis in, 1762
sudden cardiac death in, 750
systolic clicks of, 31–32, *31*
systolic crackles of, 31
transient ischemic attack in, 1830
treatment of, 1035, 1035t, 1830
ventricular tachycardia in, 682
vs. hypertrophic cardiomyopathy, 1033
Mixed connective tissue disease, 1782
pericarditis in, 1519
Mixed venous oxygen content, calculation of, 197
MLC-*ras* fusion gene, in cardiac hypertrophy, 1643
M-mode echocardiography, 54, *54*, *55*. See also *Echocardiography, M-mode.*
Mobilization, in cardiac rehabilitation, 1399
Mohr syndrome, genetic factors in, 1661t
Molsidomine, in heart failure, 475
Monitored Atherosclerosis Regression Study, in hypercholesterolemia prevention, 1132
Monoclonal antibodies, 1629
platelet-specific integrin $\alpha_{IIb}\beta_3$, 1630, *1819*, 1820
after coronary angioplasty, 1314, 1315, 1827
in PTCA-related abrupt vessel closure, 1369, 1370t, 1373
Monocytes, in adult respiratory distress syndrome, 465
in atherosclerosis, 1117–1118, *1117*, *1118*
Moricizine hydrochloride (Ethmozine), adverse effects of, 610
after myocardial infarction, 1265
dosage of, 610
electrophysiological actions of, 601t, 602t–603t, 610
hematological abnormalities with, 1804t
hemodynamic effects of, 610
in arrhythmias, 601t, 602t–603t, 610
in heart failure, 505
in renal failure, 1930t
indications for, 610
pharmacokinetics of, 610
Morphine sulfate, for anesthesia, 1757
in myocardial infarction, 1210–1211
in pediatric cardiology, 1001t
in unstable angina, 1982t
Morquio syndrome, 881t, 1669t, 1675
Motor neuropathy, 1678t
Motorcycle accident, 1535. See also *Traumatic heart disease.*
Mouse, cardiac hypertrophy in, 1640–1641, *1641*
transgenic, 1635–1637, *1635*
in atherosclerosis modeling, 1636–1637, *1636*, 1636t, *1637*
MRI. See *Magnetic resonance imaging (MRI).*
Mucocutaneous lymph node syndrome. See *Kawasaki disease (mucocutaneous lymph node syndrome).*
Mucolipidoses, 1668t

Mucopolysaccharidoses, 881t, 1668t–1669t, 1675, *1675*
Mucormycosis, myocarditis in, 1442
Mueller maneuver, with cardiac catheterization, 198
MULIBREY (*m*uscle, *li*ver, *br*ain, and *ey*e) nanism, 1498, 1666
Müller maneuver, murmur response to, 47
Müller's sign, in aortic regurgitation, 1049
Multicentre Anti-Atheroma Study, in hypercholesterolemia prevention, 1133
Multiple endocrine neoplasia, 1678t
  type 2A, 829
Multiple myeloma, heart failure in, 462
Multiple sulfatase deficiency, 1669t
Multipurpose catheters, for arteriography, 242, *243*
Multivariate analysis, in exercise stress testing evaluation, 163
Mumps, myocarditis in, 1439
Murmur(s), **35–45.** See also *Heart sound(s).*
  arterial, systolic, 40, *40*
  Austin Flint, *42*
    in aortic regurgitation, 1050
  cardiorespiratory, 45
  Carey-Coombs, 1011
  continuous, 35, 43–45, *44, 45*
    arterial, 45
    arteriovenous, 45
    pharmacological effects on, 46t, 49
    physiological effects on, 46–49, 46t
    venous, 45, *45*
  diastolic, 35, 40–43, *40*
    in aortic regurgitation, *1046*, 1050
    in mitral stenosis, 1011
    in pulmonic valve disease, 1059
    in tricuspid stenosis, *1054*, 1055
    pharmacological effects on, 46t, 49
    physiological effects on, 46–49, 46t
  early diastolic, 40–41, *40*
  early systolic, *36*, 38–39, *39*
  echocardiography of, 1042
  Graham Steell, *31*, 41
  holosystolic, 36, *36*, 38, *38*, *39*
  in anemia, 1787
  in aortic dissection, 1556
  in aortic regurgitation, *1046*, 1050
  in aortic stenosis, 1023t, 1041
  in atrial fibrillation, 1011
  in atrial septal defect, 896–897
  in children, 11
  in congenital aortic stenosis, 915, 916
  in congenital pulmonic stenosis, 925
  in coronary artery disease, 1292
  in cyanosis, 893
  in hyperthyroidism, 1892
  in hypertrophic cardiomyopathy, 1041, 1420, 1420t
  in idiopathic dilated cardiomyopathy, 1410
  in infective endocarditis, 1084–1085, 1084t, 1086
  in juxtaductal coarctation, 912
  in left atrial tumors, 1466
  in left ventricular tumors, 1467
  in mitral regurgitation, 1022–1023, 1023t
  in mitral stenosis, 1011
  in mitral valve prolapse, 1032–1033
  in myocardial infarction, 1201
  in pregnancy, 1845
  in pulmonary artery stenosis, 924
  in pulmonary hypertension, 887
  in pulmonic valve disease, 1059
  in renal failure, 1927–1928
  in right atrial tumors, 1466
  in right ventricular tumors, 1466
  in stable angina pectoris, 1292
  in supravalvular aortic stenosis, 921
  in tetralogy of Fallot, 930
  in total anomalous pulmonary venous connection, 945
  in transposition of great arteries, 937
  in tricuspid regurgitation, 1023t, 1057
  in ventricular septal defect, 1023t
  isometric exercise effects on, 48–49
  late diastolic (presystolic), *40*, 43, *43*, *44*
  late systolic, *36*, 39–40, *39*
    in mitral regurgitation, 1023
  mid-diastolic, *39*, *40*, 41–43, *42*
  midsystolic, 36–38, *36*, *37*
    in aortic sclerosis, 36–37, *37*, 38
    in aortic valve stenosis, 36–37, *37*
    in mitral regurgitation, 38
Murmur(s) *(Continued)*
    in pulmonary valve stenosis, *31*, 37
    normal, 37–38, *37*
    out-flow, 36, *36*
  Müller maneuver effect on, 47
  pansystolic, in mitral regurgitation, 1023
    in tricuspid regurgitation, 1011
  pharmacological effects on, 46t, *48*, 49
  postural effects on, 47–48, *48*
  respiration effects on, 47
  Still's, 37–38, *37*
  systolic, 35, 36–40, *36–40*
    in aortic stenosis, 1041
    in heart failure, 455
    in hypertrophic cardiomyopathy, 1033
    in mitral regurgitation, 1022–1023, 1023t
    in mitral valve prolapse, 1032, 1033
    in tricuspid regurgitation, 1011
    pharmacological effects on, 46t, *48*, 49
    physiological effects on, 46–49, 46t
    supraclavicular, 40, *40*
    Valsalva maneuver effects on, 47, *47*
Muscarinic receptors, in contraction-relaxation cycle, 374–375, *374*, 375t
Muscle bands, anomalous, in intraventricular right ventricular obstruction, 928–929
Muscle relaxants, for anesthesia, 1757
Muscular dystrophy, 880t
  Becker, 1869–1872, *1871*
  Duchenne, 1865–1869, *1866–1868*
  Emery-Dreifuss, 1872, *1872*
  limb-girdle, 1870–1871
  myotonic, 1632t, 1872–1874, *1873*, *1874*
  of Landouzy-Dejerine, 1871–1872, *1872*
Muscular subaortic stenosis. See *Cardiomyopathy, hypertrophic.*
Myasthenia gravis, 1877
  in secondary pulmonary hypertension, 801
Mycophenolate mofetil, in heart transplantation rejection, 523
Mycoplasma pneumoniae, in myocarditis, 1440
  in pericarditis, 1506
Mycotic aneurysm, in adult congenital heart disease, 974, *974*
  in infective endocarditis, 1096
Myocardial bridging, arteriography of, 258–259, *258*
Myocardial contractility, 421
  afterload and, 402, *402*
  ejection phase indices of, 430–431, *430*
  Frank-Starling mechanism in, 433, *434*
  in heart failure, 397–399, *398*
  in left ventricular function, 422
  in mitral regurgitation, 1020
  in mitral stenosis, 1009
  indices of, 429–432, 429t
  isovolumetric phase indices of, 430, *430*
  myocardial oxygen consumption and, 1162–1163
  pressure-volume relations in, 431–432, *431–433*
  ventricular dP/dt_{max} index of, 430, *430*
  V_{max} index of, 430, *430*
Myocardial contusion. See *Contusion, myocardial.*
Myocardial depression, electrocardiography in, *125*, 126
Myocardial failure. See *Heart failure.*
Myocardial glucose utilization, fluorine-18–labeled fluoro-2-deoxyglucose imaging of, 304t, 305–306, **Plate 7**
Myocardial hibernation, 388, 388t, 1176, 1215
  after coronary artery bypass surgery, 1327–1328, *1327*, 1328t
  contractile reserve in, 1327, *1327*
  detection of, 1327–1328, *1327*, 1328t
  echocardiography of, 89
  in coronary artery disease, 1299
Myocardial infarction, **1184–1266.** See also *Angina pectoris, unstable.*
  abdominal examination in, 1201
  accelerated idioventricular rhythm in, 1245t, 1246–1247
  adrenal cortex in, 1197
  adrenal medulla in, 1197
  after coronary artery bypass surgery, 1319, 1326
  after heart transplantation, 1349
  age and, 1185
  ambulatory electrocardiographic monitoring in, 1977t
Myocardial infarction *(Continued)*
  analgesia in, 1210–1211, *1211*
  anatomy of, 1192–1193, *1192*
  angiographically normal vessels and, 1194
  angiography in, 1977t
    practice guidelines for, 1950t, 1952
  anterior, *86*, 129t, 135, *135*
  anterolateral, 129t, 135, *135*
  anteroseptal, 129t, 135, *135*
  anticoagulants after, 1828, *1828*
  arrhythmias in, **1245–1257,** 1245t
    hemodynamic consequences of, 1246
    management of, 1245t
    mechanism of, 1246
    pacemakers for, 1252–1253
    ventricular, 1245t, 1246–1249, *1247*
  arterial embolism in, 1256–1257
  arteriography in, 241
  aspirin after, 1827–1828
  asystole in, 1253
  atrial, 1192–1193, 1206
  atrial fibrillation in, 1253–1254
  atrial flutter in, 1253–1254
  atrial premature contractions in, 1253
  atrioventricular block in, 1250–1251, 1251t
  atypical presentation of, 1199
  auscultation in, 1200–1201
  beta blockers in, 1211–1212, 1228–1229, *1228*, 1974t, 1978
  bifascicular block in, 1252
  blood pressure in, 1200
  blood viscosity in, 1198
  body temperature in, 1200
  bradyarrhythmias in, 1245t, 1249
  cardiac arrest in, 766–767
  cardiac catheterization in, 178–179, 178t. See also *Cardiac catheterization.*
  cardiac examination in, 1200–1201
  cardiogenic shock in, 1238–1241
    diagnosis of, 1239
    intraaortic balloon counterpulsation in, 1239
    medical management of, 1239
    pathological findings in, 1238–1239, *1238*
    pathophysiology of, 1239
    reperfusion in, 1240
  carotid pulse in, 1200
  chest examination in, 1200
  chest roentgenography in, 1206–1207
  cholesterol in, 1204
  circadian periodicity in, 1187, 1198
  circulatory regulation in, 1195, *1195*
  clinical features of, 1198–1207
  coagulation in, 1191, 1197–1198
  coagulation necrosis in, 1191
  collateral vessels in, 1175, 1192
  complications of, 1241–1245, 1241t
    computed tomography of, 336–337, *337*
    echocardiography in, 87–88, *87*, *88*
    magnetic resonance imaging of, 321, *321*
  computed tomography in, 336–337, *337*, 1206–1207
  contraction band necrosis in, 1191, *1191*
  coronary artery bypass surgery in, 1223, 1976t, 1979
  cost-effectiveness analysis in, 1750
  creatine kinase in, 1202–1203, *1202*, 1202t, 1207
  Dressler syndrome in, 1256
  during right ventricular pacing, 713–714
  dystrophic calcification in, 221
  echocardiography in, 87–90, *87–90*, 1206, *1206*, 1241, 1973t, 1977t
  electrocardiography in, 127–135, *128–135*, 129t, *147–150*, 713–714, 1189, 1202, 1205–1210, *1206*, *1209*, 1240–1241, 1725
    for monitoring, 1971, 1972t
    nondiagnostic, *1206*, 1210
    Ta segment abnormality on, 116
  electron microscopy of, *1189*, 1190, *1190*
  endocrine system in, 1197
  endothelial vasodilator dysfunction in, 1166
  evaluation after, 1976t–1977t, 1979
  exercise stress testing in, 165–167, *167*
    practice guidelines for, 1942
  expansion of, 1195, 1212, *1213*, 1238, *1238*
  extremities examination in, 1201
  false aneurysm with, 1242–1243, *1242*
    echocardiography of, 87, *87*
    magnetic resonance imaging of, 321, *321*
  fibrinolysis deficiency in, 1816

Myocardial infarction *(Continued)*
first-degree atrioventricular block in, 1250, 1251t
fourth heart sound in, 1201
free wall rupture in, 1241–1243, 1241t, *1242*
clinical characteristics of, 1242
diagnosis of, 1243
pseudoaneurysm with, 1242–1243, *1242*
funduscopic examination in, 1201
general appearance in, 1199
heart rate in, 1199–1200
hemodynamic system in, **1233–1245**
abnormalities of, 1234–1245, 1234t
cardiogenic shock as, 1238–1241, *1238*
left ventricular failure as, 1194–1195, 1235–1238, *1235*
papillary muscle rupture and, 1243–1244, *1243*
right ventricular infarction and, 1240–1241, 1240t
septal rupture and, 1243, 1244
wall rupture and, 1241–1243, 1241t, *1242*
assessment of, 1233–1235, 1233t
monitoring of, 1233–1234, 1233t, 1971, 1972t
hemorrhagic, *1191*, 1214
hyperdynamic state in, 1235
hypertension in, 815
hypotension in, 1234–1235
hypovolemic hypotension in, 1235
in diabetes mellitus, 1901
in elderly, 1697
in pregnancy, 1853–1854, *1854*
in sickle cell disease, 1788
in sudden cardiac death, 753
in women, 1710–1711, *1710*, *1711*
indium-111–labeled antimyosin imaging of, 296–297, *296*
indium-111–labeled leukocyte imaging of, 296
inferior, 129t, 135, *135*
inferolateral, 129t, 135, *135*
intraarterial pressure monitoring in, 1972t
intraventricular block in, 1251–1252
ischemic mitral regurgitation after, 1027
jugular venous pulse in, 1200
junctional rhythms in, 1254
laboratory examination in, 1202–1207, *1202*, 1202t
computed tomography in, 1206–1207
creatine kinase in, 1202–1203, *1202*, 1202t
echocardiography in, 1206, *1206*, 1241, 1973t, 1977t
electrocardiography in, 1202, 1205–1208, *1206*, *1209*, 1240–1241
hematological measurements in, 1204–1205
lactic dehydrogenase in, *1202*, 1202t, 1204
magnetic resonance imaging in, 1207
myoglobin in, *1202*, 1202t, 1203
nuclear imaging in, 1207
practice guidelines for, 1944, 1945t
roentgenography in, 1206
serum lipids in, 1204
troponins in, *1202*, 1202t, 1203–1204
lactic dehydrogenase in, *1202*, 1202t, 1204
left anterior divisional block in, 1251–1252
left bundle branch block and, electrocardiography in, 132–133, *133*
left posterior divisional block in, 1252
left ventricular aneurysm in, 1256
left ventricular dysfunction in, *746*, 747, 1194–1195, 1235–1238, *1235*
afterload reduction in, 1236–1237
amrinone in, 1237–1238
beta-adrenoceptor agonists in, 1237
digitalis in, 1237
diuretics in, 1236
hypoxemia avoidance in, 1236
milrinone in, 1237–1238
nitroglycerin in, 1236–1237
oral vasodilators in, 1237
therapeutic implications of, 1236
left ventricular ejection fraction in, 166
left ventricular thrombus in, 1256–1257, *1257*
leukocytes in, 1198
light microscopy of, *1189*, 1190–1191
magnetic resonance imaging in, 320–321, *320*, *321*, 1207
contrast agents for, 332–333
management of, **1207–1232**
afterload reduction in, 1236–1237

Myocardial infarction *(Continued)*
amrinone in, 1237–1238
analgesics in, 1210–1211, *1211*
angioplasty in, 1221–1223, *1222*
recommendations for, 1222–1223
anticoagulation in, 1974t–1975t, 1978
antiplatelet therapy in, 1225, *1225*
antithrombotic therapy in, 1223–1225, 1826, 1826t
complications of, 1224
mortality and, 1224
recommendations for, 1224–1225
aspirin in, 1210, 1225, *1225*, 1826
atropine in, 1972t
beta-adrenoceptor agonists in, 1237
beta-adrenoceptor blocking agents in, 1211–1212, 1228–1229, *1228*, 1974t, 1978
calcium channel blockers in, 1974t, 1978
changing patterns in, 1184–1185
constipation and, 1257
coronary artery bypass graft surgery in, 1223, 1976t, 1979
cost-effectiveness of, 1184, 1749–1750
diet in, 1226, 1227t
digitalis in, 501, 1237
diuretics in, 1236
emergency department, *1206*, 1208–1213, *1209*, *1210*
gender variation in, 1185
glucoprotein IIb/IIIa receptor antagonists in, 1225
heparin in, 1223–1225, 1826, 1826t, 1832–1833
hirudin in, 1224
hospital, 1226–1228, 1227t
counseling after, 1258
discharge from, 1257–1258
hypoxemia avoidance in, 1236
imaging after, 354t, 355
in women, 1711, *1711*
infarct size limitation in, 1212–1213, *1213*
intraaortic balloon counterpulsation in, 1976t, 1978–1979
lidocaine in, 1971, 1972t–1973t, 1978
limitations of, 1184–1185
milrinone in, 1237–1238
nitrates in, 1211
nitroglycerin in, 1236–1237
oral vasodilators in, 1237
outcome of, 1184, *1185*
oxygen in, 1212
pacemaker in, 707, 708t, 1252–1253, 1973t, 1978
practice guidelines for, 1964t
pain control in, 1210–1212, *1211*
percutaneous transluminal coronary angioplasty in, 1375–1376, 1975t, 1978
cost-effectiveness analysis of, 1749–1751
practice guidelines for, 1956t, 1957
pharmacological, 1228–1232
ACE inhibitors in, 1229–1230, *1230*
beta-adrenoceptor blocking agents in, 1211–1212, 1228–1229, *1228*, 1974t, 1978
calcium channel blockers in, 1231, 1974t, 1978
diltiazem in, 1231
glucose-insulin-potassium in, 1232, *1232*
lidocaine in, 1971, 1972t–1973t, *1978*
magnesium in, 1231–1232, *1231*
nifedipine in, 1231
nitrates in, 1211, 1230–1231
verapamil in, 1231
physical activity in, 1227, 1227t
practice guidelines for, 1956t, 1957, 1964t
prehospital, 1207–1208
racial variation in, 1185
reperfusion in, 1191–1192, *1191*, *1196*, 1213–1215
arrhythmias with, 1214
arterial patency and, 1215
injury with, 1213–1214
ischemic preconditioning and, 1214
prehospital, 1208
spontaneous, 1212
surgical, 1223
troponin release and, 1204
streptokinase in, 1824–1826, *1825*, 1825t
tertiary care transfer in, 1973t, 1978
therapeutic implications of, 1236

Myocardial infarction *(Continued)*
thrombolytic therapy in, *1206*, 1208–1210, *1209*, *1210*, 1215–1221, 1224, 1824–1826, *1825*, 1970–1971, 1971t
agents for, 1218–1219, 1221
angioplasty and, 1222
arterial patency and, 1215–1216
complications of, 1219–1220
contraindications to, 1210t
cost-effectiveness analysis of, 1749
door-to-needle time for, 1210t
evaluation of, 1215–1216, *1216*
intracoronary, 1215
intravascular catheterization during, 1221
intravenous, 1215, 1824–1826, *1825*, 1825t
left ventricular function and, 1219
mortality and, 1216–1218, *1216–1218*, 1218t
mortality pyramid and, 1218, *1218*
myocardial perfusion imaging after, 286–287, *287*
recommendations for, 1220–1221
TIMI frame count evaluation of, 1216
timing of, 1221, 1826
tissue-type plasminogen activator in, 1224, 1225, 1824–1826, *1825*, 1825t
ventricular assist device in, 1976t
warfarin in, 1832–1833
mechanical complications of, 1241–1245, 1241t
mitral regurgitation after, 1027
mitral valve prolapse after, 1031–1032
mortality in, *746*, 747, 1184, *1185*, 1216–1218, *1216–1218*, 1218t
age and, 1185
infarct expansion and, 1195
mural thrombus after, echocardiography of, 88, *88*
myocardial perfusion imaging in, 285–288, *285*, *286*
after thrombolytic therapy, 286–287, *287*
in emergency department, 286
myocardial viability in, positron emission tomography for, 306, 306t
myocytolysis in, 1191
myoglobin in, *1202*, 1202t, 1203
natriuretic peptides in, 1197
natural history of, echocardiography of, 88
electrocardiography of, 129–130, *130*, *131*
neuropsychiatric findings in, 1201
nitroblue tetrazolium stain in, 1190
nonatherosclerotic etiology of, 1193, 1193t
noncardiac surgery and, 1758–1761
non–Q-wave, 1185–1189, *1187*, *1188*, *1192*, 1259
nonsteroidal anti-inflammatory drugs in, 1512
nuclear imaging in, 1207
old, electrocardiography in, 132
myocardial perfusion imaging of, 288
oxyhemoglobin in, 1197
pacemaker in, 707, 708t, 1252–1253, 1973t, 1978
practice guidelines for, 1964t
pain in, 5, 1198–1199, 1254–1255
vs. angina pectoris, 1291–1292
palpation in, 1200
pancrease in, 1197
papillary muscle rupture in, 1241t, 1243–1244, *1243*
repair of, *1244*, 1245
paroxysmal supraventricular tachycardia in, 1253
pathology of, 1185–1194, *1186*, *1187*
acute plaque change in, 1185–1189, *1186–1188*
anatomy of, 1192–1193, *1192*
coagulation necrosis in, 1191, *1191*
collateral circulation and, 1193
contraction band necrosis in, 1191, *1191*
coronary artery spasm in, 1193
electrocardiography and, 1189
electron microscopy of, *1189*, 1190, *1190*
gross, *1188*, 1189–1190, *1189*
light microscopy of, *1189*, 1190–1191
nonatherosclerotic factors in, 1193, 1193t
plaque composition in, 1187, *1187*
plaque fissuring in, *1186*, 1187
plaque rupture in, 1188–1189
reperfusion in, 1191–1192, *1191*
with angiographically normal vessels, 1194

Myocardial infarction *(Continued)*
pathophysiology of, 1194–1198
circulatory regulation in, 1195, *1195*
diastolic function in, 1194–1195
endocrine system changes and, 1197
hematological system changes and, 1197–1198
infarct expansion in, 1195
pulmonary system changes and, 1196–1197
renal system changes and, 1197
systolic function in, 1194
treatment effects on, 1196, *1196*
ventricular dilatation in, 1195–1196, *1196*
ventricular remodeling in, 1195–1196, *1196*
patient history in, 1198–1199
percutaneous transluminal coronary angioplasty in, 178–179
pericardial effusion in, 1255
pericardial friction rub in, 1201
pericarditis in, 1255–1256, 1511–1512
periinfarction block and, electrocardiography in, 133, *133*
physical examination in, 1199–1201
abdominal examination in, 1201
auscultation in, 1200–1201
blood pressure in, 1200
body temperature in, 1200
cardiac examination in, 1200–1201
carotid pulse in, 1200
chest examination in, 1200
extremities examination in, 1201
funduscopic examination in, 1201
general appearance in, 1199
heart rate in, 1199–1200
jugular venous pulse in, 1200
neuropsychiatric examination in, 1201
palpation in, 1200
plaques in, 1185–1189, *1186–1188*
composition of, 1186–1187, *1187*
fissuring of, *1186*, 1187
rupture of, *1186*, 1187
platelets in, 1197
positron emission tomography in, 306, 306t
posterior, 134–135, *135*
postoperative, 1723–1725, 1724t, 1763–1764
diagnosis of, 1724, 1724t
echocardiography in, 1725
electrocardiography in, 1725
mortality with, 1725
troponin in, 1724–1725
practice guidelines for, 1942, 1970–1979, 1976t
predisposition to, 1198
premature ventricular complexes in, 677
preoperative, 1716–1718
prevention of, aspirin in, 1829, 1829t
secondary, 1263–1266
ACE inhibitors in, 1264
antiarrhythmic agents in, 1265–1266, *1266*
anticoagulants in, 1265, *1265*
antiplatelet agents in, 1264
beta-adrenoceptor blockers in, 1264, *1264*
calcium channel blockers in, 1265
estrogen replacement therapy in, 1266
life style modification in, 1263
lipid profile modification in, 1263–1264
nitrates in, 1264–1265
prodromal symptoms in, 1198
prognosis for, 1258–1263, *1259*
arterial patency in, 1260, *1260*
demographic factors in, 1258
discharge assessment in, 1260, *1260*
echocardiography of, 88–89, *89*
electrocardiography in, 1258, 1261–1263
exercise test in, 1261
hospital course in, 1258–1260
left ventricular function in, 1259–1261
myocardial perfusion imaging in, 287–288, *287*, 1261
rales classification and, 1200
pseudoaneurysm with, 1242–1243, *1242*
echocardiography of, 87, *87*
magnetic resonance imaging of, 321, *321*
pulmonary artery pressure monitoring in, 1233–1234, 1233t
pulmonary embolism in, 1256
pulmonary system in, 1196–1197
Q-wave, 128–129, 1185–1189, *1187*, *1188*, *1192*, 1205, 1259, *1259*

Myocardial infarction *(Continued)*
management of, 1208, *1209*
radionuclide angiocardiography in, 302–303, *302*
rales in, 1200, 1234t
recurrent, 1254–1255, *1255*
vs. Dressler syndrome, 1520
recurrent chest discomfort in, 1254–1255
renal function in, 1197
renin-angiotensin system in, 1197
respiration in, 1200
rest radionuclide ventriculography after, 1977t
right bundle branch block in, 1252
right heart catheterization in, 1972t
right ventricular dysfunction in, 1192, 1240–1241, 1240t
echocardiography in, 1241
electrocardiography in, 134, *134*, 1205–1206
hemodynamics in, 1241
radionuclide angiography in, 1241
treatment of, 1241
right ventricular infarction after, 88, *88*
risk stratification after, 1258–1263, *1262*
arrhythmia assessment and, 1261–1263
at hospital discharge, 1260, *1260*
hospital course and, 1258–1260, *1259*
initial presentation in, 1258, *1259*
left ventricular function in, 1260–1261
recurrent myocardial ischemia and, 1261
scar formation in, 1196
electrocardiography of, 133
second-degree atrioventricular block in, 1250, 1251t
septal, 134
septal aneurysm after, 87–88
septal defect in, 1241t, 1243, 1244, *1244*, 1245
silent, 1199
systemic hypertension in, 815
sinus tachycardia in, 1253
size of, 1207
spontaneous reperfusion in, 1212
ST alternans in, 131–132
ST segment in, 714, 1205–1206, *1206*, 1208–1210
exercise-induced changes in, 166
stenosis severity in, 269
subendocardial, *1188*, 1189–1190
supraventricular tachyarrhythmias in, 1253–1254
symptoms of, 1191, 1198–1199
syncope in, 867
systolic murmur in, 1201
T wave in, *138*, 714
Ta segment abnormality in, 116
technetium-99m–labeled Sn-pyrophosphate imaging of, 296, *296*
temporary pacing in, 706–707
third heart sound in, 1201
third-degree atrioventricular block in, 1250–1251, 1251t
thrombi in, 88, *88*, 1186–1187, *1186*, 1256–1257, *1257*
arteriography of, 265–266, *266*
thyroid gland in, 1197
transmural, *1188*, 1189–1190
magnetic resonance imaging of, 320–321, *320*
triage for, 1970–1971
triphenyltetrazolium chloride stain in, *1189*, 1190
troponins in, *1202*, 1202t, 1203–1204
tumor-related, 1798
U wave in, 132, *132*
vectorcardiography in, 135, *135*
venous thrombosis in, 1256
ventricular arrhythmias in, 1245t, 1246–1249, *1247*
ventricular assist device in, 542
ventricular dilatation in, 1195–1196, *1196*
ventricular fibrillation in, 1248–1249
ventricular premature beats in, 1245t, 1246, *1247*
ventricular pressure-volume relationships in, 404
ventricular remodeling in, 1195–1196, *1196*
ventricular septal defect in, 1241t, 1243
repair of, *1244*, 1245
vs. mitral regurgitation, 1244
ventricular tachycardia in, 1245t, 1247–1248
late potentials in, 583–584, *584*

Myocardial infarction *(Continued)*
vital capacity in, 1197
vs. aortic dissection, 1557
vs. myocardial contusion, 1538
white blood cell count in, 1204–1205
Wolff-Parkinson-White syndrome and, 126–127, *126*, *127*
Myocardial ischemia, **1161–1179.** See also *Blood flow, coronary; Myocardial infarction.*
ambulatory electrocardiography in, 1345, *1345*
practice guidelines for, 1947t, 1948
arrhythmia initiation by, 755–756
beta-adrenoceptor blocker effect on, 1304, *1305*
calcium in, 1178–1179
cardiac tamponade and, 1487
collateral vessels in, 1175
computed tomography of, 336–339, *337*
congenital coronary stenosis in, 260
consequences of, 1176–1179, *1176–1178*, 1176t, 1178t
contractile impairment in, 386–388, *386*, *387*
contracture of, 387, *387*
coronary artery fistula in, arteriography of, 259–260, *260*
coronary artery origin from aortic sinus in, 260–261
coronary artery origin from sinus of Valsalva in, 261, *261*, *262*
definition of, 1161, *1161*
demand, 386–387
diastolic current of injury in, 127, *128*
echocardiography in, 85–90, *86–90*
electrocardiography in, 127, *128*, *129*, *147*, *148*, 1295
practice guidelines for, 1947t, 1948
electrophysiology of, 561, 755–756, 1178
endothelial cell dysfunction in, 1166–1167, *1166*, *1167*
hemodynamic consequences of, 1176–1177
high-energy phosphate metabolism during, 1178, 1178t
hypertension in, 858
imaging in, 228–229, 354–355, 354t
in aortic stenosis, 1039
in cardiac rehabilitation, 1393–1394, 1396
in elderly, 1696–1697
in hypertrophic cardiomyopathy, 1418, 1419t
in pulmonary hypertension, 1610–1611
in renal failure, 1925–1926, *1925*, 1927
intermittent, 387–388
iodine-123–labeled metaiodobenzylguanidine imaging of, 303–304
left coronary artery origin from pulmonary artery in, arteriography of, 260–262, *260*
left ventricular diastolic properties in, *402*, 403
left ventricular performance in, 86–87
magnetic resonance imaging of, 320–323, *320–323*
metabolic consequences of, *1177*, 1178–1179, 1178t
noncardiac surgery and, 1758–1761
oxidative phosphorylation during, 1178
pathophysiology of, 155
practice guidelines for, 1944, 1946, 1947t, 1948
preconditioning in, 387–388, *388*
predischarge assessment of, after myocardial infarction, 1261
radionuclide imaging in, 303–304
practice guidelines for, 1944, 1946
reactive hyperemia in, 1173–1174, *1173*
recurrence of, after myocardial infarction, 1254–1255, *1255*
reperfusion injury after, *1178*, 1179
reperfusion modification of, 1191–1192, *1191*, *1196*
resting electrocardiography in, 1295
silent, 1344–1346, *1345*, *1346*
ambulatory electrocardiography in, 1345, *1345*
exercise stress testing in, 165
management of, 1345–1346
mechanisms of, 1345, *1346*
pain perception absence in, 308
prognosis for, 1345
radionuclide angiocardiography in, 302
ST segment in, 127, *127*
subendocardial, 1169–1170, *1169*, *1170*, 1177–1178, *1177*

Myocardial ischemia *(Continued)*
supply, 386–387
systolic current of injury in, 127, *128*
T wave in, *132*, 136
transient, imaging in, 354–355, 354t
transstenotic pressure gradient in, 1171–1172, *1171*, *1172*
two-dimensional echocardiography in, 85–86, *86*, *87*
ventricular pressure-volume relationships in, 404
ventricular relaxation in, 402–403, *402*
ventricular tachycardia with, 629, 631
ventricular wall stiffness in, 403, *403*, *404*
vs. acute pericarditis, 1482t
vs. postinfarction pericarditis, 1512
wavefront of, 1177–1178, *1177*
Myocardial necrosis. See also *Myocardial ischemia.*
coagulation, *1189*, 1191
contraction band, 1191, *1191*
in scleroderma, 1781
piecemeal, in cardiogenic shock, 1238
wavefront of, 1177–1178, *1177*
Myocardial oxygen consumption, 155, *1161*, 1161–1163, *1162*, 1162t
coronary blood flow and, 1163, *1163*
in contraction-relaxation cycle, 381, *381*
in heart transplantation, 517
in mitral regurgitation, 1020
in stable angina pectoris, 1293, *1293*
myocardial contractility and, 1162–1163
myocardial tension in, 1162, *1162*
Myocardial perfusion imaging, **274–295**
after heart transplantation, 520
collimation for, 275
computer acquisition for, 275
defects on, 281–282, *282*
dual-isotope, 275–276, *275*
electrocardiograph-gated, 285
energy window for, 275
gamma camera for, 275
in abdominal aortic aneurysm, 1550
in amyloidosis, 1429
in angina pectoris, 1323
in cor pulmonale, 1610
in coronary artery disease, 288–290, *288*, 289t, 290t, 307, 1296, 1323
in Duchenne muscular dystrophy, 1868
in hypertrophic cardiomyopathy, 1422
in idiopathic dilated cardiomyopathy, 1410
in infective endocarditis, 1089
in mitral valve prolapse, 1033
in myocardial contusion, 1537
in myocardial infarction, 285–288, *285–287*, 296–297, *296*
in Prinzmetal's variant angina, 1342
in sarcoidosis, 1431
in syndrome X, 293
interpretation of, 281–284, *282*
left ventricular dilation on, 282
lung uptake on, 282
of myocardial viability, 294–295, *294*, 306, 1328, 1328t
planar, 276, *276*
anterior view for, 277
artifacts on, 277–278, *279*, *280*
breast tissue on, 278, *280*
circumferential count profile for, 283, *284*
image display for, 276, *276*
in obese patients, 278
left anterior oblique view for, 277–278
left lateral view for, 278, *279*
normal, 277–279, *279*, *280*, *281*
patient positioning for, 276
quantification of, 283, *284*
preoperative, for noncardiac surgery, 1759
protocols for, 275–276, *275*
quantification of, 282–284, *284*, **Plate 5, Plate 6, Plate 7**
clinical application of, 285
radiopharmaceuticals for, 274–275, *275*, 275t
reverse redistribution on, 282
reversible defect on, 281
SPECT, artifacts on, 279, *279*, 281, *282*
breast tissue on, 279, 281
circumferential profile for, 284, **Plate 5, Plate 6, Plate 7**
normal, 279, 281, *281*
patient positioning for, 277
Myocardial perfusion imaging *(Continued)*
polar map (bull's eye display) for, 283–284
quality control for, 281
quantification of, 283–284, **Plate 5, Plate 6, Plate 7**
stress, 288–295, *288*, 289t
adenosine in, 289, 289t
after angioplasty, 294
after thrombolysis, 293
assessment of, 290, 290t
defect severity on, 291
dipyridamole in, 289, 289t
disease detection on, 291
dobutamine in, 289–290, 289t
exercise for, 288–289
for preoperative screening, 293–294
for revascularization evaluation, 294
for viability assessment, 294–295, *294*
in left bundle branch block, 293
in noncoronary artery disease, 293
in women, 293
pharmacological vasodilation for, 289–290, 289t
prognosis and, 291–294, *292*, *293*
referral bias in, 291
sensitivity of, 295
specificity of, 291, 295
technetium-99m–labeled agents in, 290–291, *291*
technetium-99m–labeled compounds for, 274–275, *275*, 275t, 290–291, *291*
kinetics of, 282–283, *283*
thallium-201 for, 274, *275*, 275t
kinetics of, 282, *283*
tomographic, 276–277, *277*
image display for, 277, *277*, *278*
orbit for, 277
patient position for, 277
value of, 295
Myocardial perfusion reserve, 200
Myocardial stunning, 388–389, 388t, *389*, 1176, *1176*
after coronary artery bypass surgery, 1327
echocardiography of, 89
Myocardial tension, myocardial oxygen consumption and, 1162, *1162*
Myocardial viability, carbon-11–labeled acetate imaging of, 306, **Plate 8**
collateral blood flow and, 1175
dobutamine echocardiography of, 1328
fluorine-18–labeled fluoro-2-deoxyglucose imaging of, 304t, 305–306, **Plate 8**
positron emission tomography of, 305–306, 307t, 354t, 355, 1327–1328, **Plate 8**
rubidium-82 imaging of, 306–307
technetium-99m–labeled sestamibi imaging of, 306
thallium-201 imaging of, 294–295, *294*, 306, 1328, 1328t. See also *Myocardial perfusion imaging.*
water-perfusable tissue index of, 307
Myocardial wall rupture, in myocardial infarction, 1241–1243, 1241t, *1242*
Myocarditis, **1435–1445**
antidepressant-induced, 1446
antimony-induced, 1447
arsenic-induced, 1448
azide-induced, 1448
bacterial, 1439–1440
carbon monoxide–induced, 1447
carnitine deficiency–induced, 1447
catecholamine-induced, 1447
chemical, 1445–1449, *1445–1447*
chloroquine-induced, 1446–1447
clinical manifestations of, 1435–1436
clostridia in, 1439–1440
cocaine-induced, 1445, *1445*, *1446*
coxsackievirus in, 988, 1437
cyclophosphamide-induced, 1448
cytomegalovirus in, 1437
diagnosis of, 1436
drug-induced, 1448–1449, 1448t
electrocardiography in, 1435–1436, 1437, 1439, 1440, 1445
emetine-induced, 1446
endomyocardial biopsy in, *1405*, 1436
etiology of, 1405t, 1435, 1435t
5-fluorouracil–induced, 1448
fungal, 1441–1442
giant cell, 1449
Myocarditis *(Continued)*
heat stroke–induced, 1449
histology of, *1405*
hydrocarbon-induced, 1447
hypersensitivity, 1448–1449, 1448t
hypocalcemia-induced, 1447
hypomagnesemia-induced, 1447
hypophosphatemia-induced, 1447
hypothermia-induced, 1449
in acquired immunodeficiency syndrome, 135, *149*, 989, 1437–1439, *1438*, 1438t
in actinomycosis, 1441
in aspergillosis, 1441, *1441*
in blastomycosis, 1441
in brucellosis, 1439
in candidiasis, 1441
in Chagas' disease, 1442–1444, *1442*, *1443*
in coccidioidomycosis, 1441
in cryptococcosis, 1441
in dengue, 1437
in diphtheria, 1440
in echinococcal cyst, 1444
in heart failure, 449
in hepatitis, 1437
in histoplasmosis, 1441–1442
in human immunodeficiency virus infection, 135, *150*, 989, 1437–1439, *1438*, 1438t
in infectious mononucleosis, 1439
in influenza, 1439
in Lassa fever, 1439
in legionnaires' disease, 1440
in leptospirosis, 1440
in Lyme disease, 1440–1441
in mucormycosis, 1442
in mumps, 1439
in myocardial infarction, 1193
in pheochromocytoma, 1898, *1899*
in poliomyelitis, 1439
in polymyositis, 1780
in psittacosis, 1440
in Q fever, 1439
in relapsing fever, 1441
in rheumatoid arthritis, 1777, *1777*
in Rocky Mountain spotted fever, 1439
in scrub typhus, 1439
in syphilis, 1441
in systemic lupus erythematosus, 1778
in trichinosis, 1445
in trypanosomiasis, 1442–1444, *1442*, *1443*
in tuberculosis, 1440
in visceral larva migrans, 1444
in Whipple disease, 1440
interferon-alpha–induced, 1445–1446
interleukin-1–induced, 1446
laboratory findings in, 1436
lead-induced, 1447
lithium-induced, 1447
Lyme, 1440–1441
management of, 1437
Meningococcus in, 1440
metazoal, 1444–1445
methyldopa-induced, 1448
methysergide-induced, 1446
Mycoplasma pneumoniae in, 1440
natural history of, *1436*
paclitaxel-induced, 1448
paraaminosalicylic acid–induced, 1449
paracetamol-induced, 1448
pathology of, 1436–1437
pediatric, 988–990
penicillin-induced, 1448
phenothiazine-induced, 1446
physical examination in, 1436
practice guidelines for, 1946
protozoal, 1442–1444, *1442*, *1443*
radiation-induced, 1449
respiratory syncytial virus in, 1439
Rickettsia in, 1439
rubella in, 988, 1439
rubeola in, 1439
Salmonella in, 1440
scorpion sting–induced, 1448
selenium deficiency–induced, 1447–1448
snake bite–induced, 1448
spider sting–induced, 1448
spirochetal, 1440–1441
Streptococcus in, 1440
streptomycin-induced, 1449

Myocarditis *(Continued)*
sudden cardiac death in, 749
sulfonamide-induced, 1448
taurine deficiency induced, 1447
tetracycline-induced, 1448
vaccinia in, 1439
varicella in, 1439
variola in, 1439
viral, 988–989, 1437–1439, *1438*, 1438t
in idiopathic dilated cardiomyopathy, 1409
pediatric, 988
wasp sting–induced, 1448
Myocytes, 360–361, 361t, *362*, *363*
calcium homeostasis in, 481, *481*
hypertrophy of, 1639–1645, *1639*
angiotensin II in, 1642, 1642t
cardiotrophin-1 in, 1642–1643
endothelin 1 in, 1642, 1642t
gene activation in, 1639–1640, 1640t
in heart failure, 399–400, *399*, *400*
in vitro assay for, 1640, 1640t
in vivo assay for, 1640–1641, *1641*
insulin-like growth factor-1 in, 1642, 1642t
intracellular signaling pathways in, 1643–1644, *1643*
structural changes of, 398, *399*
intracellular signaling pathways of, 1643–1644, *1643*
microanatomy of, 360–361, 361t
necrosis of, in heart failure, 401–402
of sinus node, 548
reperfusion injury to, 1179
Myocytolysis, 1191
Myofiber, 360, *362*
Myofibrils, 360, *362*
in heart failure, 406–407, *406*
Myogenic control, in coronary blood flow autoregulation, 1169
Myoglobin, in myocardial infarction, *1202*, 1202t, 1203
Myopotential interference, in cardiac pacing, 728, *728*
Myosin, heavy chains of, 363, 1202t
in heart failure, 406
light chains of, 363, 1202t
Myosin ATPase, in heart failure, 406
Myosin filament, 361, *364*
ATP-binding pocket of, 363, *364*, *365*
Myosin heavy chain, 363
in myocardial infarction, 1202t
Myosin light chain, 363
in myocardial infarction, 1202t
Myositis, chest pain in, 5
Myotomy-myectomy, in hypertrophic cardiomyopathy, 1426
Myotonia congenita, 1874
Myotonic muscular dystrophy, 1872–1874
cardiac manifestations of, 1873–1874, *1874*, *1973*
genetics of, 1632t, 1872–1873
pathogenesis of, 1872–1873
Myotubular myopathy, 1875
Myxedema, in hypothyroidism, 1894
pericardial effusion with, 1521–1522
Myxoma, cardiac, *1465*, 1467–1469, 1467t, 1468t, *1470*
calcifications of, *224*, 225
computed tomography of, 341–342, *341*
Cushing's syndrome and, 1896
cytogenetics of, 1469
differential diagnosis of, 1464t
early diastolic sounds in, 34
echocardiography in, 94, *94*, *95*
embolism from, 1880
embolization of, 1468–1469
familial, 1467–1468, *1468*, 1468t
genetic factors in, 1676
histogenesis of, 1469
histology of, 1468, *1469*
immunohistochemistry of, 1468
interleukin-6 in, 1464–1465
pathology of, 1468–1469, *1469*
signs of, 1464t
symptoms of, 1464t
syncope with, 867
treatment of, 1475
vs. mitral stenosis, 1011
Myxoma cells, 1468

$Na^+ \cdot Cl^-$ symport, in heart failure, 477–478, 477t
Nadolol, in arrhythmias, 610–613, 611t
in renal failure, 1931t
pharmacodynamic properties of, 487t
pharmacology of, 1307t
Nailbeds, cyanosis of, in myocardial infarction, 1201
Nail-patella syndrome, 1678t
$Na^+ \cdot K^+$-ATPase pump, cardiac glycoside effect on, 480–481
$Na^+ \cdot K^+ \cdot 2Cl$ symport, inhibitors of, in heart failure, 476–477, 477t
Naloxone hydrochloride (Narcan), in pediatric cardiology, 1001t
NAME (*n*evi, *a*trial myxoma, *m*yxoid neurofibroma, and *e*phelides) syndrome, 1468, 1676
National Heart, Lung, and Blood Institute Type II Coronary Intervention Study, in hypercholesterolemia prevention, 1129–1130
Natriuretic peptides, in heart failure, 478
Nausea, in myocardial infarction, 1199
in patient history, 10
Near-syncopal spells, in hypertrophic cardiomyopathy, 1420
Nebivelol, pharmacodynamic properties of, 487t
Necrosis, coagulation, *1189*, 1191
Needles, for cardiac catheterization, *185*
Neisseria gonorrhoeae, in infective endocarditis, 1082
Nemaline myopathy, 1877
Nembutal (pentobarbital), in pediatric cardiology, 1001t
Neomycin, digoxin interaction with, 483t
Neoplasm. See *Tumor(s).*
Neo-Synephrine. See *Phenylephrine (Neo-Synephrine).*
Nephrectomy, bilateral, 1928
Nephrons, in hypertension, *817*, 819–820
Nephropathy, contrast-induced, 1926
Nephrotic syndrome, in renal failure, 1925
Nernst equation, 555–556
Nerves, in sudden cardiac death, 753–754
of atrioventricular node, 552–553, *553*
of sinus node, 548
postoperative disorders of, 1735
Neuralgia, glossopharyngeal, 865
Neurocirculatory asthenia, chest pain in, 5
Neurofibromatosis, 1677, 1678t
Neurogenic pulmonary edema, 465, 1878
Neurologic examination, in myocardial infarction, 1201
in syncope, 872
postoperative, 1734–1735, 1736t
Neuromuscular disorders, 1865–1874. See also *Muscular dystrophy.*
in secondary pulmonary hypertension, 801
Neuronal ceroid lipofuscinosis, genetic factors in, 1661t
Neuropathy, postoperative, 1735
New York Heart Association, cardiovascular disability assessment system of, 12t, 13
Nicaladoni-Branham's sign, 460
Nicardipine (Cardene), in angina pectoris, 1309t, 1311
in hypertensive crisis, 858t
in renal failure, 1931t
pharmacokinetics of, 1309t
Nicorandil, in heart failure, 472t, 475–476
Nicotine withdrawal, in cardiac rehabilitation, 1397–1398
Nicotinic acid, in dyslipidemia, 1140–1141, 1140t
in hypercholesterolemia prevention, 1129, 1130
in renal failure, 1934t
Nifedipine (Procardia), contraindications to, 1310
digoxin interaction with, 483t
dose of, 1310
drug interactions of, 483t, 1310
in angina pectoris, 1308, 1309t, 1310, 1311–1312, 1312t
in aortic dissection, 1565
in aortic regurgitation, 1052
in heart failure, 472t
in hypertension, 855
in hypertrophic cardiomyopathy, 1425
in myocardial infarction, 1231
in pediatric cardiology, 1001t
in pregnancy, 1858

Nifedipine (Procardia) *(Continued)*
in renal failure, 1931t
in unstable angina, 1337
myocardial oxygen consumption and, 1306t
noncardiac surgery and, 1761
pharmacokinetics of, 1309t
side effects of, 1303t, 1310
Nifurtimox, in trypanosomiasis, 1444
Nimodipine, in renal failure, 1931t
Nipride. See *Nitroprusside (Nipride).*
Nitrates, after myocardial infarction, 1264–1265
doses of, 1303, 1303t
exercise stress testing effects of, 170
in angina pectoris, 1302–1304, *1302*, 1303t
in myocardial infarction, 1211, 1230–1231, 1264–1265
in pregnancy, 1859
in Prinzmetal's variant angina, 1342
in syndrome X, 1344
in unstable angina, 1336–1337, 1982t
myocardial oxygen consumption and, 1306t
noncardiac surgery and, 1761
occupational exposure to, 1349
side effects of, 1303, 1303t
tolerance to, 1304
withdrawal from, 1304, 1349
Nitrendipine, digoxin interaction with, 483t
Nitric acid, in coronary blood flow regulation, 1164, *1165*
Nitric oxide (endothelium-derived relaxing factor), *1165*
collateral vessel effects of, 1175
deficiency of, 1810
in coronary blood flow autoregulation, 1169
in pulmonary hypertension testing, 793
in systemic hypertension, 820
Nitroblue tetrazolium stain, in myocardial infarction, 1190
Nitroglycerin, coronary circulation effects of, 1302
doses of, 1303, 1303t
hematological abnormalities with, 1804t
in angina pectoris, 1302–1304, *1302*, 1303t, 1342, 1982t
in arteriography, 245
in congenital heart disease–related heart failure, 890, 891t
in coronary artery disease, 1290
in heart failure, 472t, 890, 891t
in hypertensive crisis, 858t
in myocardial infarction, 1198, 1211, *1211*, 1230–1231, 1236–1237
in pediatric cardiology, 1001t
in Prinzmetal's variant angina, 1342
in renal failure, 1932t
occupational exposure to, 1198
sublingual, 1230–1231
tolerance to, 1230, 1304
topical, 1304
with cardiac catheterization, 198–199
withdrawal from, 1304
Nitroimidazole, radiolabeled, for nuclear imaging, 304
Nitroprusside (Nipride), in aortic dissection, 1564
in congenital heart disease–related heart failure, 890, 891t
in heart failure, 472t, 474–475, 497–498, 890, 891t
in hypertensive crisis, 858t, 1003
in pediatric cardiology, 1001t
in pregnancy, 1859
in renal failure, 1932t
with cardiac catheterization, 199
Nitrous oxide, for anesthesia, 1757
Nitrovasodilators, 472t, 474–476, 497–498. See also specific agents, e.g., *Nitroprusside (Nipride).*
tolerance to, 475
Nocardia asteroides, in pericarditis, 1511
Nocturia, in heart failure, 452
in patient history, 10
Nocturnal dyspnea, paroxysmal, in heart failure, 450
Nodoventricular fibers, in Wolff-Parkinson-White syndrome, *668*, 669
Nodules, subcutaneous, in rheumatic fever, 1771
Nonbacterial thrombotic endocarditis, in infective endocarditis, 1082–1083
tumor-related, 1798

Noncardiac surgery, **1756–1766**
anesthesia for, 1756–1758
aortic regurgitation and, 981
arrhythmias after, 1764
arrhythmias and, 1763
beta blockers during, 1761
bicuspid aortic valve and, 981
calcium antagonists during, 1761
complications of, 1763–1764
conduction defects and, 1763
congenital heart block and, 981
congenital heart disease and, 981–982, 1762
contraindications to, 1764–1766, 1765t, *1766*
coronary artery disease and, 1758–1761, 1760t
cyanotic congenital heart disease and, 981–982
duration of, 1758
Ebstein's anomaly and, 981, 982
emergency, 1758
endocarditis prophylaxis and, 1762
heart failure after, 1764
heart failure and, 1762–1763
hypertension after, 1764
hypertension and, 1761
hypertrophic cardiomyopathy and, 1761–1762
ischemic heart disease and, 1758–1761, 1760t
medical consultation for, 1764–1766, 1765t, *1766*
myocardial infarction after, 1763–1764
nifedipine during, 1761
nitrates during, 1761
ostium secundum atrial septal defect and, 981
patient preparation for, 1766
permanent pacemaker and, 1763
practice guidelines for, 1946, 1989–1990, 1990t
prosthetic valves and, 982, 1066, 1762, 1835
radionuclide imaging before, 1946
risk indices for, 1764–1766, 1765t, *1766*
situs inversus with dextrocardia and, 981
valvular heart disease and, 1761–1762
ventricular function and, 982
Nonlaital, 752
Nonne-Milroy lymphedema, 1677
Nonparoxysmal atrioventricular junctional tachycardia, 659–661, *660*
clinical features of, 660–661
electrocardiography in, *650*, 659–660, *660*
in myocardial infarction, 1245t
management of, 661
Nonsteroidal anti-inflammatory drugs, in myocarditis, 1437
in uremic pericarditis, 1513
Noonan syndrome, 880t, 1660t, 1663
No-reflow phenomenon, in reperfusion injury, *1178*, 1179
Norepinephrine, atrioventricular node stimulation by, 552–553
digoxin effect on, 482
in aortic dissection, 1565
in cerebrovascular accident, 1878
in coronary blood flow regulation, 1170
in heart failure, 396, 408–410, *408*, 409–410, 412, *412*, 458, *458*, 1916t
in hypertension, 819
in myocardial infarction, 1237
pulmonary vascular effects of, 782
Norepinephrine (Levophed), in congenital heart disease–related heart failure, 891t
in pediatric cardiology, 1001t
Normodyne. See *Labetalol (Normodyne, Trandate).*
Norwood procedure, in hypoplastic left heart syndrome, 921–922
Notched T wave, 139
Novacor N-100 blood pump, 537t, 540
Nuclear cardiology, **273–308.** See also *Myocardial perfusion imaging; Positron emission tomography (PET).*
instrumentation for, 273–274
Nuclear magnetic resonance spectroscopy, after heart transplantation, 520
Nutrition. See also *Diet.*
preoperative, 1715, 1718t

Obciximob, 1820
Obesity, 1905–1907
blood pressure in, 1906
cardiac pathology in, 1905–1906, *1905, 1906*
Obesity *(Continued)*
cardiovascular hemodynamics in, 1905, *1905*
congestive heart failure in, 1906
coronary artery bypass surgery and, 1320
coronary artery disease and, 1152, 1706, 1906
hypertension and, 820–821, 1906
in elderly, 1697
pulmonary embolism and, 1583
treatment of, 1906–1907
cost-effectiveness analysis of, 1748
weight loss in, 1906, 1907
Obesity-diabetes syndrome, molecular genetics of, 1634
Obesity-hypoventilation (pickwickian) syndrome, in secondary pulmonary hypertension, 801
Ochronosis, 1668t
OKT3, in heart transplantation rejection, 523
Oliguria, in heart failure, 452
postoperative, 1734
Omeprazole, digoxin interaction with, 483t
Omniscience valve, 1061, *1062*, 1065
Ondine's curse, in cor pulmonale, 1614
Optimal care. See *Practice guidelines.*
Oral contraceptives, cardiovascular effects of, 1908
coronary artery disease and, 1707
hypertension with, 823–824
clinical features of, 823
incidence of, 823
management of, 824
mechanisms of, 824
pulmonary embolism and, 1583, 1584
Organelles, of cardiomyocytes, 360–361, 361t
Orofacial digital syndrome, genetic factors in, 1661t
Orthodromic tachycardia, 670, *672*
Orthopnea, 3
in heart failure, 450
Orthostatic hypotension, 865–866, 866t. See also *Syncope.*
treatment of, 874
Ortner's syndrome, 1010
Osborne wave, *140*, 141
Osler-Rendu-Weber disease, 16, *17*, 1676
genes for, 1632t
heart failure in, 461
Osler's nodes, 17
in infective endocarditis, 1085
Oslo Study Diet and Antismoking Trial, in hypercholesterolemia prevention, 1128
Osteoarthritis, vs. chest pain, 7
Osteoarthropathy, hypertrophic, in cyanotic congenital heart disease, 972
Osteogenesis imperfecta, 880t
genes in, 1655
Overdrive pacing, sinus node response to, 580–581, *581*
Overdrive suppression, 564
Ovine (digoxin immune Fab fragments), in pediatric cardiology, 1000t
Oxalosis, 1668t
Oxazepam, in myocardial infarction, 1226
Oxidative phosphorylation, in myocardial ischemia, 1178
Oximetry, for shunt detection, 196
Oxprenolol, in arrhythmias, 610–613, 611t
in renal failure, 1931t
pharmacodynamic properties of, 487t
Oxygen, consumption of, 155, 1161–1163, *1162*, 1162t, 1392
coronary blood flow and, 1163, *1163*
in cyanotic congenital heart disease, 973, *973*
in exercise stress testing, 439–441, *440*
in heart failure, 451–452, *452*, 509–510, 510t
in heart transplantation, 517
in mitral regurgitation, 1020
myocardial contractility and, 1162–1163
myocardial tension and, *1162*, 1162
in myocardial infarction, 1212
transport of, in chronic obstructive pulmonary disease, 1616–1617, *1618*
Oxygen saturation, in shunt defection, 196
Oxygen therapy, 1617–1619, *1618, 1619*
in chronic obstructive pulmonary disease, 1617–1619, *1618*
in cyanotic congenital heart disease, 972
in pulmonary hypertension, 792, 1613
in pulmonary parenchymal disease, 798–799
Oxygen-hemoglobin dissociation curve, in heart failure, 397

P wave, 111–112, 111t, *112*
in arrhythmias, 643
in chronic obstructive lung disease, 118–119, *118*
in faulty electrocardiography, *150*
in hyperkalemia, 141–142, *141*
in left atrial enlargement, 115–116, *115*
in right atrial enlargement, 115, *115*
P-A interval, in arrhythmias, 643, *644*
Pacemaker(s), 548, **705–731,** 708t–809t
code for, 705, 706t
discharge disorders of, 565–568, *566, 567*, 567t, *568*
exercise stress testing of, 172
in myocardial infarction, 1973t, 1978
in syncope, 874
latent, 565–566, 658
permanent, 707–709
AAI, 712, *712*, 725
AAIR, 725
AOO, 712
atrial sensing evaluation for, 729–730, *730*
atrial-based, 725
atrioventricular synchrony in, 722
automatic interval of, 712
bipolar leads for, 711
capture thresholds of, 710–711, *710, 711*
cardioversion with, 728
cardioverter-defibrillator interference with, 728
complications of, 726–729, 727t, *728*
crosstalk of, 715, *715*
DDD, *713*, 714–716, *714, 715, 717, 719, 721*, 725, *731*
tachycardia during, 720, *720*
upper rate response of, 715
DDDR, *724*, 725
DDI, 717, *719*
drug effects on, 711
dual-chamber, 714–720
endless-loop tachycardia of, 717–720, *719, 720*
multiprogrammability in, 721–722
practice guidelines for, 1966t
timing intervals of, *713*, 714–717, *714*
DVI, 716
electric interference with, 728–729
electrocardiographic evaluation of, 712–714, *713*, 1961t
electrocautery with, 728
escape interval of, 712
exit block with, 711
fixed-ratio atrioventricular block of, 715, *716*
follow-up for, 729–731, 729t, *730, 731*
hemodynamics of, 722–726
hysteresis interval of, 712
implantation methods for, 709–711, *710*, 710t, *711*
in atrioventricular block, 707–708
in bundle branch block, 707–708
in congenital atrioventricular block, 707
in congestive heart failure, 709
in hypersensitive carotid sinus syndrome, 708, 709t
in inducible atrioventricular block, 707
in myocardial infarction, 707, 1251–1252
in neurally mediated syncope, 709, 709t
in obstructive hypertrophic cardiomyopathy, 709
in sick sinus syndrome, 708, 709t
in supraventricular tachycardia, 732
in syncope, 707–708, 709, 709t
indications for, 707, 708t–709t
infection with, 726–727
intermittent wire fracture with, 728, *728*
intervals of, 712
lead design of, 711
lead displacement with, 726
lead impedance of, 711
loss of capture by, 727, 727t
lower rate timing of, 715
magnet interval of, 712
magnetic resonance imaging with, 729
malfunction of, 727–729, 727t, 1719
multiprogrammability of, 720–722, 721t

Pacemaker(s) *(Continued)*
myopotential interference with, 728, *728*, 730, *730*
noncardiac surgery and, 1763
oversensing of, 727–728
pacemaker syndrome with, 722–723
pacing rate abnormalities in, 727, 727t
pocket formation with, 726–727
pseudofusion beats with, 712–713, *713*
pulse width of, 711
Q-T interval–sensing, 723t, 725
radiation therapy with, 728–729
rate-adaptive, 723–725, 723t
respiratory-dependent, 723t, 724
selection of, 725–726, *726*, 1967
self-inhibition of, 715, *715*
sensing of, 711
signal amplitude of, 711
single-chamber, 712, *712*
multiprogrammability in, 721, 721t
practice guidelines for, 1965t–1966t
strength-duration curve of, 710–711, *711*
tachycardia-terminating, 732
telemetry follow-up of, 730–731, *731*
temperature-sensing, 723t, 724–725
thrombosis with, 726
transtelephonic monitoring of, 729
Twiddler's syndrome with, 726–727
undersensing of, 727
upper rate response of, 715
VDD, 716–717, *718*
ventricular fusion beat with, *710*, 712–713
ventricular safety pacing with, *714*, 715
VOO, *710*, 712
VVI, *710*, 712
VVIR, 723, *724*, 725
VVT, *710*, 712
Wenckebach upper rate response of, 715–716, *717*
practice guidelines for, 1963–1967, 1964t–1966t
subsidiary, 565–566
temporary, 705–707
in myocardial infarction, 706–707, 1251
indications for, 706
wandering, 647, *648*
Pacemaker current, 561
Pacemaker syndrome, 722–723
Paclitaxel, myocardial effects of, 1448
Paget's disease, heart failure in, 462
Pain. See also *Chest pain.*
in aortic dissection, 1199
in children, 888
in congenital heart disease, 888
in myocardial infarction, 1198–1199
in pulmonary embolism, 1199
pleural, 1199
Pallister-Hall syndrome, 1659t
Palmaz-Schatz stent, *1379*, 1380–1381, 1380t, *1381*
Palpation, 24–28, 24t, *26*, *27*
in myocardial infarction, 1200
of aorta, 1547
Palpitations, **9**
differential diagnosis of, 9, 9t
electrophysiological evaluation of, 582–583
practice guidelines for, 1963
in arrhythmias, 640
syncope after, 9
Pancreas, in myocardial infarction, 1197
Pancreatitis, postoperative, 1735t
vs. chest pain, 7
Pancuronium, for anesthesia, 1757
Panic disorder, syncope with, 865, 872
Papillary fibroelastoma, 1469–1470, *1470*
Papillary muscle, contractility of, experimental study of, 397–398, *398*
dysfunction of, in mitral regurgitation, 1018–1019, *1019*
post–myocardial infarction, 227, *227*
two-dimensional echocardiography in, 74
rupture of, cardiac resuscitation and, 1539
imaging of, *227*, 228
in mitral regurgitation, 1018–1019
in myocardial infarction, 1241t, 1243–1244, *1243*, *1244*
Paraaminosalicylic acid, myocardial effects of, 1449
Paracetamol, myocardial effects of, 1448
Paradoxical embolus, 1880, *1880*
in congenital heart disease, 885
Paraganglioma, 829, 1471, 1678t
Parallel conductance, calculation of, 424
Paramagnetic agents, for magnetic resonance imaging, 317, 333–334
Paramyotonia congenita, 1874
Parasystole, 693, 695, *695*
in arrhythmogenesis, 568, *569*
Parathyroid disease, 1899–1900, *1900*
Parathyroid hormone, 1899
Paroxysmal nocturnal dyspnea, 3
in heart failure, 450
Paroxysmal supraventricular tachycardia, in mitral valve prolapse, 1033
in myocardial infarction, 1245t, 1253
postoperative, 1730
Passive smoking, in coronary artery disease, 1147
Patau syndrome (trisomy 13), 881t, 1656t, 1657
Patent ductus arteriosus, *232*, 905–906, *906*, 1847
continuous murmur of, 44–45, *44*
echocardiography of, 84, *84*, *904*, 906, **Plate 4**
exercise and, 979
genetic factors in, 1660, 1660t
in adult, 966, *967*, 971
in children, 905–906
in full-term infant, 905–906
in premature infant, 905
management of, 906, *906*
pregnancy and, 975, 976
transcatheter closure of, 906, *906*
Patent ductus venosus, 884
Pectus excavatum, 24, *213*
in Marfan syndrome, 1671
Pelizaeus-Merzbacher syndrome, 1678t
Penbutolol, in arrhythmias, 610–613, 611t
in renal failure, 1931t
pharmacodynamic properties of, 487t
pharmacology of, 1307t
Penicillin, in rheumatic fever, 1773, 1773t, 1774
myocardial effects of, 1448
pericarditis with, 1519
Penn State electric ventricular assist device, *540*, 541, 545, *545*
Pentobarbital (Nembutal), in pediatric cardiology, 1001t
Peptic ulcer, pain in, 4t
vs. chest pain, 7
postoperative, 1735t
Percussion, vs. palpation, 28
Percussion wave, of arterial pulse, 21–22
Percutaneous balloon pericardiotomy, 1495–1496, *1495*
in neoplastic pericarditis, 1516
Percutaneous brachial artery technique, for cardiac catheterization, 185–186
Percutaneous radial artery technique, for cardiac catheterization, 186
Percutaneous transluminal coronary angioplasty (PTCA), **1366–1376**
abrupt vessel closure after, 1368–1370, *1369*, 1369t, 1370t
after thrombolytic therapy, 1222
collateral vessel filling during, 1175
comparative trials of, 1373–1375, 1374t
complications of, 1368–1371, *1369*, 1369t, 1370t
contraindications to, 1375, 1954
cost-effectiveness analysis of, 1749–1751
credentialing for, 1386–1387
equipment for, 1366–1367, *1367*
exercise stress testing after, 170–171
failure of, 1368
gene therapy after, 1638
hemodynamic effects of, 1367–1368, *1368*
in coronary artery disease, 1954–1957, 1955t–1956t
in elderly, 1696
in myocardial infarction, 178–179, 1221–1223, *1222*, 1375–1376, 1956t, 1957, 1975t, 1978
in Prinzmetal's variant angina, 1343
in renal failure, 1926
in stable angina, 1313–1316, *1316*, 1329–1331, *1329*, 1330t
in unstable angina, 1338–1339
in women, 1709–1710, 1710t
indications for, 1375–1376
ischemic complications of, 1368, 1370–1371, 1371t
lesion classification for, 265, 265t
myocardial perfusion imaging after, 294
Percutaneous transluminal coronary angioplasty (PTCA) *(Continued)*
occlusion after, 1827
of coronary collateral circulation, 263
outcomes of, 1371–1376, *1372*, 1373t, 1374t
physiological effects of, 1367–1368, *1368*
practice guidelines for, 1946, 1954–1957, 1955t–1956t
primary, 1221–1222, *1222*
restenosis after, 1372–1373, *1372*, 1373t
technique of, 1367
vascular smooth muscle proliferation after, gene therapy–induced inhibition of, 1638
vs. thrombolytic therapy, 1221–1222, *1222*
Percutaneous transluminal peripheral angioplasty (PTPA), 1384–1385
Pericardial biopsy, 1496
in acute pericarditis, 1484
in pericardial effusion, 1496
in tuberculous pericarditis, 1507
percutaneous, 1496
Pericardial cyst, 1522, *1523*
imaging of, 236, *236*, 340
Pericardial effusion, **1485–1496**. See also *Cardiac tamponade.*
cardiac catheterization in, 1492–1493, *1493*
chest roentgenography in, 1485–1486, *1485*
chronic, 1486
computed tomography of, 235, 340
drug-induced, 12t
echocardiography in, 93–94, *93*, 235, 1486
electrocardiography in, 1486
in Kawasaki disease, 995
in neoplastic pericarditis, 1514
in polymyositis, 1780
in pregnancy, 1846
magnetic resonance imaging in, 235, 324–325, *325*
malignant, 1797
management of, 1486
myxedematous, 1521–1522
patient history in, 1485
percutaneous balloon pericardiotomy in, 1495–1496, *1495*
pericardial biopsy in, 1496
pericardiectomy in, 1496
pericardiocentesis in, 1493–1495, *1494*
pericardioscopy in, 1496
pericardiotomy in, 1496
physical examination in, 1485
plain chest radiography in, *234*, 235
postinfarction, 1255
without cardiac compression, 1485–1486, *1485*
Pericardial fluid, 1478
evacuation of, *1492*, 1493–1495
in bacterial pericarditis, 1509
in neoplastic pericarditis, 1515
in rheumatoid arthritis, 1776
Pericardial friction rub, 1482
in Dressler syndrome, 1520
in myocardial infarction, 1201, 1511
in pericarditis, 1482, 1506
Pericardial knock, in constrictive pericarditis, 1499
Pericardial pressure, 1479–1480, *1479*. See also *Cardiac tamponade.*
Pericardial rub, 45, *49*
Pericardiectomy, contraindications to, 1505
in constrictive pericarditis, 1504–1505
in pericardial effusion, 1496
in radiation pericarditis, 1517
in tuberculous pericarditis, 1508
in uremic pericarditis, 1513
Pericardiocentesis, complications of, 1494
in acute pericarditis, 1484
in children, 1495
in effusive-constrictive pericarditis, 1505
in neoplastic pericarditis, 1515
in pericardial effusion, *1492*, 1493–1495
in radiation pericarditis, 1517
in rheumatoid arthritis–related pericarditis, 1518
in uremic pericarditis, 1513
needle insertion for, 1494–1495, *1494*
patient position for, 1494
postprocedure management in, 1495
risks of, 1494
Pericardioscopy, 1496
in tuberculous pericarditis, 1508
Pericardiostomy, in uremic pericarditis, 1513

Pericardiotomy, balloon, percutaneous, 1495–1496, *1495*
in neoplastic pericarditis, 1516
Pericarditis, **1481–1485, 1496–1523**
acute, **1481–1485**
antibiotics in, 1484
aortic dissection and, 1484
blood tests in, 1484
chest pain in, 5, 1481–1482, 1482t
chest roentgenography in, 1484
colchicine in, 1485
dyspnea in, 1482
echocardiography in, 1484
electrocardiography in, 1483–1484, *1483*, 1483t
etiology of, 1482t
friction rub in, 1482
management of, 1484
natural history of, 1484
nonsteroidal antiinflammatory agents in, 1484
patient history in, 1481–1482, 1482t
pericardial biopsy in, 1484
pericardiocentesis in, 1484
physical examination in, 1482
radionuclide scan in, 1484
recurrent, 1484–1485
vs. angina pectoris, 1292
vs. ischemia, 1482t
bacterial, 1506t, 1508–1510
clinical features of, 1509
endocarditis and, 1508–1509
in children, 1509
laboratory findings of, 1509
management of, 1509–1510
natural history of, 1509
pathology of, 1509
pericardial fluid in, 1509
calcifications in, 225
cholesterol, 1522
constrictive, **1496–1505**
angiography in, 1502–1504, *1504*
cardiac catheterization in, 1502–1504, *1502*, *1503*
chest roentgenography in, 1499–1500, *1499*
clinical features of, 1498–1502, 1498t, *1499*, *1500*, *1501*
computed tomography in, 340, *340*, 1501, *1501*
congenital, 1498
diastolic filling in, 1496, *1497*
diastolic pericardial knock in, 1499
differential diagnosis of, 1501–1502
Doppler echocardiography in, 1500, *1500*, 1503–1504, *1504*
echocardiography in, 94, 1500–1501, *1500*
electrocardiography in, 1500, *1500*
endomyocardial biopsy in, 1504
etiology of, 1498
flow velocities in, 1503–1504, *1504*
genetic factors in, 1666
in children, 1498
in rheumatoid arthritis, 1776
jugular venous pulse in, *19*, 20, 1498, *1499*
Kussmaul's sign in, 1497
magnetic resonance imaging of, 324, *325*
management of, 1504–1505
nontubercular etiology of, 1498
palpation in, 25
pathophysiology of, 1496–1498, *1497*
physical examination in, 1498–1499, *1499*
postoperative, 1498, 1521, 1734
post-traumatic, 1536
ventricular filling in, 1503, *1504*
ventricular pressure-volume relationships in, 404
vs. cardiac tamponade, 1503
vs. restrictive cardiomyopathy, 235, 1503t
vs. restrictive pericarditis, 1501, 1503, 1503t
drug-related, 12t, 1519
effusive-constrictive, 1493, 1505
computed tomography of, 340–341, *341*
fungal, 1506t, 1510–1511
histoplasmosis, 1510
in children, 990
in Churg-Strauss syndrome, 1783
in coccidioidomycosis, 1510
in CREST (calcinosis, Raynaud's, esophageal dysfunction, sclerodactylia, telangiectasia) syndrome, 1781

Pericarditis *(Continued)*
in Dressler syndrome, 1519–1520
in mixed connective tissue disease, 1519
in polymyositis, 1780
in postpericardiotomy syndrome, 1520–1521
in progressive systemic sclerosis, 1518–1519
in renal failure, 1926–1927
in rheumatoid arthritis, 1518, 1776
in sarcoidosis, 1519, *1519*
in scleroderma, 1781
in systemic lupus erythematosus, 1518, 1778
in thalassemia, 1789
in Wegener's granulomatosis, 1783
meningococcal, 1509
mycobacterial, 1506t, 1507–1508
neoplastic, 1513–1516
cardiac catheterization in, 1515
clinical features of, 1514
diagnosis of, 1514–1515
effusion in, 1514
management of, 1515–1516
natural history of, 1515
pathology of, 1513–1514, *1514*
pericardiocentesis in, 1515
noncalcific, subacute, 1497–1498, 1498t
pain in, in children, 888
vs. angina pectoris, 1292
parasitic, 1506t
patient history in, 11
postinfarction, 1255–1256, 1511–1512, 1519–1520
vs. myocardial ischemia, 1512
postoperative, 1498, 1521, 1734
post-traumatic, 1522, 1535, 1536
protozoal, 1506t
radiation, 1449, 1516–1517
clinical features of, 1517
diagnosis of, 1517
etiology of, 1516
management of, 1517
pathology of, 1516–1517
restrictive, vs. constrictive pericarditis, 1501, 1503, 1503t
rheumatic, 1517–1518
subacute, 1497–1498, 1498t
Ta segment abnormality in, *112*, 116
toxin-related, 1519
tuberculous, 1507–1508
clinical manifestations of, 1507
diagnosis of, 1507–1508
etiology of, 1507
management of, 1508
pathogenesis of, 1507
pathology of, 1507
uremic, 1512–1513
clinical features of, 1513
echocardiography in, 1513
management of, 1513
viral, 1505–1507, 1506t
antibody titers in, 1506
clinical findings in, 1506
etiology of, 1505–1506
management of, 1507
natural history of, 1506–1507
pathogenesis of, 1505–1506
pathology of, 1506
Pericardium, 1478
bronchogenic tumor extension to, 326, *326*
calcifications of, 1499, *1499*
computed tomography of, 340, *340*
plain film radiography of, *224*, 225
cardiac distention and, 1480
computed tomography of, 339–341, *340*
congenital absence of, 1522–1523, *1523*
chest pain in, 7
echocardiography in, 94
imaging of, 235–236, *235*
congenital defects of, 340, 947
cysts of, 1522, *1523*
imaging of, 236, *236*, 340
electron microscopy of, 1478
functions of, 1478–1481, *1479*, *1481*
hematoma of, 324–325, *325*
imaging of, 354t, 356
in contraction-relaxation cycle, 385
in renal failure, 1928, *1928*
layers of, 1478
magnetic resonance imaging of, 324–325, *325*
nonpenetrating trauma to, 1536, 1536t
oblique sinus of, 1478

Pericardium *(Continued)*
plain chest radiography of, 234–236, *234–236*
post-traumatic constriction of, 1535
pressures of, 1479–1480, *1479*. See also *Cardiac tamponade.*
radiation effects on, 1799
surface contact pressure of, 1479–1480
transverse sinus of, 1478
trauma to, 1522, 1536
tumors of, 1514–1516
imaging of, 236
metastatic, 1514–1516, *1514*, 1514t, 1796–1797
ventricular interdependence and, 1480
Periinfarction block, electrocardiography in, 133, *133*
Periodic paralysis, 1877
Peripartum cardiomyopathy, 1851–1852, *1851*
Peripheral arterial revascularization, 1384–1385
Peripheral balloon angioplasty, 1384–1385
Peripheral resistance units, 780
Peripheral vascular disease, coronary artery bypass surgery and, 1331
Peripheral vascular resistance, measurement of, 428
Peroneal muscular atrophy, 1875
Persistent fetal circulation, in secondary pulmonary hypertension, 800
Persistent truncus arteriosus, 907–908
cardiac catheterization in, 908
electrocardiography in, 907–908, *908*
hemodynamics of, 907
management of, 908, *908*
morphology of, 907, *907*
Personality, in cardiac rehabilitation, 1398
in coronary artery disease, 1154
in sudden cardiac death, 745
Pes cavus, in Friedreich's ataxia, *1874*
Petechiae, in infective endocarditis, 1085, *1085*
pH, in contraction-relaxation cycle, 371, *371*
in cyanosis, 893
Pharyngeal-tracheal obstruction, in secondary pulmonary hypertension, 801
Phenindione, hematological abnormalities with, 1804t
Phenobarbital, in pediatric cardiology, 1001t
Phenothiazines, myocardial effects of, 1446
Phenotype. See also *Gene(s).*
dominant, 1651, 1653, *1654*
heterogeneity of, 1655
mendelian, 1659–1663, 1660t, 1661t, *1662*
pleiotropy of, 1654
recessive, 1651, 1653, *1654*
variability in, 1654–1655
X-linked, 1653–1654, *1654*
Phenoxybenzamine, in pediatric cardiology, 1001t
in pheochromocytoma, 1898
Phentolamine (Regitine), in heart failure, 472t
in hypertensive crisis, 858t
in pediatric cardiology, 1001t
Phenylalanine, teratogenicity of, 1663t
Phenylephrine (Neo-Synephrine), auscultatory effects of, *48*, 49
in aortic dissection, 1565
in atrioventricular nodal reentrant tachycardia, 664
in pediatric cardiology, 1001t
with cardiac catheterization, 199
Phenylketonuria, teratogenicity of, 1664
Phenytoin (Dilantin), adverse effects of, 608
dosage of, 594t–595t, 608
electrophysiological actions of, 601t, 602t–603t, 608
fetal effects of, 881t
hematological abnormalities with, 1804t
in arrhythmias, 594t–595t, 601t, 602t–603t, 608
in Duchenne muscular dystrophy, 1869
in pediatric cardiology, 1001t
in renal failure, 1930t
indications for, 608
metabolism of, 608
pharmacokinetics of, 608
Pheochromocytoma, 830t, 1897–1899
cardiovascular manifestations of, 1898
diagnosis of, 829, 1898–1899
familial, 1678t
hypertension with, 829–830
laboratory confirmation of, 829–830

Pheochromocytoma *(Continued)*
localization of, 830
myocarditis with, 1898, *1899*
treatment of, 830, 1898–1899
Phlebography, in pulmonary embolism, 1589
Phlebotomy, in cor pulmonale, 1619
in cyanotic congenital heart disease, 972
Phosphate deficiency, in heart failure, 407
Phosphocreatine, in heart failure, 407
Phosphodiesterase inhibitors, in heart failure, 472t, 484–485, 502
Phospholamban, in sarcoplasmic reticulum calcium pump regulation, 368–369, *368*
Phospholipase C signal transduction, in contraction-relaxation cycle, 375, *375*
Phosphorylase kinase deficiency, 1668t, 1674
Physical activity. See also *Exercise; Exercise stress training.*
after myocardial infarction, 1227, 1227t
cost-effectiveness analysis of, 1748
in cardiac rehabilitation, 1399–1400
Physical conditioning, in cardiac rehabilitation, 1392–1394. See also *Cardiac rehabilitation.*
Physical examination, **15–23.** See also *Cardiac examination.*
appearance on, 15–17
of abdomen, 17–18
of arterial pulse, 20–23, *21*, *23*
of chest, 17–18
of extremities, 16, *17*
of eyes, 15–16, *16*
of face, 15
of fingers, 17, *17*
of head, 15
of jugular venous pulse, 18–20, *18*, *19*
of mucous membranes, 16
of skin, 16, *17*
Physical inactivity. See also *Exercise.*
in coronary artery disease, 1151, *1152*
in hypertension, 821
sudden cardiac death and, 745
Pierce-Donachy pump systems, 537t, 539, *539*, *540*
Pimobendan, in heart failure, 485
Pinacidil, in heart failure, 475–476
Pindolol, in arrhythmias, 610–613, 611t
in renal failure, 1931t
pharmacodynamic properties of, 487t
pharmacology of, 1307t
serum lipid effects of, 1306
Piretanide, in heart failure, 477t
Plaque, atherosclerotic, 1113–1114, *1113*, 1185–1189, *1186*, *1187*
complicated, 1186
composition of, 1186–1187, *1187*
fissuring of, *1186*, 1187
in unstable angina, 1335
rupture of, *1186*, 1187
stable, *1186*
vulnerable, *1186*
Plasma D-dimer, ELISA-determined, in pulmonary embolism, 1587, *1587*
Plasmin, $alpha_2$-antiplasmin inhibition of, 1816
Plasminogen, deficiency of, in venous thrombosis, 1582t
in fibrinolytic system, 1814, *1814*, *1815*
Plasminogen activator(s), recombinant, 1821–1822
tissue-type, 1218–1219, *1219*, 1814, *1815*, 1821–1822. See also *Thrombolytic therapy.*
in fibrinolysis, 1816
in myocardial infarction, 1224, 1225, 1824–1826, *1825*, 1825t
recombinant, 1821–1822
secretion of, 1816
structure of, *1815*
synthesis of, 1816
vs. streptokinase, 1220–1221
urokinase-type, 1814, 1821
receptor for, 1815
Plasminogen activator inhibitor(s), 1814–1815
in coronary artery disease, 1153
secretion of, 1816
synthesis of, 1816
Platelet(s), 1110–1111, *1111*
activation of, 1111
aggregation of, in unstable angina, 1333
growth factor formation by, 1110–1111, *1111*
in adult respiratory distress syndrome, 465
Platelet(s) *(Continued)*
in atherosclerosis, 1115, *1120*
in hemostasis, *1809*, 1810–1811, *1810*, *1811*
in myocardial infarction, *1186*, *1186*, *1188*, 1197
inhibitors of, 1818–1820, *1819*, 1819t
after coronary bypass surgery, 1321
in myocardial infarction, 1827–1828, 1827t, 1974t–1975t, 1978
in prosthetic valve replacement, 1835
nitroglycerin effects on, 1302
postoperative dysfunction of, 1731–1732, 1732t
transfusion of, 1732
Platelet-derived growth factor (PDGF), endothelial cell formation of, 1108
in atherosclerosis, 1115–1117, **Plate 9**
simian sarcoma virus protein homology with, 1117
Platelet-derived growth factor-B protein, in atherosclerosis, 1115, **Plate 9**
Platelet-specific integrin $\alpha_{IIb}\beta_3$ (GPIIb/IIIa), 1629–1630, *1629*, *1819*
blockers of, *1819*, 1820
in myocardial infarction, 1225
in unstable angina, 1333, 1823–1824
in myocardial infarction, 1187
monoclonal antibodies to, 1630, *1819*, 1820
after coronary angioplasty, 1314, 1315, 1827
in PTCA-related abrupt vessel closure, 1369, 1370t, 1373
natural inhibitors of, 1630
synthetic inhibitors of, 1630, 1820
Pleiotropy, 1654
Pleural effusion, in aortic dissection, 1558
in constrictive pericarditis, 1499–1500
in heart failure, 455
postoperative, 230
Pleural pain, 1199
Pneumatic compression, intermittent, in pulmonary embolism prophylaxis, 1598–1599
Pneumatic pulsatile ventricular assist device, 537t, 538–540, *539*, *540*
in cardiogenic shock, 541–542, 541t
Pneumatic total artificial heart, 544, *544*
Pneumonia, in children, 11
Pneumothorax, in pulmonary edema, 463t, 464
postoperative, 230
spontaneous, 5, 136
Point of maximal impulse, 25
Pokkuri, 752
Poland sequence, 1659t
Poliomyelitis, 1877
in secondary pulmonary hypertension, 801
myocarditis in, 1439
Polyarteritis nodosa, 1783
sudden cardiac death in, 747
Polychondritis, relapsing, 1783
Polycystic kidney disease, 1678t
Polycythemia, 1792–1794, *1793*
in congenital heart disease, 885
relative, 1794
secondary, 1793–1794, *1794*
Polycythemia rubra vera, 972
Polycythemia vera, 1793
in hypertension, 821
Polymer fume fever, pericarditis with, 1519
Polymyositis, 1779–1780
Polysplenia, 1659t
cardiac anomalies with, 946
Polytetrafluoroethylene (Teflon), burning of, pericarditis with, 1519
Polythiazide, in heart failure, 477–478, 477t
Pompe's disease, 880t, 992–993, *993*, 1668t, 1674
subaortic muscular hypertrophy in, 919
Porphyria, 1678t
Positive end-expiratory pressure (PEEP), right ventricular function and, 303
Positive-pressure ventilation, intraoperative, 1758
Positron emission tomography (PET), **304–308**
carbon-11–labeled acetate for, for myocardial viability assessment, 306, **Plate 8**
fluorine-18–labeled deoxyglucose for, for myocardial viability assessment, 305–306, 307t, **Plate 8**
for cholesterol assessment, 308
for myocardial blood flow assessment, 307
in coronary artery disease, 307–308, 307t
in Duchenne muscular dystrophy, 1868, *1869*
Positron emission tomography (PET) *(Continued)*
indications for, 304–305
neurocardiologic, 307–308
of myocardial viability, 305–306, 307t, 354t, 355, 1327–1328, **Plate 8**
protocols for, 304
radiopharmaceuticals for, 304, 304t
rubidium-82 for, for myocardial viability assessment, 306–307
Postextrasystolic aberration, electrocardiography in, 126
Postextrasystolic potentiation, in hypertrophic cardiomyopathy evaluation, 1423
Post–myocardial infarction syndrome (Dressler syndrome), 1256, 1511–1512, 1519–1520
plain film radiography in, 228
vs. recurrent myocardial infarction, 1520
Postpericardiotomy syndrome, 230, 990, 1520–1521, 1734
Postprandial syncope, 866
Postpump syndrome, postoperative, 1722–1723
Poststreptococcal reactive arthritis, 1771
Posture, auscultatory effects of, 47–49, *48*, *49*
Potassium, depletion of, in heart failure, *548*, 1918–1919, *1919*
efflux of, in ischemia, 386, *387*
in aldosterone secretion, 1895
in resting potential, 555
myocardial concentration of, 554t
preoperative, 1717t
serum, diuretic effects of, 479
in heart failure, *548*
Potassium channel activators, in heart failure, 475–476
Potassium chloride, in pediatric cardiology, 1001t
Potassium gluconate (Kaon) and potassium triplex, in pediatric cardiology, 1001t
Potassium supplementation, in hypertension, 845
Povidone-iodine, in post-surgical constrictive pericarditis, 1521
Power production, in myocardial oxygen uptake, 381
P-R interval, 112
in hyperkalemia, *150*
Practice guidelines, 1939–1940
for acute chest pain, 1967–1970, 1968t–1969t
for ambulatory electrocardiography, 1946–1948, 1947t
for cardiac catheterization, 1949–1954, 1949t, 1950t–1951t, 1953t
for coronary angiography, 1949–1954, 1949t, 1950t–1951t, 1953t
for coronary artery bypass graft surgery, 1957–1959, 1958t
for coronary disease prevention, 1990–1993, 1991t, *1992*, 1992t
for echocardiography, 1942–1943, 1944t–1945t
for electrocardiography, 1940–1941
for electrophysiological procedures, 1959–1963, 1960t–1962t
for exercise testing, 1941–1942, 1941t
for heart failure, 1985–1989, 1987t, *1988*
for high blood cholesterol prevention, 1991
for hypertension prevention, 1991–1993, 1991t, *1992*, 1992t, *1993*
for in-hospital cardiac monitoring, 1948
for myocardial infarction, 1970–1979, 1971t, 1972t–1977t
for noncardiac surgery, 1989–1990, 1990t
for pacemakers, 1963–1967, 1964t–1966t
for percutaneous transluminal coronary angioplasty, 1954–1957, 1955t–1956t
for radionuclide imaging, 1943–1946, 1945t
for unstable angina, 1979–1985, *1980*, 1980t, 1981t, 1982t–1983t, *1985*
Practolol, pericarditis with, 1519
Prader-Willi syndrome, 1651t
Pravastatin, in dyslipidemia, 1140t, 1141
Prazosin (Minipress), in aortic regurgitation, 1052
in congenital heart disease–related heart failure, 890, 891t
in heart failure, 472t, 890, 891t
in pediatric cardiology, 1001t
in Prinzmetal's variant angina, 1343
in renal failure, 1932t
in systemic hypertension, 852
Preconditioning, in myocardial ischemia, 387–388, *388*
Precordial leads, 110–111

Prednisone, before arteriography, 245
Preeclampsia, 830–832, 831t, 1852–1853, 1852t, 1853t
clinical features of, 831, 831t
prognosis for, 832
treatment of, 831–832
Preexcitation syndrome, **667–675.** See also *Wolff-Parkinson-White (WPW) syndrome.*
Pregnancy, **1843–1860.** See also *Congenital heart disease.*
after cardiac transplantation, 1853
amiodarone during, 1858
angiotensin-converting enzyme inhibitors during, 1859
anti-arrhythmics during, 1858
antibiotic prophylaxis during, 1846, 1859t, 1860
antithrombotic agents during, 1859–1860
aortic dissection during, 1556, 1855–1856
aortic regurgitation during, 1850
aortic valve stenosis during, 1850
arrhythmias during, 1854–1855
atenolol during, 1859
atrial fibrillation during, 1854–1855
atrial flutter during, 1854–1855
beta-adrenoceptor blockers during, 854, 1858–1859
blood pressure during, 1843–1844, *1844*
blood volume during, 1843, *1843*
calcium antagonists during, 1858
captopril during, 1852t
cardiac evaluation during, 1844–1846, 1845t
auscultation in, 1845
cardiac catheterization in, 1846
chest radiography in, 1845, 1845t
Doppler echocardiography in, 1845–1846, 1845t
electrocardiography in, 1845, 1845t
history in, 1844–1845
laboratory examinations in, 1845–1846, 1845t
magnetic resonance imaging in, 1846
physical examination in, 1844–1845, 1845t
pulmonary artery catheterization in, 1846
radionuclide imaging in, 1846
stress testing in, 1846
cardiac glycosides during, 1857–1858, 1857t
cardiac output during, 1843, 1843t, 1844
cardiac surgery during, 1856–1857
cardiomyopathies during, 1851–1852, *1851*
cardiovascular physiology during, 1843–1844, *1843*, 1843t
cesarean section in, 1844, 1846
complete heart block during, 1855
congenital heart disease and, 975–978, 975t
coronary artery disease during, 1853–1854, *1854*
counseling before, 1846
dilated cardiomyopathy during, 1665, 1851–1852, *1851*
diltiazem during, 1858
disopyramide during, 1858
diuretic agents during, 1859
drug use during, 1857–1860, 1857t
eclampsia in, 1852–1853, 1853t
exercise-mediated cardiac output during, 1844
flecainide during, 1858
heart rate during, 1843, 1843t
hemodynamic changes of, 1844
heparin during, 977, 1859
hydralazine during, 1852t
hypertension during, 830–832, 831t, 1852–1853, 1852t, 1853t
hypertrophic cardiomyopathy during, 1851
in myotonic dystrophy patient, 1873
in valve prosthesis patient, 1856–1857
labor after, 977
induction of, 1846
lidocaine during, 1858
mammary souffle of, 40, 45
Marfan syndrome in, 1672, 1850–1851, *1850*
methyldopa during, 1852t
metoprolol during, 1858–1859
mexiletine during, 1858
mitral regurgitation during, 1850
mitral stenosis during, 1849–1850, *1849*
mitral valve prolapse during, 1850
myocardial infarction during, 1853–1854, *1854*
nifedipine during, 1858
organic nitrates during, 1859
Pregnancy *(Continued)*
preeclampsia in, 1852–1853
prenatal care for, 976–977
procainamide during, 1858
propafenone during, 1858
propranolol during, 1858
prosthetic valves in, 1066
pulmonary hypertension during, 791, 1856
quinidine during, 1858
radionuclide imaging in, 1846
rheumatic heart disease during, 1848–1850, *1849*
sodium nitroprusside during, 1859
sotalol during, 1859
stroke volume during, 1843, 1843t
Takayasu's arteritis during, 1855–1856
vascular resistance during, 1843–1844
vasodilators during, 1859
venous thrombosis and, 1583, 1584
verapamil during, 1858
warfarin during, 977, 1859
Prehospital emergency services, cost-effectiveness analysis of, 1748–1749
Preload, 378, 421
in left ventricular function, 422, *422*, 428
in myocardial infarction, 1195
in myocardial oxygen uptake, 381, *381*
reduction of, in heart failure, 494–495, *495*
wall stress and, 380
Preload reserve, in young heart, 889
Premature atrial complexes, 650–652, *651*
clinical features of, 652
electrocardiography in, 650–652, *651*
interpolated, 652
management of, 652
Premature atrial contractions, in myocardial infarction, 1253
in rheumatic heart disease, 1013
Premature atrioventricular junctional complexes, 658–659, *659*
Premature excitation, electrocardiography in, 125
Premature infant. See also *Infant.*
ductus arteriosus of, 905
Premature ventricular beat (Brockenbrough maneuver), with cardiac catheterization, 198
Premature ventricular complexes, 675–677, *676*
clinical features of, 676–677
electrocardiography in, 675–676, *676*
in heart failure, 506
in myocardial infarction, 677
management of, 677
multiform, 676, *676*
Premature ventricular contractions, in sudden cardiac death, 746–747
Prenatal diagnosis, 879
Prerenal azotemia, postoperative, 1734
Pressure-volume area, in myocardial oxygen uptake, 381
myocardial oxygen consumption and, 1162, *1162*
Pressure-volume loops, for contractility measurement, 383, *383*
Pressure-work index, in myocardial oxygen uptake, 381
Prinzmetal's variant angina, 1340–1343
acetylcholine in, 1342
arteriography in, 1341–1342
clinical manifestations of, 1340–1341
electrocardiography in, 1340–1341, *1341*
ergonovine test in, 1342
hemodynamic features of, 1341–1342
hyperventilation in, 1342
management of, 1342–1343
mechanisms of, *1289*, 1340
myocardial perfusion imaging in, 1342
pathogenesis of, *1289*
precipitation of, 7
ST segment in, *137*
T wave in, *137*
Priscoline (tolazoline), in pediatric cardiology, 1002t
Probabilities, in diagnostic testing, 1743
Probucol, in coronary artery disease, 1300
in dyslipidemia, 1140t, 1142
in nonhuman primates, 1116
in renal failure, 1934t
Procainamide (Pronestyl), adverse effects of, 604
dosage of, 594t–595t, 603–604
electrophysiological actions of, 601t, 602t–603t, 603
Procainamide (Pronestyl) *(Continued)*
hematological abnormalities with, 1804t
hemodynamic effects of, 603
in arrhythmias, 594t–595t, 601t, 602t–603t, 603–604
in cardiac arrest, 766
in Duchenne muscular dystrophy, 1869
in myocardial infarction–related ventricular tachycardia, 1248
in pediatric cardiology, 1001t
in pregnancy, 1858
in renal failure, 1930t
indications for, 604
pericarditis with, 1519
pharmacokinetics of, 594t–595t, 603
Procardia. See *Nifedipine (Procardia).*
Progeria, 880t
Progestin, coronary artery disease and, 1908
Program on the Surgical Control of the Hyperlipidemias, in hypercholesterolemia prevention, 1131
Progressive systemic sclerosis, 1781–1782, *1781*, *1782*
pericarditis in, 1518–1519
sudden cardiac death in, 749
Prolonged Q-T interval syndrome, in sudden cardiac death, 750–751
Promethazine, in pediatric cardiology, 1002t
Pronestyl. See *Procainamide (Pronestyl).*
Propafenone, adverse effects of, 610
digoxin interaction with, 483t
dosage of, 610
electrophysiological actions of, 601t, 602t–603t, 609
hematological abnormalities with, 1804t
hemodynamic effects of, 609
in arrhythmias, 601t, 602t–603t, 609–610
in pregnancy, 1858
in renal failure, 1930t
indications for, 610
pharmacokinetics of, 609–610
Propranolol (Inderal), adverse effects of, 613
dosage of, 594t–595t, 612
electrophysiological actions of, 611–612
hematological abnormalities with, 1804t
hemodynamic effects of, 612
in aortic dissection, 1564
in arrhythmias, 610–613, 611t
in atrial fibrillation prophylaxis, 1720
in atrioventricular nodal reentrant tachycardia, 664
in cardiac arrest, 766
in Marfan syndrome, 1672
in myocardial infarction, 1228–1229, *1228*
in pediatric cardiology, 1002t
in pregnancy, 1858
in renal failure, 1931t
indications for, 612
oxidative metabolism of, 1306
pharmacodynamic properties of, 487t
pharmacokinetics of, 612
pharmacology of, 1307t
serum lipid effects of, 1306
Prospective Cardiovascular Münster Study, 1145
Prostacyclin (PGI_2), *1165*
collateral vessel effects of, 1175
endothelial cell production of, 1108, 1810, 1811
in pulmonary hypertension testing, 793, *794*, 795
in vasodilation, *782*, 783, *783*
side effects of, 795
Prostaglandin(s), in heart failure, 1917t
in pulmonary vascular resistance, 783
Prostaglandin E_1, in pediatric cardiology, 1002t
in pulmonic atresia with intact ventricular septum, 928
Prostaglandin H_2 (PGH_2), *1165*
Prosthetic valves, **1061–1066**
allograft, *1063*, 1065
antithrombotic therapy for, 1732, 1834–1836, *1835*, 1836t
aspirin therapy for, 1835
autograft, *1063*, 1065
caged-ball, *1062*
caged-disc, *1062*
dehiscence of, in infective endocarditis, 1094
dysfunction of, 1064, *1064*, 1066
early diastolic sounds with, 34
early systolic sounds with, 31

Prosthetic valves *(Continued)*
  echocardiography of, 78, *78*, **Plate 3**
  embolism with, 1880
    treatment of, 1835–1836
  failure of, 1064, *1064*
  hemodynamics of, 1065
  in anticoagulated patient, 1066
  in hemodialysis patient, 1066
  in mitral regurgitation, 1026–1028, *1027*
  in pregnancy, 1066, 1856–1857
  in surgical patient, 1066
  infective endocarditis of, 1079–1080, 1079t
    clinical features of, 1080
    microbiology of, 1079, 1079t
    pathology of, 1079–1080, *1080*
  mechanical, 1061–1063, *1062*
    durability of, 1062–1063
    in mitral regurgitation, 1026–1028
    thrombogenicity of, 1062–1063
  mortality rates with, 1065t, 1066
  noncardiac surgery and, 982, 1762, 1835
  porcine, 1063–1064, *1063*, *1064*
  postoperative assessment of, 231
  postoperative infection of, 1733
  renal failure and, 1928
  replacement of, 984
  selection of, 1065–1066
  sequelae of, 984
  thrombosis with, 1836
  tilting-disc, *1062*
  tissue, *1062*, 1063–1065, *1063*, *1064*
    in mitral regurgitation, 1026–1028
Protamine sulfate, contraindications to, 245
  in arteriography, 245
  in pediatric cardiology, 1002t
Protein(s), contractile, microanatomy of, 360–366, 361t, *364–366*
  G, in contraction-relaxation cycle, 372–373, *372*, 375, *375*
    in heart failure, 411–412
    in preconditioning, 387–388, *388*
  ion-channel, 553, *554*
Protein C, 1813, *1814*
  deficiency of, in pulmonary embolism, 1582–1583, 1582t
  gene mutation in, in pulmonary embolism, 1583
Protein kinase, cyclic AMP–dependent, 374
Protein kinase A, 374
Protein kinase C, in cardiac hypertrophy, 1643
Protein S, deficiency of, in venous thrombosis, 1582t
Proteinases, in atherosclerotic plaque changes, 1187
Protein-calorie malnutrition, 994, 1907–1908, 1907t
  preoperative, 1715
Proteinuria, in cyanotic congenital heart disease, 972
Proteus, in infective endocarditis, 1093
Prothrombin time, in warfarin treatment, 1818
  preoperative, 1717t
Prothrombinase, in coagulation, 1812
Protodiastolic gallop, in heart failure, 455
Prourokinase, 1220, 1821
Pseudoaneurysm, in coronary artery disease, 1347, *1347*
  in myocardial infarction, 87, *87*, 1242–1243, *1242*
  postoperative, 230, *231*
  post-traumatic, 1542
Pseudocoarctation, 911
Pseudohypertension, in elderly, 822, 1699
Pseudohypoaldosteronism, 1678t
Pseudomonas aeruginosa, in infective endocarditis, 1082, *1082*, 1092–1093, 1094
Pseudo–P pulmonale, 115
Pseudotruncus arteriosus, 929
Pseudoxanthoma elasticum, 880t, 1673, 1678t
Psittacosis myocarditis, 1440
Psychiatric illness, syncope and, 865, 872
Psychosocial factors, in coronary artery disease, 1707
  in sudden cardiac death, 745
PTCA. See *Percutaneous transluminal coronary angioplasty (PTCA).*
Pulmonary. See also *Lung(s).*
Pulmonary angiography, in pulmonary embolism, 1590–1591, *1592*
Pulmonary angioscopy, in pulmonary embolism, 1591
Pulmonary apoplexy, in mitral stenosis, 1010
Pulmonary arteriopathy, in pulmonary hypertension, 787, 787t
Pulmonary arteriovenous fistula, 924
  in adult, 967, *968*
Pulmonary artery, 1606–1607
  balloon catheter occlusion of, vascular resistance and, 781
  calcification of, in pulmonary arterial hypertension, *219*
  catheterization of, in pregnancy, 1846
  clots in, echocardiography of, 95
  diameter of, 218
  enlargement of, on plain chest radiography, 207, *207*, *208*
  in atrial septal defect, *218*
  in Eisenmenger syndrome, 800, *800*
  in pulmonary venous hypertension, 797, *797*
  in ventricular septal defect, *218*
  infarction of, in sickle cell disease, 1788
  innervation of, 1607
  left coronary artery origin from, arteriography of, 260, *260*, 909–910, *909*, *910*
    sudden cardiac death and, 747
  neonatal, *781*
  occlusion of, cardiac catheterization in, 791t
  on plain chest radiography, *205*, 207, *208*, *212*, 215–217
  sarcoma of, 1472
  stenosis of, cardiac catheterization in, 791t
    congenital, 924, *924*
      clinical findings in, 924
      diagnosis of, 924, *924*
      etiology of, 924
      morphology of, 924
    treatment of, balloon dilatation in, 1386
Pulmonary artery pressure, 188t, 189, *189*, 190t, 780
  at high altitude, 783
  in mitral stenosis, 1009
  in myocardial infarction, 1233–1234, 1233t
Pulmonary artery wedge pressure, in pulmonary edema, 465
Pulmonary blood flow, 780
Pulmonary blood flow/systemic blood flow (PBF/SBF (QP/QS) ratio), in shunt assessment, 197
Pulmonary capillaries, gravity effects on, 463, *463*
Pulmonary capillary hemangiomatosis, in pulmonary hypertension, 787–788, 787t
Pulmonary capillary wedge pressure, 188t, 189, *189*, 190t, 423
Pulmonary circulation, **780–801**
  acetylcholine effects on, 782–783
  acidosis and, 1608, *1608*
  aging and, 781
  alpha-adrenergic agonist effects on, 782
  alveolar gas tension and, 1608, *1608*
  fetal, 781, 883
  gravity in, 463, *463*
  hypoxia and, 781, 1608
  isoproterenol effects on, 782
  neonatal, 781, *781*
  neural regulation of, 781–782
  norepinephrine effects on, 782
  normal, 780–781
  physiology of, 1607–1608, *1607*
  pressure-flow relations of, 1607–1608, *1607*
  pressure-volume relations of, 1607
  vasoconstriction of, 1608
Pulmonary edema, **462–467**
  after anesthesia, 466
  after cardiopulmonary bypass, 466
  after cardioversion, 466
  alveolar-capillary membrane in, 462
  cardiogenic, 464–465
    diagnosis of, 464–465
    differential diagnosis of, 466–467, 466t
    vs. bronchial asthma, 465
  classification of, 463–466, 463t
  differential diagnosis of, 466–467, 466t
  eclampsia and, 466
  embolus-associated, 466
  gravity in, 463, *463*
  heroin overdose–associated, 465–466
  high-altitude, 465, *466*
    in secondary pulmonary hypertension, 801
Pulmonary edema *(Continued)*
  in heart failure, 457, 462–467
  in mitral valve stenosis, 798
  lymphatics in, 462
  mechanism of, 462–463
  mitral regurgitation and, 227, *228*
  neurogenic, 465, 1878
  plain film radiography of, *219*, 220–221
  postoperative, 230, 466, 1722–1723
  stages of, 463
  Starling forces in, 463t, 464
  vs. bronchial asthma, 465
Pulmonary embolism, **1582–1600**
  acquired hypercoagulable states in, 1583, 1583t
  chest pain in, 5, 1586t, 1587
  chronic, 1598, 1598t
  clinical presentation of, 1585–1586, 1585t
  deep venous thrombosis and, 1584, *1584*
  diagnosis of, 1585–1592, 1585t, 1586t, *1593*
    arterial blood gases in, 1587
    chest roentgenography in, 1588, *1588*
    computed tomography in, 344, *344*, 1591
    contrast phlebography in, 1589
    differential, 1585–1586, 1586t
    echocardiography in, 1589–1590, 1590t
    electrocardiography in, 118, *118*, 1587, 1587t
    impedance plethysmography in, 1587–1588
    integrated approach to, 1591–1592, *1593*
    intravascular ultrasound in, 1591
    lung scan in, 1589, 1589t, 1590t
    magnetic resonance imaging in, 1591
    plasma D-dimer ELISA in, 1587, *1587*
    pulmonary angiography in, 1590–1591, *1592*
    pulmonary angioscopy in, 1591
    venous ultrasonography in, 1588, *1588*
  hypercoagulable states in, 1582–1583, 1582t, 1583t
  in dilated cardiomyopathy, 1834, 1834t
  in heart failure, 449
  in secondary pulmonary hypertension, 800–801
  management of, 1592–1600, 1593t
    adjunctive measures in, 1593
    anticoagulation in, 1593–1594
    aspirin in, 1595
    dextran in, 1594
    embolectomy in, 1597–1598, *1597*
    emotional support in, 1598
    heparin in, 1593–1594
    inferior vena caval interruption in, 1595–1596, 1595t, *1596*
    thrombolysis in, 1596–1597, *1596*, 1596t
    warfarin sodium in, 1594–1595
  massive, 1586, 1586t
  moderate to large, 1586–1587, 1586t
  nonthrombotic, 1586t, 1587
  obesity and, 1583
  oral contraceptives and, 1583, 1584
  pain in, 1199
    vs. angina pectoris, 1292
  paradoxical, 1586t, 1587
  pathophysiology of, 1582–1585, 1582t, *1583–1585*, 1583t
  postoperative, 1583, 1727
  prevention of, 1598–1600, 1599t
    aspirin in, 1600
    compression stockings in, 1598
    heparin in, 1599–1600
    in pregnancy, 1600
    inferior vena caval interruption in, 1599
    intermittent pneumatic compression in, 1598–1599
    nonorthopedic surgery in, 1600
    orthopedic surgery in, 1600
    pharmacological agents in, 1599–1600
  primary hypercoagulable states in, 1582–1583, 1582t, 1583t
  pulmonary edema in, 466
  right ventricular dysfunction and, 1584
  small to moderate, 1586t, 1587
  survival with, *1583*
  syncope with, 867
  ventricular interdependency and, 1584, *1585*
  vs. pulmonary hypertension, 1586, 1586t
Pulmonary function, in myocardial infarction, 1197
  postoperative, 1722–1723, 1722t
  preoperative, 1717t
Pulmonary function testing, in dyspnea, 451
  in pulmonary hypertension, 789

Pulmonary hypertension, **783–801**
anatomical markers of, 887
clinical manifestations of, 887
familial, 1677
heart sounds in, *31*, 35, *35*
in congenital heart disease, 886–887
in hypertrophic cardiomyopathy, 1422
in infant, 886–887
in mitral stenosis, 1009
in mixed connective tissue disease, 1782
in pregnancy, 1856
in rheumatoid arthritis, 1778
in systemic lupus erythematosus, 1779
in ventricular septal defect, 903
murmur in, 887
pain in, 4–5
vs. angina pectoris, 1292
plain film radiography in, 218–219, *219*
primary, **783–796**
anorexigens in, 786
antinuclear antibodies in, 786
autonomic nervous system in, 784
cardiac catheterization in, 790–791, 791t
chemical studies in, 789
clinical features of, 788–789, *788*
differential diagnosis of, 791
echocardiography in, 789–790
electrocardiography in, 789
endothelial cells in, 784, *784*
endothelin, 784
endothelium-derived relaxing factor in, 784
etiology of, 783–787, *784*, *785*
familial, 786–787
genetic anticipation in, 786
genetic predisposition to, 785–786
hematological studies in, 789
hemodynamic findings in, 788
human immunodeficiency virus infection in, 786
laboratory findings in, 789–791, *789*
lung scan in, *789*, 790
major histocompatibility complex in, 787
mortality with, 788–789, *788*
natural history of, 788–789, *788*
pathological findings in, 787–788, 787t
physical examination in, 788, 789
portal hypertension in, 786
pulmonary angiography in, 790, *790*
pulmonary arteriopathy in, 787, 787t
pulmonary blood flow increase in, 786
pulmonary capillary hemangiomatosis in, 787–788, 787t
pulmonary function tests in, 788, 789
pulmonary veno-occlusive disease in, 787, 787t
right ventricular failure in, 789
risk factors in, 786–787
roentgenography in, 789
symptomatology of, 788–789
syncope in, 788
systemic hypertension in, 786
thrombosis in, 785, *785*
treatment of, 791–796
adenosine in, 793, *793*
anticoagulants in, 795
atrial septostomy in, 795
calcium channel blockers in, 794–795, *794*
digoxin in, 792
diuretics in, 792
heart-lung transplantation in, 795–796
lifestyle changes in, 791
lung transplantation in, 795–796, *795*
nitric oxide in, 793
oxygen in, 792
prostacyclin in, 793, 795
vasodilators in, 792–793, *793*
vascular occlusion in, 784–785, *784*
vasodilator effects in, 784, *784*
right ventricle palpation in, 27–28
right ventricular function in, 1590, 1610–1612, *1611*, *1612*
right ventricular preload augmentation in, 1612–1613
second heart sound in, 33, *33*
secondary, **796–801,** 796t
cor triatriatum in, 798
in Eisenmenger syndrome, 799–801, *800*
in high-altitude pulmonary edema, 801
in high-output cardiac failure, 801
in hypoventilation, 801
Pulmonary hypertension *(Continued)*
in intravenous drug abuse, 801
in isolated partial anomalous pulmonary venous drainage, 801
in neuromuscular disorders, 801
in obesity-hypoventilation syndrome, 801
in peripheral pulmonic stenosis, 801
in persistent fetal circulation, 800
in pulmonary parenchymal disease, 798–799
in pulmonary thromboembolism, 800–801
in sickle cell anemia, 801
in Takayasu's arteritis, 801
in tetralogy of Fallot, 801
left ventricular diastolic pressure elevation in, 797
mitral valve disease in, 797–798
mitral valve regurgitation in, 798
mitral valve stenosis in, 797–798, *798*
pulmonary vascular resistance in, 798–801, 799t
pulmonary venous drainage resistance in, 796–798, *797*
venous, plain film radiography in, 219–220, *219*, *220*
ventricular interaction in, 1611, *1612*
vs. pulmonary embolism, 1586, 1586t
Pulmonary vascular resistance, in Eisenmenger syndrome, 799
in heart transplantation, 516t
measurement of, 193
Pulmonary vasculitis, in secondary pulmonary hypertension, 799, 799t
Pulmonary veins, atresia of, 922–923
blood flow in, in ventricular diastolic filling, 438, *438*
diameter of, in pulmonary venous hypertension, 219
stenosis of, 922–923
Pulmonary veno-occlusive disease, in pulmonary hypertension, 787, 787t
Pulmonary venous drainage, resistance to, in pulmonary arterial hypertension, 796–798, *797*
Pulmonary venous pressure, 780
Pulmonary wedge angiography, in pulmonary hypertension, 887
Pulmonic regurgitation, 967, 1059, *1059*
diastolic murmur of, *48*, 49
mid-diastolic murmur of, 42–43, *43*
Pulmonic stenosis, 1059, *1059*, 1847
balloon valvuloplasty in, 1386
congenital, 924–926, 965, *965*
angiocardiography in, 926
balloon valvuloplasty in, 925
cardiac catheterization in, 926
chest roentgenography in, 926
echocardiography in, 79, *79*, 926, *926*
electrocardiography in, 925–926
exercise and, 978–979
heart sounds in, *30*
in adult, 968–969, *969*
in children, 925
in infant, 925, *925*
management of, 926, *927*
natural history of, 926
physical examination in, 925
genetic factors in, 1660t
in Noonan syndrome, 1663
in secondary pulmonary hypertension, 801
midsystolic murmur of, *31*, 37
plain chest radiography in, 233, *233*
pregnancy and, 975, 976
pressure gradients in, 194
pulmonary blood flow in, 220, *220*
systolic murmur of, 49
treatment of, 1386
Pulmonic valve, calcifications of, 221
congenital absence of, 932, *932*
congenital atresia of, 926–928
diagnosis of, 928
management of, 928
morphology of, 926–928
echocardiography of, 70, *70*, 932, *932*
in rheumatoid arthritis, 1776
Pulmonic valve disease, 1059–1060
auscultation in, 1059
carcinoid, 1059, *1059*
clinical manifestations of, 1059
echocardiography in, 1060
etiology of, 1059, *1059*
Graham Steell murmur in, 1059
Pulmonic valve disease *(Continued)*
laboratory examination in, 1059–1060, *1060*
management of, 1060
radiological findings in, 1060, *1060*
Pulsations, on chest inspection, 24
Pulse, arterial, 20–23
abnormal, 22
anacrotic, *21*, 22
dicrotic, *21*, 22
in aortic regurgitation, 22
in aortic stenosis, 1040
in atrioventricular dissociation, 22
in coarctation of aorta, 18, 22
in mitral regurgitation, 22, 1022
in mitral stenosis, 1010, 1022
in stable angina pectoris, 1292
normal, 21–22, *21*
palpation of, 20–23, *21*, 23
percussion wave of, 21–22
tidal wave of, 21–22
bisferious, *21*
in aortic regurgitation, 1049
in hypertrophic obstructive cardiomyopathy, *21*
Corrigan (water-hammer), in aortic regurgitation, 22, 1049
during palpitation, 9
Quincke's, 17, 460
in aortic regurgitation, 22, 1049
venous, 18–20
a wave of, *18*, 19–20
elevation of, 19–20, *19*
examination of, 18–20, *18*, *19*
H wave of, *18*, 19
in aortic stenosis, 1040
in arrhythmias, 641
in constrictive pericarditis, *19*, 20, 1498, *1499*
in mitral stenosis, *19*, 1010
in myocardial infarction, 1200
in tricuspid regurgitation, *18*, 20
normal, *18*
v wave of, *18*, 19
Pulse deficit, in aortic dissection, 1556–1557
Pulse wave velocity, of aging heart, 1689–1690, *1691*, *1692*
Pulse width, of pacemaker, 711
Pulsed dye laser, 1383
Pulseless electrical activity, 756
management of, 766
Pulsus alternans, 22–23, *23*
in heart failure, 455
in idiopathic dilated cardiomyopathy, 1410
Pulsus bigeminus, 23
Pulsus bisferiens, *21*, 22
in aortic regurgitation, 1049
in hypertrophic obstructive cardiomyopathy, *21*
Pulsus paradoxus, 23
in cardiac tamponade, 1488–1490, *1488*
in constrictive pericarditis, 1499
nonspecificity of, 1488–1489
reversed, 23
Pulsus parvus, 22
Pulsus parvus et tardus, 22
Pulsus tardus, *21*, 22
Purkinje cells, 552, *552*
microanatomy of, 360–361, 361t
Purkinje fibers, action potential of, 552, *552*
cable properties of, 564
terminal, 550
Purple toes syndrome, 1595
Putrescine, urinary, after heart transplantation, 520
P-wave alternans, 140
Pyelonephritis, systemic hypertension with, 824

Q fever, endocarditis with, 1439
Q wave, 111t
in AIDS myocarditis, 135, *149*
in chronic obstructive lung disease, 135–136
in cor pulmonale, 136
in diastolic overload, 117, *146*
in hypertrophic cardiomyopathy, 135, *136*, *149*, 1421
in left bundle branch block, 120, *120*
in myocardial infarction, 128–132, *130*, *131*, *147–150*

Q wave *(Continued)*
in myocardial metastasis, 135, *136*
in old myocardial infarction, 132
in pericarditis, 1483–1484, *1483*, 1483t
in septal infarction, 134, *149*
in stable angina pectoris, 1295
in Wolff-Parkisnon-White syndrome, 136
noninfarction, 135–136, *136*
transient, 135
QRS alternans, 140
QRS axis, 112–113, *113*
QRS complex, 112–114, *112*, *113*
duration of, 112
in acceleration-dependent aberrancy, 125–126, *125*
in arrhythmia evaluation, 643
in cardiac tamponade, 1490, *1490*
in hyperkalemia, *137*, 141–142, *141*
in hypertrophic cardiomyopathy, 1421
in left bundle branch block, 119–120, *120*
in myocardial infarction, 130–131, *131*
in right bundle branch block, 121
in ventricular tachycardia, 678
in Wolff-Parkinson-White syndrome, 126–127, *126*, *127*
prolongation of, ventricular late potentials in, 583–584, *584*
QRS loop, 114–115, 115t. See also *Vectorcardiography.*
Q-T interval, 114, 139–140, *140*
in chronic renal disease, *138*
in hypercalcemia, 142, *142*
in hypocalcemia, 142, *142*
prolongation of, 139–140, *140*, *151*
acquired, 751
congenital, 750–751
in sudden cardiac death, 750–751
practice guidelines for, 1963
quinidine effect on, 603
short, *151*
Q-U interval, in hypokalemia, *141*
Quadrigeminy, definition of, 676
Quality of life, in heart failure, 453, *454*
Quantitative trait linkage, in genetic research, 1679
Questran. See *Cholestyramine (Questran).*
Quinapril, first-dose effects of, 497
in heart failure, 472t
Quincke's pulse, 17, 460
in aortic regurgitation, 22, 1049
Quinethazone, in heart failure, 477–478, 477t
Quinidine, adverse effects of, 602–603
atrial flutter effect of, *653*
digoxin interaction with, 483t
dosage of, 594t–595t, 601–602
electrophysiological actions of, 601, 601t, 602t–603t
hematological abnormalities with, 1804t
hemodynamic effects of, 601
in arrhythmias, 594t–595t, 601–603, 601t, 602t–603t
in pediatric cardiology, 1002t
in pregnancy, 1858
in renal failure, 1930t
indications for, 602
intraventricular aberration and, *125*
pharmacokinetics of, 594t–595t, 601
toxicity of, 11

R wave, 111t
in chronic obstructive lung disease, 119
in exercise stress testing, 163
in myocardial infarction, 129–130, *130*, *131*, *148*, *149*
in septal infarction, 134, *148*
Radial artery technique, for cardiac catheterization, 186
Radial wall stress, of left ventricle, 426–427, *426*
Radiation pericarditis, 1516–1517
Radiation safety, in cardiac catheterization, 181
Radiation therapy, cardiac effects of, 1799, 1799t
coronary artery stenosis with, 1349
external-beam, in neoplastic pericarditis, 1516
in children, 1799
mediastinal, in myocardial infarction, 1193
myocardial effects of, 1449
pacemaker effects of, 728–729
Radiation therapy *(Continued)*
pericardial effects of, 1516–1517
toxicity of, 13
Radiofrequency catheter ablation, arrhythmia treatment with, 621–628, *621–628*
indications for, 623
pathway location for, 621–622, *621*
results of, 623
site selection for, 622, *622*
practice guidelines for, 1961t, 1963
Radiology, 204–236. See also *Chest roentgenography.*
frontal view for, 204–211, *205–211*
lateral view for, 211, *212*, *213*
left anterior oblique view for, 212–213, *216*
of acquired heart disease, 225–229, *226–228*
of cardiac calcification, 221–225, *221–224*
of pericardium, 234–235, *234–236*
of pulmonary vasculature, 215–221, *218–220*
postoperative, 229–234, *229–234*
right anterior oblique view for, 211–212, *214*, *215*
Rales, in heart failure, 453
in myocardial infarction, 1200, 1234t
Ramipril, in heart failure, 472t, 495–497, *496*
in renal failure, 1933t
Ramp protocol, for exercise stress testing, 156
Rapamycin, in heart transplantation rejection, 523
Rapid atrial pacing, in atrial flutter, 654
ras gene, in cardiac hypertrophy, 1643, *1643*
Recombinant protein therapy, 1626–1629, *1627*, *1628*
Reemployment, in cardiac rehabilitation, 1398–1399
Reentry, 569–577
anatomical, 570–571, *570*
anisotropic model of, *571*, 572, *577*
figure-of-8 model of, *571*, *572*
functional models of, 571–572, *571*
in arrhythmogenesis, 569–577, *573–577*
leading circle model of, 571–572, *571*
reflection, 572
spiral wave model of, *571*, 572
tachycardias with, 572–576, *573–577*
Regitine (phentolamine), in heart failure, 472t
in hypertensive crisis, 858t
in pediatric cardiology, 1001t
Regression Growth Evaluation Statin Study, in hypercholesterolemia prevention, 1132–1133
Regurgitant fraction, 196, 425
of left ventricle, 425
Regurgitant volume, on magnetic resonance imaging, 331
Regurgitation. See specific types, e.g., *Mitral regurgitation.*
Reiter's syndrome, 1781
aortitis in, 1575
Relapsing fever, myocardial involvement in, 1441
Relapsing polychondritis, 1783
Relaxation, in hypertension, 846
Relaxivity agents, for magnetic resonance imaging, 332–333
Renal. See also *Kidney(s).*
Renal artery, obstruction of, 825–827, 826t
classification of, 826t
diagnosis of, 826–827, 826t
mechanisms of, 826
Renal failure, 1923–1935
acute myocardial ischemia and, 1927
arrhythmias and, 1928–1929, 1929t, 1935
autonomic dysfunction in, 1935
cardiac surgery and, 1328–1329, 1925–1926, 1925t
cardiovascular calcification and, 1927, 1927t
cardiovascular drug therapy in, 1930t–1934t, 1935
coronary atherosclerosis and, 1924–1927, *1925*, 1926t
dialysis for. See *Kidney dialysis.*
heart failure and, 1923–1924, *1923*
dialysis and, 1923–1924, *1924*
management of, 1924
negative inotropic effects in, 1923
pressure overload in, 1923
renal transplantation and, 1924
volume overload in, 1923
heart murmurs and, 1927–1928
hypertrophic cardiomyopathy and, 1924
Renal failure *(Continued)*
in cholesterol embolization syndrome, 1571
myocardial oxygen demand in, 1925–1926, *1925*
myocardial oxygen supply in, 1925–1926, *1925*
oliguric, 824
pericardial disease and, 1512–1513, 1928, *1928*
postoperative, 1734
radiocontrast-induced, 245
systemic hypertension and, 824–825, 1928, *1929*
transplantation for, 1924, 1925, *1925*
valvular heart disease and, 1927–1928
Renal insufficiency, with diuretics, 480
Rendu-Weber-Osler disease, 16, *17*, 1676
genes for, 1632t
heart failure in, 461
Renin, in heart failure, *408*, 1916t
inhibitors of, 474
plasma, in hypertension, 815
Renin-angiotensin inhibitors, 473–474, *473*
in hypertension, 855–856, *855*
Renin-angiotensin system, 1895
antagonists of, 473–474, *473*
in heart failure, 413–414, *413*, 471–473
in hypertension, 819–820, *819*
in myocardial infarction, 1197
Renin-secreting tumor, 827
Renography, isotopic, in renovascular hypertension, 827
Renovascular hypertension, 825–827, 826t
classification of, 826t
diagnosis of, 826–827, 826t
mechanisms of, 826
Reperfusion injury, *1178*, 1179, 1213–1214
Repolarization, 109, *109*, 110, 139
early, ST segment in, 136, *138*
Reserpine, hematological abnormalities with, 1804t
in coronary artery disease, 1149t
in renal failure, 1932t
in systemic hypertension, 852
Residua, of congenital cardiac malformation, 982–983, 982t
Respiration, in cardiac arrest management, 763
in cyanosis, 892–893
in myocardial infarction, 1200
postoperative, 1319, 1722–1723, 1722t
Respiratory disease, digoxin in, 501
Respiratory distress, in heart failure, 450–451, 450t
Respiratory muscles, in cor pulmonale, 1614
Respiratory rate, in myocardial infarction, 1200
Respiratory syncytial virus, in myocarditis, 1439
Respiratory tract procedures, prophylactic antibiotics for, in congenital heart disease, 888t
Response-to-injury hypothesis, of atherosclerosis, 1114–1116, *1115*
Reteplase, 1821–1822
Retina, examination of, 15–16, *16*
hemorrhages of, in infective endocarditis, 1085, *1085*
Retinoic acid, teratogenicity of, 1663t, 1664
Retinopathy, 15, *16*
Retrovirus vector, for gene therapy, 1638
Rhabdomyoma, 1470
genetic factors in, 1676
Rhabdomyosarcoma, 1471
Rheumatic fever, 1769–1783
arthritis in, 1771, *1771*
Aschoff nodule in, 1770
bacterial endocarditis prophylaxis in, 1774
carditis in, 1770–1772, *1771*
chorea in, 1771, *1771*
clinical manifestations of, 1770–1772, *1771*
diagnosis of, 1770–1772, 1770t
epidemiology of, 1769
erythema marginatum in, 1771
etiologic agent of, 1769–1770, 1769t, 1772
group A streptococcus in, 1769–1770, 1769t, 1772
in pregnancy, 1848–1850, *1849*
incidence of, 1770
laboratory findings in, 1771–1772
pathogenesis of, 1769–1770, 1769t
pathology of, 1770
pericarditis in, 1517–1518
prevention of, 1772–1774, 1773t
primary prevention of, 1772–1773, 1773t

Rheumatic fever *(Continued)*
secondary prevention of, 1773–1774, 1774t
streptococcal infection in, 1772
subcutaneous nodules in, 1771
treatment of, 1772
valvulitis in, 1770–1772
Rheumatic heart disease, 1007, 1770–1771
in pregnant patient, 1848–1850, *1849*
patient history in, 11
Rheumatic valvulitis, 1770–1771
Rheumatoid arthritis, 1776–1778, 1776t
aortitis in, 1777–1778, *1777*
cardiac tamponade in, 1518
cardiomyopathy in, 1778
conduction system disease in, 1777
coronary artery disease in, 1776–1777
myocarditis in, 1777, *1777*
pericarditis in, 1518, 1776
pulmonary hypertension in, 1778
valvular disease in, 1776, *1777*
Rheumatoid factor, in infective endocarditis, 1084
Ribonucleoprotein, antibodies to, in congenital heart block, 1667
Ribs, notching of, in coarctation of aorta, 232
Rickettsia, in infective endocarditis, 1082
Right anterior oblique view, for plain chest radiography, 211–212, *214*, *215*
Right bundle branch, 550, *551*
Right bundle branch block (RBBB), 641t–642t
electrocardiography in, 121, *121*, *122*, 123, *146*, *147*
exercise stress testing in, 168–169
in myocardial infarction, 1252
left fascicular block and, *121*, *122*, 123, *147*
temporary pacing in, 706
vectorcardiography in, 121
ventricular hypertrophy in, 119
Right ventricular outflow tract obstruction, ventricular septal defect and, 903
Riley-Day syndrome, 1678t
RO43-5054, 1820
Rocky Mountain spotted fever, myocarditis with, 1439
Roller pump, 537–538, 537t
Roth spots, in infective endocarditis, 1085, *1085*
Rubella syndrome, 878, 881t, 1663t, 1664
myocarditis in, 1439
pulmonary artery stenosis in, 924
Rubeola, in myocarditis, 1439
Rubinstein-Taybi syndrome, 880t, 1659t
Rule of bigeminy, *654*
Ryanodine receptor (calcium release channel), 360, *363*
in heart failure, 405–406
of sarcoplasmic reticulum, 367–368, *367*, *368*

S wave, 111t
in hyperkalemia, 141–142, *141*
in myocardial infarction, *149*
in pulmonary venous flow velocity, 438, *438*
in right bundle branch block, 121, *121*
St. Jude valve, 1061, *1062*, 1065
St. Vitus' dance, in rheumatic fever, 1771
St Thomas' Atherosclerosis Regression Study, in hypercholesterolemia prevention, 1131
Saldino-Noonan syndrome, genetic factors in, 1661t
Salicylates, in rheumatic fever, 1772
Salmonella, in infective endocarditis, 1082
in myocarditis, 1440
Salt restriction, in hypertension, 844–845, *845*
Sanfilippo A syndrome, 1669t
Sanfilippo B syndrome, 1669t
Sanfilippo C syndrome, 1669t
Sanfilippo D syndrome, 1669t
Saphenous vein bypass graft, 1317, *1317*
angiography of, 253–254, *254*
Saphenous vein bypass graft disease, 1826–1827
Saralasin, in heart failure, 474
Sarcoidosis, arrhythmias in, 1431
pericarditis in, 1519, *1519*
restrictive cardiomyopathy in, 1431
sudden cardiac death in, 749
Sarcolemma, 360, *362*
Sarcoma, of pulmonary artery, 1472
ventricular, 326, *326*
Sarcomere, 361, *362*, 382
Sarcoplasmic reticulum, 360, *363*
Ca^{++}-ATPase of, in heart failure, 405, *405*
calcium release channel (ryanodine receptor) of, 367–368, *367*, *368*
calcium-induced calcium release from, in contraction-relaxation cycle, 366–369, *367*, *368*
calcium-pumping ATPase of, 368–369, *368*
in contraction-relaxation cycle, *363*, 366–369, *367*, *368*
in heart failure, 369
inositol triphosphate receptor of, 368, *368*
SC-5468A, 1820
Scalenus anticus (thoracic outlet) syndrome, vs. angina, 7
Scandinavian Simvastatin Survival Study, in hypercholesterolemia prevention, 1133
Scheie syndrome, 881t, 1668t, 1675
Schistosomiasis, in pericarditis, 1511
myocardial involvement in, 1444–1445
Scintillation camera, 273
Sclerae, blue, 15
Scleroderma, 1781–1782, *1781*, *1782*
cor pulmonale in, 1615
hypertension in, 824
pericarditis in, 1518–1519
Scopolamine, in syncope, 874
Scorpion fish sting, pericarditis with, 1519
Scorpion sting, myocardial effects of, 1448
Screening test. See *Practice guidelines.*
Scrub typhus, myocarditis with, 1439
Sedation, for arteriography, 244–245
Seizures, syncope in, 866
Selenium deficiency, myocardial effects of, 1447–1448
Self-efficacy, in cardiac rehabilitation, 1398
Senility, public safety and, 772
Sensitivity, of diagnostic tests, 1743
Sensitivity analysis, in cost-effectiveness analysis, 1741
Sepsis, postoperative, 1727
Septal aneurysm, echocardiography in, 58–59, *59*, 83, 87–88
in secundum-type atrial septal defect, 898
myocardial infarction–associated, 87–88
Septic aneurysm, in adult congenital heart disease, 974, *974*
Septic arteritis, in infective endocarditis, 1096
Septic shock, postoperative, 1726t, 1727
Septostomy, atrial, in congenital heart disease, 895
in pulmonary hypertension, 795
in transposition of great arteries, 939
in tricuspid atresia, 933
Septum, interatrial, lipomatous hypertrophy of, 95, 1471
tumor of, *1472*
interventricular, rupture of, in myocardial infarction, 1241t, 1243, *1244*
traumatic, 1536t, 1538, 1541, *1541*
vs. mitral regurgitation, 1244
sarcoma of, 326, *326*
Serotonin (5-hydroxytryptamine), 783, *1165*
Serratia, in infective endocarditis, 1082, 1093
Serum bactericidal titer, in infective endocarditis therapy, 1093
Serum glutamic oxaloacetic acid transferase (SGOT), in myocardial infarction, 1204
Sestamibi, technetium-99m–labeled, for myocardial perfusion imaging, 274, 275t, *280*, 290, *291*
myocardial kinetics of, 282–283, *283*
Sexual activity, in cardiac rehabilitation, 1400
in coronary artery disease, 1301
Shield chest, 24
Shock, cardiogenic. See *Cardiogenic shock.*
postoperative, 1725–1727, 1726t
septic, 1726t, 1727
vs. cardiac tamponade, 1490, 1512
Shock lung, pulmonary edema in, 465
Short rib–polydactyly syndrome, genetic factors in, 1661t
Shortness of breath, chest pain with, 7
Shoshin beriberi, 462
Shprintzen (velocardiofacial) syndrome, 881t, 1658
genetic factors in, 1660t
Shunt(s), bidirectional, 196–198
diagnosis of, indicator-dilution method for, 197, *197*
oximetric method for, 196
echocardiography of, 81–84, *82*, *83*, **Plate 3**
first-pass radionuclide angiocardiography of, 301
left-to-right, congenital, 896–911, *896–904*, *906–911*. See also specific defects, e.g., *Atrial septal defect.*
in atrial septal defect, *334*
localization of, 197–198, *197*
plain chest radiography in, 232–233, *232*
quantification of, 196–198
oximetric assessment of, 196
right-to-left, 196–198, *197*
Shy-Drager syndrome, 1678t
syncope in, 865–866
Sick sinus syndrome, 648–649, *649*
anatomical basis of, 649
exercise stress testing in, 168
management of, 649
pacemaker in, 708, 709t
syncope in, 867
Sickle cell disease, 880t, 1675, 1787–1788
cardiopulmonary manifestations of, 1788, *1788*
in secondary pulmonary hypertension, 801
pathophysiology of, 1787–1788
Signal amplitude, of pacemaker, 711
Signal transduction, in contraction-relaxation cycle, 372–376, *372–375*, 375t, *376*
Silicone, pericarditis with, 1519
Simendan, in heart failure, 485
Simian sarcoma virus, 1117
Simvastatin, in dyslipidemia, 1140t, 1141
in hypercholesterolemia prevention, 1133
Single-photon emission computed tomography (SPECT), 273–274. See also *Myocardial perfusion imaging.*
artifacts on, 279, *279*, 281, *282*
breast tissue on, 279, 281
circumferential profile for, 284, **Plate 5, Plate 6, Plate 7**
normal, 279, 281, *281*
of myocardial fatty acid metabolism, 303
patient positioning for, 277
polar map (bull's eye display) for, 283–284
quality control for, 281
quantification of, 283–284, **Plate 5, Plate 6, Plate 7**
Sinoatrial conduction time, 580–581, *581*
Sinoatrial exit block, 647, *647*
Sinoatrial node, acetylcholine stimulation of, 548, 563, *563*
in cardiac activation, 110, *110*
Sinoatrial node artery, 254
Sinus arrest, 646, *646*
Sinus arrhythmia, 646
nonrespiratory, *645*, 646
respiratory, 646
ventriculophasic, 646
Sinus bradycardia, 641t–642t, 645–646, *645*
clinical features of, 646
electrocardiography in, 645–646, *645*
in myocardial infarction, 1212–1213, 1245t, 1249
management of, 646
syncope in, 867
Sinus nodal reentry, *650*
radiofrequency catheter ablation in, 624–627
Sinus nodal reentry tachycardia, 649, *649*, *650*
Sinus node, 548, *549*
anatomy of, 548, *549*
automaticity of, 563–564
cells of, 548
dysfunction of, diagnosis of, 580–581, *581*
practice guidelines for, 1959, 1960t
pacemaker in, practice guidelines for, 1964t
innervation of, 548
Sinus node recovery time, 580, *581*
Sinus of Valsalva. See *Aortic sinus.*
Sinus rhythm, 641t–642t, *644*, 645
Sinus tachycardia, 641t–642t, 645, *645*
clinical features of, 645
electrocardiography in, 645, *645*
in Duchenne muscular dystrophy, 1868–1869
in hyperthyroidism, 1893
in myocardial infarction, 1245t, 1253
in pericarditis, 1484
management of, 598t, 624–627, *625*, 645

Sinus tachycardia *(Continued)*
  postoperative, 1764
  radiofrequency catheter ablation in, 624–627, *625*
Situational syncope, 864–865. See also *Syncope.*
Situs ambiguus, 946
Situs inversus, 946
  dextrocardia with, in adult, 966
    noncardiac surgery and, 981
Situs solitus, 946
  dextrocardia with, in adult, 966
Six-minute walk test, for exercise stress testing, 156
  in heart failure, 452, *452*
Size, cardiac, on radiograph, 215, *217*
Sjögren's syndrome, 1782
Skin, coumarin-induced necrosis of, 1818
  examination of, 16, *17*
  in cholesterol embolization syndrome, 1571
  warfarin-associated necrosis of, 1595
Sleep apnea syndrome, etiology of, 1615
  in cor pulmonale, 1614–1615
  in hypertension, 821
  management of, 1615
Sly syndrome, 1669t
Small vessel vasculitides, 1783
Smith-Lemli-Opitz syndrome, genetic factors in, 1660t
Smith-Magenis syndrome, 1651t
Smooth muscle cells, 1108–1110, *1109*
  collagen formation by, 1109, *1109*
  contractile phenotype of, 1109, *1109*
  embryogenesis of, 1109
  gene therapy–induced inhibition of, 1638
  injury to, 1109–1110
  lipid accumulation in, 1109
  phenotypes of, 1109, *1109*
  receptors of, 1109
Snake bite, myocardial effects of, 1448
Sneeze syncope, 864–865. See also *Syncope.*
Sodium, dietary, in hypertension, 844–845, *845*
  myocardial concentration of, 554t
  renal retention of, in heart failure, 1915, 1917–1918, *1918*
    in hypertension, 817–818, 817t
  serum, in heart failure, *548*
Sodium (Na^+), chloride (Cl^-) symporter, in heart failure, 477–478, 477t
Sodium (Na^+), potassium (K^+)-ATPase pump, cardiac glycoside effect on, 480–481
Sodium azide, myocardial effects of, 1448
Sodium channel, in action potential phase 0, 557–559, *557, 559*
  inactivation of, 558, *559*
  lidocaine effects on, 559, *560*
Sodium polystyrene sulfonate (Kayexalate), in pediatric cardiology, 1002t
Sodium (Na^+), potassium (K^+), chloride (2Cl) symport, inhibitors of, in heart failure, 476–477, 477t
Sodium pump, in contraction-relaxation cycle, 371–372
Sodium-bicarbonate cotransporter, in contraction-relaxation cycle, 371
Sodium-calcium exchanger, in contraction-relaxation cycle, 370–371, *370, 371*
  in heart failure, 406
Sodium-proton exchanger, in contraction-relaxation cycle, 371, *371*
Solu-Medrol (methylprednisolone), in pediatric cardiology, 1001t
Somatostatin, in acromegaly, 1887
Sones technique, for coronary artery catheterization, 185
Sotalol, adverse effects of, 616
  dosage of, 616
  electrophysiological actions of, 615–616
  hemodynamics of, 616
  in arrhythmias, 610–613, 611t, 615–616
  in elderly, 1698
  in hypertrophic cardiomyopathy, 1426
  in pregnancy, 1859
  in renal failure, 1931t
  indications of, 616
  pharmacodynamic properties of, 487t
  pharmacokinetics of, 616
Space constant, of cable, 564
Sphingolipidoses, 1669t, 1675–1676
Sphygmomanometry, for arterial pressure measurement, 20
Sphygmomanometry *(Continued)*
  for intracardiac pressure measurement, 422–423
Spider cell, of rhabdomyoma, 1470
Spider sting, myocardial effects of, 1448
Spiral wave model of reentry, *571*, 572
Spirochetes, in pericarditis, 1511
Spironolactone (Aldactone), hematological abnormalities with, 1804t
  in congenital heart disease–related heart failure, 890t
  in heart failure, 477t, 890t
  in pediatric cardiology, 1002t
  in renal failure, 1933t
Splanchnic circulation, in heart failure, 410
Spleen, abscess of, in infective endocarditis, 1095–1096
  congenital disorders of, cardiac anomalies with, 946
  enlargement of, 18
    in infective endocarditis, 1085
  examination of, 18
Splinter hemorrhages, 17
  in infective endocarditis, 1085, *1085*
Spondyloarthropathy, 1780–1781, *1780*
Springwater cysts, 1522
Sputum, in differential diagnosis, 10
Square root sign, in restrictive cardiomyopathy, 1427
Squatting posture, auscultatory effects of, 48, *48*
  in congenital heart disease, 885
ST alternans, 140
  in ischemic heart disease, 131–132
ST segment, 113, 139, 139t
  after percutaneous transluminal coronary angioplasty, 171
  digitalis effect on, 142
  during cesarean section, 854, *1855*
  in coronary artery disease, 1290
  in early repolarization, 136, *138*
  in exercise stress testing, 157–160, *157–160*, 163
  in hyperkalemia, *137*
  in ischemia, 127, *127*
  in left bundle branch block, *148*
  in left ventricular hypertrophy, 139
  in myocardial infarction, 129–131, *130, 131, 134*, 134–135, *149*, 166, 714, 1205–1206, *1206*, 1208–1210, 1256
  in pericarditis, 1483–1484, *1483*, 1483t
  in posterior left ventricular infarction, 134–135
  in Prinzmetal's variant angina, *137*, 1341
  in right bundle branch block, 121
  in right ventricular hypertrophy, 118
  in right ventricular infarction, 134, *134, 149*
  in silent myocardial ischemia, 1345, *1345*
  in unstable angina, 1334, *1334*
ST segment/heart rate slope, in exercise stress testing, 163
Standing, sudden, in hypertrophic cardiomyopathy evaluation, 1423
Staphylococcus aureus, in infective endocarditis, 1078, 1081, 1086, 1088, 1091–1092, 1092t, 1095
Staphylococcus epidermidis, in infective endocarditis, 1081
Staphylococcus lugdunensis, in infective endocarditis, 1081
Staphylococcus pneumoniae, in infective endocarditis, 1078, 1086
Staphylokinase, 1822
Stare, 15
Starr-Edwards valve, 1061, *1062*, 1065
Stenosis, coronary artery, arteriography of, 255–257, *256, 257*
  compensation for, 1172–1173, *1173*
  congenital, 260
  coronary blood flow effects of, 1171–1174, *1171–1173*
  diameter of, 1172–1173, *1172*
  eccentric, arteriography of, 256–257, *257*
  length of, 1172
  magnetic resonance imaging of, 321, *322*
  myocardial blood flow in, positron emission tomography of, 307
  pressure drop across, 1171
  radiation-induced, 1349
  severity of, 1172
 valvular. See *Aortic stenosis; Mitral stenosis; Pulmonic stenosis; Tricuspid stenosis.*
Stenosis flow reserve, 200
Stenosis resistance, 1171–1172
Stents, intracoronary, 1378–1382, *1379, 1380*, 1380t
  cost-effectiveness analysis of, 1750
  implantation of, 1381–1382, *1381*
Sternum, postoperative infection of, 1732–1733
Steroids, in rheumatic fever, 1772
  in uremic pericarditis, 1513
Still's disease, 1778
Still's murmur, 37–38, *37*
Stool hematest, preoperative, 1717t
Straight back syndrome, 24
Streinert's disease, 1872–1874, *1873, 1874*
Strength-duration curve, of pacemaker, 710–711, *711*
Streptococci, in infective endocarditis, 1080–1082, 1089–1090, 1090t
  in myocarditis, 1440
Streptococcus adjacens, 1081
Streptococcus agalactiae, 1081
Streptococcus anginosus, 1081
Streptococcus bovis, 1080, 1081, 1089–1090, 1090t
Streptococcus constellatus, 1081
Streptococcus defectivus, 1080, 1081
Streptococcus intermedius, 1081
Streptococcus milleri, 1080, 1081
Streptococcus mitior, 1080
Streptococcus pneumoniae, 1081, 1090, 1090t
Streptococcus pyogenes, 1090, 1090t
Streptococcus salivarius, 1080
Streptococcus sanguis, 1080
Streptokinase, 1218–1219, *1219*, 1821. See also *Thrombolytic therapy.*
  in myocardial infarction, 1824–1826, *1825*, 1825t, 1970–1971, 1971t
  in renal failure, 1934t
  vs. tissue-type plasminogen activator, 1220–1221
Streptomycin, myocardial effects of, 144[illegible]
Stress, in coronary artery disease, 1154, 1166
  in heart failure, 449
  in hypertension, 818–819, *818*, 819
  in myocardial infarction, 1198
  in stable angina pectoris, 1293
  reduction of, in cardiac rehabilitation, 1398
  silent ventricular dysfunction with, 302
Stress erythrocytosis, 1794
Stretch receptors, in contraction-relaxation cycle in, 376
  in heart failure, 410
Stroke, after coronary artery bypass surgery, 1319–1320
  diastolic blood pressure and, 812–813, *812*
  hypertension in, 815
  in atrial fibrillation, 655–656
  in myocardial infarction, 1198
Stroke volume, 425, 425t
  computed tomography of, 336
  in myocardial infarction, 1195, 1200
  in pregnancy, 1843, 1843t
  magnetic resonance imaging of, 331
  myocardial oxygen consumption and, 1162, *1162*
Stroke work–end-diastolic volume relation, 432, *433*
Stroke-prone spontaneously hypertensive rat, 1679
ST-T segment, 139, 139t
  in coronary artery disease, 1295
Stunned myocardium, 388–389, 388t, *389*, 1176, *1176*
  after coronary artery bypass surgery, 1327
  echocardiography of, 89
Subaortic obstruction, echocardiography in, 80, *80, 81*
Subaortic stenosis, congenital, 918–919, *919*
Subclavian artery, left, on plain chest radiography, 204, *206*
Subclavian flap arthroplasty, in juxtaductal coarctation, 913, *913*
Subcutaneous nodules, in rheumatic fever, 1771
Submaximal exercise, in exercise stress testing, 164
Submitral obstruction, echocardiography in, 81, *81*
Subpulmonic infundibular stenosis, 928
  in intraventricular right ventricular obstruction, 928

Subsarcolemmal cisternae, 360
Subungual hemorrhage, in infective endocarditis, 1085, *1085*
Subvalvular obstruction, echocardiography in, 79–81, *80*, *81*
Succinylcholine chloride (Anectine chloride), for anesthesia, 1757
  in pediatric cardiology, 1002t
Sudden cardiac death, **742–756.** See also *Cardiac arrest.*
  age and, 744
  biological risk factors for, 745, *745*
  cardiac nerves in, 753–754
  central nervous system in, 751
  cigarette smoking and, 745
  coronary artery abnormalities in, 747, 748t
  definition of, 742–743, *742*, 743t
  electrophysiological abnormalities and, 750–751, *751*
  emotional factors in, 751
  epidemiology of, 743, *745*
  etiology of, 747–752, 748t–749t, *750*, *751*
  gender and, 744–745
  hereditary factors in, 744
  hypertension and, 745
  in acute heart failure, 748–749
  in aortic stenosis, 749–750
  in arrhythmogenic right ventricular dysplasia, 749
  in Asian males, 752
  in athletes, 752
  in children, 749t, 752
  in congenital heart disease, 750
  in coronary artery disease, 752–754, 752t
  in dilated cardiomyopathy, 748–749
  in endocarditis, 750
  in hypertrophic cardiomyopathy, 747–748
  in infant, 749t, 751–752
  in mitral valve prolapse, 750
  in sudden infant death syndrome, 751–752
  in systemic disease, 749
  in valvular heart disease, 749–750
  incidence of, 743–744, *744*
  left ventricular dysfunction and, *746*, 747
  left ventricular ejection fraction and, 746
  life style factors in, 745–746
  mechanisms of, 754–756, *754*, *755*
  mimics of, 752
  model of, 754–756, *754*, *755*
  myocardial infarction and, 753
  neurohumoral factors in, 751
  onset of, 742, *742*
  pathology of, 752–756, 752t, *754*, *755*
  physical inactivity and, 745
  premature ventricular contractions and, 746–747
  previous coronary heart disease and, 746–747
  prodromes of, 742, *742*, 757
  psychosocial factors in, 746
  Q-T prolongation and, 750–751
  race and, 745
  risk for, 743–745, *744*
  specialized conducting system in, 753
  time-dependent risk of, 744, *744*
  torsades de pointes and, 751, *751*
  ventricular ectopy and, 746–747
  ventricular hypertrophy in, 747–748
Sudden death, familial syncope and, 1667
  in atherosclerosis, 1121
  in congenital aortic stenosis, 915
  in congenital heart disease, 888
  in heart failure, 504–507, 504t
  in hypertrophic cardiomyopathy, 1424–1425, 1424t
  in mitral valve prolapse, 1033
  in sarcoidosis, 1431
  in supravalvular aortic stenosis, 921
Sudden infant death syndrome, 751–752, 888
Sufentanil, for anesthesia, 1757
Sulfasalazine, digoxin interaction with, 483t
Sulfinpyrazone, after myocardial infarction, 1264
Sulfonamides, myocardial effects of, 1448
Sulmazole, in heart failure, 485
Superior vena cava syndrome, malignant cardiac tamponade and, 1515
  vs, cardiac tamponade, 1493
Supernormal conduction, 693, *694*
Supernormal excitation, 693, *694*
Superoxide dismutase, in myocardial infarction, 1214, 1232
Supravalvular aortic stenosis, 919–921, *920*, *921*
  autosomal dominant, 920
  genes for, 1632t
Supravalvular stenosing ring, 81
Supraventricular arrhythmias, exercise stress testing in, 167–168
  postoperative, *1728*, 1729–1730, *1729*
    evaluation of, 1727–1728, *1728*
    risks for, 1718–1719, *1719*
Supraventricular tachycardia, 675t. See also specific tachycardias, e.g., *Atrial tachycardia.*
  atrial reentry in, 572
  congenital, 950–951
  diagnosis of, adenosine in, 618
    electrophysiological studies in, 581–582, *582*
      practice guidelines for, 1960t, 1962
  genesis of, 572
  in hypertrophic cardiomyopathy, 1421
  paroxysmal, in mitral valve prolapse, 1033
    in myocardial infarction, 1245t, 1253
    postoperative, 1730
  sinus reentry in, 572
  surgical management of, 628–629, *629*
  vs. ventricular tachycardia, 677–678, 678t
Surgery. See also specific types, e.g., *Coronary artery bypass graft surgery.*
  antibiotic prophylaxis for, 1097–1099, 1097t, 1098t, 1099t
  noncardiac. See *Noncardiac surgery.*
Swallowing syncope, 864. See also *Syncope.*
Sweating, chest pain and, 7
Sydenham's chorea, in rheumatic fever, 1771
Sympathogonia, 829
Sympatholytics. See specific agents, e.g., *Prazosin (Minipress).*
Sympathomimetic agents. See also *Dobutamine (Dobutrex); Dopamine (Intropin).*
  digoxin interaction with, 483t
  in heart failure, 485–486, 502
Syncope, 8–9, 8t, **863–875**
  after palpitation, 9
  bundle branch block and, pacemaker in, 707–708, 708t
  cardiac, 866–867
    outcomes of, 867–868
  cardiovascular, 8
  carotid sinus, 865
  cerebrovascular, 8
  cough, 864
  defecation, 864
  diagnosis of, 868–874, 868t, *873*
    carotid massage in, 869
    differential, 8–9, 8t
    echocardiography in, 1943
    electrocardiography in, 869–870
    electrophysiological studies in, 582, 870
      practice guidelines for, 1960t, 1963
    laboratory tests in, 869
    neurological testing in, 872
    physical examination in, 868–869
    psychiatric assessment in, 872
    upright tilt testing in, 870–872, *871*, *872*, 872t
  differential diagnosis of, 8–9, 8t
  exertional, 866–867
  familial, 1667
  high-altitude, 865
  hospital admission for, 874
  in aortic dissection, 867
  in aortic stenosis, 1039–1040
  in arrhythmias, 867
  in cerebrovascular disease, 866
  in children, 9, 888
  in congenital heart disease, 888
  in elderly, 874
  in glossopharyngeal neuralgia, 865
  in heart failure, 506
  in hypertrophic cardiomyopathy, 866, 1420
  in migraine, 866
  in myocardial infarction, 867
  in patient history, 8–9, 8t
  in psychiatric illnesses, 865
  in pulmonary hypertension, 708
  micturition, 864
  neurally mediated, 863–865, *864*
    in children, 888
    mechanism of, 863, *864*
    outcomes of, 867–868
    pacemaker in, 709, 709t
    treatment of, 874
Syncope *(Continued)*
  orthostatic, 865–866, 866t
    treatment of, 874
  outcomes of, 867–868
  patient education on, 874–875
  postprandial, 866
  prevention of, 874–875
  prognosis for, 8, 873
  recurrence of, 868, 873–874
  reflex-mediated, 863–865, 863t, *864*
  situational, 864–865
  sneeze, 864–865
  swallowing, 864
  temporal lobe, 866
  treatment of, 874–875
  vasodepressor, 8
  vasovagal, 863–864
    treatment of, 874
    upright tilt testing induction of, 870–873, *871*, 872t
  with atrial myxoma, 867
  with pulmonary embolism, 867
Syndrome myxoma, 1467–1468, *1468*, 1468t
Syndrome X, *1289*, 1343–1344
  chest pain in, 1343–1344
  management of, 1344
  myocardial perfusion imaging in, 293
  prognosis for, 1344
  vs. esophageal pain, 1291
  vs. ischemic heart disease, 1343
Syphilis, aortitis in, 1193, 1441
  in thoracic aortic aneurysm, 1551
Systemic lupus erythematosus (SLE), 1778–1780, 1778t
  antiphospholipid antibody syndrome in, 1779
  cardiac tamponade in, 1518
  conduction system abnormalities in, 1779
  congenital heart block in, 1779
  coronary artery disease in, 1349, 1779
  dilated cardiomyopathy in, *227*
  endocarditis in, 1778–1779, *1779*
  maternal, 878
  myocarditis in, 1778
  pericarditis in, 1518, 1778
  pulmonary hypertension in, 1779
Systemic lupus erythematosus (SLE)–like syndrome, procainamide and, 604
Systemic sclerosis, progressive, in secondary pulmonary hypertension, 799
Systemic vascular resistance, measurement of, 193
Systemic vasculitis, 1782–1783, *1782*
Systole, 377–378, 378t
  in coronary blood flow, 1169
  in elderly, 1700
  in hypertrophic cardiomyopathy, 1415, 1415t, 1418, *1418*
Systolic click, in mitral valve prolapse, 1032
Systolic compressive forces, in coronary blood flow, 1169
Systolic current of injury, in ischemia, 127, *128*
Systolic reserve, in young heart, 889
Systolic ventricular interaction, in contraction-relaxation cycle, 385

T tubule, 360, *362*, *363*
T wave, 111t, 113–114, 139, 139t
  bifid, 139
  digitalis effect on, 142
  in acute pericarditis, 1483–1484, *1483*, 1483t
  in exercise stress testing, 157–160
  in hyperkalemia, *137*, 141–142, *141*
  in hypocalcemia, 142, *142*
  in left bundle branch block, *120*, 121, 138, *148*
  in left ventricular hypertrophy, 139
  in myocardial infarction, 129–131, *130*, *131*, *138*, *147*, 714
  in Prinzmetal's angina, *137*
  in right bundle branch block, 121
  in right ventricular hypertrophy, 118
  in ventricular aneurysm, 136, *150*
  inversion of, 136–138, *150*
  juvenile, 113, *138*, 141
  negative, *150*
  notched, 139
  of cardiac memory, 137, *150*

T wave *(Continued)*
  postextrasystolic, 138
  tented, *150*
Ta segment, 111–112
  abnormalities in, *112*, 116
Tachyarrhythmia(s), atrial reentry in, 572
  atrioventricular nodal reentry in, 572–574, *573–575*
  electrophysiological studies in, 581–582, *582*, *583*
  genesis of, 572–576, *573–575*
  in heart failure, 449
  in syncope, 582
  intraoperative, 1758
  reentry in, 572–576, *573–577*
  sinus reentry in, 572
Tachycardia, antidromic, 670, *672*
  during DDD pacing, 720, *720*
  electrophysiological evaluation of, practice guidelines for, 1960t, 1962
  endless-loop, with dual-chamber pacemaker, 717–720, *719*, *720*
  fascicular, 683, *683*
  orthodromic, 670, *672*
  pacing, with cardiac catheterization, 198
  reciprocating, accessory pathway with, 641t–642t, *650*
  reentry, 572–576, *573–577*
  reentry over concealed accessory pathway in, 665–666
  supraventricular, 675t. See also specific tachycardias, e.g., *Atrial tachycardia*.
    congenital, 950–951
  treatment of, electrical devices for, 731–736, 732t, *733–736*
    practice guidelines for, 1965t
  ventricular, 677–681. See also *Ventricular tachycardia*.
Tachycardia-dependent block, in arrhythmogenesis, 569
Tachypnea, in cyanosis, 892–893
  in newborn, 892–893
Tacrolimus (FK-506), in heart transplantation rejection, 523
Takayasu's arteritis, 1572–1573, *1572–1574*, 1575t
  aortic calcifications in, *223*, 224
  aortic regurgitation in, 1572
  clinical manifestations of, 1572
  coronary artery disease in, 1349
  diagnosis of, 1573, *1573*, *1574*, 1575t
  etiology of, 1572, *1572*
  hypertension in, 1572
  in myocardial infarction, 1193
  in pregnancy, 1855–1856
  in secondary pulmonary hypertension, 801
  natural history of, 1572–1573
  treatment of, 1573
Talc, pericarditis with, 1519
Tambocor. See *Flecainide acetate (Tambocor)*.
Tamoxifen, cardiovascular effects of, 1908
Tamponade, 1486–1495. See also *Cardiac tamponade*.
  experimental, 1488
Tangier disease, low high-density lipoprotein in, 1144
TAR (thrombocytopenia–absent radius) syndrome, 880t
Taurine deficiency, myocardial effects of, 1447
Teboroxime, technetium-99m–labeled, for myocardial perfusion imaging, 274–275, 275t, 278–279, *281*, 290–291
Temazepam, in myocardial infarction, 1226
Temperature, body, in myocardial infarction, 1200
  myocardial effects of, 1449
Temporal lobe syncope, 866
Tension pneumopericardium, cardiac tamponade and, 1490
Teratogens, in congenital heart disease, 1663–1664, 1663t
Teratoma, 1471
Terazosin, in hypertension, 852–853
  in renal failure, 1932t
Tetracycline, digoxin interaction with, 483t
  in neoplastic pericarditis, 1516
  myocardial effects of, 1448
Tetralogy of Fallot, 682, 929–932, 1847–1848
  acyanotic, 929
  axial cineangiography in, 931, *931*
  cardiac catheterization in, 930–931, *930*, *931*
Tetralogy of Fallot *(Continued)*
  clinical manifestations of, 929–930
  definition of, 929
  echocardiography in, 84, *84*, 930, *930*, 932, *932*
  exercise and, *780*, 979
  genetic factors in, 1660t
  gull-wing configuration in, 931, *931*
  heart sounds in, *31*
  hemodynamics of, 929, *929*
  in adult, 968, 970–971
  in secondary pulmonary hypertension, 801
  laboratory examinations in, 930–931, *930*, *931*
  management of, 931–932
  noncardiac surgery and, 981
  palliative surgery in, 931
  physical examination in, 930
  plain chest radiography of, *208*, 233
  postoperative complications in, 931–932
  pregnancy and, 975–976
  pulmonary artery contour in, *208*
  pulmonic valve absence with, 932
  surgical correction of, 931
  systolic murmur of, 49
Tetrodotoxin, action potential effects of, *562*
Tetrofosmin, technetium-99m–labeled, for myocardial perfusion imaging, 274, 275t
Thalassemic syndromes, 1675, 1788–1790, *1789*
  management of, 1789–1790
Thalidomide, 878, 881t
Thallium-201, 274, 295t. See also *Myocardial perfusion imaging*.
  myocardial kinetics of, 282, *283*
Theophylline, in cor pulmonale, 1619, *1619*
  in syncope, 874
Thermal balloon angioplasty, 1382
Thermodilution method, for cardiac output measurement, 191–192
  for coronary blood flow measurement, 199, *199*
Thiamine (vitamin B_1), deficiency of, 993–994
    heart failure in, 461–462, 461t
  in beriberi, 462
Thiazide diuretics, 849t
  in coronary artery disease, 1151
  in heart failure, 477–478, 477t
  in renal failure, 1933t
Thiopental, for anesthesia, 1757
Thomsen's disease, 1874
Thoracic outlet syndrome, vs. angina, 7
Thoracotomy, post-traumatic, 1540–1541, *1540*
Thoratec pump, 537t, 539–540, *539*, *540*
Thorax, deformities of, 24
  in Marfan syndrome, 1671
Three (3) sign, in juxtaductal coarctation, 912
Three-dimensional echocardiography, 59. See also *Echocardiography*.
Threshold approach, to diagnostic testing, 1743–1744
Thrills, palpation of, 28
Thrombin, *1165*
  hirudin inhibition of, 1820
  in coagulation, 1812–1813, *1813*
  inhibitors of, 1820–1821
Thrombocytopenia, drug-induced, 1805
  heparin-associated, 1594, 1805
  postoperative, 1732t
Thrombocytopenia–absent radius syndrome, genetic factors in, 1661t
Thrombocytosis, 1794
Thrombolytic therapy, 1821–1822. See also specific drugs, e.g., *Streptokinase*.
  complications of, 1219–1220
  contraindications to, 1597
  early mortality with, 1220
  in elderly, 1697
  in myocardial infarction, 1208, *1209*, *1210*, 1215–1221, *1216–1219*, 1218t, 1824–1826, *1825*, 1825t
  in pulmonary embolism, 1593, 1593t, 1596–1597, *1596*, 1596t
  in unstable angina, 1337–1338, 1824
  intracoronary, 1215
  intravenous, 1215
  mortality with, 1220
  myocardial perfusion imaging after, 286–287, *287*
  patency rates with, 1215–1216
  percutaneous transluminal coronary angioplasty after, 1222
Thrombolytic therapy *(Continued)*
  recombinant tissue plasminogen activator for, 1627–1628, *1627*
  recommendations for, 1220–1221
  survival rates after, 1216–1218, *1216–1218*, 1218t
    diabetes mellitus and, 1217, *1217*
    in elderly, 1217, *1217*
  vs. percutaneous transluminal coronary angioplasty, 1221–1222, *1222*
Thrombomodulin, 1813, *1814*
Thromboxane, receptor for, blockers of, 1819–1820
Thromboxane A_2, *1165*
  in unstable angina, 1333
Thromboxane B_2, urinary, after heart transplantation, 520
Thromboxane synthase, inhibitors of, 1819
Thrombus (thrombi), cerebral, in congenital heart disease, 885
  coronary. See also *Myocardial infarction*.
    antiplatelet therapy for, 1225, *1225*
    antithrombotic therapy for, 1223–1225, 1829–1830
    arteriography of, 265–266, *266*
    computed tomography of, 337, 342
    echocardiography of, 88, *88*, 94, *95*
    in atherosclerosis, 1121–1122
    in cardiac arrest, 753, 755
    in mitral stenosis, 1010
    in myocardial infarction, 265, *266*, 1186–1187, *1186*
    in unstable angina, 265, *266*, 268, 1333, *1333*, 1335
    magnetic resonance imaging of, 326, *326*
    mural, 1122
      in dilated cardiomyopathy, 1833–1834, 1834t
      in myocardial infarction, 88, *88*, 1256–1257, *1257*
    thrombolytic therapy for, 1215–1221, *1216–1218*, 1218t, *1219*
    venous, after myocardial infarction, 1256
      cancer and, 1584
    with ventricular assist device, 542
  pulmonary, in hypertension, 785, *785*
Thumpversion, in cardiac arrest, 762–763
  in ventricular tachycardia, 680
Thyroid gland, 1890–1895
  cancer of, 1471
    cardiac metastases from, 1794–1799, *1795*, 1795t, *1796*, 1796t
  function of, in myocardial infarction, 1197
    preoperative, 1717t
Thyroid hormones, 1891, *1892*
  cardiac effects of, 1891, *1892*
  extranuclear effects of, 1890
  nuclear effects of, 1890
  sympathetic nervous system and, 1890–1891
Thyrotoxic heart disease, 461
Thyrotoxicosis, 1893
  neonatal, 993
    heart failure in, 461
Thyroxine (T_4), digoxin interaction with, 483t
  in myocardial infarction, 1197
Ticlopidine, 1819
  in unstable angina, 1337, 1823, 1982t
Tidal wave, of arterial pulse, 21–22
Tietze syndrome, chest pain in, 5
Time constant of membrane, 564
Timolol, in arrhythmias, 610–613, 611t
  in myocardial infarction, 1228–1229, *1228*
  in renal failure, 1931t
  pharmacodynamic properties of, 487t
  pharmacology of, 1307t
Tin (Sn)-pyrophosphate, technetium-99m–labeled, for infarct imaging, 296, *296*
Tirofiban, 1820
Tissue plasminogen activator (t-PA), function of, 1628
  in myocardial infarction, 1970–1971, 1971t
  in renal failure, 1934t
  in vasodilation, *782*
  recombinant, 1627–1628, *1627*, *1628*
  structure of, 1628, *1628*
  variants of, 1627–1628, *1628*
Titin (connectin), 361, *364*
Tobacco. See *Cigarette smoking*.
Tocainide, adverse effects of, 608
  dosage of, 608

Tocainide *(Continued)*
electrophysiological actions of, 601t, 602t–603t, 607–608
hematological abnormalities with, 1804t
in arrhythmias, 601t, 602t–603t, 607–608
in renal failure, 1930t
indications for, 608
pharmacokinetics of, 608
Tolazoline (Priscoline), in pediatric cardiology, 1002t
Torsades de pointes, 684–685, *684*
antiarrhythmic agent precipitation of, 767
clinical features of, 685
early afterdepolarizations in, 567, *568*
electrocardiography in, 684–685, *684*
electrophysiological features of, 685
sudden cardiac death and, 751, *751*
treatment of, 598t, 685
triggered activity in, 577
Torsemide, in heart failure, 477t
Torulopsis glabrata, in infective endocarditis, 1082
Total alternans, 140
in heart failure, 455
Townes-Brocks syndrome, genetic factors in, 1661t
Toxin, pericarditis with, 1519
Toxoplasma gondii, in pericarditis, 1511
Toxoplasmosis, 1444
Tracheostomy, in sleep apnea syndromes, 1615
postoperative, 1723
Trandate. See *Labetalol (Normodyne, Trandate).*
Transaminase, heparin-associated levels of, 1594
Transcutaneous ventricular pacing, 705–706
Transducer, pressure, 188
Transendothelial channels, of endothelium, 1107
Transesophageal echocardiography, 57–59, *57–59*, **Plate 1.** See also *Echocardiography, transesophageal.*
Transforming growth factor-β (TGF-β), in atherosclerosis, 1115
in myocyte hypertrophy, 1640t, 1642t
Transforming growth factor-β_1 (TGF-β_1), *1165*
Transgenic mice, in genetic research, 1679
Transgenic technology, 1635–1637, *1635–1637*, 1636t
in atherosclerosis, 1636–1637, *1636*, 1636t, *1637*
insertional mutagenesis of, 1635, *1635*
Transient ischemic attacks, in myocardial infarction, 1198
Transitional cells, of atrioventricular junctional area, 550, *551*
of atrioventricular node, *551*
of sinus node, 548
Transluminal balloon angioplasty, in congenital heart disease, 895
Transplantation. See *Heart transplantation.*
Transposition of great arteries, **935–940**
angiography in, 937–938
arterial switch operation in, 939–940, *940*
atrial septostomy in, 939
cardiac catheterization in, 937–938, 941
chest roentgenography in, 937, *937*
clinical findings in, 937
congenitally corrected, 940–941
angiocardiography in, 941, *942*
clinical manifestations of, 941
laboratory examination in, 941
operative repair of, 941
physiology of, 940–941
echocardiography in, 84–85, *85*, 937, *938*, *939*
electrocardiography in, 937
embryogenesis of, 936
exercise and, 979–780
hemodynamics of, 936–937
in adult, 966, 970, *970*
interatrial communication of, 936, *936*
Lecompte procedure in, 940
magnetic resonance imaging in, 327, *327*
management of, 938–940, *940*
morphology of, 935–936, *936*
plain chest radiography of, 233, *233*
pulmonary vascular changes in, 936–937
pulmonary vascular obstructive disease and, 936
selective ventricular angiography in, 938
surgical treatment of, 939–940, *940*
Transseptal catheterization, 186
Transvenous pacing, 705
Traube's sign, in aortic regurgitation, 22, 1049
Trauma, deep venous thrombosis after, 1583
in myocardial infarction, 1198
Traumatic heart disease, **1535–1544**
imaging in, 354t, 356
nonpenetrating, 1535–1539, 1535t, 1536t, *1537–1539*, 1538t
penetrating, 1535t, 1539–1541
clinical features of, 1539–1540
diagnosis of, 1539–1540
management of, 1540–1541, *1540*, *1541*
Ta segment abnormality in, 116
Treacher Collins syndrome, genetic factors in, 1661t
Treadmill protocol, in exercise stress testing, 155–156, *156*
Trepopnea, in heart failure, 450
Treppe effect, in contraction-relaxation cycle, 380, *380*, 381, 382
Triamterene (Dyrenium), hematological abnormalities with, 1804t
in congenital heart disease–related heart failure, 890t
in heart failure, 477t, 890t
in pediatric cardiology, 1002t
in renal failure, 1933t
Triangle of Koch, *550*, *551*
Trichinosis, myocardial involvement in, 1445
Trichlormethiazide, in heart failure, 477–478, 477t
Tricuspid atresia, 932–934
angiography in, 933
balloon atrial septostomy in, 933
cardiac catheterization in, 933
clinical features of, 933, *933*
echocardiography of, 933, *933*
Fontan operation in, 933–934, *934*
management of, 933–934, *934*
morphology in, 932–933, *932*
pathophysiology of, 933
Tricuspid regurgitation, 1056–1058
angiography in, 1058, *1058*
auscultation in, 1057
clinical manifestations of, 1057
differential diagnosis of, 1023t
Doppler echocardiography in, 69–70, *69*, 1058
early systolic murmur of, 38–39
echocardiography in, 69–70, *69*, 76, *77*, 1057–1058
electrocardiography in, 1057
etiology of, 1056–1057, 1056t, *1057*
hemodynamic findings in, 1058
holosystolic murmur of, *31*, 38, *38*
in carcinoid syndrome, 1056, *1057*
laboratory examination in, 1057–1058, *1058*
murmurs in, *31*, 38, *38*, 49, 1011, 1023t
pansystolic murmur of, 1011
pathology of, 1056–1057, 1056t, *1057*
patient history in, 1057
physical examination in, 1057
radiological findings in, 1057
systolic murmur of, 49
treatment of, 1058
Tricuspid stenosis, 1054–1056
clinical manifestations of, 1054–1055, *1054*, 1055t
echocardiography in, 76, 1055, *1056*
etiology of, 1054
in hemolytic anemia, 1790
laboratory examination in, 1055, *1056*
mid-diastolic murmur of, 41
pathology of, 1054
pathophysiology of, 1054, *1054*
patient history in, 1054
physical examination in, 1054–1055, *1054*
presystolic murmur of, 43, *43*, *44*
treatment of, 1055–1056
Tricuspid valve, Ebstein's anomaly of, 934–935. See also *Ebstein's anomaly.*
in rheumatoid arthritis, 1776
infective endocarditis of, in intravenous drug abuse, 1058, 1079
lithium effect on, 878
mid-diastolic murmur across, 41–42
replacement of, in tricuspid regurgitation, 1058
thrombosis with, 1066
trauma to, 1542
Tricuspid valve prolapse, 1057
Tricyclic antidepressants, myocardial effects of, 1446
Tricyclic antidepressants *(Continued)*
toxicity of, 11
Trifascicular block, 707
electrocardiography in, 123
Trigeminy, definition of, 676
Triggered activity, in arrhythmogenesis, 566–568, *566*, *567*, 567t
in torsade de pointes, 577
Triiodothyronine (T_3), in myocardial infarction, 1197
Trimethadione, teratogenicity of, 1663t
Trimethaphan camsylate (Arfonad), in hypertensive crisis, 858t
in pediatric cardiology, 1002t
in renal failure, 1932t
Triphenyltetrazolium chloride stain, in myocardial infarction, *1189*, 1190
Triploidy, 1656t
Tris buffer (THAM; Tromethamine), in pediatric cardiology, 1002t
Trisomy 13 (Patau syndrome), 881t, 1657
Trisomy 18 (Edwards syndrome), 881t, 1656t, 1657
Trisomy 21 (Down syndrome), 881t, 1656–1657, 1656t
Tropical endomyocardial fibrosis, 994
Tropoelastin, in aortic valve stenosis, 1662
Tropomyosin, in crossbridge cycling, 362
Troponin, in myocardial infarction, *1202*, 1202t, 1203–1204
Troponin complex, of actin filament, *364*, 364–365
Troponin-C, in crossbridge cycling, 362, *364*
Troponin-I, in crossbridge cycling, 362, *365*
Troponin-M, in crossbridge cycling, 362
Troponin-T, in heart failure, *406*, 407
in unstable angina, 1335
Truncus arteriosus, embryology of, 882
partial (aorticopulmonary septal defect), 205, *208*, 906–907
persistent, 907–908, *907*, *908*
cardiac catheterization in, 908
electrocardiography in, 907–908, *908*
hemodynamics of, 907
management of, 908, *908*
morphology of, 907, *907*
second heart sound in, 33
Trypanosoma cruzi, 989
Trypanosoma rhodesiense, 989
Trypanosomiasis, acute, 1442
African, 1444
chronic, 1442–1444, *1443*
myocarditis in, 1442–1444, *1442*, *1443*
Tryptophan, pericarditis with, 1519
Tsutsugamushi disease, myocarditis with, 1439
Tuberculosis, myocarditis in, 1440
pericarditis in, 1507–1508
Tuberous sclerosis, 880t
rhabdomyoma and, 1470
Tubocurarine (curare), for anesthesia, 1757
in pediatric cardiology, 1002t
Tumor(s), calcifications of, *224*, 225, 1468, 1473
cardiac, **1464–1475**
after heart transplantation, 525
angiography in, 1474–1475
benign, 1467–1471, 1467t, *1468–1470*, 1468t
treatment of, 1475
cardiac manifestations of, 1466–1467
clinical examination in, 1472–1473
clinical presentation of, 1464–1467, *1465*
computed tomography in, 341–342, *341*, 1474
diagnosis of, 1472–1475, *1472*, *1473*
echocardiography in, 94, 95, *1472*, 1473–1474
embolization of, 1465–1466, *1465*
endocrine, 1471
incidence of, 1467t
interleukin-6 in, 1464–1465
magnetic resonance imaging in, 325–327, *326*, *1473*, 1474
malignant, 1471–1472
metastatic, 1794–1799, *1798*, *1799*
chest roentgenography in, 1797–1798
clinical manifestations of, 1795–1799
echocardiography of, 95
electrocardiography in, 135, *136*, 1797–1798
hypereosinophilic syndromes with, 1798–1799

Tumor(s) *(Continued)*
incidence of, 1794–1795, *1795*, 1795t, *1796*
myocardial infarction with, 1798
myocardial involvement in, 1797
pericardial involvement in, 236, 1796–1797
valvular effects of, 1798
treatment of, 1475
papillary, 1469–1470
radiological examination in, 354t, 356, 1473–1474
signs of, 1464t
symptoms of, 1464t
systemic findings in, 1464–1465
transesophageal echocardiography in, 1474
in secondary pulmonary hypertension, 799
of aorta, 1576, *1576*
pericarditis with, 1513–1516, *1514*, 1514t
venous thrombosis and, 1584
Tumor necrosis factor-α (TNF-α), in heart failure, 415
in portal hypertension, 786
Turner syndrome, 881t, 1656t, 1657, 1658
T-wave alternans, 138–139, *138*, 140
in arrhythmias, 579
Twiddler's syndrome, 726–727
Two-dimensional echocardiography, 54, *55*, *56*. See also *Echocardiography, two-dimensional.*
Tylenol (acetaminophen), in pediatric cardiology, 1000t
Type A behavior, in cardiac rehabilitation, 1398
in coronary artery disease, 1154
in sudden cardiac death, 745

U wave, 114
digitalis effect on, 142
in hypokalemia, 139, *141*
in ischemic heart disease, 132, *132*
negative, 139, *150*
U wave alternans, 140
Ulcer, atherosclerotic, penetrating, 1569, *1569*
Ultrasound, 53. See also *Echocardiography.*
principles of, 53–54, *53*
therapeutic, 1383
Unipolar limb leads, 110, *111*
Upright tilt testing, in arrhythmias, 584–585, 585t
in syncope, 870–873, *871*, 872t
isoproterenol for, 871
positive response in, 871, 872t
protocols for, 872t
reproducibility of, 872
sensitivity of, 871–872
Urate, metabolism of, in cyanotic congenital heart disease, 972
Uremic pericarditis, 1512–1513
Urine analysis, in infective endocarditis, 1088
Urokinase, 1220, 1821. See also *Thrombolytic therapy.*
in renal failure, 1934t
Uterus, trophoblast invasion of, in preeclampsia, 831

Vaccinia, in myocarditis, 1439
Valium (diazepam), for arteriography, 244
Valproic acid, teratogenicity of, 1663t
Valsalva maneuver, in heart failure, 456
in hypertrophic cardiomyopathy, 1423
systolic murmur response to, 47, *47*
with cardiac catheterization, 198
Valve(s), area of, *69*, 70
atresia of, 79, *80*
calcifications of, 221, *222*
closure of, palpation of, 28
function of, imaging of, 351t, 352–353
prosthetic, **1061–1066.** See also *Prosthetic valves.*
stenosis of. See *Aortic stenosis; Mitral stenosis; Pulmonic stenosis; Tricuspid stenosis.*
Valvular heart disease. See also specific types.
angiography in, 303
practice guidelines for, 1951t, 1952
Valvular heart disease *(Continued)*
cardiac catheterization in, 178t, 179. See also *Cardiac catheterization.*
exercise stress testing in, 172
imaging in, 354t, 355
in rheumatoid arthritis, 1776, *1777*
noncardiac surgery and, 1761–1762
Valvuloplasty, balloon, 1385–1386, *1385*
during pregnancy, 1849–1850
in aortic stenosis, 915, 918, 1044–1045, *1044*, 1385, *1385*, 1386
in carcinoid heart disease, 1434
in mitral stenosis, *1015*, 1016–1017, *1016*, *1017*, 1385–1386, *1385*
in pulmonic stenosis, 925, 926, *927*, 1386
Vanillylmandelic acid, in pheochromocytoma, 1898
Varicella, in myocarditis, 1439
in pericarditis, 1506
Variola, in myocarditis, 1439
Vasa vasorum, rupture of, in aortic dissection, 1554, *1555*
Vascular cell adhesion molecule-1 (VCAM-1), in atherosclerosis, 1108
Vascular compliance, in contraction-relaxation cycle, 385
Vascular endothelial growth factor (VEGF), in collateral vessel development, 1174–1175, *1175*, 1176
Vascular resistance, at birth, 883
in tetralogy of Fallot, 929
measurement of, 192–193
peripheral, aging and, 1692, *1693*
pulmonary, chemical regulation of, 782
drug effects on, 782–783, *782*, *783*
hormonal regulation of, 782
measurement of, 193
neural regulation of, 781–782
quantification of, 780
reduction in, 780–781
systemic, in pregnancy, 1843–1844, *1844*
measurement of, 193
Vascular rings, 949
Vasculitides, small vessel, 1783
Vasculitis, in giant cell arteritis, 1782
systemic hypertension in, 824
Vasoconstriction, in heart failure, 453
in stable angina, 1293
in unstable angina, 1333–1334
pulmonary, 1608
angiotensin II in, 783
hypoxia-elicited, 781, *782*, 783
serotonin in, 783
Vasodilation, endothelium-dependent, in coronary resistance vessels, 1165–1166, *1166*
in epicardial arteries, 1165, *1165*, *1166*
endothelium-derived relaxing factor in, *782*, *783*
endothelium-derived substances in, *782*
left ventricular pressure and, 1480
nitrate-induced, 1302, *1302*
pharmacological, for stress myocardial perfusion imaging, 289–290, 289t
postoperative, 1725, 1726t
prostacyclin in, *782*, 783, *783*
pulmonary, isoproterenol-induced, 782
tissue plasminogen activator in, *782*
Vasodilator therapy, collateral vessel effects of, 1175
direct, in hypertension, 855
in congenital heart disease–related heart failure, 890, 891t
in cor pulmonale, 1619–1620
in coronary artery disease, 1149t
in heart failure, **471–476,** *471*, 472t, 494–498, *495*, *496*. See also specific vasodilators, e.g., *Angiotensin-converting enzyme inhibitors.*
in idiopathic dilated cardiomyopathy, 1411
in myocardial infarction, 1236–1237
in pulmonary hypertension, 792–793, 1613
in pulmonary hypertension testing, 793, *793*
in systemic hypertension, 854–856, 854t
Vasopressin, antagonists of, in heart failure, 478
Vasopressors, in aortic dissection, 1565
Vasotec. See *Enalapril maleate (Vasotec).*
Vasovagal syncope, 863–864. See also *Syncope.*
pacemaker in, 709, 709t
Vasoxyl (methoxamine), auscultatory effects of, 49
Vasoxyl (methoxamine) *(Continued)*
in atrioventricular nodal reentrant tachycardia, 664
VATER (vertebral, ventricular septal, anal, tracheoesophageal, radial, and renal defects) association, 881t, 1659, 1659t
Vector, for gene therapy, 1638
Vectorcardiography, 114–115, *114*, 115t
in left bundle branch block, 121
in left ventricular hypertrophy, *116*, 117
in mitral stenosis, 1012
in myocardial infarction, 135, *135*
in right bundle branch block, 121
in right ventricular hypertrophy, 119, *119*
Vecuronium, for anesthesia, 1757
Vegetarian diet, in hypertension, 845
Veins, atretic, 1677
varicose, 1677
Velocardiofacial syndrome, 1658
genetic factors in, 1660t
Velocity, in myocardial contractility, 430
Vena cava, inferior, in constrictive pericarditis, 1500
in pulmonary embolism, 1595–1596, 1595t, *1596*, 1599
two-dimensional echocardiography of, 70–71, *70*
superior, obstruction of, malignant cardiac tamponade and, 1515
neoplastic disease and, 1797
vs. cardiac tamponade, 1493
on plain chest radiography, *206*
Venoconstriction, in heart failure, 397
Venous continuous murmur, 45, *45*
Venous hypertension, in heart failure, 453, 456
Venous oxygenation, in chronic obstructive pulmonary disease, 1616–1617, *1618*
Venous pressure, in heart failure, 456
Venous thrombosis, *1584*. See also *Pulmonary embolism.*
cancer and, 1584
central venous catheterization and, 1584
ischemic stroke and, 1584
oral contraceptives and, 1583, 1584
pathophysiology of, 1582–1585, 1582t, 1583t
postoperative, 1583, 1734
pregnancy and, 1583, 1584, 1600
thrombolytic therapy in, 1597
ultrasonography in, 1588, *1588*
Ventilation, in cyanotic congenital heart disease, 973, *973*
mechanical, before arteriography, 245
in pulmonary embolism, 1593
postoperative, 1722, 1722t
postoperative insufficiency of, 1723
Ventilation lung scan, in pulmonary embolism, 1589, 1589t, 1590t
Ventilation-perfusion imbalance, nitroglycerin-associated, 1303
Ventricle(s). See also at *Atrioventricular; Ventricular.*
anatomy of, 1604–1605, *1604*
embryology of, 879
function of, equilibrium radionuclide angiocardiography for, 297–300, *297–299*
first-pass radionuclide angiocardiography for, 300–301
in diabetes mellitus, 1903–1904, *1903*
magnetic resonance imaging of, 329–330, *329*
noncardiac surgery and, 982
radionuclide angiocardiography of, 297–303, *297–299*
resting, radionuclide angiocardiography for, 301–302
VEST monitoring of, 300, *300*
hypertrophy of, patterns of, 399–400, *399–401*
in cardiac malposition, 946
interaction of, in contraction-relaxation cycle, 385
in pulmonary hypertension, 1611, *1612*
pericardium and, 1480
pulmonary embolism and, 1584, *1585*
left, aneurysm of, 228
computed tomography of, 336–337, *337*
in coronary artery disease, 1347–1348, *1347*
in mitral regurgitation, 1017
in myocardial contusion, 1538, *1538*

Ventricle(s) *(Continued)*
in myocardial infarction, 136, *150*, *1242*, *1242*, 1256
palpation in, 25
post-traumatic, 1542
T wave in, 136, *150*
treatment of, 1348, *1348*, 1833
apex of, on myocardial perfusion imaging, 277
biopsy of, 187
compliance of, in heart failure, 403
delayed relaxation of, 437, *437*, *438*
diameter of, on M-mode echocardiography, *64*
diastolic function of, cardiac catheterization and, 791t
in myocardial infarction, 1194
in secondary pulmonary hypertension, 796t, 797
diastolic motion of, 25, 27
diastolic pressure of, in mitral stenosis, 1008–1009, *1009*
diastolic pressure-volume relation of, *435*, 436
diastolic properties of, *402*, 403
dilatation of, in mitral regurgitation, 1018
in myocardial infarction, 1195–1196, *1196*
on myocardial perfusion imaging, 282
on plain chest radiography, 208
Doppler echocardiography of, 67, *67*
double-inlet, 947–949, *948*
double-outlet, 944
dyskinesia of, palpation in, 25
echocardiographic performance evaluation of, 86–87
ejection fraction of, 425, 425t, 434, *434*
computed tomography of, 336
in elderly, 1694
in heart failure, 458, *459*
in myocardial infarction, 166
in sudden cardiac death, 746
ejection of, of aging heart, 1689–1690, *1691*, *1692*
end-diastolic volume of, in aortic stenosis, 1038
filling of, 436–438, *436*
abnormal pattern of, 437–438, *437*, *438*t
in heart failure, 403, *403*
normal pattern of, 437, 437t
function of, 351t, 352, 421–439, 1605–1606, *1606*
after myocardial infarction, *746*, 747
after out-of-hospital cardiac arrest, 759–760, *759*
afterload in, 428–429, *428*, *429*
cardiac catheterization and, 791t
computed tomography of, 342
contractility in, 429, 429t, *430*
equilibrium radionuclide angiocardiography for, 299, *299*
in aortic regurgitation, 1047–1048, 1052–1053, *1053*
in cardiac rehabilitation, 1392–1394, *1393*
in congenital heart disease, 342
in coronary artery disease, 1298–1299, *1322*, 1326–1328, *1326*
in hypertension, 814, *814*
in myocardial infarction, 1194–1195, *1195*, 1235–1238, *1235*
in secondary pulmonary hypertension, 796t, 797
in secundum-type atrial septal defect, 898
in unstable angina, 1335–1336
magnetic resonance imaging of, 329–330, *329*
percutaneous transluminal coronary angioplasty of, 1314–1315
preload in, 428
preoperative, 1716, 1717t
pressure-volume relations in, 431–432, *431–433*
systolic, in myocardial infarction, 1194
thrombolytic agent effect on, 1210
hypertrophy of, concentric, 25, *27*
coronary blood flow autoregulation in, 1168
electrocardiography in, 116–117, *116*, 136, 139, *150*
in aging heart, 1689, *1691*
in aortic stenosis, *210*, 1036–1037, 1039

Ventricle(s) *(Continued)*
in hypertension, 814–815, *815*
in hypertrophic cardiomyopathy, 1421
in sudden cardiac death, 747, 748t
magnetic resonance imaging of, 330, *330*
negative W waves in, *150*
sudden cardiac death and, 753
vectorcardiography in, *116*, 117
impulse of, 25–27, *27*
incomplete rupture of, in myocardial infarction, 1242–1243, *1242*
isovolumetric relaxation of, 435–436, *435*
mass of, measurement of, 425–426, 425t
on plain chest radiography, 208, *210*, 211
output of, in heart failure, 396–397, *396*, *397*
palpation of, 25–27, *26*
passive diastolic characteristics of, *435*, 436
power generation of, calculation of, 432
pressure of, direct left ventricular puncture for, 186
volume loading and, 1480
pseudohypertrophy of, in cardiac tamponade, 1491, *1491*
pseudonormalized filling of, 437, *437*, *438*
pump function of, 421, 432–439
diastolic filling in, 436–438, *436*, *437*, 437t, *438*
diastolic performance in, 434–438, *435*
isovolumetric relaxation in, 435–436, *435*
systolic performance in, 434, *435*
quantitative angiocardiography of, 423–424, *424*
relaxation of, in heart failure, 402–403, *402*, 403t
remodeling of, in myocardial infarction, 1195–1196, *1196*
restrictive filling of, 437–438, *437*
rupture of, in myocardial infarction, 1241–1243, 1241t, *1242*
size of, *64*
variation in, 1655
stiffness of, *435*, 436
in heart failure, 403
stroke volume of, 336, 425, 425t
suction effect of, 384
systolic function of, in myocardial infarction, 1194
systolic motion of, 25
thrombus of, computed tomography of, 337, 342
in myocardial infarction, 1256–1257, *1257*
magnetic resonance imaging of, 326, *326*
tumors of, 1466–1467
echocardiography of, 94–95
two-dimensional echocardiography of, 65–67, *66*
volume of, area-length calculation of, 424–425, *425*, 425t
computed tomography of, 336
measurement of, 423–427, *424*, *425*, 425t, *426–428*
wall of, motion of, 427, *427*
stresses of, 426–427, *426*
thickness of, 425t, 426
computed tomography of, 336, *336*, 337
echocardiography for, *64*, *66*, 68
in heart failure, 399–400, *401*
magnetic resonance imaging of, *329*, 330
mental stress–induced dysfunction of, 302
right, *1604*, 1605
afterload augmentation of, in pulmonary hypertension, 1613
anatomy of, *1604*, 1605
biopsy of, 186–187, *187*
cardiomyopathy of, 1413–1414, *1413*
collapse of, cardiac tamponade and, 1488
dilatation of, 1056. See also *Tricuspid regurgitation.*
double-outlet, 941–944
echocardiography in, 84
Taussig-Bing form of, 943
dysplasia of, genes for, 1632t
magnetic resonance imaging of, 324, *324*
sudden cardiac death in, 749
echocardiography of, 68
failure of, in aortic stenosis, 1040
in pulmonary hypertension, 789, 1611–1612, *1612*
postoperative, 1726–1727
function of, 796, 1605–1606, *1606*

Ventricle(s) *(Continued)*
assessment of, 438–439
computed tomography of, 342
imaging of, 351t, 352
in aortic stenosis, 1040
in congenital heart disease, 342
in pulmonary embolism, 1584, *1585*, 1589–1590, *1591*
in pulmonary hypertension, 789, 1590, 1610–1612, *1611*, *1613*
magnetic resonance imaging of, 329
positive end-expiratory pressure and, 303
preoperative, 1716, 1717t
hypertrophy of, electrocardiography in, 117–118, *117*, *146*
in cor pulmonale, 1605, *1606*
in mitral stenosis, 1011–1012
palpation in, *26*, 27
vectorcardiography in, 119, *119*
infarction of, 1192, 1205–1206, 1240–1241, 1240t
on computed tomography, 210, *210*
on plain chest radiography, 208–210, *209*
palpation of, *26*, 27–28
preload augmentation of, in pulmonary hypertension, 1612–1613
tumors of, 1466
echocardiography of, 94–95
magnetic resonance imaging of, 326, *326*
two-chambered, 928–929
volume of, measurement of, 427
rupture of, 1538–1539, *1539*
cardiac resuscitation and, 1539
silent dysfunction of, radionuclide angiocardiography in, 302
single (univentricular atrioventricular connection), 947–949, *948*
genetic factors in, 1660t
vs. ventricular septal defect, 904
Ventricular alternans, left, in aortic stenosis, 1040
Ventricular angiography, in mitral regurgitation, 1024, *1024*
in transposition of great arteries, 938
Ventricular arrhythmias, exercise stress testing in, 167, *168*
postoperative, 1730–1731, *1730*
evaluation of, 1727–1728, *1728*
Ventricular assist device, 534, 536–544, 537t
centrifugal, 537t, 538
in cardiogenic shock, 541, 541t
complications of, 542–543
electrical, 537t, 540–541, *540*
Food and Drug Administration regulation of, 537
in cardiac transplantation, 517, 542, 542t, 543–544
in myocardial infarction, 542, 1976t
in postcardiotomy cardiogenic shock, 541–542, 541t, 543
indications for, 541–542
pneumatic, 537t, 538–540, *539*, *540*
in cardiogenic shock, 541–542, 541t
roller, 537–538, 537t
Ventricular ectopy, *644*
in sudden cardiac death, 746–747
Ventricular end-diastolic volume, myocardial contractility and, 395, *395*
Ventricular fibrillation, 641t–642t, 686–687, *686*
clinical features of, 687
electrocardiography in, 686, *686*
genesis of, 572
idiopathic, 682–683
in myocardial contusion, 1537
in myocardial infarction, 1245t, 1248–1249
in Wolff-Parkinson-White syndrome, 672, *674*
management of, 687
drugs in, 598t
in myocardial infarction, 1249
postoperative, 1730–1731
prophylaxis for, in myocardial infarction, 1248–1249
reentry in, 572
Ventricular flutter, 641t–642t, 686–687, *686*
clinical features of, 687
electrocardiography in, 686, *686*
management of, 687
Ventricular fusion beats, 676, 678, *678*
with pacemaker, *710*, 712–713

Ventricular gradient, in cardiac activation, 110
Ventricular heterogeneity, in heart failure, 403
Ventricular inhibited pacing, 705
Ventricular interaction, in contraction-relaxation cycle, 385
Ventricular late potentials, in QRS complex prolongation, 583–584, *584*
Ventricular pacing, for atrioventricular nodal reentrant tachycardia, 664
  for ventricular tachycardia, 680
Ventricular premature beats, in myocardial infarction, 1245t, 1246, *1247*
Ventricular premature complex, electrophysiological evaluation of, practice guidelines for, 1960t
Ventricular premature depolarizations, postoperative, 1730
Ventricular pressure, 188t, 189, *189*, 191t
  maximum rate of rise of (dP/dt_{max}), in myocardial contractility, 430, *430*, 432
Ventricular puncture, left, direct, 186
Ventricular safety pacing, *714*, 715
Ventricular septal defect, **901–905,** 1847
  aortic regurgitation in, 903–904, *904*
  arterial pulse in, 22
  congenital, 902–903
    in adult, 967–968
  differential diagnosis of, 1023t
  early systolic murmur of, 39
  echocardiography in, 81, *82*, *83*, 901–902, **Plate 3**
  endocardial cushion defect and, 82, *83*
  exercise and, 979
  genetic factors in, 1661
  in children, 902–903
  in infant, 902
  in myocardial infarction, 1241t, 1243, *1244*
  in Noonan syndrome, 1663
  malalignment in, 901
  management of, 902, 904–905
  mid-diastolic murmur of, *42*
  morphology of, 901, *902*
  murmur in, 1023t
  paramembranous, 901
  pathophysiology of, 902
  perimembranous, 901
  plain chest radiography in, *232*, 233
  postinfarction, intraaortic balloon counterpulsation in, 535
  pregnancy and, 976
  pulmonary blood flow in, *218*
  pulmonary hypertension in, 903
  restrictive, holosystolic murmur of, 38
  right ventricular outflow tract obstruction in, 903
  subaortic stenosis in, 919
  surgical treatment of, 904–905
  systolic murmur in, *28*
Ventricular tachycardia, 641t–642t, **677–681.** See also specific types, e.g., *Arrhythmogenic right ventricular dysplasia.*
  atrioventricular dissociation in, 678
  automaticity on, 577
  bidirectional, 686
  bundle branch reentry in, 686
  clinical features of, 679–680
  dilated cardiomyopathy and, 682
  electrical induction of, 679, *679*
  electrocardiography in, 677–678, *678*, 678t, 1730, *1730*
  electrophysiological studies in, 581–582, *582*, *583*, 678–679, *679*, *680*
    practice guidelines for, 1960t, 1962t, 1963
  genesis of, automaticity in, 577
    nonreentrant mechanisms in, 576–577
    reentry in, 575–576, *577*
    triggered activity in, 577
  hypertrophic cardiomyopathy and, 682
  idiopathic, 598t, 682–683, *682*, *683*
  in heart failure, 504–507, 504t
  in hypertrophic cardiomyopathy, 1421
  in myocardial contusion, 1537
  in myocardial infarction, 1245t, 1247–1248
  in trypanosomiasis, 1443
  intraaortic balloon counterpulsation in, 536
  intraoperative mapping of, *530*, 531
  ischemia-induced, 1178
  ischemic heart disease with, 629, 631
  late potentials in, 583–584, *584*
  mapping of, intraoperative, *530*, 531
Ventricular tachycardia *(Continued)*
  mitral valve prolapse and, 682
  nonsustained, in heart failure, 506
    in hypertrophic cardiomyopathy, 1424, 1424t
  pace mapping in, 627
  pacemaker in, practice guidelines for, 1965t
  pacing termination of, 679, *680*
  postoperative, 1730, *1730*
  prevention of, 505–506, 680–681
  prognosis for, 679–680
  QRS contour in, 678
  reentry in, 575–576, *577*
  septal, left, 683, *683*
  slow-response activity in, 561, *562*
  syncope in, 867
  treatment of, 629–631, *630*, 680–681
    atrial pacing in, 680
    drugs in, 598t
    electrical cardioversion in, 620, *620*
    encircling endocardial ventriculotomy in, *529*, 531
    endocardial resection in, *529*, 531
    radiofrequency catheter ablation in, *625*, *626–628*, 627–628
  vs. supraventricular tachycardia, 677–678, 678t
Ventricular volume, equilibrium radionuclide angiocardiography for, 299
Ventriculography, direct left ventricular puncture for, 186
  left, in hypertrophic cardiomyopathy, 1423
    in idiopathic dilated cardiomyopathy, 1411
  radionuclide, in cardia tumor, 1474
    in cor pulmonale, 1610
    in hypertrophic cardiomyopathy, 1422
    in idiopathic dilated cardiomyopathy, 1411
    in myocardial contusion, 1537
    in myocardial infarction, 1977t
    in trypanosomiasis, 1443
  right, in hypertrophic cardiomyopathy, 1423
Ventriculophasic sinus arrhythmia, 646
Venules, in pulmonary venous hypertension, 797, *797*
Verapamil (Isopten), action potential effects of, *562*
  contraindications to, 1310
  digoxin interaction with, 483t
  dosage of, 594t–595t, 617
  drug interactions of, 483t, 1310
  electrophysiological actions of, 601t, 602t–603t, 616
  hemodynamic effects of, 617
  in angina pectoris, 1309t, 1310, 1311–1312, 1312t
  in arrhythmias, 594t–595t, 601t, 602t–603t, 616–618
  in atrial fibrillation prophylaxis, 1720
  in atrial flutter, 654
  in atrioventricular nodal reentrant tachycardia, 664
  in Duchenne muscular dystrophy, 1869
  in hypertension, 855, 855t
  in hypertrophic cardiomyopathy, 1425
  in myocardial infarction, 1231
  in pediatric cardiology, 1002t
  in pregnancy, 1858
  in renal failure, 1931t
  indications for, 617
  myocardial oxygen consumption effects of, 1306t
  pharmacokinetics of, 594t–595t, 617, 1309t
  preoperative, 1719–1720
  side effects of, 11, 618, 1303t
Vesnarinone, in heart failure, 472t, 485, 502
VEST monitoring, of ventricular function, 300, *300*
Video-assisted thoracoscopy, in malignant pericardial disease, 1797
Vimentin, in cardiac myxoma, 1468
Viral infection, postoperative, 1733
Viral myocarditis, 988–989, 1437–1439, *1438*, 1438t. See also *Myocarditis.*
Viral pericarditis, 1505–1507
  antibody titers in, 1506
  clinical findings in, 1506
  etiology of, 1505–1506
  management of, 1507
  natural history of, 1506–1507
  pathogenesis of, 1505–1506
  pathology of, 1506
Viridans streptococci, in infective endocarditis, 1080–1082, 1089–1090, 1090t
Virus vector, for gene therapy, 1638
Visceral larva migrans, myocarditis in, 1444
Vision, in patient history, 10
Vital capacity, in myocardial infarction, 1197
Vitamin B_1 (thiamine), deficiency of, 993–994
    heart failure in, 461–462, 461t
  in beriberi, 462
Vitamin C, in myocardial infarction, 1232
Vitamin D, teratogenicity of, 1663t
Vitamin deficiency, 1907–1908
Vitamin E, in coronary artery disease, 1154, 1300
  in myocardial infarction, 1232
Vitamin K (AquaMEPHYTON), in pediatric cardiology, 1002t
Volume loading, left ventricular pressure and, 1480
  with cardiac catheterization, 198
Volume overload, diastolic pressure-volume curve in, 403
  in renal failure, 1923
Vomiting, in myocardial infarction, 1199
  in patient history, 10
Von Hippel–Lindau syndrome, 1676, 1678t
Von Recklinghausen neurofibromatosis, 1677, 1678t
Von Willebrand factor, in cyanotic congenital heart disease, 972
Voodoo death, 751

WAGR syndrome, 1651t
Wall stress, afterload and, 380
  in contraction-relaxation cycle, 379–380, *379*
  of left ventricle, 426–427, *426*
  preload and, 380
Wallstent, 1379, *1379*
Wandering pacemaker, 647, *648*
Ward-Romano syndrome, 1667
Warfarin sodium (Coumadin), 1818
  after myocardial infarction, 1828, *1828*, 1832–1833
  complications of, 1595
  contraindications to, 1595
  in atrial fibrillation, 1831–1832, *1831*, *1832*
  in mitral stenosis, 1830
  in pediatric cardiology, 1002t
  in pregnancy, 977, 1859
  in prosthetic valve replacement, 1732, 1834–1836, *1835*, 1836t
  in pulmonary embolism, 1594–1595
  in pulmonary embolism prophylaxis, 1599t
  in pulmonary hypertension, 795
  in renal failure, 1933t
  preoperative, 1719
  teratogenicity of, 1663t, 1664
Warm-up phenomenon, in myocardial infarction, 1214
Wasp sting, myocardial effects of, 1448
Watanabe heritable hyperlipemic rabbit, for hypercholesterolemia model, 1116
Water retention, in heart failure, 1918, *1919*
Water-hammer pulse, of aortic regurgitation, 22, 1049
Water-perfusable tissue index, of myocardial viability, 307
Weakness, in heart failure, 452
Weber-Osler-Rendu syndrome, 880t
Wegener's granulomatosis, 1783
Weight loss, cardiac benefits of, 1906
  cardiac complications of, 1907
  cost-effectiveness analysis of, 1748
  in hypertension, 844
Weil disease, myocardial involvement in, 1440
West of Scotland Coronary Prevention Study, in hypercholesterolemia prevention, 1128
Westermark's sign, in pulmonary embolism, 1588, *1588*
Wheezing, in myocardial infarction, 1200, 1236
White clot syndrome, 1594
Wide QRS tachycardia, in Wolff-Parkinson-White syndrome, 673
  practice guidelines for, 1961t, 1962
Wiggers cycle, *377*
Williams syndrome, 881t, 919–921, *920*, *921*
  elfin facies of, 920, *920*
  genetic factors in, 1632t, 1662
Wilms tumor, 1678t

Wolff-Parkinson-White (WPW) syndrome, *666–667*, **667–675**
accessory pathways in, *668*, 669–672, *669–672*
atrial fibrillation in, 672, *673*
atriofascicular accessory pathways in, 669
atriohisian tracts in, *668*, 669
atrioventricular block and, 127
atrioventricular nodal reentry in, 574–575, *576*
atrioventricular reentry in, 574–575, *576*
clinical features of, 673–674
electrocardiography in, 126–127, *126*, *127*, 136, *146*, *147*, *150*, 667–669, *668*
electrophysiological studies in, *668*, 669–673, *669–674*
practice guidelines for, 1963
exercise stress testing in, 169, *169*
fasciculoventricular fibers in, *668*, 669
genetic factors in, 674
in ankylosing spondylitis, 1780
Kent bundle conduction in, 670, *671*
myocardial infarction and, 126–127, *126*, *127*
nodoventricular fibers in, *668*, 669
practice guidelines for, 1963
prevention of, 675
Q wave in, 136
sudden cardiac death in, 750
syncope in, 867
treatment of, 598t, 674–675
ventricular fibrillation in, 672, *674*
wide QRS tachycardia in, 673
Wolf-Hirschhorn syndrome, 1656t
Wolman syndrome, 1669t
Women, coronary artery bypass graft surgery in, 1328
coronary artery disease in, 1153, 1704–1711, 1908
chest pain in, 1704, 1704t
clinical features of, 1704–1706
coronary angiography in, 1706
diabetes and, 1706
diagnosis of, 1705–1706, 1705t
exercise and, 1707
hemostasis and, 1707
hormonal therapy in, 1707–1709, 1708t
breast cancer risk with, 1708–1709, 1708t
guidelines for, 1709
hypertension and, 1706–1707
lipid levels in, 1706
management of, 1709–1711
angioplasty in, 1709–1710, 1710t
bypass grafting in, 1710
medical, 1709
revascularization in, 1709–1710, 1710t
natural history of, 1705
obesity and, 1706
oral contraceptives and, 1707
prevalence of, 1704, 1704t
prognosis for, 1705
psychosocial factors in, 1707
Women *(Continued)*
risk factors for, 1706–1707
smoking and, 1707
myocardial infarction in, 1710–1711, *1710*, *1711*
mortality with, 1711
treatment of, 1711, *1711*
Wood unit, 780
in heart transplantation, 516t
Work, in myocardial oxygen uptake, 381
World Health Organization Cooperative Trial, in hypercholesterolemia prevention, 1128
Wound infection, postoperative, 1319, 1732–1733

X chromosome, in Turner syndrome, 1657
Xanthelasma, in stable angina pectoris, 1292
Xanthoma, 16, *17*
high-density lipoprotein deficiency with, 1144
Xanthoma striatum palmare, 16
Xanthoma tendinosum, 16, *17*
Xylocaine hydrochloride. See *Lidocaine (Xylocaine hydrochloride).*

Z lines, of sarcomere, 361, *362*

ISBN 0-7216-5665-X

WBS 5663-3
BRAUNWALD